ENDOCRINOLOGY & METABOLISM

fourth edition

Notice

ENDOCRINOLOGY & METABOLISM

fourth edition

Philip Felig, M.D.
Attending Physician
Senior Medical Staff
Lenox Hill Hospital
New York, New York

Lawrence A. Frohman, M.D.
Edmund F. Foley Professor and Head
Department of Medicine
University of Illinois at Chicago College of Medicine
Physician-in-Chief
University of Illinois Hospital
Chicago, Illinois

McGRAW-HILL, Inc.
Medical Publishing Division

New York Chicago San Francisco Lisbon London Madrid Mexico City
Milan New Delhi San Juan Seoul Singapore Sydney Toronto

McGraw-Hill

A Division of The ***McGraw-Hill*** *Companies*

Endocrinology and Metabolism, Fourth Edition

1 2 3 4 5 6 7 8 9 0 KGP KGP 0 9 8 7 6 5 4 3 2 1

ISBN 0-07-022001-8

This book was set in Times Roman by Progressive Information Technologies.
The editors were Martin Wonsiewicz and Susan R. Noujaim.
The production supervisor was Richard Ruzycka.
Project management was provided by Progressive Information Technologies.
The cover designer was Amiee Nordin.
Quebecor World Kingsport was the printer and binder.

This book is printed on acid-free paper.

Library of Congress Cataloging-in-Publication Data

Endocrinology and metabolism / [edited by] Philip Felig, Lawrence A. Frohman.—4th ed.
p. cm.
Includes bibliographical references and index.
ISBN 0-07-022001-8
1. Endocrinology. 2. Endocrine glands—Diseases. 3. Metabolism—Disorders.
I. Felig, Philip, 1936- II. Frohman, Lawrence A.
[DNLM: 1. Endocrine Diseases—metabolism. 2. Endocrine System—physiology. 3. Metabolic Diseases. WK 140 E559 2001]
RC648 .E464 2001
616.4—dc21

00-035134

Dedication

To our wives, children, and grandchildren:

Florence; Clifford, Minna, Noam, Yair, Daniella, and Maayan;
David, Anna, Jacob and Jordan; and Elliot.
P.F.

Barbara; Michael, Stella, Evan, and Dafni;
Marc, Susan, Alicia, Hannah and Zoe;
Erica, Aaron, and Leah; and Rena, Andrew, and Zachary.
L.A.F.

Contents

Contributors xxix
Preface xxxiii

PART I GENERAL ENDOCRINOLOGY 1

1 Introduction to the Endocrine System 3
Lawrence A. Frohman and Philip Felig
Definitions and Scope of Endocrinology 3
Types of Hormones and Their Synthesis and Release 5
Circulation of Hormones 5
Hormone Metabolism 6
Regulation of Hormone Levels 6
Hormone Uptake and Internalization 7
Mechanisms of Hormone Action 7
Regulation of Hormone Responsiveness 8
Classification of Hormone Action 8
Evolution of the Endocrine System 8
Simple and Complex Regulation 8
Origins of Hormones and Other Regulatory Ligands 8
Origin of Receptors and Other Mediators of Regulatory Ligand Actions 9
Diversification of Families of Hormones 10
Evolution of the Endocrine Glands 10
Integration of the Endocrine System 10
Integrated Actions of a Given Class of Hormone 10
Hormone Synergisms: Recruitment of Multiple Hormones for Coordinated Responses 10
Hormone Antagonism: Fine-Tuning of Metabolism 11
Mechanisms for Attenuating or Terminating the Response 11
Actions of Hormones 11
Intermediary Metabolism and Growth 11
Highly Specific Functions 11
Disorders of the Endocrine System 12
Hormone Deficiency Syndromes 12
Hormone Excess Syndromes 13
Multiple Endocrine Syndromes 14
Abnormalities of Endocrine Glands Not Associated with Hormonal Imbalance 15
Clinical Assessment of Endocrine Status 15
History and Physical Examination 15
Laboratory Testing 15
Treatment of Endocrine Diseases 17
Hormone Agonist and Antagonist Therapy of Nonendocrine Disease 17
References 17

2 The Clinical Manifestations of Endocrine Disease **19**
Lawrence A. Frohman and Philip Felig

Generalized Symptoms 19
Weakness and Fatigue 19
Weight Loss 20
Weight Gain 20
Body Temperature 20
Skin 20
Nose, Ears, Voice, and Tongue 21
Gastrointestinal System 21
Hemopoietic System 22
Cardiovascular System 23
Urinary Tract 23
Sexual Function 23
Bones and Joints 24
Central Nervous System 25
Neuromuscular Abnormalities 25
Ophthalmic Abnormalities 26

3 Biosynthesis, Secretion and Metabolism of Hormones **29**
Gordon N. Gill

Peptide Hormones 29
Biosynthesis of Messenger RNA 29
Biosynthesis of Peptide Hormones 31
Secretion, Transport, and Metabolism of Peptide Hormones 35
Steroid Hormones 37
Cholesterol Substrate for Steroid Hormone Formation 37
The Rate-Controlling Step in Steroid Hormone Synthesis 37
Pathway of Steroid Hormone Biosynthesis 39
Trophic Regulation of Steroid Hormone Synthesis 41
Transport and Metabolism of Steroid Hormones 42
Thyroid Hormone 43
Iodine Metabolism 43
Anatomy of a Distinctive Biosynthetic Pathway 44
Transport and Metabolism 45
References 46

4 Molecular Mechanisms of Hormone Action: Biology of Signal Transduction **49**
Mark M. Rasenick and Randal C. Jaffe

Introduction 49
Methods of Cell-Cell Communication 49
Classification of Hormones 49
Receptors: The Initial Step in Hormone Response 49
Methods for Receptor Analysis 50
Radioligand Binding 50
Receptor Quantitation 51
Kinetics of Receptor Binding 51
Nuclear Receptor Signaling 53
Mechanism of Action of Steroid Hormones 53
Mechanism of Action of Retinoic Acid, Vitamin D, and Thyroid Hormones 55
Biochemistry and Molecular Biology of Steroid Receptors 55
Receptors for Thyroid Hormones 55
Receptors for Retinoic Acid 56
Orphan Receptors 56
Nuclear Receptor Knockout Studies 56
Structural Organization of Nuclear Receptor Proteins 57
Mechanism of Genes Regulation by Nuclear Receptors 59

Ligand Independent Activation of Nuclear Receptors 59
Modification of Nuclear Receptor Activity by Phosphorylation 59
Chaperone Proteins 60
Signaling through G Protein-Coupled Receptors 60
Structure of G Protein-Coupled Receptors 61
Ligand Binding by G Protein-Coupled Receptors 63
Changes in Receptor Conformation upon Agonist Activation 63
Inverse Agonism 64
Regulation of Receptor Sensitivity 64
Receptor Desensitization 64
G Proteins, the Next Step in the Signaling Cascade 64
GTP Hydrolysis 65
RGS Proteins 66
Coupling of Receptor to G Protein 66
G Protein Effectors 67
Phospholipid Metabolism Mediated by G-Protein Dependent Hormone Signals 68
G Protein-Activated Ion Channels 70
G Proteins and Na/H Exchange 71
G Proteins and Changes in Cell Structure 71
Second Messenger Systems in Cellular Signaling 71
Cyclic Nucleotide Phosphodiesterase 71
The Intracellular Amplification of Extracellular Signals 72
Second Messenger-Activated Protein Kinases 72
Cyclic GMP-Dependent Protein Kinases 73
Nitric Oxide and cGMP Signaling 73
Changes in Intracellular Calcium 74
Intracellular Calcium Channels 74
Calcium Binding Proteins 74
Calmodulin 75
Ca^{2+}/Calmodulin-Dependent Protein Kinases (CaM Kinases) 75
Protein Kinase C 75
Phosphoprotein Phosphatases 76
Interplay Between Ca^{2+}/Calmodulin and cAMP Signaling 77
Receptors with Guanylyl Cyclase Activity 77
Ion Channel Receptors 78
The Nicotinic Acetylcholine Receptor 78
Glutamate Receptors 79
GABA Receptors 79
Glycine Receptors 80
The 5HT3 Serotonin Receptor 80
Growth Factor Signaling: Receptors with Tyrosine Kinase Activity 80
Receptors with Serine and Threonine Kinase Activity 80
Kinase Cascades Promoting Cell Growth 81
Protein Tyrosine Phosphatase 82
Kinase-Independent Actions of Cyclic Nucleotides 83
Ion Channels Regulated by cAMP and cGMP 83
Effects of cAMP on Gene Transcription 83
Crosstalk among Hormones or Neurotransmitters 84
Acknowledgments 84
References 84

5 Hormone Assays **91**
A. Eugene Pekary and Jerome M. Hershman
Bioassays 91
In Vivo Assays 91
In Vitro Assays 91
Cytochemical Assays 92
Complementary of In Vivo and In Vitro Assays 93
Nomenclature 93
Types of Immunoassays 93

Labeled Analyte and Reagent Limiting *93*
Reagent Excess and Labeled Antibody *93*
Free and Total Hormone Measurements *94*
Immunoassay Reagents 95
Binding Proteins *95*
Nonimmunologic Molecular Recognition Systems: Avidin/Biotin *97*
Labels *97*
Separation Systems 99
Liquid-Phase Precipitation *99*
Solid-Phase Adsorption *99*
Solid-Phase Precipitation *99*
Homogeneous Assay Systems 99
Fluorescence Polarization *99*
Phase-Modulation Fluorescence Spectroscopy *100*
Amplitude-Modulated Enzyme Assays *100*
Receptor Assays 100
Chromatographic Assays 101
Chromatography *101*
Detection *101*
Immunoassay Optimization And Validation 101
General Considerations *101*
Detection Limits *101*
Specificity *101*
Interference 102
Sample Matrix Effects *102*
Heterophilic Antibodies *102*
Complement and Rheumatoid Factors *103*
Enzyme Contaminants *103*
Drug Interference *103*
Hemodynamic Effects *103*
Quality Control 103
Future Trends 104
References 104

PART II NEUROENDOCRINOLOGY AND THE PITUITARY **109**

6 Neuroendocrinology **109**
Mark E. Molitch

General Concepts in Neuroendocrinology 111
Overview of Brain-Hypothalamic-Pituitary-Target Organ Regulation 111
Neuron-Neuron Interactions *111*
Hypophysiotropic Hormones *112*
Feedback Loops *113*
Anatomic Aspects 115
Hypothalamus *115*
Median Eminence and Hypothalamic-Pituitary Portal System *118*
Pituitary *118*
Hypophysiotropic Hormones 119
Thyrotropin Releasing Hormone *121*
Gonadotropin Releasing Hormone *124*
Somatostatin *127*
Corticotropin Releasing Hormone *130*
Growth Hormone Releasing Hormone *132*
Prolactin Inhibiting Factor *133*
Prolactin Releasing Factor *134*
Neurotransmitters 135
Biosynthesis and Metabolism of Bioaminergic Neurotransmitters *135*
Anatomic Pathways of Bioaminergic Neurotransmitters *135*
Neuropharmacology of Bioaminergic Neurotransmitters *137*

Amino Acid Neurotransmitters 137
Neuropeptides 138
Endogenous Opioid Peptides 138
Other Peptides 140
Gaseous Neurotransmitters 140
The Pineal Gland 141
Anatomy 141
Pineal Hormones and Neurotransmitters 142
Pineal and Biological Rhythms 143
CNS Rhythms and Neuroendocrine Function 143
Neuroendocrine Disease 145
Diseases of the Hypothalamus 145
Effects of Hypothalamic Disease on Pituitary Function 149
Effects of Hypothalamic Disease on Other Neurometabolic Functions 153
Neuroendocrine Alterations in Systemic Disease 156
Other CNS Disorders 158
References 159

7 Diseases of the Anterior Pituitary **173**
Peter J. Snyder

The Normal Pituitary 173
Anatomy of the Pituitary 173
Physiology of Anterior Pituitary Hormones 175
Diseases of the Anterior Pituitary 180
Causes of Anterior Pituitary Diseases 180
Clinical Presentation of Anterior Pituitary Diseases 183
Evaluation and Treatment of Mass Lesions 184
Hormonal Hypersecretion—Pituitary Adenomas 188
Hormonal Hyposecretion 204
References 208

8 Posterior Pituitary **217**
Gary L. Robertson

Normal 217
Anatomy 217
Chemistry 217
Biosynthesis and Release 217
Secretion 218
Distribution and Clearance 223
Extrahypophyseal Neurons 224
Biologic Actions 224
Thirst 226
Regulation of Water Balance 226
Pathology 228
Deficiencies of Vasopressin 228
Deficiency of Thirst 240
Excess Vasopressin 242
References 248

PART III THYROID DISEASE **259**

9 The Thyroid: Physiology, Thyrotoxicosis, Hypothyroidism, and the Painful Thyroid **261**
Robert D. Utiger

Anatomy and Physiology 261
Clinical Anatomy 261
Chemistry of Thyroid Hormones 262

Thyroid Hormone Biosynthesis 262
Thyroid Hormone Production and Metabolism 265
Regulation of Thyroid Hormone Production 266
Mechanism of Action of Thyrotropin 269
Regulation of Thyroid Secretion by Iodide 270
Regulation of Extrathyroidal Triiodothyronine Production 270
Transport and Cellular Binding of Thyroid Hormones 271
Actions of Thyroid Hormone 272
Evaluation of Thyroid Function 274
Physiological Variables Affecting Pituitary-Thyroid Function and Tests 279
Alterations in Serum Thyroid Hormone Binding 281
Nonthyroidal Illness 283
Effects of Specific Disorders on Thyroid Function 287
Effects of Drugs on Thyroid Function 288
Thyrotoxicosis 289
Pathophysiology of Thyrotoxicosis 290
Causes of Thyrotoxicosis 290
Clinical Manifestations of Thyrotoxicosis 297
Laboratory Diagnosis of Thyrotoxicosis 301
Treatment of Thyrotoxicosis 303
Special Situations 309
Extrathyroidal Manifestations of Graves' Disease 311
Hypothyroidism 315
Pathophysiology of Hypothyroidism 315
Causes of Hypothyroidism 316
Clinical Manifestations of Hypothyroidism 321
Laboratory Diagnosis of Hypothyroidism 325
Treatment of Hypothyroidism 326
Special Situations 327
The Painful Thyroid 329
Subacute Thyroiditis 329
Hemorrhage in a Thyroid Nodule 329
Radiation Thyroiditis 330
Suppurative Thyroiditis 330
References 330

10 The Thyroid: Nodules and Neoplasia 349
Barbara K. Kinder and Gerard N. Burrow
Goiter 349
Classification of Goiter and Thyroid Neoplasia 349
Historical Overview 349
Etiology of Goiter 349
Endemic Goiter 351
Sporadic Goiter 353
Nontoxic Goiter 356
Solitary Thyroid Nodules 359
Factors Predisposing to Thyroid Cancer 360
Evaluation of the Thyroid Nodule 361
Management of a Solitary Thyroid Nodule 364
Thyroid Carcinoma 366
Histologic Classification 366
Clinical Staging 366
Molecular Biology of Thyroid Neoplasms 366
Specific Primary Thyroid Carcinomas 368
Secondary Tumors 373
Surgical Treatment of Thyroid Carcinoma 373
Radioactive Iodine Treatment of Carcinomas of Follicular Cell Origin 375

Thyroid Hormone in the Treatment of Thyroid Carcinomas 376
Other Treatment Modalities 376
Follow-up of Patients with Carcinoma of the Thyroid 377
References 378

PART IV ADRENAL DISEASE **385**

11 The Adrenal Cortex **387**
Walter L. Miller and George P. Chrousos
Embryology, Anatomy, and History 387
History 387
Embryology and Development 388
Anatomy 388
Steroid Hormone Biosynthesis 389
Chemistry of Steroid Hormones 390
Cholesterol: The Precursor of Steroid Hormones 392
Cytochrome P450 395
P450scc: Conversion of Cholesterol to Pregnenolone 395
3β-Hydroxysteroid Dehydrogenase/$\Delta^5\Delta^4$ Isomerase 398
P450c17: 17α Hydroxylase/17,20 Lyase 398
P450c21: 21-Hydroxylase 400
P450c11β and P450c11AS: 11β-Hydroxylase and Aldosterone Synthase 401
Other Steroidogenic Enzymes 401
Developmental Aspects of Adrenal Steroidogenesis: The Fetal Adrenal, Adrenarche, and Adrenopause 403
Regulation of Adrenal Steroidogenesis 404
Regulation of Glucocorticoids 405
Regulation of Mineralocorticoids 411
Regulation of Adrenal Androgens 413
Plasma Steroids and Their Disposal 414
Quantities of Steroids Produced 414
Inhibitors of Adrenal Steroid Biosynthesis 414
Physical State of Steroids in Plasma 415
Metabolism of Adrenocortical Steroids 418
Variations in Steroid Metabolism 421
Molecular Mechanisms and Physiologic Actions 421
Definition of a Glucocorticoid 421
Molecular Mechanisms of Glucocorticoid Hormone Action 421
Glucocorticoid Agonists and Antagonists 422
Structure-Activity Relations of Glucocorticoids: Basis for Biological Activity 423
Definition of a Mineralocorticoid 434
Molecular Mechanisms of Mineralocorticoid Action 434
Mineralocorticoid Agonists and Antagonists 435
Physiologic Actions of Mineralocorticoids 435
Actions of Adrenal Androgens and Estrogens 437
Laboratory Evaluation of Adrenocortical Function 437
Plasma Cortisol and Related Steroids 438
Urinary Corticosteroids 439
Cortisol Production Rate 440
Dexamethasone Suppression Tests 440
Tests of Pituitary-Adrenal Reserve 441
Metyrapone Testing 443
CRH Testing 444
Insulin-Induced Hypoglycemia 444
Mineralocorticoids 444
Androgens 444

Adrenocortical Function in Children 445
Disorders of Steroid Hormone Synthesis 447
Introduction 447
21-Hydroxylase Deficiency 449
3β-Hydroxysteroid Dehydrogenase Deficiency 457
P450c17 (17α-Hydroxylase/17,20-Lyase) Deficiency 458
11β-Hydroxylase (P450c11β) Deficiency 459
P450c11AS Disorders: The "Corticosterone Methyl Oxidase" Deficiencies 459
Congenital Lipoid Adrenal Hyperplasia 460
Adrenocortical Insufficiency 461
Primary Adrenocortical Insufficiency (Addison's Disease) 461
Secondary Adrenocortical Insufficiency 469
Diagnosis 470
Treatment 472
Prognosis and Survival 474
Hypoaldosteronism 474
Adrenocortical Hyperfunction 475
Cushing's Syndrome 476
Adrenal Tumors 480
Diagnosis and Differential Diagnosis 483
Treatment of Cushing's Syndrome 487
Hyperaldosteronism 491
References 493

12 Diseases of the Sympathochromaffin System **525**
Philip E. Cryer

Sympathochromaffin Physiology 525
Biochemistry of the Catecholamines 525
Physiology of Adrenergic Axon Terminals and Chromaffin Cells 527
Biological Effects of the Catecholamines 531
Integrated Physiology of the Sympathochromaffin System 532
The Biological Roles of Epinephrine and Norepinephrine: Hormones and Neurotransmitters 535
Sympathochromaffin Pathophysiology 536
Pheochromocytoma 536
Generalized Autonomic Failure 540
Hypoglycemia 543
Diagnostic Testing 545
Measurement of Catecholamines and Their Metabolites 545
Indirect Tests of Autonomic Function 546
References 547

13 Endocrinology of Hypertension **553**
Willa A. Hsueh, Susanne B. Nicholas, Marwan Hamaty, John Baxter, and James Sowers

Epidemiology of Hypertension 555
Regulation of Blood Pressure 555
Complications of Hypertension 556
Genetic and Environmental Influences 556
Hormonal Modifiers of Blood Pressure 557
The Renin-Angiotensin System 557
Mineralocorticoids 566
Glucocorticoids 568
Estrogens, Progestins, and Androgens 569
Thyroid Hormone 569
Vasopressin 569
Erythropoietin 569

Growth Hormone 570
Calcitonin Gene-Related Peptide 570
Endothelin 570
Nitric Oxide (Endothelin-Derived Releasing Factor) 570
Endothelium-Derived Hyperpolarizing Factor (EDHF) 571
Atrial Natriuretic Peptides (ANPs) 572
Catecholamines and the Autonomic Nervous System 573
Insulin and Insulin Resistance in Hypertension 573
Evaluation of the Hypertensive Patient 579
Clinical History 579
Physical Examination 580
Laboratory Tests 580
Renovascular Hypertension 581
Prevalence 581
Causes of Renovascular Hypertension 581
Clinical Features of Renovascular Hypertension 583
Screening and Diagnostic Studies for Renovascular Hypertension 583
Selection and Sequence of Diagnostic Tests for Renovascular Hypertension 586
Management of Renovascular Hypertension 586
Summary and Recommendations 588
Disorders of the Adrenal 588
Primary Aldosteronism 588
Glucocorticoid-Remediable Hyperaldosteronism 590
Hypertension in Congenital Adrenal Hyperplasia 590
Cushing's Disease 591
Apparent Mineralocorticoid Excess (AME) 591
Pheochromocytomas 591
References 593

14 Glucocorticoid Therapy **609**
George P. Chrousos
Physiologic and Pharmacologic Actions of Glucocorticoids in Relation to Steroid Therapy 609
Therapeutic Influences 609
Adverse Influences 610
Molecular Mechanisms for Glucocorticoid-Mediated Therapeutic Influences 611
Kinetic Considerations 612
Manifestations of Iatrogenic Cushing's Syndrome 612
Comparisons with Spontaneous Cushing's Syndrome 612
Ocular Changes 613
Avascular Necrosis of Bone 613
Osteoporosis 613
Infections 614
Myopathy 614
Atherosclerosis 614
Dose and Time Dependency and Reversibility 614
Diagnosis of Iatrogenic Cushing's Syndrome 615
Determinants of Glucocorticoid Potency 615
Bioavailability 615
Distribution 616
Metabolism and Clearance 616
Concentration at Sites of Action 617
Agonist Activity 617
Overall Estimation of Glucocorticoid Potency 617
Variations in Sensitivity to Glucocorticoids: Glucocorticoid Resistance 617
Glucocorticoid Preparations 618
Steroids with Glucocorticoid Activity Available for Therapy 618
Orally and Parenterally Active Preparations 618
Intraarticular Preparations 618

Topical Preparations 619
Inhaled Corticosteroids 619
ACTH 619
Some General Principles 620
Selection of Patients 620
Need for Empirical Data 620
Short-Term Versus Long-Term 620
Testing the Sensitivity 620
Dose-Response Considerations 620
The Use of Adjunctive Therapy 621
Specific Measures to Reduce Side Effects 621
Cognizance of Objective Criteria 621
The Circadian Rhythm 621
Adjusting the Dose 621
Alternate Day Therapy 622
Special Situations 623
Pregnancy 623
Diabetes 623
Surgery 623
Psychiatry 623
Peptic Ulcer 623
Pediatrics 624
Kaposi's Sarcoma 624
Administration with Other Drugs 624
Withdrawal of Glucocorticoids and Suppression of the Hypothalamic-Pituitary-Adrenal Axis 625
Kinetics and Dosage Required for Suppression 625
Kinetics of Return to Normal Axis Function 626
Steroid Withdrawal Syndromes 627
Evaluation of Axis Function 628
Withdrawal Protocols and Indications for Steroid Coverage 628
References 629

PART V GONADAL DISEASE **633**

15 The Testis **635**
Alvin M. Matsumoto

Introduction 635
Anatomy and Development 635
Hypothalamic-Pituitary Axis and the Central Nervous System 635
Testis 636
Testicular Development 641
Fetal Testis Development 641
Testicular Descent 642
Neonatal and Pubertal Testis Development 642
Physiology 642
Hypothalamic-Pituitary-Testicular Axis 642
Physiology of Male Sexual Response 652
Male Hypogonadism 654
Clinical Manifestations and Evaluation 654
Differential Diagnosis 658
Causes of Male Hypogonadism 665
Primary Hypogonadism 668
Secondary Hypogonadism 678
Treatment of Hypogonadism 682
Precocious Puberty 688
True Precocious Puberty 688
Precocious Pseudopuberty 689
Tumors of the Testis 689

Germ Cell Cancers 689
Non-Germ Cell Tumors 690
References 690

16A The Ovary: Basic Principles and Concepts
A. Physiology **707**
Gregory F. Erickson
Anatomy 707
Morphology 707
Blood Vessels 707
Innervation 707
Histology 709
Ovarian Follicles 709
Preantral Follicles 709
Ovarian Interstitial Cells 715
Corpora Lutea 718
Biogenesis of Ovarian Hormones 720
Steroids 720
Ovarian Cytodifferentiation: Underlying Control Mechanisms 723
The Granulosa Cell 723
The Interstitial Cells 726
Follicle Development: Control Mechanisms 731
Recruitment 731
Atresia 732
Selection 732
Ovulation 734
Physiologic Correlates of Ovarian Activity with Aging 736
The Fetal Period 736
Premenarche 736
Menarche 737
Postmenarche: The Normal Menstrual Cycle 737
Menopause 738
The Concept of Ovarian Growth Factors 739
Conclusion 739
References 739

16B The Ovary: Basic Principles and Concepts
B. Clinical **745**
Henry G. Burger, David L. Healy, and Beverley J. Vollenhoven
Ovarian Disorders in Teenagers 745
Primary Amenorrhea 745
Menarcheal Menorrhagia 749
Ovarian Disorders in Young Adults 750
Secondary Amenorrhea 750
Polycystic Ovary Syndrome 754
Virilization and Hirsutism 757
Female Infertility: Diagnosis of Ovulatory Dysfunction 759
Menorrhagia and Dysmenorrhea 762
Premenstrual Syndrome 766
Ovarian Disorders in Middle Age 766
Endocrinology of the Menopause 766
Climacteric Symptoms 767
Postmenopausal Problems 768
Long-Term Hormone Replacement Therapy 769
Postmenopausal Bleeding 771
Chemical Contraception and Contragestion 771
New Progestogens 772
References 772

17 Sexual Differentiation **779**
Robert M. Couch and Jeremy S. D. Winter

Normal Sex Determination and Sexual Differentiation 779
Genetic Sex 779
Gonadal Sex 783
Differentiation of the Genital Ducts 786
Differentiation of the Urogenital Sinus and External Genitalia 787
Hormonal Sex: Differentiation of the Hypothalamic-Pituitary-Gonadal Axis 787
Abnormal Sexual Differentiation 792
Errors of Primary Sex Determination 792
Errors of Sexual Differentiation 800
Clinical Approach to Disorders of Sexual Differentiation 816
The Newborn with Abnormal Genitalia 816
Virilization During Childhood or Adolescence 817
Delayed Puberty, Amenorrhea, and Infertility 817
References 819

PART VI FUEL METABOLISM **825**

18 Diabetes Mellitus **827**
David M. Nathan, and Enrico Cagliero

Introduction 827
History 827
Endocrine Pancreas 828
Anatomy 828
Development 828
Pancreatic Hormones 830
Glucagon Chemistry and Biosynthesis 838
Somatostatin 841
Pancreatic Polypeptide 841
Islet Amyloid Polypeptide 841
Fuel Homeostasis 842
Regulatory and Counterregulatory Hormones 842
Metabolism and Energy Stores 842
The Basal State 843
Fuel Availability: The Fed State 843
Fuel Need: Starvation 844
Exercise 844
Fuel-Hormone Imbalance 844
Clinical Diabetes 845
Definition, Classification, and Diagnosis 845
Diagnosis 857
Screening 858
Therapy 858
Metabolic Emergencies—Diabetic Ketoacidosis (DKA), Hyperosmolar Hyperglycemic Nonketotic Coma (HHNKC), Hypoglycemia 887
Complications of Insulin Therapy (Hypoglycemia, Allergy, Lipodystrophy) 892
Other Complications of Insulin Treatment 893
Long-Term Complications 894
Overview 894
Pathophysiology 895
Retinopathy 896
Nephropathy 900
Neuropathy 904

Cardiovascular Disease 908
Other Complications 912
References 912

---

19 Hypoglycemia **927**
Harry Shamoon
Definition 927
Signs and Symptoms 927
Neuroglycopenia 928
Sympathoadrenal Symptoms 928
Other Symptoms and Signs 928
Tests for Evaluation of Hypoglycemia 929
Plasma Glucose 929
Plasma Insulin 929
C Peptide 929
Proinsulin 929
Supervised Prolonged Fasting 930
Oral Glucose Tolerance Test 930
Other Tests 930
Classification 931
Fasting Hypoglycemia 931
Reactive Hypoglycemias 938
Induced Hypoglycemias 939
Diagnostic and Therapeutic Approach to Fasting Hypoglycemia 940
References 941

---

20 Obesity **945**
John M. Amatruda and David L. Linemeyer
Definition and Diagnosis of Obesity 945
Prevalence and Economic Costs of Obesity 948
Medical Complications of Obesity 948
Mortality 948
Cardiovascular Disease 950
Body Fat Distribution 952
Metabolic Disorders 954
Lipid Abnormalities 955
Hypertension 955
Gallstones 955
Cancer 956
Endocrine Disorders 956
Skeletal Disorders 957
Pulmonary Disorders 957
Miscellaneous Disorders 958
Etiology of Obesity 958
Genetic Factors 958
Environmental Factors 960
Energy Expenditure 960
Food Intake 963
Endocrine Systems and the Autonomic Nervous System 966
Summary 967
Other Causes of Obesity 967
Treatment of Obesity 967
Prevention 967
Exercise 968
Behavioral Modification 970
Diet 970
Fad Diets 976

Pharmacological Treatment 976
Surgery for Morbid Obesity 978
Summary 979
References 979

21 Disorders of Lipid Metabolism **993**
P. Barton Duell, D. Roger Illingworth, and William E. Connor

The Plasma Lipoproteins 993
Lipoprotein Classification 993
Lipoprotein Composition 994
The Apoproteins 996
Lipoprotein Structure 997
Synthesis and Catabolism of Lipids and Lipoproteins 997
Lipids 997
Enzymes and Transfer Proteins Active in Lipoprotein Metabolism 998
Lipoprotein Metabolism 1000
Lipoprotein Receptors 1004
Atherogenicity of Individual Lipoprotein Particles 1006
The Hyperlipidemias 1006
Classification of Hyperlipidemias 1006
Criteria for the Diagnosis of Hyperlipoproteinemia 1007
Secondary Hyperlipidemias 1009
Hypercholesterolemia 1015
Familial Hypercholesterolemia 1015
Familial Defective Apolipoprotein B-100 1021
Combined Hypercholesterolemia and Hypertriglyceridemia 1023
Hypertriglyceridemia 1027
Disorders of High-Density Lipoproteins 1030
Familial Apolipoprotein A-I and C-III Deficiency 1031
Familial Apo-A-I, C-III, A-IV Deficiency 1031
HDL Deficiency with Planar Xanthomas 1032
Lecithin Cholesterol Acyltransferase Deficiency 1032
Fish Eye Disease 1032
Familial Apo-A-I Variants 1032
Familial Hypoalphalipoproteinemia 1032
Tangier Disease 1033
Familial Hyperalphalipoproteinemia 1034
Other Lipoprotein Disorders 1034
Abetalipoproteinemia 1034
Hypobetalipoproteinemia 1035
Chylomicron Retention Disease 1036
Familial Lecithin Cholesterol Acyltransferase Deficiency 1036
Smith-Lemli-Opitz Syndrome 1037
Sterol Storage Diseases 1037
Atherosclerosis 1037
Xanthomas 1038
Acid Cholesteryl Ester Hydrolase Deficiency 1038
Familial Diseases with Storage of Sterols Other Than Cholesterol 1039
Cerebrotendinous Xanthomatosis (CTX) 1039
Sitosterolemia and Xanthomatosis 1040
Dietary Treatment of Hyperlipidemia 1042
The Effects of Specific Nutrients on the Plasma Lipids and Lipoproteins 1042
A Phased Approach to the Dietary Treatment of Hyperlipidemia 1050
Pharmaceutical Agents for the Treatment of Hyperlipoproteinemia 1053
Bile Acid Sequestrants 1054
Nicotinic Acid 1055
HMG CoA Reductase Inhibitors 1056
Probucol 1059
Clofibrate 1059

Gemfibrozil 1060
Fenofibrate 1060
Miscellaneous Agents 1060
Future Advances 1061
The Surgical Treatment of Hyperlipoproteinemia 1062
Treatment of Special Patient Populations 1062
Hyperlipidemia in Women 1062
Hyperlipidemia in Older Patients 1063
Hyperlipidemia in Children 1063
Hyperlipidemia in Patients with Diabetes 1063
Laboratory Tests in the Diagnosis of Hyperlipidemias 1064
Collection and Handling of the Sample 1064
Lipid Determinations 1064
Lipoprotein Separations 1064
Additional Laboratory Tests 1065
References 1065

PART VII CALCIUM AND BONE METABOLISM 1077

22 Mineral Metabolism 1079
Jan M. Bruder, Theresa A. Guise, and Gregory R. Mundy
Cellular and Extracellular Calcium Metabolism 1079
Parathyroid Hormone 1081
Anatomy and Embryology of the Parathyroid Glands Anatomy 1081
Biosynthesis, Processing, and Secretion of Parathyroid Hormone Physiology of Parathyroid Hormone Secretion 1081
Metabolism of Parathyroid Hormone 1086
Assay of Parathyroid Hormone 1086
Biological Effects and Mechanism of Action of Parathyroid Hormone 1088
Calcitonin 1093
Introduction and Historical Notes 1093
Biological Effects and Mechanism of Action 1094
Biochemistry and Molecular Biology 1095
Calcitonin as a Therapeutic Agent 1098
Vitamin D 1098
Historical Introduction 1098
Biosynthesis and Chemistry 1099
Absorption, Activation, and Transport of Vitamin D 1100
Further Metabolism of $1\alpha,25\text{-}(OH)_2D$ 1103
Vitamin D Nutrition 1104
Cellular Basis of Vitamin D Action 1105
Actions of Vitamin D in Intestine, Bone, and Kidney 1105
Hypercalcemia 1109
Introduction 1109
The Defense Against Hypercalcemia 1109
Approach to the Hypercalcemic Patient 1111
Primary Hyperparathyroidism 1112
Malignancy-Associated Hypercalcemia and Osteolysis 1125
Other Hypercalcemic Disorders 1136
Hypocalcemia 1139
Clinical Features of Hypocalcemia 1140
Hyperparathyroidism 1141
Pseudohypoparathyroidism 1143
Autosomal Dominant Hypocalcemia 1147
Vitamin D Abnormalities 1148
Medications 1149
Hypocalcemia Associated with Malignant Disease 1149
Other Diseases Associated with Hypocalcemia 1150
Approach to the Hypocalcemic Patient 1150

Disorders of Phosphate Metabolism 1152
Phosphate Homeostasis 1152
Disorders Causing Hypophosphatemia 1154
Treatment 1156
Disorders Causing Hyperphosphatemia 1156
Disorders of Magnesium Metabolism 1157
Magnesium Balance 1158
Hypomagnesemia 1158
Hypermagnesemia 1159
Acknowledgments 1159
References 1159

23 Metabolic Bone Disease **1179**
Frederick R. Singer
Clinical Evaluation of Metabolic Bone Disease 1179
History and Physical Examination 1179
Routine Clinical Chemistry 1179
Biochemical Markers of Bone Turnover 1180
Radiology and Nuclear Medicine 1180
Bone Biopsy 1181
Osteomalacia and Rickets 1182
Clinical Presentation 1182
Bone Pathology 1184
Classification and Pathogenesis 1184
Vitamin D Abnormalities 1184
Hypophosphatemia 1186
Miscellaneous 1187
Treatment 1188
Osteoporosis 1189
Clinical Presentation 1189
Bone Pathology 1191
Classification and Pathogenesis 1191
Prevention of Osteoporosis 1195
Treatment of Established Osteoporosis 1196
Osteopetrosis 1198
Renal Osteodystrophy 1199
Clinical Presentation 1199
Bone Pathology 1200
Pathogenesis 1200
Treatment 1201
Hereditary Hyperphosphatasia 1201
Fibrous Dysplasia 1202
Paget's Disease of Bone 1203
Clinical Presentation 1204
Bone Pathology 1205
Pathogenesis 1206
Drug Treatment 1207
Biochemical and Radiological Monitoring of Therapy 1210
Surgery 1210
References 1210

24 Nephrolithiasis **1221**
Bruce Ettinger
Introduction 1221
Epidemiology 1221
Classification of Calculi by Clinical Presentation 1221
Classification of Calculi by Crystalline Structure 1221
Quantitating Clinical Stone Events 1222
Theories of Stone Pathogenesis 1222

Physicochemical Aspects of Stone Formation *1223*
Evaluation and Treatment *1223*
Cystinuria 1227
History *1227*
Genetics *1228*
Pathophysiology *1228*
Dependence of Cystine Solubility on Urinary pH *1228*
Dependence of Cystine Excretion on Salt Intake *1228*
Effect of Cysteine-Complexing Agents *1228*
Clinical Findings *1229*
Clinical Evaluation *1229*
Treatment *1230*
Uric Acid Stones 1231
Epidemiology *1231*
Purine Metabolism and Uric Acid Excretion *1232*
Uric Acid Solubility in Urine *1232*
Risk Factors for Uric Acid Stones *1232*
Effect of Diet on Urinary pH and Uric Acid Excretion *1232*
Gout and Uric Acid Stones *1232*
Other Clinical Disorders Associated with Uric Acid Stones *1233*
Differentiating Uric Acid from Other Purine-Related Stones *1233*
Mechanisms of the Effect of Allopurinol on Uric Acid *1233*
Efficacy of Medical Treatment of Uric Acid Lithiasis *1233*
Evaluation *1234*
Therapy *1234*
Calcium Phosphate Stones 1235
Crystalline Forms of Calcium Phosphate *1235*
Effect of pH on Solubility of Calcium Phosphate *1235*
Renal Tubular Acidosis *1235*
Pathophysiology of Stone Disease in Renal Tubular Acidosis *1235*
Incomplete Renal Tubular Acidosis *1235*
Evaluation *1236*
Treatment *1236*
Magnesium Ammonium Phosphate Stones 1236
Terminology *1236*
History and Epidemiology *1236*
Pathophysiology *1236*
Bacteriology *1237*
Clinical Risk Factors *1237*
Serious Morbidity from MAP Stones *1237*
Evaluation *1237*
Treatment *1237*
Calcium Oxalate and Mixed Calcium Stones 1238
Epidemiology *1238*
Physical Chemistry *1238*
Natural History of Calcium Oxalate Lithiasis *1239*
Risk Factors *1239*
Evaluation of Calcium Oxalate Stones *1251*
Treatment of Calcium Oxalate Nephrolithiasis *1252*
Closing Comments 1255
Acknowledgments *1256*
References 1256

PART VIII MISCELLANEOUS DISORDERS 1263

25 Disorders of Growth and Development 1265
Margaret H. MacGillivray

Biological Stages of Growth *1265*
Control of Growth Processes *1265*

Genetic Factors *1265*
Peptide Growth Factors and Hormonal Influences *1266*
Insulin-Like Growth Factors *1266*
Hormonal Regulation *1272*
Nutrition *1279*
Physiology of Skeletal Growth 1279
Developmental Stages 1280
Intrauterine Life *1280*
Infancy: Birth to 2 Years of Age *1280*
Childhood *1281*
Adolescence *1281*
Short Stature 1282
Clinical Approach to Short Stature *1282*
Causes of Short Stature *1285*
Growth Excess 1302
Normal Variants *1302*
Pathologic Overgrowth *1303*
Appendix: Details of Testing Procedures in Children 1309
Pituitary-Hypothalamic Evaluation *1309*
Adrenal Function Tests *1310*
References 1311

26 Gastrointestinal Hormones and Carcinoid Syndrome **1317**
Pradip K. Ghosh and Thomas M. O'Dorisio

Localization and Distribution of GI Peptides 1317
Regulation, Biological Actions and Clinical Applications 1319
Somatostatin *1319*
Gastrin *1322*
Cholecystokinin *1325*
Secretin *1326*
Vasoactive Intestinal Polypeptide *1327*
Gastric Inhibitory Polypeptide (Glucose-Dependent Insulinotropic Peptide) *1328*
Motilin *1329*
Pancreatic Polypeptide Family *1330*
Neurotensin *1331`*
Substance P *1332*
Galanin *1333*
Carcinoid Syndrome 1333
Pathology *1334*
Symptoms *1335*
Pathophysiology and Mediators of the Carcinoid Syndrome *1335*
Diagnosis *1337*
Differential Diagnosis *1338*
Treatment *1338*
Prognosis *1340*
Acknowledgment *1340*
References 1340

27 Multiglandular Endocrine Disorders **1355**
Leonard J. Deftos, Stephen I. Sherman, and Robert F. Gagel

Multiple Endocrine Neoplasia Type 1 (Men 1) 1355
Definition and History *1355*
Components of the Syndrome *1355*
Clinical Evaluation *1359*
Epidemiology *1360*
MEN in Other Species *1360*
Pathogenesis *1360*
Diagnosis *1361*

Relation to Other Syndromes 1362
Management 1362
Multiple Endocrine Neoplasia Type 2 (MEN 2) 1363
Individual Components of the MEN 2A Syndrome and Their Management 1365
Medullary Thyroid Carcinoma 1365
Calcitonin Gene Products and Screening for the Tumor 1366
Other Tumor Products 1367
Genetic Testing for Multiple Endocrine Neoplasia Type 2A or Familial Medullary Thyroid Carcinoma 1367
Pheochromocytomia 1368
Hyperparathyroidism 1369
Mulitple Endocrine Neoplasia Type 2A with Cutaneous Lichen Amyloidosis 1371
MEN 2A with Hirschsprung Disease 1371
Multiple Endocrine Neoplasia Type 2B 1371
Polyglandular Endocrine Insufficiency Syndromes 1373
Clinical Manifestations 1373
Genetics and Pathogenesis 1375
Diagnosis and Treatment 1375
Nonautoimmune Polyglandular Deficiency Syndromes 1376
Crow-Fukase Syndrome 1376
References 1376

28 Ectopic Hormone Production 1383
Glenn D. Braunstein
General Principles 1383
Paraneoplastic Syndromes 1383
Eutopic versus Ectopic Hormone Production 1383
Importance of Ectopic Hormone Production 1384
Criteria for Ectopic Hormone Production 1386
Frequency of Ectopic Hormone Production 1387
Etiology of Ectopic Hormone Production 1390
Therapy 1392
Hormones as Tumor Markers 1392
Specific Syndromes 1394
Hypercalcemia of Malignancy 1394
Ectopic POMC/ACTH Syndrome 1400
Syndrome of Inappropriate Antidiuresis in Cancer 1404
Hypoglycemia Associated with Malignancy 1406
Oncogenic Osteomalacia 1409
Ectopic Growth Hormone and Growth Hormone Releasing Hormone Production 1410
Ectopic Production of Placental Proteins 1412
Paraneoplastic Erythrocytosis 1413
Ectopic Production of Calcitonin 1414
Other Hormones Produced by Tumors 1414
References 1415

29 Hormone-Responsive Tumors 1427
Andrea Manni
Hormonal Influence on Normal Breast Development and Mammary Carcinogenesis 1427
Role of Growth Factors and Stromal/Epithelial Interactions 1428
Genetic Changes in Hormone-Responsive Tumors 1429
Epidemiology of Hormone-Responsive Tumors 1433
Endocrine Mechanisms Controlling the Growth of Hormone-Dependent Tumors 1434
Mechanisms of Tumor Progression 1436

Clinical Characteristics of Hormone-Responsive Cancers 1439
Breast Cancer 1439
Endometrial Cancer 1443
Prostate Cancer 1444
References 1447

30 Hormones, Aging, and Endocrine Disorders in the Elderly 1455
John E. Morley
Theories of Aging 1458
Hormonal Changes 1460
Growth Hormone and IGF-I 1460
Prolactin 1461
Hypothalamic-Pituitary-Thyroid Axis 1461
Hypothalamic-Pituitary-Adrenal Axis 1462
Sex Hormones 1463
Hormones Associated with Water Metabolism 1465
Frailty, Hormones, and Aging 1465
Growth Hormone 1466
Testosterone 1466
Estrogens 1467
Vitamin D, Type II (Age-Related) Osteopenia, and Hip Fracture 1467
Sexuality and Aging 1466
Males 1470
Females 1471
Diabetes Mellitus 1471
Hypoglycemia of Aging 1472
Should Blood Glucose Be Controlled in Older Individuals? 1472
Special Features in the Management of Older Diabetics 1472
Diet in Older Diabetics 1472
Oral Hypoglycemia Agents 1473
Insulin 1473
Monitoring Treatment 1473
Diabetes in Nursing Home Residents 1474
Summary 1474
Leptin 1474
Nutritional Disorders 1474
Conclusion 1476
References 1476

31 Hormones and Athletic Performance 1483
David C. Cumming
Energy Supply and Physical Work 1483
Evaluating Hormonal Response to Exercise and Training 1483
Effects of Physical Activity and Training on Endocrine Function 1484
Endocrine Regulation of Fluid Balance During Physical Work 1484
Arginine, Vasopressin, Exercise, and Training 1484
Aldosterone, Exercise, and Training 1484
Gastrointestinal Hormones in Training and Exercise 1485
Metabolic Control in Exercise and Training: TSH-Thyroid Axis 1485
Acute Responses 1485
Effect of Training 1485
Glucoregulation in Training and Exercise: Insulin and Glucagon in Exercise 1486
Insulin and Exercise 1486
Glucagon and Exercise 1486
Growth Hormone in Exercise 1486
ACTH-Cortisol Axis 1488
Exercise and the ACTH-Cortisol Axis 1488

The Effect of Physical Training *1488*
Physiologic Significance *1489*
Control Mechanisms *1489*
Catecholamines in Exercise 1489
Epinephrine and Norepinephrine *1489*
Control of Catecholamine Release *1489*
Dopamine Responses to Exercise *1490*
Effects of Training *1490*
Effects of Catecholamine Release *1490*
Endogenous Opiates in Exercise and Training 1490
Response to Acute Physical Activity *1490*
Physiologic Significance of the Exercise-Associated Opiate Increase *1491*
Summary *1492*
Prolactin and Exercise 1492
Effects of Training on Prolactin *1492*
Mechanisms *1493*
Exercise, Training, and the Hypothalamic-Pituitary-Gonadal Axis 1493
Acute Exercise and the HPG Axis in Men *1493*
Short-Term Exercise and the HPG Axis *1493*
Mechanism of Exercise-Associated Testosterone Increase *1494*
The Effects of Prolonged Exercise on the HPG Axis in Men *1494*
Effect of Endurance Training on thc HPG Axis in Men *1495*
Symptomatic Impairment of the HPG Axis in Men *1495*
Mechanisms of Long-Term Activity-Associated Suppression of Circulating Testosterone Levels *1495*
Exercise and the Reproductive System in Women 1496
Acute Exercise-Associated Changes in Reproductive Hormones *1496*
Reproductive Effects of Exercise in Women *1496*
The Endocrinology of Exercise-Associated Reproductive Dysfunction *1497*
Body Composition and Nutrition *1497*
Summary *1498*
Overtraining 1498
Use of Performance-Enhancing Endocrine Drugs (Doping) in Competitive and Recreational Sports Activity 1499
Mens Sana in Corpore Sano: Ethical Aspects of Doping in Sports *1499*
Androgenic-Anabolic Steroids *1500*
Other Ergogenic Aids 1504
Growth Hormone *1504*
Erythropoietin *1504*
References 1504

INDEX **1521**

Color plates appear between pages 830 & 831.

Contributors

John M. Amatruda, M.D. [20]
Vice President of Research
Bayer Corporation
Adjunct Professor of Medicine
Yale University School of Medicine
New Haven, Connecticut

John Baxter, M.D. [13]
Professor of Medicine
Chief, Division of Endocrinology
Metabolic Research Unit
Department of Medicine
University of California
San Francisco Medical Center
San Francisco, California

Glenn D. Braunstein, M.D. [28]
Professor of Medicine
University of California, Los Angeles School of Medicine
Chairman, Department of Medicine
Cedars-Sinai Medical Center
Los Angeles, California

Jan M. Bruder, M.D. [22]
Assistant Professor of Medicine
Director, Osteoporosis & Metabolic Bone Disease Clinic
University of Texas Health Sciences Center at San Antonio
San Antonio, Texas

Henry G. Burger, M.D., A.O., F.R.A.C.P., F.A.A. [16B]
Honorary Professor of Medicine
Monash University
Emeritus Director
Prince Henry's Institute of Medical Research
Monash Medical Center
Clayton, Victoria, Australia

Gerard N. Burrow, M.D. [10]
David Paige Smith Professor of Medicine
Professor of Obstetrics and Gynecology
Yale University School of Medicine
New Haven, Connecticut

Eurico Cagliero, M.D. [18]
Assistant Professor of Medicine
Harvard Medical School
Assistant in Medicine
Massachusetts General Hospital Diabetes Unit
Boston, Massachusetts

George P. Chrousos, M.D., F.A.A.P., F.A.C.P. [11, 14]
Chief, Section on Pediatric Endocrinology
Chief, Pediatric and Reproductive Endocrinology Branch
Director, Pediatric Endocrinology Training Program
National Institute od Child Health and Human Development
National Institutes of Health
Bethesda, Maryland

William E. Connor, M.D. [21]
Professor of Medicine
Oregon Health Sciences University
Portland, Oregon

Robert M. Couch, M.D., F.R.C.P. [17]
Associate Professor
Department of Pediatrics
University of Alberta
Head, Division of Pediatric Endocrinology
Stollery Children's Health Center
Edmonton, Alberta, Canada

Philip E. Cryer, M.D. [12]
Irene and Michael M. Karl Professor of Endocrinology and Metabolism
Director, Division of Endocrinology, Diabetes, and Metabolism
Washington University School of Medicine
Physician
Barne-Jewish Hospital
St. Louis, Missouri

David C. Cumming, M.B.Ch.B. [31]
Professor
Departments of Obstetrics & Gynecology and Medicine
University of Alberta
Royal Alexandria Hospital
Edmonton, Alberta, Canada

Leonard J. Deftos, M.D. [27]
Professor of Medicine
University of California, San Diego School of Medicine
La Jolla, California
San Diego Veterans Administration Medical Center
San Diego, California

P. Barton Duell, M.D. [21]
Associate Professor of Medicine
Director, Metabolic Disorders Clinic
Oregon Health Sciences University
Portland, Oregon

Gregory F. Erickson, Ph.D. [16A]
Professor
Department of Reproductive Medicine
University of California, San Diego School of Medicine
La Jolla, California

Bruce Ettinger, M.D. [24]
Clinical Professor of Medicine and Radiology
University of California, San Francisco Medical Center
San Francisco, California
Senior Investigator
Kaiser Permanente Medical Care Program
Oakland, California

Robert F. Gagel, M.D. [27]
Professor of Medicine
Head, Division of Internal Medicine (ad interim)
MD Anderson Cancer Center
Houston, Texas

Gordon N. Gill, M.D. [3]
Professor of Medicine
Department of Endocrinology and Metabolism
University of California, San Diego
La Jolla, California

Pradip K. Gosh, M.D. [26]
Research Scientist
Division of Endocrinology
Department of Internal Medicine
Ohio State University School of Medicine
Columbus, Ohio

Theresa A. Guise, M.D. [22]
Associate Professor
Department of Medicine/Endocrinology
University of Texas Health Sciences Center at San Antonio
San Antonio, Texas

Marwan Hamaty, M.D. [13]
Division of Endocrinology, Metabolism, Diabetes, and Hypertension
State University of New York
Health Sciences Center
Brooklyn, New York

David L. Healy, Ph.D., F.R.A.N.Z.C.O.G., C.R.E.I. [16B]
Chairman and Head, Reproductive Biology Unit
Monash Medical Center
Monash University
Clayton, Victoria, Australia

Jerome M. Hershman, M.D. [5]
Professor of Medicine
University of California, Los Angeles
Chief, Division of Endocrinology & Metabolism
Veterans Administration Greater Los Angeles Health Care System
Veterans Administration Medical Center
Los Angeles, California

Willa A. Hsueh, M.D. [13]
Professor of Medicine
Chief, Division of Endocrinology, Diabetes, and Hypertension
Department of Medicine
University of California, Los Angeles Medical Center
Los Angeles, California

D. Roger Illingworth, M.D., Ph.D. [21]
Division of Endocrinology
Oregon Health Sciences University
Portland, Oregon

Randal C. Jaffe, Ph.D. [4]
Professor of Physiology and Biophysics
University of Illinois at Chicago College of Medicine
Chicago, Illinois

Barbara K. Kinder, M.D. [10]
William H. Carmalt Professor of Surgery
Yale University School of Medicine
Attending Surgeon
Yale-New Haven Hospital
New Haven, Connecticut

David L. Linemeyer, Ph.D. [20]
Director, Obesity Research
Bayer Corporation
New Haven, Connecticut

Margaret H. MacGillivray, M.D. [25]
Professor of Pediatrics
School of Medicine and Biomedical Sciences
State University of New York at Buffalo
Chief, Division of Endocrinology and Diabetes
Buffalo Children's Hospital
Buffalo, New York

Andrea Manni, M.D. [29]
Department of Medicine
Section of Endocrinology, Diabetes, and Metabolism
Penn State Geisinger Health System
The Milton S. Hershey Medical Center
Pennsylvania State University College of Medicine
Hershey, Pennsylvania

Alvin M. Matsumoto, M.D. [15]
Chief of Gerontology
Professor
Department of Medicine
Veterans Administration Medical Center
Seattle, Washington

Walter L. Miller, M.D. [11]
Professor
Department of Pediatrics
University of California, San Francisco
San Francisco, California

Mark E. Molitch, M.D. [6]
Professor of Medicine
Northwestern University Medical School
Attending Physician
Center for Endocrinology, Metabolism, and Molecular Medicine
Northwestern Memorial Hospital
Chicago, Illinois

John E. Morley, M.B., Bch. [30]
Director, Division of Geriatric Medicine
St. Louis University School of Medicine
Director, Geriatrics Research Education and Clinical Center
St. Louis Veterans Administration Medical Center
St. Louis, Missouri

Gregory R. Mundy, M.D. [22]
Heyser Professor of Bone & Mineral Metabolism
Head, Division of Endocrinology
University of Texas Health Sciences Center at San Antonio
San Antonio, Texas

David M. Nathan, M.D. [18]
Professor of Medicine
Harvard Medical School
Director, Diabetes Center
Director, General Clinic Research Center
Massachusetts General Hospital
Boston, Massachusetts

Suzanne B. Nicholas, M.D., Ph. D. [13]
Assistant Professor of Medicine
Co-Director, Center for Cholesterol, Lipid, and Hypertension Management
University of California School of Medicine
Los Angeles, California

Thomas M. O'Dorisio, M.D. [26]
Professor of Medicine
Division of Endocrinology and Metabolism
University of Iowa School of Medicine
Attending Physician, Department of Medicine
Veterans Administration Medical Center
University of Iowa Hospitals
Iowa City, Iowa

A. Eugene Pekary, Ph.D. [5]
Adjunct Professor of Medicine
University of California, Los Angeles
Supervisory Research Chemist
Veterans Administration Greater Los Angeles Health Care System
Los Angeles, California

Mark M. Rasenick, Ph.D. [4]
Professor of Physiology and Biophysics
Psychiatry Director
Biomedical Neuroscience Training Program
University of Illinois at Chicago College of Medicine
Chicago, Illinois

Gary L. Robertson, M.D. [8]
Professor of Medicine and Neurology
Northwestern University Medical School
Program Director, General Clinical Research Center
Northwestern Memorial Hospital
Chicago, Illinois

Harry Shamoon, M.D. [19]
Professor of Medicine
Program Director, General Clinical Research Center, Diabetes Research Center
Albert Einstein College of Medicine
Bronx, New York

Stephen I. Sherman, M.D. [27]
Associate Professor
Chief, Section of Endocrine Neoplasia and Hormonal Disorders
MD Anderson Cancer Center
Houston, Texas

Frederick R. Singer, M.D. [23]
Director
Endocrine/Bone Disease Program
John Wayne Cancer Center Institute
Santa Monica, California
Clinical Professor of Medicine
University of California, Los Angeles
Los Angeles, California

Peter J. Snyder, M.D. [7]
Professor of Medicine
Division of Endocrinology
University of Pennsylvania School of Medicine
Philadelphia, Pennsylvania

James Sowers, M.D. [13]
Professor of Medicine and Cell Biology
Chief, Endocrinology, Metabolism, Diabetes, and Hypertension
State University of New York
Health Sciences Center
Brooklyn, New York

Robert D. Utiger, M.D. [9]
Clinical Professor of Medicine
Harvard Medical School
Attending Physician
Brigham and Women's Hospital
Deputy Editor, *The New England Journal of Medicine*
Boston, Massachusetts

Beverly J. Vollenhoven, Ph.D., F.R.A.N.Z.C.O.G., C.R.E.I. [16B]
Senior Lecturer
Department of Obetetrics and Gynecology
Monash University
Monash Medical Center
Clayton, Victoria, Australia

Jeremy S. D. Winter, M.D. [17]
Saltspring Island, British Columbia, Canada

Preface

In the six years that have elapsed since the publication of the Third Edition of *Endocrinology and Metabolism*, an enormous increase in our knowledge of basic concepts of cellular and molecular biology, genetics, and intracellular signaling mechanisms has occurred. This has resulted in a marked enhancement of our understanding of the etiology and pathophysiology of endocrine and metabolic disorders and our approach to diagnosis and treatment. The pharmacologic management of a variety of disorders has also been broadened (e.g., diabetes mellitus, polycystic ovary syndrome). This increase in our knowledge base has heightened the challenge of providing a textbook that properly balances a discussion of basic principles with the details of diagnosis and management of disease entities.

As in the previous editions, we have attempted to achieve this balance between basic science and clinical management in a manner that is useful for the clinical endocrinologist, as well as the research-oriented scholar and trainee in endocrinology. To accomplish this goal, many chapters in the present edition have been extensively revised and others have been entirely rewritten. In addition to blending basic science and clinical management in the chapters dealing with specific disorders, we have retained the format of an introductory series of chapters. These deal with general principles of the organization and the molecular and cellular biology of the endocrine system, the clinical presentations of endocrine disease, and the principles of endocrine testing.

We are grateful to our contributors for the enormity and the excellence of their efforts. We acknowledge with special thanks the contribution and support of our colleagues at McGraw-Hill, Martin Wonsiewicz, Publisher, and Susan Noujaim, Development Editor.

Philip Felig, M.D.
Lawrence A. Frohman, M.D.

PART I

General Endocrinology

CHAPTER 1

Introduction to the Endocrine System

Lawrence A. Frohman
Philip Felig

DEFINITIONS AND SCOPE OF ENDOCRINOLOGY

The endocrine system, along with the nervous system, has evolved to provide mechanisms for communication between cells and organs. Such systems have been critical for the development and function of multicellular organisms that, in higher species such as humans, have rather sophisticated control mechanisms. These systems regulate and thus permit growth and development, reproduction, metabolic homeostasis, and responses to changes in the environment such as provocative stimuli and stress.

The term *endocrine* refers to the process of the secretion of biologically active substances into the body. This contrasts with the term *exocrine*, which refers to external secretion, generally via anatomically identifiable ducts, such as into the gastrointestinal tract. As the term is ordinarily used, an endocrine gland or cell is one that secretes substances, referred to as *hormones*, that exert regulatory functions, typically in cells other than those in which they are produced. The term *hormone* is derived from a Greek verb meaning "to set in motion." In a classical sense, a hormone is a substance that is secreted by one cell and travels through the circulation, where it exerts actions on other cells (Fig. 1-1).

In order to act, hormones must interact with a docking mechanism on or in the target cell. These sites are termed *receptors* (Chap. 4). Thus, a receptor is a molecule to which the hormone binds to elicit its actions. A receptor has two functions. First, it must be able to distinguish the hormone from all the other chemicals present in the circulation and bind it. A receptor must be capable of binding the hormone with great affinity and also must not bind extraneous substances. The hormone-binding sites on receptors have evolved to include unique configurations that are complementary to the hormones they bind. In general, these hormone-receptor interactions are noncovalent in nature and are reversible. Second, the receptor must be able to transmit the information gained from the binding to trigger a cellular response. Thus, substances that bind hormones, even tightly, but do not trigger subsequent responses are not receptors; examples include *transport proteins* (discussed later in the chapter) and the enzymes involved in hormone biosynthesis or metabolism (see Chap. 3).

These simple distinctions serve to define endocrinology, receptors, and hormones in most cases. Thus, for example, insulin (Chap. 18) is secreted from an endocrine gland, the pancreatic islets; travels in the circulation; and associates with insulin receptors present on most tissues, where the interaction triggers numerous responses involved in regulating the metabolism of carbohydrates, lipids, and proteins. Parathyroid hormone (PTH) (Chap. 22) is synthesized in and released from the parathyroid glands, travels through the circulatory system, and binds to multiple target tissues, where it regulates calcium homeostasis. In addition to these clear examples, there are numerous others in which the distinctions may appear to be less precise. In most cases, however, these seeming discrepancies are more apparent than real.

A major area of overlap in terms of the function of regulatory molecules involves the nervous system, and an entire discipline—neuroendocrinology—has evolved to address the relationship between the nervous and endocrine systems (Fig. 1-1). This is discussed in detail in Chap. 6. Overall, the nervous system has evolved to release regulatory substances from nerve terminals that act across synaptic junctions on adjacent cells. These substances, or *neurotransmitters*, may travel considerable distances to act, but when they do so, this generally occurs along the axons (Fig. 1-1). Acetylcholine, enkephalins, catecholamines, and dopamine are well-known neurotransmitters.

The brain is also an endocrine gland (Chap. 6; Fig. 1-1). It is the major source of some hormones. The hypothalamic releasing hormones or factors include thyrotropin releasing hormone (TRH), corticotropin releasing hormone (CRH), growth hormone-releasing hormone (GHRH), gonadotropin releasing hormone (GnRH), somatostatin, and dopamine. All are produced in the hypothalamus and travel through the hypophysial portal system to stimulate or inhibit the synthesis and release of pituitary hormones. Some of the hormones of the anterior pituitary (Chap. 7) and all those of the posterior pituitary (Chap. 8) are also synthesized in the hypothalamus.

Because both the nervous and endocrine systems evolved to use various ligands to serve their regulatory functions, it is not surprising that the same or related ligands can function both as neurotransmitters and as hormones. Thus, both norepinephrine, secreted from nerve endings, and epinephrine, secreted from the adrenal medulla, act through adrenergic receptors (Chap. 12). Dopamine is a neurotransmitter that is also active after it travels through the circulation. The brain produces numerous other hormones (Chap. 6). Prolactin, growth hormone, pro-opiomelanocortin (POMC), renin, and atrial natriuretic factor are examples of brain hormones, though brain production probably contributes negligibly to the circulating levels of these substances. Therefore, if they exhibit biological activity (something not yet fully established), they probably play a local role in regulation. If this is true, they may serve as neurotransmitters. How can these

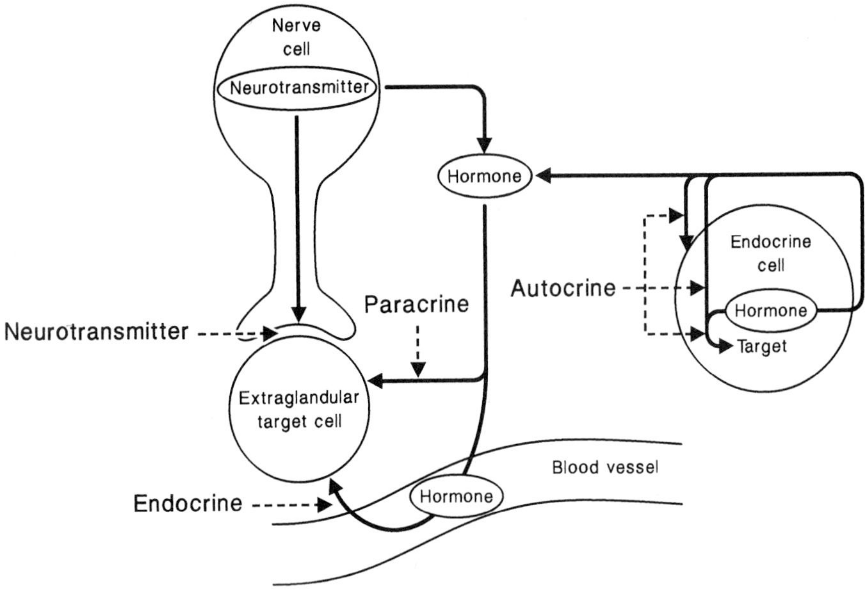

FIGURE 1-1. Distinctions between the endocrine and nervous systems and between the various types of hormone action: hormone (endocrine), neurocrine, paracrine, and autocrine. See the text for details.

overlaps be resolved in terms of definition? For the most part, the answers are simple. If a given ligand is released into the circulation to act, it is a hormone; if it is released from a nerve terminal to act locally, it is a neurotransmitter. The same substance can therefore serve as both a neurotransmitter and a hormone.

The nervous and endocrine systems are also related in other ways. In many cases the function of endocrine glands is controlled by the autonomic nervous system. Glands such as the pituitary, pancreatic islets, renal juxtaglomerular cells, and the adrenal respond to neural stimulation. Again, while the overlaps are obvious, the definitions can still be simple, and the same cell can function as both an endocrine cell and a nerve cell.

The designation of endocrine tissue has, of necessity, broadened with recent advances in the understanding of endocrinology: some tissues are specialized specifically as endocrine glands, while others also serve additional functions. Examples of the first type include the thyroid, pituitary, parathyroid, and adrenal glands and the pancreatic islets. The central nervous system, in contrast, serves other functions, and the ovaries and testes, in addition to producing hormones, also produce oocytes and sperm, respectively. The atrium of the heart produces atrial natriuretic factor (Chap. 13); the liver, insulin-like growth factor I (IGF-I; also called somatomedin C; Chap. 25) and angiotensinogen (the precursor to angiotensin II; Chap. 13); the kidney, erythropoietin[1] and the active form of vitamin D_3 (1,25-$[OH]_2$-cholecalciferol; Chap. 22); the gastrointestinal tract, gastrin, somatostatin, cholecystokinin, and others (Chap. 26); and cells of the immune system, numerous hormones such as interleukins, interferons, ACTH, and tumor necrosis factor.[2,3]

Do hormones need to travel through the circulation to act? No. Locally released hormones can act on cells in the immediate vicinity of their release (Fig. 1-1). Growth factors can be released in tissues such as bone (Chap. 23). Somatostatin is released by the pancreatic delta cells and has the potential to suppress insulin release by beta cells and glucagon release by alpha cells (Chap. 18). Prostaglandins and other eicosanoids are, in all likelihood, released to act on cells in their immediate vicinity. This type of intracellular communication has been termed *paracrine* and thus has been incorporated into the general discipline of endocrinology (Fig. 1-1).

Hormones can also act on the cells in which they are produced. This type of communication has been termed *autocrine* (Fig. 1-1). Such actions are probably important in cancer cells. Certain oncogenes encode analogs of growth factors or their receptors that enhance the progression of the malignant state.[4–6] Insulin has an inhibitory effect on its own secretion, independent of changes in blood glucose levels (Chap. 18).

Still other examples can be cited in which semantic distinctions become blurred and overlaps occur between endocrinology and other disciplines. For example, renin of renal origin is ordinarily considered a hormone, but rather than acting on other cell types, it functions as an enzyme in the bloodstream to release angiotensin I from its substrate, angiotensinogen (Chap. 13). The regulators of the immune response, such as the interleukins,[2,3] the growth factors (Chap. 25), erythropoietin,[1] and other factors, function both as hormones and in paracrine or autocrine regulation but are ordinarily not considered hormones even though they should be.

Because common clinical problems in endocrinology are due either to an excess or to a deficiency of a hormone, it is not surprising that classically, endocrinology was signal-level-oriented, with the dominant consideration being how much or how little of the hormone was present. Over time, the signal-level consideration has been expanded to include secretory reserve. For example, the diagnosis of adrenal insufficiency is based not on a random measurement of plasma cortisol in the unstressed state but on the extent to which cortisol can be released in response to provocative stimuli (Chap. 11). Increasingly, attention has also been focused on the response limb of the endocrine system. In interpreting the significance of a hormone's concentration in the blood, it is equally critical to know how sensitive the target cells are to that hormone. Some syndromes have features of hormone deficiency in the presence of elevated or normal hormone levels that are due to decreased responsiveness to hormones. Pseudohypoparathyroidism (Chap. 22), testicular feminization (Chap. 15), generalized thyroid hormone resistance (Chap. 9), vitamin D–resistant rickets (Chap. 23), Laron-type dwarfism (Chap. 25), and type II diabetes mellitus (Chap. 18) are examples. Rarely recognized are states that include features of hormone excess and normal to low hormone levels. A group of patients with the stigmata of primary aldosteronism and low plasma levels of aldosterone (Chap. 13) may fit this model. In low-renin essential hypertension, there may be an isolated feature of hormone hyperresponsiveness with increased sensitivity of adrenal glomerulosa aldosterone production to angiotensin II (Chap. 13). Normoprolactinemic galactorrhea is believed to result from increased breast sensitivity to prolactin (Chap. 7). The diseases cited are due predominantly to specific genetic defects. In addition, cellular sensitivity to hormones is extensively regulated by the same (homologous) hormone and by other factors (Chap. 4); the most common feature is negative regulation of responsiveness by the homologous hormone. It is especially important to utilize this information when one is administering hormone therapy for endocrine or other diseases.

TYPES OF HORMONES AND THEIR SYNTHESIS AND RELEASE

A number of types of molecules have evolved to regulate body processes: peptides, lipids, and amino acid analogs all serve as hormones (Fig. 1-2). Sophisticated mechanisms have also evolved to synthesize these hormones. The types of hormones that exist and the mechanisms by which they are synthesized are discussed in detail in Chap. 3 and in the chapters on specific hormonal systems. These hormones and mechanisms of synthesis are discussed here only in outline form to provide perspective.

FIGURE 1-2. Evolution of the endocrine system. Genes encoding proteins that perform critical functions were duplicated. These duplicated genes then underwent rearrangements, deletions, mutations, and insertions, leading to derivative genes that perform the biosynthetic and regulatory functions of the endocrine system.

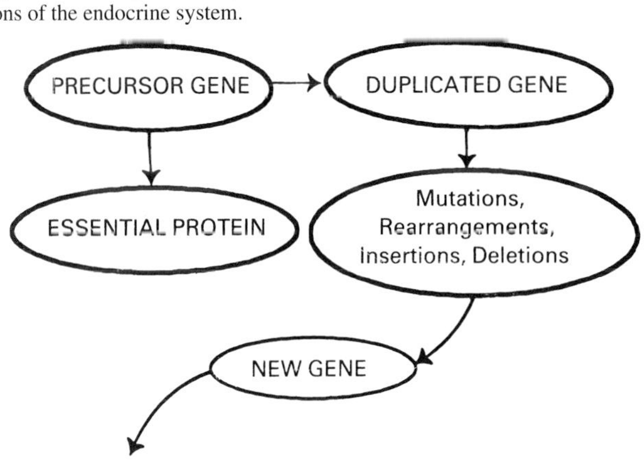

FUNCTION OF PRODUCT	EXAMPLES
Synthetic Enzyme	Cholesterol-Steroids Fatty Acids-Eiconsanoids Tyrosine-Catecholamines
Protease	Proinsulin-Insulin POMC-ACTH Thyroglobulin-Thyroxine
Hormone	Growth Hormone
Hormone Subunit	Glycoprotein Hormone α and β Subunits
Hormone Precursor	Proopiomelanocortin Prorenin
Receptor	Hormone Receptors
Modification Enzyme	Protein Kinases
Metabolizing Enzyme	Thyronine Iodinases

Peptide hormones vary in size, composition, number of chains, glycosylation, and mechanisms of production. Thus, whereas growth hormone is a single chain of 191 amino acids (Chaps. 7 and 25), TRH is a cyclized tripeptide with modified amino groups (Chaps. 3, 6, and 9). The glycoprotein hormones—thyroid stimulating hormone (TSH), luteinizing hormone (LH), follicle stimulating hormone (FSH), and chorionic gonadotropin (CG)—all have two peptide chains, one of which (α chain) is common to all, while the other (β chain) is unique for each member of the set (Chaps. 3 and 7). Insulin, in contrast, consists of two chains that are derived from a single gene product (preproinsulin) (Chaps. 3 and 18). Many hormones, such as corticotropin (ACTH; 39 amino acids), β-endorphin (29 amino acids), and insulin are proteolytic products of a larger precursor protein (Chaps. 3, 6, and 7). Some hormones (e.g., FSH) are glycosylated, whereas others (e.g., ACTH in humans) are not (Chap. 3).

The steroid hormones and prostaglandins are derived from two lipids, cholesterol and arachidonic acid, respectively (Chap. 3). They are synthesized through a series of reactions that modify their parent compounds.

The amino acid analogs include epinephrine, norepinephrine, dopamine (Chap. 12), and thyroid hormones (Chaps. 3 and 9), which are all derived from tyrosine, and 5-hydroxytryptamine, derived from tryptophan.

A variety of control mechanisms regulate hormone synthesis, release, and removal. In general, the fine-tuning of hormone levels is primarily influenced by production and release, with the removal mechanisms showing less variation. There are marked variations in the regulation of production and release. For example, the pancreatic beta cells can store several days' supply of insulin; the stimuli for insulin release (e.g., hyperglycemia) result in an early release that reflects the discharge of stored insulin, followed by a slower release associated with an increase in insulin production (Chap. 18). In contrast, there is little storage of steroid hormones, and the stimuli for release increase the production of new hormone that is released relatively rapidly (Chap. 3).

In general, the endocrine glands secrete the form of the hormone that is active in the target tissue. However, in a few instances metabolic conversion in peripheral tissues results in the final active form of the hormone. For example, testosterone, the major product of the testis, is converted to dihydrotestosterone in peripheral tissues (Chap. 15). The latter steroid is responsible for many (but not all) androgenic actions. Vitamin D, originating from the skin or diet, undergoes sequential hydroxylations in the liver and kidney to produce the final active hormone, 1,25-$(OH)_2$-cholecalciferol (Chap. 22). The major active thyroid hormone is triiodothyronine (T_3); the thyroid gland produces some T_3, but most of it is derived from monodeiodination of thyroxine (T_4) to T_3 in the peripheral tissues (Chap. 9).

CIRCULATION OF HORMONES

Released hormones may circulate in either a free or bound form (Chap. 3). Some hormones circulate predominantly free or loosely associated with other proteins, whereas others circulate mostly bound to proteins (Chap. 3). In the latter case, hormones are sequestered by transport proteins that bind them with high affinity. Thyroxine-binding globulin (TBG) binds thyroxine (Chap. 9), corticosteroid-binding globulin (CBG, or transcortin) binds cortisol (Chap. 11), sex hormone–binding globulin (SHBG) binds estradiol and testosterone (Chaps. 15 and 16), and several different IGF (insulin-like growth factor) binding proteins bind IGF (Chaps. 3 and 25). Much of the growth hormone in the circulation is bound by a growth hormone binding protein that is identical to the extracellular portion of the GH receptor (Chaps. 7 and 25). For the tightly bound hormones, >90 percent of the total hormone in the circulation is ordinarily bound. In contrast, for a hormone such as aldosterone (Chap. 11), for which there is no specific transport protein, about 50 percent of the hormone is in the circulation in a free state; the remainder is mostly loosely bound to albumin. The levels of the transport proteins can change under a variety of circumstances. For example, both TBG and CBG levels can be increased by estrogens. These changes can affect the total hormone levels, with important consequences for the clinical interpretation of measured hormone levels. Most of the other polypeptide hormones circulate predominantly in the free state (Chap. 3). A unique form of transport is observed with epidermal growth factor (EGF) and platelet-derived growth factor (PDGF), which are transported in platelets and released locally with platelet activation conditions (Chap. 3).

In general, it is the free rather than the plasma-bound hormone that is biologically active. Further, control systems that regulate hormone levels do so by adjusting the free hormone, with only secondary effects on the bound hormone. The functions of the plasma binding proteins are just beginning to be understood (Chap. 3 and individual chapters). In general, they are not required for the transport of the hormones, which are sufficiently soluble at physiologically active concentrations. An exception is cholesterol (usually not considered a hormone) that is transported in the plasma lipoproteins. The importance of hormone transport proteins is suggested by the fact that they are present in numerous species (even if their levels vary) and that, whereas genetic deficiencies in the proteins do occur, they tend not to result in a complete disappearance of the protein. Their major function may be to regulate hormone distribution to the various tissues. These proteins may also be important for the delivery of hormones to specialized sites. For example, CBG may help deliver cortisol to sites of inflammation (Chap. 11). IGF binding proteins may facilitate a continuous slow release of IGF-I that allows for its action without excessively down regulating the IGF-I receptors (Chap. 3). Plasma proteins also have a major effect in decreasing the rate of clearance of the hormone from the plasma; this may be important for stabilizing hormone levels when desired. For example, this may be advantageous with thyroxine, which has a half-life in the plasma of more than 7 days, because of its tight association with TBG (Chaps. 3 and 9).

HORMONE METABOLISM

Mechanisms for the clearance of released hormones from the circulation are critical for the regulation of hormone levels in response to various needs. Details of hormone metabolism are given in Chap. 3 and in the sections on individual hormones. The rate of clearance of different hormones varies enormously, with half-lives ranging from a few minutes for polypeptide hormones such as angiotensin II (Chap. 13), insulin (Chap. 18), ACTH (Chap. 7), and epinephrine (Chap. 12), to minutes to hours for steroid and glycoprotein hormones (Chap. 3), to days for thyroxine (Chaps. 3 and 9). The time required for reaching a new steady state in response to changes in hormone release is dependent on the half-life of the hormone in the circulation. Therefore, a sudden release of a hormone will have much more marked effects if the hormone is cleared rapidly than it will if the hormone is cleared more slowly. For example, thyroxine, with its long plasma half-life, is involved in more long-term responses than are many hormones, and it may not be advantageous for the levels of this hormone to swing widely. Conversely, hormones such as angiotensin II and the catecholamines participate in more rapid responses, and their short half-lives in plasma facilitate the ability to achieve wide swings in their levels. The peptide hormones are mostly cleared by proteolytic destruction after their uptake by cells through internalization mechanisms, but also through proteolytic cleavage in plasma (Chap. 3). Thyroid hormones, steroids, and catecholamines are metabolically altered inside tissues in which the products are recycled into general metabolic pathways (thyroid and catecholamine hormones) or excreted by the kidneys or the gastrointestinal tract (steroid hormones). Although hormone metabolism can be affected by a variety of factors, in general this is not regulated as extensively as are hormone synthesis and release. Nevertheless, such perturbations in hormone metabolism are sometimes clinically important. For example, the administration of drugs that enhance steroid metabolism, such as barbiturates, can influence the dose of administered glucocorticoid (Chap. 11), and the administration of thyroid hormone, which increases steroid clearance, can precipitate latent adrenal insufficiency (Chap. 11). Decreased clearance of insulin contributes to a decreased need for insulin in diabetes with renal failure (Chap. 18).

REGULATION OF HORMONE LEVELS

A variety of mechanisms regulate circulating hormone levels (Fig. 1-3), as discussed in the individual sections on specific hormones. Thus, there are mechanisms for (1) spontaneous, or basal, hormone release; (2) feedback inhibition by hormones of their synthesis and/or release; (3) stimulation or inhibition of hormone release by substances that may or may not be regulated by the same hormones; (4) establishment of circadian rhythms for hormone release by systems such as the brain; and (5) brain-mediated stimulation or inhibition of hormone release in response to anxiety, anticipation of a specific activity, or other sensory inputs.

In some instances complex regulatory networks are present, whereas in others the endocrine cells are more independent. The first situation is illustrated by the axis that constitutes the hypothalamus, the anterior pituitary or adenohypophysis, and the target endocrine gland (Chaps. 7 and 11). The hypothalamus produces CRH, which travels down the portal vessels through the hypothalamic stalk to the anterior pituitary, where it stimulates ACTH release. ACTH is then transported to the adrenal gland, where it stimulates the release of cortisol. Cortisol in turn inhibits both CRH and ACTH release (feedback inhibition). The brain establishes circadian rhythms and can trigger increased CRH release in response to stress. The pancreatic islets are an example of a more independent system (Chap. 18). Insulin release is regulated primarily by the levels of blood glucose, decreasing with

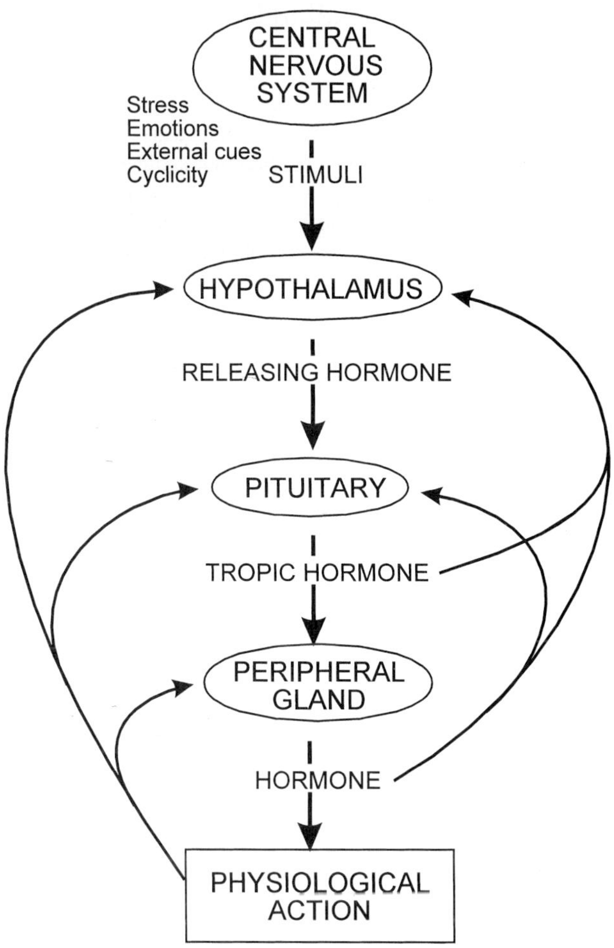

FIGURE 1-3. Organization of a set of endocrine glands, with interrelated regulatory elements. Shown is the flow of information from the central nervous system through the hypothalamus to the pituitary and then to the peripheral glands. Either the hormone product of the peripheral gland or the physiologic actions induced by the hormone can produce feedback inhibition of the stimuli to hormone release at any of several loci. As a rule, not all the potential regulatory influences operate with respect to a given set of glands, nor do all the components shown operate for all endocrine glands.

hypoglycemia and increasing with glucose ingestion. However, hormones such as gastric inhibitory peptide and other substances such as specific amino acids (e.g., arginine) can also affect insulin release, as can stress and trauma via signals from the autonomic nervous system.

HORMONE UPTAKE AND INTERNALIZATION

Various mechanisms account for the uptake of the different hormones by peripheral tissues. These mechanisms are discussed extensively in Chap. 4 and in the sections on individual hormones. The polypeptide and catecholamine hormones and the prostaglandins bind to receptors on the cell surface and are internalized. The cell surface receptor–hormone interactions initiate the actions of these hormones.

The internalization mechanism also serves to deliver some regulatory ligands into the cell for intracellular actions. Cholesterol is transported into the cell bound to lipoproteins and there inhibits further cholesterol uptake (Chap. 21). Thyroid hormones also bind to surface sites and are internalized (Chaps. 4 and 9). Once inside the cell, the hormone binds to nuclear receptors and affects the transcription of particular genes. However, it is not known whether the internalization accounts for most or all of the uptake of thyroid hormones. The question of whether polypeptide hormones are internalized to act inside the cell is a subject of active inquiry, and proof that this is the case has not been provided (Chap. 4). Steroid hormones that act inside the cell appear to be capable of readily penetrating cells and do not require a specific internalization mechanism; the hydrophobic nature of these molecules may allow them to migrate through the cell membrane and into the internal milieu of the cell.

MECHANISMS OF HORMONE ACTION

The mechanisms of hormone action are discussed in detail in Chap. 4. Peptide and catecholamine hormones and prostaglandins bind to receptors on the cell surface, where the hormone-receptor interactions affect intracellular mediators, or *second messengers.* The most extensively studied mechanism is the activation of the enzyme adenylyl cyclase by hormones such as beta-adrenergic agonists, ACTH, glucagon, and PTH. *This enzyme* catalyzes the conversion of adenosine triphosphate (ATP) to adenosine 3′,5′-monophosphate (cyclic AMP, or cAMP), which activates a particular serine and threonine kinase (protein kinase A, or PKA). Phosphorylations induced by PKA then alter the conformations of a diverse number of molecules, with consequent metabolic effects on cells. For example, such phosphorylations activate glycogenolysis through effects on specific enzymes and activate gene transcription by affecting particular transcription factors. Other hormone-receptor interactions, such as those involving insulin, alpha-adrenergic agents, and beta-endorphin, can inhibit adenylyl cyclase. Tyrosine kinase can be activated by the action of hormones such as growth hormone, EGF, and insulin. Many hormones promote an increase in intracellular calcium. This occurs with alpha-adrenergic agonists and angiotensin II. The calcium is derived either from the extracellular fluid or from intracellular stores in organelles such as mitochondria or the sarcoplasmic reticulum. The released calcium binds to and activates calmodulin and other calcium-binding proteins, inducing other metabolic effects, such as glycogenolysis, transport processes, steroidogenesis, and muscle contraction. In many instances, hormones stimulate the production and/or turnover of phospholipids. These effects can influence and cause increased calcium influx into the cytosol and can activate another serine and threonine kinase, termed protein kinase C, or PKC. Thus, these hormones utilize a variety of intracellular mediators, and a given hormone may utilize more than one pathway.

As was indicated earlier, steroid and thyroid hormones act for the most part by binding to intracellular receptors. Thyroid hormone receptors are associated with chromatin in the presence or absence of the hormone; the hormone-receptor interaction induces changes in the transcription of specific genes. Steroid receptors are either loosely associated or unassociated with chromatin in the absence of the hormone; steroid binding induces the receptor-steroid complexes to bind to specific sites on the DNA or to other transcription factors, where they affect transcription initiation of specific genes. The translation products of the steroid- or thyroid hormone–regulated mRNAs in turn have metabolic effects on the cells. For example, thyroid hormones increase the levels of beta-adrenergic receptors, with consequent effects on beta-adrenergic sensitivity, and glucocorticoids increase the levels of gluconeogenic enzymes, with subsequent increases in glucose production.

REGULATION OF HORMONE RESPONSIVENESS

Hormone responsiveness is extensively regulated. A common pattern is down regulation resulting from the homologous hormone's induction of a decrease in the levels of its own receptors; this occurs with most polypeptide hormones, catecholamine-responsive systems, and prostaglandin responses, and occurs occasionally with steroid and thyroid hormones. Less commonly, hormones may increase their own responsiveness by increasing their receptors (angiotensin II and its adrenal receptors). Hormones also regulate responsiveness by influencing postreceptor aspects of the response, and there are numerous situations in which hormones antagonize or enhance the responses to other hormones by affecting receptors or postreceptor responses. For example, estrogens increase progesterone receptors, and glucocorticoids affect the actions of epinephrine and glucagon in the liver at postreceptor loci. Thus, in the clinical assessment of a given state, not only hormone levels but also hormone responsiveness must be considered.

CLASSIFICATION OF HORMONE ACTION

Considered superficially, it might seem simple to classify hormone action. Glucocorticoid action would include all actions of glucocorticoids; insulin action would include all actions of insulin, etc. However, using these hormones as examples, it will be seen that the situation is more complex. Many glucocorticoid actions *are* typical of glucocorticoids, such as the induction of gluconeogenesis and glycogen deposition in liver, but in other cases glucocorticoids can affect sodium transport in a manner similar to aldosterone (Chap. 11). Similarly, many of the actions of insulin are typical for insulin, such as those which lower the blood sugar, but in other cases insulin can act analogously to IGF-I (Chaps. 4 and 18). These apparent paradoxes occur because cortisol can bind to the mineralocorticoid receptors that have a higher affinity for aldosterone and more typically mediate aldosterone action, and insulin can bind to IGF-I receptors that have a higher affinity for IGF-I.

Fortunately, pharmacologists have developed a simple basis for classifying drugs that is also applicable to hormones. This classification is based on the receptors rather than the hormone. A given class of action is defined as those actions that are mediated through a given type of receptor. Thus, epinephrine action, rather than including all actions mediated by epinephrine, is defined by the type of receptor that mediates the effect. Epinephrine can have actions through α_1- or α_2-adrenergic receptors or through β_1- or β_2-receptors (Chaps. 4 and 12). Similarly, cortisol can have actions mediated through glucocorticoid or mineralocorticoid receptors, and insulin can have actions mediated through insulin or IGF-I receptors.

EVOLUTION OF THE ENDOCRINE SYSTEM

The evolution of each of the various endocrine systems has involved the assimilation of a number of individual components whose functioning is coordinated in an effective manner (Fig. 1-2). These components include the hormone itself and means for regulating its concentrations and responding to it. It is likely that the roots of these systems are found in phylogenetically simpler regulatory systems. The discussions that follow, although speculative, provide a conceptual framework for considering the subject.

Simple and Complex Regulation

Tomkins classified regulation within cells as simple or complex.[7] With simple regulation, the reactants or products in a metabolic pathway regulate enzymatic or other processes important for that pathway. Such regulation is illustrated by feedback inhibition of an enzyme by products of the reaction. If regulation were limited to simple mechanisms, survival might be tenuous because the regulatory ligands themselves are important intermediaries, and large changes in their concentrations might imperil the organism. Thus, there was a need for more complex regulation involving the use of regulatory ligands that are neither reactants nor products of the processes they regulate. Such ligands therefore may not have any obvious relation to the chemicals involved in the pathway. For example, cAMP regulates the metabolism of glucose and glycogen (Chaps. 4 and 18) but differs chemically from these carbohydrates.

Origin of Hormones and Other Regulatory Ligands

Regulatory ligands of the endocrine system include hormones, second-messenger mediators of hormone-receptor interactions (Chap. 4), and extraneous factors. For a ligand to assume a role in complex regulation, its concentration should change in response to conditions that would benefit from its actions. Tomkins proposed that the concentrations of regulatory ligands such as cAMP can be varied in response to such conditions because they are byproducts rather than important intermediates.[7] As such, their production rates can vary when other factors affect the major pathways. ATP is ordinarily converted to ADP or AMP. This reaction is frequently linked to other reactions, such as the conversion of glucose to glucose-6-phosphate, and glucose deprivation might, therefore, diminish both phosphorylation of glucose and conversion of ATP to ADP. In this circumstance, more ATP might be degraded by alternative pathways, as by conversion to cAMP. As a consequence, cAMP could become a marker of insufficient glucose availability in that it would accumulate when levels of the sugar decreased.

The production of hormones may also have been first regulated in response to changes in cellular conditions.[8] For example, steroid hormone production may have been affected when cellular events altered the synthesis, metabolism, or utilization of cholesterol, which is a precursor to all the steroid hormones.[8] The incorporation of cholesterol into membranes is associated with cell growth. When growth is affected, there is altered utilization of cholesterol and potential changes in its conversion to other molecular species such as the steroid hormones. Thus steroids might have evolved into symbols for regulating cell growth. Other factors might also have increased steroid production. For instance

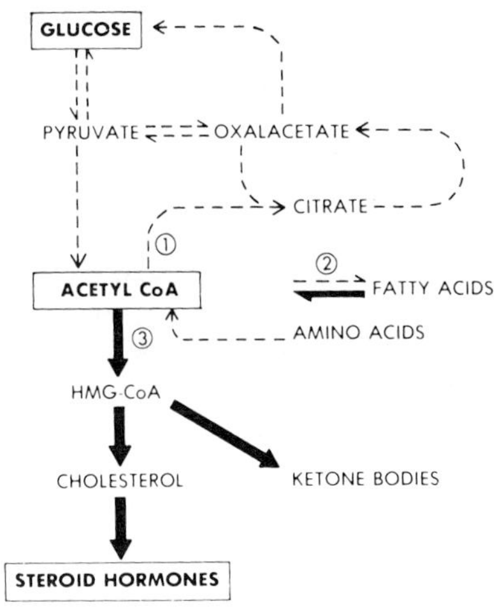

FIGURE 1-4. Metabolic interrelations of glucose, acetyl CoA, and steroid hormones. Numbers indicate the three major fates of acetyl CoA. The bold and dashed arrows indicate, respectively, the more dominant and the minor metabolic pathways under conditions of glucose deprivation. HMG CoA = hydroxymethylglutaryl CoA. [*From Baxter and Rousseau.*[8]]

(Fig. 1-4), it is possible that with decreased carbohydrate utilization and consequent decreased generation of pyruvate, there would be impaired utilization of acetyl CoA for oxidation through the citric acid cycle and for lipogenesis.[8] This might affect the pathway acetyl CoA → cholesterol → steroids. Such events might explain how glucocorticoids came to symbolize glucose deprivation and take on roles such as enhancing the production and availability of glucose (Chap. 11).

Analogous speculations can be extended to the other hormones. Thyroid and catecholamine hormones are byproducts of tyrosine (Chaps. 9 and 12), and their production may have first been regulated by circumstances that affected the metabolism of this amino acid or amino acids in general. Many of the polypeptide hormones and thyroid hormones are derived from the cleavage of large proteins, and variations in their production may have had their origins in events that affected the metabolism of proteins in general or the specific precursor proteins. The genes for these precursor proteins may have evolved from genes that encoded proteins critical for cellular structure or metabolism (Fig. 1-2). Similarly, the genes encoding polypeptide hormones that make up an entire gene may have been derived from an evolutionary precursor gene that served an essential cellular function.

Of course, not all symbols for metabolic control are regulated by simply increasing their synthesis. Ions such as Ca^{2+}, Mg^{2+}, K^{+}, and Cl^{-} are used extensively in the regulation of homeostasis (Chap. 4). In these cases, rather than creating the ions, changes in metabolism could alter their concentrations in specific cellular compartments (cytosol, mitochondria, sarcoplasmic reticulum, etc.). For instance, lack of glucose or other substrate could result in a lack of ATP or other substances, which would affect the activity of transport systems involved in the maintenance of ion-concentration gradients across membranes. The ions could then take on regulatory functions by interacting with proteins that evolved as described earlier.

Origin of Receptors and Other Mediators of Regulatory Ligand Actions

Once mechanisms were established to regulate the concentrations of a ligand by means of appropriate stimuli, there was a need for the ligand to develop means to affect the appropriate metabolic pathway(s). To do this, the ligand must interact with other molecules in the cell. Binding proteins for products such as cAMP were probably already present by the time these ligands appeared because enzymes that bound their precursors had to be present to form the ligand.[7] If these proteins could be modified to have activities that affected the metabolic pathway and if these activities were stimulated by binding of the ligand, elements for the complex regulation would be established. Genetic events such as mutation, deletion of gene sequences, and the insertion of additional gene sequences would allow the genes for such proteins ultimately to produce a molecule with the needed regulatory properties. These mechanisms are described in more detail in Chap. 3. There would be a selective advantage for any cells containing such regulatory proteins, as they would help the cell respond to overcome the original problem (e.g., glucose deprivation) that stimulated the production of the regulatory ligand. For example, in *Escherichia coli* cAMP accumulates when there is a low concentration of glucose.[7] The nucleotide binds to a regulatory protein, and the complex then stimulates the production of enzymes that metabolize other carbohydrates, such as galactose and lactose. These actions provide the organism an alternative carbohydrate source in the absence of glucose. Thus cAMP, a key mediator in hormone action and neurotransmission in humans, developed as a regulator of metabolism in much lower species.

In mammals, cAMP binds to regulatory subunits that, in the absence of cAMP, associate with and inhibit the activity of a specific protein kinase (Chap. 5). The binding of cAMP promotes dissociation of the regulatory subunits from the catalytic subunits, which are then active.

Regulatory proteins, or receptors in this case, have also evolved to bind hormones specifically and to transmit this information into postreceptor events. For example, the binding of steroid hormones to their receptors induces conformational changes that stimulate the receptors to bind to specific DNA sequences and influence the transcription of specific genes (Chap. 4).

To gain such specialized and highly specific functions, the genes encoding these proteins have had to evolve to obtain the critical structures (Chap. 3). In some cases, other genes evolved to express products that modify these proteins (e.g., through glycosylation, phosphorylation, or proteolysis). Because the evolution of genes has apparently occurred by mechanisms such as mutation of preexisting genes and recombination of pieces from different genes, some constraints are placed on the way proteins can evolve. Therefore, it has probably been simpler evolutionarily to modify preexisting structures than to create entirely new genes. It may not then be surprising that there is some homology in the amino acid sequences of diverse proteins, because their genes may have arisen by evolution from common precursor genes. Because binding sites on proteins for regulatory ligands such as cAMP and steroids or their analogues must have existed by the time these ligands appeared, as pointed out earlier, it is easy to see how modification of the genes for these proteins could result in other proteins with high binding specificity for the regulatory ligand.

Diversification of Families of Hormones

Once a given regulatory molecule became established, there was probably evolutionary pressure to preserve it. There might also be an opportunity for the molecule to extend its domain. For example, a hormone that increased in concentration in response to stress might be recruited to elicit additional responses that would relieve the stress. These responses would be recruited by mechanisms similar to those described in the preceding sections. Thus, angiotensin II stimulates not only vascular constriction but also aldosterone release, with consequent effects that conserve sodium (Chap. 11). Conversely, variants of the initial hormone might be produced, and with time they might take on one set of the responses while leaving other responses to the original hormone. Thus, cortisol and aldosterone are both released in response to stress, yet they elicit different sets of responses that help in the adjustment to stress (Chap. 11). These influences would therefore result in the diversification of hormones and their responses.

EVOLUTION OF THE ENDOCRINE GLANDS

As multicellular organisms evolved, cells began to secrete proteins and other ligands that could act on other cells. In many circumstances communication between cells in close proximity was adequate. However, as more complex forms of life evolved, the more elaborate diversification that now exists for the specialized cells of the nervous and endocrine systems became necessary; these cells release regulatory signals that act at more distant sites.

The central nervous system (CNS) has emerged as dominant in regulating and coordinating bodily functions; many processes are regulated by direct nerve-to-cell contact. In simpler forms of life (invertebrates) the CNS communicates directly with all peripheral cells.[9,10] This mechanism is, however, inadequate for survival of the more complex and highly developed species.

The next step in complexity, the release of regulatory molecules to act at more distant loci, apparently became necessary as direct nerve-to-cell contact became impractical. The first process to evolve may have been direct neurosecretion of hormones from the CNS or from specialized effectors developed as outgrowths of nerve endings. The former is represented by the direct release of neurosecretory granules from invertebrate nerve cells as described by Scharrer,[10] and the latter by cells of the posterior pituitary which secrete vasopressin (Chap. 8) and cells of the adrenal medulla that secrete epinephrine (Chap. 12). In a parallel manner, cells of neural crest origin with neurosecretory elements migrated to various other parts of the body, generally in association with the foregut and midgut and their outpouchings, resulting in CNS-like cells secreting the same neurotransmitters or peptides.[11,12] This provides an explanation for the presence of somatostatin, vasoactive intestinal peptide (VIP), neurotensin, substance P, etc., in both the CNS (Chap. 6) and the gut and pancreas (Chap. 26), the neurosecretory granule-containing Kulchitsky's cells in the bronchi, and the amine precursor uptake and decarboxylation (APUD) cells (Chap. 6).[11]

The possible need for higher concentrations of many hormones at particular locations—cortisol acting on phenylethanolamine *N*-methyl transferase (PNMT) in the adrenal medulla (Chap. 12), testosterone acting on spermatogenesis in the testis (Chap. 15), estrogen acting on corpus luteum formation (Chap. 16), and insulin and glucagon regulating hepatic glucose regulation (Chap. 18)—may have required the location of glands for their secretion in areas distant from the CNS. An additional means for the control of these glands evolved with those hormones, which could be produced near the CNS and be more readily under its control. Thus, the anterior pituitary developed in close proximity to the CNS so that its hormones could be under the control of the releasing hormones synthesized in the hypothalamus (Chaps. 6 and 7).

Two other evolutionary processes occurred which helped integrate the endocrine system. First, the appearance of portal vascular systems, hepatic (Chap. 26) and hypophysial (Chaps. 6 and 7), permitted the localization of hormone action on the basis of concentration as well as the specificity of tissue receptors. Second, varying degrees of hormone susceptibility to degradation by plasma played an important role in limiting or extending the duration of their effects (discussed previously).

INTEGRATION OF THE ENDOCRINE SYSTEM

The maintenance of homeostasis in multicellular organisms requires simultaneous and coordinated monitoring of a number of functions. For example, a fright response that may involve muscular activity requires recruitment of the musculoskeletal system. To support this, the pulmonary and cardiovascular systems must also be prepared. Energy sources must be mobilized for these responses in a manner that does not compromise critical functions. Thus, mechanisms have evolved to release glucose from glycogen, increase glucose production, stimulate alternative pathways to obtain energy (e.g., through mobilization of stored fat), and decrease glucose consumption by tissues that are not in immediate need of the substrate. The endocrine system contributes to these types of controls through (1) integrated sets of responses to each hormone, (2) coordination of simultaneous responses by several hormones, (3) counterbalancing influences by other hormones, and (4) mechanisms for terminating or attenuating the response.

Integrated Actions of a Given Class of Hormone

As discussed earlier, there may be a selective advantage for hormones to regulate simultaneously several different processes that together lead to a given result. Thus, hormones typically stimulate integrated sets of responses. Several simultaneous responses can be stimulated within a given cell, and responses can be stimulated in multiple organs, as was described previously for angiotensin II. Glucocorticoids are also illustrative in terms of their fuel-metabolizing and catabolic effects. These steroids enhance gluconeogenesis and glucose production in the liver, decrease glucose uptake in peripheral tissues, enhance protein breakdown, decrease protein synthesis in fat, muscle, and lymphoid and fibroblastic tissues, and stimulate lipolysis (Chap. 11). These actions together increase the blood glucose concentration at the expense of substrate in certain tissues. This glucose is made available for immediate use by other tissues and in particular by the brain, the continuous function of which is crucial for survival and is specifically dependent on glucose as a substrate.

Hormone Synergisms: Recruitment of Multiple Hormones for Coordinated Responses

The endocrine system has evolved so that particular stimuli can affect more than one hormone simultaneously. The actions of these hormones may be complementary. For example, several classes of hormones (e.g., epinephrine, glucagon, glucocorticoids, growth hormone) are involved in glucose conservation (Chaps. 7, 11, 12, and 18). They increase blood glucose levels by stimulating increases in glucose synthesis, decreases in glucose utilization in certain tissues, and mobilization of substrates that are precursors for glucose synthesis (e.g., glycerol and lactate) or alternative sources of energy (e.g., free fatty acids). The concerted effects of these hormones are greater than those of the individual hormones. The plasma concentrations of all these hormones are increased with severe hypoglycemia, although in ordinary physiologic circumstances the blood glucose concentration is not the major regulator of epinephrine, growth hormone, or glucocorticoid production. Catecholamines (Chap. 12), vasopressin (Chap. 8), angiotensin II (Chaps. 11 and 13), glucocorticoids (Chap. 11), mineralocorticoids (Chap. 11), and other hormones are released in response to shock. These hormones increase vascular reactivity, conserve sodium, stimulate cardiac function, and elicit other actions that are useful in compensating for the insult.

Hormone Antagonism: Fine-Tuning of Metabolism

Responses to many hormones are countered by those to other hormones. This provides capabilities in addition to those derived from the removal of a hormone. For example, insulin opposes the glucose-elevating properties of epinephrine, glucagon, glucocorticoids, alpha-adrenergic agonists, and growth hormone (Chap. 18). It stimulates glucose uptake in fat and glycogen synthesis while inhibiting glucose synthesis, lipolysis, and glycogenolysis. Further, it stimulates protein synthesis and inhibits protein breakdown. Progesterone inhibits some actions of estrogens (Chap. 16). Calcitonin tends to lower the serum Ca^{2+}, whereas PTH tends to elevate concentrations of the ion (Chap. 22).

These antagonisms do not always extend to all responses. For example, although insulin's actions are mostly antagonistic to those of the glucocorticoids, both classes of hormones tend to enhance glycogen accumulation (Chaps. 11 and 18). The α- and β-adrenergic agonists both increase glycogenolysis and gluconeogenesis, although the two classes of hormones can have opposing influences on vascular (Chap. 12), muscular (Chap. 12), and hormonal (e.g., insulin) (Chap. 18) secretory responses. The fact that two classes of hormones can be synergistic for some responses and antagonistic for others can be explained in terms of the individual needs served by the hormones.

Mechanisms for Attenuating or Terminating the Response

Responses to hormones are attenuated or terminated by a variety of mechanisms. First, most hormones, particularly stress hormones, are cleared rapidly from the circulation so that when secretion ceases, the response disappears rapidly. Second, many hormones exert feedback inhibition of their own release. These inhibitory actions occur typically through actions of other hormones secreted in response to the initial hormone (e.g., suppression of TSH release by thyroid hormone; Chap. 9) or through sequelae of the hormone's action (e.g., PTH-induced increases in Ca^{2+} levels inhibit PTH release). Third, as already discussed, hormones can induce a decrease in sensitivity to their actions. Finally, other hormones secreted simultaneously can blunt the responses; for example, a role of glucocorticoids released in stress may be to blunt the actions or secretions of other hormones (Chap. 11).

ACTIONS OF HORMONES

Hormones affect essentially all types of body processes. Several of the more prominent types of influence among the numerous actions merit particular emphasis.

Intermediary Metabolism and Growth

A number of different hormones regulate intermediary metabolism and growth. Thus, glucocorticoids, catecholamines, prostaglandin E_1, and glucagon tend to promote the availability and/or mobilization of glucose and other fuels and, in some cases, tissue catabolism (Chap. 18). Glucocorticoids (in excess) also inhibit growth (Chaps. 11 and 25). Insulin and certain growth factors, including IGFs, tend to have varying degrees of growth-promoting and fuel-storing actions (Chap. 18). Androgens, progestins, and estrogens are growth factors (Chaps. 15 and 16), although physiologic levels of progesterone can antagonize the effects of estrogens (Chap. 16). Growth hormone, prolactin, and placental lactogen are growth-promoting, although the growth responses are due in part to stimulation of the production of growth factors such as IGF-I (Chaps. 7 and 25). In addition, many actions of growth hormone and chorionic somatomammotropin, independent of those mediated secondarily by IGF-I, are of the fuel-mobilizing type, with a stimulation of hyperglycemia, increased lipolysis, etc. (Chap. 18). Interestingly, many surface-active hormones of the fuel-mobilizing group activate adenylyl cyclase, whereas those of the growth-stimulating fuel-storage group commonly do not (Chap. 4). Thus, as in bacteria, cAMP is used for mobilization of carbohydrate.

Highly Specific Functions

Tropic Actions

Integration of the endocrine system has required the evolution of hormones termed tropic hormones that specifically regulate glands specialized for the production of other hormones. Thus, TSH regulates thyroid hormone production (Chaps. 7 and 9), CG regulates progesterone production (Chap. 16), FSH regulates follicular and Sertoli cell maturation (Chaps. 15 and 16), LH regulates progesterone production in the female (Chap. 16) and testosterone production in the male (Chap. 15), ACTH regulates glucocorticoid production (Chaps. 6, 7, and 11), and angiotensin regulates aldosterone production (Chaps. 11 and 13). Although these tropic hormones may play additional roles (e.g., angiotensin II), the number of target tissues for most of these classes of hormones is restricted. In many cases these hormones activate adenylyl cyclase, but some (angiotensin II) apparently do not (Chap. 4).

Mineral and Water Metabolism

Aldosterone, vasopressin, PTH, calcitonin, and vitamin D are hormones that have the specialized functions of regulating ion and water concentrations (Chaps. 8, 11, 13, and 22). There is diversity in their mechanisms of action, and the target tissue distribution for each class of these hormones is rather restricted. However, these are not the only hormones that affect fluid and electrolyte metabolism, which is also influenced by insulin, glucagon, glucocorticoids, catecholamines, and others (Chaps. 11–13 and 18).

Cardiovascular Functions

The atrium of the heart devotes more of its protein synthetic efforts to producing a hormone, atrial natriuretic factor, than to producing any other protein, and this hormone has extensive effects on the cardiovascular system (Chap. 13). Numerous other hormones also affect cardiovascular function and blood pressure, including the catecholamines (Chaps. 12 and 13), endothelin (Chap. 13), thyroid hormone (Chaps. 9 and 13), angiotensin II (Chaps. 11 and 13), mineralocorticoids (Chaps. 11 and 13), bradykinin (Chaps. 13 and 29), and the sex steroids (Chaps. 15 and 16). Most of these hormones have other important metabolic actions for which they are predominantly known (e.g., glucocorticoids, sex steroids). The fact that they also regulate cardiovascular responses underscores the importance of the endocrine system in responding to numerous physiologic and pathologic perturbations. Further, many elements of these systems are predominantly under CNS control by catecholamines and acetylcholine released at nerve endings.

Reproductive Functions

Hormones are dominant in the control of reproductive functions, as evidenced by the lack of reproductive capacity in their absence (Chaps. 15–17). Thus, the gonadotropins of pituitary (LH, FSH; Chaps. 7, 15, and 16) or placental origin (CG; Chaps. 7 and 16) play important roles in regulating reproductive organs such as the ovary and testes, which in turn produce hormones such as the sex steroids (androgens, estrogens, and progestins). These steroids control functions critical for pregnancy and for sexual differentiation and development, and influence secondary sexual characteristics such as voice, hair, and muscular development as well as sexual behavior.

Developmental Actions

Hormones play a crucial role in extrauterine growth and development. The sex steroids (Chaps. 15 and 16); insulin (Chap. 18); other growth factors and hormones such as fibroblast growth factor (FGF), PDGF, EGF, and transforming growth factors (TGFs) (Chaps. 4, 6–12, 15, 16, 18, and 25–29); thyroid hormone (Chap. 9); and glucocorticoids (Chap. 11) are all important in this respect. Sometimes the effects are predominantly on growth, as illustrated by dwarfism due to growth hormone deficiency and gigantism due to growth hormone excess (Chaps. 7 and 25). In other cases the influences are on development, as illustrated by the pseudohermaphroditism associated with insensitivity to androgens (Chap. 17). In yet others the effects are on growth and development, as illustrated by the lack of growth and brain development in cretinism (Chaps. 9 and 25). In fact, most of the hormones mentioned here are important at some stage for development.

DISORDERS OF THE ENDOCRINE SYSTEM

Endocrinology has traditionally been signal-level-oriented, concerned largely with whether hormones are secreted appropriately or inappropriately (i.e., in excess or deficiency). Most recognizable disorders of the endocrine system are due to an excess or a deficiency of particular hormones, whether caused by abnormalities of endocrine glands, ectopic production of hormones, abnormal conversion of prohormones to their active forms, or iatrogenic factors. However, it has become increasingly evident that endocrine abnormalities may also result from changes in the responses (either enhanced or diminished) of target tissues to hormones. These disorders can occur by a variety of mechanisms (Fig. 1-5).

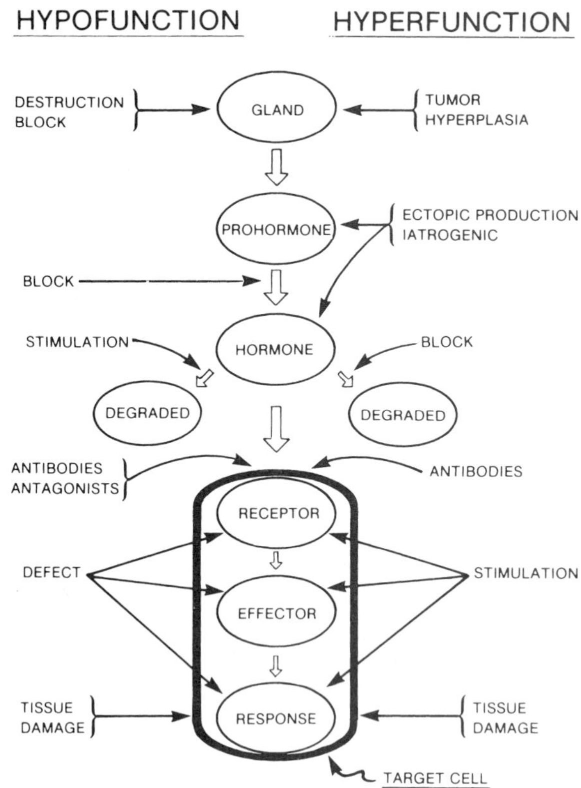

FIGURE 1-5. Causes of hypofunction or hyperfunction of the endocrine system. [*From Baxter JD, in Wyngaarden JB, Smith LH Jr (eds): Cecil's Textbook of Medicine. Philadelphia, Saunders, 1985, p. 1220.*]

Hormone Deficiency Syndromes

Hypofunction of Endocrine Glands

Endocrine glands may be damaged or destroyed by neoplasia, infections, hemorrhage, autoimmune disorders, and other causes. The destruction may be acute but is commonly chronic, with normal basal hormone production occurring until late in the disease. The gland is usually compromised in its reserve capacity before the basal level of secretion falls, and it cannot respond normally in circumstances in which an increase in hormone production is needed. Such partial defects may therefore not be detected by measurement of basal hormone levels and may require other testing of the reserve function of the gland. Because many manifestations of endocrine disease require weeks, months, or years to develop, the clinical presentation may vary over a considerable range, depending on the rapidity of glandular failure.

A deficiency of a hormone that controls the synthesis and release of another hormone may result in a syndrome, which simulates a primary deficiency of that target organ. Thus, hypothalamic lesions resulting in impaired secretion of releasing hormones may be manifested by pituitary dysfunction, which in turn may result in abnormalities in the function of its various target organs (gonads, thyroid, adrenals) (Chaps. 6 and 7).

Genetic defects can cause endocrine hypofunction, usually because of abnormalities in hormone synthesis and rarely because of the production of an abnormal hormone (as documented for insulin in rare forms of diabetes mellitus and growth hormone in rare forms of dwarfism) (Chaps. 18 and 25). These genetic defects in hormone synthesis may be partial or complete. For example, a rare form of growth hormone deficiency is due to deletion of the growth hormone gene (Chap. 25). A partial defect may be somewhat analogous to incomplete destruction of the gland; i.e., basal hormone production may be normal, but the reserve may be inadequate. In fact, genetic defects sometimes present not with the problems of hormone deficiency, but rather, with manifestations of a compensatory adaptation. For example, partial blocks in thyroid hormone biosynthesis may result in an enlarged thyroid gland (goiter) that is due to TSH hypersecretion resulting from low levels of thyroid hormone (Chaps. 9 and 10). In the 17α-hydroxylase deficiency syndrome there is defective cortisol production and consequent ACTH hypersecretion with excessive production of adrenocorticosteroids that are not 17α-hydroxylated (Chap. 11). One of these, corticosterone, substitutes for cortisol, and so manifestations of cortisol deficiency are not observed. In contrast, excessive compensatory synthesis of corticosterone and deoxycorticosterone leads to a mineralocorticoid excess syndrome with hypertension and hypokalemia.

Hormone Deficiency Secondary to Extraglandular Disorders

Extraglandular disorders can result in hormone deficiency. They may involve defective conversion of prohormones to active forms, enhanced degradation of hormones, or the production of substances (antibodies, hormone antagonists) that block the actions of hormones. Impaired conversion of a prohormone to a hormone occurs in chronic renal failure and in vitamin D dependent rickets type 1, in which there is defective conversion of 25-hydroxycholecalciferol to 1,25-$(OH)_2$-cholecalciferol (Chap. 22). A rare form of androgen deficiency is due to an abnormality in 5α-reductase, which converts testosterone to dihydrotestosterone (Chap. 17). In this condition there is only partial loss of androgenic effects because testosterone itself is weakly active in some target tissues. Rare forms of diabetes mellitus result from antibodies to the insulin receptor that block insulin action (Chap. 18). Antibodies to insulin develop during insulin therapy for diabetes; when excessive, these antibodies may affect the availability of insulin (Chap. 18). Although no primary disorders are known to be due to enhanced hormone degradation, other factors or disease states may affect the response to exogenously administered hormones; for example, phenytoin and thyroid hormone increase the metabolism of certain glucocorticoids (Chap. 11). Also, such influences may unmask or aggravate a partial hormonal deficiency; for example, the administration of thyroid hormones may unmask latent Addison's disease (Chap. 11). Finally, pharmacologic agents, given for other purposes, may impair normal hormone biosynthesis. Ketoconazole, an antifungal agent, blocks the effects of both 11α-hydroxylase and 17α-hydroxylase, leading to impaired cortisol production[13] (Chap. 11).

Hyporesponsiveness to Hormones

Hormone levels may be normal or even elevated in the presence of manifestations of endocrine deficiency. These conditions may be due to some of the problems listed previously, e.g., antibodies to the insulin receptor (Chap. 18) and abnormal conversion of testosterone to dihydrotestosterone (Chap. 17). They may also result from decreased ability of the endocrine target gland to respond to the hormone. Such disorders may be acquired or genetic and may be due to abnormalities at any step in the cascade of the hormone response from the receptor to the effect generated.

Several syndromes are associated with receptor abnormalities. The most commonly recognized abnormality of this type occurs in obese patients with type II diabetes mellitus (Chap. 18) where chronic hyperinsulinemia induced by increased food intake induces insulin resistance, in part by down regulating the concentration of insulin receptors. Recognition of this problem also affects the therapy because treatment is directed not only at correcting the hyperglycemia with insulin or other drugs but also at decreasing insulin need by means of dietary maneuvers that secondarily decrease insulin levels and, thus, restore tissue sensitivity to the hormone. This form of diabetes also exhibits an additional abnormality by which the pancreatic islets do not release insulin normally in response to glucose. In the testicular feminization syndrome there is unresponsiveness to androgens (Chap. 17). As a consequence, a female phenotype occurs in a person with a male genotype. Most persons with this X-linked disorder have a defect in the androgen receptor. Families with dwarfism have been described in which a mutation in the GHRH receptor gene leads to total insensitivity to the ligand, leading to subnormal growth hormone secretion (Chaps. 6 and 7).

Hyporesponsiveness may also be due to postreceptor abnormalities. In pseudohypoparathyroidism there is frequently an abnormality in the coupling of hormone-receptor complexes to effector mechanisms. Patients with the disorder have symptoms and chemical derangements of hypoparathyroidism associated with elevated PTH levels and insensitivity to this hormone (Chap. 22). In some of these patients this insensitivity is due to decreased levels of the guanyl nucleotide-binding regulatory protein that couples the PTH receptor complex to adenylyl cyclase because of mutations in the gene encoding the α subunit of this protein. Much of the insulin resistance of type II diabetes mellitus is due to postreceptor abnormalities.

Overall damage to the hormone target tissue may result in insensitivity to hormones. For instance, renal disease may lead to insensitivity to vasopressin (Chap. 8), and liver disease may lead to insensitivity to glucagon (Chap. 18).

Abnormal Production or Administration of Antagonists

Rarely, endogenously produced or exogenously administered substances may produce a hormone-resistant state. Antibodies to the insulin receptor may produce insulin resistance with functional insulinopenia (Chap. 18). Cimetidine given for peptic ulcer disease and spironolactone given for hypertension (Chap. 13) may act as androgen antagonists and produce an androgen-resistant state.

Hormone Excess Syndromes

Hormone excess syndromes may result from hyperfunctioning endocrine glands, from ectopic hormone production by tumors, less commonly from influences on target tissues that enhance hormone sensitivity, from autoimmune disease in which antibodies cause hypersecretion of hormones or act as hormone agonists, from defects in hormone biosynthesis in which precursor hormones produced in excess have deleterious consequences, and from the iatrogenic or therapeutic administration of hormones or substances that act like hormones.

Hyperfunction of Endocrine Glands

The most common cause of hormone excess syndromes is hyperfunction of endocrine glands secondary to tumors or hyperplasia. Hyperfunctioning tumors of endocrine glands are usually well-differentiated adenomas (although carcinomas also occur).

Hyperplasia causes hyperfunction of several endocrine glands (thyroid, adrenals, parathyroids). The most common form of thyroid hyperplasia is due to an immunologic abnormality in which antibodies stimulate the gland in a manner similar to TSH (Chap. 9). Hyperplasia of the zona fasciculata and zona reticularis of the adrenal with consequent cortisol hypersecretion is usually due to ACTH hypersecretion by a pituitary tumor or an ectopic hormone-secreting tumor (Chaps. 11 and 28). Chief cell hyperplasia of parathyroid glands with PTH hypersecretion most commonly occurs as a genetic defect of an undetermined nature (Chap. 22). The cause in other types of endocrine gland hyperplasia is less clear, as with hyperplasia of the adrenal zona glomerulosa resulting in excessive aldosterone production (Chap. 13).

Ectopic Hormone Production

Hormones may be produced in excess by cells of endocrine or nonendocrine origin that are not normally the primary source of a hormone (Chap. 28). In most instances, hormones produced ectopically by tumors are those which are derived from a single gene (e.g., ACTH, GHRH, somatostatin, calcitonin, gastrin, erythropoietin) or two genes (CG). This may be due to the fact that the synthesis of other hormones (e.g., steroids, thyroid hormones, catecholamines) requires a large number of genes not ordinarily expressed by the tumor which need to be activated for hormone biosynthesis. Although many different types of tumors can produce hormones, specific cell types are more commonly involved in this process (Chap. 28). For example, APUD-type cells are commonly associated with ectopic hormone production. These cells are found in small-cell carcinoma of the lung, carcinoid tumors, thymomas, and other tumors. Although a number of molecular mechanisms are now available to explain how genes ordinarily not expressed are activated in tumors, those actually causing ectopic hormone production are not well understood.

Hormone Administration

Hormone excess states may occur when hormones are used to treat nonendocrine diseases, hormone replacement therapy is excessive, or patients self-administer hormones (or their analogs). Patients sometimes take excessive doses of glucocorticoids (Chap. 11), androgens (Chap. 15), or thyroxine (Chap. 9) because those hormones produce a feeling of well-being. Rarely, administration of nonhormonal substances can cause hormone-like effects; licorice ingestion can produce a syndrome mimicking primary aldosteronism (Chap. 13).

Tissue Hypersensitivity

Endocrine excess syndromes caused by hypersensitivity of target tissues are uncommon. Thyroid hormones increase the catecholamine receptors in certain tissues and thus lead to excessive beta-adrenergic stimulation (Chap. 9). The hyperresponsiveness is actually part of the syndrome of hyperthyroidism. Age and gender may also modify the target tissue responsiveness to certain hormones. The dose of growth hormone appropriate for treatment of young hypopituitary patients is excessive for older individuals (Chaps. 7 and 30). Manifestations of primary aldosteronism occur in a rare syndrome with low plasma renin and aldosterone levels in which the kidney responds as if it were being excessively stimulated by aldosterone (Chap. 13). Finally, disease of the target tissue itself can render it excessively sensitive to a hormone. For instance, cardiac arrhythmias, such as atrial fibrillation in thyrotoxicosis, probably occur most frequently in an already damaged heart (Chap. 9).

A lingering question is whether subtle abnormalities in the sensitivity to hormones contribute to the pathogenesis of disease more often than is generally perceived. With more refined methods for measuring alterations in sensitivity to hormones, it may be possible to detect more subtle abnormalities. For example, are some forms of essential hypertension due to increased sensitivity to pressor substances or decreased sensitivity to vasodilator substances (Chap. 13)? Are some forms of osteoporosis due to abnormalities in sensitivity to estrogens or to calcium-regulating hormones (Chap. 23)? Why do glucocorticoids increase intraocular pressure (and even precipitate glaucoma) in some persons but not in others (Chap. 11)? Why are some women treated with estrogen more susceptible to hyperlipidemia than others (Chap. 21)?

Autoimmune Disease

In addition to endocrine deficiency states, which may be precipitated by autoimmune mechanisms (e.g., Schmidt's syndrome, discussed later in this chapter and in Chap. 11), autoimmune disease can result in the production of antibodies that act as hormones. The most frequent situation in which this occurs is thyrotoxicosis (Graves' disease; Chap. 9). Rarely, antibodies to the insulin receptor are present that have insulin-like actions (Chap. 18).

Hormone Biosynthetic or Metabolic Defects

Certain adrenal steroid biosynthetic defects (the 21α- and 11α-hydroxylase syndromes) result in overproduction of hormones proximal to the block; these syndromes are discussed in Chap. 11. A defect in the metabolism of cortisol leads to a mineralocorticoid excess state caused by excessive accumulation of cortisol with renal mineralocorticoid receptors (Chap. 13).

Secondary Hormone Hypersecretion

Hypersecretion of hormones may be due to excessive physiologic stimulation of glands that are basically normal. The secondary hyperaldosteronism of hepatic disease and ascites, congestive heart failure, the nephrotic syndrome, and other conditions is illustrative (Chap. 11). The excess aldosterone aggravates the tendency to edema in these conditions. Secondary hyperparathyroidism occurs in azotemia (Chap. 23). Secondary hyperinsulinism occurs in obesity (Chap. 18).

Multiple Endocrine Syndromes

Simultaneous involvement of more than one endocrine gland may result in syndromes of hyper- or hypofunction. The most common syndrome of multiple endocrine deficiencies may involve immunologic destruction of the pancreatic islets, thyroid, adrenals, and gonads (Chap. 27). This may result from common antigenic determinants possibly caused by a common developmental origin of the glands.

At least three syndromes of multiple endocrine hyperfunction result from hyperplasia, adenomas, or carcinomas of endocrine tissues, termed *multiple endocrine neoplasia* (MEN) types 1, 2a, and 2b (Chap. 27). Type 1, for which a tumor suppressor gene responsible for tumor susceptibility has recently been identified, is associated with hyperfunction of the parathyroids, pancreatic islets, and pituitary. In some cases more than one hormone may be produced by the tumor; islet-cell tumors can produce insulin, glucagon, gastrin, VIP, prostaglandins, ACTH, vasopressin, somatostatin, serotonin, and GHRH. Hypersecretion of GHRH can produce hyperfunction of the pituitary and acromegaly. MEN type 2a is associated with pheochromocytoma (sometimes bilateral and extra-adrenal), medullary carcinoma of the thyroid, and parathyroid hyperplasia. MEN type 2b is associated with medullary thyroid carcinoma, pheochromocytoma, and other features, such as neuromas. Mutations in the *ret* proto-oncogene have been described in both MEN 2a and MEN 2b.

Abnormalities of Endocrine Glands Not Associated with Hormonal Imbalance

Tumors, nodules, cysts, infiltrative diseases, and other abnormalities may involve endocrine glands without significantly impairing their secretory functions. For instance, nodules of the thyroid gland are common but usually nonfunctioning (Chap. 10). The major problem is that they may become malignant. Sometimes particular processes have a propensity for affecting an endocrine tissue; this is the case with tuberculosis and the adrenals (Chap. 11) and hemachromatosis and the pituitary (Chap. 7).

CLINICAL ASSESSMENT OF ENDOCRINE STATUS

The assessment of the endocrine status of a patient relies on findings from the history and physical examination and on laboratory testing. The latter may involve measurements of levels of hormones or their metabolites in plasma or urine either in the basal state or in response to provocative testing. Laboratory tests may also be used to measure abnormalities that result from derangements in hormonal secretion and to evaluate a patient's sensitivity to hormones.

History and Physical Examination

The clinical manifestations of endocrine diseases are summarized in Chap. 2 and in other individual chapters devoted to specific systems. Many syndromes of hormonal excess or deficiency display manifestations that are readily apparent at the time of initial presentation, e.g., severe thyrotoxicosis (Chap. 9) and Cushing's syndrome (Chap. 11). In other instances, the clinical presentation is more subtle and the physician must rely on laboratory testing to establish a diagnosis. This is especially true in the early stages of most endocrine problems, in elderly persons (e.g., with thyrotoxicosis or myxedema) (Chap. 9), or when the disease presents acutely and has not been present sufficiently long for chronic manifestations to develop. Because early treatment of these diseases is important, the physician must consider endocrine diseases in patients without full-blown manifestations and despite the fact that in the early stages of many of these disorders—e.g., adrenal insufficiency (Chap. 11), hypothyroidism (Chap. 9), Cushing's syndrome (Chap. 11), and hyperparathyroidism (Chap. 22)—the presenting symptoms and signs are sufficiently vague to suggest more common problems. Thus, endocrine diseases should be considered in the differential diagnosis of many common problems, such as weakness, tiredness, vague gastrointestinal discomfort, hypertension, and weight loss or gain (Chap. 2). Once the diagnosis is considered, it is usually relatively easy to establish whether the disorder is present. Because endocrine diseases may be caused by primary processes external to endocrine systems, the physician should consider these processes in taking the history and performing the physical examination. Sometimes the primary process (e.g., carcinoma of the lung producing ACTH, tuberculosis causing adrenal insufficiency) will so dominate the clinical presentation that hormonal abnormalities are not readily apparent.

Laboratory Testing

Hormone Levels

Assay of Hormones

Assays are currently available for measuring essentially all the hormones known to be important (Chap. 5). The dominant assays used are immunoassays, which take advantage of the ability to generate antibodies that bind to specific determinants on hormones with high affinity. The levels of the various hormones are measured by assessing the ability of the hormone in the sample to compete with a labeled hormone or analog for binding to the antibody. Traditionally, these labels have been radioactive, but increasingly, nonradioactive means for labeling are being used. Certain problems with an immunoassay—e.g., when inactive degraded fragments of the hormone give falsely elevated hormone levels (as can occur with PTH in renal failure; Chap. 22)—can be circumvented through the use of two different antibodies, each specific for different parts of the molecule. These assays are described in Chap. 5. Newer generations of immunoassays have markedly enhanced measurement sensitivity as well as specificity for the hormone being measured, and have shortened the assay duration from days to hours or even minutes.

Levels of Free Hormone

The level of free rather than total hormone is usually the best index of the effective hormone concentration in plasma. Problems with assessment of total hormone concentrations caused by variations in the concentrations of plasma steroid and thyroid hormone-binding proteins are emphasized earlier in this chapter and in Chaps. 3 and 5.

Levels of free hormone can be assessed by (1) physically separating the free hormone from the plasma-bound hormone and measuring the free hormone directly, (2) measuring the plasma concentration of the binding protein directly (this approach has not been used widely), and (3) assessing the saturation of the binding protein. The latter approach is now used in the case of thyroid hormone (Chap. 9). Thus, the T_3 uptake assay measures the capacity of plasma for T_3 binding, which reflects the extent of saturation of thyroid hormone-binding proteins by T_4. The free hormone concentration is estimated by combining knowledge of the total T_4 levels and the extent of saturation of the proteins (Chap. 9). Both determinations are necessary because variations in the levels of the binding protein reciprocally affect the total hormone levels and the extent of saturation of the binding proteins (Chaps. 5 and 9). The same reasoning is applied to the measurement of free testosterone used in the evaluation of hirsutism (Chap. 16). As a fourth possibility, an index of the free hormone concentration can sometimes be obtained by measuring the urinary excretion of the free hormone or that of one of its metabolites. For example, a small fraction (less than 1 percent) of the secreted cortisol is excreted unchanged into the urine (Chap. 11). A measurement of the 24-h urine free cortisol usually provides a reasonable estimate of the integrated levels of free plasma hormone. In essence, this method uses the glomerular basement membrane to separate the free from the bound hormone.

Selective Sampling

More accurate indications of a hormone excess state and the site of hormone hypersecretion can sometimes be obtained by assaying the venous effluent from a given gland or organ. For example, in renovascular hypertension, peripheral renin levels may be normal but sampling from a catheter inserted into the renal veins may reveal renin hypersecretion from one side and hyposecretion from the other (Chap. 13). Pituitary venous effluent sampling from the petrosal sinuses can be useful to determine whether ACTH hypersecretion is due to a pituitary adenoma or an ectopic site of production (Chaps. 11 and 28).

Clinical Interpretation

The clinician must remember that in both normal subjects and patients with endocrine and other diseases, hormone levels are extensively regulated, and their laboratory measurements thus must be evaluated in this context. For example, plasma insulin levels should be evaluated in relation to the plasma glucose concentration (Chap. 18) and PTH levels should be considered in relation to serum calcium levels (Chap. 22). Basal hormone secretion may not reflect the functional capacity of the gland, as considered in more detail in the Dynamic Testing section that follows.

Hormone levels should be evaluated in relation to target cell sensitivity. For example, plasma insulin levels in type II diabetes mellitus are often elevated but may still be inappropriately low in view of the associated hyperglycemia and insulin resistance (Chap. 18). Because the secretion of many hormones is pulsatile, random readings can be particularly misleading. Cortisol, for example, is released episodically (Chap. 11). In Cushing's syndrome, the number of these episodic releases may be increased. Although this commonly results in an elevation of the plasma cortisol throughout the day, morning plasma levels of this steroid may be in the normal range. Because integrated cortisol production over a 24-h period is increased in Cushing's syndrome, the 24-h urinary free cortisol provides a more accurate index of cortisol hypersecretion.

Urinary measurements can sometimes be more useful than plasma assays for obtaining an integrated assessment of the production of certain hormones (especially steroids). However, the urinary metabolites of steroids can be influenced by changes in renal function and other factors that do not affect the production of the hormone.

The significance of hormone levels can sometimes be evaluated only by the simultaneous measurement of more than one hormone. For example, with progressive damage to the thyroid gland and impaired release of thyroid hormones, secretion of TSH increases in a compensatory manner so that normal plasma levels of the thyroid hormones may be maintained (Chap. 9). When thyroid hormone levels and TSH are measured simultaneously, an indication of the compensatory response can be obtained. Such a simultaneous assessment of linked hormones can also provide an indication of the site of a primary defect. Plasma estrogens are low in ovarian failure (Chap. 16). If ovarian failure is due to disease of the ovary, plasma gonadotropins will be elevated. If ovarian failure is secondary to pituitary or hypothalamic disease, plasma gonadotropin levels will be normal or decreased.

Dynamic Testing

Provocative testing assesses the ability of a gland to respond to stimuli as an index of its reserve capacity. This is especially useful when plasma or urinary hormone measurements are borderline. It can also yield information about the site of an endocrine defect. In some cases, a hormone is administered that stimulates the release of one or more other hormones. For example, the administration of GnRH stimulates LH and FSH release (Chap. 7), and TRH stimulates TSH and prolactin release (Chap. 7). In other cases, hormone production is blocked to interrupt normal feedback inhibition. Metyrapone blocks cortisol production by inhibiting 11α-hydroxylation, thus stimulating ACTH release (Chap. 11). The elevated ACTH levels increase the release of adrenal steroids proximal to the block (e.g., 11-deoxycortisol). Sometimes a physiologic stimulus to hormone release is given. Insulin-induced hypoglycemia is used to assess the secretory ability of cells that produce ACTH and growth hormone (Chap. 7). With endocrine hyperfunction, provocative tests can assess the extent to which the normal physiologic mechanisms that control hormone release are suppressed or the degree of autonomy of the hormone-producing tumor or hyperplastic gland. In primary aldosteronism resulting from an aldosterone-producing adenoma, plasma renin levels are suppressed by excessive sodium retention and will not rise with acute postural, salt restriction, or diuretic stimuli (Chap. 13). In Cushing's syndrome resulting from ectopic secretion of ACTH by a tumor, the glucocorticoid dexamethasone ordinarily will not suppress the elevated ACTH levels (Chap. 11). In acromegaly, growth hormone secretion is not suppressed normally in response to glucose (Chap. 7).

Tests That Provide Indirect Information

Useful information can frequently be obtained from laboratory tests that provide an index of the actions of hormones (or a lack thereof) or an indication of the primary process causing the endocrine disease. Diagnosis of diabetes mellitus and assessment of therapy depend on measurement of plasma glucose rather than insulin levels (Chap. 18). It is helpful to follow the serum calcium levels in hyperparathyroidism (Chap. 22) and the serum potassium levels in primary aldosteronism (Chap. 13). Such tests often provide indices of the severity of the condition that are even more important than the hormone level. In conditions in which immunologic processes are important, assessment of antibody levels can be helpful. Other tests provide information that is more corroborative but can also be useful. For example, serum sodium is almost always greater than 139 mEq/liter in patients with an aldosterone-producing adenoma (Chap. 13), plasma cholesterol tends to be high in hypothyroidism and low in hyperthyroidism (Chap. 18), serum potassium tends to be high in Addison's disease (Chap. 11), alkaline phosphatase tends to be elevated in osteomalacia (Chap. 23), and the serum IGF-1 level is elevated in acromegaly (Chap. 7).

Evaluation of the Sensitivity of Target Cells to Hormones

Suspicion of hyposensitivity to a hormone is raised when the manifestations of a deficiency of that hormone occur in the presence of elevated hormone levels. In type II diabetes mellitus there is hyperglycemia with hyperinsulinism (Chap. 18); in pseudohypoparathyroidism, hypocalcemia is observed in the face of elevated PTH levels (Chap. 22); and pseudohermaphroditism caused by the testicular feminization syndrome is characterized by decreased androgenization with elevated plasma testosterone levels (Chap. 17). The existence of hyposensitivity can be confirmed by administering the hormone in question and determining the presence or extent of response, although it is rarely necessary to do this. In some cases, as with insulin or androgen resistance, it is possible to obtain further confirmation of the hyposensitivity state by isolating cells from the patient and measuring receptors or responses, although the techniques for this are not generally available. Conversely, hypersensitivity to hormones is characterized by low hormone levels relative to the response. In low-renin essential hypertension the adrenal glomerulosa is excessively sensitive to angiotensin II (Chap. 13). This is reflected by normal to elevated plasma aldosterone levels in the presence of low angiotensin II levels. This sensitivity can be documented by measuring the plasma aldosterone levels after an infusion of angiotensin.

TREATMENT OF ENDOCRINE DISEASES

Hormones are generally administered in endocrine deficiency syndromes to correct the deficiency. In general, the hormone that is deficient is replaced. In some cases this is not possible or expedient, and other hormones are given that help compensate for the defect. For instance, vitamin D is given instead of PTH to treat hypoparathyroidism because it can increase the extracellular Ca^{2+} (Chap. 22). In cases in which hormone resistance is present, steps are taken to alleviate the resistance when possible, such as through diet restriction in type II diabetes (Chap. 18).

In hormone-excess syndromes, a variety of approaches are used. Hyperfunctioning tumors are removed when possible, and sometimes hyperplastic glands are removed. In other cases drugs are given to block hormone production, such as propylthiouracil for thyrotoxicosis (Chap. 9), bromocriptine for prolactin-producing adenomas, and somatostatin analogs for acromegaly (Chap. 7). Antagonists such as spironolactone can sometimes be useful in primary aldosteronism due to hyperplasia (Chap. 13). More recently, hormone antagonists have been used to treat hormone-excess syndromes such as mefipristone (RU-486), a glucocorticoid and progesterone antagonist, for ectopic ACTH syndrome (Chaps. 11 and 28), and a GH antagonist for acromegaly (Chap. 7).

For both excess and deficiency syndromes adjunctive therapy is frequently important. Thus, multiple measures are used to treat the complications of diabetes mellitus, and patients with Addison's disease are cautioned to avoid stress, unless adequately pretreated (Chap. 12).

HORMONE AGONIST AND ANTAGONIST THERAPY OF NONENDOCRINE DISEASE

Finally, it should be remembered that hormones, which affect so many processes, and their analogs, are also used extensively to treat diseases that do not have a primary endocrine basis. For example, glucocorticoids are used to treat a large number of conditions (Chap. 14), analogs of releasing hormones such as GnRH are used to block gonadotropin release (Chap. 16) and treat prostate cancer (Chap. 29), steroid antagonists are used to treat hormone-responsive tumors (Chap. 29), catecholamines are used to treat shock and other cardiovascular problems (Chap. 12), and catecholamine antagonists are used to treat hypertension and other cardiovascular problems.

REFERENCES

1. Fisher JW: Erythropoietin: Physiologic and pharmacologic aspects. *Proc Soc Exp Biol Med* 216:358, 1997
2. Ihle JN, Thierfelder W, Teglund S, Stravapodis D, Wang D, Feng J, Parganas E: Signaling by the cytokine receptor superfamily. *Ann N Y Acad Sci* 865:1, 1998.
3. Curfs JH, Meis JF, Hoogkamp-Korstanje JA: A primer on cytokines: Sources, receptors, effects, and inducers. *Clin Microbiol Rev* 10:742, 1997.
4. Aaronson SA: Growth factors and cancer. *Science* 254:1146, 1991.
5. Kerr LD, Inoue J, Verma IM: Signal transduction: The nuclear target. *Curr Opinion Cell Biol* 4:496, 1992.
6. Bortner DM, Langer SJ, Ostrowski MC: Non nuclear oncogenes and the regulation of gene expression in transformed cells. *Crit Rev Oncogenesis* 4:137, 1993.
7. Tomkins GM: The metabolic code. *Science* 189:760, 1975.
8. Baxter JD, Rousseau GG: Glucocorticoids and the metabolic code, in Baxter JD, Rousseau GG (eds): *Glucocorticoid Hormone Action*. Heidelberg, Springer-Verlag, 1979, pp 613–627.
9. Bern HA, Knowles FGW: Neurosecretion, in Martini L, Ganong WF (eds): *Neuroendocrinology*, vol 1. New York, Academic, 1966, pp 139–186.
10. Scharrer E: Principles of neuroendocrine regulation: Endocrines and the central nervous system. *Assoc Res Nerv Ment Dis* 43:1, 1966.
11. Pearse AGE: The cytochemistry and ultrastructure of polypeptide hormone-producing cells of the APUD series and the embryologic, physiologic and pathologic implications of the concept. *J Histochem Cytochem* 47:303, 1969.
12. Pearse AGE: The diffuse neuroendocrine system and the APUD concept: Related "endocrine" peptides in brain, intestine, pituitary placenta and anuran cutaneous glands. *Med Biol* 55:115, 1977.
13. Sonino N: The use of ketoconazole as an inhibitor of steroid production. *N Engl J Med* 317:812, 1987.

CHAPTER 2

The Clinical Manifestations of Endocrine Disease

Lawrence A. Frohman

Philip Felig

Diseases of the endocrine-metabolic system account for some of the most common disorders encountered in humans: diabetes, obesity, hyperlipedimias, osteoporosis, and thyroid abnormalities. In recent years, a host of laboratory techniques including immunoassays, receptor methodology, recombinant DNA techniques, hormone stimulative and suppressive procedures, and advances in diagnostic imaging, have markedly enhanced diagnosis and clarified the pathophysiology of such diseases. Nevertheless, in many instances the disorder remains unrecognized until relatively late in its course; symptoms may be attributed to another disease process, and laboratory results may be confusing rather than helpful. Some of the difficulties relate to the complex clinical presentation and the multiplicity of organ systems which may be affected by a given disease process (e.g., thyrotoxicosis may masquerade as an intractable cardiac arrhythmia in an apathetic patient). A second problem concerns the nonspecific nature of some symptoms (e.g., weakness may be the major complaint in Addison's disease).

A further difficulty may arise from the laboratory tests. The striking biochemical and physiologic disturbances which occur in endocrine disease, often with only minimal anatomic changes or physical findings (e.g., diabetes, hyperparathyroidism), tend to focus the physician's attention on the laboratory results, frequently without consideration of the total clinical picture. For a patient with asymptomatic hypercalcemia due to hyperparathyroidism, early diagnosis and treatment based on an elevated serum calcium level obtained during routine multiphasic laboratory screening may prevent the subsequent development of bone disease or renal stones. However, an elevation in the serum thyroxine level of a euthyroid patient may lead to inappropriate use of antithyroid drugs if the physician fails to measure serum TSH in a patient with a history of estrogen use. Similarly, the finding of a small adrenal nodule on abdominal computed tomographic evaluation for a specific but unrelated complaint (e.g., abdominal pain) may also lead to confusion and unnecessary diagnostic or therapeutic procedures.

Consequently, the clinical approach most successful in diagnosis and management is one which combines a high index of suspicion with knowledge of the various clinical constellations in which endocrine-metabolic disorders may appear, plus an understanding of the indications, interpretations, and inherent weaknesses of various testing procedures. In this chapter the major clinical signs and symptoms which may call attention to a variety of endocrine-metabolic disorders are reviewed. Various testing procedures are considered in Chap. 5.

GENERALIZED SYMPTOMS

Hormones affect the function of all tissues and organ systems. Consequently, the symptoms and signs of endocrine disease are extremely diverse. They may vary from generalized, such as fatigue, to localized, such as weakness of the extraocular muscles. The variable nature of the clinical presentations of many endocrine disorders may result in their going unrecognized for prolonged periods (e.g., the failure to recognize, particularly in the elderly, recurrent supraventricular tachycardia or heart failure as a manifestation of hyperthyroidism). By contrast, there is a tendency (both in the general population and in the medical community) to attribute an endocrine basis to common complaints even when evidence is lacking. For example, hypoglycemia or hypothyroidism is often invoked to explain weakness and depression, obesity is frequently attributed to a "slow metabolism," and baldness is often ascribed to "glandular dysfunction." Although each of these symptoms may in fact be due to an endocrine-metabolic disorder, the diagnosis should rest not on the nature of the symptom but on rigorous clinical and laboratory evaluation.

Weakness and Fatigue

Weakness generally refers to an overall lack of strength (easy fatigability, "loss of pep") which may be persistent or episodic in nature and may be due to an actual loss of strength or only a perceived loss. Persistent weakness may reflect altered muscle function, as in some types of endocrine myopathy, or electrolyte disturbance, dehydration, or the effects of hormonal lack or excess through mechanisms which are poorly understood.

Generalized weakness is a common complaint in patients with Addison's disease or panhypopituitarism. In spontaneous or iatrogenic Cushing's syndrome, weakness secondary to steroid-induced myopathy may be observed. Both hypothyroidism and hyperthyroidism may result in fatigue, even when there is hyperactivity and nervousness in the hyperthyroid state.

Hypokalemia accompanying hyperaldosteronism, other mineralocorticoid-excess states, or Bartter's syndrome and hypercalcemia of hyperparathyroidism or malignant disease may result in a generalized decrease in strength. In a poorly controlled diabetic patient or a patient with Addison's disease dehydration may result in or worsen weakness. Furthermore, in some diabetic patients, even in the absence of severe hyperglycemia, postprandial fatigue and somnolence may be reversed by improved regulation of the blood glucose.

Patients with depression, which is common in many endocrine dysfunctions, frequently complain of fatigue or weakness. A distinction between weakness due to organic dysfunction and a feeling of fatigue due to depression can often be made. Patients with depression commonly feel "too weak" to initiate physical activity, whereas those with true weakness generally notice difficulty in the process of exertion or attempted exercise.

Episodic weakness may be caused by hypoglycemia in patients with an insulinoma. Because a marked fall in blood glucose results in a counterregulatory response which restores the blood glucose to normal or in an impairment in brain function (syncope or seizures), persistent generalized weakness lasting days to weeks cannot be ascribed to hypoglycemia. Episodic weakness may also be observed in patients with pheochromocytoma or the carcinoid syndrome as a manifestation of paroxysmal hormonal release and in thyrotoxicosis complicated by periodic paralysis.

Weight Loss

A decrease in body weight in the absence of voluntary or involuntary caloric restriction or a marked increase in exercise generally indicates the presence of an underlying disease process. From a diagnostic standpoint it is useful to differentiate weight loss associated with anorexia from that which occurs in association with hyperphagia or a normal appetite. In the absence of anorexia or diuresis, an increase in metabolic rate, abnormal losses of calorie-containing substrates in urine (e.g., glycosuria or ketonuria), or failure of gastrointestinal absorption must be present in a patient with weight loss. In hyperthyroidism and in decompensated diabetes (in which there is marked glycosuria) weight loss in the presence of hyperphagia is frequently observed. Weight loss due to increased caloric expenditure may also be observed in pheochromocytoma. In patients with severe diabetic neuropathy involving the autonomic nervous system, digestive and absorptive processes may be impaired, resulting in severe cachexia despite seemingly adequate caloric consumption.

Weight loss associated with anorexia is observed in Addison's disease and panhypopituitarism, particularly that following the postpartum state, and in severe hyperparathyroidism and other hypercalcemic states. Weight loss may occur uncommonly in the presence of hypometabolism in hypothyroidism because of accompanying anorexia. In anorexia nervosa a severe disturbance of appetite (reflecting a psychological and/or hypothalamic disturbance) may result in weight loss to the point of cachexia.

Weight Gain

An increase in body weight may reflect an accumulation of interstitial fluid (edema) or an increase in body fat (adiposity). Weight gain due to fluid retention can generally be recognized by palpable edema or rapidity of the increment in weight. A gain in weight of 1 kg or more per day invariably indicates fluid retention.

Weight gain due to an increase in adipose tissue is observed in Cushing's syndrome, where there is a characteristic truncal (rather than peripheral) distribution, a "buffalo hump" (increased fat over the lower part of the back of the neck), and large supraclavicular fat pads. In patients with insulin-producing islet-cell tumors a weight gain of 10–15 kg may be observed because of repeated bouts of hypoglycemia resulting in appetite stimulation and increased food intake. Hypometabolism due to hypothyroidism may also result in an increase in body fat. However, fluid retention may also contribute to weight gain in hypothyroidism, as reflected by fluid excess in myxedematous tissues or the presence of ascites or pleural or pericardial effusions.

Obesity is commonly observed in association with type II diabetes. However, the obesity is the predisposing factor to the development of diabetes, not the reverse. In rare circumstances, disturbances of hypothalamic satiety centers result in weight gain; this may be observed in patients with central nervous system disease (trauma, encephalitis, or tumors) or pituitary tumors with sufficient suprasellar extension to compress the ventral hypothalamus.

It should be noted that primary endocrine-metabolic disorders account for less than 5 percent of all cases of obesity (body weight 30 percent or more above ideal). Furthermore, extreme degrees of weight gain—body weight in excess of 115–135 kg (250–300 lb)—are almost never due to a primary endocrine disturbance. However, obesity may *secondarily* result in a variety of alterations in endocrine and metabolic processes. In addition, the extent to which an undefined metabolic defect contributes to the pathophysiology of at least some forms of obesity is not known.

Edema may be observed in association with cardiac failure accompanying thyrotoxicosis, myxedema, or acromegaly. In severe anorexia nervosa or in diabetic nephropathy resulting in proteinuria, edema may develop as a consequence of hypoalbuminemia. Edema is generally not observed in patients with primary hyperaldosteronism. By contrast, corticosteroids exhibiting a mineralocorticoid effect may precipitate or exacerbate fluid accumulation, particularly when administered to patients with underlying cardiac disease. Mineralocorticoids used in the treatment of Addison's disease rarely cause edema when given in excess in the absence of manifest cardiac disease.

Body Temperature

A mild increase in body temperature may be observed in thyrotoxicosis. In thyroid storm (an acute exacerbation of hyperthyroidism), a fever of 101°F or more is characteristic. Hyperpyrexia may occur in primary hypothalamic disease, in secondary disturbances of hypothalamic function after pituitary surgery, or in severely decompensated Addison's disease. Cerebral edema, a rare complication of diabetic ketoacidosis, may result in high fever. Mild increases in temperature may also be seen in untreated Addison's disease. However, caution must be exercised in attributing fever in Addison's disease or diabetic ketoacidosis to the endocrine problem because infections may be responsible for aggravating these conditions.

Hypothermia is common in hypoglycemia, particularly when induced by alcohol. Severe hypothyroidism (myxedema coma) may also be complicated by hypothermia.

SKIN

Hyperpigmentation of the skin is a characteristic finding in Addison's disease. It is accentuated in the exposed parts of the body. The knuckles, elbows, knees, areolae, genitalia, buccal mucosa, palmar creases, and recent scars are the sites of maximum pigmentation. Similar pigment changes may occur in 15–60 percent of patients who undergo bilateral adrenalectomy as treatment for Cushing's disease (bilateral adrenal hyperplasia) and are usually indicative of the presence of an ACTH (adrenocorticotropic hormone)-producing pituitary tumor (Nelson's syndrome). Ectopic production of ACTH by various neoplasms (e.g., lung and pancreas) may also lead to hyperpigmentation. An increase in pigmentation is observed in as many as 40 percent of patients with acromegaly.

Acanthosis nigricans is a syndrome in which there are localized areas of gray-brown hyperpigmentation in the posterior region of the neck and axillae. It is infrequently encountered in uncomplicated obesity, non-insulin-dependent diabetes mellitus, polycystic ovaries, Cushing's syndrome, and acromegaly. Acanthosis nigricans has also been identified in rare diabetic patients with severe insulin resistance associated with a decrease in insulin receptors or the presence of a circulating antibody to or mutation of the insulin receptor.

A generalized decrease in pigmentation occurs in panhypopituitarism. Focal areas of depigmentation (*vitiligo*) are observed in Addison's disease, thyrotoxicosis, and hypoparathyroidism.

Hirsutism, which is defined as an increase in facial hair in women beyond that which is cosmetically acceptable, is observed in a variety of androgen-excess states, including Cushing's syndrome, congenital adrenal hyperplasia, polycystic ovary syndrome, and virilizing ovarian or adrenal tumors. An increase in facial hair may also occur in acromegaly. However, in most cases of hirsutism a specific endocrine cause is not identified.

A decrease in body hair accompanying endocrine disease may be generalized (scalp, axillary and pubic areas, and extremities; *alopecia totalis*), localized to the scalp *alopecia*, or restricted to the lateral third of the eyebrow. In hypopituitarism and hypothyroidism any of these patterns may be noted. In Cushing's syndrome and virilizing ovarian or adrenal tumors frontal baldness may occur. Hair loss may also be observed in thyrotoxicosis and hypoparathyroidism. Most patients with severe alopecia, however, do not have an endocrine disease.

Coarse, dry skin is found in myxedema and in hypoparathyroidism. In myxedema the changes may be so marked as to resemble ichthyosis. In acromegaly the skin is also coarse and has a leathery texture with enlargement of the sweat glands and a true thickening of the various skin layers.

Excessive sweating occurs in thyrotoxicosis and acromegaly. Acute paroxysms of sweating accompanying adrenergic discharge are observed in pheochromocytoma, during hypoglycemic episodes in patients with insulinomas, and in insulin-treated diabetic patients who are experiencing an insulin reaction.

Acne is observed in men and women with Cushing's syndrome or androgen-producing tumors of the adrenal and in women with congenital adrenal hyperplasia, polycystic ovaries, and virilizing tumors of the ovary.

Striae, plethora, thinning of the skin, easy bruisability, and ecchymoses may be observed in spontaneous Cushing's syndrome or after glucocorticoid therapy in pharmacologic doses.

NOSE, EARS, VOICE, AND TONGUE

The hypertrophy of mucous membranes which occurs in acromegaly results in pale, boggy nasal mucosa, frequently associated with symptoms of nasal and sinus obstruction. Hyperplasia of the membranes of the eustachian tube often results in intermittent middle ear blockage and recurrent episodes of serous otitis media. Pituitary tumors may erode the floor of the sella and extend into the sphenoid sinus and even into the nose. With rupture of the dura, cerebrospinal rhinorrhea may occur. This can be diagnosed by the presence of glucose in the nasal discharge, which is detected by use of a glucose oxidase-impregnated dipstick.

Loss of olfaction (*anosmia*) can be due to a tumor in the region of the hypothalamus which destroys the olfactory nerve. It can also be seen with Kallman's syndrome, a genetic disorder associated with hypothalamic hypogonadism.

The tongue is increased in size and frequently furrowed in acromegaly. In more severe cases difficulty in articulation can be noted. The tongue, palate, and buccal and gingival mucosa are often hyperpigmented in Addison's disease and with ACTH-producing pituitary tumors, particularly after adrenalectomy (Nelson's syndrome). There are discrete patches of hyperpigmentation in each of these locations, which at times may be confluent. Tongue pigmentation may be present normally in blacks and in this case is of less diagnostic significance.

In hypothyroidism the tongue is enlarged because of myxedematous infiltration, often resulting in slurred speech. In hyperthyroidism a fine rhythmic tremor which is evident in the outstretched fingers is also present in the tongue. Fine fascicular movements of the tongue may occur in hyperparathyroidism.

In acromegaly, hypertrophy of the larynx leads to a huskiness of the voice; an increase in the paranasal sinuses tends to give the voice more resonance. Myxedematous infiltration of the larynx in hypothyroidism results in deepening of the voice and, occasionally, severe hoarseness. Laryngeal examination reveals dullness, thickening, and flabbiness of the free margins of the true vocal cords. With advanced myxedema, smooth edematous polyps may form on the vocal cords. Deepening of the voice frequently occurs in women in the presence of increased androgen secretion, as in Cushing's syndrome, congenital adrenal hyperplasia, and virilizing adrenal or ovarian tumors. In men the influence of excess androgens on the voice cannot be detected clinically unless it occurs during the prepubertal period, as in congenital adrenal hyperplasia. The voice changes do not always completely disappear upon removal of the excess androgen. Large goiters and invasive thyroid carcinomas can also produce hoarseness.

In males in whom pubertal changes fail to occur as a result of androgen deficiency due to a hypothalamic, pituitary, or gonadal disturbance, the voice remains high-pitched. However, once the voice has acquired the typical characteristics of an adult male, loss of androgen does not cause any change in quality.

GASTROINTESTINAL SYSTEM

Anorexia is often observed in primary hyperparathyroidism and other hypercalcemic conditions, Addison's disease, and diabetic ketoacidosis. A reduction in appetite may also occur in hypothyroidism, panhypopituitarism, and apathetic hyperthyroidism. Anorexia nervosa is characterized by abnormal ideation regarding body weight and food intake in addition to loss of appetite. Nausea and vomiting are often seen in diabetic ketoacidosis, hyperparathyroidism and other disorders with significant hypercalcemia, and Addison's disease.

An increase in appetite commonly accompanies hyperthyroidism, diabetes mellitus with moderate hyperglycemia, glucocorticoid therapy, and Cushing's syndrome. It is also seen in about 15 percent of patients with an insulinoma.

Oropharyngeal dysphagia may be caused by a large goiter or by a locally invasive thyroid carcinoma.

Abdominal pain occurs in a variety of endocrine disorders. Nonspecific, diffuse abdominal pain occurs frequently in children with diabetic ketoacidosis. Patients with addisonian crisis often present with diffuse abdominal pain. Less severe pain is a frequent complaint with chronic adrenal insufficiency. In thyroid storm abdominal pain may be a major complaint. However, in all these instances, the physician should consider the possibility that the pain is due to another process that has exacerbated the condition, especially if the pain is unresolved with control of the condition. Ileus with gaseous and colicky pain may be observed in myxedema. Both acute and chronic patterns of abdominal pain occur in patients with the carcinoid syndrome. In primary hyperparathyroidism abdominal pain may be due to peptic ulcer disease or to pancreatitis. In addition, a minority of patients with this disease present with a diffuse and poorly described abdominal pain of uncertain cause which resolves with surgical correction of the hyperparathyroidism. Symptoms of severe or recurrent peptic ulcer are the most characteristic features of the gastrinoma (Zollinger-Ellison) syndrome. Gastrointestinal bleeding may complicate peptic ulceration in primary hyperparathyroidism and in the gastrinoma syndrome. Patients receiving glucocorticoid therapy in combination with nonsteroidal antiinflammatory agents are at increased risk for developing peptic ulcers, and severely ill patients on high-dose glucocorticoid therapy are at increased risk for developing gastrointestinal hemorrhage.

Constipation occurs frequently in hypothyroidism and in patients with marked hypercalcemia or hypokalemia, and may occur with pheochromocytoma. Patients with diabetic autonomic neuropathy may complain of constipation alternating with diarrhea that is often nocturnal and is accompanied by fecal incontinence.

Diarrhea may be prominent in patients with metastatic medullary carcinoma of the thyroid, a metastatic carcinoid tumor, and vasoactive intestinal peptide (VIP)–producing tumors. Approximately one-third of those with the gastrinoma syndrome present with diarrhea; frank steatorrhea may be seen in both the gastrinoma and carcinoid syndromes. Hyperthyroidism is associated with an increased frequency of somewhat poorly formed stools rather than actual diarrhea. Explosive and life-threatening diarrhea dominates the clinical picture in patients with pancreatic cholera due to tumors of the pancreatic islets or other gastrointestinal neuroendocrine tumors that produce VIP.

Significant hepatic abnormalities are uncommon in endocrine disorders, but liver function tests may be abnormal in both severe thyrotoxicosis and myxedema and also in patients with far-advanced carcinoid tumors. In poorly controlled diabetic patients hepatomegaly due to fatty infiltration may be observed.

HEMOPOIETIC SYSTEM

Anemia occurs frequently in a wide variety of endocrine disorders. The anemia may be a direct consequence of the specific endocrine deficiency or hypersecretion or may result from a complication of endocrine disease such as acute blood loss anemia or iron-deficiency anemia due to peptic ulcer disease in primary hyperparathyroidism or the gastrinoma syndrome.

A mild normocytic normochromic anemia with hypoplastic bone marrow regularly accompanies panhypopituitarism and is corrected by replacement therapy with thyroid, adrenal, and gonadal hormones. Growth hormone deficiency, therefore, appears not to play a major role in the development of this anemia. The anemia may be partially masked by a coincident contraction in plasma volume.

Pernicious anemia occurs in a small percentage of patients with the polyglandular syndrome of multiple endocrine deficiencies (Schmidt's syndrome); this can result in Addison's disease, insulin-dependent diabetes mellitus, hypothyroidism, and gonadal failure.

A mild to moderate anemia is commonly noted in hypothyroidism. Thyroid hormone deficiency results in a normocytic normochromic anemia with hypoplastic bone marrow, possibly due to a decrease in erythropoietin production, and more commonly in a microcytic hypochromic anemia of iron deficiency. This is due to a high incidence of menorrhagia in female patients and the approximately 50 percent incidence of achlorhydria and iron malabsorption in patients of both sexes. A macrocytic hyperchromic anemia occurs in about 10 percent of patients with hypothyroidism and may be due to deficiency of folic acid or to classic pernicious anemia.

Hyperthyroidism is usually not accompanied by anemia, although severely thyrotoxic patients may display a mild normocytic normochromic or hypochromic anemia. Pernicious anemia with antiparietal cell antibodies occurs in approximately 3 percent of patients with Graves' disease.

Patients with adrenal insufficiency have a mild normocytic normochromic anemia which is often not readily apparent because of the concomitant decrease in plasma volume. Patients with Cushing's disease display a mild erythrocytosis with hemoglobin levels 1–2 g/dl higher than normal; this is less often observed with the administration of pharmacologic doses of exogenous steroids.

Androgens have a well-known erythropoietic effect, and pharmacologic doses are employed in treating a variety of refractory anemias. This effect contributes to the anemia in men with severe testosterone deficiency and to the higher hemoglobin values seen in sexually mature males than in females and prepubertal males. A mild elevation in hemoglobin is often seen in men treated with testosterone.

A normocytic normochromic anemia occurring in about 20 percent of patients with primary hyperparathyroidism, particularly in patients with severe hypercalcemia, resolves after surgical correction of the disease. Iron-deficiency anemia may occur in hyperparathyroidism complicated by peptic ulcer disease and gastrointestinal bleeding.

Patients with a pheochromocytoma may display a slight increase in hemoglobin values because of the concomitant contraction in plasma volume. There may also be a direct influence of catecholamines on erythropoietin production.

A relative leukopenia is frequently noted in panhypopituitarism. Approximately 10 percent of patients with thyrotoxicosis present with leukopenia and/or granulocytopenia. Failure to recognize leukopenia before instituting treatment with antithyroid drugs may lead to confusion because these drugs (e.g., propylthiouracil) may suppress the granulocyte count. The lymphocyte number is normal or slightly increased in hyperthyroid patients, leading to a relative lymphocytosis. No consistent abnormalities in leukocyte values are noted in hypothyroidism. In Cushing's syndrome, mild granulocytosis, lymphopenia, and eosinopenia are commonly observed. Lymphocytosis and eosinophilia are commonly observed in Addison's disease. The latter finding was, for many years, considered a diagnostic clue to the disorder. A leukocytosis of 15,000–30,000 cells per cubic millimeter regularly occurs in diabetic ketoacidosis, and so a leukocyte count is of little value in suggesting infection as the initiating event leading to the ketoacidosis. A marked leukocytosis is also routinely observed in hyperosmolar nonketotic coma. A minority of patients with pheochromocytoma display a mild leukocytosis.

Glucocorticoids may acutely promote a rise in platelets; thrombocytosis may also be observed with chronic glucocorticoid excess.

CARDIOVASCULAR SYSTEM

Tachycardia almost always accompanies hyperthyroidism and pheochromocytoma. Ordinarily this is of sinus origin, but occasionally there may be paroxysmal atrial tachycardia or atrial fibrillation with a rapid ventricular response, particularly in older individuals. An ectopic arrhythmia with these conditions usually signifies underlying heart disease. The tachycardia may give rise to palpitations. Tachycardia also occurs when there is dehydration, as with adrenocortical insufficiency due to destruction of the gland or 21α-hydroxylase deficiency, and in uncontrolled diabetes. There is often a bradycardia in hypothyroidism. The hypokalemia of primary aldosteronism can result in ventricular ectopy and ventricular tachycardia; rarely, patients with this disorder present with ventricular arrhythmia.

An increased incidence of myocardial infarction and stroke can be observed with any of the syndromes that result in hypercholesterolemia or hypertension. Hypercholesterolemia may be present with hypothyroidism, acromegaly, and diabetes. Hypertension is associated with acromegaly, primary aldosteronism, pheochromocytoma, Cushing's syndrome, glucocorticoid therapy (occasionally), renovascular hypertension, and renal disease (as in diabetes or hypercalcemia). The incidence of myocardial infarction, stroke, and peripheral vascular disease is increased with diabetes.

Typically, heart size is smaller than usual in Addison's disease, hypopituitarism, and hyperthyroidism. In hypothyroidism and any conditions associated with hypertension, the heart size may be increased and congestive heart failure may be present. Cardiac failure may accompany hyperthyroidism or pheochromocytoma, presumably because of the excessive demands on the heart due to the increased beta-adrenergic stimulation associated with thyroid hormone or catecholamine excess. In younger people, this rarely leads to congestive failure, but in the elderly with underlying atherosclerotic disease these conditions can lead to serious cardiac decompensation. Heart size is increased in acromegaly and can eventually lead to heart failure.

The causes of edema were discussed earlier in the section on weight gain.

Occasionally toxic reactions or resistance to the drugs used in the treatment of cardiovascular disease may signify or result in endocrine disease. For instance, digitalis toxicity may be precipitated more rapidly in hyperthyroidism and pheochromocytoma and with hypokalemia, as in primary aldosteronism. Insensitivity to the bradycardia and antianginal effects of beta-adrenergic blockers may occur with hyperthyroidism. Amiodarone used in the management of arrhythmias may result in hypothyroidism or, less commonly, hyperthyroidism.

URINARY TRACT

Frequency, polyuria, and nocturia (or enuresis in children) are classically observed in diabetes mellitus and in central or nephrogenic diabetes insipidus. Severe hypercalcemia or hypokalemia may impair renal tubular concentrating ability, and so these symptoms may also be seen in patients with primary hyperparathyroidism and other hypercalcemic disorders and in patients with primary aldosteronism and Bartter's syndrome. Patients with diabetic autonomic neuropathy may complain of frequency, incontinence, or urinary retention.

Diabetes mellitus is associated with an increased incidence of urinary tract and mycotic vaginal and vulvar infections. Patients with diabetes are also prone to the development of papillary necrosis as a complication of pyelonephritis. A number of glomerular lesions occur in diabetes mellitus that are associated with proteinuria and progressive renal impairment. The most specific and important of these lesions is nodular glomerulosclerosis. Mild proteinuria may also be observed in myxedema.

Nephrolithiasis and/or nephrocalcinosis occur in a variety of endocrine disorders. Renal stone formation is a complication of primary hyperparathyroidism. An increased incidence of stones is also observed in a number of other hypercalcemic or hypercalciuric conditions, including sarcoidosis, vitamin D intoxication, idiopathic hypercalciuria, Cushing's syndrome, and acromegaly. Nephrocalcinosis with or without a history of stone or renal impairment occurs in primary hyperparathyroidism, vitamin D intoxication, and the milk-alkali syndrome.

SEXUAL FUNCTION

Endocrine disease must be considered when there is impotence or a change in libido, but accounts for only a small proportion of these problems. Changes in libido irregularly accompany hypo- and hyperfunctioning of the adrenal cortex and the thyroid gland, hypokalemia with primary aldosteronism or Bartter's syndrome, hypercalcemia, anorexia nervosa, gonadal failure (ovarian or testicular), poorly controlled diabetes, and hypopituitarism. Impotence can be observed with gonadal failure (primary or secondary), diabetes with autonomic neuropathy, drug therapy for hypertension and hypothyroidism. Hyperprolactinemia of any etiology, but particularly that associated with pituitary tumors, results in decreased libido in both sexes and, frequently, impotence. Any severe illness, including endocrine disease, may be associated with decreased libido, although in such an illness it is unusual for this to be a prominent complaint.

Amenorrhea or oligomenorrhea can be observed in gonadal dysgenesis (e.g., Turner's syndrome), primary ovarian failure, the testicular feminizing and pseudohermaphroditic syndromes, Kallman's syndrome (gonadotropin deficiency associated with anosmia), the adrenogenital syndrome, and menopause. Menstrual disturbances generally occur in hypopituitarism, as in Sheehan's syndrome (panhypopituitarism secondary to pituitary necrosis in women who have experienced postpartum hemorrhagic shock), and in patients with prolactin-secreting pituitary tumors. Amenorrhea or oligomenorrhea may appear in women after the discontinuation of oral contraceptives, especially if they have a history of prior menstrual irregularities. These problems may also occur in Cushing's syndrome, hyperthyroidism, hypothyroidism, anorexia nervosa, or polycystic ovaries (with increased androgen production). When amenorrhea is associated with diabetes, adrenal insufficiency, or hypothyroidism, the syndrome of multiple endocrine deficiency (Schmidt's syndrome) should be considered. Most endocrinopathies in severe form can result in secondary amenorrhea.

Metrorrhagia, or bleeding between menstrual periods, can be present in hyperestrogen states resulting from a number of causes, including high-dose estrogen therapy. Spontaneous causes include anovulation secondary to diverse disorders and excess estrogen production due to tumors. For example, with anovulation associated with polycystic ovarian disease or the period just before and after the menarche, continued gonadotropin secretion results in the formation of a number of estrogen-producing nonovulatory graafian follicles. Tumors causing metrorrhagia may be of ovarian origin (e.g., thecoma, granulosa cell tumor) or of adrenal origin. Ectopic production of trophic factors (e.g., ACTH) by tumors may secondarily stimulate estrogen production, leading to metrorrhagia.

Infertility can result from any of the causes of amenorrhea or oligomenorrhea listed previously. With oligomenorrhea there may be either oligoovulation or anovulation; the distinction is important because pregnancy can occur in the former case. Infertility may result from a restricted luteal phase leading to defective support of the implantation of the fertilized egg. This situation results from deficient progesterone production due to either defective responsiveness to luteinizing hormone (LH) or inadequate LH production. The latter may result from pituitary disease or from defective hypothalamic function due to psychogenic or neurogenic problems.

In men, endocrine problems resulting in hypothalamic-pituitary or testicular failure account for only a small proportion of cases of infertility or subfertility. Prolactin-producing pituitary tumors have been implicated in some cases of male infertility.

In women, changes due to androgen excess are termed *virilization*. These changes include hirsutism (discussed earlier), male pattern baldness, deepened voice, acne, and clitoral enlargement. The excess androgens may be of ovarian or adrenal origin or may result from exogenous androgen administration. Ovarian overproduction of androgen may be due to hyperplasia (as in polycystic ovaries or ovarian androgenic dysplasia) or tumor (e.g., arrhenoblastoma, hilar cell tumor, adrenal rest tumor, or gynandroblastoma). Excess adrenal androgen production may be due to Cushing's syndrome, enzyme defects (e.g., 11- or 21-hydroxylase deficiency), or neoplasia and, in the absence of glucocorticoid excess, may account for some cases of idiopathic hirsutism.

Precocious puberty may result from a hormone-secreting tumor (most commonly ovarian but less commonly adrenal) or to constitutional, physiologic, or organic disturbances (e.g., postencephalitis, postmeningitis, postcerebral trauma, hypothalamic lesions, pinealoma or other tumors of the central nervous system). It is characterized by early breast development, axillary and pubic hair, onset of menstrual periods, and, in true precocious puberty, fertility. True cyclic menses and fertility are not, however, seen with adrenal or ovarian tumors which suppress gonadotropin secretion and cause precocious pseudopuberty. Sometimes there may be isolated precocious breast development or the appearance of pubic hair. A major problem with this syndrome is that there is premature closure of the epiphyses; as a consequence, many of the subjects are of short stature.

Gynecomastia, or abnormal breast enlargement, occurs physiologically in normal males at puberty, subsiding ordinarily during adolescence. It should be differentiated from breast enlargement due to excess fat tissue rather than ductal tissue (e.g., obesity and lipoma) and from breast tumors.

Gynecomastia may be caused by estrogen-producing tumors that are usually of adrenal origin (usually carcinomas) but may rarely be of chorionic, testicular granulosa cell, or interstitial cell origin. It may also be seen in cirrhosis, presumably because of a decrease in the metabolic clearance of circulating estrogens.

Gynecomastia may occur after estrogen, androgen, digitalis, hydralazine, phenothiazine, chorionic gonadotropin, or spironolactone therapy or marijuana use, and it may be seen in hypergonadotropic hypogonadism such as Klinefelter's syndrome or Riefenstein syndrome. Gynecomastia may signify a pituitary or ectopic tumor (usually of pulmonary origin) producing prolactin (occasionally) or gonadotropins (rarely). Gynecomastia is sometimes seen after chronic hemodialysis, in hyperthyroidism, and during recovery from severe malnutrition.

Nonpuerperal lactation (galactorrhea) may occur as a consequence of several types of pituitary disturbance. Commonly, these disturbances are associated with increased prolactin production. Galactorrhea may occur after anesthesia, thoracic surgery, exercise, nipple stimulation, sexual intercourse, chest wall trauma, infection (herpes zoster), spinal cord lesions, and several drugs (phenothiazines, methyldopa, and dopamine receptor antagonists). Galactorrhea is frequently associated with prolactin-producing pituitary adenomas. Galactorrhea is sometimes observed with acromegaly, other pituitary tumors, and destructive lesions of the hypothalamus and pituitary stalk. It may also be seen with hypothyroidism or estrogen therapy and is commonly observed in women with chronic renal failure.

BONES AND JOINTS

Decreased linear growth, dysgenetic epiphyseal centers, and ultimate dwarfing are observed in hypothyroidism that occurs in childhood. Abnormalities in linear growth are also observed in poorly controlled diabetes mellitus, panhypopituitarism, isolated growth hormone deficiency, and endogenous or exogenous glucocorticoid excess. Androgen excess produces an increased *rate* of linear growth, but premature closure of the epiphyseal centers ultimately leads to short stature. Short stature is also observed in Turner's syndrome.

Primary or secondary androgen insufficiency is associated with the development of eunuchoidal skeletal proportions. An unusual pattern of disproportionate growth of the lower extremities occurs in Klinefelter's syndrome.

Increased periosteal bone formation leads to typical facial and acral bone abnormalities in acromegaly. If the disease begins prior to epiphyseal closure, there is increased linear growth leading to gigantism. The various forms of rickets are associated with a number of bone deformities, including bowing of the limbs, frontal bossing, and beading of the ribs. Shortened fourth metacarpals occur regularly in pseudohypoparathyroidism and Turner's syndrome.

Osteoporosis or osteopenia is frequently encountered in postmenopausal women. Osteoporosis is also a feature of a variety of endocrine disorders, occurring in endogenous and exogenous hyperadrenocorticism, adult hypophosphatasia and other metabolic bone diseases, and hypogonadism (including premature ovarian failure). It is particularly severe in Turner's syndrome. Osteopenia is commonly observed in patients with long-standing hyperthyroidism or hyperprolactinemia; bone biopsies in these patients reveal a variable admixture of osteoporosis, osteomalacia, and osteitis fibrosa cystica. Severe calcium deficiency may result in osteoporosis, but there is scant evidence to suggest that calcium deficiency plays a primary role in the osteoporosis commonly encountered in the United States. Mild osteopenia has been reported in both children and adults with diabetes mellitus.

Osteomalacia with diffuse bone pain and tenderness and muscular weakness occurs in vitamin D deficiency and with vitamin D and calcium malabsorption due to a number of gastrointestinal diseases. A variety of renal tubular disorders are associated with rickets in children and osteomalacia in adults. Tumor-associated osteomalacia is an unusual and particularly severe form of the disorder which occurs in association with mesenchymal neoplasms.

Significant osteopenia is uncommonly observed in patients receiving anticonvulsant therapy in the United States. Clinically significant osteitis fibrosa cystica may occur with severe primary hyperparathyroidism; clinical or subclinical osteopenia (demonstrable by bone densitometry) in patients with less severe hyperparathyroidism may be due to osteoporosis, osteomalacia, or mild osteitis. Osteoporosis, osteomalacia, or osteitis fibrosa cystica can be present in patients with renal osteodystrophy. In the majority of patients with advanced renal insufficiency, several of these lesions coexist.

In acromegaly, bone overgrowth with distortion of the articular plate leads to degenerative arthritis, which may be severe and disabling. Chronic chondrocalcinosis (pseudogout) may occur in primary hyperparathyroidism; there are questionable associations between acute episodes of pseudogout and diabetes mellitus and between primary gout and primary hyperparathyroidism.

Increased levels of serum uric acid have been reported in primary hyperparathyroidism, myxedema, nephrogenic diabetes insipidus, Bartter's syndrome, and Paget disease. Some reports suggest that episodes of acute gouty arthritis occur with increased frequency in several of these disorders. Marked elevations in serum uric acid may accompany diabetic ketoacidosis but resolve rapidly with control of the ketoacidosis.

CENTRAL NERVOUS SYSTEM

Headache is a common finding in pituitary tumors and is caused by pressure of the expanding tumor on the dura. Headaches are particularly severe in growth hormone-secreting tumors. With rupture of the dura, the headache frequently disappears. Headache is characteristically present in pituitary apoplexy and may be present in tumors of the hypothalamus or the parasellar region. Headache also occurs in pseudotumor cerebri, hypertensive episodes associated with pheochromocytoma, and insulinomas with hypoglycemia. Headache may also be prominent in patients with the "empty sella" syndrome. Although the headaches tend to remain constant in individual patients, no characteristics are specific to the individual disease entities.

Depression, lethargy, apathy, and impaired mentation (disorientation and confusion) can be seen in hyperparathyroidism and other hypercalcemic states, hypothyroidism, hypopituitarism, hypoglycemia (irrespective of cause), Cushing's syndrome, and severe hyperglycemia (with or without ketoacidosis). Marked changes (either increases or decreases) in serum osmolality such as those seen in severe diabetes insipidus (hypernatremia) and in hyponatremic states due to inappropriately increased vasopressin also lead to a decreased sensorium. In each of these disorders, if the hormonal or metabolic disturbance is left untreated, a comatose state will develop.

Focal as well as generalized convulsions may occur in patients with severe hypoglycemia, nonketotic hyperglycemia, inappropriately increased vasopressin, Addison's disease, myxedema, hypopituitarism, and hypocalcemia associated with hypoparathyroidism. In the latter case, tetany generally precedes the onset of convulsions by a variable period of time ranging from days to years. Diabetic ketoacidosis is not accompanied by convulsions, probably because of the anticonvulsive effect of acidosis and/or ketosis.

Central nervous system effects, either direct or indirect, have been demonstrated for virtually every hormone studied. It is therefore not surprising that many abnormalities in endocrine function cause problems ranging from mild to profound depression or anxiety to profound behavioral disorders. In hypopituitarism, depression is common and psychoses are occasionally seen. In hypothyroidism, depression is frequently observed. In more severe cases, psychoses (myxedema madness) manifested by hallucinations, paranoid behavior, dementia, and even classic schizophrenic reactions can occur. In general, older patients are more prone than younger ones to develop a typical organic brain syndrome. The response to treatment is usually excellent. However, in elderly patients behavioral aberrations may persist. Hypothyroid patients are generally less aware of exteroceptive stimuli. Consequently, during the initial period of replacement therapy, behavioral problems may worsen until the patient readjusts to the new level of recognizable environmental input signals. Patients with hyperthyroidism show mood fluctuations which may progress to delirium and, as thyroid storm approaches, a florid psychosis. Patients with insulinomas that cause repeated and undiagnosed hypoglycemic episodes may develop bizarre behavioral disturbances due to impaired central nervous system metabolism. The diagnosis of a toxic psychosis is frequently made in such patients. In Addison's disease a depressive psychosis can occur. Depression and emotional lability are common in spontaneous Cushing's syndrome. Glucocorticoid therapy commonly results in euphoria. True psychotic behavior occurs uncommonly with both spontaneous and iatrogenic Cushing's syndrome.

NEUROMUSCULAR ABNORMALITIES

Neuropathy is a common long-term complication of diabetes mellitus. Symptoms of neuropathy are present in about 15 percent of diabetic patients, while abnormalities of nerve conduction are demonstrable in up to 50 percent . The spectrum of diabetic neuropathy includes (1) acute mononeuropathy of cranial or peripheral nerves, (2) mononeuropathy multiplex, (3) distal polyneuropathy, and (4) autonomic neuropathy.

In mononeuritis multiplex there is involvement of a mixed sensorimotor nerve or group of nerves, resulting in pain and focal weakness. Frequently the sites of involvement are the hip, knee, and thigh areas, with resultant pain on walking.

In diabetic polyneuropathy there is distal, symmetric involvement primarily of sensory fibers. The feet and legs are affected to a greater extent than are the hands. Numbness and paresthesias are the major complaints. There is loss of the ankle jerk and of various sensory modalities (vibration, position, light touch).

Autonomic neuropathy generally appears in patients who already have severe peripheral neuropathy. The symptoms include loss of sweating, diarrhea which is particularly severe at night and is accompanied by fecal incontinence, orthostatic hypotension, impotence, and an atonic bladder.

Polyneuropathy involving primarily sensory nerves is also occasionally observed in patients with hyperparathyroidism.

A mononeuropathy that involves the distal median nerve and is due to compression at the wrist (*carpal tunnel syndrome*) can be observed in acromegaly and hypothyroidism. This is caused by thickening of connective tissue in acromegaly or increased deposition of mucinous material between connective tissue fibers in myxedema that results in pressure on the median nerve in the carpal tunnel. The symptoms consist of numbness, tingling, and pain in the radial two-thirds of the palmar surface of the hand and fingers. Weakness of abduction and apposition of the thumb may also occur.

A prolongation of the reflex relaxation time ("hung-up reflexes") in the absence of other evidence of neuropathy is a characteristic finding in hypothyroidism. Similar findings may occur in hyponatremic states such as Addison's disease and the syndrome of inappropriate secretion of antidiuretic hormone (SIADH).

Impaired motor function due to myopathic changes may be observed in hyperthyroidism, hypothyroidism, spontaneous or iatrogenic Cushing's syndrome, and disorders of calcium and phosphorus metabolism.

In hyperthyroidism weakness is most marked in the pelvic girdle and thigh muscles and is accompanied by muscle atrophy. The shoulder and hand muscles may also show atrophy. However, tremor rather than weakness is the more prominent symptom in the upper extremities.

Myopathy may also occur in myxedema, in which patients may complain of stiffness, cramps, and aching in addition to weakness. The muscles may appear hypertrophic because of infiltration with mucinous material. Corticosteroid myopathy is characterized by weakness that is more prominent in the proximal limb and girdle musculature, resulting in difficulty in rising from a sitting position and in raising the arms.

In hypophosphatemic rickets and osteomalacia, muscle weakness and atrophy are common. In Klinefelter's syndrome, the weakness that commonly occurs is due to androgen deficiency.

Episodic weakness accompanied by hypokalemia is observed in patients with primary hyperaldosteronism or Bartter's syndrome and occasionally in patients with thyrotoxicosis. In the latter group the attacks simulate those observed in familial periodic paralysis, but a family history of episodic paralysis is lacking.

In diabetic amyotrophy, involvement of a peripheral motor nerve or nerve end plate in the neuropathic process results in focal weakness and atrophy in the absence of sensory loss, simulating primary myopathic disease.

Acromegalic neuromyopathy is occasionally seen in patients with long-standing disease. Extreme weakness, primarily of proximal musculature, is the predominant finding.

OPHTHALMIC ABNORMALITIES

Diminished vision occurs with several endocrine diseases as a consequence of pressure on the optic nerve or tract, retinal degeneration, or vascular disease. In pituitary tumors with suprasellar extension, pressure on the optic chiasm typically results in a bitemporal hemianopia, although other specific and often asymmetric field defects can occur. The visual impairment can progress to complete blindness and optic atrophy. The blindness may occur suddenly in association with hemorrhage into the tumor (pituitary apoplexy).

Pigmentary optic atrophy has been reported in association with several hereditary syndromes in which obesity, diabetes, mental retardation, and hypogonadism are components. Severe to total visual loss is frequently present. Visual loss may also occur in severe thyroid ophthalmopathy (Graves' disease) as a result of increased orbital pressure leading to compression and ischemia of the optic nerve.

Cataracts and lenticular opacities that can impair vision are seen in hypothyroidism, hypoparathyroidism, and diabetes mellitus. Transient impairment of vision with symptoms of myopia developing over days to weeks accompanies severe hyperglycemic symptoms in approximately one-third of patients with newly discovered or poorly regulated type I diabetes. Hyperopic changes are less frequent but more dramatic in onset, often appearing several days after the onset of insulin treatment. Both symptoms disappear after several weeks of therapy. Blurring of both near and distant vision may develop rapidly during episodes of hyperglycemia in diabetic patients receiving insulin therapy; the visual impairment resolves as the blood glucose concentration returns to normal. These rapid changes in visual acuity due to marked fluctuations in blood glucose must be differentiated from the more permanent and serious visual loss which may occur in diabetic retinopathy. Diabetic retinopathy, in its most severe form, results in decreased vision by fibrous scar tissue formation in the macular area in association with neovascularization and by hemorrhage into the subhyaloid space or the vitreous humor. Acute, reversible blurring of vision may also occur during attacks of hypoglycemia.

Pain in or about the eye can occur in Graves' ophthalmopathy because of increased intraorbital pressure. It is also seen in diabetes associated with ophthalmoplegia or with rubeosis iridis, a form of neovascularization of the iris which can cause a painful hemorrhagic glaucoma.

Swelling around the eyes or periorbital edema is commonly seen in patients with myxedema, in whom the eyelids and surrounding skin exhibit a nonpitting, puffy swelling which appears boggy. Chemosis and swelling of the lids and periorbital tissue are prominent features of progressive Graves' ophthalmopathy and serve to distinguish the disease from retroorbital tumors, in which these changes are not seen. Increases in lacrimal gland size as well as soft tissue swelling in the periorbital area are frequently seen in acromegaly. Periorbital edema may also occur in diabetic patients with severe renal disease and the nephrotic syndrome.

Loss of the lateral third of the eyebrow is seen in hypothyroidism and in hypopituitarism but is not diagnostic of those diseases. In long-standing hypoparathyroidism, the hair of the eyebrows and eyelids becomes thin and patchy.

Ophthalmoplegia or eye muscle weakness leading to diplopia may be seen with pituitary tumors which extend laterally into the cavernous sinus and impinge on the oculomotor nerves. Slight to moderate impairment of eye movements is extremely common in thyrotoxicosis. In its mildest form, asymptomatic symmetric impairment of elevation of the eyes without diplopia is frequently missed. Unilateral weakness of the superior rectus muscle leading to upper lid retraction may be the first manifestation of Graves' disease. With increasing ophthalmoplegia, diplopia may occur on lateral or superior gaze. Myasthenia gravis can also cause ophthalmoplegia, but ptosis is a more common finding. Diabetic ophthalmoplegia involves the third and sixth nerves with equal frequency, has a rapid onset associated with pain on the ipsilateral side of the face, and, if the third nerve is involved, characteristically spares the pupil. Improvement occurs spontaneously in a few weeks, and complete recovery is almost invariable.

Severe protrusion of the eye in Graves' exophthalmos can impair total closure of the lids (*lagophthalmos*), resulting in corneal exposure during sleep and potentially dangerous exposure keratitis. In hypothyroidism discrete gray-colored spots may occur in the central portion of the cornea but do not generally interfere with vision.

In hyperparathyroidism and other hypercalcemic states of long duration, deposition of calcium phosphate crystals, a condition referred to as *band keratopathy*, may be observed at the medial and lateral margins of the cornea close to but separate from the cornea-sclera junction. Slit-lamp examination is frequently required to demonstrate the presence of keratopathy. In hypoparathyroidism there may be severe keratoconjunctivitis. Dilatation of conjunctival venules is seen in patients with diabetes, in parallel with the changes in retinal vessels. The dilatation, which is initially reversible, eventually becomes fixed and exhibits sacculations and even exudation.

Loss of pupillary reflexes may occur with pituitary tumors which invade the cavernous sinus. In diabetic ophthalmoplegia, the pupil is generally spared.

Both flaky and crystalline lenticular opacities are occasionally seen in hypothyroidism, but they generally do not interfere with vision. In contrast, cataracts and lenticular opacities are the most common eye findings in hypoparathyroidism. They may appear as diffuse white opacities separated by fluid clefts or as small and discrete punctate opacities in the lens cortex seen only on slit-lamp examination. The opacities are usually bilateral and frequently do not interfere with vision, though in some cases mature cataracts develop and require extraction. In younger diabetic patients cataracts are classically of the "snowflake" type and appear as bilateral dense bands of white spots situated in the subcapsular region of the lens. In older diabetic patients cataracts are morphologically indistinguishable from the senile cataracts in nondiabetic individuals. Although cataracts are no more frequent in diabetic patients than in nondiabetic individuals, they mature more rapidly and require extraction at an earlier age. Long-term treatment with high-dose glucocorticoids has been associated with posterior capsular cataracts.

Retinal changes characteristic of hypertension can be seen in acromegaly, primary aldosteronism, Cushing's syndrome, pheochromocytoma, and diabetes. Diabetic patients also exhibit a specific retinopathy consisting of capillary, arteriole, and venule microaneurysms appearing as small punctate red dots along the course of small vessels. These lesions may be confused with small hemorrhages but can be differentiated with fluorescein angiography. They are almost always bilateral and tend to be most frequent in the perimacular area. Microaneurysms are seen less frequently with other diseases, such as malignant hypertension, chronic anemias, and central retinal venous thromboses. Coalescence and rupture of microaneurysms lead to hemorrhages; the leakage of protein leads to exudation.

Papilledema is seen in patients with benign intracranial hypertension (pseudotumor cerebri), often associated with the use of oral contraceptives. It also occurs in obesity and in severe Graves' exophthalmos, hypoparathyroidism, the empty sella syndrome, neuroblastoma, and severe hypertension due to pheochromocytoma. It is observed less frequently in Cushing's syndrome and pituitary tumors, and in rare instances it is seen in primary aldosteronism.

Glaucoma can be precipitated or aggravated by spontaneous or iatrogenic hypercorticism. Glaucoma is also observed with increased frequency in diabetes mellitus.

CHAPTER 3

Biosynthesis, Secretion and Metabolism of Hormones

Gordon N. Gill

Endocrinology is the study of hormones, which are allosteric effectors; hormone receptors, which are the allosteric proteins to which they bind; and the biological consequences of their interactions. Although the kinetics of the interactions between hormones and receptor proteins are complex, they can ordinarily be represented as biomolecular reactions:

$$\underset{[H]}{\text{Hormone}} + \underset{[R]}{\text{Receptor}} \underset{k_2}{\overset{k_1}{\rightleftarrows}} \underset{[HR]}{\text{Hormone} \cdot \text{Receptor}}$$

The binding of hormones to receptor proteins involves primarily hydrophobic interactions with hydrogen bonds, van der Waals forces, and salt bridges, but not covalent linkages. Thus, hormone-receptor complex formation is reversible, and allosteric regulation can be terminated quickly once the allosteric effector is reduced in concentration. In the mass action equation shown above, the formation of the active complex [HR] depends on the concentrations of both the hormone and the receptor protein as well as on the intrinsic affinity of the receptor for the hormone. Genetic and acquired endocrine diseases are ultimately expressed as an alteration from normal in one term of this equation.

Extensive control systems regulate all the components of these basic ingredients of the hormone-response system. Synthesis, secretion, transport, and metabolism of hormones determine the hormone concentration term, while synthesis, modification, and metabolism of the receptor protein determine the receptor concentration term in this equation.

Hormones have one of three major chemical structures: peptide, steroid, or amino acid analog. Although different hormones have distinct biological effects, all hormones of the peptide class and all hormones of the steroid class share common features of biosynthesis, secretion, transport, and mechanisms of action with others of the same class. These common features provide a framework in which the unique characteristics of a particular hormone can be understood and comparisons between hormones can be made. Thyroid hormones and catecholamines, which have the amino acid tyrosine as a central structural feature, are synthesized and metabolized via pathways which are unique and distinct from peptide or steroid hormones and from each other.

PEPTIDE HORMONES

Biosynthesis of Messenger RNA

Because peptide hormones are small secretory proteins, their biosynthesis and secretion occur through the same processes as those which involve larger nonhormonal secretory proteins such as immunoglobulins, albumin, pancreatic enzymes, and egg white proteins. The biosynthetic steps are general ones for all proteins with variations such as multigene families, derivation of different hormones from a common messenger RNA precursor by differential splicing, generation of multiple hormones from a common protein precursor, and synthesis of multisubunit hormones. DNA sequences whose transcripts appear in mature messenger RNA *(exons)* are interrupted by intervening sequences *(introns)*, which are transcribed, along with exon and 3′-flanking DNA sequences, into messenger RNA precursors. The intron and 3′-flanking DNA sequences are removed during the process of messenger RNA maturation before delivery of the exon-containing messenger RNA to the cytoplasm, where translation into protein occurs. Genes coding for proteins are transcribed by RNA polymerase II, a large multisubunit enzyme which begins transcription at the initiation site upstream from the first amino acid codon (corresponding to AUG) in the messenger RNA. The site of initiation, where capping occurs, is followed by a nontranslated leader sequence of variable length before the sequence which codes for AUG, the messenger RNA translation start signal.

Capping, which occurs at the site of initiation, begins early during the process of transcription by RNA polymerase II. In the capping reaction, guanylyl transferase adds a 5′-terminal GTP to form a 5′–5′ bond GpppX, and the guanosine is methylated at N_7 by N_7 methylase.[1] Capping stabilizes messenger RNA against degradation and increases the efficiency of translation. The initiator AUG codon is marked for recognition by the 40S ribosome • methionine-tRNA initiation complex by the context of surrounding nucleotides, with the preferred sequence being GCCA-C*AUG*G.[2] Secondary structure of downstream RNA may facilitate the initiation of translation, which begins at the correct AUG with remarkable fidelity.

Newly transcribed RNA is rapidly complexed with small nuclear ribonucleoproteins (snRNPs) which subsequently assemble into a spliceosome where excision of introns occurs and exons are accurately joined together.[3] Genes may contain multiple introns, and the splicing process must be extremely accurate so that the reading frame of the mature exon-containing messenger RNA is maintained.[4] The process must also be sequential to achieve correct ordering of the encoded amino acid sequence. Introns follow the general GT-AG rule that introns begin with GT and end with AG. The snRNPs contain small RNAs and proteins, with the RNAs providing part of the recognition of the splice junctions. In the spliceosome, an A residue in the 3′ end of the intron attacks the 5′ splice site which is cleaved, and the intron forms a lariat structure in which the A is linked to the 5′ end of the intron via a 2′ phosphate. The RNA is then cleaved at the 3′ splice site, and the two exons are accurately joined. The lariat intron is released and degraded in the nucleus.

Termination of transcription occurs 3′ to the final coding exon, in some cases many base pairs downstream. Poly(A) addition (tailing) occurs near points of cleavage in messenger RNA precursors and is dictated by the sequence AAUAAA, which is located 14 to 30 base pairs upstream of the poly(A) tail.[5] The sequence at the start of the poly (A) tail is similar in many genes. Poly(A) addition is catalyzed by a poly(A) polymerase enzyme. Splicing and tailing occur in the nucleus, and snRNPs remain in the nucleus when messenger RNA is transported to the cytoplasm through nuclear pores.

The expression of protein-coding genes is controlled through regulation of the rate of initiation of transcription. In many genes, the sequence TATAA is located 20 to 30 base pairs upstream of the transcription start site. This TATAA box is analogous to the Pribnow box in prokaryotes, where RNA polymerase binds. In eukaryotes a series of basal transcription factors assemble at the TATAA box to facilitate the binding of RNA polymerase II and ensure accurate initiation of transcription at a single downstream start site. The TATAA box binding protein (TBP or TFIID) binds to the DNA sequence and assembles with the general initiation factors TFIIA, TFIIB, and TFIIE.[6] RNA polymerase II selectively binds to this initial complex and, in the presence of additional factors and ATP, forms an active transcription initiation complex. A number of genes lack a TATAA sequence; many of these genes contain several copies of the sequence GGGCGG, which is recognized by the nuclear protein Sp1.[7] Fidelity of the initiation of transcription of these promoters may be less than that of promoters containing a TATAA box, but these promoters can be equally strong and regulated. Because promoters which lack a TATAA box appear to require the same group of basal initiation factors, Sp1 has been proposed to sequester the basal transcription apparatus on these TATAA-less promoters. In some genes, an initiator motif located at the transcription start site is sufficient for initiation.[8]

Changes in the rates of initiation of transcription are a major mechanism through which cells increase or decrease production of peptide hormones, hormone receptors, and enzymes of biosynthetic pathways such as steroidogenesis. Multiple signal transduction pathways transmit environmental information from outside the cell to the transcription apparatus in the nucleus. In addition to the large protein complex that assembles with RNA polymerase II at the TATAA box, multiple proteins bind to specific DNA sequence regulatory elements to control the rate of initiation of transcription. Typical binding sites for transcription factors (DNA response elements) are located in gene promoters 5′ to the TATAA box, but these may also be found in introns. Because transcriptional responses appropriate to the needs of the organism require integration of information derived from multiple inputs, the number of proteins involved in regulated transcriptional complexes is large. One group of proteins bind directly to DNA response elements, while a second group does not directly bind to DNA but assembles into regulatory complexes by binding to DNA-bound proteins. Different protein complexes may assemble onto a single DNA bound transcription factor as coactivators or corepressors depending on information received from signal transduction pathways.

Primary transcription factors contain both a DNA binding domain and an activity domain.[9,10] The modular nature of transcription factors was demonstrated by study of chimeric molecules that have altered regulatory responses. Although many transcription factors have common DNA binding structures such as zinc finger, helix-loop-helix, leucine zipper-basic region (B-zip), the specificity for DNA binding sites is high. Many bind as dimers, both homo- and heterodimers, that increase the affinity and specificity by increasing the area of DNA contacted.

Transcriptional responses depend firstly on the occupancy of the multiple DNA response elements which are present in specific organizations in each gene. The formation of gene-specific "enhancersomes" reflects the organization of *cis* active DNA response elements, the differentiated cell repertoire of transcription factors available, and their state of activity.[11] DNA binding transcription factors may be specifically transported into the nucleus in response to activating signals (Stats, NFk-B, SREBP) and may be altered by hormone binding (steroid receptors) and by covalent modification such as phosphorylation (CREB, Jun). Various response elements in genes may therefore be variably occupied by transcription factors with various conformational states and thus activities.

The conformation of the activity domain of DNA bound transcription factors determines which of the non DNA-binding cofactors assemble. In response to ligand binding, steroid receptors such as the vitamin D receptor bind a complex consisting of 13 to 16 proteins, the vitamin D receptor interacting protein or DRIP complex.[12] This is similar to a ligand-dependent thyroid hormone receptor protein (TRAP) complex[13] and nearly identical to an activator-recruited cofactor (ARC) complex that binds to the activator domain of SREBP, NFk-B, and VP16.[14] These complexes markedly enhance transcription from DNA templates assembled into chromatin, the site where regulation occurs in vivo.[15]

There are a large number of coactivators including other groups of proteins that interact with ligand-activated steroid hormone receptors. In addition, there are proteins that specifically bind to inactive transcription factors to repress transcription. The nuclear corepressor, N-CoR or SMRT, specifically binds to inactive thyroid hormone receptors but not to activated ones.[16,17] Interestingly, the N-CoR complex contains a corepressor for the Mad bHLHZ transcription factor and histone deacetylase.[18] In contrast the coactivator complex that replaces the N-CoR complex when thyroid hormone is bound contains a histone acetylase (Fig. 3-1). Acetylation of histones may be an important mechanism that enhances entry and function of core transcription factors in nucleosome-bound DNA in chromatin. Deacetylation of histone would have the opposite effect to repress the initiation of transcription.

Regulated transcription that occurs in genes in chromatin structures in the nucleus depends on regulatory complexes that assemble in *cis* both near the promoter and at considerable distances away. Multiple protein interactions are required in addition to enzyme activities such as acetyltransferase and deacetylase. Bending and folding of DNA is necessary to bring the tethered complexes into proximity with the basal transcription machinery assembled

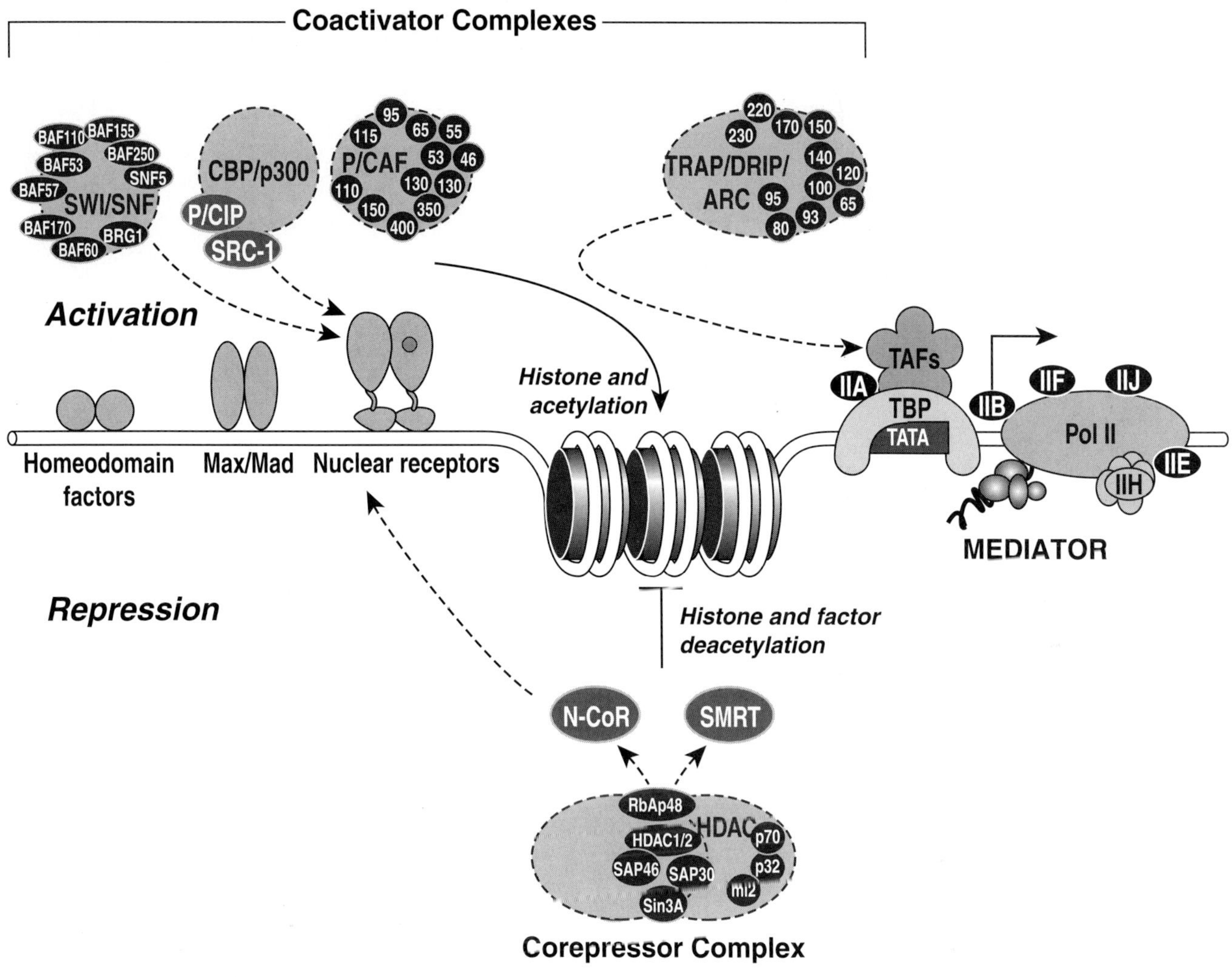

FIGURE 3-1. The action of corepressor and coactivator complexes to mediate the transcriptional effects of steroid receptors, homeodomain factors, and Mad/Max heterodimers. Binding of thyroid hormone to T_3 receptors, which are bound as heterodimers with RXR to DNA, induces a conformational change in the receptor protein that decreases binding of the corepressor complexes and increases binding of coactivator complexes. The coactivator TRAP/DRIP/ARC complex, the CBP/p300 integrator, and the SWI/SNF and p/CAF complexes each contain multiple proteins. The corepressor similarly consists of multiple proteins that integrate transcriptional responses. Changes in histone acetylation and in interactions with the basal transcription machinery provide for graded changes in the rate of initiation of transcription by RNA polymerase II. (*From Glass and Rosenfeld.*[115])

at the TATAA box.[19] Large proteins such as CBP and p300 contain binding sites for multiple transcription factors. These are proposed to function as integrators which partition to activated factors in preference to inactive DNA-bound factors.[20,21]

Biosynthesis of Peptide Hormones

Because peptide hormones are small proteins, their mature messenger RNAs frequently encode information for initial translation products which are larger than the secretory form of the peptide; the larger protein precursors are processed by a series of proteolytic cleavages to yield the final secreted peptide products. Messenger RNA translation begins at the AUG codon, specifying methionine, that lies downstream from the cap site. Because peptide hormones are secretory proteins, synthesis occurs on endoplasmic reticulum-bound polyribosomes, with vectorial movement of the growing peptide into the endoplasmic reticulum space (Fig. 3-2). A leader sequence of 15 to 25 largely hydrophobic amino acids is located at the amino terminus of the protein. When this "pre" portion emerges from the ribosome, it binds a signal recognition particle that consists of six proteins and a 7-S RNA.[23] In the absence of endoplasmic reticulum (ER) membranes, the signal recognition particle prevents further synthesis of these proteins so that presecretory proteins are not made in the cytoplasm. When the signal recognition particle · ribosome complex binds with high affinity to the integral membrane protein complex termed the *signal recognition particle receptor*,[24] the signal recognition particle is displaced from the nascent protein chain and its amino-terminal signal sequence in a GTP-dependent reaction.[25] The ribosome, with its growing peptide chain, is now bound to the endoplasmic reticulum, and the growing polypeptide chain is vectorially inserted through a large protein-conducting channel in the endoplasmic

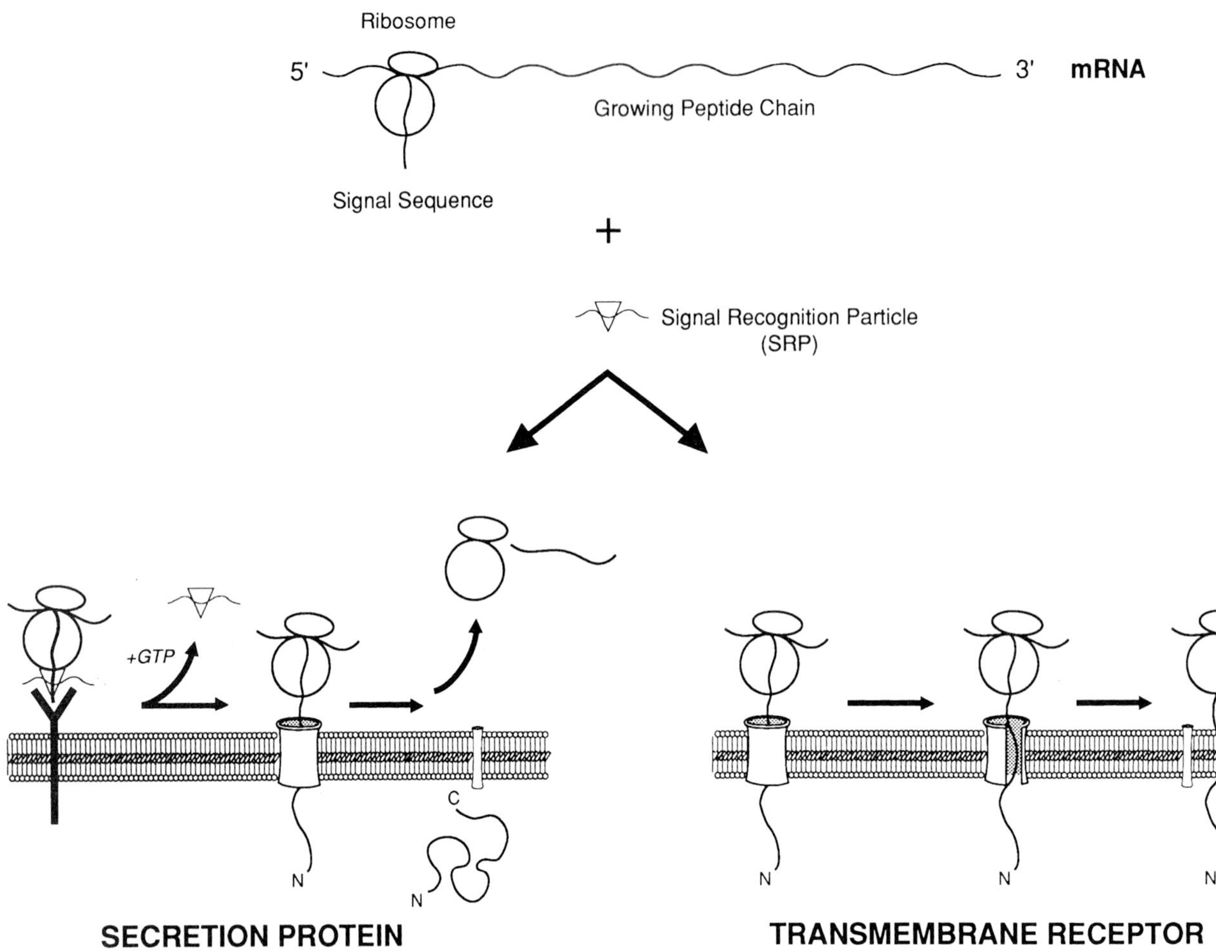

FIGURE 3-2. Synthesis of secretory proteins. The signal sequence at the amino terminus is bound by the signal recognition particle (SRP), which arrests cytoplasmic translation and delivers the complex to a recognition protein intrinsic to the endoplasmic reticulum (ER) membrane. When the SRP binds to the SRP receptor, it is displaced from the signal peptide in a GTP-dependent reaction. The growing polypeptide chain is directed into the ER space through a protein channel. When synthesis is complete, the ribosome dissociates and the protein channel closes. For synthesis of transmembrane receptor proteins, stop transfer sequences arrest vectorial synthesis, and completion of synthesis occurs in the cytoplasm. The protein channel has been proposed to open laterally to allow the exit of the transmembrane proteins. (*Modified from Simon and Blobel.*[22])

reticulum membrane to reach the endoplasmic space.[23,26] For secretory proteins such as peptide hormones, the completed peptide will ultimately be located completely within the endoplasmic reticulum space, whereas membrane-bound proteins such as hormone receptors will have their amino termini within this space (ultimately to face the outside of the cell), with a portion of the carboxy terminus of the protein remaining in the membrane and cytoplasm. Stop transfer sequences signal the cessation of transport of the growing polypeptide chain across the endoplasmic membrane, so that membrane proteins such as cell surface hormone receptors are synthesized with their ectodomains inside the endoplasmic reticulum space to ultimately face the exterior of the cell and endodomains are synthesized in the cytoplasm. These proteins must exit the protein channel in the membrane laterally; once outside the protein channel, the positively charged amino acids of the stop transfer sequence prevent protein movement into the hydrophobic membrane.[27] When synthesis is complete, the ribosomes leave the membrane and the protein channel closes. Some peptide hormones, such as epidermal growth factor, are generated by proteolytic processing from receptor-like precursors.[28]

These general mechanisms do not account for the processing of all peptide hormones and receptors. Some peptide hormones, such as fibroblast growth factor, lack a defined signal sequence but clearly act via cell surface receptors. Alternative mechanisms must exist through which signaling peptides that lack signal sequences exit the cell. Receptors that contain seven membrane-spanning segments, transporter proteins such as the glucose transporters, and enzymes which contain twelve membrane spanning segments such as adenylate cyclase must be inserted into the membrane by variations in trafficking which do not stringently depend on stop transfer sequences.

Within the endoplasmic reticulum, the precursor protein is cleaved, may be covalently modified, and is folded into the form

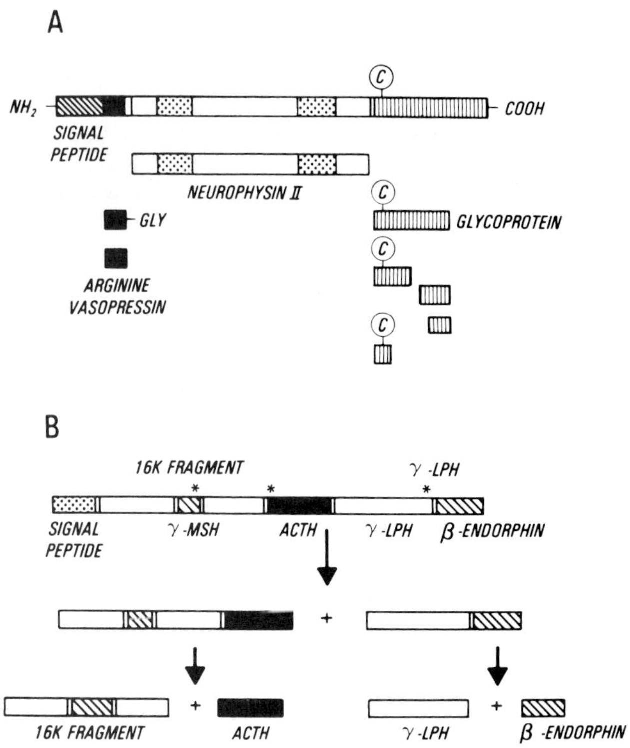

FIGURE 3-3. Proteolytic processing of precursor proteins within the endoplasmic reticulum. (*A*) Structure of the bovine antidiuretic hormone (ADH)-neurophysin II precursor and its proteolytic processing. The 19-amino acid signal peptide is followed by ADH (residues 1 to 9). Neurophysin II begins after processing signals at residue 13 and extends to residue 107; its internal homology is shown by the hatched area. The glycoprotein portion of the precursor is located at the carboxyl terminus. (*From Land et al.*[29]) (*B*) Structure of the bovine ACTH precursor and its proteolytic processing in the anterior pituitary. Reiterated MSH core sequences are indicated by an asterisk. Dibasic amino acid residues, which serve as the recognition signal for proteolytic processing, are indicated by open spaces in the bars. (*From Nakanishi et al.*[30])

which will ultimately be secreted. A membrane-bound signal peptidase first removes the "pre" or leader sequence portion of the hormone. Larger precursor "pro" hormones are then further processed within this membrane-enclosed space by proteolytic enzymes. Most of this processing involves trypsin-like proteases which recognize dibasic amino acid residues. For carboxyl-terminal amidation, glycine serves as the donor at the cleavage site.

Peptides generated during the processing of protein precursors may have a variety of functions. The precursors of antidiuretic hormone and oxytocin contain specific neurophysins which serve as carriers for these two peptides from their site of synthesis in the magnocellular nuclei in the hypothalamus to storage sites in the posterior pituitary (Fig. 3-3*A*). The ACTH precursor contains information for several peptides, which may all be involved in stress responses. Figure 3-3*B* shows the structure of the ACTH precursor molecule. The core sequence for melanocyte stimulating hormone (MSH) is reiterated within the structure of the precursor, suggesting that it arose during evolution by gene duplication. A 16,000 M_r fragment is located on the amino-terminal side, and the β-lipotropin is located on the carboxyl-terminal side of the ACTH sequence. Dibasic amino acids serve

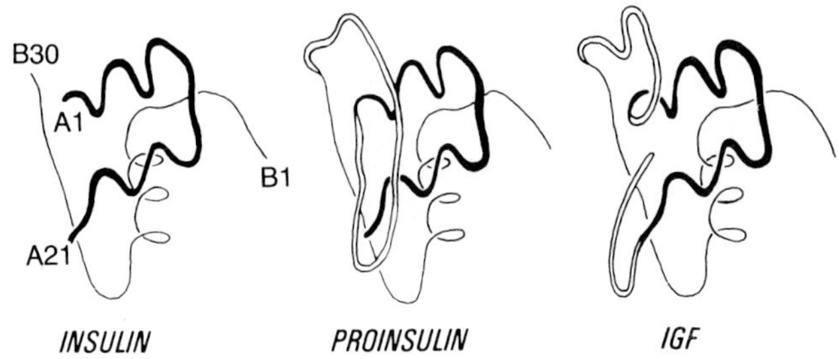

FIGURE 3-4. Schematic representation of three-dimensional structures based on x-ray analysis of insulin and on model building of proinsulin and of insulin-like growth factor 1 (IGF-1). The A chain of insulin is shown by the thickening line, the B chain by the solid line, and the connecting peptide by a double line. Disulfide bridge locations are indicated in the text. (*Modified from Blundell et al.*[31])

as recognition signals for proteolytic enzymes which cleave the precursor protein into the final hormonal products. In addition, both glycosylation and phosphorylation of the ACTH precursor occur. There is evidence for different processing of the same precursor in different cells. In the intermediate lobe of the pituitary, ACTH is processed to α-MSH, in which the amino-terminal serine is acetylated and the carboxyl-terminal valine is amidated from the adjacent glycine, and to corticotropin-like intermediate peptide (CLIP; $ACTH_{18-29}$). In the anterior pituitary, the ACTH precursor is processed as shown in Fig. 3-3*B*. The precursor to the enkephalins results in the formation of several peptides with similar activities.

The connecting peptide (C peptide) present in the insulin precursor may serve to provide correct folding and alignment of the A and B chains of insulin. The insulin precursor has the structure: hydrophobic leader sequence • B chain • C peptide • A chain. The leader sequence is rapidly removed, and the C peptide serves to fold and align the A and B chains of insulin (Fig. 3-4). The disulfide bonds between cysteines A7 and B7, A20 and B19, and A6 and A11 are required for the biological activity of insulin. If the disulfide bonds between the A and B chains of insulin and the intra-A chain disulfide bond are chemically reduced and reoxidized in vitro, random coupling of half-cysteine residues occurs and only a small fraction of biological activity is restored. However, reduced and reoxidized proinsulin (B chain • C peptide • A chain) can generate almost full biological activity.[32] The specific conformation of the proinsulin molecule presumably brings the correct pairs of half-cysteine residues into close approximation for the formation of the mature disulfide-bonded insulin. However, under defined in vitro conditions, the A and B chains can efficiently fold to yield native insulin, indicating that the overall structures can align the disulfide bonds correctly, even without the C peptide. During maturation in the endoplasmic reticulum space and Golgi complex, the C peptide, which is flanked by dibasic residues, is removed and mature insulin is secreted by the β cell with about equimolar amounts of inactive C peptide. Proinsulin has only a small fraction of the activity of the final product. A genetic variant proinsulin resistant to proteolytic processing results in the secretion of unprocessed proinsulin.[33] Active hormones may also be generated outside cells by processing from circulating precursors. The precursor for angiotensin II is a glycoprotein synthesized mainly in the liver. Renin, a proteolytic enzyme made in jux-

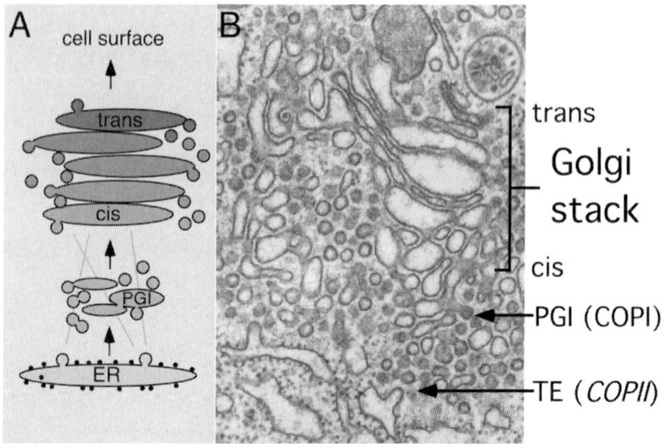

FIGURE 3-5. Biosynthetic itinerary of peptide hormones and receptors. (*A*) Proteins that are synthesized in the ER are exported in pre-Golgi intermediate (PGI) vesicles and tubular elements that deliver cargo to the Golgi along microtublar tracks. The Golgi compartment has a *cis* or entering face and a *trans* or exiting face. (*B*) Electron micrograph of the ER-Golgi region in a pancreatic acinar cell. (*Reprinted with permission from Allan BB, Balch WE:* Science *285:63, 1999.*[35] *Copyright 1999, American Association for the Advancement of Science.*)

taglomerular cells of the kidney, cleaves a decapeptide (angiotensin I) from the circulating angiotensin precursor glycoprotein. This decapeptide is then further processed to the octapeptide angiotensin II by the removal of two carboxy-terminal amino acids by a converting enzyme found in the endothelial cells of vascular beds, especially those of the lung.

Secretory and membrane proteins which are synthesized in the membrane-enclosed space of the ribosome-bound endoplasmic reticulum (RER) are vectorially transported through cell compartments where covalent modifications occur. These proteins, which always remain enclosed inside membranes, move from the ER to the Golgi complex with transport vesicles budding from each compartment and fusing with the next to deliver their load of proteins, which are progressively modified by processing enzymes such as glycosyltransferases. The itinerary between compartments is precise and consists of budding followed by the formation of coated vesicles. Vesicle formation is initiated by binding of small GTPases to the ER membranes.[34] Cargo may be selected and concentrated in a process that requires sorting determinants on the cargo that interact with proteins of the vesicle coat. Soluble cargo in the vesicle lumen may link to the proteins of the vesicle coat via sorting receptors.[35] As illustrated in Fig. 3-5, cargo from the ER is transported via pre Golgi intermediate vesicles to the *cis* Golgi, then through the Golgi stacks to the trans Golgi compartment. The coat protein complex II (COP II) is involved in export of cargo from the ER,whereas COP I is involved in return of resident components such as ER proteins, cargo receptors and Golgi enzymes to their home base. Anterograde movement of cargo is thus coupled with retrograde movement of resident proteins to maintain functional compartmentation of the pathway. The retrieval of resident proteins is a major mechanism for concentrating cargo.[36] In this process material removed by bulk flow from the ER is concentrated as selective membrane removal and recycling leaves concentrated cargo to move forward in the pathway.[37,38]

To vectorially deliver cargo, vesicles formed by fission must be transported to the next compartment, where membrane fusion occurs and cargo is transferred. These events depend on integral membrane proteins in the transport vesicle (termed v-SNAREs) that pair with receptors on the target membrane (termed t-SNAREs).[39,40] A number of soluble proteins including NSF, SNAP25, and α and γ SNAPs participate in the vesicle fusion complex where NSF hydrolysis of ATP occurs[41] (Fig. 3-6). For exocytosis SNARE complex formation and membrane fusion are triggered by Ca^{2+}.[42]

Small GTPases function both in coat formation and in vesicle targeting. These are active when GTP is bound and become inactive as GTP is hydrolyzed to GDP. ARF and SAR GTPases function in vesicle coat assembly and, when GTP hydrolysis occurs, dissociate along with the coat from vesicles.[43] Targeting and fusion of vesicle membranes is coordinated by the Rab GTPases.

Several covalent modifications may occur during this intracellular journey. Glycosylation is the major modification that affects peptide hormones such as thyroid stimulating hormone (TSH), luteinizing hormone (LH), follicle stimulating hormone (FSH), and human chorionic gonadotropin (hCG). Cell surface receptors for peptide hormones also undergo glycosylation. The initial addition of core oligosaccharide occurs within the endoplasmic reticulum. The predominant glycosylation via nitrogen linkage occurs on asparagine residues found within the sequence Asn-x-Ser-Thr. This sequence occurs in proteins which are synthesized in the endoplasmic reticulum space but is rare in cytoplasmic proteins, so that glycosylation of intracellular proteins is avoided. Less commonly, oligosaccharides are oxygen-linked via the hydroxyl side-chain group of serine, threonine, or hydroxylysine. The core *N*-linked oligosaccharide contains two *N*-acteylglucosamine residues and three mannose residues. The core oligosaccharide is first formed in the endoplasmic reticulum on an activated lipid molecule, dolichol, via a pyrophosphate bridge, and is then transferred intact to the growing polypeptide chain.[44] Complex oligosaccharides are formed within the Golgi complex, where variable numbers of glucosamine-galactose-sialic acid residues are added to the mannose core through the action of galactosyl transferase enzymes. High-mannose oligosaccharides, which contain additional mannose residues attached to the core, are donated via the dolichol pathway and are trimmed to various degrees by mannosidase enzymes present in the Golgi complex.

The α subunits of the glycoprotein hormones LH, FSH, TSH, and hCG contain two oligosaccharides of the *N*-linked complex type; β subunits contain either one or two similar oligosaccharides. The hCGβ subunit, which has a carboxyl-terminal amino acid extension, contains three additional oligosaccharides *O*-linked to serine residues in this extension. In addition to the usual oligosaccharide structures, the pituitary hormones TSH and LH contain peripheral sulfate groups. Glycosylation and sulfation occur as separate processes in Golgi compartments, with sulfation occurring late in the biosynthetic pathway. Glycosylation of secretory proteins may serve many functions. Glycosylation may favor the protein conformation necessary for optimal intracellular combination of the two subunits which are synthesized on separate messenger RNAs for hormones such as TSH, LH, FSH, and hCG. Glycosylation stabilizes hormones in the circulation. Glycoprotein hormones have circulating half-lives considerably longer than those of nonglycosylated peptide hormones, and desialylation which exposes a β-linked galactose results in a markedly reduced circulating half-life as a result of accelerated

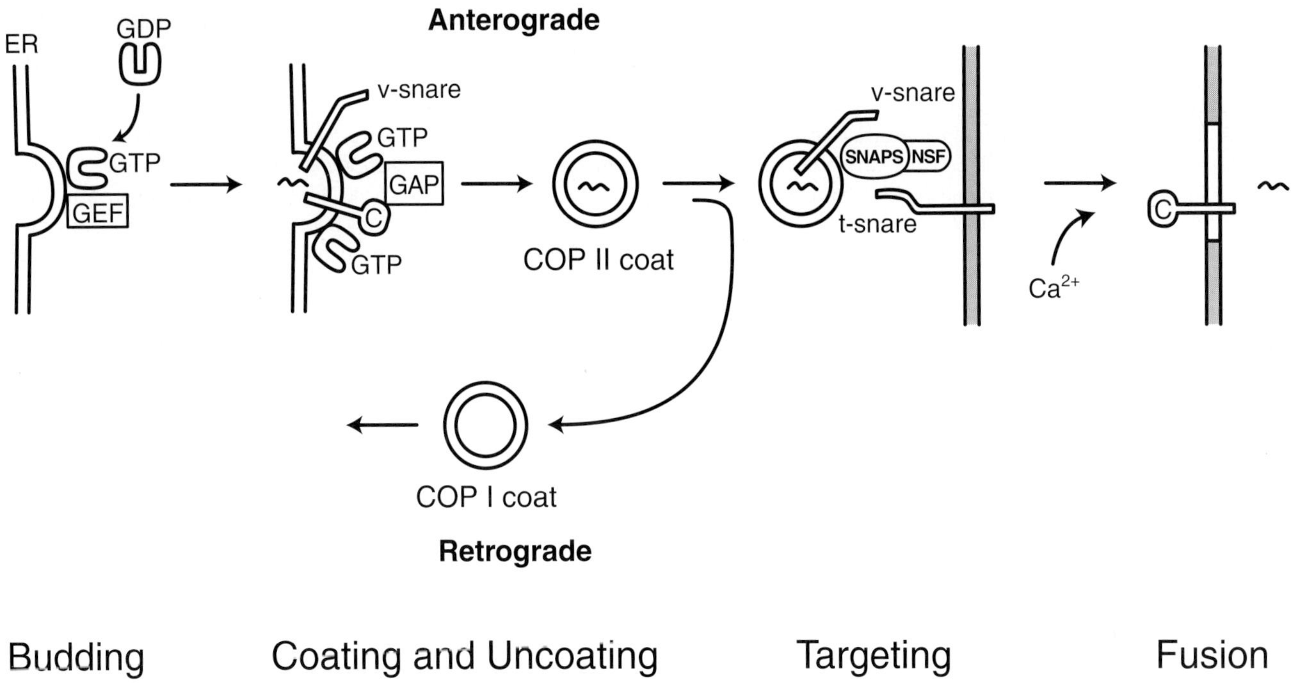

FIGURE 3-6. Subcellular transport of secretory and membrane proteins. Buds, which will pinch off as coated vesicles, are formed by recruitment of a GTPase (ARF for COPI and Sar1 for COPII vesicles) to integral membrane proteins which have guanine nucleotide exchange activity (GEF). The GTP-bound GTPase then recruits additional coat components that are specific for the origin of the vesicle. The growing bud incorporates both vesicle-SNAREs (v-SNAREs) and cargo (C); the mature vesicle buds from the parent membrane and GAP-induced hydrolysis of GTP releases the GTPase to initiate another cycle of budding. Retrieval of membranes via COP I coats markedly enhances the concentration of cargo in forward moving vesicles. Vesicles are uncoated, exposing the vesicle SNAREs that pair with specific target SNAREs (t-SNAREs) via coiled coils. A series of other proteins assembles onto the SNARE complex including NSF, SNAP-25, and α and γ SNAPs, and membrane fusion is driven by ATP hydrolysis. Exocytosis of secretory vesicles requires Ca^{2+}.

clearance via the hepatic asialoglycoprotein receptor.[45] Glycosylation may also be important in receptor recognition through effects on hormone conformation or through interaction with cellular recognition sites.

Secretion, Transport, and Metabolism of Peptide Hormones

From the trans Golgi network (TGN) peptide hormones accumulate in vesicles which lose water and form mature secretory granules. Mature secretory granules contain large amounts of stored hormone, which can be readily identified by specific immunostaining. In the absence of a secretory stimulus, such granules accumulate; conversely, intensely secreting cells have fewer secretory granules. In response to a secretory stimulus, the stored peptides are discharged by exocytosis in which the membrane of the secretory granule fuses with the cell membrane.[46] Secretion is directed, occurring at the apical part of the cell, so that the peptide hormone is discharged into the circulation. The membrane of the secretory granule is then reabsorbed into the cell by endocytosis and is reutilized. The process of exocytosis is regulated by Ca^{2+}. Proteins such as synaptotagmin which bind Ca^{2+} and interact with the SNARE complex may mediate aspects of exocytosis.[47] In neuronal cells Ca^{2+} channels are closely coupled to the SNARE exocytic complex.[48]

Cell surface hormone receptors also reach the plasma membrane via vesicle transport and fusion. In contrast to secretion, which is highly regulated, transport of cell surface proteins is constitutive. In polarized epithelial cells, receptors are asymmetrically distributed on the cell surface. Vectorial transport from the *trans* Golgi to the basolateral surface requires amino acid sequence codes in the cytoplasmic domain of the receptor[49]; in the absence of such codes receptors are transported to the apical surface. These receptor sequences resemble those which dictate clustering in clathrin coated pits at the cell surface and are thought to form a structure that specifies interaction with the adaptor complex specific to the *trans* Golgi or with other proteins. In nonpolarized cells, constitutive movement to the cell surface occurs.

Secretion of peptide hormones is regulated by specific signals, many of them hormonal, which couple the rate of secretion to the metabolic needs of the organism. A fundamental action of many hormones is to control the secretion of peptide hormones. Biosynthesis of peptide hormones is coupled to secretion, although the precise biochemical basis of this coupling is incompletely defined. Kinetically, two "pools" of hormone have been described, a rapidly releasable one which reflects hormone stored in secretory granules as well as that being synthesized and the other a slowly releasable one which reflects predominantly newly synthesized hormone.

Once they are secreted, peptide hormones have a short half-life in the circulation. Most peptide hormones, such as ACTH, parathyroid hormone (PTH), insulin, glucagon, antidiuretic hormone (ADH), thyrotropin releasing hormone (TRH), gonadotropin releasing hormone (GnRH), and corticotropin releasing hormone (CRH), act rapidly and are degraded rapidly, having circulating half-lives of 3 to 7 min. Metabolic clearance studies must be interpreted with caution because of the complexity of degrading systems for different hormones in different tissues, but several general principles operate for most peptide hormones. Although peptide hormones may be cleaved by circulating proteases, the initial step leading to the major pathway for peptide hormone degradation consists of binding to receptors in target cells. The receptor does not degrade the hormone but delivers it to degradative enzymes both in the cell membrane and in the interior of target cells. Insulin degradation, for example, is directly related to receptor binding in liver cells, quantitatively the most important site of insulin clearance.

Peptide hormone signaling is terminated and further signaling is attenuated by ligand-induced endocytosis. Inactive receptors are clustered in cholesterol-rich regions of the plasma membrane termed "rafts" that are often associated with the protein caveolin to form caveolae or "little caves" on the membrane surface.[50–52] When ligand binds and receptors are activated the complex becomes concentrated in clathrin-coated vesicles or "coated pits"[53,54] (Fig. 3-7). These form endocytic vesicles through the action of dynamin.[55] Early endocytic vesicles that contain ligand-bound receptors may continue to transmit information from inside the cell, but sorting to later endosomes where the pH is lower results in dissociation of ligand from receptor and ultimate ligand degradation in lysosomes. Receptors, which are the cargo, contain sequences that are recognized by the vesicle sorting machinery that specifies vectorial movement through the endosome compartment.[56,57] Common sequence codes in receptors consist of NPXY, dileucine, and YXXθ where X represents any amino acid and θ represents a hydrophobic residue.[58] The YXXθ code is recognized by the μ subunit of the adaptor protein 2 complex in coated pits.[59,60] Some receptors recycle to the cell surface to mediate further signaling, but some are targeted to lysosomes for degradation. Degradation of receptors attenuates further signaling. Like exocytosis, endocytosis is regulated by GTPases of the rab family and utilizes resident proteins with specific recognition properties.[61]

FIGURE 3-7. Endocytic itinerary of peptide • hormone receptor complexes. Cell surface receptors, which are clustered in cholesterol-rich regions of the cell membrane ("rafts"), leave these areas when activated by hormone binding and are internalized via clathrin-coated pits. The clathrin coats are removed early after endocytosis and endocytic vesicles move deep into the cell. Ligands dissociate as the pH is progressively lowered and are sorted to lysosomes where degradation occurs. Receptors are either recycled back to the cell surface ("Default" pathway) or are sorted through late endosomes to lysosomes. The transferrin receptor (TfR) illustrates a recycling receptor whereas the EGF receptor (EGF-R) illustrates sequence code-dependent sorting to lysosomes. (*Kindly provided by HS Wiley.*)

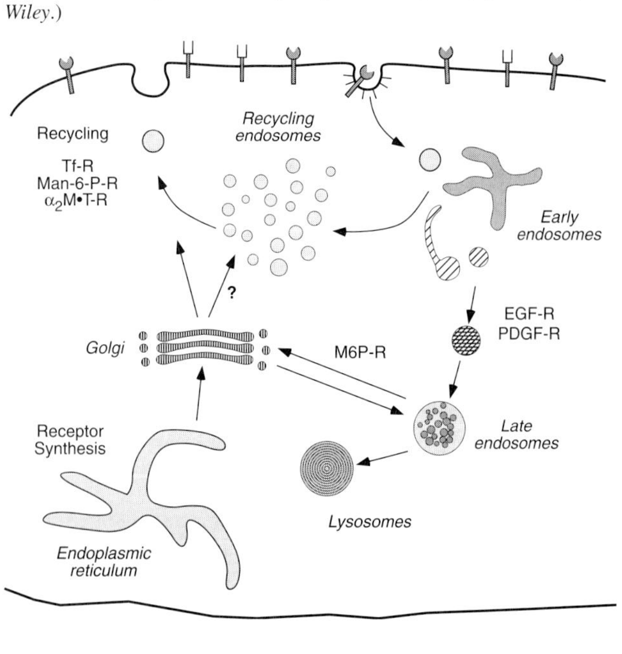

Specificities have evolved that differ for various ligand • receptor systems. Transferrin receptors release transferrin-bound iron at the lower pH of the endosome compartment but recycle with high efficiency back to the cell surface; epidermal growth factor receptors (EGFR) are sorted to lysosomes so degradation of both ligand and receptor terminate signaling (Fig. 3-7). Transferrin receptors are internalized at a high rate independently of ligand binding whereas binding of EGF increases the rate of EGFR endocytosis tenfold.[62] Seven-membrane spanning G protein-coupled receptors also undergo ligand-induced internalization. Activated β adrenergic receptors are phosphorylated by a specific kinase to increase their affinity for arrestin proteins.[63] Arrestins bind to clathrin, facilitating internalization via coated pits.

Peptide hormone degradation may also be catalyzed by cellular proteases which appear to be somewhat specific. Lysosomal enzymes contribute importantly to degradation of hormones delivered via absorptive endocytosis, but specific enzymes such as an insulin protease which cleaves insulin and glucagon, a postproline cleaving enzyme which cleaves ADH and TRH, and a pyroglutamyl aminopeptidase which cleaves TRH and GnRH may inactivate peptide hormones, which are then further degraded by other cellular proteases. Reduction of disulfide bonds may also be important for the inactivation of certain hormones, such as insulin and ADH. Some receptors may be degraded via ubiquination and the proteosome.[64,65]

Glycoprotein hormones have significantly longer circulating half-lives than do unmodified peptide hormones. HCG, the most heavily glycosylated peptide hormone, has a circulating half-life of about 4 h. Removal of the terminal sialic acid markedly shortens the half-life of circulating glycoprotein hormones because the modified proteins are now recognized and cleaved by the asialoglycoprotein receptor that is present in the liver. Although most peptide hormones circulate at low concentrations as unbound species, hormones such as the insulin-like growth factors are bound to carrier proteins in serum.[66] Such binding provides a circulating reservoir and an extended half-life. Platelet-derived growth factor and epidermal growth factor are present in platelet granules and are released locally in high concentrations when platelet activation and release reactions are triggered.[67]

The short circulating half-life of most peptide hormones provides for rapid termination of their biological actions. In normal physiology, synthesis and secretion are regulated to deliver appropriate concentrations of hormone to target tissues. Inactivation of both hormone and receptor buffers tissues against excessive responses. These buffering systems are a barrier to the clinical use of peptide hormones and, with the notable exception of insulin, have limited widespread therapeutic use of most peptide hormones.

STEROID HORMONES

The pathways for the biosynthesis of steroid hormones by the adrenal cortex, ovary, and testis are similar. Many of the biosynthetic enzymes are identical, with specialized enzymes providing modifications which give the final unique steroid structure recognized by target tissue hormone receptors. The rate-limiting step subject to acute hormone regulation is the same in adrenocortical and gonadal tissues; subcellular organization of biosynthetic enzyme pathways is also the same. Enzymes synthesizing the active form of vitamin D are similar to other steroid hydroxylases but are located in different organs (liver and kidney) rather than within a single gland. In addition, the major active androgen, dihydrotestosterone, is formed from testosterone; interconversion of precursors to estrogens occurs in peripheral tissues; and the brain has been shown to be capable of synthesizing several classes of steroid hormones.

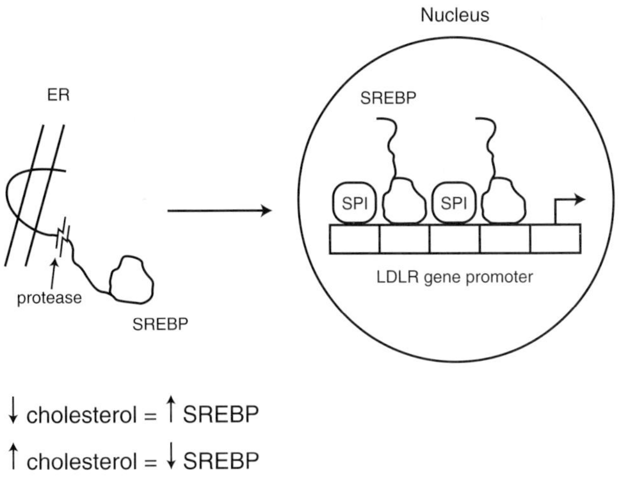

FIGURE 3-8. Maintenance of cholesterol substrate for steroid hormone synthesis. Decreases in free cholesterol due to use in steroid hormone formation are sensed in ER membranes where the sterol regulatory element binding protein (SREBP) is located. Proteolysis releases the transcriptionally active part of SREBP, which enters the nucleus to coordinately upregulate synthesis of LDL receptors and cholesterol biosynthetic enzymes.

Cholesterol Substrate for Steroid Hormone Formation

All steroid hormones are derived from cholesterol, which is provided by de novo synthesis from acetate and by uptake of circulating cholesterol synthesized in the liver and carried in low-density lipoprotein (LDL) particles. In either case, cholesterol may be used immediately for hormone biosynthesis or stored in the gland in lipid droplets as cholesterol esters. The number of LDL receptors in steroidogenic cells is higher than the number in non-steroid-secreting cells, and up to 70 percent of cholesterol utilized for steroid hormone production in the human adrenal cortex is provided from LDL cholesterol.[68] HDL cholesterol can also provide cholesterol for steroid synthesis. Although maximal ACTH-stimulated production is decreased in abetalipoproteinemia and homozygous LDL receptor deficiency, adrenal steroidogenesis is maintained in the absence of LDL and its uptake system.[69–71] The uptake of HDL cholesterol is via the class B scavenger receptor, SR-B1, which is expressed in liver and steroidogenic cells and which, like the LDL receptor, is upregulated when cholesterol stores are depleted.[72–76]

Cholesterol homeostasis is maintained by the same regulatory mechanisms present in other cells. Free cholesterol concentrations are sensed via regulated proteolysis of the sterol regulatory element binding protein (SREBP), a bHLH-Zip class transcription factor sequestered in endoplasmic reticulum membranes whose low content of cholesterol provides an environment for sensitive sensing of free cholesterol concentrations[77–79] (Fig. 3-8). When free cholesterol is decreased as a consequence of utilization in steroid hormone synthesis, enhanced release of SREBP coordinately upregulates LDL receptor synthesis to facilitate cholesterol uptake and also enhances synthesis of 3-hydroxy-3-methylglutaryl coenzyme A synthase (HMG-CoA synthase) and HMG-CoA reductase, the two rate-controlling enzymes of cholesterol synthesis. Cholesterol availability is thus tightly coupled to the metabolic requirements of steroidogenic cells.

Steroidogenic cells contain abundant lipid droplets in which cholesterol esters are stored. In response to trophic hormones, cholesterol esterase is activated via cAMP-dependent protein kinase catalyzed phosphorylation to provide free cholesterol as substrate for steroid hormone synthesis. With prolonged stimulation, lipid droplets are depleted of cholesterol, but they are subsequently replenished when stimuli are removed. With prolonged stimulation, most of the cholesterol substrate for steroidogenesis is provided by facilitated uptake of LDL cholesterol. The increased uptake, release from cholesterol ester storage depots, and de novo synthesis provide sufficient cholesterol to sustain the tenfold increase in adrenal cortisol production which occurs in response to severe stress; when basal conditions are reestablished, regulatory mechanisms reduce uptake and synthesis to levels appropriate to lower cortisol production rates (Fig. 3-9). Increased intracellular cholesterol concentrations reduce proteolytic activation of SREBP and consequently transcription of genes that enhance cholesterol production. Similar changes occur in ovarian and testicular cells stimulated by trophic hormones to produce estrogen, progesterone, and testosterone.

The Rate-Controlling Step in Steroid Hormone Synthesis

The rate-limiting step in total steroid synthesis in steroidogenic tissues is cleavage of the side chain of cholesterol to yield pregnenolone (Fig. 3-10). Cholesterol transformation and subsequent steroid hormone biosynthesis are catalyzed by cytochrome P450 enzymes and dehydrogenases. Steroid biosynthetic enzymes are named based on the carbon atom of the cholesterol ring that is modified and by the CYP nomenclature[81] (Table 3-1). Stimulation of steroidogenesis in adrenal cortex, ovary, and testis results from accelerated formation of pregnenolone because subsequent enzyme activities are present in relative excess. The cholesterol side-chain cleavage enzyme CYP11A1 is located in the inner mitochondrial membrane, and stimulation of steroid hormone formation results from increased interaction of cholesterol with this enzyme. Although hormones such as ACTH, FSH, LH, and hCG increase general cholesterol availability, regulation of the

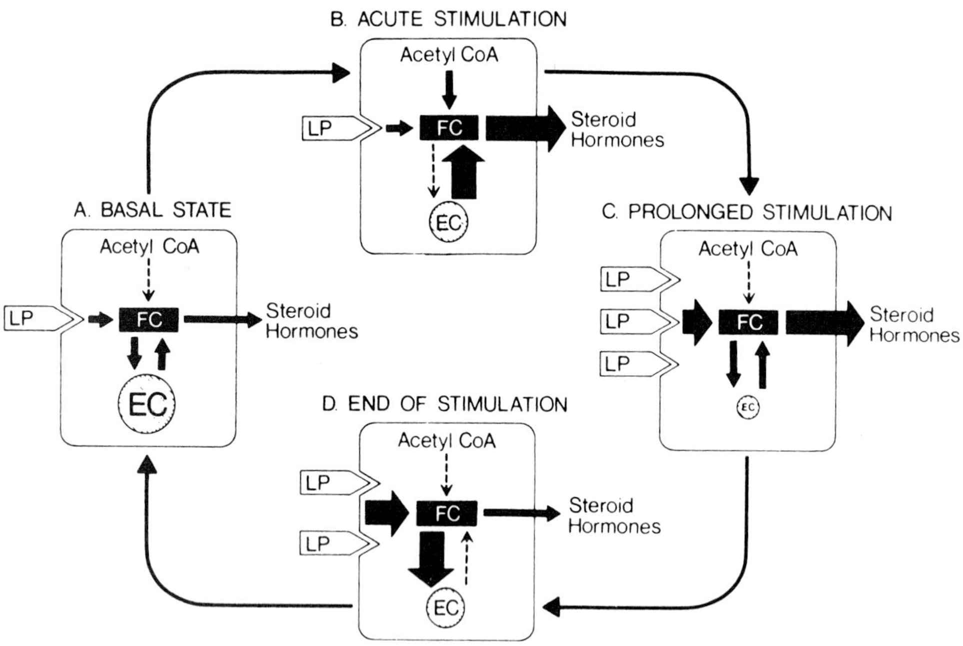

FIGURE 3-9. Provision of cholesterol for steroid hormone formation. The small metabolically active pool of free cholesterol (FC), which is the precursor of steroid hormone formation, is maintained in response to stimuli by hydrolysis of cholesterol esters (EC), de novo synthesis from acetyl CoA, and facilitated uptake from lipoproteins (LP). See text for details. (*From Brown et al.*[80])

rate of steroidogenesis depends on facilitated interaction of free cholesterol with mitochondrial CYP11A1 by transfer of cholesterol from the outer to the inner mitochondrial membrane. Because adequate active CYP11A1 and fully reduced adrenodoxin are present, the major limitation is transfer of cholesterol to the enzyme. The mechanisms through which ACTH, FSH, LH, and hCG, via their intracellular mediator cAMP, increase the interaction of cholesterol with CYP11A1 include a sterol carrier protein and the steroidogenic acute regulatory protein, StAR.[82,83] The importance of StAR, initially identified by biochemical complimentation, was provided by studies of human enzyme deficiencies that result in severe adrenal and gonadal failure.[84] Interestingly, ovarian failure occurs at puberty when the ovary is activated and cholesterol accumulates to toxic levels because it cannot be converted to steroid hormones.

The side-chain cleavage reaction catalyzed by the CYP11A1 resembles other monoxygenations of CYP enzymes, but three sequential monoxygenations are involved in the scission of the carbon-carbon bond.[85,86] Mitochondrial cytochrome P450 enzymes such as CYP11A1, involved in synthesis of adrenal and gonadal steroid hormones; CYP11B1, involved in cortisol synthesis; CYP11B2, involved in aldosterone synthesis; and, CYP1A, involved in 1,25$(OH)_2$ vitamin D synthesis; utilize a flavoprotein (adrenodoxin reductase) and an iron-sulphur protein (adrenodoxin, a form of ferrodoxin), NADPH (reduced form of nicotinamide adenine dinucleotide phosphate), and molecular oxygen. Microsomal cytochrome P450 enzymes such as CYP21A2 in adrenal cortex, CYP17 in adrenal cortex and gonads, and CYP25 in liver utilize a different flavoprotein, cytochrome P450 reductase, for electron transfer.[87]

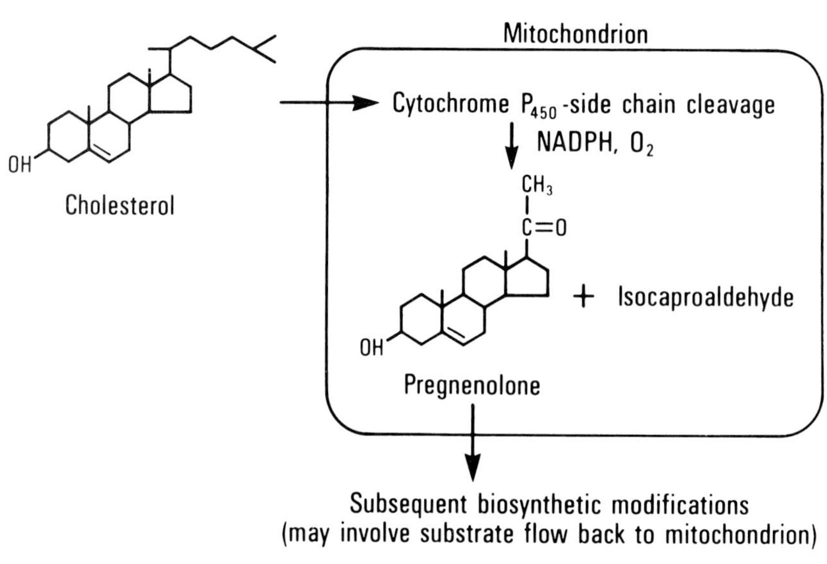

FIGURE 3-10. The rate-limiting step of steroid hormone biosynthesis.

TABLE 3-1. Nomenclature for Steroidogenic Enzymes

Trivial Name	Gene
Cytochrome P450 side chain cleavage enzyme	CYP 11A1
21-hydroxylase	CYP 21A2
11β-hydroxylase	CYP 11B1
17-hydroxylase	CYP 17
17,20-lyase	CYP 17
18-hydroxylase (corticosterone methyloxidase)	CYP 11B2
Aromatase	CYP 19
25-hydroxylase	CYP 25
1α-hydroxylase	CYP 1A

For steroid hormone biosynthesis cholesterol is first hydroxylated at C22; then it is hydroxylated at C20, and the resulting glycol is cleaved to yield the 20-ketone plus isocaproaldehyde. As in other cytochrome P450 enzymes, the active site region consists of a substrate-binding site and a heme-iron catalytic site. A general model of the reaction cycle of cytochrome P450 includes substrate binding, heme reduction, and oxygen binding (Fig. 3-11). Substrate binding occurs first, and then the iron-oxo hydroxylating complex is formed, followed by product formation. The introduction of activated oxygen into the substrate yields the hydroxylated steroid product, which is released along with a molecule of water. Abortive cycles induced by the binding of a pseudosubstrate can result in the production of oxygen-derived radicals which destroy the enzyme.[88] The large antioxidant armamentarium of steroidogenic cells presumably evolved as a protective mechanism against such abortive cytochrome P450 cycles.

Steroidogenic tissues contain large numbers of specialized mitochondria and an extensive network of smooth endoplasmic reticulum. The enzymes which progressively modify the cholesterol molecule are located in these two compartments, and substrate flows from mitochondria to endoplasmic reticulum and back to mitochondria as it is progressively modified. The movement of substrate may involve sterol carrier proteins in cytosol or movement on a membrane surface.

Pathway of Steroid Hormone Biosynthesis

Figure 3-12 shows the general pathway for steroid hormone synthesis in the adrenal cortex and other steroid-producing tissues. After cholesterol side-chain cleavage, pregnenolone flows out of mitochondria to the endoplasmic reticulum, where it is sequentially modified. In human adrenal cortex cells, pregnenolone is converted to 17α-OH pregnenolone by CYP17. 17α-OH pregnenolone is converted to 17α-OH progesterone by a 3β-hydroxysteroid dehydrogenase-$\Delta^{4,5}$-isomerase enzyme complex, which converts the 5,6 double bond of cholesterol to a 4,5 double bond and the 3-OH group to a ketone. CYP21A1 then adds a hydroxyl group to C21 of 17α-OH progesterone. The product, 11-deoxycortisol, flows back to mitochondria, where CYP11B1 catalyzes hydroxylation at C11 to yield cortisol, the final active product.

Zona glomerulosa cells contain a specific mitochondrial CYP11B2, which hydroxylates corticosterone at C18 in a double

FIGURE 3-11. Model of the cytochrome P450 reaction cycle. Electrons are transferred from NADPH via flavoprotein adrenodoxin reductase (Fp) and the iron-sulfur protein adrenodoxin (IS). Substrate (SH) binding to the enzyme brings the portion of the molecule to be modified close to the active center containing the porphyrin-bound iron-oxocomplex. The cycle is completed with production of product (SOH) and water. When a pseudosubstrate is bound, the complex breaks down to form ferric P450 and superoxide ($O_2^{\cdot}$) (center).

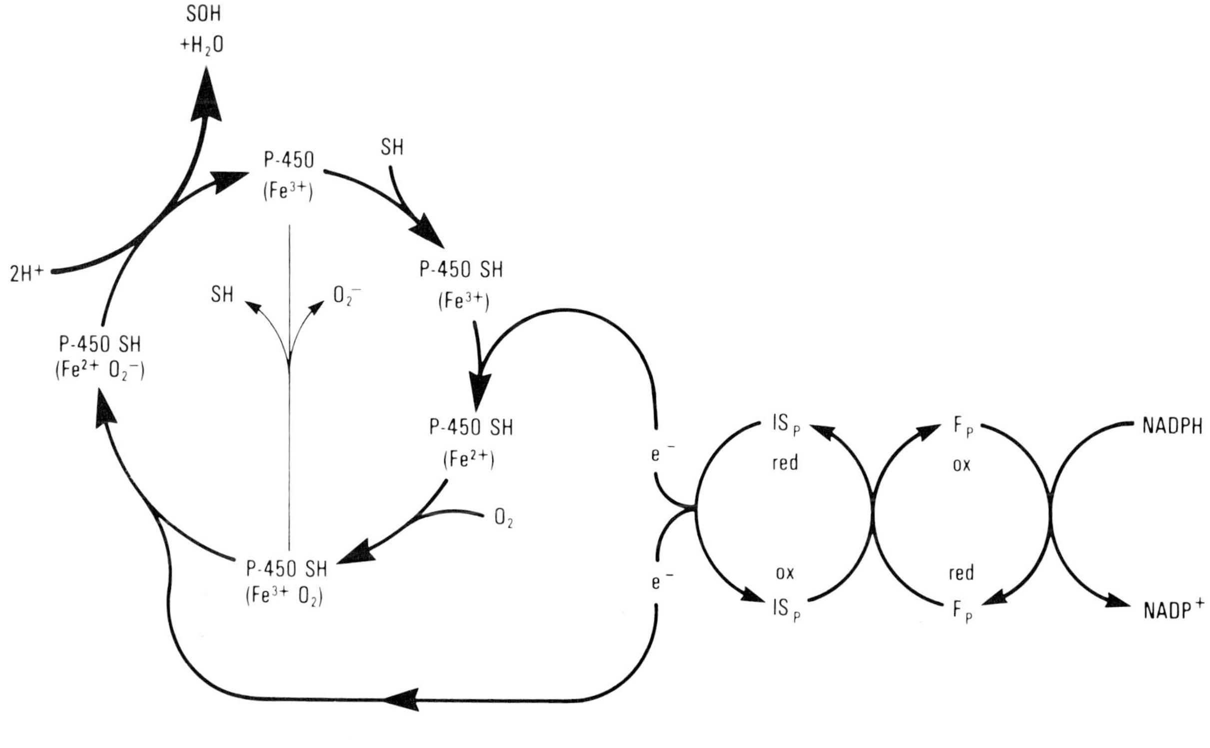

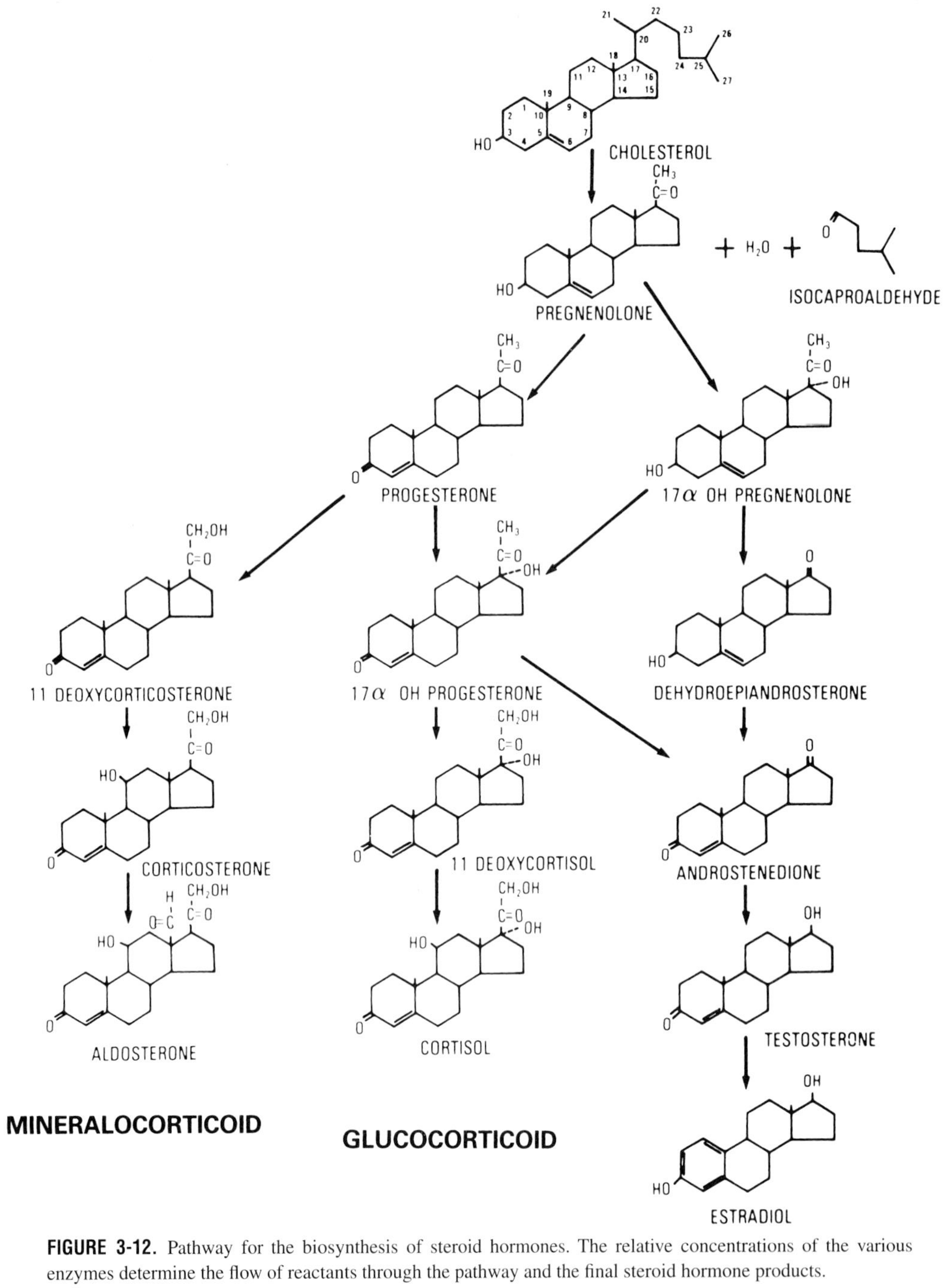

FIGURE 3-12. Pathway for the biosynthesis of steroid hormones. The relative concentrations of the various enzymes determine the flow of reactants through the pathway and the final steroid hormone products.

hydroxylation, followed by loss of water to give the aldehyde. Because zona glomerulosa cells lack CYP17, progesterone is hydroxylated at C21 to yield 11-deoxycorticosterone and then at C11 to yield corticosterone. Mitochondrial CYP11B2 then catalyze the formation of aldosterone, the active mineralocorticoid.

To produce androgens and estrogens, the C20,21 side chain must be removed. This reaction is catalyzed by C17,20-lyase, an activity intrinsic to CYP17.[89,90] This enzyme converts 17α-OH pregnenolone to dehydroepiandrosterone (DHEA) and 17α-OH progesterone to androstenedione. In the human fetal zone of the fetal adrenal cortex, 3β-hydroxysteroid dehydrogenase-$\Delta^{4,5}$-isomerase activity is low, so pregnenolone flows primarily to DHEA, which is then sulfated and transported to the placenta. The human definitive zone of the fetal adrenal cortex and the adult adrenal cortex have increased, though still low, 3β-hydroxysteroid dehydrogenase-$\Delta^{4,5}$-isomerase activity. CYP21A2 and CYP17 use the same reductase and compete for the same pool of electrons so that significant amounts of the androgen precursors, DHEA and androstenedione, are made in addition to cortisol. About half the pregnenolone formed in the human adrenal cortex is metabolized to DHEA. The adrenal cortex produces only minute amounts of testosterone and estradiol as a result of very

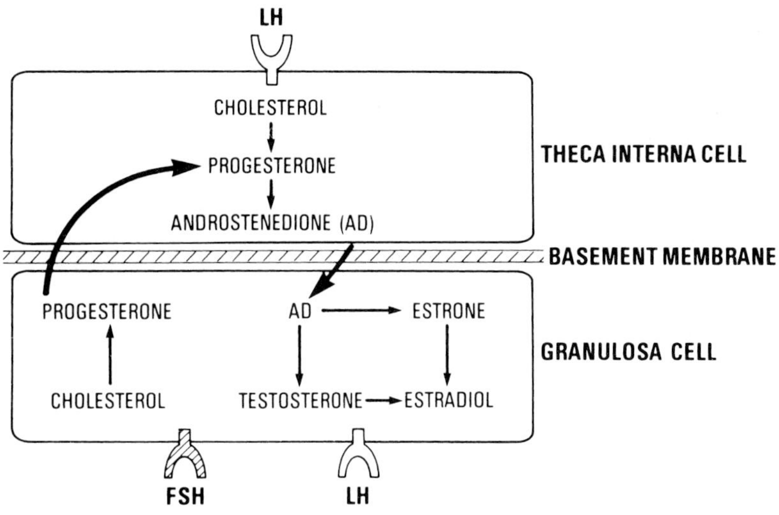

FIGURE 3-13. Two-cell, two-gonadotropin model of ovarian steroid hormone synthesis. Granulosa cells produce principally progesterone but contain aromatase, which converts androstenedione and testosterone to estrone and estradiol, respectively. Androstenedione is synthesized in theca interna cells and diffuses into adjacent granulosa cells.

low concentrations of the relevant enzymes necessary for their production.

Leydig cells of the testis lack CYP21A2 and CYP11B1 activities and thus do not produce significant quantities of mineralocorticoids and glucocorticoids. The androgen pathway shown on the right in Fig. 3-12 thus predominates. Androstenedione is converted to the active androgen, testosterone, in these cells through the actions of 17β-hydroxysteroid dehydrogenase. The testis does not produce estradiol in significant quantitites.

Estrogen and progesterone are the principal steroid products of the ovary. Granulosa cells which are converted to luteal cells during the second half of the menstrual cycle contain low levels of CYP17 and thus convert little pregnenolone or progesterone to androgens. Because these cells also lack CYP21A2 and CYP11B1, progesterone is their major steroid product. Given these enzyme deficiencies, estrogen synthesis must depend on the participation of theca cells with granulosa cells (Fig. 3-13). Theca cells produce androstenedione, which is converted to estrogen by granulosa cells. In granulosa cells, androstenedione is converted to estrogen by aromatase (CYP19), which removes C19 and catalyzes the formation of two additional double bonds in the A ring; aromatase similarly converts testosterone to estradiol. The high activity of aromatase also ensures that most of the testosterone produced is converted to estradiol and that little testosterone is released. Ovarian steroidogenesis thus depends on cooperation between two cell types, theca and granulosa, and two tropic hormones, LH and FSH.[91]

The active steroid hormone 1,25-dihydroxycholecalciferol is also synthesized from cholesterol, but the biosynthetic enzymes are located in three separate organs: skin, liver, and kidney. Initially vitamin D_3 is formed by ultraviolet irradiation of precursor 7-dehydrocholesterol present in skin (Fig. 3-14). Formation of Vitamin D_3 proceeds via a 6,7 cis isomer intermediate, previtamin D. Adequate exposure to ultraviolet light is necessary for this initial step in $1,25(OH)_2D$ formation, with more exposure being required for darker-skinned races. A dietary precursor, ergocalciferol or vitamin D_2,which differs from vitamin D_3 by a double bond between C22 and C23 and a methyl group at C24, is formed in plants from egosterol. Although most foods have only small amounts of vitamins D_2 and D_3, irradiation can convert precursors of vitamins D_2 and D_3 to vitamins D_2 and D_3. Intestinal absorption occurs principally in the ileum and requires bile salts.

Vitamins D_3 and D_2 are transported in plasma to liver via a vitamin D transport protein. This transport protein has a greater affinity for vitamin D_3 than for previtamin D, and so the latter remains in skin depots.

In the liver, vitamin D_3 is hydroxylated at C25 by a microsomal enzyme, CYP25; 25(OH)D, which is the major circulating form of vitamin D, is then transported via the α-globulin vitamin D transport protein to proximal tubule cells of the kidney, where the final modification to produce the active species occurs. In the kidney, 1α-hydroxylation of 25(OH)D is catalyzed by mitochondrial CYP, and biologically active $1,25(OH)_2D$ is secreted and transported to its sites of action.

In this unusual endocrine system with large amounts of precursor present in skin (previtamin D) and circulation [25(OH)D], the major site for synthetic regulation is at the final biosynthetic step in kidney proximal tubule cells. Elevated PTH and decreased serum phosphorus are the major factors known to stimulate CYP1A activity to increase the formation of $1,25(OH)_2D$.

Several additional modifications of the 25(OH)D nucleus occur. Hydroxylation at C24 is favored when hydroxylation at C1 is slow whereas hydroxylation at C24 is low when hydroxylation at C1 is high, suggesting that the formation of $24,25(OH)_2D$ represents a pathway for the inactivation of the steroid. Hydroxylation at C26 may also occur, with or without hydroxylation at C24 and C1.

Trophic Regulation of Steroid Hormone Synthesis

Hormones such as ACTH, FSH, LH, and hCG not only acutely stimulate steroid hormone production, but also chronically increase the synthetic capacity of their target glands by inducing synthesis of the enzymes of the biosynthetic pathway. Historically, these tropic effects were recognized from target gland atrophy with hypophysectomy before there was knowledge of the regulation of steroid hormone formation. After hypophysectomy, all the steroid-synthesizing enzymes decrease; administration of trophic hormones restores them to normal by increasing specific messenger RNAs and consequent enzyme protein biosynthesis. In adrenocortical cells, ACTH coordinately increases the synthesis of CYP11A1, CYP17, CYP21A2, CYP11B1, adrenodoxin, and

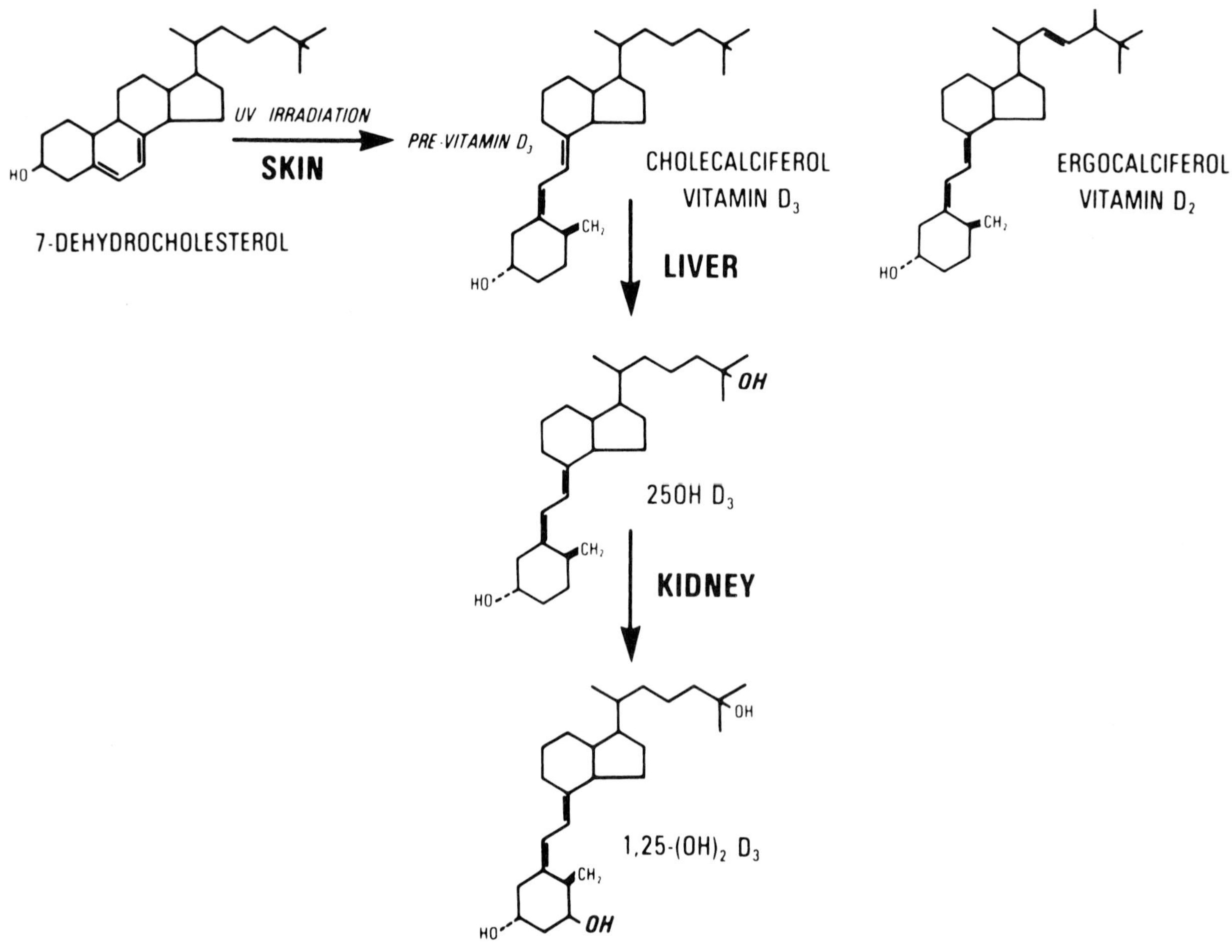

FIGURE 3-14. Biosynthesis of metabolically active $1,25(OH)_2D$.

adrenodoxin reductase; in granulosa cells, FSH induces aromatase, and increases in most other enzymes also occur. Transcriptional regulatory proteins include the cAMP response element binding protein CREB and steroidogenic factor 1 (SF1).[92,93] The DNA response element for SF1 is present in a number of CYP gene promoters although other related proteins may be relevant control elements for some CYP genes. SF1 knock-out mice lack both adrenals and gonads; additionally they have defective hypothalamic development. This member of the nuclear receptor protein family is thus essential for development of steroidogenic tissues.[94]

These trophic effects increase the capacity of the adrenal cortex to produce steroids during chronic stress and the capacity of the ovary to produce steroids during the menstrual cycle. Optimal enzyme induction requires increased protein biosynthetic capacity, which is achieved by the coordinate action of growth-promoting factors. The coordinate effects of ACTH and growth factors result in hypertrophied, hyperfunctional adrenocortical cells. The growth factors stimulate cell hypertrophy so that specific inductive effects of ACTH are maximal. ACTH does not directly stimulate cell growth; rather, it blocks cell replication. This coordinate action by two types of signal (ACTH, which induces differentiated function but inhibits replication, and growth factors such as IGF-1 and fibroblast growth factor, which increase cell growth and biosynthetic capacity) provides amplification in response to need and a return to baseline when that need is over. This method of response is well suited to hormone biosynthetic cells, which must frequently change their production capacity, because it permits large changes in this capacity without cell replication or cell death.[95] With continued stimulation, ACTH receptors down regulate, and growth factors, probably autocrine under control of ACTH, predominate; cells not only undergo hypertrophy but divide. The widely used cortrosyn stimulation test in which acute increases in $ACTH_{1-24}$-stimulated plasma cortisol are measured provides an accurate assessment of trophic maintenance of the adrenal cortex.

Transport and Metabolism of Steroid Hormones

In contrast to peptide hormones, steroid hormones are not stored but are secreted as synthesized. Increased secretion therefore directly reflects increased synthesis. After secretion into the circulation, steroid hormones are bound to transport glycoproteins which are made in the liver. Evidence that transport proteins are not essential for the activity of steroid hormones comes from patients with genetic deficiencies of binding protein who have normal endocrine function and from the observation that some synthetic analogs (e.g., dexamethasone) which are highly active bind poorly to transport proteins. Although deficiencies of steroid carrier proteins are seen in humans who are heterozygous for the protein, homozygous deficiencies are not seen, suggesting that the carrier proteins have an essential function in development and are required for viability. The plasma binding proteins provide a reservoir of hormone, protected from metabolism and renal clearance, which can be released to cells. This reservoir significantly prolongs the circulating half-life of steroid hormones, buffers increases in hormone production, and provides a source of hormone when production decreases. An important function for these proteins may be to ensure acceptable distribution to target tissues as has been shown for thyroid hormones.[96] For example, when steroid hormones circulate through tissues such as liver, the proximal portion of the tissue may take up an inappropriate proportion of hormone if it is free. By contrast, only a small amount of the total hormone can dissociate from the transport protein in the brief time period while the blood is moving through this tissue, and additional hormone will be available for entering the distal portions of the tissue. The concentration of binding proteins is regulated and affects the concentration of free active hormone.

There are three main steroid hormone transport proteins: cortisol-binding globulin (CBG), which binds cortisol and progesterone; sex hormone-binding globulin (SHBG); and vitamin D binding-globulin (DBG). CBG is a 383-amino acid glycoprotein which binds cortisol and progesterone with about equal affinity ($KD = 7.6 \times 10^{-7}\ M$). CBG has homology with the serine proteinase inhibitor superfamily.[97] CBG contains one high-affinity binding site and is normally present in concentrations sufficient to bind about 250 ng of cortisol per milliliter. When cortisol concentrations exceed this level, the hormone is weakly bound by albumin, and metabolism and excretion of the free hormone increase. Except in the third trimester of pregnancy, when high levels of progesterone occur, cortisol concentrations exceed those of progesterone about tenfold, and so most binding sites on CBG are filled by cortisol. CBG production is increased by estrogens, so by the third trimester of pregnancy, CBG concentrations are twice those of the nonpregnant state; CBG production is also increased by thyroid hormone.

The affinity of SHBG for testosterone is greater than its affinity for estradiol.[98] In males, the single binding site on the molecule is ordinarily occupied by testosterone and estradiol is weakly bound to albumin. The concentration of SHBG is increased five- to tenfold by estrogens and is decreased twofold by androgens; thyroid hormone also increases SHBG. SHBG is closely related to androgen-binding protein (ABP), which is produced in Sertoli cells and secreted into the seminiferous tubules. ABP maintains a high local androgen environment for sperm development and maturation.

The DBG glycoprotein has a single binding site with a higher affinity for 25(OH)D than for $1,25(OH)_2D$ or previtamin D_3. The relative binding affinities provide a reservoir of circulating 25(OH)D, as well as ready release of active $1,25(OH)_2D$ to target tissues. Like other steroid hormone transport proteins, DBG is synthesized in increased amounts in response to estrogen.

The small fraction of free steroid hormone, which is in equilibrium with that bound to transport protein, binds to intracellular hormone receptors to induce biological responses. The free fraction is also metabolized, principally in the liver, to inactive, water-soluble derivatives. Such metabolic steps are critical because the free hydrophobic steroids, although filtered by the kidney, are mostly reabsorbed and are largely not removed. Cortisol, for example, is inactivated by reduction of the 4,5 double bond of the A ring, and by converting less polar ketone groups such as those at C3 and C20 to hydroxyl groups. Cortisol is also inactivated by converting the 11-hydroxyl group to the ketone. 11β-OH steroid dehydrogenase is particularly important in the kidney, where it converts cortisol to cortisone. Aldosterone receptors also recognize cortisol and this local inactivation of cortisol maintains specific aldosterone responses in renal collecting duct cells and elsewhere. A specific dehydrogenase plays a role in other tissues, i.e., 20-OH steroid dehydrogenase inactivates progesterone in atretic ovarian follicles. Hydroxyl groups, especially at carbon 3, are conjugated with glucouronide and sulfate to render them more water-soluble for effective renal clearance. Hydroxylations of other steroids are also important for increasing solubility and for conjugation with glucuronic acid or sulfate. Estradiol is hydroxylated at either C2 or C16 and can be conjugated at either position; aldosterone can be conjugated via hydroxyls at either C3 or C18, and cortisol can be hydroxylated at C6. More than 50 steroid metabolites, reflecting various combinations or substitutions, have been identified, though most are produced in only small amounts.

Although most metabolic alterations of steroid hormones result in inactivation, there are several which enhance or alter biological activity. The biological activity of testosterone is increased by 5α-reductase, which converts testosterone to 5α-dihydrotestosterone, the major active species in the male reproductive tract and skin. 5α-reductase is localized in target tissues such as the prostate, so that activation of precursor testosterone occurs at the site of action. Circulating androstenedione, produced in adrenal cortex and gonads, can be converted to testosterone. Aromatase, required for estrogen production, is located in peripheral tissue cells and in producer granulosa cells in the ovary. Significant quantities of estradiol are produced in both men and women by the conversion of circulating androstenedione and testosterone to estrone and estradiol.

THYROID HORMONE

In contrast to many hormones whose concentrations fluctuate rapidly in response to environmental signals, thyroid hormone is remarkably stable. It is synthesized in the largest endocrine gland, stored in large quantities in thyroid follicles as part of the structure of a protein molecule, secreted as a prohormone, transported in the circulation bound to carrier proteins, and converted to its most active form in peripheral tissues.

Iodine Metabolism

Thyroid hormones are iodinated derivatives of the amino acid tyrosine (Fig. 3-15). Thyroxine (T_4), the major secretory product of the thyroid gland, consists of two phenyl rings linked via an ether bridge with an alanine side chain on the inner ring. Thyroxine contains four iodine atoms attached to carbons 3 and 5 of the inner ring and 3′ and 5′ of the outer ring. These substitutions impose a three-dimensional structure on the molecule so that the planes of the aromatic rings are perpendicular to each other. 3,5,3′-Triiodothyronine (T_3), the most active form of the hormone, is principally derived from T_4 by removal of one iodine from the outer ring, whereas 3,3′,5′-triiodothyronine (reverse T_3), the major inactive metabolite of T_4, results from the removal of iodine from C5 of the inner ring.

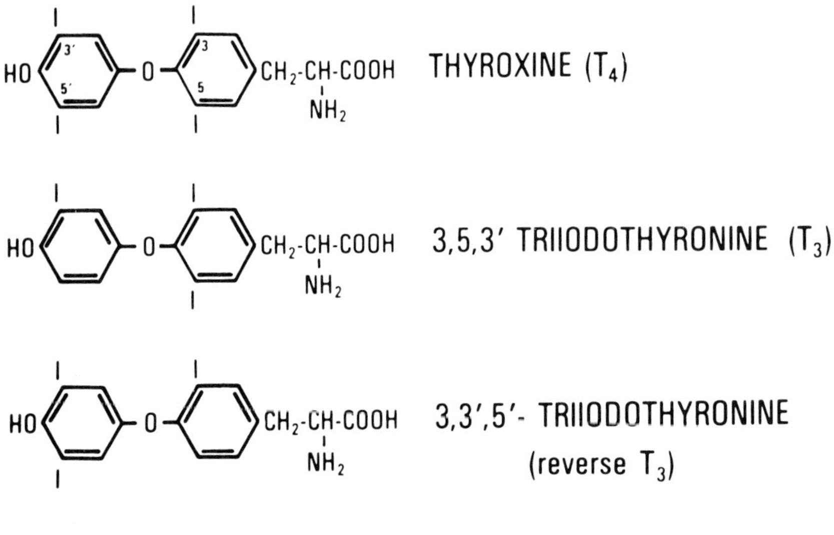

FIGURE 3-15. The major circulating thyroid hormones.

Because iodine is an essential structural component, biosynthesis of thyroid hormone depends on iodine metabolism. Dietary iodine intake in western cultures is normally about 250 μg per day but may be greater because of the use of iodized salt and iodates in bread and processed foods. In inland mountainous areas of the world iodine intake may be less than 60 μg per day. In these areas, growth of the thyroid gland and enhanced trapping of iodine may maintain a euthyroid state. Although the adaptive capacity of the gland is great, when iodine intake falls below 20 μg/day, thyroid gland compensation may be inadequate and endemic hypothyroidism and cretinism occur.

Under basal conditions, the thyroid uses about 60 μg of iodide daily for thyroid hormone biosynthesis (Fig. 3-16). Of this, 50 μg is of dietary origin and 10 μg is from hormone turnover. Iodide is concentrated from the circulation by active transport via an iodide pump located at the basal surface of the thyroid cell. The iodide transporter is a 12-membrane spanning molecule.[100] which, like thyroglobulin and thyroid peroxidase, is regulated by TSH. The concentrating mechanism requires metabolic energy from ATP and Na^+ K^+, ATPase-mediated sodium transport.[101] The transport process effectively extracts iodide from the circulation and can concentrate it more than 100-fold within the thyroid cell. Other anions, such as perchlorate and pertechnetate, are also concentrated, and these ions have been used for thyroid function tests and for imaging.

FIGURE 3-16. Average human daily iodine balance in the United States. (*From Robbins.*[99])

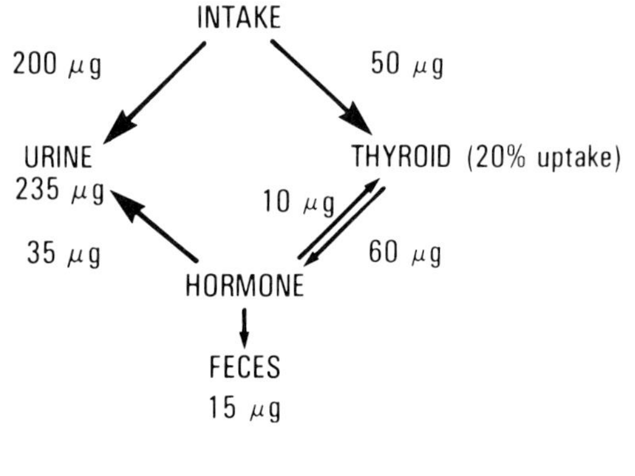

Cellular uptake of iodide is regulated by TSH and by local control mechanisms. The local autoregulatory mechanisms help provide adequate iodide for hormone synthesis when circulating levels are low and prevent excessive hormone synthesis when circulating iodide concentrations are high. In response to large quantities of iodine (2 mg or more), there is a sharp decrease in the iodination of tyrosine residues in thyroglobulin.[102] The decreased organification (Wolff-Chaikoff effect) is an acute adaptive response to high intracellular concentrations of iodide. When high iodide concentrations persist, thyroid cells adapt by decreasing active transport of iodide into the cell.[103] Increased cellular concentrations of unbound iodide are then dissipated, and the block to organification is removed. Ingestion of large amounts of iodine thus does not normally affect thyroid hormone synthesis. When these autoregulatory mechanisms are defective, dietary iodine can have marked effects on thyroid hormone synthesis. When inhibition of organification does not occur in response to increased cellular iodide, increased thyroid hormone synthesis and hyperthyroidism may occur (iod-Basedow effect). If organification is inhibited but transport of iodide does not adaptively decrease, high cellular concentrations of iodide will result in decreased thyroid hormone synthesis (iodide goiter and hypothyroidism). Damage from radioactive iodine and Hashimoto's thyroiditis impair adaptive decreases in iodide transport and predispose to iodide-induced hypothyroidism.

Anatomy of a Distinctive Biosynthetic Pathway

Thyroid cells are polarized epithelial cells that are organized into follicles with their basal surfaces exposed to the circulation and their apical surfaces facing the lumen of the central follicle, which is filled with thyroglobulin. Iodide is taken up at the basal surface and is rapidly oxidized and incorporated into tyrosine residues in thyroglobulin molecules. In the biosynthetic pathway outlined in Fig. 3-17, both the organification and coupling reactions shown occur at the apical surface of the cell, in microvilli which extend into the colloid space. Thyroid peroxidase is a membrane-bound heme-protein enzyme complex which catalyzes both organification and coupling reactions.[104–107] The proposed reaction scheme

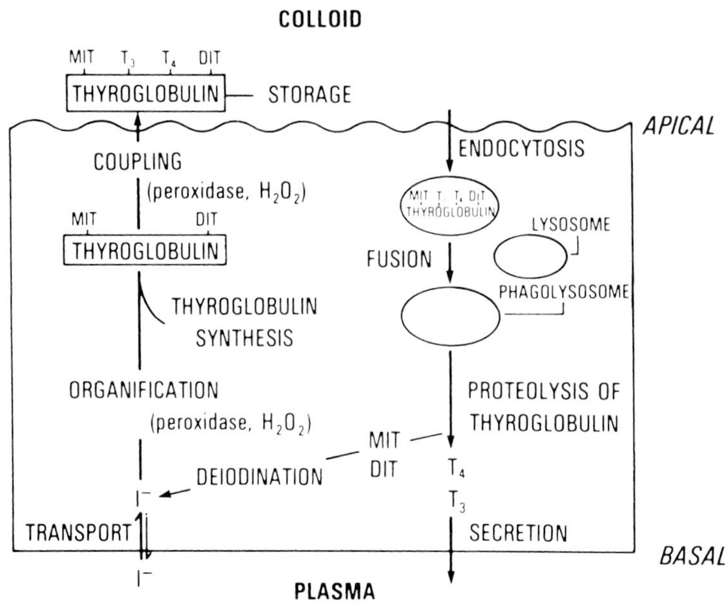

FIGURE 3-17. Pathway for the biosynthesis of thyroid hormones.

for thyroid peroxidase (E) is

(1) Organification:

$$E + H_2O_2 \xrightarrow{H_2O} EO \longrightarrow [EOI]^- \xrightarrow{+\text{ tyrosine}} \text{iodotyrosine} + OH^- + E$$

(2) Coupling:

$$E + H_2O_2 \xrightarrow{H_2O} EO \xrightarrow{+\text{ DIT (thyroglobulin)}} T_4 + E$$

The antithyroid drugs (thioureylene compounds) inhibit organification and coupling reactions by inactivating both EO and $[EOI]^-$.

The tyrosine residues which are iodinated are present in thyroglobulin, a large multisubunit glycoprotein of 660,000M_r.[108] Thyroglobulin, which accounts for about 50 percent of the total protein made by thyroid cells, has only an average content of tyrosine, but these tyrosines appear to be available for iodination both because of their location in the primary structure and because of the tertiary structure of the mature glycosylated protein. For example, specific tyrosyl residues in the amino- and carboxy termini are preferentially iodinated.[109] Thyroglobulin is transported in vesicles to the microvilli at the apical surface, where iodination, coupling, and secretion into the follicular lumen occur. Normally iodinated thyroglobulin present in lumen colloid contains about 26 atoms of iodine with 3 to 4 T_4 and 0.2 T_3 residues as well as 6 residues of monoiodotyrosine and 4 residues of diiodotyrosine.[110] Iodide availability affects the proportions of T_3 and T_4, with more T_3 being present when iodide is low.

Large amounts of thyroglobulin are stored as colloid in the lumen of thyroid follicles. The formation of active thyroid hormone requires readsorption of colloid by endocytosis and breakdown of thyroglobulin to T_4 and T_3. It is not known how endocytic vesicles containing thyroglobulin are vectorially targeted to lysosomes. Thyroglobulin may be broken down via lysosomal hydrolases, but there is also evidence for cleavage by halogens and peroxidases.[111] If the latter hypothesis is correct, the steps in thyroid hormone synthesis (organification, coupling, and proteolysis) all use one substrate, thyroglobulin, and one enzyme, thyroid peroxidase, and the cellular organization shown in Fig. 3-17 serves to segregate these various reactions.

T_4 and T_3 are secreted in a ratio of about 10:1. The iodine in mono- and diiodotyrosine is reclaimed for hormone biosynthesis by a thyroid deiodinase enzyme. This deiodination pathway reclaims about 50 percent of the iodine of thyroglobulin and is quantitatively important in thyroid gland economy, as demonstrated by the fact that congenital defects in deiodinase result in goitrous hypothyroidism.

TSH, which is the major regulator of thyroid gland function, has been reported to increase each step of the biosynthetic pathway. A rate-limiting step analogous to that for steroid hormone synthesis has not been identified, but increased availability of iodide via active transport is among the most rapid responses to TSH.

Transport and Metabolism

T_4, the major secretory product of the thyroid, circulates bound to serum proteins. The binding proteins, like those which transport steroid hormones, are made in the liver, and their synthesis is increased by estrogens and decreased by androgens. More than 99 percent of T_4 is bound to three proteins: thyroid-binding globulin (TBG), thyroid-binding prealbumin (TBPA), and serum albumin. The glycoprotein TBG, which binds about 75 percent of circulating T_4, has the highest affinity; TBPA has a lesser affinity, and serum albumin has the least affinity but the highest capacity. Protein binding provides a large protected reservoir of hormone. Because of extensive protein binding, T_4 has a circulating half-life of about 1 week, while T_3, which is bound less tightly to protein, has a half-life of 1.3 days. The roles of the thyroid hormone transport proteins appear to be similar to those for the steroid hormone transport proteins.

Thyroxine is a prohormone and is activated in target tissues via 5′-deiodination to metabolically active T_3. 5′-deiodination is catalyzed by a microsomal enzyme which requires reduced thiols for activity. The type I 5′-deiodinase contains selenocyteine in its active site.[112] Replacement with cysteine results in a less active enzyme, indicating that this unusual amino acid is important for catalytic activity. This enzyme, which is especially prominent in liver and kidney, accounts for more than 80 percent of T_3 production under normal conditions. Its activity, and thus the production of T_3, is influenced by many factors. The first site of control of thyroid hormone synthesis is the thyroid gland, where TSH regulates T_4 production. Under most conditions, conversion of T_4 to T_3 in the periphery is proportional to the concentration of substrate T_4, but a second point of control is present in target organs such as liver and kidney, where under several conditions conversion of T_4 to T_3 is decreased. Fasting, illness, cortisol, propylthiouracil, and other drugs all reduce 5′-deiodinase activity.[113] During fasting, there is a 20 percent decrease in plasma T_3 by the end of the first day and a 50 percent decrease at the end of 3 days. This decrease in T_3 production is thought to be an adaptive response contributing to a decreased metabolic rate and to conservation of body tissues when substrate is unavailable. Use of the circulating pool of prohormone T_4 is thus coupled to metabolic needs.

Type II 5′-deiodinase found in the pituitary and central nervous system differs from that in liver and kidney. It has a lower K_m for T_4, it is not inhibited by propylthiouracil, and its activity increases rather than decreases in hypothyroidism. Type II 5′-deiodinase contains cysteine rather than selenocysteine in the active site.[114] This enzyme is important in feedback effects of T_4 on TSH secretion as well as in biological effects on the nervous system. The type II 5′-deiodinase converts T_4 to T_3 in the pituitary to provide a normal hypothalamic-pituitary-thyroid axis under conditions, such as fasting, where circulating T_3 concentrations are low because of inhibition of liver and kidney 5′-deiodinase. If circulating T_3 were the major feedback regulator of TSH, the reduced circulating concentrations of T_3 in fasting and in systemic illness would remove feedback inhibition resulting in increased TSH and thus thyroid hormone production. The type II 5′-deiodinase of the pituitary allows feedback control via circulating T_4 rather than T_3 and serves to maintain normal thyroid gland production, preventing the thyroid from inappropriately compensating for the physiologically important reduction in circulating T_3 concentrations.

Deiodination of the inner ring of T_4 by 5-deiodinase yields reverse T_3 (rT_3), an inactive metabolite. About equal amounts of T_3 and rT_3 are formed from T_4, but rT_3 is cleared more rapidly, so circulating concentrations are lower. When 5-deiodinase activity is reduced, as in fasting, greater amounts of T_4 are metabolized to rT_3.

Inactivation of T_3 occurs by additional deiodinations to give 3,3′-T_2 and 3,5-T_2 and by deamination and decarboxylation of the alanine side chain and conjugation with glucuronic acid and sulfate.

REFERENCES

1. Shatkin AJ: Capping of eukaryotic mRNAs. *Cell* 9:645, 1976.
2. Kozak M: Structural features in eukaryotic mRNAs that modulate the initiation of translation. *J Biol Chem* 266:19867, 1991.
3. Sharp PA: RNA splicing and genes. *JAMA* 260:3035, 1988.
4. Staley JP, Guthrie C: Mechanical devices of the spliceosome: Motors, clocks, springs and things. *Cell* 92:315, 1998.
5. Wahle E, Keller W: The biochemistry of 3′-end cleavage and polyadenylation of messenger RNA precursors. *Annu Rev Biochem* 61:419, 1992.
6. Roeder RG: Role of general and gene-specific cofactors in the regulation of eukaryotic transcription. *Cold Spring Harbor Symposium on Quantum Biology* 63:201, 1998.
7. Gidoni D, Dynan WS, Tjian R: Multiple specific contacts between a mammalian transcription factor and its cognate promoters. *Nature* 321:409, 1984.
8. Smale ST, Baltimore D: The initiator as a transcription control element. *Cell* 57:103, 1989.
9. Pabo CO, Saver RT: Transcription factors: Structural families and principles of recognition. *Annu Rev Biochem* 61:1053, 1992.
10. Frankel AD, Kim PS: Modular structure of transcription factors: Implications for gene regulation. *Cell* 65:717, 1991.
11. Carey M: The enhanceosome and transcriptional synergy. *Cell* 92:5, 1998.
12. Rachez C, Lemon BD, Suldan Z, Bromleigh V, Gamble M, Näär AM, Erdjument-Bromage H, Tempst P, and Freedman LP: Ligand-dependent transcription activation by nuclear receptors requires the DRIP complex. *Nature* 398:824, 1999.
13. Yuan CX, Ito M, Fondell JD, Fu ZY, Roeder RG: The TRAP 220 component of a thyroid hormone receptor-associated protein (TRAP) coactivator complex interacts directly with nuclear receptors in a ligand-dependent fashion. *Proc Natl Acad Sci USA* 95:7939, 1998.
14. Naar AM, Beaurang PA, Zhou S, Abraham S, Solomon W, Tjian R: Composite co-activator ARC mediates chromatin-directed transcriptional activation. *Nature* 398:828,1999.
15. Kadonaga JT: Eurkaryotic transcription: An interlaced network of transcription factors and chromatin-modified machines. *Cell* 92:307, 1998.
16. Horlein AJ, Näär AN, Heinzel T, Torchia J, Gloss B, Kurokawa R, Ryan A, Kamei Y, Soderstrom M, Glass CK, Rosenfeld MG: Ligand-independent repression by the thyroid hormone receptor mediated by a nuclear receptor co-repressor. *Nature* 377:397, 1995.
17. Chen, JD, Evans, RM: A transcriptional co-repressor that interacts with nuclear hormone receptors. *Nature* 377:454, 1995.
18. Heinzel T, Lavinsky RM, Mullen TM, Soderstrom M, Laherty CD, Torchia J, Yang WM, Brard G, Ngo SD, Davie JR, Seto E, Eisenman RN, Rose DW, Glass CK, Rosenfeld MG: A complex containing N-CoR, mSin3 and histone deacetylase mediates transcriptional repression. *Nature* 387:43, 1997.
19. Ptashne M, Gann A: Translational activation by recruitment. *Nature* 386:569, 1997.
20. Torchia J, Rose DW, Inostroza J, Kamei Y, Westin S, Glass CK, Rosenfeld MG: The transcriptional co-activator p/CIP binds CBP and mediates nuclear-receptor function. *Nature* 387:677, 1997.
21. Xu L, Lavinsky RM, Dasen JS, Flynn SE, McInerney EM, Mullen TM, Heinzel T, Szeto D, Korzus E, Kurokawa R, Aggarwal AK, Rose DW, Glass CK, Rosenfeld, MG: Signal-specific co-activator domain requirements for Pit1 activation. *Nature* 395:301, 1998.
22. Simon SM, Blobel G: A protein conducting channel in the endoplasmic reticulum. *Cell* 65:371, 1991.
23. Walter P, Blobel G: Signal recognition particle contains a 7S RNA essential for protein translocation across the endoplasmic reticulum. *Nature* 299:691, 1982.
24. Gilmore R, Walter P, Blobel G: Protein translocation across the endoplasmic reticulum: Isolation and characterization of the signal recognition particle receptor. *J Cell Biol* 96:470, 1982.
25. Connolly T, Gilmore R: The signal recognition particle receptor mediates the GTP-dependent displacement of SRP from the signal sequence of the nascent polypeptide. *Cell* 57:599-610, 1989.
26. Matlack KES, Mothes W, Rapoport TA: Protein translocation: Tunnel vision. *Cell* 97:381, 1998.
27. Singer SJ: The structure and insertion of integral proteins in membranes. *Annu Rev Cell Biol* 6:247, 1990.
28. Grey A, Dull TJ, Ullrich A: Nucleotide sequence of epidermal growth factor cDNA predicts a 128,000-molecular weight protein precursor. *Nature* 303:722, 1983.
29. Land H, Schultz G, Schmale H, Richter D: Nucleotide sequence of cloned cDNA encoding bovine arginine vasopressin-neuropysin II precursor. *Nature* 295:299, 1982.

30. Nakanishi S, Inoue A, Kita T, Nakamura M, Chang ACY, Cohen SN, Numa S: Nucleotide sequence of clone cDNA for bovine corticotropin β-lipotropin precursor. *Nature* 278:423, 1979.
31. Blundell TL, Bedarkar S, Rinderknecht E, Humbel RE: Insulin-like growth factor: A model for tertiary structure accounting for immunoreactivity and receptor binding. *Proc Natl Acad Sci USA* 75:180, 1978.
32. Steiner DS, Clark JL: The spontaneous reoxidation of reduced beef and rat proinsulins. *Proc Natl Acad Sci USA* 60:622, 1968.
33. Gabbay KH, DeLuca K, Fisher JN Jr, Mako ME, Rubenstein AH: Familial hyperproinsulinemia: An autosomal dominant defect. *N Engl J Med* 294:911, 1976.
34. Springer S, Spang A, Schekman R: A primer on vesicle budding. *Cell* 97:145, 1999.
35. Allan BB, Balch WE: Protein sorting by directed maturation of Golgi compartments. *Science* 285:63, 1999 .
36. Martinez-Menarquez JA, Geuze HJ, Slot JW, Klumperman J: Vesicular tubular clusters between the ER and Golgi mediate concentration of soluble secretory proteins by exclusion from COP-1 coated vesicles. *Cell* 98:81, 1999.
37. Rothman JE, Wieland FT: Protein sorting by transport vesicles. *Science* 272:227, 1996.
38. Warren G, Mellman I: BULK flow redux? *Cell* 98:125, 1999.
39. Sollner T, Whiteheart SW, Brunner M, Erdjument-Bromage H, Geromanos S, Tempst P, Rothman JE: SNAP receptors implicated in vesicle targeting and fusion. *Nature* 362:318, 1993.
40. Goda Y: SNAREs and regulated vesicle exocytosis. *Proc Natl Acad Sci USA* 94:769, 1997.
41. Pfeffer SR: Transport vesicle docking: SNAREs and associates. *Annu Rev Biochem* 12:441, 1996.
42. Chen YA, Scales SJ, Patel SM, Doung YC, Scheller RH: SNARE complex formation is triggered by Ca^{2+} and drives membrane fusion. *Cell* 97:165, 1999.
43. Gonzalez L, Scheller RH: Regulation of membrane trafficking: Structural insights from a Rab/effector complex. *Cell* 96:755, 1999.
44. Hubbard SC, Ivatt RJ: Synthesis and processing of asparagine-linked oligosaccharides. *Annu Rev Biochem* 50:555, 1981.
45. Stockert RJ: The asialoglycoprotein receptor: Relationships between structure, function and expression. *Physiol Rev* 75:591, 1995.
46. Dannies PS: Protein hormone storage in secretory granules: Mechanisms for concentration and sorting. *Endo Rev* 20:3, 1999.
47. Geppert M, Goda Y, Hammer ER, Li C, Rosahl TW, Stevens CF, Südhof TC: Synaptotagmin I: A major Ca^{2+} sensor for transmitter release at a central synapse. *Cell* 79:717, 1994.
48. Mochida S, Yokoyama CT, Kim DK, Itoh K, Catterall WA: Evidence for a voltage-dependent enhancement by neurotransmitter release mediated via the synaptic protein interaction site of N-type Ca^{2+} channels. *Proc Natl Acad Sci USA* 95:14523, 1998.
49. Hunziker W, Harter C, Matter K, Mellman I: Basolateral sorting in MDCK cells requires a distinct cytoplasmic domain determinant. *Cell* 66:907, 1991.
50. Simons K, Ikonen E: Functional *rafts* in cell membranes. *Nature* 387:569, 1997.
51. Anderson RGW: The caveolae membrane system. *Annu Rev Biochem* 67:199, 1998.
52. Okamoto T, Schlegel A, Scherer PE, Lisanti MP: Caveolins, a family of scaffolding proteins for organizing "preassembled signaling complexes" at the plasma membrane. *J Biol Chem* 273:5419, 1998.
53. Schmid SL: Clathrin-coated vesicle formation and protein sorting. *Annu Rev Biochem* 66:511, 1997.
54. Musacchio A, Smith CJ, Roseman AM, Harrison SC, Kirchhausen T, Pearse BMF: Functional organization of clathrin in coats: Combining electron cryomicroscopy and x-ray crystallography. *Mol Cell* 3:761, 1999.
55. Hinshaw JE, Schmid SL: Dynamin self-assemble into rings suggesting a mechanism for coated vesicle budding. *Nature* 374:190, 1995.
56. Chang CP, Lazar CS, Walsh BJ, Komuro M, Collawn JF, Kuhn LA, Tainer JA, Trowbridge IS, Farquhar MG, Rosenfeld MG, Wiley HS, Gill GN: Ligand-induced internalization of the EGF receptor is mediated by multiple endocytic codes analogous to the tyrosine motif found in constitutively-internalized receptors. *J Biol Chem* 268: 19312, 1993.
57. Opresko L, Chang CP, Will BH, Burke PM, Gill GN, Wiley HS: Endocytosis and lysosomal targeting of epidermal growth factor receptors are mediated by distinct sequences independent of the tyrosine kinase domain. *J Biol Chem* 270:4325, 1995.
58. Kirchhausen T, Bonifacino JS, Riezman L: Linking cargo to vesicle formation: Receptor tail interactions with coat proteins. *Curr Opin Cell Biol* 9:488, 1997.
59. Owen DJ, Evans PR: A structural explanation for the recognition of tyrosine-based endocytic signals. *Science* 282:1327, 1998.
60. Nesterov A, Carter RE, Sorkina T, Gill GN, Sorkin A: Inhibition of the receptor-binding function of clathrin adaptor protein AP-2 by dominant-negative mutant $\mu 2$ subunit and its effect on endocytosis. *EMBO J* 18:2489, 1999.
61. Novick P, Brennwald P: Friends and family: The role of Rab GTPaes in vesicular traffic. *Cell* 75:597, 1993.
62. Wiley HS, Herbst JJ, Walsh BJ, Lauffenburger DA, Rosenfeld MG, Gill GN: Role of tyrosine kinase activity in endocytosis, compartmentation and downregulation of the EGF receptor. *J Biol Chem* 266:11083, 1991.
63. Pitcher JA, Freedman NJ, Lefkowitz RJ: G protein-coupled receptor kinases. *Annu Rev Biochem* 67:653, 1998.
64. Coux O, Tanaka K, Goldberg AL: Structure and functions of the 20S and 26S proteasomes. *Annu Rev Biochem* 65:801, 1996.
65. Hershko A, Ciechanover A: The ubiquitin system: *Annu Rev Biochem* 67:425, 1998.
66. Cohen P, Rosenfeld RG: Physiological and clinical relevance of the IGFβPs. *Curr Opin Pediatric* 6:462, 1994.
67. Deuel TF, Kawahara RS: Growth factors and wound healing. *Annu Rev Med* 42:567, 1991.
68. Kovanen PT, Goldstein JL, Chappell DA, Brown MS: Regulation of low density lipoprotein receptors by adrenocorticotropin in the adrenal gland of mice and rats in vivo. *J Biol Chem* 255:5591, 1980.
69. Illingworth DR, Orwoll ES, Connor WR: Impaired cortisol secretion in abetalipoproteinemia. *J Clin Endocrinol Metab* 50:977, 1980.
70. Illingworth DR, Kenny TA, Orwoll ES: Adrenal function in heterozygous and homozygous hypobetalipoproteinemia. *J Clin Endocrinol Metab* 54:27, 1982.
71. Illingworth DR, Lees AM, Lees RS: Adrenal cortical function in homozygous familial hypercholesterolemia. *Metabolism* 30:1045, 1983.
72. Acton S, Rigotti A, Landschulz KT, Hobbs HH, Krieger M: Identification of scavenger receptor SR-BI as a high density lipoprotein receptor. *Science* 271:518, 1996.
73. Wang N, Wang W, Breslow JL, Tall AR: Scavenger receptor BI (SR-BI) is up-regulated in adrenal gland in apolipoprotein A-I and hepatic lipase knock-out mice as a response to depletion of cholesterol stores *J Biol Chem* 271:21001, 1996.
74. Murao K, Terpstra V, Green SR, Kondratenko N, Steinberg D, Quehenberger O: Characterization of CLA-1, a human homologue of rodent scavenger receptor BI, as a receptor for high density lipoprotein and apoptotic thymocytes. *J Biol Chem* 272:17551, 1997.
75. Temel RE, Trigatti B, DeMattos RB, Azhar S, Krieger M, Williams DL: Scavenger receptor class B, type I (SR-BI) is the major route for the delivery of high density lipoprotein cholesterol to the steroidogenic pathway in cultured mouse adrenocortical cells. *Proc Natl Acad Sci USA* 94:13600, 1997.
76. Rigotti A, Edelman ER, Siefert P, Iqbal SN, DeMattos RB, Temel RE, Krieger M, Williams DL: Regulation by adrenocorticotropic hormone of the *in vivo* expression of scavenger receptor class B Type I (SR-BI), a high density lipoprotein receptor, in steroidogenic cells of the murine adrenal gland. *J Biol Chem* 271:33545, 1996.
77. Briggs MR, Yokoyam C, Wang X, Brown MS, Goldstein JL: Nuclear protein that binds sterol regulatory element of low density lipoprotein receptor promoter. I. Identification of the protein and delineation of its target nucleotide sequence. *J Biol Chem* 268:14490, 1993.
78. Yokoyama C, Wang X, Briggs MR, Admon A, Wu J, Hua X, Goldstein JL, Brown MS: SREBP-1, a basic-helix-loop-helix-leucine zipper protein that controls transcription of the low density lopoprotein receptor gene. *Cell* 78:187, 1993.
79. Sakai J, Rawson RB, Espenshade PJ, Cheng D, Seegmiller AC, Goldstein JL, Brown MS: Molecular identification of the sterol-regulated luminal protease that cleaves SREBPs and controls lipid composition of animal cells. *Molecular Cell* 2:505, 1998.
80. Brown MS, Kovanen PT, Goldstein JL: Receptor-mediated uptake of lipoprotein cholesterol and its utilization for steroid synthesis in the adrenal cortex. *Recent Prog Horm Res* 35:215, 1979.

81. Nelson DR, Koymans L, Kamataki T, Stageman JJ, Feyereisen R, Waxman DJ, Waterman MR, Gotoh O, Coon MJ, Estabrook RW, Gunsalus IC, Nebert DW: P450 superfamily: Update on new sequences, gene mapping, accession numbers and nomenclature. *Pharmacogen* 6:1, 1996.
82. Lind D, Sugarwara T, Strauss JF, Clark BJ, Stocco DM, Saenger P, Rogol A, Miller WL: Role of steroidogenic acute regulatory protein in adrenal and gonadal steroidogenesis. *Science* 267:1828, 1995.
83. Stocco DM: Steroidogenic acute regulatory protein. *Vit and Hormone* 55:399, 1999.
84. Bose HS, Sugawara T, Strauss JF, Miller WL: The pathophysiology and genetics of congenital *lipoid* adrenal hyperplasia. *New Engl J Med* 225:1870, 1996.
85. Hall PF, Lewes JL, Lipson ED: The role of mitochondrial cytochrome P-450 from bovine adrenal cortex in side chain cleavage of 20S, *22R dihydroxycholesterol. J Biol Chem* 250:2283, 1975.
86. Miller WL: Molecular biology of steroid hormone synthesis. *Endocrinol Rev* 9:295, 1988.
87. Gustafsson JA, Carlstedt-Duke J, Mode A, Rafter J: *Biochemistry, Biophysics and Regulation of Cytochrome P-450*. New York, Elsevier, 1980.
88. Hornsby PJ, Crivello JF: The role of lipid peroxidation and biological antioxidants in the function of the adrenal cortex. *Mol Cell Endocrinl* 30:1, 1983.
89. Barnes HJ, Arlotto MP, Waterman MR: Expression and enzyme activity of recombinant cytochrome $P450_{17}$ alpha hydroxylase in Escherichia coli. *Proc Natl Acad Sci USA* 88:5597, 1991.
90. Auchus RJ, Miller WL: Molecular modeling of human P450c17 (17α-Hydroxylase/17,20-Lyase: Insights into reaction mechanisms and effects of mutations. *Mol Endocrinol* 13:1169, 1999.
91. Hsueh AJW, Adashi EY, Jones PBC, Welsh TH Jr: Hormonal regulation of the differentiation of cultured ovarian granulosa cells. *Endocrinol Rev* 5:76, 1984.
92. Luo Y, Ikeda Y, Parker KL: A cell-specific nuclear receptor is essential for adrenal and gonadal development and sexual differentiation. *Cell* 77:481, 1994.
93. Reinhart AJ, Williams SC, Clark BJ, Stocco DM: SF1 (Steroidogenic Factor-1) and c/EBPβ (ccAAT/Enhancer binding protein-β) cooperate to regulate the murine StAR (steroidogenic acute regulatory) promoter. *Mol Endocrinol* 13:729, 1999.
94. Parker KL, Schimmer BP: Steroidogenic factor 1: A key determinant of endocrine development and function. *Endocrinol Rev* 18:361, 1997.
95. Gill GN, Crivello JF, Hornsby PJ, Simonian MH: Growth, function and development of the adrenal cortex: Insights from cell culture. *Cold Spring Harbor Conf Cell Proliferation* 9:461, 1982.
96. Mendel CM, Cavalieri RR, Weisiser RA: Uptake of thyroxine by the perfused rat liver: Implications for the free hormone hypothesis. *Am J Physiol* 255:410, 1988.
97. Hammond GL: Molecular properties of corticosteroid binding globulin and the sex-steroid binding proteins. *Endocrinol Rev* 11, 11:65, 1990.
98. Bardin CW, Musto N, Gunsalus G, Kotite N, Cheng SL, Larrea F, Becker R: Extracellular androgen binding proteins. *Endocrinol Rev* 11:54, 1990.
99. Robbins J: Iodine deficiency, iodine excess and the use of iodine for protection against radioactive iodine. *Thyroid Today* 3:1, 1980.
100. Dai G, Levy O, Carrasco N: Cloning and characterization of the thyroid iodide transporter. *Nature* 379:458, 1996.
101. Nilsson M, Björkman U, Ekholm R, Ericson LE: Iodide transport in primary cultured thyroid follicle cells: Evidence of a TSH-regulated channel mediating iodide efflux selectively across the apical domain of the plasma membrane. *Eur J Cell Biol* 52:270, 1990.
102. Wolff J, Chaikoff IL: The inhibitory action of iodide upon organic binding of iodine by the normal thyroid gland. *J Biol Chem* 17:2855, 1948.
103. Braverman LE, Ingbar SH: Changes in thyroidal function during adaptation to large doses of iodide. *J Clin Invest* 42:1216, 1963.
104. Nakamura M, Yamazaki I, Nakagawa H, Ohtaki S: Steady state kinetics and regulation of thyroid peroxidase-catalyzed iodination. *J Biol Chem* 258:3837, 1983.
105. Morrison M, Schonbaum GR: Peroxidase-catalyzed halogenation. *Annu Rev Biochem* 45:861, 1983.
106. Magnusson RP, Taurog A, Dorris ML: Mechanism of iodide-dependent catalytic activity of thyroid peroxidase and lactoperoxidase. *J Biol Chem* 259:197, 1984.
107. Magnusson B, Chazenbalk GD, Gestautas J, Seto P, Filetti S, DeGroot LJ, Rapoport B: Molecular cloning of the complementary deoxyribonucleic acid for human thyroid peroxidase. *Mol Endocrinol* 1:856, 1987.
108. Malthiery Y, Lissitzky S: Primary structure of human thyroglobulin deduced from the sequence of its 8448-base complementary DNA. *Eur J Biochem* 165:491, 1987.
109. Dunn JT, Anderson PC, Fox JW, Fassler CA, Dunn AD, Hite LA, Moore RC: The sites of thyroid hormone formation in rabbit thyroglobulin. *J Biol Chem* 62:16948, 1987.
110. Izumi M, Larsen PR: Triiodothyronine, thyroxine and iodine in purified thyroglobulin from patients with Graves' disease. *J Clin Invest* 59:1105, 1977.
111. Alexander NM: Oxidative cleavage of tryptophanyl peptide bonds during chemical- and peroxidase-catalyzed iodinations. *J Biol Chem* 249:1946, 1977.
112. Berry MJ, Banu L, Larsen PR: Type I iodothyronine deiodinase is a selenocysteine-containing enzyme. *Nature* 349:438, 1991.
113. Wartofsky L, Burman KD: Alterations in thyroid function in patients with systemic illness: The "euthyroid sick syndrome." *Endocrinol Rev* 3:164, 1982.
114. Berry MJ, Kieffer JD, Larsen PR: Evidence that cysteine, not selenocysteine, is in the catalytic site of type II iodothyronine deiodinase. *Endocrinology* 129:550, 1991.
115. Glass CK, Rosenfeld MG: The coregulator exchange in transcriptional functions of nuclear receptors. *Genes and Devel* 14:121, 2000.

CHAPTER 4

Molecular Mechanisms of Hormone Action: Biology of Signal Transduction

Mark M. Rasenick
Randal C. Jaffe

INTRODUCTION

Hormones and neurotransmitters are the molecules charged with the task of cell to cell communication. These signals can range from those which exert effects in milliseconds (neurotransmitters which open ion channels) to those which act over a period of hours to days (steroid hormones and growth factors). Although originally described as blood-borne molecules released from endocrine glands, this chapter will attempt to describe the similarities and differences of a number of molecules employed for communication among cells and the molecular mechanisms by which they act.

Methods of Cell-Cell Communication

Substances used for cell-cell communication are delivered to their targets in several ways (Fig. 4-1). Endocrine signaling involves the release of signaling molecules into the circulation where they eventually bind to cell surface receptors on target cells. Paracrine signaling involves the release of hormone or other signaling molecules by one cell and the receipt of those signals by an adjacent cell type. Autocrine signaling is closely related to paracrine signaling, but the target cell is the same as that releasing the hormone or neurotransmitter. Finally, some cells employ direct communication via gap junctions. This type of direct cellular communication need not involve diffusible molecules.

Classification of Hormones

The hormones described in this chapter fall into several classes. The simplest taxonomy involves the sorting of hormones into steroids (lipid soluble molecules which, for the most part, penetrate cell membranes; vitamin D and thyroid hormone are in this class as well) and into those hormones which exert their effects through receptors on the cell surface. These latter molecules can be derivatives of either amino acids (such as epinephrine) or peptides. Growth factors also act at the cell surface. A general scheme for the action of each of these different types is seen in Fig. 4-2.

Whether the hormone binds to a receptor on the cell exterior or passes through the membrane to bind to an intracellular receptor, the process shall be referred to as signal transduction. This process of signal transduction results in gene regulation, either directly or indirectly (as seen with the steroid class of hormones or with the growth factors, respectively), or regulation of enzymes or ion channels (as seen with the amino acid and peptide hormones). A general classification of hormones is seen in Table 4-1. This is not meant to be an exhaustive list; rather, it is designed to allow the general compartmentalization of mechanisms of hormone signaling.

Note that in each class of hormone described in Table 4-1, only a few examples are given. It is expected that this volume will give ample specifics with regard to each individual hormone or neurotransmitter (including the many not listed here). This chapter will provide the generalities that will allow the reader to appreciate the nuances of each hormone type.

RECEPTORS: THE INITIAL STEP IN HORMONE RESPONSE

Regardless of classification, each of the hormones discussed in this chapter exerts its effect by first binding to a specific receptor. Receptors are proteins (either at the cell surface or intracellular) which bind hormone agonists and begin the process of converting the hormone from extracellular signal to intracellular response. Generally, receptors for hormones are proteins that recognize a particular hormone with great specificity and high affinity. Subsequent to the binding of hormone agonist, these receptors undergo a change of conformation which shifts them into an activated state.

The concept of a hormone or neurotransmitter requiring a receptor in order to exert effects was established at the beginning of the twentieth century. At that time, receptors were conceptual entities. As of this date, the molecular structures of a great many receptors have been identified and the details of their activation are beginning to be understood. Receptors can be defined as macromolecules that exhibit highly selective properties for binding to a neurotransmitter or hormone. The term ligand can refer to any molecule that binds to a receptor, while agonist and antagonist refer to, respectively, molecules that are able to activate a receptor and molecules which bind to a receptor but evoke the inactive confirmation. Some antagonists do evoke a response, and this will be discussed later.

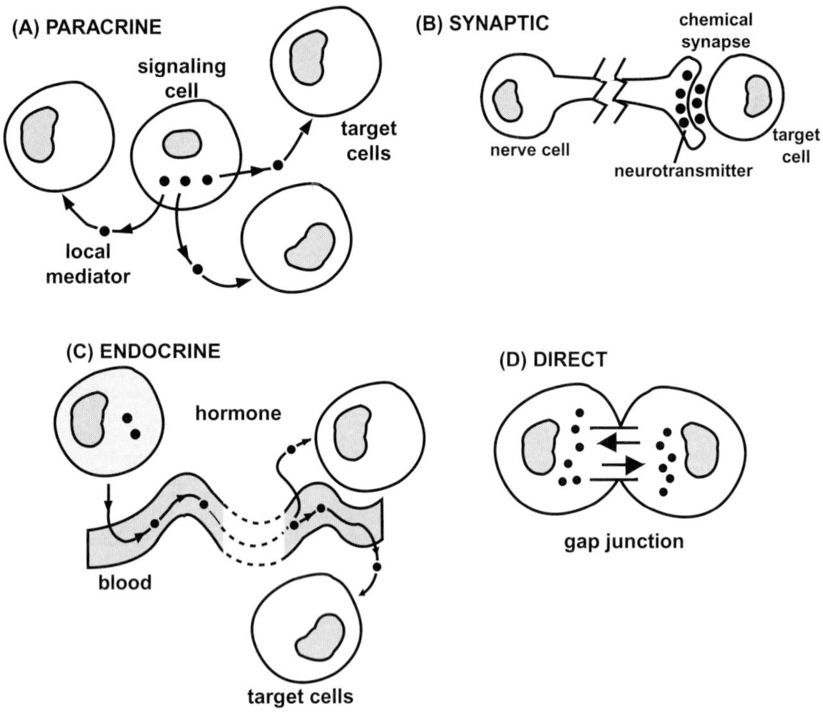

FIGURE 4-1. Forms of cellular communication through signaling molecules. In paracrine signaling (A) a cell releases a signaling molecule which is recognized by local target cells. Synaptic signaling (B) includes a similar release of a signaling molecule to an adjacent cell, but it takes place at a specialized structure known as a synapse. Endocrine signaling (C) includes the release of a signaling molecule into the circulation of an organism. Target cells recognize this signal. Finally, signaling molecules can pass from one cell to another via gap junctions (D). Similar substances may be used in each form of signaling, but the speed of onset and duration of action may differ greatly for each form. (*Modified from Alberts et al.*[313])

Methods for Receptor Analysis

There are two primary ways to study the interaction between a hormone and its receptor. One of these methods involves a biological assay. A classical biological assay utilizes an isolated organ strip, such as the guinea pig ileum, and measures changes in both the frequency and strength of contraction of the intestinal smooth muscle in response to the presence of an agonist (Fig. 4-3). Such a system allows the investigator to coordinate the dose of hormone with the strength of the response.

Radioligand Binding

Another approach to studying receptors is through radioligand binding. Hormones, neurotransmitters, or derivatives thereof have been labeled with a variety of radioactive compounds. Small amounts of membrane (or in the case of intracellular receptors, cell extract) can be assayed for their ability to bind these radioactive drugs. The radioactive compounds can be either agonist or antagonist, and through the use of these compounds, a quantitation of both the number of receptors and the affinity of those receptors for the drug can be determined.

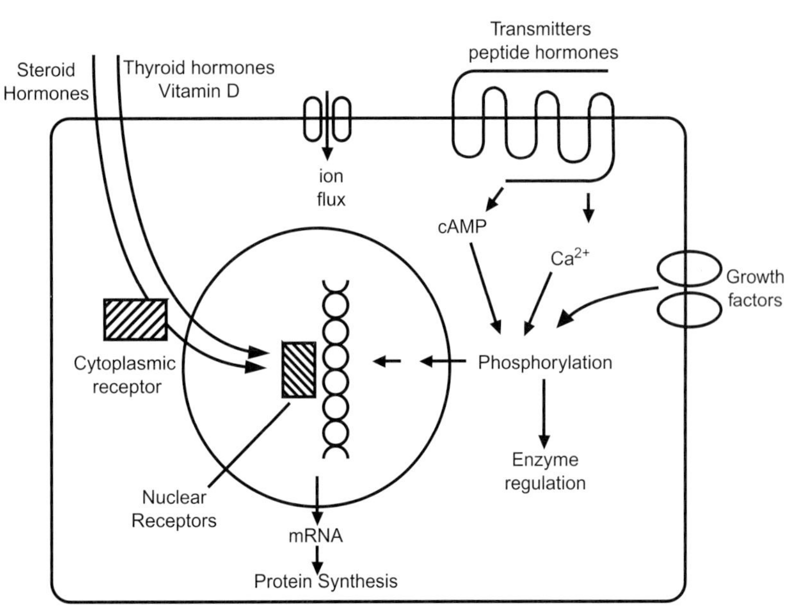

FIGURE 4-2. Mechanisms of signaling by hormones or neurotransmitters. General paradigms of cellular signaling are illustrated. Hormones which activate nuclear receptors express their effects by direct modification of gene transcription. Although the same may hold for molecules which bind to the cell surface, the route to the nucleus may be more circuitous and often involves a series of protein phosphorylations (directly, in the case of growth factors, whose receptors have kinase activity) or second messenger binding proteins. The second messengers include cAMP, cGMP, Ca^{2+}, and IP3. Further, some agents work by directly gating ion conductance through cell-surface receptors. (*Adapted from Catt.*[314])

TABLE 4-1. Hormones and Neurotransmitters—General Types

Compounds with Intracellular Receptors	Compounds Acting through G Protein-Coupled Receptors	Compounds Acting through Receptors That Are Ion Channels	Compounds Acting through Receptors That Have Protein Kinase Activity
Steroids	Peptide hormones (e.g., LH, opiates)	GABA	Insulin
Thyroid hormone	Monoamines and catecholamines	Glutamate	Growth factors (e.g., IGF, EGF, PDGF)
Vitamin D	Acetylcholine	Acetylcholine	Cytokines (e.g., TGFβ)
Retinoic acid	Eicosanoids	Serotonin	

Receptor Quantitation

Regardless of whether a bioassay or a radioligand binding assay is used, receptors can be quantified both in terms of numbers in which they are present and the affinity they show for a given hormone or neurotransmitter. Saturability and specificity can also be determined.

Saturability refers to the property of a receptor to have a limited capacity for saturation by an agonist. Any given membrane system will have a certain amount of nonspecific binding. Nonetheless, nonspecific binding will increase even past the point where specific binding has saturated. This is illustrated in Fig. 4-4A. Receptors show specific binding as well as saturability. For example, a β-adrenergic receptor will bind epinephrine and norepinephrine as well as specific β-agonists such as isoproterenol. Ligand binding is stereospecific as well. In the case of epinephrine and isoproterenol, the l-isomers are active and the d-isomers are inert. Dopamine is also capable of binding to the β-receptor, but at a much higher concentration. Radioligands designed as β-adrenergic antagonists will also bind to the β-adrenergic receptor. Many of these compounds stick to membranes or are sufficiently lipid soluble that they enter the cell. Such compounds do not show saturable binding within the concentrations likely to be used to assay their binding. Depending upon the compound, nonspecific binding of some compounds might even be observed on the glass fiber filters used to trap membrane particles that have bound radioligands.

FIGURE 4-3. Bioassay for determining potency and efficacy of a signaling agent. In this classic assay, a strip of guinea pig ileum is suspended in a chamber with oxygenated Locke's solution and the force, frequency, and duration of contraction are measured by quantifying deflections on a rotating drum. Drugs or other agents are added to the bath and washed out.

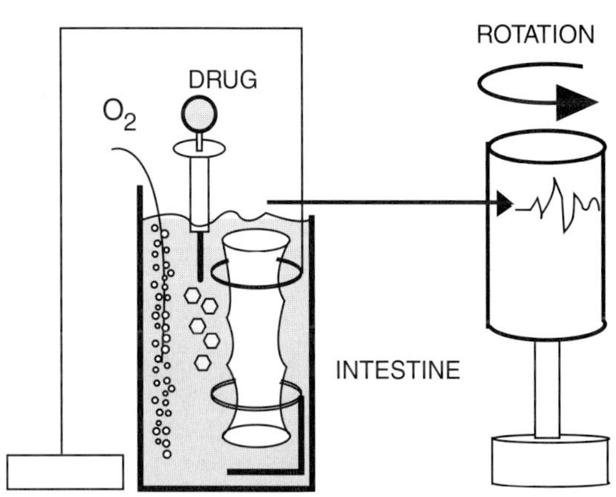

Kinetics of Receptor Binding

In order to perform radioligand binding assays, radioligands are added to plasma membranes or cell homogenates at a known concentration, and the separation of bound from free ligand allows the determination of the amount of receptor present in the reaction. The intrinsic affinity of a receptor for a given ligand can also

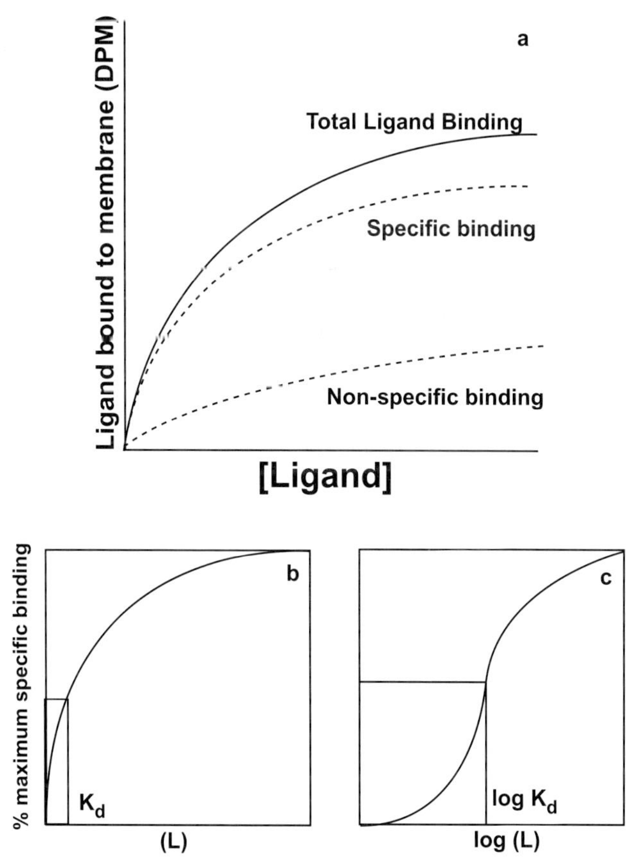

FIGURE 4-4A, B, C. Measurement of receptors using radioligand binding. Membranes (or cells) are incubated with radioactive agonist or antagonist and collected by sedimentation or filtration. Radioactivity in particulate fractions is calculated and plotted as shown. Nonspecific binding refers to that portion of the total binding which persists in the presence of an excess of unlabeled compound. Note that while specific binding is saturable, within the range of the experiment shown, nonspecific binding does not saturate. Plots of specific binding vs. ligand concentration (B) and log [ligand concentration] (C). The approximate Kd is represented by the ligand concentration at 50% saturation of specific binding.

be calculated. Receptor and ligand exist either free or bound to one another, but when saturation-binding studies are performed, the concentration of ligand varies while the concentration of receptor (membrane or homogenate) remains constant. Thus, the equation:

$$L + R \underset{k_2}{\overset{k_1}{<>}} LR \quad \text{and} \quad Kd = \frac{k_2}{k_1} = \frac{[L]\,[R]}{[LR]}$$

where

k_1 = association rate constant
k_2 = dissociation rate constant
[L] = concentration of free ligand
[R] = concentration of free receptor
[LR] = concentration of receptor/ligand complex
Kd = Dissociation equilibrium constant

The total number of receptors [Rt] = [R] + [LR] and

$$[LR] = \frac{[L]\,[Rt]}{[L] + Kd}$$

The term "r" was originally used to define *response* (when using a bioassay such as the guinea pig ileum) but is also used to describe the fraction of occupied receptors. Thus:

$$r = \text{bound ligand/total ligand} = [LR]/[Rt]$$

When measuring the binding of a radioligand to a receptor, the concentration of receptor (amount of membrane) remains constant and the amount of radioligand increases. When r vs. [L] are plotted, a classic saturation plot results (Fig. 4-4B). [L] at 50 percent of the maximal value of r (also termed n, the total number of receptors available for binding ligand) gives a good approximation of the Kd (dissociation equilibrium constant).

Occasionally, receptors may display multiple affinity states (this may not be the case for all ligands at a given receptor). This is studied by plotting the amount of bound ligand vs. the bound/free ligand (Fig. 4-5A). The result is known as a Scatchard analysis and is the most common method to determine receptor affinity or affinities.

Thus, radioligand binding studies are useful both to derive the potency of a drug and determine the maximum number of receptors on the cell surface (Bmax) which are available for binding hormone or neurotransmitter. As described earlier, these parameters can also be determined using a biological assay. Another parameter that can be obtained from biological assays, which is not learned from radioligand binding assays, is that of the efficacy of a various hormone or neurotransmitter. The efficacy refers to the ability of the hormone or neurotransmitter to actually produce a biological effect. In molecular terms, one might measure efficacy as the activation of an enzyme system linked to hormones or neurotransmitters, such as adenylyl cyclase or phospholipase C. In the bioassay described in Fig. 4-3, one might measure efficacy as the ability to increase the rate or extent of contractions versus the amount of a compound as well as the maximum amount of contraction observed in the presence of a given compound.

Some receptors are oligomers that may display cooperative binding of ligand by the subunits. This can be determined with a Hill plot. This is determined by plotting log [E/Emax-E] (where E is the effect produced and Emax is the maximal effect) vs. log [L]. The slope indicates whether cooperative ligand binding exists (Fig. 4-5B). A Hill coefficient (slope of the Hill plot) of unity indicates that binding is noncooperative. When the Hill coefficient is different from one, either positive or negative cooperativity exists in the binding of ligand. Receptors need not be preformed oligomers in order to display cooperative binding. Some receptors, which exist as monomers, might form complexes when binding agonists.[1]

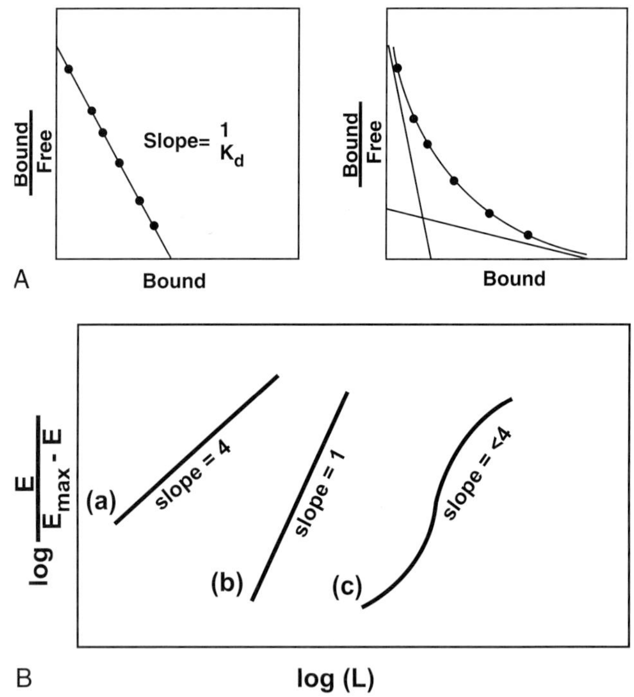

FIGURE 4-5A, B. Mechanisms for determining kinetics of ligand binding. (A) Scatchard analysis of receptor binding. The figure on the left shows a receptor with a single affinity state for the binding of ligand while that on the right shows a 2-site fit. (B) Hill plots for the determination of cooperativity in ligand-receptor binding. Three Hill plots are shown here: (a) suggests four binding sites (possibly a tetramer) because the slope = 4; (b) is representative of a single site and the slope = 1; (c) shows cooperative binding of <4 but more than one site.

"Spare Receptors"

Clark introduced a theory of drug-receptor interactions which was described as "occupation theory".[2] This theory held that the concentration of agonist should be proportional to the response. If this were the case, a plot of the agonist concentration vs. the response would yield results similar to those seen for measuring the saturation of receptor binding (Fig. 4-4). This is not usually the case. Often a maximal biological response is achieved with only a small portion of the total receptors occupied. This observation is consistent with the idea that there exist "spare receptors" (Fig. 4-6). Measures of response to agonist are also often complicated by the fact that some agonists produce a greater efficacy for the same proportion of the receptor population occupied. Agonists which produce a greater effect under such circumstances are termed to have a greater intrinsic activity.

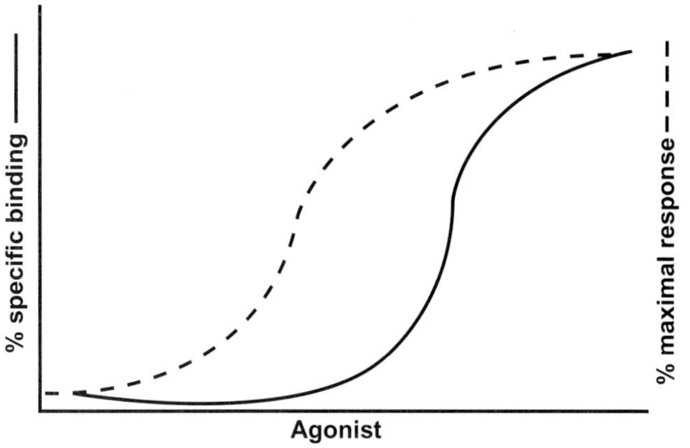

FIGURE 4-6. Effect of "spare receptors." When spare receptors are present the biological response is complete when a fraction of the receptors is occupied by agonist.

Modulation of Receptor Affinity by G Protein

G proteins will be explained in the sections to follow. It is noteworthy that several receptor types are coupled to an intracellular GTP-binding protein (G protein). G protein-coupled receptors show a significant decrease in agonist affinity following the introduction of GTP into the medium. This is demonstrated in Fig. 4-7. It is observed that the ability of isoproterenol, a β-adrenergic agonist, to displace iodocyanopindolol (a radioactive antagonist) is significantly lower in the presence of GTP. It is suggested that the complex between receptor and G protein represents the high-affinity state for agonist binding. The presence of agonist allows the active receptor to induce the G protein to bind GTP (this will be explained more completely in the section on G protein signaling), which then causes the G protein to dissociate from the receptor. This "free-receptor" has a lower affinity for agonist than does the receptor-G protein complex. Note that some antagonists also show the ability to undergo this "GTP shift." As will be noted, some antagonists also modify the conformation of certain other G protein-coupled receptors.

FIGURE 4-7. GTP decreases agonist affinity. In the experiment shown, the β-adrenergic agonist, isoproterenol, is used to displace the labeled β-adrenergic antagonist, ^{125}I-iodocyanopindolol. In the presence of GTP, significantly more isoproterenol is required in order to displace the iodocyanopindolol. This "right shift" of the binding curve indicates that, in the presence of GTP, affinity for agonist by the receptor is decreased.

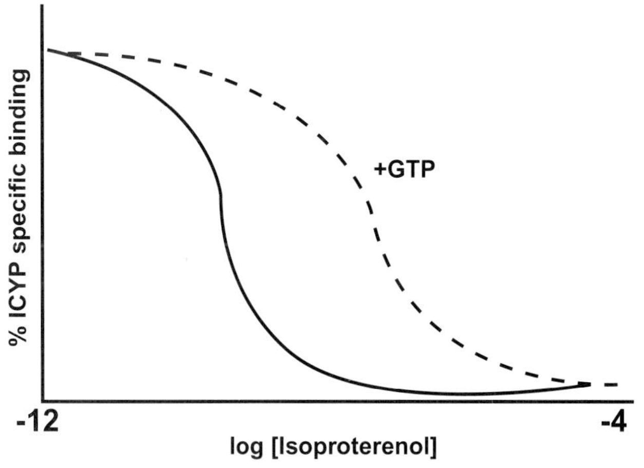

NUCLEAR RECEPTOR SIGNALING

The modern era of the investigation of the mechanism of steroid hormone action and the characterization of steroid hormone receptors began when radioactively labeled estradiol of high specific activity became available.[3] This allowed studies on the binding of the hormone within the range of the circulating levels of hormone (10^{-10}–10^{-8} M). As progestins, glucocorticoids, mineralocorticoids, and androgens of high specific activity became available, their binding was also analyzed. The basic mechanism of action for the five classes of steroid hormones was subsequently shown to be quite similar.

The cloning of the receptors for the various steroid hormones (glucocorticoids, mineralocorticoids, androgens, estrogens, and progestins), retinoic acid, thyroid hormone, and vitamin D has moved the field forward dramatically. It has been found that significant similarities exist in the sequences of all the receptors listed earlier. This has important implications as it suggests that these receptors evolved from a common ancestor. In addition, molecular studies have revealed that a number of other proteins have structural similarity to these receptors but have no known ligand; they are commonly referred to as orphan receptors. This family of steroid hormone, retinoic acid, thyroid hormone, vitamin D, and orphan receptors is often called the steroid hormone receptor superfamily. The known ligands the members of this class bind are depicted in Fig. 4-8.

Mechanism of Action of Steroid Hormones

The preponderance of the evidence indicates that steroids, which are lipophilic, enter cells by passive diffusion (Fig. 4-9). Within a target cell, the steroid binds to its receptor with high affinity. For a cell to be directly responsive to a steroid it must contain the receptor for that receptor. Before the steroid binds to the receptor, the receptor is associated with heat shock proteins (hsp). The receptor-hsp complex has a sedimentation coefficient of around 8S. Under physiological conditions, binding of steroid to the receptor dissociates the hsp. This is revealed by a change in the sedimentation coefficient of the receptor-steroid complex to 4S, which is believed to represent steroid bound to receptor monomers. The dissociation of the hsp and the acquisition of the capability to bind to DNA has been termed activation or transformation. Based upon the analysis of hormone binding in tissue compartments prepared by differential centrifugation of cell homogenates, steroid receptors were described as residing in the cytosol in the absence of steroid and becoming localized in the nucleus only after binding of hormone. Using chemical enucleation[4] and immunocytochemistry[5] it was revealed that the estradiol receptor was located in the nucleus even in the absence of steroid. Subsequently it was demonstrated that the progesterone[6,7] and androgen receptors[8] were also localized in the nucleus even in the absence of steroid. Most evidence indicates, however, that the glucocorticoid receptor is located in the cytosol in the absence of steroid.[9–14] The receptor-steroid complex can then homodimerize and bind to the hormone response element (HRE). A subsequent, yet poorly defined interaction increases (or sometimes decreases) the rate of transcription

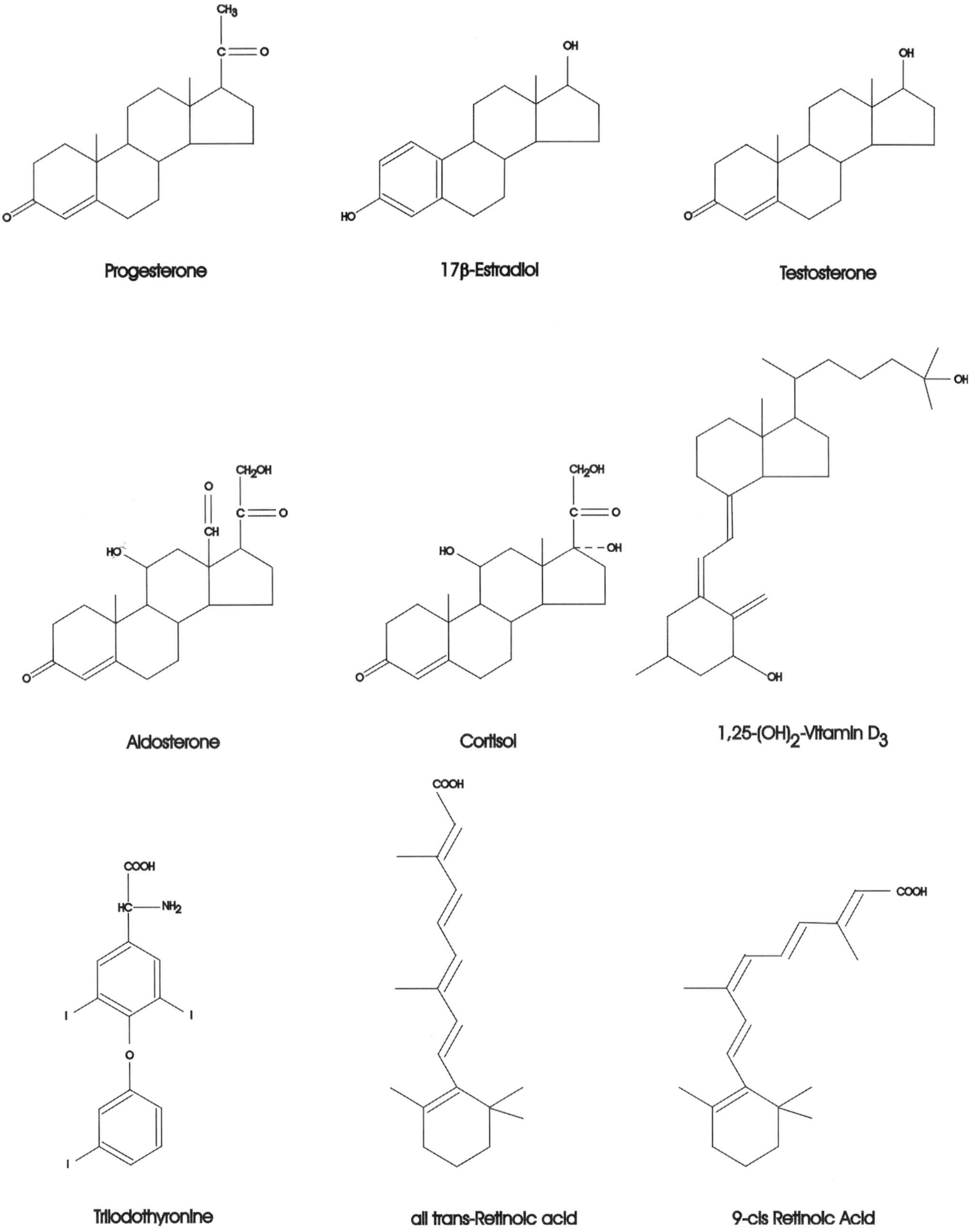

FIGURE 4-8. *See legend on opposite page.*

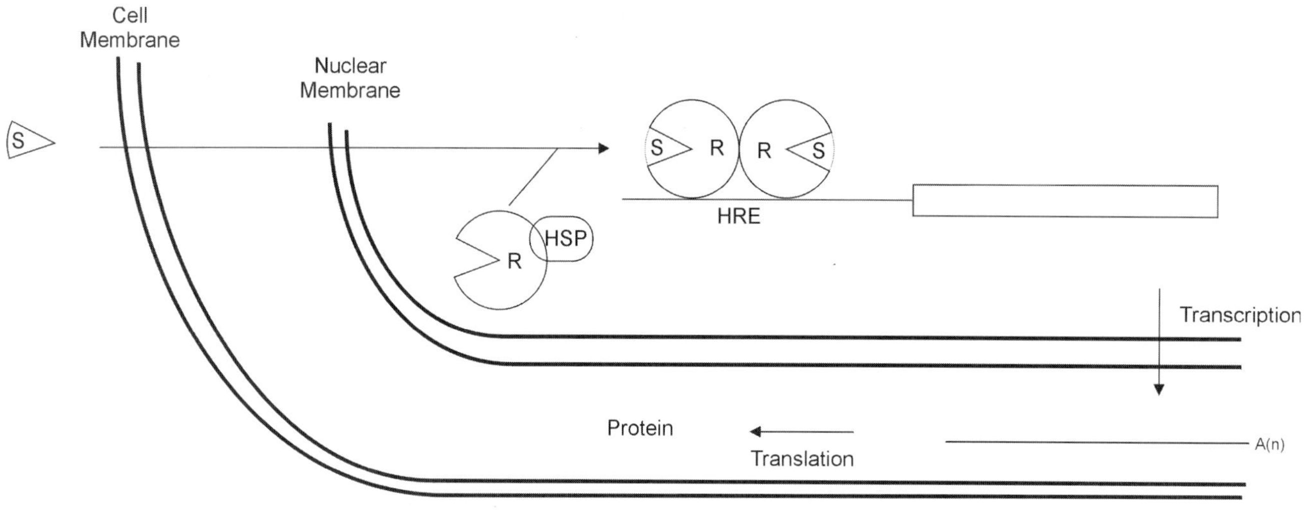

FIGURE 4-9. Mechanism of action of the steroid hormone receptors. In this schematic, the steroid (S) enters the cell by diffusion. Within the nucleus (in most cases) the steroid binds to the receptor (R)-heat shock protein (HSP) complex. Following loss of the hsp the receptor binds to its specific hormone response element (HRE) as a homodimer. This activates the transcription of its target gene. After processing, the mRNA is translated within the cytoplasmic compartment of the cell into protein.

of specific genes. Because the receptor for a given steroid is identical in all target cells yet the steroid may induce different responses in different cell types, it may be that during differentiation specific responsive elements are made accessible while others are occluded in a cell specific fashion.

Mechanism of Action of Retinoic Acid, Vitamin D, and Thyroid Hormones

The mechanism of action of the retinoic acid, vitamin D, and thyroid hormone receptors differs from the steroid hormone receptors in that they do not form complexes with the hsp and they bind to their respective response elements even in the absence of hormone.[15,16] Although homodimers can form, the preferred binding is as heterodimers with retinoid X receptors.

Biochemistry and Molecular Biology of Steroid Receptors

Gene transcripts encoding for receptors for progestins,[17–19] estrogens,[20–24] androgens,[25,26] glucocorticoids,[27–29] mineralocorticoids,[30,31] thyroid hormones,[32,33] all-transretinoic acid,[34–37] 9-cis retinoic acid (RXR),[38,39] and vitamin D[40–42] have all been cloned.

FIGURE 4-8. Structure of the major naturally occurring ligands for the nuclear hormone receptors.

Hormone	Receptor Name (abbreviation)
Progesterone	Progesterone Receptor (PR)
17β-Estradiol	Estrogen Receptor (ER)
Testosterone	Androgen Receptor (AR)
Aldosterone	Mineralocorticoid Receptor (MR)
Cortisol	Glucocorticoid Receptor (GR)
1,25-$(OH)_2$-Vitamin D_3	Vitamin D Receptor (VDR)
Triiodothyronine	Thyroid Hormone Receptor (TR)
all trans-Retinoic acid	Retinoic Acid Receptor (RAR)
9-cis Retinoic acid	Retinoid X Receptor (RXR)

One initial surprise was that these receptors are structurally related (Fig. 4-10).

There appears to be a single gene for the glucocorticoid, mineralocorticoid, androgen, progesterone, and vitamin D receptors. The two progesterone receptor forms (A and B) previously identified in functional studies arise from the use of different translation initiation sites on the same mRNA.[18,43,44] Two genes encode estrogen receptors, α[20,21] and β.[22–24] The β form of the estrogen receptor was found by cloning the product produced from PCR amplification of prostate[23] and testes[24] RNA with degenerate primers (i.e., primers designed to contain the possible nucleotides at various positions which designate the same amino acid) to highly conserved regions found in the previously cloned steroid receptors. On sequencing it was noted that there was a significant homology to the previously identified estrogen receptor and its identity as an estrogen receptor was confirmed by binding studies.

Receptors for Thyroid Hormones

The two genes for the thyroid hormone receptors were originally cloned by screening chick embryo[45] and human placenta[46] libraries with v-erbA and determining what the encoded protein bound. This avian erythroblastosis derived material was chosen because it had significant homology to the glucocorticoid receptor. The thyroid hormone receptor from the chick embryo had a higher homology to v-erbA and was designated TRα and the human placenta form TRβ. Subsequently a second β form was found which was designated TRβ2.[47] This form is derived from the same gene as TRβ1 except that an alternative first exon is used so that the N-terminal region of the protein differs. Two forms of the TRα exist and these are derived from the same gene. In this case they arise from alternative splicing at the 3′ end and thus differ at the C-terminal end of the protein. The TRα2 form does not bind thyroid hormone.[48–51] Another TRα variant, termed rev-erbAα, which also does not bind thyroid hormones arises from the noncoding DNA strand of the TRα gene.[52,53]

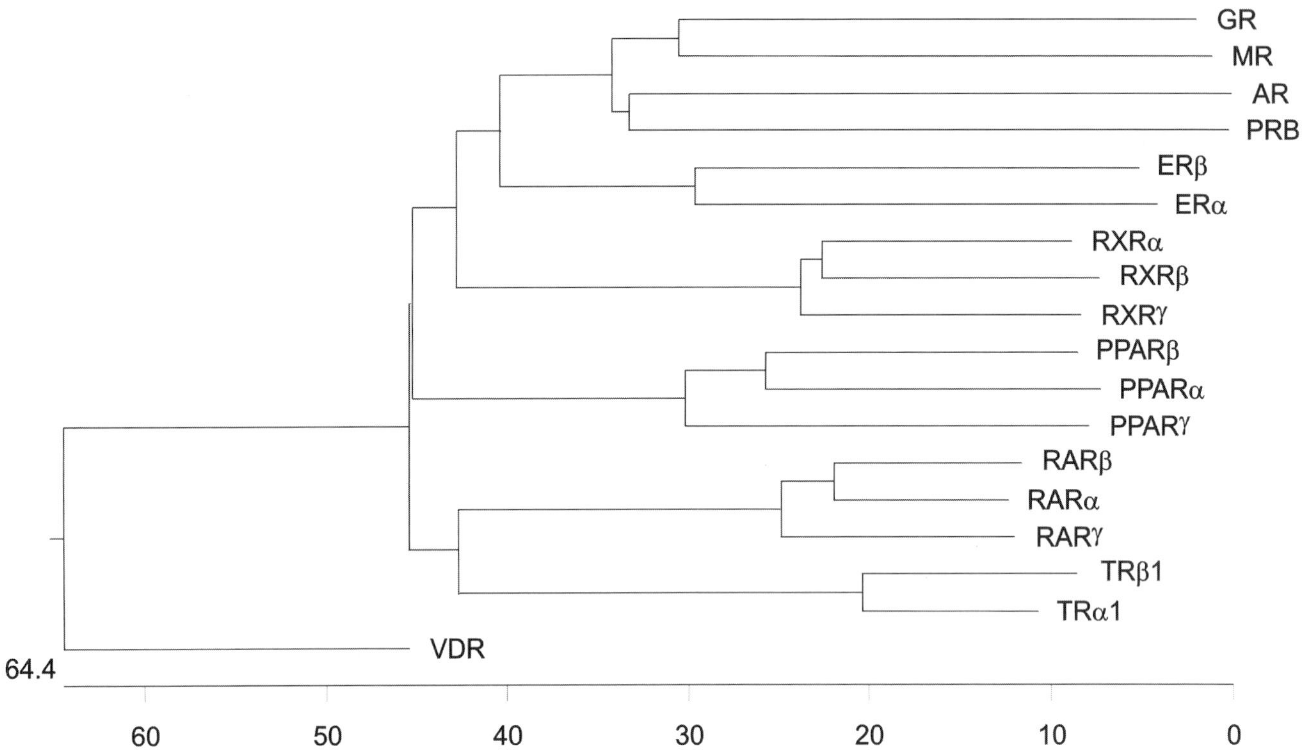

FIGURE 4-10. Evolutionary tree for the human nuclear receptor superfamily. The tree was constructed using Lasergene (DNASTAR, Inc., Madison, WI). The distance between sequence pairs is represented by the length of each pair of branches.

Receptors for Retinoic Acid

The retinoic acid receptors (RAR) were initially cloned by screening libraries with a consensus DNA-binding domain of previously sequenced steroid receptors[35] and a novel sequence which had homology to the DNA-binding domain of steroid hormone receptors.[34] Three forms of RAR (α, β, and γ) which preferentially bind all-trans retinoic acid have been identified.[34–37,54–56] A second group of receptors were subsequently found that also bound retinoids but differed in sequence and binding specificity from the RARs.[38] These are named RXR. Three forms of RXR (α, β, and γ) have been cloned thus far and they preferentially bind 9-cis retinoic acid.[39,57,58]

Orphan Receptors

A number of proteins, termed orphan receptors, have been cloned as a result of low stringency screening of libraries most frequently with the DNA binding domain of the steroid receptors. These orphan receptors have been grouped with the other members of this family because of the high degree of homology of a region to the DNA binding domain of the steroid receptors and the significant homologies of the C-terminus. The nature or identity of the ligands which bind to these orphan receptors is unknown.

Nuclear Receptor Knockout Studies

For a number of nuclear receptors further insight into their role has been obtained by producing mice completely lacking a particular receptor (knockout mice). Knockout mice provide direct testing of the importance of a hormone receptor in the response to that hormone. They have also been used to demonstrate that paracrine factors may be responsible for a particular hormonal response. That is, although a cell type may contain a receptor for a particular hormone, the response observed in this cell type may actually be due to the hormone inducing the production and release of a factor in a second cell type. Under such conditions, the second factor is responsible for inducing responses in the target cell. This type of interaction between cell types has been most extensively studied using ERα knockout (ERKO) mice. Both female[59] and male[60] ERKO mice have been shown to have a complete disruption of reproductive processes. Placing tissue from ERα knockout mice in juxtaposition to tissue from a normal mouse, it has been shown that the mitogenic effect of estradiol on uterine epithelium is mediated through the production of an ERα-stimulated stromal factor.[61] Both stromal and epithelial ERα are required for the estradiol induction of the uterine epithelial secretory proteins lactoferrin and complement component C3.[62] In vaginal tissue both stromal and epithelial ERα are required for estrogen induced cornification, normal stratification, and mucification.[63] These effects occur even in tissues where the ERβ is present. ERβ knockout mice[64] have a reduced ovarian efficiency but normal female and male sexual differentiation, fertility, and lactation.

Progesterone receptor knockout mice have the same abnormalities in reproductive function as those observed after the removal of progesterone.[65] Again, studies have indicated that some of the actions of progesterone are due to the induction of paracrine factors. By placing uterine stromal and epithelial tissue from wild type and progesterone knockout mice together in various combination, it has been shown that the uterine stromal PR is required for progesterone inhibition of estradiol-induced uterine epithelial DNA synthesis. Thus, a paracrine factor is believed to be induced in the stromal cells by progesterone.[66] In mice with a knockout of the mineralocorticoid receptor,[67] Na^+ reabsorption is significantly diminished and the functional activity of the amiloride-sensitive epithelial Na^+ channels is reduced, but there is no decrease in the mRNA for the amiloride-sensitive epithelial Na^+ channel. This suggests that the mineralocorticoid effect on amiloride-sensitive epithelial Na^+ channels is indirect and that other genes on which mineralocorticoids have direct effects bring about this action.

Studies in knockout mice have shown that there are a number of actions mediated by the α and β forms of the thyroid hormone receptor which differ. The TRβ knockout mouse[68] develops a goiter along with elevated levels of TSH. In the anterior pituitary, upregulation of TSH is not affected by the loss of TRβ in hypothyroid animals but there is only a partial suppression of TSH by thyroid hormones.[69] The effect of thyroid hormones on energy expenditure and heart rate are similar in normal and knockout mice, though thyroid hormone effects on some other thyroid hormone responsive processes (e.g., serum cholesterol, serum alkaline phosphatase, and spot 14 and malic enzyme in the liver) were affected.[70] TRα1 knockout mice, unlike TRβ knockout mice, exhibit mild hypothyroidism and a slightly slowed heart rate.[71]

Mice with a knockout of the vitamin D receptor are phenotypically normal at birth and become hypocalcemic at 21 days of age with a concomitant elevation of the parathyroid hormone levels.[72] Normalization of calcium and phosphate by dietary means prevents the development of hyperparathyroidism indicating that this is secondary to the hypocalcemia caused by the loss of vitamin D receptor-stimulated calcium uptake in the intestine.[73]

Structural Organization of Nuclear Receptor Proteins

A number of structural domains have been identified in the members of the nuclear receptor superfamily. The amino terminal region (A/B domain) has a transactivation function. This region varies in size from 24 amino acids in the vitamin D receptor to 603 amino acids in the mineralocorticoid receptor. The next domain (C) is the most highly conserved region among the members of this family. It contains two zinc fingers which encompass the DNA binding domain and dimerization domain. This region is followed by the hinge (D) region. Next comes the E region, the second most conserved region. This region plays important roles in hormone binding, transactivation, dimerization, nuclear localization, and binding to heat shock proteins.

DNA Binding by Nuclear Receptors

The most conserved sequence among the members of the nuclear receptor superfamily is the 66 to 68 amino acids of the DNA-binding domain (Fig. 4-11). This was shown to be the region involved in DNA binding using chimeric receptors constructed by inserting the DNA binding domain for the glucocorticoid receptor for the DNA binding domain of the estrogen receptor. This chimera responds to estradiol by activating a reporter gene through the glucocorticoid responsive element but not the estradiol responsive element.[74,75]

FIGURE 4-11. Alignment of the DNA binding domain of the human nuclear receptor superfamily members. Amino acids which are conserved in all members are shaded.

TRα1	CVVCGDKATGYHYRCITCEGCKGFFRRTIQKNLHPTYSCKYDSCCVIDKITRNQCQLCRFKKCIAVAM
TRβ1	CVVCGDKATGYHYRCITCEGCKGFFRRTIQKNLHPSYSCKYEGKCVIDKVTRNQCQECRFKKCIYVGM
RARα	CFVCQDKSSGYHYGVSACEGCKGFFRRSIQKNM--VYTCHRDKNCIINKVTRNRCQYCRLQKCFEVGM
RARβ	CFVCQDKSSGYHYGVSACEGCKGFFRRSIQKNM--IYTCHRDKNCVINKVTRNRCQYCRLQKCFEVGM
RARγ	CFVCNDKSSGYHYGVSSCEGCKGFFRRSIQKNM--VYTCHRDKNCIINKVTRNRCQYCRLQKCFEVGM
RXRα	CAICGDRSSGKHYGVYSCEGCKGFFKRTVRKDL--TYTCRDNKDCLIDKRQRNRCQYCRYQKCLAMGM
RXRβ	CAICGDRSSGKHYGVYSCEGCKGFFKRTIRKDL--TYSCRDNKDCTVDKRQRNRCQYCRYQKCLATGM
RXRγ	CAICGDRSSGKHYGVYSCEGCKGFFKRTIRKDL--IYTCRDNKDCLIDKRQRNRCQYCRYQKCLVMGM
VDR	CGVCGDRATGFHFNAMTCEGCKGFFRRSMKRKA--LFTCPFNGDCRITKDNRRHCQACRLKRCVDIGM
PPARα	CRICGDKASGYHYGVHACEGCKGFFRRTIRLKL-VYDKC--DRSCKIQKKNRNKCQYCRFHKCLSVGM
PPARβ	CRVCGDKASGFHYGVHACEGCKGFFRRTIRMKL-EYEKC--ERSCKIQKKNRNKCQYCRFQKCLALGM
PPARγ	CRVCGDKASGFHYGVHACEGCKGFFRRTIRLKL-IYDRC--DLNCRIHKKSRNKCQYCRFQKCLAVGM
PRB	CLICGDEASGCHYGVLTCGSCKVFFKRAMEGQH--NYLCAGRNDCIVDKIRRKNCPACRLRKCCQAGM
AR	CLICGDEASGCHYGALTCGSCKVFFKRAAEGKQ--KYLCASRNDCTIDKFRRKNCPSCRLRKCYEAGM
GR	CLVCSDEASGCHYGVLTCGSCKVFFKRAVEGQH--NYLCAGRNDCIIDKIRRKNCPACRYRKCLQAGM
MR	CLVCGDEASGCHYGVVTCGSCKVFFKRAVEGQH--NYLCAGRNDCIIDKIRRKNCPACRLQKCLQAGM
ERα	CAVCNDYASGYHYGVWSCEGCKAFFKRSIQGHN--DYMCPATNQCTIDKNRRKSCQACRLRKCYEVGM
ERβ	CAVCSDYASGYHYGVWSCEGCKAFFKRSIQGHN--DYICPATNQCTIDKNRRKSCQACRLRKCYEVGM

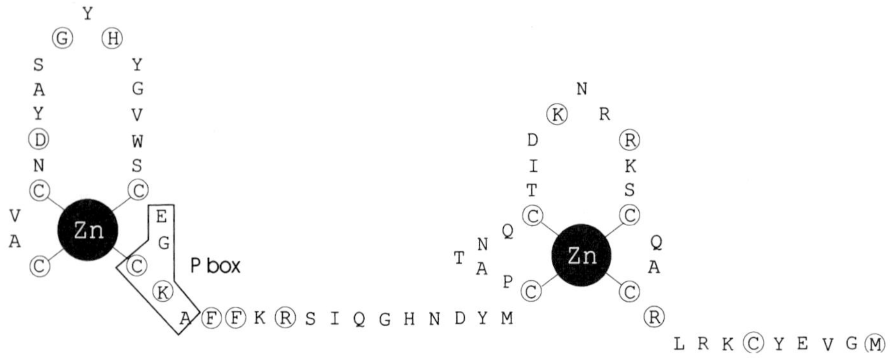

FIGURE 4-12. Structure of the DNA binding domain of the human estrogen receptor. The human estrogen receptor is shown to illustrate the coordination of the Zn^{2+} between the cysteines and the location of the P box (outlined). Amino acids conserved in all members (as shown in Fig. 4-11) are circled.

This region forms two zinc fingers with zinc ions coordinately bound by four cysteine residues (Fig. 4-12). The three-dimensional structure of the glucocorticoid[76] and estrogen[77] receptor DNA binding domains are quite similar. The importance of the first zinc finger in DNA-binding was shown by mutating different amino acids within each of the zinc fingers.[78–81] Indeed, it is a string of 5 amino acids, termed the P-box, which dictates the response element to which the receptor binds. Structural analysis with magnetic resonance imaging and X-ray crystallography[76,82–84] support the data from mutation studies, suggesting that the proximal zinc finger is the DNA-binding domain. Deletion studies have also revealed that an activation domain is in the DNA-binding region of the glucocorticoid receptors.[85] The second zinc finger appears to be involved in dimerization.[76,82–84]

Nuclear receptors bind to specific sequences (hormone response elements—HRE) which are most frequently located 5′ from the transcription start site of the target gene (Fig. 4-13). The steroid response elements have been defined primarily by deletion of the suspected element, insertion of the suspected element with a reporter gene, footprinting, and gel mobility shift assays. The first steroid response element to be defined was that for the glucocorticoid receptor in the mouse mammary tumor virus long terminal repeat[86,87] and chick lysozyme gene.[88] Subsequent analysis of other glucocorticoid response elements[89–91] allowed the definition of a consensus sequence. The same sequence was subsequently shown to be the response element for the progesterone[92,93] mineralocorticoid,[30] and androgen[94,95] receptors. The estrogen response element is also a palindrome (a replication of the nucleotide sequence, but in inverted or reverse order) with a 3-base spacer between the two half elements for both the α[96] and β[97] forms. Recently it has also been shown that the ERα and β can bind as heterodimers as well as homodimers.[97,98] Thus, for each of the steroid hormone receptors, the hormone response element consists of two 6-base pair sequences arranged as a palindrome with a 3-base pair spacer. The presence of two half sites is consistent with the binding of homodimers to the response element.

FIGURE 4-13. The response elements of the members of the nuclear receptor superfamily and their P box. For the thyroid hormone receptor the response element may be a palindrome (1), a direct repeat separated by any three nucleotides (2), or an inverse palindrome separated by any six nucleotides (3). The amino acids of the P-box are important for DNA binding.

Receptor	Response Element	P-box
GR PR AR MR	GGTACA NNN TGTTCT	GSckV
ER	AGGTCA NNN TGACCT	EGckA
TR	AGGTCA TGACCT (1) AGGTCA NNN AGGTCA (2) TGACCT NNNNNN AGGTCA (3)	EGckG
VDR	AGGTCA NNN AGGTCA	EGckG
RAR	AGGTCA NNNNN AGGTCA	EGckG

The thyroid hormone, retinoic acid, and vitamin D receptors can bind to response elements that are identical to the estrogen response element except that the two half sites are adjacent (AGGTCA TGACCT).[99,100] In addition, the same sequence as the half site (AGGTCA) in a direct repeat with spacing of 3, 4, or 5 nucleotides can serve as the response element for the vitamin D, thyroid hormone, and retinoic acid receptors, respectively.[99,100] Finally, thyroid hormone response elements have been shown to be formed by inverted palindromes with a predominant spacer of 6 nucleotides (TGACCT nnnnnn AGGTCA).[101]

The peroxisone proliferator-activated receptor (PPAR), RAR, vitamin D, and thyroid hormone receptors can also heterodimerize with RXR and bind to the same response elements as the homodimers.[102–108] The binding of thyroid hormone to the receptor homodimer decreases its affinity for the response element while not affecting binding of the heterodimer.[109] In general, the heterodimer of the various receptors with an RXR is favored over the homodimer form. The original observations that the RXR partner of the heterodimer complex binds to the upstream half site[110,111] have been confirmed for the RXR-thyroid hormone receptor heterodimer by X-ray crystallography.[84]

Hormone Binding Domains for Steroids, Retinoids, Thyroid Hormone, and Vitamin D

X-ray crystallography has revealed that the hormone-binding domain for ERα,[112] TRα,[113] RXR,[114] and RAR[115] have a similar overall architecture. The ligand-binding domain contains a number of antiparallel alpha-helices separated by short beta strands. The hydrophobic ligand-binding pocket is formed from a number of the alpha helices. In the ERα and thyroid hormone receptors the ligand is completely buried in the interior of the receptor. This implies that in the unliganded state the receptor must exist in a more open conformation which changes on binding of the ligand. This apparently occurs via the occlusion of the ligand binding domain once hormone is bound by the repositioning of alpha helix 12. In the autosomal dominant syndrome "resistance to thyroid hormone," where mutant TRβ receptors show diminished thyroid hormone binding, the mutations are clustered in regions important for direct contact between the receptor and the hormone[116,117] or for the stabilization of the bound conformation.[113]

A second region important for dimerization has been shown to reside in the hormone binding domain. Crystallographic analysis of the ligand binding domain of the TR α[113] receptor has demonstrated that the residues believed to be important for dimerization are found on the surface of helix 11. The crystallographic studies of the potential heterodimeric partner RXRα[114] show that its heterodimerization surface is contained within helices 8, 9, and 10. The steroid receptors bind to their response elements as homodimers. The crystallographic analysis of the ligand binding domain of the estrogen receptor has indicated that the residues important for the homodimerization are located on helices 8 and 11.[112] The helices 11 of two estrogen receptors intertwine while helix 8 from one molecule interacts with helices 9 and 10 of its partner.

Intracellular Localization of Nuclear Receptors

Two nuclear localization signals have been localized in the glucocorticoid receptor.[118] The steroid hormone dependent nuclear localization signal sequence is found within the steroid-binding domain. The constitutive nuclear localization signal is located at the C-terminal end of the DNA binding domain. The nuclear localization signal for the progesterone receptor is about 61 amino acids in length spanning the hinge region and second zinc finger. There is a C-terminal signal that is constitutively active and an N-terminal (second zinc finger) region that is active when the hormone is bound.[119,120]

Mechanism of Gene Regulation by Nuclear Receptors

mRNA is produced by RNA polymerase II. In order for RNA polymerase II to initiate transcription, multiple initiation complex proteins must be assembled at the TATA box. The first step in the formation of the initiation complex is the binding of transcription factor IID (TFIID). This is composed of TATA-binding protein (TBP) and more than 10 other TBP-associated factors (TAFs). TFIIB then binds to TFIID. It serves as a bridge between TBP and RNA polymerase II. The preinitiation complex is completed by the addition of TFIIA to TFIIJ.[121,122]

The estrogen,[123] progesterone,[123] thyroid hormone α[124] and β,[125] and vitamin D[126] receptors have all been shown to be capable of interacting with TFIIB. The region of the receptor reported to be important for this interaction is not the same for each receptor. Thus one possibility for gene activation by the members of this family is that they directly modulate the activity of the initiation complex.

A second possibility is that hormone binding to its receptor causes the binding of coactivators to the receptor. The coactivator, in some cases, seems capable of acetylating histones or connecting the receptor to the preinitiation complex. Acetylation of conserved lysine residues in the N-terminal domain of histones could cause the loosening of the nucleosome structure, making the DNA accessible to transcription factors.[127–129] Steroid receptor coactivator-1[130] (SRC-1) and its homologs, transcription intermediary factor 2 (TIF2)[131] which is the human homolog of glucocorticoid receptor interacting protein 1 (GRIP1),[132] receptor-associated coactivator 3 (RAC3)[133] which is identical to ACTR,[134] amplified in breast cancer 1 (AIB1),[135] p300/CBP cointegrator associated protein (p/CIP),[136] thyroid receptor activator molecule 1 (TRAM 1),[137] and cAMP response element binding protein (CREB) binding protein (CBP)[138] (and its homolog p300)[139] can serve as coactivators of the steroid receptors. They appear to be ubiquitously expressed. SRC-1,[140] RAC3,[134] and CBP[141,142] appear to be able to acetylate histones. There is also an androgen receptor-associated protein 70 (ARA70) which enhances the activity of the androgen receptor to a much greater extent than other steroid receptors.[143] There may be redundancy in the system because it was found that mice in which the SRC-1 gene was knocked out were still fertile but certain steroid target organs in both males and females exhibited a decreased growth in response to steroid hormones.[144]

One major difference between the thyroid hormone receptor and those for the steroid hormones is that in the absence of hormone the receptor can either act as a gene repressor,[145–147] for those genes upregulated by thyroid hormones, or as a gene activator,[148–150] for those genes downregulated by thyroid hormones. Two corepressor proteins have been identified, nuclear receptor corepressor (NCoR)[151,152] or retinoid X receptor (RXR)-interacting protein 13 (RIP13),[153] and silencing mediator for retinoid and thyroid hormone receptors (SMRT)[154] or T3 receptor-associating cofactor (TRAC).[155] Mutational studies have revealed that the binding of the corepressors occurs in the hinge regions between the DNA binding domain and the hormone-binding domain and the first helix of the hormone binding domain[151] The corepressor dissociates from the thyroid hormone receptor upon binding of hormone allowing coactivators to bind. The coactivator binding site is within the hormone binding domain.[156] It has been proposed that the corepressor binds to proteins with deacetylase activity (Sin3 and histone deacetylases)[157–159] which lowers the transcription rate for those genes positively regulated by thyroid hormones. On binding of hormone, the recruited coactivators cause an increase in histone acetylation which is hypothesized to make the gene more susceptible to transcription.

Ligand Independent Activation of Nuclear Receptors

Dopamine has been shown to have the capacity to activate progesterone and estrogen receptors but not glucocorticoid and mineralocorticoid receptors.[160] Dopamine appears to work through the dopaminergic D1 receptor but the second messenger system through which the activation of the steroid receptor occurs is unresolved.

8-Br-cAMP and okadaic acid, agents which activate intracellular phosphorylation by cAMP and Ca^{2+}/calmodulin dependent protein kinases, activate the progesterone receptor in the absence of ligand.[161] The growth factors IGF-1, EGR, and TGFα[162–164] have also been found to activate the estrogen receptor.

Modification of Nuclear Receptor Activity by Phosphorylation

The androgen,[165] estrogen,[166,167] glucocorticoid,[168] and vitamin D[169] receptors can undergo phosphorylation. Various studies have shown that serine and tyrosine residues can be phosphorylated by any of a number of serine and tyrosine kinases, respectively. However, the importance of the phosphorylation in the physiological function of the steroid receptors is not clear. Phosphorylation of the progesterone receptor is not required for hormone or DNA binding[170,171] but it may enhance the process.[172,173]

Chaperone Proteins

Hsp90 is the predominant heat shock protein associated with the steroid receptors, but hsp70 and 56 have also been found. Initially it was shown in the glucocorticoid receptor that the primary domain involved in the interaction of the receptor with the heat shock proteins was the steroid-binding domain.[174,175] Deletion of this region results in a receptor capable of weakly activating transcription without the steroid.[28,85,176–178] The dissociation of the hsp from the receptor in the presence of high salt activates the receptors DNA-binding activity.[179]

SIGNALING THROUGH G PROTEIN-COUPLED RECEPTORS

The discovery of G protein-mediated signal transduction can be traced to studies of Sutherland and Rall in the late 1950s.[180,181] Those studies demonstrated that epinephrine and glucagon were able to induce the production of a heat-stable intermediary com-

FIGURE 4-14. Production of cAMP from ATP by adenylyl cyclase and the subsequent hydrolysis of cAMP to 5′AMP by cAMP phosphodiesterase. (*Adapted from Alberts et al.*[313])

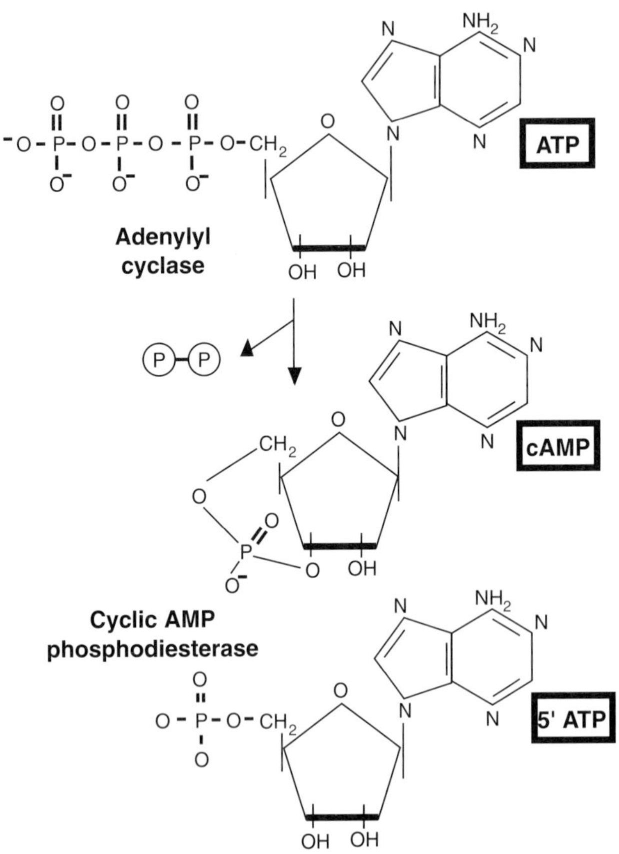

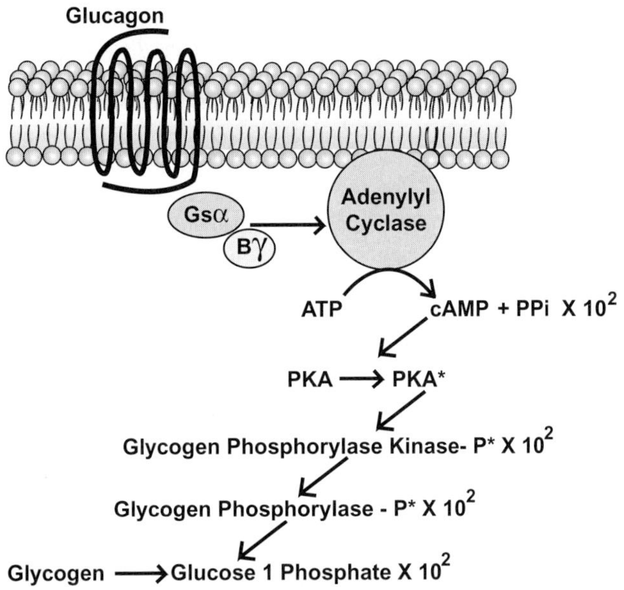

FIGURE 4-15. Amplification of hormone signals in a kinase cascade. In the illustrated case, one molecule of glucagon results in the production of 10^8 molecules of glucose-1-phosphate.

pound which caused the activation of glycogen phosphorylase. Later studies demonstrated that the intermediate was 3′5′ cyclic adenosine monophosphate (cyclic AMP or cAMP) and this compound activated a cAMP-dependent protein kinase (glycogen phosphorylase kinase kinase, now known as Protein Kinase A). It was demonstrated that epinephrine or glucagon could activate a membrane bound enzyme, adenylyl cyclase, which produced cAMP from ATP (Fig. 4-14). The resultant cascade of kinase activation allowed tremendous (10^8-fold) amplification of the initial hormone signal (Fig. 4-15).

The enzyme responsible for the conversion of ATP to cAMP is adenylyl cyclase and at this writing, nine members of the adenylyl cyclase family have been identified. Initial studies suggested that agonist increased adenylyl cyclase activity and that the activity of the enzyme in broken cell preparations was enhanced by NaF. Sutherland and Rall conceived of receptor/adenylyl cyclase as a single molecule and this notion persisted until the late 1960s.

The initial discovery of a G protein was made in the laboratory of Rodbell.[182] Adenylyl cyclase has a Km for ATP of about 250 μM. As a result, the enzyme was normally assayed in the presence of 1 mM ATP. This masked any role for GTP, as commercial preparations of ATP had sufficient GTP to satisfy requirement for this nucleotide. Pure preparations of ATP were incapable of supporting enzyme activity in the absence of GTP, suggesting that ATP served as a substrate for adenylyl cyclase, while GTP was a necessary cofactor. This eventually gave rise to the idea that some GTP-binding element was important for activation of the adenylyl cyclase enzyme. This intermediate element in signaling pathways has been expanded into the idea of the G protein and the widespread application of these proteins to the biology of hormone response.

The initial element of the G protein-signaling cascade is the receptor, and the $\beta 1$ adrenergic receptor is prototypic. This receptor was the first to be identified by molecular cloning[183] (it had

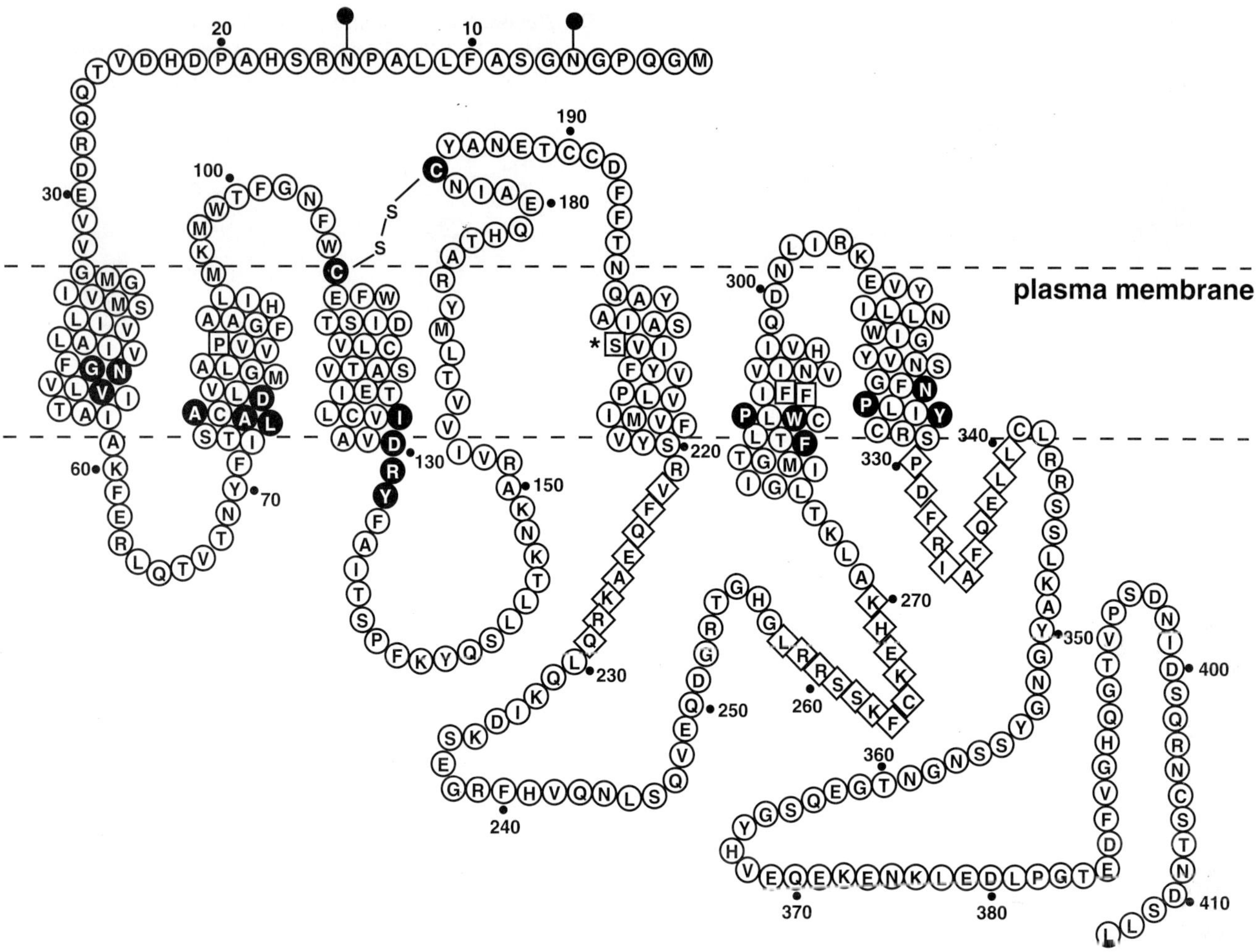

FIGURE 4-16. Model of a "classic" G protein-coupled receptor. The β_1 adrenergic receptor is shown. Highly conserved residues (among all G protein-coupled receptors) are shown in black. Boxed residues are conserved in catecholamine receptors and the serine marked with * is conserved in all G protein-coupled serotonin receptors. Diamond residues are involved in G protein coupling. (*Modified from Probst et al.*[315])

been purified by affinity chromatography and the amino acid sequence identified[184]). This receptor was the product of an intronless gene, which simplified the process of identification.

Once that identification was made, the suggested structure revealed a molecule with the amino terminus exposed to the extracellular space and the carboxy terminus in the cytosol. Seven α helical domains were identified and the receptor was thought to span the membrane seven times (a heptaspan receptor). A model is shown in Fig. 4-16.

Soon after the identification of the $\beta 1$ adrenergic receptor, a torrent of receptor cloning followed. Several different cloning strategies were employed, but most were based on the similarity seen in the amino acid sequences of the seven transmembrane segments, which were quite well conserved. It appeared that the heptaspan model provided a consistent paradigm for receptors coupled to G proteins (in excess of 1000 receptors at this point), but it was possible to demonstrate differences in the receptor structure based upon the class of ligand to which the receptor would bind. Figure 4-17 shows these classes of ligand and suggests structural paradigms for the different receptor types. Note that in addition to G protein-coupled receptors for a variety of "traditional" small molecules or peptide agonists, a class of receptors exists for odorants. This receptor family (consisting of well over 100 members) binds to molecules of odorant or pheromone. Receptors for pheromone, isolated from the vomeronasal organ of the rat, are similar to pheromone receptors which are present on the cell surface of brewer's yeast.[185] Thus, it appears that the general structure and mechanism of G protein activation has been highly conserved through eukaryote evolution.[186,187]

Structure of G Protein-Coupled Receptors

All G protein coupled receptors have a similar structure which includes 7 transmembrane domains, an extracellular amino terminus, an intracellular carboxyl terminal, 3 extracellular loops, and 3 cytosolic loops (Fig. 4-16). While each of the 7 transmembrane domains are composed of somewhere between 20 and 27 amino acids, the end terminal segments as well as either the extracellular or cytoplasmic loops can vary greatly among the different receptor types.

Rhodopsin, the visual pigment, is also a 7-transmembrane receptor linked to a G protein. Many of the paradigms used to

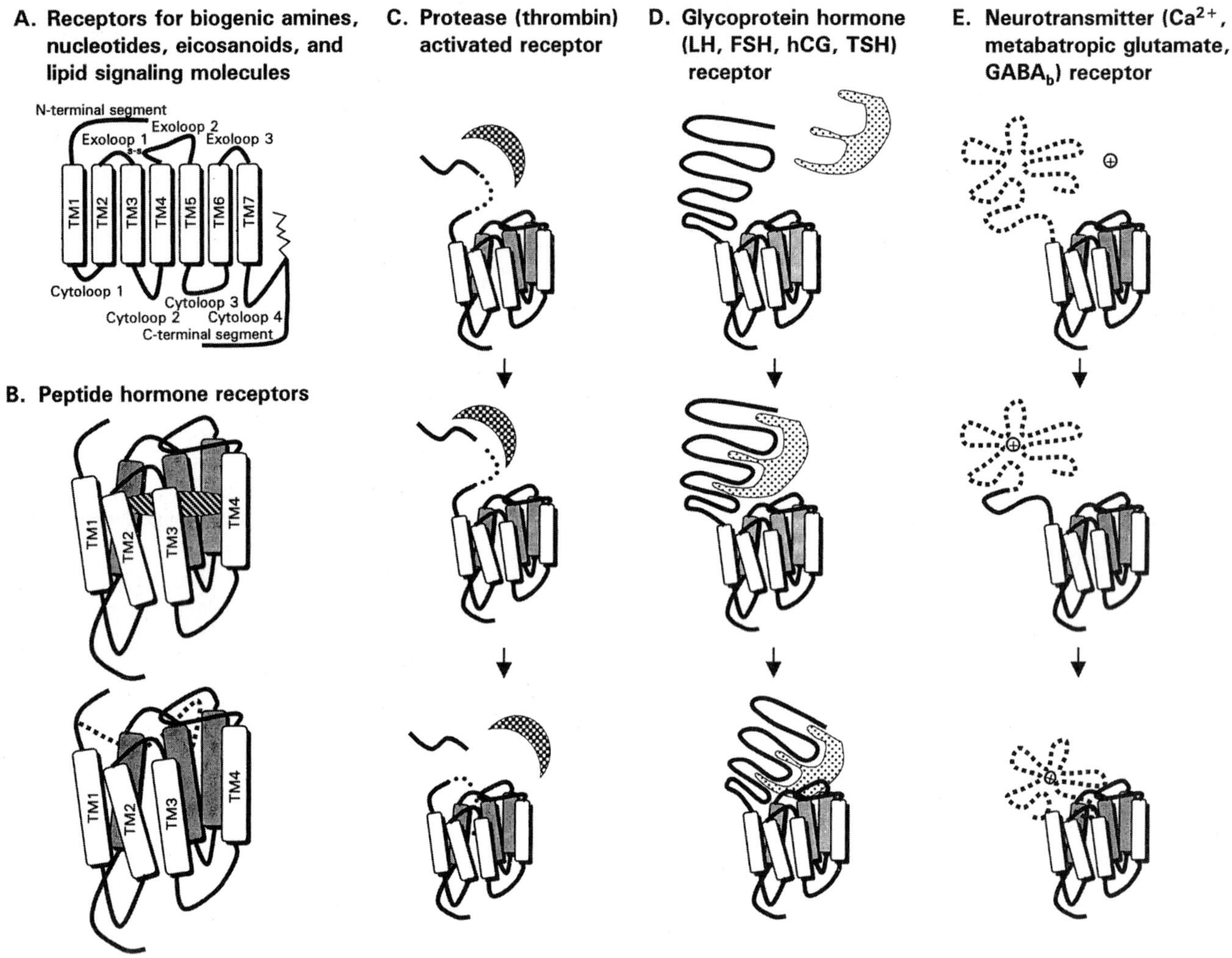

FIGURE 4-17. Different classes of G protein-coupled receptors. The figure shows the classes of ligand and suggests structural paradigms for the different receptor types. Details are given in the text. (*Modified from Ji, Grossman, Ji.*[191])

make predictions about how G protein-coupled receptors work are derived from structural studies of both rhodopsin and bacteriorhodopsin.[188,189] Although clearly both rhodopsin and bacteriorhodopsin serve functions far different from many of the other G protein-coupled receptors, the basic structural motifs dictated by studies of rhodopsin and bacteriorhodopsin are quite similar to those of the many families of G protein-coupled receptors discussed later.

The high resolution 3-dimensional structural studies of bacteriorhodopsin suggest that the transmembrane core has polar residues and perhaps has a hydrophilic rather than a hydrophobic pocket, as was originally thought.[190] Despite this, it is unlikely that the core that is formed is large enough for water or any other molecule to pass through.

Although G protein-coupled receptors show remarkable similarity, they can be classified according to the agonists which activate them. Figure 4-17 shows a division of receptors into basic structural groups and the binding of ligands will be discussed by divisions of those groups.[191]

Receptors for Biogenic Amines and Acetylcholine

Receptors for small molecule neurotransmitters are most similar to rhodopsin. These small molecule neurotransmitters bind within the transmembrane core of the G protein-coupled receptor.[192,193] Models of the receptors suggest that these small molecules form an extremely tight fit within the pocket created by the 7 transmembrane segments, and this type of tight fit could lead to the extraordinary specificity with which these receptors bind agonists. Purine nucleotides such as adenosine and ATP or ecosanoids, such as prostaglandins, prostacyclins, and thromboxanes bind in a similar manner to the biogenic amines and actylcholine.[194]

Receptors for Peptide Hormones

Peptides such as chemotactic peptide (f-met-leu-phe) and hypothalamic peptides such as corticotropin releasing hormone or growth hormone releasing hormone, angiotensin, and opioid peptides, bind to the G protein-coupled receptor in a manner somewhat different from the small molecules discussed previously. These molecules are too large to fit into the receptor core and, consequently, extracellular loops are critical for their binding. Occasionally a single amino acid from these peptide hormones fits into the core.[195,196]

Receptors for Protein Hormones

Receptors for slightly larger peptide hormones such as glucagon, vasoactive intestinal peptide, and parathyroid hormone have longer amino terminal regions which also appear to be important in ligand agonist recognition. The hormone molecules appear to bind directly to the amino terminals.[197,198]

Thrombin Receptors

Thrombin has protease activity, and this protease activity is crucial for the recognition of thrombin by its receptor. Thrombin recognizes a sequence in the amino terminal segment of the thrombin receptor and cleaves it at a precise sequence. The intact amino terminal has 74 amino acids and the cleavage results in a 33-amino acid end terminal segment, which acts as a tether ligand and binds to various groups on the segment on the cell surface in a manner similar to that seen with the peptide hormone receptors.[199,200]

Receptors for Glycoprotein Hormones

Glycoprotein hormones have another unique receptor form. The glycoproteins LH, FSH, HCG, and TSH all bind to a G protein-coupled receptor with a very long amino terminal. These amino terminals can be as long as 350 to 700 amino acids. This large amino terminal is capable of high affinity binding of the various glycoprotein hormones. It is noteworthy however, that the extracellular loops of the receptor are important to modulate the binding. In fact, it is likely that the actual signal of agonist binding is carried out by the extracellular loops of the receptor rather than by the agonist-bound amino terminal.[201]

Receptors for Calcium, Glutamate, and GABA

Metabatropic glutamate receptors, the $GABA_b$ receptor, and the calcium receptor all have an extremely long extracellular polypeptide chain (about 600 amino acids) at the amino terminal.[202] Whereas, for most of the G protein-coupled receptors, there is some rough correlation between agonist size and amino terminal length, the smallest agonist, calcium, has one of the largest amino terminals associated with its receptor. Much of the signal recognition specificity appears to be housed in the amino terminal as well.[203] The amino terminal then may contact with the extracellular loops to elicit receptor activation.

Ligand Binding by G Protein-Coupled Receptors

The formation of a complex between a receptor and agonist represents the initial step in the signal transduction process. Initially, this process was studied using a physiologic readout as a measure of the potency and efficacy of a given agonist. The contraction of intestinal smooth muscle, suspended in a bath, was a measure of norepinephrine effects (through an $\alpha 1$ adrenergic receptor). Subsequent studies with radioligands allowed a somewhat greater understanding of the nature of agonist occupancy of receptors. More recently, the ability to mutate single amino acid residues of a variety of receptors has fostered a significant understanding of the molecular determinants of receptor activation.[192]

Changes in Receptor Conformation upon Agonist Activation

Changes in molecular structure follow the activation of G protein-coupled receptors. Figure 4-18 shows a variety of mutations of different G protein-coupled receptors which have been shown to activate G proteins in the absence of agonist.[204] The importance

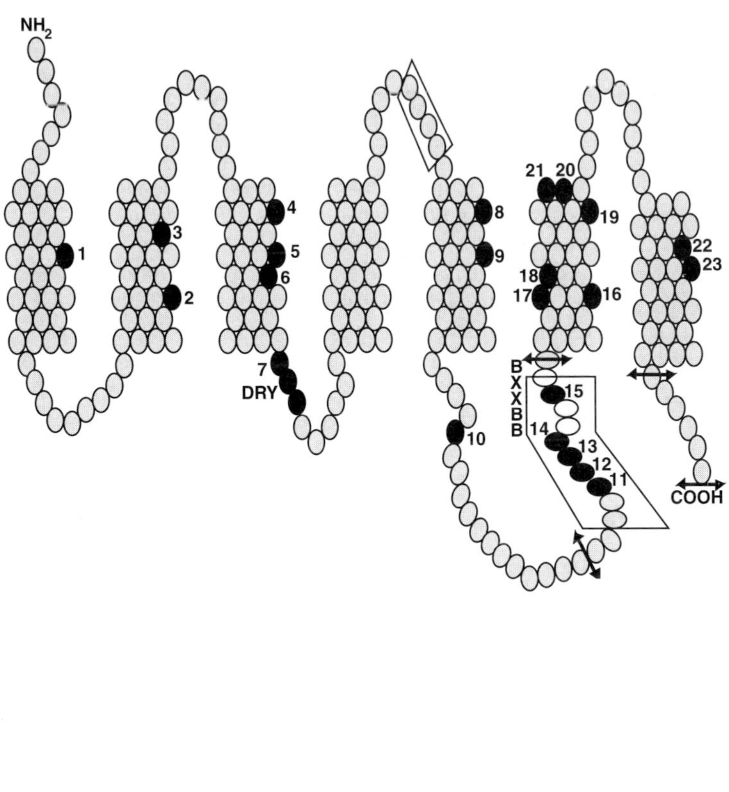

FIGURE 4-18. Mutated G-protein coupled receptors (GPCR) that yield constitutive activation. A schematic representation of a G protein-coupled receptor is shown with 7 transmembrane segments and connecting loops of arbitrary length. The numbers indicate the position of specific mutations in the following receptors, α_{1B}-adrenergic: **1** Asn63Ala; **5** Cys128Phe; **7** Asp142all amino acids (AA); **8** Ala204Val; **12** Arg2888Lys; **14** Lys290His; **15** Ala293allAA. α_{2A}-adrenergic: **15** Thr373Phe,Ala,Cys,Glu,Lys. 5-HT_{2A}: **15** Cys322 Lys,Ala,Glu. Yeast mating-pheromone α-factor: **10** Leu194Gln; **16** Pro258Leu; **17** Ser259Leu. Platelet-activating factor: **6** Asn100Ala; **11** Leu231Arg. Muscarinic m_1; **13** Glu360Ala. Rhodopsin: **2** Gly90Asp; **4** Glu113Gln; **7** Asp134Asn; **22** Ala292Glu; **23** Lys296Glu,Met,Gly. Dopamine D_1: **13** Phe264lle; **18** Leu286Ala. Luteinizing hormone: **9** lle542Leu; **19** Asp578Gly. Melanocyte-stimulating hormone: **3** Glu92Lys. Angiotensin AT1: **6** Asn111Ala. Muscarinic: m_5: **20** Ser465Tyr, Lys, Arg, Phe; 21 Thr466Pro. [open-square] represents substitution of human thrombin receptor residues 259–268 in the second extracellular loop by *Xenopus* thrombin-receptor equivalent, and substitution of β_2-adrenergic receptor residues 266–272 in the third intracellular loop (ICL) by α_{1B}-adrenergic-receptor equivalent; ↔ indicates partial deletion of the third ICL and truncation of C-terminal part of yeast mating-pheromone α-factor receptor, and truncation of C-terminal part of prostaglandin E receptor. DRY (Asp-Arg-Tyr) and BBXXB (B for basic and X for a nonbasic amino acid) represent two protein motifs involved in G-protein interaction. (*Modified from Pauwels and Wurch.*[204])

of the C-terminal portion of the third intracellular loop was demonstrated in studies on the $\alpha 1\beta$ receptor, which is linked to norepinephrine-induced activation of phosphatidylinositol metabolism. Substitution of any of the nineteen other possible amino acids at Ala293 conferred constitutive (agonist-independent) activity to the $\alpha 2$ adrenergic receptor.[205] It is likely that receptors are constrained from interacting with G proteins and that the changes brought about by agonist include a reorientation of the third intracellular loop which permits receptor-activation of G protein and the subsequent activation of the appropriate intracellular effector.[206] Studies on many receptor types have led to the postulation that a motif in the third intracellular loop, which is critical for G protein coupling, can be represented by the term BXXBB, where B is a basic amino acid (Arg, His, or Lys) and X is any other (non-basic) amino acid.[204]

Another region of heptaspan receptors that may be responsible for G protein coupling is located at the junction of the third transmembrane segment and the second intracellular loop of many G protein-coupled receptors. This region is delineated by a motif known as E/DRY (Glu/Asp-Arg-Tyr) which is highly conserved among G protein-coupled receptors, and mutations result in constitutive activation of many different receptors.[207,208]

Although the preceding studies induced mutations to study the regions on receptors that were essential to G protein coupling, some receptors are constitutively active as a result of spontaneously occurring mutations or in their normal state. Shenker and colleagues[209] have identified a mutation (Asp578Gly/Tyr) in the sixth transmembrane domain of the LH receptor which confers constitutive activation. Males carrying this mutation display precocious puberty. Although D1α dopamine receptors require the presence of agonist to activate G protein, D1β receptors show high constitutive activity, almost completely activating G protein in the absence of agonist.[210]

Inverse Agonism

The demonstration of naturally occurring constitutive activity of G protein-coupled receptors suggests that inhibition of such constitutive activity should have a functional effect. Thus, compounds exist which should block the binding of agonist (neutral antagonists) and other compounds exist which should inhibit the activity of a constitutively active receptor (inverse agonists). This was demonstrated for the δ opiate receptor in studies which revealed that the inverse agonist ICI 174864 lowered the basal activation of Gi by these receptors[211] and resulted in increased adenylyl cyclase activity (δ-opiate agonists inhibit adenylyl cyclase). Considering the model of receptor-G protein complexes presented earlier, it would be predicted that inverse agonists would show preferential binding to receptors which were not coupled to G proteins.[212] Inverse agonism has now been demonstrated at a number of receptor types.

Regulation of Receptor Sensitivity

Measures of agonist affinity often show receptors displaying multiple affinities for a single agonist (i.e., receptors bind agonist with both high and low affinity) (Fig. 4-7). The principal reason for this multiple affinity is the association of a G protein with the receptor. In fact, the addition of GTP (or a GTP analog) to these receptor binding assays shifts agonist binding completely into the low affinity state.[213] This is illustrated in Fig. 4-7. Thus, RG represents the high-affinity state for agonist binding and R + G, the low-affinity state. To complete the cycle and return to a conformation favoring the binding of G protein, agonist is released from the receptor. The receptor is then capable of "recycling" and binding agonist again.

Receptor Desensitization

Receptors are also capable of becoming desensitized. This process involves the attenuation of receptor response in the continued presence of agonist. Desensitization is either a result of continued presence of agonist specific for that receptor (homologous) or for a class of agonists working toward a "common goal" (heterologous desensitization).[214]

Heterologous Desensitization

Heterologous desensitization occurs as a result of activated kinases, either cAMP-dependent protein kinase A (PKA) or calcium/phospholipid dependent protein kinase C (PKC). Serine residues on the carboxyl terminal tail or on the third cytoplasmic loop become phosphorylated and appear to alter the conformation of the receptor such that it ceases to couple effectively to G proteins.[215] Heterologous desensitization of a β adrenergic receptor could occur either as a result of that receptor augmenting cAMP production and subsequently PKA, or of a muscarinic receptor activating phospholipase C, and the resultant activation of PKC.

Agonist-Specific Desensitization

A family of kinases, known collectively as G protein-coupled Receptor Kinases (GRK), have been identified[216–218] and six members, GRK1 through 6, have been characterized and cloned. GRK1 is also known as rhodopsin kinase and has a distribution limited to the photoreceptor where it phosphorylates light-activated rhodopsin. The other members of the GRK family have a more widespread distribution. These proteins are cytosolic and are recruited to the membrane following agonist occupancy of a receptor. Several identified regions on the C terminal tail of a variety of G protein-coupled receptors are phosphorylated and this allows the receptor to bind another protein, arrestin (the paradigm is being given for the β adrenergic receptor and may not apply to all G protein-coupled receptors). Arrestin binding prevents the receptor from coupling to G protein and allows the internalization of receptor.[219] Receptors which are mutated to remove the phosphorylation sites are not subjected to internalization. It must be cautioned that studies of receptor desensitization are often performed at concentrations of agonist many orders of magnitude in excess of those to which they would normally be exposed (Figs. 4-19 and 4-20). As such, the interplay between activation and desensitization in "normal tissue" has yet to be defined (i.e., it is unknown whether a receptor enters the desensitization cycle as a routine consequence of activation).

G Proteins, the Next Step in the Signaling Cascade

Once a receptor has attained the active conformation (whether intrinsically or by the binding of agonist), the subsequent activation of an appropriate G protein is the next step in the signaling process. Receptor-coupled G proteins are a large family of heterotrimeric

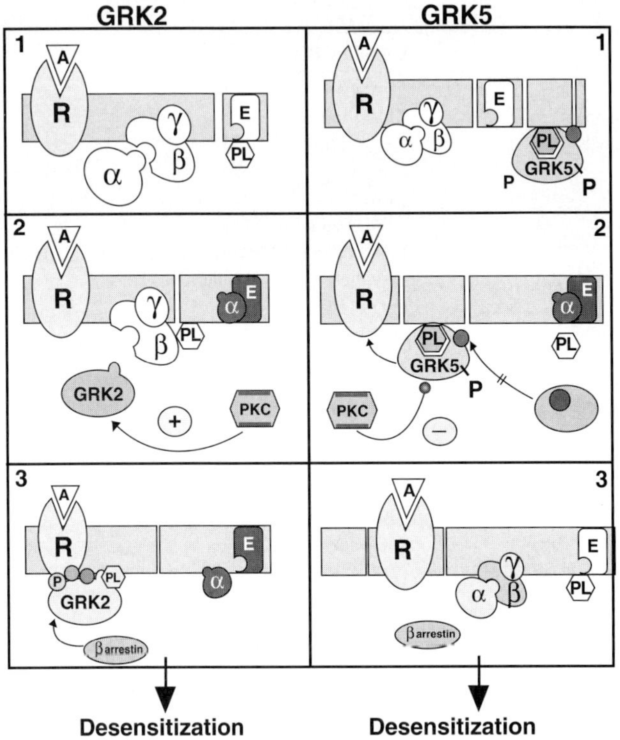

FIGURE 4-19. G protein-coupled receptor kinase (GRK)-mediated G protein-coupled receptor phosphorylation. This is schematically depicted in three arbitrary stages. Separate scenarios are depicted for GRK2 (left) and GRK5 (right). Stage 1: All signaling proteins are inactive: receptor (R), which has not yet bound agonist (A); heterotrimeric G protein (□); and effector (E) are also inactive. GRK5 adheres to the cytosolic surface of the plasma membrane and any phospholipid (PL). Phospholipid-bound GRK5 undergoes autophosphorylation (P), which is required for activation of the kinase. Stage 2 (activation): Activated by agonist, the receptor (R*) in turn activates the G protein. *G-Activated Gα and G$\beta\gamma$ subunits stimulate effector(s) (E) to produce second messenger(s), which in turn can activate protein kinase C (PKC) isoforms, among other proteins. Gβ subunits, along with PIP2, facilitate the translocation of GRK2 to the plasma membrane, where GRK2 binds to the activated receptor. Phospholipid-bound GRK5 binds to the activated receptor without requirement for G$\beta\gamma$ subunits. Phospholipid binding by GRK5 is inhibited by Ca^{2+}/calmodulin (CAM). PKC phosphorylation enhances GRK2 and inhibits GRK5. Stage 3 (signal termination): The receptor-bound GRKs phosphorylate (P) the activated receptors, which bind to a β-arrestin molecule. When bound to β-arrestin, receptor can no longer activate G proteins. (*Adapted from Pitcher et al.*[316])

proteins (α and $\beta\gamma$ subunits) which mediate many processes within the cell (Table 4-2). For reviews on G protein signaling see references[220–222] (Fig. 4-21).

All proteins that bind GTP (with the possible exception of tubulin) share significant sequence homology, especially with respect to the regions involved with the binding.[223] These regions, divided into areas binding base; ribose; and first, second, and third phosphate appear to undergo significant structural rearrangement following the binding of GTP. This has been verified by the elucidation of the crystal structures,[224,225] which appear to show multiple "switch" regions that change upon the binding of GTP and revert upon the hydrolysis of that nucleotide.[226]

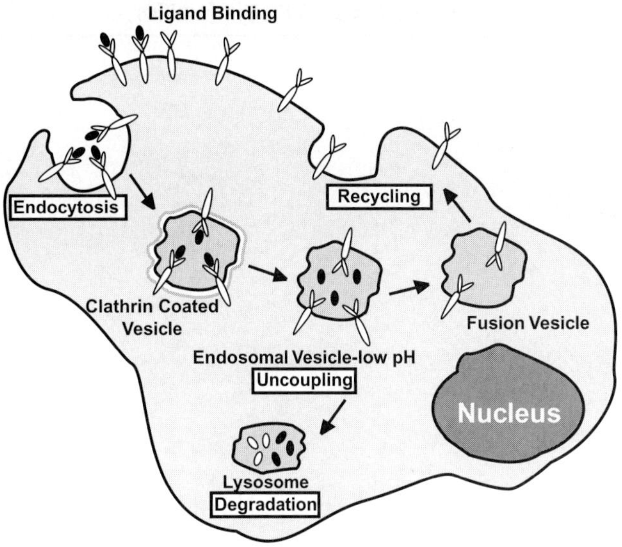

FIGURE 4-20. Receptor-mediated endocytosis. Following ligand binding, receptors rapidly move into coated pits and are internalized by endocytosis. The resulting clathrin-coated vesicles are acidified in an endosomal compartment, leading to dissociation of the ligand from the receptor. Vesicular sorting leads to a segregation of the ligand into vesicles that will fuse with primary lysosomes, resulting in the degradation or utilization of the ligand. The receptor can either be degraded, as often occurs for signaling receptors, such as the EGF and PDGF receptors, or can be recycled to the cell surface, as often occurs for transport receptors, such as the LDL (cholesterol uptake) and transferrin (iron uptake) receptors. (*Redrawn from Conn and Melmed.*[317])

GTP Hydrolysis

Heterotrimeric G protein α subunits possess intrinsic GTPase activity, and this represents one mechanism by which signals from the agonist are terminated (to be an effective signal, both an "on" and "off" mode must exist). Hydrolysis of GTP to GDP allows the reformation of a G$\alpha\beta\gamma$-receptor complex (Fig. 4-22). Inactivation of GTPase by cholera toxin maintains the G protein, Gsα, in an active state, and the resulting overproduction of cAMP by adenylyl cyclase elicits the diarrhea seen in cholera. This is a covalent modification of Gs, so the protein remains in the active state until degraded.[227] Hydrolysis-resistant GTP analogs, such as guanylylimidodiphosphate (GppNHp) or guanosinethiotriphosphate (GTPγS), have a similar effect in that the Gα binds these tightly and remains active because the GTP analog cannot be hydrolyzed by the GTPase of the G protein.

The GTPase activity of the heterotrimeric G proteins is inherent, but it is also slow (requiring several seconds to minutes). Although slow inactivation of G protein signaling may be efficient for G protein-activated enzymes such as adenylyl cyclase, it would be disastrous for G protein-activated ion channels, which must become activated and inactivated rapidly.

Small GTP binding proteins such as Ras and Arf have been known for some time to associate with GTPase activating proteins (GAPs). These GAPs were required in order to induce GTPase activity and inactivate small G proteins. Recently it has become evident that GAPs exist for heterotrimeric G proteins as well. Phospholipase Cβ1 is capable of activating the GTPase of Gqα, and it has been suggested that other G protein effectors may also have GAP activity.[228]

TABLE 4-2. G Protein Families

Subfamily		Effectors	Signaling Pathways
Gs	$G\alpha_s$	→ Adenylyl cyclase	↑ cAMP
		→ Ca^{2+} channels	↑ Ca^{2+} influx
		→ K^+ channels	↑ K^+ outflux
	$G\alpha_{olf(1\&2)}$	→ AC	↑ cAMP
Gi	G_{i1}, G_{i2}, G_{i3}	→ AC	↓ cAMP
		→ PLC	↑ IP3, DAG, Ca^{2+}
		→ PLA_2	↑ Arachidonate release
		→ K^+ channels	↑ Membrane polarization
	G_{oA}, G_{oB}	→ PLC	↑ IP3, DAG, Ca^{2+}
		→ Ca^{2+} channels	↓ Ca^{2+} influx
		→ K^+ channels	↓ K^+ channels
	Gz	→ PLC	↑ IP3, DAG, Ca^{2+}
		→ K^+ channels	↓ K^+ channels
	$Gt_{(t1\&t2)}$	→ cGMP PDE	↓ cGMP
Gq	$G\alpha_{15}$, $G\alpha_{16}$, G_{14}	→ PLC	↑ IP3, DAG, Ca^{2+}
	G_q, G_{11}	→ PLC-β	↑ IP3, DAG, Ca^{2+}
		→ PLA_2	↑ Arachidonate release
G12	$G\alpha_{12}$	→ cytoskeletal proteins?	Δ cell shape
	$G\alpha_{13}$	→ Na^+/H^+ exchanger?	↑ Na^+/H^+ exchange

This list is not meant to be comprehensive. It is a general description of G protein α subunits and their functions.

RGS Proteins

There is a recently described family of GTPase activating proteins which are now known as regulators of G protein signaling (RGS) proteins. These proteins were initially discovered in yeast and the nematode, *C. elegans*, where mutations showed a phenotype in which G proteins were "perpetually on".[229,230] These mutants failed to respond to hormonal signals because the G proteins were incapable of being modulated. A search for similar proteins in mammals yielded the first RGS protein.[231] Nine members of the RGS family have now been identified and each acts as a GAP, some with strong specificity for a certain Gα and others with a more general activity.[232] In addition to enhancing the inactivation of Gα, RGS proteins may interact with G protein effectors such as adenylyl cyclase. The number (and possible heterogenous localization) of RGS proteins lend credence to the idea that they are important participants in the regulation of signals for multiple G protein-mediated signal processing.

FIGURE 4-21. Coupling of G proteins to receptors and effectors. The activation of a G protein-coupled receptor by agonist allows activation of the G protein (the α subunits exchange GDP for GTP) and subsequent activation of an effector by Gα or Gβγ subunits. Several types of effectors are listed.

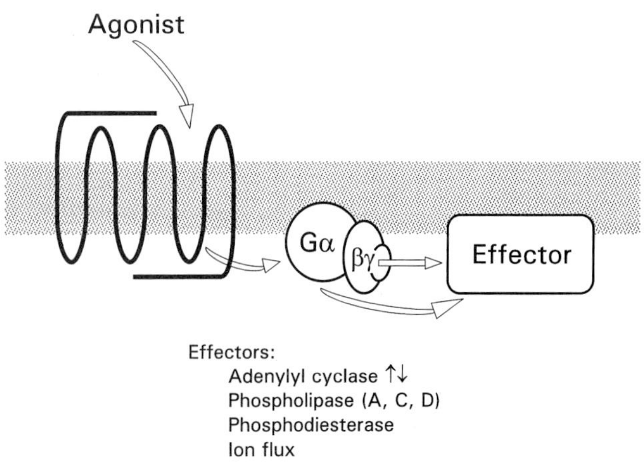

Coupling of Receptor to G Protein

GTP concentrations in most mammalian cells (100 μM) are far in excess of the Kd of most G proteins for GTP (about 10 nM).

FIGURE 4-22. The activation cycle of an heterotrimeric G protein. The activated receptor allows the exchange of GTP for GDP and this allows activated G protein α or $\beta\gamma$ subunits to combine with effector. It is not clear whether G protein subunits physically dissociate or whether there is some "tether" maintained between Gα and Gβγ subunits. Nonetheless, the hydrolysis of GTP allows an inactive Gα-GDP/βγ complex to reform and this form recouples to receptor to allow the activation process to begin again.

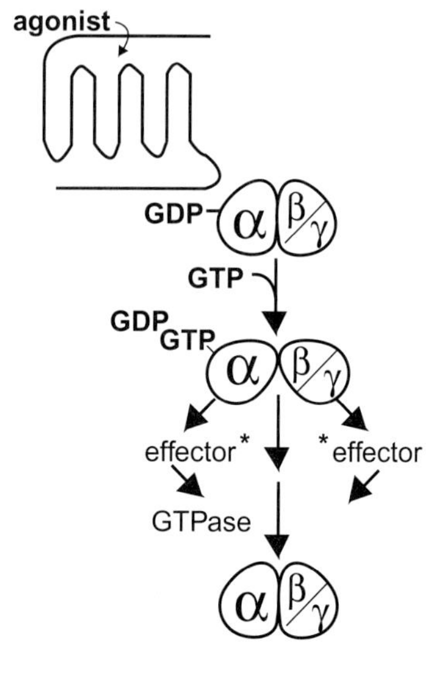

Thus, if G proteins were not "restricted" from binding GTP they would be activated without requirement for agonist. This would render hormone signaling moot (and much of endocrinology irrelevant). Coupling is the process in which the agonist-activated receptor activates the G protein by facilitating the release of GDP, which allows the G protein α subunit to bind cellular GTP (which is present at high concentrations). Studies by Cassel and Selinger[233] demonstrated that binding of agonist (isoproterenol) by the β-adrenergic receptor resulted in transient activation of adenylyl cyclase in turkey erythrocyte membranes. If hydrolysis-resistant GTP analogs were present, however, the activation of adenylyl cyclase was long-lived and was not inhibited by the subsequent addition of antagonist (propranolol) to the assay. This suggested that agonist allowed the binding of GTP (actually, the release of GDP) and subsequent steps in the cascade of effector (adenylyl cyclase in this case) activation occurred independently of receptor activation. Nonetheless, there appears to be an absolute requirement for an activated receptor (an intrinsically active receptor would fill this role as well) to activate G protein. This process is referred to as receptor-G protein coupling. Although some membrane preparations (such as the turkey erythrocyte) retain "tight coupling", many cell types lose this coupling when cells are disrupted. This allows G proteins to bind GTP directly without benefit of agonist. Initial studies of G proteins by Sutherland and Rall[181] showed that sodium fluoride was also able to activate G proteins without agonist present. Later work demonstrated that fluoride (actually aluminum fluoride[234]) elicited the same active conformation of G protein as did hydrolysis-resistant GTP analogs[235] where fluoride and aluminum bind to Gα with GDP and appear to mimic a third phosphate.[236]

Receptor-G Protein Coupling is a Bidirectional Process

Measurements of radioligand binding can be performed in the presence or absence of GTP or GTP analogs. When agonist binding is measured (either directly or by agonist displacement of radiolabeled antagonist) GTP causes a shift in the displacement curve to the right, signifying a lessened affinity (Fig. 4-7). Affinity of β receptors for antagonist is unaltered by GTP, but other receptor types may show lessened affinity for particular antagonists. The rationale for this shift in affinity is that the activation of the G protein and its subsequent dissociation from receptor results in a receptor with diminished affinity for agonist. Thus, the hormone (H), receptor (R), and G protein (G) exist as a ternary complex (HRG) with high affinity for agonist. The separation of R and G leaves R in a lower affinity state for H. This is advantageous, as it would allow R to recouple with G-GDP and permit a new cycle of response to agonist.

The physical region of Gα that appears to be critical for receptor coupling is located at the C terminal of Gα. This was demonstrated for Gs by using a peptide corresponding to the final eleven residues of that molecule. The peptide was able to block the activation of G protein or adenylyl cyclase by the β adrenergic receptor. The peptide also blocked the sensitivity of binding to GTP-induced lowering of agonist affinity previously described. The peptide mimicked Gsα in its interaction with the receptor, as it induced high-affinity agonist binding. Unlike the Gsα molecule, however, this peptide-induced high-affinity binding was insensitive to GTP. This suggested that the C terminal portion of Gsα evoked the receptor to form the high affinity agonist binding conformation.[237]

G Protein Activation

The ability to form crystals of G proteins allowed researchers to make predictions about the structures of those proteins and identification of the sites which may be responsible for interface with receptor and effector molecules.[224,225] These studies also suggested a model that described the regions of G proteins responsible for binding of GDP and GTP and the structural changes in Gα which occur upon the binding of GTP. It was suggested that three regions involved with the binding of GTP functioned as switches that promoted the formation of an ordered GTP-bound conformation of the molecule. It has been proposed that the binding of GTP to Gα promotes the formation of an activated Gα which dissociates from the $\beta\gamma$ subunit (the β and γ subunits remain tightly bound to one another under all conditions). This hypothesis originated with studies on the rod outer segment G protein (transducin) which was released from the membrane following treatment with light and GTP and a hypotonic buffer wash.[238] More recent studies, which show some common regions on Gα for the binding of effectors and G$\beta\gamma$, are consistent with the idea of subunit separation. Within the cell, however, membranes are not subjected to hypotonic wash subsequent to binding of agonist. Furthermore, although one study demonstrated overlap between binding of Gα to effectors and to G$\beta\gamma$, this overlap is incomplete and it would be possible for Gα to bind simultaneously to an effector molecule and to G$\beta\gamma$.[239] Thermodynamically, the maintenance of an association between the G protein subunits (on the membrane) is a reasonable suggestion.[240,241] A scheme for activation of Gα release of GDP, binding and hydrolysis of GTP, and subsequent change in the interaction of G$\beta\gamma$ with Gα (without a physical dissociation of the proteins) is given in Fig. 4-22.

G Protein Effectors

A vast array of cellular processes are mediated by G proteins. These molecules can either be activated or inhibited by G proteins and both α and $\beta\gamma$ subunits have been demonstrated to function as activators. A list of some of the G protein mediated events is given in Table 4-2 and Fig. 4-21.

Adenylyl Cyclase

This is the effector system that was being studied by Sutherland and Rall in their pioneering work on the activation of glycogen phosphorylase; work that led to the identification of 3′5′ cyclic adenosine monophosphate (cAMP) and the concept of intracellular messenger molecules.[180,181] Adenylyl cyclase, which generates cAMP from ATP, now appears to be a family of nine distinct enzymes, each with a different mode of regulation. A common feature of all the adenylyl cyclase enzymes is activation by Gsα and (to varying degrees) by the diterpene, forskolin. As can be seen in Table 4-3, some forms of adenylyl cyclase are inhibited by G$\beta\gamma$ while others are activated by that subunit (providing that Gα is already associated with the molecule). Although Giα (three forms of this protein exist) was called "i" because it was inhibitory to adenylyl cyclase, only a few forms of adenylyl cyclase are inhibited directly by Giα. Calcium can act to stimulate some forms of the enzyme (in conjunction with calmodulin) and can act directly to inhibit other forms. Phosphorylation may also prove to be a regulator of some forms of adenylyl cyclase.

Regardless of subtype, all adenylyl cyclase isoforms share a basic common structure. Figure 4-23 shows two similar subunits, each spanning the membrane six times and connected by a loop. The activation and inhibition processes have been elucidated in a

TABLE 4-3. Adenylyl Cyclase Isoforms and Their Regulation

Regulator	Effect	Cyclase Isoform
Gsα	Stimulatory	All
Giα	Inhibitory	I, V, VI
Goα	Inhibitory	I
Gzα	Inhibitory	I, V
G$\beta\gamma$	Inhibitory	I
G$\beta\gamma$	Stimulatory*	II, IV, VII
Forskolin	Stimulatory†	All
Ca^{2+}/calmodulin	Stimulatory	I, III, VIII
Ca^{2+}	Inhibitory	V, VI, IX‡
PKC	Stimulatory	I, II, III, V, VII
PKC	Inhibitory	IV
Calmodulin kinase	Inhibitory	III

* Enzyme must first be stimulated by Gsα.

† Very weak stimulation for type IX.

‡ Requires calcineurin.

series of experiments in which the cytoplasmic portions of adenylyl cyclase were excised, linked, and the cDNA construct expressed in *E. coli*.[242,243] Both sections must be expressed in order for the enzyme to show activity. Adenylyl cyclase generates cAMP from ATP and the substrate for the enzyme is Mg-ATP under normal cellular conditions, where Gsα serves as the activator. Mn-ATP is a substrate for the enzyme in the absence of Gsα. cAMP acts as the intracellular agent involved in transmitting the hormonal signal as explained later.

Forskolin Activation

All forms of adenylyl cyclase, with the possible exception of type IX, are activated by forskolin.[244] This diterpene extracted from the plant *Coleus forskolii* was used as a cardiotonic in India. It was suspected at that time to be an activator of adenylyl cyclase when initially isolated and this was subsequently confirmed.[245] Although forskolin binds directly to the adenylyl cyclase enzyme, it is much more potent in stimulating many, but not all, adenylyl cyclase subtypes that have been activated by Gsα.[246]

Insights To Adenylyl Cyclase From Its Crystal Structure

A homodimer of the C2 domains of adenylyl cyclase has been crystallized[247] as has a complex of Gsα-C1-C2 heterodimer (the source of C1 was type V adenylyl cyclase and C2 was from the type II form of the enzyme).[248] The crystal structure suggests a catalytic site (binding ATP) in the interface between the two cytoplasmic domains of adenylyl cyclase. Because the two halves (C1 and C2) are nearly identical, it appears that the binding sites on one domain are mirrored by those on the other. Thus, the active site of the enzyme contains the binding site for ATP and a symmetrical region binds forskolin. Furthermore, recent data suggest that a Gs binding site is mirrored by one for Gi, the latter site inhibiting the enzyme.[249]

FIGURE 4-23. Structure and regulation of adenylyl cyclase. The general structure and modes of regulation of adenylyl cyclase are shown. Note that each subtype of the enzyme enjoys a unique regulation. See Table 4-4 for a description.

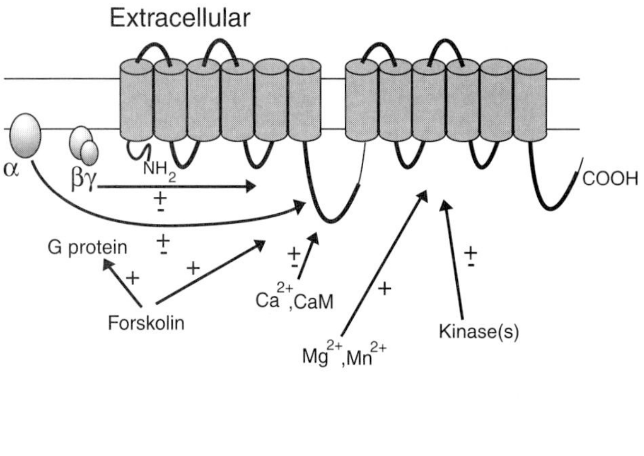

Phospholipid Metabolism Mediated by G Protein Dependent Hormone Signals

Cell membrane phospholipids are constituents of the plasma membrane and are involved in several aspects of signal transduction pathways. In response to a variety of hormones or neurotransmitters, plasma membrane phospholipids break down and the products of their breakdown, which is caused by a variety of phospholipase enzymes, are signaling molecules. The phospholipase enzymes that are responsive to G proteins fall into three families: phospholipase A, phospholipase C, and phospholipase D (Fig. 4-24).

The products of phospholipase A are metabolites of arachidonic acid and are known as eicosanoids. The eicosanoids fall into the subgroups of prostaglandins and leukotrienes. The next group of phospholipids are those that result from the breakdown of diacylglycerol and the inositol phosphates and these are the result of the actions of the phospholipase C enzymes. Finally, phospholipase D, which uses phosphatidyl choline as a substrate, can generate diacylglycerol and phosphotidic acid as well as lysophosphatidic acid. Phosphatidyl choline, the substrate for phospholipase D, constitutes as much as 60 percent of the plasma membrane lipid. Other constituents such as phosphatidyl choline, phosphatidyl ethalolamine, and phosphatidyl serine are present to lesser extents. A schema for the metabolism of the various phospholipids involved in the signaling is shown in Fig. 4-25.

Phospholipase A2

Figure 4-26 shows the action of phospholipase A2 in the synthesis of both prostaglandins and leukotrienes. These compounds act as second messengers within the cell or can act on cell surface receptors. Prostaglandins can act on cell surface receptors to engage a second messenger cascade. Thus, prostaglandins are a form of autocrine signaling. As can be seen from the figure, prostaglandins, prostacyclins, and thromboxane form a single family, and result from the breakdown of arachidonic acid by cyclooxygenase. Leukotrienes, in contrast, are formed by the action of lipogenoxygenase. It is noteworthy that the involvement of G protein signaling is at the level of phospholipase A2 which causes the generation of arachidonic acid. Phospholipase A2 can be regulated by phosphorylation as well as by the binding of calcium and phospholipid. The activation of phospholipase A2 by G proteins appears to be primarily through the $\beta\gamma$ subunits.

Phospholipase C

Inositol phospholipids are broken down into inositol trisphosphate and diacylglycerol by the phospholipase C family of enzymes. This family consists of a number of subtypes. Some, such as the phospholipase Cβ enzymes, are activated by G protein α subunits, whereas phospholipase Cγ is activated by the G protein $\beta\gamma$ subunits or by growth factors. Pathways activated by

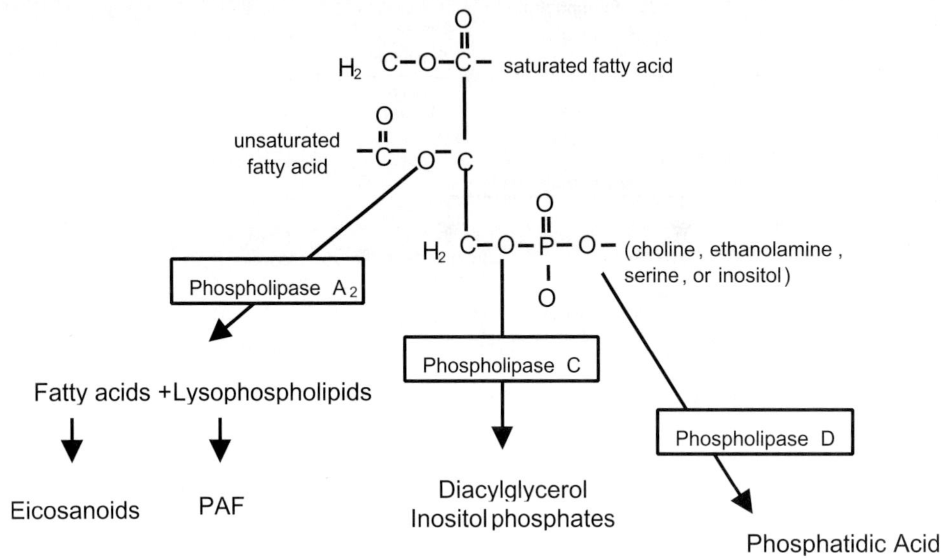

FIGURE 4-24. Substrates for and products of G protein-coupled phospholipases.

either enzyme are quite similar and are illustrated in Fig. 4-27. The 1-3-5 inositol trisphosphate generated as a result of phosphatidyl inositol breakdown binds to an intracellular receptor and elaborates or increases intracellular calcium. Diacylglycerol is also a breakdown product of the phospholipase Cβ enzymes and diacylglycerol, in the presence of calcium, is able to activate protein kinase C. The similarities and differences between the regulation of phospholipase Cβ and phospholipase Cγ are seen in Fig. 4-27. Phospholipase Cβ is activated by G protein α subunits, specifically Gq and G11, whereas phospholipase Cγ is activated by G protein $\beta\gamma$ subunits. Gq and G11 are pertussis- and cholera-toxin insensitive G proteins. Thus, G protein dependent activation of phospholipase Cβ is insensitive to disruption by bacterial toxins. However, if phospholipase Cγ is being activated by $\beta\gamma$ subunits, then the Gα which is "holding" the $\beta\gamma$ subunits must be activated by a G protein-coupled receptor, responding to agonist. This process would be sensitive to pertussis toxin if the G protein involved were Gi or Go.

Phospholipase D

Phospholipase D (PLD) catalyzes the breakdown of the membrane lipid, phosphatidylcholine, into choline and phosphatidytic acid. To date, three forms of the enzyme have been identified. Regulation of PLD occurs through G protein-coupled receptors (especially those for lipid mediators such as lysophosphatidytic acid) or via phosphorylation by protein kinase C. This latter mechanism appears to involve growth factor activation of receptor tyrosine kinases. Furthermore, several small G proteins such as ARF and Rho have been implicated in the activation of PLD.

The use of phosphatidylcholine as a substrate raises the possibility that PLD might alter the lipid composition of the plasma membrane within limited domains. PLD has been implicated in

FIGURE 4-25. Structure and enzymatic modification of three important molecules involved in phospholipase signaling. (*Modified from Alberts et al.*[313])

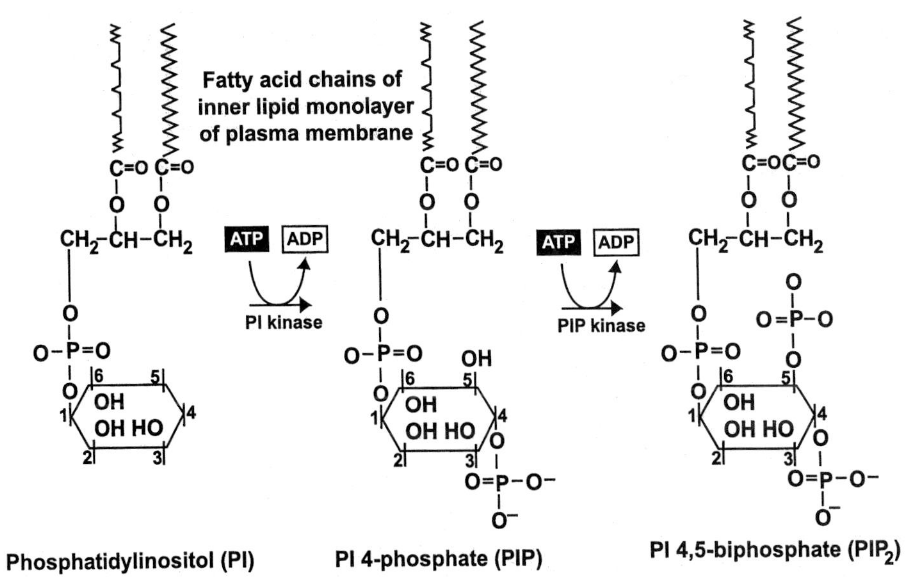

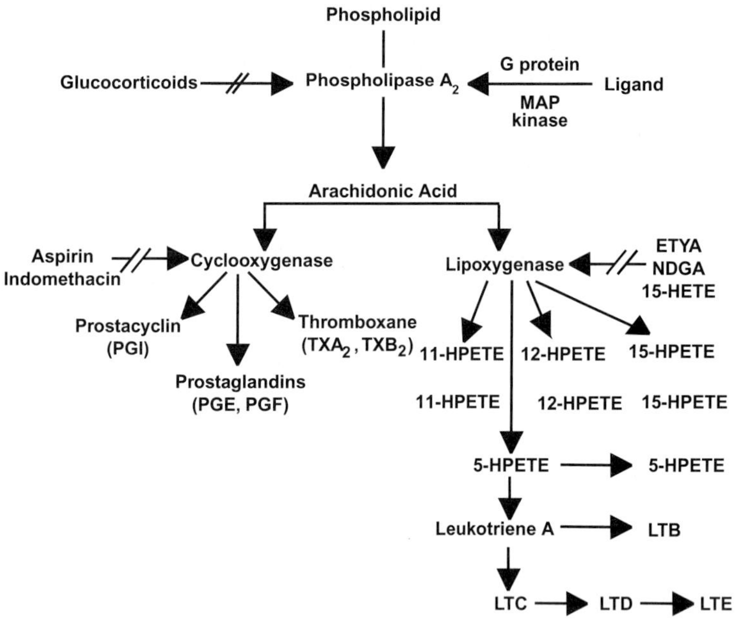

FIGURE 4-26. Phospholipase A_2 and arachidonate metabolism. The pathways for activation of phospholipase A_2 and arachidonic acid metabolites which are involved in cell signaling are shown. Classic inhibitors of these pathways are depicted by broken lines. 5-HPETE: 5-hydroperoxyeicosatetraenoic acid, NDGA: nordihydroguaiaretic acid, ETYA: eicosatrayonic acid, HETE: hydroxyarachidonic acid, TX: thromboxane, LT: leukotriene.

mitogenic signaling as well as golgi transport, but a clear function has yet to be assigned to this enzyme.[250]

G Protein-Activated Ion Channels

Heterotrimeric G proteins have been associated with the activation or inhibition of a variety of K^+ and Ca^{2+} channels as well as Na^+ channels.[251–254] Direct activation of potassium channels by G proteins is important for the agonist-induced, rapid inhibition of membrane excitability in vascular, nervous, and endocrine tissue. Five cDNAs which code for inwardly rectifying K^+ channels have been isolated and named GIRK 1-5 (GIRK = G protein-coupled inwardly rectifying K^+ channel and must be distinguished from GRK, which stands for G protein Receptor Kinase). The genes for these channels show considerable tissue-specific distribution.

Some initial studies describing the phenomenon of GIRKs suggested that they were regulated by Giα,[255] while other studies suggested that the regulation was through G$\beta\gamma$.[256] However, coexpression of GIRK1 and G$\beta\gamma$ in Xenopus oocytes produced channels that were constitutively active.[257] Direct binding of G$\beta\gamma$ to GIRKs has also been shown. There are some suggested domains on GIRK that might be involved in G$\beta\gamma$ binding, but no clear demonstration of the binding site has been made yet. Curiously, the regions on GIRK that might bind G$\beta\gamma$ are similar to those on α subunits of voltage sensitive channels. These channels appear to be regulated by G$\beta\gamma$ as well.

Even as G$\beta\gamma$ subunits appear to activate GIRKs, they inhibit voltage-dependant Ca^{2+} channels. Although several studies suggested that the α subunits of Go or Gi might be responsible for Ca^{2+} channel inhibition, the recent demonstration of binding sites

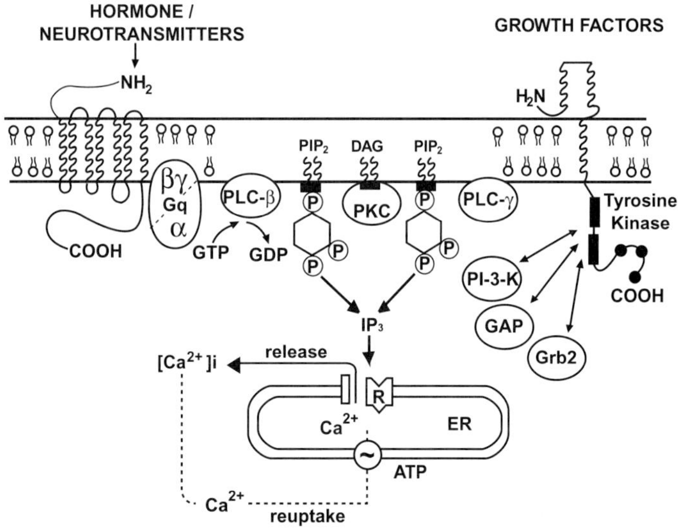

FIGURE 4-27. Activation of phospholipase C. G protein-coupled receptors which couple to Gq activate phospholipase C through the α subunits of that protein. Receptors coupling to Gi or Go show pertussis-toxin sensitive regulation of phospholipase C, and this is probably due to the activation of PLC by G$\beta\gamma$ subunits. Growth factors (tyrosine kinase) receptors also appear capable of activating PLC and stimulate the phosphoinositide-calcium signal transduction pathways. Ligands that activate G protein-coupled receptors promote coupling through a Gq of G_{ii} protein to phospholipase C, probably the β isoform of the enzyme. In contrast, growth factors that bind to tyrosine kinase-containing receptors (EGF, PDGF, FGF, and CSF-I) promote the association of the activated intracellular receptor domain with several cytoplasmic proteins, including phospholipase C-γ as well as PI-3-kinase, the GTP-activating protein of *ras* (GAP) and GRB2. These dissimilar types of stimuli cause hydrolysis of PIP_2 and generation of Ins(1,4,5)P3 and DAG, with mobilization of intracellular calcium and influx of extracellular calcium.

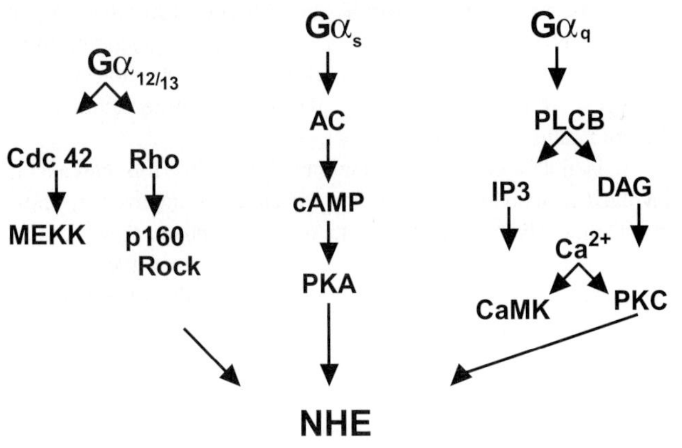

FIGURE 4-28. Suggested pathways for the regulation of Na^+-H^+ exchange (NHE). Three G protein-coupled pathways are suggested for the regulation of NHE.

for Gβγ on the cloned channel α subunits renders it likely that Gβγ binds to Ca^{2+} channels and inhibits the association of the channel subunits.[253] Preventing subunit association blocks channel function. Because these channels are often found at nerve terminals and are essential for the process of neurotransmitter release, those agonists which inhibit Ca^{2+} channels are often associated with the inhibition of the release of transmitter from those terminals. Opiate inhibition of substance P release might proceed subsequent to the binding of an opiate agonist to a μ opiate receptor. This is a G protein-mediated process.

Some atrial Ca^{2+} channels have also been suggested to be G protein activated. Norepinephrine may exert some of its cardiotonic effects by activating a Gs-linked Ca^{2+} channel.[258]

G Proteins and Na/H Exchange

The first function shown for the G proteins G12 and G13 was the regulation of Na^+/H^+ exchange proteins (NHE). Gα13 activates three forms of NHE, while Gα12 activates two forms but inhibits the third.[259,260] Although there may be direct effects of these G proteins on NHE activity, the pathways that have been identified to activate the enzymes work through protein phosphorylation. Both JNK and PKC have been implicated in this regulation. It is also likely that small G proteins such as Rho participate in the cascade which ultimately regulates NHE activity. Gsα or Gqα may also regulate NHE via Ca^{2+}/calmodulin or cAMP-dependent phosphorylation (Fig. 4-28).

G Proteins and Changes in Cell Structure

Traditional responses to agonists that activate G proteins include the activation or inhibition of the enzyme systems that generate second messengers and the direct modification of ion conductance. More recently, data have been accumulating to suggest that heterotrimeric G proteins may also modify the cytoskeleton.

G protein palmytolation may be regulated by hormone activation[261] and there is some suggestion that activated G proteins might attain a cytosolic localization.[262–264] G13 has been implicated as a protein that interacts with actin, either directly or through an actin-binding protein in the radixin, ezrin, moesin family.[265] Furthermore, G12 and G13 appear to couple to a protein, p115RhoGEF, which activates the small GTP-binding protein by promoting the exchange of GDP for GTP.[266] Increased expression of G12 or G13 clearly modifies actin fibers and the possible increase in the cytosolic distribution of the molecule could well alter actin polymerization. A hormone signal to a migratory cell (e.g., a neutrophil) could alter the chemotactic events at the membrane through such a direct modification of the cytoskeleton.

G proteins released from the membrane might also modify the microtubule cytoskeleton. G protein signals have been known, for some time, to be amplified by an increase in free tubulin dimers.[267] Further, it has been demonstrated more recently that microtubules are disrupted subsequent to the association of certain G protein α subunits with the GTP "cap" which normally stabilizes a microtubule. The G protein α subunits act as a GTPase activating protein for tubulin and destabilize microtubules by promoting hydrolysis of GTP on the "plus" end.[268] Curiously, free G protein βγ subunits stabilize microtubules.[269]

SECOND MESSENGER SYSTEMS IN CELLULAR SIGNALING

Second messengers generated as a result of G protein-coupled receptor signaling are either cAMP (generated through the activation of adenylyl cyclase) or calcium (either released from intracellular compartments or brought into the cell from the extracellular milieu). There are multiple mechanisms by which these second messengers exert their effects inside cells and these mechanisms will be considered herein. The following section also discusses the regulation and regulatory properties of those signaling molecules.

Cyclic Nucleotide Phosphodiesterase

cAMP acts as an intracellular messenger in every cell studied across the phylogenic spectrum, whether eukaryotic or prokaryotic. The cellular concentration of cAMP is normally quite low, but the intracellular concentration can rapidly be increased in response to hormonal signals. cAMP is synthesized by adenylyl cyclase and degraded by cAMP phosphodiesterase, causing cAMP to be hydrolyzed to 5′ AMP (Fig. 4-14). Initial hormonal signals are more likely to regulate cAMP by the activation or inhibition of adenylyl cyclase than they are by altering phosphodiesterase, but this is primarily because the receptors are coupled to G proteins which then directly stimulate or inhibit adenylyl cyclase.

Regulation of adenylyl cyclase has been discussed previously. The regulation of phosphodiesterases is quite complex, and much of it is due to the exquisite and unique subcellular localization of a myriad of phosphodiesterase species. Some phosphodiesterases will degrade either cyclic AMP or cyclic GMP and some are specific for one or the other. Several drugs designed for the cardiovascular system work by the inhibition of cyclic nucleotide phosphodiesterases. The relaxation of vascular smooth muscle by phosphodiesterase inhibitors can either lower blood pressure or contribute to increased blood flow in specific regions. For example, sildenafil citrate (Viagra) is a specific type 5 phosphodiesterase inhibitor.

Mammalian cells contain about 20 forms of phosphodiesterase (PDE) that are divided into five main groups. Type 1 phosphodiesterases are stimulated by Ca^{2+}/calmodulin and are activated by agonists, which results in the mobilization of calcium (e.g., muscarinic agonists that activate the phospholipase system).

These forms of phosphodiesterase are inhibited by methylxanthines such as caffeine and theophylline. Type 2 PDEs are stimulated by cyclic GMP and are activated by atrial natiuretic peptide. Type 3 PDE is inhibited by cGMP which competes with cAMP for a binding site on the catalytic subunit. These forms of phosphodiesterase are regulated by insulin or insulin-like molecules. Steroids also participate in the regulation of type 3 PDE. Type 4 PDEs are cAMP specific and can be inhibited by specific drugs such as rolipram.[270]

The genes for many PDEs have a cAMP response element; thus a sustained increase in cyclic AMP will result in the production of more phosphodiesterase and a subsequent lowering of cAMP. Furthermore, any increase in cellular calcium accompanying an increase in cAMP would activate the type 1 cyclic nucleotide PDE and cause a reduction in cellular cAMP. Thus, a cAMP signal has a specific temporal window; an increase in cAMP is followed by a decrease. This allows hormonal signals to occur in a specific timeframe.

The Intracellular Amplification of Extracellular Signals

Although the nature of signaling that occurs through G protein-coupled receptors is quite variable, there are some general principles that seem to guide most of the G protein-coupled receptor-dependent processes. One of these principles is that the extracellular signals are amplified many times prior to their intracellular effectiveness being detected.

This cascade was first illuminated by the work of Sutherland and Rall, and is diagrammed in Fig. 4-15. Note that an individual molecule of epinephrine might result in the production of 100 molecules of cAMP which would activate 100 molecules of protein kinase. Each activated protein kinase molecule would be expected to phosphorylate 100 molecules of glycogen phosphorylase kinase which further would phosphorylate 100 molecules of glycogen phosphorylase, and that each activated glycogen phosphorylase would successively phosphorylate 100 molecules of glycogen. Thus, the single molecule of epinephrine resulted in a 10^8-fold magnification of its effect.

It is noteworthy that at the same time that this cascade is involved in increasing the activity of enzymes involved in phosphorylating glycogen to yield glucose-1 phosphate, these kinases are also involved in a cascade that inactivates the enzymes responsible for glycogen synthesis. Thus, not only is there significant activation or amplification of the hormone signal, but there is also an exquisite balance to the system.

Second Messenger-Activated Protein Kinases

Common mechanisms by which cAMP and calcium exert their effects within cells are by activation of protein kinases (Fig. 4-29). The cAMP-dependent protein kinases were the initial mechanisms discovered and participate in wide-ranging signaling of a variety of different metabolic systems. Many, but not all of the actions of cAMP in vertebrates are mediated by cAMP-dependent protein kinases. In bacteria, on the other hand, most of the effects of cAMP occur directly through cAMP binding proteins which modulate gene transcription as discussed later. cAMP can also activate ion channels directly. In some systems, such as slime molds, cAMP binds to extracellular receptors for the process of cell differentiation. cAMP can also bind directly to phosphodiesterases to modulate the speed with which cAMP or cGMP are degraded.

cAMP-dependent protein kinases transfer the γ phosphate group from ATP onto serine or threonine residues of a variety of proteins. They include a variety of enzymes of glycogen metabolism, nuclear proteins involved in gene regulation, and proteins which might be involved in initiating cell division, promoting cell differentiation, or even initiating cell death.

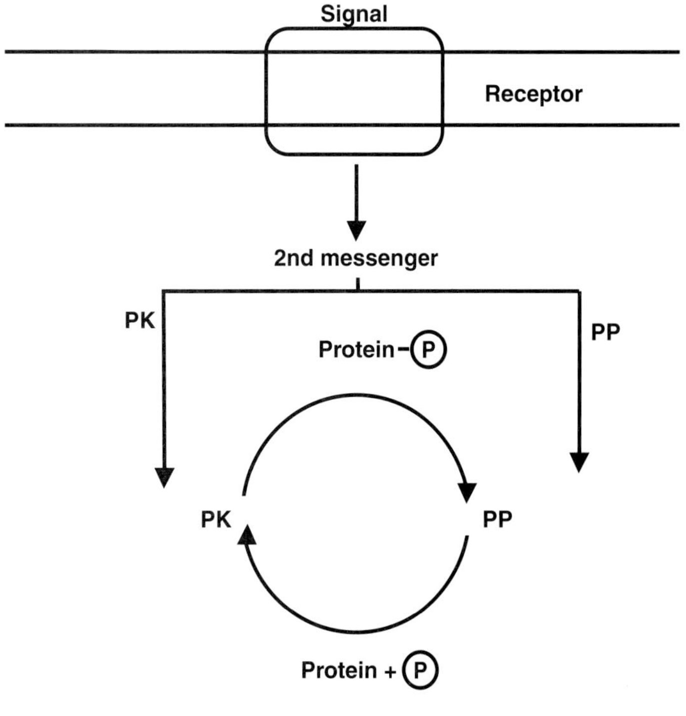

FIGURE 4-29. Regulation of protein phosphorylation. A scheme is given for the phosphorylation (protein-P) and dephosphorylation (protein + P) of proteins. Protein kinases (PK) and phosphoprotein phosphatases (PP) are both capable of responding to a variety of extracellular signals.

TABLE 4-4. Classification of Protein Kinases

Cyclic nucleotide-dependent kinases
CAMP-dependent protein kinases, types I and II
CGMP-dependent protein kinases
Calcium-dependent kinases
Calcium/calmodulin-dependent protein kinases: Types I, II, and III
Calcium/phospholipid-dependent protein kinase (protein kinase C): nine isozymes
Cyclic nucleotide- and calcium-independent kinases
Casein kinases
Pyruvate dehydrogenase kinase
Glycogen synthase kinase 3
Rhodopsin kinase; β-adrenergic receptor kinase
Tyrosine-specific kinases
Growth factor receptors
Nonreceptor tyrosine kinases

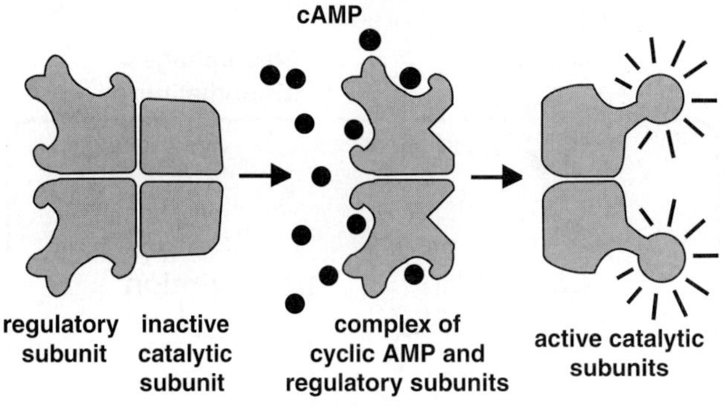

FIGURE 4-30. The activation of cAMP-dependent protein kinase (A-kinase). The binding of cAMP to the regulatory subunits induces a conformational change, causing these subunits to dissociate from the complex, thereby activating the catalytic subunits. Each regulatory subunit has two cAMP-binding sites, and the release of the catalytic subunits requires the binding of more than two cAMP molecules to the tetramer. This modifies protein phosphorylation in response to changes in cAMP concentration. There are at least two types of A-kinase in most mammalian cells: type I is mainly in the cytosol, whereas type II is bound to plasma membrane and nuclear membrane (elements of the cytoskeleton). Once the catalytic subunits (of either type) are freed and active, they can migrate into the nucleus (where they can phosphorylate gene regulatory proteins), while the regulatory subunits remain in the cytoplasm or on the membrane. (*Modified from Alberts et al.*[313])

Phosphorylation is a rapid process and allows for the activation of a variety of enzymes in short order. This also allows for the amplification of hormone signals as can be seen in Fig. 4-15. An illustration of the complexity of the numbers of kinases is given in Table 4-4.

Subcellular Localization of Protein Kinases

cAMP-dependent protein kinases are present throughout the cell and have both a cytosolic and membrane localization. A recently described family of protein kinase anchoring proteins or AKAPs allows protein kinases to attain a membrane localization and proximity to their substrates within an organized network; this facilitates cell signaling. AKAPs and localization will be discussed later. The general structure of cAMP-dependent protein kinases (PKA) is that of a regulatory subunit which contains two cAMP binding sites and a catalytic subunit which binds both ATP and the substrate, transferring a phosphate group onto the substrate. Taylor and colleagues have described the structure in great detail but the simplest explanation is that the kinases consist basically of two catalytic and two regulatory domains. When the regulatory subunits bind cAMP, the catalytic subunits are activated and phosphorylate substrate proteins.[271,272] Rapid increases in cAMP cause a rapid phosphorylation of the appropriate substrate proteins. Attempts to test the cAMP dependence of a process can be accomplished by injecting the purified cAMP-dependent protein kinase catalytic subunit. This catalytic subunit devoid of the regulatory subunits is intrinsically active (Fig. 4-30). Introducing the regulatory subunit into the cell will inhibit the enzyme while regulatory subunits of different forms of cAMP-dependent protein kinase may be divergent, catalytic subunits show marked similarity.[272]

Two major types of cAMP-dependent protein kinase have been identified and were named initially by their separation on ion exchange chromatography. Type I and type II are the terms referring to the two peaks into which they were resolved, with the type II enzyme being more acidic. Although these two forms of the enzyme are present in most tissues, type I tends to predominate in skeletal muscle and type II in cardiac muscle. Type I regulatory subunit is about 49 kDa and type II about 55 kDa. The regulatory subunits of both are about 39 kDa. The main distinguishing feature between type I and type II dependent protein kinases is the phosphorylation of the regulatory subunit of type II, but not type I. Upon phosphorylation, type II undergoes an autoregulation where its affinity for cAMP is reduced. Ostensibly this promotes the inactive form of the enzyme. Phosphorylation of type II dependent PKA also favors an inhibition of a reassociation of the associated regulatory and catalytic subunits. Thus, even though cAMP would be less likely to regulate the phosphorylated type II regulatory subunit of PKA, the free catalytic subunit would be allowed to work and would not be returned as quickly to the inactive state. Thus, cAMP could have two mechanisms for regulating the amount of active kinase in the cell at any given time.

The substrates for cAMP-dependent protein kinase contain one of two consensus amino acid sequences at their phosphorylation sites, either lys-arg-x-x-ser-x-x or arg-arg-x-ser-x-x, serine being the phosphorylated domain, and x being any amino acid. In addition to regulation by the activity of the kinase, regulation of cAMP-dependent phosphorylation depends heavily on the activation of phosphoprotein phosphatases as will be discussed later.

Cyclic GMP Dependent Protein Kinases

While cAMP- and cGMP-dependent protein kinases share a great deal of similarity, cAMP-dependent protein kinases tend to be involved more in the regulation of metabolism, whereas cGMP-dependent protein kinases are involved more in cell function. Specifically, cGMP-dependent protein kinases appear to participate in muscle tone, the vascular system, neuronal function, and platelet aggregation.

Nitric Oxide and cGMP Signaling

Nitric oxide (NO) is associated intimately with cGMP signaling. Unlike cyclic nucleotides however, NO is a gas, is degraded rapidly, and is inactivated by hemoglobin. Its diffusibility allows it to be a local signaling molecule which can easily enter most cells. It appears to be an important signaling molecule in the vascular system and the nervous system, as well as the immune

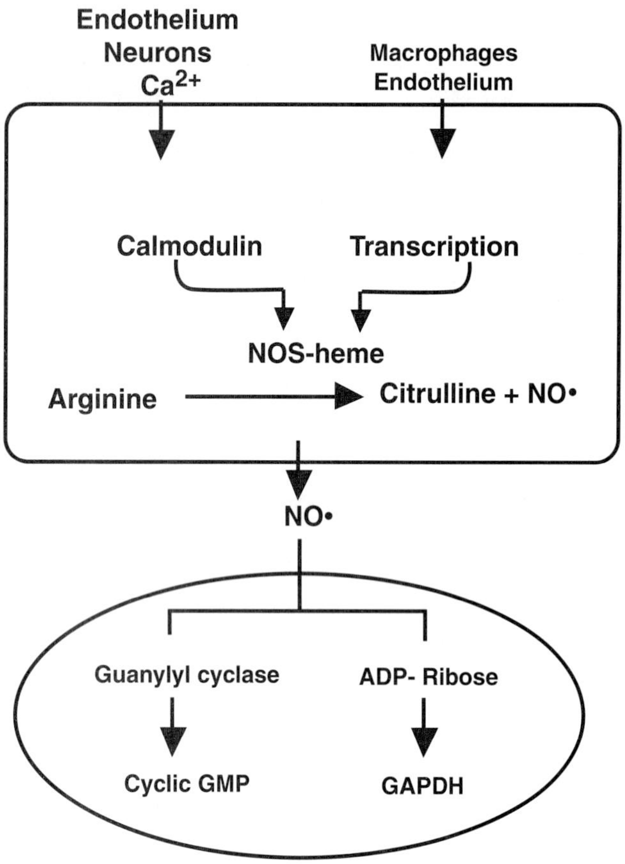

FIGURE 4-31. Cellular synthesis and effects of nitric oxide (NO). NO synthase (NOS) is activated by a variety of messengers in several cell types. It can act within cells or be released to act as a messenger for neighboring cells.

system.[273,274] NO activates soluble forms of guanylyl cyclase. In fact, it was first identified as an endothelium relaxing factor. It mediates the actions of vasodilators such as bradykinin or acetylcholine in smooth muscle. NO can also be a mediator of cytotoxicity in the immune system.

NO is formed from arginine by the enzyme nitric oxide synthase (NOS). Major isoforms of NOS exist in an endothelial form and a neural form, although the monikers endothelial and neural refer to where the forms were first isolated and not to where they exert their greatest activity (Fig. 4-31). In the nervous system the activation of NOS leads to an increase in NO and NO signals might fan out through multiple presynaptic and postsynaptic regions.

Changes in Intracellular Calcium

Calcium concentrations of most cells are quite low (from 10–100 nmol). At these concentrations, calcium does not function as an intracellular signal. When the cellular calcium concentration is elevated to between 500 and 1000 nmol, calcium functions as an intracellular messenger. Cellular calcium can be elevated by the release of calcium from intracellular stores or by the rapid transport of calcium into the cell from the outside milieu.

The calcium concentration outside of the cell is approximately 10,000-fold more than the intracellular concentration. For this reason, and the charge properties of the membrane, calcium entry from outside is a thermodynamically favored process.

Extracellular calcium enters the cell through voltage-gated calcium channels that are found primarily in the nerve terminals of excitable cells as well as in muscle and certain endocrine cells. These channels open in response to membrane depolarization and allow extracellular calcium to enter the cell. The calcium, thus entering, often functions to facilitate secretion of hormone or neurotransmitter.

Sometimes calcium influx can be due to the direct action of a receptor-mediated ion channel. These receptors, such as the NMDA-type glutamate receptor, are described elsewhere in the chapter.

Finally, calcium entry from outside the cell can be controlled by sensors which regulate the level of the intracellular calcium stores such as those found in the endoplasmic reticulum. When the endoplasmic reticulum is replete with calcium, calcium influx is inhibited. When these intracellular stores of calcium are depleted, calcium influx is activated. This process is known as capacitive calcium entry.

Intracellular Calcium Channels

Intracellular calcium stores release calcium in response to specific receptors on their surface. These receptors function as channels to allow the release of calcium from those intracellular stores. The responsible molecules consist of two basic and similar groups; one is the inositol-1-4-5-trisphosphate receptor (IP3 receptor) and the other is the ryanodine receptor. Figure 4-32 displays the actions of IP3 receptors. IP3 receptors bind IP3 as well as ATP, and have the capability for regulation by phosphorylation. IP3 activates the IP3 receptor and allows calcium to be released from the intracellular stores into the cell.

Ryanodine receptors were first isolated in skeletal muscle but appear to enjoy a wide tissue distribution as well, particularly within excitable cells. They allow for a rapid release of calcium from intracellular stores in response to cyclic ADP ribose and perhaps other intracellular messengers. Several subclasses of both IP3 receptors and ryanodine receptors are known to exist.

In addition to releasing calcium, the intracellular calcium stores must have the capability of rapidly concentrating calcium. This is important because if calcium is a diffusible messenger that delivers a discrete message, then there must be the capability of rapidly terminating the message by calcium reuptake. A variety of calcium ATP-ases are found on the plasma membrane, and these calcium ATP-ases are capable of exporting calcium from the cell into the extracellular milieu quite rapidly. These calcium ATP-ases are activated by calcium and calmodulin and in the presence of these compounds, significantly increase their sensitivity to calcium and their ability to pump it out of the cell. The calcium ATP-ases located on the endoplasmic reticulum or the sarcoplasmic reticulum likewise are able to rapidly transport calcium back into these cellular storage sites for calcium. The primary difference between these calcium pumps and those found on the plasma membrane is that the regulation by Ca^{2+}/calmodulin is not known to occur in microsomal calcium ATP-ases.

Calcium Binding Proteins

A number of calcium binding proteins have been localized to the cytosol and serve to buffer calcium once it is released from the

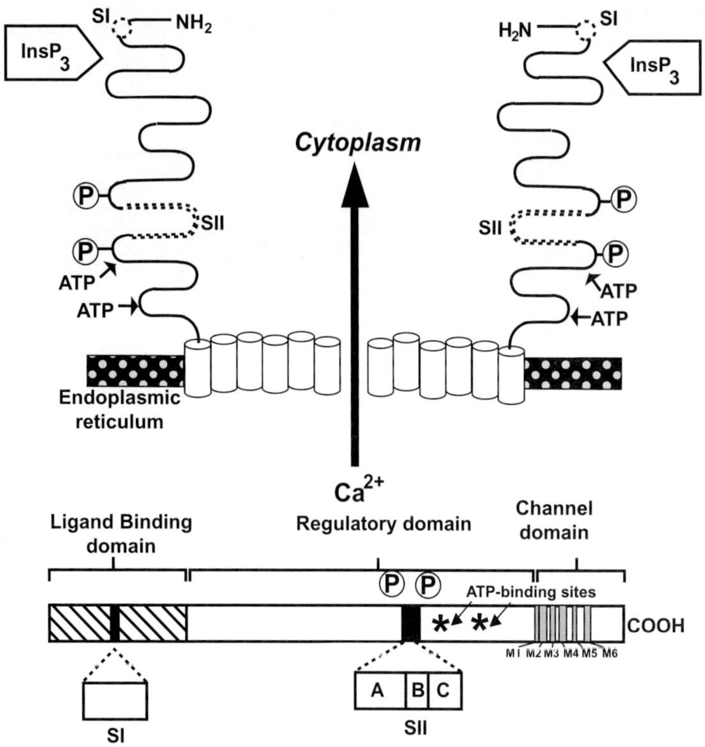

FIGURE 4-32. Structure of the Inositol(1,4,5)P_3 (IP_3) receptor protein: a ligand-regulated channel that conveys Ca^{2+} into the cytoplasm when activated by IP_3. The upper part of the figure shows a cross-section through two of the four subunits that form the receptor channel, and illustrates the several sites at which the channel is regulated. Each subunit contains an IP_3 binding site in its N-terminal region, located about 1400 amino acids away from the channel-forming transmembrane domains. The lower portion of the figure demonstrates the various domains of the IP_3 receptor protein. Sites for ATP binding and cAMP-dependent phosphorylation are located in the large region between the ligand binding site and the transmembrane domains, and regulate the opening state of the channel. RNA splicing sites (SI and SII) are indicated by the shaded areas.

intracellular stores. Examples of such proteins are parvalbumen, calretinin, and calbindin. Other proteins such as calsequestrin and calreticulin are found within the membrane of the endoplasmic reticulum and buffer calcium there. These proteins allow calcium to maintain a set concentration both in activated and inactivated states.

Calmodulin

Calmodulin was initially identified in its role as an activator of cyclic AMP phosphodiesterase. In fact, calmodulin was first known as the calcium-dependent regulator protein of phosphodiesterase. Since that time it has become clear that calmodulin is responsible for mediating the actions of calcium through a large variety of cellular processes. First among these is phosphorylation. There are a variety of Ca^{2+}/calmodulin-dependent kinases, and they phosphorylate a number of different target proteins. Calmodulin also activates calcineurin, which is a Ca^{2+}/calmodulin-sensitive protein phosphatase. Thus, once calmodulin has activated a phosphorylation event, it is capable of activating calcineurin, which dephosphorylates those proteins which have been phosphorylated by Ca^{2+}/calmodulin-dependent protein kinase, consistent with the theme of a temporally discrete event in cellular signaling.

Ca^{2+}/Calmodulin-Dependent Protein Kinases (CaM Kinases)

Many of the effects of calcium as a second messenger are exerted through the activation of CaM kinases. Some of these enzymes have extraordinary substrate specificity. Smooth muscle contraction is elicited by myosin light chain kinase and calcium activation of glycogenolysis is mediated by phosphorylase kinase. Both of these enzymes are CaM kinases along with the enzyme CaM kinase IV, which phosphorylates a 100 kDa elongation factor in mammalian cells. Of broader specificity is CaM kinase II, an enzyme of particular importance in the nervous system where it is the major protein component of the postsynaptic density.

CaM kinase II is activated initially by the binding of an activated (calcium-bound) calmodulin molecule. Enzyme activation is continued in the absence of calcium through autophosphorylation of CaM kinase II (Fig. 4-33). Such a molecular memory has proven important for many of the activities of this enzyme.[275]

Protein Kinase C

Protein kinase C (PKC) is a family of eleven enzymes, most of which are activated by diacylglycerol. As outlined elsewhere in this chapter, diacylglycerol is produced by the enzyme phospholipase C. Activated PKC appears to show a broad substrate specificity and PKC phosphorylates a huge range of proteins within the cell. As is the case with cAMP-, cGMP-, and Ca^{2+}/calmodulin-dependent protein kinases, PKC is a serine and threonine kinase. Various isozymes of phospholipase C can be activated either by ligands which act through G protein-coupled receptors or those which act through receptor tyrosine kinases. As seen in Fig. 4-34, the eleven forms of PKC can be assembled into four groups. In addition to diacylglycerol, phorbol esters represent a common mechanism which activates most species of protein kinase C. Phorbol esters can be added extracellularly, yet they affect an intracellular activation of PKC. Further, group C of the protein kinase C enzymes is activated by calcium as well as the lipid species named in Fig. 4-34.

Because protein kinase C is activated reversibly by diacylglycerol, it is likely that there is a domain for diacylglycerol binding on the enzyme. Curiously, the one family of PKC isozymes

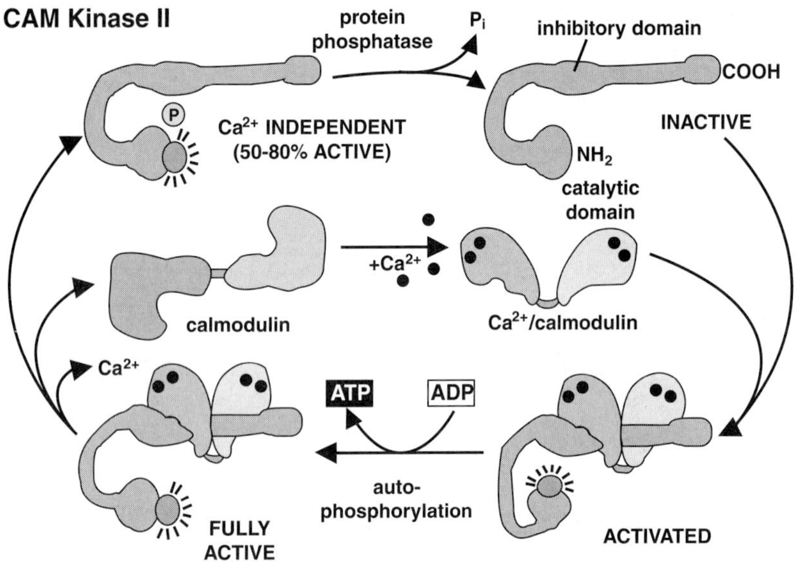

FIGURE 4-33. Activation of calmodulin (CAM) kinase II. A scheme for the activation of CAM kinase by calmodulin is shown. Ca^{2+} is represented by the small filled circles. See text for explanation. (*Adapted from Alberts et al.*[313])

that is not activated by diacylglycerol, the A family, also has within its sequence the region that has been suggested to be the diacylglycerol binding site.

Although the binding of diacylglycerol activates PKC, this alone is insufficient to achieve PKC activation in vivo. For many isozymes of PKC, it appears that phosphorylation is also required. Furthermore, the activation of PKC appears to require that the enzyme shift from a cytosolic to a membrane localization. There appear to be different select sites for the binding of different isoforms of PKC to various membrane domains.

FIGURE 4-34. Domain structure and grouping of the various isoforms of Protein Kinase C (PKC). See text for details.

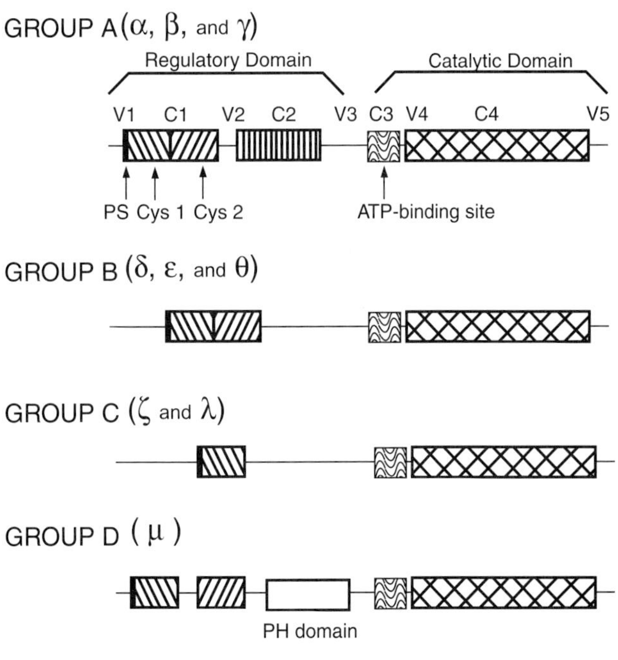

Phosphoprotein Phosphatases

Whether phosphorylation is a result of serine, threonine, or tyrosine kinases, in order for a signal to be complete it is necessary to dephosphorylate those proteins. This is accomplished by phosphoprotein phosphatases.[276]

Serine/Threonine Phosphatases

Initially, regulation of protein phosphorylation by phosphatases was assumed to be a passive process, the active phase being the signal-directed phosphorylation by kinases and dephosphorylation being something that occurred subsequent to phosphorylation but without a regulatory component. Recently, evidence has been accumulating which suggests that phosphatases are also subject to significant regulation. The number of serine/threonine phosphatase genes is enormous and may be as high as 500 in the human genome. Because serine/threonine phosphatases are made up of both regulatory and catalytic subunits, the combinatorial possibilities provide for a very large number of unique phosphatase molecules.[276]

Initial studies on phosphoprotein phosphatases identified four enzymes in mammalian tissue. They were known as PP1, PP2A, PP2B, and PP2C. While it appeared that PP1, PP2A, and PP2B were closely related, PP2C was somewhat divergent from the others. The subsequent application of molecular cloning made it obvious that there were a vast array of phosphoprotein phosphatase gene products, but this chapter will discuss only the four major types.

Phosphoprotein Phosphatase Type 1

PP1 is so named because it was the first phosphatase characterized. As with the cAMP cascade, it was the system of glycogen phosphorylation that was utilized for the study of PP1. In this system, PP1 is able to dephosphorylate the various substrates of protein kinase A. Thus, PP1 terminates the effects elicited by epinephrine or glucagon in the glycogen phosphorylase cascade. It is noteworthy that PP1 also has a specific inhibitor protein. Initially, this protein was thought to be associated exclusively with the dopamine receptor and was named DARPP-32 because it is a dopamine-receptor associated phosphoprotein of 32 kDa.[277]

Protein Phosphatase 2A

PP2A is a multiple-specificity protein kinase, as it is also able to dephosphorylate phosphotyrosine residues. Several forms of PP2A exist and some appear to be regulated both by an inhibitory protein and a specific activating protein. Furthermore, carboxymethylation of the carboxy terminal of one form of PP2A appears to be involved in its regulation. Thus, kinases could modify the activity of phosphatases, by either prolonging or diminishing their activity.

Protein Phosphatase 2B

PP2B is also known as calcineurin and it is an abundant brain protein. As described elsewhere in this chapter, PP2B is a phosphatase which dephosphorylates residues which were phosphorylated by Ca^{2+}/calmodulin-dependent protein kinase. When Ca^{2+}/calmodulin-dependent protein kinase is active, calcineurin is also active because calcineurin is activated by the binding of Ca^{2+}/calmodulin. The PP2B or calcineurin is a heterodimer consisting of a catalytic subunit and a regulatory subunit. The regulatory B subunit is homologous (but not identical) to calmodulin, as both CaM and the B subunit associate with PP2B. When both calmodulin and the regulatory B subunit are present, PP2B activity is stimulated 600-fold.

Protein Phosphatase 2C

PP2C is a monomer of about 42–45 kDa and requires magnesium for maximal activity. Unlike some of the other phosphatases, PP2C appears to contain a nuclear localization signal.

Localization of Phosphatase Signaling

It is possible that both phosphatases and kinases as well as some other regulatory enzymes enjoy a specific cellular localization which allows them to communicate readily with one another. PP2A has been localized to cellular microtubules, and it appears that A kinase anchoring proteins (or AKAPs) will bind and promote the localization of both kinase and phosphatase molecules.[278,279]

Regulation of Serine/Threonine Phosphatase Activity

The regulation of serine/threonine phosphatase activity is often accomplished by phosphorylation. This is especially true in the paradigm of the glycogen phosphorylase cascade. Protein kinase A phosphorylates and activates glycogen synthase. Thus, protein kinase A phosphorylates the enzymes involved with glycogenolysis. It also phosphorylates proteins that regulate protein phosphatase 1C, the protein phosphatase most commonly associated with this cascade. This could lead to a further increase in the breakdown of glycogen and, at the same time, an inhibition of glycogen synthesis.

Interplay Between Ca^{2+}/Calmodulin and cAMP Signaling

Cross-talk among second messengers is very important, as it allows for a variety of different hormones or neurotransmitters to modulate the effects of one another. In this regard, there are several sites of interaction between calcium signaling and cAMP signaling. As mentioned earlier, Ca^{2+}/calmodulin can activate cAMP phosphodiesterase, thus increasing the degradation of cAMP and lowering the level of that intracellular messenger. The production of cAMP can also be regulated by calcium and/or calmodulin. Types I and III adenylyl cyclase are activated by calcium and calmodulin. Thus, within some cells, cAMP is increased when calcium is elevated. Conversely, types V and VI adenylyl cyclase are inhibited when the calcium concentration is elevated within the cell. Therefore, depending upon the type of adenylyl cyclase within a cell, a calcium signal could increase or decrease the amount of cellular cAMP.

Receptors with Guanylyl Cyclase Activity

Guanylyl cyclase, the enzyme that makes cyclic GMP, can be located either in the cytosol or on the plasma membrane. The cytosolic and plasma membrane localized forms of guanylyl cyclase are quite distinct, both in regulation and in function. Receptor guanylyl cyclases are transmembane proteins with an extracellular ligand-binding domain and a cytoplasmic domain

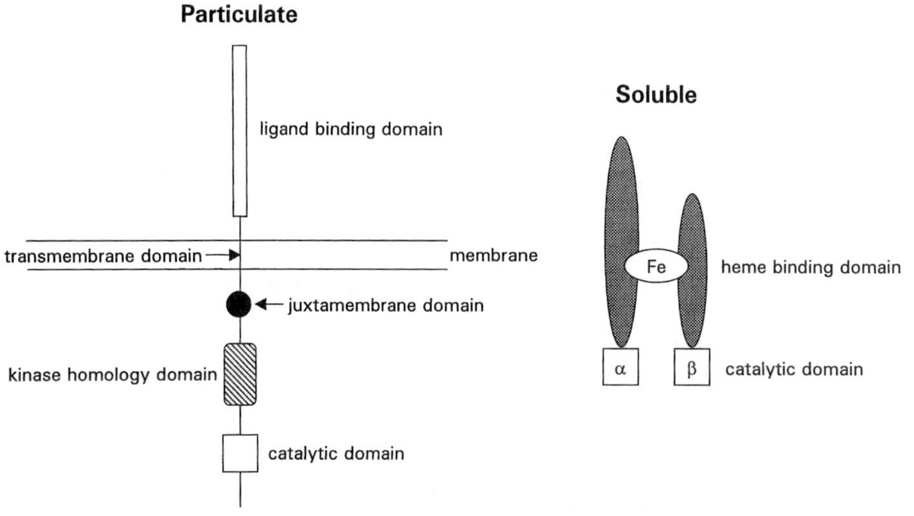

FIGURE 4-35. Typical structure of membrane binding and soluble guanylyl cyclase. Labels refer to domains within the enzyme molecules. (*Modified from Schulz and Waldman.*[280])

which resembles cyclic nucleotide-dependent protein kinase. The catalytic domain that produces cGMP from GTP is close to the carboxy terminal of membrane bound guanylyl cyclase. Six transmembrane receptor guanylyl cyclases have been cloned to date. Each is a receptor for atrial natriuretic peptide or for the similar heat-stable enterotoxin from *Escherichia coli*. Receptors that can activate the membrane-associated guanylyl cyclase also may be associated with *E. coli*[280,281] (Fig. 4-35).

Soluble guanylyl cyclase responds primarily to the intracellular signaling molecule nitric oxide (NO). In addition to NO, this enzyme might be regulated by phosphorylation. This would lead to cross-talk among signaling pathways because cAMP-dependent protein kinases appear to regulate soluble guanylyl cyclase.

ION CHANNEL RECEPTORS

Transmission in the nervous system is dependent upon rapid translocation of ions to allow rapid changes in charge distribution across the membrane. Thus, neurotransmitters should be able to affect either depolarization, hyperpolarization, or maintenance of the resting membrane potential in response to agonists within fractions of a second. Receptors that are themselves ion channels are known as ionotropic receptors. Receptors in this family all show a great deal of structural homology because much of the amino acid sequence of the receptor is devoted to the ability to translocate an ion across the plasma membrane. Transmitters that bind to and activate these receptors include acetylcholine, γ-aminobutyric acid (GABA), glutamate, and serotonin.

The ionotropic receptors usually exist as multiple subunit proteins (either tetramers or pentamers). In some cases, such as the nicotinic acetylcholine receptor, multiple molecules of agonist must bind in order to activate the receptor.

The Nicotinic Acetylcholine Receptor

The nicotinic acetylcholine receptors are located at nerve terminals and in central neurons either at synapses in ganglia or within the brain. Nicotinic receptors are quite abundant in the electric organs of electric fish or electric eels, and as such, they were easily purified and characterized.[282] Furthermore, the density of these receptors allowed for their characterization by X-ray diffraction techniques.[283] Thus, the amino acid sequence, general protein conformation, and the nature of the protein within its membrane domain have all been determined. Further, models have been suggested for the activation and adaptation of the nicotinic receptor after its interaction with acetylcholine[284,285] (Fig. 4-36).

Several genes are involved in the coding of acetylcholine receptor subunits and it appears that the combination of gene products which participate in assembling a specific receptor will dictate, to a large part, the properties of that assembled receptor in response to acetylcholine. As can be seen in Fig. 4-37, the nicotinic receptor from the neuromuscular junction has two α subunits, each of which bind agonists, plus β, γ, and δ subunits. Placed together, they form a channel that conducts both sodium and potassium. The CNS nicotinic receptor consists of α and β subunits only; however, there are several distinct genes for different α and β subunits.[286–288] Unlike neuromuscular junction nicotinic receptors, the neuronal nicotinic receptors are permeable to calcium as well. Thus, the activation of a neuronal nicotinic receptor at a nerve terminal would allow an influx of calcium and promote neurotransmitter release.

Nicotinic acetylcholine receptors appear to cluster in the plasma membrane. This clustering is often in response to a presynaptic signal, and is dependent on a cytoskeletal protein known as rapsyn.[289–291]

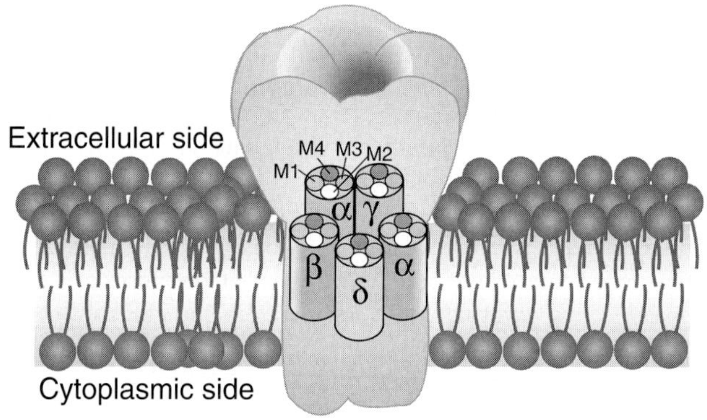

FIGURE 4-36. Topology of a nicotinic ACh receptor. Each subunit has four transmembrane domains and five subunits assemble to form the receptor. (*Modified from Kandel, Schwartz, and Jessell.*[318])

FIGURE 4-37. Activation of the nicotinic ACh receptor by agonist. This figure demonstrates the binding of one molecule of acetylcholine to each α-subunit and the subsequent opening of the ACh receptor/channel. The receptor/channel complex consists of five subunits, all of which contribute to forming the pore. When two molecules of ACh bind to portions of the α-subunits exposed to the membrane surface, the receptor-channel changes conformation. This opens a pore in the portion of the channel embedded in the lipid bilayer, and both K^+ and Na^+ flow through the open channel down their electrochemical gradients. (*Modified from Kandel, Schwartz, and Jessell.*[318])

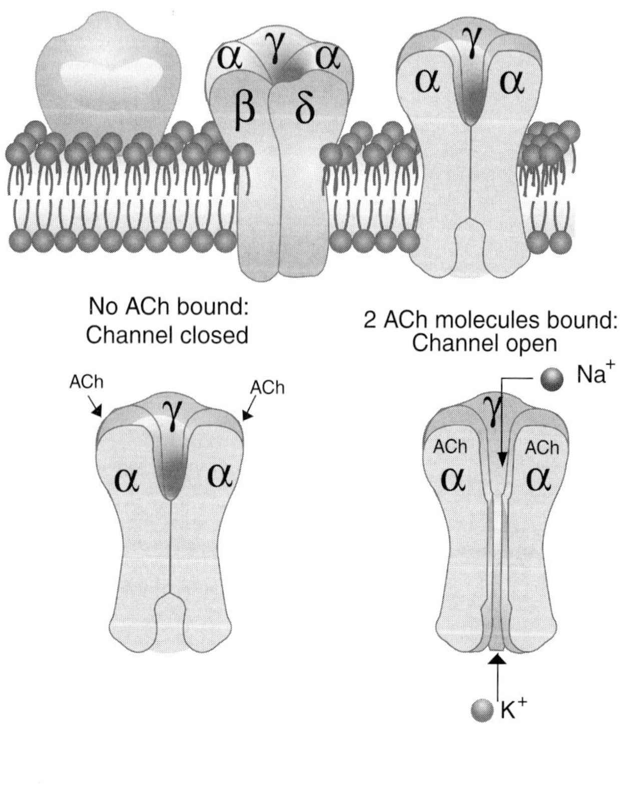

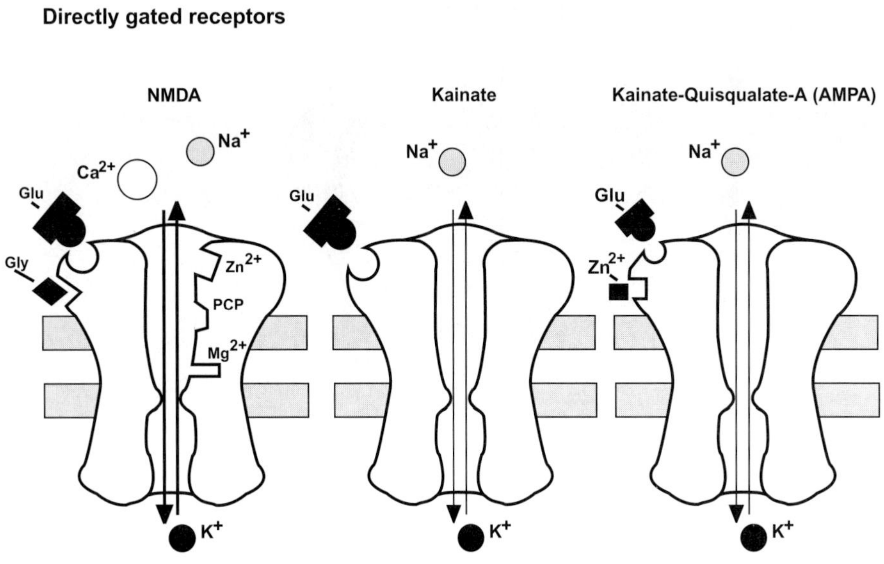

FIGURE 4-38. Glutamate receptors. Three classes of glutamate receptors regulate excitatory synaptic actions in neurons in the spinal cord and brain. Two types of ionotropic glutamate receptors directly gate ion channels. Two subtypes of non-NMDA receptors bind the glutamate agonists kainate or AMPA and regulate a channel permeable to Na^+ and K^+. The NMDA (*N*-methyl-D-aspartate) receptor regulates a channel permeable to Ca^{2+}, K^+, and Na^+ and has binding sites for glycine, Zn^{2+}, phencyclidine (PCP, or "angel dust"), MK801 (an experimental drug), and Mg^{2+}, which regulate the functioning of this channel in different ways. (*Modified from Kandel, Schwartz, and Jessell.*[318])

Glutamate Receptors

Glutamate is the major excitatory neurotransmitter in the central nervous system of all vertebrate species. Three major types of ionotropic glutamate receptors exist. They are grouped according to the specific agonists which are able to activate them. These are known as AMPA receptors (alpha amino 3-hydroxy-5-methyl-isoxazole-4-proprionate), kainate/quisqualate, and NMDA (n-methyl-d-aspartase). They are diagrammed in Fig. 4-38.

The first two receptor subtypes primarily transport sodium ions into the cell in response to activation by agonists. They appear to be tetramers composed of four similar subunits. Depending on the specific receptor subtype, small amounts of calcium can also be transported into the cell.

The NMDA receptor stands quite distinct from the AMPA and the kainate/quisqualate receptors. When the cell becomes somewhat depolarized, NMDA receptors conduct calcium into the cell. This would facilitate neurotransmission, and NMDA receptors have been implicated in the processes which may be involved with memory. The NMDA receptor also enjoys a rich regulation and several compounds of those receptors participate in the regulatory process. Glycine acts as an adjuvant for glutamate by increasing the affinity of glutamate for the receptor and in increasing the likelihood that the channels will be activated. This is illustrated in Fig. 4-38. Note that a fourth type of glutamate receptor exists. This G protein-coupled receptor is referred to as a metabotropic glutamate receptor and is coupled to the activation of phospholipase.

GABA Receptors

While glutamate is the major excitatory neurotransmitter in all vertebrates, GABA is the major inhibitory neurotransmitter. Most of the GABA neurotransmission occurs through $GABA_A$ receptors ($GABA_B$ receptors like the metabatrophic glutamate receptors, are G protein coupled and have been discussed previously). As was the case with glutamate receptors, $GABA_A$ receptors are also a multimeric complex of a putative pentameric structure. When activated, the $GABA_A$ receptor is a chloride channel. The introduction of the chloride ion into the neuron reinforces the maintenance of the resting membrane potential at the equilibrium potential for chloride. Because these two values tend to be very close to one another, the activation of a $GABA_A$ receptor makes the cell resistant to depolarization.

As is the case with the NMDA receptor, a variety of compounds bind to the $GABA_A$ receptor at sites distinct from that reserved for GABA binding. Picrotoxin interferes with the chloride channel by blocking the conductance of chloride, and as such, acts as a convulsant. Benzodiazepines such as diazepam or chlorodiazepoxide increase the likelihood that a molecule of GABA will open the chloride channel. Thus, benzodiazepines act as an adjuvant, increasing the potency of GABA at the $GABA_A$ receptor. Because GABA is inhibitory, these drugs have an anxiolytic or anticonvulsant effect. Several other drugs have binding sites at the $GABA_A$ receptor as well (Fig. 4-39).

FIGURE 4-39. Structure and function of the $GABA_A$ receptor. A model for the receptor shows binding sites for GABA as well as several compounds which affect GABA signaling. Activation of the receptor increases chloride conductance. Actions of these compounds are explained in the text. (*Adapted from Kandel, Schwartz, and Jessell.*[318])

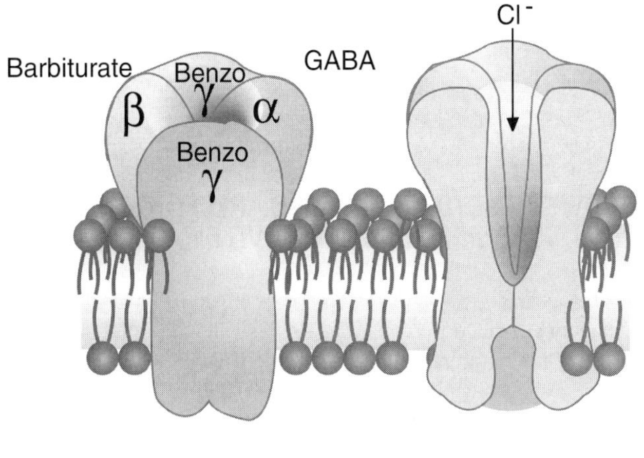

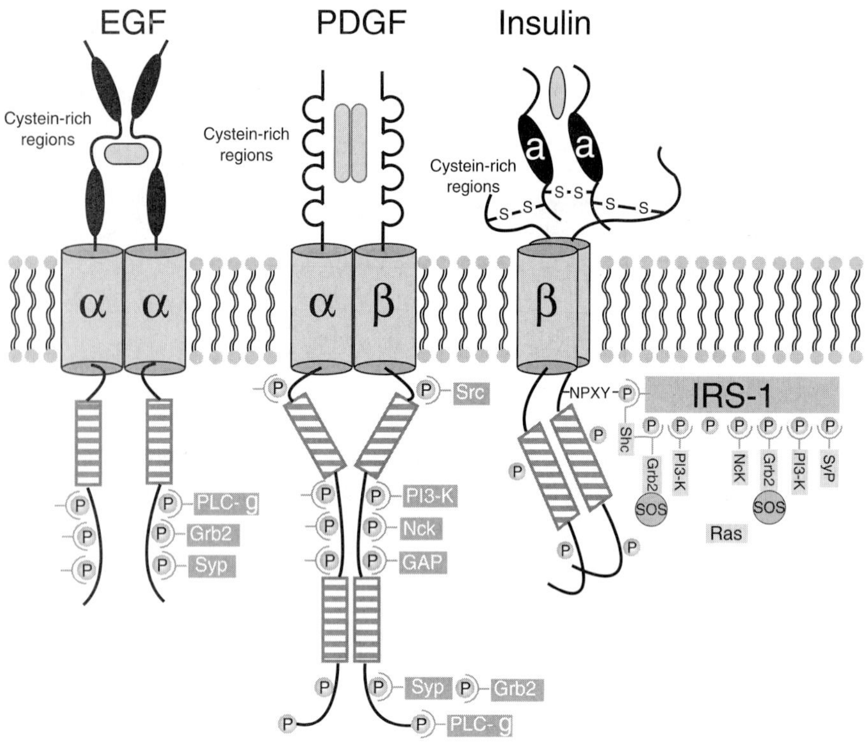

FIGURE 4-40. Receptors with tyrosine kinase activity. Receptors for epidermal growth factor (EGF), platelet derived growth factor (PDGF), and insulin are shown. Phosphorylated residues on the receptors are indicated by P and enzymatic domains are hatched. See text for abbreviations. (*Adapted from Conn and Melmed.*[317])

Glycine Receptors

Glycine is quite similar to GABA in acting as an inhibitory neurotransmitter, particularly in the spinal cord. The glycine receptor is quite similar to the $GABA_A$ receptor as is its subunit structure. Further, there is significant amino acid sequence identity between the $GABA_A$ receptor and the glycine receptor. As is the case with the $GABA_A$ receptor, the glycine receptor is also a chloride channel. The convulsant strychnine acts at the glycine receptor in a manner similar to that of picrotoxin at the $GABA_A$ receptor, binding to the channel, and preventing chloride conductance.

The 5HT3 Serotonin Receptor

More than a dozen members of several serotonin receptor families have been cloned to date. With one exception, they are all G protein-coupled receptors. The exception is the 5HT3 receptor, which is an ionotrophic receptor. The 5HT3 receptor has considerable similarity with other ligand-gated channels. Each subunit of the 5HT3 receptor has four hydrophobic transmembrane domains and a large amino terminal extracellular domain. There is also a long cytoplasmic loop between the third and the fourth membrane domains. The expressed 5HT3 receptor is a cation channel, but its precise physiological role is still unclear.

GROWTH FACTOR SIGNALING: RECEPTORS WITH TYROSINE KINASE ACTIVITY

Hormone and growth factor receptors involved in cell growth, metabolism, and differentiation possess tyrosine kinase activity. Some of the hormones which have receptors with tyrosine kinase activity are epidermal growth factor (EGF), platelet derived growth factor (PDGF), fibroblast growth factor (FGF), nerve growth factor (NGF), hepatocyte growth factor (HGF), insulin, and the insulin-like growth factors (IGF). Models for these receptor types are seen in Fig. 4-40. Regardless of the specific receptor type, most of the members of this receptor family consist of two subunits. Sometimes receptors form a homodimer and at other times, a heterodimer. Formation of a dimer, which is a result of receptor activation, leads to autophosphorylation or transphosphorylation of the receptor within its cytoplasmic domain. Consequently, other substrates for that receptor phosphate are found and phosphorylated. Signal propagation often is a result of an activation of a series of kinase cascades and is described in Fig. 4-41.

The consequences of growth factor receptor activation can be quite broad. Receptors interact with an enormous range of effectors including phospholipase Cγ, PI3 kinase, sarc kinase, and adapter proteins such as CRK, NCK, GRB2, and SAC. This "alphabet soup" is only offered to the reader so that it might be understood how a growth factor, or compound acting through a growth factor type receptor, is able to engage in the activation of a large number of processes within the cell. It is also evident from the initials that these molecules serve to effect a dialog among a variety of signal transduction systems. Another example of the growth factor receptor types and their intracellular activation is the insulin receptor. The insulin receptor (Chap. 18) phosphorylates the insulin receptor protein or insulin receptor substrate protein (IRS) at multiple tyrosine residues creating binding sites for recruitment of a number of the effectors discussed earlier which dock with the IRS protein.

Receptors with Serine and Threonine Kinase Activity

Transforming growth factor beta (TGF-β) represents a family of hormones that includes such compounds as activin, mullerian-inhibiting substance (MIS), bone morphogenic proteins (BMP),

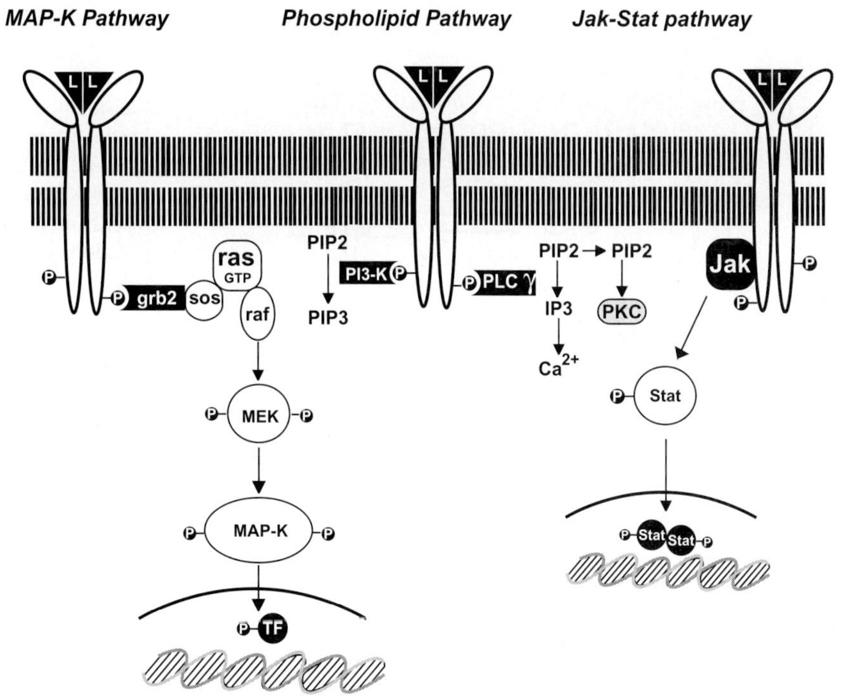

FIGURE 4-41. Signal transduction by receptor tyrosine kinases or receptors that activate cytosolic tyrosine kinases. On the left is a typical receptor protein tyrosine kinase (MAPK pathway). Hormone binding induces receptor dimerization and auto- or cross-phosphorylation on tyrosine residues. This creates binding sites for adaptor proteins, such as GRB2, or for effector enzymes, often leading to the initiation of tyrosine phosphorylation cascades. The middle segment (phospholipid pathway) shows that effector enzymes involved in phospholipid metabolism are also activated by the receptor tyrosine kinase pathway. On the right (JAK-STAT pathway) is a typical cytokine receptor superfamily protein that lacks intrinsic tyrosine kinase activity. In response to hormone binding and subunit dimerization, these receptors recruit cytoplasmic tyrosine kinases, such as the Jak kinase shown. One of several subsequent pathways leads to the activation, dimerization, and translocation to the nucleus of the Stat proteins, which are able to regulate target gene transcription directly. (*Adapted from Conn and Melmed.*[317])

and a number of other compounds. Three forms of these receptors exist, but it is not clear that the third form, type III, plays a role in signaling. The major receptor involved in signaling is the type II receptor. The type II activin receptor has been cloned; it consists of a transmembrane protein with a relatively short extracellular domain and a cytoplasmic domain which appears to contain the kinase activity.[292] Type I receptors do not appear to be able to bind ligand on their own. However, when coexpressed in vitro with a type II receptor, they appear to act as an adjuvant, a somewhat lower affinity compound which can convey signal in the presence of higher concentrations of agonist. Several type I receptors have now been cloned and they all interact similarly with the type II receptors. It is likely that the types I and II TGF β receptors form a noncovalent heteromeric complex and that both type I and type II receptors are required to complete the TGF-β signaling process. A diagram of this type of signaling is given in Fig. 4-42.

The substrates of the TGF β receptor kinases are a family of proteins known as Smad, which relay the signals from the cell-surface kinases to the nucleus. Smad proteins appear to interact with several other signaling systems and may represent a point of signal convergence for cell growth and differentiation.

Kinase Cascades Promoting Cell Growth

Sequential hormone activation of kinases (protein kinase cascades) is a common mechanism of signal transduction which allows for amplification or divergence of signaling. During the past decade several related intracellular signaling cascades, known collectively as mitogen-activated protein kinase (MAPK), have been elucidated.[293–295] Each of these signaling cascades is comprised of up to five tiers of protein kinases that display sequential activation due to protein phosphorylation. The initial step for the activation of each of these cascades is the activation of a small GTP binding protein (e.g., ras) which transmits the signal to protein kinases, commonly referred to as MAPK kinase kinase kinases (MAP4Ks) (Fig. 4-43). This initial signal is transmitted down an enzyme cascade which involves sequential phosphorylation of MAP3K-, MAPKK-, MAPK-, and MAPK-activated protein kinases (MAPKAPKs). The existence of four to five tiers in each

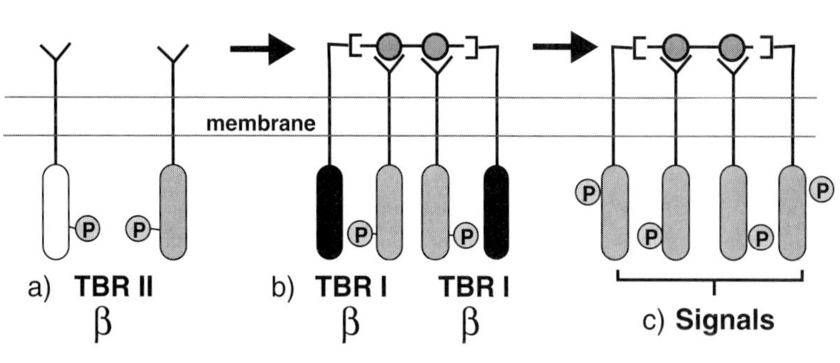

FIGURE 4-42. Signaling by TGFβ. The sequence for TGFβ signaling is shown. First (a), TGFβ binds to the phosphorylated TβRII. This allows the activated TβRII to bind TβRI (b). The activated TβRII subunits then phosphorylate TβRI (c) and the active signaling complex is complete.

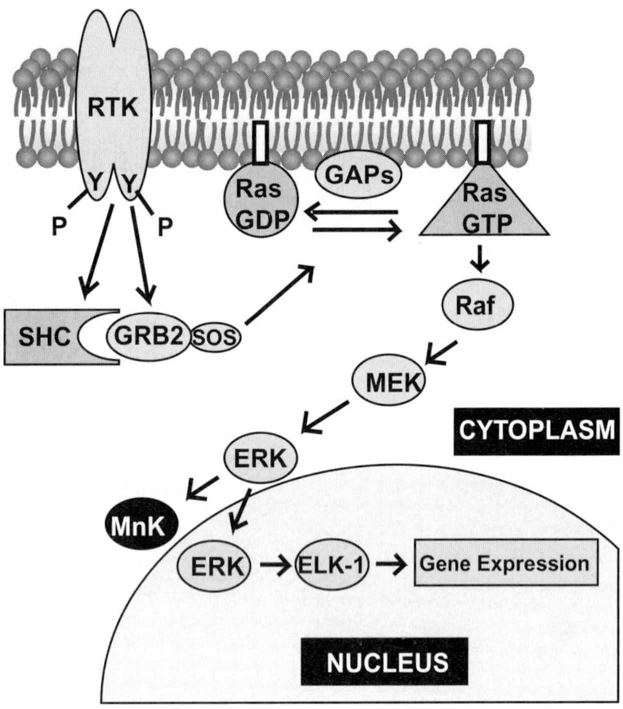

FIGURE 4-43. Ras regulation of the MAP kinase cascade. Receptor tyrosine kinases activate a series of proteins which culminate in the activation of sos (son of sevenless), an exchange factor which allows Ras-GDP to bind GTP. The activated Ras-GTP activates a series of serine/threonine kinases which culminate in the activation of transcription factors such as Elk. (*Adapted from Vojtek and Der.*[228])

of the MAPK cascades is probably essential for signal amplification, spatial and temporal signal specificity, and tight regulation of the transmitted signal. The four distinct MAPK cascades that are currently known are named according to the subgroup of their MAPK components (the ERK, JNK, SPK, p38MAPK, and BMK (ERK5) cascades). These MAPK cascades cooperate to transmit signals to their intracellular targets and thus to initiate cellular processes, such as proliferation, differentiation, development, stress response, and apoptosis.

The ERK (extracellular response kinase) cascade was the first MAPK cascade elucidated.[293] This cascade is initiated by the small G-protein Ras, which upon stimulation, causes membrane translocation and activation of the protein serine/threonine kinase, Raf1. Once activated, Raf1 continues the transmission of the signal by phosphorylating two regulatory serine residues located in the activation loop of MEK, thus, effecting full activation of the enzyme. Other kinases that can also activate MEK are A-Raf, B-Raf, Mos TPL2, and MEKK2, all of which phosphorylate the same regulatory residues of MEK. Activated MEK is a dual specificity (tyrosine and serine/threonine) protein kinase, which appears to be the only kinase capable of specifically phosphorylating and activating the next kinase in this cascade, ERK. ERK activation requires phosphorylation of two regulatory residues, threonine and tyrosine.[296] Phosphorylation of both threonine and tyrosine residues is essential for the activation of all MAPKs, but in the other cascades the identity of the middle amino acid in the TXY motif of the MAPK is different, which probably determines the specificity of the signal. In addition to activating the MAP kinase cascade, ERK appears to phosphorylate cytosolic proteins such as PLA2 or proteins which can phosphorylate nuclear targets and effect gene regulation (ELK 1 or MAKAP).[297,298] Although the activation of the ERK cascade was initially implicated in the transmission and control of mitogenic signals, this cascade is now known to be important for differentiation, development, stress response, learning and memory, and morphology determination.

ERKs are activated primarily by mitogenic signals, whereas other MAPK cascades, referred to as stress-activated protein kinase (SAPK) cascades, are activated by cellular stresses such as heat shock, UV irradiation, ischemia, and cytokines.[299] Other stress-activated MAP kinases are the c-Jun NH2-terminal kinases (JNKs; also named SAPK1) which comprise a third MAPK subgroup. As is the case with the other MAPK cascades, the JNK cascade is triggered by Rac and CDC42, which are small GTP binding proteins.[300]

No cytosolic targets have been identified for JNKs, but these enzymes appear to be major regulators of nuclear processes and, in particular, transcription. Shortly after activation, JNKs translocate to the nucleus where they bind to and activate their target transcription factors (cJun, ATF, ELK, etc.).

All the pathways mentioned are activated to some extent by distinct extracellular agents and, as a result of their action in an elaborate network, determine the outcome of each stimulation. The full dimensions of this network, the mode of regulation of its components, and the mechanism by which these cascades determine cell fates in response to various stimuli have yet to be fully elucidated. It is noteworthy, however, that in addition to activation of these kinase cascades by growth factors and the receptor kinases to which they bind and activate, several heterotrimeric G proteins have been implicated in the regulation of cell growth and proliferation. This appears to occur through the activation of PKA or PKC through Gs or Gq as well as direct interactions of Ras with $G\beta\gamma$. The possibility also exists that G12 and G13 interact directly with a number of small G proteins to activate cell growth.[301]

The Ras/MAPK pathways are normally thought to be associated with a mitogenic response. It is noteworthy, however that neurons respond to nerve growth factor (NGF) through its receptor, TRK, a receptor tyrosine kinase. Activation of TRK by NGF triggers the Ras/MAPK pathway, which results in neurite outgrowth rather than cell proliferation. Constitutive expression of activated mutants of MAPK and MEK also promote outgrowth of cellular processes.[302] This suggests that this mitogenic signaling pathway might be adapted for other purposes in nonmitotic cell types.

Protein Tyrosine Phosphatase

Protein tyrosine phosphatases such as the serine/threonine phosphatases dephosphorylate proteins which have become phosphorylated on a tyrosine residue as a result of receptor tyrosine kinases. A variety of protein tyrosine kinases have now been identified. Some are cytosolic and others appear to be transmembrane proteins. Although some cytosolic protein tyrosine phosphatases may be associated with the cytoskeleton, those which are transmembrane proteins are likely to serve both as receptors and as phosphatases. It is not clear yet which ligands actually activate these phosphatases. Nonetheless, some interesting observations have been made concerning these enzymes. For example, one form of transmembrane phosphoprotein phosphatase increases its expression in cells approaching confluence in growth. This phosphatase then inhibits cell growth by triggering a net dephosphorylation of many tyrosine residues which are often intimately involved in growth cascades as explained elsewhere in this chapter.

KINASE-INDEPENDENT ACTIONS OF CYCLIC NUCLEOTIDES

Originally, it had been suggested that all effects of cAMP and cGMP in vertebrates were due to protein phosphorylation as the result of activation of cAMP- and cGMP-dependent protein kinases. Two distinct families of cyclic nucleotide binding proteins have been identified which demonstrate functions of cAMP and cGMP independent of protein phosphorylation. These are cAMP response element binding protein (CREB) and the cAMP- and cGMP-gated ion channels.

Ion Channels Regulated by cAMP and cGMP

In vertebrate photoreceptor cells, levels of cGMP are quite high in the dark. There is also a constant depolarization, which is due to open Na^+ channels. Light-isomerization of 11-cis retinal and the attendant activation of rhodopsin causes the activation of transducin, a retinal G protein. Activated transducin binds to a portion of a retinal cGMP phosphodiesterase which, in turn, activates that enzyme and lowers cGMP in the photoreceptor. cGMP binds to the Na^+ channel and activates it. Thus, when cGMP levels are reduced, the Na^+ current is attenuated, completing the light-activation cycle. This hyperpolarizes the photoreceptor cell.[303,304]

Several analagies exist among sensory systems, and cyclic nucleotide-gated ion channels are found in other sensory systems as well. In the olfactory system, certain odorants can activate adenylyl cyclase through the Gs-like protein, G_{olf}. The cAMP produced activates a Na^+channel (Fig. 4-44). In this case, the opening of the channel and resultant depolarization of the olfactory cells represents the initial step in odorant detection.[305,306]

cAMP- and cGMP gated ion channels share structural homology with voltage-gated ion channels, but they lack voltage sensitivity. The cAMP and cGMP binding sites are not unlike those found on kinases and a single site is found on each channel subunit. Four or five of the subunits make up a cAMP- or cGMP-gated channel and the binding of nucleotide opens the channel. Increasing the number of cAMP or cGMP molecules bound facilitates ion conductance. The channels found in photoreceptors are less sensitive to cGMP (which is present at high concentrations) than the channels of the olfactory epithelium are to cAMP (which is present at very low concentrations, even in the stimulated state).

FIGURE 4-44. A cyclic nucleotide-dependent cation channel. A model of the photoreceptor channel is shown, but similar cAMP gated channels are found in olfactory and gustatory tissue.

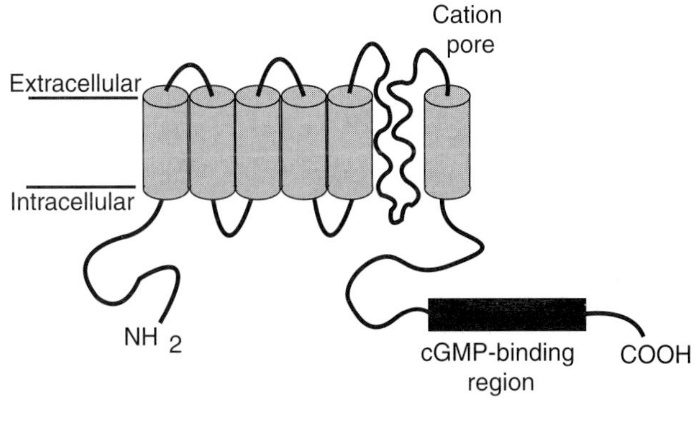

Effects of cAMP on Gene Transcription

While initial studies of cAMP signaling in vertebrates suggested that the actions of cAMP were mediated only through protein phosphorylation, the role for cAMP initially described in bacteria was to serve as a mediator of gene transcription in response to the need to induce genes required to transport and metabolize lactose.[307] This ability of cAMP to serve as a regulator of transcription is seen in eukaryotes as well. Genes stimulated by cAMP are induced through a cAMP response element (CRE). Several proteins bind to this CRE; the first to be identified was a protein called CREB (cAMP response element binding protein). CREB must be phosphorylated at ser 133 in order to be active (and bind to a CRE); the basis for this is that phosphorylated CREB binds to an accessory binding protein called CBP (CREB binding protein). The phosphorylation of CREB is due to the activated catalytic subunit of PKA, which translocates into the nucleus. It is noteworthy that a MAPK substrate, p90rsk, also phosphorylates CREB. This provides a locus for interaction between heterotrimeric G proteins and receptor tyrosine kinases.[308]

The CRE binding protein CREM is a similar cAMP-responsive transcription factor to CREB. CREM is also activated by cAMP-dependent phosphorylation. In addition to ser 133, CREM has regulatory sites which are phosphorylated by Ca^{2+}/calmodulin-activated protein kinases. Unlike CREB, several forms of CREM are produced by alternative RNA splicing, and some of these are antagonistic to transcription. One of those alternatively spliced CREM gene products is a cAMP-inducible early repressor ICER. The production of ICER and CREM from the same gene allows for a dual regulation of hormone or neurotransmitter-induced gene transcription (Fig. 4-45). Further regulation of this process is provided by the activation of specific phosphatases, which dephosphorylate, and thereby inactivate CREB and CREM.

FIGURE 4-45. Activation of cAMP response element binding protein (CREB). cAMP activates PKA and the activated catalytic subunits (or CAM Kinase) phosphorylate CREB. Activated CREB binds to a cAMP response element (CRE) and initiates transcription. Further details are provided in the text.

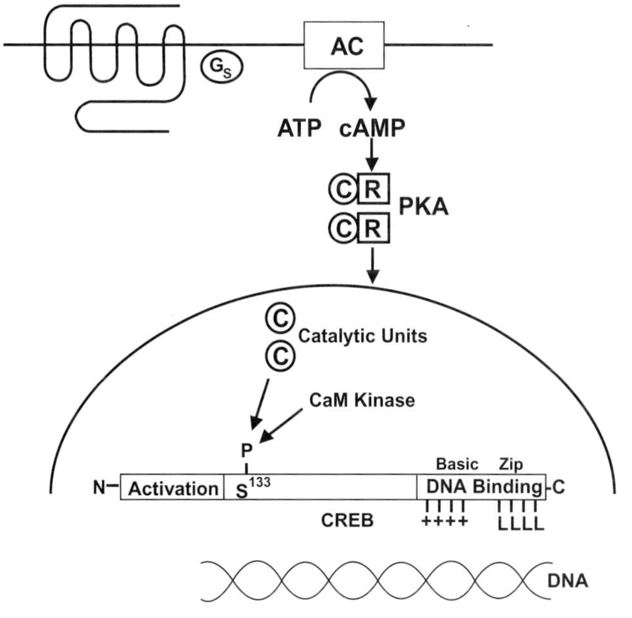

While the expression of CREB is relatively constant and widely distributed among tissues, the products of the CREM gene show distinct developmental and tissue specific regulation.[308] This allows for unique regulation of gene transcription. For example, genes involved in biological rhythms appear to use CREM/ICER to achieve their unique periodic expression and disappearance.[308]

CROSSTALK AMONG HORMONES OR NEUROTRANSMITTERS

This chapter has alluded continually to the interaction among the various signaling systems. This allows for a rich, varied, and pristine regulation of response to any given hormone or neurotransmitter. A cell that responds to a steroid hormone (including a nerve cell) is likely to possess receptors on its surface for growth factors as well as receptors for agonists which couple to G proteins.

Nuclear receptors are modified by cAMP- or Ca^{2+}/calmodulin-dependent protein kinases. Pathways normally associated with cell growth can respond to agents (e.g., opioid peptides or catecholamines) which are not normally thought to regulate those pathways.[309,310] Receptors that couple to G proteins are modified by phosphorylation induced by agonists which do not bind to those receptors. Calcium and cAMP modify the enzymes which regulate the level of cAMP or calcium in the cell. Thus calcium and cAMP feed back or feed forward to modify hormone response. Finally, in addition to G proteins modifying the cytoskeleton, elements of the cytoskeleton appear to modify G protein signaling.[267,311,312] The possibility that some continuum exists between cell form and cell function adds another layer of embroidery to this already elaborate tapestry of endocrine regulation.

Acknowledgments Thanks to Karin Riggs for making the majority of the figures and to Jane Guttman for invaluable assistance in assembling this chapter.

REFERENCES

1. Zawarynski P, Tallerico T, Seeman P, et al: Dopamine D2 receptor dimers in human and rat brain. *FEBS Lett* 441:383, 1998.
2. Clark AJ: General pharmacology, in: Heffter H (ed): *Handbuch der Experimental. Pharmakologie*, Berlin, Springer, 1937.
3. Jensen EV, Jacobson HI: Basic guides to the mechanism of hormone action. *Recent Prog Horm Res* 18:387, 1962.
4. Welshons WV, Lieberman ME, Gorski J: Nuclear localization of unoccupied oestrogen receptors. *Nature* 307:747, 1984.
5. King WJ, Greene GL: Monoclonal antibodies localize oestrogen receptor in the nuclei of target cells. *Nature* 307:745, 1984.
6. Perrot-Applanat M, Logeat F, Groyer-Picard MT, et al: Immunocytochemical study of mammalian progesterone receptor using monoclonal antibodies. *Endocrinology* 116:1473, 1985.
7. Gasc JM, Renoir JM, Radanyi C, et al: Progesterone receptor in the chick oviduct: An immunohistochemical study with antibodies to distinct receptor components. *J Cell Biol* 99:1193, 1984.
8. Sar M, Lubahn DB, French FS, et al: Immunohistochemical localization of the androgen receptor in rat and human tissues. *Endocrinology* 127:3180, 1990.
9. Antakly T, Eisen HJ: Immunocytochemical localization of glucocorticoid receptor in target cells. *Endocrinology* 115:1984, 1984.
10. Bernard PA, Joh TH: Characterization and immunocytochemical demonstration of glucocorticoid receptor using antisera specific to transformed receptor. *Arch Biochem Biophys* 229:466, 1984.
11. Wikstrom AC, Bakke O, Okret S, et al: Intracellular localization of the glucocorticoid receptor: Evidence for cytoplasmic and nuclear localization. *Endocrinology* 120:1232, 1987.
12. Brink M, Humbel BM, De Kloet ER, et al: The unliganded glucocorticoid receptor is localized in the nucleus, not in the cytoplasm. *Endocrinology* 130:3575, 1992.
13. Cidlowski JA, Bellingham DL, Powell-Oliver FE, et al: Novel antipeptide antibodies to the human glucocorticoid receptor: Recognition of multiple receptor forms in vitro and distinct localization of cytoplasmic and nuclear receptors. *Mol Endocrinol* 4:1427, 1990.
14. Welshons WV, Krummel BM, Gorski J: Nuclear localization of unoccupied receptors for glucocorticoids, estrogens, and progesterone in GH3 cells. *Endocrinology* 117:2140, 1985.
15. Dalman FC, Koenig RJ, Perdew GH, et al: In contrast to the glucocorticoid receptor, the thyroid hormone receptor is translated in the DNA binding state and is not associated with hsp90. *J Biol Chem* 265:3615, 1990.
16. Dalman FC, Sturzenbecker LJ, Levin AA, et al: Retinoic acid receptor belongs to a subclass of nuclear receptors that do not form "docking" complexes with hsp90. *Biochemistry* 30:5605, 1991.
17. Conneely OM, Sullivan WP, Toft DO, et al: Molecular cloning of the chicken progesterone receptor. *Science* 233:767, 1986.
18. Gronemeyer H, Turcotte B, Quirin-Stricker C, et al: The chicken progesterone receptor: Sequence, expression and functional analysis. *EMBO J* 6:3985, 1987.
19. Misrahi M, Atger M, d'Auriol L, et al: Complete amino acid sequence of the human progesterone receptor deduced from cloned cDNA. *Biochem Biophys Res Commun* 143:740, 1987.
20. Koike S, Sakai M, Muramatsu M: Molecular cloning and characterization of rat estrogen receptor cDNA. *Nucleic Acids Res* 15:2499, 1987.
21. Walter P, Green S, Greene G, et al: Cloning of the human estrogen receptor cDNA. *Proc Natl Acad Sci USA* 82:7889, 1985.
22. Tremblay GB, Tremblay A, Copeland NG, et al: Cloning, chromosomal localization, and functional analysis of the murine estrogen receptor beta. *Mol Endocrinol* 11:353, 1997.
23. Kuiper GG, Enmark E, Pelto-Huikko M, et al: Cloning of a novel receptor expressed in rat prostate and ovary. *Proc Natl Acad Sci USA* 93:5925, 1996.
24. Mosselman S, Polman J, Dijkema R: ER beta: Identification and characterization of a novel human estrogen receptor. *FEBS Lett* 392:49, 1996.
25. Chang CS, Kokontis J, Liao ST: Molecular cloning of human and rat complementary DNA encoding androgen receptors. *Science* 240:324, 1988.
26. Lubahn DB, Joseph DR, Sullivan PM, et al: Cloning of human androgen receptor complementary DNA and localization to the X chromosome. *Science* 240:327, 1988.
27. Hollenberg SM, Weinberger C, Ong ES, et al: Primary structure and expression of a functional human glucocorticoid receptor cDNA. *Nature* 318:635, 1985.
28. Miesfeld R, Rusconi S, Godowski PJ, et al: Genetic complementation of a glucocorticoid receptor deficiency by expression of cloned receptor cDNA. *Cell* 46:389, 1986.
29. Murray JC, Smith RF, Ardinger HA, et al: RFLP for the glucocorticoid receptor (GRL) located at 5q11-5q13. *Nucleic Acids Res* 15:6765, 1987.
30. Arriza JL, Weinberger C, Cerelli G, et al: Cloning of human mineralocorticoid receptor complementary DNA: Structural and functional kinship with the glucocorticoid receptor. *Science* 237:268, 1987.
31. Patel PD, Sherman TG, Goldman DJ, et al: Molecular cloning of a mineralocorticoid (type I) receptor complementary DNA from rat hippocampus. *Mol Endocrinol* 3:1877, 1989.
32. Thompson CC, Weinberger C, Lebo R, et al: Identification of a novel thyroid hormone receptor expressed in the mammalian central nervous system. *Science* 237:1610, 1987.
33. Benbrook D, Pfahl M: A novel thyroid hormone receptor encoded by a cDNA clone from a human testis library. *Science* 238:788, 1987.
34. Giguere V, Ong ES, Segui P, et al: Identification of a receptor for the morphogen retinoic acid. *Nature* 330:624, 1987.
35. Petkovich M, Brand NJ, Krust A, et al: A human retinoic acid receptor which belongs to the family of nuclear receptors. *Nature* 330:444, 1987.

36. Zelent A, Krust A, Petkovich M, et al: Cloning of murine alpha and beta retinoic acid receptors and a novel receptor gamma predominantly expressed in skin. *Nature* 339:714, 1989.
37. Krust A, Kastner P, Petkovich M, et al: A third human retinoic acid receptor, hRAR-gamma. *Proc Natl Acad Sci USA* 86:5310, 1989.
38. Mangelsdorf DJ, Ong ES, Dyck JA, et al: Nuclear receptor that identifies a novel retinoic acid response pathway. *Nature* 345:224, 1990.
39. Mangelsdorf DJ, Borgmeyer U, Heyman RA, et al: Characterization of three RXR genes that mediate the action of 9-cis retinoic acid. *Genes Dev* 6:329, 1992.
40. Hughes MR, Malloy PJ, Kieback DG, et al: Point mutations in the human vitamin D receptor gene associated with hypocalcemic rickets. *Science* 242:1702, 1988.
41. McDonnell DP, Mangelsdorf DJ, Pike JW, et al: Molecular cloning of complementary DNA encoding the avian receptor for vitamin D. *Science* 235:1214, 1987.
42. Baker AR, McDonnell DP, Hughes M, et al: Cloning and expression of full-length cDNA encoding human vitamin D receptor. *Proc Natl Acad Sci USA* 85:3294, 1988.
43. Conneely OM, Maxwell BL, Toft DO, et al: The A and B forms of the chicken progesterone receptor arise by alternate initiation of translation of a unique mRNA. *Biochem Biophys Res Commun* 149:493, 1987.
44. Kastner P, Krust A, Turcotte B, et al: Two distinct estrogen-regulated promoters generate transcripts encoding the two functionally different human progesterone receptor forms A and B. *EMBO J* 9:1603, 1990.
45. Sap J, Munoz A, Damm K, et al: The c-erb-A protein is a high-affinity receptor for thyroid hormone. *Nature* 324:635, 1986.
46. Weinberger C, Thompson CC, Ong ES, et al: The c-erb-A gene encodes a thyroid hormone receptor. *Nature* 324:641, 1986.
47. Hodin RA, Lazar MA, Wintman BI, et al: Identification of a thyroid hormone receptor that is pituitary-specific. *Science* 244:76, 1989.
48. Izumo S, Mahdavi V: Thyroid hormone receptor alpha isoforms generated by alternative splicing differentially activate myosin HC gene transcription. *Nature* 334:539, 1988.
49. Mitsuhashi T, Tennyson GE, Nikodem VM: Alternative splicing generates messages encoding rat c-erbA proteins that do not bind thyroid hormone. *Proc Natl Acad Sci USA* 85:5804, 1988.
50. Lazar MA, Hodin RA, Darling DS, et al: Identification of a rat c-erbA alpha-related protein which binds deoxyribonucleic acid but does not bind thyroid hormone. *Mol Endocrinol* 2:893, 1988.
51. Nakai A, Seino S, Sakurai A, et al: Characterization of a thyroid hormone receptor expressed in human kidney and other tissues. *Proc Natl Acad Sci USA* 85:2781, 1988.
52. Miyajima N, Horiuchi R, Shibuya Y, et al: Two erbA homologs encoding proteins with different T3 binding capacities are transcribed from opposite DNA strands of the same genetic locus. *Cell* 57:31, 1989.
53. Lazar MA, Hodin RA, Chin WW: Human carboxyl-terminal variant of alpha-type c-erbA inhibits trans-activation by thyroid hormone receptors without binding thyroid hormone. *Proc Natl Acad Sci USA* 86:7771, 1989.
54. Brand N, Petkovich M, Krust A, et al: Identification of a second human retinoic acid receptor. *Nature* 332:850, 1988.
55. Benbrook D, Lernhardt E, Pfahl M: A new retinoic acid receptor identified from a hepatocellular carcinoma. *Nature* 333:669, 1988.
56. Ishikawa T, Umesono K, Mangelsdorf DJ, et al: A functional retinoic acid receptor encoded by the gene on human chromosome 12. *Mol Endocrinol* 4:837, 1990.
57. Heyman RA, Mangelsdorf DJ, Dyck JA, et al: 9-cis retinoic acid is a high affinity ligand for the retinoid X receptor. *Cell* 68:397, 1992.
58. Levin AA, Sturzenbecker LJ, Kazmer S, et al: 9-cis retinoic acid stereoisomer binds and activates the nuclear receptor RXR alpha. *Nature* 355:359, 1992.
59. Lubahn DB, Moyer JS, Golding TS, et al: Alteration of reproductive function but not prenatal sexual development after insertional disruption of the mouse estrogen receptor gene. *Proc Natl Acad Sci USA* 90:11162, 1993.
60. Eddy EM, Washburn TF, Bunch DO, et al: Targeted disruption of the estrogen receptor gene in male mice causes alteration of spermatogenesis and infertility. *Endocrinology* 137:4796, 1996.
61. Cooke PS, Buchanan DL, Young P, et al: Stromal estrogen receptors mediate mitogenic effects of estradiol on uterine epithelium. *Proc Natl Acad Sci USA* 94:6535, 1997.
62. Buchanan DL, Setiawan T, Lubahn DB, et al: Tissue compartment-specific estrogen receptor-a participation in the mouse uterine epithelial secretory response. *Endocrinology* 140:484, 1999.
63. Buchanan DL, Kurita T, Taylor JA, et al: Role of stromal and epithelial estrogen receptors in vaginal epithelial proliferation, stratification, and cornification. *Endocrinology* 139:4345, 1998.
64. Krege JH, Hodgin JB, Couse JF, et al: Generation and reproductive phenotypes of mice lacking estrogen receptor beta. *Proc Natl Acad Sci USA* 95:15677, 1998.
65. Lydon JP, DeMayo FJ, Funk CR, et al: Mice lacking progesterone receptor exhibit pleiotropic reproductive abnormalities. *Genes Dev* 9:2266, 1995.
66. Kurita T, Young P, Brody JR, et al: Stromal progesterone receptors mediate the inhibitory effects of progesterone on estrogen-induced uterine epithelial cell deoxyribonucleic acid synthesis. *Endocrinology* 139:4708, 1998.
67. Berger S, Bleich M, Schmid W, et al: Mineralocorticoid receptor knockout mice: Pathophysiology of Na^+ metabolism. *Proc Natl Acad Sci USA* 95:9424, 1998.
68. Forrest D, Hanebuth E, Smeyne RJ, et al: Recessive resistance to thyroid hormone in mice lacking thyroid hormone receptor beta: Evidence for tissue-specific modulation of receptor function. *EMBO J* 15:3006, 1996.
69. Weiss RE, Forrest D, Pohlenz J, et al: Thyrotropin regulation by thyroid hormone in thyroid hormone receptor beta-deficient mice. *Endocrinology* 138:3624, 1997.
70. Weiss RE, Murata Y, Cua K, et al: Thyroid hormone action on liver, heart, and energy expenditure in thyroid hormone receptor beta-deficient mice. *Endocrinology* 139:4945, 1998.
71. Wikstrom L, Johansson C, Salto C, et al: Abnormal heart rate and body temperature in mice lacking thyroid hormone receptor alpha 1. *EMBO J* 17:455, 1998.
72. Li YC, Pirro AE, Amling M, et al: Targeted ablation of the vitamin D receptor: An animal model of vitamin D-dependent rickets type II with alopecia. *Proc Natl Acad Sci USA* 94:9831, 1997.
73. Li YC, Amling M, Pirro AE, et al: Normalization of mineral ion homeostasis by dietary means prevents hyperparathyroidism, rickets, and osteomalacia, but not alopecia in vitamin D receptor-ablated mice. *Endocrinology* 139:4391, 1998.
74. Green S, Chambon P: Oestradiol induction of a glucocorticoid-responsive gene by a chimaeric receptor. *Nature* 325:75, 1987.
75. Kumar V, Green S, Stack G, et al: Functional domains of the human estrogen receptor. *Cell* 51:941, 1987.
76. Hard T, Kellenbach E, Boelens R, et al: Solution structure of the glucocorticoid receptor DNA-binding domain. *Science* 249:157, 1990.
77. Schwabe JW, Neuhaus D, Rhodes D: Solution structure of the DNA-binding domain of the oestrogen receptor. *Nature* 348:458, 1990.
78. Green S, Kumar V, Theulaz I, et al: The N-terminal DNA-binding 'zinc finger' of the oestrogen and glucocorticoid receptors determines target gene specificity. *EMBO J* 7:3037, 1988.
79. Mader S, Kumar V, de Verneuil H, et al: Three amino acids of the oestrogen receptor are essential to its ability to distinguish an oestrogen from a glucocorticoid-responsive element. *Nature* 338:271, 1989.
80. Danielsen M, Hinck L, Ringold GM: Two amino acids within the knuckle of the first zinc finger specify DNA response element activation by the glucocorticoid receptor. *Cell* 57:1131, 1989.
81. Umesono K, Evans RM: Determinants of target gene specificity for steroid/thyroid hormone receptors. *Cell* 57:1139, 1989.
82. Luisi BF, Xu WX, Otwinowski Z, et al: Crystallographic analysis of the interaction of the glucocorticoid receptor with DNA. *Nature* 352:497, 1991.
83. Lee MS, Kliewer SA, Provencal J, et al: Structure of the retinoid X receptor alpha DNA binding domain: A helix required for homodimeric DNA binding. *Science* 260:1117, 1993.
84. Rastinejad F, Perlmann T, Evans RM, et al: Structural determinants of nuclear receptor assembly on DNA direct repeats. *Nature* 375:203, 1995.
85. Hollenberg SM, Giguere V, Segui P, et al: Colocalization of DNA-binding and transcriptional activation functions in the human glucocorticoid receptor. *Cell* 49:39, 1987.
86. Payvar F, Wrange O, Carlstedt-Duke J, et al: Purified glucocorticoid receptors bind selectively in vitro to a cloned DNA fragment whose transcription is regulated by glucocorticoids in vivo. *Proc Natl Acad Sci USA* 78:6628, 1981.

87. Scheidereit C, Geisse S, Westphal HM, et al: The glucocorticoid receptor binds to defined nucleotide sequences near the promoter of mouse mammary tumour virus. *Nature* 304:749, 1983.
88. Renkawitz R, Schutz G, von der Ahe D, et al: Sequences in the promoter region of the chicken lysozyme gene required for steroid regulation and receptor binding. *Cell* 37:503, 1984.
89. Strahle U, Klock G, Schutz G: A DNA sequence of 15 base pairs is sufficient to mediate both glucocorticoid and progesterone induction of gene expression. *Proc Natl Acad Sci USA* 84:7871, 1987.
90. Danesch U, Gloss B, Schmid W, et al: Glucocorticoid induction of the rat tryptophan oxygenase gene is mediated by two widely separated glucocorticoid-responsive elements. *EMBO J* 6:625, 1987.
91. Scheidereit C, Westphal HM, Carlson C, et al: Molecular model of the interaction between the glucocorticoid receptor and the regulatory elements of inducible genes. *DNA* 5:383, 1986.
92. Cato AC, Miksicek R, Schutz G, et al: The hormone regulatory element of mouse mammary tumour virus mediates progesterone induction. *EMBO J* 5:2237, 1986.
93. von der Ahe D, Janich S, Scheidereit C, et al: Glucocorticoid and progesterone receptors bind to the same sites in two hormonally regulated promoters. *Nature* 313:706, 1985.
94. Parker MG, Webb P, Needham M, et al: Identification of androgen response elements in mouse mammary tumour virus and the rat prostate C3 gene. *J Cell Biochem* 35:285, 1987.
95. Ham J, Thomson A, Needham M, et al: Characterization of response elements for androgens, glucocorticoids and progestins in mouse mammary tumour virus. *Nucleic Acids Res* 16:5263, 1988.
96. Klein-Hitpass L, Tsai SY, Greene GL, et al: Specific binding of estrogen receptor to the estrogen response element. *Mol Cell Biol* 9:43, 1989.
97. Pettersson K, Grandien K, Kuiper GG, et al: Mouse estrogen receptor beta forms estrogen response element-binding heterodimers with estrogen receptor alpha. *Mol Endocrinol* 11:1486, 1997.
98. Cowley SM, Hoare S, Mosselman S, et al: Estrogen receptors alpha and beta form heterodimers on DNA. *J Biol Chem* 272:19858, 1997.
99. Umesono K, Murakami KK, Thompson CC, et al: Direct repeats as selective response elements for the thyroid hormone, retinoic acid, and vitamin D3 receptors. *Cell* 65:1255, 1991.
100. Naar AM, Boutin JM, Lipkin SM, et al: The orientation and spacing of core DNA-binding motifs dictate selective transcriptional responses to three nuclear receptors. *Cell* 65:1267, 1991.
101. Williams GR, Zavacki AM, Harney JW, et al: Thyroid hormone receptor binds with unique properties to response elements that contain hexamer domains in an inverted palindrome arrangement. *Endocrinology* 134:1888, 1994.
102. Yu VC, Delsert C, Andersen B, et al: RXR beta: A coregulator that enhances binding of retinoic acid, thyroid hormone, and vitamin D receptors to their cognate response elements. *Cell* 67:1251, 1991.
103. Leid M, Kastner P, Lyons R, et al: Purification, cloning, and RXR identity of the HeLa cell factor with which RAR or TR heterodimerizes to bind target sequences efficiently. *Cell* 68:377, 1992.
104. Marks MS, Hallenbeck PL, Nagata T, et al: H-2RIIBP (RXR beta) heterodimerization provides a mechanism for combinatorial diversity in the regulation of retinoic acid and thyroid hormone responsive genes. *EMBO J* 11:1419, 1992.
105. Kliewer SA, Umesono K, Mangelsdorf DJ, et al: Retinoid X receptor interacts with nuclear receptors in retinoic acid, thyroid hormone and vitamin D3 signalling. *Nature* 355:446, 1992.
106. Kliewer SA, Umesono K, Noonan DJ, et al: Convergence of 9-cis retinoic acid and peroxisome proliferator signalling pathways through heterodimer formation of their receptors. *Nature* 358:771, 1992.
107. Zhang XK, Hoffmann B, Tran PB, et al: Retinoid X receptor is an auxiliary protein for thyroid hormone and retinoic acid receptors. *Nature* 355:441, 1992.
108. Bugge TH, Pohl J, Lonnoy O, et al: RXR alpha, a promiscuous partner of retinoic acid and thyroid hormone receptors. *EMBO J* 11:1409, 1992.
109. Yen PM, Darling DS, Carter RL, et al: Triiodothyronine (T3) decreases binding to DNA by T3-receptor homodimers but not receptor-auxiliary protein heterodimers. *J Biol Chem* 267:3565, 1992.
110. Kurokawa R, Yu VC, Naar A, et al: Differential orientations of the DNA-binding domain and carboxy-terminal dimerization interface regulate binding site selection by nuclear receptor heterodimers. *Genes Dev* 7:1423, 1993.
111. Zechel C, Shen XQ, Chen JY, et al: The dimerization interfaces formed between the DNA binding domains of RXR, RAR and TR determine the binding specificity and polarity of the full-length receptors to direct repeats. *EMBO J* 13:1425, 1994.
112. Brzozowski AM, Pike AC, Dauter Z, et al: Molecular basis of agonism and antagonism in the oestrogen receptor. *Nature* 389:753, 1997.
113. Wagner RL, Apriletti JW, McGrath ME, et al: A structural role for hormone in the thyroid hormone receptor. *Nature* 378:690, 1995.
114. Bourguet W, Ruff M, Chambon P, et al: Crystal structure of the ligand-binding domain of the human nuclear receptor RXR-alpha. *Nature* 375:377, 1995.
115. Renaud JP, Rochel N, Ruff M, et al: Crystal structure of the RAR-gamma ligand-binding domain bound to all-trans retinoic acid. *Nature* 378:681, 1995.
116. Kopp P, Kitajima K, Jameson JL: Syndrome of resistance to thyroid hormone: Insights into thyroid hormone action. *Proc Soc Exp Biol Med* 211:49, 1996.
117. Collingwood TN, Wagner R, Matthews CH, et al: A role for helix 3 of the TR beta ligand-binding domain in coactivator recruitment identified by characterization of a third cluster of mutations in resistance to thyroid hormone. *EMBO J* 17:4760, 1998.
118. Picard D, Yamamoto KR: Two signals mediate hormone-dependent nuclear localization of the glucocorticoid receptor. *EMBO J* 6:3333, 1987.
119. Guiochon-Mantel A, Loosfelt H, Lescop P, et al: Mechanisms of nuclear localization of the progesterone receptor: Evidence for interaction between monomers. *Cell* 57:1147, 1989.
120. Ylikomi T, Bocquel MT, Berry M, et al: Cooperation of proto-signals for nuclear accumulation of estrogen and progesterone receptors. *EMBO J* 11:3681, 1992.
121. Tjian R, Maniatis T: Transcriptional activation: A complex puzzle with few easy pieces. *Cell* 77:5, 1994.
122. Buratowski S: The basics of basal transcription by RNA polymerase II. *Cell* 77:1, 1994.
123. Ing NH, Beekman JM, Tsai SY, et al: Members of the steroid hormone receptor superfamily interact with TFIIB (S300-II). *J Biol Chem* 267:17617, 1992.
124. Hadzic E, Desai-Yajnik V, Helmer E, et al: A 10-amino-acid sequence in the N-terminal A/B domain of thyroid hormone receptor alpha is essential for transcriptional activation and interaction with the general transcription factor TFIIB. *Mol Cell Biol* 15:4507, 1995.
125. Baniahmad A, Ha I, Reinberg D, et al: Interaction of human thyroid hormone receptor beta with transcription factor TFIIB may mediate target gene derepression and activation by thyroid hormone. *Proc Natl Acad Sci USA* 90:8832, 1993.
126. Blanco JC, Wang IM, Tsai SY, et al: Transcription factor TFIIB and the vitamin D receptor cooperatively activate ligand-dependent transcription. *Proc Natl Acad Sci USA* 92:1535, 1995.
127. Getzenberg RH, Pienta KJ, Ward WS, et al: Nuclear structure and the three-dimensional organization of DNA. *J Cell Biochem* 47:289, 1991.
128. Adams CC,Workman JL: Nucleosome displacement in transcription. *Cell* 72:305, 1993.
129. Wolffe AP, Pruss D: Targeting chromatin disruption: Transcription regulators that acetylate histones. *Cell* 84:817, 1996.
130. Onate SA, Tsai SY, Tsai MJ, et al: Sequence and characterization of a coactivator for the steroid hormone receptor superfamily. *Science* 270:1354, 1995.
131. Voegel JJ, Heine MJ, Zechel C, et al: TIF2, a 160 kDa transcriptional mediator for the ligand-dependent activation function AF-2 of nuclear receptors. *EMBO J* 15:3667, 1996.
132. Hong H, Kohli K, Trivedi A, et al: GRIP1, a novel mouse protein that serves as a transcriptional coactivator in yeast for the hormone binding domains of steroid receptors. *Proc Natl Acad Sci USA* 93:4948, 1996.
133. Li H, Gomes PJ, Chen JD: RAC3, a steroid/nuclear receptor-associated coactivator that is related to SRC-1 and TIF2. *Proc Natl Acad Sci USA* 94:8479, 1997.
134. Chen H, Lin RJ, Schiltz RL, et al: Nuclear receptor coactivator ACTR is a novel histone acetyltransferase and forms a multimeric activation complex with P/CAF and CBP/p300. *Cell* 90:569, 1997.

135. Anzick SL, Kononen J, Walker RL, et al: AIB1, a steroid receptor coactivator amplified in breast and ovarian cancer. *Science* 277:965, 1997.
136. Torchia J, Rose DW, Inostroza J, et al: The transcriptional coactivator p/CIP binds CBP and mediates nuclear-receptor function. *Nature* 387:677, 1997.
137. Takeshita A, Cardona GR, Koibuchi N, et al: TRAM-1, A novel 160-kDa thyroid hormone receptor activator molecule, exhibits distinct properties from steroid receptor coactivator-1. *J Biol Chem* 272: 27629, 1997.
138. Kwok RP, Lundblad JR, Chrivia JC, et al: Nuclear protein CBP is a coactivator for the transcription factor CREB. *Nature* 370:223, 1994.
139. Eckner R, Ewen ME, Newsome D, et al: Molecular cloning and functional analysis of the adenovirus E1A-associated 300-kD protein (p300) reveals a protein with properties of a transcriptional adaptor. *Genes Dev* 8:869, 1994.
140. Spencer TE, Jenster G, Burcin MM, et al: Steroid receptor coactivator-1 is a histone acetyltransferase. *Nature* 389:194, 1997.
141. Bannister AJ, Kouzarides T: The CBP co-activator is a histone acetyltransferase. *Nature* 384:641, 1996.
142. Ogryzko VV, Schiltz RL, Russanova V, et al: The transcriptional coactivators p300 and CBP are histone acetyltransferases. *Cell* 87:953, 1996.
143. Yeh S, Chang C: Cloning and characterization of a specific coactivator, ARA70, for the androgen receptor in human prostate cells. *Proc Natl Acad Sci USA* 93:5517, 1996.
144. Xu J, Qiu Y, DeMayo FJ, et al: Partial hormone resistance in mice with disruption of the steroid receptor coactivator-1 (SRC-1) gene. *Science* 279:1922, 1998.
145. Brent GA, Dunn MK, Harney JW, et al: Thyroid hormone aporeceptor represses T3-inducible promoters and blocks activity of the retinoic acid receptor. *Nature New Biol* 1:329, 1989.
146. Zhang XK, Wills KN, Graupner G, et al: Ligand-binding domain of thyroid hormone receptors modulates DNA binding and determines their bifunctional roles. *Nature New Biol* 3:169, 1991.
147. Yen PM, Wilcox EC, Hayashi Y, et al: Studies on the repression of basal transcription (silencing) by artificial and natural human thyroid hormone receptor-beta mutants. *Endocrinology* 136:2845, 1995.
148. Lezoualc'h F, Hassan AH, Giraud P, et al: Assignment of the beta-thyroid hormone receptor to 3,5,3′-triiodothyronine-dependent inhibition of transcription from the thyrotropin-releasing hormone promoter in chick hypothalamic neurons. *Mol Endocrinol* 6:1797, 1992.
149. Hollenberg AN, Monden T, Flynn TR, et al: The human thyrotropin-releasing hormone gene is regulated by thyroid hormone through two distinct classes of negative thyroid hormone response elements. *Mol Endocrinol* 9:540, 1995.
150. Chin WW, Carr FE, Burnside J, et al: Thyroid hormone regulation of thyrotropin gene expression. *Recent Prog Horm Res* 48:393, 1993.
151. Horlein AJ, Naar AM, Heinzel T, et al: Ligand-independent repression by the thyroid hormone receptor mediated by a nuclear receptor co-repressor. *Nature* 377:397, 1995.
152. Kurokawa R, Soderstrom M, Horlein A, et al: Polarity-specific activities of retinoic acid receptors determined by a co-repressor. *Nature* 377:451, 1995.
153. Lee JW, Ryan F, Swaffield JC, et al: Interaction of thyroid-hormone receptor with a conserved transcriptional mediator. *Nature* 374:91, 1995.
154. Chen JD, Evans RM: A transcriptional co-repressor that interacts with nuclear hormone receptors. *Nature* 377:454, 1995.
155. Sande S, Privalsky ML: Identification of TRACs (T3 receptor-associating cofactors), a family of cofactors that associate with, and modulate the activity of, nuclear hormone receptors. *Mol Endocrinol* 10:813, 1996.
156. Feng W, Ribeiro RC, Wagner RL, et al: Hormone-dependent coactivator binding to a hydrophobic cleft on nuclear receptors. *Science* 280:1747, 1998.
157. Alland L, Muhle R, Hou H, Jr., et al: Role for N-CoR and histone deacetylase in Sin3-mediated transcriptional repression. *Nature* 387:49, 1997.
158. Heinzel T, Lavinsky RM, Mullen TM, et al: A complex containing N-CoR, mSin3 and histone deacetylase mediates transcriptional repression. *Nature* 387:43, 1997.
159. Nagy L, Kao HY, Chakravarti D, et al: Nuclear receptor repression mediated by a complex containing SMRT, mSin3A, and histone deacetylase. *Cell* 89:373, 1997.
160. Power RF, Mani SK, Codina J, et al: Dopaminergic and ligand-independent activation of steroid hormone receptors. *Science* 254:1636, 1991.
161. Denner LA, Weigel NL, Maxwell BL, et al: Regulation of progesterone receptor-mediated transcription by phosphorylation. *Science* 250:1740, 1990.
162. Aronica SM, Katzenellenbogen BS: Stimulation of estrogen receptor-mediated transcription and alteration in the phosphorylation state of the rat uterine estrogen receptor by estrogen, cyclic adenosine monophosphate, and insulin-like growth factor-I. *Mol Endocrinol* 7:743, 1993.
163. Ignar-Trowbridge DM, Nelson KG, Bidwell MC, et al: Coupling of dual signaling pathways: Epidermal growth factor action involves the estrogen receptor. *Proc Natl Acad Sci USA* 89:4658, 1992.
164. Ignar-Trowbridge DM, Teng CT, Ross KA, et al: Peptide growth factors elicit estrogen receptor-dependent transcriptional activation of an estrogen-responsive element. *Mol Endocrinol* 7:992, 1993.
165. Golsteyn EJ, Graham JS, Goren HJ, et al: Phosphorylation status of nuclear and cytosolic androgen receptors in the rat ventral prostate. *Prostate* 14:91, 1989.
166. Auricchio F, Migliaccio A, Castoria G, et al: Phosphorylation of estradiol receptor on tyrosine and interaction of estradiol and glucocorticoid receptors with antiphosphotyrosine antibodies. *Adv Exp Med Biol* 231:519, 1988.
167. Auricchio F, Migliaccio A, Castoria G, et al: Direct evidence of in vitro phosphorylation-dephosphorylation of the estradiol-17 beta receptor. Role of Ca^{2+}-calmodulin in the activation of hormone binding sites. *J Steroid Biochem* 20:31, 1984.
168. Grandics P, Miller A, Schmidt TJ, et al: Phosphorylation in vivo of rat hepatic glucocorticoid receptor. *Biochem Biophys Res Commun* 120:59, 1984.
169. Hsieh JC, Jurutka PW, Galligan MA, et al: Human vitamin D receptor is selectively phosphorylated by protein kinase C on serine 51, a residue crucial to its trans-activation function. *Proc Natl Acad Sci USA* 88:9315, 1991.
170. Sheridan PL, Francis MD, Horwitz KB: Synthesis of human progesterone receptors in T47D cells. Nascent A- and B-receptors are active without a phosphorylation-dependent post-translational maturation step. *J Biol Chem* 264:7054, 1989.
171. Bailly A, Le Page C, Rauch M, et al: Sequence-specific DNA binding of the progesterone receptor to the uteroglobin gene: Effects of hormone, antihormone and receptor phosphorylation. *EMBO J* 5:3235, 1986.
172. Edwards DP, Kuhnel B, Estes PA, et al: Human progesterone receptor binding to mouse mammary tumor virus deoxyribonucleic acid: Dependence on hormone and nonreceptor nuclear factor(s). *Mol Endocrinol* 3:381, 1989.
173. Denner LA, Weigel NL, Schrader WT, et al: Hormone-dependent regulation of chicken progesterone receptor deoxyribonucleic acid binding and phosphorylation. *Endocrinology* 125:3051, 1989.
174. Howard KJ, Holley SJ, Yamamoto KR, et al: Mapping the HSP90 binding region of the glucocorticoid receptor. *J Biol Chem* 265: 11928, 1990.
175. Pratt WB, Jolly DJ, Pratt DV, et al: A region in the steroid binding domain determines formation of the non-DNA-binding, 9 S glucocorticoid receptor complex. *J Biol Chem* 263:267, 1988.
176. Giguere V, Hollenberg SM, Rosenfeld MG, et al: Functional domains of the human glucocorticoid receptor. *Cell* 46:645, 1986.
177. Godowski PJ, Rusconi S, Miesfeld R, et al: Glucocorticoid receptor mutants that are constitutive activators of transcriptional enhancement. *Nature* 325:365, 1987.
178. Rusconi S, Yamamoto KR: Functional dissection of the hormone and DNA binding activities of the glucocorticoid receptor. *EMBO J* 6:1309, 1987.
179. Nemoto T, Mason GG, Wilhelmsson A, et al: Activation of the dioxin and glucocorticoid receptors to a DNA binding state under cell-free conditions. *J Biol Chem* 265:2269, 1990.
180. Rall TW, Sutherland EW, Berthet J: The relationship of epinephrine and glucagon to liver phosphorylase IV. Effect of epinephrine and glucagon on the reactivation of phosphorylase in liver homogenates. *J Biol Chem* 224:463, 1957.
181. Rall T, Sutherland E: Formation of a cyclic adenine ribonucleotide by tissue particles. *J Biol Chem* 232:1065, 1958.

182. Rodbell M, Birnbaumer L, Pohl SL, et al: The reaction of glucagon with its receptor: Evidence for discrete regions of activity and binding in the glucagon molecule. *Proc Natl Acad Sci USA* 68:909, 1971.
183. Frielle T, Collins S, Daniel KW, et al: Cloning of the cDNA for the human beta 1-adrenergic receptor. *Proc Natl Acad Sci USA* 84:7920, 1987.
184. Shorr RG, Lefkowitz RJ, Caron MG: Purification of the beta-adrenergic receptor. Identification of the hormone binding subunit. *J Biol Chem* 256:5820, 1981.
185. Dulac C, Axel R: Expression of candidate pheromone receptor genes in vomeronasal neurons. *Chem Senses* 23:467, 1998.
186. Dohlman HG, Thorner J, Caron MG, et al: Model systems for the study of seven-transmembrane-segment receptors. *Annu Rev Biochem* 60:653, 1991.
187. Rasenick MM: G's (a poem). *Trends in Biochemical Science* 17:71, 1992.
188. Altenbach C, Marti T, Khorana HG, et al: Transmembrane protein structure: Spin labeling of bacteriorhodopsin mutants. *Science* 248:1088, 1990.
189. Hubbell WL, Fung BK: The structure and chemistry of rhodopsin: Relationship to models of function. *Soc Gen Physiol Ser* 33:17, 1979.
190. Lanyi JK: Understanding structure and function in the light-driven proton pump bacteriorhodopsin. *J Struct Biol* 124:164, 1998.
191. Ji TH, Grossmann M, Ji I: G protein-coupled receptors. I. Diversity of receptor-ligand interactions. *J Biol Chem* 273:17299, 1998.
192. Gether U, Kobilka BK: G protein-coupled receptors. II. Mechanism of agonist activation. *J Biol Chem* 273:17979, 1998.
193. Strader CD, Fong TM, Tota MR, et al: Structure and function of G protein-coupled receptors. *Annu Rev Biochem* 63:101, 1994.
194. Funk CD, Furci L, Moran N, et al: Point mutation in the seventh hydrophobic domain of the human thromboxane A2 receptor allows discrimination between agonist and antagonist binding sites. *Mol Pharmacol* 44:934, 1993.
195. Perez HD, Vilander L, Andrews WH, et al: Human formyl peptide receptor ligand binding domain(s). Studies using an improved mutagenesis/expression vector reveal a novel mechanism for the regulation of receptor occupancy. *J Biol Chem* 269:22485, 1994.
196. Fay SP, Domalewski MD, Sklar LA: Evidence for protonation in the human neutrophil formyl peptide receptor binding pocket. *Biochemistry* 32:1627, 1993.
197. Stroop SD, Nakamuta H, Kuestner RE, et al: Determinants for calcitonin analog interaction with the calcitonin receptor N-terminus and transmembrane-loop regions. *Endocrinology* 137:4752, 1996.
198. Unson CG, Cypess AM, Wu CR, et al: Antibodies against specific extracellular epitopes of the glucagon receptor block glucagon binding. *Proc Natl Acad Sci USA* 93:310, 1996.
199. Vu TK, Hung DT, Wheaton VI, et al: Molecular cloning of a functional thrombin receptor reveals a novel proteolytic mechanism of receptor activation. *Cell* 64:1057, 1991.
200. Lerner DJ, Chen M, Tram T, et al: Agonist recognition by proteinase-activated receptor 2 and thrombin receptor. Importance of extracellular loop interactions for receptor function. *J Biol Chem* 271:13943, 1996.
201. Grossmann M, Weintraub BD, Szkudlinski MW: Novel insights into the molecular mechanisms of human thyrotropin action: Structural, physiological, and therapeutic implications for the glycoprotein hormone family. *Endocr Rev* 18:476, 1997.
202. Takahashi K, Tsuchida K, Tanabe Y, et al: Role of the large extracellular domain of metabotropic glutamate receptors in agonist selectivity determination. *J Biol Chem* 268:19341, 1993.
203. Kubo Y, Miyashita T, Murata Y: Structural basis for a Ca^{2+}-sensing function of the metabotropic glutamate receptors. *Science* 279:1722, 1998.
204. Pauwels PJ, Wurch T: Review: Amino acid domains involved in constitutive activation of G-protein-coupled receptors. *Mol Neurobiol* 17:109, 1998.
205. Kjelsberg MA, Cotecchia S, Ostrowski J, et al: Constitutive activation of the alpha 1B-adrenergic receptor by all amino acid substitutions at a single site. Evidence for a region which constrains receptor activation. *J Biol Chem* 267:1430, 1992.
206. Lefkowitz RJ, Cottechia S, Samama P, et al: Constitutive activity of receptors coupled to guanine nucleotide regulatory proteins. *Trends in Pharm. Sci.* 14:303, 1993.
207. Scheer A, Fanelli F, Costa T, et al: Constitutively active mutants of the alpha 1B-adrenergic receptor: Role of highly conserved polar amino acids in receptor activation. *EMBO J* 15:3566, 1996.
208. Cohen GB, Yang T, Robinson PR, et al: Constitutive activation of opsin: Influence of charge at position 134 and size at position 296. *Biochemistry* 32:6111, 1993.
209. Shenker A, Laue L, Kosugi S, et al: A constitutively activating mutation of the luteinizing hormone receptor in familial male precocious puberty. *Nature* 365:652, 1993.
210. Tiberi M, Caron MG: High agonist-independent activity is a distinguishing feature of the dopamine D1B receptor subtype. *J Biol Chem* 269:27925, 1994.
211. Costa T, Herz A: Antagonists with negative intrinsic activity at sigma opioid receptors coupled to GTP-binding proteins. *Proc Natl Acad Sci* 86:7321, 1989.
212. Samama P, Cotecchia P, Costa T, et al: A mutation-induced activated state of the $\beta 2$ adrenergic receptor: Extenting the ternary complex theory. *J Biol Chem* 268:4625, 1993.
213. Rodbell M, Krans HM, Pohl SL, et al: The glucagon-sensitive adenyl cyclase system in plasma membranes of rat liver. IV. Effects of guanylnucleotides on binding of ^{125}I-glucagon. *J Biol Chem* 246:1872, 1971.
214. Benovic JL, Bouvier M, Caron MG, et al: Regulation of adenylyl cyclase-coupled β-adrenergic receptor. *Annu Rev Cell Biol* 4:405, 1988.
215. Benovic JL, Pike LJ, Cerione RA, et al: Phosphorylation of mammalian β-adrenergic receptor by cyclic AMP-dependent protein kinase: Regulation of the rate of receptor phosphorylation and dephosphorylation by agonist occupancy and effects on coupling of the receptor to the stimulatory guanine nucleotide regulatory protein. *J Biol Chem* 260:7094, 1985.
216. Krupnick JG, Benovic JL: The role of receptor kinases and arrestins in G protein-coupled receptor regulation. *Annu Rev Pharmacol Toxicol* 38:289, 1998.
217. Hosey MM, DebBurman SK, Pals-Rylaarsdam R, et al: The role of G-protein coupled receptor kinases in the regulation of muscarinic cholinergic receptors. *Prog Brain Res* 109:169, 1996.
218. Benovic JL, Onorato JJ, Caron MG, et al: Regulation of G protein-coupled receptors by agonist-dependent phosphorylation. *Soc Gen Physiol Ser* 45:87, 1990.
219. Barak LS, Warabi K, Feng X, et al: Real-time visualization of the cellular redistribution of G protein-coupled receptor kinase 2 and beta-arrestin 2 during homologous desensitization of the substance P receptor. *J Biol Chem* 274:7565, 1999.
220. Gilman AG: G-proteins: Transducers of receptor-generated signals. *Annu Rev Biochem* 56:615, 1987.
221. Neer EJ, Clapham DE: Roles of G protein subunits in transmembrane signalling. *Nature* 333:129, 1988.
222. Rodbell M: The role of hormone receptors and GTP-regulatory proteins in membrane transduction. *Nature* 284:17, 1980.
223. Halliday KR: Regional homology in GTP-binding proto-oncogene products and elongation factors. *J Cyclic Nucleo Prot Phos Res* 9:435, 1984.
224. Noel JP, Hamm HE, Sigler PB: The 2.2 Å crystal structure of transducin-α complexed with GTPγS. *Nature* 366:654, 1993.
225. Mixon MB, Lee E, Coleman DE, et al: Tertiary and quaternary structural changes in Gia1 induced by GTP hydrolysis. *Science* 270:954, 1995.
226. Hamm HE: The many faces of G protein signaling. *J Biol Chem* 273:669, 1998.
227. Gill DM, Meren R: ADP-ribosylation of membrane proteins catalyzed by cholera toxin: Basis of the activation of adenylate cyclase. *Proc Natl Acad Sci USA* 75:3050, 1978.
228. Vojtek AB, Der CJ: Increasing complexity of the ras signaling pathway. *J Biol Chem* 273:19925, 1998.
229. Dohlman HG, Thorner J: RGS proteins and signaling by heterotrimeric G proteins. *J Biol Chem* 272:3871, 1997.
230. Koelle MR, Horvitz HR: EGL-10 regulates G protein signaling in the C. elegans nervous system and shares a conserved domain with many mammalian proteins. *Cell* 84:115, 1996.
231. De Vries L, Mousli M, Wurmser A, et al: GAIP, a protein that specifically interacts with the trimeric G protein G alpha i3, is a member of a protein family with a highly conserved core domain. *Proc Natl Acad Sci USA* 92:11916, 1995.

232. Berman DM, Gilman AG: Mammalian RGS proteins: Barbarians at the gate. *J Biol Chem* 273:1269, 1998.
233. Cassel D, Selinger Z: Catecholamine-stimulated GTPase activity in turkey erythrocyte membranes. *Biochim Biophys Acta* 452:538, 1976.
234. Sternweis PC, Gilman AG: Aluminum: A requirement for activation of the regulatory component of adenylate cyclase by fluoride. *Proc Natl Acad Sci USA* 79:4888, 1982.
235. Stein PJ, Halliday KR, Rasenick MM: Photoreceptor GTP binding protein mediates fluoride actvation of phosphodiesterase. *J Biol Chem* 260:9081, 1985.
236. Bigay J, Deterre P, Pfister C, et al: Fluoroaluminates activate transducin-GDP by mimicking the gamma-phosphate of GTP in its binding site. *FEBS Lett* 191:181, 1985.
237. Rasenick MM, Watanabe M, Lazarevic MB, et al: Synthetic peptides as probes for G protein function: Carboxyl terminal Gas peptides mimic Gs and evoke high affinity agonist binding to b-adrenergic receptors. *J Biol Chem* 269:21519, 1994.
238. Kuhn H, Hall S, Wilden U: Light-induced binding of 48-kDa protein to photoreceptor membranes is highly enhanced by phosphorylation of rhodopsin. *FEBS Lett* 176:473, 1984.
239. Ford CE, Skiba NP, Bae H, et al: Molecular basis for interactions of G protein betagamma subunits with effectors. *Science* 280:1271, 1998.
240. Basi NS, Okuya S, Rebois RV: GTP binding to Gs does not promote subunit dissociation. *Cell Signal* 8:209, 1996.
241. Rebois RV, Warner DR, Basi NS: Does subunit dissociation necessarily accompany the activation of all heterotrimeric G proteins? *Cell Signal* 9:141, 1997.
242. Tang WJ, Krupinski J, Gilman AG: Expression and characterization of calmodulin-activated (type I) adenylyl cyclase. *J Cell Biol* 266:8595, 1991.
243. Taussig R, Quarmby LM, Gilman AG: Regulation of purified type I and type II adenylylcyclases by G protein bg subunits. *J Biol Chem* 268:9, 1993.
244. Seamon KB, Daly JW: Forskolin: Its biological and chemical properties. *Adv Cyclic Nucl Prot Phos Res* 20:1, 1986.
245. Seamon KB, Padgett W, Daly JW: Forskolin: Unique diterpene activator of adenylate cyclase in membranes and in intact cells. *Proc Natl Acad Sci USA* 78:3363, 1981.
246. Sutkowski EM, Tang W, Broome CW, et al: Regulation of forskolin interactions with Type I, II, V and VI adenylyl cyclases by Gsa. *Biochemistry* 33:12852, 1994.
247. Zhang G, Liu Y, Ruoho AE, et al: Structure of the adenylyl cyclase catalytic core. *Nature* 386:247, 1997.
248. Tesmer JJ, Sunahara RK, Gilman AG, et al: Crystal structure of the catalytic domains of adenylyl cyclase in a complex with Gsalpha.GTPgammaS. *Science* 278:1907, 1997.
249. Dessauer CW, Tesmer JJ, Sprang SR, et al: Identification of a Gi alpha binding site on type V adenylyl cyclase. *J Biol Chem* 273:25831, 1998.
250. Exton JH: New developments in phospholipase D. *J Biol Chem* 272:15579, 1997.
251. Brown AM, Birnbaumer L: Direct G protein gating of ion channels. *Am J Physiol* 254:H401, 1988.
252. Sui JL, Chan K, Langan MN, et al: G protein gated potassium channels. *Adv Sec Mess Phos Res* 33:179, 1999.
253. Zamponi GW, Snutch TP: Modulation of voltage-dependent calcium channels by G proteins. *Curr Opin Neurobiol* 8:351, 1998.
254. Neer EJ, Clapham DE: Roles of G protein subunits in transmembrane signalling. *Nature* 333:129, 1988.
255. Yatani A, Mattera R, Codina J, et al: The G protein-gated atrial K^+ channel is stimulated by three distinct Gi alpha-subunits. *Nature* 336: 680, 1988.
256. Logothetis DE, Kurachi Y, Galper J, et al: The beta gamma subunits of GTP-binding proteins activate the muscarinic K^+ channel in heart. *Nature* 325:321, 1987.
257. Reuveny E, Slesinger PA, Inglese J, et al: Activation of the cloned muscarinic potassium channel by G protein beta gamma subunits. *Nature* 370:143, 1994.
258. Yatani A, Imoto Y, Codina J, et al: The stimulatory G protein of adenylyl cyclase, Gs, also stimulates dihydropyridine-sensitive Ca^{2+} channels. Evidence for direct regulation independent of phosphorylation by cAMP-dependent protein kinase or stimulation by a dihydropyridine agonist. *J Biol Chem* 263:9887, 1988.
259. Lin X, Voyno-Yasenetskaya TA, Hooley R, et al: G alpha12 differentially regulates Na^+-H^+ exchanger isoforms. *J Biol Chem* 271: 22604, 1996.
260. Voyno-Yasenetskaya TA: G proteins and $Na^+/H+$ exchange. *Biol Signals Recept* 7:118, 1998.
261. Linder M, Middleton P, Hepler J, et al: Lipid modifications of G proteins: A subunits are palmitoylated. *Biochemistry* 90:3675, 1993.
262. Ransas LA, Svoboda JR, Jaspar JR, et al: Stimulation of β adrenergic receptors of S49 lymphoma cells redistributes the a subunit of the stimulatory G protein between cytosol and membranes. *Proc Natl Acad Sci USA* 86:7900, 1989.
263. Milligan G, Mullaney I, Unson CG, et al: GTP analogues promote release of the alpha subunit of the guanine nucleotide binding protein, Gi2, from membranes of rat glioma C6 BU1 cells. *J Biochem* 254:391, 1988.
264. Levis MJ, Bourne HR: Activation of the alpha subunit of Gs in intact cells alters its abundance, rate of degradation, and membrane avidity. *J Cell Biol* 119:1297, 1992.
265. Lankes WT, Furthmayr H: Moesin: A member of the protein 4.1-talin-ezrin family of proteins. *Proc Natl Acad Sci USA* 88:8297, 1991.
266. Kozasa T, Jiang X, Hart MJ, et al: p115 RhoGEF, a GTPase activating protein for G alpha12 and G alpha13. *Science* 280:2109, 1998.
267. Rasenick M, Stein P, Bitensky M: The regulatory subunit of adenylate cyclase interacts with cytoskeletal components. *Nature* 294:560, 1981.
268. Roychowdhury S, Panda D, Wilson L, et al: G protein alpha subunits activate tubulin GTPase and modulate microtubule polymerization dynamics. *J Biol Chem* 274:13485, 1999.
269. Roychowdhury S, Rasenick MM: G protein beta1gamma2 subunits promote microtubule assembly. *J Biol Chem* 272:31576, 1997.
270. Yamazaki A, Yamazaki M, Tsuboi S, et al: Regulation of G protein function by an effector in GTP-dependent signal transduction. An inhibitory subunit of cGMP phosphodiesterase inhibits GTP hydrolysis by transducin in vertebrate rod photoreceptors. *J Biol Chem* 268:8899, 1993.
271. Huang LJ, Taylor SS: Dissecting cAMP binding domain A in the RI alpha subunit of cAMP- dependent protein kinase. Distinct subsites for recognition of cAMP and the catalytic subunit. *J Biol Chem* 273:26739, 1998.
272. Smith CM, Radzio-Andzelm E, Madhusudan, et al: The catalytic subunit of cAMP-dependent protein kinase: Prototype for an extended network of communication. *Prog Biophys Mol Biol* 71:313, 1999.
273. Jaffrey SR, Snyder SH: Nitric oxide: A neural messenger. *Annu Rev Cell Dev Biol* 11:417, 1995.
274. Snyder SH, Jaffrey SR, Zakhary R: Nitric oxide and carbon monoxide: Parallel roles as neural messengers. *Brain Res Rev* 26:167, 1998.
275. Schulman H, Heist K, Srinivasan M: Decoding Ca^{2+} signals to the nucleus by multifunctional CaM kinase. *Prog Brain Res* 105:95, 1995.
276. Cohen PT: Novel protein serine/threonine phosphatases: Variety is the spice of life. *Trends Biochem Sci* 22:245, 1997.
277. Walaas SI, Greengard P: DARPP-32, a dopamine- and adenosine 3′:5′-monophosphate-regulated phosphoprotein enriched in dopamine-innervated brain regions. I. Regional and cellular distribution in the rat brain. *J Neurosci* 4:84, 1984.
278. Lester LB, Scott JD: Anchoring and scaffold proteins for kinases and phosphatases. *Recent Prog Horm Res* 52:409, 1997.
279. Sontag E, Nunbhakdi-Craig V, Bloom GS, et al: A novel pool of protein phosphatase 2A is associated with microtubules and is regulated during the cell cycle. *J Cell Biol* 128:1131, 1995.
280. Schulz S, Waldman SA: The guanylyl cyclase family of natriuretic peptide receptors. *Vitam Horm* 57:123, 1999.
281. Drewett JG, Garbers DL: The family of guanylyl cyclase receptors and their ligands. *Endocrinol Rev* 15:135, 1994.
282. Changeux JP, Devillers-Thiery A, Galzi JL, et al: The acetylcholine receptor: A model of an allosteric membrane protein mediating intercellular communication. *Ciba Found Symp* 164:66, 1992.
283. Unwin N: Nicotinic acetylcholine receptor at 9 A resolution. *J Mol Biol* 229:1101, 1993.
284. Toyoshima C, Unwin N: Ion channel of acetylcholine receptor reconstructed from images of postsynaptic membranes. *Nature* 336:247, 1988.

285. Unwin N, Toyoshima C, Kubalek E: Arrangement of the acetylcholine receptor subunits in the resting and desensitized states, determined by cryoelectron microscopy of crystallized Torpedo postsynaptic membranes. *J Cell Biol* 107:1123, 1988.
286. Lewis TM, Harkness PC, Sivilotti LG, et al: The ion channel properties of a rat recombinant neuronal nicotinic receptor are dependent on the host cell type. *J Physiol (London)* 505:299, 1997.
287. Campos-Caro A, Smillie FI, Dominguez del Toro E, et al: Neuronal nicotinic acetylcholine receptors on bovine chromaffin cells: Cloning, expression, and genomic organization of receptor subunits. *J Neurochem* 68:488, 1997.
288. Colquhoun LM, Patrick JW: Pharmacology of neuronal nicotinic acetylcholine receptor subtypes. *Adv Pharmacol* 39:191, 1997.
289. Fuhrer C, Gautam M, Sugiyama JE, et al: Roles of rapsyn and agrin in interaction of postsynaptic proteins with acetylcholine receptors. *J Neurosci* 19:6405, 1999.
290. Wang ZZ, Mathias A, Gautam M, et al: Metabolic stabilization of muscle nicotinic acetylcholine receptor by rapsyn. *J Neurosci* 19:1998, 1999.
291. Yoshihara CM, Hall ZW: Increased expression of the 43-kD protein disrupts acetylcholine receptor clustering in myotubes. *J Cell Biol* 122:169, 1993.
292. Massague J: TGF-beta signal transduction. *Annu Rev Biochem* 67:753, 1998.
293. Seger R, Krebs EG: The MAPK signaling cascade. *FASEB J* 9:726, 1995.
294. Kyriakis JM, Avruch J: Sounding the alarm: Protein kinase cascades activated by stress and inflammation. *J Biol Chem* 271:24313, 1996.
295. Robinson MJ, Cobb MH: Mitogen-activated protein kinase pathways. *Curr Opin Cell Biol* 9:180, 1997.
296. Canagarajah BJ, Khokhlatchev A, Cobb MH, et al: Activation mechanism of the MAP kinase ERK2 by dual phosphorylation. *Cell* 90:859, 1997.
297. Marais R, Wynne J, Treisman R: The SRF accessory protein Elk-1 contains a growth factor-regulated transcriptional activation domain. *Cell* 73:381, 1993.
298. Fukunaga R, Hunter T: MNK1, a new MAP kinase-activated protein kinase, isolated by a novel expression screening method for identifying protein kinase substrates. *EMBO J* 16:1921, 1997.
299. Woodgett JR, Kyriakis JM, Avruch J, et al: Reconstitution of novel signalling cascades responding to cellular stresses. *Philos Trans R Soc Lond B Biol Sci* 351:135, 1996.
300. Crespo P, Schuebel KE, Ostrom AA, et al: Phosphotyrosine-dependent activation of Rac-1 GDP/GTP exchange by the vav proto-oncogene product. *Nature* 385:169, 1997.
301. Dhanasekaran N, Prasad MV: G protein subunits and cell proliferation. *Biol Signals Recept* 7:109, 1998.
302. Cowley S, Paterson H, Kemp P, et al: Activation of MAP kinase kinase is necessary and sufficient for PC12 differentiation and for transformation of NIH 3T3 cells. *Cell* 77:841, 1994.
303. Bitensky M, Rasenick M, Shinozawa T, et al: Altered cyclic nucleotide metabolism and the pathogenesis of hereditary retinal dystrophies. *Adv Cyclic Nucleo Res* 12:227, 1980.
304. Bitensky MW, Yamazaki A, Wheeler MA, et al: The mechanism of activation of light-activated phosphodiesterase and evidence for homology with hormone-activated adenylate cyclase. *Adv Cyclic Nucleotide Protein Phosphorylation Res* 17:227, 1984.
305. Kaupp UB: The cyclic nucleotide-gated channels of vertebrate photoreceptors and olfactory epithelium. *Trends Neurosci* 14:150, 1991.
306. Dhallan RS, Yau KW, Schrader KA, et al: Primary structure and functional expression of a cyclic nucleotide-activated channel from olfactory neurons. *Nature* 347:184, 1990.
307. Pastan I, Perlman R: Cyclic adenosine monophosphate in bacteria. *Science* 169:339, 1970.
308. Sassone-Corsi P: Coupling gene expression to cAMP signalling: Role of CREB and CREM. *Int J Biochem Cell Biol* 30:27, 1998.
309. Ignatova EG, Belcheva MM, Bohn LM, et al: Requirement of receptor internalization for opioid stimulation of mitogen-activated protein kinase: Biochemical and immunofluorescence confocal microscopic evidence. *J Neurosci* 19:56, 1999.
310. Daaka Y, Luttrell LM, Ahn S, et al: Essential role for G protein-coupled receptor endocytosis in the activation of mitogen-activated protein kinase. *J Biol Chem* 273:685, 1998.
311. Wang N, Yan K, Rasenick MM: Tubulin binds specifically to the signal-transducing proteins, Gs alpha and Gi alpha 1. *J Biol Chem* 265:1239, 1990.
312. Popova JS, Johnson GL, Rasenick MM: Chimeric G alpha s/G alpha i2 proteins define domains on G alpha s that interact with tubulin for beta-adrenergic activation of adenylyl cyclase. *J Biol Chem* 269:21748, 1994.
313. Alberts B, Bray D, Lewis J, et al: *Molecular Biology of the Cell*. New York: Garland Publishing, Inc., 1994.
314. Catt K: Molecular mechanisms of hormone action: Control of target cell function by peptide and catecholamine hormones, in Felig P, Baxter J, Frohman L (eds): *Endocrinology and Metabolism,* 3rd ed. New York, McGraw-Hill, Inc., 1995, p 92.
315. Probst WC, Snyder LA, Schuster DI, et al: Sequence alignment of the G-protein coupled receptor superfamily. *DNA Cell Biol* 11:1, 1992.
316. Pitcher JA, Freedman NJ, Lefkowitz RJ: G protein-coupled receptor kinases. *Annu Rev Biochem* 67:653, 1998.
317. Conn P, Melmed S: *Endocrinology: Basic and Clinical Principles*. Totowa: Humana Press, 1997.
318. Kandel E, Schwartz J, Jessell T: *Principles of Neural Science*. New York: McGraw-Hill, Inc., 1991.

CHAPTER 5

Hormone Assays

A. Eugene Pekary
Jerome M. Hershman

It is difficult to review in one chapter the vast literature describing the enormous array of hormonal assays now available for both clinical and research applications. We have consequently selected representative examples based on their heuristic value and their current and anticipated future applicability. Automation utilizing a broad range of these new immunoassay technologies has become commonplace, particularly in large clinical laboratories.[1] This process should accelerate as the cost of labor and quality control rise. Safety and environmental concerns will also influence future assay developments.[2] Noteworthy conceptual developments that have been reported since the last version of this chapter[3] include the combined use of monoclonal antibodies and recombinant receptors to produce an *immunofunctional assay*. These assays that coselect for both immunoreactivity and ability to bind to the physiologic receptor are particularly important for the glycoprotein hormones, which have extraordinary structural heterogeneity.[4,5] For example, disease states and therapeutic interventions have been identified that can suppress the ratio of bioactivity to immunoreactivity (B/I) of FSH by 90 percent. Low B/I isoforms of FSH, isolated from prostate cancer patients on gonadotropin suppression therapy, proved to be very effective antagonists of high B/I forms of FSH obtained from control subjects.[4] The opportunities as well as needs for future refinements in hormone assays are currently very expansive.

BIOASSAYS

Results from hormone assays performed in different laboratories must be reported in terms of a common standard. Bioassay results are usually reported in units of an *international standard* distributed by the World Health Organization. They may also be reported in units of a *reference preparation* distributed to laboratories over a more restricted geographic area.[6] Conversion factors for units of reference and units of established international standards should be provided along with assay results. Although polypeptide hormones are highly purified, small but significant contamination of reference preparations may occur and can obviate the reporting of bioassay or other assay results in terms of mass of hormone. The increasing availability of hormonal preparations derived from recombinant DNA expression in bacteria or mammalian cells should greatly simplify the development and maintenance of international protein hormone standards.[7]

Bioassays may be carried out in vivo or in vitro, using graded doses of an appropriate reference preparation or standard against which one interpolates the physiologic effect induced by the hormone contained in an unknown sample.[8]

In Vivo Assays

The McKenzie mouse bioassay exemplifies an in vivo bioassay for thyroid-stimulating activity. Mice are maintained on a low-iodine diet for 10 days to enhance their uptake of radioiodine and then are injected with $Na^{125}I$ and thyroxine or triiodothyronine.[9] On day 14, the mice receive varying doses of the thyrotropic standards and unknown preparations intravenously. Two hours later, blood is drawn for measurement of ^{125}I. Note the enhancement of the sensitivity of the assay by T_3, compared with T_4 treatment shown in Fig. 5-1. Thyrotropin, a pituitary hormone, and human chorionic gonadotropin (hCG), a placental hormone, both stimulate the release of ^{125}I-labeled thyroid hormones from the thyroid glands of these mice, although the thyrotropic activity of hCG is only one one-thousandth that of thyrotropin.

The dose-response curves of the reference preparation and unknown samples must be parallel to achieve valid assay results. Because the slopes of the thyroid stimulating hormone (TSH) and hCG dose-response curves may vary considerably from bioassay to bioassay, even for the same hormone preparation, statistical analysis for parallelism between the slopes and the homogeneity of variance of the dose-response curve for the assay standard and the unknown is imperative for each assay.[10] This TSH bioassay can detect elevated TSH concentrations in the sera of patients with myxedema, but it is not sufficiently sensitive for the measurement of normal serum TSH levels.

In vivo bioassays remain important tools in basic and pharmaceutical laboratory research.[11] They are generally very labor-intensive, however, in part because of the complexities of preparing the animal subjects and administering the test substance, perhaps in divided doses over several days or weeks, along with the large number of replications needed to compensate for the substantial variability of the response. More recently developed in vitro bioassays are usually more precise, sensitive, and specific and require less test substance.

In Vitro Assays

Graded doses of a characterized reference preparation are used to produce a standard curve relative to which the response produced by an unknown substance can be compared for homogeneity of variance, parallelism, and potency. The stimulation of cyclic

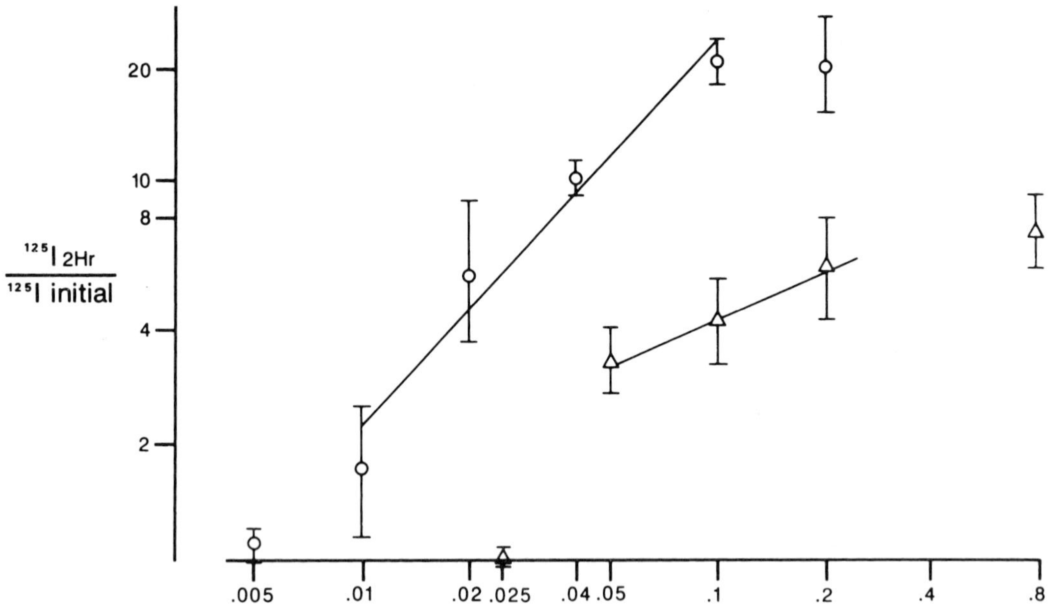

FIGURE 5-1. Dose-response curves of bovine TSH in the McKenzie bioassay using mice pretreated with T_3 (open circles) and T_4 (open triangles). Note the greater sensitivity with the former method. (*From Hershman et al.*[9])

AMP generation by FRTL-5 rat thyroid cells in response to thyrotropin (TSH) is an example of an in vitro bioassay.[12,13] FRTL-5 cells require TSH-containing media for growth in vitro. After these cells become nearly confluent, they are maintained in TSH-free media for 7 days. During this period, the number of TSH receptors on the plasma membrane of these cells increases, resulting in an increased biological response when TSH or a TSH-like substance is reintroduced into the culture medium. The cyclic AMP released in response to TSH is measured by radioimmunoassay (RIA). This assay is currently used for measuring the thyroid-stimulating immunoglobulin in patients with Graves' hyperthyroidism.[14] Several other biological responses of normal thyroid cells to TSH are retained by FRTL-5 cells, including iodide uptake, incorporation of [^{3}H]-thymidine into DNA, activation of protein kinases, and synthesis of prostaglandin E_2. These effects can also be used with FRTL-5 cells for bioassays of TSH (Fig. 5-2). A further enhancement of this in vitro bioassay has been achieved by using CHO cells stably expressing the human TSH receptor (CHO-JP09 cells).[15]

Cytochemical Assays

The cytochemical assay is a variant of the bioassay. Cytochemical bioassay responses are quantitated from histologic sections using a microdensitometer.[16] Histologic sections are prepared from specific hormone responsive tissues or cells previously exposed to graded concentrations of a standard hormone and unknowns. Several cytochemical assays are based on the chromogenic reaction resulting from a change in redox state that is induced by hormone stimulation. Histologic stains that are sensitive to those changes are used for quantitation.[17] A cytochemical bioassay for TSH has been described which quantifies the endocytosis of colloid by thyroid follicle cells.[18] The colloid vesicles fuse with lysosomes, resulting in an increase in the permeability of the lysosomal membrane. The lysosomes are then able to take up the added leucyl-β-naphthylamine substrate which is hydrolyzed by the lysosomal enzymes. The tissue segments are chilled in *n*-hexane at $-70°C$, cryostat sections are cut, and the visible reaction product is quantified by scanning densitometry.[19] Cytochemical assays are not practical

FIGURE 5-2. Effect of TNF-α on ^{125}I uptake by FRTL-5 cells stimulated by incubation with bovine TSH ($\pm$SD of triplicate wells). Levels of this and other cytokines can be greatly elevated in tissues, blood and other biological fluids during pathological processes such as cerebral malaria. (*From Pang, Hershman, Mirell, and Pekary, Endocrinology 125:76, 1989.*)

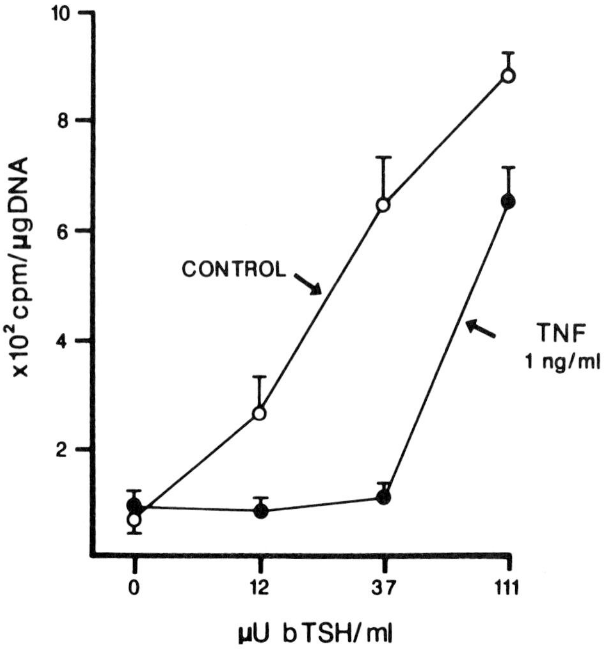

for routine clinical purposes and serve primarily as sensitive research tools.

Complementarity of In Vivo and In Vitro Assays

Comparison of in vivo and in vitro bioassays of a given hormonal substance can provide information about its in vivo transport, clearance, and enzymatic transformation prior to binding to its cellular receptor.[20,21] Comparison of the ratio of biological to immunologic activity of a hormonal preparation to that of a well-characterized hormonal standard is useful for the detection of chemical or conformational alterations which can in principle affect these two measurements independently.[22] Some hormones are released into the circulation in a precursor form and acquire a biologically active form only after enzymatic modification in either the circulation or the peripheral tissues. The conversion of T_4 to T_3 by 5′-deiodination in the liver and other tissues is an example. While T_3 has at least 10 times the thyromimetic effect of T_4 as measured with in vitro bioassays,[23] its clearance from the circulation is much faster than that of T_4.[20] This pattern of a relatively stable prohormone or transport form that is enzymatically modified either before or upon release, during circulatory transport, or after binding with a receptor, producing a derivative hormone with altered specific biological activity, is shared by other hormones.

For example, glycoprotein hormones such as TSH undergo major alterations in the composition of glycosylated side chains during biosynthesis and secretion in response to hormonal stimulation. The glycosylation reaction promoted by thyrotropin releasing hormone (TRH) apparently enhances the ratio of biological to immunologic activity of the secreted TSH.[24] Rapid changes in pH, ionic strength, and the activity of associated proteolytic enzymes accompany the exocytosis of hormone containing secretory granules. These secretion-associated events may explain the observation that the high-molecular-weight precursor form of atrial natriuretic polypeptide (ANP) is found only inside cells while the processed form is entirely extracellular.[25] After secretion, further intravascular modifications of circulating hormones may occur. Parathyroid hormone, for example, is cleaved to smaller forms during passage through the kidney.[26] Most peptide hormones require alpha-amidation of a C-terminal amino acid residue for biological activity. While this reaction occurs predominantly within the secretory vesicle, significant alpha-amidation of TRH-Gly, a TRH precursor peptide, occurs after secretion.[27]

NOMENCLATURE

Immunoassay nomenclature consists of combinations and permutations of a small number of prefixes which designate the type of label used, such as radioactive (*radio*), enzyme (*enzymatic*), fluorometric (*fluoro*), and chemiluminescent (*lumino*), and the labeling of the analyte (e.g., *radioimmuno*) or antibody (e.g., *immunoradio*). Acronyms are also used to identify types of assays, such as ELISA (*e*nzyme-*l*inked *i*mmuno*s*orbent *a*ssay), which utilizes antibody-coated microtiter plates and an enzyme-labeled reporter antibody. Because of the large number of available reagents and their possible combinations for hormone measurement, the nomenclature has become confused. Reference to relevant commercial or scientific literature is the only certain way to determine the methodologic details for any given assay.

TYPES OF IMMUNOASSAYS

Labeled Analyte and Reagent Limiting

Immunoassays using labeled antigen or hapten are equivalent to the classical RIA.[28] They require a very dilute high-affinity antibody which can be immobilized on the surface of a test tube, polystyrene bead, or paramagnetic particle or left in solution for later precipitation with a second antibody.[29] The hormone-antibody reaction can be represented by the following reactions:

$$\mathrm{Ag} + \mathrm{Ab} \underset{k_{-1}}{\overset{k_1}{\rightleftharpoons}} \mathrm{AgAb} \qquad {}^*\mathrm{Ab} + \mathrm{Ab} \underset{k_{-1}}{\overset{k_1}{\rightleftharpoons}} {}^*\mathrm{AgAb}$$

$$K_a = k_1/k_{-1} \qquad k_d = 1/K_a$$

where

Ag = antigen or hormone
Ab = antibody to the antigen or hormone
*Ag = radiolabeled antigen or hormone
k_1 = association rate constant
k_{-1} = dissociation rate constant
K_a = equilibrium association constant
K_d = equilibrium dissociation constant

The labeled hormone may differ substantially from the hormone being measured, particularly if radioiodine, a radioiodinated "tagging" compound, an enzyme, or a fluorescent or chemiluminescent derivative of the analyte is used.[30] The attendant structural modifications can be avoided through the use of the naturally occurring hormone labeled with ^3H or ^{14}C. However, the maximum specific activities attainable with these long half-life isotopes is very low, resulting in self-displacement of the tracer when the total mass of the label added to each tube is high enough for accurate counting. The detection limit can be improved by adding the label some time after the mixing of the analyte and antibody, the so-called nonequilibrium assay.[28,31] The approach to equilibrium of binding between the antibody, the analyte, and the tracer is slowed by the use of the minimum concentration of antibody required for maximum assay sensitivity. Free label and antibody-bound label are separated, and usually the bound fraction is quantitated. The plot of bound label on a linear scale versus the total antigen concentration on a log scale gives a sigmoid-shaped standard curve with negative slope values.[28] Another representation frequently used in reagent limiting assays is the log-logit plot, which usually produces a linear profile for the standard curve. Unknown results are more readily obtained with linear least-squares analysis of this form of the standard curve than with the sigmoidal form, which is shown in Fig. 5-3 superimposed on the corresponding log-logit plot.

Reagent Excess and Labeled Antibody

The advent of monoclonal antibodies[32] made feasible the "sandwich" assay methodology.[33] With this technique, one monoclonal antibody is adsorbed or chemically bonded to a solid surface such as a test tube or a polystyrene bead. Hormone standards or serum samples are then added, followed by a labeled antibody with binding specificity for a region of the hormone analyte which is different from that of the immobilized antibody.[34] The amount

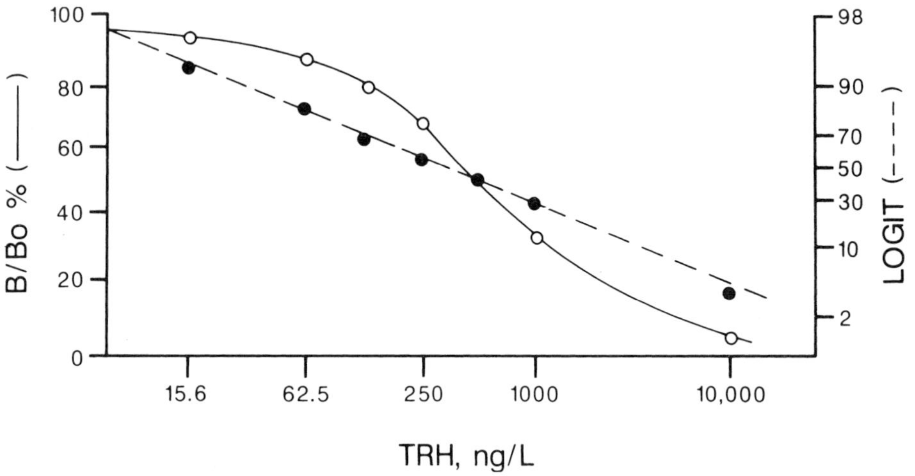

FIGURE 5-3. Standard curve for the thyrotropin releasing hormone radioimmunoassay. Comparison of the sigmoidal and linear log-logit representations.

of the labeled antibody that binds to the solid phase should be proportional to the amount of hormone in the sample resulting from the formation of the sandwich complex:

$$SP\text{-}Ab\text{-}Ag\text{-}Ab^*$$

where

SP-Ab = solid-phase antibody
Ag = hormone analyte
Ab* = labeled antibody

The addition of a large excess of the immobilized antibody can lead to nearly quantitative binding of any available analyte. A high concentration of a second, labeled "reporter" monoclonal antibody binds in direct proportion to the total analyte concentration. The advantage of this type of assay is that the minimum detectable dose is not limited by the affinity constants of the antibodies used.[35] The only limits on sensitivity are the detectability of the tracer and the extent to which the reporter antibody that is nonspecifically bound to the surfaces of the reaction tube and separation matrix can be minimized by the washing procedure. The analyte must be large enough that two antigen determinants can be bound simultaneously by two different antibody molecules without steric interference.[36] Such a requirement excludes simple steroids and small peptides with fewer than 15 to 20 amino acid residues.

The binding affinity and specificity of the large, stable, bivalent monospecific immunoglobulin molecule are not usually perturbed significantly by the attachment of tracer molecules, whether radioactive, enzymatic, fluorescent, or chemiluminescent. Labeled antibody generally has a greater storage stability than do many labeled polypeptide hormones.[37]

Free and Total Hormone Measurements

Serum contains binding or transport proteins for thyroid, steroid, and some peptide hormones. The free hormone hypothesis states that the biological action of a hormone is proportional to the concentration of the unbound (free) hormone. The trend in assays for these hormones has been to develop methods which can measure the free hormone directly. A controversy has arisen concerning the participation of the hormone-binding proteins in hormone transport across the capillary endothelium and the underlying mechanisms of this transport. Both experimental and theoretical aspects of hormone transport have been reviewed.[38] The concept that only the free fraction of plasma hormones is bioavailable and is regulated by negative feedback was based on the observation that free thyroid hormone levels were normal in euthyroid subjects who either lacked the high-affinity thyroxine-binding globulin (TBG deficiency) or had excess serum TBG as a result of a genetic defect, with very low or very high total thyroid hormone levels, respectively.[39]

Ekins has pointed out that in the case of very rapid tissue uptake, the free hormone concentration along the endothelial cell surface may be depleted. Rapid dissociation of hormones from the binding proteins would have the effect of increasing the diffusional flux of the hormone into cells.[40] Pardridge has proposed an alternative model called the *enhanced dissociation hypothesis* in which the dissociation constant of the serum binding proteins increases within the capillary epithelium and thus facilitates the transit of their bound hormones.[41] While the debate concerning the mechanisms that facilitate hormone transport continues, autoradiographic experiments with liver lobules subjected to a single-pass perfusion with radiolabeled T_4, in the absence of thyroid hormone-binding proteins, have emphasized their physiologic significance. Virtually all the T_4 in the perfusate was taken up by the first cells with which it came in contact and was unavailable to cells farther along the sinusoid.[42] When the perfusion was carried out in the presence of thyroid hormone-binding proteins, the fractional extraction was decreased and uniform uptake of T_4 was observed in all the cells of the lobule.

A number of commercial assays for free thyroid hormone are available. They may be divided into three general categories: analog, competitive binding, and ultrafiltration or equilibrium dialysis (ED) combined with immunoassay.[40] The analog assays use a labeled T_4 derivative which is designed to minimize binding to the major thyroid hormone-binding proteins, TBG and thyroxine-binding prealbumin (TBPA); however, the analog does bind to the corresponding thyroid hormone antibody. The assumption is made that the thyroid hormone antibody and the analog tracer added in vitro to the serum sample do not perturb the concentrations of free thyroid hormone. If this assumption is not valid, the measured free hormone value may not correspond to the in vivo concentration, particularly if the thyroid hormone-binding proteins are abnormal. Abnormal free T_4 (FT_4) values are sometimes obtained with this assay method in samples from pregnant women, for example, as a result of the estrogen-induced elevation of TBG values.[43]

The competitive FT_4 assay uses a high-specific-activity labeled monoclonal antibody to T_4 and a suspension of magnetizable particles with T_4 ligands attached. The FT_4 concentration determines the proportion of labeled T_4 antibody precipitated by the magnetic particles. Again, the assumption is made that FT_4 concentration is not affected by the added T_4 antibody and ligand-containing particles.

Equilibrium dialysis has been considered the gold standard for determining free hormone levels. This method, however, has also produced results, particularly for diluted serum samples from patients with nonthyroid illness,[44] which are difficult to interpret, in part because of a postulated inhibitor of T_4 binding that has not been characterized.[40] In principle, the dilution of serum before or during ED should not have a significant effect on the dializable or "free" T_4 level because 99.97 percent of the total T_4 level should be in the bound form. The decrease in ED-measured FT_4 in the serum of severely ill patients with dilution has been attributed to high free fatty acid (FFA) levels. The in vitro addition of FFA to levels several times higher than those seen in even the most severe illness is not sufficient to affect ED values.[38] In vitro artifacts such as heparin-induced release of FFA from frozen plasma during ED may explain some of the discrepant results.[45]

Measurement of total thyroid hormone values by immunoassay requires that all these hydrophobic molecules be displaced from their serum binding proteins. This is usually done by means of the in vitro addition of sodium salicylate or 8-anilino-1-naphthalenesulfonic acid.[46]

Most steroid hormones are associated with serum binding proteins. These include corticosteroid-binding globulin (CBG), which is the major binding protein for progesterone, cortisol, and other glucocorticoids, and sex hormone-binding globulin (SHBG), which binds the gonadal steroids, testosterone and estradiol, with high affinity.[38] These binding proteins interfere with immunoassay measurements. Solvent extraction is a dependable but labor-intensive method for eliminating the effects of steroid-binding proteins prior to immunoassay. Methods have been developed for the direct assay of progesterone, for example, which use acidification and displacing compounds such as cortisol to reduce the binding of label and hormone by CBG.[47]

Assays for the direct measurement of growth hormone (GH) have been available for many years. The variability of GH secretion, however, has limited its diagnostic value. Insulin-like growth factor-I (IGF-I), which is a major effector of GH action, is relatively stable in the circulation because >75% of IGF-I is bound to a 150-kDa ternary complex consisting of IGF binding protein-3 (IGFBP-3) and a unique leucine-rich, acid-labile subunit. Smaller proportions of IGF-I are associated with the other IGFBPs and <1% of serum IGF-I is in an unbound form. The high levels of association with IGFBPs complicate the routine measurement of IGF-I because the IGFBPs mask reactive epitopes or complete with antibodies in an immunoassay. The combination of acid-ethanol extraction with a noncompetitive ELISA assay provide an optimal combination of accuracy and convenience for quantifying this diagnostically important growth factor.[48]

The immunoassay field remains exceedingly active, with new technologies being rapidly incorporated into commercial "kit" assays with improved speed, sensitivity, safety, and reproducibility.

TABLE 5-1. Commercial Hormone Assays Listed in the College of American Pathologists (CAP) Ligand Assay Series 1 and 2 for 1999

Peptide	Thyroid	Steroid
FSH (23)*	T_4 (25)	Aldosterone (4)
Gastrin (4)	FT_4 (18)	Androstenedione (3)
Growth hormone (10)	T_3 (15)	Cortisol (14)
hCG (20)	FT_3 (8)	Deoxycortisol (2)
Insulin (8)	T_3 uptake (27)	Dehydroepiandrosterone sulfate (9)
LH (21)		Estradiol (23)
Parathyroid hormone (10)		Estriol (2)
Prolactin (26)		Estriol (unconjugated) (5)
Renin (4)		17-Hydroxyprogesterone (9)
TSH (26)		Progesterone (19)
		Testosterone (16)

*The numbers in parentheses represent the total number of all kits for each hormone listed in the surveys.

The commercial assays, listed by hormonal category, that are currently on the College of American Pathologists Ligand Assay Surveys 1 and 2, are listed in Table 5-1.

IMMUNOASSAY REAGENTS

Binding Proteins

Production of Antibodies

The Nature and Structure of Antibodies

Antibodies belong to the class of immunoglobulins and are predominantly gamma globulins (IgG). The IgG molecule is composed of four polypeptide chains: two heavy chains and two light chains symmetrically arranged and covalently bound by disulfide bonds. The molecule is shown schematically in Fig. 5-4.

The interaction of antigen or ligand with antibody may be considered a "lock and key" arrangement. The shape of the antibody combining site is complementary to that of the antigen. The antigen-antibody interaction is a combination of electrostatic, hydrogen-binding, van der Waals, and hydrophobic interactions.[49,50]

FIGURE 5-4. Schematic representation of a gamma globulin (antibody) molecule. The hormone recognition sites contain the variable amino acid regions of the light and heavy immunoglobulin chains. The light chains are covalently linked to the heavy chains through a disulfide bond(s), and a single disulfide bond exists between the two heavy chains. The immunoglobulin molecule assumes a Y conformation, with the antibody combining sites occupying the top portions of the Y.

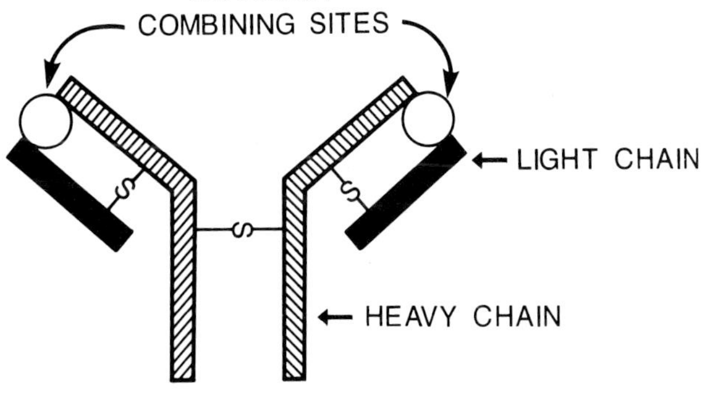

The amino acid sequence of the binding portion of the IgG molecule determines the "shape" of the binding site and, consequently, the affinity and specificity of the combining site for the desired antigen.[51]

The immune response can be divided into the primary and secondary phases. After the first exposure to a given immunogen and a relatively long lag period, IgM antibodies begin to appear in serum. A second exposure to the immunogen results in a much stronger response, consisting primarily of IgG antibodies, which declines more slowly. Moreover, antibodies of the secondary response generally have much higher affinities for the immunogen.[33] The IgM-IgG transition involves IgG class switching in which the gene coding for the immunogen-recognizing segment of the antibody—the paratope—is combined with the gene coding for the rest of the IgG molecule. With repeated immunization, the affinity of the antiserum may increase. This involves the selection of B cell clones producing antibodies with high affinity for the immunogen. This process is usually facilitated by increasing the interval between immunizations so that the time-averaged tissue concentration of the immunogen is low enough to result in the occupation of only those B-cell–associated antibodies with the highest affinity constant for the antigen.

Polyclonal Antibodies Polyclonal antisera contain a very heterogeneous mixture of antibodies, only a small fraction of which may be specific for the antigen or hapten of interest. Rabbits, guinea pigs, sheep, and goats are generally used for polyclonal antibody production. The volume of antiserum required, the quantity of immunogen available, and the degree of structural difference between the endogenous hormone and the immunogen are relevant criteria for selecting the species to be immunized.[52]

Hormonal immunogens generally fall into three antigenic classes: large proteins, small peptides, and steroids. The glycoprotein hormones, such as TSH, luteinizing hormone (LH), follicle stimulating hormone (FSH), and hCG, if foreign to the immunized animal and available in purified form, will suffice as immunogens without further modification.[53] Small peptide hormones such as TRH, by contrast, are not intrinsically immunogenic because of their small size and ubiquitous occurrence in vertebrate and invertebrate species.[54] For these small polypeptides (haptens) to be rendered immunogenic, they must be chemically linked to larger, highly immunogenic proteins such as keyhole limpet hemocyanin, bovine serum albumin, or thyroglobulin.[55] The chemistry used for this coupling reaction is determined in large measure by the available reactive groups on the polypeptide or its derivative that will be used as a haptenic group for the carrier protein. The ratio of hapten to carrier protein is important because it has a substantial influence on the overall antigenicity of the conjugate.[56] If a small haptenic peptide is derived from an exposed region of a larger protein, the resulting polyclonal antibodies will generally cross-react with the corresponding epitope in the intact protein, providing an alternative to the epitope-specific monoclonal antibody.

Similar recognition constraints apply to the conjugation of steroid haptens to proteins. The cross-linking reagent bridging the hapten with the carrier protein will influence the specificity of the resulting antibody.[57] If appropriate sites for cross-linking to the peptide hapten for iodination are not available, solid-phase synthesis of an analog with the desired characteristics is a convenient option. The judicious combination of coupling chemistry and iodinatable haptenic analogs has facilitated the development of steroid RIAs, such as that for cortisol, that use conveniently detected ^{125}I tracers.[58,59]

Multiple Antigenic Peptides Multiple antigenic peptides (MAPs) are an alternative approach to raising antipeptide antibodies. MAPs show many advantages over traditional methods, including the elimination of the conjugation step, which is time consuming and can result in a random product mixture. With MAPs, a known amount of peptide can be used for immunization each time, giving greater control over experimental conditions. MAPs have also been shown to induce higher antibody titers than their corresponding protein-conjugated haptens.[60,61] In addition, by enhancing the coating capacity and avidity of synthetic peptides, MAPs provide increased sensitivity and reliability for the use of synthetic peptides in studies of antigen-antibody interactions in solid phase immunoassays.[62]

The MAP-immunogen is composed of multiple copies of a single epitope attached to a small, nonimmunogenic, polylysine core. The MAP design maximizes the antigen concentration, with synthesized peptide-antigen accounting for up to 95 percent of the total weight of the final product. Because it introduces multiple copies of the peptide antigen, the MAP-immunogen produces higher antibody titers. The resulting antibodies are also more specific than those raised against peptide-protein conjugates, since the MAP-immunogen contains only one antigenic sequence.

Multiple antigenic peptide resins typically have four or eight peptide arms branching out from the alpha- and epsilon-NH_2 groups of a polylysine core matrix (Fig. 5-5).

In general, an immunogen of at least 10,000 Da is desirable. Therefore, the four-branch MAP resin is used for peptides containing more than 20 residues and the eight-branch MAP resin for peptides of 15 residues or less. Immunogens containing 16–20

FIGURE 5-5. Cascade designs of core matrices or templates for branched peptide. A: cascade and asymmetrical MAP with branching lysine; B: cascade and symmetrical MAP with branching Lys-β-Ala. Striped bars denote peptide antigen. (*Permission to reprint from reference 62 granted by author.*)

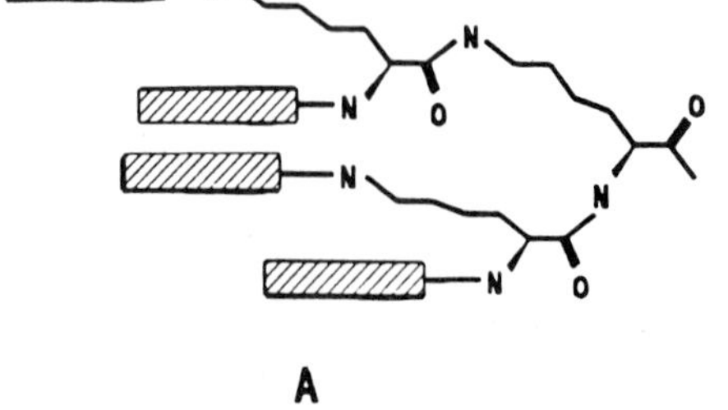

A

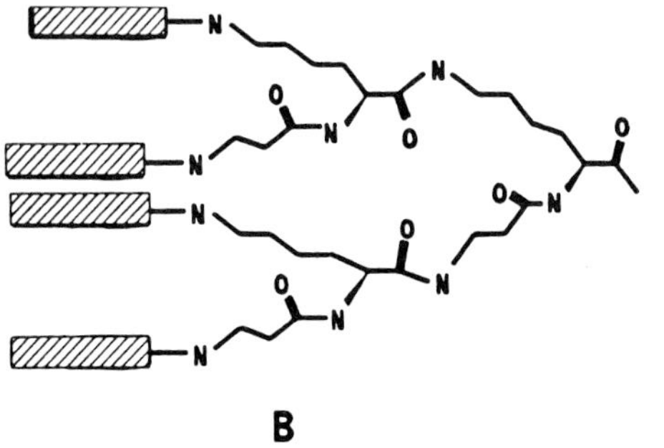

B

residues can be synthesized on either the four- or eight-branch resin. MAPs can be analyzed by reverse-phase HPLC, capillary electrophoresis, peptide sequencing, amino acid analysis, or mass spectrometry, but the results can be difficult to interpret based on the sequence.

Multiple antigenic peptides are macromolecules, often exceeding 15,000 Da, making their synthesis by the stepwise solid-phase methods and subsequent purification to high homogeneity challenging. An alternative method for obtaining highly purified MAPs for clinical purposes is through orthogonal ligation, which joins purified unprotected peptide segments to the core matrix. The modular synthesis by orthogonal ligation has the advantage that the MAP products are easily purified by conventional methods, and offer the flexibility of incorporating several types of epitopes to form di- or triepitope MAPs, as well as the option of choosing their orientation to be attached to the core matrix. Two general methods based on thiol and carbonyl chemistries have been developed to ligate unprotected peptides to form MAPs with nonpeptide bonds.[63] Lipidated MAPs do not require adjuvant for antibody production, making them potentially useful for the design of novel vaccines. MAPs can be used for the production of both polyclonal and monoclonal antibodies.

Hexahistidine Tagged Peptides A novel method for using small synthetic peptides with 6 histidyl residues attached to the N- or C-terminus as haptens for immunization of rabbits or chickens has recently been reported.[64] The hexahistidine tag binds with high affinity under a variety of conditions to the nitrilotriacetic acid chelator attached to resin. The proportion of hapten bound to resin is readily varied by changing the ratio of hapten and resin during the binding procedure. Immunization with the peptide-resin complex is then carried out using standard methods.

Monoclonal Antibodies Monoclonal antibodies are usually produced in mice or rats through in vitro transformation of antibody-producing B cells by oncogenic viruses or, more commonly, by fusion of antibody-producing cells with mutant myeloma cells (hybridomas) to confer immortality on the B cells.

A frequently used technique for generating antibody-producing hybridomas relies on the use of myeloma cells that lack hypoxanthine guanine phosphoribosyltransferase (HGPRT). HGPRT-deficient myeloma cells are selected by growing them in media containing 6-thioguanine or 8-azaguanine. Cells expressing HGPRT integrate these base analogs into DNA, resulting in a lethal interference with transcription, while HGPRT-deficient cells can produce nucleic acids only by de novo synthesis.[33]

Lymphocytes do not multiply in vitro but contain the enzymes for both the de novo and salvage pathways for DNA base synthesis. The folic acid antagonist aminopterin, which blocks the de novo synthesis pathway, is used to select for myeloma cells that have fused with lymphocytes. The salvage pathway of the surviving hybridoma cells is stimulated by the addition of hypoxanthine and thymidine [hypoxanthine, aminopterin, and thymidine (HAT) medium]. Only a small proportion of the hybridoma cells will produce useful antibodies. Unless proper precautions are taken, such cells will be rapidly overgrown by more rapidly dividing but nonproducing (revertant) cells. Feeder cells are needed during the first few days of the culture to increase the survival rate of the newly produced hybridomas. Revertant cells can be eliminated by culturing the hybridomas two to three times per year in 8-azaguanine.[30,33]

Immunization for the production of monoclonal antibodies may be carried out either in vitro or, more commonly, in vivo. The advantages of in vitro immunization are a short (5 days) immunization time and the ability to use self antigens; also, the immunogen concentration can be regulated, and antibody production can be monitored conveniently. The principal disadvantage is that only a primary (IgM) immune response can be elicited unless a complex protocol is followed involving the addition of factors for growth and differentiation so as to elicit 10 to 20 percent IgG-producing hybridomas.[65]

Monoclonal antibodies have lower apparent affinity constants because they can bind only to a single region, or epitope, of the antigen; therefore, they are less useful for reagent limiting assays. Polyclonal antibodies, by contrast, can bind to a multitude of different antigenic sites simultaneously and, as a result of the bivalent nature of the IgG molecule, can form complex, highly cooperative interactions.[66] Mixtures of two or more monoclonal antibodies with different binding specificities for a given large antigen can also result in the formation of complexes involving two (or more) antibody molecules and two (or more) antigens in highly cooperative circular or chainlike arrays.

A hybrid sandwich assay or immunofunctional hormone assay that combines the epitope specific binding of a monoclonal antibody with the physiologically important binding of a recombinant extracellular domain of a cognate hormone receptor has recently been described for growth hormone.[67]

Nonimmunologic Molecular Recognition Systems: Avidin/Biotin

Avidin, a 4-subunit protein derived from egg white, has an exceptionally high affinity for biotin ($k_a = 10^{15}\ M^{-1}$), one of the water-soluble components of the vitamin B complex. Four binding sites for biotin arranged as two pairs of closely juxtaposed, deeply penetrating binding sites occur in avidin.[68] Each paired binding site can accept only a single biotin molecule because of steric effects which perturb the neighboring binding site. The avidin/biotin system has been used for the development of new nonradioisotopic methods for hormone assay. Avidin is a very basic glycoprotein (pI = 10.5) that is stable over a wide range of pH and temperature and is resistant to proteolytic enzymes. Analogs or small fragments of biotin such as urea, glycol, tetrahydrofuran, and caproic acid may bind to or compete in the interaction with avidin. The most advantageous use of avidin is as a bridge between two biotinylated molecules such as a biotinylated enzyme and a biotinylated immunoreactant.

Labels

Radioactive Tracers

The convenience of radiochemical iodination and gamma spectrometer detection of ^{125}I-labeled peptide and protein hormones is being outweighed by the increasingly stringent regulatory burden which accompanies the use of radioisotopes. Nonradioactively labeled tracers for immunoassays are generally obtained as part of commercially prepared kit assays because their preparation generally involves the use of proprietary methods. For clinical applications, the high cost per tube of such assays is offset by the maintenance of appropriate quality controls in the manufacturing process and the savings in technician time and labor achieved by using automated assay systems.

Iodination

Oxidation of $Na^{125}I$ to form $^{125}I_2$ through the use of the oxidizing agent chloramine-T remains the most popular method for radiochemically labeling peptides and proteins.[69] The molecular iodine spontaneously reacts with tyrosyl and histidyl residues on the exposed surfaces of proteins. The major drawbacks to this method are that chloramine-T may cause oxidative damage to the substrate protein and that the reactive $^{125}I_2$ is volatile, necessitating the use of specialized fume hoods to minimize the biohazard. An enzymatic method for producing reactive $^{125}I_2$ involves the use of lactoperoxidase and hydrogen peroxide. This method generally results in less oxidative damage to the substrate protein and greater preservation of its initial biological and immunologic potency, provided that reaction-limiting amounts of hydrogen peroxide are used.[69] Because of their electronegativity and large size, iodine atoms incorporated into peptides and proteins alter their chemical and steric properties. The introduction of more than one iodine atom per host polypeptide also accelerates radiolytic damage during storage. Optimization of the conditions used for storing and repurification of iodinated proteins, which are particularly susceptible to radiolytic damage, may be as important as the method selected for the initial iodination to maintain tracer binding for several weeks or months.[31] Iodogen, a water-insoluble form of chloramine-T, was developed as another method for minimizing the exposure of proteins to the damaging effects of this oxidizing agent during the radioiodination procedure.[70] A less popular method of ^{125}I labeling proteins involves the radioiodination of the Bolton-Hunter reagent, 3-(*p*-hydroxyphenyl) propionic acid *N*-hydroxysuccinimide ester, which then is reacted with the amino groups of the polypeptide hormone.[71] Iodination with ^{131}I is infrequently used because of its short half-life of 8 days, compared with 59 days for ^{125}I, and its hazardous, high-energy gamma emission.

[^{3}*H*] *Labeling*

Small antigens, such as steroid hormones, generally cannot accommodate large iodo groups incorporated during radiochemical iodination without a substantial change in their antibody-binding specificity.[58] The incorporation of [^{3}H] into the substrate molecule does not change any chemical or immunologic properties but does necessitate the use of beta counting methods, which are more labor-intensive than the direct gamma counting of ^{125}I. The preparation of [^{3}H]-labeled antigens for immunoassay requires specialized facilities and is usually carried out in a radiolabeling facility on a contract basis if the labeled compound is not commercially available. Environmental concerns connected with the disposal of scintillation vials make this a costly alternative.

Nonradioactive Tracers

Enzyme

Enzyme immunoassays (EIA) may be broadly subdivided into two categories: activity amplification assays and activity modulation assays. Activity amplification assays and activity modulation assays are analogous to reagent excess and reagent limiting immunoassays, respectively. A large excess of immunoreactant is used in activity amplification assays to obtain a maximum signal for the analyte to be tested. From the law of mass action, which states that the rate of complex formation is proportional to the product of the analyte and antibody concentrations, a rapid and nearly quantitative reaction of all the available analyte molecules will occur in an activity amplification assay.[33] A description and examples of activity modulation enzymes assays are given in homogeneous assay systems that follow.

Fluorescence

A photon of appropriate energy (wavelength) can excite an atom, molecule, or fluorescent labeling group from its ground state to a higher electronic state. The return to the ground state may occur through nonradiative processes or emission of light at a longer wavelength. The difference between the incident (excitation) wavelength and the emission wavelength is known as the Stokes shift.[72] In fluorescence polarization assays, the path of the filtered or monochromated incident light beam is directed at right angles to the frequency-selected light path to the detector.[73] To minimize the amount of the excitation light which reaches the detector as a result of light scattering from molecules (Rayleigh scattering), particles (Tyndall scattering), and the rotational and vibrational energy of the solvent molecules (Raman scattering), a fluorescent label with a large Stokes shift is selected.[72,74]

One of the advantages of fluorometric methodology is the large dynamic range of the measured response. Endogenous fluorophores of serum, especially hemoglobin and bilirubin, however, interfere with the detection of commonly used fluorescent tags such as fluoroscein, which have similar emission wavelengths. The quantum yield (ratio of emitted to incident quanta) of fluorescent probes is also sensitive to changes in temperature, pH, and solvent polarity and to trace oxidizing agents or dissolved oxygen. Interactions of the fluorophore with quenching agents such as tryptophan, iodine-containing molecules, specific antibody, or nonspecific albumin binding can also reduce the quantum yield.[72,74]

Time-resolved fluorescence spectroscopy has been developed to eliminate the interfering endogenous fluorescence of serum. When europium chelates are used as the labeling reagent, with a fluorescence lifetime longer than that of hemoglobin or bilirubin, the start of fluorescence detection can be delayed or "gated" until these serum fluorophores have decayed completely.[72,74]

Luminescence

The fluorescence phenomenon, as described previously, is photo-induced luminescence: the transiting of an electron from a high-energy orbital of an atom or molecule, induced by an initial absorption of electromagnetic radiation, to a lower-energy orbital with the release of a photon of light.[72] *Chemiluminescence*—the excitation of a molecule to a higher-energy state by a chemical reaction followed by the release of a photon—has the potential to be as sensitive as radiochemical labeling without the radiation hazard.[75] Unlike fluorescent compounds, which can be excited repeatedly, chemiluminescent molecules can be activated only once, though all molecules are potentially available for detection. The immunochemiluminometric assay is increasingly popular because of its inherent sensitivity, but instrumental and triggering modes may jeopardize it. A new immunoelectrochemiluminometric assay (IECMA) has recently been commercialized.[76] It is based on electrogenerated chemiluminescence that, aiming to avoid the instability of luminophores, does not proceed in free solution but on the surface of a platinum electrode. The Elecsys 2010 immunoanalyzer (Boehringer Mannheim Canada, Laval, Quebec, Canada) is based on a new detection technology that uses an electrochemiluminescence label. This label, ruthenium(II) tris(bipyridyl)$_3^{2+}$ [$Ru(bpy)_3^{2+}$], can undergo multiple oxidation-reduction cycles when immobilized at the surface of an electrode in the presence of a coreactant included in the assay buffer. The coreactant, tripropylamine (TPA), when oxidized at the electrode, produces a radical cation, which acts as a reducing agent. After the release of a proton, a TPA radical is formed that reacts with the oxidized form of the label to generate $Ru(bpy)_3^{2+}$ in an excited state. After emission of a photon, the label can undergo another cycle and, therefore, generates multiple photons for each labeled molecule. Immobilization of the labeled complex is obtained by using magnetic microparticles coated with streptavidin, which binds to biotin linked covalently to reaction antibodies. A magnet immobilizes the bound fraction at the electrode to allow elimination of the unbound label before proceeding to the electrochemiluminescent detection.[77] Available hormone assays using the Elecsys 2010 immunoanalyzer include TSH (third generation), T_4, T uptake, free T_4, T_3, free T_3, hCG, FSH, LH, prolactin, progesterone, estradiol, and testosterone. Future hormone assays will include insulin and cortisol (Boehringer Mannheim Elecsys Menu).

Particle

Latex particle agglutination assays, which were most frequently used in qualitative kits for pregnancy and serology testing, have evolved into fully automated, high-sensitivity quantitative methods for measuring a variety of hormones. Antibody-coated latex particles are mixed with serum or another body fluid sample, resulting in sample antigen-induced aggregation of some of the particles. The mixture is passed through a particle counter, which counts the number of unagglutinated particles remaining. The expanding use of this method has resulted from rapid improvements in its sensitivity and reproducibility, elimination of specific and nonspecific self agglutination, and extension of the range of application, most importantly to the measurement of small molecules.[78]

Vesicle

Vesicle assays consist of lipid bilayer spheres (micelles) which encapsulate a solution of reporter molecules. Incorporated into the micelle are antigenic molecules that have been chemically combined with phospholipids which "anchor" the antigen to the bilayer surface. The solutions within the micelles may include dyes, fluorescent compounds, hemoglobin, spin-labeled molecules, or enzymes. Because of the high turnover rate of enzymes, amplification of a spectrophotometric or fluorescent signal produced by vesicle lysis is possible. Competitive, reagent excess, two-phase, and homogeneous assay methodologies have been reported.[79,80] A vesicle assay for digoxin uses digoxin antibody-coated tubes which bind either the free digoxin in the patient serum and assay standards or the digoxin-coated micelle. After incubation and washing, the vesicles that remain attached to the test tube are ruptured with detergent and the optical density of the released dye is measured spectrophotometrically.[79]

Multianalyte

Simultaneous measurement of several analytes in the same serum sample has also become an established technique.[81–83] The use of radioactive or nonradioactive tracers which can be detected separately because of differences in spectral energy of emission or absorption saves both sample and labor costs. Simplification of the assay methodology not only saves expense but improves accuracy because each manipulation represents a potential source of error. Examples are commercial kits for the simultaneous measurement of TSH and FT_4 through the use of ^{125}I and ^{51}Cr labels[81] and for the measurement of LH and FSH.[83]

SEPARATION SYSTEMS

Most assay systems require measurement of the proportion of the total hormonal analyte which is bound or free. Usually this determination is made after the hormone-antibody complex has been separated from the unbound hormone.

Liquid-Phase Precipitation

The addition of nonimmune IgG and anti-IgG antiserum (second antibody) is still a very common method for separating the bound and free hormone fractions, particularly in RIAs.[84,85] This reaction can be greatly accelerated by the addition of polyethylene glycol.[86] The kinetics of this acceleration, however, is highly dependent on the concentration and type of protein in the reaction mixture.

Solid-Phase Adsorption

The RIA, which is a reagent limiting, labeled antigen type of hormone assay, initially dominated the immunoassay field. Adsorption of the first antibody to the assay test tube greatly simplified the separation of the bound hormone but required long incubation times because of the slow kinetics for the antigen-antibody interaction. The use of monoclonal antibodies adsorbed to plastic test tubes, macroporous polystyrene beads with a large surface area, microwells, dipsticks, slides, electrodes, or fiber filters in reagent excess immunoradiometric assays has solved the kinetic limitations of the solid-phase adsorption method for separating the bound and free hormone fractions.[87]

Solid-Phase Precipitation

Another rapid separation method, which allows a large amount of a first or second antibody to maintain intimate contact with the analyte-containing sample, utilizes antibody-coated magnetizable particles. After binding of the hormone is complete, the tray of assay tubes is placed in a special, permanently magnetized rack which draws the particles toward the sides or bottom of the test tube. The supernatant can then be aspirated or decanted.[88] Clinical assays for cortisol, TSH, LH, FSH, hCG, T_4, FT_4, T_3 and FT_3, progesterone, and unconjugated estriol which utilize this method of separation are widely available.

HOMOGENEOUS ASSAY SYSTEMS

If the bound fraction of a hormone can be measured in the presence of the free fraction, physical separation is not necessary. Such homogeneous assays avoid separation error, one of the major sources of experimental variability in immunoassays.

Methods for the detection of antigen-antibody complexes without the addition of a second antibody, centrifugation, and separation of the pellet and supernatant continue to proliferate. Fluorescence polarization and amplitude-modulated immunoenzymatic assays are strategies for minimizing the errors in determining the bound/free ratio.

Fluorescence Polarization

Molecules in solution rotate in response to collisions with the surrounding solvent molecules which are undergoing rapid, chaotic movements termed *Brownian motion*. The average rotational rate for a given molecule is proportional to 1/V, where V is the volume of the molecule. If a small fluorescent-labeled hormone is excited with a polarized beam of light, the excited molecule will rotate through a large angle relative to the orientation of the incident beam before the polarized excitation is reemitted as a polarized fluorescence. If some of the fluorescent hormones are bound to large antibody molecules, these complexes will rotate much more slowly and will reemit their polarized fluorescence at nearly the same angle as the incident beam. If the emitted light is detected with a polarizer alternating between the parallel orientation and the perpendicular orientation of the incident beam, more emitted light will be detected in the parallel orientation as the extent of binding of labeled hormone to antibody increases. The potential sensitivity of this method depends on the difference in hydrodynamic mobility of the bound hormone and the free hormone. For this reason, fluorescence polarization can be utilized only for small molecules, such as steroid and thyroid hormones, medications and drugs of abuse.[89]

Phase-Modulation Fluorescence Spectroscopy

A homogenous competitive model immunoassay by multifrequency phase modulation fluorescence has been described.[90] Using a nonradiative energy transfer transduction mechanism, B-phycoerythrin conjugated to antigen is the energy donor and a carboxymethylindocyanine dye conjugated to antibody is the energy acceptor. Energy transfer from B-phycoerythrin to the acceptor results in a decreased lifetime and/or phase angle. The fluorescence lifetime change reflects the extent of energy transfer. In the competitive immunoassay format, the donor-antigen conjugate and a sample containing analyte compete for acceptor-antibody binding sites, resulting in a phase angle change which is dependent on the amount of analyte in the sample. Dose-response curves of phase angle versus analyte concentration are comparable to steady-state intensity curves. Because phase-modulation lifetime measurements are largely independent of total signal intensity, sources of optical interference are minimized. The potential for whole blood measurements exists because energy transfer lifetime method can be extended to longer wavelengths.

Amplitude-Modulated Enzyme Assays

Amplitude-modulated assays can lead to either activation or inhibition of the end product signal, depending on the enzymatic reaction which is modulated and the epitopic specificity of the antibodies used. The first of this general class of assays (Fig. 5-6*A*) was developed by Rubenstein et al.[91] for the detection of morphine, using an enzyme-hapten conjugate. The activity of the conjugated enzyme was modulated by antihapten antibody through steric hindrance or allosteric alteration of the enzyme. Free hapten decreased this modulatory effect by competitively binding with antibody. This method is known by the commercial name EMIT (Syva Co., Palo Alto, CA). If substrate is conjugated to antigen, the reaction of antibody to this conjugate will block the use of the substrate by the enzyme. The addition of free antigen as the standard or unknown leaves some conjugate free to enter the active site of the enzyme (Fig. 5-6*B*). Conjugation of antigen to an enzyme cofactor results in a third type of amplitude-modulated assay (Fig. 5-6*C*). The addition of free antigen leads to an increase in cofactor availability for the enzyme. Enzyme may also be conjugated directly to antibody so that substrate access

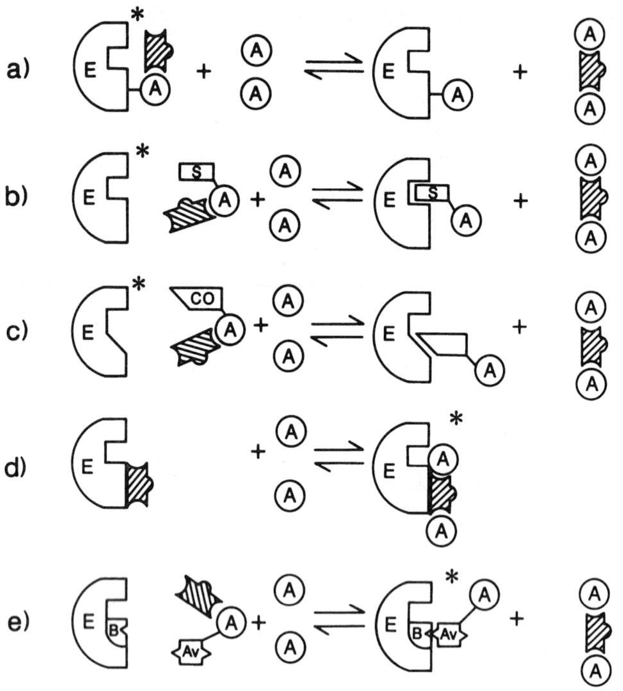

FIGURE 5-6. Competitive, homogeneous (separation-free) enzymatic immunoassays. E = enzyme; A = antigen or hapten; S = substrate; CO = enzyme cofactor; Av = avidin; B = biotin. Enzymes with an asterisk have "modulated" (increased or decreased) activities. (*From Tijssen,*[33] *by permission of Elsevier Science Publishers.*)

to the enzyme active site is blocked by antigen binding (Fig. 5-6*D*). The high affinity of avidin-conjugated hapten for biotinylated enzyme has also been utilized for hormone assay (Fig. 5-6*E*). Binding of antibody to hapten sterically hinders access of the avidin to the biotinylated enzyme. The addition of free hapten results in increased avidin/biotin complex formation and enzyme inactivation.[33]

RECEPTOR ASSAYS

The principles underlying receptor assays are very similar to those underlying immunoassays. Instead of antibody molecules, specific hormone receptors from the plasma membranes or nuclei of hormonally responsive tissues are used to bind labeled and unlabeled hormone. Receptors for peptide and protein hormones are found on the cellular plasma membrane,[92] while the steroid, thyroid, and retinoic acid receptors, which are members of the same supergene family,[93] occur in or are translocated to the nucleus, where they associate with chromosomal DNA and other nuclear proteins.[94] Purified plasma membrane receptors tend to be unstable in the absence of bound hormone and detergent or other stabilizing factors.[95] Another problem that occurs with many receptor assays is heterogeneity in the binding characteristics of the receptor, which complicates dose interpolation from the standard curve.[96]

The major protein, peptide, steroid, 1,25-dihydroxyvitamin D_3, thyroid, and retinoic acid receptors have been cloned, sequenced, and overexpressed in bacterial or mammalian cell systems.[92,97,98] Detailed structural information should lead to the availability of homogeneous, stable high-affinity–constant receptors in quantities useful for basic research and clinical assays.

CHROMATOGRAPHIC ASSAYS

Advances in chemical separation technology for peptides, biogenic amines, and steroids combined with immunoassay or physical chemical detection have greatly increased the specificity of hormone assay methods. Although many closely related compounds may cross-react with a given antibody or receptor, these molecules can usually be separated according to differences in their tendency to bind to various chromatographic media. Quantitation of the resulting chromatographic fractions allows the measurement of several hormones within the same clinical sample. The combined use of chromatography and immunoassay or direct detection methods has been reported for the simultaneous measurement of serum prednisone, prednisolone, and cortisol[99]; unconjugated estriol and estradiol[100]; glucocorticoids[101]; adrenal delta 4-steroids[102]; testosterone in female patients[103]; dehydroepiandrosterone sulfate[104]; and catecholamines, vitamin D, opioid peptides, and gastrointestinal hormones.[105]

Chromatography

The chromatographic method used most frequently in conjunction with hormone measurement is high-pressure liquid chromatography (HPLC). The chromatographic medium usually consists of microspheres of silica gel which have been chemically modified to render them hydrophobic (lipophilic). Molecules are separated on this "reverse-phase" column using a high-pressure flow of an aqueous solution with an increasing concentration of an organic solvent such as acetonitrile.[105,106] Exclusion HPLC, which separates according to effective molecular size, and ion-exchange HPLC, which separates according to the electric charge on the hormone, can also be used.

Detection

A variety of detection methods are being used to quantitate serum and tissue hormones as they emerge from the HPLC column. These include immunoassays, refractometry, electrochemical conductance, light scattering, ultraviolet spectrometry, fluorometry, chemiluminescence, and mass spectrometry.[105]

IMMUNOASSAY OPTIMIZATION AND VALIDATION

General Considerations

The trend in hormone assays has been toward progressive improvement in detection limits, labor costs, reagent stability, and assay variability. A parallel development has been the institution of laboratory quality assessment programs which distribute pooled or fully characterized samples for interlaboratory comparison. These two processes tend toward the ultimate but never fully attainable goal of providing absolutely precise and reproducible measurement of clinically important hormonal substances.[107]

Detection Limits

Detection and precision limits for competitive or reagent limiting assays are a function of the affinity constant for the antigen-antibody reaction. Selection of the optimal concentrations for the antibody and tracer concentrations and tracer specific activity on a trial-and-error basis is extremely tedious. Graphic representations of RIA detection and precision limits as a function of antibody concentration and affinity constant, labeled antigen concentration, and specific activity have been reported.[108] These representations provide valuable insights into the appropriate adjustments to be made in the reagent parameters to provide the greatest assay sensitivity and precision. The important point that optimal assay sensitivity can often be attained at initial binding (B_0/T) values <30 to 50 percent if a labeled antigen of high specific activity is used has been well illustrated. For competitive assays, the detection limit is proportional to $1/K_a$.[28] Selection of the antiserum with the highest K_a value is made by comparison of Scatchard plots for each antiserum obtained in the same assay (Fig. 5-7).

Specificity

Many hormonal analytes have similar or identical antigenic binding sites or epitopes. A good example is the α subunit of the glycoprotein hormones LH, FSH, TSH, and hCG, which is the product of a single gene.[109] Polyclonal antibodies produced

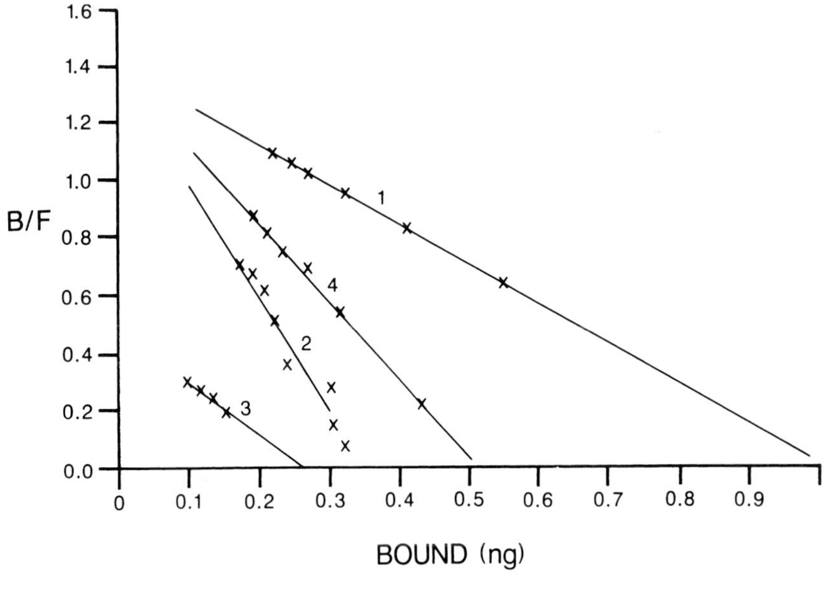

FIGURE 5-7. Scatchard plot comparison of four different rabbit antisera against human TSH. Curve 2 has the steepest slope (equal to $-k_a$) and should provide the most sensitive reagent limiting immunoassay after proper assay optimization. (*From Pekary and Hershman, unpublished results.*)

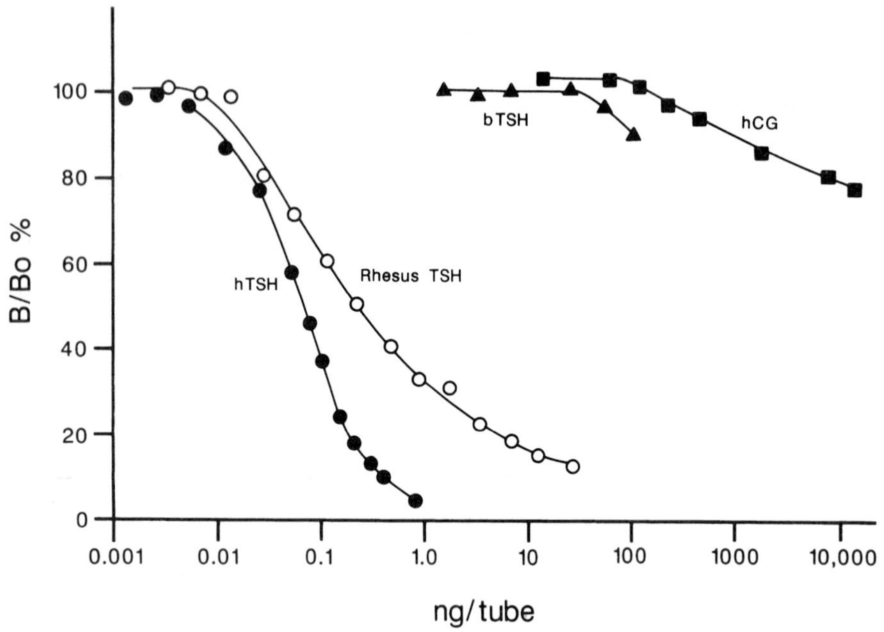

FIGURE 5-8. Saturation curves for the "high-affinity" (curve 2 in Fig. 6-6) human TSH antibody: human chorionic gonadotropin, 2980 IU/mg (solid squares); bovine TSH, 40 mU/μg (solid triangles); Rhesus monkey pituitary homogenate (units in terms of wet weight of tissue/tube are 10^4 times the indicated ng/tube) (open circles); and the 68/38 human TSH standard assuming 10 μU = 1 ng (solid circles). (*From Pekary, Hershman, and Parlow.*[31])

against any one of these hormones will produce antibodies which will cross-react with the α subunit of other glycoprotein hormones of the same species and possibly related species. One method for suppressing this cross-reactivity is to add a great excess of one of the glycoprotein hormones which is not being analyzed, such as hCG, resulting in nearly complete saturation of the α-subunit–reacting antibodies and greatly reduced cross-reaction with additional hCG (Fig. 5-8).[31] With the advent of monoclonal antibodies, much greater selectivity of the epitopic sites being recognized is possible. Any given protein hormone analyte may in fact represent a large family of chemically distinct but highly cross-reactive species produced by alternative splicing of the corresponding mRNA, variations in posttranscriptional glycosylation, acetylation, methylation, sulfation, and partial enzymatic fragmentation by serum- and membrane-associated enzymes. The biological activity of each analyte may vary from totally inactive to greatly increased effectiveness as assessed by a bioassay. This heterogeneity in the ratio of biological to immunologic activity (B/I ratio) may contribute significantly to such puzzling phenomena as the normal TSH levels in patients with hypothalamic hypothyroidism. Lack of TRH results in secretion of TSH with altered glycosylation and reduced bioactivity.[24] A number of approaches have proved useful in minimizing the interference of biologically irrelevant but highly cross-reactive species in hormonal assays. These include chromatographic separation, protein binding, ultrafiltration, protein precipitation, change in incubation time or temperature, selection of antibodies specific for epitopes unique to the relevant hormonal species, and the use of dual-site assays.[110]

INTERFERENCE

Sample Matrix Effects

The antigen-antibody reaction is very rapid, being limited only by the rate of diffusion of the reacting species. The effective diffusion rate, however, can be greatly reduced if other macromolecules occur in the same reaction mixture. Hormone assay measurements are most often made in undiluted, unextracted human serum or plasma in which serum proteins such as albumin, gamma globulins, lipoproteins, α_2-macroglobulin, and fibrinogen (plasma) occur in great excess compared to the trace levels of the hormonal analyte of interest. Because of the complex structure of proteins that have many different classes of interactive chemical groups exposed on their surfaces, complexes of these proteins with hormonal analyte and antibody, with widely varying stabilities, inevitably form. These interactions greatly retard the diffusional processes leading to the formation of the hormone-antibody complex and reduce the apparent affinity constant of hormone-antibody binding at equilibrium. For competitive or reagent limiting assays, these effects are manifested by a retarded forward rate constant for antigen-antibody binding and a reduction in the tracer bound/total (B/T) ratio for serum-containing samples compared to equivalent samples in protein-free buffer.[31,111] This "serum" or "matrix" effect can usually be compensated for by using the same amount of hormone-free serum to prepare the assay calibrators.

Heterophilic Antibodies

Mouse monoclonal antibodies are sometimes used in various therapeutic modalities, resulting in the production of human antibodies to mouse gamma globulins. The mixing of serum from such patients with the mouse monoclonal antibodies commonly used in commercial kit assays may result in a significant interference with the monoclonal antibody-hormone reaction.[112] Such interfering antibodies can also occur in "naive" (untreated) patients[113] and should be considered as a possible explanation for unexpected assay results. The direction of bias caused by the presence of patient antibodies reacting with some component of the assay system can lead to either high or low values depending on the assay method and the specificity of the heterophilic antibody. Inappropriately elevated levels of TSH in a reagent excess assay were traced to patient antibodies to mouse IgG which sandwiched between the immobilized and labeled monoclonal antibodies of the assay, leading to a diagnosis of hypothyroidism and inappropriate therapy.[114]

Complement and Rheumatoid Factors

Immunoassays that use a second antibody for the separation of bound and free antigen can fail because the complement-fixation reaction enzymes in the serum sample destroy the complexes of the first and second antibodies.[115,116] Rheumatoid factor is an IgM molecule which can also fix and activate complement. This potential problem is usually prevented by the addition of a calcium chelator such as edetic acid (ethylenediaminetetraacetic acid, or EDTA) which binds the ionized calcium that is essential for the complement-fixation reaction.[31,115–117]

Enzyme Contaminants

Microbial growth in blood or serum samples may result from an infection in the patient or improper handling and storage of the specimen. In vitro degradation of one or more of the assay reagents or of the analyte itself by the proteolytic enzymes of the contaminated sample may result in a serious measurement error. The addition of a bacteriostatic agent, such as sodium azide, to all hormonal assay reagents retards this process. Rapid sample processing and storage in a $-20°C$ freezer is usually sufficient to avoid this problem. Many hormones, such as β-endorphin, glucagon, and ACTH may be rapidly degraded by proteases in normal serum. The addition of proteolytic enzyme inhibitors such as aprotinin (Trasylol) or benzamidine combined with special handling of the samples is required for the accurate measurement of these hormones.[118]

Drug Interference

Drug therapy has the potential for biasing the results of a hormone assay. An example is the effect of heparin on the measurement of free T_4; heparin can stimulate the release of FFA in vivo and in vitro, leading to the displacement of T_4 from the thyroid hormone-binding proteins of serum.[44] A number of therapeutic drugs cross-react in hormone assays. For example, prednisolone may cross-react with hydrocortisone and spironolactone may cross-react with aldosterone. Insulin and growth hormone therapy can lead to hormone-specific antibody production which can interfere in the corresponding immunoassays.[113,119] The sera of such patients have high levels of hormone bound to the corresponding antibodies. Autoantibodies to insulin can occur spontaneously. Growth hormone-binding proteins occur normally in patient sera. The affinity constants for these proteins have been shown to be much lower than those for typical monoclonal or polyclonal antibodies used in commercial assays, resulting in dissociation of growth hormone from these binding proteins during incubation and minimal interference.[119] Hormone autoimmunity presents two major complications in immunoassay measurements: (1) the high levels of antibody-associated hormone present in the serum and (2) the competition of the antibodies derived from the patient serum with those of the assay for binding to the corresponding serum hormone. A method for high-performance protein-G affinity chromatography for quantitating hormonal antibodies in patient sera has been reported.[120]

Hemodynamic Effects

A substantial increase in blood pressure occurs in normal subjects during the transition from the supine, resting position to normal upright activity. Changes in blood pressure between supine and upright postures may cause fluid shifts that result in changes of blood volume and concentration of hormones which are not freely diffusible across the capillary endothelium. A substantial (one-third) increase in serum T_4 values was measured in subjects engaged in normal activity compared with a 3-h baseline study involving the drawing of blood at 15-min intervals while the subjects were completely supine and motionless. This increase, which would be clinically significant in evaluating borderline T_4 levels, was almost quantitatively abolished by dividing each serum T_4 value by its corresponding total serum protein concentration to normalize for fluid shifts related to physical activity.[121]

QUALITY CONTROL

The standardization of hormonal assay measurements is a complex problem because the substance being measured may be structurally and functionally heterogeneous and may occur in an extremely complex mixture of other compounds whether the source is blood, urine, cerebrospinal fluid, saliva, semen, or tissue.[122] Additional problems have arisen because of a lack of universally accepted and widely available reference preparations and the rapidly increasing variety of assay methodologies to be compared. The advent of legislatively mandated participation in interlaboratory quality control programs has discouraged the clinical use of unique "in-house" assays which do not have an equivalent at other institutions. However, the reliance on commercial kit assays leaves the clinical laboratory dependent on the manufacturer's quality control department and field representatives when problems with assay performance cannot be traced to instrumentation problems or reagent deterioration.[107]

The development of an effective intralaboratory quality control program begins with proper selection and validation of the commercial assay methodology. This process should be influenced strongly by the reputation of the assay and its manufacturer for long-term stability and dependability. The complexity of the assay, the number of "hands-on" manipulations, accuracy, sensitivity, reproducibility, safety, and the cost of the instrumentation and reagents are all relevant to the selection process. The trend toward full automation of the assay methodology, which permits much better control of pipetting accuracy and the temperature and time of incubation, along with computerized diagnosis of instrument and reagent problems, has been driven by high personnel costs and the increasingly stringent regulatory environment.[1]

An understanding of the distinction between the statistical concepts of accuracy and precision is essential to the maintenance of hormone assay performance. Using the analogy of a person firing a rifle at a target with concentric circles, if the bullet holes on the target are widely but evenly distributed about the bull's-eye, we say that the shooter is accurate (unbiased) but imprecise. If the bullet holes are tightly clustered but away from the target center, then the shooter is precise but inaccurate (biased). The goal of a quality control program is to maintain both the accuracy and the precision of hormone assay results. This requires the accumulation of data which characterize the assay standard curve—maximum binding, nonspecific counts, dose at 50 percent curve displacement, and slope—and interassay controls which monitor assay performance across the useful measurement range of the assay standard curve. Criteria for the rejection of both individual data and entire assays must be set. A variety of models for intralaboratory quality control have been proposed.[107,123]

Because of the large number of commercial hormone assays available (Table 5-1) and the continuing introduction of "new and improved" versions of these assays, decisions about when to convert to a new methodology must frequently be faced. Improvements in accuracy and reproducibility should be the first criterion when one is considering a change, given the increasingly stringent regulatory environment and the relatively mature state of current assay methodology and support by manufacturers. An improvement in assay sensitivity should be considered as a selection factor only if it is clinically relevant, as it is for TSH measurements in patients who are receiving thyroid hormone suppressive therapy. Labor and materials costs should not be considered unless the new assay is at least comparable to the current assay in all other performance categories.

Frequent changes in methodology should be discouraged because diagnostic cutoff values are dependent on the selection criteria used for the normal population and on the characteristics of the assay used for determining these values. The development and dissemination of these values are time-consuming and must be revised with every significant change in assay procedure. A committee consisting of clinical and laboratory staff members should supervise the introduction of new and replacement assays to facilitate communication between clinic and laboratory when unexpected results arise with the new method.

Maintenance of hormonal assay quality control is challenging, particularly if different personnel are involved due to shift changes or personnel rotation. Controls, calibrators, and kit reagents are consumed or become outdated. Some clinical samples, controls, or calibrators, may contain very high concentrations of analyte which might carry over into the following assay tubes. Unknown interfering substances sometimes occur in clinical specimens. Large numbers of samples require either the set up of multiple independent assays, which contributes interassay variability to the results, or intra-assay drift may occur in very large assays. A practical approach for assessing the total analytical error of hormonal assays has been described by Sadler et al.[124] Their approach recognizes the constraints of time, reagent, and personnel costs by developing a simple assay protocol which can be accessed by glancing at a wall-mounted chart. A detailed example and a MS-DOS computer program that orthogonalizes up to 80 explanatory variables can be obtained on request from the first author.

FUTURE TRENDS

Recombinant DNA technology will have a major impact on the development of future hormone assays. Recombinant proteins will be designed for binding to unique epitopes on specific hormones.[125] Structural characterization of hormones in solution[126] should lead to the development of reagents and assay conditions which further reduce between-assay variability. Genetically-engineered fragments of enzymes such as *E. coli* β-galactosidase will be used to optimize homogeneous immunoassays.[127] Kinetic analyses of complex multicomponent hormone-receptor interactions, activation, and second messenger signaling will be feasible.[128] Laboratory safety issues will be resolved. For example, a reported assay system employing a pH-sensitive photo-induced current detection system uses urea as the substrate and carbon dioxide and ammonia as the reaction products.[129] Biosensors are currently under development,[130,131] with the potential for continuous endocrine monitoring of ambulatory patients or experimental subjects. In situ measurement of hormones will have many important advantages, including the avoidance of sample storage and processing artifacts, the avoidance of immobilization and venipuncture stress, and the ability to correlate from moment to moment the signal inputs and physiologic responses to hormone secretion.[132]

REFERENCES

1. Flore M, Mitchell J, Doen T, Nelson R, Winter G, Grandone C, Zeng K, Haraden R, et al: The Abbott IMx™ automated benchtop immunochemistry analyzer system. *Clin Chem* 34:1726, 1988.
2. Patrick JW: Radiation safety in the performance of radioimmunoassay, in Abraham GE (ed): *Handbook of Radioimmunoassay*. New York, Dekker, 1977, pp 1–25.
3. Pekary AE, Hershman JM: Hormone assays, in: Felig P, Baxter JD, Frohman L (eds.): *Endocrinology and Metabolism*, 3rd ed. McGraw-Hill, New York, 1995, pp 201–218.
4. Dahl KD, Stone MP: FSH isoforms, radioimmunoassays, bioassays, and their significance. *J Androl* 13:11, 1992.
5. Norman RJ, Buck R, Medeiros SF: Measurement of human chorionic gonadotrophin (hCG): Indications and techniques for the clinical laboratory. *Ann Clin Biochem* 27:183, 1990.
6. Bangham DR: Standardization and standards, in Thorell JI (ed): *Radioimmunoassay Design and Quality Control*. Oxford, Pergamon, 1983, pp 59–67.
7. Wittliff JL, Wenz LL, Dong J, Nawaz Z, Butt TR: Expression and characterization of an active human estrogen receptor as a ubiquitin fusion protein from *Escherichia coli*. *J Biol Chem* 265:22016, 1990.
8. Pekary AE: Parallel line and relative potency analysis of bioassay and radioimmunoassay data using a desk top computer. *Comput Biol Med* 9:355, 1979.
9. Hershman JM, Kenimer JG, Kojima A, Saunders RL: Thyroid-stimulating hormone, in Antoniades HN (ed): *Hormones in Human Blood*. Cambridge, Harvard University Press, 1976, pp 464–487.
10. Finney DJ: *Statistical Method in Biological Assay*. London, Charles Griffin, 1964.
11. Bangham DR: What's in a bioassay? in Chayen J, Bitensky L (eds): *Cytochemical Bioassays*. New York, Dekker, 1983, pp 7–43.
12. Vitti P, Rotella CM, Valente WA, Cohen J, Aloj SM, Laccetti P, Ambesi-Impiombato FS, Grollman EF, et al: Characterization of the optimal stimulatory effects of Graves' monoclonal and serum immunoglobulin G on adenosine 3′,5′-monophosphate production in FRTL-5 thyroid cells: A potential clinical assay. *J Clin Endocrinol Metab* 57:782, 1983.
13. Pang X-P, Hershman JM, Smith VP, Pekary AE, Sugawara M: The mechanism of action of tumour necrosis factor-α and interleukin 1 on FRTL-5 rat thyroid cells. *Acta Endocrinol (Copenh)* 123:203, 1990.
14. Morris JC, III, Hay ID, Nelson RE, Jiang N-S: Clinical utility of thyrotropin-receptor antibody assays: Comparison of radioreceptor and bioassay methods. *Mayo Clin Proc* 63:707, 1988.
15. Van Sande J, Raspe E, Perret J, Lejuene C, Maenhaut C, Vassart G: Thyrotropin activates both the cyclic AMP and the PIP_2 cascades in CHO cells expressing the human cDNA of TSH receptor. *Mol Cell Endocrinol* 74:R1, 1990.
16. Loveridge N: The techniques of cytochemical bioassays, in Chayen J, Bitensky L (eds): *Cytochemical Bioassays: Techniques and Clinical Applications*. New York, Dekker, 1983, pp 45–82.
17. Chayen J, Bitensky L: General introduction to cytochemical bioassay, in Chayen J, Bitensky L (eds): *Cytochemical Bioassays: Techniques and Clinical Applications*. New York, Dekker, 1983, pp 1–6.
18. Dohler K-D, von zur Muhlen A, Wagner TOF, Lucke C, Weitzel HK, Hashimoto T: Thyroid-stimulating hormone, in Chayen J, Bitensky L (eds): *Cytochemical Bioassays: Techniques and Clinical Applications*. New York, Dekker, 1983, pp 107–134.
19. Petersen V, Smith BR, Hall R: A study of thyroid stimulating activity in human serum with the highly sensitive cytochemical assay. *J Clin Endocrinol Metab* 41:199, 1975.
20. DiStefano JJ III, Feng D: Comparative aspects of the distribution, metabolism, and excretion of six iodothyronines in the rat. *Endocrinology* 123:2514, 1988.

21. DiStefano JJ III, Sternlicht M, Harris DR: Rat enterohepatic circulation and intestinal distribution of enterally infused thyroid hormones. *Endocrinology* 123:2526, 1988.
22. Grossmann M, Leitolf H, Weintraub BD, Szkudlinski MW: A rational design strategy for protein hormone superagonists. *Nat Biotechnol* 16:871, 1998.
23. Shibata H, Spencer TE, Onaate SA, Jenster G, Tsai SY, Tsai MJ, O'Malley BW: Role of co-activators and co-repressors in the mechanism of steroid/thyroid receptor action. *Recent Prog Horm Res* 52:141, 1997.
24. Yamada M, Saga Y, Shibusawa N, Hirato J, Murakami M, Iwasaki T, Hashimoto K, Satoh T, Wakabayashi K, Taketo MM, Mori M: Tertiary hypothyroidism and hyperglycemia in mice with targeted disruption of the thyrotropin-releasing hormone gene. *Proc Natl Acad Sci USA* 94:10862, 1997.
25. Vuolteenaho O, Arjamaa O, Ling N: Atrial natriuretic polypeptides (ANP): Rat atria store high molecular weight precursor but secrete processed peptides of 25-35 amino acids. *Biochem Biophys Res Commun* 129:82, 1985.
26. D'Amour P, Lazure C, Labelle F: Metabolism of radioiodinated carboxy-terminal fragments of bovine parathyroid hormone in normal and anephric rats. *Endocrinology* 117:127, 1985.
27. Pekary AE, Stephens R, Simard M, Pang X-P, Smith V, DiStefano JJ III, Hershman JM: Release of thyrotropin and prolactin by a thyrotropin-releasing hormone (TRH) precursor, TRH-Gly: Conversion to TRH is sufficient for in vivo effects. *Neuroendocrinology* 52:618, 1990.
28. Feldman H, Rodbard D: Mathematical theory of radioimmunoassay, in Odell WD, Daughaday WH (eds): *Principles of Competitive Protein Binding Assay*. Philadelphia, Lippincott, 1971, pp 158–203.
29. Ratcliffe JG: Requirements for separation methods in immunoassay, in Hunter WM, Corrie JET (eds): *Immunoassays for Clinical Chemistry*, 2nd ed. Edinburgh, Churchill Livingstone, 1983, pp 135–138.
30. Hunter WM: The preparation and assessment of labelled antigen: Outline of requirements, in Hunter WM, Corrie JET (eds): *Immunoassays for Clinical Chemistry*, 2nd ed. Edinburgh, Churchill Livingstone, 1983, pp 263–266.
31. Pekary AE, Hershman JM, Parlow AF: A sensitive and precise radioimmunoassay for human thyroid-stimulating hormone. *J Clin Endocrinol Metab* 41:676, 1975.
32. Kohler G, Milstein C: Continuous culture of fused cells secreting specific antibody. *Nature* 256:495, 1975.
33. Tijssen P: *Practice and Theory of Enzyme Immunoassay*, Vol. 15: *Laboratory Techniques in Biochemistry and Molecular Biology*. Amsterdam, Elsevier, 1985.
34. Pekary AE, Turner LF Jr, Hershman JM: New immunoenzymatic assay for human thyrotropin compared with two radioimmunoassays. *Clin Chem* 32:511, 1986.
35. Ekins R, Chu F, Biggart E: Fluorescence spectroscopy and its application to a new generation of high sensitivity, multimicrospot, multianalyte, immunoassay. *Clin Chim Acta* 194:91, 1990.
36. Wide L: Labelled ligand versus labelled ligate and competitive versus non-competitive binding assays, in Thorell JI (ed): *Radioimmunoassay Design and Quality Control*. Oxford, Pergamon, 1983, pp 37–44.
37. Hunter WM, Bennie JG, Budd PS, van Heyningen V, James K, Micklem RL, Scott A: Immunoradiometric assays using monoclonal antibodies, in Hunter WM, Corrie JET (eds): *Immunoassays for Clinical Chemistry*, 2nd ed. Edinburgh, Churchill Livingstone, 1983, pp 531–544.
38. Mendel CM: The free hormone hypothesis: A physiologically based mathematical model. *Endocrinol Rev* 10:232, 1989.
39. Refetoff S: Inherited thyroxine-binding globulin abnormalities in man. *Endocrinol Rev* 10:232, 1989.
40. Ekins R: Measurement of free hormones in blood. *Endocrinol Rev* 11:5, 1990.
41. Pardridge WM: Plasma protein-mediated transport of steroid and thyroid hormones (editorial review). *Am J Physiol* 252:E157, 1987.
42. Mendel CM, Weisiger RA, Jones AL, Cavalieri RR: Thyroid hormone-binding proteins in plasma facilitate uniform distribution of thyroxine within tissues: A perfused rat liver study. *Endocrinology* 120:1742, 1987.
43. Ain KB, Mori Y, Refetoff S: Reduced clearance of thyroxine-binding globulin (TBG) with increased sialylation: A mechanism for estrogen induced elevation of serum TBG concentration. *J Clin Endocrinol Metab* 65:689, 1987.
44. Nelson JC, Wilcox RB: Analytical performance of free and total thyroxine assays. *Clin Chem* 42:146, 1996.
45. Wang YS, Hershman JM, Smith V, Pekary AE: Effect of heparin on free thyroxine as measured by equilibrium dialysis and ultrafiltration. *Clin Chem* 32:700, 1986.
46. Larsen PR: Quantitation of triiodothyronine and thyroxine in human serum by radioimmunoassay, in Antoniades HN (ed): *Hormones in Human Blood*. Cambridge, Harvard University Press, 1976, pp 679–697.
47. Ratcliffe WA: Direct (non-extraction) serum assays for steroids, in Hunter WM, Corrie JET (eds): *Immunoassays for Clinical Chemistry*, 2nd ed. Edinburgh, Churchill Livingstone, 1983, pp 401–409.
48. Khosravi MJ, Diamandi A, Mistry J, Lee PDK: Noncompetitive ELISA for human serum insulin-like growth factor-I. *Clin Chem* 42:1147, 1996.
49. Braden BC, Goldman ER, Mariuzza RA, Poljak RJ: Anatomy of an antibody molecule: Structure, kinetics, thermodynamics and mutational studies of the antilysozyme antibody D1.3. *Immunol Rev* 163:45, 1998.
50. Mylvaganam SE, Paterson Y, Getzoff ED: Structural basis for the binding of an anti-cytochrome c antibody to its antigen: Crystal structures of FabE8-cytochrome c complex to 1.8 A resolution and FabE8 to 2.26 A resolution. *J Mol Biol* 281:301, 1998.
51. Fotinou C, Beauchamp J, Emsley P, deHaan A, Schielen WJ, Box E, Isaacs NW: Structure of a Fab fragment against a C-terminal peptide of hCG at 2.0 A resolution. *J Biol Chem* 273:22515, 1998.
52. Adrian TE: Production of antisera using peptide conjugates. *Methods Mol Biol* 73:239, 1997.
53. Vaitukaitis JL: Radioimmunoassay of human choriogonadotropin. *Clin Chem* 31:1749, 1985.
54. Pekary AE, Sharp B, Briggs J, Carlson HE, Hershman JM: High concentrations of p-Glu-His-Pro-NH_2 (thyrotropin-releasing hormone) occur in rat prostate. *Peptides* 4:915, 1983.
55. Visser TJ, Klootwijk W, Docter R, Hennemann G: A new radioimmunoassay of thyrotropin-releasing hormone. *FEBS Lett* 83:37, 1977.
56. Corrie JET: Production of anti-hapten sera in rabbits, in Hunter WM, Corrie JET (eds): *Immunoassays for Clinical Chemistry*, 2nd ed. Edinburgh, Churchill Livingstone, 1983, pp 469–472.
57. Webb WA, Brooks RV: Some factors influencing antiserum specificity, in Hunter WM, Corrie JET (eds): *Immunoassays for Clinical Chemistry*, 2nd ed. Edinburgh, Churchill Livingstone, 1983, pp 474–486.
58. Thorell JI, Ekman R, Malmquist M: Technical aspects of the production and application of iodinated steroids for radioimmunoassay, in *Radioimmunoassay and Related Procedures in Medicine 1982*. Vienna, International Atomic Energy Agency, 1982, pp 147–160.
59. Sugii A, Ogawa N, Kawanishi T, Umeda T, Sato T: One-step synthesis of a cortisol derivative for radioiodination and application of the ^{125}I-labeled cortisol to radioimmunoassay. *Chem Pharm Bull (Tokyo)* 35:5000, 1987.
60. Tam JP: Synthetic peptide vaccine design: Synthesis and properties of a high-density multiple antigenic peptide system. *Proc Natl Acad Sci USA* 85:5409, 1988.
61. McLean GW, Owsianka AM, Subak-Sharpe JH, Marsden HS: Generation of anti-peptide and anti-protein sera. Effect of peptide presentation on immunogenicity. *J Immunol Methods* 137:149, 1991.
62. Tam JP, Zavala F: Multiple antigen peptide. A novel approach to increase detection sensitivity of synthetic peptides in solid-phase immunoassays. *J Immunol Methods* 124:53, 1989.
63. Tam JP: Recent advances in multiple antigen peptides. *J Immunol Methods* 196:17, 1996.
64. Sheibani N, Frazier WA: Direct use of synthetic peptides for antiserum production. *Biotechniques* 25:28, 1998.
65. Moller SA, Borrebaeck CAK: Development of an in vitro immunization technique for the production of murine monoclonal antibodies using small amounts of antigen and weak immunogens, in Borrebaeck CAK (ed): *In Vitro Immunization in Hybridoma Technology. Progress in Biotechnology*, vol. 5. Amsterdam, Elsevier, 1988, pp 3–22.
66. Ehrlich PH, Moyle WR: Cooperative immunoassays: Ultrasensitive assays with mixed monoclonal antibodies. *Science* 221:279, 1983.

67. Strasberger CJ, Dattani MT: New growth hormone assays: Potential benefits. *Acta Paediatr Suppl* 423:5, 1997.
68. Wilchek M, Bayer EA: Avidin-biotin mediated immunoassays: Overview. *Methods Enzymol* 184:467, 1990.
69. Brown NS, Abbott SR, Corrie JET: Some observations on the preparation, purification and storage of radioiodinated protein hormones, in Hunter WM, Corrie JET (eds): *Immunoassays for Clinical Chemistry*, 2nd ed. Edinburgh, Churchill Livingstone, 1983, pp 263–266.
70. Thean ET: Comparison of specific radioactivities of human alphalactoalbumin iodinated by three different methods. *Anal Biochem* 188:330, 1990.
71. Bolton AE, Hunter WM: The labelling of proteins to high specific radioactivity by conjugation to a ^{125}I-containing acylating agent: Application to radioimmunoassay. *Biochem J* 133:529, 1973.
72. Kricka LJ: *Ligand-Binder Assays*. New York, Dekker, 1985.
73. Watanabe F, Miyai K: Fluorescence polarization immunoassay: Theory and application, in Ngo TT (ed): *Nonisotopic Immunoassay*. New York, Plenum, 1988, pp 199–209.
74. Soini E, Lovgren T: Time-resolved fluoroimmunoassay, in Ngo TT (ed): *Nonisotopic Immunoassay*. New York, Plenum, 1988, pp 231–243.
75. Kricka LJ, Thorpe GHG: Bioluminescent and chemiluminescent detection of horseradish peroxidase labels in ligand binder assays, in Van Dyke K, Van Dyke R (eds): *Luminescence Immunoassay and Molecular Applications*. Cleveland, CRC Press, 1990, pp 77–98.
76. Sotorrio P, Quiros A, Izquierdo JM: New immunoelectrochemiluminometric assay to measure serum thyrotropin. *Clin Chem* 43:2428, 1997.
77. Forest JC, Masse J, Lane A: Evaluation of the analytical performance of the Boehringer Mannheim Elecsys 2010 immunoanalyzer. *Clin Biochem* 31:81, 1998.
78. Wilkins TA, Brouwers G, Mareschal JL, Limet J, Masson PL: Immunoassay by particle counting, in Collins WP (ed): *Complementary Immunoassays*. Chichester, Wiley, 1988, pp 227–240.
79. O'Connell JP, Campbell RL, Fleming BM, Mercolino MD, Johnson MD, McLaurin DA: A highly sensitive immunoassay system involving antibody-coated tubes and liposome-entrapped dye. *Clin Chem* 31:1424, 1985.
80. Canova-Davis E, Redemann CT, Vollmer YP, Kung VT: Use of a reversed-phase evaporation vesicle formulation for a homogeneous liposome immunoassay. *Clin Chem* 32:1687, 1986.
81. Smith VP, Pekary AE, Hershman JM: Evaluation of a simultaneous TSH and free T4 radioimmunoassay. *J Clin Immunoassay* 10:50, 1987.
82. Ekins RP: Ligand assays: From electrophoresis to miniaturized microarrays. *Clin Chem* 44:2015, 1998.
83. Ekins RP, Chu F: Developing multianalyte assays. *Trends Biotechnol* 12:98, 1994.
84. Coxon RE, Rae C, Gallagher G, Landon J: Development of a simple fluoroimmunoassay for paraquat. *Clin Chim Acta* 175:297, 1988.
85. Power MJ, Gosling JP, Fottrell PF: Radioimmunoassay of osteocalcin with polyclonal and monoclonal antibodies. *Clin Chem* 35:1408, 1989.
86. Edwards R: The development and use of PEG assisted second antibody as a separation technique in RIA, in Hunter WM, Corrie JET (eds): *Immunoassays for Clinical Chemistry*, 2nd ed. Edinburgh, Churchill Livingstone, 1983, pp 139–146.
87. Rasmussen SE: Solid phases and chemistries, in Collins WP (ed): *Complementary Immunoassays*. Chichester, Wiley, 1988, pp 43–55.
88. Forrest GC, Rattle SJ: Magnetic particle radioimmunoassay, in Hunter WM, Corrie JET (eds): *Immunoassays for Clinical Chemistry*, 2nd ed. Edinburgh, Churchill Livingstone, 1983, pp 147–162.
89. Williams ATR: Fluorescence polarization immunoassay, in Collins WP (ed): *Complementary Immunoassays*. Chichester, Wiley, 1988, pp 135–147.
90. Ozinskas AJ, Malak H, Joshi J, Szmacinski H, Britz J, Thompson RB, Koen PA, Lakowicz JR: Homogeneous model immunoassay of thyroxine by phase-modulation fluorescence spectroscopy. *Anal Biochem* 213:264, 1993.
91. Rubenstein KE, Schneider RS, Ullman EF: "Homogeneous" enzyme immunoassay: A new immunochemical technique. *Biochem Biophys Res Commun* 47:846, 1972.
92. Drmota T, Gould GW, Milligan G: Real time visualization of agonist-mediated redistribution and internalization of a green fluorescent protein-tagged form of the thyrotropin-releasing hormone receptor. *J Biol Chem* 273:24000, 1998.
93. Shibata H, Spencer TE, Onate SA, Jenster G, Tsai SY, Tsai MJ, O'-Malley BW: Role of co-activators and co-repressors in the mechanism of steroid/thyroid receptor action. *Recent Prog Horm Res* 52:141, 1997.
94. Ribeiro RC, Apriletti JW, Waganer RL, West BL, Feng W, Huber R, Kushner PJ, Nilsson S, Scanlan T, Fletterick RJ, Schaufele F, Baxter JD: Mechanisms of thyroid hormone action: Insights from X-ray crystallographic and functional studies. *Recent Prog Horm Res* 53:351, 1998.
95. Evans SJ, Moore FL, Murray TF: Solubilization and pharmacological characterization of a glucocorticoid membrane receptor from an amphibian brain. *J Steroid Biochem Mol Biol* 67:1, 1998.
96. Wheadon H, Devereux S, Khwaja A, Linch DC: Granulocyte-macrophage colony stimulating factor receptor alpha and beta chain complexes can form both high and intermediate affinity functional receptors. *Br J Haematol* 98:809, 1997.
97. Forman BM, Evans RM: Nuclear hormone receptors activate direct, inverted, and everted repeats. *Ann NY Acad Sci* 761:29, 1995.
98. Mangaaelsdorf DJ, Evans RM: The RXR heterodimers and orphan receptors. *Cell* 83:841, 1995.
99. McBride JH, Rodgerson DO, Park SS, Reyes AF: Rapid liquid-chromatographic method for simultaneous determination of plasma prednisone, prednisolone, and cortisol in pediatric renal-transplant recipients. *Clin Chem* 37:643, 1991.
100. Kondo Z, Makino T, Iizuka R: Measurement of serum unconjugated estriol and estradiol by high-performance liquid chromatography. *J Clin Lab Anal* 4:410, 1990.
101. Takeda M, Maeda M, Tsuji A: Chemiluminescence high performance liquid chromatography of corticosteroids using lucigenin as post-column reagent. *Biomed Chromatog* 4:119, 1990.
102. Saisho S, Shimozawa K, Yata J: Changes of several adrenal delta 4-steroids measured by HPLC-UV spectrometry in neonatal patients with congenital adrenal hyperplasia due to 21-hydroxylase deficiency. *Horm Res* 33:27, 1990.
103. Oka K, Hirano T, Noguchi M: Changes in the concentration of testosterone in serum during the menstrual cycle, as determined by liquid chromatography. *Clin Chem* 34:557, 1988.
104. Shackleton CH, Kletke C, Wudy S, Pratt JH: Dehydroepiandrosterone sulfate quantification in serum using high-performance liquid chromatography/mass spectrometry and a deuterated internal standard: A technique suitable for routine use or as a reference method. *Steroids* 55:472, 1990.
105. Makin HLJ, Newton R (eds): *High Performance Liquid Chromatography in Endocrinology. Monographs on Endocrinology*, vol. 30. Berlin, Springer-Verlag, 1988.
106. Pekary AE, Lukaski HC, Mena I, Smith SM, Bhasin S, Hershman JM: Testosterone increases TRH biosynthesis in epididymis but not heart of zinc-deficient rats. *Peptides* 14:315, 1993.
107. Jeffcoate SL: *Efficiency and Effectiveness in the Endocrine Laboratory*. London, Academic, 1981.
108. Ezan E, Tiberghien C, Dray F: Practical method for optimizing radioimmunoassay detection and precision limits. *Clin Chem* 37:226, 1991.
109. Merz WE: Biosynthesis of human chorionic gonadotropin: A review. *Eur J Endocrinol* 135:269, 1996.
110. Iitaka M, Kawasaki S, Sakurai S, Hara Y, Kuriyama R, Yamanaka K, Kitahama S, Miura S, Kawakami Y, Katayama S: Serum substances that interfere with thyroid hormone assays in patients with chronic renal failure. *Clin Endocrinol* 48:739, 1998.
111. Berzofsky JA, Berkower IJ: Antigen-antibody interaction, in Paul WE (ed): *Fundamental Immunology*. New York, Raven, 1984, pp 595–644.
112. Boscato LM, Stuart MC: Heterophilic antibodies: A problem for all immunoassays. *Clin Chem* 34:27, 1988.
113. Wasada T, Eguchi Y, Takayama T, Yao K, Hirata Y: Reverse phase high performance liquid chromatographic analysis of circulating insulin in the insulin autoimmune syndrome. *J Clin Endocrinol Metab* 66:153, 1988.
114. Kahn BB, Weintraub BD, Csako G, Zweig MH: Factitious elevation of thyrotropin in a new ultrasensitive assay: Implications for the use of monoclonal antibodies in "sandwich" immunoassay. *J Clin Endocrinol Metab* 66:526, 1988.

115. Brown EJ, Joiner KA, Frank MM: Complement, in Paul WE (ed): *Fundamental Immunology*. New York, Raven, 1984, pp 645–668.
116. Klein J: *Immunology: The Science of Self-Nonself Discrimination*. New York, Wiley, 1982.
117. Buckler JMH: A comparison of the effects of human serum in two double antibody radioimmunoassay systems for the estimation of luteinizing hormone, in Kirkham KE, Hunter WM (eds): *Radioimmunoassay Methods*. Edinburgh, Churchill Livingstone, 1971, pp 273–283.
118. Mitchell R, Lambert A, Crosby SR, White A, Robertson WR: ACTH adrenal cell bioassay: Improved sensitivity (12 ng/L) achieved by immunoextraction of ACTH from human plasma by a monoclonal antibody. *Ann Clin Biochem* 27:59, 1990.
119. Baumann G, Shaw M, Amburn K, Jan T, Daavila N, Mercado M, Stolar M, MacCart J: Heterogeneity of circulating growth hormone. *Nucl Med Biol* 21:369, 1994.
120. Riggin A, Regnier FE, Sportman JR: Quantitation of antibodies to human growth hormone by high-performance protein-G affinity chromatography with fluorescence detection. *Anal Chem* 63:468, 1991.
121. Azukizawa M, Pekary AE, Hershman JM: Plasma thyrotropin, thyroxine, and triiodothyronine relationships in man. *J Clin Endocrinol Metab* 43:533, 1976.
122. Seth J: Laboratory management and quality control, in Hunter WM, Corrie JET (eds): *Immunoassays for Clinical Chemistry*, 2nd ed. Edinburgh, Churchill Livingstone, 1983, pp 3–24.
123. Ekins RP: The precision profile: Its use in assay design, assessment and quality control, in Hunter WM, Corrie JET (eds): *Immunoassays for Clinical Chemistry*, 2nd ed. Edinburgh, Churchill Livingstone, 1983, pp 76–105.
124. Sadler WA, Smith MH, Murray LM, Turner JG: A pragmatic approach to estimating total analytical error of immunoassays. *Clin Chem* 43:608, 1997.
125. Moore GP: Genetically engineered antibodies. *Clin Chem* 35:1849, 1989.
126. Kay LE, Clore GM, Bax A, Grovenborn A: Four-dimensional heteronuclear triple-resonance NMR spectroscopy of interleukin-1β in solution. *Science* 249:411, 1990.
127. Coty WA, Loor R, Bellet N, Khanna PL, Kaspar P, Baier M: CEDIA-Homogeneous immunoassays for the 1990s and beyond. *Weiner Klinische Wochenscrift Suppl* 1991:5, 1992.
128. Ward LD, Hammacher A, Howlett GJ, Matthews JM, Fabri L, Moritz, RL, Nice EC, Weinstock J, Simpson RJ: Influence of interleukin-6 (IL-6) dimerization on formation of the high affinity hexameric IL-6 receptor complex. *Biol Chem* 271:20138, 1996.
129. Briggs J, Kung VT, Gomez B, Kasper KC, Nagainis PA, Masino RS, Rice LS, Zuk RF, Ghazarossian VE: Sub-femtomole quantitation of proteins with Threshold®, for the biopharmaceutical industry. *Biotechniques* 9:598, 1990.
130. Barnard SM, Walt DR: Chemical sensors based on controlled-release polymer systems. *Science* 251:927, 1991.
131. Graff G. Polymer scientists work to beef up biosensors. *Science* 253:1097, 1991.
132. O'Byrne KT, Thalabard J-C, Grosser PM, Wilson RC, Williams CL, Chen M-D, Ladendorf D, Hotchkiss J, Knobil C: Radiotelemetric monitoring of hypothalamic gonadotropin-releasing hormone pulse generator activity throughout the menstrual cycle of the rhesus monkey. *Endocrinology* 129:1207, 1991.

PART II

Neuroendocrinology and the Pituitary

CHAPTER 6

Neuroendocrinology

Mark E. Molitch

GENERAL CONCEPTS IN NEUROENDOCRINOLOGY

Neuroendocrinology refers to the general area of endocrinology in which the interactions of the nervous system with the endocrine system are studied. As both systems transmit information from one part of the body to another, their integration links aspects of cognitive and noncognitive neural activity with metabolic and hormonal homeostatic activity. This linkage involves the direct and indirect neural regulation of hormone secretion, the effects of hormones on neuronal action, and the interaction between the two systems in regulating how the body interacts with the environment. Some of the distinctions between the neural and endocrine systems are blurring, however, as we discover the wide range of what were formerly thought of exclusively as hormones (substances secreted directly into the blood) serving as *neurotransmitters* (substances that mediate the synaptic interaction between two neurons). Similarly, classical neurotransmitters may also function as hormones. Furthermore, neurons may have hormone receptors distinct from the area of the synapse, so that neuropeptide hormones may function in a neuromodulatory role. Adding to this complexity is the discovery of the presence of these hormones and neurotransmitters in a wide variety of tissues not thought to be either endocrine or neural, such as the gastrointestinal tract, lung, placenta, and thymus, and the subsequent discovery that the functions of these substances may vary widely depending on the tissue in which they are found.

The primary neuroendocrine interface is that of the hypothalamus and the pituitary. Of critical importance in the early understanding of this interface was the recognition and demonstration by Scharrer and Scharrer of neural cells that can secrete hormones (i.e., *neurosecretory cells*).[1] These cells can propagate action potentials and can be influenced by other neurons with their neurotransmitters, hormones, and metabolites. As such, they serve as the final common pathway linking the brain with the endocrine system. The two types of neurosecretory cells involved in hypothalamic-pituitary regulation are (1) the *neurohypophyseal* neurons, which originate from the paraventricular and supraoptic nuclei, traverse the hypothalamic-pituitary stalk, and release vasopressin and oxytocin from nerve endings in the posterior pituitary (see Chap. 8), and (2) the *hypophysiotropic* neurons, which also originate from hypothalamic nuclei and release their peptide and bioamine products into the median eminence capillaries of the hypothalamic-pituitary portal vessels (Fig. 6-1).

OVERVIEW OF BRAIN-HYPOTHALAMIC-PITUITARY-TARGET ORGAN REGULATION

Neuron-Neuron Interactions

The primary neuron-to-neuron interaction occurs at the *synapse*. Bioamine or peptide neurotransmitters that have been synthesized within the cell body and transported down the axon are stored in synaptic vesicles for release by exocytosis upon depolarization (Fig. 6-2). The bioamines are synthesized enzymatically, a process that often involves several steps, but the peptide neurotransmitters are synthesized in standard fashion for proteins, often necessitating cleavage from larger precursors. The neurotransmitters bind to specific receptors on the postsynaptic neuron, and any neurotransmitter remaining in the synapse is rapidly inactivated by enzymatic degradation or, for bioamines, reuptake by the proximal neuron or uptake into other surrounding neurons or glial tissue.[2] These receptors are specific for the neurotransmitter, and several have been sequenced and cloned, including the cholinergic muscarinic, the α and β adrenergic, the serotoninergic, the dopaminergic, and the γ-aminobutyric acid (GABA) receptors.[3,4] Binding studies have demonstrated a number of different receptor subtypes, such as the muscarinic and nicotinic cholinergic subtypes and the α and β adrenergic receptors, which can be further divided into α_{1a}, α_{1b}, α_{1c}, α_{1d}, and α_{2a}, α_{2b}, α_{2c}, and β_1, β_2, and β_3 subtypes. Similarly, for peptidergic receptors, a number of receptor subtypes have been found with varying affinities for the endogenous ligand and varying specificities for pharmacologic variations of the ligand, such as at least five subtypes of the somatostatin receptor.[5,6] The recognition of these multiple receptor subtypes has resulted in advances in our knowledge of neural regulation and has allowed the development of neuroactive medications which are highly selective in their actions, thus avoiding adverse effects.[2] In addition, it has been found that certain receptor subtypes are more important in some areas of the brain than they are in others. For example, the D_2 dopamine receptor is the primary type in the pituitary lactotrophs that responds to the hypophysiotropic bioamine dopamine, whereas it is primarily the D_1 dopamine receptor that is active in the nigrostrital system.

The precise nature of the mechanisms that transduce the signal sent by the occupied receptor, such as activation of sodium and calcium ion channels, the adenylate cyclase–cAMP cascade, the phosphoinositide–protein kinase C systems, and the calcium-calmodulin system, are currently under investigation (see Chap. 4). The transduction mechanisms for most neurotransmitters are

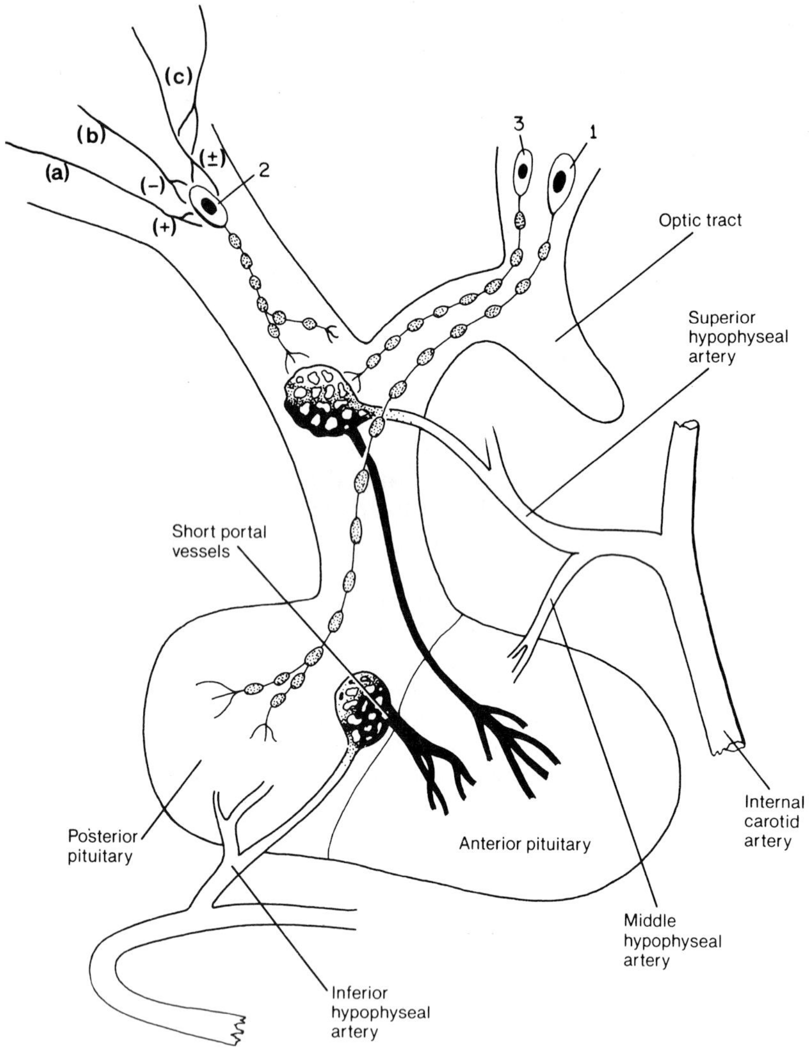

FIGURE 6-1. Neuroendocrine organization of the hypothalamus and pituitary gland. The posterior pituitary is fed by the inferior hypophyseal artery and the hypothalamus is fed by the superior hypophyseal artery, both of which are branches of the internal carotid artery. A small portion of the anterior pituitary also receives arterial blood from the middle hypophyseal artery. Most of the blood supply to the anterior pituitary is venous by way of the long portal vessels, which connect the portal capillary beds in the median eminence to the venous sinusoids in the anterior pituitary. Hypophysiotropic neuron 3 in the parvocellular division of the paraventricular nucleus and neuron 2 in the arcuate nucleus are shown to terminate in the median eminence on portal capillaries. These neurons of the tuberoinfundibular system secrete hypothalamic releasing and inhibiting hormones into the portal veins for conveyance to the anterior pituitary gland. Neuron 2 is innervated by monoaminergic neurons. Note that the multiple inputs to such neurons, using neuron 2 as an example, can be (a) stimulatory, (b) inhibitory, or (c) neuromodulatory, in which another neuron may affect neurotransmitter release. Neuron 1 represents a peptidergic neuron orig-inating in the magnocellular division of the paraven-tricular nucleus or supraoptic nucleus and projects directly to the posterior pituitary by way of the hypothalamic-neurohypophyseal tract. (*Courtesy of Ronald M. Lechan, M.D., and modified from Lechan*[31] *with permission.*)

multiple and often redundant and may involve both stimulatory (G_s) and inhibitory (G_i) guanine nucleotide-binding proteins.

A given neuron may have multiple inputs via multiple synapses with different neurotransmitters at each synapse and therefore may have potential for considerable interaction of transduction mechanisms. These multiple inputs can be synergistic or antagonistic (Fig. 6-1). These types of interactions have the potential for a rapid on-off dynamic regulatory system.[3] The same neuron may have its neurotransmitter output modulated by other neurons at a location near the synapse of its axon, an effect referred to as *neuromodulation*. A neuromodulator may augment or block release of the neurotransmitter or alter its turnover. In addition, neuron-to-neuron-signaling may occur through the diffusion of transmitters out of synaptic clefts to reach distant target receptors, a method of transmission referred to as volume transmission and via cytoplasmic gap junctions which are formed by connexin proteins.[4] The supporting glial cells, which maintain intercellular homeostasis in the CNS, also take up neurotransmitters via specific receptors, synthesize them, and even release them.[4]

A single neuron may also secrete more than one neurotransmitter, and the effects of the two neurotransmitters are usually synergistic or complementary. This type of combination generally involves a bioamine and a neuropeptide. Examples include parasympathetic nerves that control the sweat glands and contain both acetylcholine and vasoactive intestinal polypeptide (VIP); the released acetylcholine causes sweat production, while VIP increases blood flow. Conversely, sympathetic nerves to the salivary glands contain norepinephrine and neuropeptide Y; neuropeptide Y causes direct vasoconstriction and potentiates norepinephrine-evoked vasoconstriction.[7] However, two peptides may also be released, such as the corticotropin releasing hormone (CRH) and vasopressin released by neurons of the paraventricular nucleus in times of stress.[8] In this circumstance, this axon terminal is not in the posterior pituitary but rather is in the median eminence, where it releases both substances, which then have synergistic action in stimulating the secretion of adrenocorticotropic hormone (ACTH) from the pituitary.

Hypophysiotropic Hormones

Although it has been known since the beginning of this century that the hypothalamus is involved in hormone regulation, the precise nature of this involvement was not appreciated until the work of Harris[9] and others in the 1940s and 1950s. In 1901, Fröhlich

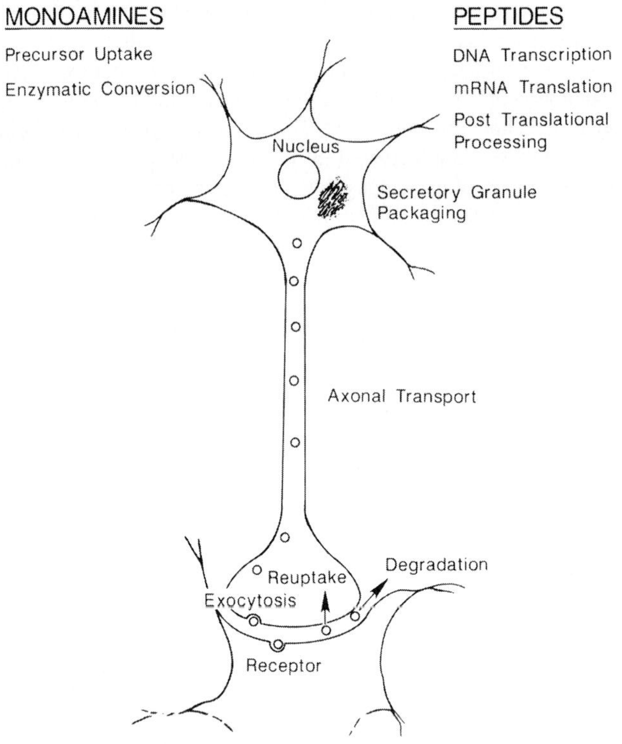

FIGURE 6-2. Schematic diagram of the neuron. For monamines, there is uptake of precursors into the neuronal cell body (perikarya) with subsequent enzymatic conversion into the active monoamine neurotransmitter. Biosynthesis of peptide neurotransmitters includes initial DNA transcription, mRNA translation, and posttranslational processing. The final products are packaged into neurosecretory granules in the cell body. The neurotransmitter reaches the nerve terminal via axonal transport. At the nerve terminal, depolarization results in fusion of the secretory granule membrane with the synaptic membrane and exocytosis with liberation of the neurotransmitter into the synaptic cleft. This liberated neurotransmitter binds to specific receptors on the postsynaptic neuron, with extra neurotransmitter being degraded by enzymes or taken back up into the proximal nerve terminal by specific reuptake mechanisms.

reported a patient with adiposogenital dystrophy due to a pituitary tumor compressing the optic chiasm and hypothalamus.[10] Shortly thereafter, Erdheim reported that obesity and hypogonadism can be caused by hypothalamic lesions that do not involve the pituitary.[11] The hypothalamic-pituitary connection was clarified in a number of experiments in which pituitary function could be enhanced by electric stimulation of the hypothalamus[9] and pituitary function was shown to cease after transplantation to other locations in the body but to remain intact after transplantation to beneath the median eminence.[12,13]

The innervation of the anterior pituitary is negligible.[14] Popa and Fielding initially described the presence of the hypothalamic-pituitary portal vessels but reported that the primary route of blood flow is from the pituitary to the hypothalamus.[15] Subsequent experiments showed that the primary flow of blood is from the hypothalamus to the pituitary,[14,16] although later experiments confirmed that there is a small amount of reverse flow that may carry hormones from the pituitary to the hypothalamus.[17,18] In 1947, on the basis of their physiologic experiments and studies of pituitary stalk blood flow, Green and Harris wrote, "It is suggested that the central nervous system regulates the activity of the adenohypophysis by means of a humoral relay through the hypophysial portal vessels."[14]

Although many experiments conducted during the next two decades confirmed this neurohumoral hypothesis and although extensive efforts were made to isolate these substances, it was not until 1969 that laboratories led by Schally and Guillemin simultaneously elucidated the structure of thyrotropin releasing hormone (TRH).[19,20] During the subsequent 20 years it was determined that the hypothalamus controls the pituitary not only through neurosecretory substances that stimulate the release of pituitary hormones, but also through substances that inhibit the release of pituitary hormones. The releasing hormones not only stimulate release but also stimulate gene transcription and new synthesis of pituitary hormones, as documented by a demonstration of the incorporation of precursors and the stimulation of the production of specific mRNAs.

The releasing and inhibitory hormones have been referred to as *hypophysiotropic hormones* for many years, dating back to a time when it was not known that the hypothalamus also contains specific inhibitory substances. However, this name has persevered and is used to refer to both hormone types. Another convention widely adopted for these substances is that a releasing or inhibiting substance is referred to as a factor until it is structurally characterized, after which it is referred to as a hormone. Thus, TRF became TRH, etc.

The hypophysiotropic hormones are synthesized in specific neuronal cell groups (nuclei) within the hypothalamus, and their axons project inferiorly to abut the proximal capillary plexus of the portal vessels in the median eminence (Fig. 6-1). Neurons from other nuclei within the hypothalamus and other parts of the brain influence pituitary hormone secretion by interacting with these specific hypophysiotropic neurons. Pituitary hormone secretion thus is regulated by the release of one or more of these hypophysiotropic hormones into the portal system.

Feedback Loops

One of the major functions of the endocrine system as a whole and of the neuroendocrine system in particular is to help maintain body homeostasis in the face of changes in the environment. This is done in part through a series of feedback loops that control pituitary and target organ hormone levels rather precisely (Fig. 6-3). Physiologic feedback systems require a controller function (in this case the pituitary hormone) and a controlled function (the target organ hormone level). The feedback loops are adjusted to maintain this target organ hormone level within a narrow range. This relation between the pituitary stimulating hormone and the target organ hormone is often referred to as the set point. This set point is analogous to setting the temperature on a thermostat. When the ambient temperature falls, the lower temperature activates the thermostat, which then causes the furnace to go on, raising the ambient temperature level. Similarly, the circulating levels of the target hormone constitute a negative feedback on the pituitary. Therefore, when the target organ hormone level falls, production and secretion of the specific pituitary hormone increase, stimulating additional production and secretion of the target organ hormone. This system is made more complex, however, by the imposition of another controller—the hypothalamus—which in turn controls the pituitary. Target organ hormones can feed back at both the hypothalamic and pituitary levels to complete the loop, and efferent controller factors from the hypothalamus may include both stimulatory and inhibitory substances.

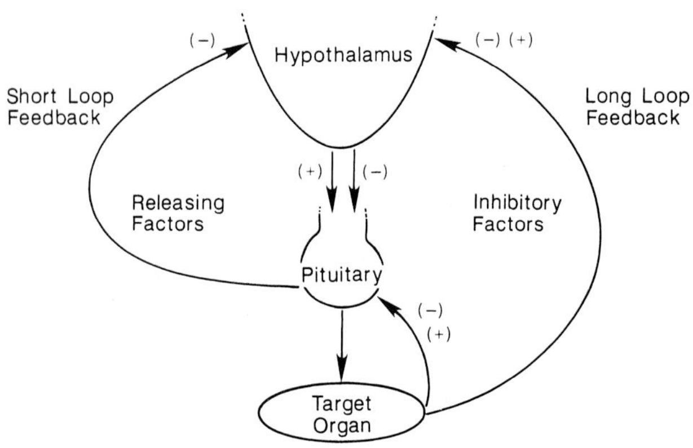

FIGURE 6-3. The hypothalamic-pituitary-target organ feedback loop. The hypothalamus influences pituitary hormone secretion via releasing and inhibiting factors. The pituitary hormone in turn stimulates target organ hormone secretion. The target organ hormone can feed back at both the pituitary and hypothalamic levels, and such feedback can be both negative and positive. The feedback may affect the secretion of the releasing factors as well as the inhibiting factors. The pituitary hormone can also feed back negatively on the hypothalamus, decreasing the secretion of releasing hormone and/or increasing the secretion of inhibiting hormone, a process referred to as short-loop feedback.

An example of how these feedback loops work is primary thyroid failure due to chronic thyroiditis: A fall in blood thyroxine (T_4) levels results in less negative feedback, causing an increase in thyroid stimulating hormone (TSH) release into the circulation. This increase in TSH then stimulates the failing thyroid gland, resulting in thyroid enlargement (goiter) and an increase in thyroid hormone levels, which may only be temporary if the gland continues to fail. TSH itself is stimulated by TRH and is inhibited by another hypophysiotropic hormone, somatostatin. Lowered thyroid hormone levels affect not only feedback on the pituitary, increasing its sensitivity to TRH in the hypothalamic-pituitary portal blood, but also feedback at the level of the hypothalamus to increase TRH production.[21] Furthermore, the low levels of thyroid hormone decrease hypothalamic somatostatin release.[22] The thyroid hormone responsible for this negative feedback at the intracellular nuclear locus in the hypothalamus and pituitary is triiodothyroinine (T_3), which is derived from plasma T_3 and intracellular deiodination from T_4.[23] The reverse happens if thyroid hormone levels are increased in the circulation as a result of the administration of exogenous thyroid hormone or the autonomous production of thyroid hormone by the thyroid itself (Graves disease). Thus, for a given hormonal axis such as the hypothalamic-pituitary-thyroidal axis, there are multiple feedback loops with considerable built-in redundancy.

Each pituitary hormone has unique aspects to its regulation (Table 6-1). Luteinizing hormone (LH) and follicle stimulating hormone (FSH) have as target organs the ovary in the female and the testes in the male, and their feedback loops are complex. The gonads produce steroid hormones which in the male feed back negatively but in the female feed back both negatively and positively, depending on the phase of the menstrual cycle. In addition, the gonads produce peptides, some of which inhibit (inhibin, follistatin) and some of which stimulate (activin) LH and FSH release. However, there is only one *established* releasing hormone—gonadotropin releasing hormone (GnRH)—and no hypophysiotropic inhibitory hormones for LH and FSH. The differential release of LH and FSH during various phases of the menstrual cycle depends on the interactive feedback effects of these steroid and peptide feedback loops at both the pituitary and hypothalamic levels. Although evidence exists for separate FSH releasing factors in some species[24] and in some experimental paradigms, as yet there is no firm evidence for such in humans.

ACTH has two releasing hormones, CRH and vasopressin, but no established inhibitory hormone in humans, although there is some evidence in mice that a portion of the precursor to TRH (prepro-TRH-[178-199]) has ACTH inhibitory properties.[25] Its primary feedback loop involves the adrenal glucocorticosteroid cortisol (hydrocortisone), which has inhibitory effects at both the pituitary and hypothalamic levels.

Growth hormone (GH) and prolactin (PRL) are different in that they have no target organs to supply feedback hormones.

TABLE 6-1. Components of the Feedback Loops for Pituitary Hormones

Hypophysiotropic Hormone	Pituitary Effect	Pituitary Hormone	Target Organ Hormone	Feedback Effect
TRH	+	TSH	T_4, T_3	−
Somatostatin	−			
GnRH	+	LH	Estradiol	−, +
			Testosterone	−
GnRH	+	FSH	Inhibin	−
			Activin	+
			Follistatin	−
CRH	+	ACTH	Cortisol	−
Vasopressin	+		Androgens	
GHRH	+	GH	IGF-I	−
Somatostatin	−			
Dopamine	−	PRL	?	?
GAP (?)	−			
TRH	+			
VIP	+			

However, GH does stimulate the production of insulin-like growth factor-I (IGF-I, also known as somatomedin C), a 7000-dalton protein, from a number of tissues. As discussed in Chap. 7, IGF-I mediates many of the GH's growth-stimulating actions. IGF-I feeds back negatively on GH production,[26,27] and there are both stimulatory [growth hormone releasing hormone (GHRH)] and inhibitory (somatostatin) hypophysiotropic hormones that regulate GH. PRL, unlike other anterior pituitary hormones, has a primary neural stimulus in the form of suckling by the neonate. However, in the absence of a suckling stimulus, PRL levels are maintained at fairly stable levels, though the feedback loops necessary for this maintenance are unknown. Unlike all the other pituitary hormones, the primary influence of the hypothalamus on PRL secretion is inhibitory rather than stimulatory. Therefore, if the hypothalamus and pituitary are disconnected, PRL levels rise while the levels of other pituitary hormone levels fall.

The feedback loops discussed so far are designated as long-loop feedback, referring to the long-distance nature of the target organ feedback. Short-loop feedback involves direct action of the pituitary hormones on hypophysiotropic hormone production or direct action on their own production. Although there is considerable experimental evidence for the existence of short-loop feedback in animal models, evidence for such feedback in humans is only indirect for hormones other than GH.[28]

The feedback loops for the various hormones maintain hormone levels within a narrow range. The loops can be perturbed in a number of ways, resulting in temporary or prolonged alterations of set points. One of the most fundamental of these perturbations is the change in hormone levels that occurs during the course of the day: circadian periodicity. These circadian rhythms are quite regular, resulting in highly reproducible changes in hormone levels at similar times from day to day. The sensitivity of each feedback loop can vary from day to day and even hour to hour and can even switch from negative to positive. This complex type of changing feedback loop is operative for the gonadotropins LH and FSH in women, in whom there is negative feedback by estrogen through most of the menstrual cycle but a switch to positive feedback at the time of the midcycle ovulatory surge of gonadotropins. Yet another type of long-term alteration of the set point has been postulated to occur at the time of puberty, when an increase in the gonadotropin set point results in increased gonadotropin and sex steroid levels.

Stress, nutritional status, and systemic illness are other factors which may perturb the system, resulting in both acute and chronic changes in hormone levels that are not related to specific organ dysfunction. Acute physical stress may result in an increase in ACTH, GH, and PRL, along with epinephrine and glucagon. Malnutrition may cause suppression of the hypothalamic-pituitary-thyroid and hypothalamic-pituitary-gonadal axes. Diseases such as renal failure and hepatic cirrhosis may increase GH levels through interruption of the GH-IGF-I axis, increase PRL levels, and alter the TRH-TSH-thyroid axis; this is referred to as the euthyroid sick syndrome.[29] Often the precise alterations in neurotransmitter and hypothalamic hypophysiotropic hormones that engender such changes are not known.

ANATOMIC ASPECTS

Hypothalamus

The hypothalamus is the most ventral portion of the diencephalon, located beneath the thalamus and subthalamus (Fig. 6-4). Anteriorly, it is bounded by the optic chiasm, lamina terminalis, and anterior commissure. Posteriorly, it is bounded by the midbrain and

FIGURE 6-4. Anatomic relations of the human hypothalamus. The MRI scan and the diagram of the midline human hypothalamus are seen in sagittal orientation. The lamina terminalis and anterior commissure constitute the anterior boundary; the posterior commissure and midbrain, the posterior boundary; and the thalamus, the dorsal boundary. (*Courtesy of Ronald M. Lechan, M.D., and reproduced from Lechan[31] with permission.*)

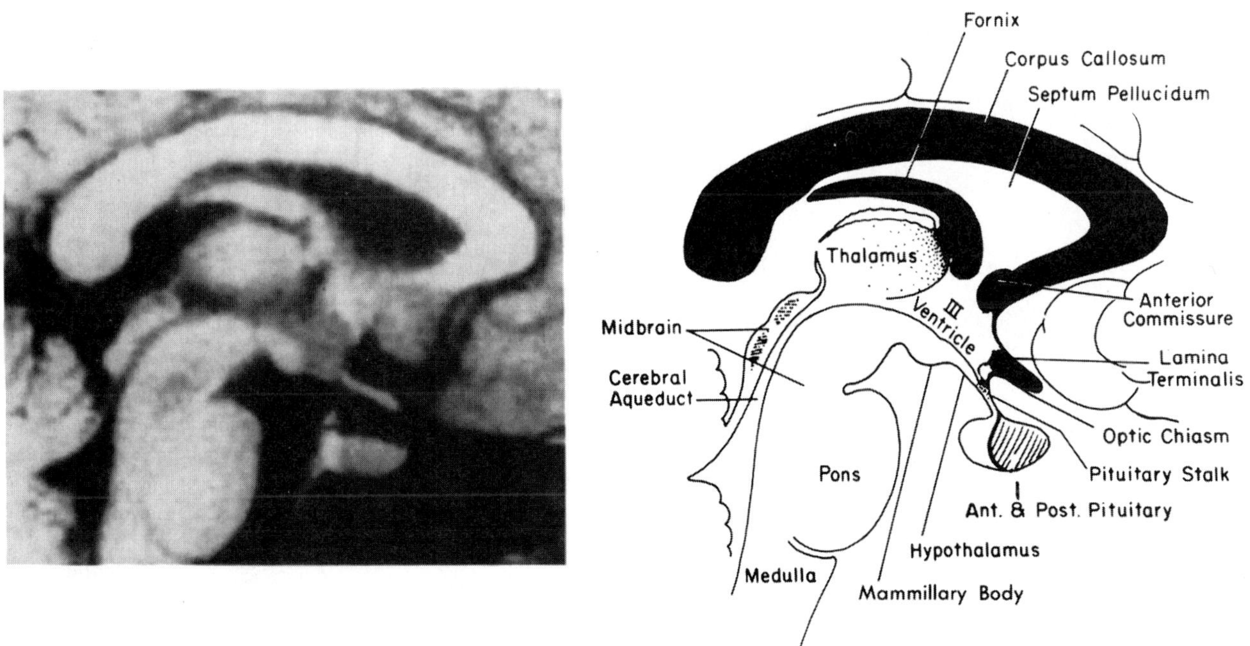

the posterior commissure. Laterally, it is bounded by the optic nerves, the sulci formed with the temporal lobes, and the internal capsule. When viewed from the inferior aspect, several features are apparent. Posteriorly are the mammillary bodies, which contain the mammillary nuclei. They are so named because of their resemblance to miniature mammary glands. Anterior to the mammillary bodies is a bulging of the hypothalamus known as the tuber cinereum, and arising from it in the midline is the median eminence, which becomes the infundibulum, or the proximal part of the hypothalamic-pituitary stalk (Fig. 6-5). The third ventricle extends ventrally into the middle of the hypothalamus and projects into the hypothalamus above the optic chiasm (supraoptic recess) and down into the infundibulum (infundibular recess).

The fornix, a neuronal fiber bundle that passes through the hypothalamus, divides the hypothalamus into medial and lateral areas (Fig. 6-6). The lateral area contains few neuronal cell bodies (perikarya) and many fibers that connect the hypothalamus and midbrain to the limbic system. The medial area contains many neuronal perikarya clustered together into nuclei, only a small portion of which subserve a neuroendocrine function. Most of the cells of the hypothalamus are involved in other functions, including memory, temperature regulation, sleep, regulation of food intake, sexual behavior, cardiovascular function, and emotions.[30,31] There are a number of connections between the medial and lateral hypothalamic areas which connect hypothalamic nuclei to the rest of the limbic system. The anterior and middle portions of the medial hypothalamus are important areas in neuroendocrine regulation.

Within the anterior portion of the medial area of the hypothalamus are the preoptic, suprachiasmatic, and supraoptic nuclei. The preoptic area and portions of the basal hypothalamus are the sites of neurons which synthesize GnRH[32] and project to the median eminence as part of the tuberoinfundibular tract (discussed later). The suprachiasmatic nuclei, which are located just above the optic chiasm, are important in regulating the circadian rhythms of the body, receiving neural input from the retina via the retinohypothalamic tract, and sending neuronal output to many areas of the hypothalamus.[33] The supraoptic nuclei are located just above the optic tracts and just behind the chiasm, and most of their neurosecretory magnocellular (large) neurons make vasopressin, although a small number make oxytocin (see Chap. 8).

The midportion of the medial hypothalamus contains the majority of the nuclei that give rise to the tuberoinfundibular tract, that is, the neurons whose axons project to the external zone of the median eminence.[31,34] This system has been defined by injecting a lectin such as wheat germ agglutinin into the external zone of the median eminence and, because of retrograde transport along axons, determining the neuronal perikarya from which these axons originate.[35] As the various hypophysiotropic hormones were characterized and antihormone antibodies were developed, their immunoreactive neuronal pathways were elucidated and compared with the results of earlier retrograde transport studies. Important nuclei contributing axons to the tuberoinfundibular tract include the ventromedial, arcuate, periventricular, dorsomedial, and the parvocellular (small) division of the paraventricular nucleus. These nuclei contain an ever-expanding list of peptides, not all of whose functions are understood (Table 6-2). Within each of the nuclei, the specific peptides that are secreted are organized into separate regions. For example, in the paraventricular nucleus the somatostatin-containing neurons are grouped medially, the CRH-containing neurons are found laterally, and the TRH-containing neurons are located between these neurons[31] (Fig. 6-7). The specific hypophysiotropic hormone distribution among these nuclei will be discussed later. These nuclei also receive input from a variety of other neuronal areas of the brain, including brainstem

FIGURE 6-5. The ventral surface of the brain showing the tuber cinereum of the hypothalamus and pituitary stalk bordered by the optic chiasm anteriorly, the uncus of the temporal lobes laterally, and the mammillary bodies and the midbrain posteriorly. The location of the neurovascular zone, or median eminence, is shown. *(Courtesy of Ronald M. Lechan, M.D., and reproduced from Lechan[31] with permission.)*

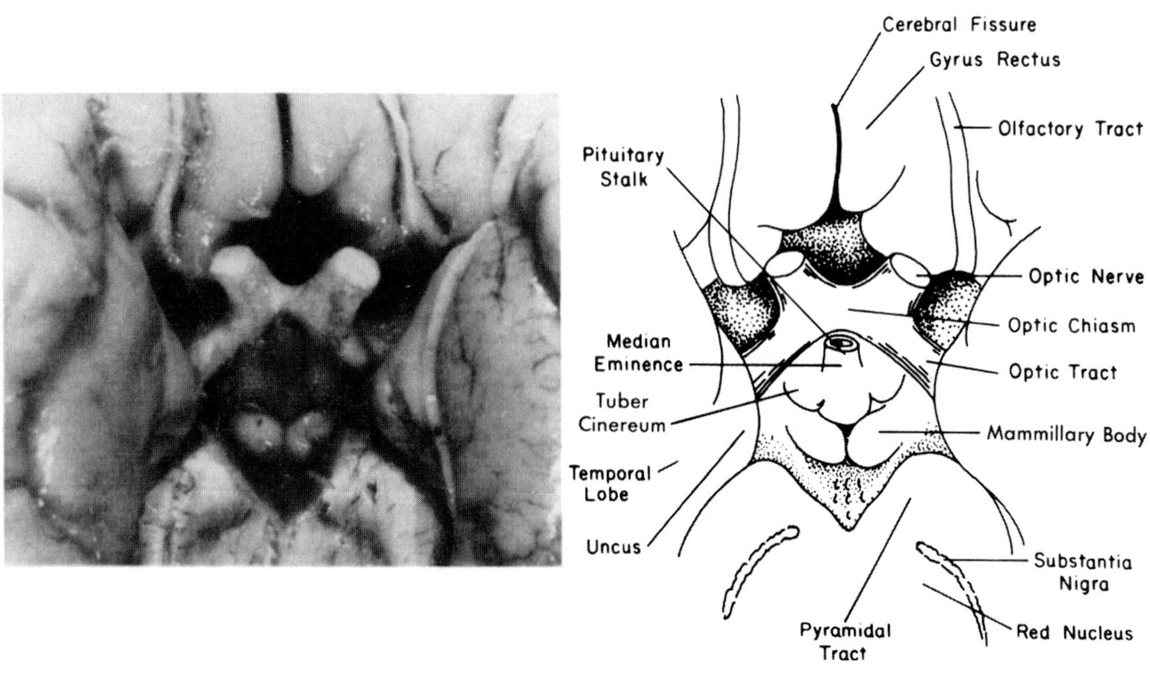

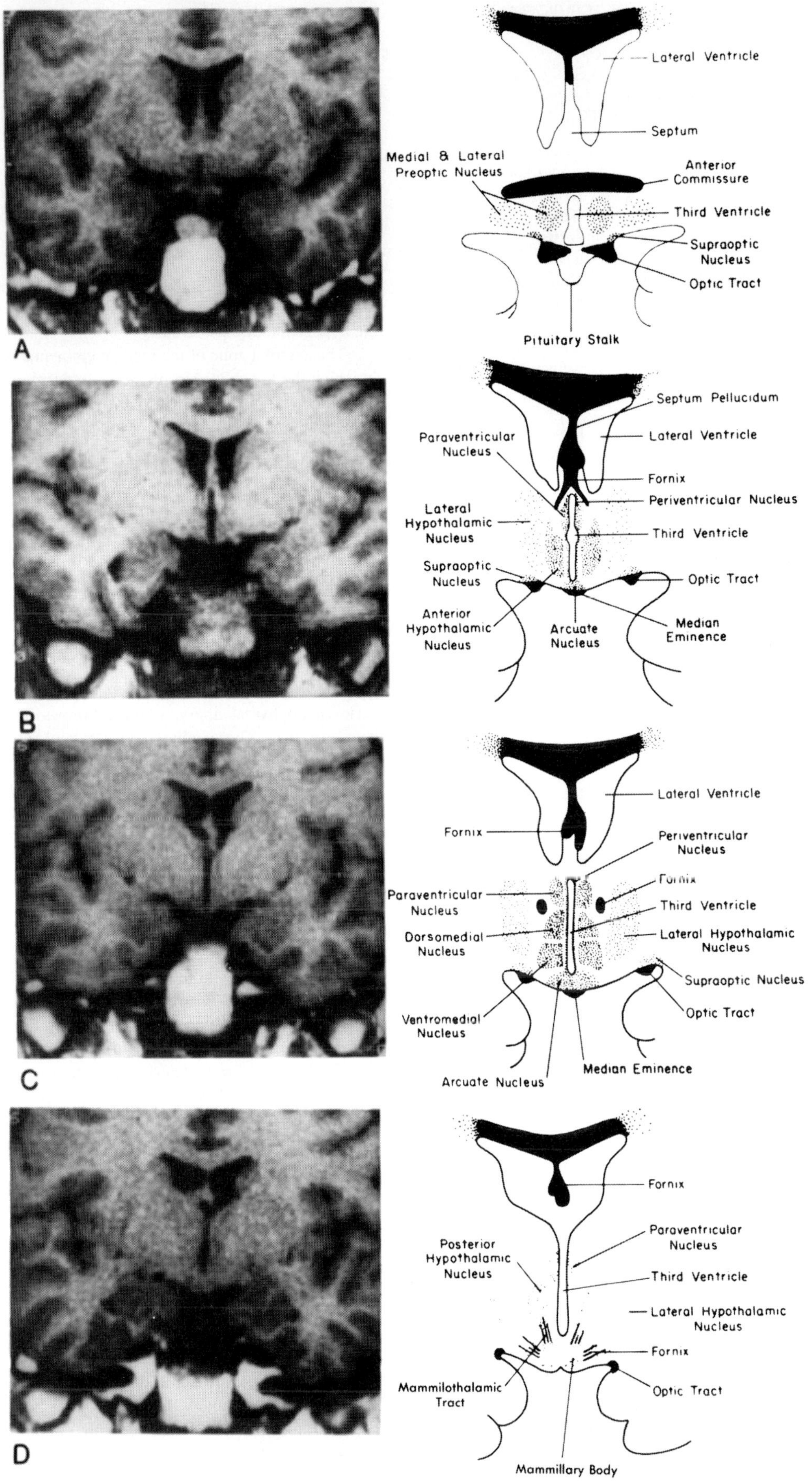

FIGURE 6-6. MRI scans and diagrams of coronal sections through the human hypothalamus. The approximate locations of the hypothalamic nuclear groups and fiber tracts are shown in the illustrations. (*Courtesy of Ronald M. Lechan, M.D., and reproduced from Lechan*[31] *with permission.*)

TABLE 6-2. Neuroactive Substances in Paraventricular and Arcuate Nucleus Neurons

Paraventricular nucleus	Arcuate nucleus
Magnocellular division	Acetylcholine
Angiotensin II	Dopamine
Cholecystokinin	Galanin
Glucagon	GABA
Oxytocin	GHRH
Peptide 7B2	Neuropeptide Y
Proenkephalin B (dynorphin, rimorphin, α-neoendorphin)	Neurotensin
Parvocellular division	Pancreatic polypeptide
Angiotensin II	Proenkephalin A (met-enkephalin, leu-enkephalin)
Atrial natriuretic peptide	Prolactin
Cholecystokinin	Pro-opiomelanocortin (ACTH, β-LPH, β-endorphin)
CRH	Somatostatin
Dopamine	Substance P
GABA	
Galanin	
Glucagon	
Neuropeptide Y	
Neurotensin	
Peptide 7B2	
Proenkephalin A (met-enkephalin, leu-enkephalin)	
Somatostatin	
TRH	
VIP/PHM	

Source: Modified from Lechan.[26]

autonomic centers, and thus mediate the effects of the extrahypothalamic brain on neuroendocrine function.[36]

Median Eminence and Hypothalamic-Pituitary Portal System

The median eminence constitutes the medial portion of the tuber cinereum and, as the infundibulum, constitutes the beginning of the pituitary stalk. Located just below the third ventricle, it can be considered a circumventricular organ and is an interface between the cerebrospinal fluid (CSF) and the blood. The median eminence is outside the blood-brain barrier, and systemic hormones and other substances pass freely into the periventricular extracellular space.[35,37] However, there are tight junctions between the tanycyte processes serving as a blood-brain barrier between the lateral margin of the median eminence and the adjacent portions of the basal hypothalamus.[35,37] The location of this barrier has obvious functional significance in that peptides secreted by neurosecretory cells into the perivascular space in the median eminence cannot diffuse out to affect other areas of the hypothalamus.[35]

The median eminence is divided into an internal ependymal zone, a middle internal zone (zona interna), and an external zone (zona externa) (Fig. 6-8). The ependymal cells form the lining of the third ventricle and have microvilli but not cilia on the ventricular surface.[38] Some of these ependymal cells, called tanycytes, are specialized in that they have long cytoplasmic processes on the inner surface that extend into the internal zone of the median eminence. Tight junctions connect the ependymal cells, preventing direct diffusion of substances between the CSF and the interior of the median eminence. The extent to which tanycytes provide a route of neuroendocrine communication between the CSF and the neurosecretory tuberoinfundibular, and hypothalamic-neurohypophyseal tracts is unknown.[38] The internal zone consists primarily of supportive structures and neurons in passage from the hypothalamus to the posterior pituitary, that is, the magnocellular hypothalamic-neurohypophyseal tract, or to the capillary plexus of the external zone of the median eminence, that is, the hypophysiotropic neurons.

The external zone of the median eminence is the contact zone in which the hypophysiotropic neurosecretory axons terminate on or near the capillaries which form the proximal portion of the hypothalamic-pituitary portal vessels. As was discussed previously, some axon terminals may end near other axon terminals, playing a neuromodulatory role. The nerve endings are rich in secretory granules, which, upon stimulation, are released into the external zone to be taken up through the fenestrations in the capillaries. True neuron-neuron synapses are not present. The axon terminals containing a given hypophysiotropic peptide tend to cluster in a specific region: GnRH and GHRH axon terminals are present in lateral portions of the median eminence, and TRH and somatostatin are present in both the medial and lateral portions (Fig. 6-9).[31]

The median eminence receives its blood supply from the superior hypophyseal artery, which arborizes into a rich capillary bed (Fig. 6-1). The capillary loops extend into the internal and external zones of the median eminence and coalesce to form the long portal veins that traverse the pituitary stalk and end in the pituitary.[14,16,39] Within the external zone the capillary walls are "fenestrated," allowing the entry of peptides secreted by the axon terminals. These fenestrations stop at the level where the blood-brain barrier is reconstituted lateral to the median eminence. At the pituitary end of the stalk the portal vessels again branch to form an extensive capillary plexus. In addition to these *long* portal vessels there is a similar *short* portal system between the posterior and anterior lobes, with the direction of flow being primarily posterior to anterior.[14,39] The resultant blood flow to the anterior pituitary is the highest of any organ in the body, being on the order of 0.7 ml/g per min.[39] By far the predominant direction of blood flow is from the hypothalamus to the pituitary, but at least in some species, there is evidence of retrograde flow.[17,39] Using direct observation or Doppler flow studies, no retrograde flow has been demonstrable in pigs[40] or rhesus monkeys,[41] and no direct observations have been made in humans. High concentrations of pituitary hormones have been found in the portal vessels in rats,[18] presumably as a result of such retrograde flow. Such flow might be a route for short-loop negative feedback in addition to the systemic circulation.

Pituitary

The pituitary will be discussed in detail in Chaps. 7 and 8. It is located within a bony pocket in the sphenoid bone referred to as the sella turcica. The pituitary (hypophysis) has two lobes: a glandular anterior lobe (also known as the anterior pituitary or adenohypophysis) and a neural posterior lobe (also known as the posterior pituitary or neurohypophysis). Embryologically, the anterior lobe originates from Rathke's pouch, which is an ectodermal structure that results from an outpouching of the oropharynx. The posterior

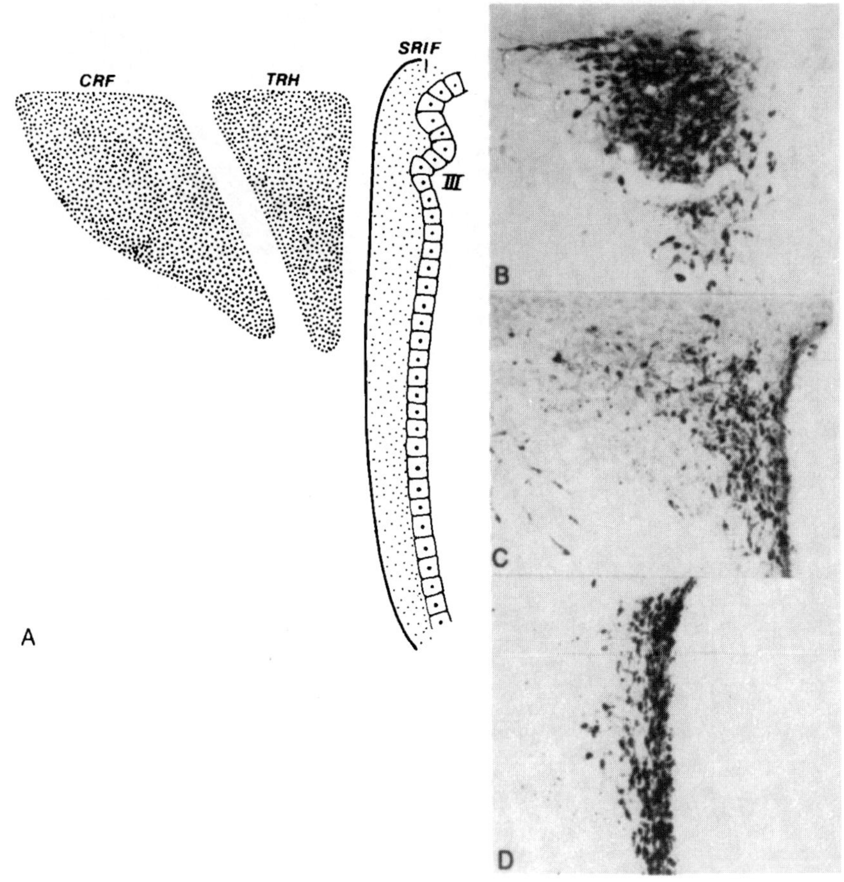

FIGURE 6-7. Organization of hypophysiotropic neurons in the medial parvocellular division of the paraventricular nucleus. (*A*) Schematic illustration of the relative distribution of neurons containing corticotropin releasing hormone (CRH), thyrotropin releasing hormone (TRH), and somatostatin (SRIF). Each of these peptides is shown by immunocytochemical techniques in *B* through *D* (*B* = CRH; *C* = TRH; *D* = SRIF). III = third ventricle. (*Courtesy of Ronald M. Lechan, M.D., and reproduced from Lechan*[31] *with permission.*)

pituitary is essentially neural tissue and is an extension of the hypothalamus; it is the site of the nerve terminals of the hypothalamic-neurohypophyseal tract.

Even during embryologic development, there is hypothalamic-pituitary interaction. During the formation of Rathke's pouch, the ectodermal primordial cells of the anterior and intermediate lobes of the pituitary make contact with the neuroectoderm of the floor of the diencephalon, and experimental studies have shown inductive interactions between these tissues that are necessary for their subsequent interdependent development.[42] Elegant studies using a series of targeted mutations have shown that there is a whole host of homeodomain transcription factors that are sequentially expressed in the developing hypothalamus and pituitary that lead to the final determination of the five mature pituitary cell types and the functional integration of the hypothalamic-pituitary system.[42,43]

Specialized cell types in the anterior lobe produce the various pituitary hormones. A number of other peptides are present in the pituitary, such as gastrin, renin, angiotensin, human chorionic gonadotropin (hCG), and proteins without clearly defined functions, such as neuromedin B, chromogranin A, and galanin. The physiologic roles of these additional substances are unknown. Interestingly, some substances primarily thought of as hypophysiotropic hormones, such as TRH and VIP, are also produced by the pituitary.[44,45] This fact raises the interesting question of the relative roles of hypothalamic vs. pituitary hypophysiotropic hormones and endocrine vs. paracrine or even autocrine effects. At present, the pituitary production of such hormones is of uncertain significance.

In addition to the hypothalamic-neurohypophyseal tract containing vasopressin and oxytocin, a number of other neural pathways from the mediobasal hypothalamus also project to the posterior pituitary and contain a variety of peptides, including GnRH, TRH, somatostatin, CRH, neurotensin, and dopamine.[31] In various experimental preparations, some of these peptides have been shown to affect vasopressin secretion, but their roles in humans are unknown. As was mentioned earlier, there are short portal vessels between the anterior and posterior lobes. It has been postulated that the posterior lobe may play a role in the regulation of anterior pituitary hormone secretion either by means of vasopressin and oxytocin or by means of the additional peptides mentioned above.[31,39] This is separate from and in addition to the known effects of vasopressin on ACTH secretion mediated by vasopressinergic neurons whose axons pass directly from the paraventricular nucleus to the external zone of the median eminence to release vasopressin there.[8] At present, the precise role of the posterior pituitary in the regulation of anterior pituitary hormone secretion is unknown.

HYPOPHYSIOTROPIC HORMONES

The elucidation of the structure of TRH in 1969[19,20] was a major milestone in the development of neuroendocrinology and was the

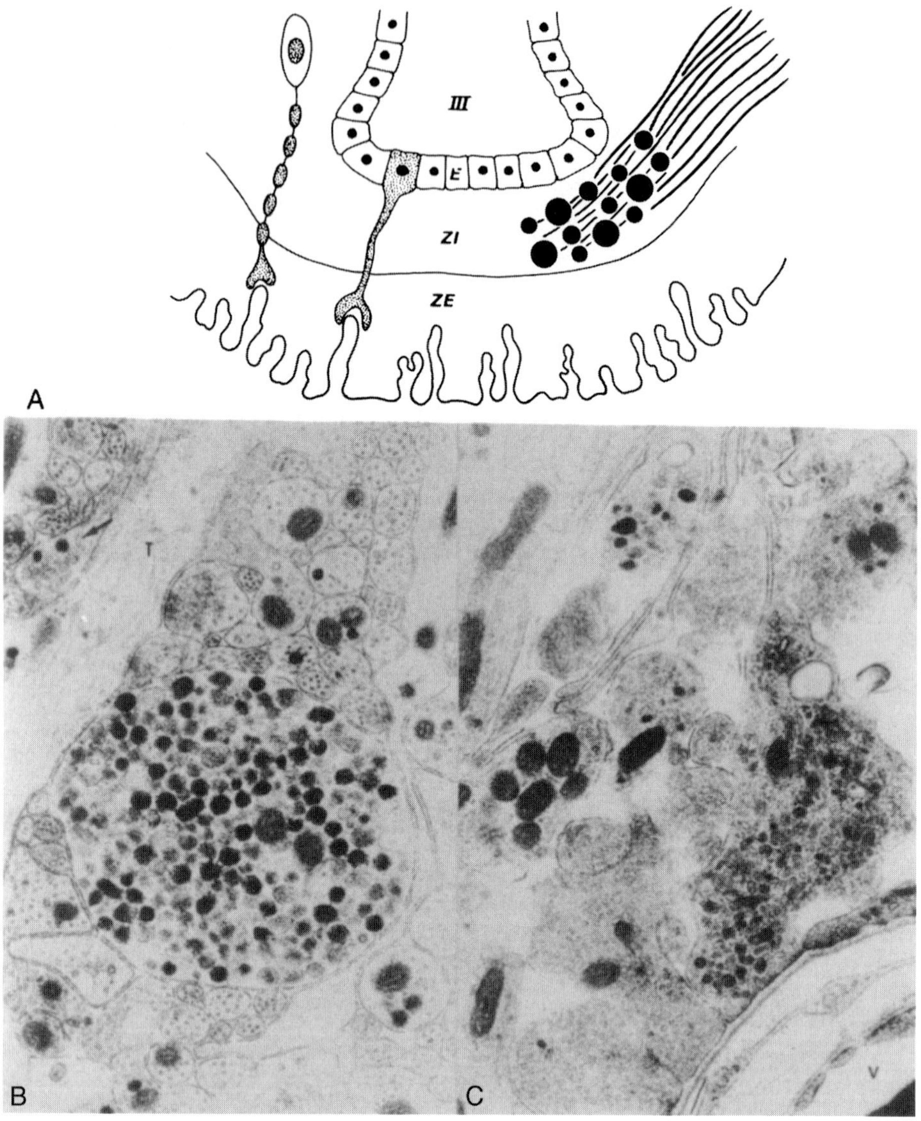

FIGURE 6-8. Diagram of the median eminence showing the location of its three major zones: the ependymal zone (E), the internal zone (ZI), and the external zone (ZE). The ZE is invaginated by portal capillaries which are contacted by axon terminals of the tuberoinfundibular system and by processes of specialized ependymal cells, tanycytes. The ZI contains numerous axons of the hypothalamic neurohypophyseal tract en route to the posterior pituitary. (*B*) Electron micrograph of the ZI showing a Herring body containing neurosecretory granules surrounded by axons of passage. Some of these axons contain dense-core vesicles (arrow) that are considerably smaller than the neurosecretory granules. T = tanycyte process. (*C*) Electron micrograph of the ZE showing axon terminals containing dense-core vesicles and small, clear vesicles abutting a fenestrated capillary of the portal system (v). (*Courtesy of Ronald M. Lechan, M.D., and reproduced from Lechan*[31] *with permission.*)

culmination of years of effort by many investigators. Guillemin has estimated that it took 270,000 sheep hypothalami weighing 50 tons to yield 1 mg of pure TRH.[46] Interestingly, the subsequent characterization of the entire 255-amino acid precursor was performed with an expression library prepared from only 65 rat hypothalami,[47] a testimony to technological progress. Subsequently, the structures of GnRH, somatostatin, CRH, and GHRH were determined (Fig. 6-10) and their roles in the regulation of the various pituitary hormones were investigated. These investigations have shown that the regulation of each pituitary hormone, as well as the effects of each hypophysiotropic hormone, is unique. Furthermore, other peptides within the hypothalamus, such as VIP, have hypophysiotropic functions under physiologic circumstances, and simple neurotransmitters such as dopamine also serve as hypophysiotropic factors.

The regulation of the pituitary hormones by the hypophysiotropic hormones is quite complex, in part because of the multiplicity of substances present in the hypothalamus that can affect pituitary hormone secretion and in part because of the redundancy and overlapping nature of the feedback loops alluded to above. In addition, some of these hypophysiotropic hormones exert effects on more than one pituitary hormone. While it seems appropriate for GnRH to stimulate the release of LH and FSH, it has also been found that TRH stimulates not only TSH but also PRL and that somatostatin inhibits not only GH but also TSH. Furthermore, a 56-amino acid portion of the precursor to GnRH, referred to as GnRH-associated peptide (GAP), both stimulates gonadotropins and inhibits PRL.

Some of the hypophysiotropic hormones are also found elsewhere in the body, particularly in the gastrointestinal tract and placenta, where they may have significant physiologic functions. For example, somatostatin is present in the pancreatic islets, where it inhibits the secretion of insulin and glucagon. It is also present in the stomach, where it inhibits gastric acid and gastrin secretion. In contrast, VIP, which is thought of primarily as a gut hormone, may serve as a physiologic stimulator of PRL release.

All the hypophysiotropic hormones are also present in the extrahypothalamic brain and subserve different functions as neurotransmitters. For some, such as TRH and GnRH, there may be behavioral effects, but in general, their physiologic functions as

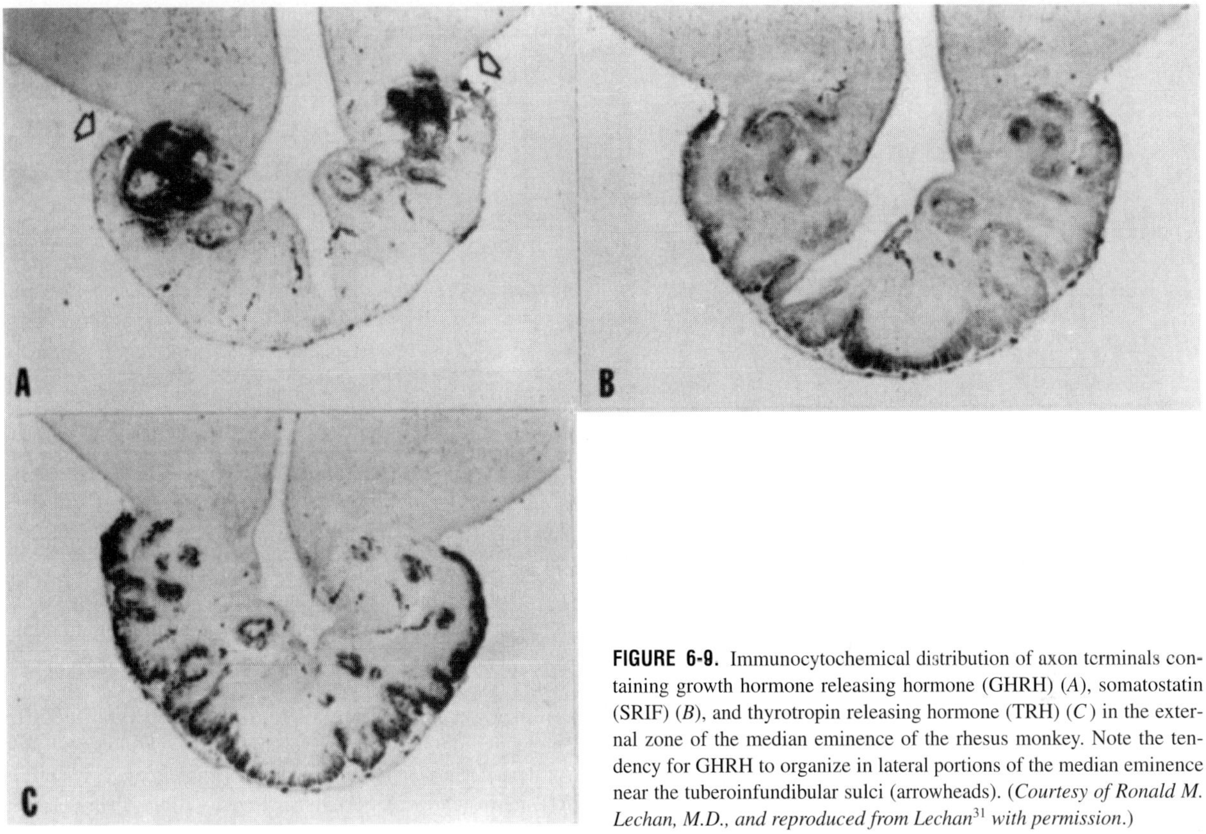

FIGURE 6-9. Immunocytochemical distribution of axon terminals containing growth hormone releasing hormone (GHRH) (*A*), somatostatin (SRIF) (*B*), and thyrotropin releasing hormone (TRH) (*C*) in the external zone of the median eminence of the rhesus monkey. Note the tendency for GHRH to organize in lateral portions of the median eminence near the tuberoinfundibular sulci (arrowheads). (*Courtesy of Ronald M. Lechan, M.D., and reproduced from Lechan*[31] *with permission.*)

neurotransmitters are unknown. The highest concentrations of all these hormones are within the hypothalamus.[48] Several hormones can occur in the same hypothalamic nucleus and even within the same secretory granule of a single cell.[48]

Thyrotropin Releasing Hormone

As was mentioned earlier, TRH was the first of the hypophysiotropic hormones to be identified.[19,20] It is a tripeptide (Glu-His-Pro) in which the N-terminal glutamine is cyclized and the proline is amidated via the donation of an amide group from the adjacent glycine in the precursor. These latter two posttranslational changes result in the final product, pyroGlu His-ProNH_2, which has a molecular weight of 362. The TRH precursor and gene structure were initially characterized partially in the frog,[49] fully in the rat,[47] and finally in the human,[50] where the preproTRH gene has been found to encode six copies of the TRH sequence and has a predicted peptide structure of 242 amino acids (Fig. 6-11). Ultrastructural analysis has shown that the processing of precursor to mature TRH occurs within the neuronal perikarya, and it is TRH rather than proTRH that is transported to axon terminals.[47]

TRH is metabolized and inactivated rapidly. One of the metabolites, cycloHis-Pro-diketopiperazine (His-Pro-DKP), has been found to inhibit PRL secretion and reverse ethanol-induced sleep.[51] However, the concentrations of TRH and His-Pro-DKP vary considerably anatomically,[47] and it is possible that His-Pro-DKP arises, at least in part, separately from TRH degradation. The biological significance of His-Pro-DKP is uncertain.[51]

The primary areas containing the TRH neuronal perikarya that project to the median eminence are the anterior, medial, and periventricular regions of the paraventricular nucleus and the anterior portion of the periventricular nucleus.[47,52] However, TRH-containing neuronal cell bodies are also abundant in the suprachiasmatic subdivision of the preoptic nucleus, the dorsomedial nucleus, and the perifornical region and basolateral hypothalamus.[47,52] TRH-containing fibers may be found not only in the median eminence but also in the organum vasculosum of the lamina terminalis (OVLT), in the posterior pituitary, and scattered throughout other portions of the brain.[47,52] In humans, substantial amounts of immunoreactive TRH are found in the thalamus and cerebral cortex.[53] Indeed, more than 70 percent of brain TRH is extrahypothalamic.[47]

Specific binding sites for TRH have been found in adult human brains in high quantities in the amygdala and hippocampus and in lesser quantities in the cortex, basal ganglia, hypothalamus, and cerebellum,[54] suggesting that this extrahypothalamic TRH is biologically active. The location of TRH receptors contrasts with the location of TRH itself. Low levels of receptors are present in the hypothalamus, which has the highest TRH concentrations, and high levels of receptors are present in the amygdala and hippocampus, which have low TRH concentrations.[54] The human TRH receptor has been cloned[55] and is a typical seven-transmembrane-domain G protein-coupled receptor whose gene is located on chromosome 8.[56]

Interestingly, a number of areas of the brain stain immunohistochemically for proTRH but not for TRH, including the reticular nucleus of the thalamus, portions of the hippocampus, the preoptic area, the supraoptic nucleus, the caudate-putamen complex, the substantia nigra, the periaqueductal gray matter, the pontine nuclei, and the dorsal motor nucleus of the vagus.[47] In situ

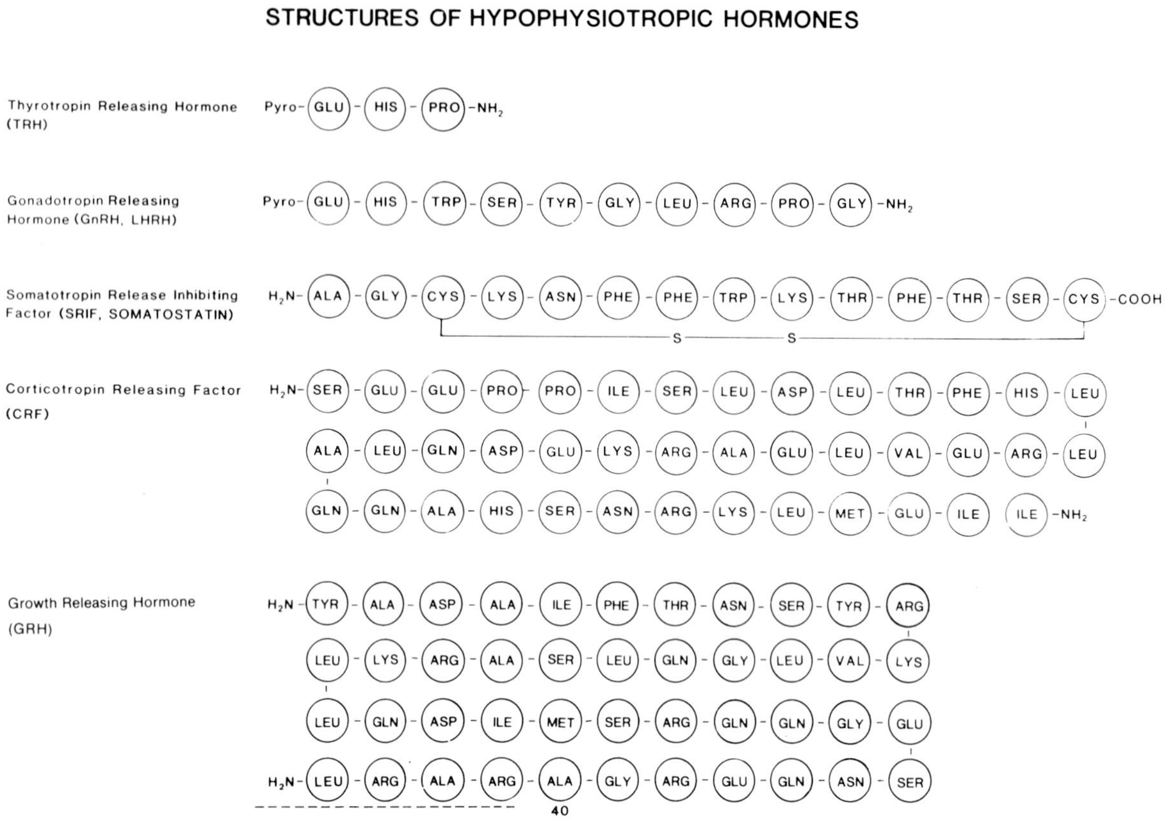

FIGURE 6-10. Structures of hypothalamic releasing and inhibiting hormones. The sequence of TRH, GnRH, and somatostatin are identical in all mammalian species studied. The sequence of human CRH, as shown in the figure, differs by 7 amino acids from ovine CRH. Two forms of GHRH have been identified which differ only by the additional COOH-terminal tetrapeptide indicated by the broken line. Porcine and rat GHRH differ by 3 and 14 amino acids, respectively.

hybridization histochemistry using RNA probes complementary to proTRH mRNA and antisera directed against putative peptides coded for by proTRH confirmed these findings, suggesting a role for both TRH and other non-TRH peptides coded for by the TRH precursor elsewhere in the brain.[47] In some areas, it appears that proTRH is processed preferentially to non-TRH peptides.[47]

TRH is also present in many areas outside the brain. Within the spinal cord, TRH-containing axons descending from the raphe nuclei are found in association with motor nuclei in the ventral gray and preganglionic sympathetic neurons in the intermediolateral column.[57] TRH is present in the mucosa of the gastrointestinal (GI) tract,[58] pancreatic islets,[59] retina,[60] placenta,[61] milk,[62] and

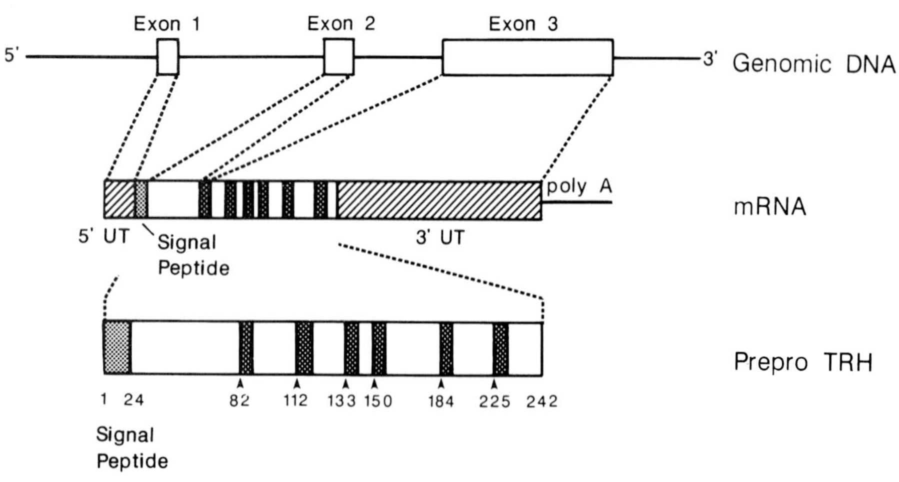

FIGURE 6-11. Schematic diagram of the structures of the human TRH gene, mRNA, and precursor peptide. Note that six copies of TRH are generated from the precursor. The sites of cleavage of each copy are indicated by arrows in the precursor structure. 5′ UT = 5′ untranslated region; 3′ UT = 3′ untranslated region.

prostate, testes, epididymis, and seminal vesicles.[63] All these tissues contribute to peripheral blood and urine TRH levels, making these levels inaccurate with respect to reflecting concentrations in the hypothalamic-pituitary portal vessels.

The primary neuroendocrine function of TRH is to stimulate the synthesis and release of TSH and PRL. Intracellular transduction mechanisms that mediate this function include activation of phosphoinositide–protein kinase C pathways and increasing intracellular calcium through the mobilization of intracellular stores and transport across calcium channels[64] (see Chap. 4). TSH is secreted in small-amplitude pulses by the pituitary, presumably as a result of the release of TRH from the hypothalamus in a pulsatile fashion.[65] It has been estimated that a single molecule of TRH, through its TSH-releasing effect, induces the release of more than 100,000 molecules of thyroxine from the thyroid.[66]

The fundamental role of TRH in stimulating TSH secretion was shown initially in hypothalamic ablation studies in which the paraventricular nucleus, the primary source of TRH, was lesioned, resulting in hypothyroidism.[67] Electric stimulation of this area causes a rapid release of TSH.[67] More specific experiments have shown that the administration of anti-TRH antibodies results in decreased basal and electrically stimulated TSH levels acutely and in decreased levels of TSH, T_4, and T_3 levels chronically.[68–71] In mice, targeted disruption of the TRH gene (TRH ko) causes hypothyroidism with elevated levels of TSH with reduced biological activity.[71a]

A number of different experimental approaches have failed to clarify the physiologic role of TRH as a PRL-releasing factor, however. The smallest dose of TRH that releases TSH also releases PRL in humans.[72] Immunoneutralization of endogenous TRH with TRH antisera caused a suppression of basal PRL levels in rats in some studies[68] but not in others and in the TRH ko mouse PRL levels are not affected.[71a] Such immunization also does not affect the PRL response to electric stimulation of the paraventricular nucleus or suckling,[71] and it delays but does not affect the magnitude of the spontaneous surge of PRL at proestrus.[73] Active, chronic immunization of ewes with TRH conjugated to albumin results in only minimal decreases in PRL levels basally and after stimulation by stress, suckling, and estrus, although reductions in TSH and thyroid hormone levels are more marked.[70]

Suckling causes an increase in hypothalamic proTRH mRNA levels and hypothalamic and portal vessel TRH levels as well as a decrease in dopamine (DA) levels.[74,75] If TRH mediates the PRL response to suckling even in part, it ought to be accompanied by an increase in TSH unless there is a concomitant increase in somatostatin. Studies of serum levels of PRL and TSH after suckling in humans have not shown any elevations of TSH.[76,77] Very small doses of TRH given systemically were effective in releasing PRL and TSH in lactating women, however, and so it is unlikely that the failure to show a rise in TSH was due to an increase in somatostatin. On the other hand, suckling also induces a mild increase in corticosterone in rats and that increase appears to be sufficient to block the TSH release induced by the rise in TRH during suckling.[75]

In hypothyroidism, TRH synthesis is increased[21] and the amount of TRH in the median eminence is increased.[78] In addition, pituitary TRH binding is increased because of an increased number of TRH receptors, but it is not clear whether there is also an effect on binding affinity.[79] Basal TSH and PRL levels are increased in human hypothyroidism, as are their responses to injected TRH.[80] Correction of the hypothyroidism with thyroid hormones decreases both the elevated TSH and PRL levels and their responses to TRH, although the decrease is more rapid for TSH.[80] Conversely, in hyperthyroidism, portal vessel TRH levels are decreased,[81] basal and TRH-stimulated TSH levels are markedly suppressed, and basal PRL levels are not low, but the PRL response to TRH is markedly blunted and returns to normal with correction of the hyperthyroidism.[80] Interestingly, in the euthyroid sick syndrome, in which there are low T3, T4, and TSH levels, TRH release into the portal blood and proTRH mRNA levels in the paraventricular nuclei of rats have also been found to be decreased[82] as has been the level of hypothalamic TRH mRNA.[83] The feedback effects of thyroid hormones therefore occur at the level of both the hypothalamus and the pituitary though the latter appears to be the more important site.[84]

These conflicting data from passive immunization studies, observation of TSH levels during lactation, and examination of PRL levels in various thyroid states support a role for TRH as a physiologic PRL releasing factor, albeit not the primary one.

In addition to the feedback effects of thyroid hormones on TRH release, somatostatin, which inhibits TSH secretion directly (described later), also inhibits TRH secretion.[85] The roles of various hypothalamic bioamines on TRH secretion alone are difficult to determine in vivo as they also have effects on somatostatin release and direct effects on the pituitary thyrotrophs. Dopamine decreases the TSH and PRL responses to TRH, implicating action at the pituitary level, although there may be some effect in decreasing TRH secretion.[86] Alpha-adrenergic agonists and serotonin stimulate, and GABA suppresses, TRH and TSH secretion.[87,88]

In various disease states, the stimulatory effect of administered TRH in humans is not limited to TSH and PRL. TRH can stimulate GH secretion in patients with acromegaly and in several states in which there is decreased IGF-I feedback on GH secretion, such as hepatic cirrhosis, renal insufficiency, anorexia nervosa, poorly controlled insulin-dependent diabetes mellitus, and malnutrition.[29] However, such responses are also seen in patients with depression and schizophrenia, which may be associated with disordered central bioaminergic regulation.[29] TRH can also stimulate FSH secretion in most patients with gonadotrope cell adenomas but not in normal individuals.[89] Obviously, somatotrope and gonadotrope cells must have TRH receptors, but there is "activation" of such receptors, which may involve alteration of intracellular transduction mechanisms, only in special circumstances.

In addition, TRH has a number of nonendocrine effects. As a neurotransmitter, TRH has generally been found to be excitatory, causing increased motor activity, tremor, arousal, and peripheral sympathetic neural activity with shivering, hypertension, tachycardia, diaphoresis, and nausea.[51] Early reports suggesting a beneficial effect of TRH on depression have not been confirmed.[51] Because of the association of TRH nerve terminals with motor neurons, TRH has been tried as therapy for amyotrophic lateral sclerosis. Despite early provocative results, subsequent studies have not shown definitive benefit with either intramuscular or intrathecal administration.[51] Early reports also suggested that TRH may be beneficial in septic shock and spinal cord shock after spinal cord trauma, but the role of TRH in the treatment of these conditions is uncertain despite several trials.[51] With the advent of very sensitive TSH assays, there is no longer any particular utility of the TRH test in diagnosing hyperthyroidism. Although TRH testing should, in theory, be useful in pinpointing the site of the defect in patients with central hypothyroidism, in fact the results of such testing are nonspecific.[90] Thus, at present, there are no clinical uses for TRH.

Gonadotropin Releasing Hormone

GnRH was the second hypophysiotropic hormone to be characterized; it consists of 10 amino acids with a molecular weight of 1182.[91] The single gene encoding the sequence for GnRH was subsequently isolated from human placenta and hypothalamus and was found to be on chromosome 21. It encodes a 92-amino acid precursor which contains a 23-amino acid signal peptide, the 10-amino acid GnRH, followed by a Gly-Lys-Arg sequence necessary for enzymatic processing and carboxy-terminal amidation of GnRH, and a 56-amino acid peptide that has been termed GAP (Fig. 6-12).[92,93] Although the gene for a similar peptide known as GnRH-II has been found to be located on chromosome 20 and expressed in humans, it is found primarily in the kidney, bone marrow, and prostate and its physiologic function remains unknown.[94] In contrast to TRH, in which the processing of the precursor occurs in the neuronal perikarya, the processing of the GnRH precursor occurs in the axonal processes and terminals, and both GnRH and GAP are located in nerve terminals.[95]

Immunohistochemical studies have localized GnRH-containing neurons to three major areas: (1) the preoptic/lamina terminalis area with projections to the OVLT (2) the mediobasal hypothalamus just anterior to the mammillary bodies and extending toward the infundibulum with axonal projections to the median eminence (tuberoinfundibular tract) and posterior pituitary, and (3) neurons in the septum, the pericommissural area, and the rostral mesencephalon with projections toward the extrahypothalamic brain, especially to portions of the limbic system such as the amygdala and hippocampus.[32,96] Studies in which the preoptic area and the mediobasal hypothalamic GnRH area have been surgically interrupted in rats resulted in loss of the midcycle surge of LH and FSH, which is thought to be in part caused by positive estrogen feedback but not negative steroid feedback.[97] Destruction of the anterior hypothalamic area in rhesus monkeys, however, does not abolish this midcycle surge, and it appears that in primates the arcuate nucleus is the primary structure involved in positive feedback[98] and is the primary source of GnRH released into the portal system.

Anatomic embryologic studies performed in mice suggest that GnRH neurons originally develop in the epithelium of the medial part of the olfactory placode, including the part that forms the anlage of the vomeronasal organ. During fetal development, these cells migrate across the nasal septum, enter the forebrain with the nervus terminalis and vomeronasal nerves, travel medial to the olfactory bulbs, and eventually enter the septal-preoptic region of the hypothalamus.[99] This demonstration of the origin of GnRH-producing neurons from olfactory epithelia is of clinical interest with respect to Kallmann's syndrome, in which gonadotropin deficiency due to GnRH deficiency is associated with anosmia caused by agenesis of the olfactory bulbs[100] (discussed later). The orphan nuclear receptor designated steroidogenic factor 1 (SF-1) that regulates the cytochrome P450 steroid hydroxylases in adrenal and gonadal tissues also appears to be important embryologically in the formation of functioning GnRH neurons through actions in the ventromedial hypothalamus.[101]

GnRH is also found in significant quantities in the placenta, where its synthesis has been demonstrated,[93] and in milk.[62] GnRH-like substances but not GnRH itself have been found in testicular interstitial cells [102] and ovaries.[103]

The primary function of GnRH is to stimulate the secretion of LH and FSH through binding to the GnRH receptor, a seven-transmembrane-domain G protein-coupled protein.[104] The transduction mechanisms that mediate the action of GnRH involve the phos-

FIGURE 6-12. Schematic diagram of the structures of the human GnRH gene, mRNA, and precursor peptide. Both GnRH and GnRH-associated peptide (GAP) are generated from the precursor. 5′ UT = 5′ untranslated region; 3′ UT = 3′ untranslated region.

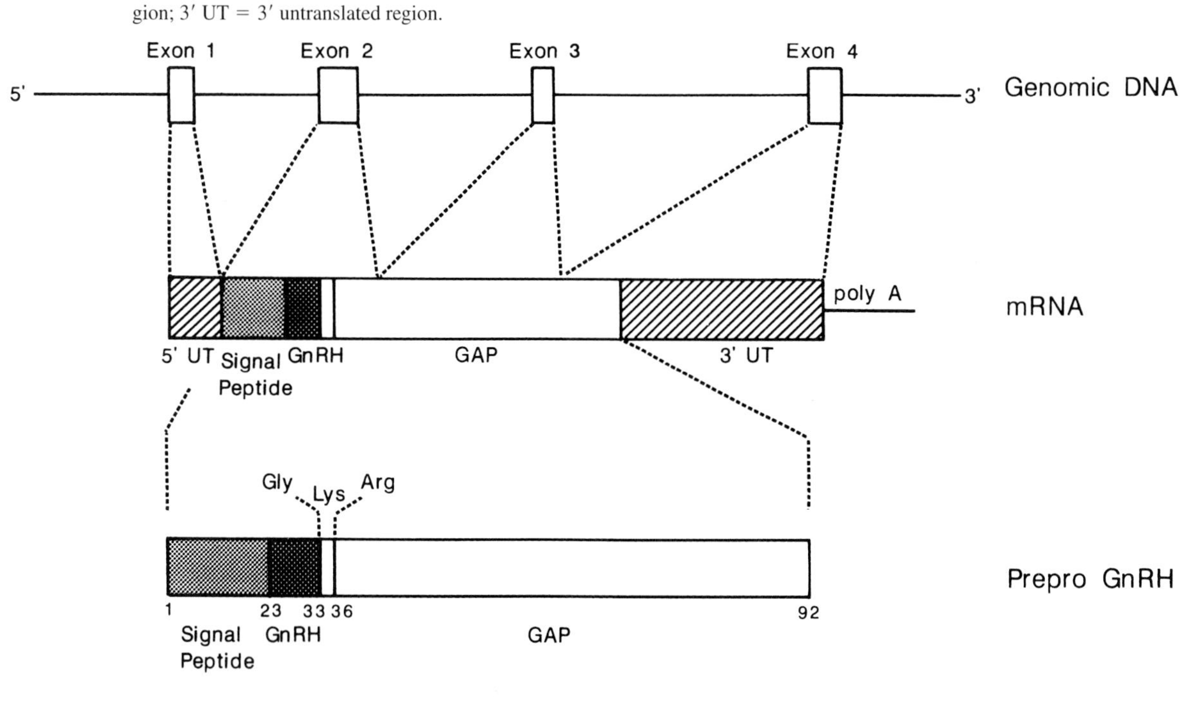

phoinositide–protein kinase C pathway as well as increases in intracellular calcium via mobilization from intracellular calcium stores and subsequent entry through a voltage-dependent calcium channel[105] (see Chap. 7). GnRH also directly up regulates its own receptors (i.e., it causes an increase in GnRH receptor number), a function shared with estradiol.[106] By contrast, continuous administration of GnRH is associated with down regulation of gonadotropin synthesis and secretion as a result of decreased receptor numbers as well as postreceptor mechanisms.[106]

Although early studies suggested the presence of separate LH and FSH releasing factors,[107] it appears that there is only one GnRH and that the differential secretion of LH and FSH is due to variations in sensitivity of the feedback effects of steroid and peptide hormones and variations in sensitivity to GnRH. For example, slower GnRH pulse frequencies result in a greater FSH/LH ratio,[97,108] inhibin has a much greater inhibitory effect on FSH than on LH,[109] and there is a more marked positive feedback effect of estrogen on LH compared to FSH.[97] When endogenous GnRH is immunoneutralized, the pulsatile secretion of LH is eliminated, but FSH secretion is maintained in the short term and decreases in the long term.[108]

The concept that exposure to a stimulating hormone in a pulsatile or episodic compared to a continuous manner results in increased target organ response was initially demonstrated for GnRH and gonadotropin secretion.[110] In experiments in rhesus monkeys in which the ovaries had been removed and hypothalamic lesions had been placed, GnRH was given in equal quantities either continuously intravenously or via pulses once per hour. Only the pulsatile administration of GnRH resulted in a reestablishment of normal gonadotropin secretion (Fig. 6-13).[110] The human pituitary secretes gonadotropins in frequent (every 15 min) pulses of small amplitude when cultured in vitro[111] and frequent sampling can detect these pulses in vivo as well.[112] The pulsatile release of GnRH then superimposes pulses of LH and FSH secretion of larger amplitude about every 70 to 96 min in humans.[113] The fact that these latter pulses are due to GnRH has been shown by means of simultaneous measurement of pituitary portal blood GnRH and peripheral blood LH and FSH concentrations in animals (Fig. 6-14).[114,115] Whether the more frequent pulses of smaller amplitude are due to GnRH or to the intrinsic secretory ability of the pituitary is not clear.[116] The exposure to pulsatile (every 1 h) vs. continuous GnRH also has effects on gonadotropin synthesis and release. Recent studies in rat pituitaries showed that α subunit mRNA increases with either mode but that FSHβ subunit mRNA increases only with pulsatile GnRH and is suppressed with continuous GnRH.[117] The actual generation of GnRH pulses appears to be an intrinsic property of the GnRH neuronal network in which there is extensive intracellular contact by both synaptic and gap junctions.[118]

Steroid hormone feedback regulation of the hypothalamic-pituitary-gonadal axis occurs at both the pituitary and hypothalamic levels. Gonadectomy results in increased GnRH secretion into the portal system[119] as well as an increase in the pituitary responsiveness to GnRH. As estrogen receptors on GnRH neurons are

FIGURE 6-13. Suppression of plasma LH and FSH concentrations after the initiation on day 0 of continuous GnRH (1 μg/min) in an ovariectomized rhesus monkey with a radiofrequency lesion in the hypothalamus; gonadotropin secretion had been reestablished before the intermittent (pulsatile) administration of the decapeptide (1 μg/min for 6 min once per h). The inhibition of gonadotropin secretion was reversed after reinstitution of the intermittent mode of GnRH stimulation on day 20. The vertical lines beneath the LH data points on days 10 and 13 of the continuous infusion regimen indicate values below the sensitivity of the radioimmunoassay. (*Reproduced with permission from Belchetz et al.*[110])

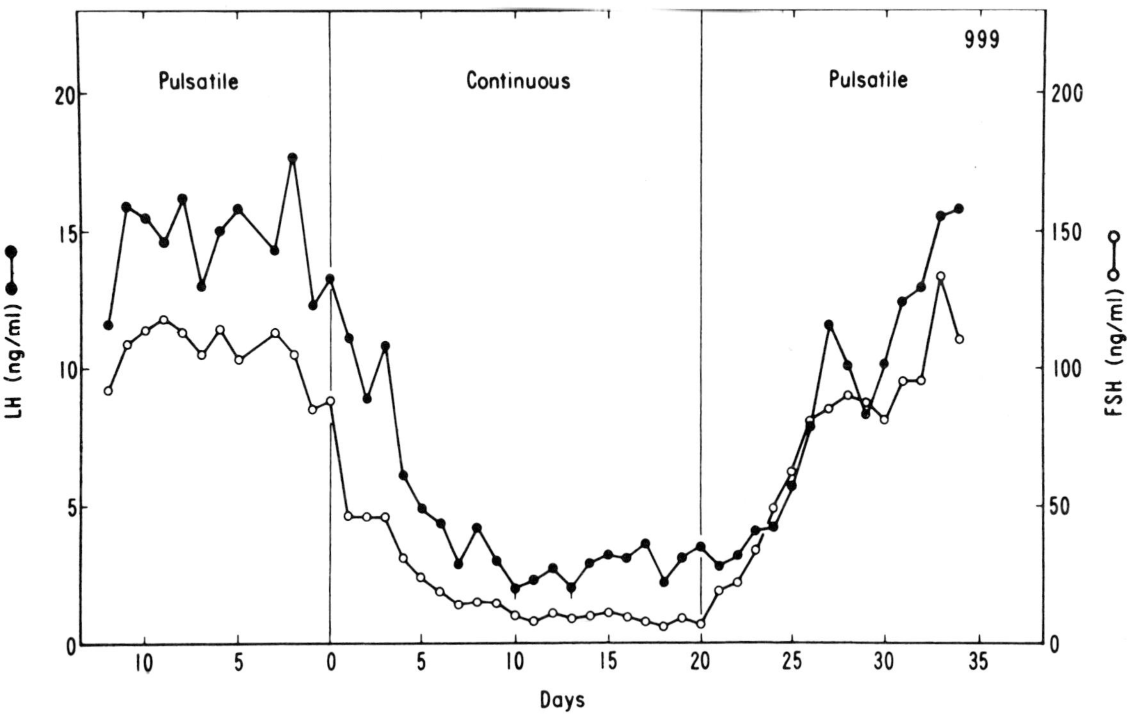

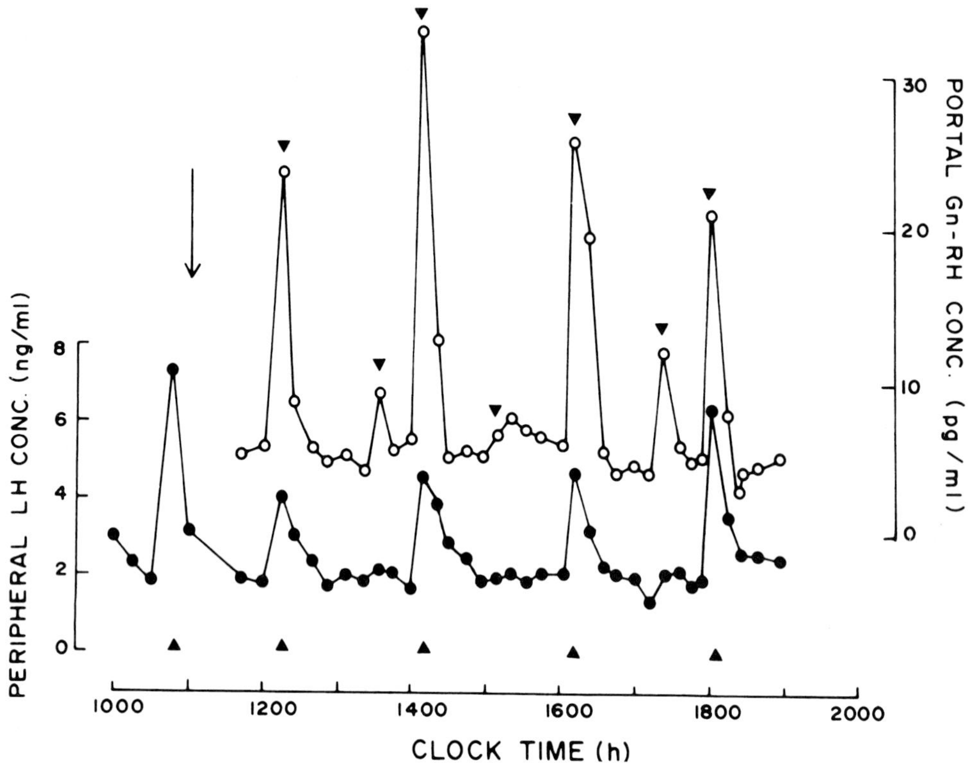

FIGURE 6-14. Concentrations of GnRH in the hypothalamo-hypophyseal portal plasma and LH in the jugular venous (peripheral) plasma of an ovariectomized ewe. The arrow indicates the time at which the portal vessels were cut. Pulsatile secretory episodes (▲ for LH and ▼ for GnRH) were defined as having occurred when the value in a given sample exceeded that of the previous sample by three times the standard deviation of the previous sample. No LH pulses occur without concomitant GnRH pulses, although GnRH pulses sometimes occur without any change in LH secretion. (*Reproduced with permission from Clark and Cummins.*[114])

quite sparse, it is likely that the effect of estrogen on GnRH release is mediated through effects on other neurotransmitter-containing neurons that have synaptic contact with GnRH neurons.[120] Estrogens have a variable feedback effect in vivo, with short-term administration causing an initial decrease in response to GnRH, longer-term administration causing a positive feedback effect, and chronic administration also causing a negative feedback effect.[120] In pituitary cell cultures, estradiol suppresses the gonadotropin response to GnRH added to the medium.[121] However, other studies have shown that short-term incubation of pituitary cell cultures with estradiol in the absence of GnRH results in no effect on transcription of α subunit or FSHβ genes, though LHβ mRNA synthesis is increased.[122] This suggests that at least part of the positive feedback effect of estrogen that occurs at midcycle may be due to a direct effect at the pituitary level, but as other studies have shown increased GnRH levels in portal blood at the time of the ovulatory gonadotropin surge,[122,123] part of the positive feedback effect of estrogen also occurs at the hypothalamic level. The negative effects of estrogen probably occur at both the hypothalamic and pituitary levels, with the hypothalamic effects being the reduction of GnRH pulse amplitude and frequency and the pituitary effects being the modulation of the gonadotropin response to GnRH.[120,122]

Progesterone also has both stimulatory and inhibitory effects on gonadotropin release through effects at both the pituitary and hypothalamic levels,[120,122,124] with the differences probably due to concurrent estrogen levels and the phase of the cycle, as the early preovulatory rise in progesterone augments the ovulatory gonadotropin surge while the later rise of progesterone in the luteal phase is inhibitory.[120] Although many experiments have suggested that testosterone can inhibit gonadotropin secretion directly, without first having to be aromatized to estrogen by acting at both the hypothalamic and pituitary levels,[125,126] recent reports show that men with aromatase deficiency, which blocks all conversion of testosterone to estradiol, had elevated LH and FSH levels, indicating that at least some of the inhibitory effect of testosterone is mediated by its conversion to estradiol.[127,128]

The negative feedback effects of inhibin are predominantly on FSH and predominantly on the pituitary and it appears to be inhibin B (α-β_B) rather than inhibin A that is the physiologically relevant inhibin in the human.[129] Inhibin causes a dose-related decrease in the sensitivity of gonadotropes to GnRH, which may involve a decrease in the number of GnRH receptors[130] as well as a direct effect on the synthesis of FSH, as shown by demonstrating effects on α subunit and FSHβ but not LHβ subunit mRNA levels in a pituitary cell culture system.[131] However, the administration of crude inhibin preparations into the dorsal anterior hypothalamus also suppresses FSH levels, and so there may also be a hypothalamic site of action.[132] The related ovarian protein, activin, stimulates FSH release from the pituitary as well as synthesis.[109,131] It appears to bind to a receptor separate from the GnRH receptor and acts additively to GnRH in stimulating FSH release.[109] Another gonadal peptide, follistatin (see Chaps. 15 and 16), also inhibits the postoophorectomy rise and the GnRH-induced rise in FSH selectively, with a molar potency 20 percent that of inhibin.[109] Again, this effect occurs not only on release but on synthesis.[109] It is now thought that the biological activity of follistatin stems primarily from its ability to bind to and inactivate activin.[109] These ovarian peptides are also found in the pituitary and activin has been found in regions of the hypothalamus in which GnRH neurons are found; therefore, these peptides may have additional neuroendocrine paracrine or even autocrine effects on gonadotropin secretion.[109]

The regulation of gonadotropin secretion is thus quite complex, involving the stimulatory effect of GnRH on its own receptors as well as LH and FSH synthesis and secretion, the positive and negative feedback effects of estrogen, the negative feedback effects of progesterone, the negative feedback effects of inhibin and follistatin, and the positive feedback effect of activin. Furthermore, the sites of feedback—the hypothalamus and pituitary—are incompletely understood, and positive and negative feedback effects at these different sites may interact.

Other neurotransmitters and hormones have an influence on GnRH secretion, although for some the data are contradictory. Neuropeptide Y, a 36-amino acid peptide expressed in the arcuate and other areas of the hypothalamus, is released into the median eminence and portal blood, where it stimulates the release of GnRH from nerve terminals and also enhances the response of gonadotroph cells to GnRH.[133] The neurotransmitter glutamate stimulates GnRH release and gene expression and may be important in the control of the onset of puberty.[134] Although most in vivo experiments suggest that dopaminergic neural input is inhibitory,[135] exposure of hypothalamic cultures to dopamine results in an increase in GnRH release.[136] It may be that the presence of other influences on GnRH secretion, such as exposure to estrogen, may modulate the response to dopamine and other neurotransmitters under differing physiologic conditions. Alpha-adrenergic and cholinergic inputs are stimulatory, and endogenous opioid peptidergic input is inhibitory.[97] Hyperprolactinemia results in decreased GnRH synthesis[137] and pulsatile release, causing decreased gonadotropin pulse amplitude.[138]

In addition to stimulating LH and FSH release from the pituitary, GnRH also has direct actions on the gonad in rats, including inhibitory effects on ovarian and testicular steroid production and a facilitating role in ovulation.[139] Such effects have not been demonstrated conclusively in humans, however.

Human placental GnRH has been demonstrated to stimulate the release of hCG from placental cultures, an effect inhibited by estrogen and progesterone.[140] The effect of GnRH on placental estrogen and progesterone production is not clear, however.[140] Furthermore, inhibin reduces GnRH release from placental cultures and inhibits the action of GnRH on hCG production; conversely, activin augments GnRH-induced release of hCG.[140] The clinical importance of these intraplacental interactions is not known.

GAP, the 56-amino acid peptide that is a portion of the precursor to GnRH, also appears to have an endocrine function, at least in the rat. Initial studies have suggested that it also is stimulatory to LH and FSH release, albeit at equal potency to GnRH for FSH and at about 20 percent of the molar potency of GnRH for LH.[141] Subsequent studies have suggested that this gonadotropin-releasing potency of GAP is considerably weaker and variable, depending on experimental conditions,[142] and that the first 13 amino acids of the peptide contains most of the gonadotropin-releasing properties.[143] Limited in vitro studies of GAP_{1-13} in baboon and human pituitary cell cultures have confirmed a gonadotropin stimulatory effect.[143] The physiologic importance of GAP in gonadotropin regulation in humans remains to be defined. GAP also has PRL inhibitory properties (discussed later).

The past decade has witnessed an explosive growth in the use of GnRH as a therapeutic agent in a variety of conditions. GnRH has been administered with great success in a pulsatile fashion to individuals with hypogonadotropic hypogonadism due to GnRH deficiency, resulting in restoration of normal sexual function and fertility.[106] Long-acting GnRH agonists have been used to down regulate gonadotropin secretion in a variety of conditions, including precocious puberty, prostate cancer, breast cancer, uterine fibroids, and endometriosis.[106] Recently, direct GnRH antagonists that compete for the GnRH receptor were explored for similar conditions.[106] These specific uses of GnRH and its agonists and antagonists are discussed in Chaps. 7, 15, 16, and 29.

Somatostatin

Most studies of GH regulation in the 1950s and 1960s focused on the essential stimulatory role of the hypothalamus on GH secretion.[144] In the course of trying to isolate and purify GHRH, Krulich et al. found a fraction of hypothalamic extract that inhibited GH secretion.[145] However, it was not until 1973 that the tetradecapeptide structure of somatostatin [also known as GH inhibitory factor or somatotropin release inhibiting factor (SRIF)] was elucidated.[146] Subsequently, a 28-amino acid precursor to somatostatin-14, referred to as somatostatin-28, was characterized[147] and was found to have GH inhibitory properties similar to those of the originally described peptide.[148] Thus, this 28-amino acid peptide (molecular weight of 3149) may function as a prohormone to somatostatin-14 (molecular weight of 1638) but also has biological activity itself. Yet a third peptide, somatostatin-28_{1-12}, has also been found in the rat hypothalamus and other tissues in which somatostatin is found (discussed later).[149] Somatostatin-14 is the major form in the hypothalamus and other neural structures while somatostatin-28 is the major form in the gastrointestinal tract.[84] The human somatostatin gene codes for a preprosomatostatin of 116 amino acids with a 24-amino acid leader sequence and a prosomatostatin structure of 92 amino acids (Fig. 6-15).[150] The amino acid sequence of human preprosomatostatin has only four amino acids different from that of the rat somatostatin precursor, indicating marked conservation of the entire structure during evolution.[151] Prosomatostatin is found not only in neuronal perikarya but also in axon terminals in the median eminence and other areas of the brain, suggesting conversion to somatostatin during transport or in nerve terminals.[152] Secretion of intact prohormone and other prohormone-derived peptides occurs at nerve terminals, including those which secrete into portal vessels.[153] The conservation of structure across species and the presence of other prohormone-derived peptides in nerve terminals and portal vessel blood suggest that peptides derived from the precursor may be of major biological importance.

Somatostatin is found throughout the brain and spinal cord, with the highest concentrations occurring in the hypothalamus.[154] Somatostatin that is present in the extrahypothalamic brain is not derived from hypothalamic neurons,[155] and cerebral cortex cells have been shown to synthesize somatostatin in vitro.[156] Immunohistochemical studies show that the somatostatin neuronal perikarya which project to the median eminence are located

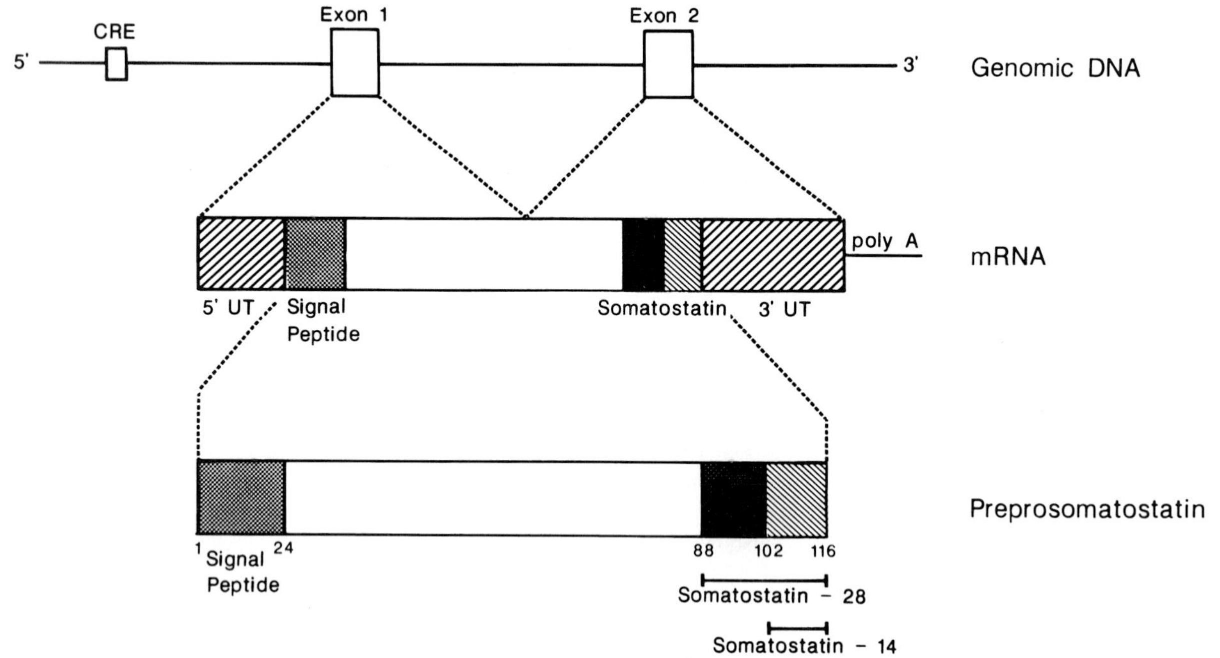

FIGURE 6-15. Schematic diagram of the structures of the human somatostatin gene, mRNA, and precursor peptide. Both somatostatin-14 and somatostatin-28 are generated from the precursor by cleavage at amino acid positions 88 and 102. 5′ UT = 5′ untranslated region; 3′ UT = 3′ untranslated region.

primarily in the preoptic nucleus, the anterior periventricular nucleus, and the parvocellular subdivision of the paraventricular nucleus.[157] Electric stimulation of these areas results in the release of somatostatin into the portal vessels,[158] and lesions in this area cause a depletion of median eminence somatostatin content and an elevation of basal serum GH levels.[159] The somatostatin-producing cells of the cortex, the amygdala, and other brain areas do not project to the median eminence,[160] but both the 14- and 28-amino acid forms are present in all areas, although the relative proportions vary.[161] About one-quarter of cells that produce somatostatin as a neurotransmitter also produce acetylcholine.[162]

Somatostatin is also present in large quantities in a number of other tissues, in many of which it plays a very important physiologic role. It is present in the D cells of the pancreatic islets and the gut mucosa as well as the myenteric neural plexus. Via paracrine and endocrine actions, it suppresses the secretion of insulin, glucagon, cholecystokinin, gastrin, secretin, VIP, and other GI hormones as well as such functions as gastric acid secretion, gastric emptying, and splanchnic blood flow (see Chaps. 18 and 26). In addition, it has also been found in the retina,[163] neurohypophysis,[164] C cells of the thyroid,[165] prostate,[166] and testis, epididymis, and semen.[167] Cerebrospinal fluid somatostatin levels can be elevated in a variety of neurologic diseases, probably as a result of nonspecific leakage from damaged neural tissue, and therefore reflect the production of somatostatin by the entire central nervous system (CNS) rather than just the hypothalamus.[168] Blood somatostatin levels reflect somatostatin produced by the GI tract and pancreas rather than that produced by the brain.

Somatostatin receptors are distributed throughout the brain, including the circumventricular organs, which are areas outside the blood-brain barrier through which interaction of peripheral blood-borne substances with the CNS may occur.[169] Recent studies have shown that tumors of cells of glial and neuroblastic origin in humans, such as meningiomas, astrocytomas, and medulloblastomas, retain somatostatin receptors.[170] The five human somatostatin receptor subtypes are all G protein-coupled receptors with seven-transmembrane domains and their genes are located on different chromosomes.[171] Receptor subtype 2 has long and short isoforms (A and B) generated through alternative splicing.[171] The receptors are associated with different G proteins and vary in their ability to inhibit adenylyl cyclase and other transduction mechanisms.[171] All five subtypes are expressed in the hypothalamus and other brain areas.[172] Receptor subtypes 1–4 have similar affinities for somatostatin-14 and -28, but subtype 5 has a greater affinity for somatostatin 28.[171] The primary subtypes expressed in normal human pituitaries are 1, 2 and 5, while GH-producing adenomas express subtypes 1, 2, 3, and 5.[6,173]

After somatostatin was discovered, its subsequent characterization was based on its ability to inhibit GH secretion.[145,146] When somatostatin is given to humans, it blocks the rise in GH that occurs with all stimuli in a dose-dependent fashion.[174,175] Active immunization against somatostatin or the administration of antisomatostatin antiserum eradicates endogenous somatostatin activity, resulting in a rise in basal and stimulated GH levels in rats and baboons,[176,177] and restores the pulse amplitude of GH that has been decreased by stress[178] or starvation.[179]

The interaction of somatostatin and GHRH on GH secretion is complex. Both somatostatin and GHRH are secreted episodically into the portal system in rats and sheep in an independent manner in which the secretory bursts are often asynchronous.[180] Thus, GH secretory episodes are associated with increased GHRH secretion accompanied by low somatostatin levels and basal or trough GH levels associated with low GHRH levels and more elevated somatostatin levels (Fig. 6-16).[177,180,181] Furthermore, somatostatin

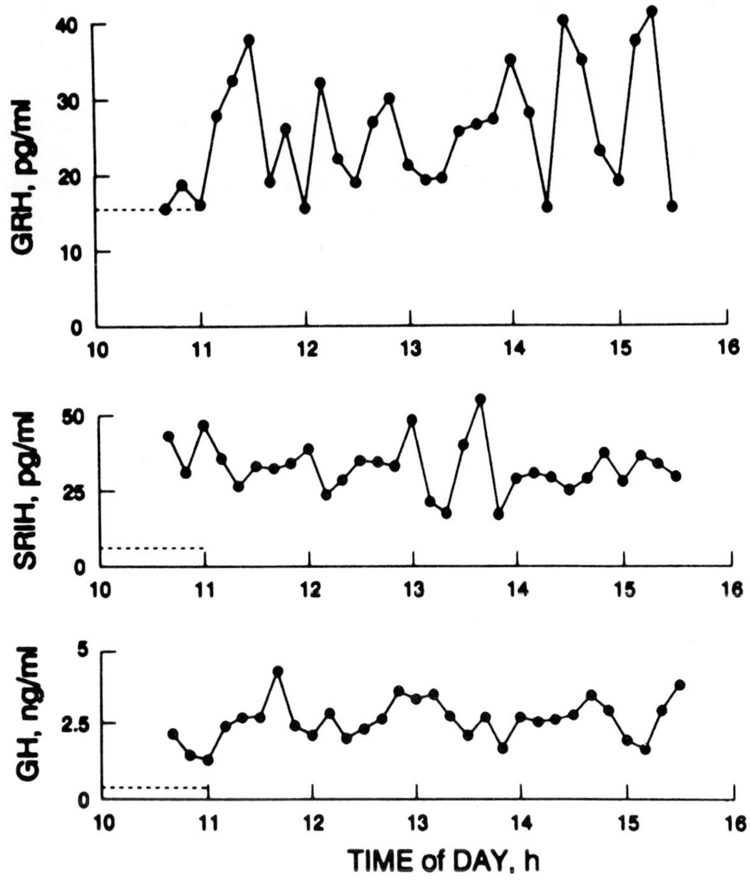

FIGURE 6-16. GHRH (GRH) and somatostatin (SRIH) levels in the hypothalamic-pituitary portal plasma and GH levels in the jugular plasma of an unanesthetized ovariectomized ewe. The interrupted horizontal lines indicate the least detectable value for each assay. Although there is an association between GHRH and GH secretory peaks, there is no association between GHRH and somatostatin secretion or between somatostatin and GH secretion. These data in sheep are compatible with independent neural rhythmicity of GHRH and somatostatin secretion, with a primary role of GHRH in determining pulsatile GH secretion. (*Reproduced with permission from Frohman et al.*[181])

may also partially inhibit GHRH secretion, and somatostatin receptors have been found on GHRH neuronal perikarya in the arcuate nucleus.[159,182] Conversely, GHRH may stimulate somatostatin release.[183] The persistence of varying GH responses to exogenous GHRH is indirect evidence for periodic hypothalamic somatostatin secretion in humans.[184]

The second major neuroendocrine function of somatostatin is the inhibition of basal and stimulated TSH secretion.[174] In the rat, somatostatin-depleting lesions which increase GH secretion also increase TSH secretion.[185] Neutralization of endogenous somatostatin by means of the administration of antisomatostatin serum raises basal and stimulated TSH levels, as it does with GH levels, as indicated previously.[186] Thyroid hormone levels also feed back positively on hypothalamic somatostatin secretion[22,186] just as they feed back negatively on TRH secretion and the TSH response to TRH, integrating the hypothalamic-pituitary-thyroid feedback loop. Somatostatin has even been found to inhibit directly the release of TRH from rat hypothalamic cultures.[85] Despite this evidence, questions remain about the physiologic role of somatostatin as an inhibitor of TSH secretion. Careful dose-response studies in humans, using somatostatin infusions that achieved serum somatostatin levels in the range reported in rat portal vessels, have shown that GH is about tenfold more sensitive to inhibition by somatostatin than is TSH.[175,187] On the basis of these studies, it has been suggested that if there is a role of somatostatin in inhibiting TSH secretion, it is limited to conditions associated with marked somatostatin-mediated suppression of GH.[187]

Hypothalamic somatostatin is itself subject to feedback regulation as well as regulation by a number of bioaminergic and peptidergic neurotransmitters. Growth hormone can itself directly increase somatostatin secretion, as can its target hormone, IGF-I.[26] Experiments which have addressed the issue of the specific regulation of somatostatin secretion and not just GH secretion have by necessity been quite unphysiologic, depending on in vitro hypothalamic explant or culture systems or intraventricular injections and measuring somatostatin in severed portal vessels. Such studies have found that dopamine, norepinephrine, and acetylcholine stimulate somatostatin secretion,[188] as do glucagon,[189] neurotensin,[190] VIP and the closely related peptide-histidine-isoleucine (PHI),[191] interleukin-1β,[192] and the amino acid taurine,[193] although it is thought that arginine causes a decrease in somatostatin release.[194] By contrast, serotonin,[188] substance P, β-endorphin, and met-enkephalin[190] had no effects on somatostatin secretion when injected intraventricularly, but β-endorphin and met-enkephalin decreased K^+-induced somatostatin release from perfused hypothalami in vitro.[195]

One of the intracellular transduction messengers responsible for somatostatin gene transcription is cAMP. In fact, it is in the somatostatin gene system that the interaction of the cAMP response element (CRE) with a specific CRE *trans*-activating binding protein (CREB) was initially elucidated.[196,197] In this system, a stimulus activates adenylate cyclase, generating cAMP, which activates cAMP-dependent protein kinase A, which then phosphorylates CREB, which binds to the CRE of the 5′-flanking region of the somatostatin gene, thus stimulating somatostatin gene transcription. The rise in cAMP also stimulates the release of somatostatin. There is also some evidence that voltage-gated calcium channels may be involved in somatostatin secretion, but this requires further definition.

Little is known about the regulation or function of somatostatin in the rest of the brain. In general, somatostatin appears to have an inhibitory function.[170] The number of receptors for somatostatin and somatostatin content are decreased in the cortex of patients with Alzheimer's disease,[198] but somatostatin is increased in the basal ganglia in patients with Huntington's disease.[199] Whether such changes are part of the pathogenesis of these disorders or are merely epiphenomena is not known.

Recently, analogs of somatostatin have been developed for the treatment of acromegaly (see Chap. 7). One analog, octreotide, is in current clinical use and has been found to have efficacy in a wide number of areas besides GH-secreting tumors, including the treatment of carcinoid tumors, VIP-secreting tumors, TSH-secreting tumors, islet-cell tumors, and diarrhea of a number of etiologies (see Chaps. 7 and 26).

Corticotropin Releasing Hormone

CRH was the first of the hypophysiotropic hormones for which evidence of bioactivity was demonstrated in hypothalamic extracts[200,201] and one of the last to be completely characterized. It was initially characterized in sheep and was found to have 41 amino acids (molecular weight of 4670).[202] Subsequent studies have shown that human CRH has seven amino acids different from those of ovine CRH[203] and that rat CRH is identical to human CRH. The human gene for CRH, on chromosome 8, has been characterized, and the deduced sequence of preproCRH consists of 192 amino acids with a 24-amino acid leader sequence (Fig. 6-17).[203]

Immunoreactive CRH is found throughout the human hypothalamus, with the highest concentrations in the paraventricular, supraoptic, and infundibular (arcuate) nuclei.[204] However, immunohistochemical studies have shown that most human CRH neuronal perikarya are located in the parvocellular region of the paraventricular nucleus and that most neurons project to the median eminence, where CRH is released into the portal plexus, although a few also project to the posterior pituitary.[205] CRH has been demonstrated in hypothalamic-hypophyseal portal blood in concentrations known to stimulate ACTH from pituitaries in vitro.[206] In rats, lesions of the paraventricular nucleus result in a marked decrease in median eminence CRH and in ACTH released by ether stress.[207] Similarly, mice with CRH gene knockouts have markedly reduced activity of the pituitary-adrenal axis.[208] CRH has been found in the human thalamus, cortex, cerebellum, pons, medulla, and spinal cord,[209] where it can be released by depolarizing agents, suggesting a functional role as a neurotransmitter in those areas.[210] It is also present in the adrenal cortex and medulla, lung, liver, stomach, duodenum, pancreas, and placenta, but its functions in these tissues are poorly understood.[136,209,211] CRH in peripheral blood is derived from both hypothalamic and extrahypothalamic sources[212] and is bound to a binding protein.[213]

CRH receptors have been demonstrated in normal and adenomatous pituitary corticotrope cells[214] and, in rats at least, are widely distributed in the CNS.[215] The cloned CRH receptor is of the seven-transmembrane domain G protein-coupled type that acts primarily through adenylyl cyclase and is related to the GHRH/VIP/calcitonin receptor family.[216] A second CRH receptor has been cloned which exists in brain and peripheral loci that do not overlap with CRH; there are three isoforms of the CRH_2 receptor that differ in their amino termini.[216,217]

CRH releases ACTH, β-endorphin, β-lipotropin, melanocyte stimulating hormone (MSH), and other peptides generated from pro-opiomelanocortin (POMC) in equimolar amounts without releasing other pituitary hormones.[211] There is no difference in the ACTH response between repetitive and continuous administration of CRH, unlike the desensitization seen with GnRH.[218]

The physiologic role of CRH in the regulation of ACTH has been established by the finding that the immunoneutralization of endogenous CRH by anti-CRH antibodies blocks the ACTH

FIGURE 6-17. Schematic diagram of the structures of the human CRH gene, mRNA, and precursor peptide. 5′ UT = 5′ untranslated region. 3′ UT = 3′ untranslated region.

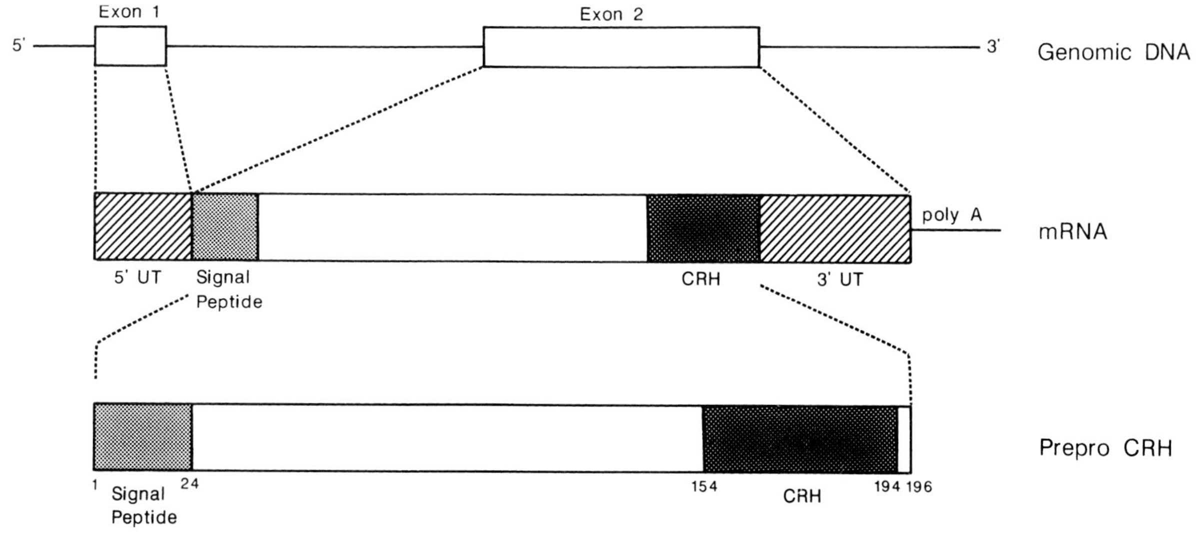

response to stress by 75 percent.[219] Furthermore, immunoneutralization studies of endogenous CRH show that CRH is responsible for the augmentation of the amplitude of an underlying CRH-independent rhythm that results in the nocturnal rise in blood ACTH levels.[220] In rats, insulin-induced hypoglycemia causes not only a release of CRH from the median eminence in parallel with the increase in ACTH secretion by the pituitary but also an increase in hypothalamic CRH mRNA levels, implying increased CRH gene transcription.[221] The remaining 25 percent of stress-induced secretion is primarily due to vasopressin, which also has very potent ACTH-releasing activity.[222] CRH and vasopressin appear to have synergistic effects on ACTH release[223] (Fig. 6-18). In fact, CRH and vasopressin coexist in about half the CRH-containing parvocellular and paraventricular neurons and even in the same neurosecretory granules.[8,224] Elegant studies in conscious sheep have shown parallel secretion of CRH and vasopressin into the portal circulation coinciding with the release of the POMC peptides ACTH, β-endorphin, and α-MSH into the systemic circulation.[225] CRH and vasopressin are not always released coordinately, however, and stress has been shown to selectively activate the vasopressin-containing subset of CRH neurons.[8] Furthermore, at least in the rat, not all pituitary cells that respond to CRH also respond to vasopressin.[226] In contrast to CRH, which uses the adenylate cyclase–cAMP system for signal transduction, vasopressin appears to use the phosphotidylinositol–diacylglycerol (DAG)–protein kinase C system for signal transduction.[211,216,227]

FIGURE 6-18. Net change ($\pm$SE) of ACTH and cortisol concentrations in six women in response to the administration of CRH (CRF), vasopressin (VP), or CRH with vasopressin at time 0. Note the marked synergistic effects of CRH and vasopressin on ACTH release. (*Reproduced with permission from Liu et al.*[223])

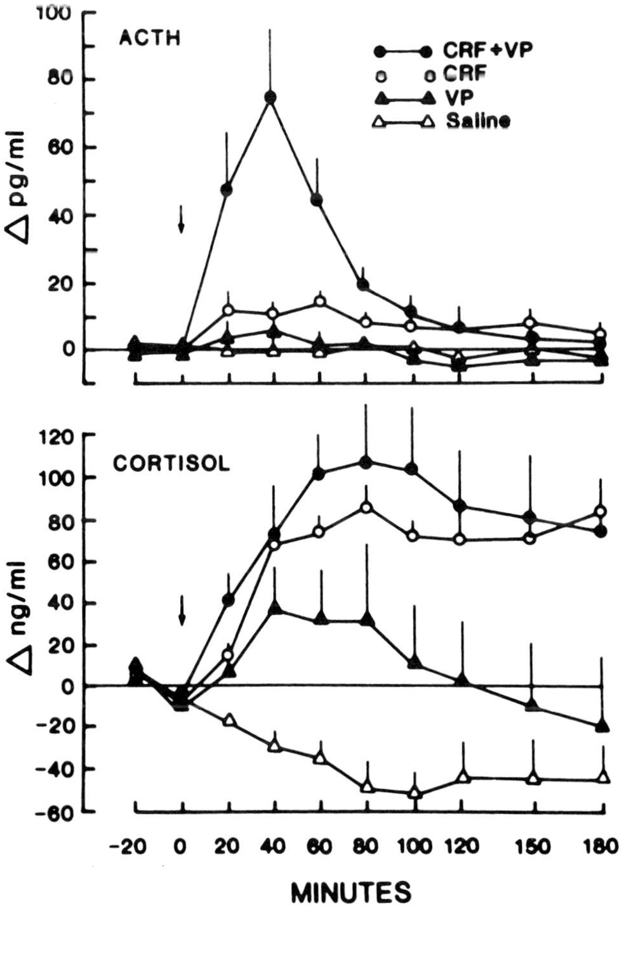

Glucocorticoid negative feedback also does not affect all the CRH neurons equally. Adrenalectomy causes an increase in the number of neurons containing both CRH and vasopressin and a decrease in the number containing only CRH,[228] an increase in paraventricular nucleus CRH mRNA[229] (implying increased gene transcription), an increase in portal vessel CRH and vasopressin levels, and an increase in peripheral ACTH levels.[230] All these effects are blocked by concomitant glucocorticoid replacement. Adrenalectomy has no effect on CRH mRNA levels in CRH-producing cells elsewhere in the brain.[229] Glucocorticoids can also inhibit the hemorrhage-induced release of CRH into the portal vessels[231] as well as the CRH-induced rise in intracellular cAMP and ACTH release from pituitary cells in vitro.[232] The more direct products of CRH stimulation also exert negative feedback. ACTH may feed back negatively on its own secretion,[233] at least in part by decreasing CRH release by the hypothalamus.[234] Another product of POMC processing, β-endorphin, also feeds back negatively on ACTH secretion.[235] Although the results from animal studies have been conflicting, morphine suppresses the ACTH response to CRH in humans,[236] presumably acting through opioid μ receptors (discussed later).

Central bioamines and peptides also influence CRH secretion. Norepinephrine and epinephrine stimulate hypothalamic CRH secretion via α_1 and α_2 receptors and both adenylate cyclase and protein kinase C second messenger systems.[237–240] Norepinephrine and epinephrine also stimulate pituitary ACTH secretion directly and are additive to the stimulatory effect of CRH.[239] Serotonin and acetylcholine also stimulate CRH secretion, the latter via both muscarinic and nicotinic receptors,[239,240] and dopamine has a mild stimulatory effect[238] whereas GABA is inhibitory.[237,238,240] Under various experimental circumstances, angiotensin II, cholecystokinin, VIP, oxytocin, and atrial natriuretic peptide all have ACTH-releasing properties, but their interactions with CRH are unknown.[240]

Monokines released by inflammatory tissue also exert effects on CRH and ACTH secretion. Interleukin 1 (IL-1, previously known as endogenous pyrogen), a product of mononuclear phagocytes that mediates many of the inflammatory responses, stimulates the synthesis and release of CRH from the hypothalamus and the release of ACTH by the pituitary.[240–243] Although it had been thought that IL-1 exerts its influence on CRH after entry into the hypothalamus via one of the circumventricular organs, the OVLT,[242] recent studies have found nerve fibers that stain immunohistochemically for IL-1β in the magnocellular and parvocellular parts of the human paraventricular nucleus, the preoptic, supraoptic, and arcuate nuclei; and the external zone of the median eminence.[244] It is not clear whether it is these IL-1–containing neurons or other neurons that mediate the CRH-releasing and other central effects of systemic IL-1 that enters via the OVLT.[242–244] Other cytokines, such as IL-2, IL-6, and tumor necrosis factor α (TNFα), have also been found to elicit secretion of ACTH, but their mechanisms of action have not been clarified.[241,242] ACTH and other POMC-derived peptides are produced by monocytes, but it is not known whether they interact with the central IL-1–CRH–ACTH system.[241]

A number of actions of extrahypothalamic CRH have been postulated. In particular, CRH has been proposed to activate biological systems within the brain in response to stress. For example, CRH administered to dogs via intracerebroventricular cannulae causes increased plasma levels of epinephrine, norepinephrine, glucagon, and glucose and an increase in heart rate and mean arterial blood pressure.[245] In addition, CRH may have central effects of suppressing the release of LH and GH, gastric acid secretion, sexual activity, and feeding activity while stimulating respiration and behavioral arousal even to the point of seizures.[246] CRH is decreased in the cerebral cortex of patients with Alzheimer's disease and in the basal ganglia in patients with Huntington's disease.[211]

Both ovine and human CRH have been given to humans in a variety of experimental paradigms, and CRH has been approved by the U.S. Food and Drug Administration for commercial use. These preparations have been found to be of use in stimulating ACTH secretion alone or in combination with dexamethasone and during petrosal sinus sampling in the differential diagnosis of Cushing's disease vs. ectopic ACTH syndrome[247,248] (see Chaps. 7 and 11). In patients with hypothalamic hypopituitarism, the ACTH response to CRH is increased and somewhat delayed and prolonged, but the response is markedly blunted in patients with the defect clearly localized to the pituitary, as in Sheehan's syndrome[246] (see Chap. 7). CRH testing has also been used diagnostically in psychiatric disorders in a fashion similar to the dexamethasone suppression test, but the responses have not been highly specific.[246]

Growth Hormone Releasing Hormone

Although GH-releasing activity had been found in hypothalamic extracts since 1964,[249] GH releasing hormone (GHRH or GRH) was finally isolated and characterized in 1982 in two separate laboratories virtually simultaneously not from the hypothalamus but from two pancreatic tumors that produced this substance ectopically, resulting in acromegaly.[250,251] The two peptides isolated from these tumors differed in their lengths, however, one having a length of 44 amino acids and an amidated COOH terminus[252] and the other having a length of 40 amino acids and a free COOH terminus[253]; their molecular weights are 5040 and 4545, respectively. Subsequent analysis of hypothalamic extracts confirmed the presence of both moieties, with about two-thirds being the 1-44 moiety and the remaining one-third being 1-40.[254] A 1-37-amino acid GHRH exists in significant quantities in some pancreatic tumors but is not present in significant quantities in the hypothalamus.[254] Bioactivity resides in the first 27 amino acids.[252] Structurally, GHRH belongs to the secretin-VIP-glucagon family.[253]

The gene for human GHRH has been characterized[255,256] and codes for two mRNAs which differ slightly in the splice site of the fifth exon, resulting in two GHRH precursors of 107 and 108 amino acids, respectively, that vary in the presence or absence of a serine near the 3′ end. The precursors consist of a 20-amino acid signal peptide, a 10-amino acid N-terminal peptide, a 44-amino acid GHRH, and a 30- or 31-amino acid C-terminal peptide[255,256] (Fig. 6-19). GHRH is inactivated quickly in the circulation by a dipeptidylpeptidase, which cleaves the amino terminal two peptides, resulting in a bioinactive $GHRH_{3-44}$.[257]

Early studies with large lesions of the medial basal hypothalamus showed that this region is crucial for growth of rats, and it is thought to be the source of GHRH.[144] In subsequent studies, rats with lesions confined to the ventromedial nucleus had reduced

FIGURE 6-19. Schematic diagram of the structures of the GHRH gene, mRNA, and precursor peptide. The gene codes for two mRNAs which differ slightly in the splice site of the fifth exon (denoted by the arrow in the mRNA structure), resulting in two GHRH precursors of 107 and 108 amino acids, respectively, that vary in regard to the presence or absence of a serine at position 103. Both $GHRH_{1-40}$ and $GHRH_{1-44}$ are generated from the precursor. 5′ UT = 5′ untranslated region; 3′ UT = 3′ untranslated region.

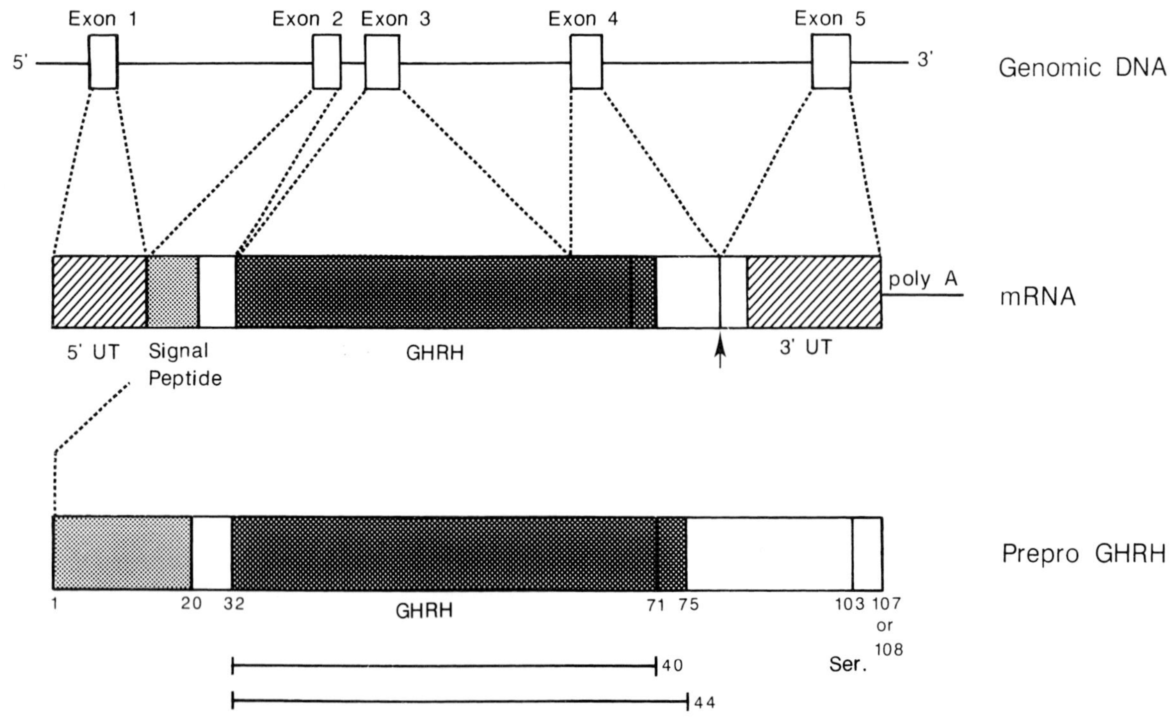

growth and lower pituitary and plasma GH levels.[258] Conversely, electric stimulation of the ventromedial and arcuate area resulted in a pronounced surge of GH.[259] Radioimmunoassays using specific GHRH antibodies have confirmed that very high concentrations of GHRH are found in the median eminence and the infundibular (arcuate) and lower portions of the ventromedial nuclei in the rat and the human, with smaller amounts elsewhere in the hypothalamus and virtually no GHRH in the extrahypothalamic brain.[260,261] Immunohistochemical studies of monkey and human brains have shown GHRH immunoreactive perikarya in the arcuate and ventromedial nuclei with most axonal projections terminating in the median eminence.[262] GHRH has also been found in a number of other tissues in humans, including the pancreas, thyroid, lung, stomach, duodenum, ileum, colon, adrenal, and kidney.[260] Although GHRH has been found in mouse and rat placentas, it has not been identified in the human placenta.[140] Plasma GHRH levels rise with meals at a time when GH levels are suppressed, even in subjects with idiopathic GH deficiency, suggesting that circulating plasma GHRH is largely gut-derived and is not reflective of hypothalamic function.[263]

$GHRH_{1-40}$ and $GHRH_{1-44}$ are essentially equipotent in stimulating GH secretion in humans in a dose-dependent fashion, with the GH rise beginning within about 5 min and with peak levels occurring about 30 to 60 min after injection.[264,265] Although many studies found GHRH to be specific for releasing only GH, other studies found that in some individuals GHRH is capable of eliciting a small increase in PRL as well.[266] Prolonged infusion of GHRH results in a gradual decrease in the amount of GH released despite maintenance of GHRH levels in the blood (i.e., somatotroph desensitization), which is thought to be due to down regulation of GHRH binding sites or to a depletion of a readily releasable pool of GH.[266] With repetitive administration every 3 h, GHRH can cause the release of sufficient GH in children with GHRH deficiency to result in an increase in IGF-I levels and an acceleration of growth.[267] Not only does GHRH stimulate release, it also stimulates GH gene transcription.[268] The critical importance of GHRH to normal GH secretion and growth was demonstrated when monoclonal antibodies to GHRH were shown to inhibit the pulsatile secretion of GH[269] and somatic growth in rats.[270] Studies using selective GHRH antagonists have shown that endogenous GHRH is required for the generation of GH pulses in humans as well.[271] The primary transduction mechanism mediating the stimulatory effect of GHRH on GH secretion is the adenylyl cyclase–cAMP system, but GHRH also stimulates the influx of calcium via calcium channels with activation of the intracellular calcium-calmodulin system.[272]

Considerable evidence in rats has documented the existence of negative feedback regulation of both IGF-I and GH in GH secretion mediated by both a decrease in GHRH synthesis and secretion and an increase in somatostatin synthesis and secretion.[26–28,273–275] In rats, the large increases in GH that occur with each spontaneous GHRH-mediated episodic surge may serve to stimulate somatostatin release, contributing to the trough of GH that follows the surge.[274] Thus, this GH "autoregulation" may prevent somatotroph desensitization.[274] In humans, GH administered acutely can block the GHRH-induced rise of GH.[28] IGF-I is also important, as documented by the high circulating GH levels that occur in IGF-I-deficient states, such as Laron dwarfism (see Chaps. 7 and 25), renal insufficiency, and cirrhosis.[29] Interactions between GHRH and somatostatin neurons within the hypothalamus have been documented in the rat, but these interactions have not been established in humans. GH short-loop negative feedback may have additional clinical importance in that some children who are GH-deficient and receive exogenous GH may develop hypothyrotropic hypothyroidism with a blunting of the TSH response to TRH.[276] It was hypothesized that this was due to an increase in hypothalamic somatostatin generation with subsequent inhibition of TSH secretion, but later studies found a normal TSH response to TRH with short-term GH infusions in normal humans.[275] However, it is likely that GH is considerably more sensitive to the inhibitory effects of somatostatin compared to TSH[175,187] so that small acute changes in somatostatin may have differential effects but long-term changes may have effects on both hormones.

In addition to these negative effects of GH and IGF-I on GHRH secretion, other factors influence GHRH secretion. Adrenergic $\alpha 2$ receptor agonists and serotonin activate GHRH and GH secretion,[277] but GABA inhibits GHRH secretion.[278] The transduction mechanism mediating GHRH secretion is primarily activation of the adenylyl cyclase–cAMP system.[278]

GHRH has been used clinically as a test to help determine the GH secretory reserve and the site of the defect in patients who are GH-deficient,[279] although the specificity of GHRH testing in this regard has not been fully established. As was mentioned earlier, GHRH can cause somatic growth in humans when given chronically,[267] but a clear benefit over standard GH therapy in this regard has not been established.

Peptides other than GHRH have also been shown to release GH and have been termed GH releasing peptides (GHRPs). Based on the knowledge that met-enkephalin can cause GH release, Bowers and colleagues investigated of number of met-enkephalin analogues for their GH releasing ability, finding that the best was a hexapeptide with the structure His-D-Trp-Ala–Trp-D-Phe-Lys-NH_2 (GHRP-6).[280] In a series of experiments it was found that the mechanism of action of GHRP-6 was not to bind to the GHRH receptor or to block somatostatin from binding to its receptor.[281] A specific receptor for the GHRPs has been cloned and is a G protein-coupled seven-transmembrane domain protein that is distinct from and unrelated to the GHRH receptor.[282] The GHRP receptor is expressed in the pituitary and in the arcuate, ventromedial, and infundibular hypothalami of humans and swine.[282] In contrast to GHRH, which acts primarily through activation of adenylyl cyclase, the GHRP receptor transduction mechanisms include activation of calcium and potassium channels and phospholipase C.[281] The GHRPs have much weaker GH releasing activity than does GHRH *in vitro,* but the GHRPs have true synergistic effects on GHRH in releasing GH. Furthermore, the GH releasing activity of GHRPs is greater in hypothalamic-pituitary preparations than in pituitary preparations, suggesting an effect on the hypothalamic GHRP receptor.[281] Recently, the 28-amino acid peptide that binds specifically to the GHRP receptor has been isolated from rat stomach and human stomach that differ by 2 amino acids.[281a] Whether these are the true endogenous hypothalamic physiologic ligands for the GHRP receptor remains to be seen. A number of orally active peptides and nonpeptide substances which act via the GHRP receptor are also in development and may prove clinically useful.[281]

Prolactin Inhibiting Factor

It was found more than 35 years ago that the luteotropic properties of the pituitary (caused by PRL) were increased when pituitaries were transplanted to beneath the renal capsule, a site distant from regulation by the hypothalamus, thus demonstrating the predominance of the inhibitory component of hypothalamic regulation of PRL secretion.[283] Subsequent experiments showed initially that hypothalamic extracts suppress PRL secretion from pituitaries in vitro[284] and then that DA can suppress PRL release from pituitaries in vitro.[285] A number of experiments have firmly established that DA is the predominant physiologic prolactin inhibiting factor (PIF), including the demonstration that the concentration of DA found in the pituitary stalk plasma is sufficient to decrease PRL levels in rats and is 5 to 10 times higher than levels found in peripheral plasma[286] and the finding that stimuli which result in an acute release of PRL usually also result in an acute decrease in portal vessel DA levels.[287] However, in many experiments it has been found that the PRL increase obtained by simply reducing DA is considerably lower than the elevation of PRL achieved by means of simultaneous stimulation by a substance with PRL-releasing activity [PRL releasing factor (PRF)]; similarly, the PRL level achieved with stimulation by a PRF simultaneously with the reduction in DA is usually greater than that achieved by a PRF alone.[288] It is likely that in most physiologic circumstances that cause a PRL rise, such as lactation, there is a simultaneous fall in DA along with a rise in a PRF, such as VIP.[289]

Although much of the direct evidence of DA in hypothalamic-pituitary portal vessels and of the effects of DA on PRL release in vitro are derived from animals, it is clear that DA is the primary PIF in humans as well. Infusion of DA causes a rapid suppression of basal PRL levels that can be reversed by metoclopramide, a DA receptor blocker.[290] Dopamine also blocks the increase in PRL release induced by such stimuli as hypoglycemia,[291] arginine,[292] and TRH.[293] Studies with low-dose DA infusions in humans have shown that DA blood concentrations similar to those found in rat and monkey hypothalamic-pituitary portal blood[285,294] are able to suppress PRL secretion.[295] Blockade of endogenous DA receptors by a variety of drugs, including phenothiazines, butyrophenones, metoclopramide, and domperidone, causes a rise in PRL.[296]

The axons responsible for the release of DA into the median eminence originate in perikarya in the dorsomedial portion of the arcuate nucleus and the inferior portion of the ventromedial nucleus of the hypothalamus.[31,297] This pathway is known as the tuberoinfundibular DA (TIDA) pathway, and DA axon terminals constitute about a third of all axon terminals in the zona externa of the median eminence.[297] Some TIDA neurons do not terminate in the median eminence but project to the posterior and intermediate lobes.[297]

The DA that traverses the TIDA pathway binds to DA D_2 receptors[298] on the lactotroph cell membrane.[299] Activation of this receptor results in (1) inhibition of adenyl cyclase with lowered intracellular cAMP levels, (2) inhibition of phosphoinositide metabolism, and (3) decreased intracellular calcium mobilization and inhibition of calcium transport through calcium channels. These different actions of DA may be mediated by multiple similar D_2 receptors that are produced by alternative RNA splicing.[300]

A number of experiments have suggested that there may be other peptide PIFs in addition to DA. The primary candidate for this putative PIF appears to be GAP, the 56-amino acid portion of the precursor to GnRH that was discussed previously. In initial studies, GAP was found to have a potency on a molar basis four times that of DA with respect to PIF activity.[137] Immunization of rabbits against GAP results in neutralization of endogenous GAP and a rise in basal PRL levels.[137] GAP_{1-13} also has minimal PRL-lowering properties in the rat.[138] Studies in sheep show no effect of GAP on either gonadotropin or PRL secretion.[301] Limited in vitro studies of GAP_{1-13} in baboon and human pituitary cell cultures have shown no PRL inhibitory effect.[139,302] Whether GAP or a metabolic product is the peptidergic PIF long postulated to exist remains to be determined, and its physiologic importance in PRL regulation in humans has not been defined.

Another potential candidate for PIF activity is GABA. GABA and muscimol, a GABA receptor agonist, have been shown to inhibit PRL synthesis and release in vitro in rats, but blockade of this inhibition with GABA receptor antagonists such as picrotoxin and bicuculline has given variable results.[303,304] A tuberoinfundibular GABAergic system has been described, with perikarya located in the arcuate nucleus and nerve endings demonstrated in the median eminence.[305] GABA is also present in portal blood.[306]

Studies of the GABA system in humans have yielded conflicting results in studies with widely differing experimental designs. Bioactive metabolites of GABA, such as γ-hydroxybutyric acid and γ-amino-β-hydroxybutyric acid and muscimol, cause modest increases in PRL levels when injected into humans.[307,308] However, GABA itself causes a modest decrease in PRL levels when given to humans for several days,[309] and activation of the endogenous GABAergic system with sodium valproate causes a suppression in the PRL rise induced by mechanical breast stimulation in puerperal women.[310] The physiologic role of GABA, like that of GAP, remains to be fully elucidated in humans as well as in various animal species.

Prolactin Releasing Factor

The role of TRH as a PRF is discussed extensively above. A number of other peptides have also been shown to have PRF activity in a variety of experimental situations. VIP stimulates PRL release.[311] VIP neuronal perikarya are present in the parvocellular region of the paraventricular nucleus and suprachiasmatic nucleus with axons terminating in the external zone of the median eminence.[312] Its effects are selective for PRL and additive to TRH[313] at concentrations found in hypothalamic-pituitary portal blood.[314] In addition to stimulating PRL release, VIP increases pituitary PRL mRNA content and PRL synthesis.[315] In conditions of increased PRL synthesis, such as lactation, hypothalamic VIP mRNA levels are also increased.[316] In addition to these studies in rats, intravenously administered VIP has been shown to increase PRL levels in humans[317] at serum levels similar to those demonstrated in rat portal blood.

A number of experiments have been performed using passive immunoneutralization techniques to determine the physiologic role of VIP as a PRF. Anti-VIP antisera administered to rats have been shown to inhibit partially the PRL responses to suckling, ether-induced stress,[289] and estrogen administration[318] and to suppress PRL pulsatile secretion in dopamine receptor–blocked rats.[319]

Within the 20-kDa 170-amino acid VIP precursor is another similarly sized peptide known as peptide histidine methionine (PHM).[320] VIP has 28 amino acid residues, and PHM has 27. The terminal amino acid in the porcine equivalent of PHM is isoleucine, and therefore the peptide of porcine origin is known as PHI. PHM and VIP colocalize in the hypothalamus and median eminence.[321] Interestingly, PHI is of similar potency to VIP in releasing PRL from rat pituitaries in vitro and in vivo.[322] Furthermore, passive immunoneutralization with anti-PHI plus anti-VIP antisera causes a greater suppression of the PRL responses to the serotonin precursor 5-hydroxytryptophan and ether than does either anti-PHI or anti-VIP antiserum alone.[323] PHM given to humans has caused increases in PRL levels in some experiments[321] but not in others.[317] Further complicating the role of VIP as a PRF is the finding that VIP is actually synthesized by anterior pituitary tissue.[45] Antisera to VIP inhibit basal PRL secretion from dispersed pituitary cells in vitro,[324] suggesting a local "autocrine" role for VIP in PRL regulation within the pituitary. The physiologic role of VIP as a PRF appears to be warranted by the experimental data. The precise roles of VIP vs. PHM and hypothalamic VIP vs. pituitary VIP are not clear. How VIP and PHM interact with other PRFs such as TRH are additional areas requiring clarification.

A number of other peptides have PRF activity in various experimental situations, including GHRH, the opioid peptides, oxytocin, vasopressin, GnRH, angiotensin II, neurotensin, substance P, cholecystokinin, secretin, gastrin, bombesin, epidermal growth factor, fibroblast growth factor, and galanin. However, their importance in regulating PRL in humans has not been established. Recently, an 87-amino acid peptide isolated from the human hypothalamus has been found to bind to specific receptors on the human pituitary and to cause a release of PRL from rat pituitary cell cultures.[325] Bovine, rat, and human cDNAs for this peptide have been isolated from the brains of these species; the putative peptide sequences were highly conserved among the species and the peptide has been designated as prolactin releasing peptide.[325]

NEUROTRANSMITTERS

Neurotransmitters may be simple amino acids, bioamines, peptides, gases, or other substances, such as cytokines and adenosine. As was noted previously, neurotransmitters may function differently in the synapses of one neuron compared with another, depending on the stage of activity of the cell, other neural inputs, and other hormonal influences, including the feedback effects of target hormones. For example, the inhibitory effect of dopamine on pituitary lactotrophs may be considerably altered by the estrogen milieu at that particular point in time; a high estrogen state, such as pregnancy, causes a considerable blunting of this inhibition. Furthermore, as can be seen from the previous discussions about the nature of neuron-neuron interactions and the characteristics of the specific hypophysiotropic hormones, various neurotransmitters can affect pituitary hormone secretion by direct action at the pituitary and indirect action through modulation of the actions of the various hypophysiotropic hormones, which themselves may be stimulatory or inhibitory. Thus, pituitary hormone secretion reflects the integration of all these inputs.

Biosynthesis and Metabolism of Bioaminergic Neurotransmitters

Bioaminergic neurotransmitters are synthesized within the neuronal perikarya. After initial uptake of specific amino acid precursors, enzymatic synthesis occurs and the monoamines are stored in neurosecretory granules (Fig. 6-2). Upon release into the synapse after neuronal depolarization, the neurotransmitter generally either binds to the specific receptor on the postsynaptic neuron or is inactivated by degradation or uptake into neuronal tissue. However, neurotransmitters may diffuse out of the synaptic cleft to reach distant target receptors, a process termed volume transmission.[4] The specific biochemical steps for the synthesis and degradation of the major bioaminergic neurotransmitters are shown in Fig. 6-20.

Anatomic Pathways of Bioaminergic Neurotransmitters

Dopamine

As was discussed earlier, the TIDA originates in the arcuate and ventromedial nuclei, and axons project inferiorly to the median eminence. Some of these axons also project to the intermediate and posterior lobes.[297,326] It is important to stress that the tuberoinfundibular dopaminergic system so important for neuroendocrine regulation is quite separate from the nigrostriatal (mesolimbic) dopaminergic system involved in Parkinson's disease and the cortical (mesocortical) dopaminergic system that has been postulated to be involved in schizophrenia. Nonetheless, medications which are dopaminergic agonists and antagonists may affect all these systems, causing unwanted side effects in one and therapeutic effects in another. For example, dopamine receptor blockers such as the phenothiazines, which may be quite beneficial in the treatment of the psychosis of schizophrenia, commonly block the inhibitory effect of dopamine on PRL, resulting in hyperprolactinemia. The dopamine receptor is of the seven-transmembrane domain G protein-coupled type, and there are at least five subtypes.[300,327]

Norepinephrine

Hypothalamic norepinephrine originates in specific brainstem regions, the locus coeruleus, the ventrolateral medulla, and the dorsal vagal complex, which includes the nucleus of the solitary tract.[326,328] Axons project to the hypothalamus via the ventral noradrenergic bundle.[326,328] Because the nucleus of the solitary tract is the major recipient of primary visceral afferent information carried by the vagus and glossopharyngeal nerves, this noradrenergic projection to the hypothalamus is important in the integration of neuroendocrine and autonomic responses to visceral stimuli.[328] All hypothalamic nuclei contain noradrenergic fibers and terminals, especially the paraventricular and supraoptic nuclei.[328] However, noradrenergic fibers project only to the internal zone, not the external zone, of the median eminence.[329] Thus, noradrenergic neurons serve an integrative function, coupling neuroendocrine with autonomic systems rather than playing a direct role at the pituitary level.

Epinephrine

The cells of origin of adrenergic neural fibers are located primarily in the lateral reticular nucleus of the medulla and the nucleus of the solitary tract,[329] although some are also located within the hypothalamus.[326] They project to the dorsomedial and arcuate nuclei and the medial parvocellular portion of the paraventricular nucleus.[329] Few fibers are found in the external zone of the median eminence,[329] but there is some evidence for direct adrenergic influence on the pituitary, including the presence of beta$_2$-adrenergic receptors of pituitary cell membranes[330] and a stimulatory effect of epinephrine on GH secretion from pituitary cell cultures.[331]

Serotonin

Most serotoninergic neuronal perikarya are in the dorsal and median raphe nuclei of the pons and upper medulla, and their

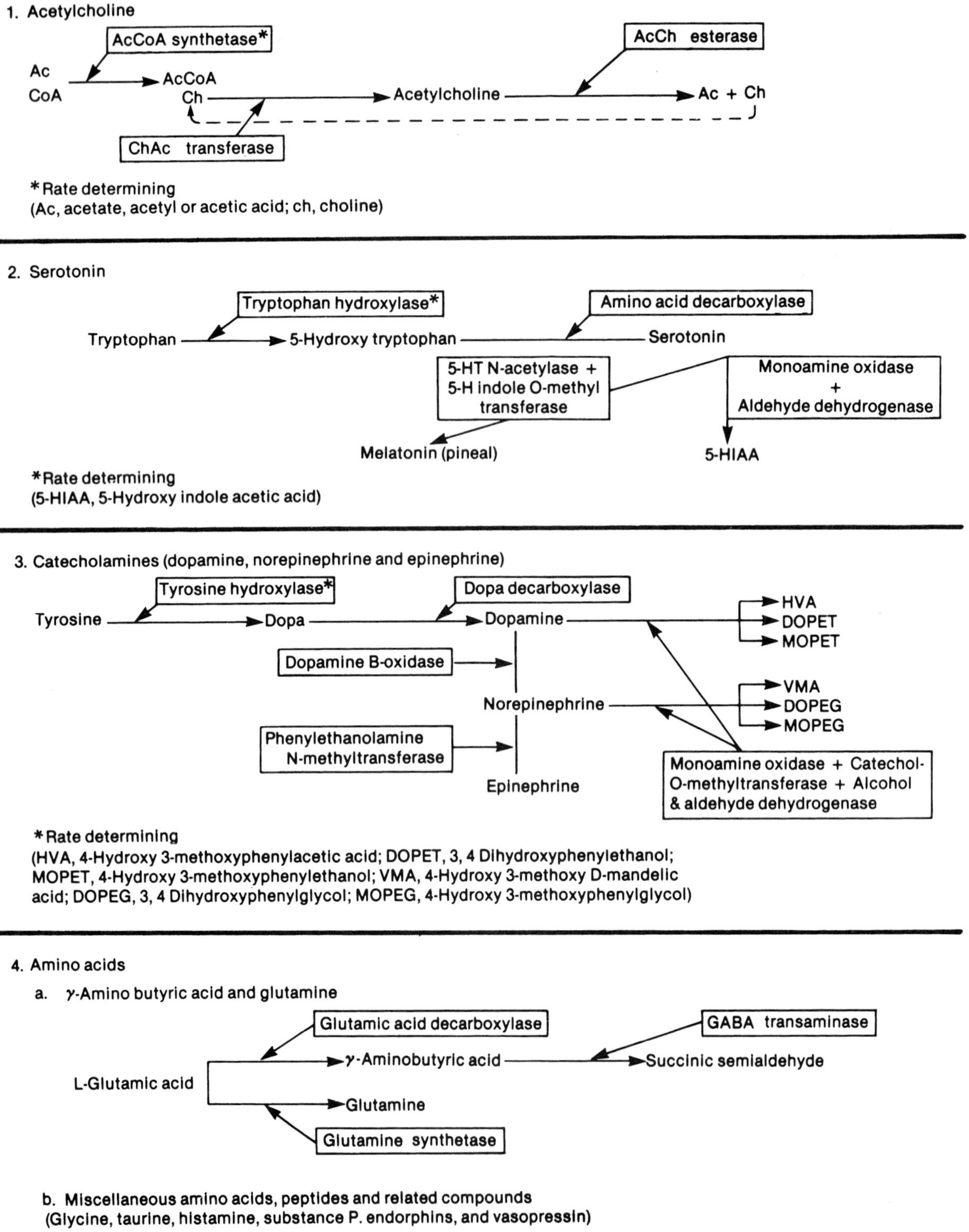

FIGURE 6-20. Neurotransmitters in the mammalian brain and their associated enzymes and major brain metabolites. (*From Samorajski T, J Am Geriatr Soc 25:337, 1977.*)

axons project forward to the hypothalamus and other limbic and cortical areas.[332] The hypothalamic area most heavily innervated with serotoninergic fibers is the suprachiasmatic nucleus, suggesting a role for serotonin in the generation of circadian rhythms.[332] Because hypothalamic serotonin is reduced by only 60 percent when all afferent nerve fibers are cut, it is likely that a considerable amount of this neurotransmitter is also generated within the hypothalamus, although the specific sites are not known.[332] Serotonin is also present within the anterior pituitary.[333] The pituitary contains tryptophan hydroxylase, the rate-limiting enzyme in serotonin synthesis,[333] suggesting in situ synthesis. The serotonin receptor is of the seven-transmembrane domain G protein-coupled type and there are at least seven subtypes.[334] High affinity S_2 serotonin receptors are present in the anterior pituitary,[335] and uptake of labeled serotonin has been demonstrated.[336] The results of direct tests of the effects of serotonin on pituitary hormone release, however, have been conflicting.

Acetylcholine

Acetylcholine, acetylcholinesterase, and choline acyltransferase are all present in the hypothalamus, with the highest concentrations occurring in the median eminence.[329] However, the neuronal perikarya and their fiber distribution within the hypothalamus are not known.[337] Acetylcholine has also been found within the pituitary,[338] but its functional significance there is uncertain.

γ-Aminobutyric Acid

Recent studies suggest that GABA is numerically the dominant neurotransmitter in the hypothalamus, being present in half of all synapses.[339] This fact alone emphasizes the importance of inhibitory circuits in neuroendocrine regulation, as GABA is primarily an inhibitory neurotransmitter. GABA fibers are widely distributed throughout the hypothalamus and are also present in the median eminence and the posterior pituitary.[305] GABA neuronal perikarya are located primarily in the arcuate nucleus and the posterior hypothalamus, although small numbers are found in many other areas of the hypothalamus.[305] The posterior hypothalamic GABAergic neurons also project to the cortex.[340] Short GABAergic interneurons also exist within all brain areas and act locally as inhibitors within neural circuits unrelated to projections from the hypothalamus.[341]

Histamine

Histamine neuronal perikarya are present in the posterior hypothalamic region, and axons project to almost all the nuclei of the hypothalamus as well as the median eminence.[342] Both H_1 and H_2 receptors are present in the brain,[325] and agonists and antagonists of these receptors can alter hormone secretion in some circumstances.

Neuropharmacology of Bioaminergic Neurotransmitters

Bioaminergic neurotransmitters can affect pituitary hormone secretion via direct action on the pituitary or indirectly via effects on the releasing and inhibiting factors that affect that hormone's secretion. An example of the complexity of this interaction is provided by an examination of the components that result in dopamine stimulating GH secretion: (1) Dopamine appears to inhibit somatostatin secretion in indirect experiments in humans,[343] (2) the GH rise induced by L-dopa is accompanied by increased GHRH levels in plasma, implying that GHRH is the intermediary,[344] (3) dopamine causes an increase in somatostatin release and a decrease in GHRH release from rat hypothalamic slices in vitro,[345] (4) dopamine alone stimulates GH secretion in pituitary cell cultures,[346] and (5) dopamine inhibits the GH response to GHRH in pituitary cell cultures.[346] Table 6-3 lists the overall composite effects of the bioaminergic neurotransmitters on the various pituitary hormones as generally understood. However, depending on the hormonal status and metabolic milieu at any point in time, other effects can be seen. Furthermore, pharmacologic agents which are claimed to be specific for one class of effects on bioamines rarely are so and, depending on the hormonal and metabolic status, may have different effects at different times (Fig. 6-21).

TABLE 6-3. Neurotransmitter Regulation of Pituitary Hormone Secretion

Neurotransmitter	GH	PRL	LH/FSH	TSH	ACTH
Norepinephrine	↑	0	↑	↑	⇅
Dopamine	↑	↓	↓	↓	↓?
Serotonin	↑	↑	↓?	⇅	↑
GABA	↑	↓	↑	0	↓
Histamine	0	↑	↑	↑	↑
Acetylcholine	↑	⇅	↑	0	↑

↑ = increase; ↓ = decrease; 0 = no effect; ⇅ = increase or decrease in different circumstances.

Amino Acid Neurotransmitters

Glutamate functions as an excitatory neurotransmitter in synapses throughout the mediobasal hypothalamus, including the magnocellular and parvocellular regions of the paraventricular nucleus

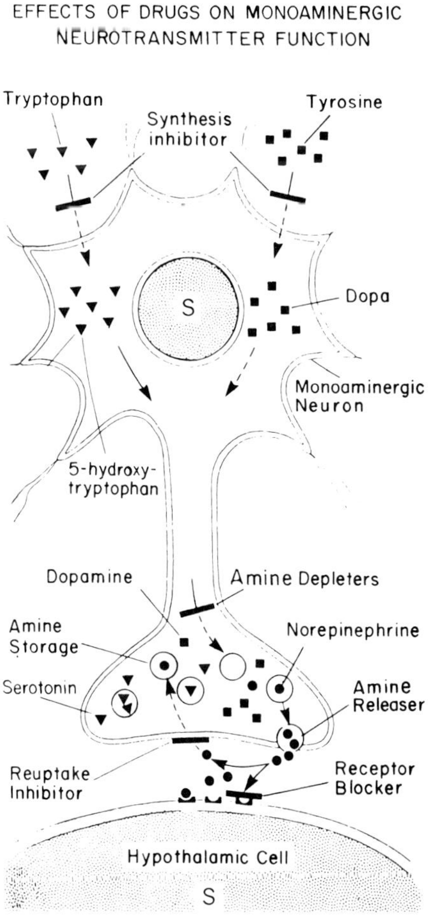

FIGURE 6-21. Schematic showing sites and modes of actions of various categories of drugs (including many agents used therapeutically) that alter neurotransmitter function. Depending on a particular drug's mode of action, the result is a net increase or decrease in the secretion of a releasing or inhibiting factor by the hypothalamic cell. (*Modified from Frohman L, Hosp Pract 10:54, 1975.*)

and the supraoptic and arcuate nuclei.[347] Glutamate and aspartate are also present in the hippocampus, cerebellum, auditory nerve, and spinal cord.[341] Ionotropic glutamate receptors include the N-methyl-D-aspartate (NMDA) receptor, which is important in the control of neuron excitability and which is also activated by serine and glycine.[348] The role of the second class of glutamate receptors, termed the metabotropic receptors, is uncertain.[348] Glycine functions as an inhibitory neurotransmitter in the brainstem, the spinal cord, and possibly the hypothalamus.[341] Despite the widespread presence of amino acids as neurotransmitters, little is known about their possible roles in neuroendocrine regulation.

Neuropeptides

Vasoactive Intestinal Peptide

VIP is synthesized by hypothalamic and cerebrocortical tissue[349] and the pituitary[45] and can be found throughout the cortex, amygdala, striatum, hippocampus, midbrain, spinal cord, and sympathetic ganglia and in autonomic nerves such as the vagus.[350] In addition to its effects as a PRF, it stimulates the release of ACTH and GH and has variable effects on LH and FSH, though it has no effect on TSH secretion.[350,351] In other areas of the brain, VIP is excitatory, causing cerebrovascular vasodilatation and stimulating adenylyl cyclase.[350,351]

Substance P

Substance P–containing nerve terminals are abundant in the substantia nigra, amygdala, and hypothalamus, including the median eminence, but their site of origin is not known.[352] Little is present in the cortex or cerebellum.[352] Substance P stimulates PRL release in some experimental situations but not in others[353,354] and inhibits CRF- or vasopressin-stimulated but not basal ACTH release.[355] Its effects on TSH and gonadotropin secretion are not known. The major known physiologic action of substance P is as a sensory neurotransmitter for pain in peripheral nerves and in the spinal cord, and some studies suggest a role in stimulating behavioral arousal.[352] Depletion of substance P with capsaicin, the irritant isolated from hot peppers, results in decreased pain, and this substance has been used therapeutically to treat painful diabetic peripheral neuropathy with varying success.[356]

Neurotensin

Neurotensin causes vasodilation, hypotension, and increased vascular permeability after systemic injection.[357] Within the brain, the highest concentrations are in the hypothalamus, thalamus, preoptic area, interpeduncular nucleus, and brainstem, with little in the cortex or cerebellum.[358] Within the hypothalamus, neurotensin can be found in the arcuate nucleus, parvocellular division of the paraventricular nucleus, and in the periventricular nucleus and neurotensin fibers project to the median eminence for release into portal blood.[359] However, most neurotensin is located in the endocrine cells of the GI tract mucosa.[357] Neurotensin receptors are found in both lobes of the pituitary and in many areas of the hypothalamus, with high densities in both the parvo- and magnocellular parts of the paraventricular nucleus and the suprachiasmatic nucleus.[359] In experimental studies, hormonal effects vary with variations in the method of administration. For example, intracerebroventricular administration results in increased somatostatin in portal blood and decreased secretion of GH and PRL, but peripheral injection increases the secretion of GH and PRL.[360] In contrast to these results in rats, intravenous administration of neurotensin to humans has no effect on PRL, GH, LH, or TSH levels.[361] However, it is likely that most effects that neurotensin may have on pituitary hormone secretion probably occur centrally and data support a stimulatory effect on CRH, dopamine, GnRH, and somatostatin either directly or through interneurons.[359] The neurotensin released into portal blood may serve to stimulate PRL secretion directly and, as neurotensin is actually synthesized in gonadotroph and thyrotroph cells, there may be additional paracrine or autocrine effects.[359] Other central effects of neurotensin include hypothermia, antinociception, and antidopaminergic activity.[357] An important peripheral hormonal effect of neurotensin is its ability to increase glucagon secretion, causing hyperglycemia.[357]

Renin-Angiotensin System

Renin, angiotensinogen, and angiotensin converting enzyme (ACE) are present in the thalamus, basal ganglia, cortex, cerebellum, hypothalamus, median eminence, and pituitary.[362,363] Renin and angiotensinogen mRNAs have been found in some of these areas, implying local synthesis.[360] In situ hybridization studies have shown that angiotensinogen mRNA is present in the magnocellular neurons of the hypothalamic paraventricular nucleus.[364] Angiotensin II receptors are present in all pituitary cell types except gonadotrophs.[363] In the human pituitary, renin, ACE, and angiotensinogen have been detected in normal lactotroph cells and in PRL-secreting adenomas.[365] However, when the generation of endogenous angiotensin II is blocked in humans by inhibition of ACE with enalapril, basal levels of PRL, GH, and ACTH and the ACTH response to hypoglycemia are unaffected and the PRL response to hypoglycemia is decreased only minimally.[366] It is therefore unlikely that the endogenous renin-angiotensin system of the hypothalamus and pituitary has significant physiologic effects on pituitary hormone regulation in humans. Angiotensin has also been found in various experimental preparations to have pressor effects, thirst-stimulating capabilities, and vasopressin-releasing properties,[367] but its role in these effects in humans is not well understood.

Cholecystokinin

Cholecystokinin is present in the cortex, thalamus, basal ganglia, and hypothalamus. It increases PRL release in vitro in the rat[313,368] but not from human pituitary cultures.[313] Intravenous administration in rats has provided both positive[368] and negative results[369] with respect to PRL stimulation. Intracerebroventricular cholecystokinin administration results in a marked PRL release that can be antagonized with antisera to VIP,[369] implying that its action may require the activation of VIPergic systems. The reasons for these varying results and their relevance to humans are unknown. Cholecystokinin has also been implicated in causing satiety, possibly by augmenting vagal afferent neural signals, and studies in humans have shown that intravenous infusions of cholecystokinin result in decreased eating.[370]

Endogenous Opioid Peptides

In the mid-1970s, the discovery of the opiate receptors and the fact that some of the endogenous opioid peptide ligands for those receptors are present within the precursor to ACTH, POMC, prompted widespread speculation about the importance of this system in neuroendocrine regulation as well as the interactions of neuroendocrinology, mental illness, and opiate addiction. Most data now suggest, however, at most a modest role for the endogenous opioid peptides in neuroendocrine regulation.[371]

There are three major opioid peptide receptors, all of the seven-transmembrane G protein-coupled receptor class, and three major groups of opioid peptides, but the correspondence is not one for one. The μ receptor mediates most of the endocrine effects and analgesia; morphine is its prototypic agonist, and naloxone is its prototypic antagonist. The primary peptide ligand for the μ receptor is β-endorphin, which is derived from POMC, although β-endorphin also binds to the δ receptor and the enkephalins also can bind to the μ receptor. The δ receptor mediates behavioral, analgesic, and some endocrine effects and has as its primary peptide ligands met- and leu-enkephalins, which are derived from proenkephalin A. It is much less well blocked by naloxone than is the μ receptor. The κ receptor mediates sedation and ataxia and binds primarily dynorphin and the neoendorphins, which are derived from proenkephalin B (prodynorphin). A fourth receptor has recently been described which has considerable sequence homology with the δ receptor and binds to an endogenous 17-amino acid peptide called nociceptin (also known as orphanin FQ).[372]

The β-endorphin opioid system has been the most intensively studied neuroendocrinologically because of the derivation of β-endorphin from POMC. POMC is a 31,000-dalton precursor peptide which contains ACTH, β-lipotropin (β-LPH), and β-endorphin; the last corresponds to the C-terminal 31 amino acids of β-lipotropin (Fig. 6-22). POMC undergoes tissue-specific posttranslational processing: In the anterior pituitary, the major cleavage products are β-LPH and ACTH, with a significant proportion of β-LPH being further processed to β-endorphin, but in the pituitary intermediate lobe, the major products are α-MSH, corticotropin-like intermediate peptide (CLIP), β-endorphin, and γ-LPH.[373] Brain POMC, however, is processed primarily to β-endorphin, γ-LPH, and ACTH, with most of the ACTH being further processed to CLIP and α-MSH.

All neuronal perikarya containing POMC-derived peptides are located in the arcuate nucleus, from which fibers containing β-endorphin and α-MSH project to the median eminence and the ventromedial, dorsomedial, paraventricular, and periventricular nuclei of the hypothalamus, as well as to the amygdala, preoptic area, periaqueductal gray matter, reticular formation, stria terminalis, locus coeruleus, striatum, and hippocampus.[373] The projection to the median eminence results in significant quantities of β-endorphin in portal blood.[373] POMC-derived peptides are also found in the placenta, thyroid C cells, pancreas, testes, ovaries, adrenal medulla, gastric antrum, and macrophages.[373] Anterior pituitary β-endorphin is secreted with ACTH after CRH and vasopressin stimulation (described previously), but the only factors known to decrease hypothalamic β-endorphin are dopamine and estradiol.[373]

The pentapeptide enkephalins are derived from the 28K precursor, proenkephalin A, which contains six copies of the met-enkephalin sequence and one copy of the leu-enkephalin sequence.[374] Other extended cleavage products with biological activity may also exist, and the ratio of met-enkephalin to leu-enkephalin ranges between 5:1 and 10:1 in various brain regions, possibly reflecting differences in tissue-specific cleavage and/or degradation. Neuronal perikarya containing the enkephalins are widely distributed throughout the brain, as are fiber networks.[374,375] Most enkephalinergic neurons are short, having the characteristics of interneurons.[374] Rich enkephalinergic neural fiber networks can be found in the globus pallidus, amygdala, and midbrain, with specific areas of innervation including the origin of the central noradrenergic system, the locus coeruleus, the origin of the central serotoninergic system, the raphe nuclei, and the origin of the striatal dopaminergic system, the substantia nigra.[375] Enkephalinergic neurons in the magnocellular portion of the paraventricular and supraoptic nuclei project to the posterior pituitary.[375] Within the pituitary, enkephalins have been detected primarily in the posterior pituitary.[374] Enkephalins have also been found in the adrenal medulla, gut, sympathetic ganglia, vagus, and retina.[374]

Dynorphin is a 17-amino acid peptide derived from a 28K

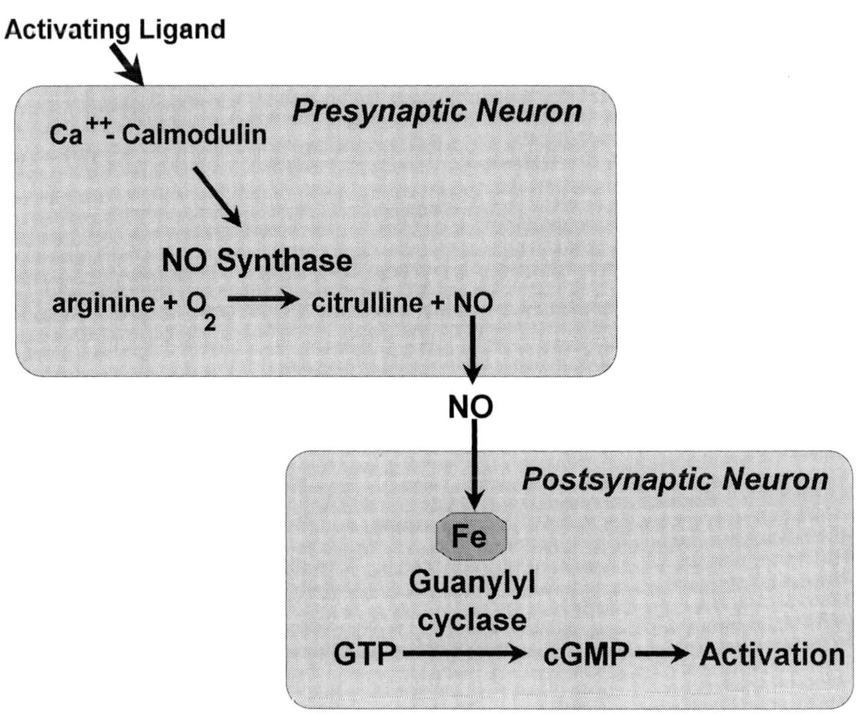

FIGURE 6-22. Structures of the precursors of the endogenous opioid peptides. Prepro-opiomelanocortin (POMC) generates several peptides, including β-lipotropin (β-LPH), β-endorphin, ACTH, α-MSH, β-MSH, γ-MSH, and corticotropin-like intermediate lobe peptide (CLIP). Preproenkephalin A generates six copies of methionine enkephalin (met-enk) and one copy of leucine enkephalin (leu-enk). Preproenkephalin B (preprodynorphin) generates α- and β-neoendorphins; dynorphins 108, 1–17, and 1–32; and rimorphin. Preprononociceptin generates the 17-amino acid peptide, nociceptin.

precursor called proenkephalin B or prodynorphin. Shorter peptides termed α- and β-neoendorphin, with 10 and 9 amino acids, respectively, have also been isolated.[374] These peptides react almost exclusively with the κ receptor. Dynorphin-containing cells also project from the magnocellular neurons of the paraventricular nucleus to the posterior pituitary. Other tissues containing dynorphin include the gut, lungs, and adrenal medulla.[374]

Nociceptin is a 17-amino acid peptide derived from a precursor called pronociceptin.[376] High concentrations of nociceptin and its receptor are present in the hypothalamus as well as in other areas of the brain that serve as the sources of monoamine neurotransmitters, including the locus coeruleus, dorsal raphe, substantia nigra, and ventral tegmental area.[372] In general, nociceptin appears to have an "anti-opioid" or "anti-nociceptive" effect.[372] When injected into the ventromedial hypothalamus of satiated rats, nociceptin stimulates feeding behavior and hyperpolarizes GnRH containing and dopamine containing neurons in the arcuate nucleus, but more detailed experiments involving neuroendocrine regulation have not yet been done.[372]

The μ receptors are located predominantly in the thalamus, hippocampus, periaqueductal gray matter, and neocortex, and the δ receptors are located primarily in the amygdala, nucleus accumbens, septum, and hypothalamus.[374] Dynorphin receptors have been localized to the cerebral cortex, the thalamus, and the caudate nucleus.[374] The anterior pituitary itself is poor in opioid receptors, but the hypothalamus is quite rich, and it has been suggested that the effects of opioid peptides on anterior pituitary hormone secretion occur via modulation of hypothalamic bioamines and hypophysiotropic factors.[374,375]

The specific functions of the various opioid peptides and opioid receptors are not completely understood, although evidence links them to a number of bodily functions, including stress, mental illness, narcotic tolerance and dependence, eating, drinking, GI function, learning, memory, cardiovascular responses, respiration, thermoregulation, seizures, brain electric activity, locomotor activity, pregnancy, and neuroimmune activity.[377] More specific functions on neuroendocrine regulation have been documented, however. In general, endogenous opioids have an inhibitory influence on gonadotropin secretion through their action on GnRH secretion, probably by inhibiting noradrenergic neuronal input.[371] Exogenous β endorphin and enkephalin analogs increase serum GH and PRL levels,[371] but blockade of endogenous opioid pathways with naloxone does not alter basal or stimulated GH and PRL levels.[371,378] Opioids feed back negatively on ACTH and β-endorphin secretion, and naloxone can increase basal and stimulated ACTH levels.[235,271] Opioids have virtually no effect on TSH secretion.[371] Overall, the effects of the endogenous opioids on normal physiologic regulation of the various pituitary hormones appear to be minimal. It is possible that increased opioid peptidergic tone is present in some states of pathologic gonadotropin dysfunction, but this appears to be somewhat inconsistent.

Other Peptides

Atrial natriuretic peptide (ANP) is a 28-amino acid peptide derived from a 126-amino acid precursor originally isolated from cardiac tissue and found to stimulate renal water and salt excretion, stimulate vasodilation, and inhibit vasopressin and aldosterone secretion (see Chap. 13). Atrial natriuretic peptide (ANP) or a cleaved derivative is present in a number of areas of rat brain, with the highest concentrations in the hypothalamus and septum.[379] Substantial numbers of neuronal perikarya are found in the parvocellular part of the paraventricular nucleus with projections to the median eminence, but cell bodies and fibers also occur elsewhere in the brain. Central ANP appears to be active in inhibiting thirst and vasopressin and CRH release, and ANP reaching the pituitary may inhibit ACTH release but stimulate gonadotropin release.[379] A related but separate peptide, *brain natriuretic peptide* (BNP), is present at higher concentrations in the brain than ANP but exists at only 2 percent of the concentration of ANP in cardiac atria.[380] Both peptides have equal affinity for the same receptors. Intravenous infusion of BNP causes a suppression of plasma renin activity and aldosterone secretion, with an increase in urinary sodium excretion.[380]

Galanin is a 29-amino acid peptide of the gut and brain, with neuronal perikarya in the supraoptic, paraventricular, and arcuate nuclei of the hypothalami and fiber projections to the medial basal hypothalamus.[381] Galanin releases GH by means of an effect on GHRH in the hypothalamus.[381] Although galanin augments the GH response to GHRH, suggesting an effect on somatostatin in humans,[382] it has no effect on somatostatin secretion from hypothalamic slices.[381] Galanin inhibits basal and stress-induced ACTH secretion[383] and is localized to corticotroph cells in human pituitaries.[384] Galanin is also important in modulating GnRH secretion with respect to both episodic secretion and the ovulatory surge of LH.[385]

Endothelins are 21-amino acid vasoconstrictor peptides produced by endothelial cells that are also produced by the supraoptic and paraventricular nuclei, with projections to the posterior pituitary.[386] Water deprivation results in a depletion of neurohypophyseal endothelin.[386] Endothelins also stimulate gonadotropin secretion[387] and inhibit PRL secretion[388] from pituitary cell cultures. Another vasoactive neuropeptide, *neuropeptide Y* (NPY), is important in the regulation of central catecholaminergic mechanisms involved in blood pressure and temperature regulation and food intake. NPY axons innervate portions of the parvocellular division of the paraventricular nucleus in contact with TRH-containing neurons,[389] and central NPY administration reduces serum TSH levels.[390] NPY also enhances the LH-releasing effects of GnRH (as described previously).[133,385]

Gaseous Neurotransmitters

Nitric Oxide

During the past several years, it has become apparent that at least two gases, nitric oxide (NO) and carbon monoxide (CO), serve as important neurotransmitters.[391] NO is made by nitric oxide synthase (NOS) in a reaction that converts arginine and oxygen into citrulline and nitric oxide (Fig. 6-23).[391] Constitutive NOS isoforms in neuronal and endothelial cells are activated by an increase in intracellular calcium with the subsequent transient formation of small amounts of NO; phosphorylation of NOS decreases its activity.[391] There may be additional regulatory proteins which decrease NOS activity that are not yet well characterized.[392] As a neurotransmitter, NO diffuses out of the cell generating it and goes to a target cell where it binds to the iron in the heme group of guanylyl cyclase, thereby activating it and producing cyclic guanosine monophosphate (cGMP) which then activates other processes.[391] Glutamate appears to be the most important regulator of NOS in the brain and hypothalamus, acting through the N-methyl-D-aspartate (NMDA) subtype receptor, which possesses a calcium channel that permits calcium to enter.[391,392]

Neuronal NOS has been found in the olfactory bulb, amygdala,

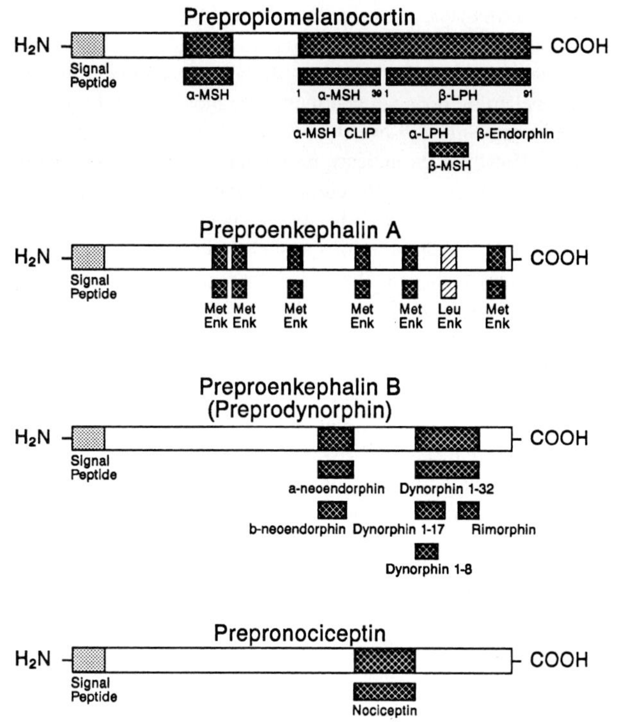

FIGURE 6-23. Nitric oxide as a neurotransmitter. An initial ligand binds to its receptor on a neuron, activating calcium channels with an increase in intracellular calcium. The calcium binds to calmodulin, activating nitric oxide synthase (NOS), which converts arginine plus oxygen to citrulline and nitric oxide (NO). Nitric oxide diffuses out of the presynaptic neuron into the postsynaptic neuron, activating guanylyl cyclase by binding to the iron in its heme group. The increase in cyclic guanosine monophosphate (cGMP) causes activation of additional transduction pathways.

cerebellum, cortex, hippocampus striatum, locus coeruleus, and hypothalamus, where it is ubiquitous.[392,393] NO appears to have a direct stimulatory effect on GnRH neurons as well as an indirect effect mediated by increased neuropeptide Y[392] or by increased GABA.[393] NOS is also present in the gonadotrophs and folliculo-stellate cells of the pituitary where it may turn off the LH response to GnRH.[392] The stimulatory effects of cytokines on CRH secretion may be mediated, in part by NO.[393] Although arginine can stimulate the release of GH and PRL, whether this is due to increased NO production is unclear.[392] There is evidence for a role of NO in a number of other hypothalamic functions as well, including sexual behavior, aggressive behavior, feeding, learning and memory.[393] Because of effects of NO at both the hypothalamic and pituitary levels, it is difficult to identify a primary role for NO in the regulation of pituitary hormone release. Rather, it appears to function as an intermediary neurotransmitter, partially mediating the effects of other stimulating and suppressing substances.

Carbon Monoxide

Carbon monoxide (CO) as a neurotransmitter has been studied for a shorter period of time than has NO and less is known about its functions. CO is formed by the action of heme oxygenase which degrades heme to biliverdin and CO.[392] The isoform heme oxygenase-2 (HO-2) is present in brain and the hypothalamus has one of the highest CO production rates in the brain.[392] HO-2 mRNA is highly expressed in the preoptic area and the mediobasal hypothalamus, but the specific regulators of HO-2 activity are unknown.[392] Like NO, CO activates guanylyl cyclase, resulting in the increased production of cGMP.[392] Studies so far have shown stimulatory effects of CO on GnRH release but both stimulatory and inhibitory effects on CRH production, perhaps due to different experimental paradigms.[392]

THE PINEAL GLAND

Anatomy

The pineal belongs to the family of *circumventricular organs* of the brain that provide a blood-brain barrier–free interface between the brain, the cerebral circulation, and the CSF of the ventricular system; these organs also include the median eminence, the OVLT, the subcommissural organ, the subfornical organ, and the neurohypophysis. Embryologically, the pineal arises as an outgrowth of the roof of the third ventricle and is an epithalamic structure that is attached to the posterior roof of the third ventricle, between the posterior commissure and the dorsal habenular commissure, sitting on top of and between the superior colliculi.[394] It is derived phylogenetically from photoreceptor cells that were photosensitive and could generate electric activity. However, these properties have been lost in mammals.[394] Its arterial supply is via the posterior choroidal arteries, and the venous drainage is via the internal cerebral veins.[394]

After birth, the pineal loses almost all direct neural connections with the brain. Although it has no photoreceptor activity, it still receives photosensory information through a very indirect route (Fig. 6-24). Light perceived by the retinal photoreceptors is transduced to electric impulses which go to the suprachiasmatic nucleus (SCN) via the retinohypothalamic tract, although some of these impulses reach the SCN by way of the primary optic tract via the lateral geniculate bodies.[394] From the SCN, this informa-

FIGURE 6-24. Neural innervation of the mammalian pineal gland. RHT = retinohypothalamic tract; SCN = suprachiasmatic nuclei; MFB = medial forebrain bundle; SCG = superior cervical ganglion. (*Reproduced with permission from Erlich and Apuzzo.*[394])

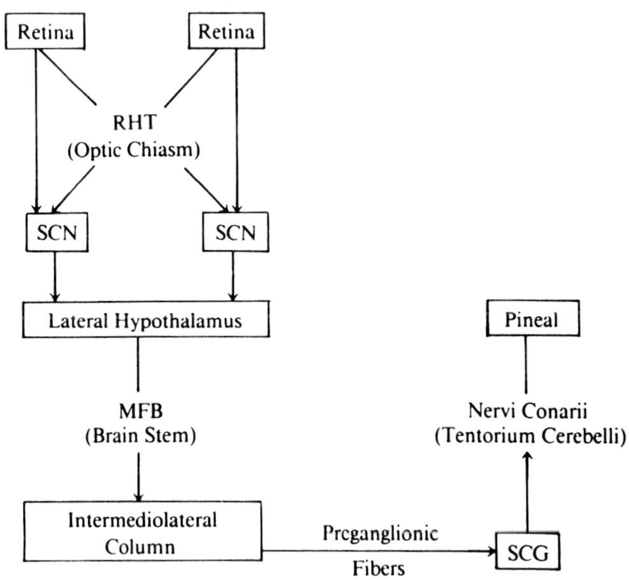

tion travels to the lateral hypothalamus and then down through the brainstem via the median forebrain bundle and through the intermediolateral column of the cervical spinal cord, eventually reaching the superior cervical ganglion. Postganglionic noradrenergic fibers from the superior cervical ganglion enter the pineal via the nerviconarii.[394] An undetermined amount of neural input may also arise from the habenular and posterior commissures and sympathetic pathways.[394]

There are two major cell types within the pineal: the parenchymal cell, or pinealocyte; and interstitial cells, which are probably glial. The sympathetic postganglionic nerve fiber terminals end freely in the parenchyma or in the pericapillary spaces rather than in true synapses, so that norepinephrine reaches the pinealocytes by way of diffusion.[394]

Pineal Hormones and Neurotransmitters

Melatonin is the major secretory product of the pineal. It is synthesized from tryptophan through a series of steps, including serotonin (Fig. 6-25). The enzyme *N*-acetyltransferase, which converts serotonin to *N*-acetylserotonin, is the rate-limiting step.[395] The last step—conversion to melatonin—is mediated by hydroxyindole-*O*-methyltransferase. The absence of light (i.e., darkness), rapidly activates the series of neural steps outlined. The final step is the adrenergic activation of adenylyl cyclase in the membranes of the pinealocytes, which causes an increase in *N*-acetyltransferase activity and melatonin synthesis. Melatonin is not stored but is immediately secreted into the blood and possibly also in the CSF, where it crosses into the blood via the choroid plexus.[394,395] Because of this lack of storage and the rapid activation of synthesis, melatonin levels change twofold to tenfold in blood in synchrony with the dark–light cycle.[395] In humans, increased production of melatonin does not continue throughout the dark cycle but gradually begins to fall over time so that low levels are found by daylight. However, an increase in the duration of the dark period increases the duration of the elevated melatonin levels. The signal that melatonin conveys to other tissues is dependent on both the amplitude and the duration of the melatonin pulse. Furthermore, this signal may change as the dark–light signal changes over days to weeks. In addition, there may be varying sensitivity of organs to melatonin that changes with the dark–light signal.[395]

The receptors for melatonin are of the seven-transmembrane domain G protein-coupled type; binding to the high affinity receptor (ML1) causes an inhibition of adenylyl cyclase and binding to the low affinity receptor (ML2) stimulates phosphoinositide hydrolysis.[396] Melatonin high affinity receptors are located in the suprachiasmatic nucleus, the pars tuberalis of the pituitary, the retina, elsewhere in the brain, the gut, the ovaries, and in blood vessels.[396] Melatonin has also been localized to the retina, the optic nerve, the SCN, and throughout the GI tract. The primary endocrine action of melatonin is antireproductive, although the site of this activity is not certain. Melatonin is able to suppress the LH response to GnRH in pituitary cell cultures, but antigonadotropic effects via modulation of central dopaminergic, serotoninergic, and GABAergic neurotransmission have also been postulated.[395] The exact site of action of melatonin and the importance of melatonin in the human in this regard are not known with certainty.[395] Although increased nocturnal melatonin

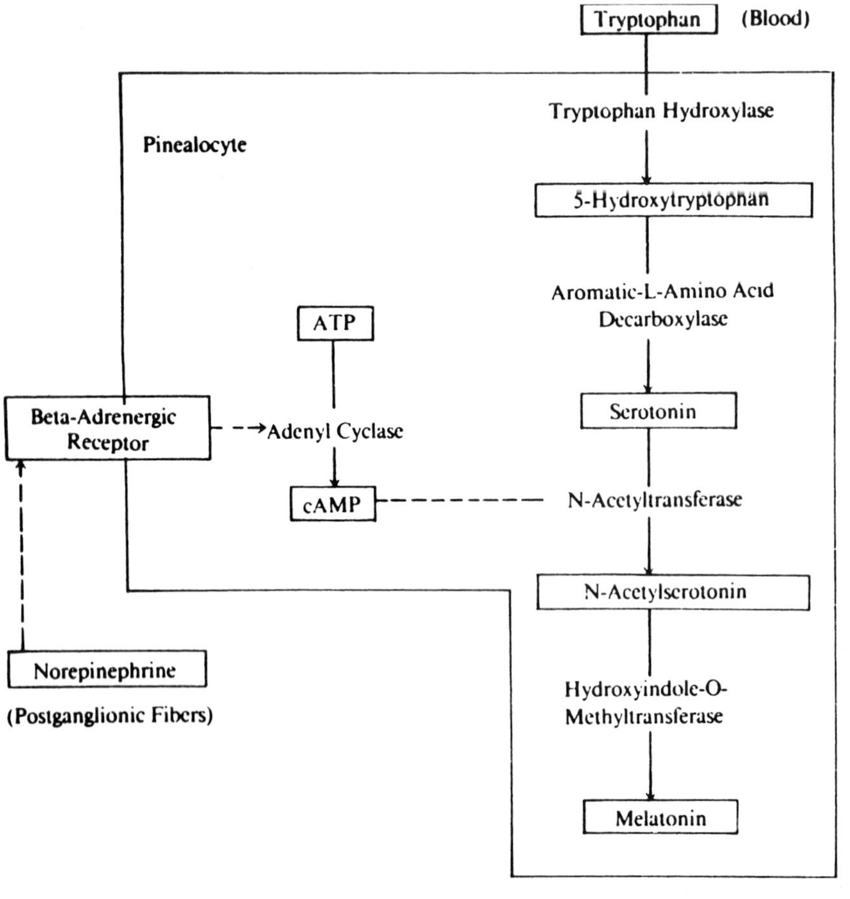

FIGURE 6-25. Stages of melatonin synthesis. ATP = adenosine triphosphate; cAMP = cyclic adenosine 3′,5′-monophosphate. (*Reproduced with permission from Erlich and Apuzzo.*[394])

levels have been observed in patients with hypothalamic amenorrhea, anorexia nervosa, delayed puberty, stress, and excessive exercise and decreased melatonin levels have been found in some patients with depression, schizophrenia, manic-depressive illness, and delayed sleep phase syndrome, the importance of melatonin changes in these disorders has not been established.[395] In addition to possible endocrine effects, melatonin is thought to serve as an antioxidant scavenger of toxic hydroxyl radicals, but this effect likely occurs only at pharmacologic levels.[396]

Other nonmelatonin pineal substances have also been postulated to be of importance in regulating the reproductive axis, including vasotocin, a nonapeptide which differs from vasopressin in that isoleucine is substituted for phenylalanine and differs from oxytocin in that arginine is substituted for leucine. However, none of these other substances have been proved to have more effects on reproduction or other endocrine function than has melatonin.[397] Somatostatin, TRH, and GnRH are also present in the pineal, but there is no evidence for their synthesis there and their functions there are unknown.

Melatonin and the pineal have also been investigated for other neuroendocrine activities. Although melatonin inhibits glucocorticoid secretion at the hypothalamic/pituitary and adrenal levels, GH secretion, and TSH secretion,[397] it is not clear that these actions of melatonin are significant in humans. The effects of melatonin and the pineal on PRL secretion have been quite variable in animal models, although oral melatonin has been shown to cause an increase in PRL levels.[398]

Pineal and Biological Rhythms

The retinal-SCN-pineal link probably serves as the primary mechanism by which light–dark cycles synchronize the reproductive axis on both a short- and a long-term basis.[394] Variations in exposure to light result in variations in the amount, duration, and phase of the daily melatonin signal, which then alters other functions, especially reproduction; on a long-term basis, this can coordinate seasonal breeding cycles.[394,395] In animals, other physiologic changes may also be similarly coordinated, such as changes in body weight and coat color.[394,395] Experimental alteration of the melatonin signal by means of pinealectomy, superior cervical ganglionectomy, or implantation of melatonin constant-release capsules results in a loss of synchronization of reproductive function with the environment. The timing of puberty may also be affected. In animals blinded from birth, there is a delay in the onset of puberty, but in humans, data are conflicting.[399] Generally, the levels of cortisol are normal in blind individuals, but there is loss of diurnal variation with a free-running cortisol rhythm being present.[399] Prepubertal blind boys have been shown to have low FSH and LH levels but individuals blinded during adult life have normal gonadotropin and testosterone levels.[399] However, studies with newer methods of documenting gonadal function, such as gonadotropin pulse analysis, have not been performed.

CNS RHYTHMS AND NEUROENDOCRINE FUNCTION

Pituitary hormones are secreted in a pulsatile fashion, with a number of rhythms superimposed. When samples are obtained every 1 to 5 min, frequent pulses of secretion may be detected using computerized algorithms which discriminate secretory pulses that exceed a threshold related to measurement error.[112] Critical to the interpretation of such pulse analyses are the necessity of sampling frequently enough and the use of a hormone assay with sufficient sensitivity to eliminate "undetectable" samples. As has been demonstrated for GH, conventional assays with a lower limit of sensitivity of about 0.5 ng/ml reveal only 4 to 6 pulses of GH per day, whereas an assay with a sensitivity of 10 pg/ml reveals 12 to 14 pulses of GH per day.[400] With sensitive assays and frequent sampling, most analyses reveal that virtually all the hormone is released with each secretory burst and that almost none is released "tonically" between secretory bursts.[401] The actual sustained level of hormone achieved is dependent on the amplitude of the secretory burst, the frequency of the secretory bursts, and the metabolic clearance rate of the hormone. The pulse amplitude of a pituitary hormone reflects the amount of releasing hormone as well as factors that may alter the cell's responsivity to that releasing hormone. Thus, the amplitude can be altered by the presence of inhibitory factors (e.g., GHRH vs. somatostatin), nutritional factors, feedback effects of target organ hormones, and prior stimulation that might have depleted a readily releasable pool of hormone.[401] The frequency is generally governed by the frequency of release of the hypophysiotropic factor, which is regulated by the hypothalamic pulse generator system (described later).

The pituitary appears to have an intrinsic rhythm of small amplitude with a frequency of 2 to 10 min, as discerned from in vitro studies using a flow-through system.[402] Superimposed on this intrinsic rhythm is the rhythm that is due to the pulsatile release of hypophysiotropic releasing factors, with or without the withdrawal of a corresponding inhibiting factor. For LH, the pulses that are detected every 20 to 25 min have a 1:1 correspondence with GnRH released by the hypothalamus, as determined by simultaneous sampling from portal and peripheral vessels.[114,115] By contrast, the pulses of GH, at least in the rat and probably in the human, are due to an increase in GHRH which often coincides with a decrease in somatostatin.[180,181] Rhythms which are shorter than a day are referred to as *ultradian* rhythms.

The next layer of rhythmicity is the *circadian* rhythm (i.e., rhythms with approximately 24-h periodicity). These rhythms are usually synchronized with the 24-h period by a periodic environmental cue, such as the dark–light cycle. This external cue has been referred to as a *zeitgeber* (time giver). The SCN is the "internal clock" which functions as a circadian pacemaker[33] in most mammals, including humans. Experiments in which the SCN is ablated result in a loss of circadian rhythms.[33] The SCN has extensive projections to and receives projections from multiple hypothalamic nuclei involved in hypophysiotropic hormone production. The SCN will give an approximate 24-h rhythm without the influence of a zeitgeber, but it may vary as much as 3 h from the 24-h periodicity. To maintain a 24-h periodicity, it must synchronize with the zeitgeber. This involves the transmission of light-induced electrical impulses from the retina to the SCN via the retinohypothalamic tract and the transmission of electrical impulses from the SCN to the pineal and then conversion of those impulses into hormonal signals (Fig. 6-24) (see the previous section).

The molecular elements of the circadian clock in the SCN are now in process of being determined. It appears that an autoregulatory program of periodic gene expression is central to generation of the circadian rhythm.[403] In such a program the clock is based on negative feedback loops that involve the rhythmic expression of RNA that encode proteins that act to shut off the genes that encode them.[404] The loops close through transcriptional steps and posttranslational processes (e.g., phosphorylation, nuclear translocation) are responsible for the kinetics of the loop.[404] Specific genes for the circadian clock have been identified in drosophila (the PER gene) and in the mouse (the CLOCK gene and the mPER gene)[405,406] and a similar gene appears to have been identified in the human (the hPER gene).[406,407] As discussed later, all the pituitary hormones have circadian rhythms, but the methods by which increases and decreases in hormone levels occur differ. The circadian increase in all hormone levels is caused by an increase in the amplitude of the secretory pulses; however, for TSH and GH there is also an increase in the frequency of secretory pulses, though this is not true for ACTH, PRL, or LH.[401]

The zeitgeber for a rhythm with a periodicity longer than 24 h (i.e., an *infradian* rhythm), may be the gravitational influence of the moon, which gives rise to a menstrual cycle of approximately the duration of the moon rotating around the earth. Longer-term cycles include responses to seasonal changes such as hibernation and breeding cycles, the timing of the onset of puberty, and perhaps death. Obviously, these rhythms operate differently in different species, and humans may be less tied to these rhythms for some bodily functions than are lower species. Humans have no specific breeding season, for example. However, the menstrual cycle clearly is a monthly rhythm, and the pituitary hormones generally have a well-defined circadian rhythm.

A number of factors may influence circadian and infradian rhythms. One of the most important is the sleep–wake cycle. GH, TSH, PRL, pubertal LH, and ACTH secretion are all entrained more to the sleep–wake cycle than to the dark–light cycle (Fig. 6-26). Each has an increase and a maximal level that occur at specified times after sleep onset. For all but ACTH, shifting the time of onset of sleep immediately shifts the hormone peak. This shift also occurs for ACTH, but not until 5 to 10 days after the shift.[408] Sleep onset itself, however, appears to be synchronized loosely with the light–dark cycle and the release of melatonin. When melatonin is given orally, it advances the time of sleep onset and waking.[396] Obviously, this cue to the internal clock can be overridden voluntarily.

One of the most striking pituitary rhythms is that of ACTH. Levels rise in the early morning hours to peak at about 0700 to 0800 hours, assuming a sleep time from midnight to 0730 hours.[408] Levels then gradually fall over the course of the day and evening, only to begin rising again 2 to 4 h after the onset of sleep.[408] Cortisol levels follow the ACTH levels with minimal lag time. This ACTH-cortisol rhythm persists despite considerable perturbation of the normal endogenous and exogenous environment, including sleep deprivation, fasting, continuous feeding, constant glucose infusion, and constant lighting.[408] The profound diurnal variation of cortisol and ACTH is often used as an index of the "normality" of the system. Loss of this diurnal rhythm occurs with disordered regulation of CRH, which may be due to endogenous depression or excessive alcohol intake, as well as with autonomous secretion of ACTH in Cushing's disease. In fact, this loss of diurnal rhythm of cortisol has been used as a diagnostic test for Cushing's syndrome (see Chap. 7).

TSH secretion is generally low throughout the day but then may double, with the rise occurring at about 2000 hours, substantially before sleep onset. These levels stay elevated through the night and then fall at about 0800 hours.[65,408]

Interesting changes in gonadotropin secretion occur as a child passes through puberty into adulthood. Before puberty, the amplitude of the gonadotropin pulses is low. Early in puberty, the amplitude of the pulses increases during sleep at night, especially for LH, but in adulthood, this nocturnal rise is lost.[409] Testosterone lev-

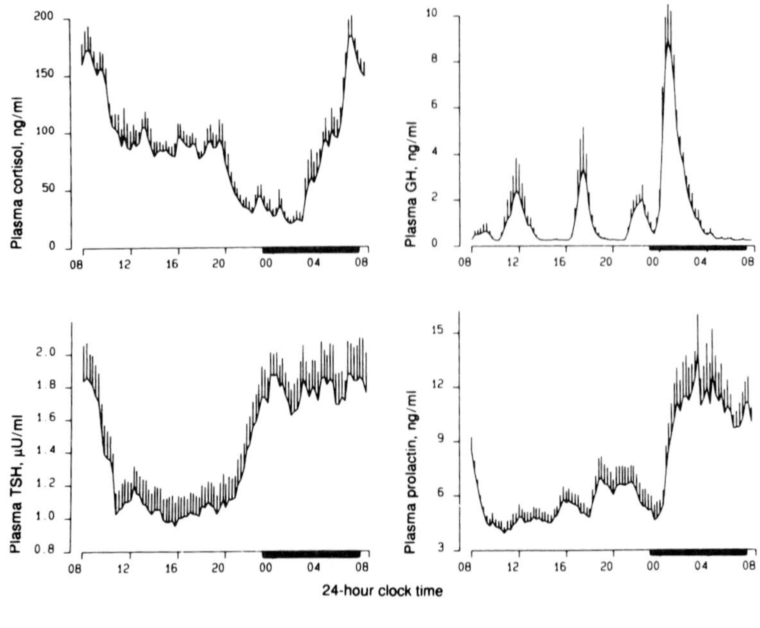

FIGURE 6-26. Mean (± SEM) profiles of plasma levels of ACTH, cortisol, TSH, testosterone, GH, and PRL from a group of 8 to 12 normal men studied at 15-min intervals for 24 h. The sleep times are indicated by black bars. (*Reproduced with permission from Van Cauter.*[408])

els tend to rise at night as well.[408] In patients with anorexia nervosa, the pattern of gonadotropin secretion often reverts to this pubertal pattern, only to deviate from the pattern again with weight gain.[409] This suggests that body composition may in some way affect the regulation of the pulsatile secretion of the gonadotropins. In fact, the percentage of body composition that is fat has been proposed to be important in the timing of the onset of puberty.[410]

Although it once was thought that there are only 2 to 6 secretory episodes of GH per day, more sensitive assays have revealed that there are 12 to 14 episodes per day with a large nighttime surge.[400] The largest nighttime surge occurs shortly after the onset of sleep, in association with the first phase of slow-wave sleep.[408] Most episodes of GH secretion correlate with the onset of periods of slow-wave sleep, but later episodes of slow-wave sleep may not be associated with GH release.[409] Although this synchronization with sleep is very strong for GH, the experimental introduction of a 5-h delay in sleep onset results in a rise in GH during wakefulness within 1 h of the expected bedtime in most shifted nights.[408] This implies a circadian rhythm that is independent of sleep per se. Episodic secretion during sleep occurs even in blind individuals, suggesting that entrainment of GH secretion with the light-dark cycle is not very important.[409]

Prolactin shows a similar pattern to GH in that there is a substantial rise with sleep and 13 to 14 peaks per day.[411] An increase in the amplitude of the PRL secretory pulses begins about 60 to 90 min after the onset of sleep; the secretory pulses increase with non-REM sleep and fall before the next period of REM sleep.[411] When subjects are kept awake to reverse the sleep–wake cycle, PRL levels do not rise until sleep begins.[412] Thus, the diurnal variation of PRL secretion is not an inherent rhythm but depends on the occurrence of sleep. Interestingly, the diurnal variation of PRL with the sleep-induced rise persists despite powerful physiologic influences such as breast-feeding.[413]

Endocrine rhythms appear to reflect a rather primitive organizing influence that helps animals adapt to the environment. The circadian synchronization with the light–dark cycle and sleep and the infradian synchronization with seasonal changes are present very early phylogenetically. Even at the top of the evolutionary scale, in humans, these rhythms are of fundamental importance in the maintenance of normal hormonal function. However, because humans are able to alter the light–dark cycle, they are less tied to environmental changes. This has led to new problems with these rhythms, such as jet lag, which involves the rapid resynchronization of the rhythms with several-hour time-zone displacements and shift-work. Because not all rhythms resynchronize at the same rates, some of the disorientation and other symptoms associated with jet lag and shift work may be due to abnormal phase relations of various body rhythms with each other and with the dark–light cycle. Efforts are now beginning to try to resynchronize these out of phase rhythms by giving melatonin and other melatonin derived compounds.[414]

NEUROENDOCRINE DISEASE

Diseases of the Hypothalamus

Diseases may affect the hypothalamus by being localized to the hypothalamus, by being part of more generalized CNS disease such as neurosarcoidosis, or by indirect means, such as by causing hydrocephalus. Furthermore, hormonal changes may occur in a variety of psychiatric disorders and are mediated by alterations in hypothalamic regulation.

The locations of the neuronal perikarya whose axons project to the median eminence and contain the various hypophysiotropic factors are well established. Most are concentrated in the basal portion of the hypothalamus in the area surrounding the third ventricle, and their axonal pathways all come together in the medial basal hypothalamus as they converge on the median eminence. Thus, lesions within this final common pathway might be expected to cause significant impairment of the hypothalamic regulation of pituitary function for all the pituitary hormones. Other functions of the hypothalamus are more diffuse, such as the regulation of temperature, which occurs in a large region of the preoptic anterior hypothalamus. Hypothalamic dysfunction can be grouped into three major categories: (1) anterior pituitary dysfunction, (2) neurohypophyseal dysfunction, and (3) nonpituitary dysfunction, including disorders of temperature regulation, thirst, eating behavior, sleep, autonomic nervous system regulation, memory, emotional behavior, and cognition.

Symptoms due to hypothalamic dysfunction are related to size of the lesion and, consequently, the area of the hypothalamus involved as well as the rapidity of increase in the size of the lesion. Tumors in this area, such as pituitary adenomas and craniopharyngiomas, can often grow quite large (8 to 10 cm in diameter) over many years with few symptoms. Slowly growing lesions tend to cause problems of hormone dysregulation rather than present with dramatic symptoms. However, a hemorrhage into even a small tumor of 1-cm diameter that causes it to increase rapidly to a 2- to 3-cm diameter can cause major disruption of hypothalamic function, including decreased levels of consciousness, temperature dysregulation, and disturbance of cardiovascular function. Large, slowly growing lesions can cause more acute problems, however, when a slight increment in growth results in the elimination of remaining vestiges of vasopressin or ACTH secretion or completely occludes the aqueduct of Sylvius or the foramen of Monro, causing hydrocephalus. Rarely, such tumors may cause mental dysfunction and symptoms and signs due to increased intracranial pressure, such as nausea, vomiting, headache, and papilledema.

A large number of disorders can affect the hypothalamus. The frequency of these disorders varies with age (Table 6-4). Because anterior pituitary regulation is incompletely developed at birth, certain types of hypothalamic damage that affect pituitary function may not be clinically recognized in the newborn. Magnetic resonance imaging (MRI) with gadolinium enhancement currently represents the best way of discerning lesions that affect the hypothalamus and any consequent distortion of other hypothalamic structures.[415,416] The relation of the hypothalamus, pituitary, and infundibulum (stalk) to routine MRI are shown in Fig. 6-4. Computed tomographic (CT) scanning with intravenous contrast is also quite effective in delineating these lesions. Formal visual field testing may discern an impingement of the optic nerves and chiasm by hypothalamic lesions, including the suprasellar extension of a pituitary tumor. The lack of a visual field defect does not exclude suprasellar disease, however, and very large lesions may be present which can be documented to distort the chiasm on MRI scan but may not cause visual field defects. Detailed testing of hypothalamic-pituitary function (see Chaps. 7 and 8) may reveal evidence of functional hypothalamic disruption with great sensitivity.

Congenital Embryopathic Disorders

The most common embryopathic disorders that affect the hypothalamus are the midline cleft syndromes, which cause varying degrees of defects of midline structures, especially the optic and

TABLE 6-4. Etiology of Hypothalamic Disease

Neonates
Intraventricular hemorrhage
Meningitis: bacterial
Tumors: glioma, hemangioma
Trauma
Hydrocephalus, hydranencephaly, kernicterus
1 month–2 years
Tumors: glioma, especially optic glioma, histiocytosis X, hemangiomas
Hydrocephalus, meningitis
"Familial" disorders: Laurence-Moon, Barder-Biedel, Prader-Labhart-Willi, etc.
2–10 years
Tumors: craniopharyngioma, glioma, dysgerminoma, hamartoma, histiocytosis X, leukemia, ganglioneuroma, ependymoma, medulloblastoma
Meningitis: bacterial, tuberculous
Encephalitis: viral and demyelinating, various viral encephalitides and exanthematous demyelinating encephalitides, disseminated encephalomyelitis
"Familial" disorders: diabetes insipidus, etc.
Damage from nasopharyngeal radiation therapy
10–25 years
Tumors: craniopharyngioma, pituitary tumors, glioma, hamartoma, dysgerminoma, histiocytosis X, leukemia, dermoid, lipoma, neuroblastoma
Trauma
Subarachnoid hemorrhage, vascular aneurysm, arteriovenous malformation
Inflammatory diseases: meningitis, encephalitis, sarcoid, tuberculosis
Associated with midline brain defects: agenesis of corpus callosum
Chronic hydrocephalus or increased intracranial pressure
25–50 years
Nutritional: Wernicke's disease
Tumors: glioma, lymphoma, meningioma, craniopharyngioma, pituitary tumors, angioma, plasmacytoma, colloid cysts, ependymoma, sarcoma, histiocytosis X
Inflammatory: sarcoid, tuberculosis, viral encephalitis
Subarachnoid hemorrhage, vascular aneurysms, arteriovenous malformation
Damage from pituitary radiation therapy
>50 years
Nutritional: Wernicke's disease
Tumors: sarcoma, glioblastoma, lymphoma, meningioma, colloid cysts, ependymoma, pituitary tumors
Vascular: infarct, subarachnoid hemorrhage, pituitary apoplexy
Inflammatory: encephalitis, sarcoid, meningitis

Source: Adapted from Plum and Van Uitert.[25]

olfactory tracts, the septum pellucidum, the corpus callosum, the anterior commissure, the hypothalamus, and the pituitary. The clinical presentation of patients with midline cleft defects varies in severity from cyclopia to cleft lip. Patients with severe lesions such as holoprosencephaly (failure of cleavage of the prosencephalon into two lateral ventricles) have been reported to have defective hypothalamic structures and absent pituitaries.[417] The combination of an absent septum pellucidum and optic nerve hypoplasia is referred to as septo-optic dysplasia; several patients with these findings have been reported with abnormalities of hypothalamic and other diencephalic structures and varying degrees of anterior and posterior pituitary deficiency.[418] Some patients with septo-optic dysplasia and hypothalamic hypopituitarism have sexual precocity, presumably caused by a lack of inhibitory influences from other parts of the hypothalamus on intact GnRH-producing structures.[419]

Mutations responsible for these developmental defects are the subject of active investigation. One possible mutation that has been found is in the *Hesx1* gene (also called *Rpx*, for Rathke's pouch homeobox[420]), which is a member of the paired-like class of homeobox genes expressed in the thickened layer of oral ectoderm which gives rise to Rathke's pouch.[421] Dattani et al. found that targeted mutation of the *Hesx1* gene in mice results in fetal mice with reduction of telencephalic vesicles, eyes, olfactory placodes, and frontonasal mass.[421] Because this mouse syndrome resembled septo-optic dysplasia in humans, Dattani et al. then cloned, mapped, and sequenced the human *Hesx1* gene and found a C → T substitution in one position that resulted in substitution of cysteine for a highly conserved arginine in the homeodomain of *Hesx1* in one kindred in which two siblings (both homozygous for the mutation) had agenesis of the corpus callosum and panhypopituitarism; they did not find the mutation in a number of familial and sporadic cases with a variety of other midline defects.[421] Many other transcription factors have been described that are expressed sequentially during embryogenesis in Rathke's pouch that are important in the ultimate development of the normal pituitary cell lineages.[43] Mutations have been found in two other homeobox transcription factor genes, *Pit-1*, which causes hypoplasia of somatotrophs, lactotrophs, and thyrotrophs,[422,423] and *Prop-1*, which causes hypoplasia of these same cell populations and, in addition, gonadotropes[424–426] (see also Chap. 7). Combined pituitary hormone deficiency has an incidence of about 1 in 8000 births and about 10 percent have an affected relative; it appears that more than half of these are due to *Pit-1* or *Prop-1* deficiencies.[426]

Children with very mild midline cleft defects consisting of just a cleft lip or palate or both have been found to have a markedly increased risk of having GH and other pituitary hormone deficiencies.[427] Recent evaluations of children with "idiopathic" growth hormone deficiency with MR scanning show that in about 50 percent the neurohypophysis (which shows as a bright spot) is adjacent to the median eminence, the pituitary volume is decreased, and there is an absence of the infundibulum (Fig. 6-27). Most of those with an absent infundibulum also have other pituitary hormone deficiencies.[428,429] It is possible that this group of patients has a very mild variant of the midline cleft syndrome.[428,429]

Congenital defects in the base of the skull that result in herniation of the pituitary and stalk through the floor of the sella (basal encephalocele) can also cause hypopituitarism and diabetes insipidus.[430] In these cases, such dysfunction could be due to the distortion of the normal hypothalamic-pituitary structures rather than to primary abnormalities of the hypothalamus.[430] However, some of these patients also have evidence of other midline facial defects (cleft lip and palate) and optic nerve abnormalities,[430] so these dysfunctions may also be considered to be variants of the midline cleft syndrome.

Kallmann's syndrome is a condition characterized by anosmia or hyposmia and hypogonadotropic hypogonadism (see Chap. 15). Studies in familial cases show several types of inheritance, including x-linked, autosomal recessive, and autosomal dominant, suggesting genetic heterogeneity.[100,431] The x-linked form is now known to be due to gene (*KAL*) mutations that result in a defective

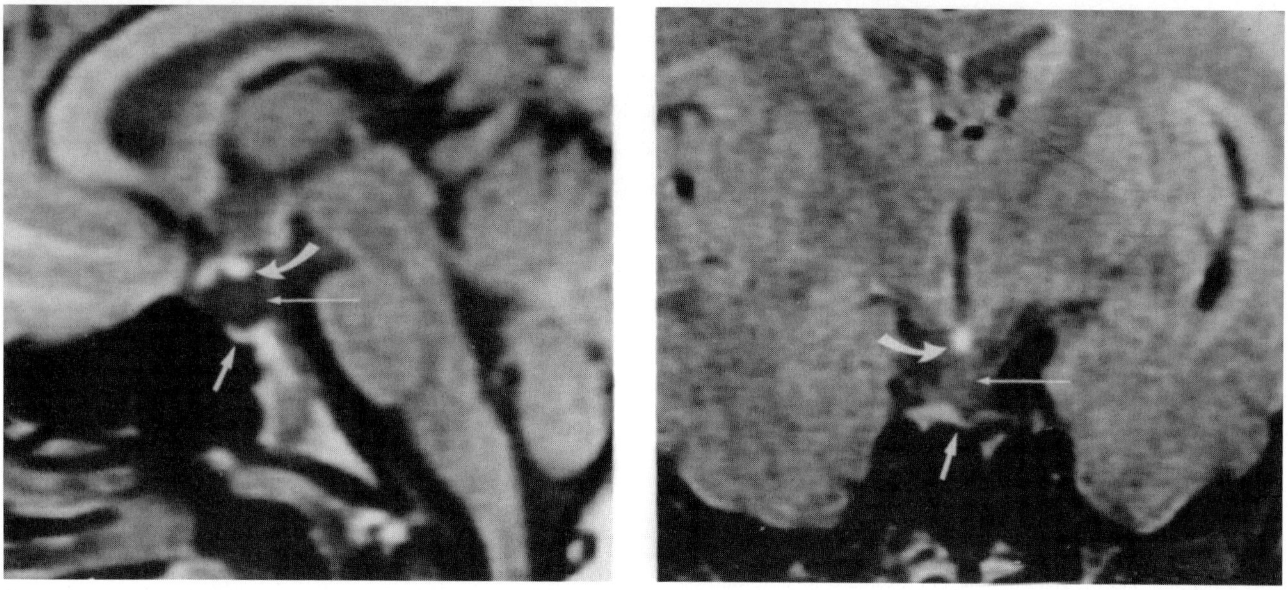

A B

FIGURE 6-27. Small anterior pituitary gland associated with an ectopic neurohypophysis in a patient with idiopathic growth hormone deficiency. (*A* and *B*) Sagittal (*A*) and coronal (*B*) MR images show the absence of the infundibulum (long arrow) and an area of bright signal in the median eminence (curved arrow) which is the ectopic neurohypophysis. (*Reproduced with permission from Abrahams et al.*[428])

protein (*anosmin*) normally responsible for facilitating the migration of the GnRH and olfactory neurons from the olfactory placode to their final positions during embryogenesis.[99,100,431] Anosmin has properties of serine protease inhibitors that modulate axonal growth, pathfinding, and target recognition as well as those of cell adhesion proteins that facilitate axonal extension.[432] MR scanning reveals partial to complete absence of the olfactory sulci.[431] The pituitary is usually intact, and treatment with pulsatile GnRH therapy or gonadotropins results in spermatogenesis and normal gonadal function.[100,106,431] In some patients, other neurologic abnormalities may be present, including cerebellar ataxia, nerve deafness, color blindness, cleft lip and palate, and mental retardation.[433] Furthermore, in a series of seven subjects with Kallmann's syndrome, three had abnormalities of thirst, one had a decreased osmotic threshold for vasopressin release, and one had an increased osmotic threshold for vasopressin release.[434] Whether these additional defects represent defects in anosmin-mediated neuronal migration or other developmental defects is unknown at present.

Tumors

The most common tumors affecting the hypothalamus are pituitary adenomas that have a significant suprasellar extension. These tumors can cause varying degrees of hypopituitarism by compressing the normal pituitary or, more commonly, by affecting the pituitary stalk and mediobasal hypothalamus; diabetes insipidus is rare.[435,436] Hyperprolactinemia occurs in about half of these tumors, caused primarily by disinhibition by the hypothalamus, with decreased dopamine reaching the pituitary.[436,437] Evidence that hypopituitarism results from pituitary compression includes a low serum PRL level and a lack of TSH response to TRH; pituitary function in such cases usually does not improve after treatment.[435] In patients with normal or elevated PRL levels, pituitary function often returns after therapy.[435] Specific treatments for the different types of pituitary tumors are discussed in Chap. 7.

Craniopharyngiomas are the next most common tumors that affect the hypothalamus. Microscopically, craniopharyngiomas consist of cysts alternating with stratified squamous epithelium. The cyst fluid is usually thick and dark, and the material is often calcified. It is thought that the craniopharyngiomas arise from remnants of Rathke's pouch. A variant or closely related lesion is the Rathke's cleft cyst, which develops from the space between the anterior and rudimentary intermediate lobes. Rathke's cleft cysts are lined with cuboidal as opposed to squamous epithelium, and the cyst fluid is usually a white mucoid fluid.[438] Clinically, the distinction is often impossible, although craniopharyngiomas are more commonly found in a suprasellar location while Rathke's cleft cysts are usually intrasellar but may have suprasellar extension; both may recur.[438–441] However, craniopharyngiomas sometimes recur postoperatively, while Rathke's cleft cysts uncommonly recur.[438,440] Craniopharyngiomas most commonly present during childhood but also occur in adults and even in the elderly.[440] These tumors present because of mass effects, including headache, vomiting, visual disturbance, seizures, hypopituitarism, and polyuria. Careful endocrine testing reveals varying degrees of hypopituitarism in 50 to 75 percent and modest hyperprolactinemia in 25 to 50 percent.[437–439,442] Some patients present with galactorrhea, amenorrhea, and hyperprolactinemia, suggestive of a prolactinoma.[443] Surgical extirpation of craniopharyngiomas commonly causes a worsening of pituitary function, often resulting in complete panhypopituitarism and diabetes insipidus because of stalk section.[440,444] Irradiation of craniopharyngiomas may be helpful and recently, focused "gamma knife" radiotherapy has been found to be particularly beneficial.[445]

Suprasellar dysgerminomas are said to arise from primitive germ cells that have migrated to the CNS during fetal life and structurally are identical to germ cell tumors of the gonads.[446,447] They usually present in children, in whom they most commonly cause decreased growth because of hypopituitarism, diabetes insipidus, and visual problems.[447] Hyperprolactinemia occurs in >50 percent, and 10 percent have precocious puberty caused by the production of hCG by the tumor.[447] As opposed to craniopharyngiomas, these tumors are very radiosensitive, and radiotherapy is the preferred treatment.[448]

Other tumors and space-occupying lesions that occur in the suprasellar area include arachnoid cysts, meningiomas, gliomas, astrocytomas, chordomas, infundibulomas, cholesteatomas, neurofibromas, lipomas, and metastatic cancer (particularly of the breast and lung).[441] These lesions may present with varying degrees of hypopituitarism, diabetes insipidus, and hyperprolactinemia; surgical therapy often worsens the hormonal deficit.

Hamartomas

A hypothalamic hamartoma is a nodule of growth of hypothalamic neurons attached by a pedicle to the hypothalamus between the tuber cinereum and the mammillary bodies and extending into the basal cistern. Asymptomatic hamartomas may be present in up to 20 percent of random autopsies.[449] Rarely, these lesions may enlarge, causing disruption of hypothalamic function because of compression of adjacent tissue. A variant of the hamartoma consisting of similar tissue present within the anterior pituitary but without a neural attachment to the hypothalamus is called a choristoma or gangliocytoma.[450] These neuronal tumors are of particular endocrine interest because they can produce hypophysiotropic hormones.

A number of cases associated with precocious puberty in which hamartomas produce GnRH have been reported. Electron microscopy with immunohistochemistry reveals GnRH to be present in secretory granules in the nerve endings.[451] Within the abnormal tissue, the neurons surround blood vessels which have a fenestrated capillary endothelium, enabling the released GnRH to enter the blood vessels and eventually be transported to the pituitary by vessels of the tuber cinereum.[451] The fact that these lesions cause precocious puberty suggests that the regulation of GnRH and gonadotropins is not normal, and several studies have recorded failure of appropriate negative feedback suppression of gonadotropins or stimulation with clomiphene.[451] Successful treatment has been reported with surgery[452] and with the administration of a long-acting GnRH analog which suppresses gonadotropin secretion but does not affect the tumor.[452,453] Medical therapy with a GnRH analog appears to be the best choice, if the hamartoma does not cause other problems from mass effects as surgery can be noncurative or even fatal.[452,453]

Some gangliocytomas have been reported which produce GHRH and acromegaly.[450] In some of these tumors, there is direct contact between the gangliocytoma GHRH-containing neuronal cells and pituitary GH-secreting cells, suggesting a paracrine effect.[450] Similarly, patients with Cushing's disease due to intrasellar gangliocytomas producing CRH and causing corticotrope cell hyperplasia have been reported.[450]

Inflammatory Disorders

Sarcoidosis

CNS involvement in sarcoidosis occurs in 1 to 5 percent of patients as determined on clinical grounds and in up to 16 percent of cases at autopsy.[454] Isolated CNS sarcoidosis is quite uncommon, however.[454] When sarcoidosis does involve the CNS, the hypothalamus is involved in 10 to 20 percent of cases.[454] Sarcoid granulomas can involve the hypothalamus, stalk, or pituitary[455] and may be infiltrative or present as a mass lesion.[456] The most common endocrine findings are varying degrees of hypopituitarism, diabetes insipidus, and hyperprolactinemia.[454,457] Obesity due to hypothalamic involvement by sarcoidosis has also been reported.[458] In patients with isolated CNS sarcoidosis, the diagnosis may be extremely difficult. Examination of the CSF usually shows elevated protein levels, low glucose levels, and a pleiocytosis. Biopsy is often necessary. Although corticosteroid therapy has been reported to reverse the thirst disorders at least partially, anterior pituitary hormone deficits usually do not respond to this therapy.[455,457]

Langerhans-Cell Histiocytosis (Histiocytosis X)

Langerhans-cell histiocytosis (histiocytosis X or eosinophilic granuloma) is a clonal neoplastic disorder[459] that may infiltrate the hypothalamus and pituitary stalk, causing diabetes insipidus, varying degrees of hypopituitarism, and hyperprolactinemia.[460] This infiltration usually appears on CT or MRI as a thickened stalk[461] (Fig. 6-28) but can rarely present as a mass in the hypothalamus or pituitary.[462] Osteolytic lesions may be present in the jaw or mastoid, and x-rays of the jaw are a worthwhile part of the diagnostic evaluation of an unknown suprasellar mass or diabetes insipidus for this reason. Therapy consists of local surgery, focal irradiation, or chemotherapy with alkylating agents and high-dose corticosteroids.

Other Inflammatory Lesions

A number of other inflammatory lesions can rarely cause hypothalamic dysfunction, including abscesses,[441,463] viral meningoencephalitis,[464] and tuberculous meningitis.[465] Chronic inflammation of the parasellar areas, including the cavernous sinus, may extend to the sella and suprasellar areas causing hypopituitarism.[466] One variety of these chronic inflammatory disorders of uncertain etiology, termed lymphocytic infundibulohypophysitis is associated with lymphocytic infiltration of the infundibulum and neurohypophysis, causing a thickened stalk on MRI and diabetes insipidus clinically with sparing of anterior pituitary function.[467]

Vascular Disease

Enlarging aneurysms may present as a mass lesion of the hypothalamic-pituitary area and may cause hypopituitarism and visual field defects.[441] Obviously, the distinction must be made before surgery. Tumors and aneurysms may also coexist, and careful radiologic evaluation with MRI is necessary to discern this. Hypothalamic disease due to vascular infarction is extremely rare.

Trauma

Head trauma can cause defects ranging from isolated ACTH deficiency to panhypopituitarism with diabetes insipidus.[468] Within the first 72 h of trauma, GH, LH, ACTH, TSH, and PRL levels may be elevated in blood, perhaps as a result of an acute release.[469] With more prolonged observation, these levels fall and patients either return to normal or develop hypopituitarism, except for a persistent PRL elevation in many cases.[468] These patients may or may not have associated loss of consciousness, but other neurologic abnormalities are common, such as blindness and cranial nerve palsies.[468] In patients dying of head injury, anterior pituitary infarction has been found in 16 percent of cases, posterior pituitary hemorrhages in 34 percent, and hypothalamic hemorrhages or infarction in 42 percent.[470] The paraventricular and supraoptic nuclei and median eminence are particularly in-

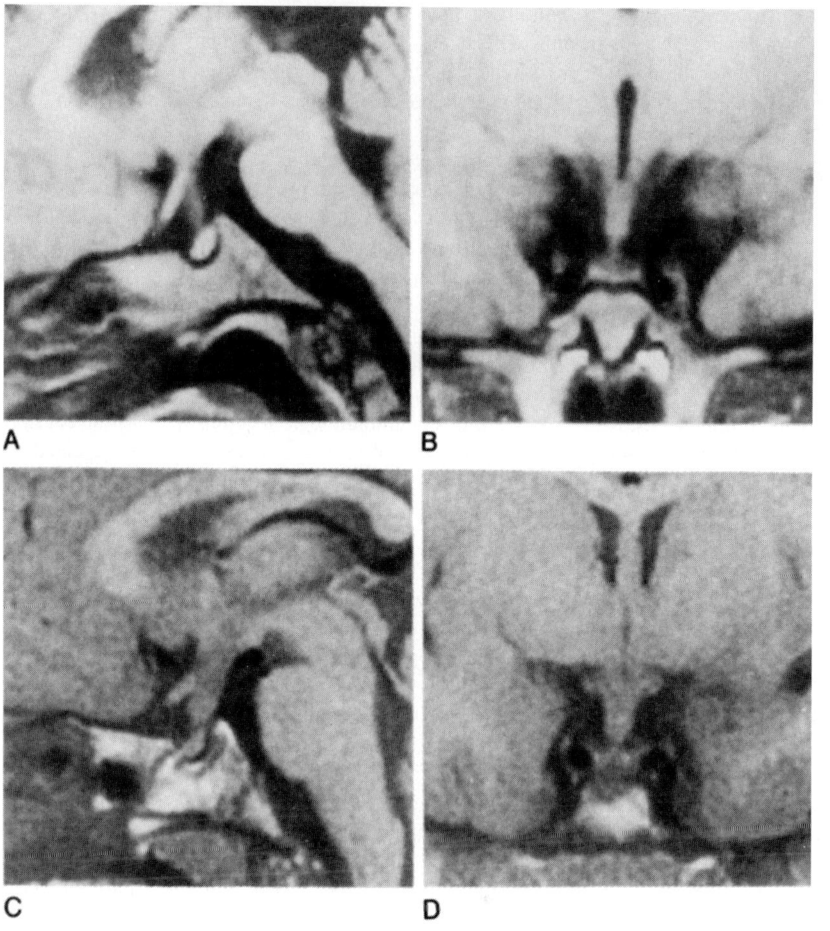

FIGURE 6-28. MR scan in a patient with diabetes insipidus due to hypothalamic infiltration with histiocytosis X. (*A* and *B*) Sagittal (*A*) and coronal (*B*) T_1-weighted images show a symmetric, slightly thickened pituitary stalk and the absence of normal high signal intensity in the posterior pituitary lobe. (*C* and *D*) Sagittal (*C*) and coronal (*D*) T_1-weighted images two years later reveal a more markedly thickened pituitary stalk and the absence of high signal intensity in the posterior pituitary lobe. (*Reproduced with permission from Tien et al.*[461])

volved with microhemorrhages, resulting in a high frequency of panhypopituitarism with diabetes insipidus.[470] With frontal injuries, the brain travels backward but the pituitary cannot move, and so the pituitary stalk becomes avulsed, with interruption of the portal vessels.[468] Most patients with head injury are hyperprolactinemic, confirming clinically that the hypothalamus and/or stalk is the primary site of injury.[468]

Irradiation

Whole-brain irradiation for intracranial neoplasms commonly results in hypothalamic dysfunction with varying degrees of hypopituitarism. In one large series, 28 percent of patients so irradiated had selective loss of thyroid, gonadal, or adrenal function or hyperprolactinemia; 25 percent had abnormalities in two axes, 25 percent had abnormalities in three axes, and 12 percent had abnormalities in all four axes.[471] When radiotherapy is targeted to the hypothalamic area, hypopituitarism occurs even more frequently. Thus, in patients receiving radiotherapy for nasopharyngeal carcinoma, impairment of pituitary function is common and progressive; 19 percent of these patients become hypopituitary within 2 years, and 100 percent have hyperprolactinemia.[472] When radiotherapy is targeted to the pituitary, by 10 years clinically significant losses of function are quite high: 50–75 percent for gonadotropins and ACTH, and 30–50 percent for TSH.[473–476] These frequencies of loss of pituitary function are so high that all patients who have had their pituitary and hypothalamic areas irradiated must be followed closely to detect these deficits when they occur.

Polyostotic Fibrous Dysplasia (McCune-Albright Syndrome)

A number of endocrine disorders have been associated with polyostotic fibrous dysplasia, the most common being precocious puberty and acromegaly associated with hyperprolactinemia.[477,478] In these cases, pituitary histology has shown mammosomatotrope cell hyperplasia or a normal pituitary.[478] A few other patients have had goiters, and one has had Cushing's syndrome due to bilateral micronodular hyperplasia.[479] Recent studies have demonstrated an activating missense mutation of the gene for the α subunit of the guanine nucleotide binding G protein that stimulates cAMP formation in the endocrine and other tissues of these patients.[480] The mutation results in a substitution of Arg^{201} with either Cys or His, thereby inhibiting the GTPase activity of $Gs\alpha$ and leads to the inappropriate stimulation of adenylyl cyclase.[480] This is the same activating mutation found in about 40 percent of GH-producing adenomas that are found in patients with acromegaly[481] (see Chap. 7).

Effects of Hypothalamic Disease on Pituitary Function

Hypothalamic disease can cause pituitary hyperfunction and hypofunction in varying degrees of severity. Although severe disease can cause absolute deficiencies of the various hormones, milder disease may cause a subtle alteration of feedback loops and timing such that, for example, the integration of signals necessary for menstrual cycling is lost, resulting in "hypothalamic" amenorrhea. Furthermore, the hypothalamic defects may be interrelated, so that the rather common finding of hyperprolactinemia occurring with hypothalamic dysfunction causes a hypogonadotropic hypogonadism that is reversible when the elevated PRL levels are brought down to normal. Detailed testing of hypothalamic-pituitary function now can detect such hormonal abnormalities with greater sensitivity and precision and at earlier points in the course of disease compared with early descriptions of hypothalamic disease, which were limited to detecting precocious puberty, hypogonadism, and diabetes insipidus. Whenever hypothalamic lesions are suspected, detailed evaluation of hypothalamic-pituitary function is indicated. Often, however, dynamic testing of pituitary function will not differentiate between the hypothalamus and the pituitary as the specific primary locus of the defect, and neuroradiologic imaging with MRI or CT is almost always necessary.[415,416]

Growth Hormone

Growth Hormone Deficiency

Loss of normal GH secretion is reported as the most common hormonal defect that occurs with structural hypothalamic disease.[435,442,447,468] However, hypogonadotropic hypogonadism follows closely behind, so that most subjects with hypothalamic disease who are found to be GH-deficient also have deficient levels of sex steroid hormones. An adequate level of sex steroids is necessary for a normal GH response, at least in children,[482] and sex hormone replacement was not performed in these series before GH testing, so that the prevalence of GH deficiency may have been overestimated. Furthermore, because only about 60 to 80 percent of normal individuals have an adequate GH response to most traditional stimuli of GH secretion and as multiple stimulation tests were not performed in these series, the frequency of GH deficiency may have been overestimated for this reason also. Therefore, it is not known whether GH deficiency is truly the most common hormone deficiency in patients with hypothalamic disease.

As was discussed previously, patients with obvious as well as subtle midline cleft defects often have GH deficiency. Among children with no obvious structural disease (i.e., patients thought to have idiopathic growth hormone deficiency (IGHD)), recent studies using MR scanning have found that about 50 percent have an absent infundibulum with a small to normal anterior pituitary and a posterior pituitary adjacent to the median eminence[428,429] (Fig. 6-22). Such patients often have abnormalities of other pituitary hormone function[428,429] as well and should be regarded as having congenital structural defects rather than IGHD. The remaining patients with IGHD studied with MRI had normal infundibula, small to normal anterior pituitaries, and normal posterior pituitaries.[428,429]

It is likely that IGHD is a heterogeneous disorder that consists of hypothalamic and pituitary defects. Between 3 and 30 percent of IGHD patients have an affected relative, and thus their defect is thought to have a genetic basis.[483] The familial forms of IGHD have subgrouped into autosomal recessive types (Type IA due to gene deletions, frame-shift and nonsense mutations, Type IB due to splice site mutations), autosomal dominant types (Type II due to splice site mutations) and X-lined forms (Type III), which are discussed further in Chap. 7.[483] When congenital GH loss is found to be combined with loss of TSH and PRL, mutations in the Pit-1 and Prop-1 transcription factors should be suspected (as previously discussed).

A preliminary RFLP linkage analysis of the GHRH gene in children with IGHD has not revealed any abnormalities.[484] However, an inactivating mutation in the GHRH receptor causing dwarfism has recently been described.[485]

The etiology of the GH deficiency in nongenetic cases of IGHD is not known, but it is thought in most cases to be due to disordered hypothalamic regulation, such as a neurotransmitter abnormality. In many children with IGHD, stimulation with GHRH results in varying GH responses, implying that their pituitaries are capable of producing GH and responding to GHRH, and in some of these patients repeated injections of GHRH can cause greater increases.[266] The initial GH response to a single dose of GHRH and the later response to repetitive doses of GHRH occur primarily in children with documented hypothalamic lesions as the cause of their GH deficiency. However, a prolonged course of repeated injections of GHRH in such children can restore a normal growth pattern in only some cases.[267] Stimulation of GH secretion by dopamine agonists such as bromocriptine has been found to result in normal growth in some patients, implying a possible underlying defect in dopaminergic neurotransmission.[486] Similarly, some studies[487] but not others[488] have found that clonidine, an α-adrenergic agonist, can stimulate normal growth in some children, implying a defect in noradrenergic neurotransmission. Interestingly, almost half of adults diagnosed as GH deficient in childhood and treated with GH are found to have normal GH responses to various stimuli when retested as adults[489]; whether this is due to unreliability of diagnostic tests used during childhood or the presence of a reversible, functional defect of GH secretion remains unknown.

Children with IGHD begin to manifest decreased growth after the first year of life. Prompt treatment with human GH injections usually results in close to normal growth (see Chap. 25). GH deficiency acquired during adult life from hypothalamic tumors, irradiation, etc. has been associated with a loss of lean body mass, an increase in fat mass, osteopenia, and variable, nonspecific symptoms of loss of energy and fatigue.[490] Treatment of adult GH deficiency with daily GH injections has been approved by the U.S. Food and Drug Administration (FDA) and can result in improved lean body and fat mass and bone mineral density, but the improvement in exercise capacity and muscle strength is limited[490] (see Chap. 7).

Growth Hormone Excess

GH excess results in gigantism if it occurs before puberty and in acromegaly if it occurs after epiphyseal closure. As was discussed earlier, these conditions may develop from a specific lesion, a GHRH-producing gangliocytoma.[450] The role of the hypothalamus in the etiology of the usual pituitary GH-secreting adenoma is discussed fully in Chap. 7. Depending on the interpretation of the data, conclusions can be reached on both sides of this issue.[491]

Gonadotropins

Hypothalamic Hypogonadism

The primary defect in this group of disorders is thought to involve the secretion of GnRH, with resultant impairment in pituitary gonadotropin secretion and gonadal function. The disorders causing these conditions may be primary (congenital defects) or acquired. Depending on the time of onset, they present either as delayed puberty, interruption of pubertal progression, or loss of adult gonadal function. The lesions causing these disorders may cause a loss of other hormones or may be isolated to GnRH. Loss of gonadotropin secretion as a result of hypothalamic structural damage is the second most common defect after GH deficiency.[435,442,447,468] However, a substantial number of these defects are due to hyperprolactinemia and are reversible with correction of the hyperprolactinemia. Thus, estimates of hypogonadotropic hypogonadism may be excessive.

Prepubertal

Lesions presenting prepubertally result in failure of the onset of puberty or incomplete progression of puberty if the defect is partial. If the disorder is limited to GnRH and the gonadotropins, prior growth and development will be normal. However, the growth spurt occurring at puberty will be lost.

The most common congenital lesion causing prepubertal GnRH deficiency is Kallmann's syndrome, which is seen in about 50 percent of males and females who present with isolated gonadotropin deficiency.[492,493] In Kallmann's syndrome, there is hyposmia or anosmia due to hypoplasia of the olfactory bulb along with absent GnRH secretion, as previously described. Most patients with idiopathic hypogonadotropic hypogonadism have normal GnRH genes[100] but some have the KAL gene mutation that causes Kallmann's syndrome, but without olfactory defects. Undescended testes and microphallus occurs in a small proportion of cases with GnRH deficiency, but up to 30 percent of cases of microphallus in neonates can be due to GnRH deficiency due to absence of gonadotropins during fetal development.[100,492] In some patients, GnRH pulsatile secretion is markedly impaired but sufficient to stimulate sufficient Leydig cell production of testosterone to support spermatogenesis yet insufficient to virilize the patient, a phenotype formerly known as the "fertile eunuch" syndrome.[100] Some patients may progress partially through puberty but then have a permanent arrest of sexual development and are found to have apulsatile GnRH activity (described later).[100] As some family members with this last phenotype have delayed puberty, it is possible that delayed puberty itself may represent the mildest form of GnRH deficiency.[100] Among women with primary amenorrhea due to GnRH deficiency, about one-third have an associated anosmia and, therefore, have Kallmann's syndrome.[100]

Although the GnRH gene itself is normal in most patients with idiopathic GnRH deficiency,[494] indirect measures of functional GnRH secretion have shown that it is not secreted normally. Detailed study of LH pulsatile secretion in such patients shows that more than 90 percent have no detectable LH pulsations, some have episodic LH secretion only during sleep (similar to that described for pubertal subjects),[409] some have normal pulse frequency but decreased amplitude, and some have normal pulse amplitude but decreased frequency.[100,495] These patterns are consistent within families with more than one affected sibling.[100,495] Stimulation with a single dose of GnRH causes a minimal rise in gonadotropins in individuals with absolutely no pubertal development but a normal rise in those with some pubertal development, presumably reflecting prior GnRH exposure.[100,495]

The ideal therapy for patients with GnRH deficiency consists of the replacement of GnRH. In males, the subcutaneous administration of 25 to 200 ng/kg of GnRH every 2 h with a portable pump causes a rapid rise in the LH and FSH responses to the GnRH, a rise in testosterone to normal, and the development of normal spermatogenesis.[495] Similar studies in women have revealed ovulatory cycles in 80 percent.[495] In men, comparable results can be obtained with exogenous gonadotropins given three times per week.[496] However, replacement with testosterone alone does not result in an increase in testicular size or in spermatogenesis.

In addition to defects in GnRH secretion, mutations in the GnRH receptor can also cause hypogonadotropic hypogonadism. In two of 46 patients with idiopathic hypogonadotropic hypogonadism screened, missense mutations were found that resulted in decreased receptor expression but minimal effects on receptor affinity.[497] Hypogonadism due to mutations in the beta subunits of LH[498] and FSH[499,500] have also been described, as have mutations in the receptors for these hormones.[501] Treatment could consist of gonadotropins and/or steroid hormone replacement in the former but only steroid hormone replacement in the latter. Activating mutations of the LH receptor can cause gonadotropin independent precocious puberty in males.[501]

Hyperprolactinemia can cause a decrease in GnRH secretion and gonadotropin pulsatile secretion.[137,138] When it occurs before puberty, it can prevent the onset of puberty, and it must always be looked for in this setting.

Postpubertal

Loss of formerly normal GnRH secretion may be due to structural hypothalamic damage such as a tumor, a functional change unassociated with a detectable lesion, or hyperprolactinemia. Structural disease must be excluded in such patients by means of CT or MR scanning.

Most but not all cases of functional hypogonadotropic hypogonadism occur in women, with the most common causes being weight loss, excessive exercise, and psychogenic stress.[410,502,503] In some cases, exercise results in a loss of body fat not detected with total body weight measures, and it is unclear whether the hypogonadism is directly due to the loss of body fat or to the exercise per se.[410,503] Changes in levels of leptin may be involved. Studies of pulsatile gonadotropin secretion in such patients reveal absent pulses.[495] Usually there is a normal gonadotropin response to injected GnRH. Regain of weight and cessation of the exercise result in a resumption of normal gonadal function.[410,502,503] The neurotransmitter mediation of this functional state is not known with certainty, although responses to naloxone and dopamine antagonists suggest that excessive opioid peptidergic and dopaminergic tone may be involved.[504] An irreversible form of adult onset idiopathic GnRH deficiency has also been described in men.[505] Such men have a history of normal puberty and sexual maturation who subsequently present with loss of libido, infertility, and impotence with no known contributing factors and with normal olfaction. Frequent LH sampling in these men showed that they had apulsatile secretion with low serum testosterone levels and a restoration of the gonadal function with pulsatile GnRH replacement.[505]

As was indicated earlier, hyperprolactinemia can decrease GnRH and the pulsatile secretion of LH and FSH.[137,138] Because gonadotropin responses to GnRH are normal in hyperprolactinemia, it appears that elevated PRL levels act at the hypothalamic level.[506] Hyperprolactinemia also inhibits positive estrogen feedback.[507] Whether these are direct effects of the elevated PRL levels or are mediated via a PRL-induced increase in central dopaminergic tone via short-loop feedback is unknown. This inhibitory effect of PRL on GnRH secretion occurs in both sexes.

Therapy should be directed at the underlying process, if possible. Efforts at weight gain and restriction of exercise should be made when appropriate. In patients with idiopathic functional hypogonadotropic amenorrhea, there are two goals, restoration of normal estrogen status to promote well-being and prevent osteoporosis, and facilitation of ovulation to achieve fertility. The former can generally be achieved with cyclic estrogen and progesterone, while the latter may require clomiphene, GnRH, or gonadotropin therapy. Men with idiopathic, acquired hypogonadotropic hypogonadism respond well to GnRH.[505]

Hypothalamic Hypergonadism (Precocious Puberty)

Precocious puberty is defined as the onset of puberty before age 8 in girls and age 9 in boys.[508] "True" precocious puberty is due to central causes with increased gonadotropins. "Pseudo" precocious puberty is due to peripheral (gonadal or adrenal) causes (see Chap. 25). Central "true" or GnRH-dependent precocious puberty is characterized by hormonal changes similar to those which occur at the time of normal puberty: an increase in the pulsatile release of LH, an increase in the gonadotropin response to GnRH, and an increase in gonadal steroid secretion.[508] Conceptually, the normal prepubertal childhood condition can be viewed as a "restraint" of the GnRH pulse generator, and puberty can be viewed as a lifting of that restraint so that GnRH secretion increases, with a resultant increase in gonadotropin secretion. GnRH-dependent precocious puberty therefore represents a premature activation of this GnRH pulse generator by a variety of lesions; it may also be idiopathic.

Less than one-quarter of cases of central precocious puberty occur in boys, but boys tend to have more serious underlying disease. In boys with central GnRH-dependent precocious puberty, hypothalamic hamartomas account for 38 percent of cases, other CNS lesions represent 31 percent, familial disease accounts for 23 percent, and idiopathic disease accounts for only 8 percent.[509] The picture is quite different in girls, however, as hypothalamic hamartomas account for only 15 percent of cases, other CNS lesions represent 14 percent, the McCune-Albright syndrome (polyostotic fibrous dysplasia) accounts for 6 percent, and fully 65 percent are idiopathic.[509] CNS lesions other than GnRH-secreting hamartomas that have been reported to trigger precocious puberty include neurofibromatosis, astrocytomas, gliomas, arachnoid cysts, hydrocephalus, neuroblastomas, head trauma, subdural hematomas, and cranial irradiation.[509,510] Dysgerminomas in the suprasellar or pineal region can produce hCG, which acts like LH in stimulating gonadal function.[447] Such tumors usually cause increased sex steroid formation but fail to cause ovulation.

Therapy for central GnRH-dependent precocious puberty consists of surgical removal of the tumor or medical therapy with a long-acting GnRH analog. The latter can suppress gonadotropin and sex steroid hormone levels and cause a stabilization or even regression of secondary sex characteristics and a slowing of growth and bone maturation in most cases with the exception of the McCune-Albright syndrome.[509,510] When therapy is discontinued at the normal time of puberty, sex steroid levels increase, secondary sexual characteristics again develop, growth increases, and regular menses develop spontaneously.[510] Thus, GnRH analogs have turned out to be an ideal therapy in that they can turn off abnormal precocious puberty for years and then allow puberty to resume at the normal time when they are discontinued. For patients who do not respond to the GnRH analogs, treatment with medroxyprogesterone acetate, testolactone, an aromatase inhibitor, or ketoconazole, which blocks the synthesis of testosterone (and cortisol) at a number of steps, may be indicated.[508,511]

Prolactin

Hypothalamic Hyperprolactinemia

As was discussed previously, PRL is under tonic inhibition by the hypothalamus. Thus, structural or infiltrative lesions of the hypothalamus such as those discussed earlier can affect hypothalamic function causing modest hyperprolactinemia. PRL elevations caused by such lesions rarely rise to greater than 150 ng/ml and usually are below 100 ng/ml.[437] Similar elevations are also seen in patients with an empty sella.[437] It is very important to differentiate nonsecreting pituitary adenomas with extensive suprasellar extension causing PRL elevations in this range from PRL-secreting adenomas which, when of such a large size, usually cause PRL elevations 5 to 50 times higher,[437,512] as the therapy is quite different (see Chap. 7). It is interesting that PRL levels can be increased in patients with hypothalamic lesions while other hypothalamic-pituitary function (i.e., ACTH and TSH) is normal, although GH levels and gonadotropin levels are also often suppressed.[437] This means that there is enough destruction or distortion of the stalk and/or mediobasal hypothalamus to cause a deficiency of dopamine while permitting sufficient CRH and TRH secretion.

Some patients with hypothalamic lesions have PRL levels over 100 ng/ml that fall to levels in the range of 35 to 50 ng/ml after surgery to remove the lesion has caused a complete stalk section.[437] Thus, the degree of PRL elevation may depend not only on the degree of defect of dopamine but also on whether the PRL-releasing activity of the hypothalamus (caused by VIP, TRH, etc.) is intact or perhaps even increased. Evidence in favor of possible increased PRL-releasing activity in such patients includes the finding that normal individuals who are given a pharmacologic blockade of dopamine activity with medications such as neuroleptics and who have intact prolactin-releasing activity have PRL elevations only in the range of 30 to 60 ng/ml.[296]

Therapy is generally directed at the underlying cause. The hyperprolactinemia itself may impair gonadal function and so efforts may also be made to lower PRL levels with bromocriptine or another dopamine agonist. PRL levels usually fall readily in such patients. Restoration of gonadal function is not automatic, however, as the primary hypothalamic lesion may also directly impair the release of GnRH. In that circumstance, sex steroid replacement may be necessary.

Idiopathic Hyperprolactinemia

Idiopathic hyperprolactinemia is defined as hyperprolactinemia that occurs in the absence of any recognized pituitary, hypothalamic, or other cause; that is, it is a diagnosis of exclusion. PRL levels in this condition are usually below 100 ng/ml. In such cases, small pituitary or hypothalamic tumors can exist that are beyond the resolution of current imaging techniques. Long-term followup of such patients shows that in about one-third, PRL levels return to normal, in 10 to 15 percent there is a rise in PRL levels to >50 percent over baseline, and in the remaining patients prolactin levels remain stable.[513,514] Over a 2–6 year follow-up of 199 patients, only 23 developed evidence of microadenomas and none developed macroadenomas.[513–517] Idiopathic hyperprolactinemia can cause amenorrhea, galactorrhea, impotence, infertility, and loss of libido, as occurs with hyperprolactinemia of other causes, and therefore may need to be treated. Premature osteoporosis related to the estrogen deficiency may also occur.[518] The only possible treatment is bromocriptine or another dopamine agonist, and these agents are successful in more than 90 percent of cases.[506] When fertility is not an issue, simple replacement regimens of estrogen and progestin have proved effective and safe.[519]

Galactorrhea can occur with normal PRL levels and with normal menses and has been attributed to increased sensitivity of the breast to normal circulating levels of PRL.[506] Lowering of the normal PRL levels to very low levels with a dopamine agonist is generally successful in eliminating the galactorrhea.

TSH

Hypothalamic Hypothyroidism

This disorder is also referred to as tertiary hypothyroidism and is usually due to a central lesion that impairs the secretion of TRH.[90] It occurs considerably less commonly than do hypothalamic GH and gonadotropin deficiency and with a frequency similar to that of ACTH deficiency.[435,442,447,468] TSH levels in this syndrome generally are normal or even slightly elevated, and the response to TRH is delayed, peaking at 60 to 120 min rather than at 20 to 30 min.[90,520] TSH in these patients is biologically less active than normal and binds to the TSH receptor less well.[521] The defective bioactivity and the receptor-binding activity appear to be due to altered glycosylation as a result of the TRH deficiency.[522] Isolated, acquired TSH deficiency is designated as being idiopathic if thyroid hormone levels are low, there is no or minimal response of TSH to TRH, and no structural lesion is found on MRI.[90] Congenital causes of central hypothyroidism include inactivating mutations in the TRH receptor gene,[523] the TSH beta subunit,[524] and the TSH receptor[525] as well as in combination with loss of the GH and PRL function with mutations in Pit-1 and Prop-1 (previously described). In all circumstances, treatment is with L-thyroxine and the dose is adjusted clinically rather than against TSH levels.

ACTH

Hypothalamic ACTH Deficiency

ACTH deficiency due to hypothalamic lesions occurs less frequently than do GH or gonadotropin deficiencies and with a frequency similar to that of TSH deficiency.[435,442,447,468] It may also appear rarely as an isolated deficiency. In the absence of CNS lesions or a history of trauma, most cases of isolated ACTH deficiency appear to have a pituitary autoimmune basis[526,527] (see Chap. 7). Patients without hypothalamic disease do not respond to either hypoglycemia or single or repetitive injections of CRH.[529] However, in patients with hypothalamic disease as the etiology, basal ACTH levels are low and the ACTH response to injected CRH may be prolonged and exaggerated,[528] much as is the case with the TSH response to TRH.[520] In most cases of isolated ACTH deficiency, the ACTH responses to hypoglycemia and CRH are decreased, compatible with the previously mentioned concept that the primary disorder is in autoimmune destruction of corticotropes.

Cushing's Disease

As was discussed earlier, Cushing's disease may develop from a CRH-producing gangliocytoma.[450] The role of the hypothalamus in the etiology of the usual pituitary ACTH-secreting adenoma is discussed fully in Chap. 7.

Vasopressin

Diabetes insipidus can develop as a result of destructive lesions in the supraoptic and paraventricular nuclei or in the mediobasal hypothalamus in the path of neural fibers containing vasopressin that terminate in the posterior pituitary. Irritative lesions can trigger the release of vasopressin in an unregulated fashion, resulting in the syndrome of inappropriate ADH (vasopressin) secretion (SIADH). These entities are discussed in Chap. 8.

Effects of Hypothalamic Disease on Other Neurometabolic Functions

A number of functions that affect the internal milieu as well as anterior and posterior pituitary function are regulated, at least in part, by the hypothalamus, including temperature regulation, behavior, consciousness, memory, sleep, food intake, and carbohydrate metabolism. Furthermore, the hypothalamus affects cardiovascular, gastrointestinal, pulmonary, and renal function through the autonomic nervous system. Although clinically obvious disturbances of these functions which occur with lesions of the hypothalamus are far less common than disturbances of hypothalamic-pituitary function, detailed evaluations of subclinical defects in these functions have not been performed to ascertain their frequency and effects on the quality of life.

Alterations in Food Intake

Body weight is kept relatively constant in nonobese individuals through an integration of a number of factors relating to the intake of nutrients, including the total amount of food eaten and the composition of that food and the output of energy, which is affected by hormonal, environmental, and genetic factors[529,530] (see Chap. 20). As with the regulation of hormone secretion, the regulation of food intake can be conceptually regarded as an adjustment of food intake and energy expenditure around set points which may be different for body weight, total body fat, lean body mass, etc.[529–531]

A number of areas of the hypothalamus are involved in the regulation of energy balance. It has long been known that destruction of the ventromedial nucleus (VMN) inhibits satiety and results in hyperphagia and hypothalamic obesity, implying a critical role for the medial hypothalamus in controlling food intake.[532,533] At present the interactions of a variety of brain peptides with their receptors and with each other in the hypothalamus with respect to the regulation of food intake and energy balance are just being worked out (see Chap. 20), and there are many possible explanations for why medial basal hypothalamic lesions cause obesity. One possibility relates to the role of leptin in regulating food intake, as this area of the brain has a high expression of leptin receptors[534] and its destruction could lead to a localized loss of leptin action.[533] Leptin reduces food intake (possibly by stimulating CRH, which is anorexic), enhances the sympathetic drive to a number of tissues, including brown adipose tissue, thereby increasing thermogenesis, and inhibits insulin secretion and action.[531,535] Its lack of action due to hypothalamic destruction would cause an increase in food intake, a decrease in sympathetic output and thermogenesis, and hyperinsulinemia.[533] The ventromedial nucleus also contains a high number of melanocortin receptors (MC4-R type) which mediate the satiety-inducing action of melanocyte stimulating hormone (MSH),[535] and targeted disruption of the murine MC4-R receptor has been shown to cause obesity.[536] Because leptin stimulates arcuate POMC production with resultant MSH production,[537] destruction of the medial basal hypothalamus could decrease MSH production as well as the MC4-R receptor. Normally, the VMN exerts an inhibitory effect

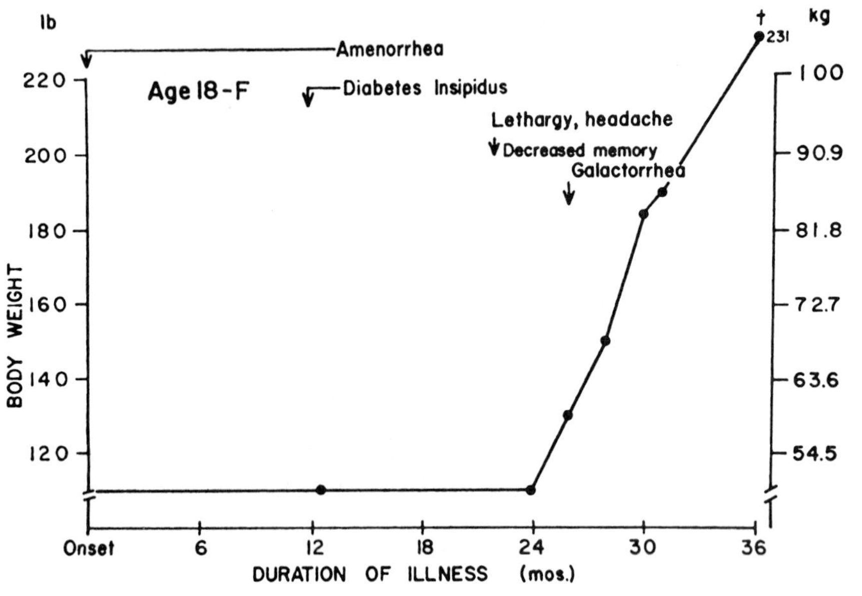

FIGURE 6-29. Clinical sequence in an 18-year-old woman with hypothalamic tuberculosis which progressed despite antituberculosis therapy. Her initial endocrine symptom was amenorrhea, which was followed over several months by the development of diabetes insipidus, lethargy, headache, decreased memory, and galactorrhea and culminated in a massive weight gain during the year before death. (*Reproduced with permission from Bray and Gallagher.*[539]) *Sources:* Adapted from Edwards et al,[542] Plum and Van Uitert,[30] Bray et al,[540] and McKusick VA: Mendelian Inheritance in Man: Catalogs of Autosomal Dominant, Autosomal Recessive, and X-Linked Phenotypes. Baltimore, The Johns Hopkins University, 1975.

on efferent impulses from the dorsal motor nucleus of the vagus, but when the VMN is destroyed, this inhibition is lost and vagal activity is increased.[533] Vagotomy reverses the obesity in VMN-lesioned rats that are fed a chow diet but not a palatable diet.[533]

Lesions of the lateral hypothalamus, which destroy the nigrostriatal dopaminergic fibers that pass through this area, produce hypophagia along with an increase in the peripheral norepinephrine turnover and metabolic rates.[535] However, in addition, neurons of the lateral hypothalamus produce melanin-concentrating hormone (MCH), which stimulates feeding through unidentified receptors, and orexins, which stimulate feeding behavior through specific orexin receptors.[535,538] Thus, destruction of the lateral hypothalamus bilaterally might result in decreases in MCH and orexins, resulting in decreased food intake. Dopamine, epinephrine, and norepinephrine have inhibitory effects on food intake at a site in the lateral hypothalamus.[532] Medications that release or enhance the synthesis of endogenous catecholamines, such as amphetamines, are more effective at this lateral site than they are in the PVN, resulting in a decrease in food intake.[537] Serotonin has inhibitory effects at the PVN in opposition to the effects of norepinephrine.[532] Cholecystokinin and CRH also have inhibitory actions on food intake at the PVN.[370,532] In addition, peripheral glucocorticoids appear to up regulate hypothalamic noradrenergic receptors, potentiating PVN norepinephrine, decreasing CRH release, and resulting in increased food intake.[532]

Hypothalamic Obesity

Destruction of the ventromedial area of the hypothalamus results in obesity in humans as well as in animals. Because the mediobasal hypothalamus is the final common pathway for the hypophysiotropic factors that travel to the median eminence and for the fibers that go to the posterior pituitary, such lesions commonly also produce hypopituitarism and diabetes insipidus. In one series of eight patients with well-characterized hypothalamic obesity, the lesions included trauma, dermoid tumor, tuberculosis, chordoma, lipoma, craniopharyngioma, aneurysm, and meningioma.[539] Seven of these patients had hypogonadotropic hypogonadism and decreased GH levels, one was also hypothyroid and hypoadrenal, and another had diabetes insipidus and galactorrhea. As the lesion grows, various hypothalamic abnormalities may appear sequentially (Fig. 6-29). In patients with hypothalamic obesity, the weight gain tends to be rapid and eventually stabilizes, with the total gain usually being <50 kg and the final body weight usually being <140 kg.[539] The weight gain is due to hypertrophy of existing adipocytes rather than to hyperplasia. The basal metabolic rate and the rate of lipolysis are not different from those of other obese patients or normal individuals. However, patients with hypothalamic obesity are even more insulin-resistant than are idiopathic obese patients, though it is not clear whether this is of pathogenetic importance.[539]

There are a number of rare syndromes in which obesity is a major component and for which a hypothalamic etiology has been postulated (Table 6-5). Prader-Willi syndrome is the most common of these syndromes, occurring in 1 in 25,000 births. It is characterized by hypotonia, obesity, short stature, mental deficiency, hypogonadism, and small hands and feet.[540,541] About 70 percent of these patients have a chromosome 15 deletion (15q11-q13) on the paternally derived chromosome. The short stature is associated with low basal and stimulated GH levels along with an absent pubertal growth spurt.[540,541] The hypogonadism is due to gonadotropin insufficiency that is unresponsive to standard GnRH stimulation tests. However, if patients are pretreated with clomiphene, the gonadotropin responses normalize.[541] Thyroid and adrenal functions are normal.[540] In the few cases studied at autopsy, no discernible hypothalamic lesions were detected.[541] In the other syndromes listed in Table 6-5, no specific hypothalamic lesions have been found.[30,542]

Hypothalamic Anorexia

This syndrome is very rare, probably owing to the requirement for bilateral lesions. As opposed to a midline lesion, that could easily damage both ventromedial nuclei, a single lesion damaging both sides of the hypothalamus in its lateral aspects would have to be very large and cause a great deal of other hypothalamic dysfunction, including panhypopituitarism in most cases.[30] The hormonal changes that occur in anorexia nervosa all

TABLE 6-5. Syndromes of Hypothalamic Obesity

Syndrome	Clinical Features	Etiology
Babinski-Froehlich	Obesity and hypogonadism	Craniopharyngioma or other tumor involving the ventromedial hypothalamus and median eminence
Kleine-Levin	Episodic hyperosmia, hyperphagia, hyperactivity when awake, hypersexuality	Preceding viral infection in some patients; disorder seen primarily in teenage males; usually disappears by mid-twenties; no histologic examinations performed; possible paroxysmal limbic system or hypothalamic disease
Laurence-Moon	Pigmentary retinal degeneration, mental deficiency, spastic paraplegia, hypogonadism, obesity	Autosomal dominant inheritance; no gross or microscopic lesions of hypothalamus seen
Bardet-Biedl	Pigmentary retinopathy, mental deficiency, polydactylism, hypogonadism, obesity	No anatomic lesions seen
Allstrom-Hallgren	Pigmentary retinopathy, hypogonadism, deafness, obesity, diabetes	No anatomic lesions seen
Edwards	Pigmentary retinopathy, hypogonadism, gynecomastia, mental retardation, deafness, obesity, diabetes	Autosomal recessive inheritance; no histologic examinations performed
Prader-Willi	Hypogonadism, diabetes, short stature, obesity, temperature intolerance, loss of diurnal rhythms	No anatomic lesions seen

Sources: Adapted from Edwards et al,[472] Plum and Van Uitert,[25] Bray et al,[472] and McKusick VA: Mendelian Inheritance in Man: Catalogs of Autosomal Dominant, Autosomal Recessive, and X-Linked Phenotypes. Baltimore, The Johns Hopkins University, 1975.

appear to be secondary to the weight loss, and there is no evidence for a primary hypothalamic disorder in this syndrome.

Diencephalic Syndrome

This syndrome consists of a diencephalic tumor associated with emaciation and minimal neurologic signs and symptoms occurring in infants and children.[543] In most cases the tumor is located in the third ventricle, but some are optic nerve gliomas and others occur in the fourth ventricle. Most of these tumors are gliomas and astrocytomas, although a small number of dysgerminomas have been reported. Although the characteristic clinical feature is emaciation with normal or slightly reduced caloric intake, these children appear inappropriately alert, hyperactive, and even euphoric.[543] The alert appearance is due to lid retraction rather than true alertness. In addition to these features, a number of neurologic signs may be present if looked for carefully, including nystagmus, optic pallor, irritability, tremor, and excessive sweating. Endocrine features include a loss of cortisol diurnal variation, an increase in basal GH levels, a paradoxic rise of GH with a glucose load and diabetes insipidus.[543] Many children die of the primary tumor or its recurrence and treatment consists of surgery and/or irradiation.[544] In those who live longer, there may be a progression of the primary symptoms of emaciation and wasting[543] or there may rarely be a reversal to hypothalamic obesity.[545] These tumors do not specifically affect the lateral hypothalamus and, if anything, tend to cause destruction of the mediobasal hypothalamus. Why the immature ventromedial area should respond differently to destruction compared to that of older individuals with regard to the regulation of food intake is not known.[30]

Hyperglycemia

Hypothalamic activation as part of the generalized response to stress can cause a release of GH, PRL, and ACTH, which serve as counterregulatory hormones with respect to insulin. These hormones serve to promote lipolysis, gluconeogenesis, and insulin resistance, resulting in glucose elevation (see Chaps. 18 and 19). Of more importance in the acute response to stress, this hypothalamic response results in sympathetic activation with release of catecholamines which inhibit insulin secretion and stimulation of glycogenolysis. In rare circumstances of acute hypothalamic injury from trauma, stroke, or infection, severe hyperglycemia can occur; it is similar to the hyperglycemia seen in animals when the floor of the fourth ventricle is pricked with a needle, a phenomenon referred to as "piqûre" diabetes by Bernard.[546]

Temperature Regulation

The anterior hypothalamus and preoptic area contain temperature-sensitive neurons that respond to internal temperature changes by initiating certain thermoregulatory responses necessary to restore a constant temperature.[547] Measures that dissipate heat include cutaneous vasodilation, sweating, panting, and behavioral changes which result in attempts to alter the environment. Measures that increase body heat include increasing metabolic heat production, shivering, cutaneous vasoconstriction, and similar behavioral changes.[547] In humans, much of the increase in metabolic heat production occurs via sympathetic activation. The thermosensitive neurons are affected by endogenous pyrogens and drugs which alter thermoregulation as well as by input from thermoreceptors in the skin and spinal cord.[547]

Rare patients have been reported with anterior hypothalamic

lesions that caused sustained hypothermia as a result of failure of heat generation by shivering and vasoconstriction but who had intact heat dissipation[548] or a resetting (lowering) of the temperature set point.[549] Paroxysmal hypothermia lasting for minutes to days caused by the sudden onset of sweating, vasodilation, and a fall in core temperature has been reported in a number of patients in association with lesions such as tumors and agenesis of the corpus callosum. Some of these patients had evidence of other hypothalamic dysfunction, including diabetes insipidus, hypogonadism, and precocious puberty.[550] Cases of idiopathic periodic hypothermia without structural abnormalities or evidence of other hypothalamic dysfunction have also been reported.[551]

Fever is uncommon as a manifestation of hypothalamic disease but has been reported in relation to trauma or bleeding into the region of the anterior hypothalamus.[30] Such fevers rarely persist more than 2 weeks.[30] Paroxysmal hyperthermia due to hypothalamic dysfunction also occurs. One patient had episodes of fever that recurred in regular 3-week cycles.[552] Some cases of paroxysmal hypo- and hyperthermia respond to anticonvulsant medications, suggesting that the neuronal discharges that cause the temperature changes are seizure-like.[30]

Poikilothermia results from the inability to dissipate or generate heat to keep the body temperature constant in the face of varying ambient temperatures. This condition results from bilateral lesions in the posterior hypothalamus and rostral mesencephalon, which are the areas responsible for the final integration of thermoregulatory neural efferents.[30] Patients with this condition do not feel discomfort with temperature changes and are unaware of having a problem. Depending on the ambient temperature, they may present with life-threatening hypo- or hyperthermia. Poikilothermia is normally present in infants and frequently occurs in elderly individuals.

Neuroendocrine Alterations in Systemic Disease

Systemic diseases have widespread effects on neuroendocrine regulation. In most cases, the only knowledge available is of alterations in pituitary function which reflect the integration of combined stimulatory and inhibitory hypothalamic influences. In many systemic illnesses reported changes in pituitary function have not been distinguished satisfactorily from the changes known to be associated with "stress" due to the illness, and so the effects of such illnesses may be considered nonspecific. In very few circumstances have the alterations in neurotransmitters that cause the changes in hormone secretion been demonstrated.

Stress

Since the early studies of Hans Selye, stress has been known to play an important role in modifying the hormonal regulation of the internal milieu. Although a distinction can be made between physical and mental stress, it is clear that when physical stress occurs, there is a considerable emotional component that must also be considered. The nature of the stress may have other complexities, including those due to infections with release of cytokines and activation of the immune system and those due to concurrent caloric deprivation. Furthermore, some changes due to acute stress/infection may change as stress becomes more chronic.

Acute Physical Stress and Illness

ACTH and cortisol levels rise within 15 min of the onset of a severe physical stress such as surgery and return to normal 8 to 10 h after surgery.[553] The corticosteroid production rate increases tenfold during surgery,[553] giving rise to the common clinical practice of administering exogenous steroids in doses 10 times normal during surgery or other severe stress in patients with adrenal insufficiency. It is the triggering of neural afferents to the hypothalamus by the surgery that is responsible for the output of ACTH and cortisol; in patients with spinal cord transection, surgery below the level of the cord lesion does not produce a rise in steroid levels.[553] If the stress is maintained, cortisol secretion stays modestly elevated for as long as the patient is ill but ACTH levels are low, suggesting an alternative pathway for cortisol release, possibly involving endothelin.[554–556] Both cholinergic and serotoninergic pathways probably mediate the release of CRH during acute stress, and the endogenous opioid pathways probably have little influence in this regard.[378] In addition, activation of the sympathetic nervous system is important, as CRH stimulates the secretion of norepinephrine and norepinephrine stimulates the secretion of CRH.[241] With acute infections, the cytokines tumor necrosis factor α (TNFα), interleukin-1, and interleukin-6 released by the inflammation stimulate CRH production by the hypothalamus,[241,242] stimulate hypothalamic noradrenergic activity,[557] and may also have direct stimulatory effects on the pituitary to release ACTH.[241] Peripherally generated cytokines likely reach the hypothalamus via several possible mechanisms, including crossing at leaky areas in the blood brain barrier, such as the circumventricular organs, active transport across the blood brain barrier, and through receptors expressed in cerebral blood vessels with subsequent activation of second messengers such as NO and prostaglandins.[242,557]

Severe illness also causes a rise in GH and PRL levels,[558] but more persistent, less acute illness does not, despite a persistent increase in cortisol.[554] The stress-induced rise in GH is probably mediated by noradrenergic pathways, resulting in an increase in GHRH, as alpha-adrenergic blockade can inhibit this response.[558] However, with more prolonged illness IGF-1 levels fall and the GH levels increase due to decreased feedback[29,556,559] while PRL levels return to normal.[556] By contrast, stress results in a reduction of TSH levels as part of the euthyroid sick syndrome acutely and chronically[560] (see Chap. 9).

Gonadotropin levels are also suppressed.[561] These hormonal changes may be viewed teleologically as beneficial in that they increase vascular tone, provide increased energy substrate, decrease the basal metabolic rate, and shunt energy away from temporarily unneeded activities. The rise in CRH and β-endorphin have direct inhibitory effects on GnRH secretion and elevated cortisol levels inhibit GnRH, the LH response to GnRH, and the gonadal response to LH.[562]

Psychological Stress

Acute psychological stress can raise ACTH, GH, and PRL levels and a number of changes in pituitary hormones occur with chronic psychiatric diseases such as depression and schizophrenia.

Metabolic Disorders

Fasting and Malnutrition

Short-term dieting can cause a reduction in gonadotropin levels sufficient to cause amenorrhea, but the LH and FSH responses to GnRH are normal, implying a hypothalamic site of action.[502] A similar blunting of basal and TRH-stimulated TSH secretion occurs.[502,560] With such dieting, basal GH levels become modestly elevated but there is no change in ACTH or PRL levels.[502] Although prolonged protein-calorie malnutrition results in decreased cortisol production, the metabolic clearance rate is also reduced, so that serum cortisol levels are minimally elevated and are only partially suppressible with dexamethasone.[563] Basal GH levels are elevated and IGF-I levels are decreased in protein-calorie malnutrition but not in marasmus,[564] suggesting that it is the decreased IGF-I feedback that causes the increased GH levels. Thyroid hormone levels remain low in protein-calorie malnutrition and basal TSH levels are normal, but the response to TRH is delayed and sometimes exaggerated.[565] With prolonged malnutrition, amenorrhea persists. The hormonal changes in patients with anorexia nervosa are similar to those in patients with simple weight loss. Again, these hormonal changes may be regarded as being adaptive to conserve energy, as with physical stress. Many of these changes may be due to starvation-induced decreases in serum leptin levels.[566] Leptin administration can reverse the starvation-induced suppression of the thyroid and reproductive axes and activation of the hypothalamic-pituitary-adrenal axis.[566,567]

Obesity

ACTH and cortisol levels are usually normal in obesity, but the normal diurnal rhythm may be disrupted and the cortisol production rate may be altered.[568,569] Although the overnight dexamethasone suppression test may not fully suppress morning cortisol levels in obese patients, a full 2-day low-dose test usually will do so.[568] Basal GH levels are low to normal in the obese, and the GH response to a variety of stimuli such as hypoglycemia, L-dopa, arginine, and exercise, as well as GHRH itself, are all markedly blunted.[568,569] This blunting of the GH response appears to be due to a defect of cholinergic tone, resulting in an excess of somatostatin, because treatment with the cholinesterase inhibitor pyridostigmine restores most of these responses.[570] Basal PRL and TSH levels and the PRL and TSH responses to TRH are usually normal.[568]

The onset of menarche frequently occurs at a younger age in obese girls than in girls of normal weight. It has been proposed that puberty and menstruation are initiated in females when body weight or the percentage of body fat reaches a critical level[410] (see Chap. 25). It has been hypothesized that the signal to the hypothalamus mediating this percentage of body fat is leptin.[571] Obese women often show menstrual irregularity. Analysis of the pattern of hormone secretion during the course of the cycle in obese women reveals that FSH levels do not rise normally during the midfollicular phase and that there is deficient progesterone secretion by the corpus luteum, resulting in a short luteal phase.[568] The mechanisms underlying these changes are not clear and gonadotropin pulsatile secretion and responses to GnRH are normal in obesity.[568]

It is clear, however, that these hormonal alterations are consequent to and in no way causative of the obesity because experimental studies have shown that they do not exist prior to the obesity.[572] The hormonal and other consequences of obesity are discussed in Chap. 20.

Diabetes Mellitus

In poorly controlled diabetes mellitus of all types, intracellular glucose metabolism is disrupted. Basal and stimulated GH levels are increased and return toward normal with improved control.[573] The elevated GH levels are associated with decreased GH binding protein and low IGF-I levels in some studies.[574] The increased GH levels are at least in part mediated by a decrease in somatostatinergic tone. Treatment with the cholinergic agonist pirenzepine, which increases central somatostatin release, causes the elevated GH levels to return to normal.[575] Few data are available on other hormone levels.

Cirrhosis

Cirrhosis of all etiologies may cause abnormalities of neuroendocrine function.[576] However, most of the information has been obtained in patients with Laënnec's cirrhosis, and in many circumstances, the effects of cirrhosis are difficult to separate from the changes induced by the alcohol.

About 25 percent of patients with chronic alcoholism have reduced cortisol responses to insulin-induced hypoglycemia.[577] However, alcoholic patients may uncommonly present with Cushingoid features and may have elevated cortisol levels that do not suppress normally in response to dexamethasone within the first few days of admission but return to normal over subsequent weeks.[578]

In patients with cirrhosis, GH levels are elevated both basally and after stimulation with arginine, hypoglycemia, and GHRH.[579,580] GH responses to TRH are found in about 75 percent of such patients.[579,580] IGF-I levels are decreased, presumably causing the increased GH levels through decreased feedback.[579,580] Basal PRL levels are increased in 15 to 20 percent of patients with alcoholic cirrhosis and 5 to 15 percent of those with nonalcoholic cirrhosis.[581] TSH levels, in contrast, are usually normal or decreased despite low to normal thyroid hormone levels, a pattern compatible with the euthyroid sick syndrome.[582]

Cirrhosis of all causes has long been known to cause androgen and estrogen deficiency with altered steroid metabolism and a defect in the testicular generation of testosterone.[583] However, despite this apparent primary testicular defect, gonadotropin levels are not usually elevated and the response to GnRH is low to normal and is not increased.[583,584] The gonadotropin response to clomiphene is markedly blunted in men with Laënnec's cirrhosis even after abstention from alcohol for several weeks, implying that the defect is at the hypothalamic level. LH pulse analysis shows a decrease in the frequency and amplitude of LH pulses.[583]

Excessive alcohol intake in normal volunteers initially causes a decrease in testosterone levels with a rise in LH but not FSH levels. After 1 to 2 weeks of heavy alcohol intake, the testosterone levels remain low, the LH levels become subnormal, but there is no change in FSH levels.[584] Thus, in alcoholic cirrhosis the effects of alcohol and cirrhosis may be additive.

Renal Failure

Basal cortisol levels in renal failure have been reported to be both normal[585] and high.[586] Although ACTH levels are high, the ACTH response to CRH is blunted and the suppression of cortisol by dexamethasone is impaired.[586] Treatment with erythropoietin causes a return to normal of elevated ACTH and cortisol levels.[587] After treatment, these levels are lower than in patients not treated with erythropoietin, but the hematocrits are similar.[587] Thus, the erythropoietin-caused changes are not due exclusively to an improvement in the anemia.

Basal GH levels are increased in patients with chronic renal failure.[588] The GH response to GHRH is increased,[588] and there are paradoxic GH responses to TRH and glucose. Serum IGF-I levels are normal if uremic samples are processed with acid-ethanol extraction and acid chromatography,[589] but uremic children are short and bioassayable IGF-I levels tend to be low, suggesting that the IGF-I has a decreased ability to stimulate mitogenic pathways in growth plate chondrocytes.[589] It has been postulated that there are low-molecular-weight compounds that interfere with the biological activity of IGF-I.[590] If the elevated GH levels are due to decreased feedback of IGF-I, this decreased biological activity of IGF-I also pertains to the feedback effects. As with ACTH, treatment with erythropoietin causes a reduction in GH levels, with at least some of the reduction being independent of the correction of the anemia.[587]

Hyperprolactinemia occurs in 73 to 91 percent of women and 25 to 57 percent of men with end-stage renal disease.[591,592] PRL suppression by dopamine infusion is decreased,[591] but this may be at least in part a result of delayed degradation of PRL in renal failure because the long-term use of bromocriptine results in suppression of PRL levels. Although PRL metabolism is reduced in renal failure, there is also increased production.[593] Therefore, there is disordered regulation of PRL secretion and possibly short-loop feedback, although the exact nature of the defect has not been defined. About one-quarter of individuals with renal insufficiency who do not require dialysis (serum creatinine 2.0 to 12.0 ng/ml) have PRL levels in the range of 25 to 100 ng/ml.[592] When such patients take medications known to alter hypothalamic regulation of PRL, such as methyldopa and metoclopramide, PRL levels may rise to over 2000 ng/ml.[592] Correction of the renal failure with transplantation causes a return of PRL levels to normal.[591,592]

Hyperprolactinemia contributes to the hypogonadism of chronic renal failure but probably does not explain all the abnormalities in every case. Return of normal menses has occurred in some women and correction of impotence has occurred in some men treated with bromocriptine,[591] but reports of restored ovulation are rare.[591]

Basal levels of TSH are low or normal, TSH responses to TRH are blunted, and thyroid hormone levels are low, compatible with the euthyroid sick syndrome.[594] After renal transplantation, thyroid hormone levels and TSH levels return to normal, but the TSH response to TRH remains blunted, presumably because of corticosteroid administration.[594]

In renal failure there is a primary gonadal failure, but gonadotropin levels are inappropriately low for the degree of hypogonadism.[595] The gonadotropin response to GnRH is normal, but the lack of an exaggerated response suggests blunted pituitary responsiveness.[595] Negative estrogen feedback is preserved, as shown by normal responses to clomiphene, but positive estrogen feedback is impaired. With renal transplantation, ovulatory cycles return in 60 percent of women.[596] Even without transplantation, occasional women with endstage renal disease on chronic dialysis will ovulate irregularly and may become pregnant.[597]

Other CNS Disorders

Pineal Region Tumors

There are a number of different types of pineal region tumors. The term *pinealoma* is incorrect, and tumors should be referred to by their specific tissue types. Tumors of the pineal parenchyma are called pineocytomas or pineoblastomas, depending on the maturity of the cells. Tumors of the supporting pineal glial tissue are gliomas, astrocytomas, or ependymomas. Pineal cell and glial tumors account for nearly 50 percent of these tumors.[598] The most common tumor, called a germinoma, arises from primitive, undifferentiated germ cells.[598] These germ cells appear to migrate aberrantly from the yolk sac to this region during early embryonic development.[446] About one-third of germinomas produce hCG, leading to precocious puberty,[598] and about 10 percent metastasize via the CSF. Some germinomas can affect the hypothalamus by direct infiltration, but others arise there, as previously discussed. The germinomas that arise in the suprasellar area were referred to as ectopic pinealomas in the past. A small portion of germ cell tumors are true teratomas, containing cell types originating from each of the three layers that differentiate to form various somatic structures, such as hair and teeth. These teratomas can be benign or malignant, giving rise to choriocarcinomas which can secrete hCG. Among a total of 389 intracranial germ cell tumors, 65 percent were germinomas, 18 percent were teratomas, 5 percent were embryonal carcinomas, 7 percent were endodermal sinus tumors, and 5 percent were choriocarcinomas.[599] Thus, intracranial germ cell tumors are similar to those which occur in the mediastinum and other locations. Overall, about one-third of pineal tumors are benign and the remainder malignant.[600]

Symptoms depend on the site of presentation of the tumor. Suprasellar germinomas classically present with the triad of diabetes insipidus, visual disturbance, and hypogonadism. Pineal region tumors can compress the aqueduct of Sylvius, giving rise to hydrocephalus with associated headaches, vomiting, and loss of consciousness. Pineal region tumors may also compress the quadrigeminal plate, interrupting fibers passing from the cortex to the superior colliculi, giving rise to Parinaud's syndrome (paralysis of conjugate upward gaze and ptosis).[598,599]

Pineal region tumors have long been associated with the syndrome of precocious puberty. However, it is now known that these tumors account for only a small percentage of such cases (as described earlier), and only a small percentage of pineal region tumors cause precocious puberty. Most cases of precocious puberty associated with pineal region tumors occur because of reasons similar to those for other intracranial neoplasms causing precocious puberty (i.e., a disinhibition of GnRH secretion).[508] Because the pineal tumors that cause precocious puberty are mostly nonparenchymal, destruction of the pineal may result in a decrease of a pineal antigonadotropin substance such as melatonin or another peptide.[601] Some hCG-secreting tumors may produce enough hormone to mimic puberty, and this probably accounts for a number of the cases of precocious puberty associated with pineal region tumors.[602]

HCG or α fetoprotein produced by tumors is often detectable in the CSF and allows an easy diagnosis; α fetoprotein is specific for malignant teratomas.[602] Occasionally, malignant cells in the CSF may stain positively for these substances. The germinomas tend to be radiosensitive, and radiotherapy can be given if such markers are found.[602] Otherwise biopsy is necessary, and surgery or radiotherapy may be needed, depending on the tissue type.[600,603] Chemotherapy may be indicated in some tumors of germ cell origin.[602,603] Overall, five-year survival rates are 86 percent for mature teratomas, 86 percent for pineocytomas, 80 percent for germinomas, 67 percent for immature teratomas, 49 percent for pineal parenchymal tumors, 38 percent for mixed germ cell tumors, and 17 percent for other germ cell histologies.[603]

Pseudotumor Cerebri

In this condition there is a chronic increase in intracranial pressure, giving rise to headache as the most common presenting feature, although visual symptoms may also occur. These symptoms mimic those of an intracranial tumor, although no tumor is present—thus the name and the alternative name, *benign intracranial hypertension*. An association with endocrine disease has been suggested in some cases, as it may occur with pregnancy, oral contraceptive use, hypoparathyroidism, or Addison's disease, after glucocorticoid withdrawal and the cure of Cushing's syndrome and after the institution of thyroid hormone replacement in hypothyroidism.[604] However, pseudotumor cerebri itself causes no hormonal deficit, although GH responses may be decreased, as is expected in a syndrome in which patients are overweight.

In some patients, however, there is an associated partially empty sella. About 10 to 15 percent of patients with pseudotumor cerebri have empty sellas, and 25 to 50 percent of patients with empty sellas who present because of headaches or visual symptoms are found to have increased intracranial pressure. In this circumstance, there is usually a defect in the diaphragma sella with transmission of the increased intracranial pressure to the sella. Varying degrees of hypopituitarism and hyperprolactinemia have been found in patients with empty sellas, and so a brief screening evaluation is usually necessary[605] (see Chap. 7).

Cerebral Gigantism

This rare syndrome is associated with an increased early growth rate, mild mental retardation, and dilated cerebral ventricles unaccompanied by increased GH levels.[606] Other clinical features include a typical facies characterized by hypertelorism, prominent supraorbital ridge, high-arched palate, and prognathism; large hands and feet; advanced bone age; and nonprogressive cerebral dysfunction. The enlarged head is due initially to increased volume of the cerebral tissue but subsequently is due to retention of cerebrospinal fluid in the ventricles and subarachnoid spaces.[607] In addition to the normal GH levels, bioactive IGF-I levels are also normal. The mean birth weight is between the 75th and 97th percentiles, and the mean birth length is at the 97th percentile, suggesting that the process started during gestation.[607] The children display moderate psychomotor retardation and behavioral difficulties.[606,607] The etiology of the condition is not known and no identifiable endocrine abnormalities have been found.

REFERENCES

1. Scharrer E, Scharrer B: Secretory cells within the hypothalamus, in *The Hypothalamus. Res Publ Assoc Res Nerve Ment Dis*, vol. XX. New York, Hafner, 1940, p 170.
2. Snyder SH: Drug and neurotransmitter receptors in the brain. *Science* 224:22, 1984.
3. Bloom FE: Neurotransmitters: Past, present, and future directions. *FASEB J* 2:32, 1988.
4. Vanhatalo S, Soinila S: The concept of chemical neurotransmission—variation on the theme. *Ann Med* 30:151, 1998.
5. Patel YC, Srikant CB: Subtype selectivity of peptide analogs for all five cloned human stomatostatin receptors (hsstr 1-5). *Endocrinology* 135:2814, 1994.
6. Shimon I, Taylor JE, Dong JZ, et al: Somatostatin receptor subtype specificity in human fetal pituitary cultures. Differential role of SSTR2 and SSTR5 for growth hormone, thyroid-stimulating hormone, and prolactin regulation. *J Clin Invest* 99:789, 1997.
7. Håkanson R, Bättcher G, Ekblad E, Grunditz T, Sundler F: Functional implications of messenger coexpression in neurons and endocrine cells, in Schwartz TW, Hilsted LM, Rehfeld JF (eds): *Neuropeptides and Their Receptors*. Copenhagen, Munksgaard, 1990, p 211.
8. Whitnall MH: Stress selectively activates the vasopressin-containing subset of corticotropin-releasing hormone neurons. *Neuroendocrinology* 50:702, 1989.
9. Harris GW: Neural control of the pituitary gland. *Physiol Rev* 28:139, 1948.
10. Fröhlich A: Ein Fall von Tumor der Hypophysis ceribri ohne Akromegalie. *Klin Rundsch* 15:883, 1901.
11. Erdheim J: Uber hypophysenganggeschwulste and Hirncholesteratome. *Sitzber Akad Wien* 113:537, 1904.
12. Harris GW, Jacobsohn D: Functional grafts of the anterior pituitary gland. *Proc R Soc London* 139:263, 1952.
13. Nikitovitch-Winer M, Everett JW: Functional restitution of pituitary grafts retransplanted from kidney to median eminence. *Endocrinology* 63:916, 1958.
14. Green JD, Harris GW: The neurovascular link between the neurohypophysis and adenohypophysis. *J Endocrinol* 5:136, 1947.
15. Popa G, Fielding U: A portal circulation from the pituitary to the hypothalamic region. *J Anat* 65:88, 1930.
16. Wislocki GB, King LS: The permeability of the hypophysis and hypothalamus to vital dyes, with a study of the hypophyseal vascular supply. *J Anat* 58:421, 1936.
17. Török B: Structure of the vascular connections of the hypothalamo-hypophysial region. *Acta Anat (Basel)* 59:84, 1964.
18. Oliver C, Mical RS, Porter JC: Hypothalamic-pituitary vasculature: Evidence for retrograde blood flow in the pituitary stalk. *Endocrinology* 101:598, 1977.
19. Bøler J, Enzmann F, Folkers K, Bowers CY, Schally AV: The identity of chemical and hormonal properties of the thyrotropin releasing hormone and pyroglutamyl-histidyl-proline amide. *Biochem Biophys Res Commun* 37:705, 1969.
20. Burgus R, Dunn T, Desiderio D, Guillemin R: Structure moleculaire du facteur hypothalamique hypophysiotrope TRF d'origine ovine: Mise en evidence par spectrometre de masse de la sequence PCA-His-Pro-NH_2. *CR Acad Sci (Paris)* 269:1870, 1969.
21. Segerson TP, Kauer J, Wolfe HC, Mobtaker H, Wu P, Jackson IMD, Lechan RM: Thyroid hormone regulates TRH biosynthesis in the paraventricular nucleus of the rat hypothalamus. *Science* 238:78, 1987.
22. Berelowitz M, Maeda K, Harris S, Frohman LA: The effect of alterations in the pituitary-thyroid axis on hypothalamic content and *in vitro* release of somatostatinlike immunoreactivity. *Endocrinology* 107:24, 1980.
23. Larsen PR, Berry MJ: Nutritional and hormonal regulation of thyroid hormone deiodinases. *Ann Rev Nutr* 15:323, 1995.
24. Yu WH, Karanth S, Walczewska A, Sower SA, McCann SM: A hypothalamic follicle-stimulating hormone-releasing decapeptide in the rat. *Proc Natl Acad Sci USA* 94:9499, 1997.
25. Redei E, Hilderbrand H, Aird F: Corticotropin release-inhibiting factor is preprothyrotropin-releasing hormone-(178-199). *Endocrinology* 136:3557, 1995.
26. Berelowitz M, Szabo M, Frohman LA, Firestone S, Chu L: Somatomedin-C mediates growth hormone negative feedback by effects on both the hypothalamus and the pituitary. *Science* 212:1279, 1981.
27. Abe H, Molitch ME, Van Wyk JJ, Underwood LE: Human growth hormone and somatomedin C suppress the spontaneous release of growth hormone in unanesthetized rats. *Endocrinology* 113:1319, 1983.
28. Rosenthal SM, Hulse JA, Kaplan SL, Grumbach MM: Exogenous growth hormone inhibits growth hormone-releasing factor-induced growth hormone secretion in normal men. *J Clin Invest* 77:176, 1986.
29. Molitch ME, Hou SH: Neuroendocrine alterations in systemic disease. *Clinics Endocrinol Metab* 12:825, 1983.
30. Plum F, Van Uitert R: Nonendocrine diseases and disorders of the hypothalamus, in Reichlin S, Baldessarini RJ, Martin JB (eds): *The Hypothalamus*. New York, Raven Press, 1978, p 415.
31. Lechan RM: Neuroendocrinology of pituitary hormone regulation. *Endocrinol Metab Clin North Am* 16:475, 1987.
32. King JC, Anthony ELP, Fitzgerald DM, Stopa EG: Luteinizing hormone-releasing hormone neurons in human preoptic/hypothalamus: Differential intraneuronal localization of immunoreactive forms. *J Clin Endocrinol Metab* 60:88, 1985.
33. Reuss S: Components and connections of the circadian timing system in mammals. *Cell Tissue Res* 285:353, 1996.
34. Hoffman GE, Phelps CJ, Khachaturian H, Sladek JR Jr: Neuroendocrine projections to the median eminence. *Curr Top Neuroendocrinol* 7:161, 1986.
35. Wiegand SJ, Price JL: Cells of origin of the afferent fibers to the median eminence in the rat. *J Comp Neurol* 192:1, 1980.
36. Swanson LW, Sawchenko PE: Paraventricular nucleus: A site for the integration of neuroendocrine and autonomic mechanisms. *Neuroendocrinology* 31:410, 1980.

37. Krisch B, Leonhardt H, Buchheim W: The functional and structural border of the neurohemal region of the median eminence. *Cell Tissue Res* 192:327, 1978.
38. McKinley MJ, McAllen RM, Mendelsohn FAO, Allen AM, Chai SY, Oldfield BJ: Circumventricular organs: Neuroendocrine interfaces between the brain and the hemal milieu. *Front Neuroendocrinol* 11:91, 1990.
39. Page RB: Pituitary blood flow. *Am J Physiol* 243:E427, 1982.
40. Page RB: Directional pituitary blood flow: A microcinephotographic study. *Endocrinology* 112:157, 1983.
41. Antunes JL, Muraszko K, Stark R, Chen R: Pituitary portal blood flow in primates: A doppler study. *Neurosurgery* 12:492, 1983.
42. Treier M, Rosenfeld MG: The hypothalamic-pituitary axis: Co-development of two organs. *Curr Opin Cell Biol* 8:833, 1996.
43. Treier M, Gleiberman AS, O'Connell SM, et al: Multistep signaling requirements for pituitary organogenesis in vivo. *Genes Dev* 12:1691, 1998.
44. Le Dafniet M, Lefebvre P, Barret A, Mechain C, Feinstein MC, Brandi AM, Peillon F: Normal and adenomatous human pituitaries secrete thyrotropin-releasing hormone *in vitro*: Modulation by dopamine, haloperidol, and somatostatin. *J Clin Endocrinol Metab* 71:480, 1990.
45. Arnaout MA, Garthwaite TL, Martinson DR: Vasoactive intestinal polypeptide is synthesized in anterior pituitary tissue. *Endocrinology* 119:2052, 1986.
46. Guillemin R: Biochemical and physiological correlates of hypothalamic peptides: The new endocrinology of neuron, in Reichlin S, Baldessarini RJ, Martin JB (eds): *The Hypothalamus.* New York, Raven Press, 1978, p 155.
47. Jackson IMD, Lechan RM, Lee SL: TRH prohormone: Biosynthesis, anatomic distribution, and processing. *Front Neuroendocrinol* 11:267, 1990.
48. Palkovits M: Neuropeptides in the brain, in Martini L, Ganong WF (eds): *Frontiers in Neuroendocrinology.* New York, Raven Press, 1988, vol. 10, p. 1.
49. *Richter K, Kawashima E, Egger R, Kreil G: Biosynthesis of thyrotropin releasing hormone in the skin of Xenopus laevis: Partial sequence of the precursor deduced from cloned cDNA.* EMBO J 3:617, 1984.
50. Yamada M, Radovick S, Wondisford FE, Nakayama Y, Weintraub BD, Wilber JF: Cloning and structure of human genomic DNA and hypothalamic cDNA encoding human prepro thyrotropin-releasing hormone. *Mol Endocrinol* 4:551, 1990.
51. O'Leary R, O'Connor B: Thyrotropin-releasing hormone. *J Neurochem* 65:953, 1995.
52. Guldenaar SEF, Veldkamp B, Bakker O, Wiersinga WM, Swaab DF, Fliers E: Thyrotropin-releasing hormone gene expression in the human hypothalamus. *Brain Res* 743:93, 1996.
53. Koch Y, Okon E: Localization of releasing hormones in the human brain. *Int Rev Exp Pathol* 19:45, 1979.
54. Manaker S, Eichen A, Winokur A, Rhodes CH, Rainbow TC: Autoradiographic localization of thyrotropin releasing hormone receptors in human brain. *Neurology* 36:641, 1986.
55. Duthie SM, Taylor PL, Anderson L, Cook J, Eidne KA: Cloning and functional characterisation of the human TRH receptor. *Mol Cell Endocrinol* 95:R11, 1993.
56. Yamada M, Monden T, Konaka S, Mori M: Assignment of the human thyrotropin-releasing hormone receptor gene to chromosome 8. *Somat Cell Mol Genet* 19:577, 1993.
57. Lechan RM, Snapper SB, Jacobson S, Jackson IMD: The distribution of thyrotropin-releasing hormone (TRH) in the rhesus monkey spinal cord. *Peptides* 5:185, 1984.
58. Dolva LO, Hanssen KF, Aadland E, Sand T: Thyrotropin-releasing hormone immunoreactivity in the gastrointestinal tract of man. *J Clin Endocrinol Metab* 56:524, 1983.
59. Kawano H, Daikoku S, Saito S: Location of thyrotropin-releasing hormone-like immunoreactivity in rat pancreas. *Endocrinology* 112:951, 1983.
60. Schaeffer JM, Brownstein MJ, Axelrod J: Thyrotropin-releasing hormone-like material in the rat retina: Changes due to environmental lighting. *Proc Natl Acad Sci USA* 74:3579, 1977.
61. Shambaugh G III, Kubek M, Wilber JF: Thyrotropin-releasing hormone activity in the human placenta. *J Clin Endocrinol Metab* 48:483, 1979.
62. Amarant T, Fridkin M, Koch Y: Luteinizing hormone-releasing hormone and thyrotropin-releasing hormone in human and bovine milk. *Eur J Biochem* 127:647, 1982.
63. Pekary AE, Meyer NV, Vaillant C, Hershman JM: Thyrotropin-releasing hormone and a homologous peptide in the male rat reproductive system. *Biochem Biophys Res Commun* 95:993, 1980.
64. Gershengorn MC: Mechanism of thyrotropin releasing hormone stimulation of pituitary hormone secretion. *Annu Rev Physiol* 48:515, 1986.
65. Greenspan SL, Klibanski A, Schoenfeld D, Ridgway EC: Pulsatile secretion of thyrotropin in man. *J Clin Endocrinol Metab* 63:661, 1986.
66. Martin JB, Reichlin S: *Clinical Neuroendocrinology,* 2nd ed. Philadelphia, Davis, 1987.
67. Reichlin S, Martin JB, Mitnick M, Boshans R, Grimm-Jorgensen Y, Bollinger J, et al: The hypothalamus in pituitary-thyroid regulation. *Recent Prog Horm Res* 28:229, 1972.
68. Koch Y, Goldhaber G, Fireman I, Zor U, Shani J, Tal E: Suppression of prolactin and thyrotropin secretion in the rat by antiserum to thyrotropin-releasing hormone. *Endocrinology* 100:1476, 1977.
69. Szabo M, Kovathana N, Gordon K, Frohman LA: Effect of passive immunization with an antiserum to thyrotropin (TSH)-releasing hormone on plasma TSH levels in thyroidectomized rats. *Endocrinology* 102:799, 1978.
70. Fraser HM, McNeilly AS: Effect of chronic immunoneutralization of thyrotropin-releasing hormone on the hypothalamic-pituitary-thyroid axis, prolactin, and reproductive function in the ewe. *Endocrinology* 111:1964, 1982.
71. Sheward WJ, Fraser HM, Fink G: Effect of immunoneutralization of thyrotrophin-releasing hormone on the release of thyrotrophin and prolactin during suckling or in response to electrical stimulation of the hypothalamus in the anaesthetized rat. *J Endocrinol* 106:113, 1985.
71a. Yamada M, Saga Y, Shibusawa N, et al: Tertiary hypothyroidism and hyperglycemia in mice with targeted disruption of the thyrotropin-releasing hormone gene. *Proc Natl Acad Sci USA,* 94:10862, 1997.
72. Noel GL, Dimond RC, Wartofsky L, Earll JM, Grantz AG: Studies of prolactin and TSH secretion by continuous infusion of small amounts of thyrotropin-releasing hormone (TRH). *J Clin Endocrinol Metab* 39:6, 1974.
73. Horn AM, Fraser HM, Fink G: Effects of antiserum to thyrotrophin-releasing hormone on the concentrations of plasma prolactin, thyrotrophin and LH in the pro-oestrous rat. *Endocrinology* 104:205, 1985.
74. De Greef WJ, Visser TJ: Evidence for the involvement of hypothalamic dopamine and thyrotrophin-releasing hormone in suckling-induced release of prolactin. *J Endocrinol* 91:213, 1981.
75. Van Haasteren GAC, van Toor H, Klootwijk W, Handler B, Linkels E, van der Schoot P, et al: Studies on the role of TRH and corticosterone in the regulation of prolactin and thyrotrophin secretion during lactation. *J Endocrinol* 148:325, 1996.
76. Gautvik KM, Tashjian AH Jr, Kourides IA, Weintraub BD, Graeber CT, Maloof F, et al: Thyrotropin-releasing hormone is not the sole physiologic mediator of prolactin release during suckling. *N Engl J Med* 290:1162, 1974.
77. Jeppsson S, Rannevik KON, Wide L: Influence of suckling and of suckling followed by TRH or LH-RH on plasma prolactin, TSH, GH and FSH. *Acta Endocrinol (Copenh)* 82:246, 1976.
78. Mori M, Yamada M: Thyroid hormones regulate the amount of thyrotrophin-releasing hormone in the hypothalamic median eminence of the rat. *J Endocrinol* 114:443, 1987.
79. Perrone MH, Hinkle PM: Regulation of pituitary receptors for thyrotropin releasing hormone by thyroid hormones. *J Biol Chem* 253:5168, 1978.
80. Snyder PJ, Jacobs LS, Utiger RD, Daughaday WH: Thyroid hormone inhibition of the prolactin response to thyrotropin-releasing hormone. *J Clin Invest* 52:2324, 1973.
81. Rondeel JMM, DeGreef WJ, Schoot PVD, Karels B, Klootwijk W, Visser TJ: Effect of thyroid status and paraventricular area lesions on the release of thyrotropin-releasing hormone and catecholamines into hypophyseal portal blood. *Endocrinology* 123:523, 1988.
82. Blake NG, Eclsand DJA, Foster OJF, Lightman SL: Inhibition of hypothalamic thyrotropin-releasing hormone messenger ribonucleic acid during food deprivation. *Endocrinology* 129:2714, 1991.
83. Fliers E, Guldenaar SEF, Wiersinga WM, Swaab DF: Decreased hypothalamic thyrotropin-releasing hormone gene expression in pa-

tients with nonthyroidal illness. *J Clin Endocrinol Metab* 82:4032, 1997.
84. Rondeel JMM, Jackson IMD: Molecular biology of the regulation of hypothalamic hormones. *J Endocrinol Invest* 16:219, 1993.
85. Hirooka Y, Hollander CS, Suzuki S, Ferdinand P, Juan S-I: Somatostatin inhibits release of thyrotropin releasing factor from organ cultures of rat hypothalamus. *Proc Natl Acad Sci USA* 75:4509, 1978.
86. Scanlon MF, Rodriguez-Arnao MD, Pourmand M, Shale DJ, Weightman DR, Lewis M, Hall R: Catecholaminergic interactions in the regulation of thyrotropin (TSH) secretion in man. *J Endocrinol Invest* 3:125, 1980.
87. Terry CL: Regulation of thyrotropin secretion by the central epinephrine system. *Neuroendocrinology* 42:102, 1986.
88. Smythe GA, Bradshaw JE, Cai WY, Symons RG: Hypothalamic serotoninergic stimulation of thyrotropin secretion and related brain-hormone and drug interactions in the rat. *Endocrinology* 111:1181, 1982.
89. Daneshdoost L, Gennarelli TA, Bashey HM, Savino PJ, Sergott RC, Bosley TM, et al: Recognition of gonadotroph adenomas in women. *N Engl J Med* 324:589, 1991.
90. Samuels MH, Ridgway EC: Central hypothyroidism. *Endocrinol Metab Clin N Amer* 21:903, 1992.
91. Matsuo H, Baba Y, Nair RMG, Arimura A, Schally AV: Structure of the porcine LH- and FSH-releasing hormone: I. The proposed amino acid sequence. *Biochem Biophys Res Commun* 43:1334, 1971.
92. Adelman JP, Mason AJ, Hayflick JS, Seeburg PH: Isolation of the gene and hypothalamic cDNA for the common precursor of gonadotropin-releasing hormone and prolactin release-inhibiting factor in human and rat. *Proc Natl Acad Sci USA* 83:179, 1986.
93. Radovick S, Wondisford FE, Nakayama Y, Yamada M, Cutler GB Jr, Weintraub BD: Isolation and characterization of the human gonadotropin-releasing hormone gene in the hypothalamus and placenta. *Mol Endocrinol* 4:476, 1990.
94. White RB, Eisen JA, Kasten TL, Fernald RD: Second gene for gonadotropin-releasing hormone in humans. *Proc Natl Acad Sci USA* 95:305, 1998.
95. Rubin BS, King JC, Millar RP, Seeburg PH, Arimura A: Processing of luteinizing hormone-releasing hormone precursor in rat neurons. *Endocrinology* 121:305, 1987.
96. Standish LJ, Adams LA, Vician L, Clifton DK, Steiner RAL: Neuroanatomical localization of cells containing gonadotropin releasing hormone messenger ribonucleic acid in the primate brain by in situ hybridization histochemistry. *Mol Endocrinol* 1:371, 1987.
97. Chappel SC: Neuroendocrine regulation of luteinizing hormone and follicle stimulating hormone: A review. *Life Sci* 36:97, 1985.
98. Plant TM, Krey LC, Moossy J, McCormack JT, Hess DL, Knobil E: The arcuate nucleus and the control of gonadotropin and prolactin secretion in the female rhesus monkey (Macaca mulatta). *Endocrinology* 102:52, 1978.
99. Schwanzel-Fukuda M, Pfaff DW: Origin of luteinizing hormone-releasing hormone neurons. *Nature* 338:161, 1989.
100. Seminara SB, Hayes FJ, Crowley WF Jr: Gonadotropin-releasing hormone deficiency in the human (idiopathic hypogonadotropic hypogonadism and Kallmann's syndrome): pathophysiological and genetic considerations. *Endocrine Revs* 19:521, 1998.
101. Ikeda Y, Luo X, Abbud R, Nilson JH, Parker KL: The nuclear receptor steroidogenic factor 1 is essential for the formation of the ventromedial hypothalamic nucleus. *Mol Endocrinol* 9:478, 1995.
102. Paull WK, Turkelson CM, Thomas CR, Arimura A: Immunohistochemical demonstration of a testicular substance related to luteinizing hormone-releasing hormone. *Science* 213:1263, 1981.
103. Aten RF, Ireland JJ, Weems CW, Behrman HR: Presence of gonadotropin-releasing hormone-like proteins in bovine and ovine ovaries. *Endocrinology* 120:1727, 1987.
104. Kakar SS: Molecular structure of the human gonadotropin-releasing hormone receptor gene. *Eur J Endocrinol* 137:183, 1997.
105. Naor Z, Harris D, Shacham S: Mechanism of GnRH receptor signaling: Combinatorial cross-talk of Ca^{2+} and protein kinase C. *Front Neuroendocrinol* 19:1, 1998.
106. Clayton RN: Gonadotrophin-releasing hormone: Its actions and receptors. *J Endocrinol* 120:11, 1989.
107. McCann SM, Mizunuma H, Samson WK, Lumpkin MD: Differential hypothalamic control of FSH secretion: A review. *Psychoneuroendocrinology* 8:299, 1983.
108. McNeilly AS: The control of FSH secretion. *Acta Endocrinol (Copenh)* 288:31, 1988.
109. Knight PG: Roles of inhibins, activins, and follistatin in the female reproductive system. *Front Neuroendocrinol* 17:476, 1996.
110. Belchetz PE, Plant TM, Nakai Y, Keogh EJ, Knobil E: Hypophysial responses to continuous and intermittent delivery of hypothalamic gonadotropin-releasing hormone. *Science* 202:631, 1978.
111. Gambacciani M, Liu JH, Swartz WH, Tueros VS, Yen SSC, Rasmussen DD: Intrinsic pulsatility of luteinizing hormone release from the human pituitary in vitro. *Neuroendocrinology* 45:402, 1987.
112. Veldhuis JD, Evans WS, Johnson ML, Wills MR, Rogol AD: Physiological properties of the luteinizing hormone pulse signal: Impact of intensive and extended venous sampling paradigms on its characterization in healthy men and women. *J Clin Endocrinol Metab* 62:881, 1986.
113. Filicori M, Santoro N, Merriam GR, Crowley WF: Characterization of the physiological pattern of episodic gonadotropin secretion throughout the human menstrual cycle. *J Clin Endocrinol Metab* 62:1136, 1986.
114. Clarke IJ, Cummins JT: The temporal relationship between gonadotropin releasing hormone (GnRH) and luteinizing hormone (LH) secretion in ovariectomized ewes. *Endocrinology* 111:1737, 1982.
115. Van Vugt DA, Diefenbach WD, Alston E, Ferin M: Gonadotropin-releasing hormone pulses in third ventricular cerebrospinal fluid of ovariectomized rhesus monkeys: Correlation with luteinizing hormone pulses. *Endocrinology* 117:1550, 1985.
116. Murdoch AP, Diggle PJ, Whites MC, Harris M, Kendall-Taylor P, Dunlop W: Luteinizing hormone in women is secreted in superimposed pulse patterns. *Clin Sci* 76:125, 1989.
117. Weiss J, Jameson JL, Burrin JM, Crowley WF Jr: Divergent responses of gonadotropin subunit messenger RNAs to continuous versus pulsatile gonadotropin-releasing hormone *in vitro*. *Mol Endocrinol* 4:557, 1990.
118. López FJ, Merchenthaler IJ, Moretto M, Negro-Vilar A: Modulating mechanisms of neuroendocrine cell activity: The LHRH pulse generator. *Cell Mol Neurobiol* 18:125, 1998.
119. Carmel PW, Araki S, Ferin M: Pituitary stalk portal blood collection in rhesus monkeys: Evidence for pulsatile release of gonadotropin-releasing hormone (GnRH). *Endocrinology* 99:243, 1976.
120. Brann DW, Mahesh VB: Regulation of gonadotropin secretion by steroid hormones. *Front Neuroendocrinol* 12:165, 1991.
121. Frawley LS, Neill JD: Biphasic effects of estrogen on gonadotropin-releasing hormone-induced luteinizing hormone release in monolayer cultures of rat and monkey pituitary cells. *Endocrinology* 114:659, 1984.
122. Gharib SD, Wierman ME, Shupnik MA, Chin WW: Molecular biology of the pituitary gonadotropins. *Endocrionol Rev* 11:177, 1990.
123. Clarke IJ, Cummins JT: Increased gonadotropin-releasing hormone pulse frequency associated with estrogen-induced luteinizing hormone surges in ovariectomized ewes. *Endocrinology* 116:2376, 1985.
124. Steele PA, Judd SJ: Positive and negative feed-back effect of progesterone on luteinizing hormone secretion in post-menopausal women. *Clin Endocrinol (Oxf)* 20:1, 1988.
125. Santen RJ: Is aromatization of testosterone to estradiol required for inhibition of luteinizing hormone secretion in men? *J Clin Invest* 56:1555, 1975.
126. Sheckter CB, Matsumoto AM, Bremner WJ: Testosterone administration inhibits gonadotropin secretion by an effect directly on the human pituitary. *J Clin Endocrinol Metab* 68:397, 1989.
127. Morishima A, Grumbach MM, Simpson ER, Fisher C, Kenan Q: Aromatase deficiency in male and female siblings caused by a novel mutation and the physiological role of estrogens. *J Clin Endocrinol Metab* 80:3689, 1995.
128. Carani C, Qin K, Simoni M, Faustini-Fustini M, Serpente S, Boyd J, et al: Effect of testosterone and estradiol in a man with aromatase deficiency. *N Engl J Med* 337:91, 1997.
129. Hayes FJ, Hall JE, Boepple PA, Crowley WF Jr: Differential control of gonadotropin secretion in the human: Endocrine role of inhibin. *J Clin Endocrinol Metab* 83:1835, 1998.
130. Wang QF, Farnworth PG, Findlay JK, Burger HG: Effect of purified 31K bovine inhibin on the specific binding of gonadotropin-releasing hormone to rat anterior pituitary cells in culture. *Endocrinology* 123:2161, 1988.
131. Carroll RS, Corrigan AZ, Gharib SD, Vale W, Chin WW: Inhibin, ac-

tivin, and follistatin: Regulation of follicle-stimulating hormone messenger ribonucleic acid levels. *Mol Endocrinol* 3:1969, 1989.
132. Condon TP, Leipheimer RE, Curry JJ: Preliminary evidence for a CNS site of action for ovarian inhibin. *Life Sci* 32:1691, 1983.
133. Freeman ME: Neuropeptide Y: A unique member of the constellation of gonadotropin-releasing hormones. *Endocrinology* 133:2411, 1993.
134. Gore AC, Roberts JL: Regulation of gonadotropin-releasing hormone gene expression *in vivo* and *in vitro*. *Front Neuroendocrinol* 18:209, 1997.
135. Lachelin GCL, Leblanc H, Yen SSC: The inhibitory effect of dopamine agonists on LH release in women. *J Clin Endocrinol Metab* 44:728, 1977.
136. Rasmussen DD, Liu JH, Wolf PL, Yen SSC: Gonadotropin-releasing hormone neurosecretion in the human hypothalamus: *In vitro* regulation by dopamine. *J Clin Endocrinol Metab* 62:479, 1986.
137. Selmanoff M, Shu C, Petersen SL, Barraclough A, Zoeller RT: Single cell levels of hypothalamic messenger ribonucleic acid encoding luteinizing hormone-releasing hormone in intact, castrated, and hyperprolactinemic male rats. *Endocrinology* 128:459, 1991.
138. Stevenaert A, Beckers A, Vandalem JL, Hennen G: Early normalization of luteinizing hormone pulsatility after successful transsphenoidal surgery in women with microprolactinomas. *J Clin Endocrinol Metab* 62:1044, 1986.
139. Hsueh AJW, Jones PBC: Gonadotropin releasing hormone: Extrapituitary actions and paracrine control mechanisms. *Annu Rev Physiol* 45:83, 1983.
140. Petraglia F, Volpe A, Genazzani AR, Rivier J, Sawchenko PE, Vale W: Neuroendocrinology of the human placenta. *Front Neuroendocrinol* 11:6, 1990.
141. Nikolics K, Mason AJ, Szönyi E, Ramachandran J, Seeburg PH: A prolactin-inhibiting factor within the precursor for human gonadotropin-releasing hormone. *Nature* 316:511, 1985.
142. Yu WH, Seeburg PH, Nikolics K, McCann SM: Gonadotropin-releasing hormone-associated peptide exerts a prolactin-inhibiting and weak gonadotropin-releasing activity *in vivo*. *Endocrinology* 123:390, 1988.
143. Millar RP, Wormald PJ, de L Milton RC: Stimulation of gonadotropin release by non-GnRH peptide sequence of the GnRH precursor. *Science* 232:68, 1986.
144. Reichlin S: Growth and the hypothalamus. *Endocrinology* 67:760, 1960.
145. Krulich L, Dhariwal APS, McCann SM: Stimulatory and inhibitory effects of purified hypothalamic extracts on growth hormone release from rat pituitary *in vitro*. *Endocrinology* 83:783, 1968.
146. Brazeau P, Vale W, Burgus R, Ling N, Butcher M, Rivier J, Guillemin R: Hypothalamic polypeptide that inhibits the secretion of immunoreactive pituitary growth hormone. *Science* 179:77, 1972.
147. Böhlen P, Brazeau P, Esch F, Ling N, Guillemin R: Isolation and chemical characterization of somatostatin-28 from rat hypothalamus. *Regul Pept* 2:359, 1981.
148. Rodriguez-Arnao MD, Rainbow SJ, Comaru-Schally AM, Meyers CA, Gomez-Pan A, Woodhead S, et al: Effects of prosomatostatin on growth hormone and prolactin response to arginine in man. *Lancet* 1:353, 1981.
149. Benoit R, Ling N, Bakhit C, Morrison JH, Alford B, Guillemin R: Somatostatin-28(1-12)-like immunoreactivity in the rat. *Endocrinology* 111:2149, 1982.
150. Shen LP, Rutter WJ: Sequence of the human somatostatin I gene. *Science* 224:168, 1984.
151. Goodman RH, Aron DC, Roos BA: Rat pre-prosomatostatin. *J Biol Chem* 258:5570, 1983.
152. Lechan RM, Goodman RH, Rosenblatt M, Reichlin S, Habener JF: Prosomatostatin-specific antigen in rat brain: Localization by immunocytochemical staining with an antiserum to a synthetic sequence of preprosomatostatin. *Proc Natl Acad Sci USA* 80:2780, 1983.
153. Charpenet G, Patel YC: Characterization of tissue and releasable molecular forms of somatostatin-28_{1-12}-like immunoreactivity in rat median eminence. *Endocrinology* 116:1863, 1985.
154. Patel YC, Reichlin S: Somatostatin in hypothalamus, extrahypothalamic brain, and peripheral tissues of the rat. *Endocrinology* 102:523, 1978.
155. Epelbaum J, Willoughby JO, Brazeau P, Martin JB: Effects of brain lesions and hypothalamic deafferentation on somatostatin distribution in the rat brain. *Endocrinology* 101:1495, 1977.
156. Delfs J, Robbins R, Connolly JL, Dichter M, Reichlin S: Somatostatin production by rat cerebral neurones in dissociated cell culture. *Nature* 283:676, 1980.
157. Alpert LC, Brawer JR, Patel YC, Reichlin S: Somatostatinergic neurons in anterior hypothalamus: Immunohistochemical localization. *Endocrinology* 98:255, 1976.
158. Chihara K, Arimura A, Kubli-Garfias C, Schally A: Enhancement of immunoreactive somatostatin release into hypophysial portal blood by electrical stimulation of the preoptic area in the rat. *Endocrinology* 105:1416, 1979.
159. Katakami H, Downs TR, Frohman LA: Inhibitory effect of hypothalamic medial preoptic area somatostatin on growth hormone-releasing factor in the rat. *Endocrinology* 123:1103, 1988.
160. Ishikawa K, Taniguchi Y, Kurosumi K, Suzuki M, Shinoda M: Immunohistochemical identification of somatostatin-containing neurons projecting to the median eminence of the rat. *Endocrinology* 121:94, 1987.
161. Pierotti AR, Harmar AJ: Multiple forms of somatostatin-like immunoreactivity in the hypothalamus and amygdala of the rat: Selective localization of somatostatin-28 in the median eminence. *J Endocrinol* 105:383, 1985.
162. Delfs JR, Zhu CH, Dichter MA: Coexistence of acetylcholinesterase and somatostatin-immunoreactivity in neurons cultured from rat cerebrum. *Science* 223:61, 1984.
163. Rorstad OP, Senterman MK, Hoyte KM, Martin JB: Immunoreactive and biological active somatostatin-like material in the human retina. *Brain Res* 199:488, 1980.
164. Van Leeuwen FW, de Raay C, Swaab DF, Fisser B: The localization of oxytocin, vasopressin, somatostatin and luteinizing hormone releasing hormone in the rat neurohypophysis. *Cell Tissue Res* 202:189, 1979.
165. Sundler F, Alumets J, Håkanson R, Bjõrklund L, Ljungberg O: Somatostatin-immunoreactive cells in medullary carcinoma of the thyroid. *Am J Pathol* 88:381, 1977.
166. Di SantAgnese PA, de Mesy Jensen KL: Somatostatin and/or somatostatin like immunoreactive endocrine-paracrine cells in the human prostate gland. *Arch Pathol Lab Med* 108:693, 1984.
167. Sasaki A, Yoshinaga K: Immunoreactive somatostatin in male reproductive system in humans. *J Clin Endocrinol Metab* 68:996, 1989.
168. Patel YC, Rao K, Reichlin S: Somatostatin in human cerebrospinal fluid. *N Engl J Med* 296:529, 1977.
169. Patel YC, Baquiran G, Srikant CB, Posner BI: Quantitative *in vivo* autoradiographic localization of [^{125}I-Tyr^{11}] Somatostatin-14-and [Leu^{8}, D-trp^{22}-^{125}I-tyr^{25}] somatostatin-28-binding sites in rat brain. *Endocrinology* 119:2262, 1986.
170. Reubi JC, Lang W, Maurer R, Koper JW, Lamberts SWJ: Distribution and biochemical characterization of somatostatin receptors in tumors of the human central nervous system. *Cancer Res* 47:5758, 1987.
171. Reisine T, Bell GI: Molecular biology of somatostatin receptors. *Endocrine Revs* 16:427, 1995.
172. Breder CD, Yamada Y, Yasuda K, Seino S, Saper CB, Bell GI: Differential expression of somatostatin receptor subtypes in brain. *J Neurosci* 12:3920, 1992.
173. Panetta R, Patel YC: Expression of mRNA for all five human somatostatin receptors (hsstr1-5) in pituitary tumors. *Life Sci* 56:333, 1995.
174. Reichlin S: Somatostatin. *N Engl J Med* 309:1495, 1983.
175. Skamene A, Patel YC: Infusion of graded concentrations of somatostatin in man: Pharmacokinetics and differential inhibitory effects on pituitary and islet hormones. *Clin Endocrinol (Oxf)* 20:555, 1984.
176. Wehrenberg WB, Ling N, Böhlen P, Esch F, Brazeau P, Guillemin R: Physiological roles of somatocrinin and somatostatin in the regulation of growth hormone secretion. *Biochem Biophys Res Comm* 109:562, 1982.
177. Plotsky PM, Vale W: Patterns of growth hormone-releasing factor and somatostatin secretion into the hypophysial-portal circulation of the rat. *Science* 230:461, 1985.
178. Terry LC, Willoughby JO, Brazeau P, Martin JB: Antiserum to somatostatin prevents stress-induced inhibition of growth hormone secretion in the rat. *Science* 192:565, 1976.
179. Tannenbaum GS, Epelbaum J, Colle E, Brazeau P, Martin JB: Anti-

serum to somatostatin reverses starvation-induced inhibition of growth hormone but not insulin secretion. *Endocrinology* 102:1909, 1978.
180. Tannenbaum GS, Ling N: The interrelationship of growth hormone (GH)-releasing factor and somatostatin in generation of the ultradian rhythm of GH secretion. *Endocrinology* 115:1952, 1984.
181. Frohman LA, Downs TR, Clarke IJ, Thomas GB: Measurement of growth hormone-releasing hormone and somatostatin in hypothalamic-portal plasma of unanesthetized sheep. *J Clin Invest* 86:17, 1990.
182. Epelbaum J, Moyse E, Tannenbaum GS, Kordon C, Beaudet A: Combined autoradiographic and immunohistochemical evidence for an association of somatostatin binding sites with growth hormone-releasing factor-containing nerve cell bodies in the rat arcuate nucleus. *J Neuroendocrinol* 1:109, 1989.
183. Aguila MC, McCann SM: Evidence that growth hormone-releasing factor stimulates somatostatin release *in vitro* via β-endorphin. *Endocrinology* 120:341, 1987.
184. Martha PM Jr, Blizzard RM, McDonald JA, Thorner MO, Rogol AD: A persistent pattern of varying pituitary responsivity to exogenous growth hormone (GH)-releasing hormone in GH-deficient children: Evidence supporting periodic somatostatin secretion. *J Clin Endocrinol Metab* 67:449, 1988.
185. Urman S, Critchlow V: Long term elevations in plasma thyrotropin, but not growth hormone, concentrations associated with lesion-induced depletion of median eminence somatostatin. *Endocrinology* 112:659, 1983.
186. Arimura A, Schally AV: Increase in basal and thyrotropin-releasing hormone (TRH)-stimulated secretion of thyrotropin (TSH) by passive immunization with antiserum to somatostatin in rats. *Endocrinology* 98:1069, 1976.
187. Williams TC, Kelijman M, Crelin WC, Downs TR, Frohman LA: Differential effects of somatostatin (SRIH) and a SRIH analog, SMS 201-995, on the secretion of growth hormone and thyroid-stimulating hormone in man. *J Clin Endocrinol Metab* 66:39, 1988.
188. Chihara K, Arimura A, Schally AV: Effect of intraventricular injection of dopamine, norepinephrine, acetylcholine, and 5-hydroxytryptamine on immunoreactive somatostatin release into rat hypophyseal portal blood. *Endocrinology* 104:1656, 1979.
189. Abe H, Kato Y, Chiba T, Taminato T, Fujita T: Plasma immunoreactive somatostatin levels in rat hypophysial portal blood: Effect of glucagon administration. *Life Sci* 23:1647, 1978.
190. Abe H, Chihara K, Chiba T, Matsukura S, Fujita T: Effect of intraventricular injection of neurotensin and other various bioactive peptides on plasma immunoreactive somatostatin levels in rat hypophysial portal blood. *Endocrinology* 108:1939, 1981.
191. Tapia-Arancibia L, Reichlin S: Vasoactive intestinal peptide and PHI stimulate somatostatin release from rat cerebral cortical and diencephalic cells in dispersed cell culture. *Brain Res* 336:67, 1985.
192. Scarborough DE, Lee SL, Dinarello CA, Reichlin S: Interleukin-1β stimulates somatostatin biosynthesis in primary cultures of fetal rat brain. *Endocrinology* 124:549, 1989.
193. Aguila MC, McCann SM: Stimulation of somatostatin release from median eminence tissue incubated *in vitro* by taurine and related amino acids. *Endocrinology* 116:1158, 1985.
194. Alba-Roth J, Müller OA, Schopohl J, von Werder K: Arginine stimulates growth hormone secretion by suppressing endogenous somatostatin secretion. *J Clin Endocrinol Metab* 67:1186, 1988.
195. Drouva SV, Epelbaum J, Henry M, Tapia-Arancibia L, Laplante E, Kordon C: Ionic channels involved in the LHRH and SRIF release from rat mediobasal hypothalamus. *Neuroendocrinology* 32:155, 1981.
196. Montminy MR, Sevarino KA, Wagner JA, Mandel G, Goodman RH: Identification of a cyclic-AMP-responsive element within the rat somatostatin gene. *Proc Natl Acad Sci USA* 83:6682, 1986.
197. Andrisani OM, Dixon JE: Somatostatin gene regulation. *Annu Rev Physiol* 52:793, 1990.
198. Beal MF, Mazurek MF, Tran VT, Chattha G, Bird ED, Martin JB: Reduced numbers of somatostatin receptors in the cerebral cortex in Alzheimer's disease. *Science* 229:289, 1985.
199. Aronin N, Cooper PE, Lorenz LJ, Bird ED, Sagar SM, Leeman SE, et al: Somatostatin is increased in the basal ganglia in Huntington disease. *Ann Neurol* 13:519, 1983.
200. Guillemin R, Rosenberg B: Humoral hypothalamic control of anterior pituitary: A study with combined tissue cultures. *Endocrinology* 57:599, 1955.
201. Saffran M, Schally AV, Benfey BG: Stimulation of the release of corticotrophin from the adenohypophysis by a neurohypophysial factor. *Endocrinology* 57:439, 1955.
202. Vale W, Spiess J, Rivier C, Rivier J: Characterization of a 41-residue ovine hypothalamic peptide that stimulates secretion of corticotropin and β-endorphin. *Science* 213:1394, 1981.
203. Shibahara S, Morimoto Y, Furutani Y, Notake M, Takahashi H, Shimizu S, et al: Isolation and sequence analysis of the human corticotropin-releasing factor precursor gene. *EMBO J* 2:775, 1983.
204. Favrod-Coune CA, Gaillard RC, Langevin H, Jaquier MC, Doci W, Muller AF: Anatomical localization of corticotropin-releasing activity in the human brain. *Life Sci* 39:2475, 1986.
205. Ohtani H, Mouri T, Sasaki A, Sasano N: Immunoelectron microscopic study of corticotropin-releasing factor in the human hypothalamus and pituitary gland. *Neuroendocrinology* 45:104, 1987.
206. Gibbs DM, Vale W: Presence of corticotropin releasing factor-like immunoreactivity in hypophysial portal blood. *Endocrinology* 111:1418, 1982.
207. Bruhn TO, Plotsky PM, Vale WW: Effect of paraventricular lesions on corticotropin-releasing factor (CRF)-like immunoreactivity in the stalk-median eminence: Studies on the adrenocorticotropin response to ether stress and exogenous CRF. *Endocrinology* 114:57, 1984.
208. Muglia L, Jacobson L, Majzoub JA: Production of corticotropin-releasing hormone-deficient mice by targeted mutation in embryonic stem cells. *Ann NY Acad Sci* 780:49, 1996.
209. Suda T, Tomori N, Tozawa F, Mouri T, Demura H, Shizume K: Distribution and characterization of immunoreactive corticotropin-releasing factor in human tissues. *J Clin Endocrinol Metab* 55:861, 1984.
210. Smith MA, Bissette G, Slotkin TA, Knight DL, Nemeroff CB: Release of corticotropin-releasing factor from rat brain regions *in vitro*. *Endocrinology* 118:1997, 1986.
211. Linton EA, Lowry PJ: Corticotrophin releasing factor in man and its measurement: A review. *Clin Endocrinol (Oxf)* 31:225, 1989.
212. Sasaki A, Sato S, Murakami O, Go M, Inoue M, Shimizu Y, et al: Immunoreactive corticotropin-releasing hormone present in human plasma may be derived from both hypothalamic and extrahypothalamic sources. *J Clin Endocrinol Metab* 65:176, 1987.
213. Behan DP, Linton EA, Lowry PJ: Isolation of the human plasma corticotrophin-releasing factor-binding protein. *J Endocrinol* 122:23, 1989.
214. Grino M, Guillaume V, Boudouresque F, Margioris AN, Grisoli F, Jaquet P, et al: Characterization of corticotropin-releasing hormone receptors on human pituitary corticotroph adenomas and their correlation with endogenous glucocorticoids. *J Clin Endocrinol Metab* 67:279, 1988.
215. Souza EB, Insel TR, Perrin MH, Rivier J, Vale WW, Kuhar MJ: Corticotropin-releasing factor receptors are widely distributed within the rat central nervous system: An autoradiographic study. *J Neurosci* 5:3189, 1985.
216. Vale W, Vaughan J, Perrin M: Corticotropin releasing factor (CRF) family of ligands and their receptors. *The Endocrinologist* 7:3S, 1997.
217. Kostich WA, Chen A, Sperle K, Largent BL: Molecular identification and analysis of a novel human corticotropin-releasing factor (CRF) receptor: The $CRF_{2\gamma}$ receptor. *Mol Endocrinol* 12:1077, 1998.
218. Schopohl J, Hauer A, Kaliebe T, Stalla GK, von Werder K, Müller OA: Repetitive and continuous administration of human corticotropin releasing factor to human subjects. *Acta Endocrinol (Copenh)* 112:157, 1986.
219. Rivier C, Rivier J, Vale W: Inhibition of adrenocorticotropic hormone secretion in the rat by immunoneutralization of corticotropin-releasing factor. *Science* 218:377, 1982.
220. Carnes M, Lent SJ, Goodman B, Mueller C, Saydoff J, Erisman S: Effects of immunoneutralization of corticotropin-releasing hormone on ultradian rhythms of plasma adrenocorticotropin. *Endocrinology* 126:1904, 1990.
221. Suda T, Tozawa F, Yamada M, Ushiyama T, Tomori N, Sumitomo T, et al: Insulin-induced hypoglycemia increases corticotropin-releasing factor messenger ribonucleic acid levels in rat hypothalamus. *Endocrinology* 123:1371, 1988.
222. Plotsky PM, Bruhn TO, Vale W: Hypophysiotropic regulation of adrenocorticotropin secretion in response to insulin-induced hypoglycemia. *Endocrinology* 117:323, 1985.
223. Liu JH, Muse K, Contreras P, Gibbs D, Vale W, Rivier J, et al: Aug-

mentation of ACTH-releasing activity of synthetic corticotropin releasing factor (CRF) by vasopressin in women. *J Clin Endocrinol Metab* 57:1087, 1983.
224. Whitnall MH, Mezey E, Gainer H: Co-localization of corticotropin-releasing factor and vasopressin in median eminence neurosecretory vesicles. *Nature* 317:248, 1985.
225. Engler D, Pham T, Fullerton MJ, Ooi G, Funder JW, Clarke IJ: Studies of the secretion of corticotropin-releasing factor and arginine vasopressin into the hypophysial-portal circulation of the conscious sheep. *Neuroendocrinology* 49:367, 1989.
226. Jia LG, Canny BJ, Orth DN, Leong DA: Distinct classes of corticotropes mediate corticotropin-releasing hormone and arginine vasopressin-stimulated adrenocorticotropin release. *Endocrinology* 128:197, 1991.
227. Oki Y, Nicholson WE, Orth DN: Role of protein kinase-C in the adrenocorticotropin secretory response to arginine vasopressin (AVP) and the synergistic response to AVP and corticotropin-releasing factor by perifused rat anterior pituitary. *Endocrinology* 127:350, 1990.
228. Whitnall MH, Key S, Gainer H: Vasopressin-containing and vasopressin-deficient subpopulations of corticotropin-releasing factor axons are differentially affected by adrenalectomy. *Endocrinology* 120:2180, 1987.
229. Beyer HS, Matta SG, Sharp BM: Regulation of the messenger ribonucleic acid for corticotropin-releasing factor in the paraventricular nucleus and other brain sites of the rat. *Endocrinology* 123:2117, 1988.
230. Plotsky PM, Sawchenko PE: Hypophysial-portal plasma levels, median eminence content, and immunohistochemical staining of corticotropin-releasing factor, arginine vasopressin, and oxytocin after pharmacological adrenalectomy. *Endocrinology* 120:1361, 1987.
231. Plotsky PM, Vale W: Hemorrhage-induced secretion of corticotropin-releasing factor-like immunoreactivity into the rat hypophysial portal circulation and its inhibition by glucocorticoids. *Endocrinology* 114:164, 1984.
232. Bilezikjian LM, Vale WW: Glucocorticoids inhibit corticotropin-releasing factor-induced production of adenosine 3′,5′-monophosphate in cultured anterior pituitary cells. *Endocrinology* 113:657, 1983.
233. Haláasz B, Szentáagothai: Control of adrenocorticotrophic function by direct influence of pituitary substance on the hypothalamus. *Acta Morphol Hung* 9:251, 1960.
234. Suda T, Yajima F, Tomori N, Sumitomo T, Nakagami Y, Ushiyama T, et al: Inhibitory effect of adrenocorticotropin on corticotropin-releasing factor release from rat hypothalamus *in vitro*. *Endocrinology* 118:459, 1985.
235. Taylor T, Dluhy RG, Williams GH: β-endorphin suppresses adrenocorticotropin and cortisol levels in normal human subjects. *J Clin Endocrinol Metab* 57:592, 1983.
236. Rittmaster RS, Cutler GB Jr, Sobel DO, Goldstein DS, Koppelman MCS, Loriaux DL, et al: Morphine inhibits the pituitary-adrenal response to ovine corticotropin-releasing hormone in normal subjects. *J Clin Endocrinol Metab* 60:891, 1985.
237. Plotsky PM, Otto S, Sutton S: Neurotransmitter modulation of corticotropin releasing factor secretion into the hypophysial-portal circulation. *Life Sci* 41:1311, 1987.
238. Calogero AE, Gallucci WT, Chrousos GP, Gold PW: Catecholamine effects upon rat hypothalamic corticotropin-releasing hormone secretion *in vitro*. *J Clin Invest* 82:839, 1988.
239. Tsagarakis S, Holly JMP, Rees LH, Besser GM, Grossman A: Acetylcholine and norepinephrine stimulate the release of corticotropin-releasing factor-41 from the rat hypothalamus *in vitro*. *Endocrinology* 123:1962, 1988.
240. Itoi K, Seasholtz AF, Watson SJ: Cellular and extracellular regulatory mechanisms of hypothalamic corticotropin-releasing hormone neurons. *Endocrine J* 45:13, 1998.
241. Chrousos GP: The hypothalamic-pituitary-adrenal axis and immune-mediated inflammation. *N Engl J Med* 332:1351, 1995.
242. Sternberg EM: Neural-immune interactions in health and disease. *J Clin Invest* 100:2641, 1997.
243. Suda T, Tozawa F, Ushiyama T, Sumitomo T, Yamada M, Demura H: Interleukin-1 stimulates corticotropin-releasing factor gene expression in rat hypothalamus. *Endocrinology* 126:1223, 1990.
244. Breder CD, Dinarello CA, Saper CB: Interleukin-1 immunoreactive innervation of the human hypothalamus. *Science* 240:321, 1988.
245. Lenz HJ, Raedler A, Greten H, Brown MR: CRF initiates biological actions within the brain that are observed in response to stress. *Am J Physiol* 21:34, 1987.
246. Taylor AL, Fishman LM: Corticotropin-releasing hormone. *N Engl J Med* 319:213, 1988.
247. Cutler GB Jr: Corticotropin-releasing hormone (CRH): Clinical studies and use. *The Endocrinologist* 7:10S, 1997.
248. Findling JW: Differential diagnosis of Cushing's syndrome. *The Endocrinologist* 7:17S, 1997.
249. Deuben RR, Meites J: Stimulation of pituitary growth hormone release by a hypothalamic extract in vitro. *Endocrinology* 74:408, 1964.
250. Thorner MO, Perryman RL, Cronin MJ, Rogol AD, Draznin M, Johanson A, et al: Somatotroph hyperplasia: Successful treatment of acromegaly by removal of a pancreatic islet tumor secreting a growth hormone-releasing factor. *J Clin Invest* 70:965, 1982.
251. Sassolas G, Chayvialle JA, Partensky C, Berger G, Trouillas J, Berger F, et al: Acromégalie, expression clinique de la production de facteurs de libération de l'hormone de croissance (G.R.F.) par une tumeur pancréatique. *Ann Endocrinol (Paris)* 44:347, 1983.
252. Guillemin R, Brazeau P, Böhlen P, Esch F, Ling N, Wehrenberg WB: Growth hormone-releasing factor from a human pancreatic tumor that caused acromegaly. *Science* 218:585, 1982.
253. Rivier J, Spiess J, Thorner M, Vale W: Characterization of a growth hormone-releasing factor from a human pancreatic islet tumour. *Nature* 300:276, 1982.
254. Sasaki A, Sato S, Yumita S, Hanew K, Miura Y, Yoshinaga K: Multiple forms of immunoreactive growth hormone-releasing hormone in human plasma, hypothalamus, and tumor tissues. *J Clin Endocrinol Metab* 68:180, 1989.
255. Gubler U, Monahan JJ, Lomedico PT, Bhatt RS, Collier KJ, Hoffman BJ, et al: Cloning and sequence analysis of cDNA for the precursor of human growth hormone-releasing factor, somatocrinin. *Proc Natl Acad Sci USA* 80:4311, 1983.
256. Mayo KE, Cerelli GM, Lebo RV, Bruce BD, Rosenfeld MG, Evans RM: Gene encoding human growth hormone-releasing factor precursor: Structure, sequence, and chromosomal assignment. *Proc Natl Acad Sci USA* 82:63, 1985.
257. Frohman LA, Downs TR, Chomczynski P, Brar A, Kashio Y: Regulation of growth hormone-releasing hormone gene expression and biosynthesis. *Yale J Biol Med* 62:427, 1989.
258. Frohman LA, Bernardis LL: Growth hormone and insulin levels in weanling rats with ventromedial hypothalamic lesions. *Endocrinology* 82:1125, 1968.
259. Frohman LA, Bernardis LL, Kant KJ: Hypothalamic stimulation of growth hormone secretion. *Science* 162:580, 1968.
260. Shibasaki T, Kiyosawa Y, Masuda A, Nakahara M, Imaki T, Wakabayashi I, et al: Distribution of growth hormone-releasing hormone-like immunoreactivity in human tissue extracts. *J Clin Endocrinol Metab* 59:263, 1984.
261. Leidy JW, Robbins RJ: Regional distribution of human growth hormone-releasing hormone in the human hypothalamus by radioimmunoassay. *J Clin Endocrinol Metab* 62:372, 1986.
262. Bloch B, Baillard RC, Brazeau P, Lin HD, Ling N: Topographical and ontogenetic study of the neurons producing growth hormone-releasing factor in human hypothalamus. *Regul Pept* 8:21, 1984.
263. Kashio Y, Chihara K, Kita T, Okimura Y, Sato M, Kadowaki S, et al: Effect of oral glucose administration on plasma growth hormone-releasing hormone (GHRH)-like immunoreactivity levels in normal subjects and patients with idiopathic GH deficiency: Evidence that GHRH is released not only from the hypothalamus but also from extrahypothalamic tissue. *J Clin Endocrinol Metab* 64:92, 1987.
264. Rosenthal SM, Schriock EA, Kaplan SL, Guillemin R, Grumbach MM: Synthetic human pancreas growth hormone-releasing factor ($hpGRF_{1-44}$-NH2) stimulates growth hormone secretion in normal men. *J Clin Endocrinol Metab* 57:677, 1983.
265. Thorner MO, Spiess J, Vance ML, Rogol AD, Kaiser DL, Webster JD, et al: Human pancreatic growth-hormone-releasing factor selectively stimulates growth-hormone secretion in man. *Lancet* 1:24, 1983.
266. Goldman JA, Molitch ME, Thorner MO, Vale W, Rivier J, Reichlin S: Growth hormone and prolactin responses to bolus and sustained infusions of GRH-1-40-OH in man. *J Endocrinol Invest* 10:397, 1987.

267. Ross RJ, Tsagarakis S, Grossman A, Preece MA, Rodda C, Davies PS, et al: Treatment of growth-hormone deficiency with growth-hormone-releasing hormone. *Lancet* 1:5, 1987.
268. Barinaga M, Yamonoto G, Rivier C, Vale W, Evans R, Rosenfeld MG: Transcriptional regulation of growth hormone gene expression by growth hormone-releasing factor. *Nature* 306:84, 1983.
269. Wehrenberg WB, Brazeau P, Luben R, Böhlen P, Guillemin R: Inhibition of the pulsatile secretion of growth hormone by monoclonal antibodies to the hypothalamic growth hormone releasing factor (GRF). *Endocrinology* 111:2147, 1982.
270. Wehrenberg WB, Bloch B, Phillips BJ: Antibodies to growth hormone-releasing factor inhibit somatic growth. *Endocrinology* 115:1218, 1984.
271. Jaffe CA, Friberg RD, Barkan AL: Suppression of growth hormone (GH) secretion by a selective GH-releasing hormone (GHRH) antagonist. Direct evidence for involvement of endogenous GHRH in the generation of GH pulses. *J Clin Invest* 92:695, 1993.
272. Lussier BT, French MB, Moor BC, Kraicer J: Free intracellular CA^{2+} concentration and growth hormone (GH) release from purified rat somatotrophs: III. Mechanism of action of GH-releasing factor and somatostatin. *Endocrinology* 128:592, 1991.
273. Chomczynski P, Downs TR, Frohman LA: Feedback regulation of growth hormone (GH)-releasing hormone gene expression by GH in rat hypothalamus. *Mol Endocrinol* 2:236, 1988.
274. Sato M, Chihara K, Kita T, Kashio Y, Okimura Y, Kitajima N, et al: Physiological role of somatostatin-mediated autofeedback regulation for growth hormone: Importance of growth hormone in triggering somatostatin release during a trough period of pulsatile growth hormone release in conscious male rats. *Neuroendocrinology* 50:139, 1989.
275. Kelijman M, Frohman LA: β-adrenergic modulation of growth hormone (GH) autofeedback on sleep-associated and pharmacologically induced GH secretion. *J Clin Endocrinol Metab* 69:1187, 1989.
276. Lippe BM, Van Herle AJ, LaFranchi SH, Uller RP, Lavin N, Kaplan SA: Reversible hypothyroidism in growth hormone-deficient children treated with human growth hormone. *J Clin Endocrinol Metab* 40:612, 1975.
277. Conway S, Richardson L, Speciale S, Moherek R, Mauceri H, Krulich L: Interaction between norepinephrine and serotonin in the neuroendocrine control of growth hormone release in the rat. *Endocrinology* 126:1022, 1990.
278. Baes M, Vale WW: Growth hormone-releasing factor secretion from fetal hypothalamic cell cultures is modulated by forskolin, phorbol esters, and muscimol. *Endocrinology* 124:104, 1989.
279. Schriock EA, Hulse JA, Harris DA, Kaplan SL, Grumbach MM: Evaluation of hypothalamic dysfunction in growth hormone (GH)-deficient patients using single versus multiple doses of GH-releasing hormone (GHRH-44) and evidence for diurnal variation in somatotroph responsiveness to GHRH in GH-deficient patients. *J Clin Endocrinol Metab* 65:1177, 1987.
280. Bowers CY, Momany FA, Reynolds GA, Hong A: On the in vitro and in vivo activity of a new synthetic hexapeptide that acts on the pituitary to specifically release growth hormone. *Endocrinology* 114:1537, 1984.
281. Camanni F, Ghigo E, Arvat E: Growth hormone-releasing peptides and their analogs. *Front Neuroendocrinol* 19:47, 1998.
281a. Kojima M, Hosada H, Date Y, Nakazato M, Matsuo H, Kangawa K: Gh relin is a growth-hormone-releasing acetylated peptide from stomach. *Nature* 402:656, 1999.
282. Howard AD, Feighner SD, Cully DF, Arena PP, Liberator PA, Rosenblum CI, et al: A receptor in pituitary and hypothalamus that functions in growth hormone release. *Science* 273:974, 1996.
283. Everett JW: Luteotrophic function of autografts of the rat hypophysis. *Endocrinology* 54:685, 1954.
284. Pasteels JL: Administration d'extraits hypothalamiques à l'hypophyse de rat *in vitro* dans le but d'en controler la secretion de prolactine. *C R Acad Sci Paris* 254:2664, 1962.
285. Birge CA, Jacobs LS, Hammer CT, Daughaday WH: Catecholamine inhibition of prolactin secretion by isolated rat adenohypophyses. *Endocrinology* 86:120, 1970.
286. Gibbs DM, Neill JD: Dopamine levels in hypophysial stalk blood in the rat are sufficient to inhibit prolactin secretion *in vivo*. *Endocrinology* 102:1895, 1978.
287. De Greef WJ, Plotsky PM, Neill JD: Dopamine levels in hypophysial stalk plasma and prolactin levels in peripheral plasma of the lactating rat: Effects of a simulated stimulus. *Neuroendocrinology* 32:229, 1981.
288. Mogg RJ, Samson WK: Interactions of dopaminergic and peptidergic factors in the control of prolactin release. *Endocrinology* 126:728, 1990.
289. Abe H, Engler D, Molitch ME, Bollinger-Gruber J, Reichlin S: Vasoactive intestinal peptide is a physiological mediator of prolactin release in the rat. *Endocrinology* 116:1383, 1985.
290. Quigley ME, Judd SJ, Gilliland GB, Yen SC: Functional studies of dopamine control of prolactin secretion in normal women and women with hyperprolactinemic pituitary microadenoma. *J Clin Endocrinol Metab* 50:994, 1980.
291. Leebaw WF, Lee LA, Woolf PD: Dopamine affects basal and augmented pituitary hormone secretion. *J Clin Endocrinol Metab* 47:480, 1978.
292. Bansal S, Lee LA, Woolf PD: Dopaminergic modulation of arginine mediated growth hormone and prolactin release in man. *Metabolism* 30:649, 1981.
293. Burrow GN, May PB, Spaulding SW, Donabedian RK: TRH and dopamine interactions affecting pituitary hormone secretion. *J Clin Endocrinol Metab* 45:65, 1977.
294. Neill JD, Frawley S, Plotsky PM, Tindall GT: Dopamine in hypophysial stalk blood of the rhesus monkey and its role in regulating prolactin secretion. *Endocrinology* 108:489, 1981.
295. Serri O, Kuchel O, Nguyen BU, Somma M: Differential effects of a low dose dopamine infusion on prolactin secretion in normal and hyperprolactinemic subjects. *J Clin Endocrinol Metab* 56:255, 1983.
296. Langer G, Sachar EJ: Dopaminergic factors in human prolactin regulation: Effects of neuroleptics and dopamine. *Psychoneuroendocrinology* 2:373, 1977.
297. Ben-Jonathan N: Dopamine: A prolactin-inhibiting hormone. *Endocrinol Rev* 6:564, 1985.
298. Creese I, Sibley DR, Leff SE: Agonist interactions with dopamine receptors: Focus on radioligand-binding studies. *Fed Proc* 43:2779, 1984.
299. Brown GM, Seeman P, Lee T: Dopamine/neuroleptic receptors in basal hypothalamus and pituitary. *Endocrinology* 99:1407, 1976.
300. Monsma FJ Jr, McVittie LD, Gerfen CR, Mahan LC, Sibley DR: Multiple D_2 dopamine receptors produced by alternative RNA splicing. *Nature* 342:926, 1989.
301. Thomas GB, Cummins JT, Doughton BW, Griffin N, Millar RP, de L Milton RC, Clarke IJ: Gonadotropin-releasing hormone associated peptide (GAP) and putative processed GAP peptides do not release luteinizing hormone or follicle stimulating hormone or inhibit prolactin secretion in the sheep. *Neuroendocrinology* 48:342, 1988.
302. Wormald PJ, Abrahamson MJ, Seeburg PH, Nikolics K, Millar RM: Prolactin-inhibiting activity of GnRH associated peptide in cultured human pituitary cells. *Clin Endocrinol (Oxf)* 30:149, 1989.
303. Schally AV, Redding TW, Arimura A, DuPont A, Linthicum GL: Isolation of gamma-aminobutyric acid from pig hypothalami and demonstration of its prolactin release-inhibiting (PIF) activity in vivo and in vitro. *Endocrinology* 100:681, 1977.
304. Grossman A, Delitala G, Yeo T, Besser GM: GABA and muscimol inhibit the release of prolactin from dispersed rat anterior pituitary cells. *Neuroendocrinology* 32:145, 1981.
305. Vincent SR, Hokfelt T, Wu JY: GABA neuron systems in the hypothalamus and the pituitary gland. *Neuroendocrinology* 34:117, 1982.
306. Mulcahey JJ, Neill JD: Gamma-aminobutyric acid (GABA) levels in hypophyseal stalk plasma of rats. *Life Sci* 32:453, 1982.
307. Tamminga CA, Neophytides A, Chase TN, Frohman LA: Stimulation of prolactin and growth hormone secretion by muscimol, a gamma aminobutyric acid agonist. *J Clin Endocrinol Metab* 47:1348, 1978.
308. Fioretti P, Melis GB, Paoletti AM, Pardo G, Caminiti F, Corsini GU, Martini L: Gamma-amino-β-hydroxy butyric acid stimulates prolactin and growth hormone release in normal women. *J Clin Endocrinol Metab* 47:1336, 1978.
309. Cavagnini F, Benetti G, Invitti C, Ramella G, Pinto M, Lazza M, et al: Effect of gamma aminobutyric acid on growth hormone and prolactin secretion in man: Influence of pimozide and domperidone. *J Clin Endocrinol Metab* 51:789, 1980.
310. Melis GB, Fruzzetti F, Paoletti AM, Mais V, Kemeny A, Striginy F, et al: Pharmacological activation of γ-aminobutyric acid-system blunts prolactin response to mechanical breast stimulation in puerperal women. *J Clin Endocrinol Metab* 58:201, 1984.
311. Kato Y, Iwasaki Y, Iwasaki J, Abe H, Yanaihara N, Imura H: Pro-

lactin release by vasoactive intestinal polypeptide in rats. *Endocrinology* 103:554, 1978.
312. Mezey E, Kiss JZ: Vasoactive intestinal peptide-containing neurons in the paraventricular nucleus may participate in regulating prolactin secretion. *Proc Natl Acad Sci USA* 82:245, 1985.
313. Malarkey WB, O'Dorisio TM, Kennedy M, Cataland S: The influence of vasoactive intestinal polypeptide and cholecystokinin on prolactin release in rat and human monolayer cultures. *Life Sci* 28:2489, 1981.
314. Said SI, Porter JC: Vasoactive intestinal polypeptide: Release into hypophyseal portal blood. *Life Sci* 24:227, 1979.
315. Carrillo AJ, Pool TB, Sharp ZD: Vasoactive intestinal peptide increases prolactin messenger ribonucleic acid content in GH_3 cells. *Endocrinology* 116:202, 1985.
316. Gozes I, Shani Y: Hypothalamic vasoactive intestinal peptide messenger ribonucleic acid is increased in lactating rats. *Endocrinology* 119:2497, 1986.
317. Yiangou Y, Gill JS, Chrysanthou BJ, Burrin J, Bloom SB: Infusion of prepro-VIP derived peptides in man: Effect on secretion of prolactin. *Neuroendocrinology* 48:615, 1988.
318. Lasaga M, Debeljuk L, Afione S, Aleman IT, Duvilanski B: Effects of passive immunization against vasoactive intestinal peptide on serum prolactin and LH levels. *Neuroendocrinology* 49:547, 1989.
319. Lopez FJ, Dominguez JR, Sanchez-Franco F, Negro-Vilar A: Role of dopamine and vasoactive intestinal peptide in the control of pulsatile prolactin secretion. *Endocrinology* 124:527, 1989.
320. Itoh N, Obata K, Yanaihara N, Okamoto H: Human preprovasoactive intestinal polypeptide contains a novel PHI-27-like peptide, PHM-27. *Nature* 304:547, 1983.
321. Sasaki A, Sato S, Go M, Shimizu Y, Murakami O, Hanew K, et al: Distribution, plasma concentration, and in vivo prolactin-releasing activity of peptide histidine methionine in humans. *J Clin Endocrinol Metab* 65:683, 1987.
322. Ohta H, Kato Y, Tojo H: Further evidence that peptide histidine isoleucine (PHI) may function as a prolactin releasing factor in rats. *Peptides* 6:708, 1985.
323. Kaji H, Chihara C, Abe H, Kita T: Effect of passive immunization with antisera to vasoactive intestinal polypeptide and peptide histidine isoleucine amide on 5-hydroxy-l-tryptophan-induced prolactin release in rats. *Endocrinology* 117:1914, 1985.
324. Hagen TC, Arnaout MA, Scherzer WJ, Martinson DR: Antisera to vasoactive intestinal polypeptide inhibit basal prolactin release from dispersed anterior pituitary cells. *Neuroendocrinology* 43:641, 1986.
325. Hinuma S, Habata Y, Fujii R, Kawamata Y, Hosoya M, Fukusumi S, et al: A prolactin-releasing peptide in the brain. *Nature* 393:272, 1998.
326. Palkovits M: Catecholamines in the hypothalamus: An anatomical review. *Neuroendocrinology* 33:123, 1981.
327. Seeman P, Van Tol HH: Dopamine receptor pharmacology. *Trends Pharmacol Sci* 15:264, 1994.
328. Sawchenko PE, Swanson LW: Central noradrenergic pathways for the integration of hypothalamic neuroendocrine and autonomic responses. *Science* 214:685, 1981.
329. Hökfelt TH, Elde R, Fuxe K, Johansson O, Ljungdahl Å, Goldstein M, et al: Aminergic and peptidergic pathways in the nervous system with special reference to the hypothalamus, in Reichlin S, Baldessarini RJ, Martin JB (eds): *The Hypothalamus.* New York, Raven Press, 1978, p 69.
330. De Souza EB: Beta-2 adrenergic receptors in pituitary: Identification, characterization, and autoradiographic localization. *Neuroendocrinology* 41:289, 1985.
331. Perkins SN, Evans WS, Thorner MO, Gibbs DM, Cronin MJ: β-adrenergic binding and secretory responses of the anterior pituitary. *Endocrinology* 177:1818, 1985.
332. Palkovits M, Saavedra JM, Jacobowitz DM, Kizer JS, Záborszky L, Brownstein MJ: Serotonergic innervation of the forebrain: Effect of lesions on serotonin and tryptophan hydroxylase levels. *Brain Res* 130:121, 1977.
333. Saavedra JM, Palkovits M, Kizer JS, Brownstein M, Zivin JA: Distribution of biogenic amines and related enzymes in the rat pituitary gland. *J Neuroendocrinol* 25:257, 1975.
334. Hoyer D, Clarke DE, Fozard JR, et al: International union of pharmacology classification of receptors for 5-hydroxytryptamine (serotonin). *Pharmacol Rev* 46:157, 1994.
335. De Souza EB: Serotonin and dopamine receptors in the rat pituitary gland: Autoradiographic identification, characterization and localization. *Endocrinology* 119:1534, 1986.
336. Johns MA, Azmitia EC, Krieger DT: Specific *in vitro* uptake of serotonin by cells in the anterior pituitary of the rat. *Endocrinology* 110:754, 1982.
337. Armstrong DM, Saper CB, Levey AI, Wainer BH, Terry RD: Distribution of cholinergic neurons in rat brain: Demonstrated by the immunocytochemical localization of choline acetyltransferase. *J Comp Neurol* 216:53, 1983.
338. Carmeliet P, Denef C: Synthesis and release of acetylcholine by normal and tumoral pituitary corticotrophs. *Endocrinology* 124:2218, 1989.
339. Decavel C, Van Den Pol AN: GABA: A dominant neurotransmitter in the hypothalamus. *J Comp Neurol* 302:1019, 1990.
340. Vincent SR, Hökfelt T, Skirboll LR, Wu JY: Hypothalamic γ-aminobutyric acid neurons project to the neocortex. *Science* 220:1309, 1983.
341. Fagg GE, Foster AC: Amino acid neurotransmitters and their pathways in the mammalian central nervous system. *Neuroscience* 9:701, 1983.
342. Knigge UP: Histaminergic regulation of prolactin secretion. *Dan Med Bull* 37:109, 1990.
343. Vance ML, Kaiser DL, Frohman LA, Rivier J, Vale WW, Thorner MO: Role of dopamine in the regulation of growth hormone secretion: Dopamine and bromocriptine augment growth hormone (GH)-releasing hormone-stimulated GH secretion in normal man. *J Clin Endocrinol Metab* 64:1136, 1987.
344. Chihara K, Kashio Y, Kita T, Okimura Y, Kaji H, Abe H, Fujita T: L-Dopa stimulates release of hypothalamic growth hormone-releasing hormone in humans. *J Clin Endocrinol Metab* 62:466, 1986.
345. Kitajima N, Chihara K, Abe H, Okimura Y, Fujii Y, Sato M, et al: Effects of dopamine on immunoreactive growth hormone-releasing factor and somatostatin secretion from rat hypothalamic slices perifused *in vitro. Endocrinology* 124:69, 1989.
346. Serri O, Deslauriers N, Brazeau P: Dual action of dopamine on growth hormone release *in vitro. Neuroendocrinology* 45:363, 1987.
347. Van Den Pol AN, Wuarin JP, Dudek FE: Glutamate, the dominant excitatory transmitter in neuroendocrine regulation. *Science* 250:1276, 1990.
348. Brann DW, Mahesh VB: Excitatory amino acids: Function and significance in reproduction and neuroendocrine regulation. *Front Neuroendocrinol* 15:3, 1994.
349. Lorenzo MJ, Sànchez-Franco F, de los Frailes MT, Reichlin S, Fernandez G, Cacicedo L: Synthesis and secretion of vasoactive intestinal peptide by rat fetal cerebral cortical and hypothalamic cells in culture. *Endocrinology* 125:1983, 1989.
350. Said SI: Vasoactive intestinal peptide. *J Endocrinol Invest* 9:191, 1986.
351. Rostène WH: Neurobiological and neuroendocrine functions of the vasoactive intestinal peptide (VIP). *Prog Neurobiol* 22:103, 1984.
352. Iversen LL: Substance P. *Br Med Bull* 38:277, 1982.
353. Rivier C, Brown M, Vale W: Effect of neurotensin, substance P and morphine sulfate on the secretion of prolactin and growth hormone in the rat. *Endocrinology* 100:751, 1977.
354. Arisawa M, Snyder GD, Yu WH, Palatis LRD: Physiologically significant inhibitory hypothalamic action of substance P on prolactin release in the male rat. *Neuroendocrinology* 52:22, 1990.
355. Jones MT, Gillham B, Homes MC, Hodges JR, Buckingham JC: Influence of substance P on hypothalamo-pituitary-adrenocortical activity in the rat. *J Endocrinol* 76:183, 1978.
356. Chad DA, Aronin N, Lundstrom R, McKeon P, Ross D, Molitch M, et al: Does capsaicin relieve the pain of diabetic neuropathy? *Pain* 43:387, 1990.
357. Brown DR, Miller RJ: Neurotensin. *Br Med Bull* 38:239, 1982.
358. Kataoka K, Mizuno N, Frohman LA: Regional distribution of immunoreactive neurotensin in monkey brain. *Brain Res Bull* 4:57, 1979.
359. Rostène WH, Alexander MJ: Neurotensin and neuroendocrine regulation. *Front Neuroendocrinol* 18:115, 1997.
360. Maeda K, Frohman LA: Dissociation of systemic and central effects of neurotensin on the secretion of growth hormone, prolactin, and thyrotropin. *Endocrinology* 103:1903, 1978.
361. Blackburn AM, Fletcher DR, Adrian TE, Bloom SR: Neurotensin infusion in man: Pharmacokinetics and effect on gastrointestinal and pituitary hormones. *J Clin Endocrinol Metab* 51:1257, 1980.
362. Moffett RB, Bumpus FM, Husain A: Cellular organization of the brain renin-angiotensin system. *Life Sci* 41:1867, 1987.

363. Sernia C, Zeng T, Kerr D, Wyse B: Novel perspectives on pituitary and brain angiotensinogen. *Front Neuroendocrinol* 18:174, 1997.
364. Aronsson M, Almasan K, Fuxe K, Cintra A, Härfstrand A, Gustafsson JÅ, Ganten D: Evidence for the existence of angiotensinogen mRNA in magnocellular paraventricular hypothalamic neurons. *Acta Physiol Scand* 132:585, 1988.
365. Saint-Andre J, Rohmer V, Alhenc-Gelas F, Menard J, Bigorgne J-C, Corvol P: Presence of renin, angiotensinogen, and converting enzyme in human pituitary lactotroph cells and prolactin adenomas. *J Clin Endocrinol Metab* 63:231, 1986.
366. Winer LM, Molteni A, Molitch ME: Effect of angiotensin-converting enzyme inhibition on pituitary hormone responses to insulin-induced hypoglycemia in humans. *J Clin Endocrinol Metab* 71:256, 1990.
367. Phillips MI: Biological effects of angiotensin in the brain, in Gross F, Vogel G (eds): *Enzymatic Release of Vasoactive Peptides.* New York, Raven, 1980, p 335.
368. Vijayan E, Samson WK, McCann SM: In vitro and in vivo effects of cholecystokinin on gonadotropin, prolactin, growth hormone and thyrotropin release in the rat. *Brain Res* 172:295, 1979.
369. Tanomoto K, Tamminga CA, Chase TN: Intracerebroventricular injection of cholecystokinin octapeptide elevates plasma prolactin levels through stimulation of vasoactive intestinal polypeptide. *Endocrinology* 121:127, 1987.
370. Gibbs J, Smith GP: Satiety: The roles of peptides from the stomach and intestine. *Fed Proc* 45:1391, 1986.
371. Morley JE: Neuroendocrine effects of endogenous opioid peptides in human subjects: A review. *Psychoneuroendocrinology* 8:361, 1983.
372. Darland T, Heinricher MM, Grandy DK: Orphanin FQ/nociceptin: A role in pain and analgesia, but so much more. *Trends Neurosci* 21:215, 1998.
373. Smith AI, Funder JW: Proopiomelanocortin processing in the pituitary, central nervous system, and peripheral tissues. *Endocrinol Rev* 9:159, 1988.
374. Beaumont A: Putative peptide neurotransmitters: The opioid peptides. *Int Rev Exp Pathol* 25:279, 1983.
375. Bloom FE: The endorphins: A growing family of pharmacologically pertinent peptides. *Ann Rev Pharmacol Toxicol* 23:151, 1983.
376. Mollereau C, Simons MJ, Soularue P, Liners F, Vassart G, Meunier JC, et al: Structure, tissue distribution, and chromosomal localization of the prepronociceptin gene. *Proc Natl Acad Sci USA* 93:8666, 1996.
377. Olson GA, Olson RD, Kastin AJ: Endogenous opiates: 1996. *Peptides* 18:1651, 1997.
378. Spiler IJ, Molitch ME: Lack of modulation of pituitary hormone stress response by neural pathways involving opiate receptors. *J Clin Endocrinol Metab* 50:516, 1980.
379. Ma LY, Zhang ML, Yang XD, Tian DR, Qi JS, Zhang DM: Neuroendocrinology of atrial natriuretic polypeptide in the brain. *Neuroendocrinology* 53:12, 1991.
380. McGregor A, Richards M, Espiner E, Yandle T: Brain natriuretic peptide administered to man: Actions and metabolism. *J Clin Endocrinol Metab* 70:1103, 1990.
381. Kitajima N, Chihara K, Abe H, Okimura Y, Shakutsui S: Galanin stimulates immunoreactive growth hormone-release factor secretion from rat hypothalamic slices perifused in vitro. *Life Sci* 47:2371, 1990.
382. Davis TME, Burrin JM, Bloom SR: Growth hormone (GH) release in response to GH-releasing hormone in man is 3-fold enhanced by galanin. *J Clin Endocrinol Metab* 65:1248, 1987.
383. Hooi SC, Maiter DM, Martin JB, Koenig JI: Galaninergic mechanisms are involved in the regulation of corticotropin and thyrotropin secretion in the rat. *Endocrinology* 127:2281, 1990.
384. Vrontakis ME, Sano T, Kovacs K, Friesen HG: Presence of galanin-like immunoreactivity in nontumorous corticotrophs and corticotroph adenomas of the human pituitary. *J Clin Endocrinol Metab* 70:747, 1990.
385. Kalra SP, Kalra PS: Nutritional infertility: The role of the interconnected hypothalamic neuropeptide Y-galanin-opioid network. *Front Neuroendocrinol* 17:371, 1996.
386. Yoshizawa T, Shinmi O, Giaid A, Yanagisawa M, Gibson SJ, Kimura S, et al: Endothelin: A novel peptide in the posterior pituitary system. *Science* 247:462, 1990.
387. Stojilkovic SS, Merelli F, Iida T, Krsmanovic LZ, Catt KJ: Endothelin stimulation of cytosolic calcium and gonadotropin secretion in anterior pituitary cells. *Science* 248:1663, 1990.
388. Samson WK, Skala KD, Alexander BD, Steven Huang FL: Pituitary site of action of endothelin: Selective inhibition of prolactin release in vitro. *Biochem Biophys Res Commun* 169:737, 1990.
389. Toni R, Jackson IMD, Lechan RM: Neuropeptide-Y-immunoreactive innervation of thyrotropin-releasing hormone-synthesizing neurons in the rat hypothalamic paraventricular nucleus. *Endocrinology* 126:2444, 1990.
390. Härfstrand A: Brain neuropeptide Y mechanisms: Basic aspects and involvement in cardiovascular and neuroendocrine regulation. *Acta Physiol Scand* 131:565, 1987.
391. Lowenstein CJ, Dinerman JL, Snyder SH: Nitric oxide: A physiologic messenger. *Ann Intern Med* 120:227, 1994.
392. Brann DW, Bhat GK, Lamar CA, Mahesh VB: Gaseous transmitters and neuroendocrine regulation. *Neuroendocrinology* 65:385, 1997.
393. Nelson RJ, Kriegsfeld LJ, Dawson VL, Dawson TM: Effects of nitric oxide on neuroendocrine function and behavior. *Front Neuroendocrinol* 18:463, 1997.
394. Erlich SS, Apuzzo MLJ: The pineal gland: Anatomy, physiology, and clinical significance. *J Neurosurg* 63:321, 1985.
395. Reiter RJ: Pineal melatonin: Cell biology of its synthesis and of its physiological interactions. *Endocrinol Rev* 12:151, 1991.
396. Brzezinski A: Melatonin in humans. *N Engl J Med* 336:186, 1997,
397. Relkin R: Pineal-hormonal interactions, in Relkin R (ed): *The Pineal Gland.* New York, Elsevier, 1983, p 225.
398. Waldhauser F, Leberman HR, Lynch HJ, Waldhauser M, Herkner K, Frisch H, et al: A pharmacological dose of melatonin increases PRL levels in males without altering those of GH, LH, FSH, TSH, testosterone or cortisol. *Neuroendocrinology* 46:125, 1987.
399. Bellastella A, Pisano G, Iorio S, Pasquali D, Orio F, Venditto T, et al: Endocrine secretions under abnormal light-dark cycles and in the blind. *Horm Res* 49;153, 1998.
400. Winer LM, Shaw MA, Baumann G: Basal plasma growth hormone levels in man: New evidence for rhythmicity of growth hormone secretion. *J Clin Endocrinol Metab* 70:1678, 1990.
401. Veldhuis JD, Iranmanesh A, Johnson ML, Lizarralde G: Twenty-four-hour rhythms in plasma concentrations of adenohypophyseal hormones are generated by distinct amplitude and/or frequency modulation of underlying pituitary secretory bursts. *J Clin Endocrinol Metab* 71:1616, 1990.
402. Stewart JK, Clifton DK, Koerker DJ, Rogol AD: Pulsatile release of growth hormone and prolactin from the primate pituitary *in vitro.* *Endocrinology* 116:1, 1985.
403. Turek FW: Circadian rhythms. *Horm Res* 49:109, 1998.
404. Dunlap JC: Genetic and molecular analysis of circadian rhythms. *Annu Rev Genet* 30:579, 1996.
405. King DP, Zhao Y, Sangoram AM, Wilsbacher LD, Tanaka M, Antoch MP, et al: Positional cloning of the mouse circadian *Clock* gene. *Cell* 89:641, 1997.
406. Tei H, Okamura H, Shigeyoshi Y, Fukuhara C, Ozawa R, Hirose M, et al: Circadian oscillation of a mammalian homologue of the *Drosophila period* gene. *Nature* 389:512, 1997.
407. Sun ZS, Abrecht U, Zhuchenko O, Bailey J, Eichele G, Lee CC: *RIGUI,* a putative mammalian ortholog of the *Drosophila period* gene. *Cell* 90:1003, 1997.
408. Van Cauter E: Diurnal and ultradian rhythms in human endocrine function: A minireview. *Horm Res* 34:45, 1990.
409. Weitzman ED, Boyar RM, Kapen S: The relationship of sleep and sleep stages of neuroendocrine secretion and biological rhythms in man. *Recent Prog Horm Res* 31:399, 1975.
410. Frisch RE: Body fat, menarche, and reproductive ability. *Semin Reprod Endocrinol* 3:45, 1985.
411. Veldhuis JD, Johnson L: Operating characteristics of the hypothalamo-pituitary-gonadal axis in men: Circadian, ultradian, and pulsatile release of prolactin and its temporal coupling with luteinizing hormone. *J Clin Endocrinol Metab* 67:116, 1988.
412. Sassin JF, Frantz AG, Kapen S, Weitzman ED: The nocturnal rise of human prolactin is dependent upon sleep. *J Clin Endocrinol Metab* 37:436, 1973.
413. Stern JM, Reichlin S: Prolactin circadian rhythm persists throughout lactation in women. *Neuroendocrinology* 51:31, 1990.
414. Van Reeth O: Sleep and circadian disturbances in shift work: Strategies for their management. *Horm Res* 49:158, 1998.

415. Donovan JL, Nesbit GM: Distinction of masses involving the sella and suprasellar space: Specificity of imaging features. *AJR* 167:597, 1996.
416. Naidich MJ, Russell EJ: Current approaches to imaging of the sellar region and pituitary. *Endocrine Metab Clin N Amer* 28:45, 1999.
417. Hintz RL, Menking M, Sotos JF: Familial holoprosencephaly with endocrine dysgenesis. *J Pediatr* 72:81, 1968.
418. Masera N, Grant DB, Stanhope R, Preece MA: Diabetes insipidus with impaired osmotic regulation in septo-optic dysplasia and agenesis of the corpus callosum. *Arch Dis Child* 70:51, 1994.
419. Huseman CA, Kelch RP, Hopwood NJ, Zipf WB: Sexual precocity in association with septo-optic dysplasia and hypothalamic hypopituitarism. *J Pediatr* 92:748, 1978.
420. Hermesz E, Mackem S, Mahon KA: *Rpx*: A novel anterior-restricted homeobox gene progressively activated in the prechordal plate, anterior neural plate, and Rathke's pouch of the mouse embryo. *Development* 122:41, 1996.
421. Dattani MT, Martinez-Barbera J-P, Thomas PQ, Brickman JM, Gupta R, Mårtensson I-L, et al: Mutations in the homeobox gene *HESX1/Hesx1* associated with septo-optic dysplasia in human and mouse. *Nat Genet* 19:125, 1998.
422. Radovick S, Nations M, Du Y, Berg LA, Weintraub BD, Wondisford FE: A mutation in the POU-homeodomain of Pit-1 responsible for combined pituitary hormone deficiency. *Science* 257:1116, 1992.
423. Pfäffle RW, DiMattia GE, Parks JS, Brown MR, Wit JM, Jansen M, et al: Mutation of the POU-specific domain of Pit-1 and hypopituitarism without pituitary hypoplasia. *Science* 257:1118, 1992.
424. Sornson MW, Wu W, Dasen JS, Flynn SE, Norman DJ, O'Connell SM, et al: Pituitary lineage determination by the *Prophet of Pit-1* homeodomain factor defective in Ames dwarfism. *Nature* 384:327, 1996.
425. Wu W, Cogan JD, Pfäffle RW, Dasen J, Frisch H, O'Connell SM, Flynn SE, et al: Mutations in *PROP1* cause familial combined pituitary hormone deficiency. *Nat Genet* 18:147, 1998.
426. Cogan JD, Wu W, Phillips JA III, Arnhold IJP, Agapito A, Fofanova OV, et al: The PROP1 2-base pair deletion is a common cause of combined pituitary hormone deficiency. *J Clin Endocrinol Metab* 83:3346, 1998.
427. Rudman D, Davis GT, Priest JH, Patterson JH, Kutner MH, Heymsfield SB, et al: Prevalence of growth hormone deficiency in children with cleft lip or palate. *J Pediatr* 93:378, 1978.
428. Abrahams JJ, Trefelner E, Boulware SD: Idiopathic growth hormone deficiency: MR findings in 35 patients. *AJNR* 12:155, 1991.
429. Triulzi F, Scotti G, diNatale B, Pellini C, Lukezic M, Scognamiglio M, et al: Evidence of a congenital midline brain anomaly in pituitary dwarfs: A magnetic resonance imaging study in 101 patients. *Pediatrics* 93:409, 1994.
430. Lieblich JM, Rosen SW, Guyda H, Reardan J, Schaaf M: The syndrome of basal encephalocele and hypothalamic-pituitary dysfunction. *Ann Intern Med* 89:910, 1978.
431. Quinton R, Duke VM, deZoysa PA, Bouloux P-MG: The neurobiology of Kallmann's syndrome. *Hum Reprod* 11:121, 1996.
432. DiMeglio LA, Pescovitz OH: Disorders of puberty: Inactivating and activating molecular mutations. *J Pediatr* 131:S8, 1997.
433. Lieblich JM, Rogol AD, White BJ, Rosen SW: Syndrome of anosmia with hypogonadotropic hypogonadism (Kallmann syndrome). *Am J Med* 73:506, 1982.
434. Hochberg Z, Moses AM, Miller M, Benderli A, Richman RA: Altered osmotic threshold for vasopressin release and impaired thirst sensation: Additional abnormalities in Kallmann's syndrome. *J Clin Endocrinol Metab* 55:779, 1982.
435. Arafah BM: Reversible hypopituitarism in patients with large nonfunctioning pituitary adenomas. *J Clin Endocrinol Metab* 62:1173, 1986.
436. Molitch ME: Natural history and diagnosis of clinically non-functioning adenomas, in Webb SM (ed): *Pituitary Tumors: Epidemiology, Pathogenesis and Management.* BioScientifica, Ltd., Bristol, U.K., 1998, pp 15–27.
437. Molitch ME, Reichlin S: Hypothalamic hyperprolactinemia: Neuroendocrine regulation of prolactin secretion in patients with lesions of the hypothalamus and pituitary stalk, in MacLeod RM, Thorner MO, Scapagnini U (eds): *Prolactin Basic and Clinical Correlates.* Padua, Italy, Liviana Press, 1985, p 709.
438. Mukerjee JJ, Islam N, Kaltsas G, Lowe DG, Charlseworth M, Afshar F, et al: Clinical, radiological and pathological features of patients with Rathke's cleft cysts: Tumors that may recur. *J Clin Endocrinol Metab* 82:2357, 1997.
439. El-Mahdy W, Powell M: Transsphenoidal management of 28 symptomatic Rathke's cleft cysts, with special reference to visual and hormonal recovery. *Neurosurgery* 24:7, 1998.
440. Bülow B, Awwewell R, Hagmar L, Malmström P, Nordström C-H, Erfurth EM: Postoperative prognosis in craniopharyngioma with respect to cardiovascular mortality, survival and tumor recurrence. *J Clin Endocrinol Metab* 83:3897, 1998.
441. Freda PU, Wardlaw SL, Post KD: Unusual causes of sellar/parasellar masses in a large transsphenoidal surgical series. *J Clin Endocrinol Metab* 81:3455, 1996.
442. DeVile CJ, Grant DB, Hayward RD, Stanhope R: Growth and endocrine sequelae of craniopharyngioma. *Arch Dis Child* 75:108, 1996.
443. Kapcala LP, Molitch ME, Post KD, Biller BJ, Prager RJ, Jackson I, et al: Galactorrhea, oligo/amenorrhea, and hyperprolactinemia in patients with craniopharyngiomas. *J Clin Endocrinol Metab* 51:798, 1980.
444. Landolt AM, Zachmann M: Results of transsphenoidal extirpation of craniopharyngiomas and Rathke's cysts. *Neurosurgery* 28:410, 1991.
445. Prasad D, Steiner M, Steiner L: Gamma knife surgery for craniopharyngioma. *Acta Neurochir* 134:167, 1995.
446. Chaganti RSK, Rodriguez E, Mathew S: Origin of adult male mediastinal germ-cell tumours. *Lancet* 343:1130, 1994.
447. Sklar CA, Grumbach MM, Kaplan SL, Conte FA: Hormonal and metabolic abnormalities associated with central nervous system germinoma in children and adolescents and the effect of therapy: Report of 10 patients. *J Clin Endocrinol Metab* 52:9, 1981.
448. Huh SJ, Shin KH, Kim IH, Ahn YC, Ha SW, Park CI: Radiotherapy of intracranial germinomas. *Radiother Oncol* 38:19, 1996.
449. Sherwin RP, Grassi JE, Sommer SC: Hamartomatous malformation of the posterolateral hypothalamus. *Lab Invest* 11:89, 1962.
450. Puchner MJA, Lüdecke DK, Saeger W, Riedel M, Asa SL: Gangliocytomas of the sellar region—a review. *Exp Clin Endocrinol* 10:129, 1995.
451. Judge DM, Kulin HE, Page R, Santen R, Trapukdi S: Hypothalamic hamartoma: A source of luteinizing-hormone-releasing factor in precocious puberty. *N Engl J Med* 296:7, 1977.
452. Stewart L, Steinbok P, Daaboul J: Role of surgical resection in the treatment of hypothalamic hamartomas causing precocious puberty. *J Neurosurg* 88:340, 1998.
453. Mahachoklertwattana P, Kaplan SL, Grumbach MM: The luteinizing hormone-releasing hormone-secreting hypothalamic hamartoma is a congenital malformation: Natural history. *J Clin Endocrinol Metab* 77:118, 1993.
454. Chapelon C, Ziza JM, Piette JC, Levy Y, Raguin G, Wechsler B, et al: Neurosarcoidosis: Signs, course and treatment in 35 confirmed cases. *Medicine (Baltimore)* 69:261, 1990.
455. Stuart CA, Neelon FA, Lebovitz HE: Hypothalamic insufficiency: The cause of hypopituitarism in sarcoidosis. *Ann Intern Med* 88:589, 1978.
456. Guoth MS, Kim J, deLotbinere ACJ, Brines ML: Neurosarcoidosis presenting as hypopituitarism and a cystic mass. *Am J Med* Sci 315:220, 1998.
457. Stuart CA, Neelon FA, Lebovitz HE: Disordered control of thirst in hypothalamic-pituitary sarcoidosis. *N Engl J Med* 303:1078, 1980.
458. Vesely DL: Hypothalamic sarcoidosis: A new cause of morbid obesity. *South Med J* 82:758, 1989.
459. Willman CL, Busque L, Griffith B, Favara Be, McClain KL, Duncan MH: Langerhans-cell histiocytosis (histiocytosis X)-clonal proliferative disease. *N Engl J Med* 331:154, 1994.
460. Kaltsas GA, Powles TB, Evanson J, et al: Hypothalamo-pituitary abnormalities in adult patients with Langerhans cell histiocytosis: clinical, endocrinological, and radiological features, and response to treatment. *J Clin Endocrinol Metab* 85:1370, 2000.
461. Tien RD, Newton TH, McDermott MW, Dillon WP, Kucharczyk J: Thickened pituitary stalk on MR images in patients with diabetes insipidus and Langerhans cell histiocytosis. *AJNR* 11:703, 1990.
462. Goodman RH, Post KD, Molitch ME, Adelman LS, Altemus LR, Johnston H: Eosinophilic granuloma mimicking a pituitary tumor. *Neurosurgery* 5:723, 1979.
463. Mohr PD: Hypothalamic-pituitary abscess. *Postgrad Med J* 51:468, 1975.

464. Lichtenstein MJ, Tilley WS, Sandler MP: The syndrome of hypothalamic hypopituitarism complicating viral meningoencephalitis. *J Endocrinol Invest* 5:111, 1982.
465. Lam KSL, Sham MMK, Tam SCF, Ng MMT, Ma HTG: Hypopituitarism after tuberculous meningitis in childhood. *Ann Intern Med* 118:701, 1993.
466. Hama S, Arita K, Kurisu K, Sumida M, Kurihara K: Parasellar chronic inflammatory disease presenting Tolosa-Hunt syndrome, hypopituitarism and diabetes insipidus: A case report. *Endocrine J* 43:503, 1996.
467. Imura H, Nako K, Shimatsu A, Ogawa Y, Sando T, Fujisawa I, et al: Lymphocytic infundibuloneurohypophysitis as a cause of central diabetes insipidus. *N Engl J Med* 329:683, 1993.
468. Edwards OM, Clark JDA: Post-traumatic hypopituitarism. *Medicine (Baltimore)* 65:281, 1986.
469. King LR, Knowles HC Jr, McLaurin RL, Brielmaier J, Perisutti G, Piziak VK: Pituitary hormone response to head injury. *Neurosurgery* 9:229, 1981.
470. Crompton MR: Hypothalamic lesions following closed head injury. *Brain* 94:165, 1971.
471. Constine LS, Woolf PD, Cann D, Mick G, McCormick K, Raubertas RF, et al: Hypothalamic-pituitary dysfunction after radiation for brain tumors. *N Engl J Med* 328:87, 1993.
472. Huang KE: Assessment of hypothalamic-pituitary function in women after external head irradiation. *J Clin Endocrinol Metab* 49:623, 1979.
473. Snyder PJ, Fowble BF, Schatz NJ, Savino PJ, Gennarelli TA: Hypopituitarism following radiation therapy of pituitary adenomas. *Am J Med* 81:457, 1986.
474. Littley MD, Shalet SM, Beardwell CG et al: Hypopituitarism following external radiotherapy for pituitary tumours in adults. *Quart J Med* 70:145, 1989.
475. Brada M, Rajan B, Traish D et al: The long-term efficacy of conservative surgery and radiotherapy in the control of pituitary adenomas. *Clin Endocrinol* 38:571, 1993.
476. Hansen LK, Molitch ME: Postoperative radiotherapy for clinically nonfunctioning pituitary adenomas. *The Endocrinologist* 8:71, 1998.
477. Albright F, Butler AM, Hampton AO, Smith P: Syndrome characterized by osteitis fibrosa disseminata, areas of pigmentation and endocrine dysfunction, with precocious puberty in females. *N Engl J Med* 216:727, 1937.
478. Cuttler L, Jackson JA, Uz-Zafar MS, Levitsky LL, Mellinger RC, Frohman LA: Hypersecretion of growth hormone and prolactin in McCune-Albright syndrome. *J Clin Endocrinol Metab* 68.1148, 1989.
479. Hall R, Warrick C: Hypersecretion of hypothalamic releasing hormones: A possible explanation of the endocrine manifestations of polyostotic fibrous dysplasia (Albright's syndrome). *Lancet* 1:1313, 1972.
480. Weinstein LS, Shenker A, Gejman PV, Merino MJ, Friedman E, Spiegel AM: Activating mutations of the stimulatory G protein in the McCune-Albright syndrome. *N Engl J Med* 325:1688, 1991.
481. Landis CA, Masters SB, Spada A, Pace AM, Bourne HR, Vallar L: GTPase inhibiting mutations activate the a chain of G_x and stimulate adenylyl cyclase in human pituitary tumours. *Nature* 340:692, 1989.
482. Lippe B, Wong SLR, Kaplan SA: Simultaneous assessment of growth hormone and ACTH reserve in children pretreated with diethylstilbestrol. *J Clin Endocrinol Metab* 33:949, 1971.
483. Phillips JA III, Cogan JD: Molecular basis of familial human growth hormone deficiency. *J Clin Endocrinol Metab* 78:11, 1994.
484. Mullis P, Patel M, Brickell PM, Brook CGD: Isolated growth hormone deficiency: Analysis of the growth hormone (GH)-releasing hormone gene and the GH gene cluster. *J Clin Endocrinol Metab* 70:187, 1990.
485. Maheshwari HG, Silverman BL, DuPuis J, Baumann G: Phenotype and genetic analysis of a syndrome caused by an inactivating mutation in the growth hormone-releasing hormone receptor: Dwarfism of Sindh. *J Clin Endocrinol Metab* 83:4065, 1998.
486. Huseman CA, Hassing JM: Evidence for dopaminergic stimulation of growth velocity in some hypopituitary children. *J Clin Endocrinol Metab* 58:419, 1984.
487. Pintor C, Cella SG, Loche S, Puggioni R, Corda R, Locatelli V, Muller EE: Clonidine-treatment for short stature. *Lancet* 1:1226, 1987.
488. Pescovitz OH, Tan E: Lack of benefit of clonidine treatment for short stature in a double-blind, placebo-controlled trial. *Lancet* 2:874, 1988.
489. Longobardi S, Merola B, Pivonello R, DiRella F, DiSomma C, Colao A, et al: Reevaluation of growth hormone (GH) secretion in 69 adults diagnosed as GH-deficient patients during childhood. *J Clin Endocrinol Metab* 81:1244, 1996.
490. Newman CB, Kleinberg DL: Adult growth hormone deficiency. *The Endocrinologist* 8:178, 1998.
491. Molitch ME: Pathogenesis of pituitary tumors. *Endocrinol Metab Clin North Am* 16:503, 1987.
492. Van Dop C, Burstein S, Conte FA, Grumbach MM: Isolated gonadotropin deficiency in boys: Clinical characteristics and growth. *J Pediatr* 111:684, 1987.
493. Waldstreicher J, Seminara SB, Jameson JL, Geyer A, Nachtigall LB, Boepple PA, et al: The genetic and clinical heterogeneity of gonadotropin-releasing hormone deficiency in the human. *J Clin Endocrinol Metab* 81:4388, 1996.
494. Weiss J, Crowley WF Jr., Jameson JL: Normal structure of the gonadotropin-releasing hormone (GnRH) gene in patients with GnRH deficiency and idiopathic hypogonadotropic hypogonadism. *J Clin Endocrinol Metab* 69:299, 1989.
495. Santoro N, Filicori M, Crowley WF Jr: Hypogonadotropic disorders in men and women: Diagnosis and therapy with pulsatile gonadotropin-releasing hormone. *Endocrinol Rev* 7:11, 1986.
496. Liu L, Banks SM, Barnes KM, Sherins RJ: Two-year comparison of testicular responses to pulsatile gonadotropin-releasing hormone and exogenous gonadotropins from the inception of therapy in men with isolated hypogonadotropic hypogonadism. *J Clin Endocrinol Metab* 67:1140, 1988.
497. Layman LC, Cohen DP, Jin M, Xie J, Li Z, Reindollar RH, et al: Mutations in gonadotropin-releasing hormone receptor gene cause hypogonadotropic hypogonadism. *Nat Genet* 18:14, 1998.
498. Weiss J, Axelrod L, Whitcomb RW, Harris PE, Crowley WF, Jameson JL: Hypogonadism caused by a single amino acid substitution in the β subunit of luteinizing hormone. *N Engl J Med* 326:179, 1992.
499. Layman LC, Lee E-J, Peak DB, Namnoum AB, Vu KV, van Lingen RL, et al: Delayed puberty and hypogonadism caused by mutations in the follicle stimulating hormone β-subunit gene. *N Engl J Med* 337:607, 1997.
500. Phillip M, Arbelle JE, Segev Y, Parvari R: Male hypogonadism due to a mutation in the gene for the β-subunit of follicle-stimulating hormone. *N Engl J Med* 338:1729, 1998.
501. Conway GS: Clinical manifestations of genetic defects affecting gonadotrophins and their receptors. *Clin Endocrinol* 45:657, 1996.
502. Vigersky RA, Andersen AE, Thompson RH, Loriaux DL: Hypothalamic dysfunction in secondary amenorrhea associated with simple weight loss. *N Engl J Med* 297:1141, 1977.
503. Shangold MM: Causes, evaluation, and management of athletic oligo/amenorrhea. *Med Clin North Am* 69:83, 1985
504. Quigley E, Sheenan KL, Casper RF, Yen SSC: Evidence for increased dopaminergic and opioid activity in patients with hypothalamic hypogonadotropic amenorrhea. *J Clin Endocrinol Metab* 50:949, 1980.
505. Nachtigall LB, Boepple PA, Pralong FP, Crowley WF Jr: Adult-onset idiopathic hypogonadotropic hypogonadism—a treatable form of male infertility. *N Engl J Med* 336:410, 1997.
506. Molitch ME: Disorders of the pituitary lactotroph, in EY Adashi, JA Rock, Z Rosenwaks (eds): *Reproductive Endocrinology, Surgery, and Technology*. Lippincott-Raven Publishers, Philadelphia, 1996, pp 1303–1324.
507. Glass MR, Shaw RW, Butt WR, Edwards RL, London DR: An abnormality of oestrogen feedback in amenorrhoea-galactorrhoea. *Br Med J* 3:274, 1975.
508. Styne DM: New aspects in the diagnosis and treatment of pubertal disorders. *Pediatric Clin N Amer* 44:505, 1997.
509. Pescovitz OH, Comite F, Hench K, Barnes K, McNemar A, Foster C, et al: The NIH experience with precocious puberty: Diagnostic subgroups and response to short-term luteinizing hormone releasing hormone analogue therapy. *J Pediatr* 108:47, 1986.
510. Manasco PK, Pescovitz OH, Feuillan PP, Hench KD, Barnes KM, Jones J, et al: Resumption of puberty after long term luteinizing hormone-releasing hormone agonist treatment of central precocious puberty. *J Clin Endocrinol Metab* 67:368, 1988.

511. Merke DP, Cutler GB Jr: Evaluation and management of precocious puberty. *Arch Dis Child* 75:269, 1996.
512. Bevan JS, Burke CW, Esiri MM, Adamas CBT: Misinterpretation of prolactin levels leading to management error in patients with sellar enlargement. *Am J Med* 82:29, 1987.
513. Martin TL, Kim M, Malarkey WB: The natural history of idiopathic hyperprolactinemia. *J Clin Endocrinol Metab* 60:855, 1985.
514. Sluijmer AV, Lappöhn RE: Clinical history and outcome of 59 patients with idiopathic hyperprolactinemia. *Fertil Steril* 58:72, 1992.
515. Pontiroli AE, Falsetti L: Development of pituitary adenoma in women with hyperprolactinaemia: Clinical, endocrine, and radiological characteristics. *Br Med J* 288:515, 1984.
516. Schlechte J, Dolan K, Sherman B, et al: The natural history of untreated hyperprolactinemia: A prospective analysis. *J Clin Endocrinol Metab* 68:412, 1989.
517. Rjosk HK, Fahlbusch R, von Werder K: Spontaneous development of hyperprolactinaemia. *Acta Endocrinol* 100:333, 1982.
518. Klibanski A, Biller BMK, Rosenthal DI, Schoenfeld DA, Saxe V: Effects of prolactin and estrogen deficiency in amenorrheic bone loss. *J Clin Endocrinol Metab* 67:124, 1988.
519. Corenblum B, Donovan L: The safety of physiological estrogen plus progestin replacement therapy and with oral contraceptive therapy in women with pathological hyperprolactinemia. *Fertil Steril* 59:671, 1993.
520. Faglia G, Peccoz PB, Ambrosi B, Ferrari C, Neri V: Prolonged and exaggerated elevations in plasma thyrotropin (HTSH) after thyrotropin releasing factor (TRF) in patients with pituitary tumors. *J Clin Endocrinol Metab* 33:999, 1971.
521. Beck-Peccoz P, Amr S, Menezes-Ferreira MM, Faglia G, Weintraub BD: Decreased receptor binding of biologically inactive thyrotropin in central hypothyroidism. *N Engl J Med* 312:1085, 1985.
522. Taylor T, Weintraub BD: Altered thyrotropin (TSH) carbohydrate structures in hypothalamic hypothyroidism created by paraventricular nuclear lesions are corrected by in vivo TSH-releasing hormone administration. *Endocrinology* 125:2198, 1989.
523. Collu R, Tang J, Castagné J, LaGacé G, Masson N, Hout C, et al: A novel mechanism for isolated central hypothyroidism: Inactivating mutations in the thyrotropin-releasing hormone receptor gene. *J Clin Endocrinol Metab* 82:1361, 1997.
524. Hayashizaki Y, Hiraoka Y, Tatsumi K, et al: Deoxyribonucleic acid analyses of five families with familial inherited thyroid stimulating hormone deficiency. *J Clin Endocrinol Metab* 71:792, 1990.
525. De Roux N, Misrahi M, Brauner R, Houang M, Carel JC, Granier M, et al: Four families with loss of function mutations of the thyrotropin receptor. *J Clin Endocrinol Metab* 81:4229, 1996.
526. Orme SM, Belchetz PE: Isolated ACTH deficiency. *Clin Endocrinol* 35:213, 1991.
527. Yamamoto T, Fukuyama J, Hasegawa K, Sugiura M: Isolated corticotropin deficiency in adults. Report of 10 cases and review of literature. *Arch Intern Med* 152:1705, 1992.
528. Tsukada T, Nakai Y, Koh T, Tsujii S, Inada M, Nishikawa M, et al: Plasma adrenocorticotropin and cortisol responses to ovine corticotropin-releasing factor in patients with adrenocortical insufficiency due to hypothalamic and pituitary disorders. *J Clin Endocrinol Metab* 58:758, 1984.
529. Rosenbaum M, Leibel RL, Hirsch J: Obesity. *N Engl J Med* 337:396, 1997.
530. Woods SC, Seeley RJ, Porte D Jr, Schwartz MW: Signals that regulate food intake and energy homeostasis. *Science* 280:1378, 1998.
531. Wilding J, Widdowson P, Williams G: Neurobiology. *Br Med Bull* 53:286, 1997.
532. Leibowitz SF: Brain monoamines and peptides: Role in the control of eating behavior. *Fed Proc* 45:1396, 1986.
533. Bray GA, York DA: Leptin and clinical medicine: A new piece in the puzzle of obesity. *J Clin Endocrinol Metab* 82:2771, 1997.
534. Schwartz MW, Seeley RJ, Campfield LA, Burn P, Basking DG: Identification of targets on leptin action in rat hypothalamus. *J Clin Invest* 98:1101, 1996.
535. Flier JS, Maratos-Flier E: Obesity and the hypothalamus. Novel peptides for new pathways. *Cell* 92:437, 1998.
536. Huszar D, Lynch CA, Fairchild-Huntress V, Dunmore JH, Fang Q, Berkenmeier LR, et al: Targeted disruption of the melanocortin-4 receptor results in obesity in mice. *Cell* 88:131, 1997.
537. Thornton JE, Chueng CC, Clifton DK, Steiner RA: Regulation of hypothalamic proopiomelanocortin mRNA by leptin in ob/ob mice. *Endocrinology* 138:5063, 1997.
538. Sakurai T, Amemiya A, Ishii M, Matsuzaki I, Chimelli RM, Tanaka H, et al: Orexins and orexin receptors: A family of hypothalamic neuropeptides and G-protein-coupled receptors that regulate feeding behavior. *Cell* 92:573, 1998.
539. Bray GA, Gallagher TF Jr: Manifestations of hypothalamic obesity in man: A comprehensive investigation of eight patients and a review of the literature. *Medicine (Baltimore)* 54:301, 1975.
540. Bray GA, Dahms WT, Swerdloff RS, Fiser RH, Atkinson RL, Carrel RE: The Prader-Willi syndrome: A study of 40 patients and a review of the literature. *Medicine (Baltimore)* 62:59, 1983.
541. Butler MG: Prader-Willi syndrome: Current understanding of cause and diagnosis. *Am J Med Genet* 35:319, 1990.
542. Edwards JA, Seihi PK, Scoma AJ, Bannerman RM, Frohman LA: A new familial syndrome characterized by pigmentary retinopathy, hypogonadism, mental retardation, nerve deafness and glucose intolerance. *Am J Med* 60:23, 1975.
543. Burr IM, Slonim AE, Danish RK, Gadoth N, Butler IJ: Diencephalic syndrome revisited. *J Pediatr* 88:439, 1976.
544. Poussaint TY, Barnes PD, Nichols K, Anthony DC, Cohen L, Tarbell NJ, et al: Diencephalic syndrome: Clinical features and imaging findings. *Am J Neuroradiol* 18:1499, 1997.
545. Gemstorp I, Kjellman B, Palmgren B: Diencephalic syndrome of infancy. *J Pediatr* 70:383, 1967.
546. Bernard C: Chiens rendus diabetiques. *Compt Rend Soc Biol* 1:60, 1849.
547. Boulant JA: Hypothalamic mechanisms in thermoregulation. *Fed Proc* 40:2843, 1981.
548. Fox RH, Davies TW, Marsh FP, Urich H: Hypothermia in a young man with an anterior hypothalamic lesion. *Lancet* 2:185, 1970.
549. Johnson RH, Delahunt JW, Robinson BJ: Do thermoregulatory reflexes pass through the hypothalamus? Studies of chronic hypothermia due to hypothalamic lesion. *Aust N Z J Med* 20:154, 1990.
550. Shapiro WR, Williams GH, Plum F: Spontaneous recurrent hypothermia accompanying agenesis of the corpus callosum. *Brain* 92:423, 1969.
551. Kloos RT: Spontaneous periodic hypothermia. *Medicine* 74:268, 1995.
552. Wolff SM, Adler RC, Buskirk ER, Thompson RH: A syndrome of periodic hypothalamic discharge. *Am J Med* 36:956, 1964.
553. Hume DM, Bell CC, Bartter F: Direct measurement of adrenal secretion during operative trauma and convalescence. *Surgery* 52:174, 1962.
554. Korpassy A, Stoeckel H, Vecsei P: Investigation of hydrocortisone secretion and aldosterone secretion in patients with severe prolonged stress. *Acta Anaesthesiol Scand* 16:161, 1972.
555. Vermes I Bieshuizen A, Hampsink RM, Haanen C: Dissociation of plasma adrenocorticotropin and cortisol levels in critically ill patients: Possible role of endothelin and atrial natriuretic hormone. *J Clin Endocrinol Metab* 80:1238, 1995.
556. Van den Berghe G, de Zegher F, Bouillon R: Acute and prolonged critical illness as different neuroendocrine paradigms. *J Clin Endocrinol Metab* 83:1827, 1998.
557. DeSimoni MG, Imeri L: Cytokine-neurotransmitter interactions in the brain. *Biol Signals Recept* 7:33, 1998.
558. Molitch ME: Pituitary response to stress: Growth hormone and prolactin, in Ober KP (ed): *Endocrinology of Critical Disease.* Totowa, NJ: Humana Press, 1997, pp 67–86.
559. Ross R, Miell J, Freeman E, et al: Critically ill patients have high basal growth hormone levels with attenuated oscillatory activity associated with low levels of insulin-like growth factor 1. *Clin Endocrinol* 35:47, 1991.
560. Wartofsky L, Burman KD: Alterations in thyroid function in patients with systemic illness: The 'euthyroid sick syndrome.' *Endocrinol Rev* 3:164, 1982.
561. Turner HE, Wass JAH: Gonadal function in men with chronic illness. *Clin Endocrinol* 47:379, 1997.
562. Chrousos GP, Torpy DJ, Gold PW: Interactions between the hypothalamic-pituitary-adrenal axis and the female reproductive system: Clinical implications. *Ann Intern Med* 129:229, 1998.
563. Smith SR, Bledsoe T, Chhetri MK: Cortisol metabolism and the pituitary adrenal axis in adults with protein-caloric malnutrition. *J Clin Endocrinol Metab* 40:43, 1975.
564. Mohan PS, Jaya RKS: Plasma somatomedin activity in protein calorie malnutrition. *Arch Dis Child* 54:62, 1979.

565. Pimstone B, Becker D, Hendricks A: TSH response to synthetic thyrotropin-releasing hormone in human protein-calorie malnutrition. *J Clin Endocrinol Metab* 36:779, 1973.
566. Flier JS: What's in a name? In search of leptin's physiologic role. *J Clin Endocrinol Metab* 83:1407, 1998.
567. Schwartz MW, Seeley RJ: Neuroendocrine responses to starvation and weight loss. *N Engl J Med* 336:1802, 1997.
568. Glass AR, Burman KD, Dahms WT, Boehm TM: Endocrine functions in human obesity. *Metabolism* 30:89, 1981.
569. Björntorp P: Endocrine abnormalities in obesity. *Diabetes Revs* 5:52, 1997.
570. Cordido F, Dieguez C, Casanueva FF: Effect of central cholinergic neurotransmission enhancement by pyridostigmine on the growth hormone secretion elicited by clonidine, arginine, or hypoglycemia in normal and obese subjects. *J Clin Endocrinol Metab* 70:1361, 1990.
571. Magoffin DA, Huang CTF: Leptin and reproduction. *The Endocrinologist* 8:79, 1998.
572. Sims EAH, Danforth E Jr, Horton ES, Bray GA, Glennon JA, Salans LB: Endocrine and metabolic effects of experimental obesity in man. *Recent Prog Horm Res* 29:457, 1973.
573. Schaper NC: Growth hormone secretion in type I diabetes: A review. *Acta Endocrinol (Copenh)* 122:7, 1990.
574. Mercado M, Molitch ME, Baumann G: Low plasma growth hormone binding protein in IDDM. *Diabetes* 41:605, 1992.
575. Martina V, Maccario M, Tagliabue M, Corno M, Camanni F: Chronic treatment with pirenzepine decreases growth hormone secretion in insulin-dependent diabetes mellitus. *J Clin Endocrinol Metab* 68:392, 1989.
576. Bayraktar M, Van Thiel DH: Endocrine changes in liver disease. *The Endocrinologist* 5:403, 1995.
577. Merry J, Marks V: Hypothalamic pituitary adrenal function in chronic alcoholics, in Gross MM (ed): *Alcohol Intoxication and Withdrawal: Experimental Studies. Advances in Experimental Medicine and Biology.* New York, Plenum, 1973, p 167.
578. Rees LH, Besser GM, Jeffcoate WJ, Goldie DJ, Marks V: Alcohol-induced pseudo-Cushing's syndrome. *Lancet* 1:726, 1977.
579. Van Thiel DH, Gavaler JS, Wight C, Smith WI Jr, Abuid J: Thyrotropin-releasing hormone (TRH)-induced growth hormone (HGH) responses in cirrhotic men. *Gastroenterology* 75:66, 1978.
580. Salerno F, Locatelli V, Müller EE: Growth hormone hyperresponsiveness to growth hormone-releasing hormone in patients with severe liver cirrhosis. *Clin Endocrinol (Oxf)* 27:183, 1987.
581. Morgan MY, Jakobovits AW, Gore MBR, Wills MR, Sherlock S: Serum prolactin in liver disease and its relationship to gynecomastia. *Gut* 19:170, 1978.
582. Chopra IJ, Solomon DH, Chopra U, Young RT, Chua Teco GN: Alterations in circulating thyroid hormones and thyrotropin in hepatic cirrhosis: Evidence for euthyroidism despite sub-normal serum triiodothyronine. *J Clin Endocrinol Metab* 39:501, 1974.
583. Bannister P, Handley T, Chapman C, Losowsky MS: Hypogonadism in chronic liver disease: Impaired release of luteinising hormone. *Br Med J* 293:1191, 1986.
584. Gordon GG, Southren AL, Liever CS: The effects of alcoholic liver disease and alcohol ingestion on sex hormone levels: Alcoholism. *Clin Exp Res* 2:259, 1978.
585. Luger A, Lang I, Kovarik J, Stummvoll HK, Templ H: Abnormalities in the hypothalamic-pituitary-adrenocortical axis in patients with chronic renal failure. *Am J Kidney Dis* 9:51, 1987.
586. Wallace EZ, Rosman P, Toshav N, Sacerdote A, Balthazar A: Pituitary-adrenocortical function in chronic renal failure: Studies of episodic secretion of cortisol and dexamethasone suppressibility. *J Clin Endocrinol Metab* 50:46, 1980.
587. Kokot F, Wiecek A, Grzeszczak W, Klin M: Influence of erythropoietin treatment on function of the pituitary-adrenal axis and somatotropin secretion in hemodialyzed patients. *Clin Nephrol* 33:241, 1990.
588. Bessarione D, Perfumo F, Giusti M, Ginevri F, Mazzocchi G, Gusmano R, et al: Growth hormone response to growth hormone-releasing hormone in normal and uraemic children: Comparison with hypoglycaemia following insulin administration. *Acta Endocrinol (Copenh)* 114:5, 1987.
589. Powell DR, Rosenfeld RG, Baker BK, Liu F, Hintz RL: Serum somatomedin levels in adults with chronic renal failure: The importance of measuring insulin-like growth factor I (IGF-I) and IGF-II in acid-chromatographed uremic serum. *J Clin Endocrinol Metab* 63:1186, 1986.
590. Phillips LS, Fusco AC, Unterman TG, DelGreco F: Somatomedin inhibitor in uremia. *J Clin Endocrinol Metab* 59:764, 1984.
591. Lim VS, Kathpalia SC, Frohman LA: Hyperprolactinemia and impaired pituitary response to suppression and stimulation in chronic renal failure: Reversal after transplantation. *J Clin Endocrinol Metab* 48:101, 1979.
592. Hou SH, Grossman S, Molitch ME: Hyperprolactinemia in patients with renal insufficiency and chronic renal failure requiring hemodialysis or chronic ambulatory peritoneal dialysis. *Am J Kidney Dis* 6:245, 1985.
593. Sievertsen GD, Lim VS, Nakawatase C, Frohman LA: Metabolic clearance and secretion rates of human prolactin in normal subjects and in patients with chronic renal failure. *J Clin Endocrinol Metab* 50:846, 1980.
594. Lim VS, Fang VS, Katz AI, Refetoff S: Thyroid dysfunction in chronic renal failure: A study of the pituitary-thyroid axis and peripheral turnover kinetics of thyroxine and triiodothyronine. *J Clin Invest* 60:522, 1977.
595. Lim VS, Henriquez C, Sievertsen G, Frohman LA: Ovarian function in chronic renal failure: Evidence suggesting hypothalamic anovulation. *Ann Intern Med* 93:21, 1980.
596. Bierman M, Nolan GH: Menstrual function and renal transplantation. *Obstet Gynecol* 49:186, 1977.
597. Okundaye I, Abrinko P, Hou S: Registry of pregnancy in dialysis patients. *Am J Kidney Dis* 31:766, 1998.
598. DeGirolami U, Schmidek H: Clinicopathological study of 53 tumors of the pineal region. *J Neurosurg* 39:455, 1973.
599. Jennings MT, Gelman R, Hochberg F: Intracranial germ-cell tumors: Natural history and pathogenesis. *J Neurosurg* 63:155, 1985.
600. Bruce JN, Stein BM: Surgical management of pineal region tumors. *Acta Neurochir* 134:130, 1995.
601. Kitay JI: Pineal lesions and precocious puberty: Review. *J Clin Endocrinol Metab* 14:622, 1954.
602. Jooma R, Kendall BE: Diagnosis and management of pineal tumors. *J Neurosurg* 58:654, 1983.
603. Schild SE, Scheithauer BW, Haddock MG, Wong WW, Lyons MK, Marks LB, et al: Histologically confirmed pineal tumors and other germ cell tumors of the brain. *Cancer* 78:2564, 1996.
604. Donaldson JO: Endocrinology of pseudotumor cerebri. *Neurol Clin* 4:919, 1986.
605. Molitch ME: The empty sella, in Bardin CW (ed): *Current Therapy in Endocrinology and Metabolism*, 4th ed. Philadelphia, B.C. Decker, Inc., 1991, p 32.
606. Sotos JF, Dodge PR, Muirhead D, Crawford JD, Talbot NB: Cerebral gigantism in childhood: A syndrome of excessively rapid growth with acromegalic features and a nonprogressive neurologic disorder. *N Engl J Med* 271:109, 1964.
607. Aoki N, Oikawa Akihiro, Sakai T: Serial neuroimaging studies in Sotos' syndrome (cerebral gigantism syndrome). *Neurol Res* 20:149, 1998.

CHAPTER 7

Diseases of the Anterior Pituitary

Peter J. Snyder

THE NORMAL PITUITARY

Anatomy of the Pituitary

The location of the pituitary, in close juxtaposition to the hypothalamus, is crucial to its function. The anterior pituitary consists of several distinct cell types, each of which secretes one or two hormones (Table 7-1). Many of the same factors that control the function of the differentiated cell types also control the differentiation of these cell types embryologically.

Gross Anatomy

The pituitary gland rests in a shallow bony cavity, the sella turcica (Turkish saddle) at the base of the skull just below the brain (Fig. 7-1). The sella turcica is part of the sphenoid bone, and below the sella turcica is the sphenoid sinus. The sella is lined by dura mater and is covered superiorly by a portion of dura called the diaphragma sella, which separates the pituitary from the CSF and the brain above.

The size of the pituitary gland varies with age, sex, and physiologic state. The average size is 6 mm vertically, 13 mm anterioposteriorly, and 10 mm across,[1–6] and the average weight is 600 mg. The size is a little larger in women than in men, and yet larger during pregnancy than in the nonpregnant state. The size decreases with increasing age.

The anterior pituitary receives its blood supply from two sources: a hypophyseal portal system, which is a local circulation bringing blood from the hypothalamus to the pituitary, and arterioles, which bring blood directly from the systemic circulation.[7] The hypophyseal portal system is far greater both in blood flow and physiologic importance. The portal system arises from hypophyseal arteries, which are branches of the internal carotid arteries. The hypophyseal arteries penetrate the hypothalamic-pituitary stalk and then form plexuses and capillaries which carry hormones from the hypothalamus through the posterior pituitary lobe to the anterior lobe. There is evidence that blood may also flow retrograde from the anterior pituitary toward the hypothalamus, but whether this flow is of physiologic significance is not yet certain. Venous blood drains from the anterior pituitary into the cavernous sinuses.

Microscopic Anatomy

By light microscopy the anterior pituitary is seen to consist of a central median wedge flanked by two lateral wings. The basic architectural pattern in all three sections is acinar.[8] Acini of relatively uniform size are surrounded by a continuous basement membrane and supplied by abundant capillaries. The cells that comprise the acini vary by location within the pituitary. Most of the corticotroph and thyrotroph cells reside in the median wedge, and most of the somatotroph cells reside in the lateral wedges. The lactotroph and gonadotroph cells are generally distributed.[8] Specific cell type can be recognized best by techniques that are specific for the hormonal secretory products of the cells (e.g., immunocytochemistry, immunoelectron microscopy, or in situ hybridization). Conventional electron microscopy may also be helpful in identifying specific cell types, but overlap among cell types in cell size and shape and in number and size of secretory granules make this technique better for obtaining ancillary information than for primary identification of specific cell type. Conventional hematoxylin and eosin staining is of very little value in determining cell type.

Somatotroph Cells

Somatotroph cells, which secrete growth hormone, are the most prevalent cell type in the anterior pituitary, comprising about 50 percent of the overall cell population and the majority of that in the lateral wings.[8] The number appears to be independent of age and gender but increases markedly in the rare patients with ectopic secretion of growth hormone releasing hormone (GHRH).[9]

Lactotroph Cells

Lactotroph cells, which secrete prolactin, comprise about 10 percent of the cell population in men and nulliparous women and as much as 30 percent in multiparous women.[10] During pregnancy the percentage increases to as high as 50 percent, and the size of the individual cells increases.[11] They are distributed diffusely throughout the lateral wings, with some predominance near the posterior and lateral edges. Granulation is usually sparse in the adult but greater in children and more so during states of prolactin hypersecretion. The cytoplasmic volume of the nonadenomatous lactotrophs decreases in response to prolactin hypersecretion by an adenoma or administration of a dopamine agonist.[8]

Corticotroph Cells

Corticotroph cells, which synthesize proopiomelanocortin (POMC), which is processed to ACTH and other peptides, are found predominantly in the median wedge, and comprise about 15 to 20 percent of anterior pituitary cells.[8] These cells usually contain numerous secretory granules but most characteristically contain bundles of cytokeratin filaments. The bundles of filaments increase markedly when they are exposed to excessive glucocorticoid, either endogenously or exogenously, and account for the Crooke's hyaline change known for many years by light microscopy.

TABLE 7-1. Cells of the Anterior Pituitary and Their Hormones

Cell	Synthesized Products	Secreted Hormone	Amino Acids	Carbohydrate
Somatotroph	Growth hormone	Growth hormone	191	
Lactotroph	Prolactin	Prolactin	198	
Corticotroph	Proopiomelanocortin	ACTH	39	
Gonadotroph	FSHβ	FSH	204	5%
	LHβ	LH	204	1%
	α			
Thyrotroph	TSHβ	TSH	201	1%
	α			

Gonadotroph Cells

Gonadotroph cells, which secrete both FSH and LH, comprise about 10 percent of pituitary cells and are found diffusely throughout the pituitary. The number and size of these cells increase in response to gonadal failure, giving rise to the term "gonadal failure cells." Secretory granules appear to exhibit sexual dimorphism; men have smaller granules and women have larger ones.[8]

Thyrotroph Cells

Thyrotroph cells, which secrete TSH, comprise only about 5 percent of the cells of the anterior pituitary and are located primarily in the median wedge. They have a characteristic shape, which is elongated and angular.[8] Thyroidal failure results in enlargement, giving rise to the term "thyroidectomy cells."

Pleurihormonal Cells

Pleurihormonal cells are found most commonly in certain pituitary adenomas but occasionally in the nonadenomatous pituitary. As in pituitary adenomas, the most common pleurihormonal cell is the mammosomatotroph, which secretes both prolactin and growth hormone. They are distributed throughout the anterior pituitary and resemble somatotrophs. Other pleurihormonal cells appear to synthesize various combinations of growth hormone, prolactin, glycoprotein α subunit, and TSH.[8]

Folliculostellate Cells

Folliculostellate cells, unlike all of the types of cells described previously, do not have an endocrine function. Instead, they appear to play a supportive function, perhaps by paracrine activity. They contain S-100 protein, as do glial cells.[12]

Embryology

Origin of the Anterior Pituitary

The anterior pituitary arises from Rathke's pouch, an endodermal structure. Rathke's pouch forms as an invagination of the roof of the oropharynx beginning at the third week of gestation, and by the sixth week has separated from it completely. By then Rathke's pouch is adjacent to the hypothalamus and is beginning to be enclosed by the developing sphenoid bone.[13]

Differentiation of Anterior Pituitary Cells as Observed Morphologically

The differentiation of the specific cell types of the anterior pituitary can be observed by immunocytochemistry and electron microscopy of pituitaries of human fetuses of various ages[14,15]

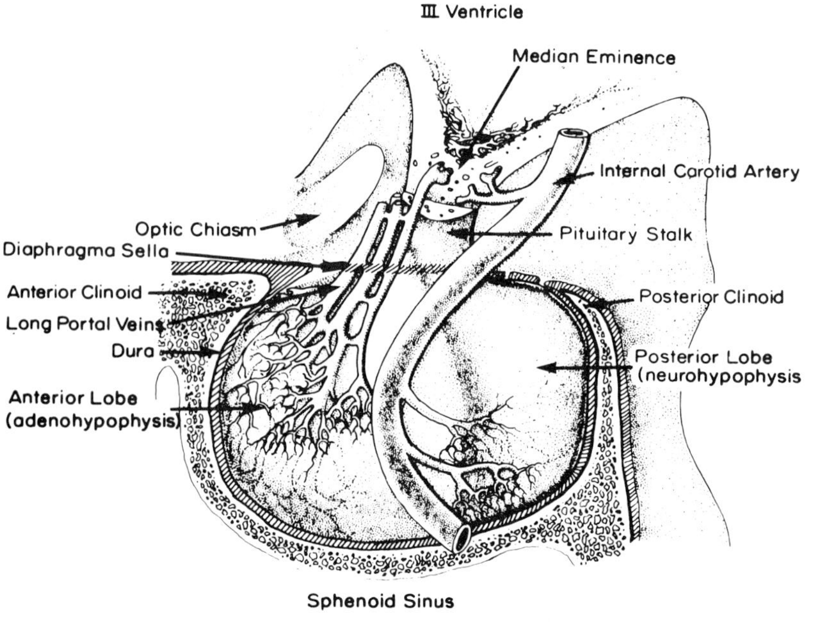

FIGURE 7-1. Schematic representation of the pituitary gland in relation to surrounding structures. The pituitary gland is shown situated within the sella turcica, bounded by the sella's anterior and posterior clinoid processes. The floor of the sella is also the roof of the sphenoid sinus. The sella is covered superiorly by a reflection of dura, called the diaphragma sella, through which pass blood vessels and neurons from the median eminence of the hypothalamus via the pituitary stalk.

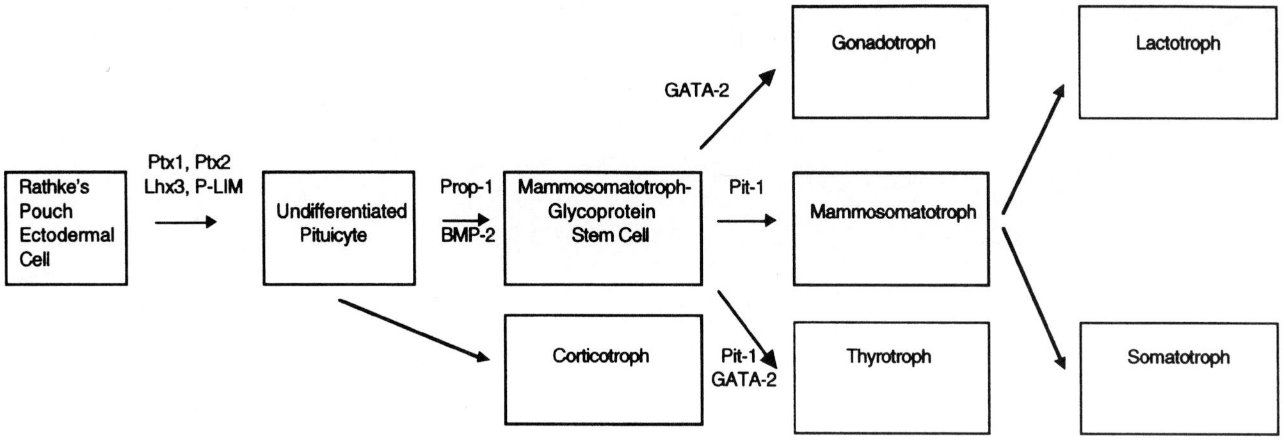

FIGURE 7-2. Schematic view of the differentiation of the cells of the anterior pituitary during embryogenesis and some of the transcription factors that play important roles.

(Fig. 7-2). Corticotrophs are the first cells that can be recognized, at about 8 weeks of gestation, by ACTH immunoreactivity and by type I microfilaments. Somatotroph cells can be identified at 8 to 9 weeks of gestation, and demonstrate hormonal secretory activity at 10 weeks. Mammosomatotroph cells can be identified at 12 weeks, but lactotroph cells cannot be identified until 23 weeks and are not numerous until 35 weeks. Cells containing glycoprotein α subunit can be identified at 9 weeks, and gonadotroph and thyrotroph cells can be identified at 12 weeks.

Mechanism of the Differentiation of Anterior Pituitary Cells

The mechanisms by which anterior pituitary cells differentiate are still being elucidated, but some information is now available. Development and differentiation requires the timely expression, and often the timely extinction, of several transcription factors in a cascade.

Earliest Development of the Pituitary Several transcription factors have been identified that are necessary for the development of the anterior pituitary prior to the differentiation of specific pituitary cell types. These include pituitary homeobox factors 1 and 2 (Ptx1 and 2),[16,17] LIM homeobox genes Lhx3 and 4[18] and P-LIM,[19] and the Rathke's pouch homeobox (Rpx) gene.[20] Targeted disruption of any of these genes usually results in failure of differentiation of all specific anterior pituitary cell types.

Anterior Pituitary Cell Differentiation Corticotroph cells differentiate the earliest, perhaps influenced by leukemia inhibitory factor (LIF), which has been shown to influence corticotroph cell differentiation in a cell line. Addition of LIF to cultured AtT20 cells inhibited their division but increased their secretion of ACTH.[21]

Differentiation of all other anterior pituitary cell types requires expression of (prophet of pit-1 PROP-1). Inactivating mutations of PROP-1 lead to a failure of the differentiation of somatotrophs, lactotrophs, thyrotrophs, and gonadotrophs and deficiencies of their corresponding secretory products. Such mutations cause the Ames dwarf mouse[22,23] and combined anterior hormone deficiency in humans.[24–26] PROP-1 is also necessary for the activation of pit-1 expression. Pit-1 is then required for the differentiation of somatotroph and lactotroph cells, and, with GATA-2, of thyrotroph cells.[27,28] The necessity of pit-1 for the expression of these three hormones has been illustrated by finding deficiencies of growth hormone, prolactin, and TSH and the corresponding clinical syndrome of short stature, prolactin deficiency, and hypothyroidism in rodents and humans who have pit-1 mutations.[29,30]

The expression of GATA-2, and the absence of expression of pit-1, appears to be responsible for the differentiation of gonadotroph cells from adenohypophyseal stem cells.[28] Steroidogenic factor-1 (SF-1) is important in gonadotroph cell function, but does not appear to be essential for its differentiation. Disruption in mice of the FTZ-F1 gene, which codes for SF-1, leads to gonadotroph hypoplasia,[31] but treatment of FTZ-F1–disrupted mice with GnRH restores gonadotroph cell function.[32] The implication is that SF-1 is important for the secretion of GnRH but not for gonadotroph cell differentiation.

Based on the temporal course of anterior pituitary cell differentiation and on the transcription factors required, a schematic view of anterior pituitary cell differentiation can be proposed (Fig. 7-2).

Physiology of Anterior Pituitary Hormones

Growth Hormone

Synthesis

Growth hormone synthesis is directed by the hGH-N gene, which is one of five genes that constitute the human growth hormone gene cluster on chromosome 17; the others are hCS-L, hCS-A, hGH-V, and hCS-B.[33] Of these five only hGH-N is expressed in the human pituitary; the others are expressed in the placenta. hGH-N expression in the somatotroph cell results in the synthesis of growth hormone. The cell-specific expression of hGH-N depends on the transcription factor pit-1, as demonstrated by the absence of growth hormone secretion and short stature that result from mutations of the pit-1 gene.[30,34] Pit-1 appears to act by binding to the proximal promoter.[35] Pit-1 mutations that result in growth hormone deficiency also result in absence of prolactin and TSH secretion,[30,34] however, so other factors also must control the expression of hGH-N in the somatotroph cell. This view is

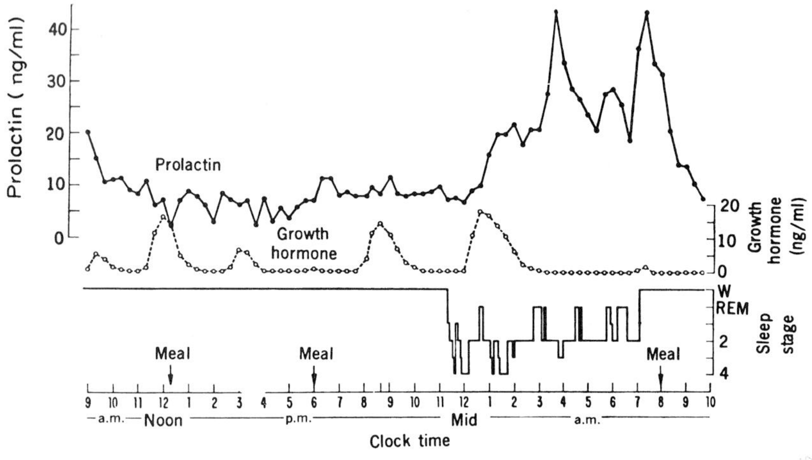

FIGURE 7-3. Pulsatile secretion in growth hormone and prolactin during the course of a 24-h period. The increase in growth hormone during sleep corresponds to the onset of deep (EEG stages III and IV) sleep. The increase in prolactin during sleep occurs at the end of sleep or shortly after awakening. (*From Sassin et al: Science 177:1205, 1972.*)

supported by the demonstration that hGH-N is not expressed in the pituitaries of transgenic mice that carry hGH-N and only its proximal promoter.[33] These other factors appear to bind upstream of the proximal promoter and to have the properties of a locus control region.[33]

Ninety percent of the mRNA transcribed by the hGH-N gene leads to an mRNA that encodes the principal growth hormone molecule, a 22 kDa single chain peptide. The other 10 percent of the hGH-N transcripts are alternatively spliced to form an mRNA that encodes a 20 kDa variant.[33]

Secretion

Growth hormone secretion is principally under the stimulatory influence of the hypothalamus via growth hormone-releasing hormone, but the hypothalamus also synthesizes somatostatin, which inhibits growth hormone secretion. Growth hormone-releasing hormone bids to a growth hormone receptor on the somatotroph and acts by stimulating adenylyl cyclase, which not only stimulates growth hormone secretion but also increases somatotroph cell division.[36] Somatostatin bids to five receptors on the somatotrophs, two of which (SSTR2 and SSTR5) act to decrease growth hormone secretion.[37] Growth hormone secretion is pulsatile (Fig. 7-3), and several physiologic and pharmacologic factors that influence these pulses are known (Table 7-2). Which factors act via growth hormone-releasing hormone, which via somatostatin, and which act directly on the somatotroph cell is uncertain. (See Chap. 6.)

Age Growth hormone secretion is relatively stable during childhood, increases during adolescence, and decreases gradually during adulthood. The values during old age are considerably lower than during childhood, but not as low as in patients with hypopituitarism.

Stimulation Deep sleep (i.e., stages III and IV) is a potent stimulus of growth hormone secretion, but REM sleep is not[38] (Fig. 7-3). Hypoglycemia[39,40] and the fasting state[41] stimulate growth hormone secretion, as do many amino acids, especially arginine.[42] Synthetic growth hormone-releasing hormone is also a potent stimulus of secretion[43] and, presumably, so is the native form, as judged by subnormal growth hormone secretion in patients with hypothalamic disease. Physical and emotional stress, including exercise and trauma,[44] increase growth hormone secretion. Drugs that stimulate growth hormone secretion include α-adrenergic agonists,[45] β-adrenergic antagonists,[46] dopamine agonists,[47] and cholinergic agonists.

Inhibition Growth hormone secretion is inhibited by conditions and drugs that have opposing actions to the stimuli described above, such as hyperglycemia, β-adrenergic agonists etc., and by serotonin antagonists.[48] Growth hormone secretion is also inhibited by somatostatin and IGF-1. Increasing age, obesity, hyperthyroidism, hypothyroidism, and pharmacologic amounts of glucocorticoids impair the response to any of the stimuli listed previously.

Transport

Growth hormone is bound to a high-affinity growth hormone–binding protein, which is the extracellular domain of

TABLE 7-2. Stimuli and Suppressors of Growth Hormone Secretion

Stimuli	Suppressors
	Physiologic
Growth hormone-releasing hormone	Hyperglycemia
Sleep, stages III and IV	Somatostatin?
Exercise	Old age
Stress, physical or psychological	
Hypoglycemia	
Fasting	
Hyperaminoacidemia	
	Pharmacologic
Hypoglycemia	Somatostatin analogs
Estrogens	IGF-1
α Adrenergic agonists	Glucocorticoids
β-Adrenergic antagonists	α Adrenergic antagonists
Dopamine agonists	β-Adrenergic agonists
Cholinergic antagonists	Dopamine antagonists
	Cholinergic agonists
	Pathologic
Starvation	Obesity
Anorexia nervosa	Hypothyroidism
Chronic renal failure	Hyperthyroidism
TRH (in acromegaly only)	Dopamine agonists (in acromegaly only)
GnRH (in acromegaly only)	

the growth hormone receptor.[49] In Laron dwarfism, which is characterized by lack of expression of the growth hormone receptor, growth hormone binding protein is absent[50] or mutated. The biological role of growth hormone binding protein, however, is not known. Growth hormone is also bound with low affinity to an α_2-macroglobulin.[51]

Actions

Growth hormone acts on virtually all tissues of the body. Some of the actions occur within minutes and others not for several hours. Some of the actions are direct and others are mediated via IGF-1.

Mechanism of Growth Hormone Action Growth hormone acts by binding to the extracellular portion of a specific growth hormone receptor. The intracellular portion of the receptor activates JAK2 tyrosine kinase, which stimulates a phosphorylation cascade in the signal transducing activators of transcription (STAT) pathway, which in turn leads to binding of STAT proteins to DNA and protein synthesis.[52]

Growth Hormone Stimulation of IGF-1 Some effects of growth hormone, most notably on bone, are mediated via IGF-1. The principal site of circulating IGF-1 appears to be the liver, but many other tissues also synthesize IGF-1, and it is uncertain to what degree the tissue effects of IGF-1 result from the circulating hormone and to what degree from that synthesized locally.

Bone Growth hormone stimulates epiphyseal bone growth and also maintenance of bone after epiphyseal closure. The evidence that this effect of growth hormone is mediated via IGF-1 was provided decades ago by the demonstration that cartilage from hypophysectomized rats could not be stimulated by growth hormone in vitro but could be stimulated by serum from growth hormone-treated, hypophysectomized rats.[53] The intermediate in serum was eventually identified to be IGF-1.

Muscle Growth hormone is anabolic for muscle. In vitro it stimulates the incorporation of amino acids into muscle.[54] In vivo it increases lean mass, presumably muscle, in patients with growth hormone deficiency.[55,56]

Carbohydrate and Fat Metabolism Growth hormone stimulates lipolysis,[57] and as a consequence, decreases body fat[55,56] and increases gluconeogenesis. Growth hormone also causes resistance to the action of insulin,[58,59] which along with gluconeogenesis, makes growth hormone diabetogenic (i.e., it exacerbates diabetes in susceptible individuals).

Prolactin

Synthesis

There is only one prolactin gene, in contrast to the cluster of growth hormone genes. Like hGH-N in the pituitary, however, expression of the prolactin gene requires the transcription factor pit-1.[33]

Secretion

Alone among pituitary hormones, prolactin is predominantly under inhibition from the hypothalamus. The hypothalamic inhibitory hormone is probably dopamine, which accounts for the effect of many of the known stimuli and inhibitors of prolactin secretion. For example, any drug which inhibits dopamine synthesis, secretion, or binding to its receptors will increase prolactin secretion and cause hyperprolactinemia, as described in detail later under cases of hyperprolactinemia. Conversely, several drugs have been designed as dopamine agonists to treat lactotroph adenomas, as described later under treatment of lactotroph adenomas. In addition, the effect of any of the stimuli is augmented by estrogen and hypothyroidism. Administration of synthetic thyrotropin releasing hormone dramatically stimulates prolactin secretion,[60] but it is uncertain if endogenous thyrotropin-releasing hormone has a physiologic role in stimulating prolactin secretion.

Actions

The principal recognized action of prolactin in man is stimulation of milk production by the mammary gland. This effect appears to require prior stimulation of the gland by estrogen and progesterone, as well as the permissive effects of insulin, thyroxine, and hydrocortisone. The increasingly high serum concentrations of prolactin, estrogen, and progesterone that occur as pregnancy progresses appear to account for milk production by the time of delivery.

Prolactin may also have a role in the immune system. Prolactin causes clonal expansion of T lymphocytes, which have prolactin receptors, in animal models.[61] It is not yet clear, however, if this effect occurs in humans, if it is mediated by prolactin exclusively of T lymphocyte origin or partly by that of pituitary origin, and if it is essential.

ACTH and Other Proopiomelanocortin Products

Synthesis

ACTH is a 39-amino acid single chain peptide that results from posttranslational processing of the 241-amino acid POMC molecule. POMC is a single-chain peptide synthesized and cleaved in the corticotroph cell to produce the 89-amino acid β-lipotropin as well as ACTH[62] (Fig. 7-4).

Secretion

ACTH secretion is pulsatile and circadian (Fig. 7-5). The circadian rhythm dictates that the magnitude of the pulses is greatest around the time of arising and lowest around the time of retiring. In response to a chronic change in the sleep-wake cycle, this pattern changes in one to two weeks.[63] Secretion is stimulated by corticotropin-releasing hormone (CRH) from the hypothalamus and physical and emotional stress of all kinds. CRH acts by binding to a cell-surface receptor, which activates adenylyl cyclase. Vasopressin potentiates the action of CRH[64] but does not stimulate ACTH itself.[65] Secretion is inhibited by endogenous cortisol and by all exogenous glucocorticoids acting directly on the corticotroph cell.

Actions

ACTH acts on the adrenal gland by binding to a cell-surface receptor, the melanocortin 2 receptor,[66] which results in adenylyl cyclase activation and an increase in the synthesis of all of the enzymes necessary for adrenal steroidogenesis. ACTH also binds to the melanocyte 1 receptor on melanocytes[67] and in supraphysiologic amounts causes hyperpigmentation.

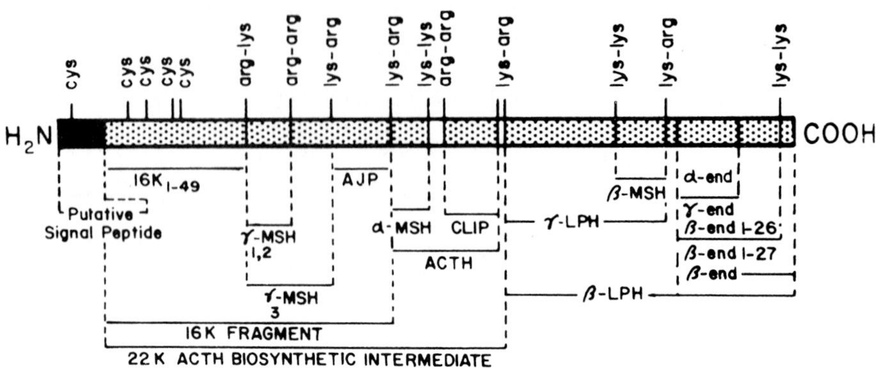

FIGURE 7-4. Schematic representation of proopiomelanocortin showing the peptides that result from proteolytic cleavage, including ACTH. (*From Smith and Funder, Endocrine Reviews 9:159, 1988.*[62])

FSH and LH

Synthesis

The gonadotropins, FSH and LH, are each dimers of a common α subunit and a distinct β subunit. Both subunits are glycoproteins, which consist of single peptide chain with one β or two α N-linked carbohydrate chains. The carbohydrate chains are variably processed and have different amounts of terminal sulfates and sialic acids, which contribute to variable acidity and clearance. The two subunits are noncovalently bound. Synthesis of both FSH and LH is stimulated by GnRH from the hypothalamus.

Secretion

GnRH is also the principal stimulus of FSH and LH secretion, and gonadal steroids and inhibin are the principal inhibitors. Both LH and FSH secretion are pulsatile (Fig. 7-6),[68] although LH pulses are easier to demonstrate, because the half-life of LH is only 30 minutes whereas that of FSH is three hours. The frequency and magnitude of the pulses of both gonadotropins appears to be controlled by the frequency of GnRH pulses.

Stimulation GnRH stimulates gonadotropin secretion by first binding to a specific G protein-coupled receptor on the gonadotroph cell surface, which in turn triggers a cascade of intracellular signaling pathways, beginning with phospholipase C.[69] GnRH secretion is normally pulsatile, and this pulsatility is essential for normal LH secretion because GnRH secretion that is either absent or continuous results in subnormal LH secretion.[69–71]

FIGURE 7-5. Pattern of plasma cortisol concentrations during 24-h periods in a normal subject. This pattern, which was subsequently shown to reflect ACTH secretion, illustrates both the episodic nature of ACTH and cortisol secretion and the highest plasma concentrations around the time of awakening. (*From Weitzman et al, J Clin Endocrinol Metab 33:14, 1971.*[366])

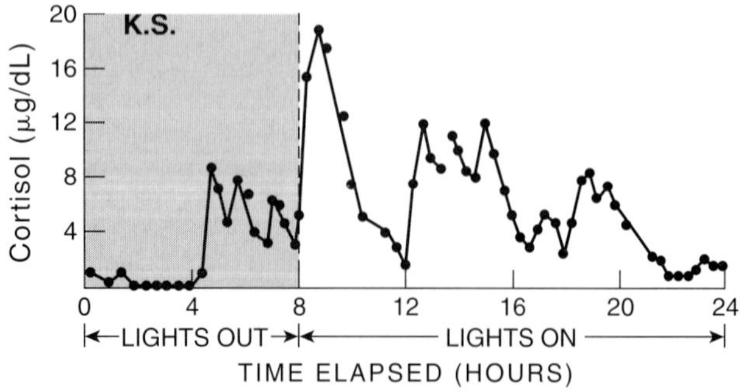

Inhibition The gonadal steroids, testosterone and estradiol in men and estradiol and progesterone in women, inhibit the secretion of LH and FSH. Inhibin selectively inhibits the secretion of FSH.

In men, testosterone appears to act directly on the gonadotroph cell to decrease LH secretion, although it also does so by inhibiting GnRH secretion by the hypothalamus. This effect appears to be mediated partially via the conversion of testosterone to estradiol, because the rare men who lack the aromatase enzyme and therefore cannot convert testosterone to estradiol[72,73] or who do not express the estrogen receptor[74] have high-normal to high serum LH concentrations. Inhibin also appears to act directly on the gonadotroph cell to suppress FSH secretion, whereas the inhibitory effect of testosterone on FSH secretion appears to be mediated solely via inhibition of GnRH secretion.[75] The inhibitory effect of testosterone on FSH secretion also appears to require conversion to estradiol.[72–74]

In women, estradiol is the principal inhibitor of FSH and LH secretion, but inhibin also inhibits FSH secretion and progesterone also inhibits LH secretion. Testosterone inhibits gonadotropin secretion in women when it is secreted excessively in pathologic states.

Actions

The gonadotropins stimulate the testes in men and the ovaries in women. In men, LH stimulates the Leydig cells to synthesize testosterone, and FSH stimulates the Sertoli cells to make several compounds thought to be involved in spermatogenesis, including inhibin and androgen binding protein. In women, FSH stimulates the recruitment of a follicle to develop, and when the follicle has developed sufficiently, an LH surge causes the ovum to be released from the follicle. After ovulation LH also stimulates the remainder of the follicle, the corpus luteum, to secrete sufficient estradiol and progesterone to maintain the endometrium ready for implantation of the fertilized ovum.

TSH

Synthesis

TSH, like FSH and LH, is a heterodimer of an α subunit that is common to all three, and a β subunit that is specific.[76] The human α subunit contains 92 amino acids and the β subunit contains 110 amino acids. Both subunits are glycosylated, the α subunit

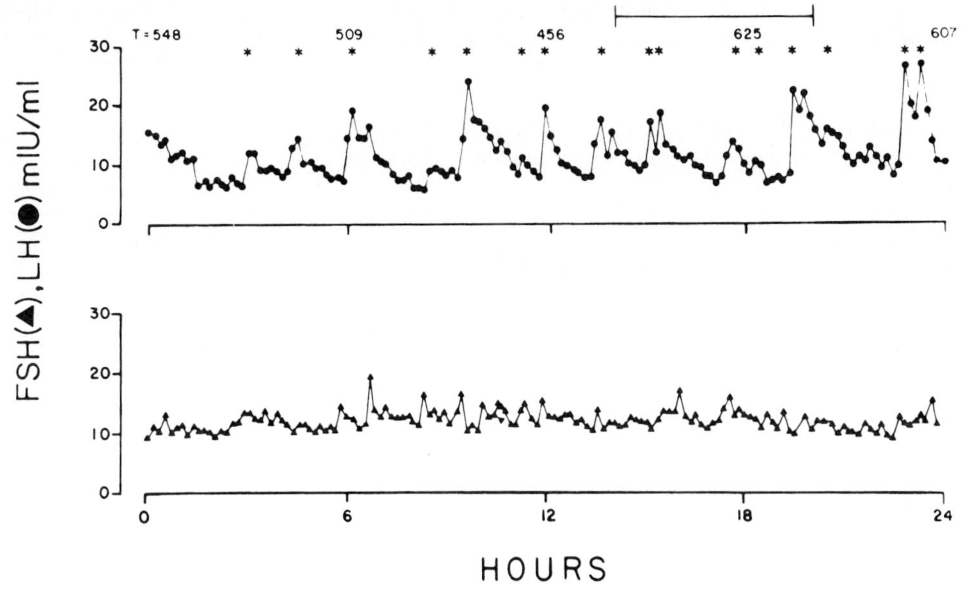

FIGURE 7-6. Pulsatile LH and FSH secretion in a normal young man during the course of 24 h. (*From Crowley et al, Recent Progress in Hormone Research 1:473, 1985.*[68])

containing two asparagine-linked carbohydrate chains and the β subunit containing one.[77] Glycosylation increases the biologic activity and increases the metabolic clearance rate.[77] Control of glycosylation appears to be exerted by TRH. When hypothalamic lesions creating hypothyroidism were produced in rats, TSH from the hypothyroid rats exhibited less mature glycosylation.[78] This phenomenon may also occur in humans and affect biologic activity. In seven patients who had hypothalamic hypothyroidism, TSH receptor binding and biologic activity was decreased compared to controls, repetitive TRH administration increased both receptor binding and biologic activity.[79]

Synthesis of TSH is stimulated by TRH and inhibited by thyroid hormones via regulation of the expression of the α and TSHβ subunits. TRH increases the expression of both subunits.[80] The effect of TRH on TSHβ expression results from its interaction with the transcription factor, pit-1.[81] Inactivating mutations of pit-1, in fact, lead to hypothyrotropic hypothyroidism.[82,83] Agents that stimulate cyclic AMP also increase TSHβ expression in vitro.[84] Thyroid hormones diminish the expression of TSHβ to a greater degree than α.[85] Thyroid hormone acts via the thyroid hormone receptor at the TSHβ promoter.[86] Consequently, individuals who have thyroid hormone resistance exhibit elevated serum TSH concentrations.

Secretion

TSH secretion is pulsatile and circadian,[87] although the magnitude of both is less than with some other pituitary hormones, such as growth hormone and ACTH. Pulses occur approximately every 1–2 hours. The circadian maximum occurs before the beginning of sleep.

Stimulation TRH secreted by the hypothalamus is the principal physiologic stimulus of TSH secretion, as demonstrated by the subnormal serum thyroxine concentration, as well as the lack of elevated serum TSH concentration, in patients who have hypothalamic disease. In addition, administration of a single bolus dose of TRH to these patients causes an acute rise of TSH, and repeated administration of TRH causes an increase in serum thyroxine concentration to normal.[88]

Inhibition The principal physiologic inhibitor of TSH secretion is thyroid hormone (Fig. 7-7). The principal mechanism is that thyroxine in the peripheral circulation is deiodinated in the pituitary to triiodothyronine,[89] which binds to the thyroid hormone receptor, which in turn inhibits the TSHβ gene.[86] The physiologic significance of this effect is demonstrated both by the common occurrence of supranormal serum TSH concentrations in patients who have subnormal serum thyroxine concentrations due to damage to the thyroid gland and the uncommon occurrence of supranormal serum TSH concentrations due to mutations of the thyroid hormone receptor.[90]

FIGURE 7-7. The inverse relationship between serum concentrations of T_4 and TSH as illustrated by patients with primary hypothyroidism before and during treatment with thyroxine. (*From Reichlin and Utiger, J Clin Endocrinol Metab 27:251, 1967.*)

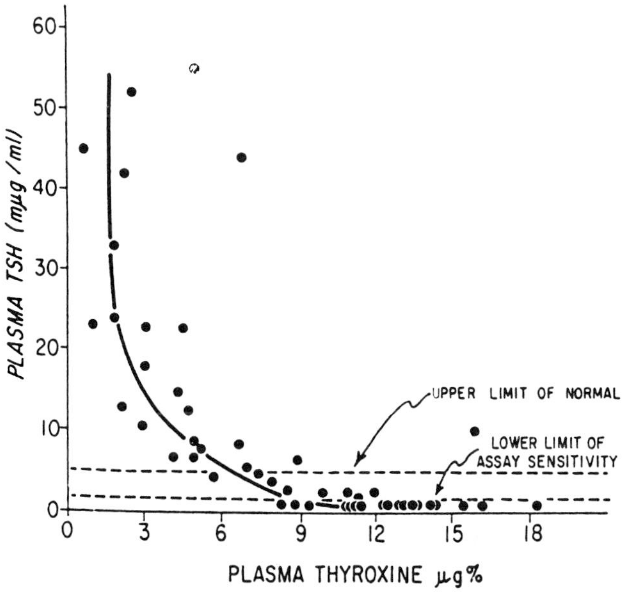

Pharmacologic doses of somatostatin[91] and dopamine[92] also inhibit TSH, but it is uncertain if they play a physiologic role.

Actions

TSH acts by binding to specific receptors on the thyroid follicular cell.[93] Mutations of these receptors result in congenital hypothyroidism.[90]

DISEASES OF THE ANTERIOR PITUITARY

Causes of Anterior Pituitary Diseases

Several different types of pathologic processes can affect the pituitary, either directly or via affecting hypothalamic hormonal secretion. The latter diseases are described in Chapter 6.

Mass Lesions

Adenomas that arise from one of the cells of the anterior pituitary are the most common mass lesions of the pituitary, but many other disease processes also cause enlargement of the pituitary, and nonpituitary mass lesions may occur in or adjacent to the pituitary (Table 7-3).

TABLE 7-3. Causes of Pituitary Enlargement

- Physiologic enlargement
  - Lactotroph hyperplasia of pregnancy
  - Thyrotroph hyperplasia of primary hypothyroidism
  - Gonadotroph hyperplasia of primary hypogonadism
- Benign tumors
  - Pituitary adenomas
  - Craniopharyngiomas
  - Meningiomas
- Malignant tumors
  - Primary malignancies
    - Ectopic pinealomas
    - Sarcomas
    - Chordomas
    - Pituitary carcinomas
  - Metastatic malignancies
- Cysts
  - Rathke's cleft
  - Dermoid
  - Arachnoid
- Lymphocytic hypophysitis
- Granulomatous hypophysitis
- Abscess

Pituitary Adenomas

Most pituitary tumors that arise from pituitary tissue itself are benign (i.e., adenomas). Because they are monoclonal, they are likely true neoplasms, which arise from a somatic mutation in one pituitary cell which then undergoes clonal expansion.[94,95] Adenomas are classified by size and the cell from which they arise. Adenomas that are less than 1 cm in diameter are called microadenomas, and those that are larger are called macroadenomas. Somatotroph adenomas usually hypersecrete growth hormone and cause acromegaly. Lactotroph adenomas usually hypersecrete prolactin, which causes hypogonadism in men and women. Corticotroph adenomas usually hypersecrete ACTH, which causes Cushing's disease. Gonadotroph adenomas may hypersecrete intact gonadotropins or their subunits but usually present because of the neurologic consequences of a mass lesion. Thyrotroph adenomas may hypersecrete TSH and cause hyperthyroidism, but more commonly secrete only free α subunit and present because of the neurologic consequences of a mass lesion. Each of these lesions is described in more detail under hormonal hypersecretion.

The pathogenesis of pituitary adenomas is still incompletely understood, but it now appears that pituitary adenomas are true, albeit benign, neoplasms. The major piece of evidence that supports this view is that each type of pituitary adenoma is monoclonal, i.e., it probably arose from a single somatic cell after early embryogenesis. When women who have a pituitary adenoma are also heterozygous for the gene for hypoxanthine phosphoribosyltransferase (HPRT) or phosphoglycerol kinase (PGK), their peripheral leukocytes have both alleles of HPRT or PGK, but their adenomas have only one allele or the other, suggesting that each of the adenomas arises from a single somatic mutation, which then expands clonally (Fig. 7-8).[94] Histologic evidence also supports the view that pituitary adenomas are true neoplasms. Pituitary adenomas are composed of sheets of similar pituitary cells, rather than a mixture of

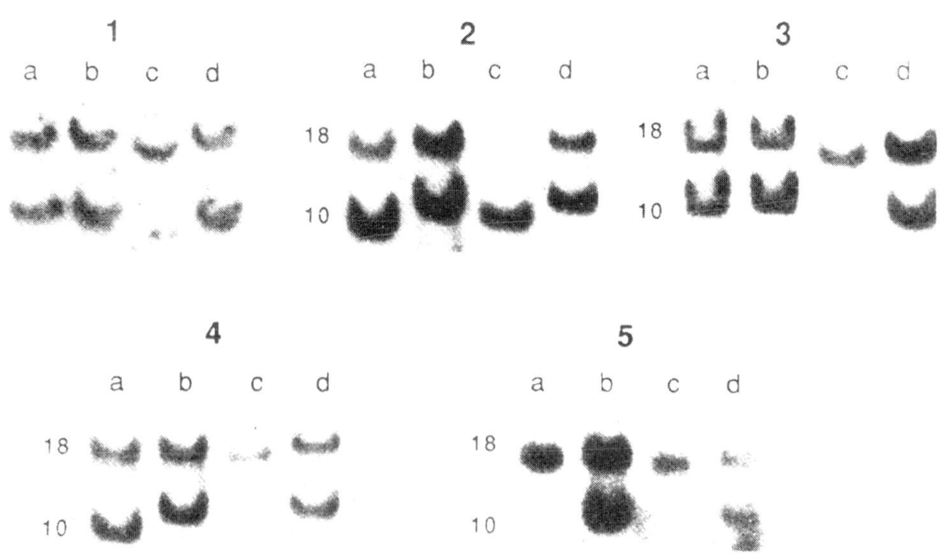

FIGURE 7-8. Demonstration of the apparent monoclonality of five pituitary adenomas. The bands represent DNA fragments of the HPRT gene from the peripheral leukocytes (lanes a and b) and pituitary adenomas (lanes c and d) of five women known to be heterozygous for the HPRT gene and to have pituitary adenomas. The leukocytes of each patient show both alleles of the HPRT gene (lane a), but each adenoma shows only one allele (lane c), supporting the hypothesis that these adenomas arose from clonal expansion of a single cell. (*From Alexander et al, J Clin Invest 86:336, 1990.*[94])

various pituitary cell types arranged a sinusoidal pattern, as occurs in the normal pituitary. Hyperplasia of one kind of pituitary cell, in contrast, is manifest by an increase in that type of cell but not an effacement of the normal pituitary sinusoidal architecture or absence of pituitary cell types. Although hypersecretion of a hypothalamic releasing hormone, such as growth hormone–releasing hormone, can cause the development of an adenoma in rodents, in man it appears to cause only somatotroph hyperplasia. Similarly, although thyroid ablation can cause a thyrotroph adenoma in rodents, in humans it causes only thyrotroph hyperplasia.

The specific mutations that cause adenoma development are not known for most kinds of pituitary adenomas, but there is evidence that some somatotroph adenomas may result from an activating mutation of the $G_s\alpha$ gene. In about 40 percent of somatotroph adenomas, adenylyl cyclase activity is much higher than in nonadenomatous pituitary tissue, and in other somatotroph adenomas, and growth hormone-releasing hormone does not stimulate adenylyl cyclase activity, as it does in nonadenomatous pituitary tissue and in other somatotroph adenomas.[96] These same somatotroph adenomas possess one of two point mutations in the $G_s\alpha$ gene, both of which cause constitutive activation of adenylyl cyclase.[97] That growth hormone-releasing hormone also stimulates adenylyl cyclase in the pituitary, and that mice transgenic for growth hormone-releasing hormone develop somatotroph adenomas[98] support the hypothesis that the activating mutation of the $G_s\alpha$ gene causes the development of somatotroph adenomas.

Mutations of the MEN/gene also cause pituitary adenomas. This gene, located on chromosome 11q13, codes for the 610 amino acid tumor suppressor protein, menin.[98] Inactivating mutations of this gene lead to underexpression of or a functionally impaired menin and to the autosomal dominant disorder, multiple endocrine neoplasia type I syndrome, which includes pituitary, parathyroid, and islet tumors. (See Chap. 27.) Few, if any, sporadic pituitary adenomas, however, appear to result from mutations of the MEN1 gene.[99,100]

Investigators have searched for many other mutations that might be causally related to the development of other pituitary adenomas, including genes that express c-Myc, c-fos, c-myb,[101] ras,[102,103] retinoblastoma suppressor,[104–106] IL-6,[107] pituitary adenylate cyclase activating peptides,[108] protein kinase C,[109] basic fibroblast growth factor,[110] epidermal growth factor,[111] transforming growth factor β,[112] and pituitary tumor transforming gene,[113] but none has been clearly associated with the pathogenesis of any pituitary adenomas.

Physiologic Enlargement of the Pituitary

Two forms of physiologic enlargement of the pituitary are well recognized: hyperplasia of the lactotroph cells during pregnancy, and hyperplasia of the thyrotroph or gonadotroph cells associated with primary hypothyroidism or hypogonadism, respectively. Lactotroph hyperplasia increases throughout pregnancy due to increasing estrogen concentrations and is paralleled by increasing overall size of the pituitary and increasing serum prolactin concentrations. The average size of the pituitary is usually only slightly increased compared to the nonpregnant state, but occasionally it is large enough, coupled with a prolactin concentration of 200–400 ng/dl, to be mistaken for a lactotroph adenoma. Primary hypothyroidism[114] and primary hypogonadism[115] cause readily recognizable enlargement of the pituitary usually only when the target gland deficiency is both severe and untreated for several years. Treatment of the hypothyroidism with thyroxine or the hypogonadism with gonadal steroids will decrease the size of the pituitary to normal. In one case, an enlarged pituitary due to thyrotroph hyperplasia in a patient with primary hypothyroidism was perceptibly smaller after one month of thyroxine treatment[114] (Fig. 7-9).

Other Benign Tumors

Several other benign tumors can arise within or near the sella. They can therefore be mistaken for a pituitary adenoma and can cause deficiencies of pituitary hormones by pressure on the stalk or on the pituitary itself. The most common of these tumors are craniopharyngiomas and meningiomas.

Craniopharyngiomas These are solid or mixed cystic-solid tumors of epithelial cells that arise from remnants of Rathke's pouch

FIGURE 7-9 Enlargement of the pituitary due to thyrotroph hyperplasia in a patient with primary hypothyroidism (*A*) and decrease in size only one month after institution of treatment with thyroxine (*B*). (*From Beck-Peccoz et al, Endocrine Rev 17:610, 1996.*[114])

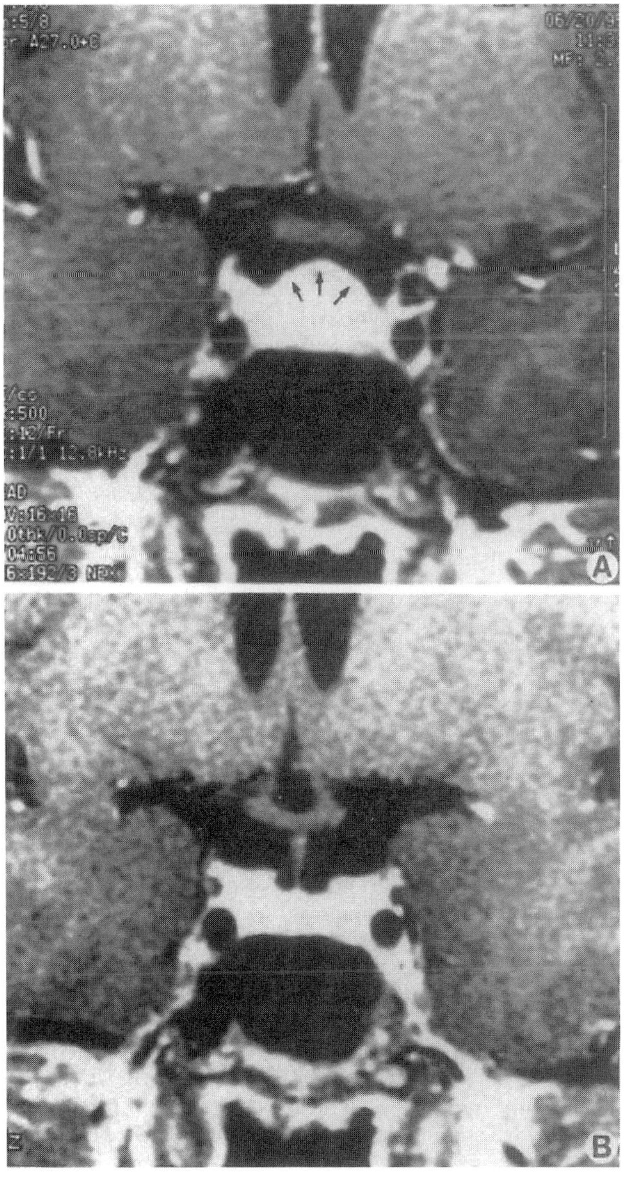

along a line from the nasopharynx to the diencephalon. There are two histologic types. The adamantinomatous type tends to produce keratin, calcify, and have both cystic and solid components. The squamous papillary type is almost entirely solid and does not produce keratin or calcify. The histologic type, however, does not appear to influence the clinical features of craniopharygiomas.[116] Most craniopharyngiomas occur either within or above the sella. About 50 percent occur before age 20 and 50 percent after, sometimes not until age 70 or 80. They present with deficiencies of anterior pituitary hormones and vasopressin, neurologic symptoms, such as visual impairment and headache, and, in children, growth retardation.

Meningiomas These are usually benign tumors that can arise from the meninges anywhere in the head. Because the meninges cover the sella, they can arise within or near the sella. They cause neurologic symptoms, such as visual impairment and headache, and deficiencies of anterior pituitary hormones.

Malignant Tumors

Primary malignancies can arise within or near the sella, and other malignancies metastasize to this area, especially to the cavernous sinuses.

Primary Malignancies These include germ cell tumors, sarcomas, chordomas, and carcinomas of anterior pituitary cells. Germ cell tumors, which are also called ectopic pinealomas, occur within the first three decades of life and present with symptoms of hydrocephalus, diabetes insipidus, and deficiencies of anterior pituitary hormones. Imaging usually demonstrates a mass in the third ventricle, and the serum concentration of human chorionic gonadotropin (hCG) is detectable. These tumors are highly malignant and metastasize readily, but are also highly radiosensitive. Chordomas are locally aggressive tumors that can also metastasize. They often arise in the clivus and present because of headaches, visual impairment, and anterior pituitary hormonal deficiencies. Pituitary carcinomas, recognizable by their ability to metastasize both intra- and extracranially,[117] are very rare. They may arise from any anterior pituitary cell, although those of lactotroph and corticotroph origin have been reported more commonly than others.

Metastases Metastases to the sellar area may occur within the sella, in a cavernous sinus, or to the hypothalamus (the last are described in Chap. 6). They can originate from many kinds of malignancies, including breast and lung. The presentation depends on the location of the metastasis; those within the sella present with hypopituitarism,[118] and those in a cavernous sinus present with unilateral periorbital pain, diplopia, and ptosis.[119]

Cysts

Several histologic types of cysts occur within the sella, including Rathke's cleft, arachnoid, and dermoid cysts. They may cause visual impairment and deficiencies of any of the anterior pituitary hormones by their mass effect.

Lymphocytic Hypophysitis

This is an apparently autoimmune condition that most often presents in women in late pregnancy or early postpartum period, although it may occur at other times in women and rarely in men. Although the pituitary gland is usually large at the time of presentation, the degree of headache is often of a greater severity than would be expected for other mass lesions of the same size. Later in the course of the disease the pituitary cells are destroyed and hypopituitarism occurs. Deficiencies of any anterior pituitary hormones may occur, but deficiency of ACTH is more common relative to deficiencies of other anterior pituitary hormones than typically occurs in patients who have other mass lesions.[120] Lymphocytic hypophysitis is associated with other autoimmune endocrine abnormalities, including chronic thyroiditis, with hypothyroidism, and Graves' disease.[121] Diabetes insipidus has also been associated.[121]

Granulomatous Hypophysitis

Giant cell, or granulomatous, hypophysitis appears to be histologically distinct from lymphocytic hypophysitis, but has many similarities in clinical presentation, including severe headache.[122]

Abscess

Abscesses are rare causes of mass lesions in the pituitary. Like cysts, the central area does not enhance following administration of gadolinium.[123]

Arteriovenous Fistula of the Cavernous Sinus

These lesions are also rare. Pituitary size returns to normal after the fistula is blocked.[124]

Pituitary Surgery

Surgery to excise a pituitary adenoma or other mass lesion in the sella can inadvertently result in removal of sufficient normal pituitary tissue to cause partial or complete hypopituitarism. This result is by no means inevitable, because often an experienced pituitary surgeon can distinguish between the lesion and normal pituitary tissue and can spare the latter, leaving pituitary function intact. In fact, if the mass lesion had caused hypopituitarism and the surgeon removes the mass and leaves the nondiseased pituitary, pituitary function may return to normal afterwards.[125]

Radiation

Radiation therapy for a pituitary adenoma often leads to hypopituitarism. One study of 22 patients who received supervoltage radiation following surgery showed that more than 50 percent developed new deficiencies of adrenal, thyroid, and gonadal function during the subsequent four years.[126] Other studies have shown similar results.[127,128] Deficiencies can become manifest for at least 10 years after radiation, so yearly monitoring of pituitary function is necessary for at least that period of time.

Infiltrative Lesions

In addition to lymphocytic hypophysitis, described previously, other infiltrative disease may affect the pituitary and cause hypopituitarism. The best recognized is hemochromotosis, which results in iron deposition in pituicytes. The most common hormonal deficiency is of gonadotropins, but other deficiencies may occur.[129] Repeated phlebotomy to remove the iron may reverse the hypogonadism.[130] Sarcoidosis usually causes hypopituitarism by infiltrating the hypothalamus, but may also cause hypopituitarism by infiltrating the pituitary directly.[131]

Infarction

Infarction of the pituitary following substantial blood loss during childbirth has been recognized as a cause of hypopituitarism since its description by Sheehan.[132,133] The mechanism is likely hypotension in the setting of highly vascular lactotroph hyperplasia. The cause of the bleeding does not seem to matter, since gastric hemorrhage in the third trimester has also been reported to cause infarction.[134] Although Sheehan's syndrome is well-recognized and methods of monitoring women during delivery have improved considerably, it still occurs. When infarction causes severe panhypopituitarism, it is manifest during the first days or weeks after delivery by the development of severe lethargy, anorexia, weight loss, and inability to lactate. Less severe damage to the pituitary causes less severe and more variable hypopituitarism, which may not be recognized for several years after the episode of hypotension. Diabetes insipidus may occasionally occur.[135–137]

Apoplexy

Sudden hemorrhage into the pituitary gland, called pituitary apoplexy, usually occurs spontaneously into a pituitary adenoma, but it may also occur when no pituitary adenoma either was previously known or can be demonstrated afterwards and may occur immediately after the injection of GnRH,[138] GnRH agonist,[139] or TRH[140] to patients with pituitary adenomas. In its most extreme form, it causes the sudden onset of excruciating headache, oculomotor nerve impairment resulting in diplopia, and hypopituitarism. The sudden onset of severe cortisol deficiency may be life-threatening. Both the hypopituitarism and diplopia may improve after surgical decompression,[141] but both may also improve spontaneously, as the blood is resorbed over the course of several weeks.[142]

Genetic Diseases

Congenital deficiencies of one or more pituitary hormones have been recognized for many years. Recently, the mutations responsible for two forms of congenital hypopituitarism have been identified, and both kinds of mutations are of transcription factors necessary for pituitary cytodifferentiation during embryogenesis. One group of mutations involves the transcription factor pit-1, which is necessary for the differentiation of the somatotrophs, lactotrophs, and thyrotrophs. Mutations of this gene result in congenital deficiencies of the secretion of growth hormone, prolactin, and TSH, and, consequently, in short stature and hypothyroidism.[82,83] Another group of mutations involves the transcription factor prop-1, which is expressed earlier in embryogenesis than pit-1 and is necessary for the differentiation of the gonadotrophs as well as of the somatotrophs, lactotrophs, and thyrotrophs. Consequently, mutations of this gene lead to short stature, hypothyroidism, and failure to undergo pubertal development.[143,144]

The mutations responsible for the majority of patients who have isolated growth hormone deficiency have not yet been identified, but a few patients have been described who mutations of the growth hormone-releasing hormone receptor,[145,146] leading to diminished growth hormone secretion, and one patient has been reported to have a mutation in the growth hormone gene, resulting in a biologically inactive hormone.[147]

Mutations have also been described in the genes encoding the thyrotropin-releasing hormone and gonadotropin-releasing hormone receptors,[148–150] leading to hypothryoidism and hypogonadism, respectively.

Empty Sella

The term empty sella refers to a sella turcica, sometimes enlarged, that is not entirely filled with pituitary tissue as in the normal case. There are two types of empty sella. In the secondary type, a mass, such as a pituitary adenoma, enlarges the sella, but then is diminished by surgery, radiation, or infarction. In this situation, hypopituitarism may occur as a consequence of the mass itself, its treatment, or spontaneous infarction. In the primary type, a tear in the diaphragm sella is thought to allow CSF pressure to enlarge the sella. There is no convincing evidence that this type of empty sella is associated with hypopituitarism or any hormonal syndrome.

Clinical Presentation of Anterior Pituitary Diseases

Anterior pituitary diseases can present clinically due to neurologic symptoms of a mass lesion in the sellar region, manifestations of hyposecretion of anterior pituitary hormones, manifestations of hypersecretion of those hormones, or some combination. Masses in the sellar region can also be first recognized as an incidental finding by radiologic imaging.

Neurologic Signs and Symptoms

Any of the mass lesions in the sellar region described above can cause neurologic symptoms, including visual impairment, headaches, diplopia, and cerebrospinal fluid rhinorrhea.

Visual Impairment

This is the most common symptom of a sellar mass lesion and is caused by suprasellar extension of the mass to elevate and compress the optic chiasm. The most characteristic pattern of visual impairment is diminished vision in the temporal fields, called bitemporal hemianopsia (Fig. 7-10). This pattern occurs as a result of pressure of the mass on the center of the optic chiasm, where the nerve fibers cross that innervate the nasal retinae, which view the temporal fields. Several variations of this pattern may occur. Initially, only the superior portion of the temporal fields may be affected; this condition is called superior temporal quadrantopsia. One or both fields may be affected, to variable degrees. Diminished visual acuity occurs when the optic chiasm is more severely compressed. Other patterns of visual loss may also occur, so an intrasellar lesion should be suspected whenever there is any unexplained pattern of visual loss.

Headaches

Headaches occur presumably due to expansion of the sella turcica. The pattern of headaches is extremely variable; there is no one pattern that is characteristic of a sellar mass.

FIGURE 7-10. Bitemporal hemianopsia in a patient with a pituitary macroadenoma markedly stretching the optic chiasm upward. The dark areas are the parts of the normal visual fields that the patient cannot see.

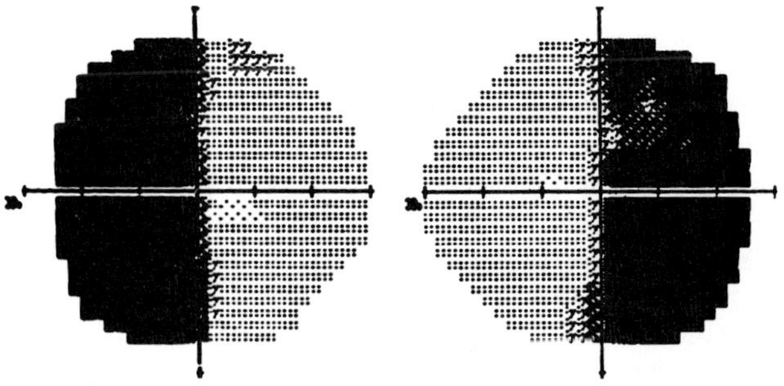

Diplopia

Extension of a sellar mass into one or both cavernous sinuses may compress the oculomotor nerves, impair oculomotor muscle function, and cause diplopia.

Cerebrospinal Fluid Rhinorrhea

Extension of a sellar mass, especially a pituitary adenoma, into the sphenoid sinus can cause cerebrospinal fluid rhinorrhea, which predisposes to meningitis.

Signs and Symptoms of Hormonal Abnormalities

Pituitary diseases frequently cause signs and symptoms due to hormonal abnormalities. Any disease of the pituitary gland or any sellar mass lesion can damage anterior pituitary cells and thereby cause deficient secretion of any or all anterior pituitary gland hormones. Only adenomas that arise from anterior pituitary cells, however, can cause hormonal hypersecretion. The signs and symptoms of pituitary hormonal hyposecretion and hormonal hypersecretion are described in subsequent sections.

Evaluation and Treatment of Mass Lesions

Evaluation

The purposes of evaluating mass lesions in the sellar area are to diagnose the type of lesion and to determine its anatomic extent and its visual and hormonal consequences.

Radiologic Evaluation

Radiologic evaluation can determine the anatomic extent of a sellar mass and can often provide some information about the possible type of lesion. The single best imaging procedure for most sellar masses is magnetic resonance imaging, and usually no other imaging procedure is needed. Magnetic resonance imaging can be performed both before and after the administration of gadolinium. Basally, normal pituitary tissue emits a signal that is similar or slightly greater than that of central nervous system tissue. Normal pituitary tissue takes up gadolinium more than central nervous system tissue, and so after the administration of gadolinium, normal pituitary tissue emits a brighter signal than does central nervous system tissue.

Anatomic Evaluation The first anatomic consideration is whether the pituitary gland is of normal size and emits a relatively homogenous signal both before and after the administration of gadolinium. In young adults the pituitary gland is usually no more than 6–7 mm tall, but in adolescents the pituitary may be as tall as 10 to 12 mm,[151] and during the last trimester of pregnancy and the first week postpartum it may be 10 mm.[152] Laterally the pituitary does not normally extend into the cavernous sinuses, and inferiorly it does not extend into the sphenoid sinus. Abnormalities of the pituitary may be manifest by a larger than normal size, extension outside the usual boundaries, or a focal increase or decrease in signal.

Diagnostic Specificity Magnetic resonance imaging may not only demonstrate the presence of a lesion in the sellar area, but may also narrow the diagnostic possibilities. Usually, though, no magnetic resonance imaging result is diagnostic of any one kind of mass (Fig. 7-11). If a sellar lesion can be seen as separate from the normal pituitary, whether on unenhanced or, more commonly, enhanced imaging, the lesion is not of pituitary tissue (i.e., not a pituitary adenoma or pituitary hyperplasia). Cystic lesions, such as Rathke's cleft cysts, often emit a low intensity signal on T1-weighted images, but craniopharyngiomas and even pituitary adenomas may be partially cystic and also emit low intensity signals. When the protein or lipid concentration of a cyst is high, however, the signal intensity on T1-weighted images will be high. On T2-weighted images, cysts may emit a high intensity image. Hemorrhage into the pituitary gland results in a high intensity signal on both T1- and T2-weighted images. Several sellar lesions take up gadolinium, including pituitary adenomas, craniopharyngiomas, and meningiomas, although often not to quite the degree of the normal pituitary, so after the administration of gadolinium these lesions emit a brighter signal than does central nervous system tissue. Cysts, however, do not take up gadolinium and so emit the same signal afterward as before. Microadenomas typically take up gadolinium to a lesser degree than does the normal pituitary.

Pituitary Incidentaloma Abnormalities in the pituitary are commonly detected as incidental findings when magnetic resonance imaging of the head is performed because of a symptom such as headache. When the lesion is clearly distinct from the pituitary or is within the pituitary and ≥1 cm in diameter, it should be evaluated for hormonal and visual abnormalities as any other mass lesion. If the lesion is within the pituitary, is <1 cm, and is not associated with any symptoms of hormonal hypersecretion, the most cost-effective approach is to measure only a serum prolactin concentration.[153] If the prolactin is normal, no further evaluation is necessary unless symptoms develop. The rationale for this approach is that these pituitary incidentalomas are very common, occurring in as many as 40 percent of young adults,[154] but rarely are associated with detectable hormonal abnormalities. It is currently thought that very few ever increase appreciably in size in subsequent years, although a significant number of such patients have not yet been followed for several years.

Visual Evaluation

All patients who have a sellar mass that elevates the optic chiasm should be evaluated by a neuroophthalmologist for visual acuity and visual fields. The latter should include evaluation by the Humphrey instrument.

Hormonal Evaluation

All patients who have a sellar mass should be evaluated for hormonal hypersecretion and hyposecretion. An exception is the incidentally discovered lesion <1 cm, as discussed previously. In patients whose clinical presentation suggests hypersecretion of one particular pituitary hormone, evaluation of hypersecretion should focus on that hormone. In patients whose clinical presentation does not suggest hypersecretion of any one pituitary hormone, evaluation for hypersecretion should include a prolactin, IGF-1, 24-h urine cortisol, FSH, LH, glycoprotein α subunit, and TSH. All patients who have a pituitary mass lesion should be evaluated for hormonal hyposecretion by measurement of serum T_4, early morning cortisol, testosterone in men, and estradiol in women of premenopausal age. If surgery is not planned for the near future and if the morning cortisol is <18 μg/dl, the test should be repeated, and if still <18 μg/dl, a test of ACTH reserve should be performed.

Treatment of Pituitary Mass Lesions

Surgery is the usual first treatment for most types of sellar masses that are causing neurologic symptoms, but there are

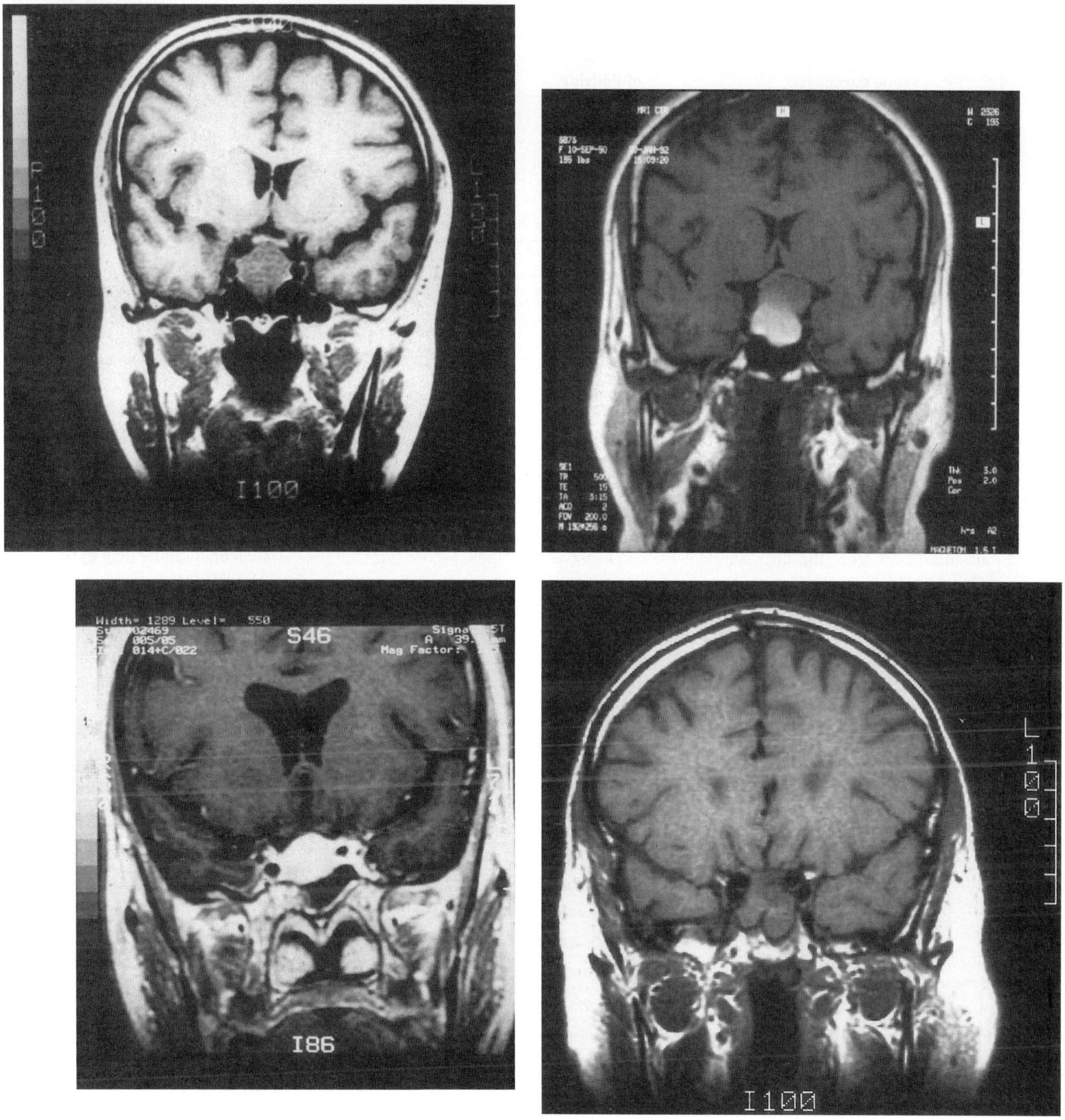

FIGURE 7-11. Magnetic resonance images of sellar masses, demonstrating the similarities in the appearances of the masses by this technique and therefore the difficulty in using this technique to differentiate one kind of sellar mass from another. Upper left, pituitary adenoma. Upper right, craniopharyngioma. Lower left, lymphocytic hypophysitis. Lower right, metastasis to the sellar region.

exceptions. One notable exception is a lactotroph adenoma, for which a dopamine agonist is the best initial treatment even when the lesion is causing neurologic symptoms. Radiation therapy may have an adjunctive role when surgery is not curative or if a mass lesion recurs. Radiation may also be appropriate for treatment of clinically nonfunctioning pituitary adenomas that are not causing neurologic symptoms but are large enough that symptoms are expected to occur eventually. Observation may be an appropriate course if there are no neurologic symptoms or deleterious effects of hormonal hypersecretion.

Surgery

Surgical Approaches to Sellar Masses The procedure most commonly used to approach sellar masses is transsphenoidal surgery via an operating microscope, but some surgeons are beginning to use a transsphenoidal endoscopic approach. When residual mass remains after transsphenoidal surgery and causes clinically important symptoms, a transcranial approach may be considered to remove additional tissue. A transcranial approach is used initially if the lesion is thought to originate superior to the diaphragma sella.

TABLE 7-4. Efficacy of Transsphenoidal Surgery for Pituitary Macroadenomas

Visual Parameter	Number of Patients	*Percent of Patients Whose Vision was* Better	Unchanged	Worse
Acuity				
Normal before surgery	181	NA	99	1
Abnormal before surgery	104	50	49	1
Fields				
Normal before surgery	71	NA	99	1
Abnormal before surgery	214	76	20	4

Source: Adapted from Trautmann and Laws.[158]

The transsphenoidal approach first gained widespread acceptance in the antibiotic era after Hardy introduced the use of the operative microscope.

An endoscopic approach to sellar masses has been reported by some surgeons recently.[155–157] This approach, which appears to be evolving, employs an endoscope in a similar fashion to endoscopic surgery of the sinuses. Some patients with hormonally active pituitary adenomas appear to have been cured by this procedure and others have not been cured. Some of the same complications that occur from the microsurgical technique have been reported.

Efficacy of Surgery Transsphenoidal surgery is usually effective in removing at least some of the sellar mass and thereby reducing or eliminating neurologic symptoms, such as visual impairment or headache. In one series of 104 patients with pituitary adenomas that extended above the sella and whose visual acuity was abnormal before transsphenoidal surgery for a pituitary adenoma, acuity improved in 50 percent, remained the same in 49 percent, and became worse in 1 percent (Table 7-4).[158] In the 214 patients in the same series whose visual fields were abnormal before transsphenoidal surgery, the fields improved in 76 percent, remained the same in 20 percent, and worsened in 4 percent. In a series of 113 pituitary adenomas that extended beyond the sella, 81 percent of those with visual field defects before surgery experienced improvement in fields after surgery, 19 percent remained the same, and none worsened.[159]

Transsphenoidal surgery is usually also successful in reducing, and less frequently in curing, hormonal hypersecretion from clinically functioning pituitary adenomas. Success rate is inversely related to adenoma size. Surgery may also be successful in correcting hypopituitarism.[125,160]

Complications of Surgery An indication of the kinds of complications of transsphenoidal surgery and their frequency can be ascertained from a survey in which neurosurgeons were asked to report their own experience (Table 7-5).[161] The complications reported by the 958 respondents included some that were serious, including carotid artery injury (1.1%), central nervous system injury (1.3%), loss of vision (1.8%), ophthalmoplegia (1.4%), hemorrhage or swelling of the residual tumor (2.9%), cerebrospinal fluid leak (3.9%), meningitis (1.5%), and death (0.9%). The chances of anterior pituitary insufficiencies (19.4%) and diabetes insipidus (17.8%) were higher. The incidence of each complication was higher among neurosurgeons who were less experienced. For example, among neurosurgeons who reported performing fewer than 200 transsphenoidal procedures, 1.2 percent of procedures resulted in death, but among neurosurgeons who reported performing more than 500 procedures, only 0.2 percent resulted in death. Although these results are based on retrospective self-reporting via questionnaire, they provide a broader assessment of complications of transsphenoidal surgery than that provided by the most experienced pituitary surgeons,[162–164] whose complication rates are closer to those of the most experienced group.[161]

Complication rates are greater in patients who have had prior pituitary surgery than in those who had not and even greater in those whose prior surgery was via craniotomy than in those whose prior surgery was transsphenoidal.[165]

Transsphenoidal surgery for other sellar masses, such as infradiaphragmatic craniopharyngiomas, appears to have similar degrees of efficacy in restoring vision and of complications as for pituitary adenomas.[166–168]

Preoperative Management Preoperative management of a sellar mass should include ascertaining the nature of the mass, assessing visual status, identifying a hormonal marker by which to judge the efficacy of the surgery if the lesion is a pituitary adenoma, identifying a very experienced pituitary surgeon, and ensuring the patient's hormonal stability. The nature of the mass is ascertained, as well as possible, by the radiologic and hormonal means described previously. If a pituitary adenoma hypersecretes an intact hormone or subunit, that can be used as a marker to judge the efficacy of any subsequent treatment. As described, the chance of

TABLE 7-5. Complications of Transsphenoidal Surgery in Relationship to the Experience of the Surgeon

Complication	*# of Previous Operations (% of Operations Resulting in Complication)* <200	20–500	>500
Carotid artery injury	1.4	0.6	0.4
Central nervous system injury	1.6	0.9	0.6
Hemorrhage into tumor bed	2.8	4.0	0.8
Loss of vision	2.4	0.8	0.5
Ophthalmoplegia	1.9	0.8	0.4
Cerebrospinal fluid leak	4.2	2.8	0.5
Meningitis	1.9	0.8	0.5
Nasal septum perforation	7.6	4.6	3.3
Anterior pituitary insufficiency	20.6	14.9	7.2
Diabetes insipidus	19.0	NA	7.6
Death	1.2	0.6	0.2

Data were collected from participating surgeons by questionnaire.

Source: Adapted from Ciric et al.[161]

complications decreases as the experience of the pituitary surgeon increases, so identifying the most experienced surgeon is essential. It is important to determine if the patient is hypothyroid prior to surgery because hypothyroidism increases the risk of respiratory arrest following postoperative administration of narcotics or barbiturates. Hypothyroidism, therefore, should be corrected preoperatively or these agents should be used in lower than usual doses. It is not necessary to test for cortisol deficiency preoperatively because all patients will be treated with high-dose glucocorticoid during the procecure unless a delay of more than a month until surgery is anticipated.

Immediate Postoperative Management In the week after surgery, diabetes insipidus, hyponatremia due to the inappropriate secretion of vasopressin, or both can occur. In one report of 92 patients, 25 percent became hyponatremic within the week after surgery and 20 percent had diabetes insipidus, at least transiently.[169] The serum sodium concentration and urine specific gravity and osmolality should therefore be monitored closely in the week after surgery. Patients who develop polyuria due to diabetes insipidus should be treated with aqueous vasopressin, either as subcutaneous bolus doses or as a continuous intravenous infusion. DDAVP should be avoided at this time because it is longer acting and therefore could cause hyponatremia if the diabetes insipidus suddenly remits, especially if it is followed by inappropriate vasopressin secretion. If diabetes insipidus is still present at the time of hospital discharge, DDAVP should be prescribed. A replacement dose of hydrocortisone should be prescribed at the time of discharge.

Short-Term Postoperative Management Four to six weeks after surgery the patient should be evaluated for the amount of residual mass, visual function by acuity and fields, and hormonal hypofunction. A crude estimate of the amount of residual mass can be made by magnetic resonance imaging, but artifacts of surgery may obscure the actual amount for several months. A better estimate of residual tissue, if the lesion is a hormonally-active pituitary adenoma, is measurement of the serum concentration of the adenoma product.

Evaluation for hypopituitarism should be made regardless of whether pituitary function was normal or abnormal before surgery, because surgery can result in damage to the normal pituitary[161–163] or in removal of a mass that had been compressing the normal pituitary and correction of hypopituitarism.[125,160] Thyroid function should be assessed by measurement of the serum thyroxine concentration. Adrenal function should be assessed by measurement of the serum cortisol concentration early in the morning. Values repeatedly less than 5 μg/dl indicate hypoadrenalism, and any value of 18 or above indicates normal adrenal function. Intermediate values require a test of ACTH reserve such as a metyrapone test. Measurement of serum cortisol 60 minutes after the administration of cosyntropin, whether 1 μg or 250 μg, should not be used in this setting because it may give a falsely normal result.[170–173] Gonadal function should be assessed by measurement of testosterone in men and estradiol in women. Vasopressin secretion should be assessed initially by measurement of 24-h urine volume if the patient has significant nocturia. A water deprivation test should be performed if the urine volume is greater than 3 liters per day; values above 6 liters are usually due to diabetes insipidus. Hormonal deficiencies should be treated, as described in the section on Hormonal Hyposecretion.

Long-Term Postoperative Management Long-term management should include evaluation every 6 to 12 months initially to detect regrowth of residual tissue and the adequacy of hormonal treatment. Evaluation for regrowth of residual tissue should include measurement of whatever serum marker was elevated before surgery, magnetic resonance imaging, and tests of vision. Detection that a clinically nonfunctioning pituitary adenoma has begun to regrow suggests the need to consider adjunctive treatment, such as radiation.

Radiation

Techniques of Radiation Radiation therapy has been used to treat pituitary adenomas for half a century. The technique used during most of this period has employed a supervoltage source to deliver a total of 45–50 Gy in daily 2-Gy doses via three external portals. Other techniques have recently been utilized which employ various radiation sources delivered stereotactically in an attempt to minimize the amount of radiation to which the brain is exposed (Table 7-6). One group of techniques, collectively called stereotactic radiosurgery, involves stereotactic administration of a large single dose of radiation from one of several possible sources, including protons from a cyclotron, high energy x-rays from a linear accelerator, or gamma radiation from a ^{60}Co source ("gamma knife"). Another technique, called "conformal radiation," involves administration of supervoltage radiation in fractionated doses, as in conventional radiotherapy, but from multiple portals and guided by a computer-generated model so that the radiation conforms to boundaries of the lesion.

Efficacy of Radiation When conventional radiation is administered following surgery for a pituitary macroadenoma, it is usually effective in preventing regrowth of the adenoma.[174–176] In one study of men who had conventional radiation therapy following surgery for clinically nonfunctioning pituitary macroadenomas, only 7 percent of the 63 patients who received radiation following surgery developed new visual impairment requiring additional treatment during the subsequent 15 years, but 66 percent of the 63 who did not receive radiation developed new visual impairment.[176] The efficacy of stereotactic methods of radiation delivery on preventing recurrence of pituitary adenomas and other sellar tumors remains to be determined.

Complications of Radiation There are both short-term and long-term side effects of conventional radiation. The short-term side effects include nausea, lethargy, loss of taste and smell, and loss of hair at the radiation portals. The first two remit within two months, and the latter two usually remit within six months but may be permanent. The most common long-term side effect is loss of one or more of the anterior pituitary hormones that had been normal prior

TABLE 7-6. Techniques of Radiation Therapy to the Pituitary

Technique	Radiation Source	Portals
Conventional	Supervoltage	Three
Conformal	Supervoltage	Multiple (computer generated)
Stereotactic radiosurgery		
Proton beam	Cyclotron	Multiple
	Linear accelerator	Multiple
Gamma knife	^{60}Co	Multiple

to radiation.[126,177,178] The chances are approximately 50 percent that at least one hormone that had been normal before surgery will be subnormal within five years afterward.[126] Neurological side effects occur less commonly. Blindness occurring due to optic neuritis,[179,180] brain tumors, and cerebrovascular accidents attributed to accelerated local atherosclerosis have been reported as case reports and in some series,[181,182] but other series that have evaluated possible neurologic sequellae have found none.[183] Because the various stereotactic techniques for administering radiation to the sella area are designed to expose the structures surrounding the sella and the brain to less radiation than does the conventional technique, it is possible that some of these may not be as likely to cause neurologic sequellae as does the conventional technique, but it is too soon to know if this hope will be realized. The larger amount of radiation given per dose during stereotactic radiosurgery, however, poses a potentially greater risk of optic neuritis than does conventional radiation. In fact, radiation-induced optic neuritis has already been reported following this procedure.[184]

Management of Patients after Radiation Following any kind of radiation for a pituitary adenoma, patients should be monitored for the development of hypopituitarism at 6 and 12 months and then once a year. Hormonal deficiencies should be treated as they are detected.

Medications

Dopamine agonist treatment is the first choice for reducing the size of lactotroph adenomas, no matter how large, as described later. Increasing evidence suggests that somatostatin analogs might be considered for reducing the size of somatotroph adenomas, also described in a later section. High-dose glucocorticoid treatment might be helpful in reducing the size of sarcoid lesions in the sella. Although medications have been occasionally reported to reduce the size of other kinds of pituitary adenomas and other sellar masses, none appears to do so with sufficient frequency to be worth using.

Observation

Mass lesions in the sella need not be treated to reduce their size if they are not causing visual impairment or other neurologic symptoms; if they are not, however, their size and their effect on vision and hormonal secretion should be monitored periodically. Masses of 1 cm or more in diameter should be reevaluated by magnetic resonance imaging in 6 to 12 months, and if no increase in size is seen in that time, less frequently thereafter. Hormonal secretion should be reevaluated at similar intervals.

Hormonal Hypersecretion—Pituitary Adenomas

Although any mass lesion in the sella area can lead to deficient secretion of anterior pituitary hormones by exerting pressure on the hypothalamus, stalk, or the pituitary itself, only adenomas of the anterior pituitary can secrete anterior pituitary hormones and thereby cause elevated serum concentrations of those hormones. Which hormone is hypersecreted by an adenoma depends on the cell type from which the adenoma arose.

Somatotroph Adenoma and Acromegaly

Somatotroph adenomas usually secrete growth hormone excessively and thereby cause the clinical syndrome of acromegaly. Rarely somatotroph adenomas do not secrete growth hormone sufficiently to cause acromegaly and can therefore be considered to be clinically silent.[185,186] Conversely, the cause of acromegaly is usually a somatotroph adenoma; rarely, excessive growth hormone-releasing hormone from the hypothalamus[187] or an ectopic source[188,189] causes somatotroph hyperplasia and excessive growth hormone secretion, and even more rarely growth hormone may be secreted by a somatotroph carcinoma.[190] Acromegaly has an annual incidence of three to four per million people.[191,192] Somatotroph adenomas represent about 25 percent of clinically recognized pituitary adenomas and are the cause of more than 99 percent of cases of acromegaly.

Causes of Acromegaly

The most common cause of acromegaly is excessive growth hormone secretion by a somatotroph adenoma. Less commonly, the cause is an adenoma that secretes both growth hormone and prolactin. Most somatotroph adenomas occur sporadically, but rarely they are familial.[193,194] Most are not associated with other abnormalities, but rarely they are associated with multiple endocrine neoplasia type I,[195] the McCune Albright syndrome,[196] or the Carney complex.[197] Somatotroph adenomas are among adenomas that have been shown to be monoclonal.[95] About 40 percent of somatotroph adenomas have an activating mutation of the $G_s\alpha$ gene, as described previously, including those with the McCune Albright syndrome.[196] Somatotroph carcinomas are extremely rare.[190] Acromegaly may rarely be caused by growth hormone hypersecretion stimulated by excessive secretion of growth hormone-releasing hormone from a hypothalamic tumor[187] or, more likely, from an ectopic source, such as a pancreatic islet tumor or a bronchial carcinoid.[188,189]

Pathology

Grossly, the majority of somatotroph adenomas are confined to the sella when the diagnosis is first made, principally in one of the lateral wings of the anterior pituitary. A substantial minority, however, especially those that secrete less efficiently, extend beyond the sella. The general histologic picture of a somatotroph adenoma is typical of pituitary adenomas, with sheets or nests of pituitary cells with more or less stroma, instead of the sinusoidal pattern of the nonadenomatous pituitary. Reticulin staining shows that the normal sinusoidal reticulin pattern is disrupted. A majority of the adenoma cells can readily be shown to be somatotroph cells by immunospecific staining for growth hormone. Adenomas that secrete both growth hormone and prolactin may be shown by immunospecific staining to be comprised of separate somatotroph and lactotroph cells[198] or of mammosomatotroph cells that contain both prolactin and growth hormone.[199] The histologic picture of the pituitary in patients who have acromegaly due to excessive secretion of growth hormone-releasing hormone is one of somatotroph hyperplasia. Somatotroph cells appear more numerous than normal, but the normal sinusoidal pattern of the anterior pituitary is preserved and other anterior pituitary cells are seen scattered among the somatotroph cells.[189] With progression of the disease, foci of adenomas are also seen.

Clinical Features

Acromegaly is the clinical syndrome caused by excessive growth hormone secretion. Thus, by definition, the clinical manifestations of acromegaly are due to excessive growth hormone secretion. When acromegaly results from a somatotroph

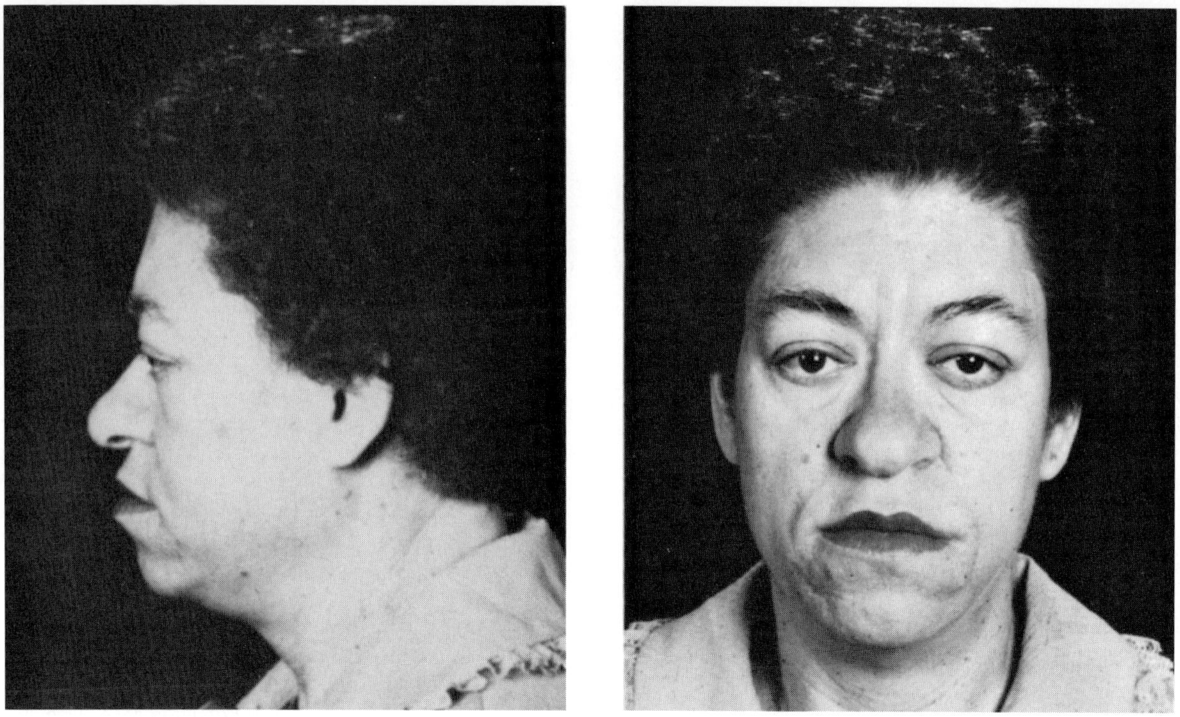

FIGURE 7-12. Severe acromegaly in a 43-year-old woman whose disease had been apparent for about 15 years. Marked soft tissue overgrowth is seen in the nose and around the eyes and mouth.

macroadenoma, the patient may also have any of the endocrinology or neurologic symptoms that a sellar mass lesion can cause, as described earlier. Excessive growth hormone secretion in adulthood causes growth of all soft tissues and stimulates the growth of cartilage and the thickness of all bones. Excessive growth hormone secretion prior to epiphyseal closure also increases the length of long bones and thereby causes gigantism, but it does not increase the length of long bones after epiphyseal closure.

Acral Enlargement Acral enlargement occurs due to growth of soft tissues, cartilage, and bone. The hands and feet become wider due to growth of soft tissues and cartilage. The nose and ears become large because of cartilaginous growth. The mandible lengthens because of the growth of cancellous bone, resulting in an underbite and increased spacing of the teeth. Growth of the maxillae leads to prominent cheekbones, and growth of the frontal bones leads to frontal bossing (Figs. 7-12 and 7-13).

FIGURE 7-13. Mild acromegaly in a woman 20 years before the diagnosis was made and before the disease was clinically apparent (*A*), when it was clinically apparent (*B*), and one year after transsphenoidal surgery and restoration of her serum growth hormone concentration to normal (*C*). Notice the subtle widening of the nose from (*A*) to (*B*) and reversal in (*C*).

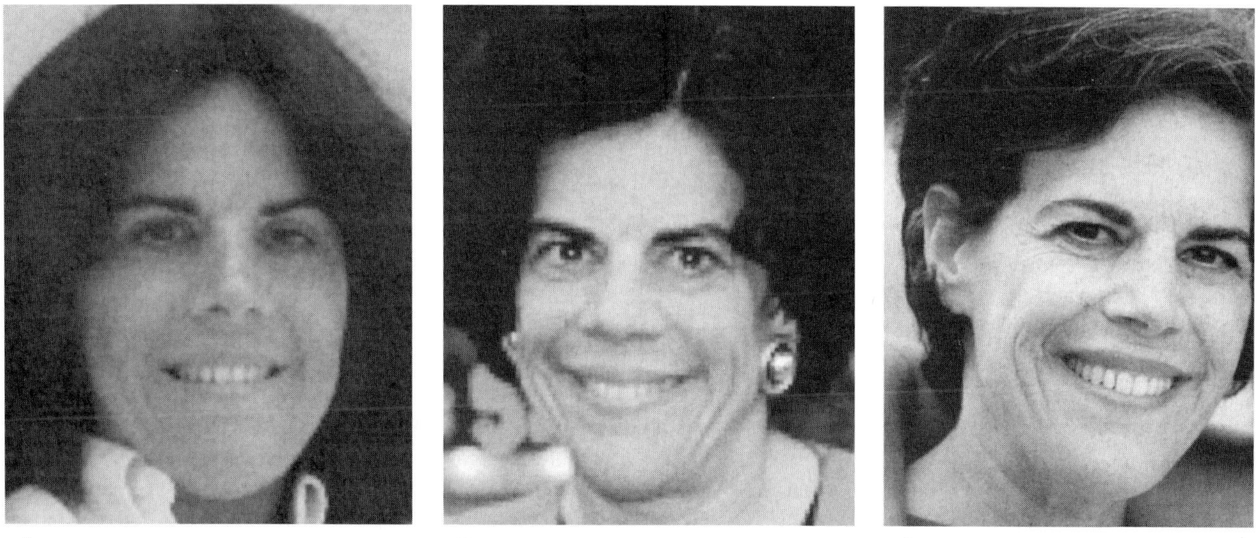

A B C

Arthritis Osteoarthritis is a common feature of acromegaly. Among a group of 500 patients with acromegaly, approximately 25 percent had moderate or severe osteoarthritis.[200] In another group of 90 patients, 76 percent had arthralgias, the majority of whom had the onset after the diagnosis of acromegaly.[201] Excessive growth of cartilage and overgrowth of the ends of the long bones may contribute to this condition. In one study of the thickness of joint cartilage as measured by ultrasonography, patients with active acromegaly had greater thickness of the cartilage of the shoulder, wrist, and knee than patients with inactive acromegaly or healthy subjects.[202]

Cancer Increased incidence of various kinds of cancer have been suspected in acromegaly, but most studies have been uncontrolled. In a retrospective cohort study of 1,362 acromegalic patients in the United Kingdom, the incidence of colon cancer was not quite of statistical significance ($P = .06$), and that of other cancers was not significant.[203] Mortality from colon cancer and from cancer overall, however, was significantly greater than expected, but not if the posttreatment growth hormone concentration was <2.5 ng/ml. If colon cancer is more prevalent in acromegalics than in nonacromegalics, it may well be related to the increased incidence of colonic polyps in acromegaly. In a prospective study of 103 acromegalic patients who were compared to 138 nonacromegalic patients with irritable bowel syndrome by colonoscopy, colonic polyps were more prevalent in acromegalic men (28.6%) than in nonacromegalic men (5.5%), but were not more prevalent in acromegalic women than in nonacromegalic women.[204] Other characteristics of the polyps in the acromegalics were that they were more likely to be multiple and more likely to be proximal to the splenic flexure than in nonacromegalics. Other studies have suggested an association between colonic polyps and multiple skin tags in acromegaly.[205,206]

Cardiovascular Disease Several cardiovascular abnormalities have long been reported anecdotally in patients with acromegaly, including hypertension, arteriosclerotic heart disease, and cardiomyopathy. Recent controlled studies confirm impaired cardiac performance in acromegalics and improved function following growth hormone reduction. In a study in 26 acromegalics and 15 nonacromegalics matched for age and gender, ventricular filling rates at rest and ejection fractions during exercise were reduced in the acromegalics.[207] Several studies have demonstrated that both cardiac enlargement and function are improved by lowering the serum growth hormone concentration by administration of octreotide.[208–210]

Diabetes Mellitus Diabetes mellitus is more common in acromegalics than in nonacromegalics, presumably because growth hormone antagonizes the effects of insulin.

Muscle Changes Increased growth hormone increases muscle mass, and early in the course of the disease may increase muscle strength. Later in the course of the disease, however, acromegalics may experience myopathy,[211] which may be the cause of muscular weakness reported in a third of patients.[200]

Neurological Symptoms The most common neurological symptoms in acromegaly are headaches and symptoms due to neuropathies. In a study of 500 acromegalics, more than 50 percent noted headaches.[200] In acromegalics, headaches may occur even in the absence of macroadenomas, and they are rapidly relieved when the serum growth hormone concentration is lowered by administration of a somatostatin analog, suggesting that they may be due to the supranormal serum growth hormone concentration. Median neuropathy due to compression of the nerve at the wrist, known as carpal tunnel syndrome, is much more common in acromegalics than in nonacromegalics, presumably as a consequence of soft tissue swelling. In one study of 100 acromegalics, 35 had carpal tunnel syndrome.[212] In the study of 500 patients, a third were affected, although only about half of them to a moderate or severe degree.[200] Peripheral neuropathy has also been reported[213] and may occur in as many as 50 percent of patients.[200]

Skin Diseases The most common skin manifestations of acromegaly are skin tags, excessive perspiration, and, in women, hirsutism. Skin tags are usually of concern because they appear to be correlated with colonic polyps,[205,206] which predispose to colon cancer. Excessive perspiration is bothersome in itself and because it predisposes to excessive body odor. In a study of 500 acromegalics, more than 70 percent noted excessive perspiration.[200]

Sleep Apnea Sleep apnea has long been noted to be more common in acromegaly than in nonacromegalics. In a study of 21 patients with a history of acromegaly, 4 of the 10 patients who were judged to have active disease were found to have sleep apnea, but none of the 11 patients judged to have inactive disease did.[214] Three of the 4 patients had only obstructive sleep apnea, and one had mixed central and obstructive disease. In another study of 43 acromegalics who had sleep apnea, two-thirds had obstructive and one-third had central sleep apnea.[215] Obstructive sleep apnea is presumably due to enlargement of the tongue and soft tissues of the pharynx, but the reason for central sleep apnea is not clear. Sleep apnea may be a reason that approximately 15 percent of acromegalics reported moderate to severe daytime somnolence.[200]

Viscera All of the viscera increase in size in acromegaly, including the heart, lungs, and kidneys. The size of the thyroid and testes also increases. The effects on the functions of these organs are mixed. Cardiomegaly, as described above, is often associated with impaired function. Increased size of the lungs is associated with a marked increase in vital capacity. Increased creatinine clearance in acromegaly may be associated with increased kidney size or with increased muscle mass.

Weight It is not surprising that acromegaly is associated with increased weight because all tissues increase in size. This increase is associated with an increase in lean body mass and a decrease in fat mass.

Mortality Several studies demonstrate increased mortality in acromegalic patients compared to what is expected for the nonacromegalic population. In a study of 194 acromegalic patients who were referred to five hospitals in the United Kingdom between 1937 and 1967, 55 died, almost twice the number expected in the general population matched for age and gender.[216] In a retrospective study of 79 acromegalic patients identified in a review of records from a 24-year period in one center in the United Kingdom, 28 had died, more than twice the number expected for the general population.[217] The increased number of deaths was due to cardiovascular and respiratory diseases in men and to cerebrovascular and respiratory diseases in women. Deaths due to

TABLE 7-7. Increased Mortality in Acromegaly Compared to the General Population

	Number of Acromegalics	Observed Deaths	Expected Deaths	Ratio Observed To Expected	P
Men	29	14	5.5	2.6	.002
Women	50	14	4.9	2.8	.001
Total	79	28	10.4	2.6	<.001

Source: Bates et al, *Quarterly Journal of Medicine* 86:293, 1993.

malignancies were greater only in women 65–74 years old. The cause of death was cardiovascular in 57 percent of the cases, and those who died had higher growth hormone concentrations than those who lived. The survival of the 39 percent who had posttreatment growth hormone concentrations <2.5 ng/ml was no different from that in the general population. In a retrospective multicenter cohort study of 1,362 patients with acromegaly in the United Kingdom, the overall mortality rate was greater than expected for acromegalics whose serum growth hormone concentrations after treatment were >2.5 ng/ml, but was not increased for those whose serum growth hormone concentrations were <2.5 ng/ml (Table 7-7).[203] Mortality rates in the acromegalic patients were higher due to cardiovascular disease and colon cancer.

Diagnosis

The diagnosis of acromegaly begins with recognition of the clinical features described previously and continues with establishing a history of growth during adult life, demonstrating excessive growth hormone secretion, establishing its cause, determining its consequences, and, if the patient has a somatotroph macroadenoma, discovering if the adenoma has any endocrinologic consequences or any neurologic consequences.

Clinical Diagnosis The most difficult aspect of diagnosing acromegaly is suspecting it. Although the clinical features of acromegaly are distinctive, at least when the disease has been present for many years, the diagnosis of acromegaly usually is not made for an average of 10 years after it is clinically apparent.[218] There are likely several reasons for this long delay. One reason is that many of the manifestations of acromegaly, such as an increase in hand size, are not recognized by the patient as representing a disease. Another reason is that physicians and patients usually do not recognize the linkage between the various clinical findings, such as increased hand size and daytime somnolence due to sleep apnea. A third reason is that the clinical manifestations of acromegaly occur so insidiously that those who see the patient frequently, both family members and physicians, are often not aware that they have occurred at all. For all of these reasons, the diagnosis is often first suspected by a physician who sees the patient for the first time.

Once the diagnosis has been suspected, the next steps are clear. First is to document growth during adult life, by obtaining a history of a clear increase in ring and/or shoe size and by examining old photographs, sometimes as many as several decades old.

Demonstrating Excessive Growth Hormone Secretion The next step is to demonstrate excessive growth hormone secretion. One way is to measure the serum growth hormone concentration 1–2 h after an oral glucose load, when the growth hormone concentration should be <2 ng/ml (radioimmunoassay) or <1 ng/ml (immunoradiometric or chemiluminescent assay) in a nonacromegalic person (Fig. 7-14). Measurement of a random growth hormone concentration is usually not of diagnostic value because it fluctuates so much spontaneously.

A more practical way to confirm the diagnosis is by measuring the serum IGF-1 concentration, which is relatively stable and so can be measured at any time. This test is also of value because there is little overlap between values of acromegalics and nonacromegalics (Fig. 7-15).[219,220] IGF-1 assays, however, should be performed only in those few commercial laboratories known to perform the test reliably. In addition, the results must be compared to age-adjusted ranges of normal because the serum IGF-1 concentration during postpubertal adult life normally decreases with increasing age.

Other tests that confirm the diagnosis but are usually not necessary are measurement of IGFBP-3 and the growth hormone response to hypothalamic releasing hormones. IGFBP-3 is an IGF-1 binding protein, and, like IGF-1, its serum concentration is growth hormone-dependent. Consequently, its serum concentration is usually higher than normal in acromegaly.[221] However, measurement of IGFBP-3 does not distinguish acromegalics from nonacromegalics better than does IGF-1,[220] so its measurement usually adds little to the diagnosis. Somatotroph adenomas, like

FIGURE 7-14. Incomplete suppression of the serum growth hormone concentration by glucose in acromegaly. Following an oral glucose load, 35 normal individuals (*left*) had a serum glucose concentration of <2 ng/ml (radioimonunoassay) two hours later, but none of nine acromegalics did. (*From Federman, Pituitary, in Dale and Federman (eds), Scientific American Medicine, Scientific American, Inc. New York, 1999.*)

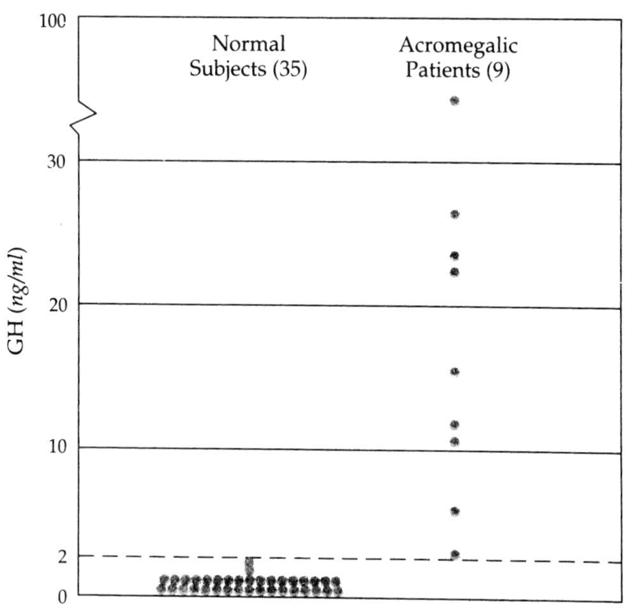

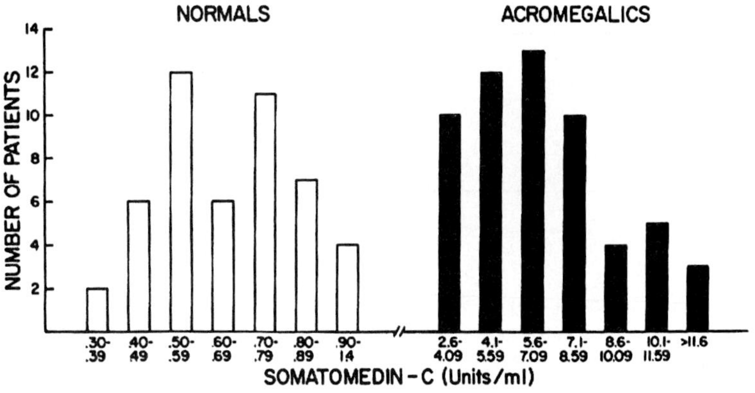

FIGURE 7-15. Serum IGF-1 (previously called somatomedin-C) concentrations in acromegalic patients compared to normal subjects, showing the usually clear separation between the two groups. (*From Clemmons et al, N Engl J Med 301:1138, 1979.*[219])

other pituitary adenomas, express receptors for hypothalamic releasing hormones and therefore respond to administration of a bolus dose of thyrotropin-releasing hormone[222] or gonadotropin-releasing hormone by secreting growth hormone. Such responses occur in only about 50 percent of somatotroph adenomas, however, so this test does not replace measurement of IGF-1. A positive test could support the diagnosis of a somatotroph adenoma in the unusual situation where the clinical evidence is equivocal and the serum IGF-1 concentration and growth hormone response to glucose are borderline.

Establishing the Cause of Excessive Growth Hormone Secretion Once the clinical suspicion of acromegaly has been confirmed by finding excessive growth hormone secretion, the next step is to look for evidence that the cause of the excessive growth hormone is a somatotroph adenoma by magnetic resonance imaging. If imaging demonstrates a clearly delineated pituitary lesion, that lesion can be assumed to be the cause. If imaging does not demonstrate a clearly delineated lesion, the chance is increased that the cause is excessive growth hormone–releasing hormone from an ectopic source. In such patients the serum concentration of growth hormone-releasing hormone should be measured. Growth hormone-releasing hormone should also be measured if transsphenoidal surgery is performed on the assumption that the cause of acromegaly is a somatotroph adenoma but pathologic examination reveals somatotroph hyperplasia.

Determining the Consequences of Excessive Growth Hormone Secretion Pretreatment evaluation of acromegaly should include determination not only of the cause but also the consequences. Some are direct consequences of excessive growth hormone secretion, as described earlier. For most of the potential consequences, it is sufficient to make an initial evaluation clinically and base further evaluation on the results. If, for example, loud snoring and daytime somnolence are reported, polysomnography should be performed to evaluate the possibility of sleep apnea. Colonic polyps, however, are usually asymptomatic, so colonoscopy should be performed in most newly discovered acromegalic patients and certainly in those who have more than three skin tags.

Discovering the Consequences of a Macroadenoma If magnetic resonance imaging demonstrates a macroadenoma, the possibility of both endocrinologic and neurologic consequences should be evaluated, as previously described under sellar mass lesions. Endocrinologic consequences include deficiencies of ACTH, TSH, and gonadotropins. Neurologic consequences include, principally, impairment of vision.

Treatment

The goals of treating acromegaly are to reduce the serum growth hormone concentration to normal, to preserve other pituitary hormone function and, for patients who have a macroadenoma neurologic symptoms, to remove enough adenoma tissue to relieve those symptoms. A current definition of what constitutes a normal serum growth hormone concentration was enunciated at a recent consensus conference as a value less than 2 ng/ml by radioimmunoassay or less than 1 ng/ml by immunoradiometric assay or chemiluminescent assay after a glucose load or a serum IGF-1 concentration within the normal range for age.[223] Most previous studies of the effect of treatment of acromegaly, however, have reported the percentage of patients who have achieved growth hormone values of less than 10 or 5 ng/ml, rather than less than 2 ng/ml, so it is difficult to tell what percentage of patients have been cured by the different kinds of treatment.

For many years the usual initial treatment for acromegaly has been transsphenoidal surgery, and the usual adjunctive treatment, if surgery was not entirely successful, has been radiation of the residual adenoma. The recent introduction of somatostatin analogs and the demonstration that they lower the serum growth hormone concentration of acromegalics, often to normal, has led to greater use of these medications as the usual adjunctive treatment and increasingly as the initial treatment.

Surgery Transsphenoidal surgery is usually successful in removing at least part of a somatotroph adenoma, lowering the serum growth hormone concentration, and ameliorating the acromegaly, but usually it is not curative. The chance of a cure depends on the size of the adenoma and on the extent of cavernous sinus invasion, as well as on the experience of the surgeon. In one series of 224 patients with acromegaly, 72 percent of patients with microadenomas and 33 percent of patients with macroadenomas had postglucose serum growth hormone values ≤ 2 ng/ml within days after transsphenoidal surgery.[225] In another series of 254 consecutive patients with acromegaly, 76 percent had basal serum growth hormone concentrations <5 ng/ml within 30 days after transsphenoidal surgery; patients with smaller, more localized adenomas were more likely to have lower values.[228] A third series also showed that patients who had smaller adenomas prior to surgery had lower growth hormone concentrations afterwards (Table 7-8).[224]

TABLE 7-8. Results of Transsphenoidal Surgery for Acromegaly Related to Adenoma Size

		Serum Growth Hormone after a Glucose Load					
		<1 ng/mL		*<2.5 ng/mL*		*<10 ng/mL*	
Size of Adenoma	**Number of Patients**	**n**	**%**	**n**	**%**	**n**	**%**
Micro (<1 cm)	25	16	64	21	84	22	88
Macro (>1 cm), within sella	18	13	72	18	100	18	100
Macro, with suprasuprasellar extension	19	5	26	10	53	14	74
Macro, with lateral and downward extension	14	3	21	9	64	10	71

Source: Adapted from Osman et al.[224]

Normal serum growth hormone and IGF-1 concentrations following transsphenoidal surgery, however, do not necessarily indicate a permanent cure, because some patients who have normal values at this time develop elevations in subsequent years. In one of the series described above, of the 193 patients who had an apparent remission within 30 days after surgery, nine subsequently developed elevations of growth hormone.[228]

Side effects of surgery for somatotroph adenomas are similar to those for other sellar mass lesions.

Radiation Radiation therapy of somatotroph adenomas is usually successful in reducing the serum growth hormone concentration, but often not entirely to normal, and the maximum effect, however much it is, often takes 10 to 15 years. In one study of 47 acromegalic patients who received 40 to 50 Gy of supervoltage radiation and were followed for 2 to 10 years, 69 percent had values ≤5 ng/ml 10 years after treatment and 43 percent had values ≤2 ng/ml (Fig. 7-16).[229] In another study of 38 patients who received 45 to 50 Gy, 89 percent had serum growth hormone concentrations <5 ng/ml at an average of 6.8 years after treatment, but only 5 percent had serum IGF-1 concentrations within the normal range.[230] Insufficient time has elapsed since the introduction of the newer forms of radiation to know if the results with them will differ from those with conventional forms.

Pharmacotherapy Two classes of drugs may decrease the serum growth hormone concentration in an acromegalic: dopamine agonists and somatostatin analogs. The action of each is dependent on the presence of the corresponding receptors on the somatotroph adeoma. The inhibitory effect of dopamine agonists in acromegalic patients is paradoxical, because they stimulate growth hormone secretion in normal people. The obvious advantage of these agents is the oral route of administration. In one series of 31 acromegalic patients, 10–20 mg/day of bromocriptine for six to nine months decreased the serum growth hormone to some degree in 74 percent, but to normal in only 3 percent.[231] The response of IGF-1 was similar. In a double-blind cross-over study of 18 acromegalic patients, up to 20 mg/day of bromocriptine for three months did not lower the serum growth hormone or IGF-1 concentrations any more than did placebo.[232] In a study of 64 patients treated with 1.0–1.75 mg/day of cabergoline, the serum growth hormone concentration decreased to ≤2 ng/ml in 64 percent of the 16 who had adenomas secreting growth hormone and prolactin and in 47 percent of adenomas secreting only growth hormone.[233] Side effects of dopamine agonists are described under treatment of lactotroph adenomas. In a study of 34 patients with acromegaly, the dopamine agonist CV 205-502 appeared to decrease the serum growth hormone concentration in a higher percentage of patients than did bromocriptine or cabergoline, although no direct comparison among the three drugs was made.[234]

Somatostatin analogs also suppress the serum growth hormone concentration in acromegalic patients. Octreotide, the preparation originally introduced, requires administration by subcutaneous injection every eight hours, but long-acting preparations of octreotide and another somatostatin analog, lanreotide require injection only once every 2–4 weeks. In one study of 115 acromegalic patients treated with 100 to 250 μg/8 h of the short-acting form of octreotide for six months, the mean serum growth hormone concentration was reduced to <5 ng/ml in approximately 50 percent of the subjects, and the serum IGF-1 concentration was reduced to normal in approximately 60 percent (Fig. 7-17).[235] When 103 of

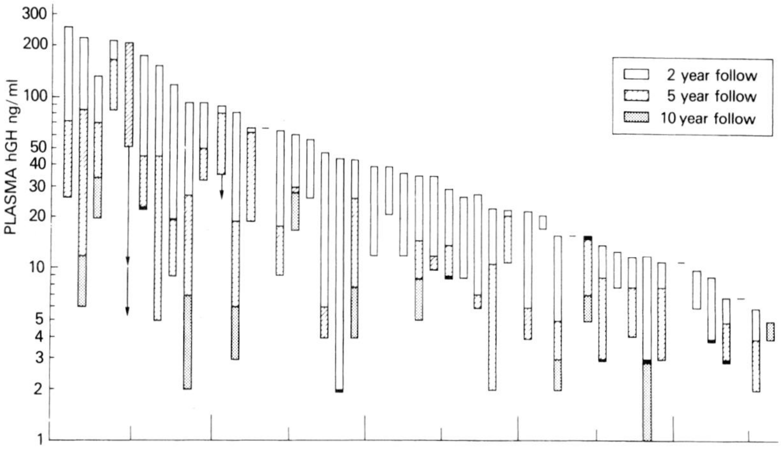

FIGURE 7-16. Serum growth hormone concentrations before and after radiation therapy in 47 acromegalic patients. Each bar represents the growth hormone concentrations in a single patient. The top each bar represents the pretreatment growth hormone concentration, the bottom of the clear area the value 2 years after radiation, the bottom of the hatched area the value 5 years after radiation, and the bottom of the stippled area the value 10 years after radiation. (*From Eastman et al, J Clin Endocrinol Metab 48:931, 1979.*[229])

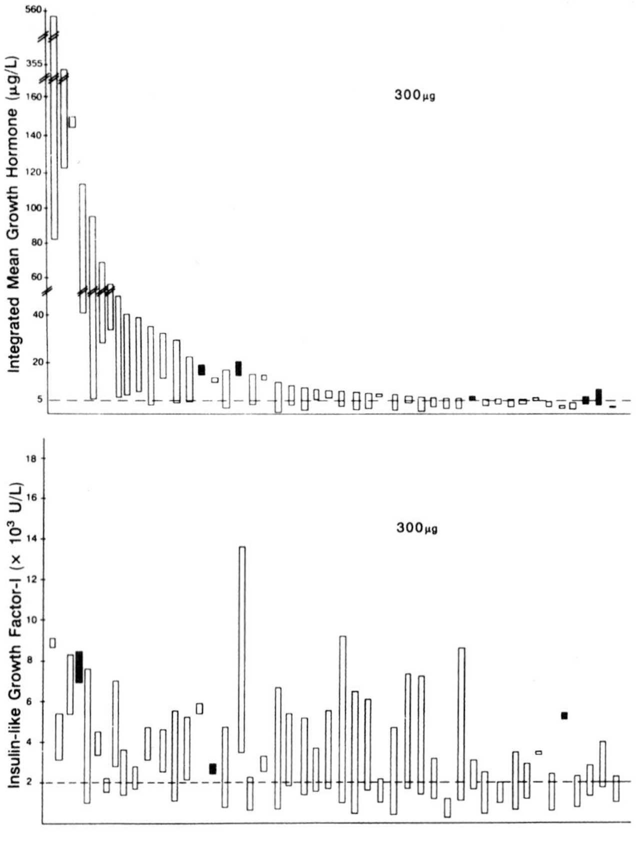

FIGURE 7-17. Serum growth hormone and IGF-1 concentrations before and during octreotide therapy of 47 acromegalic patients treated with 300 μg of octreotide a day (100 μg every eight hours) for six months. The top of each bar represents the pretreatment value and the bottom represents the value at the end of six months of treatment. (*From Ezzat et al, Ann Intern Med 117:711, 1992.*[235])

the same patients were followed for two years, the serum IGF-1 was within the normal range at least half of the times it was assessed in 64 percent of the patients.[236]

Long-acting forms of octreotide and lanreotide are at least as effective in lowering the serum growth hormone and IGF-1 concentrations as their short-acting forms and are more convenient to administer. The long-acting form of octreotide, which is administered once a month, lowered the mean serum growth hormone in a group of eight acromegalics from >10 ng/ml to <3 ng/ml.[237] A long-acting form of lanreotide lowered the serum growth hormone concentration after one year to normal in only 2 of 22 acromegalic patients, but reduced the IGF-1 to normal in 11 of 22.[238]

Side effects of the administration of octreotide or lanreotide include short-term gastrointestinal side effects, such as nausea and abdominal cramps, and long-term side effects, such as gallstones,[236,239] which occur in as many as 20 percent of patients. Nausea and cramps occur in a majority of patients immediately after the medication is begun, but usually remit within one to two weeks. These medications predispose to gallstone formation by impairing gallbladder contractility.[240,241]

Lactotroph Adenoma and Other Causes of Hyperprolactinemia

Lactotroph adenomas are the most common cause of clinically significant hyperprolactinemia and are the pituitary adenomas that are most likely to be amenable to pharmacologic treatment. However, because they are not the only cause of hyperprolactinemia, the cause must first be identified before treatment can be undertaken.

Causes of Hyperprolactinemia

Prolactin is secreted only by the lactotroph cells, so hyperprolactinemia is always caused by increased prolactin secretion by these cells. The causes can be physiologic or pathologic (Table 7-9).

Physiologic Causes of Hyperprolactinemia The most common physiologic cause is pregnancy. The serum prolactin concentration increases gradually during pregnancy until delivery. In one study the mean value at delivery was about 200 ng/ml, and the highest value was 600 ng/ml.[242] By six weeks postdelivery, the serum prolactin had returned to nonpregnant values. The likely cause of the hyperprolactinemia is the increased serum estradiol concentrations.

Another physiologic cause of hyperprolactinemia is nipple stimulation, presumably by a neural mechanism. The magnitude of the elevation is directly proportional to the preexisting status of the lactotroph cell. At the end of pregnancy, when the lactotroph cells are hyperplastic as the consequence of the high estradiol concentrations of pregnancy, the increase is as much as a few hundred ng/ml above baseline. Several months after delivery, the increase is only about 10 ng/ml above baseline. The increase in men is minimal or nil.

Stress, physical or psychologic, is yet another cause of hyperprolactinemia, although usually of small magnitude. The post stress values usually do not exceed 40 ng/ml.

TABLE 7-9. Causes of Hyperprolactinemia

Physiologic
Pregnancy
Nursing
Exercise
Physical and psychological stress
Sleep
Pharmacologic
Dopamine receptor antagonists
phenothiazines, haloperidol, metaclopramide, sulpiride, risperidone
Catecholamine inhibitors
reserpine
alpha-methyldopa
Verapamil
H_2 antagonists (e.g., cimetidine)
TRH
Estrogens
Opiates
Pathologic
Lactotroph adenomas
Other pituitary adenomas and nonpituitary lesions in the sella or hypothalamus
Hypothyroidism
Chest wall injury
Chronic renal failure
Other
Idiopathic
"Big" prolactin

Pathologic Causes of Hyperprolactinemia Pathologic causes of hyperprolactinemia include tumors of the lactotroph cell and several diseases which result in lactotroph hyperplasia.

Lactotroph Adenomas Virtually all tumors of the lactotroph cell are adenomas, although rarely they are carcinomas.[243] Lactotroph adenomas, like other pituitary adenomas, are true neoplasms, arising from a somatic mutation of a cell which then undergoes monoclonal expansion. What mutation(s), however, is not yet known. These adenomas are relatively common, accounting for 30 to 40 percent of all pituitary adenomas. Most occur sporadically, but a small proportion are associated with the multiple endocrine neoplasia type I syndrome.[244] A typical feature of lactotroph adenomas is efficiency; a microadenoma (<1 cm in diameter) usually secretes sufficient prolactin to cause hyperprolactinemia. Another typical feature is rough proportionality of the elevation of the prolactin concentration to the size of the adenoma: adenomas <1 cm are usually associated with serum prolactin concentrations of <200 ng/ml; adenomas of 1 to 2 cm with prolactin concentrations of 200 to 1000 ng/ml; and adenomas >2 cm with concentrations >1000 ng/ml.

Lactotroph Hyperplasia Continuous stimulation or decreased inhibition of prolactin secretion can cause lactotroph hyperplasia and, consequently, prolactin hypersecretion. One mechanism by which this occurs is decreased dopamine inhibition of the lactotroph cell in one of several ways. Diseases of the hypothalamus and pituitary may interfere with the secretion of dopamine from the hypothalamus or its delivery to the lactotroph cells. Tumors, both benign and malignant, and infiltrative diseases of the hypothalamus may damage the hypothalamic neurons that synthesize and secrete prolactin. Transsection of the hypothalamic-pituitary stalk, as by head trauma, or pressure on the stalk, as by a pituitary adenoma, prevents dopamine from reaching the pituitary. Several drugs antagonize D2 receptors, including neuroleptic drugs (phenothiazines, haloperidol),[245] metoclopramide,[246] sulpiride, domperidone, and respiridol. In addition, methyldopa inhibits dopamine synthesis,[247] and reserpine inhibits dopamine storage.[248]

Estrogen also causes lactotroph hyperplasia, and does so proportionately to the degree of estrogenization. The higher physiologic concentrations of estrogen in women explain why they have a greater prolactin response to most physiologic stimuli than do men.[249]

Hypothyroidism also predisposes to hyperprolactinemia. The basal serum prolactin concentration is normal in most hypothyroid patients, but it is elevated in a few, and in those it falls to normal when the hypothyroidism is treated.[250,251] The combination of primary hypothyroidism and hyperprolactinemia, which may also be associated with an enlarged pituitary gland, may be mistaken for a lactotroph adenoma.

Other Causes of Hyperprolactinemia Two other causes of hyperprolactinemia are unrelated to lactotroph adenoma or hyperplasia. One is chronic renal failure, in which the serum prolactin concentration is elevated because prolactin clearance is impaired, and following renal transplantation returns to normal.[252,253] Another cause is when the predominant prolactin is a glycosylated form which aggregates; the aggregates are called "big" prolactin.[254]

Pathology

Grossly, lactotroph adenomas are frequently <1 cm in diameter if the patient is a premenopausal woman who presents because of symptoms of hypogonadism, such as amenorrhea, or >1 cm if the patient is postmenopausal or a man who does not present until the adenoma becomes so large as to cause neurologic symptoms. Small adenomas are usually present in one of the lateral wings of the anterior pituitary. Large adenomas are often partly necrotic and/or hemorrhagic. Histologically, the cells are arranged in sheets or nests with a variable amount of stromal tissue rather than in the normal sinusoidal pattern. Reticulin staining confirms the breakdown of the sinusoidal pattern. Immunocytochemical staining usually readily demonstrates staining for prolactin, and in mammosomatotroph adenomas[199] and mixed lactotroph and somatotroph adenomas[198] demonstrates staining for growth hormone as well. Dopamine agonist treatment shrinks the size of individual lactotroph adenoma cells, but does not reduce the number of adenoma cells, resulting in a denser cell population.[255] Lactotroph carcinomas, recognizable by distant metastases, occur rarely.[117]

Clinical Features of Hyperprolactinemia

Hyperprolactinemia causes symptoms in premenopausal women and in men, but not in postmenopausal women.

Premenopausal Women The most common manifestation of hyperprolactinemia in premenopausal women is hypogonadotropic hypogonadism, due to inhibition of LH secretion. The degree of the hypogonadism is directly proportional to the magnitude of the hyperprolactinemia. For example, serum prolactin concentration >100 ng/ml typically cause pronounced hypogonadism,[256,257] including decreased estradiol secretion and failure of ovulation, which leads to amenorrhea, infertility, hot flashes, vaginal dryness, and bone loss.[257,258] Prolactin concentrations of 50 to 100 ng/ml usually cause amenorrhea or oligomenorrhea. Prolactin concentrations of 20 to 50 ng/ml usually cause oligomenorrhea or only decreased progesterone secretion, which is manifested by a short luteal phase and infertility.[259,260]

Another manifestation of hyperprolactinemia is galactorrhea,[261] although it is much less common, occurring in only about 10 to 15 percent of women with hyperprolactinemia. Only a minority of women who have galactorrhea have hyperprolactinemia and abnormal menses.

Postmenopausal Women Because postmenopausal women are already hypogonadal and have no menses, hyperprolactinemia causes no change in menstrual status and no galactorrhea. Consequently, lactotroph adenomas are not recognized in these women unless and until they become so large as to cause neurologic symptoms.

Men Hyperprolactinemia causes hypogonadotropic hypogonadism in men, as it does in premenopausal women, resulting in decreased libido and infertility.[262,263] Hyperprolactinemia in men also causes impotence and, infrequently, galactorrhea.[262] The mechanism by which hyperprolactinemia causes impotence may be different than that by which it causes hypogonadism, because correcting the hypogonadism by lowering the serum prolactin concentration increases the serum testosterone concentration and also restores potency, but correcting the hypogonadism by administering testosterone does not restore potency.

Diagnosis

The diagnosis of a lactotroph adenoma begins with finding hyperprolactinemia and continues by excluding other possible causes.

Serum Prolactin Concentration Serum prolactin concentration should be measured in any woman who has amenorrhea, oligomenorrhea, or galactorrhea and in any man who has decreased libido or potency. The serum prolactin concentration should also be measured in anyone who is found to have a sellar mass. A value that is only slightly high (e.g., 20–40 ng/ml) should be repeated because it could be the result of a physiologic stimulus, such as emotional or physical stress, exercise, or breast stimulation. A value >200 ng/ml in a man or a nonpregnant woman usually indicates a lactotroph adenoma, but a value between 20 and 200 ng/ml could result from any cause, including a lactotroph adenoma. If the value is 20–200 ng/ml, a search should be made for the cause by history, physical examination, and laboratory tests.

History and Physical Examination The history should include inquiry about medications that can cause hyperprolactinemia, including estrogens, neuroleptic drugs, metoclopramide, cimetidine, methyldopa, reserpine, verapamil, and abuse of opiates and cocaine. The history should also include inquiring about headaches, visual symptoms, symptoms of hypothyroidism, and renal disease.

Tests Tests should be performed to evaluate the possibility of hypothyroidism and renal disease. Magnetic resonance imaging should be performed to determine if a sellar or suprasellar mass exists. If so, the secretion of other pituitary hormones should be evaluated.

Treatment

The two principal reasons to consider treatment of a lactotroph adenoma are to correct hypogonadism and to reduce the size of the adenoma. Correction of hypogonadism is important in premenopausal women and in men. Reduction of adenoma size is important if the adenoma is >1 cm and especially if it is causing neurologic symptoms. Dopamine agonists usually decrease the size of lactotroph adenomas, in addition to decreasing their secretion of prolactin, so one of these agents should be the initial treatment. For the minority of adenomas that do not respond to dopamine agonists other treatment is required.

Dopamine Agonists Several dopamine agonists have been approved in many countries for treating lactotroph adenomas. They include cabergoline, bromocriptine, pergolide, and quinoglide. They are all effective in reducing prolactin secretion and adenoma size in a majority of patients, and all have similar side effects. Cabergoline, however, appears to be more effective than the others (Figs. 7-18 and 7-19) and less likely to cause side effects.

Efficacy Dopamine agonists bind to lactotroph cell-surface receptors and thereby reduce prolactin secretion and cell size.[264] The result in vivo is a reduction in serum prolactin concentration and in adenoma size. A review of 13 studies showed that bromocriptine reduced the serum prolactin concentration to normal in 229 of 280 women (82%).[265] In 12 of the studies, bromocriptine lowered the prolactin to normal in 66 of the 92 patients (71%) with macroadenomas. The reduction in adenoma size is more readily apparent in patients with macroadenomas (Fig. 7-20). In one study, bromocriptine reduced adenoma size in all 27 patients studied.[266] Dopamine agonist treatment may also restore visual function and correct hypopituitarism. Vision may begin to improve within days of the institution of treatment.[266,267] Women may recover menses and fertility, and men may recover testosterone secretion and fertility.[265] Patients who have macroadenomas and are hypothyroid and hypoadrenal may recover those functions.[268]

FIGURE 7-18. Serum prolactin concentrations before and during treatment of women with hyperprolactinemia with either cabergoline or bromocriptine for 24 weeks. (*From Webster et al, N Engl J Med 331:904, 1994.*[269])

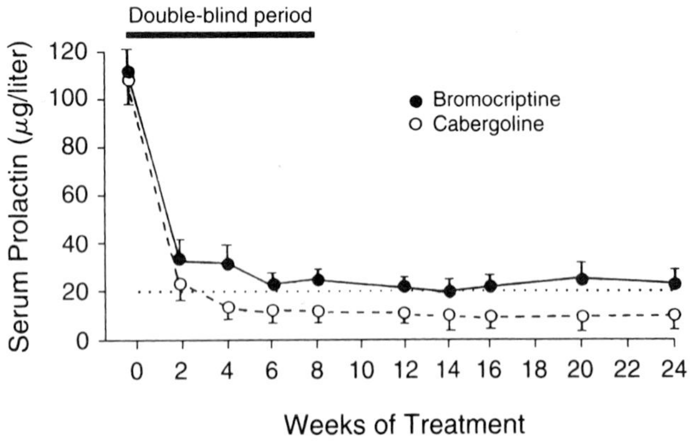

FIGURE 7-19. Decrease in the size of lactotroph adenomas in response to treatment with cabergoline for 24 months. Adenoma volume was estimated from magnetic resonance images by the formula, height × length × width × $\pi/6$. (*From Colao et al, J Clin Endocrinol Metab 82:876, 1997.*[367])

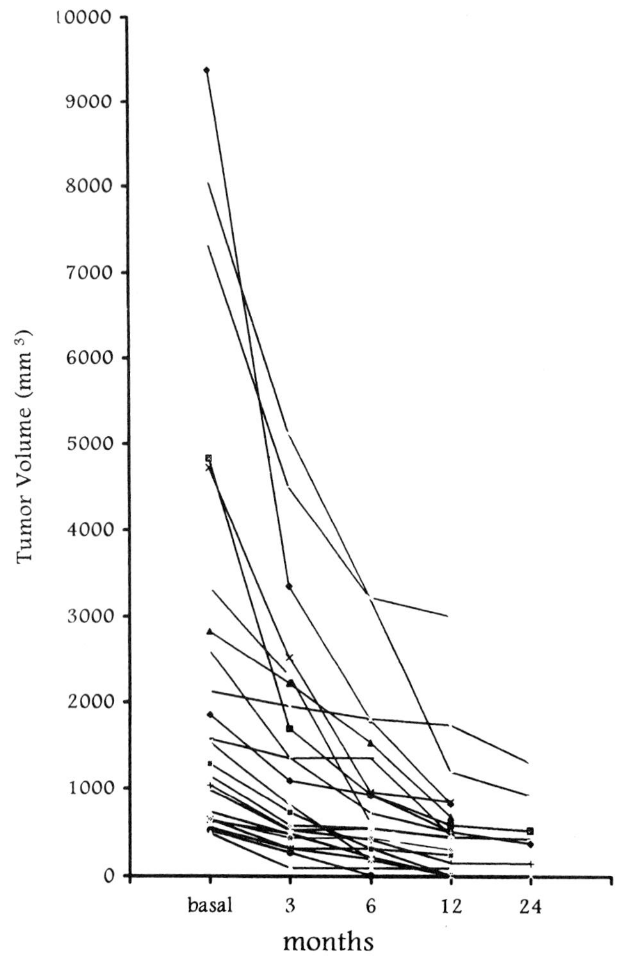

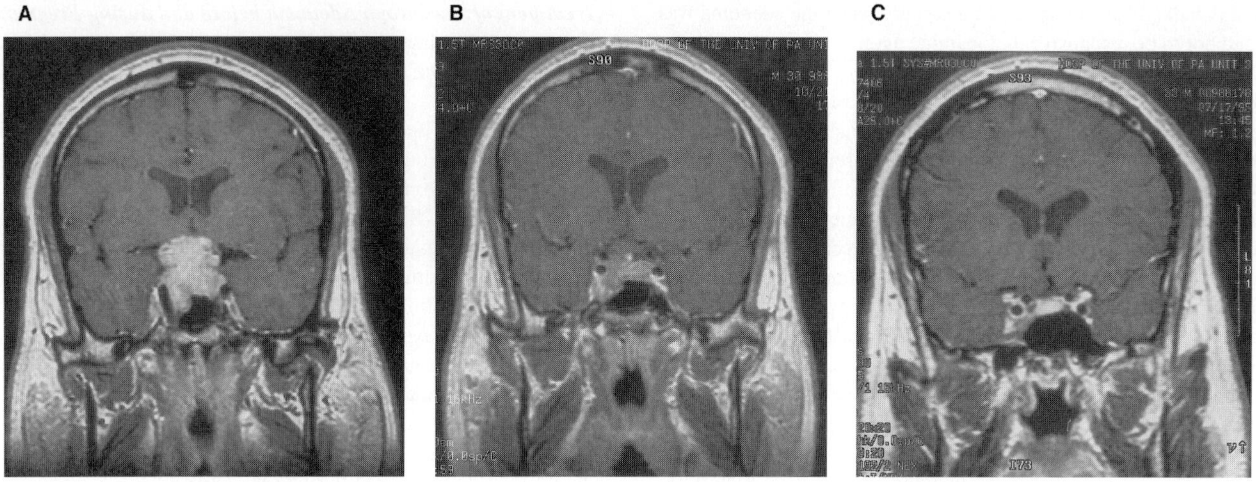

FIGURE 7-20. Magnetic resonance images of a lactotroph macroadenoma before treatment (a) and after six months (b) and three years (c) treatment with bromocriptine.

Cabergoline appears to be superior to bromocriptine in lowering the serum prolactin concentration. In a study of 459 women with hyperprolactinemic amenorrhea who had microadenomas or idiopathic hyperprolactinemia and were treated with either bromocriptine or cabergoline, 83 percent of those treated with cabergoline experienced reductions of prolactin to normal but only 52 percent of those treated with bromocriptine did (Fig. 7-18).[269] In another study of 27 patients with hyperprolactinemia resistant to bromocriptine and quinagolide, cabergoline reduced the serum prolactin concentration to normal in 15 of the 19 patients who had macroadenomas and in all 8 of the patients who had microadenomas.[270] Some lactotroph adenomas, however, both micro- and macro-, are resistant to all available dopamine agonists.

Side Effects The most common side effects of dopamine agonists are nausea and postural hypotension. Less common side effects include nasal stuffiness, mental fogginess, depression, Raynaud's phenomenon, and constipation. Side effects are more likely to occur when the medication is initiated or the dose increased; they tend to diminish when a dose is maintained. Cabergoline is less likely to cause nausea than is bromocriptine.[269]

Treatment Regimen For lactotroph microadenomas, treatment should be initiated with cabergoline at a dose of 0.5 mg once a week or 0.25 mg twice a week, and the patient should be evaluated in a month for response, both in efficacy, judged principally by a reduction in serum prolactin concentration, and possible side effects. If the initial response is satisfactory, the dose can be continued. Larger doses are not likely to be any more effective for microadenomas. Occasional patients who do not respond to cabergoline may respond to bromocriptine or pergolide. Whatever medication is successful must usually be continued indefinitely, although some patients who have idiopathic hyperprolactinemia maintain a normal serum prolactin concentration when the medication is discontinued. Patients who do not respond to any dopamine agonist and do not wish to become pregnant can be treated with an estrogen and progestin. Those who do wish to become pregnant can be treated by ovulation induction with gonadotropins or by transsphenoidal surgery.

For lactotroph macroadenomas, the initial dose is also 0.5 mg once a week or 0.25 mg twice a week. If the serum prolactin is clearly lower after a month, the dose can either be continued, or, if there are no side effects and the prolactin still markedly elevated, increased. The dose can be increased, if necessary, to as much as 1.5 mg twice a week. Magnetic resonance imaging should be repeated in 6 to 12 months to determine if the size is also decreasing.[102] Treatment should be continued indefinitely.

Surgery Transsphenoidal surgery is usually successful in reducing the size of, and prolactin secretion by, a lactotroph adenoma, and it is relatively safe when performed by an experienced transsphenoidal surgeon.[271,272]

The chance that surgery will reduce the serum prolactin concentration to normal depends on the size of the adenoma. In one report of 100 patients with lactotroph adenomas, 88 percent of those who had serum prolactin concentrations below 100 ng/ml had normal values after surgery, but only 50 percent of those who had prolactin concentrations above 100 ng/ml had normal values after surgery.[273] Even when the serum prolactin concentration is normal following transsphenoidal surgery, however, it may rise to become supranormal again within the next several years. In two studies that examined the results of 55 patients whose serum prolactin returned to normal after transsphenoidal surgery for a microadenoma, hyperprolactinemia recurred in 50 percent within four years in one study[272] and in 39 percent within five years in the other study.[274] Potential side effects are the same as might occur during surgery for any pituitary adenoma.

The role of transsphenoidal surgery for lactotroph adenomas is secondary treatment for those relatively few macroadenomas that do not respond to dopamine agonist medications. Microadenomas that do not respond to dopamine agonist medications are better treated by estrogen replacement.

Radiation Radiation therapy decreases lactotroph adenoma size and prolactin secretion, but the decrease in prolactin secretion is slow and often incomplete.[275,276] In one study of 34 patients with lactotroph or lactotroph-somatotroph adenomas treated by radiation, most still had supranormal serum prolactin concentrations 10 years later.[275] Complications of radiation therapy of lactotroph adenomas are the same as complications of pituitary adenomas of any kind. The role of radiation therapy in the treatment of lactotroph adenomas is to prevent regrowth of macroadenomas that were debulked by transsphenoidal surgery when the adenoma was found not to be responsive to dopamine agonist treatment.

Estrogen Estrogen replacement, with progestin, can be used to treat the hypogonadism caused by hyperprolactinemia in women who have lactotroph microadenomas that are not responsive to dopamine agonists and who do not desire to become pregnant soon. Although the chance of an increase in adenoma size is small with this treatment, the serum prolactin concentration should be monitored once every 6–12 months, and magnetic resonance imaging should be performed if the prolactin increases substantially. Estrogen and a progestin can be administered separately or in the form of an oral contraceptive. The former combination is more physiologic, but the latter may be preferable in a woman whose serum prolactin concentration is <100 ng/ml and who does not wish to become pregnant. Estrogen replacement should not be used as the primary treatment in women who have lactotroph macroadenomas because estrogen will not reduce adenoma size.

Lactotroph Adenoma and Pregnancy

Lactotroph adenomas, via hyperprolactinemia, impair ovulation and therefore fertility, but dopamine agonists usually lower the prolactin to normal and thereby usually allow ovulation and fertility.

Risks of Lactotroph Adenoma during Pregnancy There are potential risks to both the mother and the fetus.

Risks to the Mother The principal risk to the mother is an increase in the size of the adenoma that causes neurologic symptoms. The basis for this concern is that hyperestrogenemia causes hyperplasia of the lactotroph cells. In a study of 32 pregnant women without a known lactotroph adenoma, the size of the pituitary nearly doubled during the course of pregnancy.[277] Patients who have lactotroph microadenomas and become pregnant are unlikely to experience an increase in size of the adenomas. Twenty-five physicians, surveyed in 1979, reported that they had seen a total of 91 pregnancies in 85 women with lactotroph adenomas during pregnancy and that only five had experienced neurologic symptoms.[278] In two subsequent reviews, 4 of 246 (1.6%) patients experienced symptoms in one study,[279] and none of 56 in the other study did.[280]

The risk to the mother is greater if she has a lactotroph macroadenoma. In the 1979 survey, neurologic symptoms (headaches, visual impairment, diabetes insipidus) occurred in 20 of 56 pregnancies in 46 women with macroadenomas.[278] In two other series, neurologic symptoms occurred in 6 of 45 (279) and visual impairment occurred in all four women.[280]

Risks to the Fetus When bromocriptine is used to reduce the serum prolactin concentration and is not discontinued until the first month of pregnancy, the risk of congenital malformation is no greater than in the general population, but insufficient data are available to make this statement about other dopamine agonists. When physicians known to prescribe bromocriptine were surveyed, they reported the results of 1,410 pregnancies in 1,335 women who took the medication during pregnancy, mostly in the first month. The incidence of spontaneous abortions and major and minor malformations were comparable to those in the general population.[281] Similar results were reported in 226 pregnancies in women who took cabergoline.[282]

Treatment of Lactotroph Adenoma before and during Pregnancy Treatment of a lactotroph adenoma during pregnancy depends upon the size of the adenoma prior to pregnancy.

Microadenoma Because a microadenoma is not likely to increase in size during pregnancy, there is no reason to discourage pregnancy in a woman who has a microadenoma and wishes to become pregnant. She should be treated with a dopamine agonist to decrease the prolactin concentration to normal and restore ovarian function to normal in order to permit pregnancy. Bromocriptine is probably still the preferred agent for this purpose for most patients because experience with it is greater than with the other agents, but cabergoline may be better for women who are intolerant of bromocriptine. Whichever the agent, it should be discontinued as soon as pregnancy is confirmed because the safety of these agents has not been determined after the first trimester. The patient should then be monitored during the course of the pregnancy for headaches and visual changes. If neither occurs, dopamine agonist treatment can be resumed after delivery and after nursing has been completed.

Macroadenoma A woman who has a macroadenoma should be advised of the risk of a clinically significant increase in size during pregnancy. If the adenoma is not so large as to elevate the optic chiasm prior to surgery, treatment with a dopamine agonist prior to surgery should decrease the size sufficiently to reduce the chance of a clinically significant increase during pregnancy.[278,283] Once a substantial decrease has occurred, the patient can attempt to become pregnant. The dopamine agonist should be discontinued when pregnancy has been confirmed. Monitoring during pregnancy should be similar to that described above. If the patient perceives a change in vision, she should be examined by a neuroophthalmologist. If a visual field abnormality consistent with a chiasmal lesion is found, magnetic resonance imaging should be performed. If the adenoma has increased to a degree that could explain the visual abnormality, the dopamine agonist should be resumed for the remainder of the pregnancy and can be expected to decrease the size of the adenoma and relieve the symptoms.[284,285] In the unlikely situation that the adenoma does not respond and vision is severely compromised, transsphenoidal surgery should be performed during the second trimester. During the third trimester, surgery should be postponed until after delivery, if possible.

If, in the nonpregnant state, a lactotroph macroadenoma elevates the optic chiasm, pregnancy should be discouraged until the patient has had transsphenoidal surgery that greatly decreases the size of the adenoma. If residual adenoma tissue is demonstrated, radiation therapy should be considered. If the adenoma is sensitive to dopamine agonists, they should be employed to lower the prolactin to allow ovarian function. If substantial adenoma tissue remains and is not responsive to dopamine agonists, pregnancy should be discouraged because medical treatment would not be available if the adenoma enlarged during pregnancy.

Corticotroph Adenoma

Corticotroph adenomas usually secrete ACTH and thereby cause excessive cortisol secretion and Cushing's syndrome. By definition, they are the cause of the form of Cushing's syndrome called Cushing's disease. For a discussion of all forms of Cushing's syndrome, see Chapter 11. Most corticotroph adenomas secrete ACTH quite efficiently, and ACTH causes Cushing's syndrome, so most of these adenomas are recognized when they are small. A minority of corticotroph adenomas secrete inefficiently and may not cause Cushing's syndrome at all or until they are large.[286,287]

Etiology

Corticotroph have been shown to be monoclonal in origin,[95,288,289] but no specific mutations have yet been identified that cause this kind of adenoma.

Pathology

Grossly, most corticotroph adenomas are small when first recognized and excised, because most secrete efficiently and come to clinical attention because of Cushing's syndrome. These are found in the midline of the anterior pituitary. Occasional corticotroph adenomas secrete inefficiently. These may not cause Cushing's syndrome until they are very large or may present because of neurologic symptoms. Histologically, the typical small adenomas exhibit sheets of cells that immunocytochemically stain for ACTH. Large adenomas exhibit cells in sheets or nests with variable stroma that immunocytochemically stain less well for ACTH.

Clinical Presentation

Most corticotroph adenomas secrete ACTH efficiently, and ACTH causes excessive cortisol secretion, which results in Cushing's syndrome. The clinical manifestations of cortisol excess due to ACTH secretion from a corticotroph adenoma are generally no different from those due to cortisol excess from any cause. They include a round and red face, centripetal distribution of fat, muscle wasting, thin skin that is predisposed to striae and ecchymoses, hypertension, osteoporosis, impaired immune response, and glucose intolerance.

Diagnosis

Diagnosis of a corticotroph adenoma usually begins with the recognition that the patient has Cushing's syndrome and proceeds to documentation that the patient is secreting cortisol excessively, the excessive cortisol secretion is ACTH-dependent, and the pituitary is the source of the ACTH. Less commonly, a corticotroph adenoma first manifested itself as a sellar mass, the nature of which is recognized either by excessive cortisol secretion and inappropriately high serum ACTH or only by immunocytochemical staining of excised adenoma tissue.

Documentation of Excessive Cortisol Secretion The best single test to document excessive cortisol secretion is measurement of the amount of cortisol excreted in 24 hours. An elevated or borderline value should be confirmed several times. When the results are repeatedly borderline, a dexamethasone-corticotropin–releasing hormone stimulation test is the most helpful in distinguishing between ACTH-dependent excessive cortisol secretion and normal cortisol secretion.[290] The corticotropin-releasing hormone stimulation test without prior administration of dexamethasone is much less useful.[291]

Documentation that the Excessive Cortisol Secretion is ACTH Dependent When the 24-h urine cortisol excretion is repeatedly elevated, finding a plasma ACTH concentration in a immunoradiometric assay that is not suppressed suggests an ACTH-dependent cause, while finding a suppressed value suggests an ACTH-independent cause, namely, an adrenal tumor. If the plasma ACTH value is low but not entirely suppressed, a corticotropin-releasing hormone stimulation test should distinguish between an ACTH-dependent cause and an adrenal cause.

Documentation that the Pituitary is the Source of the ACTH If the excessive cortisol secretion is found to be dependent on ACTH, the next step is to determine if the source of the ACTH is pituitary or ectopic. If magnetic resonance imaging of the pituitary shows a mass >1 cm in diameter, the chances are high that the patient has a corticotroph macroadenoma. If imaging shows a signal abnormality of <1 cm, the abnormality could represent a corticotroph microadenoma or an incidental lesion. The best single test to distinguish between the two is petrosal sinus catheterization, performed in an institution with considerable experience in this technique, and measurement of the ACTH concentration in the petrosal sinuses and simultaneously in a peripheral vein before and after the administration of corticotropin-releasing hormone. A concentration of ACTH in the petrosal sinus more than twice that in the peripheral circulation basally and more than three times after corticotropin-releasing hormone administration is very strong evidence for a pituitary source (Fig. 7-21).[292,293] A concentration in one petrosal sinus several times that of the other side suggests that a corticotroph adenoma is on that side, but the reliability of this test for localization is not nearly as good as its reliability in distinguishing a pituitary from a nonpituitary source of ACTH.[294–296]

A decrease in the 24-h urine cortisol excretion to <50 percent of baseline in response to high-dose dexamethasone suppression, 2 mg four times a day for two days, also suggests that the source of the excessive ACTH secretion is a corticotroph adenoma. However, because some ectopic lesions that secrete ACTH respond to a high dose of dexamethasone, this test is not as good as petrosal sinus catheterization in distinguishing between pituitary and ectopic sources of excessive ACTH.

Treatment

The best initial treatment of a corticotroph adenoma is transsphenoidal surgery, but if this treatment does not result in a

FIGURE 7-21. Plasma ACTH concentrations in the right and left petrosal sinuses and the peripheral circulation before and after injection of corticotropin-releasing hormone in a patient with a right-sided corticotroph adenoma.

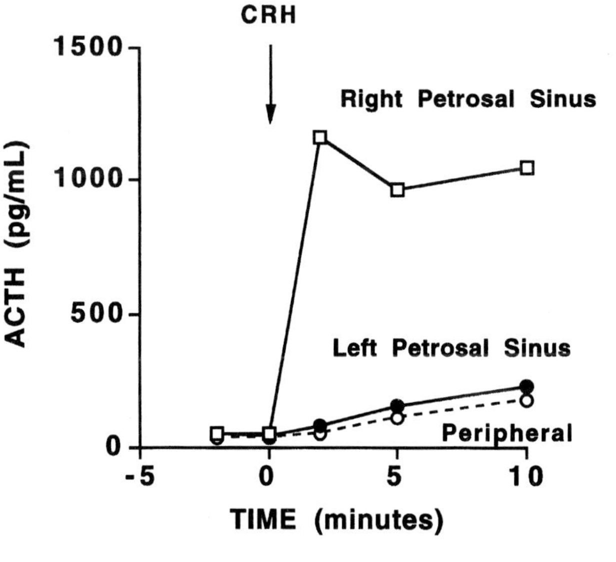

cure, radiation therapy and total bilateral adrenalectomy should be considered.

Transsphenoidal Surgery Transsphenoidal surgery offers the only means of curing a corticotroph adenoma, so it should be the initial treatment. Surgery is curative only about 75 percent of the time, however, even when an experienced pituitary surgeon performs the procedure,[297,298] and much less when a less experienced surgeon does so. Even when surgery corrects hypercortisolism initially, recurrence may occur.[299] The reasons for the less than optimal success rate are quite different from those for other pituitary adenomas. Corticotroph adenomas are often too small to see by magnetic resonance imaging, and they are often more friable than other pituitary adenomas, so they are difficult to remove entirely. When initial surgery has been unsuccessful in curing a corticotroph adenoma, a second transsphenoidal procedure can be considered.

Radiation Therapy Radiation therapy does not act nearly as quickly as surgery or adrenalectomy in reducing cortisol secretion to normal in patients who have a corticotroph adenoma, but it does do so faster than it decreases growth hormone secretion to normal in acromegalic patients. In one study of 30 adults, 83 percent experienced a remission from 6 to 60 months after the radiation, most within 24 months, and none who experienced a remission had a recurrence.[300] Consequently, this treatment should be considered in a patient who has not been cured by transsphenoidal surgery or even as primary treatment in a patient who has mild cortisol excess. Radiation, however, may lead to hypopituitarism.[300]

Adrenalectomy If transsphenoidal surgery is not successful in curing Cushing's disease, adrenalectomy should be considered, especially if the effects of cortisol excess are severe. Adrenalectomy itself, however, has its own risks, especially in the typical patient with hypercortisolism who is immunocompromised, but the risks are less if a laparoscopic approach can be employed.[301]

Pharmacotherapy Several medications, such as metyrapone, aminoglutethamide, and ketoconazole, block cortisol production in the adrenal cortex and thereby tend to reduce cortisol secretion. These medications, however, are generally ineffective in treating the hypercortisolism caused by a corticotroph adenoma because these adenomas respond to a decrease in plasma cortisol concentration by increasing ACTH secretion, thereby overcoming the block and raising the cortisol concentration again.

Gonadotroph Adenoma

Adenomas that arise from the gonadotroph cells generally differ from other pituitary adenomas in that they secrete less efficiently and what they do secrete does not usually cause a distinctive clinical syndrome. Consequently, they do not become clinically apparent until they increase in size sufficiently to cause neurologic symptoms, especially visual impairment. These adenomas comprise the majority of clinically nonfunctioning adenomas.

Etiology

Gonadotroph adenomas are among the adenomas that have been found to be monoclonal.[94] Clues to what mutation(s) might be causally related to the development of these adenomas have been sought by investigating the expression of activin,[302,303] follistatin,[304,305] somatostatin receptors,[306] and gonadotropin-releasing hormone and its receptor,[307,308] but as yet no abnormality has clearly been linked to the pathogenesis of these adenomas.

The possibility that excessive secretion of gonadotropin-releasing hormone or excessive responsiveness to it could be pathogenetically related to the development of gonadotroph adenomas was explored indirectly by administering an antagonist of gonadotropin-releasing hormone, Nal-Glu GnRH, to five patients with gonadotroph adenomas and supranormal serum concentration of FSH. Treatment for six months decreased their serum FSH concentrations to normal or below but did not change the size of the adenomas at all.[309] The implication of this result is that FSH secretion by these adenomas is dependent on endogenous gonadotropin-releasing hormone but that adenoma size (i.e., adenoma growth) is not.

Pathology

Grossly, most gronadotroph adenomas are much larger than 1 cm when they first come to clinical attention because of a neurologic symptoms and extend well beyond the sella. They often exhibit areas of necrosis and/or hemorrhage. Histologically, the cells are arranged in sheets or nests with a variable amount of stromal tissue rather than in the normal sinusoidal pattern. Reticulin staining confirms the breakdown of the sinusoidal pattern. Immunocytochemically, they often show staining for one or more of the gonadotropin subunits, but the staining is qualitatively variable and quantitatively less strong than for somatroph, lactotroph, and corticotroph adenomas.

Secretory Abnormalities

Secretion by gonadotroph adenomas differs from that by the majority of other pituitary adenomas in being less efficient and less likely to involve the entire complement of normal secretory products. Secretory abnormalities can usually be recognized, but with greater difficulty than in other kinds of adenomas. The abnormalities can be recognized in some patients by measurement of basal serum concentrations of the secretory products of the gonadotroph cell, but in other patients only by stimulation tests (Table 7-10) and in yet others only by in vitro tests.

Basal Secretion The intact hormone secreted most commonly is FSH, but in a maximum of 25 percent of patients,[310] and usually to no more than five times the upper limit of normal. The serum concentration of intact LH is usually not substantially supranormal[310] and rarely sufficiently high to raise the serum testosterone

TABLE 7-10. Hormonal Criteria for the Diagnosis of Gonadotroph Adenoma*

Men	Women
Supranormal basal serum concentrations of	
FSH	FSH but not LH
α, LHβ, or FSHβ subunits	Any subunit relative to intact FSH and LH
LH and testosterone	
Supranormal response to TRH of	
FSH	FSH
LH	LH
LHβ (most common)	LHβ (most common)

*Assuming the patient has a pituitary macroadenoma.

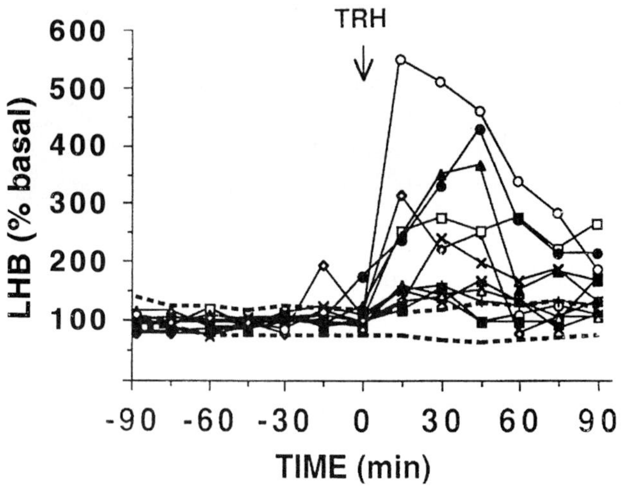

FIGURE 7-22. LHβ subunit responses to TRH in women with gonadotroph adenomas. (*From Daneshdoost et al, N Engl J Med 324:589, 1991.*[318])

concentration above normal in a man.[311,312] The serum concentrations of uncombined gonadotropin subunits—α, LHβ, and FSHβ—may also be higher than normal.[310,313–319]

Stimulated Secretion Gonadotroph adenomas, like other pituitary adenomas, respond to bolus doses of hypothalamic releasing hormones to which the normal cell type from which the adenoma arose, in this case the gonadotroph cell, does not respond. The majority of gonadotroph adenomas, both in men and in women, release LHβ subunit in response to thyrotropin-releasing hormone, (Fig. 7-22), and a minority release intact FSH, intact LH, and/or α subunit.[310,318,320]

In vitro A large majority of adenomas that appear to be clinically nonfunctioning in vivo can be recognized as being of gonadotroph cell origin when they are examined in vitro by secretion of intact gonadotropins and their subunits from the cultured adenoma cells, immunocytologic staining, or expression of mRNAs.[11,321–324] Regardless of which of these methods is used, about 85 percent of clinically nonfunctioning adenomas can be shown to be of gonadotroph cell origin, 10 percent of thyrotroph cell origin, and the remainder originating from all other pituitary cell types.

Diagnosis

The diagnosis of a gonadotroph adenoma comes from suspecting the possibility based on the clinical presentation and then by confirming the diagnosis hormonally.

Clinical Presentation The most common presentation of a gonadotroph adenoma is by a neurologic symptom, such as visual impairment or headaches, which leads to magnetic resonance imaging that shows a sellar mass (Table 7-11). A less common presentation is when a sellar mass, representing a gonadotroph adenoma, is found incidentally by magnetic resonance imaging performed for a reason unrelated to the adenoma. The least common presentation is by a clinical syndrome related to hormonal hypersecretion by the adenoma. One syndrome is precocious puberty caused by hypersecretion of intact LH in a boy.[325,326]

TABLE 7-11. Clinical Presentations of Gonadotroph Adenoma

Neurologic symptoms (most common)
Visual impairment
Headache
Other (diplopia, seizures, CSF rhinorrhea, etc.)
Incidental finding
When magnetic resonance imaging is performed because of an unrelated symptom
Hormonal symptoms (least common)
Oligo- or amenorrhea in a premenopausal woman
Premature puberty when intact LH is secreted in a prepubertal boy
Symptoms resulting from anterior pituitary hormonal deficiencies (commonly occur but uncommonly are the presenting symptoms)

Another syndrome is ovarian hypersecretion caused by hypersecretion of intact FSH in a premenopausal woman.[327,328] Hormonal hyposecretion caused by the large mass of the lesion is a frequent occurrence in patients who have gonadotroph adenomas, as with other large sellar masses, but these symptoms usually do not bring the patient to a physician.

Hormonal Confirmation Both basal and stimulated serum concentrations of gonadotropins and their subunits may be helpful in recognizing that a sellar mass is a gonadotroph adenoma.

Basal Concentrations When a large sellar mass is found, the next step is to determine if it represents a pituitary adenoma and, if so, what kind. If patient does not appear acromegalic or Cushingoid, and if the serum prolactin concentration is <100 ng/ml, a clinically nonfunctioning adenoma or a nonpituitary lesion become the most likely possibilities. In a man, elevated basal serum concentrations of intact FSH or free α or LHβ or FSHβ subunits likely mean that the sellar mass is a gonadotroph adenoma. In a postmenopausal woman, basal serum gonadotropin concentrations are usually not helpful, because the source of elevated serum concentrations of intact FSH and LH could as well be normal postmenopausal gonadotroph cells as a gonadotroph adenoma. A few combinations of intact gonadotropins and subunits in a postmenopausal woman, however, probably indicate that an associated sellar mass is a gonadotroph adenoma: an elevated serum concentration of free α subunit associated with premenopausal FSH and LH values, and a markedly elevated intact FSH in the presence of a subnormal intact LH.[318] In a premenopausal woman who has a sellar mass and is hypogonadal, an elevated intact FSH and/or free α subunit suggests that the mass is a gonadotroph adenoma.[318]

Stimulated Concentrations An increase in the LHβ subunit concentration of more than 40 percent above baseline in response to the intravenous injection of a bolus dose of TRH in a man or woman who has a sellar mass suggests that the mass is a gonadotroph adenoma. Approximately 60 percent of women and 40 percent of men who have gonadotroph adenomas have such a response. A much smaller percentage of patients who have gonadotroph adenomas exhibit intact FSH responses to TRH, although the presence of such a response is equally diagnostic. Finding that a clinically nonfunctioning sellar mass is a gonadotroph adenoma is helpful clinically because it indicates that the mass is a pituitary adenoma and not one of the many other lesions that can look the same by magnetic resonance imaging. This

TABLE 7-12. Comparison of Gonadotroph Adenoma with Gonadotroph Hyperplasia Due to Primary Hypogonadism

	Gonadotroph Adenoma	Primary Hypogonadism
Puberty incomplete	Normal	Often
Fertility history	Normal	Subnormal
Testicular size	Normal	Small
Serum testosterone	Low to high	Low to normal
Testosterone response to hCG	Marked to normal	Subnormal
Serum FSH	High	High
Serum LH	Usually normal, rarely high	High if testosterone is low
α Subunit	Normal to very high	High
FSH response to TRH	Present in 33% of patients	Absent
LHβ response to TRH	Present in 66% of patients	Absent

information can be helpful in planning the surgical approach to the mass because pituitary adenomas should be approached transsphenoidly, whereas others, such as meningiomas and craniopharyngiomas that arise above the diaphragma sella, should be approached transcranially.

Differentiation of Gonadotroph Adenomas from Gonadotroph Hyperplasia Due to Primary Hypogonadism Because longstanding, untreated primary hypogonadism in men and women can cause gonadotroph cell hyperplasia and pituitary enlargement, as well as elevated serum gonadotropin concentrations, gonadotroph adenomas must be distinguished from primary hypogonadism. Usually the distinction is not difficult (Table 7-12). Gonadotroph adenomas usually secrete inefficiently, so very large sellar masses are associated with modest elevations of serum gonadotropins, and usually not both FSH and LH.[329] Hyperplastic gonadotroph cells, in contrast, secrete efficiently, so only a slightly enlarged pituitary is associated with marked elevations of both FSH and LH.[115] Secretion by gonadotroph adenomas responds to TRH, but that by gonadotroph hyperplasia does not.[320]

Treatment

Treatment of gonadotroph adenomas generally is the same as treatment of any sellar mass lesion, as described previously. Adenomas that are causing neurologic symptoms should be treated by transsphenoidal surgery, and residual adenoma tissue that is immediately threatening or is relapsing should be treated by radiation therapy.

Dopamine Agonists and Somatostatin Analogs Several pharmacologic treatments have been tried, but none are routinely successful. Dopamine agonists, mostly bromocriptine, have been reported to reduce secretion of intact gonadotropins and α subunit in several patients and to improve vision in one, but not to reduce adenoma size.[330–334] The somatostatin analog, octreotide, has been reported to improve vision to a small degree and to reduce adenoma size to a small degree in occasional patients,[335,336] but the low frequency and modest degree of reported improvement, the lack of correlation between reduction in size and improvement in vision, and the lack of controls do not recommend using this medication as a routine treatment for gonadotroph adenomas.

GnRH Analogs Several superactive GnRH analogs have been administered to patients with gonadotroph adenomas because when these analogs are administered to subjects who have normal gonadotroph cells, they down regulate GnRH receptors and cause decreased secretion of LH and FSH. Administration of these analogs to patients who have gonadotroph adenomas, however, generally causes either an agonist or no effect on hormonal secretion and no effect on adenoma size.[337–340]

Administration of the pure GnRH antagonist, Nal-Glu GnRH, to six men with gonadotroph adenomas and supranormal serum concentrations of FSH for an average of six months reduced the serum FSH concentration to normal or below but did not decrease adenoma size at all.[309]

Thyrotroph Adenoma

Adenomas that arise from thyrotroph cells are not uncommon, as judged by immunocytochemical staining for TSHβ subunit[324] or by expression of TSHβ mRNA,[321] but most of these adenomas do not secrete intact TSH and are therefore clinically nonfunctioning. Thyrotroph adenomas that do secrete sufficient intact TSH to result in hyperthyroidism are uncommon, but are readily recognized.

Etiology

Thyrotroph adenomas, like other pituitary adenomas, appear to be monoclonal,[114] but no specific mutations have been identified. Mutations of the Gαs, pit-1, and thyroid hormone receptor genes, among others, have been sought but not found.[114]

Pathology

Grossly, thyrotroph adenomas are usually large when detected and are often fibrous, so they are difficult to excise surgically.[114] They are well- or poorly-differentiated by light microscopy. The cells are large, polymorphous, and often arranged in cords, and they have large and irregular nucleoli.[341] The thyrotroph nature of the cells can be demonstrated by immunocytochemical staining for TSHβ subunit.[341] Immunocytochemical staining also demonstrates glycoprotein α subunit and may demonstrate the presence of other pituitary hormones, especially if the adenoma is associated with the secretion of those hormones. A thyrotroph carcinoma has been reported.[342]

Secretory Abnormalities

The hormonal secretory patterns of thyrotroph adenomas are highly variable but, like gonadotroph adenomas, their secretion is usually relatively inefficient, so they are not recognized clinically until they become very large. Some adenomas eventually secrete sufficient intact and biologically active TSH to cause excessive thyroxine hypersecretion and readily recognizable hyperthyroidism. At the other end of the spectrum are adenomas that secrete so little intact and biologically active TSH that serum TSH and T_4 concentrations are normal even when the adenomas are very large, and the only way that the thyrotroph nature of the adenoma can be recognized is by in vitro techniques.[321,324] As a consequence of this variability, both the serum TSH and T_4 concentrations in patients with thyrotroph adenomas vary from normal to supranormal.[114] Approximately 80 percent of thyrotroph adenomas that can be recognized in vivo have a supranormal serum α subunit concentration, and 30 percent have supranormal serum concentrations of growth hormone and/or prolactin.[114] The serum TSH concentration virtually never responds to a bolus dose of thyrotropin-releasing hormone, but occasionally the α subunit concentration does. The serum TSH concentration increases dramatically, however, to a decrease in the serum T_4 concentration, as occurs when a patient with a thyrotroph adenoma is erroneously diagnosed as having Graves' disease and treated with radioactive iodine. Although these adenomas express somatostatin receptors variably,[343] they usually respond to somatostatin analog administration by some decrease in TSH secretion.

Clinical Presentation

Thyrotroph adenomas that secrete intact TSH may present either with symptoms of hyperthyroidism or neurologic symptoms from a sellar mass, but thyrotroph adenomas that do not secrete intact TSH present only with symptoms of a sellar mass. Occasionally the presentation results from a cosecreted hormone, for example, acromegaly in a patient whose adenoma secretes intact TSH and growth hormone. The symptoms of hyperthyroidism are present but often have existed for many years before the diagnosis is made. In a review of 246 patients reported in the literature, approximately one-third of patients had previously been diagnosed as having Graves' disease and had been treated with radioactive iodide before the correct diagnosis was made.[114] Neurologic symptoms are those typically caused by any sellar mass, such as visual impairment and headache.

Diagnosis

The diagnosis of a thyrotroph adenoma in vivo can be relatively easy if it is a macroadenoma and is associated with a supranormal serum T_4 concentration and a TSH that is not suppressed, but the diagnosis can be difficult if it is a macroadenoma that is not associated with an elevated serum T_4 or a microadenoma. The in vivo diagnosis begins with the finding of an elevated serum T_4 concentration and a serum TSH concentration that is not suppressed. An elevated free T_4 concentration, as determined by dialysis, and an undetectable TSH concentration by an ultrasensitive method will demonstrate that the patient has thyroidal hyperthyroidism, whereas a normal free T_4 and a TSH by an ultrasensitive method will demonstrate euthyroid hyperthyroxinemia, as caused by dysalbuminemia. An elevated free T_4 and a detectable TSH, even by an ultrasensitive method, will confirm the diagnosis of inappropriate TSH secretion. The two causes of inappropriate TSH secretion are a thyrotroph adenoma and thyroid hormone resistance. Several tests help to distinguish between these two, although no one test does so with certainty (Table 7-13). An elevated serum α subunit/serum TSH ratio, elevated serum SHBG concentration, and a sellar mass >1 cm in diameter all tend to confirm the diagnosis of a thyrotroph adenoma, whereas the opposite results and hyperthyroxinemia and detectable TSH concentrations in family members all tend to confirm the diagnosis of thyroid hormone resistance. The finding of a sellar mass <1 cm could represent either the unusual situation of a thyrotroph microadenoma[344] or an incidental lesion; in that situation the distinction between a thyrotroph adenoma and thyroid hormone resistance must be made on the basis of the other tests.

TABLE 7-13. Comparison of Hyperthyroxinemia Due to Thyrotroph Adenoma and Thyroid Hormone Resistance

Parameter	Thyrotroph Adenoma	Thyroid Hormone Resistance
Serum thyroxine	Elevated	Elevated
Serum free thyroxine	Elevated	Elevated
Serum TSH	Not suppressed	Not suppressed
Serum α subunit	Elevated*	Normal
α Subunit/TSH ratio	Elevated*	Normal
TSH response to TRH	Subnormal*	Normal
Serum SHBG	Elevated*	Normal
Sellar mass >1 cm	Yes*	No

* Typical, but not inevitable, findings in patients who have thyrotroph adenomas.

The pituitary gland can also be enlarged in patients who have thyrotroph hyperplasia due to primary hypothyroidism. The distinction between this situation and a thyrotroph adenoma is usually made readily by finding a subnormal serum T_4 concentration in the patients with primary hypothyroidism. In addition, pituitary enlargement due to primary hypothyoidism is readily corrected by treatment with replacement doses of thyroxine.

Treatment

Surgery, radiation therapy, and somatostatin analogs all have a role in the treatment of thyrotroph adenomas, but some of these adenomas are resistant to all treatments.

Surgery Surgical excision of a thyrotroph adenoma is often more difficult than of other pituitary adenomas because thyrotroph adenomas are often large, invasive, and more fibrotic.[114,345,346] Nonetheless, in a review of 177 patients who underwent surgery, about one-third of thyrotroph adenomas were apparently cured by surgery and another one-third were improved.[114]

Radiation Therapy In the same review, the percentage of patients who were apparently cured or improved after a combination of surgery and radiation therapy was not appreciably different from the percentage cured or improved after surgery alone.[114]

Somatostatin Analogs Thyrotroph adenomas often express somatostatin receptors[343] and respond to the administration of somatostatin analogs, octreotide and lanreotide, by decreasing their secretion of TSH[347–350] and sometimes decreasing in size.[350] These responses make somatostatin analogs, especially the long-acting formulations that need be administered only once or twice a month, worthy of consideration, especially for adenomas whose invasiveness makes them unlikely to be cured surgically. Of 73 patients with thyrotroph adenomas treated with octreotide, 95 percent experienced a long-term decrease in thyroid hormone concentration (Table 7-14).[114]

Antithyroid Drugs Antithyroid drugs, such as methimazole or propylthiouracil, reduce hyperthyroxinemia in patients with

TABLE 7-14. Effects of Treating Thyrotroph Adenomas with Octreotide

Parameter	Percent of Patients Who Improved
Reduction of TSH	92
Normalization of TSH	79
Normalization of thyroid hormone	95
Reduction of adenoma mass	52
Improvement in vision	75
Tachyphylaxis	22
True escape	10
Discontinuation of medication due to side effects	7

A compilation of the results from 73 patients who were treated with 50 to 750 μg of octreotide 2 to 3 times a day.

Source: Adapted from Beck-Peccoz et al.[114]

thyrotroph adenomas and are therefore useful in making a patient euthyroid prior to transsphenoidal surgery or after surgery and radiation while waiting for the radiation to work. However, because antithyroid drugs do not treat thyrotroph adenomas directly, and because thyrotroph adenomas respond to a decrease in the serum thyroxine concentration by increasing TSH secretion and perhaps by an increase in adenoma size, antithyroid drugs should be used only to make a patient euthyroid prior to surgery or as adjuvant therapy following radiation.

Hormonal Hyposecretion

Most diseases that affect the pituitary, and many that affect the hypothalamus, can cause decreased secretion of any anterior pituitary hormone. Although certain generalizations can legitimately be made about anterior pituitary hormone deficiencies, such as the greater likelihood that a disease of the anterior pituitary will cause deficiencies of growth hormone or gonadotropins than of TSH or ACTH, many exceptions occur. Consequently, the status of a pituitary hormone can be known only by specific testing for that hormone.

ACTH Deficiency

The only significant consequence of ACTH deficiency is cortisol deficiency, and the manifestations, diagnosis, and treatment of cortisol deficiency due to ACTH deficiency are similar in most ways to those due to cortisol deficiency resulting from adrenal disease though there are some notable exceptions.

Symptoms and Signs

Mild cortisol deficiency may cause no symptoms at all or cause lassitude and anorexia. More severe cortisol deficiency causes more severe lassitude, postural hypotension, and eventually death from hypotension. The lassitude may be exacerbated by severe hyponatremia due to the inability to excrete a water load in the face of cortisol deficiency. Cortisol deficiency due to ACTH deficiency, unlike that due to primary adrenal disease, does not cause hyperpigmentation.

Diagnosis

The diagnosis of cortisol deficiency due to ACTH deficiency in a patient who has known pituitary or hypothalamic disease can be made in one of two ways. If an early morning serum cortisol concentration is clearly subnormal (e.g., <5 μg/dl), especially if that value is confirmed by a similar result on another morning, the diagnosis of cortisol deficiency is made. An ACTH concentration that is not elevated in blood drawn at the same time indicates that ACTH deficiency is the cause of the hypocortisolism. A cortisol value ≥18 μg/dl suggests that cortisol secretion is probably normal. Cortisol values between 5 and 18 μg/dl do not distinguish between normal and partially subnormal ACTH secretion. To make that distinction, a test of ACTH reserve, such as a metyrapone (Fig. 7-23)[351] or insulin tolerance test,[39] must be performed.

Administration of cosyntropin and measurement of cortisol 30 or 60 minutes later should not be used to make the diagnosis of secondary adrenal insufficiency because both the standard dose (250 μg) and low dose (1 μg) tests frequently produce a normal cortisol response in patients who have ACTH deficiency, especially if the deficiency is partial or of recent onset.[171–173]

Unlike cortisol deficiency due to primary adrenal disease, that due to ACTH deficiency does not cause hyperkalemia because ACTH deficiency does not result in a clinically significant decrease in aldosterone secretion.

Treatment

Cortisol deficiency should be treated by replacement with hydrocortisone (hydrocortisone is a synonym for cortisol). The dose should be approximately 20 mg for someone who weighs about 120 lbs and 30 mg for someone who weighs about 180 lbs, given

FIGURE 7-23. Testing ACTH reserve by the metyrapone (Metopirone®) test. After the administration of 750 mg of metyrapone every four hours for 24 h to normal individuals, the serum cortisol concentration falls to <7 μg/dl and the 11-deoxycortisol (11-DOC) concentration increases to >10 μg/dl. (*From Spark, Ann Intern Med 75:717, 1971.*[351])

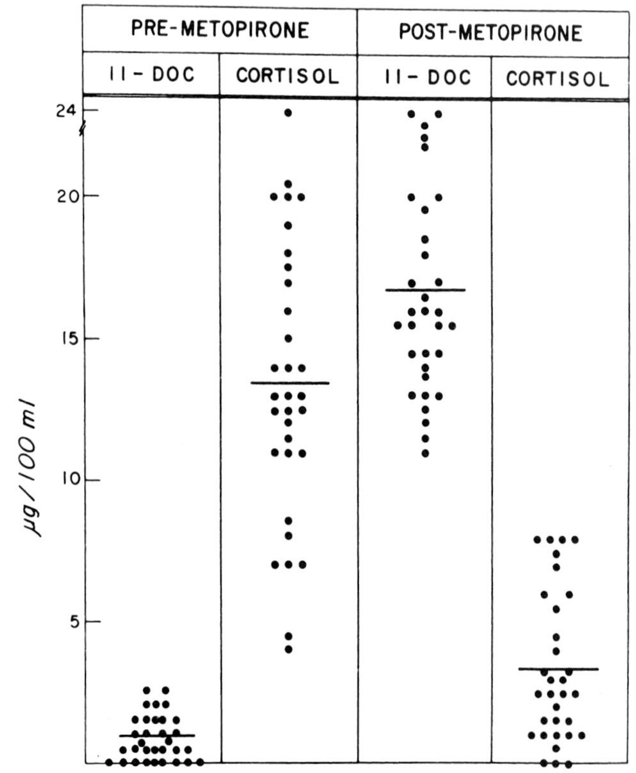

as a single dose on rising in the morning or as two-thirds of the dose on rising and one-third at noon. The dose can be increased if obvious symptoms or signs of cortisol deficiency persist or lowered if signs of cortisol excess appear, but, unfortunately, there are no good tests for monitoring the adequacy of hydrocortisone replacement. Measurement of serum or urine cortisol and plasma ACTH all give misleading results. Patients with cortisol deficiency should be instructed to increase the dose of hydrocortisone at times of physical stress and to wear identification of the deficiency on their person.

TSH Deficiency

The manifestations of thyroid hormone deficiency due to TSH deficiency are virtually the same as those due to thyroid disease, and the treatment is the same, however, unlike the situation in primary hypothyroidism, the serum TSH concentration cannot be used to make the diagnosis or to monitor the adequacy of treatment in patients who have secondary hypothyroidism.

Symptoms and Signs

The symptoms of TSH deficiency are those of the resulting thyroxine deficiency, which can vary from none to increasing degrees of lethargy, cold-sensitivity, decreased appetite, dry skin, constipation, and paresthesias. Physical examination usually does not reveal abnormalities until hypothyroidism is at least moderately severe and/or of long duration. Physical findings may include diminished sharpness of the facial features, dry skin, and delayed relaxation phase of the deep tendon reflexes.

Diagnosis

The diagnosis of TSH deficiency is made by finding a lower than normal serum thyroxine concentration and a concomitant serum TSH concentration that is not higher than normal, although occasionally it is slightly supranormal.[352] It is important to recognize that the TSH concentration is usually not subnormal. Failure of the serum TSH concentration to increase following the administration of a bolus dose TRH suggests that the cause of the TSH deficiency is due to a pituitary rather than a hypothalamic lesion, but an increase in TSH can occur in either condition.[353] This test, however, is rarely needed clinically.

Treatment

Treatment of TSH deficiency is by administration of thyroxine, similar to treatment of primary hypothyroidism, including considerations that determine the initial dose and the timing of increases in dose (see Chap. 9). There are two major differences, however, in the treatment of secondary hypothyroidism from treatment of primary hypothyroidism. One is that treatment of secondary hypothyroidism should not be initiated until the patient's adrenal status has been evaluated and treated because treatment of hypothyroidism increases the patient's metabolism, including that of cortisol. The result will be exacerbation of cortisol deficiency. The second difference is that only the serum thyroxine concentration can be used as a test of the adequacy of the thyroxine replacement dose, not the serum TSH concentration.

Gonadotropin Deficiency—Men

The clinical presentation of secondary hypogonadism in both men and women is similar to that of primary hypogonadism, but serum FSH and LH concentrations cannot be used to make the diagnosis of hypogonadism nor to follow the adequacy of treatment. Of importance is that infertility due to secondary hypogonadism is usually treatable in both men and women, whereas that due to primary hypogonadism is not.

Symptoms and Signs

The two functions of the testes are sperm production and testosterone secretion, so the clinical presentations of male hypogonadism are those of decreased sperm production, such as small testes and decreased fertility, and those of decreased testosterone secretion, which depend on when the deficiency occurs. If testosterone deficiency occurs during the first trimester in utero, male sexual differentiation is incomplete, and when it occurs during the last trimester, the phallus is small at birth. When testosterone deficiency occurs prior to the anticipated onset of puberty, the result is incomplete puberty and eunuchoid proportions. When testosterone deficiency occurs after puberty has been completed, energy and libido decrease within weeks, but sexual hair, muscle mass, and bone mineral density do not decrease for several years. If the deficiency is severe, vasomotor instability ("hot flashes") may occur.

There are several differences between the clinical presentation of secondary hypogonadism and that of primary hypogonadism. In secondary hypogonadism, testicular size does not decrease for several years after the onset of gonadotropin deficiency, whereas in primary hypogonadism testicular size decreases shortly after the testicular insult and at the same time as hypogonadism. In secondary hypogonadism the degree of the decrease in sperm production is similar to the degree of the decrease in serum testosterone concentration, whereas in primary hypogonadism degree of the decrease in sperm production is usually much greater than that in testosterone secretion. In secondary hypogonadism, gynecomastia is not as common as in primary hypogonadism.

Diagnosis

The diagnosis of secondary hypogonadism begins with recognition of the clinical presentation described and proceeds to confirmation of the diagnosis by measurement of the serum testosterone concentration. If the testosterone concentration is subnormal, the diagnosis of hypogonadism is confirmed. If the serum LH concentration is not supranormal, the hypogonadism is secondary. The serum LH concentration is usually not subnormal in secondary hypogonadism except in cases of severe deficiency of gonadotropin-releasing hormone, such as Kallmann's syndrome. Measurement of the serum LH concentration following the administration of a single bolus dose of gonadotropin-releasing hormone will not distinguish a pituitary cause from a hypothalamic cause of secondary hypogonadism, but administration of repeated doses may.[354] However, this test is rarely of clinical use.

Treatment

Choosing a treatment of secondary hypogonadism depends primarily on whether the goal is to increase the serum testosterone alone or to stimulate spermatogenesis as well.

Testosterone Treatment Several testosterone preparations can be used to increase the serum testosterone concentration to normal and cause or maintain normal virilization. These include the testosterone esters, enanthate and cypionate, and several transdermal preparations. The testosterone esters are administered by deep intramuscular injection, usually 150–200 mg every two weeks. This regimen is satisfactory to cause or maintain normal virilization in virtually all men, but has the disadvantage of requiring regular administration of an oily solution and of producing relatively wide fluctuations of the serum testosterone concentration from one dose to the next, which causes some men to experience corresponding fluctuations in energy, mood, and libido. All of the transdermal preparations currently available are patches (Testoderm, Androderm, and Testoderm TTS) and produce much steadier serum testosterone concentrations and therefore steadier energy, mood, and libido. All three result in a serum testosterone concentration within the normal range in the majority of but not all, hypogonadal men. If wearing a single body patch (Testoderm TTS and Androderm) daily does not result in a normal serum testosterone concentration, wearing two patches a day might. Androderm, by anecdotal reports, causes severe skin rashes that require discontinuation in about 25 to 33 percent of patients within the first month of administration.

The adequacy of the testosterone treatment should be monitored by measurement of the serum testosterone concentration midway between injections or any time during patch administration. The result should be in the normal range. Unlike in primary hypogonadism, measurement of the serum LH concentration is not helpful. The possibility of adverse consequences should be monitored, especially in men over 40, by the American Urologic Association symptom score for benign prostatic hypertrophy, serum concentration of prostate specific antigen, digital rectal examination, and hematocrit.

Stimulation of Spermatogenesis In stark contrast to the situation in primary hypogonadism, where spermatogenesis cannot be stimulated, spermatogenesis can usually be stimulated successfully in patients who have secondary hypogonadism. The treatment regimen for patients who have pituitary disease is by administration of gonadotropins: human chorionic gonadotropin, which acts biologically as does LH, and human menopausal gonadotropin, which contains FSH. Pulsatile administration of gonadotropin-releasing hormone, which is effective in stimulating spermatogenesis in patients who have hypothalamic disease,[355] is not effective in patients who have pituitary disease. Human chorionic gonadotropin is administered alone first because it is not as expensive as human menopausal gonadotropin and sometimes is sufficient by itself, especially if the onset of the secondary hypogonadism was postpubertal.[356] The initial dose is 2,000 units intramuscularly three times a week. If this dose does not result in a serum testosterone concentration within the normal range within two months, the dose should be adjusted, up or down, until the serum testosterone concentration is mid-normal. The full effect of this treatment on spermatogenesis may take up to two years, but usually occurs in 6 to 12 months (Fig. 7-24).[356] If treatment with human chorionic gonadotropin alone does not cause the sperm count to reach the normal range, that treatment is continued and human menopausal gonadotropin is added. The initial dose of menopausal gonadotropin is 75 units intramuscularly three times a week. If the sperm count is not normal after four to six months of combined treatment, the dose of menopausal gonadotropin can be increased to 150 units three times a week.[356] The full effect of the combined treatment usually takes at least six months and may take a year or more.

Gonadotropin Deficiency—Women

The general principals of gonadotropin deficiency in women are the same as in men as previously described.

Symptoms and Signs

The two principal functions of the ovaries are production of ova and secretion of estradiol, so the clinical presentations of hypogonadism in women are infertility and the manifestations of decreased estradiol secretion. If estradiol deficiency occurs prior to the anticipated onset of puberty, even in utero, the result is incomplete puberty. When estradiol deficiency occurs after puberty has been completed, the features are amenorrhea, reduction in breast size, a decrease in general sense of well-being and, if the deficiency is severe, vasomotor instability ("hot flashes") and vaginal dryness. These symptoms occur within days or weeks of the onset. Other manifestations take years to become obvious, including osteoporosis, increased incidence of heart disease, and poor skin texture. Sexual hair may diminish, especially in the woman who has deficiencies of both gonadotropins and ACTH.

Diagnosis

The diagnosis of secondary hypogonadism in women begins with recognition of the clinical presentation described and proceeds to confirmation of the diagnosis by establishing that estradiol secretion is subnormal. This decrease is documented by finding a subnormal serum estradiol concentration and less than normal vaginal bleeding in response to a 10-day course of medroxyprogesterone acetate. If estradiol deficiency is confirmed and the serum LH concentration is not supranormal, the hypogonadism is

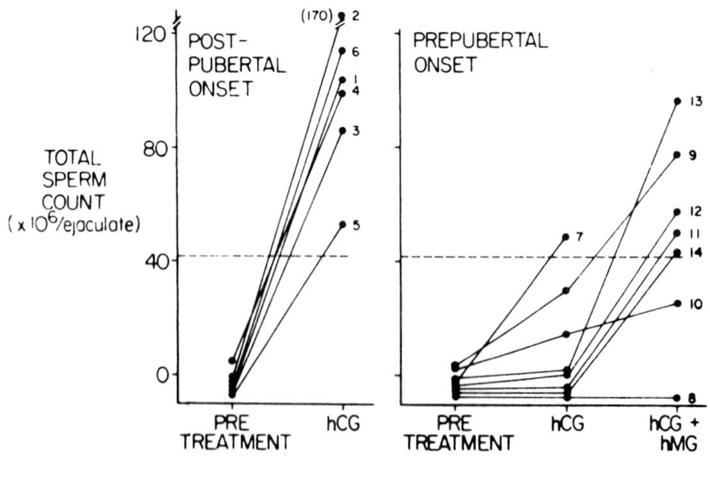

FIGURE 7-24. Stimulation of spermatogenesis in men with hypogonadotropic hypogonadism by administration of gonadotropins. Men who develop hypogonadotropic hypogonadism postpubertally require only replacement of LH, such as with human chorionic gonadotropin (hCG) to achieve normal spermatogenesis. Men who develop hypogonadotropic hypogonadism postpubertally usually require replacement of both LH and FSH, such as with human menopausal gonadotropins (hMG). (*From Finkel et al, N Engl J Med 313:651, 1985.*[356])

secondary. As in the case of men, the serum LH concentration is usually not subnormal in secondary hypogonadism except in cases of severe deficiency of gonadotropin-releasing hormone. Differentiating a pituitary from a hypothalamic cause of gonadotropin deficiency by repeated administration of gonadotropin-releasing hormone is rarely of clinical use.

Treatment

Choosing a treatment of secondary hypogonadism depends primarily on whether the goal is to replace the estrogen deficiency alone or to stimulate ovulation as well.

Estrogen Treatment Several estrogen preparations can be used to replace estrogen deficiency, including those administered orally and estradiol administered transdermally. Although the oral preparations are more commonly used, transdermal administration of estradiol by one of several commercially available patches more closely mimics estrogen secretion by the ovaries in that the estrogen is the same (estradiol); is provided continuously, rather than episodically; and is provided into the systemic circulation, rather than the portal circulation. The last feature means that transdermal administration of estradiol is not associated with increased production of thyroxine and steroid-binding proteins and blood clotting proteins and therefore should not be associated with an increased risk of thrombotic and embolic events. Another advantage of transdermal estradiol administration is that the adequacy of the treatment can be monitored by measurement of the serum estradiol concentration. This is particularly advantageous in a woman who has secondary hypogonadism, in whom the serum LH and FSH concentrations cannot be used to judge the adequacy of the dose. A progestin must be administered along with the estrogen in a woman who has a uterus no matter what the cause of the deficiency or what preparation of estrogen is used. The combination of estrogen and progestin can be given cyclically or continuously. Cyclic administration is probably preferable in women of premenopausal age with continuous administration thereafter.

The adequacy of the estradiol treatment should be monitored by measurement of the serum estradiol concentration, which should be normal at all times during patch administration. If the estrogen and progestin are administered cyclically, menses should be normal. The possibility of adverse consequences should be monitored by regular gynecologic examinations.

Androgen Treatment Women who have secondary hypogonadism, especially those who have secondary hypoadrenalism as well, have lower than normal serum testosterone concentrations. It has been hypothesized that this deficiency can cause symptoms such as a decrease in libido, but the lack of a testosterone preparation designed to provide a physiologic replacement dose for women has hindered testing this hypothesis.

Stimulation of Ovulation Ovulation can usually be induced in women who have secondary hypogonadism due to pituitary disease by administration first of an FSH preparation, such as human menopausal gonadotropin, purified urinary FSH, or recombinant human FSH, followed by human chorionic gonadotropin.[357] The FSH preparation is administered first in a regimen that is designed to attempt to produce a single dominant follicle and to avoid multiple follicles and thereby avoid multiple pregnancies, and also to avoid ovarian hyperstimulation.[357] To achieve these goals, progress is monitored by measurement of the serum estradiol concentration and by ovarian ultrasound. When a single follicle is >18 mm, indicating that the follicle has matured, human chorionic gonadotropin is administered to induce ovulation.

Growth Hormone Deficiency

For many years little attention was paid to the possibility that growth hormone deficiency in adults could have any clinical consequences. During this time the availability of growth hormone for therapeutic use was limited, so most growth hormone-deficient adults would not have been able to receive it. During the past decade, however, the results of many studies have suggested that growth hormone deficiency has adverse consequences in adults and that administration of growth hormone to such patients may reverse those consquences. However, many of the studies demonstrating effects of adult-onset growth hormone deficiency have, necessarily, been in patients who have other hormonal deficiencies as well, so it is not possible to know if the observed effects are those of growth hormone deficiency or those of the deficiencies or overtreatment of the other hormones. In addition, many of the studies reporting the effects of the administration of growth hormone have not been placebo-controlled and double-blinded. Consequently, the evidence for the effect of growth hormone on most parameters needs further substantiation.

Symptoms and Signs

The best substantiated manifestation of growth hormone deficiency in adults so far is the change it causes in body composition. Adults who have growth hormone deficiency have an increased amount of fat tissue and decreased lean tissue. When they are treated with growth hormone, fat tissue decreases and lean tissue increases.[358,359] Other potential manifestations of growth hormone deficiency are less clear. Patients who have growth hormone deficiency have lower bone mineral density than do people who do not, and several uncontrolled studies show that growth hormone treatment increases their bone mineral density, but only one controlled study, which was performed in men alone and demonstrated a 5 percent increase in spine bone mineral density in 18 months, confirms this result.[307] Growth hormone-deficient patients appear to have greater psychological abnormalities, and in a crossover placebo-controlled study, growth hormone treatment was associated with a decrease in mental distress and improvement in sense of well-being.[360] Growth hormone deficiency may impair cardiac function. In one study, growth hormone increased cardiac output and decreased peripheral resistance.[361] Growth hormone treatment does not appear to have any effects on most serum lipid concentrations.[362,363]

Diagnosis

The diagnosis of growth hormone deficiency should be suspected in anyone who has known pituitary disease that is causing deficiencies of one or more other pituitary hormones. A subnormal serum concentration of IGF-1 further increases the suspicion, but patients with growth hormone deficiency may have normal serum IGF-1 concentrations.[364] The diagnosis should be confirmed by finding a subnormal response (<5 ng/mL by radioimmunoassay or <2.5 ng/mL by immunoradiometric or immunoflurometric assays) of growth hormone to a standard stimulus, such as insulin-induced hypoglycemia[39] (which should not be used in elderly patients and those with a history of cardiovascular disease), propanolol and glucagon,[46] arginine,[42] or L-DOPA.[47] Because a normal person may have a subnormal response to any of these, it is customary to require a subnormal response to two of these stimuli before making the diagnosis of growth hormone deficiency. Two of the stimuli are often combined. The growth hormone response to all of these stimuli is impaired in obesity, so a subnormal response in an obese person could be due to the obesity and not growth hormone deficiency.

Treatment

The optimal regimen for administering growth hormone has not yet been determined, but at this time it appears that efficacy is best monitored by keeping the serum concentration of IGF-1 in the middle of the normal range for age. It also appears that the chance of side effects can be minimized by starting with a lower dose of growth hormone than that expected to raise the IGF-1 to normal and then increasing the dose gradually until the serum IGF-1 concentration reaches the mid-normal range. The starting dose, for example, might be 2 μg/kg body weight/day; the eventual dose will not likely be more than 12 μg/kg body weight/day. Doses required to achieve these results in women tend to be greater than in men.[365] Recognized side effects include peripheral edema, arthralgias, carpal tunnel syndrome, paresthesias, and worsening of glucose tolerance. Benign intracranial hypertension has been reported mainly in children. These effects are more likely to occur in women and in patients who are older or heavier. The suspicion has been raised but not documented that growth hormone treatment may worsen the progression of tumors.

Prolactin Deficiency

Prolactin deficiency occurs only as the result of damage to the lactotroph cells of the pituitary, not as the result of hypothalamic disease, which increases prolactin secretion.

Symptoms and Signs

The only known consequence of prolactin deficiency is failure of lactation following delivery. This situation does not occur commonly, probably because hypopituitarism of sufficient severity to cause prolactin deficiency also generally causes gonadotropin deficiency as well. However, pregnancy and then childbirth could certainly occur if ovulation is induced with gonadotropins. A well-recognized situation when prolactin deficiency leads to difficulty in lactation is following the acute onset of Sheehan's syndrome.[132]

Diagnosis

The diagnosis of prolactin deficiency can be suspected in any woman who has been documented to have deficiencies of all other pituitary hormones, and especially if she is not able to lactate following delivery. Although stimuli of prolactin secretion, such as TRH, are available, demonstration of a subnormal response is usually not of value, because no treatment is available.

Treatment

There is no prolactin preparation for replacement.

REFERENCES

1. DiChirio G, Nelson KB: The volume of the sella turcica. *AJR* 87:989, 1962.
2. Swartz JD, Russell KB, Basile BA, O'Donnell PC, Popky GL: High-resolution computed tomographic appearance of the intrasellar contents in women of childbearing age. *Radiology* 147:115, 1983.
3. Lurie SN, Doraiswamy PM, Hussain MM, Boyko OB, Ellinwood EH, Figiel GS, Krishnan KRR: In vivo assessment of pituitary gland volume with magnetic resonance imaging: The effect of age. *J Clin Endocrinol Metab* 71:505, 1990.
4. Kaufman B: Magnetic resonance imaging of the pituitary gland. *Radiol Clin North Am* 22:795, 1984.
5. Glaser B, Sheinfeld M, Benmair J, Kaplan N: Magnetic resonance imaging of the pituitary gland. *Clin Radiol* 37:9, 1986.
6. Wolpert SM, Molitch ME, Goldman JA, Wood JB: Size, shape, and appearance of the normal pituitary gland. *AJR* 143:377, 1984.
7. Stanfield JP: The blood supply of the human pituitary gland. *J Anat* 94:257, 1960.
8. Horvath E, Kovacs K: Fine structural cytology of the adenohypophysis in rat and man. *J Electron Microsc Tech* 8:401, 1988.
9. Sano T, Asa SL, Kovacs K: Growth hormone-releasing hormone-producing tumors: Clinical, biochemicl and morphological manifestations. *Endocrinol Rev* 9:357, 1988.
10. Asa SL, Penz G, Kovacs K, Ezrin C: Prolactin cells in the human pituitary. *Arch Pathol Lab Med* 106:360, 1982.
11. Scheithauer BW, Kovacs KT, Young WF, Ryan N, Randall RV: The pituitary gland in pregnancy: A clinicopathologic and immunohistochemical study of 69 cases. *Mayo Clin Proc* 65:461, 1990.
12. Hofler H, Walter GF, Denk H: Immunohistochemistry of foliculostellate cells in normal human adenohypophyses and in pituitary adenomas. *Acta Neuropathol* 40:35, 1984.
13. Falin LI: The development of human hypophysis and differentiation of cells in its anterior lobe during embryonic life. *Acta Anat* 44:188, 1961.
14. Asa SL, Kovacs K, Laszlo FA, Domokos I, Ezrin C: Human fetal Adneohypophysis. Histologic and immunocytochemical analysis. *Neuroendocrinology* 43:308, 1986.
15. Asa SL, Kovacs K, Horvath E, Losinski NE, Laszlo FA, Domokos I, Halliday WC: Human fetal adenohypophysis. Electron microscopic and ultrastructural immunocytochemical analysis. *Neuroendocrinology* 48:423, 1988.
16. Lamonerie T, Tremblay JJ, Lanctot C, Therrien M, Gauthier Y, Drouin J: Ptx1, a bicoid-related homeobox transcription factor involved in transcription of the pro-opiomelanocortin gene. *Genes Dev* 10:1284, 1996.
17. Gage PIJ, Camper SA: Pituitary homeobox 2, a novel member of the bicoid-related family of homeobox genes, is a potential regulator of anterior structure formation. *Hum Mol Genet* 6:457, 1997.
18. Sheng HZ, Zhadanov AB, Mosinger B Jr, Fujii T, Bertuzzi S, Grinberg A, Lee EJ, Huang SP, et al: Specification of pituitary cell lineages by the LIM homeobox gene Lhx3. *Science* 272:1004, 1996.
19. Bach I, Rhodes SJ, Pearse RV, Heinzel T, Gloss B, Scully KM, Sawchenki PE, Rosenfeld MG: P-Lim, a LIM homeodomain factor, is expressed during pituitary organ and cell commitment and synergizes with Pit-1. *Proc Natl Acad Sci USA* 92:2720, 1995.
20. Hermesz E, Machem S, Mahan KA: Rpx: A novel anterior-restricted homeobox gene progressively activated in the prechordal plate, anterior neural plate and Rathke's pouch of the mouse embryo. *Development* 122:41, 1996.
21. Stefana B, Ray DW, Melmed S: Leukemia inhibitory factor induces differentiation of pituitary corticotroph function: An immunoneuroendocrine phenotypic switch. *Proc Natl Acad Sci USA* 93:12502, 1996.
22. Gage PJ, Brinkmeier ML, Scarlett LM, Knapp LT, Camper SA, Mahan KA: The Ames dwarf gene, df, is required early in pituitary ontogeny for the extinction of Rpx transcription and initiation of lineage-specific cell proliferation. *Mol Endocrinol* 10:1570, 1996.
23. Sornson MW, Wu W, Dasen JS, Flynn SE, Norman DJ, O'Connell SM, Gukovsky I, Carriere C, et al: Pituitary lineage determination by the Prophet of Pit-1 homeodomain factor defective in Ames dwarfism. *Nature* 384:327, 1996.
24. Wu W, Cogan JD, Pfaffle RW, Dasen JS, Frisch H, O'Connell SM, Flynn SE, Brown MR, et al: Mutations in PROP1 cause familial combined pituitary hormone deficiency. *Nat Genet* 18:147, 1998.
25. Fofanova O, Takmura N, Kinoshita E, Parks JS, Brown MR, Peterkova VA, Evgrafov OV, Goncharov NP, et al: Compound heterozygous deletion of the prop-1 gene in children with combined pituitary hormone deficiency. *J Clin Endocrinol Metab* 83:2601, 1998.
26. Cogan JD, Wu W, Phillips JA III, Arnhold IJP, Agapito A, Fofanova OV, Osorio MGF, Bircan I, et al: The PROP1 2-base pair deletion is a common cause of combined pituitary hormone deficiency. *J Clin Endocrinol Metab* 83:3346, 1998.

27. Andersen B, Rosenfeld MG: Pit-1 determines cell types during development of the anterior gland. *J Biol Chem* 269:29336, 1994.
28. Dasen JS, O'Connell SM, Flynn SE, Treoer M, Gleiberman AS, Szeto DP, Hooshmand F, Aggarwai AK, Rosenfeld MG: Reciprocal interactions of Pit1 and GATA2 mediate signaling gradient-induced determination of pituitary cell types. *Cell* 97:587, 1999.
29. Ohta K, Nobukuni Y, Mitsubuchi H, Fujimoto S, Matsuo N, Inagaki H, Endo F, Matsuda I: Mutations in the Pit-1 gene in children with combined pituitary hormone deficiency. *Biochem Biophys Res Commun* 189:851, 1992.
30. Radovick S, Nations M, Du Y, Berg LA, Weintraub BD, Wondisford FE: A mutation in the POU-homeodomain of pit-1 responsible for combined pituitary hormone deficiency. *Science* 257:1115, 1992.
31. Ingraham H, Lala D, Ikeda Y, Luo X, Shen W-H, Nachtigal M, Abbud R, Nilson J, Parker K: The nuclear receptor steroidogenic factor 1 acts as at multiple levels of the reproductive axis. *Genes Dev* 8:2302, 1994.
32. Ikeda Y, Luo X, Abbud R, Nilson J, Parker KL: The nuclear receptor steroidogenic factor 1 is essential for the formation of the ventromedial hypothalamic nucleus. *Mol Endocrinol* 9:478, 1995.
33. Cooke NE, Liebhaber SA: Molecular biology of the growth hormone-prolactin gene system. *Vitamins and Hormones* 50:385, 1995.
34. Pfaffle RW, DiMattia GE, Parks JS, Brown MR, Wit JM, Jansen M, van der Nat H, van den Brande JL, et al: Mutation of the POU-specific domain of pit-1 and hypopituitarism without pituitary hypoplasia. *Science* 257:1118, 1992.
35. Nelson C, Albert VR, Elsholz HP, Lu LIW, Rosenfeld MG: Activation of cell-specific expression of rat growth hormone and prolactin genes by a common transcription factor. *Science* 239:1400, 1988.
36. Frohman LA, Jannson J: Growth hormone-releasing hormone. *Endocrinol Rev* 7:717, 1986.
37. Shimon I, Taylor JE, Dong JZ, et al: Somatostatin receptor subtype specificity in human fetal pituitary cultures: Differential role of SSTR2 and SSTR5 for growth hormone, thyroid-stimulating hormone and prolactin regulation. *J Clin Invest* 99:789, 1997.
38. Sassin J, Weitzman ED, Kapen S: Human prolactin: 24-hour pattern with increased release during sleep. *Science* 177:1205, 1973.
39. Greenwood FC, Landon J, Stamp TCB: The plasma sugar, free fatty acid, cortisol, and growth hormone response to insulin. I. In control subjects. *J Clin Invest* 45:429, 1966.
40. Roth J, Glick SMY, Berson S: Hypoglycemia: A potent stimulus to secretion of growth hormone. *Science* 10:987, 1963.
41. Ho KY, Veldhuis JD, Johnson ML, et al: Fasting enhances growth hormone secretion and amplifies the complex rhythms of growth hormone secretion in man. *J Clin Invest* 81:968, 1988.
42. Merimee TJ, Rabinowitz D, Riggs L, Burgess JA, Rimoin DL, McKusick VA: Plasma growth hormone after arginine infusion. *N Engl J Med* 276:434, 1967.
43. Rivier J, Spiess J, Thorner M, et al: Characterization of a growth hormone-releasing factor from a human pancreatic islet tumor. *Nature* 300:276, 1982.
44. Carey LC, Clothier CT, Lowery BD: Growth hormone and adrenal cortical response to shock and trauma in the human. *Ann Surg* 174:451, 1971.
45. Gil-Ad I, Topper E, Laron Z: Oral clonidine as a growth hormone stimulation test. *Lancet* 2:278, 1979.
46. Mitchell ME, Suvunrungsi P, Sawin CT: Effect of propranolol on the response of serum growth hormone to glucagon. *J Clin Endocrinol Metab* 32:470, 1971.
47. Boyd A, Lebovitz HE, Pfeiffer JB: Stimulation of human-growth secretion by L-DOPA. *N Engl J Med* 283:1425, 1970.
48. Bivens CH, Lebovitz HE, Feldman JM: Inhibition of hypoglycemia-induced growth hormone secretion by the serotonin antagonists cyproheptidine and methysergide. *N Engl J Med* 289:236, 1973.
49. Leung DW, Spencer SA, Cachianes G, Hammonds RG, Collins C, Henzel WJ, et al: Growth hormone receptor and serum binding protein: Purification, cloning, and expression. *Nature* 330:537, 1987.
50. Baumann GA, Shaw MA, Winter RJ: Absence of the plasma growth hormone binding protein in Laron-type dwarfism. *J Clin Endocrinol Metab* 65:814, 1987.
51. Kratzsch J, Selisko T, Birkenmeier G: Identification of transformed alpha 2-macroglobulin as a growth hormone-binding protein in human blood. *J Clin Endocrinol Metab* 80:585, 1995.
52. Carter-Su C, Smit LS: Signaling via JAK tyrosine kinases: Growth hormone receptor as a model system. *Recent Prog Hormone Res* 53:61, 1998.
53. Salmon WD Jr, Daughaday WH: A hormonally controlled serum factor which stimulates sulfate incorporation by cartilage in vitro. *J Lab Clin Med* 49:825, 1957.
54. Kostyo JL, Hotchkiss J, Knobil E: Stimulation of amino acid transport in isolated diaphragm by growth hormone added in vitro. *Science* 130:1653, 1959.
55. Salomon F, Cuneo RC, Hesp R, Sonksen PH: The effects of treatment with recombinant human growth hormone on body composition and metabolism in adults with growth hormone deficiency. *N Engl J Med* 321:1797, 1989.
56. Baum HBA, Biller BMK, Finkelstein JS, Canistraro KB, Oppenheim DS, Schoenfeld D, et al: Effects of physiologic growth hormone therapy on bone density and body composition in patients with adult-onset growth hormone deficiency. *Ann Intern Med* 125:883, 1996.
57. Fain JN, Kovacev VP, Scow RO: Effect of growth hormone and dexamethasone on lipolysis and metabolism in isolated fat cells of the rat. *J Biol Chem* 240:3522, 1965.
58. Weaver JU, Monson JP, Noonan K, John WG, Edwards A, Evans KA, Cunningham J: The effect of low dose replacement recombinant human growth hormone replacement on regional fat distribution, insulin sensivity, and cardiovascular risk factors in hypopituitary adults. *J Clin Endocrinol Metab* 80:153, 1995.
59. Beshayah SA, Henderson A, Niththyananthan R, Skinner E, Anyaoku V, Richmond W, Sharp P, Johnston DG: The effects of short and long term growth hormone replacement therapy in hypopituitary adults on lipid metabolism and carbohydrate tolerance. *J Clin Endocrinol Metab* 80:356, 1995.
60. Jacobs LS, Snyder PJ, Utiger RD, Daughaday WH: Prolactin response to thyrotropin-releasing hormone in normal subjects. *J Clin Endocrinol Metab* 36:1069, 1973.
61. Clevenger CV, Freier DO, Kline JB: Prolactin receptor signal transduction in cells of the immune system. *J Endocrinol* 157:187, 1998.
62. Smith AI, Funder JW: Proopiomelanocortin processing in the pituitary, central nervous system, and peripheral tissues. *Endocrinol Rev* 9:159, 1988.
63. Desir D, Van Cauter E, Fang VS: Effects of "jet lag" on hormonal patterns. I. Procedures, variations, and disruption of adrenocorticotropin-cortisol periodicity. *J Clin Endocrinol Metab* 52:628, 1981.
64. DeBold CR, Sheldon WR, DeCherney GS, et al: Arginine vasopressin potentiates adrenocorticotropin release induced by ovine corticotropin-releasing factor. *J Clin Invest* 73:533, 1984.
65. Canny BJ, Li-Guo J, Leong DA: Corticotropin-releasing factor, but not arginine vasopressin, stimulates concentration-dependent increases in ACTH secretion from a single corticotrope. *J Biol Chem* 267:8325, 1992.
66. Mountjoy KG, Robbins LS, Mortud MT: The cloning of a family of genes that encode the melanocortin receptors. *Science* 257:1248, 1992.
67. Suzuki I, Cone RD, Im S, et al: Binding of melanotropic hormones to the melanocortin receptor MC1R on human melanocytes stimulates prolferation and melanogenesis. *Endocrinology* 137:1627, 1996.
68. Crowley WF Jr, Filicori M, Spratt DI, Santoro NF: The physiology of gonadotropin-releasing hormone (GnRH) secretion in men and women. *Recent Prog in Hormone Res* 41:473, 1985.
69. Conn PM, Crowley WF Jr: Gonadotropin-releasing hormone and its analogs. *N Engl J Med* 324:93, 1991.
70. Belchetz PE, Plant TM, Nakai Y, Keogh EJ, Knobil E: Hypophyseal responses to continuous and intermittent delivery of hypothalamic gonadotropin-releasing hormone. *Science* 202:631, 1978.
71. Crowley WF Jr, Filicori M, Spratt DI, Santoro NF: The physiology of gonadotropin-releasing hormone (GnRH) in men and women. *Recent Prog Hormone Res* 41:473, 1985.
72. Bilezekian JP, Morishima A, Bell J, Grumbach MM: Increased bone mass as a result of estrogen therapy in a man with aromatase deficiency. *N Engl J Med* 339:599, 1998.
73. Carani C, Qin K, Simoni M, Faustini-Fustini M, Serpente S, Boyd J, et al: Effect of testosterone and estradiol in a man with aromatase deficiency. *N Engl J Med* 337:91, 1997.
74. Smith EP, Boyd J, Frank GR, et al: Estrogen resistance caused by a mutation in the estrogen-receptor gene in a man. *N Engl J Med* 331:1056, 1994.

75. Majundar SS, Mikuma N, Ishwood PC, Winters SJ, Attardi BJ, Perara AD, Plant TM: Replacement with recombinant human inhibin immediately after orchidectomy in the hypophysiotropically clamped male rhesus monkey (Macaca mulatta) maintains follicle stimulating hormone (FSH) secretion and FSH beta messenger ribonucleic acid levels at precastration values. *Endocrinology* 136:1969, 1995.
76. Wondisford FE, Radovick S, Moates JM, Usula SJ, Weintraub BD: Isolation and characterization of the human thyrotropin β-subunit gene. *J Biol Chem* 263:12538, 1988.
77. Magner JA: Thyroid-stimulating hormone: Biosynthesis, cell biology, and bioactivity. *Endocrinal Rev* 11:354, 1990.
78. Taylor T, Weintraub BD: Altered thyrotropin (TSH) carbohydrate structures in hypothalamic hypothyroidism created by paraventricular nuclear lesions are corrected by in vivo TSH-releasing hormone administration. *Endocrinology* 125:2198, 1989.
79. Beck-Peccoz P, Amr S, Menezes-Ferreira MM, Faglia G, Weintraub BD: Decreased receptor binding of biologically inactive thyrotropin in central hypothyroidism. *N Engl J Med* 312:1085, 1985.
80. Shupnik MA, Greenspan SL, Ridgway EC: Transcriptional regulation of thyrotropin subunit genes by thyrotropin-releasing hormone and dopamine in pituitary cell culture. *J Biol Chem* 261:12675, 1986.
81. Steinfelder HJ, Hauser P, Nakayama Y, Radovick S, McClaskey JH, Taylor T, et al: Thyrotropin-releasing hormone regulation of human TSHβ expression: Role of a pituitary-specific transcription factor (pit-1/GHF-1) and potential interaction with a thyroid hormone-inhibitory element. *Proc Natl Acad Sci USA* 88:3130, 1991.
82. Pellegrini-Bouller I, Belicar P, Barlier A: A new mutation of the gene encoding the transcription factor pit-1 is resonsible for combined pituitary hormone deficiency. *J Clin Endocrinol Metab* 81:2790, 1996.
83. Pfaffle RW, DiMattia GE, Parks JS: Mutation of the POU-specific domain of pit-1 and hypopituitarism without pituitary hypoplasia. *Science* 257:1118, 1992.
84. Kim DS, Ahn SK, Yoon JH: Involvement of a cAMP-responsive DNA element in mediating TRH responsiveness of the human thyrotropin alpha-subunit gene. *Mol Endocrinol* 8:528, 1994.
85. Chin WW, Shupnick MA, Ross DS: Regulation of the alpha and thyrotropin beta-subunit messenger ribonucleic acids by thyroid hormones. *Endocrinology* 116:873, 1985.
86. Wondisford FE, Farr EA, Radovick S, Steinfelder HJ, Moates JM, McClaskey JH, Weintraub BD: Thyroid hormone inhibition of human thyrotropin beta-subunit gene expression is mediated by a cis-acting element located in the first exon. *J Biol Chem* 264:14601, 1989.
87. Brabant G, Frank K, Ranft U: Physiologic regulation of circadian and pulsatile thyrotropin secretion in normal man and woman. *J Clin Endocrinol Metab* 70:403, 1990.
88. Snyder PJ, Utiger RD: Repetitive administration of thyrotropin-releasing hormone results in small elevations of serum thyroid hormones and in marked inhibition of thyrotropin response. *J Clin Invest* 52:2305, 1973.
89. Silva JE, Larsen PR: Pituitary nuclear 3,5,3′-triiodothyronine and thyrotropin secretion: An explanation for the effect of thyroxine. *Science* 198:617, 1977.
90. Sunthornthepvarakul T, Gottschalk ME, Hayashi Y, Refetoff S: Brief report: Resistance to thyrotropin caused by mutations in the thyrotropin-receptor gene. *N Engl J Med* 332:155, 1995.
91. Weeke J, Hansen AAP, Lundbaeke K: Inhibition by somatostatin of basal levels of serum thyrotropin (TSH) in normal men. *J Clin Endocrinol Metab* 41:168, 1975.
92. Spaulding SW, Burrow GN, Donabedian R, Van Woert M: L-Dopa suppression of thyrotropin releasing hormone response in man. *J Clin Endocrinol Metab* 35:182, 1972.
93. Paschke R, Ludgate M: The thyrotropin receptor in thyroid diseases. *N Engl J Med* 337:1675, 1997.
94. Alexander JM, Biller BMK, Bikkal H, Zervas NT, Arnold A, Klibanski A: Clinically nonfunctioning pituitary tumors are monoclonal in orgin. *J Clin Invest* 86:336, 1990.
95. Herman V, Fagin J, Gonsky R, Kovacs K, Melmed S: Clonal orgin of pituitary adenomas. *J Clin Endocrinol Metab* 71:1427, 1990.
96. Vallar L, Spada A, Giannattasio G: Altered G_s and adenylate cyclase activity in human GH-secreting pituitary adenomas. *Nature* 330:566, 1987.
97. Landis CA, Masters SB, Spada A, Pace AM, Bourne HR, Vallar L: GTPase inhibiting mutations activate the α chain of G_s and stimulate adenylate cyclase in human pituitary tumors. *Nature* 340:692, 1989.
98. Asa SL, Kovacs K, Stefaneanu L, Horvath E, Billestrup N, Gonzalez-Manchon C, Vale W: Pituitary adenomas in mice transgenic for growth hormone-releasing hormone. *Endocrinology* 131:2083, 1992.
99. Tanaka C, Kimura T, Yang P, Moritani M, Yamaoka T, Yamada S, et al: Analysis of loss of heterozygosity on chromosome 11 and infrequent inactivating of the MEN1 gene in sporadic pituitary adenomas. *J Clin Endocrinol Metab* 83:2631, 1998.
100. Asa SL, Somers K, Ezzat S: The MEN-1 gene is rarely down-regulated in pituitary adenomas. *J Clin Endocrinol Metab* 83:3210, 1998.
101. Woloschak M, Roberts JL, Post K: c-Myc, c-fos, and c-myb gene expression in human pituitary adenomas. *J Clin Endocrinol Metab* 79:253, 1994.
102. Cai WY, Alexander JM, Hedley-Whyte ET, Scheithauer BW, Jameson JL, Zervas NT, Klibanski A: Ras mutations in human prolactinomas and pituitary carcinomas. *J Clin Endocrinol Metab* 78:89, 1994.
103. Pei L, Melmed S, Scheithauer B, Kovacs K, Prager D: H-ras mutations in human pituitary carcinoma metastases. *J Clin Endocrinol Metab* 78:842, 1994.
104. Cryns VL, Alexander JM, Klibanski A, Arnold A: The retinoblastoma gene in human pituitary tumors. *J Clin Endocrinol Metab* 77:644, 1993.
105. Zhu J, Leon SP, Beggs AH, Busque L, Gilliland DG, Black PM: Human pituitary adenomas show no loss of heterozygosity at the retinoblastoma gene locus. *J Clin Endocrinol Metab* 78:922, 1994.
106. Ikeda H, Beauchamp RL, Yoshimoto T, Yandell DW: Detection of heterozygous mutation in the retinoblastoma gene in a human pituitary adenoma using pcr-sscp analysis and direct sequencing. *Endo Path* 6:189, 1995.
107. Jones TH, Daniels M, James RA, Justice SK, McCorkle R, Price A, et al: Production of bioactive and immunoreactive interleukin-6 (IL-6) and expression of IL-6 messenger ribonucleic acid by human pituitary adenomas. *J Clin Endocrinol Metab* 78:180, 1994.
108. Robberecht P, Vertongen P, Velkeniers B, DeNeef P, Vergani P, Raftopoulos C, et al: Receptors for pituitary adenylate cyclase activating peptides in human pituitary adenomas. *J Clin Endocrinol Metab* 77:1235, 1993.
109. Alvaro V, Levy L, Dubray C, Roche A, Peillon F, Querat B, Joubert D: Invasive human pituitary tumors express a point-mutated alpha-protein kinase-C. *J Clin Endocrinol Metab* 77:1125, 1993.
110. Ezzat S, Smyth HS, Ramyar L, Asa SL: Heterogenous in vivo and in vitro expression of basic fibroblast growth factor by human pituitary adenomas. *J Clin Endocrinol Metab* 80:878, 1995.
111. LeRiche V, Asa SL, Ezzat S: Epidermal growth factor and its receptor (EGF-R) in human pituitary adenomas: EGF-R correlates with tumor aggressiveness. *J Clin Endocrinol Metab* 81:656, 1996.
112. Ezzat S, Walpola IA, Ramyar L, Smythe HS, Asa SL: Membrane-anchored expression of transforming growth factor alpha in human pituitary adenoma cells. *J Clin Endocrinol Metab* 80:534, 1995.
113. Prezant TR, Kadioglu P, Melmed S: An intronless homolog of human proto-oncogene *hPTTG* is expressed in pituitary tumors: Evidence for *hPTTG* family. *J Clin Endocrinol Metab* 84:1149, 1999.
114. Beck-Peccoz P, Brucker-Davis F, Persani L, Smallridge RC, Weintraub BD: Thyrotropin-secreting pituitary tumors. *Endocrinol Rev* 17:610, 1996.
115. Samaan NA, Stephans AV, Danziger J, Trujillo J: Reactive pituitary abnormalities in patients with Klinefelter's and Turner's syndromes. *Arch Intern Med* 139:198, 1979.
116. Weiner HL, Wisoff JH, Kupersmith MJ, Cohen H, Zagzag D, Shiminski-Maher T, et al: Craniopharyngiomas: A clinicopathological analysis of factors predictive of recurrence and functional outcome. *Neurosurgery* 35:1001, 1994.
117. Pernicone PJ, Scheithauer BW, Sebo TJ, Kovacs KT, Horvath E, Young WF, et al: Pituitary carcinoma. A clinicopathologic study of 15 cases. *Cancer* 79:804, 1996.
118. Schubiger O, Haller D: Metastases to the pituitary-hypothalamic axis. *Neuroradiology* 34:131, 1992.
119. Post MJD, Mendez DR, Kline LB, Acker JD, Glaser JS: Metastatic disease to the cavernous sinus: Clinical syndrome and CT diagnosis. *J Comput Assist Tomogr* 9:115, 1985.
120. Cosman F, Post KD, Holub D, Wardlaw S: Lymphocytic hypophysitis: Report of 3 new cases and review of the literature. *Medicine* 68:240, 1989.

121. Thodou E, Asa SL, Kontogeorgos G, Kovacs K, Horvath E, Ezzat S: Lymphocytic hypophysitis: Clinicopathologic findings. *J Clin Endocrinol Metab* 80:2302, 1995.
122. Honegger J, Fahlbusch R, Hensen J, Buchfelder M, Muller M, Nomikos P: Lymphocytic and granulomatous hypophysitis: Experience with nine cases. *Neurosurgery* 40:713, 1997.
123. Wolansky LJ, Gallagher JD, Heary RF: MRI of pituitary abscesses: Two cases and review of the literature. *Neuroradiology* 39:499, 1997.
124. Sato N, Putman CM, Chaloupka JC: Pituitary gland enlargement secondary to dural arteriovenous fistula in the cavernous sinus: Appearance at MR imaging. *Radiology* 203:263, 1997.
125. Arafah BM: Reversible hypopituitarism in patients with large nonfunctioning pituitary adenomas. *J Clin Endocrinol Metab* 62:1183, 1986.
126. Snyder PJ, Fowble B, Schatz NJ, Savino PJ, Gennarelli TA: Hypopituitarism following radiation therapy of pituitary adenomas. *Am J Med* 81:457, 1986.
127. Littley MD, Shalet SM, Beardwell CG: Hypopituitarism following external radiotherapy for pituitary tumors in adults. *Q J Med* 70:145, 1989.
128. Eastman RC, Gordon P, Roth J: Conventional supervoltage irradiation is an effective treatment for acromegaly. *J Clin Endocrinol Metab* 48:931, 1979.
129. Charbonnel B, Chupin B, LeGrand A, Guillon J: Pituitary function in idiopathic haemochromocytosis: Hormonal study in 36 male patients. *Acta Endocrinol (Copenh)* 98:178, 1981.
130. Kelly TM, Edwards CQ, Meikle AW: Hypogonadism in hemochromatosis: Reversal with iron depletion. *Ann Intern Med* 101:629, 1984.
131. Missler U, Mack M, Nowack G, Muller-Esch G, Reusche E, Borgis KJ, et al: Pituitary sarcoidosis. *Klinische Wochenschrift* 68:342, 1990.
132. Sheehan HL: Simmonds's disease due to post-partum necrosis of the anterior pituitary. *Q J M* 32:277, 1939.
133. Sheehan HL, Stanfield JP: The pathogenesis of post-partum necrosis of the anterior lobe of the pituitary gland. *Acta Endocrinol (Copenh)* 37:479, 1961.
134. Taylor DS: Massive gastric haemorrhage in late pregnancy followed by hypopituitarism. *Obstet Gynaecol* 79:476, 1972.
135. Tulandi T, Yusuf N, Posner BI: Diabetes insipidus: A postpartum complication. *Obstet Gynecol* 70:492, 1987.
136. Aguilo F Jr, Vega LA, Haddock L, Rodriguez O Jr: Diabetes insipidus syndrome in hypopituitarism of pregnancy. Case report and a critical review of the literature. *Acta Endocrinol (Copenh)* 60:Suppl 137:1, 1969.
137. Barbieri RL, Randall RW, Saltzman DH: Diabetes insipidus occurring in a patient with Sheehan's syndrome during a gonadotropin-induced pregnancy. *Fertil Steril* 44:529, 1985.
138. Arafah B, Taylor HC, Salazar R, Saadi H, Selman WR: Apoplexy of a pituitary adenoma after dynamic testing with gonadotropin-releasing hormone. *Am J Med* 87:103, 1989.
139. Chanson P, Schaison G: Pituitary apoplexy caused by GnRH-agonist treatment revealing gonadotroph adenoma. *J Clin Endocrinol Metab* 80:2267, 1995.
140. Drury PL, Belchetz PE, McDonald WI, Thomas DGT, Besser GM: Transient amaurosis and headache after thyrotropin releasing hormone. *Lancet* 1:218, 1982.
141. Arafah B, Harrington F, Madhoun ZT: Improvement of pituitary function after surgical decompression for pituitary tumor apoplexy. *J Clin Endocrinol Metab* 71:323, 1990.
142. Maccagnan P, Macedo CLD, Kayath MJ, Nogueira RG, Abucham J: Conservative management of pituitary apoplexy: A prospective study. *J Clin Endocrinol Metab* 80:2190, 1995.
143. Wu W, Cogan JD, Pfaffle RW: Mutations in prop-1 cause familial combined pituitary hormone deficiency. *Nat Genet* 18: 147, 1998.
144. Deladohey J, Fluck C, Buyukgebiz A, Kuhlmann BV, Eble A, Hindmarsh PC, et al: "Hot spot" in the PROP-1 gene responsible for combined pituitary hormone deficiency. *J Clin Endocrinol Metab* 84:1645, 1999.
145. Netchine I, Talon P, Dastot F, Vitaux F, Goossens M, Amselem S: Extensive phenotypic analysis of a family with growth hormone (GH) deficiency caused by a mutation in the GH-releasing hormone receptor gene. *J Clin Endocrinol Metab* 83:432, 1998.
146. Maheshwari HG, Silverman BL, Dupuis J, Baumann G: Phenoype and genetic analysis of a syndrome caused by an inactivating mutation in the growth hormone-releasing hormone receptor: Dwarfism of Sindh. *J Clin Endocrinol Metab* 83:4065, 1998.
147. Takahashi Y, Kaji H, Okimura Y, Goji K, Abe H, Chihara K: Short stature caused by a mutant growth hormone. *N Engl J Med* 334:432, 1996.
148. Collu R, Tang J, Castagne J, Lagace G, Masson N, Huot C, et al: A novel mechanism for isolated central hypothyroidism: Inactivating mutations in the thyrotropin-releasing hormone receptor gene. *J Clin Endocrinol Metab* 82:1561, 1997.
149. deRoux N, Young J, Brailly-Tabard S, Misahi M, Milgrom E, Schaison G: The same molecular defects of the gonadotropin-releasing hormone receptor determine a variable degree of hypogonadism in affected kindred. *J Clin Endocrinol Metab* 84:567, 1999.
150. deRoux N, Young J, Misrahi M, Genet R, Chason P, Schaison G, Milgrom E: A family with hypogonadotropic hypogonadism and mutations in the gonadotropin-releasing hormone receptor. *N Engl J Med* 337:1597, 1997.
151. Elster AD, Chen MYM, Williams DW III, Key LL: Pituitary gland: MR imaging of physiologic hypertrophy in adolescence. *Radiology* 174:681, 1990.
152. Elster AD, Sanders TG, Vines FS, Chen MYM: Size and shape of the pituitary gland during pregnancy and post partum: Measurement with MR imaging. *Radiology* 181:531, 1991.
153. King JT, Justice AC, Aron DC: Management of incidental pituitary microadenomas. *J Clin Endocrinol Metab* 82:3625, 1997.
154. Chong BW, Kucharczyk W, Singer W, George S: Pituitary gland MR: A comparative study of healthy volunteers and patients with microadenomas. *Am J Neuroradiol* 15:675, 1994.
155. Sethi DS, Pillay PK: Endoscopic management of lesions of the sella turcica. *J Laryngol Otol* 109:956, 1995.
156. Jho H-D, Carrau RL: Endoscopic endonasal transsphenoidal surgery: Experience with 50 patients. *J Neurosurg* 87:44, 1997.
157. Yaniv E, Rappaport H: Endoscopic transseptal transsphenoidal surgery for pituitary tumors. *Neurosurgery* 40:944, 1997.
158. Trautmann JC, Laws ER Jr: Visual status after transsphenoidal surgery at the Mayo Clinic. *Am J Ophthalmol* 96:200, 1983.
159. Black PM, Zervas NT, Candia G: Management of large pituitary adenomas by transsphenoidal surgery. *Surg Neurol* 29:4434, 1988.
160. Arafah BM, Kailani SH, Nekl KE, Gold RS, Selman WR: Immediate recovery of pituitary function after transsphenoidal resection of pituitary macroadenomas. *J Clin Endocrinol Metab* 79:348, 1994.
161. Ciric I, Ragin A, Baumgartner C, Pierce D: Complications of transsphenoidal surgery: Results of a national survey, review of the literature, and personal experience. *Neurosurgery* 40:225, 1997.
162. Wilson CB: A decade of pituitary microsurgery. *J Neurosurg* 61:814, 1984.
163. Black PM, Zervas NT, Candia GL: Incidence and management of complications of transsphenoidal operations for pituitary adenomas. *Neurosurgery* 20:920, 1987.
164. Barrow DL, Tindall GT: Loss of vision afer transsphenoidal surgery. *Neurosurgery* 27:60, 1990.
165. Laws ER Jr, Fode NC, Redmond MJ: Transsphenoidal surgery following unsuccessful prior therapy. *J Neurosurg* 63:823, 1985.
166. Laws ER Jr: Transsphenoidal microsurgery in the management of craniopharyngioma. *J Neurosurg* 52:661, 1980.
167. Baskin DS, Wilson CB: Surgical management of craniopharyngiomas. A review of 74 cases. *J Neurosurg* 65:22, 1986.
168. Honegger J, Buchfelder M, Fahlbusch R, Daubler B, Dorr HG: Transsphenoidal microsurgery for craniopharyngioma. *Surg Neurol* 37:189, 1992.
169. Olson RR, Gumowski J, Rubino D: Pathophysiology of hyponatremia after transsphenoidal surgery. *J Neurosurg* 87:499, 1997.
170. Streeten DHP, Anderson GH Jr, Bonaventurea MM: The potential for serious consequences from misinterpreting normal responses to the rapid adrenocorticotropin test. *J Clin Endocrinol Metab* 81:285, 1996.
171. Streeten DH, Anderson GH, Bonaventura M: The potential for serious consequences from misinterpreting normal responses to the rapid adrenocorticotropin test. *J Clin Endocrinol Metab* 81:285, 1996.
172. Soule SG, Fahle-Wilson M, Tomlinson S: Failure of the short ACTH test to unequivocally diagnose long-standing symptomatic secondary hypoadrenalism. *Clin Endocrinol* 44:137, 1996.
173. Mayenknecht J, Diederich S, Bahr V, Plockinger U, Oelkers W: Com-

parison of the low and high dose corticotropin stimulation tests in patients with pituitary disease. *J Clin Endocrinol Metab* 83:1558, 1998.

174. Zaugg M, Adamman O, Pescia R, Landolt AM: External irradiation of macroinvasive pituitary adenomas with telecobalt: A retrospective study with long-term follow-up in patients irradiated with doses mostly of between 4045 Gy. *I J Radiat Oncol Biol Phys* 32:671, 1995.
175. McCord MW, Buatti JM, Fennel EM, Mendenhall WM, Marcus RM Jr, Rhoton AL, et al: Radiotherapy for pituitary adenoma: Long-term outcome and sequellae. *Int J Radiat Oncol* 39:437, 1997.
176. Gittoes NJL, Bates AS, Tse W, Bullivant B, Sheppard MC, Clayton RN, Stewart PM: Radiotherapy for non-functioning pituitary adenomas. *Clin Endocrinol* 48:331, 1998.
177. Littley MD, Shalet SM, Beardwell CG, Lillehei KO: Hypopituitarism following external radiotherapy for pituitary tumours in adults. *Q J Med* 145:160, 1970.
178. Nelson P, Goodman M, Flickenger J, Richardson D, Robinson A: Endocrine function in patients with large pituitary tumors treated with operative decompression and radiation therapy. *Neurosurgery* 24:398, 1989.
179. Schatz NJ, Lichenstein S, Corbett JJ: Delayed radiation necrosis of the optic nerves and chiasm. *Neuro-ophthalmol* 8:131, 1975.
180. Millar JL, Spry NA, Lamb DS, Delahunt J: Blindness in patients after external beam irradiation for pituitary adenoma: Two cases occurring after small daily fractional doses. *Clin Oncology* 3:291, 1991.
181. Brada M, Ford D, Ashley S, Bliss JM, Crowley S, Mason M, et al: Risk of second brain tumour after conservative surgery and radiotherapy for pituitary adenoma. *Br Med J* 304:1343, 1993.
182. Fisher BJ, Gaspar LE, Noone B: Radiation therapy of pituitary adenoma: Delayed sequelae. *Radiology* 187:843, 1993.
183. Dowsett RJ, Fowble B, Sergott RC, Savino PJ, Bosley TM, Snyder PJ, Gennarelli TA: Results of radiotherapy in the treatment of acromegaly: Lack of ophthalmologic complications. *I J Radiat Oncol Biol Phys* 19:453, 1990.
184. Girkin CA, Comey CH, Lunsford LD, Goodman ML, Kline LB: Radiation optic neuropathy after stereotactic radiosurgery. *Ophthalmopathy* 104:1634, 1997.
185. Klibanski A, Zervas NT, Kovacs K, Ridgway EC: Clinically silent hypersecretion of growth hormone in patients with pituitary tumors. *J Neurosurg* 66:806, 1987.
186. Yamada S, Sano T, Stefaneanu L, Kovacs K, Aiba T, Sawano S, Shishiba Y: Endocrine and morphological study of a clinically silent somatotroph adenoma of the human pituitary. *J Clin Endocrinol Metab* 76:352, 1993.
187. Asa SL, Scheithaurer BW, Bilbai JM, Horvath E, Ryan N, Randall RV, Laws ER Jr, et al: A case for hypothalamic acromegaly: A clinicopathological study of six patients with hypothalamic gangliocytomas producing growth hormone-releasing factor. *J Clin Endocrinol Metab* 58:796, 1984.
188. Frohman LA, Szabo M, Berelowitz M, Stachura ME: Partial purification and characterization of a peptide with growth hormone-releasing activity from extrapituitary tumors in patients with acromegaly. *J Clin Invest* 65:43, 1980.
189. Thorner MO, Perryman RL, Cronin MJ, Rogol AD, Draznin M, Johanson A, et al: Somatotroph hyperplasia. Successful treatment of acromegaly by removal of a pancreatic islet tumor secreting a growth hormone-releasing factor. *J Clin Invest* 70:965, 1982.
190. Asai A, Matsutani M, Funada N, Takakura K: Malignant growth hormone-secreting pituitary adenoma with hematogenous dural metasis: Case report. *Neurosurgery* 22:1091, 1988.
191. Alexander L, Appleton D, Hall R: Epidemiology of acromegaly in the Newcastle region. *Clin Endocrinol* 12:71, 1980.
192. Bengtsson BA, Eden S, Ernest I: Epidemiology and long-term survival in acromegaly. *Acta Med Scand* 223:327, 1988.
193. McCarthy MI, Noonan K, Wass JAH, Monson JP: Familial acromegaly: Studies in three families. *Clin Endocrinol* 32:719, 1990.
194. Gadhela MR, Prezant TR, Une KN, Glick RP, Moskal SF, Vaisman M, et al: Loss of heterozygosity on chromosome 11q13 in two families with acromegaly/gigantism is independent of mutations in multiple endocrine neoplasia type 1 gene. *J Clin Endocrinol Metab* 84:249, 1999.
195. Corbetta S, Pizzocaro A, Piracchi M, Beck-Pecoz P, Faglia G, Spada A: Multiple endocrine neoplasia type 1 in patients with recognized pituitary tumours of different types. *Clin Endocrinol* 47:507, 1997.
196. Weinstein LS, Shenker A, Gejman PV, Merino MJ, Friedman E, Spiegel AM: Activating mutations of the stimulatory G protein in the McCune-Albright syndrome. *N Engl J Med* 325:1688, 1991.
197. Carney JA, Gordon H, Carpenter PC, Shenoy BV, Go VL: The complex of myxomas, spotty pigmentation, and endocrine overactivity. *Medicine* 64:270, 1985.
198. Corenblum B, Sirek AMT, Horvath E, Kovacs K, Ezrin C: Human mixed somatotrophic and lactotrophic pituitary adenomas. *J Clin Endocrinol Metab* 42:857, 1976.
199. Horvath E, Kovacs K, Killinger DW, Smyth HS, Weiss MH, Ezrin C: Mammosomatotroph cell adenoma of the human pituitary. *Virchows Archiv* [*A*] 398:277, 1983.
200. Ezzat S, Forster MJ, Berchtold P, Redelmeier DA, Boerlin V, Harris AG: Acromegaly. Clinical and biochemical features in 500 patients. *Medicine* 73:233, 1994.
201. Dons RF, Rosselet P, Pastakia B, Doppman J, Gordon P: Arthropathy in acromegalic patients before and after treatment: A long-term follow-up study. *Clin Endocrinol* 28:515, 1988.
202. Colai A, Marzullo P, Vallone G, Marino V, Anneccheno M, Ferone D, et al: Reversibility of joint thickening in acromegalic patients: An ultrasonographic study. *J Clin Endocrinol Metab* 83:2121, 1998.
203. Orme SM, Mcnally RJQ, Cartwright RA, Belchetz PE: Mortality and cancer incidence in acromegaly: A retrospective cohort study. *J Clin Endocrinol Metab* 83:2730, 1998.
204. Delhougne B, Deneux C, Abs R, Chanson P, Fierens H, Laurent-Puig P, et al: The prevalence of colonic polyps in acromegaly: A colonoscopic and pathological study in 103 patients. *J Clin Endocrinol Metab* 80:3223, 1995.
205. Klein I, Parveen G, Gavaler JS, Van Thiel DH: Colonic polyps in patients with acromegaly. *Ann Intern Med* 97:27, 1982.
206. Ezzat S, Strom C, Melmed S: Colon polyps in acromegaly. *Ann Intern Med* 114:754, 1991.
207. Fazio S, Cittadini A, Cuocolo A, Merola B, Sabatini D, Colao A, et al: Impaired cardiac performance is a distinct feature of uncomplicated acromegaly. *J Clin Endocrinol Metab* 79:441, 1994.
208. Thuesen L, Christensen SE, Weeke J, Orskov H, Henningsen P: The cardiovascular effects of octreotide treatment in acromegaly: An echocardiographic study. *Clin Endocrinol (Oxf)* 30:619, 1989.
209. Chanson P, Timsit J, Masquet C, Warnet A, Guillausseau PJ, Birman P, et al: Cardiovascular effects of the somatostatin analog octreotide in acromegaly. *Ann Intern Med* 113:921, 1990.
210. Merola B, Cittadini A, Colao A, Ferone D, Fazio S, Sabatini D, et al: Chronic treatment with somatostatin analog octreotide improves cardiac abnormalities in acromegaly. *J Clin Endocrinol Metab* 77:790, 1993.
211. Mastaglia FL, Barwick DD, Hall R: Myopathy in acromegaly. *Lancet* 2:907, 1970.
212. O'Duffey JD, Randall RV, MacCarty CS: Median neuropathy (carpal tunnel syndrome) in acromegaly. A sign of endocrine overactivity. *Ann Intern Med* 78:379, 1973.
213. Low PA, McCleod JG, Turtle JR, Donnelly P, Wright RG: Peripheral neuropathy in acromegaly. *Brain* 97:139, 1974.
214. Hart TB, Radow SK, Blackard WG, Tucker HS, Cooper KR: Sleep apnea in active acromegaly. *Arch Int Med* 145:865, 1985.
215. Grunstein RR, Ho KY, Sullivan CE: Sleep apnea in acromegaly. *Ann Intern Med* 115:527, 1991.
216. Wright AD, Hill DM, Lowy C, Fraser TR: Mortality in acromegaly. *Q J Med* 39:1, 1970.
217. Bates AS, Van't Hoff W, Jones JM, Clayton RN: An audit outcome of treatment in acromegaly. *Q J Med* 86:293, 1993.
218. Nabarro JDN: Acromegaly. *Clin Endocrinol* 481:512, 1987.
219. Clemmons DR, Van Wyk JJ, Ridgway EC: Evaluation of acromegaly by radioimmunoassay of somatomedin-C. *N Engl J Med* 301:1138, 1979.
220. Stoffel-Wagner B, Springer W, Bidlingmaier R: A comparison of different methods for diagnosing acromegaly. *Clin Endocrinol* 46:531, 1997.
221. Grinspoon S, Clemmons D, Swearingen G, Klibanski A: Serum insulin-like growth factor-binding protein-3 levels in the diagnosis of acromegaly. *J Clin Endocrinol Metab* 80:927, 1995.
222. Irie M, Tsushima T: Increase of serum growth hormone concentration following thyrotropin-releasing hormone injection in patients with acromegaly or gigantism. *J Clin Endocrinol Metab* 35:97, 1972.
223. Melmed S, Jackson I, Kleinberg D, Klibanski A: Current treatment guidelines for acromegaly. *J Clin Endocrinol Metab* 83:2646, 1998.
224. Osman IA, James RA, Chatterjee S, Mathias D, Kendall-Taylor P:

Factors determining the long-term outcome of surgery for acromegaly. *Q J Med* 87:617, 1994.
225. Fahlbusch R, Honegger J, Buchfelder M: Surgical management of acromegaly. *Endocrinol Metab Clin North Am* 21:669, 1992.
226. Swearingen B, Barker FG, Katznelson L, Biller BMK, Grinspoon S, Klibanski A, et al: Long-term mortality after transsphenoidal surgery and adjunctive therapy for acromegaly. *J Clin Endocrinol Metab* 83:3419, 1998.
227. Freda PU, Wardlaw SL, Post KD: Long-term endocrinological follow-up evaluation in 1125 patients who underwent transsphenoidal surgery for acromegaly. *J Neurosurg* 89:353, 1998.
228. Abosch A, Tyrell JB, Lamborn KR, Hannegan LT, Applebury CB, Wilson CB: Transsphenoidal microsurgery for growth hormone-secreting pituitary adenomas: Initial outcome and long-term results. *J Clin Endocrinol Metab* 83:3411, 1998.
229. Eastman RC, Gordon P, Roth J: Conventional supervoltage irradiation is an effective treatment for acromegaly. *J Clin Endocrinol Metab* 48:931, 1979.
230. Barkan AL, Halasz I, Dornfeld KJ, Jaffe CA, Friberg RD, Chandler WF, Sandler HM: Pituitary radiation is ineffective in normalizing plasma insulin-like growth factor I in patients with acromegaly. *J Clin Endocrinol Metab* 82:3187, 1997.
231. Nortier JWR, Croughs RJM, Thijssen JHH, Schwarz F: Bromocriptine therapy in acromegaly: Effects on plasma GH levels, somatomedin-C levels and clinical activity. *Clin Endocrinol* 22:209, 1985.
232. Lindholm J, Riishede J, Vestergaard S, Hummer L, Faber O, Hagen C: No effect of bromocriptine in acromegaly. *N Engl J Med* 304:1450, 1981.
233. Abs R, Verhelst J, Maiter D, Van Acker K, Nobels F, Coolens J, et al: Cabergoline in the treatment of acromegaly: A study in 64 patients. *J Clin Endocrinol Metab* 83:374, 1998.
234. Colao A, Ferone D, Marzullo P, DiSarno A, Cerbone G, Sarnacchiaro F, et al: Effect of different dopaminergic agents in the treatment of acromegaly. *J Clin Endocrinol Metab* 82:518, 1997.
235. Ezzat S, Snyder PJ, Young WF, Boyajay LD, Newman C, Klibanski A, et al: Octreotide treatment of acromegaly. A randomized, multicenter study. *Ann Intern Med* 117:711, 1992.
236. Newman CB, Melmed S, Snyder PJ, Young WF, Boyajay LD, Levy R, et al: Safety and efficacy of long term octreotide therapy of acromegaly: Results of a multicenter trial in 103 patients—A clinical research center study. *J Clin Endocrinol Metab* 80:2768, 1995.
237. Stewart PM, Kane KF, Stewart SE, Lancranjan I, Sheppard MC: Depot long-acting somatostatin analog (Sandostatin-LAR) is an effective treatment for acromegaly. *J Clin Endocrinol Metab* 80:3267, 1995.
238. Caron P, Morange-Ramos I, Cogne M, Jaquet P: Three year follow-up of acromegalic patients treated with intramuscular slow-release lanreotide. *J Clin Endocrinol Metab* 82:18, 1997.
239. Giusti M, Gussoni G, Cuttica CM, Giordano G: Effectiveness and tolerability of slow release lanreotide treatment in active acromegaly: Six-month report on an Italian mulitcenter study. *J Clin Endocrinol Metab* 81: 2089, 1996.
240. Weins DL, Javaid A, Coskeran PB, Shah S, Butler J, Deprez PH, et al: Assessment of gall bladder dynamics, cholecystokinin release and the development of gallstones during octreotide therapy for acromegaly. *Q J Med* 300:295, 1992.
241. Hopman WPM, Van Liessum PA, Pieters GFFM, Jansen JBMJ, Lamers CBHW, Smals AGH, et al: Postprandial gallbladder motility and plasma cholecystokinin at regular time intervals after injection of octreotide in acromegalics on long-term treatment. Dig Dis Sci 37:1685, 1992.
242. Tyson JE, Ito P, Guyda H: Studies of prolactin in human pregnancy. *Am J Obstet Gynecol* 113:14, 1972.
243. Walker JD, Grossman A, Anderson JV: Malignant prolactinoma with extracranial metastases: A report of three cases. *Clin Endocrinol* 38:411, 1993.
244. Prosser PR, Karam JH, Townsend JJ: Prolactin-secreting pituitary adenomas in multiple endocrine adenomatosis type I. *Ann Intern Med* 91:41, 1979.
245. DeRivera JL, Lal S, Ettigi P: Effect of acute and chronic neuroleptic therapy on serum prolactin levels in men and women of different age groups. *Clin Endocrinol* 5:273, 1976.
246. McCalum RW, Sowers JR, Hershman JM: Metaclopramide stimulates prolactin secretion in man. *J Clin Endocrinol Metab* 42:1148, 1976.
247. Steiner J, Cassar J, Mashiter K: Effect of methyldopa on prolactin and growth hormone. *Br Med J* 1:1186, 1976.
248. Lee PA, Kelly MR, Wallin JD: Increased prolactin levels during reserpine treatment of hypertensive patients. *JAMA* 235:2316, 1976.
249. Frantz AG: Prolactin. *N Engl J Med* 298:201, 1979.
250. Groff TR, Shulkin BL, Utiger RD, Talbert LM: Amenorrhea-galactorrhea, hyperprolactinemia, and suprasellar pituitary enlargement as presenting features of primary hypothyroidism. *Obstet Gynecol* 63:86S, 1984.
251. Grubb MR, Cakeres D, Malarkey WB: Patients with primary hypothyroidism presenting as prolactinomas. *Am J Med* 83:765, 1987.
252. Lim VS, Kathpalia SC, Frohman LA: Hyperprolactinemia and impaired pituitary response to suppression and stimulation in chronic renal failure. *J Clin Endocrinol* Metab 48:101, 1979.
253. Sievertsen GD, Lim VS, Nakawatase C, Frohman LA: Metabolic clearance and secretion rates of human prolactin in normal subjects and patients with chronic failure. *J Clin Endocrinol Metab* 50:846, 1980.
254. Carlson HE, Markoff E, Lee DW: On the nature of serum prolactin in two patients with macroprolactinemia. *Fertil Steril* 58:78, 1992.
255. Tindall GT, Kovacs K, Horvath E, Thorner MO: Human prolactin-producing adenomas and bromocriptine: A histological, immunocytochemical, ultrastructural, and morphometric study. *J Clin Endocrinol Metab* 55:1178, 1982.
256. Gomez F, Reyes RI, Faiman C: Nonpuerperal galactorrhea and hyperprolactinemia. Clinical findings, endocrine features and therapeutic responses in 56 cases. *Am J Med* 62:648, 1977.
257. Schlechte J, Sherman B, Halmi N: Prolactin-secreting pituitary tumors in amenorrheic women: A comparative study. *Endocrinol Rev* 1:295, 1980.
258. Biller BMK, Baum HBA, Rosenthal DI: Progressive trabecular osteopenia in women with hyperprolactinemic amenorrhea. *J Clin Endocrinol Metab* 75:692, 1992.
259. Seppala M, Hirvonen E, Ranta T: Hyperprolactinemia and luteal insufficiency. *Lancet* 1:229, 1976.
260. Corenblum B, Fairaudeau N, Shewchux AB: Prolactin hypersecretion and short luteal phase defects. *Obstet Gynecol* 47:486, 1976.
261. Kleinberg DL, Noel GL, Frantz AG: Galactorrhea: A study of 235 cases, including 48 with pituitary tumors. *N Engl J Med* 296:589, 1977.
262. Carter JN, Tyson JE, Tolis G: Prolactin-secreting tumors and hypogonadism in 22 men. *N Engl J Med* 299:847, 1978.
263. Segal S, Yaffe H, Laufer N: Male hyperprolactinemia: Effects on fertility. *Fertil Steril* 32:56, 1979.
264. Tindall GT, Kovacs K, Horvath E, et al: Human prolactin-producing adenomas and bromocriptine: A histological, immunocytochemical, ultrastructural, and morphometric study. *J Clin Endocrinol Metab* 55:1178, 1982.
265. Vance ML, Evans WS, Thorner MO: Bromocriptine. *Ann Intern Med* 100:78, 1984.
266. Molitch ME, Elton RL, Blackwell RE, et al: Bromocriptine as primary therapy for prolactin-secreting macroadenomas: Results of a prospective multicenter study. *J Clin Endocrinol Metab* 60: 698, 1985.
267. Moster ML, Savino PJ, Schatz NJ, et al: Visual function in prolactinoma patients treated with bromocriptine. *Ophthalmology* 92:1332, 1985.
268. Warfield A, Finkel DM, Schatz NJ, et al: Bromocriptine treatment of prolactin-secreting pituitary adenomas may restore pituitary function. *Ann Intern Med* 101:783, 1984.
269. Webster J, Piscitelli MD, Polli A, et al: A comparison of cabergoline and bromocriptine in the treatment of hyperprolactinemic amenorrhea. *N Engl J Med* 331:904, 1994.
270. Colao A, Di Sarno A, et al: Prolactinomas resistant to standard dopamineagonists respond to chronic cabergoline treatment. *J Clin Endocrinol Metab* 82:876, 1997.
271. Feigenbaum SL, Downey DE, Wilson CB, et al: Transsphenoidal pituitary resection for preoperative diagnosis of prolactin-secreting adenoma in women: Long term follow-up. *J Clin Endocrinol Metab* 81:1711, 1996.
272. Serri U, Rasio E, Beauregard H, et al: Recurrence of hyperprolactinemia after selective transsphenoidal adenomectomy in women with prolactinoma. *N Engl J Med* 309:280, 1983.
273. Randall RV, Laws ERJ, Abboud CF, et al: Transsphenoidal microsurgical treatment of prolactin-producing pituitary adenomas: Results in 100 patients. *Mayo Clin Proc* 58:108, 1983.

274. Schlechte JA, Sherman BM, Chapler FK, et al: Long-term follow-up of women with surgically treated prolactin-secreting pituitary tumors. *J Clin Endocrinol Metab* 62:1296, 1986.
275. Littley MD, Shalet SM, Reid H, et al: The effect of external pituitary irradiation on elevated serum prolactin levels in patients with pituitary macroadenomas. *Q J Med* 81: 985, 1991.
276. Tsagarakis S, Grossman A, Plowman PN, et al: Megavoltage pituitary irradiation in the management of prolactinomas: Long-term follow-up. *Clin Endocrinol* 34:399, 1991.
277. Gonzales JG, Elizondo G, Saldivar D, et al: Pituitary gland growth during normal pregnancy. *Am J Med* 85:217, 1988.
278. Gemzell C, Wand CF: Outcome of pregnancy in women with pituitary adenoma. *Fertil Steril* 31:363, 1979.
279. Molitch ME: Pregnancy and the hyperprolactinemic woman. *N Engl J Med* 312:1365, 1985.
280. Kupersmith MJ, Rosenberg C, Kleinberg D: Visual loss in pregnant women with pituitary adenomas. *Ann Intern Med* 121:423, 1994.
281. Turkalj I, Braun P, Krupp P: Surveillence of bromocriptine in pregnancy. *JAMA* 247:1589, 1982.
282. Robert E, Musatti L, Piscitelli G, et al: Pregnancy outcome after treatment with the ergot derivative, cabergoline. *Reprod Toxicol* 10:333, 1996.
283. Ahmed M, Al-Dossar E, Woodhouse NJY: Macroprolactinomas with suprasellar extension: Effect of bromocriptine withdrawal during one or more pregnancies. *Fertil Steril* 58:492, 1992.
284. Konopka P, Raymond JP, Merceron RE, Seneze J: Continuous administration of bromocriptine in the prevention of neurological complications in pregnant women with prolactinomas. *Am J Obstet Gynecol* 146:935, 1983.
285. Van Roon E, van der Vijver JC, Gerretsen G, et al: Rapid regression of a suprasellar extending prolactinoma after bromocriptine treatment during pregnancy. *Fertil Steril* 36:173, 1981.
286. Nagaya T, Seo H, Kuwayama A, Sakurai T, Tsukumoto N, Nakane T, et al: Pro-opiomelanocortin gene expression in silent corticotroph adenoma and Cushing's disease. *J Neurosurg* 72:262, 1990.
287. Horvath E, Kovacs K, Killinger DW, Smyth HS, Platts ME, Singer W: Silent corticotropic adenomas of the human pituitary gland. A histologic study, immunocytologic, and ultrastructural study. *Am J Pathol* 98:617, 1980.
288. Biller BMK, Alexander JM, Zervas NT, Hedley-White ET, Arnold A, Klibanski A: Clonal origins of adrenocorticotropin-secreting pituitary tissue in Cushing's disease. *J Clin Endocrinol Metab* 75:1303, 1992.
289. Gicquel C, LeBouc Y, Luton J-P, Girard F, Bertagna X: Monoclonality of corticotroph macroadenomas in Cushing's disease. *J Clin Endocrinol Metab* 75:472, 1992.
290. Yanovski JA, Cutler GB Jr, Chrousos GP, Nieman LK: Corticotropin-releasing hormone stimulation test following low-dose dexamethasone administration. *JAMA* 269:2232, 1993.
291. Yanovski JA, Cutler GB Jr, Doppman JL, Miller DL, Chrousos GP, Oldfield EH, Nieman LK: The limited ability of inferior petrosal sinus sampling with corticotropin-releasing hormone to distinguish Cushing's disease from pseudo-Cushing states or normal physiology. *J Clin Endocrinol Metab* 77:503, 1993.
292. Oldfield EH, Doppman JL, Nieman LK, Chrousos GP, Miller DL, Katz DA, et al: Petrosal sinus sampling with and without corticotropin-releasing hormine for the differential diagnosis of Cushing's syndrome. *N Engl J Med* 325:897, 1991.
293. Findling JW, Kehoe ME, Shaker JL, Raff H: Routine inferior petrosal sinus sampling in the differential diagnosis of adrenocorticotropin (ACTH)-dependent Cushing's syndrome: Early recognition of the occult ectopic ACTH syndrome. *J Clin Endocrinol Metab* 73:408, 1991.
294. Miller DL, Doppman JL, Nieman LK, Cutler GB Jr, Chrousos GP, Loriaux DL, Oldfield EH: Petrosal sinus sampling: Discordant lateralization of ACTH-secreting pituitary microadenomas before and after stimulation with corticotropin-releasing hormone. *Radiology* 176:429, 1990.
295. de Herder WW, Uitterlinden P, Pieterman H, Tanghe HLJ, Kwekkeboom KJ, Pols HAP, et al: Pituitary tumour localization in patients with Cushing's disease by magnetic resonance imaging. Is there a place for petrosal sinus sampling? *Clin Endocrinol* 40:87, 1994.
296. Lopez J, Barcelo B, Lucas T, Salame R, Alameda C, Boronat M, et al: Petrosal sinus sampling for diagnosis of Cushing's disease: Evidence for false negative results. *Clin Endocrinol* 45:147, 1996.
297. Chandler WF, Schteingart DE, Lloyd RV, McKeever PE, Ibarra-Perez G: Surgical treatment of Cushing's disease. *J Neurosurg* 66:204, 1987.
298. Mampalan TJ, Tyrell JB, Wilson CB: Transphenoidal surgery for Cushing's disease: A report of 216 cases. *Ann Intern Med* 109:487, 1988.
299. Bochicchio D, Losa M, Buchfelder M: Factors influencing the immediate and late outcome of Cushing's disease treated by transsphenoidal surgery: A retrospective study by the European Cushing's disease survey group. *J Clin Endocrinol Metab* 80:3114, 1995.
300. Estrada J, Boronat M, Mielgo M, Magallon R, Millan I, Diez S, et al: The long-term outcome of pituitary irradiation after unsuccessful transsphenoidal surgery in Cushing's disease. *New Engl J Med* 336:172, 1997.
301. Lanzi R, Montorsi R, Losa M, Centemero A, Manzoni MF, Rigatti P, et al: Laparoscopic bilateral adrenalectomy for persistent Cushing's disease after transsphenoidal surgery. *Surgery* 123:144, 1998.
302. Alexander JM, Bikkal HA, Zervas NT, Laws ER, Klibanski A: Tumor-specific expression and alternate splicing of messenger ribonucleic acid encoding activin/transforming growth factor-beta receptors in human pituitary adenomas. *J Clin Endocrinol Metab* 81:783, 1996.
303. Haddad G, Penabad JL, Bashey HM, Asa SL, Gennarelli TA, Cirullo R, Snyder PJ: Expression of activin/inhibin subunit messenger ribonucleic acids by gonadotroph adenomas. *J Clin Endocrinol Metab* 79:1399, 1994.
304. Alexander JM, Swearingen B, Tindall GT, Klibanski A: Human pituitary adenomas express endogenous inhibin subunit and follistatin messenger ribonucleic acids. *J Clin Endocrinol Metab* 80:147, 1995.
305. Penabad JL, Bashey HM, Asa SL, Haddad G, Davis KD, Herbst AB, et al: Decreased follistatin gene expression in gonadotroph adenomas. *J Clin Endocrinol Metab* 81:3397, 1996.
306. Miller GM, Alexander JM, Bikkal HA, Katznelson L, Zervas NT, Klibanski A: Somatostatin receptor subtype gene expression in pituitary adenomas. *J Clin Endocrinol Metab* 80:1386, 1995.
307. Alexander JM, Klibanski A: Gonadotropin-releasing hormone receptor mRNA expression by human pituitary tumors in vitro. *J Clin Invest* 93:2332, 1994.
308. Miller GM, Alexander JM, Klibanski A: Gonadotropin-releasing hormone messenger RNA expression in gonadotroph tumors and normal human pituitary. *J Clin Endocrinol Metab* 81:80, 1996.
309. McGrath GA, Goncalves RJ, Udupa JK, et al: New technique for quantitation of pituitary adenoma size: Use in evaluating treatment of gonadotroph adenomas with gonadotropin-releasing hormone antagonist. *J Clin Endocrinol Metab* 76:1363, 1993.
310. Daneshdoost L, Gennarelli TA, Bashey HM, Savino PJ, Sergott RC, Bosley TM, Snyder PJ: Identification of gonadotroph adenomas in men with clinically nonfunctioning adenomas by the LH β subunit response to TRH. *J Clin Endocrinol Metab* 77:1352, 1993.
311. Snyder PJ, Sterling FH: Hypersecretion of LH and FSH by a pituitary adenoma. *J Clin Endocrinol Metab* 42:544, 1976.
312. Peterson RD, Kourides IA, Horwith M, Vaughn ED, Saxena BB, Fraser RAR: Luteinizing hormone and ∂-subunit-secreting pituitary tumor: Positive feedback of estrogen. *J Clin Endocrinol Metab* 51:692, 1981.
313. Snyder PJ, Johnson J, Muzyka R: Abnormal secretion of glycoprotein ∂-subunit and follicle-stimulating hormone (FSH) β-subunit in men with pituitary adenomas and FSH hypersecretion. *J Clin Endocrinol Metab* 51:579, 1980.
314. Snyder PJ, Bashey HM, Kim SU, Chappel SC: Secretion of uncombined subunits of luteinizing hormne by gonadotroph cell adenomas. *J Clin Endocrinol Metab* 59:1169, 1984.
315. Ridgway EC, Klibanski A, Ladenson PW, et al: Pure alpha-secreting pituitary adenomas. *N Engl J Med* 304:1254, 1981.
316. Klibanski A, Ridgway EC, Zervas NT: Pure alpha subunit-secreting pituitary tumors. *J Neurosurg* 59:585, 1983.
317. Oppenheim DS, Kana AR, Sangha JS, Klibanski A: A prevalence of alpha subunit hypersecretion in patients with pituitary tumors clinically nonfunctioning and somatotroph adenomas. *J Clin Endocrinol Metab* 70:859, 1990.
318. Daneshdoost L, Gennarelli TA, Bashey HM, et al: Recognition of gonadotroph adenomas in women. *N Engl J Med* 324:589, 1991.
319. Katznelson L, Alexander JM, Bikkal HA, Jameson JL, Hsu DW, Klibanski A: Imbalanced follicle stimulating hormone β-subunit

biosynthesis in human pituitary adenomas. *J Clin Endocrinol Metab* 74:1343, 1992.

320. Snyder PJ, Muzyka R, Johnson J, Utiger RD: Thyrotropin-releasing hormone provokes abnormal follicle-stimulating hormone (FSH) and luteinizing hormone responses in men who have pituitary adenomas and FSH hypersecretion. *J Clin Endocrinol Metab* 51:744, 1980.
321. Jameson JL, Klibanski A, Black PM, et al: Glycoprotein hormone genes are expressed in clinically nonfunctioning pituitary adenomas. *J Clin Invest* 80:1472, 1987.
322. Mashiter K, Adams E, Van Noorden S: Secretion of LH, FSH and PRL shown by cell culture and immunocytochemistry of human functionless pituitary adenomas. *Clin Endocrinol* 15:103, 1981.
323. Asa SL, Gerne BM, Singer W, Horvath E, Kovacs K, Smyth HS: Gonadotropin secretion in vitro by human pituitary null cell adenomas and oncocytomas. *J Clin Endocrinol Metab* 62:1011, 1986.
324. Black PM, Hsu DW, Klibanski A, Kliman B, Jameson JL, Ridgway EC, et al: Hormone production in clinically nonfunctioning pituitary adenoma. *J Neurosurg* 66:244, 1987.
325. Faggiano M, Criscuolo T, Perrone I, Quarto C, Sinisi AA: Sexual prococity in a boy due to hypersecretion of LH and prolactin by a pituitary adenoma. *Acta Endocrinol* 102:167, 1983.
326. Ambrosi B, Basstti M, Ferrario R, Medri G, Giannattsio G, Faglia G: Precocious puberty in a boy with a PRL, LH- and FSH-secreting pituitary tumour: Hormonal and immunocytochemical studies. *Acta Endocrinol* 122:569, 1990.
327. Djerassi A, Coutifaris C, West VA: Gonadotroph adenoma in a premenopausal woman secreting follicle-stimulating hormone and causing ovarian hyperstimulation. *J Clin Endocrinol Metab* 80:591, 1995.
328. Christin-Maitre S, Rongieres-Frydman C, Kottler M-L, Lahlou N, Frydman R, Touraine P, Bouchard P: A spontaneous and severe hyperstimulation of the ovaries revealing a gonadotroph adenoma. *J Clin Endocrinol Metab* 83:3450, 1998.
329. Snyder PJ: Gonadotroph cell adenomas of the pituitary. *Endocrinol Rev* 6:552, 1985.
330. Berezin M, Olchovsky D, Pines A, Tadmor R, Lunenfeld B: Reduction of follicle-stimulating hormone (FSH) secretion in FSH-producing pituitary adenoma by bromocriptine. *J Clin Endocrinol Metab* 59:1220, 1984.
331. Vance ML, Ridgway EC, Thorner MO: Follicle-stimulating hormone and alpha subunit-secreting pituitary tumor treated with bromocriptine. *J Clin Endocrinol Metab* 61:580, 1985.
332. Grossman A, Ross R, Charlesworth M, et. al: The effect of dopamine agonist therapy on large functionless pituitary tumours. *Clin Endocrinol* 22:679, 1985.
333. Van Schaardenburg D, Roelfsema F, Van Seters AP, Vielvoye GJ. Bromocriptine therapy for nonfunctioning pituitary adenoma. *Clin Endocrinol* 30:475, 1989.
334. Lamberts SWJ, Verleun T, Oosterom R: The effects of bromocriptine, thyrotropin-releasing hormone, and gonadotropin-releasing hormone on hormone secretion by gonadotropin-secreting pituitary adenomas in vivo and in vitro. *J Clin Endocrinol Metab* 64:524, 1987.
335. Katznelson L, Oppenheim DS, Coughlin F, Kliman B, Schonfeld DA, Klibanski A: Chronic somatostatin analog administration in patients with alpha subunit-secreting pituitary adenomas. *J Clin Endocrinol Metab* 75:1318, 1992.
336. Warnet A, Harris AG, Renard E, Martin D, James-Deidier A, Chaumet-Riffaud P: A prospective multicenter trial of octreotide in 24 patients with visual defects caused by nonfunctioning and gonadotropin-secreting pituitary adenomas. *Neurosurgery* 41:786, 1997.
337. Roman SH, Goldstein M, Kourides IA, Comite F, Bardin CW, Kreiger DT: The luteinizing hormone-releasing hormone (LHRH) agonist d-TRT^6-PRO^9-NEt]LHRH increased rather than lowered LH and alpha subunit levels in a patient with an LH-secreting pituitary tumor. *J Clin Endocrinol Metab* 58:313, 1984.
338. Sassolas G, Lejeune H, Trouillas J, et al: Gonadotropin-releasing hormone agonists are unsuccessful in reducing tumoral gonadotropin secretion in two patients with gonadotropin-secreting pituitary adenomas. *J Clin Endocrinol Metab* 67:180, 1988.
339. Klibanski A, Jameson JL, Biller BMK, et al: Gonadotropin and alpha subunit responses to chronic gonadotropin-releasing hormone analog administration in patients with glycoprotein hormone-secreting pituitary tumors. *J Clin Endocrinol Metab* 68:81, 1989.
340. Zarate A, Fonseca ME, Mason M, et al: Gonadotropin-secreting pituitary adenoma with concomitant hypersecretion of testosterone and elevated sperm count. Treatment with LRH agonist. *Acta Endocrinol* 113:29, 1986.
341. Girod C, Trouillas J, Claustrat B: The human thyrotropic adenoma: Pathologic diagnosis in five cases and critical review of the literature. *Semin Diag Pathol* 3:58, 1986.
342. Mixson AJ, Friedman TC, Katz DA, Feuerstein IM, Taubenberger JK, Colandrea JM, et al: Thyrotropin-secreting pituitary carcinoma. *J Clin Endocrinol Metab* 76:529, 1993.
343. Bertherat J, Brue T, Enjalbert A, Gunz G, Rasolonjanahary R, Warnet A, et al: Somatostatin receptors on thryrotropin-secreting pituitary adenomas: Comparison with the inhibitory effects of octreotide upon in vivo and in vitro hormonal secretions. *J Clin Endocrinol Metab* 75:540, 1992.
344. Jackson JA, Smigiel M, Greene JF: Hyperthyroidism due to a thyrotropin-secreting pituitary microadenoma. *Henry Ford Hosp Med J* 35:198, 1987.
345. McCutcheon IE, Weintraub BD, Oldfield EH: Surgical treatment of thyrotropin-secreting pituitary adenomas. *J Neurosurg* 73:674, 1990.
346. Mindermann T, Wilson CB: Thyrotropin-producing pituitary adenomas. *J Neurosurg* 79:521, 1993.
347. Comi RJ, Gesundheit N, Murray L, Gorden P, Weintraub BD: Response of thyrotropin-secreting pituitary adenomas to a long-acting somatostatin analogue. *N Engl J Med* 317:12, 1987.
348. Beck-Peccoz P, Mariotti S, Guillausseau PJ, Medri G, Piscitelli G, Bertoli A, et al: Treatment of hyperthyroidism due to inappropriate secretion of thyrotropin with the somatostatin analog SMS 201-995. *J Clin Endocrinol Metab* 68:208, 1989.
349. Gancel A, Vuillermet P, LeGrand A, Catus F, Thomas F, Kuhn JM: Effects of a slow-release formulation of the new somatostatin analogue lanreotide in TSH-secreting pituitary adenomas. *Clin Endocrinol* 40:421, 1994.
350. Chanson P, Weintraub BD, Harris AG: Octreotide therapy for thyroid stimulating-secreting pituitary adenomas. A follow-up of 52 patients. *Ann Intern Med* 119:236, 1993.
351. Spark RF: Simplified assessment of pituitary-adrenal reserve. *Ann Intern Med* 75:717, 1971.
352. Beck-Peccoz P, Amr S, Menezes-Ferreira MM, Faglia G, Weintraub BD: Decreased receptor binding of biologically inactive thyrotropin in central hypothyroidism. *N Engl J Med* 312:1085, 1985.
353. Snyder PJ, Jacobs LS, Rabello MM, Sterling FH, Shore RN, Utiger RD, Daughaday WH: Diagnostic value of thyrotropin-releasing hormone in pituitary and hypothalamic diseases. Assessment of thyrotropin and prolactin secretion in 100 patients. *Ann Intern Med* 81:751, 1974.
354. Snyder PJ, Rudenstein RS, Gardner DF, Rothman JG: Repetive infusion of gonadotropin-releasing hormone distinguishes hypothalamic from pituitary hypogonadism. *J Clin Endocrinol Metab* 48:864, 1979.
355. Spratt DI, Finkelstein JS, O'Dea LS, Badger TM, Rao P, Campbell JD, Crowley WF Jr: Long-term administration of gonadotropin-releasing hormone in men with idiopathic hypogonadotropic hypogonadism. A model for physiologic studies of the hormone's physiologic effects. *Ann Intern Med* 105:848, 1986.
356. Finkel DM, Phillips JL, Snyder PJ: Stimulation of spermatogenesis by gonadotropins in men with hypogonadotropic hypogonadism. *N Engl J Med* 313:651, 1985.
357. Kaltsas GA, Mukherjee JJ, Plowman PN, Monson JP, Grossman AB, Besser GM: The role of cytotoxic chemotherapy in the management of aggressive and malignant pituitary tumors. *J Clin Endocrinol Metab* 83:4233, 1998.
358. Bengtsson B-A, Eden S, Lonn L: Treatment of adults with growth hormone (GH) deficiency with recombinant human GH. *J Clin Endocrinol Metab* 76:309, 1993.
359. Baum HBA, Biller BMK, Finkelstein JS, Cannistraro KB, Oppenheim DS, Schoenfeld DA, et al: Effects of physiologic growth hormone therapy on bone density and body composition in patients with adult-onset growth hormone deficiency. *Ann Intern Med* 125:883, 1996.
360. Burman P, Broman JE, Hetta J, Wiklund I, Erfurth EM, Hagg E, Karlsson FA: Quality of life in adults with growth hormone (GH) deficiency: Response to treatment with recombinant human GH in a placebo-controlled 21-month trial. *J Clin Endocrinol Metab* 80:3585, 1995.

361. Boger RH, Skamira C, Bode-Boger SM: Nitric oxide may mediate the hemodynamic effects of recombinant growth homone in patients with acquired growth hormone deficiency. A double-blind, placebo-controlled study. *J Clin Invest* 98:2706, 1996.
362. Beshyah SA, Henderson A, Niththyananthan R, Skinner E, Anyaku V, Richmond W, et al: The effects of short and long term growth hormone replacement therapy in hypopituitary adults on lipid metabolism and carbohydrate tolerance. *J Clin Endocrinol Metab* 80:356, 1995.
363. Weaver JU, Monson JP, Noonan K, Johns WG, Edwards A, Evans KA, Cunningham J: The effect of low dose recombinant human growth hormone replacement on regional fat distribution, insulin sensitivity, and cardiovascular risk factors in hypopituitary adults. *J Clin Endocrinol Metab* 80:153, 1995.
364. Svensson J, Johannsson G, Bengtsson B-A: Insulin-like growth factor-I in growth hormone-deficient adults: Relationship to population-based normal values, body composition and insulin tolerance test. *Clin Endocrinol* 46:579, 1997.
365. Hayes FJ, Fiad TM, McKenna TJ: Gender differences in the response of growth hormone (GH)-deficient adults to GH therapy. *Metabolism* 48:368, 1999.
366. Weitzman ED, Fukushima D, Nogeire C, Roffwarg H, Gallagher TF, Hellman L: Twenty-four hour pattern of the episodic secretion of cortisol in normal subjects. *J Clin Endocrinol Metab* 33:14, 1971.
367. Colao A, DiSarno A, Landi ML, et al: Long-term and low-dose treatment with cabergoline induces macroprolactinoma shrinkage. *J Clin Endocrinol Metab* 82:3574, 1997.

CHAPTER 8

Posterior Pituitary

Gary L. Robertson

NORMAL

Anatomy

The posterior pituitary or *neurohypophysis* is an elongated extension of the ventral hypothalamus that attaches to the dorsal and caudal surface of the adenohypophysis (Fig. 8-1). In adult men and women it weighs approximately 100 mg and is divided into two parts by the diaphragm of the sella. The upper part is variously referred to as the *infundibulum* or *median eminence*, and the lower part is referred to as the *infundibular process* or *pars nervosa*. The two parts are supplied with blood by branches from the superior and inferior hypophyseal arteries, which arise from the posterior communicating and intracavernous portion of the internal carotid. In the pars nervosa, the arterioles break up into localized capillary networks that drain directly into the jugular vein via the sellar, cavernous, and lateral venous sinuses. In the infundibulum, the primary capillary networks coalesce into another system, the portal veins, which perfuse the adenohypophysis before discharging into the systemic circulation.

Microscopically, the neurohypophysis appears as a densely interwoven network of capillaries, pituicytes, and large, nonmyelinated nerve fibers containing many electron-dense, neurosecretory granules.[1,2] The neurons terminate as bulbous enlargements on capillary networks scattered throughout the neurohypophysis, including the stalk and infundibulum. Those that project to the pars nervosa originate primarily in the large cells of the supraoptic and to a lesser extent the paraventricular nuclei.[2–6] Those that terminate in the median eminence originate primarily in the small cells of the paraventricular or other hypothalamic nuclei. The parvocellular divisions of the paraventricular nucleus also send neuronal projections to many other areas of brain and spinal cord.[7] These areas include the nucleus tractus solitarius, substantia gelatinosa, parabrachial nucleus, and other areas thought to be involved in regulating autonomic function,[3–8] including the lateral amygdala,[4] and the walls of the lateral and third ventricles, where the neurons probably secrete directly into the cerebrospinal fluid.[9]

Chemistry

Vasopressin and oxytocin are the only hormones known to be produced in appreciable amounts by the human neurohypophysis. Their primary structures were first established by du Vigneaud and coworkers nearly 50 years ago.[10] Each is a nonapeptide composed of a six-member disulfide ring and a three-member tail on which the carboxy-terminal group is amidated (Fig. 8-2). Vasopressin differs from oxytocin only in the substitution of phenylalanine for isoleucine at position 3 in the ring and of arginine for leucine at position 8 in the tail. These two hormones have been found in all placental mammals except the suborder *Suina*, several species of which make a variant of vasopressin containing lysine instead of arginine in position 8.[11] In marsupial and egg-laying mammals arginine and/or lysine vasopressin are also present, but oxytocin is replaced or accompanied by mesotocin which has isoleucine instead of leucine at position 8. The neurohypophysis of birds and reptiles contains mesotocin and arginine vasotocin, which has a ring identical to oxytocin and a tail identical to vasopressin. This pattern of variation in the peptide hormones and the similarties between their protein precursors strongly suggests that they evolved by duplication of a common ancestral gene nearly 300 million years ago.[11] This ancestral gene probably has an even more ancient lineage because other nonapeptides structurally similar to oxytocin/vasopressin have been detected in neural tissue of invertebrates that existed before the evolution of vertebrates more than 700 million years ago.[11]

Biosynthesis and Release

Vasopressin and oxytocin are synthesized in cell bodies of the supraoptic and paraventricular nuclei, packaged in granules, transported down the axons, and stored in terminal dilatations until their release into the systemic circulation.[2,12] In the neurosecretory granules and urine, the hormones form insoluble complexes with specific carrier proteins known as *neurophysins*.[13] Two slightly different forms of neurophysin are found in humans and most other mammals.[14] One is found exclusively in granules containing vasopressin; the other, in granules containing oxytocin. Both are single-chain polypeptides which have a basic molecular weight of approximately 10,000 daltons but readily form dimers and tetramers in concentrated solutions. Each neurophysin binds oxytocin and vasopressin equally well, indicating that the specific hormonal associations found in vivo are a function of anatomic compartmentalization. Binding of the hormones to neurophysin exhibits a pH optimum around 5.2 to 5.8 and a binding constant ($K°$) of approximately 2×10^4 M. These values favor maximum association in secretory granules but complete dissociation of the neurophysin-hormone complex in plasma. The amino acid sequences of several neurophysins have been determined and found to have a considerable degree of internal homology in a part of the molecule thought to be the hormone-binding site. Occupancy of this binding site by the N-terminal amino acids of vasopressin or oxytocin facilitates proper folding, intrachain disulfide bonding, and oligomerization of neurophysin in vitro[15] and is thought to play an important role in production of the hormones in vivo.

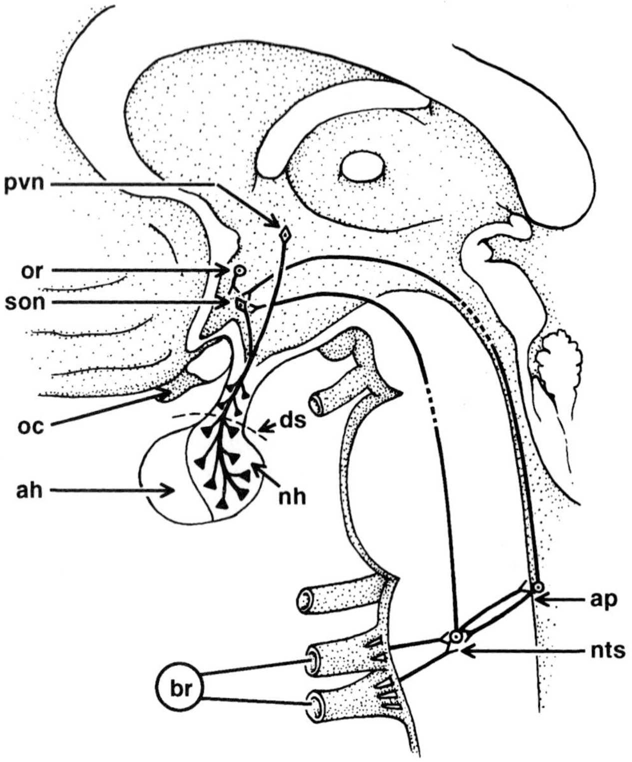

FIGURE 8-1. The neurohypophysis and its principal regulatory afferents. Key: nh = neurohypophysis; ah = adenohypophysis; ds = diaphragm of the sella; oc = optic chiasm; son = supraoptic nucleus; pvn = paraventricular nucleus; or = osmoreceptor; br = volume sensor and baroreceptor; nts = nucleus tractus solitarii; ap = area postrema (emetic center). Shading indicates areas which lack a blood-brain barrier and contain receptors for plasma insulin.

POSITION	OXYTOCIN	VASOPRESSIN	DDAVP
	NH_2	NH_2	
1	CYSTEINE	CYSTEINE	CYSTEINE
2	TYROSINE	TYROSINE	TYROSINE
3	ISOLEUCINE	PHENYLALANINE	PHENYLALANINE
4	GLUTAMINE	GLUTAMINE	GLUTAMINE
5	ASPARAGINE	ASPARAGINE	ASPARAGINE
6	CYSTEINE	CYSTEINE	CYSTEINE
7	PROLINE	PROLINE	PROLINE
8	LEUCINE	ARGININE	D-ARGININE
9	GLYCINAMIDE	GLYCINAMIDE	GLYCINAMIDE

(S–S bridge between cysteine 1 and cysteine 6 in each.)

FIGURE 8-2. The amino acid sequence of oxytocin, vasopressin, and a synthetic agonist, 1-desamino-8-D-arginine vasopressin (DDAVP).

Vasopressin and oxytocin are both synthesized via protein precursors composed of a signal peptide, the hormone moiety, a tripeptide linker, the associated neurophysin and, in the case of vasopressin, a glycosylated peptide known as copeptin (Fig. 8-3*A*).[16] The genes encoding the prohormones in several mammalian[16–18] and nonmammalian[11] species have been cloned and sequenced and found to have a considerable degree of homology. The gene for preprovasopressin in humans and other mammals has three exons that code, respectively, for (1) a signal peptide vasopressin, a tripeptide linker, and the variable, amino-terminal part of neurophysin; (2) the central, highly conserved portion of neurophysin; and (3) the variable, carboxy-terminal part of neurophysin, another linker, and copeptin (Fig. 8-3*B*). The gene for the oxytocin precursor is similar except that it lacks the part of the third exon which encodes the copeptin moiety in provasopressin. The two genes are located in close proximity on opposing strands of DNA[16,18] but are expressed exclusively in different neurons.[19] In humans, they are located on chromosome 20.[20]

Like other peptide hormones destined for secretion, the protein precursors of vasopressin and oxytocin are translocated into the endoplasmic reticulum where the signal peptide is removed by a peptidase and the prohormone folds and oligomerizes before transiting the Golgi apparatus to the neurosecretory granules. As these granules move down the neurons toward the axon terminal, the prohormone is further cleaved by endopeptidases and exopeptidases to the hormone, its neurophysin and, in the case of vasopressin, copeptin.[11,21–23] The hormone is also amidated at its c-terminus by a peptidylglycine monooxygenase and lyase,[11] packed with the other components in neurosecretory granules and stored in the nerve terminals until they are secreted by a calcium-dependent exocytotic process similar to that described for other neurosecretory systems.[24] In some unknown way, secretion increases the synthesis of vasopressin and vasopressin mRNA,[12,25] but in rats, at least, this compensatory response develops gradually and may never completely offset the increased rate of release. Consequently, a chronic stimulus such as prolonged water deprivation can severely deplete the neurohypophyseal stores of vasopressin.[26]

Secretion

Vasopressin

Osmotic Effects

Of the many variables known to influence the release of vasopressin,[27–30] the most important under physiologic conditions is the effective osmotic pressure of body water. This influence is mediated by specialized cells, known collectively as *osmoreceptors*, that are located in the anterior hypothalamus near but distinct from the supraoptic nucleus (Fig. 8-1).[31–34] This part of the brain receives a separate blood supply from small perforating branches of the anterior cerebral and/or anterior communicating arteries.[35]

The osmoregulatory mechanism functions like a discontinuous or "set point" receptor (Fig. 8-4*A*). Thus, at plasma osmolalities below a certain minimum or threshold level, plasma vasopressin is normally suppressed to low or undetectable concentrations. Above this point, plasma vasopressin rises steeply in direct proportion to plasma osmolality. The slope of this relation indicates that, on average, a change in plasma osmolality of only 1 percent will change plasma vasopressin by approximately 1 pg/ml (1 pmol/L), an amount sufficient to significantly alter urinary concentration and flow (Fig. 8-4*B*). However, owing at least partly to individual differences in the rate of hormone secretion and/or clearance, this property can differ as much as 10 fold among healthy adults.[27] These individual differences are constant over prolonged periods of time and appear to be determined largely by genetic factors.[36] However, they are not totally

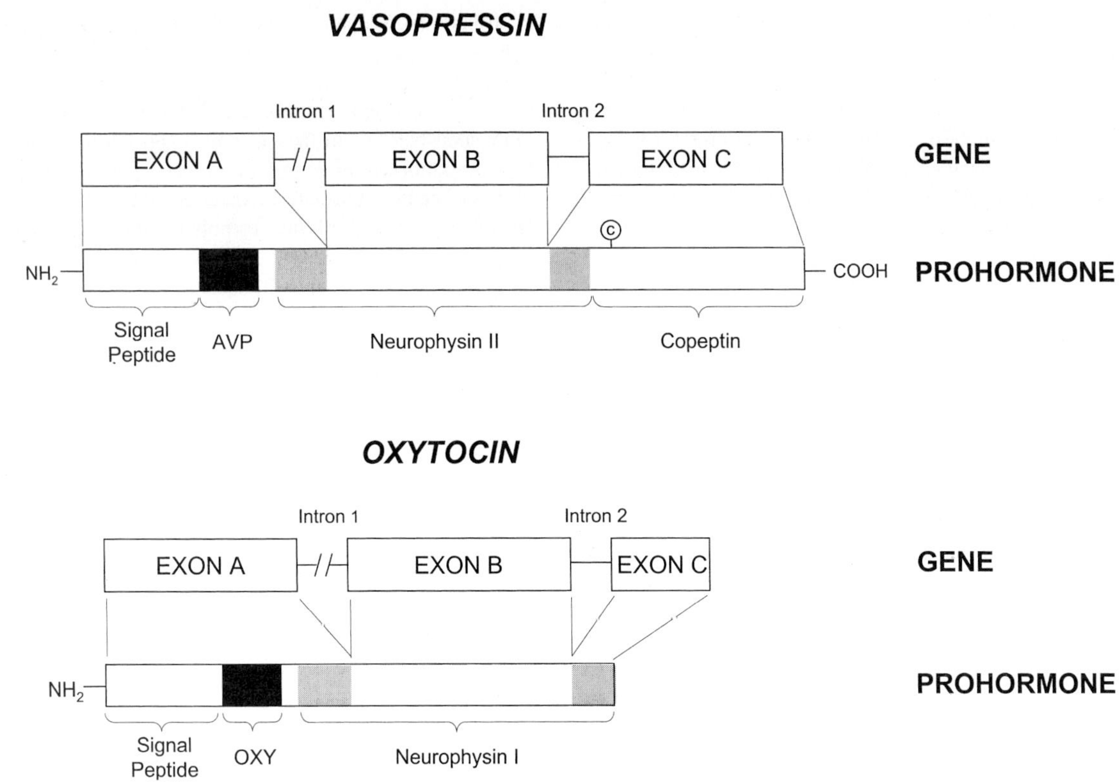

FIGURE 8-3. The structure of the vasopressin and oxytocin prohormones and the genes that encode them. © indicates the glycosylation site on the copeptin moiety.

immutable, because the slope of the plasma vasopressin-osmolality relationship can be altered reversibly by a variety of other hormones, drugs, or metabolic conditions as described later. The sensitivity of the osmoregulatory system also appears to increase with age, at least in men,[37] but it does not differ appreciably in healthy young adult men and women.[27,36]

The "set" of the osmoregulatory system also varies from person to person. In healthy adults, the osmotic threshold for vasopressin secretion ranges from 275 to 290 mosmol/kg, with an average of about 280 mosmol/kg.[36] These interindividual differences in the "set" of the osmoregulatory system are also genetically determined[36] but can vary over time, possibly as a result of changes in blood volume and/or pressure. The set of the osmoregulatory system is also reduced during pregnancy[38] and the luteal phase of the menstrual cycle.[39,40] The mechanism of these changes is unknown.

It is uncertain whether the threshold model accurately represents the operation of the osmoreceptor at its most fundamental level.[41–44] Some analyses of the relation between plasma vasopressin and osmolality suggest that it is exponential rather than

FIGURE 8-4. The relation of plasma vasopressin to plasma and urine osmolality in healthy adults in various states of hydration.

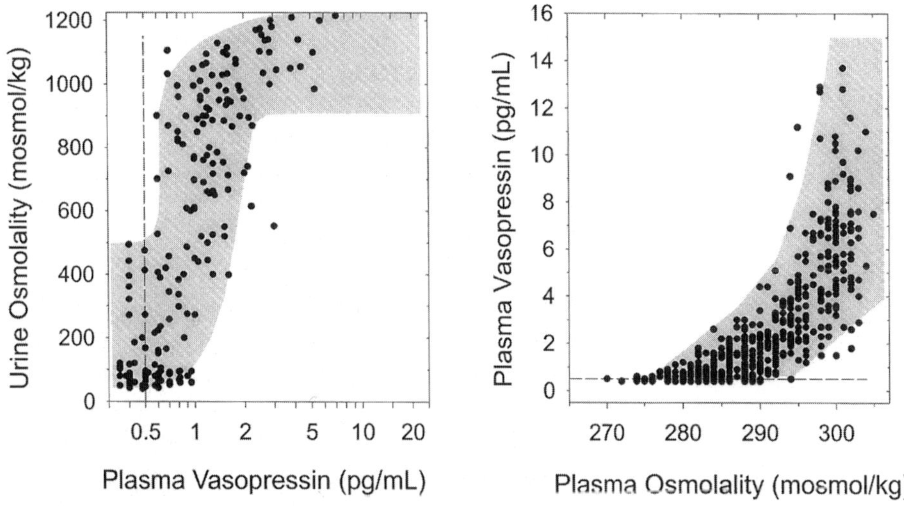

linear but others find no significant difference in the fit of the data to either model. Indeed, it is uncertain whether current methods are sufficiently precise to distinguish between the two models or, if they could, whether the distinction would be important. Moreover, there is reason to think that vasopressin secretion reflects the balance of inhibitory as well as stimulatory inputs from a bimodal system of osmoreceptors.[30] If so, both types probably have a common set or null point that corresponds closely to the normal basal effective osmotic pressure of body water. For practical purposes, however, the concept of an osmotic threshold for vasopressin secretion remains for the present a useful, if not valid, way of describing many aspects of normal and abnormal osmoregulatory function in intact animals.

It is also uncertain whether vasopressin is secreted continuously or episodically in response to osmotic stimulation. When nonosmotic stimuli such as posture, activity, and blood pressure are controlled or constant, the infusion of hypertonic saline in humans usually produces a smooth progressive rise in systemic venous plasma vasopressin that correlates closely with the rise in plasma osmolality.[30,36,43] However, when samples are obtained from animals at a point nearer the source of the hormone, for example, from the right atrium or internal jugular vein, large fluctuations in plasma vasopressin have been observed during osmotic stimulation.[44] Whether these fluctuations reflect an intrinsic property of the neurohypophysis or are artifacts of the experimental conditions is unknown. Irregular phasic firing of neurosecretory neurons has been observed by unit recording techniques,[45,46] but this activity is unlikely to be related to episodic fluctuations in plasma vasopressin because the discharge cycles have a much shorter periodicity and are not synchronized from cell to cell.

The osmoregulatory mechanism is not equally sensitive to all plasma solutes (Fig. 8-5). Sodium and its anions, which normally contribute more than 95 percent of the osmotic pressure of plasma, are the most potent solutes known in terms of their capacity to stimulate vasopressin release.[48] However, certain sugars, such as sucrose and mannitol, are also very effective when infused intravenously.[27,48,49] In fact, mannitol appears to be nearly as potent as sodium chloride on a molar basis.[48] In this respect, therefore, the control mechanism behaves like a true osmoreceptor. However, a rise in plasma osmolality due to urea or glucose causes little or no increase in plasma vasopressin in healthy adults or animals.[29,48,49] These differences in the response to various plasma solutes are independent of any recognized nonosmotic influence and are probably a property of the osmoregulatory mechanism per se. Precisely how and why the osmoreceptor discriminates so effectively between different kinds of plasma solutes is unsettled. According to current concepts, the signal which stimulates the osmoreceptor is an osmotically induced decrease in the water content of the cell.[27] If this hypothesis is correct, the ability of a given solute to stimulate vasopressin secretion ought to be inversely related to the rate at which it passes from plasma into the osmoreceptor neuron. This concept is consistent with the observed effects of solutes such as sodium, mannitol, and glucose and the rates at which they penetrate the blood-brain barrier. These experimental observations are also consistent with the view that the osmoreceptors are actually sodium receptors located within the blood-brain barrier.[50,51] However, the sodium receptor theory is difficult to reconcile with the behavior of urea, which penetrates the blood-brain barrier quite slowly yet causes little or no stimulation of thirst or vasopressin release.[48,49] This singular disparity suggests that most if not all of the osmoreceptors are located outside the blood-brain barrier and that another factor, most likely the permeability of the osmoreceptor neuron per se, determines the solute specificity of the system.

FIGURE 8-5. The relation of plasma vasopressin to elevations in plasma osmolality induced by various solutes in healthy adults. Each oblique line represents the mean regression function obtained during intravenous infusion of hypertonic solutions of the specified solutes. (*From Robertson.*[47])

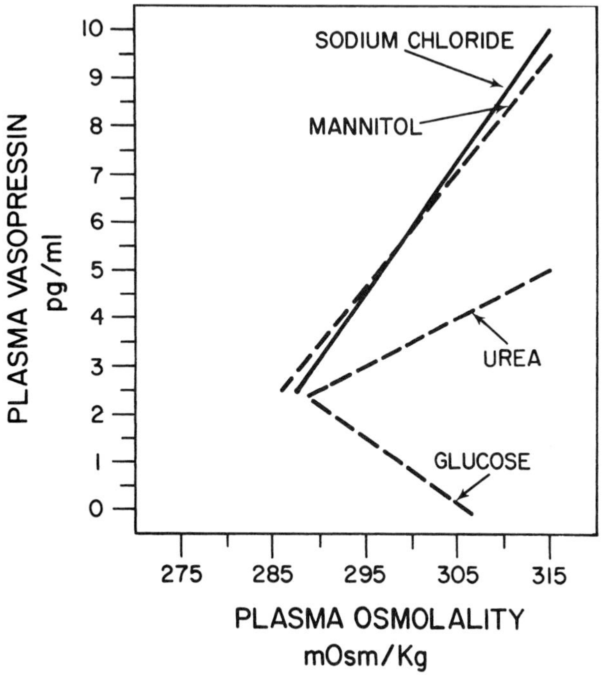

The sensitivity of the osmoreceptors to stimulation by plasma glucose appears to be critically dependent on the level of plasma insulin. Thus, hyperglycemia stimulates thirst and vasopressin secretion in patients with insulin-deficient diabetes mellitus[52] but has no effect on either variable in healthy adults[48] or in patients with insulin-treated diabetes.[53] These observations probably explain the polydipsia and some of the hypervasopressinemia that occur in patients with uncontrolled diabetes mellitus[54,55] and indicate that glucose uptake by osmoreceptor neurons is probably insulin-dependent. This concept is supported by other evidence that high-affinity receptors for plasma insulin are present in an area of the anterior hypothalamus that is thought to contain the osmoreceptors.[56]

Oropharyngeal Effects

Water intake may also inhibit the secretion of vasopressin via receptors located in the oropharynx or upper gastrointestinal tract.[57–60] This effect is rapid but transient unless it is followed by a decrease in plasma osmolality or sodium. The kind of receptor involved is unknown, and the effect may depend more on the temperature than on the tonicity of the fluid ingested.

Hemodynamic Effects

The secretion of vasopressin is also affected by changes in blood volume and/or pressure.[27,28,30] These hemodynamic influences are mediated primarily by neurogenic afferents that arise in pressure-sensitive receptors in the cardiac atria and large arteries, travel via the vagal and glossopharyngeal nerves to the nucleus of the solitary tract from whence postsynaptic pathways ascend to the lateral parabranchial nucleus, the A1 region of the ventrolateral medulla, and the paraventricular and supraoptic nuclei (Fig. 8-1).[61–69] The input from these pathways appears to be predominantly negative, or inhibitory, under basal normovolemic, normotensive conditions, since their elimination results in an acute rise in plasma vasopressin as well as arterial pressure.[70] In rats, at least, the pathways that mediate the effect of blood volume and blood pressure are distinct and appear to involve a *kappa* opioidergic projection to the lateral parabrachial nucleus.[68,71,72] An alternative pathway mediated by renal nerves may operate when the nucleus of the solitary tract is ablated.[73]

The functional properties of this baroregulatory system are exemplified in Fig. 8-6. In healthy adult humans, monkeys, and rats, acutely lowering blood pressure by any of several methods increases plasma vasopressin by an amount that is roughly proportional to the degree of hypotension achieved.[28,30,74,75] However, this stimulus-response relationship follows a distinctly exponential pattern. Thus, small decreases in blood pressure of the order of 5 to 10 percent usually have little effect on plasma vasopressin, while decreases of 20 to 30 percent result in hormone levels many times those required to produce maximum antidiuresis. The vasopressin response to changes in blood volume appears to be quantitatively and qualitatively similar to the response to blood pressure.[28,76–78] In rats, plasma vasopressin increases as an exponential function of the degree of hypovolemia.[76] Thus, little or no rise in plasma vasopressin can be detected until blood volume decreases acutely by 6 to 8 percent. Beyond that point, plasma vasopressin begins to rise at a rapidly increasing rate in relation to the degree of hypovolemia and usually reaches levels 20–30 times normal when blood volume is reduced by 20 to 30 percent. In healthy adults, plasma vasopressin is not changed appreciably by an acute decrease in blood volume of up to 7 percent, is doubled by a reduction of 10 to 15 percent, and increases markedly if the hypovolemia exceeds 20–30 percent.[76–78]

Changes in blood volume or pressure large enough to affect vasopressin secretion do not necessarily interfere with osmoregulation of the hormone. Instead, hemodynamic influences appear to lower or raise the set of the osmoregulatory system, thereby increasing or decreasing the stimulatory effect of a given level of plasma osmolality (Fig. 8-7).[29,79–84] Thus, in the presence of a hemodynamic stimulus, the capacity to osmoregulate vasopressin is preserved and the hormone can still be fully suppressed if the effective osmotic pressure of body fluids falls below the new, lower set point.[82] This interaction indicates that the osmoregulatory and baroregulatory systems, though different in location and function, ultimately converge and act on the same population of neurosecretory neurons.[29]

FIGURE 8-6. The relation of plasma vasopressin to percent fall in blood pressure in healthy adults and patients with idiopathic postural hypotension. In healthy adults, blood pressure was reduced by the infusion of trimethaphan (Arfonad) (●) or by orthostasis immediately after phlebotomy (○). In patients with orthostatic hypotension, blood pressure was reduced by tilting (triangle). (*From Robertson.*[47])

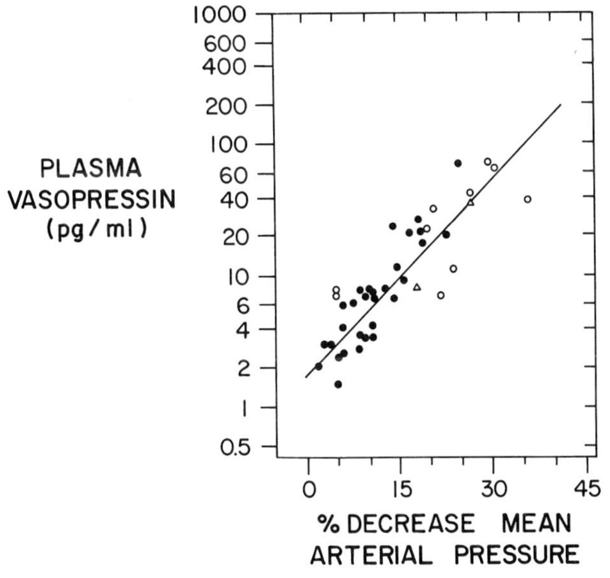

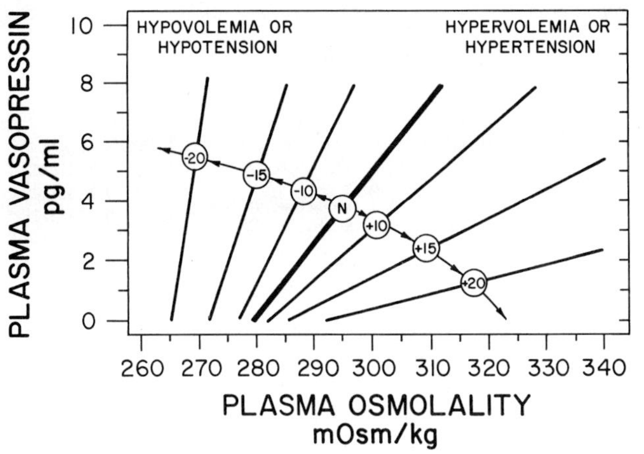

FIGURE 8-7. Schematic representation of the relation between plasma vasopressin and plasma osmolality in the presence of differing states of blood volume and/or pressure. The line labeled N represents normovolemic, normotensive conditions. Negative numbers to the left indicate percent fall and positive numbers to the right indicate percent rise in blood volume or pressure. (*From Robertson.*[47])

Emetic Effects

Nausea is an extremely potent stimulus for vasopressin secretion in humans[85–89] and monkeys.[90] The pathway that mediates this effect has not been defined but probably involves the chemoreceptor trigger zone in the area postrema of the medulla (Fig. 8-1). It can be activated by a variety of drugs and conditions, including apomorphine, morphine, nicotine, alcohol, and motion sickness. Its effect on vasopressin is instantaneous and extremely potent (Fig. 8-8). Increases of 100 to 1000 times basal levels are not unusual even when the nausea is transient and unaccompanied by vomiting or changes in blood pressure. Pretreatment with fluphenazine, haloperidol, or promethazine in doses sufficient to prevent nausea completely abolishes the vasopressin response. The inhibitory effect of these dopamine antagonists is specific for emetic stimuli because they do not alter the vasopressin response to osmotic or hemodynamic stimuli. Water loading blunts but does not abolish the effect of nausea on vasopressin release, suggesting that osmotic and emetic influences interact in a manner similar to the interaction of osmotic and hemodynamic pathways. Emesis is the only vasopressin stimulus known to exhibit a significant species difference. In rats, apomorphine has little or no effect on vasopressin but markedly stimulates oxytocin release.[86,91]

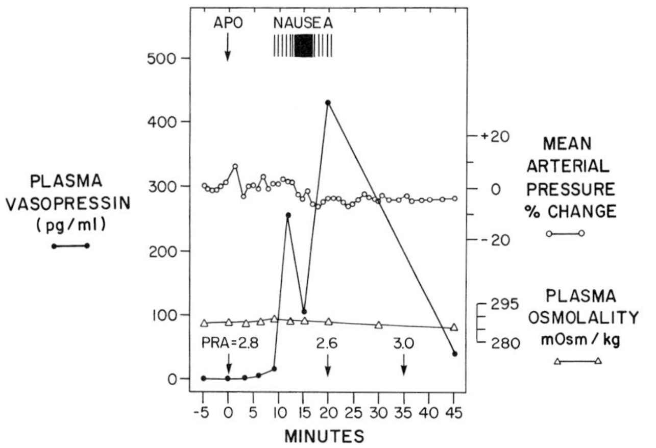

FIGURE 8-8. Relation of nausea to vasopressin secretion. Apomorphine (APO) was injected at the point indicated by the vertical arrow. Note that the rise in plasma vasopressin coincided with the occurrence of nausea and was not associated with detectable changes in plasma osmolality or blood pressure. (*From Robertson.*[47])

Glucopenic Effects

Acute hypoglycemia also stimulates vasopressin release.[92–95] The receptor and pathway that mediate this effect are unknown. However, they probably are separate from those of other recognized stimuli, as hypoglycemia stimulates vasopressin secretion in patients who have lost selectively the capacity to respond to osmotic, hemodynamic, or emetic stimuli. The effect of hypoglycemia is not due to nonspecific stress, because it can occur in the absence of symptoms and is more pronounced in rats,[93] a species in which vasopressin secretion appears to be completely unresponsive to pain and other noxious stimuli, as discussed later. The variable that actually triggers the release of vasopressin may be an intracellular deficiency of glucose or one of its metabolites, as 2-deoxyglucose is also an effective stimulus.[96,97]

The stimulus-response relations to hypoglycemia appears to be exponential.[94] Thus, in healthy adults, a drop in plasma glucose of as much as 10 to 20 percent usually has little or no effect, whereas a decrease of 50 percent increases plasma vasopressin about threefold. The rate of fall in glucose is probably the critical determinant, however, because the rise in plasma vasopressin is not sustained even when the hypoglycemia persists.[93] In addition, the vasopressin response to hypoglycemia is accentuated by dehydration and abolished by water loading.[93] Thus, glucopenic stimuli probably act in concert with osmotic influences even though the osmoreceptors per se are unnecessary for the response.

Renin-Angiotensin

The renin-angiotensin system has also been implicated in the control of vasopressin secretion.[98] The precise site and mechanism of action have not been defined, but central receptors seem likely because angiotensin is most effective when injected directly into brain ventricles or cranial arteries.[99] Moreover, intraventricular administration of angiotensin antagonists inhibits the vasopressin response to osmotic and hemodynamic stimuli.[100] The levels of plasma renin and/or angiotensin required to stimulate vasopressin release have not been determined but probably are quite high. When given intravenously, pressor doses of angiotensin increase plasma vasopressin about two- to fourfold. The magnitude of the vasopressin response may depend on the concurrent osmotic stimulus, as angiotensin has been observed to increase the sensitivity of the osmoregulatory system.[101] Hence, the effect of angiotensin on vasopressin may be imperceptible when plasma osmolality is depressed and exaggerated when plasma osmolality is high. This dependency on osmotic influences resembles that seen with glucopenic stimuli and may account for the failure of some investigators to demonstrate stimulation by exogenous angiotensin.[102]

Stress and Temperature

Nonspecific stress caused by factors such as pain, emotion, and physical exercise has long been thought to cause the release of vasopressin.[103] However, it has never been determined whether this effect is mediated by a separate pathway or is secondary to another stimulus, such as the hypotension and/or nausea that usually accompanies stress-induced vasovagal reactions.[104] In rats and humans, a variety of noxious stimuli capable of activating the pituitary adrenal axis and sympathetic nervous system do not stimulate vasopressin secretion unless they also lower blood pressure or alter blood volume.[28,105–107] The same stresses may stimulate the release of oxytocin,[107] but the role of other nonosmotic stimuli in the response has not been excluded. The marked rise in plasma vasopressin elicited by manipulation of the abdominal viscera in anesthetized dogs has been attributed to nociceptive influences,[108] but mediation by emetic pathways cannot be excluded in this setting.

Environmental temperature can also influence vasopressin secretion.[109] In healthy adults, exposure to cold for a relatively short period depresses plasma vasopressin, while a hot environment has the opposite effect. These changes occur independently of changes in plasma osmolality but cannot be disassociated from changes in effective blood volume or blood pressure. Hence, it is unclear whether there is a distinct thermoregulatory system for vasopressin secretion.

Hypoxia-Hypercapnia

Acute hypoxia and hypercapnia also stimulate vasopressin release.[110–115] In conscious humans, however, the stimulatory effect of moderate hypoxia ($Pa_{O_2} > 35$ mmHg) is inconsistent[110,111] and seems to occur only in subjects who develop nausea or hypotension.[110] In conscious dogs, more severe hypoxia ($Pa_{O_2} < 35$ mmHg) consistently increases vasopressin secretion without reducing arterial pressure.[113] Studies in anesthetized dogs suggest that the vasopressin response to acute hypoxia depends on the level of hypoxemia achieved. At a Pa_{O_2} of 35 mmHg or below, plasma vasopressin is markedly elevated even though arterial pressure is unchanged or even increased.[112,114] However, less severe hypoxemia ($Pa_{O_2} > 40$ mmHg) has no effect on vasopressin.[112] These results indicate a hypoxemic threshold for vasopressin release and suggest that severe acute hypoxemia per se may also stimulate vasopressin secretion in humans. If this is so, it may be responsible, at least in part, for the osmotically inappropriate hormonal elevations noted in some patients with acute respiratory failure.[115] In conscious or anesthetized dogs, acute hypercapnia per se, independent of hypoxia or hypotension, also increases vasopressin secretion.[112,113] It has not been determined whether this response also exhibits threshold characteristics or otherwise depends on the degree of hypercapnia. It is also unknown whether hypercapnia has similar effects on vasopressin secretion in humans or other animals.

Pharmacologic Effects

Many drugs and hormones have also been shown to influence vasopressin secretion.[116,117] Some stimulants, such as isoproterenol, nicotine, diuretics, nitroprusside, trimethaphan, and high doses of morphine, undoubtedly act at least in part by lowering blood pressure/volume or producing nausea.[116–120] Others, such as substance P, histamine, bradykinin, and prostaglandin, have not been studied sufficiently to define their mechanism of action, but probably act the same way. As discussed elsewhere, insulin and 2-deoxyglucose probably act by producing intracellular glucopenia, while angiotensin has an undefined but probably independent central effect. The stimulatory effect of cyclophosphamide may be due to its emetic effects,[119,120] while vincristine may have a direct toxic effect on the neurohypophysis or the peripheral neurons involved in the regulation of vasopressin secretion.[121] Lithium, which antagonizes the antidiuretic effect of vasopressin, also increases secretion of the hormone.[122–124] This effect is independent of changes in water balance and appears to result from an increase in the sensitivity of the osmoregulatory system.[122] Opioid antagonists selective for μ receptors may potentiate the vasopressin response to certain stimuli,[71,72] presumably by blocking the inhibitory influence of some endogenous opioid such as β-endorphin. The stimulatory effects of chlorpropamide and clofibrate are still controversial.[125–127]

Some inhibitors of vasopressin secretion such as norepinephrine and fludrocortisone undoubtedly act by raising blood pressure or volume.[116,117] Others, such as carbamazepine, inhibit vasopressin secretion by diminishing the sensitivity of the osmoregulatory system.[128–130] Dopaminergic antagonists such as fluphenazine, haloperidol, and promethazine probably act by suppressing the emetic center, as they inhibit the vasopressin response to emetic but not to osmotic or hemodynamic stimuli. When given systemically in low doses, a variety of opioids, including morphine and *kappa* agonists, inhibit vasopressin secretion in rats[131–136] and humans.[137–141] The inhibition by morphine, butorphanol, and oxilorphan is due to an increase in the osmotic threshold for vasopressin release[134,136] but is independent of changes in blood volume or pressure.[131] The mechanism of the inhibitory action of these opioids has not been completely defined but would appear to be an agonistic effect because it is blocked completely by naloxone.[131–133] The nonselective opioid antagonist diprenorphine and the *kappa-1* antagonist Mr2266Bs inhibit the vasopressin response to hypovolemic but not osmotic or hypotensive stimuli.[132] This selective inhibition occurs at least in part in the lateral parabrachial nucleus[68] and cannot be reproduced with more selective antagonists of mu or delta receptors. Presumably, therefore, it blocks synaptic transmission of some type of endogenous *kappa-1* agonist in the neuronal pathway that mediates the volume control of vasopressin secretion. The inhibitory effect of alcohol[142,143] may be mediated at least in part by endogenous opiates because it also is due to an elevation in the osmotic threshold for vasopressin release and can be blocked in part by treatment with naloxone.[144] Other drugs that are reported to inhibit vasopressin secretion include clonidine,[145,146] which appears to act via both central and peripheral adrenoreceptors; muscimol,[148] which is postulated to act as a γ-aminobutyric acid (GABA) agonist; and dizocilpine,[149] which antagonizes NMDA type glutamate receptors.

Autocrine Effects

The secretion of vasopressin may also be autoregulated by a direct feedback effect of the hormone on the neurohypophysis.[149–151] This feedback effect has been demonstrated after systemic as well as central administration and is not mediated by changes in osmotic or hemodynamic influences.[149,150] It can be blocked by pretreatment with selective vasopressin antagonists but cannot be reproduced by desamino-D-argine-vasopressin (DDAVP), an analog selective for V_2 receptors.[151] It may be mediated by a direct suppression of the excitability of neurons in the supraoptic nucleus.[152,153]

Oxytocin

The secretion of oxytocin in humans has not been extensively studied, largely because assays with the requisite simplicity and specificity have been difficult to develop. Bioassays, direct as well as indirect, have often been employed, but their specificity is suspect because vasopressin and possibly other peptides possess oxytocin activity. Radioimmunoassays have also been used but some of these findings are also open to question because some of them have been found to cross-react with one or more plasma components other than oxytocin.[154] To further complicate matters, the ovary[155] and heart[156] may also synthesize oxytocin or oxytocin-like peptides that may be the source of some of the immunoreactivity in plasma. Nevertheless, it now seems clear that nursing or mechanical/manual stimulation of the nipples triggers release of true oxytocin in women during lactation or certain phases of their menstrual cycle.[154] Insulin-induced hypoglycemia is also reported to stimulate release of small amounts of oxytocin in men as well as women.[157] Pregnancy and/or high levels of estrogen are not associated with a perceptible increase in plasma oxytocin, but they may increase the level of a novel peptide structurally related to oxytocin.[152] In rats but not in humans, oxytocin release is also stimulated by hyperosmolality and nausea.[91] Oxytocin may also have a direct feedback effect on the neurohypophysis to facilitate its own release.[158]

Distribution and Clearance

Vasopressin

The concentration of a hormone in plasma is determined by the difference between the rates of production and removal from the vascular compartment. In healthy adults, vasopressin distributes rapidly into a space roughly equivalent in size to the extracellular compartment.[28,159] This initial, or "mixing," phase has a half-life of 4 to 8 min, and is virtually complete in 10 to 15 min. The rapidity with which the hormone diffuses across capillary membranes approximates that of many other small peptides and is consistent with its lack of binding to neurophysin or other macromolecular components of plasma. The rapid mixing phase is followed by a second, slower decline that probably corresponds to the metabolic, or irreversible, phase of clearance. Studies with one immunoassay yielded mean values of 10 to 20 min by both steady-state and nonsteady-state techniques.[28,149,160,161] The rate of decline in urine osmolality after water loading is consistent with these estimates.[159] In dogs, at least, the rate of clearance is reduced by vasopressin antagonists,[162] suggesting that receptors play some role in clearance of the hormone. It should be noted that smaller animals such as the rat clear vasopressin much more rapidly than do humans because their cardiac output is much higher relative to their body weight and surface area.[159]

Although many tissues have the capacity to inactivate vasopressin in vitro, most metabolism in vivo appears to occur in the liver and kidney.[159] The enzymatic processes by which the liver and kidney inactivate vasopressin have not been established with certainty but appear to involve an initial reduction of the disulfide bridge followed by aminopeptidase cleavage of the bond between amino acid residues 1 and 2. The extent of further degradation and the peptide products, if any, that escape into plasma and urine are currently unknown. In pregnant women, the metabolic clearance of vasopressin is increased three- to fourfold because the placenta produces a vasopressinase that rapidly degrades the hormone in vivo as well as in vitro.[161]

Some vasopressin is excreted intact in the urine, but the amounts are quite small relative to total metabolic clearance. In healthy, normally hydrated adults, the urinary clearance of vasopressin ranges from 0.1 to 0.6 ml per kilogram of body weight per minute under basal conditions and has never been found to exceed 2 ml per kilogram of body weight per minute even in the presence of a solute diuresis.[28] The mechanisms involved in the excretion of vasopressin have not been defined with certainty, but the hormone is probably filtered at the glomerulus and variably reabsorbed at one or more sites along the tubule. The latter process may be linked in some way to the handling of sodium in the proximal nephron because the urinary clearance of vasopressin varies as much as 20-fold in direct relation to solute clearance.[28] Consequently, measurements of vasopressin excretion in humans do not provide a consistently reliable index of changes in plasma vasopressin and must be interpreted cautiously when glomerular filtration and/or solute clearance are inconstant or abnormal.

Oxytocin

The distribution and metabolic clearance of oxytocin appear to be similar to those of vasopressin.[159,164]

Extrahypophyseal Neurons

Relatively little is known about the biochemistry, secretory regulation, and metabolism of the vasopressin or oxytocin producing neurons that project to areas other than the pars nervosa. The parvicellular division that projects from the paraventricular nucleus to the median eminence and portal veins contains corticotropin-releasing factor (CRF), as well as vasopressin, and appears to be stimulated by general anesthesia, surgery, and glucocorticoid deficiency but not by osmolality.[164] The oxytocin-containing neurons in this pathway appear to be unaffected by adrenal insufficiency.[164] The vasopressinergic magnicellular neurons that arise in the suprachiasmatic nucleus and project to other areas of the hypothalamus also appear to be unresponsive to osmotic stimuli.[165] The vasopressin in CSF probably derives largely from direct secretion rather than diffusion from plasma.[9] However, it seems to be influenced by some, if not all, of the same variables that stimulate release from the pars nervosa because the concentrations in CSF correlate with those in plasma[9,166] and change appropriately during dehydration or rehydration, the infusion of hypertonic saline, and hemorrhage.[9,167] In humans, unlike in some lower species, CSF vasopressin does not show diurnal variation but oxytocin, which is also present, shows a distinct diurnal rhythm, with the peak occurring at about noon.[168] The function of the vasopressin in CSF is unknown, but it may play a role in regulating brain hydration,[9] thirst,[169] or intellectual function.[170] CSF vasopressin is abnormal in the syndrome of inappropriate antidiuresis,[9] diabetes insipidus,[9] dementia,[171] affective disorders,[172] and benign intracranial hypertension,[173] but the role of these abnormalties in the pathophysiology of the disorders is unknown.

Biologic Actions

Vasopressin

Renal

The most important action of vasopressin in humans is to conserve body water by reducing the rate of urine output. This antidiuretic effect is achieved by promoting the reabsorption of solute-free water in the distal and/or collecting tubules of the kidney.[174–176] In the absence of vasopressin, the luminal surfaces of the cells lining this portion of the nephron are largely impermeable to water and solutes. Hence, the relatively large volume of dilute tubular fluid issuing from the more proximal nephron passes unmodified as urine. In this condition, which is referred to as *water diuresis*, the urine is maximally dilute (osmolality less than 100 mosmol/kg) and the rate of urine flow ranges from 300 to 900 ml/h depending on the rate of solute excretion (Fig. 8-9). In the presence of vasopressin, water can penetrate the luminal surface of the principal cells in the distal and collecting tubules and passively back-diffuse down the osmotic gradient that normally exists between tubular fluid and the isotonic or hypertonic milieu of the renal cortex and medulla. Because water is reabsorbed without solute, the tubular fluid that remains to be excreted as urine is not only smaller in volume but also more concentrated. The magnitude of this antidiuretic effect varies as a direct function of the plasma vasopressin concentration (Fig. 8-4*B*). The sensitivity of this relationship differs appreciably among healthy adults but, on

FIGURE 8-9. Schematic relationship of urine flow to urine osmolality at three different rates of solute excretion, 15 (⊙), 30 (■), and 60 (●) mosmol/h. Note that (a) at any given level of urine osmolality, the rate of urine flow varies in direct proportion to the rate of solute excretion, and (b) at any given rate of solute excretion, urine flow varies as a negative exponential function of urine osmolality. Thus, the absolute changes in urine flow induced by a given change in solute load or urine osmolality is much greater when urine is dilute than when it is concentrated.

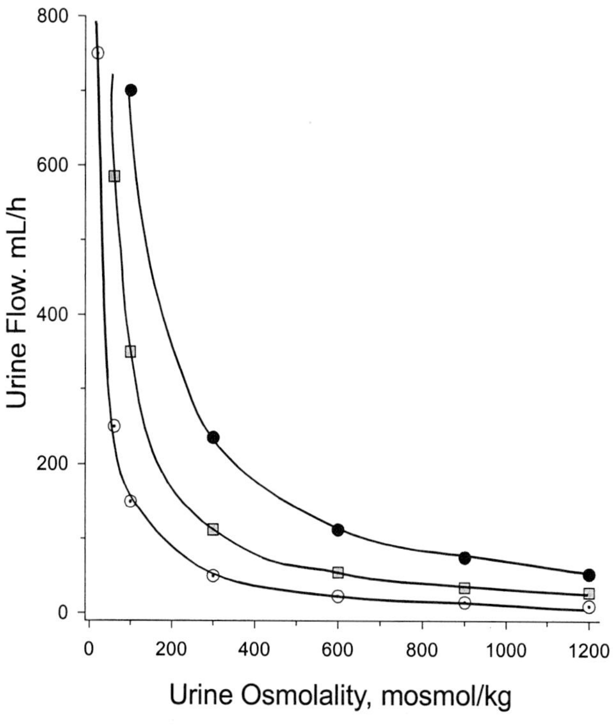

average, an increase in plasma vasopressin of 0.5 pg/ml raises urine osmolality by 150 to 250 mosmol/kg. The effect of this change on the rate of urine flow varies as an inverse curvilinear function of urine osmolality and also depends on the solute load (Fig. 8-9). Thus, it is greatest during a water diuresis and smallest when the urine is already concentrated. The maximum antidiuresis is usually achieved at a plasma vasopressin concentration between 2 to 5 pg/ml. In adults excreting normal amounts of solute (720 mosmol/day), this usually results in a urine osmolality of approximately 1,200 mosmol/kg and a urine flow of about 24 ml/h. This is the normal minimum obligatory rate of urine output and cannot be reduced further except by decreasing the solute load. Certain other species, particularly rodents, can achieve much higher levels of antidiuresis, apparently because they have longer renal papillae and correspondingly higher levels of hypertonicity in the medulla.

The cellular mechanism by which vasopressin increases the hydroosmotic permeability of the distal nephron has now been elucidated.[175–179] It results from the insertion of water channels into the luminal surface of the prinicipal cells that line the distal and collecting tubules. These water channels are formed by oligomers of a 29kD protein known as aquaporin-2. The gene that encodes aquaporin-2 in humans has been cloned and sequenced and localized to chromosome 12q13.[180] It is expressed largely if not exclusively in the distal nephron. In the absence of vasopressin, the rate of production of aquaporin-2 decreases and most of it is stored in intracellular vesicles. In the presence of vasopressin, these vesicles move rapidly to the luminal surface and fuse with the membrane, thereby increasing the hydroosmotic permeability of the cell. More prolonged stimulation by vasopressin also increases the production of aquaporin-2, which over the course of several hours further enhances urinary concentrating capacity. In addition to its effects on water channels, vasopressin also stimulates distal tubular production of a urea transporter that further enhances urinary concentrating capacity by increasing medullary hypertonicity.[181,182]

The actions of vasopressin in the distal nephron are mediated largely if not exlusively by receptors on the serosal surface of principal cells in tubular epithelia.[183] These receptors have been designated V_2 to distinguish them from those which mediate the putative extrarenal actions of vasopressin, as discussed later. The gene encoding the V_2 receptor has been cloned and sequenced and mapped to the distal long arm of the X chromosome.[184,185] The receptor has a seven-transmembrane topography characteristic of G protein-coupled receptors and uses cyclic AMP as a second messenger. Nonpeptides capable of competitively antagonizing the antidiuretic effect of vasopressin at V_2 receptors have been developed[186–188] and are undergoing testing for use in the treatment of patients with the syndrome of inappropriate antidiuresis (SIADH) and other disorders associated with excessive retention of free water.

Extrarenal

In supraphysiologic doses, vasopressin can also raise blood pressure by constricting vascular smooth muscle.[189] In dogs and some other quadrupeds, the pressor effect begins at plasma concentrations of around 50 pg/ml, which is about 10 times that required to produce maximum antidiuresis. Healthy humans are even less sensitive to the blood-pressure raising effects of vasopressin[190,191] and at high concentrations of the hormone may actually have a depressor response, at least in some vascular beds.[192] Thus, despite its common name, vasopressin probably plays little or no role in baroregulation in healthy humans. The pressor effects of vasopressin can be dissociated from its antidiuretic effects[193,194] and are mediated by a different receptor, designated V_{1A}, which is coupled to phospholipase C rather than adenyl cyclase.[183] The gene encoding the V_{1A} receptor in humans and rats has been cloned and sequenced.[195,196] It shares important homologies with the V_2 receptor and is expressed in liver and brain as well as arteries.[197] Nonpeptides that competively antagonize the actions of vasopressin at V_{1A} receptors have been developed[198,199] and tested in hypertensive or dehydrated humans[200,201] without appreciably reducing systemic arterial pressure.

Vasopressin, administered alone in high doses or in combination with CRF, also stimulates the release of ACTH.[202,203] This effect appears to be mediated at least in part by a distinct receptor on ACTH-producing cells of the anterior pituitary.[204,205] This receptor, designated V_{1B}, is also linked to phospholipase C. In addition to the anterior pituitary, it is found in the supraoptic nucleus and many other areas of brain.[206] The gene encoding the V_{1B} receptor has also been cloned and sequenced and shares many homologies with the other two vasopressin receptors.[207] The physiologic role of the V_{1B} receptor is still uncertain. It could contribute to the regulation of pituitary adrenal function because the portal veins contain high concentrations of vasopressin that probably comes from the paraventricular nucleus via a parvicellular branch that projects to the median eminence.[3,164] However, this pathway does not seem to be important for the pituitary-adrenal response to stress in rats[208,209] and may be limited to potentiating the effects of certain other stimuli, such as hypovolemia[210] or glucocorticoid deficiency.[164]

Vasopressin may also inhibit water loss from skin, lungs, and other extrarenal sites.[211] However, in humans at least, this effect cannot reduce insensible loss below a certain minimum basal level (0.2 ml/min) and is easily overridden by other factors such as an increase in ambient temperature or physical activity, which may increase water loss from skin and lungs to as high as 20 ml/min.[212] Vasopressin may also inhibit pancreatic flow,[213] stimulate hepatic glycogenolysis,[214] aggregate platelets,[215] inhibit stress-induced hyperthermia,[216] and induce nausea as well as changes in gastric motility.[217] However, like its pressor and ACTH effects, they occur only at very high concentrations of the hormone and their role in human physiology or pathology has not been determined.

Oxytocin

Mammary Gland and Uterus

The major biological action of oxytocin is to permit nursing by stimulating the contraction of myoepithelial cells in the lactating mammary gland.[218,219] Oxytocin also stimulates contraction of the uterus,[218] but this effect seems to occur only at plasma concentrations[220] above those present at initiation of normal labor. Moreover, elimination of the oxytocin gene in rats does not interfere with normal parturition,[219] indicating that the uterotonic effect of oxytocin is not essential for labor and delivery, at least in this species. The milk let-down and utertonic effects of oxytocin are mediated by a distinct receptor[221] similar to those that mediate the effects of vasopressin. Several antagonists specific for these oxytocin receptors have been developed[222,223] and some are now being evaluated as potential tocolytics for treatment of premature labor.

Other Tissues

Oxytocin may also stimulate release of atrial natriuretic peptide from heart.[224] It can also cause concentration of the urine in humans[225] as well as rats.[226] This antidiuretic effect is enhanced in patients with severe pituitary diabetes insipidus,[225] but requires plasma oxytocin concentrations 10–100 times higher than normal basal levels and is mediated by V_2 receptors.[227]

Neurophysins and Copeptin

The neurophysins have no recognized biological action apart from complexing oxytocin and vasopressin in neurosecretory granules of the neurohypophysis. Although present in plasma, they do not serve as binding or transport proteins for the hormones because the high pH and low concentration of the reactants favor complete dissociation.[14] However, the neurophysins probably do bind significant amounts of hormone in the urine.[10] Copeptin, which is coproduced and presumably cosecreted with vasopressin, has no known biologic action.

Thirst

Because the rate of urinary and insensible loss of water cannot be reduced below a certain minimum level (previously described), some mechanism to ensure adequate replacement is absolutely essential for maintaining water balance. In terrestrial animals, this indispensable role is fulfilled by the thirst mechanism.[228,229] When used in a physiologic sense, *thirst* is defined as an inner urge or desire for water. It is often associated with sensations of drymouth but the latter sensation can also result from factors such as severe anxiety or mouth breathing which have little or nothing to do with water homeostasis. Thirst also should be distinguished from other causes of drinking such as social custom or the currently fashionable belief in the therapeutic value of a high fluid intake. The efferent pathways and cortical projections that mediate the feelings of thirst have not been completely determined. As might be expected, however, the sensation is stimulated by many of the same variables and afferent mechanisms that cause the release of vasopressin.[228–239]

Dipsogenesis

Osmotic

Like vasopressin, thirst appears to be regulated primarily by plasma osmolality (Fig. 8-4*C*). In healthy adults, a rise in effective plasma osmolality of only 1 to 2 percent above basal levels usually produces a strong desire to drink. This sensation increases in intensity with further increases in plasma osmolality and is not dependent on a reduction in extracellular volume, as it is similar during the infusion of hypertonic saline and water deprivation. Thirst can also be osmotically inhibited by a sensation that is best described as "satiety."[231] In addition, water intake varies in direct proportion to changes in plasma osmolality or feelings of thirst or satiety[36,229] and can range from as high as 20 to as low as 0.5 L/day. This mechanism is so effective at maintaining water balance that it can prevent dehydration or overhydration even under conditions of maximal renal and extrarenal water loss or water retention.[232]

The neuronal pathways that mediate the osmoregulation of thirst have not been totally defined, but appear to involve osmoreceptors located in the anterior hypothalamus, near but not totally coincident with those which regulate vasopressin secretion.[233,234] The solute specificities of the two osmoreceptors also appear to be similar because plasma solutes such as urea and glucose, which have little or no effect on vasopressin secretion, are equally ineffective as dipsogens.[48,49]

Hemodynamic

Hypovolemia and/or hypotension are also dipsogenic.[228–231] The degree of hypovolemia and/or hypotension required to produce thirst has not been defined for humans, but appears to be greater even than that needed to effect vasopressin release. Thus, upright posture often induces a small but significant rise in plasma vasopressin but does not appreciably affect thirst. Hypovolemia may be a more potent dipsogen in rats, but even in that species reductions of less than 15 percent have little or no effect on water intake. The pathways by which hypovolemia and/or hypotension produce thirst are uncertain, but they are different from those that mediate osmotic dipsogenesis[235] and probably are similar if not identical to those that mediate the baroregulation of vasopressin. Hemodynamic stimuli also reset the osmotic threshold for thirst, as they do for vasopressin.[236] The effects of hypovolemia on thirst and vasopressin may also be mediated partially via the renin-angiotensin system. The latter is a potent dipsogen in rats[237,238] but has not been shown to affect thirst in humans.

Vasopressin

Thirst may also be affected by changes in plasma or CSF vasopressin and a variety of other hormones.[237,238] Because osmotic and hemodynamic stimuli cause release of vasopressin into CSF as well as plasma, the dipsogenic effect of dehydration may be mediated in part by increases in endogenous vasopressin secretion. However, the hormone probably does not play an essential or even a major role in the regulation of thirst, as dipsogenesis is normal in Brattleboro rats which lack the capacity to make vasopressin. The mechanism and site at which the various osmotic, hemodynamic, and hormonal influences are integrated to regulate thirst have not been defined.[239]

Regulation of Water Balance

Distribution, Composition, and Turnover

Water is by far the largest constituent of the human body.[240] In lean, healthy adults, it makes up 55 to 65 percent of body weight, and it accounts for an even larger proportion in infants and young children. About two-thirds of body water is intracellular. The rest is extracellular and is divided further into the intravascular (plasma) and extravascular (interstitial) compartments in a ratio of 1:3. The solute compositions of intracellular and extracellular fluid differ markedly because most cell membranes possess an array of transport systems that actively accumulate or expel specific solutes. Thus, sodium and chloride are confined largely to extracellular fluid, whereas potassium, magnesium, and various organic acids or phosphates are predominantly intracellular. Glucose, which requires an insulin-activated transport system to enter most somatic cells and is rapidly converted in those cells to glycogen or other metabolites, is present in significant amounts only in extracellular fluid. Bicarbonate is present in both compartments, but is about three times more concentrated in extracellular fluid. Urea is unique among the major naturally occurring solutes in that it diffuses freely across most cell membranes and is therefore present in similar concentrations in virtually all body fluids.

Despite marked differences in the concentration of particular solutes in extracellular and intracellular fluid, the total solute concentration is almost everywhere the same. This osmotic equilibrium is due primarily to rapid diffusion of water back and forth across most of the membranes that separate the various body compartments.[241,242] These shifts are driven by transient differences in "effective" osmotic pressure. This property is similar but not completely identical to the osmotic pressure determined by measuring the freezing point or vapor pressure of plasma or other body fluids.[243] The latter is a physicochemical property determined by the total concentration of all of the solutes present, regardless of their ability to penetrate biological membranes. The effective osmolality of a body fluid is a biological property determined by the total concentration of only those solutes that do not equilibrate freely across the membranes of living cells. Thus, sodium and chloride, which are actively excluded from the intracellular compartment, are osmotically effective, but urea is not. Normally, the difference between the effective osmolality of body fluids and that determined by freezing point or vapor pressure osmometry is too small to be important, because more than 90 percent of the solute in plasma and extracellular fluid is sodium and its anions. However, in certain situations, such as chronic renal failure, effective osmolality may be considerably less than that determined by conventional osmometry because the concentration of ineffective solutes such as urea is much higher than normal.

Because osmotic equilibrium is maintained by rapid shifts of water, any change in the concentration of an effective solute in one compartment changes the volume and osmolality of all compartments.[244] Thus, for example, a rise in extracellular concentration of sodium and its anions induced by dehydration causes water to flow from the intracellular to the extracellular compartment. As a result, the water deficit distributes evenly throughout the body, causing a proportionally equal decrease in volume and increase in osmolality in each of the compartments. Conversely, a fall in extracellular sodium and its anions induced by overhydration causes water to flow in the opposite direction, redistributing the excess to all compartments. However, if the total amount of electrolyte or other effective solute in one compartment changes (due, for example, to infusion of hypertonic saline or administration of a diuretic), the amount of water in the other compartments changes in *opposite* direction.[244] In these acute situations, the cells as a whole behave essentially like perfect osmometers; that is, the observed changes in the volume and osmolality of extracellular fluid conform closely to theoretical expectations. However, deviations from this kind of ideal behavior may occur when the disturbance in salt and water balance is particularly severe and/or prolonged. Under these conditions, many cells appear to be able to counteract osmotically induced changes in volume by reversibly activating or deactivating intracellular solute.[245] In addition, these disturbances bring into play a variety of other homeostatic mechanisms which, by altering total body content of salt and/or water, gradually restore the balance to normal, as described later.

The stability of this internal milieu is continuously threatened by unavoidable gains and losses that result from the need for nutrients, evaporation from skin and lungs, and the production of urine in amounts sufficient to carry the load of solute (mainly urea, sodium, potassium, and their associated anions) that must be excreted. The magnitude of the turnover in body fluid among healthy adults can vary from 1 to 10 percent a day depending on the choice of diet, physical activity, ambient temperature, and individual differences in the regulation of thirst and vasopressin secretion. Nevertheless, plasma osmolality and its principal determinant, the concentration of sodium and its anions, normally are maintained within a remarkably narrow range (Fig. 8-10). This stability is achieved largely by the osmoregulation of thirst and vasopressin secretion which continuously raises or lowers body water to keep it in balance with sodium. The exact level at which stabilization occurs depends on individual variations in diet, environment, and physical activity as well as genetically determined differences in the set and sensitivity of these two osmoregulatory systems.[36] On the average, however, overall intake and output come into balance at a plasma osmolality and sodium concentration around 288 mosmol/kg and 139 mEq/l, respectively. At this position, thirst and fluid intake are minimal, plasma vasopressin is maintained at levels which permit half-maximal antidiuresis, and any deviations induced by eating, drinking, or changes in insensible loss can be promptly counteracted by appropriate adjustments in thirst and vasopressin secretion.

In humans and possibly other mammals, the operation of this osmoregulatory system is subject to intermittent hemodynamic stimuli generated by changes in posture, sleep, and other activity. However, these changes in blood pressure and/or effective blood volume do not appreciably influence plasma levels of vasopressin (Fig. 8-10), probably because they are either too small (Fig. 8-6),

FIGURE 8-10. Circadian patterns of water and solute homeostasis in healthy young adults.

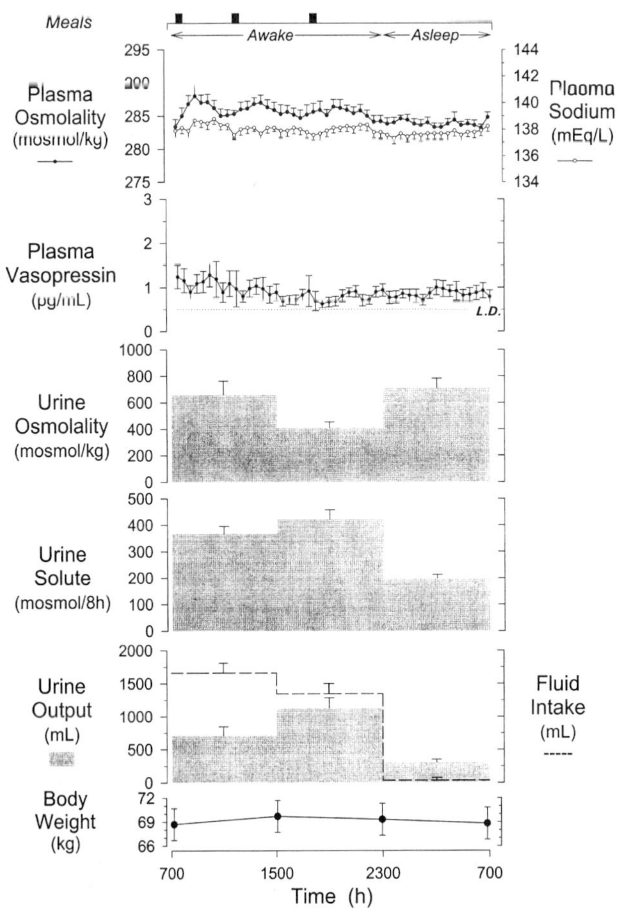

have opposing effects (as during sleep), or merely shift the set of the osmostats (Fig. 8-7). Because this resetting is probably slight and of short duration, it is unlikely to have any appreciable effect on the osmoregulation of thirst or vasopressin. It should be noted that the effects of vasopressin and thirst on the regulation of blood volume and pressure are normally trivial and occur largely as an indirect consequence of efforts to preserve osmolality. Indeed, in situations characterized by an abnormal increase in total body sodium, thirst and vasopressin act in a way that aggravates instead of ameliorates the increase in extracellular volume. The responsibility for coping with disturbances in extracellular volume per se rests primarily with those elements of the renal and endocrine systems that regulate sodium excretion. This distinction is useful to bear in mind when one is considering the role of the hypothalamic-neurohypophyseal system in the pathogenesis of clinical disorders of salt and water balance.

PATHOLOGY

Deficiencies of Vasopressin

Diabetes Insipidus

Global deficiencies in vasopressin secretion or action result in diabetes insipidus (DI), a syndrome characterized by chronic excretion of abnormally large volumes of dilute urine. The urine output typically exceeds 50 ml/kg/day in adults and older children or 75 ml/kg/day in infants and young children. In both age groups, the osmolality of the 24-h urine collection is less than 300 mosmol/kg. The polyuria usually is associated with symptoms of urinary frequency and nocturia or enuresis, especially in children. Most patients also have constant thirst and polydipsia commensurate with their polyuria. DI should be differentiated from other causes of urinary frequency in which urine output is normal but functional bladder capacity is low, and from the polyuria that results from uncontrolled diabetes mellitus or other causes of a solute diuresis. These distinctions can usually be made quite easily by means of a voiding diary, tests for urinary glucose, and estimates of 24-h urinary solute excretion. The latter, determined as the product of a 24-h urine volume and osmolality, is normally less than 1,400 mosmol/day (20 mosmol/kg/day). Higher values indicate some type of solute diuresis. DI can be subdivided into four basic types based on the cause of the antidiuretic defect.

TABLE 8-1. Causes of Pituitary Diabetes Insipidus

Acquired
Trauma
Closed
Penetrating (surgical, gunshot)
Neoplasms
Primary
Craniopharyngioma
Dysgerminoma
Meningioma
Adenoma with suprasellar extension
Metastatic (lung, breast)
Hematologic (lymphoma, granulocytic leukemia)
Granulomas
Neurosarcoid
Histiocytosis
Xanthoma disseminatum
Infectious
Chronic meningitis
Viral encephalitis
Toxoplasmosis
Inflammatory
Lymphocytic infundibuloneurohypophysitis
Wegener's granulomatosis
Lupus erythematosus
Scleroderma
Chemical toxins
Tetrodotoxin
Snake venom
Vascular
Sheehan's syndrome
Aneurysm (cavernous part of internal carotid)
Aortocoronary bypass
Generalized hypoxic encephalopathy
Idiopathic
Congenital malformations
Septooptic dysplasia
Midline craniofacial defects, holoprosencephaly
Hypogenesis, ectopia of pituitary
Genetic
Autosomal dominant (vasopressin-neurophysin gene)
Autosomal recessive (vasopressin-neurophysin gene)
Autosomal recessive-Wolfram S-(chromosome 4p—WFS 1 gene)
X-linked recessive (chromosome Xq28)
Deletion chromosome 7q

Pituitary DI

The most common type of DI is caused by a primary deficiency of vasopressin secretion. It is referred to by a variety of names including neurogenic, neurohypophyseal, pituitary, hypothalamic, central, cranial, or vasopressin-responsive DI. It is almost always due to agenesis or destruction of vasopressin-producing neurohypophyseal neurons by some developmental, acquired, genetic, or idiopathic disorder (Table 8-1).[246–250] Consequently, the hyperintense magnetic resonance signal usually emitted by the normal posterior pituitary is almost invariably absent.[251] In patients with some of the developmental or acquired forms of pituitary DI, the MRI may also reveal other abnormalities such as a congenital malformation of the forebrain, a primary or metastatic tumor in the suprasellar region, or thickening of the pituitary stalk and/or basal meninges commonly seen with many granulomatous, infiltrative, and chronic infectious diseases.

There are several forms of genetic or familial pituitary DI. The most common one is inherited in an autosomal dominant mode with virtually complete penetrance.[252–263] In these patients, the deficiency of vasopressin does not develop until several months to several years after birth, usually increases in severity throughout childhood, but is rarely, if ever, complete.[252] The loss of vasopressin secretion appears to be due to selective, postnatal degeneration of the vasopressin-producing neurons because autopsy studies in four patients showed gliosis and a marked deficiency of magnicellular neurosecretory neurons in the supraoptic and, to a lesser extent, paraventricular nuclei of the hypothalamus.[252] For unknown reasons, the DI remits spontaneously in some adults despite a continuing severe deficiency of vasopressin. Patients with the autosomal dominant form of familial pituitary DI invariably have a mutation in one allele of the gene that encodes the vasopressin-neurophysin II precursor (Fig. 8-11).[252–263] The

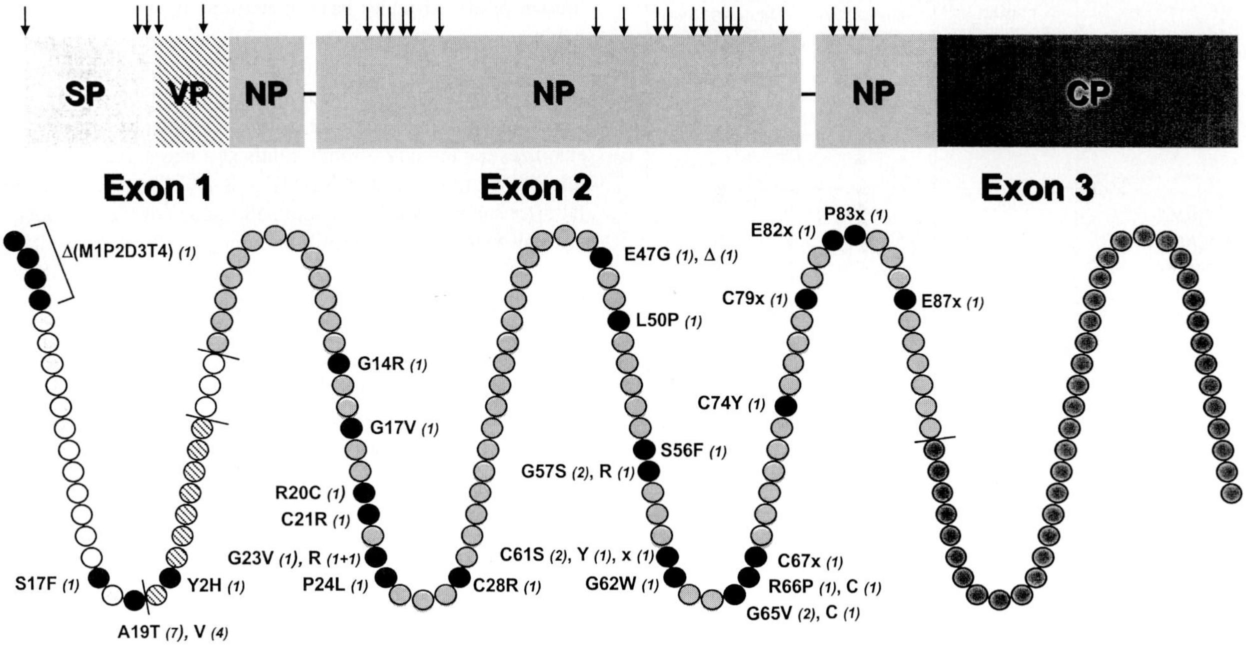

FIGURE 8-11. Mutations of the vasopressin-neurophysin 2 gene associated with the autosomal dominant form of familial pituitary diabetes insipidus. The number in parenthesis after each specific mutation indicates the number of apparently unrelated kindreds in which the mutation has been reported as of 12/99. SP = signal peptide, VP = vasopressin, NP = neurophysin, and CP = copeptin.

mutations differ widely in type and location and have been found in every area of the coding region except the part of the third exon that encodes the copeptin moiety. However, all of the mutations are expected to alter one or more amino acids known or presumed to be crucial for removing the signal peptide and/or correctly folding the prohormone in the endoplasmic reticulum. This pattern, as well as the clinical and autopsy evidence of progressive degeneration of vasopressin-producing neurons, suggests that the mutant alleles are cytotoxic because they direct the production of an abnormal precursor that cannot be folded and routed properly from the ER.[252] Expression studies in vitro support this hypothesis.[264–267]

An X-linked, recessive form of familial pituitary DI has also been reported recently.[268] In this kindred, DI and a partial deficiency of vasopressin are evident at or shortly after birth in males. These abnormalities sometimes progress in severity with time and are always associated with a very small or absent pituitary bright spot on MRI. Oxytocin production appears to be normal. Obligate female carriers are completely unaffected. The gene responsible for this form of familial pituitary DI has not been identified but appears to lie in the Xq28 region. The genes encoding the V_2 receptor and vasopressin-neurophysin II are normal.

An autosomal recessive form of familial pituitary DI has also been discovered recently.[269] In this family, asymptomatic parents who were first cousins had three children with pituitary DI. The latter were found to be homozygous for a single novel vasopressin-neurophysin II gene mutation that predicted the substitution of leucine for proline at position 7 in the vasopressin moiety. Their plasma appeared to contain high levels of immunoactive 7-leucine-vasopressin, which bound poorly to V_2 receptors in vitro. Presumably, therefore, their DI is due to production of a biologically inactive form of vasopressin rather than to destruction of their neurophypophysis. Brattleboro rats also have a form of inherited pituitary DI which is transmitted in an autosomal, semirecessive mode and results from a mutation in the vasopressin-neurophysin II gene.[16] However, the mutation in these animals affects the neurophysin portion of the gene and causes a frame shift that interferes with biosynthesis of the vasopressin precursor. It does not result in degeneration of vasopressin producing neurons or the secretion of detectable amounts of abnormal vasopressin.

Other genetic defects can also cause pituitary DI as part of a constellation of other abnormalities. These include Wolfram's syndrome, an autosomal recessive, neurodegenerative disorder that sometimes results in pituitary DI as well as diabetes mellitus, optic atrophy, deafness, and other abnormalities (DIDMOAD).[270] This disease has now been linked to mutation of a novel chromosome 4p gene that encodes a putative transmembrane protein.[271] The mechanism by which this mutation causes the disease is unknown, but it appears to result in degeneration of vasopressin-producing magnocellular neurons in the supraoptic nucleus[272] and partial to severe deficiencies of vasopressin secretion in response to nonosmotic as well as osmotic stimuli.[273] Pituitary DI can also occur in familial congenital hypopituitarism,[274] familial cerebellar ataxia,[275] and congenital midline craniofacial defects asssociated with deletion of chromosome 7q.[276] The genetic mechanisms involved are unknown.

Idiopathic forms of pituitary DI are the most common, accounting for nearly 50 percent of the total. In many cases, they probably represent the "burned-out" stage of infundibuloneurohypophysitis, a necrotizing inflammatory disorder of possible infectious or autoimmune etiology.[277–283] The few neuropathologic studies performed on patients with idiopathic pituitary DI also have shown atrophy of the pars nervosa in association with a marked deficiency of neurosecretory cells in the supraoptic nuclei.[284–286]

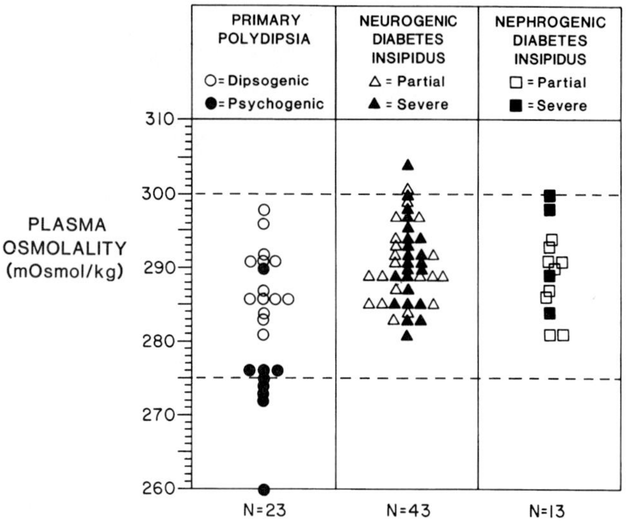

FIGURE 8-12. Basal plasma osmolality under conditions of ad libitum fluid intake in patients with untreated pituitary DI, nephrogenic DI, or primary polydipsia.

The pathogenesis and pathophysiology of pituitary DI is most thoroughly exemplified by the sequence of events following experimental section of the pituitary stalk.[287–289] During the next few weeks, the severed axons undergo retrograde degeneration leading to death of their cell bodies in the supraoptic and, to a lesser extent, the paraventricular nucleus. If the section occurs high enough to destroy more than 75 percent of magnicellular neurons (usually at the level of the infundibulum or above), the amount of vasopressin produced under basal conditions becomes insufficient to maintain urine concentration and DI develops. The increase in urine output results in a slight decrease in total body water and a rise in plasma osmolality/sodium, which stimulates thirst. The resultant increase in fluid intake restores the balance with output and stabilizes the tonicity of body fluids at a new level slightly above the osmotic threshold for thirst (Fig. 8-12). The natural history of DI after surgical section or traumatic injury of the neurohypophysis can follow any of several different patterns. In some, it develops 1–4 days after injury and never remits. In others, the DI is transient and is followed in 4 to 7 days by an increase in urine osmolality and a decline in urine volume to normal. In some of these patients, the remission lasts only a few days and is followed by return of permanent DI. The functional and anatomic basis for the triphasic pattern of response has not been established. Presumably, however, the initial phase of DI results from transient paralysis of neurohypophyseal function. It is followed by degeneration of some of these neurons with release of stored vasopressin into the circulation. The final permanent phase of DI occurs when the released vasopressin is degraded and the neurons that survive are unable to produce adequate amounts of the hormone.

It is important to note that the deficiency of vasopressin need not be complete for DI to occur (Fig. 8-13).[287,290] It is necessary only that the amount of plasma vasopressin required to concentrate the urine cannot be produced *at levels of plasma osmolality/sodium which do not stimulate thirst and polydipsia.* The extent to which secretory capacity must be reduced to produce this deficiency varies due to relatively large individual or situational differences in vasopressin metabolism, secretory reserve, and the set of the osmoregulatory system.[36,291] However, studies of cell loss in the supraoptic nuclei after pituitary surgery,[287]

FIGURE 8-13. The relationship of plasma vasopressin to plasma or urine osmolality before and during a standard fluid deprivation-hypertonic saline infusion test in patients with partial ( ) or severe (■) pituitary DI, partial (▽) or severe (▼) nephrogenic DI, or (●) primary polydipsia.

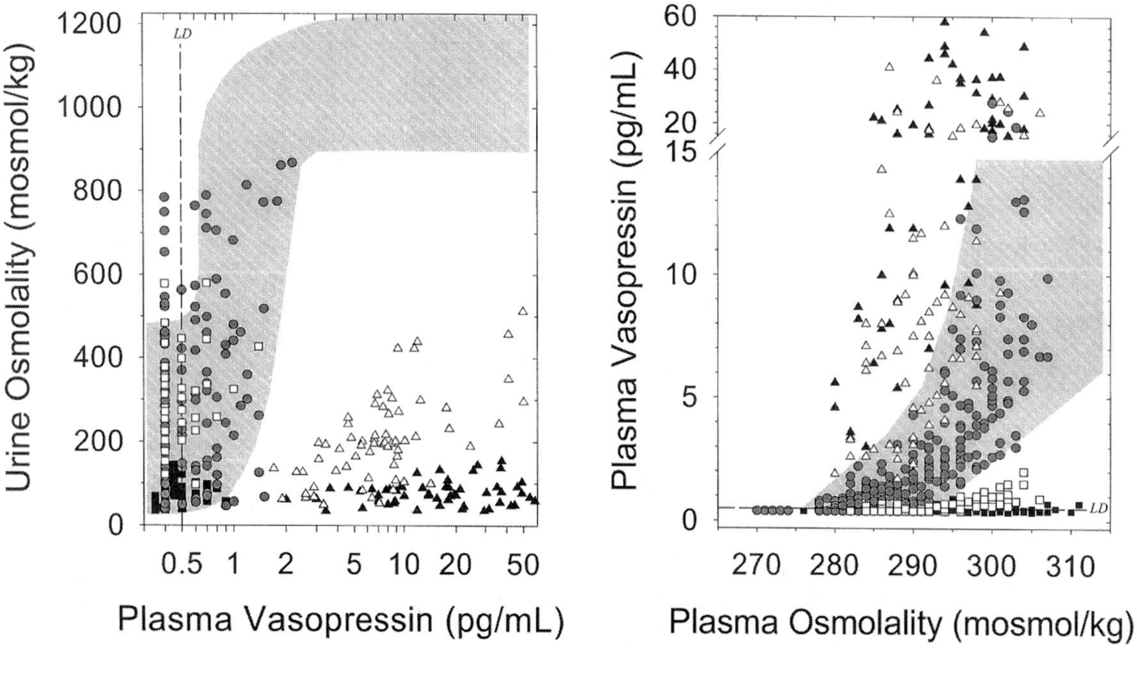

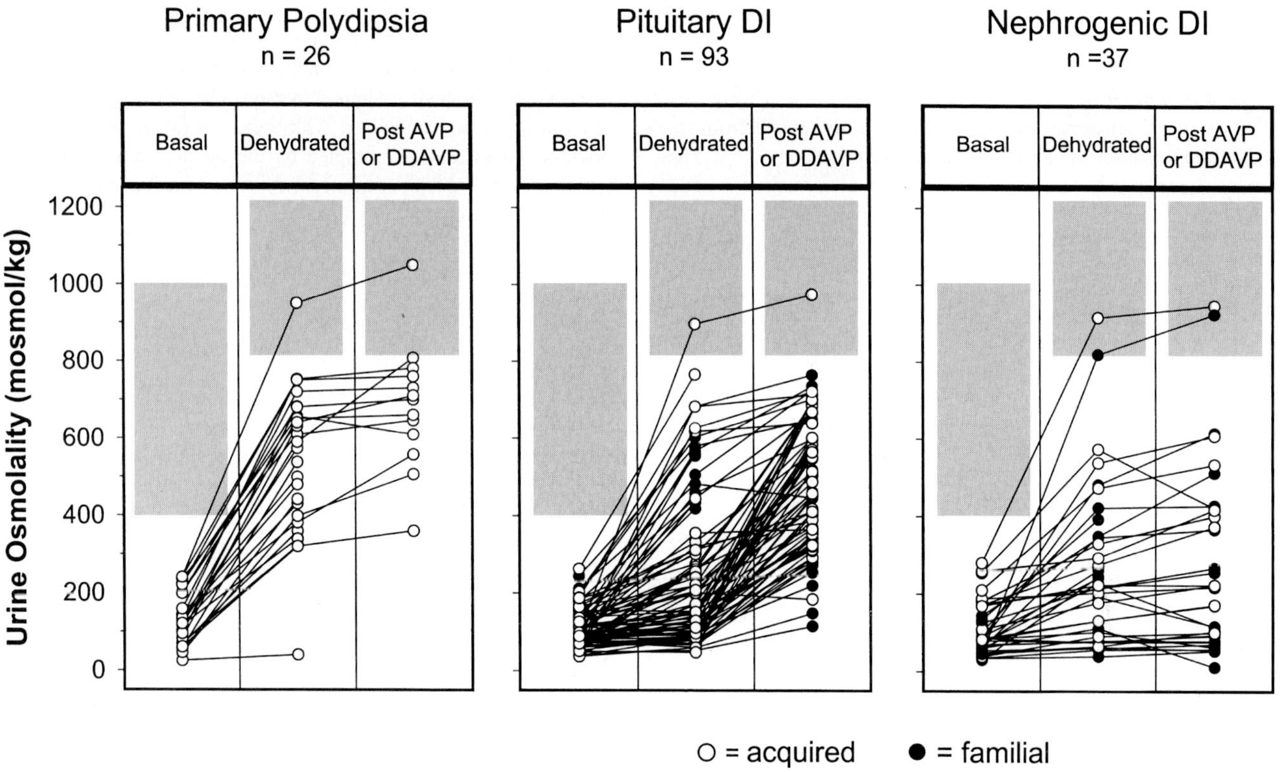

FIGURE 8-14. Urine osmolality before and after fluid deprivation or administration of antidiuretic hormone (vasopressin or DDAVP) in patients with primary polydipsia, pituitary DI, or nephrogenic DI. The shaded boxes indicate the range of values in healthy adult controls under the same conditions.

functional tests of vasopressin secretion in a large number of patients with diabetes insipidus of variable severity and etiology (Fig. 8-13),[290] and theoretical considerations[291] all indicate that DI does not develop unless secretory capacity is reduced by more than 75 percent. Thus, there are probably many patients with lesser deficiencies of vasopressin who do not develop symptomatic DI unless metabolism of the hormone is increased or some inhibitory stress is imposed.

Recognition of the fact that many patients with pituitary DI retain a limited capacity to secrete vasopressin is the key to understanding many otherwise perplexing features of the disorder. For example, restricting water intake for only a few hours will often stimulate the remaining neurohypophyseal neurons to release enough hormone to concentrate the urine (Figs. 8-13 and 8-14).[290] This response illustrates the relative nature of the vasopressin deficiency and shows that it is the compensatory increase in thirst and fluid intake that prevents these patients from using whatever residual secretory capacity they may have. Even when the vasopressin deficiency is so severe that fluid deprivation produces little or no increase in urine osmolality, a potent nonosmotic stimulus such as smoking, postural hypotension, or a vasovagal reaction may release enough hormone to concentrate the urine. Consequently, when interpreting diagnostic or therapeutic procedures in these patients, it is necessary to be circumspect about the presence of drugs or associated diseases that can modify vasopressin secretion via nonosmotic mechanisms.

Pituitary DI also alters the acute effect of vasopressin on urinary concentration. The most obvious change is a reduction in maximum concentrating capacity[290,292–295] that probably results from washout of the medullary concentration gradient[292–295] as well as suppression of aquaporin-2 production[296,297] caused by the chronic vasopressin deficiency and polyuria *per se*. The severity of this defect is proportional to the severity of the basal polyuria and is independent of its cause.[290] Because of it, the level of urinary concentration produced initially by an acute increase in plasma vasopressin is subnormal (Figs. 8-13 and 8-14).[290] However, this blunting of maximum concentrating capacity is temporary and will repair within 24 to 48 hours if the elevations in vasopressin are sustained. Moreover, in patients with pituitary DI, the defect in maximum concentrating capacity is partly offset by enhanced sensitivity to the antidiuretic effect of very low levels of plasma vasopressin (Fig. 8-13). The cause of this apparent supersensitivity is unknown, but may be upward regulation of vasopressin receptors secondary to a chronic deficiency of the hormone.

Patients with pituitary DI are also reported to have decreased bone mineral density and serum osteocalcin that is not affected by treatment of the DI with DDAVP.[298] However, there is no evidence that they have an increased incidence of bone fractures or other symptoms of osteopenia. Pituitary DI *per se* is not associated with any obvious abnormalities in baroregulation, pituitary adrenal function, clotting, or other physiologic functions linked to V_1 receptors. However, some of the diseases that cause DI can also damage one or more of these other systems. The osmoregulation of thirst is also normal in more than 90 percent of patients with pituitary DI, but a few—most notably those with a history of head trauma, pituitary-hypothalamic surgery, or a suprasellar malignancy—have either hypodipsia or hyperdipsia, apparently due to associated damage to the osmoregulatory system.

Gestational DI

A primary deficiency of vasopressin can also result from increased degradation of the hormone during pregnancy.[299–303] The increase in degradation results from overproduction of a placental vasopressinase that rapidly degrades the hormone.[301] In some patients, at least, there is also an underlying, subclinical deficiency in vasopressin secretion[302,303] that may predispose to the syndrome by limiting the capacity to compensate for the increased rate of metabolism. In some patients, a subclinical deficiency in secretion alone may be sufficient to produce the syndrome because the metabolism of vasopressin is normally increased three- to fourfold during pregnancy.[161] Gestational DI usually begins in the first trimester of pregnancy and remits within 4 to 6 weeks after delivery of the placenta. This pattern distinguishes it from pregnancy in a woman with established pituitary DI.[304,305] In both types of DI, basal plasma osmolality/sodium on ad libitum fluid intake tends to be lower because the osmotic threshold for thirst as well as vasopressin secretion is reduced during pregnancy.[38] Otherwise, the pathophysiology of gestational DI is similar to pituitary DI.

Primary Polydipsia

DI can also result from a deficiency of vasopressin secretion that is secondary to excessive intake of water. This condition is usually referred to as primary polydipsia and can be subdivided into three types depending on the cause of the excessive fluid intake (Table 8-2). One type appears to be due to a primary defect in the osmoregulation of thirst and has been referred to as dipsogenic diabetes insipidus.[306] It may result from multifocal diseases involving the hypothalamus (neurosarcoid,[306,307] tuberculous meningitis,[306] and multiple sclerosis,[307]) but is usually idiopathic. The exact location of the lesions responsible for the abnormal thirst has not been determined, but hyperdipsia can be produced experimentally in rats by lesioning the midbrain,[308] septal nuclei,[309] and nucleus medianus.[310] The second type of primary polydipsia is due to a more general cognitive defect associated with schizophrenia or other psychiatric disorders.[311,312] It is usually referred to as psychogenic polydipsia or compulsive water drinking. With rare exception, these patients do not complain of thirst and usually attribute their polydipsia to bizarre personal motives, such as a need to cleanse their system of poison. The third type of primary polydipsia is not associated with either increased thirst or overt mental illness, but is prompted by the medical advice of physicans, nurses, folk practitioners, or the lay media. It may be referred to as iatrogenic polydipsia.

TABLE 8-2. Causes of Primary Polydipsia

Acquired
Psychogenic
Schizophrenia
Obsessive-compulsive disorder
Dipsogenic (abnormal thirst)
Granulomas
Neurosarcoid
Infectious
Tuberculous meningitis
Head trauma
Closed
Penetrating (pituitary-hypothalamic surgery)
Demyelinization
Multiple sclerosis
Drugs
Lithium
Carbazepine
Idiopathic
Iatrogenic

The pathogenesis and pathophysiology of the DI produced by primary polydipsia is the opposite of that for pituitary DI. Thus, excessive intake of water slightly reduces the effective osmotic pressure of body fluids, thereby inhibiting the secretion of vasopressin. This results in a water diuresis that compensates completely for the increased intake and stabilizes the osmolality of body fluids at a new, slightly lower level approximating the osmotic threshold for vasopressin secretion. The magnitude of the DI varies from patient to patient depending on the nature and/or intensity of the stimulus to drink. In those with dipsogenic DI, the osmotic threshold for thirst appears to be reset below that for vasopressin secretion.[306] Polydipsia reduces but does not completely relieve the desire to drink because the resultant suppression of vasopressin produces a water diuresis that prevents the dilution of body water to the abnormally low level required to osmotically inhibit thirst. Thus, thirst, polydipsia, and polyuria persist at a level that is proportional to the reduction in the osmotic threshold for thirst. When the reduction is large, thirst is very intense and the rate of water intake and urine output may approximate 15 to 20 L/day.[306] In psychogenic polydipsia, the stimulus to drink is not driven by thirst. However, it may vary with the emotional state of the patient and can also reach levels exceeding 20 L/day. Iatrogenic polydipsia is usually mild and rarely results in urine outputs of more than 5 L/day.

Primary polydipsia rarely results in water intoxication unless the capacity to dilute the urine and/or mount a maximum water diuresis is also impaired. In patients with the dipsogenic form, this impairment usually results from misdiagnosis and inappropriate administration of DDAVP, but can also be caused by an increase in vasopressin secretion triggered by an acute nonosmotic stimulus such as nausea or smoking. In psychogenic polydipsia, water intoxication is much more frequent[313–315] and can be fatal.[316] It is often due, at least in part, to inappropriate secretion of vasopressin.[313–321] This defect can take any of several forms,[32] including downward resetting of the osmostat.[317,321] Patients with resetting of the vasopressin osmostat may present with hyponatremia and maximum urinary dilution, suggesting incorrectly that their water intoxication was caused by excessive drinking alone. However, if tested serially during water restriction, they begin to concentrate their urine before plasma osmolality and/or sodium return to normal.[318] Studies in rats suggest that slight downward resetting of the vasopressin osmostat could be caused by chronic polydipsia *per se*.[322] However, this does not appear to be the case in humans because it does not occur in patients with dipsogenic DI[306] or psychogenic polydipsia without a history of hyponatremia.[323] Downward resetting of the vasopressin osmostat in hyponatremic polydipsic schizophrenics also cannot be attributed to hemodynamic stimuli[321,323] or a defect in oropharyngeal influences,[324] but vasopressin release in this subgroup of schizophrenics appears to be more susceptible to stimulation by acute, drug-induced psychosis.[325] These patients may also have a vasopressin independent defect in urine dilution[321,323] and a diminution in the size of the anterior medial temporal lobe[326] of unknown cause.

Nephrogenic DI

A primary defect in the antidiuretic action of vasopressin results in a syndrome commonly referred to as *nephrogenic diabetes insipidus*. It was first recognized as a familial disorder that was inherited in an X-linked recessive or semirecessive mode.[327,328] This form has now been linked to more than 150 different mutations of the gene on chromosome Xq28 that encodes the renal V_2 receptor.[329,330] These mutations appear to impair V_2 receptor function in a variety of ways including deficient synthesis, misfolding and misrouting from the ER, increased degradation, decreased binding affinity for vasopressin, and inefficient linkage to second messenger. Recently, another form of familial nephrogenic DI that is inherited in an autosomal recessive or autosomal dominant mode has been discovered and linked to more than 15 different mutations in one or both alleles of the gene that encodes aquaporin-2,[329–333] the protein that forms the hydroosmotic water channels activated by vasopressin in renal collecting tubules. In both forms of familial nephrogenic DI, the disease is present from birth. In the X-linked type, males who inherit the mutation are always affected and female carriers usually but not always are not. Most of these mutation largely or completely abolish the antidiuretic effect of vasopressin, but a few affecting the V_2 receptor result in partial resistance[334] that is characterized by a 10-fold or greater shift to the right in the dose response curve (Fig. 8-13). As a result, they are able to concentrate their urine quite well during a fluid deprivation test (Fig. 8-14). Severe or partial nephrogenic DI can also be acquired as a result of other diseases or drugs (Table 8-3),[331,335] the most notable of which is lithium.[336] In addition to interfering with the antidiuretic action of vasopressin, this drug also increases the sensitivity of vasopressin secretion to osmotic stimulation[337] and may produce dipsogenic DI[338] by an independent effect on the thirst mechanism. Because of this and the existence of partial as well as severe forms of vasopressin deficiency, correct differentiation between the various types of DI is not always easy, as discussed later.

TABLE 8-3. Causes of Nephrogenic DI

Acquired
Drugs
Lithium
Demeclocycline
Methoxyflurane
Amphotericin B
Aminoglycosides
Cisplatin
Rifampin
Foscarnet
Metabolic
Hypercalcemia, hypercalciuria
Hypokalemia
Mechanical
Postobstruction of ureters or urethra
Vascular
Sickle cell disease and trait
Ischemia (tubular necrosis)
Granulomas
Neurosarcoid
Neoplasms
Sarcoma
Infiltration
Amyloidosis
Idiopathic
Genetic
X-linked recessive (vasopressin receptor-2 gene)
Autosomal recessive (aquaporin-2 gene)
Autosomal dominant (aquaporin-2 gene)

The pathophysiology of nephrogenic DI is similar in most respects to pituitary DI. Thus, insensitivity to the antidiuretic effect of vasopressin also results in the excretion of increased volumes of dilute urine. This loss causes a decrease in body water and a slight rise in plasma osmolality, which, by stimulating the thirst mechanism, induces a compensatory increase in water intake. As a consequence, the osmolality of body fluid stabilizes at a new and higher level which approximates the osmotic threshold for thirst. Unlike pituitary DI, however, plasma vasopressin is elevated. Moreover, for unknown reasons, this elevation is out of proportion to the relatively modest increase in plasma osmolality, and fluid deprivation produces a further increase in plasma osmolality and vasopressin to very high levels (Fig. 8-13). These large increases in vasopressin cause little or no increase in urine osmolality in most patients, but often produce very dramatic increases in urine concentration in those with partial resistance (Figs. 8-13 and 8-14). As in patients with partial pituitary DI, this residual capacity to concentrate the urine is not used under basal conditions of ad libitum fluid intake because stimulation of thirst and polydipsia prevents the patient from developing the level of hypertonic dehydration and hypervasopressinemia required to overcome renal insensitivity to the hormone. However, because infants have not yet developed the motor or verbal abilities necessary to ensure a high fluid intake, some of them may suffer chronic hypertonic dehydration and hypervasopressinemia that delays recognition of the partial defects. Unrecognized episodes of dehydration may also be responsible for the increased incidence of mental retardation in the disease. Children with untreated nephrogenic DI may also grow more slowly than normal, possibly because their thirst and polydipsia interferes with their appetite and eating. Patients with mutations of the V_2 receptor gene also lack the normal vasodepressor and coagulation factor response to DDAVP,[339] but these defects do not result in clinically appreciable defects in baroregulation or hemostasis.

Differential Diagnosis

When DI is suspected, the diagnosis should be verified by determining the volume, osmolality, and creatinine content of urine collected for 24 h under conditions of ad libitum fluid intake. Measuring the osmolality or specific gravity of a random urine collection is less reliable because it can give false positive result in an anxious patient who water loads to produce an adequate sample or a false negative result in a patient with partial pituitary or partial nephrogenic DI. Measurements of basal plasma osmolality or sodium under conditions of ad libitum fluid intake are rarely useful to verify DI because they are almost always within the normal range. However, they should be obtained because an elevated value serves to identify the occasional patient with hypodipsia who does not need and may be harmed by a fluid deprivation test. If tests of the 24-h urine are normal, no further evaluation for DI is needed unless there is reason to suspect that the disorder is being masked by a concomitant disease such as adrenal insufficiency[340,341] or adipsic hypernatremia (discussed later). In that case, the tests of a 24-h urine collection should be repeated after the associated deficiency of cortisol or water is corrected. If indicated, as in the postpartum patient with gestational DI, a hypertonic saline infusion test (see later) also may be used to determine if there is a subclinical deficiency in vasopressin secretion.

If the 24-h urine collection confirms the presence of DI and the basal plasma osmolality and sodium are not elevated, a fluid deprivation test should be performed. Because patients with a severe defect in the secretion or action of vasopressin can become severely dehydrated in only a few hours, the fluid deprivation should be performed during the day without prior restriction of eating or drinking and should be monitored closely with hourly measurements of body weight, plasma osmolality or sodium, urine output, and urine osmolality. If fluid restriction does not result in concentration of the urine (osmolality >300 mosmol/kg) before plasma osmolality and/or sodium reach 300 mosmol/kg and/or 146 mEq/l (290 mosmol/kg and/or 141 mEq/l during pregnancy), primary polydipsia as well as partial defects in vasopressin secretion or action are virtually excluded, and the distinction between severe pituitary and severe nephrogenic DI usually can be made by injecting 1–2 units of aqueous Pitressin or 1–2 μg of DDAVP and repeating the measurements of urine osmolality 1–2 h later (Fig. 8-14). In this setting, a rise in urine osmolality of more than 50 percent is virtually diagnostic of severe pituitary (or gestational) DI even though the maximum levels achieved may be markedly subnormal due to the temporary defect in renal concentrating capacity caused by the prior lack of vasopressin action.[290] Conversely, a rise in urine osmolality of <50 percent usually indicates severe nephrogenic DI.[290,342,343] However, this criterion misdiagnoses about 10 percent of patients with severe pituitary DI because their secondary defect in renal concentrating capacity is so severe that they cannot respond to DDAVP until their renal medullary hypertonicity and aquaporin production are restored. Because this repair seems to begin within an hour or two of hormone treatment, the possibility of misdiagnosing patients who fail to respond immediately can be reduced by repeating the measurements of urine osmolality at 3 to 4 h.

If fluid deprivation results in concentration of the urine, these indirect criteria are unreliable for differentiating between primary polydipsia and a partial deficiency in vasopressin secretion or action (Fig. 8-14).[290,342,343] The reason probably is that the secondary defect in renal concentrating capacity caused by the prior lack of vasopressin action[290] starts to improve almost as soon as fluid restriction begins to increase urinary concentration. Therefore, any further rise in urine osmolality that is observed after the administration of exogenous vasopressin or DDAVP can be due in whole or in part to continued improvement in the secondary defect, rather than to correction of a primary deficiency in vasopressin secretion or action. The ambiguity in interpretation that results cannot be eliminated by prolonging the initial fluid restriction because complete repair of the concentrating defect may take 24–48 h and few patients would tolerate continuing the dehydration and fasting for this length of time. The simplest and most effective way to avoid this problem is to directly measure vasopressin in aliquots of plasma and/or urine collected before and during the fluid deprivation test.[290,342–349] For maximum clarity, these values should be analyzed in relation to the concurrent plasma and urine osmolality (Fig. 8-13) and at least one measurement should be made when plasma osmolality is above the normal range. Because the requisite level of hypertonic dehydration may be difficult to achieve by fluid restriction alone once urinary concentration begins, most of these patients should also be given a supplemental infusion of hypertonic (3 percent) saline (0.1 ml/kg/min) to shorten the procedure. This infusion should be continued for 60 to 90 min or until plasma osmolality and/or sodium exceeds the upper limit of the normal range, at which point a final sample for measurement of vasopressin should be collected. With this approach, patients with partial defects in vasopressin secretion can be differentiated easily from those with partial nephrogenic DI or primary polydipsia (Fig. 8-13*A*). In most cases, the latter two disorders also can be distinguished by examining the relation of urine osmolality to the concurrent level of vasopressin during the fluid deprivation test (Fig. 8-13*B*), although this interpretation may also be clouded by secondary defects in renal concentrating capacity. In this case, the measurement of basal plasma vasopressin is usually also helpful because it is almost always elevated in patients with nephrogenic DI but is low or completely suppressed in those with primary polydipsia. In the latter group of patients, the dipsogenic, psychogenic, and iatrogenic forms can usually be differentiated on the basis of the history and the relationship of plasma osmolality to ratings of thirst[36] during the fluid deprivation/hypertonic saline infusion (Fig. 8-13).

As might be expected, most patients with pituitary DI also exhibit a subnormal rise in vasopressin secretion after hemodynamic, emetic, and glucopenic stimuli.[345] For diagnostic purposes, however, these nonosmotic tests of neurohypophyseal function do not appear to provide any particular advantage over dehydration/hypertonic saline infusion, and they are usually more stressful for the physician and the patient.

Pregnant patients with DI should be evaluated in the same manner as nonpregnant patients except that the maximum level of plasma osmolality and sodium to be achieved during the fluid deprivation/hypertonic saline infusion test should be lowered by about 10 mosmol/kg and 5 mEq/l because the osmostats for thirst and vasopressin secretion are also set lower during gestation;[38] samples for assay of plasma vasopressin should be collected directly into phenanthroline or other inhibitors of placental vasopressinase to prevent degradation of endogenous vasopressin during processing;[301,305] and the assay results should be analyzed using a special nomogram adjusted for the effects of pregnancy.[38]

Magnetic resonance imaging (MRI) of the brain is also useful in the differential diagnosis of DI.[251,350] In 80 to 90 percent of healthy children and adults, the posterior pituitary emits a hyperintense signal ("bright spot") on T_1-weighted, noninfused midsagittal images (Fig. 8-15).[351,352] The source of the signal is still uncertain, but it is usually not eliminated by fat suppression techniques[353] and may be generated by phospholipid vesicles in the neurohyphophysis.[354] In any event, this bright spot is abnormally small or absent in most[251,350] but possibly not all[355,356] patients with pituitary DI. This includes almost all patients with familial pituitary DI even though their oxytocinergic neurons are apparently normal. In contrast, the pituitary bright spot is present in 80 to 90 percent of patients with primary polydipsia. Thus, MRI is very good for ruling out pituitary DI (if the bright spot is present) but is less reliable for ruling it in (if the bright spot is absent). When used as an aid in the differential diagnosis, MRI should always be performed with fat suppression techniques to avoid confusing fat in the marrow of the dorsum sella with the posterior pituitary bright spot. Fluid filled cysts in the pars intermedia or posterior pituitary can also simulate the normal bright spot although they are usually rounder and less bean-shaped. A false positive result (absence of the bright spot) also may result if the images are more than 3 mm apart and none goes through or very near the midline of the brain.

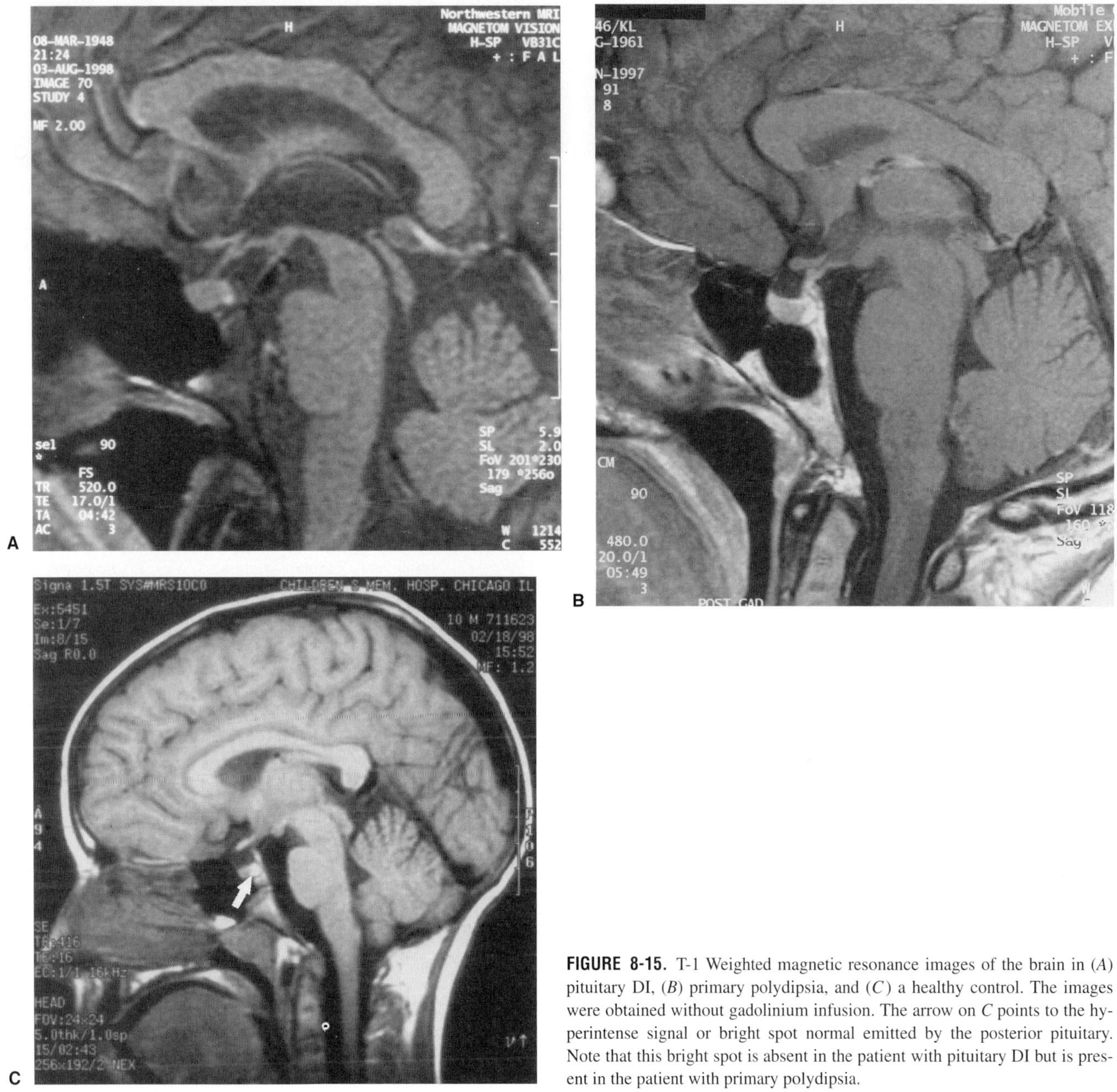

FIGURE 8-15. T-1 Weighted magnetic resonance images of the brain in (*A*) pituitary DI, (*B*) primary polydipsia, and (*C*) a healthy control. The images were obtained without gadolinium infusion. The arrow on *C* points to the hyperintense signal or bright spot normal emitted by the posterior pituitary. Note that this bright spot is absent in the patient with pituitary DI but is present in the patient with primary polydipsia.

The various types of DI can also be differentiated by their distinctive responses to a closely monitored therapeutic trial of DDAVP (see later).[342,343]

Management

Pituitary DI

The treatment of choice is a synthetic analog of vasopressin known as DDAVP (desmopressin) (Fig. 8-2).[357–362] The modifications in positions 1 and 8 of the molecule enhance its antidiuretic potency, eliminate its effects on V_1 receptors, and increase significantly its resistance to metabolic degradation. Consequently, it has a much longer duration of action than the native molecule and can be given by parenteral, intranasal, or oral routes. The most convenient mode of administration for chronic therapy is usually the nasal spray or tablet. The dose required to completely eliminate polyuria must be determined empirically, but usually ranges from 10 to 20 μg i.n. or 100 to 400 μg p.o. every 8 to 12 h in adults. It is slightly less in children. The antidiuretic effect usually begins within 60 to 90 min and is followed promptly by the retention of a small amount of water (usually about 0.5 to 1.0 kg), a slight decrease in plasma osmolality and sodium (about 1 to 2 percent) and complete cessation of thirst and polydipsia (Fig. 8-16). Consequently, water intake and urine output rapidly come back into balance and plasma osmolality/sodium stabilize within the normal range. Erratic responses to intranasal or oral DDAVP usually result from poor absorption due to sinusitis, rhinitis, or interference by food. These problems can usually be alleviated by use of nasal decongestants or taking the tablets on an empty stomach. If not, it may be necessary to take DDAVP by injection or switch to

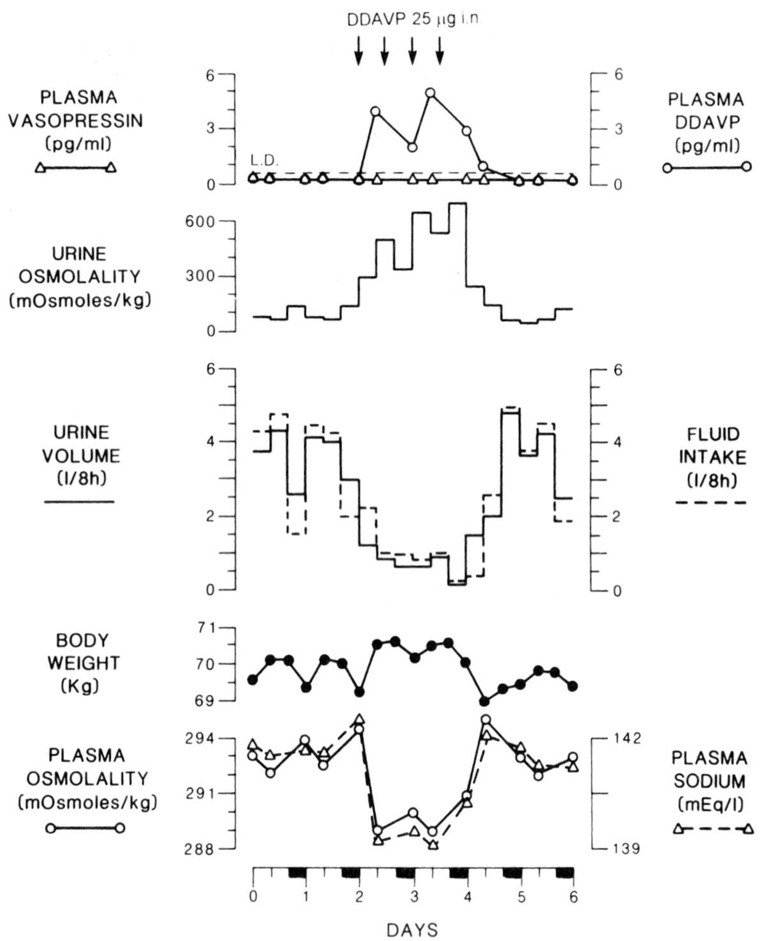

FIGURE 8-16. The effect of DDAVP on water balance in a patient with uncomplicated partial pituitary DI due to a dysgerminoma. Plasma vasopressin (AVP) was measured by an immunoassay that does not cross react with DDAVP. Plasma DDAVP was measured using an assay that cross-reacts equally with AVP and DDAVP. Note that the antidiuretic response to DDAVP was blunted during the first 8 h and did not rise to normal levels for nearly 24 h even though plasma DDAVP was near maximal levels from the beginning. Note also that discretionary fluid intake decreased as fast and as much as urine output resulting in only slight retention of water and a small decrease (1–2%) in plasma osmolality and sodium.

another form of treatment. Resistance due to antibody production has not been observed with DDAVP although it has occurred with Pitressin.[363]

During long-term treatment of uncomplicated pituitary DI, it is usually not necessary to allow periodic "escape" from the antidiuretic effect of DDAVP because the thirst mechanism normally is quite effective at down regulating fluid intake to keep it in balance with output.[229] However, it is important to educate the patient about the importance of drinking only when truly thirsty. Plasma sodium also should be checked regularly or anytime that symptoms suggestive of water intoxication occur. Two or more episodes of significant hyponatremia (plasma sodium <130 mEq/l) indicate the intake of fluid is often excessive and the reason usually can be determined from a careful interview. Sometimes there is an obvious psychogenic etiology. More often, however, the polydipsia turns out to be due to an excessive concern about the dangers of dehydration or to a defect in the osmotic suppression of thirst. If the latter appears to be present, the patient should be withdrawn from treatment and reevaluated thoroughly (see Differential Diagnosis) to verify the thirst abnormality as well as the original diagnosis of pituitary DI. If the patient proves to have the combined defect, chlorpropamide appears to be a safer form of treatment because its antidiuretic effect is reduced by overhydration (discussed later). However, if reevaluation reveals that DI is due solely to abnormal thirst (dipsogenic DI), the approach to treatment should be different.

The management of pituitary DI in infants as well as in obtunded or postoperative patients often presents special problems because DDAVP cannot be given orally or intranasally and/or water intake is not controlled by the usual physiologic variables. In this situation, the aim usually should be to inject or infuse DDAVP in doses sufficient to maintain urine output and osmolality within the normal range (15–30 ml/kg/day and 400– 800 mosmol/kg, respectively) and maintain total fluid intake at a level equal to the sum of urine output plus an appropriate amount for insensible loss (4–12 ml/kg/day when body temperature is normal). This can usually be accomplished by injecting 1–4 μg of DDAVP s.c. or i.v. every 12–24 h. If fluid intake cannot be restricted to the required level, the dose or frequency of DDAVP administration should be reduced sufficiently to allow periodic "escape" in order to prevent water intoxication. The effectiveness of the regimen should be monitored by measuring plasma osmolality or sodium at least twice a day until fluid intake can be regulated solely by thirst or other measures of physiologic need.

Pituitary DI can also be treated with chlorpropamide (Diabinese), a drug more commonly used to treat diabetes mellitus.[357,364–366] At conventional doses of 250 to 500 mg/day, it increases urine osmolality and reduces polyuria by 25 to 75 percent in patients with severe as well as partial pituitary DI.[366] This antidiuretic effect results in a small increase in body water, a commensurate decrease in plasma osmolality and sodium, and a prompt reduction in thirst and polydipsia similar to that caused by

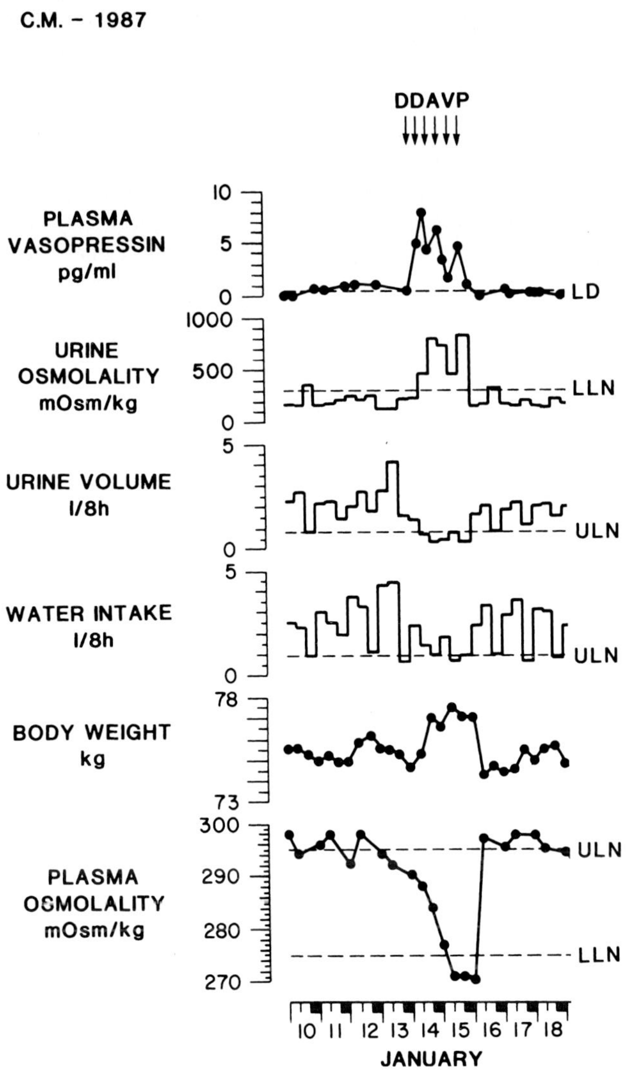

FIGURE 8-18. The effect of DDAVP on water balance in a patient with idiopathic dipsogenic DI. The values for plasma "vasopressin" were obtained with an immunoassay that cross-reacts equally well with vasopressin and DDAVP. The vertical arrows indicate the times at which 10 μg of DDAVP were taken by nasal spray. ULN and LLN indicate, respectively, the upper and lower limits of normal for the variable indicated. LD refers to the limit of detectability of the assay. Note that the antidiuretic response to DDAVP was blunted initially and did not reach normal levels for about 24 h even though plasma levels of the analogue were maximum in the first 8 h. Note also that thirst and fluid intake decreased as water was retained and plasma osmolality decreased. However, the reduction in intake was smaller than the reduction in urine output, resulting in excessive retention of water (as evidenced by the gain in weight) and decrease in plasma osmolality to subnormal levels.

of the potential hazards of nicotine and the many other drugs or illnesses that can stimulate release of endogenous vasopressin.

The management of dipsogenic DI should also include a search for the cause (Table 8-2) and possible associated defects in hypothalamic and anterior pituitary function. In addition to a history and physical focused on other symptoms and signs, this search should include an MRI of the brain and tests of baseline thyroid and adrenal function.

Nephrogenic DI

When due to a metabolic disorder or drug such as hypercalemia, hypokalemia, amphotericin B, demeclocycline, or lithium, nephrogenic DI often stops if the cause is eliminated before secondary, irreversible renal damage occurs.[385–389] However, nephrogenic DI is usually irreversible when lithium has been taken for more than a few years or it is caused by another disease or a mutation of the V_2 receptor or aquaporin-2 gene. In these patients, the nephrogenic DI cannot be eliminated completely, but it can be ameliorated by a combination of dietary sodium restriction and treatment with a thiazide diuretic,[376] amiloride,[390,391] and/or a prostaglandin synthetase inhibitor.[392–394] Used alone or in combination, these drugs will reduce polyuria by 30 to 70 percent in most patients. This antidiuretic effect is associated with a commensurate increase in urine osmolality and a slight reduction in plasma osmolality/sodium that also relieves some of the thirst and polydipsia. The thiazide diuretics work by inhibiting sodium reabsorption in the diluting segment of the nephron. The resultant reduction in body sodium causes a slight contraction of extracellular volume that stimulates increased reabsorption of glomerular filtrate in the proximal tubule, thereby decreasing delivery to the distal nephron.[376] Thus, urinary volume as well as urinary dilution are reduced by a mechanism that does not require the action of vasopressin on the distal nephron but is critically dependent on net sodium loss and contraction of the extracellular volume. The latter also produces secondary hyperaldosternism, increased excretion of potassium and hydrogen ions, and mild hypokalemia that may necessitate potassium replacement. The mechanism by which amiloride reduces DI is probably similar to thiazides except that it does not increase excretion of potassium or hydrogen and may also prevent some of the toxic effects of lithium on the renal concentrating mechanism.[390,395] The prostaglandin inhibitors are thought to act by interfering with feedback inhibition of vasopressin action within the kidney.[392] DDAVP is ineffective in severe nephrogenic DI, but it can produce urine concentration in those with partial forms of the syndrome.[334] This treatment is impractical for long-term use, however, because the doses required are high and prohibitively expensive. Chlorpropamide is ineffective in nephrogenic DI.

Other Deficiencies of Vasopressin

Enuresis and Nocturia

Enuresis and nocturia are related syndromes characterized, respectively, by involuntary or voluntary excretion of urine during sleep.[396,397] They occur most frequently in children and the elderly where they are so common as to be regarded virtually as normal stages of development or aging. However, they also afflict about 1 to 2 percent of the population between the ages of 15 and 55 years. Occasionally, enuresis or nocturia is due to DI or another form of global polyuria. More often, however, it is due to a defect in bladder function or the production of abnormally large volumes of subnormally concentrated urine during sleep.[397,398] This nocturnal polyuria appears to be due to a circadian deficiency in the secretion or antidiuretic action of vasopressin. The cause of these selective deficiencies is unknown although a genetic defect may be involved in some children with enuresis.[399]

The differential diagnosis of enuresis and nocturia includes diabetes mellitus, DI, a primary sleep disorder, defective bladder function, and idiopathic nocturnal polyuria. These various causes can be distinguished most easily by having the patient record the time and volume of each urine voided spontaneously during a 24–48-h period. If this voiding diary reveals that the total and circadian pattern of urine output is normal (Fig. 8-10), the patient probably has a primary sleep disturbance or urological defect and should be evaluated further for these abnormalities. However, if the voiding diary indicates that the total or nocturnal urine output is abnormally increased, all urine produced during three successive 8-h periods should be collected and analyzed for volume, osmolality, and creatinine to verify the accuracy of the voiding diary and determine if the global or nocturnal polyuria is due to a water diuresis or a solute diuresis. If the 24-h urine has an abnormally large volume (>50 ml/kg), a low osmolality (<300 mosmol/kg), and a normal solute excretion (<20 mosmol/kg body weight), the patient has a global water diuresis and should be evaluated to determine the type of DI before instituting appropriate treatment. However, if only the overnight urine volume is high (>4 ml/kg BW per 8 h), the patient has nocturnal polyuria and will not benefit from further evaluation of antidiuretic function. In this situation, the only therapeutically useful distinction is whether the nocturnal polyuria is due to a solute diuresis (solute excretion >3 mosmoles per kg body weight per 8 h) or water diuresis as different treatments should be used.

The treatment for enuresis or nocturia caused by a nocturnal water diuresis is a reduction in fluid intake after supper and/or administration of DDAVP at bedtime. The drug can be given by tablet, nasal insufflation, or injection, but the dose required to eliminate the enuresis or nocturia is often higher than in patients with pituitary or dipsogenic DI, possibly because nocturnal polyuria may also involve some resistance to the antidiuretic effect of the hormone. The only significant side-effect of DDAVP therapy for enuresis or nocturia is hyponatremia.[400–402] This complication seems to be unusual and may be nearly eliminated by giving the drug as a single dose at bedtime and prescreening patients to exlude those with primary polydipsia as a contributing or causative factor. If the nocturnal polyuria is due largely or wholly to a nocturnal solute diuresis, DDAVP treatment has little effect, and better results may be obtained by administering a diuretic such as furosemide in the morning in order to restablish the normal circadian pattern of salt and water excretion.

Postural Hypotension

Postural hypotension is a syndrome characterized by a significant fall in mean arterial pressure after sitting or standing (see Chap. 12). The fall in pressure may result in symptoms ranging from a mild feeling of fatigue or dizziness to syncope. It has many causes including a reduction in blood volume or a defect in autonomic activity. Some of the latter seem to be due to a lesion in the afferent or "sensing" arm of the baroregulatory system, resulting not only in a blunted rise in heart rate but also an isolated deficiency in the vasopressin response to a hypotensive stimulus.[403] These deficiencies seem particularly common in Shy-Drager disease and diabetic autonomic neuropathy. Besides localizing the lesion to the afferent arm of the baroregulatory loop, loss of the chronotropic and/or vasopressin response to hypotension may also exacerbate the orthostatic fall in blood pressure. However, they do not alter usual management because they are not correctable by any treatment now available.

Deficiency of Thirst

Hypernatremia

A prolonged reduction in water intake has little or no clinical significance if it is matched by a commensurate reduction water output. However, if the total amount of water obtained from food and beverage is less than the minimum obligatory output from the kidneys, lungs, skin, and gastrointestinal tract, total body water decreases and the solute concentration of body fluid increases. This change is evidenced by a proportionate rise in plasma osmolality and sodium. If the dehydration develops slowly, it may have no other clinically discernible effect except an increase in plasma urea, creatinine, uric acid, and sometimes thirst. The lack of effect may be due partly to adaptive increases in intracellular solute which serve to defend cell volume by counteracting the osmotically driven dehydration that would otherwise result.[404a,404b] However, if the hypertonic dehydration develops rapidly or is particularly severe, it usually results in overt clinical signs of hypovolemia and damage to the brain and other organs (described later). The causes of inadequate fluid intake are numerous and can be divided between those with and without a primary defect in the thirst mechanism.

Adipsic Hypernatremia

A global deficiency in thirst results in a syndrome characterized by chronic or recurrent episodes of severe hypertonic dehydration.[229,404a,405] Besides hypernatremia and mild to moderate signs of volume depletion (tachycardia, postural hypotension, azotemia, hyperuricemia, hypokalemia, hyperreninemia, and hyperaldosteronism), these patients report little or no thirst and usually refuse water when it is offered to them. They are often surprisingly alert and healthy in appearance. However, they may suffer a variety of complications, including chorea, confusion, coma, convulsions, paralysis, cerebral hemorrhage, rhabdomyolysis, and acute renal failure.[405–409] They may also have hyperglycemia and hyperlipidemia that requires insulin therapy until the dehydration is corrected.

The cause of deficient thirst is usually hypogenesis or destruction of the osmoregulatory system by pathology involving the anterior hypothalamus.[229,404a,405,410–420] These lesions can be induced by a variety of disorders (Table 8-4). In a few patients, no anatomic lesions have been identified. In all but one of the patients in whom it was evaluated, the osmoregulation of vasopressin has also been deficient, presumably because the cells that mediate this control are located in much the same area of the anterior hypothalamus as the thirst osmoreceptors. This deficiency is usually selective because the neurohypophysis appears normal on the MRI and vasopressin secretion responds normally or even supranormally to non-osmotic stimuli.[229,404a,405,410,411,417] Autopsy studies delineating the precise location and histologic appearance of the lesions responsible for this syndrome have not been reported, but experiments in animals have shown that similar defects in thirst and/or vasopressin secretion can be produced by lesioning areas of the anterolateral hypothalamus near the supraoptic nuclei.[33,34,233] In a few patients with adipsic hypernatremia, the neurohypophysis is also destroyed resulting in a global deficiency in vasopressin secretion.[410]

The pathogenesis and pathophysiology of adipsic hypernatremia are simple in principal. Because the thirst mechanism fails to stimulate the intake of enough water to replenish renal and extrarenal losses, total body water declines and becomes more concentrated, resulting in hypertonicity and hypernatremia.[228,229,405,410] The reduction in extracellular volume also decreases renal perfusion and increases plasma urea, plasma renin activity, and aldosterone secretion. Consequently, sodium is maximally conserved and potassium is lost, aggravating the hypernatremia and inducing

TABLE 8-4. Causes of Adipsic Hypernatremia

- Acquired
  - Vascular
    - Occlusion anterior communicating artery
  - Tumors
    - Primary
      - Craniopharyngioma
      - Pinealoma, germinoma
      - Meningioma
      - Glioma
    - Metastatic (lung, breast)
  - Granulomas
    - Neurosarcoid
    - Histiocytosis
  - Trauma
    - Closed
    - Penetrating (pituitary-hypothalamic surgery)
  - Psychogenic
    - Psychotic Depression
  - Other
    - Hydrocephalus
    - Cystic
    - Degenerative
  - Idiopathic
- Congenital
  - Midline malformation (septum & corpus callosum)
  - Microcephaly
- Genetic
  - Autosomal recessive (Schinzel-Giedion Syndrome)

hypokalemia. The hypernatremia and/or hypokalemia, in turn, sometimes result in rhabdomyolysis and myoglobinuria which, in the presence of decreased renal perfusion, may produce acute renal failure. The relationship between these changes and the severe carbohydrate intolerance and hyperlipidemia that may also occur transiently during dehydration is unknown.

In hypodipsic patients, water output need not be increased for hypertonic dehydration to develop because the amount of water in food is usually inadequate to replace even minimal obligatory urinary and insensible losses. Often, however, the development of dehydration is accelerated or exacerbated by an increase in urinary or insensible loss resulting from a deficiency of vasopressin or an increase in physical activity or ambient temperature. The deficiency of vasopressin that results from loss of osmoreceptor stimulation produces a constellation of clinical abnormalities different from that caused by a deficiency in the neurohypophysis itself. DI usually is not present when the patient presents with hypertonic dehydration because the deficiency in plasma vasopressin is not great enough to prevent concentration of the urine. However, during rehydration, plasma vasopressin and urine osmolality sometimes decrease to a level that results in DI, thereby interfering with complete correction of the dehydration. Originally, this pattern of premature urinary dilution during rehydration was attributed to upward resetting of the osmostat, an entity sometimes referred to as *essential hypernatremia*. However, regression analysis of the relation between plasma osmolality and urine osmolality or plasma vasopressin has shown that this abnormality in antidiuretic function is usually, if not always, due to a reduction in the slope or sensitivity of the osmoregulatory system (Fig. 8-19).[32,229,404a,405,410,411,418] In other patients with hypodipsic hypernatremia, forced rehydration does not result in a water diuresis even if hyponatremia develops (Fig. 8-19).[32,229,404a,405,410,416] This paradoxical defect resembles that seen in the syndrome of inappropriate antidiuresis and appears to result from two different mechanisms. One is a continuous or fixed secretion of vasopressin due to a total loss of osmoregulatory function (Fig. 8-19). In these patients, plasma vasopressin continues to circulate in small but biologically effective amounts irrespective of increases or decreases in hydration. In the other type of dilutional defect, urine osmolality remains high even when plasma vasopressin is suppressed to undetectable levels. The cause of this abnormality is unknown but may involve supersensitivity of the kidney to low levels of vasopressin.

The differential diagnosis of adipsic hypernatremia includes hypertonic dehydration due to various physical impediments such as prolonged immobilization, impaired consciousness, or an environmental deficiency of potable water, as well as from the hypernatremia that occasionally results from excessive intake or retention of sodium (Table 8-5).[404a,421,422] These distinctions can usually

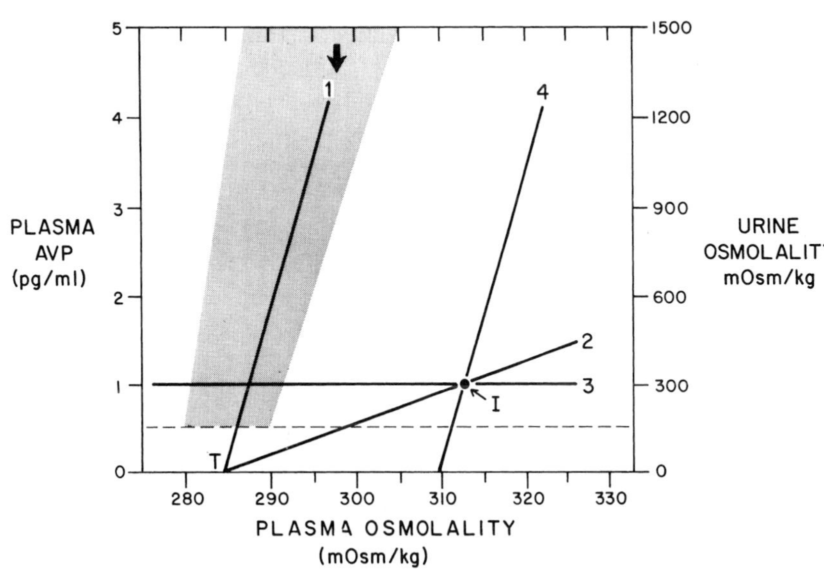

FIGURE 8-19. Schematic diagram of the relation of plasma vasopressin or urine osmolality to plasma osmolality in healthy adults and patients with hypernatremia of diverse etiology. The shaded area indicates the range of normal. Line 1 represents a typical healthy adult. Lines 2 and 3 represent patients with adipsic hypernatremia due to partial or complete destruction of the osmostat, respectively. Line 4 indicates the relation for a patient with the hypothetical entity of reset osmostat. The closed arrow indicates the osmotic threshold for thirst in the healthy adult. The level of vasopressin at which urinary dilution occurs is indicated by D. Note that dilution of the urine at inappropriately high levels of plasma osmolality can result either from partial osmoreceptor destruction or resetting of the osmostat.

TABLE 8-5. Differential Diagnosis of Hypernatremia

Deficient water intake (hypertonic dehydration)
Deficient thirst (adipsic hypernatremia)
Immobility
Stroke
Coma
Restraints
Environmental deprivation
Excessive water loss*
Pituitary or nephrogenic DI
Excessive sodium intake*
Hypertonic saline
Infant formula
Saline mouthwash
Intravenous therapy
Excessive sodium retention**
Primary hyperaldosteronism

*Transient unless associated with some deficiency in water intake.

**Depresses water intake by raising osmotic thirst threshold.

be made on the basis of the history, physical examination, and routine laboratory determinations. If a patient with physical and laboratory signs of hypertonic dehydration is conscious and mobile, a lack of thirst or desire to drink is virtually diagnostic of adipsic hypernatremia. If the patient is obtunded or otherwise unable to speak or drink on presentation the diagnosis may be made by monitoring thirst and plasma vasopressin during rehydration or a subsequent infusion of hypertonic saline.[32,229] If hypernatremia is associated with signs of extracellular volume expansion, it is probably due to an increase in total body sodium caused by excessive ingestion or retention. However, these forms of hypernatremia are usually corrected rapidly by drinking unless the patient also has a deficiency in osmotically mediated thirst or some other impediment to water intake.

The initial treatment of adipsic hypernatremia should aim to replace the water deficiency and minimize further losses by treating DI or diabetes mellitus if either is present.[404a] Hypokalemia should also be treated, particularly if it is associated with neuromuscular symptoms or hyperglycemia. The dehydration should be corrected gradually over a 24- to 48-h period. Free water should be given orally if possible, but it also can be infused intravenously either as 0.45 percent saline or 2.5 percent dextrose (if hyperglycemia is not present). The net increase in body water that must be achieved to correct the deficit can be estimated by the formula

$$\Delta H_2O = (Pna - 140/140) \times (BW)$$

where

ΔH_2O = the water deficit in liters
Pna = the plasma sodium concentration in mEq/l
BW = the body weight in kg.

If hyperglycemia is present, Pna should be corrected for dilution caused by a hydrosmotic shift from intracellular to extracellular space. This correction can be made by increasing the measured serum sodium by 1 mEq/l for every 36 mg/dl (2 mmol/l) that plasma glucose exceeds 90 mg/dl (5 mmol/l). The total amount of free water that needs to be given during a 24-h period to correct the hypernatremia can be estimated from the formula

$$\text{Total } H_2O = \Delta H_2O + \text{Uvol} + \text{IL}$$

in which Uvol and IL are, respectively, the ongoing 24-h urine output and insensible water loss, in liters. If the patient is afebrile and does not have DI or is receiving adequate amounts of DDAVP, IL and Uvol should approximate 10 and 25 ml/kg body weight, respectively. Fluid intake and urine output as well as plasma sodium, glucose, and potassium should be monitored and the treatments adjusted as necessary to normalize values by 24 to 48 h.

The long term management of patients with adipsic hypernatremia should aim to prevent or minimize recurrences of hypertonic dehydration. The keystones of this management plan should be (1) to minimize urinary water losses by treating with DDAVP or chlorpropamide if DI is present, as described previously, and (2) to ensure that fluid intake is just sufficient to replace water output. The latter objective can be quite challenging because both urinary and insensible loss can vary markedly from day to day depending on often unpredictable changes in DDAVP absorption, dietary solute load, ambient temperature, or physical activity. Moreover, too much water intake can be as dangerous as too little in these patients because their ability to excrete excess water usually is impaired by either concomitant antidiuretic therapy or a loss of the normal ability to osmotically suppress endogenous vasopressin. Hence, they are also prone to retain water and develop hyponatremia if their fluid intake is too high.[410] The best approach, therefore, is to teach the patient to drink according to a sliding scale based on daily changes in hydration as determined from changes in body weight.[229,410] The sliding scale can be made by assigning each patient a target weight that corresponds to optimum hydration (e.g., a serum sodium of 140 mEq/l) and a basal rate of water intake that approximates his or her rate of urine output and insensible loss under usual conditions of treatment, diet, temperature, and activity (e.g., 30–40 ml/kg/day). The basal rate of water intake is increased or decreased each day by an amount equal to the difference between the actual and the assigned target weight. The effectiveness of this program should be monitored by checking serum sodium every few weeks until the values stabilize and every 3–6 months thereafter. The target weight may need to be recalibrated periodically to compensate for changes in body mass. Rigorous compliance with the regimen will usually succeed in maintaining serum sodium concentration between 130 and 150 mEq/l which, in most cases, is sufficient to prevent complications and emergency readmissions to treat dehydration. However, constant reinforcement of the regimen is usually necessary because compliance tends to decline when symptoms and signs of dehydration are absent for prolonged periods.

Excess Vasopressin

A sustained increase in the secretion or action of vasopressin results in the production of smaller volumes of more concentrated urine. Normally, increasing antidiuresis has no clinically significant consequence because the resultant reduction in water loss permits a small increase in body water that, by slightly lowering plasma osmolality, induces a commensurate reduction in water intake. However, if for any reason water intake is not reduced sufficiently to match the reduction in output, the excess water accumulates and dilutes body fluids, resulting in the development of hypotonic hyponatremia. When it is mild or develops slowly, the hyponatremia usually produces few or no symptoms and may go unrecognized for long periods of time. This tolerance may be due to the fact that brain and many other cells appear to reversibly inactivate intracellular solute, thereby counteracting the osmotically driven swelling that would otherwise result from the fall in extracellular sodium concentration.[404a,423] However, if the hyponatremia develops rapidly (over 24 to 48 h) and/or is exceptionally severe (<120 mEq/l), it usually results in symptoms and signs of water intoxication which can range from mild headache or dizziness to anorexia, nausea, vomiting, confusion, coma, seizures, and occasionally death. The causes of undiminished or increased water intake in the face of increased antidiuresis are as varied as those in patients with primary polydipsia. The causes of the abnormal antidiuresis are also numerous and can be subdivided into primary and secondary disturbances in vasopressin secretion[404a] as well as several vasopressin-independent types of impaired water excretion.

Syndrome of Inappropriate Antidiuresis (SIADH)

Osmotically inappropriate antidiuresis that cannot be accounted for by any recognized nonosmotic stimulus is generally attributed to a primary abnormality in the regulation of vasopressin secretion or action. The clinical syndrome that results from this abnormality is variously referred to as SIADH, euvolemic hyponatremia, or Type IIIA hyponatremia. It was first described in two patients with bronchogenic carcinoma[424] and has since been recognized in patients with other types of tumors as well as many nonmalignant diseases or drug treatments (Table 8-6).[404a,425–435] It occurs with particular frequency and severity in patients with schizophrenia or other psychosis, probably because many of them have chronic psychogenic polydipsia that produces rapid expansion of body water and severe symptomatic hyponatremia any time that vasopressin secretion and/or urine osmolality increases sufficiently to impair even slightly a maximum water diuresis.[313–325]

Plasma vasopressin is elevated or inadequately suppressed in most patients with SIADH (Fig. 8-20).[426] In absolute terms, however, it is usually within the normal basal range. Therefore, the abnormality in vasopressin production can be identified with certainty only by measuring the hormone while plasma osmolality and sodium are subnormal. Except when the hormone is exogenous or made ectopically by a tumor,[436,437] the cause of the inappropriately high plasma vasopressin is unknown. Presumably, the hormone is released from the neurohypophysis as a result of some abnormality in the gland or one of its regulatory afferents. Several different pathogenic mechanisms probably are responsible because measurements of plasma vasopressin during treatment with hypertonic saline infusion have shown at least four distinct types of osmoregulatory dysfunction (Fig. 8-21).[404a,426,438–440] Type A is characterized by large and erratic fluctuations in plasma vasopressin which bear no relation whatever to the rise in plasma osmolality. It is found in about 25 percent of all patients with SIADH and appears to be due to a total loss of osmoreceptor control or intermittent stimulation by some unrecognized nonosmotic pathway. In the type B defect, plasma vasopressin remains fixed at

TABLE 8-6. Causes of Syndrome of Inappropriate Antidiuretic Hormone (SIADH)

- Acquired
  - Ectopic
    - Neoplasms
      - Carcinomas
        - Bronchus
        - Duodenum
        - Pancreas
        - Prostate
        - Ovary
        - Bladder, ureter
      - Thymoma
      - Mesothelioma
      - Ganglioglioma
      - Ewing's sarcoma
      - Thymoma
  - Eutopic
    - Neoplasms
      - Bronchogenic carcinoma
    - Head Trauma
      - Closed
      - Penetrating (pituitary-hypothalamic surgery)
    - Infections
      - Pneumonia, bacterial or viral
      - Abscess, lung or brain
      - Cavitation (Aspergillosis)
      - Tuberculosis, lung or brain
      - Meningitis, bacterial or viral
      - Encephalitis
    - Vascular
      - Cerebrovascular occlusions, hemorrhage
      - Cavernous sinus thrombosis
    - Neurologic
      - Guillain-Barre Syndrome
      - Multiple sclerosis
      - Delerium tremens
      - Amytrophic lateral sclerosis
      - Hydrocephalus
      - Psychosis
    - Metabolic
      - Acute intermittent porphyria
    - Pulmonary
      - Asthma
      - Pneumothorax
      - Positive pressure respiration
    - Drugs
      - Vasopressin or DDAVP
      - Oxytocin, high-dose
      - Vincristine
      - Carbamazepine
      - Nicotine
      - Phenothiazines
      - Cyclophosphamide
      - Tricyclic antidepressants
      - Monoamine oxidase inhibitors
      - Serotonin reuptake inhibitors
    - Congenital
      - Eutopic
        - Malformations
          - Agenesis corpus callosum
          - Other midline defects
            - Cleft lip/palate

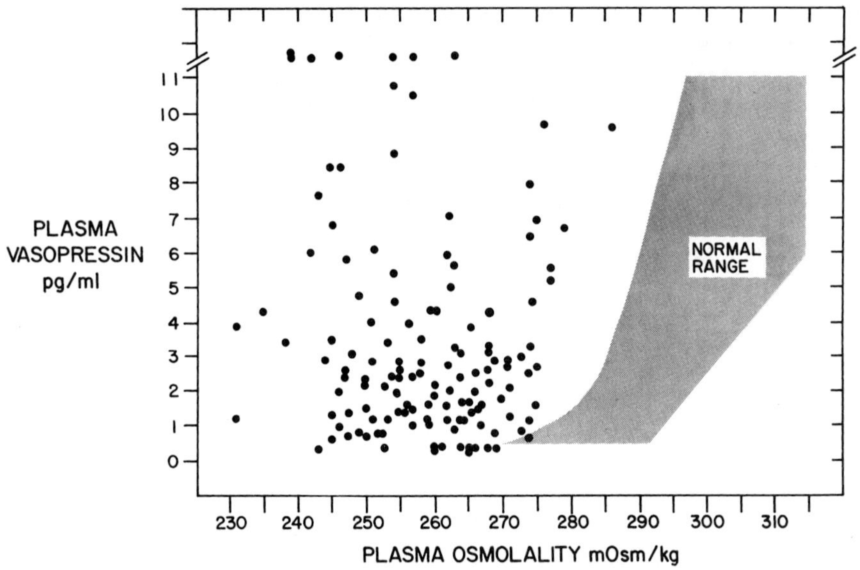

FIGURE 8-20. The relation of plasma vasopressin to plasma osmolality in the syndrome of inappropriate antidiuresis. Each value represents a single patient. (*From Robertson and Aycinena.*[405])

an inappropriately high level until plasma osmolality rises into the normal range. At that point, plasma vasopressin begins to rise appropriately in close association with a further increase in plasma osmolality. This pattern also occurs in about 25 percent of all patients with SIADH. It could reflect a constant, nonsuppressible "leak" of vasopressin or selective loss of inhibitory input in the presence of otherwise normal stimulatory component of a bimodal osmoregulatory system. The type C defect is the most common, occurring in at least 35 percent of all patients. It is characterized by increases in plasma vasopressin that correlate closely with plasma osmolality as it is raised toward normal by the saline infusion. Regression analysis of this relationship shows that the precision and sensitivity of the vasopressin response to osmolality are normal but the extrapolated threshold value is subnormal. Patients with this type of defect appear to have resetting of the osmostat

FIGURE 8-21. The relation of plasma vasopressin to osmolality during hypertonic saline infusion in four patients with the clinical syndrome of inappropriate antidiuresis. (*From Robertson.*[30])

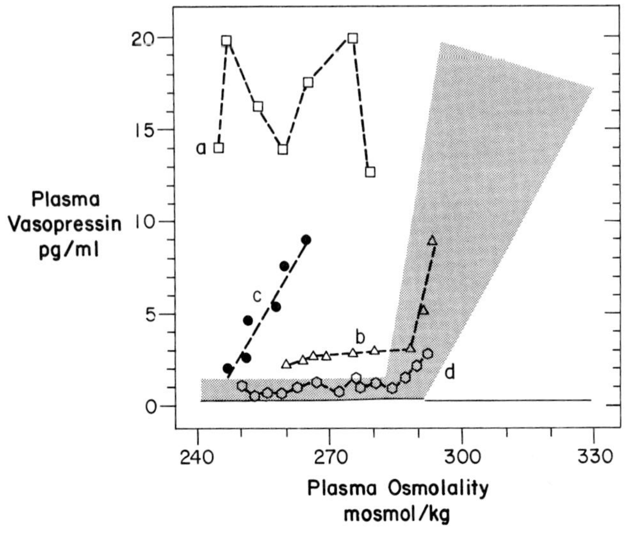

and may exhibit clinical characteristics slightly different from those found in other forms of SIADH (as noted later). Type D is much less common than the other three osmoregulatory defects and may represent a basically different abnormality in antidiuretic function. In these unusual patients, vasopressin secretion appears to be stimulated and suppressed normally, but urine osmolality remains fixed at a hypertonic level. The reason for this apparent dissociation between plasma vasopressin and urinary concentration has not been determined, but one recent study suggests that the antidiuretic effect is mediated via V_2 receptors.[441]

There appears to be no correlation between the types of osmoregulatory dysfunction and the particular diseases or drugs presumed to be responsible for the SIADH.[426] This dissociation suggests that either the cause has been misidentified or it is capable of acting by more than one mechanism. The most noteworthy example is bronchogenic carcinoma, which has been associated with every type of osmoregulatory defect, including type C, the reset osmostat.[440] Because it is highly unlikely that anaplastic cells could acquire the normally separate capacities of vasopressin synthesis and osmoregulation, many tumors probably produce the syndrome by a mechanism other than ectopic production of the hormone.

The pathophysiology of the fluid and electrolyte disturbance in SIADH is probably similar to that observed when healthy volunteers are treated with vasopressin.[232,442] If the subjects are allowed to drink ad libitum[232] or are restricted to a total intake of 1 l/day,[442] the administration of Pitressin or DDAVP in doses sufficient to maintain a fixed, maximum antidiuresis (about 10 ml/kg/day) causes little or no decrease in plasma sodium because fluid intake is also reduced or restricted to comparably low levels, thus maintaining water balance. However, if fluid intake is maintained artificially at a level greater than total output, the excess water accumulates, expanding and diluting body fluids.[442] When the expansion of body water exceeds 5–6 percent, the excretion of sodium begins to increase. This natriuresis serves to ameliorate the extracellular volume expansion but also aggravates the hyponatremia. The net result is that the hyponatremia in SIADH is due in roughly equal proportions to both a primary increase in body water and a secondary decrease in body sodium. If water intake is reduced to less than total urinary and insensible output, the entire series of events slowly reverses as body water decreases, sodium is retained, and plasma osmolality and sodium return to their original levels even though vasopressin levels remain high.[442] These observations illustrate the critical importance of fluid intake in determining the effect of vasopressin on lowering serum sodium and increasing sodium excretion. If intake is regulated normally, even high rates of vasopressin secretion will have little or no clinically appreciable effect. However, if water intake is inappropriately high, as in patients with psychogenic or dipsogenic polydipsia, even a slight increase in plasma vasopressin and urine concentration may result in profound water intoxication. In a very real sense, therefore, inappropriate secretion of vasopressin plays only a permissive role in the development of hyponatremia. This contrasts with the effects of many other hormones, such as insulin and parathormone, which occur without a concurrent abnormality in another homeostatic system.

The pathophysiology of the fluid and electrolyte imbalance in patients with SIADH appears to be similar in principal to that produced by giving vasopressin and fluid loads to normal subjects.[443–447] Total body water and the rate of sodium excretion are increased, at least during the developmental phase. Plasma renin activity and aldosterone tend to be suppressed[448] whereas atrial natriuretic peptide is elevated[449] presumably because of the volume expansion. Blood pressure is not elevated.[450] However, the patients differ from the experimental model in two important respects. One is that the excessive fluid intake in patients can be due either to inappropriate administration of fluids or to an associated abnormality in the osmoregulation of thirst. The other is that the antidiuretic defects in patients can vary enormously owing to the individual differences in the nature of their osmoregulatory defect (Fig. 8-21). The patients with downward resetting of the vasopressin osmostat (type C defect) are particularly noteworthy because they retain the capacity to maximally suppress their plasma vasopressin and dilute their urine if a high fluid intake decreases their plasma osmolality the lower set point.[451–453] Thus, unlike patients with other osmoregulatory defects, they are able to mount a maximum water diuresis and limit the severity of their hyponatremia even if their fluid intake is very high.

The major effects of hyponatremia are in the central nervous system.[447,454] They include lethargy, dizziness, confusion, headache, anorexia, pathologic reflexes, pseudobulbar palsy, coma, Cheyne-Stokes respiration, and seizures. Postmortem studies in patients who died with hyponatremia show cerebral edema, herniation of the brain, and, in a few cases, central myelinolysis.[455] The severity of the neurologic defects depends on several factors, including the degree of hyponatremia, the rate of decline, and the age of the patient.[447,454] Unless the patient has epilepsy or another preexisting brain disease, seizures and coma usually do not occur until plasma sodium falls below 120 mEq/l. If hyponatremia is chronic or slow to develop, cerebral swelling and symptoms appear to be less severe, probably because brain cells are able to inactivate or expell solute.[447]

An SIADH-like syndrome, which can be referred to as hyponatremia type IIIB, also occurs in some patients with myxedema[456,457] or secondary adrenal insufficiency.[458] In the latter, the mechanism of the impaired water excretion is complex.[458–469] It usually is associated with inappropriate levels of plasma vasopressin,[462,465–469] but the cause is uncertain. It cannot be attributed to a reduction in blood volume but may be due to hypotension, low cardiac output,[465,467] or a direct effect of cortisol deficiency on the neurohypophysis.[462,464] Cortisol deficiency can also impair water excretion without detectably increasing plasma vasopressin.[459,463,469] The mechanism of this vasopressin independent defect is also unsettled and may be due to a change in renal hemodynamics or a direct effect of glucocorticoid deficiency on the hydroosmotic permeability of the collecting tubules. As in true SIADH, the development of hyponatremia is dependent upon excessive water intake that, in some patients at least, may be due to an associated abnormality in thirst.[470] Whatever the precise mechanism of the hyponatremia, however, it is important to remember that patients with hyponatremia due to an isolated glucocorticoid deficiency do not have hyperkalemia or signs of hypovolemia and can be reliably differentiated from patients with SIAD only by measuring plasma or urinary cortisol.

Hypovolemia Hyponatremia

Osmotically inappropriate thirst and vasopressin secretion can also result from a relatively large reduction in extracellular volume. In this syndrome, which is also referred to as Type II hyponatremia, the hypovolemia is most often caused by diuretic abuse, but can also result from a number of other salt and water depleting diseases such as severe gastroenteritis, hemorrhage, renal tubular acidosis, medullary cystic disease of the kidney, and primary or secondary aldosterone deficiency.

The pathophysiology of hypovolemic hyponatremia is similar in principle to SIADH in that it results from impaired free water excretion and a relatively high fluid intake. The major differences are that the defect in water excretion caused by the increase in vasopressin is secondary to a hypovolemic stimulus and appears to be due largely, if not totally, to downward resetting of the osmostat.[82,405] Moreover, the antidiuresis is aggravated by decreased glomerular filtration and increased reabsorption of salt and water in the proximal nephron, which decrease delivery of filtrate to the distal nephron. The hypovolemia also increases plasma renin activity and aldosterone secretion, which further reduce the rate of sodium excretion and may result in potassium depletion. Thirst and fluid intake are probably also increased as a result of downward resetting of the osmostat. The net effect is that total body water is decreased rather than expanded and most, if not all, of the decrease comes from the extracellular compartment. If anything, intracellular water is slightly expanded due to an osmotically driven redistribution from the extracellular to the intracellular space.

Primary adrenal insufficiency is a special case of hypovolemic hyponatremia. The defect in water excretion also appears to be due to decreased glomerular filtration as well as increased secretion of vasopressin, but it may also involve a vasopressin-independent form of urinary concentration.[459,463,471,472] Moreover, because of the aldosterone deficiency, these patients typically develop hyperkalemia rather than hypokalemia. The abnormalities in isolated mineralocorticoid deficiency are similar.[463,473,474] As in other forms of hypovolemic hyponatremia, the increase in vasopressin secretion in isolated mineralocorticoid deficiency appears to be due to downward resetting of the osmostat.[405]

Thiazide-induced hyponatremia[475] may also be a special case of hypovolemic hyponatremia. Although this type of diuretic also decreases extracellular volume and increases plasma vasopressin,[476] both changes are relatively small. Moreover, sometimes the hyponatremia appears to be associated with net water retention and presents clinically like SIAD.[477,478] This may be due to a volume and vasopressin-independent impairment of urine dilution which results from inhibiting sodium reabsorption in the ascending limb of Henle's loop.[376] This antidilutional effect causes a relatively modest reduction in maximum free water clearance but can be used to advantage in the treatment of nephrogenic DI (discussed previously). It may also result in net water retention and hyponatremia in patients with primary polydipsia.[478]

Hypervolemic Hyponatremia

Osmotically inappropriate thirst and vasopressin secretion can also result from a marked reduction in "effective" blood volume. This syndrome, which is also referred to as hyponatremia Type I, usually occurs in patients with severe low-output congestive heart failure, advanced cirrhosis with ascites, or nephrosis.[479–485] It is thought to be due to decreased cardiac output and/or a reduction of blood volume caused by a shift of salt and water from plasma to the interstitial space. This redistribution and the associated increase in sodium retention is responsible for the formation of edema which characterizes this form of hyponatremia.

The pathophysiology of hypervolemic hyponatremia also entails impaired water excretion in association with inadequate suppression of water intake. As in hypovolemic hyponatremia, the impaired water excretion is due to a combination of decreased distal delivery of filtrate and increased secretion of vasopressin, both of which are probably secondary to a hypovolemic stimulus. The abnormal secretion of vasopressin also appears to be due to downward resetting of the osmostat.[479–483] When this marked impairment of water excretion is combined with inadequate suppression of water intake, hyponatremia develops even though total body sodium is often increased by more than 25 percent. Thus, hypervolemic hyponatremia is distinguished from the other two types of hyponatremia by the fact that total body sodium and water are markedly increased and edema is present.

Differential Diagnosis

The first step in evaluating a patient with hyponatremia is to rule out hyperglycemia as the cause. When plasma glucose or another solute such as mannitol is elevated, the effective osmotic pressure of extracellular osmotic pressure is also increased and water enters quickly from the intracellular compartment until osmotic equilibruim is reestablished. This influx of water dilutes the concentration of sodium in plasma and other extracellular compartments but does not completely reduce plasma osmolality to normal. Hence, this form of hyponatremia is not associated with hypotonicity and can be easily recognized either by correcting the sodium level for the elevation in glucose (see treatment of adipsic hypernatremia) or by measuring the osmolality of heparinized plasma. Serum or edetic acid (EDTA) plasma should not be used for these osmolality measurements because both are subject to significant artifacts caused by glucose or the anticoagulant itself.

Differentiating SIADH (hyponatremia Type IIIA) from the other forms of hypotonic hyponatremia is a process of exclusion based largely on standard clinical assessment of the extracellular volume, thyroid function, and adrenal function. Thus, patients with SIADH lack edema and postural hypotension as well as any laboratory sign of true or effective hypovolemia. Their plasma urea, creatinine, urate, and renin activity tend to be low and urinary sodium is high, at least in the developmental phase of the syndrome. Serum aldosterone may also be low and serum potassium is normal. Their thyroid function tests and morning plasma cortisol are also within normal limits, excluding the SIADH-like syndrome (hyponatremia Type IIIB). In contrast, the presence of edema in a patient with severe heart failure, advanced cirrhosis, or nephrosis is pathognomonic of hypervolemic (Type I) hyponatremia. In these patients, urinary sodium is usually low (<20 mEq/day), and plasma renin activity, aldosterone, urea, creatinine, and urate are often elevated due to a reduction in effective blood volume and glomerular filtration. Hypovolemic (Type II) hyponatremia is characterized by signs and symptoms of volume depletion *without* edema. Thus, plasma urea, creatinine, urate, and renin are usually increased. Urinary sodium is usually low unless the syndrome is caused by diuretic abuse, primary renal sodium wasting, or adrenal insufficiency in which case it may be high. Some degree of hypokalemia is the rule, except in patients with Addison's disease or isolated aldosterone deficiency, in whom serum potassium is usually elevated. Measurements of plasma vasopressin are of no help in distinguishing between the various types of hypotonic hyponatremia because they are usually elevated to the same extent in all three types.

Therapy

SIADH

The primary abnormality in vasopressin secretion can often be eliminated when the hormone is made ectopically, given exogenously, or released from the neurohypophysis in response to certain nonessential drugs such as the serotonin reuptake inhibitors. If the inappropriate secretion of vasopressin is caused by chronic or recurrent nausea (as in patients receiving some forms of chemotherapy), it can also be eliminated by treatment with standard antiemetics.[86] Most of the time, however, the abnormality in vasopressin secretion cannot be corrected and must be allowed to run its course until spontaneous recovery occurs. Fortunately, the abnormality in vasopressin is usually of short duration and remits within 2 to 3 weeks or as soon as there is significant improvement in the underlying cause. During this interval, an effort should be made to correct or prevent worsening of the hyponatremia. The standard method to do this is to restrict water intake. To be really effective, however, the *total* intake of water must be at least 500 ml a day less than the total of urinary and insensible output. Because the amount of water provided by food normally approximates insensible loss, discretionary intake of water must be kept at least 500 ml a day below urine output. In many patients, the requisite restriction is difficult to achieve because their urine is concentrated and/or their thirst is also inappropriately increased. And even if restriction is successful, the rate of decrease in body water and rise in plasma sodium is usually no greater than about 1 to 2 percent a day. Therefore, additional measures are often needed, particularly if the hyponatremia is symptomatic.

Intravenous infusion of hypertonic saline can be used for quicker correction of the hyponatremia in SIADH. When 3 percent saline is infused i.v. at a rate of 0.05 ml/kg/min, it raises plasma osmolality and sodium about 1 percent an hour. This approach is rational as well as quick as it not only corrects the sodium deficiency, but also produces a mild solute diuresis that reduces the excess body water. Many physicians believe that hypertonic saline infusion is also safe[486–488] provided the plasma sodium is raised no more than 24 mEq/l in 48 h and no higher than 130–135 mEq/l. However, others believe that raising plasma sodium more than 12 mEq/l/day runs a serious risk of producing central pontine myelinolysis,[489] a rare and often fatal neurologic disorder characterized by quadriparesis, dysphagia, and dysarthria. Therefore, hypertonic saline should be used cautiously in patients with SIADH and only to the extent necessary to raise plasma sodium to asymptomatic levels. To guard against sudden rapid increases in plasma sodium caused by remission of the abnormal vasopressin secretion, changes in urine output as well as plasma sodium should be monitored at least every 2–4 h during the infusion. These caveats apply particularly to patients in whom the hyponatremia has been present for more than 48 h because they usually have fewer symptoms and are more likely to have serious complications from too rapid correction of their hyponatremia.

Body water can also be reduced by inhibiting the antidiuretic effects of vasopressin. Among the drugs currently available in the United States for this purpose, demeclocycline (Declomycin) is probably the best.[490,491] At conventional doses of up to 1.2 g/day, it causes a reversible form of nephrogenic diabetes insipidus in almost all patients with SIADH. This effect may require a week or more to manifest. Its mechanism of action has not been defined precisely but appears to involve a step distal to the generation of cyclic AMP.[492] Because of other catabolic as well as nephrotoxic effects, it may cause a rise in plasma urea, which is reversible when the drug is stopped. Moreover, demeclocycline can have serious or potentially lethal side effects in patients with Type I and Type II hyponatremia.[493,494] Hence, its use should be monitored closely and restricted to patients with chronic SIADH that is not amenable to fluid restriction and is not associated with significant underlying cardiac, renal, or hepatic disease. Lithium carbonate also causes a form of reversible nephrogenic diabetes insipidus, but at conventional doses this effect is inconsistent and it is even more prone to produce undesirable side effects.[495] For these reasons, it is rarely used for treatment of SIADH or other forms of hyponatremia.

Recently, potent nonpeptide V_2 receptor antagonists capable of blocking the antidiuretic effect of vasopressin have been developed and tested in humans.[187–189] Preliminary clinical trials in patients with SIADH or Type I hyponatremia indicate that these antagonists are both safe and effective in promoting a water diuresis and raising the plasma sodium in a dose dependent manner.[187,485] One or more of these antagonists may soon be available in the United States for routine use in the treatment of SIADH and Type I hyponatremia.

Other measures that may be useful in the treatment of chronic SIADH include the administration of oral sodium chloride with or without furosemide.[496] This regimen works much like an osmotic diuretic in that it increases free water excretion by increasing solute load. Much the same result can be obtained by giving salt or urea per os,[497] but the latter is unpalatable and may not be well accepted by patients. Fludrocortisone (Florinef) is also quite effective in the management of chronic SIADH. At doses ranging from 0.1 to 0.2 mg twice a day, it will consistently maintain plasma sodium within the normal range. The mechanism is uncertain but may include some inhibition of fluid intake as well as increased retention of sodium. The principle side effects are hypokalemia, which can usually be avoided by dietary potassium supplements, and hypertension, which may require discontinuation of the treatment.

In patients with an SIADH-like disorder due to myxedema or secondary adrenal insufficiency (hyponatremia Type IIIB), the abnormalities in salt and water balance can be corrected completely by treatment with thyroxine or cortisol. In a hypothyroid patient, thyroxine should not be started until a codeficiency of cortisol has been excluded because the increase in metabolism caused by the treatment could provoke an adrenal crisis.

Hypovolemic (Type II) Hyponatremia

The fluid and electrolyte abnormalities in these patients can be corrected completely by correcting the cause of the hypovolemia and/or restoring extracellular volume to normal. Because their sodium deficit is relatively greater than their water deficit, the ideal combination is hypertonic (i.e., the ratio of sodium chloride to water should exceed 150 mEq/l). However, this approach is necessary only if the hyponatremia is severe and must be corrected quickly. In such a situation, an infusion of 3 percent saline at a rate of 0.1 ml/kg/min for 2 h will raise plasma sodium by almost 10 mEq/l, an amount that is usually sufficient to eliminate the threat of serious neurologic complications. In using this approach, it is important not to raise the plasma sodium too far or too fast (see treatment of SIADH). In most cases of hypovolemic hyponatremia, it is sufficient and probably preferable simply to give the salt and water by mouth or infuse isotonic saline with or without supplementary potassium. In addition, the cause of the sodium loss should be identified and, if possible, corrected. If the patient is hyperkalemic or has other signs suggestive of pituitary-adrenal dysfunction, blood for measurement of plasma cortisol, aldosterone, and renin activity should be obtained immediately and parenteral cortisol should be administered pending completion of the assays. In no case should patients with this form of hyponatremia be treated by water restriction, demeclocycline, lithium, vasopressin antagonists, or furosemide as these measures only aggravate the underlying hypovolemia and may cause cardiovascular collapse.

Hypervolemic (Type I) Hyponatremia

As expected, the impaired water excretion and hyponatremia in patients with congestive heart failure or advanced cirrhosis sometimes can be improved by increasing cardiac output[498] or shunting ascitic fluid into the vascular space.[499] Usually, however, the basic hemodynamic defect cannot be completely rectified, and other methods must be used to correct the edema and hyponatremia. Because patients in this category have a greater increase in total body water than sodium, the most rational and effective therapy is to combine fluid restriction with the administration of an osmotic or loop diuretic.[500,501] An osmotic diuresis can be produced giving mannitol i.v. However, because it increases the effective osmotic pressure of extracellular fluid, mannitol initially increases the hyponatremia and cardiac load by rapidly extracting water from the intracellular compartment. The fall in plasma sodium is inconsequential because it is more than offset by the osmotic effect of the mannitol. However, the initial expansion of the extracellular compartment is more problematic because it may further compromise cardiac function. Both effects usually disappear within a few hours when the mannitol is excreted. Preliminary clinical experience with the nonpeptide vasopressin antagonists indicates that, when combined with fluid restriction, they are also quite effective and safe in promoting a water diuresis and correcting the hyponatremia in patients with congestive heart failure or advanced cirrhosis.[485] They may soon be available in the United States for routine use in the treatment of these patients. Patients with hypervolemic hyponatremia should never be treated with hypertonic saline or fludrocortisone because they increase body sodium and worsen the edema. Demeclocycline and lithium are also contraindicated because patients with hypervolemic hyponatremia are more likely to suffer severe side effects.

REFERENCES

1. Haymaker W: Hypothalamo-pituitary neural pathways and the circulatory system of the pituitary, in Haymaker W, Anderson E, Nauta W (eds): *The Hypothalamus*. Springfield, Charles C Thomas, 1969, p 219.
2. Scharrer E, Scharrer B: Hormones produced by neurosecretory cells. *Recent Prog Horm Res* 10:183, 1954.
3. Zimmerman EA: The organization of oxytocin and vasopressin pathways, in Martin JB, Reichlin S, Bick KL (eds): *Neurosecretion and Brain Peptides*. New York, Raven, 1981, pp 63–75.
4. Sofroniew MV, Weindl A, Schrell U, Wetzstein R: Immunohistochemistry of vasopressin, oxytocin and neurophysin in the hypothalamus and extrahypothalamic regions of the human and primate brain. *Acta Histochem [Suppl]* 24:79, 1982.
5. Dierickx K, Vandesande F: Immunocytochemical localization of the vasopressinergic and the oxytocinergic neurons in the human hypothalamus. *Cell Tissue Res* 184:15, 1977.
6. Rhodes CH, Morrell JI, Pfaff DW: Immunohistochemical analysis of magnocellular elements in rat hypothalamus: Distribution and numbers of cells containing neurophysin, oxytocin and vasopressin. *J Comp Neurol* 198:45, 1981.
7. Liposits Z: Ultrastructure of hypothalamic paraventricular neurons. *Crit Rev Neurobiol* 7:89, 1993.
8. Van Zwieten EJ, Ravid R, Swaab DF: Differential vasopressin and oxytocin innervation of the human parabrachial nucleus: No changes in alzheimer's disease. *Brain Res* 711:146, 1994.
9. Luerssen TG, Robertson GL: Cerebrospinal fluid vasopressin and vasotocin in health and disease, in Wood JH (ed): *Neurobiology and Cerebrospinal Fluid*. New York, Plenum, 1980, vol 1, pp 613–623.
10. Du Vigneaud V: Hormones of the posterior pituitary gland: Oxytocin and vasopressin, in *Harvey Lectures, 1954, 1955*. New York, Academic, 1956.
11. Acher R: Neurohypophysial peptide systems: Processing machinery, hydroosmotic regulation, adaptation and evolution. *Regul Pept* 45:1, 1993.
12. Sachs H, Fawcett P, Takabatake Y, Portanova R: Biosynthesis and release of vasopressin and neurophysin. *Recent Prog Horm Res* 25:447, 1969.
13. Acher R, Chauvet J, Olivry G: Sur l'existence éventuelle d'une hormone unique hypophysaire: I. Relations entre l'oxytocine, la vasopressine et la protein de Van Dyke extraites de la neurohypophyse du boeuf. *Biochim Biophys Acta* 22:421, 1956.
14. Breslow E: The neurophysins. *Adv Enzymol* 40:271, 1974.
15. Breslow E: The conformation and functional domains of neurophysins, in Gross P, Richter D, Robertson GL (eds): *Vasopressin*. John Libbey Eurotext, 1993, pp 143–145.
16. Schmale H, Fehr S, Richter D: Vasopressin biosynthesis—from gene to peptide hormone. *Kidney Int* 32(Suppl 21):S8, 1987.

17a. Richter D: Molecular events in expression of vasopressin and oxytocin and their cognate receptors. *Am J Physiol* 255:F207, 1988.

17b. Hara Y, Battey J, Gainer H: Structure of mouse vasopressin and oxytocin genes. *Mol Brain Res* 8:319, 1990.

18. Sausville E, Carney D, Battey J: The human vasopressin gene is linked to the oxytocin gene and is selectively expressed in a cultured lung cancer cell line. *J Biol Chem* 260:10236, 1985.
19. Mohr E, Bahnsen U, Kiessling C, Richter D: Expression of the vasopressin and oxytocin genes in rats occurs in mutually exclusive sets of hypothalamic neurons. *FEBS Lett* 242:144, 1988.
20. Riddell DC, Mallonee R, Phillips JA, Parks JS, Sexton LA, Hamerton JL: Chromosomal assignment of human sequences encoding arginine vasopressin-neurophysin II and growth hormone releasing factor. *Somatic Cell Mol Genet* 11:189, 1985.
21. Dong W, Seidel B, Marcinkiewicz M, Chretien M, Seidah NG, Day R: Cellular localization of the prohormone convertases in the hypothalamic paraventricular and supraoptic nuclei: Selective regulation of PC1 in corticotrophin-releasing hormone parvocellular neurons mediated by glucocorticoids. *J Neurosci* 17:563, 1997.
22. Gainer H, Chin H: Molecular diversity in neurosecretion: Reflections on the hypothalamo-neurohypophyseal system. *Cell Mol Neurobiol* 18:211, 1998.
23. Coates LC, Birch NP: Differential cleavage of provasopressin by the major molecular forms of SPC3. *J Neurochem* 70:1670, 1998.
24. Douglass WW: How do neurons secrete peptides? Exocytosis and its consequences including synaptic vesicle formation in the hypothalamo-neurohypophyseal system. *Prog Brain Res* 39:21, 1973.
25. Carrazana EJ, Pasieka KB, Majzoub JA: The vasopressin mRNA poly (A) tract is unusually long and increases during stimulation of vasopressin gene expression in vivo. *Mol Cell Biol* 8:2267, 1988.
26. Moses AM, Miller M: Accumulation and release of pituitary vasopressin in rats heterozygous for hypothalamic diabetes insipidus. *Endocrinology* 86:34, 1970.
27. Verney EB: Antidiuretic hormone and the factors which determine its release. *Proc R Soc London [Biol]* 135:25, 1947.
28. Robertson GL: The regulation of vasopressin function in health and disease. *Recent Prog Horm Res* 33:333, 1977.
29. Robertson GL, Athar S, Shelton RL: Osmotic control of vasopressin function, in Andreoli TE, Grantham JJ, Rector FC (eds): *Disturbances in Body Fluid Osmolality*. Bethesda, American Physiological Society, 1977, p 125.
30. Robertson GL: Thirst and vasopressin function in normal and disordered states of water balance. *J Lab Clin Med* 101:351, 1983.
31. Jewell PA, Verney EB: An experimental attempt to determine the site of the neurohypophyseal osmoreceptors in the dog. *Philos Trans R Soc London [Biol]* 240:197, 1957.
32. Robertson GL: Physiopathology of ADH secretion, in Tolis G, Labrie F, Martin JB, Naftolin F (eds): *Clinical Neuroendocrinology: A Pathophysiological Approach*. New York, Raven, 1979, pp 247–260.
33. Gardiner TW, Verbalis JG, Stricker EM: Impaired secretion of vasopressin and oxytocin in rats after lesions of nucleus medianus. *Am J Physiol* 249 (*Regulatory Integrative Comp Physiol* 18):R681, 1985.
34. Thrasher TN, Keil LC: Regulation of drinking and vasopressin secretion: Role of organum vasculosum laminae terminalis. *Am J Physiol* 253 (*Regulatory Integrative Comp Physiol* 22):R108, 1987.
35. Strong OS, Elwyn A: *Human Neuroanatomy*. Baltimore, Williams & Wilkins, 1948, p 398.
36. Zerbe RL, Miller JZ, Robertson GL: The reproducibility and heritability of individual differences in osmoregulatory function in normal human subjects. *J Lab Clin Med* 117:51, 1991.
37. Helderman JH, Vestal RE, Rowe JW, Tobin JD, Andres R, Robertson GL: The response of arginine vasopressin to intravenous ethanol and hypertonic saline in man: The impact of aging. *J Gerontol* 33:39, 1978.
38. Barron WM: Water metabolism and vasopressin secretion during pregnancy. *Br J Obstet Gynaecol* 1:853, 1987.
39. Vokes TJ, Weiss NM, Schreiber J, Gaskill MB, Robertson GL: Osmoregulation of thirst and vasopressin during normal menstrual cycle. *Am J Physiol* 254 (*Regulatory Integrative Comp Physiol* 23):R641, 1988.
40. Spruce BA, Baylis PH, Burd J, Watson MJ: Variation in osmoregulation of arginine vasopressin during the human menstrual cycle. *Clin Endocrinol (Oxf)* 22:37, 1985.
41. Rodbard D, Munson PJ: Editorial comment. *Am J Physiol* 234:E340, 1978.
42. Wade CE, Bie P, Keil LC, Ramsay DJ: Osmotic control of plasma vasopressin in the dog. *Am J Physiol* 243:E287, 1982.
43. Hammer M, Ladefoged J, Olgaard K: Relationship between plasma osmolality and plasma vasopressin in human subjects. *Am J Physiol* 238:E313, 1980.
44. Weitzman RE, Fisher DA, DiStefano JH III, Bennett CM: Episodic secretion of arginine vasopressin. *Am J Physiol* 233:E32, 1977.
45. Brimble MJ, Dyball REJ: Characterization of the responses of oxytocin- and vasopressin-secreting neurones in the supraoptic nucleus to osmotic stimulation. *J Physiol (Lond)* 271:253, 1977.
46. Poulain DA: Electrophysiology of the afferent input to oxytocin- and vasopressin-secreting neurones: Facts and problems. *Prog Brain Res* 60:39, 1983.
47. Robertson GL: Regulation of vasopressin secretion, in Seldin DW, Giebisch G (eds): *The Kidney: Physiology and Pathophysiology*. New York, Raven, 1985, pp 869–884.
48. Zerbe RL, Robertson GL: Osmoregulation of thirst and vasopressin secretion in human subjects: Effect of various solutes. *Am J Physiol* 224:E607, 1983.
49. Thrasher TN, Brown CJ, Keil LC, Ramsay DJ: Thirst and vaso-

pressin release in the dog: An osmoreceptor or sodium receptor mechanism? *Am J Physiol* 238:R333, 1980.
50. McKinley MJ, Denton DA, Weisinger RS: Sensors of antidiuresis and thirst: Osmoreceptors or CSF sodium detectors? *Brain Res* 141:89, 1978.
51. Olsson K, Kolmodin R: Dependence of basic secretion of antidiuretic hormone on cerebrospinal fluid [Na]. *Acta Physiol Scand* 91:286, 1974.
52. Vokes TP, Aycinena PR, Robertson GL: Effect of insulin on osmoregulation of vasopressin. *Am J Physiol* 252 (*Endocrinol Metab* 15):E538, 1987.
53. Zerbe RL, Vinicor F, Robertson GL: The regulation of plasma vasopressin in insulin dependent diabetes mellitus. *Am J Physiol* 249(3):E317, 1985.
54. Zerbe RL, Vinicor F, Robertson GL: Plasma vasopressin in uncontrolled diabetes mellitus. *Diabetes* 28:503, 1979.
55. Walsh CH, Baylis PH, Malins JM: Plasma arginine vasopressin in diabetic ketoacidosis. *Diabetologia* 16:93, 1979.
56. Van Houten M, Posner BI, Kopriwa BM, Brawer JR: Insulin binding sites in the rat brain: In vivo localization to the circumventricular organs by quantitative radioautography. *Endocrinology* 105:666, 1979.
57. Greelen G, Keil LC, Kravik SE, Wade CE, Thrasher TN, Barnes PR, et al: Inhibition of plasma vasopressin after drinking in dehydrate humans. *Am J Physiol* 247 (*Regulatory Integrative Comp Physiol* 16):R968, 1984.
58. Seckl JR, Williams TDM, Lightman SL: Oral hypertonic saline causes transient fall of vasopressin in humans. *Am J Physiol* 251 (*Regulatory Integrative Comp Physiol* 20):R214, 1986.
59. Salata RA, Verbalis JG, Robinson AG: Cold water stimulation of oropharyngeal receptors in man inhibits release of vasopressin. *J Clin Endocrinol Metab* 65:561, 1987.
60. Thompson CJ, Burd JM, Baylis PH: Acute suppression of plasma vasopressin and thirst after drinking in hypernatremic humans. *Am J Physiol* 352 (*Regulatory Integrative Comp Physiol* 21):R1138, 1987.
61. Kirchheim HR: Systemic arterial baroreceptor reflexes. *Physiol Rev* 56:100, 1976.
62. Goetz KL, Bond GC, Bloxham DD: Atrial receptors and renal function. *Physiol Rev* 55:157, 1975.
63. de Torrente A, Robertson GL, McDonald KM, Schrier RW: Mechanism of diuretic response to increased left atrial pressure in the anesthetized dog. *Kidney International* 8:355, 1975.
64. Herbert H, Moga MM, Saper CB: Connections of the parabrachial nucleus with the nucleus of the solitary tract and the medullary reticular formation in the rat. *J Comp Neurol* 293:540, 1990.
65. Jhamandas JH, Harris KH, Krukoff TL: Parabrachial nucleus projection towards the hypothalamic supraoptic nucleus: Electrophysiological and anatomical observations in the rat. *J Comp Neurol* 308:42, 1991.
66. Ward DG: Neurons in the parabrachial nuclei respond to hemorrhage. *Brain Res* 491:80, 1989.
67. Ohman LE, Shade RE, Haywood JR: Parabrachial nucleus modulation of vasopressin release. *Am J Physiol* 258 (*Regulatory Integrative Comp Physiol* 27):R358, 1990.
68. Iwasaki Y, Gaskill MB, Fu R, Saper CB, Robertson GL: Opioid antagonist diprenorphine microinjected into parabrachial nucleus selectively inhibits vasopressin response to hypovolemic stimuli in the rat. *J Clin Invest* 92:2230, 1993.
69. Rocha MJA, Herbert H: c-fos Expression in the parabrachial nucleus following cardiovascular and blood volume changes. *J Brain Res* 37:389, 1996.
70. Thames MD, Schmid PG: Cardiopulmonary receptors with vagal afferents tonically inhibit ADH release in the dog. *Am J Physiol* 237:H299, 1979.
71. Iwasaki Y, Gaskill MB, Robertson GL: The effect of selective opioid antagonists on vasopressin secretion in the rat. *Endocrinology* 134:55, 1994.
72. Iwasaki Y, Gaskill MB, Boss CA, Robertson GL: The effect of the nonselective opioid antagonist diprenorphine on vasopressin secretion in the rat. *Endocrinology* 134:48, 1994.
73. Schreihofer AM, Hoffman GE, Sved AF: The kidneys stimulate vasopressin release during hemorrhage in rats with chronic NTS lesions. *Am J Physiol* 272:R1540, 1997.
74. Fumoux F, Czernichow P, Arnauld E, Du Pont J, Vincent JD: Effect of hypotension induced by sodium nitrocyanoferrate(III) on the release of arginine-vasopressin in the unanaesthetized monkey. *J Endocrinol* 78:449, 1978.
75. Robertson GL, Ganguly A: Osmoregulation and baroregulation of plasma vasopressin in essential hypertension. *J Cardiovasc Pharmacol* 8(Suppl 7):S87, 1986.
76. Dunn FL, Brennan TJ, Nelson AE, Robertson GL: The role of blood osmolality and volume in regulating vasopressin secretion in the rat. *J Clin Invest* 52:3212, 1973.
77. Goldsmith SR, Francis CS, Crowley AW, Cohn JN: Response of vasopressin and norepinephrine to lower body negative pressure in humans. *Am J Physiol* 243:H970, 1982.
78. Goetz KL, Wang BC, Sundet WD: Comparative effects of cardiac receptors and sinoaortic baroreceptors on elevations of plasma vasopressin and renin activity elicited by haemorrhage. *J Physiol (London)* 79:440, 1984.
79. Quillen EW Jr, Crowley AW Jr: Influence of volume changes in osmolality-vasopressin relationships in conscious dogs. *Am J Physiol* 244:H73, 1983.
80. Leimbach WN, Schmid PG, Mark AL: Baroreflex control of plasma arginine vasopressin in humans. *Am J Physiol* 247 (*Heart Circ Physiol* 16):H638, 1984.
81. Wang BC, Sundet WD, Hakumaki MOK, Geer PG, Goetz KL: Cardiac receptor influences on the plasma osmolality plasma vasopressin relationship. *Am J Physiol* 246(15):H360, 1984.
82. Weiss NM, Robertson G, Byun K: The effect of hypovolemia on the osmoregulation of thirst and AVP. *Clin Res* 32:786A, 1984.
83. Moses AM, Miller M, Streeten DHP: Quantitative influence of blood volume expansion on the osmotic threshold for vasopressin release. *J Clin Endocrinol Metab* 27:655, 1967.
84. Moses AM, Miller M: Osmotic threshold for vasopressin release as determined by saline infusion and by dehydration. *Neuroendocrinology* 7:219, 1971.
85. Coutinho EM: Oxytocic and antidiuretic effects of nausea in women. *Am J Obstet Gynecol* 105:127, 1969.
86. Rowe JW, Shelton RL, Helderman JH, Vestal RE, Robertson GL: Influence of the emetic reflex on vasopressin release in man. *Kidney Int* 16:729, 1979.
87. Eversmann T, Guttsmann M, Uhlich E, Ulbrecht G, von Werder K, Scriba PC: Increased secretion of growth hormone, prolactin, antidiuretic hormone and cortisol induced by the stress of motion sickness. *Aviat Space Environ Med* 49:53, 1978.
88. Miaskiewicz SL, Stricker EM, Verbalis JG: Neurohypophyseal secretion in response to cholecystokinin but not meal-induced gastric distention in humans. *J Clin Endocrinol Metab* 68:837, 1989.
89. Kim MS, Chey WD, Owyang C, Hasler WL: Role of plasma vasopressin as a mediator of nausea and gastric slow wave dysrhythmias in motion sickness. *Am J Physiol* 272:G853, 1997.
90. Verbalis JG, Richardson DW, Stricker EM: Vasopressin release in response to nausea-producing agents and cholecystokinin in monkeys. *Am J Physiol* 252 (*Regulatory Integrative Comp Physiol* 21):R749, 1987.
91. Verbalis JG, McHale CM, Gardiner TW, Stricker EM: Oxytocin and vasopressin secretion in response to stimuli producing learned taste aversions in rats. *Behav Neurosci* 100:466, 1986.
92. Baylis PH, Heath DA: Plasma-arginine-vasopressin response to insulin-induced hypoglycemia. *Lancet* 2:428, 1977.
93. Baylis PH, Robertson GL: Rat vasopressin response to insulin-induced hypoglycemia. *Endocrinology* 107:1975, 1980.
94. Baylis PH, Zerbe RL, Robertson GL: Arginine vasopressin response to insulin-induced hypoglycemia in man. *J Clin Endocrinol Metab* 53:935, 1981.
95. Keller-Wood ME, Wade CE, Shinsako J, Keil LC, Van Loon GR, Dallman MF: Insulin-induced hypoglycemia in conscious dogs: Effects of maintaining carotid arterial glucose levels on the adrenocorticotropin, epinephrine and vasopressin responses. *Endocrinology* 112:624, 1982.
96. Baylis PH, Robertson GL: Vasopressin response to 2-deoxy-D-glucose in the rat. *Endocrinology* 107:1970, 1980.
97. Thompson DA, Cambell RG, Lilavivat U, Welle SL, Robertson GL: Increased thirst and plasma arginine vasopressin levels during 2-deoxy-D-glucose-induced glucoprivation in humans. *J Clin Invest* 67:1083, 1981.
98. Bonjour JP, Malvin RL: Stimulation of ADH release by the renin-angiotensin system. *Am J Physiol* 218:1555, 1970.

99. Mouw D, Bonjour JP, Malvin RL, Vander A: Central action of angiotensin in stimulating ADH release. *Am J Physiol* 220:239, 1971.
100. Yamaguchi K, Sakaguchi T, Kamoi K: Central role of angiotensin in the hyperosmolality- and hypovolaemia-induced vasopressin release in conscious rats. *Acta Endocrinol (Copenh)* 101:524, 1982.
101. Shimizu K, Share L, Claybaugh JR: Potentiation of angiotensin II of the vasopressin response to an increasing plasma osmolality. *Endocrinology* 93:42, 1973.
102. Cadnapaphornchai P, Boykin J, Harbottle JA, McDonald KM, Schrier RW: Effect of angiotensin II on renal water excretion. *Am J Physiol* 228:155, 1975.
103. Rydin H, Verney EB: The inhibition of water-diuresis by emotional stress and by muscular exercise. *Q J Exp Physiol* 27:343, 1938.
104. Wiggins RC, Basar I, Slater JDH, Forsling M, Ramage CM: Vasovagal hypotension and vasopressin release. *Clin Endocrinol (Oxf)* 6:387, 1977.
105. Edelson JT, Robertson GL: The effect of the cold pressor test on vasopressin secretion in man. *Psychoneuroendocrinology* 11:307, 1986.
106. Punnonen R, Teisala K, Hakkinen V, Viinamaki O, Pystynen P: Vasopressin and prolactin as stress hormones. *Gynecol Obstet Invest* 21:76, 1986.
107. Lang RE, Heil JWE, Ganten D, Hermann K, Unger T, Rascher W: Oxytocin unlike vasopressin is a stress hormone in the rat. *Neuroendocrinology* 37:314, 1983.
108. Ukai M, Moran WH, Zimmerman B: The role of visceral afferent pathways in vasopressin secretion and urinary excretory patterns during surgical stress. *Ann Surg* 168:16, 1968.
109. Segar WE, Moore WW: The regulation of antidiuretic hormone release in man. *J Clin Invest* 47:2143, 1968.
110. Heyes MP, Farber MO, Manfredi F, Robertshaw D, Weinberger M, Fineberg N, Robertson G: Acute effects of hypoxia on renal and endocrine function in normal man. *Am J Physiol* 243:R265, 1982.
111. Baylis PH, Stockley RA, Heath DA: Effect of acute hypoxemia on plasma arginine vasopressin in conscious man. *Clin Sci Mol Med* 53:401, 1977.
112. Raff H, Shinsako J, Keil LC, Dallman MF: Vasopressin, ACTH, and corticosteroids during hypercapnia and graded hypoxia in dogs. *Am J Physiol* 244:E453, 1983.
113. Rose CE Jr, Anderson RJ, Carey RM: Antidiuresis and vasopressin release with hypoxemia and hypercapnia in conscious dogs. *Am J Physiol* 247:R127, 1984.
114. Raff H, Shinsako J, Keil LC, Dallman MF: Vasopressin, ACTH, and blood pressure during hypoxia induced at different rates. *Am J Physiol* 245:E489, 1983.
115. Farber MO, Weinberg MH, Robertson GL, Fineberg NS, Manfredi F: Hormonal abnormalities affecting sodium and water balance in acute respiratory failure due to chronic obstructive lung disease. *Chest* 85:49, 1984.
116. Miller M, Moses AM: Drug-induced states of impaired water excretion. *Kidney Int* 10:96, 1976.
117. McDonald KM, Miller PD, Anderson RJ, Berl T, Schrier RW: Hormonal control of renal water excretion. *Kidney Int* 10:38, 1976.
118. Rockhold RW, Crofton JT, Wang BC, Share L: Effect of intracarotid administration of morphine and naloxone on plasma vasopressin levels and blood pressure in the dog. *J Pharmacol Exp Ther* 224:386, 1982.
119. DeFronzo RA, Braine H, Colvin OM, Davis PJ: Water intoxication in man after cyclophosphamide therapy: Time course and relation to drug activation. *Ann Intern Med* 78:861, 1973.
120. Steele TH, Serpick AA, Block JB: Antidiuretic response to cyclophosphamide in man. *J Pharmacol Exp Ther* 185:245, 1973.
121. Robertson GL, Bhoopalam N, Zelkowitz LJ: Vincristine neurotoxicity and abnormal secretion of antidiuretic hormone. *Arch Intern Med* 132:717, 1973.
122. Gold PW, Robertson GL, Post RM, Kaye W, Ballenger J, Rubinow D, Goodwin FK: The effect of lithium on the osmoregulation of arginine vasopressin secretion. *J Clin Endocrinol Metab* 56:295, 1983.
123. Miller PD, Dubovsky SL, McDonald KM, Katz FJ, Robertson GL, Schrier RW: Central, renal and adrenal effects of lithium in man. *Am J Med* 66:797, 1979.
124. Padfield PL, Park SJ, Morton JJ, Braidwood AE: Plasma levels of antidiuretic hormone in patients receiving prolonged lithium therapy. *Br J Psychiatry* 130:144, 1977.
125. Moses AM, Howanitz J, van Gemert M, Miller M: Clofibrate-induced antidiuresis. *J Clin Invest* 52:535, 1973.
126. Moses AM, Numann P, Miller M: Mechanism of chlorpropamide-induced antidiuresis in man: Evidence for release of ADH and enhancement of peripheral action. *Metabolism* 22:59, 1973.
127. Pockracki FJ, Robinson AG, Seif SM: Chlorpropamide effect: Measurement of neurophysin and vasopressin in humans and rats. *Metabolism* 30:72, 1978.
128. Gold PW, Robertson GL, Ballenger JC, Kaye W, Chen J, Rubinow DR, et al: Carbamazepine diminishes the sensitivity of the plasma arginine vasopressin response to osmotic stimulation. *J Clin Endocrinol Metab* 57:952, 1983.
129. Stephens WP, Coe JY, Baylis PH: Plasma arginine vasopressin concentrations and antidiuretic action of carbamazepine. *Br Med J* 1:1445, 1978.
130. Thomas TH, Ball SG, Wales JK, Lee MR: Effect of carbamazepine on plasma and urine arginine-vasopressin. *Clin Sci Mol Med* 54:419, 1978.
131. Kamoi K, White K, Robertson GL: Opiates elevate the osmotic threshold for vasopressin (VP) release in rats. *Clin Res* 27:254A, 1979.
132. Miller M: Inhibition of ADH release in the rat by narcotic antagonists. *Neuroendocrinology* 19:241, 1975.
133. Van Wimersma Greidanus TB, Thody TJ, Verspaget H, deRotte GA, Goedemans HJH, Croiset G, van Ree JM: Effects of morphine and β-endorphin on basal and elevated plasma levels of α-MSH and vasopressin. *Life Sci* 24:579, 1979.
134. Summy-Long JY, Keil LC, Deen K, Severs WB: Opiate regulation of angiotensin-induced drinking and vasopressin release. *J Pharmacol Exp Ther* 217:630, 1981.
135. Leander JD: Further study of kappa opioids on increased urination. *J Pharmacol Exp Ther* 227:35, 1983.
136. Leander JD: A kappa opioid effect: Increased urination in the rat. *J Pharmacol Exp Ther* 224:89, 1983.
137. Ohnishi A, Mihara M, Yasuda S, Tomono Y, Hasegawa J, Tanaka T: Aquaretic effect of the stable dynorphin-A analog E2078 in the human. *J Pharmacol Exp Ther* 270:342, 1994.
138. Brownell J, del Pozo E, Donatsch P: Inhibition of vasopressin secretion by a met-enkephalin (FK 33-824) in humans. *Acta Endocrinol (Copenh)* 94:304, 1980.
139. Grossman A, Besser GM, Milles JJ, Baylis PH: Inhibition of vasopressin release in man by an opiate peptide. *Lancet* 2:1108, 1980.
140. Zerbe RL, Henry DP, Robertson GL: A new met-enkephalin analogue suppresses plasma vasopressin in man. *Peptides* 1:199, 1981.
141. Miller M: Role of endogenous opioids in neurohypophyseal function in man. *J Clin Endocrinol Metab* 50:1016, 1980.
142. Kleeman CR, Rubini ME, Lamdin E, Epstein FH: Studies on alcohol diuresis: II. The evaluation of ethyl alcohol as an inhibitor of the neurohypophysis. *J Clin Invest* 34:448, 1955.
143. Helderman JH, Vestal RE, Rowe JW, Tobin JD, Andres R, Robertson GL: The response of arginine vasopressin in intravenous ethanol and hypertonic saline in man: The impact of aging. *J Gerontol* 33:339, 1978.
144. Oiso Y, Robertson GL: Effect of ethanol on vasopressin secretion and the role of endogenous opioids, in Schrier R (ed): *Vasopressin*. New York, Raven, 1985, pp 265–269.
145. Reid IA, Ahn JN, Trinh T, Schackelford R, Weintraub M, Keil LC: Mechanism of suppression of vasopressin and adrenocorticotropic hormone secretion by clonidine in anesthetized dogs. *J Pharmacol Exp Ther* 229:18, 1984.
146. Roman RJ, Cowley AW Jr, Lechene C: Water diuretic and natriuretic effect of clonidine in the rat. *J Pharmacol Exp Ther* 211:385, 1979.
147. Iovino M, De Caro G, Massi M, Steardo O, Poenaru S: Muscimol inhibits ADH release induced by hypertonic sodium chloride in rats. *Pharmacol Biochem Behav* 19:335, 1983.
148. Xu Z, Herbert J: Effects of intracerebroventricular dizocilpine (MK801) on dehydration-induced dipsogenic responses, plasma vasopressin and c-fos expression in the rat. *Brain Res* 784:91, 1998.
149. Engel P, Rowe J, Minaker K, Robertson GL: Effect of exogenous vasopressin on vasopressin release. *Am J Physiol* 246:E202, 1984.
150. Wang BC, Share L, Crofton JT: Central infusion of vasopressin de-

creased plasma vasopressin concentration in dogs. *Am J Physiol* 243:E365, 1982.
151. Liu HW, Wang YX, Crofton JT, Funyu T, Share L: Central vasopressin blockade enhances its peripheral release in response to peripheral osmotic stimulation in conscious rats. *Brain Res* 719:14, 1996.
152. Kombian SB, Mouginot D, Pittman QJ: Dendritically released peptides act as retrograde modulators of afferent excitation in the supraoptic nucleus in vitro. *Neuron* 19:903, 1997.
153. Ludwig M, Leng G: Autoinhibition of supraoptic nucleus vasopressin neurons in vivo: A combined retrodialysis/electrophysiological study in rats. *Eur J Neurosci* 9:2532, 1997.
154. Amico JA, Ervin MG, Leake RD, Fisher DA, Finn FM, Robinson AG: A novel oxytocin-like and vasotocin-like peptide in human plasma after administration of estrogen. *J Clin Endocrinol Metab* 60:5, 1985.
155. Fehr S, Ivell R, Koll R, Schams D, Fields M, Richter D: Expression of the oxytocin gene in the large cells of the bovine corpus luteum. *FEBS Lett* 210:45, 1987.
156. Jankowski M, Hajjar F, Kawas SA, Mukaddam-Daher S, Hoffman G, McCann SM, Gutkowska J: Rat heart: A site of oxytocin production and action. *Proc Natl Acad Sci USA* 95:14558, 1998.
157. Nussey SS, Ang VTY, Finer N, Jenkins JS: Responses of neurohypophysial peptides to hypertonic saline and insulin-induced hypoglycaemia in man. *Clin Endocrinol (Oxf)* 24:97, 1986.
158. Moos F, Freund-Mercier MJ, Guerne Y, Guerne JM, Stoeckel ME, Richard P: Release of oxytocin and vasopressin by magnocellular nuclei in vitro: Specific facilitatory effect of oxytocin on its own release. *J Endocrinol* 102:63, 1984.
159. Lausen HD: Metabolism of the neurohypophyseal hormones, in Greep RO, Astwood EB, Knobil E, Sawyer WH, Geiger SR (eds): *Handbook of Physiology*. Washington, American Physiological Society, 1974, vol 4, pp 287–393.
160. Robertson GL, Mahr EA, Athar S, Sinha T: Development and clinical application of a new method for the radioimmunoassay of arginine vasopressin in human plasma. *J Clin Invest* 52:2340, 1973.
161. Davison JM, Sheills EA, Barron WM, Robinson AG, Lindheimer MD: Changes in the metabolic clearance of vasopressin and in plasma vasopressinase throughout human pregnancy. *J Clin Invest* 83:1313, 1989.
162. Grove L, Christensen P, Bie P: Effects of receptor blockade on metabolism and renal actions of vasopressin in conscious dogs. *Acta Physiol Scand* 163:93, 1998.
163. Amico JA, Ulbrecht JS, Robinson AG: Clearance studies of oxytocin in humans using radioimmunoassay measurements of the hormone in plasma and urine. *J Clin Endocrinol Metab* 64:340, 1987.
164. Plotsky PM, Sawchenko PE: Hypophysial-portal plasma levels, median eminence content, and immunohistochemical staining of corticotropin-releasing factor, arginine vasopressin, and oxytocin after pharmacological adrenalectomy. *Endocrinology* 120:1361, 1987.
165. Sherman TG, McKelvy JF, Watson SJ: Vasopressin mRNA regulation in individual hypothalamic nuclei: A northern and in situ hybridization analysis. *J Neurosci* 6:1685, 1986.
166. Jenkins JS, Mather HM, Ang V: Vasopressin in human cerebrospinal fluid. *J Clin Endocrinol Metab* 59:364, 1980.
167. Szczepanska-Sadowska E, Gray D, Simon-Opperman C: Vasopressin in blood and third ventricle CSF during dehydration, thirst and hemorrhage. *Am J Physiol* 245:R549, 1983.
168. Amico JA, Tenicela R, Robinson AG: Neurohypophysial hormones in cerebrospinal fluid of adults: Absence of arginine vasotocin and of a diurnal rhythm of arginine vasopressin. *J Clin Endocrinol Metab* 61:794, 1985.
169. Szczepanska-Sadowska E, Sobocinska J, Sadowski B: Central dipsogenic effect of vasopressin. *Am J Physiol* 242:R372, 1982.
170. De Wied D: Behavioral effects of intraventricularly administered vasopressin and vasopressin fragments. *Life Sci* 19:685, 1976.
171. Sorensen PS, Hammer M, Vorstrup S, Gjerris F: CSF and plasma vasopressin concentration in dementia. *J Neurol Neurosurg Psychiatry* 46:911, 1983.
172. Gold PW, Goodwin FK, Ballenger JC, Post RM, Weingartner H, Robertson GL: Central vasopressin function in affective illness. *Int J Ment Health* 9:91, 1981.
173. Sorensen PS, Hammer M, Gjerris F: Cerebrospinal fluid vasopressin in benign intracranial hypertension. *Neurology* 32:1255, 1982.
174. Berliner RW, Levinsky NG, Davidson DG, Eden M: Dilution and concentration of the urine and the action of antidiuretic hormone. *Am J Med* 24:730, 1958.
175. Hays RM: Cellular and molecular events in the action of antidiuretic hormone. *Kidney Int* 49:1700, 1996.
176. Knepper MA: Molecular physiology of urinary concentrating mechanism: Regulation of aquaporin water channels by vasopressin. *Am J Physiol* 272 (*Renal Physiol* 41):F3, 1997.
177. Knepper MA, Inoue T: Regulation of aquaporin-2 water channel trafficking by vasopressin. *Curr Opin Cell Biol* 9:560, 1997.
178. Brown D, Katsura T, Gustafson CE: Cellular mechanisms of aquaporin trafficking. *Am J Physiol* 275:F328, 1998.
179. Verkman AS, van Hoek AN, Ma T, Frigeri A, Skach WR, Mitra A, et al: Water transport across mammalian cell membranes. *Am J Physiol* 270:C12, 1996.
180. Sasaki S, Fushimi K, Saito H, Saito F, Uchida S, Ishibashi K, et al: Cloning, characterization, and chromosomal mapping of human aquaporin of collecting duct. *J Clin Invest* 93:1250, 1994.
181. Promeneur D, Bankir L, Hu MC, Trinh-Trang-Tan MM: Renal tubular and vascular urea transporters: Influence of antidiuretic hormone on messenger RNA expression in Brattleboro rats. *J Am Soc Nephrol* 9:1359, 1998.
182. Nielsen S, Terris J, Smith CP, Hediger MA, Ecelbarger CA, Knepper MA: Cellular and subcellular localization of the vasopressin-regulated urea transporter in rat kidney. *Proc Natl Acad Sci USA* 93:5495, 1996.
183. Jard S: Vasopressin receptors. A historical survey. *Adv Exp Med Biol* 449:1, 1998.
184. Lolait SJ, O'Carroll AM, McBride OW, Konig M, Morel A, Brownstein MJ: Cloning and characterization of a vasopressin V_2 receptor and possible link to nephrogenic diabetes insipidus. *Nature* 357:336, 1992.
185. Birnbaumer M, Seibold A, Gilbert S, Ishido M, Barberis C, Antaramian A, et al: Molecular cloning of the receptor for human antidiuretic hormone. *Nature* 357:333, 1992.
186. Ohnishi A, Orita Y, Okahara R, Fujihara H, Inoue T, Yamamura Y, et al: Potent aquaretic agent—A novel nonpeptide selective vasopressin 2 antagonist (OPC-31260) in men. *J Clin Invest* 92:2653, 1993.
187. Matsuhisa A, Tanaka A, Kikuchi K, Shimada Y, Yatsu T, Yanagisawa I: Nonpeptide arginine vasopressin antagonists for both V_{1A} and V_2 receptors: Synthesis and pharmacological properties of 2-Phenyl-4′-[(2,3,4,5-tetrahydro-1*H*-1-benzazepin-1-yl)carbonyl]-benzanilide derivatives. *Chem Pharm Bull* 45:1870, 1997.
188. Tahara A, Saito M, Sugimoto T, Tomura Y, Wada K, Kusayama T, et al: Pharmacological characterization of YM087, a potent, nonpeptide human vasopressin V_{1A} and V_2 receptor antagonist. *Naunyn Schmiedeberg's Arch Pharmacol* 357:63, 1998.
189. Montani JP, Liard JF, Schoun J, Mohring J: Hemodynamic effects of exogenous and endogenous vasopressin at low plasma concentrations in dogs. *Circ Res* 47:346, 1980.
190. Graybiel A, Glendy RE: Circulatory effects following the intravenous administration of pitressin in normal persons and in patients with hypertension and angina pectoris. *Am Heart J* 21:481, 1941.
191. Bussien JP, Waeber B, Nussberger J, Schaller MD, Gavras H, Hofbauer K, Brunner HR: Does vasopressin sustain blood pressure of normally hydrated healthy volunteers? *Am J Physiol* 246 (*Heart Circ Physiol* 15):H143, 1984.
192. Suzuki S, Takeshita A, Imaisumi T, Hirooka Y, Yoshida M, Ando S, Nakamura M: Biphasic forearm vascular responses to intraarterial arginine vasopressin. *J Clin Invest* 84:427, 1989.
193. Vavra I, Machova A, Holecek V, Cort JH, Zaoral M, Sorm F: Effect of a synthetic analogue of vasopressin in animals and in patients with diabetes insipidus. *Lancet* 1:948, 1968.
194. Sawyer WH, Manning M: The development of potent and specific vasopressin antagonists. *Kidney Int* 34(Suppl 26):S34, 1988.
195. Morel A, O'Carroll AM, Brownstein MJ, Lolait SJ: *Nature* 356:523, 1992.
196. Thibonnier M, Auzan C, Madhun Z, Wilkins P, Berti-Mattera L, Clauser E: *J Biol Chem* 269:3304, 1994.
197. Hurbin A, Boissin-Agasse L, Orcel H, Rabié A, Joux N, Desarménien MG, et al: The V_{1a} and V_{1b}, but not V_2, vasopressin receptor genes are expressed in the supraoptic nucleus of the rat hypothalamus, and the transcripts are essentially colocalized in the

vasopressinergic magnocellular neurons. *Endocrinology* 139:4701, 1998.

198. Ohnishi A, Ko Y, Fujihara H, Miyamoto G, Okada K, Odomi M: Pharmacokinetics, safety, and pharmacologic effects of OPC-21268, a nonpeptide orally active vasopressin V_1 receptor antagonist, in humans. *J Clin Pharmacol* 33:230, 1993.
199. Weber R, Pechére-Bertschi A, Hayoz D, Gerc V, Brouard R, Lahmy JP, et al: Effects of SR 49059, a new orally active and specific vasopressin V_1 receptor antagonist, on vasopressin-induced vasoconstriction in humans. *Hypertension* 30:1121, 1997.
200. Kawano Y, Matsuoka H, Nishikimi T, Takishita S, Omae T: The role of vasopressin in essential hypertension. Plasma levels and effects of the V_1 receptor antagonist OPC-21268 during different dietary sodium intakes. *Am J Hypertens* 10:1240, 1997.
201. Huch KM, Wall BM, Mangold TA, Bobal MA, Cooke CR: Hemodynamic response to vasopressin in dehydrated human subjects. *J Invest Med* 46:312, 1998.
202. Liu JH, Muse K, Contreras P, Gibbs D, Vale W, Rivier J, Yeu SSC: Activation of ACTH-releasing activity of synthetic corticotropin releasing factor (CRF) by vasopressin in women. *J Clin Endocrinol Metab* 57:1087, 1983.
203. Rivier C, Vale W: Interaction of corticotropin releasing factor and arginine vasopressin on adrenocorticotropin secretion in vivo. *Endocrinology* 113:939, 1983.
204. Spinedi E, Negro-Vilar A: Angiotensin II and ACTH release: Site of actin and potency relative to corticotropin releasing factor and vasopressin. *Neuroendocrinology* 37:446, 1983.
205. Jard S, Gaillard RC, Guillon G, Marie J, Schoenenberg P, Muller AF, et al: Vasopressin antagonists allow demonstration of a novel type of vasopressin receptor in the rat adenohypophysis. *Mol Pharmacol* 30:171, 1986.
206. Vaccari C, Lolait SJ, Ostrowski NL: Comparative distribution of vasopressin V_{1b} and oxytocin receptor messenger ribonucleic acids in brain. *Endocrinology* 139:5015, 1998.
207. Sugimoto T, Saito M, Mochizuki S, Watanabe Y, Hashimoto S, Kawashima H: Molecular cloning and functional expression of a cDNA encoding the human V_{1b} vasopressin receptor. *J Biol Chem* 269:27088, 1994.
208. McCann SM, Antunes-Rodrigues J, Nallar R, Valtin H: Pituitary adrenal function in the absence of vasopressin. *Endocrinology* 76:1058, 1966.
209. Arimura A, Saito T, Bowers CY, Schally AV: Pituitary adrenal activation in rats with hereditary hypothalamic diabetes insipidus. *Acta Endocrinol (Copenh)* 54:155, 1967.
210. Carlson DE, Gann DS: Effect of vasopressin antiserum on the response of adrenocorticotropin and cortisol to hemorrhage. *Endocrinology* 114:317, 1984.
211. Dicker SE, Nunn JE: The role of the antidiuretic hormone during water deprivation in rats. *J Physiol* 136:235, 1957.
212. Adolph EF: *Physiology of Man in the Desert*. New York, Hafner, 1969.
213. Schapiro H: Inhibiting action of antidiuretic hormone on canine pancreatic exocrine flow. *Am J Digest Dis* 20:853, 1975.
214. Heims DA, Whitton PD, Ma GY: Metabolic actions of vasopressin, glucagon and adrenalin in the intact rat. *Biochim Biophys Acta* 411:155, 1975.
215. Grant JA, Scrutton MC: Positive interaction between agonists in the aggregation response of human blood platelets: Interaction between ADP, adrenaline and vasopressin. *Br J Haematol* 44:109, 1980.
216. Terlouw EM, Kent S, Cremona S, Dantzer R: Effect of intracerebroventricular administration of vasopressin on stress-induced hyperthermia in rats. *Physiol Behav* 60:417, 1996.
217. Caras SD, Soykan I, Beverly V, Lin Z, McCallum RW: The effect of intravenous vasopressin on gastric myoelectrical activity in human subjects. *Neurogastroenterol Motil* 9:151, 1997.
218. Amico JA: Diabetes insipidus and pregnancy. *Front Horm Res* 13:266, 1985.
219. Nishimori K, Young LJ, Guo Q, Wang Z, Insel TR, Matzuk MM: Oxytocin is reguired for nursing but is not essential for parturition or reproductive behavior. *Proc Natl Acad Sci USA* 93:11699, 1996.
220. Amico JA, Seitchik J, Robinson AG: Studies of oxytocin in plasma of women during hypocontractile labor. *J Clin Endocrinol Metab* 58:274, 1984.
221. Rozen F, Russo C, Banville D, Zingg HH: Structure, characterization, and expression of the rat oxytocin receptor gene. *Proc Natl Acad Sci USA* 92:200, 1995.
222. Williams PD, Bock MG, Evans BE, Freidinger RM, Pettibone DJ: Progress in the development of oxytocin antagonists for use in preterm labor. *Adv Exp Med Biol* 449:473, 1998.
223. Goodwin TM, Zograbyan A: Oxytocin receptor antagonists. Update. *Clin Perinatol* 25:859, 1998.
224. Gutkowska J, Jankowski M, Lambert C, Mukaddam-Daher S, Zingg HH, McCann SM: Oxytocin releases atrial natriuretic peptide by combining with oxytocin receptors in the heart. *Proc Natl Acad Sci USA* 94:11704, 1997.
225. Kelley S, Robertson GL, Amico JA: Antidiuretic action of oxytocin in humans. *Clin Res* 40:711A, 1992.
226. Edwards BR, LaRochelle T: Antidiuretic effect of endogenous oxytocin in dehydrated brattleboro homozygous rats. *Am J Physiol* 247 (*Renal Fluid Electrolyte Physiol* 16):F453, 1984.
227. Chou CL, DiGiovanni SR, Luther A, Lolait SJ, Knepper MA: Oxytocin as an antidiuretic hormone. *Am J Physiol* 269:F78, 1995.
228. Ramsay DJ: Water: Distribution between compartments and its relationship to thirst, in Ramsay DJ, Booth DA (eds): *Thirst—Physiological and Psychological Aspects*. London, Springer-Verlag, 1990, pp 23–52.
229. Robertson GL: Disorders of thirst in man, in Ramsay DJ, Booth DA (eds): *Thirst—Physiological and Psychological Aspects*. London, Springer-Verlag, 1990, pp 453–475.
230. Rolls BJ: Physiological determinants of fluid intake in humans, in Ramsay DJ, Booth DA (eds): *Thirst—Physiological and Psychological Aspects*. London, Springer-Verlag, 1990, pp 391–398.
231. Verbalis JG: Inhibitory controls of drinking: Satiation of thirst, in Ramsay DJ, Booth DA (eds): *Thirst—Physiological and Psychological Aspects*. London, Springer-Verlag, 1990, pp 313–330.
232. Kovacs L, Rittig S, Robertson GL: Effects of sustained antidiuretic treatment on plasma sodium concentration and body water homeostasis in healthy humans on ad libitum fluid intake. *Clin Res* 40:165A, 1992.
233. McKinley MJ: Osmoreceptor for thirst, in Ramsay DJ, Booth DA (eds): *Thirst—Physiological and Psychological Aspects*. London, Springer-Verlag, 1990, pp 77–91.
234. Johnson AK, Edwards GL: Central projections of osmotic and hypovolaemic signals in homeostatic thirst, in Ramsay DJ, Booth DA (eds): *Thirst—Physiological and Psychological Aspects*. London, Springer-Verlag, 1990, pp 149–168.
235. Thrasher TN: Volume receptors and the stimulation of water intake, in Ramsay DJ, Booth DA (eds): *Thirst—Physiological and Psychological Aspects*. London, Springer-Verlag, 1990, pp 93–107.
236. Kozlowski S, Szczepanska-Sadowska E: Antagonistic effects of vasopressin and hypervolemia on osmotic reactivity of the thirst mechanism in dogs. *Pflugers Arch* 353:59, 1975.
237. Szczepanska-Sadowska E: Hormonal inputs to thirst, in Ramsay DJ, Booth DA (eds): *Thirst—Physiological and Psychological Aspects*. London, Springer-Verlag, 1990, pp 110–125.
238. Oldfield BJ: Neurochemistry of the circuitry subserving thirst, in Ramsay DJ, Booth DA (eds): *Thirst—Physiological and Psychological Aspects*. London, Springer-Verlag, 1990, pp 176–188.
239. Stricker EM: Central control of water and sodium chloride intake in rats during hypovolaemia, in Ramsay DJ, Booth DA (eds): *Thirst—Physiological and Psychological Aspects*. London: Springer-Verlag, 1990, pp 194–203.
240. Altman PL, Dittmer DS (eds): *Blood and Other Body Fluids*. Washington, American Society of Experimental Biology, 1961.
241. Leaf A, Chatillon JY, Wrong O, Tuttle EP Jr: The mechanism of the osmotic adjustment of body cells as determined in vivo by the volume of distribution of a large waterload. *J Clin Invest* 33:1261, 1954.
242. Wolf AV, McDowell ME: Apparent and osmotic volumes of distribution of sodium, chloride, sulfate and urea. *Am J Physiol* 176:207, 1954.
243. Hendry EB: Osmolarity of human serum and of chemical solutions of biologic importance. *Clin Chem* 7:156, 1961.
244. Darrow DC, Yanett H: Changes in distribution of body water accompanying increase and decrease in extracellular electrolytes. *J Clin Invest* 14:266, 1935.
245. Arieff AI, Guisado R, Lazarowitz VC: Pathophysiology of hyperosmolar states, in Andreoli TE, Grantham JJ, Rector FC (eds): *Disturbances in Body Fluid Osmolality*. Bethesda, American Physiological Society, 1977, pp 227–250.
246. Coggins CH, Leaf A: Diabetes insipidus. *Am J Med* 42:807, 1967.
247. Greger NG, Kirkland RT, Clayton GW, Kirkland JL: Central diabetes insipidus. *Am J Dis Child* 140:551, 1986.

248. Greger NG, Kirkland RT, Clayton GW, Kirkland JL: Central diabetes insipidus. 22 years' experience. *Am J Dis Child* 140:551, 1986.
249. Wang LC, Cohen ME, Duffner PK: Etiology of central diabetes insipidus in children. *Pediatr Neurol* 11:273, 1994.
250. Robertson GL: Diabetes insipidus. *Endocrinol Metab Clin North Am* 24:549, 1995.
251. Elster AD: Modern imaging of the pituitary. *Radiology* 187:1, 1993.
252. Hansen LK, Rittig S, Robertson GL: Genetic basis of familial neurohypophyseal diabetes insipidus. *Trends Endocrinol Metab* 8:363, 1997.
253. Repaske DR, Medlej R, Gültekin EK, Krishnamani MRS, Halaby G, Findling JW, Phillips JA: Heterogeneity in clinical manifestation of autosomal dominant neurohypophyseal diabetes insipidus caused by a mutation encoding $Ala^{-1} \rightarrow$ Val in the signal peptide of the arginine vasopressin/neurophysinII/copeptin precursor. *J Clin Endocrinol Metab* 82:51, 1997.
254. Gagliardi PC, Bernasconi S, Repaske DR: Autosomal dominant neurohypophyseal diabetes insipidus associated with a missense mutation encoding GLY(23)-]VAL in neurophysin II. *J Clin Endocrinol Metab* 82:3643, 1997.
255. Goking NG, Chertow BS, Robertson GL, Rittig S, Sigaard C, Pedersen EB: Familial neurohypophyseal diabetes insipidus—A novel mutation presenting with enuresis. *J Invest Med* 45:29A, 1999.
256. Heppner C, Kotzka J, Bullman C, Krone W, Müller-Wieland D: Identification of mutations in the arginine vasopressin-neurophysin II gene in two kindreds with familial central diabetes insipidus. *J Clin Endocrinol Metab* 83:693, 1998.
257. Calvo B, Bilbao JR, Urrutia I, Eizaguirre J, Gaztambide S, Castano L: Identification of a novel nonsense mutation and a missense substitution in the vasopressin-neurophysin II gene in two spanish kindreds with familial neurohypophyseal diabetes insipidus. *J Clin Endocrinol Metab* 83:995, 1998.
258. Grant FD, Ahmadi A, Hosley CM, Majzoub JA: Two novel mutations of the vasopressin gene associated with familial diabetes insipidus and identification of an asymptomatic carrier infant. *J Clin Endocrinol Metab* 83:3958, 1998.
259. Fujii H, Iida S, Moriwaki K: A novel mutation in the arginine vasopressin—neurophysin II gene associated with familial neurohy pophyseal diabetes insipidus. *80th Annual Meeting of the Endocrine Society, New Orleans,* Abstract P2-468, P347, 1998.
260. Bullmann C, Heppner C, Kotzka J, Jockenhovel F, Müller-Weiland D, Krone W: Familial central diabetes insipidus—A mutation in the arginine-vasopressin-neurophysin II gene. *Exp Clin Endocrinol Dia betes* 106:S6, 1998.
261. Kawakami A, Okamoto Y, Yamamoto T, Tatsumi Y, Miki T, Tanaka S, Fujii S: Central diabetes insipidus associated with a missense mutation in the arginine vasopressin gene that replaces Ala at the carboxyterminus of the signal peptide with Thr. *Intern Med* 37:683, 1998.
262. Rutishauser J, Kopp P, Gaskill MB, Kotlar TJ, Robertson GL: A novel mutation (R97C) in the neurophysin moiety of prepro-vasopressin-neurophysin II associated with autosomal-dominant neurohypophyseal diabetes insipidus. *Mol Genet Metab* 67:89, 1999.
263. Calvo B, Bilbao JR, Rodriguez A, Rodriguez-Arnao MD, Castaño L: Molecular analysis in familial neurohypophyseal diabetes insipidus: Early diagnosis of an asymptomatic carrier. *J Clin Endocrinol Metab* 84:3351, 1999.
264. Robertson G, Rittig S, Gu WX, Siggaard C, Jameson L, Gregersen N, Pedersen E: Pathogenesis and pathophysiology of familial neurohypophyseal diabetes insipidus. In: Saito T, Kurokawa K, Yoshida S (eds): *Neurohypophysis: Recent Progress of Vasopressin and Oxytocin Research.* Amsterdam, Elsevier Science, 1995, pp 593–603.
265. Olias G, Richter D, Schmale H: Heterologous expression of human vasopressin-neurophysin precursors in a pituitary cell line: Defective transport of a mutant protein from patients with familial diabetes insipidus. *DNA Cell Biol* 15:929, 1996.
266. Ito M, Jameson JL, Ito M: Molecular basis of autosomal dominant neurohypophyseal diabetes insipidus cellular toxicity caused by the accumulation of mutant vasopressin precursors within the endoplasmic reticulum. *J Clin Invest* 99:1897, 1997.
267. Siggaard C, Rittig S, Corydon TJ, Andreasen PH, Jensen TG, Andresen BS, et al: Clinical and molecular evidence of abnormal processing and trafficking of the vasopressin prehormone in a large kindred with familial neurohypophyseal diabetes insipidus due to a signal peptide mutation. *J Clin Endocrinol Metab* 84:2933, 1999.
268. Habiby RL, Robertson GL, Kaplowitz PB, Rittig S: A novel x-linked form of familial neurohypophyseal diabetes insipidus. *J Invest Med* 44:341A, 1996.
269. Willcutts MD, Felner E, White PC: Autosomal recessive familial neurohypophyseal diabetes insipidus with continued secretion of mutant weakly active vasopressin. *Hum Mol Genet* 8:1303, 1999.
270. Cremers CWRJ, Wijdeveld PGAB, Pinckers AJLG: Juvenile diabetes mellitus, optic atrophy, hearing loss, diabetes insipidus, atonia of the urinary tract and bladder, and other abnormalities (Wolfram syndrome). *Acta Paediatr Scand* 264:3, 1977.
271. Inoue H, Tanizawa Y, Wasson J, Behn P, Kalidas K, Bernal-Mizrachi E, et al: A gene encoding a transmembrane protein is mutated in patients with diabetes mellitus and optic atrophy (Wolfram syndrome). *Nat Genet* 20:143, 1998.
272. Gabreëls BATF, Swaab DF, de Kleijn DPV, Dean A, Seidah NG, Van de Loo JW, et al: The vasopressin precursor is not processed in the hypothalamus of wolfram syndrome patients with diabetes insipidus: Evidence for the involvement of PC2 and 7B2. *J Clin Endocrinol Metab* 83:4026, 1998.
273. Thompson CJ, Charlton J, Walford S, Baird J, Hearnshaw J, McCulloch A, et al: Vasopressin secretion in the DIDMOAD (Wolfram) syndrome. *Q J Med* 264:333, 1989.
274. Yagi H, Nagashima K, Miyake H, Tamai S, Onigata K, Yutani S, Kuroume T: Familial congenital hypopituitarism with central diabetes insipidus. *J Clin Endocrinol Metab* 78:884, 1994.
275. Robinson IC, O'Malley BP, Young ID: Familial cerebellar ataxia and diabetes insipidus. *J Neurol Neurosurg Psychiatry* 51:1576, 1988.
276. Ng PC, Lee CH, Fok TF, Lam ST, Chan YL, Wong W, et al: Central diabetes insipidus in a newborn with deletion of chromosome 7q. *J Pediatr Child Health* 33:343, 1997.
277. Imura H, Nakao K, Shimatsu A, Ogawa Y, Sando T, Fujisawa I, Yamabe H: Lymphocytic infundibuloneurohypophysitis as a cause of central diabetes insipidus. *N Engl J Med* 329:683, 1993.
278. Ahmed SR, Aiello DP, Page R, Hopper K, Towfighi J, Santen RJ: Necrotizing infundibulo-hypophysitis: A unique syndrome of diabetes insipidus and hypopituitarism. *J Clin Endocrinol Metab* 76:1499, 1993.
279. Koshiyama H, Sato H, Yorita S, Koh T, Kanatsuna T, Nishimura K, et al: Lymphocytic hypophysitis presenting with diabetes insipidus: Case report and literature review. *Endocrinol J* 41:93, 1994.
280. Nishioka H, Ito H, Sano T, Ito Y: Two cases of lymphocytic hypophysitis presenting with diabetes insipidus: A variant of lymphocytic infundibulo-neurohypophysitis. *Surg Neurol* 46:285, 1996.
281. Van Havenbergh T, Robberecht W, Wilms G, Van Calenbergh F, Goffin J, Dom R, et al: Lymphocytic infundibulohypophysitis presenting in the postpartum period: Case report. *Surg Neurol* 46:280, 1996.
282. Cemeroglu AP, Blaivas M, Muraszko KM, Robertson PL, Vazquez DM: Lymphocytic hypophysitis presenting with diabetes insipidus in a 14-year-old girl: Case report and review of the literature. *Eur J Pediatr* 156:684, 1997.
283. Maghnie M, Genovese E, Sommaruga MG, Arico M, Locatelli D, Arbustini E, et al: Evolution of childhood central diabetes insipidus into panhypopituitarism with a large hypothalamic mass: Is 'lymphocytic infundibuloneurohypophysitis' in children a different entity? *Eur J Endocrinol* 139:635, 1998.
284. Blotner H: Primary or idiopathic diabetes insipidus: A system disease. *Metabolism* 7:191, 1958.
285. Braverman LE, Mancini JP, McGoldrick DM: Hereditary idiopathic diabetes insipidus: A case report with autopsy findings. *Ann Intern Med* 63:503, 1965.
286. Green JR, Buchan GC, Alvord EC Jr, Swanson AG: Hereditary and idiopathic types of diabetes insipidus. *Brain* 90:707, 1967.
287. Maccubbin DA, Van Buren JM: A quantitative evaluation of hypothalamic degeneration and its relation to diabetes insipidus following interruption of the human hypophyseal stalk. *Brain* 46:443, 1963.
288. Randall RV, Clark EC, Dodge HW Jr, Love JG: Polyuria after operation for tumors in the region of the hypophysis and hypothalamus. *J Clin Endocrinol Metab* 20:1614, 1960.
289. Timmons RL, Dugger GS: Water and salt metabolism following pituitary stalk section. *Neurology* 19:790, 1969.
290. Zerbe RL, Robertson GL: A comparison of plasma vasopressin measurements with a standard indirect test in the differential diagnosis of polyuria. *N Engl J Med* 305:1539, 1981.

291. Robertson GL: Osmoregulation of thirst and vasopressin secretion: Functional properties and their relationship to water balance, in Schrier R (ed): *Vasopressin*. New York, Raven, 1985, pp 202–212.
292. Epstein FH, Kleeman CR, Hendrikx A: The influence of bodily hydration on the renal concentrating process. *J Clin Invest* 36:629, 1957.
293. De Wardener HE, Herxheimer A: The effect of high water intake on the kidney's ability to concentrate the urine in man. *J Physiol (Lond)* 139:42, 1957.
294. Alexander CS, Filbin DM, Fruchtman SA: Failure of vasopressin to produce normal urine concentration in patients with diabetes insipidus. *J Lab Clin Med* 54:566, 1959.
295. Harrington AR, Valtin H: Impaired urinary concentration after vasopressin and its gradual correction in hypothalamic diabetes insipidus. *J Clin Invest* 47:502, 1968.
296. Kanno K, Sasaki S, Hirata Y, Ishikawa S, Fushimi K, Nakanishi S, et al: Urinary excretion of aquaporin-2 in patients with diabetes insipidus. *N Engl J Med* 332:1540, 1995.
297. Knepper MA, Verbalis JG, Nielsen S: Role of aquaporins in water balance disorders. *Curr Opin Nephrol Hypertens* 6:367, 1997.
298. Pivonello R, Colao A, Di Somma C, Facciolli G, Klain M, Faggiano A, et al: Impairment of bone status in patients with central diabetes. *J Clin Endocrinol Metab* 83:2275, 1998.
299. Ford SM, Lumpkin HL: Transient vasopressin-resistant diabetes insipidus of pregnancy. *Obstet Gynecol* 68:726, 1986.
300. Baylis PH, Thompson C, Burd J, Tunbridge WMG, Snodgrass CA: Recurrent pregnancy-induced polyuria and thirst due to hypothalamic diabetes insipidus: An investigation into possible mechanisms responsible for polyuria. *Clin Endocrinol (Oxf)* 24:459, 1986.
301. Dürr JA, Hoggard JG, Hunt JM, Schrier RW: Diabetes insipidus in pregnancy associated with abnormally high circulating vasopressinase activity. *N Engl J Med* 316:1070, 1987.
302. Iwasaki Y, Oiso Y, Kondo K, Takagi S, Takatsuki K, Hasegawa H, et al: Aggravation of subclinical diabetes insipidus during pregnancy. *N Engl J Med* 324:522, 1991.
303. Hashimoto M, Ogura T, Otsuka F, Yamauchi T, Mimura Y, Hayakawa N, et al: Manifestation of subclinical diabetes insipidus due to pituitary tumor during pregnancy. *Endocrinol J* 43:577, 1996.
304. Amico JA: Diabetes insipidus and pregnancy. *Front Horm Res* 13:266, 1985.
305. Dürr JA: Diabetes insipidus in pregnancy. *Am J Kidney Dis* 9:276, 1987.
306. Robertson GL: Dipsogenic diabetes insipidus: A newly recognized syndrome caused by a selective defect in the osmoregulation of thirst. *Trans Assoc Am Physicians* C:241, 1987.
307. Stuart CA, Neelon FA, Lebovitz HE: Disordered control of thirst in hypothalamic-pituitary sarcoidosis. *N Engl J Med* 303:1078, 1980.
308. Coscina DV, Grant LD, Balagura S, Grossman SP: Hyperdipsia after serotonin-depleting midbrain lesions. *Nature* [*New Biol*] 235:53, 1972.
309. Blass EM, Nussbaum AI: Specific enhancement of drinking to angiotensin in rats. *J Comp Physiol Psychol* 87:422, 1974.
310. Gardiner TW, Stricker EM: Hyperdipsia in rats after electrolytic lesions of nucleus medianus. *Am J Physiol* 248 (*Regulatory Integrative Comp Physiol* 17):R214, 1985.
311. Sleeper FH, Jellinek EM: A comparative physiologic, psychologic and psychiatric study of polyuric and nonpolyuric schizophrenic patients. *J Nerv Ment Dis* 83:557, 1936.
312. Barlow ED, de Wardener HED: Compulsive water drinking. *Q J Med* 28:235, 1959.
313. Raskind MA, Orenstein H, Christopher TG: Acute psychosis, increased water ingestion and inappropriate antidiuretic hormone secretion. *Am J Psychiatry* 132:907, 1975.
314. Rosenbaum JF, Rothman JS, Murray GB: Psychosis and water intoxication. *J Clin Psychiatry* 40:287, 1979.
315. Jose CJ, Perez-Cruet J: Incidence and morbidity of self-induced water intoxication in state mental hospital patients. *Am J Psychiatry* 136:221, 1979.
316. Rendell M, McGrane D, Cuesta M: Fatal compulsive water drinking. *JAMA* 240:2557, 1978.
317. Hariprasad MK, Eisinger RP, Nadler IM, Padmanabhan CS, Nidus BD: Hyponatremia in psychogenic polydipsia. *Arch Intern Med* 140:1639, 1980.
318. Robertson GL: Psychogenic polydipsia and inappropriate antidiuresis. *Arch Intern Med* 140:1574, 1980.
319. Kirch DG, Bigelow LB, Weinberger DR, Lawson WB, Wyatt RJ: Polydipsia and chronic hyponatremia in schizophrenic inpatients. *J Clin Psychiatry* 46:179, 1985.
320. Illowsky BP, Kirch DG: Polydipsia and hyponatremia in psychiatric patients. *Am J Psychiatry* 145:675, 1988.
321. Goldman MB, Luchins DJ, Robertson GL: Mechanisms of altered water metabolism in psychotic patients with polydipsia and hyponatremia. *N Engl J Med* 318:397, 1988.
322. Verbalis JG, Dohanics J: Vasopressin and oxytocin secretion in chronically hyposmolar rats. *Am J Physiol* 261 (*Regulatory Integrative Comp Physiol* 30):R1028, 1991.
323. Goldman MB, Robertson GL, Luchins DJ, Hedeker D: The influence of polydipsia on water excretion in hyponatremic, polydipsic, schizophrenic patients. *J Clin Endocrinol Metab* 81:1465, 1996.
324. Goldman MB, Robertson GL, Hedeker D: Oropharyngeal regulation of water balance in polydipsic schizophrenics. *Clin Endocrinol (Oxf)* 44:31, 1996.
325. Goldman MB, Robertson GL, Luchins DJ, Hedeker D, Pandey GN: Psychotic exacerbations and enhanced vasopressin secretion in schizophrenic patients with hyponatremia and polydipsia. *Arch Gen Psychiatry* 54:443, 1997.
326. Luchins DJ, Nettles KW, Goldman MB: Anterior medial temporal lobe volumes in polydipsic schizophrenic patients with and without hypo-osmolemia: A pilot study. *Biol Psychiatry* 42:767, 1997.
327. Forssman H: Two different mutations of X-chromosome causing diabetes insipidus. *Am J Hum Genet* 7:21, 1955.
328. Bode HH, Crawford JD: Nephrogenic diabetes insipidus in North America—the Hopewell hypothesis. *N Engl J Med* 280:750, 1969.
329. Bichet DG, Fujiwara TM: Diversity of nephrogenic diabetes insipidus mutations and importance of early recognition and treatment. *Clin Exp Nephrol* 2:253, 1998.
330. Wildin RS, Cogdell DE, Valadez V: $AVPR_2$ variants and V_2 vasopressin receptor function in nephrogenic diabetes insipidus. *Kidney Int* 54:1909, 1998.
331. Oksche A, Rosenthal W: The molecular basis of nephrogenic diabetes insipidus. *J Mol Med* 76:326, 1998.
332. van Lieburg AF, Verdijk MAJ, Knoers VVAM, van Essen AJ, Proesmans W, Mallmann R, et al: Patients with autosomal nephrogenic diabetes insipidus homozygous for mutations in the aquaporin 2 water-channel gene. *Am J Hum Genet* 55:648, 1994.
333. Mulders SM, Bichet DG, Rijss JPL, Kamsteeg EJ, Arthus MF, Lonergan M, et al: An aquaporin-2 water channel mutant which causes autosomal dominant nephrogenic diabetes insipidus is retained in the golgi complex. *J Clin Invest* 102:57, 1998.
334. Robertson GL, McLeod JF, Zerbe RL, Baylis PH, Kovács L, Rittig S: Vasopressin function in heritable forms of diabetes insipidus, in Gross P, Richter D, Robertson GL (eds): *Vasopressin*. Paris, John Libbey Eurotext, 1993, pp 493–503.
335. Singer I, Forrest JN Jr: Drug-induced states of nephrogenic diabetes insipidus. *Kidney Int* 10:82, 1976.
336. Boton R, Gaviria M, Batlle DC: Prevalence, pathogenesis, and treatment of renal dysfunction associated with chronic lithium therapy *Am J Kidney Dis* 10:329, 1987.
337. Gold PW, Robertson GL, Post RM, Kaye W, Ballenger J, Rubinow D, Goodwin FK: The effect of lithium on the osmoregulation of arginine vasopressin secretion. *J Clin Endocrinol Metab* 56:295, 1983.
338. Weiss NM, Robertson GL: Effect of hypercalcemia and lithium therapy on the osmoregulation of thirst and vasopressin secretion, in Schrier R (ed): *Vasopressin*. New York, Raven, 1985, pp 281–289.
339. Bichet DG, Razi M, Lonergan M, Arthus MF, Papukna V, Kortas C, Barjon JN: Hemodynamic and coagulation responses to 1-desamino[8-D-arginine] vasopressin in patients with congenital nephrogenic diabetes insipidus. *N Engl J Med* 318:881, 1988.
340. Skillern PG, Corcoran AC, Scherbel AL: Renal mechanisms in coincident addison's disease and diabetes insipidus: effects of vasopressin and hydrocortisone. *J Clin Endocrinol Metab* 16:171, 1956.
341. Martin MM: Combined anterior pituitary and neurohypophyseal insufficiency. Studies of body fluid spaces and renal function. *J Clin Invest* 38:882, 1959.

342. Robertson GL: Differential diagnosis of polyuria. *Am Rev Med* 39:425, 1988.
343. Robertson GL: Diabetes insipidus. *Endocrinol Metab Clin North Am* 24:549, 1995.
344. Miller M, Moses AM: Urinary antidiuretic hormone in polyuric disorders and in inappropriate ADH syndrome. *Ann Intern Med* 77:715, 1972.
345. Baylis PH, Gaskill MB, Robertson GL: Vasopressin secretion in primary polydipsia and cranial diabetes insipidus. *Q J Med* 199:345, 1981.
346. Milles JJ, Spruce B, Baylis PH: A comparison of diagnostic methods to differentiate diabetes insipidus from primary polyuria: A review of 21 patients. *Acta Endocrinol (Copenh)* 104:410, 1983.
347. Laczi F, Iványi T, Julesz J, Janáky T, László FA: Plasma arginine-8-vasopressin responses to osmotic or histamine stimulation contribute to the differential diagnosis of central diabetes insipidus. *Acta Endocinologica (Copenh)* 113:168, 1986.
348. Labib M, McPhate G, Marks V: Post-traumatic diabetes insipidus combined with primary polydipsia. *Postgrad Med J* 63:33, 1987.
349. Iwasaki Y, Oiso Y, Yamauchi K, Takatsuki K, Kondo K, Hasegawa H, et al: Neurohypophyseal function in postpartum hypopituitarism: Impaired plasma vasopressin response to osmotic stimuli. *J Clin Endocrinol Metab* 68:560, 1989.
350. Sato N, Ishizaka H, Yagi H, Matsumoto M, Endo K: Posterior lobe of the pituitary in diabetes insipidus: Dynamic MR imaging. *Radiology* 186:357, 1993.
351. Brooks BS, Gammal TE, Allison JD, Hoffman WH: Frequency and variation of the posterior pituitary bright signal on MR images. *AJNR* 10:943, 1989.
352. Cox TD, Elster AD: Normal pituitary gland: Changes in shape, size, and signal intensity during the 1st year of life at MR imaging. *Pediatr Radiol* 179:721, 1991.
353. Mark LP, Haughton VM, Hendrix LE, Daniels DL, Williams AL, Czervionke LF, Asleson RJ: High-intensity signals within the posterior pituitary fossa: A study with fat-suppression MR techniques. *AJNR* 12:529, 1991.
354. Kucharczyk W, Lenkinski RE, Kaucharczyk J, Henkelman RM: The effect of phospholipid vesicles on the NMR relaxation of water: An explanation for the MR appearance of the neurohypophysis? *AJNR* 11:693, 1990.
355. Demerci A, Okten A, Gumele HR: Hyperintense posterior pituitary lobe in central diabetes insipidus. *Neuroradiology* 36:380, 1994.
356. Maghnie M, Genovese E, Bernasconi S, Binda S, Arico M: Persistent high MR signal of the posterior pituitary gland in central diabetes insipidus. *AJNR* 18:1749, 1997.
357. Drincic AT, Robertson GL: Treatment of diabetes insipidus in adults, in Meikle AW (ed): *Contemporary Endocrinology: Hormone Replacement Therapy*. Totowa, NJ, Humana Press, 1998, pp 21–38.
358. Harris AS: Clinical experience with desmopressin: Efficacy and safety in central diabetes insipidus and other conditions. *J Pediatr* 114:711, 1989.
359. Fjellestad-Paulsen A, Paulsen O, d'Agay-Abensour L, Lundin S, Czernichow P: Central Diabetes Insipidus: Oral treatment with DDAVP. *Regul Pept* 45:303, 1993.
360. Lam KSL, Wat MS, Choi KL, Ip TP, Pang RWC, Kumana CR: Pharmacokinetics, pharmacodynamics, long-term efficacy and safety of oral 1-deamino-8-D-arginine vasopressin in adult patients with central diabetes insipidus. *Br J Clin Pharmacol* 42:379, 1996.
361. Boulgourdjian EM, Martinez AS, Ropelato MG, Heinrich JJ, Bergada C: Oral desmopressin treatment of central diabetes insipidus in children. *Acta Paediatr* 86:1261, 1997.
362. Rittig S, Jensen AR, Jensen KT, Pedersen EB: Effect of food intake on the pharmacokinetics and antidiuretic activity of oral desmopressin (DDAVP) in hydrated normal subjects. *Clin Endocrinol (Oxf)* 48:235, 1998.
363. Vokes TJ, Gaskill MB, Robertson GL: Antibodies to vasopressin in patients with diabetes insipidus: Implications for diagnosis and therapy. *Ann Intern Med* 108:190, 1988.
364. Arduino F, Ferraz FPJ, Rodriques J: Antidiuretic action of chlorpropamide in idiopathic diabetes insipidus. *J Clin Endocrinol Metab* 26:1325, 1966.
365. Webster B, Bain J: Antidiuretic effect and complications of chlorpropamide therapy in diabetes insipidus. *J Clin Endocrinol Metab* 30:215, 1970.
366. Byun KY, Gaskill MB, Robertson GL: The mechanism of chlorpropamide antidiuresis in diabetes insipidus. *Clin Res* 32:483A, 1984.
367. Mendoza SA, Brown CF Jr: Effect of chlorpropamide on osmotic water flow across toad bladder and the response to vasopressin, theophylline and cyclic AMP. *J Clin Endocrinol Metab* 388:883, 1974.
368. Berndt WO, Miller M, Kettyle M, Valtin H: Potentiation of the antidiuretic effect of vasopressin by chlorpropamide. *Endocrinology* 86:1028, 1970.
369. Miller M, Moses AM: Potentiation of vasopressin action by chlorpropamide in vivo. *Endocrinology* 86:1024, 1970.
370. Murase T, Yoshida S: Mechanism of chlorpropamide action in patients with diabetes insipidus. *J Clin Endocrinol Metab* 36:174, 1973.
371. Ingelfinger JR, Hays RM: Evidence that chlorpropamide and vasopressin share a common site of action. *J Clin Endocrinol Metab* 29:738, 1969.
372. de Gennes JL, Bertrand C, Bigorie B, Truffert J: Etudes preliminaires de l'action antidiuretique du clofibrate (ou atromid S) dans le diabète insipide pitressonsensible. *Ann Endocrinol (Copenh)* 31:300, 1970.
373. Thompson P Jr, Earll JM, Schaaf M: Comparison of clofibrate and chlorpropamide in vasopressin-responsive diabetes insipidus. *Metabolism* 26:749, 1977.
374. Sekowski J, Samuel P: Clofibrate-induced acute muscular syndrome. *Am J Cardiol* 30:572, 1972.
375. Meinders AE, Cejka V, Robertson GL: The antidiuretic action of carbamazepine in man. *Clinical Science and Molecular Medicine* 47:289, 1974.
376. Earley LE, Orloff J: The mechanism of antidiuresis associated with administration of hydrochlorothiazide to patients with vasopressin resistant diabetes insipidus. *J Clin Invest* 41:1988, 1962.
377. Chico A, Puig-Domingo M, Martul P, De Juan M, Prats JM, Mauricio D, Webb SM: Reversible endocrine dysfunction and pituitary stalk enlargement. *J Endocrinol Invest* 21:122, 1998.
378. Martini G, Filosomi G, Valenti R, Lunghetti S, Pallavicino D, Nuti R: Central diabetes insipidus with spontaneous remission. A case report. *Recent Prog Med* 89:450, 1998.
379. Woredekal Y: Recurrent central diabetes insipidus secondary to cryptococcal meningitis. *J Assoc Acad Minor Phys* 9:22, 1998.
380. Catalina PF, Rodríguez García M, de la Torre C, Páramo C, García-Mayor RV: Diabetes insipidus for five years preceding the diagnosis of hypothalamic Langerhans cell histiocytosis. *J Endocrinol Invest* 18:663, 1995.
381. Mootha SL, Barkovich AJ, Grumbach MM, Edwards MS, Gitelman SE, Kaplan SL, Conte FA: Idiopathic hypothalamic diabetes insipidus, pituitary stalk thickening, and the occult intracranial germinoma in children and adolescents. *J Clin Endocrinol Metab* 82:1362, 1997.
382. Rosenzweig KE, Arceci RJ, Tarbell NJ: Diabetes insipidus secondary to Langerhans' cell histiocytosis: is radiation therapy indicated? *Med Pediatr Oncol* 29:36, 1997.
383. Ramelli GP, von der Weid N, Stanga Z, Mullis PE, Buergi U: Suprasellar germinomas in childhood and adolescence: Diagnostic pitfalls. *J Pediatr Endocrinol Metab* 11:693, 1998.
384. Pivonello R, Faggiano A, DiSomma C, Klain M, Filippella M, Salvatore M, et al: Effect of a short-term treatment with alendronate on bone density and bone markers in patients with central diabetes insipidus. *J Clin Endocrinol Metab* 84:2349, 1999.
385. Barbour GL, Straub KD, O'Neal BL, Leatherman JW: Vasopressin-resistant nephrogenic diabetes insipidus. *Arch Intern Med* 139:86, 1979.
386. Singer I, Rotenberg D: Demeclocycline-induced nephrogenic diabetes insipidus. *Ann Intern Med* 79:679, 1973.
387. Hayek A, Ramirez J: Demeclocycline-induced diabetes insipidus. *JAMA* 229:676, 1974.
388. Castell DO, Sparks HA: Nephrogenic diabetes insipidus due to demethylchlortetracycline hydrochloride. *JAMA* 193:137, 1965.
389. Lee RV, Jampol LM, Brown WV: Nephrogenic diabetes insipidus and lithium intoxication—Complications of lithium carbonate therapy. *N Engl J Med* 284:93, 1971.
390. Batlle DC, von Riotte AB, Gaviria M, Grupp M: Amelioration of polyuria by amiloride in patients receiving long-term lithium therapy. *N Engl J Med* 312:408, 1985.

391. Alon U, Chan JCM: Hydrochlorothiazide-amiloride in the treatment of congenital nephrogenic diabetes insipidus. *Am J Nephrol* 5:9, 1985.
392. Chevalier RL, Rogol AD: Tolmetin sodium in the management of nephrogenic diabetes insipidus. *Clin Lab Observ* 101:787, 1982.
393. Libber S, Harrison H, Spector D: Treatment of nephrogenic diabetes insipidus with prostaglandin synthesis inhibitors. *J Pediatr* 108:305, 1986.
394. Martinez EJ, Sinnott JT 4th, Rodriguez-Paz G, Oehler RL: Lithium-induced nephrogenic diabetes insipidus treated with indomethacin. *South Med J* 86:971, 1993.
395. Godinich MJ, Batlle DC: Renal tubular effects of lithium. *Kidney Int* 37(Suppl 28):S52, 1990.
396. Treatment of nocturnal enuresis, in Crawford JD (ed): Proceedings of a symposium held August 6, 1988. *J Pediatr* 114(Suppl):4, 1989.
397. Nørgaard JP: Pathophysiology of nocturnal enuresis. *Scand J Urol Nephrol Suppl* 140:7, 1991.
398. Nocturia—towards a consensus, in Mattiasson A (ed): *BJU International* 84(Suppl):1, 1999.
399. Eiberg H, Berendt I, Mohr J: Assignment of dominant inherited nocturnal enuresis (ENUR1) to chromosome 13q. *Nat Genet* 10:354, 1995.
400. Hjälmås K, Bengtsson B: Efficacy, safety, and dosing of desmopressin for nocturnal enuresis in Europe. *Clin Pediatr* (special edition):19, 1993.
401. Robson WLM, Nørgaard JP, Leung AKC: Hyponatremia in patients with nocturnal enuresis treated with DDAVP. *Eur J Pediatr* 155:959, 1996.
402. Bernstein SA, Williford SL: Intranasal desmopressin-associated hyponatremia: A case report and literature review. *J Fam Pract* 44:203, 1997.
403. Zerbe RL, Henry DP, Robertson GL: Vasopressin response to orthostatic hypotension: Etiological and clinical implications. *Am J Med* 74:265, 1983.
404a. Kovacs L, Robertson GL: Disorders of water balance—hyponatremia and hypernatremia. *Baillieres Clin Endocrinol Metab* 6:107, 1992.
404b. Star RA: Clinical consequences of hypernatremia and its correction, in Seldin DW, Giebisch G (eds): *Clinical Disturbances of Water Metabolism*. New York, Raven Press, 1993, pp 237–247.
405. Robertson GL, Aycinena P: Neurogenic disorders of osmoregulation. *Am J Med* 72:339, 1982.
406. Sparacio RR, Anziska B, Schutta HS: Hypernatremia and chorea: A report of two cases. *Neurology* 26:46, 1976.
407. Simon RP, Freedman DD: Neurologic manifestations of osmolar disorders. *Geriatrics* p 71, June 1980.
408. Opas LM, Adler R, Robinson R, Lieberman E: Rhabdomyolysis with severe hypernatremia. *J Pediatr* 90:713, 1977.
409. Han BK, Lee M, Yoon HK: Cranial ultrasound and CT findings in infants with hypernatremic dehydration. *Pediatr Radiol* 27:739, 1997.
410. Robertson GL: Abnormalities of thirst regulation. *Kidney Int* 25:460, 1984.
411. Schaff-Blass E, Robertson GL, Rosenfield RL: Chronic hypernatremia resulting from a congenital defect in osmoregulation of thirst and vasopressin. *J Pediatr* 102:703, 1983.
412. Hammond DN, Moll GW, Robertson GL, Chelmicka-Schorr E: Hypodipsic hypernatremia with normal osmoregulation of vasopressin. *N Engl J Med* 315:433, 1986.
413. Yamamoto T, Shimizu M, Fukuyama J, Yamaji T: Pathogenesis of extracellular fluid abnormalities of hypothalamic hypodipsia-hypernatremia syndrome. *Endocrinol Jpn* 35:915, 1988.
414. Fabris A, Ronco C, Pellanda MV, Gardin C, Chiaramonte S, Feriani M, La Greca G: Fluctuation of vasopressin secretion in chronic hypernatremia. *Nephron* 54:245, 1990.
415. Ben-Amitai D, Rachmel A, Levy Y, Sivan Y, Nitzan M, Steinherz R: Hypodipsic hypernatremia and hypertriglyceridemia associated with cleft lip and cleft palate: A new hypothalamic dysfunction syndrome? *Am J Med Genet* 36:275, 1990.
416. Radetti G, Rizza F, Mengarda G, Pittschieler K: Adipsic hypernatremia in two sisters. *Am J Dis Child* 145:321, 1991.
417. Sano H, Yamada K, Koyama H, Terano T, Tamura Y, Yoshida S: A case report of hypodipsic hypernatremia syndrome associated with suprasellar tumor. *Jpn J Med* 30:266, 1991.
418. Papadimitriou A, Kipourou K, Manta C, Tapaki G, Philippidis P: Adipsic hypernatremia syndrome in infancy. *J Pediatr Endocrinol Metab* 10:547, 1997.
419. Phillips MG, Gabow PA: Psychogenic adipsia in a patient with psychotic depression. *Am J Kidney Dis* 15:592, 1990.
420. Keuneke C, Anders HJ, Schlondorff D: Adipsic hypernatremia in two patients with AIDS and cytomegalovirus encephalitis. *Am J Kidney Dis* 33:379, 1999.
421. Palevsky PM: Hypernatremia. *Semin Nephrol* 18:20, 1998.
422. Conley SB: Hypernatremia. *Pediatr Clin North Am* 37:365, 1990.
423. Verbalis JG: Adaptation to acute and chronic hyponatremia: Implications for symptomatology, diagnosis, and therapy. *Semin Nephrol* 18:3, 1998.
424. Schwartz WB, Bennett W, Curelop S, Bartter FC: A syndrome of renal sodium loss and hyponatremia probably resulting from inappropriate secretion of antidiuretic hormone. *Am J Med* 25:529, 1957.
425. Kovacs L, Robertson GL: Syndrome of inappropriate antidiuresis. *Endocrinol Metab Clin North Am* 21:859, 1992.
426. Fehn M, Lohmann F, Ludecke DK, Rudorff KH, Saeger W: Ganglioglioma of the neurohypophysis with secretion of vasopressin. *Exp Clin Endocrinol Diabetes* 106:425, 1998.
427. Taskin M, Barker B, Calanog A, Jormark S: Syndrome of inappropriate antidiuresis in ovarian serous carcinoma with neuroendocrine differentiation. *Gynecol Oncol* 62:400, 1996.
428. Thiagarajan R, La Gamma E, Dey S, Blethen S, Wilson TA: Hyponatremia caused by a reset osmostat in a neonate with cleft lip and palate and panhypopituitarism. *J Pediatr* 128:561, 1996.
429. Arakawa K, Nishio T, Sunohara N: Two cases of MND/ALS developing the syndrome of inappropriate secretion of antidiuretic hormone. *Acta Neurol Scand* 96:262, 1997.
430. Girault C, Richard JC, Chevron V, Goulle JP, Droy JM, Bonmarchand G, Leroy J: Syndrome of inappropriate secretion of antidiuretic hormone in two elderly women with elevated serum fluoxetine. *J Toxicol Clin Toxicol* 35:93, 1997.
431. Bradley ME, Foote EF, Lee EN, Merkle L: Sertraline-associated syndrome of inappropriate antidiuretic hormone: Case report and review of the literature. *Pharmacotherapy* 16:680, 1996.
432. Leung VP, Chiu HF, Lam LC: Hyponatremia associated with paroxetine. *Pharmacopsychiatry* 31:32, 1998.
433. Girault C, Richard JC, Chevron V, Goulle JP, Droy JM, Bonmarchand G, Leroy J: Syndrome of inappropriate secretion of antidiuretic hormone in two elderly women with elevated serum fluoxetine. *J Toxicol Clin Toxicol* 35:93, 1997.
434. Bradley ME, Foote EF, Lee EN, Merkle L: Sertraline-associated syndrome of inappropriate antidiuretic hormone: Case report and review of the literature. *Pharmacotherapy* 16:680, 1996.
435. Leung VP, Chiu HF, Lam LC: Hyponatremia associated with paroxetine. *Pharmacopsychiatry* 31:32, 1998.
436. Amatruda TT, Mulrow PJ, Gallagher JG, Sawyer WH: Carcinoma of the lung with inappropriate antidiuresis. *N Engl J Med* 269:544, 1963.
437. George JM, Capen CC, Phillips AS: Biosynthesis of vasopressin in vitro and ultrastructure of a bronchogenic carcinoma. *J Clin Invest* 51:141, 1972.
438. Thomas TH, Morgan DB, Swaminathan R, Gall SG, Lee MR: Severe hyponatræmia: A study of 17 patients. *Lancet* I(8065):661, 1978.
439. Hammer M: Defects in osmoregulation of vasopressin secretion. *Acta Med Scand* 211:133, 1982.
440. Robertson GL: Cancer and inappropriate antidiuresis, in Rudden RW (ed): *Biological Markers of Neoplasia: Basic and Applied Aspects*. New York, Elsevier North-Holland, 1978, pp 277–293.
441. Kamoi K: Syndrome of inappropriate antidiuresis without involving inappropriate secretion of vasopressin in an elderly woman: Effect of intravenous administration of the nonpeptide vasopressin V2 receptor antagonist OPC-31260. *Nephron* 76:111, 1997.
442. Leaf A, Bartter FC, Santos RF, Wrong O: Evidence in man that urinary electrolyte loss induced by pitressin is a function of water retention. *J Clin Invest* 32:868, 1953.
443. Schwartz WB, Tassel D, Bartter FC: Further observations on hyponatremia and renal sodium loss probably resulting from inappropriate secretion of antidiuretic hormone. *N Engl J Med* 262:743, 1960.
444. Schwartz E, Fogel RL, Chokas WV, Panariello VA: Unstable osmolar homeostasis with and without renal sodium wastage. *Am J Med* 33:39, 1962.

445. Nolph KD, Schrier RW: Sodium, potassium and water metabolism in the syndrome of inappropriate antidiuretic hormone secretion. *Am J Med* 49:534, 1970.
446. Cooke CR, Turin MD, Walker WG: The syndrome of inappropriate antidiuretic hormone secretion (SIADH): Pathophysiologic mechanisms in solute and volume regulation. *Medicine* 58:240, 1979.
447. Verbalis JG: Hyponatremia: epidemiology, pathophysiology, and therapy. *Curr Opin Nephrol Hypertens* 2:636, 1993.
448. Fichman MP, Michelakis AM, Horton R: Regulation of aldosterone in the syndrome of inappropriate antidiuretic hormone secretion (SIADH). *J Clin Endocrinol Metab* 39:136, 1974.
449. Kamoi K, Ebe T, Kobayashi O, Ishida M, Sato F, Atai O, et al: Atrial natriuretic peptide in patients with the syndrome of inappropriate antidiuretic hormone secretion and with diabetes insipidus. *J Clin Endocrinol Metab* 70:1385, 1990.
450. Padfield PL, Brown JJ, Lever AF, Morton JJ, Robertson JIS: Blood pressure in acute and chronic vasopressin excess: Studies of malignant hypertension and the syndrome of inappropriate antidiuretic hormone secretion. *N Engl J Med* 304:1067, 1981.
451. Michelis MF, Fusco RD, Bragdon RW, Davis BB: Reset of osmoreceptors in association with normovolemic hyponatremia. *Am J Med Sci* 267:267, 1974.
452. DeFronzo RA, Goldberg M, Agus ZS: Normal diluting capacity in hyponatremic patients. *Ann Intern Med* 84:538, 1976.
453. Assadi FK, Agrawal R, Jocher C, John EG, Rosenthal IM: Hyponatremia secondary to reset osmostat. *J Pediatr* 108:262, 1986.
454. Arieff AI, Llach F, Massry SG: Neurological manifestations and morbidity of hyponatremia: Correlation of brain water and electrolytes. *Medicine (Baltimore)* 55:121, 1976.
455. Messert B, Ornson WW, Hawkins MJ: Central pontine myelinolysis. *Neurology* 29:147, 1979.
456. Skowsky WR, Kikuchi TA: The role of vasopressin in the impaired water excretion of myxedema. *Am J Med* 64:613, 1978.
457. De Rubertis FR, Michelis MF, Bloom ME, Mintz DU, Fidd JB, Davis BD: Impaired water excretion in myxedema. *Am J Med* 51:41, 1971.
458. Bethune JE, Nelson DH: Hyponatremia in hypopituitarism. *N Engl J Med* 272:771, 1965.
459. Kleeman CR, Maxwell MH, Rockney RE: Mechanisms of impaired water excretion in adrenal and pituitary insufficiency: I. The role of altered glomerular filtration rate and solute excretion. *J Clin Invest* 37:1799, 1958.
460. Cutler RE, Kleeman CR, Koplowitz J, Maxwell MH, Dowling JT: Mechanisms of impaired water excretion in adrenal and pituitary insufficiency: III. The effect of extracellular or plasma volume expansion, or both, on the impaired diuresis. *J Clin Invest* 41:1524, 1962.
461. Kleeman CR, Czaczkes JW, Cutler R: Mechanisms of impaired water excretion in adrenal and pituitary insufficiency: IV. Antidiuretic hormone in primary and secondary adrenal insufficiency. *J Clin Invest* 43:1641, 1964.
462. Ahmed ABJ, George BC, Gonzalez-Auvert C, Dingman JF: Increased plasma arginine vasopressin in clinical adrenocortical insufficiency and its inhibition by glucosteroids. *J Clin Invest* 46:111, 1967.
463. Green HH, Harrington AR, Valtin H: On the role of antidiuretic hormone in the inhibition of acute water diuresis in adrenal insufficiency and the effects of gluco- and mineralocorticoids in reversing the inhibition. *J Clin Invest* 49:1724, 1970.
464. Ackerman GL, Miller CL: Role of hypovolemia in the impaired water diuresis of adrenal insufficiency. *J Clin Endocrinol Metab* 30:252, 1970.
465. Boykin J, deTorrente A, Erickson A, Robertson GL, Schrier RW: Role of plasma vasopressin in impaired water excretion of glucocorticoid deficiency. *J Clin Invest* 62:738, 1978.
466. Mandell IN, DeFronzo RA, Robertson GL, Forrest JN: Role of plasma arginine vasopressin in the impaired water diuresis of isolated glucocorticoid deficiency in the rat. *Kidney Int* 17:186, 1980.
467. Linas SL, Berl T, Robertson GL, Aisenbrey GA, Schrier RW, Anderson RJ: Role of vasopressin in the impaired water excretion of glucocorticoid deficiency. *Kidney Int* 18:58, 1980.
468. Oelkers W: Hyponatremia and inappropriate secretion of vasopressin (antidiuretic hormone) in patients with hypopituitarism. *N Engl J Med* 321:492, 1989.
469. Iwasaki Y, Kondo K, Hasegawa H, Oiso Y: Osmoregulation of plasma vasopressin in three cases with adrenal insufficiency of diverse etiologies. *Hormone Res* 47:38, 1997.
470. Robertson GL: Syndrome of inappropriate antidiuresis. *N Engl J Med* 321:538, 1989.
471. Gill JR, Gann DS, Bartter FC: Restoration of water diuresis in Addisonian patients by expansion of the volume of extracellular fluid. *J Clin Invest* 41:1078, 1962.
472. Share L, Travis RH: Plasma vasopressin concentration in the adrenally insufficient dog. *Endocrinology* 86:196, 1970.
473. Ufferman RC, Schrier RW: Importance of sodium intake and mineralocorticoid hormone in the impaired water excretion in adrenal insufficiency. *J Clin Invest* 51:1639, 1972.
474. Boykin J, deTorrente A, Robertson GL, Erickson A, Schrier RW: Persistent plasma vasopressin levels in the hypoosmolar state associated with mineralocorticoid deficiency. *Miner Electrolyte Metab* 2:310, 1979.
475. Abramow M, Cogan E: Clinical aspects and pathophysiology of diuretic-induced hyponatremia. *Adv Nephrol* 13:1, 1984.
476. Clark BA, Shannon RP, Rosa RM, Epstein FH: Increased susceptibility to thiazide-induced hyponatremia in the elderly. *J Am Soc Nephrol* 5:1106, 1994.
477. Fichman MP, Vorherr H, Kleeman CR, Tefler N: Diuretic induced hyponatremia. *Ann Intern Med* 75:853, 1971.
478. Friedman E, Shadel M, Halkin H, Farfel Z: Thiazide-induced hyponatremia: Reproducibility by single dose rechallenge and an analysis of pathogenesis. *Ann Intern Med* 110:24, 1989.
479. Bichet D, Schrier RW: Water metabolism in edematous disorders. *Semin Nephrol* 4:325, 1984.
480. Takasic T, Lasker N, Shalhouh RJ: Mechanisms of hyponatremia in chronic congestive heart failure. *Ann Intern Med* 55:368, 1961.
481. Pruszczynski W, Vahanian A, Ardaillou R, Acar J: Role of antidiuretic hormone in impaired water excretion of patients with congestive heart failure. *J Clin Endocrinol Metab* 58:599, 1984.
482. Uretsky BF, Verbalis JG, Generalovich T, Valdes A, Reddy PS: Plasma vasopressin response to osmotic and hemodynamic stimuli in heart failure. *Am J Physiol* 248:H396, 1985.
483. Earley LE, Sanders CA: The effect of changing serum osmolality on antidiuretic hormone release in certain patients with decompensated cirrhosis of the liver and low serum osmolality. *J Clin Invest* 38:545, 1959.
484. Akriviadis EA, Ervin MG, Cominelli F, Fisher DA, Reynolds TB: Hyponatremia of cirrhosis: role of vasopressin and decreased 'effective' plasma volume. *Scand J Gastroenterol* 32:829, 1997.
485. Schrier RW, Fassett RG, Ohara M, Martin PY: Vasopressin release, water channels, and vasopressin antagonism in cardiac failure, cirrhosis, and pregnancy. *Proc Assoc Am Physicians* 110:407, 1998.
486. Ayus JC, Olivero JJ, Fromer JP: Rapid correction of severe hyponatremia with intravenous hypertonic saline solution. *Am J Med* 72:43, 1982.
487. Ayus JC, Krothapalli RK, Arieff AI: Treatment of symptomatic hyponatremia and its relation to brain damage. *N Engl J Med* 317:1190, 1987.
488. Cheng JC, Zikos D, Skopicki HA, Peterson DR: Long-term neurologic outcome in psychogenic water drinkers with severe symptomatic hyponatremia: The effect of rapid correction. *Am J Med* 88:561, 1990.
489. Sterns RH: The treatment of hyponatremia: First, do no harm, editorial. *Am J Med* 88:557, 1990.
490. Cherrill DA, Stote RM, Birge JR, Singer I: Demeclocycline treatment in the syndrome of inappropriate antidiuretic hormone secretion. *Ann Intern Med* 83:654, 1975.
491. deTroyer A: Demeclocycline: Treatment of syndrome of inappropriate antidiuretic hormone secretion. *JAMA* 237:2723, 1977.
492. Dousa TP, Wilson DM: Effect of demethylchlortetracycline on cellular action of antidiuretic hormone in vitro. *Kidney Int* 5:279, 1974.
493. Miller PD, Linas SL, Schrier RW: Plasma demeclocycline levels and nephrotoxicity: Correlation in hyponatremic cirrhotic patients. *JAMA* 243:2513, 1980.
494. Oster JR, Epstein M, Ulano HB: Deterioration of renal function with demeclocycline administration. *Curr Ther Res* 20:794, 1976.
495. Forrest JN, Cox M, Hong C, Morrisson G, Bia M, Singer I: Superiority of demeclocycline over lithium in the treatment of chronic syn-

drome of inappropriate secretion of antidiuretic hormone. *N Engl J Med* 298:173, 1978.

496. Decaux G, Waterlot Y, Genette F, Mockel J: Treatment of the syndrome of inappropriate secretion of antidiuretic hormone with furosemide. *N Engl J Med* 304:329, 1981.
497. Decaux G, Genette F: Urea for long term treatment of syndrome of inappropriate secretion of antidiuretic hormone. *Br Med J* 283: 1081, 1981.
498. Dzau VJ, Colucci WS, Williams GH, Curfman G, Meggs L, Hollenberg NK: Sustained effectiveness of converting enzyme inhibition in patients with severe congestive heart failure. *N Engl J Med* 302:1373, 1980.
499. Yamahiro HW, Reynolds TB: Effects of ascitic fluid infusion on sodium excretion, blood volume and creatinine clearance in cirrhosis. *Gastroenterology* 40:497, 1961.
500. Schedl HP, Bartter FC: An explanation for an experimental correction of the abnormal water diuresis in cirrhosis. *J Clin Invest* 39:248, 1960.
501. Schrier RW, Lehman D, Zacherle B, Early LE: Effect of furosemide on free water excretion in edematous patients with hyponatremia. *Kidney Int* 3:30, 1973.

PART III

Thyroid Disease

CHAPTER 9

The Thyroid: Physiology, Thyrotoxicosis, Hypothyroidism, and the Painful Thyroid

Robert D. Utiger

Thyroid hormones are the only iodine-containing compounds with biological activity. They are important determinants of normal growth and development in infants and children and of metabolic stability in adults; they therefore affect the function of virtually all organ systems. These actions require that thyroid hormone be constantly available. To maintain constant hormone availability, there are large reservoirs of thyroid hormone in both the circulation and the thyroid gland, and thyroid hormone secretion by the thyroid gland is maintained within narrow limits by a hypothalamic-pituitary regulatory mechanism that is very sensitive to small changes in circulating hormone concentrations.

Thyroid diseases are relatively common. They occur in the form of abnormalities of the size and shape of the thyroid gland (goiter) and of abnormalities of thyroid secretion. Moreover, nonthyroidal illness is accompanied by many alterations in thyroid physiology, which can complicate the evaluation of thyroid status.

ANATOMY AND PHYSIOLOGY

Clinical Anatomy

The normal thyroid gland is composed of two encapsulated lobes, one on either side of the trachea, connected by a thin isthmus that crosses the trachea anteriorly below the cricoid cartilage (Fig. 9-1). The right lobe is often somewhat larger than the left lobe. Sometimes a pyramidal lobe is found extending superiorly from the isthmus in the midline, indicating the embryologic path along which the thyroid developed. The mean thyroid weight in groups of men and women of different ages in the United States ranges from 15 to 20 g.[1] Thyroid volume, which is 10–25 ml in normal adults, is slightly greater in men than women, increases slightly with age and lean body mass, and decreases with increasing iodine intake.[2,3]

The thyroid develops as a thickening in the pharyngeal floor that elongates inferiorly as the thyroglossal duct and divides into two lobes as it descends through the neck. Rarely, one or both thyroid lobes fail to develop (thyroid hemiagenesis or agenesis).[4] The thyroid may remain at the base of the tongue (lingual thyroid), may be found at other locations between the base of the tongue and the lower neck (thyroglossal duct remnants), or may follow the developmental path of the heart into the thorax, where, decades later, it may become manifest as a substernal goiter, compressing the trachea, a recurrent laryngeal nerve, or even the superior vena cava. Some of these anomalies are shown in Fig. 9-1. The arterial supply of the thyroid is derived primarily from paired superior and inferior thyroid arteries. The venous drainage is more complex and variable, but usually there are paired superior, middle, and inferior thyroid veins. Normally, two parathyroid glands lie behind the upper and lower poles of each lobe of the thyroid. The recurrent laryngeal nerves run along the trachea, medially and behind the thyroid lobes.

Physical Examination

The thyroid gland should always be examined with the patient seated, because adequate examination is impossible when the patient is supine. The patient's neck should first be inspected from the front while the patient swallows with the head slightly extended. The thyroid lobes may be seen, and lobar enlargement or thyroid nodules may be noted. The examiner should then move behind the patient to palpate the neck. Both sides of the neck should be palpated while the patient swallows, first with the examiner's hands on the same side of the patient's neck and then with the right hand on the left side of the neck and vice versa. This maneuver allows lateral displacement of the sternomastoid muscle and thus better delineation of the outline of each lobe.

The thyroid is palpable in many normal subjects, with the lobes being up to 3 cm long. Its surface may be slightly irregular. The size and consistency of each lobe or of any nodules and the presence of tenderness should be recorded. The isthmus or a pyramidal lobe may be palpated in the midline, and other masses in addition to the thyroid lobes and abnormalities of the lobes may be palpated in the lateral neck regions (Table 9-1). Most nonthyroid masses can be distinguished from thyroid masses by either their position or their failure to move with swallowing. The sensitivity and specificity of physical examination for detection of thyroid enlargement are 70 and 83 percent, respectively, as compared with ultrasonography or postmortem examination.[5] In some patients with multinodular goiters, the goiters extend below the sternum or are mostly substernal. Raising the arms above the head may result in facial suffusion and neck vein distension, due to venous compression at the thoracic inlet (Pemberton's sign).[6]

The most practical way to determine the size of thyroid lobes and nodules is to measure their length and width based on palpation. An outline of the thyroid can be traced on thin flexible paper. Estimates based on weight or degree of enlargement are so subjective as to be of little value. The correlation between estimates of the size of thyroid lobes by palpation and by ultrasonography is poor; usually examiners overestimate the size of small goiters and underestimate the size of large goiters.[2,5]

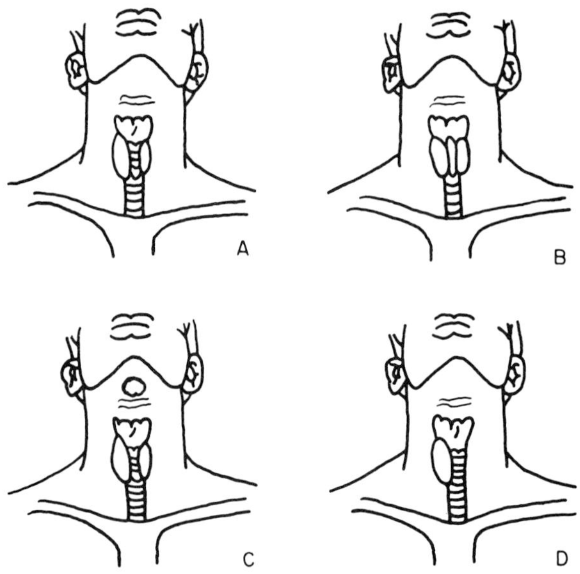

FIGURE 9-1. The normal thyroid gland and variations in thyroid anatomy. (*A*) Normal thyroid gland. (*B*) Pyramidal lobe between two normal thyroid lobes. (*C*) Thyroglossal remnant above the larynx. (*D*) Agenesis of the left lobe of the thyroid.

Histology

Microscopically, thyroid tissue consists of spherical thyroid follicles. Each follicle is composed of a single layer of cuboidal follicular cells surrounding a lumen filled with a homogeneous material called colloid. When stimulated, the follicular cells become columnar and the follicles are depleted of colloid; when suppressed, the follicular cells become flat and colloid accumulates. The luminal surface of each follicular cell is covered with microvilli extending into the colloid. The cytoplasm is filled with membrane-bound microsomes and a large Golgi apparatus. Near the apex of the cell are both exocytotic vesicles (secretory droplets) and endocytotic vesicles (colloid droplets), which are formed by the invagination of part of the luminal membrane.

Capillaries and terminals of adrenergic, cholinergic, and peptidergic nerves, including nerves containing vasoactive intestinal peptide, neuropeptide Y, and other neuropeptides, are present between the follicles. These nerve terminals abut both capillaries and follicles, and their activation may alter thyroid secretion as well as thyroid blood flow.[7] The thyroid also contains parafollicular, or C, cells in the interfollicular connective tissue and, in lesser numbers, within thyroid follicles that produce calcitonin.

TABLE 9-1. Differential Diagnosis of Neck Masses

Midline mass
Thyroid isthmus, pyramidal lobe
Thyroglossal duct cyst
Pretracheal lymph nodes
Lateral neck mass
Thyroid lobes and intrathyroidal lesions
Anterior cervical lymphadenopathy
Branchial cleft cyst
Arterial aneurysm
Carotid body tumor
Parathyroid masses

Chemistry of Thyroid Hormones

The structures of the two thyroid hormones—thyroxine (T_4) and triiodothyronine (T_3)—their precursor iodotyrosines, thyronine, and several metabolites of T_4 and T_3 are shown in Fig. 9-2. T_4, T_3, and most of their metabolites are iodinated thyronines; they are composed of a phenyl ring attached via an ether linkage to tyrosine and contain from one to four iodine atoms. T_4 is 3,5,3′,5′-tetraiodothyronine, whereas T_3 is 3,5,3′-triiodothyronine, having one less iodine atom on its outer ring. Deiodination of the inner ring of T_4 results in formation of 3,3′,5′-triiodothyronine [reverse T_3 (rT_3)]. Diiodothyronine, or T_2, can exist in three forms: two iodine atoms on the outer ring (3′,5′-T_2), two on the inner ring (3,5-T_2), or one on each ring (3,3′-T_2). Oxidative deamination and decarboxylation of T_4 result in the formation of tetraiodothyroacetic acid (tetrac); triiodothyroacetic acid (triac) is formed from T_3 in the same way. Of the compounds shown in Fig. 9-2, only T_4, T_3, tetraiodothyroacetic acid, and triiodothyroacetic acid have biological activity. The latter two are produced in such small amounts that they contribute little if at all to thyroid hormone action in vivo.

Thyroid Hormone Biosynthesis

T_4 is produced only by the thyroid gland, whereas T_3 is produced both by the thyroid and by deiodination of T_4 at extrathyroidal sites. The thyroid gland contains large amounts of T_4 and T_3, virtually all incorporated in thyroglobulin, the unique protein within which the two hormones are synthesized and stored. Because of these stores, T_4 and T_3 can be secreted rapidly without the need for new hormone synthesis. The overall process of hormone production within the thyroid gland is shown in Fig. 9-3.

Iodine Economy

An adequate supply of iodine is essential for normal thyroid function. Iodine intake varies greatly as a result of the varying iodine content of food and water and dietary preferences, and in many regions of the world is inadequate or barely adequate unless supplemented. Seafood is the richest natural source of iodine. Its content in other foods depends on the iodine content of the soil, which in general is highest near sea level and lowest in mountainous regions, and the extent to which animal feeds are supplemented with iodine. Most iodine in food is in the form of inorganic iodine, which is rapidly and completely absorbed. In the United States, some but not all salt is supplemented with potassium iodide (76 μg iodide/g). Many multivitamin preparations also contain iodide.

The recommended minimum intake of iodine is 150 μg daily, although the minimum amount required to prevent goiter due to iodine deficiency in adults is about 50 μg daily. Based on measurements of urinary iodine excretion, which closely reflect iodine intake (very little iodine is lost via the skin or gastrointestinal tract), the daily intake of iodine in the United States has declined substantially in the last 25 years. In surveys of approximately 18,000 adults, the median urinary iodine excretion was 320 μg/liter (2.6 μmol/liter) in the period 1971–74 and 145 μg/liter (1.2 μmol/liter) in the period 1988–94.[8] As a corollary to this decline the proportion of subjects with urinary iodine values less than 50 μg/liter (0.4 μmol/liter) increased from 2.6 to 11.7 percent during this interval. Estimates of intake also indicate that iodine intake in the United States has decreased recently.[9] The decrease is

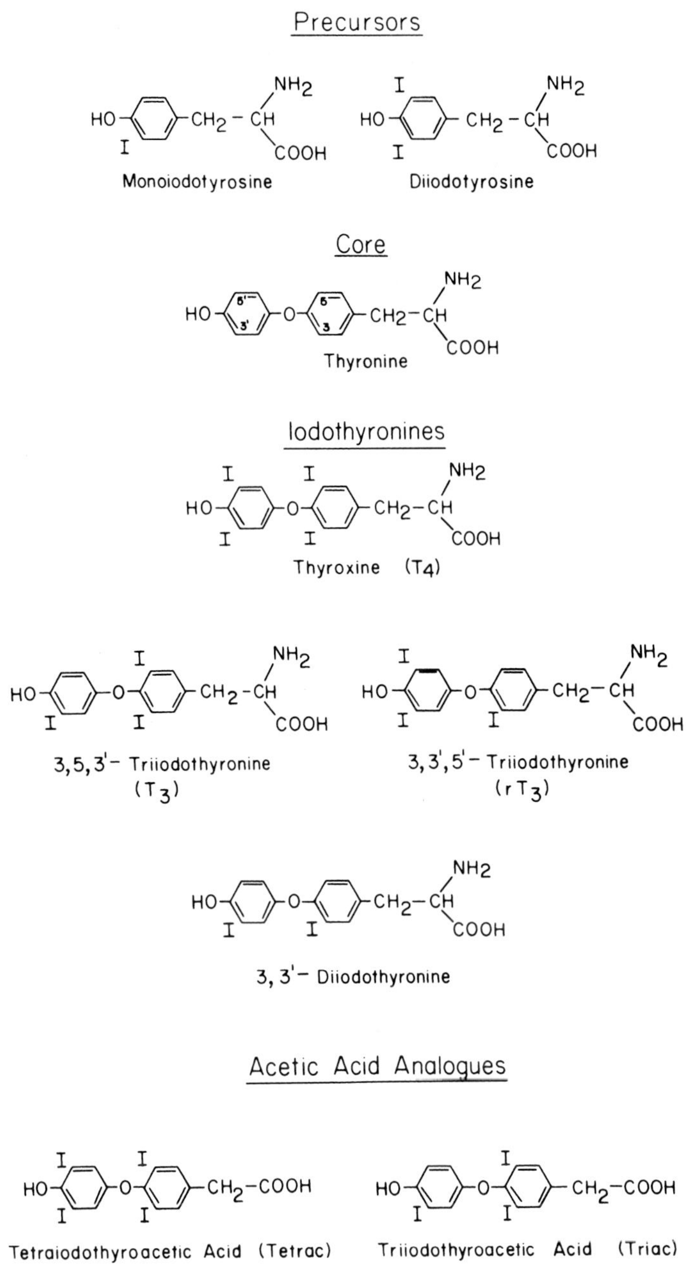

FIGURE 9-2. Structural formulas of various iodothyronines and iodothyronine analogs.

probably due to lower salt consumption and decreases in the iodine content in animal feeds and in the use of iodate in bread production. Iodine intake is lower in most of Europe, where less iodine is added to salt, and in many other countries except for those where large amounts of seafood are consumed.

Iodine that is absorbed is distributed in the extracellular fluid, in which the iodide concentration is about 1 μg/dl (0.08 μmol/liter). This pool receives not only dietary iodine, but also iodide that is released from the thyroid and iodide derived from the peripheral deiodination of iodothyronines. Iodide leaves this pool mostly by transport into the thyroid or excretion in the urine. The normal renal iodide clearance is about 30 ml/min, while thyroid clearance ranges from 10 to 20 ml/min, resulting in an absolute thyroid iodide uptake rate of about 150 μg/day. The thyroidal content of iodine is virtually all in the form of organic iodine bound to tyrosyl or thyronine residues within thyroglobulin, and varies from 10 to 15 mg.

Thyroidal Hormonogenesis

Thyroid Iodide Transport

Iodide is transported into thyroid follicular cells against a chemical and electrical gradient; it then rapidly diffuses into the follicular lumen.[10] Iodide transport is a critical step in thyroid hormonogenesis; sufficient iodide to sustain normal T_4 and T_3 synthesis cannot be provided by diffusion from the extracellular fluid. Iodide transport occurs at the basal membrane of the follicular cell, is mediated by a sodium/iodide (Na/I) cotransporter, and is energy-dependent and saturable. The transporter is a membrane-associated protein with 12 transmembrane segments.[11,11a] The rate

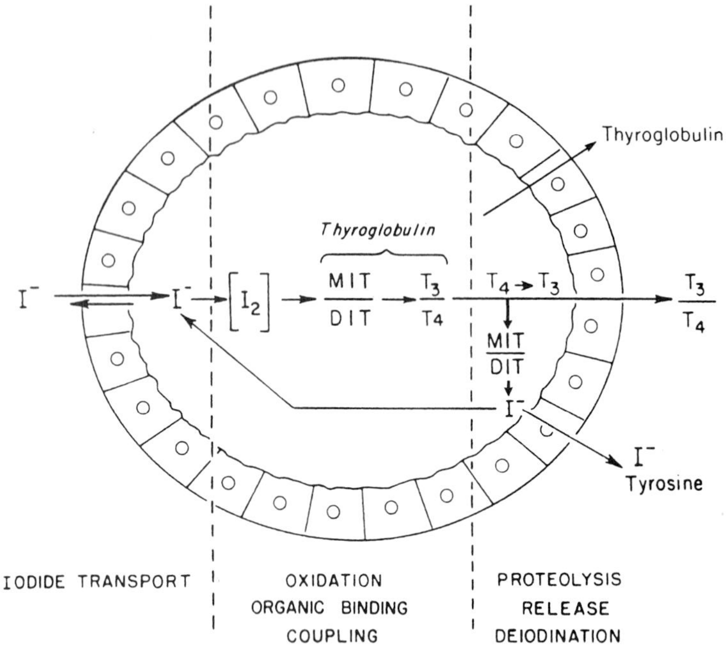

FIGURE 9-3. Outline of a thyroid follicle and the major steps in thyroid hormone biosynthesis and release. I^- denotes inorganic iodine; MIT, monoiodotyrosine; and DIT, diiodotyrosine.

of uptake of iodide is such that the intrathyroidal iodide concentration in normal subjects is 20 to 100 times that of plasma. Iodide transport is stimulated by thyrotropin (TSH). In addition, it is inhibited by excess iodide and increased by iodine deficiency, independent of TSH.

Ions of similar size, shape, and charge, such as perchlorate and pertechnetate, can serve as substrates for the transport system and therefore as competitive inhibitors of iodide transport. The ability of the thyroid to transport pertechnetate is useful clinically; $^{99m}TcO_4$, a gamma-emitting radionuclide with a short half-life, is used for thyroid scanning.

Tyrosyl Iodination and Coupling

In thyroid cells, iodide diffuses rapidly to the apical cell membrane, where it is transported to exocytotic vesicles fused with the membrane, in effect at the cell-lumen interface. This step is mediated by pendrin, a chloride-iodide transport protein.[11a,11b] In these vesicles, iodide is very rapidly oxidized and then covalently bound (organified) to some of the tyrosyl residues of thyroglobulin.[10] Iodide oxidation is catalyzed by thyroid peroxidase, a heme-containing glycoprotein that is bound to the walls of the exocytotic vesicles. The oxidized form of iodide may be iodine free radicals (I^o), iodinium atoms (I^+), or hypoiodous acid. Hydrogen peroxide is required for iodide oxidation; it is probably generated by NADPH–cytochrome c reductase. This oxidation and organification process results in mono- or diiodination of about 15 of the 134 tyrosine residues of thyroglobulin.

T_4 is formed by the coupling of two diiodotyrosyl residues and T_3 is formed by the coupling of one monoiodotyrosyl residue and one diiodotyrosyl residue within individual thyroglobulin molecules. The coupling reaction is an oxidative one, and it also is catalyzed by thyroid peroxidase.[10] The most likely mechanism involves the oxidation of two iodotyrosyl residues, followed by their ether linkage, leaving a dehydroalanyl residue at the site of the iodotyrosyl residue contributing the outer ring of the iodothyronine.

Thyroglobulin Synthesis

Thyroglobulin constitutes about 75 percent of the protein content of the thyroid gland, and almost all of it is within the follicular lumen.[12] It is a 660-kilodalton (kDa) glycoprotein composed of two identical noncovalently linked subunits and contains about 10 percent carbohydrate. A 8.5-kilobase (kb) messenger RNA (mRNA) coding for the subunit peptide has been isolated from human thyroid tissue. Thyroglobulin mRNA is translated by large polyribosomes attached to the rough endoplasmic reticulum. Glycosylation, subunit combination, and folding occur as it is chaperoned by several heat shock proteins through the endoplasmic reticulum, after which it is transferred to the Golgi apparatus and then incorporated into the exocytotic vesicles that fuse with the apical cell membrane (Fig. 9-4).[13] Only then do iodination and coupling occur. Fully glycosylated, iodinated, and iodothyronine-containing thyroglobulin is found only in the follicular lumen. Several thyroid-specific transcription factors (TTF-1, TTF-2) are necessary for thyroglobulin gene expression. TSH stimulates thyroglobulin synthesis by stimulating thyroglobulin gene expression, and it increases thyroglobulin glycosylation and shifts the pattern of iodination, increasing formation of T_3 relative to that of T_4.

FIGURE 9-4. Schematic drawing of the pathway of thyroglobulin biosynthesis and iodination in a thyroid follicular cell. The apical cell surface is at the top, and the extracellular space is at the bottom.

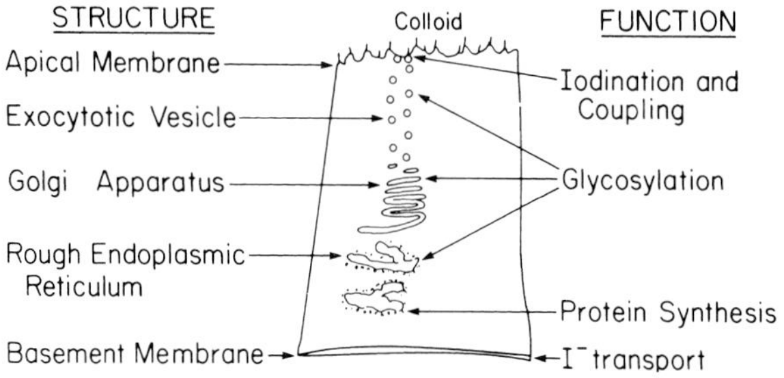

The unique feature of thyroglobulin that favors iodotyrosyl coupling is its primary structure. Its content of 134 tyrosyl residues is rather low among proteins, and tyrosyl residues in all proteins can be iodinated. However, coupling of iodotyrosyl residues occurs only in thyroglobulin. It is not random; rather, T_4 and T_3 are formed in limited domains that have unique amino acid sequences and are located near the ends of each subunit of thyroglobulin.[12]

The iodoamino acid content of thyroglobulin is dependent on iodide availability. Normal thyroglobulin contains about 8 residues of monoiodotyrosine, 5 residues of diiodotyrosine, 2 residues of T_4, and 0.4 residue of T_3 per molecule. The T_4 content of the thyroglobulin in the thyroid gland of a normal subject is about 250 μg/g of thyroid tissue[14]; therefore a person with an 18-g thyroid gland has 4500 μg stored T_4, enough to maintain normal T_4 secretion for about 45 days. In subjects with iodine deficiency, the thyroglobulin has a lower total iodide content and higher monoiodotyrosine/diiodotyrosine and T_3/T_4 ratios.[12]

Colloid Endocytosis and Hormone Release

Thyroglobulin is not only the site of formation of T_4 and T_3, but also the storage form of the two hormones. The process of T_4 and T_3 secretion requires the reuptake of thyroglobulin into the thyroid follicular cells and its enzymatic hydrolysis (Fig. 9-5). Thyroglobulin in the follicular lumen is engulfed by pinocytotic extensions of microvilli from the apical membrane, forming endocytotic vesicles (colloid droplets). These vesicles fuse with lysosomes to form phagolysosomes. As these particles migrate toward the base of the cell, the thyroglobulin is selectively cleaved by several endo- and exopeptidases to form hormone-containing peptide intermediates that are then cleaved to form the individual hormones. The T_3 and T_4 diffuse into the extracellular fluid and enter the circulation. During this process, some of the T_4 is deiodinated to form T_3, so that thyroidal T_3 secretion is greater than expected on the basis of its content in thyroglobulin.[15,16] The iodotyrosines liberated by thyroglobulin hydrolysis are rapidly deiodinated by a specific iodotyrosine deiodinase. Most of the iodide formed as a result of these deiodinations is reutilized in the thyroid, but some is released. Iodotyrosine deiodination provides more iodide for new hormone formation than does new iodide transport and thus is of critical importance in maintaining T_4 and T_3 synthesis. Thyroglobulin proteolysis and deiodination are stimulated by TSH.

FIGURE 9-5. Schematic drawing of the pathway of thyroglobulin proteolysis and T_4 and T_3 release in a thyroid follicular cell. MIT denotes monoiodotyrosine; and DIT, diiodotyrosine.

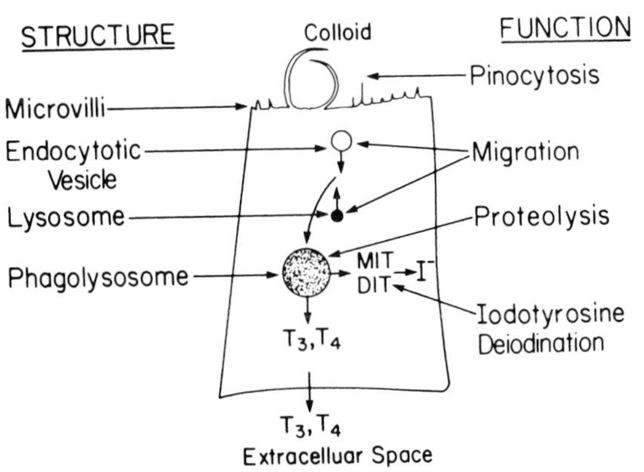

About 100 μg of thyroglobulin is released from the thyroid each day. This is a tiny fraction of the 25 mg that must be hydrolyzed to yield the 100 μg (130 nmol) of T_4 that is secreted each day. The serum half-life of thyroglobulin is 30 h.[17]

Extrathyroidal Hormonogenesis

Most of the T_3 produced each day is formed by the extrathyroidal 5′-deiodination (outer ring deiodination) of T_4. This reaction is catalyzed by T_4-deiodinase. The liver and kidney have the highest T_4-deiodinating activity per unit tissue,[18,19] and are probably the source of much of the T_3 in serum. However, deiodinating activity is widely distributed, and it is likely that multiple tissues contribute to overall extrathyroidal T_3 production. There are two T_4-5′-deiodinases (types 1 and 2 deiodinase), and one T_4-5-deiodinase (type 3 deiodinase). All three are microsomal enzymes, have selenocysteine residues at their active sites, and require reduced sulfhydryl groups as a cofactor. They are distinguished by their location, kinetic properties, sensitivity to inhibition by propylthiouracil (PTU), substrate preference, and responses to physiologic stimuli.[19–21]

Type 1 deiodinase is most prominent in the liver, kidney, thyroid, and brain. Its K_m for T_4 is high (μM), and it is PTU-sensitive. The order of substrate preference is $rT_3 > T_4 > T_3$. Type 1 deiodinase catalyzes outer ring deiodination of not only T_4 and T_3, but also T_4 and T_3 sulfates; the latter are deiodinated more efficiently than the former, but are produced only in small quantities in humans.[22]

Type 2 deiodinase is located prominently in brain, pituitary, thyroid, muscle, heart, and placenta. Its K_m for T_4 is low, it is PTU insensitive, and its order of substrate preference is $T_4 > rT_3$.[16,23]

Type 3 deiodinase catalyzes the inner ring deiodination of T_4 and T_3. It is located prominently in the brain, skin, and placenta. Its K_m for T_4 is intermediate to that of the other two deiodinases, it is PTU-sensitive, and its order of substrate preference is $T_3 > T_4$.[24,25]

Thyroid Hormone Production and Metabolism

The total daily production rate of T_4 is 80–100 μg (100–130 nmol), all derived from thyroidal secretion (Table 9-2 and Fig. 9-6). The extrathyroidal T_4 pool contains 800–1,000 μg (1,000–1300 nmol), most of which is extracellular. The T_4 turnover rate is 10 percent per day (serum half-life 6.7 days). Thus, some T_4 remains available for several weeks in the absence of any thyroidal secretion. Approximately 80 percent of the T_4 secreted each day is metabolized by deiodination, with about 40 percent being converted to T_3 and 40 percent to rT_3. The remaining 20 percent is metabolized by conjugation with sulfate and glucuronide, oxidative deamination and decarboxylation to form tetraiodothyroacetic acid, and ether-link cleavage.[19] Deiodination of T_4 to T_3 leads to increased biological activity, but the other metabolites of T_4 have little or no biological activity. The extrathyroidal conversion of T_4 to T_3 is regulated by a variety of factors, so that production of T_3, the most active thyroid hormone, may be altered independently of changes in pituitary-thyroid function.

T_3 is produced primarily (80 percent) by extrathyroidal deiodination of T_4; the remainder comes from the thyroid. The total daily production rate is 30–40 μg (45–60 nmol).[18,19] The extrathyroidal T_3 pool contains about 50 μg (75 nmol), most of which is intracellular. T_3 is much more rapidly degraded than is T_4, its turnover rate being about 70 percent per day. Hence, alterations in T_3 production rapidly alter its availability. T_3, either as

TABLE 9-2. Serum Concentrations and Production Rates of Various Iodothyronines

	Serum Concentration		*Production Rate*	
Compound	**ng/dl**	**nmol/liter**	**μg/day**	**nmol/day**
Thyroxine (T_4)	5,000–11,000	65–140	80–100	100–130
3,5,3′-Triiodothyronine (T_3)	75–200	1.1–3.0	30–40	45–60
3,3′,5′-Triiodothyronine (rT_3)	20–50	0.3–0.8	30–40	45–60
3,3′-Diiodothyronine (T_2)	1–10	0.02–0.20	25–35	48–67
3,5-Diiodothyronine (T_2)	0.5–5	0.01–0.10	2–5	4–10
3,5′-Diiodothyronine (T_2)	2–6	0.04–0.12	5–20	10–40
Tetraiodothyroacetic acid	20–50	0.26–0.65	1–2	1–4
Triiodothyroacetic acid	2–8	0.03–0.12	4–8	6–12

Conversion factors: Thyroxine, 1 nmol = 777 ng; triiodothyronine, 1 nmol = 651 ng; diiodothyronine, 1 nmol = 525 ng; tetraiodothyroacetic acid, 1 nmol = 748 ng; triiodothyroacetic acid, 1 nmol = 622 ng.

Sources: Engler,[18] Leonard,[19] and Pinna.[26]

such or after being sulfated, is metabolized primarily by deiodination to 3,3′-diiodothyronine. A small amount is deiodinated to 3,5-diiodothyronine (Fig. 9-7),[26] and the remainder (about 10 percent) is metabolized to triiodothyroacetic acid.[18]

The daily production rate of rT_3 is 30–40 μg (45–60 nmol); more than 95 percent is produced at extrathyroidal sites.[18,19] It is cleared from the circulation even more rapidly than is T_3. Most is deiodinated by type 1 deiodinase to 3,3′-diiodothyronine (Fig. 9-7), but some is deiodinated to 3,5′-diiodothyronine or metabolized by nondeiodinative pathways.

The three diiodothyronines also are very rapidly metabolized to monoiodothyronines and ultimately to thyronine, but little is known about the sites and regulation of these conversions. Table 9-2 shows the serum concentrations and production rates of most of these compounds. The serum concentrations of 3′-monoiodothyronine (T_1) and 3-monoiodothyronine (T_1) are less than 2 ng/dl (4 pmol/liter), and those of T_4 sulfate and T_3 sulfate are about 2 ng/dl (22 pmol/liter) and 5 ng/dl (66 pmol/liter), respectively.[27,28] Tetraiodothyroacetic acid, triiodothyroacetic acid, and the sulfate and glucuronide conjugates of T_4 and T_3 are metabolized largely by deiodination.

As noted earlier, a small amount of thyroglobulin is secreted by the thyroid. Monoiodotyrosine and diiodotyrosine are present in the circulation in low concentrations. They are derived from dietary sources and from the thyroid gland. Both iodotyrosines are degraded rapidly by tyrosine deiodinase in peripheral tissues.

FIGURE 9-6. Sources and production rates of circulating T_4, T_3, and rT_3 (reverse troodothyronine) in normal adults. The diagonally lined area of each bar represents production in the thyroid gland; the clear area represents production in the periphery from T_4. The daily production rates are given in μg (nmoles) and the serum concentrations in ng/dl or μg/dl (nmol/liter). The T_4/T_3 and T_4/rT_3 ratios shown at the top are those in thyroglobulin. See Table 9-2 for ranges of production rates and serum T_4, T_3, and rT_3 concentrations in normal subjects.

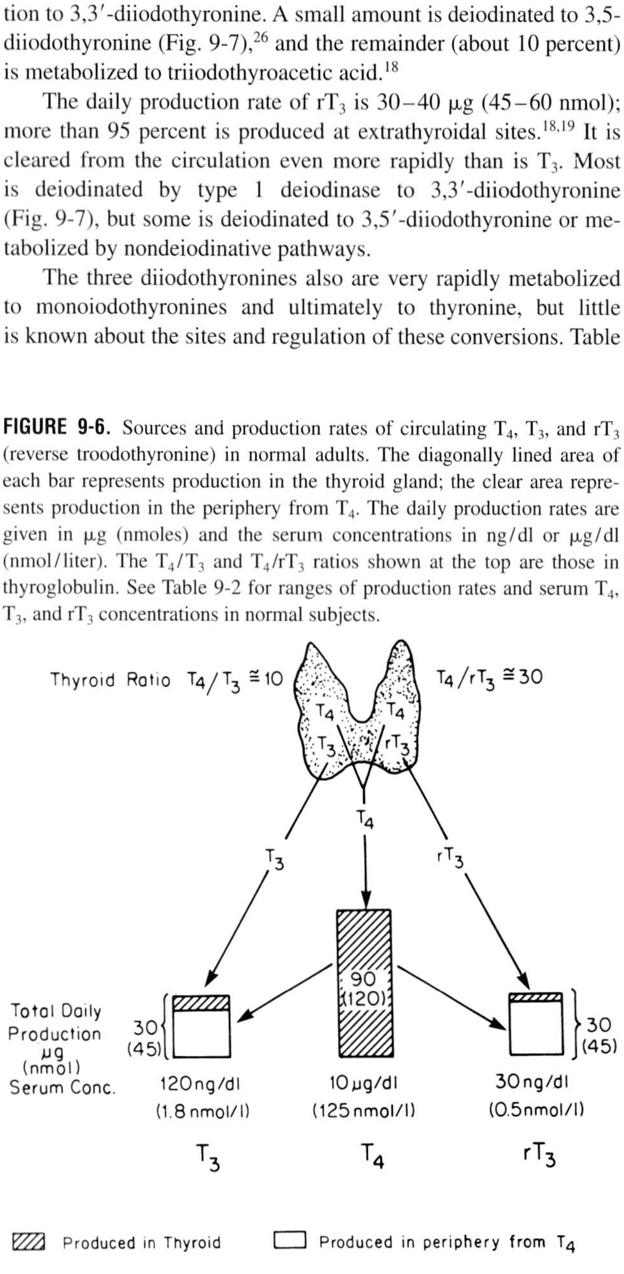

Regulation of Thyroid Hormone Production

Thyroid hormone production is regulated in two ways (Fig. 9-8). First, thyroidal T_4 and T_3 biosynthesis and secretion are stimulated by TSH. The secretion of TSH in turn is inhibited by circulating T_4 and T_3 and is stimulated by thyrotropin-releasing hormone (TRH). Second, extrathyroidal T_3 production from T_4 is regulated by a variety of nutritional, hormonal, and illness-related factors, and the effect of these regulatory factors differs in different tissues. The first mechanism provides a sensitive defense against alterations in thyroid secretion. The second provides for the rapid alterations in tissue thyroid hormone availability in response to nonthyroidal illness that probably constitute an important adaptation to illness (see section on Nonthyroidal Illness).

Control of Thyroid Secretion

Thyrotropin

Thyrotropin (TSH) is a 28-kDa glycoprotein that is synthesized and secreted by the thyrotroph cells of the anterior pituitary. It is composed of two noncovalently linked peptide subunits, an alpha subunit and a beta subunit, and contains about 15 percent carbohydrate. The alpha subunit of TSH is the same as that of luteinizing hormone, follicle-stimulating hormone, and chorionic gonadotropin. The beta subunit of TSH is unique, and therefore confers the thyroid specificity of TSH, but both subunits are required for biological activity.[29] The synthesis of each subunit is directed by separate mRNAs that are coded by separate genes on different chromosomes. After synthesis, the subunits are glycosylated and linked together to form TSH, which is then packaged

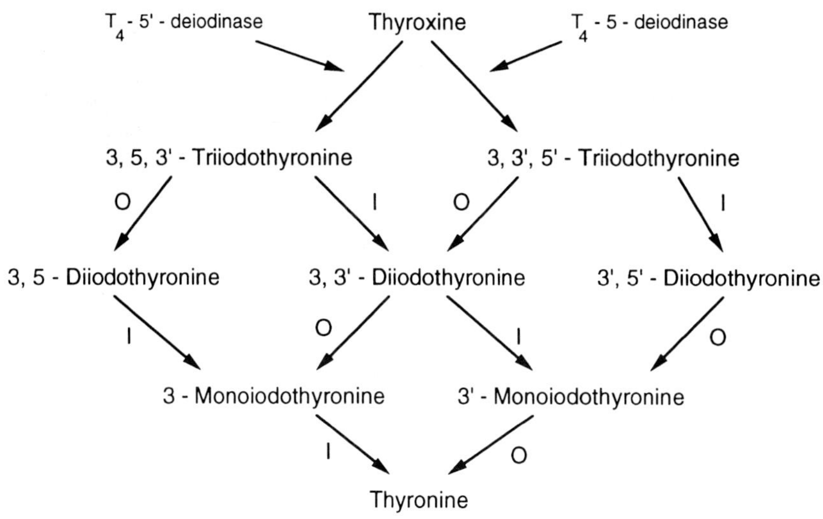

FIGURE 9-7. Pathways of deiodination of T_4 and its metabolites. O denotes outer ring deiodination (5′-deiodination); and I, inner ring deiodination (5-deiodination).

into granules. During the latter steps the carbohydrate components of the subunits are converted from components rich in mannose residues to complex oligosaccharides containing acetylated sugars, sialic acid, and sulfate.[29]

The estimated TSH secretion rate in normal subjects ranges from 75 to 150 mU/day (15 to 30 μg/day, 0.5 to 1 nmol/day). The pattern of TSH secretion is both circadian and pulsatile. Its serum half-life ranges from 50 to 80 min, and its clearance rate ranges from 40 to 60 ml/min. Small amounts of the individual subunits are found in the thyrotroph cells and in the circulation, and their secretion is regulated in the same way as is that of intact TSH.[30]

FIGURE 9-8. The hypothalamic-pituitary-thyroid axis. TSH regulates the thyroid glandular synthesis and secretion of T_4 and T_3; T_3 is also produced in many other tissues by deiodination of T_4. TSH secretion is regulated by serum T_4, serum T_3, T_3 produced from T_4 within the pituitary, and thyrotropin-releasing hormone (TRH). T_4 and T_3 also regulate TRH secretion. (−) denotes inhibitory effect, and (+), stimulatory effect.

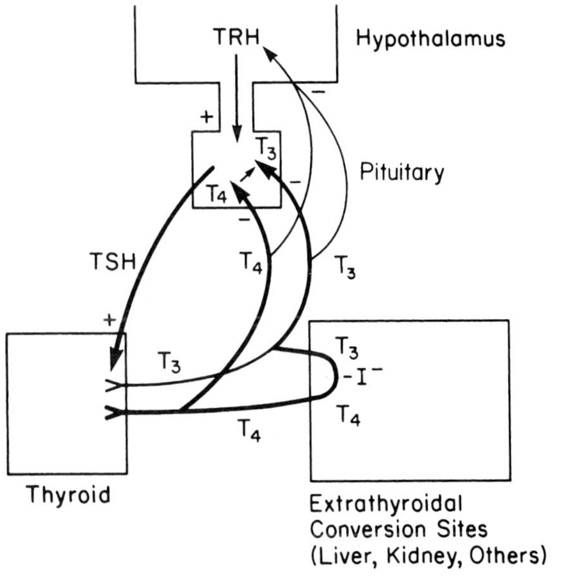

Thyroid Hormone Regulation of Thyrotropin Secretion

T_4 and T_3 directly inhibit TSH secretion, and deficiency of T_4 and T_3 increases it (Fig. 9-9). The sensitivity of the thyrotroph cells to changes in serum T_4 and T_3 concentrations is great, so that very small changes have large effects on TSH secretion, when the changes in serum T_4 and T_3 are due to changes in thyroid secretion (Fig. 9-10). Both T_4 and T_3 participate in this regulation, which serves to maintain thyroid secretion within very narrow limits. In contrast, the substantial decrease in serum T_3 concentrations that occurs in patients with nonthyroidal illness results in little change in TSH secretion (see section on Nonthyroidal Illness). The probable reason is that circulating T_4 contributes more to the nuclear T_3 content of the thyrotroph cells than it does in many other tissues because of the high deiodinase content of these cells.[19,31] The relatively smaller contribution of circulating T_3 to the cells' nuclear T_3 content allows continued TSH secretion when extrathyroidal T_3 production is decreased. It also allows increased TSH secretion

FIGURE 9-9. Factors regulating TSH secretion by the thyrotrophs of the pituitary. (−) denotes inhibitory effect; (+), stimulatory effect; and SRIH, somatostatin.

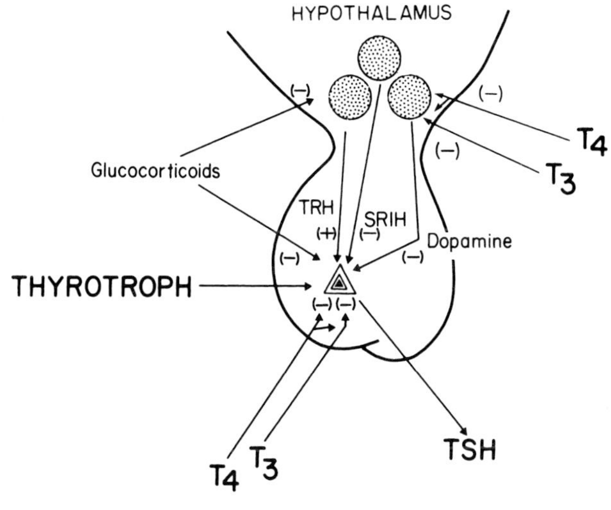

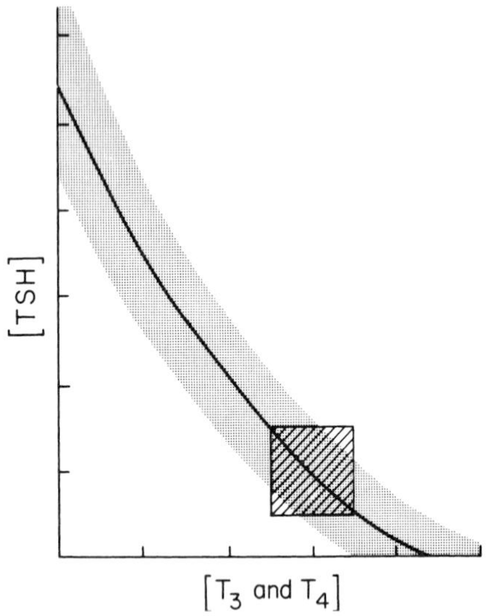

FIGURE 9-10. Diagram of the interrelation between serum TSH concentrations and serum T_4 and T_3 concentrations. The diagonally lined box encloses the respective normal ranges, and the shaded region indicates the pattern of changes in serum TSH concentrations that follow changes in thyroid secretion.

and, therefore, increased thyroid secretion in patients with abnormal thyroid glands or iodine deficiency; in these patients T_3 is produced and secreted by the thyroid in relatively more normal amounts than is T_4.[15]

T_4 and T_3 inhibit TSH secretion by decreasing both the biosynthesis and the release of TSH and, to a lesser extent, by decreasing the secretion of TRH (Fig. 9-9).[32,33] The first action is achieved primarily by thyroid hormone regulation of transcription of the TSH-subunit genes, especially that of the beta-subunit, and correlates with the extent of T_3 occupancy of the T_3 nuclear receptors.[34] Large doses of T_4 and especially T_3 reduce TSH secretion rapidly, suggesting that the hormones also directly inhibit TSH release. T_4 and T_3 also decrease the glycosylation of TSH, which reduces TSH bioactivity, and the number of thyrotroph-cell receptors for TRH.[32]

The rate and extent of inhibition of TSH secretion by T_4 and T_3 are dependent on the initial serum TSH concentration, the hormone given, and the dose.[35,36] Serum TSH concentrations decline, but not to normal, within hours after the administration of single doses of 250 to 500 μg or more of T_3 or T_4 to hypothyroid patients.[37] The maximum inhibition of TSH secretion occurs much later than the peak serum T_4 or T_3 concentration. When given in the usual therapeutic doses to patients with hypothyroidism, T_3 decreases serum TSH concentrations to normal in one to two weeks, and T_4 does so in four to six weeks. In normal subjects, even smaller doses of T_4 or T_3 inhibit TSH secretion within a few days. When given chronically, T_3 has about three times the potency of T_4 as an inhibitor of TSH secretion.[38] By contrast, recovery of suppressed TSH secretion after initiation of antithyroid treatment in patients with thyrotoxicosis or discontinuation of exogenous thyroid hormone therapy takes several weeks or longer.[39-41]

Thyrotropin-Releasing Hormone

Thyrotropin-releasing hormone (TRH) is the tripeptide pyroglutamyl-histidyl-prolineamide (see Chap. 6). The content of TRH is highest in the median eminence and paraventricular nuclei of the hypothalamus, but some TRH is found in most hypothalamic nuclei.[42] Most of the TRH entering the hypothalamic-pituitary portal circulation comes from the paraventricular nuclei, and these nuclei, therefore, are considered the thyrotrophic areas of the hypothalamus. Lesser amounts of TRH are found throughout the central nervous system and in the pituitary gland, gastrointestinal tract, pancreatic islets, parafollicular cells of the thyroid, reproductive tract, and placenta.[43] The physiologic functions of TRH in these tissues is unknown, but locally produced TRH could affect TSH secretion in the pituitary,[44] and it may serve as a local neuromodulator in other organs.

TRH is synthesized as a 26-kDa protein (proTRH) that contains five copies of the sequence glutamine-histidine-proline-glycine flanked by proteolytic cleavage sites; TRH is formed from proTRH by the action of peptidases followed by cyclization of the glutamine residue to form a pyroglutamyl residue.[45] The production of proTRH mRNA and proTRH in the paraventricular nuclei is increased in hypothyroid rats and decreases after local or systemic injection of T_3 or T_4, glucocorticoids, and fasting.[33,46-48] Presumably, TRH secretion from these neurons is regulated in a similar fashion. TRH is metabolized very rapidly; its plasma half-life is about 5 min.

TRH stimulates TSH secretion (Fig. 9-9) by binding to receptors on thyrotroph cell membranes that are linked to phospholipase C. The phosphoinositides formed by the action of this enzyme stimulate the release of calcium from intracellular storage sites; the increase in cytosol calcium concentration in turn stimulates exocytosis of TSH.[49] More chronic actions of TRH include stimulation of TSH subunit biosynthesis and TSH glycosylation; the latter action results in the secretion of TSH with increased biological activity.[29] The number of TRH receptors on the thyrotroph cells is down regulated by TRH and by thyroid hormones.[50]

TRH secretion is probably pulsatile, accounting for the pulsatility of TSH secretion, and surges of TRH secretion are responsible for the surges of TSH secretion that occur in newborn infants and during cold exposure in some subjects. More important, TRH is required for maintenance of normal TSH secretion, and it determines the set point about which thyroid hormones regulate TSH secretion.[51] In animals, administration of anti-TRH serum and lesions of the paraventricular nuclei reduce TSH and thyroid secretion. In some patients with low serum TSH concentrations and hypothyroidism, repeated TRH administration restores serum TSH, T_4, and T_3 concentrations to normal. Moreover, in patients or animals with TRH deficiency, thyroid deficiency results in smaller increases in TSH secretion, and T_4 and T_3 more readily inhibit TSH secretion than in normal subjects or animals.[52]

Exogenously administered TRH causes a dose-dependent increase in serum TSH concentrations in normal subjects.[53] TRH administered continuously for several days stimulates the release of more TSH than does the same dose given intermittently, although in both situations the initial increase in serum TSH concentrations is not sustained because the TSH-induced increase in serum T_4 and T_3 concentrations inhibits the serum TSH response to subsequent TRH administration.[54] Thus, administration of TRH for several months results in sustained increases in serum TSH concentrations of only 100 percent and in serum T_4 and T_3 concentrations of only 50 percent, providing further evidence of the ability of very small increases in serum T_4 and T_3 concentrations to inhibit TSH secretion directly.[55]

Exogenous TRH administration also stimulates prolactin release in normal subjects and most patients with hyperprolactinemia, and growth hormone secretion in elderly normal subjects and patients with several disorders, including hypothyroidism, chronic liver disease, and diabetes mellitus.[43,53] It also stimulates the release of growth hormone in some patients with acromegaly and of gonadotropins or their subunits in patients with gonadotroph adenomas or nonsecreting pituitary tumors.[56-58] However, endogenous TRH is not a physiologic regulator of the secretion of any of these hormones.

Other Factors Altering Thyrotropin Secretion

Several other factors, in addition to thyroid hormones and TRH, alter TSH secretion (Fig. 9-9). One is somatostatin. Infusions of somatostatin and its long-acting analog octreotide reduce basal serum TSH concentrations and inhibit the serum TSH response to exogenous TRH.[59,60] Both are less potent inhibitors of TSH than of growth hormone secretion, and patients receiving long-term treatment with octreotide do not become hypothyroid. Conversely, infusions of somatostatin antiserum increase basal serum TSH concentrations in animals, and hypothalamic lesions that reduce the content of somatostatin in the median eminence are accompanied by increased serum TSH concentrations. Thus, somatostatin may be a physiologically important tonic inhibitor of TSH secretion.

Dopamine also may be a physiologically important inhibitor of TSH secretion.[61] Serum TSH concentrations decline during infusions of dopamine and increase acutely after the administration of dopaminergic antagonist drugs such as metoclopramide and domperidone in both normal subjects and patients with hypothyroidism. Because domperidone does not cross the blood-brain barrier and dopamine infusions decrease TSH pulse amplitude but not pulse frequency, dopamine most likely has a direct action on the thyrotroph cells.[62]

Glucocorticoids also inhibit TSH secretion.[61] Their major action is to decrease pulsatile TSH secretion, suggesting that they inhibit TRH secretion, but they also inhibit serum TSH responses to exogenous TRH. Conversely, metyrapone-induced decreases in glucocorticoid production are accompanied by increases in serum TSH concentrations.

The long-term effect of somatostatin, dopamine, and glucocorticoids on TSH secretion is small. Transient increases in endogenous dopamine, somatostatin, or glucocorticoid secretion may transiently decrease TSH secretion. However, sustained increases in the endogenous production of these substances do not lead to inhibition of TSH secretion sufficient to cause hypothyroidism, because the direct stimulatory effect of any initial decreases in T_4 and T_3 secretion on TSH secretion overcomes the inhibition.

Mechanism of Action of Thyrotropin

TSH stimulates virtually every aspect of thyroid hormone biosynthesis and secretion. It also stimulates many steps in intermediary metabolism and the expression of many genes in thyroid tissue, and it causes thyroid hyperplasia and hypertrophy. The actions of TSH are initiated by its binding to specific plasma membrane receptors.[63] The receptor is a 100-kd glycosylated protein with an extracellular domain of approximately 400 amino acids, seven transmembrane domains of about 250 amino acids, and an intracytoplasmic domain of about 80 amino acids (Fig. 9-11).[63,64] It may exist not only as a linear protein but also in a cleaved form in which about 50 amino acids of the extracellular domain are removed; the remaining parts of the extracellular domain are linked to each other by disulfide bonds.[63] TSH binding to the extracellular domain of either form of the receptor depends primarily on the conformation of this domain, rather than the structure of any particular segment of it. The cytoplasmic domain is coupled to the alpha subunit of the stimulatory guanine-nucleotide-binding protein (Gs protein). Binding of TSH to the receptor activates the G protein, which stimulates adenylyl cyclase, increasing cyclic AMP formation, which in turn stimulates several protein kinases. How this process is linked to specific steps of intrathyroidal iodine metabolism, T_4 and T_3 synthesis, or other thyroid metabolic processes is not known. At high concentrations, TSH binding to the receptor activates a different G protein (Gq), which stimulates phospholipase C activity, increasing cytosol phosphoinositide concentrations and subsequently calcium concentrations and protein kinase C activity.[64] TSH regulates the production of its receptor in a positive way,[65] contributing to the ability of increases in TSH secretion (or production of TSH receptor-stimulating antibodies) to cause increases in thyroid gland function. Transcripts of a portion of the TSH receptor gene and receptor immunoreactivity have been detected in retroorbital and pretibial tissue, which may explain why Graves' disease affects these tissues (see section on Extrathyroidal Manifestations of Graves' Disease).[63,66,67]

TSH stimulates most if not all aspects of intrathyroidal iodide and thyroglobulin metabolism.[10,64] The stimulation of iodide transport is slow, requiring 24 hours of exposure to TSH, and is due to the production of additional transport units. The TSH-induced increase of iodothyronine formation is rapid and occurs in the absence of measurable increases in H_2O_2 production or thyroid peroxidase activity. Stimulation of colloid endocytosis and thyroglobulin proteolysis is even more rapid, occurring within minutes after TSH exposure. TSH stimulation of thyroidal deiodinase activity increases the proportion of T_3 that is secreted, thus helping to conserve iodine stores.[15] Most if not all of these TSH actions are mimicked by cyclic AMP, and the physiological importance of phospholipase C activation is not known. Physiologically, TSH stimulates the secretion of thyroglobulin as well as that of T_4 and T_3, although more slowly.[68] It is more effective in raising serum T_4 and T_3 concentrations when its secretion is pulsatile than when it is continuous.[54]

FIGURE 9-11. Schematic diagram of the TSH receptor, showing the large extracellular domain, seven transmembrane domains, and the cytoplasmic domain. Shown also are the putative sites at which the extracellular domain is cleaved to form a two-chain receptor held together by disulfide bonds (not shown), with release of a peptide from the original structure.

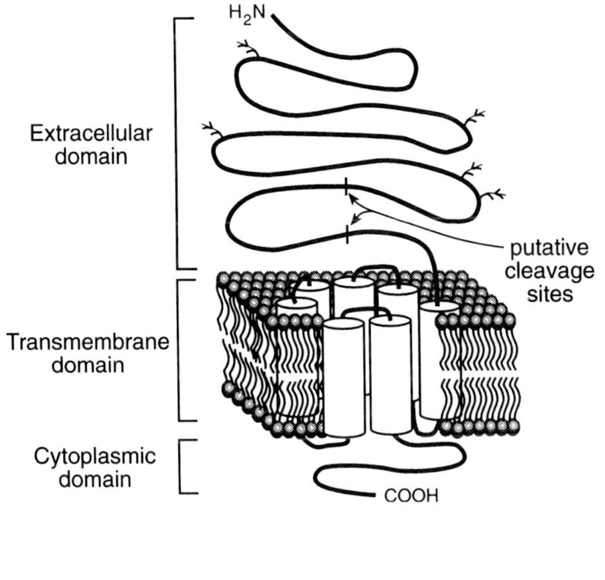

TSH stimulates many other facets of thyroid cell function.[64] It increases oxygen consumption, glucose and fatty acid utilization, and the content of NADPH, which is utilized for H_2O_2 generation as well as iodotyrosine and perhaps T_4 deiodination. A clinically obvious and important chronic action of TSH is stimulation of thyroid hypertrophy and hyperplasia, i.e., goiter formation (see Chap. 10). This growth reflects the ability of TSH to stimulate the synthesis of DNA, RNA, and structural proteins.[69]

Other factors that may be involved in the growth of the thyroid include insulin-like growth factor-I (IGF-I), epidermal growth factor (EGF), interleukin-1, and tumor necrosis factor. Thyroid cells produce and have receptors for IGF-I and EGF, and IGF-I augments the stimulatory effect of TSH on thyroidal DNA synthesis. Interleukin-1 and tumor necrosis factor, which may be produced by thyroid cells as well as by intrathyroidal mononuclear cells, stimulate thyroid cell growth but inhibit differentiated functions in thyroid cells.[70,71]

Regulation of Thyroid Secretion by Iodide

The thyroid gland utilizes iodide more efficiently when it is scarce, and less efficiently when it is abundant. Much of this regulation is achieved via changes in TSH secretion, but iodide also participates in this process.[10] When iodine intake is low, iodide transport and T_4 and especially T_3 synthesis are increased, even in the absence of TSH. With increasing iodide availability, the synthesis of T_4 rises more than does that of T_3, but high iodide concentrations inhibit iodide oxidation and organification, and therefore the synthesis of both hormones decreases. Transient increases in iodine intake therefore do not result in large increases in T_4 and T_3 synthesis. Iodine excess also inhibits thyroglobulin proteolysis and thus release of T_4 and T_3 from the thyroid. This is a rapid effect, occurring within hours, and is the principal mechanism for the antithyroid effect of inorganic iodine in patients with thyrotoxicosis.

In normal subjects, the antithyroid effect of iodine is transient, and they adapt to it in several weeks. Therefore T_4 and T_3 synthesis and secretion are not chronically inhibited. This adaptation results from inhibition of iodide transport; thus, intracellular iodide concentrations remain below those needed to maintain the block in synthesis and secretion. Adaptation does not occur in patients with a damaged thyroid gland, and therefore in them iodine administration can cause hypothyroidism (see section on Iodine Excess).

Regulation of Extrathyroidal Triiodothyronine Production

The activities of the extrathyroidal deiodinases that catalyze the conversion of T_4 to T_3 are altered by several factors (Fig. 9-12). Deiodinase activity, primarily type 1 deiodinase activity, is decreased in tissues from animals that are selenium-deficient, pointing to the key role of the selenocysteine residue in enzyme activity.[20,21,72] Type 1 deiodinase activity also is decreased in fetal animals and animals that are starved, hypothyroid, diabetic, or uremic, and those that have other nonthyroidal illnesses (Table 9-3).[18–21,73–75] It is also decreased by PTU, glucocorticoids, and beta-adrenergic antagonist drugs. Conversely, type 1 deiodinase activity is increased by thyroid hormone administration, glucose plus insulin, and a high caloric intake.[76,77]

The regulation of the type 2 deiodinase that predominates in the brain and pituitary is different (Table 9-3). Its activity is increased by thyroid deficiency, is little affected by nutritional deficiency and PTU, and is decreased by thyroid hormone excess.[18–21,78] This regulation serves to reduce the impact of thyroid deficiency in these tissues. The increase in pituitary deiodinase activity that occurs in thyroid deficiency and the decrease that occurs with thyroid hormone excess probably do not extend to the thyrotroph cells, because alterations in local T_3 production in these cells would blunt the changes in TSH secretion needed to defend against changes in thyroidal T_4 and T_3 secretion.

The biochemical mechanisms that might cause alterations in T_3 production from T_4 in extrathyroidal tissues include decreases in availability of substrate (T_4), transport of T_4 into cells, the mass or activity of one or more deiodinase, and cofactor availability. The drugs that decrease deiodinase activity bind to the enzyme, whereas starvation and nonthyroid illness probably decrease T_3 production by decreasing T_4 transport into the liver and other tis-

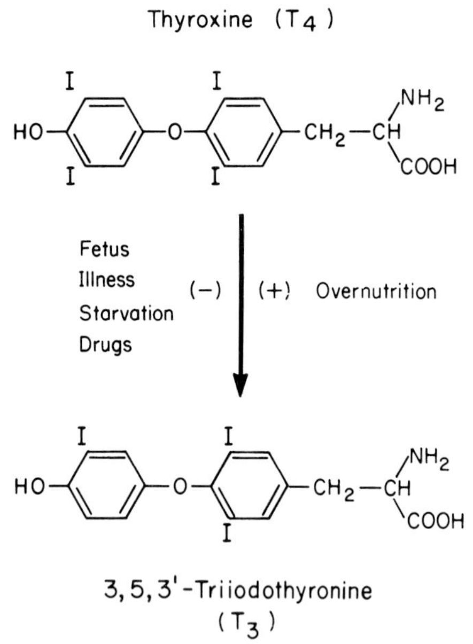

FIGURE 9-12. Effect of various nonthyroidal disorders and drugs on extrathyroidal T_4 conversion to T_3. Conversion is low in fetal tissues; is inhibited by illness, starvation, and some drugs; and is augmented by over-nutrition.

TABLE 9-3. Conditions or Drugs Altering Iodothyonine Deiodinase Activity

	*Enzyme Type Affected**	
Condition	**Type 1**	**Type 2**
Fetus	Decreased	Decreased
Hypothyroidism	Decreased	Increased
Thyrotoxicosis	Increased	Decreased
Starvation	Decreased	Normal
Diabetes mellitus	Decreased	Normal
Uremia	Decreased	Normal
Selenium deficiency	Decreased	Normal
Propylthiouracil	Decreased	Normal
Iopanoic acid	Decreased	Decreased
Amiodarone	Decreased	Decreased
Propranolol	Decreased	?

*Type 1 predominates in the liver and kidneys; type 2, in the brain and pituitary gland.

Sources: Engler,[18] Leonard,[19] Berry,[20] Larsen,[21] Chanoine,[72] Lim,[73] Grajower,[74] Kaplan,[75] Gavin,[76] Silva,[78] Meier,[79] and Shulkin.[80]

sues.[79–82] In other situations, alterations of deiodinase mass or activity are the likely causes of decreased T_3 production, but the specific nutritional, hormonal, or toxic factors or the cytokines that cause the alterations are not known.

Overall, these findings indicate that T_3 production is regulated in different ways in different tissues and that changes in thyroidal or extrathyroidal T_4 and T_3 production, as manifested by changes in their serum concentrations, are not the only, and perhaps not the major, determinants of intracellular T_3 availability. Local regulation of T_3 production may be particularly important in limiting the effects of thyroid deficiency or excess in tissues such as the brain and pituitary, and it undoubtedly leads to differences in T_3 availability in different tissues in patients with nonthyroidal illness.

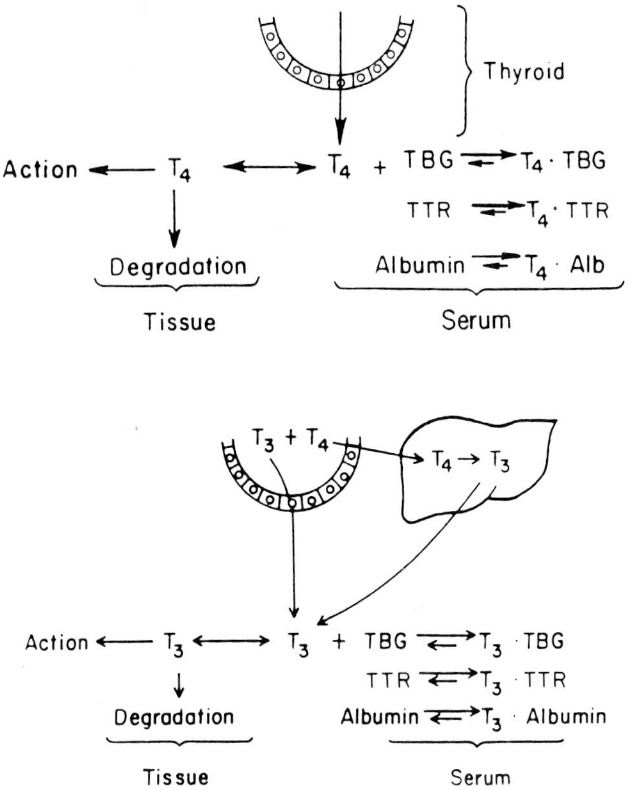

FIGURE 9-13. (*Top*) Origin, circulating forms, and degradation of T_4. (*Bottom*) Origin, circulating forms, and degradation of T_3. Only the liver is shown as a site of T_4 conversion to T_3, but the conversion occurs in many tissues. TBG denotes thyroxine-binding globulin; and TTR, transthyretin.

Transport and Cellular Binding of Thyroid Hormones

Serum Binding Proteins

Very little of the T_4 and T_3 in the circulation is free; more than 99.95 percent of the T_4 and 99.5 percent of the T_3 are bound in reversible physicochemical equilibrium to several serum proteins (Fig. 9-13).[83] These proteins are thyroxine-binding globulin (TBG), transthyretin [TTR, formerly called thyroxine-binding prealbumin (TBPA)], albumin, and lipoproteins. In normal subjects, approximately 75 percent of the T_4 in serum is bound to TBG, 10 percent to TTR, 12 percent to albumin, and 3 percent to lipoproteins. In comparison, about 80 percent of the T_3 in serum is bound to TBG, 5 percent to TTR, 10 percent to albumin, and 5 percent to lipoproteins (Table 9-4). Approximately 0.05 percent of the total serum T_4, or about 2 ng/dl (26 pmol/liter), is free; for serum T_3 the respective values are approximately 0.5 percent and 0.5 ng/dl (7 pmol/liter). Because so much of the T_4 and T_3 in serum is bound, changes in serum concentrations of binding proteins have a large effect on serum total T_4 and T_3 concentrations and fractional T_4 and T_3 metabolism, but they do not alter the serum free T_4 and T_3 concentrations or the absolute rates of T_4 and T_3 metabolism. These proteins also bind other iodothyronines, but much less avidly.[83]

It is the serum free T_4 and T_3 concentrations that determine the hormones' biological activity. The overall effect of the binding proteins is to maintain serum free T_4 and T_3 concentrations within narrow limits, yet ensure that the hormones are continuously and immediately available to tissues. They have, therefore, both storage and buffer functions. The storage function serves to facilitate the uniform distribution of T_4 and T_3 within tissues, particularly large solid organs. For example, when the liver is perfused through the portal vein with T_4 alone, the hormone is taken up only by the hepatocytes in the periportal areas; perfusion with T_4 and TBG, TTR, or albumin results in the distribution of T_4 throughout the liver.[84] In the longer term, if thyroid secretion ceases, the T_4 stored in serum serves to delay the appearance of thyroid deficiency for weeks, whereas if only free T_4 were available its supply would be exhausted within hours. Conversely, the binding proteins serve to buffer the free T_4 and T_3 concentrations in serum from sudden increases in thyroid secretion or release from extrathyroidal tissues.

Thyroxine-Binding Globulin

Thyroxine-binding globulin (TBG) is a 54-kDa glycoprotein that is synthesized in the liver. It has one binding site for T_4. While the affinity constant of TBG for T_4 is high, about 10^{10} M^{-1} (Table 9-4), the rate of dissociation is rapid ($t_{1/2}$ of 40 s). T_3 binds to TBG considerably less avidly than does T_4.[83] The carbohydrate content of TBG in serum is about 20 percent, but the content of individual TBG molecules varies, primarily as a result of differences in sialic acid content.[85] The serum TBG concentration in normal subjects is about 1.5 mg/dl (0.27 μmol/liter). This amount is capable of binding about 20 μg T_4 (26 nmol), but only about one-third of the TBG in serum normally contains T_4.

TABLE 9-4. Properties of Serum Thyroid Hormone-Binding Proteins

	Affinity Constant M^{-1}		*Serum Concentration*		*Serum Half-Life*	*T_4-Binding Capacity*		*Hormone Distribution**	
Protein	**T_4**	**T_3**	**mg/dl**	**μmol/liter**	***Days***	**μg/dl**	**nmol/liter**	**% of total T_4**	**% of total T_3**
Thyroxine-binding globulin	1×10^{10}	5×10^{8}	1.5	0.27	5	20	260	75	80
Transthyretin	7×10^{7}	2×10^{7}	25	4.6	2	200	2,600	10	5
Albumin	7×10^{5}	1×10^{5}	4,000	640	15	2,000	26,000	12	10

*Remainder bound to lipoprotein.

Source: Robbins.[83]

Transthyretin

Transthyretin (TTR) is a 55-kDa tetrameric protein composed of four identical subunits. It is synthesized in the liver, pancreatic islets, and choroid plexus. Each molecule has two identical T_4 binding sites, but occupation of one site by T_4 greatly decreases the affinity of the second site for T_4. The affinity constant of TTR for binding of T_4 is about 7×10^7 M^{-1}, its affinity for T_3 is considerably less, and the T_4-TTR complexes dissociate very rapidly (Table 9-4).[83,84] The serum concentration of TTR is about 25 mg/dl (4.6 μmol/liter), an amount capable of binding up to 200 μg T_4 (260 nmol).

TTR also binds retinol-binding protein, which in turn binds retinol (vitamin A). The binding of T_4 and of retinol-binding protein to TTR is independent, so that T_4 binding to TTR is not influenced by changes in retinol-binding protein or retinol concentrations. The serum half-life of TTR is considerably shorter than is that of TBG, so serum TTR concentrations change rapidly when its production rate changes, for example, during malnutrition.

Albumin

Albumin (66 kDa) has one strong binding site (affinity constant 7×10^5 M^{-1}) and several weaker binding sites for T_4. There are four T_4-binding albumin isoforms, and their relative affinity for T_4 and T_3 varies.[83] Because only about 12 percent of the T_4 in serum is bound to albumin, changes in serum albumin concentrations have relatively little effect on serum T_4 concentrations.

Lipoproteins

A small percentage (3–5 percent) of the T_4 and T_3 in serum is bound to lipoproteins.[83] Among them, high-density lipoproteins, mostly their apoprotein A-I component, bind the most T_4 and T_3, but some is bound to the apoprotein B-100 component of low-density and very-low-density lipoproteins.

Cellular Hormone Entry and Binding

Serum free T_4 and free T_3 are available for cellular uptake at any instant, and the rates of dissociation of T_4 and T_3 from their binding proteins are so rapid that additional T_4 and T_3 rapidly become available. The primary mechanism of cellular uptake of T_4 and T_3 in most tissues is via diffusion (Fig. 9-14), its rate being determined by the gradient in free hormone concentrations between the serum and intracellular fluid.[86] T_4 and T_3 uptake by the liver and some other tissues may be mediated by one or more ATP-dependent saturable plasma membrane transport systems; whether the uptake of T_4 and T_3 is mediated by the same or different carriers is uncertain.[87] Other factors, such as vascular flow and permeability and intracellular binding, also are important in determining T_4 and T_3 entry into cells. Ultimately, if the intracellular free hormone concentrations decline sufficiently, virtually all the protein-bound T_4 and T_3 in serum become free and may enter cells.

T_3 is also available to cells as a result of deiodination of T_4 within the cells (Fig. 9-14). Some of the locally produced T_3 must diffuse out of the cells because serum free (and total) T_3 concentrations are normal in hypothyroid patients taking T_4 in doses that raise their serum T_4 concentrations to normal. Some is not exported, however, and in many tissues local production of T_3 provides much of the T_3 that is bound to nuclear and perhaps other receptors linked to hormone action. Overall, about 90 percent of the total extrathyroidal T_3 pool of 50 μg (75 nmol) in humans is in the intracellular compartment.

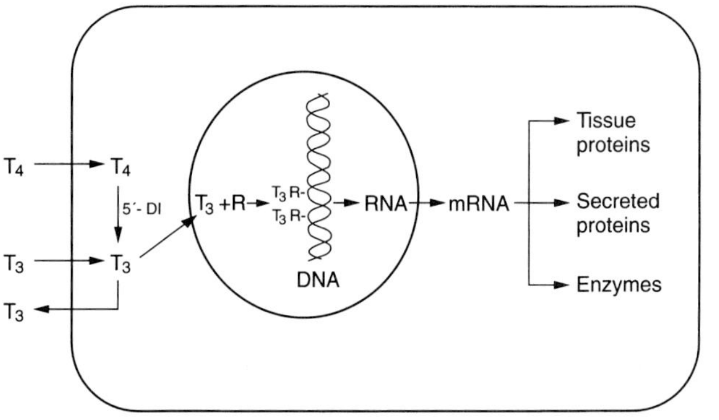

FIGURE 9-14. Schematic outline of extracellular and intracellular translocations of T_4 and T_3 and their actions in target cells. T_4 and T_3 may enter cells via concentration-dependent diffusion or active transport. T_4 is converted to T_3 in the cytosol. Cytosolic T_3 and possibly T_4 enter the nucleus by diffusion. T_3 binding to nuclear receptors and the subsequent activation of RNA synthesis results in increased synthesis of mRNAs that direct the synthesis of membrane proteins, secreted proteins, and lipogenic and other enzymes.

The distribution of T_4 and T_3 in different tissues is not uniform, because of differences in diffusion or transport of T_4 and T_3 into tissues, in the amount and type of deiodinase in the tissues, and in their storage capacity for T_4 and T_3. As a result, the fraction of the T_3 bound to its receptors that is derived from the circulation or is produced locally from T_4 varies substantially in different tissues. For example, in normal rats, locally produced T_3 accounts for about 20 percent of the nuclear T_3 in liver, 50 percent in the pituitary, and 80 percent in cerebral cortex.[31] It is therefore not surprising that optimal replacement in hypothyroid animals requires administration of both T_4 and T_3.[88,89]

T_4 and T_3 exist within cells both free and bound to cytosol, microsomes, mitochondria, and nuclei.[90] The cytosol binding proteins probably have buffering and storage functions like those of the iodothyronine-binding proteins in serum. The nature and importance of T_4 and T_3 binding to the other nonnuclear constituents are not known. Their affinity and specificity for T_4 and T_3 are lower than are those of the nuclear receptors, and their overall binding capacity is higher. Nevertheless, some may be receptors mediating hormone action.

Actions of Thyroid Hormone

T_3 Nuclear Receptors

Specific nuclear receptors in most tissues mediate most if not all of the physiologic actions of thyroid hormone.[90–93] These receptors are members of a superfamily that includes the receptors for steroid hormones, vitamin D, and retinoids; the molecular biology of this superfamily is described in Chap. 4. T_3 enters nuclei directly from the cytosol by diffusion and then binds to the receptors; no cytosol T_3-binding protein is required to facilitate entry of T_3 into nuclei. The T_3 nuclear receptors are acidic proteins that bind T_3 much more avidly than T_4, and in vivo nearly all the nuclear-bound hormone is T_3. T_4 can thus be considered largely if not completely a prohormone for T_3.

The general structure of the T_3 nuclear receptors is shown in Fig. 9-15.[90–93] The receptors are coded by two genes. One—the T_3 nuclear receptor alpha gene—is located on chromosome 17, and

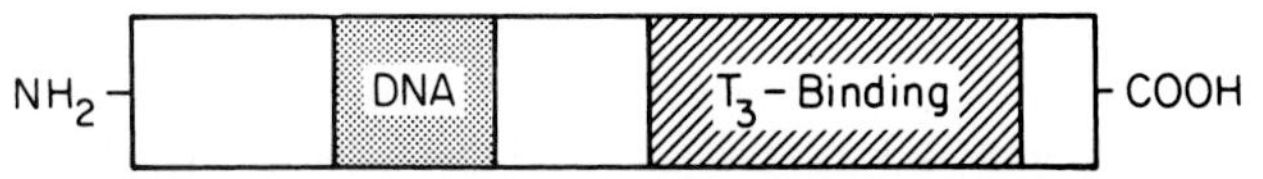

FIGURE 9-15. Schematic drawing of the structure of the T_3 nuclear receptor. NH_2 denotes the amino-terminal end of the receptor; DNA, the region of the receptor that binds to DNA; T_3 binding, the region that binds T_3; and COOH, the carboxyl-terminal end of the receptor.

the other—the T_3 nuclear receptor beta gene—is located on chromosome 3. Each of these two genes codes for mRNAs that can be alternatively spliced; thus, there are two products of the T_3 nuclear receptor alpha gene and two of the T_3 nuclear receptor beta gene. These receptors are linear polypeptides that range in molecular weight from 47 to 58 kDa; the differences among them are due to differences in both their amino- and carboxyl-terminal regions. They contain separate highly conserved DNA- and T_3-binding regions, except for the $alpha_2$ receptor. It does not bind T_3 and hence is not strictly speaking a T_3 receptor, but it binds to DNA and inhibits the action of T_3. The affinity of the $alpha_1$ receptor and the $beta_1$ and $beta_2$ receptors for T_3 is comparable.

The cell content of T_3 nuclear receptors is high in tissues that are most responsive to T_3, such as the pituitary and liver, and low in poorly responsive tissues, such as the spleen and testes. The $alpha_1$, $alpha_2$, and $beta_1$ receptors are widely distributed, although their relative abundance varies in different tissues. For example, $alpha_1$ receptors are abundant in skeletal and cardiac muscle and brain, $alpha_2$ receptors are abundant in brain and kidney, and $beta_1$ receptors are abundant in liver, kidney, and brain.[91,92] $Beta_2$ receptors are largely limited to the hypothalamus and pituitary. Alpha receptors are present early in fetal life, and beta receptors appear later.

The ultimate effects of T_3 binding to its receptors and the subsequent binding of the hormone-receptor complex to DNA are activation of transcription of some genes and inhibition of transcription of others. Most of the T_3-response elements are located a few hundred base pairs upstream of the transcription start sites of the responsive genes, but some are located near those sites or even within exons of the genes. Many of these response elements are small repeating or inverted sequences of six nucleotides separated by four to six other nucleotides, with some variation according to whether the transcriptional regulation is positive or negative[91,93]; all the response elements seem to bind the different T_3 receptors equally well. The T_3-T_3 receptor complexes bind to DNA most avidly when they are in the form of heterodimers with retinoid X receptors (Fig. 9-16), although T_3 receptor monomers and homodimers, as well as receptors containing no T_3, bind to DNA with low affinity and have some transcriptional activity. The formation of heterodimeric T_3 receptor-retinoic acid X receptor complexes, their binding to DNA, and their ability to activate transcription are augmented by several different nuclear proteins, some tissue-specific and some widely distributed, known generically as coactivators or thyroid receptor auxiliary proteins.[93,94] Conversely, the ability of unoccupied T_3 receptors to inhibit transcription is augmented by other nuclear proteins known as corepressors.

The extent to which different tissues are affected by T_3 varies widely. In some tissues many genes and therefore many cellular functions are affected, whereas in others only a few of each are affected. In some tissues, such as the pituitary and heart, there is a linear correlation between the relative saturation of these nuclear sites by T_3 and the transcriptional response.[90] In other tissues, increases in receptor occupancy result in nonlinear, amplified responses. Several factors underlie these differences in T_3 action in different tissues. They include: the diversity of the T_3 nuclear receptors themselves; the variations in their distribution and abundance among tissues; the fact that receptors containing T_3 and those not containing it have opposing biological activity, thereby broadening the range of function; the diversity in type and tissue content of the coactivator and corepressor proteins; and the presence of multiple T_3 response elements in DNA. Hence, there is an opportunity for many different alterations of gene expression, both qualitatively and quantitatively. Furthermore, there is tissue-specific regulation of production of the different forms of the T_3 nuclear receptor by thyroid hormone.[92,95] For example, in animals hypothyroidism increases and T_3 administration decreases the $beta_2$ receptor mRNA content in the pituitary, and T_3 administration decreases the $alpha_1$ receptor mRNA content in the heart and kidneys.[92,95,96] Starvation, diabetes, uremia, and partial hepatectomy decrease hepatic T_3 nuclear receptor content per cell[73,74,97]; such changes, if they occurred in humans, could serve to limit the impact of decreased T_3 production in patients with nonthyroidal illness.

Tissue Responses to Thyroid Hormones

Notwithstanding the fact that T_3 is the biologically active thyroid hormone, the effects of hypothyroidism in animals are reversed better by combinations of T_3 and T_4 than by either alone.[88,89] Similarly, in patients with hypothyroidism receiving adequate doses of T_4, substitution of 12.5 μg T_3 daily for 50 μg T_4 had beneficial effects on neuropsychological function without altering serum TSH concentrations.[98] These differences probably result from differences in cellular entry of the two hormones and differential effects on deiodinase activity. They also suggest that the small (20 percent) thyroidal contribution of T_3 to overall T_3 production is important.

FIGURE 9-16. Schematic diagram of the interactions between T_3, T_3 nuclear receptors (TR), and retinoid X receptors (RXR) with the thyroid response elements (TRE) on DNA that result in stimulation of gene expression and increased mRNA synthesis (expression of some genes is inhibited). T_3-TR homodimers have less activity than T_3-TR-RXR heterodimers, especially heterodimers containing coactivator (CoA) molecules.

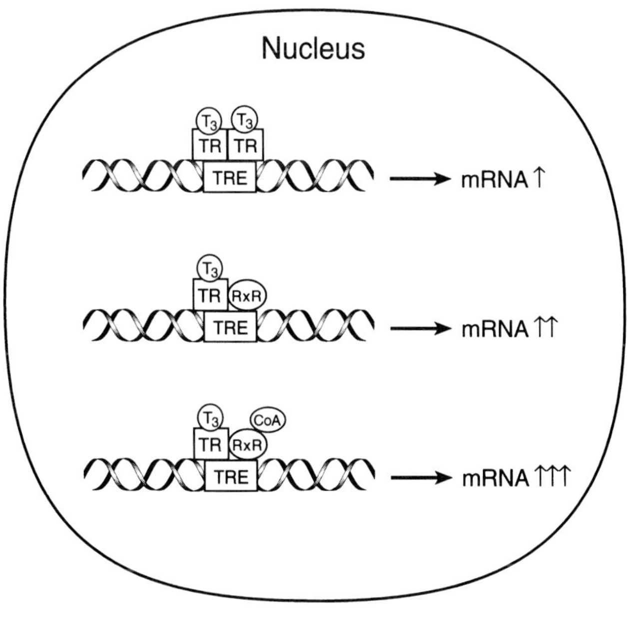

Thyroid hormones modulate a large number of metabolic processes by regulating the production and activity of many enzymes, the production and metabolism of other hormones, and the utilization of substrates, vitamins, and minerals (Fig. 9-14). Not all of these actions are due to effects on DNA transcription. Among the nonnuclear actions of thyroid hormones are stimulation of amino acid and glucose transport in lymphoid cells, calcium-ATPase activity in red blood cells, and inhibition of type 2 deiodinase activity in the pituitary and brain.[90,99,100] Thus, either T_3 nuclear receptors mediate extranuclear events or there are undetected high-affinity T_3 receptors in other cellular locations.

Effects on Protein Synthesis

T_3 stimulates the synthesis of many structural proteins, enzymes, and hormones (Table 9-5).[101] The consequences of this action are most obvious in the decreased neural and somatic growth that accompanies thyroid deficiency in infants and children. The increases in protein synthesis are due primarily to increased gene transcription, but proliferation of the ribosomal constituents involved in protein synthesis, increased translational efficiency, and perhaps increased amino acid transport may also be involved. However, not all T_3 actions on synthetic processes are stimulatory. For example, T_3 inhibits TSH secretion primarily by inhibiting the expression of the genes for its subunits,[32] and it inhibits the synthesis of glycosaminoglycan and fibronectin in fibroblasts.[102]

Thermogenic Actions

Energy released by the oxidation of substrate is stored by the formation of ATP or liberated as heat. The utilization of ATP for ion transport, synthesis of cell constituents, and muscle contraction results in the formation of ADP, and its rephosphorylation to form ATP requires an increase in mitochondrial oxidative metabolism. The single largest requirement for ATP in resting cells is for Na/K-dependent ATPase-mediated sodium transport; thus, changes in transport should have a substantial overall effect on oxidative metabolism.

Thyroid hormone stimulation of thermogenesis can be demonstrated both in vivo and in isolated tissues such as muscle, liver, and kidney.[103] The degree of stimulation correlates with the number of T_3 nuclear receptors in most tissues, except in the brain, which contains receptors but in which T_3 has no thermogenic action. There is a latent period of hours to days before oxygen consumption increases in response to T_3. The increase correlates with increased sodium transport, as measured by increases in Na/K-dependent ATPase activity, and is prevented by inhibition of ATPase activity with ouabain.[103] The increase in sodium transport results from an increase in cellular Na/K-dependent ATPase mRNA and enzyme production, i.e., an increase in sodium pump units.[104,105] Thus, thyroid hormone augmentation of thermogenesis can be explained at least in part by increased mitochondrial oxidative metabolism driven by the increase in ATP utilization that occurs as a result of increased Na/K-dependent ATPase activity. An increase in tissue concentrations of uncoupling protein-3 may contribute to the effect of T_3 on thermogenesis.[106]

TABLE 9-5. Some Genes Regulated by Thyroid Hormone

Positively regulated genes
Myelin basic protein
Fibronectin
GLUT-4 (glucose transporter)
Myosin heavy chain alpha
Malic enzyme
Fatty acid synthase
Glucokinase
Na/K-ATPase
Ca^{2+}-ATPase
Uncoupling protein
Negatively regulated genes
TSH alpha subunit
TSH beta subunit
TRH
T_3 nuclear receptor $beta_2$
Growth hormone
Myosin heavy chain beta

Cardiovascular Actions

Thyroid hormone has chronotropic and inotropic actions on the heart.[107] The increase in contractility is at least in part due to increased transcription of the myosin heavy-chain alpha gene, leading to an increase in a myosin isoform that contracts rapidly, and in calcium ATPase, which accelerates muscle relaxation.[108] T_3 also reduces peripheral vascular resistance by stimulating relaxation of vascular smooth muscle by a nongenomic action.[109]

Lipolysis and Lipogenesis

Thyroid hormones stimulate both lipogenesis and lipolysis, thereby providing increased quantities of fatty acids for oxidation to generate the ATP used for thermogenesis and other energy-consuming reactions.[110,111] The increase in lipogenesis is due to increases in lipogenic enzymes such as malic enzyme and fatty acid synthase in the liver. The increase in lipolysis is due to increases in catecholamine-sensitive lipase in adipose tissue and liver.

Effects on Carbohydrate Metabolism

The thermogenic effects of thyroid hormone are accompanied by increased peripheral and splanchnic utilization of glucose.[112,113] The increased need for glucose is balanced by an increase in hepatic glucose output, due to increases in both gluconeogenesis and glycogenolysis.[114]

Thyroid Hormone–Catecholamine Interactions

Many of the symptoms and signs of thyrotoxicosis appear to reflect increased sympathetic nervous system activity, and those of hypothyroidism decreased activity. The efficacy of beta-adrenergic antagonist drugs in ameliorating some of the clinical manifestations of thyrotoxicosis further suggests that thyroid hormone increases adrenergic activity. However, serum concentrations and production rates of norepinephrine are normal or decreased in thyrotoxicosis and increased in hypothyroidism, while those of epinephrine are not altered by either condition.[115] Thyroid hormones do have actions by which the apparent increase in sympathetic activity could be explained. They increase the number of beta-adrenergic receptors in cardiac and skeletal muscle and adipose tissue and decrease myocardial alpha-adrenergic receptors.[116] These changes do not, however, result in increased in vivo sensitivity to beta-adrenergic agonists.[117]

Evaluation of Thyroid Function

Sensitive and specific tests are available for evaluating patients suspected of having abnormalities in thyroid secretion and identifying whether the abnormality is thyroidal or hypothalamic-pituitary (central) in origin. The single most important question in an

TABLE 9-6. Strategies for Testing Thyroid Function

Subject	Possible Thyroid Dysfunction	Serum Test
Case finding		TSH
Clinically euthyroid, healthy		
Solitary nodule	Thyrotoxicosis	TSH
Multinodular goiter	Thyrotoxicosis	TSH
Diffuse goiter	Thyrotoxicosis or hypothyroidism	TSH
Clinically euthyroid, nonthyroidal illness*	Thyrotoxicosis or hypothyroidism	TSH, free T_4†
Suspected thyrotoxicosis		TSH, free T_4†
Suspected hypothyroidism		TSH, free T_4†
Thyrotoxicosis, during treatment	Thyrotoxicosis, euthyroid, or hypothyroidism	TSH, free T_4†
Hypothyroidism, during treatment		TSH

*May include patients admitted to nursing homes and psychiatric services.

†Serum free T_4 can be measured as the serum free T_4 concentration or serum free T_4 index.

individual patient is, What is the level of thyroid secretion? This question may be asked in several contexts, for example case finding, evaluating a patient with thyroid nodular disease or goiter, or evaluating a patient with symptoms and signs of thyrotoxicosis or hypothyroidism.

For case finding among patients not suspected of having any abnormality of thyroid secretion or evaluating clinically euthyroid patients with thyroid nodular disease, measurement of serum TSH is the most appropriate test (Table 9-6). Very few patients with normal serum TSH concentrations have abnormal thyroid secretion.[118,119] Thus, the standard test protocol in many practices and laboratories is to measure serum TSH. If abnormal, serum free T_4 is then measured automatically. This approach works very well and is highly cost-effective.

Measurement of the serum free T_4 index (or free T_4 concentration) is an acceptable alternative because few patients with normal values have abnormal serum TSH values.[118,119] Measurement of serum TSH is seemingly less direct; its great value lies in the fact that TSH secretion is a very sensitive indicator of changes in serum free T_4 concentrations.

Serum TSH concentrations are abnormal not only in patients with overt thyroid disease (defined as abnormal serum TSH and low or high serum free T_4 or T_3 values) but also those with subclinical thyroid disease (defined as abnormal serum TSH but normal serum free T_4 [and T_3] values). However, serum TSH values may be normal in patients with central hypothyroidism and patients with TSH-dependent thyrotoxicosis and low in patients with nonthyroid illness (Fig. 9-17). Serum free T_4 values are abnormal in patients with overt thyroid disease, but are normal, by definition, in patients with subclinical thyroid disease, and the values may be low in patients with nonthyroidal illness. Both serum TSH and free T_4 should be measured in patients strongly suspected of having thyrotoxicosis or hypothyroidism, patients with pituitary disease, and hospitalized patients with nonthyroidal illness.

Screening of newborn infants for hypothyroidism is now routine in many parts of the world because of its value for preventing cretinism. The value of screening normal adults or case finding among adults who seek medical care is debated. Among adults aged 40 years and older, about 0.4 percent have overt hypothyroidism, 4–8 percent have subclinical hypothyroidism, less than 0.1 percent have overt thyrotoxicosis, and about 2 percent have subclinical thyrotoxicosis.[120–123] Based on these data, case finding among patients seeking medical care is appropriate. Screening of all women 50 years old and older—the group with the highest frequency of abnormalities—has been recommended, but is controversial.[123–125]

Serum Thyrotropin Concentrations

Measurements of serum TSH provide a very precise indication of the availability of T_4 and T_3 to the pituitary in normal subjects and patients with thyroid disease (Fig. 9-17). Serum TSH concentrations in normal subjects range from approximately 0.3 to 3.0 mU/liter. The assays now in use have a sensitivity of about 0.02 to 0.1 mU/liter (in some instances 0.005 mU/liter), and therefore subnormal serum TSH values can be readily detected. As compared with the standard assays now available, the most sensitive assays, sometimes referred to as third generation or ultrasensitive assays, are more expensive and provide little additional information.[126] All these assays utilize two mouse monoclonal antibodies, one against an epitope of the beta subunit of TSH and the other against an epitope on the common alpha subunit of the glycoprotein hormones. To be detected, a molecule must have both epitopes, and therefore the assays are very specific. Spurious elevations are very rare, but have been found in patients given mouse monoclonal antibodies for therapeutic purposes or those who worked with rodents (and had endogenous antimouse immunoglobulin antibodies).[127,128]

FIGURE 9-17. Relationship between serum TSH and T_4 concentrations in normal subjects and patients with overt and subclinical thyrotoxicosis, overt and subclinical hypothyroidism, central hypothyroidism, and nonthyroidal illness.

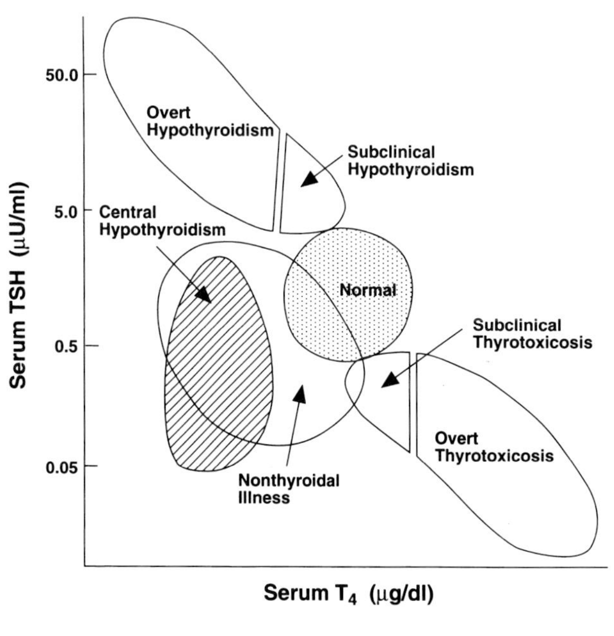

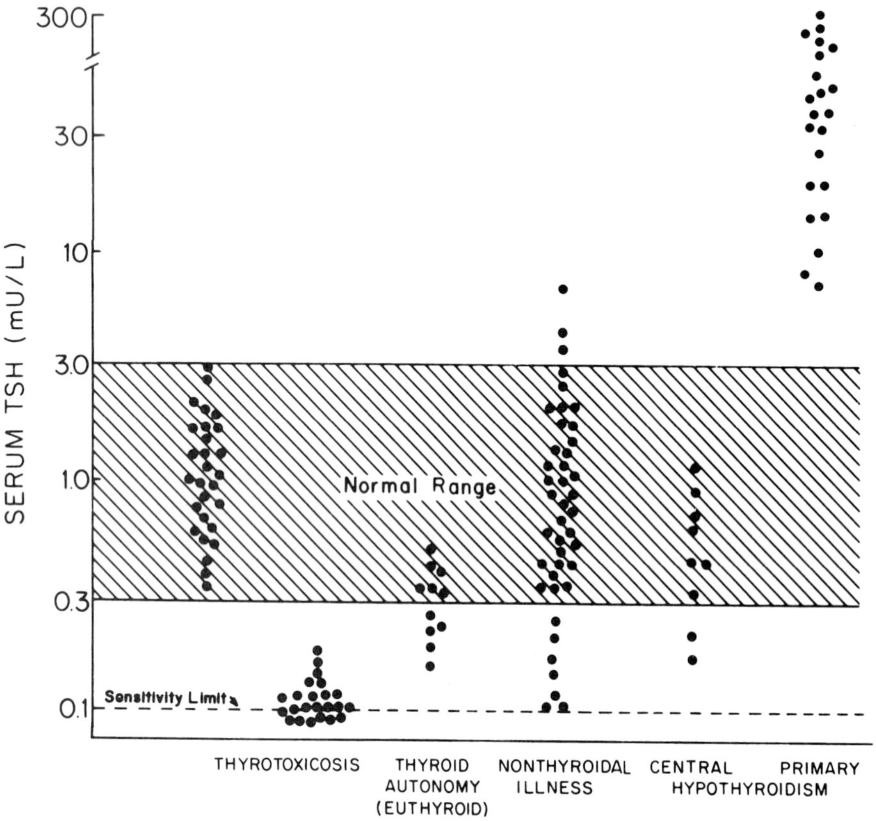

FIGURE 9-18. Serum TSH concentrations in normal subjects and patients with thyrotoxicosis, thyroid autonomy (euthyroid, some of whom have subclinical thyrotoxicosis), nonthyroidal illness, and central and primary hypothyroidism. The diagonally lined area indicates the normal range. Note the logarithmic scale of the y-axis.

In normal subjects serum TSH concentrations are not normally distributed within the normal range, but cluster in the lower part. The normal range largely encompasses the circadian and pulsatile variation in TSH secretion that occurs in normal subjects (see section on Daily Variations).

Serum TSH concentrations are high in patients with hypothyroidism when it is due to thyroid disease and are normal or low when it is due to hypothalamic or pituitary disease (central hypothyroidism) (Figs. 9-17 and 9-18). Serum TSH concentrations are low or undetectable in patients with thyrotoxicosis, excepting those few patients with TSH-dependent thyrotoxicosis. The change in serum TSH concentrations in patients with thyroid disease is continuous, so that they range from very high in patients with overt hypothyroidism to very low in patients with overt thyrotoxicosis (Fig. 9-17). Changes in serum T_4 and T_3 concentrations of as little as 15 to 25 percent caused by changes in thyroid secretion are sufficient to raise or lower serum TSH concentrations from within to outside the normal range. On the other hand, in patients with a normal thyroid gland in whom TSH secretion is not normally inhibited by excess T_4 and T_3, for example those with TSH-secreting pituitary adenomas or those with generalized resistance to thyroid hormone, serum TSH concentrations in the upper range of normal are sufficient to raise serum T_4 and T_3 concentrations to well above their respective normal ranges.

Because of the sensitivity of TSH secretion to small changes in thyroid secretion, an abnormal serum TSH concentration usually indicates the presence of an abnormality in thyroid secretion. Conversely, a normal serum TSH concentration usually provides strong evidence against the presence of any abnormality of thyroid secretion.[118,119] Serum TSH concentrations are normal in most patients with nonthyroidal illness who have decreased serum thyroid hormone concentrations, but can be either low or high (see section on Nonthyroidal Illness). Some seemingly normal subjects have low values that cannot be related to any thyroid disease and that do not persist[129,130]; whether such changes are due to wider than usual variations in pulsatile TSH secretion or to transient, clinically unrecognized nonthyroidal illness is not known.

Serum Thyroxine Concentrations

Serum total T_4 concentrations are measured by assays that use specific anti-T_4 antibodies and require the use of a compound that blocks T_4 binding to the serum thyroid hormone-binding proteins so that all the T_4 in the serum sample is available for reaction with the antibodies. The normal range in adults is about 5 to 11 μg/dl (64 to 140 nmol/liter).

The terms *hyperthyroxinemia* and *hypothyroxinemia* are used to describe values above and below this range, respectively. Serum T_4 concentrations are determined primarily by thyroid secretion of T_4 and the serum concentrations of the thyroid hormone-binding proteins. Therefore, serum T_4 concentrations are high in patients with thyrotoxicosis and those with high serum concentrations of TBG and other binding proteins (see section on Alterations in Serum Thyroid Hormone Binding) (Table 9-7). Rarer causes of high serum T_4 concentrations include the presence of autoantibodies that bind T_4 and decreases in T_4 clearance. Thus, the serum T_4 concentration can be high in patients who are euthyroid or even hypothyroid.

Conversely, serum T_4 concentrations are low in patients with hypothyroidism. They also are low in patients who have low serum concentrations of TBG and other binding proteins or who are receiving drugs that inhibit the binding of T_4 to TBG, patients receiving T_3, and those who have serious nonthyroidal illnesses (Table 9-7).

TABLE 9-7. Conditions Altering Serum Thyroxine Concentrations, Thyroid Hormone-Binding Ratios (THBR), and Serum Free Thyroxine Index Values*

	Serum T_4 Concentration	THBR	Serum Free T_4 Index
Thyrotoxicosis	High	High	High
Increased serum TBG†	High	Low	Normal
Familial dysalbuminemic hyperthyroxinemia	High	Normal	High
Hypothyroidism	Low	Low	Low
Decreased serum TBG	Low	High	Normal
Inhibitors of TBG binding	Low	High	Normal
T_3 treatment	Low	Low	Low
Nonthyroidal illness	Normal, low or high	Normal or high	Normal, low or high

*High and low indicate values higher and lower, respectively, than in the average normal subject, but not necessarily above or below the respective ranges of normal.

†TBG denotes thyroxine–binding globulin.

Misinterpretation usually can be avoided by simultaneous determination of serum thyroid hormone-binding capacity or direct measurement of serum free T_4.

Serum Thyroid Hormone-Binding Capacity (Thyroid Hormone-Binding Ratio) and Free Thyroxine Index

Because nearly all the T_4 in serum is bound to TBG or other proteins, the extent of protein binding must be determined to interpret the results of serum T_4 measurements properly. This is done most simply by determination of the thyroid hormone-binding ratio (THBR), also known as the T_3-resin uptake. This test measures the number of unoccupied protein-binding sites for T_4. It is done by mixing T_3 that is labeled with ^{125}I or in some other way with serum, adding a resin or another particulate substance, and then determining the amount of radiolabeled T_3 bound to the resin (Fig. 9-19). In normal serum, the unoccupied protein-binding sites, primarily TBG, take up about 55 to 75 percent of the labeled T_3, and 25 to 45 percent is bound to the resin, that is, the T_3-resin uptake, depending on the amounts of serum and particulate substance used. The results also may be expressed as the ratio of the amount of labeled T_3 bound to the resin in the presence of the test serum to that bound in the presence of normal serum (normal range, 0.80–1.20). The THBR determination is not a measurement of serum T_3. Moreover, because the affinity of TBG for T_3 is low in comparison with its affinity for T_4, the results are altered little by alterations in serum T_3 concentrations. Serum TBG can be measured directly, but this is necessary only when the specific cause of a binding abnormality is being sought. Serum TBG concentrations in normal subjects range from 1 to 2 mg/dl.

There are three ways in which the number of unoccupied T_4-binding sites in serum may be decreased, resulting in a high THBR: (1) when more binding sites are occupied with T_4, as in thyrotoxicosis, (2) when the binding sites are occupied by a ligand that competes with T_4 for binding to TBG, such as salicylate, and (3) when there is a decrease in the number of binding sites, as occurs when serum concentrations of TBG or another binding protein are low (Table 9-7). There are two ways in which the

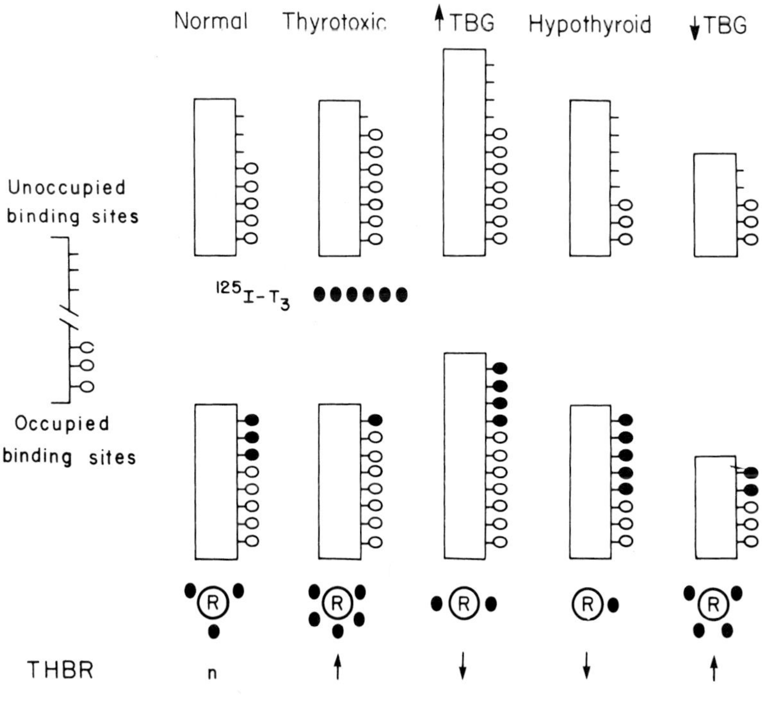

FIGURE 9-19. The thyroid hormone-binding ratio (THBR) test (T_3-resin uptake test). For clarity of representation, the proportion of the total number of binding sites occupied by endogenous hormone is underrepresented in this figure. R = resin or other inert substance added to bind the [^{125}I] T_3 that is not bound to serum protein.

number of unoccupied T_4-binding sites in serum may be increased, resulting in a low THBR: (1) when fewer binding sites are occupied by T_4, as in hypothyroidism, and (2) when there is an increase in the number of binding sites, as occurs when the serum concentration of TBG or another binding protein is high.

Thus, a serum T_4 value must be interpreted in conjunction with the THBR. If both the THBR and the serum T_4 concentration are high or if both are low, thyroid secretion is altered. If the two results are discordant, an abnormality of binding protein is likely. The product of the serum T_4 value and THBR is the serum free T_4 index (Table 9-7). Serum free T_4 index values usually correlate well with the values obtained by direct measurement of serum free T_4, but they may underestimate the degree of abnormality in protein binding in patients with nonthyroidal illness, those with very high or low serum TBG concentrations, and those with familial dysalbuminemic hyperthyroxinemia, as discussed later.

Serum Free Thyroxine Concentrations

Serum free T_4 concentrations can be measured directly by equilibrium dialysis, ultrafiltration, and immunoassay. Normal values range from 0.8 to 2.5 ng/dl (10 to 32 pmol/liter). Although the first two methods are thought to provide the closest approximation to the serum free T_4 concentration in vivo, they are technically difficult and not widely available. The immunoassays for serum free T_4 provide accurate estimates of serum free T_4 concentrations in patients with thyroid disease, but the results may not be accurate in patients with nonthyroidal illness and those with abnormalities in binding proteins, particularly those that use a T_4 analog that may not bind to the abnormal binding protein.[131–133] Measurements of serum free T_4 by radioimmunoassay are gradually replacing measurements of serum free T_4 index in clinical laboratories. As a practical matter, these measurements in general provide information comparable to that provided by serum free T_4 index measurements, but they are more expensive.

Serum Triiodothyronine Concentrations

Serum T_3 concentrations are measured by immunoassay. The normal range is 75–200 ng/dl (1.1–3.0 nmol/liter). Serum T_3 concentrations, like those of T_4, are altered by changes in thyroid secretion and changes in serum thyroid hormone–binding proteins. In patients with thyrotoxicosis, serum T_3 concentrations usually are increased to a greater degree than are serum T_4 concentrations; in patients with hypothyroidism, they are more often within the normal range than are serum T_4 concentrations. Serum T_3 concentrations are low in most patients with nonthyroidal illness (see section on Nonthyroidal Illness). The major, if not only, indication for measurement of serum T_3 is in patients with clinical manifestations of thyrotoxicosis who have normal serum T_4 concentrations.

Serum free T_3 concentrations can be measured directly or indirectly (as the serum free T_3 index) in the same ways as are used to measure serum free T_4 concentrations.[134] Measurement of serum free T_3 is rarely indicated in clinical practice.

Serum Reverse Triiodothyronine Concentrations

Serum reverse T_3 (rT_3) concentrations, also measured by immunoassay, range from 20 to 50 ng/dl (0.3 to 0.8 nmol/liter) in normal subjects. Serum rT_3 concentrations depend primarily on the level of T_4 secretion because virtually all the rT_3 in serum is produced from T_4 at extrathyroidal sites. Changes in serum thyroid hormone–binding proteins have little effect on serum rT_3 concentrations because the affinity of TBG and other binding proteins for rT_3 is low. Serum rT_3 concentrations are often high, or at least high in relation to serum T_4 concentrations, in patients with nonthyroidal illness. Serum rT_3 measurements are not useful clinically because they provide little information about thyroid secretion and because of the wide variations that occur in patients with nonthyroidal illness.[135]

Serum Thyroglobulin Concentrations

Thyroglobulin is present in small amounts (2–25 μg/liter) in the circulation of virtually all normal subjects. Thyroglobulin antibodies interfere with the measurement of thyroglobulin; therefore, serum thyroglobulin cannot be measured accurately in patients with these antibodies.[136]

Thyroglobulin secretion is TSH-dependent.[36] Serum thyroglobulin concentrations are high in patients with thyrotoxicosis, except patients with thyrotoxicosis caused by exogenous thyroid hormone administration, in whom the concentrations are low. Thus, measurements of serum thyroglobulin can be used to differentiate spontaneously occurring from exogenous thyrotoxicosis. Serum thyroglobulin concentrations also are high in some patients with endemic goiter, multinodular goiter, and benign and malignant thyroid tumors, and they may increase transiently after needle-aspiration biopsy of thyroid nodules. In hypothyroid patients, measurements of serum thyroglobulin can be used to distinguish those who have no thyroid tissue from those in whom thyroid hormonogenesis is abnormal but thyroid tissue is present, for example, to distinguish infants with thyroid agenesis from those with enzymatic or other defects in thyroid hormone production.

Serum thyroglobulin measurements are most useful in the follow-up of patients with thyroid carcinoma who have undergone thyroidectomy and radioiodine ablation of any remaining thyroid tissue. A value of 5 to 10 μg/liter or more in such a patient provides strong evidence of tumor recurrence (see Chap. 10).

Tests for Antithyroid Antibodies in Serum

Antibodies to thyroid peroxidase, formerly known as thyroid microsomal antigen, are present in high concentrations in the serum of most patients with chronic autoimmune thyroiditis, especially those with the goitrous form of the disease (Hashimoto's disease) and many patients with Graves' disease. Low concentrations of these antibodies also are found in patients with most other thyroid diseases; patients with other autoimmune diseases, such as pernicious anemia, idiopathic Addison's disease, and type 1 diabetes mellitus; and in normal subjects, particularly elderly women.[137–139] All these people probably have some chronic autoimmune thyroiditis, and some have high serum TSH concentrations. The principal value of tests for these antibodies is to confirm a suspected diagnosis of chronic autoimmune thyroiditis.

Antibodies to thyroglobulin are also found in the serum of many patients with autoimmune thyroid disease, and less often in patients with other thyroid diseases and normal subjects.[138] Tests for antithyroglobulin antibodies have little clinical value.

Antibodies that bind to and activate the TSH receptor or block the action of TSH are discussed in the sections on Graves' disease and chronic autoimmune thyroiditis, respectively.

Thyrotropin-Releasing Hormone Stimulation Test

TRH testing is usually done by intravenous administration of 400 or 500 μg. In normal subjects, serum TSH concentrations in-

TABLE 9-8. Radiation Exposure from Radionuclides Used for Thyroid Studies

				Radiation Exposure			
		Usual Scanning Dose		*Total Body*		*Thyroid**	
Isotope	**Half-Life**	**uCi**	**Mbq**	**mrad**	**Gy**	**rads**	**Gy**
^{123}I	13 h	200	7.4	6	0.0006	2.6	0.026
^{131}I	8 d	50	1.8	36	0.0036	65	0.65
$^{99}mTcO_4$	6 h	3000	110	15	0.0015	1	0.01

* Based on 25 percent 24-h uptake.

^{123}I and ^{131}I are given orally, and $^{99m}TcO_4$ is given intravenously.

Bq denotes Becquerel, and Gy, Gray.

crease two- to eightfold, to peak values of 5 to 25 mU/liter, 20–30 min after TRH administration.[53] The intravenous injection of TRH often causes transient nausea and an urge to urinate and occasionally hypertension. The serum TSH response to TRH is characteristically increased in patients with primary hypothyroidism and is subnormal, delayed, or both in those with TSH or TRH deficiency; the test cannot be used to distinguish between TSH deficiency and TRH deficiency. The response is inhibited by very small increases in serum T_4 and T_3 concentrations, so that TRH fails to increase serum TSH concentrations in euthyroid patients with autonomous thyroid secretion as well as in patients with thyrotoxicosis. Several drugs, notably dopamine and glucocorticoids, and nonthyroidal illnesses also result in subnormal serum TSH responses to TRH.

The serum TSH response to TRH correlates directly with the basal serum TSH concentration. Therefore TRH stimulation tests provide no information beyond that obtained by measurements of the basal serum TSH.

Thyroid Radionuclide Tests

The major radionuclides useful for thyroid studies and their characteristics are shown in Table 9-8. As discussed in detail in Chap. 10, the higher radiation exposure from ^{131}I-iodine makes ^{123}I-iodine the iodine isotope of choice for nearly all clinical tests.

Measurement of thyroid radioiodine uptake as the proportion of the administered dose concentrated in the thyroid per unit of time can occasionally be useful as an index of thyroid function. In the United States, the thyroid radioiodine uptake in normal subjects is usually given as 5 to 15 percent 4 h and 10 to 30 percent 24 h after oral administration of the isotope, but the values may be slightly higher now as a result of the recent decline in iodine intake (see section on Iodine Economy). The values are low in hypothyroid patients; they are high in thyrotoxic patients, except those who have some type of thyroiditis or exogenous thyrotoxicosis.

The most common cause of a low radioiodine uptake is not hypothyroidism but an expanded extracellular iodine pool resulting from oral, parenteral, or cutaneous use of inorganic iodine or iodine-containing drugs. To obtain reliable measurements of radioiodine uptake, the test should not be done for at least a week after use of inorganic iodine, two or more weeks after the use of water-soluble organic iodine compounds, and four or more weeks after the use of lipid-soluble organic iodine compounds. Radionuclides should not be administered to pregnant women.

Thyroid radionuclide imaging (scan) studies are useful for the detection of anatomic variations and ectopic location of thyroid tissue and for assessing regional function within the thyroid gland. In patients with nodular thyroid disease, scans determine whether nodules can concentrate the radionuclide and the extent to which the function of extranodular tissue is suppressed. Imaging may be done with either ^{123}I-iodine or pertechnetate-99m ($^{99m}TcO_4$), with comparable results. The latter, like iodine, is transported into the thyroid, but unlike iodine, it is not organified and diffuses back into the circulation rapidly. The peak pertechnetate uptake, therefore, is 20–30 min after its administration. Although it must be given intravenously, it has favorable detection and safety features, costs less, and is more convenient for the patient because the thyroid scan can be done soon after administration. In contrast, peak radioiodine uptake occurs 18–24 h after its administration, so a second visit is required. All these features make pertechnetate the radionuclide of choice for thyroid imaging in most patients. In either instance, proper interpretation of the scan requires that both the patient's thyroid gland and the scan be examined at the same time.

Ultrasonography and Needle Biopsy

These tests may be useful in evaluating patients with thyroid nodular disease and thyroid carcinoma (see Chap. 10). CT or MR imaging can occasionally provide useful information in patients with complicated cervical or retrosternal goiters.

Tests of Thyroid Hormone Action in Tissue

Thyroid hormones alter the function of many tissues, and measurements reflecting their impact on tissues might be expected to be useful adjuncts for the diagnosis of thyrotoxicosis or hypothyroidism. However, the tests available for this purpose, such as measurements of serum cholesterol or sex hormone-binding globulin and basal metabolic rate and tests of myocardial contractility and relaxation, are neither sensitive nor specific indicators of the impact of thyroid hormones on their target tissues.

Physiological Variables Affecting Pituitary-Thyroid Function and Tests

Daily Variations

TSH secretion is pulsatile, with 8 to 14 secretory episodes per 24 h (Fig. 9-20). The pulse frequency is similar during the day and night, but the pulse amplitude increases in the late evening, is greatest just before the onset of sleep, and declines after the onset of sleep.[62,140–142] There is therefore a circadian pattern of TSH secretion, so that mean serum TSH concentrations throughout the night are 50–100 percent higher than during the day. The nocturnal increase in TSH secretion is exaggerated if sleep is delayed.[142] Infants older than one month and children have a similar nocturnal increase in TSH secretion, but it is diminished in elderly subjects.[143] The normal pattern of nocturnal TSH secretion per-

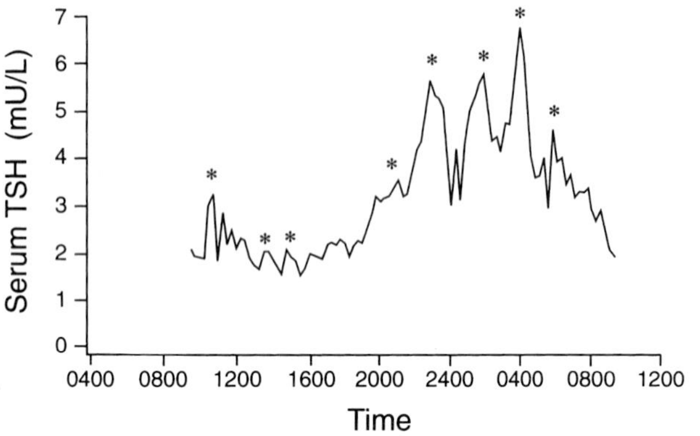

FIGURE 9-20. Serum TSH concentrations measured at frequent (15-min) intervals for 24 h in a normal young adult. The asterisks at the top indicate pulses of TSH secretion as detected by the computer program Cluster. (*Reproduced with modification from J Clin Endocrinol Metab 78:211, 1994, with permission of the publisher.*)

sists in patients who have small increases in serum TSH concentrations, but may be blunted in those with large increases.[144] There is no circadian variation in serum T_4 and T_3 concentrations.

Pregnancy

Serum T_4 and T_3 concentrations increase progressively throughout the first trimester of pregnancy to values 30–50 percent higher than those in nonpregnant women and in men, and then remain constant during the second and third trimesters (Fig. 9-21*A*).[145,146] This increase is due primarily to a 75–100 percent increase in serum TBG concentrations. Serum free T_4 and T_3 concentrations rise transiently, to near or just above the upper limit of their respective normal ranges, at 10 to 12 weeks, and then decline to the lower-normal range. The rises coincide with the period of highest serum chorionic gonadotropin concentrations and are due to its weak thyroid-stimulating activity.[146,147] Serum TSH concentrations decrease slightly, by about 30 to 40 percent, when the serum free T_4 and T_3 concentrations rise, and a few pregnant women have serum TSH values below the normal range at that time. The serum TSH concentrations then gradually increase, within the normal range, during the remainder of gestation. Serum TBG and therefore T_4 and T_3 concentrations fall to their respective normal ranges 4–6 weeks after delivery. In women with multiple gestations, peak serum chorionic gonadotropin concentrations are higher and they remain higher for longer than in women with single gestations, and therefore thyroid secretion tends to be higher and remain high longer.[148]

Pregnancy increases the need for iodine, because maternal thyroid hormone synthesis and renal iodide clearance are increased and some iodide is lost to the fetus. Thyroid size changes little in pregnant women whose iodine intake is adequate, but it increases slightly (and serum T_4 concentrations rise less) in those whose iodine intake is low; the changes are prevented by iodine supplementation.[149,150] Given the need for more iodine during pregnancy, and the declining intake of iodine in the United States[8] and the lower intake elsewhere, all pregnant women should receive supplemental iodine.

Fetal Thyroid Function

Thyroid tissue is identifiable anatomically at 7 to 8 weeks of gestation, and can be detected by ultrasonography at 20 weeks. The volume increases progressively from 0.1 ml at that time to 0.6 to 0.8 ml at term.[151] Thyroid function begins at about 10 weeks, and T_4 secretion begins soon afterward.[152,153] Fetal serum T_4 concentrations, initially very low, rise progressively so that at term the concentrations are similar to those in maternal serum (Fig. 9-21B). The pattern of increase in serum free T_4 concentrations is similar, but the increment is somewhat greater because serum TBG concentrations increase less than does T_4 secretion. Therefore, serum free T_4 concentrations in term infants are slightly higher than are those in maternal serum, whereas serum TBG concentrations are lower (although higher than in normal subjects). In keeping with this pattern of maturation, premature infants have lower serum total and free T_4 concentrations than do term infants.[154]

The progressive rise in serum free T_4 concentrations is due to a progressive rise in TSH secretion and to maturation of the fetal thyroid. TSH can be detected in serum by 12 weeks, and its serum concentration rises progressively to between 5 and 12 mU/liter at term.[152,153] This increase, in the face of increasing serum free T_4

FIGURE 9-21. Schematic diagrams of the changes in thyroid function in pregnant women and fetuses. (*A*) Serum T_4, free T_4, TSH, and chorionic gonadotropin (CG) concentrations during pregnancy. At about 10 weeks, coincident with the maximal serum CG concentrations, serum free T_4 concentrations transiently increase to near the upper limit of the normal range or slightly above it, and serum TSH concentrations decrease to near the lower limit of its normal range or just below it. These changes occur against a background of gradually rising serum T_4 concentrations, which are the result of gradually rising serum thyroxine-binding globulin (TBG) concentrations; the line for serum TBG concentrations closely parallels that for serum T_4 concentrations. (*B*) Serum T_4, free T_4, T_3, and TSH concentrations in fetuses during pregnancy and the first weeks after delivery. There is a progressive but not synchronous increase in the fetal values during gestation, and transient abrupt increase in the values in the first day after birth.

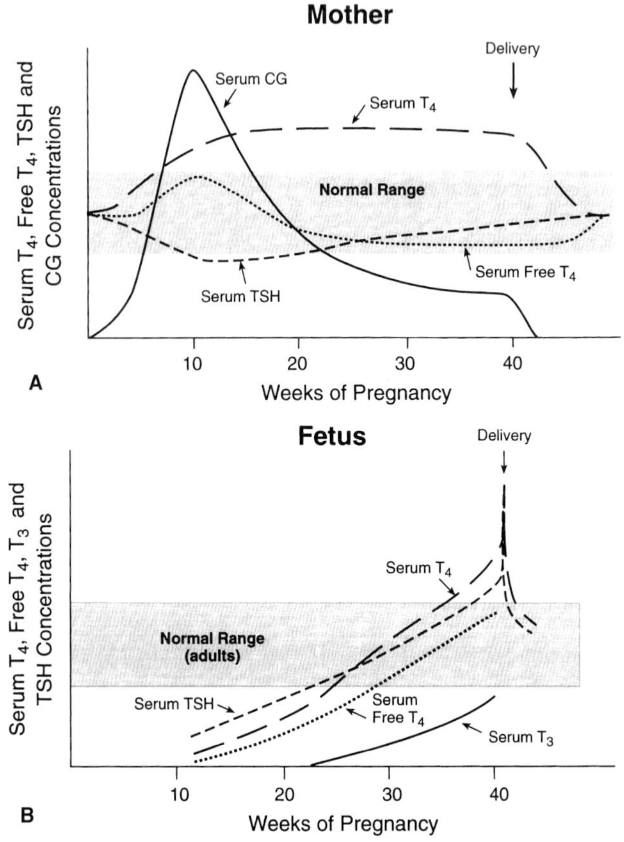

concentrations, indicates pituitary insensitivity to inhibition by T_4 during fetal life. TRH is detectable in the hypothalamus in the first trimester, but its role in fetal pituitary-thyroid function is limited. The pituitary in the fetus responds in a qualitatively normal way to hypothyroidism and thyrotoxicosis with increases and decreases, respectively, in TSH secretion.

In contrast to serum T_4, fetal serum T_3 concentrations are low because fetal tissues have little type 1 deiodinase activity and placental tissue is rich in type 3 deiodinase activity.[19,25] Therefore, little T_3 is produced, and what is produced is rapidly deiodinated. The high placental type 3 deiodinase activity also results in rapid conversion of maternal and fetal T_4 to rT_3, so that fetal serum rT_3 concentrations are high.

Iodide crosses the placenta freely. Some maternal T_4 also crosses the placenta; infants who cannot synthesize any T_4 have serum T_4 concentrations at birth that are about 25 to 40 percent of those of normal infants.[155] This is enough T_4 to allow some T_3 production in fetal tissues, particularly the central nervous system, via type 2 deiodinase activity (which increases during hypothyroidism), and therefore to provide some protection against hypothyroidism.[156] Maternal T_3 does not reach the fetus in appreciable amounts, presumably because of the high placental type 3 deiodinase activity. Similarly, little maternal TSH or TRH reaches the fetus, although maternal administration of large doses of TRH does raise fetal serum TSH concentrations transiently.[153]

Amniotic fluid contains small amounts of T_4, T_3, and TSH and large amounts of rT_3. The concentrations vary widely, and amniotic fluid measurements have not proved useful for the diagnosis of fetal thyroid disease.[157]

Infants and Children

Serum TSH concentrations increase abruptly soon after birth, reaching 40–70 mU/liter 30–60 min after delivery, and then decline to near adult values by the third or fourth day of life (Fig. 9-21B).[153] Thereafter, they decline very gradually, reaching adult values by mid-childhood or later.[158,159] The neonatal surge in TSH secretion results in an increase in T_4 secretion, so that serum total and free T_4 concentrations increase 1.5- to 2.5-fold during the first day of life. Serum T_3 concentrations increase even more at the same time because of increases in both thyroid secretion and extrathyroidal T_3 production. Both serum T_4 and T_3 concentrations then fall gradually, reaching adult values at the end of puberty.[160,161] The fall throughout childhood is a result of falling serum TBG concentrations; serum free T_4 and T_3 concentrations are similar to those of adults after the neonatal period. Serum rT_3 concentrations decline rapidly after birth, presumably as a result of rapid maturation of 5′-deiodinating pathways.

The clearance of T_4 and T_3 is more rapid in children than in adults and slows progressively throughout childhood. Thus, the production rates of T_4 and T_3 per kilogram of body weight are higher in children, and adequate treatment of hypothyroidism requires relatively larger doses of T_4 in children as compared with adults.

Sex

There are no differences in pituitary-thyroid function between women and men with regard to thyroid secretion, extrathyroidal thyroid hormone metabolism, or serum thyroid hormone-binding proteins. Thus, their serum T_4, T_3, and TSH concentrations are similar. Although serum TBG concentrations are increased by excess estrogen and decreased by excess androgen (see section on Alterations in Thyroid Hormone Binding), serum TBG concentrations are similar in normal men and premenopausal and postmenopausal women despite the disparities in gonadal steroid hormone production among them.

Aging

Thyroid gland volume increases slightly with age.[2] Serum total and free T_4 concentrations are similar in young and elderly adults, including among the latter subjects over 100 years old.[162–164] Serum total and free T_3 concentrations may decline very slightly with age; any change is more likely caused by poor nutrition or subtle nonthyroidal illness than by an age-related decrease in extrathyroidal T_4 conversion to T_3 or thyroidal secretion of T_3. There is no overall age-related change in serum binding of T_4 and T_3, although serum TBG concentrations gradually increase and those of TTR gradually decrease (mean decrease and increase, respectively, of about 20 percent from the fourth to seventh decade),[165] or in tissue sensitivity to T_4 or T_3. Daytime serum TSH concentrations also are similar in young and elderly subjects, but the amplitude of the nocturnal pulses of TSH secretion is less in the latter, and therefore their 24-h mean serum TSH concentrations are lower.[143] The clearance and production rates of T_4 and T_3 decrease with age, but in parallel, explaining why serum T_4 concentrations do not change even though TSH secretion decreases.[164]

The range of serum TSH concentrations in apparently healthy subjects widens with age. Reports from the United States and the United Kingdom that describe somewhat higher serum TSH concentrations in the elderly, especially elderly women, probably reflect the inclusion of subjects with mild autoimmune thyroiditis.[120,139] The subjects with high serum TSH concentrations often have high serum antithyroid peroxidase antibody concentrations and histologic evidence of thyroiditis. The frequency of low serum TSH concentrations also seems to be higher in elderly subjects[163,166]; such low values may reflect some thyroid autonomy, a lower set point for TSH secretion, or the need for less thyroid secretion because of the decrease in T_4 clearance.

Smoking

Cigarette smoking may have small effects on the thyroid in normal subjects, in addition to being a risk factor for Graves' thyrotoxicosis and especially ophthalmopathy (see section on Graves' Disease). They include mild thyroid enlargement, small increases in serum T_3 and thyroglobulin concentrations, and small decreases in serum TSH concentrations.[167]

Environmental Factors

Serum T_4, T_3, and TSH concentrations vary little when measured at regular intervals for several months. Small variations in serum T_4 and TSH concentrations do occur as a result of climatologic variation, with serum T_4 concentrations being slightly lower and serum TSH concentrations higher in the winter than in the summer in temperate regions.[168] Serum TSH concentrations increase in cold-exposed infants, and the abrupt rise in serum TSH concentrations in the first hour after birth is due to cold exposure. Cold exposure in adults has lesser effects, but can raise serum TSH and T_4 concentrations slightly, for example among subjects who swim in cold water (20°C) or work in cold-storage plants.[169,170] Physical stresses such as acute or chronic physical exertion are not accompanied by changes in pituitary-thyroid function.[171]

Alterations in Serum Thyroid Hormone Binding

Changes in serum thyroid hormone-binding proteins are important causes of both hyperthyroxinemia and hypothyroxinemia (Table 9-9), but they do not result in abnormal serum free T_4 (or T_3) concentrations or free T_4 index values. The most important alterations in binding are those due to changes in serum TBG concentrations, because so much of the T_4 and T_3 in serum is bound to it.

If TBG or another binding protein is added to serum in vitro, the physicochemical equilibrium between free and bound T_4 is altered so that more of the T_4 is bound. The serum free T_4 concentration therefore falls, but the serum total T_4 concentration does not change. In vivo, however, the fall in serum free T_4 concentration that follows an increase in serum TBG concentration results in a transient increase in pituitary-thyroid function and a transient decrease in T_4 clearance, so that the serum free T_4 concentration returns to normal. Once a new steady state is reached, the serum total T_4 concentration is increased, but the serum free T_4 concentration is normal. Total daily production and clearance of T_4 are normal, but the fractional daily clearance of T_4 is decreased.

The opposite changes occur when the serum TBG concentration decreases. Initially, the serum free T_4 concentration increases. Then, TSH secretion falls and T_4 clearance transiently increases, so that the serum free T_4 concentration returns to normal. Once a new steady state is reached, the serum total T_4 concentration is low, but the serum free T_4 concentration is normal. Total daily clearance and production of T_4 are normal, but the fractional daily clearance of T_4 is increased.

Increased Serum Binding

Increased serum binding of thyroid hormone may occur as a result of increased production of thyroid hormone-binding protein, production of binding protein that has increased affinity for T_4 or is slowly cleared from the circulation, or production of antibodies that bind T_4 (Table 9-9).

The most common cause of increased serum TBG concentrations is estrogen excess, whether due to pregnancy, the administration of estrogen alone or in combination with a progestin, or estrogen-secreting tumors. The increase is due to production of TBG that is more heavily glycosylated and therefore is cleared from the circulation more slowly than is the TBG produced by normal subjects, and also to an overall increase in TBG production.[172] The increase in serum TBG in response to exogenous estrogen begins within days and reaches a steady state in four to six weeks and is dose-dependent. For conjugated estrogens, the maximal dose is 1.25 mg daily; it results on average in a 50 percent increase in serum TBG concentration and a 30 percent increase in serum T_4 concentration.[173] With ethinyl estradiol, 20-μg doses have comparable effects; 50-μg doses raise serum TBG concentrations nearly 100 percent and serum T_4 concentrations 60 percent.[174] Serum TBG concentrations return to normal in about four weeks after the termination of estrogen therapy. Women taking oral contraceptives, which contain 20–35 μg ethinyl estradiol or its equivalent plus a progestin, have the expected increases in serum T_4 concentrations, but they are blunted if the progestin has some androgenic activity (e.g., norethisterone, as compared with levonorgestrel). In contrast, vaginal and transdermal estrogen preparations have little effect on serum TBG concentrations, nor do pure progestins. Like estrogens, the partial estrogen antagonists tamoxifen and raloxifene raise serum TBG concentrations.[175] Other drugs that raise serum TBG concentrations are methadone, mitotane, clofibrate, and 5-fluorouracil.[85,176,177]

Patients with several liver diseases have increases in serum TBG concentrations. The frequency and magnitude of the increases are greatest in patients with acute hepatitis, but increases also occur in patients with chronic hepatitis, biliary cirrhosis, and hepatoma. Human immunodeficiency virus infection is another cause of high serum TBG concentrations (see section on Effects of Specific Disorders on Thyroid Function). Small increases in serum TBG concentrations also occur in patients with acute intermittent porphyria and hypothyroidism.

Increased TBG production occurs as an X-linked inherited disorder.[178] Hemizygous affected males (about 1 in 30,000 newborn boys, based on the results of neonatal screening programs) have a two- to fourfold increase in serum TBG concentrations and therefore high serum T_4 concentrations; heterozygous affected females have a 1.5- to 2-fold increase in serum TBG concentrations and lesser increases in serum T_4 concentrations. The basic abnormality is increased production of TBG that is structurally normal, due at least in some families to gene duplication.[179] The production of other transport proteins such as cortisol- and sex hormone–binding globulin is not increased in these subjects.

Increased serum T_4 concentrations also occur as a result of increased production of other binding proteins. One such syndrome is familial dysalbuminemic hyperthyroxinemia.[180,181] It is the most common inherited cause of increased T_4 binding (1 in 10,000). The

TABLE 9-9. Causes of Hyperthyroxinemia and Hypothyroxinemia

- **Hyperthyroxinemia**
  - Thyrotoxicosis
  - Increased T_4 binding in serum
    - Increased thyroxine-binding globulin (TBG) binding
      - Pregnancy
      - Endogenous and exogenous estrogen excess
      - Tamoxifen and raloxifene
      - Drugs: methadone, mitotane, clofibrate, 5-fluorouracil
      - Acute and chronic hepatitis, hepatoma
      - Human immunodeficiency virus infection
      - Inherited TBG excess
    - Increased albumin binding
      - Familial dysalbuminemic hyperthyroxinemia
    - Increased transthyretin binding
      - Familial increase in transthyretin binding
      - Islet-cell carcinoma
    - Antibodies binding T_4
  - Nonthyroidal illness
    - Psychiatric illness
    - Medical illness
  - Drug-induced hyperthyroxinemia
    - Drugs slowing T_4 clearance
      - Amiodarone
      - Oral cholecystographic agents
      - Propranolol
  - Generalized thyroid hormone resistance
- **Hypothyroxinemia**
  - Hypothyroidism
  - Decreased T_4 binding in serum
    - Decreased thyroxine-binding globulin (TBG) binding
      - Inherited TBG deficiency
      - Exogenous androgen and anabolic steroid hormone excess
      - Glucocorticoid excess
      - Drugs: asparaginase, nicotinic acid
      - Nonthyroidal illness
    - Decreased transthyretin binding
      - Nonthyroidal illness
      - Familial amyloidotic polyneuropathy
    - Decreased albumin binding
      - Nonthyroidal illness
    - Drug-related inhibition of binding
      - Salicylates
      - Furosemide

affected subjects, who are euthyroid and have normal serum TSH concentrations, have albumin gene mutations that result in production of albumin molecules with increased affinity for T_4 and to a much lesser extent T_3.[182,183] As a result, their serum T_4 concentrations are high, whereas their serum T_3 concentrations are normal or only slightly high. Serum free T_4 (and T_3) concentrations are normal, but serum free T_4 index values are high. (The serum free T_4 index is high because the serum T_4 concentration is high, but the THBR is normal. The THBR is normal because the labeled T_3 used in the test binds poorly to the abnormal albumin, so that the increased number of unoccupied binding sites is not detected.) This disorder is inherited as an autosomal dominant trait.

Increases in TTR binding of T_4 are rare. They occur on a familial basis (autosomal dominant inheritance) and in some patients with islet-cell carcinoma of the pancreas.[184,185] The biochemical findings are similar to those in patients with familial dysalbuminemic hyperthyroxinemia; they include normal serum T_3 concentrations and normal THBR test values because of the limited binding of T_3 to TTR. The familial cases are due to TTR mutations that result in production of TTR molecules with increased affinity for T_4.[184,186] The islet-cell carcinoma patients, by contrast, had high serum TTR concentrations. The diagnosis of familial dysalbuminemic hyperthyroxinemia and of disorders of TTR transport can be confirmed by the use of labeled T_4 instead of labeled T_3 in a resin-uptake test; in these patients, the resin uptake of labeled T_4 is low because of the increased albumin or TTR binding of labeled T_4.[187]

Hyperthyroxinemia is occasionally due to serum autoantibodies that bind T_4, T_3, or both.[188,189] These antibodies raise serum total T_4 or T_3 concentrations (as measured in most assays) and slow the clearance of the hormones; they serve in effect as a binding protein. They are polyclonal antithyroglobulin antibodies for which the immunogenic thyroglobulin epitopes include T_4, T_3, or both, and are found most often in patients with autoimmune thyroid disease. Most of the patients are euthyroid, but they may be hypothyroid or thyrotoxic.

Decreased Serum Binding

Decreased serum binding of thyroid hormones may occur as a result of decreased production of binding protein, production of binding protein with decreased affinity for T_4, or competitive interactions of drugs with T_4 binding to TBG or the other proteins (Table 9-9).

The lowest serum TBG concentrations occur in subjects with inherited complete TBG deficiency (X-linked).[178,190] Hemizygous affected males have no detectable serum TBG (<0.05 percent of normal), whereas heterozygous affected females have serum TBG concentrations that are 50 percent of normal (unless there is selective inactivation of the normal X-chromosome allele).[191] The disorder occurs in about 1 in 10,000 newborn boys; the cause is usually a mutation in the TBG gene that leads to production of truncated TBG molecules that do not bind T_4 or cannot be secreted.[192–194] Other, more common heritable forms of TBG deficiency result in varying reductions in serum TBG and therefore T_4 concentrations, due either to decreased rates of TBG synthesis or to the production of TBG that has decreased affinity for T_4 or is cleared from the circulation more rapidly than is normal TBG.[178,190] Most are the result of single amino acid substitutions or deletions.

Serum TBG concentrations fall by about 50 percent (and serum T_4 concentrations fall by about 35 percent) in four to eight weeks in women given large doses of androgen,[195] and about as much in androgen-treated men. Serum TBG concentrations are slightly low in patients with acromegaly, Cushing's syndrome, and thyrotoxicosis. They are also low in patients receiving anabolic steroids, chronic high-dose glucocorticoid therapy, nicotinic acid, and L-asparaginase.[85,196–198]

Variant forms of TTR are found in patients with familial amyloidotic polyneuropathy, in whom the TTR is an important component of the amyloid fibrils.[85] Some of these forms of TTR have a reduced affinity for T_4, and so affected subjects may have slightly low serum T_4 concentrations.

Patients with many acute and chronic nonthyroidal illnesses have low serum T_4 and T_3 concentrations (see section on Nonthyroidal Illness). Among the causes of these changes are decreased serum TBG, TTR, and albumin concentrations.[199] Serum TTR concentrations decrease transiently in patients with most acute illnesses and are low in many chronically ill patients, although the effect on serum T_4 concentrations is small because of the relatively small contribution of TTR to overall T_4 binding in serum. The reduction in serum TBG concentrations that occurs in nonthyroidal illnesses also is usually small. Some of the TBG in these patients may be poorly sialylated, which reduces its affinity for T_4, and therefore the serum T_4 concentration is disproportionately lower than the serum TBG concentration.[200] Patients with nonthyroidal illness also often have hypoalbuminemia, which may contribute slightly to the decrease in serum T_4 concentrations. Several drugs inhibit T_4 binding to TBG or other serum proteins (as noted later), raising the possibility of endogenous inhibitors of T_4 binding in patients with nonthyroidal illness. Whatever the specific causes or the degree of deficiency of the various thyroid hormone–binding proteins, there is little doubt that many patients with severe acute or chronic nonthyroidal illness have overall decreases in serum thyroid hormone binding and therefore high THBR values. In these patients, the dialyzable fraction of T_4 is often relatively increased, so that their serum free T_4 concentrations are usually normal even if their serum free T_4 index values are low.[132,134,201,202] The same considerations apply to T_3, and its binding to TBG may be affected more by these inhibitors because its affinity for TBG is lower than that of T_4.[134]

If substances that compete with T_4 for binding to TBG or other binding proteins are present in sufficient concentration, they alter the equilibrium between free T_4 and bound T_4. The result is an initial increase in serum free T_4 concentrations, which then return toward normal as a result of transient decreases in thyroid secretion, increases in T_4 clearance, or both. Thus, the patients have low serum T_4 concentrations and high THBR values, like those with low serum TBG concentrations. Drugs that competitively inhibit T_4 binding to TBG or TTR include salicylates, salasalate (partly converted to salicylate), fenclofenac, and furosemide.[187,203–206] Phenytoin and phenylbutazone also inhibit T_4 binding, but not at the concentrations achieved when they are used therapeutically. Other substances that inhibit T_4 binding to TBG or albumin in vitro include high concentrations of free fatty acids and heparin.[203,207,208] Few if any patients have serum free fatty acid concentrations high enough to decrease T_4 binding. The effect of heparin is largely due to its ability to raise serum free fatty acid concentrations by activating lipoprotein lipase, and it is mostly an in vitro effect because it can be blocked by the in vitro addition of protamine, a heparin inhibitor.[208–210]

Nonthyroidal Illness

A wide variety of reversible abnormalities of pituitary-thyroid function, serum thyroid hormone binding, and extrathyroidal thyroid hormone metabolism occur in patients with nonthyroidal illness. These abnormalities result in decreases in serum T_3 concentrations, less often in decreases in serum T_4 concentrations, and occasionally in decreases in serum free T_4 concentrations. In general, the degree and extent of the abnormalities correlate with the severity of the nonthyroidal illness, and the nature of the illness is of secondary importance. The changes in serum hormone concentrations are accompanied by changes in T_4 metabolism, in particular by changes in extrathyroidal T_4 conversion to T_3, and less often by changes in TSH and thyroid secretion. In addition, illness-related decreases in T_3 nuclear receptors and postreceptor actions of T_3 have been identified in animals.

The two most common abnormalities in patients with nonthyroidal illness are decreased serum T_3 concentrations and decreased serum T_3 and T_4 concentrations; the latter abnormalities thus mimic those of hypothyroidism. These abnormalities are frequently referred to as the euthyroid sick syndrome, a term that is inappropriate for several reasons. First, the spectrum of the abnormalities is broad, and no single set of abnormalities can be designated the euthyroid sick syndrome. Second, although the patients have no overt clinical manifestations of hypothyroidism, the actions of thyroid hormone in some tissues may be diminished. It is more likely that these changes represent adaptive forms of hypothyroidism, serving to reduce the availability and action of thyroid hormones and lessen the physiologic impact of the nonthyroidal illness. The changes therefore are probably beneficial adaptations to illness. The fact that no overt manifestations of thyroid deficiency occur may be due to the transient nature of the abnormalities, their lack of equal impact in all tissues because of variations in local T_3 production and action, and the modifying effects of the nonthyroidal illness on the responsiveness of different tissues to thyroid deficiency. To confuse matters further, some patients with nonthyroidal illnesses have high serum T_4 concentrations. Many of these changes have been attributed to the production of cytokines, and some experimental and correlational data support this possibility, as will be noted later.

These abnormalities are shown schematically in Fig. 9-22, and the derangements that contribute to them are listed in Table 9-10. Each will be discussed in more detail below. Among outpatients with nonthyroidal illness, a substantial fraction have low serum T_3 concentrations but the results of other tests are usually normal, although abnormalities may be found in patients with some particular disorders or those taking certain drugs (see section on Effects of Specific Disorders on Thyroid Function and Effects of Drugs on Thyroid Function).

The frequency of abnormalities of thyroid function in hospitalized patients is high. In one study of 264 patients admitted to a medical service, 19 percent had low serum T_3 concentrations, 8 percent had low serum T_4 concentrations, and 1 percent had low serum TSH concentrations (about 1 percent had high serum T_4 concentrations).[211] In another study of 270 patients, 34 percent had low serum T_3 concentrations and 33 percent had low serum T_4 concentrations.[212] In a study of 1,580 patients, 17 percent had abnormal serum TSH concentrations (12 percent low and 6 percent high), 12 percent had abnormal serum T_4 concentrations and 8 percent had abnormal serum free T_4 index values (89 per-

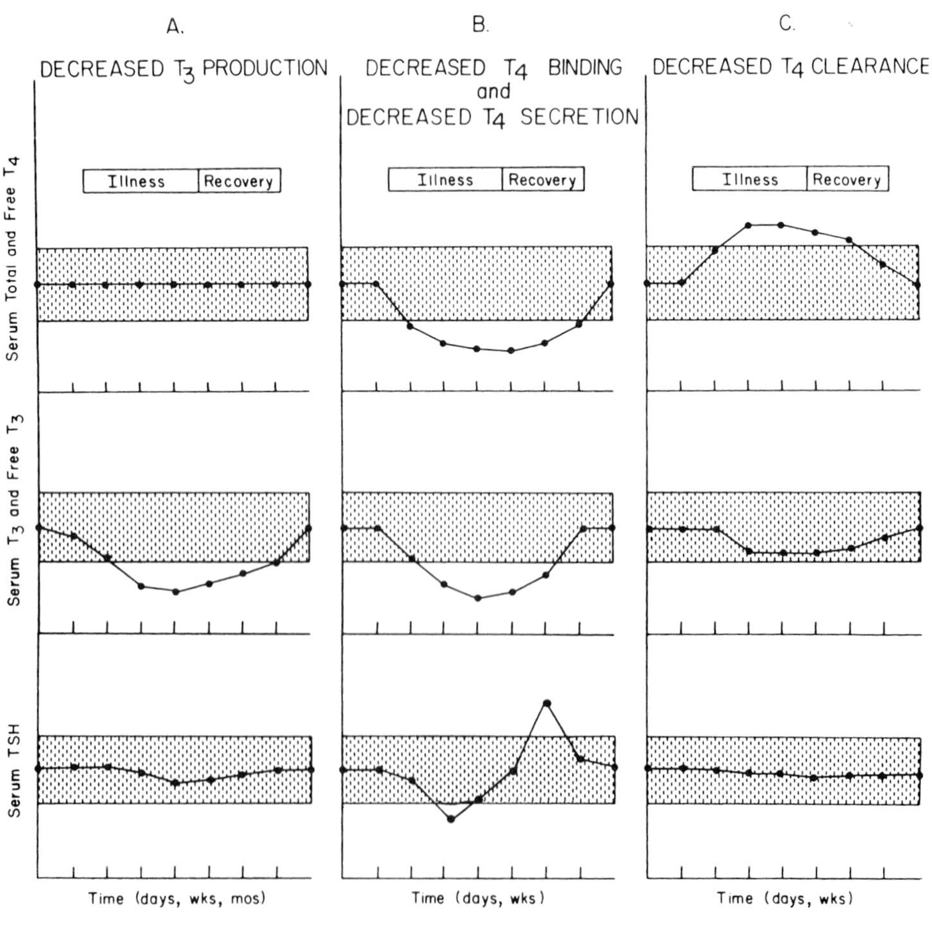

FIGURE 9-22. Patterns of the three major types of abnormalities of pituitary-thyroid function that occur in patients with nonthyroidal illness. (*A*) Decreased extrathyroidal T_3 production. (*B*) Decreased T_4 binding and decreased TSH secretion. (*C*) Decreased T_4 clearance. The shaded areas indicate the normal ranges.

TABLE 9-10. Alterations in Hypothalamic-Pituitary-Thyroid Function in Nonthyroidal Illness

Alteration	Site	Cause
Decreased serum T_3 concentrations	Extrathyroidal tissue	Decreased iodothyronine deiodinase activity
Decreased serum total T_4 concentrations	Extrathyroidal tissue	Decreased serum binding of T_4
Decreased serum free T_4 concentrations	Thyroid	Decreased TSH secretion
Decreased serum TSH concentrations	Pituitary	Decreased TRH secretion, increased dopamine, somatostatin, or cortisol secretion
Decreased T_3 action	Extrathyroidal tissue	Decreased cell uptake of T_3, decreased T_3 receptors, decreased postreceptor actions of T_3
Increased serum T_4 concentrations	Thyroid, extrathyroidal tissue	Increased TSH secretion, decreased T_4 clearance

cent of which were low).[213] The frequency of abnormal test results is even higher in patients admitted to emergency departments or intensive care units, and there is an inverse correlation between serum T_4 and T_3 concentrations and survival among patients admitted to intensive care units.[202,214] These abnormalities do not occur in isolated forms, and their extent varies widely in individual patients. Their occurrence also means that it can be difficult to identify thyrotoxicosis or hypothyroidism in patients who have nonthyroidal illness.

Low Serum Triiodothyronine Concentrations

Low serum T_3 concentrations occur in patients with virtually all acute and chronic illnesses (Fig. 9-22A). The illnesses include acute infections, which need not be severe; myocardial infarction; pulmonary embolism; sudden decreases in caloric intake; and trauma, burns, and surgery. Serum T_3 concentrations also are low in patients with chronic illnesses such as poorly controlled diabetes mellitus; chronic liver, renal, cardiac, pulmonary, and rheumatologic diseases; cancer; and chronic malnutrition. Caloric deficiency undoubtedly contributes to the decline in serum T_3 concentrations that occurs in many of these illnesses, but is not the sole explanation. Drugs such as glucocorticoids and propranolol may also cause decreases in serum T_3 concentrations (see section on Effects of Drugs on Thyroid Function).

The decrease in serum T_3 concentrations in these situations is caused by decreased extrathyroidal conversion of T_4 to T_3 and decreased serum protein binding of T_3. Extrathyroidal T_3 production may decrease by up to 50 percent, and serum T_3 concentrations may decrease more, but serum free T_3 concentrations are more normal because of decreased serum protein binding of T_3.[134,202] Serum T_3 concentrations can fall within a day after the onset of an acute illness, but usually the fall is more gradual. Recovery can occur within 24 to 48 h, depending on the cause of the nonthyroidal illness and the rapidity of its reversal. For example, in patients who have an acute myocardial infarction, serum T_3 concentrations fall by about 40 percent in 3 to 4 days and return to baseline in about 14 days.[215]

The particular organs in which T_3 production is impaired are not known, but they presumably include the liver and kidneys, because these organs are prominent sources of circulating T_3. Among 12 patients with fatal illnesses, the T_3 concentrations were lower in the liver, kidney, and brain, and higher in the heart and skeletal muscle, as compared with 10 patients with fatal injuries.[216] The decrease in T_3 production could result from decreases in cellular uptake of T_4, cofactor availability or enzyme production, or inhibition of enzyme activity (see section on Regulation of Extrathyroidal Triiodothyronine Production). Possible causative factors include the increases in circulating (or locally produced) cytokines that accompany many illnesses. Serum concentrations of interleukin-6 and tumor necrosis factor are inversely correlated with serum T_3 concentrations in patients with nonthyroidal illness,[212,217,218] and infusions of tumor necrosis factor and interleukin-6 lower serum T_3 concentrations slightly in normal subjects.[219–222] Serum from patients with nonthyroidal illnesses contains substances that inhibit T_4 uptake by tissues and inhibit T_4 conversion to T_3 in liver.[82,223,224]

The patients usually have normal serum total and free T_4 concentrations. Their serum rT_3 concentrations are high, as a result of decreased extrathyroidal 5′-deiodination of rT_3; rT_3 production from T_4 is not increased.[202,225] The lack of change in serum T_4 concentrations, despite the decrease in T_4 conversion to T_3 and the lack of change in T_4 conversion to rT_3, indicates that more T_4 is metabolized by conversion to tetraiodothyroactic acid or by sulfation or glucuronidation.

Serum TSH concentrations are usually within the normal range, although they may be slightly decreased, and the nocturnal surge in TSH secretion may be diminished.[226,227] The lack of increase in serum TSH in the face of decreased serum T_3 concentrations is probably due to the continuing availability of T_4 for T_3 generation in the thyrotroph cells of the pituitary; other possibilities include increased T_3 transport into the thyrotroph cells and increased thyrotroph-cell sensitivity to T_3 as a result of decreased TRH or increased somatostatin production.

The administration of exogenous T_3 during fasting in normal subjects and to patients with uremia in doses that prevent decreases in serum T_3 concentrations increased urinary nitrogen excretion in some but not all studies.[228–231] T_3 administration did not alter the serum glucose, fatty acid, or ketoacid responses to fasting, but did increase hepatic glucose output. The decrease in serum T_3 concentrations that occurs during illness or fasting may therefore reduce protein catabolism and serve to conserve nitrogen stores; it may also reduce the generation of free radicals, facilitating the repair of injured tissue. The decrease is accompanied by some tissue responses indicative of decreased T_3 action, for example, reductions in cardiac contractility and rate that are reversed by small doses of T_3. In animals, illness-related reductions in extrathyroidal T_3 production and T_3 nuclear receptor content are accompanied by decreased production of some liver enzymes and of cardiac beta-adrenergic receptors and myosin ATP isoenzymes, and administration of T_3 reverses these changes.[73,232,233] All these responses could serve to conserve substrate and maintain tissue integrity, although some could impair organ function.

Low Serum Thyroxine Concentrations

Many severely ill patients with systemic infections; cardiac, pulmonary, hepatic or renal diseases; severe burns; or extensive trauma have low serum T_4 concentrations (Fig. 9-22B). The rate at which their serum T_4 concentrations decline varies from hours to weeks, depending on the speed of onset and severity of the illness. Often, only serum total T_4 concentrations are low, and serum free T_4 concentrations are normal or even high.[134,201,202] These changes are due to decreased serum T_4 binding resulting from decreased serum concentrations of TBG, TTR, and albumin or to illness-related metabolites or drugs that inhibit T_4-binding in serum (see section on Alterations in Serum Thyroid Hormone Binding). The clearance rate of T_4 is therefore increased, and the rate of production of T_4 is normal or slightly low.[234] These patients have very low serum T_3 concentrations not only because of decreased serum binding of T_3, but also because their illness is always sufficiently severe to inhibit extrathyroidal T_4 conversion to T_3.

Some severely ill patients have low serum free T_4 index values, and a few have low serum free T_4 concentrations.[134,234,235] In these patients TSH secretion is decreased; serum TSH concentrations are low-normal or low, little TSH is secreted at night, serum TSH responses to TRH are low or absent,[212,226,236–238] and the TSH that is secreted may have decreased biological activity.[239,240] Many of the patients are receiving dopamine or glucocorticoids, both of which inhibit TSH secretion; in others TSH secretion is low as a result of pituitary dysfunction, decreased TRH secretion,[241] or increased endogenous dopamine, somatostatin, or cortisol secretion. Candidate causes include tumor necrosis factor and interleukin-1, which lower serum TSH concentrations in humans and animals and hypothalamic TRH content in animals.[219,220,222] These substances may also inhibit thyroidal responses to TSH. The prognosis in patients with severe nonthyroidal illnesses who have low serum T_4 values is poor; in one study, for example, 30 percent died.[202]

The changes in thyroid function in patients with severe nonthyroidal illness are indicative of a greater degree of thyroid deficiency than occurs in less ill patients, in whom the major change is low serum T_3 concentrations. Presumably, the greater reduction in thyroid hormone availability confers some additional benefit beyond that resulting from decreased extrathyroidal T_4 conversion to T_3.

These patients are often confused or obtunded, puffy, or hypothermic. They may have poor respiratory function, inappropriately slow pulse rates, and sluggish deep tendon reflexes. These clinical findings could be caused either by the nonthyroidal illness or by thyroid hormone deficiency; it is not usually possible to distinguish between the two at the bedside. Their biochemical findings mimic those of central hypothyroidism, with the addition of decreased serum binding of T_4 and T_3. With respect to T_3 action in other tissues, the patients have normal serum sex hormone-binding globulin and osteocalcin but low angiotensin-converting enzyme concentrations; all of these are low in hypothyroidism.[242,243]

The practical question raised by these findings in an individual patient is, Could the patient have central hypothyroidism that predated the illness and should treatment with T_4 be initiated? Nearly always the answer is no, especially in patients who are receiving dopamine or a glucocorticoid, for several reasons. First, low serum TSH and T_4 concentrations are expected in such patients, and the abnormalities disappear during recovery. Second, their serum free T_4 values, whether measured directly or indirectly, are not as low as are their serum T_4 values or are normal, whereas in patients with hypothyroidism the converse is true. Third, central hypothyroidism is rare, whereas illness-related decreases in serum TSH and T_4 concentrations are not. Even so, it is often appropriate to evaluate pituitary-adrenal function (see Chap. 11) to provide assurance that cortisol secretion is adequate and further evidence that the patient does not have hypothalamic-pituitary disease. With respect to treatment, the administration of T_4 to patients in an intensive care unit or of T_3 to patients with extensive burns who had these biochemical abnormalities did not lower mortality.[244,245]

When recovery begins, serum TSH concentrations may rise transiently above the normal range for several days (Fig. 9-22B). The peak values usually range from 5 to 20 mU/liter[235]; higher values suggest that the patient has hypothyroidism.[246] The transient increase in serum TSH concentrations indicates that the illness impaired the ability of the thyrotroph cells to respond to low serum free T_4 concentrations; with recovery that ability returns. The rise in serum TSH is followed by a rise in serum T_4 and T_3 concentrations that is due not only to the action of TSH on the thyroid gland but also to increases in serum binding proteins and in extrathyroidal T_3 production. Sometimes the first recorded serum TSH value in a seriously ill patient is high[213]; this finding may mean that recovery from the illness has already begun or that the patient has primary hypothyroidism. Reevaluation several days later should provide the information needed to distinguish between these possibilities.

High Serum Thyroxine Concentrations

A few patients with nonthyroidal illnesses have high serum T_4 and free T_4 concentrations (Fig. 9-22C). These findings have been reported most often in patients with psychiatric disorders, although their frequency in groups of such patients varies widely (see section on Effects of Specific Disorders on Thyroid Function). They also occur in patients with acute medical illnesses and in patients who have received drugs such as amiodarone, oral cholecystographic agents, and propranolol (see section on Effects of Drugs on Thyroid Function). Their serum T_3 concentrations are usually slightly low or normal, and their serum TSH concentrations are usually normal but may be high or low. These patients have few or no clinical manifestations of thyrotoxicosis, and their serum T_4 concentrations decline to normal within one or two weeks as they recover from the illness (longer in the case of amiodarone).

One cause of these elevations in serum total and free T_4 concentrations is decreased clearance of T_4,[18,79] combined with less than normal inhibition of TSH secretion. This is clearly the case when one of the drugs listed in the preceding paragraph was given. A second cause is a transient increase in TSH and therefore thyroid secretion. This mechanism may be operative in patients with psychiatric disease. A common additional abnormality is decreased extrathyroidal T_3 production.

In general, patients with high serum T_4 concentrations caused by nonthyroidal illness are not severely ill. The diversity of the illnesses and the transient nature of the abnormalities have made prospective study difficult, and the physiologic importance of the changes, if any, is not known. The practical importance, however, is clear: the diagnosis of thyrotoxicosis in patients who are ill must be based on clinical evidence and low serum TSH values, not merely on high serum T_4 and free T_4 values.

Effects of Specific Disorders on Thyroid Function

Caloric Restriction and Fasting

In normal or obese subjects who eat 600 calories or less a day serum T_3 concentrations fall by approximately 40 percent and serum rT_3 concentrations increase by 100 percent in two to four days.[247] The abnormalities persist until the subjects are fed carbohydrate or protein. Similar changes occur in patients with protein-calorie malnutrition and short bowel syndromes. The changes are due to decreases in extrathyroidal conversion of T_4 to T_3 and of rT_3 to T_2; serum T_4 concentrations do not change. Basal serum TSH concentrations and nocturnal TSH secretion decline slightly,[227] but not sufficiently to decrease T_4 production. The thyrotroph cells remain sensitive to increased amounts of T_3; maintaining normal (fed) serum T_3 concentrations during starvation by exogenous T_3 administration decreases TSH secretion.[228]

Cardiac Disease

Serum T_3 concentrations fall by 30 to 40 percent in three to five days in patients who have a myocardial infarction, as noted above, whereas their serum T_4 and TSH concentrations change little.[215] Similarly, many patients with congestive heart failure have low serum T_3 and normal serum T_4 and TSH concentrations; in them low serum T_3 concentrations are associated with poorer cardiac function and increased mortality.[248] Both serum T_3 and T_4 concentrations may be low in cardiac-arrest patients immediately after resuscitation,[249] and they decline within hours after coronary bypass operations in patients with coronary artery disease[250]; these changes are probably due more to dilutional effects than altered thyroid hormone metabolism. Administration of supraphysiological doses of T_3 to patients with coronary artery disease immediately after bypass surgery or patients with advanced congestive heart failure results in prompt increases in cardiac output and decreases in peripheral resistance, as compared with placebo; these changes support the idea that T_3 has nongenomic actions on vascular tissue.[251–253]

Renal Disease

Patients with stable chronic renal insufficiency and those treated with hemodialysis or peritoneal dialysis usually have normal or low serum T_4, normal free T_4, low T_3, and normal TSH concentrations.[254,255] The serum T_4 values are lower than those in normal subjects because serum T_4 binding is decreased by the presence of inhibitors of binding or abnormal forms of TBG; serum TBG concentrations are normal. Extrathyroidal production of T_3 from T_4 is decreased. Serum rT_3 concentrations are normal rather than high as in most patients with nonthyroidal illness because extravascular binding of rT_3 is increased, a phenomenon apparently unique to renal disease.[256] Patients with acute renal failure have similar abnormalities, but of greater magnitude. Serum T_4 and especially T_3 concentrations are more normal after transplantation; any persisting abnormalities are likely to be due to the glucocorticoid these patients receive for immunosuppression.

Patients with the nephrotic syndrome may excrete substantial amounts of T_4 and TBG as well as albumin in their urine.[257] Their serum TBG has a decreased affinity for T_4, and when proteinuria is massive, serum TBG concentrations may be low. Serum T_4 concentrations are often low, whereas serum free T_4 values are normal, indicating decreased T_4 binding. Serum T_3 concentrations are low because of decreases in both T_3 binding and extrathyroidal T_3 production. The loss of T_4 in the urine may be large enough to result in increased TSH secretion.[258]

Liver Disease

Patients with acute hepatitis have high serum TBG and therefore high T_4 concentrations.[259] Their serum T_3 concentrations are often normal, reflecting the counterbalancing effects of decreased extrathyroidal T_3 production and high serum TBG concentrations. These changes disappear with recovery. The increase in serum TBG concentrations may be due to the release of preformed TBG, slowed clearance of TBG, or increased hepatic synthetic function.

Serum TBG concentrations are high in some patients with chronic active hepatitis, primary biliary cirrhosis, and hepatoma. In patients with portal cirrhosis, serum T_4 binding is variably decreased, so that serum T_4 concentrations tend to be low, T_3 concentrations are low, and rT_3 concentrations are high.[260] Patients with hepatic coma have the usual findings of severe nonthyroidal illness: low serum T_4 and T_3 concentrations and free T_4 index values and normal or low serum TSH concentrations.

Human Immunodeficiency Virus Infection

Some patients with human immunodeficiency virus (HIV) infection have moderate increases in serum TBG concentrations. The concentrations may be increased not only in patients who are HIV-seropositive but otherwise healthy, but also in those with the acquired immune deficiency syndrome.[261,262] Possible explanations for the increase include coincident illness, for example subclinical liver disease, and an increase in glycosylation of TBG, leading to an increase in its affinity for T_4, slowing of TBG clearance, or both. In general, the patients' serum free T_4 concentrations are less elevated than are those of T_4, and some have slightly high serum TSH concentrations.[263]

As their illness progresses and opportunistic infections develop, these patients have the abnormalities of thyroid function characteristic of nonthyroidal illness described previously. *Pneumocystis carinii* infections are common in these patients, and this organism can cause local or generalized thyroid infection and hypothyroidism.[264]

Psychiatric Disease

Surveys of patients who are hospitalized for the treatment of acute psychiatric illness have often revealed abnormalities of thyroid function. The most common abnormality is a high serum T_4 concentration, but the frequency varies widely. In several large series of such patients, 0–33 percent had high serum T_4 concentrations and 0–18 percent had high serum free T_4 values.[265–269] Serum T_3 concentrations were high less often, and serum TSH concentrations were usually normal, but sometimes slightly high or slightly low. Hyperthyroxinemia, when present, usually subsides in a week or so.

The simplest explanation for these findings is that acute psychiatric illness results in a transient increase in TSH and therefore thyroid secretion. The greater frequency of high serum T_4 as compared with high free T_4 or T_3 values argues for the presence of some slowing of T_4 clearance or the mobilization of T_4 from extrathyroidal stores. The abnormalities are not diagnosis-specific, because they occur in patients with all forms of acute psychosis, nor can they be related to therapy with psychotropic drugs.

Abnormalities of TSH secretion are found in 20 to 30 percent of patients with depression.[270,271] The most common abnormalities are small decreases in daytime and in the nocturnal increase in serum TSH concentrations and decreases in serum TSH responses to TRH.[272,273] Serum T_4 and T_3 concentrations are normal or high-normal. The impaired TSH secretion may be due to increased corticotropin (ACTH) and cortisol secretion, although the correlation between decreased serum TSH responses to TRH and abnormal pituitary-adrenal responses to dexamethasone in depressed patients is poor. Patients with alcoholism, anorexia nervosa, and bulemia may have low serum T_3 concentrations, presumably due to nutritional deficiency.

Effects of Drugs on Thyroid Function

Dopamine

Infusions of dopamine in doses of 5 to 7.5 μg/min result in a prompt reduction of TSH secretion, which persists as long as the infusion is continued.[234,274] Dopamine reduces the amplitude of pulsatile TSH secretion, so that nocturnal TSH secretion decreases more than daytime TSH secretion.[62] Daytime serum TSH concentrations decrease by 50 percent or more, sufficient to decrease thyroid secretion and serum T_4 and T_3 concentrations in 48 to 72 hours in normal subjects and patients with nonthyroidal illness; prolonged infusions would be expected to result in overt central hypothyroidism. Dopamine is widely used in very sick patients in intensive care units, and its use contributes substantially to the abnormalities in thyroid function that are found in these patients.[275] Short-term infusions of dobutamine in doses of 20 to 50 μg/kg/m also decrease serum TSH concentrations, but not to below the normal range.[275a] None of the other drugs given to increase blood pressure or cardiac output in critically ill patients are known to alter TSH or thyroid secretion.

Glucocorticoids

Endogenous or exogenous glucocorticoids have multiple effects on pituitary-thyroid function, and increased endogenous cortisol production may account for some of the changes that occur in patients with nonthyroidal illness. Small or moderate doses of glucocorticoid inhibit pulsatile TSH secretion, the nocturnal surge in serum TSH concentrations, and serum TSH responses to exogenous TRH, indicating inhibition of both TSH and TRH secretion.[276–279] High doses inhibit extrathyroidal T_3 production and increase extrathyroidal rT_3 production and therefore decrease serum T_3 concentrations and increase rT_3 concentrations, respectively, within several days.[280] Finally, chronic glucocorticoid excess decreases serum TBG and increases serum TTR concentrations. The net result of these actions of glucocorticoids in patients with spontaneous or iatrogenic Cushing's syndrome is low-normal serum T_4, normal free T_4, low T_3, high rT_3, and low-normal TSH concentrations. (Glucocorticoids also directly inhibit thyroid radioiodine uptake and thyroidal T_4, T_3, and thyroglobulin release in patients with hyperthyroidism caused by Graves' disease.[281])

Some patients with adrenal insufficiency have overt or subclinical hypothyroidism that resolves when they are treated with replacement doses of cortisol.[282,283] The improvement suggests that cortisol may be a physiological regulator of TSH secretion or that the patients have mild chronic autoimmune thyroiditis that is ameliorated by cortisol.

Adrenergic Antagonist Drugs

When given in doses of 80 mg/day or more, propranolol causes a 20–30 percent fall in serum T_3 concentrations in seven to ten days in both normal subjects and patients with thyrotoxicosis. The fall is due to inhibition of extrathyroidal conversion of T_4 to T_3.[284] Serum T_4 concentrations increase slightly in an occasional patient given very high doses. Other beta-adrenergic antagonist drugs reduce serum T_3 concentrations to a lesser extent or not at all. All these drugs inhibit T_3 production from T_4 in rat liver homogenates, but propranolol is the most potent.[80] Their ability to inhibit T_3 production is not related to their adrenergic antagonist properties, because D-propranolol, which is not an adrenergic antagonist, is equally active as an inhibitor of 5′-deiodination of T_4.[284]

Methimazole and Propylthiouracil

Methimazole and propylthiouracil (PTU) are commonly used antithyroid drugs. Both inhibit thyroid hormone biosynthesis (see section on Treatment of Thyrotoxicosis). In addition, PTU inhibits type 1 deiodinase activity.[19,79] It therefore inhibits the extrathyroidal conversion of T_4 to T_3 and slows the clearance of T_4. When large doses of PTU are given to T_4-treated hypothyroid patients, serum T_3 concentrations fall by about 30 percent in 24 h and stay at that level until the drug is discontinued.[285] Serum TSH concentrations increase slightly, providing evidence that PTU has little effect on T_4 deiodination in the thyrotroph cells.

Iodine Excess

The administration of iodine or iodide formed in vivo by the deiodination of iodine-containing drugs, antiseptic agents, and radiographic contrast agents alters thyroid hormone production in several ways (see section on Regulation of Thyroid Secretion by Iodide). Inorganic iodine in doses of 0.5 mg daily or more, in addition to usual dietary iodine intake, has a weak, transient antithyroid action in normal subjects.[286–288] Their serum T_4 concentrations fall by 10 to 15 percent and their serum TSH concentrations rise by about 50 percent in two weeks, after which the values return toward normal. The administration of similar or larger doses of iodine can induce overt hypothyroidism in patients who have damaged thyroid glands, for example patients who were previously treated with ^{131}I or surgery for hyperthyroidism or who have chronic autoimmune thyroiditis.[287] Conversely, exogenous iodine may cause thyrotoxicosis in patients with iodine deficiency or those with autonomously functioning thyroid tissue that concentrates iodine poorly (see section on Iodine-Induced Thyrotoxicosis).

Amiodarone

The antiarrhythmic drug amiodarone is an iodine-containing drug that has many effects on pituitary-thyroid function.[289–291] It is an inhibitor of both type 1 and type 2 deiodinase and may also inhibit the binding of T_3 to its nuclear receptors. In normal subjects, it causes persistent slowing of T_4 clearance and inhibition of both extrathyroidal T_3 production and rT_3 deiodination, so that serum T_3 concentrations decrease and those of rT_3 increase. During the first several weeks and months of treatment, serum TSH concentrations increase, and thyroidal iodine uptake and T_4 secretion increase. Therefore, serum total and free T_4 concentrations increase, sometimes to above the normal range.[292] Subsequently, serum TSH and T_4 concentrations remain above baseline, although usually within their respective normal ranges, and serum T_3 concentrations remain low or low-normal, as long as the drug is given and for several months afterward, because it is stored in adipose tissue and metabolized or excreted very slowly.

Amiodarone contains 37 percent iodine and is in part metabolized by deiodination. The iodide that is formed can cause either thyrotoxicosis or hypothyroidism in appropriately susceptible persons. Thyrotoxicosis may occur at any time during amiodarone therapy, but hypothyroidism usually occurs during the first several months of therapy.[289] Amiodarone may also initiate thyroid autoimmune disease.

There are two types of amiodarone-induced thyrotoxicosis, iodide-induced thyrotoxicosis and amiodarone-induced thyroiditis with thyrotoxicosis (see section on Iodine-Induced Thyrotoxicosis and Drug-Induced Thyrotoxicosis).[290,291,293] It may be difficult to confirm a suspected diagnosis of thyrotoxicosis in a patient taking amiodarone because some increase in serum T_4 concentrations is a regular occurrence in patients taking the drug; reliance must be placed on measurement of serum TSH. Patients with amiodarone-induced hypothyroidism have the typical biochemical findings of hypothyroidism: low-normal or low serum T_4 and high TSH concentrations.

Iodinated Radiographic Contrast Agents

The water soluble iodinated contrast agents used for arteriography, pyelography, and computed tomography do not regularly alter pituitary-thyroid function. These agents contain very large amounts of organic iodine (up to 400 mg/ml), they are usually given in large doses (40–200 ml), and they are to some extent deiodinated in vivo; thus substantial quantities of iodine circulate for a few days after they are injected. Any of the changes in thyroid secretion that can be induced by iodine in appropriately susceptible patients (see previous discussion) may occur transiently after their use. In prospective studies of 861 patients who received one of these agents, 6 percent developed overt or, more often, subclinical thyrotoxicosis.[294,294a]

Iodinated radiographic agents that are used for oral cholecystography, such as iopanoic acid, have effects that are similar to those of amiodarone, except that the effects are short-lived, because only single doses are given and the drugs are not stored as is amiodarone. They reduce serum T_3 and raise serum rT_3 concentrations for up to 2 weeks, and serum TSH and T_4 concentrations increase, sometimes to slightly above the normal range.[295]

Lithium

Lithium is concentrated by the thyroid and inhibits the formation and release of thyroid hormones. Among patients receiving chronic lithium carbonate therapy, about 10 percent have goiter, 20 percent have subclinical hypothyroidism, and 5 percent have overt hypothyroidism (but with wide variations in different studies).[296–299] Decreases in thyroid secretion are most likely to occur in patients receiving prolonged therapy and in those with high serum antithyroid peroxidase antibody concentrations, who presumably also have autoimmune thyroid disease, whether preexisting or induced by lithium.[300] Lithium also slows the rate of T_4 degradation, but it does not decrease extrathyroidal T_3 production.

Phenytoin, Carbamazepine, and Rifampin

Phenytoin, carbamazepine, and rifampin accelerate the nondeiodinative clearance of T_4 and, to a lesser extent, of T_3 because of their ability to increase the activity of hepatic microsomal oxidative enzymes.[79,301,302] This effect alone does not cause changes in serum T_4 and T_3 concentrations in normal subjects. However, phenytoin and carbamazepine also have central inhibitory actions.[303,304] As a result, in patients taking these two drugs serum T_4 and free T_4 concentrations decline by about 25 percent, while serum T_3 concentrations decline somewhat less; serum TSH concentrations are normal.

Interferon Alfa

From 10 to 40 percent of patients with chronic hepatitis or tumors treated with interferon alfa have high serum concentrations of antithyroid peroxidase antibodies, and about 10 percent have thyroid dysfunction.[305–308] The latter is most often painless (silent) thyroiditis, but a few patients have permanent hypothyroidism, presumably due to chronic autoimmune thyroiditis, or Graves' thyrotoxicosis. Patients with high serum antithyroid peroxidase antibody concentrations at baseline are more likely to develop thyroid dysfunction, and among patients with chronic hepatitis it is more likely to occur in those with hepatitis C than hepatitis B infections, probably because they are treated with larger doses.[307] Similar changes in thyroid function occur in patients treated with interleukin-2 or granulocyte colony-stimulating factor.[309–311] In contrast, thyroid dysfunction does not occur in patients treated with interferon-beta or interferon-gamma.

THYROTOXICOSIS

Thyrotoxicosis is the clinical, physiologic, and biochemical syndrome that results when tissues are exposed to excessive concentrations of thyroid hormones. The term *hyperthyroidism*, although often used synonymously with *thyrotoxicosis*, refers to excessive T_4 and T_3 synthesis and secretion by the thyroid gland and is used in this context here. Hence, hyperthyroid patients have thyrotoxicosis, but thyrotoxicosis has causes other than hyperthyroidism.

Thyrotoxicosis is usually categorized as overt or subclinical. *Overt thyrotoxicosis* is defined as high serum T_4 and T_3 concentrations and low serum TSH concentrations; most patients have symptoms and signs of thyrotoxicosis. *Subclinical thyrotoxicosis* is defined as normal serum T_4 and T_3 concentrations and low serum TSH concentrations; most patients have no symptoms or signs of thyrotoxicosis (Fig. 9-17). Thyrotoxicosis may develop suddenly or gradually, it may be transient or persistent, and it may be of little importance or life-threatening. The diagnosis may be obvious and may be confirmed readily by a few simple laboratory tests, or difficult, requiring repeated investigation or prolonged observation.

Thyrotoxicosis is a rather common disorder. Community and clinic surveys in the United States and Europe have revealed overall prevalence rates of overt and subclinical thyrotoxicosis of about 0.5 to 1 and 10 to 40 per 1000 people, respectively.[120–123,139,312] These rates are based on studies done both in the community and in clinics among patients seeking medical care. Within the ranges cited, the rates are higher in older persons, especially women, and they are lower in community-based screening programs.

Among patients with overt thyrotoxicosis, women outnumber men by 4 to 8 to 1, largely independent of the cause. The cause is Graves' disease in 60 to 85 percent of patients, toxic nodular goiter in 10 to 30 percent, toxic thyroid adenoma in 2 to 20 percent, and some type of thyroiditis in the remainder.[313–316] The frequency of toxic multinodular goiter and toxic adenoma varies the most, being higher in areas of lower (but not truly deficient) iodine intake.[313,316] Most patients with Graves' disease are 30–60 years old, whereas those with toxic multinodular goiters or toxic thyroid adenomas are 40–70 years old.[316]

Pathophysiology of Thyrotoxicosis

Thyrotoxicosis is caused by the unregulated release of T_4 and T_3 from the thyroid gland or the ingestion of excessive amounts of T_4, T_3, or both. It may be caused by increased T_4 and T_3 synthesis and release due to in trinsic thyroid disease, excessive TSH or theoretically excessive TRH secretion, or the production of other thyroid-stimulating hormones, such as TSH receptor-stimulating autoantibodies and chorionic gonadotropin. It also may be caused by destruction of thyroid tissue, with release of stored T_4 and T_3. These situations are all characterized by unregulated hormone release, and thyrotoxicosis, whether overt or subclinical, cannot occur in its absence. Compensatory increases in T_4 and T_3 secretion (what might be called secondary hyperthyroidism) may occur in patients who have accelerated degradation or increased urinary excretion of T_4 and T_3 or peripheral resistance to the actions of T_4 and T_3, but they do not have thyrotoxicosis. Increased extrathyroidal T_4 conversion to T_3 should not cause thyrotoxicosis, because any substantial increase in extrathyroidal T_3 production would be expected to decrease TSH secretion and therefore decrease thyroidal T_4 and T_3 secretion.

Most patients with thyrotoxicosis have increased production of both T_4 and T_3 and increased serum T_4 and T_3 concentrations. The increases in the production rate of T_3 and serum T_3 concentrations are characteristically greater than are those in T_4. Figure 9-23 shows a schematic summary of these findings. In one study of patients with thyrotoxicosis, the mean T_4 production rate was increased 3.5-fold, whereas the mean T_3 production rate was increased more than sevenfold.[317] The disproportionate increase in T_3 production is due to a disproportionate increase in synthesis of T_3, as manifested by an increased ratio of T_3/T_4 in thyroglobulin, and increased rates of both thyroidal and extrathyroidal T_4 conversion to T_3.

Some patients with thyrotoxicosis have high serum T_3 concentrations but normal serum T_4 concentrations. This is called T_3 thyrotoxicosis; in these patients T_3 production is increased relative to that of T_4 even more than is the case in the usual patient with thyrotoxicosis. There are no characteristic clinical manifestations of T_3 thyrotoxicosis. It is most common in patients whose thyrotoxicosis is due to a toxic thyroid adenoma or recurrent Graves' disease, but it may be due to hyperthyroidism of any cause. T_3 thyrotoxicosis is rare in the United States, but is more common in regions where iodine intake is limited. The abnormality responsible for it is probably relative intrathyroidal iodide deficiency.

A few patients with thyrotoxicosis have high serum T_4 but normal T_3 concentrations (T_4 thyrotoxicosis).[18,318] In addition to thyrotoxicosis, these patients have another serious illness or have recently received a drug that inhibits extrathyroidal conversion of T_4 to T_3. The biochemical findings of T_4 thyrotoxicosis therefore are a result of excessive thyroidal T_4 and T_3 secretion and concomitantly impaired extrathyroidal conversion of T_4 to T_3.

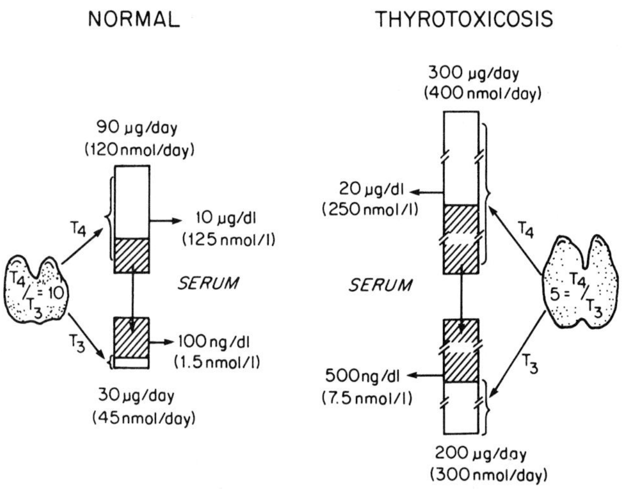

FIGURE 9-23. Diagram of thyroidal T_4/T_3 ratios, thyroidal and extrathyroidal production rates of T_4 and T_3, and serum T_4 and T_3 concentrations in normal subjects and patients with thyrotoxicosis. The diagonally lined areas in the T_4 (upper) rectangles indicate the proportion of T_4 converted to T_3 at extrathyroidal sites, and the diagonally lined areas in the T_3 (lower) rectangles indicate the proportion of T_3 formed from T_4 at extrathyroidal sites.

Causes of Thyrotoxicosis

The causes of thyrotoxicosis are listed in Table 9-11. An attempt should always be made to distinguish among these causes, because their natural history and therapy differ. The cause of thyrotoxicosis usually can be identified with reasonable certainty by history and physical examination. The most important findings concern the duration of symptoms, the degree and pattern of thyroid enlargement, and the presence or absence of thyroid pain and tenderness and of the extrathyroidal manifestations of Graves' dis-

TABLE 9-11. Causes of Thyrotoxicosis

Graves' disease
Thyroiditis
Subacute thyroiditis
Painless (silent) thyroiditis
Postpartum thyroiditis
Radiation-induced thyroiditis
Exogenous thyrotoxicosis
Thyroid hormone-induced thyrotoxicosis
Iodine-induced thyrotoxicosis
Drug- and cytokine-induced thyrotoxicosis
Toxic uninodular goiter (toxic thyroid adenoma)
Toxic multinodular goiter
Autosomal dominant and sporadic thyrotoxicosis
McCune-Albright syndrome
Ectopic thyrotoxicosis (struma ovarii)
Thyroid carcinoma
Thyrotropin-dependent thyrotoxicosis
Pregnancy-related thyrotoxicosis
Gestational thyrotoxicosis
Trophoblastic tumors

ease. Laboratory procedures such as measurements of thyroid radioiodine uptake, thyroid imaging, and serum thyroid antibody tests are rarely necessary and should not be done routinely.

Graves' Disease

Graves' disease is by far the single most common cause of thyrotoxicosis. It most often occurs in women 30–60 years old, but may occur in children and in adult men and women of any age. It is not fundamentally a thyroid disease, but rather an autoimmune disorder consisting of one or more of the following: hyperthyroidism (and thyrotoxicosis), diffuse thyroid enlargement, infiltrative ophthalmopathy (exophthalmos), localized myxedema (dermopathy), and thyroid acropachy. The clinical features and treatment of the extrathyroidal manifestations of Graves' disease are described later in this chapter (see section on Extrathyroidal Manifestations of Graves' Disease). Most patients with Graves' disease have both thyrotoxicosis and diffuse goiter, and many have ophthalmopathy as well, whereas localized myxedema and especially thyroid acropachy are rare. The extrathyroidal manifestations of Graves' disease can occur in the absence of thyroid disease.

The major gross anatomic abnormality in patients with Graves' thyrotoxicosis is diffuse thyroid enlargement. Microscopic examination reveals hypertrophy and hyperplasia of the thyroid follicular cells. The thyroid follicles are small and contain decreased quantities of colloid, and the follicular cells that line them are columnar, with increased numbers of mitochondria, a hypertrophic Golgi apparatus, and increased microvilli on the apical surface. The interfollicular spaces are richly vascular, and often contain foci of lymphocytes and occasionally lymphoid germinal centers.

Thyrotropin Receptor-Stimulating Antibodies in Graves' Disease

Hyperthyroidism in patients with Graves' disease is caused by autoantibodies that stimulate thyroid hormone synthesis and secretion (Table 9-12). These antibodies are IgG immunoglobulins that bind to the extracellular domain (and perhaps some extracellular portions of the transmembrane domain) of the TSH receptors on thyroid follicular cells (Fig. 9-11), thereby activating the receptors; they are therefore TSH receptor-stimulating antibodies that cause hyperthyroidism by mimicking the action of TSH.[319] They are not monoclonal antibodies, but their clonality is restricted, so that in an individual patient the antibodies usually belong to a single class of IgG and have a single type of light chain.[320] Peripheral blood and thyroid lymphocytes from patients with Graves' disease produce TSH receptor-stimulating antibodies in vitro.[321]

TSH receptor-stimulating antibodies can be detected in serum by bio- and receptor assays. The bioassays are based on the ability of the antibodies to stimulate adenylyl cyclase activity, iodide uptake, and T_4 and T_3 synthesis and release in animal or human thyroid cells.[322] The receptor assays are based on the ability of the antibodies to inhibit the binding of TSH to its receptors on thyroid cells or other cells containing recombinant TSH receptors[323,324]; this activity is referred to as TSH receptor-binding inhibitory activity. Patients with chronic autoimmune thyroiditis also have serum antibodies that inhibit the binding of TSH to its receptors, but they block the biological activity of TSH rather than mimicking it. Receptor assays are easier to perform, but they are less specific.

TSH receptor-stimulating antibodies can be detected in the serum of nearly all patients with Graves' thyrotoxicosis, and they may be detected in thyroid tissue even when not detected in serum.[319,324,325] Their presence correlates well with the presence of thyrotoxicosis in untreated patients with Graves' disease, and with the presence of thyroid autonomy, as reflected by low serum TSH concentrations, in patients receiving antithyroid therapy. Similarly, their presence in the serum of newborn infants of mothers with Graves' disease correlates well with the presence of thyrotoxicosis in the infants. The antibodies can be detected in some patients before they develop thyrotoxicosis, and in others who are euthyroid after completing a course of antithyroid drug therapy.[319,326] Therefore, their presence does not invariably indicate the presence of thyrotoxicosis; they can be produced in amounts just sufficient to substitute for normal amounts of TSH.

TSH receptor-stimulating antibodies stimulate thyroid growth as well as thyroid function, acting via receptors linked to adenylyl cyclase.[319,322] Some of the antibodies also stimulate the phospholipase C-phosphoinositide pathway in thyroid cells; patients whose serum activates this pathway tend to have larger goiters than those whose serum does not.[327] Other determinants of goiter size in patients with Graves' thyrotoxicosis are the extent of lymphocytic infiltration and the numbers of lymphoid germinal centers in the thyroid gland.

Many patients with Graves' thyrotoxicosis have high serum concentrations of other antithyroid antibodies (Table 9-12). They include antibodies against thyroid peroxidase, thyroglobulin, and the Na/I cotransporter[137,328]; the presence of these antibodies is indicative of widespread thyroid autoimmunity, but they have no functional importance. In terms of quantity of antibody protein, the concentrations of TSH receptor-stimulating antibodies are much lower than the concentrations of antithyroid peroxidase antibodies.[329]

TABLE 9-12. Types of Thyroid Autoantibodies Found in Patients with Graves' Disease and Chronic Autoimmune Thyroiditis

Antibody	Biological Activity of Antibody	Graves' Disease	Chronic Autoimmune Thyroiditis
TSH receptor-stimulating	Activates TSH receptors	Present*	Absent*
TSH receptor-blocking	Blocks TSH action	Absent	Present
TSH binding-inhibiting	Inhibits TSH receptor-binding†	Present	Present
Thyroid peroxidase	Inhibits peroxidase activity	Present	Present
Thyroglobulin	No activity on thyroid cells	Present	Present
Na/I cotransporter	Inhibits iodide transport	Present	Present
Cytotoxic	Cytotoxic to thyroid cells	Absent	Present

*Present means the antibody is often but not always found, and absent means the antibody is usually but not always not found.

†Based on inhibition of binding of radiolabeled TSH to TSH receptors. Antibodies detected in this way can mimic or block the action of TSH.

Pathogenesis of Graves' Thyrotoxicosis

What factors initiate and maintain the production of TSH receptor-stimulating antibodies? One possibility is their production is initiated by an injury that alters the structure of the extracellular domain of the TSH receptor, for example by modifying a carbohydrate component of the receptor, so that it becomes antigenic and therefore serves as a stimulus for production of the antibodies. No known thyroid injury, however, whether due to an infectious agent, a toxin, or a drug, is followed by sustained production of TSH receptor-stimulating antibodies and Graves' hyperthyroidism, with the possible exception of radiation injury[330,331]; and no structural abnormality of thyroid tissue unique to Graves' disease has been found. (There are polymorphisms of the extracellular domain of the receptor, but none has been linked to Graves' disease.[332,333]) Thyroid tissue from patients with Graves' thyrotoxicosis becomes morphologically and functionally normal after transplantation into nude mice.[334] Finally, like TSH binding, TSH receptor-stimulating antibody binding depends on the conformation of the extracellular domain of the TSH receptor, although T cells from different patients are sensitized to different peptide components (epitopes) of the domain.[63,319,335–338] Taken together, these findings argue against the hypothesis that Graves' disease is initiated by some thyroid abnormality or injury.

Another possibility is an infectious or other agent that has epitopes that induce production of antibodies that cross-react with thyroid tissue.[319,320,339] The most-studied candidate agent is *Yersinia enterocolitica*. Some subtypes of this organism have membrane-binding sites for TSH, and some patients with Graves' disease have anti-*Yersinia* antibodies, but the association is weak. Graves' disease does not often follow *Yersinia* infections, and there is little evidence that anti-*Yersinia* antibodies are present before the onset of Graves' disease.

A third possibility is that TSH receptor-stimulating antibody production results from the activation of B lymphocytes that were not clonally deleted in utero, a possibility supported by the limited structural heterogeneity of the antibodies.

However the B cells acquire the capability to produce the antibodies, they must be stimulated to expand and differentiate into antibody-secreting cells and then persistently stimulated so that antibody production is maintained. The activation, expansion, and persistence of B cells probably results from stimulation by interleukins and other cytokines produced by T_{H2} cells, the category of T cells that provides help to B cells.

T cells expand and produce cytokines when activated by the binding of complexes of HLA (human leukocyte antigen) class II molecules and peptides (antigens) processed within the HLA-bearing cells to the antigen receptors on the T cells. HLA class II molecules are expressed on thyroid cells from patients with Graves' disease but not on normal thyroid cells; TSH and interferon-gamma and other cytokines can induce the expression of class II molecules on normal thyroid cells.[319,340] By acquiring these molecules, thyroid cells can present peptides or glycopeptides derived from their own components, such as portions of the TSH receptor, to T cells, without the components being released into the interstitial fluid and taken up, processed, and presented by the 'professional' antigen-processing cells (macrophages and some lymphocytes) that normally express class II molecules and carry out these functions. The binding of class II molecule-thyroid antigen complexes on thyroid cells to the antigen receptors on T cells and the consequent T-cell activation is augmented by adhesion and costimulatory molecules, provided either by the thyroid cells or 'professional' antigen-presenting cells.[341]

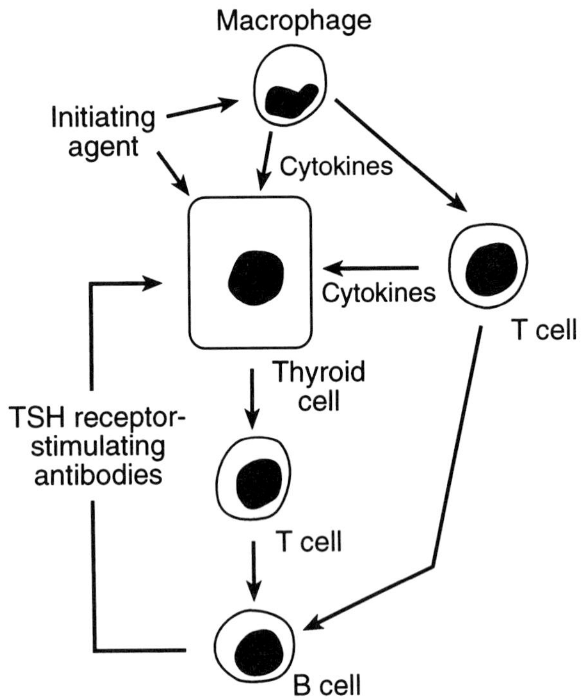

FIGURE 9-24. Hypothetical scheme for the development of Graves' disease and hyperthyroidism. In a subject with inherited susceptibility to the disease, an exogenous initiating agent (virus or toxin) activates macrophages (or intrathyroidal T cells) to secrete cytokines such as interferon, which then induce the expression of HLA class II molecules on the thyroid cells. The agent may also affect thyroid cells directly so that components of the TSH receptor are processed as antigen. The class II molecules and TSH receptor antigens form complexes that bind to the antigen receptors of T helper cells, inducing them to secrete other cytokines. These cytokines stimulate B cells to expand and secrete TSH receptor-stimulating antibodies that bind to and activate the TSH receptors of thyroid cells, thus inducing thyroid hypersecretion. T-cell function may be increased by T_4 and T_3.

Figure 9-24 shows a hypothetical scheme for the development of Graves' thyrotoxicosis based on these considerations. The disorder could be initiated in a susceptible host by some exogenous agent, perhaps a low-grade viral infection or toxin, that localizes in the thyroid gland and induces secretion of interferon-gamma or other cytokines by macrophages or lymphocytes, which in turn induce the expression of HLA class II molecules and stimulate processing of nascent TSH receptors in thyroid cells. The class II molecule–TSH receptor antigen complexes then bind to the antigen receptors of T helper cells, with the aid of costimulatory molecules, thereby activating the T cells. The cytokines produced by the activated T cells stimulate B cells that were not clonally deleted to produce the antibodies. The thyroid cells cannot be injured by the initiating agent (or T cells activated by the process) to the point wherein their function and growth capacity are impaired. The process could also be initiated by presentation by macrophages of an exogenous antigen that shared epitopes with the TSH receptor (molecular mimicry) or a fragment of the extracellular domain of the TSH receptor released from thyroid cells in response to some injury, in conjunction with HLA class II molecules and the costimulatory molecules normally expressed on macrophages, to T helper cells.[341] The process does not persist indefinitely, however, because production of TSH receptor-stimulating antibodies ceases and hyperthyroidism disappears in some patients. T_4 and T_3 may help perpetuate the autoimmune process by augmenting T-cell activation.[342]

Although the overall numbers of B and T cells in peripheral blood are normal in patients with Graves' thyrotoxicosis, variable decreases in the proportion of T suppressor cells have been reported. The thyroid tissue of these patients contains increased numbers of both B and T cells. The latter include both T_{H2} cells, some sensitized to the TSH receptor, and T_{H1} cells; the latter are generally thought to promote cell-mediated hypersensitivity, but they also secrete cytokines capable of stimulating B cells.[319,343] The antigen receptors of these intrathyroidal T cells are less structurally diverse than are those of circulating T cells, suggesting that they accumulate in response to specific stimuli originating in the thyroid.[344] The central role of T cells is supported by reports of Graves' thyrotoxicosis in recipients of bone marrow transplants from donors who had or later developed Graves' thyrotoxicosis.[345,346]

Risk Factors for Graves' Thyrotoxicosis

There are several risk factors for Graves' thyrotoxicosis. One is female sex, the disorder being 3–6 times more common in women than men, whereas among prepubertal children girls and boys are equally affected. A second is heredity.[347] The concordance rate in monozygotic twins is high (22 vs. 0 percent in dizygotic twins in one recent study[348]), and the concordance rates are about 5 percent and 1 percent, respectively, in first-degree female and male relatives of patients with Graves' thyrotoxicosis.[347] Family members also are more likely to have thyroid antibodies, abnormalities in thyroid regulation, and chronic autoimmune thyroiditis than are unrelated people. The pattern of inheritance is undoubtedly polygenic. Graves' thyrotoxicosis has been linked with certain HLA haplotypes, coded by genes on chromosome 6, but the specific haplotype linkages vary among different ethnic groups. It has also been linked to the CLTA-4 (cytotoxic lymphocyte antigen 4) locus on chromosome 2, and to loci on chromosomes 14 and 20 and the X chromosome.[347,349,350] TSH receptor peptides may bind to and thus be presented preferentially to T cells by particular HLA molecules, but how the products of other gene loci might affect susceptibility to the disease is not known. The occurrence of Graves' disease in the spouses of patients points to the existence of environmental factors in causation.[351]

Other risk factors for Graves' thyrotoxicosis are smoking and perhaps stressful life events and iodine intake.[319,352–356] Cigarette smoking increases the risk about 1.5- to twofold, and that of Graves' ophthalmopathy about sevenfold.[167,352,353] Patients with Graves' thyrotoxicosis have a history of stressful life events, particularly negative ones such as divorce and loss of job, more often than do control subjects, but the increase in these events could be a result of thyrotoxicosis than a cause of it.[354,355] With respect to iodine intake, Graves' thyrotoxicosis is more common in areas in which iodine intake is high, as compared with areas in which it is lower (but not deficient).[316]

Natural History of Graves' Thyrotoxicosis

The natural history of Graves' thyrotoxicosis varies considerably in different patients (Fig. 9-25). Some patients have a single episode of thyrotoxicosis (and Graves' disease) that subsides spontaneously in a few months or years. Other patients have life-long thyrotoxicosis, and still others have repeated remissions and relapses. In patients who are treated with an antithyroid drug, the occurrence of a remission of Graves' disease means that prolonged therapy is not required.

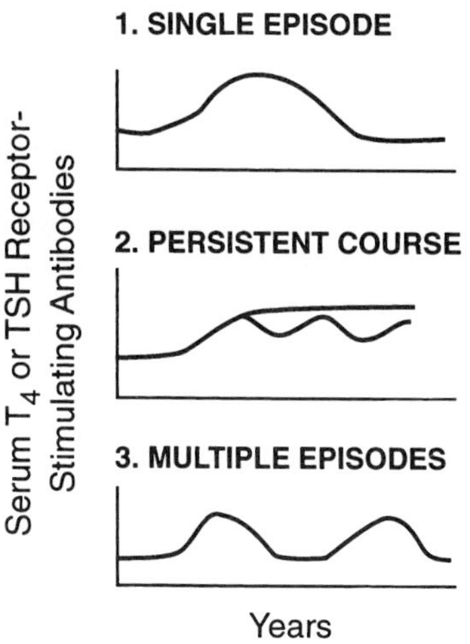

FIGURE 9-25. Variations in the natural history of Graves' disease as exemplified by variations in either serum TSH receptor-stimulating antibody concentrations or serum T_4 concentrations. (*Top panel*) Single episode of production of TSH receptor-stimulating antibodies and, therefore, of increased serum T_4 concentrations and thyrotoxicosis followed by disappearance of the antibodies and decline of the serum T_4 concentration to normal. (*Middle panel*) Persistent production of TSH receptor-stimulating antibodies and, therefore, persistently increased serum T_4 concentrations and persistent thyrotoxicosis. (*Bottom panel*) Multiple episodes of production of TSH receptor-stimulating antibodies and increased serum T_4 concentrations with an intervening remission.

A patient may have a remission of Graves' disease, with disappearance of both TSH receptor-stimulating antibodies and thyrotoxicosis, or a remission of thyrotoxicosis alone, with persistent antibody production, but in quantities too small to cause excessive T_4 and T_3 secretion. In the latter patients the Graves' disease has decreased in severity but has not disappeared; the patients might be said to have subclinical Graves' disease.[357] This is an important conceptual difference, but has no practical clinical importance, because either way the patient no longer needs antithyroid drug therapy. Because of the difficulty of measuring TSH receptor-stimulating antibodies, and the persistence of positive tests for these antibodies in some patients who remain euthyroid after drug treatment,[326,327] most studies of remission are studies of remission of thyrotoxicosis, not studies of remission of Graves' disease.

The proportion of patients who have a remission of a first episode of Graves' thyrotoxicosis varies widely, ranging from 30 to 70 percent, occasionally even higher (see section on Treatment of Thyrotoxicosis). Possible explanations for this variability include the patient's age, genetic susceptibility to Graves' disease, severity of Graves' disease (and thyrotoxicosis), and duration and type of therapy. Assessment of the importance any of these factors is confounded by the fact that the patients being studied must be treated with an antithyroid drug (methimazole, carbimazole, or

PTU), which certainly reduces thyroid secretion and may also have immunosuppressive actions. Either action could contribute to the occurrence of remissions, but remissions also could be due to the passage of time alone, because they also occur in patients treated with propranolol[358] or not treated in any way.

Among patients who remain euthyroid after discontinuation of antithyroid drug therapy, some develop hypothyroidism or at least chronic autoimmune thyroiditis years later, suggesting that Graves' disease can evolve into chronic autoimmune thyroiditis.[359,360] Conversely, hypothyroidism occasionally precedes the development of hyperthyroidism due to Graves' disease, indicating that the converse evolution can occur.[361]

TSH receptor-stimulating antibodies usually gradually disappear from the serum of patients treated with radioactive iodine or subtotal thyroidectomy, although there are transient increases in the first several weeks after thyroidectomy and more prolonged increases, lasting up to a year, after radioiodine therapy.[362] The increases indicate that thyroid injury can result in transient autoimmunization, and the decreases indicate that autoimmunization does not lead to sustained production of TSH receptor-stimulating antibodies and also that Graves' disease tends to subside with time.

Pathogenesis of Ophthalmopathy and Localized Myxedema

The causes of the extrathyroidal manifestations of Graves' disease—ophthalmopathy, localized myxedema, and thyroid acropachy—are poorly understood. The most prominent pathologic abnormality in patients with ophthalmopathy is enlargement of the extraocular muscles. The muscle cells usually appear normal; the enlargement is caused by edema, infiltration of activated T cells and B cells, and proliferation of fibroblasts and their differentiation into adipocytes.[363,364] The enlargement of the extraocular muscles displaces the eyes anteriorly, causing proptosis, the characteristic clinical finding of ophthalmopathy; and can impair venous drainage and compress the optic nerves.

The inflammatory process may begin with the accumulation of T cells sensitized to antigens shared by orbital connective tissue or muscle cells and thyroid cells.[365] A likely antigen is the TSH receptor. Most patients with ophthalmopathy have TSH receptor-stimulating antibodies, which cause their thyroid disease; orbital fibroblasts from patients with ophthalmopathy contain TSH receptor mRNA; and portions of the TSH receptor have been detected both in these cells and on their surface.[66,67,366,367] Ophthalmopathy might begin with the binding of TSH receptor-stimulating antibodies or circulating T_{H1} and T_{H2} cells sensitized to TSH receptor peptides to the fibroblasts, followed by release of cytokines capable of mediating both cell- and antibody-mediated immunity.[368] These cytokines may then damage the fibroblasts or muscle cells, causing inflammation and edema; stimulation of the synthesis of glycosaminoglycans by the fibroblasts; and stimulation of fibroblast proliferation and differentiation into adipocytes. The cytokines also may induce the fibroblasts to express class II molecules, rendering them capable of presenting antigen and therefore of increasing and perpetuating the activation of T cells, and to produce heat shock proteins, which have immunomodulatory actions.[365]

The retroorbital inflammatory process may be increased by the actions of systemically or locally produced autoantibodies to fibroblast or muscle cell antigens released in response to cytokine-induced cellular injury. The local production of these antibodies could be augmented by the stimulatory action on B cells of the cytokines secreted by the activated T cells. Antibodies that have been found in the serum of patients with ophthalmopathy include antibodies that react with eye muscle cells and their plasma membranes, antibodies that are cytotoxic to eye muscle cells, and antibodies that react with orbital fibroblasts and stimulate not only the synthesis of glycosaminoglycans and protein by these cells but also their proliferation.[369–371] Like the thyroid disease, therefore, the pathogenesis of Graves' ophthalmopathy probably involves abnormalities in cell- and antibody-mediated immunity, and at least initially the antibodies and sensitized T cells are probably primarily thyroid-directed.

Very little is known about the pathogenesis of localized myxedema and thyroid acropachy, although they too probably have an autoimmune basis. The basic pathologic abnormalities of localized myxedema are proliferation of fibroblasts and subcutaneous accumulation of glycosaminoglycans, mostly in the pretibial region.[372] The simplest explanation for localized myxedema is that it is caused by antibodies, presumably primarily thyroid-directed, that react with an antigen shared with pretibial fibroblasts, stimulating both their function and their proliferation. In support of this explanation TSH receptor-like immunoreactivity has been detected on these cells.[67] Furthermore, the serum of patients with localized myxedema contains thyroid-directed antibodies, including TSH receptor-stimulating antibodies, but the evidence that their serum stimulates glycosaminoglycan or protein synthesis by pretibial fibroblasts is conflicting.[373,374] The predilection for the pretibial region is unexplained.

Thyroiditis

The thyrotoxicosis that occurs in all the forms of thyroiditis (Table 9-11) is caused by T_4 and T_3 released from thyroglobulin as a result of thyroid inflammation and disruption of thyroid follicles. Because the stores of thyroglobulin are limited and new T_4 and T_3 synthesis ceases, the thyrotoxicosis is transient.

Subacute Thyroiditis

Approximately 50 percent of patients with subacute (granulomatous) thyroiditis have clinical manifestations of thyrotoxicosis, and many others have high serum T_4 and T_3 concentrations.[375] The illness, however, is dominated by the nonspecific systemic manifestations of inflammation, such as fever, malaise, and myalgia, and by thyroid pain and tenderness, both of which may be severe. About half of the patients have a history of a recent upper respiratory infection. The thyroid is usually moderately enlarged. The thyroid pain and tenderness and any manifestations of thyrotoxicosis are usually short-lived, lasting 4–6 weeks or less. The inflammatory and thyrotoxic phase may be followed by transient hypothyroidism, but permanent hypothyroidism is rare (Fig. 9-26). This disorder is discussed in more detail in the section on the Painful Thyroid.

Painless (Silent) Thyroiditis and Postpartum Thyroiditis

Thyrotoxicosis caused by thyroid inflammation in the absence of thyroid pain and tenderness is known as painless or silent thyroiditis, and also as subacute lymphocytic thyroiditis. It is an uncommon cause of thyrotoxicosis. It occurs in nearly equal numbers of men and women, unlike Graves' disease. In contrast, among postpartum women (defined as those in whom a pregnancy ended within the previous year), painless thyroiditis with thyro-

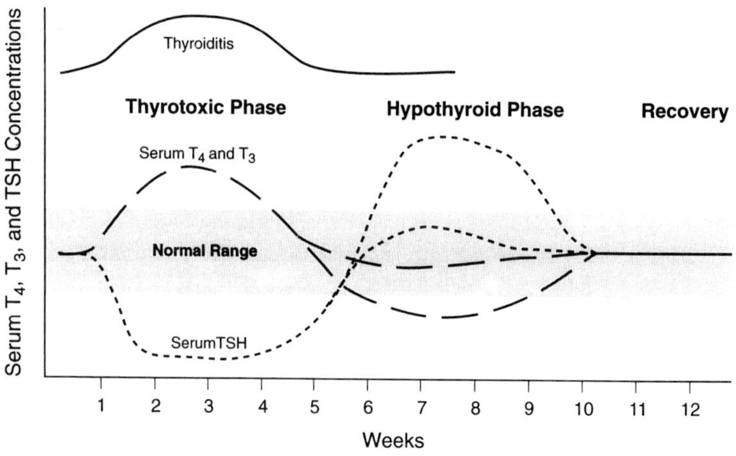

FIGURE 9-26. Schematic diagram of the course of subacute thyroiditis, painless (silent) thyroiditis, and postpartum thyroiditis. As thyroid inflammation develops, there is unregulated release of T_4 (and T_3). Serum T_4 concentrations increase, and serum TSH concentrations decrease. As the thyroid inflammation subsides, serum T_4 and TSH concentrations may return to normal. Alternatively, there may be a period of transient hypothyroidism during which serum T_4 concentrations decline to below normal and serum TSH concentrations rise to above normal for several weeks before returning to normal.

toxicosis can be detected by clinical examination in about 1 percent and by regular biochemical testing 2–6 months postpartum in 2 to 3 percent (mostly as subclinical thyrotoxicosis).[376] In men, women, and postpartum women alike the thyrotoxicosis is characteristically of recent onset and is mild, and there is no recent history of upper respiratory infection. The thyroid gland is not painful or tender and is not enlarged or is only slightly enlarged. There are none of the extrathyroidal manifestations of Graves' disease. The thyroid radioiodine uptake is low, and serum antithyroid antibody concentrations are normal or minimally elevated (in about 50 percent), except in women with postpartum thyroiditis, among whom about 75 percent have high serum antithyroid antibody concentrations. The thyrotoxicosis lasts 2–6 weeks and is followed by either recovery or transient hypothyroidism that lasts 2–8 weeks (Fig. 9-26). About 50 percent of the patients later develop goitrous autoimmune thyroiditis, hypothyroidism, or both. Painless thyroiditis with thyrotoxicosis is most likely a variant form of chronic autoimmune thyroiditis (see section on Transient Hypothyroidism in Autoimmune Thyroiditis).

The syndrome of painless thyroiditis and thyrotoxicosis can also occur in patients treated with amiodarone and several cytokines (see section on Exogenous Thyrotoxicosis).

Other Types of Thyroiditis

Radiation-induced thyroid follicular necrosis and inflammation occur regularly after ^{131}I therapy, and occasionally are sufficiently intense to cause exacerbations of thyrotoxicosis, with or without thyroid pain and tenderness. These complications of ^{131}I therapy are most likely to occur 1–2 weeks after treatment, last a week or two, and then subside. Transient thyrotoxicosis with thyroid pain and tenderness has also been reported after thyroid trauma, thyroid surgery, and tumor infiltration.[377,378]

Exogenous Thyrotoxicosis

Thyroid Hormone-Induced Thyrotoxicosis

Thyrotoxicosis can occur as a result of the prescription of high doses of thyroid hormone by physicians, the ingestion of high doses by patients on their own initiative, and rarely by accident (Table 9-11).[379] It is likely to occur in patients chronically taking T_4 in doses of 0.2 mg/day or more, T_3 in doses of 0.075 mg/day or more, or desiccated thyroid in doses of 180 mg/day or more (or the equivalent as combinations of synthetic T_4 and T_3). Smaller doses can cause subclinical and occasionally overt thyrotoxicosis, especially in patients with autonomous (TSH-independent) thyroid function.

Thyroid hormone-induced thyrotoxicosis is especially likely to occur when T_3 alone or combinations of T_4 and T_3 (as desiccated thyroid or combinations of synthetic T_4 and T_3) are used, and treatment is monitored by measurements of serum T_4, because the results underestimate the total dose of thyroid hormone administered. It should not occur if therapy is monitored by measurements of serum TSH, and furthermore nearly all patients now are treated with T_4.

Subclinical and sometimes overt thyrotoxicosis is sometimes deliberately induced in patients with thyroid carcinoma or, less appropriately, patients with nodular goiter. More often it occurs because patients with hypothyroidism receiving thyroid therapy are given too high a dose or they raise the dose on their own initiative to alleviate symptoms thought to be due to hypothyroidism or in an effort to lose weight or treat menstrual irregularities. Other patients, particularly health care workers, surreptitiously take large doses of thyroid hormone because of psychological disturbances; they usually deny use and decline psychiatric care.[380] Ingestion of single very high doses, for example, 0.5 mg/kg of T_4 or more, accidentally by children or with suicidal intent by adults can cause transient thyrotoxicosis, although others tolerate similar doses very well.[379,381,382]

Exogenous thyrotoxicosis has occurred as a result of improper meat-packing practices that resulted in the inclusion of thyroid tissue in neck muscle that was removed for consumption as ground meat.[383,384] Some nutritional supplements contain extracts of animal thyroid tissue, and therefore they too can cause thyrotoxicosis.[385,386]

Important clues to the presence of exogenous thyrotoxicosis are the absence of thyroid enlargement, or the failure of thyroid enlargement to regress much if the treatment was given for this purpose; and normal or low serum T_4 concentrations if the patient is taking T_3 or preparations containing T_3. Most patients with exogenous thyrotoxicosis also have low thyroid radioiodine uptake values and low serum thyroglobulin concentrations.

Iodine-Induced Thyrotoxicosis

Iodine supplementation decreases the size of the goiter and improves thyroid function in most residents of regions of endemic goiter. In some, however, it induces thyrotoxicosis[387]; in some endemic goiter regions the incidence of thyrotoxicosis transiently increased several-fold after supplementation was introduced. For it to occur, the patient must have a preexisting thyroid abnormality that causes autonomous thyroid secretion, for example, Graves' disease or, more commonly, a nodular goiter, but insufficient iodine intake to permit excessive production of T_4 and T_3.

Iodine-induced thyrotoxicosis also occurs in nonendemic goiter regions.[387] Most of these patients have autonomously functioning thyroid tissue, such as a multinodular goiter or a thyroid adenoma, that transports iodide poorly. They become thyrotoxic several weeks or months after receiving pharmacologic doses of inorganic iodine,[388] iodine-containing radiographic contrast agents,[294,389] or iodine-containing drugs. Whatever the source of iodine, serum iodide concentrations must increase sufficiently that enough iodide can enter the thyroid by diffusion to allow excessive thyroid hormone synthesis and secretion by the autonomously functioning thyroid tissue.

Drug- and Cytokine-Induced Thyrotoxicosis

Amiodarone, because it contains iodine, can cause iodine-induced thyrotoxicosis in patients with nodular goiter.[290,291,293] Amiodarone can also cause painless thyroiditis that is sufficiently severe to cause thyrotoxicosis, apparently due to a direct toxic effect of the drug (or a metabolite); it differs from other types of painless thyroiditis in being more prolonged. In a cohort of amiodarone-treated patients followed for up to 54 months, 12 percent developed thyrotoxicosis.[289] Distinguishing between the two types of amiodarone-induced thyrotoxicosis can be difficult. Amiodarone-treated patients with iodine-induced thyrotoxicosis usually have nodular goiters, become thyrotoxic during the first year of treatment, and have normal or high thyroid radioiodine uptake values and normal serum interleukin-6 concentrations. In contrast, those with amiodarone-induced thyroiditis have little or no thyroid enlargement, can become thyrotoxic at any time after the initiation of therapy, and have low thyroid radioiodine uptake values and high serum interleukin-6 concentrations (an indicator of inflammation).[291,390,391] The former require antithyroid therapy, whereas the latter respond to prednisone.[293]

Among patients treated with interferon-alfa, about 2 percent develop thyrotoxicosis, caused mostly by painless thyroiditis (and therefore transient) but sometimes by Graves' disease.[305–308] The thyrotoxicosis is more often subclinical than overt. It usually begins after three months of therapy, and can occur as long as treatment is continued. Interleukin-2 can also cause painless thyroiditis and thyrotoxicosis[309,310] (see also the section on Effects of Drugs on Thyroid Function).

Toxic Uninodular Goiter (Toxic Thyroid Adenoma)

Toxic uninodular goiters (toxic thyroid adenomas) are autonomously functioning thyroid adenomas. Among patients with these adenomas, about 20 percent have overt and 20 percent have subclinical thyrotoxicosis at the time of diagnosis.[392,393] These adenomas are a rather common cause of thyrotoxicosis in regions where iodine intake is marginal, but are rare in the United States. Although they occur in adults of all ages and occasionally in children, most patients with thyrotoxicosis are in the older age groups. In patients with normal thyroid function or subclinical thyrotoxicosis at diagnosis who are not treated, overt thyrotoxicosis occurs in about 4 percent/year.[393,394] It may also occur transiently as a result of hemorrhagic infarction of an adenoma.[395]

The characteristic finding in patients with a toxic thyroid adenoma is a solitary nodule, which is usually 3 cm or more in diameter. Thyroid radionuclide imaging reveals intense uptake of radionuclide in the location of the palpable nodule and nearly complete absence of uptake in the remainder of the thyroid gland. Pathologically, these lesions are well-encapsulated masses of hyperplastic thyroid tissue. At a molecular level, they are monoclonal tumors; from 20 to 80 percent have somatic activating (gain-of-function) mutations of the TSH receptor gene, and a few others have somatic activating mutations of the gene for the alpha subunit of G protein.[396–400] Most of the TSH receptor-gene mutations have been in the transmembrane domains of the receptor (Fig. 9-11). These mutations activate adenylyl cyclase, and some also activate phospholipase C.[401]

Toxic Multinodular Goiter

Thyrotoxicosis can occur late in the natural history of multinodular goiter, usually in women 50 years old or older. The typical patient has a long history of gradually increasing thyroid enlargement and insidiously develops subclinical and then overt thyrotoxicosis. Among euthyroid patients with a multinodular goiter, thyroid volume correlates positively with age and duration of goiter, and negatively with serum TSH concentrations[402,403]; in one study 9 percent of initially euthyroid patients developed overt thyrotoxicosis in 1 to 7 years.[404] These patients have no ophthalmopathy or localized myxedema and no spontaneous remissions; thyrotoxicosis persists until the autonomous thyroid tissue is destroyed.

In patients with toxic multinodular goiters the number of palpable nodules varies from one to many, and sometimes the thyroid seems to be diffusely enlarged. Not all the nodules are hyperfunctioning; some contain hyperplastic but functionally inactive thyroid tissue, atrophic follicles, or fibrous tissue. This process probably starts as diffuse thyroid hyperplasia, from which evolve foci of thyroid follicular cells capable of autonomous iodine metabolism. Some of these nodules are polyclonal and others monoclonal; some of the monoclonal nodules have activating mutations of the TSH receptor gene similar to the mutations found in toxic uninodular goiters.[405–407] As the nodules capable of producing T_4 and T_3 grow, they account for an increasing proportion and eventually all thyroid secretion, and therefore TSH secretion gradually declines.[408] Such a formulation explains the very slow development of toxic nodular goiter, the fact that most patients with multinodular goiter do not become thyrotoxic, and the varied pathology of the disorder.

Autosomal Dominant and Sporadic Nonautoimmune Thyrotoxicosis

Nonautoimmune thyrotoxicosis is characterized by diffuse goiter and thyrotoxicosis, and is caused by germline activating mutations in the TSH receptor gene. The mutations, like those in toxic adenomas (see section on Toxic Uninodular Goiter), are in the transmembrane domains of the receptor (Fig. 9-11).[409–412] This syndrome has been described in families with autosomal dominant inheritance, and it can also occur sporadically as a new mutation. Within affected families, goiter size and severity of the thyrotoxicosis have varied substantially, and age at diagnosis has ranged from birth to middle age.[409,412,413] In contrast, most of the sporadic cases have been in neonates, and their thyrotoxicosis was severe. In both groups the thyrotoxicosis is lifelong, and recurrence rates are high after destructive therapy, unless it is nearly complete.

Another form of sporadic nonautoimmune thyrotoxicosis is that which occurs in patients with the McCune-Albright syndrome. This syndrome is characterized by polyostotic fibrous dysplasia, cutaneous hyperpigmentation, and hyperfunction of the ovaries (precocious puberty) and other endocrine glands. The endocrine hyperfunction is caused by activating mutations of the gene for the alpha subunit of G protein in some cells of the affected gland, and therefore there is mosaicism within the gland.[414] Not all patients with this syndrome have thyroid disease; among those who do it is manifested by diffuse and later multinodular goiter, and subclinical and sometimes overt thyrotoxicosis.[415,416]

Ectopic Thyrotoxicosis (Struma Ovarii)

The only recognized causes of thyrotoxicosis due to excessive ectopic thyroid hormone secretion are dermoid tumors and teratomas of the ovary. Most of the rare patients with substantial amounts of thyroid tissue in their tumors (struma ovarii) who have thyrotoxicosis have Graves' disease or a multinodular goiter.[417] Thus, they have one of the common causes of thyrotoxicosis, affecting both the thyroid gland and the ectopic thyroid tissue within the ovarian tumor. The ovarian tumor is the sole source of excessive thyroid hormone only when it contains a toxic thyroid adenoma[418] or the patient has Graves' disease and most of the thyroid gland was removed earlier.

Thyroid Carcinoma

Many differentiated (papillary or follicular) thyroid carcinomas synthesize thyroglobulin, but very few can transport iodide, and therefore they cannot synthesize T_4 and T_3. For this reason, thyrotoxicosis is extremely rare in patients with thyroid carcinoma; the few affected patients have had widespread well-differentiated carcinomas.[419]

Thyrotropin-Dependent Thyrotoxicosis

Excessive TSH secretion is a rare cause of thyrotoxicosis. Affected patients have thyrotoxicosis, diffuse goiter, and sometimes symptoms attributable to a pituitary mass, but no ophthalmopathy. The majority of patients have a macro- or microadenoma of the pituitary.[420,421] Their serum TSH concentrations may be normal or high, indicating that the biological activity of the TSH that is secreted varies. There may be concomitant hypersecretion of growth hormone, prolactin, or other pituitary hormones. A minority of patients have pituitary resistance to thyroid hormone. They have germline mutations in the beta form of the T_3 nuclear receptor similar to the mutations found in patients with generalized resistance to thyroid hormone[421]; why only their pituitary and not other tissues are resistant to thyroid hormone is not known.

The tumoral and nontumoral forms of TSH-dependent thyrotoxicosis are best distinguished by radiological rather than biochemical studies. Characteristically, patients with a TSH-secreting pituitary tumor have high serum TSH and especially glycoprotein hormone alpha subunit concentrations, so that the ratio of alpha subunit to TSH is high. In contrast, patients with pituitary resistance usually have normal or only slightly high serum TSH and alpha subunit concentrations, so that the molar ratio of the alpha subunit to TSH is normal.[420] Patients with TSH-secreting tumors should have the tumors removed surgically.[422] If that is not possible or there is no tumor, treatment with octreotide, lanreotide, or occasionally bromocriptine may be effective.[423,424] Those with pituitary resistance can be given one of these drugs, or treated in the same way as are patients with Graves' thyrotoxicosis (see section on Treatment of Thyrotoxicosis).

Pregnancy-Related Thyrotoxicosis

Most pregnant women who have thyrotoxicosis have Graves' disease, but in others thyrotoxicosis is associated with pregnancy (see section on Thyrotoxicosis during Pregnancy) or with trophoblastic disease.

Gestational Thyrotoxicosis

A small percentage of pregnant women (2 percent in one survey[146]) have transient thyrotoxicosis during the latter part of the first trimester of pregnancy. As a group, they have few symptoms and signs of thyrotoxicosis and no thyroid enlargement, but some have nausea, vomiting, and weight loss. The latter are sometimes severe, and if a woman loses 5 percent or more of body weight she is said to have hyperemesis gravidarum. As compared with normal pregnant women, women with gestational thyrotoxicosis have higher serum free T_4 and lower serum TSH concentrations; their serum T_3 concentrations may be high or normal. There are three explanations for the thyroid stimulation that occurs in these women, all related to the fact that chorionic gonadotropin binds weakly to the TSH receptor. They are an excessive increase in serum chorionic gonadotropin concentrations,[425] secretion of chorionic gonadotropin that is less glycosylated and has more thyroid-stimulating activity than does normal chorionic gonadotropin,[426] and mutations in the TSH receptor gene that increase the sensitivity of the receptor to chorionic gonadotropin (but not TSH), so that normal amounts of chorionic gonadotropin cause thyrotoxicosis.[427] Whatever the explanation, the thyrotoxicosis usually subsides in 4 to 8 weeks as chorionic gonadotropin secretion declines from its peak at 10 to 12 weeks of pregnancy.[428] The nausea and vomiting may be caused by excessive estrogen secretion or thyrotoxicosis, although these symptoms are not a feature of thyrotoxicosis in nonpregnant women and men.

Trophoblastic Tumors

Women with tumors of trophoblastic origin—hydatidiform moles and choriocarcinomas—and rarely men with germ cell tumors may have thyrotoxicosis caused by tumor secretion of chorionic gonadotropin.[429,430] These patients usually have serum chorionic gonadotropin concentrations greater than 300×10^3 units/liter, values higher than are found in euthyroid patients with the same tumors,[429] and there is a rough correlation between the chorionic gonadotropin concentration and the bioassayable thyroid-stimulating activity in the serum of these patients. Other patients with these tumors, while not overtly thyrotoxic, have high serum T_4 and T_3 concentrations and decreased TSH secretion. The lack of overt thyrotoxicosis may be due to the short duration of excess thyroid secretion or masking of the symptoms and signs of thyrotoxicosis by those of the trophoblastic disease.

Clinical Manifestations of Thyrotoxicosis

Thyrotoxicosis is usually first suggested because of the presence of symptoms and signs of either increased thyroid hormone action on one or more organ systems or the inability of an organ to meet the demands imposed by excess thyroid hormone action. However, it may be discovered coincidentally in patients who seek care for thyroid enlargement or ophthalmopathy. The common symptoms and signs are listed in Table 9-13.[431–435] Their frequency and

TABLE 9-13. Common Symptoms and Signs of Thyrotoxicosis

	Frequency in Thyrotoxic Patients, %
Symptoms	
Nervousness	35–99
Increased sweating	45–95
Heat intolerance	22–92
Palpitations	22–89
Fatigue and weakness	27–88
Weight loss	50–85
Dyspnea	41–81
Increased appetite	10–65
Hyperdefecation	4–36
Signs	
Tachycardia (>90 beats/min)	50–100
Thyroid enlargement	37–100
Tremor	32–97
Lid retraction	34–80
Hyperactivity	39–80
Atrial fibrillation	3–38

Sources: Oddie,[431] Davis,[432] Nordyke,[433] Martin,[434] Trivalle.[435]

severity vary substantially among patients, and clinical severity is poorly correlated with serum T_4 and T_3 concentrations. None is specific for thyrotoxicosis, although the combination of increased appetite and weight loss is nearly so.

Factors that influence the clinical severity of thyrotoxicosis include the rate of onset, the age of the patient, and the vulnerability of different organ systems to excess thyroid hormone action. The symptoms tend to be less severe when the onset is gradual, and are often tolerated well, particularly by younger patients. Indeed, some patients may feel better than when they were euthyroid; for example, they have more energy, can eat more without gaining weight, and are more comfortable in cool weather. Careful questioning usually reveals undesirable changes such as tremor, muscle weakness, emotional lability, fatigue on exertion, and decline in work or school performance. Thyrotoxicosis is fundamentally a catabolic disorder, and if not present initially more disabling manifestations are likely to occur if it persists. The symptoms and signs in children and adolescents are similar to those in young adults, except that children are more likely to gain weight and their linear growth may be accelerated.

Compared with younger adults, older adults tend to have fewer symptoms and signs. For example, increased appetite, heat intolerance, hyperactivity, emotional lability and tremor are less common; in contrast, weight loss, atrial fibrillation, and apathy are more common.[432,433,435] The terms *apathetic thyrotoxicosis* and *masked thyrotoxicosis* are sometimes used in describing older patients because of their lack of the symptoms and signs of neural activation, but there is no evidence that apathetic or masked thyrotoxicosis is pathophysiologically different from "ordinary" thyrotoxicosis, and careful evaluation will often elicit the presence of the symptoms and signs of neural activation. Death is usually due to cardiac failure.[436] The most life-threatening form of thyrotoxicosis—thyroid storm—is discussed later.

General Appearance

Figure 9-27 shows a woman with thyrotoxicosis. Her appearance alone should suggest the diagnosis. She appears to have lost weight and has a pained or apprehensive expression. Her skin is shiny and smooth, her eyelids are retracted, and her goiter is obvious. She is probably unable to sit quietly and talk calmly, but is restless, unable to concentrate, and speaks rapidly.

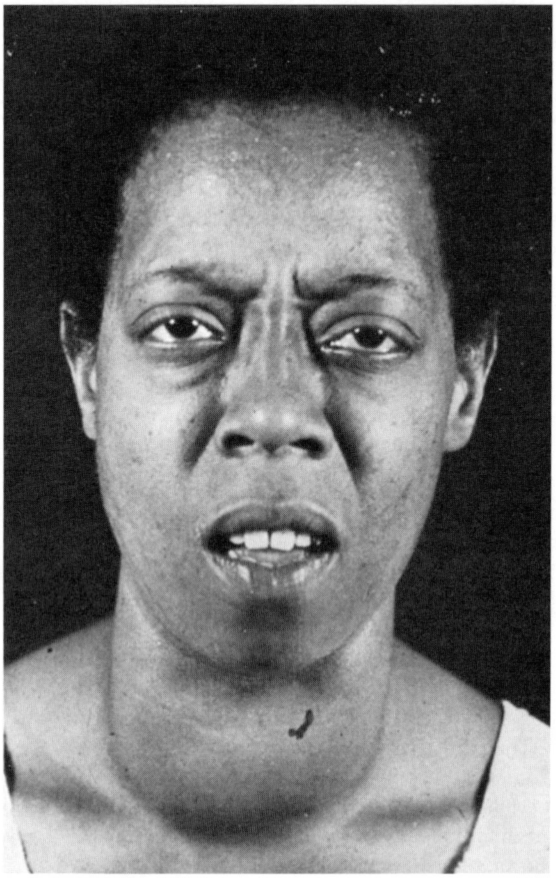

FIGURE 9-27. Photograph of a woman with thyrotoxicosis and ophthalmopathy caused by Graves' disease. Note the anxious expression, prominent eyes, periorbital edema, and diffuse goiter.

Skin and Appendages

The skin is warm and moist, and its texture is smooth or velvety; erythema and pruritis may be present. Perspiration is increased. The hair may become thin and fine in texture, and excess hair loss may be noted. The nails may be soft and separated from the nail bed (onchyolysis). Occasional findings are hyperpigmentation and vitiligo, the latter occurring mostly in patients with Graves' disease. Localized myxedema, not a manifestation of thyrotoxicosis per se, is described in the section on Extrathyroidal Manifestations of Graves' Disease.

Eyes

Two types of ocular abnormalities occur in thyrotoxic patients: noninfiltrative and infiltrative. The noninfiltrative signs of lid retraction and lid lag occur in patients with thyrotoxicosis of any cause. Usually the upper lids are symmetrically retracted so that some sclera is visible above the iris, but lid retraction may be asymmetric or may involve the lower lids as well. Lid retraction results in apparent but not in actual protrusion of the eyes (proptosis) and is often accompanied by symptoms of conjunctival irritation. Lid lag is a common but less reliable finding. Infiltrative ophthalmopathy is discussed in the section on Extrathyroidal Manifestations of Graves' Disease.

Thyroid Gland

Thyroid enlargement of some type is common. It may be the initial or only clue to the presence of thyrotoxicosis, and it usually indicates its cause. In Graves' disease, both thyroid lobes are usually diffusely and more or less symmetrically enlarged; the right lobe tends to be slightly larger, as it is in normal subjects. The goiter is usually moderate; that is, the thyroid is two to four times enlarged (average 30–60 ml).[437,438] It tends to be larger in younger patients, but about 30 percent of all patients do not have a goiter.[439] The thyroid is sometimes slightly tender, its consistency varies from soft to firm, and the surface is usually smooth, although it can be irregular or lobulated. There may be a thyroid bruit or thrill caused by greatly increased thyroid blood flow.

Painless and postpartum thyroiditis usually results in slight diffuse thyroid enlargement; the thyroid is larger and tender in subacute thyroiditis. Toxic multinodular goiters tend to be large, asymmetric, and uneven in consistency; a few extend below the sternum or are largely substernal. A thyroid adenoma causing thyrotoxicosis is usually at least 3 cm in diameter, and no other thyroid tissue should be palpable.

Nervous System and Muscle

Most thyrotoxic patients have symptoms of central nervous system dysfunction. Common complaints are nervousness, physical hyperactivity, emotional lability, anxiety, and irritability. Lability of mood is often striking; these patients are easily angered and prone to episodes of anxiety or even paranoia. They often are restless, are unable to remain still for any length of time, and sleep fitfully. Their ability to concentrate decreases, and complaints of memory loss are common. Objective testing may show some impairment of cognitive function. These changes often result in impairment of work or school performance and disturbances in home and family life. Most of the patients are aware of these changes, but their extent often becomes more clear when a family member or friend is interviewed. At the other extreme, apathy, depression, and withdrawal may occur in older patients. These striking clinical findings occur in the absence of gross abnormalities of cerebral oxygen consumption or substrate utilization.

The most prominent neuromuscular symptoms are tremor and muscle weakness. The tremor is usually limited to the hands and fingers and is most evident when the hands are extended, but it may involve the arms, legs, tongue, and head. The movements are rapid and uniform and of low amplitude. Performance of skills requiring fine coordination, such as threading a needle and writing, may become difficult. The pathophysiology of the thyrotoxic tremor is unclear. It is not a manifestation of muscle weakness, although that may aggravate it, and it is decreased by propranolol and other beta-adrenergic antagonist drugs. Rare patients have choreiform movements rather than tremor.

Most thyrotoxic patients have muscle weakness, and in some it is the predominant complaint (thyrotoxic myopathy). It usually develops gradually and varies from mild to severe; it is due to both muscle wasting and decreased efficiency of muscle contraction.[440] The strength and endurance of both proximal and distal muscles are decreased, thus causing difficulty in reaching above the head, rising from a lying or sitting position, and gripping objects.[441] Deep tendon reflexes are hyperactive, with both contraction and relaxation phases being accelerated despite the muscle weakness, and unsustained clonus may be present. The myopathy can also involve the respiratory and oropharyngeal musculature, causing difficulty in swallowing or hoarseness. Ophthalmoplegia, most commonly limitation of upward gaze, may occur but is a manifestation of infiltrative ophthalmopathy rather than extraocular muscle weakness caused by thyrotoxicosis. Serum concentrations of creatine kinase and myoglobin are normal or low.

A syndrome of periodic muscle weakness that is clinically and pathophysiologically very similar to familial hypokalemic periodic paralysis occurs in occasional patients with thyrotoxicosis. The attacks of paralysis may be the first manifestation of thyrotoxicosis. Nearly all the patients are men, and most are Asian.[442,443] As in hypokalemic periodic paralysis, the attacks may follow exercise or may be induced by food or alcohol ingestion. The weakness improves in response to therapy with potassium and also propranolol. The attacks invariably cease after antithyroid treatment. These patients have no family history of periodic paralysis.

Cardiovascular System

Heart rate, cardiac contractility, stroke volume, and cardiac output are all increased in thyrotoxicosis, and peripheral resistance is decreased.[107,444] These changes are due both to direct inotropic and chronotropic effects of thyroid hormone and to an increased need for peripheral oxygen delivery. Although cardiac output is increased, regional blood flow is not uniformly increased; skin, muscle, cerebral, and coronary flow are increased, whereas hepatic flow is not. Another adaptive mechanism augmenting peripheral oxygen delivery is an increase in red blood cell mass.[445]

These changes in cardiovascular function may result in palpitations, tachycardia, atrial fibrillation and other atrial arrhythmias, exertional dyspnea and impaired exercise capacity, and congestive heart failure. The pulse pressure is increased, arterial pulsations are bounding, and systolic hypertension may be present. Patients with angina pectoris may have an increase in the frequency of chest pain, or it may first appear as the patient becomes thyrotoxic. Examination of the heart reveals a prominent apical impulse, accentuated heart sounds, systolic ejection or other murmurs, and occasionally cardiac enlargement. A jugular venous hum may be heard. Other than disturbances of rhythm, electrocardiographic changes are limited to nonspecific ST- and T-wave abnormalities. Noninvasive studies reveal shortened systolic and diastolic time intervals, increased systolic and diastolic function, increased ventricular mass, and reduction in the left ventricular ejection fraction during exercise.[107,444,446]

Atrial fibrillation occurs in a substantial fraction of patients with thyrotoxicosis (Table 9-13). Most are elderly, and in them it may be the sole manifestation of thyrotoxicosis; conversely, among patients with lone atrial fibrillation from 0 to 5 percent have overt or subclinical thyrotoxicosis.[107,444,447,448] With antithyroid therapy, the atrial fibrillation spontaneously reverts to sinus rhythm in about 60 percent.[449] Whether the risk of systemic embolization is increased is uncertain.[450,451]

Thyrotoxicosis can cause congestive heart failure. Most of the patients have had intrinsic heart disease; their cardiac function decompensated because of vasodilatation, increased blood volume, and rhythm-related decreases in diastolic filling. It can occur, however, often in association with atrial fibrillation, in younger patients who have no evidence of cardiac disease when studied after treatment. Dynamic studies in these patients have shown higher systemic vascular resistance both at rest and during exercise compared with patients with no cardiac symptoms, normal or increased cardiac output that does not change or decreases during exercise, and cardiac dilatation (dilated cardiomyopathy).[452,453]

Respiratory Function

Abnormalities in respiratory function described in thyrotoxicosis include decreased vital capacity, decreased pulmonary compliance, and increased minute ventilation.[454,455] Alveolar and arterial oxygen and carbon dioxide content and airway resistance are usually normal, although thyrotoxicosis can aggravate asthma.[456] Ventilatory responses to hypoxemia or hypercapnia are increased. Dyspnea during exercise is a common symptom and is probably multifactorial, caused by respiratory muscle weakness, decreased lung compliance, increased ventilation, and cardiac dysfunction.

Renal Function and Fluid and Electrolyte Metabolism

Renal blood flow, glomerular filtration rate, and renal tubular reabsorptive and secretory capacities are increased, but sodium balance and serum electrolyte concentrations are normal.[457] Plasma volume is increased. As a consequence, serum atrial natriuretic hormone concentrations are increased and aldosterone secretion is decreased. Notwithsanding the increase in plasma volume, plasma renin activity is often increased, probably as a result of adrenergic stimulation.[458] Renin, aldosterone, and renal responses to sodium restriction and volume expansion are normal.[459]

Polydipsia and polyuria may be prominent symptoms.[460] They are caused by an increase in thirst, and therefore serum osmolality tends to be low. An increase in thirst is not surprising in view of the heat sensitivity and physical and emotional lability that so often occur. Urine concentrating ability may be impaired after both dehydration and vasopressin administration.

Gastrointestinal System

The major abnormality in gastrointestinal function is more rapid small and large intestinal transit.[461] The most common symptom is increased frequency of bowel movements; in one study of 168 patients with thyrotoxicosis 45 percent had more than one bowel movement daily, as compared with 16 percent of normal subjects.[462] Some patients have steatorrhea[463]; absorption of most other nutrients is normal unless hypermotility is marked. Occasional patients have nausea, vomiting, or abdominal pain, possibly as a result of gastric stasis or chemoreceptor activation.[464]

Some abnormalities in hepatic function are found in the majority of patients. These include small increases in serum alanine and aspartate aminotransferase, alkaline phosphatase, and bilirubin concentrations; occasionally jaundice is clinically evident.[465] Liver histology is normal or shows mild hepatocellular injury.

Hematopoietic System

Both red cell mass and plasma volume tend to be increased, with the increase in plasma volume predominating.[445] Thus, some patients have a modest reduction in hematocrit and hemoglobin values, and their red cells tend to be small.[466] Red cell survival is normal or slightly shortened. Serum vitamin B_{12}, folate, and iron concentrations and iron stores may be low. Iron clearance and serum erythropoetin concentrations tend to be increased. The bone marrow shows erythroid hyperplasia and occasionally megaloblastic changes. These findings, which are indicative of increased iron utilization and increased red cell production, are the expected responses to the need for increased peripheral oxygen delivery. A few patients are truly anemic, as a result of deficiency of one or more hematopoietic nutrients. About 1 percent of patients with Graves' disease have pernicious anemia, although not necessarily in a close chronologic relation to their thyroid disease, and parietal-cell antibodies are found in about 10 percent.

Granulocyte and lymphocyte counts are usually normal, although some patients have mild lymphocytosis or granulocytopenia.[466–468] Lymphadenopathy, thymic enlargement, and splenomegaly are rare findings; whether they are manifestations of thyrotoxicosis per se or of Graves' disease is not clear. Serum concentrations of several adhesion molecules and interleukins, soluble interleukin receptors and soluble Fas are increased in patients with thyrotoxicosis; most of these studies were done in patients with Graves' disease, but some included patients with other causes of thyrotoxicosis.[469–473]

Some patients with thyrotoxicosis have easy bruising and mild thrombocytopenia; their platelets contain increased amounts of IgG and platelet aggregation is impaired.[474,475]

Energy, Nutrient, and Drug Metabolism

A major consequence of thyrotoxicosis is increased energy expenditure, and maintenance of basic physiologic functions and mechanical work are less efficient than normal. To counterbalance these changes, food intake, utilization of stored energy, and oxygen consumption all increase, with an attendant increase in heat production, manifested clinically by heat intolerance. Increases in appetite and food intake are therefore a very common feature of thyrotoxicosis. In most of the patients, however, compensation is inadequate and some weight loss occurs; both fat and lean body mass are lost.[476] The loss in weight averages 15 percent of initial weight, but the variation is large.[477] Weight loss tends to be greater in elderly patients and those who are obese. By contrast, in some young patients the increase in appetite and food intake is sufficient to cause modest weight gain; these patients probably eat to satisfy emotional needs.

Major changes occur in the metabolism of carbohydrate, lipid, and protein. The absorption of glucose is increased, as is gluconeogenesis and glycogenolysis.[112–114] Peripheral insulin sensitivity is normal or decreased, and hepatic insulin sensitivity may be decreased.[478] Hepatic glucose production and muscle, adipose tissue, and splanchnic glucose utilization are increased.[113] In animals thyrotoxicosis increases the GLUT-4 content of muscle and adipose tissue. Serum glucose and insulin responses to an oral glucose load are usually normal, but oral glucose tolerance is impaired and insulin secretory responses are inadequate in some patients.[479] Thus, thyrotoxicosis, like pregnancy and Cushing's syndrome, may uncover insulin secretory deficiency. In patients with preexisting diabetes mellitus, requirements for exogenous insulin increase because of accelerated insulin catabolism.[480]

The decrease in fat mass is accompanied by a fall in serum leptin concentrations, so that the usual relationship between them is preserved.[481,482] Lipolysis is increased, so that serum fatty acid concentrations rise, leading to an increase in ketoacid production.[110] Both the synthesis and the clearance of cholesterol are increased in thyrotoxicosis, the latter more than the former. This probably results from an increase in low-density lipoprotein (LDL) receptors. Thus, modest reductions in serum total and LDL cholesterol concentrations are the usual findings; serum high-density lipoprotein (HDL) cholesterol and lipoprotein(a) concentrations may be reduced as well.[483,484] Serum triglyceride concentrations are usually normal. Hepatic lipase activity is increased, but lipoprotein lipase activity is normal.

Protein synthesis and catabolism are also increased, the latter more than the former.[476] The net overall result is excessive protein catabolism, resulting in loss of muscle mass, negative nitrogen balance, and increased urinary amino acid excretion. Serum concentrations of proteins secreted by the liver—for example, albumin, TBG,

TTR, and some other transport proteins—are normal or slightly low. An exception is sex hormone-binding globulin. Its production is stimulated by T_3 and T_4, and serum sex hormone-binding globulin concentrations are high in thyrotoxic patients.[485,486] The serum concentrations of proteins of endothelial origin, such as fibronectin, von Willebrand factor, and angiotensin-converting enzyme, also are high.[487]

The metabolism and clearance of some drugs, including digoxin and propranolol, are increased in thyrotoxic patients, and so higher doses may be needed.[488] By contrast, thyrotoxic patients may need less warfarin, because the clearance of vitamin K-dependent clotting factors or plasma binding of warfarin is decreased.[489] The metabolism of methimazole and PTU is normal.

Endocrine System

Pituitary Hormone Secretion

Linear growth in children with thyrotoxicosis may be increased. In adults, mean 24-h serum growth hormone (GH) concentrations and growth hormone secretion rates may be increased[490]; serum GH responses to growth hormone–releasing hormone or other stimuli are normal or decreased.[491] High, normal, and low serum insulin-like growth factor-I concentrations have been reported in different studies[491,492]; the conflicting results may be due to differences in assay methods, patient nutritional status, or control subjects.

Serum prolactin concentrations are normal or slightly low.[493]

Adrenal Function

Thyrotoxicosis results in an acceleration of cortisol clearance. As a result, ACTH secretion, the number of cortisol secretory episodes, the cortisol secretion rate, and urinary 17-hydroxycorticosteroid excretion are increased.[494] Serum cortisol concentrations and urinary cortisol excretion are normal, as are serum cortisol responses to ACTH and hypoglycemia. The development of thyrotoxicosis, however, can unmask subclinical adrenal insufficiency by causing more rapid clearance of cortisol.

Serum concentrations and secretion rates of epinephrine and norepinephrine are normal.[115]

Gonadal Function

In children sexual maturation may be delayed, perhaps caused by slow gain (or loss) of weight and adipose mass. Menstrual cycles are normal in most women with thyrotoxicosis; in a study of 214 women 22 percent had some menstrual dysfunction, most commonly regular cycles with decreased flow or amenorrhea.[495] An increase in serum sex hormone-binding globulin concentrations results in increased serum total estradiol and estrone concentrations but low-normal or low serum free estradiol and estrone concentrations.[486,496] Serum luteinizing hormone (LH) and follicle-stimulating hormone (FSH) concentrations are slightly increased during most of the cycle, probably because serum free estrogen concentrations are low. The midcycle serum LH and FSH peaks are subnormal in both regularly and irregularly cycling women with thyrotoxicosis, but these peaks usually are followed by increases in serum progesterone, indicating that the cycles were ovulatory.[496] Thus, infertility should occur only in women with amenorrhea. In postmenopausal women, serum LH and FSH concentrations are appropriately elevated.

In men, thyrotoxicosis results in erectile dysfunction and occasionally loss of libido and gynecomastia. Sperm density and motility may be decreased.[497] Serum sex hormone-binding globulin concentrations are increased, resulting in high serum total testosterone concentrations; serum free testosterone concentrations are normal.[486,497,498] Extragonadal conversion of androgen to estrogen is increased, resulting in high serum total and free estradiol concentrations. The high serum estradiol concentrations cause the gynecomastia and seminiferous tubule dysfunction and may increase LH and FSH secretion slightly.

Bone-Parathyroid-Vitamin D System

Thyrotoxicosis results in bone loss by directly stimulating osteoclastic bone resorption. Bone formation increases secondarily, but less than bone resorption. Thus, both serum osteocalcin and bone-specific alkaline phosphatase concentrations, markers of increased bone formation, and urinary pyridinoline and deoxypyridinoline excretion, markers of bone resorption, are increased.[499,500] Cortical and to a lesser extent trabecular bone density may be low, and increase during and after antithyroid therapy to normal or nearly so.[501,502] Present or past thyrotoxicosis may be a risk factor for hip fracture in older women.[503] Thyroid hormone-induced bone loss can be prevented by administration of a bisphosphonate.[504]

Occasional patients have mild hypercalcemia due to the increase in bone resorption[505]; another cause should be sought if the hypercalcemia is severe. Serum phosphate concentrations are usually normal. The excess skeletal calcium mobilization inhibits parathyroid hormone secretion. Serum parathyroid hormone concentrations are therefore low, resulting in low serum 1,25-dihydroxycholecalciferol concentrations and low gastrointestinal calcium absorption.[506] Serum 25-hydroxyvitamin D concentrations are usually normal, but might be low in patients with marked nutritional deficiency or steatorrhea.

Laboratory Diagnosis of Thyrotoxicosis

The biochemical hallmarks of thyrotoxicosis are high serum total and free T_4 and T_3 concentrations and low serum TSH concentrations (Fig. 9-17). The correlation between the clinical and biochemical severity of thyrotoxicosis is poor,[507] and therefore judgment of its severity should be based on clinical findings.

Serum Thyrotropin Concentrations

Serum TSH concentrations are low not only in nearly all patients with thyrotoxicosis but also, by definition, in patients with subclinical thyrotoxicosis (Fig. 9-17). Many of the latter have some autonomous thyroid secretion or are receiving T_4 therapy, but others have no evident thyroid disease and may not have persistently low serum TSH concentrations (see section on Subclinical Thyrotoxicosis).[129,130] The serum TSH concentrations in patients with overt thyrotoxicosis are usually lower than in those with subclinical thyrotoxicosis. Serum TSH concentrations may also be low in patients with nonthyroidal illness or central hypothyroidism. The only patients with high serum free T_4 values who have normal or high serum TSH concentrations are those with familial dysalbuminemic hyperthyroxinemia, TSH-dependent thyrotoxicosis, or generalized resistance to thyroid hormone.

Serum Thyroxine and Triiodothyronine Concentrations

Serum total and free T_4 concentrations and free T_4 index values are high in most patients with thyrotoxicosis. Because serum total T_4 concentrations are high in many other patients (Table 9-9), confirmation of the diagnosis of thyrotoxicosis must be based on the finding of a high serum free T_4 index or free T_4 concentration. Even a high serum free T_4 value is not a completely specific indicator of thyrotoxicosis; serum free T_4 index values are high in patients with familial dysalbuminemic hyperthyroxinemia, and both serum free T_4 index values and serum free T_4 concentrations are high in patients with generalized resistance to thyroid hormone and some patients with nonthyroidal illness. Among patients with Graves' thyrotoxicosis serum T_4 (and T_3) concentrations tend to be higher in younger than older patients, presumably because younger patients tolerate the effects of increased thyroid secretion better.[508]

Serum total (and free) T_3 concentrations also are high in most patients with thyrotoxicosis. The values usually are more abnormal than are serum T_4 values, especially in younger patients. Serum T_3 measurements thus may help confirm or exclude a suspected diagnosis of thyrotoxicosis in patients who have serum T_4 and free T_4 index values within the normal range (T_3 thyrotoxicosis), and their principal value is for this purpose. Among thyrotoxic patients with similar serum T_4 concentrations, serum T_3 concentrations tend to be higher in those with thyroid hypersecretion, as compared with those with thyroid inflammation, probably because thyroidal and peripheral deiodinase activity is not increased in the latter.[509] Increases in serum TBG concentrations raise serum T_3 concentrations just as they raise those of T_4. Serum T_3, but not T_4, concentrations can be high in euthyroid or thyrotoxic patients who are taking T_3 or desiccated thyroid.

Conversely, some patients with thyrotoxicosis, especially elderly patients, have high serum T_4 but normal serum T_3 concentrations (T_4 thyrotoxicosis).[18,318] Its occurrence provides evidence that impaired extrathyroidal conversion of T_4 to T_3 caused by nonthyroidal illness or drugs (notably amiodarone) can impair extrathyroidal T_3 production even in thyrotoxic patients. In other patients with nonthyroidal illnesses, serum T_4 concentrations may be high and serum T_3 concentrations may be normal or low initially, but both return to normal during recovery (see section on Nonthyroidal Illness).

Thyroid Radioiodine Uptake and Imaging

Thyroid radioiodine uptake is increased in most patients with thyrotoxicosis because they have hyperthyroidism (thyroid gland hyperfunction). The exceptions are patients with subacute thyroiditis, painless thyroiditis, and exogenous thyrotoxicosis, in whom radioiodine uptake is low. Among thyrotoxic patients, thyroid radioiodine uptake measurements are indicated only to distinguish between Graves' disease and painless thyroiditis, and to confirm a suspected diagnosis of exogenous thyrotoxicosis when thyroid hormone ingestion is denied by the patient.

Thyroid radionuclide scans may be helpful in identifying a thyroid adenoma or multinodular goiter as a cause of thyrotoxicosis. In patients with diffuse thyroid enlargement, this test provides little information beyond that provided by careful palpation of the thyroid gland.

Thyrotropin Receptor-Stimulating and Other Thyroid Antibodies

Tests for TSH receptor-stimulating antibodies are not tests of thyroid function in the usual sense, but if positive serve to confirm the presence of Graves' disease as the cause of thyrotoxicosis.[319,323,324,326] However, that a thyrotoxic patient has Graves' disease is usually obvious, based on history and physical examination. Furthermore, the tests have technical limitations, and they are expensive and not widely available (nor are the results rapidly available). The use of TSH receptor-stimulating antibody assays in patients receiving antithyroid drug therapy is discussed in the section on Treatment of Thyrotoxicosis and their use in pregnant women is discussed in the section on Thyrotoxicosis during Pregnancy.

Antithyroid peroxidase antibodies are a sensitive marker of thyroid autoimmune disease, and can be measured as a surrogate for TSH receptor-stimulating antibodies. Thus, in a patient with thyrotoxicosis a high serum antithyroid peroxidase antibody concentration is strong evidence that the patient has Graves' disease.[137,508,510] Serum antithyroid peroxidase antibodies should be measured in preference to TSH receptor-stimulating antibodies in the uncommon instances in which any antibody test is indicated, for example in a patient with a relatively short duration of thyrotoxicosis, a small goiter, and no extrathyroidal manifestations of Graves' disease, who could have painless thyroiditis.

Thyrotropin-Releasing Hormone Stimulation Test

Serum TSH concentrations increase promptly after the intravenous administration of TRH in normal subjects. In thyrotoxicosis, the inhibition of TSH secretion resulting from T_4 and T_3 overproduction is accompanied by subnormal or absent serum TSH responses to TRH.[53] This is a sensitive test of pituitary suppression, but no more so than measurement of basal serum TSH (Fig. 9-18).

Summary: Laboratory Diagnosis of Thyrotoxicosis

A scheme for the evaluation of patients with suspected thyrotoxicosis is shown in Fig. 9-28. The initial step should be measurements of serum TSH and serum free T_4, either as the serum free T_4 index or serum free T_4 concentration. If the serum free T_4 value is high and the serum TSH concentration is low, the diagnosis of thyrotoxicosis is confirmed and no further tests are needed. If the serum free T_4 value is normal and the serum TSH concentration is low, the patient may have T_3 thyrotoxicosis or subclinical thyrotoxicosis. These two possibilities can be distinguished by measurement of serum T_3.

A high serum free T_4 index value and a normal serum TSH concentration indicate the presence of familial dysalbuminemic hyperthyroxinemia, TSH-dependent thyrotoxicosis, or generalized resistance to thyroid hormone. The first is probably the most common of these disorders, but all are rare. Among them, only TSH hypersecretion results in thyrotoxicosis. Patients with familial dysalbuminemic hyperthyroxinemia are euthyroid, and the diagnosis can be confirmed by finding a normal or nearly normal serum T_3 concentration, a low THBR if labeled T_4 instead of labeled T_3 is used in the test, and high serum free T_4 index values and serum T_4 concentrations and normal serum TSH concentrations in family members. Generalized resistance to thyroid hormone is discussed in the section on Hypothyroidism.

Other Laboratory Manifestations of Thyrotoxicosis or Diseases Causing Thyrotoxicosis

Many other physiologic, biochemical, and serologic abnormalities may be found in patients with thyrotoxicosis. Some result from excessive thyroid hormone action in tissues, and others reflect the various diseases that cause thyrotoxicosis. The most sen-

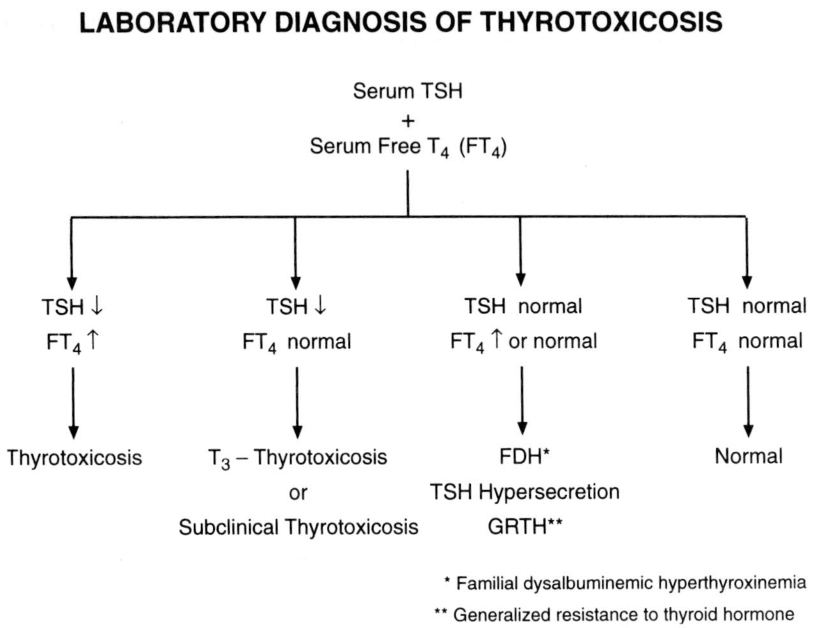

FIGURE 9-28. Diagnostic scheme for the evaluation of patients with suspected thyrotoxicosis. In familial dysalbuminemic hyperthyroxinemia, serum free T_4 values are normal if measured directly and high if measured as the serum free T_4 index. Some patients with TSH hypersecretion have high serum TSH concentrations.

sitive tests of tissue thyroid hormone action are probably measurements of cardiac rate and contractility and of serum sex hormone-binding globulin.

Tests indicative of thyroid disease include measurements of serum thyroglobulin and antithyroid antibodies. Serum thyroglobulin concentrations are high in most patients with thyrotoxicosis, except those in whom it is due to exogenous thyroid hormone administration. Serum antithyroid peroxidase antibody concentrations are high in most patients with Graves' disease, as noted previously, as are serum antithyroglobulin antibody concentrations.

Treatment of Thyrotoxicosis

The major treatments available for patients with thyrotoxicosis are listed in Table 9-14. The ideal treatment would be elimination of its cause so that the thyrotoxicosis disappears and normal pituitary-thyroid function is restored. However, for most patients, the fundamental cause of their thyrotoxicosis is not known and no truly curative treatment is available. All the available treatments ameliorate if not eliminate the symptoms and signs of thyrotoxicosis.

The following sections deal with the treatment of thyrotoxicosis caused by Graves' disease, painless (or postpartum) thyroiditis, thyroid adenoma, or multinodular goiter. The treatment of most of the rarer causes of thyrotoxicosis listed in Table 9-11 is obvious; for example discontinuing iodine therapy in patients with iodine-induced thyrotoxicosis or transsphenoidal surgery in those with a TSH-secreting pituitary tumor. For patients with any of these causes of thyrotoxicosis, concomitant therapy with drugs that decrease thyroidal production of T_4 and T_3 or drugs that ameliorate the clinical manifestations of thyrotoxicosis may be beneficial before or during more specific and permanent therapy. The considerations pertaining to the use of these drugs are the same as when they are given to patients with Graves' thyrotoxicosis, as discussed later.

TABLE 9-14. The Major Forms of Therapy for Thyrotoxicosis

Treatment of the cause of thyrotoxicosis
Antithyroid therapy
Drugs
Methimazole (carbimazole)
Propylthiouracil
Inorganic iodine
Radioactive iodine (^{131}I)
Subtotal thyroidectomy
Amelioration of thyroid hormone action
Beta-adrenergic antagonist drugs

Not all patients with overt thyrotoxicosis need treatment. In particular, it is not needed when the thyrotoxicosis is mild and can be expected to subside soon, for example, in patients with subacute thyroiditis or painless thyroiditis.

Thyrotoxicosis Caused by Graves' Disease

An antithyroid drug and radioactive iodine (^{131}I) are the two best treatments for patients with Graves' thyrotoxicosis. Both are effective, safe, and relatively inexpensive. They are treatments for hyperthyroidism rather than for Graves' disease itself, although antithyroid drugs may also have immunosuppressive actions.

The major reason to choose antithyroid drug therapy is that a spontaneous remission or at least substantial improvement of Graves' disease may occur during treatment, so that the patient remains euthyroid after it is discontinued (Fig. 9-25). Among patients treated with an antithyroid drug for one year or longer, from 30 to 70 percent (and occasionally more) have complete or partial remissions of Graves' disease, meaning that they remain euthyroid for months or years after the drug is discontinued.[468,511–526] Some clinical and treatment factors that have been associated with remissions in these or other studies are older age, recent onset, little or no thyroid enlargement, mild or moderate clinical or biochemical severity of thyrotoxicosis, low serum concentrations of TSH receptor-stimulating antibodies or other antithyroid antibodies, longer duration of treatment, higher doses of antithyroid drug, and concomitant antithyroid drug and T_4 therapy. However, in nearly

TABLE 9-15. Comparison of Features of Antithyroid Drug and ^{131}I Therapy for Hyperthyroidism Caused by Graves' Disease

	Drug Therapy	^{131}I
Dosage	Daily	Single dose
Initial response	2–6 weeks	8–12 weeks
Side effects*	Uncommon	Rare
Hypothyroidism	Uncommon	Common
Therapy inadequate	Uncommon	Rare
Need for chronic or repeated courses of therapy	Common	Rare
Change in size of thyroid	No change or decrease	Decrease
Appearance or worsening of ophthalmopathy	Rarely	Occasionally
Long-term outcome	Euthyroidism or hyperthyroidism	Hypothyroidism
Outcome dependent on continued production of TSH receptor-stimulating antibodies	Yes	No
Use during pregnancy	Acceptable	Never

* Toxic drug effects and radiation thyroiditis.

all instances the data are conflicting, and there is little agreement on the importance of any of these factors.[527]

The uncertainty concerning remission does not apply to ^{131}I therapy, because it is destructive. The hazards and expense of subtotal thyroidectomy are greater than are those of either an antithyroid drug or ^{131}I, and it is rarely indicated as primary therapy in patients of any age. The overall cost of antithyroid drug and ^{131}I therapy is roughly comparable,[528,529] but is likely to vary more among antithyroid drug-treated patients. In a Swedish study in which the patients had been randomly assigned to antithyroid drug, ^{131}I, or surgical therapy the time lost from work and overall satisfaction with treatment were similar in the three groups.[530]

The choice between an antithyroid drug and ^{131}I therapy depends on several practical and theoretical considerations. A comparison of their features is shown in Table 9-15. Antithyroid drug therapy is more rapidly effective, does not cause permanent thyroid damage, is safe, and may not have to be given indefinitely. For these reasons, an antithyroid drug is the initial treatment of choice for children and adults of all ages. If a remission does not occur and the patient tires of taking medication, or if the thyrotoxicosis is difficult to control or the drug has to be discontinued because of side effects, then ^{131}I can always be given. ^{131}I therapy is simple and safe, but is not as rapidly effective and nearly always results in hypothyroidism.

The two treatments are viewed differently by physicians and probably also patients in different countries. Antithyroid drug therapy is preferred for the "average" patient with Graves' thyrotoxicosis in Europe, Japan, and South America, whereas ^{131}I therapy is preferred in the United States.[531,532] No matter how effective either is as treatment for thyrotoxicosis, indefinite follow-up is necessary to ensure that the thyrotoxicosis does not recur, that hypothyroidism has not developed, or, if it has, that T_4 replacement therapy is continued. Whatever the physician's preference, the recommendation must be acceptable to the patient.

Antithyroid Drugs

Methimazole and Propylthiouracil

The antithyroid drugs used in the United States are methimazole (MMI) and propylthiouracil (PTU). In Europe, carbimazole, which is equipotent and rapidly metabolized to MMI, is often used instead of MMI. These drugs inhibit thyroid hormone biosynthesis by inhibiting the oxidation and organification of iodine and the coupling of iodotyrosines, reactions that are catalyzed by thyroid peroxidase.[10] PTU also inhibits the thyroidal and extrathyroidal conversion of T_4 to T_3.[79,285] Both MMI and PTU are absorbed rapidly and nearly completely from the gastrointestinal tract, and peak serum concentrations are reached about 1 hour after their ingestion.[533] MMI is metabolized more slowly than is PTU; the serum half-life of MMI is 4–6 hours, whereas that of PTU is 1–2 hours. Both drugs are concentrated in the thyroid, and intrathyroidal concentrations, especially of MMI, remain high for considerably longer than do serum concentrations.[534] The drugs are metabolized by reactions catalyzed by thyroid peroxidase, and they are less effective when iodine intake and intrathyroidal iodine stores are plentiful.[535]

MMI and PTU have immunosuppressive actions that may contribute to the occurrence of remissions of Graves' disease. Both drugs reduce the number of intrathyroidal T cells and inhibit lymphocyte function, including thyroid autoantibody production, in vitro, although the latter actions require very high concentrations.[536] In some drug-treated patients serum concentrations of TSH receptor-stimulating antibodies or other antibodies decline more rapidly than do serum T_4 and T_3 concentrations, and antithyroid drug-treated patients have remissions more often than do patients treated with propranolol, but in only a minority of studies were patients treated with high doses more likely to have a remission than those treated with lower doses.[468,516,517,519,524,527] Rather than having direct immunosuppressive actions, it is more likely that the drug-induced decreases in T_4 and T_3 production reduce the intensity of thyroid-cell activation of the immune system.[342,537]

The initial goal of antithyroid drug therapy is to inhibit thyroidal T_4 and T_3 synthesis almost completely. Even if this is achieved, release of intrathyroidal hormone stores, which may be substantial, continues until they are depleted. For most patients, the most appropriate therapy is MMI, given initially in a single daily dose of 15 to 20 mg per day. Divided doses or higher doses of MMI are only slightly more effective, and it is more rapidly effective than 10 or 20 times higher doses of PTU.[535,538–541] In a study of 420 patients in Europe, 42 percent of those treated with 10 mg MMI daily were euthyroid in 3 weeks and 77 percent were euthyroid in 6 weeks, as compared with 65 percent and 93 percent, respectively, of those treated with 40 mg MMI daily.[535] The usual initial dose of PTU should be 300–450 mg per day, given in two or three divided doses until the patient is euthyroid.[541] Higher daily doses, for example 30 mg of MMI or 600 mg of PTU, should be given to patients with severe clinical thyrotoxicosis, a large goiter, or both.

The greater potency of MMI is due to its greater accumulation and slower metabolism in thyroid tissue, and its greater potency as an inhibitor of thyroid peroxidase. In addition to its greater potency and more prolonged action, which allows once-daily administration in most patients,[535,538–540] MMI has other advantages. It is available in 5- and 10-mg tablets, whereas PTU is available only in 50-mg tablets, so that fewer tablets need be given at any one time. MMI proved superior in studies in which both drugs were compared,[541] it may have fewer adverse effects than PTU, and its adverse effects are more clearly dose-related, as described later.

Failure of antithyroid drug therapy to control thyrotoxicosis effectively may result from inadequate dosage or poor compliance with treatment, usually the latter.[542] Poor compliance can be minimized by careful explanation of the need for therapy and its goals to the patient, by prescribing once daily therapy, and by avoiding other drugs, so that the treatment regimen is simple. In some patients, thyrotoxicosis persists and the thyroid may enlarge further despite a fall in serum T_4 concentrations; these patients have persistently high serum TSH receptor-stimulating antibody and T_3 concentrations.[543] They do become euthyroid when the dose of antithyroid drug is increased, but they are unlikely to have a remission.

The patient should be reevaluated 4–6 weeks after the initiation of therapy. Some clinical and biochemical improvement is usually apparent after a week or two, and it is usually substantial after 4 to 6 weeks, especially in patients treated with MMI; many patients treated with MMI have normal serum T_4 and T_3 concentrations by this time.[535,538–540] If considerable improvement has occurred, the dose of antithyroid drug should be reduced by 25 to 50 percent. Further follow-up visits should take place at about 8-week intervals. Once the patient has become euthyroid, the goal of continued therapy is partial rather than complete inhibition of thyroid hormone biosynthesis so that hypothyroidism does not occur. Biochemical monitoring during the early months of therapy should be done by measuring serum T_4, because serum TSH concentrations remain low for several months after the initiation of antithyroid drug therapy, even if thyroid secretion falls to below normal levels, because of prior suppression of TSH secretion. One problem with antithyroid drug (and ^{131}I) treatment is that patients not only regain weight that was lost, but also gain more weight (or gain weight if they had not lost it), presumably because their appetite does not decrease as much as their energy expenditure.[477,544]

Several programs for long-term antithyroid drug therapy have been advocated. One is treatment with gradually decreasing doses, with the goal of discontinuing the drug as soon as possible. As improvement occurs, the dose of antithyroid drug is gradually reduced at approximately 8-week intervals. If the patient remains euthyroid for 8 weeks while taking 5 mg MMI or 50 mg PTU daily, the drug should be discontinued. It may be possible to discontinue treatment in as little as 4 to 6 months with such a regimen. If thyrotoxicosis recurs after the dose is reduced or the drug is discontinued, remission obviously has not occurred and the dose should be increased or treatment resumed until the patient again becomes euthyroid, at which time the dose may again be reduced. In such a pragmatic program, decisions are made largely on clinical grounds, supported when necessary during the early months of therapy by serum T_4 and less often serum TSH determinations; later, serum TSH determinations alone are sufficient. Figure 9-29 shows the results of this type of program in a patient treated with MMI who remained euthyroid after it was discontinued. A variation of this program is to continue the initial dose of antithyroid drug until the patient is clinically and biochemically euthyroid, and then stop treatment. In the study describing this program, the mean duration of therapy was 4.8 months and the sustained remission rate was 29 percent.[545]

Another program consists of treatment for a fixed time period, usually 1–2 years. Such a program requires one or more reductions in dosage during the first several months of treatment. Treatment for 18 to 24 months results in higher rates of remission than treatment for short intervals,[511,514] but even longer intervals are not associated with further benefit.[545a] This latter program of treatment for a fixed interval, usually 1–2 years, is probably the most widely used,[531,532] but some patients are treated for longer than necessary.

Prevention of hypothyroidism and further thyroid enlargement during antithyroid drug therapy are best achieved by means of judicious reduction in drug dosage. Alternatively, T_4 can be added, but then higher doses of antithyroid drug are needed and it is harder to recognize when a remission may have occurred. The results of a 1991 study done in Japan suggested that addition of T_4 increased the likelihood of remission, perhaps by keeping serum TSH concentrations low and thereby minimizing expression of

FIGURE 9-29. Serum T_3 and T_4 concentrations in a patient with thyrotoxicosis caused by Graves' disease during and after treatment with methimazole. Note the prompt fall in serum hormone concentrations after the initiation of treatment and the lack of change after treatment was discontinued.

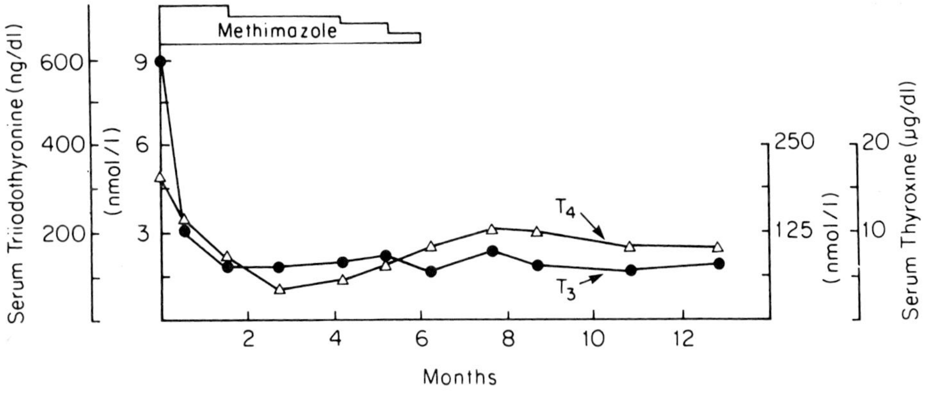

antigens on thyroid cells. Among a group of patients treated with MMI for 18 months and another group treated similarly with MMI plus 0.1 mg T_4 daily for 4 years, starting after MMI had been given for 6 months, the rates of recurrence after cessation of MMI were 37 and 2 percent, respectively.[515] However, in subsequent studies the recurrence rates were not lower among patients treated with an antithyroid drug plus T_4, as compared with the former alone.[518,520,521,525,526]

Tests proposed to determine if a patient has had a remission and therefore is likely to remain euthyroid after antithyroid drug treatment is discontinued include measurements of serum TSH receptor-stimulating antibodies or antithyroid peroxidase antibodies, serum TSH and T_3 responses to TRH stimulation, and thyroid radioiodine uptake after T_3 administration. The results of these tests tend to be normal or negative in patients who remain euthyroid after treatment is discontinued, and abnormal or positive in those who have recurrent thyrotoxicosis, but their predictive specificity and sensitivity is not high.[326,510]

Thus, whatever therapeutic program is used, it is simpler merely to discontinue the drug at the end of the initial treatment period and reexamine the patient in 6 to 8 weeks and subsequently less often if thyrotoxicosis does not recur. Many recurrences occur in the first few months after antithyroid drug therapy is discontinued, suggesting that Graves' disease had persisted, and most of the rest occur in the first two years.[513,523] The more delayed the recurrence, the more likely the patient had a true remission and then a second episode of Graves' disease. Patients with recurrent thyrotoxicosis who were previously treated effectively with low doses of an antithyroid drug may prefer to resume drug treatment, and some patients have been treated for many years.[546] However, many patients who have recurrent thyrotoxicosis choose ^{131}I therapy.

Adverse reactions to antithyroid drugs are uncommon, and probably occur with equal frequency with either MMI or PTU. Pruritis, urticaria or other rashes, arthralgia or myalgia, and fever occur in about 5 percent of patients taking either drug,[533] but at least for MMI are dose-dependent.[547] Both drugs may cause abnormal taste sensation. The most feared adverse effect is agranulocytosis [<500 granulocytes/mm^3 ($<0.5 \times 10^9$/liter)], occurring in 0.2 percent or less of patients.[548,549,549a] Very rare adverse effects include aplastic anemia, thrombocytopenia, hepatocellular (PTU) or cholestatic (MMI) hepatitis, a lupus-like vasculitis (PTU), and the insulin-autoimmune syndrome (MMI).[550–554] These adverse effects, which may be immunologic in origin, nearly always occur during the first three months of treatment, when the drug dose is higher, but they can occur later or during a subsequent course of therapy.[549] Agranulocytosis is more common in older patients and those taking higher doses (30–40 mg per day or more) of MMI, but there is no dose relation for PTU.[555,556] It usually develops rapidly, and precautionary white blood cell counts are generally thought not to be useful, although this view has been challenged.[557]

Patients must be warned about the symptoms of these adverse effects and instructed to discontinue therapy and contact the physician immediately if any symptoms occur. Hematologic, liver function, or bacteriologic studies may then be indicated. Pruritis, rash, arthralgia or myalgia, or fever may subside in a few days with no treatment, or with antihistamine or nonsteroidal anti-inflammatory drug treatment, and usually do not require discontinuation of the antithyroid drug.[547] It should be discontinued in patients in whom these adverse effects persist and those patients with any of the more serious adverse effects, including those in whom granulocyte counts fall substantially even though not to <500 cells/mm^3. All these adverse effects are reversible in nearly all patients. Patients with agranulocytosis and fever should be given antibiotic therapy and may need to be hospitalized; administration of granulocyte colony-stimulating factor provides little benefit.[558,559] Patients who have had a minor adverse effect of one antithyroid drug may be treated with another antithyroid drug, but those who have had more serious adverse effects should be treated with ^{131}I.

Inorganic Iodine

Inorganic iodine inhibits thyroid hormone secretion, primarily by inhibiting thyroglobulin proteolysis, and also inhibits thyroidal iodide transport, oxidation, and organification.[10] These actions require only a few milligrams of iodine daily, although it is usually given in far greater doses, such as 5 to 10 drops of a saturated solution of potassium iodide (about 50 mg iodide per drop) several times daily. The major limitation of inorganic iodine as an antithyroid drug is escape from its antithyroid actions. When it is given alone, serum T_4 and T_3 concentrations usually decrease by about 50 to 75 percent, reaching a nadir in 2 to 3 weeks, but may then increase.[287] Therefore, it should not be used as sole therapy. Inorganic iodine given after ^{131}I therapy results in more rapid amelioration of thyrotoxicosis, and escape does not occur. It also is often given in preparation for thyroidectomy, both for its antithyroid action and because it reduces thyroid blood flow. Inorganic iodine produced by the metabolism of organic iodine compounds has the same antithyroid actions.

There are three indications for inorganic iodine therapy: in preparation for subtotal thyroidectomy, for which it should be given for 7 to 10 days before surgery; in severe thyrotoxicosis or thyroid storm (see section on Thyroid Storm); and occasionally for several weeks or months in patients recently treated with ^{131}I. It is given in conjunction with an antithyroid drug in the first two situations and alone in the third.

Other Antithyroid Drugs

The oral cholecystographic agents sodium ipodate and iopanoic acid are iodine-rich compounds that are metabolized in part by deiodination. The iodide that is formed inhibits T_4 and T_3 secretion, and the intact compound inhibits extrathyroidal T_3 production.[79] Administration of either agent in doses of 0.5 or 1.0 g daily is therefore accompanied by prompt decreases in both serum T_4 and T_3 concentrations.[560,561] In the majority of patients, however, the benefit is not sustained and serum T_4 and T_3 concentrations do not become normal. Administration of one of these agents may be useful in the rare patients who cannot be treated with MMI, PTU, or ^{131}I.

Lithium carbonate has antithyroid actions similar to those of inorganic iodine, and has proved effective in doses of 300 mg three or four times daily.[562] Some escape from its actions occurs, and it has many side effects. It may nevertheless be useful in an occasional patient who cannot tolerate MMI or PTU and in whom ^{131}I therapy is planned but cannot be given immediately because of previous iodine exposure.

Cholestyramine binds T_4 and T_3 in the gastrointestinal tract, thus decreasing enterohepatic circulation of the two hormones. In patients with Graves' thyrotoxicosis, serum T_4 and T_3 concentrations fall slightly more rapidly in patients during treatment with MMI and cholestyramine as compared with MMI alone.[563]

Perchlorate is an inhibitor of thyroid iodide transport, and thus induces intrathyroidal iodine deficiency. Given in doses of 400 to 1000 mg daily, in conjunction with MMI, it has proven effective in patients with iodine-induced thyrotoxicosis, particularly patients in whom it is caused by amiodarone.[293]

Drugs Inhibiting Extrathyroidal T_3 Production

Drugs that inhibit extrathyroidal T_3 production decrease serum T_3 concentrations and therefore might be expected to ameliorate thyrotoxicosis. Although this is a reasonable expectation, there is little evidence that such amelioration occurs. Drugs that have both thyroidal and extrathyroidal actions, such as PTU and iopanoic acid, are little more effective clinically than is MMI, which acts only on the thyroid.

Propranolol and some beta-adrenergic antagonist drugs inhibit extrathyroidal T_4 conversion to T_3; high doses cause a 20–30 percent reduction in serum T_3 concentrations in 7 to 10 days.[284] This modest fall in serum T_3 concentrations does not explain the beneficial effects of propranolol in patients with thyrotoxicosis, and some other drugs of this class have similar clinical effects but do not lower serum T_3 concentrations.

Drugs Ameliorating Thyroid Hormone Action

The administration of propranolol, in doses of 40 to 160 mg daily in divided doses, long-acting propranolol in a dose of 60 or 80 mg daily, or more selective and long-acting beta-adrenergic antagonists such as atenolol, in a dose of 25 to 50 mg once daily, results in improvement in many of the common symptoms of thyrotoxicosis, including palpitations, increased perspiration and heat intolerance, nervousness, tremor, and weakness, within several days, but these symptoms do not disappear completely even during prolonged therapy.[284,358,564] The pulse rate slows, and myocardial contractility decreases. Nitrogen balance, oxygen consumption, and cardiac output improve but do not become normal. Thus, propranolol alone is an inadequate treatment for thyrotoxicosis, and it has no beneficial effect when given in conjunction with an antithyroid drug.[565] Other beta-adrenergic antagonist drugs have similar actions in thyrotoxic patients, although they differ in the degree of selectivity as beta-adrenergic antagonists and their duration of action. These variables are not known to be important, except that compliance may be better if a longer-acting drug is given.

Beta-adrenergic antagonist drugs should not be given routinely to patients treated with an antithyroid drug, but may be helpful in those with marked palpitations, hyperactivity, or nervousness. They also are useful for the amelioration of symptoms of thyrotoxicosis before and for several weeks after ^{131}I therapy, before subtotal thyroidectomy, in thyroiditis, and in thyroid storm.

Verapamil and diltiazem have cardiovascular effects similar to those of beta-adrenergic antagonist drugs in patients with thyrotoxicosis.[566,567]

Radioactive Iodine Therapy

The goal of ^{131}I therapy is to reduce the amount of functioning thyroid tissue, and therefore its efficacy is independent of whether a remission of Graves' disease occurs. The major advantages of ^{131}I therapy for patients with Graves' thyrotoxicosis are that usually only a single dose is needed, it reduces thyroid size to normal in most patients,[437,438] and it is safe (Table 9-15). These features make ^{131}I therapy an attractive choice for these patients, especially those with large goiters, those with recurrent thyrotoxicosis, and those who cannot tolerate or will not take an antithyroid drug. One disadvantage of this therapy is that the amelioration of thyrotoxicosis is slower than during antithyroid drug therapy; symptoms and serum T_4 and T_3 concentrations often do not change for a month or more after ^{131}I is given.

Several methods for determining ^{131}I doses have been used, most of them based on thyroid size and ^{131}I uptake; all are subject to considerable error because ^{131}I retention within the thyroid is variable and radiation sensitivity is not predictable. The most simple and appropriate approach is to administer a dose of 8 to 12 mCi (296 to 444 MBq) to nearly all patients, with small increments if thyroid radioiodine uptake is nearly normal or if thyroid enlargement is substantial.[568,569] These doses deliver approximately 100 to 200 μCi/g (3.7 to 7.4 MBq/g) estimated thyroid weight or 10,000 to 20,000 rad (100 to 200 Gy) to the thyroid. They result in clinical and biochemical improvement and reduction in thyroid size in 6 weeks to 3 months, and most patients are euthyroid, if not hypothyroid, in 4 to 6 months.[568] Other approaches are to administer repeated low doses or a single very high dose [e.g., 25 mCi (925 MBq)]. Pretreatment measurement of thyroid radioiodine uptake is not essential, but provides assurance that the patient has a high uptake and therefore has not taken iodine in some form or does not have unsuspected thyroiditis; alternatively uptake can be measured 6 h rather than the standard 24 h after administration of the test dose. Patients treated with ^{131}I should be advised to avoid nonessential close contact with partners and children for 1 to 2 weeks,[570] and premenopausal women should not become pregnant for at least 6 months.

Patients with mild or moderate thyrotoxicosis can be treated with ^{131}I immediately, with propranolol or a related drug being given to reduce bothersome thyrotoxic symptoms. Markedly symptomatic patients, however, should be treated with an antithyroid drug for 4 to 6 weeks before ^{131}I therapy because of its relatively slow action. The antithyroid drug should be discontinued 3–7 days before thyroid radioiodine uptake is determined and the therapeutic dose of ^{131}I is given. ^{131}I therapy may be less effective in patients who have received an antithyroid drug, and therefore a slightly higher dose should be given.[571,572] Iodine in any form should not be given before therapy, and care should be taken to avoid administering iodine-containing drugs or radiographic contrast agents if ^{131}I therapy is planned. Inorganic iodine administration may be beneficial after ^{131}I therapy.[573]

There are two important untoward effects of ^{131}I therapy—persistent thyrotoxicosis and hypothyroidism. Rare patients have acute temporary exacerbations of thyrotoxicosis and thyroid pain and tenderness. Both are due to radiation thyroiditis, and the risk of each is reduced by prior antithyroid drug therapy.

Persistent thyrotoxicosis results from inadequate ^{131}I therapy and, not surprisingly, is more common when lower doses of ^{131}I are given.[568,574] A recurrence of thyrotoxicosis in a patient who became euthyroid or hypothyroid after ^{131}I therapy is very rare.[575]

Hypothyroidism is not so much a complication of ^{131}I treatment as an almost inevitable consequence of it. It may occur in the first few months after therapy, in which case it may be transient,[576] or at any time thereafter. Early hypothyroidism, defined as that occurring within a year after treatment, is caused by the acute destructive effects of ^{131}I. Its frequency ranges from 40 percent to as high as 80 percent in patients treated with 8 to 12 mCi (296 to 444 MBq) ^{131}I.[569,577,578] Lower doses result in early hypothyroidism less often and persistent thyrotoxicosis more often. Therefore, higher doses are more appropriate, because the primary goal of therapy should be the permanent amelioration of thyrotoxicosis as expeditiously as possible.

After 1 year, hypothyroidism develops in additional patients (0.5–2 percent) each year for at least 10 years, whether the treatment dose was high or low.[574,578] Thus, late hypothyroidism is independent of the dose of ^{131}I given; it is due to damage to the replicative ability of thyroid follicular cells and perhaps autoimmune thyroid injury. It usually develops very slowly, with many patients having high serum TSH concentrations but normal serum T_4 and T_3 concentrations (subclinical hypothyroidism) for several years before they develop overt hypothyroidism.[579]

Some physicians have been reluctant to treat young adults and especially adolescents and children with ^{131}I. The reasons are that it might cause thyroidal or other tumors or gonadal damage, or the patient may be pregnant. ^{131}I therapy is associated with little or no increase in risk for thyroid or other tumors,[580,580a] but is associated with small increases in overall mortality, probably due to cardiovascular diseases exacerbated by thyrotoxicosis.[581] The gonadal radiation dose after ^{131}I is no more than that which results from several diagnostic radiological procedures, and follow-up of children and adolescents treated with ^{131}I has revealed neither impaired fertility nor an increase in birth defects in their offspring.[582] ^{131}I crosses the placenta and can destroy the fetal thyroid, and therefore care must be taken to ensure that any young woman about to be treated with ^{131}I is not pregnant.

Subtotal Thyroidectomy

The simplicity, safety, and lower cost of antithyroid drug and ^{131}I therapy mean that subtotal thyroidectomy is indicated only for patients with persistent or recurrent thyrotoxicosis or adverse effects of antithyroid drugs who refuse ^{131}I therapy, pregnant women in either of the above groups, and patients with large goiters. The goal of thyroidectomy, like that of ^{131}I, is reduction of the functioning mass of thyroid tissue.

Subtotal thyroidectomy has little perioperative morbidity and mortality in children and adults who receive proper preoperative care. This means antithyroid drug treatment for 4 to 6 weeks and inorganic iodide treatment for 7 to 10 days. Treatment with a beta-adrenergic antagonist drug for several weeks, with or without concomitant inorganic iodide therapy for 10 to 14 days, also has proved to be safe and effective preoperative therapy.[583] Usually, most of both thyroid lobes are removed, leaving about 3 g of tissue on each side; alternatively all of one lobe and all but 5–6 g of the contralateral lobe are removed.[584,585] The surgery can be done under local and regional anesthesia or general anesthesia, and as a day operation with discharge in the evening or an overnight hospital stay.[586]

Postoperative problems after thyroidectomy include bleeding into the neck, transient or permanent hypocalcemia, vocal cord paralysis, recurrent thyrotoxicosis, and transient or permanent hypothyroidism. The frequency of the nonthyroid complications is low. Transient hypocalcemia may be due to temporary hypoparathyroidism or healing of thyrotoxic osteopenia. Permanent vocal cord paralysis and hypoparathyroidism each occur in less than 2 percent of patients.[584]

Recurrent thyrotoxicosis occurs now in less than 10 percent of patients.[574,584,585] It usually develops years or even decades after thyroidectomy and is due to persistent Graves' disease. The long lag time reflects the time required for regrowth of sufficient thyroid tissue to secrete excessive amounts of T_4 and T_3. Patients with recurrent thyrotoxicosis should be treated with ^{131}I.

Overt or subclinical hypothyroidism may occur in the first 6–8 weeks after surgery in as many as 30 percent of patients, but in some of these patients thyroid secretion later returns to normal as a result of TSH-stimulated growth of the thyroid remnant. Therefore, a diagnosis of permanent hypothyroidism should not be made for at least 4–6 months after surgery. Currently, permanent hypothyroidism develops in the first year after surgery in about 50 percent of patients because of aggressive surgery intended to reduce the frequency of recurrent hyperthyroidism,[584,585] and thereafter, in 0.5 to 1 percent per year.[578] These data indicate that postoperative hypothyroidism is now nearly as common as is post-^{131}I hypothyroidism, and for the same reason, namely, the intent to reduce the frequency of recurrent thyrotoxicosis.

Treatment of Thyrotoxicosis Caused by Thyroiditis

The diagnosis and treatment of subacute thyroiditis are discussed in the section on The Painful Thyroid.

Painless thyroiditis is more difficult to recognize; clues to its presence were described previously (see section on Thyroiditis). Because it is transient and usually mild, most patients need no therapy. The few patients with substantial symptoms of thyrotoxicosis can be given a beta-adrenergic antagonist drug until their thyrotoxicosis subsides (see section on Drugs Ameliorating Peripheral Thyroid Hormone Action). Glucocorticoids and other, less toxic anti-inflammatory drugs reduce serum T_4 and T_3 concentrations rapidly in patients with painless thyroiditis,[587] but should not be given because of the mild nature and limited duration of thyrotoxicosis in most patients.

Glucocorticoids (20–40 mg prednisone daily for several weeks and decreasing doses thereafter) are the treatment of choice for patients with thyrotoxicosis caused by amiodarone-induced thyroiditis.[293]

Treatment of Thyrotoxicosis Caused by Thyroid Adenoma

These adenomas cause permanent thyrotoxicosis, and so the most appropriate therapy is ^{131}I. The dose used should be relatively high (15–25 mCi [555–925 MBq]) so that the adenoma decreases in size or disappears and the likelihood of persistent or recurrent thyrotoxicosis is low. With these doses, the cure rate is about 80 percent, about 10 percent of patients develop hypothyroidism and 10 percent persistent or recurrent thyrotoxicosis, and the adenoma disappears in about 50 percent.[588–590] Smaller doses may be almost as effective, but more patients have recurrent thyrotoxicosis and the nodules are less likely to disappear.[591] Transient hypothyroidism may occur until TSH secretion resumes. The risk of permanent hypothyroidism may be higher in patients treated with an antithyroid drug in whom TSH secretion has resumed at the time ^{131}I is given, because some ^{131}I may be taken up by the extranodular tissue, or in patients given very high doses of ^{131}I, in whom the extranodular radiation dose from ^{131}I taken up by the adenoma is high. Therefore, the best approach for most thyrotoxic patients with a thyroid adenoma is to give a moderately high dose of ^{131}I at the time of diagnosis, and treating symptoms of thyrotoxicosis with a beta-adrenergic antagonist drug.

These adenomas may also be surgically resected, after 4 to 6 weeks of antithyroid drug and 7 to 10 days of inorganic iodine therapy. Usually all that needs to be resected is part of the thyroid lobe containing the adenoma, thereby curing the thyrotoxicosis.

Local complications after these limited operations are rare, as is recurrent thyrotoxicosis or hypothyroidism.[590]

An alternative approach, done in some centers in Europe but rarely in the United States, is percutaneous injection of ethanol into the adenoma. Typically, 1–5 ml of 95 percent ethanol is injected 4–8 times, depending on the extent of reduction in adenoma size, at weekly or biweekly intervals. The adenomas partly or completely disappear and thyrotoxicosis disappears in most patients, and hypothyroidism and recurrent thyrotoxicosis are rare.[590,592] However, the need for multiple treatments, which nearly always cause neck pain and sometimes fever or dysphonia, make this therapy unattractive.

Treatment of Thyrotoxicosis Caused by Toxic Multinodular Goiter

^{131}I is the treatment of choice for patients with thyrotoxicosis caused by a multinodular goiter, because spontaneous remissions do not occur in this disease. High doses (e.g., 25–30 mCi (925–1,110 MBq)) are usually given because thyroid ^{131}I uptake is usually only moderately increased and the risk of persistent thyrotoxicosis should be minimized in these patients, many of whom are elderly. ^{131}I therapy effectively ameliorates thyrotoxicosis in more than 80 percent of patients, although about 10 percent require multiple doses, and from 5 to 20 percent become hypothyroid.[593,594] The goiters do not change in size during the first month after therapy, but then gradually shrink to about 60 percent of the volume before therapy at 1 year.[595-597] Because most patients with a toxic multinodular goiter are elderly and have cardiovascular manifestations of their thyrotoxicosis, treatment with an antithyroid drug for 4 to 6 weeks before administration of ^{131}I is often indicated. Such a regimen accelerates recovery, because antithyroid drugs are more rapidly effective than ^{131}I, and it minimizes the likelihood of an exacerbation of thyrotoxicosis after ^{131}I therapy.

Patients with toxic multinodular goiters can also be treated surgically, after antithyroid drug and inorganic iodine therapy. The usual operation is a bilateral subtotal thyroidectomy. Surgery is more rapidly effective than ^{131}I in ameliorating thyrotoxicosis and certainly more effective in reducing goiter size, but it is more likely to result in hypothyroidism.[594]

Special Situations

Subclinical Thyrotoxicosis

Subclinical thyrotoxicosis is defined by biochemical findings—normal serum T_4 and T_3 and low TSH concentrations (Fig. 9-17). The patients' serum TSH concentrations are low as a result of small, TSH-independent increases in thyroid secretion or slightly excessive doses of thyroid hormone. The increased thyroid secretion may be caused by any disorder that can cause overt thyrotoxicosis—a multinodular goiter, a thyroid adenoma, Graves' disease, or thyroiditis (Table 9-11). The prevalence rate of subclinical thyrotoxicosis in the community or primary care clinics ranges from 10 to 40 cases per 1,000 people.[123]

Most patients with subclinical thyrotoxicosis are asymptomatic, but some have a few, usually nonspecific, symptoms or signs compatible with thyrotoxicosis. Some have changes in cardiovascular function similar to but less marked than those that occur in patients with overt thyrotoxicosis, for example increased heart rate and increases in left ventricular function and mass,[598-601] and some, notably postmenopausal women, have slightly low trabecular or cortical bone density.[602] Other occasional findings are small increases in serum osteocalcin and sex hormone-binding globulin concentrations and small decreases in serum cholesterol concentrations.

The course of subclinical thyrotoxicosis is variable. In follow-up surveys ranging from weeks to several years about 40 percent of patients had normal serum TSH concentrations, 50 percent still had subclinical thyrotoxicosis, and 10 percent had overt thyrotoxicosis.[603] With respect to specific causes, the risk of progression to overt thyrotoxicosis is about 2 to 10 percent per year in patients with thyroid adenomas, multinodular goiters, or Graves' disease.[394,404,603] Follow-up studies have in general not revealed excessive rates of bone loss in patients with subclinical thyrotoxicosis.[604,605] With respect to cardiovascular problems, in one study the risk of atrial fibrillation during a 10-year follow-up period was increased, as compared with subjects with normal serum TSH concentrations (28 vs. 10 per 1,000 patient years).[606]

Patients with subclinical thyrotoxicosis due to exogenous thyroid hormone therapy should be treated by reduction of the dose of thyroid hormone. Those in whom it is due to a thyroid disease are not usually treated, for several reasons. First, it is a biochemical diagnosis, and the decrease in serum TSH may have been caused by thyroiditis, degeneration of a thyroid adenoma or nodule, or some unrecognized illness- or drug-induced inhibition of TSH secretion, and therefore may be transient.[129,130,579] If persistence for at least a month, and preferably longer, is confirmed, treatment may be considered if the patient has symptoms possibly attributable to thyrotoxicosis or other risk factors for cardiac arrhythmias or bone loss and has a substantial reduction in serum TSH concentration, for example it is <0.1 mU/liter (normal range 0.3–3.0 mU/liter). The appropriate treatments are ^{131}I in patients with a multinodular goiter or thyroid adenoma and low-dose MMI in those presumed to have Graves' disease. However, the benefits, if any, of treating patients with subclinical thyrotoxicosis are not known.

Thyroid Storm

Thyroid storm is severe, life-threatening thyrotoxicosis. There are no established criteria for its diagnosis, and there is little evidence that its pathophysiology differs from that of thyrotoxicosis in general; it is the combination of thyrotoxicosis and host responses to another illness. It usually occurs abruptly in a thyrotoxic patient who has an acute infection or other medical illness, an injury, or a major operation. It may also occur after ^{131}I therapy, discontinuation of antithyroid drug therapy, or spontaneously. Serum T_4 and T_3 concentrations increase in the latter group, but not in the group of patients with concomitant nonthyroidal illnesses.[607] Thyrotoxicosis may or may not have been diagnosed previously, but the symptoms usually have been present for several months.

The key clinical findings in patients with thyroid storm are fever (>38.5°C), tachycardia, and central nervous system dysfunction; some combination of these in effect define the syndrome. The central nervous system abnormalities include marked anxiety, agitation and delirium, occasionally acute psychosis or seizures, and, terminally, coma. Many patients have nausea, vomiting, abdominal pain, and diarrhea, and some have congestive failure or atrial fibrillation.[608] Signs such as fever and tachycardia may be due either to the thyrotoxicosis or to the accompanying illness. A decision concerning therapy must be made with the understanding that there are no pathognomonic symptoms or signs of thyroid storm and without waiting for the results of laboratory tests.

There also are no characteristic laboratory abnormalities in patients with thyroid storm. Serum T_4 and T_3 concentrations are high, but no more so than in ordinary thyrotoxicosis. Serum free T_4 and T_3 concentrations may be somewhat higher than in less ill patients with thyrotoxicosis,[609] because acute illness can cause decreases in TBG and TTR production, thus lowering serum binding of T_4 and T_3. Nevertheless, the increase in the availability of T_4 and T_3 to cells is probably small, suggesting that thyroid storm is not just an increase in severity of preexisting thyrotoxicosis. There is probably also adrenergic activation and a marked increase in production of proinflammatory cytokines, but the factors mediating these changes are not known.

Treatment of thyroid storm should be directed toward decreasing thyroidal production of T_4 and T_3, peripheral production of T_3, and the peripheral actions of thyroid hormone, as well as providing general supportive measures and treatment needed to deal with any coexisting illness. MMI or PTU should be given in large doses, such as 10 or 250 mg, respectively, every 6 h, by nasogastric tube or even rectally if necessary. Inorganic iodide should be given orally or by nasogastric tube in a dose of 50 to 100 mg four times daily to inhibit thyroidal release of T_4 and T_3 after the antithyroid drug is given and T_4 and T_3 synthesis is blocked. Alternatively, iopanoic acid can be given in a dose of 1,000 mg daily; it inhibits both extrathyroidal T_3 production and thyroid secretion. Propranolol given orally or intravenously is the most immediately effective treatment for the tachycardia and neuromuscular manifestations of thyroid storm. The oral dose is 20–40 mg every 4–6 h, or more if the pulse rate slows little. The initial intravenous dose is 1–2 mg given over 2 to 5 min, followed by doses of 2 to 3 mg given over 5 to 10 min every 2–4 h as needed; the patient should be continuously monitored. An alternative is esmolol, which is given by continuous intravenous infusion; the initial dose is 0.5 mg per kg given in 1 min, followed by 0.05 mg per kg per min or more if necessary.[610] A glucocorticoid is usually given in large doses, such as 50 mg hydrocortisone or 2 mg dexamethasone intravenously every 8 hours. The rationale for glucocorticoid therapy is that ACTH and cortisol secretion may not increase sufficiently to meet cortisol requirements in patients who are very sick and in whom cortisol degradation is increased. Glucocorticoids also inhibit thyroid secretion [in patients with Graves' disease[281]] and extrathyroidal T_3 production. These measures usually result in clinical improvement and some reduction in serum T_4 and T_3 concentrations in 24 to 48 h. Supportive therapy should include treatment to reduce hyperpyrexia and appropriate parenteral fluid and electrolyte therapy. Combined with aggressive treatment of any coexisting illness, these measures collectively have reduced mortality from thyroid storm.

Thyrotoxicosis during Pregnancy

The occurrence of thyrotoxicosis during pregnancy introduces additional considerations relating to the effect of the thyrotoxicosis, which is nearly always caused by Graves' disease, and its treatment on the mother and her fetus. In some women, the thyrotoxicosis precedes the pregnancy. In others, thyrotoxicosis begins during pregnancy, usually in the first trimester or early in the second. Relapses of thyrotoxicosis also occur during pregnancy in women who were in remission before becoming pregnant.[611] In general, no matter when it begins, thyrotoxicosis caused by Graves' disease tends to subside during the third trimester, and so treatment can be withdrawn in up to half of the patients.

Thyrotoxicosis may be hard to recognize in a pregnant woman because pregnancy is characterized normally by increases in oxygen consumption, heat production, and cardiovascular activity and by anxiety or nervousness. Findings particularly indicative of thyrotoxicosis are marked tachycardia, muscle weakness, tremor, weight loss, and thyroid enlargement. Thyrotoxicosis is usually tolerated well by pregnant women, as it is by nonpregnant women of the same age, and there is no increase in maternal mortality or morbidity in untreated patients.[612]

The situation with regard to the fetus is different. If the mother is not treated, there is an increase in congenital anomalies and increased fetal loss resulting from spontaneous abortion and premature delivery.[612,613] These are probably direct effects of maternal thyrotoxicosis, as they do not occur in mothers who receive antithyroid treatment. Some fetuses have thyrotoxicosis manifested by growth retardation, tachycardia (pulse rate greater than 160 beats/min), and hyperactivity.[614] The most conspicuous findings in fatal cases are cardiac and thyroid enlargement and congestion of the viscera.[615] Fetal thyrotoxicosis is caused by the transplacental passage of TSH receptor-stimulating antibodies and perhaps also of T_4 and T_3 from the mother. It also occurs in mothers who have these antibodies but are euthyroid as a result of earlier ^{131}I therapy or thyroidectomy. It can be proved by measurements of serum T_4 in blood samples collected by cordocentesis.[616] Treatment of the mother with an antithyroid drug reduces fetal tachycardia, and this therapy may very occasionally be indicated even in mothers with previously treated Graves' disease who are euthyroid.

The diagnosis of thyrotoxicosis in a pregnant woman is confirmed by the finding of an unequivocally low serum TSH concentration; a serum total T_4 concentration that is above the normal range for pregnancy, which is about 50 percent higher than normal; and a high serum free T_4 concentration or index value. If the diagnosis is not established by these tests, the wisest course is continued observation. Women with hyperemesis gravidarum tend to have higher serum T_4, T_3, and chorionic gonadotropin and slightly lower TSH concentrations than normal pregnant women at comparable stages of gestation. They do not have thyroid enlargement, there is no evidence that antithyroid therapy is beneficial, and their serum T_4 concentrations decline as the hyperemesis subsides.[428]

Pregnant women with thyrotoxicosis should be treated with an antithyroid drug. Both MMI and PTU cross the placenta, and their fractional transplacental transfer rates are similar.[617] Furthermore, the relation between maternal and fetal serum T_4 concentrations at delivery in mothers treated with either drug is the same.[618,619] Whichever drug is used, only doses sufficient to ameliorate the clinical manifestations of thyrotoxicosis and lower the serum free T_4 value to near or just within the normal range should be given. An appropriate initial dose is 10–15 mg MMI or 150–200 mg PTU daily. The patient should be evaluated at 3- to 4-week intervals and the dose reduced as necessary to maintain this level of thyroid secretion, and repeated attempts should be made to discontinue therapy. The rationale for this approach is that pregnant women tolerate mild thyrotoxicosis well and that the fetus is exposed to as little antithyroid drug as possible consistent with preventing overtly symptomatic thyrotoxicosis in the mother. However, pregnant women with severe thyrotoxicosis should be treated vigorously because serious maternal illness threatens fetal development and survival. T_4 should not be given with the antithyroid drug, because little reaches the fetus and the mother may need more antithyroid drug.

Both PTU and MMI may cause fetal goiter, hypothyroidism, or both, which subside soon after birth.[620] Infants exposed to these drugs do not have an increase in congenital anomalies,[613,620,621] with the possible exception of aplasia cutis (congenital absence of the skin) in the infants of mothers given MMI.[620,622,623] The lesions of aplasia cutis are usually small (<3 cm), solitary, on the scalp, and heal spontaneously; they probably occur during the first trimester. The presumed relationship with MMI is based on case reports; no cases were noted among 243 infants of mothers given MMI in Japan and the risk was not increased in a case-control study in the Netherlands.[613,622] The postnatal growth and development of infants of mothers who received an antithyroid drug are normal.[624] The fetal thyroid is sensitive to the antithyroid actions of iodine, but small (5–40 mg) doses may be used safely.[625] Propranolol should not be administered to pregnant women with thyrotoxicosis, because it may cause fetal loss.[626]

Pregnant women with thyrotoxicosis can be treated by subtotal thyroidectomy, but it should be done only when the previously mentioned adverse effects of antithyroid drugs preclude their continuation. Surgery is safe only after a period of drug treatment. This may have been achieved with MMI or PTU before the adverse effects developed or may necessitate short-term treatment with inorganic iodine and propranolol. Additional hazards of subtotal thyroidectomy during pregnancy include abortion, premature labor, and fetal anoxia. ^{131}I therapy is absolutely contraindicated in pregnant women.

T_4 and T_3 are present in breast milk in low concentrations. The normal breast milk iodide concentration is about 10 μg/dl (0.8 μmol/liter), which is higher than that in most infant formulas.[627] The concentrations of MMI in milk are similar to those in serum, whereas the concentrations of PTU in milk are lower than those in serum. Limited data indicate that milk does not contain enough of either drug to cause hypothyroidism in a nursing infant.[628,629] Therefore, a mother taking an antithyroid drug who wishes to nurse may do so, but the infant's thyroid function should be evaluated periodically.

Neonatal Graves' Disease

Neonatal Graves' disease, manifested primarily as thyrotoxicosis, occurs in a small fraction (<10 percent) of the infants of mothers with Graves' disease. It is caused by the transplacental passage of TSH receptor-stimulating antibodies. It occurs only in infants whose mothers have high serum concentrations of the antibodies late in pregnancy,[630] indicating that the extent of transplacental passage is limited. The mothers of about half of these infants have a history of thyrotoxicosis during the pregnancy; the others are euthyroid, having received antithyroid therapy earlier.

Those neonates who will be affected by Graves' disease have high cord serum concentrations of TSH receptor-stimulating antibodies.[631] They may or may not be thyrotoxic at birth, depending on whether the mother was taking an antithyroid drug at the time of delivery. If so, the thyrotoxicosis begins a few days later. Because it is caused by passive transfer of antibodies, which ceases at birth, it disappears within weeks. The duration is a function of the initial concentration of the antibodies and their rate of metabolism, which is about 3 to 4 percent/day (half-life 10 to 15 days).

Cord serum should be obtained for measurement of TSH and T_4 in all infants of mothers with Graves' disease, to determine if they are thyrotoxic or are likely to become so, for example if their serum TSH concentration is low even if their serum T_4 concentration is not high. The results of serum TSH and T_4 measurements in neonates must be interpreted in relation to norms that differ from adult values and change rapidly after birth (see section on Physiological Variables Affecting Pituitary-Thyroid Function and Tests).

Neonates with thyrotoxicosis tend to be small for gestational age and are hyperactive, tremulous, and irritable. Other problems include tachycardia, tachypnea, hyperphagia, feeding problems, diarrhea, cardiac failure, thyroid enlargement, and proptosis. They have high serum T_4 and T_3 concentrations and low serum TSH concentrations. They should be treated with an antithyroid drug, for example, 5 mg MMI daily. If the thyrotoxicosis is clinically severe, inorganic iodine and propranolol should be given as well. The drugs subsequently should be gradually withdrawn as indicated by clinical evaluation and serum T_4 measurements. Therapy can usually be discontinued within 8 to 15 weeks and is rarely followed by recurrence, but subsequent intellectual and physical development may be subnormal.

Postpartum Thyrotoxicosis

Thyrotoxicosis may occur in the first several months after delivery. Three forms of postpartum thyrotoxicosis are recognized.[376,611] One is the new development of Graves' hyperthyroidism. A second is recurrence of Graves' hyperthyroidism, which may be persistent or transient. In these patients, thyroid radioiodine uptake is high. Third, and most often, thyrotoxicosis occurs as part of the syndrome of postpartum thyroiditis.

Postpartum thyroiditis is a clinically heterogeneous disorder; some women have only transient thyrotoxicosis, others have transient thyrotoxicosis followed by transient hypothyroidism, and still others have only transient hypothyroidism.[376] It occurs in 1 to 6 percent of postpartum women of whom about half have thyrotoxicosis. The characteristics of the thyrotoxic phase of this syndrome are similar to those of the thyrotoxic phase of painless thyroiditis as it occurs in men and in women who did not recently deliver a baby. The thyrotoxicosis is mild and transient, there is little or no thyroid enlargement, and thyroid radioiodine uptake is low. Indeed, many patients have no symptoms; slightly high serum T_4 concentrations and subclinical thyrotoxicosis are the only abnormalities. The thyrotoxicosis usually develops 2–6 months postpartum, lasts 2–6 weeks, and in about half of patients is followed by transient hypothyroidism (Fig. 9-26). Because postpartum thyrotoxicosis is mild as well as transient, most patients need no treatment. Propranolol may be useful in patients with many symptoms. Postpartum thyroiditis is discussed further in the section on Hypothyroidism.

Extrathyroidal Manifestations of Graves' Disease

Infiltrative Ophthalmopathy

Clinical evidence of ophthalmopathy is present in 20 to 40 percent of patients with hyperthyroidism caused by Graves' disease at some time during their illness, but measurements of orbital protrusion and orbital imaging studies indicate that it is present to some degree in 75 to 80 percent.[632,633] It develops concurrently with thyrotoxicosis or during the year before or after it in most patients.[634] There is little correlation between the severity of the thyrotoxicosis and that of the ophthalmopathy, and some euthyroid

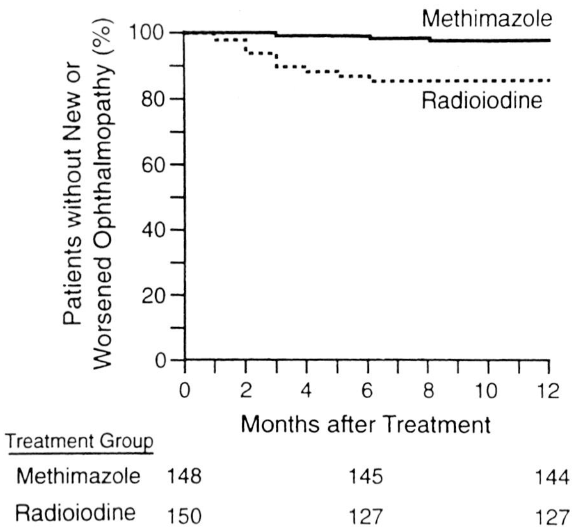

FIGURE 9-30. Kaplan-Meier plots of the development or the progression of ophthalmopathy in patients with Graves' thyrotoxicosis treated with ^{131}I or methimazole. The numbers below the graph show the numbers of patients in each group at baseline and after 6 and 12 months. *(Reproduced with modification from Bartalena L, Marcocci C, Bogazzi F, et al., N Engl J Med 338:73, 1998, with permission of the publisher.)*

and even hypothyroid patients have ophthalmopathy that is clinically indistinguishable (euthyroid Graves' disease). For this reason, the disorder is also called thyroid-associated ophthalmopathy.

The pathogenesis of infiltrative ophthalmopathy is poorly understood (see section on Pathogenesis of Ophthalmopathy and Localized Myxedema). It tends to be more severe in men and in older patients.[635] One risk factor for ophthalmopathy is smoking.[352,353,636] Another is inadequate or overtreatment of thyrotoxicosis.[637] Among the antithyroid treatments, ^{131}I therapy is more likely to be followed by the development or worsening of ophthalmopathy than antithyroid drug or surgical therapy. This was not evident from retrospective studies,[638] but was in the two studies in which patients were randomly assigned to different antithyroid therapies. In one, of 114 patients followed for 2 years or longer, ophthalmopathy developed or worsened in more patients treated with ^{131}I than in patients treated with MMI or surgery (33 vs. 10 vs. 16 percent, respectively).[639] In the other, of 271 patients followed for 1 year, ophthalmopathy developed or worsened in 15 percent of the patients treated with ^{131}I, as compared with 5 percent of those treated with MMI (Fig. 9-30).[640] The difference might be explained by formation of eye-reactive antibodies to thyroid antigen(s) released after ^{131}I-induced thyroid injury, or by a higher frequency of at least transient hypothyroidism in the ^{131}I-treated patients.

Clinical Manifestations

The clinical manifestations of Graves' ophthalmopathy reflect the fact that the eye nearly fills the orbital cavity, so that a small increase in the contents of the cavity, particularly enlargement of the eye muscles, results in forward displacement of the eye, known as proptosis or exophthalmos. Concomitantly, venous drainage is impaired, resulting in periorbital and conjunctiva edema and inflammation, and extraocular muscle function may be impaired and optic neuropathy occur (Table 9-16).[641]

TABLE 9-16. Clinical Classification of Eye Changes of Infiltrative Ophthalmopathy (NOSPECS)*

Class	Finding
0	No symptoms or signs
1	Only thyrotoxic signs and mild proptosis (<2 mm)
2	Soft tissue involvement
3	Proptosis
4	Extraocular muscle involvement
5	Corneal involvement
6	Sight loss

*Useful as a reminder of the clinical manifestation of ophthalmopathy, but not for evaluating severity or the efficacy of therapy.

Source: Werner.[641]

The most common complaint among patients with ophthalmopathy is proptosis. Other symptoms that may be present include periorbital puffiness, eye discomfort or pain, a gritty or burning sensation in the eyes, excessive tearing, and photophobia.[642] There also may be intermittent or persistent diplopia and blurring or loss of vision. The onset is usually gradual but may be abrupt. Even when asymptomatic, ophthalmopathy may be very distressing to the patient for cosmetic reasons.

The major sign is the proptosis, which is usually bilateral and symmetric, although the extent of protrusion can vary by several millimeters. It is important to distinguish proptosis from lid retraction, which is caused by thyrotoxicosis itself. Lid retraction gives the appearance of proptosis and may be accompanied by tearing, eye discomfort, conjunctival injection, and photophobia. Lid retraction and proptosis can be distinguished with an exophthalmometer, a device that measures the distance from the lateral orbital notch to the anterior surface of the cornea. True proptosis—exophthalmometer readings greater than 18 mm in Asians, 20 mm in whites, and 22 mm in blacks—is thus distinguished from apparent proptosis caused by lid retraction alone.

The other principal signs of ophthalmopathy are periorbital edema, conjunctival congestion and edema (chemosis), and limitation of ocular mobility (Fig. 9-31). Extraocular muscle involvement most often results in limitation of upward gaze, but it may limit movement in any direction. It is due more to inflammatory restriction of the muscles than muscle weakness. Interstitial keratitis and corneal ulceration caused by marked proptosis and decreased visual acuity and visual field defects due to optic neuropathy from compression of the optic nerve are fortunately rare. Finally, intraocular pressure may be increased.

The diagnosis of infiltrative ophthalmopathy when thyrotoxicosis is or was present is usually not difficult. Except when it is minimal, the patient should have a complete ophthalmologic examination. Orbital computed tomography (or magnetic resonance imaging) should be done in patients with severe proptosis, loss of vision, or marked asymmetry in proptosis. The characteristic finding is enlargement of the extraocular muscles (Fig. 9-32), and the retroorbital fat content may also be increased.

Euthyroid Graves' Disease

This term is applied to patients who are euthyroid and have no history of thyrotoxicosis but who have infiltrative ophthalmopathy that is clinically and pathologically indistinguishable from that occurring in thyrotoxic patients with Graves' disease. Patients with euthyroid Graves' disease account for only a small fraction of all patients with ophthalmopathy, but it may be more severe than in those who have or have had thyrotoxicosis.[635] Although the pa-

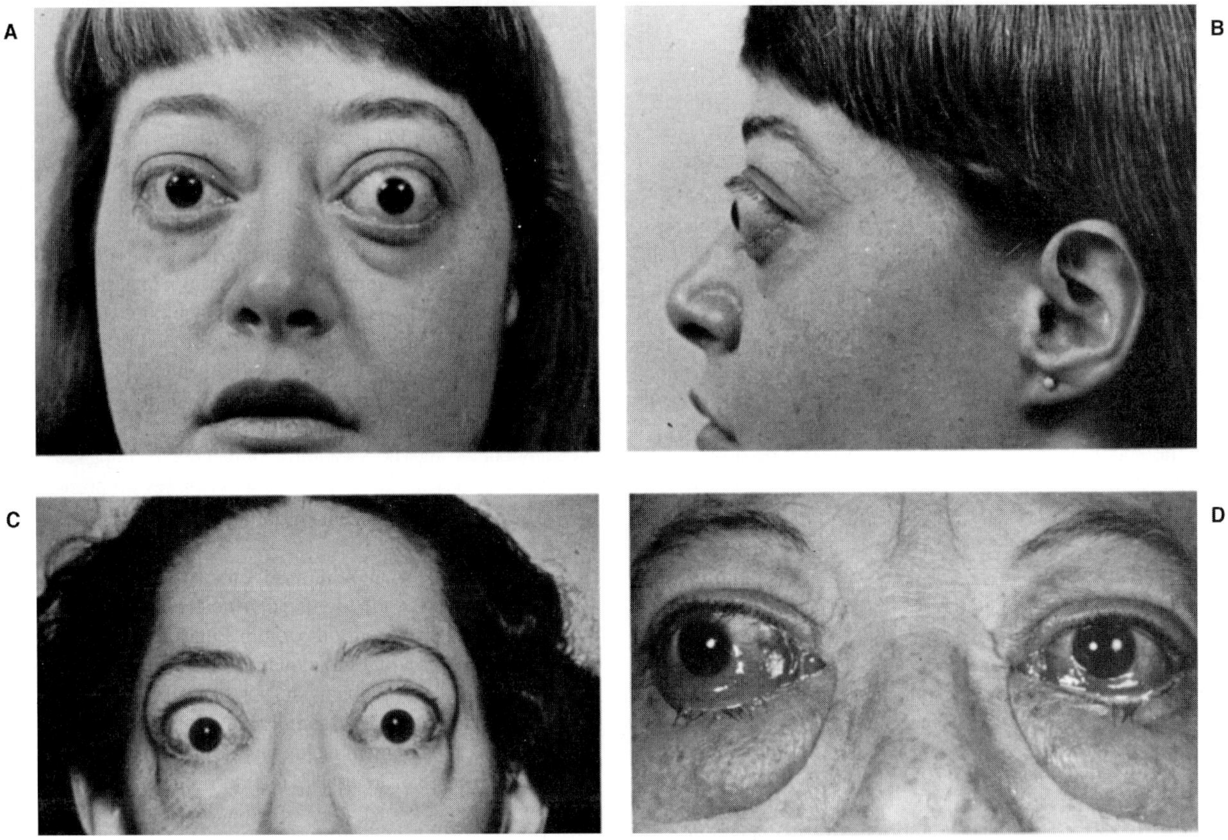

FIGURE 9-31. Photographs of three patients with ophthalmopathy caused by Graves' disease. (*A, B*) A young woman with moderate asymmetric proptosis and marked retraction of the left eyelid. This patient has few manifestations of ocular inflammation. (*C*) A young woman with marked periorbital edema, bilateral lid retraction, and proptosis. (*D*) A middle-aged woman with marked infraorbital edema, conjunctival injection and chemosis, and muscle restriction of the right eye but little proptosis.

tients are by definition euthyroid and have little or no thyroid enlargement, nearly all have some biochemical evidence of thyroid dysfunction or autoimmune thyroid disease, and a few have overt chronic autoimmune thyroiditis and hypothyroidism. Their serum TSH concentrations may be either low (subclinical thyrotoxicosis) or high (subclinical hypothyroidism), and many have high serum concentrations of antithyroid peroxidase or other antithyroid antibodies.[643] Hence, they have many manifestations of Graves' thyroid disease; they are euthyroid because they do not produce much TSH receptor-stimulating antibody or because they have some other thyroid problem, so that thyroidal responsiveness to TSH receptor-stimulating antibodies is limited.

The diagnosis of Graves' ophthalmopathy is less certain in these euthyroid patients even when the clinical manifestations, as described earlier, are characteristic of it. Their evaluation should include measurement of serum TSH to confirm that they are

FIGURE 9-32. Computed tomography of the orbits. (*A*) A normal subject. (*B*) A patient with ophthalmopathy caused by Graves' disease. Note the enlarged medial rectus muscle in *B*.

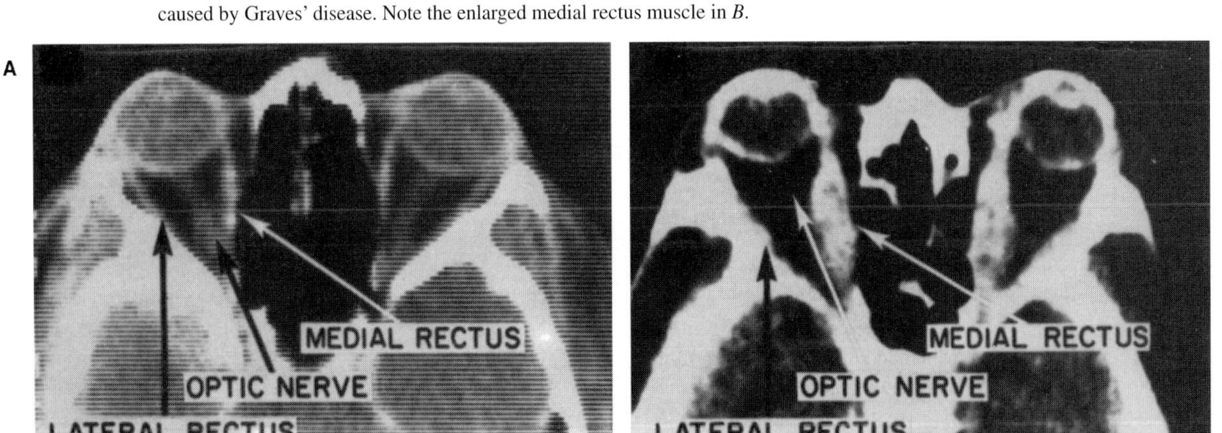

euthyroid, a complete ophthalmologic examination, and orbital computed tomography. The imaging procedure will not only confirm the presence of Graves' ophthalmopathy but also exclude other causes of bilateral ophthalmopathy, such as pseudotumor of the orbit, orbital myositis, histiocytosis X, granulomatous diseases (sarcoidosis, Wegener's granulomatosis), leukemia, and lymphoma. Tumors, vascular abnormalities, and pseudotumor of the orbit are the usual causes of unilateral ophthalmopathy.

Course and Management

The natural history of Graves' ophthalmopathy is characterized by stabilization and then gradual disappearance of the symptoms and signs of ocular inflammation but persistence of proptosis, but in a few patients it worsens.[636–640,644,645] Restoring and maintaining normal thyroid secretion contributes to a favorable course. The course is largely independent of the type of antithyroid treatment that is given, except for the increase in risk of worsening after ^{131}I therapy as noted earlier. This makes an antithyroid drug an even better choice for thyrotoxic patients with ophthalmopathy than it is for patients with thyrotoxicosis alone. The worsening of ophthalmopathy that occurs after ^{131}I can be prevented by glucocorticoid therapy,[640] but routine therapy is not warranted.

Patients can be told that their ophthalmopathy is not likely to worsen; that control of thyrotoxicosis should result in the disappearance of lid retraction and some eye symptoms, so that their eyes are likely to look and feel better; and that their conjunctival and periorbital edema should slowly subside later. The importance of careful follow up with respect to both their thyroid function and eyes should be stressed. Given reassurance that worsening is unlikely, many patients need no or only symptomatic treatment for their eyes.

Simple measures that can be used to relieve eye discomfort, reduce periorbital and conjunctival edema, and provide protection for the eyes include the use of dark glasses and methylcellulose eye drops, sleeping with the head elevated, cessation of smoking, and occasionally diuretic therapy.[642,646] Mild diplopia often can be corrected with prism lenses. These measures, and the passage of time, will often suffice. The few patients with severe, progressive ophthalmopathy can be treated with glucocorticoids, orbital radiation, or surgical decompression of the orbits. The indications for the use of these treatments are not clearly defined but include severe symptomatic periorbital and conjunctival inflammation, severe proptosis, threatened or actual corneal injury, and, less often, optic neuropathy with threatened or actual loss of vision. Their efficacy must be considered in the context of the usual course of ophthalmopathy, which is stabilization and regression, and the side effects of the treatments.

Glucocorticoid therapy is effective in ameliorating periorbital and conjunctival inflammation and edema, so that eye discomfort, tearing, and photophobia diminish, sometimes within several days after the initiation of therapy, in 50 to 70 percent of patients. Proptosis may diminish slightly, and optic neuropathy and vision may improve, but diplopia is not usually altered.[646] The usual initial dose is 60–80 mg per day of prednisone for one to two weeks, followed by gradual reduction in dosage and discontinuation of treatment in 8 to 12 weeks. Unfortunately, the ophthalmopathy often worsens when the dose of prednisone is reduced or discontinued. Short courses of very high doses of glucocorticoids given intravenously and retrobulbar injections of glucocorticoids have proven beneficial in some patients. Other immunosuppressive drugs, intravenous immunoglobulin and somatostatin analogues have had variable efficacy in small studies.[647]

Orbital radiation may be used in patients who do not respond to glucocorticoids, have intolerable glucocorticoid-related side effects, or relapse after reduction or discontinuation of glucocorticoid therapy. Radiotherapy results in improvement in periorbital and conjunctival edema in 50 to 70 percent of patients,[646,648] but its effect is slower than that of glucocorticoids. It does not often affect proptosis or diplopia or result in improvement in visual acuity, and can cause retinopathy.[649] It is a second-line anti-inflammatory therapy, and is not suitable for patients with threatened or actual loss of vision. The dose of radiation is usually 20 Gy (2,000 rads), given in a 2-week period and delivered so as to spare the lens and to some extent the retina.

Surgical decompression of the orbits is the treatment of choice for any patient in whom vision is threatened or impaired by optic neuropathy or who has corneal disease or severe proptosis.[646] It relieves periorbital and conjunctival edema and may be indicated for those problems alone in patients who do not respond to or relapse after glucocorticoid therapy.[542] It is also done for cosmetic reasons alone.[650] The orbit may be surgically decompressed by transantral, transfrontal, or lateral approaches; transantral decompression is the most satisfactory. Proptosis usually diminishes by 3 to 5 mm; diplopia may worsen. Other surgical procedures done occasionally are tarsorrhaphy to protect the cornea from exposure and muscle operations to correct diplopia.

Localized Myxedema and Thyroid Acropachy

Localized (pretibial) myxedema is rare, occurring in perhaps 2 percent of patients with Graves' disease. It usually occurs several years after treatment for thyrotoxicosis in patients who also have severe ophthalmopathy, but can occur much later.[372] Localized myxedema consists of circumscribed areas of accumulation of glycosaminoglycans in the dermis, with fragmentation of collagen and obliteration of lymphatics. The lesions are usually painless, but they may be pruritic, and are nontender, and take several forms. The majority of patients have diffuse nonpitting edema of the pretibial regions with hyperkeratosis and red, brown or orange discoloration of the skin, which has an orange-peel appearance. Other patients have erythematous or hyperpigmented, slightly scaly indurated 1–5 cm plaques or nodules in the same region (Fig. 9-33). Although often unilateral when first detected, the lesions usually become bilateral and more or less symmetric. They can enlarge, further disrupting lymph flow and causing an elephantiasis-like appearance of the ankles and feet, or become bullous or ulcerated. Very rare patients have diffuse or nodular lesions on the trunk, arms and hands, or face. In most patients the lesions of localized myxedema ultimately regress, although rarely completely.[372]

Most of the patients have localized pretibial lesions and require no therapy. For those with extensive or highly pruritic lesions, and especially those with bullous or ulcerated lesions, topical application of 0.1 or 0.2 percent fluocinolone or another fluorinated glucocorticoid cream covered by an occlusive dressing has proved effective.[651] It should initially be used nightly or every other night, but when improvement occurs, the applications can be reduced to once weekly or biweekly.

Thyroid acropachy is the rarest manifestation of Graves' disease. Nearly all reported patients have had extensive localized myxedema as well as thyrotoxicosis (usually previously treated) and ophthalmopathy. Its manifestations are clubbing of the fingers and toes, subcutaneous edema and fibrosis of the hands and feet, and periosteal

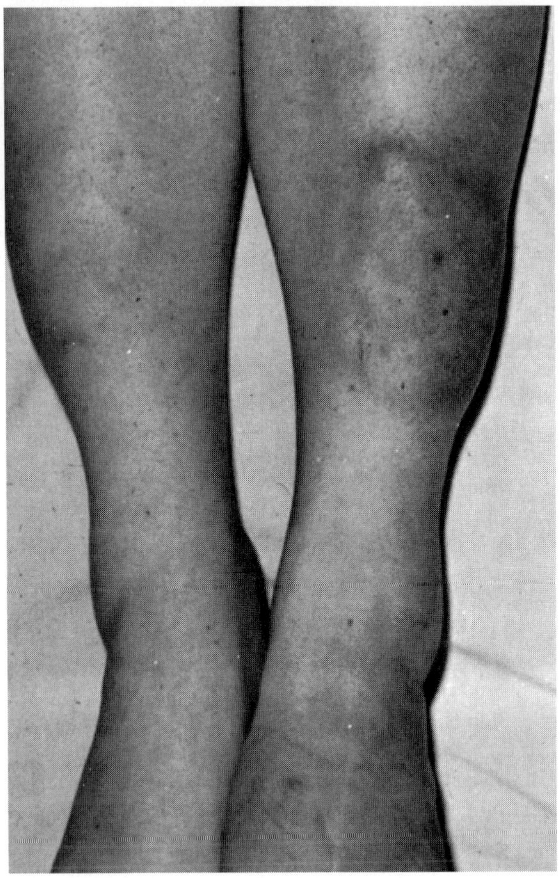

FIGURE 9-33. Photograph of localized myxedema. Note the raised, slightly hyperpigmented plaques on both anterolateral pretibial regions.

bone formation involving the phalanges and metacarpal and metatarsal bones. It usually causes no symptoms, but the hands and feet may become stiff and contractures may occur. The pathogenesis is not known, and there is no effective therapy.

HYPOTHYROIDISM

Hypothyroidism is the clinical, physiologic, and biochemical syndrome that results from decreased thyroid hormone production by the thyroid gland. The term *illness-related or adaptive hypothyroidism* is used (see section on Nonthyroidal Illness) to describe the reductions in extrathyroidal T_3 and, less often, thyroidal T_4 and T_3 production that occur in patients with nonthyroidal illness. Although illness-related hypothyroidism results from decreased thyroid hormone production, it is transient and is not accompanied by clinical manifestations of hypothyroidism, and therefore thyroid hormone treatment is not indicated. This section is devoted to a discussion of the causes, symptoms and signs, diagnosis, and management of hypothyroidism as traditionally defined.

Hypothyroidism is usually categorized as overt or subclinical. *Overt hypothyroidism* is defined as low serum T_4 and T_3 concentrations and, in nearly all patients, high serum TSH concentrations; the exception is patients with central hypothyroidism. Most patients with overt hypothyroidism have symptoms and signs of hypothyroidism. *Subclinical hypothyroidism* is defined as normal serum T_4 and T_3 concentrations and high serum TSH concentrations; most of these patients have no symptoms or signs of hypothyroidism (Fig. 9-17). Hypothyroidism may develop suddenly or gradually, it may be transient or persistent, and it may be of little importance or life-threatening (myxedema coma).

Hypothyroidism is common. The prevalence rate of overt hypothyroidism is about 1 per 1,000 in community surveys and 2 to 5 per 1,000 in patients seeking medical care.[123] The prevalence rate of subclinical hypothyroidism is 20–100 per 1,000 persons in the community.[120,122,123,139] The higher rates occur in older women, most of whom have high serum antithyroid peroxidase antibody concentrations.[120,139] The ratio of women to men with either overt or subclinical hypothyroidism ranges from 2 to 8 to 1 and increases with age.

Pathophysiology of Hypothyroidism

A comparison of thyroidal and extrathyroidal production of T_4 and T_3 in normal subjects and patients with hypothyroidism is shown in Fig. 9-34. The daily rate of T_4 production in patients with overt hypothyroidism is about 25 percent of normal. The daily production rate of T_3 is decreased less, and the proportion of T_3 that originates in the thyroid is increased and the proportion that originates in extrathyroidal sites is decreased.[317,652]

There are several defenses against hypothyroidism. The most important is TSH. Its secretion increases in response to very small decreases in thyroid secretion (Fig. 9-10). In patients with little thyroid damage or iodine deficiency, the increase in TSH secretion

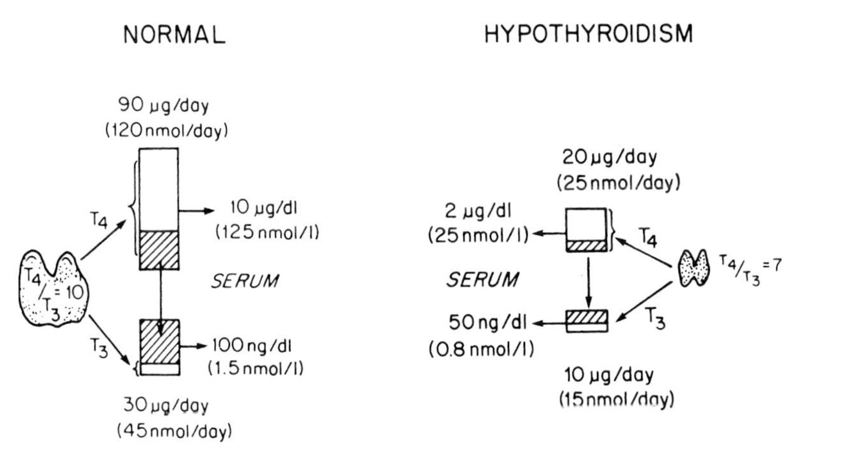

FIGURE 9-34. Diagram of thyroidal T_4/T_3 ratios, extrathyroidal production rates of T_4 and T_3, and serum T_4 and T_3 concentrations in normal subjects and patients with hypothyroidism. The diagonally lined areas in the T_4 (upper) rectangles indicate the proportion of T_4 converted to T_3 at extrathyroidal sites, and the diagonally lined areas in the T_3 (lower) rectangles indicate the proportion of T_3 formed from T_4 at extrathyroidal sites. (*Reproduced with modification from DeGroot LJ (ed): Endocrinology, 3rd ed. Philadelphia, Saunders, 1995, p 753, with permission of the publisher.*)

TABLE 9-17. Causes of Hypothyroidism

Primary (thyroidal) hypothyroidism
Insufficient functional thyroid tissue caused by
Chronic autoimmune thyroiditis*
^{131}I therapy
External neck radiation
Thyroidectomy
Infiltrative disease*
Congenital and hereditary hypothyroidism
Thyroid agenesis and dysgenesis
Hereditary defects in thyroid hormone biosynthesis*
Hereditary defects in thyroid hormone action (thyroid hormone resistance)
Acquired defects in thyroid hormone synthesis
Iodine deficiency*
Antithyroid agents*
Iodine excess
Increased degradation of thyroid hormone
Central (hypothyrotropic) hypothyroidism
Pituitary hypothyroidism (TSH deficiency)
Hypothamic hypothyroidism (TRH deficiency)

*Goiter often present.

may restore thyroid hormone secretion to normal or near normal, in so doing causing only thyroid enlargement. TSH stimulates the secretion of T_3 in preference to that of T_4 in two ways; it stimulates the synthesis of T_3 more than that of T_4, and it stimulates thyroidal deiodinase activity.[15,653] Therefore, thyroidal T_3 secretion decreases less than that of T_4, and the thyroidal contribution to overall T_3 production increases. Other mechanisms that minimize the development of hypothyroidism include an increase in the fraction of T_4 that is converted to T_3 at extrathyroidal sites, particularly in tissues rich in type 2 deiodinase.[654] All these changes serve to limit the decrease in the availability of T_3, the more efficiently produced and more active thyroid hormone, and therefore to minimize the impact of thyroid deficiency.

Causes of Hypothyroidism

Hypothyroidism is caused by thyroid disease (primary hypothyroidism) in more than 95 percent of patients, but it can be caused by pituitary or hypothalamic disease (central hypothyroidism). The major causes of hypothyroidism are listed in Table 9-17. An attempt should always be made to distinguish among them, because hypothyroidism may be the predominant or only manifestation of hypothalamic or pituitary disease. History and physical examination alone are usually sufficient for this purpose, with particular attention being paid to whether the patient has had thyroid disease or has received antithyroid treatment, current drug history, the presence of symptoms of a hypothalamic or pituitary mass lesion, and palpation of the thyroid gland.

The single most common cause of hypothyroidism worldwide is undoubtedly iodine deficiency. Where it is not a problem, the most common causes are chronic autoimmune thyroiditis and previous thyroid surgery or ^{131}I therapy.

Chronic Autoimmune Thyroiditis

Chronic autoimmune thyroiditis is the most common cause of hypothyroidism in persons living in regions of iodine sufficiency.[319] It is most common in women in the fourth decade or later but can occur in men and children. Also known as chronic lymphocytic thyroiditis, it exists in an atrophic (nongoitrous) form and a goitrous form. The atrophic form has also been called idiopathic hypothyroidism, primary myxedema, or primary thyroid atrophy, and the goitrous form Hashimoto's disease. The two forms differ clinically only in the presence or absence of goiter. Pathologically, the atrophic form is characterized by thyroid follicular atrophy, lymphocytic infiltration, and fibrosis and the goitrous form by thyroid follicular hyperplasia, lymphocytic and plasma–cell infiltration, lymphoid germinal centers, and fibrosis.

Patients with either atrophic or goitrous autoimmune thyroiditis may be euthyroid or have subclinical or overt hypothyroidism; the hypothyroidism is usually but not always permanent.[655,656] The extent of thyroid enlargement, when present, varies greatly. Painless thyroiditis with thyrotoxicosis and postpartum thyroiditis are part of the spectrum of autoimmune thyroiditis.

All forms of chronic autoimmune thyroiditis probably result from both antibody- and cell-mediated thyroid dysfunction and destruction.[319] When transplanted into nude mice, in which foreign T and B cells are destroyed, thyroid tissue from patients with the disease becomes histologically normal; in contrast, when transplanted into mice with combined immunodeficiency, in which foreign T and B cells survive, the tissue becomes histologically more abnormal.[657]

The antibodies that have been found in these patients and their possible biological activities are listed in Table 9-12. The information concerning biological activity is based largely on in vitro tests, and single antibody molecules may or may not have several different biological actions. For example, among antibodies with cytotoxic properties, some but not all react with thyroid peroxidase,[658,659] and not all antithyroid peroxidase antibodies or antibodies against the Na/I cotransporter inhibit thyroid-cell function in vitro.[328,660,661] Some antibodies that inhibit TSH biological activity in vitro have biological activity in vivo, because some newborn infants of mothers with chronic autoimmune thyroiditis have TSH receptor-blocking antibodies in their serum and are hypothyroid, and they become euthyroid when the maternal antibodies disappear.[662] Similarly, in some adult patients with hypothyroidism the presence and disappearance of TSH receptor-blocking antibodies correlate with the patient's need for T_4 therapy.[655]

Among patients with either form of chronic autoimmune thyroiditis, nearly all have high serum antithyroid peroxidase antibody concentrations, and most have thyroglobulin and Na/I cotransporter antibodies.[137,328,661] About 25 percent of patients with atrophic autoimmune thyroiditis, but only about 5 percent of those with goitrous autoimmune thyroiditis, have TSH receptor-blocking antibodies.[655,663] With respect to antibodies with biological activity, and in the absence of thyroid-cell cytotoxicity, variations in the types and amounts of antibodies produced must be important determinants of the degree of thyroid dysfunction, the degree to which the thyroid gland is atrophic or enlarged, and the natural history of the disorder.

Like Graves' disease, thyroid cells from patients with goitrous autoimmune thyroiditis express HLA class II molecules. Therefore, the thyroid cells, along with other antigen-presenting cells, may activate T helper cells, which then stimulate B cells to produce the different antibodies described earlier.

The permanent thyroid injury that occurs in most patients with autoimmune thyroiditis most likely results from disordered cellular immunity. The patients have activated intrathyroidal B and T cells, although the nature of the T cells is uncertain; increased proportions of suppressor-cytotoxic, helper-inducer, and

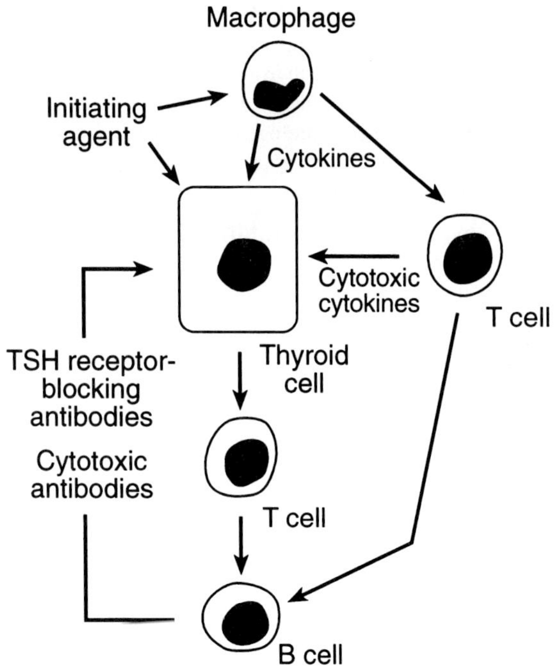

FIGURE 9-35. Hypothetical scheme for the development of chronic autoimmune thyroiditis. In a subject with inherited susceptibility to the disease, an exogenous initiating agent (virus or toxin) activates macrophages (or intrathyroidal T cells) to secrete cytokines, which then induce expression of HLA class II molecules on thyroid cells. The exogenous agent also affects the thyroid cells so that TSH receptors and other thyroid proteins are processed as antigens. The HLA class II molecules and antigens form complexes that bind to the antigen receptors of T helper cells, inducing them to secrete other cytokines. These cytokines stimulate B cells to expand and secrete antibodies that inhibit the receptor binding and action of TSH, so that thyroid secretion declines, or antibodies that are cytotoxic, so that the thyroid cells are destroyed. The same exogenous agent induces the processing of other thyroid proteins to form antigens that bind to constitutively expressed HLA class I molecules. The binding of these antigen-HLA class I complexes to the antigen receptors of T suppressor-cytotoxic cells stimulates the cells to differentiate into natural killer cells or secrete cytokines that damage or kill thyroid cells.

natural-killer T cells have been described in different studies.[319,664] Antigens are presented to T suppressor-cytotoxic cells in combination with HLA class I molecules, which are expressed constitutively on thyroid as on most other cells. Once activated by the binding of complexes of HLA class I molecules and thyroid antigens to their antigen receptors, in conjunction with several costimulatory molecules, the T cells secrete cytokines such as interleukin-2 that have direct cytotoxic actions on thyroid cells; cytokines such as interleukin-1 that stimulate expression of Fas molecules on thyroid cells, to which constitutively expressed Fas ligand molecules bind, thereby causing apoptosis; or the T cells differentiate into natural killer cells.[319,665] Thus, cytokines, cytotoxic T cells, or both are probably responsible for the thyroid injury that occurs in chronic autoimmune thyroiditis.

Figure 9-35 shows an outline of the processes by which antibody- and cell-mediated immune mechanisms, once activated, might result in chronic autoimmune thyroiditis. The initiating factors are not known but could be an infectious agent or toxin, as in Graves' disease (see section on Graves' Disease). Exogenously administered interleukin-2 and interferon alfa, but not interferon-gamma, can cause chronic autoimmune thyroiditis as well as painless thyroiditis.[305-310]

There are several known risk factors for autoimmune thyroiditis.[319] One is female sex; a second is heredity. Among twins, the concordance rate is higher in monozygotic than dizygotic twins.[665a] Thyroid autoantibodies are found in up to 50 percent of the siblings of patients and with lesser but still substantial frequency in other relatives; the frequency of Graves' disease in siblings and relatives may be increased.[347] A predominance of certain HLA haplotypes has been reported in some ethnic groups.[347,666] Patients with chronic autoimmune thyroiditis and their relatives may have autoantibodies to other endocrine tissues and occasionally other hormonal deficiency syndromes indicative of the presence of the type 2 autoimmune polyglandular syndrome (see Chap. 27). The incidence of chronic autoimmune thyroiditis is increased in patients with congenital rubella infection, Down's syndrome, Turner's syndrome, and type 1 diabetes mellitus.[667-669] A high iodine intake may also be a risk factor for chronic autoimmune thyroiditis, as manifested by high serum antithyroid peroxidase antibody concentrations, in addition to having an antithyroid action in patients with established disease.

The natural history of chronic autoimmune thyroiditis is variable. Among patients with atrophic autoimmune thyroiditis and subclinical hypothyroidism, overt hypothyroidism occurs in 5 to 20 percent per year, but in a few patients serum antithyroid antibody and TSH concentrations decline to normal spontaneously.[130,139,670] Hypothyroidism also develops in time in the majority of patients with goitrous autoimmune thyroiditis who are not hypothyroid initially.[670]

Treatment with T_4 results in decreases in goiter size in about half of patients with chronic autoimmune thyroiditis, and serum antithyroid peroxidase antibody concentrations may decline substantially.[671,672] Among patients in whom T_4 therapy is stopped after a year or more, a few remain euthyroid, and Graves' disease has occurred later in a few,[361] but most become as hypothyroid or more severely hypothyroid than they were originally.[655,656] Thus, either form of chronic autoimmune thyroiditis tends to cause progressive, persistent thyroid failure. Chronic autoimmune thyroiditis is a major risk factor for thyroid lymphoma.[673]

Transient Hypothyroidism in Autoimmune Thyroiditis

Transient hypothyroidism is an integral part of the syndromes of painless (lymphocytic) thyroiditis with thyrotoxicosis and postpartum thyroiditis. Among patients with painless thyroiditis, about 50 percent become hypothyroid several weeks after the thyrotoxic phase subsides. The hypothyroid phase is usually asymptomatic and lasts 2–8 weeks (Fig. 9-26), but some patients have permanent hypothyroidism or develop it later.[674]

Postpartum thyroiditis occurs in 1 to 6 percent of women after pregnancy.[376] About 80 percent have hypothyroidism, preceded in about half by thyrotoxicosis (see section on Postpartum Thyrotoxicosis). Whether preceded by thyrotoxicosis or not, the hypothyroidism usually develops 4–8 months after delivery and lasts 2–8 weeks. The patient may have a small diffuse goiter, and the hypothyroidism is often subclinical. This syndrome may be associated with postpartum depression.[675] It tends to recur after subsequent pregnancies, and from 25 to 50 percent of women eventually develop chronic autoimmune thyroiditis.[676,677]

Painless thyroiditis with thyrotoxicosis and postpartum thyroiditis appear to be variant forms of chronic autoimmune thyroiditis. The thyroid inflammation and injury are more intense than in chronic autoimmune thyroiditis, but thyroid follicular cells are not destroyed. Immune activation seemingly develops more rapidly, but tolerance is regained more quickly. Thyroid biopsies show lymphocytic thyroiditis, but the cellular infiltration is less intense than in chronic autoimmune thyroiditis, and there are no germinal centers or fibrosis. Painless thyroiditis and postpartum thyroiditis differ in that women with postpartum thyroiditis more often have high serum antithyroid antibody concentrations before, during, and after their thyroid illness and are more likely to have recurrences and develop chronic autoimmune thyroiditis.[674,676,677]

Hypothyroidism after Radioiodine Therapy for Thyrotoxicosis and External Radiotherapy

Hypothyroidism occurs within a year after therapy in a substantial number of patients treated with ^{131}I for thyrotoxicosis (see section on Treatment of Thyrotoxicosis), and thereafter it occurs at a rate of 0.5 to 2 percent per year.[568,569,574,577,578] Its occurrence within the first year, but not later, is dependent on the dose of ^{131}I. Late hypothyroidism is preceded by a long period of subclinical hypothyroidism,[579] attesting to the ability of TSH hypersecretion to maintain nearly adequate thyroid secretion if the thyroid is not badly damaged. Thus, among patients with subclinical hypothyroidism after ^{131}I therapy, only about 5 percent become hypothyroid each year. Late post-^{131}I hypothyroidism probably occurs because the thyroid follicular cells that survive acute radiation injury can maintain their function but cannot replicate; it may be exacerbated by autoimmune thyroid injury. Among patients with toxic uninodular or multinodular goiter treated with ^{131}I, hypothyroidism occurs in 5 to 20 percent.[590,593,594,597]

External neck irradiation therapy in doses of 25 Gy (2,500 rads) or more, as is given for the treatment of patients with lymphoma, laryngeal carcinoma, and carcinoma of the head and neck, also causes hypothyroidism in children and adults.[330,678] Its effect is dose-dependent; about 50 percent of patients who receive 40 Gy (4,000 rads) ultimately develop hypothyroidism. Hypothyroidism also occurs in patients with posterior fossa tumors who are treated with radiation, and in patients who receive total body radiation for bone marrow transplantation.[679] External irradiation-induced overt hypothyroidism, like that occurring 1 or more years after ^{131}I therapy, is usually preceded by months or years of subclinical hypothyroidism.

Postoperative Hypothyroidism

Total thyroidectomy results in an increase in serum TSH concentrations within 1 week and overt hypothyroidism within 1 month.[680] Unilateral thyroid lobectomy results in small decreases in serum T_4 concentrations and small increases in serum TSH concentrations, usually within the normal range, for several months, after which the concentrations of both hormones return to baseline.[681]

The frequency of hypothyroidism after subtotal thyroidectomy for Graves' thyrotoxicosis is high, being about 50 percent in the first year after surgery.[584,585] This high rate of postoperative hypothyroidism is a result of aggressive surgery undertaken to reduce the frequency of recurrent thyrotoxicosis after surgery. Hypothyroidism developing in the first months after subtotal thyroidectomy is not invariably permanent; in some patients, the remaining thyroid mass grows sufficiently to maintain normal thyroid secretion after a period of stimulation by TSH. Hypothyroidism also may develop later than 1 year after surgery for Graves' thyrotoxicosis, at a rate of about 0.5 to 1 percent per year.[578] Late postoperative hypothyroidism is probably due to destruction of the thyroid remnant by an autoimmune process, because it is more likely to occur in patients whose excised thyroid tissue had histological evidence of autoimmune thyroiditis.

Hypothyroidism Due to Infiltrative Disease of the Thyroid

Several infiltrative diseases may rarely result in thyroid damage sufficient to cause hypothyroidism. They include amyloidosis, sarcoidosis, scleroderma, cystinosis, iron deposition, leukemia, fibrous invasive thyroiditis (Riedel's thyroiditis), and infections, including fungal and pneumocystis infections.[682] Most of these patients have diffuse goiters, and the goiter may be slightly tender.

Congenital and Hereditary Hypothyroidism

Thyroid Agenesis and Dysgenesis (Nongoitrous Cretinism)

Developmental defects of the thyroid gland are the most common cause of hypothyroidism in the newborn (Table 9-17). About 40 percent of these infants have virtually complete absence of the thyroid (thyroid agenesis), but in the remainder some thyroid tissue is detectable by thyroid radionuclide imaging (thyroid dysgenesis).[683] The thyroid tissue may be located in the midline anywhere from the base of the tongue to below the thyroid cartilage, or on one side of the neck, or on both sides of the neck in the normal position. The cause(s) of these abnormalities, most of which are not inherited, is for the most part unknown, but 10–20 percent occur as a result of inherited defects in thyroid hormone synthesis.

One of the latter is loss-of-function mutations of the TSH receptor, usually in the extracellular domain of the receptor.[684–686] The mutations therefore result in decreased TSH binding to the receptor and unresponsiveness to TSH of varying severity. Most affected patients have had overt hypothyroidism detected by neonatal screening, but a few have had subclinical hypothyroidism; the thyroid is absent or hypoplastic. These mutations are inherited as autosomal recessive traits; in some families parents or other family members who were heterozygous for the mutation had mild subclinical hypothyroidism. TSH unresponsiveness, and hypothyroidism, also occurs in patients with pseudohypoparathyroidism, as a result of mutations in the alpha subunit of the G protein that reduce signal transduction (see Chap. 4).[687]

Transplacental passage of TSH receptor-blocking antibodies causes transient but not permanent neonatal hypothyroidism.[662,688] These antibodies have been found only in infants whose mothers had chronic autoimmune thyroiditis. Congenital hypothyroidism could be caused by transplacental passage of cytotoxic antibodies, also found in mothers with chronic autoimmune thyroiditis, but these antibodies are found with similar frequency in normal and hypothyroid neonates.[689]

Inherited Biosynthetic Defects in Thyroid Hormonogenesis

Thyroid hormone biosynthesis and secretion depend on the availability of iodine and the ability of thyroid tissue to carry out the multiple reactions needed to synthesize and secrete T_4 and T_3. It is not surprising, therefore, that there are genetic and therefore hereditary defects in the different steps of thyroid hormone production. Although rare, these defects have provided insight into the normal mechanisms of thyroid hormone biosynthesis and release. Most of these disorders are inherited as autosomal recessive traits. In homozygotes, hypothyroidism is severe and becomes apparent early in life. The compensatory increase in TSH secretion leads to thyroid enlargement, which may be minimal early in life but becomes marked in childhood or later if the disorder is not detected and treated earlier. In presumed heterozygotes, the abnormality is usually mild and results only in a moderate degree of thyroid enlargement.

Iodide Transport Defect

This rare abnormality is characterized by partial or complete lack of ability of thyroid tissue to transport iodide, and is caused by mutations in the Na/I cotransporter.[690,691] Thus, thyroid radioiodine uptake is very low despite the presence of goiter. Treatment with inorganic iodine in doses of 5 mg or more daily restores thyroid hormone secretion to normal as a result of passive diffusion of iodide into the thyroid, but treatment with T_4 is more convenient.

Iodide Organification Defects

Several different defects in iodine oxidation and organification have been described.[692] They include mutations in thyroid peroxidase, resulting in decreased or absent enzyme activity, qualitative abnormalities in the enzyme resulting in defective binding of heme prosthetic groups to it and abnormal intracellular localization of the enzyme, and deficient hydrogen peroxide generation. Thyroid iodide transport is increased, but little further intrathyroidal iodide metabolism occurs, so that iodide accumulates in the thyroid. This accumulation can be detected by a perchlorate discharge test; when iodide transport is inhibited by perchlorate, the outward diffusion (discharge) of inorganic iodide that has accumulated can be detected. Perchlorate discharge tests are done by administration of 500 mg $KClO_4$ 1 h after a tracer dose of ^{123}I; a fall in thyroid radioactivity of 10 percent or more 1 hour after $KClO_4$ administration indicates defective iodide oxidation and organification.

In some families, goiter, usually with subclinical hypothyroidism, occurs along with congenital sensorineural deafness caused by malformation of the inner ear (Pendred's syndrome).[693] The patients have a positive perchlorate discharge test, and therefore they are considered to have an organification defect. However, when studied in vitro, their thyroid tissue usually has normal peroxidase activity and ability to synthesize iodotyrosines, but not T_4 and T_3. The deafness usually precedes the development of goiter and may occur in patients with no thyroid abnormality. The gene that is defective in these patients codes for a cell-membrane protein, pendrin, is found mostly in thyroid tissue and is thought to transport iodide from thyroid cells to exocytotic vesicles in the lumen of thyroid follicles.[11a,11b]

Thyroglobulin Biosynthetic Defects

Thyroglobulin production may be inadequate even though its structure is normal. It may be produced in adequate quantities but may be structurally abnormal, so that organification of iodide or iodotyrosyl coupling within it is poor or it cannot be secreted into the thyroid follicular lumen.[694] The latter abnormalities may result from synthesis of thyroglobulin that is abnormal in either amino acid or carbohydrate composition. At the genetic level, thyroglobulin defects may result from mutations in thyroid transcription factors as well as in thyroglobulin.[695]

Iodotyrosine Deiodinase Defect

Thyroid iodotyrosine deiodinase plays an important role in the recirculation of iodide and thus in its conservation. Deiodinase deficiency results in the release of large quantities of mono- and diiodotyrosine from the thyroid gland. Because extrathyroidal iodotyrosine deiodinase also is lacking in these patients, the iodotyrosines are excreted in the urine. Thus, iodide that normally becomes available for reuse within the thyroid is lost, resulting in secondary iodine deficiency.

These disorders can be differentiated in a general way by the presence or absence of goiter, measurements of serum thyroglobulin and thyroid radioiodine uptake, and perchlorate discharge testing. The identification of specific defects requires detailed in vitro studies of thyroid iodine metabolism or thyroglobulin structure, or DNA analysis.

Inherited Defects in Thyroid Hormone Action (Thyroid Hormone Resistance)

Generalized resistance to thyroid hormones is a rare hereditary disorder characterized by few or no symptoms and signs of thyroid dysfunction, diffuse goiter, high serum total and free T_4 and T_3 concentrations, and normal or slightly high serum TSH concentrations.[696,697] It is caused by mutations in the T_3 nuclear receptor. Some patients have had physical findings, such as deafness, stippled epiphyses, and short stature, indicative of hypothyroidism in infancy. Others have had tachycardia or hyperactivity suggestive of excessive thyroid hormone action, presumably because the receptors mediating these actions of thyroid hormone are normal. The clinical manifestations are not only varied, even among patients with the same mutation, but also can vary over time in an individual patient.[697,698] Hypothyroidism may be evident in patients mistakenly treated for thyrotoxicosis by ^{131}I or surgical therapy; recurrent goiter in a hypothyroid or euthyroid patient with such a history is a clue to the presence of generalized thyroid hormone resistance.

Most reported patients have been adolescents or adults, but the disorder can be recognized soon after birth.[699] Males and females are affected in equal numbers. The pattern of inheritance is autosomal recessive in most families and autosomal dominant in a few.[696] These patients are euthyroid because they produce large amounts of T_4 and T_3; the pituitary is resistant to the same extent as other tissues, and the resistance is not complete in any tissue. Additional thyroid hormone evokes little additional response unless very high doses are given.[700]

A variety of defects in T_3 nuclear receptors have been identified in families with this syndrome, mostly point mutations of the gene for the beta form of the receptor on chromosome 3 that resulted in amino acid substitutions in the T_3-binding region of the receptor (see section on Biochemical Actions of Thyroid Hormones), but large segments of the gene were deleted in another family.[696] Defects in the alpha form of the receptor have not been found. The mutant receptors may have not only reduced affinity for T_3, but also may inhibit the actions of the normal receptors on the T_3 response elements of DNA, thus explaining the dominant effect of the mutation (dominant recessive mutation). The differences in phenotype among the patients with this syndrome are probably due to differences in the tissue distribution of the mutated receptors and the extent to which they interact with the normal receptors and interfere with the actions of the latter.

Acquired Defects in Thyroid Hormone Synthesis

Iodine Deficiency

The presence of goiter in many and cretinism in some inhabitants of regions where iodine deficiency is endemic has long been recognized. Most subjects with goiter also have abnormalities in thyroid iodine metabolism, decreased T_4 and to a lesser extent T_3 secretion, and high serum TSH concentrations. The frequency of these abnormalities varies greatly, depending on the degree of iodine deficiency. An iodine intake of 25 to 50 μg daily or less is associated with a goiter prevalence of 15 to 30 percent; when intake is lower, the prevalence of goiter is higher and overt hypothyroidism occurs frequently. Other variables such as dietary and water-borne goitrogens and selenium deficiency are important contributory factors in some regions.[701,702] Iodine deficiency persists worldwide, not just in underdeveloped areas, despite the fact that it can be readily prevented by supplementation of salt or other foods with iodine or by yearly oral or parenteral administration of iodized oil. Furthermore, continued monitoring after supplementation is introduced is vital. In the United States, iodine intake has decreased by about 50 percent in the last 20 years, and about 10 percent of people are now considered to have iodine deficiency (intake <50 μg daily).[8]

Cretinism is classically subdivided into neurological cretinism, characterized by mental retardation, spasticity, and deaf-mutism, and myxedematous cretinism, characterized by mental retardation, short stature, and hypothyroidism (neurological cretinism).[703] The differences are more apparent than real; both types of cretinism are caused by iodine deficiency, and both disappear when iodine supplementation is adequate.

Antithyroid Agents

A variety of inorganic and organic compounds, both naturally occurring and synthetic, have antithyroid actions. These compounds inhibit thyroidal T_4 and T_3 synthesis and secretion, usually by inhibiting iodide transport or iodide organification and iodotyrosine coupling, and therefore can cause both hypothyroidism and goiter. PTU and MMI are the most potent antithyroid drugs; their use should usually be evident. The most commonly used drugs that may cause hypothyroidism and goiter probably are lithium carbonate (see section on Effects of Drugs on Thyroid Function) and aminoglutethimide.[704] Many other drugs, chemicals, and constituents of naturally occurring foodstuffs have antithyroid actions and occasionally have been implicated as the cause of hypothyroidism or goiter in individual patients.[682] They are not, however, important causes of hypothyroidism. Most have very weak antithyroid actions and probably cause hypothyroidism only in patients with preexisting subclinical thyroid disease. Furthermore, other than lithium carbonate, none are widely used.

Interferon-alpha and interleukin-2 can induce autoimmune thyroiditis and hypothyroidism.[305–310]

Iodine Excess

Iodine excess also may cause subclinical or overt hypothyroidism. The iodine may be used as either inorganic iodine or organic iodine compounds in the form of dietary supplements, drugs, radiographic contrast agents, or skin and water-system disinfectants. Supranormal iodine intake has minor antithyroid actions in normal subjects; patients susceptible to iodide-induced hypothyroidism are those who have damaged thyroid glands as a result of chronic autoimmune thyroiditis or previous ^{131}I or surgical therapy for Graves' thyrotoxicosis. In them, escape from the antithyroid action of iodide does not occur as it does in normal subjects and untreated patients with Graves' hyperthyroidism, and thus the action of iodine is sustained until use is stopped or the contrast agent is excreted (see section on Effects of Drugs on Thyroid Function).

Increased Degradation of Thyroid Hormone

Hypothyroidism has been reported in infants with large hemangiomas of the liver.[704a] The tumors contained very high levels of type 3 deiodinase activity, causing very rapid deiodination of T_4 to rT_3 and T_3 to T_2, and therefore low serum T_4 and T_3 concentrations and high serum rT_3 concentrations. In one patient, very high doses of T_3 were needed to raise the serum T_3 concentration and lower TSH secretion. Thyroid gland function seems to be increased, but thyroid hormone degradation is so rapid that full compensation cannot occur.

Central (Hypothyrotropic) Hypothyroidism

Pituitary Hypothyroidism

TSH is required for normal thyroid secretion, and TSH deficiency results in decreased thyroid secretion and thyroid atrophy. This condition is much less common than is primary (thyroidal) hypothyroidism. TSH deficiency may be caused by destruction of the thyrotrophs by hormone-secreting or nonsecreting pituitary adenomas (see Chap. 7). Nearly all patients with pituitary microadenomas are euthyroid, whereas 10 to 25 percent of those with macroadenomas are hypothyroid. If not present initially, TSH deficiency may result from surgical or radiation therapy for pituitary tumors,[705] or conversely some initially hypothyroid patients with pituitary tumors may become euthyroid after resection of their tumors.[706] TSH deficiency may also result from postpartum pituitary necrosis (Sheehan's syndrome), craniopharyngioma, carotid aneurysm, trauma, cranial radiation therapy, hemochromatosis, and infiltrative processes such as lymphocytic hypophysitis, metastatic cancer, tuberculosis, and histiocytosis. In any of these situations, TSH deficiency may occur in association with other tropic hormone deficiencies or as an isolated abnormality. Isolated TSH deficiency can also occur in patients treated with bexarotene, a selective retinoid X receptor ligand developed for treatment of lymphomas and other tumors that probably act by mimicking the inhibitory action of T_3 in the thyrotroph cells.[706a] In infants and children, TSH deficiency may be caused by many of the same diseases, and also by mutations in the beta subunit of TSH[707,708] and, in combination with other pituitary hormone deficiencies, by mutations in several pituitary transcription factors.[709]

Pituitary enlargement and hypothyroidism do not invariably indicate the presence of a primary pituitary tumor and pituitary hypothyroidism, because pituitary enlargement occurs in rare patients with severe, longstanding primary hypothyroidism.[710,711] They have compensatory hyperplasia and hypertrophy of the thyrotroph cells sufficient to cause radiologically and even clinically evident pituitary enlargement, even visual field defects.[712] Recognition that pituitary enlargement can occur in patients with primary hypothyroidism is very important so that they do not undergo unnecessary pituitary surgery. The serum TSH concentrations in patients with secondary pituitary enlargement are usually very high (200–600 mU/liter). The concentrations decline during thyroid hormone therapy, indicating that TSH secretion is not autonomous, and the pituitary gland diminishes in size.[711]

Hypothalamic Hypothyroidism

TRH deficiency also causes hypothyroidism. TRH deficiency may be isolated or may coexist with other hypothalamic hormone deficiencies. Hypothalamic hypothyroidism occurs predominantly in children, in whom it is not usually accompanied by any anatomic abnormality; one cause is mutation in the TRH receptor.[713] In children and adults it may occur as a result of cranial radiation therapy; traumatic, infiltrative, and neoplastic diseases of the hypothalamus; or pituitary lesions that interrupt the hypothalamic-pituitary portal circulation.

Thyrotropin Secretion in Central Hypothyroidism

Most hypothyroid patients with pituitary or hypothalamic disease have low or normal serum TSH concentrations (Fig. 9-17). Even when the concentrations are normal, nocturnal TSH secretion is usually decreased.[144,714,715] Characteristically, there is little increase in serum TSH after TRH administration in patients with pituitary hypothyroidism and a normal or delayed response in those with hypothalamic hypothyroidism, but the responses are too variable for this test to be useful in an individual patient.[53] Rare patients with central hypothyroidism have high basal serum TSH concentrations.[239,240] Their TSH is immunoreactive but biologically inactive, and its biological activity increases when they are given TRH, probably because of changes in TSH glycosylation.

Clinical Manifestations of Hypothyroidism

The clinical manifestations of hypothyroidism are highly variable, depending on its cause, duration, and severity. The spectrum of hypothyroidism extends from subclinical hypothyroidism to overt hypothyroidism to myxedema coma. The characteristic change in organ system function in hypothyroid patients is slowing; thus, there is slowing of physical and mental activity and of the function of most organ systems.

TABLE 9-18. Symptoms and Signs of Hypothyroidism

	Frequency in Overtly Hypothyroid Patients, %
Symptoms	
Dry skin	60–100
Cold intolerance	35–95
Weakness and fatigue	52–90
Hoarseness	28–75
Weight gain	50–75
Mental slowness	45–68
Constipation	32–65
Decreased sweating	10–65
Paresthesia	18–60
Decreased hearing	5–30
Signs	
Coarse skin and hair	70–100
Slow movements	70–90
Cold skin	70–90
Periorbital puffiness	40–90
Slow reflex relaxation	24–77
Bradycardia	10–58

Sources: Billewicz,[716] Doucet,[717] Zulewski,[718] Samuels.[719]

The symptoms and signs of overt hypothyroidism and their frequency are listed in Table 9-18.[716–719] Some of these data are from older studies, and the frequency of these symptoms and signs in patients with hypothyroidism now is probably at the lower end of the ranges shown in the table. Among them, the most discriminating are dry skin, decreased sweating, hoarseness, paresthesia, periorbital edema, and delayed reflexes.[718] Older patients have fewer symptoms and signs,[717] and in both young and old the correlation between clinical and biochemical manifestations of hypothyroidism is poor. The presence of hypothyroidism may also be suggested by a history of events related to its causes, such as previous ^{131}I therapy, thyroid surgery, or treatment with iodine-containing drugs or lithium carbonate.

Spontaneously occurring hypothyroidism (e.g., that due to chronic autoimmune thyroiditis) usually develops very slowly, and as thyroid secretion declines, the resulting rise in TSH secretion limits further decline in thyroid secretion. Thus, the symptoms and signs of hypothyroidism usually develop very slowly. When hypothyroidism develops more rapidly, for example soon after ^{131}I therapy or subtotal thyroidectomy in patients with Graves' thyrotoxicosis, the symptoms appear sooner and are more pronounced, and symptoms such as muscle cramps and paresthesia are more prominent. The onset of symptoms is even more rapid, occurring within 4 weeks, among patients who become hypothyroid very rapidly, for example previously treated thyroid cancer patients in whom T_4 therapy is discontinued abruptly.[720] Hypothyroidism due to hypothalamic or pituitary disease is less likely to be associated with periorbital and peripheral edema, hoarseness, and weight gain.

The characteristic pathologic finding in patients with hypothyroidism is the accumulation of glycosaminoglycans, primarily hyaluronic acid, in interstitial tissue. These substances accumulate because their synthesis is increased, and, as a consequence of their hydrophilic properties, they lead to the mucinous edema that is characteristic of the disorder. This is myxedema. Mucinous edema of the dermis causes some of the most obvious clinical manifestations of hypothyroidism, and in fatal cases, mucinous edema has been found in the interstitial tissue of most organ systems.[721]

General Appearance

A patient with hypothyroidism may appear normal, have obvious myxedema of the face and extremities, or be comatose. The major presenting manifestations are mostly subjective, and are vague and nonspecific. The patient complains of weakness and lack of energy, tiring easily, and being mentally slow and sleepy. Too often, these symptoms are attributed to aging by the patient or the patient's relatives. Cold intolerance may be marked, with the patient using extra clothing even in the summer.

Skin and Appendages

The characteristic but now rare appearance of a patient with overt hypothyroidism (Fig. 9-36) is primarily a reflection of nonpitting periorbital and peripheral mucinous edema. The facial features are coarse, blepharoptosis is present, and the skin becomes rough, scaly, and thickened. More often the patient's appearance is less altered. The skin is dry and scaly, but it is not thickened or particularly rough, and periorbital and peripheral edema is mild. At times, the edema is pitting, particularly in the legs; such a finding need not indicate the presence of cardiac or other disease. There is often pallor caused by the thickened dermis and epidermis, decreased cutaneous blood flow, and sometimes anemia. The yellowish hue of carotinemia may be evident. The skin feels cold as a result of both thickening and decreased blood flow.

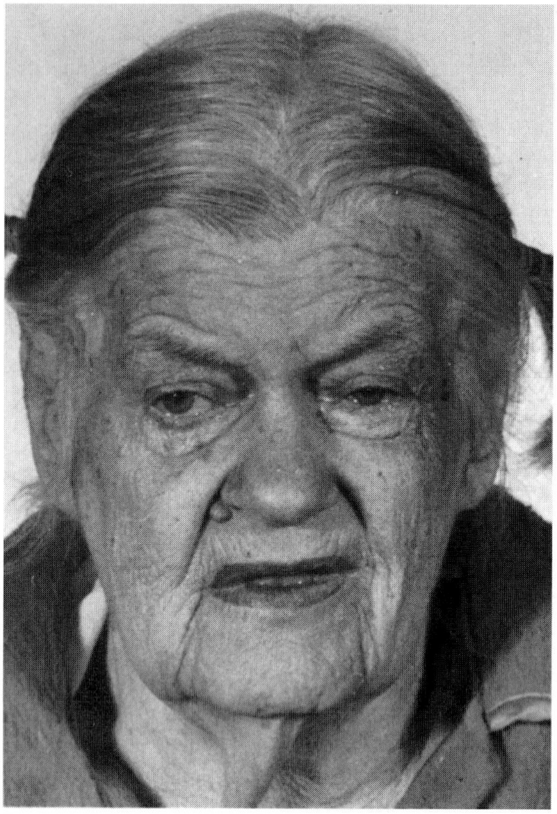

FIGURE 9-36. Photograph of a woman with severe chronic hypothyroidism, showing facial puffiness and periorbital edema.

Decreased sebaceous and sweat gland secretions add to the dryness of the skin. The hair may be coarse, dry, and brittle, and hair growth may slow or cease. Hair may be lost on the scalp, the extremities, or the eyebrows. The nails also grow slowly and may be thickened and brittle.

Thyroid Gland

The size of the thyroid may provide a valuable clue to the cause of hypothyroidism and even to its presence, because thyroid enlargement may be the first objective sign of hypothyroidism. Goitrous autoimmune thyroiditis is characterized by painless nontender diffuse thyroid enlargement, although the surface may be irregular or even nodular. The consistency of the thyroid gland is often described as firm or rubbery. The thyroid gland also is diffusely enlarged in patients with hypothyroidism caused by iodine deficiency, congenital defects in thyroid hormone biosynthesis, any antithyroid drug or any infiltrative disorder, but in all these situations it becomes irregular or nodular years or decades later. In all these conditions, the thyroid may be slightly painful or tender if the enlargement was rapid. The thyroid is small or not palpable in atrophic autoimmune thyroiditis or central hypothyroidism.

Nervous System

Hypothyroid patients have many symptoms of mental dysfunction. Although central nervous system glucose and oxygen consumption are normal, cerebral vascular resistance is increased and cerebral blood flow is reduced in proportion to the decrease in cardiac output. The reduced delivery of oxygen to tissue utilizing it at a normal rate should result in some degree of cerebral hypoxia.

The psychological and behavioral symptoms of hypothyroidism include lethargy and fatigue, decreased attention span, loss of ambition, slowing of movement and thought, and memory loss. The patient becomes complacent, less alert, mentally slow, and physically clumsy. Speech is slow and hesitant as well as hoarse. There may be some cognitive impairment,[722,723] and occasional patients have overt dementia. Changes in mood include inappropriate cheerfulness, anxiety and agitation ("myxedema madness"), and depression. Headache and hearing loss may be prominent complaints. The patient may sleep longer at night or fall asleep often during the day.

Hypothyroid patients often complain of paresthesia, but few have objective neurologic findings other than slow deep tendon reflexes. Both the contraction and relaxation phases of the reflexes are prolonged, the latter more than the former. Several neurologic syndromes that are reversible may occur; they include the carpal tunnel syndrome due to mucinous edema of the flexor retinaculum of the wrist, a symmetric sensorimotor polyneuropathy, and cerebellar dysfunction with signs such as ataxia, intention tremor, and nystagmus.

Musculoskeletal System

Myalgia, cramps, and stiffness occur in many hypothyroid patients, and may be the predominant symptoms.[724,725] Weakness, clumsiness, and fatigability are other common symptoms, and there may be objective muscle weakness. Rarely, chronic hypothyroid myopathy results in increased muscle mass (pseudohypertrophy), muscle spasms, and pseudomyotonia. High serum creatine kinase (MM fraction) concentrations are common in hypothyroidism, even in the absence of any symptoms of muscle dysfunction.[726] The increase is due to release from skeletal muscle, presumably as a result of increased cell permeability, and slowed clearance. Serum lactate dehydrogenase and aminotransferase concentrations may be high as well. Muscle biopsies show interstitial edema and muscle fiber enlargement, loss of striations, and sarcoplasmic degenerative changes.

Hypothyroid patients may complain of arthralgia and joint stiffness. Some have synovial thickening and synovial effusions, usually of the knees.

Cardiovascular-Pulmonary System

Hypothyroidism results in decreases in the rate and force of cardiac contractility and in peripheral oxygen needs.[727] Peripheral resistance increases, and cerebral, cutaneous, and renal blood flow and blood volume are decreased. Cardiac output is decreased, but ventricular end-diastolic pressure and peripheral arteriovenous oxygen differences are normal. During exercise, cardiac output increases and peripheral resistance decreases appropriately, indicating normal cardiac reserve. In fatal cases, the myocardial fibers are edematous and vacuolated.[721]

The symptoms and signs of cardiovascular dysfunction include bradycardia, evidence of poor peripheral circulation such as pallor and cold skin, dyspnea on exertion, decreased exercise tolerance, fatigability, and distant heart sounds. The lethargy, puffiness, edema, and diminished cardiac activity may suggest cardiac failure, but this is rare. When cardiac failure occurs, it is most likely due to the hemodynamic changes of hypothyroidism superimposed on preexisting cardiac disease, but cardiomyopathy that disappeared during T_4 therapy has been described.[728] There may be clinical and radiographic evidence of cardiac enlargement, and a few patients have a pericardial effusion.[729] The electrocardiogram shows bradycardia and low-amplitude P waves and QRS complexes and, less often, conduction disturbances and nonspecific QRS and T-wave abnormalities. Echocardiography may reveal pericardial effusion, varying degrees of septal and wall thickening, and diminished myocardial relaxation.[729,730]

About 20 percent of hypothyroid patients have hypertension. In most it is coincidental, but is aggravated by the increase in peripheral resistance that occurs in hypothyroidism. In a few patients hypertension is more closely related to hypothyroidism, and disappears with T_4 treatment.[731]

The coexistence of angina pectoris and hypothyroidism in some patients warrants special mention. Although hypothyroid patients may have hypercholesterolemia and hyperhomocysteinemia, there is little evidence that hypothyroidism is accompanied by accelerated atherogenesis. The development of hypothyroidism may ameliorate angina pectoris, whether directly because cardiac work and thus myocardial oxygen requirements are reduced or simply because the patient becomes less active. Hypothyroid patients should not be denied T_4 treatment because of the possibility that they might have symptoms of ischemic heart disease, but should be treated cautiously. Among 55 patients with angina and hypothyroidism, the angina improved or disappeared during thyroid hormone therapy in 21 patients, did not change in 25, and worsened in 9.[732] Among about 1,400 other hypothyroid patients, new-onset angina appeared in 6 patients during the first month of thyroid therapy, in another 6 within the first year, and in 23 after that. Antianginal therapy can be added if necessary, and coronary revascularization, if otherwise indicated, can be done safely in hypothyroid patients.[733,734]

Complaints referable to the airways and respiratory system include chronic nasal congestion, hoarseness, shortness of breath, and sleep apnea. Nasal congestion and hoarseness are due to mucinous edema of the nasal mucosa and larynx, respectively. Shortness of breath may reflect cardiac disease, the presence of pleural effusion, or impairment of pulmonary function.

Most hypothyroid patients have normal lung volumes, vital capacity, and arterial P_{O_2}, P_{CO_2}, and pH values. Maximum breathing capacity, compliance, and ventilatory drive may be reduced,[735,736] because of respiratory muscle weakness or respiratory-center depression. Some hypothyroid patients have symptomatic obstructive sleep apnea, and it can be demonstrated by polysomnography in others. It is due largely to enlargement of the tongue and pharyngeal muscles, but has a central component in some patients.[737,738] Pleural effusions may be present without other evidence of lung disease.[739]

Fluid and Electrolyte Metabolism and Renal Function

Hypothyroid patients often appear puffy or even edematous, and total body water and sodium content are increased as a result of the accumulation of hydrophilic glycosaminoglycans in extravascular tissue, increased vascular permeability, and decreased lymph flow.[740] Plasma volume is decreased, and serum atrial natriuretic hormone and aldosterone concentrations and plasma renin activity are normal or slightly decreased.[445,458]

In regard to renal function, renal blood flow is reduced in proportion to the decrease in cardiac output. The glomerular filtration rate is slightly reduced, and serum creatinine and urea nitrogen concentrations may be slightly increased.[741] Hyperuricemia and modest proteinuria may be present. Free water clearance is decreased, as is the ability to excrete a water load. Hyponatremia has been described in severely hypothyroid patients, and has usually been attributed to excess vasopressin secretion; however, vasopressin secretion, basally and in response to saline infusion or water loading, is normal in most patients.[742–744] Furthermore, in one large survey hyponatremia was no more common in hypothyroid patients than in other patients.[745]

Gastrointestinal System

The tongue is often enlarged. Decreased gastric emptying may result in nausea and vomiting, and decreased intestinal motility may result in constipation and abdominal distension.[462] Hypomotility may be severe enough to cause paralytic ileus or megacolon, with the clinical picture of intestinal obstruction. Liver size and function are usually normal, although the high serum creatine kinase, lactate dehydrogenase, and aminotransferase concentrations mentioned previously may be due in part to reduced hepatic enzyme clearance. Ascites is occasionally present; it is probably due to abnormal capillary permeability and reduced hepatic lymph flow. The gallbladder may be dilated and empty poorly.

Intestinal absorption is usually normal. Gastric atrophy and achlorhydria can occur and may be associated with vitamin B_{12} malabsorption. About 20 percent of patients with chronic autoimmune thyroiditis have antiparietal cell antibodies. Defects in gastric acid secretion and vitamin B_{12} malabsorption are more frequent in patients with this type of hypothyroidism, some of whom have or later develop pernicious anemia.

Hematopoietic System

A substantial proportion of hypothyroid patients have a low red cell mass because of decreased oxygen requirements and therefore decreased erythropoietin secretion.[445] Some of these patients are truly anemic, but the anemia is in part masked by a fall in plasma volume. Therefore, hematocrit values are rarely below 35 percent. The anemia is usually normocytic.[746] Serum iron, iron binding capacity, and vitamin B_{12} and folate concentrations usually are normal. The bone marrow is hypocellular, and kinetic studies indicate slowed iron clearance and incorporation. Occasionally patients have iron, folic acid, or vitamin B_{12} deficiency, with the appropriate peripheral blood and bone marrow findings. Iron deficiency may result from excessive menstrual bleeding or poor iron absorption secondary to decreased gastric acid production. Megaloblastic anemia may be due to malabsorption of folic acid or vitamin B_{12} caused by hypothyroidism or by pernicious anemia in patients with chronic autoimmune thyroiditis.

Leukocyte, lymphocyte, and platelet counts are normal in hypothyroidism. Platelet function or aggregation may be abnormal, bleeding time may be prolonged, and the concentrations of some clotting factors, notably factor VIII and von Willebrand factor, may be slightly decreased.[475,744,747] Some patients may bruise easily, but the abnormalities in platelet function and clotting factors do not correlate well with clinical bleeding.

Energy, Nutrient, and Drug Metabolism

The decrease in energy expenditure and oxygen consumption in hypothyroidism is accompanied by decreased utilization of a variety of substrates. The result is decreased heat production, probably the major cause of the cold intolerance that is characteristic of hypothyroidism. Decreased metabolic activity and substrate utilization, as well as physical inactivity and mental depression, also result in decreased appetite and food intake. Body weight may increase slightly, but marked increases in weight are unusual. When it occurs, weight gain is due more to retention of salt and water in interstitial tissue than to fat deposition. Serum leptin concentrations are normal or slightly reduced in relation to body fat mass.[481,482] Most hypothyroid patients lose several kg after treatment is begun, but often gain weight thereafter.[477]

Patients with hypothyroidism have normal carbohydrate tolerance, although glucose absorption may be delayed and peak serum glucose concentrations may be lower than in normal subjects. Serum glucose concentrations do not fall excessively in the postabsorptive state, and hepatic glycogen stores are normal. Overall glucose utilization is normal, as is insulin sensitivity. Insulin responses to oral glucose are appropriate for the rise in serum glucose concentrations that occur. Glucose administered intravenously is utilized more slowly than normal because of decreased insulin secretion. In patients with insulin-dependent diabetes, exogenous insulin is degraded more slowly than normal; thus, sensitivity to exogenous insulin may increase.

The synthesis of secreted, functional, and structural proteins in many tissues is decreased,[744] most obviously in hypothyroid children, in whom growth is poor (see section on Hypothyroidism in Newborn Infants and Children). Protein catabolism also is decreased. For several proteins, such as lipoproteins and albumin, degradation is decreased more than is synthesis. Serum albumin concentrations are normal, and the excess albumin is largely in the interstitial space.

Serum homocysteine concentrations are high in some patients with hypothyroidism, both basally and in response to a methionine load.[747a,747b] The increases are due to decreased conversion of homocysteine to methionine or cysteine, or both.

The serum concentrations of total and LDL cholesterol and, less often, triglycerides and lipoprotein(a) are high in many patients with primary and central hypothyroidism.[748,749] The synthesis of triglycerides is decreased, but so is their metabolism, because the activity of adipose tissue lipase and probably hepatic lipase is decreased. The increase in serum LDL cholesterol concentrations and those of its apoprotein B constituent are due primarily to decreases in the concentration of LDL receptors and consequently in receptor-mediated clearance and conversion of cholesterol to bile acids. Serum HDL cholesterol concentrations are usually normal but may be slightly increased or decreased.[749] They do not change in a consistent way in response to T_4 treatment, whereas serum LDL cholesterol concentrations decrease. Carotene also is transported by LDL, and thus carotinemia may occur.

The absorption of drugs may be impaired, reducing drug action, or their metabolism or renal clearance may be slowed, prolonging or exaggerating action.[488,750] Phenytoin, digoxin, and morphine and related drugs are in the latter group, and thus hypothyroid patients should be given lower doses. The action of warfarin may be decreased because of poor absorption or slow turnover of vitamin K-dependent clotting factors.[751]

Endocrine System

Hypothyroidism results in changes in the dynamics of other endocrine systems and in some patients causes clinically important abnormalities in endocrine function. Rates of hormone degradation are decreased, resulting in compensatory decreases in rates of hormone secretion; thus, serum hormone concentrations usually are normal.

Pituitary Function

Nocturnal growth hormone secretion and growth hormone responses to provocative stimuli such as growth hormone-releasing hormone, insulin-induced hypoglycemia, and arginine infusion are reduced. Serum insulin-like growth factor-I values are low but increase normally in response to exogenous growth hormone.[752–754] These data suggest that hypothyroid patients have decreases in 24-hour growth hormone secretion sufficient to decrease insulin-like growth factor-I production, partially explaining the short stature that occurs in hypothyroid children. Serum concentrations of insulin-like growth factor-binding protein-1 and -3 are low.[754] In addition, thyroid deficiency directly impairs bone formation.

Basal serum prolactin concentrations are normal or slightly high but may be as high as 200 μg/liter.[493,755] Hyperprolactinemia is most likely to occur in patients with long-standing hypothyroidism and may result in amenorrhea and galactorrhea, as it does in other women with hyperprolactinemia.

These abnormalities of pituitary hormone secretion are functional ones and are reversed by treatment of hypothyroidism. Trophic hormone deficiencies may also occur as a result of any of the hypothalamic or pituitary diseases that cause hypothyroidism.

Adrenal Function

Twenty-four-hour mean serum cortisol concentrations may be slightly increased.[756] Cortisol clearance is slowed, but cortisol production is nearly normal, suggesting that the sensitivity of ACTH secretion to inhibition by cortisol is decreased. The urinary excretion of cortisol is normal, whereas that of steroid metabolites tends to be low. Pituitary-adrenal responses to metyrapone, insulin-induced hypoglycemia, corticotropin-releasing hormone, and ACTH are normal or slightly impaired, or in the case of corticotropin-releasing hormone, slightly increased.[757,758] Serum cortisol concentrations increase normally in hypothyroid patients who have other illnesses.

Hypothyroidism due to chronic autoimmune thyroiditis and adrenal insufficiency due to autoimmune adrenalitis may occur in the same patient (autoimmune polyglandular syndromes).[282,759] High serum TSH concentrations and sometimes overt hypothyroidism also can occur in patients with ACTH deficiency.[283] Glucocorticoid replacement alone may result in restoration of normal thyroid function, indicating that cortisol is a physiological regulator of TSH secretion or that the patients have coexisting mild chronic autoimmune thyroiditis that is ameliorated by normal amounts of cortisol.

Serum concentrations and production rates of norepinephrine are increased, whereas those of epinephrine are normal.[115]

Gonadal Function

Women with hypothyroidism tend to have low serum estradiol concentrations, because hepatic production of sex hormone–binding globulin is decreased,[486] but their serum free estradiol concentrations are normal. The secretion of estradiol and progesterone is decreased, as is their clearance. Pulsatile FSH and LH secretion is usually normal,[760] but there is no ovulatory surge. The women therefore tend to have anovulatory and irregular cycles, infertility, and excessive menstrual bleeding. In postmenopausal women, serum FSH and LH concentrations may be somewhat lower than expected.

In men, serum testosterone concentrations may be low because production of sex hormone–binding globulin is decreased. Serum free testosterone, FSH, and LH concentrations are usually normal, but may be low.[761,762] Little is known about reproductive capacity, but erectile dysfunction, probably not due specifically to hypothyroidism, is common.

Parathyroid-Vitamin D-Bone System

Serum calcium and phosphate concentrations are normal, whereas those of parathyroid hormone and 1,25-dihydroxyvitamin D may be high.[763] Calcium absorption is decreased, as are bone formation and resorption, suggesting the presence of some resistance to the actions of parathyroid hormone and 1,25-dihydroxyvitamin D. Further supporting the presence of resistance are reports of delayed recovery from induced hypocalcemia and amelioration of primary hyperparathyroidism by hypothyroidism. Calcitonin deficiency also would be expected because of the destruction or removal of thyroid parafollicular cells, and recovery from induced hypercalcemia is slowed in hypothyroid patients.

Lumbar, femoral, and radial bone density is normal.

Pregnancy in Hypothyroidism

Fertility is decreased in women with hypothyroidism. Among women with overt hypothyroidism who do become pregnant, the frequency of preeclampsia, placental abruption, and postpartum hemorrhage is increased, and the risks of abortion, stillbirth, or premature delivery are increased.[146,764,765] In successful pregnancies, the growth of the fetus and the subsequent growth and development of the child may be slowed if the mother was not treated.[766,767,767a] The frequency of subclinical hypothyroidism and high serum antithyroid peroxidase antibody concentrations among pregnant women in the first trimester is about 2 percent, similar to that among women of the same age who are not pregnant.[768] High serum antithyroid peroxidase antibody concentrations alone early in pregnancy may be a risk factor for spontaneous abortion.[769]

Illness and Surgery in Hypothyroid Patients

The extent to which hypothyroidism alters the course or outcome of nonthyroidal illness is not known. Serum T_3 concentrations decline in hypothyroid patients who have nonthyroidal illness as they do in normal subjects.[770] Serum TSH concentrations change little during mild nonthyroidal illness, but they fall during more severe illnesses, especially if a glucocorticoid or dopamine is given.[234,246] This change could make it more difficult to diagnose hypothyroidism.

The overall morbidity or mortality of surgery do not appear to be increased in hypothyroid patients, although some complications of surgery, such as hypotension, cardiac failure, and gastrointestinal dysfunction, may be more common.[771,772] Nonetheless, hypothyroid patients should be given anesthetic, analgesic, and sedative drugs very cautiously.

Laboratory Diagnosis of Hypothyroidism

Serum Thyrotropin and Thyroid Hormone Concentrations

Measurement of serum TSH is an indispensable test for the recognition of primary hypothyroidism and the differentiation of primary from central hypothyroidism, whether caused by pituitary or hypothalamic disease (Fig. 9-17). Serum TSH concentrations are high in all patients with overt primary hypothyroidism and, by definition, in all patients with subclinical hypothyroidism (Fig. 9-18). The high values are due primarily to increased TSH secretion, although TSH clearance is decreased. Rare patients with central hypothyroidism have high serum TSH concentrations, and transient increases (rarely to more than 20 mU/liter) occur in some patients recovering from nonthyroidal illness.

In contrast, serum TSH concentrations are normal or low in most patients with hypothyroidism due to pituitary or hypothalamic disease (see section on TSH Secretion in Central Hypothyroidism). Measurement of serum TSH therefore is not only an exquisitely sensitive test for the recognition of primary hypothyroidism, but also may provide the first evidence that hypothyroidism in a patient is due to pituitary or hypothalamic disease, indicating the need for neuroradiological studies and other tests of pituitary function. Moreover, even if the patient has manifestations of pituitary disease or enlargement, such as hyperprolactinemia, sellar enlargement, and visual impairment, serum TSH must be measured because all those findings may result from primary hypothyroidism and improve with T_4 therapy alone.[710–712] Serum TSH concentrations also are normal or low in patients with severe nonthyroidal illness who have low serum T_4 and T_3 concentrations (adaptive hypothyroidism),[211–214] so that measurements of serum TSH cannot be used to differentiate between central hypothyroidism and illness-related decreases in TSH secretion.

Most patients with symptomatic hypothyroidism have low serum total T_4 concentrations. The results of THBR (T_3-resin uptake) tests are low, indicating an increased number of unoccupied T_4-binding sites in serum, and serum free T_4 concentrations and serum free T_4 index values are also low. However, low serum total T_4 concentrations do not invariably indicate the presence of hypothyroidism. Serum total T_4 concentrations may be low as a result of decreased production of TBG or treatment with drugs such as salicylate that competitively inhibit the binding of T_4 to TBG or other binding proteins (see section on Alterations in Serum Thyroid Hormone Binding). In these two situations, the results of THBR (T_3-resin uptake) tests are high, indicating decreased numbers of unoccupied T_4 binding sites; therefore, serum free T_4 concentrations and free T_4 index values are normal. Low serum total T_4 and sometimes free T_4 concentrations also occur in patients who are seriously ill as a result of nonthyroidal illness (see section on Nonthyroidal Illness).

Because most of the T_3 in serum is produced as a result of extrathyroidal deiodination of T_4, serum T_3 concentrations are usually low in patients with hypothyroidism. However, measurement of serum T_3 is neither a specific nor a sensitive test for hypothyroidism. About 20 to 30 percent of patients with hypothyroidism and low serum T_4 concentrations have normal serum T_3 concentrations,[773] as a result of both TSH-induced stimulation of thyroidal T_3 secretion and an increase in the fractional conversion of T_4 to T_3 at extrathyroidal sites. Conversely, serum T_3 concentrations are low in patients with most if not all nonthyroidal illnesses and those receiving various drugs who are euthyroid and have normal serum T_4 and TSH concentrations (see section on Nonthyroidal Illness).

Summary: Laboratory Diagnosis of Hypothyroidism

A scheme for the evaluation of patients with clinically suspected hypothyroidism is shown in Fig. 9-37. The initial step should be measurements of serum TSH and free T_4 index or serum free T_4. If the serum TSH concentration is high and the serum free T_4 value is low, the diagnosis of overt primary hypothyroidism is confirmed. If the serum TSH concentration is normal or low and the serum free T_4 value is low, the diagnosis is central hypothyroidism or nonthyroidal illness. Reliable differentiation between these conditions in a seriously ill patient at any one time may be

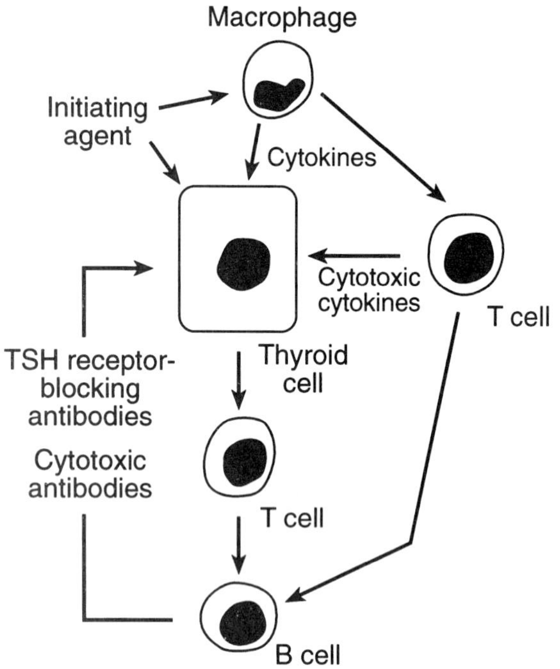

FIGURE 9-37. Diagnostic scheme for the evaluation of patients with suspected hypothyroidism.

impossible. The distinction must be based on the presence or absence of symptoms and signs of hypothyroidism and of hypothalamic or pituitary disease, the results of assessment of pituitary-adrenal function (normal in nonthyroidal illness and often decreased in hypothalamic-pituitary disease), and the results of THBR measurements (low in hypothyroidism and normal or high in nonthyroidal illness), plus the fact that central hypothyroidism is rare.

Other Laboratory Procedures

Most patients with hypothyroidism have normal or low serum thyroglobulin concentrations, but they may be increased in patients with goitrous hypothyroidism or may be artifactually high because of the presence of antithyroglobulin antibodies. High serum concentrations of antithyroid peroxidase or other autoantibodies indicate the presence of autoimmune thyroiditis but provide no information about thyroid secretion. Thyroidal radioiodine uptake is low in most patients with hypothyroidism, but can be normal or supranormal in patients with chronic autoimmune thyroiditis, iodine deficiency, and inherited defects of thyroid hormone biosynthesis.

Among other tests, the most common abnormalities are high serum total and LDL cholesterol and creatine kinase concentrations. These results should be regarded as clues to the presence of hypothyroidism, not tests for it.

Treatment of Hypothyroidism

Treatment of hypothyroidism is simple and effective. Occasionally, all that is required is discontinuation of iodine, lithium, or another drug. Consideration also should be given to the possibility that hypothyroidism is transient (see section on Causes of Hypothyroidism). For most patients, however, lifelong thyroid hormone replacement therapy is required. The general principle is simple: to restore and maintain the euthyroid state. Besides the prescription of medication, patients must be educated about the need for lifelong treatment and periodic follow-up to evaluate the response, confirm compliance, and reinforce the need for it.

L-Thyroxine (T_4) is the proper treatment. The initial dose should be 0.075–0.1 mg/day given orally once daily in young or middle-aged adults (treatment of infants and children is discussed below). For elderly patients, the initial dose should be smaller, 0.05 mg/day, because of the small risk of angina, cardiac arrhythmia, or cardiac failure, and it should be 0.025 mg/day if the patient has ischemic heart disease or a cardiac arrhythmia. Increases in well-being and pulse rate and diuresis occur within 1 to 2 weeks. An appropriate time for the first follow-up visit is 4 to 6 weeks. The dose should not be increased sooner, because this period of time is needed for an individual oral dose to become fully effective; even this period may not be sufficient to obtain the full effect on TSH secretion if the baseline serum TSH concentration was very high. Most symptoms and signs of hypothyroidism disappear within 4 to 8 weeks, although some neuropsychological and biochemical abnormalities may persist for 4 to 6 months.

About 75 percent of an oral dose of T_4 is absorbed.[774,775] In chronically treated patients serum T_4 concentrations transiently increase by 10 to 25 percent and serum TSH concentrations transiently decrease by 25 to 40 percent after each daily dose of T_4.[776] The bioavailability of different brand and generic preparations of T_4 is similar, and the generic ones cost less.[776] When taken with food, T_4 absorption is slightly lower and may be delayed,[777] In practice it is prudent to advise patients to take their dose at the same time each day, to interpret the results of serum TSH measurements done later in the day in relation to that time, and to measure serum TSH 4–6 weeks later if the brand of T_4 is changed. Occasional lots of T_4 are defective,[778,779] and a very rare patient has cutaneous allergy to T_4 or more likely to the dye used to color the tablets.[780]

Adequate replacement, as determined by normal serum TSH concentrations, in most adults requires a daily oral dose of 0.075 to 0.15 mg T_4 (1.5–1.7 μg/kg). Several factors may alter the dose needed for adequate replacement. Among them, the most obvious are body mass and the severity of hypothyroidism; heavier patients and those with higher serum TSH concentrations usually need more T_4.[781] Many pregnant women require slightly higher doses of T_4 to compensate for increased TBG production and loss of T_4 to the fetus.[782,783] Patients with gastrointestinal disorders and those taking some drugs and fiber supplements that bind T_4 within the gastrointestinal tract also may need higher doses because of decreased absorption; the drug-T_4 interactions may be avoided by separating the times of administration of the different medications.[784–789] Other conditions associated with need for higher or lower doses of T_4 are listed in Table 9-19.[790–797]

Patients receiving chronic T_4 therapy should be seen at 6- to 12-month intervals. Assessment of the adequacy of therapy should be based on the clinical response and the serum TSH concentration. No other objective measurement is as sensitive for detecting under- or overtreatment. The goal of treatment is to maintain both well-being and normal serum TSH concentrations (0.3–3.0 mU/liter). A high serum TSH concentration indicates that the dose of T_4 is inadequate or that compliance is poor. In the former situation, the serum T_4 concentration should be low. In the case of poor compliance, the serum T_4 concentration may be either low or

TABLE 9-19. Factors Altering Thyroxine (T_4) Dosage Needed for Adequate Replacement Therapy in Patients with Hypothyroidism

- Increased dosage requirement
  - Increased T_4 production
    - Obesity
    - Pregnancy
  - Decreased gastrointestinal absorption of T_4
    - Malabsorption and short bowel syndromes
    - Therapy with drugs that bind T_4 in the gastrointestinal tract: aluminum hydroxide, bile acid–sequestering drugs, calcium carbonate, ferrous sulfate, sucralfate
- Increased T_4 clearance
    - Younger age
    - Therapy with phenytoin, carbamazepine, rifampin
  - Decreased extrathyroidal T_4 conversion to T_3
    - Therapy with amiodarone
  - Apparent increase in dosage requirement (pseudomalabsorption)
    - Noncompliance
  - Mechanism unknown
    - Therapy with sertraline
- Decreased dosage requirement
  - Decreased T_4 clearance
    - Older age
  - Presence of autonomous thyroid tissue
    - Graves' disease
    - Toxic multinodular goiter

Sources: Mandel,[782] Kaplan,[783] Liel,[784] Shakir,[785] Singh,[786] Campbell,[787] Chiu,[788] Sherman,[789] Sawin,[790] Aanderud,[791] Blackshear,[792] Isley,[793] Figge,[794] Ain,[795] McCowen,[796] Bearcroft.[797]

high depending on whether the patient had taken little or no T_4 or a large dose, for example, 0.6–0.8 mg, just before visiting the physician.[798] A low serum TSH concentration indicates that treatment is excessive. In patients with central hypothyroidism one must rely on clinical assessment and measurements of serum T_4.

How important is it to maintain normal serum TSH concentrations in a hypothyroid patient? In considering this question, it should be noted that in several surveys the proportion of patients with hypothyroidism who were under- or overtreated approached 50 percent,[799–801] yet morbidity or mortality among patients treated with thyroid hormone for many years is not increased.[802,803] Therefore, while persistent overt hypothyroidism and overt thyrotoxicosis should be avoided, by appropriate increases or decreases in dosage of T_4, it appears that subclinical hypothyroidism and subclinical thyrotoxicosis are of little consequence (see also sections on Subclinical Hypothyroidism and Subclinical Thyrotoxicosis). Furthermore, hypothyroid patients feel better when they are slightly overtreated.[804] Therefore, the dose of T_4 need not be changed just because the patient has a slightly abnormal serum TSH concentration, for example, 6–10 mU/liter or 0.07–0.2 mU/liter (normal range 0.3–3.0 mU/liter). Not only is there little clinical benefit, but also frequent changes in the dose are inconvenient and lead to overzealous testing.

In one study of T_4-treated patients, substitution of 0.0125 mg T_3 for 0.05 mg T_4 had beneficial effects on mood and other psychological symptoms, without changing serum TSH concentrations.[98] It would be premature to adopt this approach, but it should be studied further.

Patients who are extremely noncompliant may be treated with 0.5 to 1 mg T_4 given every 7 days, which may allow therapy to be directly observed by another person.[805] In patients who cannot take T_4 orally, for example, because of illness or an operation, T_4 can be omitted for 5 to 7 days. If oral treatment cannot then be resumed, 50–75 percent of the usual T_4 dose should be given intravenously each day.

Other thyroid hormone preparations are available for the treatment of hypothyroidism.[379] They include T_3, a 4 to 1 combination of T_4 and T_3, and desiccated thyroid. Serum T_3 concentrations fluctuate widely in patients treated with T_3, while serum T_4 concentrations remain low; similar although less marked changes in serum T_3 concentrations occur in patients receiving the other preparations. Treatment with these preparations can be monitored with serum TSH measurements.

Special Situations

Subclinical Hypothyroidism

Patients with subclinical hypothyroidism have normal serum T_4 (and T_3) and high TSH concentrations (Fig. 9-17). Their serum TSH concentrations are rarely higher than 20 mU/liter, because the decrease in thyroid secretion is small. The most common causes of subclinical hypothyroidism are inadequate treatment of overt hypothyroidism (of any cause), chronic autoimmune thyroiditis, and previous ^{131}I therapy for thyrotoxicosis, but it may be caused by any of the disorders that cause overt hypothyroidism (Table 9-17).

Some of the patients have thyroid enlargement, and they may have some nonspecific symptoms of hypothyroidism, such as fatigue and loss of energy, but the frequency of these symptoms is only slightly higher in patients with subclinical hypothyroidism than in normal subjects.[122,806] The patients may also have neurobehavioral abnormalities, decreased hearing, slightly high serum total and LDL cholesterol and creatine kinase concentrations, and minor changes in cardiac and skeletal muscle function.[719,726,773]

Whether patients with subclinical hypothyroidism should be treated is controversial. Treatment is not necessary just to forestall the development of overt hypothyroidism, because progression to it is slow (5–20 percent per year).[139,379,670] It is most likely to occur in patients who have high serum antithyroid peroxidase antibody concentrations.[139] The risk of ischemic heart disease is not increased.[807] Treatment may reduce thyroid enlargement. It may also improve nonspecific symptoms; in controlled trials these symptoms improved slightly more often during therapy with T_4 than with placebo.[808–810] Serum cholesterol concentrations usually decrease slightly; the average decrease in several studies was 16 mg/dl (0.4 mmol/liter).[811]

These considerations lead to the conclusion that T_4 therapy is indicated for patients with subclinical hypothyroidism who have symptoms of hypothyroidism, however nonspecific those symptoms may be, or thyroid enlargement. Patients with high serum concentrations of both TSH and antithyroid peroxidase antibodies should also be treated, because of their higher risk of overt hypothyroidism.

Thyroid Hormone Withdrawal

Patients receiving thyroid hormone therapy or their physicians may question whether the therapy is needed because documentation of hypothyroidism is not available or the hypothyroidism is thought to have been transient. Assuming that the patient's serum TSH concentration is not high, the question can be answered only by discontinuation of therapy. In normal subjects pituitary and thyroid function are normal 1 month after discontinuation of T_4 or other thyroid hormone therapy, although they may have symptoms of hypothyroidism and subnormal serum T_4 concentrations for a few weeks after treatment is discontinued.[39,40] In contrast, virtually all patients who are hypothyroid develop symptoms and unequivocal biochemical evidence of the condition within 1 month. Assessment of the thyroidal response to exogenous administration of recombinant TSH offers a potential alternative approach to evaluation of the need for thyroid hormone therapy,[68] but no protocol has yet been devised to do this, and even if one was available it would likely be simpler and less expensive to stop therapy and follow the patient.

Hypothyroidism in Newborn Infants and Children

Hypothyroidism in neonates may result in respiratory difficulty, cyanosis, persistent jaundice, umbilical hernia, lethargy, somnolence, poor feeding, hoarse crying, constipation, or the presence of large anterior or open posterior fontanels. More often, however, their appearance and behavior are normal, even in neonates with severe biochemical hypothyroidism.[683,812] Because hypothyroidism during the first months of life is so hard to recognize yet results in irreversible mental and physical retardation, newborn screening to detect it is now widespread; this is usually done by measuring T_4 in blood collected on filter paper in the first 1 to 4 days of life, followed by measurement of TSH in the samples with T_4 concentrations in the lowest 10th or 20th percentile of a particular assay run. Within 14 days, infants with positive screening results should be evaluated clinically, have measurements of serum TSH and T_4, and be treated, unless the screening results were equivocal.[813] Thyroid radionuclide imaging with ^{123}I or $^{99m}TcO_4$ should be done to determine if thyroid tissue is present and its location; ultrasonography is less satisfactory for identifying dysgenetic or small but normally located thyroid tissue.[814] Should the screening results not be confirmed, therapy can be discontinued. If there is any doubt about the diagnosis the infant should be treated until about age 3 years, when treatment can be discontinued and the infant evaluated a month later.

About 1 in 4,000 infants in North America have congenital hypothyroidism[812]; additional infants have transient hypothyroidism due to maternal antithyroid drug therapy or transplacental passage of maternal TSH receptor-blocking antibodies.[620,662,688] Properly run screening programs miss few infants later found to have hypothyroidism in the first year or so of life, indicating that it rarely develops within this period. In general, infants identified by screening who are treated promptly develop and grow well, but those with thyroid agenesis and severe hypothyroidism may have some developmental and growth delay.[815–817]

When hypothyroidism develops later in infancy or childhood, little permanent mental or physical retardation results. These older children have some form of acquired hypothyroidism, usually chronic autoimmune thyroiditis. Their symptoms and signs of hypothyroidism are similar to those in adults; they also have impaired skeletal growth and development and delayed epiphyseal maturation and dental development. Both growth hormone and insulin-like growth factor-I production are decreased.[752,753] The age of onset of hypothyroidism may be dated by determining when growth slowed from school or other records and by the appearance of the epiphyses; those formed before its onset are normal, whereas those appearing after its onset are delayed or abnormal in appearance (epiphyseal stippling). Sexual maturation in both boys and girls may be accelerated, with serum gonadotropin concentrations being increased in relation to maturational if not chronologic age.[762,818] In other children, however, sexual maturation is delayed because gonadotropin secretion is decreased.

Hypothyroid infants and children also should be treated with T_4, with the recognition that inadequate treatment is hazardous because it may result in some impairment of mental and physical growth even in the absence of symptoms of hypothyroidism. The goal of therapy should be slightly low serum TSH concentrations and serum T_4 concentrations greater than 12 μg/dl (154 nmol/liter). The clearance rate of T_4 is several times higher in infants and children than in adults, and therefore the dose of T_4 should be relatively higher. Newborn infants should be treated with 10 to 15 μg/kg/day, with gradual reduction in the μg/kg/day dose throughout infancy and childhood, reaching 1.5 to 2.0 μg/kg/day by adolescence.[812,813]

Myxedema Coma

The occurrence of mental obtundation or coma in a patient with primary or central hypothyroidism is a life-threatening emergency. It occurs most often in the winter in older patients. Coma may develop spontaneously as the end stage of severe prolonged hypothyroidism, as a result of progressive respiratory depression or decreases in cardiac output and cerebral blood flow. It also may be precipitated by cold exposure, infection, cardiovascular or respiratory disease, and inappropriate administration of narcotic and analgesic drugs.[819,820]

Patients with myxedema coma usually have overt hypothyroidism. In addition to progressive stupor and coma, many have hypothermia, and they may also have seizures, hypoventilation with hypercapnia and respiratory acidosis, hyponatremia, hypotension, and hypoglycemia. The hypothermia is due to severe hypometabolism and may precede the development of coma; any situation that hastens heat loss will hasten the development of coma. Hypoventilation may be caused by respiratory muscle weakness, upper airway obstruction from the large tongue and thickened oropharyngeal mucosa, or impairment in respiratory center function. Hyponatremia and water intoxication are due to excess vasopressin secretion or a direct renal effect of thyroid hormone deficiency. Hypoglycemia suggests the presence of accompanying cortisol deficiency, but may result from impaired gluconeogenesis caused by the severe hypothyroidism alone. In a survey of medical departments in Germany between 1993 and 1995 in which 24 patients with myxedema coma or precoma were identified, the mean age was 73 years, 15 patients (62 percent) were not known to have thyroid disease, 21 percent had a temperature $<35°C$, 80 percent had hypoxia or hypercapnia, and 25 percent died.[821]

Patients with myxedema coma should be treated aggressively with T_4 and other measures. Blood for measurement of serum T_4, TSH, and cortisol should be obtained, and T_4 should be given promptly. Although the administration of large doses can be hazardous, the high mortality of myxedema coma justifies aggressive therapy. The initial dose should be 0.3 or 0.4 mg given intravenously, followed by 0.1 mg daily, because of the possibility of gastric retention or malabsorption. The initial dose should rapidly raise the serum T_4 concentration to normal, and substantial quantities of unbound T_4 thus should be available to the tissues.[37] With the use of high doses of T_4, pulse rate, blood pressure, and temperature increase and mental status improves within 24 h.[820] T_3 has been advocated because it acts more rapidly and because extrathyroidal conversion of T_4 to T_3 is decreased in such seriously ill patients. However, there is some evidence that high doses of T_3 ($\geq$0.075 mg) and also of T_4 ($\geq$0.5 mg) are more likely to be accompanied by a fatal outcome.[819,819a] Hydrocortisone or a synthetic glucocorticoid should be given intravenously because the patient may have concomitant adrenal insufficiency due to hypopituitarism or adrenal disease, or impaired ACTH or adrenal responses to stress as a result of severe primary hypothyroidism.

Supportive therapy is as important as hormonal treatment. Ventilatory assistance may be required. Infection should be sought and treated appropriately. Fluid replacement may be needed but should be given cautiously, as insensible loss is decreased and water loads are excreted poorly. Water intoxication and hyponatremia, if present, should be treated by fluid restriction. Further heat loss should be prevented by adequate covering, but active rewarming is unwise because it may result in vasodilatation and vascular collapse. These measures result in the recovery of a substantial proportion of patients with myxedema coma.

THE PAINFUL THYROID

The thyroid is an encapsulated organ; therefore, acute thyroid enlargement results in pain and tenderness in the thyroid region. The pain may be confined to the thyroid region or referred to the ears, throat, jaws, or laterally in the neck. The thyroid diseases that cause these findings characteristically develop rapidly and include subacute thyroiditis, hemorrhage into a thyroid nodule, radiation thyroiditis, and acute (suppurative) thyroiditis; rare causes are thyroiditis caused by tumor infiltration and surgical trauma[377,378] and vigorous palpation of the thyroid. Patients with many other thyroid diseases, such as Graves' disease, chronic autoimmune thyroiditis, and thyroid carcinoma, occasionally complain of discomfort in the thyroid region and have some thyroid tenderness. However, in these patients thyroid pain and tenderness are usually mild, their illnesses (and thyroid enlargement) usually do not develop rapidly, and the predominant clinical manifestations are those of thyroid dysfunction or a mass lesion rather than inflammation. A variety of nonthyroid diseases, such as musculoskeletal disorders, pharyngeal and laryngeal inflammatory diseases, and globus hystericus, also cause neck pain and tenderness, but these disorders do not cause localized thyroid pain or tenderness or thyroid enlargement.

Subacute Thyroiditis

Subacute thyroiditis, also known as granulomatous thyroiditis, de Quervain's thyroiditis, and acute or subacute nonsuppurative thyroiditis, is the most common cause of thyroid pain and tenderness. Its onset is usually sudden and is accompanied by malaise, myalgia, fatigue, and fever.[822] About half of the patients have had a recent upper respiratory infection. The pain typically radiates to the upper neck, ears, throat, or jaws. Slight to moderate thyroid enlargement is nearly always present; the goiter is commonly diffuse, but the enlargement, pain, and tenderness may be confined to one thyroid lobe or may shift from one lobe to the other during the course of the illness. The thyroid is usually firm in consistency and may be quite hard. Cervical lymphadenopathy is rare. Although serum T_4 and T_3 concentrations are high in nearly all the patients, only about half have clinical manifestations of thyrotoxicosis,[375] and they are usually overshadowed by the thyroid pain and tenderness. The thyroid radionuclide uptake is low, and ultrasonography reveals thyroid hypoechogenecity.[823] The thyroid pain and tenderness and thyrotoxicosis usually subside within 4 to 6 weeks (Fig. 9-26), but in some patients thyroid pain and tenderness persist for several months. There may be a transient (2–8 weeks) period of subclinical or occasionally overt hypothyroidism after the inflammation subsides, but permanent hypothyroidism is rare. Occasional patients have second or even third episodes years later.[824]

Considerable indirect evidence suggests that subacute thyroiditis is a viral illness, but conclusive proof is lacking. The disease has been associated with mumps and with influenza, adenovirus, and other viral infections, and small epidemics of subacute thyroiditis have been reported.[339] About 50 percent of patients have increases in the serum titers of several antiviral antibodies after recovery.[825] These increases in antibody titers, however, are probably anamnestic responses rather than responses to specific infection. The disease is closely associated with HLA-Bw35 or HLA-B67,[826] suggesting that these molecules react uniquely with antigens from one or more viruses to initiate the thyroiditis.

Pathologically, subacute thyroiditis is characterized by disruption of thyroid follicles; infiltration of polymorphonuclear, mononuclear, and giant cells; microabscess formation; and fibrosis. This process results in thyroid follicular disruption and thyroglobulin proteolysis and therefore increased serum T_4, T_3, thyroglobulin, and iodide concentrations and increased urinary iodide excretion. Thyroid radioiodine uptake is low early in the illness as a result of the follicular damage, decreased TSH secretion, and increased serum iodide concentrations. Other common laboratory findings are mild anemia, a high erythrocyte sedimentation rate, and high serum interleukin-6 concentrations[827]; leukocytosis is uncommon. Serum antithyroid peroxidase and antithyroglobulin antibody concentrations may increase transiently during the latter stages of the illness or after recovery, but subacute thyroiditis does not result in persistent autoimmunization.

Both the inflammatory and the thyrotoxic components of subacute thyroiditis may be so mild and transient that no therapy is necessary. More often, thyroid pain and tenderness result in sufficient discomfort to warrant anti-inflammatory therapy.[822,828] Salicylates in doses of 2.4 to 3.6 g daily or high doses of other nonsteroidal anti-inflammatory drugs usually provide effective relief. Patients with severe thyroid pain and tenderness and those who do not improve rapidly with one of these drugs should be treated with prednisone in a dose of 40 mg daily for 3 to 4 weeks, after which it should be gradually reduced and then discontinued to minimize the likelihood of recurrence. Adequate anti-inflammatory therapy not only promptly relieves the symptoms of subacute thyroiditis, but also probably reduces thyroid hormone release, thus accelerating recovery from thyrotoxicosis. The thyrotoxicosis usually requires no therapy, but patients with many thyrotoxic symptoms can be given a beta-adrenergic drug for 1 to 2 weeks. When hypothyroidism occurs during the recovery phase, it is usually mild as well as transient and rarely requires therapy.

Hemorrhage in a Thyroid Nodule

The sudden development of pain, tenderness, and a localized thyroid mass is indicative of hemorrhage into a thyroid nodule, and the local symptoms may be accompanied by transient thyrotoxicosis.[395] The nodule may or may not have been recognized previously. The distinction between this process and subacute thyroiditis may be difficult, but findings localized to the region of a nodule and lack of the systemic manifestations of inflammatory disease and of thyrotoxicosis favor the former diagnosis. Thyroid radionuclide imaging will show little uptake in the region of the painful nodule but some uptake elsewhere. The pain and swelling may subside spontaneously or require that the nodule be aspirated.

Radiation Thyroiditis

Clinically important thyroiditis, with or without exacerbation of thyrotoxicosis, is a rare complication of ^{131}I therapy for hyperthyroidism. It develops 1–2 weeks after therapy and then subsides spontaneously.

Suppurative Thyroiditis

Bacterial, fungal, and protozoal infections of the thyroid are rare. The routes of entry of organisms into the thyroid include the circulation, a persistent thyroglossal duct, a fistula from the piriform sinus, and direct trauma.[829,830] The thyroidal infection may develop acutely or gradually, depending on the organism, and usually is asymmetric. Staphylococcal, streptococcal, and anaerobic species are the organisms most commonly recovered from thyroid tissue, but mycobacteria, other bacteria, or fungi may be found; *Pneumocystis* infections have been identified in several patients with the acquired immune deficiency syndrome.[264,831]

Patients suspected of having suppurative thyroiditis should undergo immediate ultrasonography and needle aspiration of any regions that contain fluid. In patients with no evidence of systemic infection, and particularly in those with recurrent thyroid infections, a search for a piriform sinus fistula should be undertaken.[832]

REFERENCES

1. Pankow BG, Michalak J, McGee MK: Adult human thyroid weight. *Health Phys* 49:1097, 1985.
2. Hegedus L: Thyroid size determined by ultrasound. *Dan Med Bull* 37:249, 1990.
3. Wesche MFT, Wiersinga WM, Smits NJ: Lean body mass as a determinant of thyroid size. *Clin Endocrinol (Oxf)* 48:701, 1998.
4. Melnick JC, Stemkowski PE: Thyroid hemiagenesis (hockey stick sign): A review of the world literature and a report of four cases. *J Clin Endocrinol Metab* 52:247, 1981.
5. Siminoski K: Does this patient have a goiter? *JAMA* 273:813, 1995.
6. Wallace C, Siminoski K: The Pemberton sign. *Ann Intern Med* 125:568, 1996.
7. Ahren B: Regulatory peptides in the thyroid gland—a review on their localization and function. *Acta Endocrinol (Copenh)* 124:225, 1991.
8. Hollowell J, Staehling NW, Hannon WH, et al: Iodine nutrition in the United States. Trends and public health implications: Iodine excretion data from National Health and Nutrition Examination Surveys I and II (1971–1974 and 1988–1994). *J Clin Endocrinol Metab* 83:3401, 1998.
9. Pennington JAT, Schoen SA, Salmon GD, et al: Composition of core foods of the U.S. food supply, 1982–1991. *J Food Comp Anal* 8:171, 1995.
10. Taurog A: Hormone synthesis: Thyroid iodine metabolism, in Braverman LE, Utiger RD (eds): *The Thyroid: A Fundamental and Clinical Text*, 8th ed. Philadelphia, Lippincott Williams and Wilkins, 2000, p 61.
11. Dai S, Levy O, Carrasco N: Cloning and characterization of the thyroid iodide transporter. *Nature* 379:458, 1996.

11a. Spitzweg C, Heufelder AE, Morris JC: Thyroid iodine transport. *Thyroid* 10:321, 2000.

11b. Scott DA, Wang R, Kreman TM, et al: The Pendred syndrome gene encloses a chloride-iodide transport protein. *Nat Genet* 21:440, 1999.

12. Dunn JT, Dunn AD: Thyroglobulin: Chemistry, biosynthesis, and proteolysis, in Braverman LE, Utiger RD (eds): *The Thyroid: A Fundamental and Clinical Text*, 8th ed. Philadelphia, Lippincott Williams and Wilkins, 2000, p 91.
13. Arvan P, Kim PS, Kuliawat R, et al: Intracellular protein transport to the thyrocyte plasma membrane: Potential implications for thyroid physiology. *Thyroid* 7:89, 1997.
14. Larsen PR: Thyroidal triiodothyronine and thyroxine in Graves' disease: Correlation with presurgical treatment, thyroid status and iodine content. *J Clin Endocrinol Metab* 41:1098, 1975.
15. Laurberg P: Mechanisms governing the relative proportions of thyroxine and 3,5,3′-triiodothyronine in thyroid secretion. *Metabolism* 33:379, 1984.
16. Salvatore D, Tu H, Harney JW, et al: Type 2 diodinase is highly expressed in human thyroid. *J Clin Invest* 98:962, 1996.
17. Izumi M, Kubo I, Taura M, et al: Kinetic study of immunoreactive human thyroglobulin. *J Clin Endocrinol Metab* 62:410, 1986.
18. Engler D, Burger AG: The deiodination of the iodothyronines and of their derivatives in man. *Endocr Rev* 5:151, 1984.
19. Leonard JL, Koehrle J: Intracellular pathways of iodothyronine metabolism, in Braverman LE, Utiger RD (eds): *The Thyroid: A Fundamental and Clinical Text*, 8th ed. Philadelphia, Lippincott Williams and Wilkins, 2000, p 136.
20. Berry MJ, Larsen PR: The role of selenium in thyroid hormone action. *Endocr Rev* 13:207, 1992.
21. Larsen PR, Berry MJ: Nutritional and hormonal regulation of thyroid hormone deiodinases. *Ann Rev Nutr* 15:323, 1995.
22. Visser TJ: The role of sulfate in thyroid hormone sulfation. *Eur J Endocrinol* 134:12, 1996.
23. Croteau W, Davey JC, Galton VA, et al: Cloning of the mammalian type II iodothyronine deiodinase. *J Clin Invest* 98:405, 1996.
24. Salvatore D, Low SC, Berry M, et al: Type 3 iodothyronine deiodinase: Cloning, in vitro expression and functional analysis of the placental selenoenzyme. *J Clin Invest* 96:2421, 1995.
25. Koopdonk-Kool JM, de Vijlder JJM, Veenboer GJM, et al: Type II and II deiodinase activity in human placenta as a function of gestational age. *J Clin Endocrinol Metab* 81:2154, 1996.
26. Pinna G, Meinhold H, Hiedra L, et al: Elevated 3,5-diiodothyronine concentrations in the sera of patients with nonthyroidal illness and brain tumors. *J Clin Endocrinol Metab* 82:1535, 1967.
27. Chopra IJ, Santini F, Hurd RE, et al: A radioimmunoassay for measurement of thyroxine sulfate. *J Clin Endocrinol Metab* 76:145, 1993.
28. Santini F, Chiovato L, Bartalena L, et al: Study of serum 3,5,3'-triiodothyronine sulfate concentration in patients with systemic nonthyroidal illness. *Eur J Endocrinol* 134:45, 1996.
29. Grossmann M, Weintraub BD, Szkudlinski MW: Novel insights into the molecular mechanisms of human thyrotropin action: Structural, physiological and therapuetic implications for the glycoprotein hormone family. *Endocr Rev* 18:476, 1997.
30. Kourides IA, Re RN, Weintraub BD, et al: Metabolic clearance and secretion rates of subunits of human thyrotropin. *J Clin Invest* 59:508, 1977.
31. Larsen PR, Silva JE, Kaplan MM: Relationships between circulating and intracellular thyroid hormones: Physiological and clinical implications. *Endocr Rev* 2:87, 1981.
32. Shupnik MA, Ridgway EC, Chin WW: Molecular biology of thyrotropin. *Endocr Rev* 10:459, 1989.
33. Dyess EM, Segerson TP, Liposits Z, et al: Triiodothyronine exerts direct cell-specific regulation of thyrotropin-releasing hormone gene expression in the hypothalamic paraventricular nucleus. *Endocrinology* 123:2291, 1988.
34. Shupnik MA, Ardisson LJ, Meskell MJ, et al: Triiodothyronine (T_3) regulation of thyrotropin subunit gene transcription is proportional to T_3 nuclear receptor occupancy. *Endocrinology* 118:367, 1986.
35. Spencer CA, LoPresti JS, Nicoloff JT, et al: Multiphasic thyrotropin responses to thyroid hormone administration in man. *J Clin Endocrinol Metab* 80:854, 1995.
36. Sydow K, Emrich D, Gefeller O, et al: Quantification of the nega-

tive feedback mechanism between pituitary and thyroid in subjects with normal thyroid function. *Eur J Endocrinol* 135:316, 1996.

37. Ridgway EC, McCammon JA, Benotti J, Maloof F: Acute metabolic responses in myxedema to large doses of intravenous L-thyroxine. *Ann Intern Med* 77:549, 1972.
38. Sawin CT, Hershman JM, Chopra IJ: The comparative effect of T_4 and T_3 on the TSH response to TRH in young adult men. *J Clin Endocrinol Metab* 44:273, 1977.
39. Vagenakis AG, Braverman LE, Azizi F, et al: Recovery of pituitary thyrotropic function after withdrawal of prolonged thyroid-suppression therapy. *N Engl J Med* 293:681, 1975.
40. Krugman LG, Hershman JM, Chopra IJ, et al: Patterns of recovery of the hypothalamic-pituitary-thyroid axis in patients taken off chronic thyroid therapy. *J Clin Endocrinol Metab* 41:70, 1975.
41. Uy HL, Reasner CA, Samuels MH: Pattern of recovery of the hypothalamic-pituitary-thyroid axis following radioactive iodine therapy in patients with Graves' disease. *Am J Med* 99:173, 1995.
42. Kubek M, Wilber JF, George JM: The distribution and concentration of thyrotropin-releasing hormone in discrete human hypothalamic nuclei. *Endocrinology* 105:537, 1979.
43. Jackson IMD: Thyrotropin-releasing hormone. *N Engl J Med* 306:145, 1982.
44. Bruhn TO, Rondeel JMM, Jackson IMD: Thyrotropin-releasing hormone gene expression in the anterior pituitary. IV. Evidence for paracrine and autocine regulation. *Endocrinology* 139:3416, 1998.
45. Wu P, Lechan RM, Jackson IMD: Identification and characterization of thyrotropin-releasing hormone precursor peptides in rat brain. *Endocrinology* 121:108, 1987.
46. Kakucska I, Rand W, Lechan RM: Thyrotropin-releasing hormone gene expression in the hypothalamic paraventricular nucleus is dependent upon feedback regulation by both triiodothyronine and thyroxine. *Endocrinology* 130:2845, 1992.
47. Kakucska I, Qi Y, Lechan RM: Changes in adrenal status affect hypothalamic thyrotropin-releasing hormone gene expression in parallel with corticotropin-releasing hormone. *Endocrinology* 136:2795, 1995.
48. Legradi G, Emerson CH, Ahima RS, et al: Leptin prevents fasting-induced suppression of prothyrotropin-releasing hormone messenger ribonucleic acid in neurons of the hypothalamic paraventricular nucleus. *Endocrinology* 138:2569, 1997.
49. Gershengorn MC: Mechanism of thyrotropin releasing hormone stimulation of pituitary hormone secretion. *Annu Rev Physiol* 48:515, 1986.
50. Schomberg L, Bauer K: Thyroid hormones rapidly and stringently regulate the messenger RNA levels of the thyrotropin-releasing hormone (TRH) receptor and the TRH degrading ectoenzyme. *Endocrinology* 136:3480, 1995.
51. Greer MA, Sato N, Wang X, et al: Evidence that the major physiological role of TRH in the hypothalamic paraventricular nuclei may be to regulate the set-point for thyroid hormone negative feedback on the pituitary thyrotroph. *Neuroendocrinology* 57:569, 1993.
52. Aizawa T, Kobayashi M, Komiya I, et al: Increased sensitivity of the thyrotroph to thyrotropin-releasing hormones in rats with hypothalamic hypothyroidism. *Endocrinology* 114:8, 1984.
53. Utiger RD: Tests of thyroregulatory mechanisms, in Ingbar SH, Braverman LE (eds): *The Thyroid: A Fundamental and Clinical Text*, 5th ed. Philadelphia, Lippincott, 1986, p 522.
54. Shulkin BL, Pruitt RE, Utiger RD: TSH and thyroidal responses to continuous and intermittent TRH administration, in Medeiros-Neto G, Gaitan E (eds): *Frontiers in Thyroidology*. New York, Plenum, 1986, p 285.
55. Kaplan MM, Taft JA, Reichlin S, et al: Sustained rises in serum thyrotropin, thyroxine and triiodothyronine during long term, continuous thyrotropin-releasing hormone treatment in patients with amyotrophic lateral sclerosis. *J Clin Endocrinol Metab* 63:808, 1986.
56. Hulting A-L, Theodorsson E, Werner S: Thyrotropin-releasing hormone increases serum levels of growth hormone-releasing hormone and growth hormone in patients with acromegaly. *J Intern Med* 232:229, 1992.
57. Daneshdoost L, Gennarelli T, Baskey H, et al: Recognition of gonadotroph adenomas in women. *N Engl J Med* 324:589, 1990.
58. Popovic V, Damjanovic S: The effect of thyrotropin-releasing hormone on gonadotropin and free α-subunit secretion in patients with acromegaly and functionless pituitary tumors. *Thyroid* 8:935, 1998.
59. Williams TC, Kelijman M, Crelin WC, et al: Differential effects of somatostatin (SRIH) and a SRIH analog, SMS 201-995, on the secretion of growth hormone and thyroid-stimulating hormone in man. *J Clin Endocrinol Metab* 66:39, 1988.
60. Colao A, Merola B, Ferone D, et al: Acute and chronic effects of octreotide on thyroid axis in growth hormone-secreting and clinically nonfunctioning pituitary adenomas. *Eur J Endocrinol* 133:189, 1995.
61. Scanlon MF, Toft AD: Regulation of thyrotropin secretion, in Braverman LE, Utiger RD (eds): *The Thyroid: A Fundamental and Clinical Text*, 8th ed. Philadelphia, Lippincott Williams and Wilkins, 2000, p 234.
62. Brabant G, Prank K, Hoang-Vu C, et al: Hypothalamic regulation of pulsatile thyrotropin secretion. *J Clin Endocrinol Metab* 72:145, 1991.
63. Rapoport B, Chazenbalk GD, Jaume C, et al: The thyrotropin (TSH) receptor: Interaction with TSH and autoantibodies. *Endocr Rev* 19:673, 1998.
64. Vassart G, Dumont JE: The thyrotropin receptor and the regulation of thyrocyte function and growth. *Endocr Rev* 13:596, 1992.
65. Huber GK, Weinstein SP, Graves PN, et al: The positive regulation of human thyrotropin (TSH) receptor messenger ribonucleic acid by recombinant human TSH is at the intranuclear level. *Endocrinology* 130:2858, 1992.
66. Paschke R, Metcalfe A, Alcalde L, et al: Presence of nonfunctional thyrotropin receptor variant transcripts in retroocular and other tissues. *J Clin Endocrinol Metab* 79:1234, 1994.
67. Stadlmayr W, Spitzweg C, Bichlmair A-M, et al: TSH receptor transcripts and TSH receptor-like immunoreactivity in orbital and pretibial fibroblasts of patients with Graves' ophthalmopathy and pretibial myxedema. *Thyroid* 7:3, 1997.
68. Ramirez L, Braverman LE, White B, et al: Recombinant human thyrotropin is a potent stimulator of thyroid function in normal subjects. *J Clin Endocrinol Metab* 82:2836, 1997.
69. Dumont JE, Lamy F, Roger P, et al: Physiological and pathological regulation of thyroid cell proliferation and differentiation by thyrotropin and other factors. *Physiol Rev* 72:667, 1992.
70. Kawabe Y, Eguchi K, Shimomura C, et al: Interleukin-1 production and action in thyroid tissue. *J Clin Endocrinol Metab* 68:1174, 1989.
71. Sato K, Satoh T, Shizume K, et al: Inhibition of ^{125}I organification and thyroid hormone release by interleukin-1, tumor necrosis factor-α, and interferon-γ in human thyrocytes in suspension culture. *J Clin Endocrinol Metab* 70:1735, 1990.
72. Chanoine J-P, Safran M, Farwell AP, et al: Selenium deficiency and type II 5′-deiodinase regulation in the euthyroid and hypothyroid rat: Evidence of a direct effect of thyroxine. *Endocrinology* 130:479, 1992.
73. Lim VS, Passo C, Murata Y, et al: Reduced triiodothyronine content in liver but not pituitary of the uremic rat model: Demonstration of changes compatible with thyroid hormone deficiency in liver only. *Endocrinology* 114:280, 1984.
74. Grajower MM, Surks MI: Effect of decreased hepatic nuclear L-triiodothyronine receptors on the response of hepatic enzymes to L-triiodothyronine in tumor-bearing rats. *Endocrinology* 104:697, 1979.
75. Kaplan MM, Utiger RD: Iodothyronine metabolism in rat liver homogenates. *J Clin Invest* 61:459, 1978.
76. Gavin LA, Cavalieri RR, Moeller M: Glucose and insulin reverse the effects of fasting on 3,5,3′-triiodothyronine neogenesis in primary cultures of rat hepatocytes. *Endocrinology* 121:858, 1987.
77. Danforth E, Horton ES, O'Connell M, et al: Dietary-induced alterations in thyroid hormone metabolism during overnutrition. *J Clin Invest* 64:1336, 1979.
78. Silva JE, Leonard JL: Regulation of rat cerebrocortical and adenohypophyseal type II 5′-deiodinase by thyroxine, triiodothyronine and reverse triiodothyronine. *Endocrinology* 116:1627, 1985.
79. Meier CA, Burger AG: Effects of drugs and other substances on thyroid hormone synthesis and metabolism, in Braverman LE, Utiger RD (eds): *The Thyroid: A Fundamental and Clinical Text*, 8th ed. Philadelphia, Lippincott Williams and Wilkins, 2000, p 265.
80. Shulkin BL, Peele ME, Utiger RD: β-Adrenergic inhibition of he-

patic 3′,3,5-triiodothyronine production. *Endocrinology* 115:858, 1984.

81. Van der Heyden JTM, Docter R, van Toor H, et al: Effects of caloric deprivation on thyroid hormone tissue uptake and generation of low-T_3 syndrome. *Am J Physiol* 251:E156, 1986.
82. Vos RA, de Jong M, Bernard BA, et al: Impaired thyroxine and 3,5,3′-triiodothyronine handling by rat hepatocytes in the presence of serum of patients with nonthyroidal illness. *J Clin Endocrinol Metab* 80:2364, 1995.
83. Robbins J: Thyroid hormone transport proteins and the physiology of hormone binding, in Braverman LE, Utiger RD (eds): *The Thyroid: A Fundamental and Clinical Text*, 8th ed. Philadelphia, Lippincott Williams and Wilkins, 2000, p 105.
84. Mendel CR, Weisiger RA, Jones AL, et al: Thyroid hormone-binding proteins in plasma facilitate uniform distribution of thyroxine within tissues: A perfused rat liver study. *Endocrinology* 120:1742, 1987.
85. Bartalena L: Recent achievements in studies on thyroid hormone-binding proteins. *Endocr* Rev 11:47, 1990.
86. Mendel CR, Weisiger RA: Thyroxine uptake by perfused rat liver: No evidence for facilitation by five different thyroxine-binding proteins. *J Clin Invest* 86:1840, 1990.
87. Hennemann G, Everts ME, de Jong M, et al: The significance of plasma membrane transport in the bioavailability of thyroid hormone. *Clin Endocrinol (Oxf)* 48:1, 1998.
88. Escobar-Morreale HF, Obregon MJ, Escobar del Rey F, et al: Replacement therapy for hypothyroidism with thyroxine alone does not ensure euthyroidism in all tissues, as studied in thyroidectomized rats. *J Clin Invest* 96:2828, 1995.
89. Escobar-Morreale HF, Escobar del Rey F, Obregon MJ, et al: Only the combined treatment with thyroxine and triiodothyronine ensures euthyroidism in all tissues of the thyroidectomized rat. *Endocrinology* 137:2490, 1996.
90. Anderson GW, Mariash CN, Oppenheimer JH: Molecular actions of thyroid hormone, in Braverman LE, Utiger RD (eds): *The Thyroid: A Fundamental and Clinical Text*, 8th ed. Philadelphia, Lippincott Williams and Wilkins, 2000, p 174.
91. Lazar MA: Thyroid hormone receptors: Multiple forms, multiple possibilities. *Endocr Rev* 14:184, 1993.
92. Brent GA: The molecular basis of thyroid hormone action. *N Engl J Med* 331:847, 1994.
93. Ribeiro RCJ, Apriletti JW, Wagner RL, et al: Mechanisms of thyroid action: Insights from x-ray crystallographic and functional studies. *Rec Progr Horm Res* 53:351, 1998.
94. Koenig RJ: Thyroid hormone receptor coactivators and corepressors. *Thyroid* 8:703, 1998.
95. Hodin RA, Lazar MA, Chin WW: Differential and tissue-specific regulation of the multiple rat c-erbA messenger RNA species by thyroid hormone. *J Clin Invest* 85:101, 1990.
96. Childs GV, Taub K, Jones KE, et al: Triidothyronine receptor β-2 messenger ribonucleic acid expression by somatropes and thyrotropes: Effect of propylthiouracil-induced hypothyroidism in rats. *Endocrinology* 129:2767, 1991.
97. Jolin T: Diabetes decreases liver and kidney nuclear 3,5,3′-triiodothyronine receptors in rats. *Endocrinology* 120:2144, 1987.
98. Bunevicius R, Kazanavicius G, Zalinkevicius R, et al: Comparative effects of thyroxine plus triiodothyronine in patients with hypothyroidism. *N Engl J Med* 340:424, 1999.
99. Davis PJ, Davis FB: Nongenomic actions of thyroid hormone. *Thyroid* 6:497, 1996.
100. Kim S-W, Harney JW, Larsen PR: Studies of the hormonal regulation of type 2 5′-iodothyronine deiodinase messenger ribonucleic acid in pituitary tumor cells using semiquantitative reverse transcription-polymerase chain reaction. *Endocrinology* 139:4895, 1998.
101. Jameson JL, De Groot LJ: Mechanisms of thyroid hormone action, in De Groot LJ (ed): *Endocrinology*, 3rd ed. Philadelphia, WB Saunders, 1995, p 583.
102. Smith TJ, Murata Y, Horwitz AL, et al: Regulation of glycosaminoglycan synthesis by thyroid hormone in vitro. *J Clin Invest* 70:1066, 1982.
103. Guernsey DL, Edelman IS: Regulation of thyroid thermogenesis by thyroid hormones, in Oppenheimer JH, Samuels HH (eds): *Molecular Basis of Thyroid Hormone Action*. New York, Academic Press, 1983, p 293.
104. Chaudhury S, Ismail-Beigi F, Gick GG, et al: Effect of thyroid hormone on the abundance of Na,K-adenosine triphosphatase a-subunit messenger ribonucleic acid. *Mol Endocrinol* 1:83, 1987.
105. Desi-Yajnik V, Zeng J, Omori K, et al: The effect of thyroid hormone treatment on the gene expression and enzyme activity of rat liver sodium-potassium dependent adenosine triphosphatase. *Endocrinology* 136:629, 1995.
106. Gong DW, He Y, Karas M, et al: Uncoupling protein-3 is a mediator of thermogenesis regulated by thyroid hormone, $beta_3$-adrenergic agonists, and leptin. *J Biol Chem* 272:24129, 1997.
107. Klein I, Ojamaa K: Thyrotoxicosis and the heart. *Endocrinol Metab Clin North Am* 27:51, 1998.
108. Ojamaa K, Klein I: In vivo regulation of recombinant cardiac myosin heavy chain gene expression by thyroid hormone. *Endocrinology* 132:1002, 1993.
109. Ojamaa K, Klemperer JD, Klein I: Acute effects of thyroid hormone on vascular smooth muscle. *Thyroid* 6:505, 1996.
110. Beylot M, Martin C, Laville M, et al: Lipolytic and ketogenic fluxes in human hyperthyroidism. *J Clin Endocrinol Metab* 73:42, 1991.
111. Freake HC, Schwartz HL, Oppenheimer JH: The regulation of lipogenesis by thyroid hormone and its contribution to thermogenesis. *Endocrinology* 125:2868, 1989.
112. Sandler MP, Robinson RP, Rabin D, et al: The effect of thyroid hormones on gluconeogenesis and forearm metabolism in man. *J Clin Endocrinol Metab* 56:479, 1983.
113. Moller N, Nielsen S, Nyholm B, et al: Glucose turnover, fuel oxidation and forearm substrate exchange in patients with thyrotoxicosis before and after medical treatment. *Clin Endocrinol (Oxf)* 44:453, 1996.
114. Karlander S-G, Khan A, Wajngot A, et al: Glucose turnover in hyperthyroid patients with normal glucose tolerance. *J Clin Endocrinol Metab* 68:780, 1989.
115. Levey GS: Catecholamine-thyroid hormone interactions and the cardiovascular manifestations of hyperthyroidism. *Am J Med* 88:642, 1990.
116. Bilezikian J, Loeb JN: The influence of hyperthyroidism and hypothyroidism on α- and β-adrenergic receptor systems and adrenergic responsiveness. *Endocr Rev* 4:378, 1983.
117. Liggett SB, Shah SD, Cryer PE: Increased fat and skeletal muscle β-adrenergic receptors but unaltered metabolic and hemodynamic sensitivity to epinephrine in vivo in experimental human thyrotoxicosis. *J Clin Invest* 83:803, 1989.
118. Bauer DC, Brown AN: Sensitive thyrotropin and free thyroxine testing in outpatients. Are both necessary? *Arch Intern Med* 156:2333, 1996.
119. Nordyke RA, Reppun TS, Madanay LD, et al: Alternative sequences of thyrotropin and free thyroxine assays for routine thyroid function testing. Quality and cost. *Arch Intern Med* 158:266, 1998.
120. Tunbridge WMG, Evered DC, Hall R, et al: The spectrum of thyroid disease in a community: The Whickham survey. *Clin Endocrinol (Oxf)* 7:481, 1977.
121. Schaaf L, Pohl T, Schmidt R, et al: Screening for thyroid disorders in a working population. *Clin Invest* 71:126, 1993.
122. Canaris GJ, Manowitz NR, Mayor G, et al: The Colorado thyroid disease prevalence study. *Arch Intern Med* 160:526, 2000.
123. Helfand M, Redfern CC: Screening for thyroid disease: An update. *Ann Intern Med* 129:144, 1998.
124. Danese MD, Powe NR, Sawin CT, et al: Screening for mild thyroid failure at the periodic health examination. A decision and cost-effectiveness analysis. *JAMA* 276:285, 1996.
125. American College of Physicians: Screening for thyroid disease. *Ann Intern Med* 129:141, 1998.
126. Franklyn JA, Black EG, Betteridge J, et al: Comparison of second and third generation methods for measurement of serum thyrotropin in patients with overt hyperthyroidism, patients receiving thyroxine therapy, and those with nonthyroidal illness. *J Clin Endocrinol Metab* 78:1368, 1994.
127. Wood JM, Gordon DL, Rudinger AN, et al: Artefactural elevation of thyroid-stimulating hormone. *Am J Med* 90:261, 1991.
128. Zweig MH, Csako G, Reynolds JC, et al: Interference by iatrogenically induced anti-mouse IgG antibodies in a two-site immunometric assay for thyrotropin. *Arch Pathol Lab Med* 115:164, 1991.

129. Eggertsen R, Petersen K, Lundberg P-A, et al: Screening for thyroid disease in a primary care unit with a thyroid stimulating hormone assay with a low detection limit. *Br Med J* 297:1586, 1988.
130. Parle JV, Franklyn JA, Cross KW, et al: Prevalence and follow-up of abnormal thyrotropin (TSH) concentrations in the elderly in the United Kingdom. *Clin Endocrinol (Oxf)* 34:77, 1991.
131. Sheehan CP, Christofides ND: One-step, labeled-antibody assay for measuring free thyroxin. II. Performance in a multicenter trial. *Clin Chem* 38:19, 1992.
132. Docter R, van Toor H, Krenning EP, et al: Free thyroxine assessed with three assays in sera of patients with nonthyroidal illness and of subjects with abnormal concentrations of thyroxine-binding proteins. *Clin Chem* 39:1668, 1993.
133. Nelson JC, Nayak SS, Wilcox RB: Variable underestimates by serum free thyroxine (T_4) immunoassays for free T_4 concentrations in simple solutions. *J Clin Endocrinol Metab* 79:1373, 1994.
134. Chopra IJ: Simultaneous measurement of free thyroxine and free 3,5,3′-triiodothyronine in undiluted serum by direct equilibrium dialysis/radioimmunoassay: Evidence that free triiodothyronine and free thyroxine are normal in many patients with the low triiodothyronine syndrome. *Thyroid* 8:249, 1998.
135. Burmeister LA: Reverse T_3 does not reliably differentiate hypothyroid sick syndrome from euthyroid sick syndrome. *Thyroid* 5:435, 1995.
136. Spencer CA, Takeuchi M, Kazarosyan M, et al: Serum thyroglobulin autoantibodies: Prevalence, influence on serum thyroglobulin measurement, and prognostic significance in patients with differentiated carcinoma. *J Clin Endocrinol Metab* 83:1121, 1998.
137. Mariotti S, Caturegli P, Piccolo P, et al: Antithyroid peroxidase autoantibodies in thyroid disease. *J Clin Endocrinol Metab* 71:661, 1990.
138. Szabolcs I, Bernard W, Horster FA: Thyroid autoantibodies in hospitalized chronic geriatric patients: Prevalence, effects of age, nonthyroidal clinical state, and thyroid function. *J Am Geriatr Soc* 43:670, 1995.
139. Vanderpump MPJ, Tunbridge WMG, French JM, et al: The incidence of thyroid disorders in the community: A twenty-year follow-up of the Whickham survey. *Clin Endocrinol (Oxf)* 43:55, 1995.
140. Brabant G, Prank K, Ranft U, et al: Physiological regulation of circadian and pulsatile thyrotropin secretion in normal man and woman. *J Clin Endocrinol Metab* 70:403, 1990.
141. Samuels MH, Luther M, Henry P, et al: Effects of hydrocortisone on pulsatile pituitary glycoprotein secretion. *J Clin Endocrinol Metab* 78:211, 1994.
142. Allan JS, Czeisler CA: Persistence of the circadian thyrotropin rhythm under constant conditions and after light-induced shifts of circadian phase. *J Clin Endocrinol Metab* 79:508, 1994.
143. Greenspan SL, Klibanski A, Rowe JW, et al: Age-related alterations in pulsatile secretion of TSH: Role of dopaminergic regulation. *Am J Physiol* 260:E486, 1991.
144. Adriaanse R, Romijn JA, Endert E, et al: The nocturnal thyroid-stimulating hormone surge is absent in overt, present in mild primary and equivocal in central hypothyroidism. *Acta Endocrinol (Copenh)* 126:206, 1992.
145. O'Leary PC, Boyne P, Atkinson G, et al: Longitudinal study of serum thyroid hormone levels during normal pregnancy. *Int J Gynecol Obstet* 38:171, 1992.
146. Glinoer D: The regulation of thyroid function in pregnancy: Pathways of endocrine adaptation from physiology to pathology. *Endocr Rev* 18:404, 1997.
147. Tomer Y, Huber GK, Davies TF: Human chorionic gonadotropin (hCG) interacts directly with recombinant human TSH receptors. *J Clin Endocrinol Metab* 74:1477, 1992.
148. Grun J-P, Meuris S, De Nayer P, et al: The thyrotrophic role of human chorionic gonadotrophin (hCG) in the early stages of twin (versus single) pregnancies. *Clin Endocrinol (Oxf)* 46:719, 1997.
149. Glinoer D, De Nayer P, Delange F, et al: A randomized trial for the treatment of mild iodine deficiency during pregnancy: Maternal and neonatal effects. *J Clin Endocrinol Metab* 80:258, 1995.
150. Berghout A, Wiersinga W: Thyroid size and thyroid function during pregnancy: An analysis. *Eur J Endocrinol* 138:536, 1998.
151. Ho SSY, Metreweli C: Normal fetal thyroid volume. *Ultrasound Obstet Gynecol* 11:118, 1998.
152. Thorpe-Beeston JG, Nicolaides KH, Felton CV, et al: Maturation of the secretion of thyroid hormone and thyroid-stimulating hormone in the fetus. *N Engl J Med* 324:532, 1991.
153. Thorpe-Beeston JG, Nicolaides KH, McGregor AM: Fetal thyroid function. *Thyroid* 2:207, 1992.
154. Adams LM, Emery JR, Clark SJ, et al: Reference ranges for newer thyroid function tests in premature infants. *J Pediatr* 126:122, 1995.
155. Vulsma T, Gons MH, de Vijlder JJM: Maternal-fetal transfer of thyroxine in congenital hypothyroidism due to a total organification defect or thyroid agenesis. *N Engl J Med* 321:13, 1989.
156. Calvo R, Obregon MJ, de Ona CR, et al: Congenital hypothyroidism, as studied in rats: Crucial role of maternal thyroxine but not of 3,5,3′-triiodothyronine in the protection of the fetal brain. *J Clin Invest* 86:889, 1990.
157. Hollingsworth DR, Alexander NM: Amniotic fluid concentrations of iodothyronines and thyrotropin do not reliably predict fetal thyroid status in pregnancies complicated by maternal thyroid disorders or anencephaly. *J Clin Endocrinol Metab* 57:349, 1983.
158. Penny R, Spencer CA, Frasier SD, et al: Thyroid-stimulating hormone and thyroglobulin levels decrease with chronological age in children and adolescents. *J Clin Endocrinol Metab* 56:177, 1983.
159. Nelson JC, Clark SJ, Borut DL, et al: Age-related changes in serum free thyroxine during childhood and adolescence. *J Pediatr* 123:899, 1993.
160. Fisher DA, Sack J, Oddie TH, et al: Serum T_4, TBG, T_3 uptake, T_3, reverse T_3, and TSH concentrations in children 1 to 15 years of age. *J Clin Endocrinol Metab* 45:191, 1977.
161. Dunger DB, Perkins JA, Jowett TP, et al: A longitudinal study of total and free thyroid hormones and thyroxine-binding globulin during normal puberty. *Acta Endocrinol (Copenh)* 123:305, 1990.
162. Hershman JM, Pekary AE, Berg L, et al: Serum thyrotropin and thyroid hormone levels in elderly and middle-aged euthyroid persons. *J Am Geriatr Soc* 41:823, 1993.
163. Mariotti S, Barbesino G, Caturegli P, et al. Complex alteration of thyroid function in healthy centenarians. *J Clin Endocrinol Metab* 77:1130, 1993.
164. Mariotti S, Franceschi C, Cossarizza A, et al: The aging thyroid. *Endocr Rev* 16:686, 1995.
165. Franklyn JA, Ramsden DB, Sheppard MC: The influence of age and sex on tests of thyroid function. *Ann Clin Biochem* 22:502, 1985.
166. Sawin CT, Geller A, Kaplan MM, et al: Low serum thyrotropin (thyroid-stimulating hormone) in older persons with hyperthyroidism. *Arch Intern Med* 151:165, 1991.
167. Bertelsen JB, Hegedus L: Cigarette smoking and the thyroid. *Thyroid* 4:327, 194.
168. Konno N, Morikawa K: Seasonal variation of serum thyrotropin concentration and thyrotropin response to thyrotropin-releasing hormone in patients with primary hypothyroidism on constant replacement dosage of thyroxine. *J Clin Endocrinol Metab* 54:1118, 1982.
169. Solter M, Brkic K, Petek M, et al: Thyroid hormone economy in response to extreme cold exposure in healthy factory workers. *J Clin Endocrinol Metab* 68:168, 1989.
170. Deligiannis A, Karamouzis M, Kouidi E, et al: Plasma TSH, T_3, T_4 and cortisol responses to swimming at varying water temperatures. *Br J Sports Med* 27:247, 1993.
171. Alen M, Pakarinen A, Hakkinen K: Effects of prolonged training on serum thyrotropin and thyroid hormones in elite strength athletes. *J Sports Sci* 11:493, 1993.
172. Ain KB, Mori Y, Refetoff S: Reduced clearance rate of thyroxine-binding globulin (TBG) with increased sialylation: A mechanism for estrogen-induced elevation of serum TBG concentration. *J Clin Endocrinol Metab* 65:689, 1987.
173. Geola FL, Frumar AM, Tataryn IV, et al: Biological effects of various doses of conjugated equine estrogens in postmenopausal women. *J Clin Endocrinol Metab* 51:620, 1980.
174. Mandel FP, Geola FP, Lu JKH, et al: Biologic effects of various doses of ethinyl estradiol in postmenopausal women. *Obstet Gynecol* 59:673, 1982.
175. Kostoglu-Athanassiou I, Ntalles K, Markopoulos C, et al: Thyroid function in postmenopausal women with breast cancer on tamoxifen. *Eur J Gynaecol Oncol* 19:150, 1998.

176. English TN, Ruxton D, Eastman CJ: Abnormalities in thyroid function associated with chronic therapy with methadone. *Clin Chem* 35:1807, 1989.
177. Beex L, Ross A, Smals A, et al: 5-Fluorouracil-induced increase in total serum thyroxine and triiodothyronine. *Cancer Treat Rep* 61:1291, 1977.
178. Refetoff S: Inherited thyroxine-binding globulin abnormalities in man. *Endocr Rev* 10:275, 1989.
179. Mori Y, Miura Y, Takeuchi H, et al: Gene amplification as a cause of inherited thyroxine-binding globulin excess in two Japanese families. *J Clin Endocrinol Metab* 80:3758, 1995.
180. Ruiz M, Rajatanavin R, Young RA, et al: Familial dysalbuminemic hyperthyroxinemia: A syndrome that can be confused with thyrotoxicosis. *N Engl J Med* 306:635, 1982.
181. Heufelder AE, Klee GG, Wynne AG, et al: Familial dysalbuminemic hyperthyroxinemia: Cumulative experience in 29 consecutive patients. *Endocr Pract* 1:4, 1995.
182. Petersen CE, Scottolini AG, Cody LR, et al: A point mutation in the human albumin gene results in familial dysalbuminemic hyperthyroxinaemia. *J Med Genet* 31:355, 1994.
183. Wada N, Chiba H, Shimizu C, et al: A novel missense mutation in codon 218 of the albumin gene in a distinct phenotype of familial dysalbuminemic hyperthyroxinemia in a Japanese kindred. *J Clin Endocrinol Metab* 82:3246, 1997.
184. Moses AC, Rosen HN, Moller DE, et al: A point mutation in transthyretin increases affinity for thyroxine and produces euthyroid hyperthyroxinemia. *J Clin Invest* 86:2025, 1990.
185. Rajatanavin R, Liberman C, Lawrence GD, et al: Euthyroid hyperthyroxinemia and thyroxine-binding prealbumin excess in islet cell carcinoma. *J Clin Endocrinol Metab* 61:17, 1985.
186. Refetoff S, Marinov VSZ, Tunca H, et al: A new family with hyperthyroxinemia caused by transthyretin Val^{109} misdiagnosed as thyrotoxicosis and resistance to thyroid hormone—a Clinical Research Center study. *J Clin Endocrinol Metab* 81:3335, 1996.
187. Stockigt JR: Serum thyrotropin and thyroid hormone measurements and assessment of thyroid hormone transport, in Braverman LE, Utiger RD (eds): *The Thyroid: A Fundamental and Clinical Text*, 8th ed. Philadelphia, Lippincott Williams and Wilkins, 2000, p 376.
188. Sakata S, Nakamura S, Miura K: Autoantibodies against thyroid hormones or iodothyronine. Implications in diagnosis, thyroid function, treatment, and pathogenesis. *Ann Intern Med* 103:579, 1985.
189. Sakata S, Matsuda M, Ogawa T, et al: Prevalence of thyroid hormone autoantibodies in healthy subjects. *Clin Endocrinol (Oxf)* 41:365, 1994.
190. Bartalena L: Studies on thyroxine-binding globulin. *J Endocrinol Invest* 16:353, 1993.
191. Okamoto H, Mori Y, Tani Y, et al: Molecular analysis of females manifesting thyroxine-binding globulin (TBG) deficiency: Selective X-chromosome inactivation responsible for the difference between phenotype and genotype in TBG-deficient females. *J Clin Endocrinol* 81:2204, 1996.
192. Mori Y, Takeda K, Charbonneau M, et al: Replacement of Leu^{227} by pro in thyroxine-binding globulin (TBG) is associated with complete TBG deficiency in three of eight families with this inherited defect. *J Clin Endocrinol Metab* 70:804, 1990.
193. Miura Y, Kambe F, Yamamori I, et al: A truncated thyroxine-binding globulin due to a frameshift mutation is retained within the rough endoplasmic reticulum: A possible mechanism of complete thyroxine-binding globulin deficiency in Japanese. *J Clin Endocrinol Metab* 78:283, 1994.
194. Carvalho GA, Weiss RA, Refetoff S: Complete thyroxine-binding globulin (TBG) deficiency produced by a mutation in acceptor splice site causing frameshift and early termination of translation (TBG-Kankakee). *J Clin Endocrinol Metab* 83:3604, 1998.
195. Arafah BM: Decreased levothyroxine requirement in women with hypothyroidism during androgen therapy for breast cancer. *Ann Intern Med* 121:247, 1994.
196. Deyssig R, Weissel M: Ingestion of androgenic-anabolic steroids induces mild thyroidal impairment in male body builders. *J Clin Endocrinol Metab* 76:1069, 1993.
197. Shakir KMM, Kroll S, Aprill BS, et al: Nicotinic acid decreases serum thyroid hormone levels while maintaining a euthyroid state. *Mayo Clin Proc* 70:556, 1995.
198. Yeung S-CJ, Chiu AC, Vassilopoulou-Sellin R, et al: The endocrine effects of nonhormonal antineoplastic therapy. *Endocr Rev* 19:144, 1998.
199. Sapin R, Schlienger J-L, Kaltenbach G, et al: Determination of free triiodothyronine by six different methods in patients with nonthyroidal illness and in patients with amiodarone. *Ann Clin Biochem* 32:314, 1995.
200. Reilly CP, Wellby ML: Slow thyroxine binding globulin in the pathogenesis of increased dialysable fraction of thyroxine in nonthyroidal illnesses. *J Clin Endocrinol Metab* 57:15, 1983.
201. Chopra IJ, Van Herle AJ, Chua Teco GN, et al: Serum free thyroxine in thyroidal and nonthyroidal illnesses: A comparison of measurements by radioimmunoassay, equilibrium dialysis, and free thyroxine index. *J Clin Endocrinol Metab* 51:135, 1980.
202. Docter R, Krenning EP, de Jong M, et al: The sick euthyroid syndrome: Changes in thyroid hormone serum parameters and hormone metabolism. *Clin Endocrinol (Oxf)* 39:499, 1993.
203. Davies PH, Franklyn JA: The effects of drugs in tests of thyroid function. *Eur J Clin Pharmacol* 40:439, 1991.
204. Bishnoi A, Carlson HE, Gruber BL, et al: Effects of commonly prescribed nonsteroidal anti-inflammatory drugs in thyroid hormone measurements. *Am J Med* 96:235, 1994.
205. Surks MI, Sievert R: Drugs and thyroid function. *N Engl J Med* 333:1688, 1995.
206. Wang R, Nelson JC, Wilcox RB: Salsalate administration—a potential pharmacological model of the sick euthyroid syndrome. *J Clin Endocrinol Metab* 83:3095, 1998.
207. Chopra IJ, Chua Teco GN, Mead JF, et al: Relationship between serum free fatty acids and thyroid hormone binding inhibitor in nonthyroid illnesses. *J Clin Endocrinol Metab* 60:980, 1985.
208. Mendel CM, Frost PH, Cavalieri RR: Effect of free fatty acids on the concentration of free thyroxine in human serum: The role of albumin. *J Clin Endocrinol Metab* 63:1394, 1986.
209. Mendel CM, Frost PH, Kunitake ST, et al: Mechanism of the heparin-induced increase in the concentration of free thyroxine in plasma. *J Clin Endocrinol Metab* 65:1259, 1987.
210. Jaume JC, Mendel CM, Frost PH, et al: Extremely low doses of heparin release lipase activity into the plasma and can thereby cause artifactual elevations in the serum-free thyroxine concentration as measured by equilibrium dialysis. *Thyroid* 6:79, 1996.
211. Gow SM, Elder A, Caldwell G, et al: An improved approach to thyroid function testing in patients with non-thyroidal illness. *Clin Chim Acta* 158:49, 1986.
212. Davies PH, Black EG, Sheppard MC, et al: Relation between serum interleukin-6 and thyroid hormone concentrations in 270 hospital in-patients with non-thyroidal illness. *Clin Endocrinol (Oxf)* 44:199, 1996.
213. Spencer CA, Eigen A, Shen D, et al: Specificity of sensitive assays of thyrotropin (TSH) used to screen for thyroid disease in hospitalized patients. *Clin Chem* 33:1391, 1987.
214. Jarek MJ, Legare EJ, McDermott MT, et al: Endocrine profiles for outcome prediction from the intensive care unit. *Crit Care Med* 21:543, 1993.
215. Faber J, Kirkegaard C, Lumholtz IB, et al: Variations in serum T_3, rT_3, 3,3′-diiodothyronine and 3′,5′-diodothyronine induced by acute myocardial infarction and propranolol. *Acta Endocrinol (Copenh)* 94:341, 1980.
216. Arem R, Wiener GJ, Kaplan SG, et al: Reduced tissue thyroid hormone levels in fatal illness. *Metabolism* 42:1102, 1993.
217. Chopra IJ, Sakane S, Chua Teco GN: A study of the serum concentration of tumor necrosis factor-α in thyroidal and nonthyroidal illnesses. *J Clin Endocrinol Metab* 72:1113, 1991.
218. Boelen A, Platvoet-Ter Schiphorst MC, Wiersinga WM: Association between serum interleukin-6 amd serum 3,5,3′-triiodothyronine in nonthyroidal illness. *J Clin Endocrinol Metab* 77:1695, 1993.
219. Stouthard JML, van der Poll T, Endert E, et al: Effects of acute and chronic interleukin-6 administration on thyroid hormone metabolism in humans. *J Clin Endocrinol Metab* 79:1342, 1994.
220. Corssmit EPM, Heyligenberg R, Endert E, et al: Acute effects of interferon-α administration on thyroid hormone metabolism in healthy men. *J Clin Endocrinol Metab* 80:3140, 1995.
221. Spath-Schwalbe E, Hansen K, Schmidt F, et al: Acute effects of recombinant human interleukin-6 on endocrine and central nervous system sleep functions in healthy men. *J Clin Endocrinol Metab* 83:1573, 1998.

222. Bartalena L, Bogazzi F, Brogioni S, et al: Role of cytokines in the pathogenesis of the euthyroid sick syndrome. *Eur J Endocrinol* 138:603, 1998.
223. Chopra IJ, Huang T-S, Beredo A, et al: Evidence for an inhibitor of extrathyroidal conversion of thyroxine to 3,5,3′-triiodothyronine in sera of patients with nonthyroidal illnesses. *J Clin Endocrinol Metab* 60:666, 1985.
224. Everts ME, de Jong M, Lim C-F, et al: Different regulation of thyroid hormone transport in liver and pituitary: Its possible role in the maintenance of low T_3 production during nonthyroidal illness and fasting in man. *Thyroid* 6:359, 1996.
225. De Groot LJ: Dangerous dogmas in medicine: The nonthyroidal illness syndrome. *J Clin Endocrinol Metab* 84:151, 1999.
226. Adriaanse R, Romijn JA, Brabant G, et al: Pulsatile thyrotropin secretion in nonthyroidal illness. *J Clin Endocrinol Metab* 77:1313, 1993.
227. Samuels MH, Kramer P: Differential effects of short-term fasting on pulsatile thyrotropin, gonadotropin, and α-subunit secretion in healthy men–a Clinical Research Center study. *J Clin Endocrinol Metab* 81:32, 1996.
228. Gardner DF, Kaplan MM, Stanley CA, et al: Effect of triiodothyronine replacement on the metabolic and pituitary responses to starvation. *N Engl J Med* 300:579, 1979.
229. Burman KD, Wartofsky L, Dinterman RE, et al: The effect of T_3 and reverse T_3 administration on muscle protein catabolism during fasting as measured by 3-methylhistidine excretion. *Metabolism* 28:805, 1979.
230. Lim VS, Tsalikian E, Flanigan MJ: Augmentation of protein degradation by L-triiodothyronine in uremia. *Metabolism* 38:1210, 1989.
231. Byerley LO, Heber D: Metabolic effects of triiodothyronine replacement during fasting in obese subjects. *J Clin Endocrinol Metab* 81:968, 1996.
232. Lim VS, Henriquez C, Seo H, et al: Thyroid function in a uremic rat model: Evidence suggesting tissue hypothyroidism. *J Clin Invest* 66:946, 1980.
233. Dillmann WH, Berry S, Alexander NM: A physiological dose of triiodothyronine normalizes cardiac myosin adenosine triphosphatase activity and changes myosin isoenzyme distribution in semistarved rats. *Endocrinology* 112:2081, 1983.
234. Kaptein EM, Spencer CA, Kamiel MB, et al: Prolonged dopamine administration and thyroid hormone economy in normal and critically ill subjects. *J Clin Endocrinol Metab* 51:387, 1980.
235. Hamblin PS, Dyer SA, Mohr VS, et al: Relationship between thyrotropin and thyroxine changes during recovery from severe hypothyroxinemia of critical illness. *J Clin Endocrinol Metab* 62:717, 1986.
236. Arem R, Deppe S: Fatal nonthyroidal illness may impair nocturnal thyrotropin levels. *Am J Med* 88:258, 1990.
237. Custro N, Scafidi V, Gallo S, et al: Deficient pulsatile thyrotropin secretion in the low-thyroid-hormone state of severe non-thyroidal illness. *Eur J Endocrinol* 130:132, 1994.
238. Van den Berghe G, de Zegher F, Bouillon R: Acute and prolonged critical illness as different neuroendocrine paradigms. *J Clin Endocrinol Metab* 83:1827, 1998.
239. Beck-Peccoz P, Persani L: Variable biological activity of thyroid-stimulating hormone. *Eur J Endocrinol* 131:331, 1994.
240. Persani L: Hypothalamic thyrotropin-releasing hormone and thyrotropin biological activity. *Thyroid* 8:941, 1998.
241. Fliers E, Guldenaar SEF, Wiersinga WM, et al: Decreased hypothalamic thyrotropin-releasing hormone gene expression in patients with nonthyroidal illness. *J Clin Endocrinol Metab* 82:4032, 1997.
242. Seppel T, Becker A, Lippert F, et al: Serum sex hormone-binding globulin and osteocalcin in systemic nonthyroidal illness associated with low thyroid hormone concentrations. *J Clin Endocrinol Metab* 81:1663, 1996.
243. Brent GA, Hershman JM: Serum angiotensin-converting enzyme in severe nonthyroidal illnesses associated with low serum thyroxine concentrations. *Ann Intern Med* 100:680, 1984.
244. Becker RA, Vaughan GM, Ziegler MG, et al: Hypermetabolic low triiodothyronine syndrome of burn injury. *Crit Care Med* 10:870, 1982.
245. Brent GA, Hershman JM: Thyroxine therapy in patients with severe nonthyroidal illnesses and low serum thyroxine concentration. *J Clin Endocrinol Metab* 63:1, 1986.
246. Brent GA, Hershman JM, Braunstein GD: Patients with severe nonthyroidal illness and serum thyrotropin concentrations in the hypothyroid range. *Am J Med* 81:463, 1986.
247. O'Brian JT, Bybee DE, Burman KD, et al: Thyroid hormone homeostasis in states of relative caloric deprivation. *Metabolism* 29:721, 1980.
248. Hamilton MA: Prevalence and clinical implications of abnormal thyroid hormone metabolism in advanced heart failure. *Ann Thorac Surg* 56:S48, 1993.
249. Longstreth WT Jr, Manowitz NR, DeGroot LJ, et al: Plasma thyroid hormone profiles immediately following out-of-hospital cardiac arrest. *Thyroid* 6:649, 1996.
250. Holland FW II, Brown PS, Weintraub BD, et al: Cardiopulmonary bypass and thyroid function: A "euthyroid sick syndrome." *Ann Thorac Surg* 52:46, 1991.
251. Klemperer JD, Klein I, Gomez M, et al: Thyroid hormone treatment after coronary-artery bypass surgery. *N Engl J Med* 333:1522, 1995.
252. Bennett-Guerrero E, Jimenez JL, White WD, et al: Cardiovascular effects of intravenous triiodothyronine in patients undergoing coronary artery bypass graft surgery. A randomized, double-blind, placebo-controlled trial. *JAMA* 275:687, 1996.
253. Hamilton MA, Stevenson LW, Fonarow GC, et al: Safety and hemodynamic effects of intravenous triiodothyronine in advanced heart failure. *Am J Cardiol* 81:443, 1998.
254. Lim VS, Fang VS, Katz AI, Refetoff S: Thyroid function in chronic renal failure: A study of the pituitary-thyroid axis and peripheral turnover kinetics of thyroxine and triiodothyronine. *J Clin Invest* 60:522, 1977.
255. Kaptein EM: Thyroid hormone metabolism and thyroid diseases in chronic renal failure. *Endocr Rev* 17:45, 1996.
256. Kaptein EM, Feinstein EI, Nicoloff JT, et al: Serum reverse triiodothyronine and thyroxine kinetics in patients with chronic renal failure. *J Clin Endocrinol Metab* 57:181, 1983.
257. Gavin LA, McMahon FA, Castle JN, et al: Alterations in serum thyroid hormones and thyroxine-binding globulin in patients with nephrosis. *J Clin Endocrinol Metab* 46:125, 1978.
258. Fonseca V, Thomas M, Katrak A, et al: Can urinary thyroid hormone loss cause hypothyroidism? *Lancet* 338:475, 1991.
259. Gardner DF, Carithers RL Jr, Utiger RD: Thyroid function tests in patients with acute and resolved hepatitis B virus infection. *Ann Intern Med* 96:450, 1982.
260. Caregaro L, Alberino F, Amodio P, et al: Nutritional and prognostic significance of serum hypothyroxinemia in hospitalized patients with liver cirrhosis. *J Hepatol* 28:115, 1998.
261. LoPresti JS, Fried JC, Spencer CA: Unique alterations of thyroid hormone indices in the acquired immunodeficiency syndrome (AIDS). *Ann Intern Med* 110:970, 1989.
262. Lambert M, Zech F, De Nayer P: Elevation of serum thyroxine-binding globulin (but not of cortisol-binding globulin and sex hormone-binding globulin) associated with the progression of human immunodeficiency virus infection. *Am J Med* 89:748, 1990.
263. Hommes MJT, Romijn JA, Endert E, et al: Hypothyroid-like regulation of the pituitary-thyroid axis in stable human immunodeficiency virus infection. *Metabolism* 42:556, 1993.
264. Battan R, Mariuz P, Raviglione MC, et al: *Pneumocystis carinii* infection of the thyroid in a hypothyroid patient with AIDS: Diagnosis by fine needle aspiration biopsy. *J Clin Endocrinol Metab* 72:724, 1991.
265. Spratt DI, Pont A, Miller MB, et al: Hyperthyroxinemia in patients with acute psychiatric disorders. *Am J Med* 73:41, 1982.
266. Kramlinger KG, Gharib H, Swanson DW, et al: Normal serum thyroxine values in patients with acute psychiatric illness. *Am J Med* 76:799, 1984.
267. Chopra IJ, Solomon DH, Huang T-S: Serum thyrotropin in hospitalized psychiatric patients: Evidence for hyperthyrotropinemia as measured by an ultrasensitive thyrotropin assay. *Metabolism* 39:538, 1990.
268. Nader S, Warner MD, Doyle S, et al: Euthyroid sick syndrome in psychiatric patients. *Biol Psychiatry* 40:1288, 1996.
269. Woolf PD, Nichols D, Porsteinsson A, et al: Thyroid evaluation of hospitalized psychiatric patients: The role of TSH screening for thyroid dysfunction. *Thyroid* 6:451, 1996.
270. Loosen PT: Thyroid function in affective disorders and alcoholism. *Endocrinol Metab Clin North Am* 17:55, 1988.

271. Jackson IMD: The thyroid axis and depression. *Thyroid* 8:951, 1998.
272. Bartalena L, Placidi GF, Martino E, et al: Nocturnal serum thyrotropin (TSH) surge and the TSH response to TSH-releasing hormone: Dissociated behavior in untreated depressives. *J Clin Endocrinol Metab* 71:650, 1990.
273. Kirkegaard C, Faber J: The role of thyroid hormones in depression. *Eur J Endocrinol* 138:1, 1998.
274. Van den Berghe G, de Zegher F, Lauwers P: Dopamine and the sick euthyroid syndrome in critical illness. *Clin Endocrinol (Oxf)* 41:731, 1994.
275. Faber J, Kirkegaard C, Rasmussen B, et al: Pituitary-thyroid axis in critical illness. *J Clin Endocrinol Metab* 65:315, 1987.
275a. Lee E, Chen P, Rao H, et al: Effect of acute high-dose dobutamine administration on serum thyrotrophin (TSH). *Clin Endocrinol (Oxf)* 50:487, 2000.
276. Benker G, Raida M, Olbricht T, et al: TSH secretion in Cushing syndrome: Relation to glucocorticoid excess, diabetes, goitre, and the "sick euthyroid syndrome." *Clin Endocrinol (Oxf)* 33:777, 1990.
277. Bartalena L, Martino E, Petrini L, et al: The nocturnal serum thyrotropin surge is abolished in patients with adrenocorticotropin (ACTH)-dependent or ACTH-independent Cushing's syndrome. *J Clin Endocrinol Metab* 72:1195, 1991.
278. Hangaard J, Andersen M, Grodum E, et al: Pulsatile thyrotropin secretion in patients with Addison's disease during variable glucocorticoid therapy. *J Clin Endocrinol Metab* 81:2501, 1996.
279. Samuels MH, McDaniel PA: Thyrotropin levels during hydrocortisone infusions that mimic fasting-induced cortisol elevations: A Clinical Research Center study. *J Clin Endocrinol Metab* 82:3700, 1997.
280. Gamstedt A, Jarnerot G, Kagedal B: Dose related effects of betamethasone on iodothyronines and thyroid hormone-binding proteins in serum. *Acta Endocrinol (Copenh)* 96:484, 1981.
281. Williams DE, Chopra IJ, Orgiazzi J, Solomon DH: Acute effects of corticosteroids on thyroid activity in Graves' disease. *J Clin Endocrinol Metab* 41:354, 1975.
282. Topliss DJ, White EL, Stockigt JR: Significance of thyrotropin excess in untreated primary adrenal insufficiency. *J Clin Endocrinol Metab* 50:52, 1980.
283. Shigemasa C, Kouchi T, Ueta Y, et al: Evaluation of thyroid function in patients with isolated adrenocorticotropin deficiency. *Am J Med Sci* 304:279, 1992.
284. Wiersinga WM: Propranolol and thyroid hormone metabolism. *Thyroid* 1:273, 1991.
285. Saberi M, Sterling FH, Utiger RD: Reduction in extrathyroidal triiodothyronine production by propylthiouracil in man. *J Clin Invest* 55:218, 1975.
286. Chow CC, Phillips DIW, Lazarus JH, et al: Effect of low dose iodide supplementation on thyroid function in potentially susceptible subjects: Are dietary iodide levels in Britain acceptable? *Clin Endocrinol (Oxf)* 34:413, 1991.
287. Phillipou G, Koutras DA, Piperingos G, et al: The effect of iodide on serum thyroid hormone levels in normal persons, in hyperthyroid patients, and in hypothyroid patients on thyroxine replacement. *Clin Endocrinol (Oxf)* 36:573, 1992.
288. Namba H, Yamashita S, Kimura H, et al: Evidence of thyroid volume increase in normal subjects receiving excess iodide. *J Clin Endocrinol Metab* 76:605, 1993.
289. Trip MD, Wiersinga W, Plomp TA: Incidence, predictability, and pathogenesis of amiodarone-induced thyrotoxicosis and hypothyroidism. *Am J Med* 91:507, 1991.
290. Harjai KJ, Licata AA: Effects of amiodarone on thyroid function. *Ann Intern Med* 126:63, 1997.
291. Newman CM, Price A, Davies DW, et al: Amiodarone and the thyroid: A practical guide to the management of thyroid dysfunction induced by amiodarone therapy. *Heart* 79:121, 1998.
292. Melmed S, Nadenanee K, Reed AW, et al: Hyperthyroxinemia with bradycardia and normal thyrotropin secretion after chronic amiodarone therapy. *J Clin Endocrinol Metab* 53:997, 1981.
293. Bartalena L, Brogioni S, Grasso L, et al: Treatment of amiodarone-induced thyrotoxicosis, a difficult challenge: Results of a prospective study. *J Clin Endocrinol Metab* 81:2930, 1996.
294. Conn JJ, Sebastian MJ, Deam D, et al: A prospective study of the effect of nonionic contrast media on thyroid function. *Thyroid* 6:107, 1996.
294a. Hintze G, Blombach O, Fink H, et al: Risk of iodine-induced thyrotoxicosis after coronary angiography: An investigation in 788 unselected patients. *Eur J Endocrinol* 140:264, 1999.
295. Suzuki H, Noguchi K, Nakahata M, et al: Effect of iopanoic acid in the pituitary-thyroid axis: Time sequence of changes in serum iodothyronines, thyrotropin, and prolactin concentrations and responses to thyroid hormones. *J Clin Endocrinol Metab* 53:79, 1981.
296. Emerson CH, Dyson WL, Utiger RD: Serum thyrotropin and thyroxine concentrations in patients receiving lithium carbonate. *J Clin Endocrinol Metab* 36:338, 1973.
297. Perrild H, Hegedus L, Baastrup PC, et al: Thyroid function and ultrasonically determined thyroid size in patients receiving long-term lithium treatment. *Am J Psychiatry* 147:1518, 1990.
298. Bocchetta A, Cherchi A, Loviselli A, et al: Six-year follow-up of thyroid function during lithium treatment. *Acta Psychiatr Scand* 94:45, 1996.
299. Lazarus JH: The effects of lithium therapy on thyroid and thyrotropin-releasing hormone. *Thyroid* 8:909, 1998.
300. Wilson R, McKillop JH, Crocket GT, et al: The effect of lithium therapy on parameters thought to be involved in the development of autoimmune thyroid disease. *Clin Endocrinol (Oxf)* 34:357, 1991.
301. Smith PJ, Surks MI: Multiple effects of 5,5′-diphenylhydantoin on the thyroid hormone system. *Endocr Rev* 5:514, 1984.
302. Curran PG, De Groot LJ: The effect of hepatic enzyme-inducing drugs on thyroid hormones and the thyroid gland. *Endocr Rev* 12:135, 1991.
303. Surks MI, Ordene KW, Mann DW, et al: Diphenylhydantoin inhibits the thyrotropin response to thyrotropin-releasing hormone in man and rat. *J Clin Endocrinol Metab* 56:940, 1983.
304. Isojarvi JIT, Pakarinen AJ, Myllula VV: Thyroid function with antiepileptic drugs. *Epilepsia* 33:142, 1992.
305. Ronnblom LE, Alm GV, Oberg KE: Autoimmunity after alpha-interferon therapy for malignant carcinoid tumors. *Ann Intern Med* 115:178, 1991.
306. Watanabe U, Hashimoto E, Hisamitsu T, et al: The risk factor for develpoment of thyroid disease during interferon- therapy for chronic hepatatis C. *Am J Gastroenterol* 89:399, 1994.
307. Preziati D, La Rosa L, Covini G, et al: Autoimmunity and thyroid function in patients with chronic active hepatitis treated with recombinant interferon alpha-2a. *Eur J Endocrinol* 132:587, 1995.
308. Fernandez-Soto L, Gonzalez A, Escobar-Jimenez F, et al: Increased risk of autoimmune thyroid disease in hepatitis C vs hepatitis B before, during and after discontinuing interferon therapy. *Arch Intern Med* 158:1445, 1998.
309. Schwartzentruber DJ, White DE, Zweig MH, et al: Thyroid dysfunction associated with immunotherapy for patients with cancer. *Cancer* 68:2384, 1991.
310. Vialettes MB, Guillerand MA, Viens P, et al: Incidence rate and risk factors for thyroid dysfunction during recombinant interleukin-2 therapy in advanced malignancies. *Acta Endocrinol (Copenh)* 129:31, 1993.
311. De Luis DA, Romero E: Reversible thyroid dysfunction with filgastrim. *Lancet* 348:1595, 1996.
312. Okamura K, Nakashima T, Ueda K, et al: Thyroid disorders in the general population of Hisayama Japan, with special reference to prevalence and sex differences. *Int J Epidemiol* 16:545, 1987.
313. Williams I, Ankrett VO, Lazarus JH, et al: Aetiology of hyperthyroidism in Canada and Wales. *J Epidemiol Comm Health* 37:245, 1983.
314. Berglund J, Borup Christensen S, Hallengren B: Total and age-specific incidence of Graves' thyrotoxicosis, toxic nodular goitre and solitary toxic adenoma in Malmo 1970–74. *J Intern Med* 227:137, 1990.
315. Brownlie BEW, Wells JE: The epidemiology of thyrotoxicosis in New Zealand: Incidence and geographical distribution in North Canterbury, 1983–1985. *Clin Endocrinol (Oxf)* 33:249, 1990.
316. Reinwein D, Benker G, Konig MP, et al: The different types of hyperthyroidism in Europe: Results of a prospective survey of 924 patients. *J Endocrinol Invest* 11:193, 1988.
317. Nicoloff JT, Low JC, Dussault JH, et al: Simultaneous measurement of thyroxine and triiodothyronine peripheral turnover kinetics in man. *J Clin Invest* 51:473, 1972.

318. Caplan RH, Pagliara AS, Wickus G: Thyroxine toxicosis: A common variant of hyperthyroidism. *JAMA* 244:1934, 1980.
319. Weetman AP, McGregor AM: Autoimmune thyroid disease: Further developments in our understanding. *Endocr Rev* 15:788, 1994.
320. Weetman AP, Yateman ME, Ealey PA, et al: Thyroid-stimulating antibody activity between different immunoglobulin G subclasses. *J Clin Invest* 86:723, 1990.
321. McLachlan SM, Pegg CAS, Atherton MC, et al: TSH receptor antibody synthesis by thyroid lymphocytes. *Clin Endocrinol (Oxf)* 24:223, 1986.
322. Rees Smith B, McLachlan SM, Furmaniak J: Autoantibodies to the thyrotropin receptor. *Endocr Rev* 9:106, 1988.
323. Kakinuma A, Chazenbalk GD, Jaume JC, et al: The human thyrotropin (TSH) receptor in a TSH binding inhibition assay for TSH receptor autoantibodies. *J Clin Endocrinol Metab* 82:2129, 1997.
324. Costagliola S, Morgenthaler NG, Hoermann R, et al: Second generation assay for thyrotropin receptor antibodies has superior diagnostic sensitivity for Graves' disease. *J Clin Endocrinol Metab* 84:90, 1999.
325. Sugenoya A, Kobayashi S, Kasuga Y, et al: Evidence of intrathyroidal accumulation of TSH receptor antibody in Graves' disease. *Acta Endocrinol (Copenh)* 126:416, 1992.
326. Feldt-Rasmussen U, Schleusener H, Carayon P: Meta-analysis evaluation of the impact of thyrotropin receptor antibodies on long term remission after medical therapy of Graves' disease. *J Clin Endocrinol Metab* 78:98, 1994.
327. Di Cerbo A, Di Paola R, Bonati M, et al: Subgroups of Graves' patients identified on the basis of the biochemical activities of their immunoglobulins. *J Clin Endocrinol Metab* 80:2785, 1995.
328. Morris JC, Bergert ER, Bryant WP: Binding of immunoglobulin G from patients with autoimmune thyroid disease to rat sodium-iodide symporter peptides: Evidence for the iodide transporter as an autoantigen. *Thyroid* 7:527, 1997.
329. Jaume JC, Kakinuma A, Chazenbalk GD, et al: Thyrotropin receptor autoantibodies in serum are present at much lower levels than thyroid peroxidase autoantibodies: Analysis by flow cytometry. *J Clin Endocrinol Metab* 82:500, 1997.
330. Hancock SL, Cox RS, McDougall IR: Thyroid diseases after treatment of Hodgkin's disease. *N Engl J Med* 325:599, 1991.
331. Nygaard B, Knudsen JH, Hegedus L, et al: Thyrotropin receptor antibodies and Graves' disease, a side-effect of ^{131}I treatment in patients with nontoxic goiter. *J Clin Endocrinol Metab* 82:2926, 1997.
332. De Roux N, Shields DC, Misrahi M, et al: Analysis of the thyrotropin receptor as a candidate gene in familial Graves' disease. *J Clin Endocrinol Metab* 81:3483, 1996.
333. Kotsa KD, Watson PF, Weetman AP: No association between a thyrotropin receptor gene polymorphism and Graves' disease in the female population. *Thyroid* 7:31, 1997.
334. Leclere J, Bene MC, Duprez A, et al: Behavior of thyroid tissue from patients with Graves' disease in nude mice. *J Clin Endocrinol Metab* 59:175, 1984.
335. Nagayama Y, Rapoport B: Thyroid stimulatory autoantibodies in different patients with autoimmune thyroid disease do not all recognize the same components of the human thyrotropin receptor: Selective role of receptor amino acids Ser25-Glu30. *J Clin Endocrinol Metab* 75:1425, 1992.
336. Graves PN, Vlase H, Davies TF: Folding of the recombinant human thyrotropin (TSH) receptor extracellular domain: Identification of folded monomeric and tetrameric complexes that bind TSH receptor autoantibodies. *Endocrinology* 136:521, 1995.
337. Soliman M, Kaplan E, Yanagawa T, et al: T-cells recognize multiple epitopes in the human thyrotropin receptor extracellular domain. *J Clin Endocrinol Metab* 80:905, 1995.
338. Seetharamaiah G, Wagle NM, Morris JC, et al: Generation and characterization of monoclonal antibodies to the human thyrotropin (TSH) receptor: Antibodies can bind to discrete conformational or linear epitopes and block TSH binding. *Endocrinology* 136:2817, 1995.
339. Tomer Y, Davies TF: Infection, thyroid disease, and autoimmunity. *Endocr Rev* 14:107, 1993.
340. Migita K, Eguchi K, Otsubo T, et al: Cytokine regulation of HLA on thyroid epithelial cells. *Clin Exp Immunol* 82:548, 1990.
341. Matsuoka N, Eguchi K, Kawakami A, et al: Lack of B7-1/BB1 and B7-2/B70 expression on thyrocytes of patients with Graves' disease. Delivery of costimulatory signals from bystander professional antigen-presenting cells. *J Clin Endocrinol Metab* 81:4137, 1996.
342. Volpe R, Karlsson A, Jansson R, et al: Evidence that antithyroid drugs induce remissions in Graves' disease by modulating thyroid cellular activity. *Clin Endocrinol (Oxf)* 25:453, 1986.
343. Mullins RJ, Cohen SBA, Webb LMC, et al: Identification of thyroid stimulating receptor-specific T cells in Graves' disease thyroid using autoantigen-transfected Epstein-Barr virus-transformed B cell lines. *J Clin Invest* 96:30, 1995.
344. Davies TF: Preferential use of T-cell receptor V genes in human autoimmune thyroid disease. *Autoimmunity* 13:11, 1992.
345. Holland FJ, McConnon JK, Volpe R, et al: Concordant Graves' disease after bone marrow transplantation: Implication for pathogenesis. *J Clin Endocrinol Metab* 72:837,1991.
346. Thomson JA, Wilson RM, Franklin IM: Transmission of thyrotoxicosis of autoimmune type by sibling allogeneic bone marrow transplant. *Eur J Endocrinol* 133:564, 1995.
347. Brix TH, Kyvik KO, Hegedus L: What is the evidence of genetic factors in the etiology of Graves' disease? A brief review. *Thyroid* 8:627, 1998.
348. Brix TH, Christensen K, Holm NV, et al: A population based study of Graves' disease is Danish twins. *Clin Endocrinol (Oxf)* 48:397, 1998.
349. Barbesino G, Tomer Y, Concepcion E, et al: Linkage analysis of candidate genes in autoimmune thyroid disease: 1. Selected immunoregulatory genes. *J Clin Endocrinol Metab* 83:1580, 1998.
350. Barbesino G, Tomer Y, Concepcion ES, et al: Linkage analysis of candidate genes in autoimmune thyroid disease. 2. Selected gender-related genes and the X-chromosome. *J Clin Endocrinol Metab* 83:3290, 1998.
351. Ebner SA, Badonnel M-C, Altman LA, et al: Conjugal Graves' disease. *Ann Intern Med* 116:479, 1992.
352. Prummel M, Wiersinga WM: Smoking and risk of Graves' disease. *JAMA* 269:479, 1993.
353. Winsa B, Mandahl A, Karlsson A: Graves' disease, endocrine ophthalmopathy and smoking. *Acta Endocrinol (Copenh)* 128:156, 1993.
354. Winsa B, Adami H-O, Bergstrom R, et al: Stressful life events and Graves' disease. *Lancet* 338:1475, 1991.
355. Radosavljevic VR, Jankovic SM, Marinkovic M: Stressful life events in the pathogenesis of Graves' disease. *Eur J Endocrinol* 134:699, 1996.
356. Paunkovic N, Paunkovic J, Pavlovic O, et al: The significant increase in incidence of Graves' disease in Eastern Serbia during the civil war in the former Yugoslavia. *Thyroid* 8:37, 1998.
357. Murakami M, Koizumi Y, Aizawa T, et al: Studies of thyroid function and immune parameters in patients with hyperthyroid Graves' disease in remission. *J Clin Endocrinol Metab* 66:103, 1988.
358. Codaccioni JL, Orgiazzi J, Blanc P, et al: Lasting remissions in patients treated for Graves' hyperthyroidism with propranolol alone: A pattern of spontaneous evolution of the disease. *J Clin Endocrinol Metab* 67:656, 1988.
359. Hirota Y, Tamai H, Hayashi Y, et al: Thyroid function and histology in forty-five patients with hyperthyroid Graves' disease in clinical remission more than ten years after thionamide drug treatment. *J Clin Endocrinol Metab* 62:165, 1986.
360. Tamai H, Kasagi K, Takaichi Y, et al: Development of spontaneous hypothyroidism in patients with Graves' disease treated with antithyroidal drugs: Clinical, immunological, and histological findings in 26 patients. *J Clin Endocrinol Metab* 69:49, 1989.
361. Takasu N, Yamada T, Sato A, et al: Graves' disease following hypothyroidism due to Hashimoto's disease: Studies of eight cases. *Clin Endocrinol (Oxf)* 33:687, 1990.
362. Aizawa Y, Yoshida K, Kaise N, et al: Long-term effects of radioiodine on thyrotrophin receptor antibodies in Graves' disease. *Clin Endocrinol (Oxf)* 42:517, 1995.
363. Stover C, Otto E, Beyer J, et al: Cellular immunity and retrobulbar fibroblasts in Graves' ophthalmopathy. *Thyroid* 4:161, 1994.
364. Sorisky A, Pardesani D, Gagnon A, et al: Evidence of adipocyte differentiation in human orbital fibroblasts in primary culture. *J Clin Endocrinol Metab* 81:3428, 1996.

365. Bahn RS, Heufelder AE: Pathogenesis of Graves' ophthalmopathy. *N Engl J Med* 329:1468, 1993.
366. Burch HB, Sellitti D, Barnes SG, et al: Thyrotropin receptor antisera for the detection of immunoreactive protein species in retroocular fibroblasts obtained from patients with Graves' ophthalmopathy. *J Clin Endocrinol Metab* 78:1384, 1994.
367. Bahn RS, Dutton CM, Natt N, et al: Thyrotropin receptor expression in Graves' orbital adipose/connective tissues: Potential autoantigen in Graves' ophthalmopathy. *J Clin Endocrinol Metab* 83:998, 1998.
368. McLachlan SM, Prummel MF, Rapoport B: Cell-mediated or humoral immunity in Graves' ophthalmopathy? Profiles of T-cell cytokines amplified by polymerase chain reaction from orbital tissues. *J Clin Endocrinol Metab* 78:1070, 1994.
369. Perros P, Kendall-Taylor P: Antibodies to orbital tissues in thyroid-associated ophthalmopathy. *Acta Endocrinol (Copenh)* 126:137, 1992.
370. Kubota S, Gunji K, Stolarski C, et al: Reevaluation of the prevalences of serum autoantibodies reactive with "64-kd eye muscle proteins" in patients with thyroid-associated ophthalmopathy. *Thyroid* 8:175, 1998.
371. Gunji K, Kubota S, Swanson J, et al: Role of the eye muscles in thyroid eye disease: Identification of the principal autoantigens. *Thyroid* 8:553, 1998.
372. Fatourechi V, Pajouhi M, Fransway AF: Dermopathy of Graves' disease (pretibial myxedema). Review of 150 cases. *Medicine (Baltimore)* 73:1, 1994.
373. Shishiba Y, Imai Y, Odajima R, et al: Immunoglobulin G of patients with circumscribed pretibial myxedema of Graves' disease stimulates proteoglycan synthesis in human skin fibroblasts in culture. *Acta Endocrinol (Copenh)* 127:44, 1992.
374. Metcalfe RA, Davies R, Weetman AP: Analysis of fibroblast-stimulating activity in IgG from patients with Graves' dermopathy. *Thyroid* 3:207, 1993.
375. Christiansen NJ, Siersboek-Nielsen K, Hansen J, et al: Serum thyroxine in the early phase of subacute thyroiditis. *Acta Endocrinol (Copenh)* 64:359, 1970.
376. Gerstein HC: How common is postpartum thyroiditis? A methodologic overview of the literature. *Arch Intern Med* 150:1397, 1990.
377. Calle RA, Cohen KA: Transient thyroiditis due to surgical trauma. *Am J Med* 95:546, 1993.
378. Samuels MH, Launder T: Hyperthyroidism due to lymphoma involving the thyroid gland in a patient with acquired immunodeficiency syndrome: Case report and review of the literature. *Thyroid* 8:673, 1998.
379. Cohen JH III, Ingbar SH, Braverman LE: Thyrotoxicosis due to ingestion of excess thyroid hormone. *Endocr Rev* 10:113, 1989.
380. Gorman CA, Wahner HW, Tauxe WH: Metabolic malingerers. *Am J Med* 48:708, 1970.
381. Litovitz TL, White JD: Levothyroxine ingestions in children: An analysis of 78 cases. *Am J Emerg Med* 3:297, 1985.
382. Lewander WJ, Lacouture PG, Silva JE, et al: Acute thyroxine ingestion in pediatric patients. *Pediatrics* 84:262, 1989.
383. Hedberg CW, Fishbein DB, Janssen RS, et al: An outbreak of thyrotoxicosis caused by the consumption of bovine thyroid gland in ground beef. *N Engl J Med* 316:993, 1987.
384. Kinney JS, Hurwitz ES, Fishbein DB, et al: Community outbreak of thyrotoxicosis: Epidemiology, immunogenetic characteristics, and long-term outcome. *Am J Med* 84:10, 1988.
385. Sawin CT, London MH: 'Natural' desiccated thyroid. A 'health-food' preparation. *Arch Intern Med* 149:2117, 1989.
386. Eliason BC, Doenier JA, Nuhlicek DN: Desiccated thyroid in a nutritional supplement. *J Fam Pract* 38:287, 1994.
387. Stanbury JB, Ermans AE, Bourdoux P, et al: Iodine-induced hyperthyroidism: Occurrence and epidemiology. *Thyroid* 8:83, 1998.
388. Vagenakis AG, Wang C-A, Burger A, et al: Iodide-induced thyrotoxicosis in Boston. *N Engl J Med* 287:523, 1972.
389. Martin FIA, Tress BW, Colman PG, et al: Iodine-induced hyperthyroidism due to nonionic contrast radiography in the elderly. *Am J Med* 95:78, 1993.
390. Martino E, Aghini-Lombardi F, Lippi F, et al: Twenty-four hour radioactive iodine uptake in 35 patients with amiodarone associated thyrotoxicosis. *J Nucl Med* 26:1402, 1985.
391. Bartalena L, Grasso L, Brogioni S, et al: Serum interleukin-6 in amiodarone-induced thyrotoxicosis. *J Clin Endocrinol Metab* 78:423, 1994.
392. Hamburger JI: Evolution of toxicity in solitary nontoxic autonomously functioning thyroid nodules. *J Clin Endocrinol Metab* 50:1089, 1980.
393. Burch HB, Shakir F, Fitzsimmons TR, et al: Diagnosis and management of the autonomously functioning thyroid nodule: The Walter Reed Army Medical Center experience, 1975–1996. *Thyroid* 8:871, 1998.
394. Sandrock D, Olbricht T, Emrich D, et al: Long-term follow-up in patients with autonomous thyroid adenoma. *Acta Endocrinol (Copenh)* 128:51, 1993.
395. Hamburger JI, Taylor CL: Transient thyrotoxicosis associated with acute hemorrhagic infarction of autonomously functioning thyroid nodules. *Ann Intern Med* 91:406, 1979.
396. Russo D, Arturi F, Suarez HG, et al: Thyrotropin receptor gene alterations in thyroid hyperfunctioning adenomas. *J Clin Endocrinol Metab* 81:1548, 1996.
397. Parma J, Duprez L, Van Sande J, et al: Diversity and prevalence of somatic mutations in the thyrotropin receptor and $G_s\alpha$ genes as a cause of toxic thyroid adenomas. *J Clin Endocrinol Metab* 82:2695, 1997.
398. Krohn K, Fuhrer D, Holzapfel H-P, et al: Clonal origin of toxic thyroid nodules with constitutively activating thyrotropin receptor mutations. *J Clin Endocrinol Metab* 83:130, 1998.
399. Fuhrer D, Holzapfel H-P, Wonerow P, et al: Somatic mutations in the thyrotropin receptor gene and not in the $G_3\alpha$ protein gene in 31 toxic thyroid nodules. *J Clin Endocrinol Metab* 82:3885, 1997.
400. Paschke R, Ludgate M: The thyrotropin receptor in thyroid disease. *N Engl J Med* 337:1675, 1997.
401. Van Sande J, Parma J, Tonacchera M, et al: Somatic and germline mutations of the TSH receptor gene in thyroid disease. *J Clin Endocrinol Metab.* 80:2577, 1995.
402. Berghout A, Wiersinga WM, Smits NJ, et al: Interrelationships between age, thyroid volume, thyroid nodularity and thyroid function in patients with sporadic nontoxic goiter. *Am J Med* 89:602, 1990.
403. Rieu M, Bekka S, Sambor B, et al: Prevalence of subclinical hyperthyroidism and relationship between thyroid hormonal status and thyroid ultrasonographic parameters in patients with non-toxic nodular goiter. *Clin Endocrinol (Oxf)* 39:67, 1993.
404. Elte JWF, Bussemaker JK, Haak A: The natural history of euthyroid multinodular goiter. *Postgrad Med J* 66:186, 1990.
405. Kopp P, Kimura ET, Aeschimann S, et al: Polyclonal and monoclonal thyroid nodules coexist within human multinodular goiters. *J Clin Endocrinol Metab* 79:134, 1994.
406. Holzapfel H-P, Fuhrer D, Wonerow P, et al: Identification of consitutively activating somatic thyrotropin receptor mutations in a subset of toxic multinodular goiters. *J Clin Endocrinol Metab* 82:4229, 1997.
407. Tonacchera M, Chiovato L, Pinchera A, et al: Hyperfunctioning thyroid nodules in toxic multinodular goiter share activating thyrotropin receptor mutations with solitary toxic adenomas. *J Clin Endocrinol Metab* 83:492, 1998.
408. Studer H, Derwahl M: Mechanisms of nonenoplastic endocrine hyperplasia—a changing concept: A review focused on the thyroid gland. *Endocr Rev* 16:411, 1995.
409. Duprez L, Parma J, Van Sande J, et al: Germline mutations in the thyrotropin receptor gene cause non-autoimmune autosomal dominant hyperthyroidism. *Nature Genetics* 7:396, 1994.
410. Fuhrer D, Wonerow P, Willgerodt H, et al: Identification of a new thyrotropin receptor germline mutations ($Leu^{629}Phe$) in a family with neonatal onset of autosomal dominant nonautoimmune hyperthyroidism. *J Clin Endocrinol Metab* 82:4234, 1997.
411. Holzapfel H-P, Wonerow P, von Petrykowski W, et al: Sporadic congenital hyperthyroidism due to a spontaneous germline mutation in the thyrotropin receptor gene. *J Clin Endocrinol Metab* 82:3879, 1997.
412. Gruters A, Schoneberg T, Biebermann H, et al: Severe congenital hyperthyroidism caused by a germ-line *neo* mutation in the extracellular portion of the thyrotropin receptor. *J Clin Endocrinol Metab* 83:1431, 1998.
413. Thomas J-L, Leclere J, Hartemann P, et al: Familial hyperthyroidism without evidence of autoimmunity. *Acta Endocrinol (Copenh)* 100:512, 1982.

414. Weinstein LS, Shenker A, Gejman PV, et al: Activating mutations of the stimulatory G protein in the McCune-Albright syndrome. *N Engl J Med* 325:1688, 1991.
415. Feuillan PP, Shawker T, Rose SR, et al: Thyroid abnormalities in the McCune-Albright syndrome: Ultrasonography and hormonal studies. *J Clin Endocrinol Metab* 71:1596, 1990.
416. Mastoroakos G, Mitsiades NS, Doufas AG, et al: Hyperthyroidism in McCune-Albright syndrome with a review of thyroid abnormalities sixty years after the first report. *Thyroid* 7:433, 1997.
417. Bayot MR, Chopra IJ: Coexistence of struma ovarii and Graves' disease. *Thyroid* 5:469, 1995.
418. Brown WW, Shetty KR, Rosenfeld PS: Hyperthyroidism due to struma ovarii: Demonstration by radiodine scan. *Acta Endocrinol (Copenh)* 73:266, 1973.
419. Salvatori SM, Salatnich I, Rufini V, et al: Severe thyrotoxicosis due to functioning pulmonary metastases of well-differentiated thyroid cancer. *J Nucl Med* 39:1202, 1998.
420. Beck-Peccoz P, Brucker-Davis F, Persani L, et al: Thyrotropin-secreting pituitary tumors. *Endocr Rev* 17:610, 1996.
421. McDermott MT, Ridgway EC: Central hyperthyroidism. *Endocrinol Metab Clin North Am* 27:187, 1998.
422. Losa M, Giovanelli M, Persani L, et al: Criteria of cure and follow-up of central hyperthyroidism due to thyrotropin-secreting pituitary adenomas. *J Clin Endocrinol Metab* 81:3084, 1996.
423. Chanson P, Weintraub BD, Harris AG: Octreotide therapy for thyroid-stimulating hormone-secreting pituitary adenomas. A follow-up of 52 patients. *Ann Intern Med* 119:236, 1993.
424. Kuhn JM, Arlot S, Lefebrve H, et al: Evaluation of the treatment of thyrotropin-secreting pituitary adenomas with a slow release formulation of the somatostatin analog lanreotide. *J Clin Endocrinol Metab* 85:1487, 2000.
425. Goodwin TM, Montoro M, Mestman JH, et al: The role of chorionic gonadotropin in transient hyperthyroidism of hyperenesis gravidarum. *J Clin Endocrinol Metab* 75:133, 1992.
426. Kimura M, Amino N, Tamaki H, et al: Gestational thyrotoxicosis and hyperemesis gravidarum: Possible role of hCG with higher stimulating activity. *Clin Endocrinol (Oxf)* 38:345, 1993.
427. Rodien P, Bremont C, Sanson M-LR, et al: Familial gestational hyperthyroidism caused by a mutant thyrotopin receptor hypersensitive to human chorionic gonadotropin. *N Engl J Med* 339:1823, 1998.
428. Goodwin TM, Montoro M, Mestman JH: Transient hyperthyroidism and hyperemesis gravidarum: Clinical aspects. *Am J Obstet Gynecol* 167:648, 1992.
429. Desai RK, Norman RJ, Jialal I, et al: Spectrum of thyroid function abnormalities in gestational trophoblastic neoplasia. *Clin Endocrinol (Oxf)* 29:583, 1988.
430. Giralt SA, Dexeus F, Amato R, et al: Hyperthyroidism in men with germ cell tumors and high levels of beta-human chorionic gonadotropin. *Cancer* 69:1286, 1992.
431. Oddie TH, Boyd CM, Fisher DA, et al: Incidence of signs and symptoms in thyroid disease. *Med J Aust* 2:981, 1972.
432. Davis PJ, Davis FB: Hyperthyroidism in patients over the age of 60 years. *Medicine (Baltimore)* 53:161, 1974.
433. Nordyke RA, Gilbert FI Jr, Harada ASM: Graves' disease: Influence of age on clinical findings. *Arch Intern Med* 148:626, 1988.
434. Martin FIR, Deam DR: Hyperthyroidism in elderly hospitalised patients. Clinical features and treatment outcomes. *Med J Australia* 164:200, 1996.
435. Trivalle C, Doucet J, Chassagne P, et al: Differences in the signs and symptroms of hyperthyroidism in older and younger patients. *J Am Geriatr Soc* 44:50, 1996.
436. Parker JLW, Lawson DH: Death from thyrotoxicosis. *Lancet* 2:894, 1973.
437. Nygaard B, Hegedus L, Gervil M, et al: Influence of compensated radioiodine therapy on thyroid volume and incidence of hypothyroidism in Graves' disease. *J Intern Med* 238:491, 1995.
438. Chiovato L, Fiore E, Vitti P, et al: Outcome of thyroid function in Graves' patients treated with radioiodine: Role of thyroid-stimulating and thyrotropin-blocking antibodies and of radioiodine-induced damage. *J Clin Endocrinol Metab* 83:40, 1998.
439. Hegedus L, Hansen JM, Karstrup S: High incidence of normal thyroid gland volume in patients with Graves' disease. *Clin Endocrinol (Oxf)* 19:603, 1983.
440. Zurcher RM, Horber FF, Grunig BE, et al: Effect of thyroid dysfunction on thigh muscle efficiency. *J Clin Endocrinol Metab* 69:1082, 1989.
441. Olson BR, Klein I, Benner R, et al: Hyperthyroid myopathy and the response to treatment. *Thyroid* 1:137, 1991.
442. Ober KP: Thyrotoxic periodic paralysis in the United States: Report of 7 cases and review of the literature. *Medicine (Baltimore)* 71:109, 1992.
443. Ko GTC, Chow CC, Yeung VTF, et al: Thyrotoxic periodic paralysis in a Chinese population. *Q J Med* 89:463, 1996.
444. Woeber KA: Thyrotoxicosis and the heart. *N Engl J Med* 327:94, 1992.
445. Das KC, Mukherjee M, Sarkar TK, et al: Erythropoiesis and erythropoietin in hypo- and hyperthyroidism. *J Clin Endocrinol Metab* 40:211, 1975.
446. Mintz G, Pizzarello R, Klein I: Enhanced left ventricular diastolic function in hyperthyroidism: Noninvasive assessment and response to treatment. *J Clin Endocrinol Metab* 73:146, 1991.
447. Giladi M, Aderka D, Zeligman-Melatzki L, et al: Is idiopathic atrial fibrillation caused by occult thyrotoxicosis? A study of one hundred consecutive patients with atrial fibrillaton. *Int J Cardiol* 30:309, 1991.
448. Krahn AD, Klein GJ, Kerr CR, et al: How useful is thyroid function testing in patients with recent-onset atrial fibrillation? *Arch Intern Med* 156:2221, 1996.
449. Nakazawa HK, Sakurai K, Hamada N, et al: Management of atrial fibrillation in the post-thyrotoxic state. *Am J Med* 72:903, 1982.
450. Petersen P, Hansen JM: Stroke in thyrotoxicosis with atrial fibrillation. *Stroke* 19:15, 1988.
451. Presti CF, Hart RG: Thyrotoxicosis, atrial fibrillation, and embolism, revisited. *Am Heart J* 117:976, 1989.
452. Wilson BE, Newmark SR: Thyrotoxicosis-induced congestive heart failure in an urban hospital. *Am J Med Sci* 308:344, 1994.
453. Umpierrez GE, Challapalli S, Patterson C: Congestive heart failure due to reversible cardiomyopathy in patients with hyperthyroidism. *Am J Med Sci* 310:99, 1995.
454. Siatakas NM, Milona I, Salesiotou V, et al: Respiratory muscle strength in hyperthyroidism before and after treatment. *Am Rev Resp Dis* 146:1025, 1992.
455. Kahaly GJ, Nieswandt J, Wagner S, et al: Ineffective cardiorespiratory function in hyperthyroidism. *J Clin Endocrinol Metab* 83:4075, 1998.
456. White NW, Raine RI, Bateman ED: Asthma and hyperthyroidism: A report of 4 cases. *S Afr Med J* 78:750, 1990.
457. Ford HC, Lim WC, Chisnall WN, et al: Renal function and electrolyte levels in hyperthyroidism: Urinary protein excretion and the plasma concentrations of urea, creatinine, uric acid, hydrogen ion and electrolytes. *Clin Endocrinol (Oxf)* 30:293, 1989.
458. Hauger-Klevene JH, Brown H, Zavaleta J: Plasma renin activity in hyper- and hypothyroidism: Effect of adrenergic blocking agents. *J Clin Endocrinol Metab* 34:625, 1972.
459. Cain JP, Dluhy RG, Williams GH, et al: Control of aldosterone secretion in hyperthyroidism. *J Clin Endocrinol Metab* 36:365, 1973.
460. Harvey JN, Nagi DK, Baylis PH, et al: Disturbance of osmoregulated thirst and vasopressin secretion in thyrotoxicosis. *Clin Endocrinol (Oxf)* 35:29, 1991.
461. Wegener W, Wedmann B, Langhoff T, et al: Effect of hyperthyroidism on the transit of a calorie solid-liquid meal through the stomach, the small intestine, and the colon in man. *J Clin Endocrinol Metab* 75:745, 1992.
462. Baker JT, Harvey RF: Bowel habit in thyrotoxicosis and hypothyroidism. *Br Med J* 1:322, 1971.
463. Goswami R, Tandon RK, Dudha A, et al: Prevalence and significance of steatorrhea in patients with active Graves' disease. *Am J Gastroenterol* 93:1122, 1998.
464. Harper MB: Vomiting, nausea and abdominal pain: Unrecognized symptoms of thyrotoxicosis. *J Fam Pract* 29:382, 1989.
465. Fong T-L, McHutchinson JG, Reynolds TB: Hyperthyroidism and hepatic dysfunction. A case series analysis. *J Clin Gastroenterol* 14:240, 1992.
466. Reddy J, Brownlie BEW, Heaton DC, et al: The peripheral blood picture in thyrotoxicosis. *N Z Med J* 93:143, 1981.
467. Iitaka M, Noh JY, Kitahama S, et al: Elevated serum granulocyte

colony-stimulating factor levels in patient with Graves' disease. *Clin Endocrinol (Oxf)* 48:275, 1998.
468. Grebe SKG, Feek CM, Ford HC, et al: A randomized trial of short-term treatment of Graves' disease with high-dose carbimazole plus thyroxine versus low-dose carbimazole. *Clin Endocrinol (Oxf)* 48:585, 1998.
469. Fukazawa H, Yoshida K, Kaise N, et al: Intercellular adhesion molecule 1 (ICAM-1) in the sera of patients with Graves' disease: Correlation with disease activity and treatment status. *Thyroid* 5:373, 1995.
470. Salvi M, Girasole G, Pedrazzoni, et al: Increased serum concentrations of interleukin-6 (IL-6) and soluble IL-6 receptor in patients with Graves' disease. *J Clin Endocrinol Metab* 81:2976, 1996.
471. Lakatos P, Foldes J, Horvath C, et al: Serum interleukin-6 and bone metabolism in patients with thyroid function disorders. *J Clin Endocrinol Metab* 82:78, 1997.
472. Koukkou K, Panayiotidis P, Alevizou-Terzaki V, et al: High levels of serum soluble interleukin-2 receptors in hyperthyroid patients: Correlation with serum thyroid hormones and independence from the etiology of the hyperthyroidism. *J Clin Endocrinol Metab* 73:771, 1991.
473. Shimaoka Y, Hidaka Y, Okumura M, et al: Serum concentrations of soluble Fas in patients with autoimmune thyroid disease. *Thyroid* 8:43, 1998.
474. Hynes K, Blum M, Lackner H, et al: Easy bruising, thrombocytopenia, and elevated platelet immunoglobulin G in Graves' disease and Hashimoto's thyroiditis. *Ann Intern Med* 94:27, 1981.
475. Hofbauer LC, Heufelder AE: Coagulation disorders in thyroid disease. *Eur J Endocrinol* 136:1, 1997.
476. Lovejoy JC, Smith SR, Bray GA, et al: A paradigm of experimentally induced mild hyperthyroidism: Effects on nitrogen balance, body composition, and energy expenditure in healthy young men. *J Clin Endocrinol Metab* 82:765, 1997.
477. Hoogwerf BJ, Nuttall FQ: Long-term weight regulation in treated hyperthyroid and hypothyroid subjects. *Am J Med* 76:963, 1984.
478. Shen D-C, Davidson MB, Kuo S-W, et al: Peripheral and hepatic insulin antagonism in hyperthyroidism. *J Clin Endocrinol Metab* 66:565, 1988.
479. Bech K, Damsbo P, Eldrup E, et al: β-Cell function and glucose and lipid oxidation in Graves' disease. *Clin Endocrinol (Oxf)* 44:59, 1996.
480. Cooppan R, Kozak GP: Hyperthyroidism and diabetes mellitus: An analysis of 70 patients. *Arch Intern Med* 140:370, 1980.
481. Sreenan S, Caro JF, Refetoff S: Thyroid dysfunction is not associated with alterations in serum leptin levels. *Thyroid* 7:407, 1997.
482. Korbonits M: Leptin and the thyroid—a puzzle with missing pieces. *Clin Endocrinol (Oxf)* 49:569, 1998.
483. Kung AWC, Pang RWC, Lauder I, et al: Changes in serum lipoprotein(a) and lipids during treatment of hyperthyroidism. *Clin Chem* 41:226, 1995.
484. O'Brien T, Katz K, Hodge D, et al: The effect of the treatment of hypothyroidism and hyperthyroidism on plasma lipids and apolipoproteins AI, AII and E. *Clin Endocrinol (Oxf)* 46:17, 1997.
485. Aoki N, Maruyama Y, Imamura M, et al: Studies of sex hormone-binding plasma protein (SBP) in Graves' disease before and under antithyroid drug therapy. *Acta Endocrinol (Copenh)* 113:249, 1986.
486. Brenta G, Schnitman M, Gurfinkiel M, et al: Variations in sex hormone-binding globulin in thyroid dysfunction. *Thyroid* 9:273, 1999.
487. Graninger W, Pirich KR, Speiser W, et al: Effect of thyroid hormones on plasma protein concentrations in man. *J Clin Endocrinol Metab* 63:407, 1986.
488. O'Connor P, Feely J: Clinical pharmacokinetics and endocrine disorders: Therapeutic implications. *Clin Pharmacokinet* 13:345, 1987.
489. Chute JP, Ryan CP, Sladek G, et al: Exacerbation of warfarin-induced anticoagulation by hyperthyroidism. *Endocr Pract* 3:77, 1997.
490. Iranmanesh A, Lizarralde G, Johnson ML, et al: Nature of altered growth hormone secretion in hyperthyroidism. *J Clin Endocrinol Metab* 72:108, 1991.
491. Ramos-Dias JC, Yateman M, Camacho-Hubner C, et al: Low circulating IGF-I levels in hypothyroidism are associated with decreased GH response to GH-releasing hormone. *Clin Endocrinol (Oxf)* 43:583, 1995.
492. Miell JP, Taylor AM, Zini M, et al: Effects of hypothyroidism and hyperthyroidism on insulin-like growth factors (IGFs) and growth hormone- and IGF-binding proteins. *J Clin Endocrinol Metab* 76:950, 1993.
493. Snyder PJ, Jacobs LS, Daughaday WH, et al: Thyroid hormone inhibition of the prolactin response to thyrotropin-releasing hormone. *J Clin Invest* 52: 2324, 1973.
494. Dluhy RG: The adrenal cortex in thyrotoxicosis, in Braverman LE, Utiger RD (eds): *The Thyroid: A Fundamental and Clinical Text*, 8th ed. Philadelphia, Lippincott Williams and Wilkins, 2000, p 637.
495. Krassas GE, Pontikides N, Kaltsas T: Menstrual disturbances in thyrotoxicosis. *Clin Endocrinol (Oxf)* 40:641, 1994.
496. Akande ED, Hockaday TDR: Plasma concentration of gonadotropins, oestrogen, and progesterone in thyrotoxic women. *Br J Obstet Gynaecol* 92:541, 1975.
497. Abalovich A, Levalle O, Hermes R, et al: Hypothalamic-pituitary-testicular axis and seminal parameters in hyperthyroid males. *Thyroid* 9:857, 1999.
498. Ford HC, Cooke RR, Keightley EA, et al: Serum levels of free and bound testosterone in hyperthyroidism. *Clin Endocrinol (Oxf)* 36:187, 1992.
499. Siddiqi A, Burrin JM, Noonan K, et al: A longitudinal study of markers of bone turnover in Graves' disease and their value in predicting bone mineral density. *J Clin Endocrinol Metab* 82:753, 1997.
500. Jodar E, Munoz-Torres M, Escobar-Jimenez F, et al: Antiresorptive therapy in hyperthyroid patients: Longitudinal changes in bone and mineral metabolism. *J Clin Endocrinol Metab* 82:1989, 1997.
501. Langdahl BL, Loft AGR, Eriksen EF, et al: Bone mass, bone turnover, body composition, and calcium homeostasis in former hyperthyroid patients treated by combined medical therapy. *Thyroid* 6:161, 1996.
502. Langdahl BL, Loft AGR, Eriksen EF, et al: Bone mass, bone turnover, body composition, and calcium homeostasis in surgically and radioiodine-treated former hyperthyroid patients. *Thyroid* 6:169, 1996.
503. Wejda B, Hintze G, Katschinski B, et al: Hip fractures and the thyroid: A case-control study. *J Intern Med* 237:241, 1995.
504. Rosen HR, Moses AC, Gundberg C, et al: Therapy with parenteral pamidronate prevents thyroid hormone-induced bone turnover in humans. *J Clin Endocrinol Metab* 77:664, 1993.
505. Daly JG, Greenwood RM, Himsworth RL: Serum calcium concentration in hyperthyroidism at diagnosis and after treatment. *Clin Endocrinol (Oxf)* 19:397, 1983.
506. Peerenbbom H, Keck E, Kruskemper HL, et al: The defect of intestinal calcium transport in hyperthyroidism and its response to therapy. *J Clin Endocrinol Metab* 59:936, 1984.
507. Trzepacz PT, Klein I, Roberts M, et al: Graves' disease: An analysis of thyroid hormone levels and hyperthyroid signs and symptoms. *Am J Med* 87:558, 1989.
508. Aizawa T, Ishihara M, Hashizume K, et al: Age-related changes of thyroid function and immunologic abnormalities in patients with hyperthyroidism due to Graves' disease. *J Am Geriatr Soc* 37:944, 1989.
509. Shigemasa C, Abe K, Taniguchi S-I, et al: Lower serum free thyroxine (T_4) levels in painless thyroiditis compared with Graves' disease despite similar serum total T_4 levels. *J Clin Endocrinol Metab* 65:359, 1987.
510. Davies TF, Roti E, Braverman LE, et al: Thyroid controversy—stimulating antibodies. *J Clin Endocrinol Metab* 83:3777, 1998.
511. Tamai HT, Nakagawa T, Fukino O, et al: Thionamide therapy in Graves' disease: Relation of relapse rate to duration of therapy. *Ann Intern Med* 92:488, 1980.
512. Young ET, Steel NR, Taylor JJ, et al: Prediction of remission after antithyroid drug treatment in Graves' disease. *Q J Med* 66:175, 1988.
513. Hedley AJ, Young RE, Jones SJ, et al: Antithyroid drugs in the treatment of hyperthyroidism of Graves' disease: Long-term follow-up of 434 patients. *Clin Endocrinol (Oxf)* 31:209, 1989.
514. Allannic H, Fauchet R, Orgiazzi J, et al: Antithyroid drugs and Graves' disease: A prospective randomized evaluation of the efficacy of treatment duration. *J Clin Endocrinol Metab* 70:675, 1990.
515. Hashizume K, Ichikawa K, Sakurai A, et al: Administration of thyroxine in treated Graves' disease: Effects on the level of antibodies

to thyroid-stimulating hormone receptors and on the risk of recurrence of hyperthyroidism. *N Engl J Med* 324:947, 1991.
516. Edmonds CJ, Tellez M: Treatment of Graves' disease by carbimazole: High dose with thyroxine compared to titration dose. *Eur J Endocrinol* 131:120, 1994.
517. Weetman AP, Pickerill AP, Watson P, et al: Treatment of Graves' disease with the block-replace regimen of antithyroid drugs: The effect of treatment duration and immunogenetic susceptibility on relapse. *Q J Med* 87:337, 1994.
518. McIver B, Rae P, Beckett G, et al: Lack of effect of thyroxine in patients with Graves' disease who are treated with an antithyroid drug. *N Engl J Med* 334:220, 1996.
519. Wilson R, Buchanan L, Fraser WD, et al: Do higher doses of carbimazole improve remission in Graves' disease? *Q J Med* 89:381, 1996.
520. Pfeilschifter J, Ziegler R: Suppression of serum thyrotropin with thyroxine in patients with Graves' disease: Effects on recurrence of hyperthyroidism and thyroid volume. *Eur J Endocrinol* 136:81, 1997.
521. Lucas A, Salinas I, Rius F, et al: Medical therapy of Graves' disease: Does thyroxine prevent recurrence of hyperthyroidism? *J Clin Endocrinol Metab* 82:2410, 1997.
522. Glaser NS, Styne DM: Predictors of early remission of hyperthyroidism in children. *J Clin Endocrinol Metab* 82:1719, 1997.
523. Vitti P, Rago T, Chiovato L, et al: Clinical features of patients with Graves' disease undergoing remission after antithyroid drug treatment. *Thyroid* 7:369, 1997.
524. Benker G, Reinwein D, Kahaly G, et al: Is there a methimazole dose effect on remission rate in Graves' disease? Results from a long-term prospective study. *Clin Endocrinol (Oxf)* 49:451, 1998.
525. Rittmaster RS, Abbot EC, Douglas R, et al: Effect of methimazole with or without L-thyroxine, on remssion rates in Graves' disease. *J Clin Endocrinol Metab* 83:814, 1998.
526. Pujol P, Osman A, Grabar S, et al: TSH suppression combined with carbimazole for Graves' disease: Effect on remission and relapse rates. *Clin Endocrinol (Oxf)* 48:635, 1998.
527. Leech NJ, Dayan CM: Controversies in the management of Graves' disease. *Clin Endocrinol (Oxf)* 49:273, 1998.
528. Levetan C, Wartofsky L. A clinical guide to the management of Graves' disease with radioactive iodine. *Endocr Pract* 1:205, 1995.
529. Ljunggren J-G, Torring O, Wallin G, et al: Quality of life aspects and costs in treatment of Graves' hyperthyroidism with antithyroid drugs, surgery, or radioiodine: Results from a prospective, randomized study. *Thyroid* 8:653, 1998.
530. Torring O, Tallstedt L, Wallin G, et al: Graves' hyperthyroidism: Treatment with antithyroid drugs, surgery, or radioiodine—a prospective, randomized study. *J Clin Endocrinol Metab* 81:2986, 1996.
531. Wartofsky L, Glinoer D, Solomon B, et al: Differences and similarities in the diagnosis and treatment of Graves' disease in Europe, Japan, and the United States. *Thyroid* 1:129, 1991.
532. Romaldini JH: Case selection and restrictions recommended to patients with hyperthyroidism in South America. *Thyroid* 7:225, 1997.
533. Cooper DS: Antithyroid drugs for the treatment of hyperthyroidism caused by Graves' disease. *Endocrinol Metab Clin North Am* 27:225, 1998.
534. Jansson R, Dahlberg PA, Johansson H, et al: Intrathyroidal concentrations of methimazole in patients with Graves' disease. *J Clin Endocrinol Metab* 57:129, 1983.
535. Benker G, Vitti P, Kahaly G, et al: Response to methimazole in Graves' disease. *Clin Endocrinol (Oxf)* 43:257, 1995.
536. Weetman AP: The immunomodulatory effects of antithyroid drugs. *Thyroid* 4:145, 1994.
537. Volpe R: Evidence that the immunosupressive effects of antithyroid drugs are mediated through actions on the thyroid cell, modulating thyrocyte-immunocyte signalling: A review. *Thyroid* 4:217, 1994.
538. Shiroozu A, Okamura K, Ikenoue H, et al: Treatment of hyperthyroidism with a small single daily dose of methimazole. *J Clin Endocrinol Metab* 63:125, 1986.
539. Messina M, Milani P, Gentile L, et al: Initial treatment of thyrotoxic Graves' disease with methimazole: A randomized trial comparing different dosages. *J Endocrinol Invest* 10:291, 1987.
540. Mashio Y, Beniko M, Ikota A, et al: Treatment of hyperthyroidism with a small single daily dose of methimazole. *Acta Endocrinol (Copenh)* 119:139, 1988.
541. Okamura K, Ikenoue H, Shiroozu A, et al: Reevaluation of the effects of methylmercaptoimidazole and propylthiouracil in patients with Graves' hyperthyroidism. *J Clin Endocrinol Metab* 65:719, 1987.
542. Cooper DS: Propylthiouracil levels in hyperthyroid patients unresponsive to large doses: Evidence of poor patient compliance. *Ann Intern Med* 102:328, 1985.
543. Takamatsu J, Sugawara M, Kuma K, et al: Ratio of serum triiodothyronine to thyroxine and the prognosis of triiodothyronine-predominant Graves' disease. *Ann Intern Med* 100:372, 1984.
544. Jansson S, Berg G, Lindstedt G, et al: Overweight—a common problem among women treated for hyperthyroidism. *Postgrad Med J* 69:107, 1993.
545. Bouma DJ, Kammer H, Greer MA: Follow-up comparison of short-term versus one year antithyroid drug therapy for the thyrotoxicosis of Graves' disease. *J Clin Endocrinol Metab* 55:1138, 1982.
545a. Maugendre D, Gatel A, Champion L, et al: Antithyroid drugs and Graves' disease—prospective randomized assessment of long-term treatment. *Clin Endocrinol (Oxf)* 50:127, 1999.
546. Slingerland DW, Burrows BA: Long-term antithyroid treatment in hyperthyroidism. *JAMA* 242:2408, 1979.
547. Reinwein D, Benker G, Lazarus JH, et al: A prospective randomized trial of antithyroid drug dose in Graves' disease therapy. *J Clin Endocrinol Metab* 76:1516, 1993.
548. International Agranulocytosis and Aplastic Anaemia Study: Risk of agranulocytosis and aplastic anaemia in relation to use of antithyroid drugs. *Br Med J* 297:262, 1988.
549. Tamai H, Takaichi Y, Morita T, et al: Methimazole-induced agranulocytosis in Japanese patients with Graves' disease. *Clin Endocrinol (Oxf)* 30:525, 1989.
549a. Sheng W-H, Hung C-C, Chen Y-C, et al: Antithyroid drug-induced agranulocytosis complicated by life-threatening infections. *Q J Med* 92:455, 1999.
550. Escobar-Morreale HF, Bravo P, Garcia-Robles R, et al: Methimazole-induced severe aplastic anemia: Unsuccessful treatment with recombinant granulocyte-moncyte colony-stimulating factor. *Thyroid* 7:67, 1997.
551. Liaw Y-F, Huang M-J, Fan K-D, et al: Hepatic injury during propylthiouracil therapy in patients with hyperthyroidism. A cohort study. *Ann Intern Med* 118:424, 1993.
552. Arab DM, Malatjalian DA, Rittmaster RS: Severe cholestatic jaundice in uncomplicated hyperthyroidism treated with methimazole. *J Clin Endocrinol Metab* 80:1083, 1995.
553. Williams CV, Nayak S, Becker D, et al: Fifty years experience with propylthiouracil-associated hepatoxicity: What have we learned? *J Clin Endocrinol Metab* 82:1727, 1997.
554. Gunton JE, Stiel J, Caterson RJ, et al: Anti-thyroid drugs and antineutrophil cytoplasmic antibody positive vasculitis: A case report and review of the literature. *J Clin Endocrinol Metab* 84:13, 1999.
555. Cooper DS, Goldminz D, Levin AA, et al: Agranulocytosis associated with antithyroid drugs: Effects of patient age and drug dose. *Ann Intern Med* 98:26, 1983.
556. Meyer-Gebner M, Benker G, Lederbogen S, et al: Antithyroid drug-induced agranulocytosis: Clinical experience with ten patients treated at one institution and review of the literature. *J Endocrinol Invest* 17:29, 1994.
557. Tajiri J, Noguchi S, Murakami T, et al: Antithyroid drug-induced agranulocytosis: The usefulness of routine white blood cell count monitoring. *Arch Intern Med* 150:621, 1990.
558. Tamai H, Mukuta T, Matsubayashi S, et al: Treatment of methimazole-induced agranulocytosis using recombinant human granulocyte colony-stimulating factor (rhG-CSF). *J Clin Endocrinol Metab* 77:1356, 1993.
559. Fukata S, Kuma K, Sugawara M: Granulocyte colony-stimulating factor (G-CSF) does not improve recovery from antithyroid drug-induced agranulocytosis: A prospective study. *Thyroid* 9:29, 1999.
560. Shen D-C, Wu S-Y, Chopra IJ, et al: Long term treatment of Graves' hyperthyroidism with sodium ipodate. *J Clin Endocrinol Metab* 61:723, 1985.
561. Wang Y-S, Tsou C-T, Lin W-H, et al: Long term treatment of

Graves' disease with iopanoic acid (Telepaque). *J Clin Endocrinol Metab* 65:679, 1987.

562. Kristensen O, Andersen HH, Pallisgaard G: Lithium carbonate in the treatment of thyrotoxicosis: A controlled trial. *Lancet* 1:603, 1976.
563. Mercado M, Mendoza-Zubieta V, Bautista-Zubieta R, et al: Treatment of hyperthyroidism with a combination of methimazole and cholestyramine. *J Clin Endocrinol Metab* 81:3191, 1996.
564. Klein I, Trzepacz PT, Roberts M, et al: Symptom rating scale for assessing hyperthyroidism. *Arch Intern Med* 148:387, 1988.
565. Kvetny J, Frederikesen PK, Jacobsen JG, et al: Propranolol in the treatment of thyrotoxicosis: A randomized double-blind study. *Acta Med Scand* 209:389, 1981.
566. Nordin H, Galloe AM, Ladeoged SD, et al: The effects of propranolol and verapamil on hyperthyroid heart symptoms and function, assessed by systolic time intervals. *Acta Endocrinol (Copenh)* 128:297, 1993.
567. Kelestimur A, Basar E, Almis AD, et al: Propranolol, diltiazem and cardiac and thyroid functions in hyperthyroidism. *Clin Endocrinol (Oxf)* 39:123, 1993.
568. Nordyke RA, Gilbert FI Jr: Optimal iodine-131 dose for eliminating hyperthyroidism in Graves' disease. *J Nucl Med* 32:411, 1991.
569. Peters H, Fischer C, Bogner U, et al: Treatment of Graves' hyperthyroidism with radioiodine: Results of a prospective randomized study. *Thyroid* 7:247, 1997.
570. Beckers C: Regulations and policies on radioiodine ^{131}I therapy in Europe. *Thyroid* 7:221, 1997.
571. Hancock LD, Tuttle RM, LeMar H, et al: The effect of propylthiouracil on subsequent radioactive iodine therapy in Graves' disease. *Clin Endocrinol (Oxf)* 47:425, 1997.
572. Imesis RE, Van Middlesworth L, Massie JD, et al: Pretreatment with propylthiouracil but not methimazole reduces the therapeutic efficacy of iodine-131 in hyperthyroidism. *J Clin Endocrinol Metab* 83:685, 1998.
573. Ross DS, Daniels GH, De Stefano P, et al: Use of adjunctive potassium iodide after radioactive iodine (^{131}I) treatment of Graves' hyperthyroidism. *J Clin Endocrinol Metab* 57:250, 1983.
574. Sridama V, McCormick M, Kaplan EL, et al: Long-term follow-up study of compensated low-dose ^{131}I therapy for Graves' disease. *N Engl J Med* 311:426, 1984.
575. Tan GH, Gharib H: Recurrent hyperthyroidism after radioiodine-induced hypothyroidism: Report of two cases and literature review. *Endocr Pract* 1:158, 1995.
576. Aizawa Y, Yoshida K, Kaise N, et al: The development of transient hypothyroidism after iodine-131 treatment in hyperthyroid patients with Graves' disease: Prevalence, mechanism and prognosis. *Clin Endocrinol (Oxf)* 46:1, 1997.
577. Cunnien AJ, Hay ID, Gorman CA, et al: Radioiodine-induced hypothyroidism in Graves' disease: Factors associated with the increasing incidence. *J Nucl Med* 23:978, 1982.
578. Franklyn JA, Daykin J, Droic Z, et al: Long-term follow-up of treatment of thyrotoxicosis by three different methods. *Clin Endocrinol (Oxf)* 34:71, 1991.
579. Davies PH, Franklyn JA, Daykin J, et al: The significance of TSH values measured in a sensitive assay in the follow-up of hyperthyroid patients treated with radioiodine. *J Clin Endocrinol Metab* 74:1189, 1992.
580. Ron E, Doody MM, Becker DV, et al: Cancer mortality following treatment for adult hyperthyroidism. *JAMA* 280:347, 1998.
580a. Franklyn JA, Maisonneuve P, Sheppard M, et al: Cancer incidence and mortality after radioiodine treatment for hyperthyroidism: A population-based cohort study. *Lancet* 353:2111, 1999.
581. Franklyn JA, Maisonneuve P, Sheppard MC, et al: Mortality after treatment of hyperthyroidism with radioactive iodine. *N Engl J Med* 338:712, 1998.
582. Rivkees SA, Sklar C, Freemark M: The management of Graves' disease in children, with special emphasis on radioiodine treatment. *J Clin Endocrinol Metab* 83:3767, 1998.
583. Peek CM, Sawers JSA, Irvine WJ, et al: Combination of potassium iodide and propranolol in preparation of patients with Graves' disease for thyroid surgery. *N Engl J Med* 302:883, 1980.
584. Menegaux F, Ruprecht T, Chigot JP: The surgical treatment of Graves' disease. *Surg Gynecol Obstet* 176:277, 1992.
585. Patwardhan NA, Moront M, Rao S, et al: Surgery still has a role in Graves' hyperthyroidism. *Surgery* 114:1108, 1993.
586. Schwartz AE, Clark OH, Ituarte P, et al: Therapeutic controversy: Thyroid surgery—the choice. *J Clin Endocrinol Metab* 83:1097, 1998.
587. Nikolai TF, Coombs GJ, McKenzie AK, et al: Treatment of lymphocytic thyroiditis with spontaneously resolving hyperthyroidism (silent thyroiditis). *Arch Intern Med* 142:2281, 1982.
588. Nygaard B, Jarlov AE, Hegedus L, et al: Long-term follow-up of thyroid scintigraphies after ^{131}I therapy of solitary autonomous thyroid nodules. *Thyroid* 4:167, 1994.
589. Clerc J, Dagousset F, Izembart M, et al: Radioiodine therapy of the autonomous thyroid nodule in patients with and without visible extranodular activity. *J Nucl Med* 36:217, 1995.
590. Ferrari C, Reschini E, Paracchi A: Treatment of the autonomous thyroid nodule: A review. *Eur J Endocrinol* 135:383, 1996.
591. Nygaard B: Changes in the thyroid technetium-99m scintigram after antithyroid and subsequent radioiodine treatment for solitary adenomas. *Thyroid* 8:223, 1998.
592. Monzani F, Caraccio N, Goletti O, et al: Five-year follow-up of percutaneous ethanol injection for the treatment of hyperfunctioning thyroid nodules: A study of 117 patients. *Clin Endocrinol (Oxf)* 46:9, 1997.
593. Huysmans DAKC, Hermus ARMM, Corstens FHM, et al: Long-term results of two schedules of radioiodine treatment for toxic multinodular goitre. *Eur J Nucl Med* 20:1056, 1993.
594. Erickson D, Gharib H, Li H, et al: Treatment of patients with toxic multinodular goiter. *Thyroid* 8:277, 1998.
595. Huysmans DAKC, Hermus ARMM, Corstens FHM, et al: Large, compressive goiters treated with radioiodine. *Ann Intern Med* 121:757, 1994.
596. Nygaard B, Faber J, Hegedus L: Acute changes in thyroid volume and function following ^{131}I therapy of multinodular goitre. *Clin Endocrinol (Oxf)* 41:715, 1994.
597. Hermus AR, Huysmans DA: Treatment of benign nodular thyroid disease. *N Engl J Med* 338:1438, 1998.
598. Biondi B, Fazio S, Cuocolo A, et al: Impaired cardiac reserve and exercise capacity in patients receiving long-term thyrotropin suppressive therapy with levothyroxine. *J Clin Endocrinol Metab* 81:4224, 1996.
599. Shapiro LE, Sievert R, Ong L, et al: Minimal cardiac effects in asymptomatic athyreotic patients chronically treated with thyrotropin-suppressive doses of L-thyroxine. *J Clin Endocrinol Metab* 82:2592, 1997.
600. Biondi B, Fazio S, Palmieri EA, et al: Effects of chronic subclinical hyperthyroidism from levothyroxine on cardiac morphology and function. *Cardiologia* 44:443, 1999.
601. Mercuro G, Panzuto MG, Bina A, et al: Cardiac function, physical exercise capacity, and quality of life during long-term thyrotropin-suppressive therapy with levothyroxine: Effect of individual dose tailoring. *J Clin Endocrinol Metab* 85:159, 2000.
602. Faber J, Galloe AM: Changes in bone mass during prolonged subclinical hyperthyroidism due to L-thyroxine treatment: A meta-analysis. *Eur J Endocrinol* 130:350, 1994.
603. Marqusse E, Haden ST, Utiger RD: Subclinical thyrotoxicosis. *Endocrinol Metab Clin North Am* 27:37, 1998.
604. Marcocci C, Golia F, Bruno-Bossio G, et al: Carefully monitored levothyroxine suppressive therapy is not associated with bone loss in premenopausal women. *J Clin Endocrinol Metab* 78:818, 1994.
605. Bauer DC, Nevitt MC, Ettinger B, et al: Low thyrotropin levels are not associated with bone loss in older women: A prospective study. *J Clin Endocrinol Metab* 82:2931, 1997.
606. Sawin CT, Geller A, Wolf PA, et al: Low serum thyrotropin concentrations as a risk factor for atrial fibrillation in older persons. *N Engl J Med* 331:1249, 1994.
607. McDermott MT, Kidd GS, Dodson LE Jr, et al: Radioiodine-induced thyroid storm: Case report and literature review. *Am J Med* 75:353, 1983.
608. Burch HB, Wartofsky L: Life-threatening thyrotoxicosis. Thyroid storm. *Endocrinol Metab Clin North Am* 22:263, 1993.
609. Brooks MH, Waldstein SS: Free thyroxine concentrations in thyroid storm. *Ann Intern Med* 93:694, 1980.
610. Brunette DD, Rothong C: Emergency department management of thyrotoxic crisis with esmolol. *Am J Emerg Med* 9:232, 1991.

611. Amino N, Tanizawa O, Mori H, et al: Aggravation of thyrotoxicosis in early pregnancy and after delivery in Graves' disease. *J Clin Endocrinol Metab* 55:108, 1982.
612. Davis LE, Lucas MJ, Hankins CDV, et al: Thyrotoxicosis complicating pregnancy. *Am J Obstet Gynecol* 160:63, 1989.
613. Momotani N, Ito K, Hamada N, et al: Maternal hyperthyroidism and congenital malformation in the offspring. *Clin Endocrinol (Oxf)* 20:695, 1984.
614. Wallace C, Couch R, Ginsberg J: Fetal thyrotoxicosis: A case report and recommendations for prediction, diagnosis, and treatment. *Thyroid* 5:125, 1995.
615. Page DV, Brady K, Mitchell J, et al: The pathology of intrauterine thyrotoxicosis: Two case reports. *Obstet Gynecol* 72:479, 1988.
616. Wenstrom KD, Weiner CP, Williamson RA, et al: Prenatal diagnosis of fetal hyperthyroidism using funipuncture. *Obstet Gynecol* 76:513, 1990.
617. Mortimer RH, Cannell GR, Addison RS, et al: Methimazole and propylthiouracil equally cross the perfused human term placenta. *J Clin Endocrinol Metab* 82:3099, 1997.
618. Wing DA, Millar LK, Koonings PP, et al: A comparison of propylthiouracil versus methimazole in the treatment of hyperthyroidism in pregnancy. *Am J Obstet Gynecol* 170:90, 1994.
619. Momotani N, Noh JY, Ishikawa N, et al: Effects of propylthiouracil and methimazole on fetal thyroid status in mothers with Graves' hyperthyroidism. *J Clin Endocrinol Metab* 82:3633, 1997.
620. Mandel SJ, Brent GA, Larsen PR: Review of antithyroid drug use during pregnancy and report of a case of aplasia cutis. *Thyroid* 4:129, 1994.
621. Khoury MJ, Becerra JE, d'Almada PJ: Maternal thyroid disease and risk of birth defects in offspring. A population-based case-control study. *Pediatr Perinat Epidemiol* 3:402, 1989.
622. Van Dijke CP, Heydendael RJ, De Kleine MJ: Methimazole, carbimazole, and congenital skin defects. *Ann Intern Med* 106:60, 1987.
623. Vogt T, Stolz W, Landthaler M: Aplasia cutis congenita after exposure to methimazole: A causal relationship? *Br J Dermatol* 133:994, 1995.
624. Messer PM, Hauffa BP, Olbricht T, et al: Antithyroid drug treatment of Graves' disease in pregnancy: Long-term effects on somatic growth, intellectual development and thyroid function of the offspring. *Acta Endocrinol (Copenh)* 123:311, 1990.
625. Momotani N, Hisaoka T, Noh J, et al: Effects of iodine on thyroid status of fetus versus mother in treatment of Graves' disease complicated by pregnancy. *J Clin Endocrinol Metab* 75:738, 1992.
626. Sherif IH, Oyan WT, Bosairi S, et al: Treatment of hyperthyroidism in pregnancy. *Acta Obstet Gynecol Scand* 70:461, 1991.
627. Ares S, Quero J, Duran S, et al: Iodine content of infant formulas and iodine intake of premature babies: High risk of iodine deficiency. *Arch Dis Child Fetal Neonatal Ed* 71:F184, 1994.
628. Momotani N, Yamashita R, Yoshimoto M, et al: Recovery from foetal hypothyroidism: Evidence for the safety of breast-feeding while taking propylthiouracil. *Clin Endocrinol (Oxf)* 31:591, 1989.
629. Azizi F: Effect of methimazole treatment of maternal thyrotoxicosis on thyroid function in breast-feeding infants. *J Pediatr* 128:855, 1996.
630. Mortimer RH, Tyack SA, Galligan JP, et al: Graves' disease in pregnancy: TSH receptor binding inhibiting immunoglobulins and maternal and neonatal thyroid function. *Clin Endocrinol (Oxf)* 32:141, 1990.
631. Skuza KA, Sills IN, Stene M, et al: Prediction of neonatal hyperthyroidism in infants born to mothers with Graves' disease. *J Pediatr* 128:264, 1996.
632. Forbes G, Gorman CA, Brennan MD, et al: Ophthalmopathy of Graves' disease: Computerized volume measurements of the orbital fat and muscle. *Am J Neuroradiol* 7:651, 1986.
633. Villadolid MC, Yokoyama N, Izumi M, et al: Untreated Graves' disease patients without clinical ophthalmopathy demonstrate a high frequency of extraocular muscle (EOM) enlargement by magnetic resonance. *J Clin Endocrinol Metab* 80:2830, 1995.
634. Marcocci C, Bartalena L, Bogazzi F, et al: Studies on the occurrence of ophthalmopathy in Graves' disease. *Acta Endocrinol (Copenh)* 120:473, 1989.
635. Perros P, Crombie AL, Matthews JNS, et al: Age and gender influence the severity of thyroid-associated ophthalmopathy: A study of 101 patients attending a combined thyroid-eye clinic. *Clin Endocrinol (Oxf)* 38:367, 1993.
636. Bartalena L, Marcocci C, Tanda ML, et al: Cigarette smoking and treatment outcomes in Graves' ophthalmopathy. *Ann Intern Med* 129:632, 1998.
637. Prummel MF, Wiersinga WM, Mourits MPh, et al: Effect of abnormal thyroid function of the severity of Graves' ophthalmopathy. *Arch Intern Med* 150:1098, 1990.
638. Sridama V, DeGroot LJ: Treatment of Graves' disease and the course of ophthalmopathy. *Am J Med* 87:70, 1989.
639. Tallstedt L, Lundell G, Torring O, et al: Occurrence of ophthalmopathy after treatment for Graves' hyperthyroidism. *N Engl J Med* 326:1733, 1992.
640. Bartalena L, Marcocci C, Bogazzi F, et al: Relation between therapy for hyperthyroidism and the course of Graves' ophthalmopathy. *N Engl J Med* 338:73, 1998.
641. Werner SC: Modification of the classification of the eye changes of Graves' disease: Recommendations of the ad hoc committee of the American Thyroid Association. *J Clin Endocrinol Metab* 44:203, 1977.
642. Burch HB, Wartofsky L: Graves' ophthalmopathy: Current concepts regarding pathogenesis and management. *Endocr Rev* 14:747, 1993.
643. Salvi M, Zhang Z-G, Haegert D, et al: Patients with endocrine ophthalmopathy not associated with overt thyroid disease have multiple immunological abnormalities. *J Clin Endocrinol Metab* 70:89, 1990.
644. Perros P, Crombie AL, Kendall-Taylor P: Natural history of thyroid associated ophthalmopathy. *Clin Endocrinol (Oxf)* 42:45, 1995.
645. Bartley GB, Fatourechi V, Kadrmas EF, et al: Long-term follow-up of Graves' ophthalmopathy in an incidence cohort. *Ophthalmology* 103:958, 1996.
646. Bartalena L, Pinchera A, Marcocci C: Management of Graves' ophthalmopathy: Reality and perspectives. *Endocr Rev* 21:168, 2000.
647. Prummel MF, Wiersinga WM: Immunomodulatory treatment of Graves' ophthalmopathy. *Thyroid* 8:545, 1998.
648. Prummel MF, Mourits MPh, Blank L, et al: Randomised double blind trial of prednisone versus radiotherapy in Graves' ophthalmopathy. *Lancet* 342:949, 1993.
649. Nygaard D, Specht L. Transitory blindness after retrobulbar irradiation of Graves' ophthalmopathy. *Lancet* 351:725, 1998.
650. Fatourechi V, Garrity JA, Bartley GB, et al: Graves' ophthalmopathy. Results of transantral orbital decompression performed primarily for cosmetic reasons. *Ophthalmology* 101:938, 1994.
651. Kriss JP, Pleshakov V, Rosenblum A, et al: Therapy with occlusive dressings of preribial myxedema with fluocinolone acetonide. *J Clin Endocrinol* 27:595, 1967.
652. Bianchi R, Pilo A, Mariani G, et al: Comparison of plasma and urinary methods for the direct measurement of the thyroxine to 3,5,3′-triiodothyronine conversion rate in man. *J Clin Endocrinol Metab* 58:993, 1984.
653. Ishii H, Inada M, Tanaka K, et al: Induction of outer and inner ring monodeiodinases in human thyroid gland by thyrotropin. *J Clin Endocrinol Metab* 57:500, 1983.
654. Lum SM, Nicoloff JT, Spencer CA, et al: Peripheral tissue mechanism for maintenance of serum triiodothyronine values in a thyroxine-deficient state in man. *J Clin Invest* 73:570, 1984.
655. Takasu N, Yamada T, Takasu M, et al: Disappearance of thyrotropin-blocking antibodies and spontaneous recovery from hypothyroidism in autoimmune thyroiditis. *N Engl J Med* 326:513, 1992.
656. Comtois R, Faucher L, Lafleche L: Outcome of hypothyroidism caused by Hashimoto's thyroiditis. *Arch Intern Med* 155:1404, 1995.
657. Akasu F, Morita T, Resetkova E, et al: Reconstitution of severe combined immunodeficient mice with intrathyroidal lymphocytes of thyroid xenografts from patients with Hashimoto's thyroiditis. *J Clin Endocrinol Metab* 76:223, 1993.
658. Bogner U, Kotulla P, Peters H, et al: Thyroid peroxidase/microsomal antibodies are not identical with thyroid cytotoxic antibodies in autoimmune thyroiditis. *Acta Endocrinol (Copenh)* 123:431, 1990.
659. Rodien P, Madec A-M, Ruf J, et al: Antibody-dependent cell-mediated cytotoxicity in autoimmune thyroid disease: Relationship to antithyroperoxidase antibodies. *J Clin Endocrinol Metab* 81:2595, 1996.

660. Endo T, Kaneshige M, Nakazato M, et al: Autoantibody against thyroid iodide transporter in the sera of patients with Hashimoto's thyroiditis possesses iodide transport inhibitory activity. *Biochem Biophys Res Comm* 228:199, 1996.
661. Raspe E, Costagliola S, Ruf J, et al: Identification of the thyroid Na^+/I^- cotransporter as a potential autoantigen in thyroid autoimmune disease. *Eur J Endocrinol* 132:399, 1995.
662. McKenzie JM, Zakarija M: Fetal and neonatal hyperthyroidism and hypothyroidism due to maternal TSH receptor antibodies. *Thyroid* 2:155, 1992.
663. Chiovato L, Vitti P, Santini F, et al: Incidence of antibodies blocking thyrotropin effect *in vitro* in patients with euthyroid or hypothyroid autoimmune thyroiditis. *J Clin Endocrinol Metab* 71:40, 1990.
664. Del Prete GF, Maggi E, Mariotti S, et al: Cytolytic T lymphocytes with natural killer activity in thyroid infiltrate of patients with Hashimoto's thyroiditis: Analysis at a clonal level. *J Clin Endocrinol Metab* 62:52, 1986.
665. Giordano C, Stassi G, De Maria R, et al: Potential involvement of Fas and its ligand in the pathogenesis of Hashimoto's thyroiditis. *Science* 275:960, 1997.
665a. Brix TB, Kyvik KO, Hegedus L: A population-based study of chronic autoimmune thyroiditis in Danish twins. *J Clin Endocrinol Metab* 85:536, 2000.
666. Cho BY, Chung JH, Shong YK, et al: A strong association between thyrotropin receptor-blocking antibody-positive atrophic autoimmune thyroiditis and HLA-DR8 and HLA-DQB*0302 in Koreans. *J Clin Endocrinol Metab* 77: 611, 1993.
667. Ivarsson SA, Ericsson UB, Gustafsson J, et al: The impact of thyroid autoimmunity on children and adolescents with Down syndrome. *Acta Pediatr* 86:1065, 1997.
668. Chiovato L, Larizza D, Bendeinelli G, et al: Autoimmune hypothyroidism and hyperthyroidism in patients with Turner's syndrome. *Eur J Endocrinol* 134:568, 1996.
669. Alvarez-Marfany M, Roman SH, Drexler AJ, et al: Long-term prospective study of postpartum thyroid dysfunction in women with insulin dependent diabetes mellitus. *J Clin Endocrinol Metab* 79:10, 1994.
670. Maagoe H, Reintoft I, Christensen HE, et al: Lymphocytic thyroiditis: II. The course of the disease in relation to morphologic, immunologic and clinical findings at the time of biopsy. *Acta Med Scand* 202:469, 1977.
671. Rieu M, Richard A, Rosiliio M, et al: Effects of thyroid status on thyroid autoimmunity expression in euthyroid and hypothyroid patients with Hashimoto's thyroiditis. *Clin Endocrinol (Oxf)* 40:529, 1994.
672. Romaldini JH, Biancalana MM, Figueiredo DI, et al: Effect of L-thyroxine administration on antithyroid antibody levels, lipid profile, and thyroid volume in patients with Hashimoto's thyroiditis. *Thyroid* 6:183, 1996.
673. Holm L-E, Blomgren H, Lowhagen T: Cancer risks in patients with chronic lymphocytic thyroiditis. *N Engl J Med* 312:601, 1985.
674. Nikolai TF, Coombs GJ, McKenzie AK: Lymphocytic thyroiditis with spontaneously resolving hyperthyroidism and subacute thyroiditis. Long-term follow-up. *Arch Intern Med* 141:1455, 1981.
675. Harris B, Othman S, Davies JA, et al: Association between postpartum thyroid dysfunction and thyroid antibodies and depression. *Br Med J* 305:152, 1992.
676. Nikolai TF, Turney SL, Roberts RC: Postpartum lymphocytic thyroiditis. Prevalence, clinical course, and long-term follow-up. *Arch Intern Med* 147:221, 1987.
677. Othman S, Phillips DIW, Parkes AB, et al: A long-term follow-up of postpartum thyroiditis. *Clin Endocrinol (Oxf)* 32:559, 1990.
678. Turner SL, Tiver KW, Boyages SC: Thyroid dysfunction following radiotherapy for head and neck cancer. *Int J Radiat Oncol Biol Phys* 31:279, 1995.
679. Al-Fiar FZ, Colwill R, Lipton JH, et al: Abnormal thyroid stimulating hormone (TSH) levels in adults following allogeneic bone marrow transplants. *Bone Marrow Transplant* 19:1019, 1997.
680. Tamai H, Suemastu H, Kurokawa N, et al: Alterations in circulating thyroid hormones and thyrotropin after complete thyroidectomy. *J Clin Endocrinol Metab* 48:54, 1979.
681. Matte R, Ste-Marie LG, Comtois R, et al: The pituitary-thyroid axis after hemithyroidectomy in euthyroid man. *J Clin Endocrinol Metab* 53:377, 1981.
682. Singer P: Primary hypothyroidism due to other causes, in Braverman LE, Utiger RD (eds): *The Thyroid: A Fundamental and Clinical Text*, 8th ed. Philadelphia, Lippincott Williams and Wilkins, 2000, p 755.
683. Law WY, Bradley DM, Lazarus JH, et al: Congenital hypothyroidism in Wales (1982–1993): Demographic features, clinical presentation and effects on early neurodevelopment. *Clin Endocrinol (Oxf)* 48:201, 1998.
684. De Roux N, Misrahi M, Brauner R, et al: Four families with loss of function mutations of the thyrotropin receptor. *J Clin Endocrinol Metab* 81:4229, 1996.
685. Abramowicz MJ, Duprez L, Parma J, et al: Familial congenital hypothyroidism due to inactivating mutation of the thyrotropin receptor causing profound hypoplasia of the thyroid gland. *J Clin Invest* 99:3018, 1997.
686. Biebermann H, Schoneberg T, Krude H, et al: Mutations of the human thyrotropin receptor gene causing thyroid hypoplasia and persistent congenital hypothyroidism. *J Clin Endocrinol Metab* 82:3471, 1997.
687. Mallet E, Carayon P, Amr S, et al: Coupling defect of thyrotropin receptor and adenylate cyclase in a pseudohypoparathyroid patient. *J Clin Endocrinol Metab* 54:1028, 1982.
688. Brown RS, Bellisario RL, Botero D, et al: Incidence of transient congenital hypothyroidism due to maternal thyrotropin receptor-blocking antibodies in over one million babies. *J Clin Endocrinol Metab* 81:1147, 1996.
689. Dussault JH, Letarte J, Guyda H, et al: Lack of influence of thyroid antibodies on thyroid function in the newborn infant and on a mass screening program for congenital hypothyroidism. *J Pediatr* 96:385, 1980.
690. Pohlenz J, Rosenthal IM, Weiss RE, et al: Congenital hypothyroidism due to mutations in the sodium/iodide symporter. Identification of a nonsense mutation producing a downstream cryptic 3′ splice site. *J Clin Invest* 101:1028, 1998.
691. Kosugi S, Sato Y, Matsuda A, et al: High prevalence of T354P sodium/iodide symporter gene mutation in Japanese patients with iodide transport defect who have heterogeneous clinical pictures. *J Clin Endocrinol Metab* 83:4123, 1998.
692. Medeiros-Neto GA, Billerbeck AEC, Wajchenberg BL, et al: Defective organification of iodide causing hereditary goitrous hypothyroidism. *Thyroid* 3:143, 1993.
693. Kopp P: Pendred's syndrome: Identification of the genetic defect a century after its recognition. *Thyroid* 9:65, 1999.
694. Medeiros-Neto G, Targovnik HM, Vassart G: Defective thyroglobulin synthesis and secretion causing goiter and hypothyroidism. *Endocr Rev* 14:165, 1993.
695. Acebron A, Aza-Blanc P, Rossi DL, et al: Congenital human thyroglobulin defect due to low expression of the thyroid-specific transcription factor TTF-1. *J Clin Invest* 96:781, 1995.
696. Refetoff S, Weiss RE, Usala SJ: The syndromes of resistance to thyroid hormone. *Endocr Rev* 14:348, 1993.
697. Brucker-Davis F, Skarulis MC, Grace MB, et al: Genetic and clinical features of 42 kindreds with resistance to thyroid hormone. The National Institutes of Health prospective study. *Ann Intern Med* 123:572, 1995.
698. Beck-Peccoz P, Chatterjee VKK: The variable clinical phenotype in thyroid resistance syndrome. *Thyroid* 4:225, 1994.
699. Weiss RE, Balzano S, Scherberg NH, et al: Neonatal detection of generalized resistance to thyroid hormone. *JAMA* 264:2245, 1990.
700. Sarne DH, Refetoff S, Rosenfield RL, et al: Sex hormone-binding globulin in the diagnosis of peripheral tissue resistance to thyroid hormone: The value of changes after short term triiodothyronine administration. *J Clin Endocrinol Metab* 66:740, 1988.
701. Vanderpas JB, Contempre B, Duale NL, et al: Iodine and selenium deficiency associated with cretinism in northern Zaire. *Am J Clin Nutr* 52:1087, 1990.
702. Boyages SC: Iodine deficiency disorders. *J Clin Endocrinol Metab* 77:587, 1993.
703. Boyages SC, Halpern J-P, Maberly GF, et al: A comparative study of neurological and myxedematous cretinism in Western China. *J Clin Endocrinol Metab* 67:1262, 1988.
704. Figg WD, Thibault A, Sartor AO, et al: Hypothyroidism associated with aminoglutethimide in patients with prostate cancer. *Arch Intern Med* 154:1023, 1994.
704a. Huang SA, Tu HM, Harney JW, et al: Severe hypothyroidism

caused by type 3 iodothyronine deiodinase in infantile hemangiomas. *N Engl J Med* 343:185, 2000.
705. Littley MD, Shalet SM, Beardwell CG, et al: Radiation-induced hypopituitarism is dose-dependent. *Clin Endocrinol (Oxf)* 31:363, 1989.
706. Arafah BM: Reversible hypopituitarism in patients with large nonfunctioning pituitary adenomas. *J Clin Endocrinol Metab* 62:1173, 1986.
706a. Sherman SI, Gopal J, Haugen BR, et al: Central hypothyroidism associated with retinoid X receptor-selective ligands. *N Engl J Med* 340:1075, 1999.
707. Medeiros-Neto G, Herodotou DT, Rajan S, et al: A circulating, biologically inactive thyrotropin caused by a mutation in the beta subunit gene. *J Clin Invest* 97:1250, 1996.
708. Doeker BM, Pfaffle RW, Pohlenz J, et al: Congenital central hypothyroidism due to a homozygous mutation in the thyrotropin β-subunit gene follows an autosomal recessive inheritance. *J Clin Endocrinol Metab* 83:1762, 1998.
709. Pernasetti F, Milner RDG, Al Ashwal AAZ, et al: Pro239Ser: A novel recessive mutation of the pit-1 gene in seven middle eastern children with growth hormone, prolactin and thyrotropin deficiency. *J Clin Endocrinol Metab* 83:2079, 1998.
710. Katevuo K, Valimaki M, Ketonen L, et al: Computed tomography of the pituitary fossa in primary hypothyroidism: Effect of thyroxine treatment. *Clin Endocrinol (Oxf)* 22:617, 1985.
711. Sarlis NJ, Brucker-Davis F, Doppman JL, et al: MRI-demonstrable regression of a pituitary mass in a case of primary hypothyroidism after a week of acute thyroid hormone therapy. *J Clin Endocrinol Metab* 82:808, 1997.
712. Yamamoto K, Saito K, Takai T, et al: Visual field defects and pituitary enlargement in primary hypothyroidism. *J Clin Endocrinol Metab* 57:283, 1983.
713. Collu R, Tang J, Castagne J, et al: A novel mechanism for isolated central hypothyroidism: Inactivating mutations in the thyrotropin-releasing hormone receptor gene. *J Clin Endocrinol Metab* 82:1361, 1997.
714. Adriaanse R, Brabant G, Endert E, et al: Pulsatile thyrotopin release in patients with untreated pituitary disease. *J Clin Endocrinol Metab* 77:205, 1993.
715. Abucham J, Castro V, Maccagnan P, et al: Increased thyrotrophin levels and loss of the nocturnal surge in Sheehan's syndrome. *Clin Endocrinol (Oxf)* 47:515, 1997.
716. Billewicz WZ, Chapman RS, Crooks J, et al: Statistical methods applied to the diagnosis of hypothyroidism. *Q J Med* 38:255, 1969.
717. Doucet J, Trivalle C, Chassagne P, et al: Does age play a role in clinical presentation of hypothyroidism? *J Am Geriatr Soc* 42:984, 1994.
718. Zulewski H, Muller B, Exer P, et al: Estimation of tissue hypothyroidism by a new clinical score: Evaluation of patients with various grades of hypothyroidism and controls. *J Clin Endocrinol Metab* 82:771, 1997.
719. Samuels MH: Subclinical thyroid disease in the elderly. *Thyroid* 8:803, 1998.
720. Ladenson PW, Braverman LE, Mazzaferri EL, et al: Comparison of administration of recombinant human thyrotropin with withdrawal of thyroid hormone for radioactive iodine scanning in patients with thyroid carcinoma. *N Engl J Med* 337:888, 1997.
721. Douglas RC, Jacobson SD: Pathologic changes in adult myxedema: Survey of 10 necropsies. *J Clin Endocrinol* 17:1354, 1957.
722. Osterweil D, Syndulko K, Cohen SN, et al: Cognitive function in non-demented older adults with hypothyroidism. *J Am Geriatr Soc* 40:325, 1992.
723. Dugbartey AT: Neurocognitive aspects of hypothyroidism. *Arch Intern Med* 158:1413, 1998.
724. Khaleeli AA, Griffith DG, Edwards RHT: The clinical presentation of hypothyroid myopathy and its relationship to abnormalities in structure and function of skeletal muscle. *Clin Endocrinol (Oxf)* 19:365, 1983.
725. Rodolico C, Toscano A, Benvenga S, et al: Myopathy as the persistently isolated symptomatology of primary autoimmune hypothyroidism. *Thyroid* 8:1033, 1998.
726. Beyer IW, Karmall R, Demeester-Mirkine N, et al: Serum creatine kinase levels in overt and subclinical hypothyroidism. *Thyroid* 8:1029, 1998.
727. Klein I, Ojamaa K: The cardiovascular system in hypothyroidism, in Braverman LE, Utiger RD (eds): *The Thyroid: A Fundamental and Clinical Text*, 8th ed. Philadelphia, Lippincott Williams and Wilkins, 2000, p 777.
728. Ladenson PW, Sherman SI, Baughman KL, et al: Reversible alterations in myocardial gene expression in a young man with dilated cardiomyopathy and hypothyroidism. *Proc Natl Acad Sci USA* 89:5251, 1992.
729. Kabadi UM, Kumar SP: Pericardial effusion in primary hypothyroidism. *Am Heart J* 120:1393, 1990.
730. Shenoy MM, Goldman JM: Hypothyroid cardiomyopathy: Echocardiographic documentation of reversibility. *Am J Med Sci* 294:1, 1987.
731. Streeten DH, Anderson GH Jr, Howland T, et al: Effects of thyroid function on blood pressure. Recognition of hypothyroid hypertension. *Hypertension* 11:78, 1988.
732. Keating FR Jr, Parkin TW, Selby JB, et al: Treatment of heart disease associated with myxedema. *Prog Cardiovasc Dis* 3:364, 1961.
733. Becker C: Hypothyroidism and atherosclerotic heart disease: Pathogenesis, medical management, and the role of coronary artery bypass surgery. *Endocr Rev* 6:432, 1985.
734. Sherman SI, Ladenson PW: Percutaneous transluminal coronary angioplasty in hypothyroidism. *Am J Med* 90:367, 1991.
735. Zwillich CW, Pierson DJ, Hofeldt FD, et al: Ventilatory control in myxedema and hypothyroidism. *N Engl J Med* 292:662, 1975.
736. Duranti R, Gheri RG, Gorini M, et al: Control of breathing in patients with severe hypothyroidism. *Am J Med* 95:29, 1993.
737. Rajagopal KR, Abbrecht PH, Derderian SS, et al: Obstructive sleep apnea in hypothyroidism. *Ann Intern Med* 101:491, 1984.
738. Grunstein RR, Sullivan CE: Sleep apnea and hypothyroidism: Mechanisms and management. *Am J Med* 85:775, 1988.
739. Gottehrer A, Roa J, Stanford GG, et al: Hypothyroidism and pleural effusions. *Chest* 98:1130, 1990.
740. Parving HH, Hansen JM, Nielsen SL, et al: Mechanism of edema formation in myxedema–increased protein extravasation and relatively slow lymphatic drainage. *N Engl J Med* 301:460, 1979.
741. Montenegro J, Gonzalez O, Saracho R, et al: Changes in renal function in primary hypothyroidism. *Am J Kidney Dis* 27:195, 1996.
742. Skowsky WR, Kikuchi TA: The role of vasopressin in the impaired water excretion of myxedema. *Am J Med* 64:613, 1978.
743. Iwasaki Y, Oiso Y, Yamauchi K, et al: Osmoregulation of plasma vasopressin in myxedema. *J Clin Endocrinol Metab* 70:534, 1990.
744. Arnaout MA, Awidi AS, El-Najdawi AM, et al: Arginine-vasopressin and endothelium-associated proteins in thyroid disease. *Acta Endocrinol (Copenh)* 126:399, 1992.
745. Croal BL, Blake AM, Johnston J, et al: Absence of relation between hyponatraemia and hypothyroidism. *Lancet* 350:1402, 1997.
746. Lee GR: The anemias associated with renal disease, liver disease, endocrine disease, and pregnancy, in Lee GR, Paraskevas F, Foerster J, Greer JP, Lukens J, Rodgers GM (eds): *Wintrobe's Clinical Hematology*, 10th ed. Baltimore, Williams & Wilkins, 1998, p 1497.
747. Myrup B, Bregengard C, Faber J: Primary haemostasis in thyroid disease. *J Intern Med* 238:59, 1995.
747a. Hussein WI, Green R, Jacobsen DW, et al: Normalization of hyperhomocysteinemia with L-thyroxine in hypothyroidism. *Ann Intern Med* 131:348, 1999.
747b. Catargi B, Parrot-Roulaud F, Cochet C, et al: Homocysteine, hypothyroidism, and the effect of thyroid hormone replacement. *Thyroid* 9:1163, 2000.
748. O'Brien T, Dinneen SF, O'Brien PC, et al: Hyperlipidemia in patients with primary and secondary hypothyroidism. *Mayo Clin Proc* 68:860, 1993.
749. Pazos F, Alvarez JJ, Rubies-Prat J, et al: Long term thyroid replacement therapy and levels of lipoprotein(a) and other lipoproteins. *J Clin Endocrinol Metab* 80:562, 1995.
750. Kushnir M, Weistein R, Landau B, et al: Hypothyroidism and phenytoin intoxication. *Ann Intern Med* 102:341, 1985.
751. Stephens MA, Self TH, Lancaster D, et al: Hypothyroidism: Effect on warfarin anticoagulation. *South Med J* 82:1585, 1989.
752. Valcavi R, Dieguez C, Preece M, et al: Effect of thyroxine replacement therapy on plasma insulin-like growth factor I levels and growth hormone responses to growth hormone releasing factor in hypothyroid patients. *Clin Endocrinol (Oxf)* 27:85, 1987.
753. Chernausek SL, Turner R: Attenuation of spontaneous, nocturnal growth hormone secretion in children with hypothyroidism and its

correlation with plasma insulin-like growth factor I concentrations. *J Pediatr* 114:968, 1992.

754. Miell JP, Zini M, Quin JD, et al: Reversible effects of cessation and recommencement of thyroxine treatment on insulin-like growth factors (IGFs) and IGF-binding proteins in patients with total thyroidectomy. *J Clin Endocrinol Metab* 79:1507, 1994.
755. Contreras P, Generini G, Michelsen H, et al: Hyperprolactinemia and galactorrhea: Spontaneous versus iatrogenic hypothyroidism. *J Clin Endocrinol Metab* 53:1036, 1981.
756. Iranmanesh A, Lizarralde G, Johnson ML, et al: Dynamics of 24-hour endogenous cortisol secretion and clearance in primary hypothyroidism assessed before and after partial thyroid hormone replacement. *J Clin Endocrinol Metab* 70:155, 1990.
757. Kamilaris TC, DeBold CR, Pavlou SN, et al: Effect of altered thyroid hormone levels on hypothalamic-pituitary-adrenal function. *J Clin Endocrinol Metab* 65:994, 1987.
758. Bakiri F, Benmiloud M: Fonction hypothalamo-hypophyso-surrenalienne au cours de l'hypothyroidie primaire. *Presse Med* 23:320, 1994.
759. Candrina R, Giustina G: Addison's disease and corticosteroid-reversible hypothyroidism. *J Endocrinol Invest* 10:523, 1987.
760. Tomasi PA, Fanciulli G, Zini M, et al: Pulsatile gonadotrophin secretion in hypothyroid women of reproductive age. *Eur J Endocrinol* 136:406, 1997.
761. Jannini EA, Ulisse S, D'Armiento M: Thyroid hormone and male gonadal function. *Endocr Rev* 16:443, 1995.
762. Donnelley P, White C: Testicular dysfunction in men with primary hypothyroidism: Reversal of hypogonadotrophic hypogonadism with replacement thyroxine. *Clin Endocrinol (Oxf)* 52:197, 2000.
763. Benker G, Breuer N, Windeck R, et al: Calcium metabolism in thyroid disease. *J Endocrinol Invest* 11:61, 1988.
764. Davis LE, Leveno KJ, Cunningham FG: Hypothyroidism complicating pregnancy. *Obstet Gynecol* 72:108, 1988.
765. Wasserstrum N, Anania CA: Perinatal consequences of maternal hypothyroidism in early pregnancy and inadequate replacement. *Clin Endocrinol (Oxf)* 42:353, 1995.
766. Glinoer D, Soto MF, Bourdoux P, et al: Pregnancy in patients with mild thyroid abnormalities: Maternal and neonatal repercussions. *J Clin Endocrinol Metab* 73:421, 1991.
767. Liu H, Momotani N, Noh JY, et al: Maternal hypothyroidism during early pregnancy and intellectual development of the progeny. *Arch Intern Med* 154:785, 1994.
767a. Haddow JE, Palomaki GE, Allan WC, et al: Maternal thyroid deficiency during pregnancy and subsequent psychological development of the child. *N Engl J Med* 341:549, 1999.
768. Klein RZ, Haddow JE, Faix JD, et al: Prevalence of thyroid deficiency in pregnant women. *Clin Endocrinol (Oxf)* 35:41, 1991.
769. Stagnaro-Green A, Roman SH, Cobin RH, et al: Detection of at-risk pregnancy by means of highly sensitive assays for thyroid autoantibodies. *JAMA* 264:1422, 1990.
770. Shulkin BL, Utiger RD: Caloric restriction does not alter thyrotropin secretion in hypothyroidism. *J Clin Endocrinol Metab* 60:1076, 1985.
771. Weinberg AD, Brennan MD, Gorman CA, et al: Outcome of anesthesia and surgery in hypothyroid patients. *Arch Intern Med* 143:893, 1983.
772. Ladenson PW, Levin AA, Ridgway EC, et al: Complications of surgery in hypothyroid patients. *Am J Med* 77:261, 1984.
773. Staub J-J, Althaus BU, Engler H, et al: Spectrum of subclinical and overt hypothyroidism: Effect on thyrotropin, prolactin, and thyroid reserve, and metabolic impact on peripheral target tissues. *Am J Med* 92:631, 1992.
774. Fish LH, Schwartz HL, Cavanaugh J, et al: Replacement dose, metabolism, and bioavailability of levothyroxine in the treatment of hypothyroidism: Role of triiodothyronine in pituitary feedback in humans. *N Engl J Med* 316:764, 1987.
775. Hays MT, Nielsen KRK: Human thyroxine absorption: Age effects and methodological analyses. *Thyroid* 4:55, 1994.
776. Dong BJ, Hauck WW, Gambertoglio JG, et al: Bioequivalence of generic and brand-name levothyroxine products in the treatment of hypothyroidism. *JAMA* 277:1205, 1997.
777. Benvenga S, Bartolone L, Squadrito S, et al: Delayed intestinal absorption of levothyroxine. *Thyroid* 5:249, 1995.
778. Copeland PM: Two cases of therapeutic failure associated with levothyroxine brand interchange. *Ann Pharmacother* 29:482, 1995.
779. Peran S, Garriga MJ, Morreale de Escobar G, et al: Increase in plasma thyrotropin levels in hypothyroid patients during treatment due to a defect in the commercial preparation. *J Clin Endocrinol Metab* 82:3192, 1997.
780. Magner J, Gerber P: Urticaria due to blue dye in Synthroid tablets. *Thyroid* 4:341, 1994.
781. Kabadi UM, Jackson T: Serum thyrotropin in primary hypothyroidism. A possible predictor of optimal daily levothyroxine dose in primary hypothyroidism. *Arch Intern Med* 155:1046, 1995.
782. Mandel SJ, Larsen PR, Seely EW, et al: Increased need for thyroxine during pregnancy in women with primary hypothyroidism. *N Engl J Med* 323:91, 1990.
783. Kaplan MM: Monitoring thyroxine treatment during pregnancy. *Thyroid* 2:147, 1992.
784. Liel Y, Sperber AD, Shany S, et al: Nonspecific intestinal adsorption of levothyroxine by aluminum hydroxide. *Am J Med* 97:363, 1994.
785. Shakir KMM, Michaels RD, Hays JH, et al: The use of bile acid sequestrants to lower serum thyroid hormones in iatrogenic hyperthyroidism. *Ann Intern Med* 118:112, 1993.
786. Singh N, Singh PN, Hershman JM: Effect of calcium carbonate on the absorption of levothyroxine. *JAMA* 283:2822, 2000.
787. Campbell NRC, Hasinoff BB, Stalts H, et al: Ferrous sulfate reduces thyroxine efficacy in patients with hypothyroidism. *Ann Intern Med* 117:1010, 1992.
788. Chiu AC, Sherman SI: Effects of pharmacological fiber supplements in levothyroxine absorption. *Thyroid* 8:667, 1998.
789. Sherman SI, Tielens ET, Ladenson PW, et al: Sucralfate causes malabsorption of L-thyroxine. *Am J Med* 96:531, 1994.
790. Sawin CT, Herman T, Molitch ME, et al: Aging and the thyroid. Decreased requirement for thyroid hormone in older hypothyroid patients. *Am J Med* 75:2206, 1983.
791. Aanderud S, Myking OL, Strandjord RE: The influence of carbamazepine on thyroid hormones and thyroxine binding globulin in hypothyroid patients substituted with thyroxine. *Clin Endocrinol (Oxf)* 15:247, 1981.
792. Blackshear JI, Schultz AL, Napier JS, et al: Thyroxine replacement requirements in hypothyroid patients receiving phenytoin. *Ann Intern Med* 99:341, 1983.
793. Isley WL: Effect of rifampin therapy on thyroid function tests in a hypothyroid patient on replacement L-thyroxine. *Ann Intern Med* 107:517, 1987.
794. Figge J, Dluhy RG: Amiodarone-induced elevation of thyroid stimulating hormone in patients receiving levothyroxine for primary hypothyroidism. *Ann Intern Med* 113:553, 1990.
795. Ain KB, Refetoff S, Rein HG, et al: Pseudomalabsorption of levothyroxine. *JAMA* 266:2118, 1991.
796. McCowen KC, Garber JR, Spark R: Elevated serum thyrotropin in thyroxine-treated patients with hypothyroidism given sertraline. *N Engl J Med* 337:1010, 1997.
797. Bearcroft CP, Toms GC, Williams SJ, et al: Thyroxine replacement in post-radioiodine hypothyroidism. *Clin Endocrinol (Oxf)* 34:115, 1991.
798. England ML, Hershman JM: Serum TSH concentration as an aid to monitoring compliance with thyroid hormone therapy in hypothyroidism. *Am J Med Sci* 292:264, 1986.
799. Parle JV, Franklyn JA, Cross KW, et al: Thyroxine prescription in the community: Serum thyroid stimulating hormone level assays as an indicator of undertreatment or overtreatment. *Br J Gen Pract* 43:107, 1993.
800. DeWhalley P: Do abnormal thyroid stimulating hormone level values result in treatment changes? A study of patients on thyroxine in one general practice. *Br J Gen Pract* 45:93, 1995.
801. Watsky JG, Koeniger MA: Prevalence of iatrogenic hyperthyroidism in a community hospital. *J Am Board Fam Pract* 11:175, 1998.
802. Petersen K, Bengtsson C, Lapidus L, et al: Morbidity, mortality, and quality of life for patients treated with levothyroxine. *Arch Intern Med* 150:2077, 1990.
803. Leese GP, Jung RT, Guthrie C, et al: Morbidity in patients on L-thyroxine: A comparison of those with a normal TSH to those with a suppressed TSH. *Clin Endocrinol (Oxf)* 37:500, 1992.
804. Carr D, McLeod DT, Parry G, et al: Fine adjustment of thyroxine replacement dosage: Comparison of the thyrotropin releasing hor-

mone test using a sensitive assay with measurement of free thyroid hormones and clinical assessment. *Clin Endocrinol (Oxf)* 28:325, 1988.
805. Grebe SKG, Cooke RR, Ford HC, et al: Treatment of hypothyroidism with once weekly thyroxine. *J Clin Endocrinol Metab* 82:870, 1997.
806. Bemben DA, Hamm RM, Morgan L, et al: Thyroid disease in the elderly. Part 2. Predictability of subclinical hypothyroidism. *J Fam Pract* 38:583, 1994.
807. Vanderpump MPJ, Tunbridge WMG, French JM, et al: The development of ischemic heart disease in relation to autoimmune thyroid disease in a 20-year follow-up study in an English community. *Thyroid* 6:155, 1996.
808. Cooper DS, Halpern R, Wood LC, et al: L-Thyroxine therapy in subclinical hypothyroidism: A double-blind, placebo-controlled trial. *Ann Intern Med* 101:18, 1984.
809. Nystrom E, Caidahl K, Fager G, et al: A double-blind cross-over 12-month study of L-thyroxine treatment of women with "subclinical" hypothyroidism. *Clin Endocrinol (Oxf)* 29:63, 1988.
810. Jaeschke R, Guyatt G, Gerstein H, et al: Does treatment with L-thyroxine influence health status in middle-aged and older adults with subclinical hypothyroidism? *J Gen Intern Med* 11:744, 1996.
811. Tanis BC, Westendorp RGJ, Smelt AHM: Effect of thyroid substitution on hypercholesterolaemia in patients with subclinical hypothyroidism: A reanalysis of intervention studies. *Clin Endocrinol (Oxf)* 44:643, 1996.
812. Foley TP Jr: Congenital hypothyroidism, in Braverman LE, Utiger RD (eds): *The Thyroid: A Fundamental and Clinical Text*, 8th ed. Philadelphia, Lippincott Williams and Wilkins, 2000, p 977.
813. American Academy of Pediatrics AAP Section on Endocrinology and Committee on Genetics, and American Thyroid Association Committee on Public Health: Newborn screening for congenital hypothyroidism. Recommended guidelines. *Pediatrics* 91:1203, 1993.
814. De Bruyn R, Ng WK, Taylor J, et al: Neonatal hypothyroidism: Comparison of radioisotope and ultrasound imaging in 54 cases. *Acta Pediatr Scand* 79:1194, 1990.
815. New England Congenital Hypothyroidism Collaborative: Elementary school performance of children with congenital hypothyroidism. *J Pediatr* 116:27, 1990.
816. Tillotson SL, Fuggle PW, Smith I, et al: Relation between biochemical severity and intelligence in early treated congenital hypothyroidism: A threshold effect. *Br Med J* 309:440, 1994.
817. Kooistra L, Laane C, Vulsma T, et al: Motor and cognitive development in children with congenital hypothyroidism: A long-term evaluation of the effects of neonatal treatment. *J Pediatr* 124:903, 1994.
818. Buchanan CR, Stanhope R, Adlard P, et al: Gonadotropin, growth hormone and prolactin secretion in children with primary hypothyroidism. *Clin Endocrinol (Oxf)* 29:427, 1988.
819. Hylander B, Rosenqvist U: Treatment of myxoedema coma—factors associated with fatal outcome. *Acta Endocrinol (Copenh)* 108:65, 1985.
819a. Yamamoto T, Fukuyama J, Fujiyoshi A: Factors associated with mortality of myxedema coma: Report of eight cases and literature survey. *Thyroid* 9:1167, 1999.
820. Arlot S, Debussche X, Lalau J-D, et al: Myxoedema coma: Response of thyroid hormones with oral and intravenous high-dose L-thyroxine treatment. *Intensive Care Med* 17:16, 1991.
821. Reinhardt W, Mann K: Incidence, clinical picture and treatment of hypothyroid coma. Results of a survey. *Med Klin* 92:521, 1997.
822. Ross DS: Syndromes of thyrotoxicosis with low radioactive iodine uptake. *Endocrinol Metab Clin North Am* 27:169, 1998.
823. Bennedaek FN, Hegedus L: The value of ultrasonography in the diagnosis and follow-up of subacute thyroiditis. *Thyroid* 7:45, 1997.
824. Iitaka M, Momotani N, Ishii J, et al: Incidence of subacute thyroiditis recurrences after a prolonged latency: 24-year survey. *J Clin Endocrinol Metab* 81:466, 1996.
825. Volpe R, Row VV, Ezrin C: Circulating viral and thyroid antibodies in subacute thyroiditis. *J Clin Endocrinol* 27:1275, 1967.
826. Ohsako N, Tamai H, Sudo T, et al: Clinical characteristics of subacute thyroiditis classified according to human leukocyte antigen typing. *J Clin Endocrinol Metab* 80:3653, 1995.
827. Yamada T, Sato A, Aizawa T: Dissociation between serum interleukin-6 rise and other parameters of disease activity in subacute thyroiditis during treatment with corticosteroid. *J Clin Endocrinol Metab* 81:577, 1996.
828. Volpe R: The management of subacute (DeQuervain's) thyroiditis. *Thyroid* 3:253, 1993.
829. Berger SA, Zonszein J, Villamena P, et al: Infectious diseases of the thyroid gland. *Rev Infect Dis* 5:108, 1983.
830. Miyauchi A, Matsuzuka F, Kuma K, et al: Piriform sinus fistula: An underlying abnormality common in patients with acute suppurative thyroiditis. *World J Surg* 14:400, 1990.
831. Drucker DJ, Bailey D, Rotstein L: Thyroiditis as the presenting manifestation of disseminated extrapulmonary *Pneumocystis carinii* infection. *J Clin Endocrinol Metab* 71:1663, 1990.
832. Cases JA, Wenig BM, Silver CE, et al: Recurrent acute suppurative thyroiditis in an adult due to a fourth branchial pouch fistula. *J Clin Endocrinol Metab* 85:953, 2000.

CHAPTER 10

The Thyroid: Nodules and Neoplasia

Barbara K. Kinder
Gerard N. Burrow

Interest in the thyroid gland has centered on goiter and nodule formation. Goiter may be defined as a thyroid gland that is twice normal size, or about 40 g for an adult. Endemic goiter is the major thyroid disease worldwide, probably affecting more than 200 million people. Many goitrous glands contain one or more nodules.[1] The use of iodized salt has eliminated goiter as a medical problem in developed countries, although it continues to be a major problem in developing countries whose geographic location makes them susceptible to iodine deficiency. In North America and other developed areas, sporadic nodular goiter and the possibility of associated thyroid carcinoma cause problems in diagnosis and management. The concern about "lumps" and cancer seems particularly acute with respect to the thyroid, where a nodule is easily palpable and is often observable by the patient.

GOITER

Classification of Goiter and Thyroid Neoplasia

To bring order out of chaos in the classification of goiter, the American Thyroid Association has suggested the terminology in Table 10-1 for nontoxic goiter. This system of classification is based on whether the goiter is diffuse or nodular. Goiters are further subdivided according to whether they are endemic, sporadic, or compensatory and, if nodular, whether they are uninodular or multinodular and functional or nonfunctional.

Historical Overview

The thyroid gland was first described in detail by Vesalius in the sixteenth century. Thomas Wharton (1614–1673) named the gland from the Greek word *thureos* ("shield"). He noted: It contributes much to the rotundity and beauty of the neck filling up the vacant spaces around the larynx and making its protuberant parts almost to subside, and become smooth, particularly in females to whom for this reason a larger gland has been assigned, which renders their necks more even and beautiful.[2]

Goiter once was prevalent in Switzerland, Austria, and southern Germany as well as in northern Spain, southernmost France, and northern Italy. As a consequence, some of the earliest descriptions of goiter and cretinism came from these regions.[3]

Endemic cretinism was described by the Swiss German physician Paracelsus (1493–1541) in the region around Salzburg.[4] Paracelsus pointed out that cretinism occurred together with endemic goiter. Felix Platter (1536–1614), a Swiss physician who was a professor of medicine in Basel, also described cretinism and associated mental deficiency and noted that affected individuals "frequently have a struma at the throat."

Swellings of the neck, particularly those caused by the thyroid and glandular tuberculosis, had been treated for centuries with iodine-containing substances such as seaweed and burned sponge. In 1817, Bernard Courtois, a French manufacturer of saltpeter, discovered iodine. Subsequent research on iodine and iodine compounds led Jean François Coindet to introduce tincture of iodine for the treatment of goiter. In 1820, Coindet reported to the Swiss Scientific Society that he had administered an iodine solution to 150 goiter patients without ill effects. Coindet's work strongly influenced other physicians, among them J. G. A. Lugol, who used an aqueous solution of iodine and potassium iodide which later was named for him. Awareness of the potential problems associated with iodine eventually led to the limitation of its use, especially after 1910, when Kocher described the production of toxic goiter (iod-Basedow) in goitrous patients treated with iodine. Marine popularized the use of iodized salt in North America for the prevention of simple endemic goiter beginning in 1917.[5]

Sporadic cretinism, as opposed to the endemic form, was described by Fagge, a physician at Guy's Hospital in London, before the Royal Medical and Surgical Society in 1871. Fagge expressed the view that sporadic cretinism is caused by absence of a thyroid gland.

Etiology of Goiter

In 1924, Marine first developed the concept that periods of iodide deficiency and repletion result in cyclic hyperplasia and involution of thyroid follicular cells, with the eventual development of nodular hyperplasia.[5]

Whatever the specific cause, goitrogenesis involves the generation of new follicular epithelial cells and new follicles. Goitrogenic stimuli occurring over a long period produce the macroscopic, microscopic, and functional heterogeneity characteristic of simple goiter.[6] In contrast, a more short-term potent goitrogenic stimulus can result in follicular hypertrophy with less generation of new follicular cells and follicles (i.e., Graves' goiters).

The suggestion has also been made that thyroid nodules are caused by the shunting of blood to a particular area of the thyroid, with a subsequent increase in tissue growth. Thyroid follicles are bound together to form a lobule; a single artery supplies each lobule. In long-standing goiters, the blood supply may be greatly increased.

TABLE 10-1. Classification of Nontoxic Goiter

Nontoxic diffuse goiter
Endemic, induced by
Iodine deficiency
Iodine excess
Dietary goitrogens
Sporadic, caused by
Congenital defect in thyroid hormone biosynthesis
Chemical agents (e.g., lithium, thiocyanate, *p*-aminosalicylic acid)
Iodine deficiency
Compensatory, following subtotal thyroidectomy
Nontoxic nodular goiter caused by causes listed above
Uninodular or multinodular
Functional and/or nonfunctional

Source: Modified from Werner SC: *J Clin Endocrinol* 29:860, 1969.

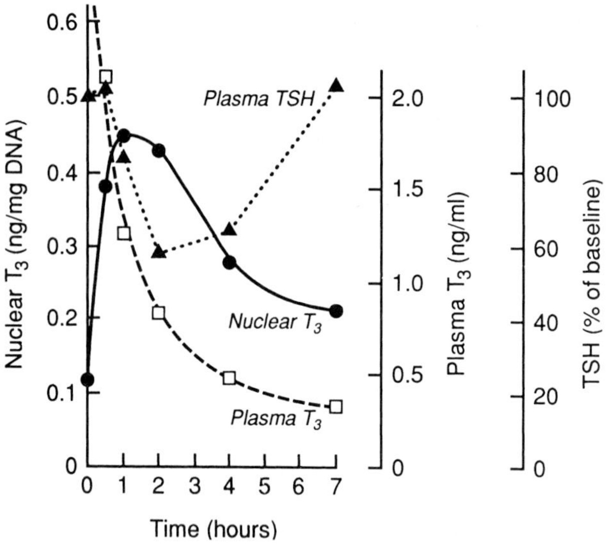

FIGURE 10-1. Time course of changes in pituitary nuclear T_3 and plasma T_3 and TSH levels. A single intravenous dose of T_3 was administered to thyroidectomized rats. The data suggest that the rapid inhibitory effect of T_3 on pituitary TSH release occurs through T_3 binding to receptors with kinetics similar to those of nuclear receptor binding. (*From Silva JE, Larsen PR: Science 198:617, 1977.*)

There has been increasing interest in the idea that growth factors in addition to thyroid stimulating hormone (TSH) play a role in the etiology of goiter.[7] The insulin-like growth factors are pleiotropic growth factors that affect DNA synthesis and differentiated cellular function in thyroid cells in culture and are produced by thyroid cells.[8,9] Epidermal growth factor (EGF) may affect the thyroid gland.[10] Immunoglobulin fractions capable of stimulating thyroid growth in a cytochemical assay based on DNA determinations have been reported in patients with nontoxic goiter.[11,12] In addition to growth factors, there are also inhibitory factors. Transforming growth factor (TGF) has an inhibitory action on thyroid cell growth and is also produced by the thyroid.[13] Interleukin 1 (IL-1) may suppress responsiveness to TSH.[14] Further, it has been suggested that iodine stimulates TGF production, which could partially explain the effect of iodine on the size of goiter.[15]

TSH Secretion

As discussed in more detail in Chap. 9, TSH secretion is controlled by the serum thyroid hormone concentration. As the concentration of thyroid hormone falls, TSH secretion increases; TSH secretion declines as the thyroid hormone concentration rises. Feedback control of TSH secretion by thyroid hormone occurs at the level of the pituitary. The hypothalamus modulates information from the rest of the central nervous system and provides the set point for TSH secretion in response to thyrotropin releasing hormone (TRH)[16] and other hormones, including estrogens, dopamine, and somatostatin (see Chap. 9).

Each individual appears to possess his or her own unique TSH set point that may be anywhere in the normal range. With the advent of second- and third-generation sensitive TSH assays, TSH responses to TRH have been found to be proportional to the basal value, with an approximate tenfold increase.[17]

There appear to be substantial variations between individuals in the relations of serum thyroid hormone concentration to TSH concentration; these variations may reflect variations in the cellular sensitivity of the pituitary to thyroid hormone, the degree of TRH release, or other factors.

As discussed in Chap. 9, the actions of thyroid hormone appear to be due to triiodothyronine (T3); thyroxine (T4) serves as a prohormone. This function is particularly important in the case of the pituitary, where T4 5-deiodinase is most active.[18] This feature allows the gland to respond more readily to changes in T4 release than do peripheral tissues (Fig. 10-1).

TSH Stimulation of Thyroid Gland

TSH is essential for the maintenance of normal thyroid hormone synthesis, although hypophysectomized animals secrete thyroid hormone to a very limited degree. The secretion of thyroid hormone is particularly sensitive to TSH and is proportional to the dose of administered TSH over a particular range. Under most physiologic conditions, TSH secretion maintains a stable serum concentration of thyroid hormone. However, the growth response of the thyroid to TSH has fixed limits; the thyroid is not capable of enlarging infinitely, and eventually a growth plateau is reached.

Evidence that goiter can be due to increased TSH stimulation has come mainly from studies of endemic goiter. In a study of 285 patients from endemic goiter regions of New Guinea, mean serum TSH concentrations were found to be increased [16 units per milliliter (U/ml)] compared with normal values in North America (1.2 U/ml).[19] However, within the group from the endemic goiter region, there was no difference in serum TSH concentration between goitrous and nongoitrous patients, suggesting that a factor in addition to TSH contributes to goitrogenesis. Perhaps that factor is the differential sensitivity of the cells of the thyroid gland to TSH.[6] In endemic goiter areas of Brazil, serum TSH concentrations were higher in goitrous patients from iodine-deficient areas than in goitrous patients from iodine-replete areas.[20] Furthermore, there was a higher peak TSH response to TRH (see Chap. 9) in the iodine-deficient goitrous group. The authors suggested that there may have been an increase of the set point so that TSH secretion continued at a higher level. However, studies from Greece, another endemic goiter area, suggested that an iodine-deficient thyroid is more sensitive to the stimulatory effect of TSH.[21,22] All these studies were done before the introduction of the sensitive TSH assay.

Studies of sporadic nontoxic goiter are even more complicated because the etiology is so diverse, ranging from thyroiditis to goitrogen ingestion. Serum TSH concentrations have been found to be increased slightly, and patients with sporadic nontoxic

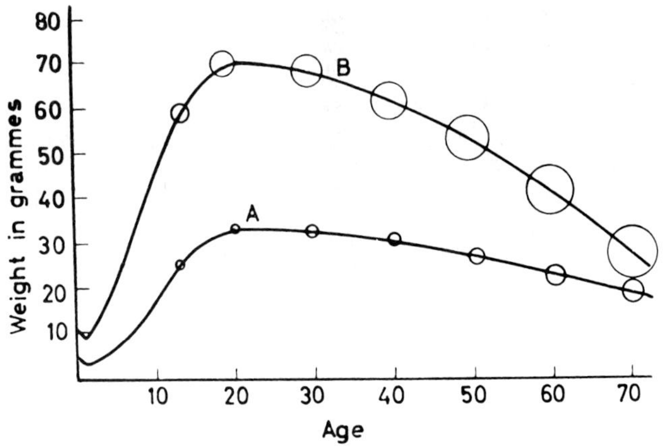

FIGURE 10-2. Goiter formation as a function of age. The size of the thyroid in grams is shown as a function of age for both nonendemic goiter areas (*A*) and endemic goiter areas (*B*). The circles represent the relative size of thyroid nodules throughout life in both groups. (*From Farris, in Deficiency Diseases. Springfield, IL, Charles C Thomas, 1958.*)

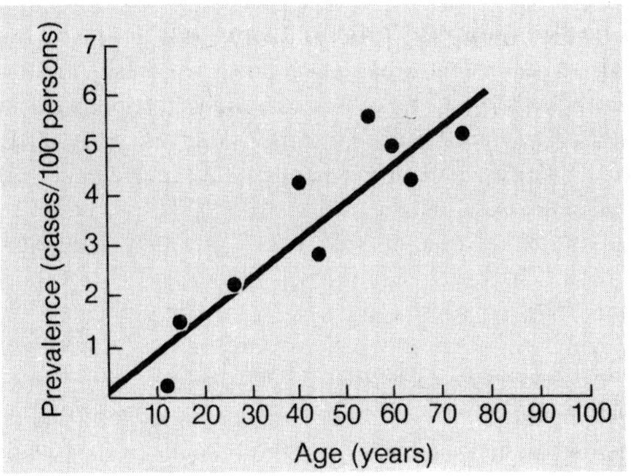

FIGURE 10-3. Prevalence of thyroid nodules with age. (*After Maxon HR, et al.*[98])

goiter often have an increased TSH response to TRH.[23] Patients with nodular goiter more often have an impaired or absent response to TRH compared with those with diffuse goiter. This impaired TSH response may indicate that there are areas of autonomy in the nodular gland, so that some thyroid hormone production is not under pituitary control; this would act to suppress the sensitivity of the pituitary to TRH. Serum TSH concentrations were higher in individuals who had goiters for less than a year.[24] Growth of the thyroid is more rapid early in life; the gland actually regresses later on (Fig. 10-2). TSH values also increase during the early decades of life. Subsequently, TSH secretion and reserve progressively decrease.[25] The prevalence of thyroid nodules, however, may increase with age (Fig. 10-3).

The variability in TSH concentrations associated with goiter may be explained by the natural progression of the disease. Over all, in the early stages of goiter formation there may be a relative thyroid hormone deficiency; this results in increased TSH release, which then stimulates thyroid hypertrophy and hyperplasia. Enlargement in thyroid size augments the ability of the gland to produce thyroid hormone, which in turn results in a suppression of TSH levels toward normal. Further, in some cases, serum TSH stimulation may result in relatively autonomous foci of thyroid hormone-producing tissue within the gland, which could lead to depressed TSH levels. Thus, depending on the stage of the disease, TSH levels can be elevated, normal, or depressed.[19–25] However, individual variations in the sensitivity of the gland to TSH and other growth or inhibitory factors may be capable of stimulating thyroid gland growth[11,26,27] and may also participate in these variations.

Endemic Goiter

When the incidence of goiter in a population rises above 10 percent, the goiter becomes "endemic." Clearly, this is not a stringent criterion. However, there is an implication that an environmental factor is the causative agent. Worldwide, iodine deficiency is the major cause of goiter, but other goitrogens have been described which affect entire populations, usually in association with iodine deficiency.

Geography, Diet, and Iodine Abundance

Although Noah might have saved the animals from extinction, the flood left their descendants susceptible to goiter. In areas subjected to flooding or intense glaciation in the last ice age, iodine was leached out of the soil. Newly formed soils are relatively iodine-deficient, although they are enriched by airborne iodine, the major source of which is seawater deposited in rain.[28]

Although individual requirements vary, most people require more than 50 g of iodine daily to replace iodine excreted in the urine (Table 10-2).[29] Diets that do not supply this amount of iodine are most often found in areas where the soil is poor in iodine. Individuals who live in villages in these areas and eat predominantly local food have iodine-deficient diets. Iodine deficiency is less likely in larger cities because the food there comes from a much wider geographic area. Similarly, members of upper socioeconomic classes are less apt to have goiter because they eat a more varied diet. In developed countries, iodine added to salt makes a major contribution to the iodine intake. With the exception of saltwater fish, there is relatively little iodine in natural food.

TABLE 10-2. Urinary Iodide Content, Goiter, and Development

Severity of Goiter	Urinary Iodide Excretion, μg/g Creatinine	Percent with Palpable Goiter	Clinical Spectrum
Mild	>50	10–20	Normal
Moderate	25–50	20–30	Occasional deafness and retardation; serum TSH elevated in 10–20%
Severe	<25	40–90	Cretinism in 1–10%; elevated serum TSH in 30–50%

Source: Modified from Ibbertson.[29] Represents approximate relations in endemic goiter areas.

Development of Endemic Goiter

The development of endemic goiter presumably follows the pattern of goiter in general. Decreased concentrations of circulating thyroid hormone resulting from iodine deficiency lead to increased TSH secretion and hyperplasia of the gland. As was discussed previously, factors other than TSH (such as cellular sensitivity to TSH and growth factors) also play a role in goiter formation.[30] It is necessary to invoke these factors to explain, for instance, why goiter is present only in certain individuals in areas of endemic goiter and the heterogeneity of the follicles within a goitrous gland (see later discussion). There is no characteristic histologic picture that distinguishes endemic goiter. With the initial stimulation, hypertrophy of the follicular cells occurs, followed by hyperplasia of the follicles and a concomitant increase in the vascularity of the gland. All the follicles in an endemic goiter are not affected equally; radioautographic studies have shown an unequal distribution of radioiodine within the individual follicles.[31] This heterogeneity, combined with an overall increase in the size of the gland, may explain why some endemic goiters contain a higher than average total amount of iodine.[32] Also, some of this thyroidal iodine may be outside the hormonally active pool. Nodular goiter may therefore be considered an extreme variant of this heterogeneity. Part of the thyroid irregularity leading to nodule formation may be due to the accumulation of connective tissue, which, during periods of further stimulation, may serve as a focus of retraction and may hinder the function of adjacent follicles.[6]

The human thyroid is limited in its ability to adapt to iodine deficiency compared with iodine excess. In severe iodine deficiency, there is an inability of the thyroid to compensate completely for the low plasma inorganic iodide concentration by proportionally increasing the iodide clearance rate.[33] In a euthyroid patient with endemic goiter, total thyroid iodine stores may be normal, although the iodine concentration in the hormonally active pool is low. With less iodine, less iodothyronine is synthesized. Iodine deficiency also increases the monoiodotyrosine/diiodotyrosine ratio. These changes do not occur early in goiter formation but are often found in nodular glands. Iodine deficiency and perhaps the increased stimulation from TSH also result in a high T3:T4 ratio in these goiters. This adaptive effect results in the production of the more potent T3 despite a deficiency of iodine.

Clinical Findings in Endemic Goiter

In areas of severe iodine deficiency, virtually everyone is goitrous regardless of gender or age. In less severely affected areas, surveys have shown that the thyroid gland may be moderately enlarged in early childhood but that the incidence of goiter is usually at its height in pubertal children. The goiter of puberty is one of the more sensitive indicators of iodine lack in a particular region. A difference in gland size between the two sexes appears during puberty. After puberty, the thyroid gland frequently diminishes in size in males but not in females. Why females are more affected than males is not clear. In the endemic goiter area of New Guinea, thyroid enlargement was found to be related to breast development but not to pregnancy, lactation, or parity.[34] The thyroid gland is more difficult to palpate in men, which may account for part of the discrepancy. However, all thyroid disease is more common in females, and the difference does not appear to be due solely to estrogens. The diagnosis and treatment of goiter are discussed later in this chapter.

Relation to Thyroid Cancer

Despite continuing long-term interest in the problem, the relation between endemic goiter and thyroid cancer remains unclear. After the introduction of iodine prophylaxis, the incidence of both nodular goiter and certain adenocarcinomas and sarcomas of the thyroid decreased. Appreciation of this change was complicated by an increase in the incidence of papillary carcinoma of the thyroid. However, when the geographic pattern of goiter prevalence was compared with the geographic patterns of mortality from thyroid cancer, there was no convincing evidence for an association between the two diseases.[35] In contrast, the comparison of the occurrence of goiter with that of hyperthyroidism showed the two to be highly significantly correlated.

Hyperfunction

Although data are not available, hyperthyroidism appears to be more common in areas of endemic goiter, especially after iodine therapy (iod-Basedow). Toxic nodular goiter (Plummer's disease) is common in association with endemic goiter; this may provide an explanation of the iod-Basedow phenomenon.[36] These hyperfunctioning nodules are avid for iodine and respond with a greatly increased production of thyroid hormone.

Cretinism

In areas of mild iodine deficiency, the inhabitants are usually euthyroid. With more profound iodine depletion, hypothyroidism may occur. A much more severe problem is the occurrence of cretinism in this population. Cretinism has been defined as permanent neurologic and skeletal retardation resulting from an inadequate supply of thyroid hormone during fetal and neonatal life, in this case caused by iodine deficiency.[29,32] Endemic cretins may present with neurologic defects, particularly spastic diplegia and mental retardation, deafness, mutism, dwarfism, and hypothyroidism in varying combinations, depending on the locale. Hypothyroidism can be diagnosed clinically by retarded linear growth and maturation of body proportions, myxedematous skin, and a marked delay in sexual development (see Chap. 9).

The various symptoms and signs of cretinism vary with the region. In central Africa, most cretins are athyrotic and myxedematous, while in the Andes, New Guinea, and the Himalayan foothills, the "nervous" type of cretinism predominates. For example, the "myxedematous" type is characterized by hypothyroidism, dwarfism, and epiphyseal dysgenesis consistent with deficient hormone production. In contrast, the "nervous" type is characterized by mental retardation and deaf-mutism. Both groups may have goiter. The prevalence of cretinism observed in these regions also varies markedly, from 1 percent in Zaire to almost 6 percent in endemic goiter districts in Nepal. The clinical picture of endemic cretinism represents a spectrum of clinical and metabolic signs reflecting varying degrees of impairment of the nervous system and thyroid function.[37,38]

The clinical features of endemic cretinism appear to result from the combined effects of hypothyroidism in utero and postnatally.[39] Fetal hypothyroidism during the first half of pregnancy affects the developing nervous system predominantly, whereas postnatal hypothyroidism results in manifestations of myxedema. Congenital hypothyroidism which persists causes stunting of growth and the other characteristic somatic abnormalities. Strict adherence to the classification of myxedematous or neurologic cretinism may obscure the spectrum of abnormalities caused by combined fetal and neonatal hypothyroidism.

Etiology of Cretinism and Iodine Deficiency

Endemic cretinism occurs only in areas where long-standing, severe endemic goiter is present. The prevalence of cretinism appears to be related to the severity of iodine deficiency. However, comparable states of iodine deficiency may be accompanied by cretinism in some areas but not in others.[40] The intrauterine period is important for the development of cretinism,[41] but this can be prevented by means of iodine administration to mothers. In a severely iodine-deficient area in Africa, 40 percent of newborns had elevated TSH concentrations more than 2.5 standard deviations (SD) above those of controls whose mothers had received iodine.[42] In 6 of 34 iodine-deficient neonates, definite biochemical signs of hypothyroidism were encountered.

Endemic Goiter Due to Other Causes

Although iodine deficiency represents the major cause of endemic goiter, genetic factors and dietary goitrogens may also participate in endemic goiter formation. For example, a striking difference in the incidence of goiter was found between the inhabitants of two regions of an isolated island in Kivu Lake in Zaire, although the iodine intake in the two areas was the same and the two groups were ethnically similar.[42] Subsequent studies indicated that goiter in this population was related to the consumption of cassava, which, like several other chemical substances, can impair the utilization of iodine by the thyroid gland. However, cassava appears to be active as a goitrogen only in the presence of severe iodine deficiency, as data from Vietnam indicate that the goitrogenic effect of this substance is easily overcome by supplementary iodine.[43]

Protein-calorie malnutrition (PCM) often is present in iodine-deficient areas and may contribute to thyroid abnormalities. Malnutrition causes various alterations in the structure and function of the thyroid gland; a defective thyroid iodine concentration has been found despite adequate hormone secretion, which would further deplete iodine stores.[44] These abnormalities can be corrected by means of adequate protein and calorie intake. Studies from Senegal have suggested that PCM may cause goiter by resulting in defective formation of the mannosyl retinene phosphate complex necessary for normal glycosylation of thyroglobulin.[45] Experimental data suggest that glycosylation is obligatory for the processing of thyroglobulin, including iodination and subsequent thyroid hormone production.[46]

Prophylaxis of Endemic Goiter

One of the strongest pieces of evidence in support of the contention that endemic cretinism is due to iodine deficiency is the disappearance of cretinism when iodine is added to the diet. Supplements of iodine to the daily diet have been widely employed since their efficacy was demonstrated by Marine and Kimball in 1917.[5,47] Similar results have been duplicated throughout the world, but the total impact so far has been small compared with the magnitude of the goiter problem. This apathetic approach may be partly due to the complexity of the etiologic aspects of endemic goiter; for example, the persistent endemic goiter which affects about 20 percent of schoolchildren in Colombia has been attributed to a goitrogenic agent in well water. However, despite these natural goitrogens and the possibility of genetically determined metabolic defects of thyroid hormone, studies have indicated that iodine is a highly effective agent for the prevention of goiter.

Iodizing salt has been the most satisfactory method so far developed to provide populations with an adequate supply of iodine. Iodination of the water supply is effective but requires that everyone use a particular water supply. Iodized oil has been used successfully as an injectable form of goiter prophylaxis that lasts for 3 or more years. This form of prophylaxis is particularly useful in less developed areas of endemic goiter, where the distribution of iodized salt is difficult. The excreted iodine may be recycled in less developed areas.

Iodine is more effective in preventing the development of goiter than in suppressing an already enlarged thyroid gland. Early diffuse hyperplastic goiters may involute, but enlarged glands that have formed nodules and undergone cystic degeneration usually do not. After a diagnosis of cretinism has been made, thyroid hormone therapy ensures an adequate hormone concentration, but the patient may not improve in growth or mentation and his or her behavior pattern may deteriorate.

Surgery may be indicated for large goiters (see "Nontoxic Goiter") (Fig. 10-4). The most important indication for surgery is the presence of pressure symptoms, which rarely occur in a goiter situated high up in the neck. Goiters that are low in the neck, intrathoracic goiters, and goiters that encircle the trachea are the most likely to produce pressure symptoms.

Sporadic Goiter

Sporadic goiter can perhaps best be defined as goiter occurring in a nonendemic goiter region. Although a number of known goitrogens and errors in thyroid hormone biosynthesis may cause goiter, most cases of sporadic goiter have no known etiology. The pathophysiology of sporadic goiter formation is presumably identical to that of endemic goiter. Population studies have indicated that approximately 4 percent of individuals in a nonendemic area have thyroid nodules.[48] In autopsy studies of unselected patients over

FIGURE 10-4. Large goiter in a cretin. (*From Merke F: Geschichte von Fropf und Kretinismus. Bern, Hans Huber, 1971.*)

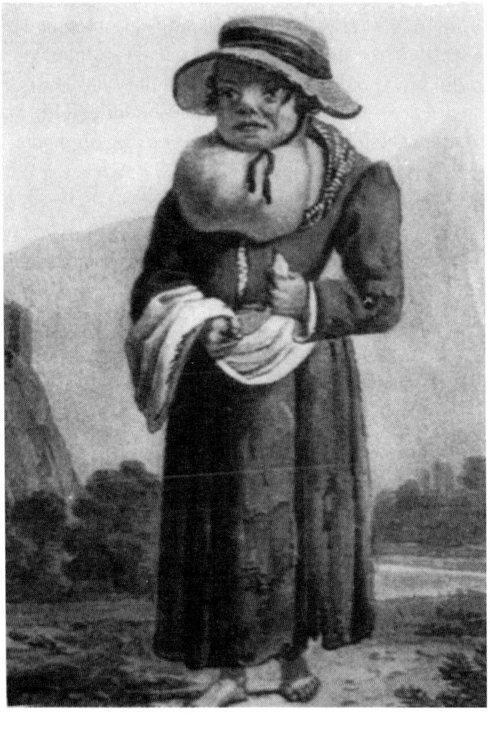

20 years of age, the incidence of nodules 1 cm or larger rose to 50 percent when the thyroid gland was sectioned serially.[49]

Sex and Age in Relation to Goiter

Most types of thyroid dysfunction are approximately four to five times more common in females than in males, and goiter formation is no exception. Estrogens are an obvious source of this difference, but there is no convincing evidence to support this possibility. In an effort to determine the reasons for this sex difference, systematic comparisons were made of the development of the pituitary-thyroid axis in male and female rats.[50] The serum TSH concentration in adult male rats is 2.8 times higher than in females, but the serum T4 concentration in males is 28 percent lower. Whether these findings are pertinent to the sex differences in human thyroid dysfunction remains to be determined.

Sporadic goiter does not usually occur before puberty. In endemic areas, the highest incidence of goiter is found between ages of 10 and 50; the incidence decreases in later decades. In contrast, the incidence of sporadic goiter has no age peak. Frequently, the thyroid gland increases rapidly in size at the time of puberty, especially in girls. Whether this "physiologic" goiter represents relative thyroid hormone deficiency caused by the stress of puberty is not clear, but the goiter tends to disappear subsequently without thyroid hormone therapy.

Goiter During Pregnancy

A physiologic increase in the size of the thyroid appears to occur during some pregnancies. Histologic examination of the typical thyroid gland during gestation reveals large follicles with abundant well-stained colloid and frequent vacuolation. Papillary infolding of thyroid follicles can be seen in 25 percent of cases, and the thyroid follicular cells are columnar rather than flat. All these findings reinforce the impression of thyroid hyperplasia. This histologic picture is one of active formation and secretion of thyroid hormone.

In a study of pregnant women in Scotland, goiter was considered to be present if the thyroid gland was both palpable and visible.[51] By these criteria, 70 percent of pregnant women had goiter, compared with 38 percent of nonpregnant women. The prevalence of goiter did not appear to be affected by previous parity because goiter occurred in 39 percent of nulliparous women and 35 percent of nongravid parous women. Thyroid enlargement occurred in each trimester with the same frequency, suggesting that goiter appears early and persists during pregnancy. When the same study was repeated in Iceland, no increase in goiter was found during pregnancy.[52] The difference in goiter incidence during pregnancy between the two countries was attributed to differences in dietary iodine content. Renal clearance of iodine is increased during pregnancy as a consequence of the increased glomerular filtration rate. The plasma inorganic iodine concentration decreases because more iodine is excreted in the urine and less is available for thyroid hormone biosynthesis. To compensate, the thyroid gland may enlarge and clear more plasma of iodine to ensure adequate thyroid hormone biosynthesis. Therefore, in areas of marginal iodine intake, pregnancy is more likely to lead to goiter formation.

In a study done in Belgium, an area of marginal iodine intake, there was a progressive increase in thyroid volume during pregnancy.[53] An analysis of 552 ultrasound tests indicated that 73 percent of pregnant women had a significant increase in thyroid volume, with an average increase of 18 percent. True goiter, defined as a total thyroid volume greater than 33 ml, was found in 9 percent of the women in the study at the time of delivery. A study done in the United States did not find a significant difference in iodine balance between pregnant and nonpregnant women.[54] The high-iodine diet in North America may vitiate the increased iodine loss during pregnancy, and goiter is apparently not significantly more common during pregnancy.[55]

Genetic Influences on Goiter Formation

It has been suggested that even in endemic goiter areas, individuals who develop goiter are genetically distinct from nongoitrous individuals from the same area. In an endemic goiter region of Greece, a uniformly high thyroidal uptake of radioiodine occurred, but only certain individuals were goitrous.[56] Because these goiters were grouped within particular families, genetic factors may play a role in goiter formation. Goiter prevalence was compared in monozygotic and dizygotic twin pairs of like sex to obtain an index of the importance of inheritance in the etiology of goiter in healthy people.[57] The data suggested that a genetically determined tendency toward thyroid growth may exist. The suggestion that the goiter of puberty and pregnancy is a consequence of an increased requirement for thyroid hormone during a period of stress does not explain why only a minority of individuals develop this goiter. Nor does this hypothesis explain the results of radioiodine studies or the abundance of colloid found in most goiters of puberty.[58] The familial occurrence of thyroid disease in adolescents with the goiter of puberty again suggests a genetic predisposition.

Specific Inherited Defects in Thyroid Hormone Biosynthesis

The clearest examples of genetic influences on thyroid function and goiter formation are found in a small group of individuals with hypothyroidism and goiter. These persons have inherited specific autosomal recessive defects in hormone synthesis (Fig. 10-5). These defects lead to inadequate thyroid hormone production, which results in prolonged stimulation of TSH release, in some cases leading to an enlarged sella. The hypersecretion of TSH leads to intense thyroid gland hyperplasia and goiter; the hyperplasia can be mistaken for a malignancy. In fact, thyroid malignancy appears to be no more common in these patients.[59] These conditions apparently occur because of genetic defects of single enzymes or other proteins, presumably corresponding to each step in thyroid hormone biosynthesis (see Chap. 9).

As indicated in Fig. 10-6, there are five major recognized defects in thyroid hormone biosynthesis, but it is almost certain that there are many more:

1. There may be a defect in the ability of the thyroid gland to trap iodine.
2. A defect may exist in the ability of the gland to convert inorganic iodide to an organic form, as an iodotyrosine. This defect is characterized by precipitate discharge of radioactive iodine from the thyroid after the administration of thiocyanate or perchlorate; it may be associated with deafness. This is a heterogeneous group of defects related to the peroxidase system and associated with the various steps in organification.
3. Thyroid hormone is synthesized within the interstices of the very large thyroglobulin molecule. Defects in thyroglobulin synthesis lead to inadequate or absent thyroid hormone synthesis. This probably reflects a large, heterogeneous group of defects. Although no proof exists, a number of cases of sporadic goiter may in fact represent minor defects in thyroglobulin synthesis.

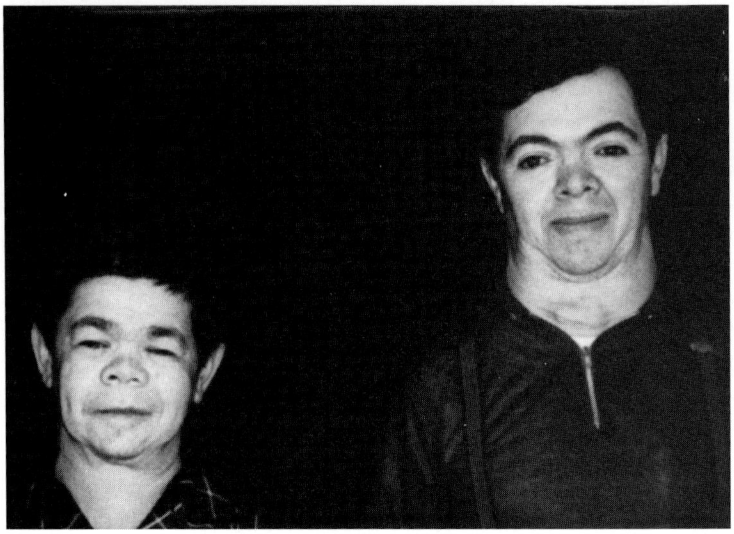

FIGURE 10-5. Two brothers with goitrous cretinism caused by a defect in thyroglobulin synthesis.

4. There may be coupling defects resulting from a variety of defects which impair iodothyronine formation.
5. The iodotyrosine deiodinase defect results in iodine loss from the gland. The enzyme usually deiodinates iodotyrosines which have not coupled to form iodothyronines, allowing the iodine to be reused within the gland.

In addition to the defects listed above, there may be an impaired tissue response to TSH or to thyroid hormones (see Chap. 9). However, the former condition would not cause goiter. Whatever the specific defect, genetic influences lead to inadequate thyroid hormone production and goiter formation. Whether similar but less well-defined genetic influences play a role in sporadic goiter remains to be determined.

Specific Goitrogens

Any substance that interferes with the biosynthesis of thyroid hormone can be a goitrogen.[60] This includes a number of chemical compounds that inhibit specific steps of thyroid hormone biosynthesis as well as dietary goitrogens in which the active compound is unknown.

Dietary Goitrogens

The development of antithyroid drug therapy began with the observation that rabbits that were fed cabbage developed goiters and the later finding that goiters developed in rats fed seeds of brassicas (cabbage, turnips, Brussels sprouts, rutabagas, etc.).[61] This finding led to the appreciation of thiourea as a goitrogen and eventually to the introduction of thioamides as valuable therapeutic agents in the treatment of hyperthyroidism. The quantity of the goitrogen and perhaps the quality of the vegetables containing the goitrogen are such that the chance of significant goiter formation in human beings is rare. Soybean milk has been observed to pro-duce goiter in infants. The goitrogenic substance in soybean flour has not been identified, but supplemention of the diet with iodide eliminates the problem. Foods such as cassava contain compounds that on hydrolysis release free cyanide. After ingestion, the cyanide is converted to thiocyanate. Cassava has been suggested as a cause of endemic goiter in central Africa.[42] In Colombia, sulfur-containing compounds found in the water supply, which are derived from sedimentary rocks, are thought to be goitrogenic.[62]

FIGURE 10-6. Defects in thyroid hormone biosynthesis.

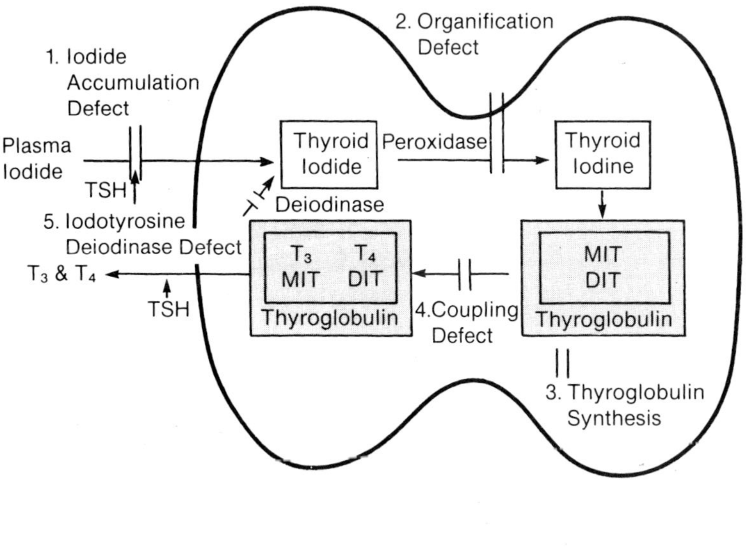

TABLE 10-3. Chemical Goitrogens

- Effect within the thyroid
- Modifiers of iodine transport: complex anions: technetium perchlorate, thiocyanate (active ingredient in *Brassica* spp. and cassava)
- Modifiers of iodination of thyroglobulin
    - Thioamides: propylthiouracil, methimazole, carbimazole
    - Thiocyanate
    - Aniline derivatives: sulfonamides, *p*-aminosalicylic acid, amphenone B, aminoglutethimide, phenylbutazone
- Effects on iodothyronine formation
    - Thioamides
    - Sulfonamides
- Influences on secretion of thyroid hormone
    - Iodide
    - Lithium
- Effect on peripheral disposal of thyroid hormone
- Hormone deiodination: propylthiouracil, iopanoic acid, ipodate, amiodarone
- Intestinal absorption of hormones: soy flour, resins (e.g., cholestyramine)
- Hormone inactivation: inducers of hepatic drug-metabolizing enzymes (e.g., phenobarbital)

Chemical Goitrogens

Various chemical goitrogens, ranging from salts and minerals to complex nitrogen-containing heterocyclic compounds, interfere with the synthesis of thyroid hormone (Table 10-3). The salts and minerals of interest here include lithium, which has an inhibitory effect on the release of thyroid hormone, and cobalt, the action of which is unclear. Type I iodothyronine deiodinase is a selenocysteine-containing enzyme, and selenium is essential for the conversion of T4 to T3.[63]

Selenium deficiency occurs in areas of iodine deficiency and may contribute to the development of myxedematous endemic cretinism.[64] The more complex chemical compounds which interfere with thyroid function by blocking iodination and the coupling reaction have some common structural features. None of the nitrogen heterocyclics are as potent as the thioamides (e.g., propylthiouracil), but there is no apparent fundamental difference in their antithyroid action.

Environmental Goitrogens

Pollution of drinking water is known to precipitate goiter in low-iodine areas. McGarrison noted that goiter prevalence increased downstream from the water supply in the group of villages which make up Gilgit in the foothills of the Himalayas.[65] Goiter occurred in 12 percent of the inhabitants at the source, and the prevalence increased to 45 percent at the terminus of the river, which had served as a drinking channel and open sewer for the villages on its banks. McGarrison was able to produce goiter in himself and his colleagues by ingesting suspended matter from those goiter-producing waters.[65] The goiter did not occur if the water was boiled first. In subsequent studies, low urinary iodine excretion (4–6 g/L) was found in residents of this area, but equally low levels were found in both goitrous and nongoitrous individuals.

Nontoxic Goiter

Whatever the cause, both endemic and sporadic goiters present clinically as nontoxic goiter and, depending on duration, may be either diffuse or nodular. Some goiters which may be associated with hyperthyroidism were considered in Chap. 9. More frequently, some of the nodules may be autonomous; that is, they release hormone constitutively and are no longer responsive to normal pituitary-thyroid regulation.

Incidence

The incidence of nontoxic goiter varies widely depending on whether goiter is endemic in the area. The discussion here centers on nonendemic areas such as North America. The occurrence of goiter has been determined in both autopsy and clinical studies. In an unselected autopsy series of 1,000 patients over 20 years old, the prevalence of goiter was 5 percent. When they were sectioned, half the thyroids contained nodules that were at least 1 cm across and would have been palpable if they had been anterior and superficial.[49] The study was carried out in Minnesota, which was an endemic goiter region before the introduction of iodine, and goiter may still be more common in these regions. However, similar results were found in Connecticut, a nonendemic goiter area.[66]

Presentations and Complications

Nontoxic goiter is usually discovered during a routine examination. Occasionally the patient will have noticed a lump in the throat. Rarely, the goiter may be symptomatic and cause pressure symptoms such as coughing, wheezing, dyspnea, dysphagia, and hoarseness. Hoarseness is only rarely caused by benign conditions, and its presence should raise the question of malignant invasion of the recurrent laryngeal nerve in the neck or in the chest. Obstructive[67] symptoms of the aerodigestive tract, in the absence of carcinoma, are more likely to occur in a long-standing goiter, particularly with a substernal or intrathoracic component. Most frequently,[68] however, goiter is diagnosed by the discovery of tracheal deviation on a routine chest film in an otherwise asymptomatic patient. Complaints of a "lump in the throat" are most often due to globus hystericus, an anxiety reaction characterized by a constrictive feeling in the throat. This feeling is heightened by the presence of a nontoxic goiter, presenting a difficult problem for physicians. Patients frequently describe fluctuation in goiter size, often related to periods of emotional stress or to the menstrual cycle, but these changes are almost impossible to document. The position and irregular shape of the thyroid have made it difficult to estimate the size of the gland accurately over a period of time. The thyroid does have a rich blood supply, and changes in blood flow may change the volume of the gland. The ancient Romans are reputed to have believed that the thyroid gland swells with sexual excitement; they used to measure a bride's neck to prove that the marriage had been consummated.[69]

Risk of Carcinoma in Multinodular Goiter

One of the undesirable side effects of cancer education programs is that the discovery of a "lump" frequently means cancer to the patient. Thus, a patient with a multinodular goiter is often very anxious, and this may make the physician anxious enough to recommend biopsy or surgery. If the patient demands that the physician guarantee that the thyroid nodule is not malignant, this can be done only if the nodule(s) is excised and examined histologically. The decision to pursue a tissue diagnosis is thus a result of both the patient's anxiety and the physician's anxiety. Because as many as 50 percent of thyroid glands in adults may harbor a nodule 1 cm or greater, physicians must know exactly how suspicious they should be about the possibility of carcinoma occurring in a nontoxic multinodular goiter. (Solitary thyroid nodules are considered separately later.)

The question to be answered is: Does the presence of a nontoxic goiter increase the risk of thyroid carcinoma over that expected for the population at large?

In two separate series of unselected autopsies, thyroid carcinoma was found in approximately 3 percent of the patients.[48,65] More recently, autopsy studies in Japan and Minnesota indicated a prevalence of small histologic malignancies in the thyroid as high as 13 percent when serial sections were carefully examined.[70,71] In contrast, the frequency of clinical thyroid cancer is about 39 cases diagnosed annually per 1 million population, or 0.0004 percent.[72] The reason for the marked discrepancy between histologic and clinically apparent thyroid carcinoma can be explained by reference to the concept that cancer is a multistep process. The histologic diagnosis of small thyroid malignancies (minimal papillary thyroid carcinoma) does not appear to correlate with true invasiveness, which is compatible with this concept. Similar relations have been found with prostatic carcinoma, with which the incidence is much higher at autopsy than is clinically apparent during life.

The important question is, then, whether the presence of a nontoxic goiter increases the incidence of clinically important thyroid cancer. Several epidemiologic studies bear on this question. The mortality rate for thyroid carcinoma was found to be 10 times higher in Switzerland, where goiter is endemic, than in England.[73] Furthermore, as the use of iodized salt increased in Switzerland, deaths from thyroid carcinoma decreased. The difficulty with this type of study is that a higher rate of thyroid surgery with careful pathologic examination might have resulted in the increased diagnosis of thyroid cancer. If the prevalence of goiter is based on medical examinations of draftees for World War I and World War II, and this difference is compared with the prevalence of thyroid carcinoma and hyperthyroidism, an estimate of the effect of goiter on thyroid carcinoma can be made.[35] The reduction in goiter prevalence between World War I and World War II was associated with the introduction of iodized salt. Despite the decrease in goiter frequency, the death rate for thyroid carcinoma changed very little during this period. Hyperthyroidism mortality rates increased immediately after the introduction of iodized salt, perhaps owing to the Jod-Basedow phenomenon, and then decreased in parallel with the decrease in goiter. The comparison of goiter prevalence with hyperthyroidism strongly supports the hypothesis that endemic goiter is an important factor in the pathogenesis of hyperthyroidism. In contrast, there is not convincing epidemiologic evidence for the existence of an association between thyroid carcinoma and goiter. However, the presence of a dominant nodule within an otherwise typical multinodular goiter carries a risk of malignancy similar to that of a solitary nodule (see later text) and should be similarly evaluated.

Laboratory Evaluation

When a patient presents with a goiter, the first question to be asked is whether the goiter is toxic or nontoxic. If the goiter is nontoxic, is thyroiditis the cause? Is the goiter diffuse or nodular, and is the nodule solitary or multiple? If the gland is nodular, are the nodules autonomous?

Evaluation of thyroid function is described in detail in Chap. 9. Patients with goiter should have a sensitive TSH determination, a serum T4 determination, a measurement of thyroxine-binding antibodies, and an assay for thyroid antibodies to determine the functional thyroid state and the presence of thyroiditis. If the thyroid function tests reveal evidence of hyperthyroidism, hypothyroidism, or thyroiditis, the patient should be managed as described in Chap. 9. A radioisotopic thyroid scan or ultrasound may be helpful in defining nodularity and confirming the presence of a dominant nodule. A nuclear scan also assesses functionality of the thyroid tissue and may help predict which patients, such as those with large hot nodules, are likely to develop hyperthyroidism in the future. In many instances, treatment decisions can be made without obtaining imaging studies.

Medical Therapy

Is the presence of goiter in a euthyroid patient a sufficient indication for thyroid hormone suppressive therapy? All goiters probably should be suppressed with thyroid hormone, with the exception of self-limited conditions such as the goiters of puberty and of pregnancy and the goiters of some elderly patients who have an increased risk of osteoporosis and cardiac disease (described later). Thyroid hormone therapy has a relatively low cost (only pennies per day) and is relatively nontoxic when the dose is adjusted properly.

To decrease the size of the thyroid gland, sufficient thyroid hormone has to be given to suppress TSH secretion without inducing hyperthyroidism. Therapy with L-triiodothyronine results in markedly elevated serum levels of the hormone for several hours after ingestion. Although there is no evidence that transient serum elevations of triiodothyronine in an otherwise healthy individual are harmful, it seems best to avoid these elevations if possible. Triiodothyronine is also less effective in maintaining TSH suppression.[18] Consequently, L-thyroxine should be used, because the hormone is slowly converted to triiodothyronine and elevated serum concentrations of T3 do not occur. Studies of TSH concentrations in hypothyroid women receiving L-thyroxine indicated that 90 percent of the patients were optimally managed, as indicated by normal serum TSH (by second-generation assay) concentration, with the daily administration of 100 to 200 mcg of L-thyroxine.[74]

With the introduction of the third-generation sensitive TSH assay, it has become clear that TSH suppression is a relative, not an absolute, phenomenon.[17] For benign, nontoxic nodular or diffuse goiter, replacement thyroxine therapy, which usually consists of 0.10 mg/day or less, is appropriate. The goal of therapy should be to use the minimal dose of thyroxine to keep the plasma TSH levels as low as possible without inducing the symptoms of hyperthyroidism. It appears reasonable to attempt to suppress the sensitive TSH value to the range of 0.1 to 0.3 U/ml.

Initial follow-up after the institution of therapy should be done at 6 to 8 weeks, with repeat thyroid function tests to exclude the possibility of autonomous functioning of the goiter with resultant hyperthyroidism. Once the dose has been adjusted, the patient generally can be followed annually, at which time the status of the goiter and of overall thyroid function can be assessed.

Results

Despite the large number of patients receiving thyroid hormone suppression, relatively few large, controlled studies have examined the efficacy of such treatment carefully. Two hundred thirty patients with nontoxic goiter were treated with 180 mg of desiccated thyroid and were observed at intervals of 1 to 3 months.[75–79] The goiter was regarded as diffuse if the entire gland was enlarged, even if the two lobes differed in size, or if there was considerable irregularity in the shape of the gland. The goiter was called nodular only when conspicuous nodules were prominent or

TABLE 10-4. Response of Nontoxic Goiter to Thyroid Hormone Therapy

Author	Year	No. Patients	Assessment	% Response
Astwood	1969			
Diffuse goiter		115	Palpation	67
Nodular goiter		78	Palpation	76
Badillo*		21	Palpation	57
Berghout*		78	Ultrasound	58

* Placebo controlled

Source: Astwood et al.,[75] Cooper DS. Thyroxine suppression therapy for benign nodular disease. *J Clin Endocrinol Metab* 80:331, 1995.

when a single nodule was found in an enlarged thyroid. A single nodule was diagnosed when there was an isolated nodule in an otherwise normal gland. Regression of the goiter with therapy was considered complete when the thyroid decreased to its normal size. The response to therapy was called "moderate" for any unequivocal regression short of a complete response. The results shown in Table 10-4 indicate that in one-fourth of patients with nodular goiter complete regression occurred and that in one-half there was moderate regression. Because of these data and the potential for adverse effects of thyroid hormone suppression, treatment of multinodular goiter should be individualized.[80–82] For example, a meta-analysis of the effects of long-term thyroid hormone suppression on bone density in postmenopausal women revealed 5–9 percent differences at the lumbar spine, the proximal femur and the radius over a 12-year period.[83] Similarly doses of thyroid hormone which suppress TSH result in a tripling of the risk of atrial fibrillation in patients over 60 years of age.[84] Adjusting the dose of thyroid hormone to achieve the maximal growth control while maintaining the TSH within the low normal range may avoid undesirable side effects.[85]

In addition to the cardiac and skeletal issues outlined earlier, some patients are not good candidates for L-thyroxine therapy. Unless the TSH level is elevated, large symptomatic multinodular goiters do not respond significantly to thyroid hormone replacement and are best managed by other modalities.

Radioiodine Therapy

Radioiodine treatment has been reported to give good results in the treatment of large symptomatic (including substernal) goiters. Patients have been treated with 20 to 100 mCi of ^{131}I with resolution of symptoms and decrease in size of the gland and with minimal complications.[82] Figure 10-7 shows the effect on thyroid volume and tracheal compression of ^{131}I therapy in 19 patients with large multinodular goiters.

Surgical Treatment

Alternatively, patients with large goiters which do not respond to suppressive therapy and/or are very symptomatic may require surgical resection. Usually these are goiters with an intrathoracic component. A routine chest film in such a patient will reveal a mediastinal soft tissue mass with or without evidence of tracheal deviation. Tracheal compression is usually seen only in individuals with a substernal component to the goiter. Maximal narrowing characteristically occurs at the thoracic inlet as seen in Fig. 10-8. Performance of pulmonary function tests and flow volume loops will clarify the extent to which mechanical upper airway obstruction due to goiter is contributing to a patient's respiratory symptoms.[67] Such obstruction is potentially dangerous because tracheitis with edema or hemorrhage into a thyroid nodule can result in an acute respiratory emergency.[68]

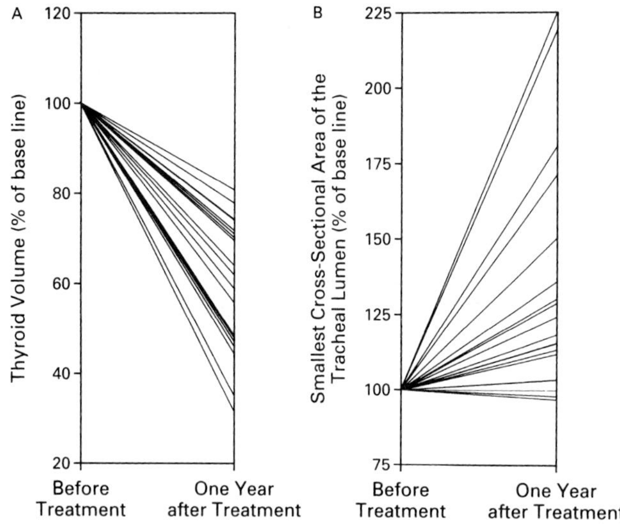

FIGURE 10-7. Thyroid volume (*A*) and smallest cross-sectional area of the tracheal lumen (*B*) by MRI before and after radioiodine therapy for goiter. (*From Hermes AR, Huysmans DA.*[82])

Most substernal goiters can be removed via a cervical incision, even in the reoperative situation, as they are only secondarily intrathoracic and their blood supply is cervical, from the superior and inferior thyroidal vessels. Primary intrathoracic goiters, derived from accessory thyroid parenchyma developing embryologically in association with the aortic sac are extremely rare (0.2–0.3 percent of cases),[86] and require thoracotomy as their blood supply is from intrathoracic vessels.[87] Establishment of an adequate airway by endotracheal intubation is of paramount importance in the safe performance of surgery for large goiters. Although tracheal deviation may be impressive in these circumstances, it does not usually pose a problem for intubation. Of more potential consequence is the tracheal narrowing that characteristically occurs at the thoracic inlet as the goiter descends into the mediastinum. Patients who exhibit stridor in the supine position or flushing of the skin and dilation of the external jugular veins on elevating the arms above the head (Pemberton's sign) can be expected to have significant tracheal narrowing. Assessment of the diameter of the airway and extent and location of the goiter by CT scan with contrast should be obtained in patients undergoing surgery for substernal goiter. MRI should be used instead of CT scan if the goiter is suspected of harboring a malignancy that might require postoperative ^{131}I therapy. Figure 10-8 shows a typical substernal goiter with tracheal deviation and maximal tracheal narrowing at the level of the thoracic inlet. Awake fiberoptic intubation is rarely necessary. Division of the middle and superior thyroidal vessels bilaterally permits mobilization of the gland. An intracapsular dissection is carried out, following the course of the gland as it descends into the mediastinum. In this way the recurrent laryngeal nerves and parathyroids are usually excluded from the dissection compartment, though care should be taken to identify them. Intrathoracic goiters that descend into the posterior mediastinum derive from the lateral and posterior aspects of the thyroid, displacing the recurrent nerves and inferior thyroid arteries *anteriorly* and the esophagus medially; the recurrent nerves are particularly vul-

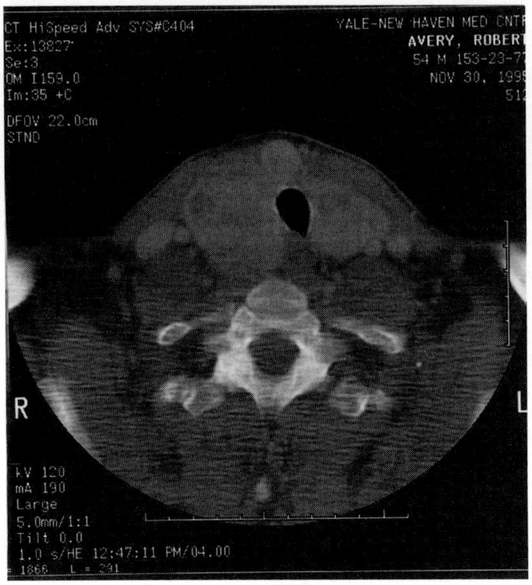

A

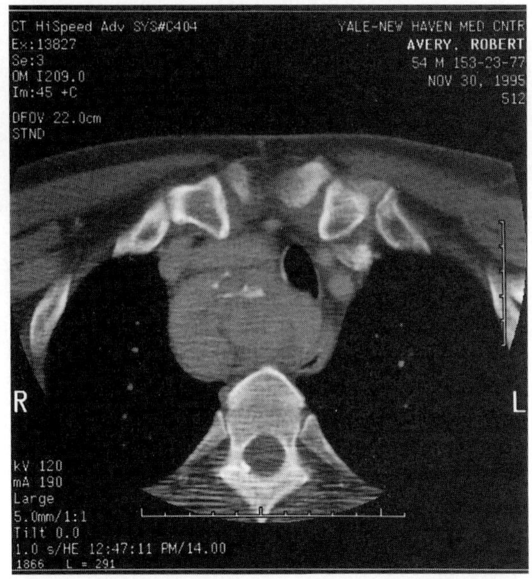

B

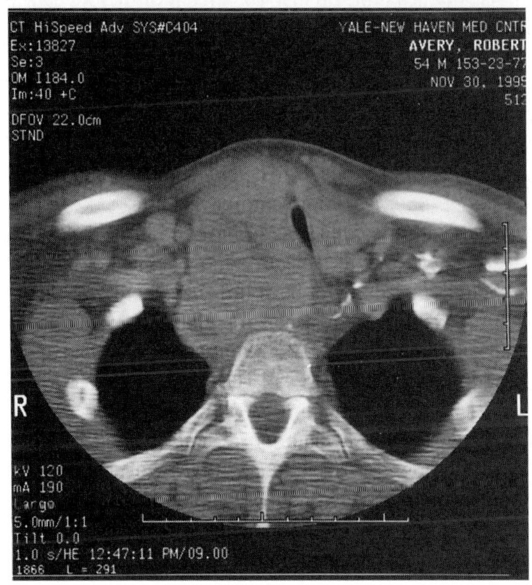

C

FIGURE 10-8. Substernal Goiter
A. Nodularity of gland and tracheal deviation in neck
B. Posterior extension of goiter and tracheal deviation at clavicular heads
C. Maximal compression of trachea at thoracic inlet

nerable in this setting.[87] Even very large intrathoracic goiters can be coaxed out of the mediastinum, although rarely a goiter must be removed piecemeal ("morcellization"). Tracheomalacia can be detected intraoperatively and provisions for more prolonged intubation for 24 to 48 hours or very rarely, tracheostomy, instituted. In most series tracheomalacia is extremely rare, even in patients with longstanding, circumferential goiters. Postoperative mortality is close to zero as are instances of hypoparathyroidism and vocal cord paresis; these procedures are well tolerated even by the infirm elderly and afford often dramatic improvement in symptoms related to obstruction of the aerodigestive systems.

SOLITARY THYROID NODULES

Although the risk of thyroid carcinoma does not appear to be increased in patients with a multinodular goiter without a dominant nodule, the risk is increased with a solitary thyroid nodule. In a series of 300 unselected autopsies of adults, 19 single thyroid nodules (6 percent) were found after sectioning of the gland.[66] The chance that a solitary thyroid nodule in this series would be a benign or malignant neoplasm was almost three times higher than was the case with a multinodular goiter. The frequency of thyroid carcinoma in single nodules was almost four times the frequency in the entire series of unselected thyroid glands. Thus, despite the difficulty in separating single from multiple thyroid nodules clinically, thyroid cancer has been found more frequently in a solitary thyroid nodule. Because thyroid carcinoma usually does not concentrate radioiodine as well as normal tissues does, malignant thyroid nodules commonly appear as hypofunctioning or nonfunctioning ("cold") areas on a radioactive iodine scan of the thyroid gland.[88] However, it must be emphasized that thyroid carcinoma also occurs in functioning nodules and that most benign nodules are also "cold" on scan. In a series of 202 patients with solitary thyroid nodules, there was an overall prevalence of thyroid carcinoma of 29 percent.[89] If cold solitary thyroid nodules had been the sole criterion for selection for surgery, 40 percent of the carcinomas would have been missed.

Factors Predisposing to Thyroid Cancer

If there is an increased risk of malignancy in solitary cold thyroid nodules, are there criteria available to select patients who are at higher risk?

Gender

As was mentioned earlier, most forms of thyroid disease are more common in females; this is true of thyroid malignancy as well. However, females have a higher incidence of nontoxic nodular goiter than males do. As a consequence, a solitary thyroid nodule occurring in a male is three times more likely to be malignant than is a solitary nodule occurring in a female.

Age

Epidemiologic studies indicate that 10 percent of thyroid cancers occur in patients under 21 years of age and represent approximately 1.5–2 percent of all pediatric malignancies.[90] The overall incidence of thyroid nodules in 5,179 children aged 11–18 years was reported by Rallison in 1975 to be around 1.8 percent. The nodularity represented adolescent goiter in 34 children and thyroiditis in 31. Only two thyroid cancers were found, which raised the question whether all thyroid nodules in children should be removed surgically. The risk of malignancy in childhood thyroid nodules has declined from 70 percent in the 1950s to around 20 percent between 1963 and 1990 coincident with the discontinuation of radiation treatment of benign conditions in this age group (see later discussion).[91]

Although the current recommendation is that all cold nodules in children should be removed, more widespread use of fine needle aspiration biopsy may permit more selective surgery, particularly in patients without a history of radiation. In a multicenter study evaluating FNAB in children by Raab et al,[92] the incidence of carcinoma was found to be 18 percent. Nodules that proved to be neoplasms were usually discrete, solitary, and of firm consistency and were not associated with changes in the rest of the thyroid.

Previous Irradiation of the Head and Neck

Previous irradiation of the head and neck markedly increases the chances of malignancy in a thyroid nodule. The observation in 1950 that 9 of 28 children with carcinoma of the thyroid had received radiotherapy to the thymus in infancy first highlighted this association, which was confirmed in prospective studies.[93,94] Most instances of thyroid malignancy after neck irradiation were reported within 10 years after radiation therapy. However, follow-up studies indicate a continuing increased incidence of thyroid nodules and carcinoma in individuals 25 years or more after radiation exposure of the head and neck[95,96] Thus, although irradiation therapy for benign diseases of infancy and childhood was discontinued many years ago, radiation-associated thyroid carcinoma continues to occur following therapy for malignancy and after environmental exposure. The risk of malignancy varies directly with radiation dose and inversely with the age at exposure.[97]

There is a linear relation between the dose of radiation to the thyroid and the incidence of thyroid cancer without a clear threshold up to about 1,000 rads (Fig. 10-9). Whether the relation remains linear at very low doses and at high doses is not clear.

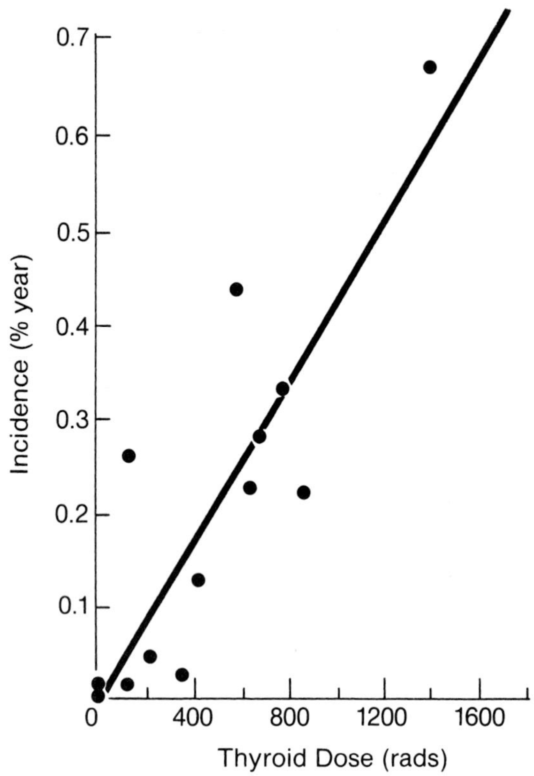

FIGURE 10-9. Incidence of thyroid cancer as a function of the dose of external radiation. (*After Maxon HR, et al.*[98])

When data from several studies were combined, the absolute risk for thyroid cancers was found to be 1.5 cases per million patients per rad per year.[98,99] Doses of external radiation as low as 50 rad have been associated with an increased risk of thyroid carcinoma, and it is likely that any amount of radiation represents an increased risk. Because low doses of radiation may induce thyroid carcinoma, the use of ^{131}I for routine thyroid scans should be discouraged. On the other hand, therapeutic doses of ^{131}I given for hyperthyroidism result in the delivery of 5,000 to 8,000 rad to the thyroid and have not been associated with the subsequent development of thyroid carcinoma.[100] The failure of therapeutic doses of ^{131}I to result in an increased risk for thyroid carcinoma may be due to destruction of thyroid cells or by the slow radiation dose rate which might provide time for repair mechanisms to work.

Considerable information about the effects of environmental exposure has been derived from the effects of the Chernobyl accident in the former USSR. Four years after the event, a dramatic increase in the frequency of thyroid cancer in children was noted in Belarus with 424 new cases diagnosed between 1986 and 1995.[28] The incidence of pediatric thyroid carcinomas was proportional to the level of radioiodine contamination in particular areas. The mechanism of age-related susceptibility to radiation-associated thyroid carcinoma is unknown, but may relate to the relatively larger dose received by the pediatric population. Histologically, more than 95 percent of the tumors have been papillary carcinomas and have been associated with a high prevalence of solid pattern growth and with a ret/PTC3 gene rearrangement. Characteristically, radiation-associated thyroid carcinoma is multicentric. In one series, multicentric thyroid cancer was found in 55 percent of operated cases compared with 22 percent in nonirradiated controls.[101]

Despite direct questioning, few patients with a thyroid nodule were able to give a history of irradiation during infancy. Public awareness increased dramatically after the relation was featured in a television drama. This increased awareness was largely due to the fact that mothers are more knowledgeable than their children about medical history. (Perhaps all patients, regardless of age, should bring their mothers with them for the initial visit to the physician's office!)

The most appropriate approach to the clinical surveillance of the irradiated thyroid is controversial. Laboratory studies have not been useful in general, although TSH should be measured, particularly in patients who have received high-dose radiation treatment for head and neck malignancies and Hodgkin's disease to rule out hypothyroidism. Because hyperparathyroidism also occurs with increased frequency in patients with a prior history of radiation treatment, a fasting serum calcium should be obtained. As an elevated serum thyroglobulin is associated with an increased incidence of thyroid nodules in irradiated patients, thyroglobulin determination, in the absence of interfering antithyroglobulin antibodies, may identify patients who require closer follow-up. Antithyroid antibodies are frequently elevated in patients who have had radiation exposure, but do not predict the occurrence of malignancy or neoplasia. Measurement of calcitonin is not indicated as there is no increase in the incidence of medullary thyroid cancer in irradiated patients.

The role of imaging studies in the routine follow-up of patients exposed to radiation is controversial, particularly in a patient with a clinically normal physical examination. The use of ultrasound in follow-up of such patients may reveal abnormalities of questionable clinical significance. In a recent study half of the nodules 1.5 cm or larger seen on routine ultrasonography were not palpable and 25 percent of those 1 cm or larger were not visualized by nuclear scan.[96]

Similarly, the use of thyroid hormone replacement in irradiated individuals either to prevent the development of nodular disease or to decrease postoperative recurrence of thyroid nodules continues to be debated. Existing evidence, however, suggests that recurrence of benign nodular disease in the irradiated patient after thyroid surgery is decreased by at least 25 percent by administration of thyroid hormone and is inversely related to the extent of thyroid resection.[102] The occurrence of malignant disease in this study was not influenced by thyroid hormone suppression, and thus new nodules in the remaining lobe in a patient receiving hormone replacement are suspicious for carcinoma. The use of FNA in the selection of patients for surgery is of less utility in this group due to the fact that carcinoma when found in the irradiated thyroid is frequently elsewhere in the gland other than in the clinically evident nodule. Given these data, it may be reasonable to consider near total thyroidectomy rather than lobectomy alone in individuals presenting with significant new or enlarging nodular disease, particularly if they are receiving thyroid hormone. In experienced hands near total thyroidectomy is a safe and effective means of treatment and prophylaxis for radiation-associated thyroid carcinoma, permits pathologic analysis of all the thyroid tissue, simplifies clinical follow-up, and permits the administration of replacement rather than suppressive doses of thyroid hormone.

Evaluation of the Thyroid Nodule

Physical Characteristics

Clinical history and physical examination of the thyroid can be extremely helpful in determining the likelihood of malignancy. Local symptoms such as dysphagia, dyspnea, or changes in voice quality should make the examiner suspicious of malignancy. Rapid growth of a nodule, particularly if painful, is usually due to hemorrhage into a benign adenoma and is not a hallmark of a thyroid malignancy.

Palpation of the thyroid should be done with particular attention to how regular and hard the nodule is, whether it is solitary, fixed to surrounding structures, or associated with palpable regional lymph nodes.The most important physical sign of thyroid malignancy is the presence of a hard, irregular thyroid nodule. Extreme hardness may be due to hemorrhage into a cyst with subsequent calcification. If the thyroid cancer has spread beyond the capsule and invaded surrounding structures, fixation to the strap muscles, trachea, or larynx may be easily detected on physical examination. Involvement of the recurrent laryngeal nerve by tumor may result in hoarseness. Some benign conditions may mimic the clinical presentation of thyroid cancer. Riedel's struma (see Chap. 9) can also extend beyond the gland and appear fixed to surrounding tissues, and the thyroid affected by Hashimoto's thyroiditis is characteristically indurated and often irregular.

In one study, a group of 53 patients with thyroid nodules were first classified clinically as to whether their nodules were benign or malignant, and these results were compared with the findings at surgery.[103] Thyroid cancer was found in 76 percent of cases thought to be malignant nodules clinically and in 12 percent of cases thought to be benign clinically but symptomatic as indicated by pain, recent change in goiter size, or dysphagia. Underscoring the reliability of the clinical signs of malignancy, carcinoma was found in only 3 percent of patients whose nodules were thought to be benign and who were asymptomatic.

Laboratory Diagnosis

The presence of a solitary thyroid nodule raises the question of thyroid malignancy, and the predisposing factors discussed above may strengthen or allay suspicions about an individual patient. The next step in the evaluation of a solitary thyroid nodule is to use the laboratory to further discriminate which nodules may be malignant and which may be benign. Most patients with thyroid nodules and thyroid carcinoma are euthyroid; measurement of the TSH will identify the patient with hyperthyroidism due to a functioning adenoma or the patient with diffuse Hashimoto's thyroiditis and hypothyroidism. Determination of thyroglobulin and calcitonin levels are not useful in the initial evaluation of the patient with a thyroid nodule unless other risk factors such as a family history which includes medullary carcinoma or a physical exam consistent with well-differentiated carcinoma are present.

Fine Needle Aspiration Cytology (FNA)

Although various diagnostic procedures may heighten suspicion that a particular solitary thyroid nodule is malignant, only a tissue diagnosis can ultimately diagnose or exclude thyroid cancer. In recent years fine needle aspiration biopsy of thyroid nodules for cytologic evaluation has emerged as the most sensitive and specific diagnostic test for thyroid malignancies. Although there are special thyroid biopsy sets, a 10-ml syringe with a 22- to 25-gauge needle works well. After the patient is reclining with a pillow under the shoulders to hyperextend the neck, the nodule is palpated and the area is prepped with alcohol. Local anesthesia is usually not required. The needle is inserted and moved back and forth within the nodule while maintaining gentle vacuum in the syringe. At the first evidence of blood in the needle hub, suction is released and the syringe and needle withdrawn, taking care not to allow the aspirate contents to enter the needle hub. The aspirate is placed on a frosted glass slide, and the two slides are "pulled." It is usually possible to identify the presence of cellular contents on the slide at this point. Slides are placed immediately into 95 percent alcohol and sent for cytologic interpretation. The syringe is rinsed with 75 percent ethanol, which is then processed for cell block. The key issues in FNA diagnosis are obtaining an adequate specimen and the expertise of the cytopathologist.

Results of FNA are characterized as satisfactory in 85 to 90 percent of cases and unsatisfactory in the remainder. Diagnostic categories are "benign," "malignant," and "suspicious" or "indeterminate." Aspiration cytology of a benign nodule will reveal bland follicular cells, hemosiderin-laden macrophages, and admixed small lymphocytes typical of a degenerative process. Many benign nodules (but some papillary carcinomas) have a substantial cystic component, which makes obtaining an adequate cellular sample difficult. Performing FNA under ultrasound guidance in these cases will enhance the chances of retrieving a representative cellular specimen.[104] A skilled cytopathologist can usually identify the characteristic nuclear features of papillary carcinoma such as nuclear grooves or intranuclear cytoplasmic inclusions. Colloid is often scant or absent, but when present may have a smeared appearance termed "bubble-gum."[105] Psamomma bodies and papillary structures may also be seen (Fig. 10-10). The cells of medullary thyroid cancer have a characteristic plasmacytoid appearance and can be immunostained for the presence of calcitonin if clinical suspicion dictates. Thyroid lymphoma and anaplastic carcinoma are more common in older patients and present in a similar manner with the history of rapid growth of a thyroid nodule and often accompanying subjective respiratory compromise and stridor. Prompt differential diagnosis is critical here as immediate chemotherapy is rapidly beneficial in the case of lymphoma, whereas surgery is usually required to establish an adequate airway in the patient with anaplastic carcinoma. Fortunately the cytologic data can resolve this diagnostic dilemma and can also differentiate large cell from lymphoplasmacytic type lymphomas, though the latter may require additional studies to subtype. A major limitation in the usefulness of FNA is in the management of follicular neoplasms. The cells comprising follicular adenomas and carcinomas rarely have distinctive cytologic features, and the final differential diagnosis depends upon the identification of capsular or vascular invasion of surrounding normal thyroid on permanent section assessment of the resected lobe containing the nodule. When a cytologic diagnosis of follicular neoplasm has been rendered, a thyroid scan (described later) may be useful, as a warm or hot nodule is much less likely to be malignant.

FIGURE 10-10. A fine-needle biopsy aspirate of papillary carcinoma of the thyroid, demonstrating papillary configuration.

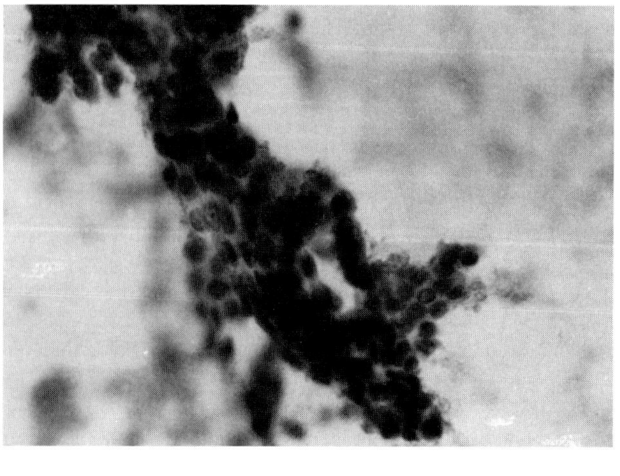

A recent summary of 7 large series of FNA biopsies by Gharib and Goellner reported that the sensitivity of FNA varies from 65 to 98 percent (mean 83 percent) with a specificity of 72 to 100 percent (mean 92 percent).[106]

Several studies have indicated that the use of FNA to identify thyroid lesions that can be safely followed clinically has reduced purely diagnostic thyroid surgery by 50 percent and increased the yield of thyroid cancers removed at surgery twofold.[107] If an adequate cytological specimen has been obtained and there has been no clinical change in the nodule, repeated FNA exams have not been found to contribute additional management information.[107] Nodules that increase in size during the clinical followup period, those in which the initial biopsy was nondiagnostic, or those that are clinically suspicious but benign cytologically should be reaspirated.[108] Despite early concerns about the theoretical risk of needle tracking of tumor, FNA has been shown to be safe, accurate, and cost-effective as the initial step in the evaluation of thyroid nodular disease in more than 15,000 biopsies at one institution.[108]

Ultrasound

Ultrasound using high resolution (5–10 MHz) transducers has largely replaced scintigraphy as the primary imaging modality in the evaluation of thyroid nodules. Because of the different acoustic properties of fluid and solid matter, ultrasound is particularly useful in differentiating cystic and solid nodules. Ultrasound can resolve cystic structures of 2 mm diameter and solid nodules of 3–4 mm.[109] True cysts of the thyroid are rare, perhaps 1 percent of all thyroid lesions. Most cystic lesions are degenerating thyroid adenomas or colloid nodules, but 0.5–3 percent of carcinomas may be predominately cystic.[110] Ultrasound permits accurate evaluation of nodule size and volume for future follow-up and identifies other nodular disease within the gland. Ultrasound differentiates intra- from extrathyroidal masses and permits accurate fine needle aspiration of non palpable and partially cystic lesions (Fig. 10-11). Although the typical ultrasound features of a benign thyroid nodule include a large cystic component with a peripheral sonolucent halo, peripheral calcification, and a hyperechoic texture,[111] malignant tumors have been less frequently found to exhibit these features. More typically the malignant thyroid nodule is an irregular, poorly defined solid mass that is hypoechoic.

Ultrasound may be used to guide nonsurgical treatment of thyroid cysts. Successful sclerosis of a recurrent thyroid cyst with injected tetracycline has been reported but is not indicated in the great majority of cases.[112] Retrotracheal and retrosternal lesions cannot be adequately assessed by ultrasound.

Radioisotopic Scan of the Thyroid

Scintigraphy of the thyroid after the administration of a tracer dose of radioactive iodine or technetium 99m is the standard method for functional imaging of the thyroid. Nodules may have

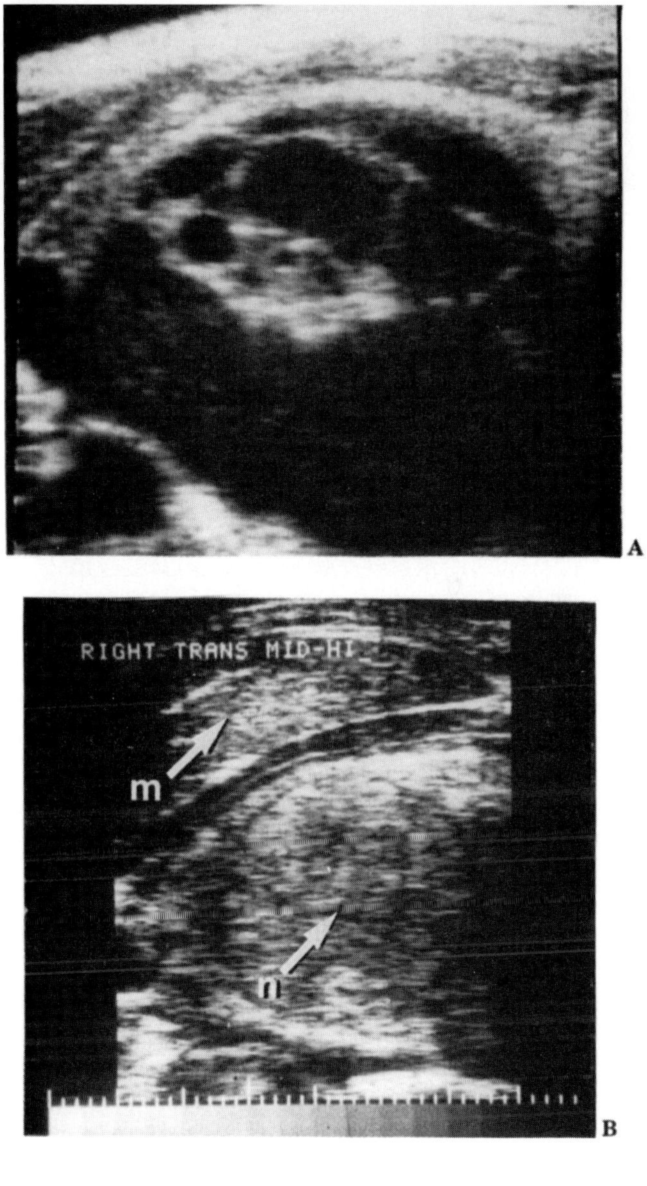

FIGURE 10-11. (*A*) A transverse ultrasound scan of the thyroid showing a 2-cm mass which has numerous septations and a mixture of cystic and solid elements. (*B*) A transverse ultrasound scan of the right lobe of the thyroid. Arrow n indicates a solid nodule that is well defined by its echo-free capsule. Arrow m indicates the sternocleidomastoid muscle. (*Reprinted from Chapter 11, Endocrinology and Metabolism, 3rd edition, Fig. 11-8.*)

decreased (cold) (Fig. 10-12), similar (warm) or increased (hot) uptake compared to surrounding normal thyroid tissue. Because even well-differentiated thyroid carcinomas do not concentrate these isotopes as efficiently as the normal thyroid does, relatively hypofunctioning thyroid nodules have been considered to carry a greater risk of malignancy. However, the majority of clinically significant thyroid nodules, benign or malignant, are less functional than the extranodular thyroid tissue.[113]

Nodules may be nonvisualized because they have the same uptake as the surrounding tissue, are too small to be seen, or despite being hypofunctional, overlie an area of normal tissue. The demonstration of a cold thyroid nodule is thus significant but nonspecific. Both iodine and technetium isotopes are used for functional imaging of the thyroid. Iodine is more physiologic as it is both trapped and organified by the thyroid. Iodine 131 has been the radionuclide most widely used for thyroid imaging. ^{131}I decays to release a medium energy β-particle and a high-energy gamma ray. The energy of the gamma ray is less suitable for imaging than that of ^{123}I, but the β-particle emission and longer half-life permits use of the isotope for treatment. Radiation exposure attendant on ^{131}I imaging has prompted given information on the delayed effects of neck irradiation on thyroid neoplasia.[114] The administration of 100 Ci of ^{131}I for a thyroid scan can result in a dose of 80 rads to the thyroid.[115] Because several scans will raise the dose of radiation delivered to the thyroid to a level which has been associated with subsequent thyroid cancer, alternative methods of thyroid imaging are highly desirable.

Iodine 123 is perhaps the ideal isotope for in vivo diagnostic studies of thyroid function and structure. It emits gamma of a single energy and has excellent imaging characteristics. Its short half-life of 13.3 h is suitable for routine uptake tests. Scans superior in resolution to those afforded by 99mTc or ^{131}I can be obtained with a radiation dose 1/85 that for a comparable ^{131}I study. On the other hand, the short half-life, the necessity for cyclotron production, and its relative expense limit the use of ^{123}I for imaging.

Technetium 99m is probably the most readily available isotope of choice for thyroid scanning at present. Technetium 99m

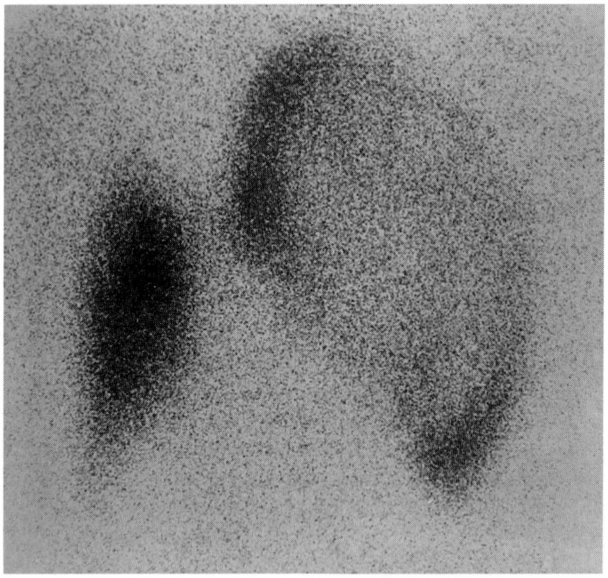

FIGURE 10-12. A radioisotopic scan shows a nonfunctioning solitary nodule in the lower pole of the right lobe of the thyroid.

delivers about 0.6 rad to the thyroid during a scanning procedure. Because the pertechnetate ion (99mTc04) is rapidly trapped by the thyroid but is not organically bound, some nodules present a discordant image, being warm on technetium but cold on iodine scan due to a defect in organification. Such nodules may have an increased risk of malignancy.[116]

The findings in most studies have been consistent with the physiologic considerations discussed earlier. Most thyroid cancers were found to be cold, but benign thyroid nodules are also predominantly cold. This lack of discrimination makes it difficult to use a thyroid scan to differentiate between benign and malignant thyroid nodules.[117] Certainly no patient with a solitary thyroid nodule should be either selected for surgery or screened from surgical consideration by a thyroid scan, although the scan can be helpful in eliminating the minority of solitary nodules with increased radioisotope uptake from serious consideration of malignancy.

Other Imaging Techniques

Thyroid imaging techniques other than radioisotopic scan and ultrasound are available, but are rarely used in the initial evaluation of thyroid nodular disease. The high Z number (i.e., radiographic density) of the thyroid has facilitated the use of the CT scan with or without prior loading with stable iodine.[111] CT and MRI are less sensitive than ultrasound in the identification of intrathyroidal nodular disease, but are superior in the assessment of mediastinal thyroid extension and in the evaluation of potential airway involvement. CT with contrast and especially MRI are useful in determining preoperatively the extent of thyroid carcinoma and in identifying nodal involvement.[109] In this setting the use of MRI is appropriate in that it avoids the use of contrast materials that will compromise use of ^{131}I treatment in the short term.

Management of a Solitary Thyroid Nodule

The results of the various diagnostic techniques for assessing the likelihood of cancer in thyroid nodular disease can be expressed according to Bayes' theorem to give the predictive value of a positive test (Fig. 10-13).[118] In this analysis, three strategies were studied for the diagnosis of thyroid nodules. Two began with a radioisotopic thyroid scan, followed, if the scan was positive, by either aspirate biopsy or ultrasound; the third began with aspiration biopsy followed by a scan.[118] The last strategy was the most cost-effective. Fine-needle aspiration biopsy was the most successful of the available tests when applied alone. Neither radioisotopic scan of the thyroid nor ultrasound has high specificity. Combining the two procedures yields the highest sensitivity but does not improve specificity.

A decision tree for management is outlined in Fig. 10-14. Solitary thyroid nodules occurring in children, in patients with prior radiation treatment to the head and neck, clinically malignant nodules, and those resulting in a suspicious or positive FNA should undergo surgical resection.

Thyroid Hormone Suppression

If the clinical evaluation including fine needle aspiration biopsy is consistent with a benign process, a trial of thyroid hormone may be undertaken. The rationale for thyroid suppressive therapy is that TSH is the primary regulator of thyroid growth and

FIGURE 10-13. Probability of disease based on test results calculated according to Bayes' theorem. Open bars represent missed malignancies; solid bars represent the percentage of surgeries in which malignancies were found. (*Modified from Van Herle AJ, et al.*[118])

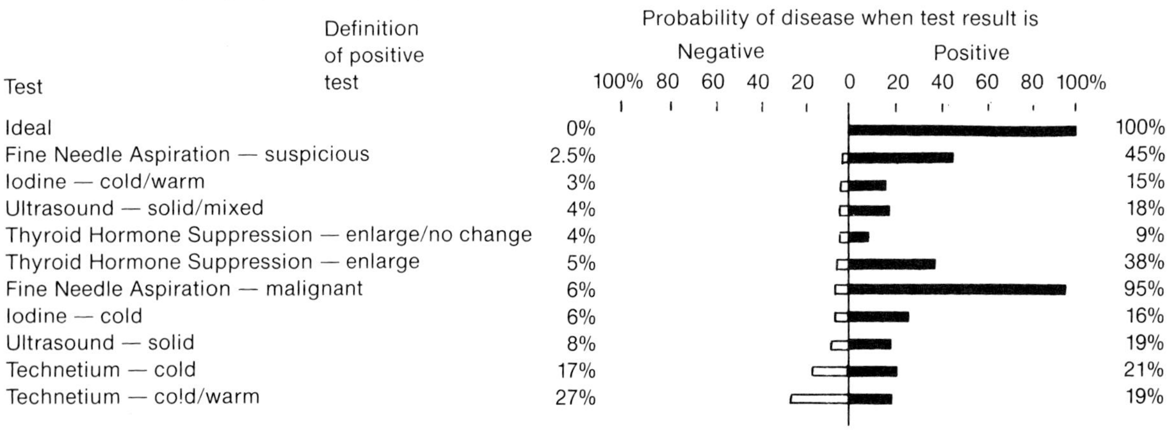

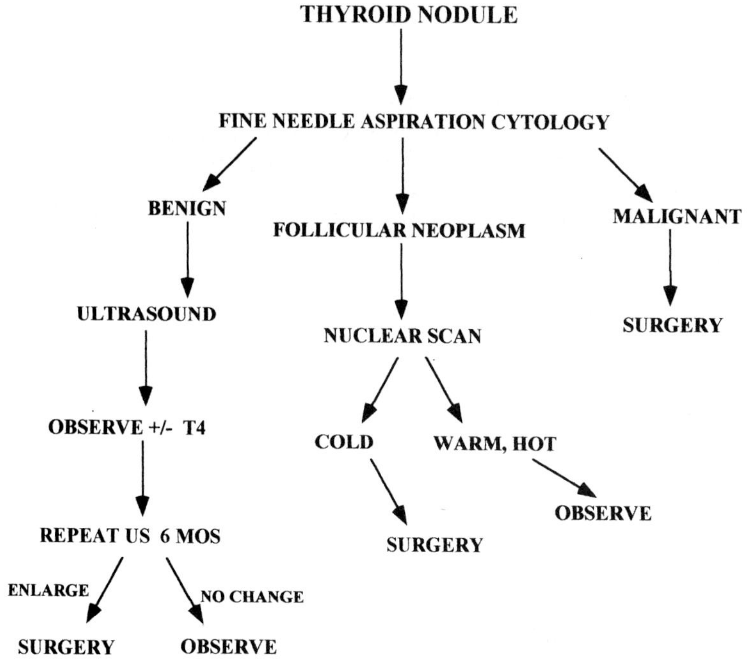

FIGURE 10-14. Management of a solitary thyroid nodule.

that in its absence nodules with physiologic characteristics (i.e, benign) will tend to regress. Despite evidence from uncontrolled studies in the 1950s and 60s that this treatment was effective, recent prospective controlled randomized trials have not conclusively supported the use of thyroid hormone to suppress nodular disease[82,119–121] (Table 10-5). However, a 5-year trial comparing levothyroxine treatment versus nontreatment of benign cold nodules showed that although TSH suppression resulted in volume reduction in only a subgroup of nodules, it did prevent the appearance of new lesions.[122] In this study nodule reduction was seen more frequently in patients with TSH levels constantly suppressed below 0.1 mU/L than in those with incomplete suppression. On the other hand, data from Kuma et al indicated that in patients with cytologically benign nodules followed over a decade without treatment, 43 percent of nodules decreased in size, 23 percent increased, and 33 percent remained stable.[123] Thus it seems that most benign nodules do not enlarge.

Given the lack of demonstrable efficacy of thyroid hormone in suppressing the growth of thyroid nodules, what are the risks of treatment? A metaanalysis of reports published between 1982 and 1994 on the effects of long-term thyroid hormone on bone density revealed decreases from 5 to 9 percent at the lumbar spine, the proximal femur, and the radius in postmenopausal women.[83] No effect was seen in men or in premenopausal women and the negative effect on bone density could be ameliorated by estrogen replacement.[124]

A threefold increased risk of atrial fibrillation has been reported in patients on thyroid hormone over the age of 60 who have a low TSH level.[84] Other studies have not clearly shown that appropriate thyroid hormone administration is associated with cardiac dysfunction.[82]

On balance, it appears difficult to justify routine or prolonged hormone suppression for all thyroid nodules. At least, when hormone treatment is elected, it should be prescribed for a definite period of time with a specific therapeutic goal.

Although there is debate about the duration of the treatment period, a trial of at least 6 months of thyroid hormone seems reasonable. If the nodule remains unchanged or shrinks, as measured by comparison of a baseline and 6-month follow-up thyroid ultrasound, suppression may be either discontinued or continued for

TABLE 10-5. Thyroxine Therapy for Benign, Solitary Thyroid Nodules: Results in Five Randomized Prospective Trials

				*% Pts with Shrinkage**		*% Pts with Growth†*	
Author	No. Patients	Duration (months)	Assessment	Rx	Control	Rx	Control
Gharib	53	6	Ultrasound	14	20	NA	NA
Reverter	40	11	Ultrasound	20	15	NA	NA
Papini	101	12	Ultrasound	20	6	14	22
La Rosa	45	12	Ultrasound	39	0	0	14
Cheung	75	18	Palpation	38	35	8	17

*Nodule shrinkage defined as >50% decrease in nodule volume

†Nodule growth defined as >50% increase in nodule volume

Source: Hermus AR, Huysmans DA. Treatment of benign nodular thyroid disease. *N Engl J Med*, 338:1441, 1998.

some defined period. Permanent suppressive therapy of presumed benign thyroid nodules is probably unwise in elderly and primarily female population, given the potential long-term skeletal and cardiac effects of thyroid hormone discussed earlier.

If the nodule enlarges during suppressive therapy, surgery is indicated. Very rarely a patient may be such a prohibitive operative risk that consideration should be given to treatment of a cold benign nodule by percutaneous ethanol injection.[125]

THYROID CARCINOMA

The biological behavior of thyroid cancer may vary markedly. Minimal papillary thyroid carcinoma is considered to have a negligible biological risk, while anaplastic carcinoma of the thyroid is one of the most malignant human tumors.

Histologic Classification

Nearly all thyroid tumors arise from the follicular or parafollicular cells. These epithelial tumors of the thyroid are shown in the classification system in Table 10-6. Thyroid carcinoma may be follicular, forming recognizable thyroid follicles, or these follicular cells may form papillary structures, either pure or mixed with follicles. Tumors of follicular cell origin may also exhibit oncocytic, clear, squamous, or mucinous features.[105] Alternatively, the follicular cells may be largely undifferentiated and appear as giant spindle cells or small cells. The higher the grade of follicular cell tumors, the less important become other classification categories such as papillary or follicular characterization. Carcinomas arising from parafollicular cells have different histologic subtypes, but these types have no definite clinical significance; all are called medullary. Classification based on the histology of the tumor does have biological significance. In a 5- to 30-year follow-up, 11 percent of patients with papillary carcinoma died of the disease, compared with 25 percent of patients with follicular carcinoma, 50 percent of patients with sporadic medullary carcinoma, and 90 percent of patients with undifferentiated carcinoma.

TABLE 10-6. Classification of Thyroid Tumors

- Primary tumors
  - Epithelial tumors
    - Tumors of follicular cells
      - Benign: Follicular adenoma
        - Conventional
        - Variants
      - Malignant: Carcinoma
        - Differentiated
          - Follicular carcinoma
          - Papillary carcinoma
        - Poorly differentiated
          - Insular carcinoma
          - Others
        - Undifferentiated
  - Tumors of C (and related neuroendocrine) cells
    - Medullary carcinoma
    - Others
  - Tumors of follicular and C cells
- Sarcomas
- Malignant lymphoma (and related hemotopoietic neoplasms)
- Miscellaneous
- Secondary tumors

Source: Rosai J, Carcangiu ML, DeLellis RA: *AFIP Fascicle Electronic Version* 2. Armed Forces Institute of Pathology, Washington DC, 1995.

TABLE 10-7. AJCC Stage Groupings for Thyroid Carcinoma

Stage	Papillary or (age <45)	Follicular (age >45)	Medullary (any age)	Anaplastic (any age)
I	MO	T1	T1	—
II	M1	T2–T3	T2–T4	—
III	—	T4 or N1	N1	—
IV	—	M1	M1	Any

Source: Beahrs, et al.[132]

Clinical Staging

Thyroid carcinoma may also be classified in regard to biological behavior. Papillary thyroid cancers occur in all age groups and tend to metastasize to lymph nodes, follicular carcinomas tend to have blood-borne metastases and occur in older age groups, and undifferentiated thyroid cancers occur predominantly in older patients and usually kill by local invasion. Although at present there is no completely satisfactory system for staging thyroid cancer (Table 10-7), certain pathologic characteristics relate to therapy and prognosis. The following prognostic factors for papillary and follicular thyroid carcinomas are thought to be of importance: (1) histologic type, (2) age of patient, (3) extent of primary tumor, (4) distant metastases, (5) size of tumor, (6) blood vessel invasion, (7) presence of multiple foci, and (8) gender of patient.[126] In particular, age, size, and invasiveness of tumor (Fig. 10-15) though not nodal involvement (Fig. 10-16) have been shown to be predictive of outcome in well-differentiated thyroid carcinoma.[127] Clinical staging of thyroid carcinoma has also been attempted. At least 10 scoring systems have been promoted in an effort to identify clinical characteristics which predict prognosis. These include the AGES system (age, grade, extent, size) and MACIS (metastasis, age, competeness of resection, invasion, and size),[128] AMES (age, metastases, extent, size)[129,130] EORTC from European Thyroid Cancer Cooperative Group),[131] the TMN classifcation from the American Joint Committee on Cancer,[132] the Ohio system of Mazzaferri and Zhiang,[133] clinical classification of DeGroot,[134] and those of Noguchi,[135] Shaha,[136] Asklen,[137] and Brierley.[138] Comparison of these staging systems indicates that they are essentially equivalent in identifying a low risk group (approximately 85 percent of patients) with an excellent outcome regardless of treatment and a high risk group (15 percent of patients) whose tumors are likely to follow a more aggressive course (Fig. 10-17).[138,127]

Molecular Biology of Thyroid Neoplasms

In addition to the clinical staging systems currently utilized, molecular biological techniques are being brought to bear on understanding the pathogenesis and predicting outcome of thyroid tumors. Nuclear DNA content as measured by flow cytometry has been used as a prognostic factor,[139] with nondiploid tumors associated with a higher risk of mortality. In general these more aggressive tumors could be predicted by application of the above staging systems.[139–141]

The recognition that cancer occurs as a result of mutations that affect the structural integrity of genes involved in the regulation of

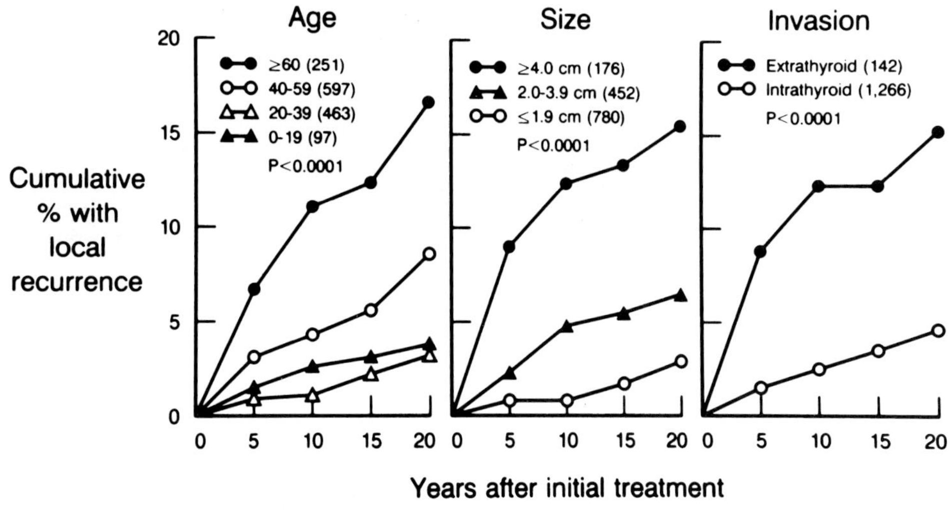

FIGURE 10-15. Cumulative risk of local recurrence in papillary carcinoma as a function of age of patient and size and invasiveness of tumor. Data from 1,408 patients. (*From Hay ID.*[127])

cell growth or differentiation has had a profound influence on the way we view the disease and offers new strategies for treatment. In the development of both benign and malignant thyroid neoplasms, a series of mutational events is believed to take place, each leading to a clonal expansion of genetically modified cells. The genes subject to mutations in cancer can be classified as oncogenes or tumor suppressor genes based on their mechanism of action. Some mutational changes leading to the development of cancer are inherited through the germline, but most are acquired or somatic in nature. Early genetic events in oncogenesis are characteristically seen in both benign and malignant tumors.

Two sites susceptible to mutation important in early oncogenesis are the TSH receptor and the ras oncogene. The adenyl cyclase/protein kinase A pathway regulated via Gs• by the TSH receptor is important for differentiated thyroid cell function and growth. Mutations of Gs• have been described in autonomous thyroid nodules and appear to be characteristic of benign as opposed to malignant thyroid tumors. TSH receptor mutations have been described in both benign tumors[142] and differentiated thyroid cancers.[143] Ras is a GTPase that regulates the interaction between tyrosine kinase receptors and a cascade of protein kinases that result in the induction of transcription factors. Activating mutations of Ras result in the unregulated growth characteristic of carcinomas. All three Ras genes have been shown to be targets of point mutations in thyroid tumors. The mutations were found primarily in H- and N-ras, in follicular neoplasms both benign and malignant, especially in those from iodine deficient regions. Ras mutations in papillary carcinomas appear to occur late in tumorigenesis.[144] Activation or overexpression of three tyrosine kinase receptors (RET, TRK, and MET) have been identified in papillary thyroid cancers. At least five types of RET rearrangements have been found in human thyroid cancer, each transposing a cellular gene adjacent to the tyrosine kinase domain of RET. Termed RET/PTC 1-5, these rearrangements have been described in up to 45 percent of papillary thyroid cancers depending on geographic location.[142,145] Other thyroid cancers and benign lesions do not express RET.[146] The

FIGURE 10-16. Lack of influence of nodal status at initial operation on cumulative mortality from papillary thyroid cancer in 1,277 patients with intrathyroidal tumors and 191 patients with locally invasive (extrathyroidal) tumors with and without distant metastases (DM). (*From Hay ID.*[127])

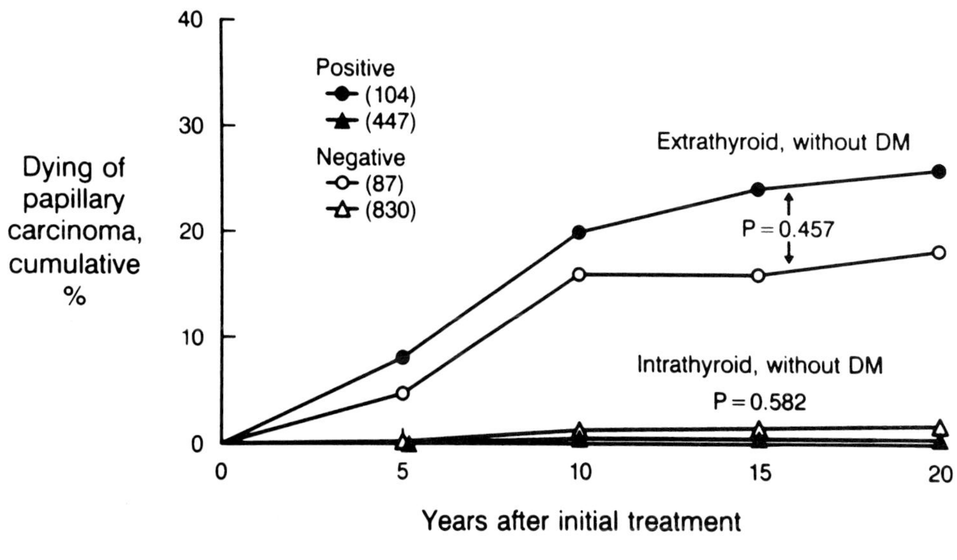

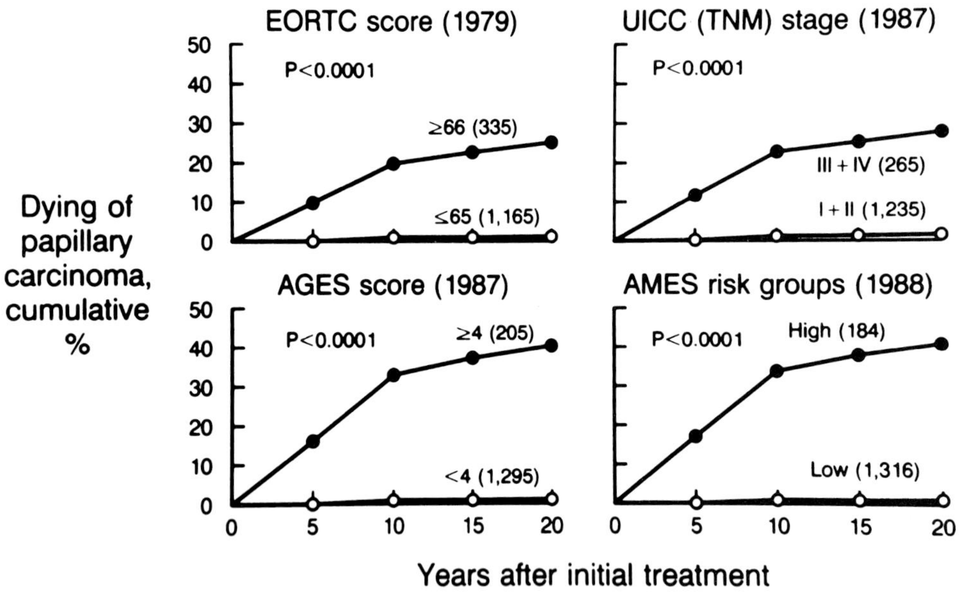

FIGURE 10-17. Cumulative mortality from papillary carcinoma in 1,500 patients in low- and high-risk groups defined by different scoring systems. (*From Hay ID.*[127])

presence of RET rearrangements in occult thyroid carcinomas support the concept that these mutations occur early in the development of papillary carcinoma. Susceptibility to RET rearrangement may be genetically conferred, as in circumstances of p53 nonsense mutations or environmentally acquired as during exposure to radiation. Papillary carcinomas occurring in childhood are more likely to be associated with RET rearrangement than are those of adults. TRK oncogenes are created by rearrangement of the NTRK1 gene which encodes a receptor for nerve growth factor and is activated in 20 percent of papillary cancers. Like RET, it is seen more frequently in younger patients and in a setting of radiation exposure.[147–149] The MET oncogene is the receptor for hepatocyte growth factor, a paracrine mitogenic factor that stimulates cell motility, invasion, and morphogenesis. Not normally expressed in thyroid follicular cells, recent data suggest that MET overexpression may be specific for papillary carcinoma and may be correlated to multicentricity and, interestingly, negatively associated with angioinvasiveness.[150]

Rearrangement of the nuclear transcription factors c-myc and c-fos does not appear to play a role in the pathogenesis of thyroid tumors benign or malignant.

In addition to oncogene formation, loss of tumor suppressor gene function has also been identified in thyroid malignancies. Mutations of both retinoblastoma and P53 suppressors, regulators of the cell cycle, have been implicated in thyroid neoplastic development. In one study deletions of the Rb gene were found in 55 percent of malignant tumors but not in benign thyroid neoplasms,[151] and were particularly prominent in metastatic lesions. P53 is a transcription factor with many functions directed toward maintaining the integrity of the genome. Thus its effects are felt on cell cycle regulation, DNA repair, and initiation of apoptosis when cellular damage is irreparable. A number of types of mutations of P53 at a variety of codons have been described in malignant but not benign thyroid tumors. Mutations were more common in carcinomas with nodal metastases and in less differentiated neoplasms.[142,152] Different point mutations have been described in childhood papillary carcinoma occurring in the setting of radiation exposure than in those tumors found in children and adults without a history of radiation.[153] Mutations, deletions, and overexpression of several of the cyclins and cyclin inhibitors have been reported in thyroid tumors,[142,154] emphasizing the importance of cell cycle regulation abnormalities in the pathogenesis of thyroid neoplasms. Although the information is far from complete, evidence to date indicates distinct genetic pathways are involved in the development of papillary and follicular carcinomas. Less clear are which changes promote the progression from benign follicular adenoma to carcinoma. Recently Zhang et al. identified a smallest common deleted region (SCDR) which was found commonly in follicular carcinomas, rarely in adenomas and in none of the papillary carcinomas studied. They suggested that this area, 7q31.2, might be a tumor suppressor gene whose somatic inactivation is important for the transition to malignant neoplasm.[155] Molecular insights have begun to offer opportunities for the design of new treatment strategies (discussed later).

Specific Primary Thyroid Carcinomas

Papillary Carcinoma

Papillary carcinoma is the most common form of thyroid carcinoma, accounting for about 75 percent of clinically evident thyroid tumors in adults and 90 percent of carcinomas in children. Much of the confusion about the incidence of thyroid carcinoma is due to the presence of minimal papillary thyroid cancer, which can be defined as a tumor less than 1.5 cm in size. The prevalence of these small tumors has been reported to be as high as 28 percent in Japan and 13 percent in the United States.[156] Because the biological risk of minimal papillary carcinoma is probably negligible, these tumors rarely are a cause of death. As a consequence, they are responsible for the disparity between thyroid cancer as a cause of death and thyroid cancer prevalence in some surgical series. The reported prevalence varies widely because diagnosis is exquisitely sensitive to the method of pathologic examination of the thyroid gland. These thyroid tumors may be occult and hence not grossly visible; as many as 300–900 slides per gland must be prepared to avoid missing the smallest tumor. If all thyroids were studied in this manner, as many as 10–30 million North Americans might be found to have minimal papillary thyroid carcinoma.[156] The magnitude of this problem is overwhelming but, from the patient's point of view, probably biologically unimportant. Papillary carcinoma is three times more common in females than in males and represents the greater majority of thyroid cancers in childhood. Although papillary carcinoma has a better prognosis in women and children compared with men, overall fewer than 10 percent of patients die of papillary thyroid cancer in prolonged follow-up, and only 25 percent have a recurrence.[134] Papillary carcinoma diagnosed during pregnancy has the same favorable prognosis as that occurring in nonpregnant women of the same age; treatment can be safely delayed until after delivery even in the presence of cervical metastases.[157]

Histologically, papillary carcinoma is an often unencapsulated tumor exhibiting papillary and/or follicular structures with characteristic nuclear features such as grooves, intranuclear cytoplasmic inclusions, and clearing of nuclear chromatin resulting in a ground glass or "orphan annie eyes" appearance (Fig. 10-18). These distinctive nuclear features are well seen in paraffin embedded specimens and in cytologic preparations, but often not in frozen sections of the same material. The presence of a follicular pattern with colloid-filled vesicles does not alter the behavior of the tumor, which is still classified as papillary. Approximately 40 percent of cases of papillary carcinoma contain laminated calcific spherules called psammoma bodies. These bodies can sometimes be identified as finely stippled calcifications on a properly exposed x-ray of the neck.[158] Although not completely specific for papillary carcinoma, their presence in benign thyroid conditions is so unusual that the diagnosis of carcinoma must be suspected when they are identified in thyroid or nodal tissue. Psammoma bodies may also be seen in other tumors including those metastatic to the thyroid.[159] In most cases, particularly in younger patients, the tumor is slow-growing and usually of low-grade malignancy, which means that long follow-up periods are necessary.[127] Spread occurs characteristically to the cervical lymph nodes; patients may actually present with enlarged cervical nodes rather than with a mass in the thyroid. Such nodes often undergo cystic degeneration and may be mistaken for branchial cleft cysts on clinical and microscopic evaluation. Thyroglobulin staining of epithelial elements within the pathological specimen will clarify the diagnosis.[105] Interestingly, the presence of metastases to the cervical nodes seems to have little deleterious effect on mortality.[160,161] Vascular invasion occurs, though less commonly than with follicular carcinoma. Metastases to lung may present a miliary or nodular appearance on chest radiographs, but also may be revealed only on radioiodine scanning after thyroid ablation. Response of pulmonary metastases to ^{131}I is best in young patients and in those with normal chest radiographs. Multifocal involvement of the thyroid gland is a characteristic of papillary tumors. Debate exists as to whether this is intraglandular lymphatic spread or true neoplastic transformation of follicular cells or perhaps both. Recent studies of RET/PTC profiles in multifocal papillary thyroid carcinoma suggest that in most cases the individual tumors arise independently in a background of genetic susceptibility.[145] Extrathyroidal extension is one of the most important (except for dedifferentiation) morphologic signs of an aggressive tumor and is associated with a sixfold increase in mortality.[162] Papillary carcinomas may remain indolent for long periods even with widespread metastases or may have more aggressive properties. In the latter case, the progression is often associated with a change to a more malignant type of thyroid cancer.

Several variants of papillary carcinoma are associated with a more aggressive clinical course. One subtype, the tall cell variant, is so named because the cells covering the papillae are twice as tall as they are wide. Such tumors tend to occur in older patients, are larger, have more mitoses, and a more aggressive clinical course.[163] Another subtype of papillary carcinoma exhibiting more aggressive behavior is the columnar cell variant. Nuclei of cells in this tumor are stratified and may lack the usual features of papillary carcinoma.[105] The diffuse sclerosing subtype of papillary carcinoma is associated with an increased incidence of lymph node involvement and pulmonary metastases and a decreased probability of disease free survival. The diffuse nature of glandular involvement may clinically mimic thyroiditis delaying diagnosis. Despite the incidence of pulmonary metastases, mortality rates are low, perhaps due to the young age of most patients with this variant.[164] Finally it appears that there is a 5–10 percent incidence of well-differentiated thyroid carcinoma (usually papillary) in patients with surgically treated Grave's disease.[165] These tumors tend to behave more aggressively, presumably due to the presence of

FIGURE 10-18. Papillary carcinoma of the thyroid. The papillary bandlike structure is lined by low columnar cells. In the lower panel, optically clear "Orphan Annie nuclei" are seen.

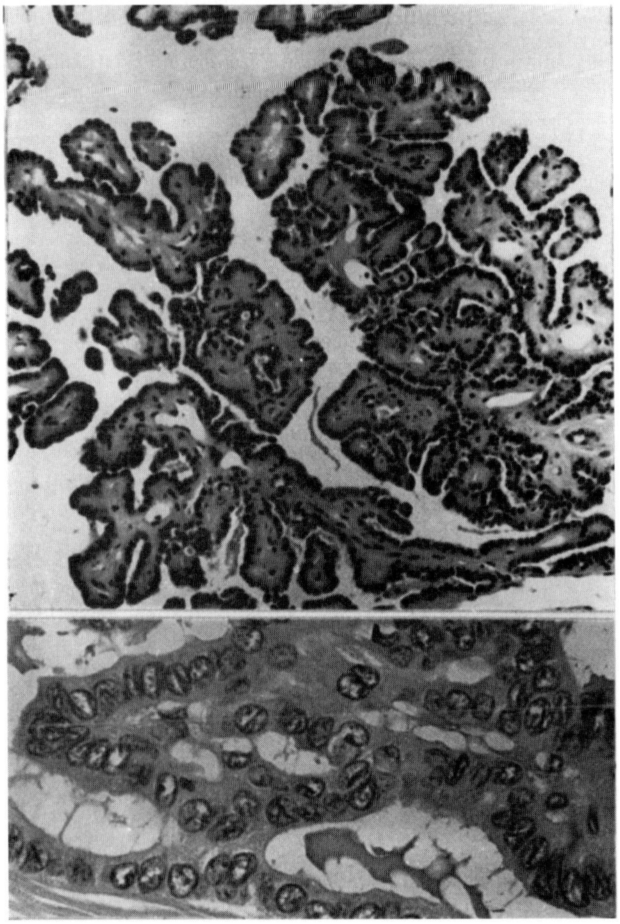

thyroid stimulating immunoglobulins which promote tumor growth.[166,167] Patients with cold nodules in the setting of Grave's disease should accordingly be considered for thyroidectomy rather than radioiodine as treatment of their hyperthyroidism. If carcinoma is indeed found, postoperative ^{131}I ablation is indicated.

Follicular Carcinoma

Follicular carcinoma accounts for up to 30 to 40 percent of carcinomas in iodine deficient regions and between 5 and 15 percent of thyroid carcinomas in iodine replete areas.[168] Like papillary carcinoma, follicular tumors are three times more common in women than in men. However, this tumor occurs less frequently in children; it is more a disease of the middle and later years. Advancing age, extrathyroidal invasion, and distant metastases are associated with a poorer prognosis.[169] Follicular carcinomas are usually nonfunctional clinically and "cold" on radionuclide scanning, though hyperthyroidism may be caused by functioning tumors and/or metastases.[170] Histologically, the tumor is characterized both by the formation of acinar structures with varying colloid content and by the absence of papillary elements (Fig. 10-19). Because of the relatively normal morphology, the tumor may be very difficult to distinguish from follicular adenomas; usually invasion of the capsule, the adjacent thyroid, or blood vessels must be demonstrated. The initial appearance of follicular carcinoma may be as a distant metastasis with no thyroid lesion clinically evident. These tumors tend to metastasize through the bloodstream or invade adjacent structures rather than spread to local lymph nodes.

The prognosis depends on the extent of tumor invasion at the time of surgery. From a morphologic and prognostic point of view these tumors can be separated into minimally invasive and widely invasive groups.[105] Follicular carcinomas that show minimal invasion and appear grossly similar to adenomas have a very high cure rate. Minimally invasive follicular carcinomas are those that have capsular invasion alone or fewer than two to three microscopic foci of vascular invasion with exhaustive sectioning of the capsule.[171,172] The widely invasive type of follicular carcinoma has extensive areas of invasion at gross and microscopic levels; these are prominent enough that the differential of follicular adenoma is not entertained.[105] With more extensive invasion, the prognosis becomes progressively poorer. In a study of 18 cases in which the patient died from follicular carcinoma of the thyroid, 56 percent had lung metastases, 89 percent had lymph node metastases, and 17 percent had skeletal, liver, or brain metastases.[173] The development of metastases may be delayed as long as 10–20 years.

FIGURE 10-19. Follicular carcinoma of the thyroid. The follicles are of uniform size and are distinctly different from the normal follicles in the upper part of the micrograph. The carcinoma is surrounded by a well-defined capsule without signs of invasion in this instance.

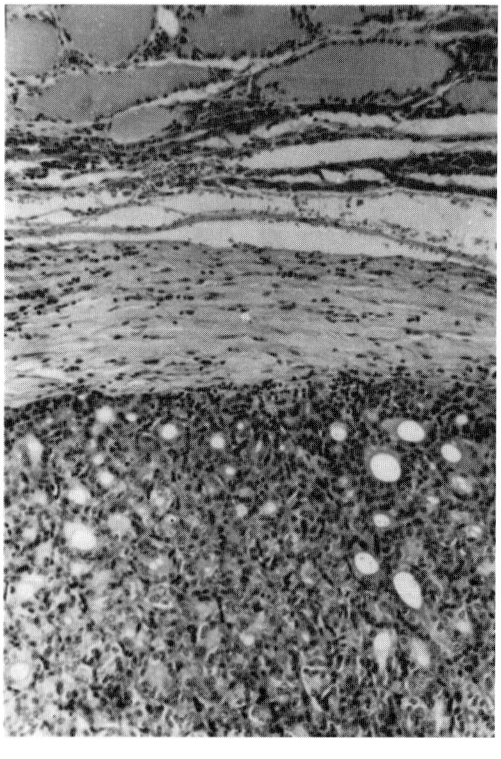

Poorly Differentiated Carcinoma

A histologically distinctive neoplasm appears to occupy a clinical niche between well differentiated and anaplastic carcinomas. "Insular" or poorly differentiated carcinoma can be identified by the presence of nests or "insulae" of monotonous round cells, sometimes forming follicles. Tumor necrosis is common. The presence of insular carcinoma even if focal within an otherwise well differentiated neoplasm portends a more aggressive course. Although the mean age at diagnosis of this tumor is 55 years, insular carcinoma may account for many of the "low risk" young patients who have aggressive papillary and follicular tumors.[174]

Anaplastic Carcinoma

Anaplastic carcinomas are highly malignant tumors that appear undifferentiated by light microscopy but in which epithelial characteristics can be discerned using immunocytochemical or ultrastructural techniques (Fig. 10-20).

These are predominately tumors of older patients with a mean age at diagnosis between 60 and 65. Unlike other thyroid tumors, anaplastic carcinoma is only slightly more common in women than in men. Clinically, patients present with a history of a rapidly enlarging neck mass, often associated with dyspnea, dysphagia, and hoarseness. A history of preexisting thyroid disease, particularly of well-differentiated thyroid carcinoma, is not uncommon. An association between ^{131}I treatment of well-differentiated thyroid cancer

FIGURE 10-20. Anaplastic carcinoma of the thyroid. The cells are bizarre and pleomorphic. The mitotic rate is high.

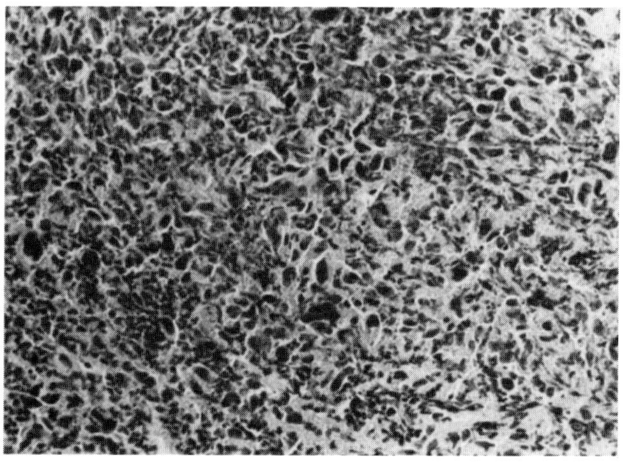

and the subsequent development of anaplastic carcinoma has been suggested but is extraordinarily rare.[175] Microscopically three distinct morphologic patterns are seen though often admixed within the same tumor. These are designated squamoid, spindle cell, and giant cell.[162] Features common to all three types are high mitotic activity, large foci of necrosis, and marked degree of invasiveness. In a small percentage of cases the mesenchymal component of the tumors exhibits heterologous features such as cartilage or bone and is sometimes referred to as *carcinosarcoma*; biologically the behavior of such lesions is indistinguishable from the other undifferentiated carcinomas.[105] Historically, a third type of aggressive thyroid tumors were grouped in the undifferentiated category as *small cell carcinoma*. It is now believed that all such tumors were actually malignant lymphomas or in some cases medullary carcinoma, insular carcinoma, or neuroendocrine malignancies[105] which can be expected to follow a different clinical course and should be considered separately.

FNA can differentiate anaplastic carcinoma from lymphoma, which it clinically resembles, as well as from other aggressive thyroid cancers, by a combination of morphology and the use of immunocytochemical and ultrastructural analysis.

Anaplastic carcinomas grow rapidly, infiltrate neck structures, and spread to regional lymph nodes, lungs, bones, and liver. Death often occurs as a result of rapid local spread before distant metastases appear. For almost all patients, anaplastic carcinoma of the thyroid has progressed beyond the possibility of cure when they are first seen. For this reason radical surgery has no role in the treatment of anaplastic carcinoma. Nonetheless, an attempt at surgical resection, including tracheostomy, for palliation is appropriate and may be necessary in order to establish an adequate airway. An occasional patient with late recurrence of anaplastic carcinoma limited to the neck may be salvaged by aggressive local resection such as laryngectomy, pharyngectomy, and gastric pull-up. In most cases, however, patients with anaplastic carcinoma die of metastatic disease.

External radiotherapy may be given in a dose of 4,000 to 5,000 rad to the neck and upper mediastinum through a variety of ports. Shrinkage of the tumor may occur rapidly (hyperfractionation of the radiation dose, 100 rad qid at 3-h intervals), caused complete tumor regression in 6 of 14 patients,[176] but recurrence is the rule. The aim of radiotherapy in these cases is to prevent obstruction, ulceration, and hemorrhage. Rarely, an anaplastic carcinoma of the thyroid takes up enough ^{131}I to make therapy possible.[177]

Chemotherapy has not been very helpful in the treatment of these very aggressive tumors but could be considered an alternative to radiation therapy.[178] A partial remission associated with subjective improvement was achieved in 5 of 19 patients with anaplastic carcinoma treated with doxorubicin (Adriamycin).[179] The most significant toxicity encountered was Adriamycin-induced cardiomyopathy. Bleomycin is another antibiotic that has been suggested to be effective in treating thyroid cancer.[180] Despite multimodality therapy the mean survival in one series was 7 months.[181]

Although traditional chemotherapeutic agents have not been useful in the treatment of anaplastic carcinoma, addition of new molecular biologic approaches hold promise. In in vitro studies, introduction of wild type P53 into anaplastic thyroid carcinoma cell lines by infection with a P53-expressing adenovirus resulted in expression of P53 downstream regulators and increased sensitivity to adriamycin.[182]

Medullary Carcinoma of the Thyroid

Although medullary carcinoma accounts for only 5 to 10 percent of all thyroid malignancies, there has been intense interest in this tumor because it has a number of unique properties. Medullary carcinoma of the thyroid (MCT) differs from other thyroid carcinomas in that the cell of origin is the parafollicular or "C" cell, which is of neural crest origin. MCT occurs over an age range from 5 to 80 years without a particular predilection for age or sex. MCT is intermediate in malignancy between follicular carcinoma and anaplastic carcinoma; the 5-year survival rate is 70–80 percent.[183] Characteristically, the tumor runs a slow but progressive course; neck structures are invaded, and metastases go both to cervical lymph nodes and to distant sites. MCT may be sharply demarcated from surrounding normal thyroid or may infiltrate the adjacent thyroid. Smaller tumors are almost invariably located in the upper, posterior portion of the thyroid lobes.

Microscopically, the tumor is distinguished by clusters of polyhedral, neoplastic cells (Fig. 10-21) arranged in compartments separated by hyaline amyloid-containing stroma, which is

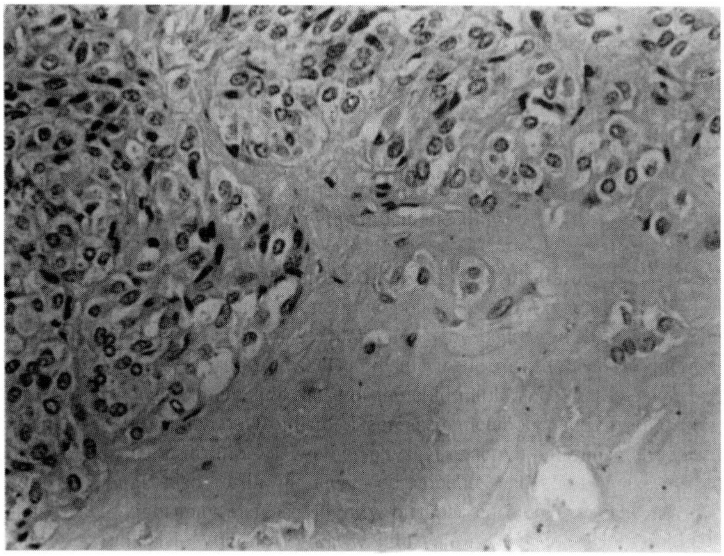

FIGURE 10-21. Medullary carcinoma of the thyroid. Pleomorphic cells are in clumps separated by amyloid.

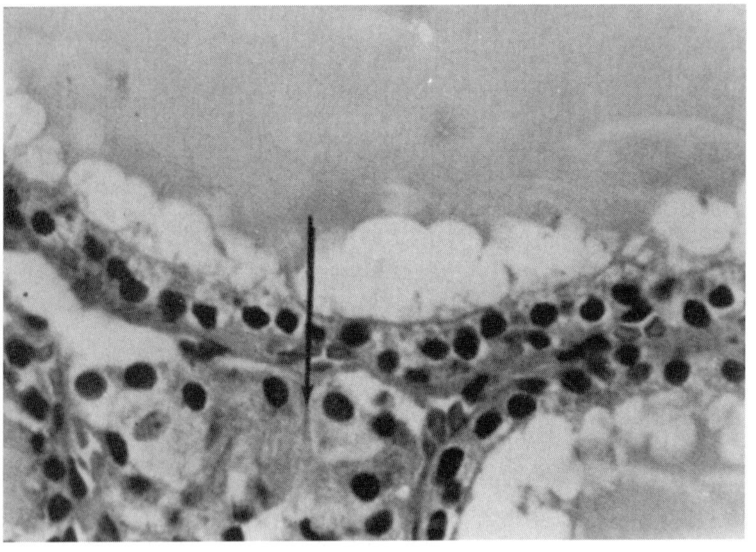

FIGURE 10-22. C cell hyperplasia. Clusters of polygonal to spindle-shaped C cells are seen in a parafollicular location. (*From Tashjian AH Jr, Wolfe HJ, Voelkel EF. Human Calcitonen. Immunologic assay, cytologic localization and studies on medullary thyroid carcinoma. Am J Med 56:840, 1974.*)

formed by the tumor cells. This organization, together with the absence of neoplastic follicles and papillary elements, is the diagnostic microscopic feature.

In contrast to the faint homogeneous calcification seen in other thyroid tumors, MCT has a tendency to calcify with a characteristic dense, irregular distribution of calcium throughout the tumor mass in both thyroid primary lesions and metastases.

Most of these malignancies are apparently sporadic, in which case the tumors are usually unifocal and are not associated with other endocrine lesions or with concomitant C cell hyperplasia (Fig. 10-22). However, in approximately 20 percent of patients the disease is familial, transmitted as an autosomal dominant trait and characterized by complete penetrance and variable expressivity. The familial form occurs as Sipple's syndrome or multiple endocrine neoplasia (MEN) types 2A and 2B and familial non-MEN MCT (see Chap. 27) and below.

Because the parafollicular cells secrete the polypeptide hormone, calcitonin, the measurement of this peptide either as a basal determination or after secretory stimulation by calcium and pentagastrin infusion, is used as a marker for the presence of MCT, particularly after surgical treatment. The pentagastrin stimulation test is performed by administering 0.5 g/kg of pentagastrin intravenously and measuring the plasma calcitonin levels at 0, 1.5, 5, 10, and 15 min. Normal ranges vary in different laboratories, but basal calcitonin levels are ordinarily less than 24.5 pmol/liter (91 pg/ml) in males and less than 19.2 pmol/liter (71 pg/ml) in females. A positive response is a 1.5-min level of 51.4 pmol/liter in a male or 21.6 pmol/liter in a female.

Normal individuals have low circulating calcitonin levels because of a small number of calcitonin-producing C cells in the normal thyroid. Higher levels of calcitonin may be seen under circumstances of physiologic (as opposed to neoplastic) C cell hyperplasia. Thus calcitonin levels per se may be misleading and should not be used as part of the routine evaluation of the patient with a thyroid nodule.

MEN 2A is characterized by the combination of MCT, bilateral adrenal pheochromocytomas, and hyperparathyroidism. In addition to MCT and pheochromocytoma, patients with MEN 2B have a generalized neural hypertrophy with mucosal neuromas of the lips and tongue and a characteristic physical appearance (Fig. 10-23).[184]

In 1993 it was shown that mutations in the RET protooncogene are associated with MEN 2A,B, and FMTC.[185,186] Medullary thyroid carcinoma occurs in all affected patients and is the most common cause of death in these individuals. The biologic behavior of MCT varies depending on the clinical setting with aggressive, early onset MTC seen in MEN2B and late onset and indolent MTC in patients with FMTC. In the kindreds with MEN2A, the clinical course is variable but may be aggressive in

FIGURE 10-23. Typical facies of a patient with MEN 2b syndrome. (*From Khari MRA, et al.*[184])

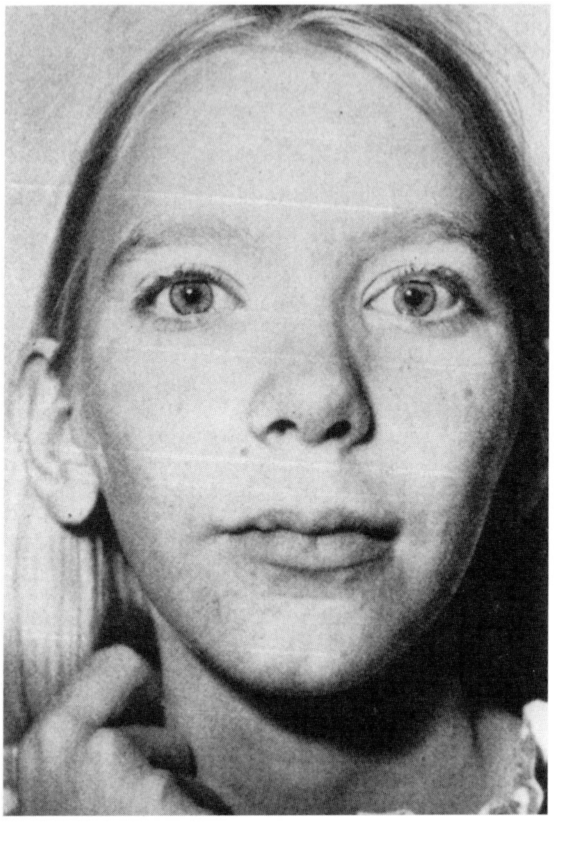

some.[187] Identification of gene carriers in known kindreds by direct DNA testing has permitted presymptomatic treatment of C cell hyperplasia and MTC in these individuals and exclusion of nonaffected family members from cumbersome and costly follow-up.[187] Unlike screening for MTC by calcitonin testing, there have been no false positive or negative results using direct DNA evaluation.[188] Wells and Skinner recently reported on follow-up of the first group of 18 patients who had prophylactic thyroidectomy for MEN2A based on DNA diagnosis. Patients ranged in age from 6 to 21 years. Microscopic or gross MTC was present in 78 percent, none of the patients had regional node involvement, and at three years after resection there was no evidence of residual disease on stimulated calcitonin testing.[187] In experienced hands successful thyroid resection can be carried out in young children with no operative complications.[187,189] Wells' group routinely performs total parathyroidectomy with autotransplantation on MEN2A (only) patients undergoing prophylactic thyroidectomy. Because the development of hyperparathyroidism may occur only in patients with specific RET mutations, it may be possible to limit parathyroid resection to those at risk for parathyroid disease.[190]

Thyroid Lymphoma

Thyroid lymphoma is uncommon, representing less than 5 percent of all thyroid malignancies. The most common type of thyroid lymphoma is the diffuse large cell type with immunoblastic lymphoma next in frequency. Thyroid lymphoma is more common in females and there is a recognized association with Hashimoto's thyroiditis which is often found elsewhere within the gland. Most low grade lymphomas of the thyroid appear to belong to the MALT (mucosa-associated lymphoid tissue) category, and nearly all are of B-cell origin.[191] Clinical presentation is frequently indistinguishable from that of anaplastic carcinoma. FNA is critical in making this differential diagnosis. Although the diagnosis of large cell lymphoma is usually straightforward, differentiation between lymphoplasmacytoid lymphoma and extensive Hashimoto's thyroiditis may be problematic. In such cases immunophenotypic evidence of light chain restriction is conclusive evidence of lymphoma as lymphocytes in Hashimoto's thyroiditis should express both types of light chains.

Unless the process is clearly confined to the thyroid, lymphoma is not primarily a surgical disease.[192] The use of multimodality chemotherapy and radiation therapy results in dramatic tumor shrinkage and rapid resolution of airway compromise. Overall 5 year survival is around 70 percent with variability based on stage and histologic type.[193,194]

Miscellaneous Tumors

Primary squamous cell carcinoma accounts for approximately 1 percent of thyroid cancers. The tumor occurs in older patient, often in males with a long history of thyroid goiter. Patients may present with systemic symptoms of hypercalcemia, fever, and leukocytosis, perhaps mediated by interleukin-1. The cellular source of squamous cell carcinoma is controversial.[195] Squamous metaplasia of follicular thyroid cells is known to occur, particularly in the setting of chronic thyroid disease. Squamous carcinoma is thought to arise by malignant transformation of benign metaplastic squamous cells.[196] Metastasis from another site of squamous carcinoma must be excluded. This is an aggressive tumor which is locally invasive and frequently metastatic at the time of diagnosis to lungs, liver, and locoregional nodes.

Secondary Tumors

The thyroid gland may be involved by direct extension or lymphatic spread from malignancies of the upper aerodigestive tract. Most such tumors are squamous cell in nature and the primary site evident on clinical grounds.[197]

Blood-borne metastases from widespread malignant tumors may be present in as many as 10 percent of cases analyzed at autopsy.[198] Most commonly seen are malignant melanoma, and carcinomas of the lung, gastrointestinal tract, breast, and kidney. Fewer than a quarter of these are clinically significant in terms of causing thyroid enlargement or dysfunction. However, renal cell carcinomas may present as significant thyroid nodules while the primary tumor is still clinically occult or long after nephrectomy.[199] Hyperthyroidism as a result of tumor destruction of thyroid follicles and release of hormone has been described.[200] Immunocytochemical and ultrastructural techniques may be required in order to identify the tissue of origin in some cases.[105]

Surgical Treatment of Thyroid Carcinoma

The goal of surgical treatment of thyroid carcinoma is the removal of all tumor from the neck, the minimization of the chance for recurrence, and facilitation of postoperative follow-up. Although the extent of surgery for well-differentiated thyroid carcinoma, particularly papillary carcinomas less than 1–1.5 cm in size in young female patients, is controversial, near total thyroidectomy is the most straightforward treatment for most patients with significant papillary or follicular carcinoma, as well as for those with poorly differentiated and medullary carcinomas.[201] In one study, residual cancer would have persisted in remaining thyroid tissue in two-thirds of the patients if only a lobectomy had been performed.[202] In a study of 576 patients with carcinoma of the thyroid, there was a significant inverse correlation between the extent of surgery and recurrence of the tumor (Table 10-8).[160,161] The tumor recurred with twice the frequency after subtotal thyroidectomy compared with nearly total thyroidectomy, and the proportion of deaths from thyroid cancer was greater. Similar results have been reported in other,[133,134,203,204] though not all, series.[205,206] In addition, the presence of a normal thyroid lobe af-

TABLE 10-8. Influence of Initial Treatment on Recurrence and Survival in Thyroid Papillary Carcinoma

	Recurrence, %	Deaths, %
Surgical therapy		
Thyroidectomy		
Subtotal	19.2	0.6
Total	10.9*	1.5
Lymphadenectomy		
None	12.3	0.8
Simple	17.9	1.7
Excision	14.7	0.7
Medical therapy after surgery		
None	40.0	10.0
Thyroid	13.1†	0.2
^{131}I and thyroid hormone	6.4	0.9

*The difference in recurrence frequency between patients with total thyroidectomy vs. subtotal thyroidectomy was statistically significant ($p < .01$).

†The difference between patients with thyroid therapy and patients who received no therapy was statistically significant ($p < .001$).

Source: Mazzaferri and Young [161]

ter subtotal thyroid resection makes use of thyroglobulin as a tumor marker unreliable and radioactive iodine for diagnosis or treatment of residual disease impossible. Although the primary argument for performing a lobectomy and isthmusectomy only for differentiated thyroid carcinoma relates to concern about potential bilateral damage to parathyroids and recurrent laryngeal nerves with a more extensive procedure, in fact with proper technique such problems are unusual.[207]

Technical Issues

Successful and safe thyroid surgery requires an appreciation for the normal anatomic relationships of the thyroid and parathyroid glands, the recurrent and superior laryngeal nerves, and the inferior thyroid arteries as well as their common embryologic variations.[208,209] Critical to the success of the operation is the maintenance of meticulous homeostasis throughout in order to visualize critical anatomic structures.

In the vast majority of cases, thyroid surgery is performed using general anesthesia. Patients carrying a diagnosis of medullary thyroid carcinoma or individuals with a thyroid nodule and a family history suggestive of an MEN syndrome should be screened for pheochromocytoma preoperatively. The presence of a pheochromocytoma takes precedence in terms of treatment to the thyroid tumor. The relatively short duration of most thyroid procedures, and the lack of significant fluid shifts and hemodynamic changes aid in making them very well tolerated, even in elderly patients with significant medical disabilities. General endotracheal anesthesia is most commonly used, although laryngeal mask anesthesia (LMA)[210] is an excellent choice, particularly in cases where functional identification of the recurrent laryngeal nerves is required and in instances where it is desirable to avoid the local trauma to the cords of intubation, such as in vocalists. Neuromuscular blockade should be avoided until the external branch of the superior laryngeal nerve has been identified, or in the case of the use of the LMA, the recurrent nerve is seen. Loco/regional anesthesia may also be used, although there is much less experience with this approach. LoGerfo recently reported on a personal series of 1,275 patients over a 9-year period who underwent thyroid surgery using a bilateral C2-C3 superficial cervical block and conscious sedation.[211] A postoperative patient questionnaire revealed high level of satisfaction with this technique.

For thyroid surgery, a transverse skin incision is made along defined skin lines in order to maximize the cosmetic outcome of the procedure. This incision can be extended laterally and superiorly along the lateral border of the sternocleidomastoid muscle to give excellent access for a lymph node dissection, if indicated. Dissection proceeds through the platysma muscle and subplatysmal skin flaps are raised to the level of the superior aspect of the thyroid cartilage and inferiorly to the sternal notch. In most cases the strap muscles do not need to be divided, although sectioning the sternothyroid muscle alone may provide easier access to the superior thyroidal vessels.

The strap muscles are dissected off the thyroid gland and the middle thyroid vein divided in order to mobilize the thyroid lobe out of the tracheoesophageal groove. In cases of thyroid malignancy, if the lesion appears to be invading the strap muscles, they are resected en bloc with the thyroid lobe. The inferior parathyroid is often identified during mobilization of the gland, close to the inferolateral border of the thyroid gland or in the thyrothymic tissue inferiorly. The primary nodal drainage of the thyroid gland are the Delphian nodes superior to the isthmus, the superoanterior mediastinal nodes, and those in the tracheoesophageal groove. Enlarged nodes identified early in the dissection should be forwarded to the pathologist and assessed for evidence of metastatic disease. Recognition that malignant thyroid disease is present directs the remainder of the procedure. As the potential space between the carotid sheath and the thyroid gland is further developed, the inferior thyroid artery should be sought. This anatomic landmark aids in the identification of the recurrent laryngeal nerve.

The recurrent laryngeal nerve is most easily identified in the low neck, where it is more laterally located. The nerve frequently divides above the level of the inferior thyroid artery to send a sensory branch superiorly to anastomose with the internal branch of the superior laryngeal nerve. Both branches must be protected, as it is usually not clear which is the motor branch. The nerve may be nonrecurrent on the right, passing directly from the vagus nerve in the carotid sheath or recurring around the inferior thyroid artery. Use of the laryngeal mask airway permits functional identification of the recurrent nerve: electrical stimulation of the nerve causes contraction of the vocal cord apparatus which can be visualized by fiberoptic bronchoscopy.[210] Mobilization of the thyroid lobe continues superiorly, freeing the lateral aspect of the gland at the level of the superior pole vessels by entering the surgical capsule of the thyroid gland. At this point the superior parathyroid gland often is visualized and left in situ with its vascular supply intact. Before dividing the superior pole vessels, care should be taken to preserve the external branch of the superior laryngeal nerve, which may be intertwined with the superior thyroidal vessels en route to the cricothyroid muscle. This nerve provides innervation of the cricothyroid muscle, and its division will result in a change in vocal timbre, vocal fatigue, and an inability to sing high pitches. Fortunately, the identity of the external branch of the recurrent nerve can be readily confirmed by using a nerve stimulator and observing contraction of the cricothyroid muscle. The thyroid lobe is further dissected off the trachea, keeping the recurrent nerve in view at all times, until the isthmus has been freed up. The isthmus is cross-clamped and the specimen sent to pathology for touch preparation and frozen section evaluation. It is advantageous for the surgeon to review the gross and microscopic data with the pathologist intraoperatively, as the additional clinical perspective may be helpful in arriving at a diagnosis of carcinoma, in which case the other lobe may need to be resected. Contralateral resection is carried out in a similar fashion with careful attention to identification of the nerves and parathyroid glands. Because of the multifocal nature of familial MCT, total thyroidectomy is required. All parathyroids should be preserved if this is consistent with gross removal of tumor. Parathyroids with doubtful viability should be locally autotransplanted. The incidence of permanent hypoparathyroidism is less than 1 percent in experienced hands.

If nodes in the central compartment are positive for carcinoma, they should be resected, taking care to protect the recurrent laryngeal nerve along which the nodes in the tracheoesophageal groove are located. Cervical lymph node metastases found at initial surgery for papillary carcinoma are associated with higher recurrence rates but not higher mortality rates.[134,212] Complete removal of involved locoregional nodes is particularly important in the treatment of medullary carcinoma as nodal metastatic disease is usually present, especially in sporadic cases, at the time of diagnosis, and other antitumor treatments are not available. If palpable jugular chain nodes are identified, a functional neck dissection is performed. A supraomohyoid disection is not required as these nodes are only rarely involved.[213,214] Characteristic sites of nodal

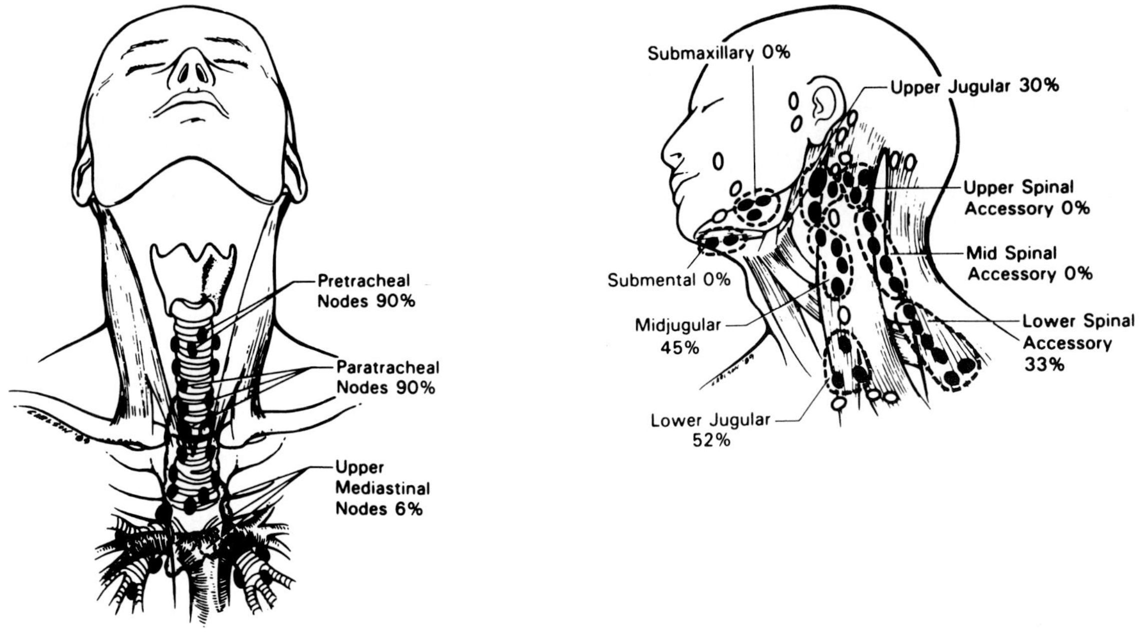

FIGURE 10-24. Primary areas of nodal involvement in papillary carcinoma of the thyroid. (*From Jossart and Clark.*[213])

involvement in thyroid carcinoma are shown in Fig. 10-24. Radical neck dissection is not indicated in the treatment of well-differentiated thyroid carcinoma, but may be required in locally aggressive, poorly differentiated, or some medullary thyroid cancers.

Thyroid carcinoma may directly invade the aerodigestive tract, particularly the trachea or larynx. Outcome of treatment of these patients depends upon the extent of invasion and the ability to achieve negative margins by concomitant resection of the involved segment of the aerodigestive tract. Complete resection of thyroid tumors offers prolonged palliation, improved local control, and opportunity for cure in selected patients with well-differentiated tumors.[215,216] Fig. 10-25 is a CT scan of a 55-year-old male who presented with airway obstruction due to tracheal compression and invasion by papillary carcinoma. An endotracheal tube is in place. He was treated by thyroidectomy, tracheal sleeve resection, postoperative radioiodine, and TSH suppression. He has had no local recurrence, but subsequently developed pulmonary metastases requiring additional ^{131}I administration. Patients with superficial invasion only may be treated successfully with cartilage shave procedures and adjuvant external beam radiotherapy.[217]

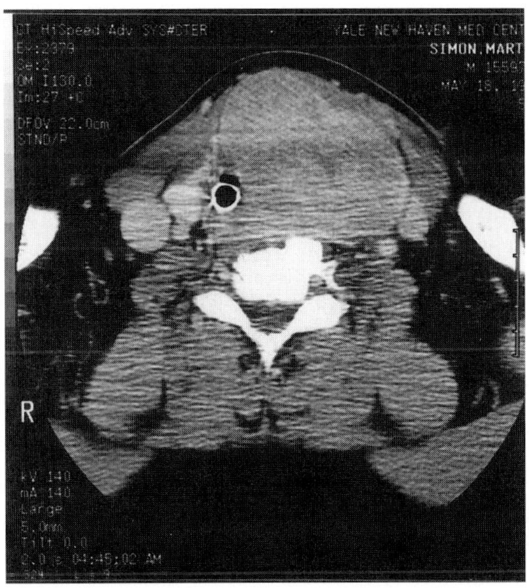

FIGURE 10-25. CT scan from a patient with papillary carcinoma invading the trachea. Urgent endotracheal intubation was required to establish an airway prior to surgical resection.

Patients are usually discharged on the day following surgery. LoGerfo[211] has reported on his experience with outpatient management of patients undergoing thyroidectomy. In his protocol, patients are observed for six hours following surgery and discharged if there is no evidence of swelling in the neck to suggest postoperative bleeding. He found that 85 percent of patients who were operated on early in the day could be discharged after the 6-hour observation period. There were no readmissions to the hospital, but two patients required reoperation while in the hospital. Although the majority of patients who experience a significant bleeding episode will have evidence of this within six hours, there are some who bleed later within a 24-h period and who might experience substantial morbidity or mortality if the condition were not treated immediately. The exact role of outpatient management for thyroid conditions is still unclear.[201]

Radioactive Iodine Treatment of Carcinomas of Follicular Cell Origin

Radioactive iodine is used after surgery for well-differentiated thyroid carcinoma in patients judged to be at risk for recurrent or metastatic disease. Postoperative treatment with ^{131}I has two effects: ablation of remaining normal thyroid tissue so that thyroglobulin can be used as a marker of tumor growth, and secondly, the eradication of potential residual or metastatic disease. Because the normal thyroid gland is so avid for iodine, particularly compared with tumor tissue, radioactive iodine will not be taken up by metastatic tumor until the thyroid remnant has been ablated. Therefore, surgical removal of most of the gland or radioablation of the gland before ^{131}I treatment of the metastases is required. If the thyroid remnant is small, as in the case of a near total thyroidectomy, it can be ablated with a low 30 mCi outpatient dose of ^{131}I.[218,219] Ablation of a whole lobe, as may be required when the diagnosis of carcinoma is rendered only on review of the permanent pathologic sections of the tumor in a patient judged to be at risk for recurrence, will require a substantially larger radioactive iodine dose. Such treatment can contribute to the radiation dose imposed on the patient without significantly affecting the cancer and can also result in neck edema syndrome.

A variety of approaches have been utilized to prepare the patient for radioiodine treatment. In a recent survey of clinical members of the American Thyroid Association, a majority of respondents recommended withholding thyroid hormone for varying periods after surgery[220] and proceeding with ablation at that point. Usually withholding hormone for 3 weeks with or without a low iodine diet can be relied upon to raise the TSH level to greater than 30 U/ml, sufficient to stimulate uptake by thyroid tissue capable of concentrating iodine.[221] Although not all endocrinologists surveyed obtained pretreatment thyroglobulin levels or radioiodine uptake determinations, these studies are useful. The thyroglobulin determination serves as a baseline assessment of the amount of thyroid tissue remaining after surgical resection. Thyroid scan with uptake using ^{123}I may be preferable to even scanning doses of ^{131}I as the latter delivers an increased radiation dose to thyroid tissue which may result in sublethal treatment or "stunning" of tumor cells.[222,223] Determination of the dose of ^{131}I to be administered is arrived at by consultation between the surgeon, endocrinologist, and nuclear medicine physician. It is based upon the ^{123}I uptake, data from surgical and pathological analysis, and overall assessment of the patient's status and future risk of recurrence. Patients with presumed or known residual disease usually receive around 200 mCi of ^{131}I unless there is evidence of pulmonary metastases, in which case the dose may be reduced to minimize the risk of radiation pneumonitis.[224] Remnant ablation in patients (without known residual disease but judged to be at risk for recurrence based on clinical staging and who have undergone a near-total or total thyroidectomy) can usually be achieved by doses of ^{131}I between 30 and 100 mCi. A posttreatment body scan is performed one week after therapy and may visualize foci of tumor not seen on the scanning dose, which usually detects only the normal thyroid remnant. Total ablation can be confirmed by total body scanning at 10 to12 months after treatment.

Thyroid Hormone in the Treatment of Thyroid Carcinomas

Hormone dependence of certain well-differentiated carcinomas of the thyroid is well established. As shown in Fig. 10-26, TSH suppression with thyroid hormone significantly influenced survival and recurrence.[161] The recurrence rate after thyroid hormone therapy was significantly less than that with no therapy but was significantly greater than that with ^{131}I plus thyroid hormone therapy. The appropriate dose of thyroid hormone that can provide maximal tumor suppression while minimizing cardiac and skeletal effects has been the focus of recent debate.[220] Seventy-eight percent of physician members of the American Thyroid Association surveyed indicated they would strive for a dosage of thyroxine that

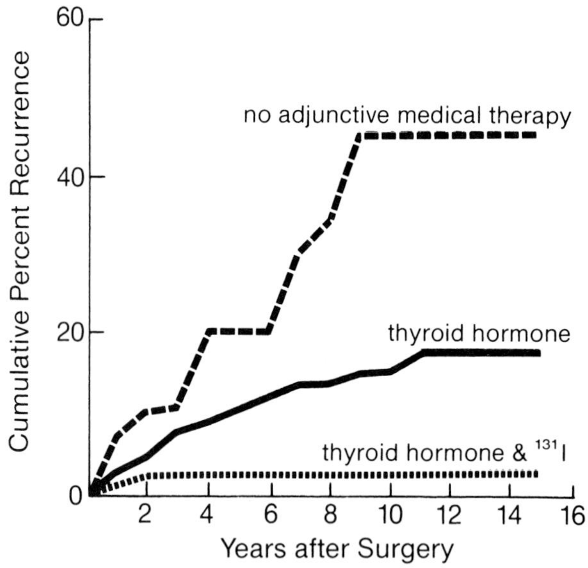

FIGURE 10-26. Recurrence of papillary thyroid carcinoma after surgery with and without adjunctive medical therapy. (*From Mazzaferri EL, et al.*[161])

would place the TSH level within a detectable range between 0.01–0.5 μg IU/ml using a third generation assay. In other studies the dose required to effect this response in patients who had had thyroid ablation for carcinoma was found to be between 2.0 and 2.7 μg/kg/day.[225-227] Thyroglobulin determinations in patients with known metastatic disease document indicate that below a certain level of TSH suppression, higher doses of thyroid hormone are unlikely to produce further reduction in thyroglobulin levels. Thus, most patients will obtain maximal benefit in terms of tumor suppression at TSH levels at or slightly below the lower range of normal. Such thyroxine doses should also be well-tolerated physiologically.[225]

Other Treatment Modalities

External Beam Irradiation

External irradiation at a moderate dose can eradicate microscopic papillary and follicular carcinoma; gross tumor also responds favorably, but the regression rate is slow.[222] At present, external irradiation is indicated only in patients in whom surgical excision is incomplete or impossible and in those whose tumors do not take up ^{131}I.[226]

Contribution of Molecular Biology to the Treatment of Thyroid Carcinoma

Loss of morphological differentiation in thyroid tumors is associated with decreased radioiodine uptake and TSH-responsiveness. Recently redifferentiation therapy with 13-cis-retinoic acid has been undertaken. Simon and colleagues reported on such therapy in a series of 10 patients with advanced differentiated thyroid carcinoma. After 6 weeks of treatment renewed uptake of iodine was seen in four of ten patients.[228] Characterization of the Na^+/I^- symporter responsible for iodide uptake into thyroid follicular cells offers new opportunities for understanding and manipulating thyroid physiology.[229] Comparative immunohistochemical analysis of the expression of the symporter in human thyroid tissues is seen in

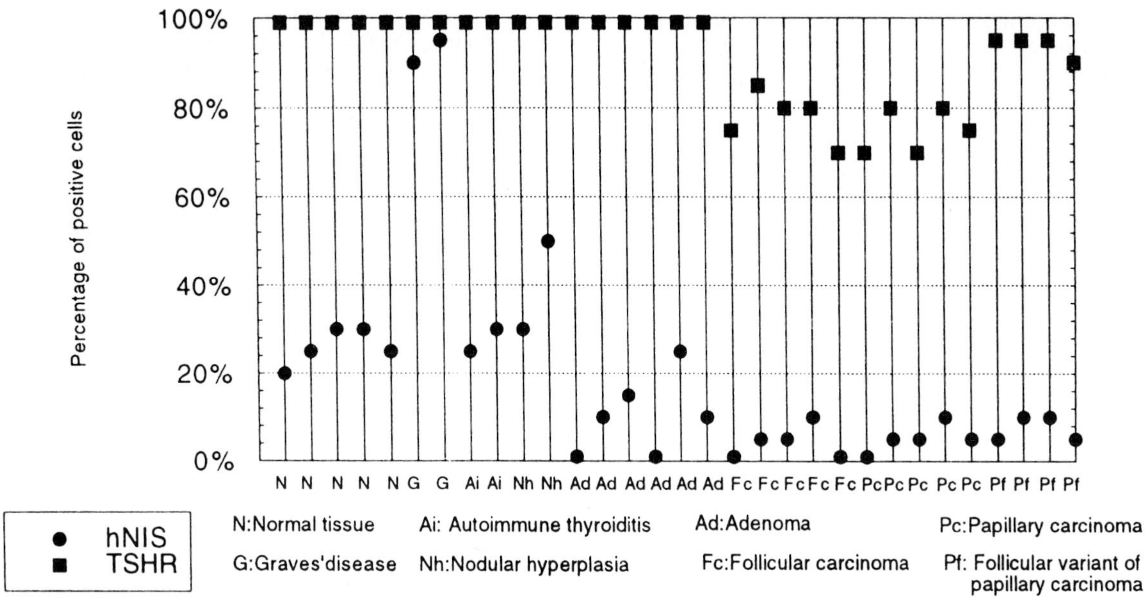

FIGURE 10-27. Comparative immunohistochemical staining for human Na/I symporter (hNIS) and TSH receptor (TSHR) in thyroid tissue specimen. (*From Caillou B, et al.*[230])

Fig. 10-27. Expression of the symporter was less in malignant cells than in normal thyroid cells and correlated with clinical uptake of radioiodine on nuclear scan.[230] Assessment of the status of symporter expression in thyroid tumors may predict therapeutic radioiodine uptake, and ultimately techniques of increasing its expression, perhaps via somatic gene transfer,[231] could facilitate treatment. Similarly, retrovirus-mediated gene therapy specifically targeting thyroglobulin expressing cells has been reported in thyroid cell lines in vitro.[232]

Follow-up of Patients with Carcinoma of the Thyroid

Well-Differentiated Tumors

Long-term follow-up of patients after initial treatment for well-differentiated carcinoma should be individualized with respect to the risk classification of the patient at time of diagnosis.[220,226,233] In patients with low risk of recurrence who are treated with lobectomy and isthmusectomy alone, clinical follow-up would include thyroid hormone administration guided by TSH determination, annual physical examination, neck ultrasound, and thyroglobulin measurement, although the presence of a remaining thyroid lobe makes this measurement less informative. In higher risk patients treated with near total thyroidectomy and ^{131}I ablation, the intensity of follow-up is dictated by the surgical, pathologic, and imaging data. In these patients clinical exam and thyroglobulin determinations guide further evaluation. Because the glycoprotein thyroglobulin is produced only by normal or neoplastic follicular cells, it should not be detectable in patients who have undergone total thyroid ablation by surgery and ^{131}I. The production of thyroglobulin is regulated in part by TSH, so measurement of thyroglobulin when the patient's TSH is elevated is a more sensitive indicator of the presence of residual or recurrent disease. Levels of thyroglobulin may be falsely elevated or suppressed by the presence of antithyroglobulin antibodies, which occur in up to 15 percent of patients with carcinoma of the thyroid. Serum samples should be routinely screened for such antibodies prior to performing thyroglobulin assays. Patients with undetectable thyroglobulin levels off thyroid hormone suppression are most likely free of disease; whereas those with TG levels >10 ng/mg on suppression or >40 ng/ml after hormone withdrawal are usually found to have detectable disease on ^{131}I treatment.[226,234,235]

Much debate exists regarding the use of treatment doses of radioactive iodine in patients who have elevated thyroglobulin levels but have negative iodine scans. Two important issues are concerns about the potential hazards of larger doses of radioiodine[222] and the inconvenience[236] and possible risk of tumor growth[237] in patients with extremely TSH-sensitive tumors during thyroid hormone withdrawal. These latter issues may be resolved by the use of human recombinant TSH to stimulate thyroid follicular cell function for scanning and treatment purposes.[237–239] Although a safe and effective treatment, radioiodine is not without short- and long-term risks. The development of leukemias and solid organ tumors is rare but dose-related.[222] Acute and chronic salivary gland dysfunction may be modulated by having patients suck on lemons during the treatment period to increase salivary flow.[240] No increases in the incidence of congenital anomalies was found in the offspring of patients who had received radioiodine for thyroid cancer, but high doses of ^{131}I may rarely have fertility consequences when administered to younger patients.[222] It is thus important to make every effort to identify treatable disease before proceeding with ^{131}I administration in scan-negative patients. Common causes of false negative studies include inadequate TSH elevation, stable iodine contamination, and dedifferentiation of tumor such that it no longer takes up iodine. In the patient with rising thyroglobulin levels, other imaging modalities may clarify the sites of residual disease.[241] Nuclear imaging with ^{201}thallium and various 99m-technetium agents have shown promise in imaging locally recurrent and metastatic thyroid carcinoma.[233] Positron emission tomography (PET) scanning with 18-fluorodeoxyglucose (FDG-PET) has also been useful in identifying thyroid carcinoma in ^{131}I-negative patients.[242] Similarly, somatostatin receptor scintigraphy with octreotide may offer advantages in selected patients with differentiated carcinoma.[243,244] Proof of the existence of metastatic tumor may also be obtained by the identification of circulating products of thyroid follicular cells using reverse-transcriptase-polymerase chain reaction (RT-PCR) analytic techniques.[245–247] Although its role in the treatment of patients with well-differentiated thyroid carcinoma is as yet unclear, intraoperative identification, using a gamma probe, of residual tumor in patients given a preoperative dose of ^{131}I has recently been described.[248]

Medullary Thyroid Cancer

Follow-up of patients with MTC is facilitated by the use of basal and stimulated calcitonin measurement to identify persistent and recurrent disease. Historically, many patients with MTC presenting with a mass have been found to have persistent hypercalcitonemia postoperatively. Depending on the extent and invasiveness of the disease and the adequacy of the initial surgical treatment, perhaps half of these patients will develop progressive disease and some will eventually die of local or metastatic tumor.[249,250] Selection of patients who are most likely to benefit from reoperative neck dissection has been recently reviewed by Moley et al.[249] In their most recent series, patients were selected for reoperation after a systematic metastatic work-up including computerized tomography or magnetic resonance imaging of the neck, chest, and abdomen, selective venous catheterization of the neck for calcitonin, and routine liver laparoscopy and biopsy. Laparoscopic assessment of the liver identified metastatic disease in 10 patients, 9 of whom had normal CT or MRI imaging. In 7 patients with metastatic liver disease reoperation was performed for bulky local disease threatening the airway or great vessels; those patients had no recurrence of their local disease, although one died of hepatic metastases. Forty-five patients were operated on with curative intent; the mean decrease in postoperative stimulated calcitonin in these patients was 73 percent, with 38 percent within the normal range. There were no deaths and minimal complications in this series from this very experienced group, and in 10 of 12 patients evaluated at 1 year, calcitonin levels remain normal. The exact role of reoperative surgery in the patient with hypercalcitonemia alone is still undergoing evaluation by these workers and other groups, but the addition of laparoscopic liver evaluation in the assessment of the patient with MTC is an important contribution to clinical management.

REFERENCES

1. Kelly FC, Snedden WW: Prevalence and geographical distribution of endemic goitre. *Bull WHO* 18:5, 1958.
2. Wharton T: *Adenographia: Sive, Glandularum Totius Corporis Descriptio*. London, 1656.
3. Burgi H, Supersaxo Z, Selz B: Iodine deficiency diseases in Switzerland one hundred years after Theodor Kocher's survey: A historical review with some new goitre prevalence data. *Acta Endocrinol (Copenh)* 123:577, 1990.
4. Rolleston HD: *The Endocrine Organs in Health and Disease*. London, Oxford University Press, 1936.
5. Marine D: Etiology and prevention of simple goiter. *Medicine (Baltimore)* 3:453, 1924.
6. Studer H, Ramelli F: Simple goiter and its variants: Euthyroid and hyperthyroid multinodular goiters. *Endocr Rev* 3:40, 1982.
7. Eggo MC, Bachrach LK, Fayet G, Errick J, Cohen MF, Kudlow JE, Burrow GN: The effects of growth factors and serum on DNA synthesis and differentiation in thyroid cells in culture. *Mol Cell Endocrinol* 38:141, 1984.
8. Bachrach LK, Eggo MC, Hintz RL, Burrow GN: Insulin-like growth factors in sheep thyroid cells: Action, receptors and production. *Biochem Biophys Res Commun* 154:861, 1988.
9. Maciel RMB, Moses AC, Villone G, Tramontano D, Ingbar SH: Demonstration of the production and physiological role of insulin-like growth factor II in rat thyroid follicular cells in culture. *J Clin Invest* 82:1546, 1988.
10. Tseng Y-CL, Burman KD, Schaudies P, Ahmann AJ, D'avis J, Geelhoed GW, Wartofsky L: Effects of epidermal growth factor on thyroglobulin and adenosine 3′,5′-monophosphate production by cultured human thyrocytes. *J Clin Endocrinol Metab* 69:771, 1989.
11. Drexhage HA, Bottazzo GF, Doniach D, Bitensky L, Chayen J: Evidence for thyroid-stimulating immunoglobulins in some goitrous thyroid diseases. *Lancet* 2:287, 1980.
12. Meinkoth JL, Goldsmith PK, Spiegel AM, Feramisco JR, Burrow GN: Inhibition of TSH-induced DNA synthesis in thyroid follicular cells by microinjection of an antibody to the stimulatory G protein of adenylyl cyclase, G_s. *J Biol Chem* 267:13239, 1992.
13. Grubeck-Loebenstein B, Buchan G, Sadeghi R, Kissonerghis M, Londei M, Turner M, Pirich K, Roka R, et al: Transforming growth factor beta regulates thyroid growth: Role in the pathogenesis of nontoxic goiter. *J Clin Invest* 83:764, 1989.
14. Tetsuya T, Sugawa H, Kosugi S, Inoue D, Toru M, Hiroo I: Prolonged effects of recombinant human interleukin-1α on mouse thyroid function. *Endocrinology* 127:2322, 1990.
15. Yuasa R, Eggo MC, Meinkoth J, Dillmann WH, Burrow GN: Iodine induces transforming growth factor beta 1 (TGF-β1) mRNA in sheep thyroid cells. *Thyroid* 2:141, 1992.
16. Bowers CY, Lee KL, Schally AV: A study on the interaction of the thyrotropin-releasing factor and L-triiodothyronine: Effects of puromycin and cycloheximide. *Endocrinology* 82:75, 1968.
17. Spencer CA, LoPresti JS, Patel A, Guttler RB, Eigen A, Shen D, et al: Applications of a new chemiluminometric TSH assay to subnormal measurement. *J Clin Endocrinol Metab* 70:453, 1990.
18. Larsen PR: Thyroid-pituitary interaction: Feedback regulation of thyrotropin secretion by thyroid hormones. *N Engl J Med* 306:23, 1982.
19. Chopra IJ, Hershman JM, Hornabrook RW: Serum thyroid hormone and thyrotropin levels in subjects from endemic goiter regions of New Guinea. *J Clin Endocrinol Metab* 40:326, 1975.
20. Medeiros-Neto GA, Penna M, Monteiro K, Kataoka K, Imai Y, Hollander C: The effect of iodized oil in the TSH response to TRH in endemic goiter patients. *J Clin Endocrinol Metab* 41:504, 1976.
21. Koutras DA, Alexander WD, Buchanan WW, Crooks J, Wayne EJ: Stable iodine metabolism in non-toxic goitre. *Lancet* 2:784, 1960.
22. Vagenakis AG, Koutras DA, Burger A, Malamos B, Ingbar SH, Braverman LE: Studies of serum triiodothyronine, thyroxine and thyrotropin concentrations in endemic goiter in Greece. *J Clin Endocrinol Metab* 37:485, 1973.
23. Dige-Petersen H, Hummer L: Serum thyrotropin concentrations under basal conditions and after stimulation with thyrotropin-releasing hormone in idiopathic non-toxic goiter. *J Clin Endocrinol Metab* 44:1115, 1977.
24. Young RL, Harvey WC, Mazzaferri EL, Reynolds JC, Hamilton CR Jr: Thyroid-stimulating hormone levels in idiopathic euthyroid goiter. *J Clin Endocrinol Metab* 41:21, 1975.
25. Bachtarzi H, Benmiloud M: TSH-regulation and goitrogenesis in severe iodine deficiency. *Acta Endocrinol (Copenh)* 103:21, 1983.
26. Brown RS, Jackson IMD, Pohl SL, Reichlin S: Do thyroid-stimulating immunoglobulins cause non-toxic and toxic multinodular goitre? *Lancet* 1:904, 1978.
27. Valente WA, Vitti P, Rotella CM, Vaughan MM, Aloj SM, Grollman EF, et al: Antibodies that promote thyroid growth: A distinct population of thyroid-stimulating autoantibodies. *N Engl J Med* 309:1028, 1983.
28. Hetzel BS, Maberly GF: Iodine, in Mertz W (ed): *Trace Elements in Human and Animal Nutrition*, Vol 2. New York, Academic, 1986, p 139.
29. Ibbertson HK: Endemic goitre and cretinism. *J Clin Endocrinol Metab* 8:97, 1979.

30. Van Herle AJ, Chopra IJ, Hershman JM, Hornabrook RW: Serum thyroglobulin in inhabitants of an endemic goiter region of New Guinea. *J Clin Endocrinol Metab* 43:512, 1976.
31. Pitt-Rivers R, Niven JSF, Young MR: Localization of protein-bound radioactive iodine in rat thyroid glands labelled with ^{125}I or ^{131}I. *Biochem J* 90:205, 1964.
32. Stanbury JB, Querido A: Genetic and environmental factors in cretinism: A classification. *J Clin Endocrinol Metab* 16:1522, 1956.
33. Dumont JE, Ermans AM, Bastenie PA: Thyroid function in a goiter endemic: V. Mechanism of thyroid failure in the Uele endemic cretins. *J Clin Endocrinol Metab* 23:847, 1963.
34. McCullagh SF: The Huon Peninsula endemic: III. The effect in the female of endemic goitre of reproductive function. *Med J Aust* 1:844, 1963.
35. Pendergrast WJ, Milmore BK, Marcus SC: Thyroid cancer and thyrotoxicosis in the United States: Their relation to endemic goiter. *J Chronic Dis* 13:22, 1961.
36. Studer H, Hunziker HR, Ruchti C: Morphologic and functional substrate of thyrotoxicosis caused by nodular goiters. *Am J Med* 65:227, 1978.
37. Delange F, Costa A, Ermans AM, Ibbertson HK, Querido A, Stanbury JB: A survey of the clinical and metabolic patterns of endemic cretinism, in Stanbury JB, Kroc RL (eds): *Human Development and the Thyroid Gland: Relation to Endemic Cretinism*. New York, Plenum, 1972, p 175.
38. Editorial: Endemic goitre and cretinism. *Lancet* 2:1165, 1979.
39. Eastman CJ, Phillips DIW: Endemic goitre and iodine deficiency disorders—aetiology, epidemiology and treatment. *Baillieres Clin Endocrinol Metab* 2:719, 1988.
40. Patel YC, Pharoah POD, Hornabrook RW, Hetzel BS: Serum triiodothyronine, thyroxine and thyroid-stimulating hormone in endemic goiter: A comparison of goitrous and nongoitrous subjects in New Guinea. *J Clin Endocrinol Metab* 37:783, 1973.
41. Pretell EA: Role of the placenta and of plasma hormone binding in the pathogenesis of cretinism, in Stanbury JB, Kroc RL (eds): *Human Development and the Thyroid Gland: Relation to Endemic Cretinism*. New York, Plenum, 1972, p 449.
42. Thilly CH, Delange F, Lagasse R, Bourdoux P, Ramioul L, Berquist H, Ermans AM: Fetal hypothyroidism and maternal thyroid status in severe endemic goiter. *J Clin Endocrinol Metab* 47:354, 1978.
43. Hershman JM, Due DT, Sharp B, My L, Kent JR, Binh LN, et al: Endemic goiter in Vietnam. *J Clin Endocrinol Metab* 57:243, 1983.
44. Gaitan JE, Mayoral LG, Gaitan E: Defective thyroidal iodine concentration in protein-calorie malnutrition. *J Clin Endocrinol Metab* 57:327, 1983.
45. Ingenbleek Y, Luypaert B, De Nayer PH: Nutritional status and endemic goitre. *Lancet* 1:388, 1980.
46. Eggo MC, Burrow GN: Glycosylation of thyroglobulin—its role in secretion, iodination, and stability. *Endocrinology* 113:1655, 1983.
47. Kimball OP: The prevention of simple goiter in man. *Am J Med Sci* 163:634, 1922.
48. Vander JB, Gaston EA, Dawber TR: The significance of nontoxic thyroid nodules. *Ann Intern Med* 69:537, 1968.
49. Mortensen JD, Bennett WA, Woolner LB: Incidence of carcinoma in thyroid glands removed at 1000 consecutive routine necropsies. *Surg Forum* 5:659, 1955.
50. Kieffer JD, Mover H, Federico P, Maloof F: Pituitary-thyroid axis in neonatal and adult rats: Comparison of the sexes. *Endocrinology* 98:295, 1976.
51. Crooks J, Aboul-Khair SA, Turnbull AC, Hytten FE: The incidence of goitre during pregnancy. *Lancet* 2:334, 1964.
52. Crooks J, Tulloch MI, Turnbull AC, Davidsson D, Skulason T, Snaedal G: Comparative incidence of goitre in pregnancy in Iceland and Scotland. *Lancet* 2:625, 1967.
53. Glinoer D, De Nayer P, Bourdoux P, Leome M, Robyn C, Van Steirteghem A, et al: Regulation of maternal thyroid during pregnancy. *J Clin Endocrinol Metab* 71:276, 1990.
54. Dworkin HJ, Jacquez JA, Beierwaltes WH: Relationship of iodine ingestion to iodine excretion in pregnancy. *J Clin Endocrinol Metab* 26:1329, 1966.
55. Levy RP, Newman DM, Rejali LS, Barford DAG: The myth of goiter in pregnancy. *Am J Obstet Gynecol* 137:701, 1980.
56. Malamos B, Miras K, Kostamis P, Mantzos J, Kralios AC, Rigopoulos G, et al: Epidemiologic and metabolic studies in the endemic goiter areas of Greece, in Cassano C, Andreoli M (eds): *Current Topics in Thyroid Research*. New York, Academic, 1965, p 851.
57. Greig WR, Boyle JA, Duncan A, Nicol J, Gray MJB, Buchanan WW, McGirr EM: Genetic and non-genetic factors in simple goitre formation: Evidence from a twin study. *Q J Med* 36:175, 1967.
58. Nilsson LR: Adolescent colloid goitre. *Acta Paediatr Scand* 55:49, 1966.
59. Vickery AL: The diagnosis of malignancy in dyshormonogenic goiter. *J Clin Endocrinol Metab* 10:317, 1981.
60. Gaitan E: Goitrens. *Baillieres Clin Endocrinol Metab* 2:683, 1988.
61. Chesney AM, Clawson TA, Webster B: Endemic goitre in rabbits: I. Incidence and characteristics. *Bull Johns Hopkins Hosp* 43:261, 1928.
62. Gaitan E, Wahner HW, Correa P, Bernal R, Jubiz W, Gaitan JE, Llanos G: Endemic goiter in the Cauca Valley: I. Results and limitations of twelve years of iodine prophylaxis. *J Clin Endocrinol Metab* 28:1730, 1968.
63. Berry MJ, Banu L, Larsen PR: Type 1 iodothyronine deiodinase is a selenocysteine-containing enzyme. *Nature* 349:438, 1991.
64. Goyens P, Golstein J, Nsombola B, Vis H, Dumont JE: Selenium deficiency as a possible factor in the pathogenesis of myxedematous endemic cretinism. *Acta Endocrinol (Copenh)* 114:497, 1987.
65. McGarrison R: *The Thyroid Gland in Health and Disease*. London, Bailliere, Tindall and Cox, 1917.
66. Silverberg SG, Vidone RA: Carcinoma of the thyroid in surgical and postmortem material. *Ann Surg* 164:291, 1966.
67. Jauregui R, Lilker ES, Bayley A: Upper airway obstruction in euthyroid goiter. *JAMA* 238:2163, 1977.
68. Cady B: Management of tracheal obstruction from thyroid diseases. *World J Surg* 6:696, 1982.
69. Medvei UC: *A History of Endocrinology*. Lancaster, United Kingdom, MTP, 1982.
70. Sampson RJ, Key CR, Buncher CR, Iijima S: Thyroid carcinoma in Hiroshima and Nagasaki: I. Prevalence of thyroid carcinoma at autopsy. *JAMA* 209:65, 1969.
71. Sampson RJ: Prevalence and significance of occult thyroid cancer, in DeGroot LJ (ed): *Radiation-Associated Thyroid Carcinoma*. New York, Grune & Stratton, 1977, p 45.
72. Cutler SJ, Young JL (eds): *Third National Cancer Survey: Incidence Data*. National Cancer Institute Monograph 41, U.S. DHEW publication (NIH) 75-787, Bethesda, MD, 1975, pp 107, 111.
73. Taylor S, Goolden AWG: Thyroid and thymus, in Kunkler PB, Rains AJH (eds): *Treatment of Cancer in Clinical Practice*. Edinburgh, E & S Livingstone, 1959, p 410.
74. Stock JM, Surks MI, Oppenheimer JH: Replacement dosage of L-thyroxine in hypothyroidism. *N Engl J Med* 290:529, 1974.
75. Astwood EB, Cassidy CE, Aurbach GD: Treatment of goiter and thyroid nodules with thyroid. *JAMA* 174:459, 1960.
76. Lamberg BA, Hernberg CA, Hakkila R: Treatment of nontoxic goitre with thyroid preparations. *Acta Endocrinol (Copenh)* 33:584, 1960.
77. Shimaoka K, Sokal JE: Suppressive therapy of nontoxic goiter. *Am J Med* 57:576, 1974.
78. Hansen JM, Kampmann J, Madsen SH, Skovsted L, Solgaard S, Grytter C, et al: L-thyroxine treatment of diffuse nontoxic goitre evaluated by ultrasonic determination of thyroid volume. *Clin Endocrinol (Oxf)* 10:1, 1979.
79. Clark OH: TSH suppression in the management of thyroid nodules and thyroid cancer. *World J Surg* 5:39, 1981.
80. Gharib H: Changing concepts in the diagnosis and management of thyroid nodules. *Endo and Metab Clin of North America* 26:777, 1997.
81. Mazzaferri EL: Management of a solitary nodule. *N Engl J Med* 328:553, 1998.
82. Hermus AR, Huysmans DA: Treatment of benign nodular thyroid disease. *N Engl J Med* 388:1438, 1998.
83. Uzzan B, Campos J, Cucherat M, Nony P, Boissel J-P, Perret GY: Effects on bone mass of long term treatment with thyroid hormone: A meta-analysis. *J Clin Endo* 81:4278, 1996.
84. Sawin CT, Geller A, Wolf PA, Belanger AJ, Baker E, Bacharach P, et al: Low serum TSH concentrations as a risk factor for atrial fibrillation in older persons. *N Engl J Med* 331:1249, 1994.
85. Wartofsky L: Levothyroxine therapy and osteoporosis. An end to the controversy? *Arch Int Med* 155:1130, 1995.
86. Newman E, Shaha AR: Substernal goiter. *J of Surg Onc* 60:207, 1995.

87. Mack E: Management of patients with substernal goiter. *Surg Clin NA* 75:377, 1995.
88. Shimaoka K, Sokal JE: Differentiation of benign and malignant thyroid nodules by scintiscan. *Arch Intern Med* 114:36, 1964.
89. Hoffmann GL, Thompson NW, Heffron C: The solitary thyroid nodule. *Arch Surg* 105:379, 1972.
90. McClennan DR, Francis GL: Thyroid cancer in children, pregnant women and patients with Graves'Disease. *Thyroid Cancer II* 25:27, 1996.
91. Gorlin R: syndromes of the head and neck. Oxford University Press, New York, p 385, 1990.
92. Raab SS, Sliverman JF, Elsheikh TM, Thomas PA, Wakely PE: Pediatric thyroid nodules: disease demographics and clinical management as determined by fine needle aspiration biopsy. *Pediatrics* 95:46, 1995.
93. Duffy BJ Jr, Fitzgerald PJ: Cancer of the thyroid in children: A report of 28 cases. *J Clin Endocrinol Metab* 10:1296, 1950.
94. Pifer JW, Hempelmann LH: Radiation-induced thyroid carcinoma. *Ann NY Acad Sci* 114:838, 1964.
95. Schneider AB, Ron E, Lubin J, Stovall M, Gierlowski TC: Dose-response relationships for radiation-induced thyroid cancer and thyroid nodules: Evidence for the prolonged effects of radiation on the thyroid. *J Clin Endocrinol Metab* 77:362,1993.
96. Schneider AB, Bekerman C, Leland J, et al: Thyroid nodules in the follow up of irradiated individuals: Comparison of thyroid ultrasound with scanning and palpation. *J Clin Endocrinol Metab* 82:4020, 1997.
97. Sarne D, Schneider AB: External radiation and thyroid neoplasia. *Thyroid Cancer II* 25:181, 1996.
98. Maxon HR, Thomas SR, Saenger EL, Buncher CR, Kereiakes JG: Ionizing irradiation and the induction of clinically significant disease in the human thyroid gland. *Am J Med* 63:967, 1977.
99. Maxon HR, Saenger EL, Thomas SR, Buncher CR, Kereiakes JG, Shafer ML, McLaughlin CA: Clinically important radiation-associated thyroid disease: A controlled study. *JAMA* 244:1802, 1980.
100. Holm L-E, Dahlqvist I, Israelsson A, Lundell G: Malignant thyroid tumors after iodine-131 therapy: A retrospective cohort study. *N Engl J Med* 303:188, 1980.
101. Schneider AB: Radiation-induced thyroid tumors. *Endocrinol Metab Clin North Am* 19:495, 1990.
102. Fogelfeld L, Wiviott MBT, Shore-Freedman E, Blend M, Bekerman C, Pinsky S, Schneider AB: Recurrence of thyroid nodules after surgical removal in patients irradiated in childhood for benign conditions. *N Engl J Med* 320:835, 1989.
103. Bowens OM, Vander BJ: Thyroid nodules and thyroid malignancy. *Ann Intern Med* 57:245, 1962.
104. Carmeci D, Jeffrey RB, McDougall IR, Nowels KW, Weigel RJ: Ultrasound-guided fine-needle aspiration biopsy of thyroid masses. *Thyroid* 8:283,1998.
105. Rosai J, Carcangiu M-L, DeLellis R: Tumors of the thyroid gland. Armed Forces Institute of Pathology, Electronic Fascicle: V.2.0, Washington, DC, 20306-6000, 1995
106. Gharib H, Goellner JR, Johnson DA: Fine needle aspiration cytology of the thyroid: A 12-year experience with 11,000 biopsies. *Clin Lab Med* 13:699, 1993.
107. Gharib H: Fine-needle aspiration biopsy of thyroid nodules: Advantages, limitations and effect. *Mayo Clin Proc* 69:44, 1994.
108. Gharib, H: Changing concepts in the diagnosis and management of thyroid nodules. *Endo and Metab Clin of North America* 26(4):777, 1997.
109. Naik KS, Bury RF: Imaging the thyroid. *Clin Radiology* 53:630, 1998.
110. Clark OH, Okerlund MD, Cavalieri RR, et al: Diagnosis and treatment of thyroid, parathyroid and thyroblossal duct cysts. *J Clin Endocrinol Metab* 48:983, 1979.
111. Gharib H, Goellner JR: Evaluation of nodular thyroid disease. *Endocrinol Metab Clin North Am* 17:511, 1988.
112. Treece GL, Georgitis WJ, Hofeldt FD: Resolution of recurrent thyroid cysts with tetracycline instillation. *Arch Intern Med* 143:2285, 1983.
113. Miller JM, Hamburger JI, Mellinger RC: The thyroid scintigram: II. The cold nodule. *Radiology* 85:702, 1965.
114. DeGroot LJ, Hoye K, Refetoff S, Van Herle AJ, Asteris GT, Rochman H: Serum antigens and antibodies in the diagnosis of thyroid cancer. *J Clin Endocrinol Metab* 45:1220, 1977.
115. Esser PD: Absorbed radiation doses in adults, in Freeman LM, Johnson PM (eds): *Clinical Scintillation Imaging*, 2nd ed. New York, Grune & Stratton, 1975, p 799.
116. Keyes JW, Thrall JH, Carey JE: Technical considerations in in vivo thyroid studies. *Semin Nucl Med* 8:43, 1978.
117. McNeil BJ, Keeler E, Adelstein SJ: Primer on certain elements of medical decision making. *N Engl J Med* 293:211, 1975.
118. Van Herle AJ, Rich P, Ljung B-ME, Ashcraft MW, Solomon DH, Keeler EB: The thyroid nodule. *Ann Intern Med* 96:221, 1982.
119. Gharib H, James EM, Charboneau JW, et al: Suppressive therapy with levothyroxine for solitary thyroid nodules: A double-blind controlled clinical study. *N Engl J Med* 317:70,1987.
120. La Rosa GL, Lupo L, Giuffrida D, et al: Levothyroxine and potassium iodide are both effective in treating benign solitary solid cold nodules of the thyroid. *Ann Intern Med* 122:1,1995.
121. Mainini E, Martinelli I, Morandi G, et al: Levothyroxine suppressive therapy for solitary thyroid nodule. *J Endo Invest* 18:796, 1995.
122. Papini E, Petrucci L, Guglielmi R, Panunzi C, Rinaldi R, Bacci V, et al: Long-term changes in nodular goiter: A 5-year prospective randomized trial of levothyroxine suppressive therapy for benign cold thyroid nodules. *J Clin Endocrinol Metab* 83:780, 1998.
123. Kuma K, Matsuzuka F, Yokozawa T, et al: Fate of untreated benign thyroid nodules: Results of long-term follow-up. *World J Surg* 18:495, 1994.
124. Schneider DL, Barrett-Connor EL, Morton DJ: Thyroid hormone use and bone mineral density in elderly women: Effects of estrogen. *JAMA* 271:1245, 1994.
125. Zingrillo M, Collura D, Ghiggi MR, Nirchio V, Trischitta V: Treatment of large cold benign thyroid nodules not eligible for surgery with percutaneous ethanol injection. *J Clin Endocrinol and Metab* 83:3905, 1998.
126. Meissner WA: The pathologic classification and staging of thyroid cancer, in DeGroot LJ (ed): *Radiation-Associated Thyroid Carcinoma*. New York, Grune & Stratton, 1977, p 45.
127. Hay ID: Papillary thyroid carcinoma. *Endocrinol Metab Clin North Am* 19:545, 1990.
128. Hay ID, Bergstralh EJ, Goellner JR, et al: Predicting outcome in papillary thyroid carcinoma: Development of a reliable prognostic scoring system in a cohort of 1,799 patients surgically treated at one institution during 1940 through 1989. *Surgery* 114:1050,1993.
129. Cady B, Rossi: An expanded view of risk-group definition in differentiated thyroid carcinoma. *Surg* 104:947, 1988.
130. Sanders LE, Cady B: Differentiated thyroid cancer: Reexamination of risk groups and outcome of treatment. *Arch Surg* 133:419, 1998.
131. Byar DP, Green SB, Dor P, Williams ED, Colon J, van Gilse HA, et al: A prognostic index for thyroid carcinoma. A study of the E.O.R.T.C. thyroid cancer cooperative group. *Eur J Cancer* 15: 1033, 1979.
132. Beahrs O, Henson DE, Hutter RVP, Kennedy BJ, (eds): Manual for staging of cancer, 3rd edition. Philadelphia, JB Lippincott Co., 1988.
133. Mazzaferri EL, Jhiang SM: Long-term impact of initial surgical and medical therapy on papillary and follicular thyroid cancer. *Am J Med* 97:418, 1994.
134. DeGroot LJ, Kaplan EL, McCormick M, Straus FH: Natural history, treatment, and course of papillary thyroid carcinoma. *J Clin Endocrinol Metab* 71:414, 1990.
135. Noguchi S, Murakami N, Kawamoto H: Classification of papillary cancer of the thyroid based on prognosis. *World J Surg* 18:552, 1994.
136. Shaha AR, Sha JP, Loree TR: Risk group stratification and prognostic factors in papillary carcinoma of thyroid. *Ann Surg Oncol* 3:534, 1996.
137. Asklen LA: Prognostic importance of histologic grading in papillary thyroid carcinoma. *Cancer* 72:2680, 1993.
138. Brierly JD, Panzarella T, Tsang RW, Gospodarowicz MK, O'Sullivan B: A comparison of different staging systems predictability of patient outcome: Thyroid carcinoma as an example. *Cancer* 79:2414, 1997.
139. Smith SA, Hay ID, Goellner JR, Ryan JJ, McConahey WM: Mortality from papillary thyroid carcinoma: A case-control study of 56 lethal cases. *Cancer* 62:1381, 1988.
140. Cohn KH, Backdahl M, Forsslund G, et al: Prognostic value of nuclear DNA content in papillary thyroid carcinoma. *World J Surg* 8:474, 1984.
141. Flynn S, Kinder BK: Histologic, flow cytometric, and genetic criteria in endocrine surgery. *Curr Opin Gen Surg* 115, 1993.

142. Farid NR: Molecular pathogenesis of thyroid cancer: The significance of oncogenes, tumor suppressor genes, and genomic instability. *Exp Clin Endocrinol Diabetes* 104:1, 1996.
143. Russo D, Arturi F, Schlumberger M, et al: Activating mutations of the TSH receptor in differentiated thyroid carcinomas. *Oncogene* 11:1907, 1995.
144. Farid NR, Shi Y, Zou M: Molecular basis of thyroid cancer. *Endocrinol Rev* 15:202, 1994.
145. Sugg SL, Ezzat S, Rosen IB, Freeman JL, Asa SL: Distinct multiple *RET*/PTC gene rearrangements in multifocal papillary thyroid neoplasia. *J Clin Endocrinol Metab* 83:4116, 1998.
146. Livolsi V, Lam A, Montone K: Ret oncogene activation in papillary thyroid carcinoma: prevalence and implication on the histological parameters. *Human Pathol* 29:565, 1998.
147. Bongarzone I, Fugazzola L, Vigneri P, et al: Age-related activation of the tyrosine kinase receptor protooncogenes RET and NTRK1 in papillary thyroid carcinoma. *J Clin Endocrinol Metab* 81:2006, 1996.
148. Fugazzola L, Pilotti S, Pinchera A, et al: Oncogenic rearrangements of the RET proto-oncogene in papillary thyroid carcinomas from children exposed to the Chernobyl nuclear accident. *Cancer Res* 55:5617,1995.
149. Nikiforov YE, Rowland JM, Bove KE, Monforte-Munoz H, Fagin JA: Distinct pattern of ret oncogene rearrangements in morphological variants of radiation-induced and sporadic thyroid papillary carcinomas in children. *Cancer Res* 57:1690, 1997.
150. Belfiore A, Gamgemi P, Santomocito MG, et al: Prognostic value of c-MET expression in papillary thyroid carcinoma. *Thyroid* 5 (suppl 1):5, 1995.
151. Zou M, Shi Y, Farid NR: Frequent inactivation of the retinoblastoma gene in human thyroid carcinoma. *Endocrine J* 2:193, 1994.
152. Fagin JA, Matsuo K, Karmakar A, et al: High prevalence of mutations of the p53 gene in poorly differentiated human thyroid carcinomas. *J Clin Invest* 91:179, 1993.
153. Smida J, Zitzelsberger H, Kellerer AM, Lehmann L, Minkus G, Negele T, et al: p53 mutations in childhood thyroid tumours from Belarus and in thyroid tumours without radiation history. *Int J Cancer* 73:802, 1997.
154. Elisei R, Shiohara M, Koeffler HP, Fagin JA: Genetic and epigenetic alterations of cyclin-dependent kinase inhibitors $p15^{INK4b}$ and $p16^{INK4a}$ in human thyroid carcinoma cell lines and primary thyroid carcinomas. *Cancer* 83:2185, 1998.
155. Zhang JS, Nelson M, McIver B, Hay ID, Goellner JR, Grant CS, et al: Differential loss of heterozygosity at 7q31.2 in follicular and papillary thyroid tumors. *Oncogene* 17:789, 1998.
156. Sampson RJ: Prevalence and significance of occult thyroid cancer, in DeGroot LJ (ed): *Radiation-Associated Thyroid Carcinoma*. New York, Grune & Stratton, 1977, p 45.
157. Moosa M, Mazzaferri EL: Outcome of differentiated thyroid cancer diagnosed in pregnant women. *J Clin Endocrinol Metab* 82:2862, 1997.
158. Margolin FR, Steinbach HL: Soft tissue roentgenography of thyroid nodules. *AJR* 102:844, 1968.
159. Satoh Y, Sakamoto A, Yamada K, Dasai N: Psammoma bodies in metastatic carcinoma to the thyroid. *Mod Pathol* 3:267, 1990.
160. Mazzaferri EL, Young RL, Oertel JE, Kemmerer WT, Page CP: Papillary thyroid carcinoma: The impact of therapy in 576 patients. *Medicine (Baltimore)* 56:171, 1977.
161. Mazzaferri EL, Young RL: Papillary thyroid carcinoma: A 10-year follow-up report of the impact of therapy in 576 patients. *Am J Med* 70:511, 1981.
162. Carcangiu ML, Zampi G, Pupi A, Castagnoli A, Rosai J: Papillary carcinoma of the thyroid A clinicopathologic study of 241 cases treated at the University of Florence, Italy. *Cancer* 55:805, 1985.
163. Johnson TL, Lloyd RV, Thompson NW, Beierwaltes WH, Sisson JC: Prognostic implications of the tall cell variant of papillary thyroid carcinoma. *Am J Surg Pathol* 12:22, 1988.
164. Fujimoto Y, Obara T, Ito Y, Kodama T, Aiba M, Yamaguchi K: Diffuse sclerosing variant of papillary carcinoma of the thyroid. *Cancer* 66:2306, 1990.
165. Mazziferri EL: Thyroid cancer and Graves' disease. *J Clin Endocrinol Metab* 70:826, 1990.
166. Belfiore A, Garofalo MR, Guiffrida D, Runello F, Filetti S, Fiumara A, et al: Increased aggressiveness of thyroid cancer in patients with Graves' disease. *J Clin Endocrinol Metab* 70:830, 1990.
167. Pellegriti G, Belfiore A, Giuffrida D, Lupo L, Vigneri R: Outcome of differentiated thyroid cancer in Graves' patients. *J Clin Endocrinol Metab* 83:2805, 1998.
168. Hofstadter F: Frequency and morphology of malignant tumours of the thyroid before and after the introduction of iodine prophylaxis. *Virchows Arch* [*A*] 385:263, 1980.
169. Simpson WJ, McKinney SE, Carruthers JS, Gospodarowicz MK, Sutcliffe SB, Panzarella T: Papillary and follicular thyroid cancer: Prognostic factors in 1578 patients. *Am J Med* 83:479, 1987.
170. Paul SJ, Sisson JC: Thyrotoxicosis caused by thyroid cancer. *Endo Metab Clin North Am* 19:593, 1990.
171. Van Heerden JA, Hay ID, Goellner JR, Salamao D, Ebersold JR, Bergstralh EJ, Grant CS: Follicular thyroid carcinoma with capsular invasion alone: A nonthreatening malignancy. *Surgery* 112:1130, 1992.
172. Lang W, Choritz H, Hundeshagen H: Risk factors in follicular thyroid carcinomas. A retrospective follow-up study covering a 14-year period with emphasis on morphological findings. *Am J Surg Path* 10:246, 1986.
173. Silliphant WM, Klinck GH, Levitin MS: Thyroid carcinoma and death: A clinicopathological study of 193 autopsies. *Cancer* 17:513, 1964.
174. Rosai J, Carcangiu, M, Delellis R: Tumors of the thyroid gland. In: *Atlas of tumor pathology*. 3rd series. Fasicle 5. Washington, D.C.: Armed Forces Institute of Pathology, 1992.
175. Kapp D, LiVolsi VA, Sanders MM: Anaplastic carcinoma following well-differentiated thyroid cancer etiological considerations. *Yale J Biol Med* 55:521, 1982.
176. Simpson WJ: Anaplastic thyroid carcinoma: A new approach. *Can J Surg* 23:25, 1980.
177. Smithers D (ed): *Tumours of the Thyroid Gland*. Edinburgh, E & S Livingstone, 1970.
178. Shimaoka K: Adjunctive management of thyroid cancer: Chemotherapy. *J Surg Oncol* 15:283, 1980.
179. Gottlieb JA, Hill CS Jr: Chemotherapy of thyroid cancer with Adriamycin. *N Engl J Med* 290:193, 1974.
180. Harada T, Nishikawa Y, Suzuki T, Ito K, Baba S: Bleomycin treatment for cancer of the thyroid. *Am J Surg* 122:53, 1971.
181. Venkatesh YS, Ordonez NG, Schultz PN, Hickey RC, Goepfert H, Samaan NA: Anaplastic carcinoma of the thyroid. A clinicopathologic study of 121 cases. *Cancer* 66:321, 1990.
182. Blagosklonny MV, Giannakakou P, Wojtowicz M, Romanova LY, Alli KB, Bates SE, Fojo T: Effects of p53-expressing adenovirus on the chemosensitivity and differentiation of anaplastic thyroid cancer cells. *J Clin Endocrinol Metab* 83:2516, 1998.
183. Hill CS Jr, Ibanez ML, Samaan NA, Ahearn MJ, Clark RL: Medullary (solid) carcinoma of the thyroid gland: An analysis of the M.D. Anderson Hospital experience with patients with the tumor, its special features, and its histogenesis. *Medicine (Baltimore)* 52:141, 1973.
184. Khari MRA, Dexter RN, Burzynski NJ, Johnston CC Jr: Mucosal neuroma, heochromocytoma and medullary thyroid carcinoma: Multiple endocrine neoplasia type 3. *Medicine (Baltimore)* 54:89, 1975.
185. Donis-Keller H, Dou S, Chi D, et al: Mutations in the RET proto-oncogene are associated with MEN 2A and FMTC. *Hum Mol Genet* 2:851, 1993.
186. Mulligan LM, Kwok JBJ, Healey CS, et al: Germline mutations of the RET proto-oncogene in multiple endocrine neoplasia type 2A. *Nature* 363:458, 1993.
187. Wells SA, Skinner MA: Prophylactic thyroidectomy, based on direct genetic testing, in patients at risk for the multiple endocrine neoplasia type 2 syndromes. *Exp Clin Endocrinol Diabetes* 106:29, 1998.
188. Lips C, Landsvater R, Hoppener J: Clinical screening as compared with DNA analysis in families with multiple endocrine neoplasm Type 2A. *N Engl J Med* 331:828, 1994.
189. Lallier M, St-Vil D, Giroux M, Huot C, Gaboury L, Oligny L, Desjardins JG: Prophylactic thyroidectomy for medullary thyroid carcinoma in gene carriers of MEN2 syndrome. *J Ped Surg* 33:846, 1998.
190. Eng C, Mulligan LM, Healey CS, et al: Heterogeneous mutation of the RET proto-oncogene in subpopulations of medullary thyroid carcinoma. *Cancer Res* 56:167, 1996.
191. Chetty R, O'Leary JJ, Biddolph SC, Gatter KC: Immunohistochemical detection of p53 and Bcl-1 proteins in Hashimoto's thyroiditis and primary thyroid lymphomas. *J Clin Path* 48:239, 1995.

192. Devine RM, Edis AJ, Banks PM: Primary lymphoma of the thyroid: A review of the Mayo Clinic experience through 1978. *World J Surg* 5:33, 1981.
193. Doria R, Jekel JF, Cooper DL: Thyroid lymphoma. The case for combined modality therapy. *Cancer* 73:200, 1994.
194. Chak LY, Hoppe RT, Burke JS, Kaplan HS: Non-Hodgkin's lymphoma presenting as thyroid enlargement. *Cancer* 48:2712, 1981.
195. Nicolaides AR, Rhys Evans P, Fisher C: Adenosquamous carcinoma of the thyroid gland. *J Laryngol Otol* 103:978, 1989.
196. Burman KD, Ringel MD, Wartofsky L: Unusual types of thyroid neoplasms. *Thyroid Cancer II* 25:49, 1996.
197. Harrison DF: Thyroid gland in the management of laryngopharyngeal cancer. *Arch Otolaryngol* 97:301, 1973.
198. Shimaoka K, Sokal JE, Pickren JW: Metastatic neoplasms in the thyroid gland. *Cancer* 15:557, 1962.
199. Green LK, Ro JY, Mackay B, Ayala AG, Luna MA: Renal cell carcinoma metastatic to the thyroid. *Cancer* 63:1810, 1989.
200. Tibaldi JM, Shapiro LE, Mahadevia PS: Thyroiditis mimicked by metastatic carcinoma to the thyroid [Letter]. *Mayo Clin Proc* 61:399, 1986.
201. Schwartz AE, Clark O, Ituarte P, LoGerfo P: Therapeutic controversy. Thyroid surgery—the choice. *J Clin Endocrinol Metab* 83:1097, 1998.
202. Clark OH: Total thyroidectomy: The treatment of choice for patients with differentiated thyroid cancer. *Ann Surg* 196:361, 1982.
203. Degroot LJ, Kaplan EL, Straus FH: Does the method of management of papillary thyroid carcinoma make a difference in outcome? *World J Surg* 18:123, 1994.
204. Samaan NA, Maheshwari YK, Nader S, Hill CS Jr, Schultz PN, Haynie TP, et al: Impact of therapy for differentiated carcinoma of the thyroid: An analysis of 706 cases. *J Clin Endocrinol Metab* 56:1131, 1983.
205. Hay ID, Grant CS, Taylor WF, McConahey WM: Ipsilateral lobectomy versus bilateral lobar resection in papillary thyroid carcinoma: A retrospective analysis of surgical outcome using a novel prognostic scoring system. *Surgery* 102:1088, 1987.
206. Shaha AR, Sha JP, Loree TR: Low-risk differentiated thyroid cancer: The need for selective treatment. *Ann Surg Oncol* 4:328, 1997.
207. Demeure MJ, Clark OH: Surgery in the treatment of thyroid cancer. *Endocrinol Metab Clin North Am* 19:663, 1990.
208. Thompson N, Eckhauser F, Harness J: The anatomy of primary hyperparathyroidism. *Surgery* 92:297, 1982.
209. Hershman JM, Edwards CL: Serum thyrotropin (TSH) levels after thyroid ablation compared with TSH levels after exogenous bovine TSH: Implications for ^{131}I treatment of thyroid carcinoma. *J Clin Endocrinol Metab* 34:814, 1972.
210. Hobbiger HE, Allen JG, Greatorex RG, et al: The laryngeal mask airway for thyroid and parathyroid surgery. *Anesthesia* 51:972, 1996.
211. LoGerfo P: Local/regional anesthesia for thyroidectomy: Evaluation as an outpatient procedure. *Am Assoc Endo Surg 19th Annual Mtg*, paper #9, 1998.
212. Mazzaferri EL: Papillary thyroid carcinoma: Factors influencing prognosis and current therapy. *Semin Oncol* 14:315, 1987.
213. Jossart GH, Clark OH. Wells SA (ed): Well-differentiated thyroid cancer. *Current Problems in Surgery*, Mosby, St. Louis, MO, 1994 p 935.
214. Frankenthaler RA, Sellin RV, Cangir A, Goepfert H: Lymph node metastasis from papillary-follicular thyroid carcinoma in young patients. *Am J Surg* 160:341, 1990.
215. Shin DH, Mark EJ, Suen HC, Grillo HC: Pathologic staging of papillary carcinoma of the thyroid with airway invasion based on the anatomic manner of extension to the trachea: A clinicopathologic study based on 22 patients who underwent thyroidectomy and airway resection. *Human Pathol* 24:866, 1993.
216. Bayles SW, Kingdom TT, Carlson GW: Management of thyroid carcinoma invading the aerodigestive tract. *Laryngoscope* 108:1402, 1998.
217. McCarty TM, Kuhn JA, Williams WL, Ellenhorn JDI, O'Brien JC, Preskitt JT, et al: Surgical management of thyroid cancer invading the airway. *Ann Surgical Oncol* 4:403, 1997.
218. DeGroot LJ, Reilly M: Comparison of 30- and 50-mCi doses of iodine-131 for thyroid ablation. *Ann Intern Med* 96:51, 1982.
219. Beierwaltes WH: The treatment of thyroid carcinoma with radioactive iodine. *Semin Nucl Med* 8:79, 1978.
220. Solomon, BL, Wartofsky L, Burman KD: Current trends in the management of well differentiated papillary thyroid carcinoma. *J Clin Endocrinol Metab* 81:333, 1996.
221. Edmonds CJ, Hayes S, Kermode JC, et al: Measurement of serum TSH and thyroid hormones in the management and treatment of thyroid carcinoma with radioiodine. *Br J Radiol* 50:799, 1977.
222. Maxon HR, Smith HS: Radioiodine-I131 in the diagnosis and treatment of metastatic well differentiated thyroid cancer. *Endocrinol Metab Clin North Am* 19:685, 1990.
223. Muratet JP, Daver A, Minier JF, Larra F: Influence of scanning doses of iodine-131 on subsequent first ablative treatment outcome in patients operated on for differentiated thyroid carcinoma. *J Nucl Med* 39:1546, 1998.
224. Leeper RD, Shimaoka K: Treatment of metastatic thyroid cancer. *Clin Endocrinol Metab* 9:383, 1980.
225. Burmeister LA: Thyroid hormone in the treatment of thyroid cancer. *Thyroid Today* XVII, 1:1, 1994.
226. Schlumberger MJ: Papillary and follicular thryoid carcinoma. *N Engl J Med* 338:297, 1998.
227. Pujol P, Daures J-P, Nsakal N, Baldet L, Bringer J, Jaffiol C: Degree of thyrotropin suppression as a prognostic determinant in differentiated thyroid cancer. *J Clin Endocrinol Metab* 74:98, 1996.
228. Simon D, Koehrle J, Reiners C, Boerner AR, Schmutzler C, Mainz K, Goretzki PE, Roeher HD: Redifferentiation therapy with retinoids: Therapeutic option for advanced follicular thyroid carcinoma. *World J Surg* 22:569, 1998.
229. Ryu, K, Tong Q, Jhiang SM: Promoter characterization of the human Na^+/I^- symporter. *J Clin Endocrinol Metab* 83:3247, 1998.
230. Caillou B, Troalen F, Baudin E, Talbot M, Filetti S, Schlumberger M, Bidart JM: Na^+/I^- symporter distribution in human thyroid tissues: An immunohistochemical study. *J Clin Endocrinol Metab* 83:4102 1998.
231. Zeiger MA, Takiyama Y, Bishop JO, Ellison AR, Saji M, Levine MA: Adenoviral infection of thyroid cells: A rationale for gene therapy for metastatic thyroid carcinoma. *Surgery* 120:921, 1996.
232. Braiden V, Nagayama Y, Iitaka M, Namba H, Niwa M, Yamashita S: Retrovirus-mediated suicide gene/prodrug therapy targeting thyroid carcinoma using a thyroid-specific promoter. *Endocrinology* 139:3996, 1998.
233. Wartofsky L, Sherman SI, Gopal J, Schlumberger M, Hay ID: The use of radioactive iodine in patients with papillary and follicular thyroid cancer. *J Clin Endocrinol Metab* 83:4195, 1998.
234. Pacini F, Lippi F, Formica N, et al: Therapeutic doses of iodine-131 reveal undiagnosed metastases in thyroid cancer patients with detectable serum thyroglobulin levels. *J Nucl Med* 28:1888, 1987.
235. Pineda JD, Lee T, Ain K, Reynolds JC, Robbins J: Iodine-131 therapy for thyroid cancer patients with elevated thyroglobulin and negative diagnostic scan. *J Clin Endocrinol Metab* 80:1488, 1995.
236. Dow KH, Ferrell BR, Anello C: Quality-of-life changes in patients with thyroid cancer after withdrawal of thyroid hormone therapy. *Thyroid* 7:613, 1997.
237. Ladenson PW, Braverman LE, Mazzaferri EL, Brucker-Davis F, Cooper DS, Garber JR, et al: Wondisford FE, Davies TF, DeGroot LJ, Daniels GH, Ross DS, Weintraub BD: Comparison of administration of recombinant human thyrotropin with withdrawal of thyroid hormone for radioactive iodine scanning in patients with thyroid carcinoma. *N Engl J Med* 337:888, 1997.
238. Meier CA, Braverman LE, Ebner SA, et al: Diagnostic use of human recombinant thyrotropin in patients with thyroid carcinoma (phase I/II study). *J Clin Endocrinol Metab* 78:188, 1994.
239. Ringel MD, Ladenson PW: Diagnostic accuracy of ^{131}I scanning with recombinant hyman thyrotropin versus thyroid hormone withdrawal in a patient with metastatic thyroid carcinoma and hypopituitarism. *J Clin Endocrinol Metab* 81:1724, 1996.
240. Alexander C, Bader JB, Schaefer A, Finke C, Kirsch CM: Intermediate and long-term side effects of high-dose radioiodine therapy for thyroid carcinoma. *J Nucl Med* 39:1551, 1998.
241. Galloway RJ, Smallridge RC: Imaging in thyroid cancer. *Thyroid Cancer II* 25:93, 1996.
242. Dietlein M, Scheidhauer K, Voth E, et al: Follow up of differentiated thyroid cancer: what is the value of FDG and sestamibi in the diagnostic algorithm? *Nuklearmedizin* 37:12, 1998.

243. Baudin E, Schlumberger M, Lumbroso J, et al: Octreotide scintigraphy in patients with differentiated thyroid carcinoma: contribution for patients with negative radioiodine scan. *J Clin Endocrinol Metab* 81:2541, 1996.
244. Garin E, Devillers A, LeCloirec J, Bernard AM, Lescouarc'h J, Herry JY, et al: Reubi JC, Bourguet P: Use of indium-111 pentetreotide somatostatin receptor scintigraphy to detect recurrent thyroid carcinoma in patients without detectable iodine uptake. *Euro J Nucl Med* 25:687, 1998.
245. Ditkoff BA, Marvin MR, Yemul S, Shi YJ, Chabot J, Feind C, LoGerfo P: Detection of circulating thyroid cells in peripheral blood. *Surgery* 120:959, 1996.
246. Tallini G, Ghossein RA, Emanuel J, Gill J, Kinder B, Dimich AB, et al: Detection of thyroglobulin, thyroid peroxidase, and *RET*/PTC1 mRNA transcripts in the peripheral blood of patients with thyroid disease. *J Clin Oncol* 16:1158, 1998.
247. Ringel MD, Ladenson PW, Levine MA: Molecular diagnosis of residual and recurrent thyroid cancer by amplification of thyroglobulin messenger ribonucleic acid in peripheral blood. *J Clin Endocrinol Metab* 83:4435, 1998.
248. Travagli JP, Cailleux AF, Ricard M, Baudin E, Caillou B, Parmentier C, Schlumberger M: Combination of radioiodine (^{131}I) and probe-guided surgery for persistent or recurrent thyroid carcinoma. *J Clin Endocrinol Metab* 83:2675, 1998.
249. Moley JF, Debenedetti MK, Dilley WG, Tisell LE, Wells SA: Surgical management of patients with persistent or recurrent medullary thyroid cancer. *J Intern Med* 243:521, 1998.
250. Van Heerden J, Grant CS, Gharib H, Hay ID, Ilstrup DM: Longterm course of patients with persistent hypercalcitoninemia after apparent curative primary surgery for medullary thyroid carcinoma. *Ann Surg* 212:F395, 1990.

PART IV

Adrenal Disease

CHAPTER 11

The Adrenal Cortex

Walter L. Miller

George P. Chrousos

EMBRYOLOGY, ANATOMY, AND HISTORY

The adrenal cortex produces three principal categories of steroid hormones. The *mineralocorticoids,* of which aldosterone is most important, regulate renal sodium retention and thus are key components in regulating sodium, potassium, blood pressure, and intravascular volume. Mineralocorticoid excess can cause hypertension and hypokalemia; mineralocorticoid deficiency can cause hyponatremia, hyperkalemia, hypotension, and shock. The *glucocorticoids,* of which cortisol is most important, are named for their role in maintaining serum glucose and regulating carbohydrate metabolism, but also play key regulatory roles in a wide variety of physiologic processes, including development, growth, immune responses, cardiovascular function, and responses to stress. Glucocorticoid excess can cause weight gain, moon facies, striae, growth arrest, weakness, easy bruisability, and glycosuria; glucocorticoid deficiency causes anorexia, anergia, fatigue, weight loss, hypoglycemia, and hypotension. There is no established role for the *adrenal androgens,* although they mediate some female secondary sexual characteristics, and there are claims that they can exert a panoply of salutory effects. Overproduction of adrenal androgens leads to acne, hirsutism, virilism, ovarian dysfunction, and infertility. Thus, the physiology and biochemistry of the adrenal cortex are of general interest in medicine and biology because of the numerous and varied effects of the secretions of the cortex. The adrenal cortex secretes dozens of steroids; although many of them are precursors or metabolites of the principal hormones, most have some biological activity. Knowledge about the actions of the various steroids in health and disease also facilitates an understanding of the actions of synthetic steroid hormones (e.g., prednisone, dexamethasone, and contraceptive steroids) widely used as pharmacotherapeutic agents.

Diseases of the adrenal cortex are being recognized with increasing frequency. Addison's disease, Cushing's syndrome, and Conn's (primary aldosteronism) syndrome, which are traditionally regarded as the three principal disorders of the adrenal cortex, are together less common than genetic disorders of steroid hormone synthesis, which are among the most common inborn errors of metabolism and are now being recognized with increasing frequency, especially among adult patients.[1] As the signs and symptoms of adrenal dysfunction are often relatively nonspecific, adrenal disorders must be considered in the differential diagnosis of many common complaints. Furthermore, because synthetic steroids are widely used to treat nonadrenal disorders, physicians often encounter syndromes of iatrogenic steroid excess. This chapter deals with the biochemistry and physiology of steroid hormone synthesis and the disorders of the adrenal cortex. Chap. 14 discusses steroid hormone therapy, and Chap. 13 deals with the roles of steroid hormones in hypertension in detail.

History

The history of medical and scientific study of the adrenal cortex closely parallels general advances in medicine, physiology, biochemistry, and molecular biology, and has been reviewed in detail.[2] The adrenals were first described by Bartolomeo Eustacchio (better known for the discovery of the eustachian tube of the ear) in 1563, but this work was lost until Lancisi republished it in 1714.[3,4] Scientific interest in the adrenals began with the description by Thomas Addison in 1849 and 1855 of the classic features of adrenocortical deficiency, which included "general languor and debility, remarkable feebleness of the heart's action, irritability of the stomach and a peculiar change in the colour of the skin." In 1856, Brown-Sequard showed that adrenalectomy is incompatible with life, supporting Addison's idea. The syndrome of glucocorticoid excess had been well described in association with adrenal tumors by the turn of the century, long before Harvey Cushing attributed the syndrome that bears his name to "pituitary basophilism."[5]

The roles of the specific products of the adrenal were elucidated with improved surgical approaches to adrenalectomy and hypophysectomy and were clarified further by the development of adrenal extracts that could replace lost function. A role for the adrenal in regulating carbohydrate metabolism was slowly elucidated between 1908 and 1940. Hypoglycemia in adrenal insufficiency was known by 1910, and in 1927 Cori and Cori showed that adrenalectomy decreases hepatic glycogen.[6] Britton and Silvette proposed that the loss of an adrenal carbohydrate-regulating property can cause the debility and mortality in adrenal insufficiency,[7] and Long and associates reported correction of hypoglycemia and decreased hepatic glycogen in adrenalectomized animals that were given adrenal extracts.[8] Additional roles for the adrenal in nitrogen excretion, gluconeogenesis, and lipid metabolism were recognized concurrently.[2,3]

The role of the adrenals in salt and water balance was appreciated somewhat later. In 1927 Banmann and Kurland reported that adrenalectomy causes hyponatremia, hypothermia, and hyperkalemia,[9] and in 1933, Loeb showed that saline can extend the survival of patients with Addison's disease.[10] By 1937, it was understood that sodium is necessary but not sufficient to maintain the life of adrenalectomized rats as these animals were also susceptible to toxins, trauma, infection, strenuous exercize, drugs, and other forms of stress. In 1946, Hans Selye coined the terms *glucocorticoid* and *mineralocorticoid,* emphasizing that both functions of the adrenal are needed for survival and for responses to stress.[11]

A role for the pituitary in regulating the adrenal was suspected by about 1925 (see Refs. 2 and 3), and by 1930 it was known that hypophysectomy causes adrenal atrophy. Adrenal feedback on pituitary function was reported in 1937, but it was correctly deduced that not all adrenal function is pituitary-dependent because survival after hypophysectomy was longer than survival after adrenalectomy. ACTH was purified in 1943 and its structure was known by 1956, but the origin of ACTH as a proteolytic cleavage product from a larger protein (proopiomelanocortin) was not established until the late 1970s (see Chap. 7).

Hypothalamic regulation of ACTH release was hypothesized in the late 1940s. Vasopressin stimulation of ACTH release was reported in 1954,[12] and this was quickly followed by studies showing that another factor is also involved.[13,14] However, another sixteen years passed before the structure of corticotrophin releasing hormone (CRH) was determined.[15]

An understanding of the functional significance of adrenal zonation, the role of the zona glomerulosa in electrolyte balance, and the independence of the glomerulosa from pituitary regulation emerged in the late 1940s. Aldosterone was identified and characterized in the 1950s,[16] and Conn described hypertension and hypokalemia with aldosterone excess in 1955.[17]

Edward Kendall and Tateus Reichstein independently purified and crystallized the first known glucocorticoid–corticosterone,[18] determined the chemical structures of numerous steroids, and synthesized these steroids, including the first known mineralocorticoid, deoxycorticosterone (DOC).[19] When Philip Hench administered cortisone to 14 arthritic patients in 1949, the results were dramatic.[20] The impact of the discovery that steroids can ameliorate the symptoms of rheumatoid arthritis made cortisone a household word. Kendall, Hench, and Reichstein were awarded the Nobel Prize in December 1950.

The availability of cortisone led immediately to its use in treating congenital adrenal hyperplasia by Wilkins[21] and Bartter.[22] The success of this experiment stimulated great interest in studying inborn errors of steroid synthesis, leading to our contemporary understanding of the pathways of steroidogenesis. The association of cytochrome P450 with 21-hydroxylase was made in 1965,[23] leading to an active era of enzymologic study. Most of the steroidogenic enzymes were ultimately isolated in the 1970s and 1980s, and their genes were cloned in the 1980s and 1990s.[24] At the same time, studies of steroid hormone action led to the identification of steroid hormone receptors in the 1960s, but it was not until they were cloned and studied in the 1980s and 90s that their biology was understood clearly.[25]

Embryology and Development

The adrenal cortex derives from the embryonic mesoderm, in contrast to the ectodermal origin of the medulla.[26,27] Between the fifth and sixth weeks of fetal development, the gonadal ridge, a proliferation of cells in the developing peritoneal epithelium at the base of the dorsal mesentary, develops near the cranial end of the mesonephros. These cells give rise to the steroidogenic cells of both the adrenal cortex and the gonads. The precursors of the adrenal and gonadal cells separate, with the adrenal anlage penetrating the retroperitoneal mesenchyme to form the primitive cortex while the gonadal anlage migrates caudally. The primitive adrenal soon becomes enveloped by a thick layer of more compactly arrayed cells to become the adrenal cortex. Soon thereafter, between the seventh and eighth weeks, the adrenal cortex is invaded by sympathetic neural cells that form the adrenal medulla. By the end of the eighth week, the adrenal has become encapsulated and has taken up residence on the cranial pole of the kidney, which at this time is much smaller than the developing adrenal.[26,27]

The fetal adrenal cortex consists of three zones: The subcapsular "definitive" zone, an ill-defined transitional zone, and the large fetal zone. Recent data suggest that these three fetal zones have steroidogenic potentials analogous to the zonae glomerulosa, fasciculata, and reticularis, respectively.[28] The fetal zone, which accounts for the overwhelming majority of fetal adrenal cells, makes androgenic precursors (principally dehydroepiandrosterone) that are used as substrates for placental synthesis of estrogens. Recent studies have suggested that placental CRH stimulates adrenal androgen secretion by the fetal adrenal zone and may play a role in trophically sustaining this zone. The adrenal is relatively huge in the fetus and newborn. At birth, the adrenals weigh about 8 to 9 g, about twice the weight of adult adrenals, and represent 0.5 percent of total body weight, compared with 0.005 percent in the adult. However, after birth, the fetal zone involutes. By the second week after birth adrenal weight has decreased by one-third, and the fetal zone is no longer detectable by age 1 year. The definitive zone of the fetal adrenal simultaneously develops into the adult adrenal cortex. However, the zona glomerulosa and zona fasciculata are not fully developed until about 3 years of age, and the zona reticularis may not be fully grown until the third decade of life.

Anatomy

The adrenal glands are extraperitoneal, at the upper poles of the kidneys (Fig. 11-1). They are located on the posterior parietal wall, on each side of the vertebral column, lateral to the eleventh thoracic and the first lumbar vertebrae. The average adult gland weighs 4 g irrespective of an individual's sex or size, and is 2- to 3-cm wide and 4- to 6-cm long.[29] It enlarges in response to ACTH and becomes smaller when ACTH production decreases. The gland is variably corrugated and nodular; it is surrounded by areolar tissue and a thick fibrous capsule. Unlike the kidneys, the adrenals are not displaced by changes in respiration or posture.[26,29] The right gland tends to be higher and more lateral than the left, which frequently overlaps the abdominal aorta.

The adrenal arteries and veins do not run in parallel (Fig. 11-1), as do those of most other organs. Blood is supplied by several short arteries that are terminal branches of the inferior phrenic artery; the superior, middle, and inferior adrenal arteries; and occasionally the ovarian or left spermatic artery.[26] Because there are several arteries, adrenal infarction is unusual. Arterial blood enters a sinusoidal circulation in the cortex and drains toward the medulla so that medullary chromaffin cells are bathed in very high concentrations of steroid hormones. The adrenal vein empties directly into the vena cava on the right and into the renal vein on the left.[26]

The innervation of the adrenal gland is autonomic.[26] Sympathetic preganglionic fibers are the axons of neurons in the lower thoracic and upper lumbar segments, whereas the parasympathetic fibers come from the celiac branch of the posterior vagal trunk; the latter may relay in ganglia in or near the adrenal. Most of the nerves are contained in an adrenal (suprarenal) plexus along the medial border of the adrenal gland, enter it as bundles near the

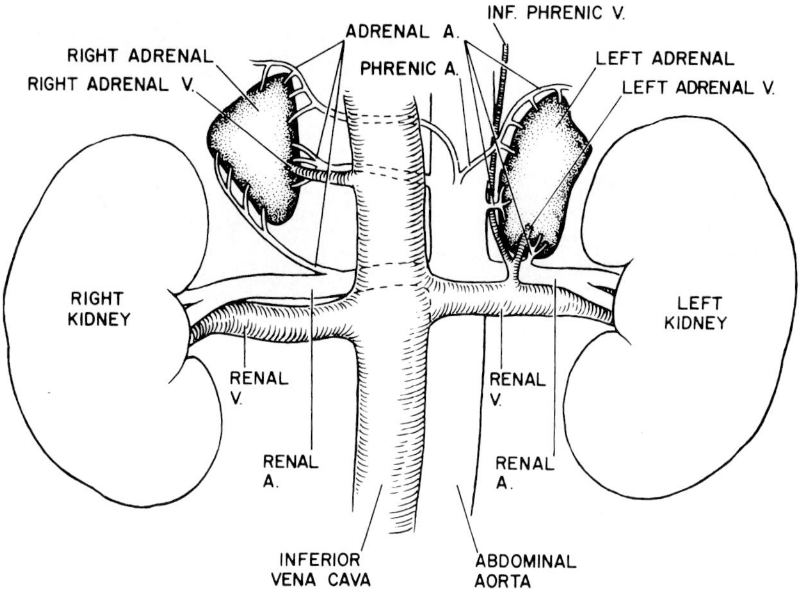

FIGURE 11-1. Location and blood supply of the adrenal glands.

hilus, and run through the cortex to the medulla. This innervation may participate in the control of adrenocortical growth and steroid secretion, and an afferent neural pathway from the adrenal to the hypothalamus mediates stress-induced feedback inhibition of ACTH secretion[30]; however, there is no clear physiologic disorder or syndrome associated with denervation of the adrenal.

In adults, the cortex makes up about 90 percent of the adrenal and surrounds the centrally located medulla.[29] The cortex consists of three histologically distinct zones: the zonae glomerulosa, fasciculata, and reticularis. The zona glomerulosa produces aldosterone but not cortisol. It is located under the capsule in ill-defined foci that constitute about 15 percent of the cortex (Fig. 11-2).[29] Glomerulosa cells have a relatively small cytoplasmic volume, with small amounts of lipid. The zona fasciculata produces cortisol but not aldosterone (Fig. 11-2). It is located between the zona glomerulosa and the zona reticularis and constitutes about 75 percent of the cortex. Its cells contain more cholesterol and cholesterol esters, giving them a vacuolated or "clear" appearance on stained sections.[29] The zona reticularis also produces cortisol (albeit at a much lower rate than do the fasciculata cells) and the major adrenal C-19 steroids dehydroepiandrosterone (DHEA), DHEA-sulfate (DHEA-S), and Δ^4-androstenedione. These three steroids are often termed "adrenal androgens," but they have little if any inherent andogenic capacity; rather, they are precursors converted to androgens and estrogens by enzymes in peripheral tissues. Cells of the zona reticularis are relatively free of lipids and have a granular, compact appearance.[29] The zonae fasciculata and reticularis also produce most of the DOC and 18-hydroxydeoxycorticosterone (18-OH-DOC) secreted by the adrenal. The three zones of the adrenal cortex cannot be dissected from one another cleanly, as each zone projects "fingers" of cells into the neighboring zones.[31,32]

ACTH has a dramatic effect on the adrenal.[29,30] Within 2 to 3 min after its administration, adrenal blood flow increases and cortisol is released. Within hours, adrenal weight increases; ultimately, the adrenal can double in size. The clear cells at the junction of the zonae fasciculata and reticularis lose their lipid content and become compact. This conversion gradually extends outward, broadening the zona reticularis, which may reach the zona glomerulosa. Meanwhile, the zona fasciculata aquires ultrastructural features of zona reticularis cells. Thus, the two inner zones appear to function as a unit; whereas by light microscopy there appears to be an abrupt structural change between the two zones, electron microscopy reveals cells with intermediate ultrastructural features. Prolonged stimulation by ACTH causes both hypertrophy and hyperplasia,[30] possibly as a result of the actions of insulin-like growth factors,[33–35] basic fibroblast growth factor,[36,37] and epidermal growth factor,[37] which decrease the concentration of apoptotic cells within these zonae. The adrenal also can regenerate.[30,33,34] This has been observed after enucleation of the rat adrenal[30] and after incomplete adrenalectomy for Cushing's disease. By contrast, ACTH deficiency leads to atrophy of the zonae fasciculata and reticularis and an increase in the concentration of apoptotic cells. Similarly, when concentrations of angiotensin II and potassium ion are elevated, there is hyperplasia of the zona glomerulosa, and when their levels are decreased, there can be atrophy.

Accessory adrenal glands composed of cortical tissue occasionally occur[26]; more rarely, such accessory glands contain both cortical and medullary tissue. By contrast, nests of adrenal "rest cells" are common in the testis (reviewed in Ref. 38). Adrenal tissue may be present in the celiac plexus, kidney, spleen, or retroperitoneal area below the kidneys; along the aorta, pelvis, spermatic cord, or broad ligament of the uterus; or attached to the uterus. One adrenal gland may occasionally be absent, but bilateral agenesis is rare.

STEROID HORMONE BIOSYNTHESIS

In the past, studies and discussions of steroid hormone synthesis emphasized the complex structural organic chemistry of these hormones. The understanding of their structures led to the determination of precursor-product relation and an understanding of both the pathways of steroidogenesis and of the structural requirements for the various steroidal activities. This traditional chemical approach has been supplanted by molecular and cellular biological approaches, yet familiarity with both is needed to un-

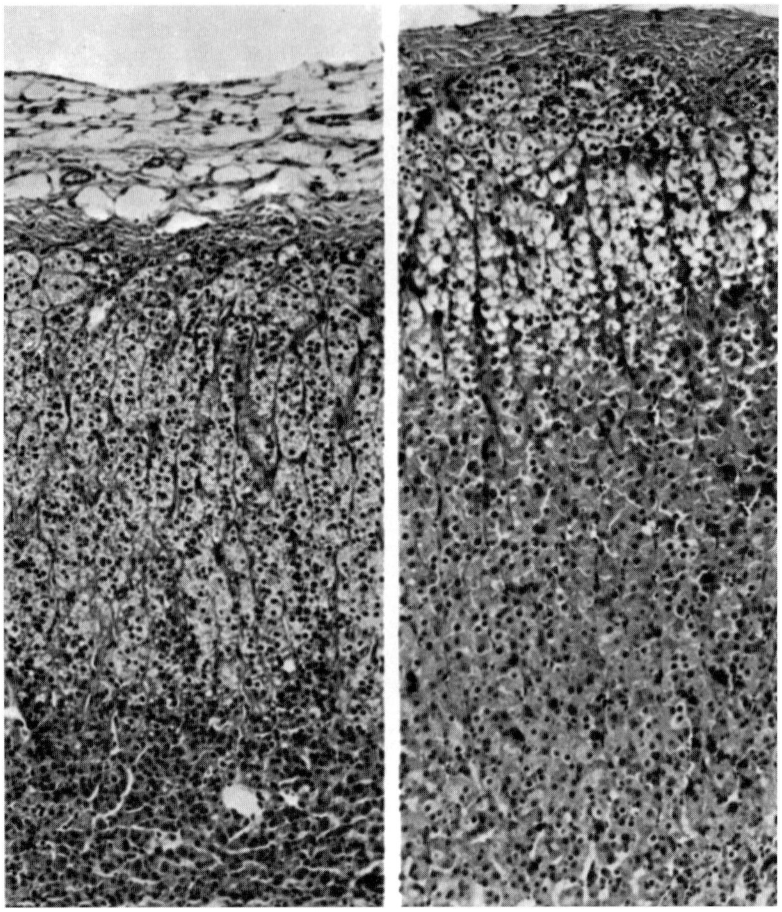

FIGURE 11-2. Normal adrenal cortex *(left)* before and *(right)* after ACTH stimulation. The focal zona glomerulosa under the capsule contains cells with a relatively small cytoplasmic volume. The zona fasciculata in the center contains clear cells, and the zona reticularis at the bottom contains compact cells separated by a clearly demarcated undulating border. After ACTH stimulation, only a narrow rim of clear cells of the fasciculata remains on the outer aspect of the glands; the remainder consists of compact cells. Hematoxylin and eosin stain; 104X. (*From Neville and Mackay.*[27])

derstand the synthesis, regulation, and pathologic disorders of steroid hormones (see also Chap. 3).

Chemistry of Steroid Hormones

All steroid hormones are derived from pregnenolone, whose structure is shown in Fig. 11-3. Pregnenolone and all its naturally occurring mineralocorticoid and glucocorticoid products contain 21 carbon atoms and hence are termed C-21 steroids (Fig. 11-4). The numbering of each carbon atom facilitates an understanding of how each step in steroid hormone synthesis alters the steroid molecule. 17α-hydroxypregnenolone, a C-21 steroid, can be cleaved to the C-19 steroid DHEA, which is the precursor of sex steroids. With the exception of the estrogens, which are characterized by an aromatic A ring, all steroid hormones have a single unsaturated carbon-carbon double bond. In pregnenolone and other so-called Δ^5 steroids, this double bond connects carbons 5 and 6 in the B ring (Fig. 11-3). The action of 3β-hydroxysteroid dehydrogenase/isomerase moves this double bond to the A ring between carbons 4 and 5, forming so-called Δ^5 steroids.

A rigorous, logically systematic, and unambiguous chemical terminology has been formulated to describe the structure of the steroid hormones and all their conceivable derivatives. However, this terminology is extremely cumbersome; for example, cortisol is 11β,17α,21-trihydroxypregn-4-ene-3,20-dione, and dexamethasone is 9α-fluoro-11β,17α,21-trihydroxy-16α-methypregna-1,4,-diene-3,20 dione. Therefore, we shall use the standard "trivial"

FIGURE 11-3. Structure of pregnenolone. The carbon atoms are indicated by numbers and the rings are designated by letters in accordance with standard convention. Pregnenolone is derived from cholesterol, which has a 6-carbon side chain attached to carbon 21. Pregnenolone is "Δ^5 compound," having a double bond between carbons 5 and 6; the action of 3β-hydroxysteroid dehydrogenase/isomerase moves this double bond from the B ring to carbons 4 and 5 in the A ring, forming Δ^4 compounds. All the major biologically active steroid hormones are Δ^4 compounds.

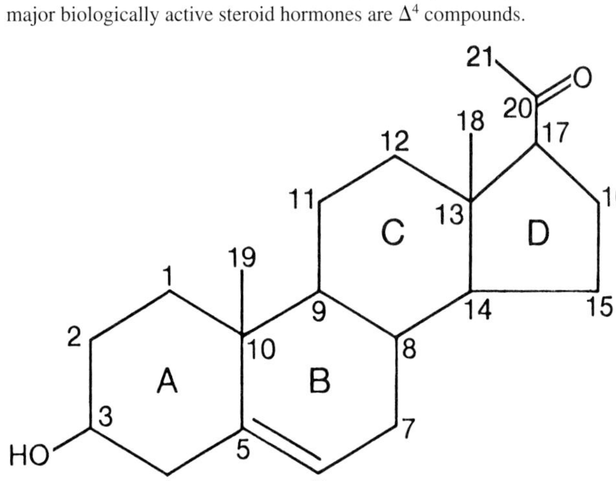

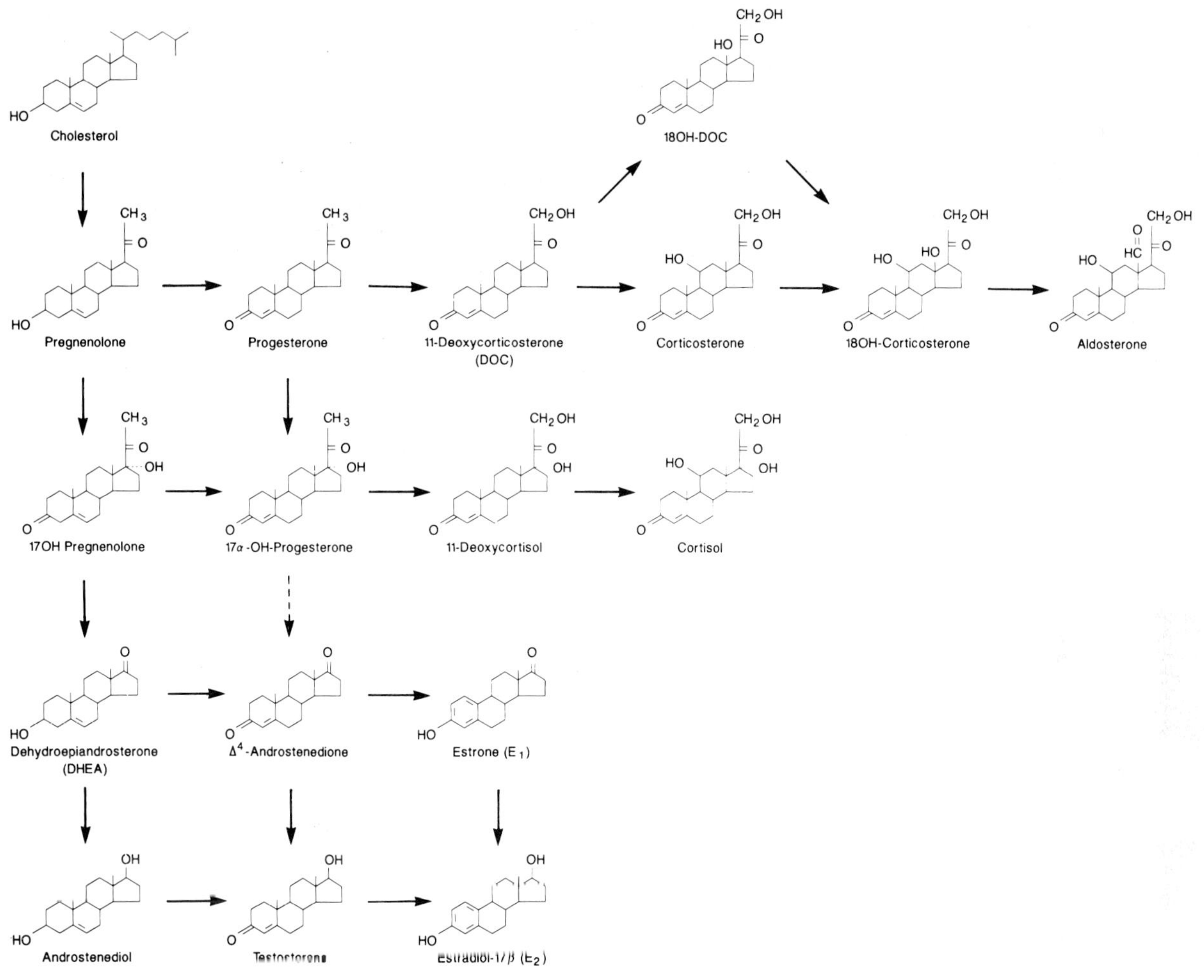

FIGURE 11-4. The principal pathways of adrenal steroidogenesis, showing the structures of the most important steroidal products and intermediates. The enzymes mediating the steroidal inter-conversions are shown in Fig. 11-7. The steroids in the left vertical column (cholesterol, pregnenolone, 17-OH pregnenolone, DHEA, and androstenediol) are all Δ^5 steroids that have double bond between carbons 5 and 6 (see Fig. 11-3). All the other nonaromatic steroids shown are Δ^4 compounds, having a double bond between carbons 4 and 5. The top horizontal row of compounds, showing the pathway from pregnenolone to aldosterone, is the mineralocorticoid pathway found almost exclusively in the zona glomerulosa; all these compounds have 21 carbon atoms (C-21 steroids). The second row of compounds showing the pathway from 17-hydroxypregnenolone to cortisol is the glucocorticoid pathway, found in the zona fasciculated and, to a lesser extent, the zona reticularis. These are all 17-hydroxy C-21 steroids. The third and fourth rows show the sex steroid pathway, found principally in the gonads but also in the zona reticularis. The 17,20 lyase activity of P450c17 has cleaved off carbon atoms 20 and 21 to yield C-19 steroids. While this activity can convert 17-hydroxyprogesterone to Δ^4 androstenedione in rodents and cattle, the human enzyme catalyzes this reaction very poorly, so that virtually all sex steroids are made from DHEA. Very little aromatase activity is found in the adrenal; estrone and estradiol are largely synthesized by peripheral conversion of androstenedione and testosterone in the liver and adipose tissues, but are shown here for clarity and completeness.

names in this chapter. The trivial and systematic names of many important steroids are given in Table 11-1. The chemical nomenclature system lists in order the hydroxyl groups, the aldehyde groups, the core ring structure (pregnane, pregnene, androstane, androstene), and the ketones, with the number of the carbon to which each is attached. In the case of carbon-carbon double bonds, the numbers of the two carbons are given with the lower number first; the presence of a double bond is alternatively indicated by the uppercase Greek delta (Δ), with a superscript indicating the lower-numbered carbon atom of the bond. A saturated ring structure is indicated by -ane (as in pregnane or androstane), and an unsaturated ring structure is indicated by -ene (as in pregnene or androstene). The core ring structure for the C-21 steroids is termed *pregnane,* C-19 steroids are *androstanes,* C-18 steroids *estranes,* and C-27 steroids are *cholestanes.*

Before the structures of the various steroid hormones were known, Reichstein, Kendall, and others identified them as spots on paper chromatograms and referred to them as unknown compounds A, B, C, etc. Unfortunately, some physicians persist in using this obsolete and arcane terminology more than half a century after these structures were determined, so that corticosterone may be referred to as "compound B," cortisol as "compound F,"

TABLE 11-1. Trivial and Systematic Names of Some Commonly Encountered Naturally Occurring and Synthetic Steroids

Trivial Name	Systematic Name
Aldosterone	11β,21-Dihydroxy-3,20-dioxopregn-en-18-al
Androsterone	3α-Hydroxy-5α-androstan-17-one
Corticosterone (compound B)	11β-21 Dihydroxypregn-4-ene-3,20-dione
Cortisol (hydrocortisone, compound F)	11β-17α,21-trihydroxypregen-4-ene-3,20-dione
Cortisone (compound E)	17α,21-Dihydroxypregn-4-ene-3,1-20-trione
Cortol	5β-Pregnane-3α,11β,17α,20,21-pentol
Cortolone	3α,17α,20α,21-Tetrahydroxy-5β-pregnan-11-one
Dehydroepiandrosterone (prasterone, DHEA)	3β-Hydroxyandrost-5-en-17-one
11-Deoxycorticosterone (DOC)	21-Hydroxypregn-4-ene-3,20-dione
11-Desoxy-17-hydroxycorticosterone (11-deoxycortisol, cortexolone, compound S)	17α,21-Dihydroxypregn-4-ene-3,20-dione
Dexamethasone	9α-Fluoro-11β,17α,21-trihydroxy-16α-methylpregna-1,4-diene-3,20-dione
Estradiol	Estra-1,3,5(10)-triene-3,17β-diol
Etiocholanolone	3α-Hydroxy-5β-androstan-17-one
Fludrocortisone (9α-fluorocortisol)	9α-Fluoro-11β,17α,21-trihydroxypregn-4-ene-3,20-dione
17α-Hydroxypregnenolone	3β,17α-Dihydroxy-5β-pregnen-20-one
17α-Hydroxyprogesterone	17α-Hydroxypregn-4-ene-3,20-dione
Betamethasone	9α-Fluoro-11β,17α,21-trihydroxy-16β-methylpregna-1,4-diene-3,20-dione
Prednisone	17α,21-Dihydroxypregna-1,4-diene-3,11,20-trione
Prednisolone	11β,17α,21-Trihydroxypregna-1,4-diene-3,20-dione
Pregnanediol	5β-Pregnane-3α,20α-diol
Pregnanetriol	5β-Pregnane-3α,17α,20α-triol
Pregnenetriol	Pregn-5-ene-3β,17α,20α-triol
Pregnenolone	3β-Hydroxypregn-5-en-20-one
Progesterone	Preg-4-ene-3,20-dione
Testosterone	17β-Hydroxyandrost-4-en-3-one
Tetrahydroaldosterone	3α,11β,21-Trihydroxy-20-oxo-5β-pregnan-18-al
Tetrahydrocortisol	3α,11β,17α,21-Tetrahydroxy-5β-pregnan-20-one
Tetrahydrocortisone	3α,17α,21-Trihydroxy-5β-pregnane-11,20-dione
Triamcinolone	9α-Fluoro-11β,16α,17α,21-tetrahydroxypregna-1,4-diene-3,20-dione

Source: *Biochem J* 113:5, 1969; modified from Brooks.[571]

and 11-deoxycortisol as "compound S." This frivolous, outmoded, nonscientific terminology obscures the precursor-product relations among the steroids and must be abandoned.

The biological activities of the various steroid hormones are determined by several factors: the class (or classes) of steroid hormone receptors to which they bind and the affinity of that binding, the plasma proteins to which they bind and the affinity of that binding, their metabolic half-lives, and "peripheral" enzymes that metabolize steroid hormones in target tissues. These variables are influenced by the various side groups attached to the four-member cyclopentanophenanthrene ring and the extent of angulation among these four component rings. This angulation is determined by the saturation of the carbon atoms and attached groups. The cyclopentanophenanthrene ring can be visualized as an irregular plane, with groups projecting below the plane (α position) or above it (β position) (Fig. 11-5).

Cholesterol: The Precursor of Steroid Hormones

Cholesterol Synthesis and Uptake

Pregnenolone and all other steroids are made exclusively from cholesterol. The adrenal readily synthesizes cholesterol from acetyl CoA.[39–41] in response to tropic stimulation by ACTH. The activity of 3-hydroxy-3-methylglutaryl coenzyme A reductase (HMGCoA reductase), the rate-limiting enzyme in cholesterol synthesis, generally parallels steroidogenic activity. HMGCoA reductase is inactivated by phosphorylation and is activated by dephosphorylation in response to intracellular cAMP elicited by the binding of ACTH to its receptor. However, endogenous synthesis is an important source of cholesterol only in transient situations or during profound stimulation.[39] Similarly, cholesterol stored as intracellular cholesterol esters is a relatively minor source of the cholesterol used for steroidogenesis.[40]

About 80 percent of the cholesterol used for steroid hormone synthesis derives from dietary cholesterol transported in the plasma as low density lipoprotein (LDL) particles synthesized in the liver.[39,40] Rats and members of some other species principally employ high density lipoproteins (HDL) for this purpose,[40,42] and human ovarian granulosa cells also may be able to take up HDL particles that contain apolipoprotein E,[43] but a clear role for HDL in human adrenal steroidogenesis has not been established as HDL does not stimulate or sustain human adrenal steroidogenesis.[40,42,43] In abetalipoproteinemia, in which LDL particles are absent, the cortisol response to ACTH is blunted, but basal cortisol concentrations are normal and symptomatic adrenal insufficiency does not occur.[44] Thus, in these patients, endogenous synthesis of cholesterol and/or uptake of HDL provides an alternative source of cholesterol.

Adrenal uptake of LDL is regulated coordinately with steroid synthesis. Adequate concentrations of LDL will suppress HMG-

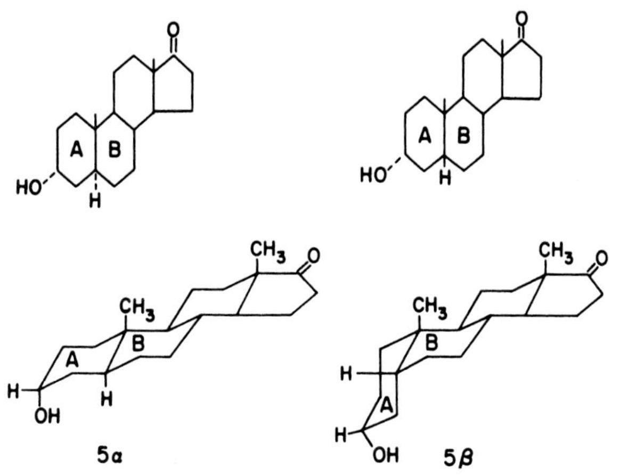

FIGURE 11-5. Effect of the hydrogen at position 6 on the conformation of the steroid molecule. The 5α-hydrogenated molecule is androsterone, and the 5β-hydrogenated molecule is etiocholanolone. The usual outline structural formulas are shown at the top, and the perspective views are shown at the bottom. (*From Bondy.*[414])

CoA reductase activity,[45] and blockade of cholesterol synthesis with HMGCoA reductase inhibitors will not suppress the secretion of cortisol in response to ACTH.[46] ACTH stimulates the activity of HMGCoA reductase, LDL receptors, and the uptake of LDL cholesterol.[47] LDL uptake is rapid; radiotracer studies show that plasma LDL cholesterol is nearly equilibrated with the intracellular pool of steroidogenic sterols.[48] In fact, imaging studies of steroidogenic tissues with radiolabeled analogs of cholesterol are not especially effective and are possible only because of the voracious appetite of steroidogenic tissues for plasma cholesterol.[48]

LDL uptake principally entails receptor-mediated endocytosis (Fig. 11-6); less than 10 percent of LDL enters the cell by a receptor-independent mechanism.[39,40] Specific "B-E receptors," which recognize apolipoproteins B and E, are located on microvilli and, upon binding of LDL, become concentrated in "coated pits" at the base of the villi. The coating of these pits is composed of clathrin; changes in the array of clathrin molecules result in the closure of the pit into a vesicle, thus internalizing the LDL. The receptors are separated from the LDL and are recycled back to the cellular surface, while the vesicles bearing LDL fuse with lysosomes.[39,40] Lysosomal proteases degrade the protein moieties, and lysosomal acid lipase cleaves the cholesterol esters to free cholesterol (Fig. 11-6). By contrast, the uptake of HDL entails receptor-independent mechanisms.[49]

Intracellular Cholesterol Storage and Transport

The regulation of the flux of cholesterol into adrenal mitochondria to initiate steroidogenesis is an active area of current research, and several factors have been associated with this action. Free sterols, including cholesterol, may be esterified by acyl coenzyme A cholesterol acyltransferase (ACAT), which is found in the rough endoplasmic reticulum,[43] Sterol esters accumulate and bud off as lipid droplets from the endoplasmic reticulum. The esterification entails linkage of polyunsaturated fatty acids such as linolenic, arachidonic, docosapentanoic, and docosahexanoic acids derived from the circulation, or synthesized de novo.[43] It is not clear how the specific unsaturated fatty acids are chosen for esterification, but in ovarian cells the patterns change with the functional status of the cell, suggesting different metabolic roles for each one.[43] Such fatty acid esters are generally hydrolyzed to free cholesterol by cholesterol esterase (sterol ester hydrolase). However, pregnenolone may be reesterified in the mitochondria to pregnenolone fatty acid esters,[50] which form biosynethic intermediates in the synthesis of corresponding adrenal steroids.[50] In the uterus, such fatty acid esters are involved in the synthesis of long-acting lipoidal derivatives of estradiol.[51]

FIGURE 11-6. The LDL pathway of cholesterol uptake by the adrenal. LDL binds to receptors that are internalized in coated vesicles and is then separated from its receptor, which is recycled back to the plasma membrane. LDL then travels in noncoated vesicles to the vicinity of the Golgi apparatus, where lysosomal hydrolases are induced. Acid proteinases degrade LDL apolipoproteins to amino acids, and acid lipase frees cholesterol from esters. Free cholesterol then diffuses out of lysosomes and may be transferred to organelles by sterol carrier proteins (SCP). (*From Strauss and Miller.*[40])

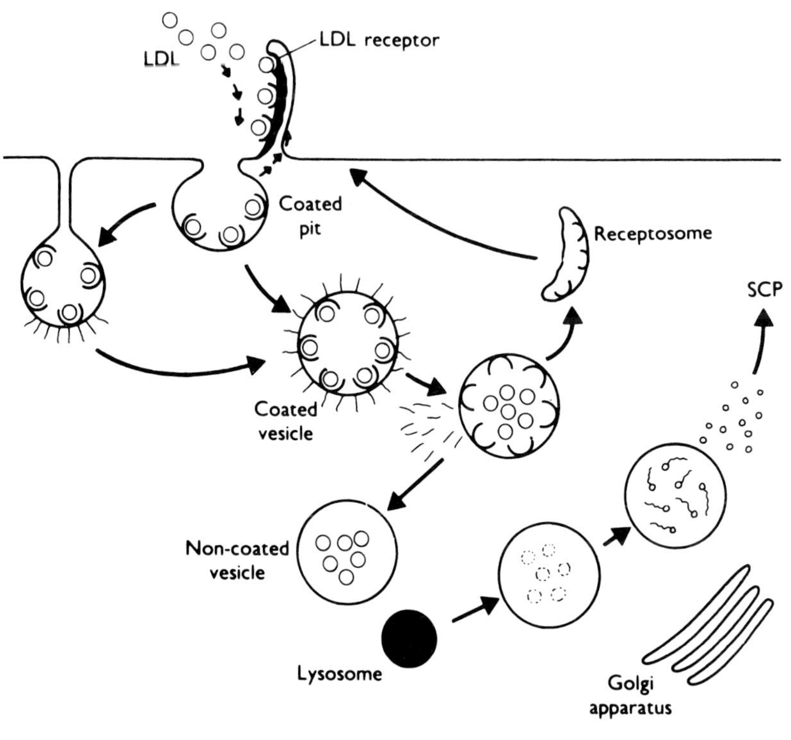

Cholesterol storage as cholesterol esters in lipid droplets is controlled by the action of two opposing enzymes: cholesterol ester synthetase and cholesterol ester hydrolase (cholesterol esterase). ACTH or other tissue-specific tropic hormones [e.g., luteinizing hormone (LH) and angiotensin II] stimulate the esterase and inhibit the synthetase, thus increasing the availability of free cholesterol for steroid hormone synthesis.[52,53] The esterase, which is encoded by a gene on chromosome 10,[54] is a soluble protein that is similar to gastric and lingual lipases,[54] and is activated by phosphorylation of serine residues by a cAMP-dependent protein kinase.[55] The synthetase, ACAT, is insoluble and is confined to the membrane of the endoplasmic reticulum. In addition to ACTH, γ_3-MSH (melanocyte stimulating hormone) may also activate the esterase by a cAMP-independent mechanism.[56]

Free cholesterol, which is nearly insoluble in the aqueous cytosol, may bind to sterol carrier protein 2 (SCP-2), a 13-kDa basic protein in the cytosol.[57,58] Another 11.3-kDa protein, sometimes termed sterol carrier protein 1 (SCP-1), apparently functions principally in fatty acid binding and hence is not truly a sterol carrier protein.[57,59] These two proteins have been found in the mitochondria, cytosol, and endoplasmic reticulum of steroidogenic tissues, and their synthesis responds to tropic hormone stimulation.[59,60] SCP-2 may facilitate the flux of cholesterol more by its action of removing cholesterol from membranes than by acting as a directed transport protein. SCP-2 promotes the flux of cholesterol from lipid droplets to mitochondria and increases pregnenolone synthesis in cell-free systems[59]; SCP-2 can also stimulate steroidogenisis by adrenal mitochondria in vitro[58,61,62] and cotransfection of COS-7 cells with vectors expressing SCP-2 and the cholesterol side-chain cleavage enzyme system promotes a 2.5-fold increase in steroidogenesis.[63] Furthermore, antibodies to SCP-2 partially but incompletely inhibit steroidogenesis.[60] Thus, SCP-2 apparently carries free cholesterol to the mitochondria and loads this cholesterol into the outer mitochondrial membrane, but SCP-2 does not enter the mitochondria. The role of SCP-1 is unclear; because SCP-1 is found within the mitochondria and mitochondria generate ATP by oxidizing fatty acids, SCP-1 may promote steroidogenesis by providing fuel for the steroidogenic machinery.

StAR and the Acute Regulation of Steroidogenesis

Whereas the chronic regulation of steroidogenesis by tropic hormones such as ACTH is at the level of gene transcription[64,65] the acute regulation, such as the production and release of cortisol within minutes of a 'fight-or-flight' stimulus, is at the level of cholesterol access to the P450scc enzyme on the inner mitochondrial membrane. When either steroidogenic cells or intact rats are treated with inhibitors of protein synthesis such as cycloheximide, the acute steroidogenic response is eliminated, suggesting that a short-lived, cycloheximide-sensitive protein acts at the level of the mitochondrion[66] as the specific trigger to the acute steroidogenic response.[67,68] Several candidate factors were proposed for this acute trigger, including the so-called steroidogenesis activator peptide (SAP), SCP-2, the peripheral benzodiazepine receptor complex (PBR), and its endogenous ligand, endozepine (also termed diazepaen binding inhibitor, DBI) (for review see Ref. 69). The role of the PBR/endozepine system remains uncertain; substantial data indicate that this system particpates in the slow, chronic delivery of cholesterol to the inner mitochondrial membrane (for review see Ref. 70), but it is now well-established that the acute trigger is the steroidogenic acute regulatory protein (StAR).[69]

StAR was first identified by two-dimensional gel electrophoresis as a cluster of short-lived, cycloheximide-sensitive 30- and 37-kDa phosphoproteins that was rapidly synthesized by steroidogenic cells stimulated with tropic hormones.[71–76] Mouse StAR was then cloned from Leydig MA-10 cells in 1994 and could induce steroidogenesis when transfected back into MA-10 cells.[77] The central role of StAR was definitively proven by showing that it promoted steroidogenesis in nonsteroidogenic COS-1 cells cotransfected with StAR and the cholesterol side chain cleavage enzyme system, and by finding that mutations of StAR caused congenital lipoid adrenal hyperplasia.[78] Thus StAR is the acute trigger that is required for the rapid flux of cholesterol to the inner mitochondrial membrane that is needed for the acute response of aldosterone to angiotensin II, of cortisol to ACTH, and of sex steroids to an LH pulse.

Some steroidogenesis is independent of StAR: nonsteroidogenic cells transfected with StAR and the P450scc system convert cholesterol to pregnenolone at about 14 percent of the StAR induced rate.[78,79] Furthermore, some steroidogenic tissues, including the placenta and brain, utilize mitochondrial P450scc to initiate steroidogenesis but do not express StAR.[80] The mechanism of StAR-independent steroidogenesis is unknown. It is possible that it occurs spontaneously, without any triggering protein, or some other protein may exert StAR-like activity to promote cholesterol flux, but without StAR's rapid kinetics. A protein termed MLN64, cloned from metastatic breast carcinoma tissue, has StAR-like sequence motifs[81] and StAR-like fragments of MLN64 can promote steroidogenesis in transfected cells.[82,82a] This protein is expressed in virtually all tissues that fail to express StAR, and is cleaved by the placenta to a StAR-like fragment,[82a] hence it is an attractive candidate for a factor involved in StAR-independent steroidogenesis. Although no physiologic role for MLN64 has been established, the determination of its structure has helped to visualize the structure of StAR.[82b] Thus it is clear that StAR is needed only for the rapid production of large amounts of steroid hormones, but is not needed for chronic, low levels of steroidogenesis (for review see Ref. 83).

The mechanism of StAR's action is unclear and remains an active area of investigation. Electron microscopy of acutely stimulated steroidogenic cells shows increased numbers of 'contact sites,' where the outer and inner mitochondrial membranes come into direct contact, transiently bridging the aqueous intracisternal space, thus it has been suspected that these contact sites permit cholesterol to flow down a simple concentration gradient from the outer to inner mitochondrial membrane. It initially was suggested that StAR created these contact sites by the simple act of traversing the mitochondrial membranes by virtue of its mitochondrial lender peptide.[77,84] This was inconsistent with the observation that deletion of only 28 carboxy-terminal residues ablated StAR-activity.[78] In fact, up to 62 amino-terminal residues of StAR can be deleted resulting in a protein (N-62 StAR) that does not enter the mitochondria, but still retains all of its biological activity.[85,86] Thus StAR acts on the outer mitochondrial membrane, and is fully active without entering the mitochondria. Recent studies have indicated that N-62 StAR can promote the transfer of cholesterol to numerous different intracellular membranes,[82] indicating that the principal role of the mitochondrial lender peptide is to target StAR to the outer mitochondrial membrane and increase its local concentration at this site, rather than to direct StAR to proceed into the mitochondrial matrix.[87] This lack of membrane specificity for StAR's action suggests that there is no StAR receptor protein on the outer mitochondrial membrane. Consistent with this, physical chemical studies show that StAR must become partially unfolded into a 'molten globule' to achieve activity, and that the central portion of the StAR molecule functions as a mitochondrial 'stop-transfer' sequence thus increasing the residency time (and hence the biological activity) of the carboxy terminus on the outer mitochondrial membrane.[88] StAR binds cholesterol,[82b] and the x-ray crystal structure of the StAR-like domain of MLN64 suggests that StAR forms a tunnel for cholesterol,[82b] but the exact mode of action remains unknown.

The flux of cholesterol from lipid droplets to the outer mitochondrial membrane and the subsequent flux of pregnenolone from the mitochondria to the endoplasmic reticulum may be facilitated by changes in the cytoskeleton.[89,90] Agents that disrupt microfilaments and microtubules inhibit cholesterol flux and steroidogenesis. Such agents include cytochalasins, which inhibit polymerization of microfilaments; vinblastine, which disrupts microtubules; and antibodies to actin. An intact cytoskeleton may simply maintain the various intracellular organelles in their proper spatial arrangement, or it could actively direct the movement of SCP-2 or other factors that promote steroidogenesis.

Cytochrome P450

Most steroidogenic enzymes are members of the cytochrome P450 superfamily of oxidases.[24,91] Cytochrome P450 is a generic term for a large number of oxidative enzymes, all of which have about 500 amino acids and contain a single heme group. They are termed P450 (pigment 450) because they all exhibit a characteristic shift in the Soret absorbance peak from 420 to 450 nm when they are reduced with carbon monoxide.[92] All cytochrome P450 enzymes reduce atmospheric O_2 with electrons donated by NADPH according to the general reaction:

$$\text{NADPH} + \text{H}^+ + \text{O}_2 + \text{RH} \xrightarrow{\text{P450}} \text{R-OH} + \text{H}_2\text{O} + \text{NADP}^+$$

The electrons from NADPH reach the P450 via one or two electron transport intermediates, (redox partners) one of which is always flavoprotein. There is a modest degree of amino acid sequence conservation at the heme-binding and redox-partner binding sites of most P450 enzymes but these enzymes otherwise have tremendous sequence diversity.

Some steroidogenic reactions have been termed "P450-dependent" but this is a misnomer, as it implies a generic P450 cofactor to a substrate-specific enzyme. The P450 *is* the enzyme that binds the steroidal substrate and mediates the steroidal conversion on an active site associated with the heme group. Most cytochrome P450 enzymes are found in the endoplasmic reticulum of the liver, where they metabolize endogenous and exogenous toxins, drugs, xenobiotics, and environmental pollutants.[91,93,94] Despite this huge variety of substrates, it appears that there are only about 200 distinct cytochrome P450 enzymes.[91,93,94] Thus, most, if not all, P450 enzymes can metabolize multiple substrates, catalyzing a broad array of oxidations (for review see Ref. 94). This theme recurs with each adrenal P450 enzyme. The size and complexity of the cytochrome P450 superfamily led to many conflicting systems of nomenclature; however, a consensus system has found widespread acceptance: the genes for these enzymes are termed CYP__, and the encoded protein may also be termed CYP__ or P450__.[95] To avoid confusion, the term CYP is generally used to name the genes and P450 to name the proteins.

Six distinct P450 enzymes are involved in steroidogenesis (Fig. 11-7). P450scc, which is found in mitochondria, is the cholesterol side-chain cleavage enzyme that mediates the series of reactions formerly mis-termed "20,22 desmolase." Two forms of P450c11, P450c11β and P450c11AS (aldosterone synthase), are also found in mitochondria; both can catalyze 11-hydroxylase activity, while P450c11AS also has 18-hydroxylase and 18-methyl oxidase activities. The vitamin D biosynthetic enzymes are also mitochondrial forms of cytochrome P450 that are closely related to P450scc and P450c11.[96–98] P450c17, which is found in the endoplasmic reticulum, catalyzes both 17α-hydroxylase and 17,20 lyase activities, and P450c21 catalyzes the 21-hydroxylation of both glucocorticoids and mineralocorticoids. In the gonads (and elsewhere), P450aro in the endoplasmic reticulum catalyzes the aromatization of androgens to estrogens; this enzyme is not a normal component of adrenocortical steroidogenesis but can be found in some adrenocortical malignancies.[99]

Present structural knowledge of steroidogenic cytochromes P450 is based on amino acid and nucleotide sequencing data. Because these enzymes exist in membrane lipid environments, they have not been crystallized; hence, their nascent three-dimensional structures have not been determined. However, several prokaryotic P450 enzymes have been crystallized and their structures determined, providing substantial information about the common structural and topological features of all cytochrome P450 enzymes.[100] These bacterial P450 structures have permitted the construction of computer-graphic models of human steroidogenic P450 enzymes,[101–103] providing structural and mechanistic insights into human steroidogenesis.

P450scc: Conversion Of Cholesterol to Pregnenolone

Enzymology

The conversion of cholesterol to pregnenolone in mitochondria is the first and rate-limiting step in the synthesis of steroid hormones (for review see Refs. 24, 43, and 104). This involves three distinct chemical reactions: 20α-hydroxylation, 22-hydroxylation, and scission of the cholesterol side-chain to yield pregnenolone and isocaproic acid. Early studies suggested that three separate and distinct enzymes were involved: a 20-hydroxylase, a 22-hydroxylase, and a 20,22-lyase. However, protein purification studies and in vitro reconstitution of enzymatic activity showed that a single protein, termed P450scc (scc refers to the side-chain cleavage of cholesterol), is responsible for catalyzing all the steps between cholesterol and pregnenolone[66,105–108] on a single active site[109] that is in contact with the hydrophobic bilayer membrane.[92] Although some have suggested that there might be pathways to pregnenolone synthesis that do not involve P450scc,[110] human beings have only one P450scc gene[24,111] and the abscence of any steroid hormone synthesis in rabbits lacking the single gene for P450scc[112,113] proves that P450scc is mandatory for all steroidogenesis.

Mechanism of Action

The cholesterol side-chain cleavage reaction consists of three catalytic cycles; the first two hydroxylate the carbon atoms at positions C-22 and C-20, and the third results in cleavage of the bond connecting these two carbons. Each catalytic cycle requires one molecule of NADPH and one molecule of O_2, such that the overall stoichiometry is cholesterol + 3 NADPH + $3H^+$ + $3O_2$ → pregnenolone + isocapraldehyde + $4H_2O$ + $3NADP^+$.[92] One cholesterol molecule is converted to pregnenolone by a single molecule

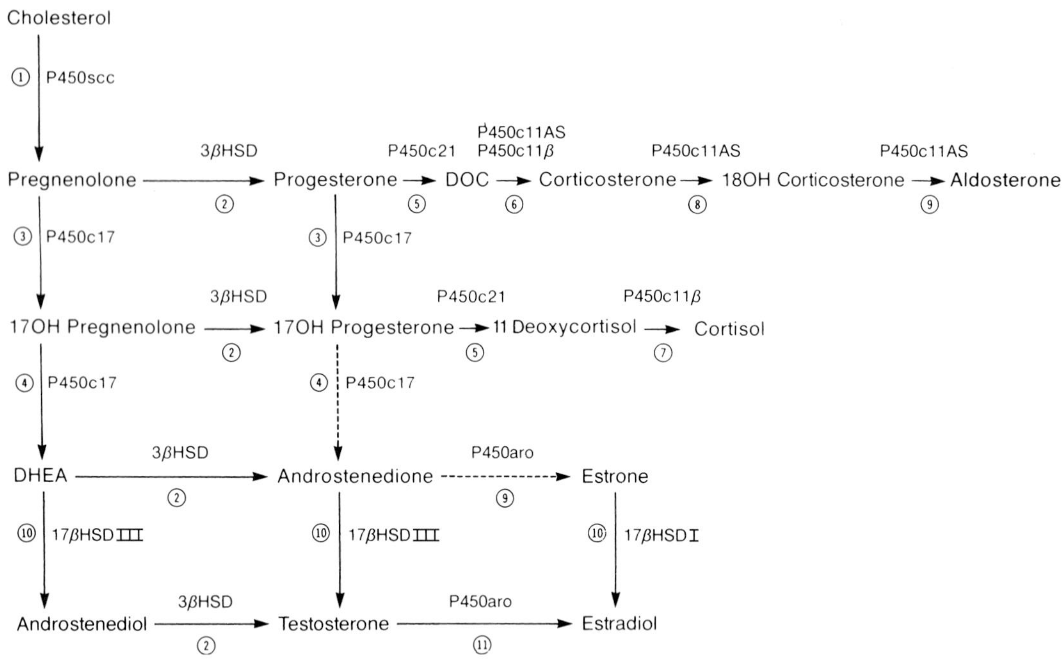

FIGURE 11-7. Principal pathways of human adrenal steroid hormone synthesis. The structures of the steroids named are shown in Fig. 11-4. Other quantitatively and physiologically minor steroids are also produced. The names of the enzymes are shown by each reaction, and the traditional names of the enzymatic activities correspond to the circled numbers. Reaction 1: Mitochondrial cytochrome P450scc mediates 20α-hydroxylation, 22-hydroxylation, and scission of the C20-22 carbon bond, a set of reactions traditionally termed 20,22-desmolase. Reaction 2: 3β-HSD, a non-450 enzyme bound to the endoplasmic reticulum, mediate 3β-hydroxysteroid dehydrogenase and isomerase activities, converting Δ^5 steroids to Δ^4 steroids. Reaction 3: P450c17 catalyzes the 17α-hydroxylation of pregnenolone to 17-OH-pregnenolone and, that of progesterone to 17-OH-progesterone. Reaction 4: The 17,20-lyase activity of P450c17 converts 17-OH-pregnenolone to DHEA; clinical evidence suggests that some 17-OH-progesterone is similarily converted to Δ^4 androstenedione, but this reaction is not catalyzed by human P450c17. Reaction 5: P450c21 catalyzes the 21-hydroxylation of progesterone to DOC and that of 17-OH-progesterone to 11-deoxycortisol. Reaction 6: DOC is converted to corticosterone by the 11-hydroxylase activity of P450c11AS in the zona glomerulosa and by P450c11β in the zona fasciculata. Reaction 7: 11-Deoxycortisol is 11-hydroxylated by P450c11 to produce cortisol in the zona fasciculata. Reactions 8 and 9: The 18-hydroxylase and 18-oxidase activities of P450c11AS convert corticosterone to 18-OH-corticosterone and aldosterone, respectively, in the zona glomerusola. Reactions 10 and 11 are found principally in the testes and ovaries: 17β-HSD, a reversible non-P450 enzyme of the endoplasmic reticulum, mediates both 17-ketosteroid reductase and 17β-hydroxysteroid dehydrogenase activities. Reaction 10: 17β-HSD Type III converts DHEA to androstenediol and androstenedione to testosterone, while 17β-HSD Type I converts estrone to estradiol. Reaction 11: Testosterone may be converted to estradiol by P450aro (10), another P450 enzyme of the endoplasmic reticulum mediating the aromatization of the A ring of the steroid nucleus.

of P450scc; the sterol substrate remains bound to the single active site on cytochrome P450scc because of the tight binding of the reaction intermediates. The K_d for the binding of cholesterol is about 5,000 nM, whereas the K_d for (22R) 22-hydroxycholesterol and (20R, 22R) 20,22-dihydroxycholesterol are 4.9 and 81 nM, respectively. Thus, once cholesterol is bound to the enzyme, it is committed to completing the reaction sequence. The estimated K_d for pregnenolone is 2,900 nM, which permits the dissociation of the final reaction product from the enzyme.[92]

P450scc is the rate-limiting step in steroidogenesis and is one of the slowest enzymes known, with a V_{max} of $\sim$1 mol cholesterol/mol enzyme per second.[108] The slowest component of this complex reaction is the entry and binding of cholesterol to the active site,[114–116] but even when the role of StAR is circumvented by providing soluble hydroxysterols as substrate, the action of P450scc to produce pregnenolone is very slow, probably because of the need to complete three distinct catalytic cycles. The composition of the inner mitochondrial membrane may influence the binding of cholesterol, as cardrolipin increases the affinity of purified P450scc for cholesterol. Molecular models derived from the study of cholesterol analogs and purified P450scc suggest that carbon 22 of the cholesterol molecule lies within 0.4 Å of the heme iron of P450scc and that carbon 20 lies 1.54 Å further away.[117] The first hydroxylation probably occurs at carbon 22 because of its proximity to the heme iron. The introduction of the 22R hydroxyl group may move the substrate slightly to bring carbon 20 closer to the heme iron, thus permitting the second hydroxylation reaction. The third step is the cleavage of the 20,22 dihydroxy cholesterol to yield pregnenolone and isocapraldehyde; this does not involve incorporation of oxygen into either product, but oxygen is required for the reaction.

Genetics

Molecular cloning studies, beginning with the cloning of bovine P450scc cDNA,[118] have revealed much about P450scc. The human genome contains only a single gene encoding P450scc.[119,120] That gene, termed CYP11A, is about 20 kb long, is divided into nine exons,[111] is located on band q23 or q24 of chromosome 15,[120,121] and encodes an mRNA of 2.0 kb. The encoded 521-amino acid protein is protolytically cleaved to 482 amino acids[120] by an endoprotease[122] that removes the 39-amino acid leader peptide that directs the protein to the mitochondria. This single gene is expressed in all the conventional tissues that make steroid hormones, including the adrenal cortex, testis, ovary, and placenta.[35,119,120,123–125] Extraglandular synthesis of various steroids has been described, and P450scc has been demonstrated in rat kidney,[126] brain,[127,128] and gut,[129] and at least in the brain, the biosynthesis of steroids by this extraglandular P450scc has been demonstrated.

Transcription of the P450scc gene is regulated by ACTH in the adrenal, by gonadotropins in the testes and ovaries, and by unknown factors in the placenta, all functioning through cAMP as the intracellular second messenger (see Chap. 4).[65,130–135] By contrast, angiotensin II stimulates P450scc gene transcription in the zona glomerusa through the calcium/protein kinase C system.[132,136] Although experiments in bovine adrenal cells suggested that cAMP stimulates the synthesis of a protein that stimulates the transcription of the P450scc gene,[130] other work in rat and human systems indicates this is not true for all species.[125,131,132,137,138] The action of ACTH can be rapid, stimulating preexisting steroidogenic machinery by StAR-mediated increases in cholesterol flow, but the effects on transcription, while rapid at the molecular level, have a fairly slow and persistent effect and account for the chronic response of the adrenal to ACTH. For example, in Cushing disease, chronic stimulation of the adrenal by ACTH results in increased transcription of the genes for P450scc and for all of the other steroidogenic enzymes so that the adrenal steroidogenic capacity is greatly increased. Angiotensin II also stimulates the adrenal acutely, working through alterations in intracellular calcium and activation of protein kinase C.[136] However, prolonged stimulation with angiotensin II or with agents that activate the protein kinase C pathway represses the quantities and activities of steroidogenic enzymes in cultured adrenal cells.[139–141] This same short-term stimulation followed by long-term repression can be demonstrated at the level of the P450scc gene.[132] The details of the transcriptional regulation of the human P450scc gene differ substantially between the adrenal and the placenta[134,142,143] and there are substantial differences in the activity of the human P450scc promoter when it is expressed in human versus rodent cell lines.[144] These data indicate that different cells, employing different nuclear proteins, utilize the promoters of various genes in a tissue-specific fashion (for review, see Ref. 65).

Transport of Electrons to P450scc: Adrenodoxin Reductase and Adrenodoxin

P450scc functions as the terminal oxidase in a mitochondrial electron transport system. Electrons from NADPH are accepted by a flavoprotein—adrenodoxin reductase—that is loosely associated with the inner mitochondrial membrane.[145–147] Adrenodoxin reductase transfers the electrons to an iron/sulfur protein termed adrenodoxin, which is found either in solution in the mitochondrial matrix[145–148] or loosely associated with the inner mitochondrial membrane.[149] Adrenodoxin then transfers the electrons to P450scc (Fig. 11-8). Adrenodoxin reductase and adrenodoxin serve as generic electron transport proteins for all mitochondrial P450s, not just those involved in steroidogenesis; hence, these proteins are also termed ferredoxin reductase and ferredoxin.

Adrenodoxin Reductase

Adrenodoxin reductase is transcribed from a single copy gene located on band q24 or q25 of chromosome 17.[121,150,151] The primary RNA transcript of this gene can be alternately spliced into two forms of mRNA that differ by 18 bases.[150] Both forms of this mRNA are expressed in all tissues[152] but the protein encoded by the longer form is inactive in steroidogenesis.[153]

FIGURE 11-8. Electron transport to mitochondrial forms of cytochrome P450. Adrenodoxin reductase (AdRed), a flavoprotein loosely bound to the inner mitochondrial membrane, accepts electrons (e^-) from NADPH, converting it to $NADP^+$. These electrons are passed to adrenodoxin (Adx^+), an iron-sulfur protein loosely associated with the inner mitochondrial membrane that functions as a freely diffusable electron shuttle mechanism. Electrons from charged adrenodoxin (Adx^-) are accepted by any available cytochrome P450, such as P450c11 or P450scc, shown here. The uncharged adrenodoxin (Adx^+) may then be again bound to adrenodoxin reductase to receive another pair of electrons. For P450scc, three pairs of electrons must be transported to the P450 to convert cholesterol to pregnenolone. The inner and outer mitochondrial membranes may become more closely opposed during active steroidogenesis, facilitating the flux of hydrophobic steroid molecules.

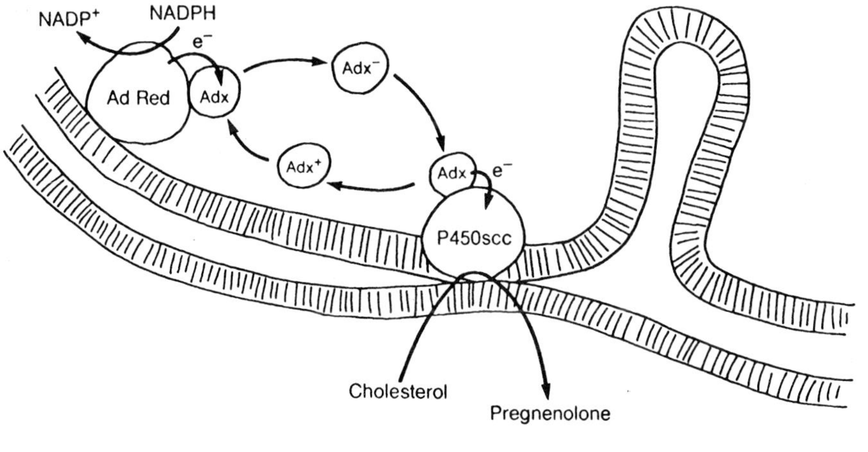

The adrenodoxin reductase gene is unique among the genes that encode steroidogenic enzymes in two respects. First, it lacks the conventional TATA and CAAT sequences typical of most eukaryotic promoters and instead has six copies of the sequence GGGCGGG, which appear to bind transcription factor Sp-1.[151] Such promoter structures are common in so-called housekeeping genes that are expressed ubiquitously without tissue specificity. Second, cAMP regulates the abundance of adrenodoxin reductase mRNA posttranscriptionally but does not regulate the transcription of the gene.[152] Adrenodoxin reductase is expressed in all human tissues, but its level is 100-fold greater in steroidogenic tissues.[152] By contrast, the gene for adrenodoxin is also expressed ubiquitously and always functions with adrenodoxin reductase, yet it has a classical promoter structure.

Adrenodoxin

Adrenodoxin is a small, soluble ion-sulfur protein that forms a 1 : 1 complex with adrenodoxin reductase, then dissociates, and subsequently reforms an analogous 1 : 1 complex with P450scc or P450c11, thus functioning as an indiscriminate diffusable electron shuttle mechanism.[109,154–160] Each adrenodoxin molecule contains two iron atoms tetrahedrally coordinated with the thiols of two cysteine residues and two labile sulfur atoms to form an Fe_2S_2 center.[158,159] The complete structure of bovine adrenodoxin has been determined at 1.85 Å resolution by x-ray crystallography, showing how the iron atoms coordinate electron transport.[161] There are one[162] or two[163] functional adrenodoxin genes encoding indistinguishable mRNAs and proteins[138] lying on band q11 of chromosome 11 and two nonexpressed pseudogenes on band q11 or q12 of chromosome 20.[121,164] There are multiple species of human adrenodoxin mRNA ranging from 1.0 to 1.8 kb in length that arise by the use of three or four different polyadenylylations sites in the 3′ untranslated region.[138,165] A role for this 3′ untranslated region in regulating adrenodoxin mRNA half-life has been ruled out.[166] Adrenodoxin mRNA is found in all human tissues[138] and accumulates in response to tropic stimulation of cultured adrenal cells with ACTH or cAMP or of cultured ovarian granulosa cells with FSH, human chorionic gonadotropin (hCG), or cAMP,[126,167] as does the mRNA for P450scc.

Interactions of P450scc, Adrenodoxin, and Adrenodoxin Reductase

P450scc, adrenodoxin, and adrenodoxin reductase are associated with the inner mitochondrial membrane.[149] Adrenodoxin reductase first accepts electrons from NADPH and then forms a 1 : 1 complex with adrenodoxin reductase, which catalyzes the reduction of adrenodoxin. Reduced adrenodoxin dissociates from the adrenodoxin reductase and may then form a 1 : 1 complex with P450scc or with any other available mitochondrial cytochrome P450, such as one of the isozymes of adrenal P450c11. Upon binding to P450scc, the adrenodoxin is oxidized and then discharged, making it available to bind again to adrenodoxin reductase and to repeat the cycle. Adrenodoxin reductase has a greater affinity for oxidized adrenodoxin than for reduced adrenodoxin, favoring productive interactions between these two proteins. Similarly, the binding of cholesterol to P450scc causes a 20-fold increase in the affinity of P450scc for reduced adrenodoxin. These differences in binding affinities promote the flux of electrons from NADPH to P450scc. These three components of the cholesterol side-chain cleavage system appear to be present in varying molar ratios in different tissues,[149] but the different and sensitive control of the transcription of each gene suggests that these ratios can be changed easily. P450scc, adrenodoxin, and adrenodoxin reductase apparently do not form a ternary complex in vivo, because the same surface of the adrenodoxin molecule interacts with both adrenodoxin reductase and P450scc.[161,168,169] However, a covalently linked trimolecular complex of these three components is functional with an increased V_{max}[170]; this fusion protein has greatly facilitated studies of StAR's action.[78,171]

3β-Hydroxysteroid Dehydrogenase/ $\Delta^5\Delta^4$ Isomerase

Once pregnenolone is produced from cholesterol, it may be converted to progesterone by 3β-hydroxysteroid dehydrogenase (3β-HSD). This single microsomal enzyme catalyzes both the 3β-hydroxysteroid dehydrogenation and the isomerization of the double bond from the B ring (Δ^5 steroids) to the A ring (Δ^4 steroids).[172–174] Both 3β HSD and isomerase activities are found in a single 42 kDa protein,[172] and expression of the cloned cDNA in COS-1 cells confers both activities to the cells.[174,175] Thus, it is clear that both the hydroxysteroid dehydrogenase and isomerase activities lie in a single protein. 3β-HSD is a typical short-chain dehydrogenase/reductase.[176]

There are two forms of human 3βHSD, encoded by different genes. The 3βHSD Type I gene is expressed in the placenta, skin, mammary gland, and possibly other peripheral tissues,[173–175,177] while the distinct 3βHSD Type II gene is expressed in the adrenals and gonads.[175,178] Unlike the P450 enzymes, where a single gene typically encodes a protein with multiple enzymatic acitivities, 3βHSD and the other short-chain dehydrogenases are encoded by multiple genes producing closely related enzymes with overlapping or identical activities. The 3βHSD genes and several related psuedogenes are localized on band p13 of chromosome 1.[175,177–180] Electron microscopy has localized 3β-HSD to multiple cellular compartments, including the cytosol, the endoplasmic reticulum adjacent to mitochondria, and within the mitochondria themselves,[181] facilitating the rapid metabolism of pregnenolone produced by P450scc.[182] It is not clear whether the distribution of the 3βHSD enzyme among these subcellular compartments is regulated, but it could clearly have an effect on whether steroidogenesis follows one pathway over another. The single human adrenal 3βHSDII enzyme catalyzes the conversion of pregnenolone to progesterone, of 17OH-pregnenolone to 17OH-progesterone, and of DHEA to androstenedione.[175] Each of these reactions occurs with similar kinetics, having a K_m of 5.2 to 5.5 μM and a V_{max} of 0.34 to 0.56 pmol of steroid per min per μg of protein.[183] Despite this widespread expression and concentrated activity in steroidogenic glands, the human fetal adrenal gland has relatively little 3βHSD activity as a result of very low levels of 3βHSD mRNA.[184] This permits the fetal adrenal to make very large quantities of the Δ^5 steroid DHEA and its sulfate, which are then metabolized to estrogens by the placenta. Even the widespread expression of multiple forms of 3β-HSD may not explain all extraglandular 3β-HSD/$\Delta^5\Delta^4$ isomerase activity. In the rabbit, such 3β-HSD activity has been found to be associated with hepatic cytochrome P450IIC5,[185] an enzyme which has 21-hydroxylase activity but is structurally unrelated to the adrenal 21-hydroxylase P450c21 (see 21-hydroxylase, later).

P450c17: 17α Hydroxylase/17,20 Lyase

Genetics and Enzymology

Both pregnenolone and progesterone may undergo 17α-hydroxylation to 17α-hydroxypregnenolone and 17α-hydroxyprogesterone

(17-OHP), respectively. These 17-hydroxylated C21 steroids may then theoretically undergo scission of the C-17,20 carbon bond to yield the C19 steroids DHEA and androstenedione, respectively. These four reactions are all mediated by a single enzyme, cytochrome P450c17, although conversion of 17-OHP to androstenedione by human P450c17 is very inefficient and biologically insignificant.[186,187] P450c17 is bound to the smooth endoplasmic reticulum, where it accepts electrons from a flavoprotein termed P450 oxidoreductase (OR), which is different from the adrenodoxin reductase in mitochondria, and without the need of an intermediary iron/sulfur protein such as adrenodoxin. As P450c17 has both 17α-hydroxylase activity and C-17,20 lyase activity, it is the key branch point in steroid hormone synthesis, directing pregnenolone to mineralocorticoids (neither activity), glucocorticoids (17α-hydroxylation but not C-17,20 cleavage), or sex steroids (after both 17α-hydroxylation and C-17,20 cleavage) (Figs. 11-4 and 11-7).

It was originally thought that 17α-hydroxylase and 17,20 lyase activities were catalyzed by two separate enzymes. The adrenals of prepubertal children synthesize ample cortisol but virtually no C19 steroids (i.e., have 17α-hydroxylase activity but not 17,20 lyase activity). At about age 7 to 9, adrenarche, a somewhat mysterious event that slightly precedes puberty but is independent from the GnRH-gonadotropin-gonadal axis, initiates production of adrenal androgens (i.e., appears to turn on 17,20 lyase activity).[188,189] Furthermore, patients had been described who lack 17,20 lyase activity but retain normal 17α-hydroxylase activity,[190,191] again suggesting that 17,20 lyase activity can be separated from 17α-hydroxylase activity. However, purification of pig testicular microsomal P450c17 and in vitro reconstitution of enzymatic activity clearly proved that both 17α-hydroxylase and 17,20 lyase activities reside in a single protein, P450c17.[192–195] Any residual doubts about this fact have been dispelled by two definitive genetic experiments. First, when vectors expressing bovine, human, or rat P450c17 cDNA are put into COS-1 cells or yeast, these cells acquire both 17α-hydroxylase and 17,20 lyase activities.[196–199] Second, severe mutations in the single human gene encoding P450c17 destroy all 17α-hydroxylase and 17,20 lyase activity in both the adrenals and the gonads.[199–201] Thus, differences in 17α-hydroxylase and 17,20 lyase activities are functional and physiologic but not genetic.

The single human gene encoding P450c17, formally termed CYP17, is located on band q24.3 of chromosome 10[121,202] and shows a striking similarity to the CYP21 gene for P450c21.[203,204] The close similarity between the intron/exon organization of the genes for P450c17 and P450c21 indicates that they diverged more recently in evolution than did either of these genes from those for other microsomal forms of P450.[204] The expression of P450c17 is primarily regulated by ACTH in the adrenals and LH in the gonads,[123,124] both operating through cAMP to promote gene transcription,[205] but having no effect on mRNA half-life.[99] Human CYP17 gene transcription also can be suppressed by phorbol esters[205] but the physiological significance of this is not clear. Elements required for adrenal expression are located between bases −63 and −220.[144,206] Computer-graphic analyses also suggest that the P450c17 and P450c21 proteins are structurally very similar, despite having only 28.9 percent amino acid sequence identity.[101,103,203,204] This is not entirely surprising, as both enzymes catalyze hydroxylation reactions on at least one common substrate, progesterone.

Several factors appear to be involved in determining whether a steroid molecule will remain on the single active site of P450c17 and undergo 17,20-bond scission after 17α-hydroxylation or whether it will leave the enzyme as a 17α-hydroxy C-21 steroid. Enzymologic analysis indicates that human P450c17 prefers Δ^5 substrates for 17,20-bond scission,[187] consistent with the large amounts of DHEA secreted by both the fetal and adult adrenal. Furthermore, the 17α-hydroxylase reaction occurs more readily (at lower K_m and faster V_{max}) than does the 17,20 lyase reaction.[187] However, more important than the relative concentrations of steroids and competing enzymes are factors regulating electron transport to P450c17.[186,187,207]

Electron Transport to P450c17: P450 Reductase and Cytochrome b_5

The membrane-bound flavoprotein P450 oxidoreductase (OR) appears to transfer electrons from NADPH to all of the various microsomal forms of P450, as it appears that there is only one species of OR, encoded by a single gene on chromosome 7.[208] The OR protein is 677 amino acids long and contains a molecule of flavin mononucleotide (FMN) and a molecule of flavin adenine dinucleotide (FAD).[208] OR receives a pair of electrons from NADPH and transfers them one at a time to the various forms of cytochrome P450 found in the endoplasmic reticulum.[209] In the adrenal, this includes P450c17 and P450c21; in other steroidogenic tissues, such as the ovary or placenta, this includes P450aro (aromatase); and in the liver, it includes most of the enzymes involved in drug metabolism (Fig. 11-9). The first electron is transferred more rapidly than is the second. The three-dimensional structure of rat OR has been determined by x-ray crystallography, showing that the FAD binding domain is bound to the endoplasmic reticulum and is connected by a protein hinge to the FMN domain in the cytoplasm.[210] Following the receipt of electrons from NADPH, the FMN domain must rotate about 90° on the hinge to extend the FMN moiety out from the concave cleft of OR to approach the concave redox-partner binding site of the P450.[210] The endoplasmic reticulum in the adrenal contains many more molecules of P450c17 and P450c21 than molecules of OR; thus, it

FIGURE 11-9. Electron transport to microsomal cytochromes P450. P450 oxidoreductase (OR), a flavoprotein distinct from adrenodoxin reductase, accepts electron pairs from NADPH via the FAD moiety and transfers them to the FMN moiety. These electrons are then passed directly to a cytochrome P450, such as P450c17, shown here. Transfer of the second electron from P450 reductase is slow; the transfer of this second electron may be facilitated by the allosteric action of cytochrome b5.

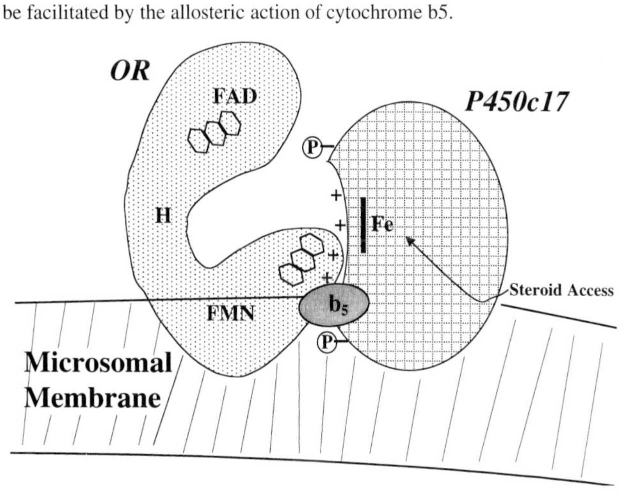

appears that these P450s compete with one another for the reducing equivalents provided by the reductase. Phospholipids may facilitate the formation of complexes of P450, OR and cytochrome b_5, thus increasing the transfer of electrons and consequently increasing enzymatic activity,[211,212] but the most important factor in determining whether the 17,20 lyase reaction follows the 17α-hydroxylase reaction appears to be the presence of cytochrome b_5.

The availability of reducing equivalents from OR determines whether 17-OH pregnenolone will undergo 17,20 bond-cleavage to DHEA. Because P450c17 catalyzes the conversion of 17-OH progesterone to adrostenedione very inefficiently[187] there is no competition between P450c17 and P450c21 for the 17-OH substrate, and virtually all 17-OHP is converted to 11 deoxycortisol, consistent with the observation that antibodies to P450c21 do not increase the conversion of 17-OHP to androstenedione.[207] The testis normally contains three to four times more P450 reductase activity than does the adrenal, consistent with its need for greater 17,20 lyase activity to produce C-19 androgens. Furthermore, increasing the ratio of P450 reductase to P450c17 in vitro[208] or in transfected cells[186] increases the 17,20 lyase activity relative to 17α-hydroxylase activity.

Until recently, it was thought that cytochrome b_5 could serve as an alternative to OR for donation of the second (but not the first) electron in the P450 reaction cycle.[24] This was based on evidence that b_5 can function in this fashion with some other microsomal forms of P450.[213,214] However, careful analysis of the enzymology of human P450c17 expressed in genetically engineered yeast shows that cytochrome b_5 promotes 17,20 lyase activity as an allosteric facillitator but not as an electron donor.[187] Thus the conversion of 17-OH pregnenelone to DHEA involves a complex of four simultaneously interacting components: steroid, P450, OR, and b_5.

Understanding of this complex has been facilitated by the construction and testing of a detailed computer-graphic model of human P450c17 that appears to fulfill all known criteria for an accurate representation of P450c17.[103] In conjunction with the crystallographic data for OR[210] it appears that the surface of the FMN domain of OR that interacts with P450c17 contains a cluster of acidic residues that interact with basic residues in the redox-partner binding-site of P450c17. However, these interactions are weak and indirect because the surfaces of the two proteins remain several Ångstroms apart, and the electron transfer actually occurs at a nearby site, but not at the interface of the charged residues of the two proteins. The stereochemical requirement for electron transfer is more stringent for the 17,20 lyase reaction than for the 17α-hydroxylase reaction, possibly due to conformational changes in P450c17 when 17-OH pregnenolone rather than pregnenolone occupies the active site. This more stringent stereochemistry requires the action of b_5 to optimize the positioning of P450c17 and OR, thus permitting electron transfer and catalysis of the 17,20 lyase reaction. The key role of cytochrome b_5 as an allosteric facilitator for the 17,20 lyase reaction is shown by the demonstration that mutations of P450c17 that selectively eliminate 17,20 lyase activity but not 17α-hydroxylase activity do not affect steroid binding but do disrupt the interaction of the P450c17 • OR complex with b_5.[215]

Human P450c17 is phosphorylated on serine and threonine, but not tyrsosine residues, by an as-yet unidentified cAMP-dependent protein kinase.[216] When P450c17 prepared from human adrenals is dephosphorylated with alkaline phosphatase, the enzyme loses 17,20 lyase activity, but the 17α-hydroxylase activity, and the enzyme's ability to bind 17α-hydroxypregnenolone is unaffected. The basis for this behavior is not yet established, but it appears likely that the phosphorylation of certain residues facilitates the interaction with b_5 and OR, thus favoring 17,20 lyase activity. Thus the 17,20 lyase activity of P450c17 can be regulated by both extrinsic factors (b_5) and intrinsic factors (phosphorylation), but in both cases the mechanism is by facilitating the interaction with OR.

P450c21: 21-Hydroxylase

After the synthesis of progesterone and 17-OHP, these steroids are hydroxylated at carbon 21 to yield DOC and 11-deoxycortisol, respectively (Fig. 11-7). The nature of the 21 hydroxylating step has been of great clinical interest because congenital adrenal hyperplasia (CAH) resulting from 21-hydroxylase deficiency is an extremely common inborn error of metabolism, as discussed later. The clinical manifestations of CAH can vary greatly, and in the most severe form, decreased synthesis of cortisol and aldosterone leads to sodium loss, hypotension, cardiovascular collapse, and, if untreated, death within the first month of life. Decreased cortisol synthesis in utero leads to overproduction of ACTH and consequent stimulation of adrenal steroid synthesis; as the 21-hydroxylase step is impaired, precursor steroids are converted to androstenedione and testosterone, resulting in severe prenatal virilization of female fetuses (for reviews, see Refs. 217 and 218). CAH has been studied extensively at both the clinical and molecular genetic levels. Variations in the manifestations of the disease, especially the presence of many patients without apparent defects in mineralocorticoid activity ("simple virilizing CAH" and "nonclassical CAH"), led to the belief that there are two seperate 21 hydroxylating enzymes that are differentially expressed in the zona glomerulosa and zonae fasciculata and reticularis of the adrenal, specifically synthesizing aldosterone or cortisol, respectively. However, characterization of the P450c21 protein from the endoplasmic reticulum and cloning of the gene have shown that there is only one 21-hydroxylase. P450c21 employs the same P450 oxidoreductase used by P450c17 to transport electrons from NADPH. Isolation of P450c21 from bovine adrenals showed a single species of protein that could 21-hydroxylate both progesterone and 17-OHP,[219] but it was not until the cDNAs and genes were cloned that it was proved that there is only one functional adrenal 21-hydroxylase gene in human beings.[220–222]

21-Hydroxylase Genes

There are two 21-hydroxylase genes, termed CYP21A and CYP21B, or P450c21A and P450c21B. Each overlaps a pair of genes termed X[223] and Y[224]; the XB gene encodes the novel extracellular matrix protein tenascin-X[225] but XA and the Y genes are nonfunctional. This CYP21/X/Y complex was duplicated with the adjacent C4A and C4B loci encoding the fourth component of serum complement; this cluster in turn lies in the midst of the HLA locus on human chromosome 6p21.3 (for review see Refs. 226 and 227). The genetic structures of the 21 hydroxylase genes are unusual as a result of the very high rate of crossover and genetic exchange between the two 21-hydroxylase genes.[226,227] As a detailed understanding of the genetics of this locus is required to understand congenital adrenal hyperplasia, the structure and genetics of these genes are discussed in disorders of steroid hormone synthesis, later, in conjunction with the clinical disorders of steroid hormone synthesis.

Extraadrenal 21-Hydroxylase

21-hydroxylase activity is found in a broad range of extraadrenal tissues, especially in the fetus and the pregnant woman.[228,229] However, this extraadrenal 21-hydroxylation is not mediated by the P450c21 enzyme found in the adrenal,[230] and this activity persists in congenital adrenal hyperplasia. The nature of the enzyme(s) responsible for extraadrenal 21-hydroxylation remain unknown. In the rabbit, hepatic 21-hydroxylase activity is mediated by P450IIC5,[160] but the human homologue of this enzyme lacks significant 21-hydroxylase acitvity. By contrast, authentic P450c21 mRNA is found in mouse liver,[231] in bovine testis,[232] and in a human testicular tumor.[38] However, human P450c21 mRNA is not found in normal human extraadrenal tissues.[230] The presence of such other 21-hydroxylating enzymes complicates the phenotypic presentation and clinical understanding of 21-hydroxylase deficiency, because even patients homozygous for a P450c21 gene deletion may still synthesize some 21-hydroxylated steroids.[233]

P450c11β and P450c11AS: 11β-Hydroxylase and Aldosterone Synthase

The enzymologic basis for the conversion of DOC to aldosterone has been studied and debated with vigor. Clinical studies suggested that at least three enzymes, 11β-hydroxylase, 18-hydroxylase, and one or more corticosterone methyl oxidases were involved,[234,235] but studies in cattle indicated that a single enzyme, P450c11, mediates all steps in the conversion of DOC to aldosterone as well as converting 11-deoxycortisol to cortisol.[236] Although a single bovine enzyme does indeed possess all of these activities,[237] the biology of the human and rodent enzyme systems is somewhat differerent.[238,239] Two isozymes of P450c11, like P450scc, are found in the inner mitochondrial membrane and, like P450scc, use adrenodoxin reductase and adrenodoxin as electron transport intermediates to receive electrons from NADPH.[240] However, unlike P450scc, the genetics of P450c11 are complex. P450c11 and P450scc share 39 percent amino acid identity and are encoded by evolutionarily related genes that have essentially identical intron/exon structures that is shared by all mitochondrial P450 enzymes.[97] The human genome has two P450c11 genes[241,242] located on chromosome 8q21-22.[243] These genes encode two P450c11 proteins that have 93 percent amino acid sequence identity. The gene generally termed CYP11B1 is expressed at high levels in the zonae fasciculata and reticularis and encodes an enzyme, generally termed P450c11β, that only has 11β hydroxylase activity and which converts 11-deoxycortisol to cortisol. The closely related CYP11B2 gene is expressed solely in the zona glomerulosa, and at very low levels. It encodes an enzyme generally termed P450c11AS (for aldosterone synthase), which has 11β-hydroxylase, 18-hydroxylase, and 18-oxidase activities, and hence is the sole enzyme needed to convert DOC to aldosterone.[244–248] This enzyme has also been called P450c11aldo, P450c11cmo, P450c18, and P450c11B. As expected, the CYP11B1 gene that encodes the P450c11β needed for cortisol synthesis is induced by ACTH and supressed by dexamethasone, while the CYP11B2 gene that encodes the P450c11AS needed for aldosterone synthesis is induced by angiotensin II and potassium and suppressed by salt.[248] Patients with classical 11β-hydroxylase deficiency have defects in their genes for P450c11β,[249] while patients with the so-called CMOI and CMOII (18-hydroxylase and 18-oxidase) deficiencies that disrupt aldosterone synthesis have defects in their genes for P450c11AS.[250–252] Thus, the molecular characterization of these genes and their encoded products has greatly clarified this formerly confusing area of steroidogenesis.

Rats have four closely linked CYP11B genes[253,254]; one is nonfunctional, and two correspond to human CYP11B1 and CYP11B2 and encode P450c11β and P450c11AS, respectively. The rat also has the novel CYP11B3 gene that is expressed only in the fetal adrenal and encodes a P450c11 isozyme that has both 11β-hydroxylase and 18-hydroxylase activities, but no aldosterone synthase activity.[255,256] Mutations in rat P450c11AS increase aldosterone synthase activity in the salt-resistant Dahl rat model of hypertension[257] and when the corresponding amino acid changes are introduced into human P450c11AS, aldosterone synthase activity is substantially increased.[258] A survey of patients with low-renin hypertension found only that human P450c11AS has a naturally occurring polymorphism where either lysine or argenine can be found at residue 173, but these two forms of P450c11AS had equivalent aldosterone synthase activity shown by measurement of their K_m and V_{max} values.[259] A survey of Japanese patients with idopathic hyperaldosteronism also found no mutations in P450c11AS, but did find evidence for increased P450c11AS expression, suggesting the possibility of promoter mutations.[260] Thus the P450c11 genes remain a potentially important locus in studies of heritable forms of hypertension.

Other Steroidogenic Enzymes

Several other enzymes are involved in synthesizing and metabolizing various steroids. These enzymes are especially important in the production of sex steroids and in regulating mineralocorticoid activity. However, as their roles are somewhat peripheral to adrenal steroidogenesis, they are considered in less detail here.

17β-Hydroxysteroid Dehydrogenase/17-Ketosteroid Reductase

A series of 17β-hydroxysteroid dehydrogenases (17β-HSD), often also referred to as 17-ketosteroid reductases (17KSR), is responsible for the production of Δ^5 androstenediol from DHEA, testosterone from Δ^4 androstenedione and estradiol from estrone. Several such enzymes have been isolated, cloned, and characterized. Although these enzymes are not expressed in the adrenal, they are of substantial interest as potential targets for pharmacologic intervention as there are distinct enzymes involved in the biosynthesis of estrogens and androgens. Nonetheless, this remains the most complex and confusing step in steroidogenesis because: (1) there are several different 17β-HSDs, (2) some are preferential oxidases, and others are preferential reductases, (3) they exhibit differences in their tissue distribution of expression and substrate preference, (4) there is inconsistent nomenclature among the human and rat enzymes, and (5) some of these proteins have inconsequential 17β-HSD activity, and are principally involved in other functions. The 17β-HSD enzymes are short-chain dehydrogenases, but their sequences show substantial differences.[176] The various forms of 17β-HSD are designated by Roman numerals designating their sequence of chronologic discovery rather than their biology. Type I 17β-HSD (17β-HSD-I) is a soluble, cytoplasmic enzyme that was first isolated and cloned from the placenta, where it produces estriol, and is also expressed in ovarian granulosa cells, where it produces estradiol.[173,261–263] 17β-HSD-I is also known as estrogenic 17β-HSD[263] and functions as a dimer using NADPH as its cofactor to catalyze its reductase activity.

17β-HSD-I is also found in the endometrium, liver, prostate, testis, and adipose tissue.[263–267] 17β-HSD-I is encoded by a small gene on chromosome 17p21 that is closely linked to an inactive pseudogene.[268,269] The three-dimensional structure of human 17β-HSD-I has been determined by x-ray crystallography.[270,271] No genetic deficiency syndrome for 17β-HSD-I has been described.

17β-HSD-II is a microsomal oxidase that uses NAD^+ to convert estradiol to estrone and testosterone to Δ^4 androstenedione, thus serving to inactivate sex steroids. 17β-HSD-II, encoded by a gene on chromosome 16q24[272] is found in the placenta, liver, small intestine, prostate, secretory endometrium and ovary.[264,267,273–275] In contrast to 17β-HSD-I, which is found in placental syncytiotrophoblast cells, 17β-HSD-II is expressed in endothelial cells of placental intravillous vessels, consistent with its apparent role in defending the fetal circulation from transplacental passage of maternal estradiol or testosterone.[267] No deficiency state for 17β-HSD-II has been reported.

17β-HSD-III, also known as the androgenic from of 17β-HSD, is a microsomal enzyme encoded by a gene on chromosome 9q22 that is apparently expressed only in the testis.[276] This is the enzyme that is disordered in the classic syndrome of male pseudohermaphroditism that is often termed 17-ketosteroid reductase deficiency.[276–279]

An enzyme termed 17β-HSD-IV was initially identified as an NAD^+-dependent oxidase with activities similar to 17β-HSD-II.[280–282] However, it appears that the 17β-HSD activity of this peroxisomal protein is a side reaction, and that its principal activities are enoyl-CoA hydratase and 3-hydroxyacyl-CoA dehydrogenase.[283,284] The mutation G16S in this enzyme selectively deletes the 3-hydroxyacyl-CoA dehydrogenase activity in peroxisomes, resulting in a unique variant of Zellweger syndrome.[284]

17β-HSD-V, originally cloned as a 3α-hydroxysteroid dehydrogenase[285] is a labile enzyme that is abundantly expressed in the prostate and catalyzes the reduction of Δ^4 androstenedione to testosterone.[286,287] The precise role of this enzyme is unclear, and no deficiency state has been described, but its abundant expression in the prostate suggests a role in androgen-induced prostatic hypertrophy. Types VI and VII 17β-HSD enzymes have been described in rodents, but it is not clear if there are human homologues to these enzymes.[288,289]

P450aro: Aromatase

The aromatization of C-18 estrogenic steroids from C-19 androgens is mediated by P450aro, which is found in the endoplasmic reticulum.[290,291] P450aro converts androgens to estrogens by two hydroxylations at the C-19 methyl group and a third hydroxylation at C-2, resulting in the loss of carbon 19 and consequent aromatization of the A ring of the steroid (Fig. 11-4).[292,293] This series of reactions requires three pairs of electrons donated by three molecules of NADPH through P450 reductase, and all occur on a single active site.[294] P450aro, a typical microsomal P450 enzyme, has been purified and cloned.[295–300] Although the enzyme has not been crystallized, a useful three-dimensional computer-graphic model of its structure has been published, providing novel insight into the probable chemical mechanisms of each step in the aromatase reaction.[102] The single gene for human aromatase termed CYP19 is located on chromosome 15q21.2[297] and encodes two mRNAs that differ in the lengths of their 3′ untranslated regions.[298,301] Expression of human P450aro cDNA in COS-1 cells[299] or yeast[300] shows that all the successive oxidation reactions that are needed to aromatize androgens to estrogens are catalyzed by this single enzyme. The CYP19 gene encoding P450aro is quite large, encompassing over 75 kb.[302] Transcription can be initiated from any one of five alternative untranslated first exons which permit different segments of DNA to function as the regulatory sequences in a tissue-specific fashion in the placenta, ovary, and adipose tissue.[303] Thus, the same enzyme is produced in different tissues under different regulatory control. Aromatase deficiency is not a disorder of adrenal steroidogenesis, but, provides substantial information about the role of this enzyme. Homozygous disruption of the human aromatase gene results in masculization of affected female fetuses, hypogonadotropic hypogonadism with multicystic ovaries following the age of puberty, and a striking delay in the advancement of bony maturation which supports a direct role of estrogens in epiphyseal fusion.[291,304–306]

5α-Reductase

Testosterone is converted to the more potent androgen dihydrotestosterone by 5α-reductase, a membrane-bound non-P450 enzyme found primarily in peripheral target tissues such as genital skin and hair follicles rather than in the adrenal or testis.[307] There are two distinct isozymes of human 5α-reductase.[308,309] The type I enzyme is a hydrophobic protein of about 29 kDa encoded by an mRNA of about 2.4 kb encoded by a large gene of about 35 kb divided into five exons that is located on the gene of chromosome 5p15.[310] This gene encodes the enzyme found in the scalp, sebaceous glands, and liver, but does not encode the enzyme required for male sexual differentiation.[310,311] The type 2 enzyme is encoded by a gene on chromosome 2p23 that has the same intron/exon structure as the gene for the type 1 enzyme.[312] The syndrome of 5α-reductase deficiency is a rare autosomal recessive disorder that causes incomplete differentiation of male genitalia but is phenotypically silent in females.[307,313,314] A wide variety of mutations have been described in the type 2 gene that cause the classical syndrome of 5α-reductase deficiency.[312] The type 1 and 2 genes show an unusual pattern of developmental regulation of expression. The type 1 gene is not expressed in the fetus, then is expressed briefly in the skin of the newborn, and then remains unexpressed until its activity and protein are again found after puberty. The type 2 gene is expressed in fetal genital skin, in the normal prostate, and in prostatic hyperplasia and adenocarcinoma. Thus, the type 1 enzyme may be responsible for the pubertal virilization seen in patients with classic 5α-reductase deficiency, and the type 2 enzyme may be involved in male pattern baldness.[312]

Steroid Sulfotransferase and Sulfatase

Steroid sulfates may be synthesized directly from cholesterol sulfate or may be formed by the sulfation of steroids by cytosolic sulfotransferases. Steroid sulfates may also be hydrolyzed to the native steroid by steroid sulfatase. An estrogen sulfotransferase has been cloned from bovine placenta[315] and guinea pig adrenal,[316] and it appears there are other steroid sulfotransferases as well. The human steroid sulfatase gene on chromosome Xp22.3 has been cloned and studied in detail, because deletions of this gene are a common cause of steroid sulfatase deficiency with X-linked icthyosis.[317,318] The regulation of steroid sulfatase is important because it regulates the abundance of DHEA that can be converted to sex steroids in peripheral tissues. In the fetal adrenal and placenta, diminished or absent sulfatase deficiency reduces the pool of free DHEA available for placental conversion to estrogen. The accumulation of steroid sulfates in the stratum corneum of the skin causes the icthyosis. Steroid sulfatase is also expressed in the fetal brain, possibly converting peripherally supplied DHEA-S to active DHEA.[319,320]

11β-Hydroxysteroid Dehydrogenase

The oxidation of cortisol to cortisone is mediated by 11β-hydroxysteroid dehydrogenase (11βHSD) and the reverse reaction is mediated by an 11-oxidoreductase activity. There are two 11βHSD enzymes, each of which has both the oxidase and the reductase activity, depending on the co-factor available.[321] The type I enzyme (11βHSD-I), sometimes called the 'hepatic form,' is a protein of 292 amino acids encoded by a gene on chromosome 1 that consists of six exons spanning about 7 kb.[322,323] Assays of enzymatic activity, protein blotting, and RNA blotting all show that this enzyme is widely distributed in many tissues.[322–326] 11βHSD-I is NAD(H)-dependent and favors the reduction of cortisone to cortisol (and of prednisone to prednisolone), and hence is primarily an activating enzyme in tissues where NADPH is abundant, such as the liver or lung. Consistent with this, mice lacking 11βHSD-I have a diminished capacity to mount glucocorticoid-induced responses such as activation of gluconeogenic enzymes,[327] although a human 11βHSD-I deficiency state has not yet been described. However, in tissues where $NADP^+$ is abundant, such as the placenta, 11βHSD-I functions primarily as an oxidase to inactivate steroids. 11βHSD-I metabolizes steroids present in high concentrations: its K_m for the reduction of cortisone to cortisol is 0.14 μM and for the oxidation of cortisol to cortisone its K_m is 1.6 μM.[323,328] The type II enzyme (11βHSD-II), sometimes called the 'renal form,' is only 14 percent identical to the type I enzyme and is encoded by a gene on chromosome 16p22 that consists of five exons spanning 6.2 kb.[329,330] 11βHSD-II is NAD^+-dependent and functions only as an oxidase, converting cortisol to cortisone (and prednisolone to prednisone) and hence is an inactivating enzyme. 11βHSD-II has a very high affinity for cortisol, having a K_m of ~50 nM[331–333] and hence inactivates steroids even at low concentrations.

Although glucocorticoids and mineralocorticoids have been distinguished functionally for 50 years,[11] the cloning of the glucocorticoid and mineralocorticoid receptors raised a logical conundrum since the human mineralocorticoid (Type I) receptor bound aldosterone, corticosterone, and cortisol with equal affinities.[334,365] Thus, it was unclear how mineralocorticoids could exhibit tissue-specific effects when the circulating concentrations of cortisol were 100 to 1,000 times greater. The explanation for the apparent physiologic specificity of the mineralocorticoid receptor in the presence of molecular non-specificity of the receptor came from studies of two disorders of 11βHSD. In the syndrome of apparent mineralocorticoid excess,[335–337] there is a genetic defect in 11βHSD-II so that cortisol is not inactivated to cortisone.[338,339] Similarly, in licorice poisoning, glyceyrrhizic acid and its metabolite glyceyrrhetinic acid inhibit 11βHSD-II activity, resulting in sodium retention and hypertension.[337,340,341] Both conditions lead to high intrarenal cortisol concentrations that then occupy the mineralocorticoid receptor. Thus 11βHSD-II "protects" the mineralocorticoid receptor from the action of glucocorticoids.[326,366] This action of 11βHSD-II appears to apply to the placenta[342] and to a variety of human fetal tissues as well[343]; thus in the placenta, both 11βHSD-I and 11βHSD-II serve to protect the fetus from high maternal concentrations of glucocorticoids.

Developmental Aspects of Adrenal Steroidogenesis: The Fetal Adrenal, Adrenarche, and Adrenopause

Adrenal steroidogenesis begins early in embryonic life, probably by the eighth week of gestation. In fetuses affected with genetic disorders of steroidogenesis such as 21-hydroxylase deficiency, the dysfunctional fetal adrenal can produce enough testosterone to virilize a female fetus to a male appearance (closure of the urogenital sinus, with a urethra traversing part or all of the clitoral phallic shaft).[217,218,313] Testosterone has such effects only between the eighth and thirteenth weeks,[313] indicating that the fetal adrenal is already steroidogenically active during this period. Experimental suppression of fetal adrenal steroidogenesis in 21-hydroxylase deficiency requires administration of suitable glucocorticoids to the mother before the seventh week of pregnancy (for reviews see Refs. 344, 345). Thus, fetal adrenal steroidogenesis begins early.

The fetal adrenal consists of a thin subcapsular 'definitive zone' that make glucocorticoids and mineralocorticoids, and the large fetal zone, which produces DHEA and DHEA-S. These zones are separated by a thin layer of nonsteroidogenic cells that appear to be the progenitors of both zones.[346] Fetal adrenal growth depends on IGF-II,[33,35] basic fibroblast growth factor,[36] and epidermal growth factor[37] (for review see Ref. 347). The involution of the fetal zone following birth appears to involve apoptosis, possibly stimulated by activin A and/or transforming growth factor β,[348] and probably involving the withdrawal of IGF-II, which is abundant in fetal circulation, then decreases rapidly at birth.

Fetal adrenal steroidogenesis differs from that in older children or adults. The thin definitive zone of the fetal adrenal produces cortisol, corticosterone, DOC, progesterone, aldosterone, and androstenedione according to the pathways shown in Figs. 11-4 and 11-7.[349] However, this accounts for only about 65 percent of circulating fetal cortisol; the remainder comes from direct placental transfer of cortisol and from fetal conversion of placentally produced cortisone back to cortisol. The placenta has abundant 11β-dehydrogenase activity such that about 85 percent of maternally produced cortisol crossing the placenta is inactivated by conversion to cortisone; the fetus can convert only very small amounts of this cortisone back to cortisol.[350] As a result, fetal blood concentrations of cortisol are only about 15 percent of those found in the mother, despite similar levels of corticosteroid binding globulin[351]; thus normal human fetal development occurs in an environment of relative glucocorticoid privation, and normal development can occur in a nearly complete absence of steroid hormones.[352]

The large fetal zone of the fetal adrenal is steroidogenically very active but has very little 3β-hydroxysteroid dehydrogenase (3βHSD) activity because of the barely detectable amounts of 3βHSD mRNA.[184] The fetal zone also has a relatively high ratio of 17,20 lyase to 17α-hydroxylase activity of P450c17, favoring abundant production of DHEA, and also has considerable sulfotransferase activity but little steroid sulfatase activity favoring conversion of the DHEA to DHEA-S. The resulting DHEA-S cannot be a substrate for 3βHSD activity and must undergo the sulfatase reaction in the placenta. Placental estrogens also inhibit adrenal 3βHSD activity, providing a feedback system that further promotes the production of DHEA-S.[353] As a result, the fetal adrenal produces tremendous quantities of DHEA and DHEA-S. These steroids are converted to 16α-OH-DHEA and 16α-OH-DHEA-S in the liver and other tissues and then are converted by placental 3βHSD-I, 17βHSD-I, and aromatase to estriol after removal of the sulfate by placental sulfatase activity. Alternatively, placental 3βHSD-I and aromatase can act on DHEA to produce estrone, or 3βHSD, aromatase, and 17βHSD-I can act on DHEA to produce estradiol. Fetal adrenal DHEA and DHEA-S account for about 90 percent of the estriol and about 50 percent of the estrone and estradiol in the maternal circulation. Thus, measurement of circulating maternal estriol constitutes a useful assay of the health of the fetoplacental unit. However, despite the massive production of estrogens by the feto-placental unit, they are not essential for pregnancy. Fetuses (and placentas) lacking StAR, P450c17, and P450aro are incapable of making estrogens, and fetuses lacking the estrogen receptor are incapable of responding to estrogens, yet such fetuses develop normally, reach term gestation, and undergo normal parturition.[352]

Although the newborn adrenal is able to make cortisol, circulating cortisol concentrations are difficult to assess because much of the adrenal's cortisol production is rapidly converted to cortisone, which will not be detected by contemporary HPLC-based assays. Furthermore, the typical diurnal variation of ACTH and cortisol are not established until 6–12 months of age. Thus, the establishment of a diagnosis of adrenal insufficiency in the newborn requires an ACTH test. The newborn adrenal is able to make substantial quantities of aldosterone. The newborn and child are remarkably resistant to aldosterone, and its circulating concentrations are normally much higher than in adults (Fig. 11-10).

Following birth, the fetal zone of the adrenal involutes and the definitive zone grows. Thus circulating concentrations of DHEA and DHEA-S fall rapidly following birth due to involution of the fetal zone and reach the low levels typical of childhood by about 1 year of age, then remain low until the onset of adrenarche at about 7 to 10 years of age. Adrenarche is defined as the onset of adrenal DHEA and DHEA-S secretion. The mechanisms triggering the onset of adrenarche remain unknown. The adrenal zona reticularis, where DHEA and DHEA-S are produced in the adult adrenal, does not become morphologically distinct until after about 3 years of age, and possibly later. The onset of adrenarche generally preceeds the onset of puberty (defined by increase GnRH pulsatility and the appearance of nighttime pulses of LH) by about two years. The slow onset of adrenarche and its consequent temporal overlap with puberty has been the cause of substantial misunderstanding, but it is clear that adrenarche is independent of GnRH, gonadotropins, the gonads, and gonadal steroids, as it occurs in individuals with Turner Syndrome and other disorders of the hypothalamic/pituitary/gonadal axis.[189] Although adrenarche begins before puberty, it finishes later, as peak concentrations of DHEA-S are not reached until about 25 years of age.[188] Thereafter, the circulating concentrations of DHEA-S and DHEA fall slowly, eventually reaching early or pre-adrenarchal levels in the eighth decade (adrenopause) (Fig. 11-11). Although substantial indirect data have been reported indicating that DHEA replacement therapy has a variety of salutary effects during aging,[354] this remains controversial and unresolved. A clear syndrome of DHEA deficiency in adrenalectomized individuals receiving adequate glucocorticoid and mineralocorticoid replacement therapy has not been defined. Furthermore, it is not possible to separate the potential effects of DHEA from the potential effects of its metabolism to androgens and estrogens, as such metabolism may occur directly in target tissues, so that biologically effective production of sex steroids may not be reflected by alterations in circulating concentrations of these steroids.

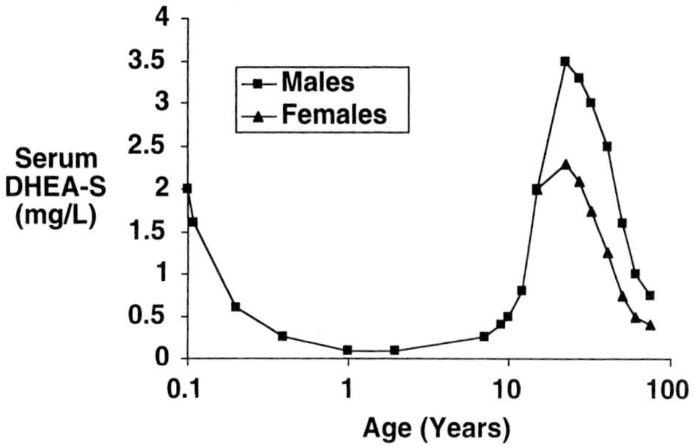

FIGURE 11-11. Serum concentrations of DHEA-S as a function of age (note the logarithmic x-axis). Data from Orentreich et al.[359] and from the reported normal values of several commercial laboratories.

FIGURE 11-10. Serum concentrations of aldosterone as a function of age. Data are pooled from the reported normal values of several commercial laboratories.

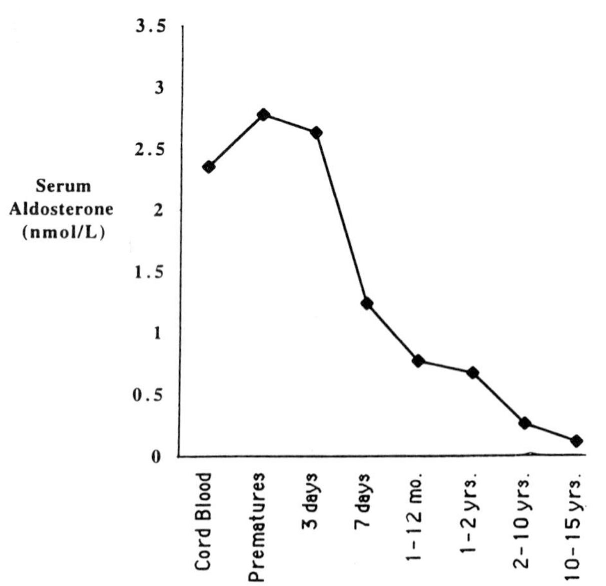

REGULATION OF ADRENAL STEROIDOGENESIS

Steroidogenic tissues do not store appreciable amounts of steroid hormones; therefore, the regulation of steroid hormone secretion occurs primarily at the level of steroid hormone synthesis. The principal regulator of glucocorticoid synthesis is the hypothalamic-pituitary-adrenal axis, and the principal regulator of adrenal mineralocorticoid synthesis is the renin-angiotensin system. The mechanisms regulating adrenal androgens are controversial but clearly involve both ACTH and other factors. The classical physiologic interrelations among the various tissues and factors regulating steroid hormone synthesis, uptake, and metabolism are shown in Fig. 11-12. This complex homeostatic balance allows rapid and sensitive control of the circulating concentrations of steroid hormones in a broad range of normal and abnormal physiologic states.[355–366]

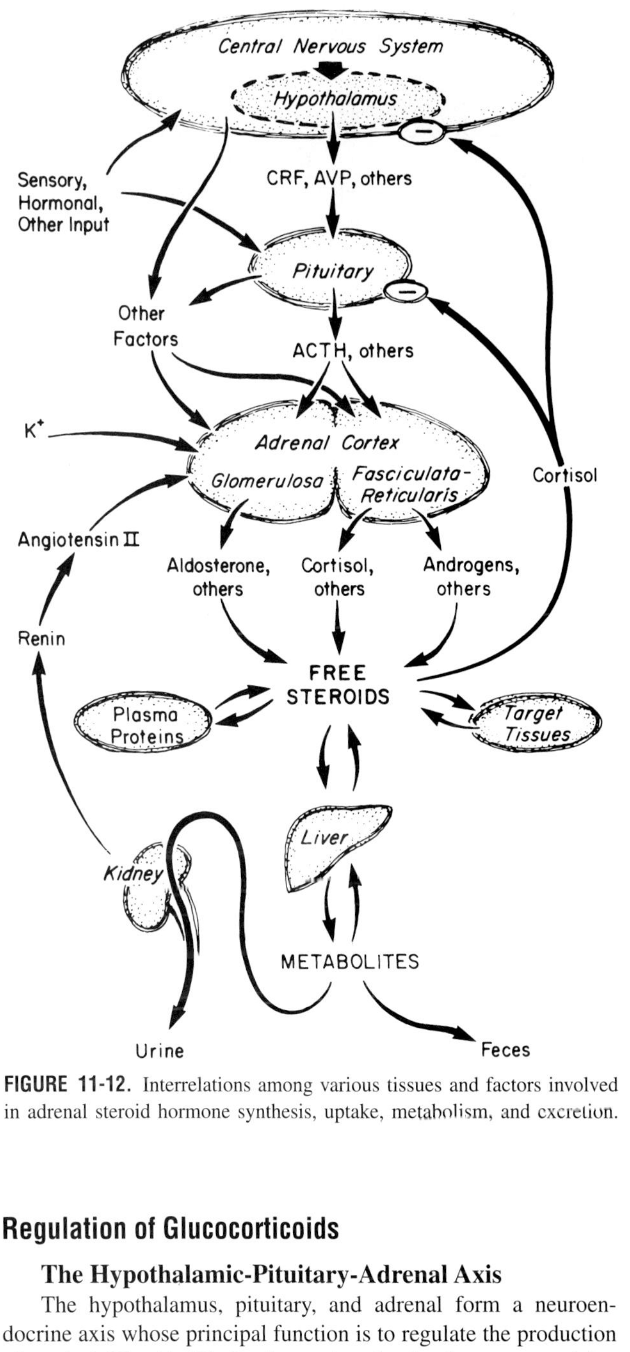

FIGURE 11-12. Interrelations among various tissues and factors involved in adrenal steroid hormone synthesis, uptake, metabolism, and excretion.

Regulation of Glucocorticoids

The Hypothalamic-Pituitary-Adrenal Axis

The hypothalamus, pituitary, and adrenal form a neuroendocrine axis whose principal function is to regulate the production of cortisol (Fig. 11-12). Corticotropin-releasing hormone, arginine vasopressin (AVP), and possibly other factors are secreted by the hypothalamus into the hypothalamic portal veins, thus exposing the anterior pituitary to high concentrations of those hypothalamic factors before they are diluted by entry into the general circulation. These factors stimulate the synthesis and release of corticotropin (ACTH) into the general circulation. ACTH in turn stimulates the synthesis and release of adrenal steroids, principally cortisol. The synthesis and release of adrenal steroids may also be mediated centrally by adrenal innervation.[355,356]

Hypothalamus: CRH and AVP

Two hypothalamic peptides—CRH and AVP—are the principal but not the sole regulators of ACTH synthesis and release. CRH is a 41-amino acid peptide synthesized primarily by the paraventricular nucleus.[367] Neuronal bodies in the paraventricular nucleus also produce AVP [also known as antidiuretic hormone (ADH)], which is also produced in the supraoptic nucleus.[368,369] Both CRH and AVP are proteolytically cleaved from larger precursors. Prepro-CRH contains no other peptides with a known function. The precursor to AVP, however, also gives rise to neurophysin II, the AVP-binding protein. The gene encoding AVP/neurophysin II is structurally very similar to the gene for oxytocin; these two evolutionarily duplicated genes lie in a tandemly duplicated tail-to-tail arrangement on chromosome 20 (for a review, see Ref. 370). Both CRH and AVP travel through neurons to the median eminence,[369] which releases them into the pituitary portal circulation, which in turn carries them to the anterior pituitary in high concentrations. These peptides normally occur at undetectably low concentrations in the general venous circulation, except during pregnancy.[371] CRH and AVP stimulate the synthesis and release of ACTH by different mechanisms. CRH acts, at least in part, by interacting with receptors linked to the protein kinase A pathway, stimulating the production of intracellular cyclic AMP.[372] AVP appears to act through other messengers, principally calcium ion.[372] When administered together, CRH and AVP act additively or synergistically, as would be predicted from their independent mechanisms of action,[373–375] and also induce hyperplasia of the ACTH-producing corticotropes.[376]

CRH and its receptor are found throughout the body, notably in the brain and gastrointestinal tract.[377,378] In the brain, CRH is an excitatory neurotransmitter that may be epileptogenic[379]; it stimulates sympathetic outflow and may modulate blood pressure.[368,380] Thus, CRH appears to be involved in responses to stress; concentrations of CRH in the cerebrospinal fluid (CSF) are increased during depression.[381]

CRH is probably the most important physiologic stimulator of ACTH. CRH is pharmacologically more potent than AVP in vivo and in vitro,[375,382] even though maximally effective doses of AVP can release an equivalent amount of ACTH.[374,375] Antibodies to CRH decrease ACTH release in rats in response to ether, stress, formalin, CRH, or AVP.[375,383–387] The release of CRH can be increased by AVP[388] and decreased by CRH[384] in short feedback loops.[389]

Pituitary release of ACTH is not totally dependent on CRH. Antibodies to CRH or CRH receptor antagonists block the rise in ACTH only in response to various stimuli; they mildly block basal ACTH release.[356,390] Similarly, AVP can act alone or act synergistically with CRH. Other factors also appear to be important. Oxytocin, which is structurally related to AVP, does not stimulate or inhibit the release of human ACTH, although it does this in some animals.[391] Both α- and β-adrenergic stimuli, inflammatory cytokines, angiotensin II, opioid peptides, and somatostatin may be involved in the regulation of ACTH synthesis and release; however, their importance remains to be established.[392]

Pituitary: POMC and ACTH

ACTH is made primarily in the anterior pituitary, although it is also synthesized in the brain, placenta, and testes. These extrapituitary sources make negligible (if any) contributions to circulating concentrations of immunoreactive ACTH, although huge amounts of "ectopic" ACTH can be produced by some malignancies. This ectopic ACTH derives from pro-opiomelanocortin (POMC) and is identical to pituitary ACTH.[393]

ACTH is a 39-amino acid peptide proteolytically cleaved from a larger 241-amino acid precursor geneally termed POMC.

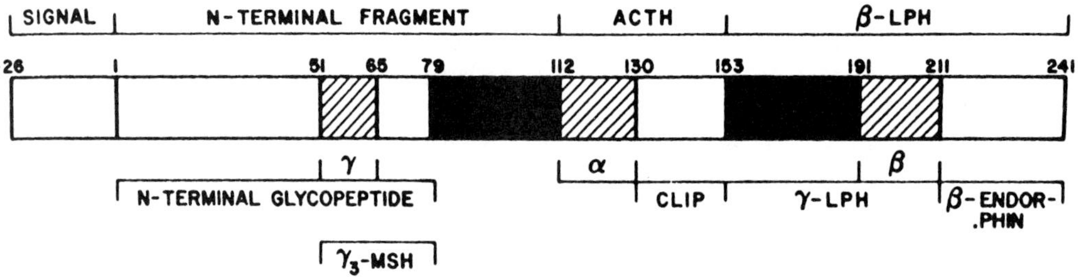

FIGURE 11-13. Structure of human prepro-opiomelanocortin. The numbers refer to amino acid positions, with 1 assigned to the first amino acid of POMC after the 26-amino acid signal peptide. The α-, β- and γ-MSH regions, which characterize the three "constant" regions, are indicated by diagonal lines; the "variable" regions are solid. The amino acid numbers shown refer to the N-terminal amino acid of each cleavage site; because these amino acids are removed, the numbers do not correspond exactly with the amino acid numbers of the peptides as usèd in the text. (*From Miller et al.*[395])

POMC is an unusual polyhormonal precursor that is differentially cleaved in various tissues into several hormonally active peptides (Fig. 11-13).[394,395] ACTH consists of amino acids 112 through 150 of POMC. The N-terminal glycopeptide can stimulate steroidogenesis and may function as an adrenal-specific mitogen.[396] POMC 112-126 and POMC 191-207 constitute α- and β-MSH, respectively; POMC 210-241 is β-endorphin, and corticotropin-like intermediate peptide (CLIP) is POMC 129-150. The earlier proposal that all or part of the POMC 79-109 region may function as an adrenal androgen stimulating hormone has been rejected convincingly.[361–363] ACTH can stimulate lipolysis in fat cells,[397] an action that may be related to the historical but technically inaccurate naming of the carboxy-terminal POMC peptides POMC 153-241 and POMC 153-191 as β- and γ-LPH (lipotrophic hormone), respectively.

Both ACTH and MSH appear to have neurotransmitter functions. They affect learning and behavior in rats and influence opioid action (see Chap. 7). The melanocyte-stimulating properties of α-, β-, and γ-MSH appear to derive from their activities within ACTH, γ-LPH, and the N-terminal glycopeptide, respectively, because free MSH peptides have not been found in human circulation with the exception of the pregnant state.[398] Most MSH activity appears to come from the α-MSH region of ACTH, as α-MSH (in ACTH) is four times more potent than β-MSH (in LPH) and because ACTH and LPH are present in approximately equimolar concentrations. CLIP can stimulate pancreatic exocrine function,[399] and α-MSH may play a minor natriuretic role.[400] Several physiologic roles have been established for αMSH in the regulation of body temperature and appetite. ACTH can be modified further by phosphorylation and, in rats, by glycosylation, but glycosylation of human ACTH is negligible.[393,401]

Only the amino-terminal half of the ACTH molecule is needed for biological activity, and the first 24 amino acids are identical among all mammals studied to date (Fig. 11-14). ACTH 1-24, 1-23, and 1-20 are all equipotent on a molar basis compared to ACTH 1-39, but the circulating half-life and duration of adrenal stimulation decrease as the molecule is shortened. As a result, synthetic ACTH 1-24 is widely used in diagnostic tests of adrenal function.

ACTH circulates unbound to other proteins and is quickly cleared from the circulation, with a half-life of about 10 min.[402] Biological activity disappears from the circulation even more rapidly than does immunoassayable activity, suggesting that the biologically most important regions, the 10 amino-terminal amino acids, are attacked early, leaving immunoactive but biologically inert peptides. ACTH is catabolized in many tissues, principally the liver and kidneys, and is not excreted in the urine in significant amounts.[402]

Actions of ACTH

ACTH stimulates the synthesis and release of steroids by interacting with cell-surface ACTH receptors that stimulate the production of intracellular cAMP. This increased cAMP in turn mediates both acute and chronic effects on steroidogenesis.

Acute Actions

ACTH acutely increases cortisol synthesis and release within 2 to 3 min, principally by stimulating the activity of cholesterol esterase and inhibiting cholesterol ester synthetase.[364,403] ACTH stimulates StAR to facilitate the transport of cholesterol across the mitochondrial membranes (see steroid hormone biosynthesis, earlier), the binding of cholesterol to P450scc, and the release of newly synthesized pregnenolone from mitochondria. Although the concentration of cortisol and other steroids is 100 to 1,000 times higher in the adrenal than in the circulation, this constitutes a nearly insignificant reservoir,[404] and the release of preformed steroids is relatively unimportant. The presense of high intraadrenal steroid concentrations suggests an active mechanism to regulate release, but little is known about this subject. ACTH also facilitates the release of adrenal androgens and mineralocorticoids as well as stimulating the release of various steroidal intermediates. By contrast, when ACTH concentrations fall, steroidogenesis decreases rapidly.

Receptors

ACTH receptors are found on the surface of adrenal cortical cells, where they bind ACTH with a K_d (equilibrium dissociation constant) of about 10^{-9} *M*.[405,406] ACTH receptors belong to the seven-transmembrane domain G protein-coupled receptor superfamily and form a family with the other melanocortin receptors.[407] The ACTH receptor gene resides on chromosome 18.[408–410] The ACTH receptor, also known as the melanocortin 2 receptor (MC2-R) is one of a family of five related receptors that bind various peptides derived from pro-opiomelanocortin.[409] The α-MSH

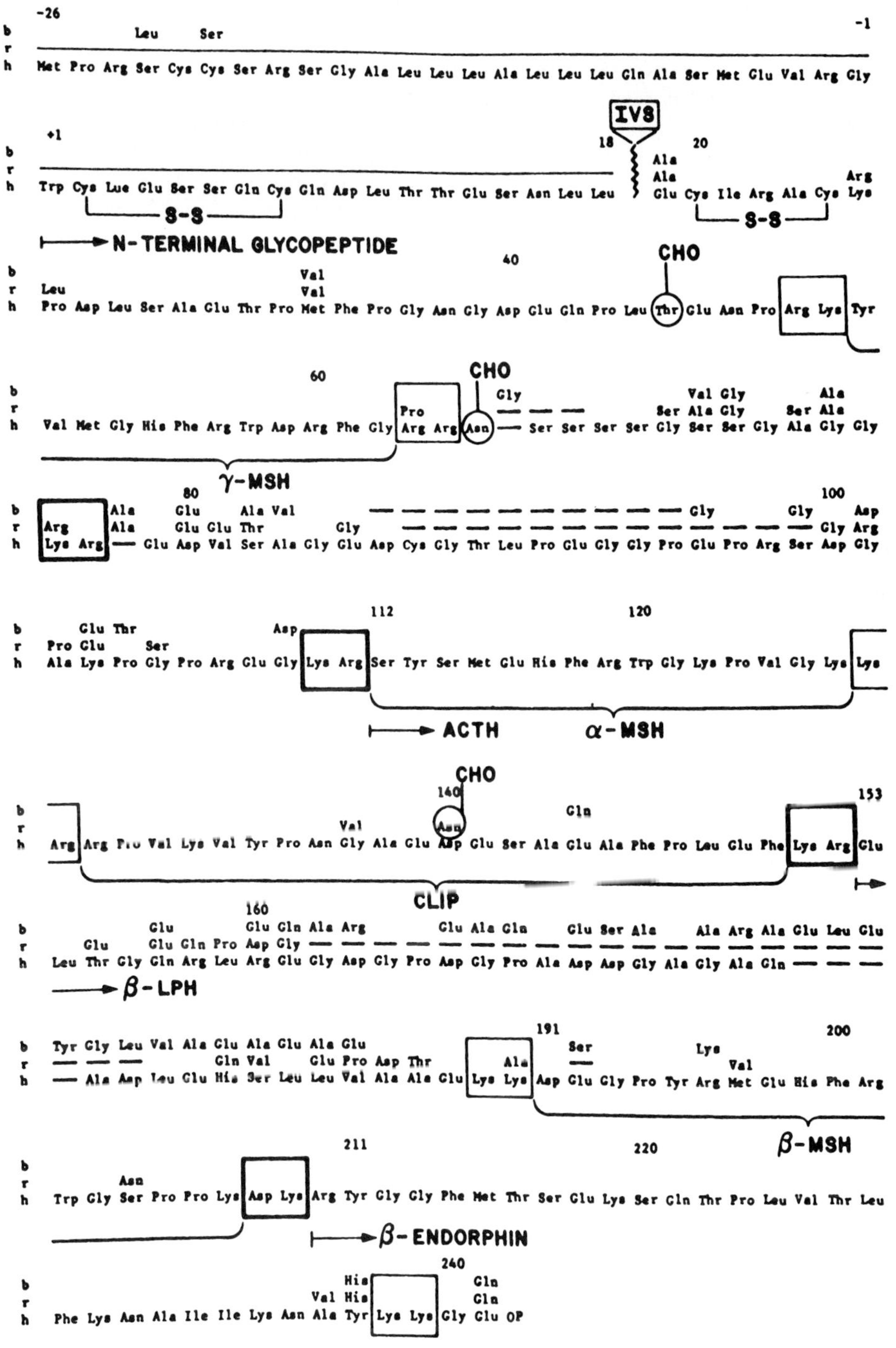

FIGURE 11-14. Bovine, rat, and human POMC. Amino acid sequences were taken from the established gene sequences. Only the complete sequence of human pre-POMC is shown. For the bovine and rat sequences, the amino acids that differ from the human sequence are shown; those which are the same are represented as blanks. Where a sequence lacks a corresponding amino acid, the gap is indicated as a dash. The amino acid numbers correspond only to the human sequence. The various known glycosylation sites are encircled and indicated by "CHO." The pairs of basic amino acids that represent major cleavage sites are enclosed in heavy boxes; other possible cleavage sites are enclosed in light boxes. (*From Miller et al.*[395])

moiety of POMC binds to MC1-R on melanocytes, where it stimulates pigmentation, to MC4-R in the brain, where it participates in appetite regulation, and to MC5-R in numerous tissues, where it influences exorcrine gland function. The MC3 receptor in the brain, placenta, and macrophages binds γ-MSH preferentially to α-MSH, and may play a role in appetite and sex drive. The abundance of ACTH receptors can be suppressed by ACTH.[405,406] Binding of ACTH to its receptor activates adenylate cyclase.[364,402,408] This increases intracellular concentrations of cAMP, which in turn activates a number of protein kinases, but it is not known which specific proteins are phosphorylated in response to ACTH or precisely how they promote steroidogenesis. However, accumulation of cAMP does precede steroidogenesis, and binding of cAMP to the regulatory subunit of protein kinase A correlates well with stimulation of steroidogenesis.[411]

Chronic Actions

ACTH exerts chronic actions on both adrenal architecture and steroidogenesis. Prolonged stimulation with ACTH increases adrenal protein and DNA synthesis and net growth.[30] There is both cellular hypertrophy (increased cell size) and hyperplasia (increased cell number). It has been claimed that adrenal cellular hypertrophy and hyperplasia are promoted by distinct regions of the N-terminal glycopeptide of POMC,[396] but synthetic ACTH 1-24 is sufficient by itself to increase the adrenal mass severalfold.[30] The mechanisms by which ACTH promotes adrenal growth are not clear. Antibodies to ACTH inhibit steroidogenesis but do not inhibit adrenal growth in animals,[412] and in primary cultures of animal or human fetal adrenal cells, ACTH inhibits rather than promotes growth. ACTH chronically increases steroidogenesis by promoting the transcription of genes for StAR and steroidogenic enzymes (see later discussion), an action apparently not linked to adrenal growth. Physiologic concentrations of ACTH also directly stimulate the synthesis and accumulation of insulin-like growth factor-II (IGF-II) mRNA[33,35,37] and consequently IGF-II peptide.[413] ACTH also promotes the synthesis of basic fibroblast growth factor and epidermal growth factor, which may act with IGF-II to stimulate adrenal growth.[36,37] However, IGF-II mRNA is unchanged in rat adrenals induced to grow by unilateral adrenalectomy and decreases in rat adrenals induced to grow by ACTH.[34]

Conversely, when ACTH concentrations are chronically low, as in hypopituitarism or when suppressed by glucocorticoid therapy, adrenal protein content, steroidogenic activity, and mass decrease substantially. After such long-term privation of ACTH and adrenal atrophy, the adrenal will recover when treated with ACTH. However, stimulation of steroidogenesis may take 24 h, full activity may take 3 days, and recovery of the ability to mount a stress-induced hypercortisolemic response may take weeks to months.

Chronic actions of ACTH on steroidogenesis occur principally by promoting the transcription of the genes that encode steroidogenic enzymes and other factors. Although most experiments in vitro and in cell culture systems show transcriptional responses to ACTH and cAMP within 1 or 2 h, the net effects on steroidogenic capacity are longer. Thus, one can conceptualize the acute action of ACTH as turning on the existing steroidogenic machinery to maximum capacity, while the chronic action increases that capacity by producing more steroidogenic machinery. ACTH increases the transcription of the genes for StAR, P450scc, P450c17, P450c21, P450c11, adrenodoxin reductase, and adrenodoxin[130–135,152,205,248] (see steroid hormone biosynthesis). Because P450scc is the rate-limiting step in steroidogenesis, much attention has been focused on it. ACTH in the adrenal and gonadotropins in the gonads stimulate the accumulation of human P450scc mRNA and human P450scc activity[123,124] (for a review, see Ref. 414), yet ACTH and cAMP increase the transcription of both the P450scc and P450c17 genes about equally.[132,205] Some but not most of the actions of ACTH (or other tropic peptides) in stimulating steroidogenesis may be blocked by the inhibition of protein synthesis.[125,126,131,138,360] It appears likely that the effects of inhibiting protein synthesis occur largely by inhibiting the synthesis of various factors involved in the transport of cholesterol to the P450scc enzyme rather than by affecting factors that regulate the transcription of the genes that encode the steroidogenic enzymes. Calcium is also important for ACTH- or cAMP-induced steroidogenesis, as it can be blocked by inhibitors of calmodulin,[92] yet calcium ionophores suppress P450scc mRNA accumulation and transcription of the P450scc gene.[132]

ACTH also chronically stimulates LDL uptake and metabolism and the synthesis and accumulation of LDL receptor and HMGCoA reductase and their mRNAs. Furthermore, ACTH also stimulates cholesterol esterase,[52,357] SCP-2,[415] endozepine,[358] and StAR so that it has general tropic effects on all known early steps in steroidogenesis (see steroid hormone biosynthesis).

A role for newly synthesized phospholipids in mediating the chronic actions of ACTH has been proposed. The reported actions can be mimicked by cAMP, require calcium, and are blocked by inhibitors of protein synthesis.[403,408,416,417] The mechanism of action of such phospholipids is unknown but may be related to promoting the flux of free cholesterol across the mitochondrial membranes to P450scc.[89,364,403,416]

Although chronic treatment with glucocorticoids clearly suppresses the hypothalamic-pituitary axis, thus suppressing the adrenal indirectly through ACTH privation, a direct action of glucocorticoids on the adrenal cortex has also been proposed. Glucocorticoids can inhibit steroidogenesis in primary cultures of human adrenal cells in vitro,[418] and a direct action of suppressing the transcription of the human P450c17 gene has been suggested.[205] However, such direct feedback probably plays a minor role in human physiology, as the hypercortisolism found in syndromes of ACTH excess does not effectively reduce steroidogenesis, and the administration of dexamethasone does not inhibit ACTH-induced cortisol secretion.[419]

Direct Patterns of ACTH and Cortisol Synthesis and Release

Plasma concentrations of ACTH and cortisol tend to be high in the morning and low in the evening. Peak ACTH levels are usually seen at 6–7:30 A.M., and peak cortisol levels follow at about 8 A.M. Both ACTH and cortisol are released episodically in pulses every 20 to 30 min throughout the day, but the amplitude of these pulses are much greater in the morning.[384,420–427] Each pulse of cortisol release is characterized by a very rapid rise in circulating cortisol concentration, followed by a slower, generally smooth decline. Large pulses of cortisol release may occur when basal cortisol concentrations are either high or low, resulting in very widely and rapidly fluctuating serum cortisol concentrations. During periods of minimal secretion, especially in the late evening, cortisol can decrease to levels that are unmeasurable in most assays. Large pulses of cortisol release occur more frequently in the early morning hours, leading to the characteristic diurnal rhythm of cortisol secretion. The basis of this diurnal rhythm is complex and poorly understood. At least four factors appear to be involved in the rhythm of ACTH and cortisol: (1) intrinsic rhythmicity of the synthesis and secretion of CRH and AVP by the hypothalamus, (2) feeding cycles, (3) light/dark and activity/rest cycles, and (4) rhythmicity in the adrenal, possibly mediated by adrenal innervation.

Rhythmicity of Hypothalamic CRH

Both static measures of CRH and AVP content and dynamic measures of CRH and AVP synthesis show a diurnal rhythm that appears to be inherent in the hypothalamic cell bodies. The diurnal pattern of hypothalamic CRH and AVP content persists in hypophysectomized animals that are deprived of ACTH and glucocorticoid feedback.[421] Furthermore, this diurnal pattern is maintained in humans even when CRH is infused continuously, revealing the pulsatile and diurnal pattern of AVP secretion by parvicellular neurons of the paraventricular nucleus of the hypothalamus.[384,426,427] Thus hypothalamic rhythmicity appears to be neuronal or intrinsic but not hormonal.

Feeding Cycles

Although diurnal rhythms are generally associated with light/dark cycles, increasing evidence points to a major role for feeding schedules in the diurnal patterns of ACTH and cortisol. Concentrations of cortisol are highest before breakfast, and additional peaks appear to be coincident with lunch and to a lesser extent supper,[422,423] although there is great individual variability in these patterns (Fig. 11-15). In rats, the feeding schedule appears to be more important than light/dark cycles in determining the diurnal rhythm of glucocorticoid release.[424,428] However, if rats are fed only during hours of light, the circadian pattern slowly changes so that after about 10 days maximal glucocorticoid concentrations coincide with the start of feeding.

Less is known about the effect of eating patterns on human patterns of ACTH and cortisol release. Although preprandial peaks of cortisol are common,[422,423] they are quite variable and do not occur in subjects whose normal patterns of activity do not include these meals.[423]

Light/Dark Cycles

The simplest correlation with the circadian rhythms of ACTH and cortisol is light/dark cycles. Nocturnal secretory episodes increase between the third and fifth hours of sleep, followed by the main secretory bursts in the sixth to eighth hours of sleep and the first several hours of wakefulness. Infants do not have entrained diurnal rhythms of sleep or feeding, a behavioral phenomenon that is well known to all parents. However, infants acquire their behavioral rhythms and learn to sleep through the night, presumably in response to their environment. The diurnal rhythm of ACTH and cortisol does not appear fully established until after the first year of life.[421] However, once it is established, this rhythm is not changed easily and persists after prolonged bed rest, continuous feeding, and 2- to 3-day periods of sleep deprivation.[421] It remains unchanged in people who work night shifts but maintain conventional hours on weekends. When individuals shift sleep/waking, light/dark, and feeding schedules congruently, such as by moving to a distant time zone, the circadian rhythm of ACTH and cortisol changes over the course of 3 to 5 days.[421]

Adrenal Rhythmicity and Other Factors

Adrenal activity appears to exhibit some diurnal rhythmicity that is independent of CRH, AVP, and ACTH; this may reflect inherent rhythmicity or may be regulated via adrenal innervation. Glucocorticoid rhythms are seen in hypophysectomized animals that are given continuous nondiurnal infusions of ACTH.[30]

FIGURE 11-15. Plasma cortisol values of normal subjects for 24-h periods of study. Samples were obtained every 20 min. "Lights out" indicates the period available for sleep. LC1 and LC2 refer to studies done on the same subject in two different 24-h periods. (*From Weitzman et al.*[420])

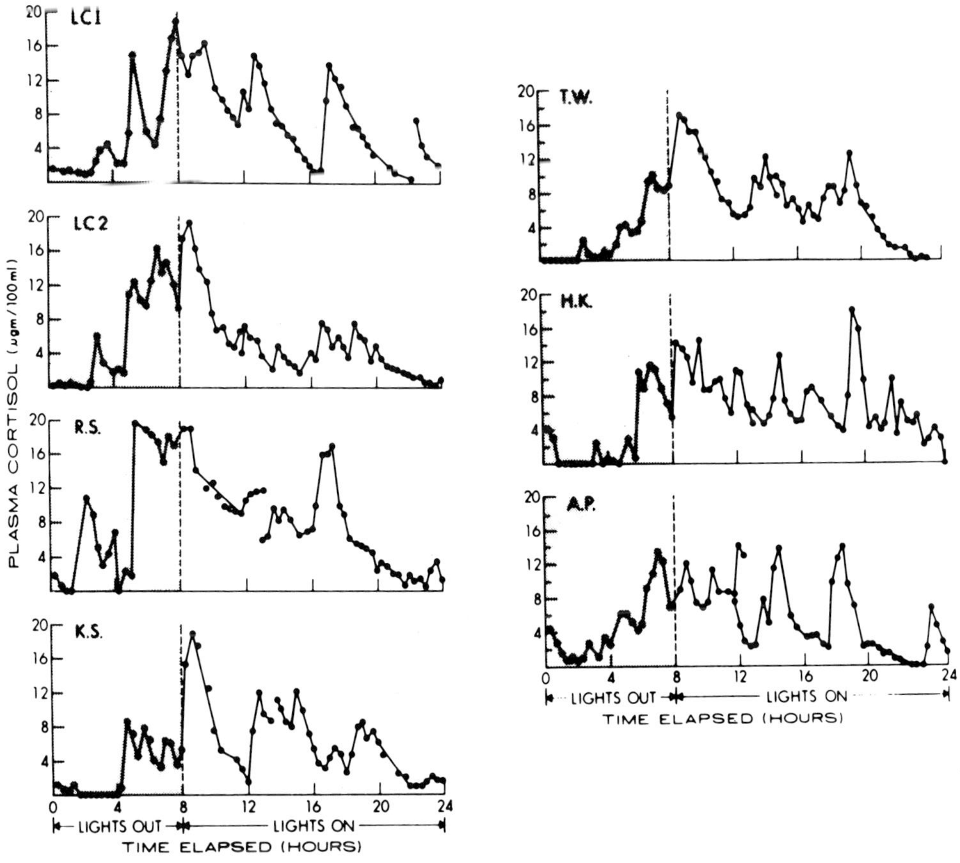

Furthermore, spinal transsection above the level of adrenal innervation or autotransplantation of adrenals freed of neural input abolish the rhythm.[30] These experiments suggest a direct effect of adrenal innervation on adrenal steroidogenesis or sensitivity to ACTH. A role for factors other than ACTH is indicated by the occasional dissociation between peaks of ACTH and cortisol[421,425] and by the frequent lack of proportionality between the magnitudes of ACTH peaks and cortisol peaks.[425,429]

Changes in the Diurnal Rhythm of Cortisol

A wide variety of physical and psychological factors can alter the complex control of the diurnal variation of ACTH and cortisol secretion. These factors appear to be mediated largely by the central nervous system (CNS).[392] Age does not appear to alter integrated 24-h adrenal function, but maximal and minimal concentrations of cortisol occur somewhat earlier in the day in aged subjects.[430] Seemingly mild fear or psychological stress, such as anticipation of venipuncture,[431] or more severe stress, such as preparation for cardiac surgery,[432] can increase the secretion of cortisol, as can anticipation of athletic competition or university examinations.[426,433]

Major physical stresses such as severe trauma, major surgery, severe illness, hypoglycemia, fever, burns, exposure to cold, irradiation, hypotension, dehydration, smoking tobacco, and moderate to intensive exercise can increase the secretion of ACTH and cortisol.[426,433,434] The response to surgery is illustrated in Fig. 11-16; such stress can increase cortisol production up to sixfold,[435] and the need for administration of increased doses of glucocorticoids to addisonian patients undergoing surgery is well known. However, minor illnesses such as upper respiratory infections and minor surgery[435,436] have little influence on cortisol secretion.

Chronic illnesses also alter the diurnal rhythm of ACTH and cortisol.[437] Congestive heart failure and primary liver disease alter cortisol disposal, and hypothalamic and limbic system disorders directly affect central control.[438] Patients with major depression have increased basal cortisol, and urinary steroid excretion as a result of a blunting of the diurnal rhythm of ACTH and cortisol similar to that seen in Cushing's disease.[439] CRH concentrations are increased in the CSF of depressed patients,[381] and the hypothalamic-pituitary-adrenal axis of such patients is less sensitive to suppression by exogenously administered glucocorticoids. Spinal fluid CRH and circulating cortisol are increased and diurnal variation and sensitivity to dexamethasone are decreased in anorexia nervosa.[440] However, many common drugs, including atropine, phenobarbital, reserpine, chlordiazepoxide, meprobamate, chlorpromazine, and phenytoin, have no detectable affect on the circadian rhythm of cortisol secretion,[421] although cyproheptadine, a serotonin antagonist, can inhibit rises in ACTH and cortisol induced by hypoglycemia or metyrapone.[441,442]

Glucocorticoid Feedback on ACTH Release

The hypothalamic-pituitary-adrenal axis is a classic example of an endocrine feedback system. ACTH increases the production of cortisol, and cortisol in turn decreases the production of both CRH/AVP and ACTH.[434,437,439–444] Disruption of this homeostatic system by adrenal insufficiency can raise concentrations of ACTH 10 to 20 times above normal, yet these profoundly elevated concentrations of ACTH can be suppressed by replacement with physiologic doses of glucocorticoids. Similarly, plasma concentrations of ACTH and ACTH responses to CRH and stress are suppressed by high concentrations of glucocorticoids.

Glucocorticoid feedback on ACTH has been described as consisting of fast, intermediate, and slow components,[443] but as in most physiologic systems, there is a continuum of responses. When patients with Addison's disease are given intravenous cortisol, the concentration of circulating ACTH decreases within 15 min and is substantially suppressed to about 10 percent of the initial value by 90 to 120 min (Fig. 11-17). This initial fast feedback blunts the ACTH response to some stimuli, such as histamine, but not the response to strong stimuli such as endotoxin and major surgery. This initial fast phase of glucocorticoid feedback appears to be exerted more at the level of hypothalamic CRH release than at the level of the pituitary, although both appear to be involved.[445,446] Both fast feedback and intermediate feedback appear to be mediated by inhibition of the release of existing CRH and ACTH rather than by inhibition of their synthesis. Fast feedback and intermediate feedback are distinguished in animals by the effects of certain agents in overcoming glucorticoid suppression[443]

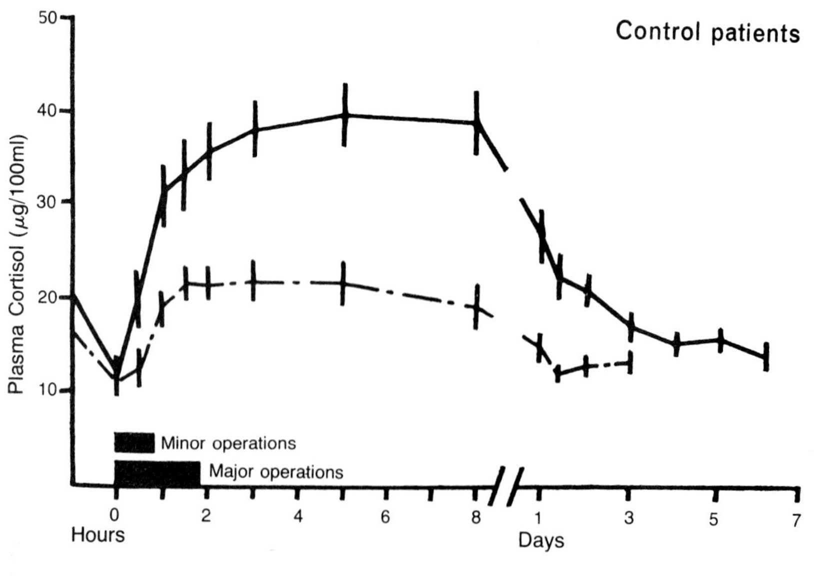

FIGURE 11-16. Plasma cortisol responds to major surgery (continuous line) and minor surgery (broken line) in normal subjects. Mean values and standard errors are shown for 20 patients in each case. (*From Plumpton et al.*[435])

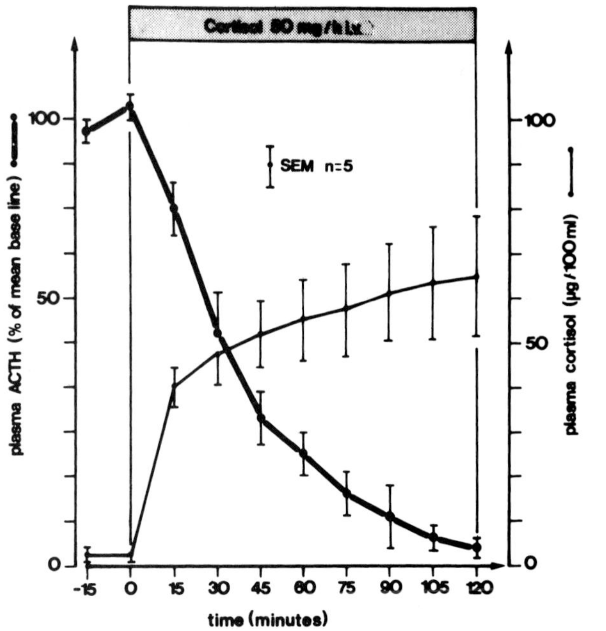

FIGURE 11-17. Time course of ACTH concentrations in response to cortisol constantly infused at 50 mg/h in patients with Addison's disease. ACTH values are given as a percentage of the individual mean starting levels. The difference between ACTH values at 15 min and the starting value was significant ($p < 0.025$). (*From Fehm et al.*[445])

and possibly by a requirement for protein synthesis to maintain intermediate feedback. Increased concentrations of glucocorticoids accelerate the progression from fast to slow feedback. Slow feedback is characterized by decreased or absent synthesis of ACTH, complete suppression of POMC gene transcription, and unresponsiveness to the administration of CRH. Glucocorticoids decrease the hypothalamic content of CRH[447] and AVP[368] and also decrease CRH and AVP mRNA content.[448,449] With increasing dose and duration of glucocorticoid exposure (such as in long-term Cushing's disease and long-term pharmacologic glucocorticoid therapy), the pituitary becomes completely unresponsive even to extreme stimuli.[436,437,443] When glucocorticoid concentrations return to normal, the recovery of the hypothalamic-pituitary axis may be slow and, depending on the dose and duration of glucocorticoid exposure, recovery of fully normal function may take months (see Chap. 15).

Regulation of Mineralocorticoids

Secretion of aldosterone from the zona glomerulosa accounts for more than half of mineralocorticoid activity in human plasma. Cortisol and several glomerulosa steroids secreted in small quantities, such as DOC, 18-OH DOC, 18-OH-corticosterone, 18-OH-cortisol, and 19-oxo-cortisol, also have mineralocorticoid activity. The secretion of the glomerulosa steroids is regulated primarily by the renin-angiotensin system and by potassium ion and, to a lesser degree, by ACTH, sodium ion, and other factors. The zona fasciculata, under the control of ACTH, secretes appreciable quantities of DOC.[449] Extraadrenal production of DOC can also contribute appreciable mineralocorticoid activity, especially in the fetus and during pregnancy.[228–230]

The Renin-Angiotensin System

Renin

Renin is a serine protease enzyme synthesized largely by the juxtaglomerular cells of the kidney; this accounts for virtually all circulating renin activity. Renin is also produced in a variety of other tissues, including the glomerulosa cells of the adrenal cortex,[450] and adrenal renin appears to act as a paracrine factor regulating expression of the gene that encodes P450c11AS but not P450c11β.[450,451] Renin is initially synthesized as a preproprotein of 406 amino acids[452] that is cleaved to 386-amino acid prorenin and then to the mature 340-amino acid form of renin. Both prorenin and renin can be found in the circulation. Hypotension, upright posture, sodium depletion, vasodilatory drugs, kallikrein, opiates, and β-adrenergic stimulation all promote the release of renin from the renal juxtaglomerular cells. Of these, serum sodium concentration is most important (Fig. 11-18). Renin enzymatically attacks angiotensinogen, the renin substrate, in the circulation. Angiotensinogen is a highly glycosolated protein and therefore has a highly variable molecular mass, ranging from 50,000 to 100,000 daltons. This renin substrate is regulated in part by estrogens and hence is elevated in pregnancy and in women taking oral contraceptives. Renin proteolytically releases the amino-terminal 10 amino acids of angiotensinogen, referred to as angiotensin I. This decapeptide is biologically inactive until its two carboxy-terminal amino acids are cleaved by the action of converting enzyme to become the octapeptide, angiotensin II. Converting enzyme is found principally in the lungs and blood vessels. Because converting enzyme is a metalloenzyme containing zinc, it can be inhibited by chelating agents and certain metals. However, the only therapeutically useful inhibitors of converting enzyme are analogs of its substrate, angiotensin I, such as captopril. Such agents are useful in the diagnosis and treatment of hyperreninemic hypertension. For a detailed discussion of the renin-angiotensin system, see Chap. 13.

Angiotensin II

The octapeptide angiotensin II (and in some species its amino-terminally cleaved heptapeptide derivative, angiotensin III) has two principal actions, both of which increase blood pressure. It directly stimulates arteriolar vasoconstriction within a few seconds and stimulates the synthesis and secretion of aldosterone within minutes.[136,453] Angiotensin II binds to receptors on the surface of glomerulosa cells with an affinity of about 0.5 n*M*.[454] The number of these receptors increases in response to angiotensin II and potassium ion and decreases in hypokalemia. Angiotensin does not work through cAMP and the protein kinase A pathway[455] but acutely stimulates mineralocorticoid production by hydrolysis of phosphatidyl inositol, mobilization of intracellular Ca^{2+}, influx of extracellular Ca^{2+}, and activation of protein kinase C.[136] Short-term stimulation of adrenal cells with angiotensin II or other activators of protein kinase C will stimulate the production of aldosterone and the enzymes needed for its synthesis. However, prolonged stimulation will repress the production of those enzymes and aldosterone.[139–141,456] It appears that much, if not all, of this biphasic response to angiotensin II is mediated directly at the level of transcription of the genes for the steroidogenic enzymes, especially of the gene for P450scc.[132,457] When the promoter of the human P450scc gene is transfected into mouse adrenal Y-1 cells, both the transfected human promoter and the endogenous mouse P450scc promoter can be stimulated acutely by calcium ionophore and phorbol ester, which are agonists of the protein kinase C

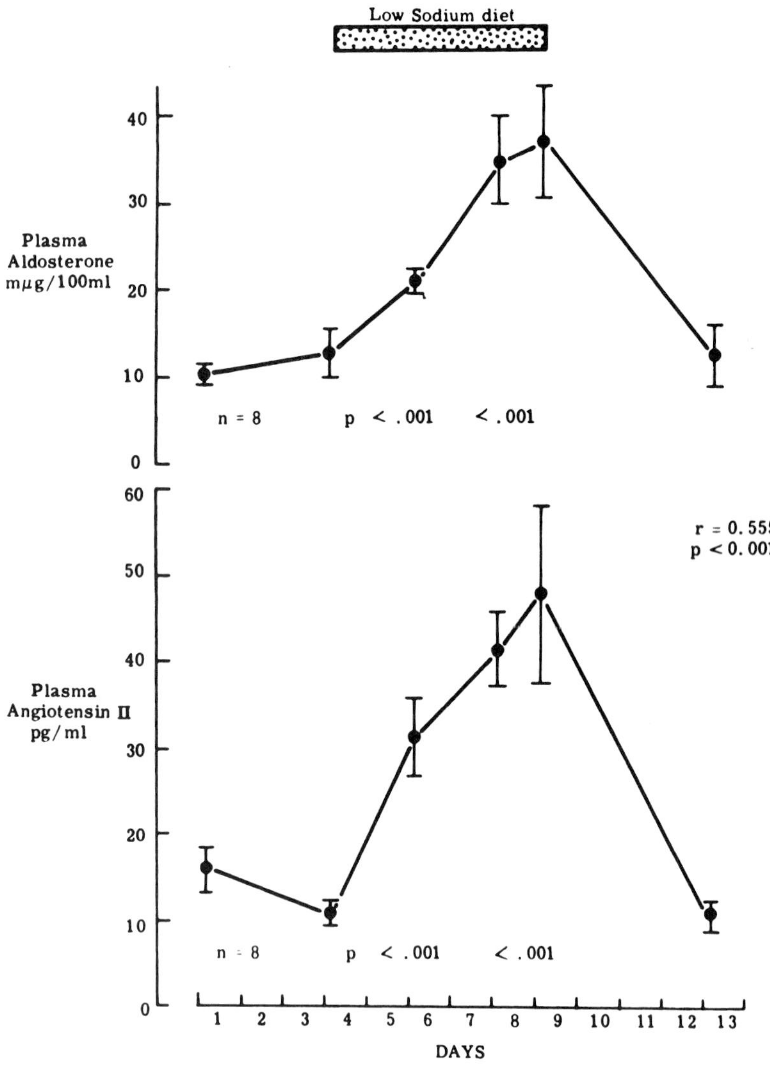

FIGURE 11-18. Effect of a low-sodium diet on plasma angiotensin II and aldosterone concentrations in normal subjects. (*From Brown et al.*[474])

pathway. The action of these two agents on P450scc gene transcription is synergistic, rapid, and biphasic, so that prolonged exposure represses transcription of the P450scc gene to levels substantially below baseline.[132] These actions appear to be mediated by several regions of the P450scc gene promoter, but these are clearly different from those that mediate induction by cAMP (stimulated by ACTH).[132] Thus, the hormonal regulation of glucocorticoids (cortisol) and mineralocorticoids (aldosterone) is clearly distinct at all levels: the circulating hormonal stimuli, the intracellular second messengers, and the DNA sequences conferring the regulation to the gene for P450scc.

The potential role of angiotensin II in stimulating the late steps in the synthesis of aldosterone is not clear. Because 18-hydroxylase and 18-methyl oxidase activities are specifically associated with mineralocorticoid production, the potential role of angiotensin II in regulating these activities has been of interest. As was discussed in steroid hormone biosynthesis, earlier, these activities are mediated by P450c11AS, a glomerulosa-specific enzyme encoded by one of the two duplicated genes for P450c11. The transcriptional regulation of the gene encoding P450c11β has been studied in the mouse,[458–461] showing inducibility by cAMP and both P450c11β and P450c11AS can be induced by cAMP in human adrenal NCI-H295 cells,[457] but the transcriptional regulation of the human gene for P450c11AS has not been studied in detail. Similarly, the potential actions of angiotensin II on the earliest steps of steroidogenesis (production of cholesterol and its flux to the mitochondria) have not been studied in detail.

Potassium Ion

Increases in plasma K^+ stimulate aldosterone production, and decreased plasma K^+ decreases aldosterone production and blunts its response to hyponatremia.[462–465] The zona glomerulosa is sensitive to very small changes in K^+, independent of the concentrations of Na^+ and angiotensin II. Prolonged hyperkalemia, prolonged exposure to angiotensin II, and chronic hyponatremia will cause hypertrophy of the adrenal zona glomerulosa and increase its sensitivity to hormonal induction. Although hyperkalemia decreases renin release, its action to stimulate aldosterone secretion predominates.[465] These divergent actions correspond to the different intracellular actions of potassium and angiotensin II on steroidogenesis. Potassium ion probably acts by depolarizing the glomerulosa cell membrane, facilitating increased uptake of extracellular calcium ion. As in the actions of angiotensin II, increased intracellular calcium increases hydrolysis of phosphoinositides. Thus, the similar actions of K^+ and angiotensin II differ in that K^+ primarily stimulates the uptake of calcium ion with secondary effects of decreasing the formation of phosphatidic acid and phosphoinositides, while angiotensin II initially affects the hydrolysis of phosphatidyl inositol. Thus, angiotensin II and potassium work at different levels of the same intracellular second messenger pathway, but they differ fundamentally from the action of ACTH. As with angiotensin II, however, the potential action of potassium on the late steps in aldosterone synthesis has not been studied in depth.

ACTH and Other Factors

POMC Peptides

ACTH and other peptides derived from POMC can influence aldosterone production, although to a much lesser degree than can angiotensin II and potassium ion. Neither acute hypophysectomy nor long-term administration of dexamethasone will lower basal aldosterone secretion or its responsiveness to sodium depletion. However, some patients with long-term hypopituitarism have blunted aldosterone responses, and decreased aldosterone production has been described in isolated ACTH deficiency.[465,466] The effects of ACTH on aldosterone are variable in different species, with relatively lesser effects in human beings, and may be permissive. Alternatively, they may reflect less than complete functional distinction between the zona glomerulosa and the zona fasciculata. Other POMC peptides, such as β-endorphin,[467] β-MSH,[468] and portions of the N-terminal glycopeptide such as γ3-MSH,[469] have all been reported to stimulate mineralocorticoid synthesis. Although there is no definitive evidence that POMC peptides regulate aldosterone production, it appears that cAMP, the second messenger of ACTH action, stimulates the production of the P450c11AS enzyme required for the late steps in aldosterone synthesis.[457]

Sodium Ion, ANP, and Other Factors

Hyponatremia increases and hypernatremia decreases aldosterone secretion, principally by the effects of intravascular volume and sodium ion on the renin-angiotensin system (Fig. 11-16). Small changes in sodium concentration can also have a substantial effect on the angiotensin-induced or potassium-induced secretion of aldosterone. These actions appear to be independent of the osmotic effects of sodium, possibly accounting for blunted aldosterone responses during water deprivation.[470]

Other factors can also influence aldosterone secretion. Ammonium ion can stimulate plasma aldosterone,[471] but it is not clear if this effect is direct or secondary to the effects of acidosis on renin and potassium. Dopamine appears to inhibit the stimulation of aldosterone secretion by other factors,[467,472] possibly by affecting late steps in the mineralocorticoid pathway, but the physiologic relevance of this is unclear, as dopamine infusion does not diminish circulating concentrations of aldosterone or their response to angiotensin II.

Atrial natriuretic peptide (ANP) appears to be a potent inhibitor of aldosterone synthesis but has no detectable effect on cortisol synthesis.[473] ANP is synthesized and possibly secreted by a wide variety of tissues in addition to cardiocytes, including the adrenal medulla, but is not produced by the adrenal cortex.[474] The biologically active 28-amino acid peptide increases with increased intravascular volume and serum sodium[475] and inhibits aldosterone secretion. However, although glucocorticoids regulate ANP secretion,[476,477] no role has been established for mineralocorticoids in ANP regulation.

Regulation of Adrenal Androgens

ACTH is the principal agent regulating adrenal androgen synthesis. Plasma concentrations of DHEA and androstenedione follow the patterns of circadian and episodic secretion of cortisol closely, rise in response to the administration of ACTH, and fall when ACTH secretion is inhibited by glucocorticoids. Concentrations of DHEA-S, which is quantitatively the principal secretory product of the human adrenal, do not follow this pattern as clearly because of its very long plasma half-life, yet DHEA-S is increased by chronic elevations of ACTH and suppressed by chronic ACTH deficiency.

Adrenarche

The term *adrenarche,* which was first coined by Fuller Albright,[478] refers to the onset of increased "adrenal androgen" secretion in children at about 8 years of age. As discussed previously, the so-called adrenal androgens (DHEA, DHEA-S, and androstenedione) have minimal capacity to bind to and activate the androgen receptor, hence these adrenal C-19 steroids are actually androgen precursors. Circulating plasma concentrations of DHEA-S are a simple effective index of adrenarche[189]; DHEA-S has a long plasma half-life and exhibits little diurnal variation.[479–481] Although the gonads produce DHEA and androstenedione as precursors to testosterone and estrogens, they secrete negligible amounts of DHEA and DHEA-S. More than 90 percent of circulating DHEA-S derives either from direct adrenal secretion[482–484] or from peripheral sulfation of DHEA secreted by the adrenals.[482–484] The concentrations of DHEA-S as a function of age in males and females are shown in Fig. 11-11. After reaching maximal values in young adulthood, DHEA-S concentrations fall steadily (adrenopause), even though cortisol secretion remains relatively constant. The fall in concentrations of DHEA in the elderly has stimulated substantial interest and study of DHEA replacement therapy.[354]

Because the effects of adrenal C-19 steroids are mild and because the onset of adrenarche is usually followed by the onset of puberty within 2 years, endocrinologists often fail to understand that adrenarche is independent of gonadarche, i.e. the onset of gonadal axis function. Whereas gonadarche is defined as the activation of the hypothalamic-pituitary-gonadal axis [and hence begins with increased secretion of hypothalamic gonadotropin releasing hormone (GnRH)], adrenarche is independent of GnRH and gonadotropins. Children under age 6 years with true central precocious puberty have increased responses of gonadotropins to GnRH and increased serum concentrations of gonadotropins and sex steroids but have DHEA-S concentrations indistinguishable from those of age-matched controls.[189] Similarly, patients with gonadal dysgenesis (Turner's syndrome) have increased responses of gonadotropins to GnRH and increased circulating gonadotropin concentrations but have DHEA-S concentrations indistinguishable from those of age-matched controls.[189] Thus, the increased secretion of adrenal androgens at adrenarche is not regulated by the hypothalamic-pituitary-gonadal axis and is not associated with increased secretion of ACTH or cortisol.

Studies of the biological basis of adrenarche are especially difficult because adrenarche is only seen in human beings and chimpanzees.[485,486] The existance of a circulating polypeptide hormone that would specifically stimulate the zona reticularis, in a fashion analogous to the action of angiotensin II on the glomerulosa and ACTH on the fasciculata, has been suggested.[189,487]

However, careful searches for such a factor have been uniformly unsuccessful.[361–363] CRF may exert important actions to stimulate DHEA secretion by the fetal adrenal,[488,489] but there is no present evidence that CRF plays a role in adrenarche. Many recent studies of adrenarche have focused on intraadrenal events, especially the roles of 3β-HSD and P450c17 (for review, see Ref. 490). The activity and abundance of 3β-HSD mRNA and protein in the zona reticularis decrease at the onset of adrenarche, favoring production of Δ^5 steroids.[491–494] Furthermore, the production of cytochrome b_5, which strongly fosters the 17,20 lyase activity of P450c17 (Ref. 187), is almost exclusively confined to the zona reticularis.[495,496] Both of these features of the cell biology of the zona reticularis favor the production of DHEA. Premature, exaggerated adrenarche has been found in association with insulin resistance,[497,498] suggesting that premature adrenarche is an early sign of the polycystic ovary syndrome. This association has now been traced back to intrauterine events.[499]

Adrenal versus Ovarian Sex Steroids

Plasma concentrations of androstenedione, testosterone (T), and dihydrotestosterone (DHT) vary during the menstrual cycle as a result of ovarian secretion of androstenedione and its peripheral conversion to T and DHT.[500,501] Plasma androstenedione averages 125 ng/dl and testosterone averages 25 ng/dl during the early follicular phase, and these values rise to 200 ng/dl and 50 ng/dl, respectively, during midcycle.[500] During the follicular phase, the adrenal accounts for about 67 percent of the testosterone, about 50 percent of the DHT (via peripheral conversion of testosterone), 55 percent of the androstenedione, 80 percent of the DHEA, and 96 percent of the DHEA-S.[500] During midcycle, the adrenal contribution to testosterone and androstenedione drops to 40 percent and 30 percent respectively.[500] Small amounts of estradiol and estriol are also synthesized by the adrenal, but most of the adrenal contribution to circulating estrogens is due to conversion of androstenedione to estrone by 17-KSR in peripheral tissues. In postpubertal males, the adrenal contribution to circulating androgens is quantitatively similar to that in females but is biologically negligible because of the 10- to 20-fold higher levels of testosterone produced by the testes.

Adrenal androgens play no known essential role. However, as was described earlier, the adrenal contributes most of the circulating androgens in women. These adrenal androgens are thus important in the development of the partial virilization that accompanies development of normal female secondary sexual characteristics. Thus, the development of pubic and axillary hair, body odor, and comedones in pubertal females is due primarily to synergism between ovarian estrogens and adrenal androgens. Furthermore, adrenal androgens may participate in the generation of female libido.

PLASMA STEROIDS AND THEIR DISPOSAL

Quantities of Steroids Produced

Several techniques have been devised to estimate the secretion rates of the steroid hormones,[502,503] and despite methodologic problems, reasonable estimates have been obtained[503–509] (Table 11-2). Cortisol is the adrenal steroid secreted in the greatest quantity, and its production has generally been estimated to be 8 to 25 mg/day.[503,506,507] However, in a recent study using stable isotope infusion, the cortisol production rate in normal adult volunteers was considerably lower at 9.9 $\pm$ 2.7 mg/24 h (5.7 mg/m^2 per day).[510] A second study using the same method showed virtually identical results in male and female children and adolescents; i.e., the cortisol production rate was 9.5 $\pm$ 2.5 mg/day or 6.8 $\pm$ 1.9 mg/m^2 per day.[511] An additional study using deconvolution analysis in normal adolescent males demonstrated a cortisol production rate of 5.7 $\pm$ 0.3 mg/m^2 per day.[512] The only other major glucocorticoid, corticosterone, has a secretion rate of 1 to 4 mg/24 h.[503,506,507] The adrenal production of cortisone is only about 4 percent that of cortisol.[503] Adrenal production of DHEA-S is also high (i.e., 6 to 8 mg/day); the adrenals secrete 90 percent of this steroid in females[513] and an even greater percentage in males. This gland also makes appreciable quantities of androstenedione (50 percent of the production in females and a higher percentage in males)[513] and its 11-oxygenated derivatives, 11-ketoandrostenedione and 11β-hydroxyandrostenedione.[504,514] Androstenedione is converted to testosterone more readily than is DHEA or DHEA-S (Fig. 11-4). Adrenal testosterone accounts for only a minor fraction of total production in men (Chap. 15). In women, the adrenals and ovaries each contribute about 25 percent of total testosterone by direct secretion.[515] The remaining 50 percent is derived from peripheral conversion of androstenedione and, to a lesser extent, DHEA.[513,515] 17α-hydroxypregnenolone and progesterone are produced in small quantities by the normal adrenal cortex and in much higher quantities in various pathologic states.[504] Negligible quantities of estradiol are produced by the adrenal. Aldosterone is produced in small quantities, but this steroid is active at low concentrations. Significant quantities of DOC are also produced.

Inhibitors of Adrenal Steroid Biosynthesis

A number of compounds inhibit adrenal steroid biosynthesis by enzymatic inhibition or through a cytotoxic effect on adrenocortical cells (for reviews, see Refs. 514 and 516–522). These compounds have been useful for research and in the diagnosis and treatment of adrenal disorders (discussed later).[520–523]

Mitotane (*o,p'*-DDD) is a derivative of DDT that was first noted to cause adrenal insufficiency in dogs.[521] The compound inhibits the mitochondrial enzymes P450c11β, P450c11AS, and P450scc, leading to decreased synthesis of glucocorticoids and DHEA in the zona fasciculata and zona reticularis.[521–524] There are relatively minor effects on the zona glomerulosa, and aldosterone production usually remains normal. Mitotane also causes structural damage to mitochondria and thus causes necrosis of the inner two zones of the cortex. It also alters hepatic metabolism of cortisol, leading to decreased urinary excretion of 17-hydroxycorticosteroids.[519,521,523,524] Mitotane is used to treat patients with adrenocortical carcinoma and, to a lesser extent, patients with Cushing's disease (discussed later).

Metyrapone in the usual doses administered to humans is a selective inhibitor of both isozymes of P450c11 in all zones of the adrenal cortex.[521,523] Thus, there is inhibition of both cortisol and aldosterone secretion and a secondary rise in ACTH and renin production. Steroids proximal to the inhibited steps increase, leading to increased levels of 11-deoxycortisol, DOC (hypertension and hypokalemia), and adrenal androgens (hirsutism). Metyrapone is useful in the diagnosis and therapy of Cushing's syndrome.[525]

Aminoglutethimide, which was developed as an anticonvulsant, inhibits P450scc, thus blocking the synthesis of all adrenal steroids.[521–523,526] This drug also blocks the conversion of adrenal

TABLE 11-2. Secretion Rates and Plasma Concentrations of Various Steroids*

Steroid	Secretion Rate, mg/24 h	Ref.	Plasma Concentration, ng/ml	Ref.
Aldosterone	0.15	506	0.15 – 0.17	Chap. 13
Androstenedione	2.5 (F)	503	1.80 ± 0.21 (F)	504
	2.2 (M)	503	1.14 ± 0.21 (M)	504
Corticosterone	1–4	503, 506, 507	2.4 ± 1.5 (F)†	508
			5.4 ± 2.2 (M)†	508
Cortisol	8–25	503, 506, 507	85 (20 – 140) (F)	509
	9.9 ± 2.7	510–512	116 (40 – 180) (M)	509
11-Deoxycorticosterone (DOC)	0.6	503, 506, 507	0.15 – 0.17	Chap. 13
11-Deoxycortisol	0.4	506	0.95 – 2.5	506
DHEA	0.7 (F)	506	5.34 ± 1.57 (F)	504
	3.0 (M)	504	5.53 ± 1.78 (M)	504
DHEA-S	6–8	503, 504	1130 ± 280 (F)	504
			1260 ± 340 (M)	504
Etiocholanolone sulfate	—	—	17 ± 6 (F)	504
			15 ± 4 (M)	504
Etiocholanolone glucuronide			15 ± 5 (F)	504
			18 ± 7 (M)	504
Progesterone (M)			0.2 ± 0.09 (F)‡	508
			11.8 ± 7.00 (F)§	508
			0.18 ± 0.10 (M)	508
17α-Hydroxyprogesterone			0.58 ± 0.26 (F)‡	508
			1.96 ± 0.75 (F)	508
			0.18 ± 0.06 (M)	508
Testosterone	0.23 (F)	504	0.48 ± 0.14 (F)	504
			5.59 ± 1.51	504

*Values are for adults and are given as mean values alone, with ranges, or ± SD. F and M denote females and males, respectively. Data on 18-hydroxycorticosterone and 18-hydroxydeoxycorticosterone can be found in Chap. 13. For many of the steroids, plasma concentrations vary with the time of day and, in females, with the menstrual cycle. Levels also change with growth and development and with aging. Estradiol and estrone production in males is extremely low and is not listed. The selection of literature sources is somewhat arbitrary; values vary in different report.

† Samples taken 8 to 9 A.M.

‡ Follicular phase of the menstrual cycle.

§ Luteal phase of the menstrual cycle.

androgens to estrogens and is used to inhibit estrogen synthesis in patients with breast carcinoma.[527]

Cyanoketone and trilostane are inhibitors of 3β-hydroxysteroid dehydrogenase and thus decrease the production of all classes of adrenocortical steroids.[521] Cyanoketone has not been used in humans, and there are conflicting reports of the efficacy of trilostane in Cushing's syndrome.[522,528,529]

Ketoconazole, an imidazole antifungal agent, is an inhibitor of cytochrome P450 enzymes.[520,530,531] This inhibition accounts for both its antifungal effects and its inhibition of steroidogenesis. In the adrenal, ketoconazole inhibits P450c11 and P450scc.[520,531] These effects decrease cortisol production when doses greater than 600 mg/day are utilized in the treatment of fungal infections.[520] When doses of 600 to 1,200 mg/day are utilized in patients with Cushing's syndrome, the majority have normalization of cortisol secretion.[520,530,531]

Etomidate, an imidazole anesthetic agent, also inhibits P450c11 and, to a lesser extent, P450scc.[520,521,532,533] Etomidate impairs cortisol and aldosterone secretion and inhibits the response of these hormones to ACTH.[520] Its prolonged use to sedate patients in the intensive care unit was associated with increased mortality.[520,532] In one study, parenterally administered etomidate was shown to rapidly reduce the hypercortisolism of Cushing's syndrome.[533]

A number of other compounds also inhibit adrenal steroid biosynthesis. Heparin can inhibit aldosterone biosynthesis in vivo but not in vitro.[516,517] This effect requires several weeks and sometimes occurs with heparin therapy.[534] Spironolactone can block aldosterone biosynthesis,[518,535] predominantly at the 11β-hydroxylation and 18-dehydrogenation steps.[527,535] This may contribute to the antimineralocorticoid actions of this compound (in addition to its antagonist actions, as discussed later) and may explain why the plasma aldosterone response to renin is blunted after spironolactone therapy (see Chap. 13).[535]

Physical State of Steroids in Plasma

Cortisol and Other Glucocorticoids

The cortisol released by the adrenal gland is free. However, approximately 90 to 97 percent of the circulating cortisol is bound by plasma proteins (see also Chap. 3).[536–543] About 90 percent of this binding is with corticosteroid-binding globulin [(CBG), also termed transcortin], which binds cortisol specifically and with a high affinity (i.e., it is saturable at moderately low concentrations of cortisol) (Fig. 11-19). A lesser quantity of cortisol is bound by albumin, and a negligible amount by other plasma proteins (Fig. 11-19).

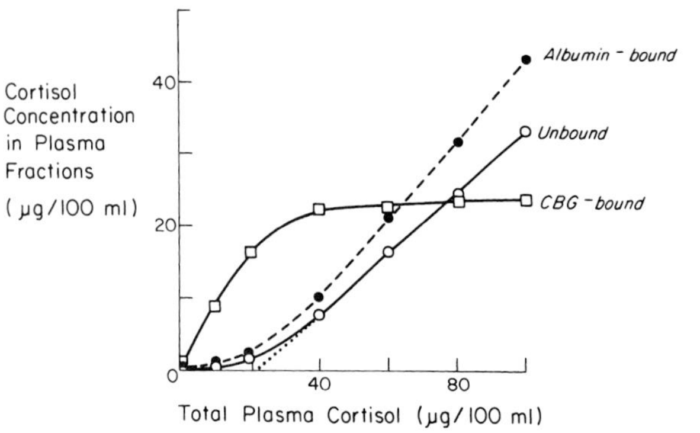

FIGURE 11-19. Distribution of cortisol in plasma. (*From Ballard.*[536])

Corticosteroid-Binding Globulin

Some properties of CBG are listed in Table 11-3. This protein has been detected in all species examined, although the levels vary from about 1 μg/dl in the sheep to 100 μg/dl in the iguana and the squirrel.[536] CBG is produced primarily in the liver,[536,543–547] but it has also been found in a number of other tissues, including brain, pituitary, lung, kidney, muscle, and uterus, and in lymphocytes.[543,544,547,548] Human CBG is a 383-amino acid glycoprotein with a molecular weight of approximately 58,000.[536,543,545] Recent studies have shown that CBG is not structurally related to other steroid-binding proteins or to steroid hormone receptors. However, it is similar to several members of the serine protease inhibitor (SERPIN) superfamily.[545,546] It is most closely related to α1-proteinase inhibitor (A1-PI), α1-chymotrypsin (A1-ACT), and thyroxine-binding globulin (TBG).[545,546] This similarity with the SERPIN family has led to speculation that CBG plays a role in delivering cortisol to sites of inflammation.[545–547,549,550]

At the usual concentrations in humans, CBG can bind up to 25 μg/dl of cortisol[536] at physiologic conditions (Fig. 11-19). Cortisol binds to and dissociates rapidly from CBG.[536–540,551] Its affinity for cortisol ($K_d \approx$ 13 to 30 n*M*)[536–540,551] is such that at a total plasma cortisol of 10 μg/dl, CBG is 50 percent saturated, and it is more than 90 percent saturated at a total cortisol concentration of 40 μg/dl. Because CBG is the major cortisol-binding protein, the free cortisol in plasma is almost linearly related to the total cortisol at normal concentrations. However, when the total cortisol concentration rises above 25 μg/dl, CBG becomes more saturated with cortisol, and the proportion of the total cortisol that is free increases in a nonlinear fashion (Fig. 11-19). Thus, at a total plasma cortisol concentration of 40 μg/dl, the free cortisol (≈10 μg/dl) would be 10-fold higher than it would be at a total plasma cortisol concentration of 10 μg/dl (free cortisol concentration ≈1 μg/dl).

A number of other endogenous and synthetic steroids also bind to CBG (Table 11-4).[536,541,546,552] However, considering their affinity for CBG and/or their plasma concentrations, the extent of this binding in physiologic circumstances is ordinarily minor and almost all the CBG-bound steroid is cortisol. One exception is third-trimester pregnancy, in which increased progesterone accounts for about 25 percent of the total CBG-bound steroid.[536,538] Also, in congenital adrenal hyperplasia (discussed later), several steroids can be elevated enough to occupy CBG to a major extent. These include corticosterone, 17α-hydroxyprogesterone, progesterone, 11-deoxycortisol, DOC, and 21-deoxycortisol. Most of the synthetic glucocorticoids used in therapy (prednisolone is an exception) have a low affinity for CBG (Table 11-5) and therefore bind to it negligibly (see also Chap. 14). Whereas prednisone and cortisone bind weakly, these compounds are converted to prednisolone and cortisol, which bind tightly.

The CBG concentrations in plasma vary between individuals and are also regulated by hormones and other factors.[543,546,547,550] Circulating glucocorticoids at supraphysiologic concentrations decrease CBG concentrations.[547,550] Estrogens increase CBG, and elevated concentrations are seen in pregnancy and with estrogen therapy and oral contraceptive use.[536,540] In pregnancy, CBG levels gradually rise and are twice normal in the third trimester.[538] Postpartum they gradually return to normal during a 6-week period.[398,539] With estrogen treatment, the effect is maximal in about 3 to 5 days, and CBG levels return to normal 2 to 3 weeks after the cessation of therapy.[538] Thyroid hormone increases CBG synthesis[540]; CBG levels are reduced in hypothyroidism and increased in hyperthyroidism.[540] Elevated CBG levels in some cases may have a genetic basis and can be associated with certain HLA types.[540,553,554] Elevated levels also occur in diabetes, chronic active hepatitis,[553,555] and certain hematologic disorders.[553] CBG levels are subnormal in liver disease (decreased protein production), multiple myeloma, obesity, and the nephrotic syndrome (urinary loss of protein).[536,538,546,547,550,556] Complete absence of CBG has not been substantiated, but there is a familial condition in which CBG levels are about 50 percent of normal with normal plasma free cortisol concentrations and no clinical symptoms.[550,557,558]

Albumin and Other Cortisol-Binding Proteins

Cortisol binding to albumin has different characteristics. The kinetics of cortisol association with and dissociation from albumin are much more rapid than is the case with CBG. The affinity of al-

TABLE 11-3. General Properties of Corticosteroid-Binding Proteins in Human Serum

	CBG	Albumin	α_1 Acid Glycoprotein
Molecular weight	58,000	69,000	39,000
Concentration, μ*M*	0.71	550	18
Concentration, g/liter	0.037	38	0.18
Cortisol-binding capacity, μg/dl	25	>20,000	630
Equilibrium dissociation constant for cortisol at 37°C (K_d), *M*	3×10^{-8}	2×10^{-4}	8.5×10^{-6}
Cortisol-binding sites per molecule	1	1–20	1
Relative distribution of cortisol at 37°C, percent	77.3	15.0	0

Source: Modified from Ballard.[536]

TABLE 11-4. Relative Affinities of Steroids for CBG, Cytoplasmic Glucocorticoid Receptor, and Albumin in Humans

	CBG	Relative Affinity for Receptor*	Albumin
Cortisol	100	100	100
Fluocinolone acetonide	<1	1350	
Methylprednisolone	<1	1190	74
Dexamethasone	<1	710	>100
Betamethasone	<1	540	>100
Fluorometholone	<1	400	
9α-Fluorocortisol	<1	350	
Triamcinolone acetonide	<1	190	
Corticosterone	94	85	100
Prednisolone	58	220	61
Aldosterone	6	38	34
11-Deoxycorticosterone (DOC)	45	39	221
11-Deoxycortisol	77	19	
Progesterone	27	11	244
17α-Hydroxyprogesterone	70	>1	225
Prednisone	6	5	68
Cortisone	6	1	128
Testosterone	5	2	232
Pregnenolone	<1		
Estradiol	<1	5	1600
Estrone	<1		800
Androstenedione	<1	<1	223
Dehydroepiandrosterone (prasterone, DHEA)	<1		506

Note: Data for CBG and receptor obtained at 2°C; however, the relative binding at 37°C is similar overall.

*Human fetal lung.

Source: Ballard.[536]

bumin for cortisol is much lower, but the capacity is more than 1,000-fold higher than that of CBG (Table 11-3).[536,540] At cortisol concentrations below 20 μg/dl, about 7 percent of the plasma cortisol is albumin-bound.[541] With an increasing cortisol level, CBG becomes saturated, and a larger proportion of the plasma-bound steroid is associated with albumin (Fig. 11-17).[536]

Synthetic glucocorticoids are bound by albumin with an affinity similar to or slightly exceeding that of cortisol.[536] For instance, 55 percent of the total prednisolone, 62 percent of the betamethasone, and 77 percent of the dexamethasone are bound by human plasma.[536]

Although the proportion of free steroid bound by albumin is relatively independent of the steroid concentration, it is affected by the plasma albumin concentration.[536] Thus, in premature infants and in hypoalbuminemia, the proportion of non-CBG-bound steroid that is free is increased.[536,541] The α_1 acid glycoprotein that binds progesterone and other steroids also binds cortisol (Table 11-4), but this appears to be of minor importance.[536]

Physiologic Role of Plasma Binding

Despite much speculation and intense interest, the precise functions of CBG and other steroid-binding proteins remain obscure.[546,547,550] One theory is that these proteins serve as a reservoir to sequester steroids in an inactive form, thus influencing the availability of steroids to tissues, their receptors, and steroid-metabolizing enzymes. However, these plasma-binding proteins have not been proved to be essential for transporting steroids in the circulation, as these steroids are sufficiently water-soluble at biologically active concentrations.[536] Further, humans with low CBG levels and animals such as sheep with extremely low CBG levels show no decrement in their responsiveness to glucocorticoids.[536,540,543]

Steroids are inactive when bound by plasma protein.[536,543,551] For example, when tissue culture cells are incubated with cortisol and either CBG or albumin, the glucocorticoid dose response is reduced concomitantly to the extent of cortisol binding.[536,551] Further, the physiologic mechanisms that control the plasma cortisol concentration respond to free rather than total cortisol levels, so that with variations in CBG levels, free cortisol concentrations do not change, even though total cortisol levels do.[536] The CBG-bound cortisol and, to a lesser extent, the albumin-bound cortisol are also protected from metabolic degradation, and when CBG levels are increased, the rate of cortisol clearance is decreased.[536] Thus, these plasma proteins serve as a reservoir to sequester active steroids.

Whereas in any equilibrium situation the plasma-bound steroids are sequestered in an inactive state, they can become active through dissociation from the proteins. This can occur rapidly. Cortisol can dissociate from albumin with a $t_{1/2}$ of around 5 s at 37°C.[542]

Thus, as the free and protein-bound steroid circulates through the various tissues, the free steroid binds specifically to receptors, steroid-metabolizing enzymes, and other proteins and binds nonspecifically to a number of cellular components. This reduces the free steroid concentration and shifts the equilibrium toward dissociation of plasma protein-steroid complexes. The dissociated steroid is then free for further tissue uptake. Current data indicate that tissue uptake of cortisol can be accounted for entirely by the pool of free cortisol; there is no need to postulate other protein or receptor mechanisms.[539,560] This available fraction depends on both the extent of tissue uptake that shifts the equilibrium and the time of transport.[561] Because the rate of dissociation from albumin

TABLE 11-5. Urinary Steroid Metabolites of Intravenously Administered Radioactive Cortisol*

Steroid	Percent in Extract
Cortols (α and β)	7
Cortolones (α and β)	17
Allocortols and allocortolones	2
Tetrahydrocortisol	14
Tetrahydrocortisone	18
Allotetrahydrocortisol	6
Cortisol	1
6β-Hydroxycortisol	1
Cortisone	1
11β-hydroxyetiocholanolone	4
11-Ketoetiocholanolone	2
11β-Hydroxyandrosterone	<1
Cortoic acids	10

*The data are taken from Peterson[570] and Monder and Bradlow.[572] The percentages of Peterson that did not include the cortoic acids were reduced by 25 percent (and rounded off) to include the contribution of the cortoic acids calculated from the data of Monder and Bradlow as based on the percentage of total cortoic acid relative to the sum of tetrahydrocortisol and tetrahydrocortisone. The numbers reported by different workers show considerable variation, and this table is intended to serve only as a rough estimate. It is also stressed that all the known metabolites have not been included and that there are probably other, unidentified metabolites.

is more rapid than that from CBG, steroid bound by albumin is a more readily available source. As the capillary transit time through liver is slower (around 5 s) than it is in brain (around 1 s), lives can extract a larger proportion of the cortisol.[561] In fact, brain uptake of corticosterone in the rat approximates the non-CBG-bound (free plus albumin-bound) steroid, whereas in liver it exceeds this fraction by three times and includes CBG-bound steroid.[542,543]

By sequestering the relevant steroid and releasing it more gradually, plasma binding may also serve to dampen the swings in cortisol levels in plasma caused by episodic pulsatile release. This could protect cortisol from metabolic degradation and render changes in receptor occupancy more gradual.

A major role of hormone-binding proteins in plasma may be to ensure uniform delivery and distribution of the hormone to the individual cells of a target tissue.[560,562] Thus, in studies with thyroxine infusion into the perfused rat liver, the absence of binding globulin or prealbumin leads to nonuniform distribution, with the major proportion being rapidly taken by the first cells encountered. Conversely, when the thyroxine was infused with its binding proteins, there was uniform uptake and distribution within hepatic cells.[560,562]

CBG is synthesized in the liver.[536,544] However, other tissues have substantial concentrations of CBG or CBG-like proteins, and it is not clear whether these proteins are synthesized locally or taken up from the circulation.[542,546,548]

Additional physiologic roles of CBG are also possible. It has been demonstrated that CBG binds specifically to plasma membranes and leads to increased intracellular cAMP. This binding occurred only when CBG was bound to either cortisol or progesterone.[547,550] The relevance of these observations is unclear. Also, the knowledge that CBG has a structure homologous to that of the SERPIN superfamily led to the observation that the CBG-cortisol complex is cleaved by neutrophil-derived elastase at sites of inflammation.[546,547,549,550] Thus, a possible physiologic role for CBG could be to facilitate the delivery of glucocorticoids to sites of infection and inflammation.[546,547,549,550]

Aldosterone

Aldosterone does not bind to a specific or high-affinity protein, but binds weakly to albumin, CBG,[538,541,561,563,564] and red cells.[565] At 37°C, about 20 percent of the total aldosterone in plasma is bound to CBG and about 40 percent is bound to other proteins.[541,561] Although high concentrations of cortisol can decrease the total plasma binding of aldosterone slightly, the percentage of free aldosterone in plasma is relatively invariant even with wide fluctuations in the concentrations of this and other steroids.[566]

Although CBG binding of aldosterone is minor relative to total plasma aldosterone, changes in aldosterone binding by CBG can affect the metabolic clearance rate of aldosterone.[563] This occurs, for instance, when cortisol concentrations are low. This greater influence of CBG compared with that of other proteins presumably results from the slower rate of dissociation of aldosterone from CBG than from other plasma-binding proteins, resulting in more of the CBG-bound aldosterone surviving passage through the liver.

Deoxycorticosterone

About 97 percent of circulating DOC is bound by plasma proteins.[541] About 60 percent and 36 percent are associated with albumin and CBG, respectively.[541] The extent of DOC binding by plasma varies little over a wide range of concentrations of this steroid (2 to 200 ng/dl).[566]

Adrenal Androgens and Estrogens

The adrenal C-19 steroids (DHEA, DHEAS, and Δ^4-androstenedione) and their 11β-hydroxylated derivatives, are bound extensively to plasma proteins, mostly to albumin.[505,536,541,543,561,567–569] About 98 percent of the testosterone circulating in plasma is bound both to albumin and to a specific testosterone-estradiol-binding globulin (TeBG) whose plasma concentration is increased by estrogens (as in pregnancy) and in hyperthyroidism and is decreased by testosterone and in acromegaly (see laboratory evaluation of adrenocortical function, later, and Chap. 15). Plasma binding of estrogens is discussed in Chap. 16.

Metabolism of Adrenocortical Steroids

The continuous dynamic control of plasma concentrations of the adrenal steroids requires mechanisms for their removal from the body. The hydrophobic steroids are filtered by the kidney but are actively reabsorbed (e.g., about 95 percent of cortisol and 86 percent of aldosterone)[570] and are therefore not excreted into the urine. Thus, the steroids undergo enzymatic modifications that transform them into inactive substances with increased water solubility that can be removed more readily.[570–573] The modifications result largely in the conversion of some of the less polar ketone groups to hydroxyl groups and of the C-21 groups to acid forms. The hydroxyl groups can then be conjugated with glucuronide or sulfate groups, rendering them even more water-soluble. The liver is the major site of metabolic conversion, although most mammalian tissues, including the adrenal, metabolize steroids to some extent, and in pregnancy the placenta is quite active in the metabolism of steroids (see steroid synthesis in the fetal adrenal).[570] These metabolized compounds are then excreted. The renal clearance of a major cortisol metabolite, tetrahydrocortisone glucuronide, is around 70 percent of the creatinine clearance.[570] In most cases, the kidney accounts for more than 90 percent of the excretion of metabolized steroids (DOC and corticosterone are exceptions); the remainder are lost in the gut. Most of the metabolized steroids excreted into the gut are reabsorbed; in addition, especially with aldosterone, there can be further metabolism by the intestinal flora before absorption.

More than 50 different metabolites of cortisol and aldosterone have been detected (Fig. 11-20).[570–572] These metabolites are generated by a limited number of metabolic conversions. Because many of the structural differences among the various steroid hormones are eliminated during metabolism, it is often difficult to identify the true precursor(s) of a given metabolite.

Cortisol

Cortisol is cleared with a half-time of 80 to 120 min in various studies (Chap. 14).[570] If radioactively labeled cortisol is given, 70 percent of the radioactivity appears in the urine within 24 h and more than 90 percent appears by 72 h (Table 11-5).[570] Approximately 3 percent is recovered in the feces.[574] Almost all the radioactivity is present as cortisol metabolites; less than 1 percent appears as unchanged cortisol (Table 11-5).

Cortisol may be modified by several different enzymes. The most important initial reaction is the reduction of the 4,5 double bond by at least two Δ^4-reductases. This reaction is irreversible, in-

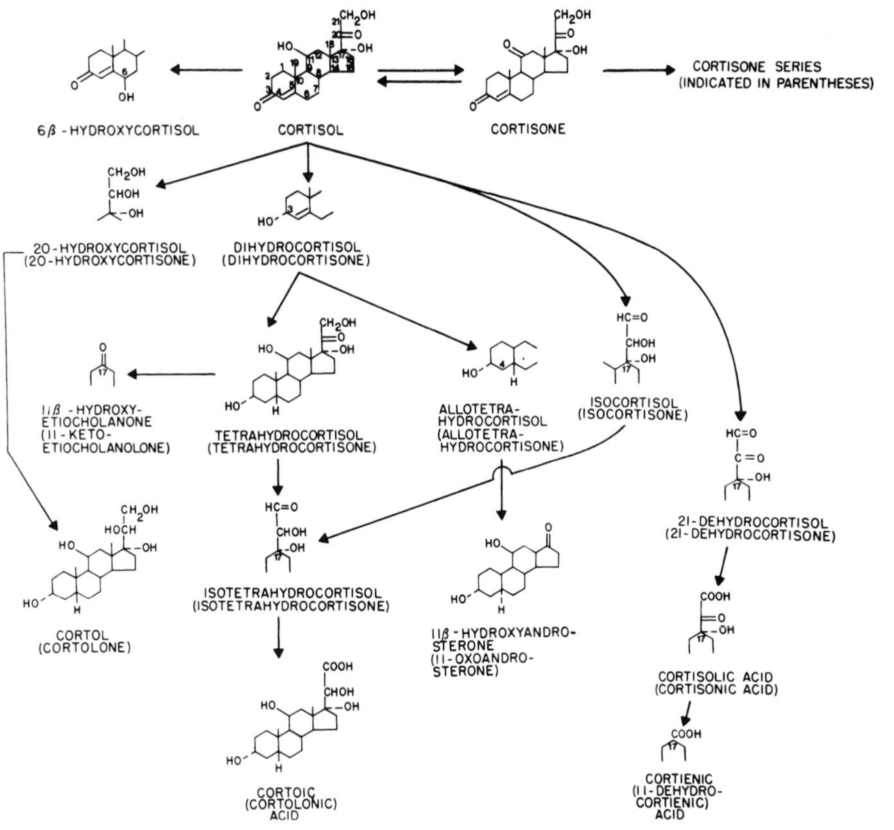

FIGURE 11-20. Pathways of cortisol and cortisone metabolism. Cortisol and cortisone are interconvertible. The steps shown are for cortisol metabolism; however, the metabolism of cortisone is similar. Thus, the name of the 11-keto metabolite resulting from cortisone metabolism is shown in parentheses for each cortisol metabolite. In many cases, only the portion of the steroid affected by the particular metabolic step is shown.

activates the molecule, and results in dihydrocortisol, which may be an α or a β form depending on the orientation of the hydrogen in the 5 position; the $5\alpha/5\beta$ ratio is about 5:1.[570] Dihydrocortisol is rapidly converted by a 3-hydroxysteroid dehydrogenase to tetrahydrocortisol (Table 11-5). Cortisol can be oxidized at the 11β-hydroxyl group by 11β-HSD to form the ketone (cortisone); this reaction does not occur after the A ring has been reduced.[570] As discussed earlier, both 11β-HSD-I and 11β-HSD-II have both oxidase and reductase activities, depending on the nature of the available co-factors. The role of the abundant hepatic 11β-HSD-I (which normally serves to activate cortisone to cortisol), in the degredative metabolism of cortisol is not clear. Cortisone is in general metabolized similarly to cortisol by 11β-HSD-I and therefore is also converted via the dihydro derivative to the tetrahydro metabolite. The net result is that roughly similar quantities of unaltered cortisol and cortisone and their metabolites are excreted (Table 11-5).[572] Cortisol, cortisone, and their tetrahydro derivatives can also be reduced to the cortols and cortolones, respectively, via hydroxy-steroid dehydrogenases (Fig. 11-14). There can also be oxidation at C-21 to form cortolic and cortolonic acids (Fig. 11-16) and conversion of the C-17 side chain to the C-20 acid.[572] The conversion to the acidic derivatives renders the steroids even more water-soluble.[572] Reduction of the C-20 keto group of cortisol or cortisone to 20-hydroxycortisol also occurs to a lesser extent. 6β-hydroxylated or 16α-hydroxylated metabolites of cortisol and other steroids ordinarily are formed in small quantities.[570] However, the 6β-hydroxylation pathway can be of major importance in infants in whom the esterification mechanisms are not fully developed, in some disease states, and after treatment with certain drugs (discussed later).[570,576–578] The 16α-hydroxylation pathway can be important for the conversion of estradiol to estriol. Finally, there can be some oxidative cleavage of the C-17 side chain to C-19 11-oxygenated 17-ketosteroids (5 to 10 percent).[570]

About 96 percent of the C-19 and C-21 metabolites of cortisol and cortisone are excreted as conjugates of cortisol, and less than 1 percent as unchanged cortisol (Table 11-5)[570]; 60 to 70 percent appears as conjugates at the 3α-hydroxyl position with glucuronic acid. A smaller amount of conjugates is formed with the sulfate through the C-21 hydroxyl.[579] The conjugation with glucuronide is due to the glucuronyl transferase, and the glucuronide donor is uridine diphosphoglucuronic acid. Glucuronyl transferase is so active that reduced steroids are almost completely esterified when they leave the liver.[580] This enzyme system differs from that responsible for conjugating bilirubin, because patients defective in the latter enzyme system have a much lesser defect in steroid conjugation.[581]

There are marked variations in cortisol metabolism in various tissues. As was discussed in steroid hormone biosynthesis, there is extensive metabolism of cortisol to cortisone in the kidney by the

11β-hydroxysteroid dehydrogenases.[321–343] This inactivation is of major physiologic significance because it protects the mineralocorticoid receptor from occupancy by cortisol and thus prevents cortisol from causing a mineralocorticoid excess state.[321–343] The quantitative role of the renal enzyme in total cortisol metabolism is unknown, but plasma cortisone levels are reduced in patients with renal disease.[576,581] By contrast, when cortisone or prednisone (both also have an 11-keto group and no intrinsic glucocorticoid activity) is administered, they are almost completely converted to cortisol and prednisolone in the liver, both of which have 11-hydroxyl groups and thus are biologically active.[321–343]

Corticosterone, 11-Deoxycortisol, and 11-Deoxycorticosterone

The metabolism of corticosterone, 11-deoxycortisol, and DOC is generally similar to that of cortisol except for minor quantitative differences.[570,572] For instance, more corticosterone than cortisol is excreted as the 21-conjugate,[570] its half-time of disappearance is shorter, C-19 metabolites have not been found,[570] and more of the metabolites are excreted into the gut.[572] A much greater proportion of DOC (perhaps 50 percent) is excreted into the gut.[572]

Aldosterone

Aldosterone turns over rapidly,[570,582] with a half-time of 15 min or less; it is almost completely removed by one passage through the liver, and less than 0.5 percent appears in urine in the free state.[570,571,582] About 35 percent of the aldosterone is excreted as tetrahydroaldosterone glucuronide (3 position; see the earlier discussion on cortisol metabolism); up to 20 percent appears as the glucuronide (18 position).[570] This metabolite is termed either the acid-labile conjugate (because free aldosterone can be released from it by hydrolysis at pH 1)[583] or the 3-oxo conjugate (because the 3-oxo group is intact). Determinations of urinary aldosterone usually measure the concentration of this metabolite. The remainder of the aldosterone is metabolized to a variety of other compounds, including a number of polar derivatives such as carboxylic acid and hydroxylated metabolites, and 21-deoxytetrahydroaldosterone.[582] This steroid is probably produced in the gut (after biliary excretion of tetrahydroaldosterone), reabsorbed, and excreted into the urine.[582] There is less metabolic modification of the 11β-hydroxy group of aldosterone than is the case in cortisol because this is protected by the steroid's cyclic 11,18-hemiacetyl form.[571] In the rat, there are significant sex differences in aldosterone metabolism, with a greater proportion of various metabolites being present in male than in female tissues; also, aldosterone metabolism can be affected by both potassium ion and spironolactone.[582]

Androgens and Estrogens

The androgens are excreted predominantly as conjugates in the urine; a small fraction is excreted into the gut.[505] More than 80 percent of the androstenedione is removed from the circulation after one passage through the liver.[541] By contrast, only 44 percent of the testosterone is removed.[505] DHEA-S of adrenal origin can be excreted unchanged; DHEA-S is also formed in liver and kidney. Both of these compounds can be metabolized further by either hydroxylation at positions 7 and 16 or transformation of the 17-keto group into a 17β-hydroxyl group[541] (Fig. 11-21). DHEA is also irreversibly converted to androstenedione. As mentioned earlier, androstenedione is converted to testosterone (mostly by extrahepatic tissues) or its 4,5 double bond is reduced, resulting in androsterone or etiocholanolone (Fig. 11-21). These steroids can be further reduced, respectively, to androstenediol and etiocholanediol (Fig. 11-21).[505] Testosterone is also converted in the androgen target tissues to DHT (Chaps. 16 and 18); DHT is reversibly inactivated, mainly by 3α-reduction to 3α-androstenediol[584,585]; a lesser amount is reversibly converted to 5α-androstenedione (Fig. 11-21). Both of these compounds can be converted to androsterone. All these

FIGURE 11-21. Major pathways in androgen metabolism. Most of the steps shown are involved in androgen degradation. However, the 5α reduction of testosterone occurs in androgen target tissues to yield the highly active 5α-dihydrotestosterone.

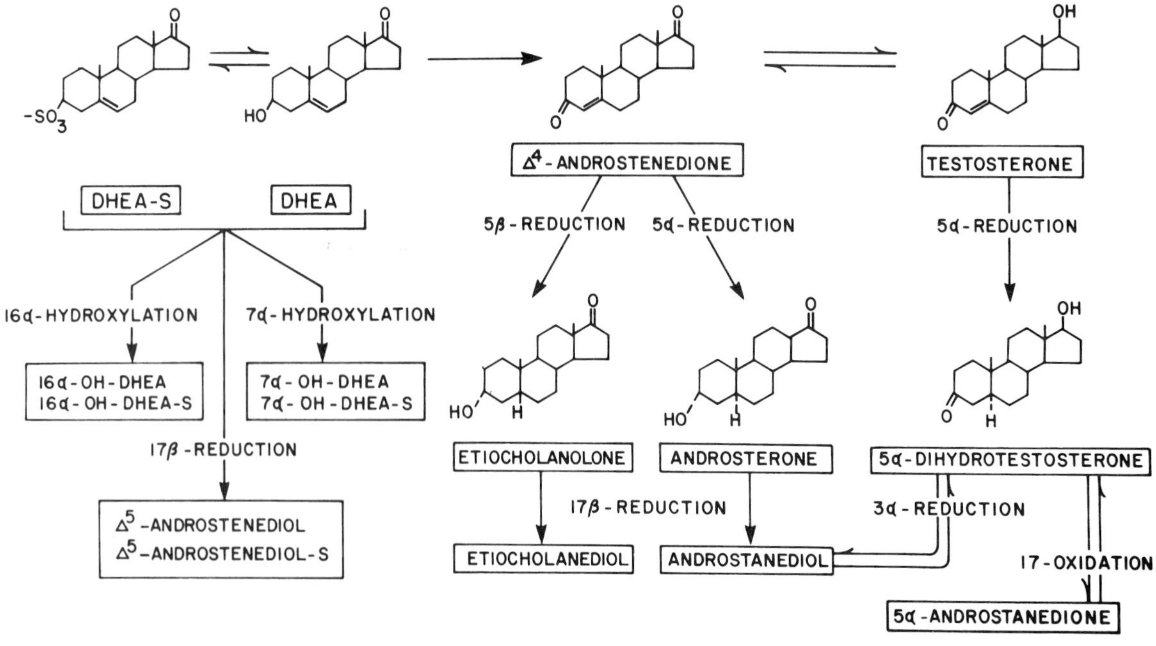

metabolites are further conjugated to glucuronides, and compared with cortisol metabolites, a larger proportion of them are converted to the sulfate derivatives (mostly through the 3 position). The sulfate conjugates are more slowly cleared because they bind more extensively to plasma proteins and are not filtered as well as are the glucuronides.

Testosterone and androstenedione are cleared two to three times more rapidly from plasma in men than in women.[505] Apparently, this is due to an effect of the androgens on their own metabolism, as values more similar to those of females are observed in the testicular feminization syndrome, in which plasma androgen concentrations tend to be elevated and there is peripheral insensitivity to androgens.[505]

Variations in Steroid Metabolism

The rate of metabolism of adrenal steroids is affected by a number of diseases, drugs, and other hormones. Agents that increase plasma CBG levels also decrease the rate of cortisol clearance.[536,570] Plasma binding also decreases aldosterone clearance.[563]

In chronic liver disease, the metabolism of cortisol and estrogens is decreased.[570] These effects are relatively specific, as the metabolism of a number of other steroids (e.g., aldosterone, cortisone, and certain cortisol metabolites) is unaffected or minimally affected. This influence may be due to changes in specific metabolizing enzymes and does not result from alterations in hepatic circulation or CBG levels. The decreased metabolism of cortisol tends to decrease cortisol secretion, presumably by feedback inhibition of ACTH release. Thus, urinary excretion of the metabolites of cortisol and other ACTH-dependent steroids (e.g., urinary 17-ketosteroids) is also low in chronic liver disease. However, plasma cortisol is normal unless CBG levels fall. By contrast, the decreased metabolism of estrogens in chronic liver disease results in elevated plasma estrogen concentrations, producing the feminizing features of cirrhosis.

The metabolism of cortisol, aldosterone, and several other adrenal steroids is increased in hyperthyroidism and decreased in hypothyroidism.[570] This apparently is a specific effect of thyroxine on biotransformation rather than on conjugation, and is not due to hypermetabolism per se, as the increase is not observed in other hypermetabolic states. There is also increased secretion of cortisol and aldosterone in hyperthyroidism and decreased secretion in hypothyroidism; these are felt to be compensatory effects on ACTH and renin release that maintain normal plasma steroid levels. They are also reflected by increased urinary 17-hydroxycorticosteroid (17-OHCS) excretion in hyperthyroidism and decreased excretion in hypothyroidism. The metabolism of progesterone and estrogens is much less affected by alterations in thyroid function, whereas the clearance of the androgens is, if anything, decreased.

The metabolism of corticosteroids is also altered in several other circumstances. Although renal disease affects the clearance of cortisol metabolites, it does not have a major effect on the hepatic metabolism of cortisol.[570] In congestive heart failure, there can be decreased clearance of aldosterone.[570] In general, there are no major differences in cortisol or aldosterone metabolism in chronic diseases, obesity, starvation, stress, anxiety, or depression.[570] In some of these cases, changes in steroid production can alter the amount of steroid excreted.[570] There can also be minor sex differences in the relative metabolic pathways.[582] The clearance of cortisol is decreased in the extremes of old age and infancy[514] but otherwise changes little throughout life.[570] Drugs such as mitotane (*o,p'*-DDD), phenytoin, rifampin, aminoglutethimide, and barbiturates result in differences in the patterns of urinary steroid secretion, including an increase in 6β-hydroxycortisol, but have only a minor influence on the total rate of disappearance of infused cortisol.[514] However, these drugs increase the clearance of synthetic glucocorticoids such as dexamethasone and prednisolone, possibly by affecting the 6β-hydroxy modification and conjugation, which are more important in the metabolism of these steroids.[570,580] The 6β-hydroxycortisol pathway is also increased in patients with liver disease,[578] in hyperestrogenic states,[578] and in cancer or prolonged terminal illness.[577] The antihypertensive agent minoxidil (unlike hydralazine) increases aldosterone clearance, possibly by hemodynamic influences.[587] In pregnancy, the cortisol clearance rate is lowered, probably as a result of increased CBG levels.[570] Finally, there can be some impairment in cortisol clearance in anorexia nervosa and protein-calorie malnutrition.[588]

MOLECULAR MECHANISMS AND PHYSIOLOGIC ACTIONS

Definition of a Glucocorticoid

The term *glucocorticoid* was coined to denote the glucose-regulating properties of these steroids.[589,590] However, glucocorticoids have many actions that do not involve carbohydrate metabolism. Thus, it seems preferable to define adrenal steroid actions in terms of the receptors that mediate them.[590] Thus, a glucocorticoid effect is one that is mediated through a class of receptors termed glucocorticoid receptors. In addition, certain glucocorticoids can act by binding to other classes of receptors, for instance, through mineralocorticoid receptors, in which case the action is termed mineralocorticoid.

Molecular Mechanisms of Glucocorticoid Hormone Action

The molecular events in glucocorticoid hormone action are similar to those of other classes of steroid hormones (Chap. 4).[591–595] In the absence of glucocorticoids, the receptors are predominantly localized in the cytosol. The receptors are encoded by a single gene, have a molecular weight of about 90,000, and are phosphorylated.[596,597] There are from 5,000 to 100,000 cytoplasmic receptors per cell.[596] They bind cortisol with an affinity constant (K_d) of around 10 to 20 n*M*; this value is close to the free cortisol concentration in plasma, suggesting that saturation of the receptors is probably ordinarily in the range of 10 to 70 percent and that increases or decreases in plasma cortisol will change the receptor occupancy and thus the physiologic responses. These receptors bind a variety of glucocorticoids in proportion to their biological activities.[591]

As described in Chap. 4, the glucocorticoid receptor gene is a member of a much larger family of genes that encode the other steroid hormone receptors, vitamin D receptors, retinoic acid and retinoid X receptors, and a number of other transcription factors. These receptors contain an amino-terminal activation domain that is larger for the glucocorticoid receptor than that of most of the other members of the family, a centrally located DNA-binding domain, and a carboxy-terminal glucocorticoid-binding domain.

This receptor and the receptor-glucocorticoid complex probably mediate almost all the actions of the glucocorticoids on transcription (Chap. 4).[594,599–602] These include both physiologic actions and those in glucocorticoid therapy. However, there are at least two exceptions. First, the fast feedback suppression of ACTH by glucocorticoids occurs too rapidly to be explained by effects on transcription (Fig. 11-5)[603–607]; second, the effects of high-dose glucocorticoids in spinal cord trauma appear to be mediated through other mechanisms (Chap. 14).

Glucocorticoids can also bind to and activate mineralocorticoid receptors.[325,326,365,366,608–610] In the kidney, this effect is blocked by the inactivation of glucocorticoids by 11β-hydroxysteroid dehydrogenase.[321–343,611,612] Mineralocorticoid receptors are also present in certain regions of the brain and in the rat are occupied by corticosterone.[334,365] These receptors mediate certain effects of the steroid on brain cell metabolism, serotoninergic neurotransmission, and behavioral adaptation.[609,610] In fact, the affinity of corticosterone for these mineralocorticoid receptors is so high that in the brain they are nearly fully occupied at basal levels of corticosterone.[610] An analogous situation probably occurs in human beings, although most glucocorticoid effects in the brain are mediated through the classic glucocorticoid receptors.

As described in Chap. 4, the unliganded glucocorticoid receptors are associated with at least two heat shock proteins and perhaps with other proteins. Hormone binding induces a conformational change in the receptors termed *activation* (or *transformation*), which results in a dissociation of the heat shock proteins from the receptors. This exposes nuclear translocation sequences on the receptors, resulting in their uptake into the nucleus. It also results in the formation of receptor dimers and exposes DNA- and protein-binding sites on the receptors so that 50 to 70 percent of the hormone-receptor complexes then bind to sites in the chromatin of the nucleus formerly called *acceptors*.[594]

The receptor-glucocorticoid complexes bind to either DNA sites in the nucleus termed hormone response elements (HREs)[594,595] or proteins involved in transcriptional stimulation. It is of interest that the HREs for the glucocorticoid, mineralocorticoid, progesterone, and androgen receptors are identical (for review, see Refs. 613 and 614). Thus, the specificity of individual hormone action appears to be conveyed by the presence of the receptor and the interaction of the HREs with other factors to form composite response elements.[613,614] The HREs contain specific sequences that have a much higher affinity for binding the receptor-glucocorticoid complexes than does random DNA. The proteins to which glucocorticoid binding has been most extensively studied is the *jun* component of the *jun* and *fos* complex termed AP1 and the Rel A component of NF-KB.

Binding of receptor-glucocorticoid complexes to HREs or proteins affects the transcription of nearby genes. The effects can either be to stimulate or inhibit transcription. Thus, the HRE functions as a regulated enhancer element and can function either upstream (with respect to transcription) or downstream (e.g., in an intron), in either orientation, and at a considerable distance away from the promoter for transcriptional initiation.[594,597,615,616] The mechanisms by which these effects occur are not understood, but two types of phenomena are being deciphered. First, different portions of the receptors interact with proteins associated with the proximal promoter and its associated essential transcription factors. This could occur directly or through other proteins termed coregulators, and ultimately could stimulate (coactivators) or inhibit (corepressors), directly or indirectly, the initiation of transcription by RNA polymerases.[598] Second, binding of the receptor-glucocorticoid complex to DNA can induce rapid and local influences on chromatin structure that can result in changes in the access of other transcription factors to the DNA, thus influencing transcriptional initiation.[594,595]

Changes in the production of RNA transcripts in response to the steroid are reflected by consequent influences on the respective mature mRNAs and protein products. The steroid-regulated proteins are responsible for the steroid response. For example, these may be enzymes such as those involved in gluconeogenesis or hormone precursors such as POMC; the latter is an example in which glucocorticoids inhibit transcription.[602] Inhibitory actions can also be mediated by inducing the synthesis of proteins that block specific cellular functions.

Glucocorticoid receptors have been detected in most tissues.[594] This extensive tissue distribution of receptors contrasts with the much more restricted distribution of the receptors for other classes of steroids and is consistent with the notion that glucocorticoids affect most, if not all, mammalian tissues.

There is generally[594] but not exclusively[617] a close correlation between the relative saturation of the receptor by the hormone and the relative magnitude of the glucocorticoid hormone response, suggesting that the receptor concentration limits the magnitude of the steroid hormone response. This contrasts with polypeptide and catecholamine hormones, in which "spare" receptors are present.

A variety of factors can affect glucocorticoid responsiveness.[594,617,618] First, factors in the cell may modulate hormone-binding activity. Second, receptor numbers can be regulated by glucocorticoids (ordinarily negatively), the cell cycle, and other factors. However, glucocorticoid receptors are not as extensively regulated as are those for polypeptide hormones. Finally, responsiveness is affected by many of the interrelations with other hormones that were discussed previously.

Glucocorticoid action is rapidly reversible. When cortisol levels drop, the steroid dissociates from the receptor and the receptor dissociates from the DNA, resulting in a cessation of the effect on gene transcription. The hormone response, however, can be longer-lived because of the persistence of mRNAs and proteins whose levels were increased by the steroid.

The glucocorticoid hormone response is restricted to a small subset of the expressed genes in each cell type. For instance, in liver, the glucocorticoids affect 7 percent of 200 quantifiable proteins.[619] Further, the proteins induced are specific for each cell type; i.e., a given protein may be induced in only one or a few but not all glucocorticoid-responsive tissues. This also indicates that factors other than the presence of the glucocorticoid receptors determine whether the expression of a given gene can be under glucocorticoid hormone control, as the receptors may be similar in the various glucocorticoid-responsive tissues.

Glucocorticoid Agonists and Antagonists

Cortisol, corticosterone, aldosterone, and the synthetic steroids used in steroid therapy (prednisolone, dexamethasone, triamcinolone, etc.) are glucocorticoid agonists and therefore elicit glucocorticoid responses.[591,620] The activity of these compounds depends on their affinity for the receptors and their plasma concentrations. Cortisol and corticosterone have similar affinities for the glucocorticoid receptor (Table 11-4); however, cortisol is the more important glucocorticoid because it circulates at much higher concentrations (Table 11-2). In 17α-hydroxylase (P450c17) deficiency), corticosterone is the predominant glucocorticoid. Aldosterone is not an important glucocorticoid, even in mineralocorticoid excess states, because it does not reach high enough concentrations.

Antagonist steroids can bind to the glucocorticoid receptor, but do not elicit glucocorticoid responses[591,620–622] and can compete with agonists for binding to the receptors and thus block the agonist response. Some compounds may have partial agonist (partial antagonist) activity such that full receptor occupancy by these steroids may result in an intermediate response; when present at a sufficient concentration, they can also block agonist binding, in which case only the intermediate response of the partial agonist will be observed.

Glucocorticoid antagonists are unable to promote the conformational changes in the receptors necessary for subsequent steps in the response.[594,623] In some cases, antagonist receptor complexes do not bind to the nucleus.[594] However, in other cases they do.[623–626] Relative to cortisol, compounds that have antagonist or partial agonist activity tend to have ketone, hydrogen, or other substitutions of the 11-hydroxyl group; alterations or deletions of the side chain at C-17; C-21 substitutions; reduction of the 4,5 double bond; or bulky 9-position substitutions.[591,620,621,627] Although these substitutions have been studied most extensively in animals, RU486 (Mifepristone), which contains several changes relative to cortisol, including a (*p*-dimethylamino)phenyl substitution at C-11, has a high affinity for both the glucocorticoid and progesterone receptors,[621,622,628,629] and is active as an antiglucocorticoid.[630] It has been used to treat patients with Cushing's syndrome due to ectopic ACTH secretion or adrenal carcinomas. Cortisone and prednisone are also antagonists; however, these activities are ordinarily not significant in vivo because their affinities for the glucocorticoid receptor are too low relative to their plasma concentrations in most natural or therapeutic situations.[591]

Structure-Activity Relations of Glucocorticoids: Basis for Biological Activity

The activities of a large number of synthetic and naturally occurring glucocorticoid agonists have been examined. Several factors, such as availability for receptor binding, intrinsic agonist activity, affinity, and clearance, are important. For steroids that are useful for systemic glucocorticoid therapy, two major types of differences relative to cortisol have been found. First, some compounds are more potent than cortisol because of their increased affinity for the glucocorticoid receptors and/or a decrease in their metabolic clearance rate. Second, some compounds have less mineralocorticoid activity relative to glucocorticoid activity, probably because of enhanced glucocorticoid receptor affinity relative to mineralocorticoid receptor affinity. This property results in fewer mineralocorticoid side effects.

In the circulation, affinity is the major immediate determinant of steroid activity, and the rate of clearance determines the duration of exposure to the steroid. The overall steroid effect is a product of these two variables. For example, dexamethasone is 17-fold more potent than cortisol when its effect on the suppression of cortisol secretion was extrapolated to zero time.[631] By contrast, dexamethasone was 154 times more potent than cortisol when they were evaluated after 14 h.[631] The early time estimate reflects the intrinsic activity differences between the two steroids but underrates the long-term relative potency of dexamethasone because of the differences in cortisol and dexamethasone clearance. Such considerations must be kept in mind when evaluating reports of relative potency. Prednisolone has about a twofold higher affinity for the receptor than does cortisol (Table 11-4) and is cleared more slowly[631]; its net activity is about five times that of cortisol.

Cortisol and the synthetic steroids used in glucocorticoid therapy are readily absorbed in the gut, and their potencies after oral or parental administration are similar. Uptake is a factor, however, when glucocorticoids are given topically or in "depo" injections. The extent to which variations in the distribution of steroids within body compartments affect activity has not been determined. With the exception of prednisone and cortisone, which are converted to prednisolone and cortisol, respectively, other glucocorticoids do not require metabolic conversion in vivo to be active.

Structural features that promote glucocorticoid activity confer the ability to have agonist (rather than partial agonist or antagonist) activity, enhance the steroid's affinity for the glucocorticoid receptors, and decrease the rate of metabolic inactivation.[591,627] These structural features can be considered in terms of modifications of the progesterone skeleton (substitutions conferring antagonist or partial agonist activity are discussed in the preceding section). Features associated with higher affinity include a reduced 4,5 or 1,2 double bond; a 9α-fluoro or 6α-methyl group; a C-17 side chain; hydroxyl groups at positions 11, 17, and 21; C-3 and C-20 keto groups; and the presence of certain 16- and 17-substitutions (16α- or 16β-methyl, 16,17-acetonide, etc.).

The ways in which such changes affect activity are partly understood.[591,627] Receptor binding involves hydrophobic contact between the surface of the steroid molecule and the receptor protein; removal of hydrophilic water from the steroid via hormone-receptor interaction is perhaps the major force driving the binding reaction. Thus, an increased surface area, such as with 9α-substitution, can increase the strength of binding. Affinity is also enhanced by the presence of key hydroxyl and keto groups that form hydrogen bonds with particular amino acids in the receptor. There is a critical angle between the A and B rings; 9α-substitution and the addition of a 1,2 double bond alter the AB angle to a more optimal position and increase the affinity relative to cortisol. Other substitutions, for instance, the Δ' substitution, render the molecule more resistant to metabolic degradation and decrease its clearance rate.

Actions of Glucocorticoids

The glucocorticoids are ubiquitous physiologic regulators and play a role in differentiation and development. They are essential for survival, at least to overcome certain stressful insults. Conversely, an excess of these hormones, particularly over a prolonged period, can lead to severe adverse influences. Nevertheless, glucocorticoids given in pharmacologic doses can also have useful therapeutic effects. Some effects of these steroids are observed only with glucocorticoid excess, as occurs with spontaneous Cushing's syndrome or glucocorticoid therapy.

Intermediary Metabolism

Glucocorticoids were named for their glucose-regulating properties and have extensive influences on carbohydrate, lipid, protein, and nucleic acid metabolism. Although these steroids are secondary to insulin in regulating glucose metabolism in humans, they influence blood sugar and play a protective role against glucose deprivation.[632] This latter role provides an excellent conceptual framework for considering many of the coordinated actions of the glucocorticoids on carbohydrate, lipid, protein, and nucleic acid metabolism (Fig. 11-22).

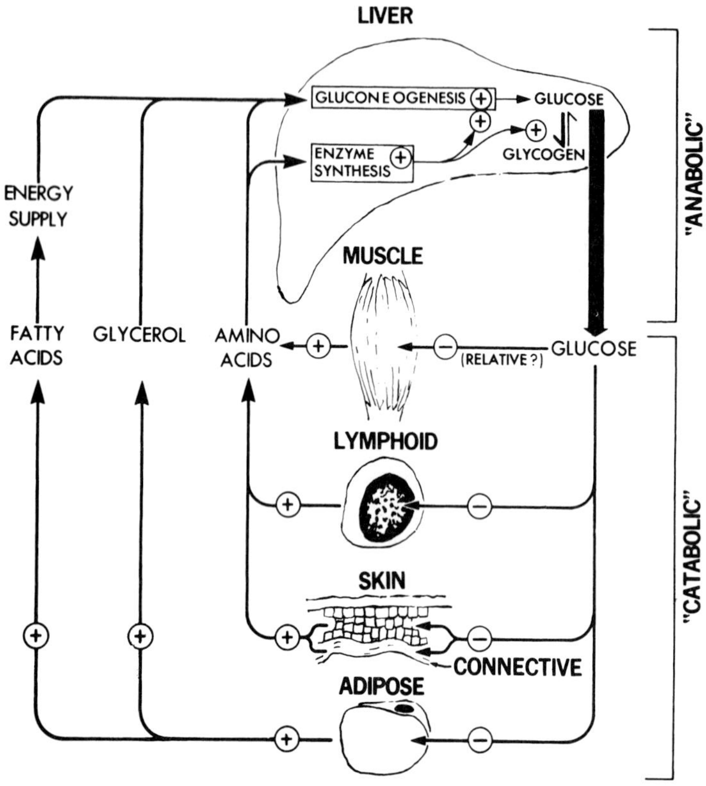

FIGURE 11-22. Glucocorticoid influences on peripheral tissues. Plus signs refer to stimulation, and minus signs to inhibitions. *(From Baxter and Rousseau.[655])*

Carbohydrate Metabolism

Glucocorticoids in excess increase hepatic glycogen and glucose production and decrease glucose uptake and utilization in peripheral tissues.[590,591,633-636] Although the relative importance of these various influences has not been clarified, they result in a tendency to hyperglycemia and decreased carbohydrate tolerance. Conversely, in glucocorticoid deficiency, there is decreased glucose production and hepatic glycogen content and an increased sensitivity to insulin that may result in hypoglycemia. The extent of these effects depends on food intake and on insulin, which opposes many glucocorticoid actions and whose secretion increases in response to steroid-mediated increases in blood glucose concentration. Thus, in a nondiabetic individual exposed to an excess of glucocorticoids, increased insulin secretion counterbalances the glucocorticoid effect so that the fasting blood sugar level, although higher on average, is usually in the normal range even though carbohydrate tolerance is impaired. In a diabetic patient with an inadequate insulin reserve, glucocorticoids in excess exacerbate the carbohydrate intolerance, resulting in an increased insulin requirement. Conversely, in an addisonian subject, feeding and a relative decrease in insulin secretion due to the lower blood sugar level blunt the tendency to hypoglycemia so that the fasting blood sugar level is commonly in the normal range.

Glucocorticoids increase glucose production by enhancing hepatic gluconeogenesis, the release of gluconeogenic substrate from peripheral tissues, and the ability of other hormones to stimulate gluconeogenesis.[634] In fed adrenalectomized animals, basal gluconeogenesis is not impaired but there is an impaired response to glucagon or catecholamines (see Chap. 18). In fasted or diabetic animals, adrenalectomy results in a net reduction in hepatic gluconeogenesis, which is reversible with cortisol administration. Thus, glucocorticoids are required to maintain gluconeogenesis in fasting and insulin deficiency but not for basal gluconeogenesis in the fed state.

It has been argued that essentially every step in the gluconeogenic pathway is increased by glucocorticoids.[633] Indeed, glucocorticoids increase total hepatic protein synthesis and increase several of the transaminases, especially alanine aminotransferase.[635,638] Glucocorticoids also increase the activity of phosphoenolpyruvate carboxykinase (PEPCK)[638] and glucose-6-phosphatase. However, the changes in PEPCK may be offset by insulin, which depresses the activity of this enzyme.[634] There is little direct information about other gluconeogenic enzymes.

Glucocorticoids also play a permissive role (discussed later) by increasing the sensitivity of the liver to the gluconeogenic actions of glucagon and the catecholamines.[591,633,634,639] For instance, the effect of glucagon or α-adrenergic stimulation on hepatic gluconeogenesis is impaired by adrenalectomy.

Several types of glucocorticoid influences result in an increased release of gluconeogenic substrate from peripheral tissues.[591,633,634,640-642] Perfused muscle from adrenalectomized rats shows a net decrease in the release of amino acids, which is reversed by glucocorticoids. Glucocorticoids decrease protein synthesis and can increase protein breakdown in several tissues, such as muscle, fat, and lymphoid, resulting in an increased release of amino acids.[591,633,634,639,641-643] In rats, the inhibition of protein synthesis can be observed in the fed and fasted states and at lower steroid doses, but an enhancement of protein breakdown is observed only in the fasted state and at higher doses.[639,641-643] Although the predominant glucocorticoid effect in muscle may be inhibition of protein synthesis,[634,639,641-643] increased proteolysis from other tissues in response to glucocorticoids may be more prominent.[634,639,641–643] These influences are accompanied by increased urinary excretion of 3-methylhistidine, nitrogen, and plasma amino acids, primarily valine, leucine, isoleucine, tyrosine, phenylalanine, and histidine.[634,639,641–643] These amino acids serve as gluconeogenic precursors, and the conversion of leucine to alanine is increased, as are plasma pyruvate levels.[643] With short exposure, many of these influences can be observed in the absence of changes in plasma insulin and glycogen concentrations.[643] With time, the secondary hyperinsulinism can attenuate the increase in total protein breakdown.[641,642] The immediate net result of glucocorticoid excess is selective increases in the levels of several amino acids[640,644]; with more prolonged exposure in the fed state, only the alanine concentration is elevated.[642] This is due to the conversion of other amino acids to alanine, which is the major gluconeogenic precursor. Glucocorticoids may also increase the amounts of amino acids available for gluconeogenesis by blocking the stimulatory effects of insulin in peripheral tissues on amino acid uptake and protein synthesis.[634]

Glucocorticoids also increase gluconeogenic substrates by increasing glycerol release from fat cells (by stimulating lipolysis) and lactate release from muscle.[634] The latter effect appears to be due to stimulation of the glycogenolytic actions of the catecholamines. The lipolysis also provides free fatty acids, which cannot themselves contribute to a net increase in gluconeogenesis but can provide energy for gluconeogenesis and spare other substrate that can be converted into glucose.

A second major effect of glucocorticoids on carbohydrate metabolism results from their inhibition of glucose uptake and metabolism in peripheral tissues (Fig. 11-23).[591,643–645] There is a direct inhibition of glucose uptake in adipose tissue,[645,646] fibroblasts,[645] certain lymphoid cells,[645,647] and fat cells.[645] In the last case, they decrease the number of glucose transporter molecules by mechanisms that require protein and RNA synthesis.[645] Even in muscle, the major site of peripheral glucose metabolism, the uptake of glucose (relative to the blood glucose concentration) may be decreased, although a direct effect on glucose uptake has not been demonstrated.[633] The decrease in glucose uptake appears to be the major early influence on carbohydrate tolerance; after cortisol infusion, the blood glucose concentration can rise with no change in glucose output (Fig. 11-21).[643,644]

FIGURE 11-23. The effect of cortisol infusion on plasma concentration and glucose kinetics in normal humans. (*From Shamoon et al.*[611])

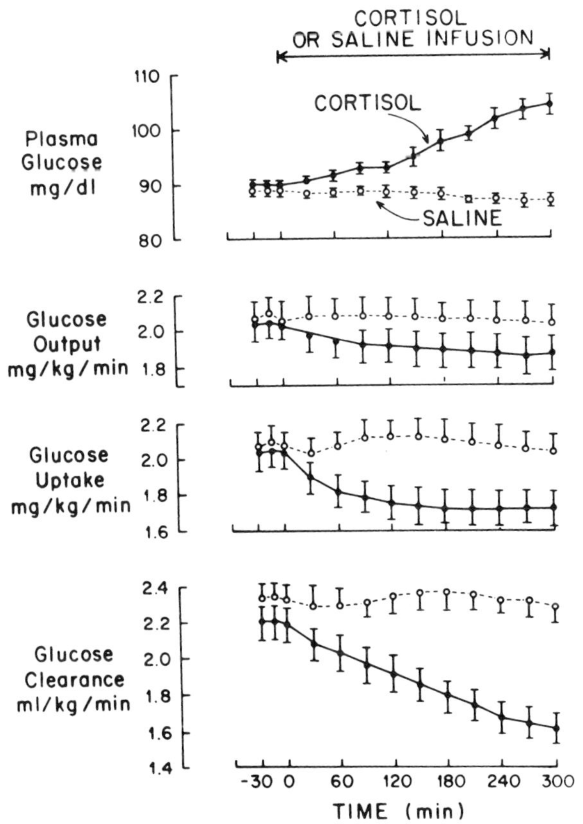

Glucocorticoids have complex effects on insulin release and action.[636] Glucocorticoid excess results in increased basal and glucose-stimulated insulin levels, and pancreatic beta cell hyperplasia occurs in the long term.[636] These effects are secondary to the glucocorticoid-induced hyperglycemia; yet, glucocorticoids have direct negative effects on the pancreatic islets whose insulin secretion is comparatively suppressed for the concurrent glucose elevations.[637] The elevated glucose and insulin levels imply that insulin resistance is present in the glucocorticoid excess states. This is due primarily to all the anti-insulin actions described earlier, which are predominantly post-insulin–receptor events.[636,648]

Glycogen Metabolism

Glucocorticoids increase glycogen deposition in the livers of both fed and fasted animals.[635] After 12 to 24 h, the glycogen content is slightly increased in muscle but not in kidney.[649] Conversely, adrenalectomy impairs hepatic glycogen synthesis; this effect is more prominent in fed than in fasted animals.[635] In this case, glucocorticoids and insulin have similar rather than opposing actions; however, the role of glucocorticoids can be perceived as protecting against long-term food deprivation by promoting glycogen storage, whereas that of insulin is more important for short-term lowering of the blood sugar level by shunting glucose into glycogen.

Glucocorticoids stimulate glycogen synthetase (UDPG-glycogen transglycosidase) by promoting its conversion from the inactive b form to the active a form[635] (Fig. 11-24). This may be a result of stimulation of glycogen synthetase phosphatase (which activates glycogen synthetase) by blocking the actions of glycogen phosphorylase a, which inhibits the phosphatase.[635] Glucocorticoids may induce a protein that inhibits the actions of phosphorylase a.[635]

A less important effect of glucocorticoids is to inhibit glycogen breakdown by the inactivation of phosphorylase a, which may occur by stimulating by unknown mechanisms its conversion to (inactive) phosphorylase b (Fig. 11-24).[635] This may occur because the phosphatase (activated by glucocorticoids) that stimulates glycogen synthetase activity (Fig. 11-24) also inactivates the enzyme that converts phosphorylase b to phosphorylase a.[635] Such an effect would favor a decrease in the amount of phosphorylase a. Glucocorticoids also stimulate glycogen production in the fetal liver.[635] In this case, in addition to the mechanisms described above, glucocorticoids may increase the amount of glycogen synthetase itself.[635]

In vivo, glucocorticoid actions on glycogen accumulation appear to be predominantly, although not exclusively, insulin-dependent, because glycogen accumulation is markedly reduced in pancreatectomized animals.[635] Glucocorticoid-stimulated increases in insulin secretion promote further glycogen accumulation.[635]

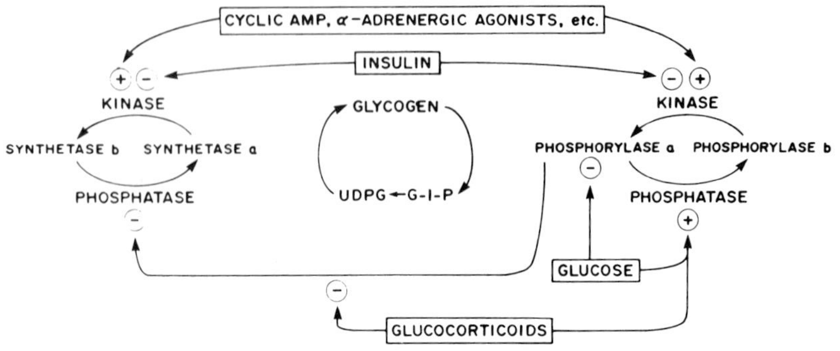

FIGURE 11-24. Actions of glucocorticoids on glycogen accumulation. The dominant effect of the steroid is to induce a factor or factors that block the inhibition by phosphorylase a of glycogen synthetase phosphatase. The steroid also decreases phosphorylase a, but this appears to be of secondary importance. Shown also are the actions of insulin, cAMP (as a mediator of glucagon action), and glucose. Plus signs refer to stimulation; minus signs refer to inhibition. UDGP = uridine diphosphoglucose; G-1-P = glucose-1-phosphate.

Lipid Metabolism

Obvious manifestations of the effects of glucocorticoids on lipid metabolism are observed in individuals with Cushing's syndrome, who have excess fat in the neck, face, and trunk and loss of fat from the extremities. Glucocorticoids also increase plasma free fatty acid, triglyceride, and cholesterol concentrations, and they increase lipolysis and hence plasma free fatty acid levels.[641,646,649] Lipolysis and free fatty acid release are increased by the glucocorticoid-induced decrease in glucose uptake and metabolism that reduces the glycerol production necessary for reesterification of fatty acids. Glucocorticoids also stimulate lipolysis by increasing the efficiency of other lipolytic factors, such as catecholamines.[646] The increase in free fatty acid release and the possible augmentation of hepatic conversion of free fatty acids to ketones by glucocorticoids cause a tendency to ketosis.[644,646] These effects are ordinarily countered by increased insulin release and glucocorticoid-stimulated gluconeogenesis. It is not known why fat is lost in some areas and increased in others. However, fat deposition in certain areas may be due to lipogenic actions (see Chap. 18) of the increased plasma insulin concentrations. This is consistent with the finding that there can be overall fat loss in diabetic patients with Cushing's syndrome.[591] Increased fat deposition may also be due to stimulation of the appetite by glucocorticoids. Fat loss may be due to direct inhibitory actions exerted on adipose tissue.[646] Thus, if different tissues vary in their relative sensitivity to glucocorticoids and insulin, there will be net fat deposition where sensitivity to insulin is dominant and fat loss where the glucocorticoid influence is dominant.

Glucocorticoids have been reported to affect the lipid content of membranes, with influences on cholesterol and sphingomyelin.[650,651] The consequences of these changes are not known, but they could influence the properties of cell membrane-localized receptors, enzymes, and other functionally important molecules.

In glucocorticoid excess states, there is an increase in very low density lipoproteins, VLDL, and LDL, but not HDL, with consequent elevations of total triglyceride and cholesterol levels.[637,652] The mechanisms for these changes are probably multifactorial, with influences on VLDL synthesis, free fatty acid production, hepatic endothelial lipase activity, and other components all possibly contributing.[652]

Protein and Nucleic Acid Metabolism

In addition to the actions of glucocorticoid-receptor complexes on the levels of particular RNAs and their protein products (discussed earlier), glucocorticoids affect protein and RNA synthesis and breakdown and/or DNA synthesis and degradation more generally in a number of tissues.[591,653,654]

The trend with protein and RNA is for glucocorticoids to stimulate synthesis in the liver, to inhibit synthesis and stimulate breakdown in many peripheral tissues, such as muscle, skin, adipose, lymphoid, and fibroblastic (Fig. 11-20); and to have a lesser general influence on brain and cardiac tissue. The general effect on DNA synthesis is inhibitory, although there are some circumstances in which DNA synthesis is stimulated, and rarely DNA breakdown can be stimulated (see later discussion). Overall, this results in net nitrogen loss in the glucocorticoid excess state.[640,643,644,653,654] This pattern may again be perceived as a general attempt by the body to provide substrate for hepatic gluconeogenesis from "less essential" tissues such as muscle and to decrease other types of substrate utilization while sparing certain critical tissues (e.g., brain and heart). However, in glucocorticoid excess states, other deleterious or beneficial effects (osteoporosis, immunosuppression, etc.) are more prominent. Many examples and more details about these effects are provided in the following sections.

Liver The liver is one of the few tissues in which there is an overall stimulatory influence of glucocorticoids on protein and RNA synthesis and in which glucocorticoids cause a slight increase in the total hepatic protein and RNA content.[591,655] Nevertheless, these effects are selective, as certain proteins (e.g., tyrosine aminotransferase and tryptophan oxygenase) are stimulated much more than are others.[591,656] The effects on other gluconeogenic enzymes and glycogen accumulation have been discussed. However, there can be inhibitory glucocorticoid actions in the liver, such as hepatic DNA synthesis.[653,654]

Muscle Glucocorticoid influences on muscle glucose and protein metabolism are important because muscle, owing to its bulk, is a major source of gluconeogenic precursors and glucose utilization. Glucocorticoids also inhibit muscle DNA and probably RNA synthesis and promote RNA breakdown.[591,633,639–642,654] These effects are partially counteracted by insulin and diet but can lead to frank muscular wasting in glucocorticoid excess states. Glucocorticoids have more pronounced influences on type 2 white glycolytic fibers than on type 1 fibers.[657] Glucocorticoids both enhance proteolysis and decrease muscle synthesis; the proteolysis is probably the more important influence and is associated with increases in certain proteolytic enzymes.[657,658]

Immune and Inflammatory Responses Glucocorticoids in excess suppress immune and inflammatory responses[591,659–674] and are used extensively to suppress excessive inflammatory or immunologic activity. These suppressive actions can also be deleterious, and infections increase in frequency and severity in spontaneous Cushing's syndrome and with corticosteroid therapy.

In contrast to the well-documented immunosuppressive and anti-inflammatory actions of corticosteroids in excess, little is known about the role of basal levels of glucocorticoids in immunologic and inflammatory responses. However, a role seems possible, as glucocorticoids can influence these responses at doses that result in steroid levels equivalent to those which occur physiologically.

The role of increased cortisol secretion during stresses such as infection is also unknown. There is evidence for immunosuppression in postsurgical patients,[663] and inflammatory reactions in these and other "stressed" patients may be blunted by the increased cortisol concentrations. It has been suggested that the increased cortisol in these circumstances may help prevent autoimmune responses to tissue antigens released by cellular injury or excessive inflammatory responses with tissue damaging potential.[663] The finding that corticosteroids can suppress autologous mixed leukocyte reactions without affecting allogenic reactions is consistent with the former role.[659,662] Nevertheless, the major role of the increased steroid levels in these circumstances may be to prevent a number of host responses recruited during the infection from becoming excessive.[665]

Many of the data on glucocorticoids and immune responses have come from animal studies. Responses vary among species; for example, the mouse, rat, and rabbit are relatively steroid-sensitive, whereas guinea pigs and humans are more steroid-resistant.[660] Nevertheless, these differences may be more quantitative than qualitative, and in various animal and human systems glucocorticoids affect nearly every step in the immunologic and inflammatory responses.[591,647,659–671,675] They affect inflammatory reactions by inhibiting (1) the production and/or activity of vasodilatory agents, (2) the movement of leukocytes to inflamed areas, and (3) the function of immunocompetent cells at the site of inflammation. The third effect includes actions on antigen processing by macrophages, specific B- and T-cell functions, antibody production and clearance, mobilization and functioning of polymorphonuclear and mononuclear cells, the liberation and actions of effector substances (prostaglandins, leukotrienes, cytokines, chemokines, kinins, proteases such as plasminogen activator, etc.) at the site of cellular injury, and the fibroblastic proliferative response. Interestingly, glucocorticoids do not cause permanent damage to the immunologic system. Thus, the precursor cells are steroid-resistant. This underscores the point that different stages in the response vary markedly in their sensitivity to glucocorticoids. The particular actions that are the most important in the observed responses are commonly unclear. In general, it appears that glucocorticoids affect human cellular processes more than humoral processes, leukocyte distribution within body compartments more than function, and macrophages more than polymorphonuclear leukocytes and are more effective if given before or concurrently with a challenge rather than later.

Effects on Vasoactive and Other Inflammatory Agents Early inflammatory changes at a site of injury result in enhanced vascular permeability and edema. These changes are mediated by a variety of inflammatory agents, including prostaglandins (PG), kinins, histamine, leukotrienes, and platelet activating factor.[665–675]

Arachidonic acid is the precursor of a number of molecules collectively called eicosanoids.[665–675] It is derived directly from the actions of phospholipase A_2 or indirectly from phospholipase C. Arachidonic acid can then be converted into prostaglandins, thromboxanes, hydroperoxyeicosatetraenoic acids (HPETE), hydroxyeicosatetraenoic acids (HETE), and leukotrienes.[667–669] A number of these compounds are relevant in inflammatory reactions, and their role is further suggested by the fact that certain nonsteroidal anti-inflammatory agents block the production of some of these substances.[667,668]

Glucocorticoids inhibit PG synthesis in a variety of cell types,[665–676] although this does not occur in all cases, and in certain conditions total prostanoid levels or excretion may not be affected.[664–676] These actions of glucocorticoids in inhibiting production and effects of phospholipase A_2 result in a more general inhibition of eicosanoid production than is the case with indomethacin and aspirin, and they may help explain the greater anti-inflammatory actions of glucocorticoids in comparison to these other molecules. Glucocorticoids block the actions of bradykinin, which may also regulate PG synthesis.[668] They also block the release of histamine, serotonin, and leukotrienes.[668]

Leukocyte Movement Glucocorticoid administration to human subjects causes a circulating lymphocytopenia, monocytopenia, and eosinopenia (Table 11-6).[659,677,678] Conversely, these cell types are increased in adrenal insufficiency.[591] The actions on lymphocytes and monocytes are maximal within 4 to 6 h and return to normal by 24 to 48 h but persist with continued steroid administration.[659,668,678] These effects are due to a redistribution of cells, with cells moving out of the circulation and into other body compartments, such as bone marrow, spleen, lymph nodes, and thoracic duct.[659,677] In other species, circulating lymphoid cells are also killed by glucocorticoids, but this appears not to be the case with humans.[591,659,660] Although there are effects on both T (thymus-derived) and B (marrow-derived) lymphocytes, the influence is much greater on the T lymphocytes, especially those with an Fc receptor for IgM (TM) compared with those with a receptor for IgG (TG).[659]

Glucocorticoid administration also increases (maximally after 4 to 6 h) the blood polymorphonuclear leukocyte concentration.[591,659,668] This is due to an accelerated release of neutrophils

TABLE 11-6. Glucocorticoid Effects on Leukocyte Movements in Humans

1. Lymphocytes
   a. Circulating lymphocytopenia caused by redistribution of cells to other lymphoid compartments
   b. Depletion of recirculating lymphocytes
   c. Selective depletion of T lymphocytes (especially T_M subset) more than B lymphocytes
2. Monocyte-macrophages
   a. Circulating monocytopenia, probably caused by redistribution
   b. Inhibition of accumulation of monocyte-macrophages at inflammatory sites
3. Neutrophils
   a. Circulating neutrophilia
   b. Accelerated release of neutrophils from the bone marrow
   c. Blocked accumulation of neutrophils at inflammatory sites, probably caused by reduced adherence
4. Eosinophils
   a. Circulating eosinopenia, probably caused by redistribution and eosinophil apoptosis
   b. Decreased migration of eosinophils into immediate hypersensitivity skin test sites

Source: Modified from Parrillo and Fauci.[659]

from the bone marrow, an increase in the half-life of circulating neutrophils, and reduced neutrophil egress from the blood.[659]

Glucocorticoids decrease markedly the number of polymorphonuclear leukocytes, monocyte-macrophages, and lymphocytes that accumulate at inflammatory sites; the effect is evident by 2 h.[591,660,663,668] Although decreases are ordinarily similar for both monocytes and polymorphonuclear leukocytes, the effects on mononuclear cells appear to be longer-lived. These actions may be due in part to the fact that glucocorticoids can inhibit chemotactic and other factors, such as plasminogen activator,[668] that affect inflammatory cell accumulation at sites of injury, and may be a major mechanism of the anti-inflammatory actions of the glucocorticoids.[659] Blood basophils are elevated in Addison's disease and depressed in Cushing's disease or with glucocorticoid therapy.[591] Presumably, the same mechanisms that regulate the levels of eosinophils are operative here.

Leukocyte Function Glucocorticoids affect lymphocyte function, and in some animals the steroids at high doses kill lymphocytes and cause involution of lymphoid tissues.[591,647] There are marked variations in the sensitivity of lymphoid cell subpopulations; for instance, in the mouse thymus, about 95 percent of the cells are killed, whereas the remaining 5 percent are steroid-resistant.[591,647] This 5 percent must contain the precursor cells for immunologic responses, as steroid treatment does not abolish certain thymic-dependent responses. Although most human lymphocytes are not killed by glucocorticoids, in some cases (e.g., cells of acute lymphocytic leukemia of childhood) there can be lymphoid cell killing.[679] The actions of glucocorticoids on lymphocytes involve stimulation (or blockade) of specific functions; even the killing activity appears to involve specific programming and is associated with an early response in which a discrete set of proteins is induced.[680] One or a few of these ultimately result in cell killing, possibly through direct or indirect actions that induce or enhance the actions of a DNase that digests the cell's DNA.[681]

A number of specific lymphocyte functions are blocked by the steroids without cell death (Table 11-7),[591,647,659,660,665,668] and there are variations in sensitivity. For instance, the lymphocyte-proliferative response to some but not other antigens can be suppressed.[659] The proliferative responses to antigens are more readily suppressed than are those to mitogens.[659] Nevertheless, blockage of some T cell mitogenic responses has been observed; this may be due to steroid actions that block the release of T-cell growth factor (interleukin 2).[665,668] This block is secondary to decreased leukotriene B_4 production resulting from the steroid-mediated inhibition of phospholipase A_2.[666] This action may help explain why glucocorticoids are more effective when given early in an immunologic response than they are later, because interleukin 2 is important for clonal expansion of cells early on but not later.[665,668] Glucocorticoids also alter macrophage functions (see later discussion) that affect T-cell function. They suppress T-lymphocyte production of interferon-γ and interleukin 12 and they inhibit natural killer cell activity.[665,668] Whereas glucocorticoids generally do not suppress antibody-dependent cell-mediated cytotoxicity of human cells, they can suppress spontaneous toxicity and cutaneous delayed hypersensitivity.[659]

TABLE 11-7. Immunologic Mediators Whose Production and/or Actions Can Be Blocked by Glucocorticoids

Bradykinin
Collagenase and other proteases
Colony-stimulating factor
Eicosanoids (prostaglandins, leukotrienes, etc.) and platelet activating factor
Histamine
γ-Interferon
Interleukins 1, 2, 6, 12
Nitric oxide
Plasminogen activator
Tumor necrosis factor α and β

Note: The inhibitions are not always observed in all tissues.

Overall, glucocorticoid effects on B-cell functions are very modest. High-dose corticosteroid therapy causes a small decrease in immunoglobulin levels as a result of both decreased synthesis and increased catabolism,[682] and anamnestic antibody responses to specific antigens ordinarily are not affected by glucocorticoids.[659] In vitro, glucocorticoids can in some cases even stimulate immunoglobulin production by cultures of B and T lymphocytes.[683] However, immunoglobulin production by B cells results from a series of steps involving early activation, later B-cell growth factor–mediated proliferation, and final differentiation to the immunoglobulin-producing state. These steps are affected by suppressor cell and helper cell functions and can be suppressed by glucocorticoids.[591,659,660,668] Studied in vitro, glucocorticoids affect substantially the early activation, have a lesser effect on the B-cell growth factor response, and do not affect the final step.[684] Because of varying sensitivities and complex accessory cell effects on B- and/or T-cell function, it is possible to observe a variety of effects, either stimulatory or inhibitory. Inhibition of suppressor cell function may explain why in sarcoidosis with anergy (that may be due in part to increased suppressor activity), glucocorticoids may increase immune responsiveness.[661]

Macrophage functions are relatively sensitive to glucocorticoid inhibitory actions.[659] Glucocorticoids induce a monocytopenia, suppress committed marrow monocyte-forming stem cells, and block the differentiation of monocytes into macrophages.[685] This may explain the effectiveness of glucocorticoids in treating many granulomatous diseases, as the monocyte is felt to be important in granuloma formation.[659] By blocking the production of interferon-γ, glucocorticoids can also decrease the levels of Fc receptors (that bind the Fc portion of immunoglobulin) on monocytes and macrophages[667]; these receptors facilitate the phagocytosis of particulate antigens and other functions of the cells in the inflammatory responses. Steroids can block the ability of the monocytes to bind to antibody-coated cells,[659] elicit bactericidal activity and cytotoxicity,[659] and release neutral proteases, including collagenase, elastase, and plasminogen activator,[668] that participate in the immunologic and inflammatory responses. Glucocorticoids suppress macrophage production of interleukin 1, which is involved in T-cell mitogenesis,[668] and of chemokines that prevent the exit of macrophages from inflammatory sites.[668] They block the production of interferon-γ and TNFα by T cells and their actions on macrophages.[665] However, glucocorticoid actions are not always inhibitory: They can increase the expression of mannose receptors in macrophages, and this has an anti-inflammatory effect by enhancing the uptake and internalization of lysosomal enzymes[671] and stimulate somatostatin secretion by peripheral nerves which also has anti-inflammatory activity.[672,673]

Actions of glucocorticoids on human neutrophil functions other than regulating their trafficking are less definite. Suppression of functions such as phagocytosis, chemotaxis, and bactericidal activity has been elicited at steroid concentrations that rarely, if ever, are achieved in vivo.[659]

Erythroid Cells and Thrombocytes A mild polycythemia frequently occurs in Cushing's syndrome, and there may be normochromic normocytic anemia in Addison's disease.[591] Glucocorticoids may acutely promote a rise in thrombocytes, but thrombocytopenia has also been reported after long-term administration.[591] The mechanisms for these influences are not known.

Fibroblastic and Epithelial Tissues The actions of glucocorticoids on fibroblastic tissues constitute a major drawback to their long-term use in therapy.[591,655,686–688] These actions probably contribute to the thinning of the bone matrix and osteoporosis. Glucocorticoids inhibit both specific matrix cell activities such as collagen and glycosaminoglycan formation and overall fibroblast function.[686–691] Inhibitory actions on fibroblasts also lead to easy bruising, poor wound healing, and a tendency to wound dehiscence after surgery. Glucocorticoids do not appear to alter the epithelialization of a wound, except indirectly through inhibition of the fibrous scar that serves as a scaffolding for the cells, but they can inhibit epidermal epithelial cell proliferation in other circumstances; this action is useful in the treatment of psoriasis.[692]

Glucocorticoid effects on fibroblast and epithelial cells can be observed in isolated cells in culture. Both stimulation and inhibition of cellular functions have been reported.[686,693] Inhibitory effects lead to decreased uptake and metabolism of glucose, decreased protein and RNA synthesis, and inhibition of DNA synthesis.[694] Glucocorticoids can also affect collagen, fibronectin, and glycosaminoglycan formation.[689–691,693] These effects can also be specific and are observed in the absence of major influences on most cellular functions. The effects on collagen involve a selective decrease in collagen mRNA, resulting in decreased collagen synthesis.[688] Glucocorticoids can also affect other enzymes involved in collagen metabolism, such as collagen galactosyltransferase and hydroxylase.[688] By contrast, stimulatory effects result in increased cell replication and incorporation of thymidine into DNA.[694] These seemingly paradoxic responses may be due to the fact that glucocorticoids can affect the actions or production of various growth factors either positively or negatively.[695] In humans, the result is predominantly inhibitory.

Cardiovascular System and Fluid and Electrolyte Balance

Glucocorticoids affect the heart, vasculature, regulators of blood pressure, water excretion, and electrolyte balance. Some of these actions are direct; others involve mineralocorticoid-like actions.

FIGURE 11-25. Effect of cortisol (hydrocortisone) on blood pressure in a patient with Addison's disease. The blood pressure had not responded to fluid replacement and other supportive measures. Cortisol was given when the diagnosis of adrenocortical insufficiency was suspected. (*From Baxter.*[591])

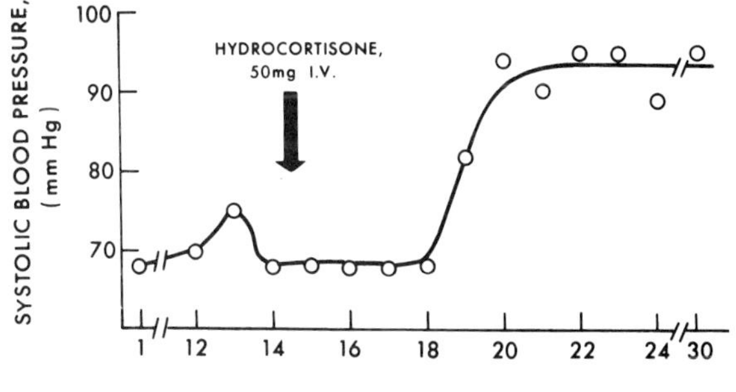

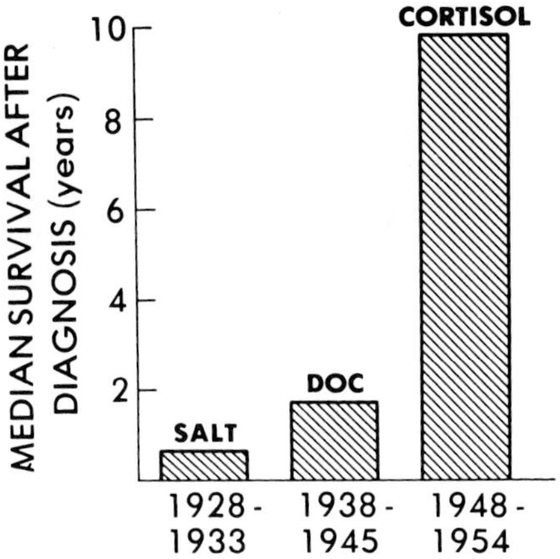

FIGURE 11-26. Median duration of survival of individual with Addison's syndrome in years after the diagnosis in relation to therapeutic advances. The specific time periods chosen were selected to avoid having patients fall into overlapping therapy categories. However, the survival in the post-cortisol era is actually greater than indicated, since most of the individuals in this group were still alive in 1963, when the data were collected, and it is not clear that all the individuals who died actually received cortisol. (*From Baxter and Rousseau*[655] *based on data from Dunlop.*[792])

In glucocorticoid-deficient states, there is hypotension with decreased responsiveness to pressor stimuli[696,697] and decreased cardiac output[696]; stresses such as surgery, infection, and trauma can precipitate an adrenal crisis with shock. This is only partly due to a loss of the mineralocorticoid functions of the adrenal steroids. However, the importance of glucocorticoids in the maintenance of normal cardiovascular function is emphasized by the finding that the hypotension seen in patients with adrenal insufficiency crisis is not reversed by correction of volume or sodium losses or by the administration of mineralocorticoids, such as DOC, that do not have glucocorticoid activity (Figs. 11-25 and 11-26).

Conversely, in glucocorticoid excess states there is hypertension, which occurs in the majority of patients with spontaneous Cushing's syndrome,[697] and enhanced responsiveness to pressors such as angiotensin II and norepinephrine.[696,697] The hypertension in spontaneous Cushing's syndrome is not accompanied by depressed plasma renin levels most likely because glucocorticoids stimulate angiotensinogen production.[697]

The mechanisms of these vascular effects are complex and multifactorial. Glucocorticoids can have direct actions on the heart and enhance the activities of vasoactive substances (as described later under synergistic and antagonistic interrelations between glucocorticoids and other hormones). They may have direct actions on vascular smooth muscle[699,700] and endothelial cells.[701] Glucocorticoids can also suppress the synthesis and actions of vasodilator and cardiac-suppressant substances that are produced in excess in adrenal insufficiency and/or in response to stress. (The role of PGs in this respect is discussed later, but this issue is addressed more comprehensively in the glucocorticoids and stress section.) Glucocorticoids can directly affect other components involved in blood pressure control such as the renin-angiotensin system.

The heart is a direct glucocorticoid target, and in isolated preparations glucocorticoids can induce cardiac protein synthesis, increase the coupling between cardiac beta-adrenergic receptors and adenylate cyclase, and have positive inotropic influences and effects on the left ventricular work index.[702] Glucocorticoids have also been reported to induce cardiac ultrastructural damage.[703] Further, they probably have mineralocorticoid-independent effects on cardiac output and stroke volume.[704]

The ability of glucocorticoids to decrease vasodilatory substances, including PGs, probably contributes to these vascular responses,[664] and although controversial[674] (see also immunologic and inflammatory responses earlier), decreased urinary PGE_2 production has been reported in glucocorticoid excess.[697] In glucocorticoid-induced hypertension in the rat, the basal and angiotensin II–stimulated release of PGE_2 from the renal medulla is diminished even though plasma and urinary PGE_2 concentrations are increased.[704] PGE_2 is a potent vasodilator and is the principal product of arachidonic acid in arteries and veins. Its production is stimulated by angiotensin II and norepinephrine.[705] Thus, glucocorticoid inhibition of the production of PGE_2 could contribute significantly to the increased vascular reactivity and blood pressure that occur in glucocorticoid excess states.[705] Conversely, overproduction of PGE_2 could result in decreased vascular reactivity and hypotension in an addisonian patient. PGE_2 also causes tachycardia, and excess PGE_2 could contribute to the presence of this sign in an addisonian individual.[705] It has been suggested that glucocorticoids stimulate the ability of mitochondria to retain calcium and thus improve vascular responses by enhancing ATP generation.[706]

Glucocorticoids can increase the levels of prorenin and renin substrate and, in isolated cells,[707] the activity of angiotensin-converting enzyme.[708] Whereas plasma renin levels are generally in the normal to high normal range in glucocorticoid excess states, this level of elevation is inappropriate in the face of hypertension.[697] Also, the hypertension in Cushing's syndrome is responsive to the administration of inhibitors of converting enzymes.[697,709] Conversely, angiotensin II generation is impaired in adrenal insufficiency in the face of elevated renin and converting enzyme levels, possibly as a result of decreased angiotensinogen, and this could contribute to the relative refractoriness of addisonian shock to therapy.[708,710]

Although glucocorticoids can affect salt and water excretion by binding to mineralocorticoid receptors, they also have other actions that are not elicited through mineralocorticoid receptors. They increase the glomerular filtration rate (GFR),[711,712] most likely due to an increase in cardiac output and increased peripheral vascular resistance.[713] Glucocorticoids can increase the levels of cardiac ANP and its mRNA,[476] and this can increase GFR. The increase in GFR can enhance the excretion of salt and water, and steroids such as dexamethasone, with much greater glucocorticoid than mineralocorticoid activity, sometimes produce natriuresis rather than sodium retention.[711,712] Glucocorticoids increase Na^+,K^+-ATPase activity in the renal outer medullary tubules,[714] erythrocytes,[715] and colon[716] and prekallikrein in the urine and on the basal membrane of distal tubular cells.[717] Although the physiologic role of these actions has not been established, they imply that glucocorticoids can have direct effects on renal hemodynamics and/or salt excretion.

Glucocorticoid deficiency results in a decreased ability to excrete water.[718] This effect is probably due both to the decreased GFR and to the elevated levels of vasopressin as a result of relative hypovolemia (decreased cardiac output and peripheral vascular resistance).[718,719] In fact, water intoxication can occur rarely in panhypopituitarism with glucocorticoid but not mineralocorticoid deficiency.[718]

Glucocorticoids also affect potassium balance.[711,712,720,721] At higher concentrations, steroids such as cortisol can produce hypokalemia through mineralocorticoid actions. However, their major effect is to produce a transient kaliuresis by increasing urine flow through increases in GRF and, possibly, protein catabolism with release of intracellular K^+. However, the plasma potassium concentration is usually normal or only slightly decreased.

Glucocorticoids can increase renal acid output. Thus, in glucocorticoid excess there is a tendency to alkalosis and in glucocorticoid deficiency there is a tendency to acidosis. These effects occur with minimal influences on urinary pH; they are due to stimulation of excretion of buffer as phosphate and ammonia by blocking tubular reabsorption of phosphate and increasing the production of ammonia.[722,723] The latter may occur as a result of a stimulation of Na^+-H^+ exchange in the proximal tubule brush border, which results in ammonia trapping.[722]

Bone and Calcium Metabolism

Glucocorticoids affect bone and calcium dynamics in a variety of ways. In Addison's disease, mild hypercalcemia can occur,[724–726] but glucocorticoid excess does not usually result in lower serum Ca^{2+} levels.[727] Serum phosphate levels are lowered and urinary Ca^{2+} and phosphorus concentrations are elevated in glucocorticoid excess states.[727] Glucocorticoid excess ultimately leads to osteoporosis, a major limitation to their long-term use. Several independent actions contribute to these effects.

Glucocorticoids partly block intestinal calcium absorption (Chap. 22).[728,729] This is a direct effect on the gut that is more prominent in the duodenum and jejunum.[730,731] Glucocorticoids apparently do not block vitamin D action in the intestine[730] and do not decrease vitamin D metabolite levels; but do increase renal vitamin D 1α-hydroxylase activity.[728,729,732] Earlier reports suggested that glucocorticoids promote a redistribution of calcium from extracellular into intracellular compartments,[706,733,734] but the significance of this is not known.

Glucocorticoids decrease renal reabsorption of calcium and phosphate and in excess cause hypercalciuria and renal calculi.[687,727,735] Hypercalciuria is a consistent effect and a major contributor to the negative calcium balance.[727,734] The glucocorticoid-induced tendency to hypocalcemia induces a secondary rise in parathyroid hormone (PTH).[687,727,736] There may also be a direct increase of PTH release[727,736]; this action explains why glucocorticoids can increase both serum calcium and PTH levels in primary hyperparathyroidism.[736] However, glucocorticoids cause hypocalcemia in parathyroidectomized animals maintained on a constant dose of PTH and are necessary for the induction of hypocalcemia in animals by thyroparathyroidectomy.[731]

Shortly after glucocorticoid administration, there is enhanced bone accretion, but with continued administration, inhibition is the predominant effect.[687] The inhibitory effects on accretion are probably due to decreased osteoblastic activity and collagen formation; inhibition of osteoblast cell proliferation and synthesis of protein, RNA, collagen, and hyaluronate has been demonstrated in vitro.[687,732,734,737] Decreased bone synthesis in glucocorticoid excess states is probably also reflected by lower blood osteocalcin (bone Gla-protein) levels.[738] Glucocorticoid excess is associated with decreased osteoclastic activity and products related to osteolysis such as the collagen N-telopeptide and pyrinidinium crosslinks.[739]

These collective actions are summarized in Fig. 11-27. The decreased calcium absorption by the gut and increased urinary calcium and phosphate loss lead to a net negative calcium balance and a tendency to hypocalcemia and hypophosphatemia. This,

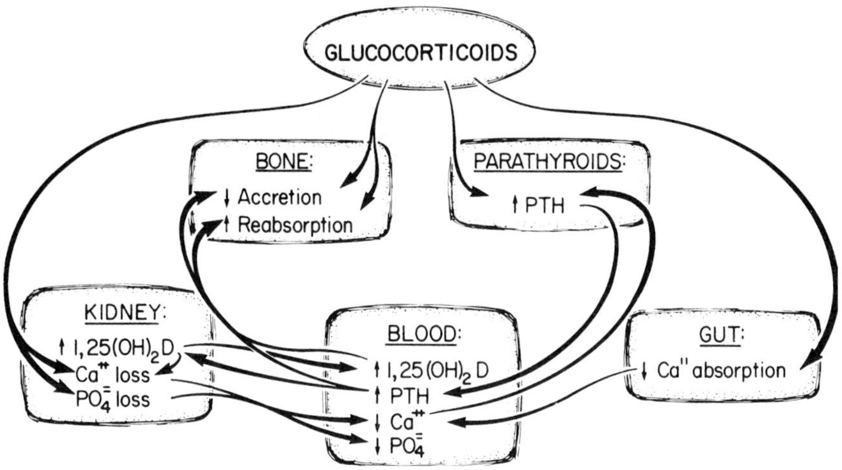

FIGURE 11-27. Effect of glucocorticoids on bone and calcium dynamics. See text.

plus direct steroid actions on the parathyroid gland, results in increased PTH release that in turn results in increased 1α,25-$(OH)_2D_3$ formation. The increased PTH and 1α,25-$(OH)_2D_3$ blunt the hypocalcemic response but also, in combination with direct glucocorticoid effects, decrease bone accretion, which even in the presence of decreased bone resorption results in an overall loss of bone mineral.[740–744]

Central Nervous System

Glucocorticoids affect behavior, mood, neural activity, and a number of specific biochemical processes.[745,746] Glucocorticoids can penetrate the blood–brain barrier; their ability to do this is inversely proportional to their polarity, which is largely dependent on the number of hydroxyl groups.[747] They can also regulate the permeability of the blood–brain barrier to other substances and are used for therapy to reduce brain edema[748]; conversely, pseudotumor cerebri is rarely associated with glucocorticoid therapy.[720]

Mood changes (and rarely psychosis) are observed with both glucocorticoid excess and glucocorticoid deficiency.[745,746] Patients receiving glucocorticoid therapy may initially have a feeling of well-being.[720,749,750] By contrast, patients with spontaneous Cushing's syndrome are commonly depressed at the time of diagnosis.[720] Patients with Addison's disease tend to be depressed, fatigued, negativistic, irritable, reclusive, and apathetic.[749] Several types of psychoses have been reported (particularly in glucocorticoid excess states); these responses frequently were not predicted by the patient's prior psychiatric history or personality traits. Patients with Addison's disease have anorexia,[750] whereas glucocorticoid excess stimulates the appetite.[720,749,750] In addition, high doses of glucocorticoids affect sleep in a major fashion: changed sleep is characterized by increased wakefulness, decreased slow wave sleep, and reducted rapid eye movement (REM) sleep with an increased latency to the first REM episode.[751]

In depressive syndromes there can be excessive glucocorticoid production with blunted circadian rhythm and a decreased ability of glucocorticoids to suppress the hypothalamic-adrenal-pituitary axis.[752,753] These abnormalities occur commonly in unipolar depression and occur particularly frequently in delusional depression.[753] They also occur in schizoaffective disorders, catatonia, borderline character disorders, chronic pain syndromes, and bulimia, but are uncommon in mania.[753] The abnormalities usually abate with clinical improvement; failure to do so is correlated with a high rate of relapse. The contribution of glucocorticoid excess to these problems and the mechanisms of its development are not understood.

Addisonian subjects can have increased sensitivity to a variety of sensory stimuli, including sound and taste, and impaired judgment and ability to discriminate sensory input.[745,749,754] In animals, bilateral adrenalectomy attenuates the circadian variations in paradoxic sleep.[745] Adrenal steroids facilitate and help consolidate addictive behaviors and potentiate anxiety behaviors. Glucocorticoids regulate a variety of developmental and other events in the brain.[746] In excess, they can have detrimental effects on brain development in animals. They regulate the catecholamine biosynthetic pathway, transsynaptic induction, the actions of nerve growth factor and epidermal growth factor on brain cells, the development of cholinergic ganglionic properties, glutamine synthetase, α-glycerophosphate dehydrogenase, myelination, γ-aminobutyric acid, and a neuron-specific phosphoprotein, protein 1.[746,756] They can affect brain cell electric activity and the EEG.[745,751] Most of these effects have been elicited at very high steroid concentrations; therefore, their importance is not understood. By contrast, certain ACTH-related peptides may have contrasting effects.[755]

Whereas most of these actions on the CNS are probably mediated by the glucocorticoid receptors, as described later, some may be mediated through mineralocorticoid receptors. In the brain, cortisol can have ready access to the receptor and in fact may keep it relatively saturated even under nonstimulated conditions.[608,609]

Adrenal Medulla

The adrenal cortex surrounds and is contiguous with the adrenal medulla, which is also involved in stress responses. The adrenal medulla receives adrenocortical venous effluent and thus is exposed to much higher cortisol concentrations than are other tissues.[746] Glucocorticoids affect adrenal chromaffin cell phenotypic characteristics and the catecholamine biosynthetic pathway.[746] In the latter, they regulate phenylethanolamine *N*-methyl transferase (PNMT), tyrosine hydroxylase, and dopamine β-hydroxylase activities.[746,757] The effects are most prominent on PNMT, which catalyzes the formation of epinephrine. Thus, resting and exercise-stimulated epinephrine levels are reduced in ACTH deficiency states.[758] Glucocorticoids can also increase adrenal medullary proenkephalin.[759] Conversely, adenomedullary products, such as CRH, POMC-derived peptides, and NPY, all under the control of the splachnic nerve, influence adrenocortical function, augmenting the sensitivity of adrenocortical cells to ACTH.[355]

Eye

Glucocorticoids in excess can increase the intraocular pressure in certain susceptible individuals, particularly patients with primary open-angle glaucoma.[591,760] This appears to be due to a glucocorticoid effect on the aqueous outflow, perhaps through actions on the trabecular meshwork.[760] The role of the endogenous glucocorticoids in determining intraocular pressure in normal individuals is not known, but the intraocular pressure tends to show a circadian variation that parallels, with about a 3-h lag, the overall fluctuations in plasma cortisol,[760] and an increase in intraocular pressure can be observed in ocular hypertensive patients about 3 h after glucocorticoid administration.[760] Glucocorticoid therapy can stimulate cataract formation after long-term high-dose therapy.[760] Interestingly, this may be due to covalent linkage of the steroid molecules to the lens crystalline proteins.[761] Glucocorticoids decrease the absorption of topical antibiotics, and therapy can result in nonspecific keratitis, refractive changes, papilledema due to intracranial hypertension, limitation of ocular movement, and changes in the aqueous and vitreous compositions.[761]

Gastrointestinal Tract

In animals, glucocorticoids at high doses inhibit DNA synthesis in gastric but not jejunal mucosa,[654] increase acid secretion in response to stimuli such as histamine,[591] and increase the incidence of gastric ulceration.[591] In humans, prolonged steroid treatment may increase acid output slightly.[762] Although the issue has been controversial,[763] the most recent data suggest that glucocorticoids in high doses do not result in an increased incidence of peptic ulcers, except in patients who are concomitantly receiving nonsteroidal anti-inflammatory agents.[764] In glucocorticoid-deficient states there can be nausea and vomiting, fever, and arthralgias and myalgias, all manifestations of the sickness syndrome observed in inflammatory states. Inflammatory cytokines are elevated in glucocorticoid-deficiency, providing a potentially causative mechanism for these manifestations.[765,766]

Growth and Development

Glucocorticoids in excess inhibit linear growth and final stature; this limits their prolonged use in children.[653,654,767] These steroids also inhibit skeletal maturation; the result is that some growth potential is maintained during and after therapy, and there can be further growth (sometimes with a growth spurt) after its withdrawal.

Glucocorticoids also inhibit growth (and cell division) in a number of individual tissues.[653,654] The effects on lymphoid, fibroblastic, epithelial, and bone cells have already been discussed. These actions are useful in steroid therapy but can also be detrimental. There are variations in sensitivity; in a growing rat, for instance, liver, heart, muscle, and kidney are more sensitive than gastric and jejunal mucosa, spleen, brain, and testis.[654]

In vitro, glucocorticoids can either stimulate or inhibit cell division of a large number of cell types.[653,654,656–658,679,688,694,695] Stimulation may occur by a steroid-induced augmentation of the actions of growth factors such as fibroblast growth factor[768] and IGF-I,[769] and glucocorticoids can also increase the levels of IGF-I receptors.[770] Conversely, inhibition could be due to actions of the steroid in blocking growth factor (e.g., PG)[695] production and/or action; it could be due to other inhibitory actions of the glucocorticoids on the cell (discussed previously in the protein and nucleic acid metabolism and carbohydrate metabolism sections).[591,649,653,660,679] The steroid-induced increase in fibronectin biosynthesis could also inhibit replication, as this extracellular glycoprotein may stimulate cell adhesion, which may inhibit cell replication.[693]

The mechanisms of inhibition of growth in the intact organism are not known.[355,653,654,767,772] They may in part be due to inhibitory influences on bone cells; for instance, chondrocyte proliferation can be inhibited by steroids. Glucocorticoids also inhibit growth hormone production, but this action probably does not explain all the growth-inhibiting effects, as they can be overcome by the administration of quite high doses of growth hormone. Although glucocorticoids do not decrease levels of IGF-I in plasma, they decrease the sensitivity of tissues to this hormone.

It is not known whether glucocorticoids at physiologic concentrations play a role in regulating growth. In animals, physiologically equivalent concentrations of glucocorticoids inhibit new cell accretion in several growing tissues.[653,767] It has also been reported that adrenalectomy increases the mitotic index in skin.[654]

Glucocorticoids accelerate developmental events in various species in several fetal and postnatal differentiating tissues, including lung (induce surfactant), liver (induce enzymes of intermediary metabolism), intestine (induce digestive enzymes), pancreas (regulate the production of insulin and induce digestive enzymes), stomach (induce pepsinogen), skin (induce epidermal proteins), retina (induce glutamine synthetase), brain (induce Na^+, K^+-ATPase), adrenal medulla (induce PNMT), placenta (induce enzymes for estrogen synthesis), mammary gland, and heart.[773] The endogenous glucocorticoids may act similarly in the developing fetus because plasma corticosteroid levels increase before term delivery, and this is associated with normal maturation of the tissues. However, any potential role of glucocorticoids in human fetal development must be minor, as anencephalic fetuses, fetuses with adrenal hypoplasia, and those born with the most severe defects in adrenal steroid synthesis, are nonetheless born at the correct stage of pregnancy and without pulmonary or hepatic metabolic disorders.[352]

Sensitivity to glucocorticoids varies during development, and various proteins may be regulated only at certain stages.[773] For instance, corticosteroids regulate surfactant synthesis in the fetal lung but not in the adult. In some instances (e.g., induction of intestinal sucrase activity) the steroid-induced changes are reversible, whereas in other instances (e.g., induction of glutamine synthetase in neural retina) the enzyme does not return to pretreatment levels after the withdrawal of the steroid.

Little is known about the importance of these developmental influences in children, but glucocorticoid effects on the fetus may prepare it for extrauterine existence.[352] For instance, the actions on hepatic enzymes and the pancreatic islets may assist in regulating glucose homeostasis, the effects on the adrenal medulla could aid in responsiveness to stress, and the surfactant-inducing actions permit the lung to carry out gas exchange.[773] Some of these functions can be induced by glucocorticoids before the normal increase in steroid levels that precedes delivery. For example, treatment of a mother in spontaneous premature labor increases fetal surfactant levels and reduces the incidence and/or severity of the respiratory distress syndrome (hyaline membrane disease) associated with premature birth.

Production and Clearance of Other Hormones

Glucocorticoids can affect the production and/or clearance of other classes of hormones. In the liver, these glucocorticoids induce a specific cytochrome P450 that could participate in oxidative reactions involving a variety of drugs, steroids, bile acids, and other compounds.[774] The influences on ACTH, angiotensin II, vasopressin, IGF-I growth hormone, insulin, glucagon, PTH, vitamin D, epinephrine, and PGs have been mentioned. Glucocorticoids in excess inhibit pancreatic polypeptide production,[775] basal and metoclopramide-stimulated prolactin release,[775] and basal and stimulated gastrin secretion.[775] They can stimulate the production of calcitonin and related peptides.[776]

Glucocorticoids affect thyroid stimulating hormone (TSH) release and thyroxine (T_4) metabolism. In glucocorticoid excess states, there is a blunted TSH response to thyrotropin releasing hormone (TRH).[777] Plasma T_4 concentrations are generally in the low-normal range in glucocorticoid excess states, but triiodothyronine (T_3) levels can be subnormal[777] because of decreased conversion of T_4 to T_3 and increased conversion of T_4 to reverse T_3.[778] Glucocorticoids also increase the thyroid hormone-binding prealbumin concentration.[778]

Reproductive Function

The effects of glucocorticoids on reproductive function are predominantly inhibitory, are observed at high glucocorticoid levels, and may be part of an overall mechanism that delays reproductive function in times of stress. In men, glucocorticoid therapy and spontaneous Cushing's syndrome decrease the plasma testosterone concentration.[779,780] This is probably due both to an inhibition of LH release and to direct actions on the testis.[780,781] In the short term, there can be a decrease in the testosterone concentration without a change in LH levels, whereas long-term testosterone levels are better correlated with depressed LH (but not FSH) levels.[780,782] Glucocorticoids may also increase the ability of testosterone to block gonadotropin release by feedback inhibition.[779] They may also regulate factors that delay the onset of puberty.[783] In females, glucocorticoids in excess suppress basal and gonadotropin releasing hormone–stimulated LH (but not FSH) levels, plasma estrogen and progestin concentrations (variably), ovulation, and the onset of puberty. They result in a slight increase in testosterone clearance and have selective effects on FSH action.[783–785] In fat cells, they increase the levels of aromatase, which converts androgens to estrogens.[786]

Synergistic and Antagonistic Interrelations between Glucocorticoids and Other Hormones

Glucocorticoids can positively or negatively alter cellular sensitivity to other hormones by shifting the dose-response curve or influencing the maximal response obtained.[591,656,787,788] In some cases, the cellular response to another hormone is amplified by the glucocorticoid and vice versa, effects termed by Ingle "permissive."[591,656,787] Tissue synergistic and antagonistic actions can occur by influencing receptors for the other hormones or, more typically, through post-receptor mechanisms. Influences of glucocorticoids on receptors mediating the actions of insulin and immunologic mediators and on the postreceptor steps in these processes have been discussed. Other permissive actions may explain glucocorticoid effects on blood pressure in addisonian individuals,[591] lipolysis,[646] and PTH action.[740,741] Many of the synergisms occur with hormones that activate adenylate cyclase (epinephrine, glucagon, PTH).[591,787] Occasionally, glucocorticoids increase cAMP levels by decreasing levels of the phosphodiesterase that degrades cAMP.[785] Conversely, cAMP can modulate glucocorticoid receptor action.[789] Glucocorticoids can affect β-adrenergic receptors. In adipocytes, they promote a loss in β_1- and an increase in β_2-adrenergic receptors[790]; in human neutrophils, glucocorticoids induce a tightened coupling of β-adrenergic receptors and adenylate cyclase and attenuate isoproterenol-induced uncoupling between receptors and cyclase activation.[791] Glucocorticoids increase β-adrenergic receptor density in several other cell types.[791] These actions may contribute to glucocorticoid effectiveness in treating asthma.[791]

Glucocorticoids and Stress

The survival rate in patients with untreated adrenocortical insufficieny is decreased (Fig. 11-26).[792] Therapy with mineralocorticoids alone [e.g., with DOC (Fig. 11-26)] increases life expectancy only slightly.[792] However, survival is increased markedly when cortisol is given.[792] Decompensation is usually precipitated by a stressful insult (surgery, infection, injury, etc.) and is associated with a variety of derangements, including an inability to maintain a normal blood pressure (Fig. 11-25). Thus, it appears that glucocorticoids are required to cope with stress, but it is generally thought that glucocorticoid levels higher than basal are required to combat stress. This would be consistent with the fact that glucocorticoid production is generally increased in stress and with the occasional finding of a patient in addisonian crisis who has a normal random plasma cortisol concentration.

The actions of glucocorticoids inhibiting the production of mediators active on vascular and other systems may be especially critical in the response to stress.[665] One of the important physiologic functions of glucocorticoids during stress may be protection against the harmful effects of the body's defense mechanisms and the products produced by those mechanisms.[647,665,668] The specific case with prostaglandins was discussed previously (see the cardiovascular system and fluid and electrolyte balance sections). In addition, many stressful stimuli, such as serious infections, result in an increased production of numerous mediator substances, including kinins such as bradykinin; lymphokines such as γ-interferon, which stimulates the release of other inflammatory mediators; serotonin; histamine; collagenase and other proteases, which cause tissue damage; plasminogen activator, which in excess can cause blood vessel leakage and hemorrhage; catecholamines; immunologic mediators; fever-producing substances such as endogenous pyrogen (interleukin 1); PGs and related substances; vasopressin; myocardial depressant factor; TNFα, which has been implicated in endotoxin-induced shock[675]; and other vasoactive substances. It is possible that the actions of these substances are so profound that they can be harmful if left unchecked. Indeed, these substances could result in excessive vasodilatation, cardiac suppression, edema, fever, hemorrhage, and other deleterious effects. Glucocorticoids suppress the production and/or actions of most of the mediators listed.

Other specific effects may also contribute to the stress response.[665] For example, the increase in GFR may facilitate the clearance of toxic products and combat excessive fluid retention. The induction of glutamine synthetase in the brain may help lower concentrations of the potentially toxic glutamate and ammonia, which are elevated in stress. The induction of hepatic cytochrome P450 may help remove toxic foreign chemicals. The induction of metallothionein may help in the elimination of toxic metals such as zinc.

Definition of a Mineralocorticoid

Because both glucocorticoids and mineralocorticoids affect salt balance, it is important to define the term *mineralocorticoid.* As already mentioned, there is a class of binding proteins that appear to mediate the actions of these steroids on ion movement, and these receptors can be distinguished from glucocorticoid receptors. Thus, analogous to the case with glucocorticoids, "mineralocorticoid" actions are referred to as those mediated through these receptors. This would also apply to actions of glucocorticoids on these receptors, for instance, in the brain and pituitary, as described. Also, it is possible that other receptors mediating the actions of sodium-retaining steroids will be found.

Molecular Mechanisms of Mineralocorticoid Action

The early molecular events in aldosterone action are similar to those of other classes of steroids (see Fig. 11-28). Thus, specific mineralocorticoid receptors (MR) that bind aldosterone are present in the cytosol of mineralocorticoid-responsive tissues; they have been best characterized in kidney and toad bladder.[793–797] They are similar to glucocorticoid receptors but can be distinguished from them by some differences in their binding characteristics. For example, they have a much higher affinity for mineralocorticoids such as aldosterone and DOC than do glucocorticoid receptors[793] and have a low affinity for certain glucocorticoid receptor–specific compounds, such as RU 26988.[798] As discussed earlier, they have a relatively high affinity (although lower than that for aldosterone and DOC) for certain "classic" glucocorticoids, such as cortisol and corticosterone.[797] In the kidney, these receptors are located in the branched collecting tubules, the cortical collecting tubules, and the outer medullary collecting tubules.[796] In intact cells, they bind aldosterone and DOC with a K_d of around 0.6 to 1 n*M* and cortisol with a K_d of around 50 n*M*,[797] although in isolated kidney preparations the relative affinity for cortisol is higher.[608–610] Aldosterone enters the cell and binds to the specific receptor proteins; the receptor-mineralocorticoid complex is then translocated to the nucleus and binds to either specific DNA sequences (HREs) or to other transcription factors.[793]

The various steroid receptors share a common HRE. Thus, specificity of mineralocorticoid action is not solely dependent on binding of the MR to DNA, as the other steroid receptors bind equally well. Specificity is multifactorial and is dependent on (1) the presence of the receptor in specific tissues, (2) the ability of certain tissues to inactivate other steroids that bind to the MR, e.g., cortisol inactivation by 11β-HSD-II in the kidney, and (3) the interaction of steroid-receptor complexes with "composite response elements," which results in differential transcriptional effects of the MR and glucocorticoid receptors (GR).[613,614] This results in an increase (or decrease) in the transcription of particular genes.[795] Presumably, the protein products of these mineralocorticoid-regulated mRNAs then mediate the mineralocorticoid hormone responses.

The kidney is also a glucocorticoid target organ and contains both glucocorticoid and mineralocorticoid receptors. The free cortisol concentrations in plasma are 100–1,000 times those of aldosterone; thus, left unchecked, cortisol would be the major occupant of the mineralocorticoid receptor. The 50- to 100-fold lower apparent affinity for cortisol relative to aldosterone is due to

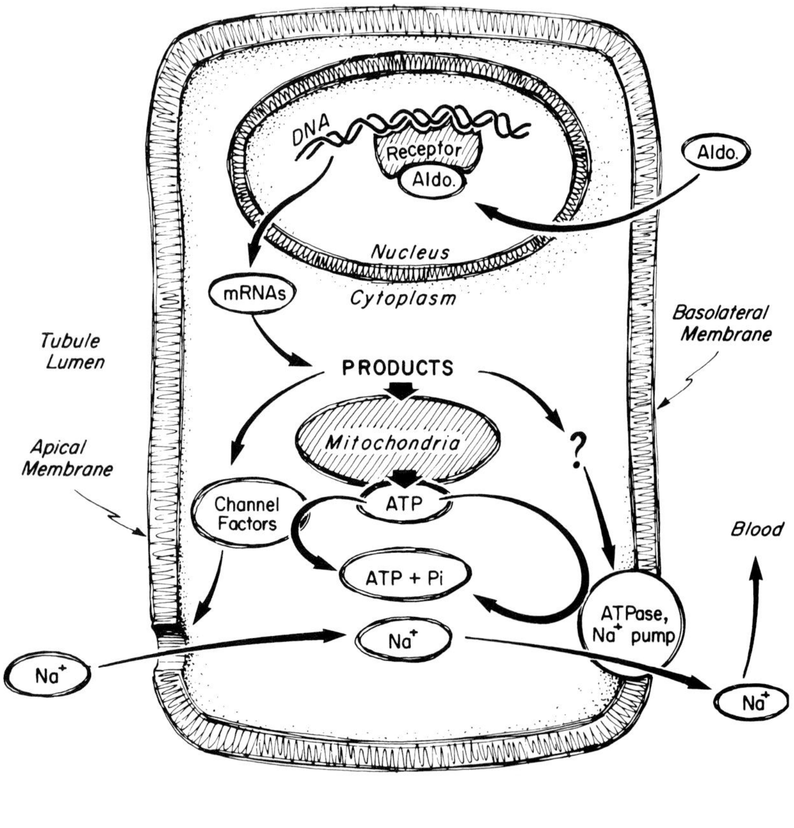

FIGURE 11-28. Steps in mineralocorticoid action. Illustrated are the early molecular events leading to the association of the aldosterone (Aldo)-receptor complex with DNA with consequent induction of mRNA's that encode proteins that comprise or affect the amiloride-sensitive sodium channel, ATP generation, and Na^+ pumping activity.

the fact that cortisol is metabolized to cortisone[321–343]; thus, aldosterone is more available for receptor occupancy and mineralocorticoid actions. Nevertheless, cortisol may occupy the mineralocorticoid receptor to some extent, especially at very high levels.[797]

Sodium bathing the luminal surface passively enters the renal cell through channels in the apical membrane. The intracellular sodium ions are then pumped into the interstitial fluid on the serosal side of the cell by an Na^+, K^+-dependent ATPase. ATP is required to drive the pump and for maintenance of the Na^+ channels in the apical membrane. Aldosterone may act in three ways (Fig. 11-24)[582,793,795]: (1) by increasing the cellular permeability to Na^+ by affecting channels in the apical membrane, (2) by affecting the energy-generating system and thus increasing cellular energy, and (3) by affecting the pump.

Mineralocorticoids increase the number of specific apical membrane amiloride sensitive sodium channels,[793,795] with an increase in the conductance of the apical membrane and an increased number of conducting sodium channels.[799] An aldosterone-regulated protein recruits these channels from a pool of nonconducting channels. This may be the earliest and primary effect. In the toad bladder, aldosterone stimulates phospholipase activity, fatty acid synthesis, and acetyltransferase activity.[793] These actions may affect membrane phospholipids and ion transport and may thus mediate aldosterone action.

Aldosterone increases the renal NADH/NAD^+ ratio and the activities of mitochondrial enzymes involved in ATP generation, in particular citrate synthase,[793,800–802] and, in the toad bladder, cellular ATP levels.[803] Thus, the effect of aldosterone in increasing the potential to generate ATP may both drive the Na^+ pump and affect the number of active Na^+ channels. Aldosterone also increases the incorporation of riboflavin into renal flavin nucleotides, and analogues of riboflavin that inhibit this incorporation also block the antinatriuretic effects of aldosterone.[582]

Aldosterone also increases the Na^+,K^+-ATPase activity of the basolateral membranes of the cortical collecting tubule.[793,800,801,804–807] This may be due to an augmentation of the activity of pump sites rather than an increase in Na^+,K^+-ATPase synthesis. Whether it involves the direct actions of an aldosterone-induced protein or is a secondary effect that occurs after initial effects on the apical membrane and possibly mediated by the increased sodium entry is controversial. Nevertheless, this influence would further enhance sodium transport. These changes in the cortical collecting tubules are also associated with aldosterone-regulated increases in the basolateral cell membrane areas in which the Ka^+,K^+-ATPase enzyme unites are located.

Thus, several aldosterone-regulated proteins appear to act in a coordinated manner to stimulate sodium transport. Several other aldosterone-regulated proteins have also been identified,[793] and some of them could also affect energy generation, the apical channels, or other processes.

Much less is known about the way aldosterone stimulates potassium or hydrogen ion secretion. The Na^+,K^+-ATPase action affects K^+ excretion by exchanging K^+ for Na^+. However, because effects on Na^+ can occur in the absence of influences on K^+, there might also be effects on a potassium pump or on the permeability of the luminal membrane to K^+.[793]

The effects on hydrogen ion appear to be exerted predominantly in the medullary collecting tubule and in this respect are independent of effects on Na1, although the factors mentioned above are operative.793 Suggested targets for aldosterone effects on hydrogen ion include effects on glutamine entry into or exit from mitochondria, on mitochondrial glutaminase, and on cytoplasmic PEPCK.[793]

Mineralocorticoid Agonists and Antagonists

Natural and synthetic steroids have mineralocorticoid agonist activity. Aldosterone, the predominant mineralocorticoid, contains an aldehyde at position 18 that is in equilibrium with the 11-hydroxyl function, forming a cyclic 11,18-hemiacetyl (Fig. 11-29). Cortisol, corticosterone, DOC, 19-nor-DOC, 19-OH-androstenedione, and other 18- and 19-substituted derivatives of these steroids have mineralocorticoid agonist activities. The synthetic steroid fludrocortisone (9α-fluorocortisol) is extremely potent and ordinarily is the steroid chosen for replacement mineralocorticoid therapy. Aldosterone and DOC are not useful for oral therapy, as they are rapidly degraded by the liver after absorption.

A number of compounds have mineralocorticoid antagonist activity. Progesterone, the most potent naturally occurring antagonist, plays a minor physiologic role, except possibly during the third trimester of pregnancy, when progesterone concentrations are extremely high (see Chap. 16). Spironolactone, a steroid analogue, is used clinically as a mineralocorticoid antagonist. Mineralocorticoid antagonists competitively inhibit the binding of agonists by the receptors.[793]

Almost all the mineralocorticoid activity of human plasma can be accounted for by aldosterone and cortisol.[808,809] The role of cortisol is limited by its metabolism to cortisone. The extent to which cortisol, DOC, 18- and 19-substituted derivatives of these steroids, and 19-OH androstenedione contribute to mineralocorticoid activity has not been clarified. DOC circulates at concentrations similar to those of aldosterone and has equal affinity for mineralocorticoid receptors.[809] However, because less than 5 percent of circulating DOC is free compared with 45 percent of aldosterone,[810] DOC contributes negligibly to mineralocorticoid action under physiologic circumstances. The physiologic importance of 19-nor-DOC and 19-OH-androstenedione is controversial and is potentially significant. Because 19-nor-DOC is produced in the kidney, its plasma concentrations may not reflect its levels in the renal target tissue.[811–813] 19-OH-androstenedione is present in the circulation in concentrations about half those of aldosterone, although its plasma binding has not been reported.[811]

Physiologic Actions of Mineralocorticoids

Mineralocorticoid actions are predominantly due to aldosterone, although cortisol and occasionally DOC may play roles. Mineralocorticoids regulate sodium and potassium balance and act on

FIGURE 11-29. The two forms of aldosterone.

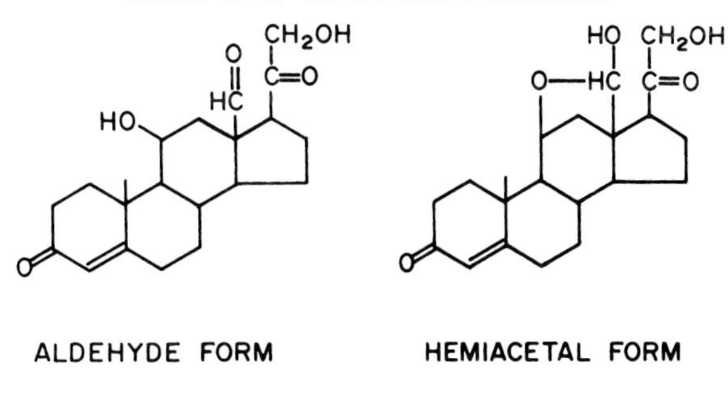

fewer tissues than do glucocorticoids because of the limited tissue distribution of 11β-HSD-II. Mineralocorticoid-responsive tissues include the kidney, gut, salivary glands, sweat glands, vascular endothelium, brain, and possibly mammary gland and pituitary.[582,793,794,798,814,815] The major effect of these actions is to conserve sodium and eliminate potassium and hydrogen ions.

Kidney

The kidney is the most important known site of mineralocorticoid action. Most, if not all, of the physiologically relevant effects occur in the connecting segment, cortical collecting tubules, and medullary collecting tubules.[582,793] Mineralocorticoids promote the reabsorption of sodium and the secretion of potassium in the cortical collecting tubules and possibly the connecting segment and hydrogen ion secretion in the medullary collecting tubules.[582,793,796,804–807] Aldosterone also has a permissive effect on the osmotic water flux response to vasopressin in the cortical collecting tubule.[793,816] These effects can be observed after a lag of about 30 min to 2 h and require protein and RNA synthesis.[793] In mineralocorticoid deficiency states, there is sodium loss, potassium retention, and decreased renal acid excretion, leading to dehydration, hyponatremia, hyperkalemia, and metabolic acidosis.[817] Conversely, in mineralocorticoid excess states, there is an increase in total body sodium, hypertension, hypokalemia, and a tendency to metabolic alkalosis.[795]

Only a fraction of the filtered sodium is reabsorbed in response to aldosterone, but this fraction can have marked influences on electrolyte balance. The magnitude of the response to aldosterone is dependent on the amount of solute delivered to the kidney.[795] The amount of sodium retention that can occur in response to an excess of mineralocorticoids in subjects with normal cardiac and renal function is limited[795,813,819]; i.e., such patients do not usually develop edema.[818] Thus, in primary mineralocorticoid excess states, after an initial period of positive sodium balance, the body adjusts to the excess sodium (the "escape" phenomenon) by reabsorbing less of the filtered sodium. This decrease occurs mostly in the proximal tubule, so that sodium intake ultimately equals excretion.[818] Patients with heart failure, cirrhosis of the liver, or nephrosis cannot respond normally and do not escape[819]; thus, secondary aldosteronism contributes to the fluid retention and edema. The mineralocorticoid influence on potassium excretion does not show this escape phenomenon.[818,819]

The escape phenomenon may in part be mediated through secondary increases in ANP levels, which produce natriuresis. ANP levels increase in response to volume expansion, as occurs after mineralocorticoid treatment, and increase in dogs under conditions of escape.[820] Cardiac output also increases under these conditions; this can increase GFR with secondary increases in sodium excretion.[820] A volume increase caused by sodium retention also depresses proximal sodium reabsorption, although this is partly compensated by distal tubular reabsorption.[818] This effect can be independent of increases in GFR[818] and may be due in part to an increase in renal interstitial pressure that lowers the tubular capacity for sodium reabsorption.[818] Urinary PGs and kallikrein increase in concentration after mineralocorticoid administration, have natriuretic actions, and may also participate in escape.[818] Although escape can occur in the absence of afferent and efferent neural pathways, it is conceivable that the increased vascular volume stimulates volume receptors that decrease renal adrenergic activity and that this decreases sodium transport directly and through renal vasodilatory mechanisms.[818]

Stimulation of potassium loss by mineralocorticoids depends largely on sodium intake.[793,795,819,820] The sodium reabsorbed by the distal tubule increases the electronegativity of the lumen in relation to the peritubular fluid; this is important for passive diffusion of potassium ion into the tubule from which it is excreted. Thus, when there is sufficient delivery of sodium to the distal tubules, a kaliuretic effect of aldosterone is readily observed. By contrast, when sodium intake is restricted, there is minimal delivery of sodium to the distal tubule, as it is mostly reabsorbed in the proximal tubule. In this case, the necessary electronegativity is not generated and potassium excretion is not stimulated. This lack of a prominent kaliuretic effect can be apparent when aldosterone is present in excess in patients with cardiac failure, nephrosis, or cirrhosis who have a decreased GFR and increased proximal tubular reabsorption of sodium.

Changes in sodium and potassium concentrations do not always parallel each other, and there is not a stoichiometric relation between sodium reabsorption and potassium excretion.[793,820] Potassium excretion may increase before there is an effect on sodium, and vice versa.[793]

In addition to their role in the ordinary maintenance of potassium balance, mineralocorticoids participate in the defense against chronic hyperkalemia.[793,819,821] Increased aldosterone secretion in response to hyperkalemia increases potassium excretion.

Several factors account for the effects of mineralocorticoids on renal acid production. First, aldosterone produces a net decrease in urinary pH and, therefore, an increase in urinary acidification without much change in titratable acid.[723,822] This effect is due to an increase in the tubular fluid-to-blood pH gradients across the distal nephron, predominantly across the inner stripe of the outer medulla.[723,822] These effects on hydrogen ion can occur independently of those on sodium and potassium ions. Second, some of the sodium reabsorbed in response to aldosterone is exchanged for hydrogen ion, and this accelerates urinary loss of acid.[822,823] Thus, hydrogen ion loss due to mineralocorticoid excess can be decreased by reducing the intake of sodium and thus its delivery to the distal nephron.[822,823] Third, there is some movement of hydrogen ions into cells in exchange for the potassium lost in the urine.[822,823] Fourth, the potassium deficiency increases hydrogen ion excretion by increasing ammonia production and decreasing the exchange of Na^+ for K^+ that enhances the exchange of Na^+ for H^+.[822,823] The production of alkalosis is blunted by the increased extracellular volume that suppresses bicarbonate reabsorption.[822,823] In adrenal insufficiency, the opposite effect occurs and there are increases in bicarbonate removal and urinary pH and decreased excretion of titratable acid and ammonia.[823]

Mineralocorticoids also influence magnesium and calcium ion excretion.[819] In primary aldosteronism, there is increased urinary excretion of both magnesium and calcium but normal plasma levels are maintained.[819] This effect is probably secondary to sodium retention, which decreases proximal tubular resorption of these ions.

Mineralocorticoids do not directly affect water excretion, GFR, renal plasma flow, or renin production. However, their effects on sodium and water retention with increased extracellular fluid volume indirectly increase GFR and renal plasma flow and suppress the plasma renin concentration. In addition, these steroids (and also glucocorticoids) enhance vasopressin actions, increasing water permeability.[793]

Mineralocorticoids increase the levels of urinary kallikrein, the enzyme that cleaves bradykinin from kininogen. The urinary kallikrein level is increased in primary aldosteronism but not in most other forms of hypertension. Although the role of this influence is not known, bradykinin generated as a result of kallikrein action may block sodium reabsorption and serve to blunt aldosterone action.[824]

Extrarenal Tissues

Mineralocorticoid actions on extrarenal tissues also contribute to sodium retention and potassium excretion. Mineralocorticoids decrease sodium excretion and enhance potassium loss in the ileum, colon, skin, and salivary glands.[819,825] Thus, patients with primary aldosteronism lose potassium in the stool, have a decreased level of stool sodium, have an increased potential difference across the colonic epithelium, and have a decreased salivary Na^+/K^+ ratio. In arterial smooth muscle, mineralocorticoids stimulate passive and sodium pump–dependent transmembrane movements.[813]

Actions of Adrenal Androgens and Estrogens

The adrenal C-19 steroids, DHEA, DHEA-S, and androstenedione, have little inherent androgen action, as they bind poorly to the androgen receptor. However, these adrenal C-19 steroids provide an important pool of circulating precursor steroids that can be converted to active androgens and estrogens in the peripheral tissues where they act. Thus, the principal C-19 steroids secreted by the adrenal, DHEA and DHEA-S, have no sex steroid action whatsoever, but DHEA-S can be acted upon by steroid sulfatase to produce DHEA, and DHEA can be converted to androstenedione in the liver, kidney, brain, breast, placenta, and other "peripheral" tissues. This conversion of DHEA to androstenedione is catalyzed by 3β-HSD-I, which is enzymatically equivalent to the 3β-HSD-II expressed in the adrenals and gonads, but is encoded by a distinct gene.[173–177] Androstenedione is a very weak androgen, but it can be activated to testosterone by 17β-HSD-III in the testis,[276] and probably by 17β-HSD-V, which is widely expressed in many tissues. It is likely that this, or a closely related mechanism involving other isozymes of 17β-HSD in target tissues, is responsible for the action of adrenal C-19 steroids to foster the development of pubic and axillary hair in hypogonadal women.

Circulating androstenedione and testosterone can also be converted to esterone and estradiol, respectively, by the action of P450aro (aromatase) in peripheral target tissues. P450aro is widely expressed, especially in "gynecoid" adipose tissue,[290,291] where it apparently accounts for many of the changes in body fat distribution seen in aging. P450aro is also expressed in the epiphyses of growing bones, so that it is the action of estrogen locally produced from circulating C-19 steroids that accounts for the rapid growth and epiphyseal fusion of adolescence.[291] Thus, many of the actions of the so-called adrenal androgens are, in fact, mediated by their conversion to conventional androgens and estrogens at their sites of action.

In addition to the actions of adrenal C-19 steroids as precursors to classical sex steroids, a developing body of evidence suggests that these steroids, particularly DHEA, may exert actions through other mechanisms. The fall in circulating concentrations of DHEA and DHEA-S during aging (Fig. 11-11) has stimulated substantial interest in a potential role for a DHEA deficiency state in aging. Several studies have reported that administration of DHEA to normal elderly men and women has increased muscular strength, bone density, a sense of well-being, and sexuality.[354,826–829] The psychological effects were seen at relatively low doses (50 mg/d), at which the conversion to testosterone and estradiol was negligible.[354,829] Whether or not the claimed benefits of DHEA replacement therapy are real remains a controversial area of continuing investigation. However, as recent data indicate that DHEA is also made in the brain,[830–832] and has an action as a neocortical organizer in the fetal rodent brain,[833] it is reasonable to consider a broad range of potential non-classical endocrine actions of this steroid.

LABORATORY EVALUATION OF ADRENOCORTICAL FUNCTION

Specific plasma assays allow the precise determination of adrenal hormones, including the major glucocorticoids, mineralocorticoids, androgens, and estrogens, and the trophic hormones, i.e., ACTH, angiotensin, and renin, that control adrenal secretion. In many instances, these assays have simplified the evaluation of adrenal dysfunction and have supplanted determinations of urinary metabolites. However, some urinary assays and, in particular, measurement of the 24-h urinary free cortisol, are quite useful. The plasma steroid methods measure the total hormone concentration; therefore, alterations in plasma-binding proteins must be considered in their interpretation. The plasma concentrations of the adrenal hormones and their trophic factors vary widely in normal individuals and in both endocrine and nonendocrine disorders. Thus, isolated plasma measurements are frequently not reliable in establishing definitive diagnoses and must be interpreted with regard to the time of the sample and the clinical situation. In general, more precise information is obtained by determining integrated assessments of hormone production and the responses of those hormones to appropriate stimulation and suppression tests (Fig. 11-30).

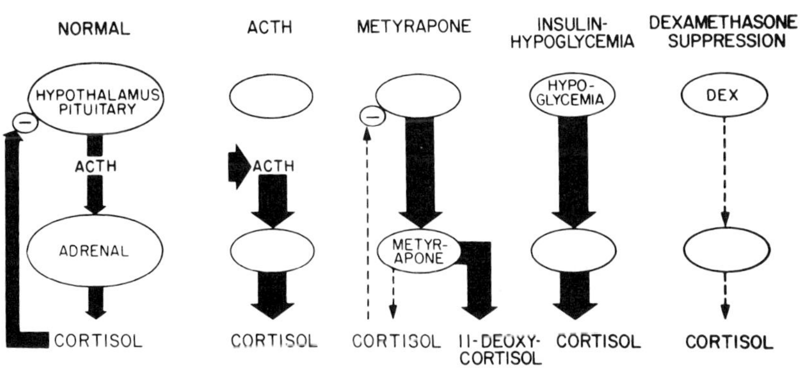

FIGURE 11-30. Tests used to evaluate the hypothalamic-pituitary-adrenal axis. The thickness of the arrow indicates the relative quantities of compounds present if the test is normal. Dotted lines show a blocked pathway. See text for details.

Plasma Cortisol and Related Steroids

Determination of the plasma cortisol concentration is essential in the evaluation of adrenal function. The current method of choice is high-performance liquid chromatography (HPLC)[836,837] cortisol can also be determined by radioimmunoassay[834,835] and by competitive protein-binding radioassay[838,839] but these methods generally fail to distinguish cortisol from cortisone.

Cortisol

Liquid Chromatography (HPLC)

High performance liquid chromatography (HPLC) has replaced immunoassay for cortisol, but not other steroids in modern hospital laboratories. Cortisol is separated from other steroids by liquid chromatography and the concentration of the eluted cortisol is then measured by spectrophotometry or fluorimetry.[836,837] This assay is not interfered with by drugs and medications and does not detect prednisone, prednisolone, cortisone, dexamethasone, or other common natural and synthetic steroids.[837] Generally, cortisol levels measured by HPLC are lower than those measured by RIA, as a result of some nonspecificity of the RIA.

Radioimmunoassay

Radioimmunoassay is also widely used to assay plasma cortisol. Currently available antibodies have limited cross-reactivity with other steroids.[835,844,845] Earlier antisera varied greatly in specificity and exhibited cross-reactivity with 11-deoxycortisol, 21-deoxycortisol, 17α-hydroxyprogesterone, corticosterone, DOC, progesterone, cortisone, prednisone, and prednisolone.[816,835,846] Commonly used drugs and medications also do not interfere with the radioimmunoassay.

Competitive Protein-Binding Radioassay

This assay is similar to radioimmunoassay except that CBG is used instead of an antibody to cortisol.[838,839] This assay usually provides a valid estimate of plasma cortisol except when levels of steroids that also have a high affinity for CBG are elevated, e.g., pregnancy (progesterone), congenital adrenal hyperplasia (17α-hydroxyprogesterone, progesterone, corticosterone, DOC, 21-deoxycortisol, or 11-deoxycortisol), and adrenal carcinoma (11-deoxycortisol). The synthetic steroids prednisolone and methylprednisolone also cross-react in this assay system. Modifications of this method to separate the various steroids can circumvent these problems.[838,847] This assay is not interfered with by other hormones and commonly used drugs and medications.[838]

Salivary Cortisol Measurement

The estimation of cortisol in saliva accurately reflects the plasma free cortisol[848] and has been measured by both radioimmunoassay and competitive protein binding.[849,850] This method has proved useful in the assessment of adrenocortical function because of the ease of sample collection and because it allows the collection of multiple or frequent samples in ambulatory outpatients.[850] In one study, normal volunteers had values of 5.6 ± 0.3 ng/ml at 8 A.M. and 1.4 ± 0.1 at 10 P.M., showing the expected normal diurnal variation.[850] Values were markedly elevated after stimulation with ACTH (18.9 ± 0.8) and were suppressed after the administration of 1 mg dexamethasone (0.8 ± 0.4).[850]

Basal salivary cortisol was subnormal in adrenal insufficiency with deficient responses to ACTH administration. In primary adrenal insufficiency, basal salivary cortisol was 1.3 ± 0.2 ng/ml and there was no response to ACTH stimulation (1.5 ± 0.3 ng/ml). In secondary adrenal insufficiency, basal levels were equally low (1.8 ± 0.3 ng/ml); however, in these patients there was an increase (although inadequate) to 3.62 ± 0.8, indicating partial ACTH deficiency and partial adrenal atrophy.[850] In Cushing's syndrome, both 8 A.M. and 10 P.M. salivary cortisol levels were elevated (11.5 ± 1.9 and 13.0 ± 1.8, respectively), demonstrating elevated basal secretion and abnormal diurnal variation. There was no overlap in this series between 10 P.M. salivary cortisol values in normals (range, 0.8 to 1.5 ng/ml) and in patients with Cushing's syndrome (range, 3.3 to 23.9 ng/ml). In addition, patients with Cushing's syndrome had subnormal suppression of salivary cortisol values (range, 2.1 to 24.2 ng/ml) after 1 mg dexamethasone, and there was no overlap with normal subjects (range 0.6 to 1.1 ng/ml). Salivary cortisol levels are also elevated in third trimester pregnancy but maintain a normal diurnal variation.[851]

Interpretation of Plasma Cortisol Determinations

Variations in plasma cortisol levels due to circadian changes, episodic release, and stimulation of the hypothalamic-pituitary-adrenal axis must be considered in evaluating plasma cortisol determinations, and limit the usefulness of single measurements.[420,852–854] Subnormal or elevated levels should arouse suspicion of adrenal hypo- or hyperfunction, but in general, more specific testing of the hypothalamic-pituitary-adrenal axis is required. Plasma cortisol levels are not altered with advancing age.[855]

The method used must be considered in interpreting the results of plasma cortisol determinations. Morning (8 A.M.) plasma cortisol levels measured by either radioimmunoassay or competitive protein binding average 10 to 12 μg/dl with a range of 3 to 20 μg/dl,[834,847,854] and values at 4 to 6 P.M. approximate 50 percent of morning levels. In one study using the competitive protein-binding assay, values were 10.4 ± 4 (mean ± SD) at 8 A.M. compared to 4.0 ± 2.0 at 8 P.M. and were less than 3 μg/dl between 10 P.M. and 2 A.M.[854]

Plasma cortisol is appropriately elevated with acute illness, trauma, or surgery,[432,435,856] and levels tend to be elevated in patients with depression, alcoholism, severe anxiety, starvation, anorexia nervosa, and chronic renal failure.[431–433,440,857–860] Because most assays measure total plasma steroid levels, the cortisol concentration is elevated in conditions with increased CBG levels, such as pregnancy and estrogen (including oral contraceptive) therapy.[536,540,857,861] In these instances, plasma cortisol levels may be as high as 40 to 60 μg/dl and may take several weeks to return to normal after delivery or the cessation of estrogen therapy.[538,857] CBG levels may also be increased congenitally and in hyperthyroidism, diabetes, and certain hematologic disorders[540,553]; decreased CBG levels also occur congenitally and in hypothyroidism, liver disease, nephrotic syndrome, multiple myeloma, and obesity.[536–540] CBG binding capacity may be measured in plasma.[536]

Determination of Other Plasma Steroids

The precursors of both cortisol and aldosterone can be assayed in plasma. These steroids include pregnenolone, 17α-hydroxypregnenolone, progesterone, 17α-hydroxyprogesterone, DOC, corticosterone, and 11-deoxycortisol. The steroids are first separated by solvent extraction and/or chromatography, and their concentrations are then measured by either competitive protein binding or radioimmunoassay[838,847,862,863]; their levels can also be measured by HPLC. Precursors to cortisol include pregnenolone, 17α-hydroxypregnenolone, 17α-hydroxyprogesterone, and 11-deoxycortisol. Steroids of the mineralocorticoid pathway include pregnenolone, progesterone, DOC, and corticosterone as well as 18-hydroxy DOC and 18-hydroxy corticosterone (see Figs. 11-4 and 11-7).

Measurements of these steroids are required in the diagnosis of congenital enzymatic defects of adrenal steroid biosynthesis. Normal ranges and responses to ACTH stimulation are described later in the sections on adrenocortical function testing in children and disorders of steroid hormone biosynthesis. Many of these steroids are elevated in patients with adrenocortical carcinoma, and plasma 11-deoxycortisol is measured in assessing the adrenal response to metyrapone, as discussed later.

Plasma ACTH and Related Peptides

Assays of plasma ACTH have simplified the diagnosis of pituitary-adrenal dysfunction.[864,865] ACTH is unstable in plasma, is inactivated at room temperature, and adheres strongly to glass. Careful sample collection and preparation are essential; specimens must be collected with EDTA in plastic or siliconized tubes on ice, centrifuged in the cold within an hour of collection, and then frozen until assayed. Antisera have been produced that react with the NH_2-terminal or COOH-terminal sequences or against the entire molecule.[866,867] In general, an antiserum that reacts with the biologically active 1-24 sequence of human ACTH should be used to reduce the detection of biologically inactive fragments.

A radioimmunoassay using a sensitive and highly specific antibody that binds to ACTH (5-18) but not to other fragments or precursors can be performed in unextracted plasma and has a lower limit of detection of 5 pg/ml.[868] In addition, "two-site" or "sandwich" immunoradiometric assays (IRMA) have been developed[869–873] and are commercially available.[869–873] These methods utilize two antibodies directed at the N- and C-terminal portions of ACTH (1-39) and thus have excellent sensitivity and specificity. These assays can be performed on unextracted plasma, and the detection limit is 2 to 4 pg/ml.[869–873] Generally, two-site IRMAS measure less ACTH than IRAs because they do not interact with some ACTH fragments, although some of these fragments have ACTH bioactivity.

When one is evaluating and interpreting ACTH levels, the status of adrenal secretion must be compared and factors, such as episodic secretion and circadian variation, must also be considered. The normal range of plasma ACTH concentration with specific radioimmunoassay is 10 to 40 pg/ml in the morning.[868] With the IRMA, the normal range is 5 to 30 pg/ml in the morning; at 4:30 P.M., mean values are 5–10 pg/ml.[869–873]

Plasma ACTH levels are of the greatest diagnostic utility in the differential diagnosis of spontaneous adrenal disorders. In patients with adrenal insufficiency proved by stimulation testing with exogenous ACTH, elevated plasma ACTH levels confirm primary adrenal insufficiency. In these patients, ACTH levels are usually greater than 200 pg/ml, and can be as high as 1,000 to 2,000 pg/ml. Conversely, plasma ACTH levels below 20 pg/ml are suggestive but not diagnostic of secondary hypoadrenalism (ACTH deficiency).[869–873]

In Cushing's syndrome, a suppressed plasma ACTH level (less than 8 pg/ml) is diagnostic of a primary glucocorticoid-producing adrenal tumor or the rare forms of ACTH-independent micro- or macronodular hyperplasia. In contrast, patients with pituitary ACTH hypersecretion have plasma ACTH levels in the normal to moderately elevated range (20 to 200 pg/ml); in general, patients with the ectopic ACTH syndrome have markedly elevated plasma ACTH concentrations (200 to >1,000 pg/ml).[874,875] However, plasma ACTH levels do not always correctly differentiate pituitary from ectopic sources of ACTH hypersecretion, as a considerable overlap occurs in the range of 100 to 200 pg/ml.[875]

Sensitive bioassays have also been described, but they are technically difficult and have been restricted largely to research use. These bioassays measure plasma ACTH concentration by radioreceptor assay,[876] steroid response of dispersed adrenal cells, or an extremely sensitive cytochemical bioassay.[877]

Radioimmunoassays have also been developed for human β-lipotropin (β-LPH); normal concentrations are 20 to 200 pg/ml.[878–880] β-LPH and ACTH are secreted simultaneously; thus, the circadian variations of β-LPH follow those of ACTH.[880,881] β-LPH levels also respond to hypoglycemia, dexamethasone, and other factors that influence ACTH secretion.[880,881] β-LPH has a longer half-life and greater stability in plasma than does ACTH; in addition, immunoassays are less difficult than those for ACTH. However, this assay is not in general use, and it is not clear that it has any specific advantage over the measurement of plasma ACTH concentration. Similarly, radioimmunoassays for plasma β-endorphin have been developed, but their clinical utility is unknown, and β-LPH cross-reacts with all these assays.[882,883] Thus, precise measurement of the β-endorphin concentration requires prior separation of the peptides by chromatography. An IRMA which measures the ACTH precursors POMC and pro-ACTH has also been described.[884]

Urinary Corticosteroids

Several methods measure urinary cortisol and its metabolites. Traditionally, these methods have involved 24 h urine collections, a feature that can be a disadvantage because of the difficulty of obtaining complete collections. However, these methods provide an integrated assessment of the amount of cortisol produced during a 24-h period, and the problems of episodic release that are present with plasma assays can be bypassed. The 24-h urine sample is collected in a suitable preservative and is then stable when refrigerated. The utility of spot and shorter collections is described later.

Free Cortisol

In spite of the fact that less than 1 percent of the total cortisol secreted by the adrenal is excreted unchanged in the urine (see the section on variations in steroid metabolism),[885] a measurement of this fraction can yield useful information. It is especially helpful when cortisol secretion is increased because the unbound plasma cortisol is elevated more than the total level since the capacity of CBG is exceeded.

Urinary free cortisol (UFC) is measured by extraction of the urine and assay of the extract by radioimmunoassay,[834] competitive protein-binding radioassay,[886,887] or HPLC.[888] These assays are rapid and suitable for routine clinical use but have the same limitations of specificity described for plasma cortisol. In 24-h urine collections, normal values range from 20 to 100 μg/24 h when measured by radioimmunoassay and from 10 to 50 μg/24 h by HPLC.[874,887,888] Elevated UFC is nearly always found in spontaneous Cushing's syndrome. In contrast to urinary 17-OHCS, the UFC excretion is not elevated in obesity,[886] and this greatly enhances the diagnostic usefulness of this test in Cushing's syndrome; correction of 17-OHS value excretion per gram creatinine excreted, however, makes this assay equivalent to that of UFC in the differentiation between Cushing's syndrome and obesity, with the limitations described later. UFC levels are increased in acute illness and during the other stressful situations discussed and are elevated in the latter part of pregnancy.

In addition, 1-h or 4-h urine collections for free cortisol measurement are useful in assessing dynamic adrenocortical function.[889,890] In one study in normal subjects, urine collections from 7 to 8 A.M. and 10 to 11 P.M. demonstrated normal diurnal variation and suppressibility in response to dexamethasone. In contrast, patients with Cushing's syndrome had absent diurnal variability and lack of suppression with dexamethasone,[889] whereas patients with adrenal insufficiency had very low values in both the morning and evening.[889] In another study, urine cortisol collected from 8 P.M. to 12 midnight clearly separated normal controls from patients with Cushing's syndrome.[890] However, there was some overlap between markedly obese subjects (those >50 percent above normal weight) and patients with Cushing's syndrome.[890] Thus, spot and shorter urine collections and the estimation of salivary cortisol are useful methods for assessing free cortisol in ambulatory subjects.

17-Hydroxycorticosteroids and 17-Ketogenic Steroids

Measurements of urinary 17-OHCS and 17-ketogenic steroids (17-KGS) were previously of major importance in the evaluation of adrenal function; these tests also provide an integrated assessment of adrenal function. The response of urinary 17-OHCS to stimulation or suppression does have clinical utility; however, determination of urinary free cortisol and measurement of plasma cortisol with the rapid dynamic tests discussed later are preferred. However, urinary 17-KGS determinations are no longer used.

Urinary 17-OHCS are assayed by the Porter-Silber reaction, which is specific for steroids with a 17,21-dihydroxy-20-keto configuration.[840,841] The method ordinarily measures levels of the major urinary metabolites of cortisol and cortisone (discussed earlier), but with inhibition of 11β-hydroxylase, as with metyrapone testing (described later), it determines the metabolites of 11-deoxycortisol. The normal adult excretion rate of urinary 17-OHCS is 3 to 10 mg/24 h. Total urinary excretion is elevated in obesity, but this elevation can be compensated for by comparing the result to urinary creatinine excretion (normal range, 2.0 to 6.5 mg per gram of creatinine).[874,891] Urinary 17-OHCS may be decreased in starvation, renal failure, liver disease, pregnancy, and hypothyroidism and may be increased in hyperthyroidism.[891–896] Drugs that induce hepatic microsomal enzymes, such as phenytoin, primidone, phenobarbital, and mitotane, reduce urinary 17-OHCS excretion by increasing steroid metabolism via the 6β-hydroxylation pathway to metabolites that are not measured by the Porter-Silber method.[857,897,898] Other drugs cause direct interference with urinary 17-OHCS determinations, including spironolactone, chlordiazepoxide, hydroxyzine, meprobamate, phenothiazines, quinine, and troleandomycin.[899,900]

The 17-ketogenic steroids are those that are converted to 17-ketosteroids by oxidation and then measured colorimetrically by the Zimmerman reaction (discussed in the section on urinary androgens later).[901] Such steroids include the 17-OHCS (cortisol, cortisone, 11-deoxycortisol), the cortols and cortolones, steroids without a hydroxyl at position 21 (17α-hydroxyprogesterone and 21-deoxycortisol), pregnanetriol, and certain of their metabolites. In addition, the assay measures levels of the endogenous 17-ketosteroids. However, these levels can be determined separately, and the values can be subtracted from the total of ketogenic steroids to yield the actual level of 17-KGS. Normal values are 6 to 20 mg/24 h in most laboratories. The assay of 17-KGS does not have any advantages over the other tests and has several disadvantages.[514,899,900] Basal measurements are not reliable in the diagnosis of adrenal insufficiency, Cushing's syndrome, or CAH, and drug interference is common. Thus, this method is no longer used in most centers.

Cortisol Production Rate

Several methods are available for determining the production or secretory rate of cortisol.[503] However, technical complexity has largely limited their use to research situations.[503,504] Early studies estimated that cortisol production ranges from 8 to 25 mg/day, and most studies have given results in the higher range.[503,504] In recent studies using more specific methods, the cortisol production rate was about 10 mg/day (5.7 to 6.8 mg/m^2 per day) in normal adult volunteers and normal children and adolescents.[510–512] In adult patients with Cushing's syndrome, the cortisol production rate was 30.7 $\pm$ 9.3 mg/day (18.1 mg/m^2 per day). These studies indicate that the usual cortisol replacement dose of 20 to 30 mg/day used in adrenal insufficiency is too high if more than 50 percent of the oral dose is absorbed. Cortisol production is increased in obesity, pregnancy, hyperthyroidism, and other circumstances; it is decreased in adrenal insufficiency and hypothyroidism.[504]

Dexamethasone Suppression Tests

Low-Dose Tests

Low-dose tests are used in the diagnosis of Cushing's syndrome and assess the integrity of negative feedback control by glucocorticoids on the hypothalamic-pituitary-adrenal axis (see earlier discussion). Dexamethasone is used because in the small amounts utilized, it is not measured in the plasma and urine corticosteroid assays employed. Thus, in normal individuals, dexamethasone inhibits pituitary ACTH release and consequently adrenal cortisol secretion. In patients with Cushing's syndrome (in whom feedback control is abnormal), secretion is rarely normally suppressible with these tests.[857,874,902–905] These low-dose tests diagnose Cushing's syndrome but do not define the specific etiology.

Overnight Test

The overnight dexamethasone suppression test is a reliable screening test for adult Cushing's syndrome and requires only one plasma specimen. Dexamethasone (1.0 mg orally) is administered at 11 P.M., and plasma cortisol is measured at 8 A.M. the following morning. A plasma cortisol level below 5 μg/dl excludes Cushing's syndrome with rare exceptions, and patients with Cushing's syndrome usually have plasma cortisol levels above 10 μg/dl.[874] If the response is abnormal, Cushing's syndrome should be suspected and confirmed with other diagnostic tests.

Less than 2 percent of patients with Cushing's syndrome show normal suppressibility, and only 1.1 percent of outpatient controls have false-positive results.[874] Thus, this test is valuable for outpatient screening. It is less useful in obese individuals, as 13 percent fail to show suppression, and it is of minimal usefulness in hospitalized or chronically ill patients, among whom approximately 25 percent have false-positive results.[874] False-positive responses may also occur in acutely ill patients; in those with severe depression, anorexia nervosa, anxiety, alcoholism, or chronic renal failure; and in high-estrogen states (pregnancy, estrogen therapy, and oral contraceptive administration).[857] Lack of suppression can also occur when accelerated metabolism of dexamethasone caused by phenytoin, barbiturates, or other anticonvulsants results in failure to achieve plasma levels sufficient to suppress ACTH secretion.[857]

Two-Day Test

This test, introduced by Liddle in 1960,[905] has been used extensively in the diagnosis of Cushing's syndrome and provides the same information that the overnight 1-mg test provides. In its original form, the test is performed by collecting a 24-h urine sample for baseline determination. Dexamethasone is then given in a dose of 0.5 mg every 6 h for 2 days, with concurrent 24-h urine collections. Although the test can be performed on an outpatient basis, hospitalization may be required to ensure adequate urine collections. A normal urinary 17-OHCS response is suppression to less than 2.5 mg per day on the second day of dexamethasone administration.[874,905]

When these criteria are used, approximately 94 percent of patients with Cushing's syndrome have lack of suppression, and false-positive responses in controls are rare.[874] False-positive results occur rarely in obesity or high-estrogen states,[857,891,906,907] but as is the case with the overnight 1-mg test, false positives occur with acute and chronic illness, depression, alcoholism, and phenytoin therapy.[857,908,909] Because some patients with Cushing's syndrome show normal suppression with this dose, a modification of the test was introduced in which dexamethasone is given in a dose of 20 μg per kilogram of body weight per day.[891] In this study, normal and obese controls had urinary 17-OHCS excretion of less than 1 mg per gram of creatinine whereas none of 15 patients with Cushing's syndrome displayed this degree of suppression.[891]

The response of the urinary free cortisol excretion to the 2-day low-dose dexamethasone test was assessed in two studies; the lower limit was 19 to 25 μg/24 h on the second day.[906,907] Using these criteria, 95.6 percent of patients with Cushing's syndrome failed to suppress normally, and the frequency of false-positive responses in control subjects was 3 percent.[874] In one study, plasma cortisol fell to less than 5 μg/dl in normal subjects in response to low-dose dexamethasone.[910]

High-Dose Tests

High-dose dexamethasone tests are helpful in differentiating Cushing's disease from other types of hypercortisolism once the presence of Cushing's syndrome has been confirmed. These tests depend on the characteristic finding that the hypothalamic-pituitary axis in patients with Cushing's disease is suppressible with glucocorticoids, although pharmacologic doses are required. Thus, ACTH and cortisol secretion decrease when large amounts of dexamethasone are administered.[874,905,911] In contrast, in patients with hypercortisolism secondary to autonomous adrenal tumors or the ectopic ACTH syndrome, high-dose dexamethasone characteristically fails to suppress cortisol hypersecretion, as it is not under the control of the hypothalamic-pituitary axis. Although it is extremely useful, a number of exceptions occur in the use of the high-dose dexamethasone suppression test. These are discussed later (in the diagnosis and differential diagnosis and determining the etiology and tumor localization subsections in the section on Cushing's syndrome) and include Cushing's syndrome with periodic hormonogenesis, nonsuppressible pituitary Cushing's disease, occasional ectopic ACTH-secreting tumors that are suppressible, and nodular adrenal hyperplasia.[857,874]

Overnight 8-mg Test

The overnight high-dose dexamethasone suppression test is more reliable and easier to perform than the standard 2-day test described later (Fig. 11-31). A baseline morning cortisol specimen is obtained, and a single dose of dexamethasone (8.0 mg) is administered orally at 11 P.M. Plasma cortisol is then measured at 8 A.M. the following morning.[912] Among 60 patients with Cushing's disease, plasma cortisol levels were suppressed below 50 percent of baseline in 55 (92 percent), whereas no patient with either the ectopic ACTH syndrome or glucocorticoid-producing adrenal tumors ($N = 16$) had this degree of suppression. This test had a sensitivity of 92 percent, a specificity of 100 percent, and a diagnostic accuracy of 93 percent.[912] This single-dose test was more reliable than the 2-day test when compared in the same patients because in only 75 percent of patients with Cushing's disease was urinary 17-OHCS excretion suppressed with the 2-day test.[912] This overnight 8-mg high-dose dexamethasone suppression test is the procedure of choice because of its simplicity and reliability.

Two-Day High-Dose Test

This test first reliably differentiated Cushing's disease from other types of endogenous hypercortisolism.[874,905] A baseline 24-h urine sample is collected, and then dexamethasone (2.0 mg every 6 h for 2 days) is administered with concurrent 24-h urine collection. Again, hospitalization may be required for accurate urine collection. The test is best standardized for urinary 17-OHCS or UFC; patients with Cushing's disease show suppression of urinary 17-OHCS or UFC to below 50 and 90 percent of baseline levels, respectively.[905,912,914] In patients with adrenal tumors or the ectopic ACTH syndrome, there is usually no decrease in urinary corticosteroid excretion.

The diagnostic accuracy of this procedure is limited because 15 to 30 percent of patients with pituitary-dependent Cushing's disease do not adequately suppress urinary 17-OHCS or UFC excretion.[857,874,912,913] The response of urinary free cortisol has been less extensively studied, but in two series, 16 percent of patients with Cushing's disease did not display 50 percent suppression.[906,907] Measurement of plasma cortisol does not increase diagnostic reliability,[906,907] and measurement of urinary 17-KGS excretion is less reliable than that of urinary 17-OHCS.[874,907]

When the responses of both urinary free cortisol and urine 17-OHCS to the 2-day high-dose test were compared, urine cortisol was more profoundly suppressed than was urine 17-OHCS.[914] Thus, suppression of urinary cortisol by >90 percent or suppression of urine 17-OHCS by >64 percent correctly established a diagnosis of pituitary disease, and with these criteria no patient with the ectopic ACTH syndrome or an adrenal tumor was incorrectly classified.[914] The sensitivity was 83 percent, the specificity was 100 percent, and the diagnostic accuracy was 86 percent. The disadvantage is that 17 to 31 percent of patients with Cushing's disease do not suppress to this extent and will not be correctly identified.

Tests of Pituitary-Adrenal Reserve

Tests of pituitary-adrenal reserve assess the functional capacity of the hypothalamic pituitary-adrenal axis, its reserve capacity, and

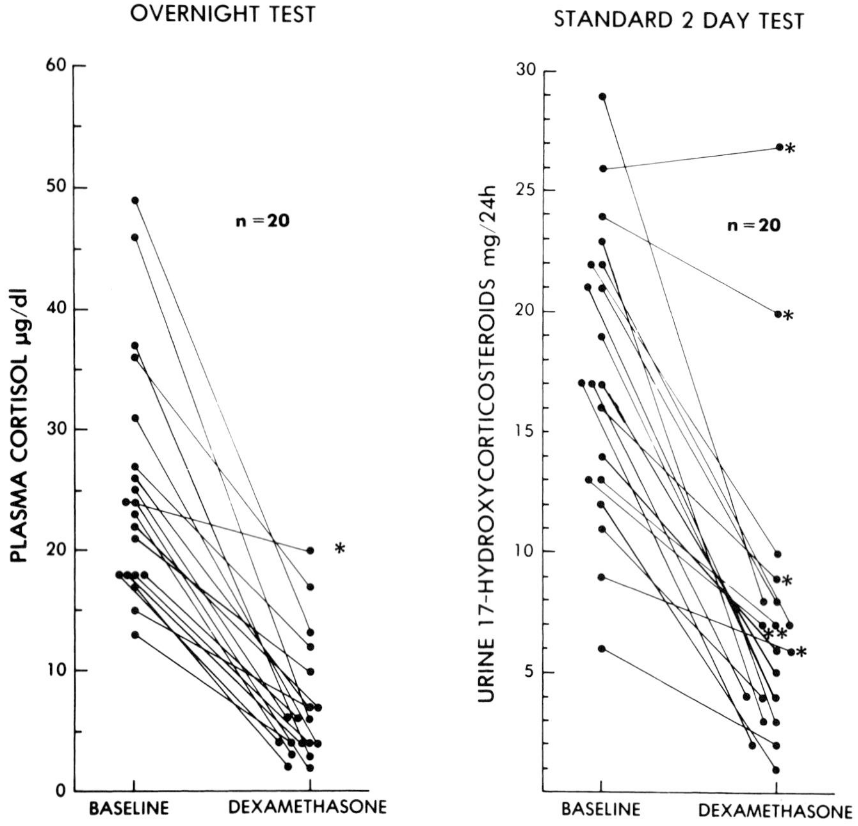

FIGURE 11-31. *(Left)* Plasma cortisol response to the overnight high-dose (8 mg) dexamethasone suppression test. *(Right)* Urinary 17-OHCS response to the standard 2-day, high-dose dexamethasone suppression test in 20 patients with Cushing's disease. Asterisks indicate tests in which the response was not suppressed to <50 percent of the baseline level. (*Based on data of Tyrrell et al.*[912])

its ability to respond to stress. The four most reliable tests use (1) ACTH, which directly stimulates adrenal glucocorticoid secretion, (2) metyrapone, which inhibits adrenal cortisol production and thus indirectly stimulates pituitary ACTH secretion, (3) human or ovine CRF to stimulate ACTH and cortisol release,[915–918] and (4) insulin-induced hypoglycemia, which acts via the pituitary to stimulate ACTH release.[919] Measurement of the adrenal and pituitary responses to these tests is thus used to establish the diagnosis of primary or secondary adrenal insufficiency.

The administration of ACTH directly stimulates adrenal cortisol secretion. In primary adrenocortical insufficiency, the adrenal cortex is destroyed and thus cannot respond. In secondary adrenocortical insufficiency, there is atrophy of the cortex; thus, there is an inadequate acute response to ACTH although cortisol secretion ultimately increases if ACTH stimulation is continued. The rapid ACTH stimulation is usually the first step in evaluating patients with suspected adrenocortical insufficiency.

Rapid ACTH Stimulation Test

This test measures the acute response to ACTH; it is useful in the diagnosis of both primary and secondary adrenal insufficiency. It can be performed on an outpatient basis at any time of the day, does not require fasting, and in emergencies requires only a 30-min delay in the institution of therapy.[920–926] The potent synthetic ACTH derivative cosyntropin (tetracosactrin) is used. It contains the first 24 amino acids of human ACTH and is preferred to previously used animal ACTH preparations, to which there is a greater incidence of allergic reactions.[920] Cosyntropin (250 µg) is administered intramuscularly (IM) or intravenously (IV), and samples for plasma cortisol determination are obtained at 30 min or 60 min after the injection (Fig. 11-32). An additional basal plasma sample is collected before the injection; this is subsequently assayed for plasma ACTH if the response to cosyntropin is subnormal (see the section on adrenocortical insufficiency).

The original normal criteria using the fluorimetric cortisol assay were a basal level of plasma cortisol >5 µg/dl, an ACTH-stimulated increment of >7 µg/dl, and a maximal level of >18 µg/dl at 30 min.[920–922] However, more recent studies have established that the best criteria for a normal response is the maximal plasma cortisol level achieved. In a retrospective study using a cortisol immunoassay, a normal response was defined as a peak cortisol of 20 µg/dl or greater regardless of the increment.[923] This study documented the frequently noted clinical finding that patients with high basal cortisol values may show no further increase in response to acute ACTH stimulation. A prospective study in 50 normal patients confirmed that the peak serum cortisol 30 min after ACTH stimulation should exceed 20 µg/dl and that the calculation of the increment is of no value.[924] Another study showed that the 30-min peak cortisol value was most useful and that the response was not related to either the time of day or the basal cortisol level.[925] In an additional study, either IM or IV administration of ACTH resulted in equal adrenal cortisol responsiveness.[926] Thus, the rapid ACTH stimulation test can be performed at any time of the day, the ACTH can be administered either IV or IM, the plasma cortisol response is best assessed at 30 min after ACTH administration, and a normal response is a peak plasma cortisol of 20 µg/dl or greater regardless of the increment. In a more recent study, the levels of cortisol after IM administration of AGTH were lower than those after IV administration by approximately 2 µg/dl.[927]

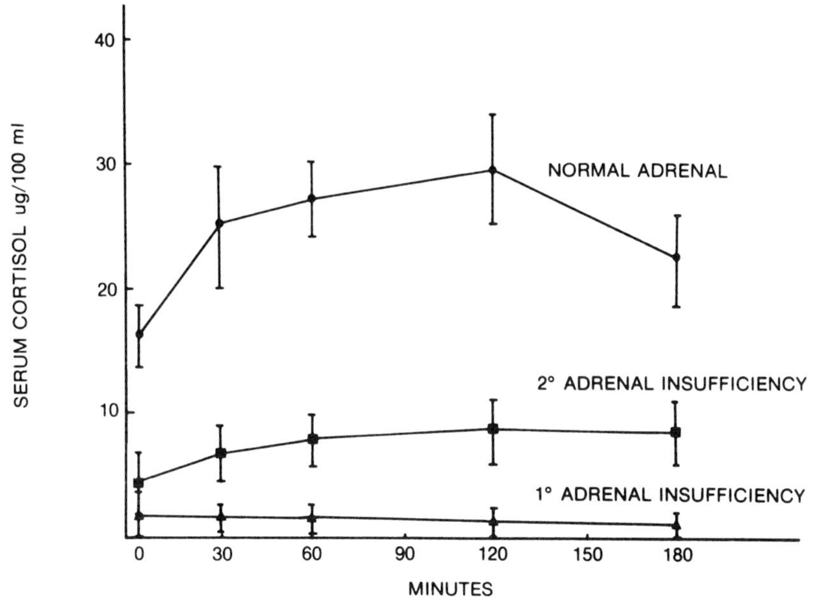

FIGURE 11-32. Serum cortisol response to 0.25 mg cosyntropin in nine normal individuals (normal adrenal), eight patients with hypopituitarism (secondary adrenal insufficiency), and seven patients with Addison's disease (primary adrenal insufficiency). (*From Speckart et al.*[921])

Subnormal responses to the rapid ACTH stimulation test establish the diagnosis of primary or secondary adrenal insufficiency. In primary adrenal insufficiency, the cortex is damaged; cortisol secretion is reduced, endogenous ACTH secretion is increased, and any remaining cortical tissue is unable to increase cortisol secretion in response to maximal stimulation with exogenous ACTH (decreased adrenal reserve). In secondary adrenal insufficiency, inadequate ACTH secretion leads to atrophy of the zonae fasciculata and reticularis and therefore to adrenal unresponsiveness to brief (but not prolonged) stimulation with exogenous ACTH. In this setting, a subnormal response to exogenous ACTH accurately predicts deficient responsiveness to insulin hypoglycemia, metyrapone, and surgical stress.[923,928–934] The cortisol determinations per se do not differentiate primary from secondary etiology; however, the plasma ACTH concentration is elevated in the primary form but depressed in the second form as described in the section on adrenocortical insufficiency later.

A normal response to the rapid ACTH stimulation test excludes the diagnosis of primary adrenal insufficiency, as it provides a direct assessment of adrenal reserve. The response is also abnormal in almost all cases of secondary adrenocortical insufficiency; however, in partial ACTH deficiency, ACTH secretion may be sufficient to maintain adrenocortical function to the extent that atrophy does not occur, and so adrenal responsiveness to exogenous ACTH stimulation remains normal or nearly normal. However, in these patients ACTH secretion is unable to increase further in response to stress because they have a decreased pituitary reserve.[931,932,934] Thus, a normal response to ACTH does not always predict a normal response to direct stimuli such as hypoglycemia and stress and cannot be used to exclude partial secondary adrenal insufficiency with an inadequate pituitary reserve.[933] Such patients are best studied with the overnight metyrapone test described later.

The rapid ACTH stimulation test can also be used to measure plasma aldosterone responsiveness. This modification can be used to differentiate primary and secondary adrenocortical insufficiency.[935] In primary adrenal insufficiency, destruction of all three zones of the cortex leads to deficient responses of both cortisol and aldosterone to exogenous ACTH. However, in most patients with secondary adrenal insufficiency, aldosterone secretion is maintained by the renin-angiotensin system. Therefore, the aldosterone response to exogenous ACTH is normal even though cortisol does not respond. Patients with secondary adrenal insufficiency have an increment in plasma aldosterone of >4 ng/dl, whereas patients with primary Addison's disease have no response.[935]

Three-Day ACTH Stimulation Tests

Three-day ACTH stimulation tests have traditionally been used in the diagnosis of adrenal insufficiency and the differentiation of the primary and secondary forms. These tests are rarely performed at present.

Metyrapone Testing

Metyrapone stimulation assesses both pituitary and adrenal reserve and thus can be used in the diagnosis of both primary and secondary adrenal insufficiency. Metyrapone inhibits adrenal P450c11β and thus blocks cortisol synthesis. The fall in circulating cortisol levels increases a release of ACTH that in turn stimulates increased production of steroids proximal to the site of enzyme inhibition. As a result, plasma levels of 11-deoxycortisol increase, as does urinary 17-OHCS excretion (due to increased excretion of the tetrahydro metabolite of 11-deoxycortisol).[928,936,937] The response to metyrapone correlates well with insulin-induced hypoglycemia,[928,930,937] and a normal metyrapone test predicts a normal response to surgical stress in virtually all patients.[931] Because of its simplicity and low risk, the overnight metyrapone test is preferred to insulin-induced hypoglycemia. This test is not used in patients with suspected primary adrenal insufficiency because the rapid ACTH stimulation test is diagnostic in virtually all patients (see earlier discussion and the section on adrenocortical insufficiency). The metyrapone test is used to evaluate patients with suspected secondary adrenal insufficiency who have normal or nearly normal responses to ACTH stimulation. In this setting, a subnormal response to metyrapone confirms secondary adrenal insufficiency, and glucocorticoid therapy is required in times of stress.

Overnight Test

The overnight test is performed by administering a single dose of metyrapone at midnight with a snack to minimize gastrointestinal upset. The dose of metyrapone is 30 mg/kg, i.e., approximately 2.0 g for patients weighing less than 70 kg, 2.5 g for patients weighing 70 to 90 kg, and 3.0 g for patients weighing more than 90 kg.[936] Blood for 11-deoxycortisol and cortisol is drawn at 8 A.M. Patients with a normal pituitary-adrenal axis have a post-metyrapone level of plasma 11-deoxycortisol >7 μg/dl, whereas patients with adrenal insufficiency do not respond.[936] Simultaneous plasma cortisol measurement is useful because 4 percent of normal subjects and patients on phenytoin have a rapid clearance or inactivation of metyrapone, and thus adequate 11β-hydroxylase inhibition does not occur.[936] An 8 A.M. plasma cortisol level of <10 μg/dl indicates adequate inhibition. A normal response to the overnight test indicates normal ACTH secretion and adrenal function, as both are required to increase plasma 11-deoxycortisol concentration. A subnormal response indicates primary or secondary adrenal insufficiency but does not differentiate between them.

Three-Day and Intravenous Tests

The original 3-day protocol of the metyrapone test and an intravenous modification are less commonly used. The overnight test described earlier provides the same information and does not require either urine collections or IV administration of the drug.

CRH Testing

Synthetic human CRH and ovine CRH are available for evaluation of the pituitary-adrenal axis.[915–918,938] Ovine CRH is more useful for testing because of its longer duration of action. CRH is given IV in a dose of 1 μg per kilogram of body weight. CRH directly stimulates pituitary secretion of the products of POMC, e.g., ACTH, β-LPH, and β-endorphin. Reported normal responses of ACTH and cortisol have varied and have to be established for individual laboratories.

Patients with primary adrenal insufficiency have high basal ACTH levels and subnormal cortisol levels. In response to CRH, ACTH levels increase but cortisol levels do not, reflecting primary adrenal damage. In secondary adrenal insufficiency, plasma cortisol also fails to respond to CRH; however, reported ACTH responses have been very variable and are probably not diagnostically reliable. In general, CRH testing is not required in patients who are being evaluated for adrenal insufficiency because adequate information can be obtained with standard ACTH stimulation and metyrapone tests.

CRH has also been used to differentiate the various etiologies of Cushing's syndrome. In general, patients with Cushing's disease have normal or exaggerated plasma ACTH and cortisol responses to CRH, although an occasional patient fails to respond. Patients with the ectopic ACTH syndrome do not respond to CRH, although exceptions do occur.[917,939] Patients with adrenal tumors causing Cushing's syndrome have suppressed ACTH levels that do not respond to CRH.

Insulin-Induced Hypoglycemia

The response to insulin-induced hypoglycemia (insulin tolerance test) is the most sensitive and accurate test of the integrity of the hypothalamic-pituitary-adrenal axis[933,934,940,941] and its ability to respond to stress. However, this test is generally limited to the evaluation of patients with suspected hypopituitarism in whom the growth hormone response can be simultaneously evaluated; the test is not commonly used at present. Hypoglycemia elicits a potent stress response via pituitary adrenergic receptors[919] and stimulates ACTH release. The test is performed after an overnight fast with measurement of plasma cortisol, glucose, and serum growth hormone levels before and at 30, 45, 60, and 90 min after the administration of IV regular insulin. The plasma glucose concentration is measured to assess the adequacy of the hypoglycemia; a value less than 40 mg/dl is considered an adequate stimulus.[933,934,940,942] The usual dose of insulin is 0.15 U/kg of body weight (0.10 U/kg in children) but must be adjusted on the basis of the patient's clinical status and suspected pituitary function. In suspected hypopituitarism or adrenal insufficiency, 0.1 U/kg of body weight is used (0.05 U/kg in children), and the usual dose of 0.15 U/kg is increased by 0.1 U/kg in patients with obesity, diabetes mellitus, Cushing's syndrome, or acromegaly, as these patients exhibit significant insulin resistance. An experienced physician must be in attendance, with careful monitoring of the patient and with IV glucose available. Most patients experience hypoglycemic symptoms, i.e., sweating, tachycardia, and hunger; the test should be terminated with IV glucose if significant symptoms of neuroglycopenia, such as confusion and disorientation, occur. The test is contraindicated in patients with seizure disorders, cardiovascular disease, and cerebrovascular disease, and in those greater than 65 years of age. It should not be performed in acutely ill patients with suspected adrenocortical insufficiency because they may be extremely sensitive to insulin. When these precautions are observed, there is little risk to the patient.

With adequate hypoglycemia, plasma cortisol levels peak 60 to 90 min after insulin injection. A normal response is an increment of plasma cortisol of >8 μg/dl and a maximum plasma cortisol level of >18 to 20 μg/dl when cortisol concentration is measured fluorimetrically.[435,934,940,942–944] Normal criteria using the competitive protein-binding assay are an increment of plasma cortisol of >5 μg/dl and a maximal level >15 μg/dl.[928]

A normal plasma cortisol response to hypoglycemia excludes adrenal insufficiency and indicates an intact hypothalamic-pituitary-adrenal axis; these patients do not require glucocorticoid supplementation for stress or surgery.[435] A subnormal response documents adrenal insufficiency and the requirement for glucocorticoid therapy.

Mineralocorticoids

The measurement of aldosterone, DOC, 18-OH-DOC, and other mineralocorticoid levels and the clinical evaluation of the renin-angiotensin-aldosterone axis are discussed in Chap. 13.

Androgens

Dynamic tests such as those described previously for studying cortisol excess or cortisol deficiency states have not been as useful in the evaluation of disorders of adrenal androgen production. Thus, greater reliance has been placed on measurement of basal plasma levels of the major adrenal androgens and the active metabolites derived from them (i.e., androstenedione, testosterone, and DHT). These steroids are assayed after extraction and chromatographic separation. Additional techniques that measure the free fraction of testosterone (and other hormones) or the binding capacity of sex hormone–binding globulin (SHBG, TeBG) improve the diagnostic usefulness of the tests. Urinary assays of androgen metabolites have been replaced by more sensitive plasma assays.

Plasma Androgens

Because of similarities in their structures, it has been difficult to assay the individual androgens in unfractionated plasma extracts.[862,863] However, DHEA-S can be measured directly because it is present in plasma in relatively high concentrations.[862] The other androgens and their precursors require separation and purification before assay. This is accomplished by solvent extraction, which fractionates steroids with differing polarity, and then chromatography.[862] After separation, the concentrations of steroids can be accurately measured by radioimmunoassay[862] or competitive protein binding.[945] With these techniques, total plasma concentrations of DHEA, DHEA-S, androstenedione, testosterone, and DHT can be measured simultaneously.[862,863] The normal plasma levels of these steroids are listed in Table 11-2.

The plasma concentration of free testosterone may also be assayed by flow dialysis, charcoal adsorption, equilibrium dialysis, steady-stage gel filtration, and ultrafiltration.[945–950] Plasma free testosterone concentrations (mean $\pm$ SD) have been reported as follows: normal females, 5.39 $\pm$ 2.13 pg/ml (1 to 1.4 percent free); pregnancy, 4.64 $\pm$ 1.70 pg/ml (0.6 percent free); hirsute females, 16.1 $\pm$ 11.7 pg/ml (1.7 to 2.2 percent free); and normal males, 128 $\pm$ 57 pg/ml (1.7 to 2.5 percent free).[945–948] These free levels more clearly reflect the biological activity of circulating testosterone than do total testosterone levels. Recent studies also have confirmed the utility of measuring plasma androstenediol and androstenediol glucuronide concentrations in disorders of androgen excess. Levels of these metabolites of DHT are elevated in the majority of women with androgen excess and provide an assessment of the tissue metabolism of androgens.[955]

The binding capacity of SHBG is estimated after its removal from plasma (by adsorption or precipitation) with the use of radiolabeled testosterone or DHT.[954,956] The SHBG binding capacity is higher in normal women than in normal men. It is increased in pregnancy, cirrhosis, and hyperthyroidism and with estrogen (including oral contraceptive) therapy.[951,954,956] SHBG binding capacity is decreased in most females with hirsutism and in acromegaly.[951,954] Recently, SHBG-specific IRAs have been developed and are gradually replacing the binding assays.

Urinary Androgens

Measurement of urinary 17-ketosteroid excretion was the first method of quantification of adrenal steroid secretion, but it is a less useful index of androgenicity than are the plasma methods described previously.[957] This method measures the levels of urinary metabolites of plasma androgens; the major contribution to urinary 17-ketosteroids is from DHEA and DHEA-S (Table 11-2). Testosterone and DHT constitute less than 1 percent of the total urinary 17-ketosteroids.[957] The ketosteroids are first extracted from urine and then measured by a colorimetric chemical assay (the Zimmerman reaction).[958] Normal excretion is generally in the range of 7 to 17 mg/24 h in males and 5 to 15 mg/24 h in females.[827] Drug interference is a disadvantage; i.e., chlorpromazine, ethinamate, meprobamate, nalidixic acid, penicillin, phenaglycodol, spironolactone, and troleandomycin falsely increase 17-ketosteroid values, and chlordiazepoxide, etryptamine acetate, progestins, propoxyphene, and reserpine decrease 17-ketosteroid values.[899]

Clinical Utility

The assays described are used in the evaluation of hyperandrogenic states. Idiopathic hirsutism and the polycystic ovary syndrome are frequently associated with elevated androgen secretion; however, androgen levels are also elevated in Cushing's syndrome, congenital adrenal hyperplasia, adrenal tumors, and ovarian tumors.

The utility of 17-ketosteroid determination is limited because this measurement is unreliable in the diagnosis of Cushing's syndrome[874,913] and androgen excess in hirsutism.[957] The diagnosis of congenital adrenal hyperplasia is best established by an assay of more specific plasma steroids. Plasma androgen assays are more useful; however, serial plasma samples and the assay of several plasma hormones may be required to document androgen excess.[949,953,957,959,960] In addition, assay of the plasma free testosterone concentration is the best single indicator of androgen excess.[945–949,951,954,961]

Adrenocortical Function in Children

Laboratory evaluation of adrenocortical function in children and adolescents should be preceded by a complete clinical evaluation. In addition, the rarity and complexity of these patients mandate referral to a pediatric endocrinologist. The laboratory evaluation must take into account the age-related changes in adrenocortical function. As stated above, precise plasma assays are tending to replace urinary steroid determinations, and as is the case with adult patients, interpretation of plasma steroid values must take into account the diurnal and episodic variability of their levels.

Plasma and Urinary Steroids

The normal plasma concentrations of glucocorticoids and mineralocorticoids in children and adolescents are shown in Table 11-8.[494] The concentrations of adrenal precursor steroids and gonadal steroids are shown in Table 11-9.[494]

Current methods include radioimmunoassay and competitive protein-binding radioassay, as discussed previously. However, cross-reactivity is a problem with these assays: in the newborn cortisone can cross-react, and in patients with CAH elevated levels of adrenal steroid precursors may cross-react. Thus, precise determination of specific steroids requires chromatographic separation procedures or specific measurement by HPLC.[494]

As discussed earlier, urinary 17-OHCS measures the major metabolites of cortisol; however, this measurement has been largely replaced by the more specific measurement of urine free cortisol. Normal excretion of free cortisol in children is 15 to 20 μg per gram of creatinine and may be up to 40 μg in obese children.[494] Urine cortisol expressed in terms of body surface area is 25 to 70 $\mu g/m^2$ per 24 h in normal children and adolescents.[962] Values above these normal ranges are found in Cushing's syndrome.

Dexamethasone Suppression Tests

In children as in adults, these tests are used to establish the diagnosis of Cushing's syndrome. A modification of the overnight

TABLE 11-8. Mean Glucocorticoid and Mineralocorticoid Concentrations

	Cortisol	DOC	Corticosterone	18-OH Corticosterone	Aldosterone	Plasma Renin Activity
Cord blood	12	180	650		85	1800
Prematures	6.5			200	100	8000
Newborns	5		230	350	95	2100
Infants	9	20	545	80	30	1200
Children (8 A.M.)						
1–2 yr	4–20			65	28	535
2–10 yr	As adults	10		45	10→30*	300
10–15 yr	As adults			25	5→20*	120
Adults (8 A.M.)	10–20	7	425	20	7→13*	100→145*
(4 P.M.)	5–10		130			

DOC = deoxycorticosterone.

All values in ng/dl plasma except cortisol (μg/dl) and plasma renin activity (ng/dl/per hr).

*Two values separated by an arrow indicate those in supine and upright posture.

Source: Reproduced with permission from Miller.[575]

screening test demonstrated that a dose of 0.3 mg/m^2 or 15 μg/kg of dexamethasone could suppress plasma cortisol in normal children.[963]

Traditional low- and high-dose dexamethasone suppression tests are extremely useful and are best performed in a hospital or metabolic ward.[494] After the collection of baseline data, dexamethasone is administered in a dose of 30 μg/kg per day (low-dose) given in divided doses every 6 h for 2 days. For the subsequent 2 days, the patient is given 120 μg/kg per day (high-dose) in divided doses every 6 h. Normal responses to the low-dose test are plasma cortisol values less than 5 μg/dl and urine 17-OHCS <1 mg per gram of creatinine. In most patients, normal responses to low-dose dexamethasone exclude Cushing's syndrome; however, some children and adolescents with Cushing's disease have

TABLE 11-9. Mean Sex Steroid Concentration in Infants and Children

	PROG	17-OHP	DHEA	DHEA-S μg/dl	Δ^4-A	E_1	E_2	*T* M	*T* F	*DHT* M	*DHT* F
Cord Blood	36,000	1900	600	235	90	1400	810	30	25	6	6
Prematures	350	250	800	400	200			120	10	30	40
Term newborns		35	570	160	150			200	40	25	10
Infants	30	30	110	30	20	<1.5	<1.5	190	<10	40	<3
Children 1–6 yr			30	10	25	<1.5	<1.5	5		<3	
6–8 yr			90	20	25	<1.5	<1.5	5		<3	
8–10 yr			160	50	25	<1.5	<1.5	5		<3	
Males											
Pubertal stage I	20	40	160	35	25	1.1	0.8	5		<3	
II	20	50	300	95	45	1.6	1.1	40		8	
III	25	60	390	120	70	2.1	1.6	190		20	
IV	35	80	400	200	80	3.3	2.2	370		35	
V	40	100	500	230	100	3.2	2.1	550		45	
Adult	35	100	450	270	115	3.0	2.0	620		50	
Females											
Pubertal stage I	20	30	160	40	25	1.3	0.8		5		<3
II	30	50	330	70	65	2.1	1.6		20		8
III	40	70	390	90	120	3.0	2.5		25		10
IV	290	90	430	120	130	3.6	4.7		25		10
V	160	110	540	150	160	6.1	11.0		30		10
Adult											
Follicular	30	45	450	150	165	6.0	5.0		30		10
Luteal	750	165	450	150	165	11.0	13.0		30		10

PROG = progesterone; 17-OHP = 17-hydroxyprogesterone; DHEA = dehydroepiandrosterone; DHEA-S = DHEA sulfate; Δ^4-A = androstenedione; E_1 = estrone; E_2 = estradiol; T = testosterone; DHT = dihydrotestosterone; M = male; F = female.

All values except DHEA-S are in ng/dl.

Data adapted from Endocrine Sciences, Tarzana, California.

Source: Reproduced with permission from Miller.[575]

normal responses to this test. In these patients, the diagnosis must be established by elevated urine cortisol values and by the demonstration of abnormal diurnal variation of plasma cortisol.[494]

The responses to high-dose dexamethasone testing are the same as those described above in adults. Patients with Cushing's disease suppress plasma or urine steroids to <50 percent of baseline; patients with adrenal tumors or the ectopic ACTH syndrome show little change in steroid levels.[494]

Plasma ACTH Levels

Plasma ACTH in children measured by sensitive radioimmunoassay or by IRMA has the same utility as in adults (described earlier). Thus, elevated levels are present in Cushing's disease, Nelson's syndrome, the ectopic ACTH syndrome, primary adrenal failure (Addison's disease), and, most important in children, CAH. Suppressed levels are present with adrenal tumors causing Cushing's syndrome and in hypopituitarism (secondary hypoadrenalism) or after exogenous glucocorticoid therapy.

Adrenal Stimulation Testing

Stimulation of the adrenal cortex with ACTH is the most direct means of testing adrenocortical function. In children, these procedures are of the greatest utility in the diagnosis of adrenocortical insufficiency (as explained earlier) and the syndromes of CAH (see the next section).

The traditional ACTH stimulation test consists of the administration of 0.5 units/kg of ACTH (1–39) given as a 4- to 6-h infusion, which results in maximal stimulation of adrenocortical steroids.[494] However, this procedure has been replaced by the plasma corticosteroid response to a single intravenous dose of synthetic ACTH (1–24). With this procedure, the response of plasma cortisol or other steroids is measured 30 and/or 60 min after ACTH injection; the usual doses are 0.1 mg in newborns, 0.15 mg in children less than 2 years of age, and 0.25 mg in older children and adults. Normal responses to this ACTH stimulation test in children are shown in Table 11-10.[494]

The greatest utility of ACTH stimulation testing in childhood is in patients with suspected CAH. In such patients, ACTH markedly stimulates steroids proximal to the enzymatic block. For example, in P450c21 deficiency, the classic and most frequent form of CAH, plasma 17-hydroxyprogesterone increases excessively. The utility of this diagnostic procedure in CAH is described in the section on disorders of steroid hormone synthesis.

Other Pituitary-Adrenal Stimulation Tests

Metyrapone

Metyrapone blocks P450c11 and cortisol secretion, thus stimulating ACTH secretion and increasing adrenal 11-deoxycortisol secretion. In children, metyrapone has been most frequently given in dose of 300 mg/m^2 orally every 4 h for six doses (total dose not to exceed 3.0 g).[494] The normal response is a peak plasma 11-deoxycortisol level of >5 μg/dl. Older children and adults can also be tested with a variation of the overnight test in which 30 mg/kg is given at midnight.[494]

Other Tests

Testing with CRH and insulin hypoglycemia has been used less extensively in the evaluation of adrenal function in childhood.

DISORDERS OF STEROID HORMONE SYNTHESIS

Introduction

Genetic abnormalities of each of the steps in the biosynthesis of steroid hormones have been described earlier in the section on steroid hormone biosynthesis. Because the same steroidogenic enzymes are involved in the synthesis of steroid hormones in both the adrenal cortex and the gonads, genetic disorders of steroidogenesis may affect both the adrenals and the gonads. Many of these disorders impair cortisol synthesis, resulting in stimulation of pituitary POMC and secretion of ACTH, which in turn causes adrenal growth. This adrenal enlargement, which was described at autopsy in the nineteenth century, is the basis of the term *congenital adrenal hyperplasia* (CAH), which refers to genetic disorders of cortisol synthesis. Disorders of 21-hydroxylation account for more than 90 percent of these genetic disorders, and thus, the term *CAH* generally implies 21-hydroxylase deficiency.

Congenital adrenal hyperplasia is often considered a rare disease; however, the incidence of severe forms of CAH is about 1 in 14,000 people[965] and the incidence of the milder forms is probably 10 times higher.[964] In addition to coming to medical attention as newborns with ambiguous genitalia and life-threatening cardiovascular collapse, patients with genetic disorders of steroid hormone synthesis may seek medical attention for infertility, impotence, hypertension, menstrual irregularity, hirsutism, and acne, and many

TABLE 11-10. Responses of Adrenal Steroids to a 60-Min ACTH Test

	Infants		*Prepubertal*		*Pubertal*	
	Basal	**Stimulated**	**Basal**	**Stimulated**	**Basal**	**Stimulated**
17-OH-Pregnenolone	225		55	320	120	800
17-OHP	25	190	50	190	60	160
DHEA	40		70	125	260	560
11-Deoxycortisol	80		60	200	60	170
Cortisol (μg/dl)	10	30	13	30	10	25
DOC	20	80	8	55	8	55
Progesterone	35	100	35	125	60	150

All values are mean values in ng/dl of plasma, except cortisol, which is μg/dl.

Data adapted from Endocrine Sciences, Tarzana, California.

Source: Reproduced with permission from Miller.[575]

children with these severe forms of CAH are now surviving to adulthood. Thus knowledge of these disorders is of increasing importance in adult as well as pediatric endocrinology.[1]

In theory, the congenital adrenal hyperplasias are easy to understand. A genetic disorder in one of the steroidogenic enzymes interferes with normal steroid hormone synthesis. The signs and symptoms of the disease derive from a deficiency of the steroidal end product and from the effects of the accumulated steroidal precursors proximal to the disordered step. Thus, reference to Figs. 11-4 and 11-7 and a knowledge of the biological actions of the various steroids permit one to deduce and predict the clinical manifestations of the disease.

In practice, the various forms of CAH can be confusing both clinically and scientifically. The principal clinical, laboratory, and therapeutic features of the major forms of CAH are shown in Table 11-11. As discussed in the section on steroid hormone biosynthesis, each steroidogenic enzyme has multiple activities, and many extraadrenal tissues contain other enzymes with similar steroidogenic activities. Thus, complete elimination of an adrenal enzyme may not result in the complete elimination of certain steroids from the circulation, making diagnosis difficult. For example, patients with severe salt-losing 21-hydroxylase deficiency can nevertheless have nearly normal levels of serum 21-hydroxylated steroids as adults[233] as a result of an extraadrenal 21-hydroxylase that is

TABLE 11-11. Clinical and Laboratory Findings in Congenital Adrenal Hyperplasia

Enzyme Deficiency	Presentation	Laboratory Findings	Theraputic Measures
StAR	Salt-wasting crisis Male pseudohermaphroditism	Low levels of all steroid hormones, with decreased/absent response to ACTH Decreased/absent response to HCG in male pseudohermaphroditism ↑ ACTH ↑ plasma renin activity (PRA)	Glucocorticoid and mineralocorticoid replacement Estrogen replacement in adolescence Gonadectomy of male pseudohermaphrodite
3β-HSD	*Classical form:* Salt-wasting crisis Male and female pseudohermaphroditism Precocious adrenarche *Nonclassical form:* Precocious adrenarche, disordered puberty, menstrual irregularity, hirsutism, acne, infertility	↑ Baseline and ACTH-stimulated Δ^5 steroids (pregnenolone, 17-OH pregnenolone, DHEA); ↑ Δ^5/Δ^4 serum steroids Suppression of elevated adrenal steroids after glucocorticoid administration ↑ ACTH ↑ PRA	Glucocorticoid and mineralocorticoid replacement Surgical correction of genitalia and sex hormone replacement as necessary, consonant with sex of rearing
P450c21	*Classical form:* Salt-wasting crisis Female pseudohermaphroditism Pre- and postnatal virilization *Nonclassical form:* Precocious adrenarche, disordered puberty, menstrual irregularity, hirsutism, acne, infertility	↑ Baseline and ACTH-stimulated 17-OHP ↑ Serum androgens and urine 17-KS Suppression of elevated adrenal steroids after glucocorticoid administration ↑ ACTH ↑ PRA	Glucocorticoid and mineralocorticoid replacement Vaginoplasty and clitoroplasty in female pseudohermaphroditism
P450c11β	Female pseudohermaphroditism Postnatal virilization in males and females Hypertension	↑ Baseline and ACTH-stimulated 11-deoxycortisol and DOC ↑ Serum androgens and urine 17-KS Suppression of elevated adrenal steroids after glucocorticoid administration ↑ ACTH, ↓ PRA, hypokalemia	Glucocorticoid administration Vaginoplasty and clitorial recession in female pseudohermaphroditism
P450c11AS	Poor growth in infancy Failure-to-thrive Weakness Salt loss	Hyponatremia, hyperkalemia ↑ Corticosterone ↓ Aldosterone, ↑ PRA	Mineralocorticoid replacement Salt supplementation
P450c17	Male pseudohermaphroditism Sexual infantilism Hypertension	↑ DOC, 18-OH-DOC, corticosterone, 18-hydroxycorticosterone Low 17α-hydroxylated steroids and poor response to ACTH Poor response to HCG in male pseudohermaphroditism ↑ ACTH ↓ PRA Hypokalemia	Glucocorticoid administration Surgical correction of genitalia and sex steroid replacement in male pseudohermaphroditism consonant with sex of rearing Sex hormone replacement in female

Source: Modified from Miller.[575]

different from adrenal P450c21.[228–230] In the past, disorders of steroidogenesis could be studied only by examining steroids in blood or urine because the disordered enzymes and the disordered genes encoding them were not available. This indirect approach, which is analogous to studying hemoglobinopathies by examining O_2 carrying capacity, led to many incorrect conclusions about the nature of the steroidogenic enzymes and their disorders. The cloning of the genes for the various steroidogenic enzymes has recently permitted direct study of these complex disorders. The current picture is substantially different from what was understood just a few years ago.

21-Hydroxylase Deficiency

21-hydroxylase deficiency is one of the most common inborn errors of metabolism. It is due to mutations in the gene encoding adrenal P450c21; recent surveys show that the incidence of the severe form is about 1 in 14,000 and that the mild nonclassical forms affect about 1 in 1,000 persons (see the section on incidence of 21-hydroxylase deficiency later). Because of increased success in diagnosis and treatment in infancy, many patients with severe forms of 21-hydroxylase deficiency now live well into the adult age group.[1] Furthermore, there is increasing recognition of the milder forms. Detailed reviews of the complex clinical physiology and molecular genetics of this disorder are available.[217,218,226,227,966,967]

Pathophysiology

For patients with complete deficiency of P450c21 (for example, a patient with homozygous gene deletion), the resulting clinical manifestations can be deduced from Fig. 11-7. Inability to convert progesterone to DOC results in aldosterone deficiency, which causes profound hyponatremia (Na^+ often below 110 mEq/liter), hyperkalemia (K^+ often above 10 mEq/liter), and acidosis (pH often below 7.1) with concomitant hypotension, shock, cardiovascular collapse, and death in an untreated newborn infant. As the control of fluids and electrolytes in the fetus can be maintained by the placenta and the mother's kidneys, this "salt-losing crisis" develops only after birth, usually during the second week of life. In addition, the inability to convert 17-OHP to 11-deoxycortisol results in cortisol deficiency; this impairs postnatal carbohydrate metabolism and exacerbates cardiovascular collapse. Cortisol also exerts a permissive effect on the pressor action of catecholamines, hence cortisol deficiency compromises vascular integrity by this mechanism as well. Cortisol deficiency is also manifested prenatally because low concentrations of fetal cortisol result in increased production and secretion of ACTH from the fetal pituitary. ACTH stimulates adrenal hyperplasia and transcription of the genes for all the steroidogenic enzymes, especially for P450scc, the rate-limiting enzyme in steroidogenesis (see the section on regulation of adrenal steroidogenesis). This increased gene transcription results in increased enzyme production and activity, with consequent accumulation of non-21-hydroxylated steroids, especially 17-OHP. 17-OHP accumulates to a massive degree because it is not readily converted to androstenedione,[186,187] and hence, in 21-hydroxylase deficiency, it is a "dead-end" steroid. The ACTH-induced increases in other steroidogenic enzymes contribute substantially to the overproduction of testosterone (Fig. 11-7).

In the male fetus, the testes produce large amounts of mRNA for the steroidogenic enzymes and concentrations of testosterone are high in early to midgestation.[968] This testosterone differentiates external male genitalia from the pluripotential embryonic precursor structures. In the male fetus with 21-hydroxylase deficiency, the additional testosterone produced in the adrenals has little, if any, demonstrable phenotypic effect. In a female fetus, the ovaries lack steroidogenic enzyme mRNAs and are steroidogenically quiescent.[968] No sex steroids or other factors are needed for differentiation of the female external genitalia (i.e., the default phenotype of the human fetus is female) (for review, see Ref. 969). In a female fetus with 21-hydroxylase deficiency, the testosterone inappropriately produced by the adrenals causes varying degrees of virilization of the external genitalia. This can range from mild cliteromegaly with or without posterior fusion of the labioscrotal folds to complete labioscrotal fusion that includes a urethra traversing the enlarged clitoris (Fig. 11-33). At birth, these female infants, who have normal ovaries, fallopian tubes, and a uterus, may have "ambiguous" genitalia or may be sufficiently virilized so that they appear to be male, resulting in errors of sex assignment at birth. This physiology leads to the other common terms for 21-hydroxylase deficiency: *virilizing adrenal hyperplasia* and *adreno-genital syndrome.*

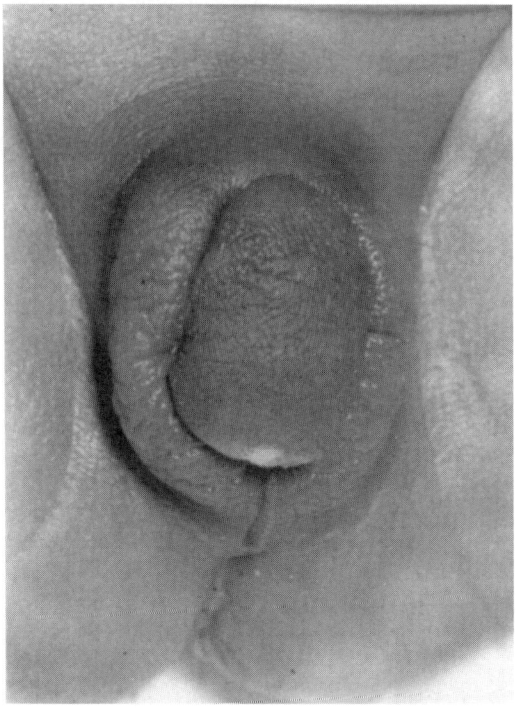

FIGURE 11-33. Genitalia of a severely virilized 2-week-old 46, XX female with severe salt-losing CAH. At birth, this infant was incorrectly thought to be a male with undescended testes and mild hypospadias. Presenting symptoms included vomiting, dehydration, Na^+ = 107 mEq/liter, K^+ = 10.1 mEq/liter, pH 7.4.

The diagnosis of 21-hydroxylase deficiency is suggested by genital ambiguity in females, a salt-losing episode in either sex, or rapid growth and virilization in males. Plasma 17-OHP is markedly elevated (>2,000 ng/dl after 24 h of age) and hyperresponsive to stimulation with ACTH (Fig. 11-34). Measurement of other steroids, such as 11-deoxycortisol, 17-OHP, DHEA, and androstenedione, is important because certain adrenal or testicular tumors can also produce 17-OHP[38] and high 17-OHP values that rise further after ACTH can also be seen in 3β-HSD and P450c11 deficiencies.[970] 17-OHP is normally high in cord blood but falls to

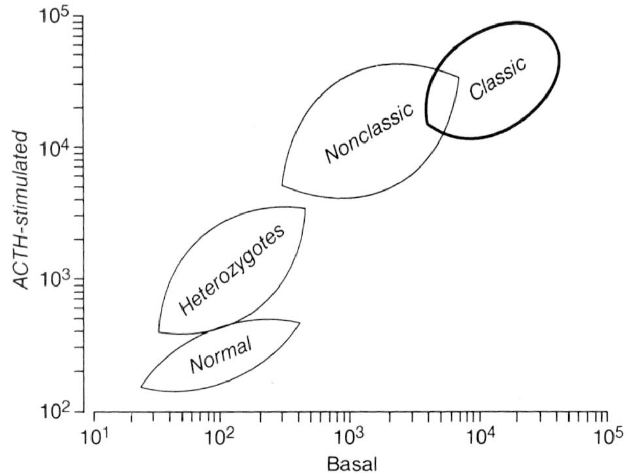

FIGURE 11-34. 17-OHP values before and after stimulation with ACTH in normals, patients with CAH, and heterozygotes. (*Redrawn from Miller.*[575])

"normal" levels in the newborn after 12 to 24 h (Fig. 11-35) so that assessment of 17-OHP levels should not be made in the first 24 h of life. Endocrinologically normal premature infants and term infants under severe stress (e.g., with cardiac or pulmonary disease) may have persistently elevated concentrations of 17-OHP with normal 21-hydroxylase.

Clinical Forms of 21-Hydroxylase Deficiency

21-hydroxylase deficiency is characterized by a broad spectrum of clinical manifestations, depending on the genetic disorders of the P450c21 alleles. Although these presentations are generally described as different diseases or different forms of 21-hydroxylase deficiency, there is a continuous spectrum of manifestations of this disease, ranging from the severe "salt-wasting form" described previously to clinically inapparent forms that may be normal variants. Thus, the disease forms listed here are mainly a clinical convenience.

Salt-Wasting CAH

The clinical phenotype described previously is that of a patient with salt-wasting 21-hydroxylase deficiency. Females with this disorder are frequently diagnosed at birth because of ambiguous development of the external genitalia. After appropriate resuscitation of the cardiovascular collapse, acidosis, and electrolyte disorders, the mineralocorticoids and glucocorticoids can be replaced orally and the ambiguous genitalia can be corrected with plastic surgical procedures. The steroidal replacement management is difficult because of the rapidly changing needs of a growing infant or child. Not only must drug doses be adjusted frequently as the child grows, there is also considerable individual variability in what constitutes "physiologic" replacement. As an underdosage of glucorticoids can be life-threatening, especially during illness, physicians have tended to err on the "safe side" and so these children usually receive inappropriately large doses of glucocorticoids. It is not possible to compensate for the growth lost during the first 2 years of life, when growth is fastest, and so these children inevitably end up shorter than predicted from their genetic potential. Female survivors may have sexual dysfunction, marry with a low frequency, and have decreased fertility, ostensibly through "imprinting" of the fetal brain by excessive adrenal androgens.[971–975] Males with this disorder generally go undiagnosed at birth and either come to medical attention during the salt-losing crisis that follows 5 to 15 days later or die, invariably with an incorrect diagnosis.

Simple Virilizing CAH

Females who are virilized with ambiguous genitalia and increased concentrations of 17-OHP but who do not suffer a salt-losing crisis have long been recognized as having the "simple virilizing" form of CAH. The existence of this clinical variant first led to the incorrect belief that there are two different adrenal 21-hydroxylases, one metabolizing progesterone in the zona glomerulosa and the other metabolizing 17-OHP in the zona fasciculata. Males with this disorder often escape diagnosis until age 3 to 7 years, when they come to medical attention because of inappropriate virilization (pubic, axillary, and facial hair, etc.). An astute physician can readily differentiate boys with sexual precocity caused by CAH from boys with true central precocious puberty: in CAH the testes remain of prepubertal size, while gonadotropic stimulation in true precocious puberty results in pubertal-sized testes. Although these children grow rapidly and are tall for age when diagnosed, their epiphyseal maturation (bone age) advances at a disproportionately rapid rate so that their ultimate adult height is invariably compromised. Untreated or poorly treated children with CAH may fail to undergo normal puberty, and boys may have small testes and azoospermia because of the feedback effects of the adrenally produced testosterone. When treatment is begun at several years of age, suppression of adrenal testosterone secretion may remove tonic inhibition of the hypothalamus, occasionally resulting in true central precocious puberty, requiring treatment with a GnRH agonist. High concentrations of ACTH in some

FIGURE 11-35. Means and ranges of 17-OHP in normal newborns. Note that values can be very high and quite variable for the first 24 h of life. (*Redrawn from Miller.*[575])

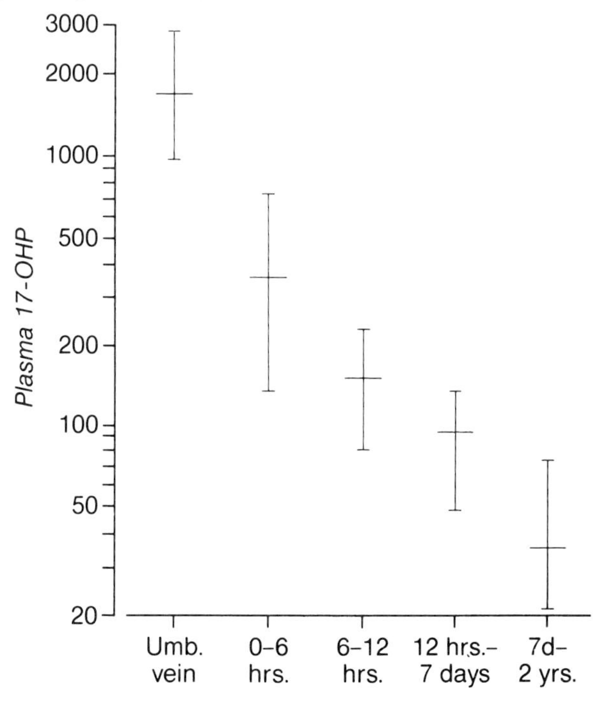

poorly treated boys may stimulate the enlargement of adrenal rests in the testes. These enlarged testes are usually nodular, unlike the homogeneously enlarged testes in central precocious puberty (for review and references, see Ref. 38). Because the adrenal normally produces 100 to 1,000 times as much cortisol as aldosterone, mild defects (point mutations) in P450c21 are much less likely to affect mineralocorticoid secretion than cortisol secretion. Thus, patients with simple virilizing CAH simply have a less severe disorder of P450c21. This is reflected physiologically by the increased plasma renin activity seen in these patients after moderate salt restriction.

Nonclassic CAH

Many people have very mild forms of 21-hydroxylase deficiency. These forms may be evidenced by mild to moderate hirsutism, virilism, menstrual irregularities, and decreased fertility in adult women (so-called late-onset CAH),[976–978] or there may be no phenotypic manifestations at all other than an elevated response of plasma 17-OHP in response to the administration of ACTH (so-called cryptic CAH).[979] Despite the minimal manifestations of this disorder, these individuals also have hormonal evidence of a mild impairment in mineralocorticoid secretion, as predicted from the existence of a single adrenal 21-hydroxylase.[980]

There has been considerable debate about how to classify patients into these three categories. The difficulty is due principally to the fact that each diagnostic category is not a specific disease but represents a typical picture in a continuous spectrum of disease. As described later, this is due to a broad spectrum of genetic lesions in the P450c21 gene. Furthermore, because many different mutant P450c21 alleles are common in the general population, most patients are compound heterozygotes, carrying a different mutation in the alleles inherited from each parent.

Incidence of 21-Hydroxylase Deficiency

The reported incidence of 21-hydroxylase deficiency varies widely. Perinatal screening for elevated concentrations of serum 17-OHP in several countries yielded an incidence of 1 in 14,000 for "classical" CAH (i.e., salt-wasting and simple virilizing CAH) and 1 in 60 for heterozygous carriers.[981] This calculation has now been confirmed through the screening of 1.9 million newborns in Texas.[965] The overall incidence found was 1 in 16,000; because of the large numbers involved, an ethnic breakdown was possible showing an incidence of 1 in 15,600 Caucasians, 1 in 14,500 Hispanics (primarily Mexican-Americans of indiginous American ancestry) and 1 in 42,300 Afro-Americans.[965]

Nonclassical CAH is clearly much more common, but these data are also variable. One group has reported very high frequencies: 1 in 27 for Ashkenazi Jews, 1 in 53 for Hispanics, 1 in 63 for Yugoslavs, 1 in 333 for Italians, and 1 in 1,000 for other whites.[982–984] These data would indicate that one-third of Ashkenazi Jews, one-fourth of Hispanics, one-fifth of Yugoslavs, one-ninth of Italians, and one-fourteenth of other whites are heterozygous carriers. However, other studies have shown carrier rates of 1.2 percent[978] to 6 percent[985,986] for white populations that were not subdivided further. The considerable differences in the reported incidences reflect differences in the small populations examined and the errors that inevitably arise when hormonal data are used to distinguish individuals with nonclassical CAH from heterozygous carriers of classical CAH. This error can be circumvented by careful measurement of 17-OHP before and after stimulation with ACTH (Fig. 11-34).[218] Furthermore, in homozygotes for both classical and nonclassical CAH, serum concentrations of 21-deoxycortisol rise in response to ACTH, but ACTH-induced 21-deoxycortisol remains normal in heterozygotes for both classical and nonclassical CAH.[987] However, all these studies have classified individuals only by hormonal phenotype; none has examined the P450c21 genes directly to establish these incidences. Therefore, the diagnosis of nonclassical CAH requires family studies, as the hormonal data (17-OHP responses to ACTH) in these individuals may be indistinguishable from those for unaffected heterozygous carriers of the more severe forms. The high incidence, lack of mortality, and lack of decreased fertility in most individuals with nonclassical CAH indicate that this is probably a variant of normal and is not a disease in the classic sense. Nevertheless, patients with nonclassical CAH may seek help for complaints of virilism and menstrual disorders.

Genetics of the 21-Hydroxylase Locus

21-Hydroxylase Genes

There are two 21-hydroxylase loci, a functional gene formally termed CYP21A2 and a nonfunctional pseudogene formally termed CYP21A1P.[95] These are generally termed P450c21B (functional gene) and P450c21A (pseudogene). These two genes are duplicated in tandem with the C4A and C4B genes encoding the fourth component of serum complement (Fig. 11-36).[988,989] The P450c21A gene cannot encode P450c21 because it has three different mutations, each of which prevents the translation of a corresponding mRNA.[220–222] However, the P450c21A locus is transcribed into two alternately spliced, adrenal-specific, polyadenylated mRNAs, but neither of these mRNAs encodes a protein.[221] Thus, only the P450c21B gene encodes adrenal 21-hydroxylase. P450c21 has a calculated molecular weight of 55,829, and Western blotting studies show a single band of this size.[991] The P450c21 genes consist of 10 exons, are about 3.4 kb long, and differ in only 87 or 88 of these bases.[220–222] This very great degree of sequence similarity indicates that these two genes are evolving in tandem (concerted evolution)[992–994] through intergenic exchange of DNA. The P450c21 genes of mice[231] and cattle[995,996] are also duplicated and linked to leukocyte antigen loci. However, while only the P450c21B gene functions in human beings, only the P450c21A gene functions in mice[997,998] and both genes function in cattle.[999] Nevertheless, sequencing of the gene duplication boundaries show that this locus duplicated after mammalian speciation,[1000] consistent with data that indicate that horses[1001] and pigs[1002] may have single P450c21 gene copies.

HLA Linkage

The diagnosis of 21-hydroxylase deficiency is greatly facilitated by the linkage of the P450c21 gene to the human major histocompatibility complex (MHC).[1003] This complex contains genes encoding three major classes of proteins: HLA-A, -B, and -C (class I); HLA-DP, -DQ, and -DR (class II); and serum complement components C2 and C4, properdin factor Bf, and tumor necrosis factors α and β (class III) (Fig. 11-36). HLA typing has been widely used for prenatal diagnosis and to identify heterozygous family members. The P450c21 locus lies about 600 kb from HLA-B and about 400 kb from HLA-DR.[1004,1005]

Statistical associations (linkage disequilibrium) are well established between CAH and certain specific HLA types. Salt-losing CAH is associated with HLA-B60 and HLA-40 in some populations[1006] and the rare HLA type Bw47 is very strongly associated with salt-losing CAH.[1007,1008] HLA-Bw51 is often associated with

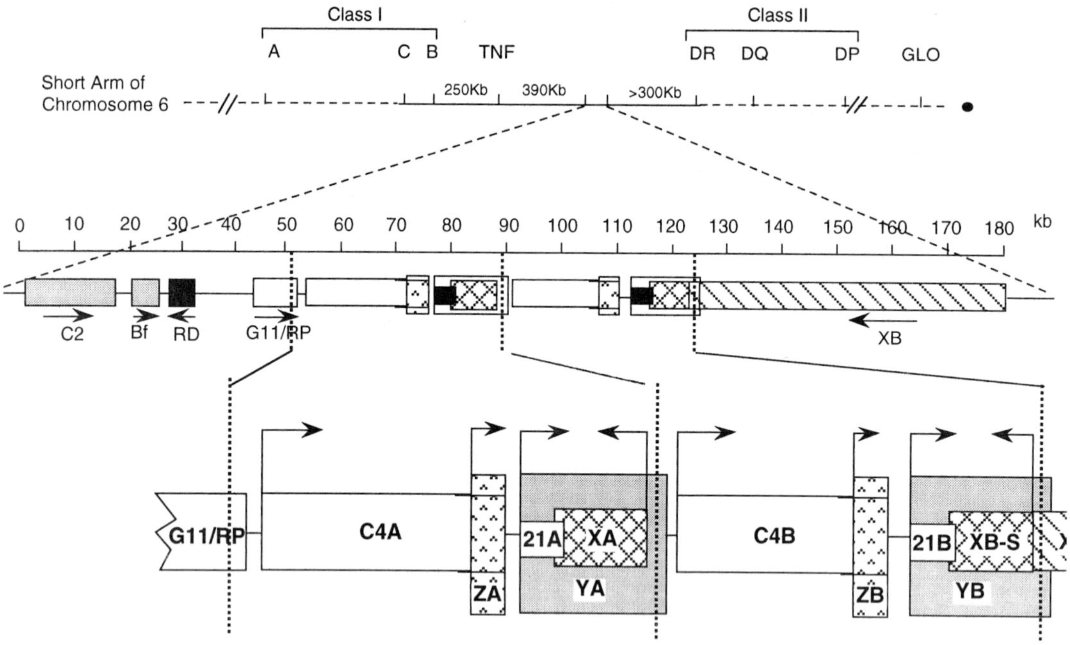

FIGURE 11-36. Genetic map of the HLA locus containing the genes for P450c21. The top line shows the p21.1 region of chromosome 6. The HLA Class III region containing the P450c21 genes lies between the Class I and II regions. The second line shows the genes for complement factor C2, properedin factor Bf, the RD and G11/RP genes of unknown function and the P450c21 locus. The scale is in kilobases (kb) and the arrows indicate transcriptional orientation. The bottom line shows the 21-hydroxylase locus on an expanded scale, including the C4A and C4B genes for the fourth component of complement, the inactive CYP21A gene (21A) and the active CYP21B gene (21B) that encodes P450c21. XA, YA, and YB are adrenal specific transcripts that lack open reading frames. The XB gene encodes the extracellular matrix protein Tenascin-X; XB-S encodes a truncated adrenal-specific form of the tenascin-X protein whose function is unknown. ZA and ZB are adrenal-specific transcripts that arise within the C4 genes and have open reading frames, but it is not known if they are translated into protein; however, the promoter elements of these transcripts are essential components of the CYP21A and CYP21B promoters. The arrows indicate transcriptional orientation. The vertical dotted lines designate the boundaries of the genetic duplication event that led to the presence of A and B regions.

simple virilizing CAH in some populations,[1009] and 30 to 50 percent of haplotypes for nonclassical CAH carry HLA-B14.[1010] HLA-B14 is often associated with a duplication of the C4B gene.[1011,1012] By contrast, all HLA-B alleles can be found linked to CAH.

Different individuals in the same family may have markedly different clinical features of CAH despite HLA identity of the affected individuals.[1013–1016] Such cases can represent extraadrenal 21-hydroxylation, de novo mutations, or multiple genetic crossover events. In one family with clinically nonconcordant HLA-identical siblings, the Southern blotting pattern of P450c21 genes digested with *Eco* RI showed a within-generation genetic rearrangement not detectable by other means.[1015]

C4 Genes

The tandemly duplicated C4A and C4B loci are both functional, and their encoded serum proteins can be distinguished functionally and immunologically, with the C4B protein having substantially more hemolytic activity despite greater that 99 percent sequence identity with C4A.[1017,1018] The C4A gene is 22 kb long and encodes a 5-kb mRNA. The C4B gene exists in a long (22 kb) form and a short (16 kb) form as a result of the presence or absence of a 6.8-kb intron at the 5′ end of the gene.[1019,1020] The 3′ ends of the C4 genes are only 2466 bp upstream from the transcriptional start sites of the P450c21 genes. Elements needed for the transcription of the human P450c21B gene lie within intron 35 of the C4B gene[1021] and also initiate the transcription of the 'Z transcripts,' which have an open reading frame, but their translational status is unclear.[1022]

Other Genes in the 21-Hydroxylase Locus

Recent studies have shown that the genetic anatomy of the 21-hydroxylase locus is complicated and crowded. In addition to the P450c21 and C4 genes, there are at least 10 and possibly more genes within 100 kb of the P450c21 gene (Fig. 11-34). The genes for complement factor C2 and properdin factor Bf lie 90 to 120 kb 5′ to the P450c21B gene and have the same transcriptional orientation (i.e., lie on the same strand of DNA). Lying just 3′ of the Bf gene is the RD gene, so called because it encodes a protein with a long stretch of alternating arginine (R) and aspartic acid (D) residues.[1023] This gene lies on the opposite strand of DNA from the complement and P450c21 genes and is expressed in all tissues, but the function of this gene and its influence, if any, on the genetics of this locus are unknown.[1024] Thirteen other putative genes have been identified lying between the gene for tumor necrosis factor (TNF) and C4A, but no functions have been ascribed to any of these genes.[1025]

A pair of genes, termed XA and XB, is duplicated with the C4 and P450c21 genes. These genes lie on the strand of DNA opposite from the C4 and P450c21 genes and overlap the 3′ end of P450c21. The last exon of XA and XB lies within the 3′ untranslated region of exon 10 in P450c21A and P450c21B, respectively.[223] Although the human XA locus was truncated during the duplication of the ancestral C4-P450c21-X genetic unit, the XA gene is abundantly transcribed in the adult and fetal adrenal.[1000] By contrast, the XB gene encodes a large extracellular matrix protein—Tenascin X—that is expressed in a wide variety of adult and fetal tissues, especially in cardiac, smooth, and striated muscle.[225,1026] The XB gene covers more than 65 kb of DNA and includes 43 exons encoding a 12 kb mRNA.[225,1027] The XB gene actually encodes two proteins, Tenascin-X and a short truncated form of Tenascin-X having unknown function and arising from an intragenic promoter.[1028] Identification of a patient with a 'contiguous gene syndrome' comprising a deletion of both the P450c21B and XB genes, demonstrated that deficiency of Tenascin-X results in Ehlers-Danlos syndrome (EDS).[1029] EDS can also be caused by mutations in collagen genes and genes for collagen-modifying enzymes; studies in cattle indicate that Tenascin-X is associated with and stabilizes collagen fibrils,[1030] thus explaining the related phenotype of mutations in Tenascin-X and collagen-associated genes. Although the various transcripts from the XA and XB genes are complementary to the mRNA for P450c21 and the other transcripts that arise from the P450c21 promoters,[224] these RNAs do not form RNA/RNA duplexes in vivo.[1031]

P450c21 Gene Lesions Causing 21-Hydroxylase Deficiency

21-hydroxylase deficiency can be caused by three general categories of mutations in the P450c21B gene: gene deletions, gene conversions, and apparent point mutations. As summarized below and reviewed in detail elsewhere,[226,227,1032] most of the point mutations described in the P450c21B gene to date are actually small gene conversion events, so gene conversions account for about 85 percent of the lesions in 21-hydroxylase deficiency. This highly unusual genetics led to controversy and confusion in this field, but authorities now agree on the nature of the various genetic lesions causing CAH. Because the P450c21 genes are autosomal, each person has 21-hydroxylase activity encoded by two different alleles, one contributed by the mother and one by the father. As is typical of any autosomal recessive disorder, the severity and clinical manifestations of 21-hydroxylase deficiency are determined by the less severely affected allele. Most patients with 21-hydroxylase deficiency are compound heterozygotes, having different lesions on their two alleles. Hence, statistical calculations about the causes of CAH must be measured in terms of the frequency of specific alleles rather than in terms of how many patients have which mutation. Because gene deletions and large conversions eliminate all P450c21B gene transcription, in the homozygous state these lesions will always cause salt-losing CAH. Some microconversions, such as those creating premature translational termination, are also associated with salt-losing CAH. Milder forms, such as simple virilizing and nonclassical CAH, are associated with various amino acid replacements in the P450c21 protein caused by other gene microconversion events. Patients with these forms of CAH are usually compound heterozygotes bearing a severely disordered allele (e.g., a gene deletion) and a mildly disordered allele (a microconversion) so that the clinical manifestations are based on the nature of the mildly disordered allele.

Mapping of P450c21 Genes in Normals and in CAH Although the P450c21B and P450c21A loci differ by only 87 or 88 nucleotides, they can be distinguished by restriction endonuclease digestion and Southern blotting. The P450c21A locus is characterized by 3.2- and 2.4-kb *Taq* I fragments and 12-kb *Bgl* II fragments, whereas the functional P450c21B gene is characterized by 3.7- and 2.5-kb *Taq* I fragments and 11-kb *Bgl* II fragments. *Eco* RI digests led to much initial confusion about this locus (for reviews, see Refs. 226 and 227) because the sites at the 3′ end of the genes are polymorphic, and the digestion is unpredictable because of variable methylation of these sites. Nevertheless, *Eco* RI digests can be highly informative in family studies.[1015] Two unusual and related features of the 21-hydroxylase locus complicate its analysis. First, although gene deletions in this locus are not rare, they are most unusual in that they extend 30 kb from a point in the middle of the P450c21A pseudogene to the precisely homologous point in the P450c21B gene. Thus, the 15 percent of alleles that have gene deletions do not yield a typical Southern blotting pattern with a band of a size different from that of one of the normal bands. This is true irrespective of the restriction endonuclease used to examine the locus, unless one uses very rarely cutting enzymes and analyzes the resulting large DNA fragments by pulsed-field gel electrophoresis.[1033–1037] With this technique, the entire gene complex extending from C4A to P450c21B can be seen as a 110-kb *Bss* HII fragment, with typical P450c21B gene deletions (which also delete C4B) appearing as 80-kb fragments. The second unusual feature of this locus is that gene conversions are extremely common.[1038,1039]

Gene Conversions The term *gene conversion* refers to a change in which a segment of gene A replaces the corresponding segment of related gene B; thus, the structure of recipient gene B is "converted" to that of donor gene A.[1040] A hallmark of gene conversion is that the number of closely related genes remains constant, while their diversity decreases. Gene conversion is thus the key mechanism in concerted evolution.[992–994] The mechanism of gene conversion is unclear, but evidence in yeast favors the creation of double-stranded breaks yielding a double-stranded gap that is repaired by copying both strands of the undamaged homologue.[1041–1043] Gene conversion–like events have been reported with a broad array of human genes.

Two types of gene conversions commonly cause 21-hydroxylase deficiency: large gene conversions that can be mistaken for gene deletions and small microconversions that resemble point mutations. When a large gene conversion causes 21-hydroxylase deficiency, the *Taq* I digestion pattern of the functional P450c21B gene is converted to that of the P450c21A pseudogene. This gene conversion changes the 5′ end of the P450c21B sequence to the 5′ end of P450c21A, as detected by Southern blotting studies,[1012,1013,1044] oligonucleotide probing,[1045] or sequencing.[1046] The relative frequency of large gene conversions versus gene deletions in CAH has been controversial,[1039,1045–1048] principally because initial studies used relatively small groups of patients from single locations or ethnic groups. A study of 68 French patients showed that 12.5 percent of the mutant alleles had large gene conversions, 12.5 percent had gene deletions, and 75 percent had microconversions.[1012] A compilation of the world literature on the genetics of CAH found that 19 percent of mutant alleles had gene deletions, 8 percent had large gene conversions, 67 percent had microconversions, and 6 percent had uncharacterized lesions (Fig. 11-37).[227] However, such statistics must be viewed with caution because there is considerable ascertainment bias in favor of the more severely affected patients[1012] and because some studies excluded

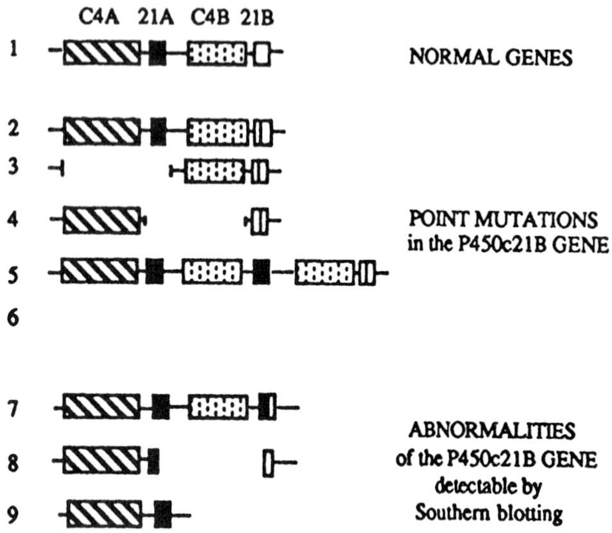

FIGURE 11-37. Classes of genetic rearrangements causing 21-hydroxylase deficiency. Deletions or duplications of the C4A and C4B genes can occur with or without associated lesions in the P450c21B gene. Note that all "point mutations" in P450c21B are actually "microconversions" (see text). (*Modified from Morel and Miller.*[227])

mildly affected patients. Thus, those statistics are weighted in favor of gene deletions and large conversions, which can only yield a phenotype of salt-wasting CAH.

Point Mutations (Microconversions) Causing CAH About 75 percent of mutated P450c21 genes appear to be structurally intact by Southern blotting and thus appear to carry point mutations.[1039] Many such mutant P450c21B genes causing CAH have been cloned and sequenced (Table 11-12), revealing that a relatively small number of mutations cause CAH, virtually all of which are also found in the P450c21A pseudogene. These observations indicate that most CAH alleles bearing apparent point mutations (as inferred from Southern blotting patterns) actually carry microconversions.[226,227,1032] Small localized gene conversions may occur more than once in a single P450c21 gene. Several mutant P450c21B genes have been described as having structures suggesting multiple crossover events, i.e., having alternating segments derived from the B and A genes.[1049,1050]

Effects of Known Point Mutations on 21-Hydroxylase Activity The biochemical consequences of microconversions on 21-hydroxylase activity have been studied by expressing the mutated genes and cDNAs transferred into various cell systems.[991,1051,1052] There are three changes in the P450c21A pseudogene that render its product nonfunctional. Each change results in an altered reading frame, with a consequent downstream in-phase translational stop codon (nonsense mutation). Each mutation can also be found in the P450c21B gene. The C→T transition at codon 318, the 8-bp deletion in exon 3, and the T insertion in exon 7 have all been found in P450c21B alleles that cause severe salt-losing CAH.[1045,1050,1053–1056] Three closely clustered base changes alter the normal amino acid sequence Ile-Val-Glu-Met at codons 236 to 239 in exon 6 to Asn-Glu-Glu-Lys in both P450c21A and a small number of genes causing CAH.[1051] The result is severe salt-losing CAH in the patient and absent assayable 21-hydroxylase activity when this gene is transfected into COS cells.

The most common lesion in classical CAH is an A→G change in the second intron, 13 bases upstream from the normal 3′ splice acceptor site of this intron.[1051] This mutation, which is found in more than 25 percent of severely affected CAH alleles, results in aberrant splicing of the P450c21 mRNA in a cryptic splice site 19 bases upstream from the 5′ end of exon 3. This changes the reading frame, destroying all P450c21 activity. However, a small portion of this mRNA may be spliced normally in some patients. Thus, the phenotypic presentation of this mutation can be somewhat variable; most such patients are salt losers, but some are more typical of non-salt-losing classic CAH. This intronic mutation, which results from another gene microconversion event, is often associated with the Ser→Thr polymorphism at codon 268; this is a true polymorphism as Ser268→Thr does not alter enzymatic activity.[1057] This intron 2 mutation is the most common lesion causing classical simple virilizing CAH in white patients, but it is rare in black and Hispanic patients.[1054,1055,1058–1060] In addition to these mutations, which grossly alter the structure of the encoded P450c21 protein, the mutation

TABLE 11-12. P450c21 Microconversions Causing 21-Hydroxylase Deficiency

Mutation	Location	Associated Phenotypes	Activity
Pro30 → Leu	Exon 1	NC/SV	30–60 percent
A → G	Intron 2	SV/SW	Minimal
8 bp deletion	Exon 3	SW	0
Ile 172 → Asn	Exon 4	SV	3–7 percent
Ile 236 → Asn Val 237 → Glu Met 239 → Lys	Exon 6	SW	0
Val 281 → Leu	Exon 7	NC	18 ± 9 percent
Gly 292 → Ser	Exon 7	SW	
T insertion @ 306	Exon 7	SW	0
Gly 318 → Stop	Exon 8	SW	0
Arg 339 → His	Exon 8	NC	20–50 percent
Arg 356 → Trp	Exon 8	SV/SW	2 percent
Pro 453 → Ser	Exon 10	NC	20–50 percent
GG → C @ 484	Exon 10	SW	0

Source: Data as compiled by Miller.[967]

Arg356→Trp, which results from a microconversion, eliminates all detectable activity,[991] apparently because it changes a residue in the binding site for P450 oxidoreductase.[103,1061,1062] This mutation is found in about 10 percent of severely affected alleles.[1057,1060] Other, extremely rare mutations have been described in single individuals.[1063–1065]

Missense Mutations Causing Simple Virilizing CAH A change of isoleucine, a nonpolar amino acid, to asparagine, a polar one, at codon 172 is the most common cause of simple virilizing CAH.[991,1049,1053] Ile 172 is conserved in the other known mammalian P450c21 genes and may contribute to the hydrophobic interactions needed to maintain the correct conformation of the enzyme. This mutation does not appear to affect the abundance or stability of P450c21 mRNA, suggesting that the resulting clinical phenotype is directly due to altered enzyme activity.[1049] When Ile 172 was changed to Asn, Leu, Gln, or His and the constructed mutants were expressed in mammalian cells, the mutant constructions yielded only 3 to 7 percent of the 21-hydroxylase activity of normal P450c21.[991,1052] Thus, Ile 172 is crucial, but its precise role has not been established.

As mentioned earlier, the common mutation causing a splicing error in intron 2 has occasionally been associated with simple virilizing CAH. The mutation Pro30→Leu is generally associated with the milder, nonclassical phenotype of CAH. However, the activity of this mutation in vitro is less than that of the common Val281→Leu mutation causing nonclassical CAH and has been reported in some patients with simple virilizing CAH. This emphasizes the fact that the distinctions among salt-losing, simple virilizing, and nonclassical CAH are matters of degree, so that some overlap is to be expected. Similarly, as the Arg356→Trp mutant retains a small degree of activity,[991,1053] it would not be surprising if it were described in simple virilizing rather than salt-wasting patients.

Missense Mutations Causing Mild, Nonclassic CAH DNA sequencing and oligonucleotide hybridization studies have established that the most common mutation causing nonclassical CAH is Val281→Leu.[1012,1057,1066] This mutation is seen in all patients with the form of nonclassical CAH linked to HLA-B14 and HLA-DR1, but is also found in patients with other HLA types, as is expected from a common gene conversion event. This mutation does not alter the affinity of the enzyme for substrate but drastically reduces its V_{max}.[1066]

The second most common mutation causing nonclassical CAH is Pro30→Leu, which is found in about 15 to 20 percent of alleles for this disorder. Both measurements of the activity of this mutant in vitro and clinical studies have suggested that this mutation is slightly more severe and may also be associated with simple virilizing CAH in some patients.[1056,1060,1067] In addition, the mutations Arg339→His and Pro453→Ser have been associated with nonclassical CAH.[1068,1069] Initial surveys of the mutations in the P450c21A pseudogene failed to reveal these mutations, suggesting that they are bona fide point mutations rather than gene microconversions.[1068,1069] However, examination of large numbers of P450c21A pseudogenes shows that at least the Pro453→Ser mutation is polymorphic in about 20 percent of P450c21A pseudogenes; hence, its rare association with CAH is probably due to a microconversion event.[1068]

Structure-Function Inferences from P450c21 Mutations Each P450c21 missense mutation appears to occur in a functional domain of P450c21. By analogy with the membrane-anchoring domain of hepatic P450IIB,[1070] amino acids 167 to 178 of P450c21, including the crucial Ile 172 residue, appear to constitute a similar domain.[991] By analogy with the computationally-inferred structure of the closely related enzyme P450c17,[103] Arg 356 may be part of the redox-partner-binding site, Val 281 appears to participate in coordinating the heme moiety, and Cys 428 is the crucial cystine residue in the heme-binding site found in all cytochrome P450 enzymes. All these mutations can arise by gene microconversions. The N-terminal region of P450c21, including Pro30, appears to be required for membrane insertion and enzyme stability.[1071]

Finding most mutations in the amino-terminal portion of P450c21 is consistent with finding most gene conversion and gene deletion events occurring in exons 1–8 of the P450c21B gene. Changes in exons 9 and 10 are very rare, probably as a result of evolutionary pressure to retain the 3′ untranslated and 3′ flanking DNA of the P450c21B gene, as this DNA also contains the 3′ end of the XB gene.[223,225]

Prenatal Diagnosis and Treatment of CAH

The prenatal diagnosis of and therapy for 21-hydroxylase deficiency are being actively pursued, but prenatal therapy remains experimental and controversial.[345,967,1072,1073] The fetal adrenal is active in steroidogenesis from very early in gestation, hence a diagnosis can be made by amniocentesis and measurement of amniotic fluid 17-hydroxyprogesterone.[1074–1076] Concentrations of Δ^4-androstenedione are also elevated in the amniotic fluid of fetuses with CAH, providing a potentially useful adjunctive assay.[1077] However, amniotic fluid concentrations of 17-hydroxyprogesterone and Δ^4-androstenedione are reliable only for identifying fetuses affected with severe salt-losing CAH, because these hormones may not be elevated above the broad range of normal in non-salt-losing or nonclassical CAH.[1078,1079]

If a fetus is known to be at risk because the parents are known heterozygotes (e.g., they have had an affected child previously), 21-hydroxylase deficiency can be diagnosed by HLA typing of fetal amniocytes or by analysis of fetal amniocyte DNA. If the fetus has the same HLA type as the previously affected child, the fetus will be affected; a fetus that shares one parent's HLA type with the index case will be a heterozygous carrier, and a fetus having both haplotypes differing from the index case will be unaffected. However, HLA typing of cultured amniocytes requires previous linkage analysis of the affected child and parents. Only HLA-A and HLA-B can be reliably determined in cultured amniocytes, but some HLA-B alleles are expressed weakly in amniocytes; and there is a relatively high incidence of HLA-B homozygosity among CAH patients. Also HLA-B loci are frequently identical between parents and patients, some HLA-B antigens may cross-react, and amniocytes do not express HLA-DR antigens, further limiting the usefulness of HLA typing. Thus HLA typing is of limited clinical utility.

Experimental prenatal treatment requires early and accurate prenatal diagnosis. Female fetuses affected with CAH begin to become virilized at about 6 to 8 weeks gestation, i.e., at the same time that a normal male fetal testis produces large amounts of testosterone, causing fusion of the labioscrotal folds, enlargement of the genital tubercle into a phallus, and the formation of the phallic urethra.[969] The adrenals of female fetuses with CAH can produce concentrations of testosterone that may approach those in a normal male, resulting in varying degrees of masculinization of the external genitalia. If fetal adrenal steroidogenesis is suppressed in a female fetus with CAH, the virilization can theoretically be reduced or eliminated. Several studies have reported the successful application of this approach through the administration of dexamethasone to the mother as soon as pregnancy is diagnosed.[344,1080–1083] This approach can be attempted only when the parents are known to be heterozygotes by having already had an affected child. However, even in such pregnancies, Mendelian genetics requires that only one in four fetuses will have CAH. Furthermore, as no prenatal treatment is needed for male fetuses affected with CAH, only one in eight pregnancies of obligate heterozygous parents would harbor a fetus that might potentially benefit from prenatal treatment.

The efficacy, safety, and desirability of such prenatal treatment remain highly controversial.[227,344,345,967,1072–1074,1083–1086] The rationale for prenatal treatment is that dexamethasone will suppress fetal ACTH and consequently suppress adrenal steroidogenesis. However, it is not known precisely when the fetal hypothalamus begins to produce CRH, when the fetal pituitary begins to produce ACTH, whether all fetal ACTH production is regulated by CRH, or whether these hormones are suppressible by dexamethasone in the early fetus. Although there is considerable evidence that pharmacologic doses of glucocorticoids do not harm pregnant women, no such data exist for the fetus. Pregnant women with diseases such as nephrotic syndrome and systemic lupus erythematosus are generally treated with prednisone, which does not reach the fetus because it is inactivated by placental 11β-HSD-I and -II. Treatment of a fetus with CAH requires the use of fluorinated steroids that escape metabolism by these enzymes, and few data are available about the long-term use of such agents throughout gestation. The available preliminary studies also indicate that the response of the fetal genital anatomy to treatment is generally good if the treatment is started very early (before week 6); thereafter, the virilization is reduced, but it may not be eliminated, so that at least one reconstructive surgical procedure may still be needed by the infant. Successful treatment requires dexamethasone doses of 20 μg/kg of maternal body weight, which is equivalent to that in the "low dose dexamethasone suppression test" (i.e. twice physiologic for the mother). However, the fetus normally develops in the presence of very low cortisol concentrations of only about 100 nmol/L (3.6 μg/dL).[351] Thus the doses used in prenatal treatment appear to achieve effective concentrations of active glucocorticoid that may be 10 times physiologic for the fetus. Treatment of pregnant rats with 20 μg/kg dexamethasone predisposes the fetuses to hypertension in adulthood,[1087] and some studies indicate that even moderately elevated concentrations of glucocorticoids can be neurotoxic.[1088–1091] Thus prenatal treatment of CAH remains an experimental and controversial therapy that is done in only a few research centers, and which will require follow-up studies of very long duration to evaluate its effects fully.

Diagnosis

As discussed earlier, genital ambiguity or a salt-losing crisis will generally alert pediatricians to most cases of severe 21-hydroxylase deficiency. Salt-losing crises generally occur in the second week of life, and the child presents with vomiting, diarrhea, dehydration, hyperkalemia, and hyponatremia. Such infants have on occasion been thought to have viral syndromes or gastrointestinal obstructions; such a failure to make the diagnosis will result in the infant's death. Similarly, boys with simple virilizing CAH often escape diagnosis until they are 3 to 7 years old, when they present with isosexual precocity, advanced bone age, and characteristically prepubertal testes. Teenage and adult females with nonclassical CAH may consult an internist, obstetrician, or dermatologist for virilism, hirsutism, menstrual irregularity, infertility, or acne.

The key diagnostic maneuver in all the various forms of 21-hydroxylase deficiency is the measurement of the 17-OHP response to intravenous synthetic ACTH (cosyntropin). The usual doses are 0.1 mg in newborns, 0.15 mg in children up to 2 years of age, and 0.25 mg in older children and adults. 17-OHP and cortisol should be measured at 0 and 60 min. Individual patient responses must be compared to age- and sex-matched data from normal children.[1092,1093] Normal responses are shown in Table 11-10 and Fig. 11-34. Both basal and stimulated levels of 17-OHP are markedly elevated in patients with salt-losing and simple virilizing forms of 21-hydroxylase deficiency. Basal levels are usually greater than 2,000 ng/dl and increase to more than 5,000 to 10,000 ng/dl after ACTH (see Fig. 11-34). Patients with the milder late-onset or cryptic forms typically have normal to mildly elevated basal levels but have supranormal responses to ACTH stimulation, i.e., 1,500 to >10,000 μg/dl.[1093,1094] The cortisol response to ACTH varies from absent to subnormal in patients with the classic severe forms of 21-hydroxylase deficiency and is normal in patients with late-onset and cryptic forms. Basal plasma ACTH levels reflect the extent of 21-hydroxylase and cortisol deficiency; i.e., they are markedly elevated in severe forms (<500 pg/ml) and may be "normal" in patients with the milder forms who are not overtly adrenal-insufficient.

Other ancillary tests are listed in Table 11-11. Urinary excretion of 17-ketosteroids will generally be elevated, but this test is more useful for monitoring the efficacy of suppressive therapy than for initial diagnosis. When urinary steroids are measured, a complete 24-h sample must be obtained, and a concomitant measurement of creatinine excretion is required to monitor the completeness of the collection. Shorter urine collections are not accurate because of diurnal variability of the steroids.

Plasma renin activity and its response to salt-restriction constitute an especially useful test. Most patients with "simple virilizing" 21-hydroxylase deficiency have high plasma renin activity that increases further on sodium restriction, confirming the fact that these patients are partially mineralocorticoid deficient and can maintain a normal serum sodium only by hyperstimulation of the zona glomerulosa. Mineralocorticoid therapy in these patients returns plasma volume to normal and eliminates the hypovolemic drive to ACTH secretion. Thus, mineralocorticoid therapy often permits the use of lower doses of glucocorticoids in patients with simple virilizing CAH, optimizing growth in children and diminishing unwanted weight gain in adults.

Long-term management is difficult to monitor and requires careful clinical and laboratory evaluation. Measurements of growth should be made at 3- to 4-month intervals in children, along with an annual assessment of bone age. Each visit should be accompanied by measurement of urinary 17-KS and serum Δ^4-androstenedione, DHEA, DHEA sulfate, and testosterone. Measurement of 3α-androstenediol glucuronide may also be useful. In general, plasma 17-OHP is not a useful indicator of therapeutic efficacy because of its great diurnal variation and hyperresponsiveness to stress (e.g., clinic visits).

Treatment

Although Wilkins[21] and Bartter[22] first demonstrated effective treatment of 21-hydroxylase deficiency with cortisone in 1950, the management of this disorder remains difficult. Overtreatment with glucocorticoids causes delayed growth even when the degree of overtreatment is insufficient to produce signs and symptoms of Cushing's syndrome. Undertreatment results in continued overproduction of adrenal androgens that hastens epiphiseal maturation and closure, again resulting in compromised growth and other manifestations of androgen excess.

Doses of glucocorticoids should be based on the expected normal cortisol secretory rate. Widely cited classical studies have reported that the secretory rate of cortisol is 12.5 ± 3 mg/m^2 per day[1095–1097] and have led most authorities to recommend doses of 10 to 20 mg of hydrocortisone (cortisol)/m^2 per day. However, the cortisol secretory rate is substantially lower, at 7 ± 2 mg/m^2/per day[1098] or even 5 to 6 mg/m^2 per day.[1099] Although no single formula can be applied to all patients and extensive experience and judgment are needed, we consider the cortisol secretory rate to be about 6 to 8 mg/m^2 per day. It must be stressed, however, that newly diagnosed patients, especially newborns, will require substantially higher initial dosages to suppress their hyperactive CRH-ACTH-adrenal access.

The glucocorticoid used is also important. Most widely used tables of glucocorticoid dose equivalencies are based on their equivalence in anti-inflammatory assays. However, the growth-suppressant equivalences of various glucocorticoids do not parallel their anti-inflammatory equivalencies.[1100] Thus, long-acting synthetic steroids such as dexamethasone have a disproportionately greater growth-suppressant effect and hence must be avoided in treating growing children and adolescents (Table 11-13). Most authorities favor the use of oral hydrocortisone or cortisone acetate in three divided daily doses in growing children. However, adults and older teenagers who already have fused their epiphyses may be managed very effectively with prednisone or dexamethasone.

Only one oral mineralocorticoid preparation, fludrocortisone (9α-fluorocortisol), is currently available. When the oral route is not available in severely ill patients, mineralocorticoid replacement is achieved through supraphysiologic doses of intravenous hydrocortisone plus sodium chloride. About 20 mg of hydrocortisone has a mineralocorticoid effect of about 0.1 mg of 9α-fluorocortisol (Table 11-13). Mineralocorticoids are unique in pharmacology in that their doses are essentially the same regardless of the size of the patient. In fact, newborns are quite insensitive to mineralocorticoids as reflected by their high serum aldosterone concentrations (Fig. 11-10), and often require larger doses than do adults (0.15 to 0.30 mg/day). In older children, the replacement dose of 9α-fluorocortisol is 0.05 to 0.15 mg daily. It must be emphasized that a mineralocorticoid is essentially useless unless adequate sodium is presented to the renal tubules. Thus, additional salt supplementation, usually 1 to 2 g NaCl/day in the newborn, is also needed. Patients with severe salt-losing congenital adrenal hyperplasia can in some cases discontinue mineralocorticoid replacement and salt supplementation as adults. Perhaps adults become more sensitive to the mineralocorticoid action of hydrocortisone via a developmental decrease in renal 11β-HSD activity, which normally inactivates cortisol to cortisone.

3β-Hydroxysteroid Dehydrogenase Deficiency

Severe deficiency of 3β-HSD activity is a rare cause of glucocorticoid and mineralocorticoid deficiency and is fatal if not diagnosed early in infancy.[1101] In its classic form, genetic females have cliteromegaly and mild virilization because the fetal adrenal overproduces large amounts of DHEA, a small portion of which is converted to testosterone by extraadrenal 3β-HSD type I. Genetic males also synthesize some androgens by peripheral conversion of adrenal and testicular DHEA, but the concentrations are insufficient for complete male genital development, so that these males have a small phallus and severe hypospadias.

There are two functional human genes for 3β-HSD: the type I gene is expressed in the placenta and peripheral tissues,[173–175,177] and the type II gene is expressed in the adrenals and gonads.[179,1102] Clinical, genetic, and endocrine studies of 3β-HSD deficiency show that both the gonads and the adrenals are affected as a result of a single mutated 3β-HSD gene expressed in both tissues. However, considerable hepatic 3β-HSD activity persists in the face of complete absence of adrenal and gonadal activity and is presumably due to the enzyme encoded by the type I gene, thus complicating the diagnosis of 3β-HSD deficiency. Not surprisingly, genetic studies have shown that the mutations causing 3β-HSD

TABLE 11-13. Potency of Various Therapeutic Steroids (Relative to the Potency of Cortisol)

Steroid	Anti-Inflammatory Glucocorticoid Effect	Growth-Retarding Glucocorticoid Effect	Salt-Retaining Mineralocorticoid Effect
Cortisol (hydrocortisone)	1.0	1.0	1.0
Cortisone acetate (oral)	0.8	0.8	0.8
Cortisone acetate (IM)	0.8	1.3	0.8
Prednisone	3.5–4.0	5	0.8
Prednisolone	4		0.8
Methyl prednisolone	5	7.5	0.5
Betamethasone	25–30		0
Triamcinolone	5		0
Dexamethasone	30	80	0
Fludrocortisone (9α-fluorocortisol)	15		200
DOC acetate*	0		20
Aldosterone†	0.3		200–1000

* No longer commercially available.

† Not commercially available. Shown for comparison.

Data compiled from various sources and Styne et al.[1100]

deficiency are all found in the type II gene.[1103–1108] Mutations have never been found in 3βHSD-I, presumably because this would prevent placental biosynthesis of progesterone, resulting in a spontaneous first-trimester abortion. Some alleles causing the severe, salt-losing form of 3β-HSD deficiency have a nonsense mutation at the position normally occupied by Trp 171. Others have point mutations, including Tyr253→Asn, Glu142→Lys, and the insertion of a single base, causing a frame shift.[1104] Patients with a milder, non-salt-losing form of 3βHSD deficiency have been reported carrying the mutations Ala245→Pro[1104] Tyr254→Asp[1109] and Asn100→Ser.[1110] The wide variety of mutations found in the small number of alleles studied to date suggests that a great variety of mutations cause 3β-HSD deficiency.[1108]

The presence of peripheral 3β-HSD activity complicates the hormonal diagnosis of this disease; i.e., affected infants should have low concentrations of 17-OHP, the steroid that is typically elevated in 21-hydroxylase deficiency. Yet some newborns with 3β-HSD deficiency have very high concentrations of serum 17-OHP, approaching those of patients with classical 21-hydroxylase deficiency. The high 17-OHP concentrations are due to extraadrenal 3β-HSD activity[970] presumably encoded by the type I 3β-HSD gene. The adrenal of a patient with 3β-HSD deficiency will secrete very large amounts of the three principal Δ^5 compounds: pregnenolone, 17-hydroxypregnenolone, and DHEA. Some of the secreted Δ^5 17-hydroxypregnenolone is then peripherally converted to 17-OHP. However, in all cases, the ratio of the Δ^5 to the Δ^4 compound is high, consistent with the adrenal and gonadal deficiency of 3β-HSD.[970] Thus, the principal diagnostic test in 3β-HSD deficiency is intravenous administration of ACTH with measurement of the three Δ^5 compounds and the corresponding Δ^4 compounds.

Mild or "partial" defects of adrenal 3β-HSD activity have been reported on the basis of high ratios of Δ^5 steroids to Δ^4 steroids following an ACTH test; these patients are typically young girls with premature adrenarche or young women with a history of premature adrenarche and complaints of hirsutism, virilism, and oligomenorrhea.[1111–1113] However, the 3β-HSD-II genes are normal in these patients, and patients with true 3β-HSD-II mutations have ratios of Δ^5 to Δ^4 steroids that exceed 8 SD above the mean.[1106,1107,1114,1115] The basis of the elevated ratios of Δ^5 to Δ^4 steroids in these hirsute individuals with normal 3β-HSD genes is unknown. However, in adult women the hirsutism can be ameliorated and regular menses can be restored by suppressing ACTH with 0.25 to 0.5 mg of dexamethasone given orally each day.

P450c17 (17α-Hydroxylase/17,20 Lyase) Deficiency

P450c17 is the single enzyme, found in both the adrenals and gonads, that has both 17α-hydroxylase and 17,20 lyase activities (see the earlier section on steroid Hormone Biosynthesis). Deficient 17α-hydroxylase activity and deficient 17,20 lyase activity have been described as separate genetic diseases, but it is now clear that they represent different clinical manifestations of different lesions in the same gene.[1116]

P450c17 deficiency is fairly rare, although more than 120 cases have been reported.[1117] Deficient 17α-hydroxylase activity results in decreased cortisol synthesis, overproduction of ACTH, and stimulation of the steps proximal to P450c17. These patients may have mild symptoms of glucocorticoid deficiency, but this is not life-threatening, as the lack of P450c17 results in the overproduction of corticosterone, which also has glucocorticoid activity. These patients typically overproduce DOC in the zona fasciculata, which causes sodium retention, hypertension, and hypokalemia and also suppresses plasma renin activity and aldosterone secretion from the zona glomerulosa. When P450c17 deficiency is treated with glucocorticoids, DOC secretion is suppressed and plasma renin activity and aldosterone concentrations rise to normal.[1118]

The absence of 17α-hydroxylase and 17,20 lyase activities in complete P450c17 deficiency prevents the synthesis of adrenal and gonadal sex steroids. As a result, affected females are phenotypically normal but fail to undergo adrenarche and puberty[1119] and genetic males have absent or incomplete development of the external genitalia (male pseudohermaphroditism).[1120] The classical presentation is that of a teenage female with sexual infantilism and hypertension.[1121] The diagnosis is made by finding low or absent 17-hydroxylated C-21 and C-19 plasma steroids and low urinary 17-OHCS and 17-KS, which respond poorly to stimulation with ACTH. Serum levels of DOC, corticosterone, and 18-OH-corticosterone are elevated, show hyperresponsiveness to ACTH, and are suppressible with glucocorticoids.

The single gene for P450c17 has been cloned[204] and localized to chromosome 10q24.3.[121,202,1122] The molecular basis of 17α-hydroxylase deficiency has been determined in several patients by cloning and sequencing of the mutated gene identifying at least 26 distinct mutations.[1116] The genetic lesions identified include twelve mutations that cause frameshifts or premature translational termination; as expected, none of these mutants has any detectable hydroxylase or lyase activity. Fourteen mis-sense and in-frame mutations have been found, most of which also eliminate all activity, while some others, such as Pro 342 Thr, reduce both activities by 80 percent.

Selective deficiency of the 17,20 lyase activity P450c17 has been reported in about a dozen cases,[1117] which initially led to the incorrect conclusion that 17α-hydroxylase and 17,20 lyase are separate enzymes. One of the original patients was studied at the genetic level, showing two wholly inactivating mutations,[1123] which led to a revised diagnosis of the patient as an adult.[1124] Thus, because both the 17α-hydroxylase and 17,20 lyase activities of P450c17 are catalyzed by the same active site, it was not clear that a syndrome of isolated 17,20 lyase deficiency could exist until two patients with genital ambiguity, normal excretion of 17OHCS, and markedly reduced production of C_{19} steroids were studied at the molecular genetic level.[1125] One patient was homozygous for the P450c17 mutation Arg 347→His, and the other was homozygous for Arg 358→Gln; both mutations changed the distribution of surface charges in the redox-partner binding site.[1125] When expressed in transfected cells, both mutants retained nearly normal 17α-hydroxylase activity but had no detectable 17,20 lyase activity.[215,1125] Enzymatic competition experiments proved that the mutations did not affect the substrate binding site.[215] When an excess of both P450 oxidoreductase and cytochrome b_5 was provided, some 17,20 lyase activity was restored, demonstrating that the loss in lyase activity was due to impaired electron transfer.[215] A third patient with similar findings has been reported with the mutation Phe 417→Cys, but the enzymology of that mutation has not been studied.[1126]

A detailed computer-graphic model of P450c17 has been built and tested by a variety of computational, enzymatic, and mutagenesis approaches, which show that the model is an excellent representation of the human enzyme.[103] This model accurately predicts the effects of all known mutations, including those with partial retention of both activities and those causing selective 17,20 lyase deficiency. The model identifies both Arg 347 and Arg 358 and a variety of other lysine and argenine residues in the redox partner binding site; mutation of these residues all cause varying degrees of selective loss of 17,20 lyase activity.[103,215,1062,1125,1127] Another example of the critical nature of redox-partner interactions comes from the sole reported case of cytochrome b_5 deficiency; although this patient was not evaluated hormonally, it was a male pseudohermaphrodite.[1128] Thus the central role of electron transfer in 17,20 lyase activity is now well-established.

11β-Hydroxylase (P450c11β) Deficiency

There are two distinct forms of 11-hydroxylase (see previous discussion of steroid hormone biosynthesis). P450c11β mediates the 11β-hydroxylation of 11-deoxycortisol to cortisol and that of DOC to corticosterone in the zonae fasciculata and reticularis. P450c11AS, or aldosterone synthase, is found only in the zona glomerulosa and mediates 11β-hydroxylation, 18-hydroxylation, and 18-oxidation; thus, it is the sole enzyme required to convert DOC to aldosterone. Deficient P450c11β activity is a rare cause of CAH in persons of European ancestry, but accounts for about 15 percent of cases in both Moslem and Jewish Middle Eastern populations.[1129] Severe deficiency of P450c11β results in decreased secretion of cortisol, causing CAH and virilization of affected females, as described previously for P450c21 deficiency. However, unlike the typical salt-losing syndrome seen in 21-hydroxylase deficiency, patients with P450c11β are able to retain sodium normally because the substrate for 11β-hydroxylation in the mineralocorticoid pathway DOC, is itself a mineralocorticoid. Although DOC is less potent than aldosterone, it is secreted at higher levels in 11β-hydroxylase deficiency, so that salt is retained and the serum sodium remains normal. Overproduction of DOC frequently leads to hypertension; as a result, 11β-hydroxylase deficiency is often termed "the hypertensive form of CAH." However, newborns often manifest mild, transient salt loss,[1129,1130] presumably as a result of the normal newborn resistance to mineralocorticoids (Fig. 11-10); this often obscures the diagnosis. Thus, there may be a poor correlation between DOC concentrations, serum potassium, and blood pressure or between the degree of virilization in affected females and the electrolyte and cardiovascular manifestations.[218] The diagnosis is established by demonstrating elevated basal concentrations of DOC and 11-deoxycortisol, which hyperrespond to ACTH; the normal or suppressed plasma renin activity is a hallmark of this disease.[1131]

The genetic lesions causing 11β-hydroxylase deficiency are in the CYP11B1 gene that encodes P450c11β. In a study of Sephardic Jews of Moroccan ancestry, 11 of 12 affected alleles bore the mutation Arg448→His.[249] In several other patients, the identified mutations include two frame shifts due to the insertion or deletion of one or two nucleotides, four premature stop codons (nonsense mutations), and five missense mutations that change amino acids: Thr318→Met, Arg374→Gln, Arg384→Gln, Val441→Gly, and Arg448→His.[1132] All these mutations appear to cluster in exons 6–8 of the CYP11B1 gene, possibly associated with frequent CpG sites.[1133]

A milder, nonclassic form of 11β-hydroxylase deficiency, analogous to non-classic 21-hydroxylase deficiency, has been reported in otherwise asymptomatic women with hirsutism, virilism, and menstrual irregularities.[1129,1134] A recent study examined the CYP11B1 gene that encodes P450c11β in five hyperandrogenemic women who had 11-deoxycortisol values more than three times higher than the 95th percentile in response to stimulation with ACTH.[1135] Mutations were found in only two women, who carried a total of three P450c11β mis-sense mutations: Pro42→Ser, Asn133→His, and Thr319→Met. When expressed in transfected cells these mutants had 15 to 37 percent of normal activity.[1135] Repeated ACTH testing in two of the three women who lacked mutations showed much lower (but still elevated) 11-deoxycortisol values. This study shows that nonclassical 11β-hydroxylase deficiency is very rare, and further shows that an abnormal steroid response to ACTH is not sufficient to diagnose a genetic lesion, similarly to the situation in patients with pseudodeficiency of 3β-HSD, as discussed previously.

P450c11AS Disorders: The "Corticosterone Methyl Oxidase" Deficiencies

P450c11AS, an isozyme of P450c11β that is 93% identical in its amino acid sequence, is expressed exclusively in the zona glomerulosa, where it has 11β-hydroxylase, 18-hydroxylase, and 18 methyl oxidase activities. Both P450c11AS and P450c11β are expressed in the human zona glomerulosa, and both can convert DOC to corticosterone, but the conversion of corticosterone to 18OH-corticosterone and subsequently to aldosterone is exclusively performed by P450c11AS (see the section on steroid hormone biosynthesis). Disorders of P450c11AS cause the so-called corticosterone methyl oxidase (CMO) deficiencies. Thus in both disorders aldosterone biosynthesis is impaired while the zona fasciculata and reticularis continue to produce corticosterone and DOC. The absence of aldosterone biosynthesis will generally result in a salt-wasting crisis in infancy at which time the normal secretory rate of DOC is insufficient to meet mineralocorticoid requirements. Thus these infants typically present with hyponatremia, hyperkalemia, and metabolic acidosis, but the salt-wasting syndrome is typically less severe than in patients with 21-hydroxylase deficiency or lipoid CAH because of the persistent secretion of DOC. These patients have been known to recover spontaneously and grow to adulthood without therapy. This probably reflects the increasing sensitivity to mineralocorticoid action with advancing age in childhood, as reflected by the normal, age-related changes in serum aldosterone (Fig. 11-10). Consistent with this, plasma renin activity is markedly elevated in affected children but may be normal in affected adults.[1136]

CMOI deficiency results from a complete loss of P450c11AS activity so that no 18-hydroxylase or 18 methyl oxidase activity persists, eliminating the biosynthesis of 18OH-corticosterone and aldosterone, while preserving the biosynthesis of corticosterone by P450c11β. Thus the usual diagnostic criterion for CMOI deficiency is an increased ratio of corticosterone to 18OH-corticosterone.[250] The described molecular defects causing CMOI deficiency include a 5 bp deletion causing a frameshift and premature stop codon in exon 1,[1137] a premature stop codon mutation[1138] and the P450c11AS missense mutation Arg384→Pro.[1139] CMOI deficiency is quite rare.

CMOII deficiency results from missense mutations in P450c11AS that selectively delete the 18 methyl oxidase activity while preserving the 18-hydroxylase activity. The usual diagnostic criterion for CMOII deficiency is an increased serum level of 18OH-corticosterone and very low concentrations of aldosterone.

CMOII deficiency is common in Sephartic Jews of Iranian origin, all of whom appear to be homozygous for two different mutations in P450c11AS: Arg181→Trp and Val385→Ala.[251] Family members who were homozygous for only one of these mutations were clinically unaffected; both mutations are required to cause disease.

The distinction between CMOI and CMOII is not always clear. One patient with the clinical history and hormonal phenotype of CMOII had two mutations on each parental allele.[252] The mother's allele carried Arg181→Trp and a deletion/frame-shift mutation that deleted all activity; the father's allele carried Thr318→Met and Val386→Ala. Thr318 is predicted to be the universally conserved Thr residue in all P450 enzymes that participates in cleavage of the dioxygen bond of O_2 to create the iron-oxy intermediate required for P450 catalysis. When the Thr318→Met and Val386→Ala double mutant was recreated in vitro there was no detectable activity.[252] These data would have predicted the CMOI phenotype instead of the patient's CMOII phenotype. Similarly, another patient was homozygous for the mis-sense mutations Glu198→Asp and Val386→Ala. When recreated in vitro the mutant enzyme behaved similarly to the mutant enzyme found in the Iranian Jewish CMOII patients, but the patient's clinical phenotype was CMOI.[1140] This patient also carried Arg173→Lys, but that is a normally occurring polymorphism that has no affect on the enzyme's K_m or V_{max}.[259] Thus the distinction between CMOI and CMOII is not precise, and these disorders should be regarded as different degrees of severity on a continuous clinical spectrum just as the various forms of 21-hydroxylase deficiency are part of a broad clinical spectrum.

Although rats have four CYP11B genes encoding three P450c11 enzymes, it is clear that there are only two CYP11B genes in the human genome, encoding P450c11β and P450c11AS.[242] This genetic anatomy is reminiscent of the P450c21A and P450c21B genes. Although gene conversion can cause CMOII deficiency,[1141] gene conversion appears to be much rarer than in the P450c21 locus. This may be due to the higher recombinational frequency in the HLA region carrying the P450c21 genes, or it may be related to the abundant antisense transcripts produced in the P450c21 locus.[224,1031]

Although gene conversion events in the P450c11 locus are rare, an unusual gene duplication causes glucocorticoid-suppressible hyperaldosteronism.[1142–1144] This homologous recombination event creates a third P450c11 gene that fuses the 5′ flanking DNA of the P450c11β gene onto a gene for P450c11AS. In two such patients the genetic crossover occurred in intron 2, and in two other patients it occurred in intron 3 or exon 4.[1143] All these hybrid genes produce a hybrid P450c11 that retains aldosterone synthase activity; however, as the hybrid gene has P450c11β regulatory regions, it is turned on by ACTH and cAMP, as is the normal P450c11β gene. Thus, these patients make P450c11AS in response to physiology that should stimulate P450c11β. The excess P450c11AS causes hyperaldosteronism and hypertension; this is then suppressible by glucocorticoid suppression of ACTH.

A potential disorder related to the tandem duplication of these two genes might involve gene conversions that insert sequences crucial for aldosterone synthase activity into the P450c11β gene. Creation of chimeric proteins in vitro has identified the residues Ser288 and Val320 as important for this activity.[1145] Similarly, activating mutations that increase the aldosterone synthase activity of P450c11AS have been created in vitro.[258] However, examination of large numbers of patients with low-renin hypertension has failed to show mutations in this gene system, other than the gene conversions described previously that cause glucocorticoid suppressible hypertension.[259,260,1146]

Congenital Lipoid Adrenal Hyperplasia

Lipoid CAH is the most severe genetic disorder of steroid hormone synthesis. This disorder is characterized by the absence of significant concentrations of all steroids, high basal concentrations of ACTH and plasma renin activity, an absent steroidal response to long-term treatment with high doses of ACTH or hCG, and grossly enlarged adrenals laden with cholesterol and cholesterol esters.[1147–1150] These findings indicate a lesion in the first step in steroidogenesis—the conversion of cholesterol to pregnenolone—and have led to other names for lipoid CAH, including *20,22-desmolase deficiency* and *P450scc deficiency*.[119,1150–1155] That view seemed logical enough, as all other errors in steroidogenesis were in steroidogenic enzymes. However, the P450scc gene is normal in these patients,[1154,1155] as are the mRNAs for adrenodoxin reductase and adrenodoxin.[1154] This finding, plus the accumulation of cholesterol esters in the affected adrenal, suggested that the lesion lay in an upstream factor that is involved in cholesterol transport to the mitochondria. Initial searches for such a factor ruled out all the candidates known at the time.[1154,1156] However, the cAMP-induced, cycloheximide-sensitive factor required for the acute steroidogenic response, termed the steroidogenic acute regulatory (StAR) protein (see earlier section on steroid hormone biosynthesis) was cloned in 1994[77] and was quickly identified as the disordered step in lipoid CAH.[78,79,1157] Thus lipoid CAH is the only disorder in steroid hormone biosynthesis that is not caused by a disrupted steroidogenic enzyme.

Lipoid CAH provided a gene knockout of nature, elucidating the complex physiology of the StAR protein.[83] Transfection of nonsteroidogenic COS-1 cells with the P450scc system with and without StAR shows that StAR promotes steroidogenesis by increasing the movement of cholesterol into mitochondria, but that in the absence of StAR steroidogenesis proceeds at about 14 percent of the StAR-induced level.[78,79,87,1157] This observation led to the two-hit model of lipoid CAH.[79] The first hit is the loss of StAR itself, leading to a loss of most, but not all steroidogenesis. This diminished steroidogenesis results in a compensatory rise in the secretion of the hopic hormones: ACTH and LH. These tropic hormones elicit the biosynthesis of intracellular cAMP, fostering increased biosynthesis of LDL receptors and consequent uptake of LDL cholesterol, as well as increased de novo synthesis of cholesterol. In the absence of StAR, this increased intracellular cholesterol accumulates, causing the second hit, which is the mitochondrial and cellular damage caused by the accumulated cholesterol and cholesterol esters, and their autooxidation products.[79]

The two-hit model explains the clinical physiology of lipoid CAH. In the fetal testis, which is steroidogenically very active under the tropic stimulation of hCG, the Leydig cells are destroyed very early in fetal life, abrogating testosterone biosynthesis so that the affected 46XY fetus does not undergo normal virilization and is born with female external genitalia and a blind vaginal pouch. The Sertoli cells remain undamaged, and hence produce Müllarian inhibitory factor, so that the phenotypically female 46XY fetus has no cervix, uterus, or fallopian tubes. The steroidogenically active fetal zone of the fetal adrenal is similarly affected, abrogating fetal adrenal DHEA biosynthesis, thus eliminating the feto-placental production of estriol, so that mid-gestation maternal and fetal estriol levels are nil.[1158] The definitive zone of the fetal adrenal, which differentiates into the zonae glomerulosa and fasciculata, normally produces very little aldosterone, as fetal salt and water metabolism are handled by the placenta. Thus stimulation of the glomerulosa by angiotensin II generally begins at birth; consistent with this, many newborns with lipoid CAH do not have a salt-wasting crisis until after several weeks of life, when chronic stimulation then leads to cellular damage.[79] However, patients with lipoid CAH born in hot, dry climates tended to develop a salt-wasting crisis very early, presumably reflecting chronic compensated hypovolemia in the mother with secondary stimulation of the fetal renin-angiotensin system, so that damage to the aldosterone-producing cells begins before birth.[79] Finally the two-hit model explains the spontaneous feminization of affected 46XX females who are treated in infancy and reach adolescence. The fetal ovary makes no steroids and contains no steroidogenic enzymes[968]; consequently the ovary remains undamaged until it is first stimulated with gonadotropins at the time of puberty. However, gonadotropins will recruit only individual follicles, which then produce some estrogen by StAR-independent steroidogenesis. Continued stimulation results in cholesterol accumulation and cellular damage, so that biosynthesis of progesterone in the latter part of the cycle is impaired. Cyclycity is determined by the hypothalamic-pituitary axis, and remains normal. With each new cycle, a new follicle is recruited and more estradiol is produced by StAR-independent steroidogenesis, leading to breast development, general feminization, monthly estrogen withdrawal, and cyclic vaginal bleeding.[79,1159] However, progesterone synthesis is disturbed so that the cycles are anovulatory. Measurements of estradiol, progesterone, and gonadotropins throughout the cycle in affected adult females with lipoid CAH confirms this model.[1160] Similarly, examination of StAR-knockout mice confirms the two-hit model.[1161] Thus examination of patients with lipoid CAH has elucidated the physiology of the StAR protein.

Genetic analysis of patients with lipoid CAH has revealed numerous mutations in the StAR gene.[79,1162–1165] These data reveal two distinct genetic clusters. As first reported by Hauffa[1150] lipoid CAH is common in Japan, and about 65–70 percent of affected Japanese alleles and virtually all affected Korean alleles carry the mutation Glu258→Stop.[78,79,1162,1162a,1163] The carrier frequency for this mutation appears to be about one in 300[79,1163] so that one in every 250,000 to 300,000 newborns in these countries is affected, for a total of about 500 patients. A second genetic cluster is found among Palestinian Arabs, most of whom carry the mutation Arg182→Leu.[79] Many other mutations have also been described.[78,79,1157,1159,1160,1162–1165] These mutations are found throughout the gene, but all amino acid replacement (mis-sense) mutations are found in the carboxy-terminal 40 percent of the protein, suggesting that this is the biologically important domain.[79,83] Spectroscopic analysis of these mutant proteins indicates that they have lost activity because they are substantially misfolded.[1166] Deletion of only 10 carboxy-terminal residues reduces StAR activity by half[85] and deltetion of 28 carboxy-terminal residues by the common Glu258→Stop mutation eliminates all activity. By contrast, deletion of up to the first 62 amino-terminal residues has no effect on StAR activity, even though this deletes the entire mitochondrial leader sequence and forces StAR to remain in the cytoplasmic compartment.[85] Physical studies and partial proteolysis indicate that residues 63–193 of StAR (i.e., the domain that lacks most of the crucial residues identified by mis-sense mutations) are protease-resistant and constitute a 'pause-transfer' sequence, which permits the bioactive loosely-folded carboxy-terminal molten globule domain to have increased interaction with the outer mitochondrial membrane.[88]

Treatment of lipoid CAH is straightforward if the diagnosis is made. Physiologic replacement with glucocorticoids, mineralocorticoids and salt will permit survival to adulthood.[1149,1150] The differential diagnosis includes 3βHSD deficiency and adrenal hypoplasia congenita.[1150,1162a,1167,1168] The glucocorticoid requirement is less than in the virilizing adrenal hyperplasias because it is not necessary to oversuppress excess adrenal androgen production. Genetic males have female external genitalia and should undergo orchiectomy and be raised as females.[79,1149,1150]

ADRENOCORTICAL INSUFFICIENCY

Impairment of adrenal function leads to deficient adrenal production of glucocorticoids and/or mineralocorticoids. Such impairment usually results from destruction of or damage to the adrenal cortex (primary adrenocortical insufficiency, Addison's disease) or is secondary to deficient pituitary ACTH secretion (secondary adrenocortical insufficiency) (Fig. 11-38). Primary adrenocortical insufficiency is an uncommon disorder. However, it must be considered in the differential diagnosis of many common conditions that present with weakness, lassitude, weight loss, anorexia, or gastrointestinal symptoms. Secondary adrenal insufficiency due to natural causes is also uncommon; however, iatrogenic secondary adrenocortical insufficiency is more frequent because of the large number of individuals who receive exogenous glucocorticoid therapy which suppresses pituitary ACTH production.

Primary Adrenocortical Insufficiency (Addison's Disease)

Adrenal destruction results from a variety of causes (Fig. 11-38 and Table 11-14); however, excluding CAH, the autoimmune or "idiopathic" atrophic type of Addison's disease (autoimmune adrenal atrophy, autoimmune adrenalitis, lymphocytic adrenalitis) accounts for approximately 75 to 80 percent of cases.[1169] These patients have disordered organ-specific immunity, a high incidence of associated immunologic and autoimmune endocrine dysfunction, and disorders of other tissues and organs (Chap. 27).[1170–1174] In addition, there are two distinct subtypes of these

FIGURE 11-38. Causes of adrenocortical insufficiency. Secondary insufficiency can be due to lesions of either the hypothalamus or the pituitary, although the most common cause (indicated by the asterisk) is iatrogenic and is due to glucocorticoid therapy. The most common cause of primary adrenocortical insufficiency is idiopathic, also indicated by an asterisk.

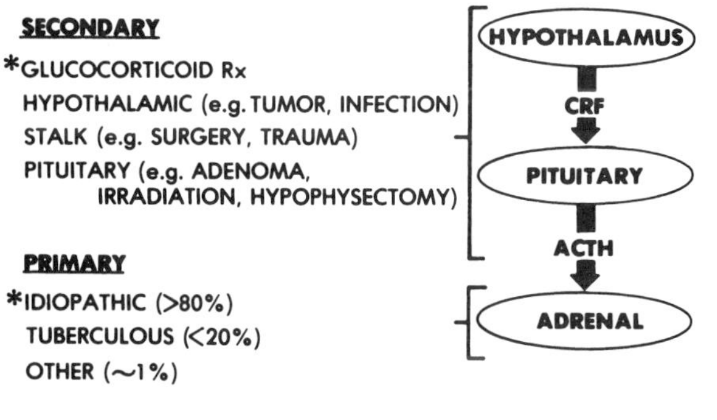

TABLE 11-14. Etiology of Primary Adrenocortical Insufficiency

Idiopathic/autoimmune (~80%)
Tuberculosis (~20%)
Miscellaneous causes (~1%)
  Vascular
    Hemorrhage: sepsis, anticoagulants, coagulopathy, trauma, surgery, pregnancy, neonate
    Infarction: thrombosis, embolism, arteritis
  Fungal infection: histoplasmosis, paracoccidioidomycosis, blastomycosis, coccidioidomycosis, cryptococcosis
  Acquired immune deficiency syndrome (AIDS)
  Metastases
  Lymphoma
  Amyloidosis
  Sarcoidosis
  Hemochromatosis
  Irradiation
  Surgery: bilateral adrenalectomy
  Enzyme inhibitors: ketoconazole, etomidate, metyrapone, aminoglutethimide, trilostane
  Cytotoxic agents: mitotane
  Congenital: adrenal hypoplasia, familial glucocorticoid deficiency, adrenal leukodystrophy

Source: Irvine et al.[817] and Irvine and Barnes.[1169]

syndromes known as the polyglandular autoimmune syndromes (PGA types I and II) (Chap. 27).[1171–1173,1175–1177]

Tuberculosis currently accounts for approximately 20 percent of cases of Addison's disease, with a higher prevalence in populations with poor control of this disease. This current distribution is a marked reversal of the relative frequency in the 1920s and 1930s, when tuberculosis was responsible for 70 to 80 percent of reported cases (Table 11-15).[817,1169,1178] Adrenal insufficiency is relatively unusual in patients with tuberculosis,[1179,1180] and even with adrenal involvement, the extent of cortical destruction may not be sufficient to impair adrenal function.[1179]

Other etiologies of primary adrenal insufficiency are distinctly unusual in larger published series (Table 11-14).[817,1169,1178] However, personal experience suggests that adrenal insufficiency due to invasive and hemorrhagic disorders is becoming more commonly diagnosed. These etiologies include many systemic disorders (e.g., infections, hemorrhagic disorders, neoplasia, trauma) that involve a number of organ systems. The most common cause of adrenal hemorrhage in adults is anticoagulant therapy or spontaneous coagulopathy,[1181–1185] and in childhood it is meningococcal and *Pseudomonas* septicemias.[1186,1187] Adrenal insufficiency may also occur in the acquired immune deficiency syndrome (AIDS); however, the exact cause and incidence are unknown.[1188]

Primary adrenocortical insufficiency due to any cause is a rare disease; the exact incidence and prevalence are unknown. Current reports may underestimate the true incidence, as patients may die in acute crisis without an established diagnosis.[1189] A prevalence of Addison's disease of 39 per 1 million inhabitants in the age group from 25 to 69 years in the United Kingdom was reported, and there were 60 cases per 1 million population in Denmark.[1178,1189] It is difficult to determine whether the dramatic alteration in the relative frequencies of autoimmune and tuberculous Addison's disease is due to an increase in the incidence of autoimmune cases or to a decrease in the number of cases secondary to tuberculosis. However, the series of Dunlop[792] suggests that the total incidence of Addison's disease is declining concomitantly with control of tuberculosis, favoring the idea that the increase in the autoimmune variety is a relative one.

Tuberculous Addison's disease occurs predominantly in male patients, but autoimmune Addison's disease is more frequent in females. Thus, in recent series, the female/male ratio approximates 1.25.[1190] In autoimmune Addison's disease, the female/male ratio is 3/1.[817]

Addison's disease is an unusual diagnosis at the extremes of life; approximately 60 to 70 percent of cases are diagnosed in the third to fifth decade.[817] The autoimmune variety occurs among all age groups, but tuberculous Addison's disease was previously diagnosed in patients over age 40 years.[1178,1190,1191] However, in more recent reports, mean ages were 34 and 38 years.[817,1178,1190]

Only isolated information is available regarding death rates. Guttman estimated in 1930 that the death rate from Addison's disease was 4 per million population in the United States,[1179] and Stuart-Mason and coworkers reported an annual death rate of 1.4 per million population in the United Kingdom in the 1960s.[1189]

Autoimmune Adrenocortical Insufficiency

Etiology, Pathogenesis, and Genetic Aspects

The etiology of the most common form of primary adrenocortical failure is autoimmune, although there is also a genetic predisposition. Early in the disease, there is lymphocytic infiltration of the adrenal. There is a high incidence of associated endocrine disorders and of pernicious anemia, vitiligo, and other disorders. Antibodies to the adrenal gland and to other potentially affected organs are commonly present, and there is evidence for abnormal cell-mediated immunity. Although circulating antibodies to adrenocortical antigens are present in up to 65 percent of patients at the time of diagnosis,[817,1170,1171] their role in the pathogenesis of Addison's disease has been obscure. In one study, serum immunoglobulins from patients with autoimmune Addison's disease were incubated with cultured adrenal cells[1192]; immunoglobulins from 23 of 25 patients blocked the ACTH-induced increases in both cortisol and DNA synthesis.[1192] Thus, such antibodies could inhibit adrenal steroidogenesis early in the course of Addison's disease, before extensive destruction of adrenocortical cells.

The nature of the antigen(s) responsible for the cytotoxic antibodies that cause the adrenocortical destruction in autoimmune Addison's disease remains unclear. Recent studies have found antibodies to the steroidogenic enzymes P450scc, P450c17, and P450c21 (especially P450c21) in the sera of adults and children with autoimmune Addison's disease.[1193–1197] However, it appears likely that these autoantibodies represent secondary markers of cellular destruction, analogous to the antibodies to insulin and glutamic acid decarboxylase found in patients with Type 1 diabetes, and are not the primary cytotoxic agents.

TABLE 11-15. Changing Patterns in Primary Adrenocortical Insufficiency

	*Percent**	
	1928–1938	**1962–1972**
Idiopathic	17	78
Tuberculous	79	21
Other	4	1

*Percent of cases with each of the three classes of adrenocortical insufficiency in each time period.

Source: Dunlop[792] and Irvine and Barnes.[1169]

Associated Disorders

In 1926, Schmidt described two patients with Addison's disease who had chronic lymphocytic thyroiditis at autopsy.[1198] In 1964, Carpenter and coworkers reviewed this association of hypoadrenalism and hypothyroidism and also noted the association of diabetes mellitus.[499] More recently, an association of Addison's disease with gonadal failure, hyperthyroidism, hypothyroidism, Hashimoto's thyroiditis, vitiligo, hypoparathyroidism, and pernicious anemia has been established (see Chap. 27).[817,1169,1178,1190,1191,1199] One or more of these clinical disorders are present in about half the patients with autoimmune Addison's disease, and the presence of organ-specific antibodies is even more common. These disorders are not associated with Addison's disease due to tuberculosis or other invasive or infiltrative processes. Although these associated disorders are common in patients with primary adrenal insufficiency, patients with more commonly occurring conditions such as diabetes mellitus and autoimmune thyroid disease rarely develop Addison's disease. Autoimmune hypoparathyroidism represents an exception, as the two disorders commonly coincide and are frequently familial (see later discussion).[817,1200,1201]

The association of Addison's disease with one or more of these conditions has been referred to as Schmidt's syndrome, autoimmune endocrine failure, the polyglandular failure syndrome, and the polyglandular autoimmune syndromes (PGA types I and II) (Table 11-16).[1171,1172,1175–1177]

PGA Type I Polyglandular autoimmune syndrome type I may occur sporadically but is more commonly familial.[1172,1173,1175–1177] It is inherited in an autosomal recessive pattern[1173,1175,1176] with a slight female preponderance, and there is no HLA association. The cardinal manifestations are hypoparathyroidism, mucocutaneous candidiasis, and adrenal insufficiency (Table 11-16).[1172] Hypoparathyroidism and mucocutaneous candidiasis occur in about 90 percent and 75 percent of patients, respectively, and are the earliest manifestations, with onset usually occurring in early childhood.[1172] The onset of adrenal insufficiency occurs later in 95 percent of patients, with a peak incidence at 10 to 15 years.[1172] The overall incidence of gonadal failure is about 45 percent of patients, but it is present in 60 percent of female patients.[1172,1173,1175–1177] Autoimmune thyroid disease occurs in 12 percent, but diabetes mellitus is rare. There is a high incidence of hypoplasia of dental enamel, dystrophic nails, and keratopathy; nonendocrine disorders such as vitiligo, alopecia, pernicious anemia, malabsorption, and chronic active hepatitis occur in 4 to 25 percent of these patients.[1173] Recently, the APECED gene, coding for a transcription factor, was found to be defective in PGA Type I.

TABLE 11-16. Polyglandular Failure Syndromes

Endocrine Disorders	Type I Prevalence, Percent	Type II Prevalence, Percent
Adrenal insufficiency	60	100
Hypoparathyroidism	89	—
Mucocutaneous candidiasis	75	—
Gonadal failure	45	5–50
Autoimmune thyroid disease	12	70
Insulin-dependent diabetes mellitus	1	50
Hypopituitarism	Rare	Rare
Diabetes insipidus	Rare	Rare
Nonendocrine Disorders		
Pernicious anemia	16	Rare
Vitiligo	4	5
Alopecia	20	Rare
Malabsorption syndrome	25	—
Chronic active hepatitis	9	—
Myasthenia gravis	—	Rare
Thrombocytopenic purpura	—	Rare
Sjögren's syndrome	—	Rare
Rheumatoid arthritis	—	Rare

Source: Modified and reproduced with permission from Leshin.[1172]

PGA Type II Polyglandular autoimmune syndrome type II is the classic prototype of these disorders and has most frequently been termed Schmidt's syndrome. This syndrome is familial in about half the patients, and its inheritance is linked to the inheritance of the HLA antigens B8 (DW3), DR3, and DR4.[1175,1176] There is a female/male ratio of 1.8/1, and the age at onset is usually in the range of 20 to 35 years.[1202] The classic manifestations are adrenal insufficiency (in 100 percent of patients) plus either autoimmune thyroid disease (70 percent) or insulin-dependent diabetes mellitus (50 percent) (Table 11-16).[1172] The incidence of gonadal failure has been variably reported (5 to 50 percent) and is rare in males.[1172,1175–1177] Ovarian and adrenal failure may occur in the same patient in the absence of thyroid disease or diabetes mellitus.[1172] Vitiligo is present in about 5 percent of patients, and other nonendocrine disorders are unusual.

Pathology

In autoimmune adrenal insufficiency, there is early lymphocytic infiltration of the adrenal cortex, thus giving rise to the term *diffuse lymphocytic adrenalitis*. Subsequently, the adrenal cortex is gradually destroyed and the adrenals are small, atrophic, and frequently difficult to locate at autopsy. The capsule is thickened, and the normal cortical architecture is destroyed; however, the adrenal medulla is preserved. The cortical cells of all three zones are largely absent, and those remaining are scattered, show degenerative change, and are surrounded by a fibrous stroma and lymphocytic infiltrates. The degree of lymphocytic infiltration is variable, but its association with the loss of cortical cells is the classic pathologic feature.[817,1179,1203]

Primary Adrenocortical Insufficiency Due to Invasive or Hemorrhagic Disorders

Adrenal insufficiency secondary to invasive or hemorrhagic disorders is a consequence of total or nearly total destruction of both glands and is often accompanied by advanced or disseminated systemic disease. Thus, destruction of the adrenal rarely occurs without involvement of other organs by the same disease process. In these conditions, the rate of development of adrenocortical insufficiency can vary markedly, depending on the nature of the primary process. With septicemia or hemorrhage, the adrenal can be destroyed rapidly, whereas with conditions such as tuberculosis, a much longer period may be required.

Invasive Disorders

Adrenal tuberculosis is a consequence of blood-borne infection of the adrenal cortex. It is virtually always accompanied or preceded by tuberculous infection elsewhere in the body, especially of the lung, gastrointestinal tract, or kidney.[1179,1180] Although the adrenals may be involved in 85 percent of patients dying of tuberculosis,[1179] the incidence of clinical adrenal insufficiency is much lower and appears to occur in only a minority of patients.[1179] In one series, adrenal insufficiency was present in 3 percent of patients with extrapulmonary tuberculosis. Because extrapulmonary tuberculosis is present in about 10 percent of all cases of tuberculosis, this would suggest an overall incidence of adrenal insufficiency of about 0.3 percent.[1180] The incidence of adrenal involvement with atypical strains of tuberculosis is unknown; however, *Mycobacterium avium-intracellulare* (MAI) was demonstrated at autopsy in the adrenals of 5 of 41 (12 percent) patients with AIDS[1204] (see later discussion).

In tuberculous Addison's disease, the adrenal glands are totally replaced by caseous necrosis with little or no remaining cortical or medullary tissue. CT scan shows adrenal enlargement in patients with tuberculous Addison's disease of less than 2 years duration,[1205] and these patients typically have a central hypodense area of caseous necrosis with contrast enhancement of the periphery of the gland.[1206] In response to therapy, the enlarged adrenals may revert to normal size or become atrophic, and in a few patients there is recovery of adrenal function.[1206] In patients with a longer duration of adrenal insufficiency, the adrenals become atrophic and calcification is radiologically evident in approximately 50 percent of cases.[1190,1205]

Fungal infections can also involve the adrenal glands and cause Addison's disease. This can occur with histoplasmosis, paracoccidioidomycosis (South American blastomycosis), North American blastomycosis, coccidioidomycosis, and cryptococcosis. Histoplasmosis in its rare disseminated form is an important cause of Addison's disease because as many as 50 percent of these patients develop adrenal insufficiency.[1207] CT scans demonstrate bilateral adrenal enlargement with central necrosis,[1208,1209] and recovery of adrenal function with therapy is unusual.[1210] Paracoccidioidomycosis is also a frequent cause of Addison's disease in endemic areas, and adrenal insufficiency may occur in as many as 10 percent of these patients.[1211] In contrast, North American blastomycosis rarely causes adrenal insufficiency, and only a few cases have been reported.[1212,1213] Coccidioidomycosis and cryptococcosis are also rare causes of Addison's disease.[1214,1215] Syphilis is an additional rare cause of adrenal destruction.[1179]

Metastases to the adrenal are quite common,[1202] but overt adrenal disease requires bilateral involvement and destruction of both cortices. Thus, Addison's disease has been relatively unusual, but more recent studies suggest that it may occur in up to 20 percent of patients with bilateral adrenal metastases[1216,1217] and may occasionally be the presenting feature of malignancy.[1218] Both Hodgkin's and non-Hodgkin's lymphoma may also cause adrenal insufficiency,[1219,1220] and an occasional patient recovers normal function after chemotherapy.[1221]

Other rare invasive etiologies of Addison's disease include amyloidosis and sarcoidosis.[1222–1225] When destruction is due to processes other than tuberculosis, the pathologic findings in the adrenal are characteristic of the particular disorder, with loss of adrenal tissue and scarring, inflammatory changes, or replacement of tissue with abscess, tumor, amyloid, etc. Adrenal calcification is less common than with tuberculosis.

AIDS

Although adrenal insufficiency occurs in only a minority, pathologic abnormalities of the adrenal glands are extremely common in patients dying of AIDS and have been demonstrated in 50 to 78 percent of these patients.[1204,1226–1229] HIV can directly infect adrenocortical cells,[1230] but it is not known if this contributes to adrenal dysfunction in AIDS. The most common abnormality at autopsy is that of involvement of the adrenal cortex by cytomegalovirus (CMV) with typical inclusion bodies and adrenalitis.[1204,1227,1228] However, the adrenal necrosis in these patients is generally not extensive enough to impair adrenal function.[1204] However, other infectious and invasive etiologies of adrenal insufficiency occur, and patients with AIDS may have adrenal involvement with *Mycobacterium tuberculosis, M. avium-intracellulare,* toxoplasmosis, cryptococcosis, Kaposi's sarcoma, and lymphoma.[1204,1226–1229] Despite this high incidence of adrenal involvement, clinically significant adrenal insufficiency occurs in only a few percent of patients.[1226] However, even this low incidence would make AIDS a more common etiology than the autoimmune and tuberculous forms.

Some patients with AIDS have elevated cortisol levels.[1226] This has been attributed to a stress response to chronic severe illness[1231] or to the development of an acquired form of glucocorticoid resistance with abnormalities of the glucocorticoid receptor.[1232] This latter report has not been confirmed, and there is no evidence that treating patients with elevated cortisol levels is beneficial.

Adrenal Hemorrhage

Bilateral adrenal hemorrhage may cause rapid and total adrenal destruction, leading to acute loss of both glucocorticoid and mineralocorticoid secretion. In adults, adrenal hemorrhage usually occurs in patients over age 50 years, and anticoagulant therapy and spontaneous coagulopathy are the most common contributing factors, being present in most patients.[1181–1185] Adrenal hemorrhage can also occur in patients with either overwhelming infection with sepsis or severe and frequently life-threatening major illnesses.[1184–1187,1233] These include coagulation disorders, adrenal vein thrombosis, adrenal metastases, trauma, major surgery, severe cardiovascular disease, congestive heart failure, pulmonary emboli, acute renal failure, local infection, leukemias, lymphomas, malignancy, trauma, and severe burns.[1184–1187,1233] In children, the most common cause of bilateral adrenal hemorrhage is fulminant meningococcemia or *Pseudomonas* septicemia.[1186–1187] Adrenal hemorrhage may also occur in a neonate after a complicated delivery or in the presence of a coagulation disorder. Adrenal hemorrhage may also occur during a complicated pregnancy or in the postpartum period.

Until recently, the diagnosis of bilateral adrenal hemorrhage was rarely made premortem and was usually established only at autopsy.[1183] However, increased awareness of this syndrome and the availability of modern imaging techniques have led to more frequent recognition.[1234] Survival with adrenal insufficiency is now being reported more frequently,[1185,1234] and recovery of adrenal function occurs in an occasional patient.[1181,1235]

The adrenal glands in this syndrome are enlarged, not infrequently to a massive degree, and the cortex may be totally destroyed.[1185,1205] The hemorrhage usually replaces the medulla and inner cortex; the outer cortex undergoes ischemic necrosis, with only a thin rim of cortical cells remaining.[1233] Venous thrombosis frequently accompanies the hemorrhage. CT and MR imaging studies demonstrate the adrenal enlargement and usually can establish the diagnosis. In surviving patients, the hematomas resolve and the adrenals atrophy and may calcify.[1181,1234]

Other Congenital and Familial Etiologies

In addition to the disorders of steroid hormone biosynthesis discussed previously, there are several inherited disorders of adrenal development and metabolism that present to the clinician as Addison's disease.

Adrenoleukodystrophy

Adrenoleukodystrophy (ALD) is a group of fairly common X-linked disorders affecting both the adrenal and the cerebral white matter in about 1 in 25000 males.[236] Affected cells accumulate very long-chain fatty acids (VLCFA), and it was initially thought that the defect was in lignoceroyl-CoA synthetase, a key enzyme in fatty acid oxidation localized to the peroxisomal matrix. However, positional cloning demonstrated that the responsible gene on Xp28a encodes a peroxisomal membrane protein with homology to the ATP-binding cassette (ABC) transporter proteins.[1237] The mechanism by which mutations in this protein cause the symptomatology of the various forms of ALD remains unclear.[1238,1239] The diagnosis is made by finding dramatically elevated ratios of serum C-26 (hexacosanoic) to C-22 (behenic) VLCFA.[1240] This test can also detect carrier females and affected fetuses.

The classic form of the disease, termed childhood cerebral ALD, generally presents with adrenal insufficiency at 2–10 years of age, generally followed by progressive neurologic dysfunction leading to a vegetative state followed by death, usually within 4 years from the diagnosis. Adolescent and adult cerebral ALD are somewhat milder allelic variants presenting in teenagers and young adults, in which the neurologic disorder is often misdiagnosed as a psychiatric disorder.[1241] Adrenomyeloneuropathy, which was previously thought to be a distinct disease, is a milder allelic variant of ALD presenting in young adults, primarily as a disorder of the spinal cord, characterized by leg weakness, altered gait, diminished vibratory sensation, loss of sphincter control, and impotence.[1241] About half of these patients have progressive cerebral dysfunction, but half can have a normal life expectancy without intellectual impairment. About 10–20 percent of ALD patients have Addison's disease only, and some may even be asymptomatic. Yet up to half of obligately heterozygous women who carry a mutant gene for ALD will have some neurologic dysfunction, which is occasionally misdiagnosed as multiple sclerosis.

Therapy for the ALD disorders consists of steroid hormone replacement and supportive measures. The demonstration that orally ingested radiolabeled C26 VLCFA accumulated in affected tissues prompted efforts at dietary therapy. However, both restricted oral intake of C26 VLCFA and efforts to interfere with synthesis of VLCFA by administration of a 4:1 mixture of glyceryl trioleate and glyceryl trierucate ("Lorenzo's oil") have been uniformly unsuccessful.[1236] Until gene therapy becomes feasible, the most promising approach appears to be bone marrow transplantation, in which transplanted hematopoetic cells enter the nervous system and degrade VLCFA.[1236]

Familial Glucocorticoid Deficiency

Familial isolated glucocorticoid deficiency (hereditary adrenocortical unresponsiveness to ACTH) is a rare type of adrenal insufficiency that is inherited as an autosomal recessive and which in many families was due to mutations in the ACTH receptor.[1242–1244] The disorder is characterized by glucocorticoid and adrenal androgen deficiency with elevated plasma ACTH levels.[1244–1246] Cortisol secretion does not respond to prolonged ACTH stimulation; however, aldosterone is usually normally responsive to posture and sodium deprivation.[1244–1246] The disorder usually presents in childhood and the presenting sign is hypoglycemic seizures in the first year of life. A related syndrome accompanied by achalasia, alacrima, and autonomic and motor neuropathy (Triple A syndrome) is not linked to the ACTH receptor but to another gene.[1243–1246]

Adrenal Hypoplasia Congenita

Adrenal hypoplasia congenita is caused by mutations on the DAX-1 gene on chromosome Xp21 (Ref. 1247). This gene encodes a nuclear transcription factor that participates in the differentiation of adrenal and gonadal tissues, as well as in gonadotropin expression,[1248] so that successfully treated children may not enter puberty.[1249] In this disorder, the definitive zone of the fetal adrenal does not develop, and the fetal zone is vaccuolated and cytomegalic. Poor function of the fetal zone results in low maternal estriol concentrations during pregnancy, but parturition is normal. Neonatal glucocorticoid and mineralocorticoid deficiencies manifest with a typical salt-wasting crisis, and respond well to replacement therapy. Deletions of the DAX-1 gene may also encompass adjacent genes, causing a contiguous gene syndrome consisting of glycerol kinase deficiency, Duchenne's muscular dystrophy, and mental retardation.[1247,1248]

Wolman Disease

Wolman disease and cholesterol ester storage disease are both caused by mutations in the secreted form of lysosomal acid lipase (cholesterol esterase), which mobilizes cholesterol esters from adrenal lipid droplets.[1250] The gene for this enzyme on chromosome 10q has been cloned and mutations causing 1 case of Wolman disease have been identified.[1251] Because insufficient free cholesterol is available to P450scc, there is adrenal insufficiency. As all cells must store and utilize cholesterol, the disease affects all cells, not just the adrenal, hence the disorder is relentless and fatal. Vomiting, steatorrhea, failure to thrive, hepatosplenomegaly, and adrenal calcification are the usual presenting findings. The diagnosis is established by bone marrow aspiration yielding foam cells containing large lysosomal vaccules engorged with cholesterol esters, and is confirmed by finding absent cholesterol esterase activity in fibroblasts, leukocytes, or marrow cells. Cholesterol ester storage disease is caused by a milder defect in the same enzyme, generally presenting in childhood or adolescence.

Pathophysiology

The development of the clinical manifestations of adrenocortical insufficiency requires the loss of more than 90 percent of both adrenal cortices. In the autoimmune and invasive types, destruction is usually gradual, leading to the manifestations of chronic adrenocortical insufficiency; however, in one-third of cases there is a more rapid course, with a symptom duration less than 3 months.[1190] In addition, approximately 25 percent of these patients are in crisis or impending crisis at the time of diagnosis.[1190] Hemorrhagic destruction of the adrenals results in an abrupt state of adrenal insufficiency with sudden loss of both glucocorticoid and mineralocorticoid secretion.

With gradual destruction, normal regulatory mechanisms are able to compensate temporarily. Decreased cortisol production results in decreased feedback at the hypothalamus and pituitary with increased release of CRH and the POMC-derived peptides ACTH, β-LPH, and the NH_2-terminal fragment. The increased ACTH level results in increased stimulation of the remaining adrenal with normal cortisol production in the early stages but inadequate production as the disease progresses. The MSH sequences within the POMC-derived peptides also lead to increased pigmentation, one of the cardinal signs of Addison's disease. In the minority of patients with more rapid adrenal destruction, prominent hyperpigmentation may not be present. The decreased mineralocorticoid production leads to sodium loss and potassium retention. The sodium loss results in stimulation of renin release and angiotensin II production. The increased potassium and angiotensin II stimulate the remaining glomerulosa to produce more aldosterone, but with progressive adrenal destruction, this mechanism also becomes inadequate.

When adrenal destruction is gradual, there is a phase characterized by normal basal steroid secretion but inability to respond to stress, i.e., a decreased adrenal reserve. This may progress to a state in which overall steroid production is diminished but enough episodic releases of cortisol occur so that basal cortisol determinations can be in the normal range. In this state of partial adrenal insufficiency, the patient may have few complaints, but a history usually discloses symptoms and most of these patients show pigmentation because of increased POMC peptide production. In this state, a crisis can be precipitated by the stress of surgery, trauma, or infection.

As destruction of the adrenal cortex progresses, mineralocorticoid and glucocorticoid secretion become inadequate and even basal cortisol levels are low, leading to all the metabolic derangements described previously (see actions of glucocorticoids and physiologic actions of mineralocorticoids). These derangements are reflected in manifestations of chronic adrenocortical insufficiency, as discussed later.

Clinical Features

The clinical presentation depends on the rate and degree of adrenocortical destruction and on extraadrenal factors that may precipitate a crisis. Thus, most cases with autoimmune or invasive etiologies are insidious in onset and gradually progressive, but a crisis may be precipitated by intercurrent stress.[1190] Adrenal hemorrhage presents with acute adrenal insufficiency. Because the presentations of these three subtypes of primary adrenocortical insufficiency differ, the clinical manifestations are discussed separately here.

Chronic Primary Adrenocortical Insufficiency

The gradual development of adrenal insufficiency may go unnoticed by the patient or physician until adrenocortical function is lost to a major extent. However, in retrospect, it is noted that the symptoms were usually present for months or even years before diagnosis or presentation.

Major clinical features and an estimate of their frequency are shown in Table 11-17.[1169,1190,1200] These features include weakness and fatigue, weight loss, anorexia, and gastrointestinal symptoms. The most distinctive physical finding is hyperpigmentation. Its presence in association with any of these other manifestations should elicit the suspicion of Addison's disease. Weakness is always present and is accompanied by fatigue and malaise. It is generalized and usually is manifested by an inability to complete routine tasks rather than being restricted to particular muscle groups. Weight loss is also very common, may vary from 2 to 15 kg, and becomes more severe as adrenal failure progresses.[792] It is largely due to tissue loss resulting from anorexia, but dehydration also contributes.

TABLE 11-17. Clinical Features of Chronic Primary Adrenocortical Insufficiency

Feature	Percent with Condition
Weakness and fatigue	100
Weight loss	100
Anorexia	100
Hyperpigmentation	92
Hypotension	88
Gastrointestinal symptoms	56
Salt craving	19
Postural symptoms	12

Source: Adapted from Nerup.[1190]

The majority of these patients have gastrointestinal symptoms. Anorexia is extremely common and contributes to the weight loss. Nausea, vague abdominal discomfort, and vomiting occur more frequently with progressive adrenal failure. Diarrhea may be present but occurs less frequently. Gastrointestinal symptoms may be pronounced as an adrenal crisis supervenes and may lead to the mistaken diagnosis of primary gastrointestinal disease. It is important for the physician to consider Addison's disease in patients with these symptoms, as radiologic studies that require enemas, cathartics, and fasting can precipitate shock and collapse.

Hypotension is common but in many patients may not be profound enough to suggest the diagnosis. Nevertheless, systolic blood pressure is <110 mmHg in more than 90 percent of these patients and is frequently associated with complaints of orthostatic dizziness and occasionally[792,1169] syncope. In patients in crisis, recumbent hypotension or shock is an almost universal finding.

Hyperpigmentation of the skin and mucous membranes is the single most distinctive sign in chronic primary adrenocortical insufficiency and can be most useful, especially in an acutely ill patient with unexplained hypotension. It may precede other manifestations of adrenal insufficiency (Fig. 11-39). It is generalized, with accentuation in sun-exposed areas and pressure points such as the elbows, knees, knuckles, and toes and around the wrist. Abnormal pigmentation should be suspected when it is present on palmar creases, nail beds, buccal mucosa, nipples, navel, areolae, and the perivaginal or perianal mucosa. Pigmentation of the buccal mucosa and gums is always accompanied by generalized hyperpigmentation.[817] Surgical scars acquired after the onset of Addison's disease are frequently hyperpigmented, whereas previous scars remain unpigmented. The increased pigmentation is frequently accompanied by the appearance of numerous black or brown freckles. In people of dark-skinned races, pigmentation of the mouth, palmar creases, vulva, and anus may be normally present and the diagnosis of hyperpigmentation is frequently difficult. Pigmentation of the tongue is probably abnormal regardless of racial background. The hyperpigmentation is commonly misinterpreted as being due to sun exposure, and the healthy appearance of the patient may lead to dismissal of other symptoms.

Vitiligo occurs in 4 to 17 percent of patients with autoimmune Addison's disease; however, it occurs rarely in those with tuberculosis.[792,1190]

Salt craving is a significant feature in approximately 20 percent of cases[1249]; some patients may actually eat salt by the spoonful despite anorexia.

Although both fasting and postprandial hypoglycemia were frequently reported in older series,[792] they are currently uncommon.[1169]

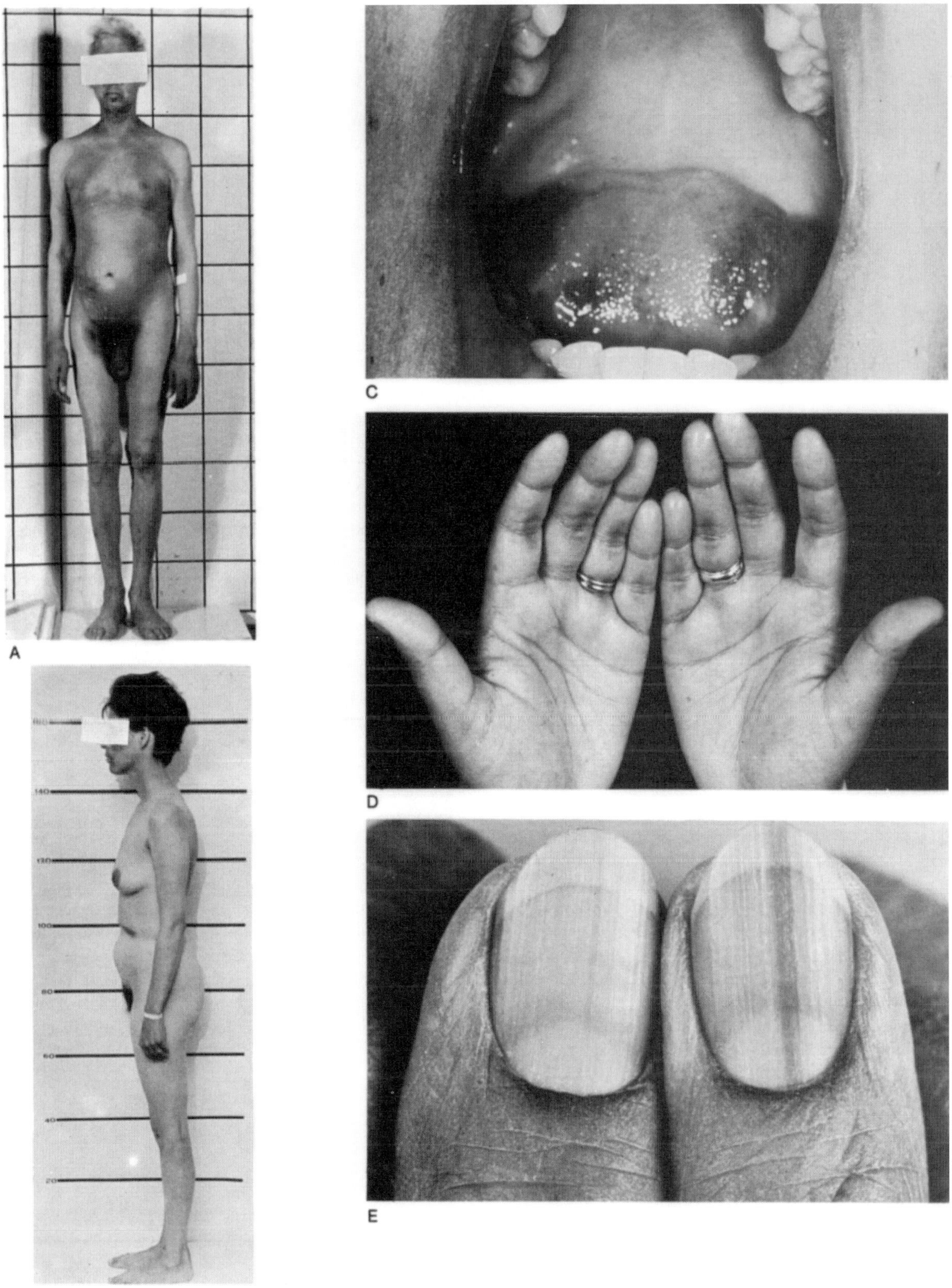

FIGURE 11-39. Abnormal pigmentation due to hypersecretion of ACTH and β-LPH. (*A*) Generalized hyperpigmentation with accentuation over exposed areas. (*B*) Pigmentation in sun-exposed areas, although the abdominal surgical scar is markedly hyperpigmented. (*C*) Hyperpigmentation of the tongue. (*D*) Hyperpigmentation is prominent in skin creases. (*E*) Hyperpigmentation of and around the nails.

The fasting blood sugar level is within the low normal range in most patients; it is unusual for a patient with Addison's disease to present with or have symptomatic complaints of hypoglycemia, and severe hypoglycemia is rare, except in children. Hypoglycemia may be provoked by fasting, fever, infection, or nausea and vomiting and may be present in acute adrenal crisis. In a patient with preceding diabetes, improvement in blood sugar control and a decrease in insulin requirement tend to occur when Addison's disease emerges.

Amenorrhea is common in untreated Addison's disease patients and may be a manifestation of weight loss and chronic illness or of primary ovarian failure from an associated immunologic cause. Loss of axillary and pubic hair occurs in a minority of female patients as a result of a loss of adrenal androgens.

Patients with autoimmune Addison's disease may also have symptoms of the associated disorders discussed earlier. Similarly, patients with tuberculosis or other invasive diseases causing adrenal insufficiency usually have involvement of other organ systems.

Acute Adrenocortical Insufficiency (Adrenal Crisis)

The most common emergency presentation of primary adrenal insufficiency is that of acute adrenal crisis in a patient with undiagnosed or treated Addison's disease who is exposed to stress such as infection, trauma, surgery, or dehydration as a result of salt deprivation, vomiting, or diarrhea. The requirement for increased glucocorticoid levels during stress has already been emphasized, although addisonian patients usually tolerate minor insults such as upper respiratory infections. Thus, an addisonian patient who does not receive therapy during these stresses may rapidly develop an acute adrenal crisis.

When acute adrenal insufficiency develops (Table 11-18), anorexia becomes profound and there is increased nausea and vomiting; this contributes to volume depletion and dehydration. Abdominal pain occurs frequently and may mimic an acute surgical abdomen. Specific localizing features are usually absent, although there may be tenderness and pain on deep palpation. The blood pressure falls farther, and hypovolemic shock develops with extreme weakness, apathy, and confusion. The patient may rapidly develop severe dehydration. Fever is common, and hypoglycemia may be present. The fever may be due either to hypoadrenalism or to a precipitating infection. Hyperpigmentation is usually present in a patient with primary adrenocortical insufficiency and is an important clinical sign. Without appropriate therapy death may occur rapidly, with coma and shock. Hyponatremia, hyperkalemia, lymphocytosis, and eosinophilia should suggest the diagnosis of adrenal crisis, and the possibility of adrenal insufficiency must be considered in any patient with unexplained shock. Because another process commonly precipitates adrenal crises, these manifestations may divert attention from the possibility of Addison's disease. For instance, in a patient with coexisting diabetes mellitus, ketoacidosis can precipitate or be caused by the crisis. In previously undiagnosed patients, it is frequently possible to obtain a history of preceding chronic adrenal insufficiency at the time of acute presentation; however, this is not always the case, because some patients may have enough basal glucocorticoid production to prevent chronic symptoms but the adrenal reserve may be decreased in response to stress.

TABLE 11-18. Clinical Features of Acute Primary Adrenocortical Insufficiency (Adrenal Crisis)

Hypotension/shock (vascular collapse)
Weakness, apathy, confusion
Nausea, vomitting, anorexia
Dehydration, hypovolemia, hyponatremia, hyperkalemia
Abdominal or flank pain
Hyperthermia
Hypoglycemia

TABLE 11-19. Clinical Features of Adrenal Hemorrhage

Features	Percent
General	
Hypotension/shock	74
Fever	59
Nausea and vomiting	46
Confusion, disorientation	41
Tachycardia	28
Cyanosis/lividity	28
Local	
Abdominal, flank, or back pain	77
Abdominal or flank tenderness	38
Abdominal distension	28
Abdominal rigidity	20
Chest pain	13
Rebound tenderness	5

Source: Adapted from Xarli et al.[1184]

Adrenal Hemorrhage Causing Acute Adrenal Insufficiency

The typical clinical picture in patients with bilateral adrenal hemorrhage and acute adrenal destruction is that of a progressively deteriorating course in an already complicated patient with a major illness (Table 11-19).[1181–1187,1233] The classic clinical features of Addison's disease—hyperpigmentation, weight loss, and preceding chronic gastrointestinal symptoms—are absent. The patients at greatest risk are those with thromboembolic disease, those with spontaneous or iatrogenic coagulopathy, and those who are postoperative.[1181–1183] The usual presenting symptoms are abdominal, flank, or chest pain with abdominal tenderness.[1184,1185] Fever, hypotension leading to shock, and electrolyte abnormalities are common, as are nausea, vomiting, confusion, and disorientation. With progression, severe hypotension, volume depletion, dehydration, hyperpyrexia, cyanosis, coma, and death may ensue.[1184,1185] The diagnosis of acute adrenal hemorrhage should be considered in a deteriorating patient with thromboembolic disease, with coagulopathy, or in the postoperative period who develops unexplained abdominal or flank pain, vascular collapse, hyperpyrexia, electrolyte abnormality, or hypoglycemia.

Laboratory Features of Primary Adrenocortical Insufficiency

The specific laboratory diagnosis of Addison's disease depends on measurement of plasma cortisol and ACTH levels (see later discussion). However, other laboratory abnormalities that are not diagnostic should suggest the diagnosis (Table 11-20).

Hyponatremia and hyperkalemia secondary to mineralocorticoid deficiency are characteristic manifestations of primary adrenal insufficiency; in the absence of chronic renal failure, their presence should suggest Addison's disease. Hyponatremia is

TABLE 11-20. Laboratory Features of Primary Adrenocortical Insufficiency

Hyponatremia (88%)*
Hyperkalemia (64%)*
Azotemia
Anemia
Increased plasma renin activity
Eosinophilia
Lymphocytosis
Hypoglycemia
Hypercalcemia

* Percent occurrence from Nerup.[1190]

present in 88 percent and hyperkalemia in 64 percent of patients at the time of diagnosis.[1178]

A normocytic normochromic anemia is common but may also be masked by dehydration and hemoconcentration. Pernicious anemia is present in 4 percent of patients with autoimmune Addison's disease.[1169] The differential white cell count shows neutropenia, a relative lymphocytosis, and eosinophilia. Elevations of blood urea nitrogen (BUN) and serum creatinine levels are ascribable to dehydration and hemoconcentration and are frequently accompanied by mild acidosis due to dehydration, hyperkalemia, and the loss of the acid-secreting properties of the mineralocorticoids. Increased plasma renin activity is a result of mineralocorticoid deficiency and the hypovolemia of the patients.

Mild to moderate hypercalcemia occurs in approximately 6 percent of patients and may be mistaken for the hypercalcemia of dehydration. Hypocalcemia and hyperphosphatemia are present in patients with associated hypoparathyroidism.

The heart can be small and vertical on x ray. Routine radiographs of the abdomen are usually normal, but adrenal calcification is present in approximately 50 percent of cases because of tuberculosis[792] and can also be present with other invasive etiologies and after hemorrhagic destruction of the gland. With CT of the abdomen, adrenal enlargement and/or calcification is demonstrated with tuberculosis, metastases, adrenal hemorrhage, and other invasive etiologies, whereas in the autoimmune form, the adrenals may be destroyed and thus are small or absent on abdominal scans.[1202,1205,1206,1223,1234]

The electrocardiogram may reveal low voltage with a vertical QRS axis. There may be nonspecific abnormalities due to electrolyte imbalance (e.g., peaked T waves due to the hyperkalemia or a shortened QT segment).

With sudden adrenal destruction, typical laboratory manifestations are usually absent. Hyponatremia and hyperkalemia occur in a minority of patients; however, their presence should suggest the diagnosis.[1184,1185,1233] Azotemia is common, whereas hypoglycemia occurs infrequently in adults.[1185,1233] Increased circulating eosinophils or an increased total eosinophil count may be present and should also arouse the suspicion of acute insufficiency.

Secondary Adrenocortical Insufficiency

Etiology

The causes of secondary adrenocortical insufficiency are reviewed in Chaps. 6 and 7. Therapy with pharmacologic doses of glucocorticoids is the most frequent cause (Chap. 14). If the steroid-treated population is excluded, tumors of the pituitary and/or hypothalamic region are the most common cause of pituitary ACTH deficiency, and surgical or radiation therapy for these tumors may also contribute to panhypopituitarism. In patients with hypothalamic or pituitary tumors, ACTH deficiency is virtually always accompanied by deficiencies of other anterior pituitary hormones as the ACTH-producing cells are more resistant to pituitary damage. Growth hormone and gonadotropins are usually lost first, followed by the loss of TSH and finally of ACTH (Chap. 7). Other, less common causes of hypothalamic-pituitary dysfunction are discussed in Chaps. 6 and 7.

Isolated ACTH Deficiency

This disorder is a rare cause of secondary adrenocortical failure. In a recent review of 76 patients, 54 percent were male and 46 percent female; the mean age at diagnosis was 50 years (range, 24 to 79 years).[1252] Thus, in most patients this is an acquired disorder. Current data suggest that the etiology of this disorder is frequently autoimmune and that in many instances it is a sequela of lymphocytic hypophysitis.[1252,1253] Thus, most women of childbearing age who have isolated ACTH deficiency develop it postpartum, and many of these patients have autoimmune thyroid disorders and positive antithyroid and antipituitary antibody titers.[1252,1254] Whether isolated ACTH deficiency in male patients is autoimmune is less clear. The idea that a primary pituitary defect is responsible in most cases is confirmed by the failure of the pituitary to respond to repeated stimulation with CRH or vasopressin.[1252,1255,1256] Other possible etiologies include congenital defects, birth trauma, and partial pituitary infarction associated with pregnancy.[1252]

Isolated ACTH deficiency is accompanied by numerous endocrine abnormalities that appear to be secondary to the glucocorticoid insufficiency. These include elevations of TSH, prolactin, and LH that are not accompanied by hypothyroidism or hypogonadism and are reversible with glucocorticoid replacement.[1252] Growth hormone secretion was impaired in about one-third of patients and was also reversible after glucocorticoid therapy.[1252]

In many patients with isolated ACTH deficiency there is decreased plasma renin activity and a decreased plasma aldosterone concentration.[466,1252,1257] These patients may be hypotensive and hyponatremic, but hyperkalemia is rare. A return to normal plasma renin activity (PRA) and plasma aldosterone concentration (PAC) has been reported after glucocorticoid therapy.[466,1252,1257] Hyponatremia in these patients with glucocorticoid insufficiency is a result of the inability to excrete a water load, a syndrome that resembles the syndrome of inappropriate secretion of ADH (SIADH), albeit in this case the increase of vasopressin secretion is compensatory rather than inappropriate.

Pathophysiology

The pathogenesis of secondary adrenal insufficiency differs from that of primary adrenocortical destruction because the predominant effect of ACTH deficiency is decreased cortisol and adrenal androgen secretion. With hypothalamic or pituitary tumors, gradual growth of the lesion compresses the normal anterior pituitary, resulting in gradual destruction of corticotrophic cells with impairment of ACTH secretion. Initially, basal ACTH levels are maintained; however, there may be impaired ACTH reserve. Basal cortisol secretion is also normal, but ACTH and cortisol levels cannot increase in response to stress. With progression, basal ACTH secretion becomes deficient, resulting in atrophy of the adrenal zonae fasciculata and reticularis and decreased cortisol secretion in the basal state. When this occurs, not only is there an impaired ability to increase ACTH secretion in response to stress, the atrophic adrenal becomes unable to increase cortisol secretion in response to acute stimulation with ACTH.

Glucocorticoid therapy also suppresses the pituitary-adrenal axis; the effect is both dose- and time-dependent (Chap. 14). Although growth hormone and gonadotropin secretion may be depressed, pituitary function is generally intact (see actions of glucocorticoids, earlier; Cushing's Syndrome, later; and Chap. 14).

The glucocorticoid deficiency present in these conditions results in manifestations similar to those seen in primary adrenocortical insufficiency except that derangements due to mineralocorticoid deficiency are usually absent. The functional status of the zona glomerulosa is initially preserved, and aldosterone secretion, controlled by the renin-angiotensin system, is normal. When ACTH deficiency is long-standing, mineralocorticoid deficiency may develop in a few patients; many of those reported have had isolated ACTH deficiency.[466,1252,1257] The majority of these patients have hyporeninemia, and the renin and aldosterone deficiencies are correctable with glucocorticoid administration.[466,1252,1257,1258]

Clinical Features

The clinical presentation of secondary adrenal insufficiency, like that of the primary type, is usually chronic. However, an acute presentation can occur in undiagnosed patients during stress and in treated patients who do not receive increased steroid dosage during infection, surgery, or trauma. Pituitary apoplexy, i.e., hemorrhagic infarction of a pituitary tumor, may be accompanied by acute secondary adrenocortical insufficiency.

The usual presentation of secondary adrenal insufficiency is similar to that of primary adrenocortical insufficiency, with two important exceptions. First, because pituitary secretion of ACTH and β-LPH is deficient, the characteristic hyperpigmentation of Addison's disease is absent. In fact, patients with hypopituitarism frequently present with pallor of the skin. Second, as discussed previously, the clinical features of mineralocorticoid deficiency are usually absent, and therefore volume depletion, dehydration, and hyperkalemia are usually absent. Hypotension is also less severe, except in acute presentations. Hyponatremia can be present and is usually due to water retention and the inability to excrete a water load rather than to sodium loss (see previous discussions of cardiovascular system and fluid and electrolyte balance under actions of glucocorticoids). Thus, the clinical features of ACTH and glucocorticoid deficiency are nonspecific and consist predominantly of weakness, lethargy, easy fatigue, anorexia, weight loss, nausea, and occasionally vomiting. Patients may also describe arthralgias, myalgias, and exacerbation of allergic responses. Hypoglycemia is occasionally the presenting feature.[1252] With acute decompensation, severe hypotension or shock may occur and be unresponsive to vasopressors unless glucocorticoids are administered.

Patients with secondary adrenal insufficiency (except those with isolated ACTH deficiency) commonly have associated historical or clinical features that suggest the diagnosis. There may be a history of glucocorticoid therapy or the presence of cushingoid features, suggestive of previous therapy (Chap. 14). Patients with hypothalamic or pituitary tumors usually have loss of other pituitary hormones; i.e., hypogonadism and hypothyroidism are common, and there may be hypersecretion of growth hormone or prolactin. Most patients also have local tumor manifestations such as visual field defects, headache, and enlargement of the sella turcica (see Chaps. 6 and 7).

Laboratory Features

Routine laboratory testing in secondary adrenal hypofunction may reveal a mild normochromic normocytic anemia, neutropenia, relative lymphocytosis, and eosinophilia. The serum sodium concentration may be low, but potassium, BUN, creatinine, and bicarbonate concentrations are usually normal. Hypoglycemia may be present. Cardiac size on x-ray is normal, as is the ECG. MRI studies of the head may reveal a hypothalamic or pituitary tumor, or other lesions, such as a granuloma, vascular malformations, etc.

Diagnosis

Although the clinical suspicion of adrenal insufficiency must be confirmed by definitive laboratory testing, therapy should not be delayed by prolonged diagnostic measures, and the patient should not be subjected to ancillary diagnostic tests that may lead to further volume loss, dehydration, and hypotension. In the acute situation, if rapid diagnostic tests are not available, therapy should be instituted and the diagnosis should be established later.

Measurement of basal levels of urine or plasma cortisol is not recommended, as partial degrees of adrenal insufficiency occur. Thus, a normal plasma cortisol level (5 to 20 μg/dl) does not exclude the diagnosis of adrenocortical insufficiency because it is not uncommon to find random cortisol determinations in the normal range with partial adrenal insufficiency. However, the finding of a basal plasma cortisol level of 20 μg/dl or greater virtually excludes the diagnosis. Conversely, if plasma cortisol is low or undetectable in a critically ill patient, adrenal insufficiency should be strongly considered. Tests that specifically measure adrenocortical reserve are needed to confirm the diagnosis (Fig. 11-40). These tests, discussed later in the context of their diagnostic utility, have been described in laboratory evaluation of adrenocortical function previously.

FIGURE 11-40. Evaluation of suspected primary or secondary adrenocortical insufficiency. Boxes enclose clinical decisions; circles enclose diagnostic tests.

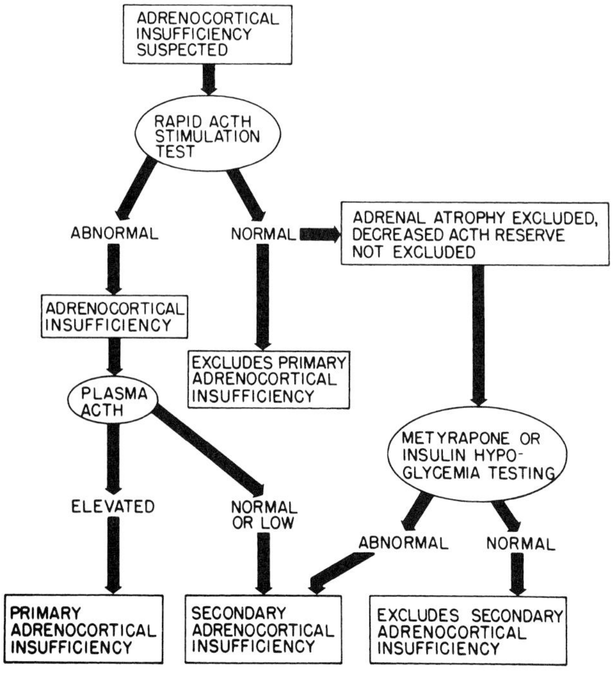

The rapid ACTH stimulation test is the procedure of choice in the assessment of patients with possible adrenal insufficiency. This test is used as the initial diagnostic step in all suspected cases, either primary or secondary.[920–922,924–926,1259] Because the procedure requires only 30 min, it usually can be performed even in acute situations. In suspected primary adrenal insufficiency, a normal response (peak plasma cortisol >20 μg/dl at 30 min after ACTH administration) excludes the diagnosis, and these patients do not require further evaluation.[924,1259] However, normal responses do not always exclude secondary adrenal insufficiency, as some patients have a decreased pituitary reserve or decreased responsiveness of the hypothalamic-pituitary-adrenal axis to stress but maintain the ability to respond to exogenous ACTH stimulation (discussed later and in the laboratory evaluation of adrenocortical function section).[920,930–932,934,1260]

Subnormal responses to the rapid ACTH stimulation test establish the diagnosis of adrenocortical insufficiency and correlate well with subnormal responsiveness of the pituitary-adrenal axis to metyrapone, insulin-induced hypoglycemia, and stress.[920,930–932,934,1260] Three-day ACTH stimulation tests were traditionally used in the diagnosis of adrenocortical insufficiency, but are usually unnecessary and give little additional diagnostic information in the presence of a subnormal response to the rapid ACTH stimulation test.

If the rapid ACTH stimulation test indicates adrenal insufficiency, primary and secondary forms are readily differentiated by measurement of the plasma ACTH level. Plasma ACTH levels in patients with untreated primary adrenal insufficiency exceed 200 pg/ml and are usually between 400 and 2,000 pg/ml (Fig. 11-41).[1261] In secondary adrenal insufficiency due to pituitary ACTH deficiency, plasma ACTH levels are inappropriately low compared to circulating cortisol levels and are less than 10 to 20 pg/ml.[868,893,1261]

If plasma ACTH assays are unavailable, the plasma aldosterone response to the rapid ACTH stimulation test or the 3-day ACTH stimulation test can be used to differentiate primary from secondary adrenal insufficiency. However, experience with the aldosterone response is less extensive than experience with measurement of plasma ACTH levels (see previous section on laboratory evaluation of adrenocortical function).

Although a subnormal response to the rapid ACTH stimulation test establishes the diagnosis of adrenal insufficiency, a normal adrenal response to ACTH stimulation does not exclude partial ACTH deficiency. This problem usually arises in patients who have been treated with glucocorticoids (Chap. 14) and patients with partial pituitary or hypothalamic dysfunction. When secondary adrenal insufficiency is still suspected in a patient with a normal response to the rapid ACTH stimulation test, more specific information regarding pituitary responsiveness can be obtained by testing with metyrapone or insulin-induced hypoglycemia. The overnight metyrapone test is preferred because of its simplicity and low risk. A normal response to either metyrapone or hypoglycemia excludes secondary adrenocortical insufficiency (see laboratory evaluation of adrenocortical function). Subnormal responses to these tests establish the diagnosis of secondary adrenal insufficiency, because in these patients the primary form has been excluded by a normal rapid ACTH stimulation test and normal or subnormal plasma ACTH levels.

In patients with primary adrenocortical insufficiency, further evaluation may be required to establish the specific etiology. If the patient has manifestations of or a family history of the PGA I or PGA II syndrome, autoimmune Addison's disease is present with rare exceptions. The presence of adrenal antibodies confirms the diagnosis, but these assays are not generally available. If autoimmune adrenal insufficiency is established, patients and their families should be screened for the associated disorders detailed previously. If other endocrine autoimmune disorders are not present and if adrenal antibodies are negative or not available, an adrenal CT scan should be performed. Absent or atrophic adrenals are most consistent with autoimmune adrenal failure, but adrenal atrophy may also occur months or years after adrenal hemorrhage or infections. Bilateral adrenal enlargement in primary adrenal failure can be due to hemorrhage or any of the infectious or invasive etiologies described earlier.[1202,1205,1206,1223,1226,1234] Hemorrhage can usually be demonstrated by current CT or MRI techniques.[1234] If hemorrhage is not present, further evaluation should be directed to determining the specific cause and a CT-guided adrenal biopsy with appropriate cytology and cultures is indicated to establish the diagnosis and direct specific therapy. Further evaluation should then be directed to determining the extent of dissemination of the primary diseas%, e.g., extrapulmonary tuberculosis, disseminated fungal infection, AIDS, or metastatic malignancy (see the section on primary adrenocortical insufficiency due to invasive or hemorrhagic disorders and Refs. 1202, 1205, 1223, and 1226).

In secondary adrenocortical insufficiency, the patient should be evaluated for other pituitary deficiencies and for the presence of a hypothalamic or pituitary space-occupying lesion (see Chap. 6). The evaluation of patients with adrenal insufficiency resulting from steroid therapy is discussed in Chap. 14.

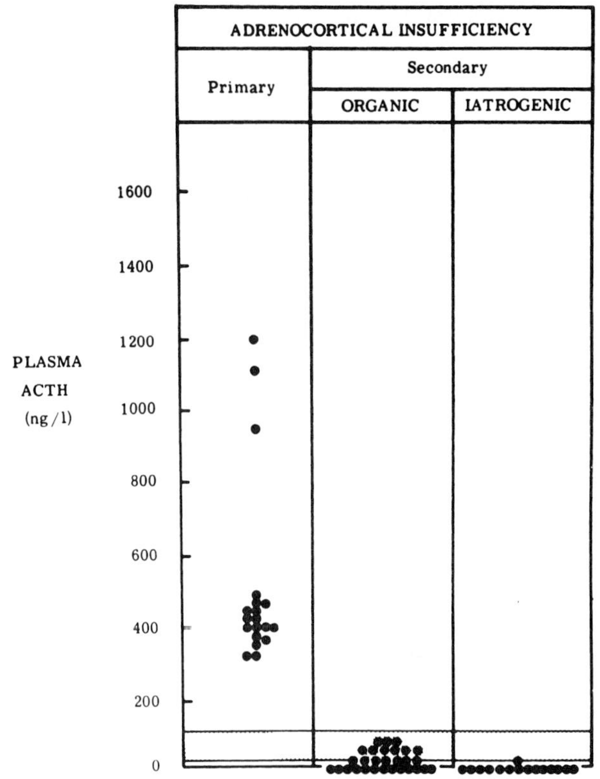

FIGURE 11-41. Basal plasma ACTH level in primary and secondary adrenocortical insufficiency. (*From Irvine et al.*[817] *based on data from Besser et al.*[1261])

In an acutely ill patient with adrenal insufficiency, it is also imperative to determine the etiology of the condition that precipitates the crisis. For example, whereas fever can be due to glucocorticoid insufficiency, it may also be a manifestation of an underlying infection or another systemic disorder.

A patient who has been treated with glucocorticoids before the establishment of a diagnosis presents a special problem, as the therapy may itself suppress the hypothalamic-pituitary-adrenal axis. This is especially true when high-dose glucocorticoids are given to an acutely ill patient. However, when the steroid is tapered and the patient is placed on maintenance cortisol, normal hypothalamic-pituitary-adrenal responsiveness should return within several weeks and the rapid ACTH stimulation test can be used (see Chap. 14). In the exceptional circumstance in which longer high-dose therapy has been given, the 3-day ACTH stimulation test can be used; the overall management and diagnostic approaches in this case are discussed in Chap. 14.

Treatment

Acute Addisonian Crisis

Therapy for acute addisonian crisis should be instituted immediately if a strong clinical suspicion is present and induces both fluid and electrolyte replacement and high dose steroids (Table 11-21). The rationale for high-dose glucocorticoids is based on the fact that the adrenal gland responds to serious illness with increased cortisol production. Therapy should include the administration of large doses of a soluble glucocorticoid preparation, the correction of hypovolemia and electrolyte abnormalities, general supportive measures, and treatment of coexisting or precipitating disorders. Because both mineralocorticoid deficiency and glucocorticoid deficiency are present in primary adrenocortical insufficiency, a preparation with sodium-retaining potency is recommended. The drug of choice is a soluble form of injectable cortisol (hydrocortisone hemisuccinate or hydrocortisone phosphate), which should be administered IV in doses of 100 mg q 6 h for the first 24 h. If the patient's progress is satisfactory and no additional complications are present, dose may be reduced to 50 mg q 6 h on the second day and then tapered gradually to oral maintenance doses by the fourth to fifth day. When severe concurrent illnesses are present, a dose of 50 to 100 mg q 6 h should be continued until the patient stabilizes. Intramuscular cortisone acetate should not be used in the treatment of acute adrenal insufficiency because there is poor absorption, failure to achieve adequate blood levels of cortisol, and inadequate biological activity, as evidenced by failure to suppress ACTH levels.[1262] Mineralocorticoid therapy is usually required when the cortisol dose is decreased below 50 to 60 mg per day (see later discussion).

TABLE 11-21. Treatment of Acute Adrenocortical Insufficiency (Adrenal Crisis)

1. Cortisol* 100 mg IV, q 6 h for 24 h. Reduce to 50 mg q 6 h if progress is satisfactory and then taper to oral maintenance dose by day 4 or 5. Maintain or increase dose to 200–400 mg/24 h if complications persist
2. IV saline and glucose
3. Correction of precipitating factors
4. General supportive measures

* As hydrocortisone phosphate or hemisuccinate.

TABLE 11-22. Treatment of Chronic Primary Adrenocortical Insufficiency

1. Cortisol, 15–20 mg in A.M. and 10 mg at 4–5 P.M.
2. 9α-fluorocortisol 0.05–0.2 mg orally in A.M.
3. Clinical follow-up: maintenance of normal weight, blood pressure, and electrolytes with regression of clinical features
4. Patient education plus identification card or bracelet
5. Increased cortisol dosage during "stress"

Because patients in adrenal crisis may have profound dehydration, volume depletion, hypotension, and hypoglycemia, adequate replacement with IV glucose and saline must be given. Severe hyperkalemia and/or acidosis may occasionally require specific therapy.

A patient with a crisis due to secondary adrenocortical insufficiency usually does not have the severe electrolyte abnormalities and volume depletion seen in patients with primary adrenocortical insufficiency. Thus, the major requirement is for glucocorticoid replacement; the regimen outlined earlier is standard, has been proved effective, and will provide adequate mineralocorticoid replacement in the few patients with impaired aldosterone production. The use of other glucocorticoids, such as prednisolone and dexamethasone, is probably equally effective.

Chronic Adrenal Insufficiency

The treatment of chronic primary Addison's disease requires maintenance therapy with both glucocorticoids and mineralocorticoids (Table 11-22). The patient must be taught that a lifetime of therapy is required and that cessation of therapy may endanger life. In the majority of patients, 20 to 30 mg of cortisol per day is sufficient, with two-thirds given in the morning and one-third in the late afternoon. The higher morning dose is given to approximate roughly the normal circadian rhythm of cortisol secretion. Cortisol is ordinarily used; it may have a theoretical advantage over some of the cortisol analogues (prednisone, prednisolone, dexamethasone, etc.), as it has greater mineralocorticoid potency and may therefore serve as partial replacement for the deficient mineralocorticoid function as well, and as it has a shorter duration of biological effect than the other synthetic steroids and hence a dminished chance of causing osteoporosis and other chronic manifestations of glucocorticoid excess. However, a very conservative equivalent dose of a steroid such as prednisone, prednisolone, or dexamethasone might be acceptable.[1263] Oral cortisone acetate is equally acceptable, as oral absorption is rapid and it is quickly converted to cortisol in the liver and other tissues.[1262]

Mineralocorticoid replacement is given using 9α-fluorocortisol 0.05 to 0.2 mg daily. A majority of these patients require mineralocorticoid therapy, although a minority do not and can be maintained on cortisol alone.[1264] The major problem with omission of the mineralocorticoid is a tendency to develop hyperkalemia. The natural steroids aldosterone and DOC are not available and are not useful because they are degraded rapidly after ingestion so that adequate plasma concentrations are not achieved.

These doses are satisfactory in the majority of patients; they are accompanied by regression of the classic clinical features, including a return of a general feeling of well-being, weight gain, maintenance of normal blood pressure, improvement in pigmentation, and a return to normal physical activity. Occasional patients who perform heavy manual labor may require up to 40 mg. Many of the subjective complaints of Addison's disease can be reversed within a few days; a somewhat longer period is required before strength returns to normal, and weeks may be required before the abnormal pigmentation subsides.

In an evaluation of the adequacy of glucocorticoid replacement, strong reliance is placed on the patient's subjective assessment. Excessive dosage is usually manifested by excessive weight gain; this is an indication to lower the dose. Because glucocorticoids given in excess can produce euphoria, occasional patients may increase the dose on their own. Such excessive glucocorticoid replacement should be avoided. Inadequate dosage results in continuing manifestations of Addison's disease, especially weakness, fatigue, and excessive pigmentation. Caution should be exercised in the administration of other drugs as those that induce hepatic microsomal enzymes, such as rifampin, may result in accelerated glucocorticoid metabolism with the induction of an adrenal crisis.[1265] This may also occur with phenytoin and phenobarbital. The timing of the doses can be varied to fit individual needs and activities; i.e., although most patients do well with twice-daily doses, some feel better with three doses. The last dose is usually given at 4 to 5 P.M. as the cortisol may cause insomnia in some patients when given later in the evening. Plasma or urinary cortisol determinations are not usually necessary or helpful, and there is no reliable biochemical method for assessing the adequacy of glucocorticoid therapy. Thus, plasma ACTH levels have not proved useful because of episodic variation in secretion and because therapy with the short-acting glucocorticoids usually does not suppress ACTH levels to normal.[1266–1268]

Adequate mineralocorticoid therapy is indicated by the maintenance of normal blood pressure and sodium, potassium, and plasma renin activity levels.[1264,1269] Excessive therapy causes hypertension and hypokalemia,[1264] and inadequate therapy may result in persisting fatigue, malaise, orthostatic hypotension, hyponatremia, hyperkalemia, and hyperreninemia.[1269] The dose may be altered using these parameters; the usual dose of 9α-fluorocortisol is 0.05 to 0.2 mg daily. Some patients may require variable doses at different times of the year, e.g., 0.1 to 0.2 mg and increased salt intake during the summer and 0.05 mg in the winter. Measurement of the plasma renin concentration is useful because an increased level suggests inadequate replacement and a suppressed level may indicate excessive mineralocorticoid therapy.[1264,1269,1270]

Every effort should be made to avoid adrenal crises. This can be achieved by patient education and an appropriate increase in steroid dosage during stress. It is therefore necessary to inform the patient fully of the nature of his or her disorder and the necessity of obtaining prompt medical assistance in the event of illness or injury. Patients should carry an identification card or bracelet to notify the treating physician of the diagnosis of Addison's disease and should be instructed to increase the dose of cortisol in the event of illness. Because it is difficult for the patient to assess the severity of illness, it is best to err on the side of overreplacement rather than underreplacement during acute minor illnesses. Thus, patients are instructed to double or triple the cortisol dose at the onset of minor illnesses such as upper respiratory and viral infections. If the illness is minor, the dose can be reduced to the usual maintenance level in 24 to 48 h; no adverse effects accompany this short-term increase. If more severe or persisting symptoms develop, the patient is instructed to continue the increased cortisol dose and contact a physician. Increased dosage of 9α-fluorocortisol is not required during minor illnesses, provided that adequate cortisol is given. Patients with vomiting, and thus an inability to take oral cortisol, must seek immediate medical attention and receive parenteral cortisol, as must those with diarrhea, who may rapidly develop dehydration, volume depletion, and hypotension. Patients who do not have rapid access to medical attention should be provided with injectable cortisol and instructed in its use (available in preloaded syringes of hydrocortisone phosphate, 100 mg).

In patients with secondary adrenal insufficiency, mineralocorticoid therapy is usually not required and the cortisol doses listed above may be given without 9α-fluorocortisol.

Patients with adrenal insufficiency due to previous high-dose glucocorticoid therapy are ordinarily maintained quite adequately on the same steroid they received for therapy (usually prednisone). The management of these patients is discussed in Chap. 14.

Steroid Coverage for Illness, Surgery, or Trauma

Patients with primary or secondary adrenocortical insufficiency who suffer trauma or an acute illness should be treated according to the protocol described above for acute addisonian crisis. In patients undergoing elective surgery (Table 11-23), electrolyte status, blood pressure, and hydration should be assessed and, if necessary, corrected before the induction of anesthesia. A regimen that has been proved effective for increased steroid coverage includes the administration of 100 mg cortisol IM on call to the operating room, 50 mg IM or IV in the recovery room, and then 50 mg q 6 h for three doses. On the second postoperative day, if the patient is progressing satisfactorily, the dose may be reduced to 25 mg q 6 h. The dose may then be tapered to normal maintenance levels over a period of 3 to 5 days. If fever, hypotension, or other complications occur or persist, the dosage should be maintained at or increased to a total of 200 to 400 mg/24 h.

This protocol, a modification of that described by others,[1271] has been used successfully for the past 20 years in patients with primary, secondary, or glucocorticoid-induced adrenal insufficiency. It is also used routinely in patients undergoing adrenalectomy or pituitary surgery. No instance of acute adrenal insufficiency has been noted, nor have complications of the glucocorticoid therapy occurred. Intramuscular cortisone acetate should not be used (see earlier discussion) because adequate plasma cortisol concentrations are not achieved even if the cortisone acetate is administered 12 to 24 h before surgery.[1262,1271] Intraoperative or postoperative shock has been reported in such patients receiving injectable cortisone acetate in preparation for surgery.[1272] Recent studies in animals suggest that such supraphysiologic doses are not required during surgical stress; however, no studies in humans are available, and thus we continue to recommend the above protocol.[1273]

TABLE 11-23. Steroid Coverage for Surgery

1. Correct electrolyte levels, blood pressure, and hydration if necessary.
2. Give cortisol,* 100 mg IM, on call to operating room.
3. Give cortisol, 50 mg IM or IV, in recovery room and q 6 h for first 24 h.
4. If progress is satisfactory, reduce dose to 25 mg q 6 h for 24 h; then taper to maintenance dose over 3–5 days. Resume previous 9α-fluorocortisol dose when patient is taking oral medications.
5. Maintain or increase cortisol dose to 200–400 mg/24 h if fever, hypotension, or other complications occur.

* As hydrocortisone phosphate or hemisuccinate.

Prognosis and Survival

Before the availability of glucocorticoid therapy, primary adrenocortical insufficiency was a rapidly and uniformly fatal illness, and most patients died within 2 years of the diagnosis (Fig. 11-26).[792] Life expectancy increased somewhat when mineralocorticoid therapy in the form of deoxycorticosterone acetate became available in the late 1930s. However, despite correction of mineralocorticoid deficiency, hypotension, and electrolyte abnormalities, life expectancy was still usually less than 5 years and these patients were still susceptible to stress.[792] The introduction of glucocorticoid therapy in the late 1940s resulted in an immediate and marked increase in survival (Fig. 11-26).[792,1189] Survival in patients with either primary or secondary adrenocortical insufficiency now approximates that of the normal population when appropriate therapy, including patient education and increased coverage for stress, is carried out.[792,1189] Deaths from adrenal insufficiency are rare in diagnosed and appropriately treated patients, and the majority of deaths occur in patients with a more rapid "acute" course, such as those with a massive bilateral adrenal hemorrhage. These patients are frequently not receiving medical care; many die without diagnosis, and the adrenocortical insufficiency is discovered only at autopsy.[1189]

Hypoaldosteronism

Hypoaldosteronism may occur selectively or in association with an impairment in the production of cortisol. Hypoaldosteronism in association with hypocortisolism due to Addison's disease, hypopituitarism, and congenital adrenal biosynthetic defects are discussed in other sections. Selective hypoaldosteronism is commonly associated with a deficiency of renin secretion by the kidney (hyporeninemic hypoaldosteronism). It can also be due to defective adrenal release of aldosterone in association with normal or elevated plasma renin levels.[1274,1275] These primary adrenal causes of selective hypoaldosteronism occur with isolated adrenal biosynthetic defects [corticosterone methyloxidase deficiency that is due to mutations in the gene for P450c11AS (see disorders of steroid hormone synthesis, earlier)], with focal dysfunction of the adrenal glomerulosa with absent responsiveness to angiotensin II (hyperreninemic hypoaldosteronism), after resection of an aldosterone-producing adenoma (see Chap. 13), in pseudohypoaldosteronism (unresponsiveness to aldosterone), after heparin administration (discussed previously in inhibitors of adrenal steroid biosynthesis[516,517,534]), and with potassium deficiency.[1274]

Hyporeninemic Hypoaldosteronism

Hyporeninemic hypoaldosteronism occurs generally in older patients with renal disease who have hyperkalemia and hyperchloremic metabolic acidosis that is disproportionately more severe than expected from the extent of renal impairment.[1274–1278] In a series of 22 patients, the mean creatinine clearance was 33 (range, 11 to 56) ml/min per 1.73 m^2 [1278]; six patients had diabetes mellitus, one had multiple myeloma, and most of the remainder appeared to have interstitial nephritis. The hypoaldosteronism is due to decreased renin release by the kidney.[1274–1278] Plasma renin levels are low and do not increase normally in response to postural changes and sodium restriction. Plasma aldosterone levels are also low and do not increase normally with postural changes and sodium restriction. However, they do increase appropriately relative to the small change in plasma renin levels, suggesting that the adrenal glomerulosa is normal.[1274,1277] In addition, angiotensin II infusion or ACTH administration results in prompt increases in aldosterone release.[1274–1278] In fact, the plasma aldosterone concentration is disproportionately high relative to the plasma renin concentration, possibly because of the associated hyperkalemia.[1274–1278] However, occasional patients with hyporeninemic hypoaldosteronism also have a defect in the late steps in adrenal aldosterone biosynthesis, and plasma aldosterone levels do not respond normally to increased renin concentration (e.g., with diuretic treatment) or ACTH.[1274,1277] This may be due to the hyperreninemic syndrome discussed later.

The pathogenesis of the hyporeninemia is not clear.[1274–1280] It is likely that the renal disease in some way impairs the ability of the kidney to release renin. This could be due to direct damage to the juxtaglomerular or macula densa cells or to an effector mechanism such as the efferent limb of the autonomic nervous supply, the functions that control exposure or responsiveness to ions, and the renal baroreceptor system (Chap. 13). It has also been speculated that there is a defect in the conversion of prorenin to renin or an inhibitor of renin. Others have proposed that increased extracellular fluid volume causes physiologic suppression; indeed, an increase in extracellular fluid volume has been found in some patients, hypertension is present in about a third of cases, and renin and aldosterone concentrations have been shown to increase progressively as the extracellular fluid volume decreases with diuretic therapy, although it is not clear that the renin level increases normally. Another postulated mediator of the hyporeninemia is ANP, which reduces renin levels and inhibits responsiveness to potassium (see previous discussion).[473,1281–1283] In addition, a deficiency of renal PG or prostacyclin production has been implicated in the renin deficiency.[1281,1284]

The major consequence of the hypoaldosteronism in these patients is hyperkalemia; the serum potassium concentration is usually between 5.5 and 6.5 mEq/liter.[1274,1277,1279] The extent of hyperkalemia is related to dietary potassium intake and, in diabetic patients, to diabetic control.[1274] Occasional patients have had third-degree heart block.[1274,1277,1278] In fact, this condition appears to be the most common cause of chronic hyperkalemia in patients without severe renal disease (e.g., creatinine clearance less than 15 mg/min per 1.73 m^2).[1274] Most patients do not lose sodium or develop dehydration; increased extracellular fluid volume and hypertension are more common.[1274] This lack of salt wasting may be due to the associated renal disease, to other primary factors, and to the fact that cortisol secretion is normal. However, hyponatremia is occasionally present.[1279]

These patients also develop hypochloremic acidosis,[1274] which is accentuated by the renal insufficiency; the extent of acidosis is related to the degree of glomerular insufficiency. The acidosis is renal in origin and can be differentiated from renal tubular acidosis type 1 by the fact that the urine is acidic and relatively bicarbonate-free during periods of acidosis; it can be distinguished from type 2 renal tubular acidosis by the fact that the extent of decreased reabsorption of bicarbonate at normal bicarbonate concentrations is not great enough to indicate defective proximal tubular dysfunction and by a lack of aminoaciduria, glucosuria, or increased renal phosphate clearance. Urinary excretion of ammonia is markedly reduced, even with an acidic urine. Thus, these changes, combined with evidence for low potassium clearance, have led to the classification of the dysfunction as type 4 renal tubular acidosis. The acidosis itself appears to be due to both the hyperkalemia that reduces renal ammonia production and the reduced hydrogen secretory capacity.

The initial differential diagnosis includes all the causes of hyperkalemia,[1274–1280] including the hypoaldosterone states mentioned earlier that have normal or elevated plasma renin levels. Pseudohypokalemia due to abnormal potassium release from clotting when elevated platelet or white blood cell counts are present can be excluded by obtaining heparinized blood with minimal turbulence and measuring the plasma K^+ concentration, which is normal in this condition. The use of drugs that elevate the serum potassium ion concentration (spironolactone, triamterene, amiloride) can be excluded by history and also by the fact that the plasma aldosterone concentration is not abnormally high in these circumstances. Also, hyporeninemic hypoaldosteronism has been reported in association with chronic and massive intake of sodium bicarbonate.[1282] Addison's disease and adrenal biosynthetic deficiency states are usually associated with a high plasma renin concentration and may have the other manifestations described above. However, as mentioned previously, occasional patients with hyperkalemia and chronic renal disease have hypoaldosteronism with normal plasma renin levels. Oliguric renal failure and other causes of severe acidosis (e.g., diabetic ketoacidosis) can be excluded by the clinical setting. There are rare syndromes with hyperkalemia and lack of responsiveness to aldosterone (pseudohypoaldosteronism; see later discussion); however, these patients have several distinguishing clinical characteristics, including high aldosterone and renin levels.

Patients with hyporeninemic hypoaldosteronism generally respond to 9α-fluorocortisol with amelioration of the hyperkalemia and acidosis.[1277–1279] Doses of around 0.2 mg per day are ordinarily required[1277–1279]; however, in some patients the kidneys appeared to be hyporesponsive to mineralocorticoids, and in these patients higher doses may be required.[1275] Mineralocorticoid replacement is not the therapy of choice in patients with hypertension and increased fluid volume. In many cases, furosemide therapy can ameliorate both the hyperkalemia and the acidosis.[1285] Further, in patients with severe hypoaldosteronism, the combination of furosemide and small doses of mineralocorticoids can be synergistic.[1279,1285] Thus, diuretics and mineralocorticoids should be used alone or in combination, and the relative doses should be individualized, depending on the clinical setting and the response. Alternative measures depending on the individual patient can include restriction of dietary potassium; oral administration of sodium polystyrene sulfonate, a resin that binds potassium ion and releases sodium ion in the gastrointestinal tract; and the oral administration of sodium bicarbonate.[1275]

Normoreninemic or Hyperreninemic Hypoaldosteronism

Normo- and hyperreninemic hypoaldosteronism appear to result from acquired dysfunction of the adrenal glomerulosa.[1275,1286–1289] This occurs most commonly in critically ill patients with hypotension[1288,1289]; it has been reported in more than 50 percent of such patients. These patients have hypoaldosteronism despite markedly increased plasma renin level; aldosterone secretion is subnormally responsive to stimulation with ACTH or angiotensin II.[1288,1289] The mechanism of impaired aldosterone production and the role of ischemia with potential anoxia and adrenal damage are not known, but the frequency of this condition should alert the physician to consider it in such patients. There has been one report of a patient with hyperkalemia and moderate renal insufficiency who had hyperreninemia and subnormal plasma aldosterone responses to ACTH, upright posture, and sodium depletion.[1286] This patient was shown to have antibodies against the zona glomerulosa, suggesting possible selective autoimmune destruction of the adrenal glomerulosa.[1287]

Pseudohypoaldosteronism (Unresponsiveness to Aldosterone)

There are rare cases in which patients do not exhibit a response to aldosterone.[1274,1275] This has been reported in infants without renal parenchymal disease and in children and adults with azotemia due to renal interstitial disease (salt-wasting nephropathy). These patients have hyperkalemia, metabolic acidosis, and renal sodium wasting with extracellular fluid depletion and hypotension despite elevated plasma aldosterone and renin levels. These abnormalities do not respond to large doses of mineralocorticoids. These patients apparently have a renal defect that leaves them unable to respond to mineralocorticoids, and treatment with sodium chloride and/or bicarbonate is ordinarily required to maintain them. This defect is usually found in one or more of the subunits of the amiloride-sensitive sodium channel and/or the mineralocorticoid receptor.[1275]

An additional rare syndrome has been termed *type 2 pseudohypoaldosteronism.*[1275,1290] It has been described in children and young adults and is characterized by hyperkalemia and hyperchloremia, metabolic acidosis with hypertension, hyporeninemia, and hypoaldosteronism. These patients differ from hyporeninemic hypoaldosteronism patients in that they have a normal GFR. As is the case with pseudohypoaldosteronism, their renal potassium excretion fails to increase normally when large amounts of mineralocorticoids are administered, but unlike the case with pseudohypoaldosteronism, pseudohypoaldosteronism type 2 patients have a normal antinatriuretic and antichloriduric response to mineralocorticoids.[1275] It has been suggested that the primary abnormality in this syndrome is a defect in the distal nephron for chloride reabsorption that increases distal NaCl reabsorption, resulting in hyperchloremia, volume expansion, and hypertension that also limits the sodium- and mineralocorticoid-dependent voltage driving force for potassium and hydrogen secretion, resulting in hyperkalemia and hypertension[1275]; the syndrome might also be explained by an isolated collecting tubule defect in potassium secretion.[1275] Restriction of dietary NaCl or administration of a chloruretic diuretic ameliorates the hyperkalemia and acidosis in these patients.[1275]

There can also be other circumstances in which selective unresponsiveness to certain actions of mineralocorticoids occurs. Thus, after several days of mineralocorticoid excess, further sodium retention does not occur (the escape phenomenon) even though responses of potassium and hydrogen loss persist (see previous discussion). The lack of response of the kaliuretic actions of the mineralocorticoids occurs in the rare hypertensive syndrome with possibly increased chloride reabsorption (see earlier discussion), and in pregnancy there is a relative resistance to the kaliuretic responses of the mineralocorticoids (discussed later).

ADRENOCORTICAL HYPERFUNCTION

Hyperfunction of the adrenal cortex can result from excessive activity of the zonae fasciculata and reticularis or the zona glomerulosa and from steroid-producing adenomas or carcinomas. Excessive stimulation of the zonae fasciculata and reticularis by ACTH is due to pituitary hypersecretion of ACTH (usually by a small pituitary adenoma), abnormal ACTH release by extrapituitary tumors (ectopic ACTH syndrome), or ACTH therapy. This results in increased secretion of cortisol, adrenal androgens, and DOC. Excessive activity of the zona glomerulosa can be due to primary aldosteronism, with adenomas or hyperplasia resulting from unknown causes, or it can be due to activation of the renin-angiotensin system by a variety of causes. Adrenal adenomas usually produce either cortisol or aldosterone and rarely androgens, whereas carcinomas frequently secrete multiple steroids.

Cushing's Syndrome

Cushing's syndrome refers to the manifestations of glucocorticoid excess without regard to specific etiology; there may also be androgen excess. It is most commonly iatrogenic, caused by glucocorticoid therapy. Cushing's *disease* refers to the disorder resulting from pituitary ACTH hypersecretion. Spontaneous Cushing's syndrome is an uncommon disorder; however, it must be considered in the differential diagnosis of such diverse entities as obesity, hypertension, diabetes, weakness, osteoporosis, hirsutism, and menstrual disorders.

Classification, Occurrence, and Age and Sex Distributions

Spontaneous Cushing's syndrome is either ACTH-dependent or ACTH-independent (Table 11-24). The ACTH-dependent types are Cushing's disease, the ectopic ACTH syndrome, and, very rarely, ectopic CRH production.[1291–1293] In these disorders, chronic ACTH hypersecretion stimulates the zonae fasciculata and reticularis, resulting in bilateral adrenocortical hyperplasia with increased secretion of cortisol, androgens, and DOC. ACTH-independent Cushing's syndrome is due to primary adrenocortical neoplasms, either adenomas or carcinomas; the resulting hypercortisolism suppresses the hypothalamic-pituitary axis. Other rare forms of Cushing's syndrome are discussed later.

Cushing's disease accounts for approximately 70 percent of adult patients in current series,[1294,1295] and the majority of these patients have pituitary microadenomas. There is a distinct female preponderance in Cushing's disease. In older series, the female/male ratio was 3:1,[1296] but it is 8:1 in current experience.[1297,1298] The age range in Cushing's disease is most frequently 20 to 40 years.[1296] Cushing's disease is being diagnosed with increasing frequency in children and adolescents, who account for 10–15 percent of cases in large centers.[1297,1309] Many young adults with Cushing's disease had the onset of disease during adolescence.

Ectopic ACTH hypersecretion is responsible for approximately 15 percent of reported cases of Cushing's syndrome. This is an underestimate of the true incidence, as many patients lack the classic features of hypercortisolism. They are thus not brought to the attention of an endocrinologist; severe hypercortisolism and rapid death are common.[1299] The tumors causing the ectopic ACTH syndrome are discussed later; oat-cell carcinoma of the lung is the most common, and ectopic ACTH secretion occurs in 0.5 to 2 percent of these patients.[1300] In addition, immunoreactive and bioactive ACTH has been demonstrated in the majority of these tumors, even when clinical evidence of ectopic ACTH hypersecretion is not present.[1301–1303] The ectopic ACTH syndrome is more common in males (female/male ratio = 1 : 3), and the peak incidence of 40 to 60 years reflects the greater incidence of malignancy in this age group.[1295,1304]

Table 11-24. Classification and Etiology of Cushing's Syndrome

	Percent
ACTH-dependent	
Cushing's disease	68
Ectopic ACTH syndrome	15
ACTH-independent	
Adrenal adenoma	9
Adrenal carcinoma	8
Micronodular adrenal disease (rare)	—
	100

Source: Huff.[1294]

ACTH-independent primary adrenal tumors cause 17 to 19 percent of cases of Cushing's syndrome, with equal frequencies of adenoma and carcinoma in adults.[1294,1295] Adrenal adenomas causing Cushing's syndrome occur more frequently in females.[1295] Adrenocortical carcinoma causing Cushing's syndrome also shows a female preponderance (approximately 66 percent of cases)[1305]; however, the prevalence of all types of adrenal carcinoma is higher in males.[1305] The overall prevalence of adrenal carcinoma is approximately 2 per 1 million population. Approximately 75 percent of cases occur after age 12, with the peak incidence in the fourth to sixth decade; the mean age at diagnosis is 38 years.[1203,1295,1305]

Cushing's syndrome in childhood is unusual. Cushing's disease is responsible for only 35 percent of cases; the majority of these patients are 10 years old or older at the time of diagnosis,[1295,1306–1309] and the incidence by sex is approximately equal.[1306–1309] Adrenal tumors account for the majority (65 percent) of cases in childhood, with carcinoma responsible for 51 percent and adenoma for 14 percent.[1295] The majority of these tumors occur in girls, and most occur between the ages of 1 and 8 years.[1295]

Pathology

Anterior Pituitary

Pituitary adenomas are found either at surgery or at autopsy in more than 90 percent of patients with Cushing's disease[1297,1310–1313] and confirm Cushing's original description of pituitary adenomas in six of his eight autopsied cases (Fig. 11-42). Approximately 80 to 90 percent of these are microadenomas (diameter less than 10 mm); 50 percent are 5 mm or less in diameter, and microadenomas less than 2 mm in diameter have been reported.[1297,1310–1313] Thus, these small adenomas do not result in sellar enlargement, although focal radiologic abnormalities may occur.[1312] The remainder of the pituitary adenomas in Cushing's disease are larger than 10 mm; these adenomas cause sellar enlargement, frequently with extrasellar extension, and invasive tendencies are common.[1314] Malignant tumors have occasionally been reported.[1314]

The adenomas of Cushing's disease are characteristically basophilic, unencapsulated, and located within the anterior pituitary.[1311,1312,1315–1317] Chromophobe adenomas may also occur.[1312] The tumors are composed of compact sheets of uniform, well-granulated cells with a sinusoidal arrangement and a high content of ACTH, β-LPH, and β-endorphin.[1318,1319] The cytoplasm usually contains abundant basophilic granules that, on immunocytochemical staining, are positive for ACTH and β-LPH. These cells frequently show a zone of perinuclear hyalinization known

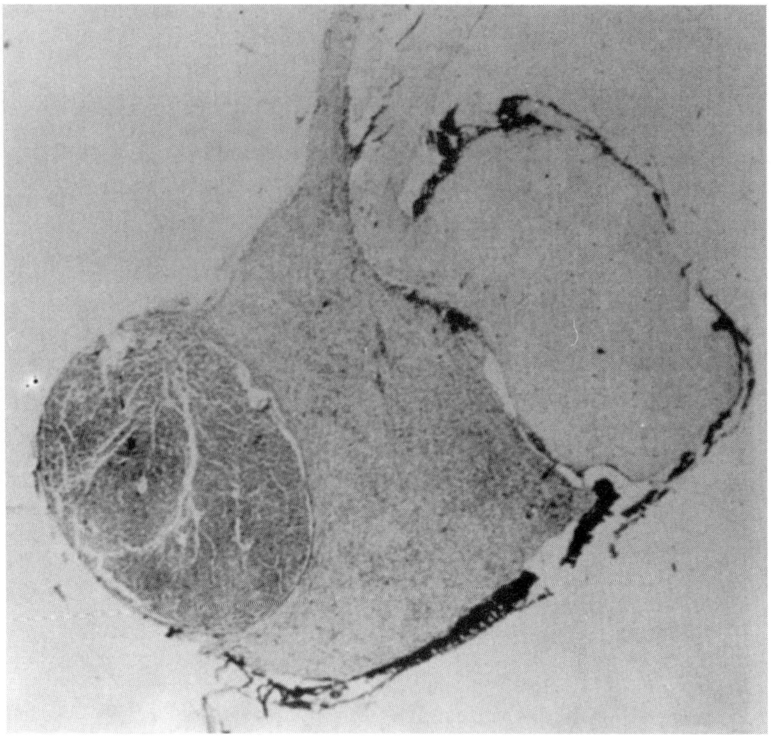

FIGURE 11-42. A basophilic anterior pituitary microadenoma from Cushing's original series. (*From Cushing.*[5])

as Crooke's changes that results from exposure of the corticotrophs to hypercortisolism.[1311] Electron microscopy demonstrates considerable heterogeneity of granule size (200 to 700 mm) and variability in the number of granules, which may be scattered throughout the cytoplasm or marginated along the cell membrane.[1311] The hyaline changes seen on light microscopy appear as bundles of perinuclear microfilaments (average 7.0 nm in diameter) that encircle the nucleus.[1311]

The portion of the anterior pituitary not involved by the adenoma has been less well studied. In most cases there is atrophy of the surrounding corticotrophs; however, paraadenomatous hyperplasia has been reported in some cases.[1320–1322] In addition, ACTH content in the paraadenomatous tissue is decreased, in contrast to the increased content in the adenoma cells themselves.[1318,1319]

Patients in the subgroup with Cushing's disease and no demonstrable pituitary adenoma may have diffuse corticotroph hyperplasia,[1317,1323,1324] although a few patients have no demonstrable pituitary abnormality.[1325,1326] Several patients with corticotroph hyperplasia have been found to have intrasellar gangliocytomas that secrete CRH,[1291] and a few additional patients have been found to have ectopic tumors that secrete CRH but not ACTH.[1292,1293,1324] Additional patients have been described with adenomatous hyperplasia postulated to be of intermediate lobe origin[1327]; however, in other series, this type of hyperplasia has been absent or rare.[1316,1328,1329]

In patients with adrenal tumors or the ectopic ACTH syndrome and in those subjected to steroid therapy, the pituitary corticotrophs show prominent Crooke's hyaline changes with perinuclear microfilaments and reduced ACTH content.

Adrenal Cortex

Adrenocortical Hyperplasia Bilateral hyperplasia of the adrenal cortex occurs in patients with ACTH hypersecretion from either pituitary or ectopic sources. Three types of hyperplasia have been described: simple, that associated with the ectopic ACTH syndrome, and bilateral nodular.[1295,1330,1331] With simple hyperplasia (usually secondary to Cushing's disease), the combined adrenal weight is between 12 and 24 g (normal weight, 8 to 10 g; see previous discussion of anatomy). The enlarged glands have a yellowish-brown color. On microscopic examination, the cortex is thickened because of approximately equal hyperplasia of the compact cells of the zona reticularis and the clear cells of the zona fasciculata, with normal ultrastructural features. The zona glomerulosa is normal.

The adrenals in the ectopic ACTH syndrome are usually much more enlarged, with combined weights of 24 to more than 100 g.[1203,1295,1304,1330,1331] The cut surface of the cortex is generally brownish. Microscopically, there is typically marked hyperplasia of the zona reticularis, with columns of hypertrophied compact cells extending to and into the zona glomerulosa. The clear cells of the zona fasciculata are markedly reduced; however, the zona glomerulosa is normal. These histologic features are consistent with the effects of the markedly elevated ACTH levels typically seen in the ectopic ACTH syndrome.[1203]

Bilateral nodular hyperplasia is present in approximately 20 percent of cases.[1295,1330,1331] The precise etiology of these pathologic subtypes is unclear, although most result from pituitary ACTH excess (see etiology and pathogenesis section, later). The adrenals are enlarged, and adrenal weight is variable, depending on the number and size of the nodules present. The cut surface reveals at least one and usually multiple macroscopic yellow nodules that are usually bilateral. The nodules resemble both nonfunctioning adenomas and those causing Cushing's syndrome and consist mainly of clear cells that are similar to those of the normal zona fasciculata. The intervening cortex shows the typical features of simple hyperplasia described earlier.[1295,1331] Rarely, this condition is associated with adrenal carcinoma.[1332]

Adrenocortical Tumors Benign hyperfunctioning adrenal adenomas causing Cushing's syndrome weigh from 10 to 70 g and range in size from 1 to 6 cm.[1295,1330,1331] They are encapsulated, with a well-delineated margin, and the cut surface is yellow with brown or red areas. Microscopically, clear cells of the zona fasciculata type predominate and make up the yellow areas, whereas the darker areas contain cells resembling those of the compact zone of the zona reticularis. Rarely, these adenomas can be black because of the presence of lipofuscin.[1203]

Adrenal carcinomas are generally quite large (over 100 g), may weigh in excess of several kilograms, and are commonly palpable as abdominal masses.[1295,1330,1331] These tumors are encapsulated; the cut surface reveals a highly vascular tumor with necrosis, hemorrhage, and cystic degeneration. Calcification is not uncommon. Adrenal carcinomas may have a benign histologic appearance with a predominance of compact cells, although variable degrees of pleomorphism occur, especially in larger tumors. The histologic features frequently do not predict the clinical behavior of the tumor.[1295,1330,1331] Thus, in many cases, a definite diagnosis of malignancy can be established only if there is vascular invasion, local extension, or metastatic spread. These carcinomas spread by local invasion of the retroperitoneum, kidney, or liver or hematogenously to the liver and lungs.[1305]

With both functioning adrenal adenomas and carcinomas there is atrophy of the cortex contiguous to the tumor and of the contralateral gland.[1330] The capsule of the uninvolved cortex is thickened, and the atrophic cortex is narrow and consists entirely of clear, lipid-containing cells. The zona reticularis is absent, and the zona glomerulosa is normal.[1304]

Etiology and Pathogenesis

Cushing's Disease

Cushing's disease is caused by pituitary ACTH hypersecretion, and pituitary adenomas are present in the great majority of patients (see the section on pathology, earlier, and treatment of Cushing's Syndrome, later). Most cases of Cushing's disease are due to spontaneous ACTH-secreting pituitary adenomas, and hypothalamic abnormalities are secondary to hypercortisolism. However, it is possible that this disorder results from a primary CNS abnormality with excessive stimulation of anterior pituitary corticotrophs by CRH or other factors with secondary adenoma formation (see Chaps. 6 and 7).[1312,1333,1334]

Several endocrine abnormalities are characteristic of Cushing's disease. First, there is hypersecretion of ACTH with bilateral adrenocortical hyperplasia and hypersecretion of cortisol (Table 11-25). Second, there is absent circadian periodicity of ACTH and cortisol release; episodic secretion persists at a higher than normal frequency but is sporadic and lacks a diurnal pattern.[1335,1336] Third, there is absent responsiveness of ACTH and cortisol to stresses such as hypoglycemia and major surgery.[875,1337] Fourth, although negative feedback regulation of ACTH secretion by glucocorticoids is present, pharmacologic concentrations are required to suppress ACTH release and there is hyperresponsiveness of ACTH release when cortisol secretion is inhibited.[875] Fifth, abnormalities of other pituitary hormones are present in most of these patients, including subnormal responsiveness of growth hormone, TSH, and gonadotropin release to a variety of stimuli.[1337–1340]

TABLE 11-25. Endocrine Abnormalities in Cushing's Disease

Hypersecretion of ACTH and cortisol
Absent circadian periodicity of ACTH and cortisol
Abnormal ACTH and cortisol responsiveness to stress (hypoglycemia, surgery)
Abnormal negative feedback regulation of ACTH secretion by glucocorticoids
Abnormal suppressibility with dexamethasone
Hyperresponsiveness to inhibition of cortisol synthesis with metyrapone
Subnormal responsiveness of growth hormone, thyrotropin, and gonadotropins to stimulation

That Cushing's disease is a primary pituitary disorder in most patients is based on the high frequency of pituitary adenomas, the response to their removal, and the interpretation of hypothalamic abnormalities as being secondary to hypercortisolism. ACTH hypersecretion from a pituitary adenoma results in hypercortisolism that suppresses the normal hypothalamic-pituitary axis and CRH release; this abolishes hypothalamic regulation of circadian variability and stress responsiveness.[1312,1341] It has been postulated that the feedback control of ACTH secretion is mediated directly on the pituitary tumor and that other pharmacologic agents, such as cyproheptadine, and bromocriptine, directly inhibit an ACTH-secreting adenoma.[1312,1341] In addition, abnormalities of growth hormone, TSH, and gonadotropin secretion are due to hypercortisolism, and not to a primary hypothalamic disorder.[1312,1341] Also, when hypersecreted in rare patients with CRH-secreting tumors or when administered to animals, CRH does not result in pituitary adenomas but instead leads to pituitary corticotroph hyperplasia.[1324,1341]

The response to pituitary microsurgery strongly supports a primary pituitary etiology. Selective removal of pituitary microadenomas by transsphenoidal microsurgery corrects ACTH hypersecretion and hypercortisolism in most patients.[1297,1308,1309,1312,1340,1342,1344–1348] This suggests that the adenoma, not generalized corticotroph hyperplasia, is responsible for ACTH excess. Postoperatively, almost all these patients have transient ACTH deficiency and secondary hypoadrenalism with preservation of other pituitary hormones,[1308,1309,1312,1340,1344–1348] demonstrating that the normal hypothalamic-pituitary axis is suppressed by the hypercortisolism. This is supported by the in vitro demonstration of markedly decreased ACTH content in nonadenomatous pituitary tissue removed from patients with active Cushing's disease.[1318,1319] In cases studied after selective surgical removal of the adenoma, there is a return to normal of (1) the circadian rhythm of ACTH and cortisol secretion, (2) the responsiveness of the hypothalamic-pituitary axis to hypoglycemic stress, (3) suppressibility of cortisol secretion by dexamethasone,[1340,1344–1348] and (4) the formerly suppressed growth hormone, TSH, and gonadotropin responses.[1340,1345–1349] Thus, in these patients, there is no evidence for a persisting hypothalamic abnormality. Recovery of ACTH and growth hormone responsiveness to hypoglycemia also occurs when patients with Cushing's disease are treated with bilateral adrenalectomy.[875,1350] The idea that these abnormalities are due to hypercortisolism rather than to a primary hypothalamic lesion is further supported by the fact that glucocorticoid administration can suppress ACTH responses to hypoglycemia as well as growth hormone, TSH, and gonadotropin responses.[777,1337,1340,1349] Thus, the hypothalamic abnormalities of Cushing's disease are reversed simply by removing the source of hypercortisolism, suggesting again that the preoperative abnormalities were due solely to the pituitary adenoma with resulting hypersecretion of ACTH and cortisol.

The postulate that suppression of ACTH and cortisol secretion by high-dose dexamethasone in Cushing's disease occurs directly at the pituitary level is supported by evidence that the pituitary is an important site of glucocorticoid feedback (see previous discussion) and by the demonstration in vitro of a direct suppressive effect of glucocorticoids on ACTH secretion by adenomas removed from patients with Cushing's disease.[1351–1353]

There is also evidence for direct effects of other pharmacologic agents at the pituitary level in Cushing's disease. Vasopressin, which stimulates ACTH release in patients with Cushing's disease and in normal individuals, also stimulates secretion in ACTH-secreting pituitary adenomas in vitro but does not release ACTH in normal nonadenomatous anterior pituitary tissue from these patients.[1351–1353] Evidence that bromocriptine, cyproheptadine, and dopamine directly suppress pituitary ACTH secretion in patients with Cushing's disease is less direct.[1354] In one pituitary adenoma from a patient with Cushing's disease, dopamine inhibited ACTH release,[1351] and in a tumor from a patient with Nelson's syndrome, dopamine and cyproheptadine inhibited ACTH secretion.[1355]

The Ectopic ACTH Syndrome

The ectopic ACTH syndrome is caused by ACTH hypersecretion from nonpituitary tumors. These tumors contain immunoreactive and bioactive ACTH; they also secrete ACTH in vitro.[1356] They contain the POMC mRNA and secrete β-LPH, β-endorphin, and both large and small ACTH fragments, indicating that the ACTH is derived from a POMC similar to that of the anterior pituitary.[393,1357–1359] Ectopic tumors may also contain CRH-like activity[1357]; the biological significance of this is unclear, as most of these tumors also contain and secrete ACTH. It is unlikely that the CRH in these cases is stimulating pituitary ACTH, as the histology of the gland in the ectopic ACTH syndrome shows Crooke's changes that are consistent with its suppression by hypercortisolism.[1359] However, as mentioned previously, several tumors have been described that secrete CRH in quantities sufficient to cause pituitary ACTH hypersecretion.[1292,1293,1324]

The majority of cases of the ectopic ACTH syndrome are due to a small number of tumor types (Table 11-26).[1358–1361] Oat-cell carcinoma of the lung is by far the most common type. Other tumors, in order of frequency, are islet-cell tumors of the pancreas; carcinoid tumors of the lung, thymus, gut, pancreas, and ovary; medullary carcinoma of the thyroid; and pheochromocytoma and its related neuroectodermal tumors.[1361] Additional miscellaneous and rare cases include prostate carcinoma, malignant melanoma, adenocarcinoma of the colon, ovarian arrhenoblastoma, parathyroid carcinoma, and nephroblastoma.[1292,1293,1358,1361,1362] Undifferentiated or poorly differentiated carcinomas in the gallbladder, parotid, ovary, and cervix have been described with the ectopic ACTH syndrome, but the exact pathologic classification and site of origin of these carcinomas are difficult to ascertain.[1361]

TABLE 11-26. Tumors Most Frequently Causing the Ectopic ACTH Syndrome

Oat-cell carcinoma of the lung
Pancreatic islet-cell carcinoma
Carcinoid tumors (lung, gut, thymus, pancreas, ovary)
Thyroid medullary carcinoma
Pheochromocytoma and related tumors

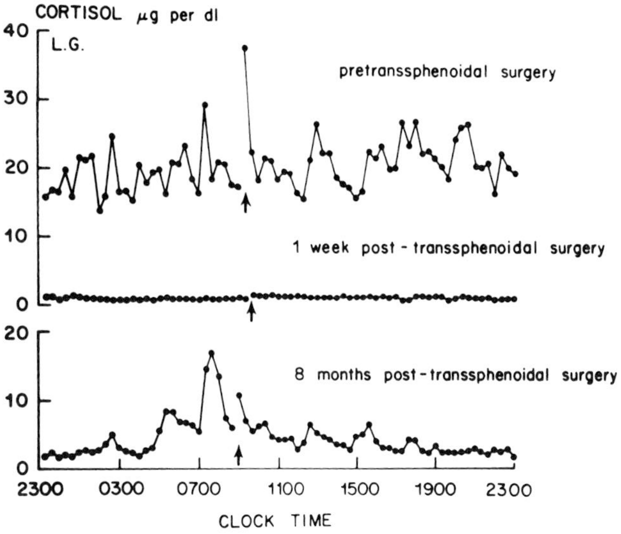

FIGURE 11-43. Twenty-four-h cortisol secretory patterns in a patient with Cushing's disease before treatment *(top)* and 1 week *(middle)* and 8 months *(bottom)* after transsphenoidal adenomectomy. Arrows denote the start of the sampling period. (*From Boyer et al.*[1347])

Adrenal Tumors

Glucocorticoid-producing adrenal tumors, whether adenoma or carcinoma, arise de novo and autonomously secrete adrenocortical steroids.[355,356] Rarely, adrenal carcinomas occur in patients with nodular adrenal hyperplasia[1332] or congenital adrenocortical hyperplasia, raising the possibility that in these special circumstances the development of carcinoma is promoted by prolonged ACTH stimulation of the adrenal. However, the majority of adrenal tumors developed spontaneously and are not associated with chronic ACTH excess.

Pathophysiology

Cushing's Disease

In Cushing's disease, pituitary adenomas release ACTH episodically without a circadian pattern,[1335,1336,1348] and because the feedback inhibition of ACTH by glucocorticoids is defective,[911] the elevated cortisol secretion does not adequately decrease ACTH secretion (Fig. 11-43). Thus, a state of glucocorticoid excess persists; it is the number and magnitude of ACTH and adrenal secretory episodes that account for the increase in total cortisol secretion. This episodic secretion results in variable plasma cortisol and ACTH levels, which may at times be moderately or markedly elevated and at other times may be within the normal range.[911,1335,1336,1348] However, measurement of cortisol production rate or urinary free cortisol excretion or multiple plasma cortisol samples over 24 h reveal cortisol hypersecretion (see later section on laboratory features and diagnosis and Refs. 361, 1336, and 1348). Thus, the major differences in plasma ACTH and cortisol in Cushing's disease occur in the afternoon and at night, when cortisol secretion is usually low in normal individuals. This overall increase in tissue exposure to glucocorticoids is sufficient to cause obvious Cushing's syndrome; however, the modest increase in ACTH secretion usually does not cause increased pigmentation. β-LPH is also hypersecreted.[878–880] In addition to ACTH hypersecretion and resistance to suppression with glucocorticoids, the axis does not respond normally to stressful stimuli such as hypoglycemia and surgery.[875,1337] This is probably due to the relative autonomy of the pituitary adenoma and suppression by glucocorticoids of the normal ability of the hypothalamic-pituitary axis to secrete CRH and ACTH.

The pathophysiologic basis for the clinical abnormalities caused by excess cortisol have already been described in the section on actions of glucocorticoids. Thus, cortisol not only inhibits normal pituitary and hypothalamic function, affecting ACTH, TSH, growth hormone, and gonadotropin release, but also causes all the peripheral effects described on most tissues of the body.

The secretion of adrenal androgens (also controlled by ACTH) is increased in patients with Cushing's disease; the extent of hypersecretion is roughly proportional to and parallels that of ACTH and cortisol. DHEA, DHEA-S, and androstenedione are all hypersecreted; they are converted peripherally to testosterone and DHT. Thus, plasma levels of these steroids are moderately increased in Cushing's disease, and a state of androgen excess develops. In the female, this causes the classic manifestations of hirsutism, acne, and amenorrhea. Amenorrhea is in part a consequence of androgen suppression of gonadotropin secretion.[1339] In a male patient with Cushing's disease, testicular production of testosterone is decreased by the glucocorticoid suppression of gonadotropin secretion.[1363] Despite increased adrenal androgen production, the net result is a lowering of circulating testosterone levels, accompanied by decreased libido and impotence.

Aldosterone production is usually not increased in Cushing's disease, and the renin-angiotensin-aldosterone axis usually remains intact. Although there is some increase in DOC production, DOC and cortisol are not elevated enough to produce a frank mineralocorticoid excess state, in contrast to the case with the ectopic ACTH syndrome (Chaps. 13 and 28).

Ectopic ACTH Syndrome

Patients with this syndrome usually have much more marked ACTH and cortisol hypersecretion than is seen in Cushing's disease. β-LPH and other POMC peptides are also secreted in excess (see Chap. 27).[1357,1358] ACTH and cortisol hypersecretion are also episodic, although at greatly elevated levels. With uncommon exceptions, the secretion of ACTH by an ectopic tumor is not suppressible even with high doses of glucocorticoids.

The marked ACTH hypersecretion results in a greater degree of hyperplasia of the zonae fasciculata and reticularis, and the secretion of cortisol, adrenal androgens, and DOC is higher than in most patients with Cushing's disease.[1295] Thus, plasma levels and urinary excretion of these steroids and their metabolites usually are markedly elevated.[735,1364] However, in spite of the marked elevations of these steroids, the classic features of Cushing's syndrome are commonly absent.[1364] This is presumably due to the rapid onset of hypercortisolism and the associated malignancy. Also, manifestations of androgen excess may not be prominent because most of these patients are male. However, the elevated DOC and cortisol concentrations frequently result in a frank mineralocorticoid excess syndrome with hypertension, hypokalemia, and suppressed plasma renin levels (Chap. 13).

Adrenal Tumors

Glucocorticoid-secreting primary adrenal tumors, whether adenomas or carcinomas, autonomously hypersecrete cortisol and suppress the hypothalamic-pituitary axis, CRH, and circulating plasma ACTH levels.[875] This results in atrophy of the zonae fasciculata and reticularis not involved by the tumor.[1295]

Adrenal adenomas causing Cushing's syndrome usually secrete only cortisol in significant excess; thus, the clinical picture is one of pure glucocorticoid excess. Cortisol secretion is again episodic, but feedback control of cortisol release is lost, and thus these tumors typically show no response to either dexamethasone or metyrapone. The adrenal secretion of androgens is usually subnormal, as manifested by low urinary 17-ketosteroid excretion or plasma DHEA-S levels.[1365]

Adrenal carcinomas frequently secrete multiple steroids in an unpredictable pattern.[1305,1305a] However, most commonly, cortisol, DOC, and androgens are secreted in excess; less commonly, there is hypersecretion of aldosterone or estrogens. Concentrations of plasma cortisol and its urinary metabolites frequently are markedly elevated in patients with adrenal carcinomas. In addition, androgen hypersecretion is frequently even more markedly elevated, with very high levels of urinary 17-ketosteroids or plasma DHEA and DHEA-S.[1305] These patients usually have severe and rapidly progressive clinical manifestations of cortisol excess; in females, androgen excess is prominent.[1305] These patients also frequently have mineralocorticoid excess due to cortisol and DOC, with resulting hypertension and hypokalemia.

Clinical and Laboratory Features

Clinical Features

The clinical manifestations of Cushing's syndrome were well described by Cushing himself[5]; the frequencies of these features are listed in Table 11-27.[735,1296] Although the frequency of presenting signs and symptoms has remained remarkably constant, the severity of the condition appears to be less in more recent series, presumably because of earlier clinical recognition and diagnosis.[735,1296]

Obesity is the most common manifestation (Fig. 11-44), and weight gain is usually the initial symptom. Weight gain is classically central, affecting mainly the face, neck, trunk, and abdomen, with relative sparing of the extremities.[1296] However, generalized obesity is equally frequent and was present in 60 percent of the

TABLE 11-27. Clinical Features of Cushing's Syndrome

Feature	Percent with Feature
Obesity	94
Facial plethora	84
Hirsutism	82
Menstrual disorders	76
Hypertension	72
Muscular weakness	58
Back pain	58
Striae	52
Acne	40
Psychological symptoms	40
Bruising	36
Congestive heart failure	22
Edema	18
Renal calculi	16
Headache	14
Polyuria/polydipsia	10
Hyperpigmentation	6

Source: Modified from Plotz et al.[1296] and Ross et al.[735]

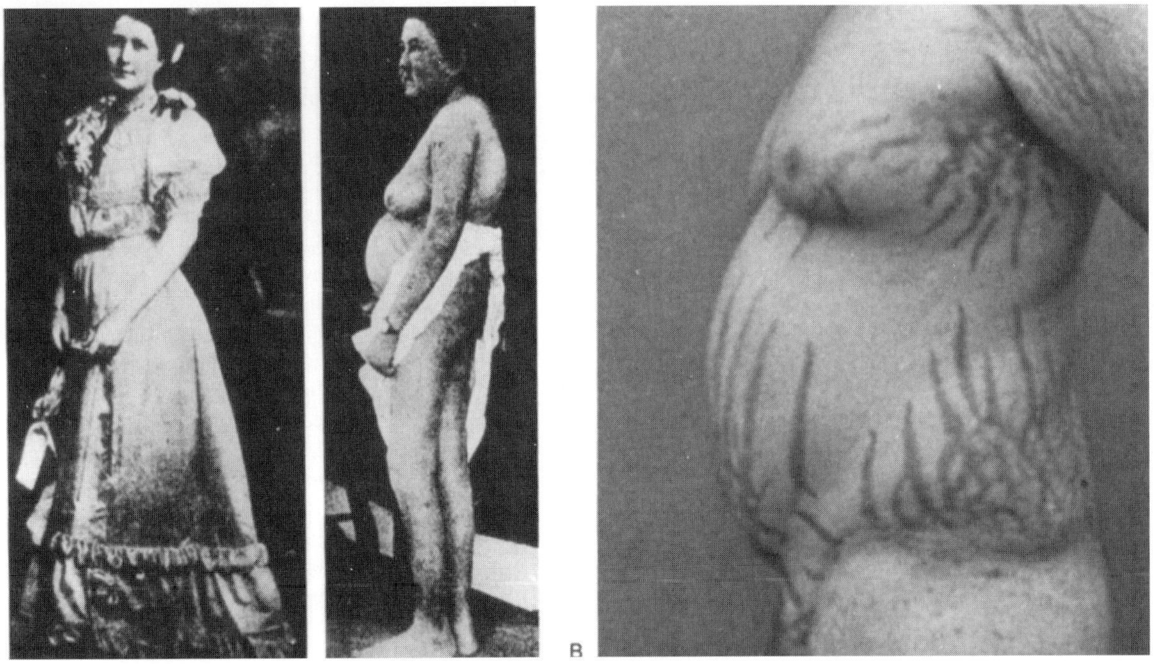

FIGURE 11-44. *(A)* Patient from Cushing's original series before and after the development of clinical features. *(B)* Marked striae in a patient with Cushing's syndrome. (*Panel A from Cushing.*[5])

cases described by Ross and associates.[735] In children with Cushing's syndrome, obesity is invariably present and is almost always generalized.[1306–1309] In addition to obesity, 85 percent of children with Cushing's syndrome have short stature and growth failure.[1306–1309]

Whether central or generalized, the obesity of Cushing's syndrome has certain features that distinguish it from simple obesity. Accumulation of fat in the face leads to the typical "moon facies," which is present in 75 percent and is accompanied by facial plethora in most patients. Fat accumulation around the neck is prominent in the supraclavicular and dorsocervical fat pads; the fat deposition in the latter is responsible for the "buffalo hump." Adipose tissue accumulates over the thorax and frequently leads to protruberance of the abdomen. A minority of the patients are not obese and do not gain weight; however, they usually have central redistribution of fat and a typical facial appearance.[1296]

Although skin changes are less common, their presence should arouse suspicion of cortisol excess. Atrophy of the epidermis and its underlying connective tissue leads to thinning and a transparent appearance of the skin in advanced cases. This also accounts for the plethoric appearance. Easy bruisability with minimal trauma is present in 40 to 60 percent of patients. Such patients on occasion have been detected after referral for a work-up of a bleeding diathesis. Purple striae occur in 50 to 70 percent of these patients; they are typically red to purple in color, depressed below the skin surface because of loss of underlying connective tissue, and wider (not infrequently 0.5 to 2.0 cm) than the pinkish-white striae seen with pregnancy or rapid weight gain. These striae are most commonly abdominal but also may occur over the breasts, hips, buttocks, thighs, and axillae. Minor wounds and abrasions frequently heal slowly and poorly, as do surgical incisions, which sometimes dehisce.[1296] Mucocutaneous fungal infections occur frequently, including tinea versicolor, involvement of the nails, and oral candidiasis. Hyperpigmentation of the skin occurs rarely in patients with Cushing's disease or adrenal tumors but is more common in the ectopic ACTH syndrome.[735,1365] Hirsutism is present in 65 to 70 percent of female patients as a result of hypersecretion of adrenal androgens; it is generally mild to moderate. Facial hirsutism is most common, but increased hair growth also may occur over the abdomen, breasts, chest, and upper thighs. Virilism is unusual except in adrenal carcinomas, in which it occurs in approximately 20 percent of patients.[1305] Acne, most frequently involving the face, and seborrhea usually accompany hirsutism.

Hypertension, a classic feature of spontaneous Cushing's syndrome, is present in 75 to 85 percent of these patients. The diastolic blood pressure is >100 mmHg in over 50 percent of patients (see Chap. 13).[735] In one series, 23 of 24 patients over age 40 were hypertensive, and of these, 11 had congestive heart failure.[735] Hypertension and its complications contribute greatly to morbidity and mortality in spontaneous Cushing's syndrome; in the series of Plotz and colleagues, 40 percent of those dying with the syndrome did so directly as a result of hypertension and/or atherosclerosis.[1296] Peripheral edema was frequently described in early series[1296,1365] but was present in only 18 percent of the patients in the series of Ross et al.[735]

Gonadal dysfunction is extremely common because of elevated levels of androgens (in females) and cortisol (in males and, to a lesser extent, females). Amenorrhea occurs in approximately 75 percent of premenopausal females and is usually accompanied by infertility.[735,1296] Patients without amenorrhea generally have a mild form of the condition and shorter duration of symptoms.[1365] Male patients frequently have decreased libido, and some have decreased body hair and soft testes.[735,1365] Gynecomastia is unusual in male patients but may be seen in patients with estrogen-producing adrenal carcinomas.

Psychological disturbances occur in approximately two-thirds of these patients.[1296] The presentation and severity of these features are extremely variable. Mild features include emotional lability and increased irritability. Increased anxiety, depression, decreased concentration, and poor memory may also be present. Some patients are euphoric and occasionally may manifest overtly manic behavior. The majority of these patients also have disordered sleep with either insomnia or early morning awakening. A minority of patients exhibit more severe psychological disorders, which may include severe depression, psychosis with delusions or hallucinations and paranoia; some have committed suicide.[1296] A patient's premorbid personality or psychiatric history has not been helpful in predicting the types of psychoses that occur. About 40 percent of children and adolescents with Cushing's disease have overachieving, compulsive behavior, which remits following surgical removal of the tumor.[1309]

Muscle weakness occurs in approximately 60 percent; it is most frequently proximal and is usually most prominent in the lower extremities.[735] Thus, patients typically first note difficulty in climbing stairs and in more severe cases may have difficulty arising from a chair.

Approximately 50 percent of these patients have clinically obvious osteoporosis, although the incidence of this probably approaches 100 percent when refined measurements are made. Back pain is an initial complaint in 40 percent.[735] Pathologic fractures occur frequently in severe cases and most often involve the ribs and vertebral bodies.[735,1365] Compression fractures of the spine are demonstrable radiographically in 16 to 22 percent and may be accompanied by loss of height and kyphosis.[735,1365]

Renal calculi occur in approximately 15 percent of these patients, and renal colic may occasionally be a presenting complaint.[735] These calculi are a consequence of glucocorticoid-induced hypercalciuria, although a few patients have had associated primary hyperparathyroidism.[735] Thirst and polyuria may also occur in an occasional patient with hypercalciuria. Thirst and polyuria ascribable to overt hyperglycemia and diabetes mellitus occur in approximately 10 percent of these patients, whereas glucose intolerance is much more common. Diabetic ketoacidosis is rare, as are diabetic microvascular complications.

Laboratory Features

Routine laboratory examinations are rarely of major diagnostic utility in the diagnosis of Cushing's syndrome, although certain abnormalities may suggest the diagnosis. The specific utility of ACTH and corticosteroid measurements is discussed here.

Patients with Cushing's syndrome frequently have high normal values of hemoglobin, hematocrit, and red cell count, but elevations into the range of polycythemia are rare.[735] The total white cell count is usually normal; however, patients have neutrophilia, the percentage of lymphocytes is below 25 in 50 percent of cases and the total lymphocyte count is subnormal in 35 percent.[735] The total eosinophil count is usually below $100/mm^3$ and is less than $10/mm^3$ in approximately 30 percent of patients. Serum sodium concentration is normal in most patients. In patients with Cushing's disease, serum potassium and bicarbonate concentrations are usually normal, but hypokalemia and alkalosis are common with the ectopic ACTH syndrome and adrenocortical carcinoma.[735,1364] The degree of hypokalemia correlates well with adrenocortical hypersecretion; thus, it is not unexpected that hypokalemic alkalosis occurs most frequently in these latter two conditions, in which steroid levels frequently are markedly elevated.[1364,1366] Renal function is normal in uncomplicated Cushing's syndrome but can be abnormal in patients with long-standing hypertension, renal stones, nephrocalcinosis, or infection. Serum calcium and phosphorus concentrations are normal; however, hypercalciuria occurs in 40 percent of these patients.[735] Fasting hyperglycemia occurs in 10 to 15 percent of cases, and glucose intolerance with associated hyperinsulinemia occurs in the majority.[735,1296,1365] Glycosuria is present in patients with fasting hyperglycemia and may also occur postprandially. Ketosis or ketoacidosis is rare; its presence suggests coexisting insulinopenic diabetes. Plasma lipoprotein (VLDL and LDL) concentrations tend to be elevated, with consequent elevations of triglyceride and cholesterol levels,[1367] especially in patients with hyperglycemia.

Routine radiographs may reveal cardiomegaly due to hypertensive or atherosclerotic heart disease; rib or spinal compression features and renal calculi may be noted. The ECG may be abnormal in patients with long-standing disease in whom hypertensive or atherosclerotic myocardial injury has occurred.

Features Suggesting a Specific Etiology

Although a definitive diagnosis of the type of Cushing's syndrome present must be established biochemically, certain features suggest a specific etiology.

Patients with Cushing's disease present with the classic clinical picture. Women predominate, the onset is generally between ages 20 and 40, and the clinical manifestations are usually slowly progressive over several years. Hyperpigmentation and hypokalemic alkalosis are rare. Cortisol and adrenal androgen secretion is increased moderately, and androgenic manifestations are generally limited to acne and mild to moderate hirsutism.[735]

In contrast, the ectopic ACTH syndrome occurs predominantly in males, with the highest incidence in the fifth to seventh decade.[1364] The primary tumor is usually apparent, but the clinical manifestations are frequently limited to weakness, hypertension, and glucose intolerance. Hyperpigmentation, hypokalemia, and alkalosis are common.[1364] Weight loss and anemia due to malignancy are also common. The features of hypercortisolism are of rapid onset. Steroid hypersecretion is frequently severe, with equally elevated levels of glucocorticoids, androgens, and DOC.[1364] Survival in these patients with both metastatic carcinoma and severe hypercortisolism is extremely limited.[1364]

A minority of patients with the ectopic ACTH syndrome have more "benign" tumors, especially bronchial carcinoids, and present with a more slowly progressive course with typical features of Cushing's syndrome. These patients may be clinically identical to those with pituitary-dependent Cushing's disease; the responsible tumor may not be apparent.[857,1368] Hyperpigmentation, hypokalemic alkalosis, and anemia are commonly absent. Further confusion may arise because a number of these patients with occult ectopic tumors may have ACTH and steroid dynamics typical of Cushing's disease (see later discussion).[939,1368,1369]

The clinical picture in patients with adrenal adenomas is usually that of glucocorticoid excess alone. Androgenic effects such as hirsutism are usually absent. The onset is gradual, and the hypercortisolism is mild to moderate. Urinary 17-ketosteroid excretion and plasma androgen concentrations are usually in the low normal or subnormal range.[1370]

With adrenal carcinomas in general, the clinical features of excessive glucocorticoid, androgen, and mineralocorticoid hypersecretion have a rapid onset and are rapidly progressive.[1305] Marked elevations of cortisol, androgens, and DOC are usual. Hypokalemia is common. Abdominal pain, palpable masses, and hepatic and pulmonary metastases are also common at the time of diagnosis.[1305]

Diagnosis and Differential Diagnosis

Diagnosis

The evaluation of Cushing's syndrome must first include a general assessment of the patient regarding the presence of other illnesses, drugs and medications, alcoholism, and depression, as these factors may lead to misleading results (see previous section on laboratory features). In suspected hypercortisolism, either the overnight 1-mg dexamethasone suppression test or the measurement of the 24-h urine cortisol may be chosen as the initial test.[1371] The overnight 1-mg dexamethasone suppression test is an excellent screening test in an outpatient setting and for many is the initial procedure of choice because of its simplicity. A normal response to the overnight test (plasma cortisol <5 ng/dl) excludes Cushing's syndrome with 98 percent accuracy (Fig. 11-45),[874] and the only exceptions have been rare patients with episodic Cushing's syndrome or abnormal dexamethasone metabolism (see later discussion). The test should not be used in patients with marked obesity, patients receiving estrogen therapy, and those who are on drugs that accelerate dexamethasone metabolism, as described later. In these patients, measurement of free urinary free cortisol is preferable.

Measurement of the 24-h urine cortisol (Fig. 11-46) is an equally acceptable initial test and is preferable in the setting of marked obesity, with estrogen therapy, or if the patient is taking drugs that accelerate dexamethasone metabolism.[874,886,906,907] Urine cortisol levels are elevated in more than 90 percent of patients with Cushing's syndrome[874] but may also be elevated in stress, depression, and alcoholism, as discussed later. An abnormal result of either test should be confirmed by the performance of the other, and if both tests are abnormal, hypercortisolism is present and the diagnosis of Cushing's syndrome is established, provided that conditions causing false-positive responses are excluded, as discussed in a later section.

In patients with equivocal or borderline results, the 2-day low-dose dexamethasone suppression test is performed, with

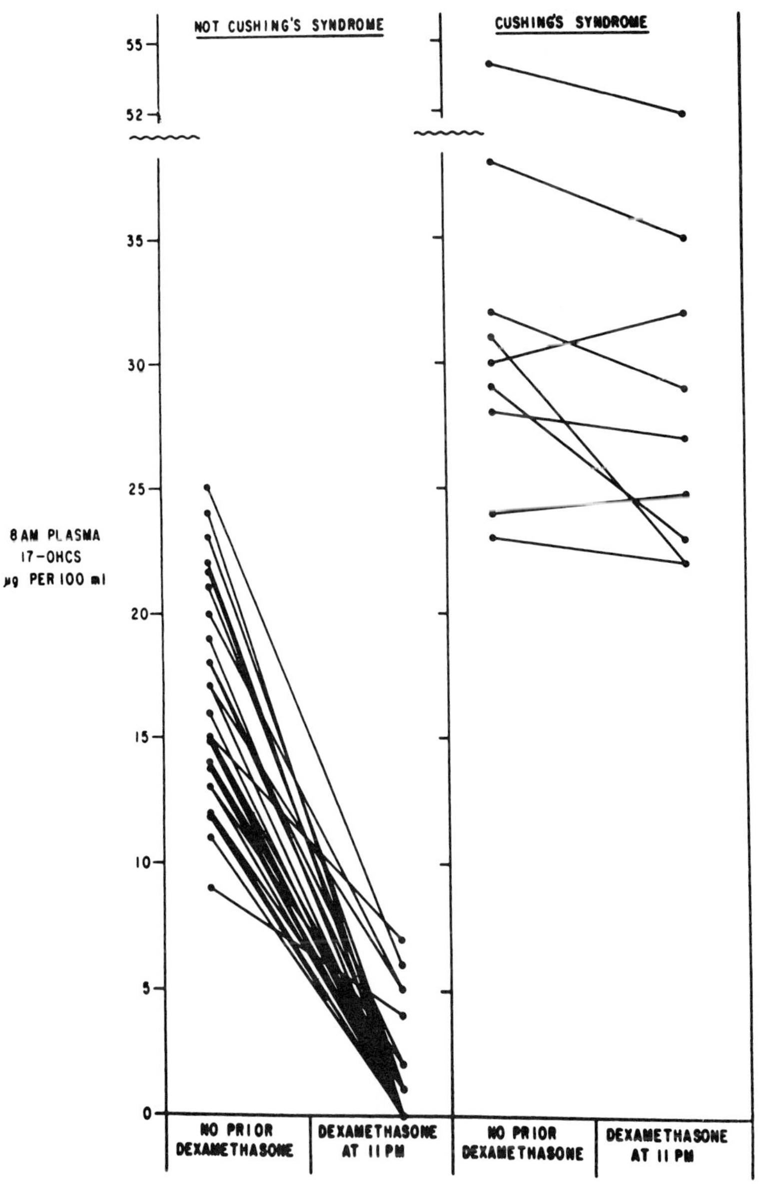

FIGURE 11-45. Plasma cortisol (8 A.M. plasma 17-OHCS) response to the low-dose dexamethasone suppression test (see text) in control subjects ("not Cushing's syndrome") and patients with Cushing's syndrome. (*From Nugent CA, et al., Arch Intern Med 116:172, 1965.*)

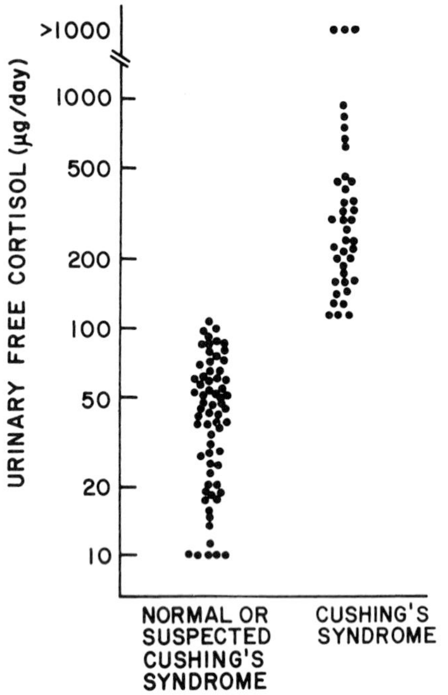

FIGURE 11-46. Urinary free cortisol excretion (measured by the competitive protein-binding assay) in normal individuals, individuals with suspected but not substantiated hypercortisolism, and patients with Cushing's syndrome. (*Based on data of Burke and Beardwell.*[907])

measurement of urinary 17-OHCS or free cortisol excretion (normal responses, 11-OHCS >2.5 mg/24 h or 1.0 mg per gram of creatinine[874,891]; free cortisol <20 μg/24 h.[874,906,907] In this setting, a normal response excludes Cushing's syndrome and abnormal suppressibility is consistent with the diagnosis, as the incidence of false-positive responses is negligible.[874]

The measurement of late evening (8 P.M. to 12 A.M.) plasma or salivary cortisol level and the cortisol production rate are also useful in the diagnosis of Cushing's syndrome,[874] but these procedures have not come into general use, as discussed in the section on laboratory features.

Other tests and procedures are less reliable in the diagnosis and are no longer recommended because there is considerable overlap between patients with and without Cushing's syndrome.[874,913] These include basal morning cortisol levels; single afternoon or early evening diurnal cortisol level; basal 24-h urinary 17-OHCS, 17-KGS, or 17-ketosteroid excretion; and responsiveness to either ACTH or metyrapone stimulation tests, as discussed in the section on laboratory evaluation of adrenocortical function.[874,913]

Problems in Diagnosis

Despite the generally clear separation of patients with and without Cushing's syndrome using a combination of the tests described, several factors may complicate the diagnosis.[857,874,1371] These include both rare false-negative results and, more commonly, false-positive results.

False-negative responses have been reported in patients with Cushing's syndrome. First, there may be normal suppression of glucocorticoid secretion with low-dose dexamethasone because of delayed clearance of the steroid and higher than usual plasma levels of dexamethasone.[857,874,902,903] The measurement of plasma dexamethasone concentrations, if available, will reveal the reason for "normal" suppressibility.[902,903] A second unusual cause of normal suppressibility is periodic or episodic hormonogenesis in Cushing's syndrome.[904,1372–1374] In these patients, hypercortisolism is either cyclic, with a regular period of days to weeks, or episodic, without a regular pattern; cortisol secretion may be normal or nearly normal between cycles or episodes.[904,1373] Thus, in these patients with spontaneously varying cortisol secretion, adrenal function may be normal at times and dexamethasone administration during phases of normal secretion may reveal normal suppressibility.[904] In these patients, repeated evaluation is required to establish the diagnosis of hypercortisolism and additional difficulties may be encountered in the differential diagnosis.

False-positive responses are more common. Patients with acute and/or chronic illnesses, especially those who are hospitalized, may have appropriately elevated glucocorticoid secretion. These patients may have elevated plasma cortisol and urinary free cortisol levels, and their adrenal function is frequently nonsuppressible with the 1-mg overnight suppression test.[874] If Cushing's syndrome is suspected, diagnostic evaluation should be repeated when the acute stress has resolved.

Obesity is the most common differential diagnostic problem because more than 15 percent of obese patients have abnormal responses to the overnight 1-mg suppression test.[874] Urinary excretion of 17-OHCS is also elevated in obese patients and is the major reason for the limited ability of this test.[857,874,1371] However, the urinary free cortisol excretion is virtually always normal in simple obesity.[886,906,907] In addition, in those with an abnormal overnight test, the 2-day low-dose suppression test will resolve the problem, as normal suppressibility is maintained in obese patients.[857,891]

High-estrogen states (pregnancy, estrogen therapy, and oral contraceptive use) that increase CBG also cause confusion because total plasma cortisol levels may be as high as 40 to 60 μg/dl[857,891] and the overnight 1-mg test may be abnormal; however, urinary free cortisol excretion is normal or slightly increased.

Patients on phenytoin, rifampin, and other anticonvulsants, including phenobarbital and primidone, can have false-positive results on low-dose dexamethasone tests. However, urinary free cortisol excretion is normal, as is the suppressibility of plasma corticosterone levels by oral hydrocortisone.[857]

A number of alcoholic patients have both clinical and biochemical features of Cushing's syndrome ("alcohol-induced pseudo–Cushing's syndrome").[857,1375] These patients have elevated basal plasma cortisol levels with abnormal circadian variation, an increased cortisol production rate, increased urinary corticosteroid excretion, and abnormal suppressibility with dexamethasone, i.e., steroid dynamics consistent with Cushing's syndrome.[857,1375] The steroid dynamics revert to normal after the cessation of alcohol intake; thus, if diagnostic test results are abnormal, testing should be repeated after abstention from alcohol for at least 4 weeks. In view of the frequency of excessive alcohol use, this possibility should be considered whenever hypercortisolism is suspected.

Similarly, obese patients with depression frequently have abnormal steroid dynamics that suggest Cushing's syndrome.[857] These patients also have increased cortisol secretion with elevated plasma levels, absence of diurnal variation, increased urinary free cortisol excretion, and impaired dexamethasone suppression.[857] The abnormal steroid dynamics revert to normal upon psychological recovery. These patients frequently cannot be differentiated from those with true Cushing's syndrome. These patients have normal cortisol responsiveness to insulin-induced hypoglycemia, whereas in patients with Cushing's syndrome, cortisol levels do not increase further during hypoglycemia.[857,875] CRH testing done

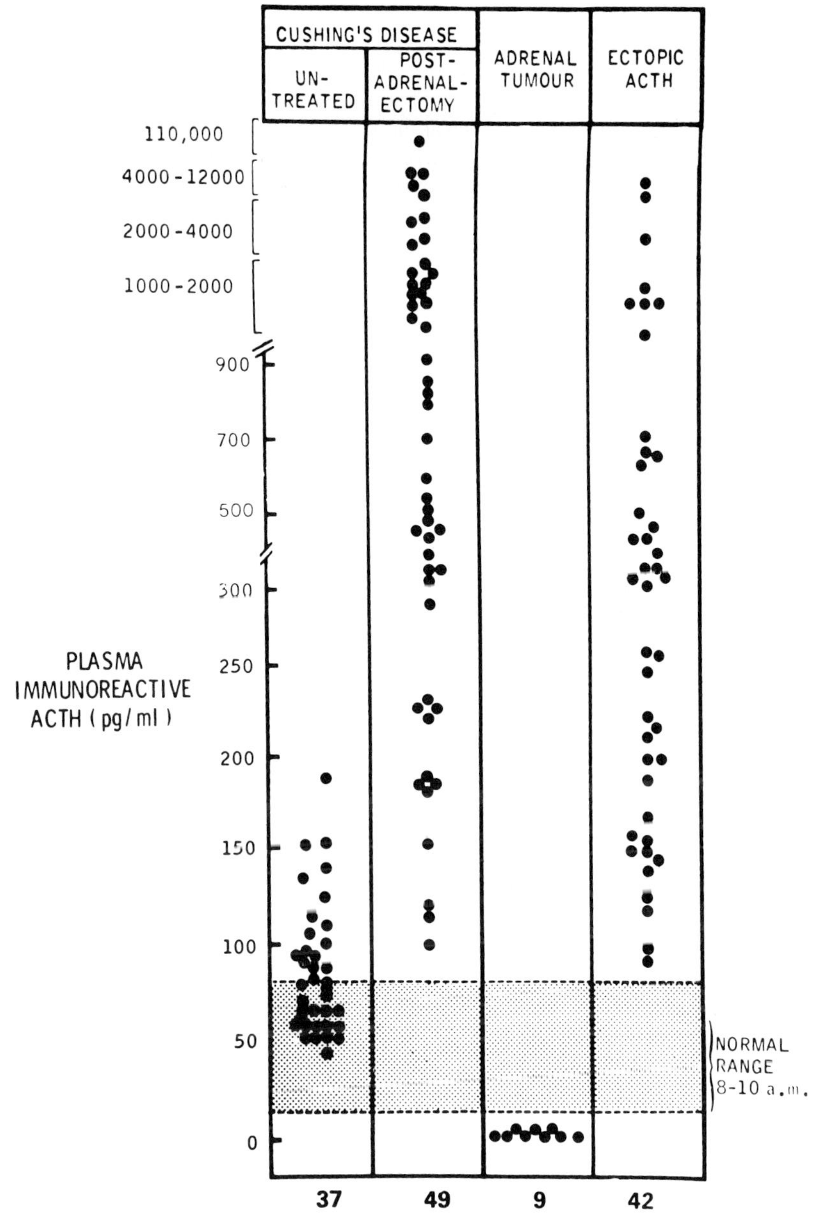

FIGURE 11-47. Basal plasma ACTH levels in patients with Cushing's disease before (untreated) and after bilateral adrenalectomy and with cortisol-producing adrenal adenomas and ectopic ACTH syndrome. (*From Besser and Edwards.*[875])

after 2 days of low dose dexamethasone appears to differentiate these etiologies adequately.[1376,1377]

Patients with anorexia nervosa also have cortisol dynamics similar to those of Cushing's disease.[440] However, these patients can be distinguished from Cushing's disease patients by their clinical presentation and from those with the ectopic ACTH syndrome by high-dose dexamethasone suppression.

Determining the Etiology and Tumor Localization

When Cushing's syndrome is present, the specific etiology must be defined, and this diagnosis cannot be completely secure until a tumor is localized and confirmed histologically. Thus, the most common etiology, pituitary ACTH hypersecretion (Cushing's disease), must be differentiated from the ectopic ACTH syndrome and primary adrenal tumors. Less common etiologies account for a few percent of patients with Cushing's syndrome, as discussed. The initial step in establishing the etiology of Cushing's syndrome is the measurement of plasma ACTH levels[874,875] basally and/or after ovine or human CRH administration (Fig. 11-47). Subsequent evaluation is directed by the ACTH levels and may consist of additional endocrine tests such as high-dose dexamethasone suppression and metyrapone (see section on laboratory features and Refs. 857, 874, 875, 915–918, 1378, and 1379) and imaging evaluations that may include CT scans of the adrenals, gadolinium-enhanced MRI of the pituitary, and venous sampling of the inferior petrosal sinuses to determine whether ACTH hypersecretion is of pituitary origin.

If the plasma ACTH level is suppressed (<5 pg/ml by IRMA or <8 pg/ml by radioimmunoassay (RIA), the patient has

ACTH-independent Cushing's syndrome.[871,873,874] In this case, the next step is to perform a CT scan of the adrenals, which will reveal a solitary adrenal tumor with rare exceptions.[1380,1381] Adrenal adenomas are homogeneous, 3 to 6 cm in diameter, and secrete only cortisol. Larger tumors, in particular those that secrete multiple steroids (especially androgens), are likely to be adrenocortical carcinomas. Measurement of DHEA-S levels is useful in this differential diagnosis; i.e., they are suppressed with adrenal adenomas and usually are elevated in patients with adrenal carcinoma.[1305,1370] If adrenal carcinoma is suspected, an evaluation for local and distant spread should be undertaken.

If the CT scan shows "normal" adrenals, the diagnostic possibilities include primary pigmented nodular adrenocortical disease (PPNAD) (described earlier) and exogenous cortisol or cortisone administration.[1382–1385] The diagnosis of PPNAD is likely if the patient is young and if there is familial Cushing's syndrome or manifestations of the Carney complex.[1381–1385] In addition, careful review of the CT scans or additional MR imaging will reveal irregularity of the adrenals consistent with micronodularity.[1382–1385] If the imaging procedures do not demonstrate nodularity of the adrenals, iodocholesterol scanning may be performed; the demonstration of bilateral function excludes exogenous glucocorticoid administration.[1382–1385]

If the CT scan demonstrates bilateral adrenal enlargement, the patient has macronodular adrenal hyperplasia, which may be either ACTH-independent or ACTH-dependent (a variant of Cushing's disease).[1369,1386–1390] The differentiation of these two entities is best substantiated by repeated plasma ACTH and cortisol determinations with CRH stimulation.[1386] The rare primary adrenal form of this disorder is characterized by repeatedly suppressed ACTH levels, failure to respond to CRH administration, and absent responses to high-dose dexamethasone. Patients with ACTH-dependent macronodular hyperplasia have variable ACTH levels; however, the levels are measurable if repeated determinations are obtained, and most of these patients have ACTH responsiveness to CRH.[1386] Responses to high-dose dexamethasone are variable; however, about 50 percent of those patients show suppression. If ACTH dependency is confirmed, further evaluation of these patients with pituitary MRI and inferior petrosal sinus sampling should follow the guidelines described later to establish a pituitary source. Ectopic tumors rarely cause macronodular hyperplasia.

If the initial ACTH determination is normal to elevated (10 to 1,550 pg/ml) but not suppressed, ACTH dependency should be confirmed by repeat ACTH determinations, CRH stimulation, and high-dose dexamethasone. These patients should next undergo CT scans of the adrenals, which may demonstrate macronodular or simple hyperplasia. Cushing's disease is the most likely etiology. However, about 5 percent of patients will have the occult ectopic ACTH syndrome, primarily as a result of small ACTH-secreting carcinoid tumors.[1368] If the CRH and high dexamethasone dose tests are positive, Cushing's disease is present with rare exceptions,[939,1306,1391–1395] and the patient should undergo an MRI study of the pituitary with gadolinium enhancement. If this study demonstrates a definite adenoma, surgery is recommended. However, caution should be exercised if the MRI study reveals only minor abnormalities; i.e., 1- to 3-mm lesions may be artifacts or incidental cysts or incidental adenomas. If the MRI is equivocal or normal, inferior petrosal sinus sampling for ACTH determinations should be performed; the demonstration of central ACTH gradients documents Cushing's disease.[1396] If the result of ACTH sampling is negative, further evaluation for an ectopic source is indicated.[1368,1397,1398] If the responses to high-dose dexamethasone and CRH are negative, the ectopic ACTH syndrome is most likely, although a few patients with Cushing's disease do not respond to these procedures. In this setting, venous sampling for ACTH should be performed; the results, if positive, confirm Cushing's disease and, if negative, direct an evaluation to localize an ectopic tumor.

In patients with initial ACTH levels greater than 200 pg/ml, the ectopic ACTH syndrome is probable. ACTH levels frequently are markedly elevated (500–10,000 pg/ml), and in most patients the tumor is either already clinically evident or readily localized by appropriate imaging studies. If no tumor is evident, venous sampling will exclude a pituitary source and CT, MRI, and octreotide scans of the chest and abdomen are employed to localize nonpituitary tumors.[1397,1398,1399]

Problems in Determining the Etiology

Although the procedures described in the preceding section can establish a specific etiology in the majority of cases, enough exceptions occur to warrant discussion.

Problems are encountered in the rare patients with periodic or episodic hormonogenesis who may have Cushing's disease, the ectopic ACTH syndrome, adrenal tumors, or PPNAD.[904,1373,1374] Thus, these patients may show normal suppression with the low-dose test if it is performed during certain periods; when studied at other times, secretion in these patients may be nonsuppressible or even show paradoxic increases during high-dose dexamethasone administration.[904,1373] Repeated evaluations and use of the localizing procedures described here may be necessary to establish the correct etiology in such patients.

About 10 to 20 percent of patients with Cushing's disease fail to suppress with high-dose dexamethasone, and an additional 10 percent do not respond to CRH stimulation; these responses falsely suggest the ectopic ACTH syndrome.[857,874,912,913,1378,1391] Thus, the diagnostic accuracy of either procedure is about 90 percent; however, if both tests are utilized, diagnostic accuracy is close to 100 percent.[1391–1395] Failure of suppression may occur with pituitary macroadenomas and in patients with macronodular adrenal hyperplasia. This variant of Cushing's disease frequently causes diagnostic difficulties because approximately 50 percent of these patients do not suppress with the standard 2-day high-dose dexamethasone suppression test[857,874,1369] and plasma ACTH levels may be low, normal, or elevated.[874,1369] In patients who do not show suppression with high-dose dexamethasone, in whom ACTH levels are not markedly elevated, and who do not have an obvious pituitary or ectopic tumor, selective venous ACTH sampling should be performed, as discussed later.[857,1369] In addition, the diagnosis is supported by the demonstration of nodular hyperplasia by CT scan of the adrenals.[857,1369]

Although the ectopic ACTH syndrome is usually easily diagnosed by markedly elevated ACTH levels and absent responses to high-dose dexamethasone and CRH in the presence of an extrapituitary tumor, there are some cases in which the tumor is occult.[939,1368] In these cases, steroid secretion may be responsive to dexamethasone, CRH, and metyrapone.[857,939,1368] In addition, the tumor may not reveal itself for a number of years after the onset of Cushing's syndrome.[857,1368] These occult tumors are usually bronchial carcinoids, and the plasma ACTH levels can be in the range of those seen with Cushing's disease.[857,1368] These findings may lead to the mistaken diagnosis of Cushing's disease and lead to inappropriate pituitary therapy. Although it is not possible to make this differentiation with certainty in all cases, certain features should increase suspicion of the presence of the ectopic ACTH syndrome; these are male sex, rapid onset, severe hypercortisolism, hypokalemia, and weight loss. If the ectopic ACTH syndrome is suspected but no tumor is obvious, selective venous ACTH sampling is helpful; the demonstration of a pituitary venous ACTH gradient establishes the diagnosis of Cushing's disease.[857,1368,1396,1400–1404] In the absence of a pituitary gradient, the ectopic ACTH syndrome is likely, and selective venous sampling may occasionally localize the ACTH-secreting ectopic tumor.[1358,1402] Additional diagnostic imaging procedures should be directed to the common sites of ACTH production: lungs, thymus, pancreas, thyroid, and adrenals.[1397,1398]

Adrenocortical tumors rarely cause diagnostic difficulties, as the ACTH levels are undetectable and the tumor is easily visualized by CT scan. Reproducible suppressibility by dexamethasone has not been documented[874] but might occur with episodic secretion.[1374] Another rare exception is that of an ACTH-secreting adrenal carcinoma.[1405]

Tumor Localization

These procedures are used to localize tumors in Cushing's syndrome and must be integrated with the biochemical tests described previously, as radiologic procedures alone can give misleading results.

In Cushing's disease, MRI of the pituitary is the procedure of choice and is used to define sellar size and anatomy and suprasellar tumor extension. In the 10 to 15 percent of patients with larger tumors (macroadenomas), MRI defines the size of the tumor and may demonstrate extrasellar extension.

The problem of tumor localization in patients with Cushing's disease who have microadenomas has not been solved, and this remains the major difficulty in the differential diagnosis of Cushing's syndrome. MRI is performed with thin sections and gadolinium enhancement, which clearly define normal sellar anatomy. The presence of a convex upper pituitary margin, increased height of the pituitary, deviation of the stalk, and focal "low-intensity" areas are the criteria on which a diagnosis of a pituitary adenoma is based. However, MRI is clearly positive in only approximately 60 percent of patients with Cushing's disease, presumably because adenomas less than 5 mm in diameter are too small to resolve with current techniques. False-positive scans may occur in patients with coincidental nonfunctional pituitary adenomas, intrapituitary cysts, or the empty sella syndrome.[1378,1391]

Selective pituitary venous ACTH sampling is helpful in patients in whom the source of ACTH hypersecretion is in doubt, i.e., when clinical features suggest the ectopic ACTH syndrome, when responses to high-dose dexamethasone or CRH are negative, or when a sellar MRI does not reveal a conclusive adenoma. In these circumstances, venous sampling will establish or exclude the pituitary as the source of ACTH.[1358,1396,1400–1402] The venous system is catheterized by the femoral route; ACTH samples are obtained simultaneously from the inferior petrosal sinuses (a major site of venous drainage of the anterior pituitary) and are compared to simultaneous peripheral vein samples. ACTH gradients are enhanced by CRH stimulation during the procedure.[1396,1403,1404] In patients with Cushing's disease, basal inferior petrosal sinus/peripheral ACTH ratios are usually greater than 2:1 and are greater than 3:1 after CRH administration.[1396,1401] In patients with the ectopic ACTH syndrome, no inferior petrosal/peripheral ACTH gradient is demonstrable. The attempt to lateralize pituitary microadenomas with venous sampling is successful in only about 65 percent of cases, and thus significant exceptions occur.[1391,1396]

CT scans are most commonly used to define adrenal pathology. However, ultrasonography and isotope scanning using radiolabeled cholesterol are also useful.[1223,1380,1381,1406,1407] In patients with ACTH hypersecretion, these procedures exclude an adrenal tumor and confirm bilateral adrenal hyperplasia or nodular adrenal hyperplasia. These procedures also effectively localize adrenal tumors in virtually all cases because these tumors are usually more than 2 cm in diameter (Fig. 11-48). However, nodular hyperplasia of the adrenals with a solitary or dominant nodule can be misinterpreted as an autonomous hyperfunctioning adenoma.[857,1369] Adrenocortical carcinomas do not take up radiolabeled cholesterol.[355,356]

Treatment of Cushing's Syndrome

The treatment of Cushing's syndrome has been improved by advances in pituitary microsurgery and sophisticated radiotherapeutic techniques. Medical therapy is also becoming more effective in controlling ACTH and/or cortisol secretion. The aim of treatment in Cushing's syndrome is to remove or destroy the basic lesion and thus correct hypersecretion of adrenal hormones without inducing permanent pituitary or adrenal deficiencies.

Cushing's Disease

Treatment of Cushing's disease is currently directed at the pituitary to control ACTH hypersecretion; available methods include microsurgery, various forms of radiation therapy, and pharmacologic inhibition of ACTH secretion. Treatment of hypercortisolism per se by surgical or medical adrenalectomy is less commonly used. Because pituitary adenomas in Cushing's disease are frequently not localized by MRI, venous sampling should be used when necessary to confirm the diagnosis.

Transsphenoidal microsurgery is the current procedure of choice for Cushing's disease in both adults and children.[1297,1306,1309,1312,1313,1344–1348] Hypertension and hyperglycemia should be controlled before surgery, and these patients should receive glucocorticoid coverage for surgery according to the protocol described above (see adrenocortical insufficiency). Because the pituitary tumors of Cushing's disease are small and are frequently within the anterior lobe tissue, an experienced surgeon and meticulous exploration of the intrasellar contents are required.[1297,1311–1313] Once identified, the micro- or macroadenoma is selectively removed, and the normal gland is left intact.

Among patients with microadenomas (less than 1 cm in diameter), selective microsurgery is successful in correcting the biochemical abnormalities in approximately 85 percent.[1297,1306,1308,1309,1311–1313,1344,1345] Surgical damage to anterior pituitary function is rare, but the majority of successfully treated patients develop transient secondary adrenocortical insufficiency, which is followed by the recovery of normal pituitary-adrenal function (see previous section on etiology and pathogenesis). In approximately 10 percent the tumor is too small to locate at surgery, and in adult patients hemihypophysectomy on the side of lateralization of the venous sampling or total hypophysectomy may be performed.[1297,1312,1313] Patients with corticotroph hyperplasia obviously do not respond to selective pituitary microsurgery and must be treated with other modalities, as is discussed later.[1324] Unfortunately, current diagnostic procedures cannot identify these patients preoperatively.

Transsphenoidal surgery is successful in only 25 percent of the approximately 10 to 15 percent of patients with Cushing's dis-

A

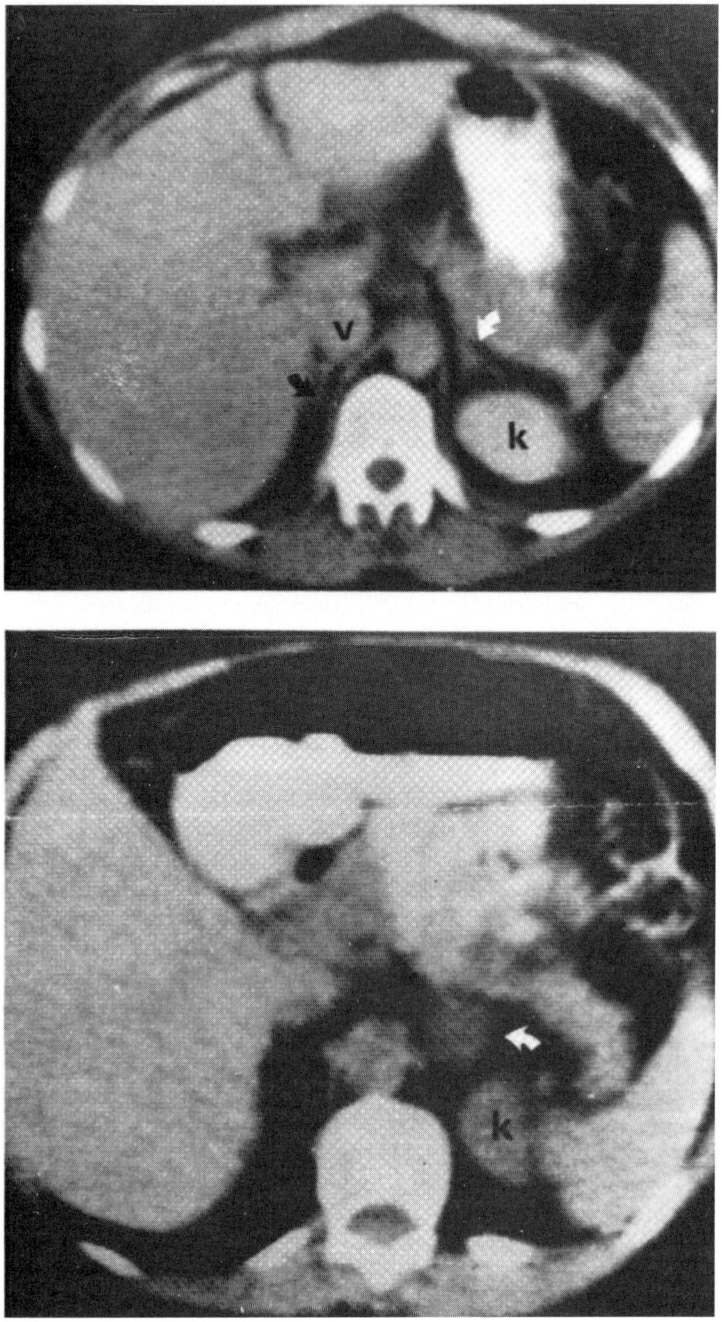

B

FIGURE 11-48. CT scans in Cushing's syndrome. *(A)* A patient with ACTH-dependent Cushing's syndrome. The adrenal glands are not detectably abnormal by this procedure. The curvilinear right adrenal (black arrow) is shown posterior to the inferior vena cava (v) between the right lobe of the liver and the right crus of the diaphragm. The left adrenal (white arrow) has an inverted Y appearance anteromedial to the left kidney (k). *(B)* A 3-cm left adrenal adenoma (white arrow) anteromedial to the left kidney (k). (*From Korobkin et al.*[1223])

ease with pituitary macroadenomas and in those with extrasellar extension of the tumor.[1297,1313,1345,1408] These patients usually require multiple therapies and frequently present difficult problems in management. Rare patients with massive tumors and suprasellar extension may require craniotomy to achieve decompression of the optic chiasm and other vital structures.[1408]

Postoperatively, steroid coverage is reduced to maintenance doses of hydrocortisone (30 mg/day) by the seventh to tenth day. In these patients, who are accustomed to cortisol excess, the steroid withdrawal syndrome (see Chap. 14) may be prominent and may necessitate increased cortisol dosage and slower tapering to maintenance levels. An oCRH stimulation test is recommended on postoperative day 7–10.[1346] It is performed in the morning, while the morning dose of hydrocortisone is withheld to be given at the end of the test. A normal ACTH response predicts a recurrence with a probability of 50 percent. The pituitary-adrenal axis is reevaluated 4 to 6 weeks after surgery to ensure that hypercortisolism has been corrected; other pituitary hormones are also reevaluated at this time. Because the majority of these patients develop transient secondary adrenal insufficiency,[1340] cortisol therapy is required until there is recovery of normal responsiveness of the pituitary-adrenal axis (see earlier section on diagnosis under adrenocortical insufficiency). The complications of selective transsphenoidal microsurgery have been surprisingly few, considering the nature of the metabolic abnormalities in these patients. Transient diabetes insipidus occurs in approximately 20 percent, and there is intra- or postoperative hemorrhage in an occasional patient.[1297,1312,1313,1341,1344,1345] Potential complications such as hypopituitarism, CSF rhinorrhea, infection, meningitis, visual impairment, and oculomotor dysfunction have not materialized in larger series.[1297,1313] Patients undergoing total hypophysectomy develop panhypopituitarism; in these patients, diabetes insipidus may persist. The subsequent management of these patients is discussed in Chaps. 6 and 7 and previously in the section on treatment under adrenocortical insufficiency. Follow-up data in patients with successful surgical removal of microadenomas, although limited, are accumulating; the majority of patients achieve persisting control of Cushing's disease, although in a minority (5–10 percent) it recurs.[1297,1308,1309,1312,1313,1340,1344–1348] Thus, transsphenoidal microsurgery is an effective therapy for Cushing's disease and corrects hypercortisolism with minimal morbidity in the majority of patients with microadenomas.

Heavy particle irradiation of the pituitary is also an effective initial therapy for Cushing's disease, although this technique is currently available in only one center in the United States.[1409] Because the size of the radiation field is limited, these methods are not applicable to patients with either suprasellar or sphenoid sinus extension of the tumor. Alpha particle radiation is effective in controlling hypercortisolism in 80 percent of patients, with an incidence of hypopituitarism of approximately one-third.[1410] Proton beam therapy is effective in 65 percent of patients, and the incidence of hypopituitarism was reported to be 13 percent, although the follow-up period was not reported.[1409] Neurologic complications, including visual loss and oculomotor paralysis, rarely occur.[1409,1410] With both of these techniques there is a lag period of 6 to 12 months before cortisol secretion returns to normal, and as the effects of radiation are prolonged, the incidence of hypopituitarism may increase with further follow-up.

Conventional pituitary irradiation has been used for many years; however, it is effective in only about 30–40 percent of adults.[1307,1402] Additional disadvantages include the prolonged period of time (often 12 to 18 months) before it is effective and the occurrence of posttreatment hypopituitarism, which is increasingly being recognized.[1411] In children, conventional irradiation has been reported to be effective in 80 percent;[1307] however, the potential for hypopituitarism and consequent growth failure must be considered. Because of the limitations of conventional radiotherapy in adults, various other maneuvers have been used to increase its efficiency. Pituitary irradiation combined with unilateral adrenalectomy increases the remission rate to 50 percent; however, this rate does not appear to justify the use of both radiation and a major surgical procedure.[1412] Radiation has also been combined with metyrapone, ketoconazole, or mitotane.[519,1402,1413,1414] These regimens have the advantage of reducing cortisol secretion more rapidly, although it appears that the ultimate response to radiation will still be unsatisfactory and prolonged drug therapy is required. Thus, conventional pituitary irradiation is not recommended as the primary therapy of Cushing's disease. However, this therapy as well as γ-irradiation therapy ("gamma knife") play a definite role in patients who have persisting pituitary hypersecretion of ACTH after transphenoidal microsurgery and those with extrasellar extension of the tumor.[1415]

Implantation of radioactive seeds within the sella turcica has been used in Cushing's disease, although experience is limited.[1308,1416] In the largest reported series, remission occurred in 65 percent of patients with no radiologic evidence of a pituitary tumor; however, in patients with possible tumors and those with definite tumors, remission occurred in only 50 percent and 14 percent, respectively.[1416,1417] Replacement hormone therapy was required in 55 percent for total or partial hypopituitarism, and 5 percent developed CSF rhinorrhea.[1416] The same group reported successful treatment of juvenile Cushing's disease with pituitary implants; remission was attained in each of nine patients, and partial or complete hypopituitarism developed in only two.[1308]

Pharmacologic inhibition of ACTH secretion in Cushing's disease has been attempted with limited success. Cyproheptadine, a serotonin antagonist, and bromocriptine, a dopamine agonist, have been reported to control both ACTH hypersecretion and hypercortisolism in a few cases.[1333,1354,1402] However, to date these agents have been successful in only a minority of patients and cannot be considered a definitive therapy as relapse occurs after their discontinuation.

Treatment of Cushing's disease by bilateral adrenalectomy by the transabdominal or flank approaches was the major form of therapy from the early 1950s until the 1970s. This method has now been largely replaced by therapy directed at the pituitary. Although bilateral adrenalectomy rapidly reverses hypercortisolism, it is accompanied by an operative mortality up to 5 percent, a high incidence of postoperative complications (poor wound healing, infection, pancreatic injury, and thromboembolism), permanent glucocorticoid and mineralocorticoid deficiency, and a recurrence rate of up to 10 percent.[1402,1418] Further, it may be followed by the development of large and progressive pituitary tumors (Nelson's syndrome; see later discussion). The potential lethality and morbidity of bilateral adrenalectomy has been almost completely eliminated with the advent of laparoscopic surgery. Still, adrenalectomy should be used only in the few patients who cannot be treated successfully by other methods.

Pharmacologic agents that inhibit adrenal cortisol secretion are useful in Cushing's disease but mainly as adjunctive therapy[520,524,526,531,1402,1414,1419] (see previous section inhibitors of adrenal steroid biosynthesis). Ketoconazole is the drug of choice and is effective in most patients in doses of 600 to 1,000 mg/day in divided doses.[520,531] Metyrapone and aminoglutethimide inhibit cortisol synthesis, although this is accompanied by increased ACTH levels that may overcome the enzyme inhibition. Adequate data are not available on the long-term use of these agents as the sole treatment of Cushing's disease; relapse occurs after discontinuation. Ketoconazole is generally well tolerated but may cause liver damage. Metyrapone is expensive and causes gastrointestinal side effects. Aminoglutethimide causes somnolence, skin rash, and goiter. Thus, these agents are ordinarily used while one is awaiting a response to therapy or in the preparation of patients for surgery.[1402,1414] More effective control of hypercortisolism with fewer side effects is obtained by the combined use of these agents.[526] The adrenolytic drug mitotane not only inhibits cortisol synthesis but also causes adrenal atrophy, predominantly of the zonae fasciculata and reticularis. It induces remissions in approximately 80 percent of patients with Cushing's disease, but 60 percent relapse after the cessation of therapy.[524] Approximately 60 percent of these patients experience gastrointestinal side effects; other side effects include somnolence, depression, and skin rash. The high rate of relapse after treatment usually necessitates more definitive therapy.[524]

Ectopic ACTH Syndrome

Therapy for the ectopic ACTH syndrome is difficult in the setting of metastatic malignancy and the accompanying severe hypercortisolism. Although therapy is directed at the primary tumor, this is usually unsuccessful and other means must be used to correct the steroid excess state. Because severe hypokalemia may be present, it may be necessary to administer potassium replacement in large doses and spironolactone to block mineralocorticoid effects. Drugs that block steroid synthesis, including ketoconazole, metyrapone, and aminoglutethimide, are more useful in this situation, as in the ectopic ACTH syndrome plasma ACTH levels usually do not increase in response to the lowered cortisol levels.[1419] Because these drugs may produce hypoadrenalism, steroid secretion must be monitored and replacement steroids must be given if necessary. In this setting, mitotane is less useful because of its slow onset of action and because several weeks may be required to control cortisol secretion. Bilateral adrenalectomy rarely may be required if hypercortisolism cannot otherwise be controlled. Lasting cure of the ectopic ACTH syndrome is usually possible only in tumors such as carcinoids or in pheochromocytomas, which are frequently benign.[939,1358,1362,1368]

Adrenal Tumors

Benign adrenal adenomas are successfully treated by unilateral adrenalectomy; the outlook is excellent. Because the hypothalamic-pituitary axis and the contralateral adrenal are suppressed by the prolonged autonomous cortisol secretion, these patients have postoperative adrenal insufficiency.[1420] Thus, they require glucocorticoid but usually not mineralocorticoid therapy both during and after surgery, until the remaining adrenal recovers. This usually requires 6 to 12 months but may take as long as 2 years.[1420]

Therapy for adrenocortical carcinoma is less satisfactory; the majority of patients have metastases at the time of diagnosis, usually to the retroperitoneum, liver, and lungs.[1305,1355,1421] Surgery is the first step in therapy and the only therapeutic modality that prolongs survival. Although surgical cure is rare, it serves to reduce the tumor mass and the degree of steroid hypersecretion. Curative surgery should be accompanied by essentially absent steroid secretion, as the hypothalamic-pituitary axis and the contralateral adrenal are suppressed. Persisting nonsuppressible steroid secretion in the immediate postoperative period indicates a residual or metastatic tumor. When metastatic or residual disease is present, mitotane is the drug of choice.[1422] It is administered in doses of 6 to 12 g per day; however, the dose must be reduced because of side effects in 80 percent of patients (diarrhea, nausea, vomiting, depression, somnolence). Approximately 60 percent of these patients display a reduction of steroid secretion, but only 35 percent show a reduction in tumor size.[1421,1422] Because mitotane elevates CBG concentrations in plasma and reduces urinary 17-OHCS excretion by altering the hepatic metabolism of cortisol, these patients should be followed up with urinary free cortisol assays. It should be noted that mitotane does not prolong survival of patients with adrenocortical cancer. Ketoconazole, metyrapone, and/or aminoglutethimide are useful in controlling steroid hypersecretion in patients who do not respond to mitotane. Radiotherapy and conventional chemotherapy have not been useful in treating this disease.

Nelson's Syndrome

Nelson's syndrome involves the appearance or clinical progression of an ACTH-secreting pituitary adenoma after bilateral adrenalectomy for Cushing's disease.[1317,1423] Because pituitary adenomas are present in the majority of patients with untreated Cushing's disease, it is presumed that the tumors of Nelson's syndrome are due to progressive growth of preexisting pituitary adenomas. It is possible that the hypercortisolism in untreated patients restrains not only ACTH secretion but also growth of the adenoma. That ACTH secretion in Cushing's disease is restrained by the circulating cortisol levels is demonstrated by its stimulation with metyrapone. Further, the tumors in Nelson's syndrome are dexamethasone-suppressible, although larger doses may be required than with untreated Cushing's disease.[911] Thus, after adrenalectomy, the suppressive effect of cortisol is no longer present, ACTH secretion increases, and the adenoma may progress. Conventional pituitary irradiation before or after adrenalectomy does not prevent the development of Nelson's syndrome, and it may rarely occur after heavy particle irradiation.[1410,1424]

The incidence of Nelson's syndrome ranges from 5 to 78 percent in reported series.[1424–1426] It is higher in series studied with immunoreactive plasma ACTH levels and more sophisticated radiologic techniques.[1425,1426] Up to 30 percent of patients adrenalectomized for Cushing's disease have been found to develop classic Nelson's syndrome. Another 50 percent develop evidence of a microadenoma without marked progression, and about 20 percent never develop a progressive pituitary tumor. The reasons for these differences in clinical behavior are unknown and have not been predictable. Thus, patients who have undergone bilateral adrenalectomy for Cushing's disease require continuous observation by means of plasma ACTH assay, sellar radiology, and visual field examinations so that pituitary tumors may be diagnosed and treated early.

The tumors in patients with classic Nelson's syndrome are among the most aggressive and rapidly growing of all pituitary tumors.[1314] These patients present with hyperpigmentation similar to but generally more severe than that seen in Addison's disease and the manifestations of an expanding intrasellar mass lesion, usually within months to 2 years after adrenalectomy. Sellar enlargement, extrasellar extension, headache, visual field defects, and hypopituitarism are common.[1314] Invasion of the cavernous sinus or cranial fossae may lead to extraocular muscle palsies and other neurologic defects.[1314] These tumors can occasionally be frankly malignant with local invasion and extracranial metastases, and there is a high incidence of pituitary apoplexy (spontaneous hemorrhagic infarction of the tumor).[1314] The diagnosis is usually obvious from the history of bilateral adrenalectomy followed by hyperpigmentation and the manifestations of an expanding pituitary tumor. Plasma ACTH levels are markedly elevated, usually to more than 1,000 pg/ml, and levels not infrequently are higher than 10,000 pg/ml.[875] MRI is used to define the extent of tumor growth and the response to therapy.

These tumors are treated by pituitary surgery and radiotherapy. Larger tumors, especially those with extrasellar extension, are frequently unresectable at surgery by either transsphenoidal or craniotomy approaches. Conventional radiation alone is satisfactory in only a minority of patients but should nonetheless be used postoperatively in patients with residual or extrasellar tumor extension, in whom it may prevent progression.

Patients adrenalectomized for Cushing's disease who develop pituitary microadenomas generally present later and usually have a slower course accompanied by mild to moderate hyperpigmentation and plasma ACTH levels in the range of 500 to 4,000 pg/ml.[1425,1426] The sella turcica is usually normal in size; however,

MRI reveals a pituitary microadenoma.[1426] Extrasellar extension, visual defects, headache, and panhypopituitarism are unusual.[1426] Spontaneous remission has occurred in such a patient ("silent pituitary apoplexy").[1427] Transsphenoidal microsurgery or irradiation is somewhat more successful in these patients with microadenomas. Although hyperpigmentation resolves, plasma ACTH levels frequently remain modestly elevated.

Patients who never manifest evidence of a progressive pituitary tumor after adrenalectomy for Cushing's syndrome do not develop hyperpigmentation or abnormal pituitary function. However, plasma ACTH levels in these patients are mildly elevated in the range of 100 to 500 pg/ml and are not normally suppressible with low doses of dexamethasone.

Prognosis

Untreated Cushing's syndrome is frequently a fatal illness. Mortality may be due to the underlying tumor itself, as in the ectopic ACTH syndrome and adrenal carcinoma. However, in many cases, death is a consequence of sustained hypercortisolism and its complications, including hypertension, cardiovascular disease, stroke, thromboembolism, and susceptibility to infection.[1296,1418] Thus, in a series reported in 1952, 50 percent of the patients died within 5 years of the onset of the disease.[1296] In a recent Spanish study, the relative risk for coronary heart disease in Cushing syndrome is elevated 5 times, predicting a loss of more than 30 years of life expectancy.

With current refinements in pituitary microsurgery and irradiation, the great majority of patients with Cushing's disease can be treated successfully and the operative mortality and morbidity that attended bilateral adrenalectomy are no longer present. Although there is currently no statistical information regarding survival in these patients, it appears that they live considerably longer. Patients with Cushing's disease who have large pituitary tumors at the time of diagnosis and those with Nelson's syndrome have a considerably less satisfactory prognosis and may die as a consequence of tumor invasion and persisting hypercortisolism.[1314]

The prognosis in adrenal adenomas is excellent.[1421] In adrenal carcinoma, the prognosis is almost universally poor and the median survival from the onset of symptoms is approximately 4 years.[1305,1421]

The prognosis is also poor in patients with ectopic ACTH syndrome due to malignant tumors. In these patients with severe hypercortisolism, survival is frequently only weeks.[1299,1364] However, a minority of patients respond to tumor resection or chemotherapy.[1362] The prognosis is better in those with benign tumors producing the ectopic ACTH syndrome.[857,939,1368]

Hyperaldosteronism

Hyperaldosteronism (aldosteronism) can occur as a "primary" adrenal problem or can be secondary to other metabolic derangements that stimulate its release.

Primary Hyperaldosteronism

Primary hyperaldosteronism (primary aldosteronism) results from adrenal tumors or from a hyperplastic adrenal glomerulosa and leads to hypertension and hypokalemia, as discussed in detail in Chap. 13.

Secondary Hyperaldosteronism

Secondary hyperaldosteronism due to stimulation of the adrenal glomerulosa by extraadrenal factors (usually the renin-angiotensin system) is classified in Table 11-28. It can be physiologic or can contribute to the pathology of disease states.

The factors that stimulate the renin-angiotensin system and the influences of aldosterone are discussed in preceding sections and in Chap. 13. The role of increased aldosterone in chronic hyperkalemia[819,821] has been discussed in the section on physiologic actions of mineralocorticoids. Secondary hyperaldosteronism can occasionally occur on an iatrogenic basis as a result of oral contraceptive use (see Chap. 13).

Extrarenal Sodium Loss and Sodium Restriction

In these circumstances (Table 11-28 and Chap. 13), activation of the renin-angiotensin-aldosterone system serves to correct the deficiency by conserving sodium ion with minimal potassium wasting.[1428]

Changes in Aldosterone during the Menstrual Cycle and Pregnancy

Modest increases in plasma renin, angiotensin, and aldosterone concentrations occur during the luteal phase of the menstrual cycle and could be due to the marked increase (10- to 20-fold) in the

TABLE 11-28. Classification of Secondary Hyperaldosteronism

Primary Abnormality	Potassium Loss	Edema	Hypertension	Effect of Sodium Load
Extrarenal sodium loss (e.g., from hemorrhage, thermal stress, or gastrointestinal loss)	Absent	Absent	Absent	Repairs deficit
Sodium restriction	Absent	Absent	Absent	Repairs deficit
Abnormal distribution of sodium excess (e.g., from congestive heart failure, nephrotic syndrome, cirrhosis with ascites, or idiopathic edema)	Present	Present	Absent	Worsens edema
Abnormal renal electrolyte loss (e.g., from salt-losing renal disease,* Bartter's syndrome, diuretic abuse, or renal tubular acidosis)	Present	Absent	Absent	Variable
Other renal lesions (e.g., renal artery stenosis, unilateral renal ischemia, accelerated hypertension, renin-secreting tumor, or chronic renal failure*)	Present	Absent	Present	May worsen hypertension
Excessive potassium intake	Present	Absent	Absent	May facilitate kaliuresis
Luteal phase of menstrual cycle and pregnancy	Absent	May be present	Usually present	Suppresses renin and aldosterone

*Exception; no potassium loss.

plasma progesterone level.[1274] The mineralocorticoid antagonist properties of progesterone block mineralocorticoid action, promoting sodium loss and in turn stimulating renin release.[1275] Levels of estrogens that induce renin substrate (Chap. 13) are also increased, but this has not been shown to be a significant factor.[1275] The increased aldosterone concentration may contribute to the pathogenesis of premenstrual edema, but this is difficult to conceive of if the increased aldosterone concentration is secondary to natriuresis. Further, there is no correlation between the severity of edema and the levels of renin and aldosterone.[1275]

Aldosterone secretion increases progressively during normal pregnancy, although its physiologic significance is not known.[1274,1429] It is of maternal origin, is increased by the fifteenth week of gestation, and reaches levels in the third trimester 10 times those of nonpregnant women. The aldosterone contributes to sodium retention as blockade of aldosterone production by heparin results in natriuresis.[1274] The increased renin levels may be due to the decrease in blood pressure that occurs in early pregnancy because of decreased systemic vascular resistance.[1429] In addition, particularly in late pregnancy, progesterone levels are high and may further increase renin release by the mechanisms discussed earlier.[1274] However, renin levels are elevated more during the first trimester, whereas plasma aldosterone levels are highest during the third trimester.[1274] This may be due to a progressive increase in the sensitivity of the glomerulosa to angiotensin II, caused by either chronic exposure to angiotensin II (Chaps. 4 and 13) or to possible or unidentified factors, such as placental αMSH. Whereas there is increased sodium retention in pregnancy, potassium loss does not occur.[1274] This suggests that a functional mineralocorticoid excess state is not present and that activation of the renin-angiotensin-aldosterone system is a compensatory response to other changes.

Because the renin-angiotensin-aldosterone axis is activated in pregnancy, there has been considerable interest in whether this contributes to the hypertension, edema, and other manifestations of toxemia.[1274] If anything, levels of the components of the renin-angiotensin-aldosterone axis are decreased rather than increased in toxemia, although this condition is associated with an increased sensitivity to angiotensin II.[1274,1429] However, certain of the changes observed in toxemia (e.g., reduced uterine blood flow) are opposite to those elicited by angiotensin II (which leads to vasodilatation and increased blood flow in the uterine circulation, in contrast to its effects in other vascular beds; Chap. 13).[1274]

Abnormal Distribution of Sodium Excess

The renin-angiotensin-aldosterone system is only one of several factors involved in the pathogenesis of edema.[1274,1428] In untreated patients with congestive heart failure, aldosterone excess is not consistently present, although it might be argued that normal aldosterone levels are inappropriate. In severe congestive failure, aldosterone excess may result from increased production as well as decreased clearance. Overall, aldosterone levels in congestive heart failure result from the counterbalancing influences of decreased renal perfusion due to decreased cardiac output that increases renin and aldosterone release and subsequent sodium retention that tends to suppress renin and aldosterone levels.

Secondary hyperaldosteronism ordinarily occurs when there is significant hypoalbuminemia and decreased plasma oncotic pressure associated with the nephrotic syndrome. Although aldosterone is only one factor, it appears to play a role in the sodium retention that occurs.

In liver disease with ascites, renin and aldosterone concentrations are commonly elevated, but this is unusual in cirrhosis without ascites. There appears to be general agreement that mineralocorticoid excess plays at most a small role in the initial development of ascites. The stimulus to renin release appears to be an effectively decreased arterial volume due to abnormal transudation of fluid from the vascular compartment. The increased renin level promotes aldosterone production; aldosterone levels rise, and this is accentuated by the decreased clearance of aldosterone in this condition. The increased aldosterone concentration further promotes sodium retention and potassium loss; the sodium retention can be more marked than in other circumstances, because escape fails to occur in these patients, probably as a result of the lack of retention of the excess sodium in the intravascular space. Thus, in this condition, the administration of aldosterone antagonists can be particularly beneficial.

Aldosterone has been implicated in the pathogenesis of idiopathic edema, a form of dependent edema that occurs in women who do not have a history of heart, liver, kidney, or venous disease. These patients have an increased incidence of impaired carbohydrate tolerance and may be emotionally disturbed or may have history of allergy, subtle abnormalities in albumin metabolism with slightly low serum albumin concentrations, capillary permeability defects, and occasionally abnormalities in the sympathetic nervous system. The diagnosis is made by exclusion of other causes of edema; these causes are commonly unveiled during the evaluation. Although aldosterone excretion is usually in the normal range, it has been argued that the values found are inappropriate relative to the increased extracellular fluid volume and that these patients do not adequately escape from the sodium-retaining actions of the mineralocorticoids. However, the syndrome has been described in addisonian patients with very low aldosterone levels and no specific mineralocorticoid replacement. Thus, this syndrome may not be a single entity, and the various defects described previously could contribute to the pathogenesis. In any event, it is unlikely that aldosterone is primarily responsible, as this syndrome differs significantly from primary aldosteronism, in which edema does not usually occur (Chap. 13). The edema ordinarily responds to conservative measures such as bed rest, use of elastic stockings, limitation of sodium intake, caloric restriction, intermittent diuretic use, and administration of aldosterone antagonists.

Abnormal Renal Electrolyte Loss

The renin-angiotensin-aldosterone system is stimulated by excessive salt loss by the kidney resulting from salt-losing nephropathy, Bartter's syndrome, excessive diuretic use, or renal tubular acidosis. In these syndromes, the compensatory increase in aldosterone level does not correct the loss, but because there is increased sodium delivery to the distal nephron, aldosterone can accelerate potassium loss.[1428]

Bartter's Syndrome

Bartter's syndrome is characterized by increased renin, angiotensin II, and aldosterone concentrations; hypokalemia and alkalosis; normal blood pressure; absence of edema; and hyperplasia of the renal juxtaglomerular cells.[1275,1430] In addition, there is decreased pressor responsiveness to angiotensin II, vasopressin-resistant impairment in urinary concentrating ability, variably decreased pressor responsiveness to IV norepinephrine, hypomagnesemia, hyperuricemia, and increased amounts of urinary PGE_2.

Other Renal Lesions

Hyperaldosteronism can occur with renal artery stenosis, unilateral renal ischemia, accelerated hypertension, and renin-secreting tumors. These disorders are associated with hypertension and are discussed in Chap. 13.

REFERENCES

1. Miller WL: Congenital adrenal hyperplasia in the adult patient. *Adv Int Med* 44:155–173, 1999.
2. Baxter JD: Cortisone and the adrenal cortex. *Trans Assoc Am Physicians* 100:clxvii, 1987.
3. Gaunt R: History of the adrenal cortex, in Greep RO, Astwood EB (eds): *Handbook of Physiology: Endocrinology. Washington DC, American Physiological Society* section 7, vol 6, p 1, 1975.
4. Fine LG: Eustachio's discovery of the renal tubule. *Am J Nephrol* 6:47, 1986.
5. Cushing H: The basophil adenomas of the pituitary body and their clinical manifestations. *Bull Johns Hopkins Hosp* 50:137, 1932.
6. Cori CF, Cori GT: The fate of sugar in the animal body: VII. The carbohydrate metabolism of adrenalectomized rats and mice. *J Biol Chem* 74:473, 1927.
7. Britton SW, Silvette H: The apparent prepotent function of the adrenal glands. *Am J Physiol* 100:701, 1932.
8. Long CNH, Katzin B, Fry EG: The adrenal cortex and carbohydrate metabolism. *Endocrinology* 26:39, 1940.
9. Banman EJ, Kurland S: Changes in the inorganic constituents of blood in supradrenalectomized cats and rabbits. *J Biol Chem* 71:281, 1927.
10. Loeb EG: Effect of sodium chloride in treatment of a patient with Addison's disease. *Proc Soc Exp Biol* 30:808, 1933.
11. Selye H: The general adaptation syndrome and the diseases of adaptation. *J Clin Endocrinol* 6:117, 1946.
12. McCann SM, Brobeck JR: Evidence for a role of the supraoptico-hypophyseal system in regulation of adrenaocorticotrophin secretion. *Proc Soc Exp Biol Med* 87:318, 1954.
13. Saffran M, Schally AV, Benfrey BG: Stimulation of the release of corticotrophin from the adenohypophysis by a neurohypophysical factor. *Endocrinology* 57:439, 1955.
14. Guillemin R, Rosenberg B: Humoral hypothalamic control of anterior pituitary: A study with combined tissue cultures. *Endocrinology* 57:599, 1955.
15. Spiess J, Rivier J, Rivier C, Vale W: Primary structure of corticotrophin-releasing factor from bovine hypothalamus. *Proc Natl Acad Sci USA* 78:6517, 1981.
16. Fasciolo JC: Historical background of the renin angiotensin system, in Genest J, Koiw E, Kuchel E (eds): *Hypertension*. New York, McGraw-Hill, 1977, p 134.
17. Conn JH: Primary aldosteronism. *J Lab Clin Med* 45:661, 1955.
18. Kendall EC, Mason HL, McKenzie BF, Myers CS, Koelsche GA: Isolation in crystalline form of the hormone essential to life from the supranetal cortex: Its chemical nature and physiologic properties. *Trans Assoc Am Physicians* 49:147, 1934.
19. Steiger M, Reichstein T: Desoxy-cortico-steron (21-oxyprogesterone) aus Δ 5-3-xoy-atio-cholensaure. *Helv Chim Acta* 20:1164, 1937.
20. Hench PS, Kendall EC, Slocumb CH, Polley HF: The effect of a hormone of the adrenal cortex (17-hydroxy-11-dehydrocorticosterone compound E) and of pituitary adrenocorticotropic hormone on rheumatoid arthritis. *Proc Staff Meet Mayo Clin* 24:181, 1949.
21. Wilkins L, Lewis RA, Klein R, Rosenberg E: The supression of androgen secretion by cortisone in a case of congenital adrenal hyperplasia. *Bull Johns Hopkins Hosp* 86:249, 1950.
22. Bartter FC, Forbes AO, Leaf A: Congenital adrenal hyperplasia associated with the adrenogenital syndrome: An attempt to correct its disordered hormonal pattern. *J Clin Invest* 29:797, 1950.
23. Cooper DY, Levin S, Narasimhulu S, Rosenthal O, Estabrook RW: Photochemical action spectrum of the terminal oxidase of mixed function oxidase systems. *Science* 145:400, 1965.
24. Miller WL: Molecular biology of steroid hormone synthesis. *Endocr Rev* 9:295, 1988.
25. Evans RM: The steroid and thyroid hormone receptor superfamily. *Science* 240:889, 1988.
26. Netter FH: Endocrine system and selected metabolic diseases, in *Ciba Collection of Medical Illustrations*. Summitt, NY, Ciba Pharmaceutical 4:77, 1965.
27. Langman J: *Medical Embryology*. Baltimore, Wilkins & Wilkins, 1963.
28. Mesiano S, Coulter CL, Jaffe RB: Localization of cytochrome P450 cholesterol side-chain cleavage, cytochrome P450 17α-hydroxylase/17,20 lyase, and 3β-hydroxysteroid dehydrogenase-isomerase steroidogenic enzymes in human and rhesus monkey fetal adrenal glands: Reappraisal of functional zonation. *J Clin Endocrinol Metab* 77:1184, 1993.
29. Neville AM, Mackay AM: The structure of the human adrenal cortex in health and disease. *Clin Endocrinol Metab* 1:361, 1972.
30. Dallman MF: Control of adrenocortical growth in vivo. *Endocr Rev* 10:213, 1985.
31. Marusic ET, Mulrow PJ: In vitro conversion of corticosterone 4-14C to 18-hydroxycorticosterone by zona fasciculata-reticularis of beef adrenal. *Endocrinology* 80:214, 1967.
32. Oshima T, Suzuki H, Hata JI, Mitani F, Ishmura Y: Zone-specific expression of aldosterone synthase cytochrome P450 and cytochrome P45011β in rat adrenal cortex: Histochemical basis for the functional zonation. *Endocrinology* 130:2971, 1992.
33. Voutilainen R, Miller WL: Coordinate tropic hormone regulation of mRNAs for insulin-like growth factor II and the cholesterol side-chain cleavage enzyme, P450scc, in human steroidogenic tissues. *Proc Natl Acad Sci USA* 84:1590, 1987.
34. Townsend S, Dallman MF, Miller WL: Rat insulin-like growth factors-I and -II mRNAs are unchanged during compensatory adrenal growth but decrease during ACTH-induced adrenal growth. *J Biol Chem* 265:22117, 1990.
35. Voutilainen R, Miller WL: Developmental and hormonal regulation of mRNAs for insulin-like growth factor and steroidogenic enzymes in human fetal adrenals and gonads. *DNA* 7:9, 1988.
36. Mesiano S, Mellon SH, Gospodarowicz D, Di Blasio AM, Jaffe RB: Basic fibroblast growth factor expression is regulated by corticotropin in the human fetal adrenal: A model for adrenal growth regulation. *Proc Natl Acad Sci USA* 88:5428, 1991.
37. Mesiano S, Mellon SH, Jaffe RB: Mitogenic action, regulation, and localization of insulin-like growth factors in the human fetal adrenal gland. *J Clin Endocrinol Metab* 76:968, 1993.
38. Solish SB, Goldsmith MA, Voutilainen R, Miller WL: Molecular characterization of a Leydig cell tumor presenting as congenital adrenal hyperplasia. *J Clin Endocrinol Metab* 69:1148, 1989.
39. Brown MS, Kovanen PT, Goldstein JL: Receptor-mediated uptake of lipoprotein-cholesterol and its utilization for steroid synthesis in the adrenal cortex. *Rec Prog Horm Res* 35:215, 1979.
40. Gwynne JT, Strauss JF III: The role of lipoproteins in steroidogenesis and cholesterol metabolism in steroidogenic glands. *Endocr Rev* 3:299, 1982.
41. Hechter O, Solomon MM, Zaffaroni A, Pincus G: Transformation of cholesterol and acetate to adrenal cortical hormones. *Arch Biochem Biophys* 46:201, 1953.
42. Ohashi M, Carr BR, Simpson ER: Binding of high density lipoprotein to human fetal adrenal membrane fractions. *Endocrinology* 109:783, 1981.
43. Strauss JF III, Miller WL: Molecular basis of ovarian steroid synthesis, in Hillier S (ed): *Ovarian Endocrinology*. Oxford, UK, Blackwell Scientific, 1991, pp 25–72.
44. Illingsworth DR, Keny TA, Orwoll ES: Adrenal function in heterozygous and homozygous hypobetalipoproteinemia. *J Clin Endocrinol Metab* 54:27, 1982.
45. Mason JI, Rainey WE: Steroidogenesis in the human fetal adrenal: A role for cholesterol synthesized de novo. *J Clin Endocrinol Metab* 64, 1987.
46. Laue L, Hoeg JM, Barnes K, Loriaux DL, Chrousos GP: The effect of mevinolin on steroidogenesis in patients with defects in the LDL receptor pathway. *J Clin Endocrinol Metab* 64:531, 1987.
47. Golos TJ, Strauss JF III: 8-bromo adenosine cyclic 3′5′ phosphate rapidly increases 3-hydroxy-3-methylglutaryl coenzyme A reductase mRNA in human granulosa cells: Role of cellular sterol balance in controlling the response to tropic stimulation. *Biochemistry* 27:3503, 1988.

48. Bolte E, Coudert W, Lefebvre Y: Steroid production from plasma cholesterol II. *In vivo* conversion of plasma cholesterol to ovarian progesterone and adrenal C19 and C21 steroids in humans. *J Clin Endocrinol Metab* 38:394, 1974.
49. Glass C, Pittman RC, Civen M, Steinberg D: Uptake of high density lipoprotein-associated apoliprotein A-I and cholesterol esters by 16 tissues of the rat *in vivo* and by adrenal cells and hepatocytes in vitro. *J Biol Chem* 260:744, 1985.
50. Mellon-Nussbaum S, Ponticorvo L, Liebermann S: Characterization of the lipoidal derivatives of prenenolone prepared by incubation of the steroid with adrenal mitochondria. *J Biol Chem* 257:5678, 1979.
51. Mellon-Nussbaum S, Ponticorvo L, Schaltz F, Hochberg RB: Estradiol fatty acid esters: The isolation and identification of the lipoidal derivative of estradiol synthesized in the bovine uterus. *J Biol Chem* 257:5678, 1982.
52. Beins DM, Vining R, Balasubramaniam S: Regulation of neutral cholesterol esterase and acyl-CoA: Cholesterol acetyltransferase in the rat adrenal gland. *Biochem J* 202:631, 1982.
53. Suckling KE, Tocher DR, Smelhe CG, Boyd GS: In vitro regulation of bovine adrenal cortical acyl-CoA: Cholesterol acyltransferase and comparison with rat liver enzyme. *Biochem J* 202:631, 1983.
54. Anderson RA, Sando GN: Cloning and expression of cDNA encoding human lysosomal acid lypase/cholesterol ester hyrolase. *J Biol Chem* 266:22479, 1991.
55. Colbran RJ, Garton AJ, Cordle SR, Yeaman SJ: Regulation of cholesterol ester hydrolase by cyclic AMP-dependent protein kinase. *FEBS Lett* 201:257, 1986.
56. Pedersen RC, Brownie AC, Ling N: Pro-adrenocorticotrophin/endorphin derived peptides: Cooridinate action on adrenal steroidogenesis. *Science* 208:1044, 1980.
57. Scallen TJ, Noland BJ, Gavey KL, Bass NM, Ockner RK, Chanderbhan R, Vahouny GV: Sterol carrier protein 2 and fatty acid-binding protein: Separate and distinct physiological functions. *J Biol Chem* 260:4733, 1985.
58. Chandebhan R, Noland BJ, Scallen TJ, Vahouny GV: Sterol carrier protein 2: Delivery of cholesterol from adrenal lipid droplets to mitochondria for pregnenolone synthesis. *J Biol Chem* 257:8928, 1982.
59. Vahouny GV, Chanderbhan RF, Kharroubi A, Noland BJ, Pastuszyn A, Scallen TJ: Sterol carrier and lipid transfer proteins. *Adv Lipid Res* 22:83, 1987.
60. Trzeciak WH, Simpson ER, Scallen TJ, Vahouny GV, Waterman MR: Studies on the synthesis of sterol carrier protein 2 in rat adrenocortical cells in monolayer culture. Regulation by ACTH and dibutyryl cyclic 3′,5′-AMP. *J Biol Chem* 262:3713, 1987.
61. Vahouny GV, Chanderbhan R, Noland BJ, Irwin D, Dennis P, Labmeth JD, Scallen TJ: Sterol carrier protein 2: Identification of adrenal sterol carrier protein 2 and site of action for mitochondrial cholesterol utilization. *J Biol Chem* 258:11731, 1983.
62. McNamara BC, Jefcoate CR: The role of sterol carrier protein 2 in stimulation of steroidogenesis in rat adrenal mitochondria by adrenal cytosol. *Arch Biochem Biophys* 275:53, 1989.
63. Yamamoto R, Calen CB, Babalola GO, Rennert H, Bilheimer JT, Strauss JF III: Cloning and expression of a cDNA encoding human sterol carrier protein 2. *Proc Natl Acad Sci USA* 88:463, 1991.
64. Moore CCD, Miller WL: The role of transcriptional regulation in steroid hormone biosynthesis. *J Steroid Biochem Mol Biol* 40:517, 1991.
65. Hum DW, Miller WL: Transcriptional regulation of human genes for steroidogenic enzymes. *Clin Chem* 39:333, 1993.
66. Simpson ER: Cholesterol side-chain cleavage, cytochrome P450, and the control of steroidogenesis. *Mol Cell Endocrinol* 13:213, 1979.
67. Ferguson JJ: Protein synthesis and adrenocorticotropin responsiveness. *J Biol Chem* 238:2754, 1963.
68. Garren LD, Ney RL, Davis WW: Studies on the role of protein synthesis in the regulation of corticosterone production by ACTH *in vivo*. *Proc Natl Acad Sci USA* 53:1443, 1965.
69. Stocco DM, Clark BJ: Regulation of the acute production of steroids in steroidogenic cells. *Endocr Rev* 17:221, 1996.
70. Papadopoulos V: Peripheral-type benzodiazepine/diazepam binding inhibitor receptor: Biological role in steroidogenic cell function. *Endocr Rev* 14:222, 1993.
71. Krueger RJ, Orme-Johnson NR: Acute adrenocorticotropic hormone stimulation of adrenal corticosteroidogenesis. *J Biol Chem* 258:10159, 1983.
72. Pon LA, Orme-Johnson NR: Acute stimulation of steroidogenesis in corpus luteum and adrenal cortex by peptide hormones. *J Biol Chem* 261:6594, 1986.
73. Pon LA, Hartigan JA, Orme-Johnson NR: Acute ACTH regulation of adrenal corticosteroid biosynthesis: rapid accumulation of a phosphoprotein. *J Biol Chem* 261:13309, 1986.
74. Alberta JA, Epstein LF, Pon LA, Orme-Johnson NR: Mitochondrial localization of a phosphoprotein that rapidly accumulates in adrenal cortex cells exposed to adrenocorticotropic hormone or to cAMP. *J Biol Chem* 264:2368, 1989.
75. Stocco DM, Sodeman TC: The 30 kDa mitochondrial protein induced by hormone stimulation in MA-10 mouse Leydig tumor cells are processed from larger precursors. *J Biol Chem* 266:19731, 1991.
76. Epstein LF, Orme-Johnson NR: Regulation of steroid hormone biosynthesis: Identification of precursors of a phosphoprotein targeted to the mitochondrion in stimulated rat adrenal cortex cells. *J Biol Chem* 266:19739, 1991.
77. Clark BJ, Wells J, King SR, Stocco DM: The purification, cloning and expression of a novel luteinizing hormone-induced mitochondrial protein in MA-10 mouse Leydig tumor cells. Characterization of the steroidogenic acute regulatory protein (StAR). *J Biol Chem* 269:28314, 1994.
78. Lin D, Sugawara T, Strauss JF III, Clark BJ, Stocco DM, Saenger P, Rogol A, Miller WL: Role of steroidogenic acute regulatory protein in adrenal and gonadal steroidogenesis. *Science* 267:1828, 1995.
79. Bose HS, Sugawara T, Strauss JF III, Miller WL: The pathophysiology and genetics of congenital lipoid adrenal hyperplasia. *N Engl J Med* 335:1870, 1996.
80. Sugawara T, Holt JA, Driscoll D, Strauss JF III, Lin D, Miller WL, Patterson D, Clancy KP, et al: Human steroidogenic acute regulatory protein (StAR): Functional activity in COS-1 cells, tissue-specific expression, and mapping of the structural gene to 8p11.2 and an expressed pseudogene to chromosome 13. *Proc Natl Acad Sci USA* 92:4778, 1995a.
81. Moog-Lutz C, Tomasetto C, Régnier CH, Wendling C, Lutz Y, Muller D, Chenard MP, Basset P, et al: MLN64 exhibits homology with the steroidogenic acute regulatory protein (StAR) and is over-expressed in human breast carcinomas. *Int J Cancer* 71:183, 1997.
82. Watari H, Arakane F, Moog-Lutz C, Callen CB, Tomasetto C, Gerton GL, Rio MC, Baker ME, et al: MLN64 contains a domain with homology to the steroidogenic acute regulatory protein (StAR) that stimulates steroidogenesis. *Proc Natl Acad Sci USA* 94:8462, 1997.
82a. Bose HS, Whittal RM, Huang MC, Baldwin MA, Miller WL: N-218 MLN64, a protein with StAR-like steroidogenic activity, is folded and cleaved similarly to StAR. *Biochemistry* 39:11722, 2000.
82b. Tsujishita Y, Hurley JH: Structure and lipid transport mechanism of a StAR-related domain. *Nature Struct Biol* 7:408, 2000.
83. Miller WL: Congenital lipoid adrenal hyperplasia: The human gene knockout of the steroidogenic acute regulatory protein. *J Mol Endocrinol* 17:227, 1997.
84. King SR, Ronen-Fuhrmann T, Timberg R, Clark BJ, Orly J, Stocco DM: Steroid production after in vitro transcription, translation, and mitochondrial processing of protein products of complementary deoxyribonucleic acid for steroidogenic acute regulatory protein. *Endocrinology* 136:5165, 1995.
85. Arakane F, Sugawara T, Nishino H, Liu Z, Holt JA, Pain D, Stocco DM, Miller WL, et al: Steroidogenic acute regulatory protein (StAR) retains activity in the absence of its mitochondrial targeting sequence: Implications for the mechanism of StAR action. *Proc Natl Acad Sci USA* 93:13731, 1996.
86. Arakane F, Kallen CB, Watari H, Foster JA, Sepuri NBV, Pain D, Stayrook SE, Lewis M, et al: The mechanism of action of steroidogenic acute regulatory protein (StAR): StAR acts on the outside of mitochondria to stimulate steroidogenesis. *J Biol Chem* 273:16339, 1998.

87. Miller WL, Strauss JF III: Molecular pathology and mechanism of action of the steroidogenic acute regulatory protein, StAR. *J Steroid Biochem Mol Biol* 69:131, 1999.
88. Bose HS, Whittal RM, Baldwin MA, Miller WL: The active form of the steroidogenic acute regulatory protein, StAR, appears to be a molten globule. *Proc Natl Acad Sci USA* 96:7250, 1999.
89. Hall PF: The role of the cytoskeleton in the supply of cholesterol for steroidogenesis in lipoprotein and cholesterol metabolism in steroidogenic tissues, in Strauss J III, Menon K (eds): Lipoprotein and Cholesterol Metabolism in Steroidogenic Tissues. Philadelphia, George F. Stickley Co., 1985, p 207.
90. Amsterdam A, Rotmensch S: Structure-function relationships during granulosa cell differentiation. *Endocr Rev* 8:309, 1987.
91. Nebert DW, Gonzalez FJ: P450 genes: Structure, evolution and regulation. *Ann Rev Biochem* 56:945, 1987.
92. Hall PF: Cytochromes P450 and the regulation of steroid syntheses. *Steroids* 48:131, 1986.
93. Black SD, Coon MJ: P-450 cytochromes: Structure and function. *Adv Enzymol Relat Areas Mol Biol* 60:35, 1987.
94. Gonzalez FJ: The molecular biology of cytochrome P450s. *Pharmacol Rev* 40:243, 1989.
95. Nebert DW, Nelson DR, Coon MJ, Estabrook RW, Feyereisen R, Fujii-Kuriyama Y, Gonzalez FJ, Guengerich FP, et al: The P450 superfamily: Update on new sequences, gene mapping, and recommended nomenclature. *DNA Cell Biol* 10:1, 1991.
96. Fu GK, Lin D, Zhang MYH, Bikle DD, Shackleton CHL, Miller WL, Portale AA: Cloning of human 25-hydroxy vitamin D-1α-hydroxylase and mutations causing vitamin D-dependant rickets type I. *Mol Endocrinol* 11:1961, 1997.
97. Fu GK, Portale AA, Miller WL: Complete structure of the human gene for the vitamin D 1α-hydroxylase, P450c1α. *DNA Cell Biol* 16:1499, 1997.
98. Wang JT, Lin CJ, Burridge SM, Fu GK, Labuda M, Portale AA, Miller WL: Genetics of vitamin D 1α-hydroxylase deficiency in 17 families. *Am J Hum Genet* 63:1694, 1998.
99. Staels B, Hum DW, Miller WL: Regulation of steroidogenesis in NCI-H295 cells: A cellular model of the human fetal adrenal. *Mol Endocrinol* 7:423, 1993.
100. Hasemann CA, Kurumbail RG, Boddupalli SS, Peterson JA, Deisenhofer J: Structure and function of cytochromes P450: A comparative analysis of three crystal structures. *Structure* 2:41, 1995.
101. Lin D, Zhang L, Chiao E, Miller WL: Modeling and mutagenesis of the active site of human P450c17. *Mol Endocrinol* 8:392, 1994.
102. Graham-Lorence S, Amarneh B, White RE, Peterson JA, Simpson ER: A three-dimensional model of aromatase cytochrome P450. *Prot Sci* 4:1065, 1995.
103. Auchus RJ, Miller WL. Molecular modeling of human P450c17 (17α-hydroxylase/17,20-lyase): Insights into reaction mechanisms and effects of mutations. *Mol Endocrinol* 13:1169, 1999.
104. Sybert DW, Lancaster JR Jr, Lambeth JD, Kamin H: Participation of the membrane in the side-chain cleavage of cholesterol. *J Biol Chem* 254:12088, 1979.
105. Shikita M, Hall PF: Cytochrome P-450 from bovine adrenocortical mitochondria: An enzyme for the side chain cleavage of cholesterol. I. Purification and properties. *J Biol Chem* 248:5596, 1973.
106. Shikita M, Hall PF: Cytochrome P-450 from bovine adrenocortical mitochondria: An enzyme for the side chain cleavage of cholesterol. II. Subunit structure. *J Biol Chem* 248:5605, 1973.
107. Kimura T: ACTH stimulation on cholesterol side chain cleavage activity of adrenocortical mitochondria. *Mol Cell Biochem* 36:105, 1981.
108. Morisaki M, Duque C, Ikekawa H, Shikita M: Substrate specificity of adrenocoritcal cytochrome P450. I. Effect of structural modification of cholesterol side chain on pregnenolone production. *J Steroid Biochem* 13:545, 1980.
109. Lambeth JD, Pember SO: Cytochrome P-450scc-adrenodoxin complex: Reduction properties of the substrate-associated cytochrome and relation of the reduction states of heme and iron-sulfur centers to association of the proteins. *J Biol Chem* 258:5596, 1983.
110. Lieberman S, Prasad VVK: Heterodox notions on pathways of steroidogenesis. *Endocr Rev* 11:469, 1990.
111. Morohashi K, Sogawa K, Omura T, Fujii-Kuriyama Y: Gene structure of human cytochrome P-450(scc), cholesterol desmolase. *J Biochem* 101:879, 1987.
112. Pang S, Yang XH, Wang M, Tissot R, Nino M, Manaligod J, Bullock LP, Mason JI: Inherited congenital adrenal hyperplasia in the rabbit: Absent cholesterol side-chain cleavage cytochrome P450 gene expression. *Endocrinology* 131:181, 1992.
113. Yang X, Iwamoto K, Wang M, Artwohl J, Mason JI, Pang S: Inherited congenital adrenal hyperplasia in the rabbit is caused by a deletion in the gene encoding cytochrome P450 cholesterol side-chain cleavage enzyme. *Endocrinology* 132:1977, 1993.
114. Lambeth JD, Xu XX, Glover M: Cholesterol sulfate inhibits adrenal mitochondrial cholesterol side-chain cleavage at a site distinct from cytochrome P450scc. Evidence for an intramitochondrial cholesterol translocator. *J Biol Chem* 262:9181, 1987.
115. Iida S, Papadopoulos V, Hall PF: The influence of exogenous free cholesterol on steroid synthesis in cultured adrenal cells. *Endocrinology* 124:2619, 1989.
116. Stocco DM, Clark BJ, Lin D, Sugawara T, Strauss JF III, Miller WL: Characterization of the protein responsible for the acute regulation of steroidogenesis in mouse Leydig tumor cells, in Desjardins C (ed): *Cellular and Molecular Regulation of Testicular Cells.* New York, Springer-Verlag, 1996, pp 311–336.
117. Heyl BL, Tyrrell DJ, Lambeth JD: Cytochrome P450scc-substrate interactions. Role of the 3β- and side-chain hydroxyls in binding to oxidized and reduced forms of the enzyme. *J Biol Chem* 261:2743, 1986.
118. Morohashi K, Fujii Kuriyama Y, Okada Y, Sogawa K, Hirose T, Inayama S, Omura T: Molecular cloning and nucleotide sequence of cDNA for mRNA of mitochondrial P450(scc) of bovine adrenal cortex. *Proc Natl Acad Sci USA* 81:4647, 1984.
119. Matteson KJ, Chung B, Urdea MS, Miller WL: Study of cholesterol side chain cleavage (20,22 desmolase) deficiency causing congenital lipoid adrenal hyperplasia using bovine-sequence P450scc oligodeoxyribonucleotide probes. *Endocrinology* 118: 1296, 1986.
120. Chung B, Matteson KJ, Voutilainen R, Mohandas TK, Miller WL: Human cholesterol side-chain cleavage enzyme, P450scc: cDNA cloning, assignment of the gene to chromosome 15, and expression in the placenta. *Proc Natl Acad Sci USA* 83:8962, 1986.
121. Sparkes RS, Klisak I, Miller WL: Regional mapping of genes encoding human steroidogenic enzymes: P450scc to 15q23-q24, adrenodoxin to 11q22; adrenodoxin reductase to 17q24-q25; and P450c17 to 10q24-q25. *DNA Cell Biol* 10:359, 1991.
122. Matocha M, Waterman MR: Synthesis and processing of mitochondrial steroid hydroxylases. *In vivo* maturation of the precursor of cytochrome P450scc, cytochrome P450 and adrenodoxin. *J Biol Chem* 260:12259, 1985.
123. Voutilainen R, Tapanainen J, Chung B, Matteson KJ, Miller WL: Hormonal regulation of P450scc (20,22-desmolase) and P450c17 (17α-hydroxylase/17,20-lyase) in cultured human granulosa cells. *J Clin Endocrinol Metab* 63:202, 1986.
124. DiBlasio AM, Voutilainen R, Jaffe RB, Miller WL: Hormonal regulation of mRNAs for P450scc (cholesterol side-chain cleavage enzyme) and P450c17 (17α-hydroxylase/17,20 lyase) in cultured human fetal adrenal cells. *J Clin Endocrinol Metab* 65:170, 1987.
125. Ringler GE, Kao LC, Miller WL, Strauss JF III: Effects of 8-bromo-cAMP on expression of endocrine functions by cultured human trophoblast cells. Regulation of specific mRNAs. *Mol Cell Endocrinol* 62:13, 1989.
126. Mellon SH, Kushner JA, Vaisse C: Expression and regulation of adrenodoxin and P450scc mRNAs in rodent tissues. *DNA Cell Biol* 10:339, 1991.
127. Mellon SH, Deschepper CF: Neurosteroid biosynthesis: Genes for adrenal steroidogenic enzymes are expressed in the brain. *Brain Res* 629:283, 1993.
128. Compagnone NA, Bulfone A, Rubenstein JLR, Mellon SH: Expression of the steroidogenic enzyme P450scc in the central and peripheral nervous systems during rodent embryogenesis. *Endocrinology* 136:2689, 1995.
129. Keeney DS, Ikeda Y, Waterman MR, Parker KL: Cholesterol side-chain cleavage cytochrome P450 gene expression in the primitive gut of the mouse embryo does not require steroidgenic factor 1. *Mol Endocrinol* 9:1091, 1995.
130. John ME, John MC, Boggaram V, Simpson ER, Waterman MR:

Transcriptional regulation of steroid hydroxylase genes by corticotropin. *Proc Natl Acad Sci USA* 83:4715, 1986.

131. Mellon SH, Vaisse C: cAMP regulates P450scc gene expression by a cycloheximide-insensitive mechanism in cultured mouse leydig MA-10 cells. *Proc Natl Acad Sci USA* 86:7775, 1989.
132. Moore CCD, Brentano ST, Miller WL: Human P450scc gene transcription is induced by cyclic AMP and repressed by 12-*O*-tetradecanolyphorbol-13-acetate and A23187 by independent *cis*-elements. *Mol Cell Biol* 10:6013, 1990.
133. Ahlgren R, Simpson ER, Waterman MR, Lund J: Characterization of the promoter/regulatory region of the bovine CYP11A (P450scc) gene. *J Biol Chem* 265:3313, 1990.
134. Moore CCD, Hum DW, Miller WL: Identification of positive and negative placental-specific basal elements, a transcriptional repressor, and a cAMP response element in the human gene for P450scc. *Mol Endocrinol* 6:2045, 1992.
135. Hum DW, Staels B, Black SM, Miller WL: Basal transcriptional activity and cyclic AMP responsiveness of the human P450scc promoter transfected into mouse Leydig MA-10 cells. *Endocrinology* 132:546, 1993.
136. Barrett PQ, Bollag WB, Isales CM, McCarthy RT, Rasmussen H: The role of calcium in angiotensin II-mediated aldosterone secretion. *Endocr Rev* 10:496, 1989.
137. Golos TJ, Soto EA, Tureck RW, Strauss JF III: Human chorionic gonadotropin and 8-bromo-adenosine 3′5′-monophosphate stimulate [125I] low density lipoprotein uptake and metabolism by luteinized human granulosa cells in culture. *J Clin Endocrinol Metab* 61:633, 1985.
138. Picado-Leonard J, Voutilainen R, Kao L, Chung B, Strauss JF III, Miller WL: Human adrenodoxin: Cloning of three cDNAs and cycloheximide enhancement in JEG-3 cells. *J Biol Chem* 263:3240, 1988.
139. Enyedi P, Szaba B, Spat A: Reduced responsiveness of glomerulosa cells after prolonged stimulation with angiotensin II. *Am J Physiol* 178:E209, 1985.
140. Mason JI, Carr BR, Rainey WE: The action of phorbol ester on steroidogenesis in cultured human fetal adrenal cells. *Endocr Res* 12:447, 1986.
141. Cozza EN, Vila MDC, Acevedo-Duncan M, Farese RV, Gomez-Sanchez CE: Treatment of primary cultures of calf adrenal glomerulosa cells with adrenocorticotropin (ACTH) and phorbol esters: A comparative study of the effects on aldosterone production and ACTH signaling system. *Endocrinology* 126:2169, 1990.
142. Hum DW, Aza-Blanc P, Miller WL: Characterization of placental-specific transcription of the human gene for P450scc. *DNA Cell Biol* 14:451, 1995.
143. Huang N, Miller WL: Cloning of factors related to HIV-inducible LBP proteins that regulate steroidogenic factor-1-independent human placental transcription of the cholesterol side-chain cleavage enzyme, P450scc. *J Biol Chem* 275:2852, 2000.
144. Rodriguez H, Hum DW, Staels B, Miller WL: Transcription of the human genes for cytochrome P450scc and P450c17 is regulated differently in human adrenal NCI-H295 cells than in mouse adrenal Y1 cells. *J Clin Endocrinol Metab* 82:365, 1997.
145. Omura T, Sanders S, Estabrook RW, Cooper DY, Rosenthal O: Isolation from adrenal cortex of a non-heme iron protein and a flavoprotein functional as a reduced triphosphopyridine nucleotide-cytochrome P-450 reductase. *Arch Biochem Biophys* 117:660, 1966.
146. Nakamura Y, Otsuka H, Tamaoki B: Requirement of a new flavoprotein and a non-heme iron-containing protein in the steroid 11β and 18 hydroxylase system. *Biochem Biophys Acta* 122:34, 1966.
147. Kimura T, Suzuki K: Components of the electron transport system in adrenal steroid hydroxylase. *J Biol Chem* 242:485, 1967.
148. Gnanaiah W, Omdahl JL: Isolation and characterization of pig kidney mitochondrial ferredoxin: NADP+ oxidoreductase. *J Biol Chem* 261:12649, 1986.
149. Hanukoglu I, Suh BS, Himmelhoch S, Amsterdam A: Induction and mitochondrial localization of cytochrome P450scc system enzymes in normal and transformed ovarian granulosa cells. *J Cell Biol* 111:1373, 1990.
150. Solish SB, Picado-Leonard J, Morel Y, Kuhn RW, Mohandas TK, Hanukoglu I, Miller WL: Human adrenodoxin reductase: Two mRNAs encoded by a single gene of chromosome 17cen→q25 are expressed in steroidogenic tissues. *Proc Natl Acad Sci USA* 71:7104, 1988.
151. Lin D, Shi Y, Miller WL: Cloning and sequence of the human adrenodoxin reductase gene. *Proc Natl Acad Sci USA* 87:8516, 1990.
152. Brentano ST, Black SM, Lin D, Miller WL: cAMP post-transcriptionally diminishes the abundance of adrenodoxin reductase mRNA. *Proc Natl Acad Sci USA* 89:4099, 1992.
153. Brandt ME, Vickery LE: Expression and characterization of human mitochondrial ferredoxin reductase in Escherichia coli. *Arch Biochem Biophys* 294:735, 1992.
154. Lambeth JD, Seybert D, Kamin H: Ionic effects on adrenal steroidogenic electron transport: The role of adrenodoxin as an electron shuttle. *J Biol Chem* 254:7255, 1979.
155. Lambeth JD, Seybert DW, Kamin H: Phospholipid vesicle-reconstituted cytochrome P450scc. Mutually facilitated binding of cholesterol and adrenodoxin. *J Biol Chem* 255:138, 1980.
156. Hanukoglu I, Jefcoate CR: Mitochondrial cytochrome P-450scc: Mechanism of electron transport by adrenodoxin. *J Biol Chem* 255:3057, 1980.
157. Hanukoglu I, Spitsberg V, Bumpus JA, Dus KM, Jefcoate CR: Adrenal mitochondrial cytochrome P450scc: Cholesterol and adrenodoxin interactions at equilibrium and during turnover. *J Biol Chem* 256:4321, 1981.
158. Cupp JR, Vickery LE: Identification of free and [Fe_2S_2]-bound cystine residues of adrenodoxin. *J Biol Chem* 263:17418, 1988.
159. Coghlan VM, Vickery LE: Expression of human ferredoxin and assembly of the [2Fe-2S] center in *Escherichia coli*. *Proc Natl Acad Sci USA* 86:835, 1989.
160. Cupp JR, Vickery LE: Adrenodoxin with a COOH-terminal deletion (des 116-128) exhibits enhanced activity. *J Biol Chem* 264:1602, 1989.
161. Müller A, Müller JJ, Müller YA, Uhlmann H, Bernhardt R, Heinemann U: New aspects of electron transfer revealed by the crystal structure of a truncated bovine adrenodoxin, Adx(4-108). *Structure* 6:269, 1998.
162. Chang CY, Wu DA, Lai CC, Miller WL, Chung B: Cloning and structure of the human adrenodoxin gene. *DNA* 7:609, 1988.
163. Chang C, Wu D, Mohandas TK, Chung B: Structure, sequence, chromosomal location, and evolution of the human ferredoxin gene family. *DNA Cell Biol* 9:205, 1990.
164. Morel Y, Picado-Leonard J, Wu DA, Chang C, Mohandas TK, Chung B, Miller WL: Assignment of the functional gene for adrenodoxin to chromosome 11q1.3→qterm and two adrenodoxin pseudogenes to chromosome 20cen→13.1. *Am Hum Genet* 42:52, 1988.
165. Okamura T, Kagimoto M, Simpson ER, Waterman MR: Multiple species of bovine adrenodoxin mRNA. Occurrence of two different mitochondrial precursor sequences associated with the same mature sequence. *J Biol Chem* 262:10335, 1987.
166. Brentano ST, Miller WL: Regulation of human P450scc and adrenodoxin mRNAs in JEG-3 cytotrophoblast cells. *Endocrinology* 131:3010, 1992.
167. Voutilainen R, Picado-Leonard J, DiBlasio AM, Miller WL: Hormonal and developmental regulation of human adrenodoxin mRNA in steroidogenic tissues. *J Clin Endocrinol Metab* 66:383, 1988.
168. Coghlan VM, Vickery LE: Site-specific mutations in human ferredoxin that affect binding to ferredoxin reductase and cytochrome P450scc. *J Biol Chem* 266:18606, 1991.
169. Coghlan VM, Vickery LE: Electrostatic interactions stabilizing ferredoxin electron transfer complexes: Disruption by "conservative" mutations. *J Biol Chem* 267:8932, 1992.
170. Harikrishna JA, Black SM, Szklarz GD, Miller WL: Construction and function of fusion enzymes of the human cytochrome P450scc system. *DNA Cell Biol* 12:371, 1993.
171. Miller WL: Mitochondrial specificity of the early steps in steroidogenesis. *J Steroid Biochem Mol Biol* 55:607, 1995.
172. Thomas JL, Myers RP, Strickler RC: Human placental 3β-hydroxy-5-ene-steroid dehydrogenase and steroid 5→4-ene-isomerase: Purification from mitochondria and kinetic profiles, biophysical characterization of the purified mitochondrial and microsomal enzymes. *Steroid Biochem* 33:209, 1989.
173. Luu-The V, Lechance Y, Labrie C, Leblanc G, Thomas JL, Strickler RC, Labrie F: Full length cDNA structure and deduced amino

acid sequence of human 3β-hydroxy-5-ene steroid dehydrogenase. *Mol Endocrinol* 3:1310, 1989.
174. Lorence MC, Murry BA, Trant JM, Mason JI: Human 3β-hydroxysteroid dehydrogenase/$\Delta^5 \rightarrow \Delta^4$ isomerase from placenta: Expression in nonsteroidogenic cells of a protein that catalyzes the dehydrogenation/isomerization of C21 and C19 steroids. *Endocrinology* 126:2493, 1990.
175. Lachance Y, Luu-The V, Labrie C, Simard J, Dumont M, de Launoit Y, Guerin S, Leblanc G, et al: Characterization of human 3β-hydroxysteroid dehydrogenase/Δ^5-Δ^4-isomerase gene and its expression in mammalian cells. *J Biol Chem* 265:20469, 1990.
176. Penning TM: Molecular endocrinology of hydroxysteroid dehydrogenases. *Endocr Rev* 18:281, 1997.
177. Lorence MC, Corbin CJ, Kamimura N, Mahendroo MS, Mason JI: Structural analysis of the gene encoding human 3β-hydroxysteroid dehydrogenase/$\Delta^5 \rightarrow \Delta^4$ isomerase. *Mol Endocrinol* 4:1850, 1990.
178. Rhéaume E, Lachance Y, Zhao HL, Breton N, Dumont M, de Launoit Y, Trudel C, Luu-The V, et al: Structure and expression of a new complementary DNA encoding the almost exclusive 3β-hydroxysteroid dehydrogenase/Δ^5-Δ^4-isomerase in human adrenals and gonads. *Mol Endocrinol* 5:1147, 1991.
179. Lachance Y, Luu-The V, Verreault H, Dumont M, Leblanc G, Labrie F: Characterization and expression of human type II 3β hydroxysteroid dehydrogenase/Δ^5-Δ^4 isomerase (3β-HSD) gene, the almost exclusive 3β-HSD speicies expressed in the adrenals and gonads. *DNA Cell Biol* 10:701, 1991.
180. Berube D, Luu-The V, Lachance Y, Gagne R, Labrie F: Assignment of the human 3β-hydroxysteroid dehydrogenase gene (HSDB3) to the p13 band of chromosome 1. *Cytogenet Cell Genet* 52:199, 1989.
181. Cherradi N, Rossier MF, Vallotton MB, Timberg R, Friedberg I, Orly J, Wang XJ, Stocco DM, et al: Submitochondrial distribution of three key steroidogenic proteins (steroidogenic acute regulatory protein and cytochrome P450scc and 3β-hydroxysteroid dehydrogenase isomerase enzymes) upon stimulation by intracellular calcium in adrenal glomerulosa cells. *J Biol Chem* 272:7899, 1997.
182. Laffargue P, Chamlian A, Adechy-Senkoel L: Localization probable en microscopie electronique de la 3B hydroxysteroide dehydrogenase, de la glucose 6 phosphate dehydrogenase, et de la NADH diaphorase dans le corps jaune ovarian de la femme. *J Microsc* 13:325, 1972.
183. Lee TC, Miller WL, Auchus RJ: Medroxyprogesterone acetate and dexamethasone are competitive inhibitors of different human steroidogenic enzymes. *J Clin Endocrinol Metab* 84:2104, 1999.
184. Voutilainen R, Ilvesmaki V, Miettinen PJ: Low expression of 3β-hydroxy-5-ene steroid dehydrogenase gene in human fetal adrenals *in vivo*; adrenocorticotropin and protein kinase C-dependent regulation in adrenocortical cultures. *J Clin Endocrinol Metab* 72:761, 1991.
185. Trant JM, Lorance MC, Johnson EF, Shackleton CHL, Mason JI, Estabrook RW: Characterization of the steroid-metabolizing capacity of the hepatic cytochrome P450II5 expressed in COS-1 cells: 3β-hydroxysteroid dehydrogenase/$\Delta^5 \rightarrow \Delta^4$ isomerase type activity. *Proc Natl Acad Sci USA* 87:9756, 1990.
186. Lin D, Black SM, Nagahama Y, Miller WL: Steroid 17α-hydroxylase and 17,20 lyase activities of P450c17: Contributions of serine[106] and P450 reductase. *Endocrinology* 132:2498, 1993.
187. Auchus RJ, Lee TC, Miller WL: Cytochrome b_5 augments the 17,20 lyase activity of human P450c17 without direct electron transfer. *J Biol Chem* 273:3158, 1998.
188. Orentreich N, Brind JL, Rizer RL, Vogelman JH: Age changes and sex differences in serum dehydroepiandrosterone sulfate concentrations throughout adulthood. *J Clin Endocrinol Metab* 59:551, 1984.
189. Sklar CA, Kaplan SL, Grumbach MM: Evidence for dissociation between adrenarche and gonadarche: Studies in patients with idiopathic precocious puberty, gonadal dysgenesis, isolated gonadotropin deficiency, and constitutionally delayed growth and adolescence. *J Clin Endocrinol Metab* 51:548, 1980.
190. Zachmann M, Vollmin JA, Hamilton W, Prader A: Steroid 17,20 desmolase deficiency: A new cause of male pseudohermaphroditism. *Clin Endocrinol* 1:369, 1972.
191. Goebelsmann U, Zachmann M, Davajan V, Israel R, Mestman JH, Mishell DR: Male pseudohermaphroditism consistent with 17,20-desmolase deficiency. *Gynecol Invest* 7:138, 1976.
192. Nakajin S, Hall PF: Microsomal cytochrome P450 from neonatal pig testis. Purification and properties of a C_{21} steroid side-chain cleavage system (17α-hydroxylase-$C_{17,20}$ lyase). *J Biol Chem* 256:3871, 1981.
193. Nakajin S, Hall PF: Testicular microsomal cytochrome P450 for C_{21} steroid side-chain cleavage. *J Biol Chem* 256:6134, 1981.
194. Nakajin S, Shively JE, Yuan P, Hall PF: Microsomal cytochrome P450 from neonatal pig testis: Two enzymatic activities (17α-hydroxylase and C17,20-lyase) associated with one protein. *Biochemistry* 20:4037, 1981.
195. Nakajin S, Shinoda M, Haniu M, Shively JE, Hall PF: C_{21} steroid side-chain cleavage enzyme from porcine adrenal microsomes. Purification and characterization of the 17α-hydroxylase/$C_{17,20}$ lyase cytochrome P450. *J Biol Chem* 259:3971, 1984.
196. Zuber MX, Simpson ER, Waterman MR: Expression of bovine 17α-hydroxylase cytochrome P450 cDNA in non-steroidogenic (COS-1) cells. *Science* 234:1258, 1986.
197. Sakaki T, Shibata M, Yabusaki Y, Murakami H, Ohkawa H: Expression of bovine cytochrome P450c17 cDNA in *Saccharomyces cerevisiae*. *DNA* 8:409, 1989.
198. Fevold HR, Lorence MC, McCarthy JL, Trant JM, Kagimoto M, Waterman MR, Mason JI: Rat P450-17α from testis: Characterization of a full-length cDNA encoding a unique steroid hydroxylase capable of catalyzing both Δ^4 and Δ^5-steroid-17,20-lyase reactions. *Mol Endocrinol* 3:968, 1989.
199. Lin D, Harikrishna JA, Moore CCD, Jones KL, Miller WL: Missense mutation Ser106→Pro causes 17α-hydroxylase deficiency. *J Biol Chem* 266:15992, 1991.
200. Yanase T: 17α-Hydroxylase/17,20 lyase defects. *J Steroid Biochem Mol Biol* 53:153, 1995.
201. Fardella CE, Zhang LH, Mahachoklertwattana P, Lin D, Miller WL: Deletion of amino acids Asp[487]-Ser[488]-Phe[489] in human cytochrome P450c17 causes severe 17α-hydroxylase deficiency. *J Clin Endocrinol Metab* 77:489, 1993.
202. Fan YS, Sasi R, Lee C, Winter JSD, Waterman MR, Lin CC: Localization of the human CYP17 gene (cytochrome P450 17α) to 10q24.3 by fluorescence *in situ* hybridization and simultaneous chromosome banding. *Genomics* 14:1110, 1992.
203. Chung B, Picado-Leonard J, Haniu M, Bienkowski M, Hall PF, Shivley JE, Miller WL: Cytochrome P450c17 (steroid 17α-hydroxylase/17,20 lyase): Cloning of human adrenal and testis cDNAs indicates the same gene is expressed in both tissues. *Proc Natl Acad Sci USA* 84:407, 1987.
204. Picado-Leonard J, Miller WL: Cloning and sequence of the human gene encoding P450c17 (steroid 17α-hydroxylase/17,20 lyase): Similarity to the gene for P450c21. *DNA* 6:439, 1987.
205. Brentano ST, Picado-Leonard J, Mellon SH, Moore CCD, Miller WL: Tissue-specific, cAMP-induced, and phorbol ester repressed expression from the human P450c17 promoter in mouse cells. *Mol Endocrinol* 4:1972, 1990.
206. Lin CJ, Miller WL: An element located at −220/−185 bp of the human gene for P450c17 (steroid 17α-hydroxylase/17,20 lyase) is essential for its transcription in human adrenal NCI-H295A cells. (submitted).
207. Yanagibashi K, Hall PF: Role of electron transport in the regulation of the lyase activity of C-21 side-chain cleavage P450 from porcine adrenal and testicular microsomes. *J Biol Chem* 261:8429, 1986.
208. Yamano S, Aoyama T, McBride OW, Hardwick JP, Gelboin HV, Gonzalez FJ: Human NADPH-P450 oxidoreductase: Complementary DNA cloning, sequence, vaccinia virus-mediated expression, and localization of the CYPOR gene to chromosome 7. *Mol Pharmacol* 35:83, 1989.
209. Oprian DD, Coon MJ: Oxidation-reduction states of FMN and FAD in NADPH-cytochrome P450 reductase during reduction by NADPH. *J Biol Chem* 257:8935, 1982.
210. Wang M, Roberts DL, Paschke R, Shea TM, Masters BSS, Kim JJP: Three-dimensional structure of NADPH-cytochrome P450 reductase: Prototype for FMN- and FAD-containing enzymes. *Proc Natl Acad Sci USA* 94:8411, 1997.
211. French JS, Guengerich FP: Interactions of cytochrome P450 NADPH-cytochrome P450 reductase, and substrate in the reconstituted liver microsomal enzyme system. *J Biol Chem* 255:4112, 1980.

212. Muller-Enoch D, Churchill P, Fleischer S, Guengerich FP: Interaction of liver microsomal cytochrome P450 and NADPH-cytochrome P450 reductase in the presence and abscence of lipid. *J Biol Chem* 259:8174, 1984.
213. Tamburini PP, Gibson GG: Thermodynamic studies of the protein-protein interactions between cytochrome P-450 and cytochrome b_5. *J Biol Chem* 258:13444, 1983.
214. Yamazaki H, Gillam EM, Dong MS, Johnson WW, Guengerich FP, Shimada T: Reconstitution of recombinant cytochrome P450 2C10(2C9) and comparison with cytochrome P450 3A4 and other forms: Effects of cytochrome P450–P450 and cytochrome P450-b5 interactions. *Arch Biochem Biophys* 342:329, 1997.
215. Geller DH, Auchus RJ, Miller WL: P450c17 mutations R347H and R358Q selectively disrupt 17,20-lyase activity by disrupting interactions with P450 oxidoreductase and cytochrome b_5. *Mol Endocrinol* 13:167, 1999.
216. Zhang L, Rodriguez H, Ohno S, Miller WL: Serine phosphorylation of human P450c17 increases 17,20 lyase activity: Implications for adrenarche and for the polycystic ovary syndrome. *Proc Natl Acad Sci USA* 92:10619, 1995.
217. Miller WL, Levine LS: Molecular and clinical advances in congenital adrenal hyperplasia. *J Pediatr* 111:1, 1987.
218. New MI, White P, Pang S, Dupont B, Speiser PW: The adrenal hyperplasias, in Scriver CR, Beaudet A, Sly S, Valle D (eds): *The Metabolic Basis of Inherited Disease.* New York, McGraw-Hill Inc., 1989, pp 1881–1917.
219. Kominami S, Ochi H, Kobayashi Y, Takemori S: Studies on the steroid hydroxylation system in adrenal cortex microsomes: Purification and characterization of cytochrome P450 specific for steroid 21 hydroxylation. *J Biol Chem* 255:3386, 1980.
220. Higashi Y, Yoshioka H, Yamane M, Gotoh O, Fujii-Kuriyama Y: Complete nucleotide sequence of two steroid 21-hydroxylase genes tandemly arranged in human chromosome: A pseudogene and genuine gene. *Proc Natl Acad Sci USA* 83:2841, 1986.
221. White PC, New MI, Dupont B: Structure of the human steroid 21-hydroxylase genes. *Proc Natl Acad Sci USA* 83:5111, 1986.
222. Rodrigues NR, Dunham I, Yu CY, Carroll MC, Porter RR, Campbell RD: Molecular characterization of the HLA-linked steroid 21-hydroxylase B gene from an individual with congenital adrenal hyperplasia. *EMBO J* 6:1653, 1987.
223. Morel Y, Bristow J, Gitelman SE, Miller WL: Transcript encoded on the opposite strand of the human steroid 21-hydroxylase/complement component/C4 gene locus. *Proc Natl Acad Sci USA* 86:6582, 1989.
224. Bristow J, Gitelman SE, Tee MK, Staels B, Miller WL: Abundant adrenal-specific transcription of the human P450c21A "pseudogene." *J Biol Chem* 268:12919, 1993.
225. Bristow J, Tee MK, Gitelman SE, Mellon SH, Miller WL: Tenascin-X. A novel extracellular matrix protein encoded by the human XB gene overlapping P450c21B. *J Cell Biol* 122:265, 1993.
226. Miller WL, Morel Y: Molecular genetics of 21-hydroxylase deficiency. *Ann Rev Genet* 23:371, 1989.
227. Morel Y, Miller WL: Clinical and molecular genetics of congenital adrenal hyperplasia due to 21-hydroxylase deficiency. *Adv Hum Genet* 20:1, 1991.
228. Casey ML, MacDonald PC: Extra-adrenal formation of a mineralocorticoid: Deoxycorticosterone and deoxycorticosterone sulfate biosynthesis and metabolism. *Endocr Rev* 3:396, 1982.
229. Casey ML, Winkel CA, MacDonald PC: Conversion of progesterone to deoxycorticosterone in the human fetus: Steroid 21-hydroxylase activity in fetal tissues. *J Steroid Biochem* 18:449, 1983.
230. Mellon SH, Miller WL: Extra-adrenal steroid 21-hydroxylation is not mediated by P450c21. *J Clin Invest* 84:1497, 1989.
231. Amor M, Tosi M, Duponchel C, Steinmetz M, Meo T: Liver cDNA probes disclose two cytochrome P450 genes duplicated in tandem with the complement C4 loci of the mouse H-2S region. *Proc Natl Acad Sci USA* 82:4453, 1985.
232. Chung B, Matteson KJ, Miller WL: Structure of the bovine gene for P450c21 (steroid 21-hydroxylase) defines a novel cytochrome P450 gene family. *Proc Natl Acad Sci USA* 83:4243, 1986.
233. Speiser PW, Agdere L, Veshiba H, White PC, New MI: Aldosterone synthesis in patients with salt-wasting congenital adrenal hyperplasia (21-hydroxylase deficiency) and complete absence of adrenal 21-hydroxylase (P450c21). *N Engl J Med* 321:145, 1991.
234. Ulick S: Diagnosis and nomenclature of the disorders of the terminal portion of aldosterone biosynthetic pathway. *J Clin Endocrinol Metab* 43:92, 1976.
235. Veldhuis JD, Kulin HE, Santen RJ, Wilson TE, Melby JC: Inborn error in the terminal step of aldosterone biosynthesis: Corticosterone methyl oxidase type II deficiency in a North American pedigree. *N Engl J Med* 303:118, 1980.
236. Yanagibashi K, Haniu M, Shively JE, Shen WH, Hall P: The synthesis of aldosterone by the adrenal cortex: Two zones (fasciculata and glomerulosa) possess one enzyme for 11-, 18-hydroxylation, and aldehyde synthesis. *J Biol Chem* 261:3556, 1986.
237. Mathew PA, Mason JI, Trant JM, Sanders D, Waterman M: Amino acid substitutions $Phe^{66}\rightarrow Leu$ and $Ser^{126}\rightarrow Pro$ abolish cortisol and aldosterone synthesis by bovine cytochrome P45011B. *J Biol Chem* 265:20228, 1990.
238. Fardella CE, Miller WL: Molecular biology of mineralocorticoid metabolism. *Ann Rev Nutrition* 16:443, 1996.
239. White PC, Curnow KM, Pascoe L: Disorders of steroid 11β-hydroxylase isozymes. *Endocrine Reviews* 15:421, 1994.
240. Chua SC, Szabo P, Vitek A, Grzeschik KH, John M, White PC: Cloning of cDNA encoding steroid 11β-hydroxylase, P450c11. *Proc Natl Acad Sci USA* 84:7193, 1987.
241. Mornet E, Dupont J, Vitek A, White PC: Characterization of two genes encoding human steroid 11β-hydroxylase (P45011β). *J Biol Chem* 264:20961, 1989.
242. Zhang G, Miller WL: The human genome contains only two CYP11B (P450c11) genes. *J Clin Endocrinol Metab* 81:3254, 1996.
243. Wagner MJ, Ge Y, Siciliano M, Wells DE: A hybrid cell mapping panel for regional localization of probes to human chromosome 8. *Genomics* 10:114, 1991.
244. Kawamoto T, Mitsuuchi Y, Ohnishi T, Ohnishi T, Ichikawa Y, Yokoyama Y, Sumimoto H, Toda K, et al: Cloning and expression of a cDNA for human cytochrome P450aldo as related to primary aldosteronism. *Biochem Biophy Res Commun* 173:309, 1990.
245. Kawamoto T, Mitsuuchi Y, Toda K, Yokoyama Y, Miyahara K, Miura S, Ohnishi T, Ichikawa Y, et al: Role of steroid 11β-hydroxylase and 18-hydroxylase in the biosynthesis of glucocorticoids and mineralocorticoids in humans. *Proc Natl Acad Sci USA* 89:1458, 1992.
246. Carnow KM, Tusie-Lung M, Pascoe L, Nataarajan R, Gu J, Nadler JL, White PC: The product of the CYP11B2 gene is required for aldosterone biosynthesis in the human adrenal cortex. *Mol Endocrinol* 5:1513, 1991.
247. Domalik LJ, Chaplin DD, Kirkman MS, Wu RC, Liu WW, Howard TA, Seldin JF, Parker KL: Different isozymes of mouse 11 beta-hydroxylase produce mineralocorticoids and glucocorticoids. *Mol Endocrinol* 5:1853, 1991.
248. Malee MP, Mellon SH: Zone-specific regulation of two distinct messenger RNAs for P450c11 (11/18-hydroxylase) in the adrenals of pregnant and non-pregnant rats. *Proc Natl Acad Sci USA* 88:4731, 1991.
249. White PC, Dupont J, New MI, Lieberman E, Hochberg Z, Rösler A: A mutation in CYP11B1 (Arg 448→His) associated with steroid 11β-hydroxylase deficiency in Jews of Moroccan origin. *J Clin Invest* 87:1664, 1991.
250. Ulick S, Wang JZ, Morton H: The biochemical phenotypes of two inborn errors in the biosynthesis of aldosterone. *J Clin Endocrinol Metab* 74:1415, 1992.
251. Pascoe L, Curnow K, Slutsker L, Rösler A, White PC: Mutations in the human CYP11B2 (aldosterone synthase) gene causing corticosterone methlyoxidase II deficiency. *Proc Natl Acad Sci USA* 89:4996, 1992.
252. Zhang G, Rodriguez H, Fardella CE, Harris DA, Miller WL: Mutation T318M in P450c11AS causes corticosterone methyl oxidase II deficiency. *Am J Hum Genet* 57:1037, 1995.
253. Mukai K, Imai M, Shimada H, Ishimura Y: Isolation and characterization of rat CYP11B genes involved in late steps of mineralo- and glucocorticoid syntheses. *J Biol Chem* 268:9130, 1993.
254. Nomura M, Morohashi K, Kirita S, Nonaka Y, Okamoto M, Nawata H, Omura T: Three forms of rat CYP11B genes: 11 beta-hydroxyalse gene, aldosterone synthase gene, and a novel gene. *J Biochem* 113:144, 1993.

255. Mellon SH, Bair SR, Monis H: P450c11B3 mRNA, transcribed from a third P450c11 gene, is expressed in a tissue-specific, developmentally and hormonally regulated fashion in the rodent adrenal, and encodes a protein with both 11-hydroxylase and 18-hydroxylase activities. *J Biol Chem* 270:1643, 1995.
256. Zhou M, Gomez-Sanchez EP, Foecking MF, Gomez-Sanchez CE: Cloning and expression of the rat adrenal cytochrome P450c11B3 (CYP11B3) enzyme cDNA. Preferential 18-hydroxylation over 11β-hydroxylation of DOC. *Mol Cell Endocrinol* 114:137, 1995.
257. Cover CM, Wang JM, St Letzin E, Kurtz TW, Mellon SH: Molecular variants in the P450c11AS gene as determinants of aldosterone synthase activity in the Dahl rat model of hypertension. *J Biol Chem* 270:16555, 1995.
258. Fardella CE, Rodriguez H, Hum DW, Mellon SH, Miller WL: Artificial mutations in P450c11AS (aldosterone synthase) can increase enzymatic activity: A model for low-renin hypertension? *J Clin Endocrinol Metab* 80:1040, 1995.
259. Fardella CE, Rodriguez H, Montero J, Zhang G, Vignolo P, Rojas A, Villaroel L, Miller WL: Genetic variation in P450c11AS in Chilean patients with low renin hypertension. *J Clin Endocrinol Metab* 81:4347, 1996.
260. Takeda Y, Furukawa K, Inaba S, Miyamori I, Mabuchi H: Genetic analysis of aldosterone synthase in patients with idiopathic hyperaldosteronism. *J Clin Endocrinol Metab* 84:1633, 1999.
261. Peltoketo H, Isomaa V, Mäenlavsta O, Vihko R: Complete amino acid sequence of human placental 17β-hydroxysteroid dehydrogenase deduced from cDNA. *FEBS Lett* 239:73, 1988.
262. Gast MJ, Sims HF, Murdock GL, Gast PM, Strauss AW: Isolation and sequencing of a complementary deoxyribonucleic acid clone encoding human placental 17β-estradiol dehydrogenase: Identification of the putative cofactor binding site. *Am J Obstet Gynecol* 161:1726, 1989.
263. Tremblay Y, Ringler GE, Morel Y, Mohandas TK, Labrie F, Strauss JF III, Miller WL: Regulation of the gene for estrogenic 17-ketosteroid reductase lying on chromosome 17cen→q25. *J Biol Chem* 264:20458, 1989.
264. Zhang Y, Word RA, Fesmire S, Carr BR, Rainey WE: Human ovarian expression of 17β-hydroxysteroid dehydrogenase types 1, 2, and 3. *J Clin Endocrinol Metab* 81:3594, 1996.
265. Sawetawan C, Milewich L, Word RA, Carr BR, Rainey WE: Compartmentalization of type 1 17β-hydroxysteroid oxidoreductase in the human ovary. *Mol Cell Endocrinol* 99:161, 1994.
266. Mäentausta O, Sormunen R, Isomaa V, Lehto VP, Jouppila P, Vihko R: Immunohistochemical localization of 17β-hydroxysteroid dehydrogenase in the human endometrium during the menstrual cycle. *Lab Invest* 65:582, 1991.
267. Takeyama J, Sasano H, Suzuki T, Iinuma K, Nagura H, Andersson S: 17β-hydroxysteroid dehydrogenase types 1 and 2 in human placenta: An immunohistochemical study with correlation to placental development. *J Clin Endocrinol Metab* 83:3710, 1998.
268. Luu-The V, Labrie C, Simard J, Lachance Y, Zhao HF, Covet J, Leblanc G, Labrie F: Structure of two in tandem human 17β-hydroxysteroid dehydrogenase genes. *Mol Endocrinol* 4:268, 1990.
269. Tremblay Y, Beaudoin C: Regulation of 3 β-hydroxysteroid dehydrogenase and 17β-hydroxysteroid dehydrogenase messenger ribonucleic acid levels by cyclic adenosine 3′,5′-monophosphate and phorbol myristate acetate in human choriocarcinoma cells. *Mol Endocrinol* 7:355, 1993.
270. Ghosh D, Pleuteu VZ, Zhu DW, Wawarzak Z, Duax WL, Plaugborn W, Labrie F, Lin SX: Structure of human estrogenic 17β-hydroxysteroid dehydrogenase at 2.2 Å resolution. *Structure* 3:503, 1995.
271. Sawicki MW, Erman M, Puranen T, Vihko P, Ghosh D: Structure of the ternary complex of human 17β-hydroxysteroid dehydrogenase type 1 with 3-hydroxyestra-1,3,5,7-tetraen-17-one (equilin) and NADP+. *Proc Nat Acad Sci USA* 96:840, 1999.
272. Wu L, Einstein M, Geissler WM, Chan HK, Ellison KO, Andersson S: Expression cloning and characterization of human 17β-hydrosteroid dehydrogenase Type 2, a microsomal enzyme possessing 20α-hydroxysteroid dehydrogenase activity. *J Biol Chem* 268:12964, 1993.
273. Andersson S, Geissler WM, Patel S, Wu L: The molecular biology of androgenic 17β-hydroxysteroid dehydrogenases. *J Steroid Biochem Mol Biol* 53:37, 1995.
274. Beaudoin C, Blomquist CH, Tremblay Y: Gene expression of 17β-hydroxysteroid dehydrogenase type 2 isozyme in primary cultures of human trophoblasts predicts different mechanisms regulating type 1 and type 2 enzymes. *Endocrinology* 136:3807, 1995.
275. Casey ML, MacDonald PC, Andersson S: 17β-Hydroxysteroid dehydrogenase type 2: Chromosomal assignment and progestin regulation of gene expression in human endometrium. *J Clin Invest* 94:2135, 1994.
276. Geissler WM, Davis DL, Wu L, Bradshaw KD, Patel S, Mendonça BB, Elliston KO, Wilson JD, et al: Male pseudohermaphroiditism caused by mutations of testicular 17β-hydroxysteroid dehydrogenase 3. *Nat Genet* 7:34, 1994.
277. Saez JM, De Peretti E, Morera AM, David M, Bertrand J: Familial male pseudohermaphroditism with gynecomastia due to a testicular 17-ketosteroid reductase defect. I. Studies in vivo. *J Clin Endocrinol Metab* 32:604, 1971.
278. Andersson S, Geissler WM, Wu L, Davis DL, Grumbach MM, New MI, Schwarz HP, Blethen SL, et al: Molecular genetics and pathophysiology of 17β-hydroxysteroid dehydrogenase 3 deficiency. *J Clin Endocrinol Metab* 81:130, 1996.
279. Boehmer AL, Brinkmann AO, Sandkuijl LA, Halley DJ, Niermeijer MF, Andersson S, de Jong FH, Kayserili H, et al: 17β-hydroxysteroid dehydrogenase-3 deficiency: Diagnosis, phenotypic variability, population genetics, and worldwide distribution of ancient and de novo mutations. *J Clin Endocrinol Metab* 84:4713, 1999.
280. Leenders F, Adamski J, Husen B, Thole HH, Jungblut PW: Molecular cloning and amino acid sequence of the porcine 17β-estradiol dehydrogenase. *Euro J Biochem* 222:221, 1994.
281. Adamski J, Normand T, Leenders F, Montae D, Begue A, Staehelin D, Jungblut PW, de Launoit Y: Molecular cloning of a novel widely expressed human 80 kDa 17β-hydroxysteroid dehydrogenase IV. *Biochem J* 311:437, 1995.
282. Carstensen JF, Tesdorpf JG, Kaufmann M, Markus MM, Husen B, Leenders F, Jakob F, de Launoit Y, et al: Characterization of 17β-hydroxysteroid dehydrogenase IV. *J Endocrinol* 150:S3, 1996.
283. Leenders F, Tesdorpf JG, Markus M, Engel T, Seedorf U, Adamski J: Porcine 80-kDa protein reveals intrinsic 17β-hydroxysteroid dehydrogenase, fatty acyl-CoA-hydratase/dehydrogenase, and sterol transfer activities. *J Biol Chem* 271:5438, 1996.
284. van Grunsven EG, van Berkel E, Ijlst L, Vreken P, De Klerk JBC, Adamski J, Lemonde H, Clayton PT, et al: Peroxisomal D-hydroxy-acyl-CoA dehydrogenase deficiency: Resolution of the enzyme defect and its molecular basis in bifunctional protein deficiency. *Proc Natl Acad Sci USA* 95:2128, 1998.
285. Lin HK, Jez JM, Schlegel BP, Peehl DM, Pachter JA, Penning TM: Expression and characterization of recombinant type 2 3α-hydroxysteroid dehydrogenase (HSD) from human prostate: Demonstration of bifunctional $3\alpha/17\beta$-HSD activity and cellular distribution. *Mol Endocrinol* 11:1971, 1997.
286. Dufort I, Rheault P, Huang XF, Soucy P, Luu-The V: Characteristics of a highly labile human type 5 17β-hydroxysteroid dehydrogenase. *Endocrinology* 140:568, 1999.
287. El-Alfy M, Luu-The V, Huang XF, Berger L, Labrie F, Pelletier G: Localization of type 5 17β-hydroxysteroid dehydrogenase, 3β-hydroxysteroid dehydrogenase, and androgen receptor in the human prostate by in situ hybridization and immunocytochemistry. *Endocrinology* 140:1481, 1999.
288. Biswas MG, Russell DW: Expression cloning and characterization of oxidative 17β- and 3α-hydroxysteroid dehydrogenases from rat and human prostate. *J Biol Chem* 272:15959, 1997.
289. Nokelainen P, Peltoketo H, Vihko R, Vihko P: Expression cloning of a novel estrogenic mouse 17β-hydroxysteroid dehydrogenase/17-ketosteroid reductase (m17HSD7), previously described as a prolactin receptor-associated protein (PRAP) in rat. *Mol Endocrinol* 12:1048, 1998.
290. Simpson ER, Mahendroo MS, Means GD, Kilgore MW, Hinshelwood MM, Graham-Lorence S, Amarneh B, Ito Y, et al: Aromatase cytochrome P450, the enzyme responsible for estrogen biosynthesis. *Endocr Rev* 15:342, 1994.
291. Grumbach MM, Auchus RJ: Estrogen: Consequences and implications of human mutations in synthesis and action. *J Clin Endocrinol Metab* 84:4677, 1999.

292. Fishman J, Goto J: Mechanism of estrogen biosynthesis: Participation of multiple enzyme sites in placental aromatase hydroxylations. *J Biol Chem* 256:4466, 1981.
293. Fishman J, Rajo MS: Mechanism of estrogen biosynthesis: Sterochemistry of C-1 hydrogen elimination in the aromatization of 2β hydroxy-19-oxoandrostenedione. *J Biol Chem* 256:4472, 1981.
294. Thompson EAJ, Siiteri PK: The involvement of human placental micorosomal cytochrome P450 in aromatization. *J Biol Chem* 249:5373, 1974.
295. Nakajin S, Shinoda M, Hall PF: Purification to homogeneity of aromatase from human placenta. *Biochem Biophys Res Commun* 134:704, 1986.
296. Evans CT, Ledesma DB, Schulz TZ, Simpson ER, Mendelson CR: Isolation and characterization of a complementary DNA specific for human aromatase-system P-450 mRNA. *Proc Natl Acad Sci USA* 83:6387, 1986.
297. Chen S, Besman MJ, Sparkes RS, Zollman S, Klisak I, Mohandas T, Hall PF, Shively JE: Human aromatase: cDNA cloning, southern blot analysis and assignment of the gene to chromosome 15. *DNA* 7:27, 1988.
298. Harada N: Cloning of a complete cDNA encoding human aromatase: Immunochemical identification and sequence analysis. *Biochem Biophys Res Commun* 156:725, 1988.
299. Corbin CJ, Graham-Lorence S, McPhaul LM, Mason JI, Mendelson CR, Simpson ER: Isolation of full-length cDNA insert encoding human aromatase system cytochrome P-450 and its expression in nonsteroidogenic cells. *Proc Natl Acad Sci USA* 85:8948, 1988.
300. Pompon D, Liu RYK, Besman MJ, Wang PL, Shively JE, Chen S: Expression of human placental aromatase in *Saccharomyces cerevisae. Mol Endocrinol* 3:1477, 1989.
301. Means GD, Mahendroo MS, Corbin CJ, Mathis JM, Powell FE, Mendelson CR, Simpson ER: Structural analysis of the gene encoding human aromatase cytochrome P-450, the enzyme responsible for estrogen biosynthesis. *J Biol Chem* 264:19385, 1989.
302. Mahendroo MS, Means GD, Mendelson CR, Simpson ER: Tissue specific expression of human P450 arom: The promoter responsible in adipose tissue is different from that utilized in placenta. *J Biol Chem* 266:11276, 1991.
303. Simpson ER, Mahendroo MS, Means GD, Kilgore MW, Corbin CJ, Mendelson CR: Tissue-specific promoters regulate aromatase cytochrom P450 expression. *Clin Chem* 39:317, 1993.
304. Shozu M, Akasofu K, Harada T, Kubota Y: A new cause of female pseudo-hermaphroditism: Placental aromatase deficiency. *J Clin Endocrinol Metab* 72:560, 1991.
305. Ito Y, Fisher CR, Conte FA, Grumbach MM, Simpson ER: Molecular basis of aromatase deficiency in an adult female with sexual infantilism and polycystic ovaries. *Proc Natl Acad Sci USA* 90:11673, 1993.
306. Conte FA, Grumbach MM, Ito Y, Fisher CR, Simpson ER: A syndrome of female pseudohermaphrodism, hypergonadotropic hypogonadism, and multicystic ovaries associated with missense mutations in the gene encoding aromatase (P450arom). *J Clin Endocrinol Metab* 78:1287, 1994.
307. Wilson JD: Disorders of androgen action. *J Pediatr* 35:1, 1987.
308. Andersson S, Russell DW: Structural and biochemical properties of cloned and expressed human rat steroid 5α-reductases. *Proc Natl Acad Sci USA* 87:3640, 1990.
309. Andersson S, Berman DM, Jenkins EP, Russell DW: Deletion of a steroid 5α-reductase 2 gene in male pseudohermaphroditism. *Nature* 354:159, 1991.
310. Jenkins EP, Anderson S, Imperato-McGinley J, Wilson JD, Russell DW: Genetic and pharmacologic evidence for more than one human steroid 5α-reductase. *J Clin Invest* 89:293, 1992.
311. Harris G, Azzolina B, Baginsky W, Cimis G, Rasmussen GH, Tolman RL, Raetz CRH, Ellsworth K: Identification and selective inhibition of an isozyme of steroid 5α-reductase in human scalp. *Proc Natl Acad Sci USA* 89:10787, 1992.
312. Thigpen AE, Silver RI, Guileyardo JM, Casey ML, McConnell JD, Russell DW: Tissue distribution and ontogeny of steroid 5α-reductase isozyme expression. *J Clin Invest* 92:903, 1993.
313. Saenger P: Abnormal sex differentiation. *J Pediatr* 104:1, 1984.
314. Johnson L, George FW, Neaves WB, Rosenthal IM, Christensen RA, Decristofo A, Scheikert H, Sauer MV: Characterization of the testicular abnormality in 5α-reductase deficiency. *J Clin Endocrinol Metab* 63:1091, 1986.
315. Nash AR, Glenn WK, Moore SS, Kerr J, Thompson AR, Thompson EOP: Oestrogen sulfotransferase: Molecular cloning and sequencing of cDNA for the bovine placental enzyme. *Aust J Biol Sci* 41:507, 1988.
316. Oeda T, Lee Y, Driscoll W, Chen H, Strott C: Molecular cloning and expression of the full-length complementary DNA encoding the guinea pig adrenocortical estrogen sulfotransferase. *Mol Endocrinol* 6:1216, 1992.
317. Yen PH, Allen E, Marsh B, Mohandas T, Shapiro LJ: Cloning and expression of steroid sulfatase cDNA and the frequent occurrence of deletions: Implications for X-Y interchange. *Cell* 49:443, 1987.
318. Ballabio A, Shapiro LJ: Steroid sulfatase deficiency and X-linked icthiosis, in Schriver CR, Beaduet AL, Sly WS, Valle D (eds): *The Metabolic and Molecular Basis of Inherited Disease.* New York, McGraw-Hill, 1995, pp 2999–3022.
319. Compagnone NA, Salido E, Shapiro LJ, Mellon SH: Expression of steroid sulfatase during embryogenesis. *Endocrinology* 138:4768, 1997.
320. Compagnone NA, Mellon SH: Dehydroepiandrosterone: A potential signalling molecule for neocortical organization during development. *Proc Natl Acad Sci USA* 95:4678, 1998.
321. White PC, Mune T, Agarwal AK: 11β-hydroxysteroid dehydrogenase and the syndrome of apparent mineralocorticoid excess. *Endocr Rev* 18:135, 1997.
322. Tannin GM, Agarwal AK, Monder C, New MI, White PC: The human gene for 11β-hydroxysteroid dehydrogenase. Structure, tissue distribution, and chromosomal localization. *J Biol Chem* 266: 16653, 1991.
323. Moore CCD, Mellon SH, Murai J, Siiteri PK, Miller WL: Structure and function of the hepatic form of 11β-hydroxysteroid dehydrogenase in the squirrel monkey, an animal model of glucocorticoid resistance. *Endocrinology* 133:368, 1993.
324. Agarwal AK, Monder C, Eckstein B, White PC: Cloning and expression of rat cDNA encoding corticosteroid 11β-dehydrogenase. *J Biol Chem* 264:18939, 1989.
325. Edwards CRW, Burt D, McIntyre MA, deKloet ER, Stewart PM, Brett L, Sutanto WS, Monder C: Localization of 11β-hydroxysteroid dehydrogenase—tissue specific protector of the mineralocorticoid receptor. *Lancet* 2:986, 1988.
326. Funder JW, Pearce PT, Smith R, Smith I: Mineralocorticoid action: Target tissue specificity is enzyme, not receptor, mediated. *Science* 242:583, 1988.
327. Kotelevtsev Y, Holmes MC, Burchell A, Houston PM, Schmoll D, Jamieson P, Best R, Brown R, et al: 11β-Hydroxysteroid dehydrogenase type 1 knockout mice show attenuated glucocorticoid-inducible responses and resist hyperglycemia on obesity or stress. *Proc Natl Acad Sci USA* 94:14924, 1997.
328. Agarwal AK, Tusie-Luna M-T, Monder C, White PC: Expression of 11β-hydroxysteroid dehydrogenase using recombinant vaccinia virus. *Mol Endocrinol* 4:1827, 1990.
329. Agarwal AK, Rogerson FM, Mune T, White PC: Gene structure and chromosomal localization of the human HSD11K gene encoding the kidney (type 2) isozyme of 11β-hydroxysteroid dehydrogenase. *Genomics* 29:195, 1995.
330. Albiston AL, Obeyesekere VR, Smith RE, Krozowski ZS: Cloning and tissue distribution of the human 11β-hydroxysteroid dehydrogenase Type II enzyme. *Mol Cell Endocrinol* 105:R11, 1994.
331. Brown RW, Chapman KE, Edwards CRW, Seckl JR: Human placental 11β-hydroxysteroid dehydrogenase: evidence for and partial purification of a distinct NAD^+-dependent isoform. *Endocrinology* 132:2614, 1993.
332. Rusvai E, Náray-Fejes-Tóth A: A new isoform of 11β-hydroxysteroid dehydrogenase in aldosterone target cells. *J Biol Chem* 268:10717, 1993.
333. Wilson R, Dave-Sharma S, Wei J, Obeyesekere V, Kevin L, Ferrari P, Krozowski Z, Shackleton C, et al: A genetic defect resulting in mild low-renin hypertension. *Proc Natl Acad Sci USA* 95:10200 1998.
334. Arriza JL, Simerly RB, Swanson LW, Evans RM: The neuronal mineralocorticoid receptor as a mediator of glucocorticoid response. *Neuron* 1:887, 1988.
335. Ulick S, Levine LS, Gunczler P, Giovanni Z, Ramirez LC, Rauh W, Rösler A, Bradlow HL, et al: A syndrome of apparent miner-

alocorticoid excess associated with defects in the peripheral metabolism of cortisol. *J Clin Endocrinol Metab* 49:757, 1979.
336. Monder C, Schackleton CHL, Bradlow HL, New MI, Stoner E, Iohan F, Lakshmi V: The syndrome of apparent mineralocorticoid excess: Its association with 11-dehydrogenase and 5-reductase deficiency and some consequences for corticosterone metabolism. *J Clin Endocrinol Metab* 63:550, 1986.
337. Stewart PM, Corrie JET, Shackleton CHL, Edwards CRW: Syndrome of apparent mineralocorticoid excess. A defect in the cortisol-cortisone shuttle. *J Clin Invest* 82:340, 1988.
338. Wilson RC, Krozowski ZS, Li K, Obeyesekere VR, Razzaghy-Azar M, Harbison MD, Wei JQ, Shackleton CHL, et al: A mutation in the HSD11B2 gene in a family with apparent mineralocorticoid excess. *J Clin Endocrinol Metab* 80:2263, 1995.
339. Mune T, Rogerson FM, Nikkila H, Agarwal AK, White PC: Human hypertension caused by mutations in the kidney isozyme of 11β-hydroxysteroid dehydrogenase. *Nat Genet* 10:394, 1995.
340. Stewart PM, Wallace AM, Valentino R, Burt D, Shakleton CHL, Edward CRW: Mineralocorticoid activity of liquorice: 11β-hydroxysteroid dehydrogenase deficiency comes of age. *Lancet* 2:821, 1987.
341. Stewart PM, Wallace AM, Atherden SM, Shearing CH, Edwards CRW: Mineralocorticoid activity of carbenoxolone: Contrasting effects of carbenoxolone and liquorice on 11β-hydroxysteroid dehydrogenase activity in man. *Clin Sci* 78:49, 1990.
342. Krozowski Z, MaGuire JA, Stein-Oakley AN, Dowling J, Smith RE, Andrews RK: Immunohistochemical localization of the 11β hydroxysteroid dehydrogenase type II enzyme in human kidney and placenta. *J Clin Endocrinol Metab* 80:2203, 1995.
343. Hirasawa G, Sasono H, Suzuki T, Takeyama J, Muramatu Y, Fukushima K, Hiwatashi N, Toyota T, et al: 11β-hydroxysteroid dehydrogenase type 2 and mineralocorticoid receptor in human fetal development. *J Clin Endocrinol Metab* 84:1453, 1999.
344. Forest MG, Morel Y, David M: Prenatal treatment of congenital adrenal hyperplasia. *Trends Endocrinol Metab* 9:284, 1998.
345. Miller WL: Prenatal treatment of congenital adrenal hyperplasia—a promising experimental therapy of unproven safety. *Trends Endocrinol Metab* 9:290, 1998.
346. Mitani F, Suzuhi H, Hata J, Ogishima T, Shimada H, Ishimura Y: A novel cell layer without corticosteroid-synthesizing enzymes in rat adrenal cortex: Histochemical detection and possible physiologic role. *Endocrinology* 135:431, 1994.
347. Mesiano S, Jaffe RB: Role of growth factors in the developmental regulation of the human fetal adrenal cortex. *Steroids* 62:62, 1997.
348. Spencer SJ, Mesiano S, Lee JY, Jaffe RB: Proliferation and apoptosis in the human adrenal cortex during the fetal and perinatal periods: implications for growth and remodeling. *J Clin Endocrinol Metab* 84:1110, 1999.
349. Sippell WG, Muller-Holve W, Dorr HG, Bidlingmaier F, Knorr D: Concentrations of aldosterone, corticosterone, 11-deoxycoritcosterone, progesterone, 17-hydroxy-pregesterone, 11-deoxycortisol, cortisol, and cortisone determined simultaneously in human amniotic fluid throughout gestation. *J Clin Endrocrinol Metab* 52:385, 1981.
350. Pasqualini JR, Nguyen BL, Uhrich F, Wiqvist N, Diczfalvay E: Cortisol and cortisone metabolism in the human fetoplacental unit at midgestation. *J Steroid Biochem* 1:209, 1970.
351. Kari MA, Raivio KO, Stenman UH, Voutilainen R: Serum cortisol, dehydroepiandrosterone sulfate, and sterol-binding globulins in preterm neonates: Effects of gestational age and dexamethasone therapy. *Pediatr Res* 40:319, 1996.
352. Miller WL: Steroid hormone biosynthesis and actions in the materno-feto-placental unit. *Clin Perinatol* 25:799, 1998.
353. Fujieda K, Faiman C, Feyes FI, Winter JSD: The control of steroidogenesis by human fetal adrenal cells in tissue culture: IV. The effects of exposure to placental steroids. *J Clin Endocrinol Metab* 54:89, 1982.
354. Arlt W, Callies F, van Vlijmen JC, Koehler I, Reincke M, Bidlingmaier M, Huebler D, Oettel M, et al: Dehydroepiandrosterone replacement in women with adrenal insufficiency. *N Engl J Med* 341:1013, 1999.
355. Bornstein SR, Chrousos GP: Adrenocorticotropin ACTH- and non-ACTH-mediated regulation of the adrenal cortex: Neural and immune inputs. *J Clin Endocrinol Metab* 84:1729, 1999.
356. Bornstein SR, Webster EL, Torpy DJ, Richman SJ, Mitsiades N, Igel M, Lewis DB, Rice KC, Joost HG, Tsokos M, Chrousos GP: Chronic effects of a nonpeptide corticotropin-releasing hormone type 1-receptor antagonist on pituitary-adrenal function, and body weight and metabolic regulation. *Endocrinology* 139:1546, 1998.
357. Suckling KE, Tocher DR, Smelhe CG, Boyd GS: *In vitro* regulation of bovine adrenal cortical acyl-CoA: Cholesterol acyltransferase and comparison with rat liver enzyme. *Biochem Biophys Acta* 753:422, 1983.
358. Yanagibashi K, Ohno Y, Kawamura M, Hall PF: The regulation of intracellular transport of cholesterol in bovine adrenal cells: Purification of a novel protein. *Endocrinology* 123:2075, 1988.
359. Orentreich N, Brind JL, Rizer RL, Vogelman JH: Age changes and sex differences in serum dehydroepiandrosterone sulfate concentrations throughout adulthood. *J Clin Endocrinol Metab* 59:551, 1984.
360. Golos TG, Miller WL, Strauss JF III: Human chorionic gonadotropin and 8-bromo cyclic adenosine monophosphate promote an acute increase in cytochrome P450scc and adrenodoxin messenger RNAs in cultured human granulosa cells by a cycloheximide-insensitive mechanism. *J Clin Invest* 80:896, 1987.
361. Mellon SH, Shively JE, Miller WL: Human proopiomelanocortin (79-96), a proposed androgen stimulatory hormone, does not affect steroidogenesis in cultured human fetal adrenal cells. *J Clin Endocrinol Metab* 72:19, 1991.
362. Penhoat A, Sanchez P, Jaillard C, Langlois D, Begeot M, Saez JM: Human proopiomelanocortin (79-96), a proposed cortical androgen stimulating hormone, does not affect steroidogenesis in cultured human adult adrenal cells. *J Clin Endocrinol Metab* 72:23, 1991.
363. Robinson P, Bateman A, Mulay S, Spencer SJ, Jaffe RB, Solomon S, Bennett HPJ: Isolation and characterization of three forms of joining peptide from adult pituitaries: Lack of adrenal androgen-stimulating activity. *Endocrinology* 129:859, 1991.
364. Jefcoate CR, McNamara BC, DeBartolomeis MS: Control of steroid synthesis in adrenal fasciculata cells. *Endocr Res* 12:35, 1986.
365. Arriza JL, Weinberger C, Cerelli G, Glaser TM, Handelin B, Housman DE, Evans RM: Cloning of human mineralocorticoid receptor complementary DNA: Structural and functional kinship with the glucocorticoid receptor. *Science* 237:268, 1987.
366. Rundle SE, Funder JW, Lakshmi V, Monder C: The intrarenal localization of mineralocorticoid receptors and 11β-dehydrogenase: Immunochemical studies. *Endocrinology* 125:1700, 1989.
367. Furutani Y, Morimoto Y, Shibahara S, Noda M, Takahashi H, Hirose T, Asai M, Inayama S, et al: Cloning and sequence analysis of cDNA for ovine corticotropin-releasing factor precursor. *Nature* 301:537, 1983.
368. Sawchenko PE, Swanson LW, Vale WW: Co-expression of corticotropin-releasing factor and vasopressin immunoreactivity in parvocellular neurosecretory neurons of the adrenalectomized rat. *Proc Natl Acad Sci USA* 81:1883, 1984.
369. Whitnall MH, Mezey E, Gainer H: Co-localization of corticotropin-releasing factor and vasopressin in median eminence neurosecretory vesicles. *Nature* 317:248, 1985.
370. Miller WL: Molecular genetics of familial central diabetes insipidus. *J Clin Endocrinol Metab* 77:592, 1993.
371. Sasaki A, Liotta AS, Luckey MM, Margioris AN, Suda T, Krieger DT: Immunoreactive corticotropin-releasing factor is present in human maternal plasma during the third trimester of pregnancy. *J Clin Endocrinol Metab* 59:812, 1984.
372. Aguilera G, Harwood JP, Wilson JX, Morell J, Brown JH, Catt KJ: Mechanisms of action of corticotropin-releasing factor and other regulators of corticotropin release in rat pituitary cells. *J Biol Chem* 258:8039, 1983.
373. Vale W, Vaughan J, Smith M, Yamamoto G, Rivier J, Rivier C: Effects of synthetic ovine corticotropin-releasing factor, glucocorticoids, catecholamines, neurohypophyseal peptides, and other substances on cultured corticotropic cells. *Endocrinology* 113:1121, 1983.
374. Lamberts SWJ, Verleun T, Oosterom R, de Jong F, Hackeng WHL: Corticotropin-releasing factor (ovine) and vasopressin exert a synergistic effect on adrenocorticotropin release in man. *J Clin Endocrinol Metab* 58:298, 1984.
375. Tilders FJH, Berkenbosh F, Vermes I, Linton EA, Smelik PG: Role of epinephrine and vasopressin in the control of the pituitary-adrenal response to stress. *Fed Proc* 44:155, 1985.

376. Westlund KN, Aquilera G, Childs GV: Quantification of morphological changes in pituitary corticotropes produced by *in vivo* corticotropin-releasing factor stimulation and adrenalectomy. *Endocrinology* 116:439, 1985.
377. Nieuwenhuijzen-Kruseman AC, Linton EA, Lowry PJ, Rees LH, Besser GM: Corticotropin-releasing factor immunoreactivity in human gastrointestinal tract. *Lancet* 2:1245, 1982.
378. De Souza EB, Perrin MH, Insel TR, Rivier J, Vale WW, Kuhar MJ: Corticotropin-releasing factor receptors in rat forebrain: Autoradiographic identification. *Science* 224:1449, 1984.
379. Baram TZ: Pathophysiology of massive infantile spasms: Perspective in the putative role of the brain-adrenal access. *Ann Neurol* 33:231, 1993.
380. Brown MR, Fisher LA, Spiess J, Rivier C, Rivier J, Vale W: Corticotropin-releasing factor: Actions on the sympathetic nervous system and metabolism. *Endocrinology* 111:928, 1982.
381. Nemeroff CB, Widerlov E, Bissette G, Walleus H, Karlsson I, Eklund K, Kilts CD, Loosen PT, et al: Elevated concentrations of CSF corticotropin-releasing factor-like immunoreactivity in depressed patients. *Science* 226:1342, 1984.
382. Gillies GE, Linton EA, Lowry PJ: Corticotropin releasing activity of the new CRF is potentiated several times by vasopressin. *Nature* 299:355, 1982.
383. Rivier C, Vale W: Interaction of corticotropin-releasing factor and arginine vasopressin on adrenocorticotropin secretion *in vivo. Endocrinology* 113:939, 1983.
384. Chrousos GP: Ultradian, circadian and stress-related hypothalamic-pituitary-adrenal axis activity: A dynamic digital-to-analog modulation (editorial). *Endocrinology* 139:437, 1998.
385. Chrousos GP, Torpy D, Gold PW: Interactions between the hypothalamic-pituitary-adrenal axis and the female reproductive system: Clinical implications. *Ann Intern Med* 129:229, 1998.
386. Rivier J, Rivier C, Vale W: Synthetic competitive antagonists of corticotropin-releasing factor: Effect on ACTH secretion in the rat. *Science* 224:870, 1984.
387. Linton EA, Tilders FJH, Hodgkinson S, Berkenbosch F, Vermes I, Lowry PJ: Stress-induced secretion of adrenocorticotropin in rats is inhibited by administration of antisera to ovine corticotropin-releasing factor and vasopressin. *Endocrinology* 116:966, 1985.
388. Plotsky PM, Bruhn TO, Vale W: Central modulation of immunoreactive corticotropin-releasing factor secretion by arginine vasopressin. *Endocrinology* 115:1639, 1984.
389. Ono N, Bedran de Castro JC, McCann SM: Ultrashortloop positive feedback of corticotropin (ACTH)-releasing factor to enhance ACTH release in stress. *Proc Natl Acad Sci USA* 82:3528, 1985.
390. Ono N, Samson WK, McDonald JK, Lumpkin MD, Bedran De Castro JC, McCann SM: Effects of intravenous and intraventricular injection of antisera directed against corticotropin-releasing factor on the secretion of anterior pituitary hormones. *Proc Natl Acad Sci USA* 82:7787, 1985b.
391. Lewis DA, Sherman BM: Oxytocin does not influence adrenocorticotropin secretion in man. *J Clin Endocrinol Metab* 60:53, 1985.
392. Mezey E, Reisine TD, Brownstein MJ, Palkovits M, Axelrod J: β-Adrenergic mechanism of insulin induced adrenocorticotropin release from the anterior pituitary. *Science* 226:1085, 1984.
393. Miller WL, Johnson LK, Baxter JD, Roberts JL: Processing of the precursor to corticotropin and beta-lipoprotein in man. *Proc Natl Acad Sci USA* 77:5211, 1980.
394. Whitfeld PL, Seeburg PH, Shine J: The human proopiomelanocortin gene: Organization, sequence, and interspersion with repetitive DNA. *DNA* 1:133, 1982.
395. Miller WL, Baxter JD, Eberhardt NL: Peptide hormone genes: Structure and evolution, in Krieger DT, Martin JB (eds): *Brain Peptides*. New York, Wiley, 1983, p 15.
396. Lowry PJ, Silas L, McLean C, Linton EA, Estivariz FE: Pro-γ-melanocyte-stimulating hormone cleavage in adrenal gland undergoing compensatory growth. *Nature* 306:70, 1983.
397. Grunfeld C, Hagman J, Sakin EA, Buckley DI, Jones DS, Ramachandran J: Characterization of adrenocorticotropin receptors that appear when 3T3-L1 cells differentiate into adipocytes. *Endocrinology* 116:113, 1985.
398. Margioris A, Grino M, Protos P, Gold PW, Chrousos GP: Corticotropin releasing hormone and oxytocin stimulate the secretion of immunoreactive -MSH, -endorphin and ACTH from the human placenta in vitro. *J Clin Endocrinol Metab* 66:922, 1988.
399. Marshall JB, Kapcala LP, Manning LD, McCullough AJ: Effect of corticotropin-like intermediate lobe peptide on pancreatic exocrine function in isolated rat pancreatic lobules. *J Clin Invest* 74:1886, 1984.
400. Lymangrover JR, Buckalew VM, Harris J, Klein MC, Gruber KA: γ-2-MSH is natriuretic in the rat. *Endocrinology* 116:1227, 1985.
401. Miller WL, Johnson LK: Synthesis and glycosylation of proopiomelanocortin by a Cushing tumor. *J Clin Endocrinol Metab* 55:441, 1982.
402. Nicholson WE, Liddle RA, Puett D, Liddle GW: Adrenocorticotrophic hormone biotransformation, clearance and catabolism. *Endocrinology* 103:1344, 1978.
403. Hall PF: Trophic stimulation of steroidogenesis: In search of the elusive trigger. *Recent Prog Horm Res* 41:1, 1985.
404. Dickerman Z, Grant DR, Faiman C, Winter JSD: Intraadrenal steroid concentrations in man: Zonal differences and developmental changes. *J Clin Endocrinol Metab* 59:1031, 1984.
405. Cheitlin R, Buckley DI, Ramachandran J: The role of extracellular calcium in corticotropin-stimulated steroidogenesis. *J Biol Chem* 260:5323, 1985.
406. Catalano RD, Stuve L, Ramachandran J: Characterization of corticotropin receptors in human adrenocortical cells. *J Clin Endocrinol Metab* 62:300, 1986.
407. Tsigos C, Arai K, Hung W, Chrousos GP: Hereditary isolated glucocorticoid deficiency is associated with abnormalities of the adrenocorticotropin receptor gene. *J Clin Invest* 92:2461, 1993.
408. Kojima I, Kojima K, Rasmussen H: Role of calcium and cAMP in the action of adrenocorticotropin on aldosterone secretion. *J Biol Chem* 260:4248, 1985.
409. Cone RD, Lu D, Koppula S, Vage DI, Klungland H, Boston B, Chen W, Orth DN, Pouton C, Kesterson RA: The melanocortin receptors: Agonists, antagonists, and the hormonal control of pigmentation. *Recent Prog Horm Res* 51:287, 1996.
410. Vamvakopoulos NC, Durkin S, Nierman W, Chrousos GP: Mapping the human adrenocorticotropin hormone (ACTHR) gene to the small arm of chromosome 18 (18p. 11.21- pter.). *Genomics* 18:454, 1993.
411. Hayashi K, Sala G, Catt KJ, Dufau ML: Regulation of steroidogenesis by adrenocorticotrophic hormone in isolated adrenal cells. *J Biol Chem* 254:6678, 1979.
412. Jagannadha Rao J, Long JA, Ramachandran J: Effects of antiserum to adrenocorticotropin on adrenal growth and function. *Endocrinology* 102:371, 1978.
413. Ramasharma K, Li CH: Human pituitary and placental hormones control human insulin-like growth factor II secretion in human granulosa cells. *Proc Natl Acad Sci USA* 84:2643, 1987.
414. Miller WL: Regulation of mRNAs for human steroidogenic enzymes. *Endocr Res* 15:1, 1989.
415. Conneely OM, Headon DR, Olson CD, Ungar F, Dempsey ME: Intramitochondrial movement of adrenal sterol carrier protein with cholesterol in response to corticotropin. *Proc Natl Acad Sci USA* 81:2970, 1984.
416. Farese RV, Sabir AM: Polyphosphoinositides: Stimulator of mitochondrial cholesterol side chain cleavage and possible identification as an adrenocorticotropin-induced, cycloheximide-sensitive, cytosolid steroidogenesis factor. *Endocrinology* 106:1869, 1980.
417. Farese RV: Phospholipids as intermediates in hormone action. *Mol Cell Endocrinol* 35:1, 1984.
418. Saito E, Ichikawa Y, Homma M: Direct inhibitory effect of dexamethasone on steroidogenesis of human adrenal *in vivo. J Clin Endocrinol Metab* 48:861, 1979.
419. Rosenfield RL, Lucky AW, Helke J: Dexamethasone preparation does not alter corticoid and androgen responses to adrenocorticotropin. *J Clin Endocrinol Metab* 60:585, 1985.
420. Weitzman ED, Fukushima D, Nogeire C, Roffwarg H, Gallagher TF, Hellman L: Twenty four hour pattern of the episodic secretion of cortisol in normal subjects. *J Clin Endocrinol Metab* 33:14, 1971.
421. Krieger DT: Rhythms in CRF, ACTH, and corticosteroids, in Krieger DT (ed): *Endocrine Rhythms*. New York, Raven, 1979, p 123.
422. Goldman J, Wajchenberg BL, Liberman B, Nery M, Achando S, Germek OA: Contrast analysis for the evaluation of the circadian

rhythms of plasma cortisol, androstenedione, and testosterone in normal men and the possible influence of meals. *J Clin Endocrinol Metab* 60:164, 1985.
423. Follenius M, Brandenberger G, Hietter B, Simqoni M, Reinhardt B: Diurnal cortisol peaks and their relationships to meals. *J Clin Endocrinol Metab* 55:757, 1982.
424. Dallman MF: Viewing the ventromedial hypothalamus from the adrenal gland. *Am J Physiol* 246:R1, 1984.
425. Fehm HL, Klein E, Holl R, Voigt FH: Evidence for extrapituitary mechanisms mediating the morning peak of plasma cortisol in man. *J Clin Endocrinol Metab* 58:410, 1984.
426. Schulte HM, Chrousos GP, Gold PW, Booth JD, Oldfield ED, Cutler GB Jr, Loriaux DL: Continuous administration of synthetic bovine corticotropin-releasing factor in man. *J Clin Invest* 75: 1781, 1985.
427. Mellon PL, Windle JJ, Goldsmith PC, Padula CW, Roberts JL, Weiner RI: Immortalization of hypothalamic GnRH neurons by genetically targeted tumorigenesis. *Neuron* 5:1, 1990.
428. Kato H, Saito M, Suda M: Effect of starvation on the circadian adrenocortical rhythm in rats. *Endocrinology* 106:918, 1980.
429. Brandenberger G, Follqnius M, Muzet A, Simqoni M, Reinhardt B: Interactions between spontaneous and provoked cortisol secretory episodes in man. *J Clin Endocrinol Metab* 59:406, 1984.
430. Sherman B, Wysham C, Pfohl B: Age-related changes in the circadian rhythm of plasma cortisol in man. *J Clin Endocrinol Metab* 61:439, 1985.
431. Davis J, Morrill F, Fawcett J, Upton V, Bondy PK, Spiro HM: Apprehension and serum cortisol levels. *J Psychosom Res* 6:83, 1962.
432. Czeister CA, Ede MCM, Regenstein QR, Kisch ES, Fang US, Ehrlich EN: Episodic 24-hour cortisol secretory patterns in patients awaiting elective cardiac surgery. *J Clin Endocrinol Metab* 42:273, 1976.
433. Sutton JR, Casey JH: The adrenocortical response to competitive athletics in veteran athletes. *J Clin Endocrinol Metab* 40:135, 1975.
434. Dallman MF: Adrenal feedback on stress-induced corticoliberin (CRF) and corticotropin (ACTH) secretion, in Jones MT, Gillham B, Dallman MF, Chattopadahyay S (eds): *Interaction within the Brain-Pituitary Adrenocortical System*. New York, Academic, 1979, p 149.
435. Plumpton FS, Besser GM, Cole PV: Corticosteroid treatment and surgery: I. An investigation of the indications for steroid cover. *Anaesthesia* 24:3, 1969.
436. Dempsher DP, Gann DS: Increased cortisol secretion after small hemorrhage is not attributable to changes in adrenocorticotropin. *Endocrinology* 113:86, 1983.
437. Parker LN, Levin ER, Lifrak ER: Evidence for adrenocortical adaptation to severe illness. *J Clin Endocrinol Metab* 60:947, 1985.
438. Krieger DT: Rhythms of ACTH and corticosteroid secretion in health and disease and their experimental modification. *J Steroid Biochem* 6:785, 1975.
439. Linkowski P, Mendlewicz J, Leclercq R, Brasseur M, Hubain P, Goldstein J, Copinschi G, Van CE: The 24-hour profile of adrenocorticotropin and cortisol in major depressive illness. *J Clin Endocrinol Metab* 61:429, 1985.
440. Hotta M, Shibasaki T, Masuda A, Imaki T, Demura H, Ling N, Shizume K: The responses of plasma adrenocorticotropin and cortisol to corticotropin-releasing hormone (CRH) and cerebrospinal fluid immunoreactive CRH in anorexia nervosa patients. *J Clin Endocrinol Metab* 62:319, 1986.
441. Plank J, Feldman JM: Modification of adrenal function by the antiserotonin agent cyproheptadine. *J Clin Endocrinol Metab* 42:291, 1976.
442. Chimara K, Kato Y, Maeda K, Matsukura S, Imura H: Suppression by cyproheptadine of human growth hormone and cortisol during sleep. *J Clin Invest* 57:1393, 1976.
443. Keller-Wood ME, Dallman ME: Corticosteroid inhibition of ACTH secretion. *Endocr Rev* 5:1, 1984.
444. Birnberg NC, Lissitzky JC, Hinman M, Herbert E: Glucocorticoids regulate pro-opiomelanocortin gene expression *in vivo* at the levels of transcription and secretion. *Proc Natl Acad Sci USA* 80:6982, 1983.
445. Fehm HL, Voigt KH, Kummer G, Lang R, Pfeiffer EF: Differential and integral corticosteroid feedback effects on ACTH secretion in hypoadrenocorticism. *J Clin Invest* 63:247, 1979.
446. Widmaier EP, Dallman MF: The effects of corticotropin-releasing factor on adrenocorticotropin secretion from perfused pituitaries *in vitro:* Rapid inhibition by glucocorticoids. *Endocrinology* 115: 2368, 1984.
447. Suda T, Tomori N, Tozawa F, Mouri T, Demura H, Shizume K: Effect of dexamethasone on immunoreactive corticotropin-releasing factor in the rat median eminence and intermediate-posterior pituitary. *Endocrinology* 114:851, 1984.
448. Davis LG, Arentzen R, Reid JM, Manning RW, Wolfson B, Lawrence KL, Baldino FJ: Glucocorticoid sensitivity of vasopressin mRNA levels in the paraventricular nucleus of the rat. *Proc Natl Acad Sci USA* 83:1145, 1986.
449. Tan SY, Mulrow PJ: The contribution of the zona fasciculata and glomerulosa to plasma 18-deoxycorticosterone levels in man. *J Clin Endocrinol Metab* 41:126, 1975.
450. Deschepper CF, Mellon SH, Cumin F, Baxter JD, Ganong WF: Analysis by immunocytochemistry and in situ hybridization of renin and its mRNA in kidney, testis, adrenal, and pituitary of the rat. *Proc Natl Acad Sci USA* 83:7552, 1986.
451. Sander M, Ganten D, Mellon SH: The role of adrenal renin in the regulation of adrenal steroidogenesis by ACTH. *Proc Natl Acad Sci USA* 91:148, 1994.
452. Hardman JA, Hort YJ, Catanzaro DF, Telloam JT, Baxter JD, Morris BJ, Shine J: Primary structure of the human renin gene. *DNA* 3:457, 1984.
453. Kramer RE, Gallant S, Brownie AC: Actions of angiotensin II on aldosterone biosynthesis in the rat adrenal cortex. *J Biol Chem* 255:3442, 1980.
454. Catt KJ, Harwood JP, Aquilera G, Dufau ML: Hormonal regulation of peptide receptors and target cell responses. *Nature* 280:109, 1979.
455. Fujita K, Aguilera G, Catt KJ: The role of cyclic AMP in aldosterone production by isolated zona glomerulosa cells. *J Biol Chem* 254:8567, 1979.
456. McAllister JM, Hornsby PJ: Dual regulation of 3β-hydroxysteroid dehydrogenase, 17α-hydroxylase, dehydroepiandrosterone sulfotransferase by adenosine 3′,5′-monophosphate and activators of protein kinase C in cultured human adrenocortical cells. *Endocrinology* 122:2012, 1988.
457. Staels B, Hum DW, Miller WL: Regulation of steroidogenesis in NCI-H295 cells: A cellular model of the human fetal adrenal. *Mol Endocrinol* 7:423, 1993.
458. Wong M, Rice DA, Parker KL, Schimmer BP: The roles of cAMP and cAMP-dependent protein kinase in the expression of cholesterol side-chain cleavage and steroid 11β-hydroxylase genes in mouse adrenocortical tumor cells. *J Biol Chem* 264:12867, 1989.
459. Mouw AR, Rice DA, Meade JC, Chua CS, White PC, Schimmer BP, Parker KL: Structural and functional analysis of the promoter region of the gene encoding mouse steroid 11β-hydroxylase. *J Biol Chem* 264:1305, 1989.
460. Rice DA, Aitkin LD, Vandenbark GR, Mouw AR, Franklin A, Schimmer BP, Parker KL: A cAMP-responsive element regulates expression of the mouse steroid 11β-hydroxylase gene. *J Biol Chem* 264:14011, 1989.
461. Bogerd AM, Franklin A, Rice DA, Schimmer BP, Parker KL: Identification and characterization of two upstream elements that regulate adrenocortical production of steroid 11β-hydroxylase. *Mol Endocrinol* 4:845, 1990.
462. Farese RV, Larson RE, Sabir MA, Gomez-Sanchez CE: Effects of angiotensin II, K^+, adrenocorticotropin, serotonin, adenosine 3′,5′-monophosphate, guanosine 3′,5′-monophosphate, A23187, and EGTA on aldosterone synthesis and phospholipid metabolism in the rat adrenal zona glomerulosa. *Endocrinology* 113:1377, 1983.
463. McKena TJ, Island DP, Nicholson WE, Liddle GW: The effects of potassium on early and late steps in aldosterone biosynthesis in cells of the zona glomerulosa. *Endocrinology* 103:1411, 1978.
464. Fraser R, Mason PA, Buckingham JC, Gordon RD, Morton JJ, Nicholls MG, Semple PF, Tree M: The interaction of sodium and potassium states, of ACTH and of angiotensin II in the control of corticosteroid secretion. *J Steroid Biochem* 11:1039, 1979.
465. Williams GH, Bailey LM: Effects of dietary sodium intake and potassium intake and acute stimulation on aldosterone output by isolated human cells. *J Clin Endocrinol Metab* 45:55, 1977.

466. Merriam GR, Baer L: Adrenocorticotropin deficiency: Correction of hyponatremia and hypoaldosteronism with chronic glucocorticoid therapy. *J Clin Endocrinol Metab* 50:10, 1980.
467. Gullner H-G, Gill JR Jr: Beta-endorphin selectively stimulates aldosterone secretion in hypophysectomized, nephrectomized dogs. *J Clin Invest* 71:124, 1983.
468. Yamakado AM, Franco-Saenz R, Mulrow PJ: Effect of sodium deficiency on β-melanocyte-stimulating hormone stimulation of aldosterone in isolated rat adrenal cells. *Endocrinology* 113:2168, 1983.
469. Seidah NG, Rochemont J, Hamelin J, Lis M, Chretien M: Primary structure of the major human pituitary pro-opiomelanocortin NH_2-terminal glycopeptide: Evidence for an aldosterone-stimulating activity. *J Biol Chem* 256:7977, 1981.
470. Scheider EG, Radke KJ, Ulderich DA, Taylor RE Jr: Effect of osmolality on aldosterone secretion. *Endocrinology* 116:1621, 1985.
471. Perez GO, Oster JR, Vaamondi CA, Katz FH: Effect of NH_4Cl on plasma aldosterone, cortisol and renin activity in supine man. *J Clin Endocrinol Metab* 45:762, 1977.
472. Sowers JR, Berg G, Martin VS, Mayes D: Dopaminergic modulation of aldosterone secretion in the rhesus monkey: Evidence that dopamine affects the late pathway of aldosterone biosynthesis by inhibiting the conversion of corticosterone to 18-hydroxycorticosterone. *Endocrinology* 110:1173, 1982.
473. Atarashi K, Mulrow PJ, Franco-Saenz R: Effect of atrial peptides on aldosterone production. *J Clin Invest* 76:1807, 1985.
474. Brown JJ, Fraser R, Lever AF, Morten JJ, Oelkeis W, Robertson JIS, Young J: Further observations on the relationship between plasma angiotensin II and aldosterone during sodium deprivation. *Excerpta Med Int Cong Ser* 302:148, 1973.
475. Yamaji T, Ishibashi M, Takaku F: Atrial natriuretic factor in human blood. *J Clin Invest* 76:1705, 1985.
476. Gardner DG, Hane S, Trachewsky D, Schenk D, Baxter JD: Atrial natriuretic peptide mRNA is regulated by glucocorticoids *in vivo. Biochem Biophys Res Commun* 139:1047, 1986.
477. Gardner DG, Gertz BJ, Deschepper CF, Kim DY: Gene for the rat atrial natriuretic peptide is regulated by glucocorticoids *in vitro. J Clin Invest* 82:1275, 1988.
478. Albright F, Smith PH, Fraser R: A syndrome characterized by primary ovarian insufficiency and decrease of stature: Report of 11 cases with digression on hormonal control of axillary and pubic hair. *Am J Med Sci* 204:625, 1942.
479. Korth-Schutz S, Levine L, New MI: Dehydroepiandrosterone sulfate (DS) levels, a rapid test for abnormal adrenal androgen secretion. *J Clin Endocrinol Metab* 42:1005, 1976.
480. Korth-Schutz S, Levine L, New MI: Serum androgens in normal prepubertal and pubertal children and children with precocious adrenarche. *J Clin Endocrinol Metab* 42:117, 1976.
481. Vaitukaitis JL, Dale SL, Melby JC: Role of ACTH in the secretion of free dehydroepiandrosterone and its sulfate ester in man. *J Clin Endocrinol Metab* 29:1443, 1969.
482. Reiter EO, Fuldauer VG, Root AW: Secretion of the adrenal androgen, dehydroepiandrosterone sulfate, during normal infancy, childhood, and adolescence, in sick infants and in children with endocrinologic abnormalities. *J Pediatr* 90:766, 1977.
483. Nieschlag E, Loriaux DL, Ruder HJ, Zucker IR, Kirschner MA, Lipsett MB: The secretion of dehydroepiandrosterone and dehydroepiandrosterone sulphate in man. *J Endocrinol* 57:123, 1973.
484. Abraham GE, Chakmakjian ZH: Serum steroid levels during the menstrual cycle in a bilaterally adrenalectomized woman. *J Clin Endocrinol Metab* 37:581, 1973.
485. Cutler GB, Glenn M, Bush M, Hodgen GD, Graham CE, Loriaux DL: Adrenarche: A survey of rodents, domestic animals and primates. *Endocrinology* 103:2112, 1978.
486. Smail PJ, Faiman C, Hobson WC, Fuller GB, Winter JSD: Further studies on adrenarche in nonhuman primates. *Endocrinology* 111:844, 1982.
487. Parker LN, Odell WD: Evidence for existence of cortical androgen-stimulating hormone. *Am J Physiol* 236:E616, 1979.
488. McLean M, Davies JJ, Woods R, Lowry PJ, Smith R: A placental clock controlling the length of human pregnancy. *Nature Med* 1:460, 1995.
489. Smith R, Mesiano S, Chan E-C, Brown S, Jaffe RB: Corticotropin-releasing hormone directly and preferentially stimulates dehydroepiandrosterone sulfate secretion by human fetal adrenal cortical cells. *J Clin Endocrinol Metab* 83:2916, 1998.
490. Miller WL: The molecular basis of adrenarche—An hypothesis. *Acta Pediatrica* 88(Suppl. 433):60, 1999.
491. Byrne GC, Perry YS, Winter JSD: Kinetic analysis of adrenal 3β-hydroxysteroid dehydrogenase activity during human development. *J Clin Endocrinol Metab* 60:934, 1985.
492. Endoh A, Kristiansen SB, Casson PR, Buster JE, Hornsby PJ: The zona reticularis is the site of biosynthesis of dehydroepiandrosterone and dehydroepiandrosterone sulfate in the adult human adrenal cortex resulting from its low expression of 3β-hydroxysteroid dehydrogenase. *J Clin Endocrinol Metab* 81:3558, 1996.
493. Gell JS, Carr BR, Sasano H, Atkins B, Margraf L, Mason JI, Rainey WE: Adrenarche results from development of a 3β-hydroxysteroid dehydrogenase-deficient adrenal reticularis. *J Clin Endocrinol Metab* 83:3695, 1998.
494. Dardis A, Saraco N, Rivarola MA, Belgorosky A: Decrease in the expression of the 3β-hydroxysteroid dehydrogenase gene in human adrenal tissue during prepuberty and early puberty: Implications for the mechanism of adrenarche. *Pediatr Res* 45:384, 1999.
495. Yanase T, Sasano H, Yubisui T, Sakai Y, Takayanagi R, Nawata H: Immunohistochemical study of cytochrome b_5 in human adrenal gland and in adrenocortical adenomas from patients with Cushing's syndrome. *Endocr J* 45:89, 1998.
496. Mapes S, Corbin C, Tarantal A, Conley A: The primate adrenal zona reticularis is defined by expression of cytochrome b_5, 17a-hydroxylase/17,20-lyase cytochrome P450 (P450c17) and NADPH-cytochrome P450 reductase (reductase) but not 3β-hydroxysteroid dehydrogenase/Δ5-4 isomerase (3β-HSD). *J Clin Endocrinol Metab* 84:3382, 1999.
497. Oppenheimer E, Linder B, DiMartino-Nardi J: Decreased insulin sensitivity in prepubertal girls with premature adrenarche and acanthosis nigricans. *J Clin Endocrinol Metab* 80:614, 1995.
498. Ibañez L, Potau N, Zampolli M, N P, Virdis R, Vicens-Calvet E, Carrascosa A: Hyperinsulinemia in postpubertal girls with a history of premature pubarche and functional ovarian hyperandrogenism. *J Clin Endocrinol Metab* 81:1237, 1996.
499. Ibañez L, Potau N, Marcos MV, de Zegher F: Exaggerated adrenarche and hyperinsulinism in adolescent girls born small for gestational age. *J Clin Endocrinol Metab* 84:4739, 1999.
500. Abraham GE: Ovarian and adrenal contribution to peripheral androgens during the menstrual cycle. *J Clin Endocrinol Metab* 39:340, 1974.
501. Carter JN, Tysen JE, Warne GJ, McNeilly AS, Faiman C, Friesen HG: Adrenocortical function in hyperprolactinemic women. *J Clin Endocrinol Metab* 45:973, 1977.
502. Siiteri PK: Qualitative and quantitative aspects of adrenal secretion of steroids, in Cristy NP (ed): *The Human Adrenal Cortex.* New York, Harper & Row, 1971, p 1.
503. Zumoff B, Fukushima DK, Hellman L: Intercomparison of four methods for measuring cortisol production. *J Clin Endocrinol Metab* 38:169, 1974.
504. Nelson DH: The adrenal cortex: Physiological function and disease, in Smith LH (ed): *Major Problems in Internal Medicine.* Philadelphia, Saunders, 1980, vol 18, p 1.
505. Migeon C: Adrenal androgens in man. *Am J Med* 53:606, 1972.
506. New MI, Seaman MP, Peterson RE: A method for the simultaneous determination of the secretion rates of cortisol, 11-deoxycortisol, corticosterone, 11-deoxycorticosterone and aldosterone. *J Clin Endocrinol Metab* 29:514, 1969.
507. Peterson RE: The miscible pool and turnover rate of adrenocortical steroids in man. *Recent Prog Horm Res* 15:231, 1959.
508. Schoneshofer M, Wagner GG: Sex differences in corticosteroids in man. *J Clin Endocrinol Metab* 45:814, 1977.
509. Zumoff B, Fukushima DK, Weitzman ED, Kream J, Hellman L: The sex difference in plasma cortisol concentration in man. *J Clin Endocrinol Metab* 39:805, 1974.
510. Esteban NV, Loughlin T, Yergey AL, Zawadzki JK, Booth JD, Winterer JC, Loriaux DL: Daily cortisol production rate in man determined by stable isotope dilution/mass spectrometry. *J Clin Endocrinol Metab* 72:39, 1991.
511. Linder BL, Esteban NV, Yergey AL, Winterer JC, Loriaux DL, Cassoria F: Cortisol production rate in childhood and adolescence. *J Pediatr* 117:892, 1990.

512. Kerrigan JR, Veldhuis JD, Leyo SA, Iranmanesh A, Rogol AD: Estimation of daily cortisol production and clearance rates in normal pubertal males by deconvolution analysis. *J Clin Endocrinol Metab* 76:1505, 1993.
513. Stearns HC, Sneeden VD, Fearl JD: A clinical and pathologic review of ovarian stromal hyperplasia and its possible relationship to common diseases of the female reproductive system. *Am J Obstet Gynecol* 119:375, 1974.
514. Bondy PK: The adrenal cortex, in Bondy PK, Rosenberg LE (eds): *Metabolic Control and Disease.* Philadelphia, Saunders, 1979, p 1427.
515. Longcope C: Adrenal and gonadal androgen secretion in normal females. *Clin Endocrinol Metab* 15:213, 1986.
516. Samuels LT, Nelson DH: Biosynthesis of corticosteroids, in Greep RO, Astood EB (eds): *Handbook of Physiology: Endocrinology.* Washington, DC, American Physiological Society, 1975, vol 6, section 7, p 55.
517. Liddle GW: Regulation of adrenocortical function in man, in Christy NP (ed): *The Human Adrenal Cortex.* New York, Harper & Row, 1968, p 41.
518. Aguilera G, Catt KJ: Loci of action of regulators of aldosterone biosynthesis in isolated glomerulosa cells. *Endocrinology* 104:1046, 1980.
519. Schteingart DE, Tsao HS, Taylor CI, McKenzie A, Victoria R, Therrien BA: Sustained remission in Cushing's disease with mitotane and pituitary irradiation. *Ann Intern Med* 92:613, 1980.
520. Feldman D: Ketoconazole and other imidazole derivatives as inhibitors of steroidogenesis. *Endocr Rev* 7:409, 1986.
521. James VHT, Few JD: Adrenocorticosteroids: Chemistry, synthesis and disturbances in disease. *Clin Endocrinol Metab* 14:867, 1985.
522. Miller JW, Crapo L: The medical treatment of Cushing's syndrome. *Endocr Rev* 14:443, 1993.
523. Schteingart DE: Cushing's syndrome. *Endocrinol Metab Clin North Am* 18:311, 1989.
524. Luton JP, Mahoudeau JA, Bouchard PH, Thiebolt PH, Hautecouverture M, Simon D, Laudat MH, Touitou Y, et al: Treatment of Cushing's disease by o,p'-DDD: Survey of 62 cases. *N Engl J Med* 300:459, 1979.
525. Verheist JA, Trainer PJ, Howlett TA, Perry L, Rees LH, Grossman AB, Wass JAH, Besser GM: Short and long-term responses to metyrapone in the medical management of 91 patients with Cushing's syndrome. *Clin Endocrinol* 35:169, 1991.
526. Child DF, Burke CW, Burley DM, Rees LH, Russell Fraser T: Drug control of Cushing's syndrome: Combined aminoglutethimide and metyrapone therapy. *Acta Endocrinol* 82:330, 1976.
527. Samojlik E, Veldhius JD, Wells SA, Santen RJ: Preservation of androgen secretion during estrogen suppression with aminoglutethimide in the treatment of metastatic breast cancer. *J Clin Invest* 65:602, 1980.
528. Dewis P, Anderson C, Bu'lock DE, Earnshaw R, Kelly WF: Experience with trilostane in the treatment of Cushing's syndrome. *Clin Endocrinol* 18:533, 1983.
529. Komanicky P, Spark RF, Melby JC: Treatment of Cushing's syndrome with trilostane (WIN 24,250), an inhibitor of adrenal steroid biosynthesis. *J Clin Endocrinol Metab* 47:1024, 1978.
530. Sonino N, Boscaro M, Merola G, Mantero F: Prolonged treatment of Cushing's disease by ketoconazole. *J Clin Endocrinol Metab* 61:718, 1985.
531. Sonino N, Boscaro M, Paoletta A, Mantero F, Ziliotto D: Ketoconazole treatment in Cushing's syndrome: Experience in 34 patients. *Clin Endocrinol* 35:347, 1991.
532. Wagner RL, White PF, Kan PB, Rosenthal MH, Feldman D: Inhibition of adrenal steroidogenesis by the anesthetic etomidate. *N Engl J Med* 310:1415, 1984.
533. Schulte HM, Benker G, Reinwein D, Sippell WG, Allolio B: Infusion of low dose etomidate: Correction of hypercortisolemia in patients with Cushing's syndrome and dose-response relationship in normal subjects. *J Clin Endocrinol Metab* 70:1426, 1990.
534. Wilson ID, Goetz FC: Selective hypoaldosteronism after prolonged heparin administration. *Am J Med* 36:635, 1964.
535. Tuck ML, Sowers JR, Fittingoff DB, Fisher JS, Berg GJ, Asp ND, Mayes DM: Plasma corticosteroid concentrations during spironolactone administration: Evidence for adrenal biosynthetic blockade in man. *J Clin Endocrinol Metab* 52:1057, 1981.
536. Ballard PL: Delivery and transport of glucocorticoids to target cells, in Baxter JD, Rousseau GG (eds): *Glucocorticoid Hormone Action.* New York, Springer-Verlag, 1979, p 25.
537. Chrousos GP, Renquist D, Brandon D, Eil C, Pugeat M, Vigersky R, Cutler GB, Loriaux DL, Lipsett MB: Glucocorticoid resistance and primate evolution: Receptor-mediated mechanisms. *Proc Natl Acad Sci USA* 179:2036, 1982.
538. Sandberg AA, Slaunwhite WR Jr: Physical state of adrenal cortical hormones in plasma, in Christy NP (ed): *The Human Adrenal Cortex.* New York, Harper & Row, 1971, p 69.
539. Magiakou MA, Mastorakos G, Rabin D, Dubbert B, Gold PW, Chrousos GP: Hypothalamic corticotropin releasing hormone suppression during the postpartum period: Implications for the increase of psychiatric manifestations during this time. *J Clin Endocrinol Metab* 81:1912, 1996.
540. Westphal U: *Steroid-Protein Interactions.* New York, Springer-Verlag, 1971.
541. Dunn JF, Nisula BC, Rodbard D: Transport of steroid hormones. Binding of 21 endogenous steroids to both testosterone-binding globulin and corticosteroid-binding globulin in human plasma. *J Clin Endocrinol Metab* 53:58, 1981.
542. Partridge WM, Sakiyama R, Judd HL: Protein bound corticosterone in human serum is selectively transported into rat brain and liver *in vivo. J Clin Endocrinol Metab* 57:160, 1983
543. Siiteri PK, Murai JT, Hammond GL, Nisker JA, Raymoure WJ, Kuhn RW: The serum transport of steroid hormones. *Recent Prog Horm Res* 38:457, 1982.
544. Wolf G, Armstrong EG, Rosner W: Synthesis *in vitro* of corticosteroid-binding globulin from rat liver messenger ribonucleic acid. *Endocrinology* 108:805, 1981.
545. Hammond GL, Smith CL, Goping IS, Underhill DA, Harley MJ, Reventos J, Musto NA, Gunsalus GL, et al: Primary structure of human corticosteroid binding globulin, deduced from hepatic and pulmonary cDNAs, exhibits homology with serine protease inhibitors. *Proc Natl Acad Sci USA* 84:5153, 1987.
546. Hammond GL: Molecular properties of corticosteroid binding globulin and the sex-steroid binding proteins. *Endocr Rev* 11:65, 1990.
547. Rosner W: Plasma steroid-binding proteins. *Endocrinol Metab Clin North Am* 20:697, 1991.
548. Perrot-Applanat M, Racodot O, Milgrom E: Specific localization of plasma corticosteroid binding globulin immunoreactivity in pituitary corticotrophs. *Endocrinology* 115:559, 1984.
549. Hammond GL, Smith CL, Paterson NAM, Sibbald WJ: A role for corticosteroid-binding globulin in delivery of cortisol to activated neutrophils. *J Clin Endocrinol Metab* 71:34, 1990.
550. Rosner W: The functions of corticosteroid-binding globulin and sex hormone-binding globulin: Recent advances. *Endocr Rev* 11:80, 1990.
551. Ogawa T, Sudea K, Matsui N: The effect of cortisol, progesterone, and transcortin on phytohemagglutinin-stimulated human blood mononuclear cells and their interplay. *J Clin Endocrinol Metab* 56:121, 1983.
552. Pugeat MM, Dunn JF, Nisula BC: Transport of steroid hormones: Interaction of 70 drugs with testosterone-binding globulin and corticosteroid-binding globulin in human plasma. *J Clin Endocrinol Metab* 53:69, 1981.
553. DeMoor P, Louwagie A, Van Baelen H, Van de Putte I: Unexplained high transcortin levels in patients with various hematological disorders and in their relatives: A connection between these high transcortin levels and HLA antigen B12. *J Clin Endocrinol Metab* 50:421, 1980.
554. Coolens JL, Heyns W: Marked elevation and cyclic variation of corticosteroid-binding globulin: An inherited abnormality. *J Clin Endocrinol Metab* 68:492, 1989.
555. Orbach O, Schussler GG: Increased serum cortisol binding in chronic active hepatitis. *Am J Med* 86:39, 1989.
556. Kawai S, Ichikawa Y, Homma M: Differences in metabolic properties among cortisol, prednisolone and dexamethasone in liver and renal diseases. Accelerated metabolism of dexamethasone in renal failure. *J Clin Endocrinol Metab* 60:848, 1985.
557. Roitman A, Bruchis S, Bauman B, Kaufman H, Laron Z: Total deficiency of corticosteroid-binding globulin. *Clin Endocrinol* 21:541, 1984.

558. Doe RP, Lohrenz FN, Seal US: Familial decrease in corticosteroid-binding globulin. *Metabolism* 14:940, 1965.
559. Mendel CM, Kuhn RW, Weisiger RA, Cavalieri RR, Siiteri PK, Cunha GR, Murai JT: Uptake of cortisol by the perfused rat liver: Validity of the free hormone hypothesis applied to cortisol. *Endocrinology* 124:468, 1989.
560. Mendel CM: The free hormone hypothesis: A physiologically based mathematical model. *Endocr Rev* 10:232, 1989.
561. Partridge WM: Transport of protein-bound hormones into tissues *in vivo*. *Endocr Rev* 2:103, 1981.
562. Mendel CM, Weisiger RA, Jones AL, Cavalieri RR: Thyroid hormone-binding proteins in plasma facilitate uniform distribution of thyroxine within tissues: A perfused rat liver study. *Endocrinology* 120:1987, 1987.
563. Zager PG, Burtis WJ, Luetscher JA, Dowdy AJ, Sood S: Increased plasma protein binding and low metabolic clearance rate of aldosterone in plasma of low cortisol concentration. *J Clin Endocrinol Metab* 42:207, 1976.
564. Zipser RD, Meidor V, Horton R: Characteristics of aldosterone binding in human plasma. *J Clin Endocrinol Metab* 50:158, 1979.
565. Chanarri M, Luetscher JA, Dowdy AJ, Ganguly A: The effects of temperature and plasma cortisol on distribution of aldosterone between plasma and red blood cells: Influences on metabolic clearance rate and on hepatic and renal extraction of aldosterone. *J Clin Endocrinol Metab* 44:752, 1977.
566. Matulich DT, Morris JA, Bartter FC, Baxter JD: Unpublished data.
567. Plager JE: The binding of androsterone sulfate, etiocholanolone sulfate and dehydroisoandrosterone sulfate by plasma protein. *J Clin Invest* 44:1234, 1965.
568. Forest MG, Rinarola MA, Migeon CJ: Percentage binding of testosterone, androstenedione and dehydroisoandrosterone in human plasma. *Steroids* 12:323, 1968.
569. Pearlman WH, Crepy O, Murphy M: Testosterone-binding levels in the serum of women during the normal menstrual cycle, pregnancy and the post-partum period. *J Clin Endocrinol Metab* 27:1012, 1967.
570. Peterson RE: Metabolism of adrenal cortical steroids, in Christy NP (ed): *The Human Adrenal Cortex.* New York, Harper & Row, 1971, p 87.
571. Brooks RV: Biosynthesis and metabolism of adrenocortical steroids, in James VHT (ed): *The Adrenal Gland.* New York, Raven, 1979, p 67.
572. Monder C, Bradlow LH: Cortoic acids: Exploration at the frontier of corticosteroid metabolism. *Recent Prog Horm Res* 36:345, 1980.
573. Bradlow HL, Monder C, Zumoff B: Metabolism of cortoic acids in man. *J Clin Endocrinol Metab* 54:296, 1982.
574. Peterson KE: The production of cortisol and corticosterone in children. *Acta Paediatr Scand* 281:2, 1980.
575. Miller WL: The adrenal cortex, in Rudolph AM, Hoffman JIE, Rudolph CR (eds): *Rudolph's Pediatrics*, 19th ed. Norwalk, Conn., Appleton & Lange, 1991, p 1584.
576. Ulstrom RA, Colle E, Burkey J, Gummelle R: Adrenocortical steroid metabolism in newborn infants: II. Urinary excretion of 6β-hydroxycortisol and other polar metabolites. *J Clin Endocrinol Metab* 20:1080, 1961.
577. Werk EE, MacGee J, Sholiton LJ: Altered cortisol metabolism in advanced cancer and other terminal illnesses: Excretion of 6β-hydroxycortisol. *Metabolism* 13:1425, 1964.
578. Katz FH, Lipman MM, Frantz AG, Jailer JW: The physiologic significance of β-hydroxycortisol in human corticoid metabolism. *J Clin Endocrinol Metab* 22:71, 1962.
579. Pasqualini JR, Jayle MR: Corticosteroid 21-sulphates in human urine. *Biochem J* 81:147, 1961.
580. Drucker WD, Sfikakis A, Borowski AJ, Christy NP: On the rate of formation of steroidal glucuronides in patients with familial and acquired jaundice. *J Clin Invest* 43:1952, 1964.
581. Whitworth JA, Stewart PM, Burt D, Atherden SM, Edwards CRW: The kidney is the major site of cortisone production in man. *Clin Endocrinol* 31:355, 1989.
582. Morris DJ: The metabolism and mechanism of action of aldosterone. *Endocr Rev* 2:234, 1981.
583. Luetscher JA, Hancock EW, Camargo CA, Dowdy AJ, Nokes GW: Conjugation of 1,2-^{3}H-aldosterone in human liver and kidneys and renal extraction of aldosterone and labeled conjugates from blood plasma. *J Clin Endocrinol Metab* 25:628, 1965.
584. Parker L: *Adrenal Androgens in Clinical Medicine.* San Diego, Academic Press, 1989.
585. Parker LN: Control of adrenal androgen secretion. *Endocrinol Metab Clin North Am* 20:401, 1991.
586. Meikle AW, Daynes RA, Araneo BA: Adrenal androgen secretion and biologic effects. *Endocrinol Metab Clin North Am* 20:381, 1991.
587. Pratt JH, Grim CE, Parkinson CA: Minoxidil increases aldosterone metabolic clearance in hypertensive patients. *J Clin Endocrinol Metab* 49:834, 1979.
588. Doehr P, Fichter M, Pirke KM, Lund R: Relationship between weight gain and hypothalamic pituitary adrenal function in patients with anorexia nervosa. *J Steroid Biochem* 13:529, 1980.
589. Gaunt R: History of the adrenal cortex, in Greep RO, Astwood EB (eds): *Handbook of Physiology: Endocrinology.* Washington, DC, American Physiological Society, 1975, section 7, vol 6, p 1.
590. Tan SY, Mulrow PJ: Aldosterone in hypertension and edema, in Bondy PK, Rosenberg LE (eds): *Metabolic Control and Disease.* Philadelphia, Saunders, 1979, p 1501.
591. Baxter JD: Glucocorticoid hormone action, in Gill GN (ed): *Pharmacology of Adrenal Cortical Hormones.* Oxford, Pergamon, 1979, p 67.
592. Bamberger CM, Schulte HM, Chrousos GP: Molecular determinants of glucocorticoid receptor function and tissue sensitivity. *Endocr Rev* 17:221, 1996.
593. Bloom E, Matulich DT, Higgins SJ, Simons SJ, Baxter JD: Nuclear binding of glucocorticoid receptors: Relations between cytosol binding, activation and the biological response. *J Steroid Biochem* 12:175, 1980.
594. Lan NC, Karin M, Nguyen T, Weisz A, Birnbaum MJ, Eberhardt NL, Baxter JD: Mechanisms of glucocorticoid hormone action. *J Steroid Biochem* 20:77, 1984.
595. Yamamoto KR: Steroid receptor regulated transcription of specific genes and gene networks. *Annu Rev Genet* 19:209, 1985.
596. Singh VB, Moudgil VK: Phosphorylation of rat liver glucocorticoid receptor. *J Biol Chem* 260:3684, 1985.
597. Moudgil VK: Phosphorylation of steroid hormone receptors. *Biochim Biophys Acta* 1055:243, 1990.
598. Chrousos GP: A new "new" syndrome in the new world: Is multiple postreceptor steroid hormone resistance due to a coregulator defect? (editorial). *J Clin Endocrinol Metab* 84:4450, 1999.
599. Duval D, Durant S, Homo-Delarche F: Non-genomic effects of steroids: Interactions of steroid molecules with membrane structures and functions. *Biochim Biophys Acta* 737:409, 1983.
600. Raghow R, Gossage D, Kang AH: Pretranslational regulation of type I collagen, fibronectin, and a 50-kilodalton noncollagenous extracellular protein by dexamethasone in rat fibroblasts. *J Biol Chem* 261:4677, 1986.
601. Fulton R, Birnie DG, Knowler JT: Post-transcriptional regulation of rat liver gene expression by glucocorticoids. *Nucleic Acids Res* 13:6467, 1985.
602. Birnberg NC, Lissitzky JC, Hinman M, Herbert E: Glucocorticoids regulate pro-opiomelanocortin gene expression *in vivo* at the levels of transcription and secretion. *Proc Natl Acad Sci USA* 80:6982, 1983.
603. Keller-Wood ME, Dallman MF: Corticosteroid inhibition of ACTH secretion. *Endocr Rev* 5:1, 1984.
604. Fehm HL, Voigt KH, Kummer G, Lang R, Pfeiffer EF: Differential and integral corticosteroid feedback effects on ACTH secretion in hypoadrenocorticism. *J Clin Invest* 63:247, 1979.
605. Widmaier EP, Dallman MF: The effects of corticotropin-releasing factor on adrenocorticotropin secretion from perfused pituitaries *in vitro:* Rapid inhibition by glucocorticoids. *Endocrinology* 115: 2368, 1984.
606. Jones MT, Gillham B: Factors involved in the regulation of adrenocorticotropic hormone/β-lipotropic hormone. *Physiol Rev* 68:743, 1988.
607. Dallman MF, Akana SF, Cascio CS, Darlington DN, Jacobson L, Levin N: Regulation of ACTH secretion: Variations on a theme of B. *Recent Prog Horm Res* 43:113, 1987.
608. Krozowski ZS, Funder JW: Renal mineralocorticoid receptors and hippocampal corticosterone binding species have identical intrinsic steroid specificity. *Proc Natl Acad Sci USA* 80:6056, 1983.

609. Reul MJH, de Kloet ER: Two receptor systems for corticosterone in rat brain: Microdistribution and differential occupation. *Endocrinology* 117:2505, 1985.
610. Beaumont K, Fanestil DD: Characterizaztion of rat brain aldosterone receptors reveals high affinity for corticosterone. *Endocrinology* 113:2043, 1983.
611. Lakshmi V, Monder C: Evidence for independent 11-oxidase and 11-reductase activities of 11β-hydroxysteroid dehydrogenase: Enzyme latency, phase transitions and lipid requirements. *Endocrinology* 116:552, 1985.
612. Lakshmi V, Monder C: Purification and characterization of the corticosteroid 11β-dehydrogenase component of the rat liver 11β-hydroxysteroid dehydrogenase complex. *Endocrinology* 123:2390, 1988.
613. Funder JW: Mineralocorticoids, glucocorticoids, receptors and response elements. *Science* 259:1132, 1993.
614. Pearce D, Yamamoto KR: Mineralocorticoid and glucocorticoid receptor activities distinguished by nonreceptor factors at a composite response element. *Science* 259:1161, 1993.
615. Ponta H, Kennedy N, Skroch P, Hynes NE, Groner B: Hormonal response region in the mouse mammary tumor virus long terminal repeat can be dissociated from the proviral promoter and has enhancer properties. *Proc Natl Acad Sci USA* 82:1020, 1985.
616. Slater EP, Rabenau O, Karin M, Baxter JD, Beato M: Glucocorticoid receptor binding and activation of a heterologous promoter by dexamethasone by the first intron of the human growth hormone gene. *Mol Cell Biol* 5:2984, 1985.
617. Rousseau GG, van Bohemen GC, Lareau S, Degelaen J: Submicromolar free calcium modulates dexamethasone binding to the glucocorticoid receptor. *Biochem Biophys Res Commun* 106:16, 1982.
618. Holbrook NJ, Bodwell JE, Munck A: Effects of ATP and pyrophosphate on properties of glucocorticoid-receptor complexes from rat thymus cells. *J Biol Chem* 258:14885, 1983.
619. Beyer HS, Carr FE, Mariash CN, Oppenheimer JH: Hepatic messenger ribonucleic acid activity profile of rats subjected to alterations in thyroidal and adrenocortical states: Evidence for significant interaction. *Endocrinology* 116:2669, 1985.
620. Rousseau GG, Baxter JD: Glucocorticoid receptors, in Baxter JD Rousseau GG (eds): *Glucocorticoid Hormone Action.* New York, Springer-Verlag, 1979, p 49.
621. Chrousos GP, Cutler GB Jr, Sauer M, Simons SS Jr, Loriaux DL: Development of glucocorticoid antagonists. *Pharmacol Ther* 20:263, 1983.
622. Healy DL, Chrousos GP, Schulte HM, Gold PW, Hodgen GD: Increased adrenocorticotropin, cortisol, and arginine vasopressin secretion in primates after the antiglucocorticoid steroid RU 486: Dose response relationships. *J Clin Endocrinol Metab* 60:1, 1985.
623. Schmidt TJ: Comparison of *in vivo* activation of triaminolone acetonide- and RU 38486-receptor complexes in the CEM-C7 and IM-9 human leukemic cell lines. *Cancer Res* 49:4390, 1989.
624. Schmidt TJ: *In vitro* activation and DNA binding affinity of human lymphoid (CEM-C7) cytoplasmic receptors labeled with the antiglucocorticoid RU38486. *J Steroid Biochem* 24:1986.
625. Gruol DJ, Wolfe KA: Transformation of glucocorticoid receptors bound to the antagonist RU 486: Effects of aldaline phosphatase. *Biochemistry* 29:7958, 1990.
626. Bourgeois S, Pfahl M, Baulieu EE: DNA binding properties of glucocorticosteroid receptors bound to the steroid antagonist RU-486. *EMBO* J 3:751, 1984.
627. Wolff ME: Structure-activity relationships in glucocorticoids, in Baxter JD, Rousseau GG (eds): *Glucocorticoid Hormone Action.* New York, Springer-Verlag, 1979, p 97.
628. Baulieu EE: The antisteroid RU486: Its cellular and molecular mode of action. *Trends Endocrinol Metab* 2:233, 1991.
629. Spitz IM, Bardin CW: Mifepristone (RU486)—a modulator of progestin and glucorticoid action. *N Engl J Med* 329:404, 1993.
630. Nieman LK, Chrousos GP, Kellner C, Spitz IM, Nisula BC, Cutler GB Jr, Merriam GR, Bardin CW, et al: Successful treatment of Cushing's syndrome with the glucocorticoid antagonist RU-486. *J Clin Endocrinol Metab* 61:536, 1985.
631. Meikle AW, Tyler FH: Potency and duration of action of glucocorticoids: Effects of hydrocortisone, prednisone and dexamethasone on human pituitary adrenal function. *Am J Med* 63:200, 1977.
632. Rousseau GG, Baxter JD: Glucocorticoids and the metabolic code, in Baxter JD, Rousseau GG (eds): *Glucocorticoid Hormone Action.* New York, Springer-Verlag, 1979, p 613.
633. Cahill GF: Action of adrenal cortical steroids on carbohydrate metabolism, in Christy NP (ed): *The Human Adrenal Cortex.* New York, Harper & Row, 1971, p 205.
634. Exton JH: Regulation of gluconeogenesis by glucocorticoids, in Baxter JD, Rousseau GG (eds): *Glucocorticoid Hormone Action.* New York, Springer-Verlag, 1979, p 535.
635. Stalmans W, Laloux M: Glucocorticoids and hepatic glycogen metabolism, in Baxter JD, Rousseau GG (eds): *Glucocorticoid Hormone Action.* New York, Springer-Verlag, 1979, p 517.
636. Lenzen S, Bailey CJ: Thyroid hormones, gonadal and adrenocortical steroids and the function of the islets of Langerhans. *Endocr Rev* 5:411, 1984.
637. Friedman TC, Mastorakos G, Newman TD, Mullen NM, Horton EG, Costello R, Papadopoulos NM, Chrousos GP: Carbohydrate and lipid metabolism in endogenous hypercortisolism: Shared features with metabolic syndrome X and noninsulin-dependent diabetes mellitus. *Endocrine J* 43:645, 1996.
638. Coufalik AH, Monder C: Stimulation of gluconeogenesis by cortisol in fetal rat liver in organ culture. *Endocrinology* 108:1132, 1981.
639. Goldberg AL, Tischler M, DeMortino G, Griffin G: Hormonal regulation of protein degradation and synthesis in skeletal muscle. *Fed Proc* 39:31, 1980.
640. Wise JK, Hendler R, Felig P. Influences of glucocorticoids on glucagon secretion and plasma amino acid concentrations in man. *J Clin Invest* 52:2774, 1973.
641. Tomas FM, Munro HN, Young VR: Effect of glucocorticoid administration on the rate of muscle protein breakdown *in vivo* in rats, as measured by urinary excretion of N-methylhistidine. *Biochem J* 178:139, 1979.
642. Odedra B, Millward D: Effect of corticosterone treatment on muscle protein turnover in adrenalectomized rats and diabetic rats maintained on insulin. *Biochem J* 204:663, 1982.
643. Simmons PS, Miles JM, Gerich JE, Haymond MW: Increased proteolysis: An effect of increased plasma cortisol within the physiologic range. *J Clin Invest* 73:412, 1984.
644. Shamoon H, Soman V, Sherwin RS: The influence of acute physiological increments of cortisol on fuel metabolism and insulin binding to monocytes in normal humans. *J Clin Endocrinol Metab* 50:495, 1980.
645. Carter-Su C, Okamoto K: Effect of glucocorticoids on hexose transport in rat adipocytes. *J Biol Chem* 260:11091, 1985.
646. Fain JN: Inhibition of glucose transport in fat cells and activation of lipolysis by glucocorticoids, in Baxter JD, Rousseau GG (eds): *Glucocorticoid Hormone Action.* New York, Springer-Verlag, 1979, p 7.
647. Munck A, Crabtree GR, Smith KA: Glucocorticoid receptors and actions in rat thymocytes and immunologically-stimulated human peripheral lymphocytes, in Baxter JD, Rousseau GG (eds): *Glucocorticoid Hormone Action.* New York, Springer-Verlag, 1979, p 341.
648. Rizza RA, Mandarino LJ, Gerich JE: Cortisol-induced insulin resistance in man: Impaired suppression of glucose production and stimulation of glucose utilization due to a post-receptor defect of insulin action. *J Clin Endocrinol Metab* 54:131, 1982.
649. Gaca G, Bernend K: Plasma glucose, insulin and free fatty acids during long term corticosteroid treatment in children. *Acta Endocrinol (Copenh)* 77:699, 1974.
650. Murray DK, Ruhmann-Wennhold A, Nelson DH: Adrenalectomy decreases the sphingomyelin and cholesterol content of fat cell ghosts. *Endocrinology* 111:452, 1982.
651. Nelson DH: Corticosteroid induced changes in phospholipid membranes as mediators of their action. *Endocr Rev* 1:180, 1980.
652. Taskinen MR, Nikkila EA, Pelkonen R, Sane T: Plasma lipoproteins, lipolytic enzymes, and very low density lipoprotein triglyceride turnover in Cushing's syndrome. *J Clin Endocrinol Metab* 57:619, 1983.
653. Baxter JD: Mechanisms of glucocorticoid inhibition of growth. *Kidney Int* 14:330, 1978.
654. Loeb JN: Corticosteroids and growth. *N Engl J Med* 295:547, 1976.
655. Baxter JD, Rousseau GG: Glucocorticoid hormone action: An overview, in Baxter JD, Rousseau GG (eds): *Glucocorticoid Hormone Action.* New York, Springer-Verlag, 1979, p 1.

656. Ernest MJ, Feigelsen P: Multihormonal control of tyrosine aminotransferase in isolated liver cells, in Baxter JD, Rousseau GG (eds): *Glucocorticoid Hormone Action.* New York, Springer-Verlag, 1979, p 219.
657. Clark AF, Vignos PJ: Experimental corticosteroid myopathy: Effect on myofibrillar ATPase activity and protein degradation. *Muscle Nerve* 2:265, 1979.
658. Clark AF, Vignos PJ: The role of proteases in experimental glucocorticoid myopathy. *Muscle Nerve* 4:219, 1981.
659. Parrillo JE, Fauci AS: Mechanisms of glucocorticoid action on immune processes. *Annu Rev Pharmacol Toxicol* 19:179, 1979.
660. Glaman NH: How corticosteroids work. *J Allergy Clin Immunol* 55:145, 1975.
661. Saxon A, Stevens RH, Ramer SJ, Clements PJ, Yu DTY: Glucocorticoids administered *in vivo* inhibit suppressor T lymphocyte function and diminish B lymphocyte responsiveness in *in vivo* immunoglobulin synthesis. *J Clin Invest* 61:922, 1978.
662. Fauci AS, Dale DC, Balow JE: Glucocorticoid therapy: Mechanisms of action and clinical considerations. *Ann Intern Med* 84:304, 1976.
663. Craddock CG: Corticosteroid-induced lymphopenia, immunosuppression and body defense. *Ann Intern Med* 88:564, 1978.
664. Casey LM, MacDonald PC, Mitchell MD: Despite a massive increase in cortisol secretion in women during parturition, there is an equally massive increase in prostaglandin synthesis. *J Clin Invest* 75:1852, 1985.
665. Munck A, Guyre PM, Holbrook NJ: Physiological functions of glucocorticoids in stress and their relation to pharmacological actions. *Endocr Rev* 5:25, 1984.
666. Goodwin JS, Atluru D, Sierakowski S, Lianos EA: Mechanism of action of glucocorticosteroids: Inhibition of T cell proliferation and interleukin 2 production by hydrocortisone is reversed by leukotriene B_4. *J Clin Invest* 77:1244, 1986.
667. Larsen GL, Henson PM: Mediators of inflammation. *Annu Rev Immunol* 1:335, 1983.
668. Fahey JV, Guyre PM, Munck A: Mechanisms of anti-inflammatory actions of glucocorticoids, in Weissman G (ed): *Advances in Inflammatory Research.* New York, Raven, 1981, vol 2, p 21.
669. Goetzl EJ: Oxygenation products of arachidonic acid as mediators of hypersensitivity and inflammation. *Med Clin North Am* 65:809, 1981.
670. Flower RJ: The mediators of steroid action. *Nature* 320:20, 1986.
671. Johnson LK, Baxter JD: The mechanism of action of adrenocorticosteroids at the molecular level, in McCarty D (ed): *Landmark Advances in Rheumatology.* New York, Contact Associates, 1985, p 13.
672. Karalis K, Mastorakos G, Chrousos GP, Tolis G: Somatostatin analogs suppress the inflammatory reaction in vivo. *J Clin Invest* 93:2000, 1994.
673. Karalis K, Mastorakos G, Sano H, Davis C, Wilder RL, Chrousos GP: Somatostatin may participate in the antiinflammatory actions of glucocorticoids. *Endocrinology* 136:4133, 1995.
674. Naray-Fejes-Toth A, Fejes-Toth G, Fischer C, Frolich JC: Effect of dexamethasone on *in vivo* prostanoid production in the rabbit. *J Clin Invest* 74:120, 1984.
675. Beutler B, Cerami A: Cachectin and tumour necrosis factor as two sides of the same biological coin. *Nature* 320:584, 1986.
676. Wallner B, Mattalino RJ, Hession L, Cate RL, Tizard R, Sinclair LK, Foeller C, Chow EP, et al: Cloning and expression of human lipocortin, a phospholipase A2 inhibitor with potential anti-inflammatory activity. *Nature* 320:77, 1986.
677. Altman LC, Hill JS, Hairfield WM, Mullarkey MF: Effects of corticosteroids on eosinophil chemotaxis and adherence. *J Clin Invest* 67:28, 1981.
678. Shoenfeld Y, Gurewich Y, Gallant LA, Pinkhas J: Prednisone-induced leukocytosis: Influence of dosage, method and duration of administration on the degree of leukocytosis. *Am J Med* 71:773, 1981.
679. Lippman ME: Glucocorticoid receptors and effects in human lymphoid and leukemic cells, in Baxter JD, Rousseau GG (eds): *Glucocorticoid Hormone Action.* New York, Springer-Verlag, 1979, p 377.
680. Maytin EV, Young DA: Separate glucocorticoid, heavy metal, and heat shock domains in thymic lymphocytes. *J Biol Chem* 258: 12718, 1983.
681. Compton MM, Cidlowski JA: Rapid *in vivo* effects of glucocorticoids on the integrity of rat lymphocyte genomic deoxyribonucleic acid. *Endocrinology* 118:38, 1986.
682. Butler WT, Rossen RD: Effects of corticosteroids on immunity in man: I. Decreased serum IgG concentration caused by 3 or 5 days of high doses of methylprednisolone. *J Clin Invest* 52:2629, 1973.
683. Grayson J, Dooley NJ, Koski IR, Blaese RM: Immunoglobulin production induced *in vitro* by glucocorticoid hormones. *J Clin Invest* 68:1539, 1981.
684. Cupps TR, Gerrard TL, Falkoff RFM, Whalen G, Fauci AS: Effects of in vitro corticosteroids on B cell activation, proliferation, and differentiation. *J Clin Invest* 75:754, 1985.
685. Bar-Shavit Z, Kahn AJ, Pegg LE, Stone KR, Teitelbaum SL: Glucocorticoids modulate macrophage surface oligosaccharides and their bone binding activity. *J Clin Invest* 73:1277, 1984.
686. Aronow L: Effects of glucocorticoids on fibroblasts, in Baxter JD, Rousseau GG (eds): *Glucocorticoid Hormone Action.* New York, Springer-Verlag, 1979, p 327.
687. Gordan GS: Drug treatment of the osteoporoses. *Annu Rev Pharmacol Toxicol* 18:253, 1978.
688. Cutroneo KR, Rokowski R, Counts DF: Glucocorticoids and collagen synthesis: Comparison of *in vivo* and cell culture studies. *Coll Relat Res* 1:557, 1981.
689. Furcht LT, Mosher DF, Wendelschafter-Crabb G, Woodbridge PA: Dexamethasone induced accumulation of a fibronectin and collagen extracellular matrix in transformed human cells. *Nature* 277:393, 1979.
690. Smith TJ: Dexamethasone regulation of glycosaminoglycan synthesis in cultured human skin fibroblasts. *J Clin Invest* 74:2157, 1984.
691. Sterling KMJ, Harris MJ, Mitchell JJ, DiPetrillo TA, Delaney GL, Cutroneo KR: Dexamethasone decreases the amounts of type I procollagen mRNAs *in vivo* and in fibroblast cell cultures. *J Biol Chem* 258:7644, 1983.
692. Hammarstrom S, Hamberg M, Duell EA, Stawiski MA, Anderson TF, Voorhees JJ: Glucocorticoid in inflammatory proliferative skin disease reduces arachidonic and hydroxyeicosatetraenoic acids. *Science* 197:994, 1977.
693. Oliver N, Newby RF, Furcht LT, Bourgeois S: Regulation of fibronectin biosynthesis by glucocorticoids in human fibrosarcoma cells and normal fibroblasts. *Cell* 33:287, 1983.
694. De Asua LJ, Carr B, Clingan D, Rudland P: Specific glucocorticoid inhibition of growth promoting effects of prostaglandin F2α on 3T3 cells. *Nature* 265:450, 1977.
695. Pratt WB, Aronow L: The effect of glucocorticoids on protein and nucleic acid synthesis in mouse fibroblasts growing *in vitro. J Biol Chem* 241:5244, 1966.
696. Christy NP: Adrenal cortical steroids in various types of hypertension, in Manger MW (ed): *Hormones and Hypertension.* Springfield, IL, CC Thomas, 1966, p 169.
697. Saruta T, Suzuki H, Handa M, Igarashi Y, Kondo K, Senba S: Multiple factors contribute to the pathogenesis of hypertension in Cushing's syndrome. *J Clin Endocrinol Metab* 62:275, 1986.
698. Grunfeld J, Eloy L, Moura A, Ganeval D, Ramos-Frendo B, Worcel M: Effects of antiglucocorticoids on glucocorticoid hypertension in the rat. *Hypertension* 7:292, 1985.
699. Nichols NR, McNally M, Campbell JH, Funder JW: Overlapping but not identical protein synthetic domains in cardiovascular cells in response to glucocorticoid hormones. *Hypertension* 2:663, 1984.
700. Nichols NR, Tracy KE, Funder JW: Glucocorticoid effects on newly synthesized proteins in muscle and non-muscle cells cultured from neonatal rat hearts. *J Steroid Biochem* 21:487, 1984.
701. Nichols NR, Lloyd CJ, Mendelsohn FAO, Funder JW: Glucocorticoid-induced proteins in bovine endothelial cells. *Mol Cell Endocrinol* 32:245, 1983.
702. Davies AO, De Lean A, Leflkowitz RJ: Myocardial beta-adrenergic receptors from adrenalectomized rats: Impaired formation of high-affinity agonist-receptor complexes. *Endocrinology* 108:720, 1981.
703. Clark AF, Tandler B, Vignos PJ: Glucocorticoid-induced alterations in the rabbit heart. *Lab Invest* 47:603, 1982.
704. Sambhi MP, Weil MH, Udhoji VN: Acute pharmacologic effects of glucocorticoids: Cardiac output and related hemodynamic

changes in normal subjects and patients with shock. *Circ Res* 31:523, 1965.

705. Axelrod L: Inhibition of prostacyclin production mediates permissive effect of glucocorticoids on vascular tone. *Lancet* 2:904, 1983.
706. White BC, Hoehner PJ, Wilson RF: Mitochondrial O_2 use and ATP synthesis: Kinetic effects of Ca^{+2} and HPO_4^{-2} modulated by glucocorticoids. *Ann Emerg Med* 2:396, 1980.
707. Friedland J, Setton C, Silverstein E: Angiotensin converting enzyme induction by steroids in alveolar macrophages in culture. *Science* 197:64, 1977.
708. Stockigt JR, Hewett MJ, Topliss DJ, Higgs EJ, Taft P: Renin and renin substrate in primary adrenal insufficiency: Contrasting effects of glucocorticoid and mineralocorticoid deficiency. *Am J Med* 66:915, 1979.
709. Nasjletti A, Erman A, Cagen LM, Baer PG, Matthews C, Killmar JT: Plasma concentrations, renal excretion, and tissue release of prostaglandins in the rat with dexamethasone-induced hypertension. *Endocrinology* 114:1033, 1984.
710. Falezza G, Santonactaso CL, Parisi T, Muggeo M: High serum levels of angiotensin-converting enzyme in untreated Addison's disease. *J Clin Endocrinol Metab* 61:496, 1985.
711. Bengele HH, McNamara ER, Alexander ER: Natriuresis after adrenal enucleation: Effect of spironolactone and dexamethasone. *Am J Physiol* 233:F8, 1977.
712. Haack D, Mohring J, Mohring B, Petri M, Hackenthal E: Comparative study on development of corticosterone and DOCA hypertension in rats. *Am J Physiol* 233:F403, 1977.
713. Udelsman R, Gallucci WT, Ramp J, Goldstein DS, Lipford R, Norton JA, Loriaux DL, Chrousos GP: Adaptation during surgical stress: A reevaluation of the role of glucocorticoids. *J Clin Invest* 77:1377, 1986.
714. Klein LE, Hsiao P, Bartolomei M, Lo CS: Regulation of rat renal (Na^+K^+)-adenosine triphosphatase activity by triiodothyronine and corticosterone. *Endocrinology* 115:1038, 1984.
715. Kaji DM, Thakkar U, Kahn T, Torelli JA: Glucocorticoid induced alterations in the sodium potassium pump of the human erythrocyte. *J Clin Invest* 68:422, 1981.
716. Bastl CP, Barnett CA, Schmidt TJ, Litwack G: Glucocorticoid stimulation of sodium absorption in colon epithelia is manifested by corticosteroid IB receptor. *J Biol Chem* 259:1186, 1984.
717. Noda Y, Yamada K, Igic R, Erdos EG: Regulation of rat urinary and renal kallikrein and prekallikrein by corticosteroids. *Proc Natl Acad Sci USA* 80:3059, 1983.
718. Boykin J, deTorrente A, Erickson A, Robertson G, Shrier RW: Role of plasma vasopressin in impaired water excretion of glucocorticoid deficiency. *J Clin Invest* 62:738, 1978.
719. Schwartz J, Keil L, Maselli J, Reid I: Role of vasopressin in blood pressure regulation during adrenal insufficiency. *Endocrinology* 112:234, 1983.
720. Christy NP: Iatrogenic Cushing's syndrome, in Christy NP (ed): *The Human Adrenal Cortex*. New York, Harper & Row, 1971, p 395.
721. Stanton B, Giebisch G, Klein-Robbenhaar G, Wade J, DeFronzo RA: Effects of adrenalectomy and chronic adrenal corticosteroid replacement on potassium transport in rat kidney. *J Clin Invest* 75:1317, 1985.
722. Freiberg JM, Kinsella J, Sacktor B: Glucocorticoids increase the Na^+-H^+ exchange and decrease the Na^+ gradient-dependent phosphate-uptake systems in renal brush border membrane vesicles. *Proc Natl Acad Sci USA* 79:4932, 1982.
723. Wilcox CS, Cemerikic DA, Giebisch G: Differential effects of acute mineralo- and glucocorticosteroid administration on renal acid elimination. *Kidney Int* 21:546, 1982.
724. Cope CL: *Adrenal Steroids and Disease*. London, Pitman, 1972.
725. Nerup J: Addison's disease—clinical studies: A report of 108 cases. *Acta Endocrinol (Copenh)* 76:127, 1974.
726. Downic WW, Gunn A, Paterson CR, Howie GF: Hypercalcaemic crisis as presentation of Addison's disease. *Br Med J* 1:145, 1977.
727. Findling JW, Adams ND, Lemann JJ, Gray RW, Thomas CJ, Tyrrell JB: Vitamin D metabolites and parathyroid hormone in Cushing's syndrome: Relationship to calcium and phosphorus homeostasis. *J Clin Endocrinol Metab* 54:1039, 1982.
728. Hahn TJ, Halstead LR, Baran DT: Effects of short term glucocorticoid administration on intestinal calcium absorption and circulating vitamin D metabolite concentrations in man. *J Clin Endocrinol Metab* 52:111, 1981.
729. Hahn TJ, Halstead LR, Teitelbaum SL: Altered mineral metabolism in glucocorticoid-induced osteopenia. *J Clin Invest* 64:655, 1979.
730. Lee DBN: Unanticipated stimulatory action of glucocorticoids on epithelial calcium absorption. *J Clin Invest* 71:322, 1983.
731. Williams GA, Peterson WC, Bowser EH, Henderson WJ, Hargis GK, Martinez NJ: Interrelationship of parathyroid and adrenocortical function in calcium homeostasis in the rat. *Endocrinology* 95:707, 1974.
732. Manolagas SC, Anderson DC, Lamb GA: Glucocorticoids regulate the concentration of 1,25 dihydroxycholecalciferol receptors in bone. *Nature* 277:314, 1979.
733. Kimura S, Rasmussen H: Adrenal glucocorticoids, adenine nucleotide translocation, and mitochondrial calcium accumulation. *J Biol Chem* 252:1217, 1977.
734. Hansen JW, Gordan GS, Purssin SG: Direct measurement of osteolysis in man. *J Clin Invest* 52:304, 1973.
735. Ross EJ, Marshall-Jones P, Friedman M: Cushing's syndrome: Diagnostic criteria. *Q J Med* 35:149, 1966.
736. Breslau NA, Zerwekh JE, Nicar MJ, Pak CYC: Effects of short term glucocorticoid administration in primary hyperparathyroidism: Comparison to sarcoidosis. *J Clin Endocrinol Metab* 54:824, 1982.
737. Chyun YS, Kream BE, Raisz LG: Cortisol decreases bone formation by inhibiting periosteal cell proliferation. *Endocrinology* 114:477, 1984.
738. Reid IR, Chapman GE, Fraser TRC, Davies AD, Surus AS, Meyer J, Huq NL, Ibbertson HK: Low serum osteocalcin levels in glucocorticoid treated asthmatics. *J Clin Endocrinol Metab* 62:379, 1986.
739. Leong GM, Mercado-Asis LB, Reynolds JC, Oldfield EH, Chrousos GP: The effect of cushing disease on bone mineral density, body composition, growth and puberty: A report of an identical adolescent twin pair. *J Clin Endocrinol Metab* 81:1905, 1996.
740. Chen TL, Feldman D: Glucocorticoid potentiation of the adenosine 3′,5′-monophosphate response to parathyroid hormone in cultured rat bone cells. *Endocrinology* 102:589, 1978.
741. Ng B, Hekkelman JW, Heersche JNM: The effect of cortisol on the adenosine 3′,5′-monophosphate response to parathyroid hormone of bone *in vitro*. *Endocrinology* 104:1130, 1979.
742. Wong GL, Kukert BP, Adams JS: Glucocorticoids increase osteoblast like bone cell response to $1{,}25(OH)_2D_3$. *Nature* 285:254, 1980.
743. Chen TL, Cone CM, Morey-Holton E, Feldman D: Glucocorticoid regulation of $I{,}25(OH)_2$-vitamin D_3 receptors in cultured mouse bone cells. *J Biol Chem* 257:13564, 1982.
744. Binstock ML, Mundy GR: Effect of calcitonin and glucocorticoids in combination in the hypercalcemia of malignancy. *Ann Intern Med* 93:269, 1980.
745. McEwen BS: Influences of adrenocortical hormones on pituitary and brain function, in Baxter JD, Rousseau GG (eds): *Glucocorticoid Hormone Action*. New York, Springer-Verlag, 1979, p 467.
746. Doupe AJ, Patterson PH: Glucocorticoids and the developing nervous system, in Ganten D, Pfaff D (eds): *Current Topics in Neuroendocrinology*. New York, Springer-Verlag, 1982, vol 2, p 23.
747. Partridge WM, Mietus LJ: Transport of steroid hormones through the rat blood-brain barrier. *J Clin Invest* 64:145, 1979.
748. Long JB, Holaday JW: Blood–brain barrier: Endogenous modulation by adrenalcortical function. *Science* 27:1580, 1985.
749. Woodbury DM: Relation between the adrenal cortex and the central nervous system. *Pharmacol Rev* 10:275, 1958.
750. Knowlton AI: Addison's disease: A review of its clinical course and management, in Christy NP (ed): *The Human Adrenal Cortex*. New York, Harper & Row, 1971, p 329.
751. Gillin JC, Jacobs LS, Fram DH, Snyder F: Acute effect of a glucocorticoid on normal human sleep. *Nature* 237:398, 1972.
752. Sachar EJ, Asnis G, Halbreich U, Nathan RS, Halpern F: Recent studies in the neuroendocrinology of major depressive disorders. *Adv Psychoneuroendocrinol* 3:313, 1980.
753. Sternberg DE: Biologic tests in psychiatry. *Psychiatry Clin North Am* 7:639, 1984.
754. Bohus B, deKloet ER: Behavioral effects of neuropeptides (endorphins, enkephalins, ACTH fragments) and corticosteroids, in Jones

MT, Gililam B, Dallman MF, Chattopadhyay S (eds): *Interaction within the Brain Pituitary-Adrenocortical System.* New York, Academic, 1979, p 7.
755. Sandman CA, George J, McCanne TR, Nolan JD, Kaswan J, Kastin AJ: MSH/ACTH 4-10 influences behavioral and physiological measures of attention. *J Clin Endocrinol Metab* 44:884, 1977.
756. Nestler EJ, Rainbow TC, McEwen BS, Greengard P: Corticosterone increases the amount of protein 1, a neuron-specific phosphoprotein in rat hippocampus. *Science* 212:1162, 1981.
757. Axelrod J, Reisine TD: Stress hormones: Their interaction and regulation. *Science* 224:452, 1984.
758. Rudman D, Moffitt SD, Fernoff PM, Blackston RD, Faraj BA: Epinephrine deficiency in hypocorticotropic hypopituitary children. *J Clin Endocrinol Metab* 53:722, 1981.
759. Naranjo JR, Mocchetti I, Schwartz JP, Costa E: Permissive effect of dexamethasone on the increase of proenkephalin mRNA induced by depolarization of chromaffin cells. *Proc Natl Acad Sci USA* 83:1513, 1986.
760. Polansky JR, Weinreb RM: Anti-inflammatory agents: Steroids as anti-inflammatory agents, in Sears ML (ed): *Handbook of Experimental Pharmacology.* New York, Springer-Verlag, 1984, vol 69, p 459.
761. Manabe S, Bucala R, Cerami A: Nonenzymatic addition of glucocorticoids to lens proteins in steroid-induced cataracts. *J Clin Invest* 74:1803, 1984.
762. Fenster FL: The ulcerogenic potential of glucocorticoids and possible prophylactic measures. *Med Clin North Am* 57:1289, 1973.
763. Conn HO, Blitzer BL: Nonassociation of adrenocorticosteroid therapy and peptic ulcer. *N Engl J Med* 294:473, 1976.
764. Messer J, Reitman D, Sacks HS, Smith H, Chalmers TC: Association of adrenocorticosteroid therapy and peptic-ulcer disease. *N Engl J Med* 309:21, 1983.
765. Chrousos GP: The stress response and immune function: Clinical implications, the 1999 Novera H. Spector lecture. Ann NY Acad Sci, 2000.
766. Papanicolaou DA, Tsigos C, Oldfield EH, Chrousos GP: Acute glucocorticoid deficiency is associated with plasma elevation of interleukin-6: Does the latter participate in the symptomatology of the steroid withdrawal syndrome and adrenal insufficiency? *J Clin Endocrinol Metab* 81:2303, 1996.
767. Daughaday WJ, Herrington AC, Phillips LS: The regulation of growth by endocrines. *Annu Rev Physiol* 37:211, 1975.
768. Gospodarowicz D, Moran J: Stimulation of division of sparse and confluent 3T3 cell populations by a fibroblast growth factor, dexamethasone and insulin. *Proc Natl Acad Sci USA* 71:4584, 1974.
769. Conover CA, Rosenfeld RG, Hintz RL: Aging alters somatomedin-C-dexamethasone synergism in the stimulation of deoxyribonucleic acid synthesis and replication of cultured human fibroblasts. *J Clin Endocrinol Metab* 61:423, 1985.
770. Bennett A, Chen T, Feldman D, Hintz RL: Characterization of insulin-like growth factor I receptors on cultured rat bone cells: Regulation of receptor concentration by glucocorticoids. *Endocrinology* 116:1577, 1984.
771. No reference.
772. Unterman TG, Phillips LS: Glucocorticoid effects on somatomedins and somatomedin inhibitors. *J Clin Endocrinol Metab* 61:618, 1985.
773. Ballard PL: Glucocorticoids and differentiation, in Baxter JD, Rousseau GG (eds): *Glucocorticoid Hormone Action.* New York, Springer-Verlag, 1979, p 493.
774. Schuetz EG, Wrighton SA, Barwick JL, Guzelian PS: Induction of cytochrome P-450 by glucocorticoids in rat liver: I. Evidence that glucocorticoids and pregnenolone 16α-carbonitrile regulate de novo synthesis of a common form of cytochrome P-450 in cultures of adult rat hepatocytes and in the liver *in vivo. J Biol Chem* 259:1999, 1984.
775. Lantiguce RL, Streck WF, Lockwood DH, Jacobs LS: Glucocorticoid suppression of pancreatic and pituitary hormones: Pancreatic polypeptide, growth hormone, and prolactin. *J Clin Endocrinol Metab* 50:298, 1980.
776. Muszynski M, Birnbaum RS, Roos BA: Glucocorticoids stimulate the production of preprocalcitonin-derived secretory peptides by a rat medullary thyroid carcinoma cell line. *J Biol Chem* 19:11678, 1983.
777. Sowers JR, Carlson HE, Brautbar N, Hershman JM: Effect of dexamethasone on prolactin and TSH responses to TRH and metoclopramide in man. *J Clin Endocrinol Metab* 44:237, 1977.
778. Burr WA, Griffiths RS, Ramsden DB, Black EG, Hoffenberg R, Meinhold H, Wenzel KW: Effect of a single dose of dexamethasone on serum concentration of thyroid hormone. *Lancet* 2:58, 1976.
779. Vreeburg JTM, de Greef WJ, Ooms MP, van Wouw P, Wever RFA: Effects of adrenocorticotropin and corticosterone on the negative feedback action of testosterone in the adult male rat. *Endocrinology* 115:977, 1984.
780. Karpas AE, Rodriguez-Rigau LJ, Smith KD, Steinberger E: Effect of acute and chronic androgen suppression by glucocorticoids on gonadotropin levels in hirsute women. *J Clin Endocrinol Metab* 59:780, 1984.
781. Sapolsky RM: Stress-induced suppression of testicular function in the wild baboon: Role of glucocorticoids. *Endocrinology* 116:2273, 1985.
782. Cumming DC, Quigley ME, Yen SSC: Acute suppression of circulating testosterone levels by cortisol in men. *J Clin Endocrinol Metab* 57:671, 1983.
783. Novotny M, Jemiolo B, Harvey S, Wiesler D, Marchlewska-Koj A: Adrenal-mediated endogenous metabolites inhibit puberty in female mice. *Science* 231:722, 1986.
784. Schoonmaker JN, Erickson GF: Glucocorticoid modulation of follicle-stimulating hormone-mediated granulosa cell differentiation. *Endocrinology* 113:1356, 1983.
785. Suter DE, Schwartz NB: Effects of glucocorticoids on secretion of luteinizing hormone and follicle-stimulating hormone by female rat pituitary cells *in vitro. Endocrinology* 117:849, 1985.
786. Simpson ER, Ackerman GE, Smith ME, Mendelson CR: Estrogen formation in stromal cells of adipose tissue of women: Induction by glucocorticosteroids. *Proc Natl Acad Sci USA* 78:5690, 1981.
787. Granner DK: The role of glucocorticoids as biological amplifiers, in Baxter JD, Rousseau GG (eds): *Glucocorticoid Hormone Action.* New York, Springer-Verlag, 1979, p 593.
788. Harris AW, Baxter JD: Variations in the cellular sensitivity to glucocorticoids: Observations and mechanisms, in Baxter JD, Rousseau GG (eds): *Glucocorticoid Hormone Action.* New York, Springer-Verlag, 1979, p 423.
789. Gruol DJ, Campbell NF, Bourgeois S: Cyclic AMP-dependent protein kinase promotes glucocorticoid receptor function. *J Biol Chem* 261:4909, 1986.
790. Lai E, Rosen O, Rubin CS: Dexamethasone regulates the β-adrenergic receptor subtype expressed by 3T3-L1 preadipocytes and adipocytes. *J Biol Chem* 257:6691, 1982.
791. Davies AO, Lefkowitz RJ: *In vitro* desensitization of beta adrenergic receptors in human neutrophils. *J Clin Invest* 71:565, 1983.
792. Dunlop D: Eighty six cases of Addison's disease. *Br Med J* 2:887, 1963.
793. Marver D, Kakko JP: Renal target sites and the mechanism of action of aldosterone. *Miner Electrolyte Metab* 9:1, 1983.
794. Claire M, Oblin ME, Steimer J, Nakane H, Misumi J, Michaud A, Corvol P: Effect of adrenalectomy and aldosterone on the modulation of mineralocorticoid receptors in rat kidney. *J Biol Chem* 256:142, 1981.
795. Ludens JH, Fanestil DD: The mechanism of aldosterone function, in Gill GN (ed): *Pharmacology of Adrenal Cortical Hormones.* New York, Pergamon, 1979, p 143.
796. Kurt Lee SM, Chekal MA, Katz AL: Corticosterone binding sites along the rat nephron. *Am J Physiol (Renal Fluid Electrolyte Physiol 13)* 244:F504, 1983.
797. Lan NC, Graham B, Bartter FC, Baxter JD: Binding of steroids to mineralocorticoid receptors: Implications for *in vivo* occupancy by glucocorticoids. *J Clin Endocrinol Metab* 54:332, 1982.
798. Quirk SJ, Gannell JE, Funder JW: Aldosterone-binding sites in pregnant and lactating rat mammary glands. *Endocrinology* 113:1812, 1983.
799. Park SC, Edelman IS: Dual action of aldosterone on toad bladder: Na^+ permeability and Na^+ pump modulation. *Am J Physiol (Renal Fluid Electrolyte Physiol 15)* 246:F517, 1984.
800. Park SC, Edelman IS: Effect of aldosterone on abundance and phosphorylation kinetics of Na-K-ATPase of toad urinary bladder. *Am J Physiol (Renal Fluid Electrolyte Physiol 15)* 246:F509, 1984.

801. El Mernissi G, Chabardes D, Doucet A, Hus-Citharel A, Imbert-Teboul M, Le Bouffant F, Montegut M, Siaume S, et al: Changes in tubular basolateral membrane markers after chronic DOCA treatment. *Am J Physiol (Renal Fluid Electrolyte Physiol 14)* 245:F100, 1983.
802. Karbowiak Al, Krozowski Z, Funder JW, Adam WR: The mechanism of mineralocorticoid action of carbenoxolone. *Endocrinology* 111:1683, 1982.
803. Cortas N, Abras E, Arnaout M, Mooradian A, Muakasah S: Energetics of sodium transport in the urinary bladder of the toad: Effect of aldosterone and sodium cyanide. *J Clin Invest* 73:46, 1984.
804. Tomita K, Pisano JJ, Knepper MA: Control of sodium and potassium transport in the cortical collecting duct of the rat. *J Clin Invest* 76:132, 1985.
805. Petty KJ, Kokko JP, Marver D: Secondary effect of aldosterone on Na-K-ATPase activity in the rabbit cortical collecting tubule. *J Clin Invest* 68:1514, 1981.
806. Mujais SK, Chekal MA, Jones WJ, Hayslett JP, Katz AI: Modulation of renal sodium-potassium-adenosine triphosphate by aldosterone. *J Clin Invest* 76:170, 1985.
807. Mujais SK, Chekal MA, Jones WJ, Hayslett JP, Katz AL: Regulation of renal Na-K-ATPase in the rat. *J Clin Invest* 73:13, 1984.
808. Speiser PW, Martin KO, Kao-Lo G, New MI: Excess mineralocorticoid receptor activity in patients with dexamethasone-suppressible hyperaldosteronism is under adrenocorticotropin control. *J Clin Endocrinol Metab* 61:297, 1985.
809. Lan NC, Matulich DT, Stockigt JR, Biglieri EG, New MI, Baxter JD: Radioreceptor assay of plasma mineralocorticoid activity. *Circ Res* 46(Suppl.):194, 1980.
810. Dunn JF, Nisula BC, Rodbard D: Transport of steroid hormones: Binding of 21 endogenous steroids to both testosterone-binding globulin and corticosteroid-binding globulin in human plasma. *J Clin Endocrinol Metab* 53:58, 1981.
811. Gomez-Sanchez CE, Gomez-Sanchez EP, Shackleton CHL, Milewick L: Identification of 19-hydroxydeoxycorticosterone, 19-oxo-deoxycorticosterone, and 19-oic-deoxycorticosterone as products of deoxycorticosterone metabolism by rat adrenals. *Endocrinology* 110:384, 1982.
812. Griffing GT, Wilson TE, Melby JC: Unconjugated and conjugated urinary 19-nor-deoxycorticosterone glucosiduronate: Elevated levels in essential hypertension. *Hypertension* 7:112, 1985.
813. Griffing GT, Dale SL, Holbrook MM, Melby JC: Relationship of 19 nor-deoxycorticosterone to other mineralocorticoids in low-renin hypertension. *Hypertension* 5:385, 1983.
814. Moura AM, Worcel M: Direct action of aldosterone on transmembrane ^{22}Na efflux from arterial smooth muscle: Rapid and delayed effects. *Hypertension* 6:425, 1984.
815. Nichols NR, Nguyen HH, Meyer WJ III: Physical separation of aortic corticoid receptors with type I an type II specificities. *J Steroid Biochem* 22:577, 1985.
816. West CD, Mahajan DK, Chavre VJ, Nabors CJ, Tyler FH: Simultaneous measurement of multiple plasma steroids by radioimmunoassay demonstrating episodic secretion. *J Clin Endocrinol Metab* 36:1230, 1973.
817. Irvine WJ, Toft AD, Feek CM: Addison's disease, in James VHT (ed): *The Adrenal Gland.* New York, Raven, 1979, p 131.
818. Knox FG, Burnett JC Jr, Kohan DE, Spielman WS, Strand JC: Escape from the sodium-retaining effects of mineralocorticoids. *Kidney Int* 17:263, 1980.
819. Forman BH, Mulrow PJ: Effect of corticosteroids on water and electrolyte metabolism, in Greep RO, Astwood EB (eds): *Handbook of Physiology: Endocrinology.* Washington, DC, American Physiological Society, 1975, vol 6, p 179.
820. Metzler CH, Gardner DG, Keil LC, Baxter JD, Ramsay DJ: Increased synthesis and release of atrial peptide during mineralocorticoid escape in conscious dogs. *Am J Physiol* 252:R188, 1987.
821. Cox M, Stevens RH, Singer I: The defense against hyperkalemia: The roles of insulin and aldosterone. *N Engl J Med* 299:525, 1978.
822. Seldin DW: Metabolic acidosis, in Brenner B, Rector F (eds): *The Kidney.* Philadelphia, Saunders, 1976, p 615.
823. Sebastian A, Sutton JM, Hulter HM, Schambelan M, Poler SM: Effect of mineralocorticoid replacement therapy on renal acid-base homeostasis in adrenalectomized patients. *Kidney Int* 18:762, 1980.
824. Lieberthal W, Oza NB, Arbeit L, Bernard DB, Levinsky NG: Effects of alterations in sodium and water metabolism on urinary excretion of active and inactive kallikrein in man. *J Clin Endocrinol Metab* 56:513, 1983.
825. Binder HJ: Effect of dexamethasone on electrolyte transport in the large intestine of the rat. *Gastroenterology* 75:212, 1978.
826. Morales AJ, Nolan JJ, Nelson JC, Yen SSC: Effects of replacement dose of dehydroepiandrosterone in men and women of advancing age. *J Clin Endocrinol Metab* 78:1360, 1994.
827. Labrie F, Diamond P, Cusan L, Gomez JL, Belanger A, Caudas B: Effect of 12-month dehydroepiandrosterone replacement therapy on bone, vagina and endometrium in postmenopausal women. *J Clin Endocrinol Metab* 82:3498, 1997.
828. Morales AJ, Haubrick RH, Huang JY, Asakura H, Yen SSC: The effect of six months treatment with a 100 mg daily dose of dehydroepiandrosterone (DHEA) on circulating sex steroids, body composition, and muscle strength in age-advanced men and women. *Clin Endocrinol (Oxf)* 49:421, 1998.
829. Baulieu EE, Thomas G, Legrain S, Lahlou N, Roger M, Debuire B, Faucounau V, Girard L, et al: Dehydroepiandrosterone (DHEA), DHEA sulfate, and aging: Contribution of the DHEAge study to a sociobiomedical issue. *Proc Natl Acad Sci USA* 97:4279, 2000.
830. Baulieu EE: Neurosteroids: A new function in the brain. *Biol Cell* 71:3, 1991.
831. Zwain IH, Yen SSC: Dehydroepiandrosterone: Biosynthesis and metabolism in the brain. *Endocrinology* 140:880, 1999.
832. Compagnone NA, Mellon SH: Neurosteroids: Biosynthesis and function of these novel neuromodulators. *Frontiers Neuroendocrinol* 21:1, 2000.
833. Compagnone NA, Mellon SH: Dehydroepiandrosterone: A potential signalling molecule for neocortical organization during development. *Proc Natl Acad Sci USA* 95:4678, 1998.
834. Ruder HJ, Guy RL, Lipsett MB: A radioimmunoassay for cortisol in plasma and urine. *J Clin Endocrinol Metab* 35:219, 1972.
835. Vecsi P: Glucocorticoids: Cortisol, corticosterone and compound S, in Jaffe BM, Behrman HR (eds): *Methods of Hormone Radioimmunoassay.* New York, Academic, 1974, p 393.
836. Kabra PM, Tsai L, Marton LJ: Improved liquid-chromatographic method for determination of serum cortisol. *Clin Chem* 25:1293, 1979.
837. Gotelli GR, Wall JH, Kabra PM, Marton LJ: Fluorometric liquid-chromatographic determination of serum cortisol. *Clin Chem* 27:442, 1981.
838. Murphy BEP: Some studies of the protein-binding of steroids and their application to the routine micro and ultramicro measurement of various steroids in body fluids by competitive protein binding radioassay. *J Clin Endocrinol Metab* 27:973, 1967.
839. Murphy BEP: Non-chromatographic radiotransinassay for cortisol: Application to human adult serum, umbilical cord serum and amniotic fluid. *J Clin Endocrinol Metab* 41:1050, 1975.
840. Porter CC, Silber RH: A quantitative color reaction for cortisone and related 17,21-dihydroxy-20-ketosteroids. *J Biol Chem* 185:201, 1950.
841. Nelson DH, Samuels LT: A method for the determination of 16-hydroxy-corticosteroids in blood: 17-Hydroxycorticosterone in the peripheral blood. *J Clin Endocrinol Metab* 12:519, 1952.
842. Mattingly D: A simple fluorimetric method for the estimation of free 11-hydroxycorticoids in human plasma. *J Clin Pathol* 15:374, 1962.
843. Nielsen E, Asfeldt VH: Studies on the specificity of fluorimetric determination of plasma corticosteroids ad modum de Moor and Steeno. *Scand J Clin Lab Invest* 20:185, 1967.
844. Dash RJ, England BG, Midgley AR, Niswender GD: A specific non-chromatographic radioimmunoassay for human plasma cortisol. *Steroids* 26:647, 1975.
845. Colburn WA: Radioimmunoassay for cortisol using antibodies against prednisolone conjugated at the 3-position. *J Clin Endocrinol Metab* 41:868, 1975.
846. Willig RP, Blunck W: Quantitation of plasma cortisol and other C21-steroids by radioimmunoassay, in Gupta D (ed): *Radioimmunoassay of Steroid Hormones.* Weinheim, Verlag-Chemie, Germany, 1975, p 135.
847. Newsome HH, Clements AS, Borum EA: The simultaneous assay of cortisol, corticosterone, 11-deoxycortisol and cortisone in human plasma. *J Clin Endocrinol Metab* 34:473, 1972.

848. Evans P, Peters J, Dyas J, Walker R, Riad-Fahmy D, Hall R: Salivary cortisol levels in true and apparent hypercortisolism. *Clin Endocrinol (Oxf)* 20:709, 1984.
849. Tunn S, Mollmann H, Barth J, Derendorf H, Krieg M: Simultaneous measurement of cortisol in serum and saliva and different forms of cortisol administration. *Clin Chem* 38:1491, 1992.
850. Laudat MH, Cerdas S, Fournier C, Guiban D, Guilhaume B, Luton JP: Salivary cortisol measurement: A practical approach to assess pituitary-adrenal function. *J Clin Endocrinol Metab* 66:343, 1988.
851. Allolio B, Hoffmann J, Linton EA, Winkelmann W, Kusche M, Schulte HM: Diurnal salivary cortisol patterns during pregnancy and after delivery: Relationship to plasma corticotropin-releasing-hormone. *Clin Endocrinol (Oxf)* 33:279, 1990.
852. Krieger DT, Allen W, Rizzo F, Krieger HP: Characterization of the normal temporal pattern of plasma corticosteroid levels. *J Clin Endocrinol Metab* 32:266, 1971.
853. Gallagher TF, Yoshida K, Roffwarg HD, Fukushima D, Weitzman ED, Hellman L: ACTH and cortisol secretory patterns in man. *J Clin Endocrinol Metab* 36:1058, 1973.
854. DeLacerda L, Kowarski A, Migeon CJ: Integrated concentration and diurnal variation of plasma cortisol. *J Clin Endocrinol Metab* 36:227, 1973.
855. Silverberg A, Rizzo F, Krieger DT: Nyctohemeral periodicity of plasma 17-OHCS levels in elderly subjects. *J Clin Endocrinol Metab* 28:1661, 1968.
856. Jacobs HS, Nabarro JDN: Plasma 11-hydroxysteroid and growth hormone levels in acute medical illnesses. *Br Med J* 2:595, 1969.
857. Aron DC, Tyrrell JB, Fitzgerald PC, Findling JW, Forsham PH: Cushing's syndrome: Problems in diagnosis. *Medicine (Baltimore)* 160:25, 1981.
858. Rao KSJ, Srikantia SG, Gopalan C: Plasma cortisol levels in protein calorie malnutrition. *Arch Dis Child* 43:356, 1968.
859. Walsh BT, Katz JL, Levin J, Kream I, Fukushima DK, Hellman LD, Weiner H, Zumoff B: Adrenal activity in anorexia nervosa. *Psychosom Med* 40:499, 1978.
860. Wallace EZ, Rosman P, Toshav N, Sacerdote A, Balthazar A: Pituitary adrenocortical function in chronic renal failure: Studies of episodic secretion of cortisol and dexamethasone suppressibility. *J Clin Endocrinol Metab* 50:46, 1980.
861. Carr BR, Parker CR Jr, Maddin JD, MacDonald PC, Porter JC: Plasma levels of adrenocorticotropin and cortisol in women receiving oral contraceptive steroid treatment. *J Clin Endocrinol Metab* 49:346, 1979.
862. Abraham GE, Manlimos FS, Garza R: Radioimmunoassay of steroids, in Abraham GE (ed): *Handbook of Radioimmunoassay.* New York, Marcel Dekker, 1977, p 591.
863. Anderson DC, Hopper BR, Iasley BL, Yen SSC: A simple method for the assay of eight steroids in small volumes of plasma. *Steroids* 28:179, 1976.
864. Berson SA, Yalow RS: Radioimmunoassay of ACTH in plasma. *J Clin Invest* 47:2725, 1968.
865. Landon J, Greenwood FC: Homologous radioimmunoassay for plasma levels of corticotrophin in man. *Lancet* 1:273, 1968.
866. Orth DN: Adrenocorticotropic hormone and melanocyte stimulating hormone (ACTH and MSH), in Jaffe BM, Behrman HR (eds): *Methods of Hormone Radioimmunoassay.* New York, Academic, 1974, p 125.
867. Ruhmann-Wennhold A, Nelson DH: Adrenocorticotropic hormone, in Antoniades HN (ed): *Hormones in Human Blood.* Cambridge, MA, Harvard University Press, 1976, p 325.
868. Nicholson WE, Davis DR, Sherrell BJ, Orth DN: Rapid radioimmunoassay for corticotropin in unextracted human plasma. *Clin Chem* 30:259, 1984.
869. Hodgkinson SC, Allolio B, Landon J, Lowry PJ: Development of a non-extracted "two-site" immunoradiometric assay for corticotropin utilizing extreme amino- and carboxy-terminally directed antibodies. *Biochem J* 218:703, 1984.
870. White A, Smith H, Hoadley M, Dobson SH, Ratcliffe JG: Clinical evaluation of a two-site immunoradiometric assay for adrenocorticotrophin in unextracted human plasma using monoclonal antibodies. *Clin Endocrinol (Oxf)* 26:41, 1987.
871. Zahradnik R, Brennan G, Hutchison JS, Odell WD: Immunoradiometric assay of corticotropin with use of avidin-biotin separation. *Clin Chem* 35:804, 1989.
872. Raff H, Findling JW: A new immunoradiometric assay for corticotropin evaluated in normal subjects and patients with Cushing's syndrome. *Clin Chem* 35:596, 1989.
873. Findling JW: Clinical application of a new immunoradiometric assay for ACTH. *The Endocrinologist* 2:260, 1992.
874. Crapo L: Cushing's syndrome: A review of diagnostic tests. *Metabolism* 28:955, 1979.
875. Besser GM, Edwards CRW: Cushing's syndrome. *Clin Endocrinol Metab* 1:451, 1972.
876. Wolfsen AR, McIntyre HB, Odell WD: Adrenocorticotropin measurement by competitive binding receptor assay. *J Clin Endocrinol Metab* 34:684, 1972.
877. Daly JR, Fleisher MD, Chambers DJ, Bitensky L, Chayen J: Application of the cytochemical bioassay for corticotrophin to clinical and physiological studies in man. *Clin Endocrinol (Oxf)* 3:335, 1974.
878. Weidemann E, Saito T, Linfoot JA, Li C: Radioimmunoassay of human β-lipotropin in unextracted plasma. *J Clin Endocrinol Metab* 45:1108, 1977.
879. Jeffcoate WJ, Rees LH, Lowry PJ, Beser GM: A specific radioimmunoassay for human β-lipotropin. *J Clin Endocrinol Mebab* 47:160, 1978.
880. Krieger DT, Liotta AS, Suda T, Goodgold A, Condon E: Human plasma immunoreactive lipotropin and adrenocorticotropin in normal subjects and in patients with pituitary-adrenal disease. *J Clin Endocrinol Metab* 48:566, 1979.
881. Mullen PE, Jeffcoate WJ, Linsell C, Howard R, Rees LH: The circadian variation of immunoreactive lipotrophin and its relationship to ACTH and growth hormone in man. *Clin Endocrinol (Oxf)* 11:533, 1979.
882. Wardlow SL, Frantz AG: Measurement of β-endorphin in human plasma. *J Clin Endocrinol Metab* 48:176, 1979.
883. Wiedemann E, Saito T, Linfoot JA, Li CH: Specific radioimmunoassay of human β-endorphin in unextracted plasma. *J Clin Endocrinol Metab* 49:478, 1979.
884. Crosby SR, Stewart MF, Ratcliffe JG, White A: Direct measurement of the precursors of adrenocorticotropin in human plasma by two-site immunoradiometric assay. *J Clin Endocrinol Metab* 67:1272, 1988.
885. Beisel WR, Cos JJ, Horton R, Chao PY, Forsham PH: Physiology of urinary cortisol excretion. *J Clin Endocrinol Metab* 24:887, 1964.
886. Murphy BEP: Clinical evaluation of urinary cortisol determinations by competitive protein-binding radioassay. *J Clin Endocrinol Metab* 28:343, 1968.
887. Beardwell CG, Burke CW, Cope CL: Urinary free cortisol measured by competitive protein binding. *J Endocrinol* 42:79, 1968.
888. Nakamura J, Yakata M: Determination of urinary cortisol and 6β-hydroxycortisol by high performance liquid chromatography. *Clin Chim Acta* 149:215, 1985.
889. Contreras LN, Hane S, Tyrrell JB: Urinary cortisol in the assessment of pituitary-adrenal function: Utility of 24-hour and spot determinations. *J Clin Endocrinol Metab* 62:965, 1986.
890. Laudat MH, Billaud L, Thomopoulos P, Vera O, Yllia A, Luton JP: Evening urinary free corticoids: A screening test in Cushing's syndrome and incidentally discovered adrenal tumours. *Acta Endocrinol (Copenh)* 119:459, 1988.
891. Streeten DHP, Stevenson CT, Dalakos TG, Nicholas JJ, Dennick LG, Fellerman H: The diagnosis of hypercortisolism: Biochemical criteria differentiating patients from lean and obese normal subjects and from females on oral contraceptives. *J Clin Endocrinol Metab* 29:1191, 1969.
892. Burke CW: Hormones in urine: Uses and misuses. *J R Coll Physicians Lond* 8:335, 1974.
893. McCann VJ, Fulton TJ: Cortisol metabolism in chronic liver disease. *J Clin Endocrinol Metab* 40:1038, 1975.
894. Peterson RE: The influence of the thyroid on adrenal cortical function. *J Clin Invest* 37:736, 1958.
895. Brown H, Englert E, Wallack S: Metabolism of free and conjugated 17-hydroxycorticosteroids in subjects with thyroid disease. *J Clin Endocrinol Metab* 18:167, 1958.
896. Hellman K, Bradlow HL, Zumoff B, Gallagher TF: The influence of thyroid hormone on hydrocortisone production and metabolism. *J Clin Endocrinol* 21:1231, 1961.

897. Garib H, Munoz JM: Endocrine manifestations of diphenyl-hydantoin therapy. *Metabolism* 23:515, 1974.
898. Bledsoe T, Island DP, Ney RK, Liddle GW: An effect of o,p'-DDD in the extraadrenal metabolism of cortisol in man. *J Clin Endocrinol Metab* 24:1303, 1964.
899. Dillon RS: *Handbook of Endocrinology,* 2nd ed. Philadelphia, Lea & Febiger, 1980.
900. Boruskek S, Gold JJ: Commonly used medications that interfere with routine endocrine laboratory procedures. *Clin Chem* 10:41, 1964.
901. Appleby JI, Gibson G, Normyberski JK, Stubbs RD: Indirect analysis of corticosteroids: I. The determination of 17-hydroxycorticosteroids. *Biochem J* 60:453, 1955.
902. Caro JF, Meikle AW, Check JH, Cohen SN: "Normal suppression" to dexamethasone in Cushing's disease: An expression of decreased metabolic clearance for dexamethasone. *J Clin Endocrinol Metab* 47:667, 1978.
903. Meikle AW: Dexamethasone suppression tests: Usefulness of simultaneous measurement of plasma cortisol and dexamethasone. *Clin Endocrinol (Oxf)* 16:401, 1982.
904. Liberman B, Wajchenberg BL, Tambascia MA, Mesquita CH: Periodic remission in Cushing's disease with paradoxical dexamethasone response: An expression of periodic hormonogenesis. *J Clin Endocrinol Metab* 43:913, 1976.
905. Liddle GW: Tests of pituitary adrenal suppressibility in the diagnosis of Cushing's syndrome. *J Clin Endocrinol Metab* 12:1539, 1960.
906. Eddy RL, Jones AL, Gilliland PF, Ibarra JD, Thompson JQ, McMurry IF: Cushing's syndrome: A prospective study of diagnostic methods. *Am J Med* 55:621, 1973.
907. Burke CW, Beardwell CG: Cushing's syndrome. An evaluation of the clinical usefulness of urinary free cortisol and other urinary steroid measurements in diagnosis. *Q J Med* 42:175, 1973.
908. Butler PWP, Besser GM: Pituitary-adrenal function in severe depressive illness. *Lancet* 1:1234, 1968.
909. Jubiz W, Meikle AW, Levinson RA, Mizutani S, West CD, Tyler FH: Effect of diphenylhydantoin on the metabolism of dexamethasone: Mechanism of the abnormal dexamethasone suppression in humans. *N Engl J Med* 283:11, 1970.
910. Ashcraft MW, Van Herle A, Vener SL, Geffner DL: Serum cortisol levels in Cushing's syndrome after low- and high-dose dexamethasone suppression. *Ann Intern Med* 97:21, 1982.
911. Cook DM, Kendall JW, Allen JP, Lagerquist LG: Nyctohemeral variation and suppressibility of plasma ACTH in various stages of Cushing's disease. *Clin Endocrinol (Oxf)* 5:303, 1976.
912. Tyrrell JB, Findling JW, Aron DC, Fitzgerald PA, Forsham PH: An overnight high-dose dexamethasone suppression test for rapid differential diagnosis of Cushing's syndrome. *Ann Intern Med* 104:180, 1986.
913. Nichols T, Nugent CA, Tyler FH: Steroid laboratory tests in the diagnosis of Cushing's syndrome. *Am J Med* 45:116, 1968.
914. Flack MR, Oldfield EH, Cutler GB Jr, Zweig MH, Malley JD, Chrousos GP, Loriaux L, Nieman LK: Urine free cortisol in the high-dose dexamethasone suppression test for the differential diagnosis of the Cushing syndrome. *Ann Intern Med* 116:211, 1992.
915. Chrousos GP, Schuermeyer TH, Doppman J, Oldfield EH, Schulte HM, Gold PW, Loriaux DL: Clinical applications of corticotropin-releasing factor. *Ann Intern Med* 102:344, 1985.
916. Chrousos GP, Schulte HM, Oldfield EH, Gold PW, Cutler GB Jr, Loriaux DL: The corticotropin releasing factor stimulation test: An aid in the evaluation of patients with Cushing's syndrome. *N Engl J Med* 310:622, 1984.
917. Lytras N, Grossman A, Perry L, Tomlin S, Wass JAH, Coy DH, Schally AV, Rees LH, et al: Corticotrophin releasing factor: Responses in normal subjects and patients with disorders of the hypothalamus and pituitary. *Clin Endocrinol (Oxf)* 20:71, 1984.
918. Pieters GFFM, Hermus ARMM, Smals AGH, Bartelink AKM, Benraad TJ, Kloppenborg PWC: Responsiveness of the hypophyseal-adrenocortical axis to corticotropin-releasing factor in pituitary-dependent Cushing's disease. *J Clin Endocrinol Metab* 57:513, 1983.
919. Mezey E, Reisine TD, Brownstein MJ, Palkovits M, Axelrod J: β-Adrenergic mechanism of insulin induced adrenocorticotropin release from the anterior pituitary. *Science* 226:1085, 1984.
920. Wood JB, Frankland AW, James VHT, Landon J: A rapid test of adrenocortical function. *Lancet* 1:243, 1965.
921. Speckart PF, Nicoloff JT, Bethune JE: Screening for adrenocortical insufficiency with cosyntropin (synthetic ACTH). *Arch Intern Med* 128:761, 1971.
922. Grieg WR, Jasani MK, Boyle JA, Maxwell JD: Corticotrophin stimulation tests. *Mem Soc Endocrinol* 17:175, 1968.
923. May ME, Carey RM: Rapid adrenocorticotropic hormone test in practice. *Am J Med* 79:679, 1985.
924. Patel SR, Selby C, Jeffcoate WJ: The short Synacthen test in acute hospital admissions. *Clin Endocrinol (Oxf)* 35:259, 1991.
925. Dickstein G, Shechner C, Nicholson WE, Rosner I, Shen-Orr Z, Adawi F, Lahav M: Adrenocorticotropin stimulation test: Effects of basal cortisol level, time of day, and suggested new sensitive low dose test. *J Clin Endocrinol Metab* 72:773, 1991.
926. Hawkins JB, Burch WM: Rapid tests of adrenocortical function: Intravenous versus intramuscular administration of synthetic ACTH. *NC Med J* 50:306, 1989.
927. Longui CA, Vottero A, Harris AG, Chrousos GP: Plasma cortisol responses after intramuscular ACTH 1-24 in healthy men. *Metabolism* 47:1419, 1998.
928. Nelson JC, Tindall DJ: A comparison of the adrenal responses to hypoglycemia, metyrapone and ACTH. *Am J Med Sci* 275:165, 1978.
929. Lindholm J, Kehlet H, Blickert-Toft M, Dinesen B, Rushede J: Reliability of the 30-minute ACTH test in assessing hypothalamic-pituitary-adrenal function. *J Clin Endocrinol Metab* 47:272, 1978.
930. Jasani MK, Boyle JA, Greig WR, Dalakos JG, Browning MCK, Thompson A, Buchanon WW: Corticosteroid-induced suppression of the hypothalamic-pituitary-adrenal axis: Observations on patients given oral corticosteroids for rheumatoid arthritis. *Q J Med* 36:261, 1967.
931. Jasani MK, Freeman PA, Boyle JA, Reid AM, Diver MJ, Buchanan WW: Studies of the rise in plasma 11-hydroxycorticosteroids (11-OHCS) in corticosteroid treated patients with rheumatoid arthritis during surgery: Correlations with the functional integrity of the hypothalamo-pituitary-adrenal axis. *Q J Med* 37:407, 1968.
932. Kehlet H, Binder C. Value of an ACTH test in assessing hypothalamic pituitary-adrenocortical function in glucocorticoid-treated patients. *Br Med J* 2:147, 1973.
933. Borst GC, Michenfelder HJ, O'Brian JT: Discordant cortisol response to exogenous ACTH and insulin-induced hypoglycemia in patients with pituitary disease. *N Engl J Med* 306:1462, 1982.
934. Landon J, Greenwood FC, Stamp TCB, Wynn V: The plasma sugar, free fatty acid, cortisol and growth hormone response to insulin, and the comparison of this procedure with other tests of pituitary and adrenal function: II. In patients with hypothalamic or pituitary dysfunction or anorexia nervosa. *J Clin Invest* 45:437, 1966.
935. Dluhy RG, Himathongkam T, Greenfield M: Rapid ACTH test with plasma aldosterone levels: Improved diagnostic discrimination. *Ann Intern Med* 80:693, 1974.
936. Spiger M, Jubiz W, Meikle AW, West CD, Tyler FH: Single-dose metyrapone test: Review of a four-year experience. *Arch Intern Med* 135:698, 1975.
937. Staub JS, Noelpp B, Girard J, Baumann JB, Graf S, Ratcliffe JG: The short metyrapone test: Comparison of the plasma ACTH response to metyrapone and insulin-induced hypoglycemia. *Clin Endocrinol (Oxf)* 10:595, 1979.
938. Orth DN: Corticotropin-releasing hormone in humans. *Endocr Rev* 13:164, 1992.
939. Malchoff CD, Orth DN, Abboud C, Carney JA, Pairolero PC, Carey RM: Ectopic ACTH syndrome caused by a bronchial carcinoid tumor responsive to dexamethasone, metyrapone and corticotropin-releasing factor. *Am J Med* 84:760, 1988.
940. Jacobs HS, Nabarro JDN: Tests of hypothalamic-pituitary-adrenal function in man. *Q J Med* 38:475, 1969.
941. Thorn GW: Adrenal cortical insufficiency, in Conn HF, Clohecy R, Conn RB (eds): *Current Diagnosis.* Philadelphia, Saunders, 1966, p 445.
942. Greenwood FC, Landon J, Stamp TCB: The plasma sugar, free fatty acid, cortisol, and growth hormone response to insulin: I. In control subjects. *J Clin Invest* 45:429, 1966.

943. Krieger DT, Glick SM: Growth hormone and cortisol responsiveness in Cushing's syndrome: Relation to a possible central nervous system etiology. *Am J Med* 52:25, 1972.
944. Donald RA: Plasma immunoreactive corticotrophin and cortisol response to insulin hypoglycemia in normal subjects and patients with pituitary disease. *J Clin Endocrinol Metab* 32:225, 1975.
945. Moll GW, Rosenfield RL: Testosterone binding and free plasma androgen concentrations under physiological conditions: Characterization by flow dialysis technique. *J Clin Endocrinol Metab* 49:730, 1979.
946. Vermeulen A, Ando S: Metabolic clearance rate and interconversion of androgens and the influence of the free androgen fraction. *J Clin Endocrinol Metab* 48:320, 1979.
947. Vermeulen A, Stoïca T, Verdonck K: The apparent free testosterone concentrations: An index of androgenicity. *J Clin Endocrinol Metab* 33:759, 1971.
948. Fisher RA, Anderson DC, Burke C: Simultaneous measurement of unbound testosterone and estradiol fractions in undiluted plasma at 37°C by steady-state gel filtration. *Steroids* 24:809, 1974.
949. Vermuelen A, Rubens R: Adrenal virilism, in James VHT (ed): *The Adrenal Gland.* New York, Raven, 1979, p 259.
950. Hammond GL, Nisker JA, Jones LA, Siiteri PK: Estimation of the percentage of free steroid in undiluted serum by centrifugal ultrafiltration-dialysis. *J Biol Chem* 255:5023, 1986.
951. Givens JR: Normal and abnormal androgen metabolism. *Clin Obstet Gynecol* 21:115, 1978.
952. Rosenfield RL: Studies of the relation of plasma androgen levels to androgen action in women. *J Steroid Biochem* 6:695, 1975.
953. Rosenfield RL: Plasma free androgen patterns in hirsute women and their diagnostic implications. *Am J Med* 66:417, 1979.
954. Anderson DC: The role of sex hormone binding globulin in health and disease, in James VHT, Serio M, Giusti G (eds): *The Endocrine Function of the Human Ovary.* London, Academic, 1976, p 141.
955. Horton R, Hawks D, Lobo R: 3α, 17β-Androstanediol glucuronide in plasma: A marker of androgen action in idiopathic hirsuitism. *J Clin Invest* 69:1203, 1982.
956. Nisula BC, Loriaux DL, Wilson YA: Solid phase method for measurement of the binding capacity of testosterone-estradiol binding globulin in human serum. *Steroids* 31:681, 1978.
957. Maroulis GB, Manlimos FS, Abraham GE: Comparison between urinary 17-ketosteroids and plasma androgens in hirsute patients. *Obstet Gynecol* 49:454, 1977.
958. Margraf HW, Weichselbaum TE: Laboratory procedures in diagnosis of adrenal cortical diseases, in Eisenstein AB (ed): *The Adrenal Cortex.* Boston, Little Brown, 1967, p 405.
959. Abraham GE, Maroulis GB, Buster JE, Chang RJ, Marshall JR: Effect of dexamethasone on serum cortisol and androgen levels in hirsute patients. *Obstet Gynecol* 47:395, 1976.
960. Abraham GE, Chakmakjian ZH: Plasma steroids in hirsutism. *Obstet Gynecol* 44:171, 1974.
961. Paulson JD, Keller DW, Wiest WG, Warren JC: Free testosterone concentrations in serum: Elevations is the hallmark of hirsutism. *Am J Obstet Gynecol* 128:851, 1977.
962. New MI, del Balzo P, Crawford C, Speiser PW: The adrenal cortex in clinical pediatric endocrinology, in Kaplan SA (ed): *Endocrinology.* Philadelphia, Saunders, 1990, p 181.
963. Hindmarsh PC, Brook CGD: Single dose dexamethasone suppression test in children: Dose relationship to body size. *Clin Endocrinol (Oxf)* 23:67, 1985.
964. Azziz R, Dewailly D, Owerbach D: Non-classic adrenal hyperplasia: Current concepts. *J Clin Endocrinol Metab* 78:810, 1994.
965. Therrell BLJ, Berenbaum SA, Manter-Kapanke V, Simmank J, Korman K, Prentice L, Gonzalez J, Gunn S: Results of screening 1.9 million Texas newborns for 21-hydroxylase-deficient congenital adrenal hyperplasia. *Pediatrics* 101:583, 1998.
966. Miller WL: The congenital adrenal hyperplasias. *Endocrinol Metab Clin North Am* 20:721, 1991.
967. Miller WL: Genetics, diagnosis, and management of 21-hydroxylase deficiency. *J Clin Endocrinol Metab* 78:241, 1994.
968. Voutilainen R, Miller WL: Developmental expression of genes for the steroidogenic enzymes P450scc (20,22 desmolase), P450c17 (17α-hydroxylase/17,20 lyase) and P450c21 (21-hydroxylase) in the human fetus. *J Clin Endocrinol Metab* 63:1145, 1986.
969. Grumbach MM, Conte FA: Disorders of sex differentiation, in Wilson JD, Foster DW, Kronenberg HM (eds): *Williams Textbook of Endocrinology,* 9th ed. Philadelphia, WB Saunders, 1998, pp 1303–1425.
970. Cara JF, Moshang T Jr, Bongiovanni AM, Marx BS: Elevated 17-hydroxy-progesterone and testosterone in a newborn with 3β-hydroxysteroid dehydrogenase deficiency. *N Engl J Med* 313:618, 1985.
971. Mulaikal RM, Migeon CJ, Rock JA: Fertility rates in female patients with congenital adrenal hyperplasia due to 21-hydroxylase deficiency. *N Engl J Med* 316:178, 1987.
972. Dittmann RW, Kappes ME, Kappes MH: Sexual behavior in adolescent and adult females with congenital adrenal hyperplasia. *Psychoneuroendocrinology* 17:153, 1992.
973. Kuhnle U, Bollinger M, Schwarz HP, Knorr D: Partnership and sexuality in adult female patients with congenital adrenal hyperplasia. First results of a cross-sectional quality-of-life evaluation. *J Steroid Biochem Mol Biol* 45:123, 1993.
973a. Kuhnle U, Bullinger M, Schwarz HP: The quality of life in adult female patients with congenital adrenal hyperplasia—A comprehensive study of the impact of genital malformations and chronic disease on female patient's life. *Eur J Pediatr* 154:708, 1995.
974. Zucker KJ, Bradley SJ, Oliver G, Blake J, Fleming S, Hood J: Psychosexual development of women with congenital adrenal hyperplasia. *Horm Behavior* 30:300, 1996.
975. Meyer-Bahlburg HFL, Gruen RS, New MI, Bell JJ, Morishima A, Shimshi M, Bueno Y, Vargas I, et al: Gender change from female to male in classical congenital adrenal hyperplasia. *Horm Behavior* 30:319, 1996.
976. Migeon CJ, Rosenwask Z, Lee PA, Urban MD, Bias WB: The attenuated form of congenital adrenal hyperplasia as an allelic form of 21-hydroxylase deficiency. *J Clin Endocrinol Metab* 51:647, 1980.
977. Kohn B, Levine LS, Pollack MS, Pang S, Lorenzen F, Levy D, Lerner A, Rondanini GF, et al: Late-onset steroid 21-hydroxylase deficiency: A variant of classical congenital adrenal hyperplasia. *J Clin Endocrinol Metab* 51:817, 1982.
978. Chrousos GP, Loriaux DL, Mann DL, Cutler GB: Late-onset 21-hydroxylase deficiency mimicking idiopathic hirsutism or polycystic ovarian disease: An allelic variant of congenital virilizing adrenal hyperplasia with a milder enzymatic defect. *Ann Intern Med* 96:143, 1982.
979. Levine LS, Dupont B, Lorenzen F, Pang S, Pollack MS, Oberfield SE, Kohn B, Lerner A, et al: Genetic and hormonal characterization of the cryptic 21-hydroxylase deficiency. *J Clin Endocrinol Metab* 53:1193, 1981.
980. Fiet J, Gueux B, Gourmelen M, Kuttenn F, Vexiau P, Cuillin P, Pham-Huu-Trung MT, Vilette JM, et al: Comparison of basal and adrenocorticotropin-stimulated plasma 21-desoxycortisol and 17-hydroprogesterone values as biological markers of late-onset adrenal hyperplasia. *J Clin Endocrinol Metab* 66:659, 1988.
981. Pang S, Wallace MA, Hofman L, Thuline HC, Dorche C, Lyon ICT, Dobbind RH, Kling S, et al: Worldwide experience in newborn screening for classical congenital adrenal hyperplasia due to 21-hydroxylase deficiency. *Pediatrics* 81:866, 1988.
982. Speiser PW, Dupont B, Rubinstein P, Piazza A, Kastelan A, New MI: High frequency of nonclassical steroid 21-hydroxylase deficiency. *Am J Hum Genet* 37:650, 1985.
983. Sherman SL, Aston CE, Morton NE, Speiser PW, New MI: A segregation and linkage study of classical and nonclassical 21-hydroxylase deficiency. *Am J Hum Genet* 42:830, 1988.
984. Dumic M, Brkljacic L, Speiser PW, Wood E, Crawford C, Plavsic V, Baniceviac M, Radmanovic S, et al: An update on the frequency of nonclassic deficiency of adrenal 21-hydroxylase in the Yugoslav population. *Acta Endocrinol* 122:703, 1990.
985. Kuttenn F, Couillin P, Girard F, Billaud L, Vincens M, Boucekkine C, Thalabard JC, Maudelonde T, et al: Late-onset adrenal hyperplasia in hirsutism. *N Engl J Med* 313:222, 1985.
986. Chetkowski RJ, DeFazio J, Shamonki I, Judd HL, Chang RJ: The incidence of the late-onset congenital adrenal hyperplasia due to 21-hydroxylase deficiency among hirsute women. *J Clin Endocrinol Metab* 58:595, 1984.
987. Gourmelen M, Gueux B, Pham-Huu-Trung MT, Fiet J, Raux-Demany MC, Girard F: Detection of heterozygous carriers for 21-hydroxylase deficiency by plasma 21-deoxycortisol measurement. *Acta Endocrinol* 116:507, 1987.

988. Carroll MC, Campbell RD, Porter RR: Mapping of steroid 21-hydroxylase genes to complement component C4 genes in HLA, the major histocompatibility locus in man. *Proc Natl Acad Sci USA* 82:521, 1985.
989. White PC, Grossberger D, Onufer BJ, Chaplin DD, New MI, Dupont B, Strominger JL: Two genes encoding steroid 21-hydroxylase are located near the genes encoding the fourth component of complement in man. *Proc Natl Acad Sci USA* 82:1089, 1985.
990. No reference.
991. Chiou SH, Hu MC, Chung BC: A missense mutation of Ile172→Asn or Arg356→Trp causes steroid 21-hydroxylase deficiency. *J Biol Chem* 256:3549, 1990.
992. Hood L, Campbell JH, Elgin SCR: The organization expression and evolution of antibody genes and other multigene families. *Ann Rev Genet* 9:305, 1975.
993. Liebhaber SA, Goossens M, Kan YW: Homology and concerted evolution at the $\alpha 1$ and $\alpha 2$ loci of human α-globin. *Nature* 290:26, 1981.
994. Miller WL, Eberhardt NL: Structure and evolution of the growth hormone gene family. *Endocr Rev* 4:97, 1983.
995. Skow LE, Womack JE, Petresh JM, Miller WL: Synteny mapping of the genes for steroid 21-hydroxylase, alpha-A-crystallin, and class I bovine leukocyte antigen (BoLA) in cattle. *DNA* 7:143, 1988.
996. Chung B, Matteson KJ, Miller WL: Cloning and characterization of the bovine gene for steroid 21-hydroxylase (P450c21). *DNA* 4:211, 1985.
997. Parker KL, Chaplin DD, Wong M, Seidman JG, Smith JA, Schimmer BP: Expression of murine 21-hydroxylase in mouse adrenal glands and in transfected Y1 adrenocortical tumor cells. *Proc Natl Acad Sci USA* 82:7860, 1985.
998. Chaplin DD, Galbraith LJ, Seidman JG, White PC, Parker KL: Nucleotide sequence analysis of murine 21-hydroxylase genes: mutations affecting gene expression. *Proc Natl Acad Sci USA* 83:9601, 1986.
999. John ME, Okamura T, Dee A, Adler B, John MC, White PC, Simpson ER, Waterman MR: Bovine steroid 21-hydroxylase: Regulation of biosynthesis. *Biochemistry* 25:2846, 1986.
1000. Gitelman SE, Bristow J, Miller WL: Mechanism and consequences of the duplication of the human C4/P450c21/Gene X locus. *Mol Cell Biol* 12:2124, 1992.
1001. Kay PH, Dawkins RL, Bowling AT, Bernoco D: Heterogeneity and linkage of equine C4 and steroid 21-hydroxylase genes. *J Immunogenetics* 14:247, 1987.
1002. Geffrotin C, Chardon P, DeAndres-Cara DR, Feil R, Renard C, Vaiman M: The swine steroid 21-hydroxylase gene (CYP21): Cloning and mapping within the swine leukocyte antigen locus. *Animal Genet* 21:1, 1990.
1003. Dupont B, Oberfield SE, Smithwick ER, Lee TD, Levine LS: Close genetic linkage between HLA and congenital adrenal hyperplasia (21-hydroxylase deficiency). *Lancet* ii:1309, 1977.
1004. Dunham I, Sargent CA, Trowsdale J, Campbell RD: Molecular mapping of the human major histocompatibility complex by pulsed-field gel electrophoresis. *Proc Natl Acad Sci USA* 84:7237, 1987.
1005. Spies T, Blanck G, Bresnarhan M, Sands J, Strominger JL: A new cluster of genes within the human major histocompatibility complex. *Science* 243:214, 1989.
1006. Partanen J, Koskimies S, Sipila I, Lipsanen V: Major histomcompatibility-complex gene markers and restriction fragment analysis of steroid 21-hydroxylase (CYP21) and complement C4 genes in classical adrenal hyperplasia patients in a single population. *Am J Hum Genet* 44:660, 1989.
1007. Dupont B, Pollack MS, Levine LS, O'Neill GJ, Hawkins BR, New MI: Congenital adrenal hyperplasia: Joint report from the eight international histocompatibility workshop, in Terasaki P (ed): *Histocompatibility Testing 1980.* Berlin, Springer Verlag, 1981, pp 693–706.
1008. Fleischnick E, Awdeh ZL, Raum D, Granados J, Alosco SM, Crigler JR Jr, Gerald PS, Giles CM, et al: Extended MHC haplotypes in 21-hydroxylase deficiency congenital adrenal hyperplasia: Shared genotypes in unrelated patients. *Lancet* i:152, 1983.
1009. Holler W, Scholz S, Knorr D, Bidlingmaier F, Keller E, Ekkehard DA: Genetic differences in the salt-wasting, simple virilizing, and nonclassical types of congenital adrenal hyperplasia. *J Clin Endocrinol Metab* 60:757, 1985.
1010. Pollack MS, Levine LS, O'Neill GL: HLA linkage and B14, DR1, BfS haplotype association with the genes for late onset and cryptic 21-hydroxylase deficiency. *Am J Hum Genet* 33:540, 1981.
1011. Speiser PW, New MI, White P: Molecular genetic analysis of nonclassical steroid 21-hydroxylase deficiency associated with HLA-B14DR1. *N Engl J Med* 319:19, 1988.
1012. Morel Y, Andre J, Uring-Lambert B, Hauptman G, Bétuel H, Tosi M, Forest MG, David M, et al: Rearrangements and point mutations of P450c21 genes are distinguished by five restriction endonuclease haplotypes identified by a new probing strategy in 57 families with congenital adrenal hyperplasia. *J Clin Invest* 83:527, 1989.
1013. Rosenbloom NR, Smith DW: Varying expression for salt-losing in related patients with congenital adrenal hyperplasia. *Pediatrics* 38:215, 1966.
1014. Stoner E, DiMartina J, Kuhnle U, Levine LS, Oberfield SE, New M: Is salt-wasting in congenital adrenal hyperplasia genetic? *Clin Endocrinol* 24:9, 1986.
1015. Morel Y, David M, Forest MG, Betuel H, Hauptman G, Andre J, Bertrand J, Miller WL: Gene conversions and rearrangements cause discordance between inheritance of forms of 21-hydroxylase deficiency and HLA types. *J Clin Endocrinol Metab* 68:592, 1989.
1016. Sinnott PJ, Dyer PA, Price DA, Harris R, Strachan T: 21-hydroxylase deficiency families with HLA identical affected and unaffected sibs. *J Med Genet* 26:10, 1989.
1017. Isenman DE, Young JR: The molecular basis for the difference in immune hemolysis activity of the Chido and Rodgers isotypes of human complement component C4. *J Immunol* 132:3019, 1984.
1018. Law SKA, Dodds AW, Porter RR: A comparison of the properties of two classes, C4A and C4B, of the human complement component C4. *EMBO J* 3:1819, 1984.
1019. Carroll MC, Campbell RD, Bentley DR, Porter RR: A molecular map of the human major histocompatibility class III region lining complement genes C4, C2 and factor B. *Nature* 307:237, 1984.
1020. Yu CY, Belt KT, Giles CM, Campbell RD, Porter RR: Structural basis of the polymorphism of the human complement components C4A and C4B: Gene size, reactivity and antigenicity. *EMBO J* 5:2873, 1986.
1021. Wijesuriya S, Zhang G, Dardis A, Miller W: Transcriptional regulatory elements of the human gene for cytochrome P450c21 (steroid 21-hydroxylase) lie within intron 35 of the linked C4B gene. *J Biol Chem* 274:38097, 1999.
1022. Tee MK, Babalola GO, Aza-Blanc P, Speek M, Gitelman SE, Miller WL: A promoter within intron 35 of the human C4A gene initiates adrenal-specific transcription of a 1kb RNA: location of a cryptic CYP21 promoter element? *Hum Mol Genet* 4:2109, 1995.
1023. Lévi-Strauss M, Carroll MC, Steinmetz M, Meo T: A previously undetected MHC gene with an unusual periodic structure. *Science* 240:201, 1988.
1024. Speiser PW, White PC: Structure of the human RD gene: A highly conserved gene in the class III region of the major histocompatibility. *DNA* 8:745, 1989.
1025. Sargent CA, Dunham I, Campbell RC: Identification of multiple HTF-island associated genes in the major histocompatibility complex class III region. *EMBO J* 8:2305, 1989.
1026. Burch GH, Bedolli MA, McDonough S, Rosenthal SM, Bristow J: Embryonic expression of tenascin-X suggests a role in limb, muscle, and heart development. *Dev Dynamics* 203:491, 1995.
1027. Speek M, Barry F, Miller WL: Alternate promoters and alternate splicing of human tenascin-X, a gene with 5′ and 3′ ends buried in other genes. *Hum Mol Genet* 5:1749, 1996.
1028. Tee MK, Thomson AA, Bristow J, Miller WL: Sequences promoting the transcription of the human XA gene overlapping P450c21A correctly predict the presence of a novel, adrenal-specific, truncated form of Tenascin-X. *Genomics* 28:171, 1995.
1029. Burch GH, Gong Y, Liu W, Dettman R, Curry CJ, Smith L, Miller WL, Bristow J: Tenascin-X deficiency is associated with Ehlers-Danlos syndrome. *Nat Genet* 17:104, 1997.
1030. Elefteriou F, Exposito J, Garrone R, Lethias C: Characterization of the bovine Tenascin-X. *J Biol Chem* 272:22866, 1997.
1031. Speek M, Miller WL: Hybridization of complementary mRNAs for (P450c21 steroid 21-hydroxylase) and Tenascin-X is prevented

by sequence-specific binding of nuclear proteins. *Mol Endocrinol* 9:1655, 1995.
1032. White PC, Speiser PW: Congenital adrenal hyperplasia due to 21-hydroxylase deficiency. *Endocr Rev* 21:245, 2000.
1033. Tokunaga K, Saueracker G, Kay PH, Christiansen FT, Anand R, Dawkins RL: Extensive deletions and insertions in different MHC supratypes detected by pulsed field gel electrophoresis. *J Exp Med* 168:933, 1988.
1034. Collier S, Sinnott PJ, Dyer PA, Price DA, Harris R, Strachan T: Pulse field gel electrophoresis identifies a high degree of variability in the number of tandem 21-hydroxylase and complement C4 gene repeats in 21-hydroxylase deficiency haplotypes. *EMBO J* 8:1393, 1989.
1035. Dunham I, Sargent CA, Dawkins RL, Campbell RD: Direct observation of the gene organization of the complement C4 and 21-hydroxylase loci by pulse field gel electrophoresis. *J Exp Med* 169:1803, 1989.
1036. Partanen J, Kere J, Wessberg S, Koskimies S: Determination of deletion sizes in human C4 and CYP21 genes using pulsed field gel electrophoresis. *Genomics* 5:345, 1989.
1037. Sinnott P, Collier S, Costigan C, Dyer PA, Harris R, Strachan T: Genesis by meiotic unequal crossover of a *de novo* deletion that contributes to steroid 21-hydroxylase deficiency. *Proc Natl Acad Sci USA* 87:2107, 1990.
1038. Miller WL: Gene conversions, deletions, and polymorphisms in congenital adrenal hyperplasia. *Am J Hum Genet* 42:4, 1988.
1039. Matteson KJ, Phillips JA III, Miller WL, Chung B, Orlando PJ, Frisch H, Ferrandez A, Burr IM: P450XXI (steroid 21-hydroxylase) gene deletions are not found in family studies of congenital adrenal hyperplasia. *Proc Natl Acad Sci USA* 84:5858, 1987.
1040. Baltimore D: Gene conversion: Some implications for immunoglobulin genes. *Cell* 24:592, 1981.
1041. Szostak J, Orr-Weaver T, Rothstein R: The double-stranded-break repair model for recombination. *Cell* 33:25, 1983.
1042. Nicolas A, Treco D, Schultes N, Szostak J: An initiation site for meiotic gene conversion in the yeast *Saccharomyces cerevisiae. Nature* 338:35, 1989.
1043. Fincham J, Oliver P: Initiation of recombination. *Nature* 338:14, 1989.
1044. Donohoue PA, Van Dop C, McLean RH, White PC, Jospe N, Migeon CJ: Gene conversion in salt-losing congenital adrenal hyperplasia with absent complement C4B protein. *J Clin Endocrinol Metab* 62:995, 1986.
1045. Higashi Y, Tanae A, Inoue H, Fujii-Kuriyama Y: Evidence for frequent gene conversions in the steroid 21-hydroxylase (P-450c21) gene: Implications for steroid 21-hydroxylase deficiency. *Am J Hum Genet* 42:17, 1988.
1046. Harada F, Kimura A, Iwanaga T, Shimozawa K, Yata J, Sasazuki T: Gene conversion-like events cause steroid 21-hydroxylase deficiency in congenital adrenal hyperplasia. *Proc Natl Acad Sci USA* 84:8091, 1987.
1047. Jospe N, Donohoue PA, Van Dop C, McLean RH, Bias W, Migeon CJ: Prevalence of polymorphic 21-hydroxylase gene (CAH21B) mutations in salt-losing congenital adrenal hyperplasia. *Biochem Biophys Res Commun* 142:798, 1987.
1048. White PC, Vitek B, Dupont B, New MI: Characterization of frequent deletions causing steorid 21-hydroxylase deficiency. *Proc Natl Acad Sci USA* 85:4436, 1988.
1049. Amor M, Parker KL, Globerman H, New MI, White PC: Mutation in the *CYP21B* gene (Ile-172-Asn) causes steroid 21-hydroxylase deficiency. *Proc Natl Acad Sci USA* 85:1600, 1988.
1050. Globerman H, Amor M, Parker PL, New MI, White PC: Nonsense mutation causing steroid 21-hydroxylase deficiency. *J Clin Invest* 82:139, 1988.
1051. Higashi Y, Tanae A, Inoue Y, Hiroshima T, Fujii-Kuriyama Y: Aberrant splicing and missense mutation cause steroid 21-hydroxylase [P-450(C21)] deficiency in humans: Possible gene conversion products. *Proc Natl Acad Sci USA* 85:7486, 1988.
1052. Hu MC, Chung B-C: Expression of human 21-hydroxylase (P450c21) in bacterial and mammalian cell—a system to characterize normal and mutant enzymes. *Mol Endocrinol* 4:893, 1990.
1053. Urabe K, Kimura A, Harada F, Iwanage T, Sasazuki T: Gene conversion in steroid 21-hydroxylase genes. *Am J Hum Genet* 46:1178, 1990.
1054. Mornet E, Crété P, Kuttenn F, Raux-Demay MC, Boué J, White PC, Boué A: Distribution of deletions and seven point mutations on CYP21B genes in three clinical forms of steroid 21-hydroxylase deficiency. *Am J Hum Genet* 48:79, 1991.
1055. Morel Y, Murena M, Forest M, Nicolino M, David M: Frequency of the 8 known deleterious point mutations of the CYP21B gene in more than 100 families with 21-hydroxylase deficiency (CAH): Implications for prenatal diagnosis. Abstracts of the 73rd Annual Meeting of the Endocrine Society 375, 1991.
1056. Speiser PW, Dupont J, Zhu D, Serrat J, Buegeleisen M, Tusie-Luna M, Lesser M, New MI, et al: Disease expression and molecular genotype in congenital adreanl hyperplasia due to 21-hydroxylase deficiency. *J Clin Invest* 90:584, 1992.
1057. Donohoue PA, Neto RS, Collins MM, Migeon CJ: Exon 7 Nco I restriction site within CYP21B (steroid 21-hydroxylase) is a normal polymorphism. *Mol Endocrinol* 4:1354, 1990.
1058. Owerbach D, Crawford YM, Draznin MB: Direct analysis of CYP21B genes in 21-hydroxylase deficiency using polymerase chain reaction amplification. *Mol Endocrinol* 4:125, 1990.
1059. Owerbach D, Ballard AL, Draznin MB: Salt-wasting congenital adrenal hyperplasia: Detection and characterization of mutations in the steroid 21-hydroxylase gene, CYP21, using the polymerase chain reaction. *J Clin Endocrinol Metab* 74:553, 1992.
1060. Higashi Y, Hiromasa T, Tanae A, Miki T, Nakura J, Kondo T, Ohura T, Ogawa E, et al: Effects of individual mutations in the P-450(C21) pseudogene on P-450(C21) activity and their distribution in patient genomes of congenital steroid 21-hydroxylase deficiency. *J Biochem* 109:638, 1991.
1061. Picado-Leonard J, Miller WL: Homologous sequences in steroidogenic enzymes, steroid receptors and a steroid binding protein suggest a consensus steroid-binding sequence. *Mol Endocrinol* 2:1145, 1988.
1062. Kitamura M, Buczko E, Dufau ML: Dissociation of hydroxylase and lyase activities by site-directed mutagenesis of the rat P450-17α. *Mol Endocrinol* 5:1373, 1991.
1063. Wedell A, Ritzen E, Haglund-Stengler B, Luthman H: Steroid 21-hydroxylase deficiency: Three additional mutated alleles and establishment of phenotype-genotype relationships of common mutations. *Proc Natl Acad Sci USA* 89:7232, 1992.
1064. Wedell A, Luthman H: Steroid 21-hydroxylase (P450c21): A new allele and spread of mutations through the pseudogene. *Hum Mol Genet* 91:236, 1993.
1065. Wedell A, Luthman H: Steroid 21-hydroxylase deficiency: Two additional mutations in salt-wasting disease and rapid screening of disease-causing mutations. *Hum Mol Genet* 2:499, 1993.
1066. Wu DA, Chung B: Mutations of P450c21 (steroid 21-hydroxylase) at Cys^{428}, Val^{281}, or Ser^{268} result in complete, partial, or no loss of enzymatic activity. *J Clin Invest* 88:519, 1991.
1067. Tusie-Luna M, Speiser PW, Dumic M, New MI, White PC: A mutation (Pro-30 to Leu) in CYP21 represents a potential nonclassic steroid 21-hydroxylase deficiency allele. *Mol Endocrinol* 5:685, 1991.
1068. Owerbach D, Sherman L, Ballard AL, Azziz R: Pro453 to Ser mutation in CYP21 is associated with non-classic steroid 21-hydroxylase deficiency. *Mol Endocrinol* 6:1211, 1992.
1069. Helmburg A, Tusie-Luna M, Tabarelli M, Kofler R, White PC: R339H and P453S: CYP21 mutations associated with nonclassic steroid 21-hydroxylase deficiency that are not apparent gene conversion. *Mol Endocrinol* 6:1318, 1992.
1070. Monier S, VanLuc P, Kreibich G, Sabatini DD, Adesbik M: Signals for incorporation and orientation of cytochrome P450 in the endoplasmic reticulum membrane. *J Cell Biol* 107:457, 1988.
1071. Hsu L, Hu M, Cheng H, Lu J, Chung B: The N-terminal hydrophobic domain of P450c21 is required for membrane insertion and enzyme stability. *J Biol Chem* 268:14682, 1993.
1072. Seckl JR, Miller WL: How safe is long-term prenatal glucocorticoid treatment? *JAMA* 277:1077, 1997.
1073. Miller WL: Dexamethasone treatment of congenital adrenal hyperplasia—an experimental therapy of unproven safety. *J Urol* 162:537, 1999.
1074. Pang SY, Clark A: Newborn screening, prenatal diagnosis, and prenatal treatment of congenital adrenal hyperplasia due to 21-hydroxylase deficiency. *Trends Endocrinol Metab* 1:300, 1990.
1075. Forest MG, Bétuel H, Couillin P, Boué A: Prenatal diagnosis of congenital adrenal hyperplasia (CAH) due to 21-hydroxylase

deficiency by steroid analysis in the amniotic fluid of mid-pregnancy: Comparison with HLA typing in 17 pregnancies at risk for CAH. *Prenatal Diagnosis* 1:197, 1981.

1076. Forest MG, Bétuel H, David M: Prenatal treatment in congenital adrenal hyperplasia due to 21-hydroxylase deficiency: Update 88 of the French multicentric study. *Endocr Res* 15:277, 1989.

1077. Pang S, Levine LS, Cederqvist LL, Fuentes M, Riccard VM, Holcombe JH, Nitowski HM, Sachs G, et al: Amniotic fluid concentrations of Δ^5 and Δ^4 steroids in fetuses with congenital adrenal hyperplasia due to 21-hydroxylase deficiency and in anencephalic fetuses. *J Clin Endocrinol Metab* 51:223, 1980.

1078. Pang S, Pollack MS, Loo M, Green O, Nussbaum R, Clayton G, Dupont B, New MI: Pitfalls of prenatal diagnosis of 21-hydroxylase deficiency congenital adrenal hyperplasia. *J Clin Endocrinol Metab* 61:89, 1985.

1079. Hughes IA, Dyas J, Riad-Fahmy D, Laurence KM: Prenatal diagnosis of congenital adrenal hyperplasia: Reliability of amniotic fluid steroid analysis. *J Med Genet* 24:344, 1987.

1080. Forest MG, David M, Morel Y: Prental diagnosis and treatment of 21-hydroxylase deficiency. *J Steroid Biochem Mol Biol* 45:75, 1993.

1081. Speiser PW, New MI: Prenatal diagnosis and management of congenital adrenal hyperplasia. *Clin Perinatol* 21:631, 1994.

1082. Mercado AB, Wilson RC, Cheng KC, Wei JQ, New MI: Prenatal treatment and diagnosis of congential adrenal hyperlasia owing to 21-hydroxylase deficiency. *J Clin Endocrinol Metab* 80:2014, 1995.

1083. Lajic S, Wedell A, Bui T-H, Ritzen E, Holst M: Long-term somatic follow-up of prenatally treated children with congenital adrenal hyperplasia. *J Clin Endocrinol Metab* 83:3872, 1998.

1084. Migeon C: Comments about the need for prenatal treatment of congenital adreanl hyperplasia due to 21-hydroxylase deficiency. *J Clin Endocrinol Metab* 70:836, 1990.

1085. Pang S, Pollack MS, Marshall RN, Immken LD: Prenatal treatment of congenital adrenal hyperplasia due to 21-hydroxylase deficiency. *N Engl J Med* 322:111, 1990.

1086. New MI, Wilson RC: Steroid disorders in children: congenital adrenal hyperplasia and apparent mineralocorticoid excess. *Proc Natl Acad Sci USA* 96:12790, 1999.

1087. Benediktsson R, Lindsay R, Noble J, Seckl JR, Edwards CRW: Glucocorticoid exposure in utero: A new model for adult hypertension. *Lancet* 341:339, 1993.

1088. Wolkowitz OM: Prospective controlled studies of the behavioral and biological effects of exogenous corticosteroids. *Psychoneuroendocrinology* 19:233, 1994.

1089. Trautman PD, Meyer-Bahlburg HFL, Postelnek J, New MI: Effects of early prenatal dexamethasone on the cognitive and behavioral development of young children: Results of a pilot study. *Psychoneuroendocrinology* 20:439, 1995.

1090. Seeman TE, McEwen BS, Singer BH, Albert MS, Rowe JW: Increase in urinary cortisol excretion and memory declines: MacArthur studies on successful aging. *J Clin Endocrinol Metab* 82:2458, 1997.

1091. Kalmijn S, Launer LJ, Stolk RP, de Jong FH, Pols HAP, Hofman A, Breteler MMB, Lamberts SWJ: A prospective study on cortisol, dehydroepiandrosterone sulfate, and cognitive function in the elderly. *J Clin Endocrinol Metab* 83:3487, 1998.

1092. Lashansky G, Saenger P, Fishman K, Gautier T, Mayes D, Berg G, DiMartino-Nardi J, Reiter E: Normative data for adrenal steroidogenesis in a healthy pediatric population: Age and sex-related changes after ACTH stimulation. *J Clin Endocrinol Metab* 73:674, 1991.

1093. New MI, Lorenzen F, Lerner AJ, Kohn B, Oberfield S, Pollack M, Dupont B, Stoner E, et al: Genotyping steroid 21-hydroxylase deficiency: Hormonal reference data. *J Clin Endocrinol Metab* 57:320, 1983.

1094. Laue L, Cutler GJ: 21-Hydroxylase deficiency: Overview of treatment. *The Endocrinologist* 2:291, 1992.

1095. Peterson K: The production of cortisol and corticosterone in children. *Acta Paediatri Scand* 281:2, 1980.

1096. Kenny F, Preeyasombat C, Migeon C: Normal infants, children and adults. *Pediatrics* 37:24, 1966.

1097. Kenny F, Taylor F, Richards C: Reference standards for cortisol production and 17-hydroxy corticosteroid excretion during growth: Variation in the pattern of excretion of radiolabled cortisol metabolites. *Metabolism* 19:280, 1970.

1098. Linder BL, Esteban NV, Yergey AL, Winterer JC, Loriaux DL, Cassorla F: Cortisol production rate in childhood and adolescence. *J Pediatr* 117:892, 1990.

1099. Kerrigan JR, Veldhuis JD, Leyo SA, Iranmanes HA, Rogol AD: Estimation of daily cortisol production and clearance rates in normal pubertal males by deconvolution analysis. *J Clin Endocrinol Metab* 76:1505, 1993.

1100. Styne DM, Richards GE, Bell JJ, Conte FA, Morishima A, Kaplan SL, Grumbach MM: Growth patterns in congenital adrenal hyperplasia—Correlation of glucocorticoid therapy with stature, in Lee P, Plotnick L, Kowarski A, Migeon C (eds): *Congenital Adrenal Hyperplasia.* Baltimore, University Park Press, 1977, pp 247–261.

1101. Bongiovanni AM: The adrenogenital syndrome with deficiency of 3β-hydroxysteroid dehydrogenase. *J Clin Invest* 41:2086, 1962.

1102. Rheaume E, Lachance Y, Zhao H, Boeton N, Dumont M, DeLaunoit Y, Trudel C, Luu-The V, et al: Structure and expression of a new cDNA encoding the major 3β-hydroxysteroid dehydrogenase/Δ^5-Δ^4 isomerase. *Mol Endocrinol* 5:1147, 1991.

1103. Rheaume E, Simard J, Morel Y, Mebarki F, Zachmann M, Forest M, New M, Labrie F: Congenital adrenal hyperplasia due to point mutations in the type II 3β–hydroxysteroid dehydrogenase gene. *Nat Genet* 1:239, 1992.

1104. Simard J, Rhéaume E, Sanchez R, Laflamme N, de Launoit Y, Luu-The V, van Seters AP, Gordon RD, et al: Molecular basis of congenital adrenal hyperplasia due to 3β-hydroxysteroid dehydrogenase deficiency. *Mol Endocrinol* 7:716, 1993.

1105. Chang YT, Kappy MS, Iwamoto K, Wang X, Pang S: Mutations in the type II 3β-hydroxysteroid dehydrogenase gene in a patient with classic salt-wasting 3β-HSD deficiency congential adrenal hyperplasia. *Pediatr Res* 34:698, 1993.

1106. Morel Y, Mébarke F, Rhéaume E, Sanchez R, Forest MG, Simard J: Structure-function relationships of 3β-hydroxysteroid dehydrogenase: Contribution made by the molecular genetics of 3β-hydroxysteroid dehydrogenase deficiency. *Steroids* 62:176, 1997.

1107. Pang S: The molecular and clinical spectrum of 3β-hydroxysteroid dehydrogenase deficiency disorder. *Trends Endo Metab* 9:82, 1998.

1108. Moisan AM, Ricketts ML, Tardy V, Desrochers M, Mebarki F, Chaussain JL, Cabrol S, Raux-Demay MC, et al: New insight into the molecular basis of 3β-hydroxysteroid dehydrogenase deficiency: Identification of eight mutations in the HSD3B2 gene eleven patients from seven new families and comparison of the functional properties of twenty-five mutant enzymes. *J Clin Endocrinol Metab* 84:4410, 1999.

1109. Sanchez R, Rheaume E, Laflamme N, Rosenfield RL, Labrie F, Simard J: Detection and functional characterization of the novel missense mutation Y254D in type II 3β-hydroxysteroid dehydrogenase (3βHSD) gene of a female patient with nonsalt-losing 3βHSD deficiency. *J Clin Endocrinol Metab* 78:561, 1994.

1110. Mébarki F, Sanchez R, Rhéaume E, Laflamme N, Simard J, Forest MG, Bey-Omar F, David M, et al: Nonsalt-losing male pseudohermaphroditism due to the novel homozygous N100S mutation in the type II 3β-hydroxysteroid dehydrogenase gene. *J Clin Endocrinol Metab* 80:2127, 1995.

1111. Rosenfield RL, Rich BH, Wolfsdorf JI, Cassorla F, Parks JS, Bongiovanni AM, Wu CH, Shackleton CHL: Pubertal presentation of congenital Δ^5-3β hydroxysteroid dehydrogenase deficiency. *J Clin Endocrinol Metab* 51:345, 1980.

1112. Pang S, Levine LS, Stoner E, Opitz JM, Pollack MS, Dupont B, New MI: Nonsalt-losing congenital adrenal hyperplasia due to 3β-hydroxysteroid dehydrogenase deficiency with normal glomerulosa function. *J Clin Endocrinol Metab* 56:808, 1983.

1113. Pang SY, Lerner AJ, Stoner E, Levine LS, Oberfield SE, Engel I, New MI: Late-onset adrenal steroid 3β-hydroxysteroid dehydrogenase deficiency. I. A cause of hirsutism in pubertal and postpubertal women. *J Clin Endocrinol Metab* 60:428, 1985.

1114. Chang YT, Zhang L, Alkaddour HS, Mason JI, Lin K, Yang X, Garibaldi LR, Bourdony CJ, et al: Absence of molecular defect in the Type II 3β-hydroxysteroid dehydrogenase (3β-HSD) gene in premature pubarche children and hirsute female patients with moderately decreased adrenal 3β-HSD activity. *Pediatr Res* 37:820, 1995.

1115. Sakkal-Alkaddour H, Zhang L, Yang X, Chang YT, Kappy M, Slover RS, Jorgensen V, Pang S: Studies of 3β-hydroxysteroid dyhydrogenase genes in infants and children manifesting premature pubarche and increased adrenocorticotropin-stimulated Δ^5-steroid levels. *J Clin Endocrinol Metab* 81:3961, 1996.
1116. Miller WL, Auchus RJ: Biochemistry and genetics of human P450c17, in Hughes IA, Clark AJL (eds): *Adrenal Disease in Childhood: Clinical and Molecular Aspects.* Basel, Switzerland, Karger, 2000, pp 63–92.
1117. Yanase T, Simpson ER, Waterman MR: 17α-hydroxylase/17,20 lyase deficiency: From clinical investigation to molecular definition. *Endocr Rev* 12:91, 1991.
1118. Scaroni C, Opocher G, Mantero F: Renin-angiotensin-aldosterone system: A long-term follow-up study in 17α-hydroxylase deficiency syndrome. *Hypertension (Clin Exp Theory Pract)* A8:773, 1986.
1119. Biglieri EG, Herron MA, Brust N: 17α-hydroxylation deficiency in man. *J Clin Invest* 15:1945, 1966.
1120. New MI, Suvannakul L: Male pseudohermaphroditism due to 17α-hydroxylase deficiency. *J Clin Invest* 49:1930, 1970.
1121. Goldsmith O, Solomon DH, Horton R: Hypogonadism and mineralocorticoid excess: The 17-hydroxylase deficiency syndrome. *N Engl J Med* 277:673, 1976.
1122. Matteson KJ, Picado-Leonard J, Chung B, Mohandas TK, Miller WL: Assignment of the gene for adrenal P450c17 (17α-hydroxylase/17,20 lyase) to human chromosome 10. *J Clin Endocrinol Metab* 63:789, 1986.
1123. Yanase T, Waterman MR, Zachmann M, Winter JSD, Simpson ER, Kagimoto M: Molecular basis of apparent isolated 17,20-lyase deficiency: Compound heterozygous mutations in the C-terminal region (Arg(496)→Cys, Gln(461)→Stop) actually cause combined 17α-hydroxylase/17,20-lyase deficiency. *Biochem Biophys Acta* 1139:275, 1992.
1124. Zachmann M, Kenpken B, Manella B, Navarro E: Conversion from pure 17,20 desmolase to combined 17,20-desmolase/17α-hydroxylase deficiency with age. *Acta Endocrinologica* 127:97, 1992.
1125. Geller DH, Auchus RJ, Mendonça BB, Miller WL: The genetic and functional basis of isolated 17,20 lyase deficiency. *Nat Genet* 17:201, 1997.
1126. Biason-Lauber A, Leiberman E, Zachmann M: A single amino acid substitution in the putative redox partner-binding site of P450c17 as cause of isolated 17,20 lyase deficiency. *J Clin Endocrinol Metab* 82:3807, 1997.
1127. Lee-Robichaud P, Akhtar ME, Akhtar M: Control of androgen biosynthesis in the human through the interaction of Arg^{347} and Arg^{358} of CYP17 with cytochrome b_5. *Biochem J* 332:293, 1998.
1128. Giordano SJ, Kaftory A, Steggles AW: A splicing mutation in the cytchrome b_5 gene from a patient with congenital methemoglobinemia and pseudohermaphrodism. *Hum Genet* 93:568, 1994.
1129. Zachmann M, Tassinari D, Prader A: Clinical and biochemical variability in congenital adrenal hyperplasia due to 11β-hydroxylase deficiency. *J Clin Endocrinol Metab* 56:222, 1983.
1130. Holcombe JH, Keenan BS, Nichols BL, Kirkland RT, Clayton GW: Neonatal salt loss in the hypertensive form of congenital adrenal hyperplasia. *Pediatrics* 65:777, 1980.
1131. Sonino N, Levine LS, Vecsci P, New MI: Parallelism of 11- and 18-hydroxylation demonstrated by urinary free hormones in man. *J Clin Endocrinol Metab* 51:557, 1980.
1132. White PC, Curnow KM, Pascoe L: Disorders of steroid 11β-hydroxylase isozymes. *Endocr Rev* 15:421, 1994.
1133. Curnow KM, Slutsker L, Vitek J, Cole T, Speiser PW, New MI, White PC, Pascoe L: Mutations in the CYP11B1 gene causing congenital adrenal hyperplasia and hypertension cluster in exons 6, 7 and 8. *Proc Natl Acad Sci USA* 90:4552, 1993.
1134. Azziz R, Boots LR, Parker CR Jr, Bradley E Jr, Zacur HA: 11β-hydroxylase deficiency in hyperandrogenism. *Fertil Steril* 55:733, 1991.
1135. Joehrer K, Geley S, Stasser-Wozak E, Azziz R, Wollmann A, Schmitt K, Kofler R, White P: CYP11B1 mutations causing nonclassic adrenal hyperplasia due to 11β-hydroxylase deficiency. *Hum Mol Genet* 6:1829, 1997.
1136. Rösler A: The natural history of salt-wasting disorders of adrenal and renal origin. *J Clin Endocrinol Metab* 59:689, 1984.
1137. Mitsuuchi Y, Kawamoto T, Miyahara K, Ulick S, Morton D, Naiki Y, Kuribayashi I, Toda K, et al: Congenitally defective aldosterone biosynthesis in the humans: Inactivation of the P-450c18 gene (CYP11B2) due to nucleotide deletion in CMO I deficient patients. *Biochem Biophys Res Commun* 190:864, 1993.
1138. Peter M, Fawaz L, Drop S, Visser H, Sippell W: Hereditary defect in biosynthesis of aldosterone: Aldosterone synthase deficiency 1964–1997. *J Clin Endocrinol Metab* 82:3525, 1997.
1139. Geley S, Jöhrer K, Peter M, Denner K, Bernhardt R, Sippell WG, Kofler R: Amino acid substitution R384P in aldosterone synthase causes corticosterone methyloxidase type I deficiency. *J Clin Endocrinol Metab* 80:424, 1995.
1140. Portrat-Doyen S, Tourniaire J, Richard O, Mulatero P, Aupetit-Faisant B, Curnow KM, Pascoe L, Morel Y: Isolated aldosterone synthase deficiency caused by simultaneous E198D and V386A mutations in the CYP11B2 gene. *J Clin Endocrinol Metab* 83:4156, 1998.
1141. Fardella CE, Hum DW, Rodriguez H, Zhang G, Barry F, Bloch CA, Miller WL: Gene conversion in the CYP11B2 gene encoding aldosterone synthase (P450c11AS) is associated with, but does not cause, the syndrome of corticosterone methyl oxidase II deficiency. *J Clin Endocrinol Metab* 81:321, 1996.
1142. Lifton R, Dluhy RG, Powers M, Rich GM, Cook S, Ulick S, Lalouel JM: A chimaeric 11β-hydroxylase/aldosterone synthase gene causes glucocorticoid-remediable aldosteronism and human hypertension. *Nature* 335:262, 1992.
1143. Pascoe L, Curnow K, Slutsker L, Connel JMC, Speiser PW, New MI, White PW: Glucocorticoid-suppressible hyperaldosteronism results from hybrid genes created by unequal crossover between CYP11B1 and CYP11B2. *Proc Natl Acad Sci USA* 89:8327, 1992.
1144. Dluhy RG, Lifton RP: Glucocorticoid-remediable aldosteronism. *J Clin Endocrinol Metab* 84:4341, 1999.
1145. Curnow KM, Mulatero P, Emeric-Blanchouin N, Aupetit-Faisant B, Corvol P, Pascoe L: The amino acid substitutions Ser288Gly and Val320Ala convert the cortisol producing enzyme, CYP11B1, into an aldosterone producing enzyme. *Nat Struct Biol* 4:32, 1997.
1146. Mulatero P, Curnow KM, Aupetit-Faisant B, Foekling M, Gomez-Sanchez C, Veglio F, Jeunemaitre X, Corvol P, et al: Recombinant CYP11B genes encode enzymes that can catalyze conversion of 11-deoxycortisol to cortisol, 18-hydroxycortisol, and 18-oxocortisol. *J Clin Endocrinol Metab* 83:3996, 1998.
1147. Sandison AT: A form of lipoidosis of the adrenal cortex in an infant. *Arch Dis Childh* 30:538, 1955.
1148. Prader A, Siebenmann RE: Nebenniereninsuffizienz bie kongenitaler Lipoidhyperplasie der Nebennieren. *Helv Paed Acta* 12:569, 1957.
1149. Kirkland RT, Kirkland JL, Johnson CM, Horning MG, Librik L, Clayton GW: Congenital lipoid adrenal hyperplasia in an eight-year-old phenotypic female. *J Clin Endocrinol Metab* 36:488, 1973.
1150. Hauffa BP, Miller WL, Grumbach MM, Conte FA, Kaplan SL: Congenital adrenal hyperplasia due to deficient cholesterol side-chain cleavage activity (20,22 desmolase) in a patient treated for 18 years. *Clin Endocrinol* 23:481, 1985.
1151. Camacho AM, Kowarski A, Migeon CJ, Brough A: Congenital adrenal hyperplasia due to a deficiency of one of the enzymes involved in the biosynthesis of pregnenolone. *J Clin Endocrinol Metab* 28:153, 1968.
1152. Degenhart HJ, Visser KHA, Boon H, O'Doherty NJD: Evidence for deficiency of 20α cholesterol hydroxylase activity in adrenal tissue of a patient with lipoid adrenal hyperplasia. *Acta Endocrinologia* 71:512, 1972.
1153. Koizumi S, Kyoya S, Miyawaki T, Kidani H, Funabashi T, Nakashima H, Nakanuma Y, Ohta G, et al: Cholesterol side-chain cleavage enzyme activity and cytochrome P450 content in adrenal mitochondria of a patient with congenital lipoid adrenal hyperplasia (Prader disease). *Clin Chim Acta* 77:301, 1977.
1154. Lin D, Gitelman SE, Saenger P, Miller WL: Normal genes for the cholesterol side chain cleavage enzyme, P450scc, in congenital lipoid adrenal hyperplasia. *J Clin Invest* 88:1955, 1991.
1155. Sakai Y, Yanase T, Okabe Y, Hara T, Waterman M, Takayanagi R, Haji M, Nawata H: No mutation in cytochrome P450 side chain cleavage in a patient with congenital lipoid adrenal hyperplasia. *J Clin Endocrinol Metab* 79:1198, 1994.
1156. Lin D, Chang YJ, Strauss JF III, Miller WL: The human peripheral benzodiazepine receptor gene. Cloning and characterization of

alternative splicing in normal tissues and in a patient with congenital lipoid adrenal hyperplasia. *Genomics* 18:643, 1993.
1157. Tee MK, Lin D, Sugawara T, Holt JA, Guiguen Y, Buckingham B, Strauss JF III, Miller WL: T→A transversion 11 bp from a splice acceptor site in the gene for steroidogenic acute regulatory protein causes congenital lipoid adrenal hyperplasia. *Hum Mol Genet* 4:2299, 1995.
1158. Saenger P, Klonari Z, Black SM, Compagnone N, Mellon SH, Fleischer A, Abrams CAL, Shackleton CHL, et al: Prenatal diagnosis of congenital lipoid adrenal hyperplasia. *J Clin Endocrinol Metab* 80:200, 1995.
1159. Bose HS, Pescovitz OH, Miller WL: Spontaneous feminization in a 46,XX female patient with congenital lipoid adrenal hyperplasia caused by a homozygous frame-shift mutation in the steroidogenic acute regulatory protein. *J Clin Endocrinol Metab* 82:1511, 1997.
1160. Fujieda K, Tajima T, Nakae J, Sageshima S, Tachibana K, Suwa S, Sugawara T, Strauss JF III: Spontaneous puberty in 46,XX subjects with congenital lipoid adrenal hyperplasia. *J Clin Invest* 99:1265, 1997.
1161. Caron K, Soo SC, Wetsel W, Stocco D, Clark B, Parker K: Targeted disruption of the mouse gene encoding steroidogenic acute regulatory protein provides insights into congenital lipoid adrenal hyperplasia. *Proc Natl Acad Sci USA* 94:11540, 1997.
1162. Nakae J, Tajima T, Sugawara T, Arakane F, Hanaki K, Hotsubo T, Igarashi N, Igarashi Y, et al: Analysis of the steroidogenic acute regulatory protein (StAR) gene in Japanese patients with congenital lipoid adrenal hyerplasia. *Hum Mol Genet* 6:571, 1997.
1162a. Bose HS, Sato S, Aisenberg J, Shalev SA, Matsuo N, Miller WL: Mutations in the steroidogenic acute regulatory protein (StAR) in six patients with congenital lipoid adrenal hyperplasia. *J Clin Endocrinol Metab* 85:3636, 2000.
1163. Yoo H, Kim G: Molecular and clinical characterization of Korean patients with congenital lipoid adrenal hyperplasia. *J Pediatr Endocrinol Metab* 11:707, 1998.
1164. Okuyama E, Nishi N, Onishi S, Itoh S, Ishii Y, Miyanaka H, Fujita K, Ichikawa Y: A novel splicing junction mutation in the gene for the steroidogenic acute regulatory protein causes congenital lipoid adrenal hyperplasia. *J Clin Endocrinol Metab* 82:2337, 1997.
1165. Katsumata N, Kawada Y, Yamamoto Y, Noda M, Nimura A, Horikawa R, Tanaka T: A novel compound heterozygous mutation in the steroidogenic acute regulatory protein gene in a patient with congenital lipoid adrenal hyperplasia. *J Clin Endocrinol Metab* 84:3983, 1999.
1166. Bose HS, Baldwin MA, Miller WL: Incorrect folding of steroidogenic acute regulatory protein (StAR) in congenital lipoid adrenal hyperplasia. *Biochemistry* 37:9768, 1998.
1167. Guo W, Burris TP, McCabe ERB: Expression of DAX-1, the gene responsible for X-linked adrenal hypoplasia congenita and hypogonadotropic hypogonadism, in the hypothalamic-pituitary-adrenal/gonadal axis. *Biochem Mol Med* 56:8, 1994.
1168. Zanaria E, Muscatelli F, Bardoni B, Strom TM, Guioli S, Guo W, Lalli E, Moser C, et al: An unusual member of the nuclear hormone receptor superfamily responsible for X-linked adrenal hypoplasia congenita. *Nature* 372:635, 1994.
1169. Irvine WJ, Barnes EW: Adrenocortical insufficiency. *J Clin Endocrinol Metab* 1:549, 1972.
1170. Doniach D, Cudworth AG, Khoury EL, Bottazzo GF: Autoimmunity and the HLA-system in endocrine disease, in O'Riordan JLH (ed): *Recent Advances in Endocrinology and Metabolism.* London, Churchill Livingstone, 1982.
1171. Muir A, Maclaren NK: Autoimmune diseases of the adrenal glands, parathyroid glands, gonads, and hypothalamic-pituitary axis. *Endocrin Met Clin North Am* 20:619, 1991.
1172. Leshin M: Southwestern internal medicine conference: Polyglandular autoimmune syndromes. *Am J Med* Sci 290:77, 1985.
1173. Ahonen P, Myllarniemi S, Sipila I, Perheentupa J: Clinical variation of autoimmune polyendocrinopathy-candidiasis-ectodermal dystrophy (apeced) in a series of 68 patients. *N Engl J Med* 322:1829, 1990.
1174. Kasperlik-Zaluska AA, Migdalska B, Czarnocka B, Drac-Kaniewska J, Niegowska E, Czech W: Association of Addison's disease with autoimmune disorders—a long-term observation of 180 patients. *Postgrad Med J* 67:984, 1991.
1175. Maclaren NK, Riley WJ: Inherited susceptibility to autoimmune Addison's disease is linked to human leukocyte antigens-DR3 and/or -DR4, except when associated with type I autoimmune polyglandular syndrome. *J Clin Endocrinol Metab* 62:455, 1986.
1176. Neufeld M, Maclaren NK, Blizzard RM: Two types of autoimmune Addison's disease associated with different polyglandular autoimmune (PGA) syndromes. *Medicine (Baltimore)* 60:355, 1981.
1177. Trence DL, Morley JE, Handwerger BS: Polyglandular autoimmune syndromes. *Am J Med* 77:107, 1984.
1178. Nerup J: Addison's disease—a review of some clinical, pathological and immunological features. *Dan Med Bull* 21:201, 1974.
1179. Guttman PH: Addison's disease: A statistical analysis of 566 cases and a study of the pathology. *Arch Pathol* 10:742, 1930.
1180. Alvarez S, McCabe WR: Extrapulmonary tuberculosis revisited: A review of experience at Boston city and other hospitals. *Medicine (Baltimore)* 63:25, 1984.
1181. Dahlberg PJ, Goellner MH, Pehling GB: Adrenal insufficiency secondary to adrenal hemorrhage. Two case reports and a review of cases confirmed by computed tomography. *Arch Intern Med* 150:905, 1990.
1182. Rao RH, Vagnucci AH, Amico JA: Bilateral massive adrenal hemorrhage: Early recognition and treatment. *Ann Intern Med* 110:227, 1989.
1183. Rao RH, Vagnucci AH: The clinical profile and management of bilateral massive adrenal hemorrhage. *Adv Endocrinol Metab* 3:213, 1992.
1184. Xarli VP, Steele AA, Davis PJ, Buescher ES, Rios CN, Garcia-Bunuel R: Adrenal hemorrhage in the adult. *Medicine (Baltimore)* 57:211, 1978.
1185. Amador E: Adrenal hemorrhage during anticoagulant therapy. *Ann Intern Med* 63:559, 1965.
1186. Migeon CJ, Kenny FM, Hung W, Voorhess ML: Study of adrenal function in children with meningitis. *Pediatrics* 40:163, 1967.
1187. Margaretten W, Nakai H, Landing BH: Septicemic adrenal hemorrhage. *Am J Dis Child* 105:346, 1963.
1188. Guenthmer EE, Rabinowe SL, Van Niel A, Naftilian A, Dluhy R: Primary Addison's disease in a patient with the acquired immunodeficiency syndrome. *Ann Intern Med* 100:847, 1984.
1189. Stuart-Mason A, Mead TW, Lee JAH, Morris JN: Epidemiological and clinical picture of Addison's disease. *Lancet* 2:744, 1968.
1190. Nerup J: Addison's disease—Clinical studies: A report of 108 cases. *Acta Endocrinol (Copenh)* 76:127, 1974.
1191. Maisey MN, Lessof MH: Addison's disease: A clinical study. *Guys Hosp Rep* 18:363, 1969.
1192. Wulffraat NM, Drexhage HA, Bottazzo GF, Wiersinga WM, Jeucken P, Van der Gaag R: Immunoglobulins of patients with idiopathic Addison's disease block the *in vitro* action of adrenocorticotropin. *J Clin Endocrinol Metab* 69:231, 1989.
1193. Krohn K, Uibo R, Aavik E, Peterson P, Savilahti K: Identification by molecular cloning of an autoantigen associated with Addison's disease as steroid 17α-hydroxylase. *Lancet* 339:770, 1992.
1194. Bednarek J, Furmaniak J, Wedlock N, Kiso Y, Baumann-Antczak A, Fowler S, Krishnan H, Craft JA, et al: Steroid 21-hydroxylase is a major autoantigen involved in adult onset autoimmune Addison's disease. *Fed Eur Biochem Soc* 309:51, 1992.
1195. Winqvist O, Karlsson FA, Kämpe O: 21-Hydroxylase, a major autoantigen in idiopathic Addison's disease. *Lancet* 339:1559, 1992.
1196. Uibo R, Aavik E, Peterson P, Perheentupa J, Aranko S, Pelkonen R, Krohn KJ: Autoantibodies to cytochrome P450 enzymes P450scc, P450c17, and P450c21 in autoimmune polyglandular disease types I and II and in isolated Addison's disease. *J Clin Endocrinol Metab* 78:323, 1994.
1197. Colls J, Betterle C, Volpato M, Prentice L, Smith BR, Furmaniak J: Immunoprecipitation assay for autoantibodies to steroid 21-hydroxylase in autoimmune adrenal diseases. *Clin Chem* 41:375, 1995.
1198. Schmidt MB: Eine biglandulare erkrankung (nebennieren und Schilddruse) bei morbus Addisonii. *Verh Dtsch Ges Pathol* 212:1926.
1199. Turkington RW, Lebovitz HE: Extra-adrenal endocrine deficiencies in Addison's disease. *Am J Med* 43:499, 1967.
1200. Irvine WJ, Barnes EW: Addison's disease, ovarian failure and hypoparathyroidism. *Clin Endocrinol Metab* 4:379, 1975.
1201. Spinner MW, Blizzard RM, Childs B: Clinical and genetic heterogeneity in idiopathic Addison's disease and hypoparathyroidism. *J Clin Endocrinol Metab* 28:795, 1968.

1202. Chodosh LA, Daniels GH: Addison's disease. *The Endocrinologist* 16:102, 1993.
1203. Symington T: *Functional Pathology of the Human Adrenal Gland.* Edinburgh and London, Livingston, 1969.
1204. Glasgow BJ, Steinsapir KD, Anders K, Layfield LJ: Adrenal pathology in the acquired immune deficiency syndrome. *Am J Clin Pathol* 84:594, 1985.
1205. Vita JA, Silverberg SJ, Goland RS, Austin JHM, Knowlton AI: Clinical clues to the cause of Addison's disease. *Am J Med* 78:461, 1985.
1206. Buxi TBS, Vohra RB, Sujatha, Byotra SP, Mukherji S, Daniel M: CT in adrenal enlargement due to tuberculosis: A review of literature with five new cases. *Clin Imaging* 16:102, 1992.
1207. Sarosi GA, Voth DW, Dahl BA, Doto IL, Tosh FE: Disseminated histoplasmosis: Results of long-term follow-up. *Ann Intern Med* 75:511, 1971.
1208. Schonfeld AD, Jackson JA, Smith DJ, Hurley DL: Disseminated histoplasmosis with bilateral adrenal enlargement: Diagnosis by computed tomography-directed needle biopsy. *J Tex Med* 87:88, 1991.
1209. Wilson DA, Muchmore HG, Tisdal RG, Fahmy A, Pitha JV: Histoplasmosis of the adrenal glands studied by CT. *Radiology* 150:779, 1984.
1210. Washburn RG, Bennett JE: Reversal of adrenal glucocorticoid dysfunction in a patient with disseminated histoplasmosis. *Ann Intern Med* 110:86, 1989.
1211. Moreira AC, Martinez R, Castro M, Elias LLK: Adrenocortical dysfunction in paracoccidioidomycosis: Comparison between plasma β-lipotrophin/adrenocorticotrophin levels and adrenocortical tests. *Clin Endocrinol (Oxf)* 36:545, 1992.
1212. Chandler PT: Addison's disease secondary to North American blastomycosis. *South Med J* 70:863, 1977.
1213. Halvorsen RA Jr, Heaston DK, Johnston WW, Ashton PR, Burton GM: CT guided thin needle aspiration of adrenal blastomycosis. *J Comput Assist Tomogr* 6:389, 1982.
1214. Maloney PJ: Addison's disease due to chronic disseminated coccidioidomycosis. *Arch Intern Med* 90:869, 1952.
1215. Walker BF, Gunthel CJ, Bryan JA, Watts NB, Clark RV: Disseminated cryptococcosis in an apparently normal host presenting as primary adrenal insufficiency: Diagnosis by fine needle aspiration. *Am J Med* 86:715, 1989.
1216. Seidenwurm DJ, Elmer EB, Kaplan LM, Williams EK, Morris DG, Hoffman AR: Metastases to the adrenal glands and the development of Addison's disease. *Cancer* 54:552, 1984.
1217. Redman BG, Pazdur R, Zingas AP, Loredo R: Prospective evaluation of adrenal insufficiency in patients with adrenal metastasis. *Cancer* 60:103, 1987.
1218. Kung AWC, Pun KK, Lam K, Wang C, Leung CY: Addisonian crisis as presenting feature in malignancies. *Cancer* 65:177, 1990.
1219. Feinmann C, Gillett R, Irving MH: Hodgkin's disease presenting with hypoadrenalism. *Br Med J* 2:455, 1976.
1220. Gamelin E, Beldent V, Rousselet M, Rieux D, Rohmer V, Ifrah N, Boasson M, Bigorgne J: Non-Hodgkin's lymphoma presenting with primary adrenal insufficiency. *Cancer* 69:2333, 1992.
1221. Carey RW, Harris N, Kliman B: Addison's disease secondary to lymphomatous infiltration of the adrenal glands. *Cancer* 59:1087, 1987.
1222. Gruhn JG, Gould VE: The adrenal glands, in Kissane JM (ed): *Anderson's Pathology.* St. Louis, Mosby, 1990, vol 2, p 1586.
1223. Korobkin M, White EA, Kressel HY, Moss AA, Montagne JP: Computed tomography in the diagnosis of adrenal disease. *AJR* 132:231, 1979.
1224. Danby P, Harris KPG, Williams B, Feehally J, Walls J: Adrenal dysfunction in patients with renal amyloid. *Q J Med* 76:915, 1990.
1225. Arik N, Tasdemir I, Karaaslan Y, Uasavul U, Turgan C, Caglar S: Subclinical adrenocortical insufficiency in renal amyloidosis. *Nephron* 56:246, 1990.
1226. Masharani U, Schambelan M: The endocrine complications of acquired immunodeficiency syndrome. *Adv Intern Med* 38:323, 1993.
1227. Bricaire F, Marche C: Adrenocortical lesions and AIDS. *Lancet* 1:881, 1988.
1228. Tapper ML, Rotterdam HZ, Lerner CW, Al Khafaji K, Seitzman PA: Adrenal necrosis in the acquired immunodeficiency syndrome. *Ann Intern Med* 100:239, 1984.
1229. Reichert CM, O'Leary TJ, Levens DL, et al: Autopsy pathology in AIDS. *Am J Pathol* 112:357, 1983.
1230. Barboza A, Castro BA, Whalen M, Moore CCD, Harkin JS, Miller WL, Gonzales-Scarano F, Levy JA: Infection of cultured adrenal cells by different strains of HIV. *AIDS* 6:1437, 1992.
1231. Parker LN, Levin ER, Lifrak ER: Evidence for adrenocortical adaptation to severe illness. *J Clin Endocrinol Metab* 60:947, 1985.
1232. Norbiato G, Bevilacqua M, Vago T, Baldi G, Chebat E, Bertora P, Moroni M, Galli M, et al: Cortisol resistance in acquired immunodeficiency syndrome. *J Clin Endocrinol Metab* 74:608, 1992.
1233. Greendyke RM: Adrenal hemorrhage. *Am J Clin Pathol* 43:210, 1965.
1234. Siu SCB, Kitzman DW, Sheedy PF II, Northcutt RC: Adrenal insufficiency from bilateral adrenal hemorrhage. *Mayo Clin Proc* 65:664, 1990.
1235. Feuerstein B, Streeten DHP: Recovery of adrenal function after failure resulting from traumatic bilateral adrenal hemorrhages. *Ann Intern Med* 115:785, 1991.
1236. Moser HW: Adrenoleukodystrophy: Phenotype, genetics, pathogenesis and therapy. *Brain* 120:1485, 1997.
1237. Mosser J, Dovar AM, Sarde CO, Kioschis P, Feil R, Moser H, Poustka HM, Mandel JL, Aubourg P: Putative X-linked adrenoleukodystrophy gene shares unexpected homology with ABC transporters. *Nature* 361:726, 1993.
1238. Ligtenberg MJ, Kemp S, Sarde CO, van Geel BM, Kleijer WJ, Barth PG, Mandel JL, van Oost BA, Bolhuis PA: Spectrum of mutations in the gene encoding the adrenoleukodystrophy protein. *Am J Hum Genet* 56:44, 1995.
1239. Watkins PA, Gould SJ, Smith MA, Braiterman LT, Wei HM, Kok F, Moser AB, Moser HW, Smith KD: Altered expression of ALDP in X-linked adrenoleukodystrophy. *Am J Hum Genet* 57:292, 1995.
1240. Watkins PA, Naidu S, Moser HW: Adrenoleukodystrophy: Biochemical procedures in diagnosis, prevention and treatment. *J Inherit Metab Dis* 10:46, 1987.
1241. Moser HW, Smith KD, Moser AB: X-linked adrenoleukodystrophy, in Scriver CR, Beaudet AL, Sly SW, Valle D (eds): *The Metabolic and Molecular Bases of Inherited Disease.* New York, McGraw Hill, 1995, pp 2325–2350.
1242. Clark AJL, McLoughlin L, Grossman A: Familial glucocorticoid deficiency associated with point mutation in the adrenocorticotropin receptor. *Lancet* 341:461, 1993.
1243. Tsigos C, Arai K, Latronico AC, DiGeorge A, Rapaport R, Chrousos GP: A novel mutation of the adrenocorticotropin receptor (ACTH-R) gene in a family with the syndrome of isolated glucocorticoid deficiency but no ACTH-R abnormalities in two families with triple A syndrome. *J Clin Endocrinol Metab* 80:2186, 1995.
1244. Clark AJL, Weber A: Adrenocorticotropin insensitivity syndromes. *Endocr Rev* 19:828, 1998.
1245. Spark RF, Etzkorn JR: Absent aldosterone response to ACTH in familial glucocorticoid deficiency. *N Engl J Med* 297:917, 1977.
1246. Moshang T, Rosenfield RL, Bongiovanni AM, Parks JS, Amrhein JA: Familial glucocorticoid insufficiency. *J Pediatr* 82:821, 1973.
1247. Zanaria E, Muscatelli F, Bardoni B, Strom TM, Guioli S, Guo W, Lalli E, Moser C, Walker AP, McCabe ERB, Meitinger T, Monaco AP, Sassone-Corsi P, Camerino G: An unusual member of the nuclear hormone receptor superfamily responsible for X-linked adrenal hypoplasia congenita. *Nature* 372:635, 1994.
1248. Merke DP, Tajima T, Baron J, Cutler GB Jr: Hypogonadotropic hypogonadism in a female caused by an X-linked recessive mutation in the DAX-1 gene. *N Engl J Med* 340:1248, 1999.
1249. Burris TP, Guo W, McCabe ER: The gene responsible for adrenal hypoplasia congenita, DAX-1, encodes a nuclear hormone receptor that defines a new class within the superfamily. *Recent Prog Horm Res* 51:241, 1996.
1250. Schmitz G, Assman G: Acid lipase deficiency: Wolman's disease and cholesteryl ester storage disease, in Scirer C, Beaudet A, Sly W, Valle D (eds): *The Metabolic Basis of Inherited Disease.* New York, McGraw-Hill, 1989, pp 1623–1644.
1251. Anderson RA, Byrum RS, Coates PM, Sando GN: Mutations at the lysosomal acid cholesteryl ester hydrolase gene locus in Wolman disease. *Proc Natl Acad Sci USA* 91:2718, 1994.
1252. Yamamoto T, Fukuyama J, Hasegawa K, Sugiura M: Isolated corticotropin deficiency in adults. *Arch Intern Med* 152:1705, 1992.

1253. Jensen MD, Handwerger BS, Scheithauer BW, Carpenter PC, Mirakian R, Banks PM: Lymphocytic hypophysitis with isolated corticotropin deficiency. *Ann Intern Med* 105:200, 1986.
1254. Sauter NP, Toni R, McLaughlin CD, Dyess EM, Kritzman J, Lechan RM: Isolated adrenocorticotropin deficiency associated with an autoantibody to a corticotroph antigen that is not adrenocorticotropin or other proopiomelanocortin-derived peptides. *J Clin Endocrinol Metab* 70:1391, 1989.
1255. Koide Y, Kimura S, Inoue S, Ikeda M, Uchida K, Ando J, Shimuzu A, Oda K, et al: Responsiveness of hypophyseal-adrenocortical axis to repetitive administration of synthetic ovine corticotropin-releasing hormone in patients with isolated adrenocorticotropin deficiency. *J Clin Endocrinol Metab* 63:329, 1986.
1256. Fukata J, Usui T, Tsukada T, Nakai Y, Koh T, Ishihara T, Tanaka I, Uchida K, et al: Effects of repetitive administration of corticotropin releasing hormone combined with lysine vasopressin on plasma adrenocorticotropin and cortisol levels in secondary adrenocortical insufficiency. *J Clin Endocrinol Metab* 71:1624, 1990.
1257. Major P, Kuchel O, Boucher R, Nowaczynski W, Genest J: Selective hypopituitarism with severe hyponatremia and secondary hyporeninism. *J Clin Endocrinol Metab* 46:15, 1978.
1258. Lieberman AH, Luetscher JA: Some effects of abnormalities of pituitary, adrenal or thyroid function on excretion of aldosterone and the response to corticotropin or sodium deprivation. *J Clin Endocrinol Metab* 20:1004, 1960.
1259. May ME, Carey RM: Rapid adrenocorticotropic hormone test in practice. *Am J Med* 79:679, 1985.
1260. Borst GC, Michenfelder HJ, O'Brian JT: Discordant cortisol response to exogenous ACTH and insulin-induced hypoglycemia in patients with pituitary disease. *N Engl J Med* 306:1462, 1982.
1261. Besser GM, Cullen DR, Irvine WJ, Ratcliffe JG, Landon J: Immunoreactive corticotrophin levels in adrenocortical insufficiency. *Br Med J* 1:374, 1971.
1262. Fariss BL, Hane S, Shinsako J, Forsham PH: Comparison of absorption of cortisone acetate and hydrocortisone hemisuccinate. *J Clin Endocrinol Metab* 47:1137, 1978.
1263. Khalid BAK, Burke CW, Hurley DM, Funder JW, Stockigt JR: Steroid replacement in Addison's disease and in subjects adrenalectomized for Cushing's disease: Comparison of various glucocorticoids. *J Clin Endocrinol Metab* 55:551, 1982.
1264. Thompson DG, Stuart-Mason A, Goodwin FJ: Mineralocorticoid replacement in Addison's disease. *Clin Endocrinol (Oxf)* 10:499, 1979.
1265. Kyriazopoulou V, Parparousi O, Vagenakis A: Rifampicin induced adrenal crisis in addisonian patients receiving corticosteroid replacement therapy. *J Clin Endocrinol Metab* 59:1204, 1984.
1266. Feek CM, Ratacliffe JG, Setil J, Gray CE, Toft AD, Irvine WJ: Patterns of plasma cortisol and ACTH concentrations in patients with Addison's disease treated with conventional corticosteroid replacement. *Clin Endocrinol (Oxf)* 14:451, 1981.
1267. Scott RS, Donald RA, Espiner EA: Plasma ACTH and cortisol profiles in Addisonian patients receiving conventional substitution therapy. *Clin Endocrinol (Oxf)* 9:571, 1978.
1268. Nickelsen T, Schultz F, Demisch K: Studies on cortisol substitution therapy in patients with adrenal insufficiency. *Exp Clin Endocrinol* 82:35, 1983.
1269. Smith SJ, Markaandu ND, Banks RA, Dorrington Ward P, MacGregor GA, Bayliss J, Prentice MG, Wise P: Evidence that patients with Addison's disease are undertreated with fluorocortisone. *Lancet* 1:11, 1984.
1270. Oelkers W, Diederich S, Bahr V: Diagnosis and therapy surveillance in Addison's disease: Rapid adrenocorticotropin (ACTH) test and measurement of plasma ACTH, renin activity, and aldosterone. *J Clin Endocrinol Metab* 75:259, 1992.
1271. Plumpton FS, Besser GM, Cole PV: Corticosteroid treatment and surgery. II. The management of steroid cover. *Anaesthesia* 24:12, 1969.
1272. Hayes MA: Surgical treatment as complicated by prior adrenocortical steroid therapy. *Surgery* 40:945, 1956.
1273. Udelsman R, Ramp J, Gallucci WT, Gordon A, Lipford E, Norton JA, Loriaux DL, Chrousos GP: Adaptation during surgical stress: A reevaluation of the role of glucocorticoids. *J Clin Invest* 77:1377, 1986.
1274. Mulrow PJ: Aldosterone in hypertension and edema, in Bondy PK, Rosenberg LE (eds): *Metabolic Control and Disease.* Philadelphia, Saunders, 1979, p 1501.
1275. Sebastian A, Hernandez RE, Schambelan M: Disorders of renal handling of potassium, in Brenner BM, Rector FC Jr (eds): *The Kidney.* Philadelphia, Saunders, 1986, p 519.
1276. Arai K, Zachman K, Shibasaki T, Chrousos GP: Polymorphisms of amiloride sensitive sodium channel subunits in five sporadic cases of pseudohypoaldosteronism: Do they have pathologic potential? *J Clin Endocrinol Metab*, 84:2434, 1999.
1277. Schambelan M, Sebastian A: Hyporeninemic hypoaldosteronism. *Adv Intern Med* 24:385, 1979.
1278. Schambelan M, Sebastian A, Biglieri EG, Brust NL, Chang BC, Hirai J, Slater KL: Prevalence, pathogenesis, and functional significance of aldosterone deficiency in hyperkalemic patients with chronic renal insufficiency. *Kidney Int* 17:89, 1980.
1279. Phelps KR, Lieberman RL, Oh MS, Caroll HJ: Pathophysiology of the syndrome of hyporeninemic hypoaldosteronism. *Metabolism* 29:186, 1980.
1280. Tuck ML, Mayes DM: Mineralocorticoid biosynthesis in patients with hyporeninemic hypoaldosteronism. *J Clin Endocrinol Metab* 50:341, 1980.
1281. Williams GH: Hyporeninemic hypoaldosteronism. *N Engl J Med* 314:1041, 1986.
1282. Oster JR, Perez GO, Rosen MS: Hyporeninemic hypoaldosteronism after chronic sodium bicarbonate abuse. *Arch Intern Med* 136:1179, 1976.
1283. Obana K, Naruse M, Naruse K, et al: Synthetic rat atrial natriuretic factor inhibits *in vitro* and *in vivo* renin secretion in rats. *Endocrinology* 117:1282, 1985.
1284. Nadler JL, Lee FO, Hsueh W, Horton R: Evidence of prostacyclin deficiency in the syndrome of hyporeninemic hypoaldosteronism. *N Engl J Med* 314:1015, 1986.
1285. Sebastian A, Schambelan M: Amelioration of hyperchloremic acidosis with furosemide therapy in patients with chronic renal insufficiency and type 4 renal tubular acidosis. *Am J Nephrol* 4:287, 1984.
1286. Williams JAJ, Schambelan M, Biglieri EG, Carey RM: Acquired primary hypoaldosteronism due to an isolated zona glomerulosa defect. *N Engl J Med* 309:1623, 1983.
1287. Carey RM, Schambelan M, Biglieri EG, Bright GM: Primary hypoaldosteronism due to zona glomerulosa defect. *N Engl J Med* 310:1395, 1984.
1288. Stern N, Bech FWJ, Sowers JR, Tuck ML, Hsueh WA, Zipser R: Plasma corticosteroids in hyperreninemic hypoaldosteronism: Evidence for diffuse impairment of the zona glomerulosa. *J Clin Endocrinol Metab* 57:217, 1983.
1289. Zipser RD, Davenport MW, Martin KL, Tucck ML, Warner NF, Swinnery RR, Davis CL, Horton R: Hyperreninemic hypoaldosteronism in the critically ill: A new entity. *J Clin Endocrinol Metab* 53:867, 1981.
1290. Schambelan M, Sebastian A, Rector FC Jr: Mineralocorticoid-resistant renal hyperkalemia without salt wasting (type II pseudohypoaldosteronism): Role of increased renal chloride reabsorption. *Kidney Int* 19:716, 1981.
1291. Asa SL, Kalman K, Tindall GT, Barrow DL, Horvath E, Vecsei P: Cushing's disease associated with an intracellular gangliocytoma producing corticotrophin-releasing factor. *Ann Intern Med* 101:789, 1984.
1292. Carey RM, Varma SK, Drake CR, Thorner MO, Kovacs K, Rivier J, Vale W: Ectopic secretion of corticotropin-releasing factor as a cause of Cushing's syndrome. *N Engl J Med* 311:13, 1984.
1293. Belsky JL, Cuello B, Swanson LW, Simmons DM, Jarrett RM, Braza F: Cushing's syndrome due to ectopic production of corticotropin-releasing factor. *J Clin Endocrinol Metab* 60:496, 1985.
1294. Huff TA: Clinical syndromes related to disorders of adrenococorticotrophic hormone, in Allen MB, Makesh VB (eds): *The Pituitary: A Current Review.* New York, Academic, 1977, p 153.
1295. Neville AM, O'Hare MJ: Aspects of structure, function and pathology, in James VHT (ed): *The Adrenal Gland.* New York, Raven, 1979, p 1.
1296. Plotz CM, Knowlton AI, Ragan C: The natural history of Cushing's syndrome. *Am J Med* 13:597, 1952.
1297. Mampalam TJ, Tyrrell JB, Wilson CB: Transsphenoidal microsurgery for Cushing disease: A report of 216 cases. *Ann Intern Med* 109:487, 1988.

1298. Findling JW, Aron DC, Tyrrell JB: Cushing's disease, in Imura H (ed): *The Pituitary Gland.* New York, Raven, 1985, p 441.
1299. Ratcliffe JG, Knight RA, Besser GM, Landon J, Stansfield AG: Tumor and plasma ACTH concentrations in patients with and without the ectopic ACTH syndrome. *Clin Endocrinol (Oxf)* 1:27, 1972.
1300. Azzopardi JG, Freeman E, Pook G: Endocrine and metabolic disorders in bronchial carcinoma. *Br Med J* 4:528, 1970.
1301. Gewirtz G, Yalow RS: Ectopic ACTH production in carcinoma of the lung. *J Clin Invest* 53:1022, 1974.
1302. Knight RA, Ratcliffe JG, Besser GM: Tumor ACTH concentrations in ectopic ACTH syndrome and in control tissues. *Proc R Soc Med* 64:1266, 1971.
1303. Bloomfield GA, Holdaway IM, Corrin B, Ratcliffe JG, Rees GM, Ellison M, Rees LH: Lung tumors and ACTH production. *Clin Endocrinol (Oxf)* 6:95, 1977.
1304. Neville AM, Symington T: The pathology of the adrenal gland in Cushing's syndrome. *J Pathol Bacteriol* 93:19, 1967.
1305. Hutter AM, Kayhoe DE: Adrenal cortical carcinoma: Clinical features of 138 patients. *Am J Med* 41:572, 1966.
1305a. McArthur RG, Cloutier MD, Hayles AB, Sprague RG: Cushing's disease in children. *Mayo Clin Proc* 47:318, 1972.
1306. Magiakou MA, Mastorakos G, Oldfield EH, Gomez MT, Doppman JL, Cutler CB Jr, Nieman LK, Chrousos GP: Cushing's syndrome in children and adolescents. Presentation, diagnosis and therapy. *N Engl J Med* 331:629, 1994.
1307. Cassar J, Doyle FH, Mashiter K, Joplin GF: Treatment of Cushing's disease in juveniles with interstitial pituitary irradiation. *Clin Endocrinol (Oxf)* 11:313, 1979.
1308. Styne DM, Grumbach MM, Kaplan SL, Wilson CB, Conte FA: Treatment of Cushing's disease in childhood and adolescence by transsphenoidal microadenomectomy. *N Engl J Med* 310:889, 1984.
1309. Devoe DJ, Miller WL, Conte FA, Kaplan SL, Grumbach MM, Rosenthal SM, Wilson CB, Gitelman SE: Long-term outcome in children and adolescents after transsphenoidal surgery for Cushing's disease. *J Clin Endocrinol Metab* 82:3196, 1997.
1310. Robert F, Pelletier G, Hardy J: Pituitary adenomas in Cushing's disease. *Arch Pathol Lab Med* 102:448, 1978.
1311. Tyrrell JB, Brooks RM, Fitzgerald PA, Cofoid PB, Forsham PH, Wilson CW: Cushing's disease: Selective transsphenoidal resection of pituitary adenomas. *N Engl J Med* 298:753, 1978.
1312. Boggan JE, Tyrrell JB, Wilson CB: Transsphenoidal microsurgical management of Cushing's disease. *J Neurosurg* 59:195, 1983.
1313. Rovitt RL, Duane TD: Cushing's syndrome and pituitary tumors: Pathophysiology and ocular manifestations of ACTH-secreting pituitary adenomas. *Am J Med* 46:416, 1969.
1314. Kovacs K, Horvath E: Pathology of pituitary tumors. *Endocrinol Metab Clin* 16:529, 1987.
1315. Lloyd RV, Chandler WF, McKeever PE, Schteingart DE: The spectrum of ACTH-producing pituitary lesions. *Am J Surg Pathol* 10:618, 1986.
1316. Grua JR, Nelson DH: ACTH-producing pituitary tumors. *Endocrinol Metab Clin North Am* 20:319, 1991.
1317. Suda T, Abe Y, Demura H, Demura R, Shizume K, Tamahashi N, Sasano N: ACTH, α-LPH and α-endorphin in pituitary adenomas of the patients with Cushing's disease: Activation of α-LPH conversion to α-endorphin. *J Clin Endocrinol Metab* 49:475, 1979.
1318. Suda T, Demura H, Demura R, Jibiki K, Tozawa F, Shizume K: Anterior pituitary hormones in plasma and pituitaries from patients with Cushing's disease. *J Clin Endocrinol Metab* 51:1048, 1980.
1318a. Miller WL, Johnson LK: Synthesis and glycosylation of proopiomelanocortin by a Cushing's tumor. *J Clin Endocrinol Metab* 55:441, 1982.
1319. Saeger W: Surgical pathology of the pituitary in Cushing's disease. *Pathol Res Pract* 187:613, 1991.
1320. Lüdecke D, Kautzky R, Saeger W, Schrader D: Selective removal of hypersecreting pituitary adenomas. *Acta Neurochir (Wien)* 35:27, 1976.
1321. Peillon F, Racador J, Oliver L, Vila-Porcile E: Microadenomas, structure and function, in Faglia G, Giovanelli MA, MacLeod RM (eds): *Microadenomas.* London, Academic, 1980, p 91.
1322. McKeever PE, Koppelman MC, Metcalf D, Quindlen E, Kornbluth PL, Strott CA, Howard R, Smith BH: Re-fractory Cushing's disease caused by multinodular ACTH cell hyperplasia. *J Neuropathol Exp Neurol* 41:490, 1982.
1323. Samuels MH: Cushing's syndrome associated with corticotroph hyperplasia. *The Endocrinologist* 3:242, 1993.
1324. Schnall AM, Kovacs K, Brodkey JS, Pearson OH: Pituitary Cushing's disease without adenoma. *Acta Endocrinol (Copenh)* 94:293, 1981.
1325. Taylor HC, Velasco ME, Brodkey JS: Remission of pituitary-dependent Cushing's disease after removal of non-neoplastic pituitary gland. *Arch Intern Med* 140:1366, 1980.
1326. Lamberts SWJ, DeLange SA, Stefanko SZ: Adrenocorticotropin secreting pituitary adenomas originate from the anterior or the intermediate lobe in Cushing's disease: Differences in the regulation of hormone secretion. *J Clin Endocrinol Metab* 54:286, 1982.
1327. McNicol AM, Teasdale GM, Beastal GH: A study of corticotroph adenomas in Cushing's disease: No evidence of intermediate lobe origin. *Clin Endocrinol (Oxf)* 24:715, 1986.
1328. Raffel C, Boggan JE, Eng LF, Davis RL, Wilson CW: Pituitary adenomas in Cushing's disease: Do they arise from the intermediate lobe? *Surg Neurol* 30:125, 1988.
1329. Neville AM, O'Hare MJ: Histopathology of the human adrenal cortex. *Clin Endocrinol Metab* 14:791, 1985.
1330. McNicol AM: The human adrenal gland: Aspects of structure, function and pathology, in James VHT (ed): *The Adrenal Gland,* 2nd ed. New York, Raven, 1992.
1331. Anderson DC, Child DF, Sutcliffe CH, Buckley CH, Davies D, Longson D: Cushing's syndrome, nodular hyperplasia and virilizing carcinoma. *Clin Endocrinol (Oxf)* 9:1, 1978.
1332. Krieger DT, Amorosa L, Linick F: Cyproheptadine-induced remission of Cushing's disease. *N Engl J Med* 293:893, 1975.
1333. Krieger DT: Physiopathology of Cushing's disease. *Endocr Rev* 4:22, 1983.
1334. Hellman L, Weitzman ED, Roffwarg H, Fukushima DK, Yoshida K, Gallagher TF: Cortisol is secreted episodically in Cushing's syndrome. *J Clin Endocrinol Metab* 30:686, 1970.
1335. Sederberg-Olsen P, Binder C, Kehlet H, Neville AM, Nielsen LM: Episodic variation in plasma corticosteroids in subjects with Cushing's syndrome of differing etiology. *J Clin Endocrinol Metab* 36:906, 1973.
1336. Von Werder K, Smilo RP, Hane S, Forsham PH: Pituitary response to stress in Cushing's disease. *Acta Endocrinol (Copenh)* 67:127, 1971.
1337. Duick DS, Wahner HW: Thyroid axis in patients with Cushing's syndrome. *Arch Intern Med* 139:767, 1979.
1338. Smals AGH, Kloppenborg PWC, Benraad TJ: Plasma testosterone profiles in Cushing's syndrome. *J Clin Endocrinol Metab* 45:240, 1977.
1339. Fitzgerald PA, Aron DC, Findling JW, Brooks RM, Wilson CB, Tyrrell JB: Cushing's disease: Transient secondary adrenal insufficiency after selective removal of pituitary tumors. Evidence for a pituitary origin. *J Clin Endocrinol Metab* 54:413, 1982.
1340. Tyrrell JB: Cushing's disease. *Present Concepts Intern Med* 13:5, 1980.
1341. Gertz BJ, Contreras LN, McComb DJ, Kovacs K, Tyrrell JB, Dallman MF: Chronic administration of corticotropin-releasing factor increases pituitary corticotroph number. *Endocrinology* 120:381, 1987.
1342. Avgerinos PC, Chrousos GP, Nieman LK, Oldfield EH, Loriaux DL, Cutler GB: The corticotropin releasing hormone test in the postoperative evaluation of patients with Cushing's syndrome. *J Clin Endocrinol Metab* 65:906, 1987.
1343. Salassa RM, Laws ER Jr, Carpenter PC, Northcutt RC: Transsphenoidal removal of pituitary microadenoma in Cushing's disease. *Mayo Clin Proc* 53:24, 1978.
1344. Bigos ST, Somma M, Rasio E, Eastman RC, Lanthier A, Johnston NH, Hardy J: Cushing's disease: Management by transsphenoidal pituitary microsurgery. *J Clin Endocrinol Metab* 50:348, 1980.
1345. Avgerinos PC, Chrousos GP, Nieman LK, Oldfield EH, Loriaux DL, Cutler GB: The corticotropin releasing hormone test in the postoperative evaluation of patients with Cushing's syndrome. *J Clin Endocrinol Metab* 65: 906, 1987.
1346. Schnall AM, Brodkey JS, Kaufman B, Pearson OH: Pituitary function after removal of pituitary microadenomas in Cushing's disease. *J Clin Endocrinol Metab* 47:410, 1978.
1347. Boyer RM, Witkin M, Carruth A, Ramsey J: Circadian cortisol rhythms in Cushing's disease. *J Clin Endocrinol Metab* 48:760, 1979.

1348. Doerr P, Pirke KM: Cortisol-induced suppression of plasma testosterone in normal adult males. *J Clin Endocrinol Metab* 43:622, 1976.
1349. Krieger DT, Gewirtz GP: Recovery of hypothalamic-pituitary-adrenal function, growth hormone responsiveness, and sleep EEG pattern in a patient following removal of an adrenal cortical adenoma. *J Clin Endocrinol Metab* 38:1075, 1974.
1350. Jaquet P, Lissitzky JC, Boudouresque F, Guibout M, Goldstein E, Grisoli F, Oliver C: Peptides lipocorticotropes dans la maladie de Cushing: Etudes *in vitro, in vivo. 23rd International Symposium on Clinical Endocrinology,* Paris, 1980, p 54.
1351. Gillies G, Ratter S, Grossman A, Gaillard R, Lowry PJ, Besser GM, Rees LH: ACTH, LPH and β-endorphin secretion from perfused isolated human pituitary tumor cells *in vitro. Horm Res* 13:280, 1980.
1352. Lüdecke DK, Westphal M, Schabet M, Hollt V: *In vitro* secretion of ACTH beta-endorphin and beta-lipotropin in Cushing's disease and Nelson's syndrome. *Horm Res* 13:259, 1980.
1353. Lamberts SWJ, Klijn JGM, De Quijada M, Timmermans HAT, Uitterlinden P, De Jong FH, Birkenhager JC: The mechanism of the suppressive action of bromocryptine on adrenocorticotropin secretion in patients with Cushing's disease and Nelson's syndrome. *J Clin Endocrinol Metab* 51:307, 1980.
1354. Ishibashi M, Yamaji T: TRH stimulation and dopaminergic and antiserotonergic inhibition of ACTH release from cultured pituitary adenoma tissues of Nelson's syndrome. *Program of the VIth International Congress of Endocrinology,* Melbourne, 1980, p 407.
1355. Orth DN: Establishment of human malignant melanoma clonal cell lines that secrete ectopic adrenocorticotropin. *Nature (New Biol)* 242:26, 1973.
1356. Hashimoto K, Takahara J, Ogawa N, Yunoki S, Ofuji T, Arata A, Kanda S, Terada K: Adrenocorticotropin, β-lipotropin, β-endorphin and corticotropin-releasing factor-like activity in an adrenocorticotropin-producing nephroblastoma. *J Clin Endocrinol Metab* 50:461, 1980.
1357. Rees LH, Bloomfield GA, Gilkes JJH, Jeffcoate WJ, Besser GM: ACTH as a tumor marker. *Ann NY Acad Sci* 297:603, 1977.
1358. Allen RG, Orwell E, Kendall JW, Herbert E, Paxton H: The distribution of forms of adrenocorticotropin and β-endorphin in normal, tumorous, and autopsy human anterior pituitary tissue: Virtual absence of 13K adrenocorticotropin. *J Clin Endocrinol Metab* 51:376, 1980.
1359. Styne DM, Isaac RM, Miller WL, Leish SJ, Connors MH, Conte FA, Grumbach MM: Endocrine, histologic and biochemical characterization of ACTH-producing islet cell carcinoma of the pancreas in childhood, with characterization of proopiomelanocortin. *J Clin Endocrinol Metab* 57:723, 1983.
1360. Azzopardi JG, Williams ED: Pathology of nonendocrine tumors associated with Cushing's syndrome. *Cancer* 22:274, 1968.
1361. Liddle GW, Nicholson WE, Island DP, Orth DN, Abe K, Lowder SC: Clinical and laboratory studies of ectopic humoral syndromes. *Recent Prog Horm Res* 25:283, 1969.
1362. Luton JP, Thieblot P, Valcke JC, Mahoudeau JA, Bicaire H: Reversible gonadotropin deficiency in male Cushing's disease. *J Clin Endocrinol Metab* 45:488, 1977.
1363. Friedman M, Marshall-Jones P, Ross EJ: Cushing's syndrome: Adrenocortical hyperactivity secondary to neoplasms arising outside the pituitary-adrenal system. *Q J Med* 35:193, 1966.
1364. Soffer LJ, Iannaccone A, Gabrilov JL: Cushing's syndrome: A study of fifty patients. *Am J Med* 30:129, 1961.
1365. Prunty FTG, Brooks RV, Dupre J, Gilmette TMD, Hutchinson JSM, McSwiney RR, Mills IH: Adrenocortical hyperfunction and potassium metabolism in patients with "non-endocrine" tumors and Cushing's syndrome. *J Clin Endocrinol Metab* 23:737, 1963.
1366. Taskinen MR, Nikkila EA, Pelkonen R, Sane T: Plasma lipoproteins, lipolytic enzymes, and very low density lipoprotein triglyceride turnover in Cushing's syndrome. *J Clin Endocrinol Metab* 57:619, 1983.
1367. Findling JW, Tyrrell JB: Occult ectopic secretion of corticotropin. *Arch Intern Med* 146:929, 1986.
1368. Aron DC, Findling JW, Tyrrell JB, Fitzgerald PA, Brooks RM, Fisher FE, Forsham PH: Pituitary-ACTH dependency of nodular adrenal hyperplasia in Cushing's syndrome. *Am J Med* 71:302, 1981.
1369. Yamaji T, Ishibashi M, Sekihara H, Itabashi A, Yanaihara T: Serum dehydroepiandrosterone sulfate in Cushing's syndrome. *J Clin Endocrinol Metab* 59:1164, 1984.
1370. Aron DC, Findling JW, Tyrrell JB: Cushing's disease. *Endocrinol Metab Clin* 16:705, 1987.
1371. Meikle AW, Stanchfield JB, West CD, Tyler FH: Hydrocortisone suppression test for Cushing's syndrome. *Arch Intern Med* 134:1068, 1974.
1372. Bailey RE: Periodic hormonogenesis—a new phenomenon: Periodicity in function of a hormone-producing tumor in man. *J Clin Endocrinol Metab* 32:317, 1971.
1373. Blau N, Miller WE, Miller ER, Cervi-Skinner J: Spontaneous remission of Cushing's syndrome in a patient with an adrenal adenoma. *J Clin Endocrinol Metab* 40:659, 1975.
1374. Lamberts SWJ, Klijn JGM, DeJong FH, Birkenhäger JC: Hormone secretion in alcohol induced pseudo-Cushing's syndrome: Differential diagnosis with Cushing's disease. *JAMA* 242:1640, 1979.
1375. Gold PW, Loriaux DL, Roy A, Kling MA, Calabrese JR, Kellner CH, Nieman LK, Post RM, et al: Responses to corticotropin-releasing hormone in the hypercortisolism of depression and Cushing's disease. *N Engl J Med* 314:1329, 1986.
1376. Yanovski JA, Cutler GB, Chrousos GP, Nieman LK: Corticotropin-releasing hormone stimulation following low-dose dexamethasone administration: A new test to distinguish Cushings syndrome from pseudo-Cushings states. *JAMA* 269:2232, 1993.
1377. Kaye TB, Crapo L: The Cushing syndrome: An update on diagnostic tests. *Ann Intern Med* 112:434, 1990.
1378. Orth DN: The old and the new in Cushing's syndrome. *N Engl J Med* 310:649, 1984.
1379. Fig LM, Gross MD, Shapiro B, Ehrmann DA, Freitas JE, Schteingart DE, Glazer GM, Francis RF: Adrenal localization in the adrenocorticotropic hormone-independent Cushing's syndrome. *Ann Intern Med* 109:547, 1988.
1380. Perry RR, Nieman LK, Cutler GB Jr, Chrousos GP, Loriaux L, Doppman JL, Travis DT, Norton JA: Primary adrenal causes of Cushing's syndrome: Diagnosis and surgical management. *Ann Surg* 210:59, 1989.
1381. Carney JA, Young WF Jr: Primary pigmented nodular adrenocortical disease and its associated conditions. *The Endocrinologist* 2:6, 1992.
1382. Young WF, Carney JA: Cushing's syndrome: Primary pigmented nodular adrenal disease, in Mazzaferi EL (ed): *Advances in Endocrinology and Metabolism.* Mosby-Year Book, St. Louis, vol 3, 1992, p 179.
1383. Doppman JL, Travis WD, Nieman L, Miller DL, Chrousos GP, Gomez MT, Cutler GB Jr, Loriaux DL, et al: Cushing syndrome due to primary pigmented nodular adrenocortical disease: Findings at CT and MR imaging. *Radiology* 172:415, 1989.
1384. Zeiger MA, Nieman LK, Cutler GB Jr, Chrousos GP, Doppman JL, Travis WD, Norton JA: Primary bilateral adrenocortical causes of Cushing's syndrome. *Surgery* 110:1106, 1991.
1385. Orloff DG, Cutler GB Jr: The spectrum of macronodular adrenal disease in Cushing's syndrome: Diagnosis and treatment, in Mazzaferi EL (ed): *Advances in Endocrinology and Metabolism.* Mosby-YearBook, St. Louis, 1992, vol 3 p 199.
1386. Doppman JL, Miller DL, Dwyer AJ, Loughlin T, Nieman L, Cutler GB Jr, Chrousos GP, Oldfield E, et al: Macronodular adrenal hyperplasia in Cushing's disease. *Radiology* 166:347, 1988.
1387. Findlay JC, Sheeler LR, Engeland WC, Aron DC: Familial adrenocorticotropin-independent Cushing's syndrome with bilateral macronodular adrenal hyperplasia. *J Clin Endocrinol Metab* 76:189, 1993.
1388. Doppman JL, Niemann LK, Travis WD, Miller DL, Cutler GB Jr, Chrousos GP, Norton JA: CT and MR imaging of massive macronodular adrenocortical disease: A rare cause of autonomous primary hypercortisolism. *J Comput Assist Tomogr* 15:773, 1991.
1389. Malchoff CD, Rosa J, DeBold CR, Kozol RA, Ramsby GR, Page DL, Malchoff DM, Orth DN: Adrenocorticotropin-independent bilateral macronodular adrenal hyperplasia: An unusual cause of Cushing's syndrome. *J Clin Endocrinol Metab* 68:855, 1989.
1390. Trainer PJ, Grossman A: The diagnosis and differential diagnosis of Cushing's syndrome. *Clin Endocrinol (Oxf)* 34:317, 1991.

1391. Grossman AB, Howlett TA, Perry L, Coy DH, Savage MO, Lavender P, Rees LH, Bessier GM: CRF in the differential diagnosis of Cushing's syndrome: A comparison with the dexamethasone suppression test. *Clin Endocrinol (Oxf)* 29:167, 1988.
1392. Hermus AR, J PG, Benraad TJ, Pieters GF, Smals AG, Kloppenborg PW: The corticotropin-releasing-hormone test versus the high-dose dexamethasone test in the differential diagnosis of Cushing's syndrome. *Lancet* 2:540, 1986.
1393. Nieman LK, Chrousos GP, Oldfield EH, Avgerinos PC, Cutler GB Jr, Loriaux DL: The ovine corticotropin-releasing hormone stimulation test and the dexamethasone suppression test in the differential diagnosis of Cushing's syndrome. *Ann Intern Med* 105:862, 1986.
1394. Hermus AR, Pieters GF, Benraad TJ, Smals AG, Kloppenborg PW: The CRH test and the high-dose dexamethasone test in the differential diagnosis of Cushing's syndrome, in Casanueva FF, Dieguez C (eds): *Recent Advances in Basic and Clinical Neuroendocrinology.* New York, Elsevier, 1989, p 351.
1395. Oldfield EH, Doppman JL, Nieman LK, Chrousos GP, Miller DL, Katz DA, Cutler GB Jr, Loriaux DL: Petrosal sinus sampling with and without corticotropin-releasing hormone for the differential diagnosis of Cushing's syndrome. *N Engl J Med* 325:897, 1991.
1396. Doppman JL: The search for occult ectopic ACTH-producing tumors. *The Endocrinologist* 2:41, 1992.
1397. Doppman JL, Nieman L, Miller DL, Pass HI, Chang R, Cutler GB Jr, Schaaf M, Chrousos GP, et al: Ectopic adrenocorticotropic hormone syndrome: Localization studies in 28 patients. *Radiology* 172:115, 1989.
1398. Torpy DJ, Chen C, Mullen N, Doppman JL, Carrasquillo J, Chrousos GP, Nieman LK: Lack of utility of ^{111}In-pentetreotide scintigraphy in localizing ectopic ACTH producing tumors: Follow-up of 18 patients. *J Clin Endocrinol Metab* 84:1186, 1999.
1399. Corrigan DF, Schaaf M, Whaley RA, Czerwinski CL, Earll JM: Selective venous sampling to differentiate ectopic ACTH secretion from pituitary Cushing's syndrome. *N Engl J Med* 296:861, 1971.
1400. Findling JW, Aron DC, Tyrrell JB, Shinsako JH, Fitzgerald PA, Norman D, Wilson CB, Forsham PH: Selective venous sampling for ACTH in Cushing's syndrome: Differentiation between Cushing's disease and the ectopic ACTH syndrome. *Ann Intern Med* 94:647, 1981.
1401. Howlett TA, Rees HL, Besser GM: Cushing's syndrome. *Clin Endocrinol Metab* 14:911, 1985.
1402. Manni A, Latshaw RF, Page R, Santen RJ: Simultaneous bilateral venous sampling for adrenocorticotropin in pituitary-dependent Cushing's disease: Evidence for lateralization of pituitary venous drainage. *J Clin Endocrinol Metab* 57:1070, 1983.
1403. Doppman JL, Oldfield E, Krudy AG, Chrousos GP, Schulte HM, Schaaf M, Loriaux DL: Petrosal sinus sampling for Cushing's syndrome: Anatomical and technical considerations. *Radiology* 150:99, 1984.
1404. Komanicky P, Spark RF, Melby JC: Treatment of Cushing's syndrome with trilostane (WIN 24,250), an inhibitor of adrenal steroid biosynthesis. *J Clin Endocrinol Metab* 47:1024, 1978.
1405. Sample WF, Sarti DA: Computed tomography and gray scale ultrasonography of the adrenal gland: A comparative study. *Radiology* 128:377, 1978.
1406. Thrall JH, Freitas JE, Beirwaltes WH: Adrenal scintigraphy. *Semin Nucl Med* 8:23, 1978.
1407. Orth DN, Liddle GW: Results of treatment in 108 patients with Cushing's syndrome. *N Engl J Med* 285:243, 1971.
1408. Miller WL, Townsend JJ, Grumbach MM, Kaplan SL: An infant with Cushing's disease due to an adrenocorticotropin-producing pituitary adenoma. *J Clin Endocrinol Metab* 48:1017, 1979.
1409. Linfoot JA: Heavy ion therapy: Alpha particle therapy of pituitary tumors, in Linfoot JA (ed): *Recent Advances in the Diagnosis and Treatment of Pituitary Tumors.* New York, Raven, 1979, p 245.
1410. Sheline GE: Role of conventional radiation therapy in the treatment of functional pituitary tumors, in Linfoot JA (ed): *Recent Advances in the Diagnosis and Treatment of Pituitary Tumors.* New York, Raven, 1979, p 289.
1411. Lamberts SWJ, DeJong FH, Birkenhager JC: Treatment of Cushing's disease by unilateral adrenalectomy followed by external pituitary irradiation, in Fahlbush R, von Werder K (eds): *Treatment of Pituitary Adenomas.* Stuttgart, Germany, Georg Thieme, 1978, p 339.
1412. Jeffcoate WJ, Rees LH, Tomlin S, Jones AE, Edwards CRW, Besser GM: Metyrapone in long-term management of Cushing's disease. *Br Med J* 2:215, 1977.
1413. Orth DN: Metyrapone is useful only as adjunctive therapy in Cushing's disease. *Ann Intern Med* 89:128, 1978.
1414. Lafferty AR, Chrousos GP: Pituitary tumors in children and adolescents. *J Clin Endocrinol Metab* 84:4317, 1999.
1415. Burke CW, Doyle FH, Joplin GF, Arnot RN, MacErlean DP, Russell Fraser T: Cushing's disease: Treatment by pituitary implantation of radioactive gold or yttrium seeds. *Q J Med* 42:693, 1973.
1416. White MC, Doyle FH, Mashiter K, Joplin GF: Successful treatment of Cushing's disease using yttrium-90 rods. *Br Med J* 285:280, 1982.
1417. Welbourn RB, Montgomery DAD, Kennedy TL: The natural history of treated Cushing's syndrome. *Br J Surg* 58:1, 1971.
1418. Schteingart DE: Cushing's syndrome. *Endocrinol Metab Clin North Am* 18:311, 1989.
1419. Graber AL, New RL, Nicholson WE, Island DP, Liddle GW: Natural history of pituitary adrenal recovery following long term suppression with corticosteroids. *J Clin Endocrinol Metab* 25:11, 1965.
1420. Bertagna C, Orth DN: Clinical and laboratory findings and results of therapy in 58 patients with adrenocortical tumors admitted to a single medical center (1951 to 1978). *Am J Med* 71:855, 1981.
1421. Hutter AM, Kayhoe DE: Adrenocortical carcinoma: Results of treatment with o,p'DDD in 138 patients. *Am J Med* 41:581, 1966.
1422. Nelson DH, Meakin JW, Dealy JB, Matson DD, Emerson K, Thorn GW: ACTH-producing tumor of the pituitary gland. *N Engl J Med* 259:161, 1958.
1423. Moore TJ, Dluhy RG, Williams GH, Cain JP: Nelson's syndrome: Frequency, prognosis and effect of prior pituitary irradiation. *Ann Intern Med* 85:731, 1976.
1424. Barwich D, Bahner P: Pituitary tumors in adrenalectomized patients with Cushing's disease, in Fahlbush R, von Werder K (eds): *Treatment of Pituitary Adenomas.* Stuttgart, Germany, Georg Thieme, 1978, p 326.
1425. Weinstein M, Tyrrell JB, Newton TH: The sella turcica in Nelson's syndrome. *Radiology* 118:363, 1976.
1426. Findling JW, Tyrrell JB, Aron DC, Fitzgerald PA, Wilson CW, Forsham PH: Silent pituitary apoplexy: Subclinical infarction of an ACTH-producing adenoma. *J Clin Endocrinol Metab* 52:95, 1981.
1427. Stockigt JR: Mineralocorticoid excess, in James VHT (ed): *The Adrenal Gland.* New York, Raven, 1979, p 197.
1428. Ferris TF: Toxemia of pregnancy: A model of human hypertension. *Cardiovasc Med* 2:877, 1977.
1429. Gill JR: Bartter's syndrome. *Annu Rev Med* 31:405, 1980.

CHAPTER 12

Diseases of the Sympathochromaffin System

Philip E. Cryer

The sympathochromaffin system is a prototype neuroendocrine system.[1,2] Its major biologically active products—the catecholamines—serve as both neurotransmitters and hormones. The sympathochromaffin system includes two components: the sympathetic nervous system and the chromaffin tissues.[2] The major clusters of chromaffin cells that persist through postnatal life constitute the adrenal medullae. The catecholamines—epinephrine, norepinephrine, and dopamine—are neurotransmitters in the central nervous system (CNS). In the periphery, epinephrine serves as a hormone.[3] Although regulated epinephrine secretion from extraadrenal chromaffin cells occurs, biologically effective plasma epinephrine levels are derived only from the adrenal medullae, at least in adults.[2] Outside the CNS, norepinephrine functions primarily as a neurotransmitter of sympathetic postganglionic neurons;[4] it may also serve a hormonal function under some conditions. The physiologic function of dopamine outside the CNS is unclear, although it may also play a neurotransmitter role.

The sympathochromaffin system is a component of the autonomic nervous system (ANS).[5] The ANS consists of afferent, CNS, and efferent elements and is divided on anatomic grounds into parasympathetic and sympathetic divisions. Parasympathetic efferents include preganglionic and postganglionic neurons; the former arise from the brainstem and sacral spinal cord and synapse with the latter in ganglia which generally lie close to the innervated organs. Both preganglionic and postganglionic parasympathetic neurons release the neurotransmitter acetylcholine. Sympathetic efferents also include preganglionic and postganglionic neurons; the preganglionic neurons arise from the thoracolumbar spinal cord. Some sympathetic preganglionic neurons innervate chromaffin cells, including the adrenal medullae; the latter can be conceptualized as postganglionic neurons without axons.[3,6,7] The adrenal medullae release epinephrine, norepinephrine, or dopamine directly into the circulation. The remaining sympathetic preganglionic neurons synapse with postganglionic neurons in ganglia that are generally remote from the innervated organs (e.g., paravertebral ganglia). Like parasympathetic neurons, sympathetic preganglionic neurons release acetylcholine. A minority of sympathetic postganglionic neurons, such as those innervating sweat glands, also release acetylcholine. However, the vast majority of sympathetic postganglionic neurons release the neurotransmitter norepinephrine. In addition to catecholamines, components of the sympathochromaffin system contain a variety of peptides of potential but undefined biological importance.

The sympathochromaffin system is a rapid communication system. Its direct neural effects are virtually instantaneous, and its hormonal effects are detectable within minutes. The rapidity of the hormonal effects is comparable to that of pancreatic hormones such as insulin and glucagon but contrasts with the more gradual onset of action of pituitary hormones such as growth hormone, the adrenocortical and gonadal steroids, and, particularly, the thyroid hormones.

It has long been appreciated that the sympathochromaffin system is critically involved in cardiovascular homeostasis and that the catecholamines have prominent metabolic effects, but the precise physiologic roles of the catecholamines in human metabolic regulation have only begun to emerge. A better understanding of their physiology will provide further insight into the pathophysiologic roles of the catecholamines.

There are three established clinical disorders of sympathochromaffin function[3]: (1) hypertension and a variety of symptoms that result from excessive catecholamine release from a pheochromocytoma, a tumor of chromaffin cells, (2) postural (orthostatic) hypotension resulting from deficient sympathetic neural norepinephrine release in various forms of autonomic failure, and (3) hypoglycemia resulting from combined deficiencies of epinephrine and glucagon secretion.

SYMPATHOCHROMAFFIN PHYSIOLOGY

Biochemistry of the Catecholamines

Amines containing a 3,4-dihydroxyphenyl (catechol) nucleus are termed *catecholamines*. These include epinephrine (adrenaline), norepinephrine (noradrenaline), and dopamine. The conventions of catecholamine nomenclature and the structures of these catecholamines are shown in Fig. 12-1.

Catecholamine Biosynthesis

Catecholamines are synthesized from the amino acid tyrosine through the sequence tyrosine → dihydroxyphenylalanine (dopa) → dopamine → norepinephrine (NE) → epinephrine (E).[8] As shown in Fig. 12-2, some systems (e.g., most cells of the adrenal medullae) express all the necessary biosynthetic enzymes and produce epinephrine as their major product. Others, such as most sympathetic postganglionic neurons and some cells of the adrenal medullae, lack the final enzyme and release norepinephrine. Various CNS neurons release dopamine, norepinephrine, or epinephrine.

Tyrosine utilized in catecholamine biosynthesis is derived from the diet or formed from phenylalanine, in the presence of phenylalanine hydroxylase, in the liver (Fig. 12-2).[9,10]

The catecholamine biosynthetic sequence is illustrated in Fig. 12-3. The initial step—conversion of tyrosine to dopa—is

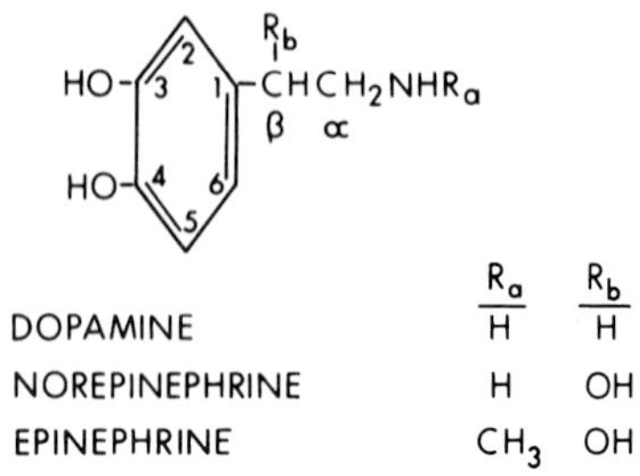

FIGURE 12-1. Conventions of catecholamine nomenclature.

catalyzed by tyrosine hydroxylase, the rate-limiting enzyme in catecholamine biosynthesis. Tyrosine hydroxylase (and phenylalanine and tryptophan hydroxylases) requires tetrahydrobiopterin as a cofactor. Tetrahydrobiopterin deficiency results in deficient catecholamine biosynthesis.[11] Tyrosine hydroxylase activity is product-inhibited. Accordingly, intracellular catecholamine depletion results in a rapid increase in enzyme activity and catecholamine biosynthesis. The activation of tyrosine hydroxylase involves phosphorylation of the enzyme;[12] both phosphorylation and activation are stimulated by acetylcholine, the preganglionic neurotransmitter. Further, prolonged sympathetic stimulation results in increased synthesis of tyrosine hydroxylase. Because of effective regulation of tyrosine hydroxylase, intracellular catecholamine stores are generally well-maintained despite a marked variation in catecholamine release.

In the presence of the relatively nonspecific enzyme aromatic L-amino acid decarboxylase, dopa is decarboxylated to form dopamine. As was noted earlier, subsequent enzymes are not

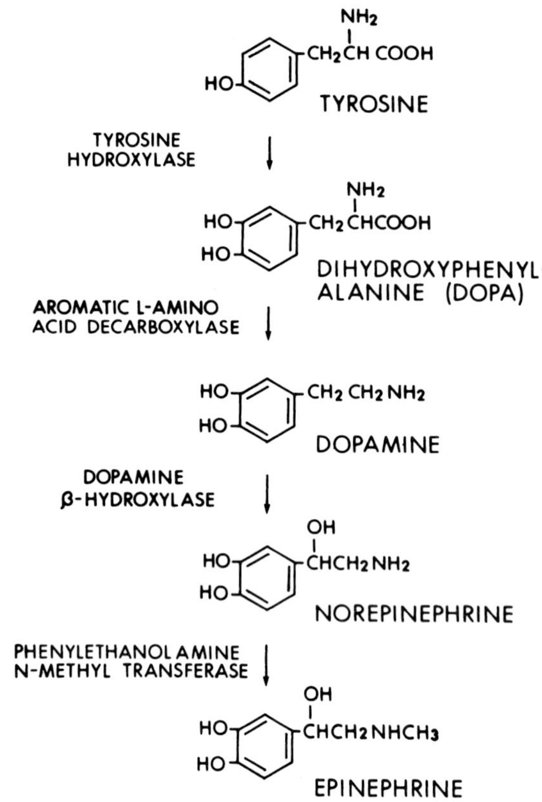

FIGURE 12-3. Catecholamine biosynthesis.

expressed in some catecholamine-forming neurons in which dopamine is the final product.

In tissues expressing dopamine β-hydroxylase, such as the adrenal medullae and most sympathetic postganglionic neurons, dopamine is hydroxylated to form norepinephrine. Norepinephrine is the final product of most sympathetic postganglionic neurons.

In chromaffin tissues, such as the adrenal medullae, norepinephrine is methylated to form epinephrine in the presence of the enzyme phenylethanolamine *N*-methyl transferase (PNMT).[13] The methyl donor is *S*-adenosyl-L-methionine. PNMT is a glucocorticoid-inducible enzyme; this may explain the persistence of high activity of the enzyme in the adrenal medullae, which receive portal blood flow from the adrenal cortex. Indeed, histochemical studies suggest that norepinephrine-releasing adrenomedullary cells are located around medullary arteries, whereas epinephrine-releasing adrenomedullary cells appear to receive most of their blood supply from corticomedullary venous sinuses. Furthermore, the glucocorticoid receptor has been localized to epinephrine-producing adrenomedullary cells.[14] Interestingly, patients with secondary adrenocortical insufficiency (ACTH deficiency) have been reported to have reduced basal and postexercise plasma epinephrine concentrations.[15]

FIGURE 12-2. Sites of catecholamine biosynthesis from tyrosine and major end products in those sites.

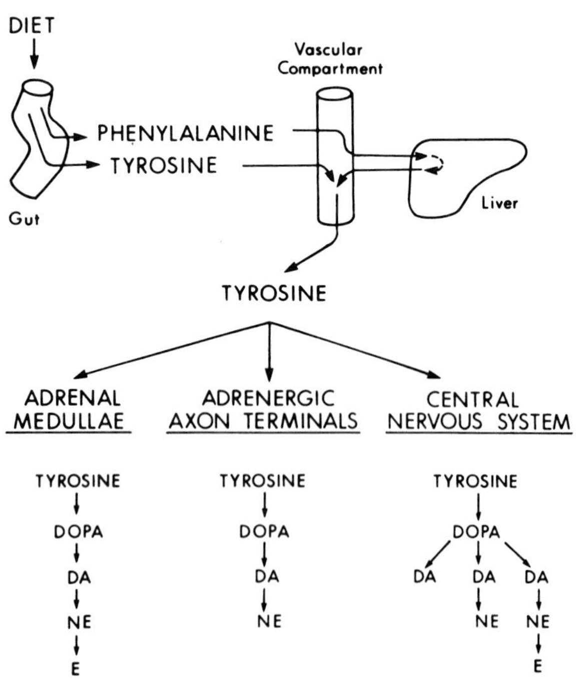

Catecholamine Degradation

The catecholamines are degraded by two principal intracellular enzyme systems, catechol-*O*-methyl transferase (COMT) and monoamine oxidase (MAO).[8] The major pathways of norepinephrine and epinephrine degradation are illustrated in Fig. 12-4.

In the presence of COMT and the methyl donor *S*-adenosyl-L-methionine, norepinephrine and epinephrine are converted to

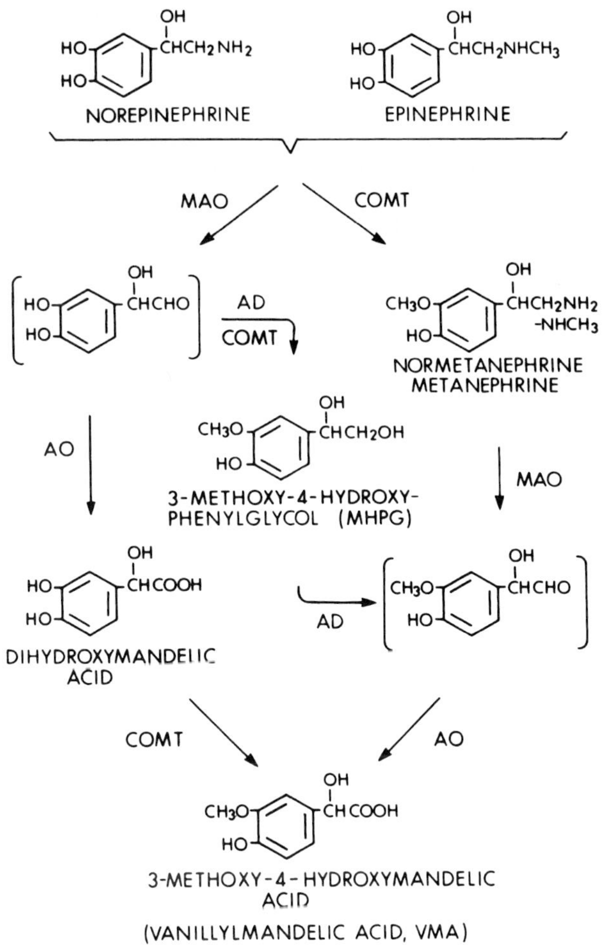

FIGURE 12-4. Catecholamine degradation. MAO = monoamine oxidase; COMT = catechol-*O*-methyl transferase; AD = alcohol dehydrogenase; AO = aldehyde oxidase.

their respective *O*-methyl metabolites, normetanephrine (NMN) and metanephrine (MN). In the presence of MAO these metabolites can be converted to an aldehyde (3-methoxy-4-hydroxymandelaldehyde), which, in the presence of an aldehyde oxidase, is converted to 3-methoxy-4-hydroxymandelic acid, better known as vanillylmandelic acid (VMA). Alternatively, norepinephrine and epinephrine can be converted in the presence of MAO to 3,4-dihydroxymandelic acid. In the presence of COMT, the latter is also converted to VMA. Thus, VMA is a major end product of catecholamine degradation.

As indicated in Fig. 12-4, an alternative fate of the oxidative intermediate 3,4-dihydroxymandelaldehyde is *O*-methylation and conversion to 3-methoxy-4-hydroxyphenylglycol (MHPG). Although MHPG was formerly thought to be a marker for CNS norepinephrine metabolism, it is now known that it is formed from catecholamines in the periphery as well as in the CNS and that nearly half the MHPG formed is further converted to VMA. It has been estimated that the brain accounts for only 30 percent of total body production of MHPG.[16] Thus, although MHPG is produced by the human brain[17] and cerebrospinal fluid (CSF) MHPG can be used as an index of CNS norepinephrine metabolism, if corrected for plasma MHPG,[18] neither urinary nor plasma MHPG can be considered a measure of CNS catecholamine metabolism.

The degradation of dopamine (not shown in Fig. 12-4) is similar to that outlined for norepinephrine and epinephrine except that the dopamine metabolites lack the hydroxyl group present on the β-carbon of norepinephrine and epinephrine metabolites. For example, dopamine is converted to 3-methoxytyramine via COMT and to 3-methoxy-4-hydroxyphenylacetic acid via MAO and COMT. Structurally, the latter compound, which is better known as homovanillic acid (HVA), corresponds to VMA except for the absence of the β-hydroxyl group.

COMT[19] is present in diverse body tissues, including the liver, kidneys, large intestine, and erythrocytes. It is involved in extraneuronal catecholamine degradation. MAO, which is also found in diverse tissues, plays an important role in intraneuronal catecholamine degradation. It exists in two forms—MAO A and MAO B—which are products of separate genes.[20]

Physiology of Adrenergic Axon Terminals and Chromaffin Cells

Organization of the Sympathochromaffin System

Afferent signals for sympathetic reflexes, which are derived primarily from the viscera, reach the CNS through a variety of visceral afferent nerves.[5] Central sympathetic connections include those in the spinal cord and medulla oblongata, where many sympathetic reflexes are mediated, and the hypothalamus, which is a principal site of autonomic integration. Efferent fibers from these central areas traverse the spinal cord and synapse with cell bodies of sympathetic preganglionic neurons in the intermediolateral columns of the eighth cervical through the second or third lumbar cord segments. The preganglionic axons leave the cord and synapse with sympathetic postganglionic neurons in the sympathetic ganglia. Preganglionic to postganglionic neurotransmission is cholinergic (mediated by acetylcholine). Neurotransmission from the axon terminals of sympathetic postganglionic neurons to effector cells is in the vast majority of instances adrenergic (mediated by norepinephrine).

The sympathetic ganglia include the paravertebral, prevertebral, and terminal ganglia. Postganglionic axons extend from the paravertebral ganglia to sympathetically innervated structures of the trunk and extremities via somatic nerves, to those of the head and neck (from the superior cervical ganglion), to the heart (from the cervical ganglia, stellate ganglia, and upper thoracic ganglia), and to the lungs and pulmonary vasculature (from the stellate ganglia and upper cervical ganglia). The major prevertebral sympathetic ganglia are the celiac (solar), aorticorenal, superior mesenteric, and inferior mesenteric ganglia. The greater splanchnic nerve carries preganglionic fibers to the adrenal medullae as well as the celiac ganglion. Sympathetic postganglionic axons from the celiac ganglion project to the liver, spleen, pancreas, stomach, small intestine, proximal colon, and kidneys. The kidneys also receive postganglionic fibers from the aorticorenal ganglion. Postganglionic fibers from the superior mesenteric ganglion extend to the distal colon, and those from the inferior mesenteric ganglion extend to the rectum, bladder, and external genitalia. Terminal sympathetic ganglia are found in the region of the bladder and rectum.

The anatomy of the sympathetic efferents facilitates progressive spreading of signals. A given preganglionic axon may traverse several vertebral ganglia before terminating and may synapse with several postganglionic neurons. The long axons of the postganglionic neurons are highly branched and studded with thousands of axon terminals that release their neurotransmitter directly at their effector cells. This anatomic arrangement does not, of course, preclude regional organization of sympathetic firing.

Chromaffin cells are widely distributed and intimately associated with the sympathetic nervous system during fetal life. Most degenerate after birth; the major residual clusters of chromaffin cells constitute the adrenal medullae. However, extraadrenal chromaffin tissues adjacent to the aorta (paraganglia), in the carotid bodies, in the viscera, and within sympathetic ganglia persist in adults.[21] The physiologic function, if any, of these extraadrenal chromaffin cells is unknown.

Catecholamine Formation, Storage, and Release

The enzymes required for catecholamine biosynthesis are synthesized in the cell bodies of chromaffin cells and postganglionic neurons. In the postganglionic neurons they are transported by axoplasmic flow to the axon terminals where the catecholamines are formed. Tyrosine is taken up from the circulation and, in the presence of the cytoplasmic enzymes tyrosine hydroxylase and aromatic L-amino acid decarboxylase, converted to dopa and then dopamine. Dopamine is transported into cytoplasmic vesicles (storage or secretion [chromaffin] granules) where, in the presence of dopamine β-hydroxylase, it is converted to norepinephrine. In chromaffin cells containing PNMT (mainly in the adrenal medullae), which is located in the cytoplasm, norepinephrine must leave the granules to be converted to epinephrine, which is then reincorporated into granules. Norepinephrine and epinephrine are taken up from the cytoplasm into granules by an energy-dependent process.

Within the chromaffin granules of adrenomedullary cells, catecholamines are concentrated to high (approximately 0.5 mmol/L) levels.[22] This uptake into vesicles is a secondary transport coupled to and driven by a transmembrane proton electrochemical gradient generated by an inwardly directed proton pump adenosine triphosphatase (ATPase) and mediated by a specific monamine transporter. This transporter has low specificity; it transports not only dopamine, norepinephrine, and epinephrine but also monamines not normally present in the adrenal medullae, including *m*-iodobenzylguanidine, which is used clinically to localize pheochromocytomas (see section on Diagnosis). It is antagonized by reserpine, which depletes catecholamines in vivo. It differs from the monamine uptake system that mediates uptake across the plasma membrane (see later discussion) in that the latter is antagonized by imipramine and guanethidine but not reserpine, is coupled to Na^+ but not to H^+ flux, and has other distinct pharmacologic properties. Despite lower catecholamine concentrations, uptake into vesicles into the axon terminals of sympathetic postganglionic neurons is thought to involve processes similar to those participating in uptake into vesicles in chromaffin cells.

The chromaffin cell vesicles contain catecholamines bound to ATP in association with specific proteins called chromogranins, forming a nondiffusible complex. Interestingly, chromogranin A has been found in a variety of peptide-producing tissues and tumors and may be a marker for peptide- as well as catecholamine-secreting cells.[23,24] Thus, chromogranins may be involved in storage mechanisms in a variety of granule-containing secretory cells. The adrenal medullae contain distinct epinephrine- and norepinephrine-containing cells that are distinguishable on the basis of differences in the electron microscopic appearance of the chromaffin granules as well as differences in biochemical composition.[25]

Catecholamine release into the extracellular fluid involves the release of the entire soluble contents of chromaffin granules (including catecholamines, dopamine β-hydroxylase, and chromogranins) through fusion and rupture of adjacent granule and plasma membranes. This release process is termed *exocytosis*. It normally results from an acetylcholine-stimulated influx of calcium from the extracellular fluid into the cytoplasm through a subset of voltage-dependent calcium channels.[26] It appears to involve cellular cytoskeletal elements and may be triggered by conformational changes in one or more fusion proteins.[27]

Norepinephrine storage and exocytotic release from axon terminals of sympathetic postganglionic neurons is similar to that of chromaffin cells, as described previously. Despite wide variations in norepinephrine release and some loss through intraneuronal oxidation (discussed later), the norepinephrine content of sympathetic axon terminals is normally well maintained. This is a result of regulated tyrosine hydroxylase activity and norepinephrine biosynthesis, as discussed earlier, and reuptake and storage of released norepinephrine, as discussed later. Because of release directly into the circulation rather than into a synaptic cleft, one might speculate that the adrenal medullae would less effectively recapture released catecholamines and therefore maintain their stores less efficiently. Indeed, depletion of adrenomedullary catecholamines occurs in some experimental models of fasting hypoglycemia.[28]

Biological Inactivation of Catecholamines

A fundamental principle of neurotransmission is the existence of a mechanism or mechanisms capable of rapidly terminating the actions of a released neurotransmitter. At cholinergic junctions, for example, the action of released acetylcholine is terminated rapidly by degradation of the neurotransmitter by acetylcholinesterase. Biological inactivation of norepinephrine released from the adrenergic axon terminals of sympathetic postganglionic neurons is accomplished by (1) axonal reuptake, (2) local metabolism, and (3) escape into the circulation.

Axonal reuptake (uptake 1) is believed to be the major route of inactivation of released norepinephrine. Axonal reuptake is blocked by tricyclic antidepressants as well as by cocaine and guanethidine. Uptake 1 recognition sites have been measured with [^{3}H]desipramine and have been found to change in parallel with changes in norepinephrine content produced by MAO inhibition (increased norepinephrine) and reserpine treatment (decreased norepinephrine).[29] Through the reuptake process, norepinephrine is returned from the synaptic cleft to the axon terminal, where it can be stored in granules (approximately 75 percent) or metabolized via MAO. MAO is associated with mitochondria in axon terminals and is the major enzyme in the initial intraneuronal degradation of norepinephrine. In contrast, COMT is an extraneuronal enzyme. It is present in cells adjacent to the synaptic cleft and mediates the initial degradation of released norepinephrine after its uptake (uptake 2) into those cells. COMT is widely distributed. Thus, both oxidized metabolites and released catecholamines are rapidly *O*-methylated. Extraneuronal (and circulating) 3,4-dihydroxyphenylglycol (DHPG) is derived from norepinephrine metabolized intraneuronally (by MAO), while extraneuronal MHPG (Fig. 12-4) is derived from norepinephrine metabolized extraneuronally and from DHPG formed within sympathetic postganglionic neurons.[30]

From the foregoing, it is apparent that catecholamine metabolites in plasma and urine reflect not only local and systemic extraneuronal metabolism of released catecholamines but also metabolic degradation of catecholamines initiated within adrenergic axon terminals (or adrenomedullary cells). It has been estimated that only 25 percent of urinary norepinephrine metabolites are derived from the extraneuronal degradation of released norepinephrine.[31]

Catecholamines are cleared rapidly from the circulation; plasma half-times are 1 to 2 min. Clearance largely results from cellular uptake and metabolism. Only 2 to 3 percent of the norepinephrine that enters the circulation is excreted unchanged in the urine.[31] Catecholamine clearance sites are widespread. Removal by the liver, kidneys, skeletal muscle, and other sites has been demonstrated in humans.

In addition to cellular uptake and metabolism, catecholamines in humans are conjugated, largely to the sulfate, at least in part in the circulation.[32] The biological importance of conjugation is unclear, but it is a potentially important route of inactivation of circulating catecholamines. Plasma concentrations of conjugates are substantial. The concentrations of the corresponding sulfate exceeds that of norepinephrine by about 50 percent and that of epinephrine about fourfold in the basal state. The ratio of the conjugated form to the unconjugated form of dopamine is so high that some have suggested that dopamine per se does not circulate in the basal state in humans. Amounts of conjugates also exceed those of catecholamines in the urine. During short-term physiologic adaptation, such as standing and exercise, changes in plasma catecholamine concentrations are not associated with corresponding changes in plasma concentrations of the conjugates.

Axonal reuptake and storage or metabolism and extraneuronal uptake and metabolism are the major processes that inactivate norepinephrine released from the axon terminals of sympathetic postganglionic neurons. Only a small fraction of released norepinephrine, estimated to be about 10 percent, escapes from synaptic clefts into the circulation.[4]

Neurally stimulated norepinephrine release from adrenergic axon terminals may be modulated by several factors acting through receptors on the axon terminals.[33] These prejunctional receptors include adrenergic receptors (see later discussion): prejunctional α_2-adrenergic receptors mediate inhibition of norepinephrine release, whereas prejunctional β-adrenergic receptors mediate stimulation of norepinephrine release. An additional compound that facilitates release through prejunctional receptors is angiotensin II. Compounds that have been reported to diminish release include acetylcholine, prostaglandins, adenosine, histamine, serotonin, and opiates, as well as dopamine. The precise physiologic relevance of these factors has not been determined.

Mechanisms of Catecholamine Action

In order to produce biological actions, hormones and neurotransmitters must first interact with target cell receptors. It is the presence of specific receptors linked to intracellular effector mechanisms that makes a given cell a target cell for a given hormone or neurotransmitter. Whereas steroid and thyroid hormones bind to intracellular receptors, the initial cellular interaction of the catecholamines (as well as acetylcholine and the peptide hormones) is at the external surface of the cell with receptors in the plasma membrane. These concepts were discussed earlier (see Chap. 5).

Adrenergic receptors[34–42] are of two broad types: α- and β-adrenergic receptors (or adrenoceptors). Each is divided into subtypes that include α_1- and α_2-adrenergic receptors and β_1-, β_2-, and β_3-adrenergic receptors. Originally classified on the basis of the potency sequence of various agonists,[42] adrenergic receptor subtypes were studied extensively with ligand-binding techniques employing various antagonists and agonists. Representative agonists and antagonists are listed in Table 12-1. The genes that code

TABLE 12-1. Adrenergic Receptors

Type	Subtype	Agonist Potency Sequence	Agonists: Selective	Agonists: Nonselective	Antagonists: Selective	Antagonists: Nonselective
Alpha	α_1	E > NE > ISP	Methoxamine	Prazosin		
			Phenylephrine			
					Phenoxybenzamine	
					Phentolamine	
				Epinephrine		
				Norepinephrine		
	α_2	E > NE > ISP	Clonidine		Yohimbine	
Beta	β_1	ISP > E ≅ NE	Prenalterol (?)		Metoprolol	
					Atenolol	
				Isoproterenol		Propranolol
				Epinephrine		Nadolol
				Norepinephrine		Timolol
						Oxprenolol
						Sotalol
						Alprenolol
						Pindolol
	β_2	ISP > E > NE	Terbutaline		Butoxamine	
			Salbutamol			
			Soterenol			
	β_3	ISP ≅ NE > E	Fenoterol	Isoproterenol	None	Metoprolol
			BRL 37344	Norepinephrine		ICI 118551
			BRL 26830A	Epinephrine		CGP 20712A

Note: E = epinephrine; NE = norepinephrine; ISP = isoproterenol.

for the four original subtypes (α_1, α_2, β_1, β_2) and for additional putative adrenergic receptors have been cloned,[34,41] permitting deduction of the amino acid sequences of the receptors and their chromosomal assignments.[36] Among the recently discovered adrenergic receptors, the β_3-adrenergic receptor (which may be only one of the so-called variant β-adrenergic receptors) is of particular interest because it may mediate stimulation of metabolic rate among other actions of the catecholamines.[41] Additional subtypes of α_1- and β_2-adrenergic receptors have been cloned.[35]

Although the receptor subtype selectivity of some adrenergic receptor antagonists (Table 12-1) is high, it is important to recognize that subtype selectivity is not absolute. For example, although metoprolol is a relatively selective β_1-adrenergic receptor antagonist, it can produce β_2-adrenergic receptor antagonism if used in a large enough dose. In addition, it has been reported to antagonize β_3-adrenergic receptors in vitro.[41]

It is fundamental to recognize that the endogenous catecholamines norepinephrine and epinephrine are mixed agonists. They interact with both α- and β-adrenergic receptors. Thus, the response of a given tissue is largely a function of the types (and subtypes) of adrenergic receptors that populate that tissue. As shown in Table 12-1, however, there are some differences between the two agonists. In general, epinephrine has a higher affinity for adrenergic receptors and exhibits greater potency than does norepinephrine in vivo as well as in vitro. Epinephrine has a particularly high affinity for β_2-adrenergic receptors relative to that of norepinephrine. Thus, β_2-mediated responses to epinephrine are more prominent than are those to norepinephrine. In contrast, norepinephrine has a higher affinity than epinephrine does for β_3-adrenergic receptors.[41]

Several adrenergic (and dopaminergic) receptors are linked, through guanine nucleotide regulatory (G) proteins, to adenylyl cyclase on the inner aspect of the plasma membrane of target cells.[34,35,41,43] Agonist occupancy of β-adrenergic receptors, through the action of a stimulatory G protein (G_s), increases adenylyl cyclase activity and, thus, levels of intracellular cyclic AMP. The latter, as well as the biochemical cascade that includes the protein kinase A activation that results from cyclic AMP elevation, mediates the cellular response. Agonist occupancy of α_2-adrenergic receptors, through the action of an inhibitory G protein (G_i), decreases adenylyl cyclase activity and, thus, intracellular cylic AMP levels. Agonist occupancy of D_1 receptors (see later discussion) increases adenylyl cyclase activity, an effect that also involves a G protein. Although also G protein-linked, transmembrane signaling following agonist occupancy of α_1-adrenergic receptors differs. It generally involves the activation of phospholipase C and the generation of messengers including diacylglycerol (which activates protein kinase C) and inositol trisphosphate (which mobilizes intracellular calcium). There is, however, evidence of other subtypes of α_1-adrenergic receptors that open calcium channels and thus permit the influx of extracellular calcium into the cell.[39]

Adrenergic receptors are dynamic, not static, and are regulated by catecholamines.[37,38] The phenomenon of *desensitization*—a diminished cellular response over time despite the continued presence of the agonist—has been studied extensively.[38] Heterologous β-adrenergic receptor desensitization, which results in decreased adenylyl cyclase responsiveness to multiple agonists, is thought to involve phosphorylation of the receptor by protein kinase A (and perhaps by protein kinase C) and a functional alteration of G_s; phosphorylation of the catalytic subunit of adenylyl cyclase may also be involved. Homologous β-adrenergic receptor desensitization, which results in decreased adenylyl cyclase responsiveness only to the agonist that induced desensitization, is thought to involve, sequentially, functional uncoupling of the receptor from adenylyl cyclase, sequestration of the receptor away from the cell surface and into an intracellular compartment, and receptor down regulation. Down regulation—a decrease in the total number of receptors per cell—involves phosphorylation of the agonist-occupied receptor by a novel kinase named, initially, β-adrenergic receptor kinase (βARK). However, βARK may well be a more general adenylyl cyclase-coupled receptor kinase; it also phosphorylates, for example, the α_2- (but not the α_1-) adrenergic receptor.

In contrast to desensitization, little is known about the mechanisms of *hypersensitization*—an increased cellular response following a period of agonist deprivation. However, an increase in the numbers of adrenergic receptors has been reported in autonomic failure, as is discussed later in this chapter.

Hormones that are not adrenergic agonists, including thyroid hormones and steroids, also regulate adrenergic receptors.[44–46] For example, an excess of thyroid hormone results in increased β-adrenergic receptor densities in mononuclear leukocytes,[45] skeletal muscle, and fat.[46] Interestingly, this is not sufficient to enhance metabolic or hemodynamic sensitivity to epinephrine in vivo.[46]

Dopamine interacts with specific dopaminergic receptors.[40,47] These are of at least two subtypes: D-1 receptors linked to stimulation of adenylyl cyclase, and D-2 receptors linked to inhibition of adenylyl cyclase or not linked to adenylyl cyclase. Dopamine is a full agonist at both D-1 and D-2 receptors. In contrast, apomorphine and dopaminergic ergots such as bromocriptine are full agonists at D-2 receptors but only partial agonists at D-1 receptors. Phenothiazines and thioxanthenes are nonselective dopaminergic antagonists, whereas butyrophenones and related drugs (spiroperiodol, haloperidol, domperidone) are relatively selective D-2 receptor antagonists; substituted benzamides such as sulpiride are also D-2 antagonists.

Adrenergic receptors can be prejunctional (on axon terminals), postjunctional (on target cells adjacent to axon terminals), or extrajunctional (on noninnervated target cells). Prejunctional (presynaptic) α_2-adrenergic receptors on the axon terminals of sympathetic postganglionic neurons mediate suppression of norepinephrine release; their blockade, as with phentolamine, results in increased norepinephrine release. Prejunctional β-adrenergic receptors mediate facilitation of norepinephrine release. Postjunctional adrenergic receptors can be of the α_1 subtype (e.g., those which mediate arterial constriction), the α_2 subtype (e.g., those which mediate suppression of insulin secretion), the β_1 subtype (e.g., those which mediate an increase in heart rate), or, perhaps, the β_3 subtype (e.g., those which mediate an increase in the metabolic rate). Extrajunctional adrenergic receptors include those of the β_2 subtype (e.g., those which mediate lactate production and vasodilatation in skeletal muscle and those on lymphocytes) and those of the α_2 subtype (e.g., those which mediate platelet aggregation).

It has been postulated that there are physiologically distinct adrenergic receptors for neurally released norepinephrine and for circulating catecholamines such as epinephrine.[48–52] It has been observed that tissues with little sympathetic innervation, such as skeletal, uterine, and tracheal muscle, are more sensitive to epinephrine than to norepinephrine and are populated predominantly by β_2-adrenergic receptors. In contrast, tissues with rich sympathetic innervation, such as the heart and large intestine, tend to be more sensitive to norepinephrine and are populated predominantly by β_1-adrenergic receptors. Thus, it has been suggested that β_2-adrenergic receptors are extrajunctional and are the β-adrenergic receptors for the hormone epinephrine (β_H- or β_E-adrenergic receptors), whereas β_1-adrenergic receptors are postjunctional and are the β-adrenergic receptors for the neurotransmitter norepinephrine (β_T- or β_{NE}-adrenergic receptors). This notion is supported by the finding that neuronal catecholamine uptake inhibition potentiates β_1- but not β_2-adrenergic responses.[50] The findings that stimulated catecholamine release activates α_1- and β_1-adrenergic receptor processes at low doses of the releasing agent and α_2- and β_2-adrenergic receptor processes only at higher doses and that the latter is prevented by bilateral adrenalectomy[51] suggest a similar pattern for α-adrenergic receptors: α_2-adrenergic receptors are extrajunctional and are epinephrine receptors (α_H- or α_E-adrenergic receptors), and α_1-adrenergic receptors are postjunctional and norepinephrine receptors (α_T- or α_{NE}-adrenergic receptors). Nonetheless, it would seem too simplistic to consider all α_2- and β_2-adrenergic receptors to be hormone receptors, as prejunctional α_2- and β_2-adrenergic receptors are probably affected by released neurotransmitter.

Biological Effects of the Catecholamines

Catecholamines produce a variety of effects in vivo. The hemodynamic effects of the catecholamines—vasoconstriction (α), vasodilatation (β_2), and an increase in the rate and force of myocardial contraction (β_1)—are well known.[53] Norepinephrine causes generalized vasoconstriction and an increase in both systolic and diastolic blood pressure. The latter effect causes reflex (parasympathetic) limitation of the increase in heart rate and cardiac output that would otherwise be expected. Epinephrine causes vasoconstriction in many vascular beds (e.g., skin, kidney, mucosae) but vasodilatation (β_2) in others (e.g., skeletal muscle). It also increases hepatic blood flow. It causes substantial increments in heart rate, cardiac output, and systolic blood pressure. Diastolic blood pressure does not change at low doses but decreases with increasing plasma epinephrine concentrations that span the physiologic range.[54] Diastolic hypertension in patients with epinephrine-secreting tumors may reflect concomitant norepinephrine release; hypotension in such patients may reflect massive epinephrine release, although other tumor products may be responsible. Dopamine increases cardiac output, an effect mediated at least partially by β_1-adrenergic receptors; the increase may result from stimulation of norepinephrine release from adrenergic axon terminals.[53] Relatively small doses reduce mesenteric and renal vascular resistance but cause vasoconstriction in other vascular beds. Thus, systolic blood pressure rises more than does diastolic blood pressure.

Other effects of catecholamines include bronchodilation (β_2), mydriasis (α), decreased gastrointestinal motility (β_1), uterine contraction (α) and relaxation (β_2), and stimulation (α) and inhibition (β) of the release of mast cell mediators.

Catecholamines produce multiple metabolic effects through both direct and indirect actions. Indirect actions result from catecholamine-induced changes in the secretion of hormones that regulate metabolic processes. For example, catecholamines both suppress (α_2) and stimulate (β_2) insulin secretion; the suppressive effect generally predominates. They also stimulate glucagon (β), growth hormone (α), and renin (β_1) secretion under some conditions. Indeed, there is evidence of adrenergic modulation of the secretion of most hormones, although the physiologic relevance of this remains to be determined in most instances.

Direct metabolic actions of catecholamines include (1) stimulation of hepatic glucose production—both glycogenolysis and gluconeogenesis—and glucose release ($\beta_2 \gg \alpha$ in humans) and limitation of extracentral nervous system glucose utilization (β_2)[4,54–61]; (2) stimulation of glycogenolysis and glycolysis with increased lactate and pyruvate release from tissues such as muscle (β_2)[4,54,62]; (3) stimulation of the release of some amino acids (e.g., alanine) from muscle (β)[63]; (4) stimulation of lipolysis (β_1 and β_3), with increased glycerol and fatty acid release, which predominates over the inhibition of lipolysis (α_2) in fat[64]; (5) stimulation of hepatic ketogenesis, largely secondary to lipolysis and increased fatty acid delivery to the liver[65]; (6) stimulation of shifts of potassium (β) and phosphate into cells, causing hypokalemia and hypophosphatemia[66]; and (7) stimulation of thermogenesis (β_3).[67,68]

The mechanisms of the hyperglycemic effect of epinephrine are complex. They involve both indirect and direct actions of the hormone and stimulation of glucose production and limitation of glucose utilization and are mediated through both β- and α-adrenergic receptors in humans.[54–62,69] These mechanisms are shown schematically in Fig. 12-5.

Limitation of insulin secretion is an important indirect hyperglycemic action of epinephrine.[61,69] α-adrenergic blockade prevents this effect of epinephrine and reduces the glycemic response[57]; in contrast, α-adrenergic blockade has little effect on the glycemic response to epinephrine when changes in insulin (and glucagon or glucose) are prevented, i.e., when only the direct hyperglycemic action is examined.[58] By contrast, there is some insulin secretion, albeit limited, during sustained epinephrine elevations,[54,57] and this is physiologically important in that it normally limits the magnitude of the glycemic response to epinephrine.[61] Thus, patients with type 1 diabetes mellitus, who are unable to release any insulin as the plasma glucose concentration rises, exhibit an enhanced glycemic response to epinephrine.[61] The role of epinephrine-stimulated glucagon secretion is less clear. In-

FIGURE 12-5. Model of the mechanisms of catecholamine-induced increments in plasma glucose concentration in humans. (*Rosen et al.*[60])

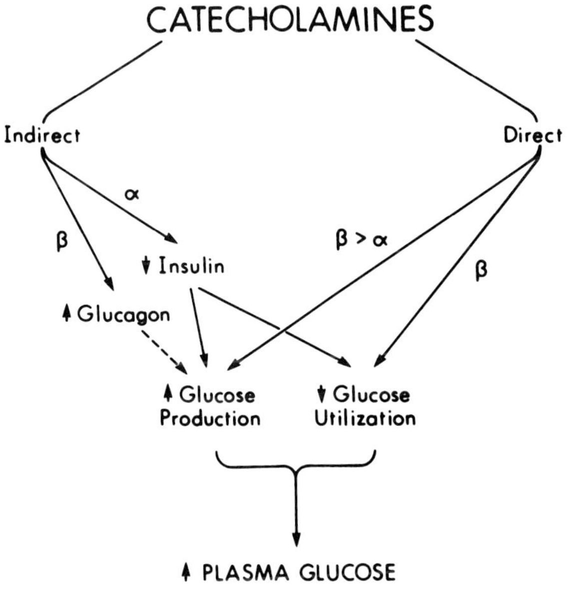

crements in plasma glucagon during epinephrine infusions have not been apparent in some studies[54,55,61] but have been observed in several studies in humans and dogs.[56,57,70] Although epinephrine-stimulated increments in glucose production clearly occur in the absence of glucagon release,[58] this does not exclude the possibility that glucagon normally mediates part of the hyperglycemic effect. However, using a somatostatin dose that suppressed glucagon secretion but not insulin secretion (as judged by peripheral insulin levels) in dogs, Gray et al. found no effect on the glycemic response to epinephrine and concluded that the effect of epinephrine on glucose production is normally independent of glucagon.[70]

The direct hyperglycemic actions of epinephrine involve both limitation of glucose utilization and stimulation of glucose production.[53,59] The first action is mediated through β_2-adrenergic mechanisms.[58,59] In humans, direct stimulation of hepatic glucose production is mediated predominantly through β_2-adrenergic mechanisms,[58] although direct α-adrenergic stimulation of glucose production can be demonstrated under some conditions.[60] However, there is also a large body of evidence indicating predominant (although not exclusive) α-adrenergic mediation in rats.[71]

The glucose concentration and kinetic responses to infused norepinephrine are similar to those during epinephrine infusion, although norepinephrine is less potent.[4,72] It is reasonable to assume that the mechanisms of the hyperglycemic effect of norepinephrine are fundamentally the same as those of epinephrine discussed previously, although this has not been studied in detail.

Infusions of norepinephrine and epinephrine in doses that result in steady-state plasma norepinephrine and epinephrine concentrations that span the physiologic range have been used to estimate plasma concentration thresholds for the hemodynamic and metabolic effects of these catecholamines in normal humans.[4,54,55,67,69] Thresholds for the metabolic actions of epinephrine are listed in Table 12-2. Those for the cardiac chronotropic and systolic pressor effects of the hormone are in the range of 410 to 680 pmol/L. It should be emphasized that these are estimates of *venous* plasma catecholamine threshold concentrations. Although they are relevant to comparisons with endogenous venous levels, they cannot be equated with biological thresholds because arterial epinephrine levels are commonly double the venous levels; venous norepinephrine concentrations tend to exceed arterial levels.[73]

It was estimated initially that plasma norepinephrine concentrations in excess of 9.0 nmol/L (~1500 pg/ml) are required to produce measurable hemodynamic and metabolic effects. At least with respect to the pressor effect, this estimate may be somewhat high. Subsequent studies have demonstrated diastolic pressor responses at venous plasma norepinephrine levels of about 6.0 nmol/L (~1000 pg/ml) or perhaps lower.[74,75] For example, Grimm et al. found that the mean extrapolated norepinephrine infusion rate that produced no change in mean arterial pressure in normal humans corresponded with plasma norepinephrine concentrations of about 4.7 nmol/L (~800 pg/ml); the rate required to produce a 20 mmHg increase in mean pressure corresponded to plasma norepinephrine concentrations of approximately 18.0 nmol/L (~3000 pg/ml).[74]

Integrated Physiology of the Sympathochromaffin System

Measurement of Catecholamines and Catecholamine Kinetics

The development of sensitive and precise methods for the measurement of catecholamines in plasma (as well as in urine and tissues) stimulated renewed interest in the study of human adrenergic physiology and pathophysiology.[76] Single-isotope-derivative (radioenzymatic) assays have become the reference methods, but high-pressure liquid chromatography (HPLC) using electrochemical detection is now used widely for measurements of catecholamines in plasma and urine.[77] Gas chromatography–mass spectroscopy (GC-MS) has also been used to measure catecholamines and their metabolites in plasma and urine.[78–80]

Venous plasma norepinephrine and epinephrine concentrations determined with a single-isotope-derivative assay in normal humans sampled in the supine and standing positions and during insulin-induced hypoglycemia are summarized in Table 12-3.

Spectrophotometric measurements of urinary catecholamine metabolites, such as metanephrines and VMA, continue to be used clinically. The clinically relevant analytic methods are discussed in more detail in Diagnostic Testing, later.

It is possible to calculate plasma appearance and plasma disappearance or clearance rates from infusions of trace amounts of radioactive catecholamines, specifically norepinephrine.[81–84] At steady state the clearance of norepinephrine is the infusion rate divided by the plasma concentration of labeled norepinephrine, and the plasma appearance rate is the infusion rate divided by the specific radioactivity of plasma norepinephrine. It should be emphasized that the plasma appearance rate is only a fraction (perhaps about 10 percent) of the rate of norepinephrine release, because released norepinephrine is largely dissipated locally, as was discussed earlier.[4] Esler et al. underscored this point by referring to the plasma appearance rate as the "spillover" rate.[82] Nonetheless, the plasma norepinephrine appearance rate should reflect the

TABLE 12-2. Venous Plasma Epinephrine Threshold Concentrations for Metabolic Effects in Humans

Metabolic Process	Parameters Measured	*Epinephrine Threshold* pmol/L	pg/ml
Lipolytic effect	↑ Glycerol, ↑ nonesterified fatty acids, ↑ palmitate turnover	410–680	75–125
Thermogenic effect	↑ Resting metabolic rate	410–680	75–125
Glycemic effect	↑ Glucose, ↑ glucose production, ↓ glucose clearance	550–1100	100–200
Ketogenic effect	↑ β-Hydroxybutyrate	550–1100	100–200
Glycolytic effect	↑ Lactate	550–1100	100–200

TABLE 12-3. Venous Plasma Norepinephrine and Epinephrine Concentrations in Normal Humans

	Supine	Standing, 10 min	Hypoglycemia
No. of subjects	165	60	26
Norepinephrine, nmol/L (pg/ml)*			
Mean	1.30 (220)	3.13 (529)	2.92 (494)
Standard deviation	0.49 (83)	1.18 (199)	1.72 (291)
Range	0.38–3.37 (65–570)	1.38–6.15 (223–1040)	1.06–6.97 (179–1180)
Epinephrine, pmol/L (pg/ml)†			
Mean	160 (30)	270 (50)	5620 (1030)
Standard deviation	90 (17)	160 (29)	5840 (1070)
Range	<50–620 (<10–113)	70–810 (12–148)	560–24940 (103–4570)
Correlations (norepinephrine with epinephrine)			
Correlation coefficient (*r*)	0.115	0.080	0.829
P Value	n.s.	n.s.	<0.001

*To convert pg/ml to nmol/L, multiply by 0.005911.

†To convert pg/ml to pmol/L, multiply by 5.458.

n.s. = not significant.

biologically relevant synaptic cleft concentration to the extent that norepinephrine is neurally derived. The sampling site affects the absolute calculated values.[81] Venous sampling has been used extensively, but because both removal and release of norepinephrine occur in an extremity, arterial sampling has been advised.[84] Because norepinephrine is extracted by the lungs, truly mixed venous (pulmonary arterial) sampling might be ideal,[84] but this is debatable. This technique assumes, reasonably, that both labeled and unlabeled norepinephrine are handled identically in the body and, more problematically, that recycling of labeled norepinephrine from sympathetic axon terminals back into the circulation is negligible.

Linares and colleagues[83] developed a compartmental model that includes a parameter considered to be the sympathetic neural norepinephrine release rate. Although this remains to be proved, the model has gained empirical support.

Despite these methodologic reservations and others not discussed here, there is rather good agreement among the various methods used to calculate catecholamine kinetics.[85] Esler and colleagues reported basal plasma appearance rates of approximately 2.9 to 8.6 ng/kg/min for norepinephrine, 2.1 to 5.0 ng/kg/min for epinephrine, and 0.4 to 1.4 ng/kg/min for dopamine in adult humans.[82] Metabolic clearance rates are similar for the catecholamines, ranging from approximately 15 to 45 ml/kg/min.

In general, plasma norepinephrine concentrations correlate with plasma norepinephrine appearance rates rather than with norepinephrine metabolic clearance rates.[81,82,83,86] However, there are several cases in which altered clearance affects the plasma norepinephrine concentration.[82] For example, patients with a degenerative disorder of the sympathetic nervous system (discussed later) exhibit decreased norepinephrine clearance because the axon terminals of sympathetic postganglionic neurons are major sites of catecholamine removal, as was discussed earlier. Thus, plasma norepinephrine appearance rates are more clearly reduced than are plasma norepinephrine concentrations in such patients. Tricyclic antidepressant drugs, such as desipramine, also decrease norepinephrine clearance into nerve terminals and tend to elevate plasma levels. β-Adrenergic antagonists such as propranolol also reduce the clearance of catecholamines (both norepinephrine and epinephrine) from the circulation.[82,87] This has little effect on basal plasma catecholamine concentrations but results in markedly elevated levels when catecholamine release is stimulated. Reduced norepinephrine clearance in patients with cardiac failure has been reported.[88] Aging and reduced caloric intake have also been reported to decrease norepinephrine clearance.[81,82]

In a study of regional norepinephrine kinetics in humans, Esler and colleagues[82] found that the kidneys and skeletal muscle each contribute approximately 25 percent of norepinephrine appearance. The liver, gastrointestinal tract, heart, and skin contribute less than 10 percent each. They also found evidence of substantial norepinephrine release from the lungs and some from the CNS, although these sources are questionable.[82]

A different approach to the estimation of norepinephrine production rates is by measurement of the quantities of norepinephrine metabolites excreted in the urine.[89,90] This method assumes that extraurinary losses are negligible, requires corrections for epinephrine-derived metabolites and adrenomedullary catecholamine production, and, if used to estimate peripheral norepinephrine production, requires corrections for CNS-derived metabolites.[89] It also includes norepinephrine that is degraded intraneuronally, a major fraction of total norepinephrine degradation.[31] Thus, the norepinephrine production rate calculated in this manner must be substantially greater than the norepinephrine release rate. Nonetheless, with this general approach it is possible to distinguish patients with degeneration of sympathetic postganglionic neurons as well as those with decreased central sympathetic outflow from normal subjects.[90]

Urinary norepinephrine and epinephrine excretion generally reflects circulating levels of these catecholamines. In contrast, dopamine in the urine is largely formed (from dopa) in the kidneys.[82] Therefore, urinary dopamine values are not a good index of circulating dopamine.

Patterns during Physiologic Adaptation

Human plasma norepinephrine and epinephrine concentrations under a variety of physiologic and pathophysiologic conditions are described in Figs. 12-6 and 12-7, respectively.[1] Note that plasma catecholamine levels vary markedly. For example, plasma norepinephrine concentrations increase two- to threefold when a subject stands. Plasma epinephrine concentrations increase up to

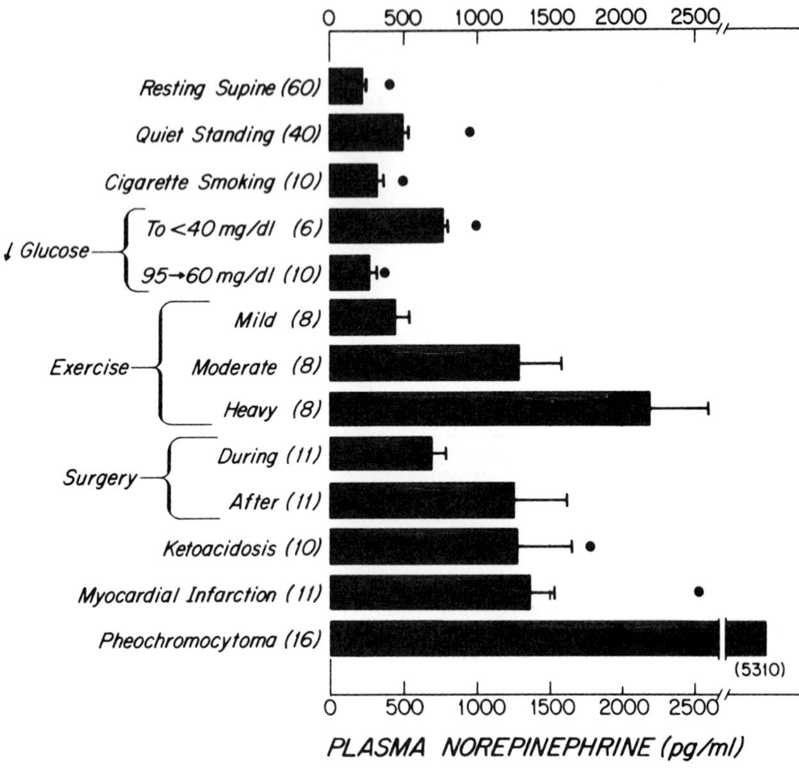

FIGURE 12-6. Mean (± SE) venous plasma norepinephrine concentrations in various physiologic and pathophysiologic states in humans. The numbers in parentheses indicate the number of subjects studied; solid circles represent the highest value observed. (*Cryer.*[1])

100-fold during hypoglycemia. The plasma levels of both catecholamines increase severalfold during vigorous exercise. Note also that plasma epinephrine concentrations commonly exceed their thresholds for the biological actions discussed earlier in this section. Plasma norepinephrine concentrations less commonly exceed their thresholds.

The sympathochromaffin system is known to be intimately involved in the maintenance of cardiovascular homeostasis during daily activities. For example, maintenance of blood pressure in the standing position requires an intact sympathetic neural reflex arc. Defects in this arc result in postural hypotension and syncope, as discussed later in this chapter. The roles of the sympathochromaf-

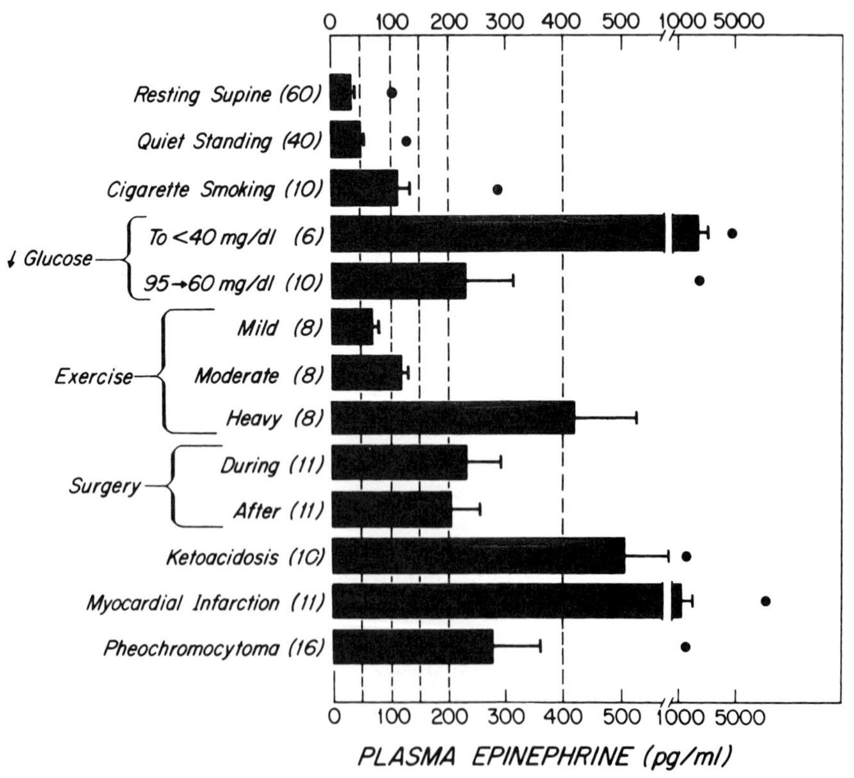

FIGURE 12-7. Mean (± SE) venous plasma epinephrine concentrations in various physiologic and pathophysiologic states in humans. The numbers in parentheses indicate the number of subjects studied; solid circles represent the highest value observed. (*Cryer.*[1])

fin system in metabolic regulation are only beginning to emerge. The importance of epinephrine, in concert with glucagon, in the prevention or correction of hypoglycemia is also discussed later in this chapter. It seems likely that epinephrine plays additional roles in the regulation of intermediary metabolism. Thus, the sympathochromaffin system can no longer be considered important only under conditions of "stress."

The Biological Roles of Epinephrine and Norepinephrine: Hormones and Neurotransmitters

The biological roles of epinephrine and norepinephrine outside of the CNS are shown schematically in Fig. 12-8. Epinephrine is a hormone of the adrenal medullae. Although regulated epinephrine secretion from extraadrenal chromaffin cells occurs, biologically effective plasma epinephrine levels are derived only from the adrenal medullae, at least in adults.[2] Thus, measurements of the plasma epinephrine concentration can be interpreted like those of other hormones—as measurements of a biologically active substance en route to its target cells and to metabolic degradation and elimination. Although it seems most reasonable to view peripheral epinephrine strictly as a hormone at the present time, it is conceivable that it also serves an autocrine, paracrine, or neurotransmitter function.

The interpretation of plasma norepinephrine measurements is less clear-cut. In the periphery, norepinephrine functions primarily as a neurotransmitter of sympathetic postganglionic neurons. Because its plasma concentrations exceed biological thresholds in some conditions, such as during vigorous exercise and in a variety of pathophysiologic states (Fig. 12-6), it may also serve a hormonal function under those conditions. Nonetheless, to the extent that norepinephrine is derived from sympathetic neurons, its neurotransmitter function must be considered primary.

Norepinephrine is released from the axon terminals of sympathetic postganglionic neurons in direct relation to postjunctional adrenergic receptors on effectors cells. Transport via the circulation is not required to explain its biological actions. As was discussed earlier, only a fraction, perhaps about 10 percent, of neurally released norepinephrine escapes into the circulation,[4,82] but it should reflect the biologically relevant synaptic cleft concentration of norepinephrine. Nonetheless, the plasma norepinephrine concentration is at best an index of sympathetic neural norepinephrine release.

FIGURE 12-8. Schematic representation of the biological roles of epinephrine (E) and norepinephrine (NE) outside the CNS.

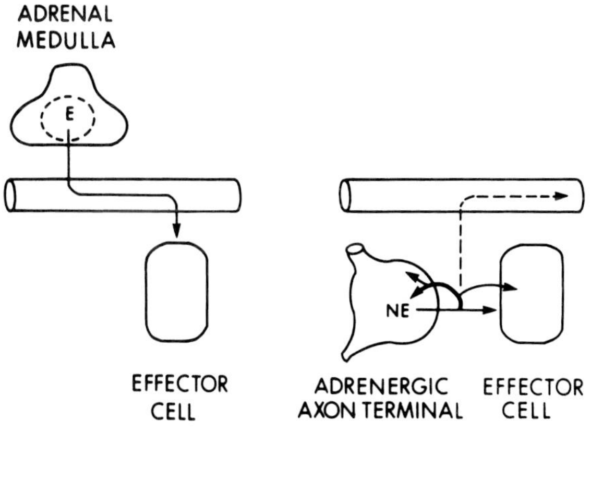

There is considerable evidence (reviewed in Refs. 4, 91, and 92) that the plasma norepinephrine concentration is a valid index of sympathetic neuronal activity under common physiologic conditions. Under basal conditions in humans, the adrenal medullae have been estimated to produce only 2–8 percent of circulating norepinephrine;[89,93,94] bilaterally adrenalectomized humans have normal basal plasma norepinephrine concentrations and exhibit normal plasma norepinephrine increments in response to upright posture.[4] Further, plasma norepinephrine and epinephrine concentrations are not correlated in normal humans sampled in the supine resting state or after 10 min of standing (Table 12-3); these findings suggest different sources (and regulation) of norepinephrine and epinephrine release. Thus, the plasma norepinephrine concentration is a reasonable index of sympathetic neuronal activity in the basal site and during ordinary upright activity. It is not, however, an optimally sensitive measure of sympathetic neuronal activity. It is conceivable that directionally different changes in sympathetic activity in different target tissues could occur with no change in the plasma norepinephrine concentration.[91] It is also clear that increments in sympathetic activity sufficient to produce measurable biological effects can be associated with small or even undetectable increments in plasma norepinephrine.[95,96] Finally, as was discussed earlier, altered norepinephrine clearance from the circulation can alter the impact of norepinephrine release on the plasma norepinephrine concentration.[82]

It cannot be assumed, however, that increments in plasma norepinephrine are derived from sympathetic neurons under all conditions. It has been estimated that the adrenal medullae contribute 30 to 45 percent of circulating norepinephrine in stressed animals,[92] and this contribution may be even greater during hypoglycemia. Some studies in animals have failed to demonstrate increased tissue (i.e., sympathetic neuronal) norepinephrine turnover during hypoglycemia despite increases in norepinephrine excretion[28,97]; such increases are prevented by adrenalectomy.[28] The capacity of the human adrenal medullae to release norepinephrine (along with large amounts of epinephrine) is well established.[93,94,98] Plasma norepinephrine and epinephrine concentrations are highly correlated during hypoglycemia in normal humans (Table 12-3), suggesting a predominant adrenomedullary source of the increases in norepinephrine. Further, in contrast to normal persons (Table 12-3), bilaterally adrenalectomized humans do not exhibit an increase in plasma norepinephrine during hypoglycemia.[2] Thus, the plasma norepinephrine response to hypoglycemia may be derived predominantly from the adrenal medullae rather than from sympathetic neurons.[97].

The origins of the increases in plasma norepinephrine (Fig. 12-6) that occur in other physiologic conditions such as exercise and in pathophysiologic states such as surgery, diabetic ketoacidosis, and acute myocardial infarction have not been established conclusively. However, because these states and conditions are often associated with substantial increases in plasma epinephrine (Fig. 12-7), the adrenal medullae probably contribute to the circulating norepinephrine pool. Thus, the plasma norepinephrine concentration is best viewed as an index of net sympathochromaffin activity under these conditions.

Despite these reservations, the plasma norepinephrine concentration correlates remarkably well with muscle sympathetic nerve activity measured directly with microneurography in humans.[99,100]

SYMPATHOCHROMAFFIN PATHOPHYSIOLOGY

Pheochromocytoma

Pheochromocytomas are catecholamine-producing tumors of chromaffin cells that typically cause hypertension.[3,101,102] They are an uncommon cause of hypertension; approximately 1 in 1,000 hypertensive patients harbors a pheochromocytoma.[103] However, for several reasons, it is important to detect a pheochromocytoma when it is present. First, hypertension due to a pheochromocytoma is often curable by means of surgical removal of the tumor. Second, patients with a pheochromocytoma are at risk for suffering a lethal hypertensive paroxysm. Third, there is an incidence, probably about 10 to 20 percent, of malignancy among pheochromocytomas, and early detection and removal can be expected to reduce the frequency of metastatic disease. Extraadrenal pheochromocytomas (paragangliomas) are more often malignant. Fourth, the presence of pheochromocytomas can be a clue to the presence of associated endocrine and nonendocrine familial disorders.

Pheochromocytomas are components of the multiple endocrine neoplasia (MEN) type 2a and type 2b syndromes (Chap. 27).[104–106] These familial disorders are inherited as autosomal dominant traits. MEN 2a (Sipple's syndrome) includes medullary carcinoma of the thyroid, primary hyperparathyroidism, and pheochromocytoma. MEN 2b includes medullary carcinoma of the thyroid, multiple mucosal neuromas, and pheochromocytoma. It is essential to exclude pheochromocytoma before neck surgery in a member of such a family, because an unrecognized pheochromocytoma can result in a fatal hypertensive paroxysm during surgery. Specific mutations of the *ret*-proto-oncogene (the MEN 2 gene) have been found to underlie each of the MEN 2 syndromes—MEN 2a, MEN 2b and medullary carcinoma of the thyroid only—and permit premorbid diagnosis.[107] Familial pheochromocytoma also occurs as an isolated disorder, in neurofibromatosis, and in some kindreds with von Hippel-Lindau disease (including hemangioblastomas of the retinas, cerebellum, and other areas of the CNS). Pheochromocytomas occur in less than 1 percent of patients with neurofibromatosis but in up to 25 percent in some kindreds with von Hippel-Lindau disease.

Clinical manifestations of pheochromocytomas generally result from released catecholamines. They often contain a variety of peptides, including enkephalins,[108] somatostatin,[109] and calcitonin.[110] The clinical relevance of these, if any, is unknown. Pheochromocytomas can, however, be a source of clinically important ectopic hormone secretion.[111]

Origin and Distribution

Pheochromocytomas arise from chromaffin cells. These cells are widespread and generally are associated with sympathetic ganglia during fetal life. Postnatally, most chromaffin cells degenerate; the major residual clusters constitute the adrenal medullae. Thus, it is not surprising that approximately 90 percent of pheochromocytomas arise from the adrenal medullae. Extraadrenal pheochromocytomas have been found in sites ranging from the carotid body to the pelvic floor. However, the majority are associated with paravertebral sympathetic ganglia or the organ of Zuckerkandl near the aortic bifurcation in the abdomen, and most of the others are associated with ganglia in the posterior mediastinum. Multiple pheochromocytomas, including bilateral adrenomedullary tumors, occur in up to 10 percent of apparently sporadic cases.

Bilateral adrenomedullary pheochromocytomas with or without extraadrenal tumors are the rule in familial pheochromocytoma associated with multiple endocrine neoplasia.[105] Bilateral adrenomedullary hyperplasia, which is thought to be a precursor to pheochromocytoma, has been found in members of such families.[106] Some have reasoned that bilateral tumors are inevitable in a member of an affected family who is found to have a pheochromocytoma and have advocated bilateral adrenalectomy at the initial operation.[105] However, at least in some patients, decades may pass between the removal of one pheochromocytoma and the emergence of a clinically apparent contralateral pheochromocytoma. Thus, a more conservative approach coupled with careful, long-term follow-up seems reasonable.

Clinical Manifestations

The vast majority of pheochromocytomas release norepinephrine, and most also release epinephrine. Rarely, a pheochromocytoma releases epinephrine predominantly or even exclusively.[112,113] The clinical manifestations of pheochromocytomas are commonly due to the effects of released catecholamines, rarely to mass effects. There is marked variation over time in catecholamine release from a given pheochromocytoma and among different pheochromocytomas. Some pheochromocytomas have been discovered at autopsy or incidentally at surgery.[103] Whether these synthesized catecholamines that were degraded within the tumor and not released, released catecholamines at rates that did not produce plasma levels sufficient to cause biological effects or caused clinical manifestations that the physician failed to recognize during the patient's life is conjectural. However, retrospective analysis of patients whose pheochromocytomas were missed often yields suggestive symptoms or signs. In one series, more than half the patients with unrecognized pheochromocytomas had hypertension.[103] Clearly, the physician must have a high index of suspicion if this generally curable disease is to be diagnosed appropriately.

The common symptoms of pheochromocytoma are headache, palpitations, and diaphoresis.[101,102] Less common symptoms include abdominal or chest pain, gastrointestinal symptoms, weakness, and visual symptoms. The symptoms are typically paroxysmal and are associated with increases in blood pressure. During a paroxysm patients are commonly pale, soaked with perspiration, and markedly hypertensive. Tachycardia is not commonly striking with norepinephrine-releasing pheochromocytomas. The paroxysms often last only a few minutes but may persist for an hour or longer. Their frequency varies greatly.

Hypertension is sometimes truly intermittent; in many cases it is sustained but exhibits marked fluctuations, with peak values occurring during symptomatic episodes. In general, these paroxysmal clinical expressions can be explained by episodic catecholamine release; plasma catecholamine levels are higher during symptomatic hypertensive episodes than they are during asymptomatic, less hypertensive, or even normotensive intervals. The event that precipitates episodic catecholamine release is usually not identifiable. However, the relation between plasma catecholamine concentrations and blood pressure is not strong.[114] This may reflect contrasting effects of norepinephrine and epinephrine but raises the possibility that hypertension in a patient with a pheochromocytoma is not exclusively the result of a direct effect of circulating norepinephrine on the cardiovascular system. Indeed, it has been suggested that hypertension may result from catecholamine release from an expanded sympathetic neuronal pool.[114] This would explain the relatively weak relation between blood pressure and the plasma norepinephrine concentration, the hypotensive response to clonidine without a decrease in plasma norepinephrine, and the occurrence of paroxysms that appear to be triggered by reflex mechanisms. However, this would require a coexistent abnormality of baroreflex regulation of sympathetic activity and conflicts with the concept of finely regulated norepinephrine stores in sympathetic neurons that was discussed earlier.

The metabolic features of pheochromocytoma include an increased metabolic rate (some patients complain of heat intolerance, weight loss, or both), limitation of insulin secretion, and an insulin-resistant state.[115] Glucose intolerance occurs, but overt diabetes is unusual and probably reflects a coexistent defect in insulin secretion (i.e., genetic diabetes mellitus).

The rare predominantly epinephrine-releasing pheochromocytomas can produce different paroxysms, including systolic hypertension, tachycardia, hypotension, noncardiac pulmonary edema, and cardiac arrhythmias.[112,113] Even with these clinical features attributable to massive overproduction of epinephrine, substantial overproduction of norepinephrine may also be present.[113]

Diagnosis

The diagnosis of pheochromocytoma is based on clinical suspicion and biochemical confirmation. Pheochromocytoma should be suspected in patients with paroxysmal symptoms; hypertension that is intermittent, unusually labile, or resistant to conventional therapy; or conditions known to be associated with pheochromocytoma. Persons with a history of familial pheochromocytoma or other components of MEN 2a or 2b should be evaluated thoroughly even if they are asymptomatic and normotensive. Radiographic studies should be used only to localize pheochromocytomas that are known or strongly suspected to be present on the basis of clinical and biochemical evidence. Nonfunctional adrenal masses are not infrequently found with modern imaging techniques (perhaps 2–4 percent of otherwise normal individuals). In the absence of other clinical clues, such lesions are rarely pheochromocytomas, although that diagnosis, as well as diagnoses of functioning adrenocortical tumors, must be considered once the lesion is detected. Members of MEN 2a or 2b families, particularly those known to have another component of the syndrome, are an exception to this general rule. In such patients an adrenal mass must be assumed to be a pheochromocytoma until proved otherwise.

Measurement of catecholamines, metanephrines, or VMA in 24-h urine collections is the traditional approach to the biochemical diagnosis of a pheochromocytoma.[116–118] Of the three, VMA determinations give a slightly higher frequency of false-negative findings. Nonetheless, the excretion of all three is substantially increased in most patients with a pheochromocytoma. For example, the urinary catecholamines were found to be more than twice the upper limit of normal in 90 percent of the patients in one large series.[116] These measurements provide somewhat different information. Catecholamine excretion provides an index of released catecholamines, whereas catecholamine degradation within the tumor also contributes to the excreted VMA and metanephrines.

With the development of sufficiently sensitive methods, specifically the single-isotope-derivative method that was discussed earlier and later HPLC methods, plasma catecholamine measurements have been effectively introduced into the diagnosis of pheochromocytoma.[3,119–121] After a direct comparison of plasma catecholamine measurements and 24-h urinary metanephrine and VMA measurements in the diagnosis of pheochromocytoma, Bravo and coworkers concluded that plasma catecholamine measurements were superior because there was less overlap in the data between affected and unaffected hypertensive patients.[121] Duncan and coworkers judged urinary norepinephrine values to be slightly superior to plasma norepinephrine values.[118] However, the two approaches yield somewhat different information. Urinary measurements provide an index of catecholamine release integrated over time. Thus, they may reflect intermittent plasma catecholamine elevations that could be missed by plasma measurements, which provide information relevant to a time frame of only a few minutes. The measurement of catecholamines in platelets is conceptually similar. Platelets take up and store circulating catecholamines. The platelet catecholamine content has been shown to be elevated in some pheochromocytoma patients whose plasma catecholamine concentrations were within the normal range.[122]

It has been suggested that measurements of plasma metanephrines are diagnostically superior because the levels of these metabolites reflect a universal feature of pheochromocytomas—degradation of catecholamines within the tumors—whereas catecholamine release is more variable.[123]

Our experience with plasma norepinephrine and epinephrine measurements in patients with proven pheochromocytomas is summarized in Fig. 12-9. As can be seen in the figure, most patients have markedly elevated values. Three points warrant emphasis, however. First, occasional patients with typical paroxysmal histories have normal plasma catecholamine concentrations when sampled during an asymptomatic, normotensive period. Second, some patients, commonly those investigated because of a family history of pheochromocytoma, have no symptoms or signs and have normal plasma catecholamine concentrations but are found to have pheochromocytomas. Measurement of epinephrine is particularly important in such patients.[106] These are not innocent tumors; lethal hypertensive paroxysms have occurred. Third, patients thought on clinical grounds to have predominantly epinephrine-secreting pheochromocytomas may also have substantial overproduction of norepinephrine.[113]

Strict attention to the details of sample collection, handling, and storage; to the sources of possible biological variation; and to the effects of drugs, as detailed later in Diagnostic Testing, is critical if diagnostic error is to be avoided in the biochemical assessment of patients with suspected pheochromocytomas. Patients should be studied in the drug-free state if possible.

When pheochromocytoma is suspected, samples for plasma norepinephrine and epinephrine should be obtained in the basal state, with the patient supine. Substantial elevations over reference values provide strong support for the diagnosis of a pheochromocytoma and are commonly found in affected patients. Samples are also obtained during symptomatic paroxysms. However, the interpretation of such values is more open to judgment because reference values cannot be defined precisely; patients without pheochromocytomas may be expected to have somewhat elevated plasma norepinephrine and epinephrine levels during these symptomatic episodes. Thus, the biochemical diagnosis of pheochromocytoma is more convincing if plasma catecholamine levels are elevated in the basal state and rise further during symptomatic episodes.

It is useful to record the blood pressure and determine whether symptoms are present when plasma samples for catecholamine measurements are drawn from a patient suspected of having a pheochromocytoma. Normal plasma or urinary catecholamine values obtained when the patient is normotensive and

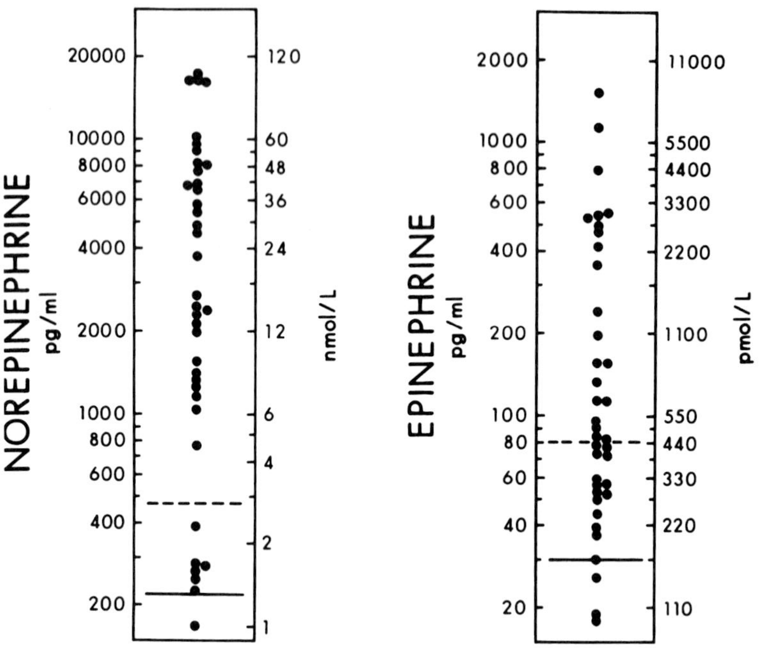

FIGURE 12-9. Plasma norepinephrine and epinephrine concentrations in the basal state (and supine position) in 38 patients with pheochromocytomas. Note the logarithmic scales. The interrupted horizontal lines are 3 SD above the mean (solid horizontal lines) of data from 165 normal humans.

free of symptoms do not exclude the presence of a pheochromocytoma. Theoretically, 24-h urinary catecholamine or metabolite measurements can detect intermittent catecholamine release missed by plasma sampling.

Because substantial plasma norepinephrine elevations are required to produce hypertension in normal humans, as was discussed earlier, and plasma epinephrine elevations within the physiologic range do not raise the diastolic blood pressure, it is reasonable to consider that normal or even minimally elevated plasma norepinephrine levels measured when the patient is hypertensive constitute strong evidence against the diagnosis of pheochromocytoma. It could be argued, however, that this reasoning is flawed if hypertension results from excessive norepinephrine release from an expanded neuronal pool rather than being a direct result of elevated circulating norepinephrine, as was discussed earlier.

It should again be emphasized that most patients ultimately found to have pheochromocytomas have distinctly elevated plasma and urinary catecholamine levels. The considerations raised in the preceding paragraphs apply to the much less frequently encountered patients in whom the diagnosis is less clear-cut and to the problem of the degree of certainty of a negative conclusion. Obviously, one can never be absolutely certain that a given patient does not have a pheochromocytoma. As in many other areas of medicine, a clinical judgment based on probability must be made.

Blood pressure changes following the administration of pharmacologic agents, for example, a precipitous fall in blood pressure after phentolamine in a hypertensive patient and an exaggerated rise in blood pressure after histamine, tyramine, or glucagon in a normotensive patient, were used in the past to test for pheochromocytoma. These tests are potentially dangerous, have unacceptably high false-positive and false-negative rates, and are not decisive. Consequently, they should not be used. Oral clonidine 0.3 mg has been reported to suppress plasma catecholamine levels in nonpheochromocytoma hypertensive patients but not in patients with a pheochromocytoma.[124] Thus, the clonidine suppression test has been suggested to separate essential hypertension patients with elevated basal plasma norepinephrine levels from patients with hypertension due to a pheochromocytoma. The utility of this test awaits further experience. False positives and negatives have been reported.[125] Further, clonidine commonly produces sedation and can produce hypotension (especially in patients treated with diuretics) or bradycardia (especially in patients treated with a β-adrenergic antagonist). Plasma chromogranin A levels are also often elevated in patients with pheochromocytomas.[126]

After biochemical confirmation of a pheochromocytoma, anatomic localization is necessary. Pheochromocytomas are rarely palpable, although those associated with the carotid body may be. The rare mediastinal pheochromocytomas are usually but not invariably seen on chest radiographs. A history of paroxysms precipitated by micturition suggests strongly that the pheochromocytoma is in or adjacent to the urinary bladder. In the absence of this history, a mass seen on chest radiographs, or a palpable neck mass, the pheochromocytoma is probably in the abdomen.

Computed tomography (CT) can localize the majority of pheochromocytomas. Virtually all adrenomedullary tumors, about 90 percent of pheochromocytomas, are seen on CT scans. Magnetic resonance (MR) imaging appears to identify adrenomedullary tumors at least as well as CT and may identify extraadrenal pheochromocytomas more effectively.[127] Furthermore, MR often produces relatively distinct images—hyperintense T_2-weighted images—of pheochromocytomas.[127] Scintigraphy using [^{131}I]-*m*-iodobenzylguanidine (MIBG) has the advantage of measuring function rather than anatomy and permits scanning of the entire trunk. It appears to be superior to CT and perhaps MR in the localization of recurrent or metastatic pheochromocytoma[127] and to CT in the localization of extraadrenal tumors. In general, CT (and presumably MR) images and MIBG scans provide complementary information.[127,128] However, the MIBG test is expensive, requires several days, and necessitates iodine administration to protect the thyroid gland. It is the author's practice to use MR imaging first and reserve MIBG scanning for difficult cases. Pheochromocytomas have also been localized with octreotide scans[129] and with [^{18}F]deoxyglucose positron emission tomography.[130]

Screening

As pheochromocytoma is a serious and generally treatable disease, it is tempting to suggest that all hypertensive patients should be screened for its presence, particularly because sensitive, noninvasive tests are available. However, given the high prevalence of hypertension in the population, the cost of screening would be appreciable. There are, of course, additional problems with screening. Screening tests require diagnostic sensitivity at the expense of specificity; false-negative tests are undesirable (because the diagnosis will be rejected), and some false-positive tests must therefore be accepted. The lower the prevalence of the disease sought in the population screened, the higher the number of false-positive tests. Clearly, the prevalence of pheochromocytoma is low (0.1–0.5 percent) in patients with hypertension.[131] Thus, screening results in a large number of false-positive tests. At the very least, these patients require repeat testing, increasing the cost. In some instances the test results can lead to more extensive diagnostic studies and perhaps unnecessary surgery, greatly increasing the monetary cost and making the human cost of screening inestimable. Thus, a high index of clinical suspicion is used to select patients in whom further testing is indicated for the diagnosis of pheochromocytoma.

Treatment

Most pheochromocytomas are benign and can be excised totally. Many believe that preoperative α-adrenergic blockade reduces surgical morbidity and mortality, although critical evidence is lacking.[102] The premises are that preoperative α-adrenergic blockade will permit reexpansion of intravascular volume, for which there is evidence,[116] and will reduce the frequency and severity of intraoperative pressor episodes. The long-acting, orally effective α-adrenergic antagonist phenoxybenzamine hydrochloride (Dibenzyline) is often used. Starting with 10 mg twice daily, the dose is increased over 7 to 10 days until the blood pressure is controlled and symptomatic paroxysms are prevented. Although total daily doses of 60 mg or more may be required, hypertension typically responds to phenoxybenzamine in patients with pheochromocytomas. The side effects include postural hypotension and occasionally the emergence of cardiac arrhythmias. The relatively selective α_1-adrenergic antagonist prazosin hydrochloride (Minipress) has also been used to prepare patients with pheochromocytomas for surgery.[102,132–134] Hypotensive responses to initial 1.0-mg oral doses of prazosin have been observed in patients with pheochromocytomas,[132–134] and an initial dose of 0.5 mg is recommended.[102] It has been suggested that prazosin may not be the preferred preoperative drug because of its inability to prevent perioperative pressor episodes.[134] However, these episodes can also occur in patients treated with phenoxybenzamine prior to surgery.

β-Adrenergic antagonists such as propranolol hydrochloride (Inderal) are generally not administered before surgery unless tachycardia or arrhythmias are or become a problem. It is generally recommended that a β-adrenergic antagonist be given only after effective α-adrenergic blockade has been established, because β-adrenergic blockade alone may result in an increase in blood pressure as a result of unopposed α-adrenergic stimulation. However, this does not occur invariably.[135] Pulmonary edema has been reported to follow the administration of propranolol to patients with pheochromocytomas.[136] Another alternative is the use of the tyrosine hydroxylase inhibitor α-methyl-L-tyrosine (Demser). However, intraoperative pressor episodes have also occurred after preparation with this drug.[137]

Pheochromocytoma surgery is high-risk surgery that requires a surgeon and an anesthesiologist who have experience with this disorder. Careful monitoring of the blood pressure and electrocardiogram is fundamental. Plasma catecholamine levels vary widely;[138] severe hypertension, arrhythmias, or both can occur during the induction of anesthesia, during manipulation of the tumor, or without obvious explanation. Pressor episodes can be treated with the rapid-acting α-adrenergic antagonist phentolamine (Regitine), among other drugs. Arrhythmias can be treated with a β-adrenergic antagonist or another antiarrhythmic agent. Given modern imaging techniques, a unilateral surgical approach is often appropriate in a patient with a sporadic adrenomedullary pheochromocytoma; indeed, laparascopic surgery has been used. Appropriate intraoperative fluid replacement is thought to reduce postoperative hypotension.[138]

Pheochromocytomas are occasionally first detected during pregnancy. Such patients have been treated to term with adrenergic antagonists, and the baby has been delivered by cesarean section, with removal of the tumor during the same operation.[139]

Given surgical and anesthesiologic experience and vigilance, the operative mortality is low, approximately 1 percent.[140] Reported surgical cure rates range from about two-thirds to 85 percent of patients. About 5 to 10 percent of patients initially thought to be cured suffer a recurrence.[140] Thus, lifelong follow-up is indicated. Probably because of postoperative stress, plasma and urinary catecholamine levels often remain elevated for about 1 week after surgery.[141] Therefore, thorough clinical and biochemical reassessment, which is fundamentally important, should be deferred until after discharge from the hospital. Persistent hypertension can be caused by a missed pheochromocytoma, a surgical complication resulting in renal ischemia,[142,143] or underlying essential hypertension. Surgery cannot be curative of malignant pheochromocytomas because this diagnosis is based on the presence of metastases; histologic criteria are not reliable.

The biochemical effects of unresectable pheochromocytomas can be treated medically with adrenergic antagonists. A tyrosine hydroxylase inhibitor, α-methyl-P-tyrosine, has also been used effectively, although it can cause side effects, including postural hypotension and CNS dysfunction.[144]

Malignant pheochromocytomas are generally resistant to radiotherapy and chemotherapy.[145] Some success has been reported with streptozocin[145] and with a combination of cyclophosphamide, vincristine, and dacarbazine.[146] Beneficial effects of [^{131}I]-*m*-iodobenzylguanidine therapy have been noted in some patients, but there were no complete remissions.[147] The clinical course of patients with metastatic pheochromocytomas is quite variable: Some die within months; others live for more than two decades. The 5-year survival rate is about 45 percent.[140]

Other Sympathochromaffin Tumors

Pheochromocytomas are tumors of differentiated neural crest cells, the chromaffin cells. Tumors of more primitive cells and of cells differentiated toward neuronal elements also occur. These include neuroblastoma,[148] a common malignant tumor of infancy and early childhood which is responsible for 15 percent of cancer deaths in children, as well as generally benign tumors such as ganglioneuromas.

Neuroblastomas arise commonly in the adrenal medullae (40 percent) or paravertebral sympathetic ganglia in the abdomen (25 percent); mediastinal, pelvic, or cervical ganglia represent less common sites of origin.[148] These tumors synthesize catecholamines commonly but generally do not release sufficient quantities of biologically active catecholamines to produce clinical manifestations. Presumably, catecholamines are degraded within the tumors, because more than 90 percent of patients excrete excessive quantities of catecholamine metabolites such as HVA and VMA. Such measurements provide prognostic as well as diagnostic information: The duration of survival is correlated directly with the VMA/HVA ratio in patients with advanced disease.[148] Measurements of catecholamine metabolites can also be used to follow the effects of therapy. Although mean plasma epinephrine, norepinephrine, and dopamine levels are increased in patients with neuroblastomas, there is considerable overlap with values from unaffected individuals.[149] In contrast, the majority of patients have elevated levels of plasma dihydroxyphenylalanine (dopa) and the enzyme aromatic L-amino acid decarboxylase.[149] These, as well as urinary VMA and HVA, appear to be useful markers for assessing the response to therapy and recurrence.

There have been notable advances in the treatment of neuroblastomas with surgery, radiation therapy, and chemotherapy.[148] A subset (about 10 percent) of patients with metastatic neuroblastomas, usually diagnosed at less than 1 year of age and with small primary tumors, is of particular interest because these patients exhibit a high spontaneous remission rate. More than 80 percent become long-term survivors with minimal or no therapy. Nonetheless, neuroblastoma is commonly a highly malignant tumor that requires aggressive therapy.

Generalized Autonomic Failure

Another established clinical disorder of sympathochromaffin function[3] is postural (orthostatic) hypotension resulting from deficient sympathetic neural norepinephrine release in various forms of autonomic failure.[150] However, mechanisms other than autonomic failure more frequently cause postural hypotension.

Assumption of the upright position causes a sharp reduction in venous return (preload) to the heart because of pooling of an estimated 500–700 ml of blood in the distensible venous system in the lower extremities and abdomen. In the absence of compensatory mechanisms, this would result in a corresponding decrease in cardiac output, arterial pressure, and CNS perfusion; cerebrovascular autoregulation notwithstanding, syncope would result from the simple act of standing. Obviously, there are effective compensatory mechanisms. The primary, if not exclusive, compensatory mechanism is a baroreceptor-initiated, CNS-mediated sympathetic neural reflex that results in norepinephrine release from axon terminals within the tissues, which in turn results in a sharp increase in systemic vascular resistance (and limitation of the fall in venous return and cardiac output) and, thus, maintenance of blood pressure in the standing position. Postural activation of this sympathetic reflex is reflected in a rapid, approximately twofold rise in plasma norepinephrine concentrations,[151] as shown in Table 12-3 and Fig. 12-10. Maximum levels are achieved within 5 min. Thus, measurement of the plasma norepinephrine response to standing provides a relatively simple means of assessing the integrity of this sympathetic reflex.

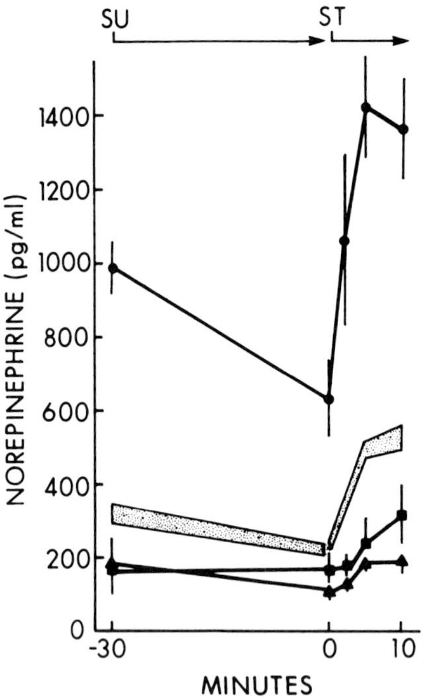

FIGURE 12-10. Mean (± SE) venous plasma norepinephrine concentrations measured in the supine (SU) and standing (ST) positions in posturally hypotensive patients with (1) severe sodium depletion (round symbols), (2) progressive autonomic failure (square symbols), or (3) diabetic adrenergic neuropathy (triangular symbols). The shaded areas encompass 1 SE around the mean for normal subjects..

Postural Hypotension

Defective postural adaptation results in a decrement in blood pressure upon standing—postural (orthostatic) hypotension. Postural hypotension is a common clinical finding, particularly in older persons.[152] Although a supine-to-standing decrement in systolic blood pressure of 30 mmHg is often used to define postural hypotension, decrements of 20 mmHg have been found to be a significant risk factor for falls and syncope and, in patients with diabetes mellitus, to be associated with an excess 5-year mortality rate.[152]

Upon standing, patients with postural hypotension note lightheadedness, blurring or even loss of vision, and a profound weakness that may culminate in syncope. The symptoms clear rapidly if the patient lies down. Postural symptoms are commonly worse in the morning, after a meal, and after exercise.

Conceptually, postural hypotension can be caused by one or more of three general mechanisms: (1) intravascular volume contraction, (2) resistance to the cardiovascular actions of norepinephrine, and (3) an afferent, central, or efferent defect in the sympathetic neural reflex arc. Patients with postural hypotension due to intravascular volume contraction or resistance to the action of norepinephrine exhibit an exaggerated plasma norepinephrine response to standing.[153,154] They have hyperadrenergic postural hypotension. In contrast, patients with postural hypotension due to a defect in the sympathetic reflex arc have a blunted plasma norepinephrine response to standing.[155–157] They have hypoadrenergic postural hypotension. These patterns are shown in Fig. 12-10.

In a posturally hypotensive patient a supine-to-standing plasma norepinephrine increment of less than 140 pg/ml—the smallest increment we have observed in normal subjects—is indicative of hypoadrenergic postural hypotension. There is considerable scatter in the responses of normal subjects (Table 12-3). In a posturally hypotensive patient a maximum plasma norepinephrine concentration during standing of more than 1,040 pg/ml—the highest value we have observed in normal subjects—is indicative of hyperadrenergic postural hypotension.

In practice, most patients with postural hypotension can be placed in the hyperadrenergic or hypoadrenergic categories on the basis of plasma norepinephrine measurements. Not infrequently, however, the plasma norepinephrine response overlaps the normal range. This may reflect the fact, discussed earlier, that plasma norepinephrine concentrations provide only an index of sympathetic activity, the scatter in the normal response, the presence of more than one mechanism of postural hypotension in a given patient, or a combination of these factors. One could reason that a normal norepinephrine response is inappropriately low and thus indicative of a hypoadrenergic component in a posturally hypotensive patient with intravascular volume contraction or resistance to norepinephrine. Obviously, this approach cannot be applied to all posturally hypotensive patients, as severely affected patients are unable to stand for any period of time.

The relative clinical utility of routine plasma norepinephrine measurements in posturally hypotensive patients who are able to stand remains to be determined; I believe these measurements are reasonable and have found them useful in individual patients. Typically, these are patients who are thought initially to have postural hypotension due to a defect in the sympathetic reflex arc, because of an associated disorder such as diabetes mellitus, or because of the absence of any other clinically apparent mechanism but are found to have a hyperadrenergic pattern caused by a potentially treatable abnormality.[154]

The heart rate and blood pressure should be recorded during supine and upright sampling for norepinephrine determinations. Although the heart rate response, which involves withdrawal of vagal tone as well as sympathetic stimulation, is not a sensitive measure for predicting the hypotensive mechanism, a marked supine-to-standing increase in the heart rate provides evidence against a defect in the sympathetic reflex arc. The forms of postural hypotension discussed here must, of course, be distinguished from bradycardic (vasovagal or vasodepressor) postural hypotension, which can occur in apparently normal persons and is generally not reproducible.

Mechanisms of Postural Hypotension

The mechanisms of hyperadrenergic postural hypotension are outlined in Table 12-4. Detailed discussion of these disorders is beyond the scope of this chapter. However, in the absence of drug administration, they most commonly result from intravascular volume contraction.[154,158,159] Clinically, they exhibit a spectrum ranging from postural symptoms without hypotension (the postural tachycardia syndrome), which can be disabling, to frank postural hypotension with recurrent syncope. This mechanism should be considered in all patients with postural symptoms and postural hypotension because it is commonly treatable. A given patient can have multiple hypotensive mechanisms, and correction of one can result in clinical improvement. For example, in a patient with relatively mild autonomic hypofunction, otherwise trivial sodium depletion can result in symptomatic postural hypotension that can be treated with sodium repletion.

TABLE 12-4. Mechanisms of Postural Hypotension

Hyperadrenergic (sympathicotonic) postural hypotension
Intravascular volume contraction (e.g., salt and water depletion, anemia)
Decreased vascular responsiveness to vasoconstrictors (e.g., vasodilator drugs, adrenocortical insufficiency, Bartter's syndrome)
Hypoadrenergic (asympathicotonic) postural hypotension-generalized autonomic failure
Primary
Secondary

Hypoadrenergic postural hypotension can result from afferent, central, or efferent lesions in the sympathetic neural arc. Diseases recognized to cause secondary hypoadrenergic postural hypotension produce lesions in the brain, spinal cord, or peripheral nerves.[150,160] These diseases are listed in Table 12-5. In the absence of such diseases, generalized autonomic failure is considered to be idiopathic or primary.

Primary autonomic failure can be divided into two clinical and pathophysiologic syndromes (Table 12-5)[150,160,161]: pure autonomic failure (idiopathic orthostatic hypotension) (PAF), and progressive autonomic failure with parkinsonism or multiple system atrophy (MSA). Because the etiology, or etiologies, of these disorders is not known, it is not clear whether these are two separate diseases or portions of a spectrum of one disease. The fact that there is overlap in the pathologic findings, such as loss of neurons from the intermediolateral columns of the spinal cord, favors the latter interpretation and provides evidence against the simple designation of PAF as a primary peripheral neural disorder and of MSA as a primary central neural disorder.[160,161] Nonetheless, there are several clinical and pathophysiologic differences between the two syndromes.

Hypofunction of both the sympathetic and parasympathetic components of the ANS in the absence of other neurologic dysfunction characterizes PAF. Sympathetic hypofunction results in hypoadrenergic postural hypotension. In addition to reduced

TABLE 12-5. Classification of Generalized Autonomic Failure

Primary autonomic failure
Pure autonomic failure (idiopathic orthostatic hypotension, Bradbury-Eggleston syndrome)
Multiple system atrophy (Shy-Drager syndrome)
Secondary autonomic failure
Metabolic disorders: diabetes mellitus, alcoholism, amyloidosis, others (porphyria, Tangier disease, Fabry's disease)
Structural CNS disorders: trauma, tumors, or vascular lesions of the brain or spinal cord
Paraneoplastic autonomic failure
Autoimmune disorders: acute and subacute dysautonomia, Guillian-Barre syndrome, pernicious anemia
CNS infections: syphilis, Chaga's disease
Others: hereditary sensory neuropathies, familial dysautonomia (Riley-Day syndrome)

Source: Modified from Bannister.[160]

TABLE 12-6. Acute Autonomic Neuropathy

Primary (? Autoimmune)
Associated with and perhaps secondary to
Antecedent viral syndrome, human immunodeficiency virus infection
Autoimmune disorders: systemic lupus erythematosus, ucerative colitis, thyroiditis
Malignancy
Secondary to
Porphyria
Botulism
Toxins: vincristine, rodenticide [pyriminil (Vacor)], podophyllin, others

Source: Modified from Hart and Kanter.[172]

plasma norepinephrine responses to standing,[155–157,162] patients with PAF, but not those with MSA, exhibit reduced resting (supine) plasma norepinephrine concentrations.[155–157,161,163] Patients with PAF, but not those with MSA, also exhibit reduced plasma norepinephrine responses to stimulation of postganglionic neurons with edrophonium (an acetylcholinesterase inhibitor).[157,164] They also excrete smaller amounts of norepinephrine metabolites than do patients with MSA.[165] Collectively, these findings suggest more prominent damage to the norepinephrine-producing sympathetic postganglionic neurons in PAF than in MSA. Parasympathetic hypofunction can cause a variety of symptoms,[151,161,166] including those referable to genitourinary (urinary frequency, incontinence or retention, impotence), gastrointestinal (diarrhea, incontinence), and respiratory (sleep apnea, stridor) dysfunction, as well as hypohidrosis. Although typically slowly progressive, the course of PAF is variable.

The clinical manifestations of autonomic hypofunction are similar in PAF and MSA. However, patients with MSA have additional neurologic disorders,[151,160,161,166] including extrapyramidal dysfunction that can resemble typical Parkinson's disease. In addition to striatonigral degeneration, olivopontocerebellar atrophy (with gait disturbance and truncal ataxia) and pyramidal dysfunction (with hyperreflexia and extensor plantar reflexes) can occur.[166] Somatic neuropathies are sometimes found.[161,166] However, intellectual function is generally preserved; dementia is not a feature of MSA. The course of MSA is progressive and debilitating. The disease is generally fatal. In one large series, death followed the onset of neurologic manifestations by an average of 4 to 5 years.[151]

Patients with primary autonomic failure have been found to have increased mononuclear leukocyte β_2-adrenergic receptor and platelet α_2-adrenergic receptor densities, probably representing receptor up regulation in response to decreased norepinephrine levels.[167] On the basis of increased cardiovascular sensitivity to agonists in vivo adrenergic, receptor up regulation is thought to be a generalized phenomenon in such patients.

Rarely, hypoadrenergic postural hypotension occurs in the absence of other evidence of autonomic hypofunction. This has been attributed to dopamine β-hydroxylase deficiency resulting in deficient norepinephrine synthesis[168–170] and to a defect in norepinephrine release.[171]

As shown in Table 12-5, there are a variety of causes of secondary autonomic failure, of which diabetic autonomic neuropathy is the most common. Although most result in chronic autonomic failure, one form of acute autonomic neuropathy often resolves completely.[172] It often occurs in young, previously healthy individuals, evolves over 1 to 3 weeks, and resolves over months, although recovery can be incomplete. Gastrointestinal symptoms (vomiting, abdominal pain, diarrhea) are common, but syncope and visual or urinary symptoms may also occur.[172] The associations and known causes of acute autonomic neuropathy are listed in Table 12-6.

Treatment of Postural Hypotension

Treatment of a patient with postural hypotension[150,152,173] begins with a search for reversible pathogenic factors such as anemia, sodium depletion, or offending drugs. This is important even if the patient has autonomic failure, as treatment of such secondary factors can result in clinical improvement even though the basic neurologic disease cannot be corrected. For example, in a patient hospitalized for the management of Parkinson's disease who becomes further incapacitated by postural hypotension, discontinuation of a diet unnecessarily low in sodium, a diuretic, or both coupled with progressive ambulation will often resolve the orthostatic problem. In the absence of reversible factors, symptomatic therapy for postural hypotension is often required.

Mechanical measures are often recommended for patients with chronic postural hypotension.[150,152,173] These include sleeping with the head of the bed elevated and the use of elastic support garments that extend from the costal margin to the feet. The premise of the first is that it reduces fluid loss from the intravascular compartment during sleep, and that of the second is that external pressure reduces venous pooling when the patient stands.

The objective of drug therapy for patients with postural hypotension is to raise the blood pressure in the upright position to a level that prevents symptoms. One does not attempt to normalize the standing blood pressure, because supine hypertension is a predictable result. Indeed, an increase in the supine blood pressure is a concomitant of most effective therapies.

Administration of the mineralocorticoid fludrocortisone (9α-fluorohydrocortisone; Florinef) 0.1–0.3 mg or more daily is the mainstay of symptomatic treatment of chronic postural hypotension.[150,152,173] This potent sodium-retaining agent often increases the standing blood pressure and relieves symptoms. If it is not adequate in itself, most physicians then add other drugs. Fludrocortisone increases plasma volume only transiently; in the long term it increases vascular resistance, perhaps by increasing vascular sensitivity to norepinephrine.[173,174] To the extent that the efficacy of fludrocortisone results from sodium retention, it is essential to ensure a liberal sodium intake, with sodium chloride tablets if necessary, and to document an initial positive sodium balance by means of serial measurements of body weight. Hypokalemia is a common complication and requires potassium supplementation. Cardiac failure is a potential but relatively uncommon complication. As with other therapies, supine hypertension occurs.[174] Administration of a β-adrenergic antagonist has been used to attempt to minimize this problem, although it can precipitate cardiac failure.

Drugs with inconsistent efficacy in the treatment of chronic postural hypotension include MAO inhibitors (e.g., pargyline), cyclooxygenase inhibitors (e.g., indomethacin), dopaminergic agonists (e.g., metoclopramide), β-adrenergic antagonists (e.g., propranolol, pindolol), indirectly acting sympathomimetics (e.g., ephedrine, amphetamines, dietary tyramine), and directly acting vasoconstrictors (e.g., phenylephrine hydrochloride). Drugs that produce venous as well as arterial constriction include midodrine, the ergotamines, and clonidine. Midodrine, an α-adrenergic agonist, appears to be effective in some patients, specifically those with less severe impairment of autonomic reflexes.[175] Aside from one report involving ergotamine tartrate,[176] oral ergotamines have not been found to be effective, although parenteral dihydroergotamine has been reported to be effective. The α_2-adrenergic agonist clonidine has been shown to raise blood pressure in severely affected patients but to lower pressure in less severely affected patients; that is, the blood pressure response was inversely related to the plasma norepinephrine level.[177] Clonidine lowers blood pressure in normal individuals by suppressing central sympathetic outflow, but it also has direct vasoconstrictive effects. The latter action appears to predominate in patients with severe autonomic failure. The α_2-adrenergic antagonist yohimbine releases norepinephrine from adrenergic axon terminals and has been shown to raise blood pressure in some patients.[177] Finally, with respect to drug treatment, the somatostatin analogue octreotide has been reported to prevent postprandial hypotension in patients with MSA but not in those with PAF.[178] Several other drugs have been used.[177]

Among other treatments, atrial pacing has been helpful in some but not all of these patients.[179] Finally, preliminary studies with a closed-loop computer-based system for blood pressure monitoring and controlled norepinephrine infusion have been reported.[180]

The preceding paragraphs have focused on supportive management of sympathetic hypofunction. Manifestations of parasympathetic hypofunction are common in patients with primary autonomic failure and are usually not treated. However, subcutaneous bethanechol chloride has been reported to improve tearing, salivation, sweating, and gastrointestinal and bladder functions.[181]

Hypoglycemia

The third established clinical disorder of sympathochromaffin function is symptomatic hypoglycemia resulting from combined, selective deficiencies of the epinephrine and glucagon secretory response to plasma glucose decrements. This has been well-documented only in patients with type 1 diabetes mellitus (T1DM).[182–184] However, because T1DM is a common disease and because deficient epinephrine and glucagon secretory responses to falling plasma glucose concentrations are common, iatrogenic hypoglycemia in T1DM is undoubtedly the most common clinical expression of abnormal sympathochromaffin function. As was mentioned in the preceding section, diabetic autonomic neuropathy[185] is the most common cause of generalized autonomic failure. However, this section describes a distinct form of hypoglycemia-associated autonomic failure that involves hypofunction of the adrenal medullae as well as the remainder of the autonomic nervous system that is limited to the stimulus of falling plasma glucose levels and is associated with a high frequency of severe iatrogenic hypoglycemia in T1DM.

Glucose is an obligate fuel for the brain under physiologic conditions. Even brief hypoglycemia can cause profound dysfunction of the brain, and prolonged severe hypoglycemia can cause brain death. Therefore, it is not surprising that mechanisms that effectively prevent or correct hypoglycemia have evolved. Indeed, because of the efficacy of these mechanisms, hypoglycemia is an uncommon clinical event except in persons receiving drugs, such as insulin, that tend to lower the plasma glucose concentration.[184] Patients with T1DM must, of course, take insulin to survive.

Hypoglycemia is the limiting factor in the management of T1DM.[184] Patients undergoing conventional therapy experience an average of one episode of symptomatic hypoglycemia per week; those undergoing intensive therapy experience an average of two such episodes per week. Ten percent of patients receiving conventional therapy and 25 percent of those receiving intensive therapy have at least one episode of severe, temporarily disabling hypoglycemia, often with seizure or coma, in a given year. Four percent of deaths of patients with T1DM have been attributed to hypoglycemia. In addition to recurrent physical morbidity and some mortality, hypoglycemia causes psychological morbidity. Many patients live in fear of hypoglycemia, and some feel guilty about that fear.

Although previously thought to be exclusively a result of imperfect insulin replacement in the setting of the variable carbohydrate intake and utilization that characterize daily life, it is now recognized that impaired defenses against plasma glucose decreases also play an important role in the pathogenesis of iatrogenic hypoglycemia in T1DM.[182–184]

Physiology of Glucose Counterregulation

The physiology of glucose counterregulation—the mechanisms that prevent or correct hypoglycemia—has been reviewed in detail[184] (see Chap. 19) and will only be summarized here. The prevention or correction of hypoglycemia involves both dissipation of insulin and activation of glucose counterregulatory (glucose-raising) systems. Whereas insulin is the dominant glucose-lowering factor, there are redundant glucose counterregulatory factors. There is also a hierarchy among the glucoregulatory factors.

Decreases in circulating insulin normally play an important role in defending against reductions in plasma glucose. However glucose recovery from hypoglycemia can occur despite a degree of peripheral hyperinsulinemia and in the absence of decreases in portal insulin levels below baseline because of the efficacy of the counterregulatory systems.[186] Among the latter, glucagon plays a primary role (Fig. 12-11). Although epinephrine is involved, it is not normally critical, but compensates partially and becomes critical when glucagon secretion is deficient (Fig. 12-11). Hypoglycemia develops or progresses when both glucagon and epinephrine are deficient and insulin is present. Thus, these three hormones stand high in the hierarchy of glucoregulatory factors. Some of the studies leading to this conclusion are summarized in Fig. 12-11.

Growth hormone and cortisol are demonstrably involved in defending against prolonged, as opposed to short-term, hypoglycemia.[187–189] However, these hormones are not critical to the prevention of hypoglycemia, at least in adults, and are not critical to recovery from even prolonged hypoglycemia.[189] There is evidence consistent with the concept that glucose autoregulation (hepatic glucose production as an inverse function of the plasma glucose concentration independent of hormonal and neural regulatory factors) is operative in humans, although only during severe hypoglycemia.[190,191] Nonetheless, these factors stand low in the hierarchy of the redundant glucose counterregulatory factors, since hypoglycemia develops or progresses when both glucagon and epinephrine are deficient and insulin is present despite normal growth hormone and cortisol secretion and intact autoregulatory mechanisms. The same reasoning applies to the potential counterregulatory roles of other hormones, neurotransmitters, and substrates other than glucose.

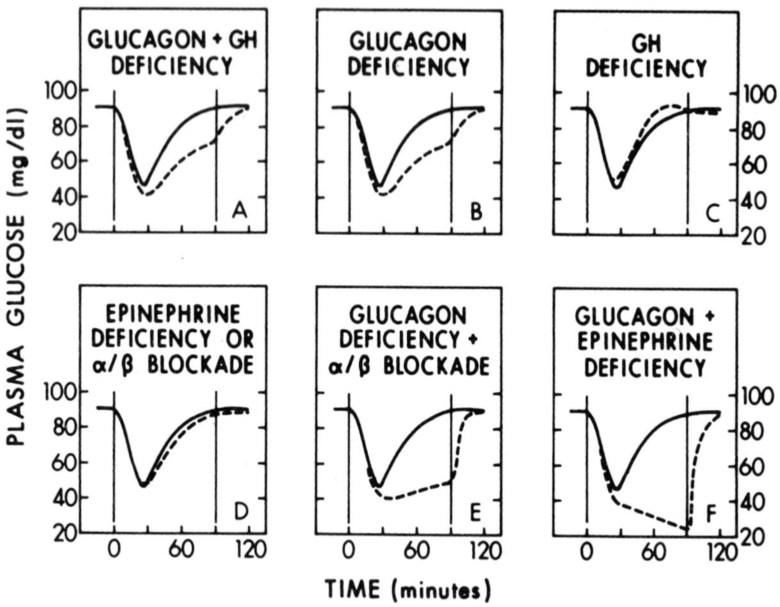

FIGURE 12-11. Plasma glucose curves following the intravenous injection of regular insulin at 0 min in human subjects during control studies (solid lines, same in all panels) and as modified (dashed lines) by (*A*) somatostatin infusion from 0 through 90 min (glucagon + GH deficiency); (*B*) somatostatin infusion with growth hormone replacement (glucagon deficiency); (*C*) somatostatin infusion with glucagon replacement (GH deficiency); (*D*) phentolamine plus propranolol infusion or studies in bilaterally adrenalectomized, glucocorticoid- and mineralocorticoid-replaced patients (α/β blockade or epinephrine deficiency); (*E*) somatostatin plus phentolamine and propranolol infusion (glucagon deficiency + α/β blockade); (*F*) somatostatin infusion in bilaterally adrenalectomized patients (glucagon + epinephrine deficiency). (*From Cryer PE: Glucose counterregulation in man.* Diabetes *30:261, 1981*).

Pathophysiology of Glucose Counterregulation in T1DM

There are three recognized hypoglycemia-associated clinical syndromes in patients with T1DM: defective glucose counterregulation, hypoglycemia unawareness, and elevated glycemic thresholds for the symptoms and activation of glucose counterregulatory systems during effective intensive therapy. Autonomic hypofunction distinct from diabetic autonomic neuropathy plays a central role in all three syndromes.

Deficient glucagon secretory responses to decreases in plasma glucose are the rule in T1DM.[183,184,192] This is an acquired defect, but it develops in the first few years of the disease. It is a selective defect in that glucagon secretory responses to other stimuli are generally normal. Its mechanism is unknown, although it is closely associated with absolute insulin deficiency. To the extent that they have deficient glucagon responses to hypoglycemia, patients with T1DM are largely dependent on epinephrine to prevent or correct hypoglycemia.[193] Thus, patients with established T1DM have altered glucose counterregulation, but this appears to be generally adequate, presumably because epinephrine compensates for deficient glucagon responses.

Most patients with T1DM also develop deficient epinephrine secretory responses to decreases in plasma glucose.[183,184] The precise mechanism of this acquired defect, which also appears to be specific to the stimulus of hypoglycemia, is unknown. Pancreatic polypeptide responses to hypoglycemia are also reduced.[194] Nonetheless, as will be discussed later, the disorder is not linked closely with diabetic autonomic neuropathy.

Patients with combined deficiencies of glucagon and epinephrine responses to plasma glucose decrements have the syndrome of defective glucose counterregulation. Compared with patients with deficient glucagon but normal epinephrine responses, patients with the combined defect have been shown in prospective studies to have a 25-fold[195] or greater[196] increased risk for developing severe iatrogenic hypoglycemia, at least during intensive therapy.

Reduced sympathochromaffin responses to falling glucose levels can increase the frequency of severe hypoglycemia in patients with T1DM not only by impairing physiologic defenses against hypoglycemia, as just discussed, but also by impairing recognition of developing hypoglycemia. Indeed, reduced sympathochromaffin (sympathetic neural as well as adrenomedullary) responses to falling glucose levels are thought to underlie the clinical syndrome of hypoglycemia unawareness.[197,198] Affected patients no longer experience the neurogenic (autonomic) warning symptoms of developing hypoglycemia (e.g., palpitations, tremor, sweating) and therefore fail to act (e.g., eat) to prevent severe hypoglycemia. The result is recurrent episodes of neuroglycopenia.[199] Although the glycemic thresholds for the release of epinephrine, and probably pancreatic polypeptide, are high—i.e., at lower plasma glucose concentrations—hypoglycemia unawareness is not associated with diabetic autonomic neuropathy, as will be discussed later.

Glycemic thresholds for both symptoms and activation of glucose counterregulatory systems are also higher during intensive therapy that effectively lowers plasma glucose concentrations. Tightly controlled patients with T1DM require lower plasma glucose concentrations to elicit these responses.[200] Although this syndrome per se has not been shown to increase the frequency of severe iatrogenic hypoglycemia, it is reasonable to suspect that it does. Certainly the frequency of severe hypoglycemia is increased during intensive therapy.[201]

The syndromes of defective glucose counterregulation, hypoglycemia unawareness, and elevated glycemic thresholds during effective therapy have much in common. First, they segregate together.[202,203] Second, they are associated with a high frequency of iatrogenic hypoglycemia.[195,196,199,200] Third, they share several pathophysiologic features, including reduced adrenomedullary epinephrine responses to a given degree of hypoglycemia (i.e., high glycemic thresholds).[195,196,198,200,202,203] Thus, these are clinically, and perhaps at least in part pathogenetically, interrelated syndromes. Therefore, it is reasonable to group them as the syndromes of hypoglycemia-associated autonomic failure.[182–184]

Hypoglycemia-associated autonomic failure (HAAF) is distinct from classical diabetic autonomic neuropathy (CDAN). First, HAAF and CDAN do not cosegregate.[195,198,199,202] Second, deficient autonomic responses are specific for hypoglycemia in HAAF but generalized in CDAN.[185] Third, whereas reduced

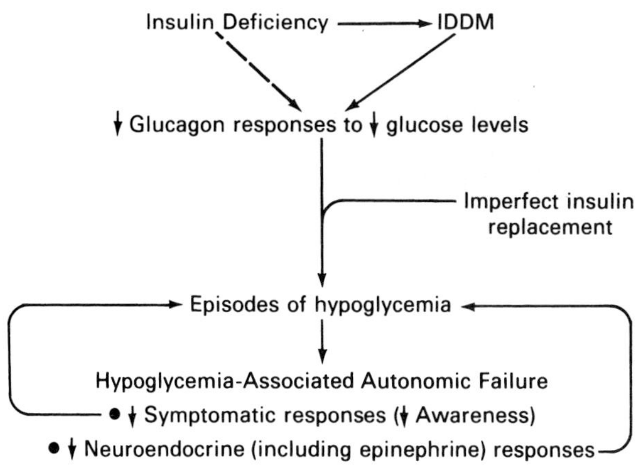

FIGURE 12-12. Pathogenesis of hypoglycemia-associated autonomic failure.

adrenomedullary responses to a given degree of hypoglycemia constitute a central feature that is undoubtedly relevant to the pathogenesis of iatrogenic hypoglycemia in the setting of deficient glucagon responses in HAAF, epinephrine responses to hypoglycemia are reduced little if at all in CDAN.[185] Fourth, HAAF is associated with a high frequency of iatrogenic hypoglycemia, but there is no evidence that CDAN per se plays a role in the pathogenesis of hypoglycemia.[185] Fifth, for reasons discussed later, HAAF may be at least in part reversible[204] while CDAN is not.[185]

A single 2-h episode of afternoon hypoglycemia reduces the symptomatic and neuroendocrine (including adrenomedullary) responses (e.g., elevates the glycemic thresholds) to hypoglycemia the following morning in normal humans.[204] It is, therefore, conceivable that recent antecedent hypoglycemia is one factor in the pathogenesis of the syndromes of HAAF. This hypothesis is illustrated in Fig. 12-12. Deficient glucagon responses to blood glucose decreases in the setting of imperfect insulin replacement result in episodes of hypoglycemia. These episodes in turn lead to reduced symptomatic responses (i.e., decreased awareness) and a reduced adrenomedullary response (i.e., further compromised glucose counterregulation) to hypoglycemia, thus creating a vicious cycle.

It is conceivable that administration of a β-adrenergic antagonist can produce HAAF. Compelling clinical evidence that this class of drugs increases the frequency or severity of clinical hypoglycemia in T1DM is lacking, but to the author's knowledge this issue has not been examined critically in the setting of intensive therapy in which hypoglycemia is particularly common. As was mentioned earlier, β-adrenergic antagonists impair recovery from experimental hypoglycemia in T1DM.[193] Furthermore, although β-adrenergic antagonism does not produce absolute unawareness of hypoglycemia, it shifts the glycemic thresholds for symptoms to lower plasma glucose concentrations.[205]

Clearly, pending the prevention or cure of T1DM, we need to learn to deliver insulin in a much more physiologic fashion or to prevent, correct, or compensate for compromised defenses against hypoglycemia if we are to achieve euglycemia safely in the majority of patients with T1DM. However, adherence to the principles of modern therapy—patient education and support, self blood glucose monitoring, flexible and more physiologic insulin regimens—coupled with prudent glycemic goals can minimize the frequency of severe hypoglycemia without compromising glycemic control completely.

DIAGNOSTIC TESTING

Measurement of Catecholamines and Their Metabolites

Measurements of catecholamines and of catecholamine metabolites are used clinically in the diagnosis of pheochromocytoma and other sympathochromaffin tumors. Measurement of the plasma norepinephrine response to standing can be used to define the mechanism of postural hypotension (hyperadrenergic vs. hypoadrenergic).

Determination of catecholamines, their metabolites, or both in urine, usually in 24-h samples, have been used clinically for decades. Older fluorometric techniques have been replaced by HPLC methods in clinical laboratories. Most HPLC methods employ electrochemical detection,[206] but other detection systems can be used.[207] These methods provide quantitative measurements of norepinephrine, epinephrine, and dopamine excretion. Normal urinary norepinephrine excretion is approximately 10–90 μ/24 h, while that of epinephrine is less than 15 μg/24 h. Urinary dopamine excretion, which is largely derived from the kidneys rather than the circulation, is generally in the range of 100 to 450 μg/24 h.

Although they were formerly determined by selective extraction and conversion to vanillin, as measured spectrophotometrically,[8] urinary MN and NMN (often reported as total metanephrines) and VMA can also be measured with HPLC methods.[206,207] Normal persons generally excrete less than 1.0 mg of total metanephrines and 7.0 mg of VMA per 24 h.

Single-isotope-derivative (radioenzymatic) methods, which are based on the conversion of the catecholamines to their respective tritiated *O*-methyl derivatives in the presence of *S*-adenosyl-L-methione containing a tritiated methyl group that is transferred to the catecholamines by the enzyme COMT, are the reference methods for measurements of catecholamines in plasma.[208,209] They provide the sensitivity, specificity, and precision needed for measurement of physiologic concentrations of epinephrine as well as norepinephrine in plasma. They can, of course, be used to measure catecholamines in urine (and tissue), but the high concentrations present in urine do not require a sensitive method.

However, isotope-derivative methods are technically demanding, time-consuming, and expensive. Most clinical laboratories now use HPLC methods to measure catecholamines, as well as precursors and metabolites, in plasma.[210–212] These methods are sufficiently sensitive to answer the clinical question: are plasma catecholamine levels elevated above normal?

Representative venous plasma norepinephrine and epinephrine concentrations in normal individuals are listed in Table 12-3. Levels in various physiologic and pathophysiologic states are shown in Figs. 12-6, 12-7, 12-9, and 12-10.

Strict attention to the details of sample collection, handling, and storage, sources of possible biological variation, and the effects of drugs is critical if diagnostic error is to be avoided in the use of catecholamine measurements. This applies to both plasma and urinary catecholamine measurements but is even more critical with plasma measurements.

Potential sources of error in the use of plasma catecholamine measurements are listed in Table 12-7. From a technical standpoint, it is important that the patient be in the supine position before and during sampling. Plasma norepinephrine and epinephrine concentrations double when a normal person stands, and the

TABLE 12-7. Potential Sources of Error in the Use of Plasma Catecholamine Measurements

1. Technical
   a. Sampling: patient in supine position
   b. Sample handling: iced, special tubes; prompt separation of plasma
   c. Sample storage: −20°C (hours to days); −70°C (longer)
   d. Analytic method: HPLC or radioenzymatic method
2. Biological variation: normally marked; increased catecholamine levels
   a. Acute stress (physical or emotional)
   b. Chronic illness
3. Drug-induced variation: increased catecholamine levels
   a. Catecholamines and related compounds: methyldopa, dopa, isoproterenol, etc.
   b. Increased catecholamine release
      (1) Sympathomimetics: epinephrine, amphetamines, tyramine, etc.
      (2) Vasodilators: nitrates/nitrites, hydralazine, minoxidil, methylxanthines, phenothiazines, calcium channel antagonists, angiotensin converting enzyme inhibitors, etc.
      (3) α-adrenergic antagonists: prazosin, phentolamine, phenoxybenzamine
      (4) Diuretics (sodium depletion)
      (5) Cigarette and marijuana smoking, caffeine ingestion
   c. Decreased catecholamine clearance
      (1) β-adrenergic antagonists: propranolol, etc.
      (2) Others: cocaine, guanethidine, reserpine

scatter in the values increases (Table 12-3). Although we have used a 30-min interval in the supine position, 10–15 min is probably sufficient. Because the stress of venipuncture elevates mean plasma catecholamine levels somewhat and increases the scatter in the values, some advocate sampling through a previously inserted indwelling intravenous needle or catheter.

Catecholamines are readily oxidized. They are most stable at low temperature, at low pH, and in the presence of an antioxidant. Furthermore, erythrocytes contain COMT. In whole blood catecholamines have been reported to degrade at a rate of approximately 30 percent per hour at room temperature,[208] although slower rates have also been reported.[213] Thus, blood samples for plasma catecholamine determinations should be drawn into iced tubes containing an anticoagulant and an antioxidant, and the plasma should be promptly separated, preferably in a refrigerated centrifuge. Many laboratories, including ours, use the calcium chelating agent EGTA and the antioxidant reduced glutathione. 1,4-Dithiothreitol, but not metabisulfite or ascorbic acid, can be substituted for reduced glutathione. Once it is separated, the plasma should be frozen quickly. Catecholamines deteriorate at a rate of approximately 5 percent per month at −20°C. At −70°C they are stable for at least 1 year.[208] At the present time only single-isotope-derivative and HPLC methods are appropriate for the measurement of catecholamines in plasma.

Biological variation in plasma catecholamine concentrations can be substantial (Table 12-3 and Figs. 12-6 and 12-7). For example, plasma epinephrine concentrations increase as much as 100-fold during hypoglycemia. Smaller but substantial increments in norepinephrine and epinephrine levels occur during common activities. Thus, scrupulous attention to sampling conditions and reluctance to attach undue importance to single measurements are required if plasma catecholamine levels are to be interpreted correctly.

Elevated plasma catecholamine levels have been well documented during acute mental and physical stress. Stable elevations also occur in several chronic diseases, such as hypothyroidism, congestive cardiac failure, chronic pulmonary disease, and duodenal ulcer. Additional physiologic factors should be kept in mind. For example, plasma norepinephrine concentrations increase slightly with age.[214] Sodium depletion due to disease, diuretics, or dietary sodium restriction (less than 3.0 g per day) elevates resting plasma norepinephrine concentrations and increases the response to standing.[98,215]

Patients should be sampled in the drug-free state if possible. Drug-induced alterations are perhaps the most common cause of erroneous interpretation of plasma catecholamine determinations. Most antihypertensive drugs, other than clonidine, and many other drugs can elevate plasma and urinary catecholamines. Some of these mechanisms are summarized in Table 12-7. If the physician is compelled to treat hypertension before measuring catecholamines, clonidine is the drug of choice because it will not produce a false-positive result.

Urine samples for catecholamine determinations are commonly collected in refrigerated containers to which 15 ml of 6*N* HCl has been added, as catecholamines are more stable at low temperature and low pH. Urine samples for metanephrines and VMA need not be acidified, but the analytic methods are compatible with this form of collection if catecholamines are also to be measured. The collection of a complete 24-h urine specimen requires careful instruction of the patient. The creatinine content should be measured in all specimens to detect major collection errors. Dietary restrictions are not necessary for specific measurements of urinary metanephrines and VMA.

Catecholamine and catecholamine metabolite excretion is subject to the same sources of biological variation that apply to plasma catecholamine levels, as was discussed earlier. However, because these variations in catecholamine release are usually brief, their effect on 24-h excretion is relatively small and sampling conditions need not be controlled rigorously. Nonetheless, major stress should be avoided during these collections, as conditions known to produce stable elevations in plasma catecholamine levels will produce corresponding elevations in urinary catecholamine and metabolite excretion.

Drug-induced alterations are also common. All the drugs that elevate plasma catecholamine levels, as discussed earlier, can be expected to increase urinary catecholamine and metabolite values. Short-term administration of the mild analgesics acetylsalicylic acid, acetaminophen, and propoxyphene or of the sedative-tranquilizers diazepam, chlordiazepoxide, diphenhydramine, and phenobarbital does not alter catecholamine excretion.[216]

Indirect Tests of Autonomic Function

Tests of cardiovascular reflexes are often used to assess autonomic function. Some relatively simple tests that can be used to document and to some extent quantitate autonomic failure[217–219] are described in Table 12-8. Measurement of blood pressure (and heart rate) in the supine and standing positions is the most widely used indirect clinical test of sympathetic function, as was discussed earlier in this chapter. Clearly, it is neither a sensitive nor a specific test of sympathetic function. Patients with other evidence of sympathochromaffin hypofunction may not have postural hypotension, and postural hypotension can result from mechanisms other than sympathetic hypofunction, as was discussed earlier. The utility of this maneuver is enhanced by the simultaneous measurement of the plasma norepinephrine response.

TABLE 12-8. Clinical Tests for Autonomic Hypofunction

Test	Normal	Borderline	Abnormal
Postural fall in blood pressure: fall in systolic blood pressure (mmHg) after 2 min standing	<11	11–29	>29
Heart rate variation: ratio of maximum to minimum heart rate (bpm) during deep breathing at 6 breaths per min	>15	11–14	<11
Heart rate response to standing: ratio of the R-R interval at approximately beat 30 to that at approximately beat 15 after initiation of standing (30:15 ratio)	>1.04	1.01–1.03	<1.01
Valsalva maneuver: ratio of longest R-R interval after to shortest R-R interval during the Valsalva maneuver (40 mmHg × 15 s) with an aneroid manometer or modified sphygmomanometer (Valsalva ratio)	>1.20	1.11–1.120	<1.11
Sustained handgrip: increase in diastolic blood pressure (mmHg) measured during 30% of maximal handgrip for up to 5 min with a handgrip dynamometer	>15	11–15	<11

Source: From Ewing.[246]

Among tests of parasympathetic function, measurements of the variation in heart rate associated with deep breathing is commonly used.[217–219] The normal variation is determined largely by vagal inputs; variation is decreased by parasympathetic hypofunction. A simple approach is to obtain an ECG recording during deep breathing at five to six cycles per minute in a resting subject.[217] R-R intervals are measured, and beat-to-beat variation is calculated as the difference between maximal and minimal heart rate and expressed as the mean of differences in five successive respirations. Values lower than 10 per minute are considered abnormal.

Acknowledgments The author is grateful for the efforts of his collaborators, whose names appear in the reference list, and for the support of U.S. Public Health Service grants DK 27085, RR 00036, and DK 20579. Particular thanks are due to Ms. Karen Muehlhauser for preparation of the manuscript.

REFERENCES

1. Cryer PE: Physiology and pathophysiology of the human sympathoadrenal neuroendocrine system. *N Engl J Med* 303:436, 1980.
2. Shah SD, Tse TF, Clutter WE, Cryer PE: The human sympathochromaffin system. *Am J Physiol* 247:E380, 1984.
3. Cryer PE: The adrenal medullae, in James VHT (ed): *The Adrenal Gland*, 2nd ed. New York, Raven Press, 1992, pp 465–489.
4. Silverberg AB, Shah SD, Haymond MW, Cryer PE: Norepinephrine: Hormone and neurotransmitter in man. *Am J Physiol* 234:E252, 1978.
5. Mayer SE: Neurohumoral transmission and the autonomic nervous system, in Gilman AG, Goodman LS, Gilman A (eds): *The Pharmacological Basis of Therapeutics*. New York, Macmillan, 1980, pp 55–90.
6. Cryer PE: Decreased sympathochromaffin activity in IDDM. *Diabetes* 38:405, 1989.
7. Trifaró J-M: Cellular and molecular mechanisms in hormone and neurotransmitter secretion. *Can J Physiol Pharmacol* 68:1, 1990.
8. Nagatsu T: *Biochemistry of the Catecholamines*. Baltimore, University Park Press, 1973.
9. Clarke JTR, Bier DM: The conversion of phenylalanine to tyrosine in man: Direct measurement by continuous intravenous tracer infusions of L-[ring$^2H_5$]phenylalanine and L-[1-^{13}C]tyrosine in the postabsorptive state. *Metabolism* 31:999, 1982.
10. Fukami MH, Haavik J, Flatmark T: Phenylalanine as a substrate for tyrosine hydroxylase in bovine adrenal chromaffin cells. *Biochem J* 268:525, 1990.
11. McInnes RR, Kaufman S, Warsh JJ, Van Loon GR, Milstein S, Kapatos G, Soldin S, Walsh P, et al: Biopterin synthesis defect. *J Clin Invest* 73:458, 1984.
12. Haycock JW: Phosphorylation of tyrosine hydroxylase *in situ* at serine 8, 19, 31 and 40. *J Biol Chem* 265:11682, 1990.
13. Kaneda N, Ichinose H, Kobayashi K, Oka K, Kishi F, Nakazawa A, Kurosawa Y, Fujita K, Nagatsu T: Molecular cloning of cDNA and chromosomal assignment of the gene for human phenylethanolamine N-methyltransferase, the enzyme for epinephrine biosynthesis. *J Biol Chem* 263:7672, 1988.
14. Ceccatelli S, Dagerlind Å, Schalling M, Wikström A-C, Okret S, Gustafsson JÅ, Goldstein M, Hökfelt T: The glucocorticoid receptor in the adrenal gland is localized in the cytoplasm of adrenaline cells. *Acta Physiol Scand* 137:559, 1989.
15. Rudman D, Moffitt SD, Fernhoff PM, Blackston RD, Faraj BA: Epinephrine deficiency in hypocorticotropic hypopituitary children. *J Clin Endocrinol Metab* 53:722, 1981.
16. Blombery PA, Kopin IJ, Gordon EK, Markey SP, Ebert MH: Conversion of MHPG to vanillylmandelic acid. *Arch Gen Psychiatry* 37:1095, 1980.
17. Maas JW, Hattox SE, Greene NM, Landis DH: 3-Methoxy-4-hydroxyphenethyleneglycol production by human brain in vivo. *Science* 205:1025, 1979.
18. Kopin IJ, Gordon EK, Jimerson DC, Polinsky RJ: Relation between plasma and cerebrospinal fluid levels of 3-methoxy-4-hydroxphenylglycol. *Science* 219:73, 1983.
19. Axelrod J, Tomchick R: Enzymatic O-methylation of epinephrine and other catechols. *J Biol Chem* 233:702, 1958.
20. Shih JC: Molecular basis of human MAO A and B. *Neuropsychopharmacology* 4:1, 1991.
21. Coupland RE: *The Natural History of the Chromaffin Cell*. London, Longmans, 1965.
22. Johnson RG: Accumulation of biological amines into chromaffin granules: A model for hormone and neurotransmitter transport. *Physiol Rev* 68:232, 1988.
23. Takiyyudin MA, Cerrenka JH, Pandian MR, Stuenkel CA, Neumann HPH, O'Connor DT: Neuroendocrine sources of chromogranin-A in normal man: Clues from selective stimulation of endocrine glands. *J Clin Endocrinol Metab* 71:360, 1990.
24. Cryer PE, Wortsman J, Shah SD, Deftos LJ: Plasma chromogranin A as a marker of sympathochromaffin activity in humans. *Am J Physiol* 260:E243, 1991.

25. Kryvi H: Comparison of the ultrastructure of adrenaline and noradrenaline storage granules of bovine adrenal medulla. *Eur J Cell Biol* 20:76, 1979.
26. Miller RJ: Multiple calcium channels and neuronal function. *Science* 235:46, 1987.
27. Almers W: Exocytosis. *Annu Rev Physiol* 52:607, 1990.
28. Young JB, Landsberg L: Sympathoadrenal activity in fasting pregnant rats: Dissociation of adrenal medullary and sympathetic nervous system responses. *J Clin Invest* 64:109, 1979.
29. Lee C-M, Javitch JA, Snyder SH: Recognition sites for norepinephrine uptake: Regulation by neurotransmitter. *Science* 220:626, 1983.
30. Eisenhofer G, Goldstein DS, Ropchak TG, Nguyen HQ, Keiser HR, Kopin JJ: Source and physiological significance of plasma 3,4-dihydroxyphenylglycol and 3-methoxy-4-hydroxyphenylglycol. *J Auton Nerv Syst* 24:1, 1988.
31. Maas JW, Benensohn H, Landis HD: A kinetic study of the disposition of circulating norepinephrine in normal male subjects. *J Pharmacol Exp Ther* 174:381, 1970.
32. Wang P-C, Buu NT, Kuchel O, Genest J: Conjugation patterns of endogenous plasma catecholamines in human and rat. *J Lab Clin Med* 101:141, 1983.
33. Starke K: Presynaptic α-autoreceptors. *Rev Physiol Biochem Pharmacol* 107:73, 1987.
34. Lefkowitz RJ, Caron MG: Adrenergic receptors. *J Biol Chem* 263:4993, 1988.
35. Insel PA: Adrenergic receptors—evolving concepts and clinical implications. *N Engl J Med* 334:580, 1996.
36. Yang-Feng TL, Xue F, Zhong W, Cotecchia S, Frielle T, Caron MG, Lefkowitz RJ, Francke U: Chromosomal organization of adrenergic receptor genes. *Proc Natl Acad Sci USA* 87:1516, 1990.
37. Mahan LC, McKernan RM, Insel PA: Metabolism of alpha- and beta-adrenergic receptors in vitro and in vivo. *Ann Rev Pharmacol Toxicol* 27:215, 1987.
38. Benovic JL, Bouvier M, Caron MG, Lefkowitz RJ: Regulation of adenyl cyclase-coupled β-adrenergic receptors. *Annu Rev Cell Biol* 4:405, 1988.
39. Minneman KP: α_1-Adrenergic receptor subtypes, inositol phosphates, and sources of cell Ca^{2+}. *Pharmacol Rev* 40:87, 1988.
40. Todd RD, Khurana TS, Sajovic P, Stone KR, O'Malley KL: Cloning of ligand-specific cell lines via gene transfer: Identification of a D_2 dopamine receptor subtype. *Proc Natl Acad Sci USA* 86:10134, 1989.
41. Emorine LJ, Marullo S, Briend-Sutren M-M, Patey G, Tate K, Delavier-Klutchko C, Strosberg AD: Molecular characterization of the human β_3-adrenergic receptor. *Science* 245:1118, 1989.
42. Ahlquist RP: A study of adrenotropic receptors. *Am J Physiol* 153:586, 1948.
43. Hall A: The cellular functions of small GTP-binding proteins. *Science* 249:635, 1990.
44. Cryer PE: Adrenergic receptors in endocrine and metabolic diseases, in Insel PA (ed): *Adrenergic Receptors in Man*. New York, Marcel Dekker, 1987, pp 285–301.
45. Ginsberg AM, Clutter WE, Shah SD, Cryer PE: Triiodothyronine induced thyrotoxicosis increases mononuclear leukocyte β-adrenergic receptor density in man. *J Clin Invest* 67:1785, 1981.
46. Liggett SB, Shah SD, Cryer PE: Increased fat and skeletal muscle β-adrenergic receptors but unaltered metabolic and hemodynamic sensitivity to epinephrine in vivo in experimental human thyrotoxicosis. *J Clin Invest* 83:803, 1989.
47. Creese I, Silbey DR, Hamblin MW, Leff SE: The classification of dopamine receptors. *Annu Rev Neurosci* 6:43, 1983.
48. Ariens EJ, Simonis AM: Receptors and receptor mechanisms, in Saxena PR, Forsyth RP (eds): *Beta-Adrenoceptor Blocking Agents*. Amsterdam, North-Holland, 1976, pp 3–27.
49. Ariens EJ: The classification of beta-adrenoceptors. *Trends Pharmacol Sci* 2:170, 1981.
50. Hawthorn MH, Broadley KJ: Evidence from use of neuronal uptake inhibition that β_1-adrenoceptors, but not β_2-adrenoceptors, are innervated. *J Pharm Pharmacol* 34:664, 1982.
51. Wilffert B, Timmermans PBMWM, van Zwieten PA: Extrasynaptic location of alpha-2 and noninnervated beta-2 adrenoceptors in the vascular system of the pithed normotensive rat. *J Pharmacol Exp Ther* 221:762, 1982.
52. Zukowska-Grojec Z, Bayorh MA, Kopin IJ: Effect of desipramine on the effects of α-adrenoceptor inhibitors on pressor responses and release of norepinephrine into plasma of pithed rats. *J Cardiovasc Pharmacol* 5:297, 1983.
53. Weiner N: Norepinephrine, epinephrine and the sympathochromimetic amines, in Gilman AG, Goodman LS, Gilman A (eds): *The Pharmacological Basis of Therapeutics*. New York, Macmillan, 1980, pp 138–175.
54. Clutter WE, Bier DM, Shah SD, Cryer PE: Epinephrine plasma metabolic clearance rates and physiologic thresholds for metabolic and hemodynamic actions in man. *J Clin Invest* 66:94, 1980.
55. Galster AD, Clutter WE, Cryer PE, Collins JA, Bier DM: Epinephrine plasma thresholds for lipolytic effects in man. *J Clin Invest* 67:1729, 1981.
56. Rizza RA, Haymond MW, Cryer PE, Gerich JE: Differential effects of physiological concentrations of epinephrine on glucose production and disposal in man. *Am J Physiol* 237:E356, 1979.
57. Rizza RA, Haymond MW, Miles JW, Verdonk CH, Cryer PE, Gerich JE: Effect of alpha-adrenergic stimulation and its blockade on glucose turnover in man. *Am J Physiol* 238:E467, 1980.
58. Rizza RA, Cryer PE, Haymond MW, Gerich JE: Adrenergic mechanisms for the effect of epinephrine on glucose production and clearance in man. *J Clin Invest* 65:682, 1980.
59. Deibert DC, DeFronzo RA: Epinephrine-induced insulin resistance in man. *J Clin Invest* 65:717, 1980.
60. Rosen SG, Clutter WE, Shah SD, Miller JP, Bier DM, Cryer PE: Direct, α-adrenergic stimulation of hepatic glucose production in postabsorptive human subjects. *Am J Physiol* 245:E616, 1983.
61. Berk MA, Clutter WE, Skor DS, Shah S, Cryer P: Enhanced glycemic responsiveness to epinephrine in insulin-dependent diabetes mellitus is the result of inability to secrete insulin. *J Clin Invest* 75:1842, 1985.
62. Chiasson J-L, Shikama H, Chu DTW, Exton JH: Inhibitory effect of epinephrine on insulin-stimulated glucose uptake by rat skeletal muscle. *J Clin Invest* 68:706, 1981.
63. Miles JM, Nissen S, Gerich JE, Haymond MW: Effects of epinephrine infusion on leucine and alanine kinetics in man. *Am J Physiol* 247:E166, 1984.
64. Fain JN, Garcia-Sainz JA: Adrenergic regulation of adipocyte metabolism. *J Lipid Res* 24:945, 1983.
65. Bahnsen M, Burrin JM, Johnston DG, Pernet A, Walker M, Alberti KGMM: Mechanisms of catecholamine effects on ketogenesis. *Am J Physiol* 247:E173, 1984.
66. Brown MJ, Brown DC, Murphy MB: Hypokalemia from beta$_2$-receptor stimulation by circulating epinephrine. *N Engl J Med* 309:1414, 1983.
67. Staten MA, Matthews DE, Cryer PE, Bier DM: Physiologic increments in epinephrine stimulate metabolic rate in humans. *Am J Physiol* 253:E322, 1987.
68. Staten MA, Matthews DE, Cryer PE, Bier DM: Epinephrine's effect on metabolic rate is independent of changes in insulin or glucagon. *Am J Physiol* 257:E185, 1989.
69. Clutter WE, Rizza RA, Gerich JE, Cryer PE: Regulation of glucose metabolism by sympathochromaffin catecholamines. *Diabetes Metab Rev* 4:1, 1988.
70. Gray DE, Lickley HLA, Vranic M: Physiologic effects of epinephrine on glucose turnover and plasma free fatty acid concentrations mediated independently by glucagon. *Diabetes* 29:600, 1980.
71. Morgan NG, Blackmore PF, Exton JH: Age-related changes in the control of hepatic cyclic AMP levels by α_1- and β_2-adrenergic receptors in male rats. *J Biol Chem* 258:5103, 1983.
72. Sacca L, Morrone G, Cicala M, Corso G, Ungaro B: Influence of epinephrine, norepinephrine and isoproterenol on glucose homeostasis in normal man. *J Clin Endocrinol Metab* 50:680, 1980.
73. Halter JB, Pflug AE, Tolas AG: Arterial-venous differences of plasma catecholamines in man. *Metabolism* 29:9, 1980.
74. Grimm M, Weidmann P, Keusch G, Meier A, Gluck Z: Norepinephrine clearance and pressor effect in normal and hypertensive man. *Klin Wochenschr* 58:1175, 1980.
75. Izzo J Jr: Cardiovascular hormonal effects of circulating norepinephrine. *Hypertension* 5:787, 1983.
76. Cryer PE: Catecholamines and metabolism. *Am J Physiol* 247:E1, 1984.
77. Hjemdahl P: Catecholamine measurements by high performance liquid chromatography. *Am J Physiol* 247:E13, 1984.

78. Wang M-T, Imai K, Yoshioka M, Tamura Z: Gas-liquid chromatographic and mass fragmentographic determination of catecholamines in human plasma. *Clin Chim Acta* 63:13, 1975.
79. Wang M-T, Yoshioka M, Imai K, Tamura Z: Gas-liquid chromatographic and mass fragmentographic determination of 3-O-methylated catecholamines in human plasma. *Clin Chim Acta* 63:21, 1975.
80. Elshisak MA, Polinsky RJ, Ebert MH, Kopin IJ: Kinetics of homovanillic acid and determination of its production rate in humans. *J Neurochem* 38:380, 1982.
81. Marker JC, Cryer PE, Clutter WE: Simplified measurement of norepinephrine kinetics: Application to studies of aging and exercise training. *Am J Physiol* 267:E380, 1994.
82. Esler M, Jennings G, Lambert G, Meredith I, Horne M, Eisenhofer G: Overflow of catecholamine neurotransmitters to the circulation: Source, fate and functions. *Physiol Rev* 70:963, 1990.
83. Linares OA, Jaquez JA, Zech LA, Smith MJ, Sanfield JA, Morrow LA, Rosen SG, Halter JB: Norepinephrine metabolism in humans: Kinetic analysis and model. *J Clin Invest* 80:1332, 1987.
84. Christensen NJ, Hilsted J, Hegedus L, Madsbad S: Effects of surgical stress and insulin on cardiovascular function and norepinephrine kinetics. *Am J Physiol* 247:E29, 1984.
85. Cryer PE: Diseases of the sympathochromaffin system, in Felig P, Baxter J, Broadus A, Frohman L (eds): *Endocrinology and Metabolism*, 2nd ed. New York, McGraw-Hill, 1987, pp 651–692.
86. Goldstein DS, Horwitz D, Keiser HR, Polinsky RJ, Koprin IJ: Plasma l-[^{3}H]norepinephrine, d-[^{14}C]norepinephrine and d,l-[^{3}H]isoproterenol kinetics in essential hypertension. *J Clin Invest* 72:1748, 1983.
87. Cryer PE, Rizza RA, Haymond MW, Gerich JE: Epinephrine and norepinephrine are cleared through β-adrenergic, but not α-adrenergic, mechanisms in man. *Metabolism* 29:1114, 1980.
88. Ghione S, Palombo C, Pellegrini M, Fommei E, Pilo A, Donato L: The kinetics of plasma noradrenaline in normal and hypertensive subjects. *Clin Sci* 55:89S, 1978.
89. Hoeldtke RD, Cilmi KM, Reichard GA Jr, Boden G, Owen OE: Assessment of norepinephrine secretion and production. *J Lab Clin Med* 101:772, 1983.
90. Kopin IJ, Polinsky RJ, Oliver JA, Oddershede IR, Ebert MH: Urinary catecholamine metabolites distinguish different types of sympathetic neural dysfunction in patients with orthostatic hypotension. *J Clin Endocrinol Metab* 57:632, 1983.
91. Folkow B, DiBona GF, Hjemdahl P, Toren PH, Wallin BG: Measurements of plasma norepinephrine concentrations in human primary hypertension. *Hypertension* 5:399, 1983.
92. Goldstein DS, McCarty R, Polinsky RJ, Kopin IJ: Relationship between plasma norepinephrine and sympathetic neural activity. *Hypertension* 5:552, 1983.
93. Brown MJ, Jenner DA, Allison DJ, Dollery CT: Variations in individual organ release of noradrenaline measured by an improved radioenzymatic technique: Limitations of peripheral venous measurements in the assessment of sympathetic nervous activity. *Clin Sci* 61:585, 1981.
94. Planz G: Adrenaline and noradrenaline concentration in blood of suprarenal and renal vein of man with normal blood pressure and with essential hypertension. *Klin Wochenschr* 56:1109, 1978.
95. Cryer PE, Haymond MW, Santiago JV, Shah SD: Norepinephrine and epinephrine release and adrenergic mediation of smoking-associated hemodynamic and metabolic events. *N Engl J Med* 295:573, 1976.
96. Mancia G, Ferrari A, Gregorini L, Leonetti G, Parati G, Picotti GB, Ravazzani C, Zanchetti A: Plasma catecholamines do not invariably reflect sympathetically induced changes in blood pressure in man. *Clin Sci* 65:227, 1983.
97. Young JB, Rose RM, Landsberg L: Dissociation of sympathetic nervous system and adrenal medullary responses. *Am J Physiol* 247:E35, 1984.
98. Cryer PE: Isotope derivative measurements of plasma norepinephrine and epinephrine in man. *Diabetes* 25:1071, 1976.
99. Wallin GB: Peripheral sympathetic neural activity in conscious humans. *Annu Rev Physiol* 50:565, 1988.
100. Rea RF, Eckberg DL, Fritsch JM, Goldstein DS: Relation of plasma norepinephrine and sympathetic traffic during hypotension in humans. *Am J Physiol* 258:R982, 1990.
101. Cryer PE: Pheochromocytoma. *West J Med* 15:399, 1992.
102. Manger WM, Gifford RW: *Clinical and Experimental Pheochromocytoma*. Cambridge, Blackwell Science, 1996.
103. Sutton MGS, Sheps SG, Lie JT: Prevalence of clinically unsuspected pheochromocytoma: Review of a 50-year autopsy series. *Mayo Clin Proc* 56:354, 1981.
104. Steiner AL, Goodman AD, Powers SR: Study of a kindred with pheochromocytoma, medullary thyroid carcinoma, hyperparathyroidism and Cushing's disease: Multiple endocrine neoplasia, type 2. *Medicine (Baltimore)* 47:371, 1968.
105. Lips KJM, Veer JVDS, Struyvenberg A, Alleman A, Leo JR, Wittebol P, Minder WH, Kooiker CJ, et al: Bilateral occurrence of pheochromocytoma in patients with the multiple endocrine neoplasia syndrome type 2a (Sipple's syndrome). *Am J Med* 70:1051, 1981.
106. DeLellis RA, Wolfe HJ, Gagel RF, Feldman ZT, Miller HH, Gang DL, Reichlin S: Adrenal medullary hyperplasia. *Am J Physiol* 83:177, 1976.
107. Thakker RV: Multiple endocrine neoplasia—Syndromes of the twentieth century. *J Clin Encrinol Metab* 83:2617, 1998.
108. Yoshimasa T, Nakao K, Li S, Ikeda Y, Suda M, Sakamoto M, Imura H: Plasma methionine-enkephalin and leucine-enkephalin in normal subjects and patients with pheochromocytoma. *J Clin Endocrinol Metab* 57:706, 1983.
109. Berelowitz M, Szabo M, Barowsky HW, Arbel ER, Frohman LA: Somatostatin-like immunoactivity and biological activity is present in a human pheochromocytoma. *J Clin Endocrinol Metab* 56:134, 1983.
110. Weinstein RS, Ide LF: Immunoreactive calcitonin in pheochromocytomas. *Proc Soc Exp Biol Med* 165:215, 1980.
111. Spark RF, Connolly PB, Gluckin DS, White R, Sacks B, Landsberg L: ACTH secretion from a functioning pheochromocytoma. *N Engl J Med* 301:416, 1979.
112. Page LB, Raker JW, Beberich FR: Pheochromocytoma with predominant epinephrine secretion. *Am J Med* 47:648, 1969.
113. Aronoff SL, Passamani E, Borowsky BA, Weiss AN, Roberts R, Cryer PE: Norepinephrine and epinephrine secretion from a clinically epinephrine-secreting pheochromocytoma. *Am J Med* 69:321, 1980.
114. Bravo EL, Tarazi RC, Fouad FM, Textor SC, Gifford RW Jr, Vidt DG: Blood pressure regulation in pheochromocytoma. *Hypertension* 4(Suppl 2):193, 1982.
115. Cryer PE: Catecholamines, pheochromocytoma and diabetes. *Diabetes Reviews* 1:309, 1993.
116. Sjoerdsma A, Engelman K, Waldmann TA, Cooperman LH, Hammond WG: Pheochromocytoma: Current concepts of diagnosis and treatment. *Ann Intern Med* 65:1302, 1966.
117. Sheps SG, Jiang NS, Klee GG, van Heerden JA: Recent developments in the diagnosis and treatment of pheochromocytoma. *Mayo Clinic Proc* 65:88, 1990.
118. Duncan MW, Compton P, Lazarus L, Smythe GA: Measurement of norepinephrine and 3,4-dihydroxyphenylglycol in urine and plasma for the diagnosis of pheochromocytoma. *N Engl J Med* 319:136, 1988.
119. Engelman K, Portnoy B, Sjoerdsma A: Plasma catecholamine concentrations in patients with hypertension. *Circ Res* 26(Suppl 1):141, 1970.
120. Geffen LB, Rush RA, Louis WJ, Doyle AE: Plasma catecholamine and dopamine β-hydroxylase amounts in phaeochromocytoma. *Clin Sci* 44:421, 1973.
121. Bravo EL, Tarazi RC, Gifford RW Jr, Stewart BH: Circulating and urinary catecholamines in pheochromocytoma. *N Engl J Med* 301:682, 1979.
122. Zweifler AJ, Julius S: Increased platelet catecholamine content in pheochromocytoma. *N Engl J Med* 306:890, 1982.
123. Eisenhofer G, Keiser H, Friberg P, Mezey E, Thanh-Truc H, Hiremagalur B, Ellingson T, Duddempudi S, Eijsbouts A, Lenders JWM: Plasma metanephrines are markers of pheochromocytoma produced by catechol-O-methyltransferase within tumors. *J Clin Endocrinol Metab* 83:2175, 1998.
124. Bravo EL, Tarazi RC, Fouad FM, Vidt DG, Gifford GW Jr: Clonidine suppression test: A useful aid in the diagnosis of pheochromocytoma. *N Engl J Med* 305:623, 1981.
125. Taylor HC, Mayes D, Anton AH: Clonidine suppression test for pheochromocytoma: Examples of misleading results. *J Clin Endocrinol Metab* 63:238, 1986.

126. Hsiao RJ, Parmer RJ, Takiyyudin MA, O'Connor DT: Chromogranin A storage and secretion: Sensitivity and specificity for the diagnosis of pheochromocytoma. *Medicine (Baltimore)* 70:33, 1991.
127. Quint LE, Glazer GM, Francis IR, Shapiro B, Chenevert TL: Pheochromocytoma and paraganglioma: Comparison of MR imaging with CT and I-131 MIBG scintigraphy. *Radiology* 165:89, 1987.
128. Shapiro B, Copp JE, Sisson JC, Eyre PL, Wallis J, Bierwaltes WH: Iodine-131 metaiodobenzylguanidine for the locating of suspected pheochromocytomas: Experience in 400 cases. *J Nucl Med* 26:576, 1985.
129. Kopf D, Bockisch A, Steinert H, Hahn K, Beyer J, Neuman PH, Hensen J, Lehnert H: Octeocide scintigraphy and catecholamine response to an octreotide challenge in malignant pheochromocytoma. *Clin Endocrinol* 46:39, 1997.
130. Arnold DR, Villamagne VL, Civelek AC, Dannals RF, Wagner HN, Udelsman R: FDG-PET: A sensitive tool for the localization of MIBG-negative pelvic pheochromocytomas. *The Endocrinologist* 8:295, 1998.
131. Mellicow MM: One hundred cases of pheochromocytoma (107 tumors) at the Columbia-Presbyterian Medical Center. *Cancer* 40:1907, 1977.
132. Cubbeddu LX, Zarate NA, Rosales CB, Zshaeck DW: Prazosin and propranolol in preoperative management of pheochromocytoma. *Clin Pharmacol Ther* 32:156, 1982.
133. Glass AR, Ballou R: Pheochromocytoma, prazosin and hypotension. *Ann Intern Med* 97:455, 1982.
134. Nicholson JP Jr, Vaugh ED Jr, Pickering TG, Resnick LM, Artusio J, Kleinert HD, Lopez-Overjero JA, Laragh JH: Pheochromocytoma and prazosin. *Ann Intern Med* 99:477, 1983.
135. Plouin P-F, Menard J, Corvol P: Noradrenaline producing pheochromocytomas with absent pressor response to beta-blockade. *Br Heart J* 42:359, 1979.
136. Wark JD, Larkins RG: Pulmonary edema after propranolol therapy in two cases of phaeochromocytoma. *Br Med J* 1:1395, 1978.
137. Ram CVS, Meese R, Hill SC: Failure of α-methyltyrosine to prevent hypertensive crisis in pheochromocytoma. *Arch Intern Med* 145:2114, 1985.
138. Feldman JM, Blalock JA, Fagraeus L, Miller JN, Farrell RE, Wells SA Jr: Alterations in plasma norepinephrine concentration during surgical resection of pheochromocytoma. *Ann Surg* 188:758, 1978.
139. Leak D, Carroll JJ, Robinson DC, Ashworth EJ: Management of pheochromocytoma during pregnancy. *Can Med Assoc J* 116:371, 1977.
140. Sheps SG, Jiang N-S, Klee GG, van Heerden JA: Recent developments in the diagnosis and treatment of pheochromocytoma. *Mayo Clin Proc* 65:88, 1990.
141. Hengstmann JH, Dengler HJ: Evidence for extratumoral storage of catecholamines in pheochromocytoma patients. *Acta Endocrinol (Copenh)* 87:589, 1978.
142. Hammerman M, Levitt R, Clutter WE, Meltzer V, Bobzein B: Persistent hypertension after resection of a pheochromocytoma. *Am J Med* 73:97, 1982.
143. Castle CH: Iatrogenic renal hypertension: Two unusual complications of surgery for familial pheochromocytoma. *JAMA* 225:1085, 1973.
144. Jones NF, Walker G, Ruthven CRJ, Sandler M: α-Methyl-p-tyrosine in the management of phaeochromocytoma. *Lancet* ii:1105, 1968.
145. Feldman JM: Treatment of metastic pheochromocytoma with streptozotocin. *Arch Intern Med* 143:1799, 1983.
146. Averbuch SD, Steakley CS, Young RC, Gelman EP, Goldstein DS, Stull R, Keiser HR: Malignant pheochromocytoma: Effective treatment with a combination of cyclophosphamide, vincristine and decarbazine. *Ann Intern Med* 109:267, 1988.
147. Krempf M, Lumbroso J, Mornex R, Brendel AJ, Wemeau JL, Delisle MJ, Aubert B, Carpentier P, et al: Use of m-[^{131}I]iodobenzylguanidine in the treatment of malignant pheochromocytoma. *J Clin Endocrinol Metab* 72:455, 1991.
148. Seeger RC, Siegel SE, Sidell N: Neuroblastoma: Clinical perspectives, monoclonal antibodies and retinoic acid. *Ann Intern Med* 97:873, 1982.
149. Boomsma F, Ausema L, Hakvoort-Cammel FGA, Oosterom R, Man in't Veld AJ, Krenning EP, Hahlen K, Schalekamp MADH: Combined measurements of plasma aromatic L-amino acid decarboxylase and DOPA as tumor markers in diagnosis and follow-up of neuroblastoma. *Eur J Cancer Clin Oncol* 25:1045, 1989.
150. Low PA (ed): *Clinical Autonomic Disorders*. Philadelphia, Lippincott-Raven, 1997.
151. Cryer PE, Santiago JV, Shah SD: Measurement of norepinephrine and epinephrine in small volumes of human plasma by a single isotope derivative method: Response to the upright posture. *J Clin Endocrinol Metab* 39:1025, 1974.
152. Lipsitz LA: Orthostatic hypotension in the elderly. *N Engl J Med* 321:952, 1989.
153. Cryer PE, Silverberg AB, Santiago JV, Shah SD: Plasma catecholamines in diabetes: The syndromes of hypoadrenergic and hyperadrenergic postural hypotension. *Am J Med* 64:407, 1978.
154. Tohmeh JF, Shah SD, Cryer PE: The pathogenesis of hyperadrenergic postural hypotension in patients with diabetes. *Am J Med* 67:772, 1979.
155. Cryer PE, Weiss S: Reduced plasma norepinephrine response to standing in autonomic dysfunction. *Arch Neurol* 33:275, 1976.
156. Ziegler MG, Lake CR, Kopin IJ: The sympathetic nervous system defect in primary orthostatic hypotension. *N Engl J Med* 296:293, 1977.
157. Leveston SA, Shah SD, Cryer PE: Cholinergic stimulation of norepinephrine release in man: Evidence of a sympathetic postganglionic axonal lesion in diabetic adrenergic neuropathy. *J Clin Invest* 64:374, 1979.
158. Fouad FM, Tadena-Thoma L, Bravo EL, Tarazi RC: Idiopathic hypovolemia. *Ann Intern Med* 104:298, 1986.
159. Streeten DHP: Pathogenesis of hyperadrenergic orthostatic hypotension. *J Clin Invest* 86:1582, 1990.
160. Bannister R: Introduction and classification, in Bannister R (ed): *Autonomic Failure*. New York, Oxford University Press, 1983, p 1.
161. Cohen J, Low P, Fealey R, Sheps S, Jiang N-S: Somatic and autonomic function in progressive autonomic failure and multiple system atrophy. *Ann Neurol* 22:692, 1987.
162. Sever PS: Plasma noradrenaline in autonomic failure, in Bannister R (ed): *Autonomic Failure*. New York, Oxford University Press, 1983, p 155.
163. Goldstein DS, Polinsky RJ, Garty M, Robertson D, Brown RT, Biaggioni I, Stull R, Kopin IJ: Patterns of plasma levels of catechols in neurogenic orthostatic hypotension. *Ann Neurol* 26:558, 1989.
164. Gemmill JD, Venables GS, Ewing DJ: Noradrenaline response to edrophonium in primary autonomic failure: Distinction between central and peripheral damage. *Lancet* i:1018, 1988.
165. Kopin IJ, Polinsky RJ, Oliver JA, Oddershede IR, Ebert MH: Urinary catecholamine metabolites distinguish different types of sympathetic neuronal dysfunction in patients with orthostatic hypotension. *J Clin Endocrinol Metab* 57:632, 1983.
166. Bannister R: Clinical features of progressive autonomic failure, in Bannister R (ed): *Autonomic Failure*. New York, Oxford University Press, 1983, p 67.
167. Davies B: Adrenergic receptors in autonomic failure, in Bannister R (ed): *Autonomic Failure*. New York, Oxford University Press, 1983, p 174.
168. Robertson D, Goldberg MR, Onrot J, Hollister AS, Wiley R, Thompson JG Jr, Robertson RM: Isolated failure of autonomic noradrenergic neurotransmission. *N Engl J Med* 314:1494, 1986.
169. Biaggioni I, Robertson D: Endogenous restoration of noradrenaline by precursor therapy in dopamine-beta-hydroxylase deficiency. *Lancet* 2:1170, 1987.
170. Man in't Veld AJ, Boomsma F, van den Meiracker AH, Schalekamp MADH: Effect of an unnatural noradrenaline precursor on sympathetic control and orthostatic hypotension in dopamine-beta-hydroxylase deficiency. *Lancet* ii:1172, 1987.
171. Nanda RN, Boyle FC, Gillespie JS, Johnson RH, Keogh HJ: Idiopathic orthostatic hypotension from failure of noradrenaline release in a patient with vasomotor innervation. *J Neurol Neurosurg Psychiatry* 40:11, 1977.
172. Hart RG, Kanter MC: Acute autonomic neuropathy. *Arch Intern Med* 150:2373, 1990.
173. Bannister R: Treatment of progressive autonomic failure, in Bannister R (ed): *Autonomic Failure*. New York, Oxford University Press, 1983, p 316.
174. Chobanian AV, Volicer L, Tifft CCP, Gavras H, Liang C-S, Faxon D: Mineralocorticoid-induced hypertension in patients with orthostatic hypotension. *N Engl J Med* 301:68, 1979.

175. Low PA, Gilden JL, Freeman R, Sheng K-N, McElliot MA, Midodrine Study Group. Efficacy of midodrine vs placebo in neurogenic orthostatic hypotension. *JAMA* 277:1046, 1997.
176. Chobanian AV, Tifft CP, Faxon DP, Creager MA, Sackel H: Treatment of chronic orthostatic hypotension with ergotamine. *Circulation* 67:602, 1983.
177. Jordan J, Shannon JR, Biaggioni I, Norman R, Black BK, Robertson D. Contrasting actions of pressor agents in severe autonomic failure. *Am J Med* 105:116, 1998.
178. Hoeldtke RD, Dworkin GE, Gaspar SR, Israel BC, Boden G: Effect of the somatostatin analogue SMS-201-995 on the adrenergic response to glucose ingestion in patients with postprandial hypotension. *Am J Med* 86:673, 1989.
179. Kristinsson A: Programmed atrial pacing for orthostatic hypotension. *Acta Med Scand* 214:79, 1983.
180. Polinsky RJ, Samaras GM, Kopin IJ: Sympathetic neural prothesis for managing orthostatic hypotension. *Lancet* i:901, 1983.
181. Khurama RK, Nelson E, Azzarelli B, Garcia JH: Shy-Drager syndrome: Diagnosis and treatment of cholinergic dysfunction. *Neurology* 30:805, 1980.
182. Dagogo-Jack S, Craft S, Cryer PE: Hypoglycemia-associated autonomic failure in insulin dependent diabetes mellitus. *J Clin Invest* 91:819, 1993.
183. Dagogo-Jack S, Rattarasarn C, Cryer PE: Reversal of hypoglycemia unawareness, but not defective glucose counterregulation, in IDDM. *Diabetes* 43:1426, 1994.
184. Cryer PE: *Hypoglycemia: Pathophysiology, Diagnosis and Treatment*. Oxford University Press, New York, 1997.
185. Hilsted J, Low PA: Diabetic autonomic neuropathy, in Low PA (ed): *Clinical Autonomic Disorders*. Philadelphia, Lippincott-Raven, 1997.
186. Heller SR, Cryer PE: Hypoinsulinemia is not critical to glucose recovery from hypoglycemia in humans. *Am J Physiol* 261:E41, 1991.
187. DeFeo P, Periello G, Torlone E, Ventura MM, Santeusanio F, Brunetti P, Gerich JE, Bolli GB: Demonstration of a role for growth hormone in glucose counterregulation. *Am J Physiol* 256:E835, 1989.
188. DeFeo P, Periello G, Torlone E, Venture MM, Fanelli C, Santeusanio F, Brunetti P, Gerich JE, Bolli GB: Contribution of cortisol to glucose counterregulation in humans. *Am J Physiol* 257:E35, 1989.
189. Boyle PJ, Cryer PE: Growth hormone, cortisol, or both are involved in defense against, but are not critical to recovery from, prolonged hypoglycemia in humans. *Am J Physiol* 260:E395–E402, 1991.
190. Bolli G, DeFeo P, Perriello G, DeCosmo S, Ventura M, Campbell P, Brunetti P, Gerich J: Role of hepatic autoregulation in defense against hypoglycemia in humans. *J Clin Invest* 75:1623, 1985.
191. Hansen I, Firth R, Haymond M, Cryer P, Rizza R: The role of autoregulation of hepatic glucose production in man. *Diabetes* 35:186, 1986.
192. Gerich J, Langlois M, Noacco C, Karam J, Forsham P: Lack of glucagon response to hypoglycemia in diabetes: Evidence for an intrinsic pancreatic alpha-cell defect. *Science* 182:171, 1973.
193. Popp DA, Shah SD, Cryer PE: The role of epinephrine-mediated β-adrenergic mechanisms in hypoglycemic glucose counterregulation and posthypoglycemic hyperglycemia in insulin dependent diabetes mellitus. *J Clin Invest* 69:315, 1982.
194. White NH, Gingerich R, Levandoski L, Cryer P, Santiago J: Plasma pancreatic polypeptide response to insulin induced hypoglycemia as a marker for defective glucose counterregulation in insulin-dependent diabetes mellitus. *Diabetes* 34:870, 1985.
195. White NH, Skor DA, Cryer PE, Bier DM, Levandoski L, Santiago JV: Identification of type 1 diabetic patients at increased risk for hypoglycemia during intensive therapy. *N Engl J Med* 308:485, 1983.
196. Bolli GB, DeFeo P, DeCosmo S, Periello G, Ventura MM, Massi-Bendetti M, Santeusanio F, Gerich J, Brunetti P: A reliable and reproducible test for adequate glucose counterregulation in type 1 diabetes mellitus. *Diabetes* 33:732, 1984.
197. Cryer PE, Binder C, Bolli GB, Cherrington AD, Gale EAM, Gerich JE, Sherwin RS: Hypoglycemia in insulin dependent diabetes mellitus. *Diabetes* 33:1193, 1989.
198. Heller SR, Herbert M, Macdonald IA, Tattersall RB: Influence of sympathetic nervous system on hypoglycaemic warning symptoms. *Lancet* ii:359, 1987.
199. Hepburn DA, Patrick AW, Eadington DW, Ewing DJ, Frier BM: Unawareness of hypoglycemia in insulin treated diabetes patients: Prevalence and relation to autonomic neuropathy. *Diabetic Med* 7:711, 1990.
200. Amiel SA, Sherwin RS, Simonson DC, Tamborlane WV: Effect of intensive insulin therapy on glycemic thresholds for counterregulatory hormone release. *Diabetes* 37:901, 1988.
201. Diabetes Control and Complications Trial: Results of feasibility study. *Diabetes Care* 10:1, 1987.
202. Ryder REJ, Owens DR, Hayes TM, Ghatei MA, Bloom SR: Unawareness of hypoglycaemia and inadequate hypoglcaemic counterregulation: No causal relation with diabetic autonomic neuropathy. *Br Med J* 301:783, 1990.
203. Clarke WL, Gonder-Frederick LA, Richards FE, Cryer PE: Multifactorial origin of hypoglycemic symptom unawareness in insulin dependent diabetes mellitus. *Diabetes* 40:680, 1991.
204. Heller SR, Cryer PE: Reduced neuroendocrine and symptomatic responses to subsequent hypoglycemia after one episode of hypoglycemia in normal humans. *Diabetes* 40:223, 1991.
205. Hirsch IB, Boyle PJ, Craft S, Cryer PE: β-adrenergic blockade shifts glycemic thresholds for symptoms to lower plasma glucose concentrations in insulin dependent diabetes mellitus. *Diabetes* 40:1177, 1991.
206. Parker NC, Levtzow CB, Wright PW, Woodard LL, Chapman JF: Uniform chromatographic conditions for quantifying urinary catecholamines, metanephrines, vanillylmandelic acid, 5-hydroxyindoleacetic acid by liquid chromatography with electrochemical detection. *Clin Chem* 32:1473, 1986.
207. Moleman P, van Dijk J: Determination of urinary norepinephrine and epinephrine by liquid chromotography with fluorescence detection and pre-column devirilization. *Clin Chem* 36:732, 1990.
208. Johnson GA, Kupiecki RM, Baker CH: Single isotope derivative (radioenzymatic) methods in the measurement of catecholamines. *Metabolism* 29(Suppl 1):1106, 1980.
209. Shah SD, Clutter WE, Cryer PE: External and internal standards in the single isotope derivative (radioenzymatic) measurement of plasma norepinephrine and epinephrine in normal humans and persons with diabetes mellitus or chronic renal failure. *J Lab Clin Med* 106:624, 1985.
210. Hjemdahl P: Catecholamine measurements in plasma by high performance liquid chromatography with electrochemical detection. *Methods Enzymol* 142:521, 1987.
211. Bouloux P, Perrett D, Besser GM: Methodological considerations in the determination of plasma catecholamines by high performance liquid chromatography with electrochemical detection. *Ann Clin Biochem* 22:194, 1985.
212. Eisenhofer G, Goldstein DS, Stull R, Keiser HR, Sunderland T, Murphy DL, Kopin IJ: Simultaneous liquid-chromatographic determination of 3,4-dihydroxyphenylglycol, catecholamines and 3,4-dihydroxyphenylalanine in plasma, and their responses to inhibition of monoamine oxidase. *Clin Chem* 32:2030, 1986.
213. Weir TB, Smith CCT, Round JM, Betteridge DJ: Stability of catecholamines in whole blood, plasma and platelets. *Clin Chem* 32:882, 1986.
214. Christensen NJ: Sympathetic nervous activity and age. *Eur J Clin Invest* 12:91, 1982.
215. Romoff MS, Keusch G, Campese VM, Wang M-S, Friedler RM, Weidman P, Massry SG: Effect of sodium intake on plasma catecholamines in normal subjects. *J Clin Endocrinol Metab* 48:26, 1978.
216. Cryer PE, Sode J: Drug interference with measurement of adrenal hormones in urine: Common analgesics and tranquilizer-sedatives. *Ann Intern Med* 75:697, 1971.
217. Hilsted J, Jensen SB: A simple test for autonomic neuropathy in juvenile diabetics. *Acta Med Scand* 205:385, 1979.
218. Ewing DJ: Practical bedside investigation of diabetic autonomic failure, in Bannister R (ed): *Autonomic Failure*. New York, Oxford University Press, 1983, p 371.
219. Johnson RH: Clinical assessment of sympathetic function in man. *Methods Find Exp Clin Pharmacol* 6:187, 1984.

CHAPTER 13

Endocrinology of Hypertension

Willa A. Hsueh
Susanne B. Nicholas
Marwan Hamaty
John Baxter
James Sowers

Hypertension is a major risk factor for cardiovascular disease (CVD). Indeed, CVD morbidity and mortality—including coronary heart disease (CHD), stroke, renal disease, left ventricular hypertrophy, and congestive heart failure—increase progressively, at higher levels of blood pressure. These relationships are strong, continuous, graded, consistent, independent, predictable and etiologically significant.[1] Table 13-1 provides current levels for defining hypertension by the level of blood pressure (Joint National Committee on Detection, Evaluation, and Treatment of High Blood Pressure [JNC VI]).[1] Hypertension is common in older Americans, the fastest growing segment of our population.[2-4] In the National Health and Nutrition Examination Survey (NHANES III), it was estimated that hypertension is present in 60 percent of elderly non-Hispanic whites, 71 percent of non-Hispanic African-Americans, and 61 percent of elderly Mexican-Americans.[1,5] Fifty percent of the United States population ≥65 years have elevated systolic blood pressure with or without elevated diastolic blood pressure. Particularly in older persons, systolic blood pressure is a better predictor of CVD morbidity and mortality than is diastolic blood pressure, as emphasized in the JNC-VI report.[1,2] The pulse pressure also correlates with target organ damage, as diastolic pressure decreases with progressive loss of arterial elasticity (hardening of the arteries).[6]

Hypertension is defined as an inappropriate elevation in resting arterial systolic blood pressure (BP) of 140 mm Hg or greater, diastolic BP of 90 mm Hg or greater. Classification of blood pressure (Table 13-1) is based on two or more blood pressure readings taken at each of two or more visits. When systolic and diastolic BP fall into different categories, the highest category is considered the patient's category of BP. These values are determined for patients with no acute illnesses and who are not taking any antihypertensive medication. The blood pressure measurement should be taken preferably by a mercury sphygnomanometer, using the appropriate cuff size, at least 30 minutes after the last coffee drink or cigarette smoking and 5 minutes after resting in a sitting position in a chair with back support and arms bared and supported at heart level. Essential hypertension is further defined according to blood pressure responses to sodium supplementation as salt-sensitive and salt-resistant hypertension. Salt-sensitive hypertensives demonstrate an increase in systolic or diastolic blood pressure by 5 mm Hg or more upon changing from low (50–80 mmol/day) to high (200–250 mmol/day) sodium diet.[7] The normal increase in parasympathetic tone in response to sodium supplementation is impaired in salt-sensitive subjects with essential hypertension, and the normal decline of blood pressure is also attenuated by high-sodium diet in these subjects.[8,9] Salt sensitivity is not affected by either race, age, sex, or weight changes.[9] Another classification refers to "modulators" or "nonmodulators" depending on their target organ response to alterations of the renin angiotensin system.[10] These classifications have implications with regard to pathophysiology and treatment. An additional classification of essential hypertension depends on plasma renin activity (PRA) compared to sodium excretion; subjects with high or normal PRA levels have increased risk of CVD compared to those with low PRA.[11] These classifications of blood pressure have been designed to identify pathophysiologic mechanisms and to design specific treatment strategies; however, these are not applied clinically.

Normally blood pressure follows a diurnal pattern with lower blood pressure during the nighttime and a rise in blood pressure in the early morning hours upon waking. These changes in blood pressure are in association with changes in autonomic nervous system activity in which the sympathetic component dominates during daytime and diminishes during the nighttime, when parasympathetic activity increases. Upon waking, parasympathetic activity is decreased and sympathetic activity dominates again.[12] Subjects, normotensive as well as hypertensive, who have failure of blood pressure lowering during nighttime (non-dippers) suffer from a higher 24-hour blood pressure load compared with those who have normal diurnal variation of blood pressure. Elevated 24-hour blood pressure load contributes to the development of left ventricular hypertrophy, which is an independent cardiovascular risk factor.[13,14] Thus, it is also helpful to use 24-hour BP monitoring in the diagnosis and evaluation of treatment of hypertension and possibly in screening subjects who have normal BP during office visits but have strong family history of hypertension, sudden death, and cardiovascular disease. Blood pressure levels sufficient for the perfusion of vital organs are controlled by interactions of multiple, complex, delicately balanced, and counterbalanced systems that facilitate adjustments to physiologic and pathologic changes in activity, posture, and volume status. Hormones, acting as endocrine,

TABLE 13-1. Classification of Blood Pressure for Adults Aged 18 Years and Older*

	Blood Pressure, mm Hg		
Category	**Systolic**		**Diastolic**
Optimal†	<120	and	<80
Normal	<130	and	<85
High-normal	130–139	or	85–89
Hypertension‡			
Stage 1	140–159	or	90–99
Stage 2	160–179	or	100–109
Stage 3	≥180	or	N≥110

*Data from the Joint National Committee on Detection, Evaluation, and Treatment of High Blood Pressure (JNC V).[1] Classification is for adults age 18 years and older. When the pressures are in more than one category, the higher category should be used.

†Optimal blood pressure with respect to cardiovascular risk is less than 120/80 mm Hg. However, unusually low readings should be evaluated for clinical significance.

‡Based on the average of 2 or more readings taken at each of 2 or more visits after an initial screening.

autocrine, and/or paracrine factors (see Chap. 1) play key roles in this control. These hormones are produced in multiple tissues including the kidneys, liver, adrenals, heart, vasculature, peripheral nerves, and brain. They display diverse mechanisms of actions and interactions. These actions are further modified by the major anions and cations, the nervous system, intravascular volume, genetics, metabolism, and other factors.

Hypertension typically is classified as "primary" (essential) or "secondary" in nature. Most hypertensive patients have essential hypertension in which the cause appears to be multifactorial involving genetics and environment. The multifactorial nature is reflected by the fact that any one type of drug is fully effective only in 30 to 50 percent of patients at best[15,16] and characterized by highly variable individual patient responses. Various factors influence renal mechanisms, the release of pressor and depressor substances, and transmembrane transport of ions such as Na^+ and Ca^{2+}. Much of the information about the mechanisms involved in essential hypertension is derived from observations of patients with both essential and secondary hypertension, experimentally produced hypertension in animals, and strains of animals that develop hypertension spontaneously. These studies have led to the realization that abnormalities in levels of, and responses to, hormones play a dominant role in essential hypertension. This chapter focuses on specific hormonal abnormalities that contribute directly to secondary forms of hypertension as well as genetic alterations that may relate or contribute to the hormonal abnormalities. Common forms of secondary hypertension are listed in Table 13-2.

It is important to identify persons with secondary forms of hypertension. Identification of a specific cause (i.e., hormonal) allows for directed correctional therapy, lessening or eliminating the need for antihypertensive drug therapy. Secondary forms of hypertension, particularly those associated with diabetes mellitus, adrenal disorders, and conditions involving the activation of the renin-angiotensin-aldosterone axis (RAS) are often referred to the endocrinologist for work-up and medical therapy. It is the pathogenesis and therapy of these hypertensive disorders that are reviewed in this chapter.

TABLE 13-2. Types of Hypertension

- Essential, primary
- Systolic hypertension
  - Diabetes mellitus
  - Aortic valvular insufficiency
  - Arteriovenous fistula, patent ductus arteriosus
  - Hyperthyroidism
  - Paget disease of bone
  - Beriberi heart disease
  - Hyperkinetic circulation
  - Complete heart block
  - Rigidity of aorta and great vessels due to atherosclerosis
- Renal
  - Parenchymal disease: glomerulonephritis, pyelonephritis, interstitial nephritis, radiation nephritis; polycystic disease; connective tissue diseases; trauma
  - Obstructive uropathies; hydronephrosis
  - Renovascular; renal arterial stenosis; extrarenal-induced renal ischemia (e.g., vasculitis, coarctation of the aorta); vasculitis
  - Primary sodium retention (Liddle's and Gordon's syndromes)
- Endocrine
  - Acromegaly
  - Adrenal cortical hormones
    - Apparent mineralocorticoid excess
    - Congenital adrenal hyperplasia
    - Cushing's syndrome
    - Deoxycorticosterone-producing tumors
    - Glucocorticoid resistance
    - Primary aldosteronism
  - Catecholamine-producing tumors
    - Glioma
    - Neurofibroma
    - Pheochromocytoma
    - Hypertension associated with diabetes
  - Hyperparathyroidism
  - Hyperthyroidism
  - Hypothyroidism
  - Renin-producing tumors
- Exogenous
  - Alcohol abuse
  - Cyclosporine
  - Erythropoietin therapy
  - Estrogen/oral contraceptives
  - Excessive salt intake
  - Glucocorticoids
  - Mineralocorticoids: licorice, carbenoxolone
  - Sympathomimetics
  - Tyramine-containing foods and monoamine oxidase inhibitors
  - Thyroid hormone
- Coarctation of the aorta
- Hypertensive disease of pregnancy
- Neurogenic
  - Acute lead poisoning
  - Acute porphyria
  - Familial dysautonomia
  - Increased intracranial pressure
    - Respiratory acidosis (CO_2 retention): lung or CNS disease (poliomyelitis)
    - Encephalitis
    - Brain tumor
  - Psychogenic
  - Spinal cord damage
- Miscellaneous
  - Polycythemia
  - Burns (extensive)

Epidemiology of Hypertension

Forty to fifty million Americans have elevated blood pressure.[1] The prevalence of hypertension may vary largely depending on the criteria used to define hypertension. He et al. have studied the incidence of hypertension during a seven-year period in 140 African-American and 237 white middle-age adults (30–54 years old). The incidence of hypertension, defined as BP $\geq 160/95$ mm Hg, was similar (25 percent) in whites and African-Americans. In this study, baseline age, blood pressure, heart rate, and gender but not race influenced the incidence of hypertension.[17] These data contrast with previous surveys that reported higher prevalence of hypertension among African-Americans. The NHANES III reported a 24 percent prevalence of hypertension among US adult population.[5] Age adjusted prevalence in non-Hispanic black, non-Hispanic white, and Mexican-American populations was 32 percent, 23 percent, and 22 percent respectively.[5] However, the incidence and prevalence of hypertension varies in different areas of the world and between urban and rural areas of the same country, implicating an important role of the environment. For example, the prevalence of hypertension in Cameroon is markedly lower in rural than urban areas using the same criteria mentioned previously for defining blood pressure.[18]

Hypertension is a major risk factor for premature death and morbidity from cardiovascular disease, stroke, and renal failure.[1-3,19] Cardiovascular morbidity and mortality increase with higher levels of the systolic blood pressure, even at levels not considered hypertensive (Fig. 13-1).[1-3,19,20] Although there is no precise dividing line between normotensive and hypertensive, it is estimated that optimal blood pressure with respect to cardiovascular risk is <120 mm Hg systolic and <80 mm Hg diastolic.[1] Mild hypertension (stage 1) is the most common form of hypertension and therefore is responsible for most of the excess morbidity, disability, and mortality attributed to hypertension.[1] Other risk factors including cigarette smoking, hyperlipidemia, glucose intolerance, and male sex amplify the risk of CV disease.

FIGURE 13-1. Annual incidence of cardiovascular disease among the Framingham group over an 18-year follow-up based on systolic blood pressure at the onset of the study. The upper and lower curves are for men and women, respectively. (*From Kannel*[19] *and Kaplan*[21])

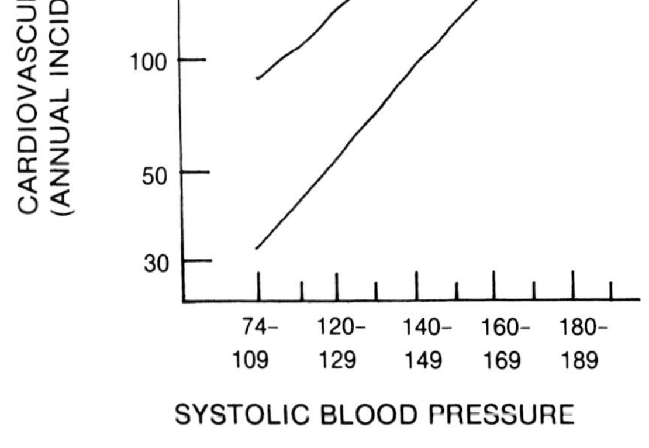

Treatment of hypertension can have a significant influence on the clinical outcome. The most impressive data are associated with malignant or accelerated hypertension, in which the reduction of mortality by drug therapy is marked.[1,21] Similarly, the data are impressive in terms of preventing the development of stroke.[22] Protection from coronary events and regression of left ventricular hypertrophy have also been demonstrated.[1-3,23,24] Because the prevalence of heart attacks is greater than that of strokes, the absolute reduction in coronary events due to treatment of hypertension is about twice that for strokes.[3] It was recently concluded that a reduction by as little as 5 to 6 mm Hg in diastolic blood pressure and of 10 mm Hg in systolic pressure can reduce stroke risk by about a third and the risk for coronary events by about a sixth.[2,3] It has also been suggested that the benefits of anti-hypertensive therapy have probably been underestimated in most of the randomized trials because of crossover of patients from placebo to active treatment, preferential inclusion of low-risk patients in trials, and the short-term duration.[2] Therapy has also been shown to slow the progression of loss of renal function significantly.[25] A major question is whether certain classes of antihypertensives provide more target organ protection than do other classes.

Hypertension occurs frequently in association with other cardiovascular risk factors such as hyperinsulinemia, glucose intolerance, diabetes mellitus, and hypertriglyceridemia. Researchers have studied extensively the possibility of a cause-effect relationship among these factors, especially the relation between hyperinsulinemia and hypertension. However, a recent epidemiologic report using the data from the Framingham study showed that there is no direct relationship among these factors and that the association of obesity with each risk factor mediates the clustering of these risk factors.[26]

Regulation of Blood Pressure

Mean arterial pressure is a function of cardiac output, systemic blood flow, and resistance to flow in the perfused organs.[27,28] These functions are regulated by hormones, neurotransmitters, and local factors and are affected by structural and functional abnormalities in the heart and vasculature that occur with chronic hypertension. Derangements in any or several of these functions can lead to hypertension, although in the long term, the increased vascular resistance is primarily responsible for the elevated blood pressure in most patients with essential and secondary hypertension. The hemodynamic derangements in hypertension vary with the etiology, duration, and severity of the disorder. In general, in patients with borderline hypertension, cardiac output, stroke volume, and heart rate are relatively high and total peripheral resistance is normal.[29] However, peripheral resistance is inappropriate for the elevated level of cardiac output and is abnormal during exercise. The plasma volume is typically normal or slightly decreased with attenuation of the microcirculation. Cardiac and renal function are normal, but myocardial contractility is increased and arterial compliance, coronary reserve, and renal blood flow are decreased. With exercise, cardiac output decreases and stroke volume does not increase sufficiently, while cardiac index and heart rate are elevated.

Patients with established or long-standing hypertension and older hypertensives characteristically have an increase in total peripheral resistance that is attributable both to structural changes in the resistance vessels and to the influence of vasoactive mediators.[6,30,31] The systolic blood pressure increases with age while the diastolic decreases, as a result of loss of arterial elasticity, thus widening the pulse pressure.[6] Systolic blood pressure and pulse pressure importantly correlate with (Fig. 13-1) cardiovascular disease.[32,33] Cardiac output and cardiac index are normal or decreased, and myocardial contractility is normal to increased. However, early left ventricular filling is delayed, left ventricular compliance is decreased, and left ventricular mass is increased. Renal blood flow is normal to decreased.

Complications of Hypertension

Hypertension is a chronic disease that normally evolves over the course of 20 to 30 years. Most patients remain asymptomatic until target organ damage is well advanced. The major complications of hypertension result from its acceleration of atherosclerosis in large elastic arteries and medium-sized muscular arteries such as the carotid, coronary, cerebral, mesenteric, aortoiliac, and renal arteries.[34–36] These changes are associated with early alterations in endothelial cell function leading to changes in vascular smooth muscle cell remodeling processes. Atherosclerosis accelerated by hypertension in turn leads to the development of thrombotic brain infarction; occlusive coronary artery disease; thromboembolic occlusive disease in the aortoiliac, mesenteric, and peripheral arteries; and aneurysm formation. Atherosclerosis also causes stiffening, decreased elasticity, and tortuosity in medium and large arteries. These changes result in altered pressure and flow relationships and further raise systolic pressure. The incidence of these events is compounded by the association of additional risk factors for atherosclerosis such as advancing age, male sex, cigarette smoking, hyperlipidemia, and glucose intolerance.[1,23]

Changes in the heart are due both to atherosclerosis and to left ventricular hypertrophy.[1–3,24] The left ventricle hypertrophies by increasing wall thickness, which maintains normal wall tension, compensates for the increased afterload, and maintains normal systolic cardiac performance. However, even mild left ventricular enlargement impairs diastolic function.[32] Left ventricular hypertrophy is an independent atherosclerotic risk factor and is a predictor of a poor prognosis among untreated patients with hypertension.[19,24] Ultimately, left ventricular systolic function can become impaired sufficiently to lead to heart failure.

In chronic hypertension, structural alterations occur in the microvascular circulation.[30] These alterations consist of increased thickness of the resistance arterioles as a result of hypertrophy and hyperplasia of smooth muscle cells and osmotic trapping of water. These changes reduce the size of the arterial lumen and increase the resistance to flow. There is also a reduction in the number of arterioles. Hypertension also accelerates the rate of endothelial cell turnover. These changes may play a role in the increased lipid transport and accumulation in the vessels of hypertensive patients.

In the cerebral circulation, chronic hypertension accelerates the development of atherosclerosis and aneurysm formation in the larger arteries and of specific degenerative changes in the small arteries.[22,23,24,36] These abnormalities can lead to ischemic infarcts of the brain, transient ischemic attacks, intracerebral hemorrhage, and dementia. Retinal changes reflect similar processes and eventually cerebral edema manifested as papilledema. In hypertensive encephalopathy, the extreme and rapid rise of blood pressure exceeds the ability of the cerebral vasculature to adapt (autoregulate), and there is segmental overdistension alternating with areas of vasoconstriction of cerebral arterioles. These responses lead to cerebral edema, hemorrhage, and herniation unless the blood pressure is reduced rapidly.

There are progressive changes in the kidneys during the course of hypertension. Renal blood flow is reduced early in many patients, with preservation of the glomerular filtration rate, resulting in an increased filtration fraction.[37–39] A hallmark of the disorder is afferent arteriolar narrowing.[40] There can also be impressive heterogeneity in this response.[40] Nephrosclerosis is common in the kidneys of hypertensives.[37] As described in the section on renovascular hypertension, atherosclerosis in the larger arteries can also contribute to renal damage, leading to renal failure[41,42] and to microalbuminuria.[43,44] An increase in serum uric acid levels reflects increased intrarenal vascular resistance and decreased glomerular filtration.[45] In the era before effective drug therapy was available, about 40 percent of hypertensives developed proteinuria and about 25 percent developed nitrogen retention.[46] Renal failure can be progressive in a poorly treated patient. An elevated albumin excretion rate or an elevated serum creatinine remains a potent independent risk factor for mortality.[47,48] Renal failure can develop rapidly with malignant hypertension and exacerbate the condition; it was the cause of death in up to 60 percent of patients before effective drug therapy was available,[21] and hypertension is still a major cause of renal failure among blacks. Overall, about 30 percent of chronic dialysis patients may have hypertension as the primary cause of their renal failure.[49]

GENETIC AND ENVIRONMENTAL INFLUENCES

The development of essential hypertension depends on the interaction of both genetic and environmental influences. The familial correlations for blood pressure range from 0.14 to 0.34 between parents and offspring and adult siblings to 0.75 with identical twins, and a positive family history is a good predictor of the development of hypertension.[50] The inherited nature of the disorder is also reflected by the differences in its prevalence in men and women and in blacks and whites, as discussed previously.[1] Relatives of hypertensives have significantly higher mean blood pressure levels at all ages than do those of normotensives.[50,51] The distribution of blood pressure in the general population is unimodal rather than bimodal, suggesting that the etiology of the elevated blood pressure is polygenic or multifactorial.[50]

Known biochemical markers of hypertension relate to hormones and to hormonal systems. Prominent among these are abnormal ion fluxes in red blood cells, with the best correlations having been established between certain subgroups of hypertensives and the Na^+-Li^+ counter-transport and possibly others.[52] There is also a correlation between an inherited tendency toward high urinary kallikrein excretion and a decreased likelihood of developing hypertension.[53]

Gene polymorphisms of the components of renin-angiotensin system are the target of intensive investigation because of the importance of this system in the control of blood pressure. Renin gene polymorphism has been shown to be associated with hypertension only in one study.[54] Angiotensinogen (AGT) gene polymorphisms affect blood pressure. In Caucasian families in France and Utah the AGT M235T genotype was associated with marked blood pressure elevations and increased circulating AGT levels.[55] This polymorphism was more prevalent among hypertensive men in France and among women who had hypertension diagnosed before age 45 years.[55] Similar results were seen in Mexican-

Americans.[56] However, a European multicenter study and a Chinese study did not show an association between angiotensinogen gene M235T polymorphism and hypertension.[57,58] Another angiotensinogen gene polymorphism was described to involve the core promoter element 1 at −20 and −18.[55] Among Japanese, the −20 genotype has a weak correlation with hypertension and plasma angiotensinogen levels.[59] However, the −18 genotype is considered a genetic risk factor for essential hypertension and is more strongly associated with hypertension compared with M235T polymorphism.[60] Although the M235T polymorphism of the AGT was not associated with blood pressure response to sodium restriction, patients homozygous for the insertion allele of the angiotensin converting enzyme (ACE) gene (II) had significantly higher BP response to high salt intake than patients with the DI or DD allele.[61]

Data about the role of ACE polymorphism as a risk factor for hypertension from different studies and different populations are conflicting, probably reflecting the interaction with different environmental factors and with other factors related to genetic background (ethnicity). In a Japanese population, the DD genotype was found to be associated with higher risk for early onset hypertension although the frequency of the alleles (DD, DI, and II) were not different between hypertensive and normotensive groups.[62] On the other hand, ACE polymorphism explains interindividual variation of blood pressure among white males, but not females, especially in the presence of a family history of hypertension. There is an increase in diastolic blood pressure in association with the DD ACE genotype.[63,64] Further, the DD ACE genotype is associated with impaired endothelium-dependent vascular relaxation.[65] On the other hand, studies from China and Taiwan did not find a relation between ACE polymorphism and hypertension.[66,67] In France, Tiret et al. also did not find any association between ACE polymorphism and hypertension.[68] However, the ACE D allele was more frequent among hypertensive patients with a parental history of stroke before age 65 years and/or parental history of myocardial infarction before age 60 years.

The genotype frequency of angII AT1 receptor gene polymorphism AT1 A-C1166 is not different in Caucasian populations between normotensive and hypertensive subjects.[69,70] However, among patients with hypertension, the C allele is associated with higher blood pressure only if increased weight and older age coexist.[70] In France, Tiret et al. had found an increased prevalence of the angiotensin receptor AT1 C1166 allele among female hypertensives but not among males.[68] On the other hand, a Japanese study showed no association between angiotensin receptor polymorphism and hypertension but rather the polymorphism of angII receptor type 1 influenced left ventricular mass.[71]

A well-defined type of genetic hypertension is Liddle's syndrome. Liddle's syndrome is a rare cause of hypertension. It is inherited as an autosomal dominant trait. Patients with Liddle's syndrome are markedly salt-sensitive because of increased activity of sodium channels in the epithelium of renal distal tubules. The defect was described originally to be the result of an abnormality in the carboxy terminus of the beta subunit of the epithelial sodium channels caused by deletion of 32 nucleotides that modifies the open reading frame and introduces a stop codon at position 582.[72] However, Liddle's syndrome seems to be caused by heterogeneous mutations such as those resulting in a truncated carboxy terminus of epithelial sodium channel gamma subunit or in deletion of the PY-motif, which is a conserved proline-rich amino acid sequence of the beta subunit (beta Arg564X mutation with premature stop codon).[72–76] Another mutation of the beta subunit, T594M mutation, is encountered with a higher frequency among hypertensive blacks who reside in London. However, the frequency of this mutation was only 8 percent among hypertensive blacks compared with 2–3 percent among normotensives. On the other hand, this mutation was highly associated with low renin (salt-sensitive) hypertension.[77] Thus the T594M mutation may explain a small but significant percentage of salt-sensitive hypertension.

Endothelial nitric oxide affects blood pressure control by several mechanisms including vasodilation, nitriuresis,[78] and modulation of renin secretion (see regulation of renin-angiotensin system later). Thus, a mutation in genes of the constitutive endothelial nitric oxide synthase (eNOS) is likely to affect blood pressure by one or more of the previously mentioned mechanisms. The eNOS4 gene has two alleles, a and b. Healthy subjects homozygous for the a allele (eNOS a/a) have about 20 percent lower concentration of plasma NO metabolites compared with those who are homozygous for the b allele (eNOS b/b)[79] and it is suggested that polymorphism of eNOS contributes to essential hypertension.[80] Uwabo et al. identified two alleles of eNOS that contain a variable number of tandem repeats in intron 4, a four-repeat allele and a five-repeat allele. The four repeat allele is more frequent in Japanese people with essential hypertension.[81]

Some investigators have considered possible abnormalities in the gene(s) that encode for one or more cytoskeletal protein. Of these, polymorphism of adducin gene is well-studied, but the association between adducin polymorphism and hypertension is weak.[82–84] On the other hand, the work by Cusi et al. has linked the polymorphism of adducin gene to salt sensitivity.[85]

Because hypertension and obesity coexist frequently, the leptin gene (OB gene) was studied for possible association with hypertension. However, available data do not support this possibility.[86] Other polymorphisms that have been linked to hypertension include beta 2-adrenergic receptor gene polymorphism among African-Caribbeans and African-Americans.[87,88] The mutation of beta3-adrenergic receptor Trp64Arg does not seem to play a role in the development of hypertension.[89] Whether gene polymorphisms accounting for some rare forms of hypertension play a role in populations with essential hypertension remains to be determined.

HORMONAL MODIFIERS OF BLOOD PRESSURE

Many hormone-regulated processes affect blood pressure. Abnormalities in the release of and/or responsiveness to hormones are important in essential and secondary hypertension. A number of these factors are discussed later in relation to essential and secondary forms of hypertension and their effects on blood pressure.

The Renin-Angiotensin System

The renin-angiotensin system (Figs. 13-2 and 13-3) is important in adaptive blood pressure responses and is involved in essential and secondary forms of hypertension. The effector substance of this system is angiotensin II (angII), an octapeptide. A glycoprotein enzyme, renin, acts on angiotensinogen, an α_2-globulin substrate, to form the decapeptide angiotensin I, the precursor to angII. The two carboxyl-terminal amino acids of angiotensin

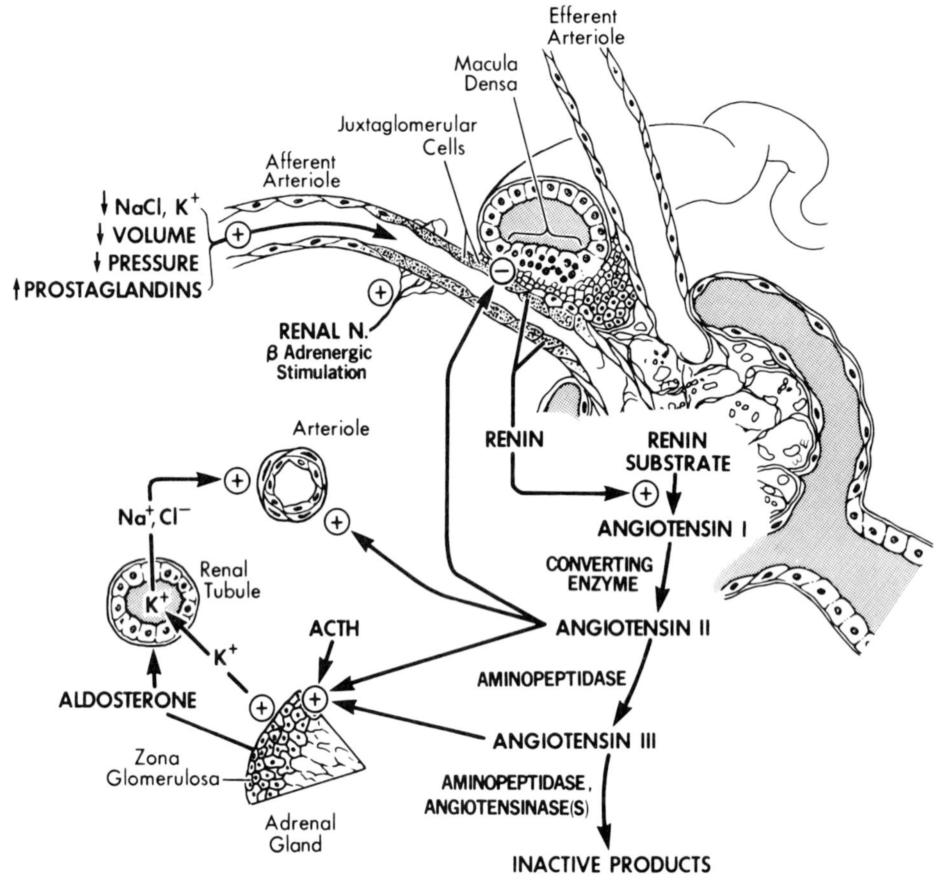

FIGURE 13-2. The renin-angiotensin system. Plus and minus signs indicate stimulation and inhibition, respectively. Only the major influences on the system are shown.

I are then cleaved in vascular beds by converting enzyme to form angII. Proteases in the circulation inactivate angII. Its activity is mediated by three angiotensin receptor subtypes: AT_1, AT_2, and AT_4. Both circulating and tissue renin-angiotensin systems contribute to its effects on blood pressure and target organ damage.

Components of the Renin-Angiotensin System

Renin and Prorenin

Renin occurs in two major forms at low concentrations in blood.[90–92] The active form of this aspartyl protease has a molecular weight of about 40,000.[91] Prorenin, the precursor of renin, has

FIGURE 13-3. Formation and metabolism of angiotensins. (*Modified from Boucher et al.*[57a])

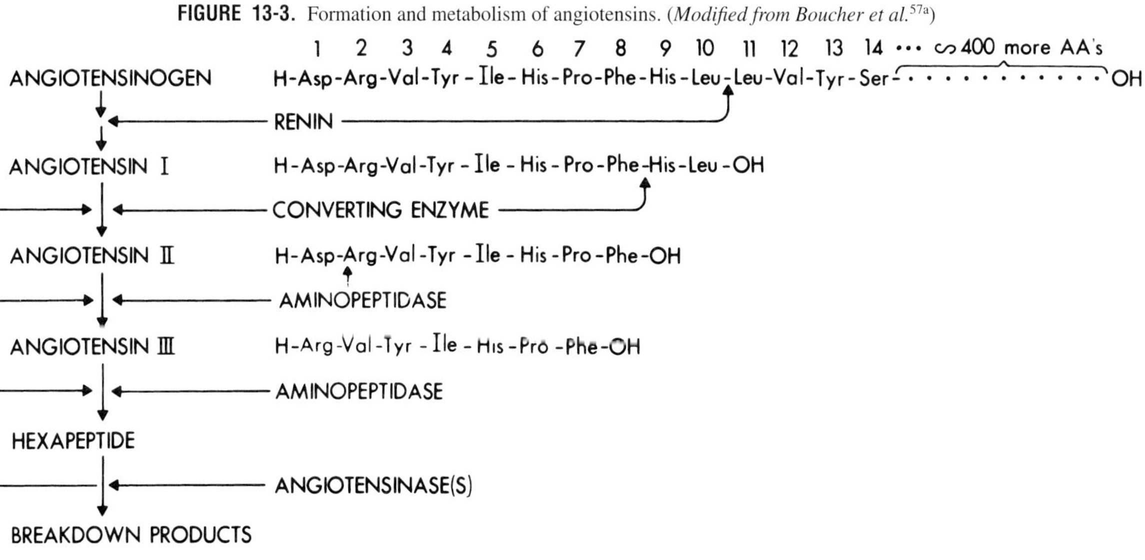

a small amount of renin activity and a molecular weight of 47,000 and can be acid- or protease-activated. Prorenin constitutes most of the renin proteins in the normal circulation.[92-95]

A single human renin gene located on chromosome 1 encodes for the 406 amino acids of preprorenin.[96-100] A 20-amino acid signal peptide is cleaved from preprorenin as it enters the rough endoplasmic reticulum to form prorenin.[101] Prorenin is then glycosylated and transported to the Golgi.[101] Renin in the circulation is variably glycosolated and exists as four to five isoenzymes with differing isoelectric points.[92] At the trans-Golgi, about half the prorenin is constitutively secreted without proteolytic processing and the other half is sorted to secretory granules, where prorenin is processed to renin by cleavage of the 46-amino acid prosegment.[91,101] Less than 5 percent of prorenin is sorted to lysosomes, where it is metabolized.[102] Cathepsin B in juxtaglomerular cell granules cleaves human prorenin to renin.[103,104] Constitutive secretion of prorenin is nonregulated, while release of renin stored in secretory granules is regulated, for example, by cAMP.[105]

Renal and Extrarenal Sources of Renin Circulating active renin arises almost exclusively from the kidney, whereas plasma prorenin can come from extrarenal sources.[106] After nephrectomy, plasma renin activity (PRA) and protein and angII concentrations drop to levels of about 6 percent of normal.[94] The prorenin levels are decreased approximately 35 to 55 percent, depending on the assay.[94,107] These data also indicate that plasma angII levels are mostly dependent on renin of renal origin, although there can be a small contribution by extrarenally produced renin and/or prorenin. Evidence for extrarenal production of prorenin and renin is supported by studies in humans and animals that have demonstrated prorenin, renin, and/or renin mRNA in pituitary, brain, vascular endothelial and smooth muscle tissue, adrenal gland, chorion, decidua, pituitary, testes, ovary, and other tissues.[107-116] The finding that most extrarenal prorenin is not processed to active renin has led to speculation that prorenin may be active locally. Prorenin has a small amount of renin activity and might also be activated locally through means that do not remove its prosegment.[117] Prorenin could also be activated locally by removal of its prosegment in the tissue; this probably occurs in the adrenal.[114]

In animals, injected renin can be taken up by the vasculature, and levels of vascular renin generally parallel those in plasma.[118] Infused prorenin in monkeys is mostly taken up by the kidneys and liver, where it is probably degraded; very little active renin enters the circulation.[119]

Nonrenin Renin-Like Enzymes Several nonrenin proteolytic enzymes can generate angiotensin I or angII from renin substrate.[113,120,121] For example, tonin can act on angiotensinogen, tetradecapeptide renin substrate, and angiotensin I to form angII.[122] Cathepsins other than cathepsin B and chymase can generate angiotensins I and II and are found in several tissues.[123,124] However, their angiotensin I or II-generating activity at physiologic pH is low. The importance of these enzymes in blood pressure regulation is unknown.

Regulation of Renal Renin Renin is rate-limiting for the cascade of events that generate angII. Renal renin is synthesized in the juxtaglomerular cells of the afferent renal arteriole (Fig. 13-2) and is stored as rhomboid-appearing granules.[125,126] It is released into both the bloodstream and the renal lymphatics in response to stimuli.[101,125-136] These stimuli act mostly through (1) renal baroreceptors, (2) adrenergic receptors, and (3) circulating factors such as ions and hormones. Renin release is stimulated by lowering the blood pressure, changing from supine to erect posture, salt depletion, β-adrenergic or CNS stimulation, vasodilating prostaglandins and hormones, opiate peptides, kallikrein, calcitonin, calcitonin gene-related peptide (CGRP), growth factors, and a high-protein diet. Renin release is inhibited by increases in blood pressure, assumption of the supine posture, salt loading, angII, vasopressin, inhibitors of prostaglandin biosynthesis, potassium, calcium, endothelin, endothelium-derived releasing factor (EDRF), adenosine, and atrial natriuretic peptide (ANP). It is also inhibited by certain antihypertensive drugs, including β-adrenergic blockers, α-methyldopa,[137] and clonidine.[138] The importance of only some of these factors is well understood.

Renin is inactivated by proteolytic enzymes in the liver, kidney, and plasma or is excreted by the kidney and in the bile. Its half-life in plasma is 10 to 20 min.[119,139]

The macula densa is a specialized segment of the distal nephron where the distal tubule contacts the afferent arteriole before it enters the glomerulus (Fig. 13-2). The macula densa has an intimate anatomic relation to the juxtaglomerular apparatus and inhibits renin release.[125,134,140-142] This inhibitory influence is inversely proportional to the renal tubular fluid NaCl concentration and may be due to release from macula densa cells of adenosine that acts through juxtaglomerular cell α_1-adenosine receptors.[140-142] The macula densa detects renal tubular fluid sodium[141] or its associated chloride concentration.[143] The concentration of NaCl may be more important than the flux.[142] NaCl may stimulate adenosine release by blocking Na^+-K^+-$2K^+$-cotransporter activity.[142] Whatever the mechanism, factors that reduce volume and/or lower the plasma [NaCl], such as dehydration or a loss of fluid or blood, stimulate renin release. The relation between plasma renin activity and sodium intake, as reflected by urinary sodium excretion, is shown in Fig. 13-4.[144] Renal baroreceptors stimulate renin release in response to decreased renal perfusion pressure.[126-128] Apparently, changes are more important than the absolute perfusion pressure, because they can influence renin release in the presence of renal arteriolar constriction or dilatation. These receptors can function independently of innervation and of the influences of NaCl delivery to the macula densa. They probably regulate renin release in response to fluid loss and decreased blood pressure.

Renal sympathetic nerves that terminate in the juxtaglomerular cells and in smooth muscle cells of renal afferent arterioles secrete norepinephrine and stimulate renin release.[126,128,131] These nerves mediate CNS stimuli and responses to posture, changes in blood pressure, and salt depletion. They can act independently of baroreceptors and salt influences on the macula densa. The activity of these nerves is stimulated primarily by low-pressure cardiopulmonary venous receptors; an independent role for arterial baroreceptors has not been established, although effects probably occur through baroreceptors in concert with those through low-pressure receptors.[145]

β-adrenergic receptors mediate catecholamine influences on renin release.[126,128,131] Thus, the effects of norepinephrine released by the sympathetic nerves are abolished by β- but not α-adrenergic blockers in most studies. Some of the efficacy of β-adrenergic blockers in treating essential hypertension may be due to blocking of renin release.[146] β-adrenergic stimulation of renin release is independent of the vasoconstrictor effects of catecholamines that affect the renal glomerular filtration rate and filtered sodium load.

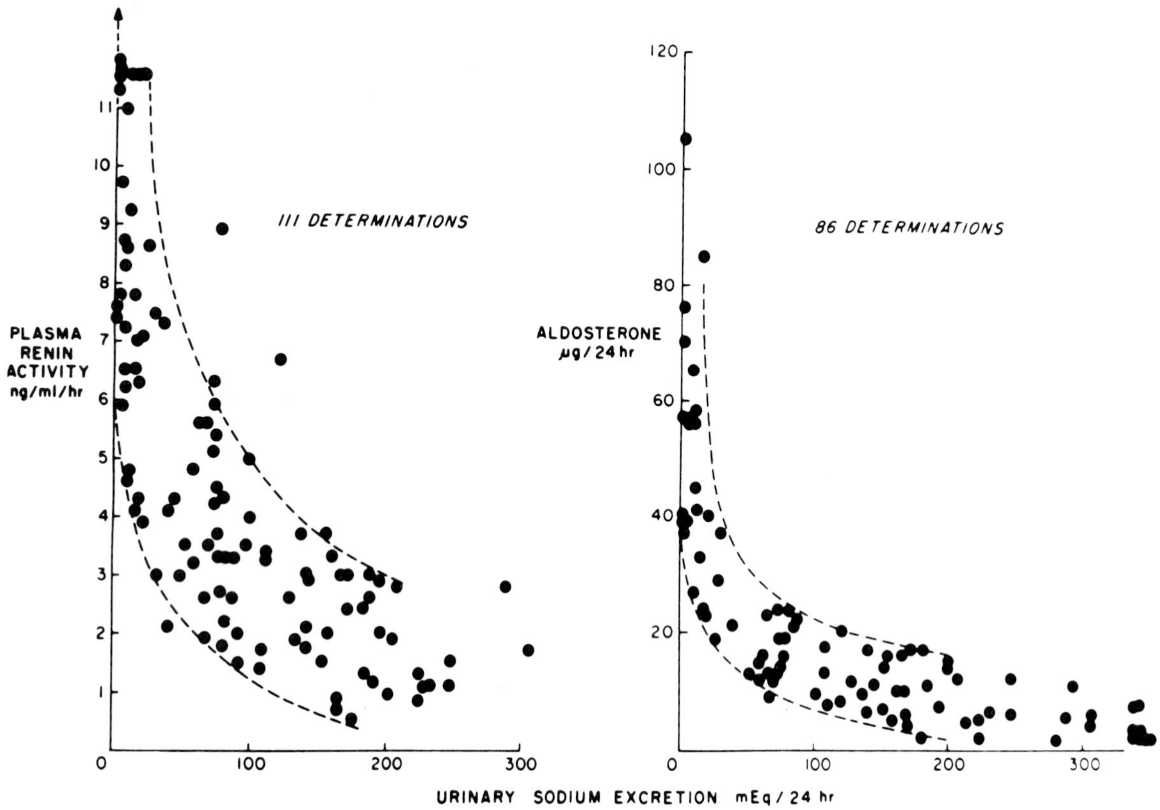

FIGURE 13-4. Relation of 4-h plasma renin activity (PRA, upright posture, *left*) or 24-h urinary aldosterone levels (*right*) to the daily rate of sodium excretion in 52 normal subjects with 111 determinations. (*From Brunner et al.*[118])

Conversely, the effects of NaCl and other influences on renin release can occur independently of β-adrenergic receptors.

AngII is a potent inhibitor of renin release.[125,147] This occurs under all conditions of sodium intake. Thus, inhibition of converting enzyme stimulates renin release even when it does not decrease blood pressure. This negative feedback inhibition appears to be calcium-dependent. Calcium-channel blockers thus enhance renin release.[148] However, these blockers also inhibit the release of aldosterone (whose production is stimulated by intracellular Ca^{2+}) and thus uncouple renin-aldosterone responses. Ca^{2+}-mediated inhibition of renin release may be mediated in part by nitric oxide.[127] Renal prostaglandins are important mediators of renal renin release and may mediate baroreceptor and macula densa signals to release renin.[128,149–152] Administration of either the prostaglandin precursor arachidonic acid or various prostaglandins increases renin secretion. The vasodilator prostacyclin (PGI_2) is the major prostaglandin produced in the human renal cortex.[149] PGI_2 stimulates renin secretion.[153] This influence is independent of changes in renal hemodynamics or the sympathetic nervous system.[151] Inhibition of prostaglandin synthesis, for example, with indomethacin, reduces renin production, decreases plasma renin levels, and can induce hyporeninemic hypoaldosteronism in some patients with renal disease (see Chap. 11).[153] Arachidonic acid precursors can form lipoxygenase products that impair renin release.[152] In patients with hyporeninemic hypoaldosteronism, renal prostacyclin production is low, while lipoxygenase products are increased.[154]

Renin release is affected by several growth factors and cytokines.[155] Tumor necrosis factor (TNF) and interleukin 1 (IL-1) stimulate renin release from rat cortical slices and suppress aldosterone secretion.[155] These changes have been implicated in hyperreninemic hyperaldosteronism with severe illness.[156] Transforming growth factor β (TGF-β) stimulates renin at a concentration of 10^{-12} M, but enhances the angII suppressive effect at 10^{-10} M. TGF-β levels are increased in the streptozotocin diabetic rat kidney[157] and may contribute to renin suppression in this model.

Acute stimulation results almost exclusively in the release of renin with either little effect on or a decrease in prorenin.[93,95] By contrast, with chronic stimulation, there is a parallel increase in both renin and prorenin.[95] During periods of relative suppression, more prorenin than renin is released, although as described previously, some of the prorenin may be derived from extrarenal sources. Nevertheless, certain stimuli probably result in a preferential processing of prorenin to renin or preferential release of renin as a result of increased shuttling of newly synthesized protein to secretory granules where the conversion of prorenin to renin occurs. It is not known whether the processing is specifically regulated. Prostaglandins may regulate prorenin to renin conversion.[158] The idea that there is control of the processing of prorenin to renin is also suggested by the finding of an increase in prorenin but not renin levels in diabetic nephropathy.[159,160]

Certain stimuli affect not only renin release and synthesis but also the number of cells that produce renin. Prolonged stimulation by salt deprivation increases the cellular content of both renin and its mRNA in the rat.[161] However, the major influence of removal of the negative effect of angII (e.g., by converting enzyme inhibitor treatment of rats) is to recruit more cells that release renin.[130]

Angiotensinogen (Renin Substrate)

Angiotensinogen is a glycoprotein synthesized predominantly in the liver, with a molecular weight of 55,000 to 100,000 that varies according to the carbohydrate content of the protein (Fig. 13-4).[139] Several molecular-weight forms are present in the circulation, and higher-molecular-weight forms are synthesized in greater quantities during pregnancy or oral contraceptive administration.[162] The protein is also synthesized at lower levels in a variety of extrahepatic tissues, including kidney (primarily the proximal convoluted tubule), brain, adrenal, aorta, heart, testis, and perivascular fat.[162,163] Release of angiotensinogen from the liver is constitutive, and regulators of angiotensinogen levels affect the synthesis of the protein. Circulating angiotensinogen levels are increased by angII, estrogens, glucocorticoids, thyroid hormone, and inflammatory mediators.[162,164,165] Angiotensinogen production is decreased by glucagon and certain prostaglandins[164] and in untreated Addison's disease.[161]

Under most circumstances, angiotensinogen appears to circulate at concentrations that do not greatly exceed the K_m for renin, that is, around 1.15 *M*, using pure human renin substrate.[91] This implies that variations in angiotensinogen levels influence the amount of angiotensin I that is generated. However, the extent to which circulating angiotensinogen is limiting for angiotensin I production in the circulation has not been resolved.[161] The finding that a RFLP in the angiotensinogen gene links to hypertension,[55] implies that levels of expression of the gene in the liver or extrahepatic tissues is an important determinant of angII generation. Genetic knockout of angiotensinogen and its overexpression in the mouse have helped to define the role of the renin-angiotensin system in blood pressure regulation and development.[166,167] The complete knockout is lethal, suggesting that the system is necessary for organ development. Levels of overexpression correlate directly with blood pressure across a spectrum of angiotensinogen levels.[167]

Angiotensin-Converting Enzyme

Expression and Actions Angiotensin-converting enzyme (ACE) is a zinc-containing glycoprotein found in lung, plasma, brush borders of the proximal renal tubule, and in endothelium of all vascular beds (Fig. 13-3).[168,169] A single gene encodes for ACE, but alternative transcription start sites generate differences in size between pulmonary and testicular ACE.[170] The enzyme is mostly membrane-bound, although there is a soluble form.[169] This enzyme removes two carboxyl-terminal amino acids from a number of peptide substrates. Its two most important actions are the inactivation of bradykinin and the conversion of angiotensin I to angII (Fig. 13-2). It can also have actions on other proteins.[169,171]

Converting enzymes have an enormous capacity for generating angII. Thus, even though in certain diseases (e.g., pulmonary disease) there can be a decrease in the plasma levels of converting enzyme, this does not noticeably affect angII generation.[172] Converting enzyme levels are increased in patients with essential and renovascular hypertension, by diuretic therapy, in some patients with diabetes mellitus, and in hyperthyroidism.[173-175] The activity of the enzyme is increased by glucocorticoids (see Chap. 11) in tissues during injury, e.g., in rat heart after aortic banding[176] and in vascular tissue after endothelial injury.[177] Ventricular ischemia and heart failure are also associated with increased cardiac angiotensin converting enzyme.[178] Thus, cardiovascular damage is associated with increased local AII production. An RFLP in the converting enzyme gene has been linked to the development of diabetic nephropathy, left ventricular hypertrophy, and myocardial infarction, but not hypertension.[178-182]

Converting Enzyme Inhibitors Converting enzyme inhibitors have great clinical utility for treating hypertension, improving hemodynamics and mortality in heart failure, inhibiting remodeling after myocardial infarction, and preventing renal failure.[140,183-189] Recently, ramipril was shown to reduce myocardial infarction, stroke, and cardiovascular death in high-risk patients as compared to placebo and to decrease the development of diabetes in this cohort.[190] They are also useful for the diagnosis and treatment of renin-dependent hypertension[140,191,192] (see also the sections on the role of the renin-angiotensin system in hypertension and on renovascular hypertension, later). Activation of the renin-angiotensin system plays a pathophysiologic role in the development of congestive heart failure, and converting enzyme inhibitors reduce afterload, increase exercise tolerance, and decrease mortality in this condition. Converting enzyme inhibition can also lessen mortality and prevent the development of severe heart failure after myocardial infarction, suggesting that angII plays a role in cardiac remodeling. Another use of converting enzyme inhibitors is in diabetic and other forms of nephropathy, where these drugs can decrease proteinuria.[186,188] Captopril was demonstrated to decrease mortality and the progression of renal disease in a large study in type I diabetic patients with 500 mg proteinuria per day.[186]

Interpretation of the actions of converting enzyme inhibitors must be made in light of the fact that the enzyme can also degrade bradykinin and other peptides.[163,171,172,184,193] This bradykinin-metabolizing activity has been termed kininase II or peptidyldipeptide hydroxylase. Bradykinin is also inactivated by another enzyme, kininase I (carboxypeptidase N).[194] Inhibitors of converting enzyme can increase bradykinin concentrations.[195] An argument for a role for increased bradykinin production in the effectiveness of converting enzyme therapy is that administration of a bradykinin antagonist can attenuate the effects of angiotensin converting enzyme inhibitors in some models.[196]

Angiotensins I, II, III, IV, and (1-7)

Production Although a significant amount of angiotensin I is produced in the circulation, more than half of it occurs in tissues.[112,121,194] Most of this angiotensin I generation appears to be due to renin of renal origin that has been taken up by these tissues because plasma angII levels are very low in anephric individuals[94] (also discussed in the section on renin). Conversely, most of the plasma angII appears to be derived in the circulation as a result of tissue-bound converting enzyme (Fig. 13-3).[197]

Actions Angiotensin I is not known to have physiologically important actions, although it can, at very large doses, stimulate the adrenal medulla to produce catecholamines and the CNS to increase blood pressure and induce thirst.[196]

AngII has multiple effects on the cardiovascular system and other systems. The actions of angII in inhibiting renin release are discussed in the preceding section (Fig. 13-2).[124,147] AngII is one of the most potent stimulators of aldosterone production by the adrenal zona glomerulosa, as described in Chap. 11. AngII also stimulates the production of its substrate, angiotensinogen.[164]

AngII has potent vasoconstrictor activity and can elevate the blood pressure through direct action on arterioles.[108,147] These blood pressure–elevating effects may be amplified by angII actions in the CNS, kidney, and by stimulation of other vasoactive substances, such as endothelin.[108,198] AngII stimulates sympathetic nervous system activity through actions on muscle sympathetic nerve activity, adrenergic nerve endings, sympathetic ganglia, and the CNS.[199] AngII acts within a few seconds, and the duration of action is a few minutes.

AngII induces a coordinated set of responses in the kidney that affect blood flow, glomerular function, and ion and solute transport. These effects are also modified by angII-mediated aldosterone release. AngII decreases renal blood flow and the glomerular filtration rate.[78,121,147,197,200,201] There is renal vasoconstriction with greater effects on efferent than afferent glomerular arterioles.[147,200,201] These influences modify glomerular filtration and sodium balance. The effects on glomerular blood flow are especially important when renal function is compromised. In this case, angII maintains the glomerular filtration rate; loss of this effect explains why converting enzyme inhibitors sometimes lead to a decrease in renal function[187] (see the section on renovascular hypertension). AngII increases the activity of the Na^+-H^+ antiporter that enhances Na^+ and Cl^- reabsorption in the proximal convoluted tubule.[202] Na^+ retention can be further increased by angII-induced vasoconstriction in the medullary circulation and in the cortical collecting tubules secondary to aldosterone actions.[202] Some renal effects of angII may be mediated through changes in the kallikrein and prostaglandin systems, endothelial-derived releasing factors, and norepinephrine release.[197,200,201]

There are a number of other effects of angII.[163,203,204] In the heart, angII can affect coronary blood flow, induce positive ionotropic effects, stimulate the development of cardiac hypertrophy, increase intracellular Ca^{2+}, and influence ion channel responses.[147] In the brain, angII stimulates dipsogenic behavior, elevates blood pressure, and stimulates the release of vasopressin, corticotropin (ACTH), prolactin, oxytocin, and luteinizing hormone (LH).[147,205] AngII stimulates a "resetting" of the baroreceptor reflex, absorption of salt and water across extrarenal epithelial tissues such as jejunum and colon, uterine smooth muscle contraction, blood coagulation, erythropoietin production, and catecholamine production from nerve endings and the adrenal medulla.[108,147] AngII also has metabolic effects to stimulate insulin-mediated glucose uptake, inhibit glucagon effects on the liver, decrease plasma fatty acids, and elevate plasma lactate levels.[206,207]

A growing list of paracrine actions of angII contribute to tissue injury in cardiovascular and renal damage (Table 13-3). AngII promotes growth of vascular smooth muscle cells (VSMC), renal mesangial and proximal tubular cells, cardiac fibroblasts and myocytes.[208–211] Whether the response is proliferative or hypertrophic depends on the origin and type of cells and the presence of other growth factors in the milieau. For example, angII is hypertrophic for VSMC from normal animals, and increases the levels of platelet-derived growth factor (PDGF-A chain), c-fos, c-myc, and TGF-β mRNAs.[212] Whereas PDGF may stimulate the growth of these cells, TGF-β inhibits their growth and thus the proliferative response to PDGF, resulting in hypertrophy.[213,214] AngII can induce hyperplasia in human fetal mesangial cells and in vascular smooth muscle cells from the spontaneously hypertensive rat (SHR).[215,216] Thus, angII may enhance growth by altering the balance of autocrine growth factors and growth inhibitors in smooth muscle cells.

TABLE 13-3. Paracrine Effects of Angiotensin II Mediating Tissue Injury

1. Cellular Growth
2. Cellular Migration
3. Inflammation
4. Thrombosis
5. Oxidation
6. Adhesion
7. Fibrosis

Increasing evidence suggests that angII is a profibrotic factor. AngII stimulates TGF-β in VSMC, mesangial cells, cardiac fibroblasts, and other cells, which mediates its effects to enhance extracellular matrix (ECM) protein production.[217–219] In addition, angII stimulates production of plasminogen activator inhibitor I (PAI-1) in several tissues; PAI-1 inhibits enzyme activity of plasmin and metalloproteases that could prevent degradation of ECM and, thus, promote its accumulation.[220,221]

AngII contributes to vascular injury not only through its effects on VSMC, but also through its proinflammatory, prothrombotic, and oxidant effects. AngII enhances cytokine production in the vasculature and enhances endothelial expression of intracellular adhesion molecule-1 (ICAM-1), vascular cell adhesion molecule (VCAM), p-selection and other adhesion receptors that enhance the attachment of monocytes and macrophages to the vessel wall.[222,223] In addition to stimulating PAI-1, angII increases platelet adhesion and thromboxane production.[224] AngII also decreases nitric oxide activity by enhancing the metabolism of nitric oxide to peroxynitrite and other species that damage vascular tissue.[225] These effects contribute to coronary artery disease by promoting the atherosclerotic process.

The concentrations of angII in plasma vary between 5 and 100 pm.[94,111,120] Tissue levels of angII are probably higher, in the nanomolar range. Physiologic stimuli may increase the plasma concentrations 10- to 25-fold. AngII may circulate partly bound by plasma proteins. It has a half-life of a very few minutes in plasma; 50 percent or more of the activity disappears in a single passage through the vascular beds.

There are other angiotensin products whose roles have not been clarified. The heptapeptide angIII (cles-Asp^1)-AngII has activity that is similar qualitatively to that of angII, but may be less quantitatively.[196] The plasma concentrations of angIII are perhaps only 20 percent of those of angII, and the former is even more susceptible to proteolytic degradation than is angII. AngIII is further metabolized to the hexapeptide angiotensin IV by amino peptidase N. AngiotensinIV binds specifically to the AT_4 receptor present in heart, vascular tissue, adrenal, and brain.[226] This receptor has been implicated in vasodilation and memory.[227,228]

Angiotensinogen may undergo an alternative processing pathway mediated by two endopeptidases, neutral endopeptidases 24.11 and prolyl-endopeptidase 24.26, to produce the heptapeptide angiotensin-(1-7). These endopeptidase are present in the circulation, vascular endothelium, kidneys, and brain.[229] A third endopeptidase, metalloendopeptidase 24.15, is present in vascular smooth muscles and can convert angiotensin I to angiotensin-(1-7).[230] Angiotensin-(1-7) has vasodilative activity, mediated by the release of nitric oxide and prostacyclin,[231–232] and enhances sodium and water excretion from the proximal tubule of the kidney.[232] Angiotensin-(1-7) seems to exert its effects through receptor(s) other than AT1 and AT2 receptors[233] and seems to regulate pressor and growth effects of angII.[234] In addition, angiotensin-(1-7) prevents ACE-mediated degradation of bradykinin by binding to ACE. Therefore, angiotensin-(1-7) is a substrate for and an inhibitor of ACE activity[235] and seems to potentiate the hemodynamic effects of bradykinin.[236] Thus, the balance between these two hormones seems to be important. Angiotensin-(1-7) is metabolized by ACE.[237] Thus, ACE activity enhances vascular tone by generating angII and degrading angiotensin-(1-7). In addition, the activity of ACE regulates blood pressure by inactivating the vasodilator bradykinin, which induces nitric oxide production from vascular endothelium.

Mechanisms of Action Angiotensin binds to specific receptors on the cell membrane (see Chaps. 4 and 11). Four types of angII receptors have been classified.[238–240] The AT_1 receptor, defined by binding to the angII antagonist losartan, has been identified in vasculature, kidney, adrenal, and heart, and appears to mediate the cardiovascular and renal effects of angII.[241] The AT_2 receptor is defined by its binding to PD123177; the specific function of this receptor is unknown, although it appears to antagonize the growth and vasoconstrictive effects of the AT_1 receptor.[242,243] It is abundant in fetal tissue.[244] In the adult, AT_2 receptors have been found in brain, heart, uterus, and adrenal medulla.[245–247] Both receptor types have seven transmembrane-spanning domains.[238–240,248,249] The AT_1 receptor is G protein-linked.[238–240] The AT_2 receptor apparently can inhibit protein tyrosine phosphatase activity.[248]

Immediate post-angII–receptor binding events involve effects on phospholipids, with increased intracellular levels of inositol 1,4,5-triphosphate (IP_3) and mobilization of intracellular Ca^{2+} (see Chaps. 4 and 11), which occur in all angII-responsive tissues.[251,252] These changes lead to aldosterone release, as described in Chap. 11. The initial events in the vasculature are similar; angII-induced increases in intracellular Ca^{2+} mobilization initiating the formation of Ca^{2+} calmodulin complexes, activation of myosin light-chain kinase phosphorylation of myosin light chain, and ultimately actin-myosin interaction and contraction.[147] Effects on prostaglandins and lipoxygenase production may also contribute, although the precise role of these systems has not been elucidated.[253] The mitogen activated protein kinase (MAPK) pathway appears to mediate many of the growth effects of AII in a variety of tissues.[254–256] It also mediates the effect of AII to stimulate cell migration.[257] The protein kinase C isoform, PKC-zeta can be activated by angII and subsequently can activate Ras to activate MAPK.[258]

Genetic knockout of the AT_1 and AT_2 receptors has been highly useful in defining the physiologic action of these receptors. Complete elimination of any of the major components of the RAS including renin angiotensinogen, angiotensin-converting enzyme, and the AT_1 receptor is generally lethal.[259,260,261] The small percent of knockout animals that survive (<10 percent) have diminished growth, thickening of renal vessels, atrophy of the inner medulla of the kidney, and lower blood pressure, compared to wild type mice.[259] When given an ACE inhibitor, animals lacking the AT_1 receptor have a paradoxical rise in blood pressure, possibly as a result of decreasing available angII to bind to the AT_2 receptor.[259] Thus, the RAS is important for somatic growth and renal development. Targeted disruption of the AT_2 receptor is associated with increased blood pressure and increased pressor sensitivity to angII.[242,243] Loss of the AT_2 receptor is also associated with central nervous system effects including decreased drinking response to water deprivation, decreased spontaneous movements, decreased exploratory behavior, and lower body temperature.

Regulation of Responsiveness to Angiotensin Cellular sensitivity to angII can vary in physiologic circumstances and disease states. Such variations occur partly through influences on cellular receptor levels (see Chap. 4).[262] In the rat, angII increases the concentration of adrenal receptors (an exception to the general case with polypeptide hormones) and decreases the concentration of uterine, vascular, and cardiac fibroblast receptors.[262] Prolonged infusion of angII increases the sensitivity of the adrenal gland to the hormone. However, in some circumstances in which plasma angiotensin concentrations are chronically low (e.g., in low-renin essential hypertension, discussed later), the sensitivity of the adrenal gland to angII is increased. Hyperkalemia and decreased sodium increase and hypokalemia and increased sodium decrease the adrenal content of angiotensin receptors.[262] The affinity of these receptors for angII can also be increased transiently by sodium restriction.[262]

AngII Receptor Antagonists These compounds have been useful in defining the subclasses of angiotensin receptors. They are also effective in treating hypertension and other conditions.[263,264] AT_1 receptor blockers inhibit angII-induced vascular mesangial smooth muscle cell migration, TGF-β and extracellular matrix production, and enhanced PAI-1 expression.[265,266] AT_1 receptor blockade is one of the newest approaches to lower blood pressure. Low-dose diuretics markedly enhance their efficacy.[263,264] Clinical trials are ongoing to test their effectiveness in heart failure, postmyocardial infarction cardiac remodeling, and diabetic nephropathy. It is likely that AT_1 receptor blockers will have different clinical effects and end points than angiotensin converting enzyme inhibitors. As discussed above, angiotensin converting enzyme inhibitors inhibit degradation of a variety of tissue and circulating peptides, such as bradykinin, which is a vasodilator and a stimulator of nitric oxide. AT_1 receptor blockade is highly specific,[267] although it may have a modest effect to stimulate bradykinin and nitric oxide.[268] In general, both approaches similarly lower blood pressure. The only available comparison study in human heart failure is the ELITE trial (Effect of Losartan in the Elderly), which demonstrated improved mortality of losartan compared to captopril in patients over age 65 with low ejection fractions and no prior use of ACE inhibitors.[269] This result was attributed to increased arrhythmias in the captopril group, as bradykinin has been shown to stimulate cardiac nerve endings.[270] However, the Elite II Trial, which studied elderly patients with heart failure who had previously been administered ACE inhibitors, showed no difference between losartan and captopril.[271] Further studies are ongoing to address this issue and to examine additive effects of angiotensin converting enzyme inhibitors and AT_1 receptor blockers.

Maintenance of Blood Pressure Information about the physiologic role of angII in blood pressure control has been provided by the development of angiotensin antagonists and converting enzyme and renin inhibitors. In sodium-replete normotensive individuals, blockade of the renin-angiotensin system does not reduce blood pressure, even with changes in posture, but it does induce a significant fall in blood pressure in volume-depleted (salt-deprived, etc.) normotensive individuals.[272,273] The failure to reduce the blood pressure in the salt-replete state probably reflects the fact that mechanisms that compensate for the angII deficiency can normalize the blood pressure under these conditions.

Role of the Renin-Angiotensin System in Hypertension

Experimental Hypertension

Studies with animal models have elucidated how the renin-angiotensin system can cause hypertension.[274–276] The two-kidney one-clip model resembles the acute stages of renovascular hypertension in humans. Plasma renin activity and blood pressure increase after the renal artery is clamped. Sodium balance is positive in the early stages and returns to normal or becomes negative in the chronic phase. The sodium balance is inversely related to the degree of hypertension. Inhibition of renin, converting enzyme, or angII action lowers blood pressure in animals with two-kidney Goldblatt hypertension.[277] Thus, in the two-kidney model, increased renin activity not only initiates but maintains the hypertension. However, with longer periods of time (e.g., 2 to 4 months), the hypertension becomes non-angII-dependent and more volume-dependent.[277] This change appears to be due to a hypertension-induced decrease in the ability of the contralateral kidney to excrete salt. At this stage, the two-kidney preparation resembles the one-kidney preparation described later.

A different sequence of events occurs in the one-kidney Goldblatt model.[278] There is a prompt increase in arterial blood pressure and an increase in plasma renin activity. During the chronic phase, hypertension persists and there is sodium retention. The sodium retention depresses renin release, and plasma renin levels return to the normal range but are slightly elevated compared with those in control nonclipped rats. The use of an angiotensin antagonist or a converting enzyme inhibitor can prevent the occurrence of hypertension early after the experimental lesion is produced, but neither is persistently effective. However, blood pressure can be reduced by inhibiting angII action if the rats are first given a low-sodium diet. The hypertension can be reversed in the chronic phase by removal of the renal artery constriction, which is accompanied by a negative sodium balance that correlates with the drop in blood pressure. Although the increase in renin activity is the primary initiating event, other factors (most likely the sodium retention) participate more in the maintenance of the hypertension. This model may be useful for understanding chronic renovascular hypertension in humans. The hypertension in this state can become volume-dependent, possibly as a result of chronic hypertensive changes in the nonstenotic kidney. The hypertension during this phase in humans is not responsive to correction of the stenosis.

Two transgenic animal models illustrate differences in the ways in which the renin-angiotensin system can generate hypertension. In a chimeric mouse model, hypertension results from the hypersecretion of human renin and angiotensinogen in the circulation.[279] Transgenic rats that overexpress the mouse renin gene in multiple tissues were discussed previously. These animals have fulminant angII-dependent hypertension[280,281] with low levels of plasma renin activity, circulating angII, and kidney renin mRNA, and high levels of plasma prorenin, adrenal renin, and plasma aldosterone. In these animals, the mouse renin gene is expressed primarily in the rat adrenal, which hypersecretes prorenin and mineralocorticoids. Adrenal-derived renin is thought to mediate the hypertension, which is lowered by treatment with converting enzyme inhibitors. This model demonstrates the role of a tissue renin angiotensin system, i.e., the adrenal, in the development and maintenance of hypertension.

Renin-Secreting Tumors

As described in the section on renovascular hypertension, there are rare renin-secreting tumors.[282,283] These tumors result in severe hypertension, hypokalemia, hyperreninemia, and markedly elevated prorenin levels. They are generally associated with the ovary or adrenal gland.

Human Renovascular Hypertension

In human renovascular hypertension, renal ischemia and hypoperfusion resulting from renal artery lesions lead to excessive renin release, with consequences similar to those in animals.[277] The overall results depend on the severity of the lesions and the functional capacity of both the contralateral kidney and the involved kidney. Functional capacity depends on both the extent of preceding renal impairment and hypertension-induced changes.[284] Plasma renin levels can be high, normal, or even low-normal and are determined by the degree of stimulus induced by the ischemic kidney and the extent to which subsequent sodium retention suppresses renin levels. Sodium retention is greatly affected by the functional capacity of the kidneys. Thus, when human renovascular hypertension occurs in the absence of a severe impairment in renal function, the hemodynamic and hormonal profile resembles more that of the two-kidney model, whereas with major impairment in renal function, there can be sodium dependency of the hypertension similar to that which occurs with the one-kidney model. This heterogeneity of clinical presentation accounts for some of the problems in the diagnosis and management of renovascular hypertension.

Accelerated Hypertension

Accelerated hypertension is characterized by marked elevation of blood pressure, decreased renal function, and severe retinopathy. Renin levels are usually extremely high and result in secondary aldosteronism.[285,286] Activation of the renin system in these patients is due predominately to altered renal hemodynamics that result in ischemia. This activation enhances further the vasoconstriction and arterial hypertension. Patients with chronic renal failure are particularly susceptible to this form of hypertension, and an increased blood volume usually aggravates the condition. This renin-dependent form of accelerated hypertension occurs in a small subgroup of hypertensive patients and is an acute disorder that requires immediate treatment.

Essential Hypertension

The renin-angiotension system appears to participate in the pathogenesis of essential hypertension. Genetic polymorphisms of angiotensinogen are associated with elevated blood pressure. As shown in Fig. 13-5, plasma renin levels show considerable variation as a function of urinary sodium excretion in patients with essential hypertension (a reflection of sodium intake) in comparison to normal subjects. This type of comparison has been the basis for classifying patients as having low-, normal-, or high-renin essential hypertension.

Normal and High-Renin Essential Hypertension The presence of normal or high plasma renin levels in essential hypertension could be taken as an abnormality, as the expected response to an elevation of blood pressure would be suppression of the plasma renin

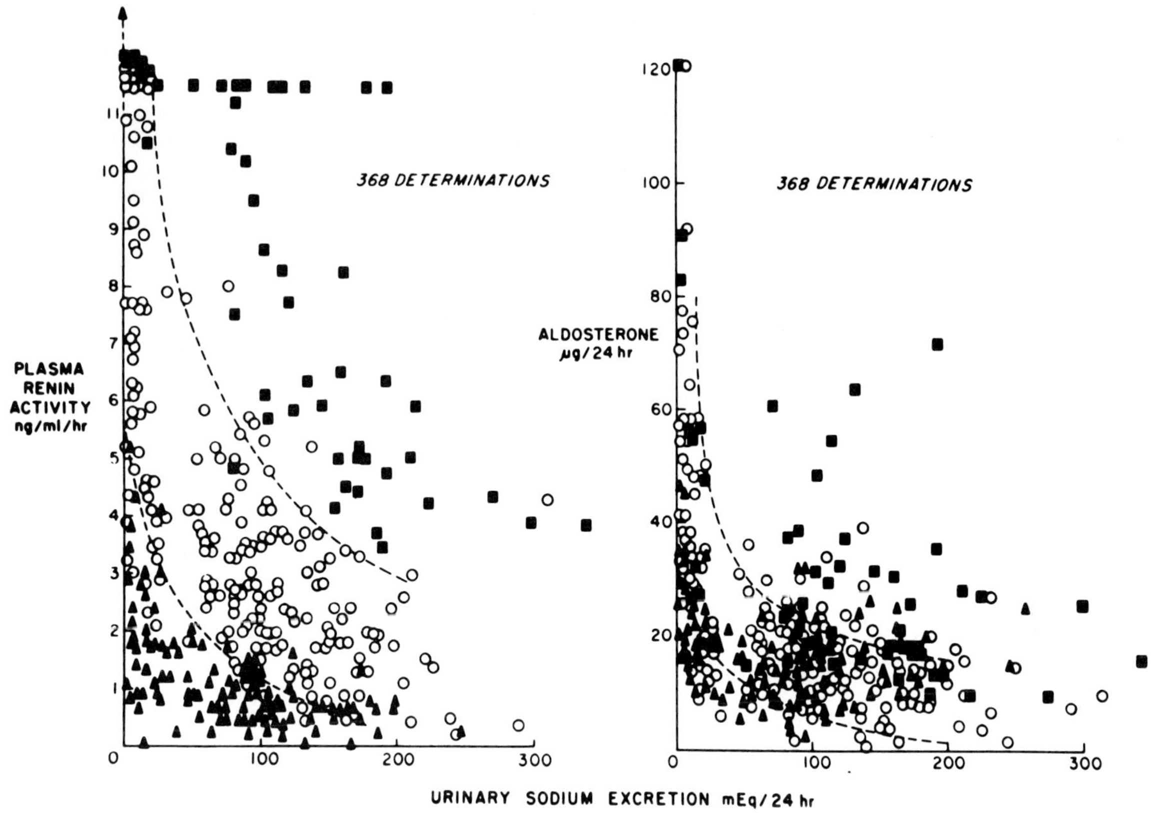

FIGURE 13-5. Plasma renin activity measured at noon after 4 h upright (*left*) and corresponding daily urinary aldosterone excretion (*right*) plotted against the concurrent daily rate of sodium excretion in 219 patients with essential hypertension. Plasma renin activity levels are indicated by triangles for low, open circles for normal, and squares for high activity. Values for 52 normal individuals are represented by the dotted line. In some cases, individual points fall outside the indicated classification. This is due to the fact that repeated samples in these patients mostly fall into another category. (*From Brunner et al.*[118])

activity. "Abnormally normal" or elevated plasma renin levels have been attributed to a primary renal abnormality with heterogeneity of the nephrons.[40] In this abnormality, some nephrons are proposed to oversecrete renin because of vasospasm, whereas in others, there is more dilatation with glomerular hyperfiltration. Renal biopsy data showing heterogeneity in afferent arteriolar narrowing support this model.[40] In essence, these patients are proposed to have a microform of renovascular hypertension. In addition, activity of the adrenergic nervous system is enhanced in essential hypertension; this would stimulate renin release and contribute to inappropriate levels of plasma renin.[287] The utility of this classification is its relationship to target organ damage. Patients with high renin hypertension have twofold increases in myocardial infarction and stroke compared to those with normal renin, who have twofold increases compared to those with low renin.[11]

Low-Renin Essential Hypertension The low-renin subgroup (Fig. 13-5) includes approximately 5 to 15 percent of patients with essential hypertension, depending on the study group.[40,288] The condition is more common in blacks and may be present in up to 50 percent of elderly patients.[40,289] These patients have salt-sensitive hypertension, a tendency toward sodium retention, blunted catecholamine responses to provocative stimuli, abnormal sensitivity to angII, and possible ion transport abnormalities.[40,288,289] The existence of low plasma renin activity in essential hypertension could reflect an attempt by the body to adapt to the hypertension. The idea is supported by findings of an inverse correlation between blood pressure and plasma renin activity in hypertensive and normotensive persons[39,40,289] and the fact that borderline hypertensive patients have greater variations in plasma renin levels than do age-matched normotensive control subjects.[290] In the normotensive offspring of hypertensive parents, there tend to be lower levels of plasma renin activity and aldosterone, with increased renal vasoconstriction, compared to the offspring of normotensive parents.[34] Although patients with low-renin essential hypertension show reduced blood pressure–lowering responses to converting enzyme inhibition compared to normal-renin and high-renin hypertensives,[40,274] these patients do respond to some extent. The responses observed in low-renin patients may be due to the fact that they are more sensitive to the low levels of circulating angII that are present than are normal-renin hypertensives (also discussed later).[274] Alternatively, the responses could reflect participation of extrarenal renin-angiotensin systems in the hypertension (discussed earlier).

The abnormal sensitivity to angII in patients with low-renin essential hypertension is observed in both the adrenal and the kidney.[10,288] In normal subjects, the response of the adrenal glomerulosa to angII varies with the level of sodium intake; sodium restriction enhances the response, while a high sodium intake enhances the renal blood flow response.[10,288,291] In patients with low-renin essential hypertension, the normally reduced response of aldosterone release to angII on a high-salt diet do not occur, and these individuals release angII that induces an inappropriately enhanced aldosterone release.[10,288] This leads to lower plasma renin levels and a tendency toward sodium retention.

The putative ion-transport abnormalities in low-renin patients involve either a Ca^{2+} leak or impaired cell membrane Ca^{2+} pumping activity.[292,293] The effect of the abnormality is to elevate intracellular [Ca^{2+}] and lower serum [Ca^{2+}] levels and to enhance blood pressure responses to calcium-channel blockers and dietary calcium supplementation (see also the section on Ca^{2+} and hypertension).[40,293] Such a defect could simultaneously affect the blood pressure and the adrenal glomerulosa response to angII.

Patients with low-renin essential hypertension do not have hypokalemia and elevated plasma and/or urinary aldosterone levels and thus differ from those with primary aldosteronism and hypokalemia, as described in the section on primary aldosteronism. However, there may be only a quantitative distinction between low-renin essential hypertension and primary aldosteronism with hyperplasia. The normal plasma aldosterone levels in patients with low-renin essential hypertension are high relative to the suppressed plasma renin levels. Thus, these patients have high plasma aldosterone/renin ratios. Their inappropriately high aldosterone levels are due to enhanced adrenal sensitivity to angII, an abnormality also present in primary aldosteronism with hyperplasia. Aldosterone and plasma renin responses to posture and other stimuli in patients with low-renin essential hypertension also resemble primary aldosteronism with hyperplasia. In fact, some patients with low-renin essential hypertension do have primary aldosteronism, as many patients with the latter disorder can have normal plasma aldosterone levels and be normokalemic. However, the proportion of low-renin hypertensive patients with occult primary aldosteronism has not been determined.

Modulators and Nonmodulators Another categorization of hypertension is modulating and nonmodulating essential hypertension, as reflected by certain abnormalities of the renin-angiotensin-aldosterone axis (Fig. 13-5).[10,288,294,295] Unlike the case with normotensives and modulating hypertensive patients, nonmodulating patients display a failure of renal blood flow to increase in response to salt loading, leading to a reduced ability to excrete a salt load, reduced responsiveness of renin and aldosterone release (in response to angII), and impaired responsiveness of ANP release. The plasma aldosterone levels in nonmodulating patients tend to be lower than those in other patients. This results in a normal to high plasma renin level. The sodium sensitivity of their blood pressures appears to arise from the sodium-dependent changes in renal blood flow mediated by endogenous angII. The abnormalities in the nonmodulators are corrected by the administration of converting enzyme inhibitors or calcium-channel blocking agents. These classes of drugs therefore constitute a specific form of therapy in these patients. As in other salt-sensitive hypertensives, nonmodulators typically have a strong family history of hypertension. They also tend to have an increase in erythrocyte Na^+-Li^+ countertransport. It has been argued that this may be the most common form of hypertension, although at present the classification of modulators vs. nonmodulators is cumbersome and restricted to research use.

Mineralocorticoids

Adrenal glucocorticoids and mineralocorticoids have been implicated in hypertension (Fig. 13-6). Glucocorticoids and mineralocorticoids are described in Chap. 11. An excess of mineralocorticoid activity can cause hypertension, and aldosterone, deoxycorticosterone (DOC), and cortisol can all lead to a mineralocorticoid excess state. Glucocorticoids can also elevate the blood pressure through mineralocorticoid receptor–independent mechanisms, as discussed in the following section. Other adrenal steroids may be capable of elevating blood pressure, but it is not known whether they contribute to human disease.

The identification of aldosterone as a mineralocorticoid that can cause hypertension was made in 1955 by Conn, who described primary aldosteronism.[296] In 1956, Eberlein and Bongiovanni identified the tetrahydro metabolite of DOC in patients with

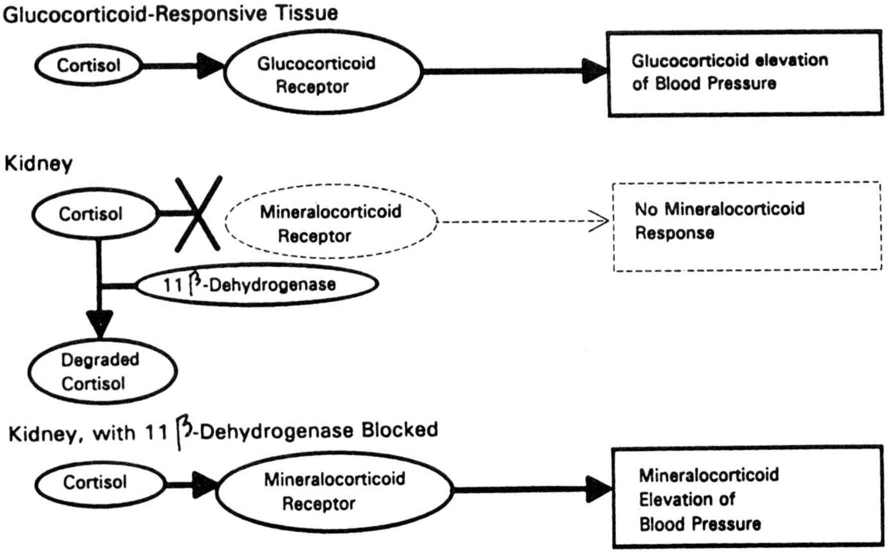

FIGURE 13-6. Actions of glucocorticoids and mineralocorticoids on the blood pressure. Glucocorticoids can elevate the blood pressure by binding to the glucocorticoid receptor. Cortisol exhibits major actions through the mineralocorticoid receptors in the kidney when its degradation is blocked. 11β-Dehydrogenase = 11β-hydroxysteroid dehydrogenase.

11β-hydroxylase deficiency.[297] Further evidence that DOC excess can lead to hypertension was reported in 1966 with the discovery of the 17α-hydroxylase syndrome.[298]

Steroids with Mineralocorticoid Activity

Aldosterone

Aldosterone is the major mineralocorticoid in humans. Regulation of synthesis and release and states of deficiency and secondary excess of aldosterone are discussed in Chap. 11. The hormone is released in response to posture or fluid loss to conserve sodium and to protect against hyperkalemia. In contrast to cortisol, aldosterone probably is not critical for maintenance of blood pressure in the sodium-replete state under normal circumstances. However, in children with mineralocorticoid deficiency and in salt-deprived adults, the sodium-retaining actions of the steroid can be critical for maintaining blood pressure. Administration of mineralocorticoids without concomitant glucocorticoid replacement does not ameliorate the hypotension in Addison's disease.

Aldosterone excess can result from primary aldosteronism (see the section on primary aldosteronism) or from secondary causes (see Chap. 11). Whereas hypersecretion of aldosterone in primary aldosteronism results in hypertension, the steroid usually does not cause hypertension in most cases of secondary aldosterone excess, such as cirrhosis and heart failure. In those states, elevations of the steroid occur in response to a perceived decrease in intravascular volume. Aldosterone excess can also occur with renin-producing tumors, renovascular hypertension, high-renin essential hypertension, and accelerated hypertension, and in these cases it aggravates the hypertension (see the discussion on the role of the renin-angiotensin system in hypertension).

Mineralocorticoid Actions of Cortisol and Other Steroids with Glucocorticoid Activity

Cortisol and other steroids with glucocorticoid activity can act as mineralocorticoids by binding to the mineralocorticoid receptor (Fig. 13-6) (see also Chap. 11).[299–302] The affinity of cortisol for the mineralocorticoid receptor is about 10 percent that of aldosterone, although some recent studies suggest the mineralocorticoid receptor can be equally activated by aldosterone and cortisol. Cortisol circulates at approximately 1,000-fold higher total concentration than does aldosterone. Thus, at levels in the normal range, cortisol would ordinarily be expected to occupy the mineralocorticoid receptor instead of aldosterone and to cause a mineralocorticoid-excess state. However, at least two mechanisms prevent this from happening in the kidney (see also Chap. 11).[299–302] First, cortisol is about 92 percent bound to plasma proteins, whereas only about 50 percent of the aldosterone is so bound. Thus, the free concentrations of cortisol are only about 200-fold those of aldosterone, and the effective concentration would be only about 20-fold higher based on the relative receptor-binding affinities of the two steroids. Cortisol access to the mineralocorticoid receptor in the kidney also may be restricted by sequestering of the steroid by renal intracellular cortisol-binding proteins. Second, in epithelial aldosterone target tissues like the kidney, 11β-hydroxysteroid dehydrogenase degrades cortisol to the inactive metabolite cortisone by converting the 11β-OH group of cortisol (and other steroids) to a keto group (Fig. 13-6).[299–302] The hemiacetyl group of aldosterone, which links its 11- and 19-positions, prevents the enzyme from degrading aldosterone. In some tissues, however, such as brain, this enzyme is not as active, and cortisol can have greater actions through the mineralocorticoid receptors. Thus, cortisol and other glucocorticoids can apparently elicit potent mineralocorticoid activities only when they are present in sufficient excess to overwhelm 11β-hydroxysteroid dehydrogenase or when this enzyme is blocked. The former mechanism may occur in patients with severe Cushing's syndrome, in the syndrome of primary glucocorticoid resistance (associated with hypertension and hyperandrogenism), or with glucocorticoid antagonist treatment when the body produces large quantities of cortisol to overcome the resistance to glucocorticoid suppression of ACTH (see the section on other low-renin hypertension syndromes later).[303,304] However, the mineralocorticoid excess could also be due to deoxycorticosterone (DOC), which is usually produced in excess in these states (see the section on other low-renin hypertension syndromes). Defective function of 11β-hydroxysteroid dehydrogenase resulting in a cortisol-induced mineralocorticoid-excess state is observed after ingestion of licorice containing glycerolitic acid or carbenoxolone which blocks the enzyme, or in a rare syndrome of apparent mineralocorticoid excess.[300,301,305–307]

Deoxycorticosterone

DOC is as potent as aldosterone in eliciting mineralocorticoid responses, but its free concentrations in plasma are normally too low to contribute substantially to plasma mineralocorticoid activity (Chap. 11). Exogenous DOC can lead to hypertension in animal models of hypertension and in humans.[308–311] Secretion of DOC is predominantly under ACTH control. States in which DOC produces mineralocorticoid-excess hypertension are described in the section on DOC-excess hypertension. These states occur with adrenal enzymatic defects, in some patients with Cushing's syndrome, and in rare patients with predominantly DOC-secreting tumors.

19-Nor-Deoxycorticosterone (19-Nor-DOC)

19-Nor-DOC is produced in the adrenals, the kidney, and aldosterone-producing adenomas from precursors synthesized in the adrenal and has mineralocorticoid activity equivalent to that of aldosterone.[308,312] Its adrenal production is regulated by ACTH.[312] It has not been detected in normal plasma,[271] but elevated levels of urinary 19-nor-DOC have been found in three rat models of hypertension[308] and in the plasma of patients with aldosterone-producing adenomas.[312] Thus, this steroid is a candidate for contributing to mineralocorticoid action in primary aldosteronism, although its importance is unknown.

Other Steroids

Several other steroids have mineralocorticoid activity, including 18-hydroxydeoxycorticosterone (18-OH-DOC), 18-hydroxycorticosterone (18-OHB), 19-nor-DOC, 18-oxo-cortisol, 18-OH-cortisol, and 18-deoxy-19-noraldosterone. 18-OH-DOC, 18-OHB, 18-oxo-cortisol, and 18-OH-cortisol have weak mineralocorticoid activity. 18-OH-DOC production is predominantly under ACTH control (Chap. 11), and its levels are elevated in ACTH-excess states.[308] Given the weak activities and low levels of 18-OH-DOC and 18-OHB, these steroids are unlikely to contribute to known mineralocorticoid-excess states.[313] 18-Deoxy-19-noraldosterone has potent mineralocorticoid antagonist activity and is synthesized in both normal and adenomatous adrenal tissue,[314] and the aldosterone metabolites dihydroaldosterone and tetrahydroaldosterone can elevate the blood pressure in rats[315]; however, the importance of these steroids is not documented.

Mechanisms of Mineralocorticoid Elevation of Blood Pressure

Mineralocorticoids regulate ion transport in secretory tissues, such as sweat glands, salivary glands, kidney, and intestinal tract, and possibly in arterial walls (see Chap. 11). These actions promote Na^+ reabsorption and secretion of K^+ and H^+.[316,317] The effects of mineralocorticoids on the kidney are quantitatively the greatest.

Mineralocorticoid excess leads to sodium retention, increased extracellular fluid volume, and increased total body sodium content. The changes are reflected by normal or elevated serum sodium ion concentrations and a reduced hematocrit.[318] The increased extracellular fluid volume suppresses plasma renin levels and abolishes the usual parallel relations between renin and aldosterone.[319] Sodium and fluid overload are essential for the initiation of mineralocorticoid hypertension,[320] although this may not be the sole mechanism.[321] Continued sodium retention increases the intracellular sodium content in tissues.[322] Excess intracellular Na^+ increases intracellular [Ca^{2+}], which enhances vascular reactivity (see the section on Ca^{2+} and hypertension later). These changes can further elevate the blood pressure. However, in some studies, intracellular [Ca^{2+}] was not found to be elevated in the platelets of patients with primary aldosteronism.[323]

Mineralocorticoid excess also leads to a depletion of potassium and magnesium. Potassium depletion results in hypokalemia, alkalosis, increased ammonia production,[324] decreased carbohydrate tolerance, and resistance to vasopressin (nephrogenic diabetes insipidus). Depletion of K^+ also causes diminished adrenergic nervous system activity, decreased catecholamine levels, abnormalities in baroreceptor functions, and postural falls in blood pressure without reflex tachycardia.[325] Baroreceptor function may also be more directly affected by aldosterone.[326] These influences enhance blood pressure dependency on intravascular volume and decrease dependency on the nervous system. Hypokalemia also creates a special problem with diuretic therapy in these patients; such therapy can precipitously lower both the blood pressure and serum K^+ concentrations to dangerously low levels. Severe hypokalemia can also lead to renal damage with scarring and the development of renal cysts.[327] The hypomagnesemia increases vascular activity (see also the section on magnesium) and perpetuates the hypertension. Mineralocorticoids can increase ouabain-sensitive Na^+-K^+-ATPase activity.[328]

A period of weeks to months is required for mineralocorticoid hypertension to develop. Short-term administration of large amounts of mineralocorticoids to normotensive subjects has modest effects on blood pressure, even though the mineralocorticoid promotes sodium retention.[329,330] The time course of the development of mineralocorticoid hypertension can be observed after withdrawal of spironolactone therapy in patients with primary aldosteronism whose blood pressures have been normalized with the drug.[330] When this antimineralocorticoid therapy is withdrawn, these patients begin to retain sodium and gain weight until the usual mineralocorticoid "escape" occurs, and they develop progressive renal potassium wasting. Their blood pressures increase only gradually over a period of weeks. The hypertension is sodium- and volume-dependent, but sodium restriction does not prevent it.[330] Thus, more slowly developing events in the arteriole, such as intracellular changes in ionic concentrations or other effects on vascular reactivity, must also take place to produce the sustained elevated blood pressure of long-term mineralocorticoid administration.

With the development of sustained hypertension, as with all forms of hypertension, the body apparently attempts to compensate by decreasing the plasma volume. Thus, even though the increased level of exchangeable sodium and extracellular fluid volume persists, patients with long-established hypertension can have normal blood volumes.[322] Under these circumstances, the hypertension may be due to a large extent to the increased peripheral vascular resistance with normal cardiac output.[321,322] Nevertheless, even in this circumstance, continued mineralocorticoid actions contribute to the hypertensive state: removal of an adenoma or treatment of hyperplasia with mineralocorticoid antagonists can ameliorate the hypertension. The hypertension can progress to a malignant phase and stimulate the kidney to release renin, resulting in a "high-renin" primary aldosteronism state.[331]

Mineralocorticoid excess also may have direct effects on organs. It can induce fibrosis in the myocardium and other tissues in excess of that expected from the hypertension alone; this can cause myocardial stiffness, cardiac hypertrophy, and cardiac arythmias.[332,333]

Glucocorticoids

The natural glucocorticoid, cortisol, and the synthetic steroids used in glucocorticoid therapy can elevate the blood pressure through their actions as glucocorticoids. These effects are independent of any mineralocorticoid activities of these steroids. Circumstances in which cortisol can cause mineralocorticoid-excess hypertension through mineralocorticoid-receptor interactions are discussed earlier and in the section on the other low-renin hypertension syndromes. The importance of glucocorticoids in maintaining normal blood pressure is demonstrated by the hypotension that occurs in adrenal insufficiency; this is correctable with glucocorticoid but not mineralocorticoid replacement (see Chap. 11).

Clinical features of hypertension in patients with spontaneous and iatrogenic Cushing's syndrome are described in the section on Cushing's syndrome. Most patients with spontaneous Cushing's syndrome have hypertension without the stigmata of frank mineralocorticoid excess.[309,334,335] It is thought that the glucocorticoid actions of cortisol in this condition are predominantly responsible for the hypertension. Additional evidence for blood pressure–elevating actions of glucocorticoids is derived from studies of responses to administered steroids. Synthetic glucocorticoids such as prednisolone, methylprednisolone, triamcinolone, and dexamethasone have much lower relative mineralocorticoid activity than does cortisol (see Chaps. 11 and 14) but can all increase the blood pressure. However, in short-term experiments, the effects are modest.[336] Estimates of the incidence of hypertension in patients treated with glucocorticoids have ranged from 17 to 69 percent.[335,337,338] The lower range of these values is not very different from the incidence of hypertension in the general population of around 20 percent.[1,2] Because hypertension in spontaneous Cushing's syndrome may be aggravated by mineralocorticoid actions of the cortisol excess, the overall influences of glucocorticoids in causing hypertension may be modest.

Glucocorticoids can increase blood pressure by acting through mineralocorticoid receptors (i.e., apparent mineralocorticoid excess) and through mineralocorticoid-independent mechanisms.[335–345] Nonmineralocorticoid actions include glucocorticoid-mediated increases in plasma angiotensinogen[335] and prorenin levels.[336] These effects may explain why plasma renin levels are not suppressed in Cushings' syndrome[335] and why hypertension in this syndrome responds well to converting enzyme inhibition.[335] Additional actions include reduced production of prostaglandins or components of the kallikrein-kinin system,[336] decreased vascular production of nitric oxide (NO),[345] and increased pressor responses to angII and norepinephrine.[337] Glucocorticoid-induced hypertension[335-339] is associated with increased cardiac output and forearm vascular responsively to norepinephrine. Glucorticoids also increase sodium retention[340] and increase Na^+ and Ca^{2+} influx into vascular smooth muscle cells.[341,344]

Estrogens, Progestins, and Androgens

Men have higher blood pressures than women at younger ages, with a crossover in which women have higher pressures in the fourth to sixth decades.[1] There are no known sex differences in children. These studies raise the issue of the role of sex steroids in hypertension.

Little is known regarding the role of testosterone in hypertension in humans. In spontaneously hypertensive rats, genetic studies have linked the Y chromosome to hypertension.[345] Castration results in a lower blood pressure. Androgen-resistant animals have lower blood pressures than controls but have higher levels than females. Thus, both androgen action and other factors could be contributory.

Most women receiving oral contraceptives experience a small but detectable increase in blood pressure within the normal range.[1] A few women also experience blood pressure rises when estrogen replacement is initiated.[1] Hypertension is more common in women who have taken contraceptives for several years, and this incidence increases with the duration of use.[1] The mechanisms are not clear.[1] Estrogens can have vasodilatory actions in pregnancy and other conditions; these actions are probably due to estrogen-mediated effects on prostacyclin synthesis.[330,331] Estrogens can also increase the levels of angiotensinogen[161] and nitric oxide synthetase.[346,347] Progestin only preparations are not known to cause hypertension.[348]

Thyroid Hormone

Abnormalities in blood pressure occur in both hyperthyroidism and hypothyroidism. In hyperthyroidism, diastolic pressure may be decreased but systolic pressure is typically either increased or normal.[348,349] Hypothyroidism has been associated with diastolic hypertension.

Systolic hypertension with hyperthyroidism is due to increased cardiac stroke volume, whereas the decreased diastolic pressure is due to peripheral vasodilation. The increased cardiac stroke volume is probably due to direct thyroid hormone actions on the heart. Thyroid hormone excess can enhance cardiac β-adrenergic responsiveness and probably has other direct effects on tension development and shortening velocity.[348] Mechanisms for decreased diastolic pressure in hyperthyroidism are less well understood; increases in metabolism or Na^+-K^+-ATPase may enhance vasodilator mechanisms in peripheral tissues.

The incidence of hypertension in patients with hypothyroidism has been difficult to document. In a survey of 688 consecutive hypertensive outpatients, 3.6 percent were found to be hypothyroid.[350] The blood pressures decreased in these patients with replacement thyroid hormone, suggesting a cause-and-effect relation. These data suggest that hypothyroidism may be one of the most common causes of secondary hypertension. Conversely, when the incidence of hypertension in patients with hypothyroidism is compared with that in the general population, an increased incidence is not evident. Changes with hypothyroidism are the converse of those with hyperthyroidism.There is increased vasoconstriction and decreased stroke volume. Patients with hypothyroidism also tend to have decreased plasma renin activity and angiotensinogen levels[348,350] and increased arginine vasopressin (AVP) levels. The significance of these changes is not known.

Vasopressin

Arginine vasopressin (AVP) is a hormone peptide that functions to regulate water balance in the kidney, but is also a potent vasoconstrictor. The peptide acts on two classes of receptors, V_1 and V_2, that have different modes of action. The V_1 type a receptors, V_{1a}, appear to mediate blood pressure and increase peripheral vascular resistance due to a direct vasopressor effect. This property has been beneficial in symptomatic improvement of orthostatic hypotension.[351] Increases in plasma levels of AVP have also been demonstrated in patients with essential hypertension and animal models of hypertension.[352,353] In chronic excess, AVP does not result in sustained hypertension in experimental animal models or in humans.[354] This illustrates the fact that while the fluid-retaining properties of AVP may lead to a rise in blood pressure, the phenomenon of "vasopressin escape" prevents the effects from remaining sustained.[356]

Erythropoietin

The anemia in patients with chronic renal failure can be partially corrected by treatment with recombinant human erythropoietin (rHuEPO). The additional benefits associated with the use of rHuEPO are numerous and include improvements in quality of life, cognitive function, exercise ability, and cardiovascular function. However, systemic hypertension can develop or become worse in 20–50 percent of patients on rHuEPO, particularly when given intravenously. In the event of an acute elevation in blood pressure, hypertensive encephalopathy, which may be associated with seizures, may occur.[357]

The cause of the rise in blood pressure, which can be seen within 2–4 weeks of starting therapy, is still not clear.[357] However, several risk factors that contribute to the development of the induced hypertension have been identified. They include preexisting hypertension,[358,359,360,361,362] a rapid rise in hematocrit,[363,364] a relatively low initial hematocrit before the start of rHuEPO treatment,[365] enhanced responsiveness to norepinephrine, intravenous administration of rHuEPO, a high dose of rHuEPO, and the presence of native kidneys.[362]

A number of mechanisms have been proposed that might contribute to the development of hypertension such as increased blood viscosity, loss of hypoxic vasodilatation, and activation of neurohumoral system. Although a direct vascular effect has also been suggested, so far no one has been able to prove that direct or indirect vasoconstriction occurs via increased cellular calcium uptake or increased endothelin-1 release.

Some simple preventive measures can be exercised that may decrease the incidence of hypertension associated with rHuEPO.

For example, the hematocrit should be increased gradually to the 30–35 percent range.[366] This target hematocrit range should achieve adequate symptomatic improvement but not significant elevation in blood pressure. Medical treatment for the hypertension should include the use of beta blockers and vasodilators, as well as sufficient fluid removal in patients on dialysis.

Growth Hormone

Patients with acromegaly usually have hypertension (Chap. 7), and growth hormone-deficient adults treated with growth hormone can develop hypertension and fluid retention.[367] Growth hormone-deficient children treated with growth hormone generally do not develop hypertension but can have transient blood pressure elevation and some fluid retention.[368] The mechanisms are unknown. Growth hormone excess causes insulin resistance, but the transient blood pressure-elevating actions of growth hormone in children precede insulin resistance.[368] Growth hormone treatment has also been reported to increase the activity of the renin-angiotensin-aldosterone axis in adults,[367] but this has not been observed in children.[368] There is no evidence implicating growth hormone in the pathogenesis of essential hypertension.

Calcitonin Gene-Related Peptide

Calcitonin gene-related peptide (CGRP) has potent vasodilator actions and can lower blood pressure in humans and animals.[369,370] CGRP is produced in the CNS, and peripheral nerves in the vascular wall, and its receptors are widely distributed in the CNS and the cardiovascular system. The peptide can also increase urinary volume and sodium excretion, inhibit angII-mediated contraction of renal mesangial cells, and increase renal blood flow and glomerular filtration. Thus, it could be an important component of the vasodilatory system. Little is known about its potential function in hypertension. Measurements of the blood levels of the peptide, which may not reflect the hormone's autocrine or paracrine functions, have shown conflicting results, with elevations or depressions of the levels in essential hypertension, for example. CGRP levels have been reported to increase with calcium supplementation and lowering of the blood pressure in patients with essential hypertension, leading to speculation that the peptide could be involved in the hypotensive effects of calcium supplementation.[370]

Endothelin

The vascular endothelium produces both vasoconstrictor and vasodilator substances. In general the vasodilators prevent interactions of the endothelium with circulating cells that lead to inflammation and thrombosis and inhibit growth and migration of underlying vascular smooth muscle cells. Nitric oxide, NO, the most well-known vasodilator, is also an antioxidant. The vasoconstrictors include angII, the endothelins, and others. They tend to promote inflammation, thrombosis, proliferation and migration of vascular smooth muscle cells, and oxidation.

The endothelins are a family of three peptides with extremely potent and sustained vasoconstrictor and vasopressor actions.[371–372] Infused endothelin induces transient vasodilation, followed by a profound and long-lasting increase in blood pressure. These peptides also potentiate the actions of vasopressors such as catecholamines, stimulate sympathetic tone, and induce the release of vasopressin and epinephrine. They also have proliferative effects on vascular smooth muscle and renal mesangial cells. Their actions can be inhibited by cGMP produced in response to vasodilators such as nitrous oxide and ANP.

Endothelin-1 predominates in the vascular endothelium and is generated from proendothelin-1 through the actions of a unique neutral metalloprotease, "endothelin-converting enzyme."[371,372] It is the most potent vasoconstrictor yet found. Certain vasoconstrictor substances, angII, catecholamines and vasopressin, and ouabain-like factors can increase endothelin production, and their actions may be mediated in part through endothelin. Hypoxia, ischemia, and insulin also stimulate endothelin. Endothelin appears to act predominantly in a paracrine manner and its release is mainly abluminal.

There are at least two distinct endothelin receptor subtypes.[373] The ET_A receptor is preferentially activated by endothelin-1, highly expressed in vascular smooth muscle, and the major receptor subtype that causes vasoconstriction. Binding of endothelin with this receptor activates phosphoinositide hydrolysis and/or calcium channels. The ET_B receptor is activated equally by all three endothelin subtypes and is present on the luminal surface of endothelial cells, where it mediates release of endothelium-dependent vasodilator substances including NO, ANP, and prostacyclins. It is also present in smooth muscle in some tissues, where it participates in vasoconstrictor actions. The existence of the ET_C subtype remains controversial. Specific endothelin receptor antagonists can inhibit pressure responses to the peptide.

The potential of endothelin to cause hypertension is suggested by the rare occurrence of hemangioendotheliomas.[373] These tumors release large amounts of endothelin into the circulation, and patients with these tumors have profound hypertension. Removal of the tumor ameloriates the hypertension and lowers plasma endothelin levels.

A role for endothelin in essential hypertension is suggested by the observation that the ET_A/ET_B antagonist, bosenten, reduced blood pressure of essential hypertensive patients equally to enalapril.[374] Although plasma concentrations of endothelin are not elevated in patients with essential hypertension,[371,372] they are elevated in conditions associated with vasoconstriction, such as heart failure, pulmonary hypertension, vasospastic disorders (Raynaud's disease, Prinzmetal's angina), and myocardial infarction. Increased tissue concentrations of and/or binding sites for endothelin-1 have been found in sustained cerebral vasospasm after subarachnoid hemmorhage. Circulating endothelin levels can be elevated with renal failure, atherosclerosis, severe hypertension with end organ complications, and disseminated intravascular coagulation. Bosentan improved hemodynamics in heart failure and primary pulmonary hyperensin and thus, may have widespread therapeutic implications in various vascular diseases.[375] In addition, cyclosporin-induced hypertension may be mediated in part through endothelin release.[371] Cyclosporin A increases plasma levels of endothelin and increases endothelin release from cells in culture. Endothelin receptor antagonists protect against cyclosporin toxicity in the rat renal circulation.

Nitric Oxide (Endothelium-Derived Releasing Factor)

The endothelium is important for vasodilator responses and is necessary for the vasodilator actions of bradykinin and acetylcholine. The endothelium releases relaxing factors termed endothelium-de-

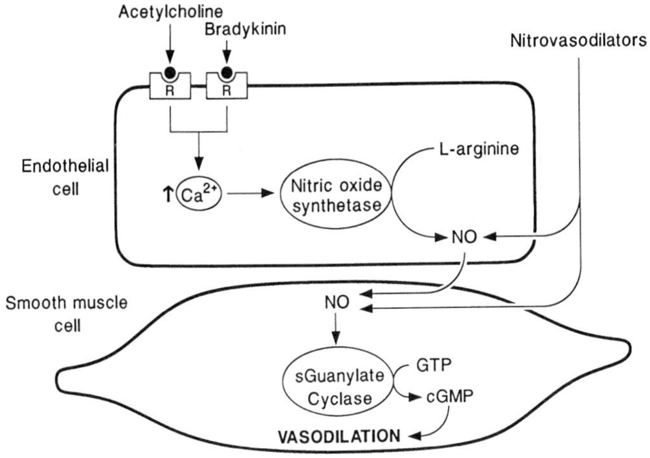

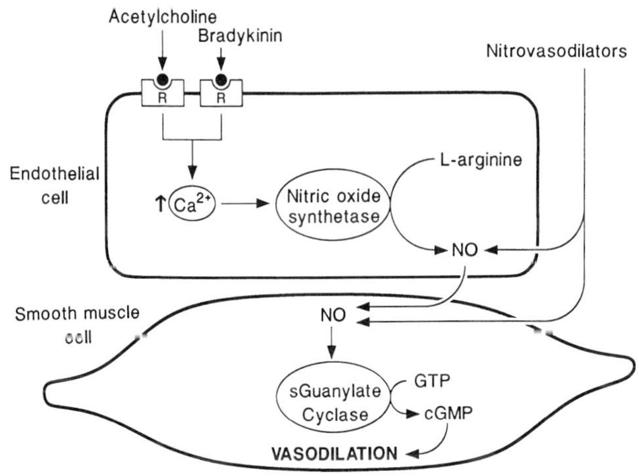

FIGURE 13-7. Synthesis and actions of nitric oxide (NO). s = soluble. The arrow next to the Ca^{2+} indicates that bradykinin and acetylcholine increase intracellar Ca^{2+}. Cytokines can induce Ca^{2+}-independent NO synthetase, and this can be blocked by glucocorticoids (not shown). (*From Moncada and Higgs.*[332])

rived relaxing factors (EDRFs). The major EDRF appears to be nitric oxide (NO), a water-soluble gas. EDRF is responsible for the vasodilator tone that is essential for the regulation of blood pressure[347] (Fig. 13-7). The molecule also regulates a number of other diverse functions, including neurotransmitter, platelet aggregation, gastrointestinal, genitourinary, respiratory, inflammatory, and immunologic processes,[347] as well as renin release[127] and cardiac hypertrophy.[128] Endogenously produced NO appears to act predominantly in a paracrine or autocrine manner.

All known NO actions are mediated by the activation of soluble guanylate cyclase. NO binds directly to a heme prosthetic group of this enzyme. Actions of the cGMP formed directly induce vasorelaxation and inhibit the production of other vasoconstrictor substances such as endothelin.[376]

Nitric oxide is produced by nitric oxide synthetases from L-arginine.[185,347] There are at least three different enzymes. A major form of the enzyme is constitutive, and its activity is dependent on calcium and calmodulin. This enzyme is activated by acetylcholine and bradykinin, which increase intracellular Ca^{2+}. Other forms are inducible, for example, with cytokines; this induction can be blocked by glucocorticoids. Estrogens can induce nitric oxide synthetase. Most of the NO is released from the vascular endothelium, although there can be some release from nonadrenergic, noncholinergic terminals. The actions of nitric oxide are mimicked by compounds such as nitroglycerin and sodium nitroprusside, which are converted to nitric oxide.

Competitive inhibitors of nitric oxide synthetase, such as N^G-monomethyl-L-arginine, have been useful for studying the role of NO in blood pressure control. These inhibitors are potent vasoconstrictors and can produce decreased forearm blood flow responses in patients with essential hypertension.[377] Inhibition of nitric oxide synthetase in animals induces hypertension, glomerular damage, and cardiac fibrosis,[378–380] exacerbates the development of cardiac hypertrophy,[381] and attenuates pressure-induced natriuresis.[382] Hypertension induced by blockade of the enzyme in Wistar rats was prevented by an angII receptor antagonist but not by sodium restriction.[383] Mice genetically lacking the eNOS gene develop significant hypertension and doubling of plasma renin concentration, confirming the importance of this system in maintenance of normal blood pressure.[383a,383b]

Endothelium-dependent relaxation may be involved in various forms of hypertension.[384–388] Acetylcholine activates NO synthetase and is a probe for endothelium-dependent relaxation. Several groups have reported that the vasodilator response to acetylcholine is decreased in patients with essential hypertension,[384–388] although these findings have been disputed.[389] These defects have not been reversed with antihypertensive therapy. This finding suggests that in essential hypertension there is defective EDRF action and that the defect, if it exists, either is primary or becomes longstanding with time.[387] The putative defect in hypertension appears to reside in the ability to synthesize NO rather than respond to it,[388] as suggested by the lack of differences in response to nitroprusside between normotensive and hypertensive subjects.[384] Overall, the data suggests that the cardiovascular system is in a state of active vasodilation but that there is defective NO action in certain forms of hypertension. However, it remains to be clarified whether the abnormalities are primary or secondary and how they are generated. Other cardiovascular risk factors, in addition to hypertension, are associated with impaired endothelial-dependent relaxation. These include hypercholesterolemia, smoking, diabetes, the postmenopausal state, and heart failure.[390–392] Administration of L-arginine has been shown to modestly improve endothelial function in heart failure.[393] Endothelial dysfunction is also associated with increased adhesion of monocytes, macrophages, and platelets to the endothelial surface due to increased expression of adhesion molecules, ICAM-1 and VCAM,[394,395] probably due to decreased NO activity.

Endothelium-Derived Hyperpolarizing Factor (EDHF)

Endothelium-derived hyperpolarizing factor (EDHF) is a vasodilator that is distinct from NO.[396] Its existence can explain endothelium-dependent vasorelaxation that is resistant to inhibition of nitric oxide synthetase and cyclooxygenase. It contributes to endothelium-dependent vasorelaxation by opening K^+ channels in the vascular smooth muscle. It can be induced by bradykinin. The identity of EDHF and its role in hypertension are unknown.

Atrial Natriuretic Peptides (ANPs)

The atrial natriuretic peptides belong to a family of hormones whose main action is to decrease blood pressure and promote sodium excretion.[397,398] Members of the natriuretic peptide family are derived from at least three genes that encode ANP, brain natriuretic peptide (BNP), and C-type natriuretic peptide (CNP). ANP is produced and stored in the heart, particularly, the atria.[399-401] It is also produced in lower concentrations in the ventricles as well as in the lung, aortic arch, pituitary, and CNS.[402,403] BNP is also produced in the ventricles, but it was initially found in the brain.[404,405] Although the level of circulating BNP is much lower than that of ANP (~20 percent), in congestive heart failure BNP levels can become much higher than ANP levels. CNP is produced in the CNS as well as the kidney and vascular endothelial cells.[406,407] Its function may involve a paracrine or autocrine role in the regulation of local blood flow.[408]

ANP and BNP have similar actions in natriuresis, diuresis, and relaxation of the vasculature.[405,409] ANP is released in response to stretching of the atria (right more than left) due to volume expansion, and from the ventricles during cardiac hypertrophy.[399-401,403,410] as well as by the action of glucocorticoid and thyroid hormone.[411] ANP has many effects on the kidney, both direct and indirect, that result in an increase in glomerular filtration rate and excretion of water, sodium, chloride, magnesium, calcium, and phosphate.[404,410,412,413] The direct effect of ANP on the kidney is seen in the inner medullar and cortical collecting ducts where it inhibits water and sodium reasbsorption, and in the juxtamedullary loop of Henle where it decreases chloride reabsorption.[413] Other effects that contribute to a lowering of blood pressure by the action of ANP include inhibition of renal artery vasoconstriction and diminished release of renin, arginine vasopressin, aldosterone, and catecholamines.[399-401,410,412,413,414] Additional actions external to the kidneys that also contribute to a decrease in blood pressure include a direct vasodilatory effect, a decrease in thirst sensation, and fluid shifts from the intravascular to the interstitial spaces.

The majority (>90 percent) of ANP action is mediated via the cell membrane natriuretic peptide receptor A, which then activates guanylate cyclase to produce cyclic GMP.[415,416] In the inner medullary collecting duct, the production of cGMP leads to closure of luminal sodium channels that usually allow sodium entry into the the tubular cells.[417,418] The ANP C receptor appears to be involved in the clearance of ANP.[419]

Levels of ANP and BNP are elevated in essential hypertension and conditions of fluid overload such as congestive heart failure and hepatic cirrhosis.[384,394,395,400,410,414,420,421] However, their importance in sodium and water excretion is unclear. Results from animal studies indicate that the absence of the ANP type A receptor can lead to hypertension and cardiac hypertrophy, whereas overexpression of the ANP gene is associated with lower blood pressure but maintained sodium balance.[422,423]

ANP has growth-inhibitory properties and blocks the actions of other growth factors in several tissues, including the adrenal glomerulosa, vascular smooth muscle, and renal glomerular mesangial cells.[424,425]

Production and Forms

Natriuretic peptides are encoded by at least three genes. These genes encode ANP, brain natriuretic peptide (BNP), and C-type natriuretic peptide (CNP). ANP is a 28-amino acid peptide (Fig. 13-8) that is derived from the carboxy terminus of a 126-amino acid precursor protein (pro-ANP) that is stored in the heart.[399-401,406,410] ANP is cleaved from pro-ANP with release of the storage vesicles and secretion of ANP.[401,406,410] The major sites of ANP production are the cardiac atria.[399,400] The right atrium produces more ANP than does the left.[399,400] ANP is produced in much lower quantities in the ventricles and in other tissues, including the lung, aortic arch, CNS, and pituitary, where the peptide probably exerts autocrine and paracrine actions.[402,403]

Urodilan contains 32 amino acids that are derived from the carboxy terminus of pro-ANP.[406,422] It is produced in the kidney and has not been detected in other tissues or in the circulation.[406] It is resistant to endopeptidase and is more stable than ANP and may be more effective than ANP in the kidney.[406]

BNP contains 32 amino acids and is cleaved from the carboxy terminus of a 108-amino acid precursor protein.[404,405] BNP was originally discovered in the brain, but the major source of the peptide is the cardiac ventricles.[404,405] BNP is highly homologous with ANP.

CNP is a 22-amino acid peptide derived from the carboxy terminus of a larger precursor protein.[404,406] It is produced predominantly in the CNS, where it acts as a neuropeptide.[406] It has also been found in the kidney and in vascular endothelial cells.[404,407]

Regulation of Release

Regulation of the release of the three peptides differs. The major control of ANP release is through stretch influences on the atria.[399,401,410] In contrast, BNP release is thought to be mostly constitutive but is also increased with left ventricular hypertrophy and in heart failure.[405,406] Little is known about the regulation of CNP.

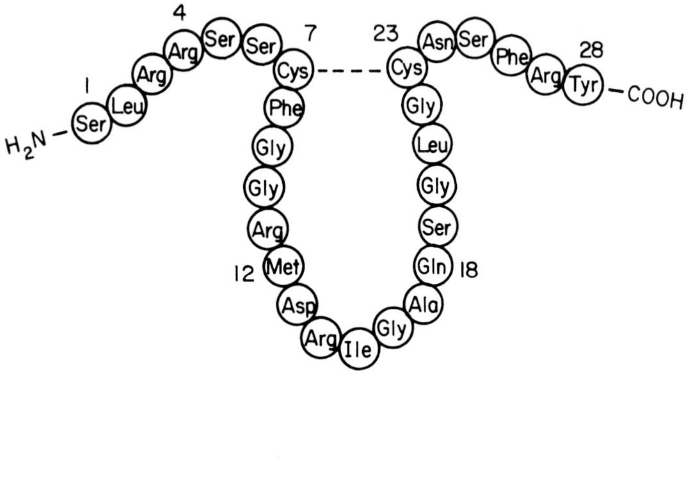

FIGURE 13-8. Structure of human atrial natriuretic peptide. (*Data from Schwartz et al.*[372] *and Greenberg et al.*[373])

Stretch influences that increase ANP release occur through stimuli such as vasopressors, volume increases, postural changes, tachycardia, and mineralocorticoid treatment.[399–401,403] ANP release also may be increased by glucocorticoid and thyroid hormones.[401] Synthesis of the peptide is also increased in the ventricles in myocardial adaptations such as heart failure and cardiac hypertrophy, along with other proteins, such as embryonic contractile protein isoforms (myosin light chain-2, α-myosin heavy chain, and skeletal α-actin)[423] and the adhesion protein oseopointin.[425] ANP has a half-life in the circulation of only a few minutes.[399] The peptide is eliminated through three routes.[426,427] First, there is loss by renal glomerular filtration. Second, elimination through the C-type "clearance" receptors (see later discussion) is the most important quantitatively. Third, ANP is cleaved at a Cys-Phe bond within its 17-member ring by a neutral endopeptidase 24.11 (NEP). This enzyme also cleaves insulin, kinins, and other peptides and is widely distributed.[426,427] This issue may become clinically relevant, as compounds that have the dual effect to inhibit ACE and NEP are being tested for treatment of hypertension and heart failure.[428] These agents are more effective at lowering blood pressure than are ACE inhibitors alone.[429] BNP is cleared more slowly than is ANP and has a plasma half-life of around 19 mins.[409]

Normal plasma levels of ANP are 6 to 8 pM and of BNP are around 4 to 6 pM, while CNP is undetectable.[406,407] Levels of ANP and BNP are increased with age, essential hypertension, primary aldosteronism, pheochromocytoma, renal failure, and heart failure.[420,430,431] ANP levels are elevated with paroxysmal atrial arrhythmias,[399–401] while BNP levels are not affected by acute atrial or ventricular pacing. BNP plasma levels are elevated in left ventricular hypertrophy.[405]

Catecholamines and the Autonomic Nervous System

Catecholamines, the autonomic nervous system, and the CNS are involved in multiple aspects of blood pressure control and essential hypertension. The synthesis, actions, and molecular actions of catecholamines are described in Chaps. 4 and 12. Hypertension due to catecholamine-producing tumors is addressed in Chap. 12. Many aspects of catecholamines relevant to blood pressure control are described in other sections of this chapter. The role of beta-adrenergic activation in regulation of renin release and that of angII in stimulating adrenergic activity are described earlier in the section on the renin-angiotensin system. The role of adrenergic mechanisms in obesity, insulin resistance and salt-sensitivity of blood pressure responses, stimulation by insulin and food intake of central adrenergic activity, and use of drugs that affect sympathetic nervous system activity are described later in the section on obesity, insulin, and insulin resistance in hypertension. The role of the sympathetic nervous system in hypertension is also reflected by the utility of drugs that affect adrenergic activity in treating essential hypertension.[146,287] Although an extensive analysis of the role of the autonomic nervous system in blood pressure control is beyond the scope of this chapter, certain comments may be useful.

The sympathetic nervous system appears overall to be overactive in essential hypertension.[146,287] Plasma norepinephrine levels are higher in young patients with essential hypertension than in control subjects and increase with age.[146,287] These increases are greater in normotensives than in hypertensives such that differences in plasma norepinephrine levels are blunted with advancing age. This may explain some of the controversy regarding differences between normotensives and hypertensives.[146,150,287] There is also enhanced regional release of norepinephrine in essential hypertension that is selective for the heart and kidneys.[146,287,432] It has been proposed that as hypertension progresses, there is a transition from hyperkinetic, sympathetic nervous system-dependent hypertension to a state of increased vascular resistance with normal sympathetic nervous system activity.[146] Plasma epinephrine levels are usually normal or elevated in essential hypertension.[146] Dopamine exerts natriuretic actions in and is produced in the kidneys.[287,433] Plasma levels of conjugated dopamine appear to be elevated, but urinary free dopamine is depressed in essential hypertension.[146,287] Decreased dopamine levels or responses could result in impaired sodium excretion.

There is also evidence for enhanced pressor sensitivity to catecholamines in essential hypertension.[146,287] β-adrenergic blockers and other sympatholytic agonists produce greater depressor responses in essential hypertensive than in normotensive subjects.[146] Blood pressure responses to these agents are correlated with plasma norepinephrine levels.[146] This enhanced responsiveness in the face of excessive norepinephrine production differs from the usual case of negative regulation of adrenergic responsiveness by catecholamines (see Chap. 4). Firing rates of sympathetic nerves are increased in young patients with essential hypertension and are normal to increased in essential hypertension in general.[146,287] There is a blunting in some essential hypertensives of baroreceptor-mediated heart rate slowing and reduced sympathetic nervous system activity in response to blood pressure increases.[51] Efferent renal nerve sympathetic activity is elevated in essential hypertension and in several animal models of hypertension.[433] This enhanced renal activity is influenced by dietary sodium and environmental stress, tends to be inherited, and influences renal sodium handling and renin release.[432]

Insulin and Insulin Resistance in Hypertension

Insulin resistance is a defect in insulin-mediated glucose uptake into target tissues such as adipose tissue and skeletal muscle. This defect is generally associated with a resultant increase in pancreatic insulin secretion. Because of its predisposition to diabetes and cardiovascular disease, it is important to recognize the insulin resistance (cardiovascular hypertension dysmetabolic syndrome), which appears more commonly in Orientals, Asian Indians, Mexican-Americans, Southwestern Indians and possibly African-Americans.[434–440] The presence of visceral adiposity occurring with hypertriglyceridemia, low HDL cholesterol, and hypertension strongly suggests the syndrome. Because of its variability, the measurement of fasting insulin is not currently recommended to diagnose the syndrome. The presence of impaired glucose tolerance or impaired fasting glucose (110–125 mg/dl) also strongly suggests the syndrome. However, all abnormalities are not consistently present in all patients; thus, several different defects may dictate the spectrum of features that are observed.[26] Other factors of the syndrome include elevated levels of small, dense LDL cholesterol suggesting increased oxidized cholesterol, and elevated levels of the prothrombotic factor, plasminogen activator inhibitor 1, PAI-1.[441,442] Both of these features are thought to play a major role in the increased cardiovascular disease associated with insulin resistance.

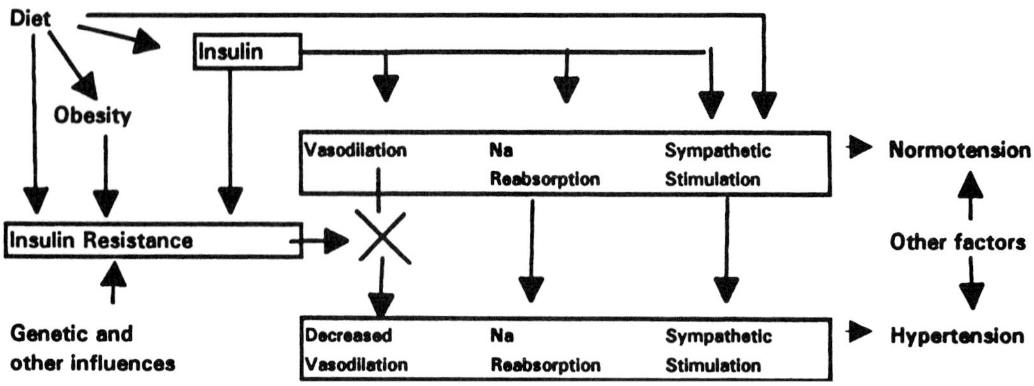

FIGURE 13-9. Representation of the development of insulin resistance and the influence of insulin and insulin resistance on blood pressure.

Actions of Insulin that Influence Blood Pressure

Insulin has a number of actions that may influence blood pressure either positively or negatively (Fig. 13-9).[434–437] Among these, vasodilator actions on peripheral blood vessels tend to lower blood pressure and influences on renal sodium handling and sympathetic activity tend to elevate blood pressure.

Actions on Blood Vessels

Insulin and insulin-like growth factor 1 (IGF-1) have direct vascular actions, which are endothelial-mediated and depend on the geographic location of the vessel.[437,443–445] In intact mesenteric artery, insulin enhances vasoconstrictor effects through the stimulation of an endothelial-dependent cyclooxygenase product. In contrast, in rat aortic ring, insulin opposes vasoconstrictor effects by stimulating endothelial nitric oxide production. Thus, the overall effect of insulin on blood pressure may be a balance between vasoconstrictor and vasodilator responses, which appears to be altered in the setting of obesity and diabetes. In normal subjects insulin increases vasodilation of skeletal muscle beds.[446] Insulin-mediated glucose uptake is enhanced in the presence of vasodilation.[206] Insulin can increase skeletal muscle blood flow,[447] decrease forearm vascular resistance, and attenuate responses to various vasoconstrictors.[448] These actions are selective for certain vascular beds. They are blunted in obesity and in type II diabetes mellitus.[447,449] Blood vessels from insulin-deficient or insulin-resistant/hyperinsulinemic rats exhibit enhanced pressor responses to vasoconstrictor substances.[450] Exogenous insulin restores normal vascular responsiveness and blunts the vasoconstrictor effects of catecholamines; higher concentrations are required for these effects in obese and insulin-resistant hypertensive rats.[450] Insulin actions on skeletal muscle blood flow can occur independent of hypoglycemia, are not secondary to insulin stimulation of glucose uptake, but probably contribute to insulin-stimulated glucose uptake.[451] A common signaling pathway, the phosphoinositol-3 kinase, PI_3K, pathway mediates both insulin mediated glucose uptake in skeletal muscle and NO production in endothelial cells (Fig. 13-10)[452]: this pathway appears to be defective in both tissues in insulin resistance.[439]

Renal

Insulin increases renal sodium reabsorption and can cause sodium retention.[434,435,452] The major mechanism for this effect appears to involve insulin stimulation of sodium reabsorption in the loop of Henle.[453] The sodium-retaining actions of insulin may be enhanced through indirect stimulatory influences on sympathetic nervous system activity and on angII-mediated aldosterone secretion.[435,454] The effects of insulin on sodium retention can occur independently of insulin-induced hypokalemia, stimulation of angII production, or decreases in prostaglandin production and of changes in the GFR.[454,455] They can be blocked by calcium-channel blockers,[453] in vasopressin deficient animals,[453] and by ANP.[456] Insulin can affect glomerular hemodynamics by increasing glomerular efferent arteriolar vasodilation and afferent arteriole vasoconstriction[455] and can increase renal plasma flow at high concentrations.[456]

Sympathetic

Insulin can increase noradrenergic sympathetic activity, plasma norepinephrine levels, urinary norepinephrine, and norepi-

FIGURE 13-10. Two pathways of insulin action. The phospatidylinositol-3 (PI-3) kinase pathway is vasculoprotective by mediating nitric oxide (NO) transport and potentially by reversing insulin resistance and, thus, components of the cardiovascular dysmetabolic phenotype. In contrast, the mitogen activated protein kinase (MAPK) pathway mediates effects in the vasculatures, which are proatherogenic. IRS = insulin receptor substrate; MEKK = MAPK kinase; PAI-1 = plasminogen activator inhibitor-1.

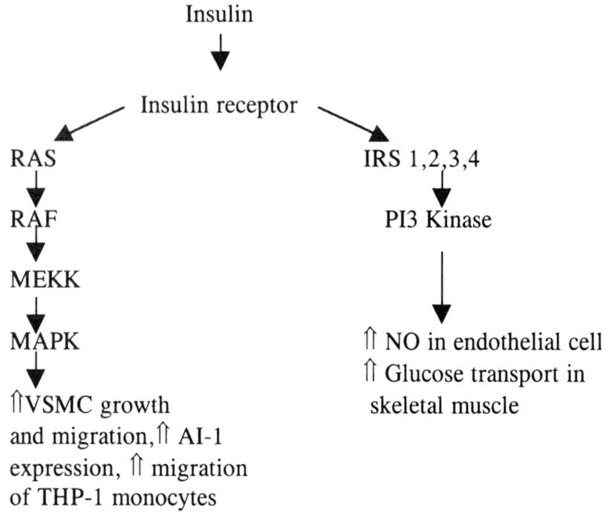

nephrine turnover.[146,434–436,451] Insulin actions in the CNS probably elicit these responses. There is regional nonuniformity in the stimulation. Thus, insulin increases lumbar but not renal or adrenal activity in rats and increases medial hypothalamic and muscle, but not skin activity in humans. Some sympathetic effects could be secondary to baroreceptor reflex responses. The effects of insulin occur in the absence of hypoglycemia (which activates the sympathetic nervous system and stimulates adrenal epinephrine release) and are independent of insulin stimulation of carbohydrate metabolism.

Vascular Structure

Insulin is a growth factor and can stimulate smooth muscle and fibroblast proliferation and migration, the uptake and esterification of lipoprotein by smooth muscle cells, and can increase PAI-1 production.[435,457,458] In physiologic concentrations, insulin enhances these effects of other growth factors such as platelet derived growth factor and angII.[459] These actions are mediated by the mitogen activated protein kinase (MAPK) pathway, which may be accelerated in insulin resistant states (Fig. 13-10).[434,460–462] These actions could accelerate the development of secondary changes in hypertension and atherosclerosis.[434]

Peroxisome Proliferator Activated Receptor Gamma (PPARγ) and Insulin Resistance

Thiazolidinediones, used to improve insulin-mediated glucose transport in patients with Type 2 diabetes, bind to the nuclear receptor, PPARγ, which is present in adipose tissue and found in lower quantities in skeletal muscle, heart, vascular smooth muscle cells, endothelial cells, monocyte/macrophages, liver, and some other tissues.[434,463,464] PPARγ regulates adipocyte differentiation.[465] The mechanism by which these ligands improve insulin's action on glucose transport is unknown. They can activate PPARγ on skeletal muscle, the major target tissue of insulin,[466] or they can attenuate fat production of free fatty acids or tumor necrosis factor alpha (TNF-α) or other substances from fat that inhibit insulin-mediated glucose transport.[467] Thiazolidinediones not only improve glucose control in type 2 diabetes, but they improve many components of the insulin resistance syndrome including high triglycerides, low HDL cholesterol, and hypertension.[434] Troglitazone, one member of the class, has also been shown to decrease both circulating PAI-1 levels and small, dense LDL cholesterol levels.[468,469] In addition, activation of vascular and macrophage receptors is associated with decreased blood pressure, inhibition of neointima formation after endothelial injury, and attenuation of atherosclerosis in animal models.[434,470,471] In contrast to effects on insulin and glucose metabolism, these effects appear to result from inhibition of nuclear effects of the MAPK pathway activated by a variety of growth factors including insulin. Recently, identification of mutations of PPARγ in man demonstrate its important role in insulin resistance, type 2 diabetes, and hypertension. Two different heterozygous mutations in the ligand-binding domain, which markedly transcriptionally impaired the receptor, were associated with the development of type 2 mellitus diabetes and hypertension at an early age in three patients.[472] None of the subjects were obese, but all had high triglycerides and low HDL cholesterol levels. In contrast, a proline to glutamine missense mutation at codon 115 in PPARγ 2 caused a gain of function that enhanced adipocyte differentiation that was associated with marked obesity in three unrelated subjects, but all had normal insulin sensitivity and blood pressure.[473] Thus, gain or loss of PPARγ function is associated with obesity or insulin resistance and hypertension, respectively. The role of PPARγ activation in blood pressure control and vascular protection in insulin resistant subjects remains to be determined.

Ion Transport Abnormalities in Diabetes and Insulin Resistance

There has been considerable interest in the role of abnormal divalent cation metabolism in the pathogenesis of hypertension, particularly as it relates to diabetes mellitus and insulin resistance. Work conducted by Draznin and colleagues[474] demonstrated that intracellular cation status is critical for optimal insulin action and that altered divalent cation metabolism is associated with a diminution in the ability of insulin to stimulate glucose uptake in insulin sensitive tissues such as adipose cells and skeletal muscle tissue. Indeed, this group has shown that an "optimal intracellular free calcium level" is necessary for optimal insulin action.[466] Levels either below or above (most commonly seen in insulin resistant states) this optimal level are associated with diminished insulin-stimulated glucose transport. Subsequent studies[475–476] demonstrated that an optimal level of intracellular free calcium $[Ca^{2+}]_i$ was also necessary for optimal insulin and IGF-1-induced glucose transport in cardiovascular tissue. In obese insulin resistant hypertensive rodents, resistance to the actions of insulin exists at the level of vascular smooth muscle cells (VSMC),[475] as well as in classical insulin responsive tissues.[477,478] This VSMC resistance to insulin-stimulated uptake of glucose is associated with abnormalities of $[Ca^{2+}]_i$ metabolism in this tissue.[475] VSMC display exaggerated VSMC $[Ca^{2+}]_i$ transients in response to vasoagonists in this resistant rodent model.[475] These data suggest that insulin resistance is associated with abnormal $[Ca^{2+}]_i$ metabolism in vascular tissue as well as in conventionally recognized insulin sensitive tissue. As the insulin resistance and abnormal cation metabolism in cardiovascular tissue likely contributes to development of hypertension and cardiovascular disease (CVD), much of this review will address the actions of insulin and insulin-like growth factors in regulation of CV cation metabolism and CV function.[479]

Insulin and IGF 1 reduce vascular tone, in part, through effects on cation metabolism (Fig. 13-11). Both peptides attenuate Ca^{2+} influx into VSMC by decreasing both receptor-mediated and voltage-operated Ca^{2+} channel currents in conjunction with VSMC contractile responses.[478–480] Insulin decreases intracellular Ca^{2+} release and efflux as well.[480–481] Both insulin and IGF-1 modulate cation transport mechanisms. These peptides have been demonstrated to increase Ca^{2+}-ATPase activity in plasma membranes and intracellular organelles.[476,480] Both peptides increase the activation of Ca^{2+} dependent potassium channels.[482] These effects appear to be mediated, in part, via increases in nitric oxide (NO) production by endothelial cells and VSMC.[482,483] Increased NO results in activation of VSMC Ca^{2+}-dependent potassium channels.[483] This activation of Ca^{2+}-dependent potassium channels is cGMP-independent, and may chemically modify sulfhydryl groups on Ca^{2+}-dependent potassium channels or other membrane constituents. This action of NO suggests an alternative pathway for the vasorelaxation of insulin/IGF-1-induced NO mediated vasorelaxation of NO in situations where cGMP activity remains unaltered. Indeed, low concentrations of arginine analogs such as L-NMMA inhibit the vasodilation mediated by ATP-sensitive potassium channels.[484]

Another potential mechanism by which insulin and IGF-1 may decrease VSMC $[Ca^{2+}]_i$/vasoconstriction is through

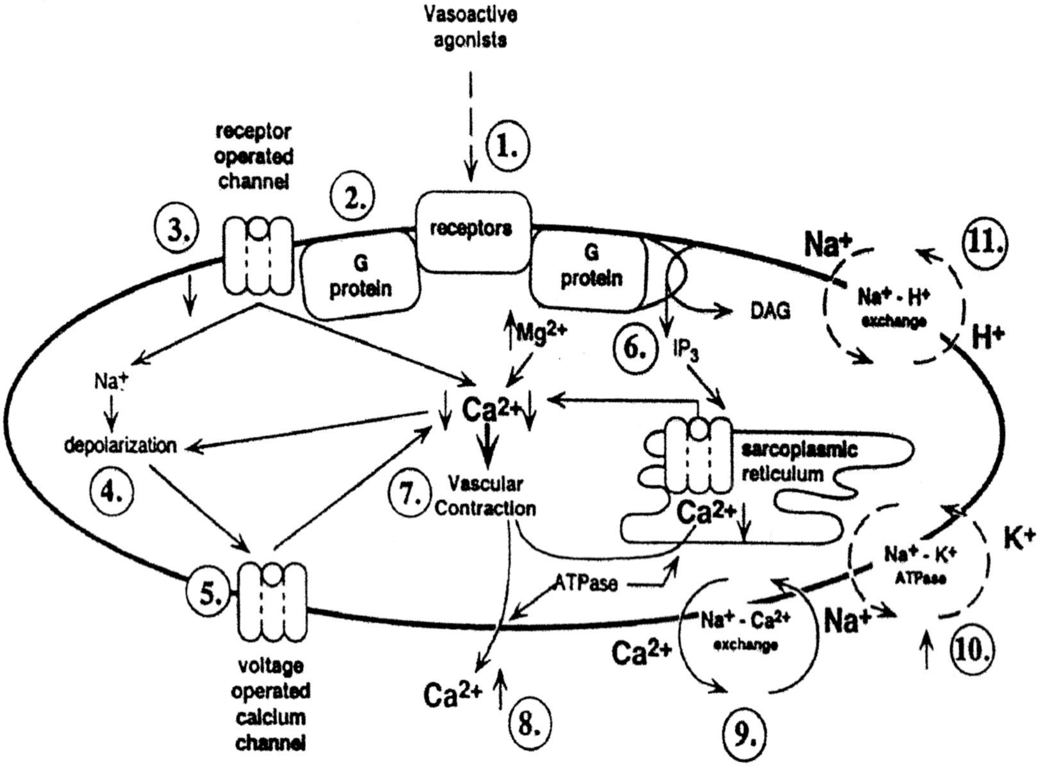

FIGURE 13-11. Effects of insulin and IGF-1 on vascular tone are mediated in part through changes in cation metabolism.

stimulation of Na^+, K^+-ATPase via changes in Na^+-Ca^{2+} exchange. Both insulin and IGF-1 increase Na^+-K^+-ATPase activity in a number of tissues including VSMC (Fig. 13-11).[476,480,485–487] Insulin has been shown to translocate alpha subunits of the heterodimeric Na^+-K^+-ATPase from intracellular stores to skeletal muscle plasma membrane,[486] as well as increasing transcription of the $\alpha2$ subunits in cultured VSMC.[487] Long-term regulation of the pump may involve either pre- or posttranslational changes in subunit synthesis and/or degradation rates or stimulation of isoform-specific expression. In contrast, more rapid regulation of pump activity may occur via covalent or noncovalent modification of the enzyme or by translocation of preformed pumps from an intracellular pool.[486] Insulin has been reported to utilize these pathways in a tissue-specific fashion: translocation of pump subunits from intracellular stores in skeletal muscle,[486] enhancement of infinity for Na^+ in adipocytes[488] stimulation of Na^+/H^+ exchanges in liver and myocytes,[489] as well as increasing transcription of catalytic subunit[483] and activation of the pump in vascular tissues.[487] Vasodilatory actions of insulin and IGF-1 are mediated, in part, through increased vascular production of nitric oxide (NO).[452,476,480,490,491] This increased NO, in turn, stimulates Na^+-K^+-ATPase activity in vascular tissue[492] suggesting another mechanism by which these growth factors may stimulate pump activity.

Increased peripheral vascular resistance is the hallmark of hypertension associated with both type 1 and type 2 diabetes mellitus. In both of these entities there are abnormalities of $[Ca^{2+}]_i$ metabolism.[493] Indeed, agonist-induced VSMC $[Ca^{2+}]_i$ and vascular reactivity are exaggerated in both the insulinopenic streptozotocin diabetic rat[493] and in the insulin-resistant Zucker obese rat.[475] The exaggerated VSMC $[Ca^{2+}]_i$ responses may be due, in part, to reduced Na^+-K^+-ATPase pump activity. Decreased activity of the Na^+ pump has been observed in insulin-resistant[476] and insulin-deficient states.[494,495] An isoform-specific decrease in the expression of the aortic $\alpha2$ catalytic subunit of the pump in conjunction with increased $[Ca^{2+}]_i$[496] and vascular tone has been observed in insulin-resistant spontaneously hypertensive rats.[475] Attenuated tissue glucose uptake has also been attributed to elevated $[Ca^{2+}]_{li}$.[476] Accordingly, increased VSMC $[Ca^{2+}]_i$ may be the underlying factor in impaired VSMC insulin and IGF-1 action and increased vascular resistance, growth, and remodeling.[476,480]

Alterations in intracellular magnesium $[Mg^{2+}]_i$ regulation may also be an important contributing factor for increased vascular resistance associated with insulin resistant states.[497–500] Under normal circumstances insulin increases cellular uptake of Mg^{2+}, and in states of decreased cellular insulin action (i.e., type 1 and type 2 diabetes mellitus), there is a reduction in $[Mg^{2+}]_i$.[497–501] Depletion of $[Mg^{2+}]_i$ leads to increased peripheral vascular resistance[495] and insulin resistance.[479] Indeed, oral Mg^{2+} supplementation has been shown to improve insulin sensitivity in animals[500] and people[501] with type 2 diabetes. Recently, using nuclear magnetic resonance imaging techniques, Dominguez et al.[502] showed that IGF-1, like insulin, increases tissue Mg^{2+} levels. Mg^{2+} protects against endothelial injury due to oxidative stress[503] and increases the production of the endothelial vasodilator prostacyclin.[504] Thus, in addition to being an important mediator of the actions of insulin/IGF-1, the divalent cation Mg^{2+} has a direct role in preventing exaggerated vasoconstriction and atherosclerosis in diabetes.

Correlations between Hypertension, Insulin Resistance, Hyperinsulinemia, and Obesity

The term *obesity* denotes an increase in adipose tissue mass and a body weight of >120 percent of the ideal.[505] The association between obesity and hypertension exists in populations (e.g., blacks and whites in the United States) that differ in the prevalence of the two disorders. The association between obesity and hypertension appears to weaken with advancing age. Body fat distribution is also related to the risk of developing hypertension; increased abdominal fat with a high waist-to-hip ratio is associated with high blood pressure and insulin resistance.[436] The correlation is even greater in subjects with increased visceral fat as measured by CT scanning.[506] There are also correlations between hypertension and obesity in diabetic patients.[460]

In addition to obesity, both hyperinsulinemia and insulin resistance have been identified as independent risk factors for predicting the development of hypertension.[435–437,507–509] Insulin resistance is a common feature shared by patients with obesity, diabetes, hypertension, and cardiovascular disease.[435,439] Insulin resistance is correlated with essential hypertension even in thin patients,[434,435,510] is greater in obese hypertensives than in obese normotensives,[437] and is present in the offspring of hypertensives before the development of either obesity or hypertension.[511,512] Insulin resistance and hypertension are correlated in Caucasians, Chinese, and in normal- or low-weight Mexican-Americans.[513–515] The issue is unclear in black populations.[513]

Insulin resistance and hyperinsulinemia are not a consequence of hypertension. For example, patients with hyperaldosteronism or renovascular hypertension have higher sensitivity to insulin than do those with essential hypertension.[516] Hypertension does not alter the suppressive effects of insulin on hepatic glucose production in obese or type II diabetic subjects.[517] Hyperinsulinemia in hypertensive subjects does not change with blood pressure control.[518] Insulin resistance and hyperinsulinemia are antecedents to hypertension. These derangements were found to predict the development of hypertension in normal weight individuals in an 8-year prospective study of Mexican-Americans[508] and to be present in 1) normotensive children of hypertensive but not normotensive patients,[512,519] 2) borderline hypertensive subjects in the Tecumseh study,[520] and 3) borderline hypertensive, but not normotensive African-American adolescents.[521]

However, the association between hypertension and insulin resistance and/or hyperinsulinemia is not universal.[522,523] Some studies have failed to show a correlation between hyperinsulinemia and hypertension in obese subjects.[522] There are a number of patients with type II diabetes mellitus and marked insulin resistance who do not have hypertension.[517] More than 40 percent of hypertensives have normal insulin-stimulated whole-body glucose uptake.[524,525] In Pima Indians and Mexican-Americans in the United States and some other groups, hypertension is uncommon but insulin resistance is common.[441,522,525] Finally, some states with clear hyperinsulinemia, for example, insulinomas, do not regularly lead to hypertension.[434]

The SNS and Renal Sodium Handling in Insulin Resistance

Excessive sympathetic nervous system activity, an enhanced tendency to sodium retention, and a greater tendency to develop hypertension seem to occur in insulin resistance.[435,446,447,454,526] The contribution of insulin to activation of the autonomic nervous system and that of renal sodium retention to insulin-resistant states has not been accurately defined. The contributions of autonomic nervous system activity and renal salt retention to the hypertension in these states are also not known. However, with insulin resistance and hyperinsulinemia, there is excessive sympathetic nervous system activity and salt sensitivity of the blood pressure. Hypertensive rats can have selective insulin resistance[435] and augmented adrenal sympathetic nerve responses to insulin compared with normotensive strains.[437] Rats made insulin-resistant with fructose also have exaggerated pressor and sympathetic responses to insulin.[437]

Increased sympathetic nervous system activity occurs in humans with insulin resistance, obesity, and hypertension.[146,436] There is a positive correlation between plasma norepinephrine levels and the abdominal form of obesity, the phenotype most commonly associated with hypertension and insulin resistance.[436] There are accentuated plasma norepinephrine responses to postural and other stimuli and to glucose ingestion in obesity.[146] Obese and salt-sensitive hypertensive subjects also have enhanced sympathetic activity.[146] Urinary norepinephrine levels are highest in those with the highest fasting levels of insulin and glucose.[436] Both insulin and food intake can stimulate the sympathetic nervous system in obesity.[146,436] The overall weight probably contributes as well.[146]

Insulin resistance is strongly correlated in obese and nonobese hypertensives with enhanced sodium sensitivity of blood pressure.[435,527,528,529] Plasma insulin levels correlate with salt-induced changes in blood pressure in obese subjects. Improvement of insulin sensitivity by means of weight reduction reduces salt sensitivity. A hyperinsulinemic response to oral glucose occurs in normotensive salt-sensitive men.[527] The blood pressure of obese adolescents is more dependent on salt than is that of nonobese adolescents; this sodium sensitivity is attenuated with weight loss.[435] Hypertension with weight gain in the dog occurs only if adequate salt is present in the diet.[435] However, plasma insulin levels were similar in salt-sensitive vs. salt-resistant hypertensives,[528] which could imply that insulin does not induce salt sensitivity in all individuals. However, the salt-retaining actions of insulin can be demonstrated in hypertensives.[454]

Weight loss has a hypotensive effect[146,436]; this is associated with decreased insulin resistance and is independent of simple energy restriction[465] or salt intake.[449] Overall, this is correlated with decreases in plasma norepinephrine levels.[146] However, there is some decrease in blood pressure before plasma norepinephrine levels fall, and this may be mediated in part by changes in sodium balance caused by decreases in plasma insulin levels and salt intake.[146] Dopamine levels may increase during caloric restriction, and this may enhance natriuresis.[146]

Genetic influences impact the interaction of the components of the insulin resistance syndrome. Genetic mutations resulting in a gain of function and loss of function of PPARγ are discussed earlier. LDL subclass patterns are correlated with an increased risk of developing coronary heart disease because of the greater oxidation of the apo B moiety on this particle and are influenced by a gene located near the LDL and insulin receptor genes.[529] Thus, it is conceivable that this allele predisposes to insulin resistance. In addition, a locus near and possibly at the lipoprotein lipase gene, which is responsible for triglyceride metabolism, links to systolic but not diastolic pressure in Taiwanese sibpairs recruited for type 2 diabetes.[530] Thus, the lipoprotein lipase gene potentially links two important components of the insulin resistance syndrome: hypertension and hypertriglyceridemia.

Hypertension and Diabetes Mellitus

About 2.5 million to 3 million Americans have both diabetes and hypertension.[460] The prevalence of hypertension in type 1 and type 2 diabetes mellitus is about twofold that in the nondiabetic population.[460] Around 30 to 40 percent of patients with type 2 diabetes mellitus are hypertensive when the diagnosis is made.[460] By the fifth decade of life, 85 percent of all diabetic individuals (most of whom have type 2 diabetes) are estimated to be hypertensive and obese.[435] The prevalence of the hypertension in type 2 diabetes increases markedly once proteinuria develops.[460] The presence of hypertension increases both morbidity and mortality in diabetic patients and accelerates the course of diabetic nephropathy and retinopathy.[460,531,532] Hypertension has been implicated in 44 percent of deaths coded to diabetes, and diabetes has been attributed to around 10 percent of deaths caused by hypertension.[460] An absence of hypertension is the usual finding in long-term survivors of diabetes.[460]

Hypertension contributes significantly to the morbidity and mortality of diabetes and appears as important as glycemic control in decreasing the incidence of both microvascular and macrovascular complications.[531] Hypertension associated with diabetes is often difficult to treat and requires multiple medications, 3.5 on average.[531] Diabetic nephropathy further worsens blood pressure control. The target of blood pressure control is lower (<130/85 mm Hg) among hypertensive patients with diabetes compared with those without diabetes because of the high risk (two- to fourfold) for cardiovascular disease among individuals with diabetes. In addition, patients with diabetes and hypertension are at higher risk of developing atherosclerotic renal artery stenosis, which is a rare cause of hypertension in nondiabetic patients. Subsequently, secondary hypertension and the risk for renal artery stenosis is markedly increased in the presence of coronary artery disease, stroke, and especially peripheral vascular disease.[533] Conlon et al. reported an incidence of significant (>50 percent) unilateral renal artery stenosis of 11 percent and bilateral renal artery stenosis of 4 percent in 1,235 patients (diabetic and nondiabetics) who underwent simultaneous cardiac catherization and abdominal aortography.[534] Diabetes mellitus carried a highly significant increase in the mortality risk ratio (1.7), second only to peripheral vascular disease (risk ratio 2.3). Renal artery stenosis is an independent mortality risk factor and its surgical correction is associated with improved survival.[534,535]

Diabetes related hypertension is often associated with salt sensitivity, a condition associated with nondipping of blood pressure during nighttime, especially if patients are on a high-sodium diet.[536] The relation between nondipping of blood pressure and salt sensitivity is not well-studied yet, although an abnormal circadian rhythm of blood pressure in patients with diabetes has been tightly linked with diabetic autonomic neuropathy. Abnormal circadian rhythm of blood pressure is associated with a higher incidence of vascular events, both fatal and nonfatal. Indeed, the pattern of the circadian rhythm of blood pressure is a more powerful predictor of fatal events than are hypertension and diabetic nephropathy.[537] A recent study has raised the concern that intensive glycemic control in patients with type 1 diabetes using multiple insulin injections was associated with elevated nighttime blood pressure, which is attributed to possible subclinical nocturnal hypoglycemia.[538] Thus, determination of the 24-hour blood pressure pattern, using ambulatory blood pressure monitoring, is particularly informative in patients with diabetes. Because of the higher incidence of orthostatic hypotension among patients with diabetic autonomic neuropathy, office blood pressure should be measured in supine, sitting, and standing positions. If orthostasis is diagnosed, the standing blood pressure is the target for pharmacological therapy.[1]

Plasma renin activity is usually normal during the early stage of diabetes. However, as the disease progresses, plasma renin activity decreases despite an elevation in total plasma renin and prorenin levels. The elevation in plasma renin and prorenin concentrations antidate the development of microalbuminuria and is considered as a predictor for microalbuminuria and nephropathy. In fact, plasma prorenin is higher in patients with diabetic complications.[539–543] Prorenin and renin are thought to participate in the vascular injury and nephropathy by providing the substrate for the rate limiting step (renin) to the vascular renin-angiotensin system; blood vessels express prorenin at very low concentration but take up circulating prorenin avidly.[544] Indirect support of this hypothesis comes from the United Kingdom Prospective Diabetes Study, which showed equal efficacy of two medications that modulate the renin-angiotensin system in reducing microvascular and macrovascular complications of type 2 diabetes mellitus: the ACE inhibitor, captopril, and the beta-adrenergic receptor blocker, atenolol.[531,532]

Therapeutic Implications

Because insulin resistance is associated with increased cardiovascular disease, early recognition of its presence and aggressive treatment of associated cardiovascular risk factors is warranted. This applies to the spectrum of patients with insulin resistance usually beginning with obesity, impaired fasting glucose and progressing to frank type 2 diabetes. Hypertension in these individuals responds especially well to caloric restriction.[146,435–437,518] Even small reductions in weight can have a significant effect on blood pressure. When obese adolescents lost weight,[435] a fall in insulin, catecholamine, and aldosterone levels correlated with the drop in blood pressure. The greatest reductions occur in individuals with the greatest fall in plasma insulin levels (a reflection of insulin sensitivity).[435] Blood pressure and insulin resistance also respond favorably to exercise.[435] Salt restriction is helpful when there is moderate caloric restriction but is less beneficial with very low calorie diets.[518]

Lowering of blood pressure in diabetes attenuates or prevents the development of both microvascular and macrovascular complications.[531,532] The Joint National Committee on Evaluation and Treatment of Blood Pressure (JNC VI) recommends lower goals (130/85 mm Hg) for patients with diabetes compared to those with essential hypertension alone (140/90 mm Hg).[1] In the presence of renal disease, goals should be even lower (125/75).[1] Because of multiple vascular and renal abnormalities, multiple antihypertensive agents (average 3.5) are needed to reach goals.[531] Reversal of insulin resistance itself with the thiazolidinedione class of insulin sensitizers has a modest, but statistically significant effect on lowering blood pressure in patients with impaired glucose tolerance[545] or type 2 diabetes.[546] Small studies comparing angiotensin converting enzyme inhibitors (ACEI) with long-acting dihydropyridine calcium channel blockers suggest ACEI provide better renal and cardiovascular protection[547,548]; thus, ACEI have been recommended as first line antihypertensive therapy in diabetes and possibly insulin resistance.[549] This recommendation is consistent with the demonstrations that AII has multiple injurious effects on the renal and cardiovascular systems in diabetes. AT_1 receptor blockers should be used if ACEI are not well tolerated;

several current studies are evaluating their role in renal and cardiovascular protection in diabetes, and they may be recommended as first line therapy in the future. The only other class of antihypertensive agents that has been demonstrated to be renal protective is the nonhydropyridine calcium channel blockers, so they may be useful to add to inhibitors of the RAS.[550] In addition, low-dose diuretics may also be added because they enhance the effects of ACEI and AT_1 receptor blockers without inducing hypokalemia, hypomagnesemia, or other metabolic alterations. Dihydropyridines effectively lower blood pressure in diabetes and can be added once the RAS is inhibited.[548] Converting enzyme inhibitors[551,552] and alpha-adrenergic blockers[553] can improve glucose tolerance, although improved insulin sensitivity has not been linked to the antihypertensive effects of these drugs.

EVALUATION OF THE HYPERTENSIVE PATIENT

Evaluation of a hypertensive patient should provide sufficient information to (1) confirm the presence and level of persistent inappropriately elevated blood pressure, (2) assess the presence and severity of secondary target organ involvement of the heart, brain, kidneys, and vasculature, (3) identify clues for secondary forms of hypertension which would lead to more extensive evaluation, (4) identify coexistent medical illnesses and other treatable risk factors for accelerated atherosclerosis, (5) determine the urgency and basis for the selection of specific antihypertensive therapy, and (6) assess previous therapy for hypertension and responses to or side effects from such therapy. This evaluation can be obtained from a careful medical history, physical examination, and selected screening laboratory studies as outlined elsewhere.[1,2,4] The evaluation should also allow the physician to decide whether further work-up should be performed to look for a secondary form of hypertension. Features from the history and physical examination that suggest secondary hypertension are provided in Tables 13-4 and 13-5.

TABLE 13-4. Features on History Suggestive of Secondary Hypertension

No family history of hypertension
Very strong family history, particularly of severe hypertension, hypertension at an early age, or a disorder such as renal disease that is associated with hypertension
Abrupt onset of hypertension
Onset of hypertension before age 20 or after age 60
Sudden acceleration of previously existing hypertension or development of malignant hypertension de novo
Rapid deterioration of renal function despite well-controlled hypertension or after treatment with converting enzyme inhibitors
Unresponsiveness to standard antihypertensive therapy (other than converting enzyme inhibitor therapy)
Rapid development of hypokalemia with standard doses of diuretics
History of renal trauma, flank pain, and hematuria, suggesting renal infarction
Sudden onset of hypertension in a patient with systemic emboli or vasculitis
Development of hypertension in association with lower-extremity ischemia, calf or buttock claudication, and erectile incompetence, abdominal angina, or aortic aneurysm
Nocturnal polyuria
Periodic paralysis or muscle weakness
Weight loss or gain; change in fat distribution
Change in menses
Change in appearance (e.g., with Cushing's syndrome, acromegaly)
Headaches
Palpitations
Tremulousness
Symptoms of postural hypertension
Skin changes (acne, excessive bruising, pigmentation, dry skin)
Muscle weakness
Edema
Excessive sweating

Clinical History

The clinical history should provide (1) information on timing of the onset and known duration of hypertension, (2) the family history, including the presence of hypertension and its complications or premature arteriosclerosis in close relatives, (3) evidence of target organ involvement manifested as symptoms or clinical episodes of ischemic cerebral, cardiac, or peripheral vascular disease or renal disease, (4) clues such as symptoms or events suggesting secondary hypertension, such as congenital, acquired, or iatrogenic endocrine diseases (Table 13-4), (5) history of coexistent systemic diseases that could influence management, such as asthma, gout, diabetes mellitus, arthritis, and thyroid disease, (6) use of substances that have the potential to raise the blood pressure, such as glucocorticoids, erythropoietin, nonsteroidal anti-inflammatory agents, estrogens, over-the-counter nasal decongestants, licorice, or recreational drugs (cocaine, tobacco, and alcohol), and (7) dietary habits (sodium, potassium, calories, and fat intake).

Secondary hypertension is suggested when the hypertension occurs in younger ($<$20 years of age) or older ($>$60 years of age) patients, when blood pressure responds very poorly to drug therapy, with accelerated or malignant hypertension in well-controlled patients whose hypertension becomes worse, and with

TABLE 13-5. Findings on Physical Examination Suggestive of Secondary Hypertension

Malignant hypertension, grade III or IV Keith Wagener retinopathy
Widespread occlusive vascular disease in the carotid, aortoiliac, or femoral arteries manifested by decreased pulses or bruits
Epigastric or flank bruit with both systolic and diastolic components
Abdominal aortic aneurysm
Positive Chvostek's or Trousseau's signs, suggesting alkalosis
Impaired autonomic reflexes; postural hypotension
Central obesity with thinning of the extremities, hirsutism, etc., suggesting Cushing's syndrome
Tremor, weight loss, etc., suggesting thyrotoxicosis
Hypertension in the upper extremities only or radiofemoral pulse disparity (suggesting coarctation)
Skin: striae, acne, sweating, café au lait spots and neurofibromas
Mumurs: interscapular late systolic murmur (coarctation of the aorta)
Radiofemoral pulse delay (coarctation of the aorta)
Abdominal fat distribution
Muscle wasting
Postural hypertension with and without reflex tachycardia
Wide swings in blood pressure levels
Abdominal or flank masses (polycystic kidneys)
Tachycardia, tremor, orthostatic hypotension, sweating, and pallor (pheochromocytoma)

sudden onset of hypertension. The diagnosis of essential hypertension is made by exclusion.

Physical Examination

Physical examination should begin with careful measurement of the blood pressure, as its level determines the diagnosis of hypertension, predicts the long-term prognosis, justifies a search for secondary hypertension, and becomes the basis for initiating therapy. Recommendations for the indirect measurement of blood pressure with a sphygmomanometer, using the Korotkoff sounds, have been recently updated by a task force of the American Heart Association.[554] To establish the diagnosis of hypertension, multiple blood pressure determination should be made. Elevated readings should be confirmed on at least two subsequent visits during one to several weeks unless hypertension is very severe (Table 13-1), in which case more immediate treatment is indicated. Normal fluctuations in blood pressure levels resulting from diurnal variations, effects of ambient temperature, activity, hospitalization, emotional factors, and so on, must be appreciated. In some patients, home blood pressure recordings or automated 24-h recordings are needed to define whether the blood pressure is elevated persistently or only in the physician's office.[1] Target organ damage is correlated better with out-of-office than with office-pressure readings.[1] Average levels of diastolic blood pressure of >90 mm Hg or of systolic of over 140 mm Hg are required for the diagnosis of hypertension (Table 13-1).[1] Blood pressure should also be measured in supine, erect, and sitting positions. A marked postural fall in blood pressure (e.g., >10 mm Hg systolic) suggests volume depletion, blunted baroreceptor reflexes, or peripheral neuropathy.[555]

The remainder of the general physical examination should include careful inspection of the skin, head, and neck, including the optic fundi; detailed cardiovascular examination with palpation and auscultation of the major vessels; determination of cardiac size, rhythm, and the presence of murmurs; examination of the chest, abdomen, and extremities; and a screening neurologic examination. Features on physical examination that suggest the presence of secondary hypertension are listed in Table 13-5.

Laboratory Tests

Laboratory tests are used to obtain clues about secondary forms of hypertension and assess end organ damage and associated risk factors. Some general tests should be performed in all hypertensive patients, as outlined. More specialized tests should be performed as necessary. The specialized tests described in this chapter to evaluate the renovascular hypertension or mineralocorticoid-excess states are described in the sections dealing with those disorders.

General tests that should be performed in all hypertensive patients are listed in Table 13-6.[1] Additional studies such as chest x-ray, echocardiogram, and treadmill exercise test should be performed if additional cardiac evaluation is suggested by the clinical findings.

TABLE 13-6. Laboratory Evaluation of the Hypertensive Patient*

Complete blood count
Urinalysis
Serum creatinine, uric acid, and electrolytes
Blood urea nitrogen
Fasting blood glucose
Fasting serum LDL and HDL cholesterol and triglycerides
Electrocardiogram

*General tests that should be performed in all hypertensive patients.

Plasma Renin Activity

PRA is measured to assess renovascular hypertension and low-renin states and has been recommended as a general screening procedure to indicate the type of hypertensive medication to be used.[156] PRA can be measured under basal conditions or after stimulatory maneuvers. It is sometimes measured in samples taken from the renal veins.

PRA is measured by its ability to generate angiotensin I from the substrate angiotensinogen.[66,214,566–570] In vivo, this reaction occurs in the circulation, within blood vessel walls, and probably within some tissues. PRA is determined by incubation of plasma at 37°C followed by radioimmunoassay (RIA) of the generated angiotensin I.[66,569–571] Thus, plasma samples for renin determination must be processed quickly on collection (usually in tubes containing EDTA) and stored frozen at temperatures <20°C until assay. Prolonged storage of plasma at temperatures just below freezing can result in a slow activation of prorenin that can invalidate the results. The incubation pH is critical. A pH around 5.7 is used by some laboratories because it is the optimum pH for the reaction between human renin and human angiotensinogen. Conversely, a neutral pH is used by others to mimic in vivo conditions and eliminate the effects of plasma proteases, which may have renin-like activity. Generation of angiotensin I at neutrality generally gives lower PRA values than generation at pH 5.7. The reactions should include angiotensinase inhibitors; the choice depends on the incubation pH. PRA is usually expressed as nanograms of angiotensin I generated per milliliter per hour and is dependent on linear angiotensin I generation with time. There is also a direct RIA for renin.[567] The values obtained with it in general correlate with the PRA values.[567]

In human plasma, the reaction between renin and angiotensinogen occurs at substrate concentrations near the K_m for renin such that the reaction rate is proportional to concentrations of both renin and substrate. Ordinarily, the plasma renin substrate concentration is quite constant. However, in some clinical conditions it may be altered, leading to a change in the measured rate of angiotensin I generation. During estrogen administration and pregnancy and in patients with glucocorticoid excess, renin substrate concentration is increased, leading to elevated PRA.[139] Renin substrate concentration is reduced in liver disease and in states of glucocorticoid deficiency.

Plasma renin concentration (PRC) is measured by generating angiotensin I in the presence of excess substrate so that the reaction between renin and angiotensinogen is not limited by the concentration of angiotensinogen (i.e., is zero-order). Except in situations in which the human substrate concentration is altered, PRA and PRC are directly proportional. PRC measurements are not generally performed, but can be useful in situations in which angiotensinogen concentration is altered or to better define a low-renin state such as primary aldosteronism.

Plasma prorenin concentrations can also be measured by assaying PRC before and after acid or protease treatment of plasma to activate prorenin to renin.[62,67] Some patients with diabetes mellitus, patients with renin-secreting tumors, and pregnant women have elevated plasma levels of prorenin (5 to 10 times normal).[72]

PRA levels fluctuate spontaneously.[4,51,63,66,87,97,104,122,135,153,156,214,250] They are influenced by sex, race, age, sodium balance, position, activity, severity of hypertension, concurrent medication such as birth control pills and antihypertensive drugs, and illnesses such as diabetes mellitus, congestive heart failure, and cirrhosis (see previous discussion).[4,51,63,66,87,97,104,122,135,153,156,214,250] Several protocols have been proposed to standardize the measurement of PRA. They include normal and low-sodium diet, pretreatment with a diuretic, and measurement of PRA after overnight recumbency before the patient arises; others measure PRA after the patient has been ambulatory and upright for 4 h. Hence, "normal" values differ from laboratory to laboratory and under different circumstances.

PRA values[4,51,63,66,87,97,104,122,135,153,156,214,250] can be more easily interpreted by comparing them with concurrent 24-h urinary sodium excretion rates after several days on a stable sodium intake and without antihypertensive medications for at least 2 weeks (Fig. 13-5).[4,156] If renal, endocrine, and cardiac functions are normal, the sodium excretion rate is a convenient marker for extracellular fluid volume. Sodium excretion and extracellular fluid volume normally are inversely related to PRA and plasma aldosterone levels. The sodium/creatinine concentration ratio in a specimen of urine collected at the same time as the blood for PRA can also be used as a marker of volume status. PRA falls with age, and normal subjects above 55 years of age have PRA values that range up to 50 percent less than in younger subjects. Patients with diabetes mellitus with and without renal failure may have lower PRA levels.

In hypertensive patients, PRA levels are low in primary aldosteronism and other mineralocorticoid-excess states (see the sections on primary aldosteronism and other mineralocorticoid-excess states). They can also be low in low-renin essential hypertension and in renal disease.[50,51,141,156,219] PRA can also be low with excessive salt loading.

To diagnose a low renin state, PRA can be measured before and after stimulation of the renin system. Stimulatory maneuvers include provision of a low-sodium diet, standing (1 to 4 h), intravenous (IV) administration of furosemide (40 to 60 mg), and oral captopril. These maneuvers are described in the section on primary aldosteronism.

In hypertensive patients, PRA values are elevated in some patients with essential hypertension, renovascular hypertension, accelerated hypertension, renin-secreting tumors, and diuretic therapy.[252,572-575] In states not associated with hypertension, they can be high with dehydration, blood loss, and diuretic therapy. In patients with renin-secreting tumors, plasma prorenin levels are also markedly elevated.[225,572] In patients with unexplained hyperkalemia, a PRA determination is necessary in the diagnosis of hyporeninemic hypoaldosteronism (see Chap. 11).

Increased PRA in renovascular hypertension is seen in 50 to 80 percent of patients subsequently improved by angioplasty.[8,573,575] Because discontinuation of medication is not possible in patients with severe hypertension, depending on the standards for the particular laboratory, up to 20 percent of patients with proven renovascular hypertension can have normal to low PRA and approximately 15 percent of patients with essential hypertension can have elevated PRA. Thus, random determination of PRA per se has limited use in screening for renovascular hypertension.[573-575] Further, in chronic renovascular hypertension, especially if both renal arteries are stenotic, extracellular fluid volume can increase and PRA can be suppressed.

Measurement of PRA after the administration of a converting enzyme inhibitor may be helpful in differentiating patients with high-renin essential hypertension from those with renovascular hypertension (see the sections on the evaluation of renovascular hypertension).[575]

RENOVASCULAR HYPERTENSION

Prevalence

Renovascular hypertension (RVHT) defines the condition in which a sustained elevation in arterial blood pressure occurs due to the presence of a stenosis, constriction, or lesion in the artery of one or both kidneys. Although essential or primary hypertension accounts for up to 95 percent of the population with hypertension, renovascular hypertension accounts for the majority of the secondary causes of hypertension. The exact prevalence and incidence of renovascular disease are not known because not all cases of renal artery stenosis are sufficiently hemodynamically significant to result in renovascular hypertension. Studies indicate that as the patient population differs, the prevalence of RVHT also differs. For example, hypertensive patients with significant cardiovascular disease or those presenting with accelerated hypertension, or hypertension and rapidly progressive renal insufficiency tend to have a higher prevalence of renovascular disease.[556,557] In fact, the prevalence of renal artery stenosis in white patients presenting with severe or malignant hypertension has been reported to be as high as 10–45 percent.[558] The prevalence of renovascular hypertension occurs less frequently in black patients with hypertension than in whites (9 percent versus 18 percent).[559] Black hypertensive patients appear to suffer more from essential hypertension. However, patients with essential hypertension may have RAS but not RVHT, as well as RAS with RVHT.

The relationship between hypertension and cardiac and renal disease was recognized in the late 1890s.[560] In 1934 Goldblatt and colleagues established the relationship between renal artery stenosis and arterial hypertension in an experimental model of hypertension.[561] They produced persistent hypertension in dogs by constricting either both renal arteries, or one artery with the other kidney removed. This laid the groundwork for establishing a mechanism of renovascular hypertension by Braun-Menendez, Pickering, and Page, who described the involvement of the renin-angiotensin system.[562,563] Increased noncollagenous protein and collagen synthesis of small arteries may play some role in the etiology of the chronic phase of hypertension in this model.[564]

Causes of Renovascular Hypertension

The stenosis that restricts blood flow in the renal arteries in renovascular hypertension may be due to a number of causes. Of these, atherosclerosis and fibromuscular dysplasia are the most common. In general, the lesions that are associated with renovascular hypertension can be classified as intrinsic or extrinsic. Intrinsic lesions include arterial cholesterol emboli, renal artery aneurysm, dissection of the renal artery or aorta, arteriovenous malformations, fistula or hemangioma, hypoplasia of the suprarenal abdominal aorta, neurofibroma, and Takayasu's arthritis. Extrinsic lesions include those that result in compression of the renal arteries such as tumor, retroperitoneal fibrosis, perirenal or subcapsular hematoma, and scarring.

Atherosclerosis

Renal artery stenosis from atherosclerosis accounts for the majority of cases of renovascular hypertension. Some reports indicate that atherosclerotic renal artery disease can account for 60–70 percent of renal arterial lesions.[565] Patients who fall into this category tend to be older and have higher systolic blood pressure and evidence of vascular disease in other sites, such as the carotids and peripheral vasculature.[566] An autopsy study of 297 patients performed by Uzu et al. determined the prevalence of atherosclerotic renal artery stenosis in patients with cardiovascular disease and documented myocardial infarction.[567] Atherosclerotic renal artery was found in 12 percent of patients. The number increased in those patients who had hypertension (19 percent), proteinuria (39 percent), and renal insufficiency (39 percent). In addition, as the number of coronary vessels with significant stenosis increased, the prevalence of renal artery stenosis also increased.

The existence of atherosclerotic renal artery stenosis heralds diffuse atherosclerotic disease and reports indicate a higher prevalence of target organ damage than that seen in essential hypertension. Assessment of left ventricular hypertrophy and ischemic heart disease by electrocardiography suggest that in patients with comparable degrees of atherosclerotic vascular disease, renovascular hypertension may be responsible for the higher prevalence of target organ damage versus that seen in essential hypertension.[568]

The atheromatous lesion that occurs in atherosclerotic renovascular hypertension mimics those seen in other muscular arteries. Typically, these lesions are in the initial one-third of both renal arteries, and can be focal or extensive. Importantly, they can be complicated by ulcerating plaques that embolize to the kidneys. The patients who present with these lesions are typically older men (whites more than blacks) with a history of cardiovascular risk factors that include hypertension, diabetes, hyperlipidemia, cigarette smoking, and visceral obesity.

More often that not, renal artery lesions are sufficiently stenotic (>75 percent) to cause renal tissue ischemia and initiate the process that culminates in renovascular hypertension.[565] These lesions tend to progress unless surgically revascularized resulting in complete occlusion. In fact, complete occlusion can occur in 10–15 percent of cases, especially in those cases with greater than 75 percent occlusion.[565,569]

Fibromuscular Dysplasia

The muscular layers of the renal artery are divided into the intima, media, and adventitia. The nonatheromatous lesions of fibromuscular dysplasia are described by the layer that undergoes proliferation to produce a stenotic lesion and are therefore, classified anatomically: intimal, medial, perimedial, and periarterial fibroplasia.[570] Fibromuscular dysplastic lesions account for 30–40 percent of renal artery lesions.

The most common form of fibromuscular dysplasia seen in adults is medial fibroplasia, accounting for 65 percent of cases.[570] The lesion more frequently observed in children is focal fibroplasia.[571] Medial fibroplasia is characterized by the appearance of a "string of beads" on arteriogram. The typical appearance results from thickening of the media interspersed by aneurysmal dilatations that are not limited to the renal arteries and can be observed in other arteries that arise from the aorta such as the carotid arteries. The lesions are typically bilateral and found in the middle and distal thirds of the primary renal arteries and intrarenal branches. The pathogenesis of these lesions is still unclear, but unlike the pattern of progression seen in atherosclerotic renal artery stenosis, medial fibroplasia progresses much less frequently, occurring in approximately one-third of all patients.[565] The incidence of complete occlusion associated with this disease is overall quite low.

Perimedial fibroplasia is the next most common form of fibromuscular dysplasia, occurring with a frequency of 25 percent. It also appears as a "string of beads" on arteriogram due to proliferation of fibrous tissue in the outer half of the media to form a stenotic collar. No aneurysms form, but because the diameter of the lesion is smaller, it can lead to complete occlusion of the artery.[572,573,574]

Medial hyperplasia has a similar angiographic appearance as intimal fibroplasia. It occurs in 1–5 percent of cases and differ in the layer and type of cells that proliferate. Smooth muscle and fibrous tissue in the media are increased in medial hyperplasia, while intimal fibroplasia is characterized by proliferation of mesenchymal cells and connective tissue within the intima.

Medial dissection occurs in approximately 5–10 percent of cases of fibromuscular dysplasia. In these lesions, the intimal elastic membrane dissects. In the case of periarterial hyperplasia, as with intimal and perimedial lesions, there may be rapid progression of the lesions. In this lesion, there is proliferation of collagen in the periarterial adventitia that can lead to severe stenosis.[570]

Other Causes of Renovascular Hypertension

A number of other intrinsic causes of renovascular hypertension are less common but deserve some mention. Aneurysms are more likely to occur with medial fibroplasia. Atheroemboli tend to occur more often following angiography or invasive aortic surgery, but can also occur spontaneously in patients with a known history of atherosclerosis. Typically, these patients may present with acute renal failure after the procedure and cutaneous lesions called Livedo reticularis, but the diagnosis may sometimes require renal biopsy that reveals cholesterol microemboli.[527,576] Takayasu's arteritis is a disorder that can also cause stenosis of large vessels such as the aorta and other major blood vessels, including the renal arteries. Stenosis of the renal arteries in Takayasu's arteritis can be reversed by angioplasty. Posttransplant renal artery stenosis is relatively common and can occur in up to 12 percent of renal transplant patients. The diagnosis should be particularly suspected in a postrenal allograft patient with polycythemia, difficult to control hypertension, impaired graft function, and a loud bruit with a diastolic component.[577]

Extrinsic compression of the renal artery has also been seen in patients with retroperitoneal fibrosis, tumors, and ureteral obstruction (Table 13-7).[578,579,580] Ptosis of the kidney, although uncommon, can occur in moving from a supine to an upright position, and can also cause stenosis of the renal artery. The diagnosis is suspected when hypertension worsens on standing.[581]

TABLE 13-7. Causes of Renovascular Hypertension

Intrinsic Lesions	Extrinsic Lesions
Atherosclerosis	Pheochromocytoma
Fibromuscular dysplasia	Tumors
Intimal	Retroperitoneal fibrosis
Medial	Scarring
Periarterial or periadventitial	Ptosis
	Ureteral obstruction

TABLE 13-8. Comparison of Features of Renovascular Hypertension and Essential Hypertension

Features	Essential Hypertension (%)	Renovascular Hypertension (%)
Age of onset >50	9	15
Family history of hypertension	71	46
Severe retinopathy (grade III or IV)		15
Abdominal bruit	9	46
Blood urea nitrogen (>20 mg/dl)	8	15
Proteinuria	32	46

(Simon N, Franklin SS, Bleifer KH, Maxwell MH: Clinical characteristics of renovascular hypertension. *JAMA* 220:1209, 1972.)

Clinical Features of Renovascular Hypertension

Typical Features

Patients suspected of having renovascular hypertension can be distinguished from those with severe essential hypertension by some of the features outlined in Table 13-8. Many of these characteristics were recognized in a study that compared the clinical features of 2,442 hypertensive patients in which 880 patients were diagnosed with renovascular hypertension.[582] Of these, 60 percent had renal artery stenosis from atherosclerosis and 35 percent had fibromuscular dysplasia. Table 13-8 shows some of their findings.

Typically, the age of onset of renovascular hypertension is younger than 30 years and older than 50 years, particularly in patients with artherosclerotic renal artery stenosis (Table 13-9). There is a less frequent family history of hypertension. Renovascular hypertension appears to be less common in blacks.[569] On physical examination, patients with renovascular hypertension more often have severe retinopathy and an abdominal bruit. An abdominal bruit, particularly one with a diastolic component is more suggestive of renovascular hypertension than a purely systolic bruit.[583]

Laboratories may reveal some renal impairment with azotemia and proteinuria that is usually mild (<1 gm/day) but can reach the nephrotic range.[584] Renovascular hypertension can also be accompanied by an elevated plasma renin concentration and unprovoked hypokalemia from hyperaldosteronism.

TABLE 13-9. Signs and Symptoms of Renovascular Hypertension

History	
	Onset of hypertension <age 30 or >age 50
	Abrupt onset of hypertension
	Hypertension refractory to an appropriate three-drug regimen
	Symptoms of atherosclerotic disease in other vascular beds
	No family history of hypertension
	Recurrent pulmonary edema
	Acutely impaired renal function following ACEI
	Undiagnosed renal failure
Physical exam	
	Abdominal bruit (particularly in diastole)
	Bruits elsewhere
	Severe retinopathy
Laboratory	
	Hypokalemia
	Proteinuria
	Unilateral small kidney
	High renin concentration

Ischemic Nephropathy

Ischemic nephropathy occurs when there is significant renal impairment marked by a reduction in glomerular filtration rate due to a hemodynamically significant reduction in renal blood flow from renal artery occlusive disease. More commonly, renoocclusive disease is unilateral, though bilateral renovascular disease has been demonstrated in up to 28 percent of patients.[585] Some clinical clues to the presence of bilateral renovascular disease include signs of generalized atherosclerosis obliterans, presumed renovascular hypertension, unilateral small kidney, unexplained azotemia, recurrent "flash" pulmonary edema, a fall in renal function with a decrease in blood pressure, and acute renal failure following angII antagonist therapy. Because surgical revascularization or angioplasty may be successful in relieving both the hypertension and progressive renal failure in patients with renovascular hypertension, recognition of the disorder is of utmost importance.

Who Should be Evaluated for RVHT?

The estimated prevalence of renovascular hypertension in the absence of clinical clues is low (0.2 percent) and the cost of unnecessary diagnostic procedures may be quite high.[586] Therefore, the selection of patients to be evaluated for RVHT should be assessed carefully. Patients in whom an extensive workup should be performed include those with a high clinical index of suspicion for renal artery stenosis and who are candidates for surgical revascularization or angioplasty. Patients with moderate index of suspicion should undergo an initial screening test while those who are considered to have a low index of suspicion of renal artery stenosis should not undergo diagnostic study. Although medical therapy with β-adrenergic blockers or antagonists of angII action may be effective in controlling blood pressure, care should be taken to pursue invasive therapy in those patients with potentially "curable" disease to prevent further progression of renal parenchymal disease.

Screening and Diagnostic Studies for Renovascular Hypertension

The gold standard for diagnosing renovascular hypertension is the renal arteriogram. There are a number of less invasive screening tests that can be performed prior to renal arteriogram, but unfortunately, none of those currently available is perfect. Two noninvasive tests, the peripheral plasma renin activity and the captopril test, are relatively inexpensive and can be done in a physician's office but do not provide information on which kidney might be involved. Other screening tests determine the relative function of both kidneys and can more reliably isolate the affected kidney. These include differential renal vein renin determination, intravenous pyelogram, digital subtraction, renal scans, the captopril renogram, magnetic resonance arteriogram, and the exercise renogram. The sensitivity and specificity of these tests vary, and the decision to use one versus another depends on patient selection, clinical suspicion of renovascular hypertension, and availability of the specific test.

Renal arteriography is performed after all screening is complete to make the final diagnosis. Even so, the truly definitive test of renovascular hypertension is retrospectively made when control of the blood pressure occurs following surgical revascularization, angioplasty, or nephrectomy.

Peripheral Plasma Renin Activity

PRA is usually elevated in patients with functionally significant renovascular hypertension. However, it can also be increased in patients with essential hypertension as well as in many other situations. In particular, 50–80 percent of patients with renovascular hypertension demonstrate increased PRA levels, whereas only 16 percent of essential hypertensives have elevated PRA levels.[586,587] It is important to remember that when measuring plasma renin activity, the following conditions should be noted: whether the patient is fasting or on a regular diet, a salt restricted diet, and/or on diuretics and whether the patient is supine or upright and the length of time ambulating prior to having the sample taken. Ideally, all medications should be discontinued for approximately one week prior to the test. Rudnick et al. (1984) showed that the sensitivity of the plasma renin activity in renovascular hypertension was 57 percent while the specificity was 66 percent.[588]

Captopril Test

The predictive value of the peripheral blood plasma renin activity in the diagnosis of renovascular hypertension can be improved by mechanisms that augment renin secretion. One method is following the administration of an angiotensin receptor blocker or ACEI.[589] A set of criteria for the correct administration of the oral captopril test was designed by Muller et al.[590] The test requires that the patient be maintained on a normal salt intake, avoid diuretics, and withhold antihypertensives for at least 3 weeks prior to the test, where possible. A baseline PRA is taken after 30 min of rest followed by oral administration of 50 mg of captopril diluted in 10 ml of water. A smaller dose of 25 mg may also be used to avoid episodes of hypotension.[590,591,592] A stimulated PRA level is measured after 1 hr.

The interpretation of a positive test is based on the following criteria: a stimulated PRA of ≥12 ng/ml/hr, an absolute increase in PRA of ≥10 mg/ml/hr, and an increase in PRA of ≥150 percent or ≥400 percent if the baseline PRA is <3 ng/ml/hr (Table 13-10). In laboratories where PRA levels are standardized, the accuracy of the captopril test can be quite high.[590] Unfortunately, the test may not be as accurate in patients with renal insufficiency, and false positive results have been observed in 2 out of 112 patients with essential hypertension and in 6 patients with secondary hypertension.[590] Additionally, a high false-positive rate may be seen in patients with elevated baseline levels of PRA. Therefore, the test is less useful in patients with renovascular hypertension who may have elevated PRA levels due to refractory hypertension and renal insufficiency. The advantage of the captopril test is that it may provide some information on reversibility of a lesion if there is a change in glomerular filtration following captopril. The test is also widely available. Furthermore, a completely positive study indicates that the hypertension is most likely due to significant vascular disease.

TABLE 13-10. Criteria for A Positive Captopril-Augmented Test

Plasma renin activity ≥12 ng/ml
Absolute increase of plasma renin activity ≥10 mg/ml
From a baseline plasma renin activity <3 ng/ml/h, the increase should be ≥400 percent
From a baseline plasma renin activity >3 ng/ml/h, the increase should be 150 percent

Differential Renal Vein Renin Determination

The purpose of measuring PRA by catheterization of both renal veins is twofold: to diagnose renovascular hypertension and to predict the outcome of surgical revascularization. The test is positive if the ratio between the renal veins is >1.5 : 1 and is 92 percent predictive of a surgically correctable lesion.[588] The results, however, can be affected in patients in whom renin levels are suppressed, such as those with a high dietary sodium or following the use of β-adrenergic agents. Differential renal renin vein levels may fail to lateralize in patients with collateral circulation to the kidney with a significant stenosis or in patients with bilateral renal artery stenosis. The predictive value of this test can be even further improved by administration of an ACEI.[593]

Bilateral renal artery stenosis can occur in 25 percent of cases of renovascular hypertension and lateralization may not be evident by the differential renin vein determination so that the diagnosis may be missed.[588] Determination of the functional significance of bilateral lesions can be assessed by comparing the renal vein renin to the systemic renin level. The renal/systemic renin index is defined as the renal vein renin minus the systemic (infrarenal vena cava) renin divided by the systemic renin. An index >0.24 is indicative of excess renin secretion.[594] A nonischemic kidney would have an index of zero. In the presence of bilateral lesions, the differential renin vein determination may not lateralize and the ratio between the two renal veins may be <1.5:1. In this case, the renal/systemic renin index will be >0.24 on both sides, indicating significant bilateral disease, which warrants further evaluation for definitive treatment.

Intravenous Pyelography

Intravenous pyelography is not used as frequently now in the diagnostic evaluation of a patient with renovascular hypertension as in the past. The criteria for an abnormal test include a delayed excretion, a difference in size ≥1.5 cm between the kidneys and a difference in the concentration of dye.[585] The sensitivity of this test is 70–80 percent. Therefore, renovascular hypertension is not reliably excluded in a negative test in 20–25 percent of cases. In addition, this method may not detect bilateral disease.[586]

Renal Scintigraphy

The renogram can be useful in screening patients suspected of having renovascular hypertension, particularly when enhanced by pretreatment with captopril (i.e., the captopril augmented renogram).[586,591,595–598] Without captopril, the percentage of false negatives is 20–25 percent.[599] A number of isotopes can be used in this test to assess the glomerular filtration rate such as diethylene triamine penta-acetic acid (DTPA), and hippuran, which can approximate the renal blood flow. The more preferred isotope, ^{99m}Tc-mercuraptoacetyl-triglycine (Mag_3), is particularly reliable in patients with renal insufficiency.[600] In general, Mag_3 is more accurate and provides less radiation exposure and more detailed images but is more costly.

The efficacy of the captopril-augmented renogram is based on the fact that the ACEI will cause a decrease in glomerular filtration rate and, therefore, a decrease in uptake of the tracer in the stenotic kidney. The isotope-labeled tracer is administered intravenously 1 hr after 25 to 50 mg of oral captopril (or 50 μg/kg of intravenous enalapril) and both static and dynamic images are used for analysis. The criteria for a positive test are decreased uptake of the isotope in one kidney relative to the other, accounting for 40 percent of the total glomerular filtration rate and delayed peak uptake of the isotope of >10 to 11 minutes. The normal peak uptake is 3 to 6 minutes.[601,602]

The sensitivity and specificity of the captopril-enhanced renogram can be 90 percent or greater, particularly in patients with significant occlusion. A study by Elliot et al. in which 100 patients were further evaluated by arteriogram showed that 59 have significant stenotic lesion. The negative predictive value of the captopril scan was 90 percent.[591]

Exercise renograms, used more in the diagnosis of essential hypertension than renovascular hypertension, appear to detect the presence of renal parenchymal disease.[603,604] Normal individuals show a prolonged tracer transit during exercise whereas individuals with essential hypertension demonstrate a much more significant delay. On the other hand, patients with renovascular hypertension demonstrate a normal exercise response. The utility of the test in renovascular hypertension is the detection of potentially irreversible parenchymal disease indicating a nonsalvageable kidney.[603,605]

Duplex Doppler Imaging

The advantage of duplex Doppler imaging is that it can directly visualize the renal arteries (B-mode) and record hemodynamic changes (Doppler), providing both anatomic as well as functional evaluation of renovascular hypertension.[606] The most reliable criteria for the diagnosis of renal artery stenosis in duplex Doppler imaging is a ratio of peak systolic velocities in the renal artery compared to the aorta of >3.5, as velocity increases across a stenotic lesion. A ratio >3.5 indicates the presence of a 60 percent or greater stenotic lesion. This corresponds to a sensitivity of 84–90 percent and a specificity of 95–97 percent.[607,608] The procedure allows the extent of stenoses present either bilaterally or unilaterally to be determined.

The disadvantage of duplex Doppler imaging is that it is very operator-dependent and time-consuming. It can also be limited by the presence of bowel gas, obesity, and other technical obstacles such as inability to identify accessory renal artery lesions and inadequate measurement of renal artery velocity because of the short length of the artery. Therefore, the sensitivity and specificity can vary. Numerous maneuvers have been applied to try to improve the results of this method, such as pretreatment with captopril[609] and color coding,[610] as well as intravascular ultrasound.[611,612] Intravascular ultrasound provides the added ability to distinguish between lesions due to atherosclerosis versus fibromuscular dysplasia. Overall, duplex ultrasound is fairly inexpensive and is suitable for comparing serial studies, but does not provide much information on renal function.

Renal Arteriography

Renal arteriography remains the gold standard for the diagnosis of renal artery stenosis. However, it must be emphasized that not all stenoses are the definitive cause of the hypertension. Indeed, renal artery stenosis may occur concurrently with essential hypertension in more than 30 percent of patients with RVHT.[613] In such cases, a renal artery stenotic lesion is more likely to cause ischemia and hypertension when the occlusion is ≥75 percent.[614,615]

Renal arteriography is an invasive procedure that uses a percutaneous catheter to deliver either ionic or nonionic contrast material. The risk of complications correlates with the experience of the arteriographer[616] but the rate of complications is lower than that seen following cardiac catheterization.[617] The incidence of nephrotoxicity from the contrast material can be reduced with the use of minimal amount of dye, adequate pre- and postprocedure hydration, and avoidance of nonsteroidal inflammatory drugs.[618]

The advantage of renal arteriography is that it allows visualization of the main renal artery as well as the presence of collateral or accessory arteries, aneurysms, poststenotic dilatations, and vascular malformation.[595,619,596,591] This visualization provides an assessment of the extent and pathologic etiology of the stenotic lesion. The accuracy of distinguishing an atherosclerotic lesion from fibromuscular disease was determined to be 82 percent following analysis of the pathologic specimen in one study.[620] However, further distinction between different classes of fibromuscular disease is not reliable and must depend on complete analysis of the pathology. The added advantage of renal arteriography is that it provides the immediate opportunity for corrective angioplasty.[621] Even so, renal arteriography alone cannot accurately identify a curable lesion and the results of a renal scan can be very useful.[622] Renal arteriography can be further supplemented with intraarterial digital subtraction, which gives more visual detail by comparing pre- and postcontrast images.

Renal Angiography

Renal angiography is a noninvasive procedure that involves intravenous, rather than percutaneous, administration of contrast material with images taken by computerized tomography (CT) or magnetic resonance (MRA). Both studies can visualize the renal arteries without the potential risks associated with arteriography.

Magnetic resonance angiography (MRA) uses gadolinium as the contrast material, which is less nephrotoxic than the contrast dyes used in arteriography. The technique has significantly improved over the years and is becoming more available as a routine noninvestigational imaging option for the diagnosis of renal artery stenosis. It provides better results than the other noninvasive screening tests, described previously, especially in patients with a high clinical suspicion for renovascular hypertension.[623] As the use of magnetic resonance has improved, newer modalities have evolved, including: two-dimensional (2-D) and three-dimensional (3-D) time-of-flight imaging with incorporation of phase-contrast and cine MR angiography techniques.[624] The breath-hold ultrafast 3D angiography, which further shortens the acquisition time of the procedure, provides a series of slices through the suspected stenotic area during a 32-second period.[625] The images are then analyzed as individual slices or collapsed into a single 3-D picture.

In a study which compared dynamic gadolinium 3-D MRA to renal arteriography, the sensitivity and specificity of MRA was 100 percent and 71 percent, respectively, for renal artery stenosis of ≥75 percent.[623] Unlike arteriography, accessory renal arteries are not visualized with MRA.

MRA can also be combined with image subtraction, which improves the quality of the imaging by visualization of the distal renal arteries.[626] This method is contraindicated in patients with any form of metallic implants and in individuals who may be claustrophobic.

Helical CT angiography, also called spiral or volumetric CT angiography, has a high degree of accuracy. It provides excellent 3-D images, but requires larger amounts of contrast material and breath holds. This technique may be suitable for transplant donor evaluation. The sensitivity and specificity in a study of 62 patients was 98 percent and 94 percent, respectively.[627] Results were compared to that of renal arteriography. Unfortunately, this accuracy falls to 93 percent (sensitivity) and 81 percent (specificity) in patients with renal insufficiency and a plasma creatinine greater than 1.7 mg/dl.

Other Procedures

Various other procedures that are no longer in use include the angiotensin infusion test and renal biopsy.[627,628] The split renal function test, which was introduced in 1953, required cystoscopy and bilateral ureteral catheterization.[629] This has been bypassed for the less invasive techniques that are currently available.

Selection and Sequence of Diagnostic Tests for Renovascular Hypertension

As described previously, there are a number of screening tests available for the complete work-up of renovascular hypertension. Investigators have reviewed and assessed many of these procedures in an attempt to assist the clinician in choosing the best test for an individual patient.

In each evaluation, the factor that will determine the route by which to proceed in the evaluation will be the level of clinical suspicion that renal artery stenosis is present and is the cause of the hypertension. The level of the patient's renal function as well as the availability of specific procedures will also be determinants. Assessment of the relative sensitivity, specificity, and predictive value of various procedures suggests that patients with poor renal function may be better served by tests such as the captopril renogram, which avoids the use of nephrotoxic contrast materials. Patients with relatively well-preserved renal function, however, can undergo effective screening with almost any screening test available.[630]

Because the overall prevalence of renovascular hypertension is relatively low, it is not cost-effective to screen patients with a low suspicion of renovascular hypertension, and these patients should be treated medically. Patients with a moderate suspicion of disease should have a captopril test, preferably combined with a renal scan as an initial test, as it also provides functional information. However, the captopril test should not be performed in patients with a creatinine clearance less than 30 ml/min, as the accuracy of the captopril test under these circumstances has not been evaluated.[631] Other tests, including duplex ultrasound spiral CT and MRA are also appropriate. As the algorithm in Fig. 13-12 illustrates, a high clinical suspicion for renovascular hypertension may be evaluated with the noninvasive intraarterial digital subtraction angiography or directly by renal arteriography because they provide the immediate opportunity for corrective angioplasty.

Management of Renovascular Hypertension

There are at least three treatment options available for the management of renovascular hypertension: medical therapy, surgical revascularization, and percutaneous transluminal angioplasty by balloon or stent placement. The ultimate goals of therapy are to cure or improve management of the hypertension and to preserve renal function. Though medical therapy can succeed in improving the hypertension, surgical revascularization and angioplasty offer a chance of cure. In rare cases of renovascular hypertension resistant to therapy, nephrectomy is performed. In every patient, the choice of therapy must be individualized. Typically, surgical revascularization is performed for bilateral renal artery atherosclerotic stenosis, while angioplasty is usually chosen for unilateral disease due to fibromuscular disease.

Medical Therapy

Medical therapy for renovascular hypertension becomes necessary for patients in whom a definite cause cannot be undertaken or in management of hypertension prior to and following partially successful or unsuccessful revascularization procedures. Although medical therapy may improve control of the hypertension, it will not avert progression of the lesion. No randomized controlled trials have compared medical therapy with surgical treatment, but a retrospective study by Hunt et al.[632] compared these two modalities. There was a 70 percent mortality rate in the medically-treated individuals versus 30 percent in the surgically-treated patients. The majority of the deaths were due to stroke and myocardial infarctions related to complications of atherosclerosis in other vascular beds. Although, the study was done prior to the improved options of therapy with ACEI, angiotensin receptor blockers (ARBs) and calcium channel blockers (CCBs), it illustrates the rate of progression of the disease and its consequences.

The appropriate drugs for treating renovascular hypertension include those directed at inhibiting the effects of the renin-angiotensin system: ACEI and ARB. The concern with these agents is that they can cause renal failure in patients with bilateral renal artery stenosis or an occlusion in the artery of a solitary kidney.[42,187,203,633,634] A study done in the two-kidney, one-clip rat model of renovascular hypertension has demonstrated the same effect of the ARB, losartan, as the ACEI, enalapril, on the structure and function of both the stenotic and non-stenotic kidney.[635] Renal blood flow and subsequently, glomerular filtration rate, is normally maintained by the angII-dependent vasoconstriction of the efferent arterioles. When there is an occlusion to the flow of blood in the glomerular afferent arterioles, renal blood flow becomes even more dependent on the action of angII. The effect of an ACEI is to decrease autoregulated intrarenal efferent arteriolar resistance to the extent that glomerular filtration is significantly compromised, necessitating discontinuation of therapy.[187] A similar reversible effect is seen with ARBs, which stimulate the angII type I receptor. This effect may also be seen with other antihypertensives, although the effect is more dramatic with inhibitors of RAS.[636] Therefore, with the use of these agents in the treatment of renovascular hypertension, renal function and serum potassium should be closely monitored. Surgical revascularization should be seriously reconsidered in the event of rapid, progressive deterioration in renal function. The presence of mild proteinuria that may accompany renovascular hypertension can be decreased with the use of ACEIs probably due to the effect on renal hemodynamics.

CCBS may also be used to control blood pressure. Renal function may deteriorate to a smaller degree because of the difference in action of CCBs, which do not preferentially vasodilate the glomerular efferent arterioles. β-blockers may also be effective in controlling hypertension in renovascular hypertension by decreasing plasma renin activity through their action of blocking sympathetic β-adrenergic receptors.[637] Unlike ACEIs and ARBs, β-blockers have little effect on altering renal blood flow.

Surgical Revascularization

Surgical revascularization refers to any surgical procedure that will alleviate the mechanical obstruction of the lesion causing renovascular hypertension. This can be achieved by various techniques including endarterectomy, resection and replacement of the

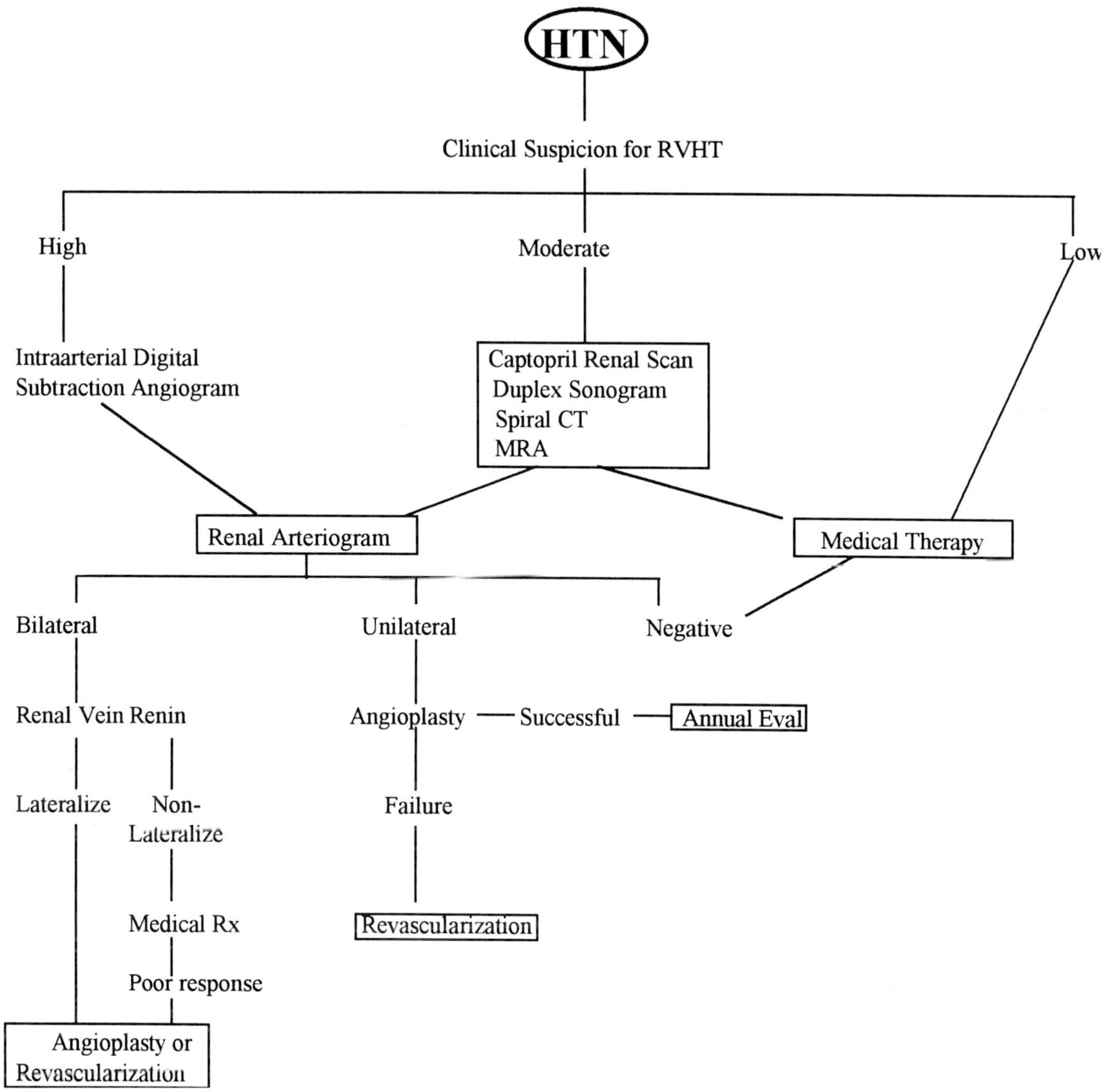

FIGURE 13-12. Algorithm for evaluation of renovascular hypertension.

occluded artery, or bypass of the lesion. The method chosen depends on the type of the lesion (unilateral or bilateral), the nature of the occlusion (atherosclerosis or fibromuscular dysplasia), and the extent and location of the lesion.

Surgical revascularization in renovascular hypertension is indicated for lesions that are considered high grade (>75 percent) because the rate of progression to total occlusion is especially high.[565] This is particularly seen in atherosclerotic disease because total occlusion in fibromuscular disease is rare, although some progression still may occur. A kidney size >9 cm, evidence of renal function on renal flow scan, and collateral filling of distal renal arteries containing total proximal occlusion predict salvageability of that kidney, and every attempt should be made to preserve its function.

The most common technique of surgical revascularization used is the aortorenal bypass, though other techniques employed include ileorenal, splenorenal, and hepatorenal bypass.[638] The benefit of surgical revascularization is 85 percent to 95 percent of appropriately chosen patients with renovascular hypertension.[613] In addition to atherosclerotic lesion, renovascular revascularization appears particularly applicable to pediatric age groups, who do not have coexisting essential hypertension and for whom surgical reconstruction of a stenotic renal artery can completely restore renal blood flow.

A retrospective study to evaluate the unilateral and bilateral surgical repair of renal artery stenosis due to fibromuscular dysplasia by Anderson et al. indicates that younger patients tend to have a better rate of hypertension cure than do older patients (age >45 years).[639] The older patients appear to have more significant involvement of branch renal arteries and coincident atherosclerosis.

In a series of 5 patients with flash pulmonary edema from renovascular hypertension, surgical revascularization was shown to be the optimal mode of treatment over medical therapy.[640] Both morbidity and mortality in this study were low and the procedure resulted in control of blood pressure and restoration of renal function as well as cure of recurrent flash pulmonary edema 57 months later. In general, most reports indicate that the mortality associated with surgical revascularization of stenotic renal arteries is 3 percent to 6 percent. Patients who are at greatest risk are those with diffuse atherosclerotic disease and congestive heart failure.[641]

Angioplasty

Percutaneous transluminal angioplasty is the treatment of choice for renovascular hypertension due to fibromuscular dysplasia. The procedure offers a low risk of complications as well as a low rate of restenosis in these patients.

Angioplasty of atherosclerotic lesions is less successful as these lesions appear to be more resistant to angioplasty than fibromuscular disease.[642] Thus, there is a much higher restenosis rate in one year (at least 16 percent) following an initial angioplasty of atherosclerotic renal artery stenosis.[643] This is due, in part, to the presence of ostial lesions that are seen in atherosclerosis.[569]

The use of stent placement has helped to improve the success rate in angioplasty of atherosclerotic occlusions, particularly in patients with ostial lesions.[644] Although stent placement appears to be necessary in atherosclerotic disease, it has also been reported in the treatment of renal artery stenosis due to fibromuscular disease that showed elastic recoil immediately following conventional angioplasty.[645]

Renal angioplasty is not limited to atherosclerotic or fibromuscular disease, but can also be used in the treatment of renal artery stenosis due to nonspecific aortoarteritis, also called Takayasu's disease. A study of 66 patients revealed that this procedure is safe and effective in the treatment of renovascular hypertension due to nonspecific aortoarteritis with a restenosis rate of 16 percent after 22 months.[646]

Percutaneous angioplasty is also the treatment of choice in posttransplant renal artery stenosis. Renal occlusion occurs in 2–12 percent of cases and causes include atherosclerosis, clamp injury, faulty suture technique, and kinking of the renal artery. Rejection of the donor artery has also been postulated as a potential cause but this has not been conclusive. The success rate following angioplasty is 60–85 percent, but restenosis can occur in 20 percent to 30 percent of cases.[577] Repair of a transplanted stenotic renal artery is technically difficult and when angioplasty fails, loss of the allograft during surgical repair can occur in up to 30 percent of cases.[647]

In general, the complications associated with transluminal balloon angioplasty of bilateral atherosclerotic renal artery disease occurs in approximately 10 percent of patients and consist of atheroemboli, arterial thrombosis, acute renal infarction, arterial spasm, and rupture of the artery.[558,648–650] As a result, surgical backup is usually required during renal artery angioplasty. Stent placement is associated with a higher rate of mortality and complications in men following stent placement for coronary disease, but this gender difference does not exist in patients undergoing stent placement of the renal artery.[651]

Nephrectomy

Nephrectomy as a treatment for renal artery stenosis is reserved for patients with a confirmed nonfunctioning kidney that continues to produce renin. In the past, renal nephrectomy for renovascular hypertension was more commonly performed for lesions that appeared to be irreparable. However, as techniques and success rates improve, even in the toughest cases, and complication rates decrease, nephrectomy is less often performed.[652] Every attempt should be made towards revascularization, even in patients with complete occlusion of the renal artery by evidence of collateral blood flow.[653]

Renin-Secreting Tumors

Although the incidence of renin-secreting tumors is low, it is important to note that a high renal vein renin level may be the result of a tumor rather than renovascular hypertension. Patients who should be suspected for having a renin-secreting tumor usually present with severe, malignant, or accelerated hypertension. The patients are typically young (age <25 years).[654] Signs and symptoms of secondary hyperaldosteronism, such as unprovoked hypokalemia, weakness, and metabolic alkalosis, are also usually present.

The renin-secreting tumors tend to be hemangiopericytomas composed of juxtaglomerular cells, but pancreatic adenocarcinomas, Wilm's tumors, and ovarian tumors have also been seen. The tumor can be detected by abdominal CT scan or MRI. The most appropriate treatment is surgical removal. However, in the event that surgical resection cannot be performed, medical therapy with angiotensin converting enzyme inhibitors, angiotensin receptor blockers, or calcium channel blockers is effective in controlling the hypertension.

Summary and Recommendations

Fig. 13-12 illustrates an algorithmic approach to the diagnosis and management of renovascular hypertension. The important point to remember is that patient selection for a complete work-up depends on the clinical index of suspicion of the disease. Following the appropriate screening tests, a renal arteriogram must be performed to confirm the diagnosis. This is usually followed by surgical revascularization for definitive therapy. When patient selection prevents surgical revascularization, other options include percutaneous transluminal angioplasty, with or without stent placement, or medical therapy with angiotensin converting enzyme inhibitors, angiotensin receptor blockers, calcium channel blockers or β-blockers to control hypertension. The presence of a renin-secreting tumor should be kept in mind.

DISORDERS OF THE ADRENAL

Although adrenal-dependent hypertension is a relatively uncommon cause of hypertension, its diagnosis provides physicians with an opportunity to more definitively treat the cause of hypertension and its attending complications.[655] Primary aldosteronism is the most common type of adrenal-dependent hypertension and thus will be reviewed in some detail.

Primary Aldosteronism

Primary aldosteronism is a syndrome resulting from the production and secretion of excessive quantities of aldosterone from the adrenal cortex, usually by a single adenoma or bilateral hyperplasia, and occasionally by variants of these two disorders.[656–659] The prevalence of primary aldosteronism in unselected patients is between 0.5 percent and 2 percent of hypertensives.[655,656] Nevertheless, pathological changes of the adrenal, including incidentally discovered adrenocortical adenoma (incidentaloma), are observed in a greater percentage of persons with hypertension than in patients without hypertension.[156,660] Indeed, it has been suggested that 1 percent of those with incidentally discovered adenomas may have aldosteronomas.[656]

Aldosteronoma is the most common cause of primary aldosteronism (60 percent).[656] Aldosteronomas are typically small (less than 2 cm in diameter), are almost always benign, and contain cells from all three adrenal zones.[656] Idiopathic aldosteronism, which is associated with bilateral micronodular or macronodular adrenal hyperplasia, is responsible for 20 to 30 percent of cases of primary aldosteronism.[656] A subgroup of patients with bilateral or unilateral adrenal hyperplasia has been described as having primary adrenal hyperplasia.[656,661] Unilateral adrenal hyperplasia has also been described.[661] In rare cases, adrenal carcinoma causes primary aldosteronism.[662] These malignant tumors are usually larger than the more common, benign aldosteronomas; they often secrete other adrenal hormones and may be locally invasive or display distant metastasis.

Aldosteronomas occur more commonly in women than in men, and are infrequent in children.[656] This disorder is more common in persons aged 30 to 50 years. Idiopathic aldosteronism is more common in men, occurs at an older age than does aldosteronoma, and may be as common as aldosteronoma in series where more patients are evaluated for primary aldosteronism.[656] In contrast to many endocrine tumors, most aldosterone-producing tumors do not have a familial basis. Nevertheless, familial aldosterone producing adenomas have been reported.[663] The ipsilateral and/or contralateral adrenal glands of patients with dominant adenomas frequently have additional small adenomas.[656] Adrenal adenomas and hyperplasia likely reflect a spectrum of adrenal abnormalities rather than two distinct entities. This is indicated by the following: (1) both adenomas and hyperplasia can be either responsive or unresponsive to stimulatory maneuvers, (2) adenomatous and hyperplastic abnormalities are often seen in the same patient, and (3) hyperplasia can be diffuse, micro- or macronodular.

Aldosterone secretion in primary aldosteronism is partially autonomous and PRA is low. Aldosterone secretion is not suppressed by volume expansion or by increased sodium intake (sodium loading). In patients with aldosteronoma, secretion is significantly regulated by corticotropin, and in most cases is unresponsive to angiotensin (i.e., upright posture), parallels the circadian rhythm of cortisol, and transiently decreases in response to glucocorticoids.[656] In patients with idiopathic aldosteronism and 20 percent of those with aldosteronomas the secretion is regulated by angII, and consequently they display a normal response to upright posture.[658,661] Thus, there are two types of aldosteronomas, approximately 80 percent are responsive to corticotropin and the rest respond to angII.

The classic clinical features of primary aldosteronism are hypertension, hypokalemia, excessive urinary potassium excretion, hypernatremia, and metabolic alkalosis.[656] The hypertension is hemodynamically characterized by an increased peripheral vascular resistance, a slightly expanded plasma volume, and an increased total body and exchangeable sodium content.[656] The pressor effects of aldosterone are related to its effects on sodium retention via its action on renal mineralocorticoid receptor.[656] The human mineralocorticoid receptor has been cloned, sequenced, expressed, and demonstrated to be equally receptive to glucocorticoids and mineralcorticoids. Relatively small concentrations of aldosterone are able to exert receptor mediated effects in the face of much higher concentrations of cortisol because of the action of the 11-beta-hydroxysteroid dehydrogenase enzyme, which converts cortisol into cortisone (without mineralocorticoid effects). The effects of excess aldosterone on renal mineralocorticoid receptors results in increased sodium reabsorption and potassium and hydrogen ion excretion (distal tubule)[656] resulting frequently in hypokalemic metabolic alkalosis as well as hypertension.

Biochemical findings suggestive of primary hyperaldosteronism include spontaneous hypokalemia with metabolic alkalosis and a serum sodium at the high normal level.[656] Increased urinary excretion of potassium (>30 mmol per 2.4 hours) in the presence of hypokalemia without extra potassium intake strongly suggests hyperaldosteronism.[656] Hypokalemia is often more striking in patients with aldosteronoma and less severe or absent in patients with idiopathic aldosteronism. Hypomagnesemia and/or glucose intolerance may also be observed.[656] Plasma renin activity is suppressed in almost all patients with untreated primary aldosteronism. However, hypokalemia and suppressed plasma renin levels are not sufficient for a diagnosis of primary hyperaldosteronism. Determination of the ratio of the plasma aldosterone to renin level is increasingly recognized as a good screening test for primary aldosteronism.[655,664] If the cutoff value of this ratio is >30, most cases of aldosteronism will be identified.[655,656,664] The conditions for this measurement includes upright posture and morning collection.[664] The captopril test, with aldosterone measurement two hours after administration, may also be helpful in making the diagnosis.

More definitive biochemical diagnosis of aldosteronism is made by inhibiting and stimulating aldosterone and renin secretion by physiological maneuvers of sodium loading and depletion, respectfully. In patients with hypertension (untreated or after medication has been discontinued for two weeks), a high urinary aldosterone excretion while on a high-salt diet for two to three days, a high plasma aldosterone after two to four hours of saline infusion, followed by a low plasma renin activity with low salt intake and furosemide establishes the diagnosis.[656] Urinary aldosterone excretion of less than 14 μg in 24 hours after salt loading rules out the diagnosis of primary aldosteronism. It should be noted that a high intake of salt can accentuate hypokalemia, and correction of hypokalemia is thus important to prevent medical problems as well as maintain the appropriate aldosterone responses. In severe hypertension, in which medications cannot be completely stopped, it is appropriate to continue antihypertensive medications that are least likely to affect renin and aldosterone responses (i.e., alpha blockers).

Tests to Differentiate Aldosteronoma from Idiopathic Hyperplasia

After a definitive biochemical diagnosis of aldosteronism, the precise etiology is then determined. A postural test helps differentiate a potentially surgically correctable disorder (aldosteronoma) from the medically-treated hyperplastic aldosteronism. In patients with aldosteronoma the aldosterone levels do not rise significantly and may decrease in patients who are maintained in an upright posture for two to four hours in the morning after overnight recumbancy.[656] Persons with idiopathic aldosteronism have a significant plasma aldosterone response to upright posture. However, about 20 percent of persons with aldosteronoma will have a positive aldosterone response to upright posture.

Measurement of plasma 18-hydroxycorticosterone (18-OHB) is often helpful in differentiating aldosteronoma from idiopathic hyperplasia.[656] Adenomas are typically composed of cell types resembling those of all three zones of the adrenal gland, including hybrid cells similar to zona glomerulosa and fasciculata cells.[655,656,661] This is reflected by increased production of certain cortisol metabolites, such as 18-OHB. A basal 8 am plasma 18-OHB level of greater than 100 ng/dl (2,800 nmol/ml), strongly supports a diagnosis of aldosteronoma.[656,661] More recently a level of 65 ng/dl has been advocated as a cut-off value.[665]

Computerized tomographic (CT) scanning detects most aldosteronomas, except those that are very small.[656,666] MRI may provide greater specificity, and continued improved technology and lesser cost may make it superior to CT.[661] However, some aldosteronomas are less than 5 mm, and CT and MRI may miss them.[656] Further, bilateral nodularity may suggest bilateral hyperplasia when a unilateral adenoma is the cause of excess aldosterone secretion.[668] Similarly, what may appear to be a solitary nodule may be the only visible aspect of diffuse hyperplasia.[669] The observation of a large adrenal lesion (>3 cm in diameter) should raise the possibility of adrenal carcinoma, and in those cases other adrenal steroids (androgens, corticosteroids, and estrogen) in the plasma or urine should be measured.[656] If the CT or MRI is not definitive, adrenal scentiscans with the isotope 6-beta-[^{131}I]-iodomethyl-19-norcholesterol (NP-59) offer good discrimination.[656,670] Following dexamethasone suppression the uptake of tracer is increased in patients with aldosteronoma and absent in those with idiopathic aldosteronism.[670] Sampling of adrenal venous blood, preferably with corticotropin stimulation, for measurement of aldosterone and cortisol is a very reliable method of definitively diagnosing the source of excessive aldosterone secretion, provided that both adrenal veins can be catheterized.[656,671] Measurement of cortisol as well as aldosterone in the adrenal effluent and in the sample from the inferior vena cava is crucial for evaluating the accuracy and success of adrenal venous sampling.[656] Patients with aldosteronomas have a high aldosterone/cortisol ratio from the affected gland as well as a lower ratio from the nonaffected gland than in the lower caval blood, (indicating contralateral suppression of aldosterone secretion). In cases with hyperplasia, the ratio from both adrenals is higher than that found in the lower caval blood.[656,672]

Treatment

The treatment of choice for aldosteronoma is surgical removal of the tumor.[656] This usually significantly improves hypertension and ameliorates hypokalemia. Spironolactone therapy for three to five weeks before surgery is helpful in minimizing postoperative hypoaldosteronism and for restoration of body potassium stores. With improved preoperative diagnosis of an adenoma, a unilateral extraperitoneal approach is preferable.[656] If bilateral hyperplasia is seen at surgery despite the diagnosis of adenoma, a unilateral adrenalectomy is indicated.[656] Laparascopic adrenalectomy is now commonly used to resect aldosteronomas and generally is associated with fewer complications and shorter hospitalization periods. Idiopathic aldosteronism is treated medically with spironolactone, triamterene, or amiloride in addition to other antihypertensive agents as necessary. Calcium antagonists and ACE inhibitors are also useful in controlling blood pressure. The utility of aldosterone antagonists is increasingly recognized as beneficial, particularly with recognition of the deleterious role of excess aldosterone on the cardiovascular system.[656,673] Excess aldosterone has been associated with myocardial extracellular collagen and other matrix deposition and, therefore, to myocardial fibrosis and left ventricular hypertrophy.[673]

Glucocorticoid-Remediable Hyperaldosteronism

Familial hyperaldosteronism type I (glucocorticoid-suppressible hyperaldosteronism), a potentially curable form of hypertension is inherited in an autosomal dominant fashion.[675-677] The underlying genetic defect is a "hybrid"/chimeric gene in which 11 beta-hydroxylase gene regulatory elements are fused to the coding region of the aldosterone synthase gene. In persons with glucocorticoid remedial aldosteronism, secretion of aldosterone (along with other adrenal corticosteroids) is regulated entirely by corticotropin because of the presence of the abnormal steroidogenic gene.[676] In persons with glucocorticoid-remedial aldosteronism, the serum potassium can be low, but it is often normal.[678-679] Because most patients with this syndrome and hypertension have normal potassium levels, the prevalence of this disorder is likely more common than previously appreciated.[678-679]

Moderately low doses of glucocorticoids (0.5 to 2 mg of dexamethasone daily) usually reverse the biochemical abnormalities and hypertension in this disorder.[678] Because the chimeric gene results in aldosterone synthase being under control of the promoter for the 11β-hydroxylase gene expressed in the zona fasciculata under the control of corticotropin, the production of aldosterone is controlled by corticotropin, and is not suppressed by usual feedback mechanisms. Other 18-hydroxylation products of steroids made in the zona fasciculata, 18-OH-cortisol and 18-oxocortisol, are also produced in excess. Accordingly, the substantial response to dexamethasone in the syndrome is due to suppression of corticotropin and thus the synthesis of these steroids.[139]

The patients with this disorder characteristically develop significant hypertension at an early age, and there is a very high incidence of early mortality from strokes.[675-679] In patients whose blood pressure and aldosterone measurements normalize with glucocorticoid treatment, family screening should be conducted, with measurements of hybrid corticosteroids (18-oxocortisol and 18-hydroxycortisol) or even by chimeric-gene analysis in referral centers.[675,676] Once a diagnosis is made, genetic counseling is recommended for patients with this genetic disorder.

Hypertension in Congenital Adrenal Hyperplasia

Deficiencies of steroid 11-beta-hydroxylase or 17 alpha-hydroxylase are hypertensive forms of congenital hyperplasia resulting from the genetically related autosomal recessive inability to synthesize cortisol.[680] These two enzymatic defects cause hypertension due to overproduction of cortisol precursors that are, or are metabolized to, mineralocorticoid agonists.[680-684] These disorders result from mutations in the CYP11B1 and CYP17 genes encoding the corresponding enzymes.[681] In the 11-beta-hydroxylase deficiency syndrome, 11-deoxycorticosterone is present in excess along with adrenal androgens,[684] and in 17 alpha-hydroxylase deficiency, there is also an excess of DOC but a deficiency of androgen production.[680,681]

The 11-beta-hydroxylase deficiency syndrome is typically recognized in infancy, as the defect results in excessive androgen production.[684] The enzyme deficit prevents the hydroxylation of 11-deoxycortisol, resulting in cortisol deficiency. The defect also prevents the conversion of DOC to corticosterone and aldosterone; the high levels of DOC result in hypertension and hypokalemia, suggestive of mineralcorticoid excess. The high levels of corticotropin result in elevated 17-hydroxyprogesterone, androstenedione, and dehydroepiandrosterone sulfate.[684] Thus, the clinical features of this syndrome include virilization of the infant as well as hypertension and hypokalemia. This disease is caused by mutations in the CYP11B1 gene, which encodes a mitochondrial cytochrome P450 enzyme. The biochemical diagnosis is based on the finding of high levels of 11-deoxycortisol and DOC in urine and plasma.[684] Glucocorticoid treatment corrects the hypertension, hypokalemia, and androgen excess. Because aldosterone synthesis is blocked, when glucocorticoid therapy is instituted, the resultant decrease in DOC production may result in excessive sodium loss.

A deficiency of 17-alpha-hydroxylase 17,20-lyase is inherited as an autosomal recessive trait[680,681]; although rare, it probably exists with twice the frequency of the 11-beta-hydroxylase deficiency. Deficient 17-alpha-hydroxylation of pregnenolone and progesterone and subsequent deficiency of the cleavage of the C-17,20 carbon bond result in the absence of sex hormone formation in both the adrenal glands and the gonads, causing hypogonadism and male pseudohermaphroditism. Though most affected males are phenotypically females, some may appear as partially virilized males at birth, probably because they have a less severe enzyme deficiency.

Elevated and glucocorticoid-suppressible levels of the 17-deoxysteroids—DOC and corticosterone—as well as their 18-hydroxylated products—18-OHDOC and 18-OHB (in addition to 19-nor-DOC)—are responsible for hypertension, hypokalemia, and renin and aldosterone suppression. Like other forms of congenital adrenal hyperplasia, treatment of 17-alpha-hydroxylase deficiency consists of replacement doses of glucocorticoid hormones (i.e., cortisol in doses of 10 to 30 mg/day) and supplemental estrogen therapy in the young adult patient. Heterozygotes may be detected by slightly exaggerated responses of some or all of the 17-deoxysteroids to ACTH stimulation, and by the elevated ratio of total urinary metabolites of corticosterone to the total metabolites of cortisol. This syndrome is typically not recognized until after the onset of puberty in girls, when sexual development does not progress in a normal manner in patients who are phenotypically female. Only about 40 cases have been diagnosed, but adolescents with hypertension, hypokalemia and abnormal sexual development should be considered to have this syndrome.

Cushing's Disease

Hypertension is present in more than 80 percent of patients with Cushing's disease, and undoubtedly contributes to the inordinately high cardiovascular disease (CVD) mortality that exists in this syndrome.[685,686] This increased cardiac mortality may be related to the high prevalence of left ventricular hypertrophy that exists in Cushing's syndrome.[687] Hypertension in Cushing's syndrome is often severe, with accompanying loss of the normal nocturnal fall in blood pressure.[688,689] both contributing to the high prevalence of CVD associated with this syndrome. Hypertension is generally salt-sensitive in Cushing's syndrome.[336,340,685,690,691] Other potential mechanisms for the pathogenesis of hypertension induced by glucocorticoid excess have been reviewed. Causes of Cushing disease are discussed in Chapter 11.

Apparent Mineralocorticoid Excess (AME)

When the human mineralocorticoid receptor was cloned and expressed in vitro, it was found to have equal binding affinity for cortisol and aldosterone.[692] However, renal tubular cell 11-beta-hydroxysteroid dehydrogenase (11-beta OHSD) enzyme normally converts the large amounts of cortisol to the inactive cortisone protecting the mineralocorticoid receptor from the potential mineralocorticoid actions of cortisol.[307] There are both congenital and acquired deficiencies of the 11-beta-OHSD enzyme so that cortisol retains its mineralocorticoid effects, resulting in a mineralocorticoid excess syndrome: potassium wasting, sodium retention, and hypertension with suppressed aldosterone and renin.[307] The congenital forms include type I AME (deficiency of 11-beta-OHSD), and type 2 AME resulting from a deficiency of the 5-beta-reductase enzyme that normally converts cortisol to the inactive tetrohydrocortisol metabolite, thereby maintaining cortisol effects on mineralocorticoid receptors in the same manner as when 11-beta-OHSD is deficient.[693] Glycyrrhetenic acid, the active ingredient in licorice extract, has been shown to cause potassium wasting sodium retention and hypertension by inhibiting the renal 11 beta-OHSD enzyme,[307] and through similar central mechanisms.[694]

Pheochromocytomas

Pheochromocytomas are relatively rare endocrine tumors associated with a wide variety of symptoms, although hypertension is the most consistent clinical sign.[694-700] Pheochromocytomas probably account for less than 0.1 percent of patients with sustained diastolic hypertension.[694-697] The majority of pheochromocytomas arise from the adrenal medulla (85 percent) and organ of Zuckerkandl (8 percent). They occur rarely in extraadrenal sites in the chest (less than 2 percent), neck (less than 0.1 percent), abdomen, and bladder. Pheochromocytomas occur at all ages, with a peak incidence in the third and fourth decades.[694-696] The tumor occurs with equal frequency in both sexes in adults, whereas 60 percent of children affected are males.[699] Multiple tumors (adrenal and extraadrenal) are more common in children (35 percent) than in adults (8 percent).[699] Less than 10 percent of pheochromoctomas are malignant[700] and the prognosis of these tumors is poor.

Approximately 10 percent of pheochromocytomas are familial, and greater than 70 percent of these are bilateral.[694] Familial tumors occur in von Hippel-Lindau disease (VHLD),[701-704] neurofibromatosis,[703] and multiple endocrine neoplasia type II.[702,703,705] In association with von Hippel Lindau kindreds, there have been described several mutations of the VHDL gene.[701-704] The identification of RET proto-oncogene mutations in multiple endocrine neoplasma-2 (MEN-2)[703,704] has provided a good screening test for MEN-2 in patients with pheochromocytoma.[706]

Pheochromocytomas are usually encapsulated, vascular tumors averaging 5 cm in diameter and weighing less than 70 grams. (Fig 13-13). No relation exists in most patients between tumor size, elevation of plasma catecholamines, and clinical manifestations.[694-697] Most pheochromocytomas secrete both norepinephrine and epinephrine, with norepinephrine being the predominant catecholamine secreted. However, some tumors secrete only norepinephrine, or rarely, some tumors secrete only epinephrine. Very rarely, dopamine is the predominant catecholamine secreted.[694-697] Chromogranin A and adrenomedullin are also secreted by pheochromocytomas.[707,708]

The clinical manifestations of pheochromocytoma are shown in Table 13-11. The most common clinical findings are sustained or paroxysmal hypertension, headache, palpitations, and sweating.[694-697] Symptomatic episodes can occur as often as 30 times a day or as infrequently as once every few months. About 74 percent of patients experience one or more attacks per week. The duration is usually less than 1 hour but some have persisted for as long as 1 week. An episode often begins with palpitations and dyspnea. Alpha-receptor-mediated peripheral vasoconstriction results in hypertension, facial pallor, and cool, moist hands and feet. Decreased heat loss and increased basal metabolism can cause a rise in temperature, flushing, and sweating. When episodes are se-

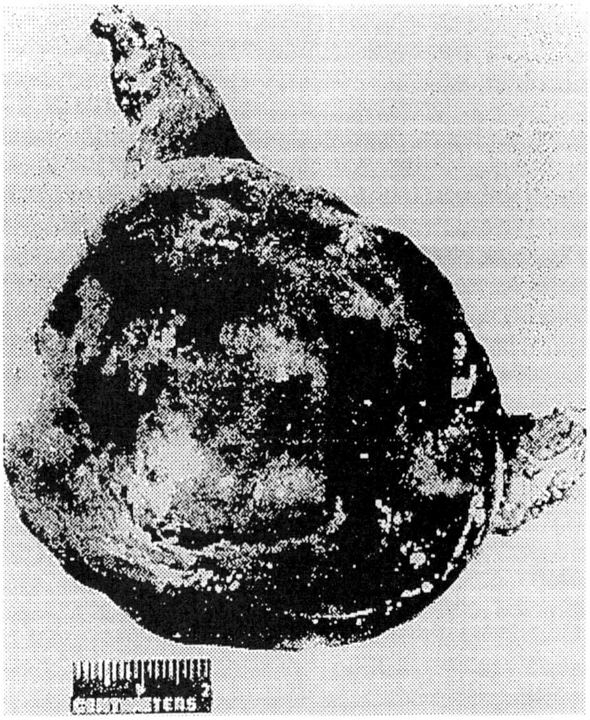

FIGURE 13-13. Pheochromocytoma of the adrenal. Tumor is well encapsulated and exhibits hemorrhagic dark mottling.

vere or prolonged, nausea, vomiting, headache, visual disturbances, abdominal and/or, paresthesias, palpitations, and seizures can occur. A sensation of fatigue often accompanies these episodes.[694-697] Pheochromocytomas are associated with a variety of EKG abnormalities, resulting from catecholamine myocarditis/cardiomyopathy, left ventricular hypertrophy, and ischemic changes.[694-697] Orthostatic hypotension may occur because of volume depletion and predominance of epinephrine/dopamine secretion.[694-697]

All patients with severe, sustained, and paroxysmal hypertension and associated symptoms (Table 13-11), particularly if resistant to antihypertensive treatment, should be screened for pheochromocytoma.[694-697] Other indications for screening include all persons with MEN-2, those with hypertensive episodes during labor, anesthesia, or radiologic procedures[694-697]; and those with incidentalomas who have suggestive symptoms.[694-697] The diagnosis of pheochromocytoma is initially established by demonstrating elevated urinary or plasma catecholamines.

Total metanephrine (metanephrine plus normotanephrine) concentration in a 24-hour urine specimen is the most reliable screening test.[694-697,709] A single void (spot) urine metanephrine level relates closely with the results of 24-hour urine collections, particularly when collected following an attack.[710] Urinary free catecholamines (norepinephrine, epinphrine, and dopamine) are measured to help confirm the diagnosis of pheochromocytoma in patients with elevated metanephrines. Measurement of fractionated catecholamines is also particularly helpful if epinephrine and dopamine are selectively secreted.[694-697] In view of the availability of these measurements in most laboratories, these are measurements of choice. Chromogranin A levels have been reported to be elevated in most pheochromocytoma patients[707,711]; however, this has not been established as a routine test.[707,711] Because of the accuracy of the urinary tests,[707] it is probably not appropriate to employ provocative or suppressive tests.[707] If urine assay results are equivocal, the clonidine suppression (if patient is hypertensive) or

TABLE 13-11. Clinical Manifestations of Pheochromocytoma

Symptoms
Common
Headache (72–92 percent)
Sweating (60–70 percent)
Palpitations with or without tachycardia (51–73 percent)
Nervousness (35–40 percent)
Weight loss (40–70 percent)
Chest or abdominal pain (22–48 percent)
Nausea with or without vomiting (26–43 percent)
Weakness or fatigue (15–38 percent)
Less Common
Visual disturbances, constipation, warmth, dyspnea, paresthesias, flushing, polyuria, polydipsia, dizziness, grand mal seizures, bradycardia (noted by patients), tightness in throat, tinnitus, dysarthria, gagging, painless hematuria
Signs
Blood pressure changes (seen in 98 percent of patients)
Sustained hypertension
Paroxysmal hypertension (which may alternate with hypotension)
Orthostatic hypotension
Hypertension induced by a physical maneuver
Paradoxical blood pressure response to some antihypertensive drugs
Marked pressor response to anesthesia
Other signs of catecholamine excess
Hyperhidrosis
Tachycardia, arrhythmia, reflex bradycardia, forceful heartbeat
Pallor of the face and upper part of the body
Anxious, frightened, troubled appearance
Hypertensive retinopathy
Dilated pupils; very rarely, exophthalmos, lacrimation, scleral pallor or injection, pupils may not react to light
Leanness or underweight
Tremor
Raynaud phenomenon or livedo reticularis; occasionally puffy, red cyanotic hands in children; skin of extremities wet, cold clammy, and pale; gooseflesh, cyanotic nail beds
Mass lesion in abdomen or neck
Signs caused by encroachment on adjacent structures or by invasions and pressure effects of metastases
Manifestations Related to Complications of Coexisting Diseases or Syndromes
Myocardial infarction
Congestive heart failure ± cardiomyopathy
Arrhythmias, tachycardia, unexplained hypotension, or cardiac arrest following induction of general anesthesia
Shock
Cerebrovascular accident
Azotemia
Hypertensive encephalopathy
Ischemic enterocolitis ± megacolon
Dissecting aneurysm
Severe preeclampsia during pregnancy; fever, shock, or sudden death pre- or postpartum
Cholelithiasis
Mucocutaneous neuromas
Thickened corneal nerves (seen only with slit lamp)
Marfanoid habitus
Alimentary tract ganglioneuromatosis
Neurofibromatosis
Cushing's syndrome

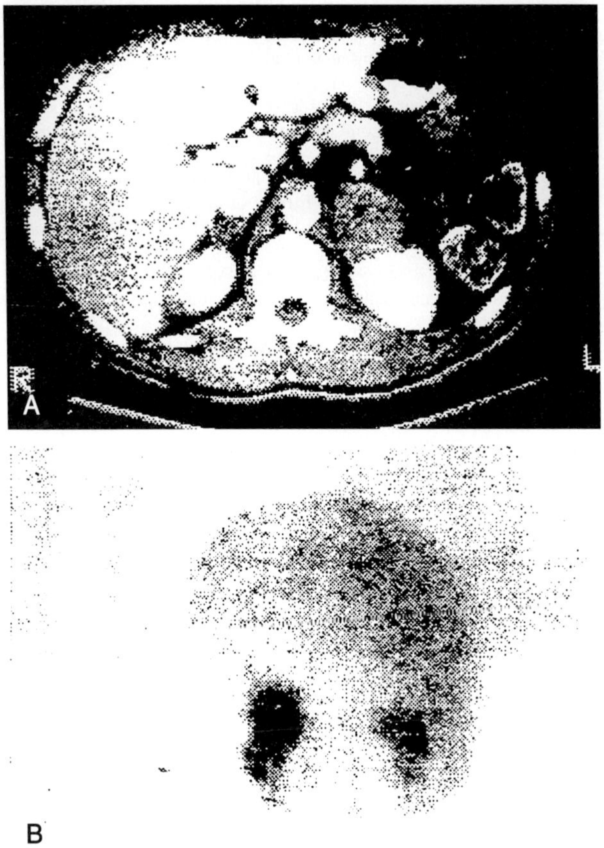

FIGURE 13-14. *A*. Demonstration of pheochromocytoma in the left adrenal by computerized tomography. ***B***. MIBG scan, posterior view, localizing the pheochromocytoma to left adrenal, this location was confirmed by renal scan (MIBG = ^{131}I meta-iodobenzylguanidine).

the glucagon provocation test (if patient is normotensive with orthostatic hypotension) may be helpful.

Most pheochromocytomas are large enough to be detected by either CT or MRI (Fig. 13-14). Both CT and MRI provide high sensitivity and negative predictive value, but only about 70 percent positive predictive value.[712,713] With MRI pheochromocytomas usually have distinctive bright signals in T_2-weighted images.[703] Both CT and MRI can also identify extraadrenal tumors[194] and metastasis from malignant pheochromocytomas.[176] The most accurate way to localize a pheochromocytoma is with metaiodobenzylguanidine (MIBG) scintigraphy.[713,714] This test has a higher positive predictive value than CT and MRI and is indicated in patients with abnormal biochemical tests and equivocal findings on CT or MRI.[714]

Medical therapy is often useful to prepare for definitive surgical treatment of pheochromocytomas. For acute treatment of a severe hypertensive episode either alpha-blockade with phentolamine or sodium nitroprusside infusion is indicated, followed by beta-adrenergic blockade once alpha blockage is accomplished. Intravascular volume repletion may also be necessary, even with adequate alpha blockade.[694-697] For longer term alpha blockade, phenoxybenzamine and prazosin are indicated.[694-697]

With adequate preoperative blood pressure control and good perioperative management, the risk of surgery is not significantly higher than for other operations.[694-697] Certain anesthetic agents are indicated and others to be avoided.[715] Patients should be monitored by EKG, arterial blood pressures, and pulmonary wedge pressure to access intravascular volume status.[694-697,715] Aggressive fluid replacement to manage intra- and postoperative hypotension is very important.[715] In the last several years, there have been increasing reports of the utility of subtotal adrenalectomy by the posterior retroperitoneoscopic approach[716] or by lapararoscopic adrenalectomy, which are safe and reduce wound complications and hospitalization.[717,718] Indeed, improvement of preoperative imaging of pheochromocytomas and paragangliomas may render laparotomy unnecessary in the operative management of these tumors unless bilateral adrenal disease or carcinoma is expected.[719] Recently, the utility of using ^{131}I MIBG in therapy of malignant pheochromocytoma has been reviewed.[720,721] This approach appears promising for even those lesions that have not responded well to chemotherapeutic therapy with cyclophosphamide, vincristine, and dacarbazine.[722] Long-term control of symptoms is often possible with alpha and beta blockade and use of metyrosine (alpha-methyl-para-tyrosine).[723]

REFERENCES

1. The sixth report of the Joint National Committee on prevention, detection, evaluation and treatment of high blood pressure. *Arch Intern Med* 157:2413, 1997.
2. National High Blood Pressure Education Program Working Group: National High Blood Pressure Education Program Working Group Report on Hypertension in the elderly. *Hypertension* 23:275, 1994.
3. Stuck SE, Siu AL, Wieland GD, et al: Comprehensive geriatric assessment: A meta-analysis of controlled trials. *Lancet* 342:1032, 1993.
4. Sowers JR, Farrow SL: Treatment of elderly hypertensive patients with diabetes, renal disease, and coronary heart disease. *Am J Geriatr Cardiol* 5:57, 1996.
5. Burt VL, Whelton P, Roccelo EJ, Brown C, Culter JA, Higgins M, Horan MJ, Labarthe D: Prevalence of hypertension in the US adult population. Results from the Third National Health and Nutrition Examination Survey, 1988–1991. *Hypertension*, 25:305, 1995.
6. Franklin SS, Gustin W, Wong ND, Larson MG, Weber MA, Kannel WB, Levy D: Hemodynamic patterns of age-related changes in blood pressure: The Farmingham Heart Study. *Circulation* 96:308, 1997.
7. Luft FC, Weinberger MH: Hetrogenous responses to changes in dietary salt intake: The salt-sensitivity paradigm. *Am J Clin Nutr* 65:612S, 1997.
8. Minami J, Kawano Y, Ishimitsu T, Takishita S: Blunted parasympathetic modulation in salt-sensitive patients with essential hypertension: Evaluation by power-spectral analysis of heart-rate variability. *J Hypertens* 15:727, 1997.
9. Chrysant SG, Weir MR, Weder AB, Mc Carron DA, Cannosa-Terris M, Cohen JD, Mennella RF, Kirkegaard LW, Lewin AJ, Weinberger MH. There are no racial, age, sex, or weight differences in the effect of salt on blood pressure in salt-sensitive hypertensive patients. *Arch Intern Med* 157:2489, 1997.
10. Williams G, Dluhy R, Lifton R, et al: Non-modulation as an intermediate phenotype in essential hypertension. *Hypertension* 20:788, 1992.
11. Alderman M, Madhavan S, Ooi W, et al: Association of the renin-sodium profile with the risk of myocardial infarction in patients with hypertension. *N Engl J Med* 324:1098, 1991.
12. Furlan R, Guzzetti S, Crivellaro W, Dassi S, Tinelli M, Baselli G, Cerutti S, Lombardi F, Pagani M, Milliani A: Continuous 24-hour assessment on the regulation of systemic arterial blood pressure and RR variabilities in ambulants subjects. *Circulation* 81:537, 1990.
13. Mayet J, Shahi M, Hughes AD, Stanton AV, Poulter NR, Sever PS, Foale RA, Thoms SA: Left ventricular structure and function in previously untreated hypertensive patients: The importance of blood pressure, the nocturnal blood pressure dip and heart rate. *J Cardiovas Risk* 2:255, 1995.

14. Bayes-Genis A, Guindo J, Vinola X, Tomas L, Elosua R, Duran I, Bayes De Luna A: Cardiac arrhythmias and left ventricular hypertrophy in systemic hypertension and their influences on prognosis. *Am J Cardiol* 76:54D, 1995.
15. Collins R, Peto R, MacMahon S, et al: Blood pressure, stroke, and coronary heart disease: II. Short term reduction in blood pressure: Overview of randomized drug trials in their epidemiological context. *Lancet* 335:827, 1990.
16. Müeller F, Laragh J: Clinical evaluation and differential diagnosis of the individual hypertensive patient. *Clin Chem* 37:1868, 1991.
17. He J, Klag MJ, Appel LJ, Charleston J, Whelton PK: Seven-year incidence of hypertension in a cohort of middle-aged African Americans and Whites. *Hypertension* 31:1130, 1998.
18. Mbanya JC, Minkoulou EM, Salah JN, Balkau B: The prevalence of hypertension in rural and urban Cameroon. *Int J Epidemiol* 27:181, 1998.
19. Kannel W: The clinical heterogenity of hypertension. *Am J Hypertens* 4:283, 1991.
20. Stokes J, Kannel W, Fwolff P, et al: Blood pressure as a risk factor for cardiovascular disease: The Framingham Study-30 year of follow-up. *Hypertension* 13:I, 1989.
21. Kaplan NM: *Clinical Hypertension*. 7th Edition, in Norman M, Kaplan MD (eds). Baltimore, Williams & Wilkins, 1978.
22. Harrington M, Kincaid-Smith P, McMichael J: Results of treatment in malignant hypertension: A seven-year experience in 94 cases. *Br Med J* 2:969, 1959.
23. Agabiti E, Muiesan M, Muiesan G: Regression of structural alterations in hypertension. *Am J Hypertens* 2:70, 1989.
24. Russel R: Pathological changes in small cerebral arteries causing occlusion and hemorrhage. *J Cardiovasc Pharmacol* 6:S691, 1984.
25. Klahr S, Levey A, Beck G, et al: The effects of dietary protein restriction and blood-pressure control on the progression of chronic renal disease. *N Engl J Med* 330:877, 1994.
26. Meigs JB, D'Agostino RB, SR, Wilson PWF, Cupples LA, Nathan DM, Singer DE: Risk variable clustering in the insulin resistance syndrome: The Framingham offspring study. *Diabetes* 46:1594, 1997.
27. Conway J: Hemodynamic aspects of essential hypertension. *Physiol Rev* 64:617, 1984.
28. Pickering T: Pathophysiology of systemic hypertension. *Am J Cardiol* 58:12, 1986.
29. Ventura H, Messerli FH, Oigman W, et al: Impaired systemic arterial compliance in borderline hypertension. *Am Heart J* 108:132, 1984.
30. Folkow B: Physiological aspects of primary hypertension. *Physiol Rev* 62:347, 1982.
31. Frohlich ED: Physiologic considerations in left ventricular hypertrophy. *Am J Med* 75:12, 1983.
32. Franklin SS, Khan SA, Wong ND, Larson MG, Levy Daniel: In pulse pressure useful in predicting risk for coronary heart disease: The Framingham Heart Study. *Circulation* 100:354, 1999.
33. Franklin SS, Khan SA, Wong ND, Larson MG, Levy D: Is pulse pressure useful in predicting risk for coronary heart disease: The Framingham Heart Study. *Circulation* 100:354, 1999.
34. Chobanian AV, Brecher PL, Haudenschild CC: Effects of hypertension and antihypertensive therapy on atherosclerosis: State of the art lecture. *Hypertension* 8:15, 1986.
35. Wang M, Wise SC, Leff T, Su TZ: Troglitazone, an antidiabetic agent, inhibits cholesterol biosynthesis through a mechanism independent of peroxisome proliferator-activated receptor-gamma. *Diabetes* 48:254, 1999.
36. Phillips S, Whisnant J: Hypertension and the brain. *Arch Intern Med* 152:938, 1992.
37. Lindeman RD, Tobin JD, Shock NW: Association between hypertension and the rate of decline of renal function. *Kidney Intl* 26:861, 1984.
38. Ledingham JGC: Early assessment of organ involvement in hypertension: *J Hypertens* 3:S33, 1985.
39. van Hooft I, Grobbee D, Derkx F, et al: Renal hemodynamics and the renin-angiotensin-aldosterone system in normotensive subjects with hypertensive and normotensive parents. *N Engl J Med* 324:1305, 1994.
40. Laragh J: The renin system and four lines of hypertension research: Nephron heterogeneity, the calcium connection, the prorenin vasodilator limb, and plasma renin and heart attack. *Hypertension* 20:267,1992.
41. Dean R, Tribble R, Kansen K, et al: Evolution of renal insufficiency in ischemic nephropathy. *Ann Surg* 213:446, 1991.
42. Hallet JJ, Schriger A, Bower T, et al: The current role of surgical revascularization for combined renovascular and renal insufficiency. *Int Angiol* 11:64, 1992.
43. Bianchi S, Bigazzi R, Baldari G, et al: Microalbuminuria in patients with essential hypertension: Effects of an angiotension converting enzyme inhibitor and of a calcium channel blocker. *Am J Hypertens* 4:291, 1991.
44. Campese VM, Bianchi S, Gigazzi R: Association between hyperlipidemia and microalbuminuria in essential hypertension. *Kidney Int* 71:S10, 1999.
45. Messerli FH, Frohlich ED, Dreslinski GR, et al: Serum uric acid in essential hypertension: An indication of renal vascular involvement. *Ann Intern Med* 93:817, 1980.
46. Perera GA: Hypertensive vascular disease: Description and natural history. *J Chronic Dis* 1:33, 1955.
47. Schulman N, Ford C, Hall W, et al: Prognostic value of serum creatinine and effect of treatment of hypertension on renal function. Results from the hypertension detection and follow-up program. *Hypertension* 13:I80, 1989.
48. Keane WF, Eknoyan G: Proteinuria, Albuminuria, Risk Assessment, Detection, Elimination (PARADE): A position paper of the National Kidney Foundation. *Am J Kidney Dis* 33:1104, 1999.
49. He J, Whelton PK: Elevated systolic blood pressure and risk of cardiovascular and renal disease: overview of evidence from observational epidemiologic studies and randomized controlled trials. *Am Heart J* 138:211, 1999.
50. Muldoon M, Terrell D, Bunker C, et al: Family history studies in hypertension research. *Am J Hypertens* 6:76, 1993.
51. Havlik R: Predictors of hypertension, population studies. *Am J Hypertens* 4:586, 1991.
52. Stutts MJ, Canessa CM, Olsen JC, Hamrick M, Cohn JA, Rossier BC, Boucher RC: CFTR as a cAMP-dependent regulator of sodium channels. *Science* 269:847, 1995.
53. Berry T, Hasstedt S, Hunt S, et al: A gene for high urinary kallikrein may protect against hypertension in Utah kindreds. *Hypertension* 13:3, 1989.
54. Chiang FT, Hsu KL, Tseng CD, Lo HM, Chern TH, Tseng YZ: Association of the renin gene polymorphism with essential hypertension in a Chinese population. *Clin Genet* 51:370, 1997.
55. Jeunmaitre X, Soubrier F, Kotelevtsev YV, Lifton RP, Williams CS, Charru A, Hunt SC, Hopkins PN, Williams RR, Lalouel JM, Corvol P: Molecular basis of human hypertension: Role of angiotensinogen. *Cell* 71:169, 1992.
56. Atwood LD, Kammere CM, Samollow PB, Hixson JE, Shade RE, MacCluer JW: Linkage of essential hypertension to the angiotensinogen locus in Mexican Americans. *Hypertension* 30:326, 1997.
57. Brand E, Chatelain N, Keavney B, Cauldfield M, Citterio L, Connell J, Grobbee D, Schmidt S, Schunkert H, Schuster H, Sharma AM, Soubrier F: Evaluation of the angiotensinogen locus in human essential hypertension: A European study. *Hypertension* 31:725, 1998.
58. Niu T, Xu X, Rogus J, Zhou Y, Chen C, Yang J, Fang Z, Schmitz C, Zhao J, Rao VS, Lindpainter K: Angiotensinogen gene and hypertension in Chinese. *J Clin Invest* 101:188, 1998.
59. Ishigami T, Umemura S, Tamura K, Hibi K, Nyui N, Kihara M, Yabana M, Watanabe Y, Sumida Y, Nagahara T, Ochiai H, Ishii M: Essential hypertension and 5′ upstream core promoter region of human angiotensinogen gene. *Hypertension* 30:1325, 1997.
60. Sato N, Katsuya T, Rakugi H, Takami S, Nakata Y, Miki T, Higaki J, Ogihara T: Association of variants in critical core promoter element of angiotensinogen gene with increased risk of essential hypertension in Japenese. *Hypertension* 30:321, 1997.
61. Giner V, Poch E, Bragulat E, Oriola J, Gonzalez D, Coca A, Alejandro De La Sierra: Renin-angiotensin system genetic polymorphisms and salt sensitivity in essential hypertension. *Hypertension* 35:512, 2000.
62. Nakano Y, Oshima T, Hiraga H, Matsuura H, Kajiyama G, Kambe M: DD genotype of the angiotensin I-converting enzyme gene is a risk factor for early onset of essential hypertension in Japanese patients. *J Lab Clin Med* 131:502, 1998.

63. Fornafe M, Amos CI, Kardia S, Sing CF, Turner ST, Boerwinkle E: Variation in the region of the angiotensin-converting enzyme gene influences interindividual differences in blood pressure levels in young white males. *Circulation* 97:1773, 1998.
64. O'Donnell CJ, Lindpainter K, Larson MG, Rao VS, Ordavos JM, Schaefer EJ, Meyers RH, Levy D: Evidence for association and genetic linkage of the angiotensin-converting enzyme locus with hypertension and blood pressure in men but not women in the Framingham Heart Study. *Circulation* 97:1766, 1988.
65. Perticone F, Ceravolo R, Maio R, Ventura G, Zingone A, Perrotti N, Mattioli PL: Angiotensin-converting enzyme gene polymorphism is associated with endothelium-dependent vasodilation in never treated hypertensive patients. *Hypertension* 31:900, 1998.
66. Chiang FT, Lai ZP, Chern TH, Tseng CD, Hsu KL, Lo HM, Tseng YZ: Lack of association of the angiotensin converting enzyme polymorphism with essential hypertension in a Chinese population. *Am J Hypertens* 10:197, 1997.
67. Chuang LM, Chiu KC, Chiang FT, Lee KC, Wu HP, Lin BJ, Tai TY: Insertion/deletion polymorphism of the angiotensin I-converting enzyme gene in patients with hypertension, non-insulin-dependent diabetes mellitus, and coronary heart disease in Taiwan. *Metabolism: Clinical and Experimental* 46:1211, 1997.
68. Tiret L, Blanc H, Ruidavets JB, Arveiler D, Luc G, Jeunmaitre X, Tichet J, Mallet C, Poirier O, Plouin PF, Cambien F: Gene polymorphism of the renin-angiotensin system in relation to hypertension and parental history of myocardial infarction and stroke: The PEGASE study. Projet d'Etude des Genes de l'Hypertension Arterielle Severe a moderre Essentielle. *J Hypertens* 16:3, 1998.
69. Schmidt S, Beige J, Walla-Friedel M, Michel MC, Sharma AM, Ritz E: A polymorphism in the gene for the angiotensin II type 1 receptor is not associated with hypertension. *J Hypertens* 15:1385, 1997.
70. Szombathy T, Szalai C, Katalin B, Palicz, T, Romics L, Csazar A: Association of angiotensin II type 1 receptor polymorphism with resistant essential hypertension. *Clinica Chimica Acta* 269:91, 1998.
71. Takami S, Katsuya T, Rakugi H, Sato N, Nakata Y, Kamitani A, Miki T, Higaki J, Ogihara T: Angiotensin II type 1 receptor gene polymorphism is associated with increase of left ventricular mass but not with hypertension. *Am J Hypertens* 11:316, 1998.
72. Hansson JH, Nelson-Williams C, Suzuki H, Schild L, Shimkets R, Lu Y, Canessa C, Iawasaki T, Rossier B, Lifton RP: Hypertension caused by a truncated epithelial sodium channel gamma subunit: Genetic heterogeneity of Liddle syndrome. *Nat Genet* 11:76, 1995.
73. Jeunemaitre X, Bassilana F, Persu A, Dumont C, Champigny G, Lazdunski M, Corvol P, Barbry P: Genotype-phenotype analysis of a newly discovered family with Liddle's Syndrome. *J Hypertens* 15:1091, 1997.
74. Malender O, Orho M, Fagerudd J, Bengtsson K, Groop PH, Mattiason I, Groop L, Hulthen UL: Mutation and variants of the epithelial sodium channel gene in Liddle's syndrome and primary hypertension. *Hypertension* 31:1118, 1998.
75. Inoue J, Iwaoka T, Tokunaga H, Takamune K, Naomi S, Araki M, Takahama K, Yamaguchi K, Tomita K: A family with Liddle's syndrome caused by a new missense mutation in the beta subunit of the epithelial sodium channel. *J Clin Endocrinol Metab* 83:2210, 1998.
76. Schild L, Lu Y, Gautschi I, Schneeberger E, Lifton RP, Rossier BC: Identification of a PY motif in the epithelial Na Channel subunits as a target sequence for mutations causing channel activation found in Liddle syndrome. *EMBO J* 15:2381, 1996.
77. Baker EH, Dong YB, Sagnella GA, Rothwell M, Onipinala AK, Markandu ND, Cappuccio FP, Cook DG, Persu A, Corvol P, Jeunmaitre X, Carter ND, MacGregor GA: Association of hypertension with T594M mutation in beta subunit of epithelial sodium channels in black people resident in London. *Lancet* 351:1388, 1998.
78. Schnackenberg C, Patel AR, Krichner KA, Granger JP: Nitric oxide, the kidney and hypertension. *Clin Exp Pharmacol Physiol* 24:600, 1997.
79. Tsukada T, Yokoyama K, Arai T, Takemoto F, Hara S, Yamada A, Kawaguchi Y, Hosoya T, Igari J: Evidence of association of the ecNOS gene polymorphism with plasma NO metabolite levels in humans. *Biochem Biophys Res Commun* 245:190, 1998.
80. Lacolley P, Gautier S, Poirier O, Pannier B, Cambien F, Benetos A: Nitric oxide synthase gene polymorphisms, blood pressure and aortic stiffness in normotensive and hypertensive subjects. *J Hypertens* 161:31, 1998.
81. Uwabo J, Soma M, Nakayama T, Kanmatsuse K: Association of a variable number of tandem repeats in the endothelial constitutive nitric oxide synthase gene with essential hypertensive in Japanese. *Am J Hypertens* 11:125, 1998.
82. Tamaki S, Iwai N, Tsujita Y, Nakamura Y, Kinoshita M: Polymorphism of alpha-adducin in Japanese patients with essential hypertension. *Hypertens Res* 21:29, 1998.
83. Castellano M, Barlassina C, Muiesan ML, Beschi M, Cinelli A, Rossi F, Rizzoni D, Cusi D, Agabiti-Rosei E: Alpha-adducin gene polymorphism and cardiovascular phenotypes in a general population. *J Hypertens* 15:1707, 1997.
84. Kato N, Sugiyama T, Nabika T, Morita H, Kurihara H, Yazaki Y, Yamori Y: Lack of association between the alpha-adducin locus and essential hypertension in the Japanese population. *Hypertension* 31:730, 1998.
85. Cusi D, Barlassina C, Azzani T, Casari G, Citterio L, Devoto M, Glorioso N, Lanzani C, Manunta P, Righetti M, Rivera R, Stella P, Troffa C, Zagato L, Bianchi G: Polymorphisms of alpha-adducin and salt sensitivity in patients with essential hypertension. *Lancet* 349;1353, 1997.
86. Rutkowski MP, Klanke CA, SU YR, Reif M, Menon AG: Genetic markers at the leptin (OB) locus are not significantly linked to hypertension in African Americans. *Hypertension* 31:1230, 1998.
87. Kotanko P, Binder A, Tasker J, DeFreitas P, Kamdar S, Clark AJ, Skrabal F, Caulfield M: Essential hypertension in African Caribbeans associates with a variant of the beta2-adrenoreceptor. *Hypertension* 30:773, 1997.
88. Svetkey LP, Chen YT, McKeown SP, Preis L, Wilson AF: Preliminary evidence of linkage of salt sensitivity in black Americans at the beta 2-adrenergic receptor locus. *Hypertension* 29:918, 1997.
89. Fujisawa T, Ikegami H, Yamato E, Hamada Y, Kamide K, Rakugi H, Higaki J, Murakami H, Shimamoto K, Ogihara T: Trp64Arg mutation of beta3-adrenergic receptor in essential hypertension: Insulin resistance and the adrenergic system. *Am J Hypertens* 10:101, 1997.
90. Yokosawa H, Holladay LA, Inagami T, et al: Human renal renin: Complete purification and characterization. *J Biol Chem* 265:3498, 1980.
91. Do YS, Shinagawa T, Tam H, et al: Characterization of pure human renal renin: Evidence for its subunit structure. *J Biol Chem* 1986:1986.
92. Sealey JE, Atlas SA, Laragh JH: Prorenin and other large molecular weight forms of renin. *Endocr Rev* 1:365, 1980.
93. Goldstone R, Horton R, Carlson EJ, et al: Reciprocal changes in active and inactive renin after converting enzyme inhibition in normal man. *J Clin Endocrinol Metab* 56:264, 1983.
94. Campbell D, Kladis A, Skinner S, et al: Characterization of angiotensin peptides in plasma of anephric man. *J Hypertens* 9:265, 1991.
95. Toffelmire E, Slater K, Corvol P, et al: Response of plasma prorenin and active renin to chronic and acute alteration of renin secretion in normal humans. *J Clin Invest* 83:679, 1989.
96. Hobart PM, Fogliano M, O'Connor BA, et al: Human renin gene: Structure and sequence analysis. *Proc Natl Acad Sci USA* 81:5026, 1984.
97. Hardman JA, Hort YJ, Catanzaro DF, et al: Primary structure of the human renin gene. *DNA* 3:457, 1984.
98. Miyazaki H, Fukamizu A, Hirose S, et al: Structure of the human renin gene. *Proc Natl Acad Sci USA* 81:5999, 1984.
99. Soubrier F, Panthier JT, Corvol P, et al: Molecular cloning and nucleotide sequence of a human renin cDNA fragment. *Nucleic Acids Res* 20:7181, 1983.
100. Imai T, Miyazaki H, Hirose S, et al: Cloning and sequence analysis of cDNA for human renin precursor. *Proc Natl Acad Sci USA* 80:7405, 1983.
101. Hsueh W, Baxter J: Human prorenin. *Hypertension* 17:469, 1991.
102. Faust P, Chirgwin J, Kornfield S: Renin, a secretory-glycoprotein, acquires phosphomannosyl residues. *J Biol Chem* 105:1947, 1987.
103. Wang PH, Do Y, Macauley L, et al: Identification of renal cathepsin B as a human prorenin processing enzyme. *J Biol Chem* 266:12633, 1991.
104. Fritz L, Hadar M, Arfsten A, et al: Human renin is correctly processed and targeted to the regulated secretory pathway in mouse pituitary AtT-20 cells. *J Biol Chem* 262:12409, 1987.

105. Pratt R, Flynn J, Hobart P, et al: Different secretory pathways of renin from mouse cells transfected with the human renin gene. *J Biol Chem* 263:3137, 1987.
106. Yan Y, Chen R, Pitarresi T, Sigmund CD, Gross KW, Sealey JE, Laragh JH, Catanzaro DR: Kidney is the only source of human plasma renin in 45-kb human renin transgenic mice. *Circ Res* 14-28;83(12):1279–88, 1998.
107. Campbell D: Extrarenal renin and blood pressure regulation: An alternative viewpoint. *Am J Hypertens* 2:266, 1989.
108. Re RN: Cellular biology of the renin-angiotensin systems. *Arch Intern Med* 144:2037, 1984.
109. Deschepper CF, Mellon SH, Cumin F, et al: Analysis by immunocytochemistry and in situ hybridization of renin and its mRNA in kidney, testis, adrenal, and pituitary of the rat. *Proc Natl Acad Sci USA* 83:7552, 1986.
110. Lou Y, Smith D, Robinson B, et al: Renin gene expression in various tissues determined by single-step polymerase chain reaction. *Clin Exp Pharmacol Physiol* 18:357, 1991.
111. Lee MA, Böhm M, Paul M, et al: Tissue renin-angiotensin systems: Their role in cardiovascular disease. *Circulation* 87:IV7, 1993.
112. Ferrario C, Barnes K, Block C, et al: Pathways of angiotension formation and function in the brain. *Hypertension* 15:I-13, 1990.
113. Danser A, van den Dorper M, Deinum J, et al: Renin, prorenin and immunoreactive renin in vitreous fluid from eyes with and without diabetic retinopathy. *J Clin Endocrinol Metab* 68:160, 1989.
114. Yamahuchi T, Franco-Saenz R, Mulrow P: Effect of angiotensin II on renin production by rat adrenal glomerulosa cells in culture. *Hypertension* 19:263, 1992.
115. Shaw KJ, Do YS, Kjos S, Anderson PW, Shinagawa T, Dubeau L, Hsueh WA: Human decidua is a major source of renin. *J Clin Invest* 83:2085, 1989.
116. Do YS, Sherrod A, Lobo R, Paulson R, Shinagawa T, Chem S, Kjos S, Hsueh WA: Human ovarian theca cells are a source of renin. *Proc Nat Acad Sci* 75:1957, 1988.
117. Sealey J, von Lutterotti N, Rubattu S, et al: The greater renin system: Its prorenin-directed vasodilator limb: Relevance to diabetes mellitus, pregnancy, and hypertension. *Am J Hypertens* 4:972, 1991.
118. Lever A: Endocrine, paracrine, or part-paracrine control of blood pressure. *Am J Hypertens* 2:276, 1989.
119. Kim S, Hosoi M, Ikemoto F, et al: Conversion to renin of exogenously administered recombinant human prorenin in liver and kidney of monkeys. *Am J Physiol* 285:E-151, 1990.
120. Rosenthal J, Thurnreiter M, Plaschke M, et al: Reninlike enzymes in human vasculature. *Hypertension* 15:848, 1990.
121. Admiraal P, Derkx F, Danser A, et al: Metabolism and production of angiotensin I in different vascular beds in subjects with hypertension. *Hypertension* 15:44, 1990.
122. Ikeda M, Sasaguri M, Maruta H, et al: Formation of angiotensin II by tonin-inhibitor complex. *Hypertension* 11:63, 1988.
123. Wintroub B, Klickstein LD, Watt KWK: A human neutrophil dependent pathway for generation of angiotensin II. *J Clin Invest* 68:484, 1981.
124. Taugner R, Yokota S, Buhrle CP, et al: Cathepsin D coexists with renin in the secretory granules of juxtaglomerular epithelioid cells. *Histochemistry* 84:19, 1986.
125. Davis JO, Freeman RH: Mechanisms regulating renin release. *Physiol Rev* 56:1, 1976.
126. Hachenthal E, Ganten P, Taugner R: Morphology, physiology and molecular biology of renin secretion. *Physiol Rev* 70:1067, 1990.
127. Beierwaltes W: Nitric oxide participates in calcium-mediated regulation of renin release. *Hypertension* 23:I-40, 1994.
128. Chuchill P: Second messengers in renin secretion. *Am J Physiol* 245:F175, 1985.
129. Rosenberg M, Chmlelewski D, Hostetter T: Effect of dietary protein on rat renin and angiotensinogen gene expression. *J Clin Invest* 85:1144, 1990.
130. Geary K, Hunt M, Peach M, et al: Effects of angiotensin converting enzyme inhibition, sodium depletion, calcium, isoproterenol, and angiotensin II on renin secretion by individual renocortical cells. *Endocrinology* 131:1588, 1992.
131. Stella GR, Zanchetti A: Neural control of renin release. *Am J Hypertens* 2:7, 1989.
132. Kurtz A, Kaissling B, Busse R, et al: Endothelial cells modulate renin secretion from isolated mouse juxtaglomerular cells. *J Clin Invest* 88:1147, 1991.
133. Kurtz A, Muff R, Born W, et al: Calcitonin gene-related peptide is a stimulator of renin secretion. *J Clin Invest* 82:538, 1988.
134. Martinez-Maldonada M, Gely R, Tapia E, et al: Role of macula densa in diuretic-induced renin release. *Hypertension* 16:261, 1990.
135. Beierwaltes W, Carretero O: Non-prostanoid endothelium-derived factors inhibit renin release. *Hypertension* 19:II-68, 1992.
136. Resnick L, Churchill M, Churchill P, et al: Effects of calcitonin analogues, and calcitonin gene-related peptide on basal in vitro renin secretion. *Am J Hypertens* 2:453, 1989.
137. Weidmann P, Hirsch D, Maxwell MH, et al: Plasma renin and blood pressure during treatment with methyldopa. *Am J Cardiol* 34:671, 1974.
138. Niarchos AP, Baer L, Radichevich I: Role of renin and aldosterone suppression in the antihypertensive mechanism of clonidine. *Am J Med* 65:614, 1978.
139. Boucher R, Rojo-Ortega JM, Genest J: Description of renin angiotensin system and methods of measurement, in Genest J, Koiw E, Kuchel O (eds): *Hypertension: Physiopathology and Treatment*. New York, McGraw-Hill, 1977, p 140.
140. Itoh S: Role of the macula densa in renin release. *Hypertension* 7:49, 1985.
141. Itoh S, Carretero OA, Murray RD: Possible role of adenosine in the macula densa mechanism of renin release in rabbits. *J Clin Invest* 76:1412, 1985.
142. Briggs J, Skatt O: Direct demonstration of macular densa-mediated renin secretion. *Science* 237:1618, 1987.
143. Kotchen TA, Galla JH, Luke RG: Contribution of chloride to the inhibition of plasma renin by sodium chloride in the rat. *Kidney Int* 13:201, 1978.
144. Brunner HR, Laragh JH, Baer L, et al: Essential hypertension: Renin and aldosterone, heart attack and stroke. *N Engl J Med* 286:441, 1972.
145. Egan BM, Julius S, Cottier C, et al: Role of cardiovascular receptors on the neural regulation of renin release in normal men. *Hypertension* 5:779, 1983.
146. Tuck M: Obesity, the sympathetic nervous system, and essential hypertension. *Hypertension* 19:I-67, 1992.
147. Timmermans P, Benfield P, Chiu A, et al: Angiotensin II receptors and functional correlates. *Am J Hypertens* 5:221, 1992.
148. Kotchen T, Guthrie G: Effects of calcium on renin and aldosterone. *Am J Cardiol* 62:41, 1988.
149. Gerber JG, Olson RD, Nies AS: Interrelationship between prostaglandins and renin release. *Kidney Int* 19:816, 1981.
150. Oates J, Whorton AR, Gerkens JF, et al: The participation of prostaglandins in the control of renin release. *Fed Proc* 38:72, 1979.
151. Patrono C, Pugliese F, Ciabattoni G, et al: Evidence for a direct stimulatory effect of prostacyclin on renin release in man. *J Clin Invest* 69:231, 1982.
152. Antonipillal I: 12-Lipoxygenase products are potent inhibitors of prostacyclin-induced renin release. *Proc Soc Exp Biol Med* 194:224, 1990.
153. Whorton AR, Misono K, Hollifield J, et al: Prostaglandins and renin release: I. Stimulation of renin release from rabbit renal cortical slices by PGI2. *Prostaglandins* 14:1095, 1977.
154. Tan SY, Shapiro R, Franco R, et al: Indomethacin induced prostaglandin inhibition with hyperkalemia: A reversible cause of hyporeninemic hypoaldosteronism. *Ann Intern Med* 90:783, 1979.
155. Antonipillal I, Wang Y, Horton R: Tumor necrosis factor and interleukin-1 may regulate renin secretion. *Endocrinology* 126:273, 1990.
156. Zipser R, Davenport M, Martin K, et al: Hyperreninemic hypoaldosteronism in the critically ill: A new entity. *J Clin Endocrinol Metab* 53:867, 1981.
157. Yamamoto T, Nakamura T, Noble N, et al: Expression of transforming growth factor β is elevated in human and experimental diabetic nephropathy. *Proc Natl Acad Sci USA* 90:1814, 1993.
158. Hsueh WA, Goldstone R, Carlson EJ, et al: Evidence that the beta-adrenergic system and prostaglandins stimulate renin release through different mechanisms. *J Clin Endocrinol Metab* 61:399, 1985.

159. Leutscher JA, Kraemer FB, Wilson DM, et al: Increased plasma inactive renin in diabetes mellitus. *N Engl J Med* 312:1412, 1985.
160. Wilson D, Leutscher J: Plasma prorenin activity and complications in children with insulin-dependent diabetes mellitus. *N Engl J Med* 323:1101, 1990.
161. Nakamura N, Soubrier F, Menard J, et al: Nonproportional changes in plasma renin concentration, renal renin content, and rat renin messenger RNA. *Hypertension* 7:855, 1986.
162. Lynd K, Peach M: Molecular biology of angiotensinogen. *Hypertension* 17:263, 1991.
163. Campbell DJ, Habener JF: Angiotensin gene is expressed and differentially regulated in multiple tissues of the rat. *J Clin Invest* 78:31, 1986.
164. Klett C, Bader M, Ganten D, et al: Mechanism by which angiotensin II stabilizes messenger RNA for angiotensinogen. *Hypertension* 23:I-120, 1994.
165. Bouhnik J, Galen FX, Clauser E, et al: The renin-angiotensin system in thyroidectomized rats. *Endocrinology* 108:647, 1981.
166. Kim H-S, Krege JH, Kluckman KD, Hagman JR, Hodgin JB: Best control of blood pressure and the angiotensinogen locus. *Proc Nat Acad Sci USA* 92:5266, 1995.
167. Smithies O: Theodore Cooper Memorial Lecture. A mouse view of hypertension. *Hypertension* 30:1318, 1997.
168. Strittmatter SM, Thiele EA, DeSouza EB, et al: Angiotensin-converting enzyme in the testis and epididymis: Differential development and pituitary regulation of isozymes. *Endocrinology* 117:1374, 1985.
169. Erdos EG, Skidgel RA: The unusual substrate specificity and the distribution of human angiotensin I converting enzyme. *Hypertension* 8:1, 1986.
170. Kumar R, Thekkumkara T, and Sen G: The mRNA's encoding the two angiotensin-converting isozymes are transcribed from the same gene by a tissue-specific choice of alternative transcription initiation sites. *J Biol Chem* 266:2854, 1991.
171. Skidgel RA, Erdos EG: Novel activity of human angiotensin I converting enzyme: Release of the NH_2- and COOH-terminal tripeptides from the luteinizing hormone-releasing hormone. *Proc Natl Acad Sci USA* 82:1025, 1985.
172. Fantone JC, Schrier D, Weingarten B: Inhibition of vascular permeability changes in rats by captopril. *J Clin Invest* 69:1207, 1982.
173. Liberman J, Sastri A: Serum angiotensin-converting enzyme: Elevations in diabetes mellitus. *Ann Intern Med* 93:825, 1980.
174. Niarchos AP, Resnick LM, Weinstein DL, et al: Angiotensin I converting enzyme activity in hypertension: Relationship to blood pressure, renin-sodium profiles, and antihypertensive therapy. *Am J Med* 79:435, 1985.
175. Silverstein E, Schussler GC, Friedland J: Elevated serum angiotensin-converting enzyme in hyperthyroidism. *Am J Med* 75:233, 1983.
176. Schunkert H, Dzau V, Tang S, et al: Increased rat cardiac angiotensin converting enzyme activity and mRNA expression in pressure overload left ventricular hypertrophy: Effects of coronary resistance, contractility and relaxation. *J Clin Invest* 86:1913, 1990.
177. Ohishi M, Ueda M, Rakugi H, Okamura A, Naruko T, Becker AE, Hiwada K, Kamitani A, Kamide K, Higaki J, Ogihara T: Upregulation of angiotensin-converting enzyme during the healing process after injury at the site of percutaneous transluminal coronary angioplasty in humans. *Circulation* 18;96(10):3328, 1997.
178. Studer R, Reinecke H, Muller B, Holtz J, Drexter H: Increased angiotensin-I converting enzyme gene expression in the failing human heart. Quantification by competitive RNA polymerase chain reaction. *J Clin Invest* 94:301, 1994.
179. Doria A, Warram J, Krolewski A: Genetic predisposition to diabetic nephropathy: Evidence for a role of the angiotensin I-converting enzyme gene. *Diabetes* 43:690, 1994.
180. Gharavi AG, Lipkowitz MS, Diamond JA, Jhang JS, Phillips RA: Deletion polymorphism of the angiotensin-converting enzyme gene is independently associated with left ventricular mass and geometric remodeling in systemic hypertension. *Am J Cardiol* 77:1315, 1996.
181. Straessen JA, Wang JG, Ginocchio G, Petrov V, Saavedra AP, Soubrier F, Vlietinck R, Fagard R: The deletion/insertion polymorphism of the angiotensin converting enzyme gene and cardiovascular-renal risk. *J Hypertens* 15:1579, 1997.
182. Kreutz R, Hubner N, Ganten D, Lindpaintner K: Genetic linkage of the ACE gene to plasma ACE activity, but not to blood pressure a quantitative trait locus confers identical complex phenotypes in human and rat hypertension. *Circulation* 92:2381, 1995.
183. Helgeland A, Strömmen R, Hagelund CH, et al: Enalapril, atenolol and hydrochlorothiazide in mild to moderate hypertension: A comparative multicentre study in general practice in Norway. *Lancet* 1:872, 1986.
184. Cachofeiro V, Sakakibara T, Nasjletti A: Kinins, nitric oxide, and the hypotensive effect of captopril and ramiprilat in hypertension. *Hypertension* 19:138, 1992.
185. Pfeifer M, Braunwald E, Moye L, et al: Effect of captopril on morbidity and mortality in patients with left ventricular dysfunction after myocardial infarction. *N Engl J Med* 327:669, 1992.
186. Lewis EJ, Hunsicker LG, Bain RP, Rodhe RD: The effect of angiotensin-converting-enzyme inhibition on diabetic nephropathy: The Collaborative Study Group. *N Engl J Med* 329:1456, 1993.
187. Hollenberg N: Renal perfusion and function: The implication of converting enzyme inhibition. *Am J Med* 84:9, 1988.
188. Kamper AL, Strandgaard S, Leyssac PP: Effect of enalapril on the progression of chronic renal failure: A randomized controlled trial. *Am J Hypertens* 5:423, 1992.
189. GISSI-3 Coordinating Centre. GISSI-3: Effects of lisinopril and transdermal glyceryl trinitrate singly and together on 6-week mortality and ventricular function after acute myocardial infarction. *Lancet* 343:1115, 1994.
190. The Heart Outcomes Prevention Evaluation Study Investigators: Effects of an angiotensin-converting-enzyme inhibitor, ramipril, on cardiovascular events in high-risk patients. *N Engl J Med* 342:145, 2000.
191. Todd PA, Heel RC: Enalapril: A review of its pharmacodynamic and pharmacokinetic properties, and therapeutic use in hypertension and congestive heart failure. *Drugs* 3:198, 1986.
192. Stansby G, Hamilton G: Atherosclerotic renal artery stenosis. *Br J Hosp Med* 49:388, 1993.
193. Campbell D, Kladis A, Duncan AM: Effects of converting enzyme inhibitors on angiotensin and bradykinin peptides. *Hypertension* 23:439, 1994.
194. Oparil S: Angiotensin I converting enzyme inhibitors and analogues of angiotensin II, in Genest J, Kuchel O, Hamet P, Cantin M (eds): *Hypertension*. New York, McGraw-Hill, 1983, p 250.
195. Mersey JH, Williams HG, Hollenberg NK, et al: Relationship between aldosterone and bradykinin. *Circ Res* 40:84, 1977.
196. Goodfriend TL: Angiotensin receptors and specific functions of angiotensins I, II and III, in Genest J, Kuchel O, Hamet P, Cantin M (eds): *Hypertension*. New York, McGraw-Hill, 1983, p 271.
197. Admiraal PJ, Danser AH, Jong MS, et al: Regional angiotensin II production in essential hypertension and renal artery stenosis. *Hypertension* 21:173, 1993.
198. Rossi GP, Sacchetto A, Cesari M, Pessina AC: Interactions between endothelin-1 and the renin-angiotensin-aldersterone system. *Cardiovasc Res* 1;43:300, 1999.
199. Matsukawa T, Mano T, Gotoh E, et al: Elevated sympathetic nerve activity in patients with accelerated essential hypertension. *J Clin Invest* 92:25, 1993.
200. Carmines P, Inscho E: Renal arteriolar angiotensin responses during varied adenosine receptor activation. *Hypertension* 23:I-114, 1994.
201. Carmines P, Flemming J: Control of the renal microvasculature by vasoactive peptides. *FASEB J* 4:3300, 1990.
202. Cogan M: Angiotensin II: A powerful controller of sodium transport in the early proximal tubule. *Hypertension* 15:451, 1990.
203. Crysant SG, Dunn M, Marples D, et al: Severe reversible azotemia from captopril therapy: Report of three cases and review of the literature. *Arch Intern Med* 143:437, 1983.
204. Gibbons GH, Dzau VJ: The emerging concept of vascular remodeling. *New Engl J Med* 330:1431, 1994.
205. Saaveda J: Brain and pituitary angiotensin. *Endocr Rev* 13:329, 1992.
206. Buchanan TA, Thawani H, Kades W, Modrall JG, Weaver FA, Laurel C, Poppiti R, Xiang A, Hsueh WA: Angiotensin II increaes glucose utilization during acute hyperinsulinemia via a hemodynamic mechnism. *J Clin Invest* 92:720, 1993.
207. Conzales-Espenosa C, Garcia Sainz JA: Hormonal modulation of c-fos expression inisolated hepatocytes. Effects of angiotensin II

and phorbol myristate acetate on transcription and mRNA degradation. *Biochem Biophys Acta* 2:1310:217, 1996.
208. Anderson P, Do Y, Hsueh W: Angiotensin II causes mesangial cell hypertrophy. *Hypertension* 21:29, 1993.
209. Norman J, badie-Dezfooly B, Nord EP, Kurta I, Schlosser J, Chaudhari A, Fine LG: EGF-induced mitogenesis in proximal tubular cells: Potentiation by angiotensin II. *Am J Physiol* 253:F299, 1987.
210. Schorb W, Booz G, Dostal D, et al: Angiotensin II is mitogenic in neonatal rat cardiac fibroblasts. *Circ Res* 72:1245, 1993.
211. Sadoshima J, Yuhui X, Slater HS, Izumo S: Autocrine release of angiotensin II mediates stretch-induced hypertrophy of cardiac myocytes in vitro. *Cell* 75:977, 1993.
212. Gelsterfer A, Peach M, Owens G: Angiotensin II induces hypertrophy, not hyperplasia, of cultured rat aortic smooth muscle cells. *Circ Res* 62:749, 1988.
213. Gibbons G, Pratt R, Dzau V: Vascular smooth muscle cell hypertrophy vs. hyperplasia: Autocrine transforming growth factor-13 expression determines growth response to angiotensin II. *J Clin Invest* 90:456, 1992.
214. Naftilan A, Pran R, Dzau V: Induction of platelet-derived growth factor A-chain and c-mycogene expressions by angiotensin II in cultured rat vascular smooth muscle cells. *J Clin Invest* 83:1419, 1989.
215. Stouffer G, Owens G: Angiotensin II-induced mitogenesis of spontaneously hypertensive rat-derived cultured smooth muscle cells is dependent on autocrine production of transforming growth factor-13. *Circ Res* 70:820, 1992.
216. Ray P, Aguilera G, Kipp J, et al: Angiotensin II receptor-mediated proliferation of cultured human fetal mesangial cells. *Kidney Int* 40:764, 1991.
217. Karami S, Border WA, Miller DE, Noble NA: Angiotensin II stimulates extracellular matrix protein synthesis through a cAMp response element. *Kidney Int* 46:1019, 1994.
218. Koichi I, Ashizawa N, Do YS, Graf K, Hsueh WA: Comparison of angiotensin II with other growth factors on Egr-1 and matrix gene expression in cardiac fibroblasts. *Am J Physiol* 270:H2100, 1996.
219. Weber KT: Extracellular matrix remodeling in heart failure. *Circulation* 96:4065, 1997.
220. Okiawa T, Freeman M, Lo W, Vaughan DE, Fogo A: Modulation of plasminogen activator inhibitor-1 in vivo: A new mechanism for the anti-fibrotic effect of renin-angiotensin inhibition. *Kidney Int* 47:1039, 1995.
221. Baricos WH, Cortez SL, El-Dahr SS, Schnaper HW: Ecm degradation by cultured human mesangial cells is mediated by a PA/plasmin/MMP-2 cascade. *Kidney Int* 47:1039, 1995.
222. Tummala PE, Chen XL, Sundell CL, Laursen JB, Hammes CP, Alexander RW, Harrison DG, Medford RM: Angiotensin II induces vascular cell adhesion molecule-1 expression in rat vasscular: A potential link between the renin-angiotensin system and atherosclerosis. *Circulation* 14;100(11):1223–9. 1999.
223. Pestore L, Tessitore A, Martinotti S, Toniato E, Alesse E, Bravi MC, Ferri C, Desideri G, Gulino A, Stanucci A: Angiotensin II stimulates intercellular adhesion molecule-1 (ICAM-1) expression by human vascular endothelial cells and increaes soluble ICAM-1 release in vivo. *Circulation* 12;100(15):1646, 1999.
224. Guerra-Cuesta JI, Monton M, Rodrequez-Feo JA, Jimenez AM, Gonzalez-Fernandez F, Ricl LA, Garcia R, Gomez J, Farre J, Casado S, Lopez-Farre A: Effect of losartan on human platelet activation. *J Hypertens* 17:447, 1999.
225. Searles CD, Harrison DG: The interaction of nitric oxide, bradykinin, and the angiotensin II type 2 receptor: Lessons learned from transgenic mice. *J Clin Invest* 104:1013, 1999.
226. Harding JW, Wright JW, Swanson GN, Hanesworth JM, Krebs LT: AT4 receptors: Specificity and distribution. *Kidney Int* 46:1510, 1994.
227. Coleman JKM, Ong B, Sardinia MI, Hading JW, Wright JW: Changes in renal blood flow due to infusion of angiotensin II (3-8) [AIV] in normotensive rats. *FASEB J* 6:A981, 1992.
228. Wright JW, Miller-Wing AV, Shaffer AV, Higginson C, Wright DE, Hanesworth JM, Harding JW: Angiotensin II (3-8) [ANG IV] hippocampal binding: Potential role in the facilitation of memory. *Brain Res Bull* 32:497, 1993.
229. Welches WR, Brosnihan KB, Ferrario CM: A comparison of properties, and enzymatic activity of three angiotensin processing enzymes: angiotensin converting enzyme, proly endopeptidase and neutral endopeptidase 24,11. *Life Sci* 52:1461, 1993.
230. Chappell MC, Tallant EA, Brosnihan KB, Ferrario CM: Conversion of angiotensin-(1-7) by thimet oligopeptidase (EC 3.4.24.15) in vascular smooth muscle cells. *J Vas Med Biol* 5:129, 1994.
231. Kohara K, Brosnihan KB, Chappell MC, et al: Angiotensin-(1-7): A member of circulating angiotensin peptides. *Hypertension* 17:131, 1991.
232. Handa RK, Ferrario CM, Strandhoy JW: Renal actions of angiotensin-(1-7): In vivo and in vitro studies. *Am J Physiol* 270:F141, 1996.
233. Benter IF, Diz DI, Ferrario CM: Cardiovascular actions of angiotensin-(1-7). Peptides 14:679.
234. Freeman EJ, Chisolm GM, Ferrario CM, Tallant EA: Angiotensin-(1-7) inhibits vascular smooth muscle cell growth. *Hypertension* 28:104, 1996.
235. Deddish PA, Marcic B, Jackman HL, Wang HZ, Skidgel RA, Erdos EG: N-domain-specific substrate and C-domain inhibitors of angiotensin-converting enzyme: Angiotensin-(1-7) and Keto-ACE. *Hypertension* 31:912, 1998.
236. Lima CV, Paula RD, Resende FL, Khosla MC, Santos RA: Potentiation of the hypotensive effect of bradykinin by short-term infusion of angiotensin-(1-7) in normotensive and hypertensive rats. *Hypertension* 30:542, 1997.
237. Chappell MC, Pirro NT, Sykes A, Ferrario CM: Metabolism of angiotensin-(1-7) by angiotensin-converting enzyme. *Hypertension* 31:362, 1998.
238. Chiu A, Herblin W, McCall D, et al: Identification of angiotensin II receptor subtypes. *Biochem Biophys Res Commun* 265:196, 1989.
239. Murphy T, Alexander R, Griendling K, et al: Isolation of a cDNA encoding the vascular type-1 angiotensin II receptor. *Nature* 351:233, 1991.
240. Sasaki K, Yamamono Y, Bardham S, et al: Cloning and expression of a complementary DNA encoding a bovine adrenal angiotensin II type-1 receptor. *Nature* 351:230, 1991.
241. Bernstein K, Alexander R: Counterpoint: Molecular analysis of the angiotensin II receptor. *Endocr Rev* 13:381, 1992.
242. Hein L, Barsh GS, Pratt RE, Dzau VJ, Kobilka BK: Behavioural and cardiovascular effects of disrupting the angiotensin II type-2 receptor in mice. *Nature* 377:744, 1995.
243. Ichiki T, Labosky PA, Shiota C, Okuuyama S, Imagawa Y, Fogo A, Niimura F, Ichikawa I, Hogan BL, Inagami T: Effects on blood pressure and exploratory behaviour of mice lacking angiotensin II type-2 receptor. *Nature* 377:748, 1995.
244. Grady E, Sechl L, Griffin C, et al: Expression of AT2 receptors in the developing rat fetus. *J Clin Invest* 88:921, 1991.
245. Sechi L, Griffin C, Grady E, et al: Characterization of angiotensin II receptor subtypes in rat heart. *Circ Res* 71:1482, 1992.
246. Millan M, Jacobowitz D, Aguilera G, et al: Differential distribution of AT1, and AT2 angiotensin II receptor subtypes in the rat brain during development. *Proc Natl Acad Sci USA* 88:11440, 1991.
247. Zwart AS, Davis EA, Widdop RE: Modulation of AT1 receptor-mediated contraction of rat uterine artery by AT2 receptors. *Br J Pharmacol* 125:1429, 1998.
248. Kambayashi Y, Bardham S, Takahashi K, et al: Molecular cloning of a noval angiotensin II receptor, type 1. *J Biol Chem* 268:24543, 1993.
249. Mukoyama M, Nakajuma M, Horiuchi M, et al: Expression cloning of type 2 angiotensin II receptor reveals a unique class of seventransmembrane receptors. *J Biol Chem* 268:24539, 1993.
250. Zhang J, Pratt RE: The AT2 receptor selectively associates with G_{in2} and G_{in3} in the rat fetus. *J Biol Chem* 271:15026, 1996.
251. Ambroz C, Catt K: Angiotensin II receptor-mediated calcium influx in bovine adrenal glomerulosa cells. *Endocrinology* 131:408, 1992.
252. Barrett P, Bollag W, Isales C, et al: Role of calcium in angiotensin II-mediated aldosterone secretion. *Endocr Rev* 10:496, 1989.
253. Diz DI, Bear PG, Nasjletti A: Angiotensin II-induced hypertension in the rat: Effects on the plasma concentration, renal excretion, and tissue release of prostaglandins. *J Clin Invest* 72:466, 1983.
254. Kawano H, Do Y, Kawano Y, Starnes V, Barr M, Law RE, Hsueh WA: Angiotensin II has multiple profibrotic effects inhuman cardiac fibroblasts. *Circulation*, 2000. In press.
255. Graf K, Xi XP, Hsueh WA, Law RE: Troglitazone inhibits an-

giotensin II-induced DNA synthesis and migrationin vascular smooth muscle cells. *FEBS Lett* 400:119, 1997.
256. Blume A, Herdegen T, Unger T: Angiotensin peptides and inducible transcription factors. *J Mol Med* 77:339, 1999.
257. Xi XP, Graf K, Goetze S, Gleck E, Hsueh WA, Law RE: Central role of the MAPK pathway in AngII-mediated DNA synthesis and migrartion in rat vascular smooth muscle cells. *Arterioscler Thromb Vasc Biol* 19:73, 1999.
258. Liao DF, Monia B, Dean N, Berk BC: Protein kinase C-zeta mediates angiotensin II activation of ERK1/2 in vascular smooth muscle cells. *J Biol Chem* 272:6146, 1997.
259. Oliverio MI, KIM HS, Ito M, LeT, Audoly L, Best CF, Hiller S, Kluckman K, Maeda N, Smithies O, Coffman TM: Reduced growth, abnormal kidney structure, and type 2 (AT2) angiotensin receptor-mediated blood pressure regulation in mice lacking both AT1A and AT1B receptors for angiotensin II. *Proc Nat Acad Sci USA* 95:1549, 1998.
260. Nimura F, Labosky PA, Kakuchi J, Okubo H, Yoshida T, Oikawa TI, Naftilan AJ, Fogo A, Inagami T, et al: Gene targeting in mice reveals a requirement of angiotensin in the development and maintenance of kidney morphology and growth factor regulation. *J Clin Invest* 96:2947, 1995.
261. Catt KJ, Harwood JP, Aquilera G, et al: Hormonal regulation of peptide receptors and target cell responses. *Nature* 280:109, 1979.
262. Lehoux JG, Bird I, Rainey W, et al: Both low sodium and high potassium intake increase the level of adrenal angiotensin-II receptor type 1, but not that of adrenocorticotropin receptor. *Endocrinology* 134:776, 1994.
263. Weber MA: Clinical experience with the angiotensin II receptor antagonist losartan: A preliminary report. *Am J Hypertens* 5:247, 1992.
264. Brunner HR, Christen Y, Munafo A, et al: Clinical experience with antiotensin II receptor antagonists. *Am J Hypertens* 5:243, 1992.
265. Fogo AB: The role of angioensin II and plasminogen activator inhibitor-1 in progressive glomerulosclerosis. *Am J Kidney Dis* 35:179, 2000.
266. Kawano Y, Nicholas SB, Kawano H, Law RE, Hsueh WA: Activation of peroxisomal proliferating activated receptors (PPARγ) attenuates plasminogen activator inhibitor-1 (PAI-1) expression in mesangial cells (MC). *Diabetes* 48: A267, 1999.
267. Wexler RR, Greenlee WJ, Irvin JD, Goldberg MR, Prendergast K, Smith RD, Timmermans PB: Nonpeptide angiotensin II receptor antagonists: The next generation in antihypertensive therapy. *J Med Chem* 39:625, 1996.
268. Bennai F, Morsing P, Paliege A, Ketteler M, Mayer B, Tapp R, Bachmann S: Normalizing the expression of nitric oxide synthase by low-dose AT1 receptor antgonism parallels improved vascular morphology in hypertensive rats. *J Am Soc Nephrol* 11:S104, 1999.
269. Pitt B, Segal R, Martinez FA, Meurers G, Cowley AJ, Thomas I, Deedwania PC, Ney DE, Snavely DB, Chang PI: Randomized trial of losartan versus captopril in patients over 65 with heart failure (Evaluation of Losartan in the Elderly Study, ELITE). *Lancet* 349:747, 1997.
270. Seyedi N, Win T, Lander HM, Levi R: Bradykinin B2-receptor activation augments norepinephrine exocytosis from cardiac sympathetic nerve endings. Mediation by autocine/paracrine mechanisms. *Circ Res* 81:774, 1997.
271. ELITE II-2000, Am Coll Cardiol Mtg (presented)
272. Haber E, Sancho J, Re R, et al: The role of the renin-angiotensin-aldosterone system in the cardiovascular homeostasis in normal man. *Clin Sci Mol Med* 48:49, 1975.
273. Noth RH, Tan SY, Mulrow PJ: Effects of angiotensin II blockade by saralasin in normal man. *J Clin Endocrinol Metab* 45:10, 1977.
274. Gavras H, Ribeiro AB, Gavras I, et al: Reciprocal relation between renin dependency and sodium dependency in essential hypertension. *N Engl J Med* 295:1278, 1976.
275. Miller EDJ, Samuels AI, Haber E, et al: Inhibition of angiotensin conversion and prevention of renal hypertension. *Am J Physiol* 228:448, 1975.
276. Carretero OA, Romero JC: Production and characteristics of experimental hypertension in animals, in Genest J, Koiw E, Kuchel O (eds): *Hypertension: Physiopathology and Treatment*. New York, McGraw-Hill, 1977, p 485.
277. Martinez-Maldonado M: Pathophysiology of renovascular hypertension. *Hypertension* 17:707, 1991.
278. Akahoshi M, Carretero O: Body fluid volume and angiotensin II in maintenance of one-kidney, one clip hypertension. *Hypertension* 14:269, 1989.
279. Fukamizu A, Sugimura K, Takimoto E, et al: Chimeric renin-angiotensin system demonstrates sustained increase in blood pressure of transgenic mice carrying both human renin and human angiotensinogen genes. *J Biol Chem* 268:11617, 1993.
280. Mullins J, Peters J, Ganten D: Fulminant hypertension in transgenic rats harbouring the mouse Ren-2 gene. *Nature* 344:541, 1990.
281. Mullins JJ, Mullins LJ: Transgenes, hypotheses, and hypertension. *Hypertension* 23:428, 1994.
282. Schambelan M, Howes ELJ, Stockigt JR, et al: Role of renin and aldosterone in hypertension due to a renin-secreting tumor. *Am J Med* 55:86, 1973.
283. Anderson P, Macaulay L, Do Y, et al: Insights into hypertension and ovarian renin production. *Medicine (Baltimore)* 68:257, 1990.
284. London G, Safr M: Renal hemodynamics in patients with sustained essential hypertension and in patients with unilateral stenosis of the renal artery. *Am J Hypertens* 2:244, 1989.
285. Brown JJ, Davies DL, Lever AF, et al: Variations in plasma renin concentration in several physiological and pathological states. *Can Med Assoc J* 90:201, 1964.
286. McAllister RGJ, Van Way CWI, Dayani K, et al: Malignant hypertension: Effect of therapy on renin and aldosterone. *Circ Res* 8:160, 1971.
287. Esler MD: Catecholamines and essential hypertension. *Baillieres Clinic Endrocrinol Metab* 7:415, 1993.
288. Williams G, Hollenberg N: Non-modulating hypertension: A subset of sodium-sensitive hypertension. *Hypertension* 17:I–81, 1991.
289. Larah J: Issues, goals, and guidelines in selecting first-line drug therapy for hypertension. *Hypertension* 13:I–103, 1989.
290. Drury P: Disorders of mineralocorticoid activity. *J Clin Endocrinol Metab* 14:175, 1985.
291. Muntzel M, Drueke T: A comprehensive review of the salt and blood pressure relationships. *Am J Hypertens* 5:1, 1992.
292. Hatton D, McCarron D: Dietary calcium and blood pressure in experimental models of hypertension; A review. *Hypertension* 23:513, 1994.
293. Resnick L, Barbagallo M, Gupta R, et al: Ionic basis of hypertension in diabetes mellitus. *Am J Hypertens* 6:413, 1993.
294. Redgrave J, Rabinowe S, Hollenberg NK, et al: Correction of abnormal renal blood flow response to angiotensin II by converting enzyme inhibition in essential hypertensives. *J Clin Invest* 75:1285, 1985.
295. Luparini R, Ferri C, Santucci A, et al: Atrial natriuretic peptide in non-modulating essential hypertension. *Hypertension* 21:803, 1993.
296. Conn JW: Presidential address: Primary aldosteronism: A new clinical syndrome. *J Lab Clin Med* 45:3, 1955.
297. Eberlein WB, Bongiovanni AM: Plasma and urinary corticosteroids in the hypertensive form of congenital adrenal hyperplasia. *J Biol Chem* 223:85, 1956.
298. Biglieri EG, Herron MA, Brust N: 17α-Hydroxylation deficiency in man. *J Clin Invest* 45:1946, 1966.
299. Ulick S: Evidence for defective functional zonation of adrenal hyperplasia syndromes in man, in Mantero F, Biglieri E, Funder J, Scoggins B (eds): *The Adrenal Gland and Hypertension*. New York, Raven Press, 1985, p 357.
300. Monder C: Corticosteroids, kidneys, sweet roots and dirty drugs. *Mol Cell Endocrinol* 78:C95, 1991.
301. Stewart P, Edwards C: The cortisol-cortisone shuttle and hypertension. *J Steroid Biochem Mol Biol* 40:501, 1991.
302. Monder C, White P: 11β-Hydroxysteroid dehydrogenase. *Vitam Horm* 47:187, 1993.
303. Lamberts S, Koper J, Biemond P, et al: Cortisol receptor resistance: The variability of its clinical presentation and response to treatment. *J Clin Endocrinol Metab* 74:313, 1992.
304. Malchoff CD, Javier EC, Malchoff DM, et al: Primary cortisol resistance presenting as sexual precocity. *J Clin Endocrinol Metab* 70:503, 1990.
305. Shackelton C, Rodriguez J, Arteaga G, et al: Congenital 11β-hydroxysteroid dehydrogenase deficiency associated with juvenile hypertension: Corticosteroid metabolite profiles of four patients and their families. *Clin Endocrinol (Oxf)* 22:701, 1985.
306. Farese RJ, Biglieri F, Schaklcton C, et al: Licorice-induced hypertension. *N Engl J Med* 325:1223, 1991.

307. Walerk BR, Edwards CR: Licorice-induced hypertension and syndromes of apparent mineralocorticoid excess. *Endocrinol Metab Clin North Am* 23:359, 1994.
308. Griffing GT, Melby JC: Adrenocortical factors in hypertension. *J Clin Pharmacol* 25:218, 1985.
309. Krakoff L, Nicolis G, Amsel B: Pathogenesis of hypertension in Cushing's syndrome. *Am J Med* 58:216, 1975.
310. Cassar J, Loizou S, Kely WF, et al: Deoxycorticosterone and aldosterone excretion in Cushing's syndrome. *Metabolism* 29:115, 1980.
311. Hogan MJ, Schambelan M, Biglieri EG: Concurrent hypercortisolism and hypermineralocorticoidism. *Am J Med* 62:777, 1977.
312. Azar S, Melby J: 19-Nor-deoxycorticosterone production from aldosterone-producing adenomas. *Hypertension* 19:362, 1992.
313. Baxter JD, Schambelan M, Matulich D, et al: Aldosterone receptors and the evaluation of plasma mineralocorticoid activity in normal and hypertensive states. *J Clin Invest* 58:579, 1976.
314. Takeda Y, Iki K, Takeda R: Formation of 18-deoxy-19- noraldosterone by a human aldosterone-producing adenoma. *Steroids* 58:282, 1993.
315. Gorsline J, Harnik M, Tresco PA, et al: Hypertensinogenic activities of ring A-reduced metabolites of aldosterone. *Hypertension* 8:187, 1986.
316. Pelletier M, Ludens JH, Fanestil DD: The role of aldosterone in active sodium transport. *Arch Intern Med* 129:248, 1972.
317. Mion DJ, Rea R, Anderson E, et al: Effects of fludrocortisone on sympathetic nerve activity in humans. *Hypertension* 23:123, 1994.
318. Biglieri EG, Forsham PH: Studies on expanded extracellular fluid and responses to various stimuli in primary aldosteronism. *Am J Med* 30:564, 1961.
319. Weinberger MH, Grim CE, Hollifield JW, et al: Primary aldosteronism: Diagnosis, localization, and treatment. *Ann Intern Med* 90:386, 1979.
320. Slaton PE, Biglieri EG: Hypertension and hyperaldosteronism renal artery stenosis: Serial observations on 54 patients treated medically. *Clin Pharmacol Ther* 6:700, 1965.
321. Tarazi RC, Ibrahim MM, Bravo EL, et al: Hemodynamic characteristics of primary aldosteronism. *N Engl J Med* 289:1330, 1973.
322. Went GJ, MarintVeld AJ, Verhoeven RP, et al: Volume-pressure relationships during development of mineralocorticoid hypertension in man. *Circ Res* 40:163, 1977.
323. Oh-hashi S, Takata M, Ueno H, et al: Cytosolic free calcium concentration in platelets in patients with renovascular hypertension and primary aldosteronism. *J Human Hypertens* 6:71, 1992.
324. Tannen RL: Potassium handling by the kidney, in Tannen RL, Massry S, Glassock RJ (eds): *Textbook of Nephrology*. Baltimore, Williams & Wilkins, 1983, p 3.
325. Miyajima E, Yamada Y, Yoshida Y, et al: Muscle sympathetic nerve activity in renovascular hypertension and primary aldosteronism. *Hypertension* 17:1057, 1991.
326. Wang W, McClain J, Zucker I: Aldosterone reduces baroreceptor discharge in the dog. *Hypertension* 19:270, 1992.
327. Torres, Young WJ, Offord KP, et al: Association of hypokalemia, aldosteronism, and renal cysts. *N Engl J Med* 322:345, 1990.
328. Smith J, Wade M, Fineberg N, et al: Sodium transport parameters in erythrocytes of patients with primary aldosteronism. *Hypertension* 11:141, 1988.
329. Funder JW, Adam WR, Mantero F, et al: The etiology of a syndrome of factitious mineralocorticoid excess: A steroid-containing nasal spray. *J Clin Endocrinol Metab* 49:842, 1979.
330. Schalekamp M, Wenting G, Man A: Pathogenesis of mineralocorticoid hypertension. *Clin Endocrinol Metab* 10:397, 1981.
331. Idewhi M, Kishikawa K, Kinoshita A, et al: High-renin malignant hypertension secondary to an aldosterone-producing adenoma. *Nephron* 54:259, 1990.
332. Brills C, Matsubara L, Wever K: Anti-aldosterone treatment and the prevention of myocardial fibrosis in primary and secondary hyperaldosteronism. *J Mol Cell Cardiol* 25:563, 1993.
333. Campbell S, Janicki J, Matsubara B, et al: Myocardial fibrosis in the rat with mineralocorticoid excess: Prevention of scarring by amiloride. *Am J Hypertens* 6:487, 1993.
334. Gomez-Sanchez CE: Cushing's syndrome and hypertension. *Hypertension* 8:258, 1986.
335. Mantero F, Boscardo M: Glucocorticoid-dependent hypertension. *J Steroid Biochem Mol Biol* 43:409, 1992.
336. Whitworth J, Gordon D, Andrew J, et al: The hypertensive effect of synthetic glucocorticoids in man: Role of sodium and volume. *J Hypertens* 7:537, 1989.
337. Sato A, Suzuki H, Murakami M, et al: Glucocorticoid increases angiotensin II type 1 receptor and its gene expression. *Hypertension* 23:25, 1994.
338. Kennedy B, Elayan H, Ziegler M: Glucocorticoid hypertension and nonadrenal phenylethanolmine N-methyltransferase. *Hypertension* 21:415, 1993.
339. Pirpiris M, Yeung S, Dewar E, et al: Hydrocortisone-induced hypertension in man: The role of cardiac output. *Am J Hypertens* 6:287, 1993.
340. Montrella-Waybill M, Clore J, Schoolwerth A, et al: Evidence that high dose cortisol-induced Na^+ retention in man is not mediated by the mineralocorticoid receptor. *J Clin Endocrinol Metab* 72:1060, 1991.
341. Kornel L, Manisundaram B, Nelson W: glucocorticoids regulate N^+ transpost in vascular smooth muscle through the glucocorticoid receptor-mediated mechanism. *Am J Hypertension* 6:736, 1993.
342. Saruta T: Mechanism of glucocorticoid-induced hypertension. *Hypertens Res* 19:1, 1996.
343. Watt G, Harrap S, Foy C, et al: Abnormalities of glucocorticoid metabolism and the renin-angiotensin system: A fur-corners approach to the identification of genetic determinants of blood pressure. *J Hypertens* 10:473, 1992.
344. Hayashi T, Nakai T, Miyabo S: Glucocorticoids increase Ca^{2+} uptake and [3H]dihydropyridine binding in A7r5 vascular smooth muscle cells. *Am J Physiol* 261:C106, 1991.
345. Radomski MW, Palmer R, Moncarda S: Glucocorticoids inhibit the expression of an inducible, but not constitutive, nitric oxide synthase in vascular endothelial cells. *Proc Natl Acad Sci USA* 87:10043, 1990.
346. Radwanska E: The role of reproductive hormones in vascular disease and hypertension. *Steroids* 58:605, 1993.
347. Moncada S, and Higgs A: The L-arginine-nitric oxide pathway. *N Engl J Med* 329:2002, 1993.
348. Polikar R, Burger AG, Scherrer U, et al: The thryoid and the heart. *Circulation* 87:1435, 1993.
349. Streeten D, Anderson G, Howland T, et al: Effects of thyroid function on blood pressure: Recognition of hypothyroid hypertension. *Hypertension* 11:78, 1988.
350. Bing R, Briggs R, Burden A, et al: Reversible hypertension and hypothyroidism. *Clin Endocrinol (Oxf)* 13:339, 1980.
351. Kochar, M: Hemodynamic effects of lysine-vasopressin in orthostatic hypotension. *Am J Kidney Dis* 6:49, 1985.
352. Padfield, P: Vasopressin in hypertension. *Am Heart J* 94:531, 1977.
353. Cowley Jr, AJ, Cushman E, et al: Vasopressin elevation in essential hypertension and increased responsiveness to sodium intage. *Hypertension Dallas* 3:93, 1981.
354. Bartter F, Schwartz W: The syndrome of inappropriate secretion of antidiuretic hormone. *Am J Med* 42:790, 1967.
355. Smith M Jr, Cowley A Jr, et al: Acute and chronic effects of vasopressin on blood pressure, electrolytes, and fluid volumes. *Am J Physiol* 249(Heart and Circulatory Physiology) 18:H1001, 1979.
356. Cowley A Jr, Liard J: Cardiovascular actions of vasopressin. *Vasopressin*. D. Gash and G. Boer. New York, Plenum: 389–433, 1987.
357. Martinez-Vea A, Bardaji A, Garcia C, et al: Long-term myocardial effects of correction of anemia with recombinant human erythropoietin in aged patients on hemodialysis. *Am J Kidney Dis* 19:353, 1992.
358. Martinez-Vea A, Bardaji A, Garcia C, et al: Long-term myocardial effects of correction of anemia with recombinant human erythropoietin in aged patients on hemodialysis. *Am J Kidney Dis* 19:353, 1992.
359. Buckner F, Eschbach J, Haley N, Davidson R, Adamson J: Hypertension following erythropoietin therapy in anemic hemodialysis patients. *Am J Hypertens* 3:947, 1990.
360. Casati S, Passerini P, Campise M, et al: Benefits and risks of protracted treatment with human recombinant erythropoietin in patients having hemodialysis. *Br Med J* 295:1017, 1987.
361. Raine A: Hypertension, blood viscosity, and cardiovascular morbidity in renal failure: implications of erythropoietin therapy. *Lancet* 1:97, 1988.
362. Samtleben W, Baldamus C, Bommer J, Fassbinder W, Nonnast-Daniel B, Gurland H: Blood pressure changes during treatment with recombinant human erythropoietin. *Contr Nephrol* 76:114, 1988.

363. Drucke T, Zins B, Naret C, et al: Utilization of erythropoietin in the treatment of anemia due to chronic renal failure. *Adv Nephr* 18:187, 1989.
364. Canadian Erythropoietin Study Group: Effect of recombinant human erythropoietin therapy on blood pressure in hemodialysis patients. *Am J Nephrol* 11:23, 1991.
365. Eschbach J, Egrie J, Downing M, Browne J, Adamson J: Correction of anemia of end-stage renal disease with recombinant human erythropoietin. *N Engl Journal Med* 316:73, 1987.
366. Nonnast-Daniel B, Frei U, Pollock M, Granolleras C, Shaldon S, Koch K: Correction of renal anemia by daily subcutaneous administration of erythropoietin: An approach to avoid the induction of hypertension. *Nephrol Dial Transplant* 5:742A, 1990.
367. Cuneo R, Salomon F, Wilmshurst P, et al: Cardiovascular effects of growth hormone treatment in growth-hormone-deficient adults: Stimulation of the renin-aldosterone system. *Clin Sci* 81:587, 1991.
368. Barton J, Hindmarshi P, Preece M, et al: Blood pressure and the renin-angiotensin-aldosterone system in children receiving recombinant growth hormone. *J Clin Endocrinol* 38:245, 1993.
369. Masuda A, Kazuaki S, Mori Y, et al: Plasma calcitonin gene-related peptide levels in patients with various hypertensive diseases. *J Hyperten* 10:1499, 1992.
370. Wimalawansa S: Antihypertensive effects of oral calcium supplementation may be mediated through the potent vasodilator CGRP. *Am J Hypertens* 6:996, 1993.
371. Lüscher T, Sco B, Bühler F: Potential role of endothelin in hypertension: Controversy on endothelin in hypertension. *Hypertension* 21:752, 1993.
372. Vanhoutte P: Is endothelin involved in the pathogenesis of hypertension. *Hypertension* 21:747, 1993.
373. Yokokawa K, Tahara H, Kohno M, et al: Hypertension associated with endothelin-secreting malignant hemangioendothelinoma. *Ann Intern Med* 114:213, 1991.
374. Krum H, Viskoper RJ, Lacourciere Y, Budde M, Charlon V: For The Bosentan Hypertension Investigators: The effect of an endothelin-receptor antagonist, bosentan, on blood pressure in patients with essential hypertension. *N Engl J Med* 338:784, 1998.
375. Clozel M, Breu V, Burri K, et al. Pathophysiological role of endothelin revealed by the first orally active endothelin receptor antagonist. *Nature* 365:759, 1993.
376. Kourembanas S, McQuillan L, Leung G, et al: Nitric oxide regulates the expression of vasoconstrictors and growth factors by vascular endothelium under both normoxia and hypoxia. *J Clin Invest* 92:99, 1993.
377. Calver A, Collier J, Moncada S, et al: Effect of local intra-arterial N^G-monomethyl-L-arginine in patients with hypertension: The nitric oxide dilator mechanism appears abnormal. *J Hypertens* 10:1025, 1992.
378. Salazar F, Alberola A, Pinila J, et al: Salt-induced increase in arterial pressure during nitric oxide synthesis inhibition. *Hypertension* 22:49, 1993.
379. Baylis C, Mitruka B, Deng A: Chronic blockade of nitric oxide synthesis in the rat produces systemic hypertension and glomerular damage. *J Clin Invest* 90:278, 1992.
380. Hou J, Kato H, Cohen RA, Chobanian AV, Brecher P: Angiotensin II-induced cardiac fibrosis in the rat is increased by chronic inhibition of nitric oxide synthase. *J Clin Invest* 96:2469, 1995.
381. Arnal JF, Armrani AI, Chatellier G, et al: Cardiac weight in hypertension induced by nitric oxide synthetase blockade. *Hypertension* 22:380, 1993.
382. Ikenaga H, Suzuki H, Ishii N, et al: Role of NO on pressure-natriuresis in Wistar-Kyoto and spontaneously hypertensive rats. *Kidney Int* 43:205, 1993.
383. Jover B, Herizi A, Ventre F, et al: Sodium and angiotensin in hypertension induced by long-term nitric oxide blockade. *Hypertension* 21:944, 1993.
383a. Shesely EG, Maeda N, Kim HS, Desai KM, Krege JH, Laubach VE, Sherman PA, Sessa WC, Smithies O. Elevated blood pressures in mice lacking endothelial nitric oxide synthase. *Proc Natl Acad Sci* 93:13176-81, 1996.
383b. Huang PL, Huang Z, Mashimo H, Block KD, Moskowitz MA, Bevan JA, Fishman MC: Hypertension in mice lacking the gene for endothelial nitric oxide synthase. *Nature* 377:239, 1995.
384. Panza J, Quyyuma A, Brush JJ, et al: Abnormal endothelium-dependent vascular relaxation in patients with essential hypertension. *N Engl J Med* 323:22, 1990.
385. Petros A, Hewletyt A, Bogle R, et al: L-arginine-induced hypotension. *Lancet* 337:1044, 1991.
386. Panza J, Casino P, Badar D, et al: Effect of increased availability of endothelium-derived nitric oxide precursor on endothelium-dependent vascular relaxation in normal subjects and in patients with essential hypertension. *Circulation* 87:1475, 1993.
387. Panza J, Quyyumi A, Callahan T, et al: Effect of antihypertensive treatment on endothelium-dependent vascular relaxation in patients with essential hypertension. *J Am Coll Cardiol* 12:1145, 1993.
388. Taddei S, Virdis A, Mattei P, et al: Vasodilation to acetylcholine in primary and secondary forms of human hypertension. *Hypertension* 21:929, 1993.
389. Cockcroft J, Chowienczyk P, Benjamin N, et al: Preserved endothelium-dependent vasodilatation in patients with essential hypertension. *N Engl J Med* 330:1036, 1994.
390. Panza JA, Casino PR, Kilcoyne CM, Quyyumi AA: Impaired endothelium-dependent vasodilation in patients with essential hypertension: Evidence that abnormality is not at the muscarinic receptor level. *J Am Cell Cardiol* 23:1610, 1994.
391. Glasser SP, Selwyn AP, Glass P: Atherosclerotic risk factors and the vascular endothelium. *Am Heart J* 131:379, 1996.
392. Hsueh WA, Law RE: Pharmacological treatment and mechanisms of insulin resistance: Impact on vascular smooth muscle cells, blood pressure, and lipids. *Ann NY Acad Sci* 827:170, 1997.
393. Rector TS, Bank AJ, Mulle KA, Tschumperlin LK, Sih R, Pillai K, Kubo SH: *Circulation* 15;93:2135, 1996.
394. Van de Stolpe A, van der Saag PT: Intercellular adhesion molecule-1. *J Mol Med* 74:13, 1996.
395. Davis MJ, Gordon JL, Gearing AHJ, Pigott R, Woolf N, Katz D, Kyriakopoulos A: The expression of the adhesion molecules ICAM-1, VCAM-1, PECAM, and E-selection I human atherosclerosis. *J Pathol* 171:223, 1993.
396. Nakashima M, Mombouli JV, Taylor A, et al: Endothelium-dependent hyperpolarization caused by bradykinin in human coronary arteries. *J Clin Invest* 92:2867, 1993.
397. Schwartz D, Geller DM, Manning PT, et al: Ser-Leu-Arg-Arg-atriopeptin III: The major circulating form of atrial peptide. *Science* 229:397, 1985.
398. Greenberg BD, Bencen GH, Seilhamer JJ, et al: Nucleotide sequence of the gene encoding human atrial natriuretic factor precursor. *Nature* 312:656, 1984.
399. De Bold AJ: Atrial natriuretic factor: A hormone produced by the heart. *Science* 230.767, 1985.
400. Cantin M, Genest J: The heart as an endocrine gland. *Sci Am* 254:76, 1986.
401. Needleman P, Greenwald JE: Atriopeptin: A cardiac hormone intimately involved in fluid, electrolyte, and blood-pressure homeostasis. *N Engl J Med* 314:828, 1986.
402. Gardner DG, Deschepper CF, Ganong WF, et al: Extra-atrial expression of the gene for atrial natriuretic factor. *Proc Natl Acad Sci USA* 83:6697, 1986.
403. Chen YF, Elton T, Oparil S: Quantitation of hypothalamic atrial natriuretic peptide messenger RNA in hypertensive rats. *Hypertension* 19:296, 1992.
404. Suga SI, Nakao K, Hosoda K, et al: Receptor selectivity of natriuretic peptide family: Atrial natriuretic peptide, brain natriuretic peptide, and c-type natriuretic peptide. *Endocrinology* 130:229, 1992.
405. Richards A, Crozier I, Espiner E, et al: Plasma brain natriuretic peptide and endopeptidase 24.11 inhibition in hypertension. *Hypertension* 22:231, 1993.
406. Jamison R, Canaan-Kuhl S, Pratt R: The natriuretic peptides and their receptors. *Am J Kidney Dis* 20:519, 1992.
407. Wei CM, Heublein D, Perrella M, et al: Natriuretic peptide system in human heart failure. *Circulation* 88:1004, 1993.
408. Mattingly M, Brandt R, et al: Presence of C-type natriuretic peptide in human kidney and urine. *Kidney Int* 46:744, 1994.
409. Richards A, Crozier I, Holmes S, et al: Brain natriuretic peptide: Natriuretic and endocrine effects in essential hypertension. *J Hypertens* 11:163, 1993.
410. Ballermann BJ, Brenner BM: Biologically active atrial peptides. *J Clin Invest* 76:2041, 1985.

411. Gardner DG, Hane S, Trachewsky D, et al: Atrial natriuretic peptide mRNA is regulated by glucocorticoids in vivo. *Biochem Biophys Res Commun* 139:1047, 1986.
412. Atlas SA: Atrial natriuretic factor: A new hormone of cardiac origin. *Rec Prog Horm Res* 42:207, 1986.
413. Nonoguchi H, Tomita K, Marumo F: Effects of atrial natriuretic peptide and vasopressin on chloride transport in long- and short-looped medullary thick ascending limbs. *J Clin Invest* 90:349, 1992.
414. Hollister A, Inagami T: Atrial natriuretic factor and hypertension, a review and metaanalysis. *Am J Hypertens* 4:2, 1991.
415. Chinkers M, Garbers D: The protein kinase domain of the ANP receptor is required for signaling. *Science* 245:1392, 1989.
416. Duda T, Goraczniak R, et al: Site-directed mutational analysis of a guanylate cyclase cDNA reveals the atrial natriuretic factor signaling site. *Proc Nat Acad Sci USA* 88:7882, 1991.
417. Zeidel M, Kikeri D, et al: Atrial natriuretic peptides inhibit conductive sodium uptake by rabbit inner medullary collecting duct cells. *J Clin Invest* 82:1067, 1988.
418. Cogan M: Atrial natriuretic peptide. *Kidney Int* 37:1148, 1990.
419. Wilkins M, Redondo J, et al: The natriuretic peptide family. *Lancet* 349:1307, 1997.
420. Musca A, Cammarella I, Ferri C, et al: Natriuretic hormones in young hypertensives and in young normotensives with or without a family history of hypertension. *Am J Hypertens* 5:592, 1992.
421. Awazu M, Ichikawa I: Biological significance of atrial natriuretic peptide in the kidney. *Nephron* 63:1, 1993.
422. Hummel M, Kuhn M, Bub A, et al: Urodilatin, a new therapy to prevent kidney failure after heart transplantation. *J Heart Transplant* 12:209, 1993.
423. McDonough P, Glembotski C: Induction of atrial natriuretic factor and myosin light chain-2 gene expression in cultured ventricular myocytes by electrical stimulation of contraction. *J Biol Chem* 267:11665, 1992.
424. Appel R: Growth-regulatory properties of atrial natriuretic factor. *Am J Physiol* 262:F911, 1992.
425. Levin E: Natriuretic peptide c-receptor: More than a clearance receptor *Am J Physiol* 264:E483, 1993.
426. Watkins R, Vemulapalli S, Chiu P, et al: Atrial natriuretic factor potentiating and hemodynamic effects of SCH 42495, a new, neutral metalloendopeptidase inhibitor. *Am J Hypertens* 6:357, 1993.
427. Wilkins M, Needleman P: Effect of pharmacological manipulation of endogenous atriopeptin activity on renal function. *Am J Physiol* 262:F161, 1992.
428. Graf K, Do YS, Ashizawa N, Meehan WP, Giachelli CM, Marboe CC, Gleck E, Hushe WA: Myocardial osteopontin expression is associated with left ventricular hypertrophy. *Circulation* 96:3063, 1997.
429. Trippodo NC, Robl JA, Asaad MM, Fox M, Panchal BC, Schaeffer TR: Effects of omapatrilat in low, normal, and high renin experimental hypertension. *Am J Hypertens* 11:363, 1998.
430. Yandle T, Richards A, Gilbert A, et al: Assay of brain natriuretic peptide (BNP) in human plasma: Evidence for high molecular weight BNP as a major plasma component in heart failure. *J Clin Endocrinol Metab* 76:832, 1993.
431. Predel HG, Schulte-vels O, Glanzer K, et al: Atrial natriuretic peptide in patients with essential hypertension: Hemodynamic, renal, and hormonal responses. *Am J Hypertens* 4:871, 1991.
432. DiBona G: Sympathetic neural control of the kidney in hypertension. *Hypertension* 19:I28, 1992.
433. Tuck ML, Corry DB: Pathophysiology and management of hypertension in diabetes. *Ann Rev of Medicine* 42:533, 1991.
434. Hsueh WA, Law RE: Cardiovascular Risk Continuum: Implications of insulin resistance and diabetes. *Am J Med* 105:4S, 1998.
435. Rocchini A: Insulin resistance and blood pressure regulation in obese and nonobese subjects. *Hypertension* 17:837, 1991.
436. Landsberg L: Hyperinsulinemia: Possible role in obesity-induced hypertension. *Hypertension* 19:61, 1992.
437. Hsueh WA, Buchanan TA: Obesity and hypertension. 23:405, 1994.
438. Reaven G: Role of insulin resistance in human disease (syndrome X): An expanded definition. *Annu Rev Med* 44:121, 1993.
439. Stern MP: Diabetes and cardiovascular disease: The "common soil" hypothesis. *Diabetes* 44:369, 1995.
440. Hamaty M, Lamberti M, Sowers JR: Diabetic vascular disease and hypertension. *Curr Opin Cardiol* 13:298, 1998.
441. Reaven G, Chen Y, Jeppesen J, et al: Insulin resistance and hyperinsulinemia in individuals with small, dense, low density lipoprotein particles. *J Clin Invest* 92:141, 1993.
442. Festa A, D'Agostino R Jr, Mykkanen L, Tracey RP, Zaccaro DJ, Hales CN, Haffner SM: *Arterioscler Thromb Vasc Biol* 19:562, 1999.
443. Saito F, Hori M, Fittingoff M, et al: Insulin attenuates agonist-mediated calcium mobilization in cultured rat vascular smooth muscle cell. *J Clin Invest* 92:1161, 1993.
444. Meehan WP, Buchanan TA, Hsueh W: Chronic insulin administration elevates blood pressure in rats. *Hypertension* 23:1012, 1994.
445. Wu HY, Jeng YY, Yue CJ, et al: Endothelial-dependent vascular effects of insulin and insulin-like growth factor I in the perfused rat mesenteric artery and aortic ring. *Diabetes* 43:1994.
446. Anderson E, Mark A: The vasodilator action of insulin: Implications for the insulinhypothesis of hypertension. *Hypertension* 21:136, 1993.
447. Baron A, Brechtel G: Insulin differentially regulares systemic and skeletal muscle vascular resistance. *Am J Physiol* 265:E61, 1993.
448. Sakai K, Imaizumi T, Masaki H, et al: Intra-arterial infusion of insulin attenuates vasoreactivity in human forearm. *Hypertension* 22:67, 1993.
449. Laakso M, Edelman SV, Brechtel G, Baron AD: Decreased effect of insulin to stimulate skeletal muscle blood flow in obese man: A novel mechanism for insulin resistance. *J Clin Invest* 85:1844, 1990.
450. Resnick L: Ionic basis of hypertension, insulin resistance, vascular disease, and related disorder. *Am J Hypertens* 6:123, 1993.
451. Vollenweider P, Tappy L, Randin D, et al: Differential effects of hyperinsulinemia and carbohydrate metabolism on sympathetic nerve activity and muscle blood flow in humans. *J Clin Invest* 92:147, 1993.
452. Zeng G, Quon MJ: Insulin-stimulated production of nitric oxide is inhibited by wortmannin: Direct measurement in vascular endothelial cells. *J Clin Invest* 98:894, 1996.
453. Gupta A, Clark R, Kirchner K: Effects on insulin on renal sodium excretion. *Hypertension* 19:I78, 1992.
454. Goodfriend T, Ball D, Elliott M, et al: Fatty acids may regulate aldosterone secretion and mediate some of insulin's effects on blood pressure. *Prostaglandins Leukot Essent Fatty Acids* 48:43, 1993.
455. Juncos L, Ito S: Disparate effects of insulin on isolated rabbit afferent and efferent arterioles. *J Clin Invest* 92:1981, 1993.
456. Miller J. Abouchacra S, Zimman B, et al: Atrial natriuretic factor counteracts sodium-retaining action of insulin in normal men. *Am J Physiol* 265:R584, 1993.
457. Imai Y, Clemmons DR: Roles of phosphatidylinositol 3-kinase and mitogen-activated protein kinase pathways in stimulation of vascular smooth muscle cell migration and deoxyribonucleic acid synthesis by insulin-line growth factor-1. *Endocrinology* 140:4228, 1999.
458. Alessi MC, Peiretti F, Morange P, Henry M, Nalbone G, Juhan-Vague I: Production of plasminogen activator inhibitor 1 by human adipose tissue: Possible link between visceral fat accumulation and vascular disease. *Diabetes* 46:860, 1997.
459. Banskota NK, Taub R, Seliner K, King GL: Insulin, insulin-like growth factor 1 and platelet-derived growth factor interact additivity in the induction of the protooncogene c-myc and cellular proliferation in cultured bovine aortic smooth muscle cells. *Mol Endocrinol* 3:1183, 1989.
460. Zhen YJ, You WL, Clemont A, Feener EP, Hein KD, Igarashi M, Yamauchi T, White MF, King GL: Characterization of selective resistance to insulin signaling in the vasculature of obese Zucher (fa/fa) rats. *J Clin Invest* 104:447, 1999.
461. XI XP, Graf K, Goetz S, Hsueh WA, Law RE: Inhibition of MAP kinase blocks insulin-mediated DNA synthesis and transcriptional activation of *c-fos* by Elk in vascular smooth muscle cells. *FEBS Lett* 417:283, 1997.
462. Goetze S, Xi XP, Kawano H, Gotlibowski T, Fleck E, Hsueh WA, Law RE: PPARγ ligands inhibit migration mediated by multiple chemoattractants in vascular smooth muscle cells. *J Cardiovasc Pharm* 33:798, 1999.
463. Desvergne B, Wahli W: Peroxisome proliferator-activted receptors: Nuclear control of metabolism. *Endocr Rev* 20:649, 1999.
464. Giguere V: Orphan nuclear receptors: From gene to function. *Endocr Rev* 20:689, 1999.

465. Tontonoz P, Hu E, Spiegelman BM: Stimulation of adipogenesis in fibroblasts by PPARγ2, a lipid-activated trasncription factor. *Cell* 79:1147, 1994.
466. Park KS, Ciaraldi TP, Lindgren K, Abrams-Carter L, Mudaliar S, Nikoulina SE, Tufari SR, Veerkamp JH, Vidal-Puig A, Henry RR: Troglitazone effects on gene expression in human skeletal muscle of type II diabetes involve up-regulation of peroxisome proliferator-activated receptor-gamma. *J Clin Endocrinol Metab* 83:2830, 1998.
467. Maggs DG, Buchanan TA, Burant CF, Cline G, Gumbiner B, Hsueh WA, Inzucchi S, Kelley D, Nolan J, Olefsky JM, Polanski KS, Silver D, Valiquett TR, Shulman GI: Metabolic effects of troglitazone monotherapy in type 2 diabetes mellitus. A randomized, double-blind, placebo-controlled trial. *Ann Intern Med* 128:176, 1998.
468. Ehrmann DA, Schneider DJ, Sobel BE, Cavaghan MK, Imperial J, Rosenfield RL, Polonsky KS: Troglitazone improves defects in insulin action, insulin secretion, ovarian steroidogenesis, and fibrinolysis in women with polycystic ovary syndrome. *J Clin Endocrinol Metab* 82:2108, 1997.
469. Tack CJ, Smits P, Demacker PN, Stalenhoef AF: Troglitazone decreases the proportion of small, dense LDL and increases the resistance of LDL to oxidation in obese subjects. *Diabetes Care* 21:796, 1998.
470. Law RE, Meehan WP, Xi XP, et al: Troglitazone inhibits vascular smooth muscle cell grwoth and intimal hyperplasia. *J Clin Invest* 98:1897, 1996.
471. Collins AR, Meehan WP, Howard-Taylor TR, Castellani LW, Palinski W, Hsueh WA, Law RE: Troglitazone attenuates atherosclerosis in low density lipoprotein receptor mice fed a high fat diet. *Diabetes* 48:A30, 1999.
472. Barroso I, Gurnell M, Crowley VEF, Agostini M, Schwabe JW, Soos MA, Maslen G, Williams TBM, Lewis H, Schafer AJ, Chatterjee VKK, O'Rahilly S: Dominant negative mutations in human PPARγ associated with severe insulin resistance, diabetes mellitus and hypertension. *Nature* 402;23/30:880, 1999.
473. Ristow M, et al: Obesity associated with a mutation in a genetic regulator of adipocyte differentiation. *N Engl J Med* 339:953, 1998.
474. Begum N, Leitner W, Reusch JE, Sussman KE, Draznin B: GLUT-4 phosphorylation and is intrinsic activity: Mechanisms of Ca^{2+}-induced inhibition of insulin-stimulated glucose transport. *J Biol Chem* 193;268:3352, 1993.
475. Zemel MB, Peuler JD, Sowers JR: Hypertension in insuln-resistant Zxucker obese rats is independent of sympathetic neural support. *Am J Physiol* 262:E368, 1992.
476. Standley PR, Ram JL, Sowers JR: Insulin attenuation of vasopressin-induced calcium responses in arterial smooth muscle from Zucker rats. *Endocrinology* 193;133:1693.
477. Jacob RJ, Sherwin RS, Greenwalt K, Shulman GI: Simultaneous insulin-like growth factor-1 and insulin resistance in obese Zucker rats. *Diabetes* 41:691, 1992.
478. Liu S, Baracos VE, Quinney HA, Bricon TH, Clandinin MT: Parallel insulin-like growth factor-1 and insulin resistance in muscles of rats fed a high fat diet. *Endocrinology* 136:3318, 1995.
479. Sowers JR: Insulin and insulin-like growth factor in normal and pathological cardiovascular physiology. *Hypertension* 29:691, 1997.
480. Standley PR, Zhang F, Ram JL, Zemel MB, Sowers JR: Insulin attenuates vasopressin-induced calcium transient and voltage-dependent calcium response in rat vascular smooth muscle cells. *J Clin Invest* 88:1230, 1991.
481. Kahn AM, Seidel CL, Allen JC, O'Neil RG, Shelat H, Song T: Insulin reduces contraction and intracellular calcium concentration in vascular smooth muscle. *Hypertension* 22:735, 1993.
482. Touyz RM, Tolloczko B, Schiffrin EL: Insulin attenuates agonist evoked calcium transients in vascular smooth muscle cells. *Hypertension* 23:123, 1994.
483. Kahn AM, Husid A, Allen JC, Seidel CL, Song T: Insulin acutely inhibits cultured vascular smooth muscle cell contraction by a nitric oxide synthase-dependent pathway. *Hypertension* 30:929, 1997.
484. Bolotina VM, Najibl JJ, Pagano PJ, Cohen RA: Nitric oxide directly activates calcium dependent potassium channels in vascular smooth muscle. Nature 368:850, 1994.
485. Kontos HA, Wei EP: Arginine analogues inhibit responses mediated by ATP-sensitive K^+ channels. *Am J Physiol* 271:H1498, 1996.
486. Ohara T, Sussman KE, Draznin: β Effect of diabetes on cytosolic free Ca^{2+} and Na^+, K^+-ATPase in rat aorta. *Diabetes* 40:1560, 1991.
487. Hundal HS, Marette A, Mitsumoto T, et al: Insulin induces translocation of the α_1 and β_1 subunits of the Na^+,K^+-ATPase from intracellular compartments to the plasma membrane in mammalian skeletal muscle. *J Biol Chem* 267:5040, 1992.
488. Standley PR, Zhang F, Zayas R, Sowers JR: IGF-1 regulation of Na^+, K^+-ATPase in rat arterial smooth muscle. *Am J Physiol* 273: E113, 1997.
489. Lytton J: Insulin affects the sodium affinity of the rat adipocyte (N^+, K^+)-ATPase. *J Biol Chem* 260:1075, 1985.
490. Rosic NK, Standaert ML, Pollet RJ: The mechanism of insulin stimulation of (Na^+, K^+)-ATPase transport activity in muscle. *J Biol Chem* 260:6206, 1985.
491. Steinberg HO, Brechtel G, Johnson A, Feneberg N, Baraon AD: Insulin-mediated skeletal muscle vasodilation in nitric oxide-dependent: A novel action of insulin to increase nitric oxide release. *J Clin Invest* 94:1172, 1994.
492. Walsh MF, Barazi M, Pete G, Muniyappa R, Dunbar JC, Sowers JR: IGF-1 diminishes in vivo and in vitro vascular contractility: Role of vascular nitric oxide. *Endocrinology* 137:1798, 1996.
493. Gupta SC, McArthur C, Grady C, Ruderman NB: Stimulation of vascular (Na^+,K^+)-ATPase activity by nitric oxide: A cGMP-independent effect. *Am J Physiol* 266:H2146, 1994.
494. Reddy S, Shehin MS, Sowers JR: Aortic calcium-45 flux and blood pressure regulation in streptozotocin-induced diabetic rats. *Vasc Biol* 2:47, 1990.
495. O'Hare T, Sussman KE, Draznin B: Effect of diabetes on cytosolic free Ca^{2+} and Na^+, K^+-ATPase in rat aorta. *Diabetes* 40:1560, 1991.
496. Herrara VLM, Chobanian AV, Ruiz-Opazo N: Isoform-specific modulation of Na^+,K^+-ATPase α subunit gene expression in hypertension. *Science* 241:221, 1988.
497. Sada T, Koike H, Ikeda M, Sato K, Ozaki H, Karaki H: Cytosolic free calcium of aorta in hypertensive rats. *Hypertension* 16:245, 1990.
498. Rayssiguier Y: Magnesium, lipids and vascular diseases; Experimental evidence in animal models. *Magnesium* 5:182, 1986.
499. Zemel PC, Zemel M, Urberg M, Douglas F, Sowers JR: Metabolic and hemodynamic effects of magnesium supplementation in patients with essential hypertension. *Am J Clin Nutr* 51:665, 1990.
500. Paolisso G, Sgambato S, Pizza G, Passariello N, Varricchio M, D'Onofrio F: Improved insulin response and action by chronic magnesium administration in aged NIDDM subjects. *Diabetes Care* 12:265, 1989.
501. Balon JTW, Gu JL, Tokuyama Y, Jasman AP, Nadler JL: Magnesium supplementation reduces development of diabetes in a rat model of spontaneous NIDDM. *Am J Physiol* E745, 1995.
502. Nadler JL, Buchanan T, Natarajan R, Antonipillai I, Bergman R, Rude R: Magnesium deficiency produces insulin resistance and increased thromboxane synthesis. *Hypertension* 21:1024, 1993.
503. Dominguez LJ, Barbagallo M, Sowers JR, Resnick LM: Magnesium responsiveness to insulin and IGF-1 in erythrocytes from normotensive and hypertensive subjects. *J Clin Endocrinol Metab* 83:4402, 1998.
504. Dickens BF, Weglicki Y, Li S, Mak IT: Magnesium deficiency in vitro enhances free radical-induced intracellular oxidation and cytotoxicity in endothelial cells. *FEBS Lett* 311:187, 1992.
505. Sipes SL, Weiner CP, Gelhaus TM, Goodspeed JD: Effects of magnesium sulfate infusion upon plasma prostaglandins in preeclampsia and preterm labor. *Hypertens Pregnancy* 13:293, 1994.
506. Caro J: Insulin resistance in obese and nonobese man. *J Clin Endrocinol Metab* 73:691, 1991.
507. Brunsell JD, Hokanson JE: Dyslipidemia of central obesity and insulin resistance. *Diabetes Care* 22:C10, 1999.
508. Haffner SM, Ferrannini E, Hazuda HP, et al: Clustering of cardiovascular risk factors in confirmed prehypertensive individuals: The San Antonio Heart Study. *Am J Epidemiol* 41:715, 1992.
509. Lissner L, Bengtsson C, Lapidus L, et al: Fasting insulin in relation to subsequent blood pressure changes and hypertension in women. *Hypertension* 20:797, 1992.
510. Ferrannini E: Metabolic abnormalities of hypertension: A lesson in complexities. *Hypertension* 18:636, 1991.
511. Grunfeld B, Balzareti M, Romo M, et al: Hyperinsulinemia in normotensive offspring of hypertensive parents. *Hypertension* 23:I12, 1994.
512. Allemann Y, Horber F, Colombo M, et al: Insulin sensitivity and

body fat distribution in normotensive offspring of hypertensive patients. *Lancet* 341:327, 1993.
513. Saad MF, Lillioja S, Nyomba BL, et al: Racial differences in the relation between blood pressure and insulin resistance. *N Engl J Med* 324:733, 1991.
514. Saad MF, Howard G, Rewers M, et al: Insulin resistance but not insulinemia is associated with hypertension: The insulin resistance atherosclerosis study. *Circulation* 89:934, 1994.
515. Stern M, Morales P, Haffner S, et al: Hyperdynamic circulation and the insulin resistance syndrome ("syndrome X"). *Hypertension* 20:802, 1992.
516. Shamiss A, Carroll J, Rosenthal T: Insulin resistance in secondary hypertension. *Am J Hypertens* 5:26, 1992.
517. Bonora E, Bonadona R, Del Prat S, et al: In vivo glucose metabolism in obese and type II diabetic subjects with or without hypertension. *Diabetes* 42:764, 1993.
518. Nilsson P, Lindholm L, Scherstein B: Hyperinsulinemia and other metabolic disturbances in well controlled hypertensive men and women: An epidemiological study of the Dalby population. *J Hypertens* 8:953, 1990.
519. Ferrari P, Weidmann P, Shaw S, et al: Altered insulin sensitivity, hyperinsulinemia, and dyslipidemia in individuals with a hypertensive parent. *Am J Med* 91:589, 1991.
520. Julius S, Jamerson K, Mejiia A, et al: The association of borderline hypertension with target organ changes and higher coronary risk. Techumseh Blood Pressure Study. *JAMA* 264:354, 1990.
521. Faulkner B, Hulman S, Tannenbaum, et al: Insulin resistance and blood pressure in young blank males. *Hypertension* 15:681, 1990.
522. Jarrett R: In defense of insulin: A critique of syndrome X. *Lancet* 340:469, 1992.
523. Dowse G, Collins V, Alberti K, et al: Insulin and blood pressure levels are not independently related in Mauritians of Asian Indian, Creole or Chinese origin. *J Hypertens* 11:297, 1993.
524. Hypertension Detection and Follow-up Program Cooperative Group: Five-year findings of the hypertension detection and follow up program: I. Reduction in mortality of persons with high blood pressure, including mild hypertension. *JAMA* 242:2562, 1979.
525. Ferranini E, Natali A, Bell P, Cavallo-Perin P, Lalic N, Mingrone G. Insulin resistance and hypersecretion in obesity. European Group for the Study of Insulin Resistance (EGIR). *J of Clin Invest* 100:1166, 1997.
526. Del Rio A, Rodriguez-Villamil JL: Metabolic effects of strict salt restriction in essential hypertensive patient. *J Intern Med* 233:409, 1993.
527. Sharma A, Schorr U, Distler A: Insulin resistance in young salt-sensitive normotensive subjects. *Hypertension* 21:273, 1993.
528. Egan BM, Stepniakowski K, Nazzaro P: Insulin levels are similar in obese salt-sensitive and salt-resistant hypertensive subjects. *Hypertension* 23:I1, 1994.
529. Nishina P, Johnson J, Naggert J, et al: Linkage of atherogenic lipoprotein phenotype to the low density lipoprotein receptor locus on the short arm of chromosome 19. *Proc Natl Acad Sci USA* 89:708, 1992.
530. Wu DA, Bu X, Warden CH, Shen DDC, Jeng CY, Sheu WHH, Fuh MMT, Katsuya T, Dzau VJ, Reaven GM, Lusis AJ, Rotter JI, Chen YDI: Quantitative trait locus mapping of human blood pressure to the lipoprotein lipase gene locus on chromosome 8p22. *J Clin Invest* 97:2111, 1996.
531. UK prospective study group: Tight blood pressure control and risk of macrovascular and microvascular complications in type 2 diabetes: UKPDS 38. *Br Med J* 317:703, 1998.
532. UK prospective diabetes study group: Efficacy of atenolol and captopril in reducing risk of macrovascular and microvascular complications in type 2 diabetes: UKPDS 39. *Gr Med J* 317:713, 1998.
533. Laakso M: Epidemiology of macrovascular disease in diabetes. *Diabetes Rev* 5:294, 1997.
534. Conlon PJ, Athirakul K, Kovalik E, Schwab SJ, Crowley J, Stack R, Mccants JR, Mark DB, Bashore TM, Albers F: Survival in renal vascular disease. *J Am Soc Nephrol* 9:252, 1998.
535. Kimberly JH, Lundberg AH, Benjamin ME, Casey WJ, Craven TE, Bleyer AJ, Dean RH: Is renal revascularization in diabetic patients worthwhile? *J Vas Surg* 24:383, 1996.
536. Higashi Y, Oshima T, Ozono R, Nakano Y, Mastuura H, Kambe M, Kajiyama G: Nocturnal decline in blood pressure is attenuated by NaCl loading in salt-sensitive patients with essential hypertention: Non-invasive 24-hour ambulatory blood pressure monitoring. *Hypertension* 30:163, 1997.
537. Nakano S, Fukuda M, Hotta F, Ito T, Ishoo T, Kitazawa M, Nishizawa M, Kigoshi T, Uchida K: Reversed circadian blood pressure rhythm is associated with occurrences of both fatal and nonfatal vascular events in NIDDM subjects. *Diabetes* 47:1501, 1998.
538. Azara ST, Birbari A: Nocturnal blood pressure elevation in patients with type 1 diabetes receiving intensive insulin therapy compared with that in patients receiving conventional insulin therapy. *J Clin Endocinol Metab* 83:3190, 1998.
539. Naruse M, Wasada T, Naruse K, Yoshimoto T, Omori Y, Demura H: Pathophysiological significance of plasma total renin and prorenin in patients with diabetes mellitus. *Endocr J* 42:225, 1995.
540. Luetscher JA, Kreamer FB, Wilson DM, Schwartz HC, Bryer-Ash M: Increased plasma inactive renin in diabetes mellitus. A marker of microvascular complications. *N Engl J Med* 312:1412, 1985.
541. Franken AA, Derkx FH, Man in't Veld AJ, Hop WC, van Rens GH. Peperkamp E, de Jong PT, Schalekamp MA. High plasma prorenin in diabetes mellitus and its correlation with some complications. *J Clin Endocrinol Metab* 71:1008, 1990.
542. Allen TJ, Cooper ME, Gillbert RE, Winikoff J, Skinni Sl, Jerums G: Serum total renin is increased before microalbuminuria in diabetes. *Kidney Int* 50:902, 1996.
543. Daneman D, Crompton CH, Balfe JW, Sochett EB, Chatzilias A, Cotter BR, Osmond DH. Plasma prorenin as an early marker of nephropathy in diabetic (IDDM) adolescents. Kidney Int 46:1154, 1994.
544. Rosendorff C: The renin-angiotensin system and vascular hypertrophy. *J Am Coll Cardiol* 28:803, 1996.
545. Nolan JJ, Ludvik B, Beerdsen P, et al: Improvement in glucose tolerance and insulin resistance in obese subjects treated with roglitaozne. *N Engl J Med* 331:1188, 1994.
546. Walker AB, Naderali EK, Chattington PD, Buckingham RE, Williams G: Differential vasoactive effects of the insulin sensitizers rosiglitazone (BRL 49653) and troglitazone on human small arteries in vitro. *Diabetes* 47:810, 1998.
547. Estacio RO, Barrett JW, Hiatt WR, Biggerstaff SL, Gifford N, Schrier RW: The effect of nisoldipine as compared with enalapril on cardiovascular outcomes in patients with non-insulin-dependent diabetes and hypertension. *N Engl J Med* 338:646, 1998.
548. Tatti P, Pahor M, Byington RP, Di Mauro P, Guarisco R, Strollo GT, Strollo F: Outcome results of the Fosinopril versus Amlodipine Cardiovascular Events randomized trial (FACET) in patients with hypertension and NIDDM. *Diabetes Care* 21:597, 1998.
549. Bakris G: Treatment of hypertension in adults with diabetes to preserve renal function: A position paper by the National Kidney Foundation Working Groups (in press, 2000).
550. Bakris GL, Copley JB, Vicknair N, Sadler R, Leurgans S: Calcium channel blockers versus other antihypertensive therapies on progression of non-insulin-dependent diabetes mellitus associated nephropathy. *Kidney Int* 56:1641, 1996.
551. Santoro D, Natali A, Palombo C, et al: Effects of chronic angiotensin coverting enzyme inhibition on glucose tolerance and insulin sensitivity in essential hypertension. *Hypertension* 20:181, 1992.
552. Pollare T, Lithell H, Berne C: A comparison of the effects of hydrochlorothiazide and captopril on glucose and lipid metabolism in patients with hypertension. *N Engl J Med* 322:776, 1990.
553. Giordano M, Matsuda M, Sanders L, Canessa ML, DeFronzo RA: Effects of angiotensin-converting enzyme inhibitors, calcium channel antagonists, and alpha-adrenergic blockers on glucose and lipid metabolism in non-insulin-dependent diabetes mellitus patients with hypertension. *Diabetes* 44:665, 1995.
554. Perloff D, Grim C, Glack J, Frohlich ED, Hill M, McDonald M, Morgenstern BZ, Writing Group: Human blood pressure determination of sphygmomanometry: Special Report. *Circulation* 88:2460, 1993.
555. Kirkendall WM, Feinleib M, Freis ED, et al: Recommendations for human blood pressure determination by sphygmomanometers. *Circulation* 62:1145, 1980.
556. Brunner H: ACE inhibitors in renal disease. *Kidney Int* 42:463, 1992.
557. Wachtell K, Ibsen H, Olsen M, et al: Prevalence of renal artery

stenosis in patients with peripheral vascular disease and hypertension. *J Hum Hypertens* 10:83, 1996.

558. Davis B, Crook J, Vestal R, Oakes J: Prevalence of renovascular hypertension in patients with grade III or IV retinopathy. *N Engl J Med* 301:1273, 1997.
559. Emovon O, Klotman P, Dunnick N, et al: Renovascular hypertension in blacks. *Am J Hypertens* 9:18, 1996.
560. Mahomed F: Chronic Bright's disease without albuminuria. *Guys Hospital Reports* 25:295, 1881.
561. Goldblatt H, Lynch J, Hanzal R, Summerville W: The production of persistent elevation of systolic blood pressure by means of renal ischemia. *J Exp Med* 59:347, 1934.
562. Braun-Menendez E, Fasciolo J Leloir F, Munoz J: La substancia hipertensionora de la sangre del rinon isquemiado. *Rev Soc Argent Biol* 15:420, 1939.
563. Pickering G: The role of the kidney in acute and chronic hypertension following renal artery constriction in the rabbit. *Clin Sci* 5:229, 1945.
564. Nakada T, Iijima Y, Kubota Y, Watanabe M, Ishigooka M, Suzuki H: Increased vascular collagen and noncollagenous protein synthesis contributes to sustain chronic phase of two-kidney, one-clip renovascular hypertension. *J Urol* 156:1180, 1996.
565. Pohl M, Novick A: Natural history of atherosclerotic and fibrous renal artery disease: Clinical implications. *Am J Kidney Dis* 5:A120, 1985.
566. Connolly J, Higgins R, Walters H, et al: Presentation, clinical features and outcome in different patterns of atherosclerotic renovascular disease. *Q J Med* 87:413, 1994.
567. UZU T, Inoue T, Fujii T, Nakamura S, Inenga T, Yutani G, Kimura G: Prevalence and predictors of renal artery stenosis in patients with myocardial infarction. *Am J Kidney Dis* 29:733, 1997.
568. Losito A, Fagugli R, Zampi I, et al: Comparison of target organ damage in renovascular and essential hypertension. *Am J Hypertens* 9:1062, 1996.
569. Greco B, Breyer J: Atherosclerotic ischemic renal disease. *Am J Kidney Dis* 29:167, 1997.
570. Luscher T, Lie J, Stanson A, et al: Arterial fibromuscular dysplasia. *Mayo Clin Proc* 62:931, 1987.
571. Stanley J: Surgical treatment of renovascular hypertension. *Am J Surg* 174:102, 1997.
572. Goncharenko V, Gerlock A, Schaff M, et al: Progression of renal artery fibromuscular dyslasia in 42 patients as seen on angiography. *Radiology* 139, 1981.
573. Harrison EJ, McCormack L: Pathologic classification of renal arterial disease in renovascular hypertension. *Mayo Clini Proc* 46:161, 1971.
574. Stanley J, Gewartz B, Boue E, et al: Arterial fibrodysplasia: Histopathologic character and current etiologic concepts. *Arch Surg* 110:561, 1975.
575. Harrington J, Sommers S, Kassirer J: Atheromatous emboli with progressive renal failure. Renal arteriography as the probable inciting factor. *Ann Intern Med* 68:152, 1968.
576. Kassirer J: Atheroembolic renal disease. *N Engl J Med* 280:812, 1969.
577. First M, Neylan J, Rocher L, et al: Hypertension after renal transplantation. *J Am Soc Nephrol* 4:S30, 1994.
578. Castle C: Iatrogenic renal hypertension: Two unusual complications of surgery for familial pheochromocytoma. *JAMA* 225:1085, 1973.
579. Restrick L, Ledermann J, Hoffbrand B: Primary malignant retroperitoneal germ cell tumor presenting with accelerated hypertension. *J Hum Hypertens* 3:243, 1992.
580. Sacks S, Aparicio S, Bevan A, et al: Late renal failure due to prostatic outflow obstruction: a preventable disease. *Br Med J* 298:156, 1989.
581. de Zeeuw D, Donker A, Burema J, et al: Nephroptosis and hypertension. *Lancet* 1:213, 1977.
582. Simon N, Franklin SS, Bleifer KH, Maxwell MH: Clinical characteristics of renovascular hypertension. *JAMA* 220:1209, 1972.
583. Turnbull J: Is listening for abdominal bruits useful in the evaluation of hypertension? *JAMA* 274:1299, 1995.
584. Kumar A, Shapiro A: Proteinuria and nephrotic syndrome induced by renin in patients with renal artery stenosis. *Arch Intern Med* 140:1631, 1980.
585. Bookstein J, Maxwell M, Abrams H, et al: Cooperative study of radiologic aspects of renovascular hypertension. Bilateral renovascular disease. *JAMA* 237:1706, 1977.
586. Mann S, Pickering T: Detection of renovascular hypertension. *Ann Intern Med* 117:845, 1992.
587. Brunner H, Laragh J, Baer L, et al: (1972): Essential hypertension: Renin and aldosterone, heart attack and stroke. *N Engl J Med* 286:441, 1972.
588. Rudnick M, Maxwell M: Limitations of renin assays, in Narins R (ed): *Controversies in Nephrology and Hypertension*. New York: Churchill Livingstone, 1984, pp 123–160.
589. Case D, Laragh J: Reactive hyperreninemia in renovascular hypertension after angiotensin blockade with saralasin or converting enzyme inhibitor. *Ann Intern Med* 91:153, 1979.
590. Muller F, Sealey J, Case D, et al: The captopril test for identifying renovascular disease in hypertensive patients. *Am J Med* 80:633, 1986.
591. Elliott W, Martin W, Murphy M: Comparison of two noninvasive screening tests for renovascular hypertension. *Arch Intern Med* 153:755, 1993.
592. Mueller F, Laragh J: Clinical evaluation and differential diagnosis of the individual hypertensive patient. *Clin Chem* 37:1868, 1991.
593. Simon G, Coleman C: Captopril-stimulated renal vein renin measurements in the diagnosis of atherosclerotic renovascular hypertension. *Am J Hypertens* 7:1, 1994.
594. Vaughn EJ: Renovascular hypertension. *Kidney Int* 27:811, 1985.
595. Davidson R, Wilcox C: Newer tests for the diagnosis of renovascular disease. *Renovascular Dis* 268:3353, 1992.
596. Dunnick N, Sfakianakis G: Screening for renovascular hypertension. *Radiol Clin North Am* 29:497, 1991.
597. Fommei E, Bellina C, Carmellini M, et al: High sensitivity of a computerized radioisotopic method to evaluate unilateral renal blood flow reduction by firstpass analysis and static imaging with 99mTc-glucoheptonate. *J Nuclear Med Allied Sci* 27:303, 1983.
598. Nally J, Chen C, Fine E, et al: Diagnostic criteria of renovascular hypertension with captopril renography. *Am J Hypertens* 4:749, 1991.
599. Cazanello W, Textor S: Noninvasive diagnosis of renovascular disease. *Mayo Clin Proc* 69:1172, 1994.
600. Derkx F, Schalekamp M: Renal artery stenosis and hypertension. *Lancet* 344:237, 1994.
601. Pedersen E: Pathophysiological, diagnostic and therapeutic aspects of renal artery stenosis. *Nephrol Dial Transplant* 9:482, 1994.
602. Setaro J, Saddler M, Chenn. C, et al: Simplified captopril renogram in diagnosis and treatment of renal artery stenosis. *Hypertension* 18:289, 1991.
603. Clorius J, Allenberg J, Hupp T, et al: Predictive value of exercise renography in presurgical evaluation of nephrogenic hypertension. *Hypertension* 10:280, 1987a.
604. Clorius J, Mann J, Schmidlin P, et al: Clinical evaluation of patients with hypertension and exercise-induced renal dysfunction. *Hypertension* 10:287, 1987b.
605. Hupp T, Clorius J, Allenberg J: Renovascular hypertension: Predicting surgical cure with exercise renography. *J Vasc Surg* 14:200, 1991.
606. Mitty H, Shapiro R, Parsons R, Silberzweig J: Renovascular hypertension. *Radiol Clin North Am* 34:1017, 1996.
607. Greene E, Avasthi P, Hodges J: Noninvasive Doppler assessment of renal artery stenosis and hemodynamics. *J Clin Ultrasound* 15:653, 1987.
608. Norris C, Pfeiffer J, Rittgers S, Barnes R: Noninvasive evaluation of renal artery stenosis and renovascular hypertension: Experimental and clinical studies. *J Vasc Surg* 1:192, 1984.
609. Rene P, Oliva V, Bui E, et al: Renal artery stenosis: Evaluation of Doppler US after inhibition of angiotensin-converting enzyme with captopril. *Radiology* 196:675, 1995.
610. Spies K, Fobbe F, El-Bedewi M, et al: Color-coded duplex sonography for noninvasive diagnosis and grading of renal artery stenosis. *Am J Hypertens* 8:1222.
611. Sheikh K, Davidson C, Newman G: Intravascular ultrasound assessment of the renal artery. *Ann Intern Med* 115:22, 1991, 1995.
612. von Birgelen C, van der Lugt A, Nicosia A, et al: Computerized assessment of coronary lumen and atherosclerotic plaque dimensions in three-dimensional intravascular ultrasound correlated with histomorphometry. *Am J Cardiol* 78:1202, 1996.

613. Stanley J: Surgical treatment of renovascular hypertension. *Am J Surg* 174:102, 1997.
614. Levin D, Beckman C, Serur J: Vascular resistance changes distal to progressive arteriolar stenosis: A critical re-evaluation of the concept of vasodilator reverse. *Invest Radiol* 14:120, 1980.
615. Shipley R, Gregg D: The effect of external constriction of a blood vessel on blood flow. *Am J Physiol* 141:287, 1944.
616. Hessel S: Complications of angiography and other catheter procedures, in Abrams H (ed): *Angiography*. Boston, Little Brown, 1983, pp 1041.
617. Steinberg E, Moore R, Powe N, et al: Safety and cost-effectiveness of high-osmolality as compared with low-osmolality contrast materials in patients undergoing cardiac angiography. *N Engl J Med* 326:425, 1992.
618. Barrett BJ, Parfrey PS, McDonald JR, Hefferton DM, Reddy ER, McManamon PJ: Nonionic low-osmolality versus ionic high-osmolality contrast material for intravenous use in patients perceived to be at risk: randomized trial. Radiology, 183:105, 1992.
619. Distler A, Spics KP: Diagnostic procedure in renovascular hypertension. *Clin Nephrol* 36:295, 1991.
620. Scott J, Rabe F, Becker G, et al: Angiographic assessment of renal artery pathology: How reliable? *Am J Radiol* 141:1299, 1983.
621. Bonelli F, McKusick M, Textor S, et al: Renal artery angioplasty: Technical results and clinical outcome in 320 patients. *Mayo Clin Proc* 70:1041, 1995.
622. Feltrin G, G R, Talenti E, et al: Prognostic value of nephrography in atherosclerotic occlusion of the renal artery. *Hypertension* 8:962, 1986.
623. Rieumont M, Kaufman J, Geller S, et al: Evaluation of renal artery stenosis with dynamic gadolinium-enhanced MR angiography. *Am J Roentgenol* 169:39, 1997.
624. Silverman J, Friedman M, Van Allan R: Detection of main renal artery stenosis using phase-contrast cine MR angiography. *Am J Radiol* 166:1131, 1995.
625. Siegelman B, Gilfeather M, Holland G, Carpenter J, Golden M, Townsend R, Schnall M: Breath-hold ultrafast three-dimensional gadolinium-enhanced MR angiography of the renovascular system. *Am J Radiol* 168:1035, 1997.
626. Leung D, Pelkonen P, Hany T, Zimmermann G, Pfammatter T, Debatin J: Value of image subtraction in 3D gadolinium-enhanced MR angiography of the renal arteries. *J Magn Reson Imaging* 8:598, 1998.
627. Kaplan N, Silah J: The angiotensin infusion test. *N Engl J Med* 271:536, 1994.
628. Vertes V, Grauel J, Goldblatt H: Renal arteriography, separate renal-function studies and renal biopsy in human hypertension. *N Engl J Med* 270:656, 1964.
629. Schaffer AJ, Stamey TA: Ureteral cathertization. *Studies Urologic Clin North Am* 2:327, 1975.
630. Blaufox M, Middleton M, Bongiovanni J, Davis B: Cost efficacy of the diagnosis and therapy of renovascular hypertension. *J Nucl Med* 37:171, 1996.
631. Wilcox C: Use of angiotensin-converting enzyme inhibitors for diagnosing renovascular hypertension. *Kidney Int* 44:1379, 1993.
632. Hunt JC, Stron CG: Renovascular hypertension mechanisms, natural history and treatment. *Am J Cardiol* 32:563, 1973.
633. Epstein M, Oster J: Beta blockers and renal function: A reappraisal. *J Clin Hypertens* 1:85, 1985.
634. Mimran A, Ribstein J, Ducailar G: Converting enzyme inhibitors and renal function in essential and renovascular hypertension. *Am J Hypertens* 4:7, 1991.
635. Imamura A, Mackenzie H, Lacy E, Hutchison F, Fitzgibbon W, Ploth D: Effects of chronic treatment with angiotensin converting enzyme inhibitor or an angiotensin receptor antagonist in two-kidney, one-clip hypertensive rats. *Kidney Int* 47:1394, 1995.
636. Textor S: Revascularization in atherosclerotic renal artery disease. *Kidney Int* 53:799, 1998.
637. Buhler F, Laragh J, Vaughan E, et al: Antihypertensive action of propranolol. Specific antirenin responses in high and normal renin forms of essential, renal, renovascular and malignant hypertension. *Am J Cardiol* 32:511, 1973.
638. Novick A: Current concepts in the management of renovascular hypertension and ischemic renal failure. *Am J Kidney Dis* 13:33, 1989.
639. Anderson C, Hansen K, Benjamin M, Keith D, Craven T, Dean R: Renal artery fibromuscular dysplasia: Results of current surgica therapy. *J Vasc Surg* 22:207, 1995.
640. Weatherford D, Freeman M, Regester R, Serrell P, SL S, MH G: Surgical management of flash pulmonary edema secondary to renovascular hypertension. *Am J Surg* 174:160, 1997.
641. Textor S: Revascularization in atherosclerotic renal artery disease. *Kidney Int* 53:799, 1998.
642. Cicuto K, McLean G, Oleaga J, et al: Renal artery stenosis: Anatomic classification for percutaneous transluminal angioplasty. *Am J Radiol* 137:599, 1981.
643. Plouin PF, Darne B, Chatellier G, et al: Restenosis after a first percutaneous transluminal renal angioplasty. *Hypertension* 21:89, 1993.
644. van de Ven P, Beutler J, Kaatee R, et al: Transluminal vascular stent for ostial atherosclerotic renal artery stenosis. *Lancet* 346:672, 1975.
645. Imamura H, Isobe M, Takenaka H, Kinoshita O, Sekiguchi M, Ohta M: Successful stenting of bilateral renal artery stenosis due to fibromuscular dysplasia assessed by use of pressure guidewire technique. *J Vasc Dis* 49:69, 1998.
646. Sharma S, Gupta H, Saxena A, Kothari S, Taneja K, Guieria S, Rajani M: Results of renal angioplasty in nonspecific aortoarteritis (Takayasu Disease). *JVIR* 9:429, 1988.
647. Merkus J, Huysmans F, Hoitsma A, et al: Treatment of renal allograft artery stenosis. *Transpl Int* 6:111, 1993.
648. Hayes J, Risius B, Novick A, et al: Experience with percutaneous transluminal angioplasty for renal artery stenosis at the Cleveland Clinic. *J Urol* 139:488, 1988.
649. Ring E, McLean G: *Interventional Radiology: Principles and Techniques*. Boston, Little Brown, 1981.
650. Rudnick M, Berns J, Cohen R, Goldfarb S: Nephrotoxic risks of renal angiography: Contrast-media associated nephrotoxicity and atheroembolism—A critical review. *Am J Kidney Dis* 24:713, 1994.
651. Harjai K, Khosla S, Shaw D, Collins T, Jenkins S, White C, Ramee: Effect of gender on outcomes following renal artery stent placement for renovascular hypertension. *Catheter Cardiovasc Diagnosis* 42:381, 1997.
652. Hansen K, Starr S, Sands R, et al: Contemporary surgical management of renovascular disease. *J Vasc Surg* 16:319, 1992.
653. Vogt P, Pairolero P, Hollier L, et al: The occluded renal artery: Durability of revascularization. *J Vasc Surg* 2:125, 1985.
654. Haab F, Duclos J, Guyenne T, et al: Renin secreting tumors: Diagnosis, conservative surgical approach and long-term results. *J Urol* 153:1781, 1995.
655. Young WF: Pheochromocytoma and primary aldosteronism: Diagnostic approaches. *Endocrinol Metabol Clin North Am* 26:801, 1997.
656. Ganguly A: Primary aldosteronism. *N Engl J Med* 339:1828, 1998.
657. Bravo EL: Primary aldosteronism: Issues in diagnosis and management. *Endocrinol Metab Clin North Am* 23:271, 1994.
658. Gordon RD: Mineralocorticoid hypertension. *Lancet* 344:240, 1994.
659. Valloton MB: P:rimary aldosteronism II. Differential diagnosis of hyperaldosteronism and pseudoaldosteronism. *Clin Endocrinol (Oxf)* 45:53, 1996.
660. Rácz K, Pinet F, Marton T, Szendi B, Gláz E, Corvol P: Expression of steroidogenic enzyme messenger ribonucleic acids and corticosteroid production in aldosterone-producing and "nonfunctioning" adrenal adenomas. *J Clin Endocrinol Metab* 77:677, 1993.
661. Irony I, Kater CE, Biglieri EG, Shackleton CHL: Correctable subsets of primary aldosteronism: Primary adrenal hyperplasia and renin responsive adenoma. *Am J Hypertens* 3:576, 1990.
662. Furge D, Chatellier G, Pagny JY, Jeunemaitre X, Plonin PF, Corvol P: Isolated clinical syndrome of primary aldosternism in four patients with adrenocortical carcinoma. *Am J Med* 83:635, 1987.
663. Gordon R, Klemm D, Tunney T: Primary aldosteronism with a genetic basis. *Lancet* 340:159, 1992.
664. Weinberger MH, Fineberg NS: The diagnosis of primary aldosteronism and separation of two major subtypes. *Arch Intern Med* 153:2125, 1993.
665. Kater CE, Biglieri EG, Brust N, Chang B, Herai J, Irony I: Stimulation and suppression of the mineralocorticoid hormones in normal

subjects and adrenocortical disorders. *Endocrinol Rev* 10:149, 1989.
666. Gross MD, Shapiro B: Scentigraphic studies in adrenal hypertension. *Semin Nucl Med* 19:122, 1989.
667. Edelman RR, Warach S: Magnetic resonance imaging. *N Engl J Med* 328:785, 1993.
668. Doppman JL, Gill JR, Miller DL, et al: Distinction between hyperaldosteronism due to bilateral hyperplasia and unilateral aldosteronoma. Reliability of CT. *Radiology* 184:677, 1992.
669. Radin DR, Manoogian C, Nadler JL: Diagnosis of primary hyperaldosteronism: Importance of correlating CT findings with endocrinologic studies. *Am J Radiol* 158:553, 1992.
670. Hattner RS: Practical considerations in the scintigraphic evaluation of endocrine hypertension. *Radiol Clin North Am* 31:1029, 1993.
671. Young WF, Stanson AW, Grant CS, Thompson GB, van Heerden JA: Primary aldosteronism: Adrenal venous sampling. *Surgery* 120:913, 1996.
672. Miller DL: Endocrine angiography and venous sampling. *Radiol Clin North Am* 31:1051, 1993.
673. Rossi GP, Sacchetto A, Pavan E, Palatini P, Graniero GR, Canali C. Remodeling of the left ventricle in primary aldosteronism due to Conn's adenoma. *Circulation* 95:1471, 1997.
674. Stowasser M, Bachmann AW, Jansson JR, Tunny TJ, Klemm SA, Gordon RD: Clinical, biochemical and genetic approaches to the detection of familial aldosteronism type 1. *J Hypertens* 13:1610, 1995.
675. Lifton RP, Dlughy RG, Powers M, et al: Hereditary hypertension caused by chimaeric gene duplications and ectopic expression of aldosterone synthase. *Nat Genet* 2:66, 1992.
676. Dlughy RG, Lifton RP. Glucocorticoid-remediable aldosteronism. *Endocrinol Metab North Am* 23:285, 1994.
677. Jamieson A, Slutsker L, Inglis GC, Fraser R, White PC, Connell JM: Glucocorticoid-suppressible hyperaldosteronism: Effects of crossover site and parental origin of chimaeric gene on phenotypic expression. *Clin Sci* 88:563, 1995.
678. Litchfield WR, Collidge C, Silva P, Lifton RP, Fallo F, Williams GH, Dluhy RG: Impaired potassium-stimulated aldosterone production: A possible explanation for normokalemic glucocorticoid-remediable aldosteronism. *J Clin Endocrinol Metab* 82:1507, 1997.
679. Rich GM, Wick S, Cook S, Wang J, Lifton RP, Dluhy RG: Glucocorticoid-remediable aldosteronism in a large kindred: Clinical spectrum and diagnosis using a characteristic biochemical phenotype. *Ann Intern Med* 116:813, 1992.
680. Kater CE, Biglieri EG: Disorders of steroid 17?-hydroxylase deficiency. *Endocrinol Metab Clin North Am* 23:341, 1994.
681. White PC: Inherited forms of mineralocorticoid hypertension. *Hypertension* 28:927, 1996.
682. Juresch S, Kornely E, Kley HK, Schlaghecke R: Adrenal incidentoloma and patients with congenital adrenal hyperplasia. *J Clin Endocrinol Metab* 74:685, 1992.
683. Helmberg A, Ausserer B, Kofler R: Frame shift by insertion of two base pairs in codon 394 of CYP11?1 causes congenital adrenal hyperplasia due to steroid 11?-hydroxylase deficiency. *J Clin Endocrinol Metab* 75:1278, 1992.
684. Burren CP, Montalto J, Young AB, Batch JA: CYP11beta1(11-beta-hydroxylase) deficiency in congenital adrenal hyperplasia. *J Pediatr Child Health* 32:433, 1996.
685. Saruta T, Suzuki H, Handa M, et al: Multiple factors contribute to the pathogenesis of hypertension in Cushing's syndrome. *J Clin Endocrinol Metab* 62:275, 1986.
686. Sugihara N, Shimizu M, Kita Y, et al: Cardiac characteristics and postoperative courses in Cushing's syndrome. *Am J Cardiol* 69:1475, 1992.
687. Fallo F, Budano S, Sonino N, Muiesan M, Agabiti-Roser E, Boscaro M: Left ventricular structural characteristics in Cushing's syndrome. *J Hum Hypertens* 8:509, 1994.
688. Imai Y, Abe K, Sasaki S, et al: Altered circadian blood pressure rhythm in patients with Cushing's syndrome. *Hypertension* 12:11, 1988.
689. Stiefel P, Gimenez J, Miranda ML, et al: Description of a new quotient that may differentiate blood pressure profiles in essential versus Cushing's syndrome-related hypertension. *J Endocrinol Invest* 18:789, 1995.
690. Montrella-Waybill M, Clore JN, Schoolwerth AC, Watlington CD: Evidence that high dose cortisol-induced Na^+ retention in man is not mediated by the mineralocorticoid receptor. *J Clin Endocrinol Metab* 72:1060, 1991.
691. Wick S, Wang JZ, Blumenfeld JD, Pickering TG: Cortisol inactivation overload; A mechanisms of mineralocorticoid hypertension in the ectopic adrenocorticotropin syndrome. *J Clin Endocrinol Metab* 75:1005, 1992.
692. Arriza JL, Weinberger C, Cerelli G: Cloning of human mineralocorticoid receptor complementary DNA: Structural and functional kinship with the glucocorticoid receptor. *Science* 237:268, 1987.
693. Ulick S, Tedde R, Wang JZ: Defective ring A reduction of cortisol as the major metabolic error in the syndrome of apparent mineralocorticoid excess. *J Clin Endocrinol Metab* 74:593, 1992.
694. Gomez-Sanchez EP, Gomez-Sanchez CE: Central hypertensinogenic effects of glycyrrhizic acid and carbenoxolone. *Am J Physiol* 263:E1125, 1992.
695. Gifford RW, Manger WM, Bravo EL: Pheochromocytoma. *Endocrinol Metab Clin North Am* 23:387, 1994.
696. Manger WM, Gifford RW: *Clinical and Experimental Pheochromocytoma*, 2nd edition. Cambridge, MA, Blackwell Science, 1998.
697. Morris DA, Sowers JR: Pheochromocytoma: An update, in Lavin N (ed): *Manual of Endocrinol and Metab* (2nd edition). Boston, MA Little Brown and Co., 13:131, 1994.
698. Faria G, Lumachi F, Polistina F, D'Amico DF: Pheochromocytoma, a rare cause of hypertension: Long-term follow-up of 55 surgically treated patients. *World J Surg* 22:689. 1998.
699. Atiyeh BA, Barakat AJ, Abumrad NN: Extra-adrenal pheochromocytoma 10:25, 1997.
700. Ein SH, Pullerits J, Creighton R, Balfe JW: Pediatric pheochromocytoma. A 36-year review. *Pediatric Surg Int* 12:595, 1997.
701. Tato A, Orto L, Diz P, Quereda C, Ortuno J, Malignant pheochromocytoma, still a therapeutic challenge. *Am J Hypertens* 10:479, 1997.
702. Atuk NO, Stole C, Owen JA, Carpenter JL, Vance ML: Pheochromocytoma in von Hippel-Lindau disease: Clinical presentation and mutation analysis in a large, multigenerational kindred. *J Clin Endocrinol Metab* 83:117, 1998.
703. Miller JA, Norton JA. Multiple endocrine neoplasis. *Cancer Treat Res* 90:213, 1997.
704. Woodward ER, Eng C, McMahon R, et al: Genetic predisposition to phaeochromocytoma: Analysis of candidate genes GDNF, RET and UHL. *Hum Mol Genet* 6:1051, 1997.
705. Garacia A, Matias-Guiu X, Cabezas R, et al: Molecular diagnosis of von Hippel-Lindau disease in a kindred with a predominance of familial phaeochromocytoma. *Clin Endocrinol* 46:359, 1997.
706. Rodien P, Jeunemaitre X, Dumont C, Beldjord C, Plonin PF: Genetic alterations of the RET proto-oncogene in familial and sporadic pheochromocytomas. *Horm Res* 47:263, 1997.
707. Bar M, Friedman E, Jakobovitz O, et al: Sporadic phaeochromocytomas are rarely associated with germline mutations in von Hippel-Lindau and RET genes. *Clin Endocrinol* 47:707, 1997.
708. Kimura N, Miura W, Noshire T, et al: Plasma chromogranin A in pheochromocytoma, primary hyperparathyrodism and pituitary adenoma in comparison with cytocholamine, parathyroid hormone and pituitary hormones. *Endocrin J* 44:319, 1997.
709. Liu J, Kahri AI, Heikkila P, Vontilainen R: Adrenomedullin gene expression and its different regulation in human adrenocortical and medullary tumors. *J Endocrinol* 155:483, 1997.
710. Eisenhofer G, Keiser H, Fribert P, et al: Plasma metanephrines are markers of pheochromocytoma produced by catechol-o-methyltransferase within tumors. *J Clin Endocrinol Metab* 83:2175, 1998.
711. Ito Y, Ohara T, Okamoto T, et al: Efficacy of single-voided urine metanephrine and normitaniphrine assay for diagnosing pheochromocytoma. *World J Surg* 22:684, 1998.
712. Stridsberg M, Husibye ES: Chromogranin A and chromogranin B are sensitive circulating markers for pheochromocytoma. *Eur J Endocrinol* 136:67, 1997.
713. Case Records of the Massachusetts General Hospital. Case 16-1991. Presentation of Case. *N Engl J Med* 324:1119, 1991.
714. Jalil ND, Patton FN, Combemale F, et al: Effectiveness and limits of preoperative imaging studies for the localization of pheochromocytomas and paragangliomas. A review of 282 cases. *Eur J Surgery* 164:23, 1998.
715. Hanson MW, Feldman JM, Beam CA, Leight CS, Coleman E: Iodine 131-labelled metaiodobenylguanidine scintigraphy and

biochemical analysis in suspected pheochromocytoma. *Arch Intern Med* 151:1397, 1991.

716. Russel WJ, Metcalfe IR, Tonkin AL, Frewin DB: The preoperative management of pheochromocytoma. *Anaesth Intensive Care* 26:196, 1998.
717. Walz MK, Peitgen K, Saller B, et al: Subtotal adrenolectomy by the posterior retroperitoneoscopic approach. *World J Surg* 22:621, 1998.
718. Gagner M, Breton G, Pharand D, Pomp A: Is laparscopic adrenalectomy indicated for pheochromocytomas? *Surgery* 120:1076, 1996.
719. Gagner M, Pomp A, Henifort BT, Pharand D, Lacroix A: Laparoscopic adrenalectomy: Lesions learned from 100 consecutive procedures. *Ann Surg* 226:337, 1997.
720. Patton FN, Combemale FP, Poirette JF, et al: Questionability of the benefits of routine laparatomy as the surgical approach for pheochromocytomas and abdominal paragangliomas. *Surgery* 20:1006, 1996.
721. Loh KC, Fitzgerald PA, Matthay KK, Yeo PP, Price DC: The treatment of malignant pheochromocytoma with iodine-131 meta-iodobenzyl-guanidine (131I-M1BG): A comprehensive review of 116 reported patients. *J Endocrinol Invest* 20:648, 1997.
722. Troncone L, Rafini V: 131I-M1BG therapy of neural chest tumors (review). *Anticancer Res* 17:1823, 1997.
723. Steinsapir J, Carr AA, Prisant LM, Bransome ED: Metyrosine and pheochromocytoma. *Arch Intern Med* 157:901, 1997.

CHAPTER 14

Glucocorticoid Therapy

George P. Chrousos

Glucocorticoids are among the most commonly used drugs. They are employed to treat many medical problems, varying from self-limited processes such as poison ivy, poison oak, and other hypersensitivity reactions, to life-threatening problems such as leukemia. A partial list of these conditions is shown in Table 14-1.[1] Christy estimated in 1971[2] that 5 million persons in the United States receive some form of steroids (Fig. 14-1) annually in therapy. The overall use has, if anything, increased with the expanding population. Because of such extensive use and the numerous conditions for which steroids are given, glucocorticoid-treated patients are encountered in all medical and surgical specialties.

Although glucocorticoids have many beneficial influences, their use is frequently accompanied by deleterious side effects. Physicians must be aware of these effects and must exercise judgment in the decision to use steroids in the first place. It is also important to be aware of methods for reducing the total dosage by manipulating the timing and route of administration while maximizing adjunctive measures. This allows maximum therapeutic benefit while minimizing adverse effects. Many of the sequelae of long-term glucocorticoid therapy are similar to those of the diseases for which steroids are given (weakness, bruising, etc.). Thus, clinicians must also know the features that can be helpful in differentiating the cause of such disturbances in glucocorticoid-treated patients.

Many endocrinologists encounter steroid-treated patients less commonly than do other specialists (e.g., nephrologists, rheumatologists, dermatologists), yet the endocrinologist commonly is asked to evaluate whether clinical stigmata are due to the steroid or to another process and to give advice on therapy or its withdrawal. An endocrinologist is also asked to evaluate the hypothalamic-pituitary-adrenal axis, which may be suppressed in glucocorticoid-treated patients, and to give advice on patient management in such situations.

Over the past 30 years, much has been learned about the pharmacokinetics of glucocorticoids and the mechanisms by which these steroids elicit their diverse effects (Chap. 11). This knowledge, although incomplete, is helping physician's formulate more rational approaches to steroid therapy. This may increase the scope of steroid use in therapy and diminish the deleterious effects.

In this chapter, the pharmacology of the glucocorticoids is reviewed with the hope of providing a rational basis for the use of these steroids in therapy. For the most part, specific clinical indications for glucocorticoid administration are avoided, as they require discussions of the particular diseases that are found in the literature about them.

PHYSIOLOGIC AND PHARMACOLOGIC ACTIONS OF GLUCOCORTICOIDS IN RELATION TO STEROID THERAPY

Therapeutic Influences

The diverse actions of the glucocorticoids and the manifestations of excessive concentrations are detailed in Chap. 11. Several different types of these actions are exploited in glucocorticoid therapy.

In most circumstances, the anti-inflammatory and/or immunosuppressive actions of the glucocorticoids are responsible for the therapeutic response. As detailed in Chap. 11, glucocorticoids can affect nearly every component involved in the inflammatory and immunologic response, although in humans some components are more sensitive than others (e.g., cell mediated more than humoral responses) (for a review, see Refs. 3 and 4). It is less clear which particular responses account for the beneficial therapeutic influences. For instance, the anti-inflammatory actions are clearly important when steroids are given topically for inflammatory conditions. Thus, certain skin diseases benefit from glucocorticoid therapy because the inflammatory response to the offending agent is excessive. In other cases (e.g., lupus erythematosus, other collagen vascular disorders, transplant rejection, and the nephrotic syndrome), it is not clear whether immunosuppressive or anti-inflammatory actions are more important. In general, glucocorticoid therapy for conditions of excessive inflammatory and/or immunologic activity does not cure the primary condition but instead ameliorates its manifestations. Sometimes this "buys time" for the body's natural defenses to cure the problem or for more definitive therapy to work.

When steroids are used to treat certain lymphoid cell malignancies, they act by killing or inhibiting the functions of lymphoid cells that mediate the response.[5,6] The different subpopulations of lymphoid cells vary markedly in their sensitivity to glucocorticoids (Chap. 11), and in humans under normal conditions (in contrast to certain animal species), glucocorticoids exhibit minimal lymphoid cell killing.[6] Thus, many leukemias are steroid-resistant. Acute lymphoblastic leukemia of childhood is the most commonly occurring steroid-sensitive leukemia, yet even this disease has a tendency to become steroid-resistant (see later discussion).[5,6]

Whereas most malignancies are steroid-resistant, one occasionally observes patients with ordinarily steroid-resistant malignancies who respond to glucocorticoids. For instance, in a study of the preleukemic syndrome (hemopoietic dysplasia), 3 of 34 patients responded favorably to glucocorticoids.[7]

TABLE 14-1. Selected Clinical Conditions for Which Glucocorticoids Are Used

Addison's disease: replacement therapy	Choroiditis
Adrenal hyperplasia due to enzymatic defects (e.g., 11β-, 17α-, and 21-hydroxylase syndromes)	Optic neuritis
Allergic diseases	Gastrointestinal diseases
Angioneurotic edema	Inflammatory bowel disease
Bee stings	Nontropical sprue
Contact dermatitis	Regional enteritis
Drug reactions	Subacute hepatic necrosis
Hay fever	Ulcerative colitis
Serum sickness	Hypercalcemia (e.g., due to sarcoidosis; most hypercalcemias not responsive)
Urticaria	Infections (occasionally helpful to suppress excessive inflammation)
Arthritis, bursitis, and tenosynovitis; inflammatory complications of a variety of types of arthritis	Malignant exophthalmos
Blood dyscrasias	Malignant hyperthermia
Acquired hemolytic anemia	Neurologic diseases
Allergic purpura	Pulmonary diseases
Autoimmune hemolytic anemia	Aspiration pneumonia
Idiopathic thrombocytopenic purpura	Bronchial asthma
Lymphoblastic leukemia	Infant and adult respiratory distress syndrome
Multiple myeloma	Sarcoidosis
Collagen vascular disorders	Renal diseases: certain nephrotic syndromes
Giant cell arteritis	Skin conditions
Lupus erythematosus	Atopic dermatitis
Mixed connective tissue syndromes	Dermatoses
Polymyositis	Lichen simplex chronicus (localized neurodermatitis)
Polymyalgia rheumatica	Mycosis fungoides
Rheumatoid arthritis	Pemphigus
Temporal arteritis	Seborrheic dermatitis
Eye diseases	Xerosis
Acute uveitis	Transplantation: prevent of rejection
Allergic conjunctivitis	

*This table is not meant to be comprehensive, nor are steroids always indicated for the condition listed.

Source: Baxter and Rousseau.[1]

The actions of glucocorticoids on cell growth may also explain how these steroids inhibit solid tumors such as juvenile hemangiomas.[8]

In certain circumstances, glucocorticoid therapy is used not to affect the primary process but to ameliorate associated problems. For example, steroids are used to treat the hemolytic anemia that occurs in association with chronic granulocytic leukemia in adults[9] and to treat the hypercalcemia associated with malignancy (Chaps. 11 and 22).

Glucocorticoids are commonly used to treat patients with severe or moderately severe asthma (Fig. 14-2)[10–14] and some patients with chronic obstructive pulmonary disease.[15,16] Pulmonary function in asthma can improve after steroid administration, although several hours must pass for this to occur.[10,17] The improvement is due to one or a combination of several effects. First, the steroid may directly promote bronchodilation by sensitizing the bronchioles to gb-adrenergic agonists (Chap. 11).[10,18] Second, glucocorticoids may also inhibit the production of bronchoconstrictor substances, such as leukotrienes, other eicosanoids (Chap. 11), and histamine,[11] generated by immunologic mechanisms. The suppression of phospholipase A_2 and cyclooxygenare II activity by glucocorticoids may be of critical importance in this respect (Chap. 11). Third, the steroid may suppress inflammatory responses in the lung and thus improve pulmonary function.[12]

There are several examples of steroid actions not strictly directed at inflammatory or immunologic responses. For instance, in sarcoidosis, the steroid ameliorates the hypercalcemia by inhibiting the conversion of 25-hydroxycholecalciferol to 1α,25-dihydroxycholecalciferol in the granuloma (Chap. 22).[19] Glucocorticoids are used to decrease brain edema in some patients with brain tumors, meningitis, and other conditions[20–22] and are also beneficial in conditions such as acute mountain sickness (which is believed to be due to cerebral edema presumably unassociated with inflammation).[23] The effectiveness of glucocorticoids in reducing damage resulting from spinal cord injury is probably not mediated by suppression of inflammation. The antiemetic actions of the steroids are sometimes useful in cancer chemotherapy.[24]

Adverse Influences

Glucocorticoids have some acute adverse influences, including insomnia, which is common, and acute psychosis or acute pancreatitis, which are rare.[25] It is their common chronic adverse influences of glucocorticoids that lead to Cushing's syndrome

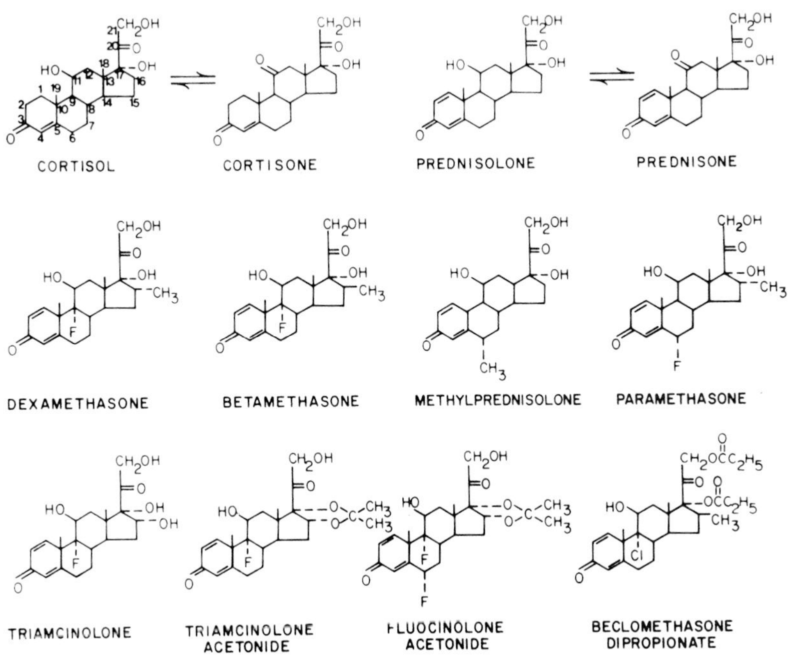

FIGURE 14-1. Structures of some steroids commonly used for glucocorticoid therapy. The numbers of the carbon atoms are shown for cortisol (upper left). Arrows indicate the interconvertibility of cortisol and cortisone and of prednisolone and prednisone. Dotted lines indicate side groups in the ga position; solid lines indicate steroids in the gb position (see also Chap. 11).

manifestations and limit their usefulness in therapy. These problems are discussed in Chap. 11 and below. The actions on immune and inflammatory responses play a major role in generating morbidity and mortality because they increase the incidence and severity of infections.[26–29] The actions on carbohydrate metabolism, fibroblasts, bone, and other tissues also produce the prominent manifestations of iatrogenic Cushing's syndrome which are responsible for significant cardiovascular morbidity and mortality.

FIGURE 14-2. Effect of hydrocortisone hemisuccinate (4 mg per kilogram of body weight, followed in some cases by 3 mg per kilogram of body weight at 3-h intervals and in other cases by a continuous intravenous infusion at 3 mg per kilogram of body weight every 6 h and of cosyntropin depot (1 mg IM) on pulmonary function (FEV_1 and FVC) in acute asthma. (*From Collins et al.*[10])

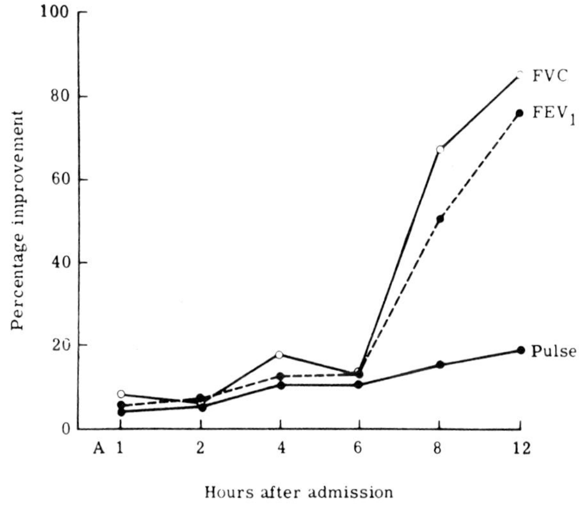

MOLECULAR MECHANISMS FOR GLUCOCORTICOID-MEDIATED THERAPEUTIC INFLUENCES

Most physiologic and pharmacologic actions of glucocorticoids are mediated through intracellular receptors, termed "glucocorticoid receptors," that bind the steroid, associate with the nucleus, and then affect transcription of specific genes (for a review see Refs. 3, 31, 12 and Chaps. 4 and 11). The relative potency of steroids in eliciting therapeutic responses correlates with receptor-binding activities. The receptors are widely distributed and are generally present in the relevant target tissues thought to be involved in both therapeutic and deleterious glucocorticoid responses. Further, with lymphoblastic leukemia cells, as discussed previously and in Chap. 11, loss of the glucocorticoid receptor is associated with unresponsiveness to glucocorticoids.[5] The existence of similar receptors in many different tissues explains how glucocorticoids can influence all these tissues.[30–32] The responses differ in the various tissues (e.g., killing in lymphoid cells and glucoconeogenesis in liver) because of postreceptor cellular differentiation (Chap. 11).

As discussed in Chaps. 4, 11, and 13, some glucocorticoid actions are mediated through "mineralocorticoid receptors." These receptors are present in several different tissues in addition to the kidneys, and they regulate transcription in a manner analogous to the glucocorticoid receptors (Chaps. 4 and 11). Mineralocorticoid receptors regulate renal sodium and potassium transport, mostly in response to aldosterone. Cortisol and other steroids with glucocorticoid activity bind tightly to the mineralocorticoid receptors (Table 14-2). However, in the kidney, many of these steroids are prevented from acting through mineralocorticoid receptors due to local reduction of the 11βDH group to a ketone by the enzyme 11-ketosteroid reductase Type II.

The sodium-retaining actions of various steroids mediated through mineralocorticoid receptors affect the selection of the steroid to be used in therapy. This selection is dictated by both the

TABLE 14-2. Affinities of Some Steroids for Human Glucocorticoid Receptors and Relative Mineralocorticoid/Glucocorticoid Receptor Affinities

Steroid	Affinity for Glucocorticoid Receptor*	Mineralocorticoid/ Glucocorticoid Receptor Affinity Ratio*
Cortisol	1.0	1.0
Fludrocortisone	3.5	11.6
Triamcinolone acetonide	1.9	
Prednisolone	2.1	0.9
Betamethasone	5.4	0.8
Dexamethasone	7.1	0.2
Fluocinolone acetonide	11.4	

*Relative to cortisol.

Source: Data for human receptor binding from Ballard PL, Carter JP, Graham BS, Baxter JD: A radioreceptor assay for evaluation of the plasma glucocorticoid activity of natural and synthetic steroids in man. *J Clin Endocrinol Metab* 41:290, 1975. Data for the ratio of affinities using rat mineralocorticoid receptors and human glucocorticoid receptors for unpublished data of Lan NC, Matulich DT, and Baxter JD.

affinities of these steroids for the mineralocorticoid receptor (Table 14-2) and the stability of the steroids to metabolic changes or degradation. The overall weaker mineralocorticoid activities of steroids such as prednisone, prednisolone, dexamethasone, and betamethasone (Chap. 11) constitute one reason why these steroids are ordinarily used in preference to cortisol.

Glucocorticoid responses usually require hours to days to be observed. These kinetics are consistent with a requirement for influences on macromolecular synthesis mediated through nuclear receptors.[30]

KINETIC CONSIDERATIONS

The actions of glucocorticoids through their specific receptors and the subsequent modulation of DNA transcription require some time before a response is observed (Chap. 11). Similarly, in terminating the response, some time is required for the steroid to leave the circulation. When this occurs, dissociation of the steroid from the receptor occurs within a few minutes,[30] resulting in the termination of further steroid action. However, some time is required for the levels of the induced mRNAs and their protein products to return to baseline before the response is terminated.[33] Further, the response may be even more prolonged because the steroid might have induced other factors that affect transcription; thus, a stimulation of transcription may occur for some time after removal of the steroid because of the period required for the concentrations of these factors to decrease to basal levels. The time required for induced mRNAs and proteins to return to basal levels depends on their rates of turnover.[33] These rates vary for different mRNAs. The rates of protein and mRNA turnover also affect the kinetics of induction (for a discussion, see Ref. 33 and Chap. 11); for steroid-regulated mRNAs and proteins that turn over with a long half-life, a longer time is required for the response to reach a maximum (and to terminate) than is the case with the more rapidly turning over macromolecules. Thus, there may be considerable variation in the time required for the onset and disappearance of various glucocorticoid responses; these variations form the basis for alternate-day steroid therapy (discussed later) and emphasize that the kinetics of each response must be determined independently in order to develop the most rational approach to glucocorticoid therapy.

MANIFESTATIONS OF IATROGENIC CUSHING'S SYNDROME

Comparisons with Spontaneous Cushing's Syndrome

The clinical features of iatrogenic Cushing's syndrome are similar to those of spontaneous Cushing's syndrome with several exceptions (Chap. 11). In fact, since many patients receive very high doses over prolonged periods, the symptoms and signs are commonly more prominent than is the case with spontaneous Cushing's syndrome. Thus, there can be weight gain with redistribution of fat to the truncal areas, "moon face," plethora, "buffalo hump," thin skin, easy bruising, osteoporosis, avascular necrosis, striae, poor wound healing, increased incidence of infections, psychiatric problems, myopathy and muscular weakness, decreased carbohydrate tolerance, negative nitrogen balance, renal calculi, and other stigmata. An extensive analysis of these and other factors and of the pathophysiology is provided in Chap. 11.

The major differences between iatrogenic and spontaneous Cushing's syndrome (unless ACTH therapy is used) relate to the presence of androgens and mineralocorticoids. Because adrenal androgen excess is not present in the iatrogenic syndrome, the hirsutism and other virilizing features are not observed. However, glucocorticoid-treated individuals develop an increase in fine lanugo hair and a noncystic form of pustular acne (steroid-induced acne) on the face and elsewhere.[34] Steroids with less mineralocorticoid potency (relative to their glucocorticoid potency) than cortisol are ordinarily used for steroid therapy (Table 14-2). Further, steroids with mineralocorticoid potency, such as 11-deoxycorticosterone (DOC), are sometimes present in excess in spontaneous Cushing's syndrome (Chaps. 11 and 13). Thus, the features of mineralocorticoid excess—hypertension and hypokalemia (Chap. 13)—are much less common in the iatrogenic syndrome. However, in iatrogenic Cushing's syndrome there is an increased frequency of hypertension (Chaps. 11 and 13), and fluid retention can be exaggerated in patients with congestive heart failure (Chap. 11).

Whereas steroid-treated patients can become euphoric or depressed, it appears that euphoria is more common in iatrogenic than in spontaneous Cushing's syndrome. In some individuals, this may be due to improvement in the disease for which steroids were given; however, others develop euphoria without any detectable beneficial effect on the primary disease.[2,21,35]

It has been reported that several other features are unique to iatrogenic Cushing's syndrome.[2,36] Some of these features are uncommon; they include benign intracranial hypertension, pancreatitis, cataracts, and vasculitis. Although it has been reported that an increased incidence of glaucoma and avascular necrosis of bone (discussed later) is unique to the iatrogenic syndrome,[2,37] glaucoma has been reported[38] and some authors have observed avascular necrosis of bone in the spontaneous syndrome. Whereas this deposition of fat in various body areas in Cushing's syndrome is well known, excessive deposition of fat around the spinal cord causing motor neuron symptoms has been reported rarely in iatrogenic Cushing's syndrome.[39,40]

Ocular Changes

Serous choroidopathy is a relatively common complication of glucocorticoids.[41]

Posterior subcapsular cataracts occur commonly in both pediatric and adult steroid-treated individuals, especially with prolonged treatment.[42–46] As discussed in Chap. 11, there is some evidence that steroid-induced cataract may be a result of the formation of covalent complexes between the steroids and lens proteins.[43,47]

Steroid-induced increases in intraocular pressure with subsequent development of glaucoma occur in a subset of patients who are susceptible to this action.[42,43] There are a significant number of these individuals,[42] and all glucocorticoid-treated patients should be monitored for changes in intraocular pressure.

Avascular Necrosis of Bone

Avascular or ischemic necrosis of bone has been reported in up to 50 percent of patients in some series and is apparently related more to the dose than to the duration of therapy.[48,49] It is also more prevalent in patients with vasculitis and Raynaud's phenomenon, although it also occurs frequently with steroid therapy in other conditions, such as in transplant recipients.[48–50] It has been proposed that this complication is due to steroid-induced enlargement of intramedullary lipocytes, with resulting pressure on the bone leading to ischemia.[48–50]

Osteoporosis

Osteoporosis is one of the major limitations of long-term glucocorticoid therapy (see also Chap. 23).[2,51,52] The precise prevalence is difficult to determine, but most patients on chronic therapy develop decreased bone density when studied by sophisticated methods.[53,54] In a study of patients with rheumatoid arthritis who were given prednisone in a mean daily dose of 7.5 mg/day for 20 weeks, bone density of the lumbar spine decreased by 8 percent, a rate that was partially reversible after discontinuation of the steroid.[53] In another study, about two-thirds of patients receiving chronic glucocorticoid therapy were classified as having osteoporosis.[54] In addition, many of these patients develop fractures. In a study of asthmatic patients who received systemic steroids for at least a year, 11 percent developed fractures, compared with none of the control patients; in a prospective study, 8 of 19 patients and none of 11 control patients had fractures.[55] The long-term steroid-treated patients also had decreased trabecular but not cortical bone density, as measured by photon absorptiometry (Fig. 14-3).[55] Further, alternate-day steroid therapy (see later discussion) did not protect them against osteoporosis.[56]

The pattern of bone loss due to glucocorticoids is similar to that seen with primary hyperparathyroidism but differs from that observed in idiopathic osteoporosis (Fig. 14-4) (see also Chap. 23). The osteoporosis is most prominent in trabecular bone, with less dramatic changes in cortical bone, which turns over more slowly.[52–56] Thus, the most pronounced bone loss occurs in the axial skeleton, such as the ribs and vertebrae, rather than in the long bones. Steroid-induced bone loss is more profound in patients with previously reduced bone mineral, such as postmenopausal or oophorectomized women; alcoholics in whom endogenous hypercortisolism may already be contributing to bone loss[57]; patients with bowel disease and decreased calcium absorption; and those with liver or renal disease and impaired vitamin D metabolism (Chap. 23). Children are also susceptible to steroid-induced osteoporosis, presumably because of their lower bone mass and higher initial bone turnover.[51,58] The mechanisms of corticosteroid-induced bone loss are discussed in Chap. 11.

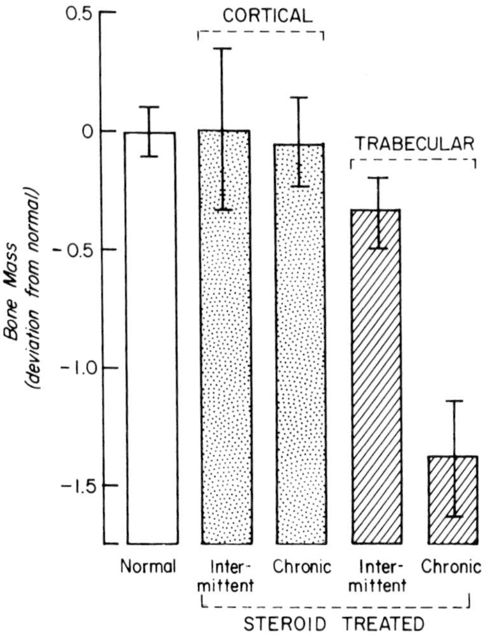

FIGURE 14-3. Trabecular and cortical bone mass in control and glucocorticoid-treated asthmatic patients. Bone mass was measured by single-photon absorption and was calculated by dividing the bone mineral content by bone width. Trabecular mass was taken from a metaphyseal site 2 cm proximal to the distal end of the ulnar styloid process, which contains a large proportion of trabecular bone. Cortical mass was taken from a diaphyseal site one-third the distance from the distal to the proximal end of the ulna, which is composed primarily of cortical bone. The bone mass is expressed as a fraction of the standard deviation of the mean of the normal value for the patient's sex and decade of age (z score). "Intermittent" refers to patients who had received intermittent courses of steroids but who did not require constant treatment for as long as a year. "Chronic" refers to patients who received daily or alternate-day corticosteroids for 1 year or more or at least eight short courses for 10 days or less of high-dose steroids for as long as a year. (*Data taken from Adinoff and Hollister.*[55])

Prevention and treatment of glucocorticoid-induced osteoporosis have been unsatisfactory and controversial.[59–62] However, several promising studies have been reported and hold promise for future long-term regimens. Bone density studies should be performed before the initiation of glucocorticoid therapy if long-term or high-dose treatment is being contemplated or if the patient has other risk factors for osteoporosis. In addition, every effort should be directed toward minimizing the dose and the duration of therapy, and if possible, compartmentalized topical or inhaled corticosteroid should be used in conjunction with other ancillary therapies.

Dietary calcium intake should be supplemented to a total intake of 1,200 to 1,500 mg of elemental calcium per day, and vitamin D should be given in a minimum dose of 400 U/day. Appropriate replacement therapy for decreased gonadal function also retards bone loss, and serial assessment of gonadal function should be undertaken as glucocorticoids in excess suppress gonadotropin secretion and gonadal function (Chap. 11).

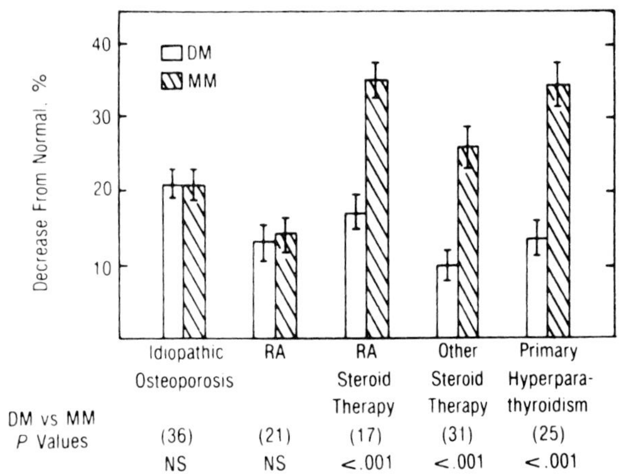

FIGURE 14-4. Decrease in bone mass (percent decrease from normal) estimated by photon absorption measurements of bone mass in the midshaft diaphyseal site (DM) and the distal metaphyseal site (MM) in patients with idiopathic osteoporosis, rheumatoid arthritis (RA) that was not treated or was treated with glucocorticoids, and primary hyperparathyroidism. Vertical bars indicate mean percent decrease from normal for age and sex (SEM). Number of patients studied is indicated in parentheses. (*From Hahn.*[58])

Treatment with pharmacologic doses of vitamin D and its active metabolites can restore intestinal calcium absorption and suppress the secondary hyperparathyroidism. The doses used have been ergocalciferol 50,000 U three times weekly,[63] calcifidiol (25-hydroxyvitamin D) 40 gmg/day,[62,63] and calcitriol (1,25-dihydroxyvitamin D) 0.5 to 1.0 gmg/day.[64] The risks of this therapy include hypercalcemia (especially with calcitriol) and hypercalcuria, which can occur with all forms of vitamin D and is correctable with thiazide diuretics.[56,62–64]

In addition, antiresorptive agents such as biphosphonates may be useful.[65] The bisphosphonates etidronate, pamidronate, and alendronate have been reported to prevent bone loss in steroid-treated patients.[65–67]

Finally, fluoride salts have been used to increase bone formation in glucocorticoid-treated patients.[62,68] However, long-term efficacy has not been established.

In summary, promising data are emerging which suggest that glucocorticoid-induced osteoporosis may be prevented and/or reversed, at least in part. However, longer-term controlled studies will be required to determine appropriate treatment regimens.

Infections

Infections are a major problem with long-term glucocorticoid therapy (Chap. 11).[2,27–29,69–71] Several types of infections can occur (Chap. 11), including bacterial, viral, fungal, and parasitic; gram-negative and fungal infections appear to be particularly prevalent.[2,27–29,70] Except in specific situations (e.g., reactivation of quiescent tuberculosis, abscesses, osteomyelitis), it is not possible to predict the organism that will cause a complicating infection,[27] and opportunistic organisms can be responsible.[70] Hepatitis B virus poses a special concern because steroids are used to treat chronic active hepatitis[72] but can be harmful when this form of hepatitis is associated with hepatitis B surface antigen positivity.[73,74] Because glucocorticoids decrease the inflammatory response, it may be particularly difficult to detect and diagnose infections in glucocorticoid-treated individuals. The incidence, severity, and frequency of serious infections increase with both the dose and duration of steroid therapy.[71,75] Infectious complications may be decreased when alternate-day steroid therapy is used.[75] The mechanisms of glucocorticoid-mediated decreased host defense against infection are discussed in Chap. 11.

The probable increase in the incidence and severity of tuberculosis in steroid-treated patients with systemic disease has been of particular concern.[27,76] Diagnosis may be difficult in the presence of the systemic disease for which the steroid is administered, and in addition, the tuberculin response may be suppressed by glucocorticoids. However, reactivation of tuberculosis does not appear to occur with increased frequency in patients on long-term steroid therapy.[76] Thus, patients receiving glucocorticoids who were tuberculin-positive prior to initiation of steroid therapy do not require antituberculosis therapy unless active disease is present.

Myopathy

Myopathy is a common manifestation of prolonged steroid therapy (Chap. 11).[2,36,77] The onset is usually gradual and often requires weeks or months to develop. It first affects the proximal muscles, although distal muscles can also be involved and muscle atrophy may be profound with prolonged high-dose therapy. Levels of serum enzymes [glutamic oxaloacetic transaminase (SGOT), creatine phosphokinase, and aldolase] are normal in glucocorticoid-induced myopathy, although they may be elevated in myopathy resulting from hypokalemia, polymyositis, or other causes.[77] However, creatine excretion is increased with glucocorticoid-induced and other myopathies, and its measurement can be useful. Muscle biopsy has not been shown to be helpful. Changes in muscle may also be monitored with the use of CT and isokinetic dynamic testing.[78] A study has suggested that glucocorticoid-induced muscle wasting can be reversed by physical training.[78] Thus, steroid-treated patients should exercise when possible.

Atherosclerosis

Although atherosclerosis has not traditionally been considered a complication of glucocorticoid therapy, a body of retrospectively obtained data suggests that atherosclerosis is more prevalent in glucocortisol-treated individuals,[79] and prednisone therapy was an independent risk factor for coronary artery disease.[80] In addition, patients with spontaneous Cushing's syndrome have an increased mortality from atherosclerotic disease.[81,82] These atherogenic effects are probably secondary effects of glucocorticoids-induced obesity, insulin resistance, dyslipidemia, and/or hypertension (metabolic syndrome X).[83,84] Thus, the potential for increasing the rate of progression of atherosclerosis should be considered in the overall decision to administer glucocorticoids on a long-term basis.

Dose and Time Dependency and Reversibility

The manifestations of iatrogenic Cushing's syndrome are generally dose- and time-dependent, although the time required to develop particular features varies considerably. Further, some complications also occur less frequently with alternate-day therapy (see later discussion). Increased appetite, euphoria, and insomnia can be observed within hours, whereas days to weeks are ordinarily required for the development of a cushingoid appearance. Effects on carbohydrate metabolism can occur within hours, although they become more pronounced with time (Chap. 11). The time required to develop an increased susceptibility to infections is not known, although it is likely that this happens within hours, as influences on leukocytes and other factors involved in inflammatory and immunologic responses occur by this time (Chap. 11). The development of frank osteoporosis[58–61,85] usually occurs after weeks or months of therapy. Occasional patients have experienced the onset of muscular weakness after a few days.[77] Psychiatric problems may develop soon after the institution of therapy or may develop later.[2,22,86–88] Other, rarer stigmata caused by glucocorticoid excess usually develop after weeks of therapy, although their appearance is unpredictable.

Most of the manifestations of glucocorticoid excess are reversible. Thus, within weeks to several months after the discontinuation of therapy, body weight can return to normal, the skin changes and cushingoid appearance disappear, and muscular strength returns. However, although most subjects regain muscle mass and lose visceral fat they do not return to the pretreatment levels. The immunosuppressive and metabolic effects (e.g., on carbohydrate tolerance) return to normal within hours to days after the discontinuation of therapy. Unfortunately, the osteoporosis is not fully reversible with current therapy, even though further steroid-mediated bone destruction ceases.

DIAGNOSIS OF IATROGENIC CUSHING'S SYNDROME

The diagnosis of iatrogenic Cushing's syndrome is usually obvious from the clinical manifestations, the history of steroid therapy, and the finding of suppression of the hypothalamic-pituitary-adrenal axis (see later discussion and Chap. 11). Thus, morning plasma cortisol and ACTH levels are low, and the rapid ACTH stimulation test result is subnormal.

DETERMINANTS OF GLUCOCORTICOID POTENCY

The potency of a steroid depends on its absorption ("bioavailability"), distribution, rate of metabolic clearance, concentration at sites of action, affinity for the glucocorticoid receptors, and ability to act as an agonist once it is bound (Chap. 11). It is important to consider each of these factors in using steroids for therapy.

Bioavailability

Most glucocorticoids are readily absorbed after oral administration. The estimates of fractional cortisol absorption expressed as bioavailability range from 0.45 to 0.8 (45 to 80 percent).[89] The absolute bioavailability of prednisolone from all forms of oral prednisone ranges from 77 to 99 percent.[89] Although glucocorticoid uptake is not impaired in most patients with intrinsic intestinal disease,[89] this can occur rarely, usually in association with severe disease.[90] Food intake does not have an appreciable effect on uptake.[89] Uptake is generally not impaired in renal or pulmonary disease.[89] Rare patients have decreased absorption of oral glucocorticoids in the absence of obvious bowel disease.

In the case of intramuscular (IM) injections, the uptake of steroids can vary markedly, depending on the preparation. For instance, triamcinolone acetonide is absorbed very slowly by the intramuscular route, and so the effect of a single injection may last for several weeks (see also Intrarticular Preparations, later).[91] Intramuscular injections of cortisone acetate do not reproducibly yield adequate blood levels of cortisol in the first 4 to 6 h after injection (Chap. 11),[92,93] although ultimately the steroid is absorbed. However, when more soluble derivatives of cortisol (e.g., hydrocortisone hemisuccinate) are injected IM, maximal cortisol levels are attained within an hour.[92,93] Thus, a physician must be aware of the properties of each preparation when the IM route is anticipated.

Inhaled glucocorticoids are highly effective in the treatment of asthma. Current preparations include beclomethasone dipropionate, triamcinolone acetonide, budesonide, and flunisolide. Their efficacy and systemic side effects vary with the method of administration and the dosage form.[12] Current types of inhaled steroid administration include metered-dose inhalers, large-volume spacer attachments, dry powder inhalers, and nebulizers. For current use, a metered-dose inhaler with a large-volume attachment is preferred because this method reduces the amount of the steroid deposited in the oropharynx and then swallowed and absorbed systemically. This method maximizes the dose delivered to the intrapulmonary airways while minimizing the total systemic dose.[12] When a steroid is inhaled, peak plasma concentrations are achieved within an hour and plasma half-life is about 2 h.[12]

Compounds topically administered to the skin must penetrate the keratin layer of the stratum corneum to reach the squamous cell layer of the epidermis; high lipid solubility favors such penetration. For instance, the more lipophilic triamcinolone acetonide is 10 times as active as triamcinolone topically but is only equiactive systemically.[94–96] However, both compounds are more active than cortisol, which penetrates very poorly. By contrast, hydrocortisone butyrate appears to have an activity similar to that of triamcinolone acetonide.[95] Nevertheless, only a small fraction of the topically applied steroid is actually absorbed.[95,96] With cortisol, only 1 percent is so taken up; the remainder rubs off, exfoliates with the stratum corneum, or washes off. Percutaneous penetration of glucocorticoids can vary in different anatomic regions. For instance, uptake by the scrotum and forehead is about 42 and 6 times, respectively, that of the forearm.[95] Absorption is enhanced when skin is damaged and when occlusive dressings are applied, particularly to open areas.[95] Uptake is affected by the vehicle; for example, ointment bases are taken up better than are creams and lotions.[95,96]

Uptake of steroids applied topically to the eyes presents a special problem in that they must penetrate both the corneal epithelium, which is hydrophobic, and the corneal stroma, which is hydrophilic.[42,43] For this reason, acetate steroid derivatives have been shown to be the most effective.[42,43] They are applied as aqueous suspensions and are most effective when applied frequently.[42,43]

Uptake in specific tissues after systemic administration can also vary. For example, in lung, the uptake of cortisol and methylprednisolone is greater than that of prednisone.[97] Dexamethasone is sometimes given to mothers at risk for premature delivery to prevent respiratory distress syndrome in the newborn.[98] In this case, the blood levels attained in the fetus are only a fraction of those reached in the mother.[98,99] Although this may be due in part to decreased uptake, there is enhanced metabolism of the drug as well.[99]

Distribution

The effect of distribution on steroid dynamics is discussed in Chap. 11; corticosteroid-binding globulin (CBG), other plasma proteins, and the peripheral tissues sequester administered steroids to a variable extent. For steroids that bind to CBG, variations in the protein affect the rate of metabolic clearance. The presence of the protein also changes the rate of clearance of prednisolone after prednisone administration; this is more rapid shortly after the dose is given than it is later[89] because at the early time the plasma prednisolone level exceeds the CBG binding capacity and more of the steroid is available for metabolic degradation or excretion. With prednisolone, it has also been reported that individual patient differences in the volume of distribution may explain in part why certain patients are more prone to develop cushingoid side effects[34]; it has been reported that patients with low serum albumin concentrations are more likely to develop cushingoid side effects.[100] Dexamethasone has only about sevenfold greater intrinsic activity than cortisol (Table 14-2) but was found in vivo to have 17 times the potency of cortisol when the data were extrapolated to zero time to eliminate any influence of clearance.[101] This greater activity may be due in part to enhanced availability of this steroid relative to cortisol because of less plasma binding.

Metabolism and Clearance

Metabolic pathways convert inactive compounds to active forms and vice versa. Although most glucocorticoids are active without metabolic alteration, two commonly used compounds—prednisone and cortisone—are themselves antagonists, although their affinities for the glucocorticoid receptor (see Chap. 11) are so low[102] that these compounds are effectively inactive. These 11-ketosteroids are, however, rapidly converted, mostly by the liver, to the 11-hydroxyl forms—prednisolone and cortisol—which have full agonist activity (Chap. 11). Ordinarily this conversion proceeds readily (Fig. 14-5); in the study shown in the figure, the concentration of prednisolone was 10 times that of prednisone even in the first 30 min after a 10-mg oral dose of prednisone.[103] However, inadequate 11-hydroxylation could explain certain clinical findings, such as the fact that cortisone, which can penetrate human skin, does not exhibit glucocorticoid activity when applied

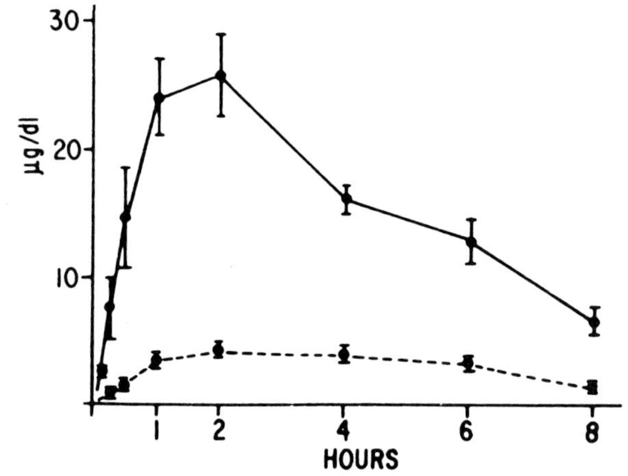

FIGURE 14-5. Plasma concentrations of prednisone (– – –) and prednisolone (—) after oral administration of 10 mg of prednisone. (*From Meikle et al.*[103])

topically[95] or injected into joints[104] and the fact that cortisone acetate injections are sometimes ineffective in the first few hours after injection[92,93] (see earlier discussion and Chap. 11). In liver disease, the conversion of cortisone to cortisol is rarely affected, although the conversion of prednisone to prednisolone can be impaired.[89] For this reason, it is generally recommended that prednisolone rather than prednisone be used in patients with liver disease.[69,89] Other than with the 11-ketosteroids, there is only a small role for metabolic conversion in the formation of more active steroids; instead, the rate of inactivation is an important determinant of biological potency. The plasma half-life is commonly used as an index of the rate of clearance of corticosteroids; this parameter has some utility. However, because both the distribution and the clearance can vary differentially for various steroids and in states where these parameters change, the use of half-life alone can sometimes be misleading and can underestimate true differences in clearance.[89]

The rates of clearance of the steroids used in therapy show considerable variation (Table 14-3), and the decreased clearance of many of the commonly used steroids (prednisone, dexamethasone, etc.) relative to cortisol is one of the most important factors explaining their enhanced potency.[89,101,105–109] To a large extent, it is the modification of the steroid molecule around the A ring and the AB ring angle that accounts for the delayed clearance, as these

TABLE 14-3. Plasma Half-Life and Glucocorticoid and Mineralocorticoid Potencies of Some Commonly Used Glucocorticoid Preparations

			Relative Potency		
Steroid	**Half Time, min**	**Ref.**	**Glucocorticoid**	**Mineralocorticoid**	**Ref.**
Cortisol	80–120	82	1.0	1.0	107–109
Cortisone			0.8	0.8	107–109
Prednisone	200–210	98	3.5–4.0		107, 108
			1.05–5.2		101
Prednisolone	120–300	82	4.0	0.8	107
Methylprednisolone	120–180	82	5.0	0.5	107
Triamcinolone			5.0	0	107
Dexamethasone	150–270	82	30.0	~0	107
			17–154		101
Betamethasone	130–330	82	25–30	~0	107

modifications decrease the ability of the liver to reduce the ring (Chap. 11). In these cases, the 6-hydroxylation/methylation and 21-conjugation pathways become more important. There also appear to be some variations in the rates of clearance of the steroids in different individuals.[110] For example, in one study the half-life for prednisolone clearance in nine subjects ranged from 134 to 342 min.[90] In another study, 11 of 54 patients had accelerated clearance of methylprednisolone.[111] Although it has been reported that the plasma clearance of prednisolone is lower in steroid-treated patients who develop cushingoid side effects than in those who do not (Fig. 14-5),[34,112] this was not confirmed in a later study.[113] However, in the latter case, in the cushingoid steroid-treated patients the plasma cortisol levels while on the steroid were higher.[113] This may imply that the hypothalamic-pituitary-adrenal axis is more resistant to suppression in cushingoid patients so that higher endogenous cortisol levels contribute to the development of side effects.

As outlined in Chap. 11, drugs and disease states can affect the clearance of administered glucocorticoids. There is impaired steroid clearance in liver disease.[89] In renal diseases, some researchers have reported that the pharmacokinetics of steroids are unchanged.[89] However, a later report suggests that the clearance and half-life of prednisolone are decreased but that those of dexamethasone are increased in renal disease.[114] Drugs such as phenytoin (diphenylhydantoin), phenobarbital, and rifampin can increase the rate of steroid clearance by inducing hepatic metabolizing enzymes.[89]

Estrogen-containing oral contraceptives and estrogen therapy in general result in decreased clearance of administered steroids.[89,115] Nonsteroidal anti-inflammatory agents may increase steroid availability, although this has not been rigorously studied.[89] It appears that the use of antacids or cimetidine does not appreciably affect steroid pharmacokinetics.[89] In general, clearance is similar in children and adults but may decrease slightly with advancing age.[89]

Concentration at Sites of Action

The potency of compounds with agonist activity, including all the major steroids used for glucocorticoid therapy (see the earlier discussions regarding the exceptions with cortisone and prednisone), is directly related to affinity for glucocorticoid receptors (see Chap. 11 and Table 14-2). Thus, once the steroid has been delivered to the target tissue, affinity is the overwhelming determinant of activity. For instance, dexamethasone and prednisolone have, respectively, about eight and two times the affinity of cortisol for the receptors.[102] Initially, this is a major determinant of the relative differences in their potencies.

Agonist Activity

Most of the steroids that are used in glucocorticoid therapy are full agonists (Chap. 11). The major exceptions are the steroids with an 11-keto group, prednisone, and cortisone (discussed earlier), which are rapidly converted in vivo to the agonists prednisolone and cortisol respectively.

Overall Estimation of Glucocorticoid Potency

Because the relative potencies of steroids vary even with the time after administration, it is an oversimplification to consider only a single set of potency ratios. Thus, whereas dexamethasone and prednisone were found to be, respectively, 154 and 5.2 times as potent as cortisol when examined at 14 h, they were only 17 and 1.05 times as potent when the data were extrapolated to zero time.[101] Because other responses have different kinetics, it is likely that the changes in relative potency with time will also differ, depending on the particular response. For all these reasons, the safest way to develop clinical protocols would be to standardize each drug for each disease, adjust the dose for each patient (see later discussion), and exercise caution when switching steroids.

Over the years, a number of estimates of relative potency have been made (Table 14-3). In spite of the inherent problems, the relative potency values serve as a rough index of relative activity; these relative activities are generally similar for various responses in a number of different tissues in animals and humans (Chap. 4).[31,101] The data have been obtained from a variety of assays in several different species, including those which quantify liver glycogen deposition and lymphocyte killing in the rat (Chap. 12), and clinical responses (e.g., cortisol suppression, antiarthritic).[36]

Variations in Sensitivity to Glucocorticoids: Glucocorticoid Resistance

Variations in intrinsic sensitivity to glucocorticoids are discussed in Chap. 11 and reviewed in Refs. 31 and 116. It is clear that marked and generalized hyposensitivity is rare; when this occurs, an androgen and/or mineralocorticoid excess syndrome occurs (Chap. 13). Similarly, there is scant evidence for a syndrome of primary increased sensitivity to glucocorticoids. Nevertheless, there are known situations in which the steroid dosage must be altered because of individual differences (discussed under Metabolism and Clearance, earlier) or therapy with other drugs (e.g., phenytoin or barbiturates) that increase the hepatic metabolism of glucocorticoids (Chap. 11). However, it is possible that there are also variations in intrinsic sensitivity between individuals and between various tissues in an individual. Individual differences in the steroid's ability to suppress the hypothalamic-pituitary-adrenal axis could explain the higher cortisol levels in the cushingoid patients in the study of Benet and associates.[113] If this is the case, it is likely that the lowered sensitivity of the axis in certain individuals is also selective for the tissues involved in axis suppression, because the presence of effects of the steroid sufficient to produce Cushing's syndrome in these individuals indicates that other target tissues are sensitive to glucocorticoids. Individual differences could also explain why only subpopulations of patients with certain diseases respond to glucocorticoid therapy; the study of patients with the preleukemic syndrome[7] quoted previously in the section Therapeutic Influences underscores this point.

The concentrations of glucocorticoid receptors, unlike those of receptors for other classes of hormones, such as the polypeptide and catecholamine hormones, are not extensively regulated; however, they can be regulated to some extent, and other factors have a pronounced effect on cellular sensitivity to glucocorticoids (Chap. 11). Although the clinical importance of these phenomena is not known, they could affect the sensitivity of selected target tissues to glucocorticoids and be of therapeutic relevance. It is possible that studies of these influences may yield information that will facilitate the design of protocols to enhance specifically the effectiveness of glucocorticoids on certain tissues while minimizing that on other tissues.

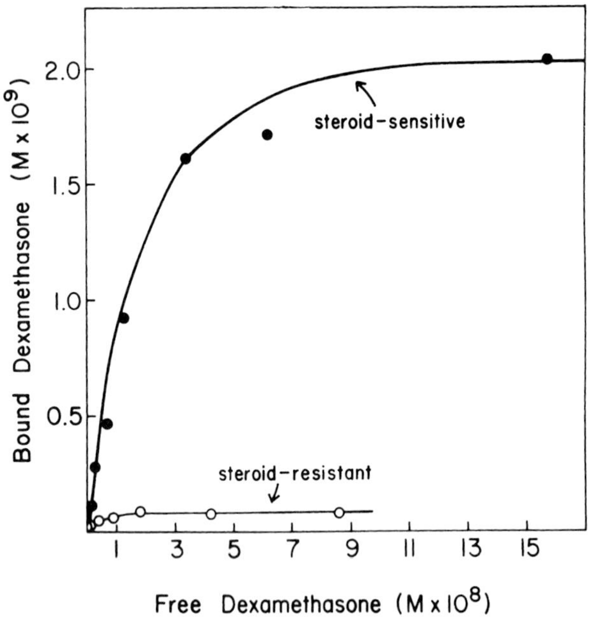

FIGURE 14-6. Binding of radioactive dexamethasone to receptors from glucocorticoid-sensitive lymphoma cells and to glucocorticoid-resistant cells selected by growing steroid-sensitive cells in the presence of dexamethasone. [*From Rosenau W, Baxter JD, Rousseau GG, Tomkins GM: Mechanism of resistance to steroids: Glucocorticoid receptor defect in lymphoma cells. Nature (New Biol) 237:20, 1972.*].

In the treatment of lymphoid leukemias, patients who initially respond can become resistant to the steroid.[6] This appears to be due to a mutation in a gene of a protein within the glucocorticoid signal transduction pathway and the selection of a clonal cell line that does not respond to the steroid (Fig. 14-6).

GLUCOCORTICOID PREPARATIONS

Steroids with Glucocorticoid Activity Available for Therapy

A great number of steroids with glucocorticoid potency are available. The structures of some of the more commonly used synthetic glucocorticoid preparations are shown in Fig. 14-1. The modifications that enhance activity are discussed earlier and in Chap. 11. The steroids may be given orally, parenterally, topically, intraarticularly, or as aerosols. The advantage of topical, intraarticular, or aerosol therapy is that certain areas (skin, joints, and the bronchial tree) can be exposed to high concentrations of glucocorticoids while systemic exposure and side effects are minimized.

Orally and Parenterally Active Preparations

In general, with oral administration, the unmodified steroid is given, because for the commonly used steroids (e.g., prednisone, prednisolone, dexamethasone, cortisol), substitutions (21-phosphate, etc.) are not needed for absorption (see Bioavailability, section).

Parenteral administration is indicated in the immediate treatment of addisonian patients in crisis (Chap. 11) and patients who cannot take oral medications. There appears to be no acute danger in giving moderate doses (1 g or less) intravenously (IV), although in general the oral route is effective. The preparations used intravenously are ordinarily compounds with C-21 substitutions to enhance solubility (Table 14-4). Intramuscular administration is described in the preceding section.

TABLE 14-4. Some Parenteral and Topical Glucocorticoid Preparations

Intravenous	Intraarticular
Hydrocortisone phosphate	Hydrocortisone acetate
Hydrocortisone hemisuccinate	Prednisolone tebutate
Prednisolone phosphate	Triamcinolone hexacetonide
Dexamethasone phosphate	Betamethasone acetate phosphate
Methylprednisolone hemisuccinate	Methylprednisolone acetate
Topical	
Lowest potency	Low potency
0.25–0.5% cortisol	0.01% flucinolone acetonide
0.04–0.1% dexamethasone	0.01% betamethasone valerate
0.5% prednisolone	0.025% fluorometholone
0.2% betamethasone	0.025% triamcinolone acetonide
Intermediate potency	High potency
0.1% betamethasone valerate	0.05% betamethasone dipropionate
0.025% halcinolone	0.5% triamcinolone acetonide
0.1% triamcinolone acetonide	0.2% fluocinolone acetonide
0.025% flucinolone acetonide	0.1% halcinonide

Source: Data on topical preparations from Robertson and Maibach.[95]

The four major considerations in selecting the particular steroid to be used are experience with prescribing it for the disease in question, duration of action, the possible need to avoid concomitant mineralocorticoid activity, and cost. Whereas in principle all the various glucocorticoids should be effective when given in equivalent doses, caution should be exercised in substituting them because the relative potencies have not been established as clearly as has generally been assumed (see earlier discussion and Chap. 11). Thus, in general, it is best to use preparations that have been shown to be effective for a particular condition. For instance, if a physician were treating an asthmatic crisis and wanted to administer the equivalent of 100 mg of cortisol, the prednisolone equivalent over the first few hours would be around 50 to 95 mg rather than the usually considered value of 20 to 25 mg (Table 14-2).[101] In the acute treatment of primary adrenocortical insufficiency cortisol is preferred because of its relatively greater mineralocorticoid activity, but in other circumstances it is generally preferable to avoid sodium-retaining actions by giving a steroid with less mineralocorticoid activity. Duration of action is particularly relevant for alternate-day steroid therapy (discussed later). Finally, physicians should be aware that the various steroid preparations vary considerably in cost, and when possible, less expensive preparations should be used.

Intraarticular Preparations

Glucocorticoids can be injected into joints for the relief of inflammation.[36,104,117] Although these measures are usually for supplemental and temporary therapy, they can provide dramatic symptomatic relief. In general, the preparations are relatively insoluble and form microcrystals. Substitution with a tert-butylacetate or a hexacetonide group has proved to be particularly effective in this respect (Table 14-4).[36,104,117] These properties retard systemic absorption, promote retention within the joint space, and lead to a longer period of clinical effect; a single injection of such a preparation can last for weeks.[97] As stated earlier, preparations containing cortisone are not effective.[36,104,117]

When intraarticular preparations are used, generalized problems caused by glucocorticoid excess, including suppression of the hypothalamic-pituitary-adrenal axis, are uncommon.[97] Intraarticular steroid administration is not, however, without risk. It is important to adhere to scrupulous aseptic technique and avoid injection into potentially infected joints, as steroids can worsen the course of such infections. Nevertheless, infections in the joint or needle tract occur infrequently in spite of strict aseptic techniques.[33] Other problems with intraarticular steroids include the infrequent occurrence of synovitis, induced presumably by the steroid-containing crystals; occasional damage to the cartilage, supporting ligaments, and surrounding bone; partial absorption of bony margins; and cutaneous atrophy at the site of injection.[33,97,110] The last condition can be minimized by avoiding overdistension of the synovial cavity and leakage along the needle track.[97]

Topical Preparations

The use of topical glucocorticoid preparations constitutes the major advance in the pharmacology of dermatology.[88,89] Some of the factors involved in topical uptake of glucocorticoids are discussed earlier in the section on Determinants of Glucocorticoid Potency. Thus, many of the cortisol analogues are much more effective than cortisol itself. Some of the commonly used steroids are listed in Table 14-4. These steroids come in ointment, cream, lotion, or aerosol vehicles and in varying strengths. The ointment bases tend to give better activity than do cream or lotion vehicles but also tend to be less acceptable cosmetically to the patient in spite of the fact that they are more soothing to dry skin.[95,96] However, hairy areas are best treated with lotions or aerosol vehicles.[95] The availability of several strengths helps a physician provide the needed dosage while minimizing excess dosage. For most indications, high-potency steroid preparations are unnecessary; they carry a higher risk of local side effects (see later discussion) and are used primarily on areas of skin that have been thickened by disease.[95,96] Although topical steroid preparations are commonly given without occlusion, they can be used (e.g., with plastic wrap, sometimes intermittently,[95] or with wet dressings[95]) to enhance penetration.[95,96] Single daily applications of an ointment are probably as effective as three daily applications.[95,96] In general, topical steroid use on ulcerated skin should be avoided. Except for circumstances under which there is markedly increased absorption, systemic toxicity, including suppression of the hypothalamic-pituitary-adrenal axis, is uncommon, although the possibility that it may develop must be kept in mind.[95] Other complications of topical therapy include exacerbation of an infection when steroids are given inappropriately, localized striae (usually in areas of increased uptake such as the groin), rosacea-like eruptions, pustules (steroid acne), and, rarely, an allergic contact dermatitis from the steroids themselves.[95]

Inhaled Corticosteroids

Corticosteroid aerosols are effective in the treatment of asthma.[12,44,118,119] Beclomethasone dipropionate, trimacinolone acetonide, budesonide, flunisolide, and betamethasone valerate are the most commonly used preparations.[12,44,118,119] These preparations are preferable to other steroids because they are not absorbed as well systematically as many other steroids, such as cortisol.[44] Inhalers that deliver higher doses of up to 250 μg of beclomethasone dipropionate per puff have been shown to have significant efficacy.[119] In general, aerosols are used for maintenance therapy for asthma and are substituted for oral or parenteral steroids after they have induced a good response.[44] In some cases, delivery of the steroid to the lower bronchial tissue is enhanced by prior administration of a bronchodilator such as albuterol.[118] Delivery can be difficult during heavy sputum production.

Although it is clear that steroids given in this way improve the ratio of therapeutic to toxic effects, this form of therapy is not without problems.[120] First, there is an increased incidence of fungal infections of the upper respiratory tract, including candidiasis of the pharynx.[120] Second, patients can experience dysphonia, which may be a steroid-induced myopathy of the phonatory muscle.[120] Although suppression of the hypothalamic-pituitary-adrenal axis with corticosteroid aerosol therapy[12,44] might occur, it is overall minor and of no clinical significance[121,122]; this can be minimized further in asthmatic patients by holding the aerosol canister outside the mouth, using the inhaler before meals, rinsing the mouth and throat after inhalation, and using a spacer or holding chamber into which the medication is delivered.[12,44] The extent to which aerosols produce atrophy of the pharynx and airways has not been determined.[44]

ACTH

ACTH can be given instead of a glucocorticoid, and such preparations are occasionally used. Cosyntropin ($ACTH_{1-24}$; see Chap. 11) is not commonly used because of its short duration of action (unless continuous intravenous ACTH is given); instead, repository ACTH preparations are available for IM injection.[37] When given in this way, the peptide is released slowly, and daily injections can be used to provide therapeutically effective steroid levels. These injections vary in composition and can include zinc or gelatin (the zinc preparations have a greater duration of action); 15 to 40 U of ACTH given in this way is roughly equivalent to 37.5 to 100 mg of cortisol.[37] However, a problem in comparing the efficacy of ACTH and glucocorticoids involves determining the equivalency of doses.[37]

ACTH stimulates the production of cortisol, adrenal androgens, and other steroids. Thus, the observed effects are due not only to cortisol but also to the other steroids and resemble spontaneous Cushing's syndrome, in which acne and hirsutism in females can be prominent.[106] Also, patients receiving ACTH appear to have a greater prevalence of hypertension than do those receiving synthetic steroids.[37] This may be due to the greater mineralocorticoid activity of cortisol compared with the other, more commonly used synthetic glucocorticoid preparations and to increased secretion of deoxycorticosterone (Chap. 13). Further, ACTH itself can cause hyperpigmentation of skin and mucosae.[37]

ACTH produces less suppression of the hypothalamic-pituitary-adrenal axis than do glucocorticoids. In almost all ACTH-treated patients, the responses to provocative testing with insulin-induced hypoglycemia are normal or only slighty impaired.[37] For instance, Daly and associates found a diminished plasma ACTH response but a normal cortisol response to insulin hypoglycemia testing.[123] These data suggest that ACTH therapy does suppress the axis to some extent but that the adrenal, when stimulated by the therapy, can respond to lower ACTH concentrations.[37] However, some patients on prolonged ACTH therapy show suppression of the hypothalamic-pituitary-adrenal axis.[124] The decreased frequency of suppression of the axis by ACTH compared with the frequency of suppression by glucocorticoids probably reflects differences in the maximal plasma glucocorticoid level attained and the duration of the effect. ACTH gel (20–40 U) given once daily results in only a moderate increase in plasma cortisol levels (maximum approximately 40–50 gmg/dl), and these levels return to normal by approximately 16 h.[124] Thus, the effect of daily ACTH injections appears to be roughly comparable to that of a single morning dose of a short-acting glucocorticoid.[37] If ACTH was given twice daily, the degree of suppression of the axis might approximate that seen with glucocorticoids given in multiple doses. The fact that glucocorticoid concentrations are only moderately elevated and are not sustained over 24 h by once-daily ACTH therapy[124] may also explain the observation that ACTH causes less suppression of linear growth in children than does daily glucocorticoid therapy.[37]

The disadvantages of ACTH therapy are the necessity for daily injection and the side effects of androgen excess and hypertension.[37] Because there is no clear advantage over oral glucocorticoids, ACTH in doses which achieve similar plasma glucocorticoid concentration is not commonly used for prolonged therapy.[125]

SOME GENERAL PRINCIPLES

Selection of Patients

The decision to use glucocorticoids implies that the benefits will outweigh the serious side effects. Thus, it should be clear that there is a reasonable chance that the patient will respond.

Need for Empirical Data

If there are no data to suggest that a given condition will respond to glucocorticoids, their use for that condition constitutes experimentation. Clearly, the decision to use corticosteroids should be based on verification that the drugs are effective.

Short-Term Versus Long-Term

The major complications of glucocorticoid therapy are ones that require a considerable time to develop (see earlier discussion). Thus, in general, the use of steroids over a short period of time is not associated with major risk.[126] If steroids will significantly benefit a patient and need be given for only a few days, they should not be withheld. For instance, severe poison oak or poison ivy or an allergic skin reaction that is not responsive to topical steroids is an indication for a short course of systemic steroids. However, short courses of glucocorticoids may induce hyperglycemia in susceptible individuals and can rarely precipitate avascular necrosis.[48,49]

The decision to initiate steroid therapy when it may involve treatment for a longer period is a more serious one. For instance, with asthma, once steroid therapy is started, it may be necessary to continue the drug for months to years. Clearly, the seriousness of the primary disease commonly mandates this, but the physician must be aware of the consequences of such long-term therapy.

Testing the Sensitivity

With many conditions (e.g., acute lymphoblastic leukemia of childhood[5] and suppression of transplant rejection[127]), most patients respond to glucocorticoids, whereas with other conditions only a subgroup of patients with the disease respond. In the latter case, it is sometimes possible to identify the patients who will respond. For instance, asthmatic patients with less fixed airway obstruction respond better than do those with a greater complement of this.[120] Thus, documentation of such factors may assist in the selection of patients who can benefit from therapy. The identification of steroid-responsive patients also may be achieved by in vitro testing. This appears to be the case with the preleukemic syndrome mentioned under Therapeutic Influences earlier. In this study, bone marrow cells of 34 patients were tested in vitro; the cells of 5 patients responded to the steroid, and 3 of these patients responded to glucocorticoid therapy.[7] In acute lymphoblastic leukemia and several other hematologic malignancies, there is a good correlation between the concentration of glucocorticoid receptors measured in the malignant cells in vitro and the responsiveness of the disease to glucocorticoid therapy.[5] In a study of T lymphocyte–mediated granulopoietic failure, prednisone-responsive patients could be identified by in vitro testing of the ability of the steroid to stimulate clonal growth of bone marrow cells.[128] It is hoped that approaches such as these will be applied to other conditions to increase the ability to detect glucocorticoid-sensitive patients.

Dose-Response Considerations

The recommended doses of glucocorticoids used in therapy are based on empirical observations; this approach is reasonable and is probably safest. As more is learned about glucocorticoid action, it will be possible to predict which doses will be required. This may facilitate the development of therapeutic trials and help optimize the dosage in order to minimize toxicity while maximizing therapeutic responses.

The application of current information about glucocorticoid receptors illustrates this point. For responses that are mediated by the receptors, doses resulting in steroid levels far in excess of those necessary to saturate the receptors will not provide greater short-term benefit than will those minimally required to do this. Such "excess" doses may, however, produce a greater effect, as higher levels of the steroid will be present longer.

As emphasized in Chap. 11, there is in general a close correlation between the relative saturation of the hormone by the receptor and the relative magnitude of the hormone response. In such cases, the effectiveness of a steroid can be calculated from its affinity for the receptor and the free concentrations of the steroid with time. However, in vitro there appear to be circumstances[116] in which the steroid achieves a maximal response at concentrations lower than those required to fully saturate the receptors. Knowledge of whether this ever occurs in therapeutic situations would be particularly important because lower than usual steroid concentrations might be used and would have fewer undesirable side effects.

With human systems, precise data on the doses of steroids required to occupy the receptors have not been collected; however, from the known binding constants, free steroid levels, and so on, it can be calculated that oral doses of 7.5 and 15 mg of prednisolone would result in blood levels 8 h after the dose that would bind the receptors to 42 and 63 percent, respectively, of saturation. Much higher doses (e.g., 100 mg or more) would be required to result in nearly complete receptor saturation for long periods. Thus, a dose this large given several times a day should stimulate nearly maximal receptor-mediated responses.

There are situations, such as acute renal transplant rejection,[127] gram-negative sepsis with shock,[20,129–131] tumors of the central nervous system,[21] and certain immune-mediated hematologic dyscrasias[132] in which the use of even larger doses of glucocorticoids has been recommended. Subsequent studies of renal transplant rejection have indicated that such large doses actually decrease survival,[127] and for this indication the trend has been toward the use of progressively lower steroid doses.[133] Studies in baboons show clear beneficial effects of high-dose glucocorticoids given early in the course of bacteria-induced shock.[134] Dexamethasone at doses of 3 to 5 mg per kilogram of body weight per day has been shown to be beneficial in patients with suspected typhoid fever who are delirious, obtunded, stuporous, comatose, or in shock.[135] Overall, it appears that glucocorticoids must be given early and in a sustained fashion to be beneficial. High, but not industrial, doses of corticosteroids should be given.[136]

The Use of Adjunctive Therapy

In the majority of conditions for which glucocorticoids are used, there are either alternative or adjunctive therapeutic modalities; these modalities must be considered and if possible used before beginning steroid therapy, as their use may be associated with a lower incidence of complications. Further, if the patient's condition can be adequately controlled by such methods, glucocorticoid therapy may not be indicated. Conversely, failure to respond to maximal utilization of conventional treatment may be an indication for the use of glucocorticoids in certain conditions.

If glucocorticoid therapy is used, adjunctive therapy should in most cases be continued, as it may be beneficial, improve the overall response to therapy, and allow the use of lower steroid doses. For instance, in rheumatoid arthritis, the use of physical therapy, braces, salicylates, and other nonsteroidal anti-inflammatory agents may obviate the need for steroids or provide additional benefit. In asthma, other bronchodilators, such as beta-adrenergic agents, are used in conjunction with steroids. Immunosuppressants in addition to a glucocorticoid may be helpful in the treatment of nephritis[137] or the prevention of renal transplant rejection.[127] Other chemotherapeutic agents can be helpful in malignancies or in conditions such as amyloidosis.[138]

Specific Measures to Reduce Side Effects

There is a growing awareness that certain specific measures may reduce side effects. The potential use of measures to reduce osteoporosis and myopathy and of insulin to control diabetes is discussed elsewhere in this chapter. An increased protein intake can reduce steroid-induced nitrogen wasting.[139] Vitamin A may decrease the steroid effect of impaired wound healing.[140]

Cognizance of Objective Criteria

In evaluating the response to steroid therapy, objective criteria should be used whenever possible because glucocorticoids can induce a sense of well-being[2,21,35,86–88] that is not necessarily accompanied by improvement in the primary disease for which the steroids are being administered. Conversely, patients on long-term therapy frequently develop symptoms of steroid withdrawal when the dose is lowered (see later discussion), and these symptoms may be misinterpreted as an exacerbation of the primary disease. For example, arthralgias and myalgias are common during steroid withdrawal and do not necessarily indicate increased activity of rheumatoid arthritis. Similarly, lowering the steroid dose in patients with inflammatory bowel disease may provoke anorexia and nausea which may not be due to an exacerbation of the gastrointestinal disorder. Thus, subjective changes may be misleading and may lead to inappropriate alterations in dosage.

Although many of the disorders for which steroids are used have no clearly identifiable chemical criteria which can be used to quantify maximal benefit or improvement, objective criteria should be used when possible. Such criteria include pulmonary function studies in patients with asthma,[141] gallium lung scanning or assay of the activity of serum angiotensin converting enzyme in sarcoidosis,[142] evaluation of serum complement levels in patients with lupus erythematosus, determination of serum Ca^2 concentrations in patients with hypercalcemia and sarcoidosis, serial creatinine clearance measurements in patients treated for renal transplant rejection, and evidence of true joint inflammation in patients with arthritis.

The Circadian Rhythm

When moderate doses of glucocorticoids are given for a short time (e.g., a few days or less), the circadian rhythm of endogenous steroid production (Chap. 11) is ignored; the transient suppression of the hypothalamic-pituitary-adrenal axis in this setting is not a problem. When it is necessary to give moderate to large doses of steroids on a daily basis for a longer period; however, suppression of the axis is unavoidable and must be considered and dealt with as described later (see Withdrawal of Glucocorticoids and Suppression of the Hypothalamic-Pituitary-Adrenal Axis).

However, there are other circumstances in which it is important to tailor glucocorticoid therapy to the circadian rhythm; this is the case with alternate-day therapy, with replacement therapy in a patient whose hypothalamic-pituitary-adrenal axis is suppressed (both discussed later), and sometimes when low doses of steroids are required. In the latter situation, a patient with lupus arthritis or asthma refractory to other therapy may sometimes respond to low doses of glucocorticoids (e.g., 5 mg or less of prednisone per day). If these doses are given in the evening, there will be suppression of the rise in plasma ACTH concentration and therefore in the cortisol level. In this case, the total additional effect will be minor because the suppression of endogenous cortisol production will offset the effect of the steroid administered. However, if the steroid is given in the morning, when ACTH levels spontaneously fall, the net effect can be additive, with a minimal influence on the body's normal rhythm of steroid secretion.

Adjusting the Dose

Once glucocorticoid therapy has been instituted, it is important to monitor the dose carefully. The major endpoint is clinical response; side effects can be minimized by decreasing the dose when the patient is responding. Alternatively, it may be necessary to increase the dose when the patient is not responding, and the literature regarding that condition suggests that higher doses may be more effective.

The factors that lead to variations in response were discussed earlier. Because variations exist in metabolism and distribution, absorption, and possibly even intrinsic sensitivity, it should be obvious that adherence to a fixed drug protocol is not ideal, although in certain situations this may be necessary because other information is not available.

It is hoped that plasma measurements of the glucocorticoids used in therapy will be used more in the future to minimize variations resulting from uptake, metabolism, and distribution. In this way, patients in whom higher drug levels develop could have their doses lowered sooner, minimizing cushingoid side effects. Conversely, patients in whom adequate blood levels are not attained could receive an increased dose (and possible improvement) sooner.

ALTERNATE DAY THERAPY

Alternate-day therapy emerged after it was found that if a single dose of glucocorticoid was given once in the morning on alternate days, certain adverse effects of the steroid could be minimized while a therapeutically beneficial response could still be obtained.[37,44,125,143,144] Conditions in which alternate-day glucocorticoid therapy has been effective include certain nephrotic syndromes (particularly in children), renal transplantation rejection and other renal diseases, ulcerative colitis, rheumatoid arthritis and some other arthritic disorders, rheumatic fever, myasthenia gravis, muscular dystrophy, sarcoidosis, alopecia areata, chronic dermatoses, asthma, and pemphigus vulgaris.[37,44,125,145,146] However, alternate-day therapy has been shown not to be effective in giant cell arteritis.[147] Thus, before the use of alternate-day steroid therapy is contemplated, the specific literature about each condition should be examined.

Based on studies in which the same dose of steroid was given once in the morning on alternate days rather than over a 48-h period, a number of glucocorticoid side effects are decreased.[37,44,125,144] These side effects include suppression of the hypothalamic-pituitary-adrenal axis, growth inhibition in children, cushingoid facies, abnormal fat deposition, obesity, excessive appetite, striae, easy bruisability, carbohydrate intolerance, infections, myopathy, and other features. The decrease in growth inhibition constitutes a major advantage of alternate-day glucocorticoid therapy in the pediatric group.[37,44,125,148]

The effect of alternate-day steroid therapy on the hypothalamic-pituitary-adrenal axis has been studied by ACTH stimulation, metyrapone testing, insulin hypoglycemia testing, and corticotropin releasing hormone (CRH) stimulation.[37,44,149,150] These studies show less suppression than with equivalent divided doses given on a daily basis, and in one study there was recovery of a suppressed axis when children were switched from daily to alternate-day therapy.[146] However, some suppression of the hypothalamic-pituitary-adrenal axis does occur with alternate-day therapy.[37,146,149–151] For example, in a study of patients receiving 5–60 mg of prednisone on alternate days, the response to CRH was markedly suppressed on the day of treatment and was mildly blunted on the day off treatment.[150] However, the cortisol response to ACTH was normal in all cases, including that enough ACTH was secreted to maintain normal adrenal function.[150]

The precise mechanisms of the effectiveness of alternate-day therapy are not known. However, when various responses to glucocorticoids are examined, some persist on the "off steroid" day of alternate-day therapy, whereas other influences are present only during the "on" day. For instance, Fauci and Dale[152] found that glucocorticoid-induced lymphocytopenia and monocytopenia returned to normal by 8 A.M. on the day off prednisone, yet at this time there was evidence that the steroid was suppressing disease activity. Considerations such as these underscore a general problem that must be faced with glucocorticoid therapy: The dose response and the kinetics of each particular beneficial and deleterious effect must be known. It might then be possible to optimize even more precisely the dose and the interval between doses. However, other dosage intervals have been tried and have not been found to be superior.[34,143,153]

TABLE 14-5. Recommendations Regarding Alternate-Day Glucocorticoid Therapy

1. Use an intermediate-acting glucocorticoid.
2. Avoid in acute situations or if only short-term therapy (e.g., <3 weeks) is anticipated.
3. Inform patient fully of the advantages, then be diligent.
4. Give special attention if there is already suppression of the hypothalamic-pituitary-adrenal axis.
5. Maximize adjuctive therapy, particularly on the "off" day.
6. Check the literature: may not be effective for certain diseases.

If alternate-day therapy is used, one of the intermediate acting glucocorticoids should be administered (Table 14-5).[37,143–145,153] These include prednisone, prednisolone, and methylprednisolone, which are cleared more rapidly from the plasma than fluorinated steroids (Table 14-3). The optimal alternate-day therapy requires that the steroid be administered in the morning (preferably before breakfast) as a single dose.[37,143,145] If the steroid is given in divided doses, the effect of the later doses may persist into the alternate day. Avoidance of late afternoon and evening doses is especially important in terms of minimizing suppression of the hypothalamic-pituitary adrenal axis (discussed later), and with the short-acting steroid, morning-only administration allows the steroid to be cleared from the circulation before the nocturnal increase in ACTH release. Steroids such as dexamethasone, betamethasone, triamcinolone, triamcinolone acetonide, and fluocinolone acetonide are cleared more slowly, are longer-acting, and should not be used for alternate-day therapy.[37,143,145]

Alternate-day therapy is best used for prolonged[146] therapy and is not in general indicated for initial treatment, especially when glucocorticoids are used for acute problems (Tables 14-1 and 14-5).[37,143,145,146] Thus, most people experienced in the use of steroids recommend that even for chronic diseases, daily therapy should be used initially. In fact, if only short-term treatment is anticipated, alternate-day therapy may not be necessary. Thus, in instituting steroid therapy, the glucocorticoid is given on a daily (or more frequent) basis and then, once there is amelioration or control, the patient is switched to alternate-day therapy. The change to alternate-day therapy should be made as soon as possible (within several weeks) after beginning steroid therapy and before there is major suppression of the hypothalamic-pituitary-adrenal axis, as the change is more difficult if the axis is suppressed.

In patients in whom the axis is not suppressed, the change can be made abruptly. In changing to alternate-day therapy, it is generally best not to reduce the total dose of steroid given.[37,143–145] In fact, sometimes it may be advantageous to increase the total dose. Thus, the overall dosage for two days used with daily therapy can be administered as a single dose on the mornings of alternate days. Then the overall dose can be reduced as indicated by the condition of the problem for which the steroid was given.

Patients on long-term daily multiple-dose therapy in whom the axis is suppressed frequently have manifestations of adrenal insufficiency and steroid withdrawal (discussed below) on the off day when switched abruptly to alternate-day therapy.[37,143–145] In these patients, the change can be made slowly; it may first require gradual reduction in the total dose, then a change to single daily doses, and finally a switch to alternate-day therapy. This can be done by gradually reducing (e.g., by 5 mg every 4–5 days) the steroid dose on alternate days and adding this dose to the one given on the other days until the transition is achieved. In making this transition, the physician should be concerned not only with an exacerbation of the primary disease but also with the problem of a lack of well-being while the patient is off the steroid. This can be due to symptoms of adrenal insufficiency in cases where the hypothalamic-pituitary adrenal axis is suppressed, to a lack of the general euphoric influences of the steroid independent of the primary disease, or to the primary disease. Thus, the patient is likely to complain on the off day, and the physician and patient must be committed to alternate-day therapy once the decision to use it has been made. In a patient who has symptoms on the off day, special attention must be given to objective criteria and to whether the therapy is ineffective or effective and whether the complaints are due to the other factors discussed previously. However, during this time, if there is a documented flare-up of the primary disease, it may be necessary to switch to daily therapy for a short time, and several attempts at conversion to alternate-day therapy may be required. In switching to alternate-day therapy, the physician should be especially aware of the use of adjunctive modalities (described earlier) that may minimize symptoms.

SPECIAL SITUATIONS

Pregnancy

There has been concern that the use of glucocorticoids in pregnancy may increase the incidence of fetal deaths or congenital abnormalities.[36,69,154–156] Indeed, glucocorticoid-treated pregnant animals have an increased incidence of spontaneous abortions and stillbirths, placental insufficiency, and congenital malformations, including cleft palate, in their offspring.[36,69,154,155] Despite these valid concerns, there are circumstances in which pregnant patients with life-threatening conditions such as asthma and systemic lupus erythematosus may require steroid therapy. Fortunately, the overall experience with glucocorticoids in pregnancy has not been as bad as expected.[36,69,154,155] For instance, during 70 pregnancies in 55 asthmatic patients, there were 71 live births, only 1 spontaneous abortion, and possibly a slight increase in premature births.[154] Further, there were no fetal, maternal, or neonatal deaths, and the incidence of toxemia, uterine hemorrhage, and congenital malformations was not increased. In a series of 260 pregnancies (reviewed in Ref. 36), seven full-term infants had disorders. One had apparent adrenocortical failure for 3 days, and there were two cases of cleft palate. Cleft palate has also been noted in a few instances in which steroids were used at the time of conception and were continued for significant periods thereafter.[36] However, cleft palate was not observed in two other series of 46 mothers who were on steroids during and after conception.[36] Thus, glucocorticoids should not be used indiscriminately during pregnancy and should be avoided especially in the first trimester. However, they should not be withheld in conditions where a steroid may ameliorate life-threatening disease.

When glucocorticoids are required in pregnant individuals, it is best to use cortisol or prednisolone because they are short-acting and are changed to their inactive 11-keto forms, cortisone and prednisone, by the placenta and thus minimize the exposure of the fetus (see Chap. 11). Steroids such as dexamethasone and betamethasone cross the placenta unchanged and thus should not be used during pregnancy (Chap. 11).

Prednisone and prednisolone administration are not contraindicated in breast-feeding women even though small amounts are excreted in breast milk.[157–159] In general, higher doses such as >20 mg/day of prednisone should be avoided in lactating women.

The use of steroid aerosols in pregnancy appears to be safe when recommended doses are used.[155]

Diabetes

Glucocorticoids alter carbohydrate metabolism by increasing gluconeogenesis, antagonizing the peripheral uptake of glucose, and inhibiting insulin secretion.[83,84] However, in glucocorticoid-treated patients without subclinical or overt diabetes, significant clinical problems with hyperglycemia are unusual (Chap. 11). Thus, in most patients, fasting blood sugar levels are usually normal or only mildly elevated, although glucose tolerance may be impaired. However, in patients with subclinical or overt diabetes, steroid therapy may provoke or worsen hyperglycemia. Steroid therapy is not contraindicated in such patients, although oral hypoglycemic agents, insulin therapy, or an increase in the insulin dose may be required. In the rare patient with insulin resistance ascribable to the development of anti-insulin antibodies, glucocorticoids may be beneficial and may reduce the insulin requirement by suppressing the immune response.[36]

Surgery

It is generally recommended that patients on prolonged high-dose glucocorticoids receive additional, perioperative steroid coverage (2–10 times replacement dose) for the stress of surgery over 24–72 h (discussed later and in Chap. 11). Patients with iatrogenic Cushing's syndrome also have an increased risk of developing serious postoperative complications. Local problems include poor healing, wound infections, and occasionally dehiscence of the incision; hematomas and abscesses may occur with abdominal or thoracic surgery. The courses of these patients may also be complicated by systemic infection. Thus, morbidity is increased and recovery is prolonged; if time allows, elective surgery should be deferred and the steroid dose should be decreased.

Psychiatry

Changes in mood and psychological state occur frequently in glucocorticoid-treated patients, and although many patients initially note a feeling of psychological well-being, depression, hypomania and several types of psychosis may also occur.[2,21,35,86–88] The type of disorder that may occur is not predictable by the patient's pretherapy condition, but it is ordinarily reversible after the discontinuation of therapy. Previous psychiatric disorders are in general not a contraindication to steroid therapy.

Peptic Ulcer

The relationship between glucocorticoid therapy and peptic ulcer disease is reviewed in Chap. 11. Recent studies have demonstrated a twofold increased risk of peptic ulcer in glucocorticoid-treated individuals,[160,161] while patients who were concomitantly receiving nonsteroidal antiinflammatory drugs (NSAIDs) had a 15-fold estimated increased risk of peptic ulcer.[161] This study also suggested that among NSAID users, both the dose and the duration of glucocorticoid therapy were associated with increased risk.[161]

Thus, caution should be observed in prescribing these drugs together, and when this is done, patients should be informed of the risk of peptic ulcer disease.

Pediatrics

In children, glucocorticoid therapy has the major additional disadvantage of causing growth failure (for a review, see Ref. 12 and Chap. 11). There tends to be a minor growth spurt after discontinuation of the steroid, as it also inhibits bone maturation (Chap. 11); however, chronic therapy leads to permanent growth retardation.[12] Nevertheless, alternate-day therapy in children results in a less inhibitory effect on growth (see previous discussion) and decreased cushingoid effects in general.[44] In addition, at the recommended doses, inhaled steroids do not inhibit growth in childhood asthma.[12]

Kaposi's Sarcoma

Kaposi's sarcoma occurs with an increased prevalence in patients who receive immunosuppressive therapy or have the acquired immune deficiency syndrome (AIDS).[162] There are several case reports of regression of their tumors in association with discontinuation of treatment with glucocorticoids.[162] Thus, glucocorticoids should be used with caution in such patients, and their use should be avoided in patients who are at a greater risk for developing Kaposi's sarcoma.

Administration with Other Drugs

Special attention is required in the concomitant use of glucocorticoids with other drugs because of potential interactions, and because some drugs may affect the metabolism of steroids and vice versa. Such interactions and effects are shown in Tables 14-6A, B, and C.

TABLE 14-6A. Interactions of Glucocorticoids With Other Drugs

Drug	Side Effect	Comments
Amphotericin B	Hypokalemia	Monitor potassium levels frequently
Digitalis glycosides	Digitalis toxicity Hypokalemia	Monitor potassium levels frequently
Growth hormone	Ineffective	—
Potassium-depleting diuretics	Hypokalemia	Monitor potassium levels frequently
Vaccines from live attenuated viruses	Severe generalized infections	—

TABLE 14-6B. Effects of Glucocorticoids on Blood Levels of Drugs

Drug	Drug Blood Levels	Comments
Aspirin	Decreased	Increased metabolism or clearance Monitor salicylate levels
Coumarin anticoagulants	Decreased	Frequent control of prothrombin levels
Cyclophosphamide	Increased	Inhibition of hepatic metabolism Adjust the dosage of the drug
Cyclosporine	Increased	Inhibition of hepatic metabolism
Insulin	Decreased	Adjust the dosage of the drug
Isoniazid	Decreased	Increased metabolism and clearance
Oral hypoglycemic agents	Decreased	Adjust the dosage of the drug

TABLE 14-6C. Effect of Drugs on Plasma Glucocorticoid Concentrations

Drug	Glucocorticoid Blood Levels	Comments
Antacids	Decreased	Possible physical adsorption to antacid
Carbamazepine	Decreased	Increased cytochrome P-450 activity
Cholestyramine	Decreased	Decreased gastrointestinal absorption of glucocorticoids
Colestipol	Decreased	Decreased gastrointestinal absorption of glucocorticoids
Cyclosporine	Increased	Inhibition of hepatic metabolism
Ephedrine	Decreased	Probably increased metabolism
Erythromycin	Increased	Impaired elimination
Mitotane	Decreased, with elevated transcortin	Total plasma cortisol unreliable Adjust glucocorticoid levels
Oral contraceptives	Increased	Impaired elimination, increased protein binding
Phenobarbital	Decreased	Increased cytochrome P-450 activity Adjust glucocorticoid dosage
Phenytoin	Decreased	Increased cytochrome P-450 activity Adjust glucocorticoid dosage
Rifampin	Decreased	Probably increased cytochrome P-450 activity Adjust glucocorticoid dosage
Troleandomycin	Increased	Partially resulting from impaired elimination

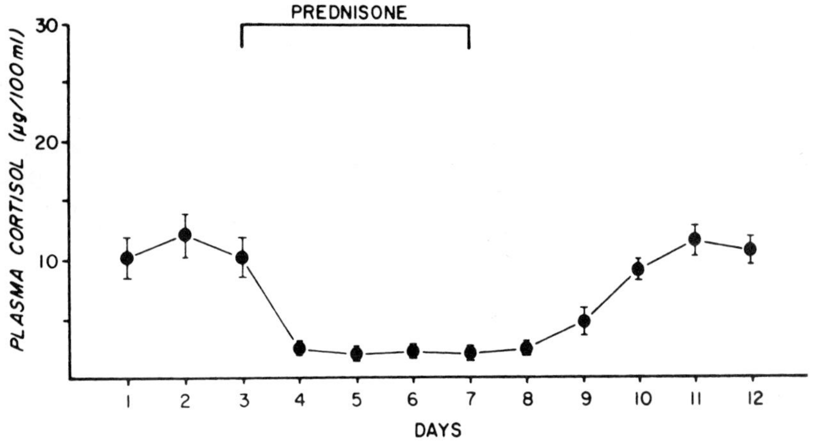

FIGURE 14-7. Fasting plasma cortisol levels (mean ± SEM) in 10 subjects before, during, and after the oral administration of prednisone, 25 mg twice daily on days 3 to 7. (*From Streck and Lockwood.*[163])

WITHDRAWAL OF GLUCOCORTICOIDS AND SUPPRESSION OF THE HYPOTHALAMIC-PITUITARY-ADRENAL AXIS

As was mentioned earlier, spontaneous Cushing's syndrome or glucocorticoid therapy can result in suppression of the hypothalamic-pituitary-adrenal axis. However, such suppression is most frequently encountered in glucocorticoid therapy because of the large number of patients receiving these steroids and must be considered in all patients who will discontinue or have discontinued glucocorticoid therapy.

Kinetics and Dosage Required for Suppression

Glucocorticoid suppression of the hypothalamic pituitary-adrenal axis is discussed in Chap. 11. Even a single dose of a glucocorticoid can, for some hours, prevent a response of the axis to a major insult such as surgery. However, with short exposure, that is, one or two doses, the axis recovers rapidly and the suppression occurs for the most part while the glucocorticoid is present in the circulation.[153] With more prolonged therapy, suppression increases with both duration and total dose. When glucocorticoids are administered for a period of days, there may be both suppression of basal cortisol levels (Fig. 14-7) if doses are sufficiently high, and decreased responsiveness of both the hypothalamic-pituitary-adrenal axis and the adrenal to stimulation.[163] Thus, in one study (Fig. 14-8), the administration of 50 mg of prednisone per day for 5 days resulted in decreased responsiveness to both insulin-induced hypoglycemia and exogenous ACTH 2 days after discontinuation of the steroid, but responses returned to normal at 5 days.[163] In another study, asthmatic children who were given high-dose prednisone (up to 2 mg/kg per day) for 5 days had normal responses to insulin hypoglycemia 10 days after discontinuing the drug.[164] In addition, on some occasions, the administration of high-dose steroids for as long as a month does not seriously impair the hypothalamic-pituitary-adrenal axis. Children with leukemia who were given high-dose prednisone (2 mg/kg per day) for 1 month had normal basal plasma cortisol 9 days after discontinuation, and this group of patients had normal clinical and plasma cortisol responses to intercurrent stress in the 3 months

FIGURE 14-8. Plasma cortisol response (mean ± SEM) to insulin-induced hypoglycemia [FA] and synthetic ACTH [FB] in 10 subjects before (Δ) and at 2 days (O) and 5 days ( ) after oral prednisone, 25 mg twice daily for 5 days. (*From Streck and Lockwood.*[163])

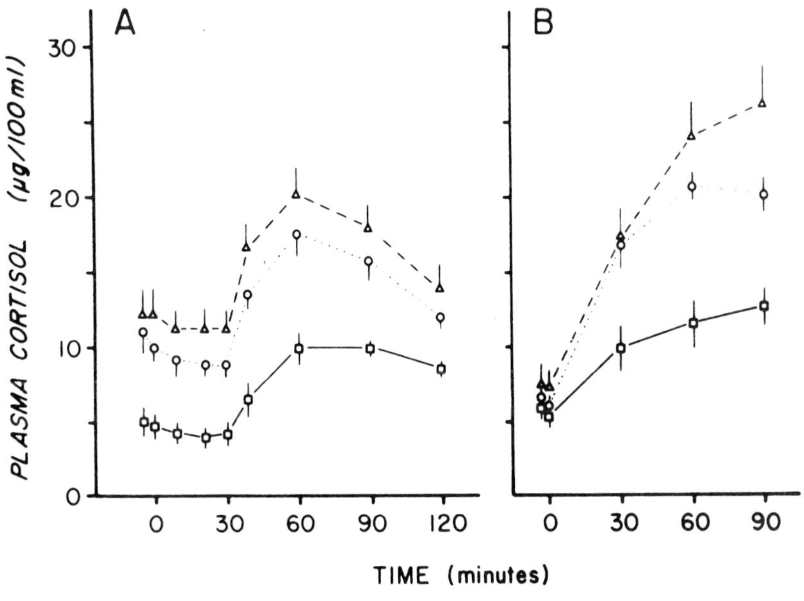

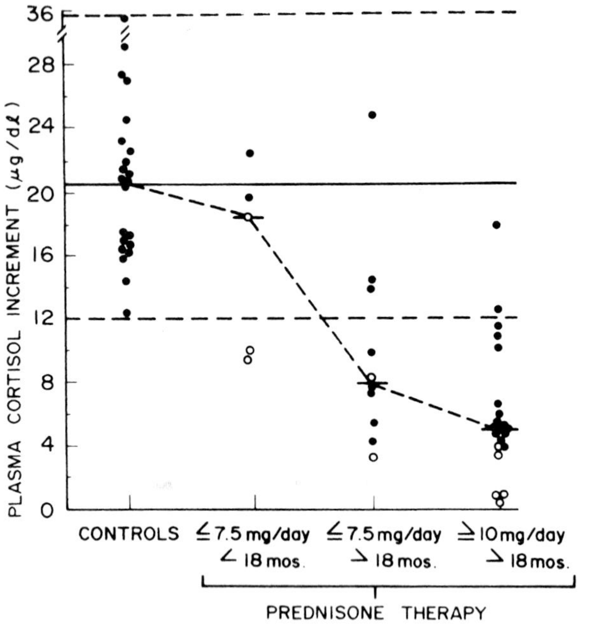

FIGURE 14-9. Plasma cortisol response (shown as the increment) after insulin hypoglycemia testing in control subjects and patients on various doses of glucocorticoids for various times. A dashed line connects median values, the solid line shows the median value for the control subjects, and the horizontal dashed lines show the upper and lower values for the control subjects. For the steroid-treated patients, open circles indicate that the test was performed while the patient was on steroids, and closed circles indicate that the test was performed 48 h after discontinuing therapy. (*Based on data from Livanou et al.*[166])

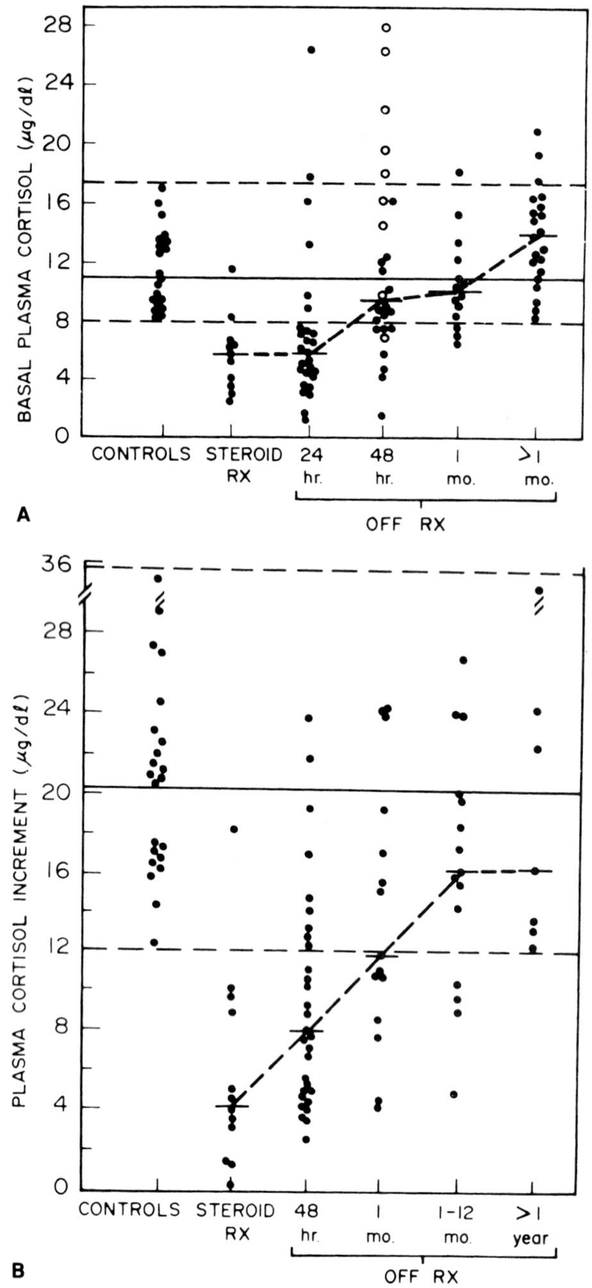

FIGURE 14-10. (*A*) Basal plasma cortisol levels in control subjects, patients on glucocorticoid therapy, and patients in whom glucocorticoid therapy had been withdrawn ("off Rx") for the indicated times. For the period 48 h after steroid withdrawal, open circles indicate the patients who had been on 7.5 mg of prednisone or less and closed circles indicate patients who had been on 10 mg of prednisone or more. (*B*) Plasma cortisol response to insulin-induced hypoglycemia testing in control subjects and patients on glucocorticoid therapy and after withdrawal of therapy for the indicated times. For both panels, heavy dashed lines connect median values. The solid line indicates the median value for the controls, and the lighter dashed line shows the upper and lower values for the control subjects. (*Based on data from Livanou et al.*[166])

after prednisone was discontinued.[165] It is important to note, however, that concurrent major stress of children may negate suppressive effect of glucocorticoids. With lower doses, there may be suppression of basal secretion but normal responsiveness of the axis to stimulation even when the steroid is given for a more prolonged period.[166] Finally, with long-term therapy, particularly in high doses, there is profound and prolonged suppression of the axis and absent responsiveness to major stimuli (Fig. 14-9).[166,167]

The degree of pituitary-adrenal suppression also depends on the timing of the dose and the steroid preparation used.[168] As previously discussed under Alternate-Day Therapy, longer-acting steroids such as dexamethasone result in greater suppression than do short or intermediate-acting compounds such as cortisol, prednisolone, and prednisone, as they are present in the circulation for a longer period.[101,110] Suppression is also greater if glucocorticoids are administered in the evening or at night rather than in the morning because this results in maximal suppression of the normal early morning circadian rise in ACTH.[169] This timing of steroid administration is essential to the success of alternate-day therapy, as described earlier.[149] Also discussed previously was the fact that therapy with ACTH, if given once daily, causes less suppression than does therapy with oral corticosteroids.[123,124]

Kinetics of Return to Normal Axis Function

The kinetics of the return of the hypothalamic-pituitary-adrenal axis are also time- and dose-dependent. Recovery of the axis may require hours to months.[163,166,167] Thus, as mentioned earlier, hypothalamic-pituitary-adrenal responsiveness remains normal after single doses and returns to normal within several days after short courses of glucocorticoids (Fig. 14-8).[163–165] When moderate doses of glucocorticoids have been continued for months to years,

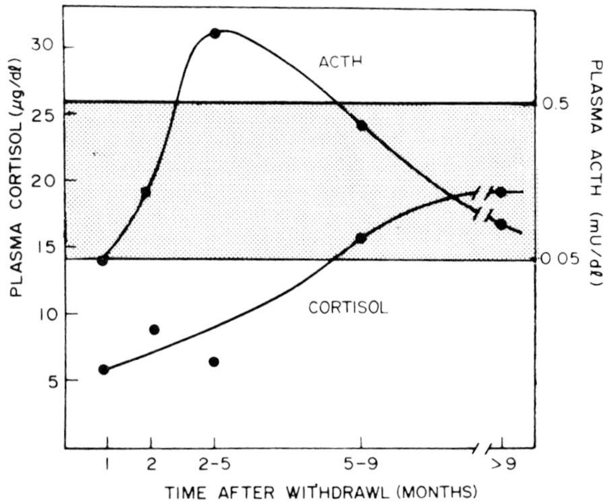

FIGURE 14-11. Median plasma cortisol and ACTH levels (at 6 A.M.) in patients after withdrawal of glucocorticoids. The shaded area indicates the range of values for control subjects. The data were obtained from eight patients with spontaneous Cushing's syndrome after removal of an adrenal tumor and from six patients on high-dose glucocorticoid therapy for 1 to 10 years. Glucocorticoids were not abruptly withdrawn in these patients but instead were tapered over periods of 1 to 4 weeks. The time after withdrawal indicates the period following complete cessation of therapy. (*Based on data from Graber et al.*[167])

recovery is prolonged in general, although considerable individual variability is present (Fig. 14-10).[166] Recovery of both basal cortisol secretion and stress responsiveness is more rapid in patients who have received lower glucocorticoid doses (7.5 mg or less of prednisone per day) and those in whom therapy was of shorter duration.[166] Basal plasma cortisol levels return to normal first, usually within 1 month of the cessation of therapy, but months may be required before the response to insulin-induced hypoglycemia returns to normal (Fig. 14-10).[166]

The kinetics of the return of the axis in patients exposed to higher glucocorticoid concentrations for more prolonged periods (i.e., 1 to 10 years) are shown in Fig. 14-11.[167] In the first month after withdrawal of glucocorticoid excess, both plasma cortisol and ACTH levels were subnormal. During the next several months, plasma ACTH levels increased to supranormal in most of these patients. Despite this, cortisol levels remained low and were subnormally responsive to stimulation with exogenous ACTH, indicating persisting adrenal atrophy.[167] However, at 5 to 9 months the plasma cortisol levels gradually increased into the normal range because of the trophic influence of ACTH, and in this study normal concentrations of plasma cortisol and ACTH were attained in all patients more than 9 months after glucocorticoid withdrawal.[167] Although suppression after more than a year is rare, the author has followed several patients with a successfully resected cortisol-producing adrenal adenoma whose axis has remained suppression for longer than 1 year[168] in spite of otherwise normal pituitary function.[168] Thus, the return of normal axis function requires sequential recovery of the hypothalamus, pituitary, and adrenal. The recovery of the suprapituitary centers is the primary and limiting determinant for recovery[169]; with recovery, ACTH levels gradually rise and stimulate the adrenal. However, they generally need to become elevated before adequate adrenal stimulation occurs with reversal of the adrenal atrophy. As plasma cortisol levels reach the normal range, the feedback inhibition by hydrocortisone begins to suppress ACTH production; as this happens, this axis returns to normal.

As mentioned in Chap. 11, administration of ACTH for 2 to 5 days can increase the responsiveness of the adrenal gland to normal or nearly normal.[166–173] It might therefore seem desirable to administer ACTH to restore such responsiveness to the adrenal. However, the limiting factor in the return of the axis is the ability of the hypothalamus to release CRH. Thus, if ACTH is administered, the subsequent increase in steroid production may in fact impair the return of the hypothalamus to normal.[172] Further, once ACTH is withdrawn, it is still necessary to wait until the hypothalamic-pituitary unit returns to normal function[172] before it can be predicted with confidence that the patient will respond to an insult requiring increased cortisol production. Thus, there is no evidence that ACTH hastens recovery of the axis[170,172,173] when given either as a single course or intermittently for months, and ACTH administration is therefore not recommended.

Steroid Withdrawal Syndromes

The response to withdrawal of steroids can vary. First, the primary disease may remain in remission, and the patient may be asymptomatic. Second, there may be a recurrence or worsening of the disease, and the patient may or may not experience other symptoms of withdrawal. Third, the patient may experience symptoms caused by adrenal insufficiency. Fourth, the patient may experience symptoms similar to those of adrenal insufficiency yet have no biochemical evidence of deficient adrenal secretion ("steroid withdrawal syndrome").[174,175] Perhaps a subclass within the last category is the case in which there is a general lack of well-being without other symptoms or signs of adrenal insufficiency.

In the first case, in which there are no symptoms and the disease for which steroids were given is quiescent, has improved, or has resolved, it is necessary only to follow the disease and the potential for a suppressed axis. Many patients can have a suppressed hypothalamic-pituitary-adrenal axis without symptoms of adrenal insufficiency, and if these patients are exposed to stress (see Chap. 11), they can develop acute adrenal insufficiency. Thus, all the precautions outlined later for the withdrawal procedures should be taken.

In the second case, where there is exacerbation of the primary disease, it may be necessary to reinstitute glucocorticoid therapy. Of course, there are times when this is not warranted. For instance, in acute lymphocytic leukemia of childhood, the development of glucocorticoid resistance precludes further glucocorticoid therapy. In other cases, serious complications of glucocorticoid therapy (e.g., compression fractures and severe osteoporosis) may be present to such an extent that further steroid administration may be more damaging than relief of the primary condition. In cases where therapy is not reinstituted, the precautions relative to hypothalamic-pituitary-adrenal axis suppression must be followed.

The symptoms of adrenal insufficiency that occur with a suppressed hypothalamic-pituitary-adrenal axis are similar to those of secondary adrenal insufficiency discussed in Chap. 11. Thus, the adrenal glomerulosa, with its electrolyte-regulating properties, is almost always intact, so that hyperkalemia is uncommon (see Chap. 11).

The steroid withdrawal syndrome is characterized by symptoms similar or identical to those of adrenocortical insufficiency in a patient who is receiving physiologic doses of glucocorticoids or has a normally responsive hypothalamic-pituitary-adrenal axis.[174,175] The syndrome occurs in patients in whom exogenous glucocorticoid doses are either reduced or withdrawn. Thus, patients may develop the syndrome even though they continue to receive "physiologic" or even supraphysiologic doses of glucocorticoids. The most prominent clinical features are lethargy, malaise, anorexia, nausea, arthralgias, myalgias, weight loss, desquamation of the skin, headache, and fever.[175] Vomiting is less common; postural hypotension may occur occasionally.[175] These symptoms are variable and may be transient.[163] For example, the reduction of the steroid dosage may be accompanied by mild to moderate symptoms that resolve within several days and permit continuation of the lower dose. However, in other patients, the symptoms may be severe and disabling; the persistence of severe symptoms for more than several days is an indication to reinstitute glucocorticoids in small doses (e.g., 10–20 mg of cortisol) or to increase the steroid dose to its former level and then to taper it by smaller decrements over a more prolonged period.

The mechanisms of the steroid withdrawal syndrome are unknown; however, there are two potential explanations. First, it is possible that the transition from higher to lower doses of glucocorticoids, even when the lower dose is "normal," causes the same type of subjective findings as those observed in adrenal insufficiency. Second, it is possible that these patients have a relative state of glucocorticoid resistance that renders them effectively hypoadrenal. However, there is no evidence that this group is in danger of developing acute adrenal insufficiency, suggesting that any resistance, if present, is not severe or complete enough to prevent certain responses to stress. In either case, plasma concentration of interleukin-6 may be elevated which may explain some of the manifestations, including lethargy, malaise, anorexia, nausea, arthralgias, myalgias, headache and fever.[176]

Evaluation of Axis Function

The same considerations discussed in Chap. 12 for evaluation of adrenal insufficiency apply in evaluating suppression of the hypothalamic-pituitary-adrenal axis. First, a normal random cortisol determination does not exclude significant suppression; however, a random plasma cortisol of 18 μg/dl or greater excludes adrenal insufficiency in virtually all circumstances. Conversely, a subnormal random cortisol level may occur during episodic cortisol secretion and thus does not prove suppression of the axis. If the plasma cortisol concentration is 1 μg/dl during an obvious major acute stress (e.g., during shock), significant suppression is likely. However, stimulation tests of the axis are usually required for verification.

The tests used to assess the integrity of the axis are discussed in Chap. 11. Among them, the rapid ACTH stimulation, metyrapone, and insulin-induced hypoglycemia tests are most frequently used. The rapid ACTH stimulation test is more commonly used because of its ease; it is a simple and safe outpatient procedure. If the cortisol response is subnormal, this test confirms suppression of the axis, as deficient cortisol responsiveness indicates adrenal atrophy secondary to ACTH deficiency. However, a normal response to this test does not necessarily predict normal pituitary responsiveness to stress in certain circumstances. These include testing of the hypothalamic-pituitary-adrenal axis within a week of an acute pituitary insult (e.g., Sheehan syndrome) or successful pituitary adenomectomy for Cushing disease. In such cases the insulin tolerance test is more appropriate than the rapid ACTH test (see Chap. 11). Thus, in usual circumstances, a normal response to the rapid ACTH test is sufficient to preclude the necessity of daily maintenance therapy. Another potential problem is the interpretation of the rapid ACTH test in patients with increased cortisol-binding globulin concentrations, including pregnant women, women on high dose estrogen or op'DDD etc. In these patients one should measure free plasma cortisol concentrations and use appropriate normal ranges.

Withdrawal Protocols and Indications for Steroid Coverage

When the status of the disease being treated permits withdrawal of glucocorticoids, both the patient and the physician must be fully aware of the tedious nature and potential difficulty of the process. The patient should be informed of the symptoms of steroid withdrawal; this knowledge may allow differentiation of these symptoms from those caused by worsening of the disease. The patient should also be aware of the potential time required for the return to normal of the axis. Patients who have undergone only short courses of steroid therapy usually do not have great difficulty during steroid withdrawal, but patients on high-dose, long-term therapy may require close monitoring for as long as a year before pituitary-adrenal function returns to normal. In assessing these patients, the physician must assess the underlying disease and the potential symptoms of steroid withdrawal and in addition must serially assess the hypothalamic-pituitary-adrenal-axis.[170]

In patients who have been on long-term glucocorticoid therapy, it is usually necessary to reduce the total dosage more gradually toward physiologic levels, as abrupt changes may precipitate exacerbation of the underlying disease and steroid withdrawal symptoms. For instance, the glucocorticoid dose may be reduced by 2.5 to 5.0 mg of prednisone (or its equivalent) per week. As the dose is being reduced, an attempt should also be made to administer the dose either once daily in the morning or on alternate days to give the hypothalamic-pituitary-adrenal axis a better chance to recover, as previously described. The dose may have to be increased if there is worsening of the underlying disease or if severe symptoms of steroid withdrawal develop. Acute flare-ups or unrelated acute illness should be managed by means of short-term administration of high-dose steroids, with a return to the previous dosage as soon as the clinical situation permits. During this period, adjunctive therapy should also be continued or increased, as this will assist in the control of the primary disorder.

When the total steroid dosage has been tapered to the equivalent of 20 to 30 mg of cortisol or 5 mg of prednisone given as a single morning dose, the function of the hypothalamic-pituitary-adrenal axis should be assessed. The simplest method is to measure basal morning cortisol levels before the daily glucocorticoid dose at 1- to 2-month intervals. When basal cortisol levels are normal (>10 μg/dl), therapy may be withdrawn, because this indicates normal basal steroid secretion. Additionally, at this point, serial assessment of the axis may be begun, also at 1- to 2-month intervals. Persisting subnormal responses to the rapid ACTH stimulation test indicate continuing suppression of the axis (Chap. 11). When normal responsiveness to ACTH occurs, the axis can be presumed to be normal in most patients.

Supplementation with high doses of glucocorticoids may be required at any point in the withdrawal process for acute illness or elective surgery. In these circumstances, increased steroid doses should be administered to patients who have (1) a continuing requirement for glucocorticoid therapy, (2) subnormal basal cortisol levels, (3) subnormal responsiveness to the rapid ACTH stimulation test. A patient who presents with an acute illness and for whom no previous data are available should empirically be covered with steroids, which may be withdrawn rapidly as the acute stress resolves. Similarly, patients undergoing surgery who have a history of prior glucocorticoid therapy may require additional steroid coverage. In these patients, a normal response to ACTH indicates normal function of the axis, and glucocorticoid therapy is not required. If time does not allow an assessment of hypothalamic-pituitary-adrenal axis function, steroid coverage should be given during surgery and the postoperative period. The doses and ancillary procedures for the treatment of acute illness and steroid coverage for surgery in these patients with secondary adrenocortical insufficiency caused by glucocorticoid suppression are detailed in Chap. 11. Generally, doses of steroids equivalent to twofold replacement are given over 24–48 h in patients with febrile illness or minor surgery and equivalent to 5- to 10-fold replacement over 48–72 h in patients with major trauma or surgery.

REFERENCES

1. Baxter JD, Rousseau GG: Glucocorticoid hormone action: An overview, in Baxter JD, Rouseau GG (eds): *Glucocorticoid Hormone Action*. New York, Springer-Verlag, 1979, p 1.
2. Christy NP: Iatrogenic Cushing's syndrome, in Christy NP (ed): *The Human Adrenal Cortex*. New York, Harper & Row, 1971, p 395.
3. Boumpas DM: Glucocorticoid therapy for immune-mediated diseases: Basic and clinical correlates. *Ann Intern Med* 119:1198, 1993.
4. Schleimer R, Claman H, Oronsky A (eds): *Anti-Inflammatory Steroid Action: Basic and Clinical Aspects*. San Diego, Academic, 1989.
5. Lippman ME: Steroids in malignant diseases: Progress in patient selection. *Hosp Pract* 19:93, 1984.
6. Cohen J: Lymphocyte death induced by glucocorticoids, in Schleimer R, Claman H, Ornonsky A (eds): *Anti-Inflammatory Steroid Action: Basic and Clinical Aspects*. San Diego, Academic, 1989, p 110.
7. Bagby GC, Gabourel JD, Linman JW: Glucocorticoid therapy in the preleukemic syndrome (hemopoietic dysplasia). *Ann Intern Med* 92:55, 1980.
8. Brennan MJ: Corticosteroids in the treatment of solid tumors, in Azarnoff DL (ed): *Steroid Therapy*. Philadelphia, Saunders, 1975, p 134.
9. Atkinson JP, Frank MN: Glucocorticoids in the treatment of hemolytic disorders, in Azarnoff DL (ed): *Steroid Therapy*. Philadelphia, Saunders, 1975, p 49.
10. Collins JV, Clark TJH, Brown D, Townsend J: The use of corticosteroids in the treatment of acute asthma. *Q J Med* 44:259, 1975.
11. Bruce C, Weatherstone R, Seaton A, Taylor WH: Histamine levels in plasma, blood and urine in severe asthma and the effect of corticosteroid treatment. *Thorax* 31:724, 1976.
12. Barnes P, Pedersen S: Efficacy and safety of inhaled corticosteroids in asthma. *Am Rev Respir Dis* 148:S1, 1993.
13. Szefler S: Glucocorticoid therapy for asthma: Clinical pharmacology. *J Allergy Clin Immunol* 88:147, 1991.
14. Corrigan C: Mechanism of glucocorticoid action in asthma: Too little, too late. *Clin Exp Allergy* 22:315, 1992.
15. Mitchell DM, Gilfeh P, Rehahn M, Diamond AH, Collins JV: Effects of prednisolone in chronic airflow limitation. *Lancet* 2:193, 1984.
16. Mendella LA, Manfreda J, Warren CPW, Anthonisen NR: Steroid response in stable chronic obstructive pulmonary disease. *Ann Intern Med* 96:17, 1982.
17. Fanta FH, Rossing TH, McFadden ER Jr: Glucocorticoids in acute asthma: A critical controlled trial. *Am J Med* 74:845, 1983.
18. Collins JV, Jones D: Corticosteroid mechanisms and therapeutic schedules, in Weiss EB (ed): *Status Asthmaticus*. Baltimore, University Park Press, 1978, p 235.
19. Frame B, Parfitt AM: Corticosteroid-responsive hypercalcemia with elevated serum 1-alpha, 25-dihydroxyvitamin D. *Ann Intern Med* 93:449, 1980.
20. Tauber MG, Khayam-Bashi H, Sande MA: Effects of ampicillin and corticosteroids on brain water content, cerebral spinal fluid pressure and lactate in experimental pneumococcal meningitis. *J Infect Dis* 151:528, 1985.
21. Ellison GW: Corticosteroids in neurological disease. *Hosp Pract* 19:105, 1984.
22. Fishman RA: Steroids in the treatment of brain edema. *N Engl J Med* 306:359, 1982.
23. Johnson TS, Rock PB, Fulco CS, Trad LA, Spark RF, Maher JT: Prevention of acute mountain sickness by dexamethasone. *N Engl J Med* 310:683, 1984.
24. Markman M, Sheidler V, Ettinger DS, Quaskey SA, Mellits ED: Antiemetic efficacy of dexamethasone: Randomized, double-blind, crossover study with prochlorperazine in patients receiving cancer chemotherapy. *N Engl J Med* 9:549, 1984.
25. Chrousos GA, Kattah JC, Beck RW, et al: Side effects of glucocorticoid treatment. Experience of the optic neuritis treatment trial *JAMA* 269:2110, 1993.
26. Baxter JD: Glucocorticoid hormone action, in Gill GN (ed): *Pharmacology of Adrenal Cortical Hormones*. Oxford, UK, Pergamon, 1979, p 67.
27. Dale DC, Petersdorf RG: Corticosteroids and infectious diseases, in Azarnoff DL (ed): *Steroid Therapy*. Philadelphia, Saunders, 1975, p 209.
28. Kass EH, Finland M: Corticosteroids and infections. *Adv Intern Med* 9:45, 1958.
29. Parrillo JE, Fauci AS: Mechanisms of glucocorticoid action on immune processes. *Annu Rev Pharmacol Toxicol* 19:179, 1979.
30. Rousseau GG, Baxter JD: Glucocorticoid receptors, in Baxter JD, Rousseau GG (eds): *Glucocorticoid Hormone Action*. New York, Springer-Verlag, 1979, p 49.
31. Bamberger CM, Schulte HM, Chrousos GP: Molecular determinants of glucocorticoid receptor function and tissue sensitivity. *Endo Rev* 17:221, 1996.
32. Chrousos GP, Detera-Wadleigh S, Karl M: Syndromes of glucocorticoid resistance. *Ann Int Med* 119:1113, 1993.
33. Baxter JD, MacLeod KM: The molecular basis for hormone action, in Bondy PK, Rosenberg LE (eds): *Metabolic Control and Disease*. Philadelphia, Saunders, 1979, p 104.
34. Gambertoglio JG, Vincenti F, Feduska NJ, Birnbaum J, Salvatierra O, Amend WJC Jr: Prednisolone disposition in cushingoid and noncushingoid kidney transplant patients. *J Clin Endocrinol Metab* 51:561, 1980.
35. Thorn GW, Jenkins D, Laidlow JC, Goetz FC, Dingman JF, Arons WL, Streeten DHP, McCraken BH. Medical progress: Pharmacological aspects of adrenocortical steroids and ACTH in man. *N Engl J Med* 248:232, 1953.
36. Cope CL: *Adrenal Steroids and Disease*, London, Pittman Medical, 1977.
37. Axelrod L: Glucocorticoid therapy. *Medicine (Baltimore)* 55:39, 1976.
38. Bayer JM, Neuner H-P: Cushing-Syndrom und erhohter Augeninnedruck. *Dtsch Med Wochenschr* 40:1791, 1967.
39. George WE Jr, Wilmot M, Greenhouse A, Hammeke M: Medical management of steroid-induced epidural lipomatosis. *N Engl J Med* 308:316, 1983.
40. Russell N, Belanger G, Benoit B, Latter D, Finestone D, Armstrong G: Spinal epidural lipomatosis: A complication of glucocorticoid therapy. *J Can Sci Neurol* 11:383, 1984.
41. Bouzas EA, Scott MH, Mastorakos SG, Gold PW, Chrousos GP, Kaiser-Kupfer MI: Central serous chorioretinopathy in endogenous hypercortisolism. *Arch Ophthalmol* 111:1229, 1993.
42. Polansky JR, Weinreb RN: Anti-inflammatory agents: Steroids as anti-inflammatory agents, in Sears ML (ed): *Handbook of Experimental Pharmacology*. Heidelberg, Springer-Verlag, 1984, vol 69, p 459.
43. Roberts AM, Leibovitz HM: Corticosteroid therapy of ophthalmologic diseases. *Hosp Pract* 19:181, 1984.
44. Ellis EF: Corticosteroid regimens in pediatric practice. *Hosp Pract* 19:143, 1984.
45. Brocklebank JT, Harcourt RB, Meadow SR: Corticosteroid induced cataracts in idiopathic nephrotic syndrome. *Arch Dis Child* 53:30, 1982.
46. Toogood J, Markov A, Baskerville J, Dyson C: Association of ocular cataracts with inhaled and oral steroid therapy during long term

treatment for asthma. *J Allergy Clin Immunol* 91:571, 1993.
47. Manabe S, Bucala R, Cerami A: Nonenzymatic addition of glucocorticoids to lens proteins in steroid-induced cataracts. *J Clin Invest* 74:1803, 1984.
48. Mankin H: Nontraumatic necrosis of bone (osteonecrosis). *N Engl J Med* 326:1473, 1992.
49. Zizic T: Osteonecrosis. *Curr Opin Rheumatol* 3:481, 1991.
50. Zizic TM, Marcoux C, Hungerford DS, Dansereau J-V, Stevens MB: Corticosteroid therapy associated with ischemic necrosis of bone in systemic lupus erythematosis. *Am J Med* 79:596, 1985.
51. Chesney RW, Mayess RB, Rose P, Jax DK: Effect of prednisone on growth and bone mineral content in childhood glomerular disease. *Am J Dis Child* 132:768, 1978.
52. Baylink DJ: Glucocorticoid-induced osteoporosis. *N Engl J Med* 309:306, 1983.
53. Laan R, van Riel P, van de Putte L, van Erning L, van't Hof M, Lemmens J: Low-dose prednisone induces rapid reversible axial bone loss in patients with rheumatoid arthritis. *Ann Intern Med* 119:963, 1993.
54. Reid I, Evans M, Stapleton J: Lateral spine densitometry is a more sensitive indicator of glucocorticoid-induced bone loss. *J Bone Mineral Res* 7:1221, 1992.
55. Adinoff AD, Hollister JR: Steroid-induced fractures and bone loss in patients with asthma. *N Engl J Med* 309:265, 1983.
56. Gluck OS, Murphy WA, Hahn TJ, Hahn B: Bone loss in adults receiving alternate day glucocorticoid therapy. A comparison with daily therapy. *Arthritis Rheum* 24:892, 1981.
57. Spencer H, Rubio N, Rubio E, Indreika M, Seitam A: Chronic alcoholism: Frequently overlooked cause of osteoporosis in men. *Am J Med* 80:393, 1986.
58. Hahn TJ: Corticosteroid-induced osteopenia. *Arch Intern Med* 138:882, 1978.
59. Lukert B, Raisz L: Glucocorticoid-induced osteoporosis: Pathogenesis and management. *Ann Intern Med* 112:352, 1990.
60. Hodgson S: Corticosteroid-induced osteoporosis. *Endocrinol Metab Clin North Am* 19:95, 1990.
61. Libanati C, Baylink D: Prevention and treatment of glucocorticoid-induced osteoporosis. *Chest* 102:1426, 1992.
62. Meunier P: Is steroid-induced osteoporosis preventable? *N Engl J Med* 328:1781, 1993.
63. Hahn T, Halstead L, Teitelbaum S, Hahn B: Altered mineral metabolism in glucocorticoid-induced osteopenia: Effect of 25-hydroxyvitamin D administration. *J Clin Invest* 64:655, 1979.
64. Sambrook P, Birmingham J, Kelly P, Kempler S, Nguyen T, Pocock N, Eisman J: Prevention of corticosteroid osteoporosis. *N Engl J Med* 328:1747, 1993.
65. Saag KG, Emkey R, Schnitzer TJ, Brown JP, Hawkins F, Goemaere S, Thamsborg G, Liberman UA, Delmas PD, Malice MP, Czachur M, Daifotis AG: Alendronate for the prevention and treatment of glucocorticoid-induced osteoporosis. Glucocorticoid-Induced Osteoporosis Intervention Study Group. *N Engl J Med* 339:292, 1998.
66. Reid I, King A, Alexander C, Ibbertson H: Prevention of steroid-induced osteoporosis with (3-amino-1-hydroxypropylidene)-1, 1-bisphonsphonate (APD). *Lancet* 1:143, 1988.
67. Mulder H, Shelder H: Effect of cyclical etidronate regimen on prophylaxis of bone loss of glucocorticoid therapy in postmenopausal women. *Bone Miner* 17:168, 1992.
68. Greenwald M, Brandli D, Spector S, Silverman S, Golde G: Corticosteroid-induced osteoporosis: Effects of a treatment with slow-release sodium fluoride. *Osteoporosis Int* 2:303, 1992.
69. Claman HN: Glucocorticosteroids: II. The clinical responses. *Hosp Pract* 18:143, 1983.
70. Graham BS, Tucker WS Jr: Opportunistic infections in endogenous Cushing's syndrome. *Ann Intern Med* 101:334, 1984.
71. Sheagren J: Glucocorticoid action: Infectious diseases, in Schleimer R, Claman H, Oronsky A (eds): *Anti-Inflammatory Steroid Action: Basic and Clinical Aspects*. San Diego, Academic, 1989, p 525.
72. Czaja AJ, Ludwig J, Baggenstoss AH, Wolff A: Corticosteroid-treated chronic active hepatitis in remission: Uncertain prognosis of chronic persistent hepatitis. *N Engl J Med* 304:5, 1981.
73. Lam KC, Lai CL, Ng RP, Trepo C, Wu PC: Deleterious effect of prednisolone in HBsAg-positive chronic active hepatitis. *N Engl J Med* 304:380, 1981.
74. Hoofnagle JH, Davis GL, Pappas C, Hanson RG, Peters M, Avigan MI, Waggoner JG, Jones EA, Seeff LB: A short course of prednisolone in chronic type B hepatitis: Report of a randomized, double-blind, placebo-controlled trial. *Ann Intern Med* 104:12, 1986.
75. Tuberculosis in corticosteroid-treated asthmatics (editorial). *Br Med J* 2:266, 1976.
76. Fauci AS, Dale DC, Balow JE: Glucocorticosteroid therapy: Mechanisms of action and clinical considerations. *Ann Intern Med* 84:304, 1976.
77. Askari A, Vignos PJ, Moskowitz RW: Steroid myopathy in connective tissue disease. *Am J Med* 61:485, 1976.
78. Horker FF, Scheidegger JR, Grunig BE, Frey FJ: Evidence that prednisone-induced myopathy is reversed by physical training. *J Clin Endocrinol Metab* 61:83, 1985.
79. Nashel DJ: Is atherosclerosis a complication of long-term corticosteroid treatment? *Am J Med* 80:925, 1986.
80. Petri M, Perez-Gutthann S, Spence D, Hochberg M: Risk factors for coronary artery disease in patients with systemic lupus erythematosus. *Am J Med* 93:513, 1992.
81. Plotz C, Knowlton A, Ragan C: The natural history of Cushing's syndrome. *Am J Med* 13:597, 1952.
82. Etxabe J, Vazquez JA: Morbidity and mortality in Cushing's Disease: An epidemiological approach. *Clin Endocrinol (Oxf)* 40:479, 1994.
83. Friedman TC, Mastorakos G, Newman TD, Mullen NH, Horton EG, Costello R, Papadopoulos NM, Chrousos GP: Carbohydrate and lipid metabolism in endogenous hypercortisolism: Shared features with metabolic syndrome X and noninsulin-dependent diabetes mellitus. *Endocrine Journal* 43:645, 1996.
84. Chrousos GP, Gold PW: A healthy body in a healthy mind and vice versa: The damaging 'power of "uncontrollable" stress' (editorial). *J Clin Endocrinol Metab* 83:1842, 1998.
85. Gordan GS: Drug treatment of the osteoporoses. *Annu Rev Pharmacol Toxicol* 18:253, 1978.
86. Litz T, Carter JD, Lewis BI, Suvratt C: Effects of ACTH and cortisone on mood and mentation. *Psychosom Med* 14:363, 1952.
87. Woodbury DM: Relation between the adrenal cortex and the central nervous system. *Pharmacol Rev* 10:275, 1958.
88. Gookler P, Schein J: Psychic effects of ACTH and cortisone. *Psychosom Med* 15:589, 1953.
89. Gustavson LE, Benet LZ: Pharmacokinetics of natural and synthetic glucocorticoids, in Anderson DC, Winter JSD (eds): *The Actual Cortex*. Cornwall, UK, Butterworth, 1985, p 235.
90. Hsueh WA, Pay-Guevara A, Bledsoe T: Studies comparing the clearance rate of 11 gb,17,21-trihydroxypreg-1,4-diene-3,20-dione (prednisolone) after oral 17,21-dihydroxypreg-1,4-diene-3,11,20-trione and intravenous prednisolone. *J Clin Endocrinol Metab* 48:748, 1959.
91. Melby JC: Clinical pharmacology of adrenal steroids, in Thorn GW (ed): *Steroid Therapy*. Kalamazoo, MI, Medcom, 1974, p 16.
92. Fariss BL, Hane S, Shinsako J, Forsham PH: Comparison of absorption of cortisone acetate and hydrocortisone hemisuccinate. *J Clin Endocrinol Metab* 47:1137, 1978.
93. Plumpton FS, Besser GM, Cole PV: Corticosteroid treatment and surgery: II. The management of steroid cover. *Anaesthesia* 24:12, 1969.
94. Wolff ME: Structure-activity relationships in glucocorticoids, in Baxter JD, Rousseau GG (eds): *Glucocorticoid Hormone Action*. New York, Springer-Verlag, 1979, p 97.
95. Robertson DB, Maibach HI: Topical corticosteroids. *Hosp Formulary* 16:1130, 1981.
96. Weston WL: Topical corticosteroids in dermatologic disorders. *Hosp Pract* 19:159, 1984.
97. Braude AC, Rebuck AS: Prednisone and methylprednisolone disposition in the lung. *Lancet* 2:995, 1983.
98. Collaborative Group on Antenatal Steroid Therapy: Effect of antenatal dexamethasone administration on the prevention of respiratory distress syndrome. *Am J Obstet Gynecol* 141:276, 1981.
99. Kream J, Mulay S, Fukushima DK, Solomon S: Determination of plasma dexamethasone in the mother and the newborn after administration of the hormone in a clinical trial. *J Clin Endocrinol Metab* 56:127, 1983.
100. Lewis GP, Jusko WJ, Burke CW, Graves L: Prednisone side effects and serum protein levels. *Lancet* 2:778, 1971.
101. Meikle AW, Tyler FH: Potency and duration of action of glucocorti-

coids: Effects of hydrocortisone, prednisone and dexamethasone on human pituitary-adrenal function. *Am J Med* 63:200, 1977.

102. Ballard PL, Carter JP, Graham BS, Baxter JD: A radioreceptor assay for evaluation of the plasma glucocorticoid activity of natural and synthetic steroids in man. *J Clin Endocrinol Metab* 41:290, 1975.
103. Meikle AW, Weed JA, Tyler FH: Kinetics and interconversion of prednisolone and prednisone studied with new radioimmunoassays. *J Clin Endocrinol Metab* 41:717, 1975.
104. Gifford RH: Corticosteroid therapy for rheumatoid arthritis, in Azarnoff DL (ed): *Steroid Therapy*. Philadelphia, Saunders, 1975, p 78.
105. Rose JQ, Yurchak AM, Jusko WJ: Dose dependent pharmacokinetics of prednisone and prednisolone in man. *J Pharmacokinet Biopharm* 9:389, 1981.
106. Bondy PK: The adrenal cortex, in Bondy PK, Rosenberg LE (eds): *Metabolic Control and Disease*. Philadelphia, Saunders, 1979, p 1427.
107. Haynes RC Jr, Murad F: Adrenocorticotropic hormone; adrenocortical steroids and their synthetic analogs: Inhibitors of adrenocortical steroid biosynthesis, in Gilman AG, Goodman LS, Rall TW, Murad F (eds): *The Pharmacological Basis of Therapeutics*. New York, Macmillan, 1985, p 1459.
108. Dluhy RG, Newmark SR, Lauler DP, Thorn GW: Pharmacology and chemistry of adrenal glucocorticoids, in Azarnoff DL (ed): *Steroid Therapy*. Philadelphia, Saunders, 1975, p 1.
109. Brooks RV: Biosynthesis of adrenocortical steroids, in James VHT (ed): *The Adrenal Gland*. New York, Raven, 1979, p 67.
110. Meikle AW, Clarke DH, Tyler FH: Cushing's syndrome from low doses of dexamethasone. *JAMA* 235:1592, 1976.
111. Hill M, Szefler S, Ball B, Bartoszek M, Brenner A: Monitoring glucocorticoid therapy: A pharmacokinetic approach. *Clin Pharmacol Ther* 48:390, 1990.
112. Kozower M, Veatch L, Kaplan MM: Decreased clearance of prednisone, a factor in the development of corticosteroid side effects. *J Clin Endocrinol Metab* 38:407, 1974
113. Benet LZ, Frey FJ, Amend JC Jr, Lozada F, Frey BM: Endogenous and exogenous glucocorticoids in cushingoid patients. *Drug Intell Clin Pharm* 16:863, 1982
114. Kawai S, Ichikawa Y, Homma M: Differences in metabolic properties among cortisol, prednisolone, and dexamethasone in liver and renal diseases: Accelerated metabolism of dexamethasone in renal failure. *J Clin Endocrinol Metab* 60:848, 1985
115. Boekenoogen SJ, Szefler SJ, Jusko WJ: Prednisolone disposition and protein binding in oral contraceptive users. *J Clin Endocrinol Metab* 56:702, 1983.
116. Harris AW, Baxter JD: Variations in cellular sensitivity to glucocorticoids: Observations and mechanisms, in Baxter JD, Rousseau GG (eds): *Glucocorticoid Hormone Action*. New York, Springer-Verlag, 1979, p 423.
117. Intra-articular steroids (editorial). *Lancet* 1:38, 1984.
118. Clark RA, Anderson PB: Combined therapy with salbutamol and beclomethasone inhalers in chronic asthma. *Lancet* 2:70, 1978.
119. High dose corticosteroid inhalers for asthma (editorial). *Lancet* 2:23, 1984.
120. McAllen MK, Kochanowski SJ, Shaw KM: Steroid aerosols in asthma: An assessment of betamethasone valerate and a twelve month study of patients on maintenance treatment. *Br Med J* 1:171, 1974.
121. Chrousos GP, Harris AG: Hypothalamic-pituitary-adrenal axis suppression and inhaled corticosteriod therapy. Part I. General principles. *Neuroimmunodulation* 5:277, 1998.
122. Chrousos GP, Harris AG: Hypothalamic-pituitary-adrenal axis suppression and inhaled corticosteroid therapy Part II. Review of the literature. *Neuroimmunodulation* 5:288, 1998.
123. Daly JR, Fletcher MR, Glass D, Chambers DJ, Bitensky L, Chayen L: Comparison of effects of long term corticotrophin and corticosteroid treatment on responses of plasma growth hormone, ACTH and corticosteroid to hypoglycemia. *Br Med J* 2:521, 1974.
124. Bacon PA, Daly JR, Myles AB, Savage O: Hypothalamo-pituitary-adrenal function in patients on long-term adrenocorticotrophin therapy. *Ann Rheum Dis* 27:7, 1968.
125. Axelrod L: Glucocorticoids, in Kelly W, Harris E, Ruddy S, Sledge C (eds): *Textbook of Rheumatology*. Philadelphia, Saunders, 1989, p 845.
126. Chrousos G, Kattah J, Beck R, Cleary P, Group ONS: Side effects of glucocorticoid treatment: Experience of the optic neuritis treatment trial. *JAMA* 269:2110, 1993.
127. Vincenti F, Amend W, Feduska NJ, Duca RM, Salvatierra JRO: Improved outcome following renal transplantation with reduction in the immunosuppression therapy for rejection episodes. *Am J Med* 69:107, 1980.
128. Bagby GC Jr, Lawrence HJ, Neerhout RC: T-lymphocyte-mediated granulopoietic failure: In vitro identification of prednisone-responsive patients. *N Engl J Med* 309:1073, 1983.
129. Schumer W: Steroids in the treatment of clinical septic shock. *Ann Surg* 184:333, 1976.
130. Sheagren JN: Septic shock and corticosteroids. *N Engl J Med* 305:456, 1981.
131. Sprung CL, Panagiota V, Caralis MD, Marcial RTT, Pierce M, Gelbard MA, Long WM, Duncan RC, et al: The effects of high dose corticosteroids in patients with septic shock. *N Engl J Med* 311:1137, 1984.
132. Jacob HS: Pulse steroids in hematologic diseases. *Hosp Pract* 20:87, 1985.
133. Morris PJ, Chan L, French ME, Ting A: Low dose oral prednisolone in renal transplantation. *Lancet* 1:525, 1982.
134. Hinshaw LB, Archer LT, Beller-Todd BK, Coalson JJ, Flournoy DJ, Passey R, Benjamin B, White GL: Survival of primates in LD_{100} septic shock following steroid/antibiotic therapy. *J Surg Res* 28:151, 1980.
135. Hoffman SL, Punjabi NH, Kumala S, Moechtar A, Pulungsih SP, Rivai AR, Rockhill RC, Woodward TE, Loedin AA: Reduction of mortality in chloramphenicol-treated severe typhoid fever by high-dose dexamethasone. *N Engl J Med* 310:82, 1984.
136. Meduri GV, Chrousos GP: Duration of glucocorticoid treatment and outcome in sepsis: Is the right drug used the wrong way? (editorial). *Chest* 114:355, 1998.
137. Felson DT, Anderson J: Evidence for the superiority of immunosuppressive drugs and prednisone over prednisone alone in lupus nephritis. *N Engl J Med* 311:1528, 1984.
138. Kyle RA, Greipp PR, Garton JP, Gertz MA: Primary systemic amyloidosis: Comparison of melphalan/prednisone versus colchicine. *Am J Med* 79:708, 1985.
139. Cogan MG, Sargent JA, Yarbrough SG, Vincenti F, Amend WJ Jr: Prevention of prednisone-induced negative nitrogen balance: Effect of dietary modification on urea generation rate in hemodialyzed patients receiving high dose glucocorticoids. *Ann Intern Med* 95:158, 1981.
140. Hunt TK, Ehrlich HP, Garcia JA, Dunphy JE: Effect of vitamin A on reversing the inhibitory effect of cortisone on healing of open wounds in animals and man. *Ann Surg* 170:633, 1969.
141. Baigelman W, Chodosh S, Pizzuto D, Cupples LA: Sputum and blood eosinophils during corticosteroid treatment of acute exacerbations of asthma. *Am J Med* 75:929, 1983.
142. Lawrence EC, Teague RB, Gottlieb MS, Jhingran SG, Liberman J: Serial changes in markers of disease activity with corticosteroid treatment in sarcoidosis. *Am J Med* 74:747, 1983.
143. Harter JG, Reddy WJ, Thorn GW: Studies on an intermittent corticosteroid dosage regimen. *N Engl J Med* 269:591, 1963.
144. Fauci AS: Corticosteroids in autoimmune disease. *Hosp Pract* 18:99, 1983.
145. Fauci AS: Alternate-day corticosteroid therapy. *Am J Med* 64:729, 1978.
146. Fleisher DS, Pellecchier P: Pituitary-adrenal responsiveness after corticosteroid therapy in children with nephrosis. *J Pediatr* 70:54, 1967.
147. Hunder GG, Sheps SG, Allen GL, Joyce JW: Daily and alternate day corticosteroid regimens in treatment of giant cell arteritis: Comparison in a prospective study. *Ann Intern Med* 82:613, 1975.
148. Foote KD, Brocklebank JT, Meadow SR: Height attainment in children with steroid-responsive nephrotic syndrome. *Lancet* 2:917, 1985.
149. Ackerman GL, Nolan CM: Adrenocortical responsiveness after alternate-day corticosteroid therapy. *N Engl J Med* 278:405, 1968.
150. Schurmeyer TH, Tsokos GC, Avgerinos PC, Balow JE, D'Agata R, Loriaux DL, Chrousos GP: Pituitary-adrenal responsiveness to corti

cotropin-releasing hormone in patients receiving chronic, alternate day glucocorticoid therapy. *J Clin Endocrinol Metab* 61:22, 1985.
151. Wyatt R, Waschek J, Weinberger M, Sherman B: Effects of inhaled beclomethasone dipropionate and alternate day prednisone on pituitary-adrenal function in children with chronic asthma. *N Engl J Med* 299:1387, 1978.
152. Fauci AS, Dale DC: Alternate day prednisone therapy and human lymphocyte subpopulations. *J Clin Invest* 55:22, 1975.
153. Harter JG: Alternate day therapy, in Thorn GW (ed): *Steroid Therapy*. Kalamazoo, MI, Medcom, 1974, p 42.
154. Schatz M, Patterson R, Zeit S, O'Rourke J, Melam H: Corticosteroid therapy for the pregnant asthmatic patient. *JAMA* 233:804, 1975.
155. Greenberger PA, Patterson R: Beclomethasone dipropionate for severe asthma during pregnancy. *Ann Intern Med* 98:478, 1983.
156. Rayburn W: Glucocorticoid therapy for rheumatic diseases: Maternal, fetal, and breast-feeding considerations. *Am J Reprod Immunol Microbiol* 28:138, 1992.
157. Committee on Drugs AAoP: The transfer of drugs and other chemicals into human breast milk. *Pediatrics* 84:924, 1989.
158. Katz F, Duncan B: Entry of prednisone into human milk. *N Engl J Med* 293:1154, 1975.
159. Ost L, Wettrell G, Bjorkhem I, Rane A: Prednisolone excretion in human milk. *J Pediatr* 106:1008, 1985.
160. Messer J, Reitman D, Sacko H, Smith H, Chalmer T: Association of adrenocorticosteroid therapy and peptic ulcer disease. *N Engl J Med* 309:21, 1983.
161. Piper J, Ray W, Daugherty J, Griffin M: Corticosteroid use and peptic ulcer disease: Role of nonsteroidal anti-inflammatory drugs. *Ann Intern Med* 114:735, 1991.
162. Real FX, Krown SE, Koziner B: Steroid-related development of Kaposi's sarcoma in a homosexual man with Burkitt's lymphoma. *Am J Med* 30:119, 1986.
163. Streck WF, Lockwood DH: Pituitary adrenal recovery following short-term suppression with corticosteroids. *Am J Med* 66:910, 1979.
164. Zora J, Zimmerman D, Carey T, O'Connell E, Yunginger J: Hypothalamic-pituitary-adrenal axis suppression after short-term, high-dose glucocorticoid therapy in children with asthma. *J Allergy Clin Immunol* 77:9, 1986.
165. Lightner E, Johnson H, Corrigan J: Rapid adrenocortical recovery after short-term glucocorticoid therapy. *Am J Dis Child* 135:790, 1981.
166. Livanou T, Ferriman D, James VHT: Recovery of hypothalamo-pituitary-adrenal function after corticosteroid therapy. *Lancet* 2:856, 1967.
167. Graber AL, Ney RL, Nicholson WE, Island DP, Liddle GW: Natural history of pituitary-adrenal recovery following long-term suppression with corticosteroids. *J Clin Endocrinol Metab* 25:11, 1965.
168. Doherty JM, Nieman LK, Culter GB, Chrousos GP, Norton J: Time to recovery of the hypothalamic-pituitary-adrenal axis following curative resection of adrenal tumors in patients with Cushing's syndrome. *Surgery* 108:1085, 1990.
169. Gomez MT, Magiakou MA, Mastorakos G, Chrousos GP: The pituitary corticotroph is not the rate limiting step in the postoperative recovery of the hypothalamic-pituitary-adrenal axis in patients with Cushing's syndrome. *J Clin Endocrinol Metab* 77:173, 1993.
170. Byyny RL: Withdrawal from glucocorticoid therapy. *N Engl J Med* 295:30, 1976.
171. Nichols T, Nugent CA, Tyler FH: Diurnal variation in suppression of adrenal function by glucocorticoids. *J Clin Endocrinol Metab* 25:343, 1965.
172. Donald RA, Espiner EA: The plasma cortisol and corticotropin response to hypoglycemia following adrenal steroid and ACTH administration. *J Clin Endocrinol Metab* 41:1, 1975.
173. Steroid therapy and the adrenals (editorial). *Lancet* 2:537, 1975.
174. Dixon RB, Christy NP: On the various forms of corticosteroid withdrawal syndrome. *Am J Med* 68:224, 1980.
175. Amatruda TT, Hurst MM, D'Esopo ND: Certain endocrine and metabolic facets of the steroid withdrawal syndrome. *J Clin Endocrinol Metab* 25:1207, 1965.
176. Papanicolaou DA, Tsigos C, Oldfield EH, Chrousos GP: Acute glycocorticoid deficiency is associated with plasma elevation of interlocking 6: Does the latter participate in the symptomatology of the steriod withdrawal syndrome and adrenal insufficiency? *J Clin Endocrinol Metab* 81:2303, 1996.

PART V

Gonadal Disease

CHAPTER 15

The Testis

Alvin M. Matsumoto

INTRODUCTION

The two major functions of the human testis are to produce the sex steroid hormone, testosterone, and mature spermatozoa. The testis plays important physiological roles during various stages of human development.[1] During embryonic development, production of testosterone and Müllerian inhibiting substance by the fetal testis is required for normal primary male sexual differentiation (see Chap. 17). At the time of puberty, increased production of testosterone by the testis is necessary for the development of normal male secondary sexual characteristics and sexual function, and the initiation of spermatogenesis, which is required for future fertility. In the adult male, continued normal production of testosterone and sperm are necessary for the maintenance of normal virilization, sexual function, and fertility. Therefore, the clinical manifestations of disorders that affect testis function will vary depending on the stage of development during which testicular dysfunction occurs.

Disorders of testicular function occur commonly and are associated with significant clinical consequences in affected men. Klinefelter syndrome, a chromosomal disorder that affects approximately one in every 400–500 males, results in permanent androgen deficiency and infertility.[2,3] Infertility due to impaired sperm production affects 5–6% of otherwise healthy men and usually results in a permanent inability to father children.[4–6] Testicular dysfunction occurs commonly in association with chronic systemic illnesses, malnutrition, wasting syndromes, the use of certain medications, and normal aging. Erectile dysfunction and gynecomastia, major manifestations of androgen deficiency, are common complaints in men, especially as they age. Finally, germ cell cancers of the testis are one of the most fatal neoplasms affecting young men.

Although most testicular disorders are not curable, they can be treated in many instances, resulting in significant improvements in the quality of life of affected men. In androgen-deficient men, testosterone replacement therapy can induce and restore secondary sexual characteristics and normal sexual functioning. With the realization that androgen deficiency occurs commonly in association with a variety of systemic illnesses, medications, and normal aging, there has been renewed interest recently in the development of new androgen formulations for therapeutic use, e.g., testosterone patches and gel. In men with testicular dysfunction due to hypogonadotopic hypogonadism, gonadotropin or pulsatile gonadotropin-releasing hormone therapy is able to stimulate the production of both testosterone and sperm production, and therefore, treat the infertility associated with these disorders. Recently, recombinant human follicle-stimulating hormone preparations have become available for clinical use, providing an alternative to the purified urinary preparations used previously. Advances in artificial reproductive technologies, specifically intracytoplasmic sperm injection, have made fertility possible in infertile men due to a variety of causes. GnRH analogues and pure antiandrogens are used routinely now to induce androgen deficiency and block androgen action, respectively, in androgen-dependent pathological states such as prostate cancer. Finally, seminomas are exquisitely sensitive to radiotherapy and curable, and multidrug chemotherapy regimens have markedly improved survival and cure rates in men with nonseminoma germ cell cancers.

ANATOMY AND DEVELOPMENT

The testis is controlled by the gonadotropins, luteinizing hormone (LH), and follicle stimulating hormone (FSH), which are secreted by the anterior pituitary gland. Pituitary gonadotropin secretion is regulated by episodic release of gonadotropin-releasing hormone (GnRH) produced by neurons in hypothalamus of the brain; feedback control by sex steroid hormones, primarily testosterone and estradiol; and peptide hormones, such as inhibin B secreted by the testis.

Hypothalamic-Pituitary Axis and the Central Nervous System

The hypothalamus is the part of the diencephalon that surrounds the inferior portion of the third ventricle at the base of the brain. It is delineated by the optic chiasm rostrally, the mammary bodies caudally, the optic tracts laterally, the hypothalamic stalk dorsally, and the infundibulum ventrally. The hypothalamic GnRH neuronal system is composed of a relatively small number of perikarya (~1,000) concentrated predominantly in the *arcuate* or *infundibular nucleus* of *medial basal hypothalamus* and forebrain areas (*medial septal area, diagonal band of Broca, medial preoptic area, lamina terminalis,*) with sparse numbers of cell bodies in anterior hypothalamic areas (*suprachiasmatic, supraoptic, and paraventricular nucleus*) and the *premamillary nucleus* caudally.[7,8]

Axons from GnRH cell bodies project to the internal and external neurovascular contact zones of the *median eminence* where they terminate directly onto capillaries of the *hypothalamic-hypophyseal portal system.*[7–9] GnRH secreted from these axon terminals into the hypothalamic capillary bed is transported through portal veins that descend in the pituitary or infundibular stalk to another capillary bed in the anterior pituitary, where it stimulates synthesis and release of LH and FSH from the gonadotropin-producing cells (gonadotrophs). GnRH fibers also project to other GnRH neurons and brain regions (e.g., *organum vasculosum of the lamina terminalis,* part of the circumventricular system) where they serve as a neuromodulator of other neurons. Because the infundibulum (Latin for "funnel") and hypophyseal portal system occupy a relatively narrow and small area, they are susceptible to pathological processes that affect the base of brain (e.g., granulomatous diseases such as sarcoidosis) and pituitary stalk damage (e.g., associated with basilar skull fracture). These disease processes often cause defects in GnRH secretion and secondary hypogonadism, in addition to loss of other anterior pituitary function and hyperprolactinemia.

Embryologically, GnRH neurons originate from outside the central nervous system in the epithelium of the olfactory pit or placode at about 4 to 6 weeks of gestation and migrate from the nose to their final destination in the forebrain and hypothalamus along nerve fibers of the terminal, olfactory, and vomeronasal nerves that are rich in neural-cell adhesion molecule (N-CAM).[10,11] *Kallmann syndrome* is a developmental disorder characterized by GnRH deficiency and anosmia or hyposmia. In X chromosome-linked forms of Kallmann syndrome, a deletion of the KAL-1 gene located on the short arm of the X chromosome (Xp22.3) and deficiency of its product, anosmin-1, an extracellular matrix adhesion protein, result in functional GnRH deficiency due to failure of migration of GnRH neurons from the olfactory placode to the hypothalamus, and anosmia or hyposmia due to dysgenesis of the olfactory bulbs.[12–14]

The negative feedback influence of testosterone and its active metabolites, estradiol and dihydrotestosterone, on gonadotropin secretion occurs both at the level of hypothalamic GnRH and pituitary gonadotropin secretion. Although sex steroid hormone receptors are present in brain areas where GnRH neurons are concentrated, GnRH neurons themselves have not been demonstrated to possess androgen or estrogen receptors.[15,16] Therefore, steroid negative feedback regulation of GnRH neurons is mediated largely through androgen and estrogen actions on neurons that secrete neurotransmitters and neuromodulators that, in turn, control GnRH synthesis and/or secretion.

GnRH neurons receive neuromodulatory inputs from a large number of neuronal systems within the central nervous system (see Chapter 6). These include neurons that produce: norepinephrine and serotonin from brainstem nuclei; dopamine from brainstem and hypothalamic nuclei; neuropeptide Y (NPY) from the arcuate nucleus; pro-opiomelanocortin (POMC) that produce the endogenous opiate, β-endorphin, and melanocortin, α-melanocyte-stimulating hormone (α-MSH), from the arcuate nucleus; corticotropin-releasing hormone (CRH) from the paraventricular nucleus; neurotensin from the arcuate and medial preoptic nucleus; and excitatory (e.g., glutamate and aspartate) and inhibitory (e.g., γ-aminobutyric acid, GABA) amino acids from a number of hypothalamic nuclei.[8,17]

GnRH released episodically from the ME into the hypophyseal portal system is carried to the anterior pituitary where it stimulates gonadotropin-producing cells (gonadotrophs), which are interspersed throughout the adenohypophysis. Gonadotrophs express cell surface GnRH receptors and most all gonadotrophs produce both LH and FSH that are secreted into the systemic circulation.[18] Only a few gonadotrophs produce LH or FSH exclusively.

Testis

Adult Testis

The normal adult human testes are paired organs that hang down within the scrotum. Each testis measures 3.5–5.5 cm in length × 2.0–3.0 cm in width, and has a volume of 15–30 mL.[19,20] The testis is composed of two structurally distinct functional compartments: the *seminiferous tubule compartment* containing Sertoli cells and developing germ cells that produce mature spermatozoa, and the *interstitial compartment* containing Leydig cells that secrete testosterone.[21,22] Seminiferous tubules comprise about 80–90% of the volume of the testis so that clinically, a very small testis size on physical examination usually indicates significantly reduced total sperm production.

Blood supply to the testis is provided primarily by the internal spermatic or testicular artery with contributions from the cremasteric and vasa deferential arteries. Under the fibrous capsule of the testis, *tunica albuginea,* the testicular artery branches initially over the lower pole of the testis.[23] Fibrous septa emanate from the tunica albuginea into the parenchyma of the testis to form lobules.

During fetal and neonatal development, the testes descend from within the abdomen into their normal scrotal position in the adult (see later discussion). Location of the testes in the scrotum exposes them to a temperature that is approximately 2°C lower than the abdomen. Furthermore, venous drainage from the testis forms a pampiniform plexus that surrounds the testicular artery with cooler venous blood and provides a countercurrent heat exchange mechanism that cools the arterial blood supply to the testis. The lower temperature of the testis is essential for normal spermatogenesis. Alterations in these cooling mechanisms such as occur with failure of normal testicular descent into scrotum (*cryptorchidism*) or varicose veins of the scrotum (*varicocele*) may result impaired sperm production and function.

Blood from the pampiniform venous plexus drains into the internal spermatic or testicular vein. On the right, the internal spermatic vein enters directly into the inferior vena cava, and on the left, it drains into the left renal vein. Absence or failure of valves in the left internal spermatic vein is thought to be responsible for the predominance of varicocele in the left scrotum. Presence of a prominent varicocele on right may indicate obstruction of venous return by tumor or lymphadenopathy, or *situs inversus.*

Interstitium

Leydig, or interstitial cells, are the steroid-producing cells of the testis. They measure 10–25 μm in size, are polygonal in shape, and contain a characteristic ovoid nucleus with a prominent nucleolus.[21,22] The adult testes contain about 430 million Leydig cells, comprising approximately 5% of the testis volume.[24] Clusters of Leydig cells are contiguous with capillaries in the interstitium (Fig. 15-1), into which they secrete sex steroids, primarily testosterone that is delivered to testicular veins and into the systemic circulation. Leydig cells are in close proximity to seminiferous tubules, facilitating delivery of the relatively high concentrations of testosterone that are required for initiation and maintenance of spermatogenesis.

Peritubular myoid cells and fibroblasts surround the seminiferous tubules. Peritubular cells are contractile and involved in transport of fluid and sperm through the seminiferous tubules.[21,22] They also contain androgen receptors and are thought to mediate some of the paracrine effects of testosterone and other factors on adjacent Sertoli and germ cells in the seminiferous tubules. Macrophages in

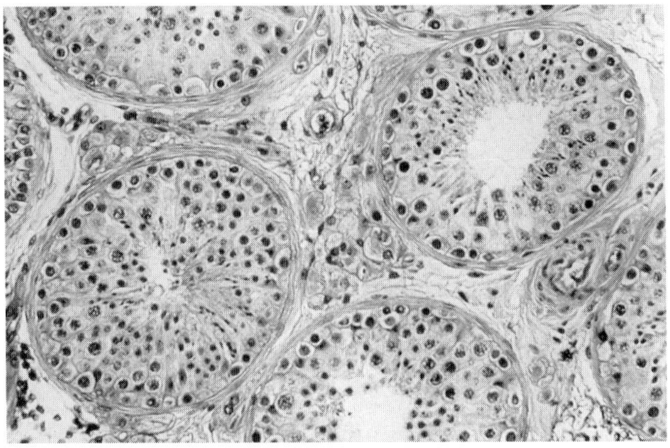

FIGURE 15-1. Light photomicrograph of the normal human testis. Note the cluster of Leydig cells (most prominent in the middle of the photomicrograph) in the interstitium between numerous seminiferous tubules at various stages of spermatogenesis. (*From Matsumoto.*[100])

the interstitial compartment may regulate testis function through local secretion of cytokines and by phagocytosis of degenerating cells. Arterioles and the rich network of capillaries in the interstitium serve to deliver the main endocrine regulators of testis function, the pituitary gonadotropins, LH, and FSH. Lymphatic vessels provide lymph drainage from the testis.

Seminiferous Tubule

Seminiferous tubules serve as the continuous conduit into which sperm are released for transport into the rete testis, efferent ducts, epididymis, and vas deferens for ultimate ejaculation. Individual tubules measure approximately 0.12–0.30 mm in diameter and up to 70 cm in length but are tightly coiled within the lobules of the testis. Therefore, histological sections of a testis biopsy reveal cross-sections of many different seminiferous tubules (Fig. 15-1).[21,22] A basal lamina composed of extracellular matrix separates seminiferous tubules from the interstitial compartment. An extracellular matrix, produced by Leydig, peritubular, and Sertoli cells, provides structural integrity to the testis and seminiferous tubules and regulates the function of cells in contact with it.

Seminiferous tubules contain columnar Sertoli cells that extend from the basal lamina to the lumen of the tubule and envelope developing germ cells (Fig. 15-2).[21,22] Sertoli cells provide developing germ cells with a structural scaffolding and secrete numerous products that support spermatogenesis. Sertoli cells are characterized by their elongated, folded, or indented nucleus containing a large, basally positioned nucleolus. Lying along the basal lamina of seminiferous tubules, stem cells known as *spermatogonia* are interspersed with Sertoli cells. Lateral cytoplasmic projections of adjacent Sertoli cells surround the spermatogonia and form specialized junctional complexes or tight junctions that impede the passage of large molecules, steroid hormones, and ions. These junctions constitute the structural basis for the blood-testis barrier. Sertoli cell tight junctions divide the seminiferous tubule into an outer *basal compartment* containing spermatogonia, and an inner *adluminal compartment* that contains developing spermatocytes undergoing meiosis and spermatids undergoing maturation (spermiogenesis) that develop within evaginations of Sertoli cell cytoplasm (Fig. 15-2). Thus, developing germ cells occupy positions within the tubule closer to the lumen as they become more differentiated. Upon completion of spermatogenesis and spermiogenesis, mature spermatozoa are released into the lumen of seminiferous tubule (spermiation).

FIGURE 15-2. (*Top*) Diagrammatic representation of a seminiferous tubule to illustrate the relation between the lining membrane structures (i.e., basal lamina and myoid cells), Sertoli cell cytoplasm, and germinal epithelial cells. (*Bottom*) As above, with deletion of germinal cells. The basal or outer compartment lies outside the tight-junction barrier formed by the Sertoli cells, whereas the adluminal compartment lies within it.

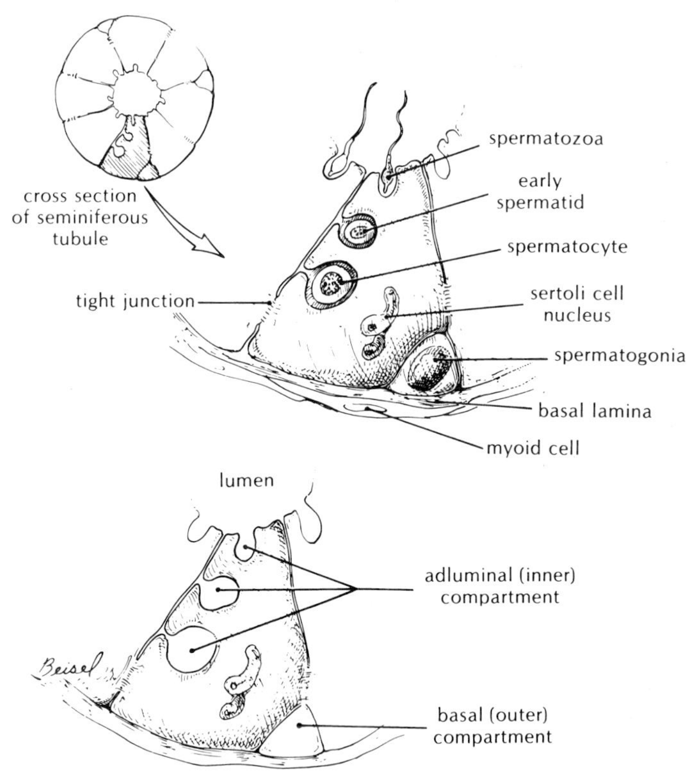

Spermatogonia present within the basal compartment of the seminiferous tubule are the only germ cells that are directly accessible to endocrine and paracrine regulatory factors from the interstitium. Because molecules from the circulation and interstitium are not directly accessible to the adluminal compartment of the seminiferous tubule, Sertoli cells synthesize and secrete a number of products and provide the appropriate microenvironment to support and regulate the processes of spermatogenesis, spermiogenesis, and spermiation.[25,26] Sertoli cells contain both FSH and androgen receptors and, therefore, mediate the endocrine effects of FSH and paracrine effects of testosterone, produced by Leydig cells in response to LH, on spermatogenesis.[27,28] Early reports of androgen receptors on spermatogonia have not been confirmed.[29] Sertoli cells also produce MIS and *inhibin B,* a glycoprotein hormone that mediates negative feedback suppression of FSH secretion from the pituitary gland.[25,26]

Germ Cell Development

The human testis produces approximately 120 million sperm daily.[30] In order to sustain this production rate, both a pool of uncommitted, undifferentiated stem cells held in reserve as well as a pool of cells committed to full differentiation are required. Spermatogenesis may be divided into three functionally distinct phases: the *proliferative phase,* during which most spermatogonia undergo mitotic division in a manner analogous to somatic cells to replenish the stem cell pool (stem cell renewal) and a minority of spermatogonia become committed to further differentiation and produce spermatocytes; the *meiotic phase,* during which spermatocytes undergo meiosis, a process unique to germinal tissue, to give rise to haploid spermatids; and *spermiogenesis,* during which immature round spermatids differentiate into elongated mature spermatozoa that are capable of motility and fertilizing an ovum (Fig. 15-3).[22,31]

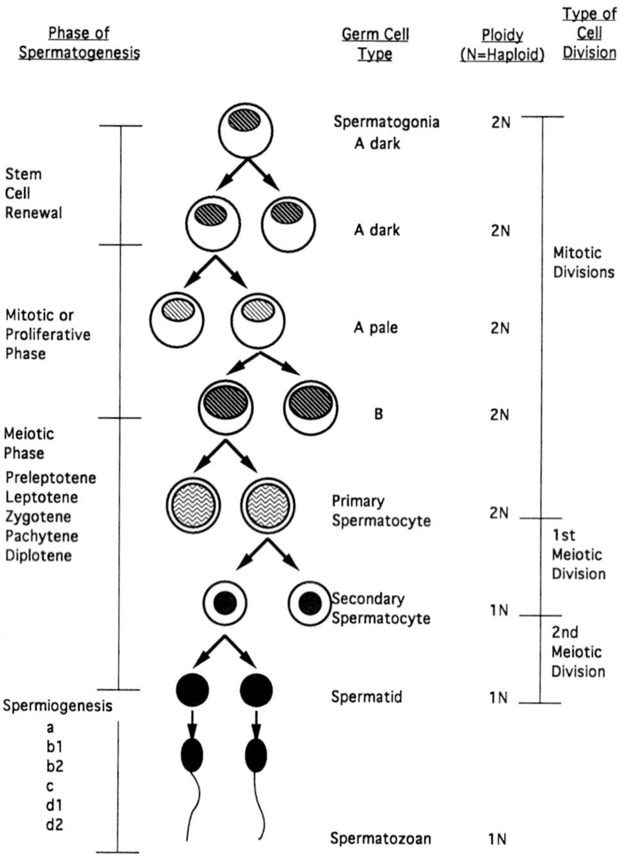

FIGURE 15-3. Schematic diagram of the phases of spermatogenesis and the corresponding germ cell types, chromosomal number or ploidy (N, haploid number), and type of cell division occurring within each phase. (*From Matsumoto.*[100])

Proliferative Phase

Spermatozoa are classified into three major types, which are distinguished by the staining and pattern of chromatin in their nucleus: A dark (A_d), A pale (A_p), and B spermatogonia (Fig. 15-3). A_d spermatogonia are characterized by darkly staining, dense chromatin with a central pale area, and their cytoplasm is closely applied to the basal lamina. Because of their low mitotic rate, they are thought to be the spermatogonial stem cells. A_d spermatogonia are relatively resistant to external insults (e.g., ionizing radiation), after which they undergo mitotic division to replenish the spermatogonial population. Complete depletion of A_d spermatogonia such as occurs with high-dose irradiation or vascular compromise causes irreversible loss of spermatogenic capacity.[32]

During the proliferative phase of spermatogenesis, some A_d spermatogonia undergo mitosis to form A_p spermatogonia, which are characterized by pale-staining, less dense chromatin with one or two nucleoli attached to the nuclear membrane. The latter undergo further mitotic division to form B spermatogonia, which have darkly staining clumps of chromatin along the rim of the nuclear membrane. In humans, the rate of mitotic division of A to B spermatogonia is relatively low, resulting in a submaximal number of B spermatogonia available to enter meiosis and limiting the efficiency of spermatogenesis.[33] B spermatogonia are the most radiosensitive germ cells and therefore are commonly reduced by external irradiation of the testis.[32]

B spermatogonia that become committed to further differentiation undergo mitotic division to produce preleptotene or resting spermatocytes, which enter a prolonged (24 days) meiotic phase. Spermatogonia do not completely separate during mitotis (incomplete cytokinesis). Groups of germ cells remain connected to each other via thin cytoplasmic bridges and undergo meiosis and further development synchronously within this syncytium.[34]

Preleptotene primary spermatocytes are slightly smaller and have fewer chromatin clumps than B spermatogonia. As a result of active DNA synthesis, preleptotene spermatocytes contain a diploid complement of chromosomes (46 chromosomes or 2N, where N is a haploid number of chromosomes). However, because each chromosome is compromised of a pair of identical sister chromatids, the total DNA content is twice the diploid content (4N) (Fig. 15-3). Preleptotene primary spermatocytes are located in the adluminal compartment and are the last germ cells to undergo DNA synthesis.

Meiotic Phase

Meiosis I After DNA synthesis and sister chromatid formation are completed, spermatocytes enter prophase (prophase I) of the first meiotic division (meiosis I), which is characteristically long in duration (Figs. 15-3 and 15-4).[22] Primary spermatocytes pass successively through five stages during prophase I: leptotene I, during which chromosomes condense but are unpaired; zygotene I, during which homologous chromosomes begin to pair (synapsis); and pachytene I, which lasts for 2 weeks and during which homologous chromosomes each composed of two sister chro-

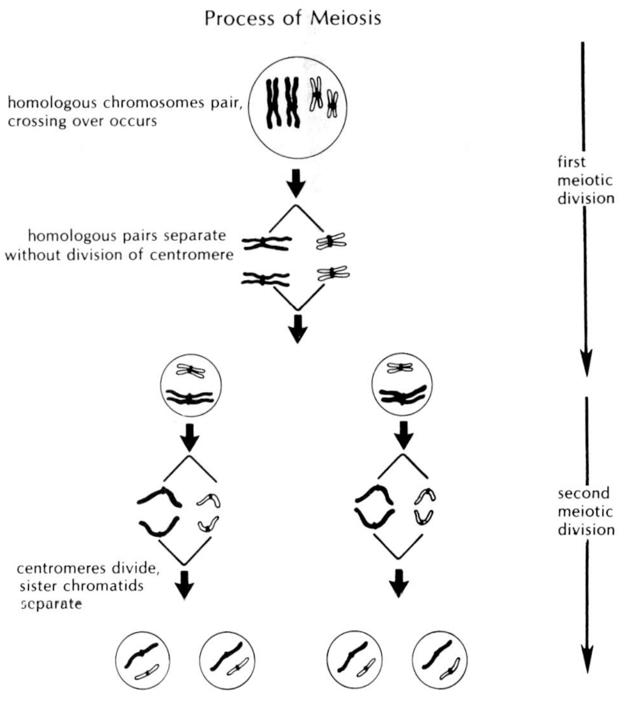

FIGURE 15-4. Diagrammatic representation of meiosis. [*Adapted from Flickinger, Brown, Kutchai, and Ogilvie.*[809]]

matids are fully paired, and exchange of genetic material occurs through crossing over between chromatids of homologous chromosomes that are linked by chiasmata. This genetic recombination is responsible for the production of germ cells that contain chromosomes with a unique combination of genetic material; diplotene I, during which homologous chromosome pairs begin to separate except at sites where chiasmata are located; and diakinesis I, during which chromosomes completely separate, shorten, condense maximally, and detach from the nuclear membrane.[31,35,36] Following the prolonged prophase I, the remaining stages of meiosis I proceed rapidly.

Prophase I is followed rapidly by metaphase I during which the nuclear membrane breaks down, paired chromosomes align themselves on the equatorial axis of the cell, and spindles form. Paired homologous chromosomes with sister chromatids attached to centromeres then separate towards opposite poles during anaphase I. Homologous chromosomes then become grouped at opposite poles during telophase I, and the cell divides to form two secondary spermatocytes, each containing a haploid complement of chromosomes (23 or 1N chromosomal number) composed of two sister chromatids each still joined together at the centromere (i.e., a 2N DNA content). Secondary spermatocytes are present for only ~8 hours and lack distinguishing histological features, making them difficult to identify.

Meiosis II After a brief interphase, secondary spermatocytes undergo the second meiotic division (meiosis II) (Figs. 15-3 and 15-4). During metaphase II, the 23 chromosomes of the secondary spermatocyte, each composed of two sister chromatids joined together at the centromere, align themselves on the equatorial axis of the cell. The centromeres then divide and the sister chromatids from each chromosome begin to separate towards opposite poles during anaphase II. Chromatids then become grouped at opposite poles during telophase II, and the cell divides to form two spermatids, each containing a haploid complement of chromosomes and now a haploid DNA content (1N chromosomal number and DNA content).

Disorders of mitotic or meiotic divisions (nondisjunction) during spermatogenesis occur commonly and contribute to the relatively high incidence of chromosomal abnormalities in humans, estimated to occur in 0.7 percent of live births and 50 percent of first trimester abortuses.[37–39] Aneuploidy, an abnormal number of chromosomes, is the most common and clinically significant chromosomal abnormality. Trisomy 21 or Down syndrome occurs in approximately 1 in 700 live births, and 5–20 percent of cases are due to paternal meiotic nondisjunction during anaphase I.[39,40] Klinefelter syndrome, which classically has a 47, XXY karyotype, and its variants occurs in about 1 in 400–500 live births, and approximately 50 percent of cases result from spermatogenic nondisjunction during meiosis I.[38,39] Finally, Turner syndrome (45, XO) occurs in approximately 1 in 9,000 births, and is due to meiotic nondisjunction in about 80 percent of the cases.[39,41]

Spermiogenesis

Spermiogenesis is the process of differentiation of spermatids both morphologically and functionally into mature spermatozoa that are capable of motility and fertilization of an ovum.[21,22,31] Major changes that occur during spermiogenesis include the formation of a flagellum that permits motility; the formation of the acrosome containing proteolytic enzymes needed for sperm penetration of the ovum; condensation of chromosomes and nucleoproteins to form the spermatozoon head; removal of excessive spermatid cytoplasm; and release of spermatozoa into the seminiferous tubule lumen (spermiation). Spermiogenesis is directed and controlled in large part by Sertoli cells that envelope spermatids during development and the major endocrine regulators of Sertoli cell function, FSH and testosterone. There are six types of spermatids, known as S_a, S_{b1}, S_{b2}, S_c, S_{d1}, and S_{d2} spermatids, which are distinguished by differences in nuclear morphology, and in the development of the acrosome and flagella.[35,36]

Germ Cell Degeneration

In humans the efficiency of spermatogenesis is relatively poor compared to that of most other species.[42] Germ cell loss as a result of degeneration that occurs throughout development and all phases of spermatogenesis is a major contributor to this relatively low spermatogenic efficiency and sperm output. Normally, germ cell loss occurs most commonly during mitotic and meiotic divisions, and rarely during spermiogenesis. In humans, prominent germ cell degeneration during the final stages of meiosis is common and accounts for the approximately 40 percent reduction in the ratio of spermatids to pachytene primary spermatocytes from the expected 4:1 ratio.[43,44] As men age, this ratio is reduced further, accounting for the decreased daily sperm production in elderly men. Degeneration of germ cells is thought to serve a quality control function by preventing abnormal germ cells from progressing further through spermatogenesis. Factors that regulate germ cell degeneration are unknown.

Organization of Spermatogenesis

In cross-sections of seminiferous tubules, germ cells at particular phases of development are associated together in six stages of spermatogenesis that constitute a complete cycle of spermatogenesis (Fig. 15-5).[22,36] In most mammals, stages of spermatogenesis are

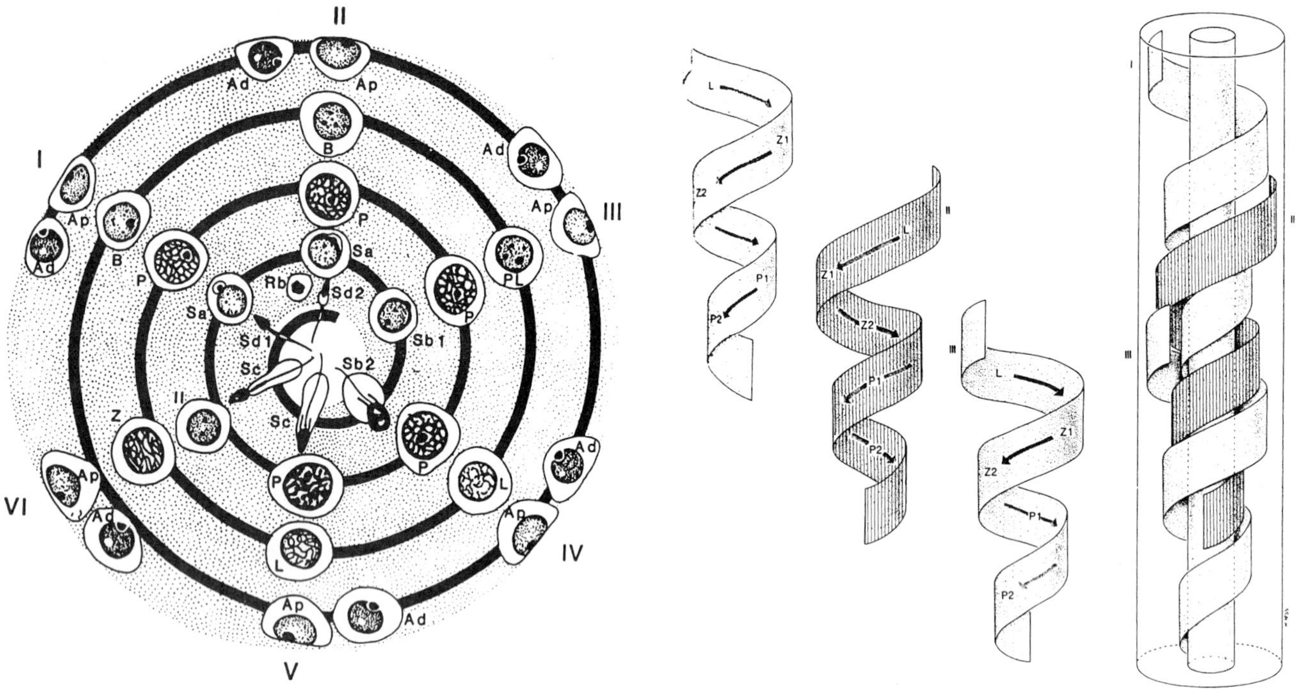

FIGURE 15-5. (*Left*) Schematic diagram of the germ cell types associated with the six stages (I-VI) of the human spermatogenic cycle demonstrating the organization of developing germ cells in a helical pattern of progressively decreasing radius. [*From Kerr.*[22]] (*Right*) Schematic model of the organization of spermatogenic stages within the human seminiferous tubule. (*From Schulze and Rehder.*[45])

arranged sequentially along the longitudinal axis of the seminiferous tubule, and each cross-section of a tubule contains the same stage of spermatogenesis. In contrast, cross-sections of seminiferous tubules from humans usually contain two to four different spermatogenic stages (Fig. 15-1). This apparently chaotic arrangement of stages is a consequence of the arrangement of successive spermatogenic stages along the length of the seminiferous tubule in a helical pattern of progressively decreasing radius, similar to an Archimedean spiral (Fig. 15-5).[45] Sequentially, stages are located external to and spiral concentrically around the helix of the preceding stage.

The duration of one cycle of spermatogenesis in humans is about 16 ± 1 days, and the entire duration of spermatogenesis from the formation A_p spermatogonia to release of S_{d2} spermatids is approximately 74 ± 4 days (4.6 spermatogenic cycles).[46] Furthermore, epididymal transit takes approximately 12–21 days in humans.[47,48] Therefore, insults to testis (e.g., irradiation) or gonadotropin deficiency that result in arrested early development of germ cells or reduced spermatogenesis may not be detected as reduced sperm counts in the ejaculate until months later.

Sperm Transport

After release from the seminiferous tubule, spermatozoa are carried via rete testis to the efferent ducts and then into the caput epididymis by peristaltic contractions, intratubular fluid flow, and some sperm movement.[48] In the epididymis, spermatozoa undergo minor morphological but important functional modifications. They acquire capacity for sustained motility and for fertilization of an ovum following the poorly understood process of capacitation in the female reproductive tract.[49]

Sperm Morphology and Motility

Most ejaculated human spermatozoa have an oval head, composed of the nucleus that contains compactly condensed chromosomes and nucleoproteins and an acrosomal cap which covers the anterior two thirds of the head (Fig. 15-6). The part of the head that is not covered by the acrosome is known as the postacrosomal region. The neck is the region where the sperm flagellum or tail implants into the head.

The flagellum is responsible for normal progressive forward motility of the spermatozoon. It is composed primarily of the *axoneme complex* of two central microtubules surrounded by nine microtubule doublets that are connected to each other by dynein arms, to the central microtubules by radial spokes, and to the axonemal membrane by Y links (Fig. 15-6).[50] Dynein arms contain a protein, dynein adenosine triphosphatase (ATPase).[51] Sperm motility is thought to involve coordinated dynein arm-mediated sliding of microtubules. The anterior portion of the flagellum, known as the middle piece, is composed of the central axoneme and stabilized by nine outer coarse fibers that run parallel and peripheral to the nine microtubular doublets. The outer coarse fibers are surrounded by a mitochondrial sheath that generate the energy for motility. In the longest, middle portion of the flagellum, known as the principal piece, the central axoneme is stabilized by two longitudinal columns that are joined together by fibrous sheath ribs. The short posterior portion of the flagellum, known as the end piece, is composed of the central axoneme alone surrounded by plasma membrane without a fibrous sheath.

In humans, sperm concentration in the ejaculate is highly variable and normally ranges from 20 to 200 million/mL of ejaculate

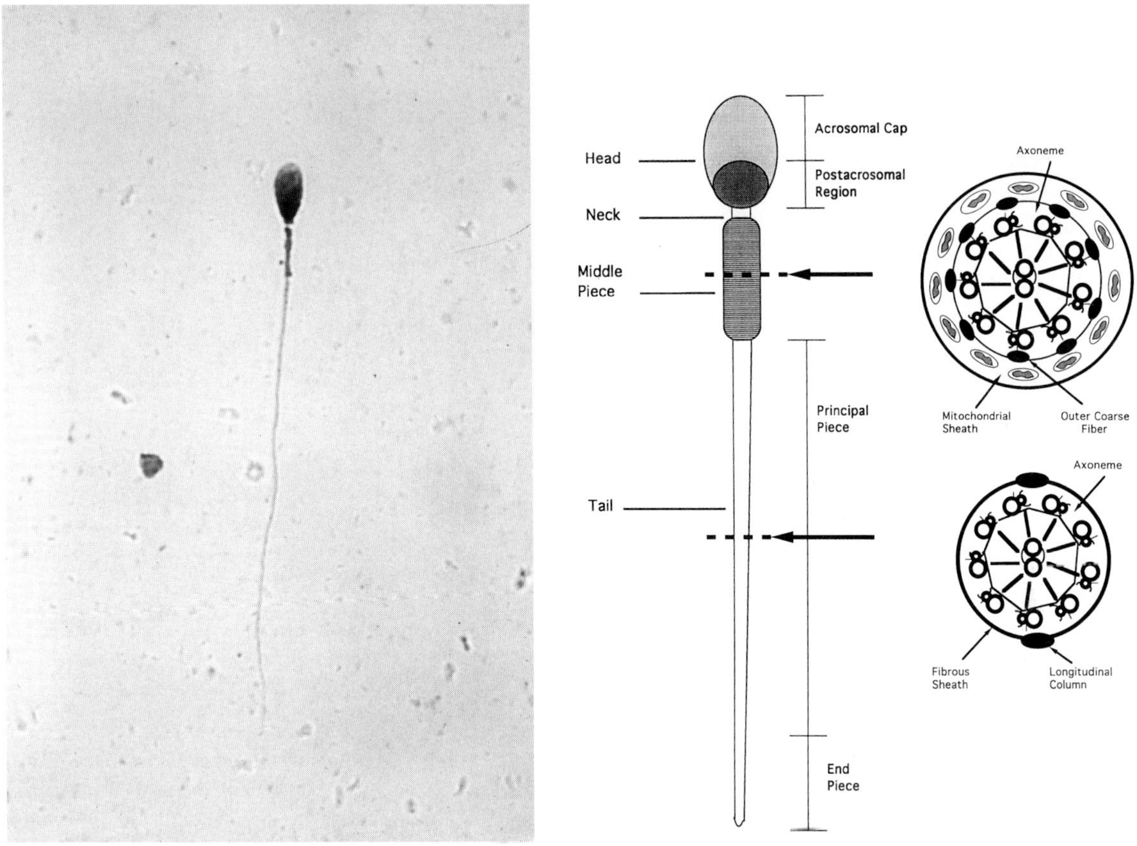

FIGURE 15-6. Light photomicrograph (*left*) of an ejaculated mature human spermatozoon and schematic diagram of its structure (*right*). (*From Matsumoto.*[100])

with more than 30 percent of the sperm exhibiting a normal oval head morphology using strict criteria, and more than 50 percent exhibiting vigorous forward motility.[52] In addition to having reductions of sperm concentration, men with infertility often exhibit abnormal sperm morphology and motility. For example, men with varicocele-associated infertility commonly exhibit sperm with tapered or amorphous head morphology and reduced motility. Mutations in the structural or functional components of the axoneme, e.g; dynein ATPase deficiency, may result in immotile cilia syndrome, underscoring the importance of the axoneme for normal sperm motility.

TESTICULAR DEVELOPMENT

Fetal Testis Development

Based on deletion mapping, the genes that are responsible for development of the testis are located on the short arm of the Y chromosome (see Chap. 17).[53] The *SRY (sex-determining region of the Y chromosome) gene,* located between the centromere and pseudoautosomal region of the Y chromosome, is thought to be the primary director of testis development from an undifferentiated anlage during embryogenesis.[53–55] This gene encodes a transcription factor, but the exact mechanism by which the SRY gene and its product are responsible for testis determination is not known. The finding of 46, XY phenotypic female without testes despite an intact SRY gene suggests that genes (e.g., SOX-9) outside this region of the Y chromosome may be important in testis determination.[55]

Primordial germ cells migrate from their origin in the yolk sac endoderm to the genital ridges where they organize with cells from the coelomic epithelium and mesenchyme (that eventually differentiate into Sertoli cells, and Leydig and peritubular myoid cells, respectively) to form the *genital blastema* by 6 weeks of gestation. Primordial germ cells that fail to reach the genital ridges may be the source of extragonadal germ cell tumors postnatally. At 6–7 weeks of gestation, sexually dimorphic gonadal differentiation occurs with the formation of *seminiferous or sex cords* (primordial germ cells surrounded by primative Sertoli cells) that will eventually develop into seminiferous tubules.

At 8 weeks of gestation, fetal Leydig cells begin to form from mesenchymal cells of the genital ridges. From 8–14 weeks of gestation under the influence of placental human chorionic gonadotropin (hCG) initially and then fetal pituitary FSH and LH secretion, immature germ cells, Sertoli cells, and Leydig cells proliferate, differentiate, and organize. Testosterone production from the latter increases progressively during this time, reaching levels comparable to those of adults.[53,56] During this period of development, MIS produced by the fetal Sertoli cell induces regression of Müllerian or paramesonephric ducts (preventing the development of the uterus and fallopian tubes) and testosterone produced by Leydig cells induces development of male internal and external genitalia. Under the action of testosterone, the epididymis, vas deferens, and seminal vesicles develop from the wolffian or mesonephric ducts. Testosterone is converted to dihydrotestosterone in the urogenital tract and the latter induces formation of the prostate and prostatic urethra from the urogenital sinus, the penis from the genital tubercle and folds, and the scrotum from the urogenital swelling. In the absence of normal testis function, and in particular, testosterone or testosterone action, internal and external genital development proceeds along female lines. Male phenotypic development is largely completed by about 15 weeks of gestation. After 17 weeks of gestation, proliferation of both germ cells and Sertoli cells continues at a markedly reduced rate and Leydig cells involute until the time of puberty.

Testicular Descent

The developing testis is attached to the *genital swellings* (that eventually differentiates into the scrotum) by a caudal ligamentous band of mesenchyme, known as the *gubernaculum,* that anchors the fetal testis to the inguinal region.[57] At the same time, the mesenchymal band cranial to the testis disappears under the influence of MIS produced by the fetal Sertoli cell. Testis development is largely complete by 3 months of gestation. At that time, a herniation of the abdominal cavity, called the *processus vaginalis,* forms along the course of the gubernaculum into the developing scrotum. Enlargement of the processus vaginalis forms the inguinal rings and canal. As the gubernaculum thickens and then degenerates, and with increasing intra-abdominal pressure associated with the development of the abdominal musculature, the testis moves from its intra-abdominal location through the inguinal canal into the scrotum. The testis is usually completely within the scrotum by 7 months of gestation. With the development of the abdominal musculature, the inguinal rings close and the processus vaginalis is obliterated to form the *tunica vaginalis,* which covers the anterolateral portion of the adult testis. Incomplete closure of the inguinal rings predisposes to the development of an inguinal hernia. Incomplete obliteration of the processus vaginalis with serous fluid accumulation results in a hydrocele. Androgen secretion is thought to play an important role in testicular descent, probably through regulation of the formation and development of the processus vaginalis and function of the gubernaculum.[57] Conditions associated with androgen deficiency during development are commonly associated with failure of normal testicular descent, i.e., cryptorchidism.

Neonatal and Pubertal Testis Development

During the first 6 months after birth in humans and nonhuman primates, the hypothalamic-pituitary-testicular axis is activated transiently, resulting in an increase in the number of germ cells and Sertoli cells and testosterone secretion by Leydig cells.[58] The physiological significance of neonatal activation of the gonadal axis is not clear. However, monkeys in whom the neonatal gonadotropin surge is inhibited by administration of a GnRH analog demonstrate reduced peripubertal increases in LH and testosterone levels, and decreased testicular size and sperm production,[59] suggesting a possible role for neonatal gonadotropins in quantitative aspects of adult testis function. After this transient neonatal surge, serum gonadotropin concentrations remain low until the time of puberty. Despite low circulating gonadotropin levels, both Sertoli cell and germ cell numbers increase during the prepubertal period, and infantile germ cells mature into spermatogonia.[53] The number of Sertoli cells and spermatogonial stem cells produced during these periods of development are thought to be the major determinants of the maximum capacity of the testis to produce sperm as an adult. Failure to develop normal numbers of Sertoli and spermatogonia as a result of gonadotropin deficiency occurring during early testicular development may explain why gonadotropin therapy in adult patients with Kallmann syndrome does not usually stimulate quantitatively normal sperm production.

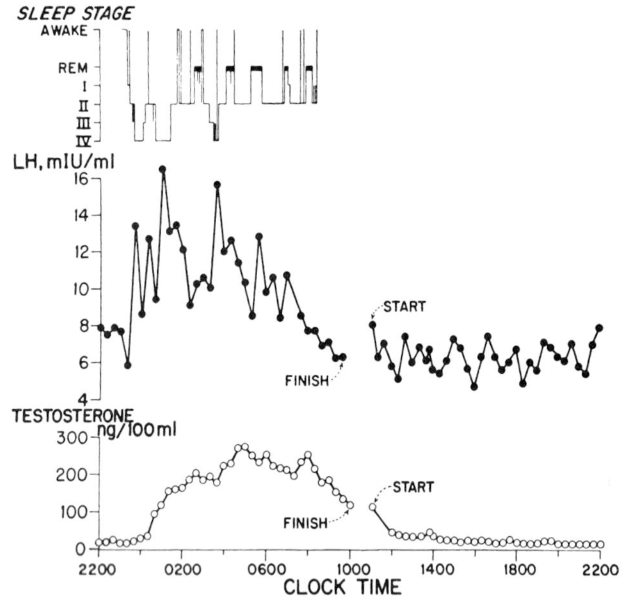

FIGURE 15-7. Levels of LH and testosterone concentration during sleep in a pubertal boy. (*From Boyar, Rosenfeld, Kapen S, et al.*[816])

With the reactivation of hypothalamic GnRH secretion at the time of puberty, serum LH and FSH increase, initially only during the evening and then throughout the entire day (Fig. 15-7).[60] Increases in LH stimulate Leydig cells to secrete increasing amounts of testosterone, which plays a vital role in the development of secondary sexual characteristics and, together with increases in FSH, the initiation of spermatogenesis. Increasing gonadotropins during puberty also cause Sertoli cells to compartmentalize germ cells within the seminiferous tubule such that spermatogonia localized at the base of the tubule are separated by Sertoli cell tight junctions from germ cells (spermatocytes) that have entered meiosis. With the onset spermatogenesis and increased germ cell numbers, the testis size increases progressively. The latter is the earliest clinical sign of the onset of puberty on physical examination. The release of spermatozoa from the seminiferous tubules and their appearance in urine (spermarche) also occurs during the early pubertal period, between 12–15 years of age.[53,60]

PHYSIOLOGY

Hypothalamic-Pituitary-Testicular Axis

Brain Regulation of GnRH Secretion

The brain plays a major role in the regulation of reproductive function. Neurons concentrated in the medial basal hypothalamus (in particular, the arcuate nucleus) synthesize a decapeptide, GnRH, that is released episodically from axon terminals in the median eminence into the hypophyseal portal system. Episodic

GnRH release stimulates the production and pulsatile secretion of LH and, to a lesser extent, FSH, from the anterior pituitary gland (Fig. 15-8).[61–64] The concentration of GnRH in the portal system is estimated indirectly to be approximately 30–300 pg/mL.[65] Because it is degraded rapidly in portal blood, little GnRH accumulates in the peripheral circulation. Compared to highly sensitive assays for gonadotropins in blood, immunoassays for GnRH and its cleavage products in serum or urine are not sufficiently sensitive for clinical use.

Pulsatile GnRH secretion is a manifestation of an intrinsic periodicity of GnRH neuronal firing. Although the precise mechanism of synchronous release from a number of separate hypothalamic GnRH neurons is not clear, the "pulse generator" that is responsible for episodic secretion of GnRH into hypophyseal portal capillaries resides within the medial basal hypothalamus.[62,66,67] Because GnRH pulses are temporally coupled with those of LH (and to a lesser extent FSH), the frequency of LH pulses as assessed by hormone measurements on blood sampled frequently (e.g., every 10 minutes for 12 to 24 hours) indirectly reflects GnRH pulse frequency and the activity of GnRH neurons in the brain. The amplitude of LH pulses, however, reflects not only the amplitude of GnRH pulses from the hypothalamus but also pituitary responsiveness to GnRH. In normal adult men, approximately 10–14 LH pulses of varying amplitude occur during the day (Fig. 15-9).[64,68] In contrast, most men with idiopathic hypogonadotropic hypogonadism (IHH), or Kallmann syndrome, who lack endogenous GnRH secretion, demonstrate an absence LH pulses or abnormalities of pulsatile LH secretion.[68] Furthermore, low-dose pulsatile GnRH administration in men with IHH stimulates normal LH and FSH release which, in turn, stimulate testicular function, emphasizing the importance of hypothalamic GnRH control of reproductive function in men.[69]

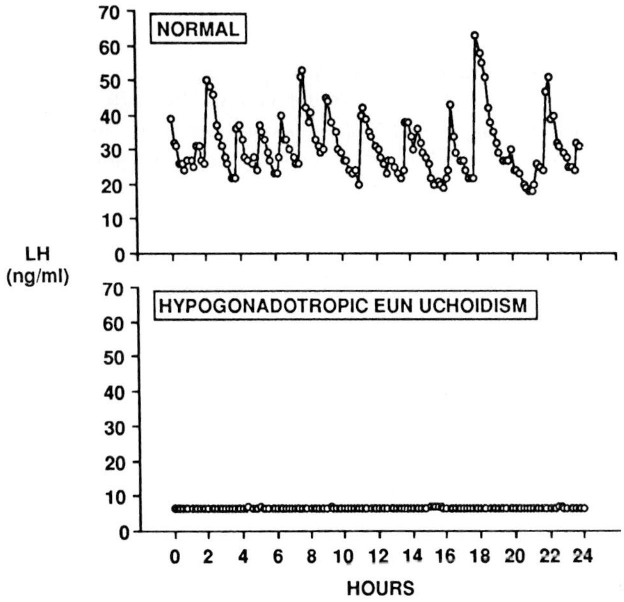

FIGURE 15-9. Pulsatile LH secretion in a normal man *(top)* and a man with hypogonadotropic hypogonadism *(bottom)*. [*From Matsumoto, Gross, Sheckter, and Bremner.*[810]]

FIGURE 15-8. Schematic diagram of the hypothalamic-pituitary-testicular axis.

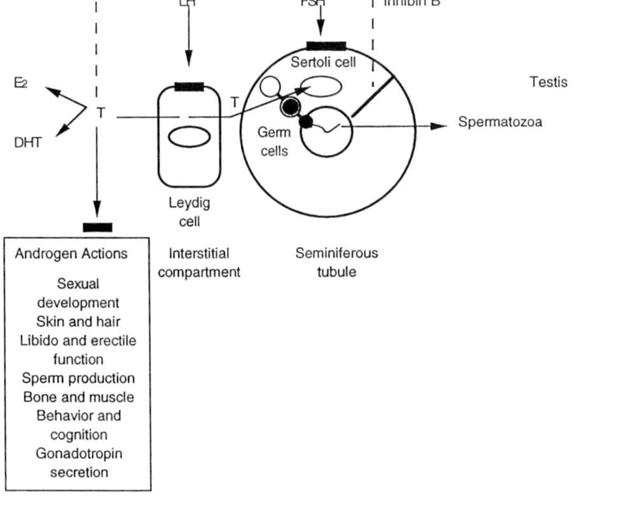

The GnRH neuronal system receives inputs from other hypothalamic and brain regions, such as the limbic system, through a number of excitatory and inhibitory neuromodulatory systems, and from testicular feedback influences, primarily from sex steroids (Fig. 15-8). Therefore, the hypothalamic GnRH system plays an important integrative role in the regulation of testicular function. The ensemble of neuroregulators that interact to control GnRH secretion is large and complex, and it includes systems that stimulate (e.g., norepinephrine, neuropeptide Y, and excitatory amino acids such as glutamate) and inhibit GnRH release (e.g., dopamine, serotonin, endogenous opiates such as β-endorphin, CRH, and inhibitory amino acids such as GABA).[8,17] Understanding of how these brain systems regulate GnRH has provided insight into the mechanisms by which stress and nutritional alterations associated with systemic illness and medications, such as opiates or drugs that alter brain neurotransmitters, may affect testicular function. To add to the complexity of GnRH regulation, animal studies indicate that the effects of most GnRH neuromodulators are influenced by androgen and/or estrogen feedback from the testis, such that the same neuromodulator may have completely opposite effects on GnRH release in an intact compared to orchidectomized animal.[70]

GnRH Regulation of Gonadotropin Secretion

GnRH released from hypothalamic neurons into the hypophyseal portal circulation is carried to the anterior pituitary, where it binds to G protein-coupled GnRH receptors on the plasma membrane of gonadotrophs.[71] Binding of GnRH to its receptor and subsequent dimerization of GnRH receptors causes G_s protein to bind and activate phospholipase C to produce 1,2 diacylglycerol and inositol 1,4,5 triphosphate. The latter mobilizes intracellular calcium that binds to the calcium-binding protein, calmodulin, and together with diacylglycerol activates protein kinase C to phosphorylate several proteins. Activation of these second messengers by GnRH binding to pituitary gonadotrophs stimulates LH and, to a lesser extent, FSH release and synthesis (Fig. 15-8).

The episodic stimulation of gonadotrophs by GnRH is essential for normal pituitary gonadotropin secretion. In GnRH-deficient men with IHH, pulsatile GnRH administration at a near physiological dose and frequency stimulates normal immunoreactive and bioactive LH and FSH concentrations.[72] In contrast, continuous infusion of the same GnRH dose increases immunoreactive but fails to stimulate bioactive LH, and fails to stimulate either immunoreactive or bioactive FSH production.[72] In normal men, continuous administration of high-dose GnRH or a potent GnRH agonist analog markedly suppresses gonadotropin (LH greater than FSH) secretion and testicular function (in particular testosterone secretion).[73] This effect, referred to as pituitary down regulation or desensitization, is used therapeutically to induce a "medical castration" in men with androgen-dependent disorders, such as metastatic prostate cancer, who are treated with long-acting potent GnRH agonists. Furthermore, the frequency of pulsatile GnRH stimulation of pituitary gonadotrophs regulates the relative secretion of LH and FSH. A slow GnRH pulse frequency favors FSH over LH secretion, whereas a rapid pulse frequency favors LH over FSH release.[74] Together with negative feedback effects of the testicular sex steroids (testosterone and its active metabolite, estradiol) and peptides (inhibin B and activins), GnRH frequency modulation of gonadotropin secretion provides interacting mechanisms by which a single hypothalamic releasing factor can regulate the relative secretion of LH and FSH, hormones that are mostly synthesized and released from the same pituitary cell.[18]

LH and FSH are members of the glycoprotein hormone family that also includes hCG and thyroid-stimulating hormone (TSH). These hormones are composed of an identical α subunit and a unique β subunit that determines their functional specificity; both subunits are needed for full biological activity.[75] The common α, LHβ, and FSHβ subunits are synthesized from separate genes that are regulated differentially. After transcription and translation, α and LHβ or FSHβ subunits combine and undergo variable degrees of glycosylation (addition of carbohydrate moieties) to form LH and FSH molecules with a high degree of microheterogeneity.[76,77] Free α subunits are produced in excess of gonadotropins and are also released into circulation in response to GnRH stimulation.

The amount of carbohydrate that is added to the primary structure of LH and FSH alters their rate of clearance from the circulation that affects their in vivo biological activity and intrinsic biological potency.[76,77] Glycosylation also alters gonadotropin immunoreactivity, which affects their recognition in radioimmunoassays (RIAs). Changes in biological activity associated with alterations in gonadotropin microheterogeneity have been demonstrated during puberty, aging, androgen deprivation, and GnRH analog administration.[76-81] Increasing circulating half-life of gonadotropins and free a subunit correlate with increasing degrees of glycosylation, with the half-life of hCG > FSH > LH > free α subunit. The initial and second phase half-life of disappearance is ~40 and 120 minutes, respectively, for LH, and ~4 hours and 70 hours, respectively, for FSH.[61,81,82]

Clinically, measurements of serum gonadotropins are made using immunoassays (e.g., immunofluorometric assays). Newer assays that utilize two monoclonal antibodies that recognize separate epitopes of the gonadotropin molecule are highly sensitive and correlate with in vitro bioassays.[83,84] Although a number of sensitive in vitro LH and FSH bioassays have been developed, they are not used clinically nor are they generally available. Except for situations in which blood sampling is difficult (e.g., patients in the pediatric age group), urinary LH and FSH radioimmunassays do not offer advantages over highly sensitive two-site monoclonal immunoassays.[85,86] Specific immunoassays for free α subunit are useful in diagnosing and monitoring gonadotropin-secreting pituitary adenomas and tumors, such as pancreatic islet cell tumors, that produce excessive amounts of free α subunit, and as an indirect marker of pulsatile GnRH secretion.[87]

Gonadotropin Control of Testicular Function

LH Regulation of Leydig Cells

LH binds to high affinity G protein-coupled plasma membrane receptors on Leydig cells.[88,89] Following binding, LH receptors aggregate, undergo a conformational change and bind G_s protein. Guanosine triphosphate (GTP) then binds to $G_{s\alpha}$ subunit, displacing guanosine diphosphate (GDP), and $G_{s\alpha}$ binds and activates adenylate cylase resulting in generation of cyclic adenosine monophosphate (cAMP). cAMP then binds to the regulatory subunits of protein kinase A, releasing activated catalytic subunits that phosphorylate a number of proteins in the Leydig cell and result in stimulation of steroidogenesis and testosterone production (Fig. 15-8).

Both LH and hCG bind to the LH receptor and administration of high concentrations of either hormone causes a decrease (down regulation) of LH receptor number and reduction in responsiveness to further stimulation by LH or hCG (desensitization).[90,91] In contrast to the suppression of pituitary LH production induced by continuous high-dosage GnRH administration, production of testosterone is not inhibited by high dosage LH or hCG administration,[92] raising questions regarding the clinical significance of LH receptor down regulation and Leydig cell desensitization.

FIGURE 15-10. Diagrammatic representation of the androgen synthetic pathway in the Leydig cells of the testis. Preferred pathways are shown by heavy arrows. Only small amounts of dihydrotestosterone are synthesized from testosterone within the Leydig cell.

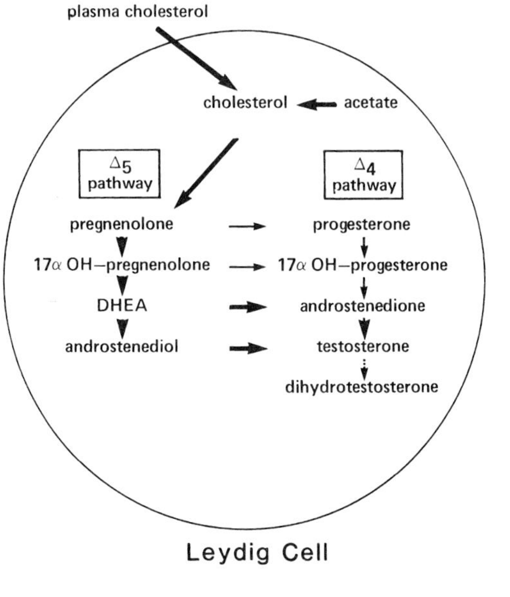

LH stimulation of Leydig cells increases testosterone production by increasing the activity of the enzyme, 20,22-desmolase (cholesterol side-chain cleavage enzyme, CYP11A1), that catalyzes the conversion of cholesterol to pregnenolone in mitochondria, the rate-limiting step in testosterone biosynthesis. In humans, cholesterol is derived both from de novo synthesis from acetate in Leydig cells and uptake of plasma cholesterol from circulating low-density lipoprotein (LDL) particles (Fig. 15-10).[93] Testosterone synthesis in the human testis proceeds via a series of enzymatic conversions, initially via the Δ^5 pathway; pregnenolone is converted to 17α hydroxy (OH)-pregnenolone by 17 α-hydroxylase (CYPc17); 17α OH-pregnenolone is converted to dehydroepiandrosterone (DHEA) by 17,20-desmolase or lyase (the same enzyme as 17α-hydroxylase, CYPc17); and DHEA is converted to Δ^5-androstanediol by 17β OH-steroid dehydrogenase. DHEA and Δ^5-androstanediol are then converted to Δ^4-androstenedione and testosterone, respectively in the Δ^4 pathway, by 3β-OH-steroid dehydrogenase. Androgen precursors and products can be sulfated, stored, and subsequently cleaved to yield free steroids for release into the circulation. The physiological significance of this *sulfate storage shunt* is not known.

Testosterone, the major androgen produced by the testis, is secreted at a rate of approximately 7,000 μg or 7 mg per day into the circulation (Fig. 15-11).[94] The testis also secretes significant amounts of 17α OH-progesterone, Δ^4-androstenedione, and pregnenolone. There is relatively little conversion of testosterone to 5α-dihydrotestosterone (DHT) and estradiol (E_2) by the enzymes 5α-reductase and aromatase, respectively, in the testis so that only small amounts of DHT (69 μg per day) and E_2 (10 μg per day) are secreted by the testis.

FIGURE 15-11. Testicular secretion rates of various androgens. T = testosterone; 17-OHP = 17α-hydroxyprogesterone; Δ^5P = pregnenolone; Δ^4A = androstenedione; P = progesterone; DHT = dihydrotestosterone. Secretion rates (SR) calculated from the arteriovenous (av) differences across the testis as measured by Hammond et al.[91] Calculations based on assumptions used by Kirchner et al.[811] for adrenal secretion rates, represented by the formula

$$\text{Secretion rate (SR)} = \frac{\text{Assumed testosterone SR}}{\text{testosterone av difference} \times \text{av difference of steroid in question}}$$

Testosterone SR assumed to be 7000 μg/day. (*From Hammond, Ruokonen, Kontturi, Koskela, and Vihko*[94]; *Kirschner, Zucker, and Jespersen.*[811])

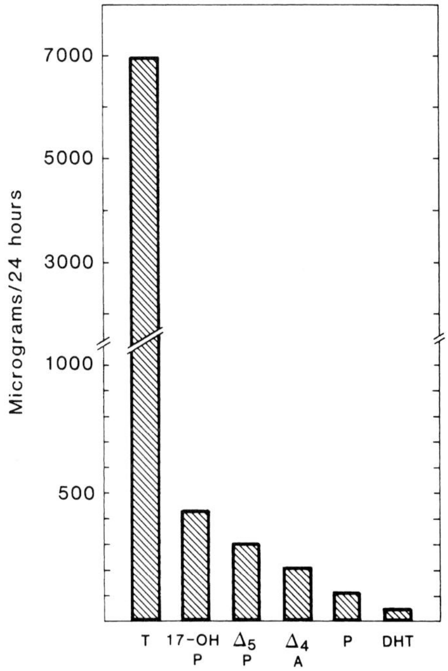

In response to LH pulses, testosterone is secreted into the spermatic vein and then into the peripheral circulation in a pulsatile manner. However, in men, testosterone pulses are less distinct with low amplitude, and there is relatively poor concordance with LH pulses.[64,95] The lack of distinct testosterone pulses is due in part to dilution of a relatively small amount of testosterone secreted per pulse into a large pool of mostly protein-bound testosterone in plasma. Also, Leydig cells respond sluggishly to LH stimulation, with only small increases in testosterone within 2–4 hours and peak increases that do not occur until 24–48 hours.[91]

In young men, testosterone levels exhibit a circadian variation of about 1.5 ng/mL with peak levels occurring at approximately 8 A.M. and nadir concentrations at approximately 8 P.M.[96] The circadian variation in testosterone levels is blunted in elderly men. The diurnal rhythm is not associated clearly with circadian variations in LH secretion. The testosterone response to hCG is greater in the morning than in the afternoon, suggesting that a diurnal variation in Leydig cell sensitivity to LH may contribute to the circadian rhythm in testosterone concentrations.[97]

FSH Regulation of Sertoli Cell Function

FSH binds to high-affinity G protein-coupled plasma membrane receptors on Sertoli cells (Fig. 15-8).[98] Signal transduction follows a pathway that is analogous to that for LH with FSH receptor binding leading to G protein activation of adenylate cyclase, generation of cAMP that activates protein kinase A, followed by protein phosphorylation. As with the regulation of LH receptors by LH or hCG, FSH administration also down regulates the number of FSH receptors on Sertoli cells, but the physiological significance of down-regulation is not known. FSH binding has also been reported in rat spermatogonia, but direct effects of FSH on these stem cells, if any, are unknown.[99]

In response to FSH stimulation, the Sertoli cell secretes a large number of proteins and other products that are important in the process of spermatogenesis.[25,26,100] However, the specific roles played by most Sertoli cell products in human spermatogenesis are unknown. Most of what is known regarding the presumed function of these products or their human homologues is derived from studies in experimental animals, mostly rodents, and experiments in vitro using Sertoli cells isolated from immature animals.

The major functions of the Sertoli cell are: *maintenance of seminiferous tubule structure; compartmentalization of the seminiferous tubule* into the basal and adluminal compartment that serves to provide an environment which is protected from external influences and the immune system; *translocation of developing germ cells* from the basal compartment to the seminiferous tubule lumen; *pinocytosis and phagocytosis* of degenerating germ cells, residual cytoplasm from late spermatids, and seminiferous tubule fluid and contents; *spermiation,* the release of spermatozoa from the seminiferous epithelium into the lumen of the tubule; *secretion of seminiferous tubule fluid* that delivers nutrients to developing germ cells and released spermatozoa, transports regulatory substances involved in cell-cell communication from the basal to apical portion of the seminiferous tubule, and transports spermatozoa from the seminiferous tubule to the rete testis, efferent ducts, and caput epididymis; *delivery of nutrients to germ cells,* including lactate, the preferred energy substrate of germ cells; and *secretion of a large number of proteins and other products* that are important for spermatogenesis.[25,26,100]

Because the adluminal compartment of the seminiferous tubule is isolated from substances in the systemic circulation by the blood-testis barrier, the Sertoli cell plays a vital role in transporting or producing essential proteins, cofactors, and nutrients to support spermatogenesis. A majority of the total protein produced by Sertoli cells is composed of *binding or transport proteins* for a variety of substances (e.g., androgens, metals, sphingolipids, vitamins, and growth factor) that serve as cofactors and modulators of germ cell development within the seminiferous tubule.[25,26,100] These include: *androgen-binding protein (ABP),* a testicular homolog of testosterone-estrogen-binding globulin (TeBG), also known as sex hormone-binding globulin (SHBG), that is encoded by the same gene; transferrin, an iron binding protein; ceruloplasmin, a copper binding protein; testibumin and clusterin, or sulfated glycoprotein 1 and 2, respectively, glycosphingolipid binding proteins; α_2-macroglobulin that serves as a binding protein for inhibin and activin; and insulin-like growth factor binding proteins (IGFBPs) that bind insulin-like growth factor-1 (IGF-1). ABP is secreted into the seminiferous tubule lumen and carried to the epididymis, where it is concentrated.[101] It is thought to play an important role in supporting spermatogenesis by maintaining high local testosterone concentrations in the seminiferous tubule and epididymis, but this has not been established conclusively.

Other Sertoli cell products include *hormones* such as: inhibin B and activin, peptide hormones that participate in the negative feedback regulation of pituitary FSH secretion as well as act as possible paracrine factors within the testis; MIS, which mediates regression of the Müllerian ducts during embryogenesis and regulates prepubertal germ cell proliferation and maturation; and estradiol that is produced in prepubertal Sertoli cells.[25,26,100] The Sertoli cell also secretes *growth factors* (e.g., IGF-1, basic fibroblast growth factor, transforming growth factor [TGF] α and β, interleukin (IL)-1α and -6, Steel factor or *c-kit ligand,* and polyamines [putrescine, spermine, spermidine]) that act as paracrine regulators of germ cell development, and Leydig and peritubular cell function, as well as autocrine modulators.[25,26,100] Finally, the Sertoli cell produces: *proteases and protease inhibitors* (e.g., plasminogen activators, type IV collagenase, cystatin, α_2-macroglobulin) that are involved in translocation of developing germ cells within the seminiferous tubule, removal of degenerating germ cells and spermiation; *energy substrates,* such as lactate and pyruvate, which are essential for germ cell development; and *extracellular matrix and junctional complex proteins* (e.g., cell adhesion molecules such as cadherins, laminin, types I and IV collagen, proteoglycans such as chondroitin, and heparin), that are important in maintaining the structural integrity of the seminiferous tubule, supporting developing germ cells, forming the blood-testis barrier, mediating cell-cell interactions, and maintaining polarized secretion of products by the Sertoli cell.

FSH regulates many of the Sertoli cell products mentioned earlier, notably ABP, transferrin, testibumin, inhibin B, TGFβ, activin, MIS, IGFBP-3, Steel factor, polyamines, plasminogen activators, lactate, and pyruvate during various periods of development.[25,26,100] Sertoli cells also possess *androgen receptors.* Therefore, in addition to FSH, testosterone secreted locally from Leydig cells (in response to LH stimulation) may regulate Sertoli cell secretion of some of its products (e.g., ABP, transferrin, inhibin B, and MIS) either directly or indirectly by stimulating peritubular myoid cell production of paracrine factors, such as P-Mod-S).[25,26,100]

Paracrine and Autocrine Regulation of Testis Function

It is clear that the major endocrine regulators of testis function are the pituitary gonadotropins, LH and FSH. There is a growing body of evidence from studies in vitro utilizing isolated cell types from experimental animals that local paracrine and autocrine factors secreted from Leydig, peritubular myoid, Sertoli, and germ cells as well as macrophages in the interstitium may play important roles in modulating testosterone production and spermatogenesis.[102] Because there is considerable variation between species, the role of paracrine factors in regulating human testis function is unclear at this time.

Transport, Metabolism and Actions of Testosterone

Testosterone Transport in Plasma Like other steroid hormones and thyroid hormones, the vast majority of testosterone secreted by Leydig cells into the circulation is bound to plasma proteins, primarily *testosterone-estrogen-binding globulin (TeBG),* also referred to as *sex hormone-binding globulin (SHBG*), and *albumin* (Fig. 15-12).[103–105] Approximately 30–40 percent of circulating testosterone is bound to SHBG with sufficiently high affinity (1.6×10^{-9} M) such that SHBG-bound testosterone is not available to target tissues. In contrast, approximately 58–68 percent of circulating testosterone is bound to albumin, but with an affinity that is several orders of magnitude less than SHBG (4×10^{-4} M). Therefore, albumin-bound testosterone is generally available for entry into target tissues, together with the approximately 2 percent of testosterone in circulation that is free, i.e., unbound to plasma proteins. The free plus albumin-bound fractions of testosterone are referred to as *bioavailable testosterone,* or non-SHBG-bound (or non-SHBG-bound) testosterone.[103,107,108] Measurement of non-SHBG-bound testosterone in blood may provide the best clinical estimate of biologically available testosterone.

A number of clinical conditions alter plasma levels of SHBG (Fig. 15-12).[106–110] Conditions that decrease SHBG concentrations include: moderate obesity; hypothyroidism; protein-wasting conditions, such as nephrotic syndrome or malnutrition; androgens or androgenic anabolic steroids; glucocorticoids or Cushing syndrome; acromegaly; and congenital SHBG deficiency. Clinical conditions in which SHBG levels are increased include: normal aging; hyperthyroidism; hepatic cirrhosis; estrogens; progestagens, such as megesterol acetate; hypogonadism; and spironolactone.

In men with an intact hypothalamic-pituitary-testicular axis, alterations in SHBG levels and protein-bound testosterone have little affect on the physiology and action of androgens in the steady state. For example, an increase in SHBG results in a transient decrease in free testosterone and negative feedback on the hypothalamic-pituitary axis. Reduced testosterone feedback causes an increase in LH secretion that stimulates Leydig cells to secrete testosterone until free testosterone concentrations are normalized. In contrast, changes in SHBG levels may have significant consequences in men with reproductive axis disorders that have altered feedback regulation of free testosterone.[109,110] Thus, the pharmacological actions of testosterone administered for replacement therapy may be altered in hypogonadal men who also have alterations in circulating SHBG concentrations.

Because the majority of circulating testosterone is bound to plasma proteins, alterations in SHBG concentrations result in

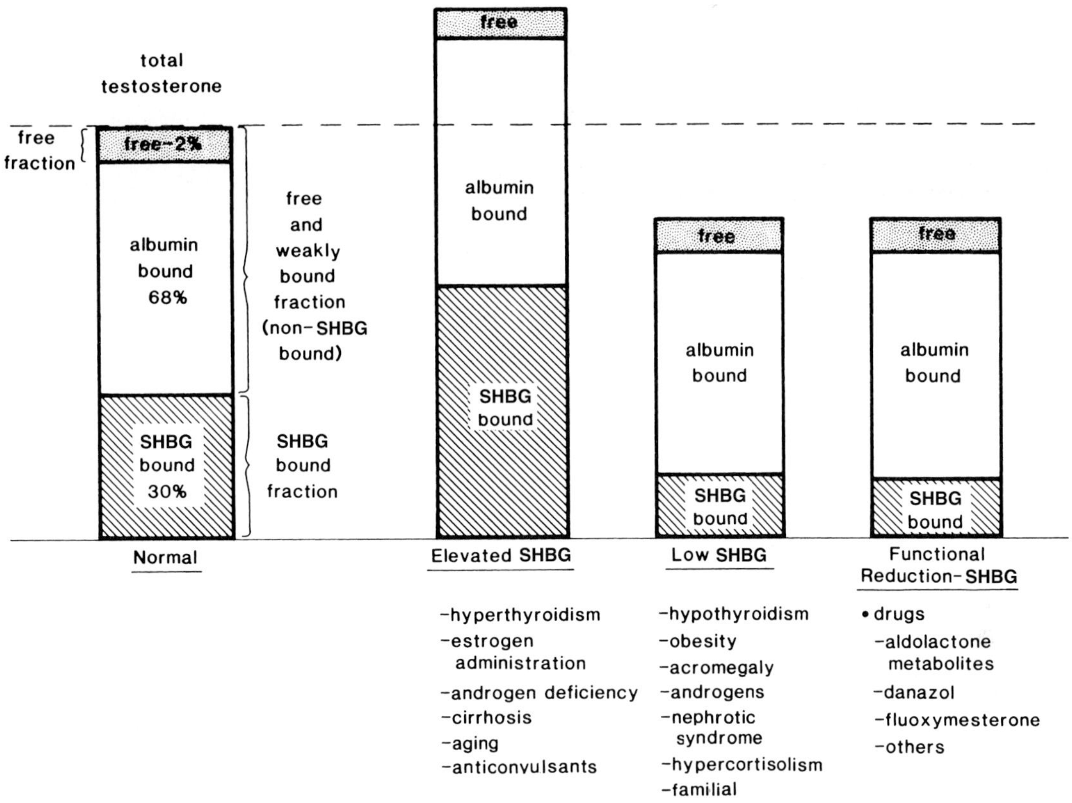

FIGURE 15-12. Fractions of bound, weakly bound, and free testosterone in normal men and in men with disorders producing high or low levels of sex hormone-binding globulin (SHBG) or testosterone estrogen binding globulin (TeBG).

changes in total testosterone measurements in the same direction, e.g., conditions that decrease SHBG concentrations in otherwise normal eugonadal men lower total testosterone levels, sometimes into the hypogonadal range. However, free and bioavailable testosterone levels are normal so that these men are eugonadal despite low total testosterone concentrations. Therefore, in clinical conditions associated with alterations in SHBG concentrations, total testosterone concentrations do not reflect bioavailable testosterone levels or gonadal status. In these situations, measurement of free or bioavailable testosterone levels should be obtained to assess gonadal Leydig cell function.

SHBG is a heterodimeric glycoprotein β-globulin that is synthesized in the liver.[111] A single gene encodes for SHBG and its testicular homolog, ABP. Structural differences in SHBG and ABP are due to different tissue-specific transcription start sites and/or modifications in a common primary transcript or its translation products. SHBG has a single competitive steroid-binding site per molecule that binds testosterone and DHT with high affinity and estradiol much less avidly. Variations in posttranslational glycosylation result in different circulating isoforms of SHBG that contribute to the differences in binding affinity of androgens and estrogens.[111] In some target tissues, SHBG-testosterone complexes may bind to plasma membrane receptors that activate cAMP and affect target organ function without binding to classical intracellular androgen receptors.[112]

Metabolism of Testosterone Metabolism of circulating testosterone to active metabolites plays an important role in mediating many of its biological actions on target tissues. Thus, testosterone serves as a prohormone, and is converted to *17β-estradiol* (estradiol) by the enzyme *aromatase* and to *5a-dihydrotestosterone (DHT)* by 5α-reductase (Fig. 15-8). These active metabolites may act locally in tissues in which they are formed or as circulating hormones at target tissues. Thus, the physiological effects of testosterone represent the combined actions of testosterone itself, and its active androgenic and estrogenic metabolites.

Aromatase, a cytochrome P450 enzyme (CYP19), catalyzes the conversion of testosterone and other C19 androgens to C18 estrogens, primarily in adipose tissue, but also in liver, muscle, brain, skin, and testis within Leydig and Sertoli cells.[113] In men, the majority of the 40–50 μg of estradiol (the most potent endogenous estrogen) that is produced daily is derived from extratesticular aromatization of testosterone and Δ^4-androstenedione to estradiol and the weak estrogen, estrone, respectively, and subsequent reduction of the latter to estradiol. Only 15–25 percent of circulating estradiol is produced by the testis, primarily in Leydig cells of adults.[114]

Aromatization of testosterone to estradiol is thought to mediate some of the effects of testosterone on bone mineral density, epiphyseal closure, pituitary gonadotropin secretion, high-density lipoprotein (HDL) cholesterol levels, and some aspects of brain function.[115,116] Aromatase activity in the testis is regulated by gonadotropins and in nontesticular tissue by increasing body adiposity.[91,92,117,118] In men, plasma estradiol levels are determined primarily by the amount of androgenic substrate that is available and aromatase activity in adipose and other peripheral tissues.[117,118]

There are two forms of the enzyme 5α-reductase (1 and 2), which convert testosterone to DHT, an androgen that is 2.5 times more potent than testosterone.[119] 5α-reductase 2 is expressed most highly in the male urogenital tract (prostate and seminal vesicles), genital skin, and the liver, while 5α-reductase 1 is found predominantly in skin (hair follicles) and liver. The majority of the 200–300 μg of DHT produced daily is derived from conversion of testosterone in peripheral tissues with little coming directly from the testis.[94]

As inferred from individuals with congenital 5α-reductase 2 deficiency, local formation of DHT is required to mediate the effects of testosterone on the normal development of male external genitalia, prostate, seminal vesicles, and male hair pattern.[120,121] In contrast, the stimulatory effects of testosterone on muscle and sexual function do not require the 5α-reduction of testosterone to DHT. Inhibitors of 5α-reductase, such as finasteride (predominantly a 5α-reductase 2 inhibitor), are used to reduce prostate size and to treat symptoms, abnormalities in urine flow and complications of benign prostatic hyperplasia, and male pattern baldness or androgenic alopecia.[122,123]

Androgens are catabolized in the liver (50–70%) and other peripheral tissues (Fig. 15-13). Testosterone is taken up effectively by the liver and converted to the inactive metabolites androsterone and etiocholanolone (both 17-ketosteroids) and to DHT, which is metabolized to 3α-androstanediol. These compounds are conjugated in the liver to glucuronide and sulfate derivatives that are released into plasma and excreted in the urine. In peripheral tissues, predominantly in skin, DHT is converted reversibly to 3α-androstanediol and subsequently to 3α-androstanediol glucuronide (3α–diol G). Blood and urine measurements of 3α–diol G have been used as markers of peripheral androgen action. In patients with 5α-reductase deficiency, 3α–diol G levels are reduced, and in those with androgen excess states associated with increased androgen metabolism in skin, levels are elevated.[124,125] The amount of acne and body hair correlates with plasma 3α–diol G levels.[126]

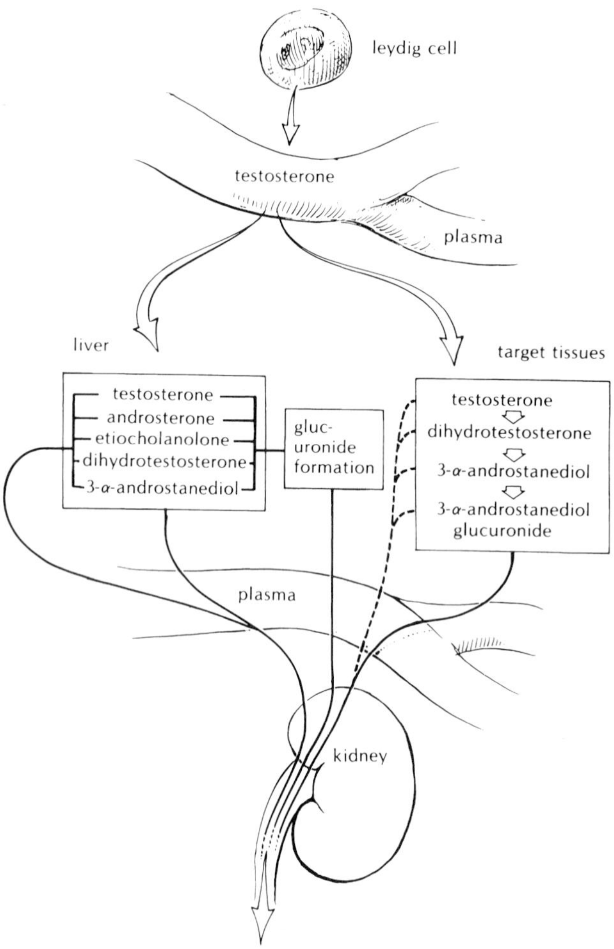

FIGURE 15-13. Diagrammatic representation of the metabolism of testosterone. After secretion by the Leydig cell, testosterone travels through the plasma to the liver or target tissues. After metabolism and conjugation, products are excreted into the urine.

Androgen Action In target tissues androgens, both testosterone and DHT, bind to the hormone-binding domain of high-affinity intracellular receptors.[127,128] The ligand-bound receptor is translocated to the nucleus, where it binds to androgen response elements (palindromic DNA sequences located in the 5' regulatory regions) of specific genes and interacts with tissue-specific transcription factors (coactivators and corepressors) to regulate gene transcription and protein synthesis, resulting in specific androgen actions.

The androgen receptor is encoded by a gene located on the long-arm of the X chromosome.[129,130] The amino acid sequence of the androgen receptor shares ~80 percent homology with progesterone, glucocorticoid, and mineralocorticoid receptors. The affinity and stability of DHT binding to the androgen receptor is greater than that of testosterone, and contributes the greater potency of DHT as an androgen.[129–131] Mutations of the androgen receptor gene that cause quantitative or qualitative abnormalities of the receptor and impair androgen action result in males with varying degrees of genital ambiguity or male pseudohermaphroditism (see Chap. 17).

Androgens exert differing actions at various stages of sexual development (Table 15-1). Therefore, the clinical consequences of androgen deficiency or reduction in androgen action (androgen resistance) depend on the developmental stage during which it occurs. During embryogenesis, testosterone secreted by the fetal testis and its conversion to DHT are essential for normal differentiation of male internal and external genitalia, so-called primary sexual characteristics. The physiological role of the neonatal surge in testosterone is not clear. However, boys with microphallus do not exhibit normal androgen-mediated growth of the penis unless androgen is administered during infancy.[132] Therefore, neonatal androgen exposure may have a potentiating or priming effect on male urogenital tract growth. Although it is postulated that neonatal androgens may play a role in subsequent male gender behavior and identity, this has not been established in humans.

During puberty, the progressive increase in testosterone and its active metabolism to estradiol and DHT are responsible for the development secondary sexual characteristics (Fig. 15-14), such as:

1. Growth and development of the penis and scrotum
2. Enlargement of the prostate gland and seminal vesicles and stimulation of secretion from these accessory sexual glands
3. Growth of hair in a male pattern of distribution (i.e., facial, external ear, chest, axillary, lower abdomen, pubic, perianal, leg, and inner thigh hair growth) and recession of frontal hair

TABLE 15-1. Clinical Actions of Testosterone

- **In Utero**
  - External genitalia development
  - Wolffian duct (internal genital organ) development
- **Neonatal**
  - Possible male behavioral effects
  - Possible priming of male urogenital tract (e.g., penis)
- **Pubertal**
  - External genitalia
    - Penis and scrotum increase in size and become pigmented
    - Rugal folds appear in scrotal skin
  - Accessory sex glands
    - Prostate and seminal vesicles enlarge and secretion begins
  - Hair growth
    - Facial (mustache and beard) hair growth develops; scalp undergoes recession
    - Pubic hair growth develops
    - Axillary, body, extremity, and perianal hair growth appears
  - Linear growth
    - Pubertal growth spurt
    - Interaction with growth hormone to increase insulin-like growth factor-1 (IGF-1)
    - Eventual closure of epiphyses (in part, via aromatization to estradiol)
  - Bone
    - Bone mineral density increases (in part, via aromatization to estradiol)
    - Peak bone mass develops
  - Muscle
    - Muscle bulk and strength increase
    - Positive nitrogen balance is demonstrable
  - Adipose tissue
    - Decrease and redistribution of body fat
  - Voice
    - Larynx enlarges and vocal cords thicken, resulting in lower-pitched voice
  - Behavior
    - Libido and erections are stimulated
    - Motivation and initiative increase; more aggressive attitudes are manifest
    - Possible cognitive effects
  - Erythropoiesis
    - Erythropoietin secretion is stimulated
    - Direct bone marrow stimulation of hematopoiesis
    - Hematocrit increases
  - Lipids
    - High-density lipoprotein cholesterol is suppressed
  - Spermatogenesis
    - Sertoli cell function is stimulated via interaction with FSH
    - Sperm production is initiated
- **Adult**
  - Accessory sex glands
    - Prostate and seminal vesicles size is maintained
    - Prostate growth continues
  - Hair growth
    - Male hair patterns (facial, axillary, body, extremity, and perianal) are maintained
    - Male pattern baldness (androgenic alopecia) may be initiated
  - Bone
    - Bone mineral density is maintained (in part, via aromatization to estradiol)
    - Bone loss and osteoporosis are prevented
  - Muscle
    - Muscle bulk and strength are maintained
  - Behavior
    - Libido and erectile function are maintained
    - Motivation and initiative are maintained
  - Erythropoiesis
    - Erythropoietin secretion and direct bone marrow stimulation are maintained
    - Hematocrit is maintained
  - Lipids
    - High-density lipoprotein cholesterol remains suppressed
  - Spermatogenesis
    - Sertoli cell function is maintained via interaction with FSH
    - Sperm production is maintained

4. Stimulation of long bone growth and eventual closure of epiphyses (in part, via aromatization of testosterone to estradiol)
5. Increase in bone mineral density and acquisition of peak bone mass
6. Increase in skeletal muscle bulk and strength, especially in the shoulder and pectoral muscles
7. Decrease and redistribution of body fat
8. Enlargement of the larynx and thickening of vocal cords, resulting in deepening of the voice
9. Prominent behavioral changes, including sexual behavior with stimulation of libido and erections, increase in motivation and aggressiveness, and possible cognitive effects, especially in the visuospatial domain
10. Stimulation of erythropoiesis and increase in hematocrit
11. Suppression of HDL cholesterol
12. Initiation of spermatogenesis and acquisition of fertility.[60]

In the adult male, continued normal testosterone secretion and its conversion to estradiol and DHT are necessary for:

1. Maintenance of prostate and seminal vesicle secretions and continued growth of the prostate gland with development of benign prostatic hyperplasia in the middle to later years of life
2. Maintenance of a male hair pattern and initiation of male pattern baldness or androgenic alopecia
3. Maintenance of bone mineral density
4. Maintenance of muscle mass and strength
5. Maintenance of sexual behavior (libido and erectile function), motivation, and initiative
6. Maintenance of hematocrit in the male range, higher than that of the female
7. Maintenance of an HDL cholesterol lower than females
8. Maintenance of normal spermatogenesis and fertility.

Some of the effects of testosterone completed during pubertal maturation are permanent. For example, once full development is completed, testosterone is not required for the maintenance of penis size, scrotal development, linear growth, or laryngeal and vocal cord size in adults.

Hormonal Control of Spermatogenesis

Both FSH and LH are important regulators of spermatogenesis in man. As described previously, the effects of FSH are mediated through direct stimulation of Sertoli cell function and those of LH are mediated indirectly through Leydig cell production of testosterone that acts on Sertoli cells either directly or through

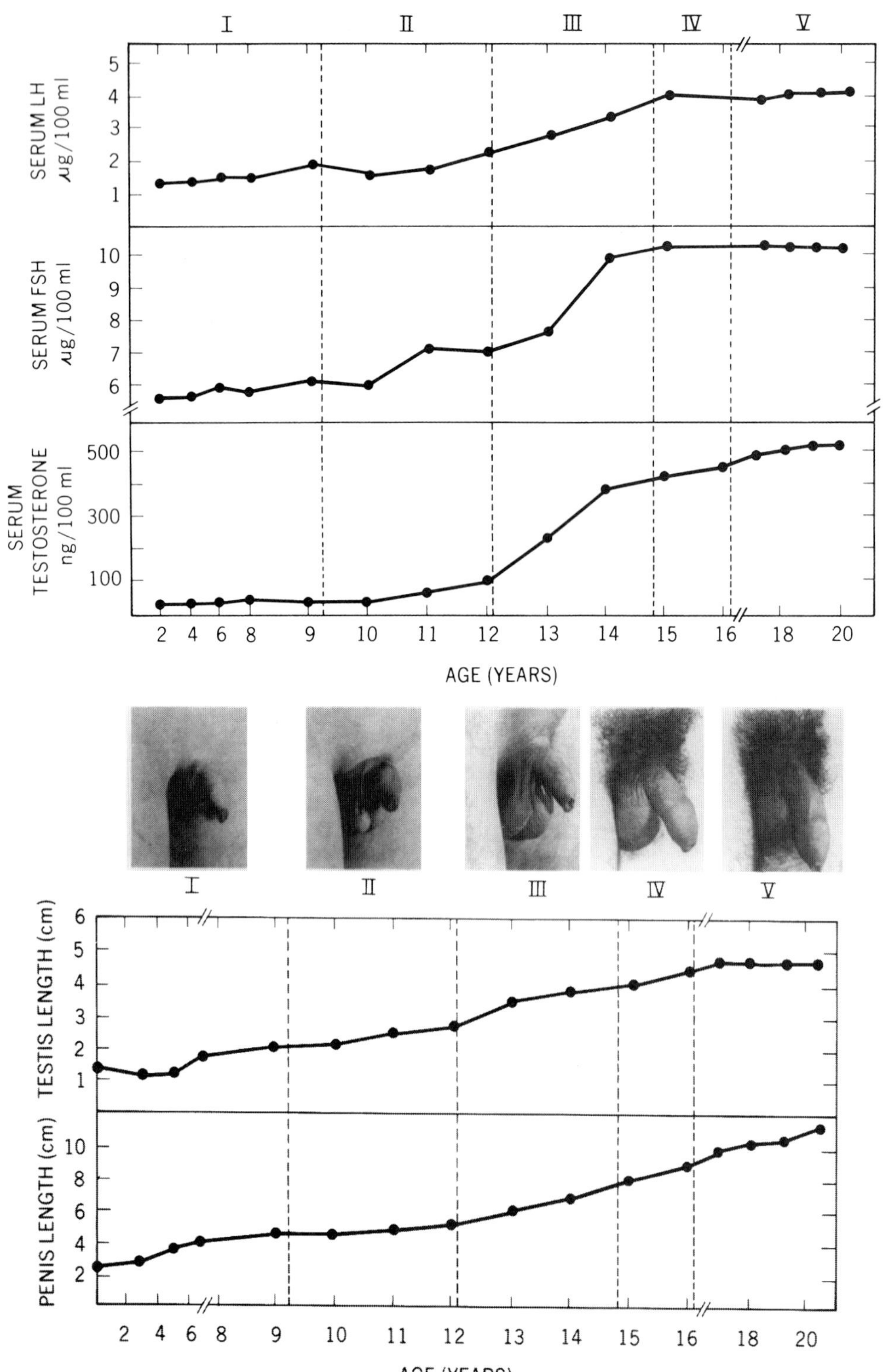

FIGURE 15-14. (*Top*) Genital changes during puberty. I to V represent the pubertal stages of Marshall and Tanner. (*Bottom*) Hormonal changes during puberty. (*From Marshall and Tanner*[812] and *Faiman and Winter.*[813])

paracrine factors released by peritubular myoid cells. The hormonal requirements necessary to initiate spermatogenesis during puberty differ from those needed to maintain sperm production in adults, and the relative roles of FSH and LH (testosterone), in particular the former, in the initiation and maintenance of spermatogenesis in humans remain controversial.

Initiation of Spermatogenesis

It is generally thought that both FSH and LH stimulation of the testis are necessary for initiation of spermatogenesis at the time of puberty.[100,133] This view has been supported by studies of gonadotropin therapy to induce sperm production in patients with prepubertal gonadotropin deficiency due to idiopathic hypogonadotropic hypogonadism (IHH) or Kallmann syndrome who lack active spermatogenesis.[134,135] It is clear that LH-stimulated testosterone secretion is necessary to initiate sperm and seminal fluid production in these patients. Treatment of these patients with FSH activity alone does not stimulate spermatogenesis.[136,137]

The role of FSH in the initiation of spermatogenesis is less clear. Although some patients with IHH produce sperm with LH or hCG treatment alone (usually those with evidence of some endogenous FSH secretion), most require both LH and FSH treatment to initiate spermatogenesis, suggesting that both FSH and testosterone stimulated by LH are necessary for initiation of sperm production.[136,138–141] However, recent reports of complete spermatogenesis in men with inactivating mutations of the FSH receptor question the absolute role of FSH.[142] Although sperm concentrations and testicular size were significantly reduced in these cases, it is not clear that FSH action was completely eliminated. These findings are similar to those in FSHβ subunit and FSH receptor knockout mice who are able to initiate complete spermatogenesis and are fertile.[143,144] In contrast, men with FSHβ gene mutations have been azoospermic but their serum testosterone has been low or low-normal with elevated LH levels, suggesting a role of FSH on Leydig cell development and/or function.[145,146] Therefore, we can conclude that stimulation of testosterone by LH is absolutely necessary, but very little, if any, FSH is required for the initiation of *qualitatively* normal spermatogenesis when normal LH (and testosterone) levels are present. However, FSH may play a very important role in initiating *quantitatively* normal spermatogenesis, perhaps by increasing the number of Sertoli cells during testicular development. Practically, most patients with prepubertal gonadotropin deficiency require both FSH and LH activity to initiate sperm production.

Maintenance of Spermatogenesis

Several lines of evidence suggest that FSH is not necessary to maintain *qualitatively* normal sperm production in humans. In men with IHH, after spermatogenesis is initiated by FSH and LH treatment, it can be maintained by LH or hCG alone.[100,147] Furthermore, in most men with acquired gonadotropin deficiency as adults, sperm production can be reinitiated and maintained by LH activity alone.[100,140] In normal men with experimental gonadotropin deficiency induced by high-dosage testosterone administration, sperm production is suppressed to zero (azoospermia) or severely low levels (oligozoospermia). Administration of either LH or hCG alone reinitiates spermatogenesis, although not to quantitatively normal levels, despite extremely low levels of FSH.[148,149] Interestingly, FSH administration alone in these men is also able to restore sperm production to a similar extent, despite markedly suppressed LH and presumably intratesticular testosterone concentrations.[150] Similarly, an hypophysectomized man with an activating mutation of the FSH receptor was able to maintain spermatogenesis despite undetectable circulating gonadotropin levels.[151] Administration of both LH and FSH activity is able to fully restore spermatogenesis quantitatively in normal men with experimentally induced gonadotropin deficiency.[152]

These findings suggest that neither normal levels of FSH nor LH are required for maintenance of *qualitatively* normal spermatogenesis but both gonadotropins are required for *quantitatively* normal sperm production. Clinically, in most men with IHH in whom spermatogenesis is initiated with gonadotropin therapy and acquired gonadotropin deficiency, spermatogenesis can be reinitiated and maintained with LH activity (i.e., hCG) alone. Because treatment using currently available FSH preparations is much more expensive than hCG, treatment with hCG alone versus regimens that include FSH translates into a considerable savings for these patients.

Although high intratesticular testosterone concentrations are produced by Leydig cells stimulated by LH, spermatogenesis can proceed in the presence of concentrations that are 10 percent of those normally present.[153] However, intratesticular testosterone levels are normally approximately 100 times those in plasma,[154] so that concentrations needed to support spermatogenesis are still much greater than those present in blood. Practically, exogenous testosterone therapy of men with gonadotropin deficiency usually does not support spermatogenesis. The role of intratesticular conversion of testosterone to DHT and estradiol in spermatogenesis is not clear.

Studies in experimental animals and some in humans have provided insight into the predominant site and mechanism of action of FSH and testosterone in supporting spermatogenesis. FSH is important in maintaining the transition of spermatogonia A to spermatogonia B; testosterone is important in the survival of primary spermatocytes and in the conversion of step 7 to 8 spermatids during spermiogenesis; and both FSH and testosterone are important in spermiation or release of spermatozoa from the seminiferous tubule.[155–158]

Feedback Regulation of Gonadotropin Secretion

Hypothalamic GnRH stimulation of pituitary LH and FSH secretion and gonadotropin stimulation of testicular testosterone and sperm production are the feed-forward components of the reproductive axis. An important aspect of hypothalamic-pituitary-testicular axis control is the negative feedback regulation of hypothalamic GnRH and pituitary gonadotropin secretion by steroid and protein hormones produced by the testis. Testosterone exerts negative feedback effects at both the hypothalamic and pituitary levels to inhibit GnRH secretion and both LH and FSH, and inhibin suppresses FSH secretion at the level of the pituitary gland (Fig. 15-8).

Hypothalamic Feedback

The *acute* negative feedback effect of testosterone on LH and FSH secretion (over hours to days) occurs exclusively by inhibition of hypothalamic GnRH secretion, specifically by suppressing GnRH pulse frequency (as reflected by a decrease in LH pulse frequency) without inhibiting pituitary responsiveness to GnRH.[63,159–163] This action of testosterone is mediated through interaction with androgen receptors present in the hypothalamus, as nonaromatizable androgens (e.g., DHT or fluoxymesterone) also inhibit and pure antiandrogens (e.g., flutamide) increase LH and GnRH pulse frequency. The more chronic negative feedback effects of testosterone involve actions at both the hypothalamic and pituitary level (see later discussion).

Aromatase is present in the hypothalamus, and conversion of testosterone to estradiol mediates some of the negative feedback effects of testosterone on GnRH secretion via interaction with estrogen receptors.[159,160,164–167] In men, administration of an antiestrogen (e.g., clomiphene citrate or tamoxifen) or an aromatase inhibitor (e.g., testolactone) increases LH (and presumably GnRH) pulse frequency and amplitude without affecting pituitary responsiveness to GnRH acutely. The enzyme 5α-reductase is also found in the hypothalamus. However, men with 5α-reductase deficiency exhibit only modest elevations in gonadotropins, and normal men treated with a 5α-reductase inhibitor, finasteride, do not demonstrate increases in LH or FSH.[168,169] These findings suggest a relatively minor role for DHT in the physiological feedback regulation of gonadotropins. The negative feedback effect of testosterone on LH and presumably GnRH pulse frequency can be blocked by μ-opiate receptor antagonists, such as naltrexone, suggesting that this effect may be mediated by endogenous opiate neuromodulatory systems, such as β-endorphin, in the hypothalamus.[170]

Pituitary Feedback

Testosterone (via conversion to estradiol) also exerts a negative feedback effect at the pituitary level by inhibiting pituitary LH responsiveness to GnRH, resulting in reduced spontaneous LH pulse amplitude.[171,172] In GnRH-deficient men treated with pulsatile GnRH therapy to restore gonadotropin secretion, the inhibition of LH and FSH levels by testosterone administration is blocked by an aromatase inhibitor, suggesting that the negative feedback effect of testosterone at the pituitary is mediated primarily by its conversion to estradiol and interaction with estrogen receptors on pituitary gonadotrophs.

Sertoli cells of the testis produce a protein hormone, inhibin, that is postulated to exert a negative feedback effect on the pituitary to selectively inhibit FSH secretion. Inhibin is a heterodimeric glycoprotein hormone composed of an α subunit and either a β_A or β_B subunit connected by a disulfide bridge to yield inhibin A or inhibin B, respectively.[173,174] In men, inhibin B appears to be the physiologically relevant inhibin species.[175] Circulating inhibin B levels decrease progressively in conditions associated with increasing degrees of germ cell damage and presumably Sertoli cell dysfunction (Fig. 15-15). Furthermore, inhibin B secretion is regulated by gonadotropins. Thus, inhibin B levels are low in men with Kallmann syndrome and are stimulated by FSH and LH, the latter presumably acting via Leydig cell production of testosterone that in turn acts on Sertoli cells.[176,177] Although studies in monkeys demonstrate that inhibin B is an important negative feedback regulator of FSH at the pituitary level,[178,179] the physiological significance of inhibin B has not been demonstrated clearly in men.

The β_A or β_B inhibin subunits also combine to form proteins called activin A (β_A-β_A homodimer), activin B (β_B-β_B homodimer), or activin AB (β_A-β_B heterodimer). In contrast to inhibin B, activins stimulate FSH secretion from the pituitary.[173,174] Although activin A circulates, its levels do not decrease following orchidectomy. Activin/inhibin subunits are produced by pituitary cells, and—based primarily on studies in vitro—activins are postulated to act as a paracrine factor that stimulates FSH secretion.[173,174] Another pituitary protein, known as follistatin, regulates activin action by binding to it and neutralizing its activity.[173,174] Activin/inhibin subunits and follistatin produced in the pituitary are regulated by GnRH, testosterone and inhibin B. Therefore, FSH secretion by the pituitary is regulated by local factors (activins and follistatin) as well as by GnRH, testosterone and inhibin B. Activin and follistatin are also produced by germ cells and Sertoli cells and may participate in local paracrine regulation of testicular function.[173,174]

FIGURE 15-15. Serum inhibin B and inactive pro-α-C levels in normal men and patients with hypogonadism. (*From Anawalt, Bebb, Matsumoto, et al.*[175])

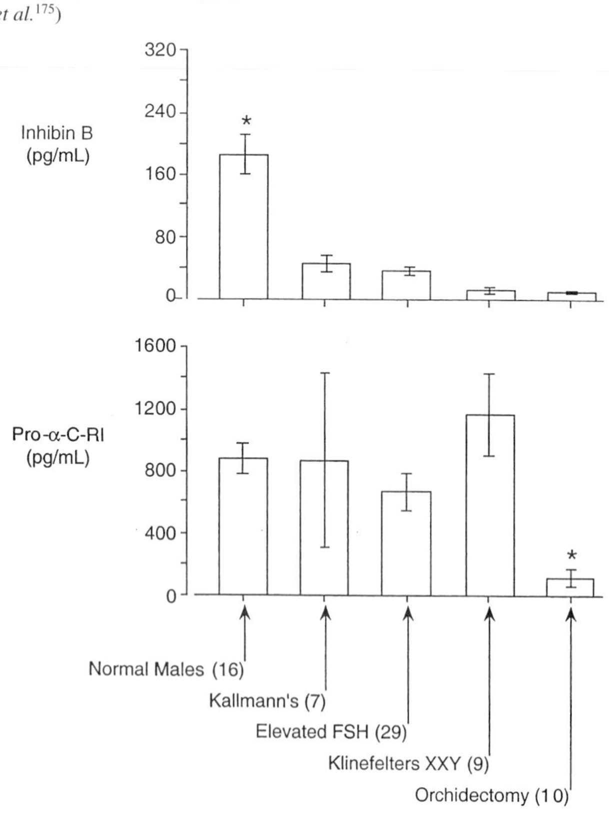

Physiology of Male Sexual Response

Normal male sexual function requires coordinated regulation of a series of physiological events: *libido; erection; ejaculation; orgasm;* and *detumescence.*[180]

Libido

Libido (sexual interest and desire) is generated by visual, tactile, imaginative, auditory, and/or gustatory erotic stimulation of the central nervous system.[180–182] These erotic stimuli are received in a number of cortical and subcortical brain regions, most notably the limbic system, and relayed via the medial preoptic and anterior hypothalamic areas to the sympathetic thoracolumbar and parasympathetic sacral spinal cord centers that regulate penile vascular smooth muscle and erection. Therefore, disturbances in libido are usually accompanied by varying degrees of erectile dysfunction.

Libido is regulated primarily by psychological factors and sex steroid hormones, in particular testosterone.[181,182] Psychological disturbances of various degrees from anxiety to major psychiatric illnesses, central nervous system disorders, drugs that affect brain function, and androgen deficiency may cause a reduction or loss of libido and erectile dysfunction. Testosterone plays an important role in maintaining normal libido and nocturnal erections, but much less of a role in erections due to erotic stimuli.[183–185] Occasionally, castrated men may maintain sexual desire and erectile function for long periods following removal of the testes, suggesting that the requirement for androgens is quite variable.[186]

Erection

Penile erection or sustained penile tumescence is primarily a vascular event involving dilatation of vascular and sinusoidal smooth muscle within the corpora cavernosa of the penis that is regulated both by the peripheral and central nervous system and modulated by psychological and hormonal factors. Penile erections are generated by two separate but synergistic mechanisms: *Reflexogenic erections* are induced by sensory stimulation of the penis and mediated through a sacral spinal reflex arc; and *psy-*

chogenic erections are induced by psychogenic stimuli from higher brain centers and are mediated by both the thoracolumbar and sacral spinal cord erection centers.[181,182]

In reflexogenic erections, sensory afferent impulses from stimulation of the penis travel via the pudendal nerve to the sacral spinal erection center (S_2 to S_4).[181,182] Efferent parasympathetic fibers return via the pelvic splanchnic nerve (nervi erigentes), which joins the pelvic plexus and reaches the penis via the cavernosal nerve. These fibers innervate the vascular and sinusoidal smooth muscles of the corpora cavernosa of the penis, causing them to dilate and resulting in an erection. Therefore, induction of a penile erection is primarily but not exclusively controlled by the parasympathetic nervous system. Efferent somatic fibers traveling in the pudendal nerve innervate the striated muscles (ischiocavernosus and bulbocavernosus) of the perineum.

Sympathetic fibers originating in the thoracolumbar spinal erection center (T_{12} to L_2) travel via the hypogastric nerve to the pelvic plexus and also reach the penis via the cavernosal nerve.[181,182] These fibers innervate the muscles of the vas deferens, seminal vesicles, prostate, and internal sphincter of the bladder, and serve to coordinate erection and antegrade ejaculation. In psychogenic erections, erotic stimuli received and integrated in the brain are relayed via descending pathways in the lateral spinal columns and regulate both the sympathetic thoracolumbar and parasympathetic sacral spinal erection centers to stimulate penile erections.

Penile erectile tissue consists of paired corpora cavernosa on the dorsum of the penis and the ventral corpus spongiosum that surrounds the urethra and forms the glans penis.[187] The corpora are composed of sponge-like, interconnected trabecular spaces lined by vascular epithelial and smooth muscle cells. Each corpus is surrounded by a thick fibrous sheath, the tunica albuginea, and all three corporal bodies are surrounded by a single dense fascia, Buck's fascia.

Activation of the spinal cord erection centers and the resulting stimulation of neurotransmission in the cavernosal nerves results in corporal smooth muscle relaxation and vasodilatation of the cavernosal arterioles (branches of the internal pudendal arteries) and vascular sinusoids within the corpora cavernosa.[187] As a result, blood flow into the trabecular spaces of the corpora increases several-fold, causing engorgement of the penis (tumescence). Expansion of the trabecular walls against the tunica albuginea compresses subtunical venular plexus and impedes venous outflow, resulting in sustained penile tumescence, i.e., an erection. Masturbation or sexual intercourse triggers the bulbocavernosus reflex and contraction of the ischiocavernosus and bulbocavernosus muscles by pudenal nerve stimulation, compressing the base of the erect penis. This increases cavernosal pressure to levels greater than systemic blood pressure, resulting in maximal penile rigidity.

Nitric oxide (NO) is probably the major neurotransmitter that mediates penile erection.[187] In response to parasympathetic cholinergic stimulation mediated via acetylcholine, NO is released both by endothelial cells and postganglionic noncholinergic, nonadrenergic nerve fibers. Within smooth muscle cells, NO activates guanylate cyclase and increases intracellular cyclic guanosine monophosphate (cGMP) levels. The latter then activates a cGMP-dependent protein kinase to phosphorylate a number of proteins and ion channels that ultimately decrease intracellular calcium, causing smooth muscle relaxation. During the flaccid state, cGMP is hydrolyzed by the enzyme phosphodiesterase type 5. A number of other neurotransmitters including prostaglandin E_1 may induce smooth muscle relaxation by activating adenylate cyclase and cAMP-dependent protein kinase.[187]

Knowledge of the neurotransmitter mechanisms involved in the regulation of penile erection has been used to design treatments for erectile dysfunction in men. By preventing the breakdown of cGMP, *sildenafil,* a type 5 phosphodiesterase inhibitor, and *papaverine,* a nonspecific phosphodiesterase inhibitor, result in sustained penile smooth muscle relaxation, usually sufficient to induce a penile erection in patients with erectile dysfunction.[187] Prostaglandin E_1 administered by injection into the corpus cavernosum or a transurethral pellet activates adenylate cylase in smooth muscle and has also been used to treat erectile dysfunction.[187]

Erectile dysfunction is a consistent inability to achieve or maintain an erection sufficient to complete intercourse.[187] It may be caused by: androgen deficiency; central and peripheral nervous system diseases; vascular disorders; and penile abnormalities. Erectile dysfunction is an important clinical manifestation of hypogonadism (see later section).

Ejaculation

Sympathetic nervous system activation from the thoracolumbar spinal cord via the hypogastric nerve and α-adrenergic receptors causes contractions of the cauda epididymis, vas deferens, accessory sex glands, and ejaculatory ducts, resulting in movement of sperm and seminal fluid into the posterior urethra (*emission*).[188–190] Sympathetic activation also stimulates closure of the internal urethral sphincter, preventing retrograde ejaculation of sperm into the bladder. Emission is followed by reflex stimulation of the sacral spinal cord erection center, which sends somatic nerve fibers to the perineum and stimulates rhythmic contractions of the ishchiocavernosus and bulbocavernosus muscles, causing expulsion of semen from the urethra, i.e., ejaculation. Like erection, the ejaculatory reflex is under considerable control by higher cerebral centers and is both voluntary and involuntary in nature.

Premature ejaculation is characterized by ejaculation that occurs before or immediately during vaginal penetration, followed by a rapid loss of erection. The majority of men with this disorder have an underlying psychological etiology, such as performance anxiety or an emotional disorder, and rarely is there an organic cause.[191,192] *Retarded ejaculation* is a psychological disorder characterized by an inability to ejaculate despite normal libido, erectile function, and stimulation that is commonly due to excessive anxiety.[193,194] *Retrograde ejaculation* into the bladder usually occurs in patients with sympathetic neuropathy (e.g., with diabetes), sympatholytic agents, or after extensive abdominopelvic or bladder neck surgery (e.g., transurethral resection of the prostate).[195–204] *Reduced or absent ejaculation* may occur with androgen deficiency; sympatholytic drugs, sympathectomy, or extensive retroperitoneal or pelvic surgery resulting in retrograde ejaculation; or urethral abnormalities.[205–208]

Orgasm

Ejaculation usually occurs simultaneously with orgasm, the pleasurable sensation associated with emission and ejaculation. Orgasm is primarily a central nervous system-mediated phenomena that is triggered, under normal circumstances, by ascending spinal cord pathways associated with ejaculation. However, orgasm can occur in the absence of erection or ejaculation (e.g., with temporal lobe lesions).[209] Conversely, normal libido, erection, and ejaculation can occur without orgasm; this is nearly always due to a psychological disorder.

Detumescence

Detumescence is mediated by α_2-adrenergic stimulation that occurs during ejaculation, resulting in relaxation of penile smooth muscle and vasoconstriction of the cavernosal arteries that reduces arterial blood flow into the penis. As a result of sympathetic nervous system activation, the trabecular spaces of the corpora collapse, the subtunical venular plexus is decompressed, venous outflow is increased, and the penis becomes flaccid. *Phentolamine,* an α-adrenergic antagonist, prevents penile smooth muscle relaxation and vasoconstriction, and delays detumescence. It is injected into the corpus cavernosum in combination with papaverine to treat men with erectile dysfunction.[187]

In many cases, premature detumescence may contribute to the pathophysiology of erectile dysfunction, e.g., venous leak or incompetence. Failure of detumescence, *priapism,* is often painful and unrelated to sexual intercourse. It is commonly idiopathic in etiology, but may be associated with spinal cord injury, sickle cell disease, chronic myelogenous leukemia, and intracorporal injection of vasodilatory substances used in the treatment of erectile dysfunction.[210,211]

MALE HYPOGONADISM

Clinical Manifestations and Evaluation

Hypogonadism is the most common disorder of testis function that is encountered in clinical practice. In the clinical evaluation of patients, it is extremely helpful to utilize knowledge of testicular development and hypothalamic-pituitary-testicular physiology both to make the diagnosis of hypogonadism and to identify the etiology of gonadal failure. The two major functions of the testis are to produce testosterone and sperm. Therefore, male hypogonadism may present with either an impairment of testosterone production or androgen deficiency, which is nearly always associated with an impairment of spermatogenesis (*deficiency of androgen and sperm production*), or an *isolated impairment of sperm production or function* with normal testosterone production.

Furthermore, because androgens exert differing actions during sexual development (see previous section), the clinical presentation of androgen deficiency (or resistance) will depend upon whether it occurs *in utero* during embryogenesis, in a child *before or during puberty,* or in a fully developed *adult.*

Finally, clinical manifestations associated with the etiology of male hypogonadism will differ depending on whether it is caused by a primary disorder of the testis (*primary hypogonadism*) or is secondary to a hypothalamic-pituitary disorder (*secondary hypogonadism*). For example, secondary hypogonadism caused by a pituitary tumor may be associated with manifestations of tumor mass effects (e.g., headaches or visual field abnormalities) and/or deficiencies or excessive secretion of other anterior pituitary hormones.

In the following sections, differences in clinical presentation depending on whether there is a deficiency of androgen and sperm production or isolated impairment of sperm production or function, and whether androgen deficiency occurs in utero, before or during puberty or as an adult are considered (Table 15-2). The signs and symptoms discussed provide the clinical clues that are necessary to consider the diagnosis, and measurements of serum testosterone and/or sperm concentrations are used to confirm the diagnosis of hypogonadism.

TABLE 15-2. Clinical Manifestations of Androgen Deficiency

- In utero androgen deficiency
  - Ambiguous genital development (male pseudohermaphroditism)
- Prepubertal hypogonadism
  - Eunuchoidism
    - Lack of genital development (infantile genitalia)
      - Small penis <3–5 cm long
      - Lack of scrotal pigmentation and rugal folds
    - Small testes <2.5 cm long or volume <5 mL
    - Small prostate gland
    - Lack of male pattern hair growth
      - Lack of facial (mustache and beard) hair
      - Sparse pubic hair, female escutcheon
      - No temporal hair recession
      - Sparse axillary, body, extremity, and perianal hair
    - Fine cross-hatched skin wrinkling (lateral to orbits and mouth)
    - Eunuchoidal skeletal proportions
      - Floor to symphysis pubis length 5 cm > symphysis pubis to crown length
      - Arm span 5 cm > height
    - Prepubertal body fat distribution
      - Hips, face, and chest
    - Muscle mass poorly developed
    - High-pitched voice
  - Failure to achieve peak bone mass
    - Increased risk of osteoporosis
  - Poor motivation and initiative
  - Decreased hematocrit (in the female range)
  - Decreased libido and erectile function
  - Infertility, failure to initiate spermatogenesis, and aspermia
  - Gynecomastia
- Adult Hypogonadism
  - Decreased libido and erectile dysfunction
  - Infertility, reduced sperm production
  - Gynecomastia
  - Decreased rate of facial hair growth and amount of axillary and pubic hair
  - Fine, cross-hatched skin wrinkling (lateral to orbits and mouth)
  - Decreased muscle bulk and strength, fatigue
  - Osteopenia, osteoporosis, bone fractures
  - Testes may be soft and small (length <3.5 cm, volume <15 mL) or normal size
  - Diminished motivation and initiative, asthenia, increased irritability
  - Hot flushes (with rapid and severe androgen deficiency)
  - Prostate may be smaller than average size
  - Mild hypoproliferative anemia (in the female range)

Deficiency in Androgen and Sperm Production

In Utero Androgen Deficiency

During early fetal development, testosterone and its active metabolite, DHT, mediate the differentiation of male internal and external genitalia. Androgen deficiency or disorders of androgen action that occur during this period of development result in varying degrees of ambiguous external genital development, or *male pseudohermaphroditism.* These disorders are discussed in greater detailed in Chap. 17.

Prepubertal Hypogonadism

During puberty, testosterone is responsible for the development of male secondary sexual characteristics, long bone growth and the eventual closure of long bone epiphyses, stimulation of libido and erectile function, and initiation of spermatogenesis. Patients who develop androgen deficiency before the onset of puberty usually present to physicians as adolescents or young adults with delayed puberty. Testosterone deficiency before puberty results in *eunuchoidism* (Fig. 15-16), which is characterized by infantile genitalia; poor accessory sexual organ development and failure to develop an ejaculate (aspermia); a lack of male pattern hair growth; excessive long bone growth due to failure of long bone epiphyseal closure; a prepubertal fat distribution predominantly in the hips, face and chest; poor muscular development and strength; and a high-pitched voice. The testes are small, usually <2 cm in length or 5 ml in volume. A eunuchoidal body habitus is characterized by excessively long arms and legs in proportion to height. Although there are racial differences in body proportions, eunuchoidal body measurements consist of a total arm span that exceeds height by >5 cm, or a distance from the floor to the symphysis pubis that exceeds the distance from the symphysis to the crown of the head by >5 cm. Patients with prepubertal androgen deficiency fail to achieve normal peak bone mass, and if prolonged, this increases the risk of osteoporosis and bone fractures in the future.[212,213] These individuals usually exhibit poor motivation and initiative. Hematocrit remains in the female range because of inadequate androgen stimulation of erythropoiesis. As with adult hypogonadal men, patients with prepubertal deficiency of androgen production usually have diminished libido and erectile dysfunction, are infertile, and may have gynecomastia (benign enlargement of breast tissue).

FIGURE 15-16. Example of features of eunuchoidism as a result of prepubertal androgen deficiency due congenital anorchia before (*A* and *C*) and after (*B* and *D*) 18 months of testosterone treatment. (*From Bardin and Paulsen.*[814])

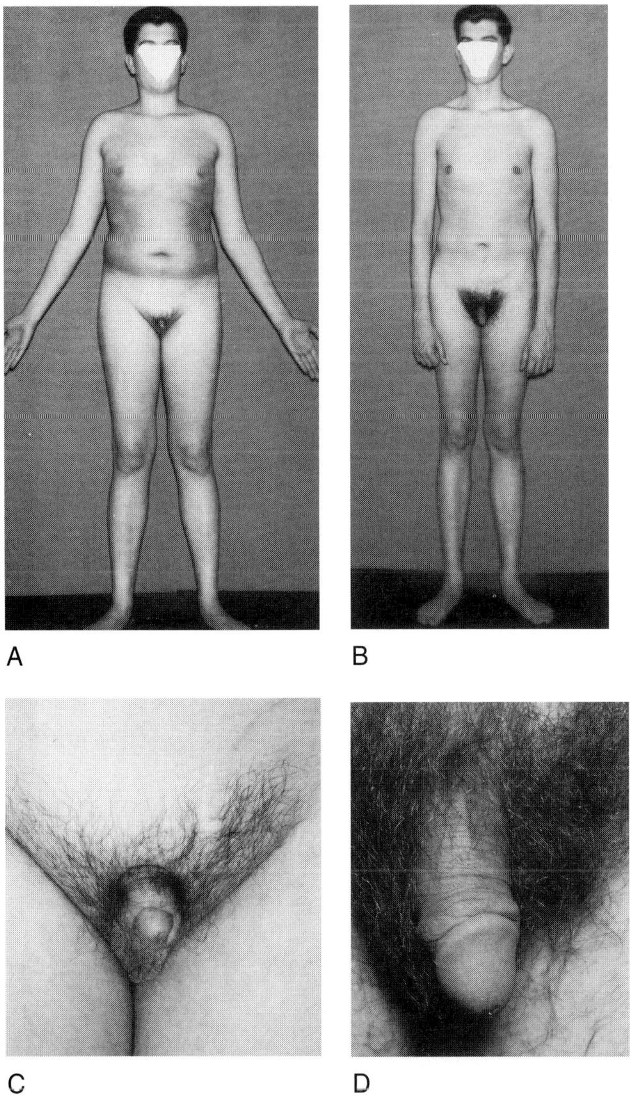

Adult Hypogonadism

In adults, testosterone maintains normal sexual function, some secondary sexual characteristics, and spermatogenesis. Men with adult hypogonadism complain primarily of poor sexual performance with diminished libido and erectile dysfunction, gynecomastia, and infertility as a result of impaired spermatogenesis. Secondary sexual characteristics do not regress to the prepubertal state. However, with long-standing androgen deficiency, there may be significant loss of hair in androgen-dependent (e.g., facial, axillary, and pubic) areas, fine cross-hatched wrinkling of skin most noticeable lateral to the eyes and mouth, diminished muscle mass and strength, increased body fat, and osteopenia or osteoporosis. Androgen deficiency is being recognized increasingly as a major cause of male osteoporosis and fractures, especially in older hypogonadal men.[214] With the greater use of dual energy x-ray absorptiometry (DEXA) to measure bone mass, osteoporosis is increasingly the major presenting complaint of men with hypogonadism.

Depending on the specific cause, severity, and duration of the disorder, testis size may be small or normal in disorders that result in androgen deficiency and impaired spermatogenesis. For example, men with recent onset of gonadotropin deficiency from a destructive pituitary tumor may have normal size testes, despite severe testosterone deficiency. In contrast, patients with Klinefelter syndrome have extremely small testes. Androgen deficiency in adults may also cause behavioral changes, such as diminished motivation and initiative, asthenia, and irritability. Rapid development of severe androgen deficiency, such as occurs following medical or surgical castration, may cause vasomotor instability or hot flushes similar to those that many women develop at the time of menopause. With long-standing androgen deficiency, the prostate gland may be smaller than average and there may be a mild normochromic, normocytic hypoproliferative anemia with hematocrits falling within the normal female range.

Isolated Impairment in Sperm Production

Men with an isolated impairment of sperm production or function usually present as adults with infertility as their chief complaint, without symptoms or signs of testosterone deficiency. Testis size may be decreased, which suggests a reduced seminiferous tubule compartment, or normal. *Cryptorchidism* (an undescended testis) or *varicocele* (dilatation of pampiniform venous plexus of the testis) may be found. The remainder of the physical examination is usually unremarkable. Sperm counts are usually low (i.e., less than 20 million/ml, *oligozoospermia*) or zero (*azoospermia*), and there may be isolated or associated abnormalities of sperm motility and/or morphology. Serum testosterone levels are normal.

History and Physical Examination

Clinical evaluation of patients with hypogonadism should begin with a careful history that includes specific inquiry regarding the presence of genital ambiguity or developmental abnormalities at birth and need for surgical correction (e.g., hypospadius, epispadius, microphallus, cryptorchidism); a family history of pubertal or reproductive disorders; the extent of sexual maturation (e.g., growth, male pattern hair growth, penis and testis size, and voice change) and need for hormonal therapy during puberty; the functional and psychological effects of delayed puberty; sexual function (e.g., sexual interest, desire and thoughts, frequency of sexual intercourse, and erectile function); fertility; breast enlargement or tenderness; rate of beard growth (frequency of shaving); loss of axillary or pubic hair; muscle strength and functional limitations; osteoporosis or minimal trauma fractures; testis size; motivation and initiative in school, work and athletics; energy; and excessive irritability or presence of a short temper.

Patients should be carefully examined for hypospadius, epispadius, microphallus, or cryptorchidism; eunuchoidal body habitus (long arms and legs) and features (e.g., small penis and testis, lack of male pattern hair growth, prepubertal fat distribution, poor muscle development); gynecomastia; testis size; absence of a testis; and the presence of a varicocele.

The presence of palpable breast tissue, or gynecomastia, is detected by using fingers to grasp the periareolar area of the breast and a pinching motion to detect glandular tissue that is firmer than surrounding adipose tissue (Fig. 15-17). The diameter of palpable breast tissue is a useful objective measurement to assess the amount of gynecomastia (see discussion later). Using a technique similar to that used to examine the female breast (i.e., using the flat part of hand to palpate the breast against the chest wall) usually fails to detect mild breast enlargement in men. Testis size is assessed either by measuring its length and width with a small ruler or calipers, or comparison with a series of ellipsoids of increasing volume, a Prader orchidometer (Fig. 15-18). Normal testis size varies with age and the population examined (Table 15-3). The normal adult testis size usually measures approximately 3.5–5.5 cm in length × 2.0–3.0 cm in width, and has a volume of 15–30 mL.[19,20] In boys or men with a retractile testis, testis may be palpable only after the patient has a warm bath or assumes a squatting position.

FIGURE 15-17. Correct method of palpation for gynecomastia.

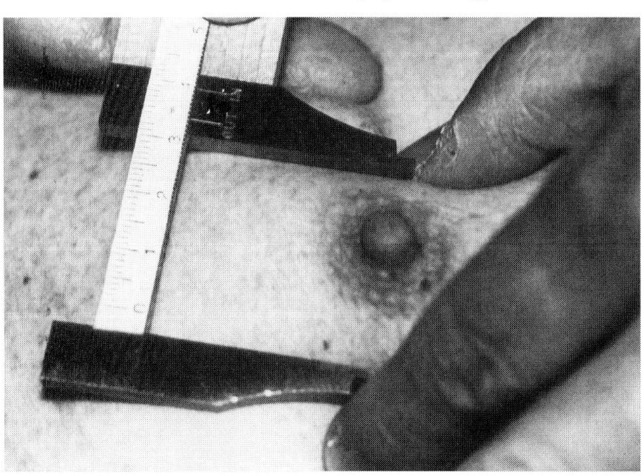

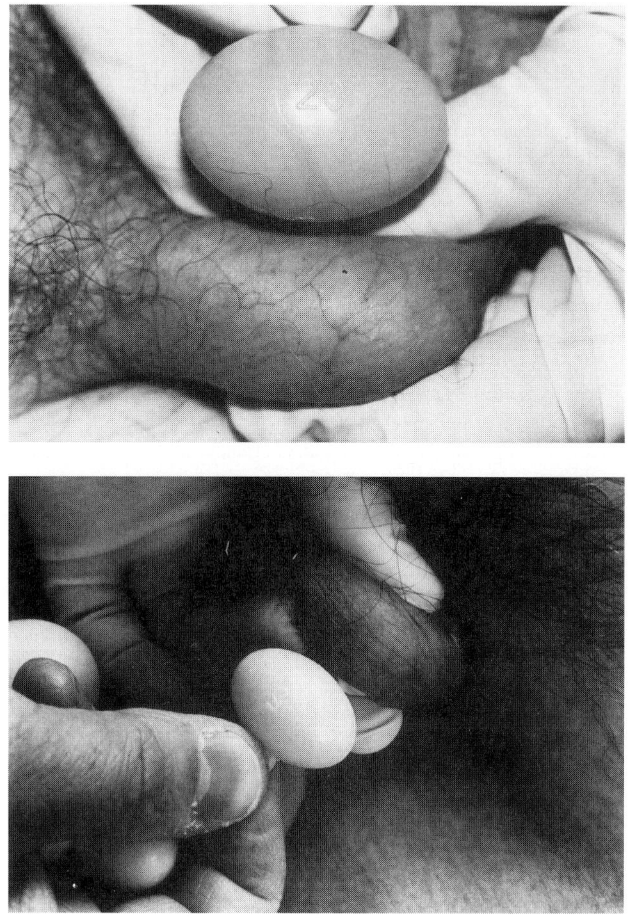

FIGURE 15-18. Assessment of testis size using a Prader orchidometer in a normal man (*above*, 20 mL testis) and man with Kallmann syndrome (*below*, 5 mL testis).

Serum Testosterone Measurement

Very sensitive and specific immunoassays for serum testosterone are generally available and are relatively inexpensive (Table 15-4). Routinely available assays measure total testosterone, i.e., all circulating fractions of testosterone (free, albumin-bound, and SHBG-bound testosterone). Although reference ranges vary with the methodology and reference population used, a clinically useful normal range for total testosterone is between 300–1,000 ng/dL (10.4–34.7 nmol/L). Testosterone levels vary diurnally with peak concentrations occurring at approximately 8 AM.[95,96] Therefore,

TABLE 15-3. Assessment of Testicular Size

Method	Prepubertal	Pubertal	Adult
Orchidometer*	1–6	8–15	20–30†
Ruler measurement‡			
Length	1.6–2.9	3.1–4.0	4.1–5.5
Width	1.0–1.8	2.0–2.5	2.7–3.2

*Measured in milliliters.

†24 ± 4 SD ml; $n = 44$.

‡Measured in centimeters.

Source: Adapted from Sherins and Howards.[20]

TABLE 15-4. Assays for Testosterone and Gonadotropins

Assay	Reference Range (SI units)	Physiological Changes	Methodological Considerations
Total testosterone (T)	300 to 1,000 ng/dL (10.4 to 34.7 nmol/L)	↓ Total T with ↓ in SHBG: moderate obesity (hyperinsulinemia) androgens hypercortisolism nephrotic syndrome malnutrition hypothyroidism acromegaly familial ↑ Total T with ↑ in SHBG: estrogens androgen deficiency hepatic cirrhosis hepatitis hyperthyroidism aging anticonvulsants Circadian variation with highest values in the morning.	Reference ranges vary with methodology and reference populations used. Some assays overestimate or underestimate T if serum is not extracted due to nonspecific serum effects.
Non-SHBG-bound T (bioavailable T)	60 to 510 ng/dL	Non-SHBG-bound T is unaltered with ↓ or ↑ SHBG. Circadian variation with highest values in the morning.	Reference ranges vary with methodology and reference populations used. Assay involves ammonium sulfate precipitation of SHBG and T assay of the supernatant fraction. Non-SHBG-bound T may also be calculated from measurements of total T, SHBG, and albumin, using affinity constants of T for SHBG and albumin. Values obtained using this calculation are similar to those obtained by ammonium sulfate precipitation and are often more reproducible.[104,214]
Free T (equilibrium dialysis)	5 to 41 ng/dL (0.18 to 1.42 nmol/L)	Free T is unaltered with ↓ or ↑ SHBG, *except* when is free T measured by solid-phase analogue kits* that varying with ↓ or ↑ SHBG levels. Circadian variation with highest levels in the morning.	Reference ranges vary with methodology and reference populations used. *Free T measured by solid phase analogue kits varies with ↓ or ↑ SHBG levels similar to total T levels.[216] Free T may also be calculated from measurements of total T, SHBG, and albumin, using affinity constants of T for SHBG and albumin. Values obtained using this calculation are similar to those obtained by equilibrium dialysis and are often more reproducible.
LH	Varies between 1–2.4 to 9–16 IU/L depending on assay and methodology	Episodic secretion with peaks approximately every 2 hours. Day-to-day variation as much as 30%.	Some assays cross-react with hCG (e.g., during therapy or secreted by germ cell tumors), or free α-subunit (e.g., secreted by gonadotropin-secreting pituitary tumors, other tumors or with reduced clearance in renal failure).

continued

TABLE 15-4. (*Continued*)

Assay	Reference Range (SI units)	Physiological Changes	Methodological Considerations
			Highly or ultrasensitive immunochemiluminescent and immunofluorimetric assays are available to measure very low levels of LH.
FSH	Varies between 0.9–1.0 to 8–15 IU/L	Episodic secretion but less prominent than LH. Day-to-day variation as much as 40%.	Some assays crossreact with free α-subunit (e.g., secreted by gonadotropin-secreting pituitary or other tumors, or with reduced clearance in renal failure). Highly or ultrasensitive immunochemiluminescent and immunofluorimetric assays are available to measure very low levels of FSH.

normal ranges should be established using morning blood samples, and attempts should be made to collect patient samples at that time. In addition to circadian variation, there are low amplitude ultradian variations in testosterone levels due mostly to pulsatile secretion by testes. Therefore, a low testosterone value should be repeated at least once before a diagnosis of androgen deficiency is made.

Because most circulating testosterone is bound to plasma proteins, total testosterone measurements are affected by clinical states that alter SHBG levels (Fig. 15-12).[106–110] Particularly problematic are clinical conditions that lower SHBG and therefore, total testosterone concentrations (e.g., moderate obesity, protein deficiency states such as nephrotic syndrome, and hypothyroidism). In these situations, the low total testosterone may lead to an erroneous diagnosis of hypogonadism. Therefore, when abnormal testosterone levels are detected, the possibility of SHBG abnormalities should be considered, and measurements of non-SHBG-bound (free plus albumin-bound) or free testosterone should specifically be determined.

Non-SHBG-bound testosterone, also called bioavailable testosterone, is determined by precipitating SHBG with ammonium sulfate, and measuring testosterone in the supernatant. Alternatively, it can be calculated from measurements of total testosterone, SHBG and albumin, and using affinity constants of testosterone for SHBG and albumin.[215] Free testosterone may also be calculated. Values of non-SHBG and free testosterone calculated in this way are similar to those obtained by the ammonium sulfate precipitation and equilibrium dialysis methods, respectively, and are often more reproducible.

Measurement of free testosterone is determined using an equilibrium or centrifugation dialysis method, or it can be calculated using separate determinations of total testosterone, SHBG, and albumin. Caution should be used in interpreting free testosterone levels determined by solid-phase analog kits that are utilized routinely by most clinical laboratories. Similar to total testosterone, free testosterone values obtained using these kits varies with the level of SHBG (Fig. 15-19).[216] In contrast, non-SHBG-bound testosterone does not correlate with SHBG concentrations.

Seminal Fluid Analysis

Impairment of sperm production is usually confirmed by low sperm counts on seminal fluid analysis. Assessment of sperm production is usually undertaken only in clinical instances in which fertility is an issue. Seminal fluid analysis is performed on semen samples obtained by masturbation, usually after 48 hours of abstinence from ejaculation (Table 15-5).[52] Normal ejaculate volume ranges from 2–6 ml. Although the normal range of sperm concentration is generally considered to be 20–200 million/ml, many men with sperm concentrations below 20 million/ml are fertile. In addition to determining sperm count, a careful microscopic examination of the seminal fluid is usually performed to assess sperm motility and morphology. Normally, ≥50 percent of spermatozoa examined within one hour after ejaculation are motile and ≥30 percent of sperm present have a normal oval head morphology, using strict criteria (≥50 percent using less stringent criteria).[52]

The minimum levels of sperm concentration, motility, and normal oval forms that are compatible with fertility are not clearly defined. In any individual, sperm counts normally exhibit extreme variability (Fig. 15-20), and are often temporarily suppressed by factors such as a febrile illness or hot tub use. Therefore, at least three seminal fluid analyses should be performed during a two- or three-month period to clinically assess sperm production. A diagnosis of oligozoospermia or azoospermia should not be made on values obtained on a single seminal fluid analysis. Functional tests of sperm penetration into cervical mucus of various mammalian species or zona pellucida-free hamster ova may be helpful in assessing fertilizing capability of spermatozoa.[217] However, these and other tests of sperm function and integrity have been difficult to standardize, and improvements in the predictive value of these tests for fertility have been marginal.

Differential Diagnosis

Erectile dysfunction, infertility, and gynecomastia are major manifestations of androgen deficiency. These complaints are encountered commonly in clinical practice. Hypogonadism is a major cause of these clinical manifestations, but there are many other causes. Therefore, it is important to be familiar with the differential diagnosis of erectile dysfunction, infertility, and gynecomastia.

Erectile Dysfunction

Erectile dysfunction is defined as the inability to achieve or maintain penile erection that is adequate for completion of satisfactory intercourse. It is a common complaint in medical practice, occurring in 10–35 percent of adult men with medical problems

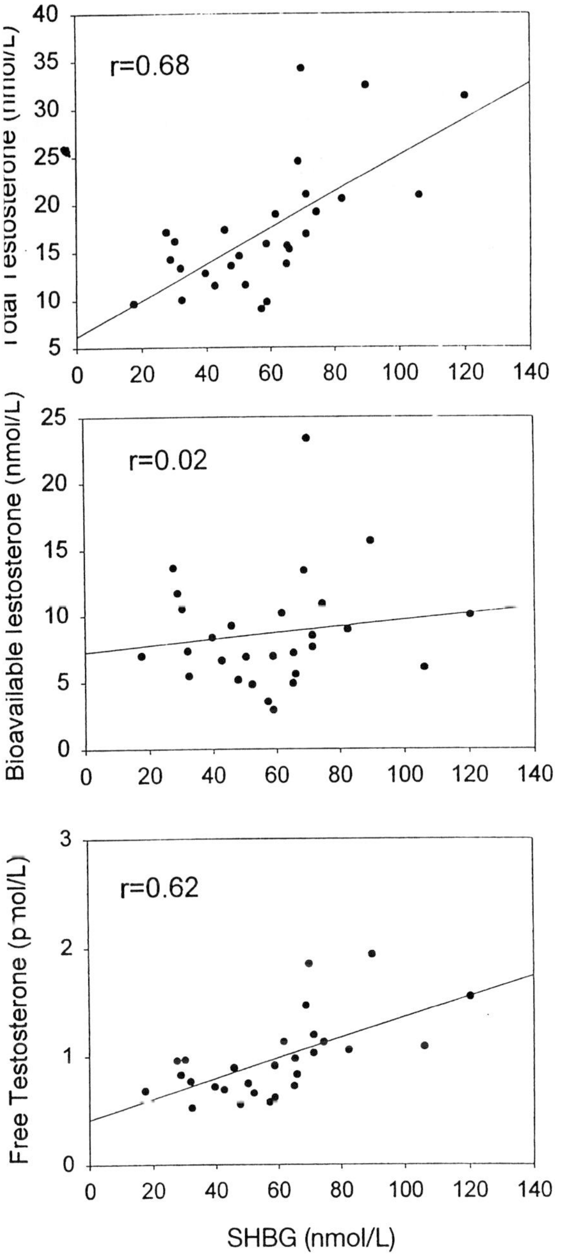

FIGURE 15-19. Correlation between serum sex hormone-binding globulin (SHBG) or TeBG and total (*top*), bioavailable (*middle*), and analog method free (*bottom*) testosterone concentrations in healthy men. (*From Winters, Kelley, and Goodpaster.*[216])

and increasing in prevalence with advancing age.[187,218] More than 50 percent of men between the ages of 40 and 60 have some degree of erectile dysfunction. Major risk factors include age, hypertension, atherosclerotic vascular disease, diabetes mellitus, medications, smoking, alcoholism, and depression.[218] Because patients and physicians are reluctant to discuss sexual issues, erectile dysfunction is often underdiagnosed. Although psychogenic causes are common, the majority of men with erectile dysfunction followed in a general medical clinic have one or more organic cause.[219] Furthermore, organic causes of erectile dysfunction often result in performance anxiety, and secondarily cause psychogenic sexual dysfunction.

Table 15-5. Normal Values for Seminal Fluid Analysis

Parameter	Normal Value
Sperm concentration	$\geq 20 \times 10^6$ spermatozoa/mL
Seminal fluid volume	$\geq$2.0 mL
Total sperm count	$\geq 40 \times 10^6$ spermatozoa/ejaculate
Motility	$\geq$50% spermatozoa with forward progression within 60 minutes of ejaculation
Morphology	$\geq$30% normal forms using strict WHO criteria [$\geq$50% normal forms using less strict criteria]

Source: World Health Organization (WHO) laboratory manual.

Causes

As described previously, a penile erection that is sufficient to complete satisfactory intercourse requires a normal *central nervous system* and thoracolumbar sympathetic and sacral parasympathetic *spinal cord* outputs to the penis; an intact vascular system, including a sufficient *arterial supply* and mechanism to prevent premature *venous drainage* of the penis; and an anatomically *normal penis.* Disorders affecting of any of these components will interfere with the normal initiation and maintenance of penile erection. It is useful to classify the causes of erectile dysfunction into disorders that affect central nervous system and spinal cord control of erection, and those that affect the peripheral erectile response (Table 15-6).

Normal central nervous system function is necessary to produce penile erections. *Libido* (sexual interest and desire) is generated by the brain, and has an important stimulatory influence on erectile function. In most central nervous system disorders that cause sexual dysfunction, reduced sexual interest and motivation is usually but not always associated with erectile dysfunction. Central nervous system causes of erectile dysfunction that are generally associated with reduced libido include varying degrees of *psychiatric disturbance,* from minor stress and performance anxiety to major psychiatric illness, such as depression[220]; debilitating *chronic systemic illness,* such as cardiac, respiratory, renal or liver failure, or malignancy[219,221]; and *drugs* that affect brain function (alcohol, centrally active antihypertensive agents, narcotics, sedatives, anticonvulsants, antidepressants, and antipsychotic drugs).[222–224] *Androgen deficiency (hypogonadism), hyperprolactinemia, glucocorticoid excess (Cushing syndrome),* and *thyroid dysfunction* are endocrine disorders that also impair libido and erectile function.[182,183,219,225–227] Hyperprolactinemia and glucocorticoid excess cause erectile dysfunction, in part, by suppressing GnRH and gonadotropin secretion and inducing androgen deficiency. However, in some men with hyperprolactinemia, erectile dysfunction may not resolve with androgen replacement therapy alone, and may require additional therapy aimed at reducing the elevated prolactin concentrations.

In contrast to these central nervous system disorders, destructive or infiltrative diseases of certain brain regions (e.g., tumor or infarction of the *temporal lobe or limbic system*)[228–231] or *spinal cord disorders* (e.g., spinal cord injury, multiple sclerosis, transverse myelitis, tumor, vascular compromise, epidural abscess, spinal stenosis, spina bifida, or syphilis)[232–234] may cause erectile dysfunction without associated loss of libido. Patients with spinal cord lesions at the thoracic or lumber level, i.e., above the sacral spinal cord erection center (S_2–S_4), generally retain the ability to have reflexogenic erections. Psychogenic erections are possible in

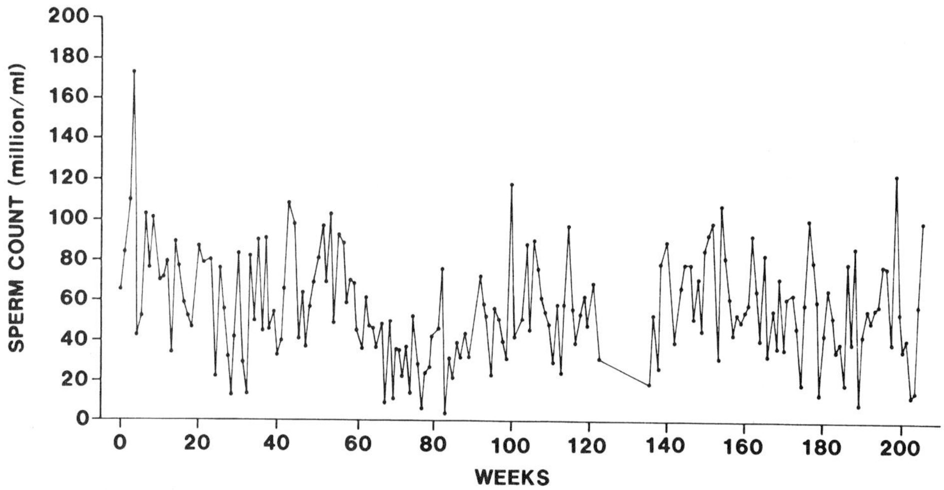

FIGURE 15-20. Example of the normal variations in sperm count in a healthy young man. (*From Bardin and Paulsen.*[814])

some men with spinal cord lesions below the thoracolumbar spinal erection center (T_{10}–L_2).

In addition to intact central nervous system functioning, normal penile erections require normal peripheral nervous system function, adequate blood flow to the penis, and normal erectile structures within the penis. *Disorders of peripheral autonomic nerve function* that cause erectile dysfunction include *drugs* that affect autonomic nerve function (anticholinergic drugs, antihistamines, antidepressants, β-adrenergic antagonists, sympathominetic agents, α-adrenergic agonists, and antihypertensive agents); *pelvic, prostate, or retroperitoneal surgery or damage* (e.g., prostatectomy, aorto-iliac bypass, abdominoperineal resection of the rectum, pelvic lymph node dissection, and lumbar sympathetectomy; and *diabetes mellitus* or *other causes of peripheral neuropathy* (e.g., amyloidosis, vasculitis, arsenic or mercury exposure, renal failure, Shy-Drager syndrome, acute intermittent porphyria).[222–224,235–242] Although agents that affect the peripheral and central autonomic function more commonly affect erectile function, all antihypertensive drugs, including diuretics, angiotensin converting enzyme inhibitors, and calcium channel antagonists, have been implicated as causes of erectile dysfunction.[222,224,242]

Atherosclerotic *peripheral vascular disease* involving the distal *aorto-iliac* arteries are common causes of vascular erectile dysfunction, especially in elderly men.[243–246] These patients usually have diminished or absent femoral pulses and may present with *Leriche's syndrome,* although claudication may be absent in some cases. Both small and large vessel atherosclerosis and peripheral neuropathy contribute to the high incidence of erectile dysfunction (~50%) in men with diabetes mellitus.[241,247–249] Other disorders that compromise aorto-iliac circulation, such as trauma, radiation, or vasculitis, are less common causes of erectile dysfunction.[250,251] In addition to being a major risk factor for atherosclerotic cardiovascular disease, *smoking,* specifically nicotine, inhibits erections directly by causing cavernosal vasoconstriction.[252,253]

Penile *venous incompetence (or leakage)* may cause premature detumescence and inability to maintain an erection.[254,255] *Penile abnormalities* such as Peyronie's disease, chordee, micropenis, microphallus, penile trauma, phimosis, and priapism may also cause erectile dysfunction.[221,252,256,257]

Evaluation

The etiology of erectile dysfunction can be strongly suspected by a thorough history and physical examination. Erectile dysfunction that occurs abruptly, and is transient, intermittent, or associated temporally with a stressful situation is usually psychogenic in origin. Men with psychogenic erectile dysfunction usually retain spontaneous nocturnal and morning erections. They are able to achieve normal erections with some partners but not with others, or with masturbation but not sexual intercourse. Patients with organic erectile dysfunction related to central or peripheral nervous system disorders, vascular disease, or penile abnormalities will usually exhibit clinical manifestations of the underlying disorder. A careful drug history may reveal offending medications that cause or are associated with erectile dysfunction.

Normal testosterone levels are necessary for maintenance of libido and erectile function. Hypogonadism resulting in androgen deficiency is a cause of erectile dysfunction in approximately 15–20 percent of men complaining of sexual dysfunction in a general medical clinic.[219] Therefore, all men with erectile dysfunction should have serum testosterone concentrations measured as part of their diagnostic work-up, especially if they are older.[258]

With the availability of relatively simple methods for treatment that do not depend upon the specific etiology, the need to do expensive and/or invasive testing to determine the specific cause of erectile dysfunction is not necessary. Measurement of nocturnal penile tumescence (NPT) and buckling resistance may be used to differentiate psychogenic from organic erectile dysfunction.[187,221,259] NPT is present in psychogenic erectile dysfunction, but absent in organic causes of erectile dysfunction. Formal evaluation is performed in a sleep laboratory with electroencephalographic monitoring in order to detect sleep disturbances that may disturb NPT. Resistance of the penis to buckling is also measured, and correlates better than NPT alone with the ability to have sexual intercourse. NPT may be detected more simply by the breakage of wires of different tensile strength in a snap gauge.[260]

The ratio of supine penile to brachial systolic blood pressure (penile/brachial index) determined by Doppler ultrasound may be used to diagnose penile vascular insufficiency, e.g., due to pelvic steal syndrome.[187,221,261] An index >0.75 is normal, and one <0.60 is suggestive of vascular erectile dysfunction, which may

TABLE 15-6. Causes and Drugs Associated with Erectile Dysfunction

- Central nervous system disorders
  - Psychiatric disorders
    - Stress, performance anxiety
    - Depression
    - Major psychiatric illness
  - Chronic systemic illness
    - Cardiac failure
    - Respiratory failure
    - Renal failure
    - Liver failure
    - Malignancy
  - Central nervous system-active drugs
    - Alcohol
    - Centrally active antihypertensive agents (α-methyldopa, reserpine, clonidine)
    - Narcotics (morphine, methadone, heroin)
    - Sedative-hypnotic drugs (barbiturates, benzodiazepines)
    - Anticonvulsants (phenytoin, carbamazepine)
    - Antidepressant drugs (monoamine oxidase inhibitors, tricyclic antidepressants, selective serotonin reuptake inhibitors)
    - Antipsychotic drugs (phenothiazines, thioridazine)
  - Endocrine disorders
    - Hypogonadism (androgen deficiency)
    - Hyperprolactinemia
    - Cushing syndrome
    - Hyperthyroidism, hypothyroidism
  - Brain disease
    - Temporal lobe disorders
    - Limbic system disease
    - Parkinson's disease
  - Spinal cord disorders
    - Trauma
    - Multiple sclerosis
    - Syphilis
    - Other spinal cord lesions
- Peripheral disorders of erectile response
  - Drugs
    - Anticholinergic drugs (atropine, butyrophenones, disopyramide, ganglionic blocking agents)
    - Antihistamines
    - Antidepressant drugs
    - β-Adrenergic antagonists (propanolol, atenolol)
    - Sympathomimetic drugs
    - α-Adrenergic agonists
    - Antihypertensive agents (thiazide diuretics, prazocin)
  - Autonomic neuropathy
    - Pelvic, prostate or retroperitoneal surgery or damage (e.g., prostatectomy, aorto-illiac bypass)
    - Diabetes mellitus
    - Other causes of peripheral neuropathy
  - Peripheral vascular disease
    - Aorto-iliac atherosclerosis, trauma, vasculitis
    - Diabetes mellitus
    - Venous incompetence (leakage)
    - Smoking
  - Penile abnormalities
    - Peyronie's disease, chordee
    - Microphallus or micropenis
    - Trauma, penectomy
    - Priapism, phimosis

be confirmed using arteriography in younger patients in whom surgical correction is being considered. Intracavernosal injection of vasodilating agents (e.g., prostaglandin E_1) with and without duplex ultrasound, or direct pressure monitoring (cavernosometry) may be used to determine the capacity to have a normal penile erection, teach patients the injection technique, and test the dose and response to vasodilator drugs.[187,221,262] Development of a sustained erection implies a normal vascular status, while a short-lived, partial, or an absent response suggests a hemodynamic abnormality. The sufficiency of corporal venoocclusion may also be evaluated by cavernosometry and cavernosography following intracavernosal injection of a vasodilating drug. In the absence of neurogenic bladder dysfunction, electromyographic determination of the bulbocavernosus reflex latency and somatosensory-evoked response of the dorsal nerve may be useful in detecting peripheral and sacral spinal cord abnormalities contributing to erectile dysfunction.

Treatment

Psychosexual education, counseling, and therapy are often useful in restoring sexual function in many men with either primary or secondary psychogenic erectile dysfunction. If possible, discontinuation of potential drugs associated with sexual dysfunction and/or use of alternative medications to the offending agent(s) is a useful initial strategy to treat erectile dysfunction. Testosterone therapy should be reserved for hypogonadal men with androgen deficiency.[187,221] Libido and erectile function may be restored with adequate androgen replacement in these men. However, in many older men with androgen deficiency, normal erectile function is not completely restored with androgen therapy alone, despite normal libido, because of concomitant vascular and/or neurological abnormalities.[187,221,262] Men with erectile dysfunction and hypogonadism due to hyperprolactinemia may require agents to lower prolactin levels (e.g., bromocriptine) as well as testosterone treatment to improve erections.

Irrespective of etiology, the majority of men with erectile dysfunction may be treated satisfactorily with nonsurgical interventions.[187,221,264] Intracavernosal injections of vasodilatory drugs (e.g., *prostaglandin E_1 [Alprostadil®]*, 2.5–20 μg, and/or a combination of *papaverine* and *phentolamine*) induce erections that are sufficient for sexual intercourse in many patients with erectile dysfunction.[187,221,264] In general, these therapies are very effective and tolerated well. However, only 50 percent of men who start treatment remain on long-term intracavernosal injection therapy because of dissatisfaction with the mechanical nature of injections and penile pain, burning, or induration. The latter is more common with papaverine and phentolamine combinations. Although less effective than intracavernosal administration, prostaglandin E_1 is also effective when it is delivered intraurethrally (Medicated Urethral System for Erection or *MUSE*). Patients with severe arterial insufficiency or venous leaks are least likely to respond to this therapy.

Sildenafil (Viagra®), a phosphodiesterase type 5 inhibitor, given at dosages between 25–100 mg orally, induces erection upon sexual arousal within about one hour following administration.[265,266] It is effective in inducing an erection in 80 percent of men with erectile dysfunction. Sildenafil is tolerated well but should be administered with caution in men with coronary heart disease. Because sildenafil may potentiate the hypotensive effects of nitrates, it is contraindicated in men on nitrate medications (e.g., nitroglycerin). Occasional patients experience headache, lightheadedness, flushing, or visual disturbances. Despite the relatively high cost of therapy, ease of use and effectiveness of sildenafil make it an attractive alternative to intracavernosal injection therapy for most men.

A variety of external vacuum devices to induce penile tumescence are available for the treatment of erectile dysfunction.[187,221,264] A cylinder is placed over the flaccid penis, and a vacuum is applied to generate negative pressure, drawing blood into the penis and resulting in an erection. A constrictive band is then placed around the base of the penis to prevent the drainage of blood from the penis, maintaining tumescence for the duration of intercourse. This is the least expensive nonsurgical treatment alternative available to treat erectile dysfunction. It is effective but may occasionally cause penile trauma or hematoma, a cold, cyanotic penis, or inability to ejaculate.

Selected younger patients with vascular erectile dysfunction are candidates for corrective surgical procedures. In patients who do not tolerate or fail noninvasive therapy, surgical implantation of a penile prosthesis offers rigidity sufficient for sexual intercourse without interfering with ejaculation or orgasm.

Infertility

Infertility is defined as the inability of a *couple* to achieve a pregnancy after one year of unprotected intercourse. Approximately 14 percent of couples are infertile, and in 40–50 percent of cases, a male factor is the sole or contributing cause of infertility.[4–6] Therefore, approximately 5–6 percent of men in the reproductive age group are infertile. Most causes of male infertility result in an abnormal sperm count and/or quality, as reflected on seminal fluid analysis.[267] About 90 percent of male infertility is caused by hypogonadism resulting in impaired spermatogenesis or sperm function, and in at least 60–70 percent of these men the etiology is unclear, i.e., *idiopathic oligozoospermia* or *azoospermia* (see later section).[268,269] Other causes of male infertility include *erectile dysfunction, coital disorders, impaired innervation of the genital tract, genital tract obstruction, disorders of accessory sexual organs,* and *ejaculatory dysfunction* (Table 15-7). Because a coexisting female factor contributes to infertility in 30 percent of couples, the female partner should undergo a diagnostic evaluation.

TABLE 15-7. Causes of Male Infertility

- Hypogonadism (impairment of sperm production)
  - Androgen deficiency
  - Isolated impairment of sperm production or function
- Erectile dysfunction
- Coital disorders
  - Defects in technique
    - Infrequent intercourse
    - Excessive intercourse with others or masturbation
    - Poor timing in relationship to ovulation
    - Premature withdrawal of penis
- Impaired sympathetic innervation of genital tract
  - Spinal cord disease
  - Sympatholytic drugs or sympathectomy
  - Retroperitoneal lymphadenectomy
  - Vasovasostomy
- Genital tract obstruction
  - Congenital defects of vas deferens, epididymides or seminal vesicles
  - Postinfectious obstruction (tuberculosis, gonorrhea, leprosy)
  - Cystic fibrosis, Young syndrome
  - Epididymal cysts, Mullerian duct cysts
  - Vasectomy
- Accessory sexual gland dysfunction
  - Androgen deficiency
  - Epididymitis, seminal vesiculitis, prostatitis
  - Immunological (sperm autoimmunity)
- Ejaculatory dysfunction
  - Premature or retarded ejaculation
  - Retrograde ejaculation
    - Prostatectomy
    - Bladder neck surgery
    - Urethrocytosplasty
  - Sympathetic nervous system dysfunction
    - Autonomic neuropathy (e.g., diabetes mellitus)
    - Sympatholytic drugs or sympathectomy
    - Retroperitoneal or abdominopelvic surgery
    - Spinal cord injury
  - Reduced ejaculation
    - Androgen deficiency or resistance
    - Sympathetic nervous system dysfunction
    - Urethral abnormalities (e.g., stricture, hypospadius, epispadius)

Erectile dysfunction from any cause may result in unsuccessful intercourse, and therefore infertility. Although uncommon, *defects in coital technique,* such as infrequent sexual intercourse, excessive intercourse with other partners or masturbation, timing of intercourse during menses, rather than at the time ovulation near mid-cycle, and premature withdrawal of the penis prior to ejaculation may contribute significantly to male infertility.[270] With proper education, these coital disorders are potentially reversible causes of infertility. In order to optimize the timing of intercourse around the time of ovulation, basal body temperature measurements or commercially-available rapid urinary LH determinations are used to estimate the timing of ovulation.

Impaired sperm transport from the testis to the urethra may result in oligozoospermia or azoospermia and infertility. This may be caused by *impaired sympathetic innervation of the genital tract,* e.g., by spinal cord disease, sympatholytic drugs or sympathectomy, retroperitoneal lymphadenectomy, or vasovasostomy.[267] Sperm transport may also be impeded by *genital tract obstruction.* Disorders that cause genital tract obstruction include congenital absence or defects of the vas deferens or seminal vesicles; congenital defects of the epididymis or vas, e.g., as a consequence of diethylstilbesterol exposure in utero; scarring as a complication of genitourinary infection, especially epididymitis (e.g., tuberculosis, gonorrhea, leprosy); *cystic fibrosis* or *Young syndrome,* in which thickened, inspissated mucous secretions block the epididymides and vas deferans; and vasectomy.[270–281]

Serum FSH levels are often helpful in differentiating azoospermia caused by genital tract obstruction versus that due to a severe defect in spermatogenesis.[282,283] Elevated FSH concentrations usually indicate severely disordered germ cell and Sertoli cell function. Normal FSH levels occur in either obstructive azoospermia or seminiferous tubule dysfunction. Although not available widely, serum inhibin B concentrations are decreased in men with germ cell failure, and normal in men with azoospermia due to genital tract obstruction.[175,285] In the latter, an ultrasound or contrast radiographic vasogram may confirm genital tract obstruction, and a testis biopsy will confirm normal spermatogenesis.[285] Evaluation of azoospermia is one of the few indications for performing a testis biopsy. Vasectomy has been used widely and successfully to induce infertility for family planning without deleterious effects on the hypothalamic-pituitary-testicular axis or general health. Earlier reports of an association of vasectomy with atherosclerotic cardiovascular disease and prostate cancer have not been substantiated.[286,287]

Accessory sexual gland dysfunction may contribute to male infertility.[267] In addition to impairing sperm production and causing erectile dysfunction, long-standing, severe androgen deficiency decreases seminal vesicle and prostate gland secretions. Infections of the epididymis, seminal vesicles, and/or prostate may contribute to infertility by affecting sperm maturation or function directly, or by inducing antisperm antibodies that, in turn, may affect sperm function.[288,289] Mycoplasma (*Ureaplasma urealyticum*) infection of genital tract has been implicated as a cause of male infertility, and a trial of tetracyline therapy has been advocated empirically in the treatment of infertility with varied results. Antisperm antibodies in the semen may cause sperm agglutination and reduce sperm motility.[290] However, the precise role of antisperm antibodies in infertility is not certain. Prednisone has been used to lower antibody titers and improve fertility. Formation of antisperm antibodies induced by vasectomy may be responsible for the discrepancy observed between the success rate for the return of sperm in the ejaculate (90%) and restoration of fertility (50%) after vasectomy reversal, or vasovasostomy.[291]

Ejaculatory dysfunction may cause or contribute to infertility by preventing the normal deposition of sperm into the female genital tract. Premature ejaculation is often treated successfully by sex therapy.[191,192] Retrograde ejaculation most commonly results from diabetic autonomic neuropathy, prostatic resection, pelvic surgery, sympatholytic drugs, or spinal cord injury.[195–204] It should be suspected if orgasm results in little or no ejaculate. The diagnosis is confirmed by the presence of large numbers of sperm in a postejaculation urine sample. Sympathomimetic drugs, imipramine, and harvesting and concentrating of sperm from the urine for artificial insemination are used to treat retrograde ejaculation and infertility.

Gynecomastia

Benign glandular enlargement of the male breast is known as *gynecomastia.* It is usually asymptomatic. However, rapid development of breast tissue may cause pain and tenderness. It is often very difficult to distinguish between true gynecomastia and increase in adipose tissue in obese boys or men, and a careful physical examination using the correct technique for palpation is needed (see earlier discussion).

A number of hormones regulate the growth and differentiation of the breast.[292–294] Estradiol stimulates cellular growth and differentiation of glandular epithelium to form ductal elements. Growth hormone, insulin, and cortisol play a permissive role for breast growth. Prolactin acts on the differentiated breast acinar cells to stimulate milk protein production. In contrast, testosterone exhibits an inhibitory effect on the growth and differentiation of breast tissue. Thyroid hormone increases SHBG and estradiol levels and, therefore, exerts indirect stimulatory effects on the breast. Both prolactin and cortisol suppress testosterone levels, diminishing its inhibitory influences on the breast.

The specific pathophysiological mechanisms that cause gynecomastia are not understood completely, but it usually occurs in a hormonal milieu of increased estrogen relative to androgen activity or concentrations, i.e., an increased estrogen to androgen ratio.[292–294] This hormonal milieu may result from either increased estrogen or decreased testosterone activity or levels. Therefore, conditions associated with androgen deficiency are major causes of gynecomastia.

Gynecomastia is usually bilateral but may be asymmetrical. In the rare instances that it is unilateral, gynecomastia must be distinguished from other benign chest wall tumors that may occur on or near the breast, e.g., lipomas, neurofibromas, and lymphomas, and most importantly, male breast cancer. In contrast to benign breast conditions, breast carcinoma is usually eccentric in location, more indurated and hard, and associated with skin or nipple retraction and bloody discharge.[295] Axillary lymphadenopathy due to metastatic disease may also be found.

Causes

Physiological Gynecomastia Gynecomastia is frequently observed in normal *physiological* situations (Table 15-8). Transient gynecomastia is usually seen in *neonatal* boys, as a result of in utero exposure to high maternal estrogen concentrations. At the time of puberty, gynecomastia >0.5 cm in diameter is observed in 60–70 percent of adolescent boys by age 14 years.[296–302] *Pubertal* gynecomastia usually lasts for months to years and does not persist into adulthood. A transient rise in the estrogen to testosterone ratio during puberty is thought to contribute to the pathogenesis of pubertal gynecomastia. Finally, small amounts of palpable breast tissue can be detected by careful examination in 40 percent of healthy normal *adult* men, increasing in prevalence with advancing age.[303–306] This gynecomastia is usually <2 cm in diameter and nearly always asymptomatic. Gynecomastia measuring 2–5 cm is present in 60–80 percent of hospitalized adults over 45 years of age, and is thought to be due to increased aromatase activity associated with increased body adiposity with aging.[305] Therefore, gynecomastia is concerning clinically when there is breast tenderness or discharge, progressive increase in breast size, or enlargement of the breast beyond the physiological range, e.g., >2–5 cm in adults.

Pathological Gynecomastia Because they result in an increased estrogen to testosterone ratio, most pathological causes of gynecomastia (Fig. 15-8) are due to disorders or drugs that cause *androgen deficiency,* including both primary testicular disorders and those secondary to gonadotropin deficiency, or *androgen resistance.*[292–294] *Drugs that cause androgen deficiency* include cytotoxic agents, spironolactone, and ketoconazole, and *drugs that interfere with androgen action* include spironolactone, pure androgen receptor antagonists (flutamide, nilutamide, bicalutamide), cimetidine, and progestagens. Causes of *hyperprolactinemia resulting in androgen deficiency* may also cause gynecomastia. Hyperprolactinemia-induced androgen deficiency is probably a major reason why central nervous system active drugs, such as certain antihypertensives, sedatives, tranquilizers, antidepressants, and amphetamines, are associated with gynecomastia.

Gynecomastia may also result from conditions that cause *absolute or relative estrogen excess.*[292–294] Excessive estrogen levels or action inhibit endogenous gonadotropin secretion resulting in reduced testosterone production. Thus, secondary hypogonadism induced by estrogens may contribute to the development of gynecomastia.[307]

Exogenous estrogen exposure in men may occur in a number of circumstances, including ingestion of estrogen-treated animal foodstuffs, use or contact with estrogen-containing creams, accidental occupational exposure, or (although rarely used anymore), diethylstilbesterol administration for metastatic prostate cancer. Certain drugs, such as marijuana and digitoxin, result in breast enlargement by interacting with the estrogen receptor. Administra-

TABLE 15-8. Causes of Gynecomastia

- Physiological
  - Neonatal
  - Pubertal
  - Adult
- Androgen deficiency or resistance
  - Hypogonadism (androgen deficiency)
  - Drugs that cause androgen deficiency
    - Cytotoxic agents (busulfan, nitrosourea, vincristine, combination chemotherapy)
    - Spironolactone
    - Ketoconazole
  - Androgen resistance syndromes
  - Drugs that interfere with androgen action
    - Spironolactone
    - Androgen receptor antagonists (flutamide, nilutamide, bicalutamide)
    - Cimetidine
    - Progestagens
- Hyperprolactinemia resulting in androgen deficiency
  - Hypothalamic lesions
  - Hypothyroidism
  - Pituitary stalk section
  - Drugs
    - Dopamine antagonists, antipsychotic drugs, antidepressants, sedative-hypnotic drugs, amphetamines, centrally-active antihypertensive drugs
  - Pituitary adenoma
  - Estrogen
  - Renal failure
  - Local chest wall trauma or irritation (Herpes Zoster)
- Absolute or relative estrogen excess
  - Estrogens or estrogen agonists
    - Estrogen administration
    - Marijuana
    - Digitoxin
    - Aromatizable androgens (testosterone, testosterone enanthate, testosterone cypionate)
  - Increased peripheral aromatase activity
    - Obesity
    - Familial
  - Estrogen-secreting tumors
    - Adrenal carcinoma
    - Testicular Leydig or Sertoli cell tumors
  - hCG-secreting tumors
    - Testicular carcinoma
    - Lung cancer
    - Liver carcinoma
  - hCG treatment
- Systemic illness and endocrine disorders
  - Hepatic cirrhosis
  - Renal failure
  - Hyperthyroidism
  - Acromegaly
  - Cushing syndrome
- Nutritional disorders
  - Refeeding
  - Recovery from chronic illness (e.g., renal failure, diabetes, pulmonary tuberculosis)
- Idiopathic
  - Persistent pubertal macromastia
  - Adult

tion of aromatizable androgens to prepubertal boys or men with long-standing, severe hypogonadism, especially in high dosages, may induce gynecomastia.[308] *Increased peripheral aromatase* activity and conversion of endogenous androgens to estrogens in adipose tissue may be the cause of mild to moderate gynecomastia observed in obese men.[308] *Familial gynecomastia* and *idiopathic increase in peripheral aromatase activity* are very rare causes of gynecomastia.[309,310]

Although the tumors are very uncommon, gynecomastia may be the initial manifestation of an *estrogen-secreting tumor* of the adrenal gland or testis. Feminizing adrenal tumors are usually malignant and present with a palpable abdominal mass. In contrast, estrogen-secreting Leydig or Sertoli cell tumors of the testis are often small and benign. Unlike many exogenous estrogen preparations that do not cross react within immunoassays for estradiol, these tumors secrete large amounts of estradiol that are detected in blood by clinically available assays.

Human chorionic gonadotropin (hCG) binds to the LH receptor on Leydig cells of the testis and has biological activities that are identical to that of LH. *hCG-secreting tumors,* such as testicular, lung, and hepatic carcinomas, may cause rapid onset of gynecomastia by stimulating excessive estrogen relative to testosterone secretion by Leydig cells.[308] Because hCG cross reacts with some routinely available LH assays, patients with hCG-secreting tumors may have elevated LH levels. Also, because LH cross reacts with some intact hCG assays, a specific hCGβ assay should be used to confirm the diagnosis of an hCG-secreting tumor. By stimulating relatively greater testicular production of estradiol compared to testosterone, *hCG treatment* of hypogonadotropic hypogonadal men may also cause gynecomastia.

Certain *systemic illnesses* are associated with benign breast enlargement. In *hepatic cirrhosis,* gynecomastia is associated with increased estrogen production, primarily by accelerated peripheral conversion of the adrenal androgen, androstenedione to estrone.[308,311] Also, serum SHBG concentrations are increased, and total and bioavailable serum testosterone levels are low, favoring an increased estrogen to androgen ratio. In patients with *renal failure,* gynecomastia is due in part to androgen deficiency, resulting from both primary and secondary testicular failure; estrogen production is not increased. High estradiol and relatively reduced bioavailable testosterone levels as a result of increased SHBG concentrations are found commonly in men with *hyperthyroidism* and contribute to the development of gynecomastia in this condition.[312] Gynecomastia in patients with *Cushing syndrome* and *acromegaly* probably result from excessive glucocorticoid and growth hormone stimulation of breast growth and androgen deficiency associated with these disorders.

Gynecomastia is often associated with nutritional repletion and weight gain after a period of starvation and weight loss, and is termed *refeeding gynecomastia.*[292–294] It was described originally in former World War II prisoners who developed tender gynecomastia following liberation and resumption of a normal diet. A similar situation may occur during recovery from any prolonged, severe *chronic illness* associated with malnutrition and weight loss. For example, refeeding gynecomastia may contribute to the breast enlargement associated with initiation of hemodialysis in men with chronic renal failure, institution of insulin treatment in men with type 1 diabetes, and drug treatment of men with tuberculosis. Malnutrition results in severe suppression of the hypothalamic-pituitary-testicular axis. Refeeding and restoration of nutrition and body weight results in resumption of normal gonadal function, a dynamic hormonal state analogous to the onset of puberty. The hormonal changes associated with this rapid restoration of gonadal function ("second puberty") may explain the gynecomastia associated with refeeding.

Some boys develop an exaggerated, persistent form of pubertal gynecomastia with breast enlargement that reaches nearly adult female size, Tanner stage III–V. The etiology of this condition, known as *persistent pubertal macromastia,* is not known.[313] It is not associated with specific hormonal or receptor abnormalities. A number of cases of adult-onset gynecomastia also remain *idiopathic.*

Evaluation

Indications for evaluation of breast enlargement include breast pain or tenderness; rapid enlargement of the breast; breast enlargement of >5 cm in obese and >2 cm in lean men; eccentric or hard irregular masses; associated galactorrhea or bloody nipple discharge; evidence of infiltration or fixation to overlying or underlying tissue, e.g., peau d'orange of overlying skin or nipple retraction; and associated axillary lymphadenopathy.

Initial clinical evaluation should include a careful history and physical examination with emphasis on evidence of androgen deficiency or resistance; review of medications and drug use; symptoms or signs of malignancy, especially in testis and lung; evidence of systemic illness (hepatic or renal disease) or other endocrine disorders (thyroid, growth hormone, or cortisol excess); and previous malnutrition and weight loss with recent recovery. Based on the initial clinical evaluation, additional laboratory tests such as testosterone, LH, FSH, prolactin, estradiol, hCGβ, and thyroxine and TSH levels, and diagnostic procedures, e.g., a chest x-ray to rule out lung cancer, may be obtained.

Treatment

Treatment of gynecomastia should be focused on the correction of the underlying disorder or withdrawal of the offending drugs. In the past, prophylactic low dose irradiation of the breast was used prior to the institution of diethylstilbesterol treatment in men with prostatic carcinoma to prevent the development of gynecomastia. Testosterone treatment of androgen deficiency may result occasionally in partial regression of breast enlargement. In general, the results of medical therapy of gynecomastia with antiestrogens to block estrogen action (e.g., tamoxifen), nonaromatizable androgens (e.g., DHT), and aromatase inhibitors (e.g., testolactone or anastrozole) have been disappointing.[314–318] Severe, long-standing gynecomastia of any cause is associated with an increase in fibrous tissue stroma. Therefore, surgical removal of breast tissue, or reduction mammoplasty, is usually necessary, especially in men with large, painful, or cosmetically disfiguring gynecomastia.

Causes of Male Hypogonadism

The diagnosis of male hypogonadism is suspected from the clinical manifestations described previously and confirmed by repeated measurements of serum testosterone level and sperm count. A low serum testosterone concentration confirms the presence of androgen deficiency and reduced sperm concentrations confirms an impairment in sperm production. The majority of hypogonadal men with androgen deficiency also have impairment in sperm production.

Once androgen deficiency is diagnosed, it is important to distinguish between disorders that result from primary disorders of the testis, i.e., *primary hypogonadism,* and those that are secondary to inadequate gonadotropin stimulation of the testis as a result of either pituitary or hypothalamic disease, i.e., *secondary hypogonadism.* In addition to helping define the specific etiology of androgen deficiency, the distinction between primary and secondary hypogonadism has important diagnostic and practical therapeutic implications.

Regardless of the specific etiology, primary hypogonadism is usually treated with androgen replacement, and in most cases, the infertility is not treatable. However, secondary hypogonadism may result, for example, from disorders that cause destruction of pituitary gonadotropin-secreting cells, e.g., a pituitary adenoma. In this instance, the presence of a pituitary tumor needs to be evaluated using imaging procedures such as magnetic resonance imaging (MRI) or computerized tomography (CT). Also, in addition to androgen deficiency, the space-occupying effects of the tumor mass on brain function, such as impairment of visual fields and cerebroventricular flow, and alterations (both increases and decreases) in the secretion of other anterior pituitary hormones, such as ACTH, TSH, growth hormone, and prolactin, need to be considered in formulating a therapeutic plan. Furthermore, because the testes usually function normally in response to adequate gonadotropin stimulation in men with secondary hypogonadism, gonadotropin or GnRH treatment may be used to stimulate sperm and androgen production, and induce fertility.

An understanding of the negative feedback relationship between gonadotropin secretion and circulating testosterone levels (Fig. 15-8) provides the physiological basis and rationale for the use of serum gonadotropin levels to distinguish between primary and secondary hypogonadism. As a result of reduced negative feedback effects of testosterone (and inhibin B) on gonadotropin secretion, men with *primary hypogonadism* resulting in a deficiency of androgen and sperm production exhibit reduced serum testosterone and elevated serum LH and FSH levels, i.e., *hypergonadotropic hypogonadism* (Fig. 15-21). A disproportionate elevation of serum FSH compared to LH levels is common, espe-

FIGURE 15-21. Schematic diagram of alterations in the hypothalamic-pituitary-testicular axis with primary hypogonadism resulting in deficiency of androgen and sperm production.

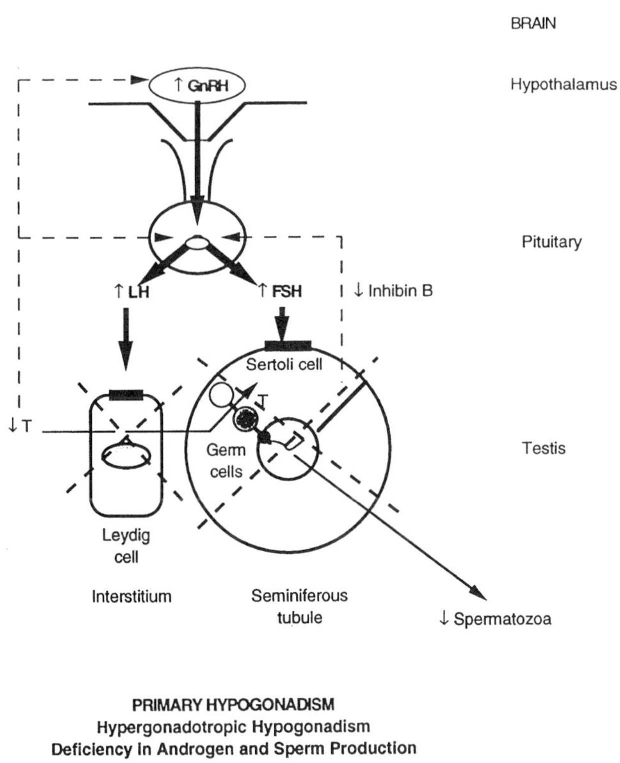

cially with severe seminiferous tubule dysfunction. However, selective elevation of serum LH levels is distinctly unusual, and should raise the possibility of the presence of a substance, such as hCG or free α-subunit, that cross reacts in the LH assay.

Men with *secondary hypogonadism* usually demonstrate a deficiency in androgen and sperm production as a result of inadequate gonadotropin stimulation of the testis, and are unable to increase gonadotropin secretion appropriately in the presence of reduced testosterone negative feedback. Therefore, these men exhibit a hormonal pattern of reduced serum testosterone and low to low-normal serum LH and FSH levels, i.e., *hypogonadotropic hypogonadism* (Fig. 15-22). Gonadotropin levels may be within the broad normal ranges for LH and FSH (usually in the lower part of the normal range) in men with secondary hypogonadism, but they are inappropriately normal in the presence of low serum testosterone levels and reduced negative feedback.

The majority of hypogonadal men with an *isolated impairment of sperm production* have primary testicular disease. They present with infertility and no clinical manifestations of androgen deficiency. Sperm counts are low, and serum testosterone and gonadotropin levels are usually normal, i.e., they are *eugonadotropic*. Therefore, hormone measurements are not obtained routinely as part of a work-up for male infertility unless clinical androgen deficiency is also present.

Infertile patients that present with no sperm in their ejaculate, i.e., *azoospermia,* may have either severe seminiferous tubule failure or obstruction of the genital tract. Measurement of serum FSH level may be helpful in evaluation of a man with azoospermia. A selective elevation of serum FSH levels with normal LH levels in a patient with azoospermia implies severe germ cell failure with loss of negative feedback influences, such as inhibin B, on the pituitary gland (Fig. 15-23). The prognosis for fertility is generally very poor in these men, and no further work-up is usually necessary. A normal serum FSH level in a patient with azoospermia leaves open the possibility of a surgically-correctable genital obstruction. In this instance, an ultrasound or contrast vasogram and testis biopsy is usually performed. In addition to severe germ cell failure, selective elevation in serum FSH levels may be observed in men with gonadotropin-secreting pituitary adenomas. Occasionally, isolated impairment of sperm production results from inadequate gonadotropin stimulation of the testis, e.g., in men taking high doses of androgenic anabolic steroids. In these instances, serum gonadotropin levels are generally reduced, and very rarely selective FSH deficiency may occur.

FIGURE 15-22. Schematic diagram of alterations in the hypothalamic-pituitary-testicular axis with secondary hypogonadism resulting in deficiency of androgen and sperm production.

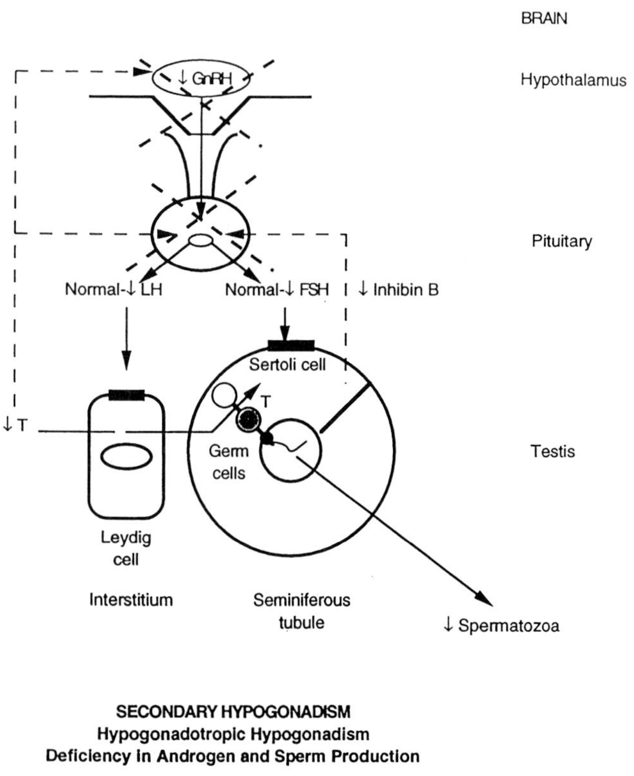

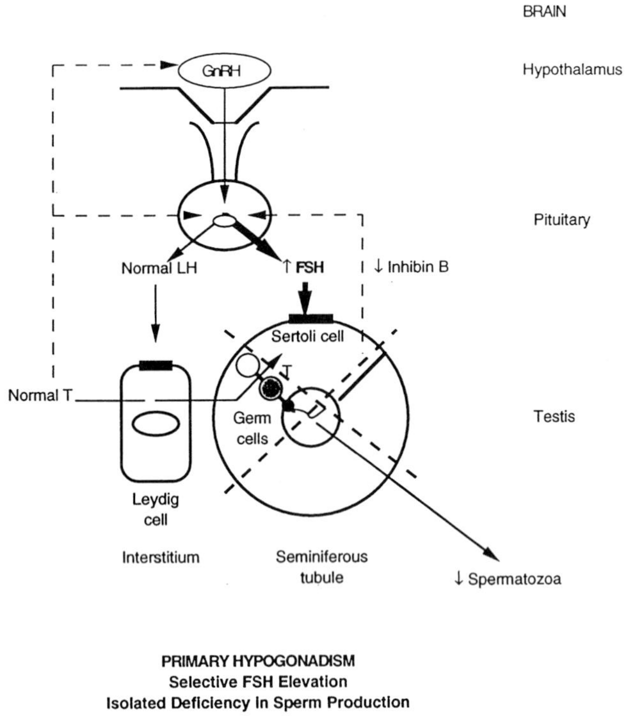

FIGURE 15-23. Schematic diagram of alterations in the hypothalamic-pituitary-testicular axis with primary hypogonadism resulting in isolated impairment of sperm production.

Patients with gonadotropin-secreting pituitary tumors may complain of erectile dysfunction and have low serum testosterone. These tumors most commonly secrete excessive amounts of FSH but may also produce both FSH and LH and/or free α and β subunits.[319–321] They rarely produce LH alone.[322] Therefore, patients with gonadotropin-secreting pituitary tumors may present with complaints and a hormonal profile consistent with primary hypogonadism. A high index of suspicion is needed to diagnose these tumors in men with symptoms or an established diagnosis of hypogonadism. Stimulation of free α-subunit with thyrotropin releasing hormone (TRH) may be a useful diagnostic test in hypogonadal men with gonadotropin-secreting tumors.[323]

The majority of adults with male hypogonadism have either primary or secondary testicular failure. Rarely, disorders of androgen action or *androgen resistance* may present in adults with a clinical picture of hypogonadism. Unlike the severe androgen resistance syndromes that present at birth with male pseudohermaphroditism (see Chapter 17), these disorders in adults are characterized by mild defects in androgen action, resulting in a nearly normal male phenotype, frequently with varying degrees of hypospadius or impairments in sperm production. Both serum testosterone and gonadotropin levels are usually elevated. Therefore, they present with a clinical and hormonal profile of hypergonadotropic hypogonadism but with high serum testosterone levels (Fig. 15-24).

LH and to a lesser extent FSH exhibit episodic fluctuations as a result of pulsatile secretion from the pituitary. Estimates of gonadotropin levels from single samples may differ by approximately ±60 percent for LH and ±20 percent for FSH.[61] Standard gonadotropin radioimmunoassays have limits of sensitivity close to the lower range of normal. Recently developed two-site monoclonal radioimmunometric, time-resolved fluorometric and chemiluminescent assays are characterized by a marked enhancement in sensitivity.[83,84] Clinically, serum LH and FSH are measured initially using highly sensitive immunoassays on a single blood sample (Table 15-4). Clearly elevated or low levels can be interpreted reliably without further measurements. If the initial values are borderline, they should be confirmed by repeated measurements. A pool of four samples taken at 20-minute intervals, or a precisely timed 3-hour urine sample integrates fluctuations in gonadotropin levels due to pulsatile secretion, and these procedures may be used to assess gonadotropins in certain circumstances, e.g., children for the latter.[85,86,324]

In summary, clinical manifestations combined with measurements of serum testosterone and gonadotropin levels and sperm counts permit a physiological classification of the causes of male hypogonadism into *primary* or *secondary hypogonadism* and further subclassification into disorders that result in *deficiency of androgen and sperm production* or those with *isolated impairment of sperm production or function* with normal androgen production (Tables 15-9 and 15-10).

FIGURE 15-24. Schematic diagram of alterations in the hypothalamic-pituitary-testicular axis with androgen resistance.

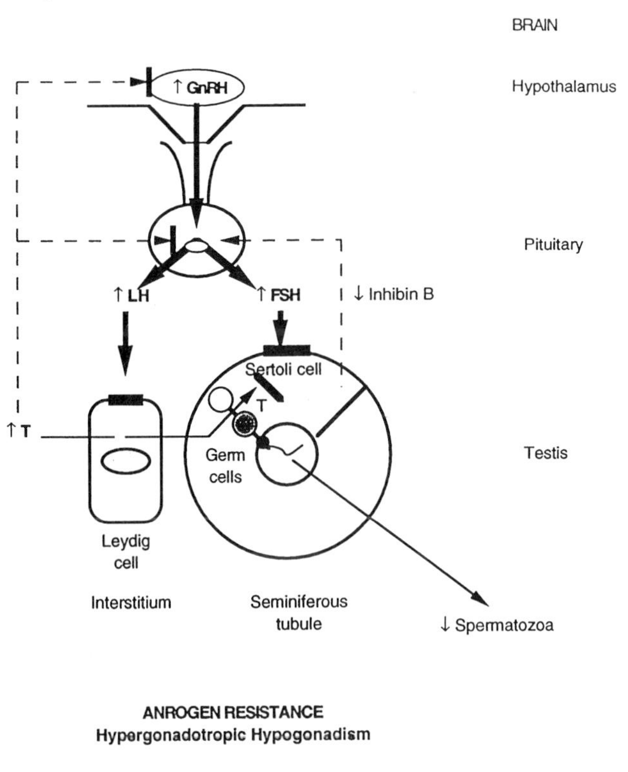

TABLE 15-9. Causes of Primary Hypogonadism in Adults

- Deficiency of androgen and sperm production [hypergonadotropic]
  - Congenital or developmental disorders
    - Klinefelter syndrome and variants
    - XYY syndrome
    - Myotonic dystrophy
    - Noonan (Bonnevie-Ullrich) syndrome
    - Polyglandular autoimmune disease
    - Functional prepubertal castrate (vanishing testes) syndrome
    - Testosterone biosynthetic enzyme defects (17-ketoreductase deficiency, 17,20-desmolase deficiency, 17α-hydroxylase deficiency)
    - Complex genetic syndromes
    - LH resistance
    - Down syndrome
  - Aging men
  - Acquired disorders
    - Surgical or traumatic castration
    - Drugs (spironolactone, ketoconazole, alcohol, marijuana, cytotoxic agents, digoxin, cimetidine, anticonvulsants)
    - Ionizing radiation
    - Orchitis (mumps, leprosy, etc)
  - Systemic illness (combined primary and secondary hypogonadism in many)
    - Chronic liver disease (hepatic cirrhosis)
    - Chronic renal failure
    - Malignancy (Hodgkin's disease, testicular cancer)
    - Sickle cell disease
    - Spinal cord injury
    - Vasculitis (polyarteritis nodosa)
    - Infiltrative disease (amyloidosis, leukemia)
- Isolated impairment of sperm production or function [hypergonadotropic or eugonadotropic]
  - Congenital or developmental disorders
    - Cryptorchidism
    - Varicocele
    - Y Chromosome microdeletions
    - Myotonic dystrophy
    - Germinal cell aplasia (Sertoli cell-only syndrome)
    - Immotile cilia syndrome (Kartagener syndrome)
    - Down syndrome
  - Acquired disorders
    - Orchitis (mumps, leprosy, etc.)
    - Ionizing radiation
    - Cytotoxic agents
    - Thermal trauma
    - Environmental toxins
  - Systemic illness
    - Acute febrile illness
    - Spinal cord injury
  - Idiopathic oligozoospermia or azoospermia
- Androgen resistance syndromes [hypergonadotropic]
  - Incomplete androgen resistance syndromes (Reifenstein, Lubs, Rosewater, and Dreyfus syndromes)
  - Idiopathic oligozoospermia or azoospermia
  - Spinal bulbar muscular atrophy (Kennedy's disease)
  - 5α-reductase type 2 deficiency
  - Androgen receptor antagonists
  - Celiac disease (gluten-sensitive enteropathy)

TABLE 15-10. Causes of Secondary Hypogonadism in Adults

- Deficiency of androgen and sperm production [hypogonadotropic]
  - Congenital or developmental disorders
    - Constitutional delayed puberty
    - Idiopathic hypogonadotropic hypogonadism and variants
      - Hypogonadotropic eunuchoidism and anosmia (Kallmann syndrome)
      - Congenital adrenal hypoplasia
      - Selective LH deficiency (fertile eunuch syndrome)
    - Hemochromatosis, transfusion-induced iron overload
    - Complex genetic syndromes
      - Prader-Willi-Labhart
      - Laurence-Moon-Biedl
      - Other (see Table 15-12)
  - Aging men
  - Acquired disorders
    - Hypopituitarism
      - Pituitary or hypothalamic tumor
        - (pituitary adenoma, craniopharyngioma, meningioma, glioma, metastatic, pinealoma, or germinoma)
      - Granulomatous or infiltrative disease
        - (sarcoidosis, tuberculosis, histiocytosis X, fungal, syphilis, lymphoma, or leukemia)
      - Vascular disorders
        - (pituitary apoplexy, infarction, vasculitis, or vascular malformations)
      - Surgical or traumatic hypophysectomy
      - Irradiation
      - Lymphocytic hypophysitis
      - Pituitary stalk section
    - Hyperprolactinemia
    - Sex steroid hormones and opiates
      - Estrogen excess
      - Progestagens
      - Androgenic anabolic steroids
      - Opiates
    - GnRH agonists
    - Systemic illness
      - Glucocorticoid excess (Cushing syndrome)
      - Acute stress or illness
      - Nutritional deficiency
        - Protein-calorie malnutrition
        - Anorexia nervosa
      - Chronic illnesses
        - AIDS
        - Malignancy
        - Chronic liver and renal disease
        - Chronic obstructive pulmonary disease
        - Diabetes mellitus
        - Spinal cord injury
      - Massive obesity
- Isolated impairment of sperm production [hypogonadotropic]
  - Androgen excess
    - Congenital adrenal hyperplasia
      - 21-hydroxylase deficiency
      - 11β-hydroxylase deficiency
    - Androgenic anabolic steroids
    - Androgen-secreting tumors
  - Hyperprolactinemia
  - Isolated FSH deficiency

Primary Hypogonadism

Deficiency of Androgen and Sperm Production

Congenital or Developmental Disorders

Klinefelter Syndrome and Variants Klinefelter syndrome is the most common cause of primary hypogonadism that results in a deficiency of both testosterone and sperm production. The fundamental chromosomal abnormality in Klinefelter syndrome and its variants is the presence of one or more extra X chromosomes. Classically, the syndrome is characterized by small, firm testes; azoospermia and infertility; gynecomastia; varying degrees of eunuchoidism and testosterone deficiency; and uniformly elevated gonadotropin levels (Table 15-11).[325–328] Klinefelter syndrome is a very common disorder, affecting 1 in 400–500 men (0.21% of infants and 0.15–0.24% of adults).[213,329] The incidence of Klinefelter syndrome increases to 5 percent when maternal age is more than 45 years.[41]

The karyotype in classical Klinefelter syndrome is 47,XXY, as a result of either maternal or paternal meiotic nondisjunction.[326] Variants of the syndrome demonstrate a variety of karyotypes, including XXYY, more than two X (poly X) plus Y, and mosaicism. Men with mosaic Klinefelter syndrome (~10%) exhibit variable cytogenetic features with combinations of normal and classical or variant karyotypes that may vary among different tissues within the same individual. In classical Klinefelter syndrome (47,XXY), the presence of an extra X chromosome is responsible for the presence of a sex chromatin or *Barr body* in the nucleus of epithelial cells obtained on a buccal smear, a normal finding in females who carry two X chromosomes.[326–328] Variant syndromes characterized by more than two X chromosomes may exhibit more than one Barr body per nucleus; the number of sex chromatin bodies always being one less than the number of X chromosomes. Although a buccal smear evaluation may be helpful in diagnosis of Klinefelter syndrome, confirmation requires karyotype analysis of lymphocytes or fibroblasts grown from the testis or other tissues.

The testes in prepubertal boys with Klinefelter syndrome are smaller than normal.[330] However, clinical features are usually not evident prior to puberty.[326–328] At puberty, the testes fail to increase in size and become firmer in consistency as a result of fibrosis and hyalinization of the seminiferous tubules and progressive loss of germ cells.[331,332] The most remarkable clinical feature of Klinefelter syndrome in adults is the very small testis size, rarely exceeding 2 cm in length, compared to a lower limit of 3.5 cm in the normal adult.[19,326–328] The small, firm testes are easily detected on examination and should alert the clinician to the possibility of Klinefelter syndrome.

Clinical androgen deficiency is usually present, but the degree of androgen deficiency and eunuchoidism is variable (Fig. 15-25).[326–328] Even though clinical manifestations are usually present, men with Klinefelter syndrome usually do not seek medical attention for signs or symptoms of androgen deficiency and, as a result, escape diagnosis. In contrast to other disorders that result in prepubertal androgen deficiency and classical eunuchoidism (see earlier discussion), Klinefelter syndrome results in a disproportionate increase in lower compared to upper extremity long bone growth.[333] Bilateral gynecomastia of varying amounts is present in about 80–90 percent of patients with Klinefelter syndrome.[326–328] The prevalence of this syndrome, in particular its variants, is significantly increased in mentally retarded individuals.[334] Although intelligence scores are below age-matched normal individuals, the majority of men with Klinefelter

TABLE 15-11. Features of Klinefelter Syndrome

		*Variant Forms**		
Parameter	**Classic Form (XXY)**	**XX**	**Mosaic Forms***	**Poly X + Y**
Incidence	1/500	1/9000	Unknown	Unknown
Clinical features	Testes <2 cm and firm	Shorter in stature	Testes may be normal-sized	Increased incidence of cryptorchism
	Eunuchoidal proportions	Hypospadias		Radioulnar synostosis
	Gynecomastia			
	Personality disorder			
	Androgen deficiency of variable degree			
Laboratory determinations	LH elevated			
	FSH extremely elevated			
	Testosterone lowered (in 50%)			
Karyotype	Barr body present 47,XXY	46,XX	XXY/XY; XXY/XX	XXXY, XXXXY, XXXXXY
Spermatogenesis	Azoospermia		Impairment less severe	
Testis biopsy	Hyalinized tubules		Less severe damage	
	Relative Leydig cell hyperlasia			

* Only divergent features are listed.

Source: Adapted from Bardin and Paulsen.[814]

syndrome are not mentally retarded.[335] Learning disabilities and character or personality disorders are common in these men, possibly related, in part, to the psychosocial consequences of androgen deficiency.[336] There is a slightly increased incidence of certain systemic diseases associated with Klinefelter syndrome, including diabetes mellitus, thyroid dysfunction, restrictive lung disease, autoimmune disorders such as systemic lupus erythematosus, and lower extremity varicose veins and venous stasis. Men with Klinefelter syndrome have a 20-fold increase in risk of breast cancer compared to normal men.[337]

The clinical manifestations of Klinefelter syndrome variants differ from those of the classical syndrome. In general, the presence of more than two extra X chromosomes results in much higher incidence of mental retardation and somatic abnormalities such as hypospadius, cryptorchidism, and bony abnormalities of the radius and ulna (e.g., radioulnar synostosis).[338–340] The majority of patients with mosaic Klinefelter syndrome exhibit less severe clinical manifestations, particularly if a normal XY cell line is present. Indeed, normal size testes and fertility has been documented in men with mosaic Klinefelter syndrome

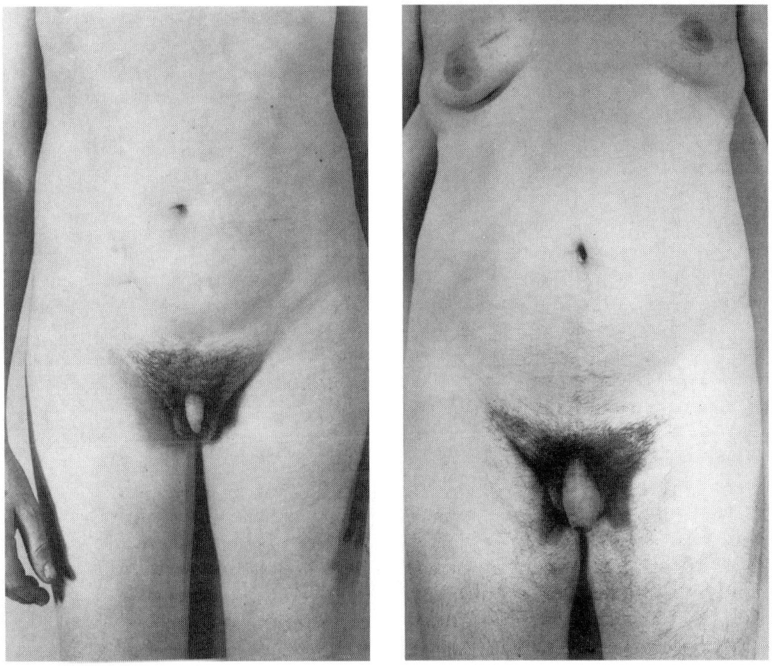

FIGURE 15-25. Two patients with untreated Klinefelter syndrome, demonstrating the variability in the degree of androgenization and gynecomastia in this disorder. (*From Bardin and Paulsen.*[814])

(XXY/XY).[341,342] Very rarely, a patient exhibits the classical features of Klinefelter syndrome with a normal (46, XY) karyotype, a so-called *mutant phenocopy.* Finally, phenotypic males with a 46, XX karyotype demonstrate the typical clinical manifestations of classical Klinefelter syndrome, except they have shorter stature and a greater (9%) incidence of hypospadius.[343–345] In most cases, the mechanism by which these individuals develop a male phenotype in the apparent absence of Y chromosome involves translocation of the small, sex-determining region of the Y chromosome, as the SRY gene is usually detectable on the X chromosome.[346,347]

Azoospermia is present in >95 percent of patients with classical Klinefelter syndrome.[348] Serum total testosterone levels are usually low, but may be in the low-normal adult range in 40–50 percent of patients (Fig. 15-26).[349–351] Serum estradiol levels are approximately twofold higher than normal in men with Klinefelter syndrome, contributing to the development of gynecomastia. As a result of increased estradiol levels, serum SHBG concentrations increase and the non-SHBG-bound and free testosterone levels are low, despite total testosterone levels within the low-normal range.[352] Serum gonadotropin levels, especially serum FSH levels, however are uniformly elevated. Occasionally, serum LH levels may fall in the high normal adult range.

Treatment of Klinefelter syndrome is aimed primarily at correction of the androgen deficiency with testosterone replacement therapy (see later discussion). The infertility is irreversible. However, recent advances in assisted reproductive technology (ART) has permitted the successful use of sperm harvested from testis biopsy for intracytoplasmic sperm injection in a patient with Klinefelter syndrome.[353] Gynecomastia may be a source of great embarrassment, and reduction mammoplasty should be performed in these cases. Patients and their spouses should be counseled regarding the clinical consequences of their diagnosis, and support groups are available, e.g., Klinefelter Syndrome and Associates.

XYY Syndrome Patients with an additional Y chromosome, the *XYY syndrome,* tend to have tall stature and severe nodular cystic acne.[3,354–356] The prevalence of this syndrome is 0.1–0.2 percent of live male births. Men with XYY syndrome exhibit reduced intellectual function, poor adjustment patterns, and extremely aggressive, antisocial behavioral abnormalities, resulting in high incidence (~45%) of convictions for criminal behavior.[334] In adults, this disorder has been identified primarily in prisoners and patients in mental hospitals. Most men with the XYY syndrome have normal testosterone and gonadotropin levels.[357,358] However, some men have been reported to have impairments in androgen and sperm production with elevated gonadotropin levels, i.e., primary hypogonadism.

Myotonic Dystrophy Myotonic dystrophy is an autosomal dominant disorder characterized by progessive weakness and atrophy of muscles, especially those of the face, neck, and distal extremities.[359] An important diagnostic feature in this disorder is the presence of myotonia, or prolonged contraction of muscles. Other characteristic findings include cataracts, cardiac arrhythmias, dysphagia, premature frontal balding, mild intellectual deterioration, and gonadal atrophy. Testicular atrophy and hypogonadism, which occurs in middle age, is found in about 80 percent of men affected by myotonic dystrophy.[360–363] The majority of these men have isolated impairment of spermatogenesis with normal androgen production. However, approximately 20 percent of men with myotonic dystrophy demonstrate varying degrees of androgen deficiency as a result of primary testicular failure. In these individuals, serum testosterone levels are moderately reduced to low-normal, and gonadotropin, in particular FSH, levels are increased. In addition to treating the manifestations of androgen deficiency, testosterone replacement therapy may help to maintain or improve muscle mass in some of these men, but it does not usually affect strength significantly.[364] Infertility is irreversible.

FIGURE 15-26. Serum FSH, LH and total testosterone in healthy normal men (shaded bars) and men with Klinefelter syndrome (dots). (*From Smyth and Bremner.*[328])

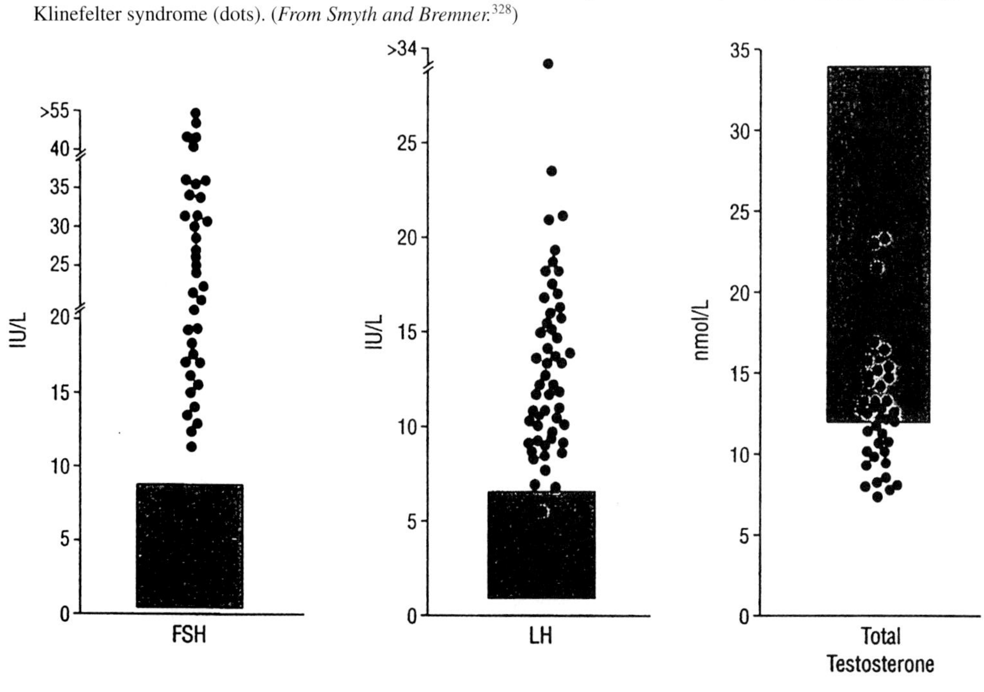

Noonan (Bonnevie-Ullrich) Syndrome This syndrome is an autosomal recessive disorder that occurs in both males and females with a normal karyotype. It is characterized by a number of clinical features that resemble those of females with Turner syndrome, and this disorder has been called male Turner syndrome.[365–367] Characteristic findings include short stature, typical Turner syndrome facial features (hypertelorism, antimongoloid eye slant, ptosis, low-set ears, micrognathia, high-arched palate, low hairline, and dental malocclusions), webbed neck, shield-like chest, pectus excavatum, cubitus valgus, mental retardation, cardiovascular anomalies (especially pulmonic stenosis), and lymphedema of hands and feet. The diagnosis is established by the presence of four or more cardinal features and a normal karyotype.

Males with Noonan syndrome exhibit primary testicular dysfunction with impairment of both androgen and sperm production and elevated serum gonadotropin levels. Cryptorchidism and a small penis are frequently present. Treatment of this disorder consists of testosterone replacement to correct the androgen deficiency, and orchiopexy for associated cryptorchidism, both for psychological reasons and to monitor the testes for malignancy.

Polyglandular Autoimmune Disease This is a group of disorders characterized by clustering of organ-specific autoimmune diseases involving several endocrine and nonendocrine organs associated with the presence of circulating auto-antibodies to these organs. Specific autoimmune disorders that occur in association with each other in patients with polyglandular autoimmune disease include Addison's disease; hypothyroidism due to Hashimoto's thyroiditis; type 1 diabetes mellitus; pernicious anemia, ovarian failure; hypoparathyroidism; vitiligo; mucocutaneous candidiasis; Grave's disease; hypopituitarism due to lymphocytic hypophysitis; and alopecia areata or totalis. Although much less common than ovarian failure, primary testicular failure associated with antitesticular antibodies directed at testis basement membrane may occur in males with this disorder, resulting in androgen deficiency or more commonly isolated impairment in sperm production.[368–370]

Functional Prepubertal Castrate Syndrome (Congenital Anorchia, Vanishing Testis Syndrome) This syndrome is characterized by bilateral absence of functioning testicular tissue, occasionally associated with absent epididymides, in a genotypic and phenotypic male.[371] Testosterone produced from the fetal testis is required for normal male internal and external genital development during the critical fetal period of 8–14 weeks. In men with this syndrome, the presence of otherwise normal male internal and external genitalia without Müllerian duct derivatives and descent of the vas and testicular blood vessels into the scrotum imply that a normally functioning testis was present during fetal and early neonatal development. It is hypothesized that testicular damage due to bilateral testicular torsion and/or vascular compromise in the fetus results in atrophy of the gonads, but evidence for this mechanism is lacking.

Patients with congenital anorchia usually present with *suspected* bilateral cryptorchidism before puberty, or with delayed puberty, eunuchoidal features, and sexual infantilism (Fig. 15-16).[371] Examination reveals an absence of palpable testes ("empty scrotum"). Palpation of the scrotum may reveal the vas deferens or small masses consisting of Wolffian duct remnants. Unlike other conditions associated with eunuchoidism, these individuals have relatively short stature. Serum testosterone remain in the prepubertal range, and during puberty, gonadotropin levels increase to castrate levels in patients with congenital anorchia.[372] Normal gonadotropin levels in a pubertal or adult patient with anorchia excludes the diagnosis of congenital anorchia and should prompt a search for bilateral cryptorchid testis.

Congenital anorchia must be distinguished from bilateral abdominal cryptorchidism, which also presents with absent scrotal testes. Because of the increased risk of malignancy, intra-abdominal testes require orchidectomy or orchiopexy. An hCG stimulation test may be helpful in distinguishing between congenital anorchia and bilateral cryptorchidism.[373,374] Individuals with congenital anorchia usually lack a serum testosterone response to administration of 1,000–2,000 IU hCG, given three times weekly for 2 weeks. In contrast, cryptorchid testes usually exhibit a testosterone response to hCG, and often descend during treatment. However, absent responses to hCG administration for 6 weeks in patients with idiopathic hypogonadotropic hypogonadism and bilateral cryptorchidism have been reported.[373,374] Ultimately, laparoscopy or surgical abdominal exploration may be necessary to confirm the diagnosis. Abdominal exploration may be avoided if patients demonstrate prepubertal testosterone levels that fail to respond to hCG and castrate gonadotropin levels, or if a blind-ending vas deferens and vascular structures are seen on laparoscopy. Treatment of this syndrome consists of androgen replacement therapy to induce full sexual maturation. Insertion of testicular prostheses may be of psychological value.

Testosterone Biosynthetic Enzyme Defects Defects in 17-ketoreductase, 17,20-desmolase or lyase, and 17α-hydroxylase result in deficiency of androgen production and elevated gonadotropin secretion (see Chap. 17). Males with severe deficiencies in these enzymes of testosterone biosynthesis present as phenotypic females with partial virilization at the time of puberty. However, incomplete defects may result in androgenized males with hypospadius, gynecomastia, and lack of complete pubertal development.[375–379] Men with 17α-hydroxylase deficiency also exhibit hypertension and hypokalemia because of increased adrenal mineralocorticoid secretion. Diagnosis of these disorders is confirmed by elevated levels of precursor steroids, i.e., an elevation in androstenedione for 17-ketoreductase deficiency, 17α-hydroxyprogesterone for 17,20-desmolase deficiency, and progesterone for 17α-hydroxylase deficiency.

Complex Genetic Disorders Primary hypogonadism may be present in a number of complex genetic disorders such as the *Alstrom, ataxia telangiectasia, Sohval-Soffer, Weinstein,* and *Werner syndromes.* Rarely, patients with Prader-Labhart-Willi and Laurence-Moon-Beidl syndromes exhibit primary hypogonadism with elevated gonadotropins rather than the more commonly associated gonadotropin deficiency.[380–382] The number of complex genetic is very large, and the best clinical approach is to consult a compendium of genetic disorders such as that written by Rimoin and Schimke[383] when unusual congenital manifestations are noted in a patient with hypogonadism.

LH Resistance Most males with inactivating mutations of the LH receptor present with male pseudohermaphroditism and female phenotype.[384] However, males with an inactivating mutations of the LH receptor have been reported who presented with descended small testis, undervirilization, and a hormone profile of primary hypogonadism (low testosterone and high LH levels).[385,386] Of note is that in one individual with an LH receptor mutation, hCG treatment induced testosterone secretion into the normal range and spermatogenesis, suggesting dissociation of LH and hCG actions on the LH receptor.[386]

Down Syndrome Patients with trisomy 21, or Down syndrome, usually have a mild degree of testicular dysfunction.[387] The defects in spermatogenesis are usually more severe than those of Leydig cell function. Histologically, the spectrum of findings includes moderate to severe reduction in all germ cell types (hypospermatogenesis), germ cell maturation arrest, or loss of all germ cells, i.e., Sertoli cell only. Serum FSH levels may be normal or elevated. Serum testosterone levels are low-normal to low with elevated LH levels.

Aging Men

Aging is associated with a decline in testicular function that affects both the seminiferous tubule and interstitial compartments. Daily sperm production, sperm motility, spermatozoa with normal morphology, Sertoli number, and serum inhibin B levels decline with aging.[388,389] Serum testosterone also declines gradually with aging, beginning at age 40–50 years, with the lowest concentrations found in men more than 70 years old.[388–391] Because SHBG levels increase with aging, serum free or non-SHBG-bound testosterone decline to a greater extent (~1% per year) than total testosterone levels (~0.4% per year). The normal circadian variation in serum testosterone is blunted and Leydig cell number and hCG-stimulated testosterone production are reduced with aging.[388,389,392] In approximately 20–30 percent of elderly men, serum total testosterone levels are below the normal range established in younger men, i.e., in the hypogonadal range.[388,389] Because testicular function and testosterone production are affected by illness, medications (e.g., glucocorticoids), malnutrition, severe obesity, and alcohol or drug abuse, a much greater proportion (>60%) of elderly men with these conditions have testosterone concentrations below the normal range.

The age-related reduction in testosterone levels is associated with increases in average concentrations of LH and FSH. Clinically, some elderly men exhibit low testosterone levels accompanied by elevated gonadotropin levels, i.e., a hormone profile consistent with a diagnosis of "primary hypogonadism." Aging is also associated with alterations in hypothalamic GnRH secretion with relatively preserved gonadotropin responsiveness to GnRH.[388,389] Both LH and FSH secretion are also suppressed by comorbid illnesses that occur and medications used commonly in aging men. For these reasons, the most common hormonal profile observed in elderly men is low testosterone levels associated with normal LH and FSH levels, consistent with a diagnosis of "secondary hypogonadism" (see later discussion).[388,389]

Aging is also associated with a number of alterations in body functions that may be androgen-dependent.[393–402] These include an increase in fat mass; a decrease in muscle mass and strength; reduction in bone mineral density and increase risk of osteoporosis and fractures; decline in sexual interest and function, including diminished libido and erectile function; changes in mood including decreased vigor and feeling of well-being, and an increase in the incidence of depressed mood; reduced cognitive function; and alterations in sleep quality. Because similar changes occur in younger hypogonadal men and are improved with androgen replacement therapy, it is possible that the age-related decline in serum testosterone levels may contribute to alterations in androgen-responsive tissues and body functions in aging men.

Short-term preliminary studies in small numbers of elderly men with low testosterone levels suggest that testosterone therapy may have beneficial effects on body composition, bone mineral density, energy, and feeling of well-being.[403–407] The only short-term adverse effect noted in a few men was excessive stimulation of erythrocytosis. Although these preliminary studies are encouraging, the potential longer-term effects of testosterone therapy in elderly men on the prostate gland, specifically on the stimulation of growth of benign prostatic hyperplasia (BPH) and subclinical prostate cancer, and on atherosclerotic cardiovascular disease risk are not known. Larger and longer-term randomized placebo-controlled studies are needed to determine the balance of potential benefits and risks of testosterone therapy in elderly men.

Acquired Disorders

Because the process of spermatogenesis involves active cellular division, it is much more sensitive to external or environmental influences, such as irradiation, cytotoxic agents, or heat than Leydig cell production of testosterone. As a result, most testicular disorders causing acquired hypogonadism result more commonly in isolated impairment of sperm production (see later discussion), than in androgen deficiency. Some acquired disorders, however, affect both androgen and sperm production.

Bilateral Surgical or Traumatic Castration Bilateral surgical or traumatic castration results in a rapid decline in testosterone levels within hours. The acute androgen deficiency syndrome that results is characterized by hot flushes and irritability, similar to symptoms that many women experience at the time of menopause.

Drugs Certain drugs produce androgen deficiency by inhibiting testosterone biosynthesis and/or by blocking androgen action. The aldosterone antagonist *spironolactone* inhibits testosterone biosynthesis by inhibiting17,20-desmolase and 17α-hydroxylase, and interferes with androgen action by competitively binding to the androgen receptor.[408] *Ketoconazole* is an antifungal agent that also inhibits testosterone biosynthesis by inhibiting17,20-desmolase and 17α-hydroxylase when given in dosages exceeding 400 mg daily.[409–411] In higher dosages, it may also inhibit adrenal steroidogenesis. *Alcohol* and *marijuana (tetrahydrocannabinol)* have direct toxic effects on both spermatogenesis and steroidogenesis in the testis, in addition to their effects on the brain.[412–417] The predominant effect in the testis is on 3β-hydroxysteroid dehydrogenase activity. A number of *cytotoxic drugs* used in cancer chemotherapy interfere with spermatogenesis and, rarely, with androgen production. In particular, combination chemotherapy for Hodgkin's disease and acute leukemias, and regimens including potent alkylating agents such as cyclophosphamide, may impair Leydig cell function.[418–423] *Digoxin* elevates serum estradiol levels, reduces serum testosterone concentrations, and interacts with both the estrogen and androgen receptor.[424] The immunosuppressive drug *cyclosporine* also inhibits testosterone production.[425] *Cimetidine* is an histamine H2 receptor antagonist that is also a weak androgen receptor antagonist.[426,427] The *anticonvulsants* phenytoin and carbamazepine may increase SHBG levels, reduce non-SHBG-bound testosterone, and raise LH levels, although the latter may be within the normal range (i.e., producing a hormonal pattern of either primary or secondary hypogonadism).[428,429]

Ionizing Radiation Irradiation of the testes commonly affect spermatogenesis (see later section) but rarely causes permanent androgen deficiency. However, exposure of the testes to very large doses, those exceeding 600–800 rads or cGy, may compromise Leydig cell function and reduce testosterone production.[32,430–435]

Orchitis *Mumps orchitis* is a very common cause of acquired primary hypogonadism and infertility.[436–438] Approximately 15–25 percent of males with mumps develop an extremely painful acute orchitis. Although mumps orchitis occurring before puberty is very uncommon, individuals usually recover completely without subsequent testicular dysfunction. However, acute mumps infection in pubertal or adult testes usually causes permanent seminiferous tubule damage and impaired spermatogenesis.[439–441] In severe cases, Leydig cell failure with androgen deficiency also occurs.[442] Although clinical mumps orchitis is usually unilateral in 60–70 percent of cases, degenerative changes are often observed in the clinically uninvolved testis. Damage to the testis results from the infection, inflammatory reaction, and ischemia from pressure induced by swelling of the testis within the tunica albuginea. Orchitis usually develops acutely within a few days of parotitis. During this acute phase, there is interstitial edema and germ cell sloughing. The acute phase is followed by progressive seminiferous tubule sclerosis, and then by testicular atrophy during the next several months. The treatment of mumps orchitis is symptomatic with bedrest, pain medications, and occasionally prednisone. The latter may reduce pain and swelling but does not prevent testicular damage.

Orchitis may complicate infections with other viruses, e.g., *echoviruses, lymphocytic choriomeningitis virus,* and *arboviruses.*[443] Uncommon causes of orchitis include *gonorrhea, leprosy, tuberculosis, brucellosis, glanders, syphilis,* and parasitic diseases such as *filariasis* and *bilharziasis.*[444] As in mumps, orchitis complicating these infections results more commonly in isolated impairment of sperm production, although in severe cases androgen production is also affected.

Systemic Illness

A number of systemic diseases cause a deficiency in androgen and sperm production, primarily by affecting testicular function directly.[445,446] It is often difficult to distinguish the effects of the illness from those related to generalized debility and malnutrition associated with these systemic disorders. The latter often also suppress the hypothalamic-pituitary axis so that secondary as well as primary testicular dysfunction occurs in most of these systemic illnesses.

Chronic Liver Disease In patients with chronic liver disease, in particular *hepatic cirrhosis,* erectile dysfunction, gynecomastia, and testicular atrophy are commonly present in 50–75 percent of affected men.[447] Total testosterone levels in blood are low or low-normal and spermatogenesis is reduced. SHBG levels are increased about twofold.[448,449] Free and non-SHBG-bound testosterone levels are low, and serum estradiol and LH levels are usually elevated, but may fall in the high-normal range.[448–452] LH secretion may be suppressed partially by the high circulating levels of estrogens and prolactin, and malnutrition that are present in cirrhotic patients.[450–452] Increased estrogen concentrations result from impaired hepatic clearance of adrenal androgens such as androstenedione. Higher adrenal androgen levels provide increased substrates for peripheral aromatization to estrone and estradiol. The increased estrogen to testosterone ratio contributes to the formation gynecomastia.[453] Treatment of androgen deficiency in patients with cirrhosis with an aromatizable androgen is usually tolerated well but may result occasionally in worsening of gynecomastia. Hormonal abnormalities associated with chronic liver disease may be partially reversed by liver transplantation.[454,455]

Chronic Renal Failure Renal failure causes reductions in both androgen and sperm production in more than 50 percent of cases.[456–458] Serum LH and FSH levels are elevated as a result of increased production as well as reduced renal clearance. The response of Leydig cell testosterone production to hCG stimulation is impaired, confirming a primary testicular defect. Hyperprolactinemia and zinc deficiency may also contribute to testicular dysfunction in uremic patients.[456–458] Alterations in LH pulse frequency suggest a concomitant disorder of hypothalamic GnRH secretion.[458,459] Hemodialysis does not significantly improve testosterone or sperm production. However, successful renal transplantation results in some improvement in testis function, which may be tempered by immunosuppressive drugs used to prevent graft rejection.[458] In addition to treating androgen deficiency, testosterone replacement therapy may also improve the anemia of renal failure and reduce erythropoietin requirements.[460,461]

Other Systemic Illnesses In some *malignancies,* androgen deficiency may be present prior to exposure to chemotherapy agents, e.g., advanced Hodgkin's disease or testicular cancer.[462–464] In many instances, androgen deficiency may be the result of generalized debilitation and malnutrition associated with the malignancy. *Sickle cell disease* often results in low serum testosterone and clinical signs of androgen deficiency, impaired spermatogenesis, testicular atrophy, and elevated serum gonadotropin levels, implying primary testicular failure.[465,466] *Spinal cord injury* causing paraplegia or quadraplegia may result in an acute reduction in testosterone and sperm production.[467–469] Although gonadotropin levels are usually suppressed, some men exhibit elevated LH and/or FSH with low testosterone. Testosterone levels usually return to normal in the chronic state, unless chronic malnutrition occurs. However, impaired spermatogenesis usually persists. Rarely, *vasculitis* and *infiltrative disease* (e.g., amyloidosis, leukemia) involving both testes may result in primary hypogonadism affecting both androgen and sperm production.[470,471] The former may present as a painless testicular mass mimicking a neoplasm of the testis.[472]

Isolated Deficiency of Sperm Production or Function

Congenital or Developmental Disorders

Cryptorchidism In cryptorchidism, the testis fails to descend normally into the scrotum and remain along the path of descent within the abdomen or inguinal canal.[473] Whether unilateral or bilateral, cryptorchidism is associated with impaired spermatogenesis and infertility and an increased risk of developing a testicular carcinoma.[474,475] In contrast, *ectopic testes* are located outside the normal pathway of testicular descent and may be located in the perineal, femoral, or superficial inguinal areas. To avoid unnecessary treatment, cryptorchidism must be distinguished from *retractile testes* (pseudocryptorchidism), which occurs more commonly. Retractile testes are located in the scrotum, but are withdrawn into the inguinal canal or abdomen with minimal stimulation. Retractile testes are usually not associated with infertility or an increased risk of cancer, but bilateral high retractile testes may exhibit disordered spermatogenesis and impaired fertility.[476,477]

The testes usually descend into the scrotum at about the eighth fetal month. Undescended testes are found in 3–4 percent of new born males, but descend during the first year in all but about 0.5 percent of infants. The prevalence of cryptorchidism in adults is ~0.3–0.4 percent.[473] Because a patent processus vaginalis is usually also present, inguinal hernia is associated with cryptorchidism in 50–80 percent of cases.[473]

Bilateral cryptorchidism may be the presenting complaint in a number of hypogonadal disorders, such as congenital anorchia, Noonan syndrome, and Reifenstein syndrome.[473,478] It is associated with many other causes of hypogonadism that result in androgen deficiency, such as idiopathic hypogoadotropic hypogonadism, idiopathic hypopituitarism, poly X plus Y variant of Klinefelter syndrome (but not classical Klinefelter syndrome), Prader-Labhart-Willi syndrome, and Laurence-Moon-Biedl syndrome.[473,478]

Cryptorchidism that does not occur in association with hypogonadal disorders usually causes isolated impairment of sperm production and rarely affects Leydig cell function. Even when cryptorchidism is unilateral, testicular dysfunction is very common, suggesting altered function in both testes.[479,480] Underlying developmental abnormalities of the testis and gubernaculum, perhaps secondary to mild gonadotropin or androgen deficiency during fetal life, are thought to contribute to the etiology of cryptorchidism in these individuals.[481,482] Azoospermia occurs in ~50 percent of men with bilateral and ~20 percent of men with unilateral cryptorchidism.[483] Rarely, normal descent is impeded by anatomical abnormalities along the path of descent, e.g., external inguinal hernias. In these cases, both testes function normally and orchiopexy before puberty usually preserves normal testicular function.

Careful physical examination of the scrotum should be performed in order to distinguish cryptorchidism from a retractile testis. Diagnosis is especially difficult in obese patients. Examination should be performed in the standing, squatting, and recumbent positions. Observation with the scrotum immersed in warm water or after a hot bath may be helpful to facilitate descent and detection of a retractile testis. The Valsalva maneuver or pressure applied to the lower abdomen is also useful. In men with a retractile testis, elicitation of a cremasteric reflex may cause a localized puckering of the scrotal skin. Failure to palpate a testis after repeated examinations suggests that the testis is within the abdomen, severely atrophic, or absent. As many as 50 percent of boys with a unilateral nonpalpable testis will have an absent rather than undescended testis.[484] In the former, the contralateral testis may be hypertrophic on examination.[485] An ultrasound or CT scan may help to locate testes that are not palpable.

As a consequence of exposure of the seminiferous tubules to higher extrascrotal temperatures at puberty, the germinal epithelium of cryptorchid testes show severe degeneration, eventually resulting in fibrosis of the tubules.[486,487] Bilateral cryptorchidism causes infertility. Sperm counts are low, and serum FSH levels are elevated selectively. Leydig cell function is usually preserved, and serum testosterone and LH concentrations remain normal. The risk of malignancy in an undescended testis is 20–40 times greater than in a scrotal testis, and the risk remains increased after orchiopexy.[488,489] Although the testicular cancer is uncommon, occurring in only 1–2 per 100,000 males, the lifetime risk is substantial. The prevalence of carcinoma in situ may be as high as 8 percent in cryptorchid testes.

Therapy for cryptorchidism should be instituted before puberty, when the degenerative changes of the germ cells occur. The exact age at which treatment should be instituted is controversial and recommendations vary between 6–18 months to just before puberty.[489–491] Administration of hCG (1,000 IU three times weekly for 6 weeks) or GnRH to prepubertal boys with cryptorchidism may cause testicular descent in some patients. Reports of the efficacy of hormonal therapy are widely discrepant, most likely because variable numbers of patients with retractile testes were included in different studies. When patients with pseudocryptorchidism are excluded, controlled studies of hormonal therapy found that only 12–24 percent of boys with unilateral cryptorchidism responded to hormones with testicular descent.[492–494] Despite these results, a trial of hormonal therapy should be attempted in boys with definite cryptorchidism on repeated examinations in order to avoid unnecessary surgery.

If hormonal therapy is unsuccessful, orchiopexy is performed in an attempt to preserve testis function, to permit palpation of the testis for malignancy, and to provide cosmetic therapy. Despite orchiopexy, fertility rates are usually reduced, particularly in patients with bilateral cryptorchidism.[480,483] At the time of orchiopexy, bilateral testis biopsies may be performed to determine the extent of testicular abnormalities. If a unilateral undescended testis is atrophic and shows extensive seminiferous tubule fibrosis, it may be removed, provided that the contralateral testis is located within the scrotum.

Varicocele Varicocele is a dilatation of the pampiniform plexus of veins surrounding the spermatic cord that is caused by retrograde blood flow into the internal spermatic vein. A palpable varicocele occurs in about 10–20 percent in the general population and in 30–40 percent of men with infertility.[268,269,495–498] To detect a varicocele, examination of the scrotum should be performed optimally with the patient standing and performing a Valsalva maneuver.

Although it is associated with infertility, approximately 50 percent of men with a varicocele exhibit normal semen parameters.[499,500] Furthermore, some men with a varicocele and abnormal seminal fluid analysis are fertile. About 90 percent of varicoceles occur on the left side as a result of valvular incompetence between the left internal spermatic and renal vein.[501] Occurrence of an isolated right-sided varicocele may be an early clue to venous obstruction by a retroperitoneal tumor or lymph nodes, or *situs inversus*. Varicoceles are thought to affect testicular function by a variety of mechanisms, including increasing testicular temperature and blood flow.[502,503]

Men with a large varicoceles and infertility usually exhibit low sperm counts with reduced motility and increased numbers of sperm with abnormal morphology, such as tapered and amorphous forms.[499,500] However, these abnormalities are not specific for varicocele. Testis size and serum testosterone, LH, and FSH levels are usually normal. Ligation of testicular veins in the inguinal canal is the standard treatment for varicocele. In infertile men, surgery has been reported to improve semen quality and fertility, but well-controlled clinical studies have not been performed.[504–507] In the absence of such studies, patients must be informed that the majority of studies indicate an improvement in fertility rate of ~20 percent in men who undergo varicocele ligation. Individuals with large varicoceles and progressive atrophy of the ipsilateral testis should probably undergo surgical treatment.[508,509]

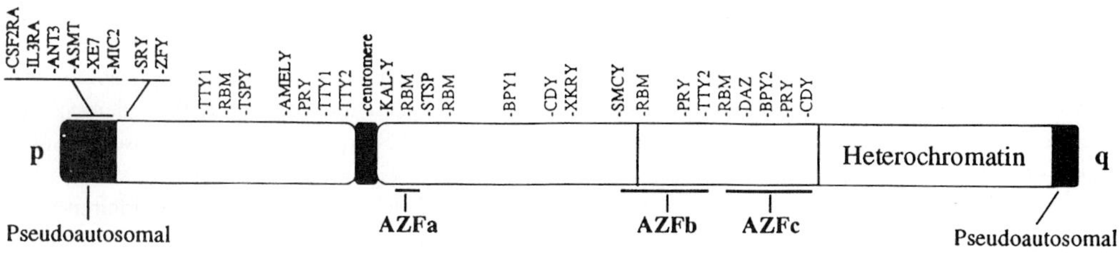

FIGURE 15-27. Diagram of the Y chromosome with relative locations of AZF regions, the DAZ gene and RBM gene family. (*From Roberts.*[510])

Y Chromosome Microdeletions More than 20 years ago it was recognized that the Y chromosome determinants were necessary for spermatogenesis. Subsequent deletion studies identified a region on the long (q) arm of the Y chromosome, called the *azoospermic factor* (AZF), that was required for spermatogenesis (Fig. 15-27).[510–512] Higher resolution mapping identified three deletion regions designated AZFa, AZFb, and AZFc that were associated with infertility and distinct histological patterns. Microdeletions of AZFa are mostly associated with Sertoli cell- only histology, AZFb with germ cell arrest at the pachytene spermatocyte stage, and AZFc with germ cell arrest at the spermatid stage.[510–512] Serum FSH levels are usually elevated selectively in men harboring these microdeletions. Y chromosome microdeletions are found in 10–15 percent of men with infertility, especially those with azoospermia and severe oligozoospermia.[510–512] Two candidate genes have been cloned from the AZF region: *RBM* (RNA Binding Motif, originally named YRRM, Y-specific gene with RNA Recognition Motif) gene, of which there are multiple copies scattered along both arms of the Y chromosome; and *DAZ* (Deleted in Azoospermia) gene located in the AZFc region, where the majority of the Y chromosome microdeletions found in infertile men reside. Microdeletion analysis should be considered in couples considering in vitro fertilization using intracytoplasmic sperm injection (*ICSI*) because Y chromosome microdeletions (and other genetic causes of male infertility) have been demonstrated to be transmitted to male offspring during ICSI.[510–514]

Myotonic Dystrophy The majority of patients with myotonic dystrophy (see earlier discussion) have isolated impairment of spermatogenesis with normal androgen production.

Germinal Cell Aplasia or Sertoli Cell-Only Syndrome This is an uncommon condition diagnosed on testis biopsy. It is characterized by seminiferous tubules devoid of germ cells and lined only with Sertoli cells with little or no tubular fibrosis.[515–517] Clinically, patients present with infertility and are normally androgenized. They have moderately small testes (2–4 cm in length or 10–20 mL in volume), azoospermia, and selectively elevated serum FSH levels, indicative of severe seminiferous tubule dysfunction.[517] Serum testosterone concentrations are normal, and LH levels are normal or occasionally elevated slightly. Leydig cell testosterone production in response to hCG stimulation may also be reduced, suggesting mild, subclinical Leydig cell dysfunction.

It is hypothesized that germinal cell aplasia is caused by congenital absence of germ cells. However, in some familial cases, germ cells are present on testis biopsy prior to puberty and subsequently lost during and after puberty.[515–517] Other disorders that cause severe germ cell damage, such as mumps orchitis, cryptorchidism, irradiation, or cytotoxic drugs, may also exhibit tubules lined with only Sertoli cells. However, in these acquired causes of Sertoli cell-only syndrome, there is usually extensive seminiferous tubule sclerosis and hyalinization, and testes are usually much smaller. Infertility in congenital germinal cell aplasia is irreversible, but may be reversible with time in some acquired cases of severe germ cell damage.

Immotile Cilia Syndrome Immotile cilia syndrome is a group of inherited disorders characterized by sinusitis, bronchiectasis, and infertility.[518–521] The association of this syndrome with *situs inversus* is known as Kartagener syndrome. Patients with immotile cilia syndrome usually suffer from chronic, recurrent respiratory infections because of impaired mucociliary clearance in the respiratory tract, leading to the development of bronchiectasis. They also produce nonmotile or poorly motile spermatozoa. Some men exhibit defects in sperm motility without involvement of the respiratory tract. A number of ultrastructural abnormalities that impair motility of cilia have been identified using electron microscopy.[522] Cilia in the respiratory tract and the sperm tail are immotile in Kartagener syndrome because they lack *dynein,* a protein that is important in microtubular filament movement. Other patients were found to have a *deficiency in protein carboxyl methylase,* an enzyme that is important in sperm motility.[523] Infertility in these disorders is irreversible, but ICSI offers hope for treatment of men with these disorders who wish to father children.

Down Syndrome Men with Down syndrome usually exhibit isolated impairment of sperm production with normal androgen production (see earlier discussion).

Acquired Disorders

The majority of adults who develop mumps *orchitis* and orchitis due to other infectious agents sustain severe germ cell damage and isolated impairment of sperm production with normal Leydig cell function (see earlier section). Seminiferous tubule function is much more sensitive to damage from external or environmental agents than Leydig cell function. Therefore, exposure of the testis to *ionizing radiation, cytotoxic agents, thermal trauma,* and *environmental toxins* often results in impairment in sperm production without androgen deficiency.

The human testis is very sensitive to *ionizing radiation.* Spermatogonia are particularly sensitive to radiation.[32,430–435] Radiation doses as little as 15 rads or cGy of x-irradiation may suppress sperm production temporarily. Doses >700 rads or cGy usually produce permanent testis damage and infertility. Despite shielding of the testis, scatter from radiation doses used to treat malignant lymphoma may cause permanent germ cell injury and infertility.[524] Spermatogenesis is also very sensitive to damage by *cytotoxic agents* used in cancer chemotherapy. Alkylating agents such as cyclophosphamide or chlorambucil are particularly toxic to the testis. The likelihood of severe seminiferous tubule damage and infertility is greater with combination chemotherapy regimens, e.g., MOPP (methotrexate, vincristine, procarbazine, and prednisone) for Hodgkin's disease or ABVD (adriamycin, bleomycin, vinblastine, and dacarbazine).[418–423] Sulfasalazine and methotrexate may cause oligozoospermia, low sperm motility, and infertility.[525,526]

Despite being very sensitive to radiation and cytotoxic drugs, the germinal epithelium has great regenerative properties, and recovery of spermatogenesis may occur despite very severe germ cell loss induced by high doses of these agents. Recovery time is dose-dependent. Return to baseline sperm counts takes about 9–18 months after 100 cGy or rads or less, 30 months after 200–300 cGy, and up to 5 years after 400–600 cGy or rads.[527] Although Leydig cell function is generally more resistant to both irradiation and cytotoxic agents, high doses (e.g., >800 cGy or rads) may produce androgen deficiency. As mentioned previously, some men with advanced Hodgkin's disease and testicular cancer have impaired testicular function (including isolated impairment in spermatogenesis) prior to chemotherapy or irradiation.[528,529] Sperm banking offers hope for fertility for those patients that may develop permanent infertility as a result of irradiation or chemotherapy for malignant disease.

Damage to the germinal epithelium has been reported in workers exposed to carbon disulfide, a solvent used in production of rayon, and dibromochloropropane, an insecticide.[530] A number of other chemical agents used in industry and laboratories have been implicated as direct testicular toxins (e.g., lead, deuterium oxide, ethyl glycol, cadmium, fluoroacetamide, nitrofurans, dinitropyrroles, diamines, and alpha-chlorhydrin).[531,532] It is postulated that environmental toxins/xenobiotics might act as antiandrogens and/or estrogens to alter reproductive function, in particular sperm production (i.e., act as "endocrine disruptors" of spermatogenesis).[533] For example, environmental agents have been implicated in contributing to declining sperm counts in normal men that has been found in some studies but not in others. Even relatively minor *thermal trauma,* such as that occurring with hot tub use, may result in suppression of sperm production.[534]

Systemic Illness

Even relatively minor *acute febrile illnesses* may result in temporary suppression of sperm production, e.g., viral upper respiratory tract infection.[534] More than 50 percent of men with *spinal cord injury* resulting in paraplegia or quadraplegia develop impaired sperm production with normal androgen production.[467–469,535] Reduced spermatogenesis may be caused by elevated scrotal temperature from loss of lumbar sympathetic innervation.

Idiopathic Oligozoospermia or Azoospermia

In the majority (60–70 percent) of men who present with infertility and isolated impairment of sperm production, no etiology can be found, leading to a "diagnosis" of *idiopathic oligozoospermia* or *azoospermia*. Because male infertility affects 5–6 percent of young men, this represents the most common cause of male hypogonadism.

Men with oligospermia or azoospermia exhibit either selective elevations in serum FSH (hypergonadotropic hypogonadism) or normal gonadotropin levels (eugonadotropic hypogonadism). About 30 percent of these individuals demonstrate exaggerated increases in FSH and/or LH in response to GnRH administration, suggesting subclinical primary hypogonadism.[536,537] Men with isolated FSH elevation have low serum inhibin B levels,[175] and some exhibit LH pulse frequencies that are slow compared to normal men.[538] The pathophysiological significance of the latter is unclear. However, administration of exogenous pulsatile GnRH at an increased frequency lowers FSH levels but does not improve sperm production consistently or improve fertility.[539–543]

Because the pathogenesis of impaired sperm production in these men is not known, therapy has been empirical. Trials of treatment with high dosage testosterone and recovery (testosterone rebound), gonadotropins, clomiphene citrate, testolactone, cortisone, thyroid hormone, caffeine, and vitamins have generally been unsuccessful in improving fertility rates greater than those achieved by untreated or placebo-treated men.[544–550] Untreated men with oligozoospermia and infertility have a 25 percent fertility rate in 1 year.[551]

In vitro fertilization using intracytoplasmic sperm injection (ICSI) of ejaculated, epididymal or testis aspiration-derived spermatozoa or spermatids has been used successfully to treat infertility in men with idiopathic oligozoospermia or azoospermia.[552,553] Fertility rates of 50–70 percent using poor quality semen have been obtained using ICSI. In men with obstructive azoospermia, near normal fertility rates are obtained using sperm aspirated from the epididymis for ICSI.[554]

Androgen Resistance Syndromes

Androgen resistance syndromes are caused by defects in androgen action (see Chap. 17).[555–557] The severity of androgen insensitivity determines the clinical presentation of these disorders. Most androgen resistance syndromes result from severely defective androgen action, and present at birth as either phenotypic females, *testicular feminization* syndrome, or with extremely ambiguous genitalia, *male pseudohermaphroditism.*

Genetic males with *complete androgen resistance* or *insensitivity* (tesicular feminization) present as phenotypic females with primary amenorrhea.[555–557] They do not present with a clinical picture of male hypogonadism. As a result of androgen resistance, they lack facial, axillary, and pubic hair and have normal appearing female external genitalia. The distal two-thirds of the vagina is well developed but the proximal vagina, uterus, and fallopian tubes are absent. Serum testosterone, estradiol, and LH are elevated, but FSH levels are usually normal.

Men with less severe, *incomplete androgen resistance syndromes* present as pubertal boys or adults with a clinical picture of mild androgen deficiency with a nearly normal male phenotype.[555–557] The spectrum of clinical presentation varies from men with severe underandrogenization to normally virilized men with infertility or minimally undervirilized men with preserved fertility. These patients undergo puberty at the appropriate age but usually fail to androgenize completely. Gynecomastia, hypospadius, a bifid scrotum, and cryptorchidism are common. These disorders encompass disorders previously named Reifenstein, Lubs, Rosewater, and Dreyfus syndromes. However, there is considerable variability in the manifestations of these syndromes. For example, most patients with Reifenstein syndrome have hypospadius, gynecomastia, undervirilization, a small prostate gland, impaired spermatogenesis, and cryptorchidism, while other men from the same family may be normally virilized and not have hypospadius.[558] Thus, it is not clinically useful to use the eponyms previously used for these syndromes of incomplete androgen resistance. Serum testosterone and LH levels are elevated and FSH levels are normal in these syndromes.

Very mild androgen resistance may present with only *idiopathic oligozoospermia* or *azoospermia* with elevated serum testosterone and LH levels, and lacking other phenotypic abnormalities.[559–564] The frequency of this disorder is controversial but recent evidence suggests that mild androgen resistance is relatively uncommon in men with idiopathic oligozoospermia or azoospermia and normal virilization.

The molecular basis for the androgen resistance syndromes described previously is a complete lack or reduced number of androgen receptors, a defect in androgen receptor function, or postreceptor defects due to mutations in the androgen receptor. In general, androgen receptor mutations may be classified into two major categories: mutations that disrupt the primary sequence of the androgen receptor, and uniformly cause complete androgen resistance; and more commonly, point mutations in the androgen receptor gene that cause single amino acid substitutions in the androgen receptor protein.[555–557] The latter cause the full spectrum of androgen resistance phenotypes, including incomplete forms of androgen insensitivity. Point mutations in the hormone binding domain of the androgen receptor are the most frequently identified mutations in patients with androgen resistance (Fig. 15-28). The degree of androgen resistance observed clinically reflects the amount of disruption of androgen receptor function rather than the specific location of the mutation.

The androgen receptor gene contains a polymorphic trinucleotide (CAG_n) repeat locus in exon 1 that encodes for a polyglutamine tract in the transactivation domain of the receptor protein. Expansion of the polyglutamine tract (≥40) in males causes a fatal neuromuscular disease, *spinal bulbar muscular atrophy*, or Kennedy's disease.[565] Men with this disease exhibit undervirilization, testicular atrophy, oligozoospermia or azoospermia, reduced fertility, a hormonal profile consistent with androgen resistance, and reduced transactivation of the androgen receptor.[565] Recently, a mutation in the CAG triplet region of the androgen receptor was found to cause complete androgen resistance in a family, suggesting that it is an important region for androgen action.[566] Moreover, long polyglutamine tracts (≥28) in the androgen receptor have been reported to be associated with a four fold increase in risk for impaired spermatogenesis.[567] It is also possible that mutations in androgen receptor co-activators or co-repressors may result in varying degrees of androgen resistance.

Another type of partial androgen resistance results from *5α-reductase deficiency*.[568–571] Individuals with this disorder present with a male pseudohermaphroditism syndrome, termed pseudovagi-

FIGURE 15-28. Schematic diagram of the structure of the androgen receptor (above) and localization and effects of androgen receptor mutations (below). (*From McPhaul and Griffen.*[556])

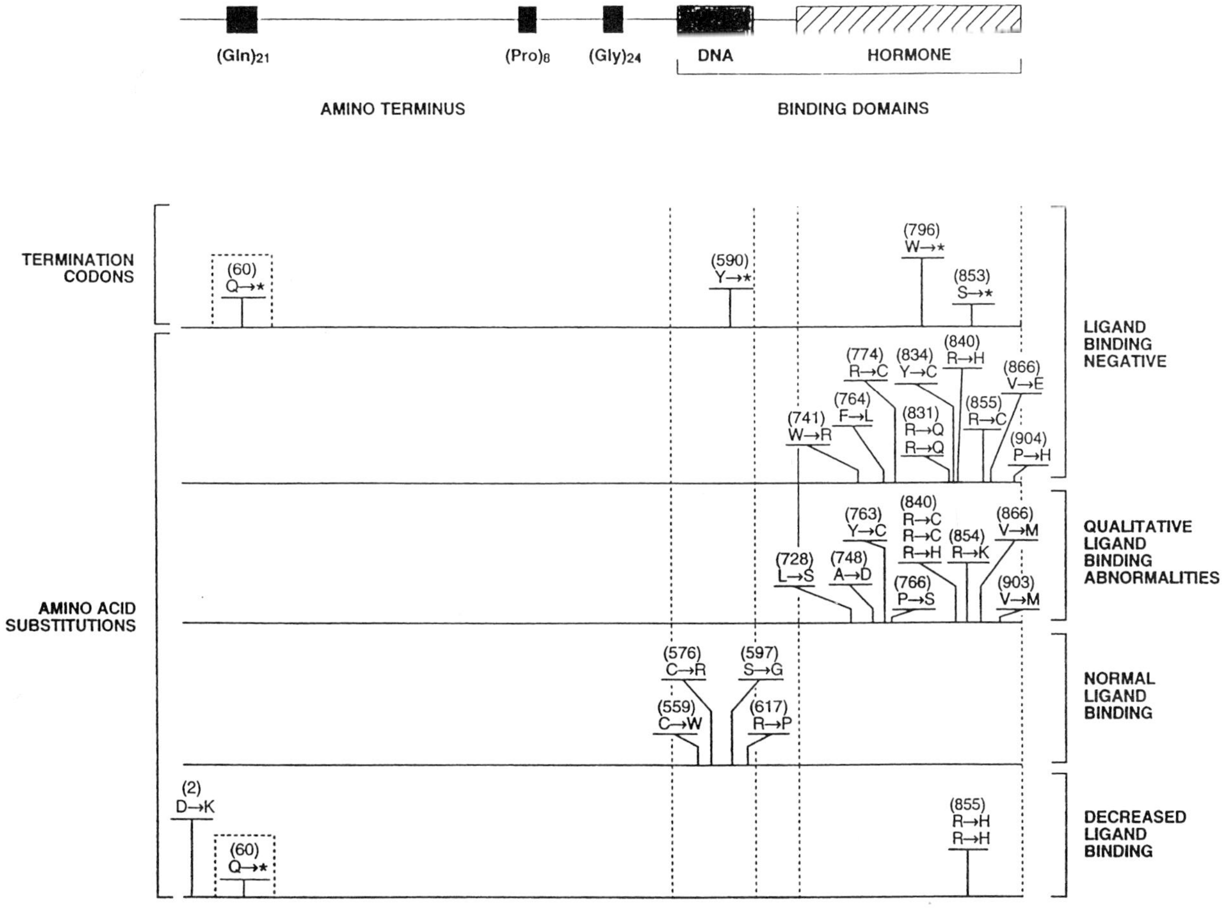

nal perineoscrotal hyospadius, and are raised as females. They have a normal male excretory duct system, including epididymides, vasa deferentiae, seminal vesicles, and ejaculatory ducts, but the latter terminate in a vagina and the external genitalia are ambiguous. With increasing testosterone secretion at puberty, partial virilization occurs with penile growth and increased muscle mass. However, they do not develop a male hair pattern or acne. In some cultures, these individuals take on a male gender role at puberty. Spermatogenesis is impaired, either as a result of inadequate DHT formation in the testis or cryptorchidism that is usually present.[571]

Androgen resistance is induced in men with prostate cancer treated with pure nonsteroidal androgen receptor antagonists, such as flutamide, bicalatamide or nilutamide (see later section). Men with celiac disease, or gluten-sensitive enteropathy, may present with a hormonal pattern consistent with androgen resistance, namely elevated serum testosterone and LH levels that may be reversible with a gluten-free diet.[572, 573]

Secondary Hypogonadism

Secondary hypogonadism is testicular failure due to inadequate gonadotropin secretion as a result of either disordered hypothalamic or pituitary function. In the majority of cases, both LH and FSH secretion are diminished, resulting in impairment of both sperm and androgen production. Rarely, patients may exhibit an isolated impairment of sperm production due to gonadotropin suppression (Table 15-10).

Deficiency of Sperm and Androgen Production

Congenital or Developmental Disorders

Constitutional Delayed Puberty In boys, puberty usually begins at age 9–13 years. With the maturation of the central nervous system mechanism that regulates GnRH production, pulsatile gonadotropin and testosterone secretion begin, initially during sleep and then throughout the day (Figs. 15-7 and 15-9).[60] The first clinical indications of the onset of puberty are an increase in the testicle size (>3 cm in length or >6 mL in volume) and development of rugal folds and pigmentation of scrotum (Fig. 15-14).[60] Subsequently, there is an increase in penile length and appearance of pubic hair, followed by increasing long bone growth and development of other secondary sexual characteristics. The increase in testis size precedes the appearance of pubic hair by about 1–2 years and peak height velocity by 3 years. There is considerable variability in the onset and duration of puberty and degree of development of secondary sexual characteristics, largely attributable to the genetic background of an individual.

Delayed puberty is suspected when there is no evidence of sexual maturation by 14 years of age. Disorders that cause primary or secondary hypogonadism, or androgen resistance, may present as delayed puberty.[574] *Severe systemic illness* (e.g., malabsorption, asthma, diabetes, and malignancy) usually associated with growth retardation and *thyroid hormone deficiency* may also cause delayed sexual maturation. However, the vast majority of boys with delayed puberty have physiological or *constitutional delayed puberty*. This is a benign, frequently familial form of delayed adolescence that represents a normal variation in the onset of puberty. These boys undergo a delayed but normal puberty and attain normal sexual maturation and height.

The diagnosis of constitutional delayed puberty can be strongly suspected in a healthy boy with retarded growth and bone age, normal growth velocity in relationship to bone age, family history of delayed adolescence, testicular volume >2 ml, and a bone age between 12 and 13 years. However, these features may not be present, and the diagnosis can be very difficult. Diagnostic evaluation to exclude organic causes of delayed puberty, i.e., hypogonadism, systemic illness, and hypothyroidism, should be performed. In the absence of anosmia or other morphological manifestations, constitutional delayed puberty can not be distinguished from idiopathic hypogonadotropic hypogonadism, or Kallmann syndrome (see later discussion).

Delayed sexual maturation often results in severe psychosocial distress in both the boy and his parents. Therefore, after exclusion of organic causes, patients with delayed puberty are usually treated with androgen therapy to induce sexual maturation. It is generally recommended that patients not be treated with androgens until after 14 years of age. However, the emotional trauma of delayed puberty often dictates early treatment, e.g., beginning at 13–14 years of age, so that sexual maturation coincides with that of his contemporaries. Androgen treatment is stopped intermittently to determine if spontaneous onset of puberty occurs (see later discussion).

Idiopathic Hypogonadotropic Hypogonadism and Variants Idiopathic hypogonadotropic hypogonadism (IHH) is a group of disorders characterized by isolated hypogonadotropic hypogonadism, in most cases of unclear etiology.[575,576] Hypogonadotropic eunuchoidism or Kallmann syndrome represents the classical form of these disorders. Kallmann syndrome is a congenital and often familial disorder (in ~35 percent) characterized by isolated hypogonadotropic hypogonadism resulting in eunuchoidal features, and anosmia or hyposmia. Gonadotropin deficiency in this disorder is caused by defect in hypothalamic GnRH synthesis, as evidenced by absent or abnormal patterns of endogenous pulsatile LH secretion (Fig. 15-29) and the ability of exogenous pulsatile GnRH administration to restore normal testis function.[69] A developmental failure of the olfactory bulbs and tract is responsible for absent or reduced sense of smell (Fig. 15-30).[577]

Classically, patients with Kallmann syndrome present with delayed pubertal maturation, eunuchoidal features, and prepubertal size testes.[575,576,578–581] An early prepubertal manifestation of this syndrome is micropenis. In addition to anosmia or hyposmia, these patients may also exhibit other developmental defects including: cleft lip, cleft palate, color blindness, renal agenesis, congenital nerve deafness, cryptorchidism, skeletal abnormalities (e.g., syndactyly, short fourth metacarpals, craniofacial asymmetry, pes cavus deformity of the feet), mirror movements (synkinesia) and eye movement abnormalities; and café-au-lait spots.[579–581] However, there is considerable variability in the clinical manifestations of IHH. Many men demonstrate isolated gonadotropin deficiency without anosmia, hyposmia, or other developmental abnormalities.[576] Family members of patients with IHH may exhibit anosmia, hyposmia, or delayed puberty in absence of other manifestations, suggesting variable expression of the disorder.[582] Recently, an adult-onset form of IHH has been described.[583]

There is also substantial genetic heterogeneity in Kallmann syndrome and other forms of IHH.[13,576,579,582,584,585] These disorders may be inherited as an autosomal dominant with male-predominant expression, autosomal recessive, or X-linked recessive conditions, or may be sporadic in nature. Individuals with an X-linked form (the least common inherited form) of Kallmann syndrome demonstrate a failure of normal migration of GnRH

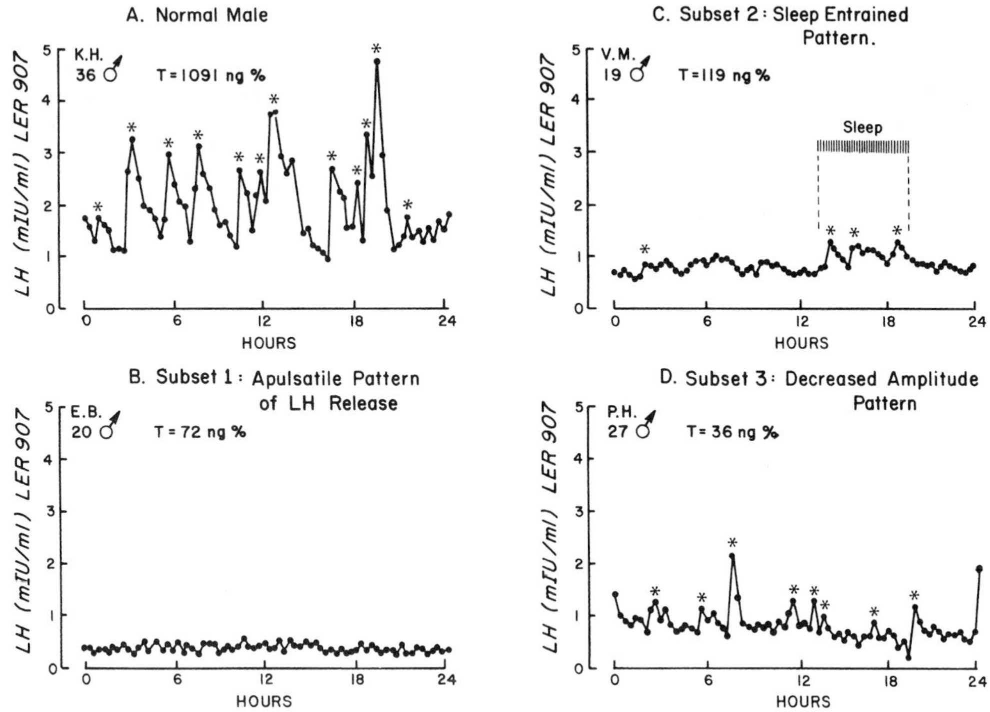

FIGURE 15-29. Patterns of endogenous LH secretion in idiopathic hypogonadotropic hypogonadal men. (*A*): LH values determined every 20 min for 24 h in a normal male displaying discrete LH pulsations occuring about every 2 h and resulting in a normal plasma testosterone concentration. (*B*) LH determinations in a male with idiopathic hypogonadotropic hypogondism displaying no detectable LH pulsations and a prepubertal testosterone level. (*C*) Sleep LH entrained pulsations have decreased amplitude associated with prepubertal testosterone levels in an 18-years-old idiopathic hypogonadotropic hypogonadal male. (*D*) LH pulsations of decreased amplitude occuring throughout sleep and wake periods in a 27-year-old idiopathic hypogonadotropic hypogonadal male. (*From Santen and Swerdloff* (eds).[817])

neurons from the olfactory placode to the hypothalamus during fetal development. This developmental failure is due to a deletion of the *KAL-1* gene on the X chromosome, and deficiency of its product, anosmin-1, an extracellular matrix adhesion protein that is thought to be important in GnRH neuronal migration.[13,14,586–588]

FIGURE 15-30. Five-mm T1-weighted axial image by MRI demonstrating hypoplastic olfactory gyri. (*From Brackett, Demers, Mamourian, et al.*[633])

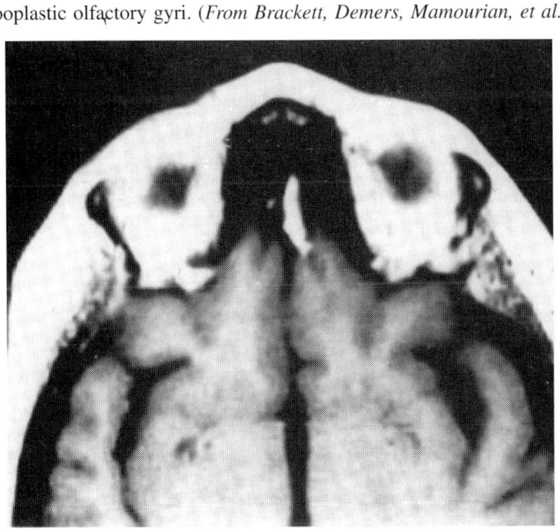

Thus, isolated gonadotropin deficiency due to functional GnRH deficiency occurs as a result of this X-chromosome deletion. However, because deletions often affect other genes on the X chromosome, gonadotropin deficiency is more commonly associated with other manifestations (e.g., congenital icthyosis) in complex genetic syndromes (see later section). Thus, KAL-1 deletions and mutations are found infrequently in classical Kallmann syndrome.

IHH associated with X-linked congenital adrenal hypoplasia is due to a mutation in the *DAX-1* (dosage-sensitive sex-reversal AHC critical region on the human X chromosome 1) gene.[589] Individuals with this disorder usually present with primary adrenal failure as infants. If diagnosed and treated appropriately, they survive and present as adults with hypogonadotropic hypogonadism. Clinically, unlike typical patients with IHH, these patients usually (but not always) fail to stimulate gonadotropin secretion in response to chronic pulsatile GnRH treatment and may manifest a combination of defects at multiple levels of the hypothalamic-pituitary-testicular axis.[589] Finally, mutations in the GnRH and GnRH receptor gene are rare causes of Kallman syndrome and IHH.[590]

Men with Kallmann syndrome are often aspermic, i.e., have no ejaculate. Serum testosterone, LH, and FSH levels are low to low-normal, while other anterior pituitary function is normal. A single dose GnRH test may not result in stimulation of gonadotropin secretion, but repeated or chronic pulsatile GnRH ad ministration will increase LH and FSH levels. Men with Kallman syndrome do not respond to administration of clomiphene citrate, an antiestrogen that normally stimulates hypothalamic GnRH, and as a result gonadotropin secretion.[591] Determination of olfactory threshold may be made using scratch and sniff cards[592] or bottles containing familiar odors (e.g., coffee grounds).

In the absence of anosmia or hyposmia, the differentiation between Kallmann syndrome and constitutional delayed puberty is very difficult, and cannot be made reliably in the prepubertal boys. A number of tests have been utilized unsuccessfully to differentiate these diagnoses, including GnRH, clomiphene citrate, GnRH agonist stimulation of gonadotropins; and thyrotropin releasing hormone (TRH), metoclopramide, chlorpromazine stimulation of prolactin.[593–600] Currently, there is no diagnostic test that can completely and reliably distinguish Kallman syndrome from constitutional delayed puberty. Usually, androgen therapy is initiated to induce sexual maturation in both of these conditions, and is intermittently discontinued to determine whether spontaneous onset of puberty occurs. Patients with Kallmann syndrome will continue to require androgen therapy to achieve and maintain sexual maturation, while patients with constitutional delayed puberty will not require treatment after spontaneous endogenous gonadotropin and testosterone secretion commence. It may be necessary to continue intermittent androgen therapy until patients are older than 18–20 years of age, as some individuals undergo spontaneous puberty even after age 20.[601]

When fertility is desired, androgen replacement treatment is discontinued and spermatogenesis may be induced with gonadotropin or pulsatile GnRH therapy (see later discussion). Previous androgen therapy does not alter the subsequent testicular response to gonadotropin therapy. Gonadotropin therapy is much less successful in men with Kallmann syndrome and a documented history of cryptorchidism, particularly if it is bilateral.[140] Uncommonly, some (~5 percent) individuals with IHH maintain gonadotropin and testicular function even after pulsatile GnRH is discontinued, perhaps as a result of a priming effect of testosterone on the hypothalamus and/or pituitary gland.[602]

The degree of gonadotropin deficiency in Kallmann syndrome may vary considerably, and some individuals demonstrate partial gonadotropin secretion with LH and FSH levels in the low-normal range and alterations in the amplitude or frequency of pulsatile LH secretion (Fig. 15-28).[68] With partial GnRH deficiency, FSH secretion may predominate and germ cell maturation may proceed to some extent. This variant form of Kallmann syndrome, *isolated LH deficiency*, which is also called the *"fertile" eunuch syndrome*, is characterized by a selective deficiency in LH secretion that results in prepubertal androgen deficiency and eunuchoidism.[603,604] FSH secretion is relatively preserved, resulting in near normal size testes in which advanced spermatogenesis may be present. However, spermatogenesis is not completely normal and these patients are not fertile, as the name of the syndrome would imply. In these men, treatment with hCG alone stimulates Leydig cell production of testosterone, ameliorates androgen deficiency, and increases spermatogenesis. Men with isolated FSH deficiency have also been reported, but the extent and nature of the defect in gonadotropin secretion has not been well-documented.[605–607]

Hemochromatosis Hemochromatosis is a very common autosomal recessive disorder in which there is parenchymal iron deposition in a variety of tissues, most prominently in the liver, skin, pancreas, and heart.[608,609] It is estimated to affect approximately 1 in every 200–300 Caucasian Americans, making it one of the most common genetic diseases. The molecular bases for hereditary hemochromatosis are point mutations in the HLA-linked iron-loading gene (*HFE*). Marked iron deposition in the pituitary gonadotrophs selectively inhibits gonadotropin production without significantly affecting the secretion of other anterior pituitary hormones.[610–612] Iron overload of the pituitary can be demonstrated by MRI.[613] The resulting hypogonadotropic hypogonadism and androgen deficiency is responsible for the common complaint of erectile dysfunction that usually precedes the diagnosis of hemochromatosis. Frequent phlebotomies or treatment with desferioxamine to decrease iron overload may restore gonadotropin secretion in some patients.[614,615] Even in the presence of significant iron overload, gonadotropin administration is able to stimulate testicular function, including inducing spermatogenesis and fertility, but gonadotropin response to GnRH is absent or markedly attenuated.[611,612,616] Parenchymal iron deposition resulting in hypogonadotropic hypogonadism may also occur in patients with conditions that require frequent blood transfusions, such as β-thalassemia (*transfusion-induced iron overload*).[617–619]

Complex Genetic Syndromes Secondary hypogonadism may be present in a number of *complex genetic syndromes*, such as *Prader-Willi-Labhart syndrome, Laurence-Moon-Biedl syndrome, RUD syndrome, Mobius syndrome, multiple lentigines (Leopard syndrome), steroid sulfatase deficiency, Lowe syndrome, CHARGE syndrome, Martsolf syndrome, Rothmund-Thompson syndrome*, and *Borjeson-Forrsman-Lehman syndrome*.[620–633] The diagnosis of these disorders is made by recognizing the characteristic congenital anomalies associated with the hyogonadotropic hypogonadism (Table 15-12). In some of these syndromes, e.g., Prader-Labhart-Willi and Laurence-Moon-Beidl syndrome, hypergonadotropic hypogonadism has also been reported.[380–382] The list of complex genetic disorders associated with a variety of congenital anomalies is encyclopedic. The clinical approach recommended is to consult a compendium of genetic disorders such as that written by Rimoin and Schimke[383] when unusual congenital malformations are noted in a patient with hypogonadism.

Aging Men As discussed earlier, elderly men commonly exhibit low serum testosterone and sperm concentrations with low-normal gonadotropin levels, a hormonal pattern consistent with secondary hypogonadism.

Acquired Disorders

Hypopituitarism Any destructive or infiltrative lesion of the hypothalamus or pituitary may cause an acquired impairment of gonadotropin secretion, either selectively or in conjunction with deficiencies in other anterior pituitary hormones.[634,635] Specific pathological conditions include *pituitary or hypothalamic tumor* (e.g., functioning or nonfunctioning pituitary adenoma, craniopharyngioma, meningioma, optic glioma or astrocytoma, metastatic carcinoma, pinealoma, or germinoma); *granulomatous or infiltrative disease* (e.g., sarcoidosis, tuberculosis, histiocytosis X, fungal infection, syphilis, lymphoma, or leukemia); *vascular disorder* (e.g., pituitary apoplexy, infarction, vasculitis, or vascular malformation); *surgical or traumatic hypophysectomy*; pituitary *irradiation*; *lymphocytic hypophysitis*; *transfusion-induced iron overload*; and *pituitary stalk section*. These are discussed in detail in Chap. 7.

Table 15-12. Clinical Features of Complex Genetic Syndromes that Cause Hypogonadotropic Hypogonadism

Syndrome	Clinical Features
Prader-Willi-Labhart	Hypomentia, hypotonia, hypogonadism,* obesity, short stature, small hands and feet, Cupid's bow mouth, diabetes mellitus
Laurence-Moon-Biedl	Retinitis pigmentosa, polydactyly, mental retardation, hypogonadism,* obesity, ataxia, nystagmus, spastic paraplegia, short stature
RUD	Mental *R*etardation, *U*nderdeveloped gonads (hypogonadism), *D*ermatoses (congenital ichthyosis), hyposmia, epilepsy
Möbius	Multiple cranial nerve abnormalities, anosmia, mental retardation, hypogonadism
Multiple lentigines (Leopard syndrome)	Multiple lentigines, sensorineural hearing loss, pulmonic stenosis, hypertelorism, short stature, hypogonadism, genital and urologic defects
Steroid sulfatase deficiency	Steroid sulfatase and arylsulfatase C deficiency, congenital ichthyosis, nystagmus, strabismus, decreased visual acuity, hypopigmentation of iris, unilateral renal hypoplasia or agenesis, hypogonadism
Lowe	Fanconi syndrome, cataracts, glaucoma, buphtalmos, hypotonia, mental retardation, hypogonadism
CHARGE	*C*oloboma, *H*eart disease, *A*tresia of choanae, *R*etarded growth and development, *G*enital hyperplasia, *E*ar abnormalities, hypogonadism
Martsolf	Short stature, severe mental retardation, hypogonadism, mainly Jewish ancestry
Rothmund-Thompson	Hypodontia, soft tissue contractures, anemia, osteogenic sarcoma, hypogonadism
Borjeson-Forssman-Lehman	Prominent supraorbital ridges, ptosis, large ears, hypotonia, severe mental retardation, hypogonadism

* Both hypogonadotropic or hypergonadotropic hypogonadism have been described.

Usually, gradually destructive or infiltrative processes involving the pituitary gland result in progressive loss of anterior pituitary function.[634,635] Gonadotropin and growth hormone secretion are the first to be affected, followed by TSH production, and finally ACTH secretion. It is particularly important to recognize combined gonadotropin and growth hormone deficiency in prepubertal children with growth retardation. In adults, clinical secondary hypogonadism may be the initial manifestation of a hypothalamic or pituitary process. Because loss of TSH and ACTH secretion are associated with greater degrees of pituitary destruction, secondary hypothyroidism and hypoadrenalism do not usually occur without associated secondary hypogonadism. Acute destructive processes of the pituitary gland (e.g., apoplexy) or stalk (e.g., traumatic sectioning) usually cause panhypopituitarism.

Patients with prepubertal gonadotropin deficiency present with delayed puberty and have eunuchoidal features and small testes, usually ≤2 cm. Children with associated growth hormone deficiency will also exhibit short stature. Adults with gonadotropin deficiency usually present with diminished libido and erectile dysfunction. Testis size may be normal initially, but with long-standing gonadotropin deficiency, they become small. In addition, men with hypopituitarism may have findings of deficiency or excess of other anterior pituitary hormones and/or tumor mass effects (e.g., headaches, visual field defects). Clinically, it is most important to have a high index of suspicion for the presence of secondary adrenal insufficiency in patients with hypothalamic or pituitary disorders, as it is a life-threatening, treatable condition that often presents with nonspecific symptoms and signs.

Serum testosterone concentration and sperm counts are low, and LH and FSH levels are low or in the low-normal adult range.[634,635] The gonadotropin response to single-dose GnRH administration does not reliably differentiate hypothalamic and pituitary causes of gonadotropin deficiency. In many instances, an acute GnRH stimulation test will fail to stimulate gonadotropin secretion in patients with hypothalamic disease, as well as stimulate gonadotropin levels in men with pituitary disease. Therefore, this test is rarely, if ever, useful clinically. Clinical evaluation of men with secondary hypogonadism should include anatomic studies, such as a MRI or CT scan and visual field examination, to determine the presence, extent, and effects of a hypothalamic or pituitary tumor, and investigation of other anterior pituitary hormone secretion.

Treatment is aimed at the underlying cause of hypopituitarism and correction of androgen deficiency with testosterone replacement therapy. When fertility is desired, androgens are discontinued and gonadotropin therapy is instituted (see later discussion).

Hyperprolactinemia Causes of high serum prolactin levels include hypothalamic lesions; hypothyroidism; pituitary stalk section; central nervous system drugs (e.g., dopamine antagonists, antipsychotic drugs, antidepressants, sedative-hypnotic drugs, amphetamines, and centrally-active antihypertensive drugs); pituitary adenoma; estrogen; renal failure; and local chest wall trauma or irritation (e.g., herpes zoster).[225] Hyperprolactinemia resulting from any of these etiologies may cause secondary hypogonadism primarily by suppressing hypothalamic GnRH secretion and causing gonadotropin deficiency.[636,637] In men, prolactin-secreting adenomas are usually large (macroadenomas) and gonadotropin deficiency may also be caused by destruction of pituitary gonadotrophs as well as pituitary cells producing other hormones.[638] Drugs that elevate serum prolactin are common causes of secondary hypogonadism.[639]

Treatment is directed at the underlying cause of hyperprolactinemia and stopping potential offending drugs. In men with prolactin-secreting macroadenomas, treatment is initiated with dopamine agonists, such as bromocriptine, pergolide, or carbergoline, alone. This is often associated with a restoration of normal gonadal function and fertility.[640] Surgery is occasionally also needed (e.g., for pituitary apoplexy or a rapidly progressive tumor mass effect, such as visual loss).[641] If hyperprolactinemia can be treated adequately, these men do respond to GnRH and gonadotropin therapy.[637,642,643] In some men with hyperprolactinemia, correction of androgen deficiency with testosterone replacement therapy does not correct erectile dysfunction. The addition of a dopamine agonist to decrease pituitary prolactin secretion may be useful in these situations.[638,644]

Sex Steroid Hormones and Opiates In men, *estrogen excess* exerts negative feedback inhibition on gonadotropin secretion and causes secondary hypogonadism[645–647] Estrogen excess may result from either exogenous administration or exposure to estrogens or estrogenic substances or endogenous secretion from an estrogen-producing neoplasm (e.g., feminizing adrenal carcinoma).[648,649] Digoxin may increase serum estradiol and suppress LH and testosterone concentrations.[424] Because the estrogen to testosterone ratio is increased, men with estrogen excess manifest gynecomastia of varying degrees (see earlier section). *Progestagens* (e.g. medroxyprogesterone acetate)[650,651] and *opiates* (e.g., morphine, methadone, and heroin)[652–654] also inhibit gonadotropin production and can cause secondary hypogonadism.[652–654]

GnRH Agonists Potent GnRH agonist analogs suppress endogenous LH and testosterone secretion and are used alone or in combination with androgen receptor antagonists to treat men with prostate cancer (see later section).

Systemic Illness *Glucocorticoid excess,* or Cushing syndrome, either as a result of endogenous causes (pituitary Cushing's disease, ectopic ACTH, or adrenal adenoma or carcinoma), or exogenous glucocorticoid administration, suppresses gonadotropin secretion, resulting in secondary hypogonadism with loss of libido, erectile dysfunction, androgen deficiency, and oligozoospermia.[655,656] Glucocorticoids may also have direct suppressive effects on the testis. During *acute stress* or *illnesses*, such as emotional stress, vigorous physical exercise, trauma, myocardial infarction, surgery, trauma, severe burns, sepsis, etc., high circulating glucocorticoid levels and CNS activation of hypothalamic CRH inhibit GnRH secretion. This may contribute to the reductions in serum testosterone, LH, and FSH levels and secondary hypogonadism observed in these clinical situations.[445,446,657–666] *Nutritional deficiency*, such as that associated with starvation, protein-calorie malnutrition, or anorexia nervosa, inhibits gonadotropin production and may cause secondary hypogonadism.[667,668] There may also be concurrent primary testicular dysfunction associated with inadequate nutrition. Malnutrition, weight loss, and wasting may contribute to the secondary testicular dysfunction associated with a number of *chronic illnesses*, such as AIDS; malignancy; chronic liver, renal, and lung disease; untreated or poorly controlled type 1 diabetes mellitus; cystic fibrosis; and chronic spinal cord injury.[445,446,457,462,463,467–469,529,669–680] Moderate obesity results in reduction in SHBG and total testosterone levels, with normal non-SHBG-bound and free testosterone levels.[681] However, some men with *massive obesity* exhibit clinical androgen deficiency with low non-SHBG-bound and free testosterone concentrations and reduced gonadotropin levels.[681,682] Increased aromatization of testosterone to estradiol may contribute to gonadotropin suppression. However, it is clearly not the only mechanism, as weight loss insufficient to lower estradiol levels is associated with normalization of testosterone levels.[682]

Isolated Impairment of Sperm Production

Androgen Excess

Congenital adrenal hyperplasia caused by either 21-hydroxylase or 11β-hydroxylase deficiency results in excessive production of adrenal androgens that can be converted to testosterone. Androgen excess suppresses gonadotropin secretion through negative feedback effects, resulting in secondary hypogonadism.[683] Androgen and sperm production by the testis is suppressed. However, excessive adrenal androgen production causes premature virilization and precocious pseudopuberty, rather than androgen deficiency. Thus, the secondary hypogonadism induced by adrenal androgen excess is manifested by isolated impairment of sperm production. Of note is that glucocorticoid therapy of some patients with congenital adrenal hyperplasia may result in true precocious puberty, with a premature activation of the hypothalamic-pituitary gonadotropin axis, and induction of normal spermatogenesis and gonadotropin levels (see later discussion).

Androgen excess caused by administration of *testosterone* or *androgenic anabolic steroids*[684] or *androgen-secreting tumors* (e.g., Leydig cell tumors of the testis)[649] also results in secondary hypogonadism presenting with isolated impairment of sperm production with normal androgenization. Administration of high dosages of testosterone in normal men has been used as strategy to suppress sperm production in male contraceptive development trials.[685–687]

Hyperprolactinemia Rarely, *hyperprolactinemia* causes an isolated impairment of sperm production with normal gonadotropin and testosterone levels.[642] Treatment with a dopamine agonist (e.g., bromocriptine) restores sperm production in these men.

Isolated FSH Deficiency Isolated FSH deficiency is an extremely rare condition. The few men that have been reported with this disorder were normally virilized and had normal serum testosterone and LH levels, and low serum FSH levels.[605–607] Spermatogenesis and fertility have not been characterized well in this disorder, although testis biopsy revealed germ cell maturation arrest at the spermatid stage in one man.

Treatment of Hypogonadism

Androgen Therapy

Male Hypogonadism

Therapeutic Goals The main indication for androgen therapy is the treatment of hypogonadism in men, due either to primary testicular or secondary hypothalamic-pituitary disease.[688–690] The goal of androgen replacement therapy in hypogonadal men is to correct or improve the clinical consequences of testosterone deficiency, and depends on whether gonadal failure occurs in prepubertal boys or adults.

In prepubertal androgen deficient boys, the aims of androgen replacement are to induce and maintain male secondary sexual characteristics, muscle and bone mass, long bone growth, erythropoiesis, libido, and erectile function without compromising adult height by inducing premature closure of long bone epiphyses.[688–690] In adults with testosterone deficiency, the objective of androgen therapy is to restore and maintain libido, erectile function, muscle and bone mass, erythropoiesis, and secondary sexual characteristics.[688–690] Androgen treatment is very successful in accomplishing these goals. However, testosterone cannot be administered in sufficiently high dosages to achieve the high intratesticular concentrations required to stimulate and support spermatogenesis. As discussed later, infertility is usually only possible in men with secondary hypogonadism using gonadotropin or GnRH therapy.

Testosterone Preparations and Regimens Currently, the long-acting parenteral, 17β-hydroxyl esters of testosterone, *testosterone enanthate* and *cypionate*, are the most effective, practical, inexpensive, and safe preparations for androgen replacement therapy in hypogonadal men.[688–690] These preparations are clinically equivalent with regard to their duration of action and therapeutic efficacy.[691,692] Although administration of these testosterone esters requires intramuscular (IM) injections, most patients are either able to perform self-administration, or have a family member or friend administer the injections, thereby avoiding frequent clinic visits.

In adult hypogonadal men, the usual replacement dosage of testosterone enanthate or cypionate is 150–200 mg IM every two weeks (Table 15-13). After injection of this dose to hypogonadal men, serum testosterone levels increase into the upper-normal range or above for 1–2 days and then gradually fall to the lower-normal range or sometimes below during the subsequent two weeks, prior to the next injection (Fig. 15-31).[691] The wide variation in testosterone levels between injections may be associated with often disturbing fluctuations in sexual desire and function, mood, and energy level. In men who experience symptoms of diminished androgen effects prior to their next injection, the dosing interval may be shortened to every 10 days. Some patients prefer treatment with injections of 100 mg IM weekly in order to reduce fluctuations in testosterone levels and symptoms. Administration of larger doses of testosterone esters, e.g., 300–400 mg every 3–4 weeks, is not be recommended. These high doses produce much larger fluctuations of serum testosterone with prolonged supraphysiological levels for several days following an injection, and levels below the normal range after three weeks (Fig. 15-31).

In some clinical situations, full androgen replacement may not be required, e.g., elderly hypogonadal men with severe BPH in whom anabolic effects of androgens on muscle and bone are the primary therapeutic goals and there is concern regarding worsening of bladder outlet obstruction. In these instances, low-dose androgen supplementation may be accomplished using testosterone enanthate or cypionate, 50–100 mg IM every 2 weeks, or less.[689,690] Alternatively, the shorter-acting, 17 β-hydroxyl testosterone ester, *testosterone propionate*, 25–50 mg IM three times weekly may be used. However, the frequent injections needed to maintain normal serum testosterone levels using this preparation make it a less desirable option to most patients. In men with severe, long-standing testosterone deficiency, the dramatic changes in sexuality, behavior and physical appearance induced by androgen replacement therapy may be distressing. Counseling of patients and their partners prior to and during androgen replacement is important in order to prevent serious adjustment problems. In these men, it is reasonable to use a lower starting dosage of testosterone ester, e.g., 100 mg IM every two weeks, for several months and gradually increasing the dosage to full androgen replacement.

The adequacy of androgen replacement is usually monitored by the patient's clinical response.[689,690] Most hypogonadal men experience an increase in sexual desire, function, and activity, energy and motivation, and improvement in feeling of well being and mood within the first few months of androgen treatment. Increases muscle mass and strength, bone mass, and body hair occur during the subsequent months to years of therapy. If the clinical response to androgen replacement is not adequate, serum testosterone measurements should be considered following an injection, either at the expected peak (1–2 days) or midpoint (5–7 days) to document inadequate absorption (e.g., in a very obese man), or at the nadir (prior to the next injection) to check the adequacy of the dosing interval.[693] Some practitioners routinely monitor testosterone levels during testosterone treatment as an indicator of the adequacy of replacement and to avoid overreplacement.

In boys with delayed puberty, androgen therapy is usually withheld until they are at least 14 years of age.[689,690] However, if the delay in sexual maturation and growth causes severe psychological distress, treatment may be started at an earlier age. In order

TABLE 15-13. Treatment of Male Hypogonadism

Condition	Treatment Goal	Drug Used	Dosage
Prepubertal hypogonadism (delayed puberty)	Stimulation of growth and puberty	Testosterone enanthate or cypionate	50–100 mg IM monthly, increasing to 50–100 mg IM every 2 weeks and then to adult replacement
		hCG	1,000–2,000 IU SC weekly, increasing to adult dosage
Adult hypogonadism Primary and secondary hypogonadism	Virilization and normal sexual function	Testosterone enanthate or cypionate	150–200 mg IM every 10–14 days (androgen replacement) 50–100 mg IM every 14 days (low-dosage androgen supplementation
		Transdermal testosterone	
		AndroGel®	50–100 mg (2–4 packets) applied once daily
		Testoderm TTS®	1 patch (5 mg) applied daily (evening)
		Androderm®	1 patch (5 mg) applied daily (evening)
		Testoderm®	1 patch (4 or 6 mg) applied to scrotum daily (morning)
Secondary hypogonadism	Initiation and maintenance of spermatogenesis and fertility	hCG	1,000–2,000 IU SC 2–3 times weekly to maintain normal testosterone for 6–12 months
		Then continued hCG administration at the same dosage plus:	
		hMG, hFSH, or rhFSH	75–300 IU SC 3 times weekly for 6–18 months
		GnRH	2–40 μg SC every 2 hours by programmable infusion pump for 6–30 months

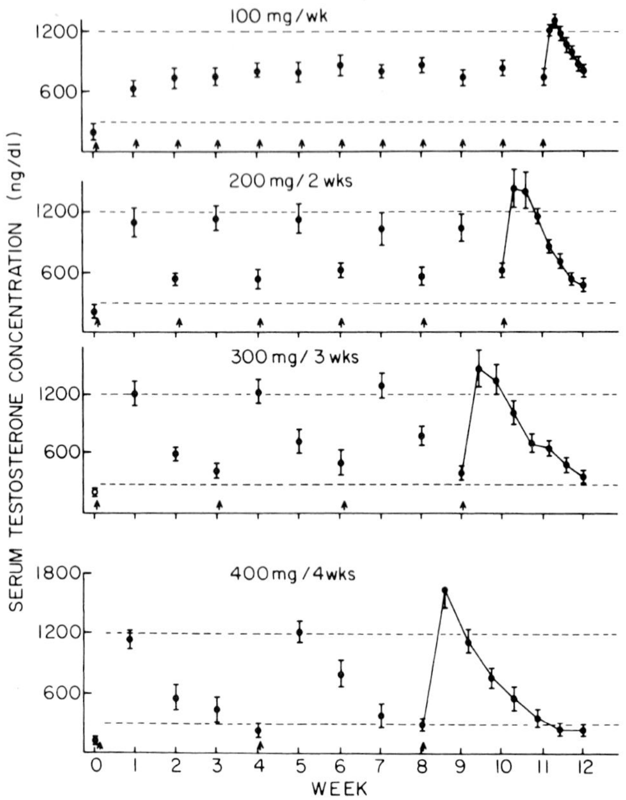

FIGURE 15-31. Serum testosterone level during testosterone replacement therapy in adult primary hypogonadal men. Testosterone enanthate was administered by intramuscular injections for 12 weeks in four dosage regimens: 100 mg weekly; 200 mg every 2 weeks; 300 mg every 3 weeks; and 400 mg every 4 weeks. (*From Snyder and Lawrence.*[691])

to prevent premature closure of long bone epiphyses and compromise of adult height potential, androgen therapy in boys is usually initiated using a very low dose of a testosterone ester, usually 50–100 mg IM monthly. This dosage is sufficient to stimulate long bone growth and induce some virilization, but does not usually interfere with spontaneous pubertal onset. During the next several years, the dosage is increased to 50–100 mg IM every two weeks and then to full adult replacement doses. Because permanent hypogonadism causing gonadotropin deficiency may not be distinguishable from constitutional delayed puberty, androgen therapy in prepubertal boys is intermittent. Treatment is continued for periods of about 3–6 months and then stopped for 3–6 months to determine if spontaneous pubertal onset and progression will occur, as evidence clinically by an increase in testis size to >8 mL in volume.

Four *transdermal testosterone* delivery systems are available as safe and effective alternatives to injectable testosterone esters for androgen replacement therapy of hypogonadal men.[694] They are particularly useful in men who prefer to not administer or are unable to tolerate IM injections. Transdermal testosterone systems provide more physiological serum testosterone levels than testosterone ester injections. All of these systems require daily application and are more expensive than therapy using injections of testosterone ester. None are approved for use in boys with delayed puberty.

The *scrotal testosterone patch* (Testoderm®, ALZA, Palo Alto, CA) contains testosterone within the matrix of the patch and does not utilize permeation enhancers. Long-term daily morning application of the scrotal testosterone patch in hypogonadal men maintains physiological serum testosterone levels, mimicking the normal circadian variation of testosterone, and improves clinical manifestations of androgen deficiency.[695,696] This patch is generally well tolerated with minor skin irritation, but use of this patch requires an adequate size, clean, shaven, and dry scrotal surface area for optimal adhesion. Furthermore, serum DHT levels increase above the normal range, presumably as a result of high 5 α-reductase activity in genital skin.[695,696] The clinical significance of chronic exposure to high circulating DHT levels is unclear.

The *permeation-enhanced nonscrotal testosterone patch* (Androderm®, Watson, Corona, CA) is composed of a central reservoir containing testosterone and permeation-enhancers within an adhesive patch. Long-term nightly application of this nonscrotal testosterone patch in hypogonadal men also maintains serum testosterone within the physiological range with a normal diurnal variation, and improves the clinical manifestations of androgen deficiency.[697–699] A single (44 cm^2) patch that delivers 5.0 mg of testosterone daily is available for use in androgen replacement therapy of hypogonadal men. This patch is generally tolerated well, but local skin irritation can be a significant problem in ~20 to 30 percent of patients.[700] Pretreatment with triamcinolone acetonide 0.1 percent cream under the drug reservoir reduces the severity and incidence of skin irritation.[701] In contrast to the scrotal patch, serum DHT levels remain in the normal range with this transdermal system.

A *non-permeation-enhanced, nonscrotal testosterone patch* (Testoderm TTS®, ALZA, Palo Alto, CA) that is composed of a relatively large reservoir containing an alcohol-based testosterone gel within a lightly adhesive patch and, notably, does not contain permeation enhancers is available for androgen therapy. Initial studies demonstrate that this patch delivers similar amounts of testosterone and causes much less skin irritation than the permeation-enhanced nonscrotal patch.[702–704]. However, reliable adhesion to the skin may be problematic.

Recently, a transdermal *testosterone gel* formulation (AndroGel®, UNIMED/Solvay, Deerfield, IL) became available for androgen replacement in hypogonadal men.[705–707] In hypogonadal men, daily application of 100 mg of testosterone in a 1 percent hydroalcoholic gel (at either one or four skin sites) for 7 days produces steady-state serum testosterone and DHT levels at the upper limit of the normal range (Fig. 15-32).[705] Long-term, daily application of 50, 75, or 100 mg of testosterone gel in androgen deficient men produces relatively constant serum testosterone levels in mid- to upper-normal range throughout the entire day and improves manifestations of androgen deficiency.[706,707] By comparison, nightly application of the permeation-enhanced nonscrotal testosterone patch produced testosterone levels that demonstrated a normal circadian variation in the lower normal range. Compared to the nonscrotal patch, testosterone gel caused relatively little skin irritation and was associated with better compliance. However, it did cause a disproportionate increase in serum DHT levels, probably because of the large surface area of skin containing 5α-reductase on which it is applied.

Currently, all oral androgen preparations available in the United States are 17α-alkylated derivatives of testosterone. The bioavailability of oral androgens is relatively low and they are weak androgens. Therefore, even with three times daily administration, it is difficult to achieve full androgen replacement with 17α-alkylated androgens.[688–690,693] In addition to being less effec-

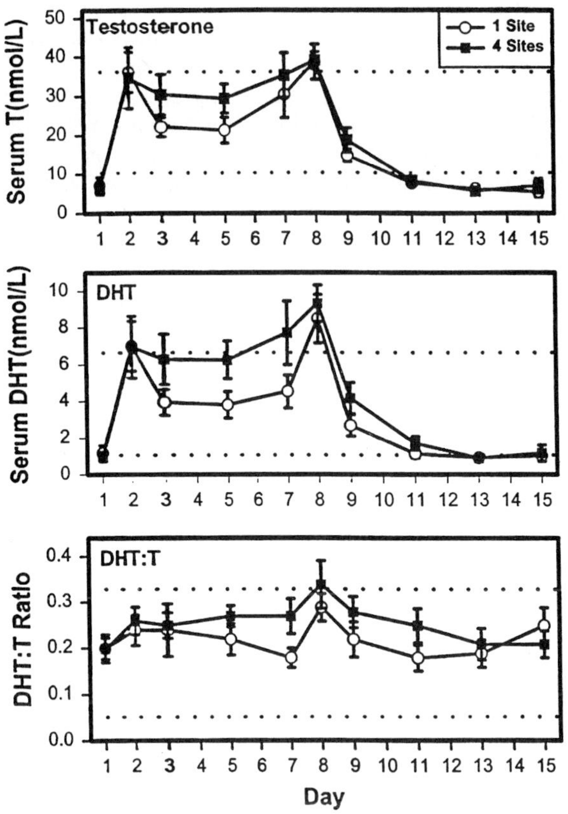

FIGURE 15-32. Serum testosterone (top) and DHT (middle) levels, and the ratio of DHT/testosterone before, during (day 1 to 7) and after (day 8 to 15) daily application of testosterone gel 100 mg daily at one (○) or four (■) skin sites for 7 days in hypogonadal men. (*From Wang, Berman, Longstreth, et al.*[705])

tive, they are also more expensive than other testosterone preparations. Most importantly, 17α-alkylated androgens have the potential to cause serious hepatotoxicity (cholestasis, jaundice, peliosis hepatis, and benign and malignant hepatic tumors).[708] They also significantly lower HDL and higher LDL cholesterol.[709] Because they have less therapeutic benefits and carry greater risks compared to either testosterone esters or transdermal testosterone formulations, oral 17α-alkylated androgens should not be used for androgen replacement therapy of hypogonadal men.

Risks and Side Effects Androgen treatment is contraindicated in men with prostate or breast cancer. These are androgen-responsive malignancies, and testosterone administration may stimulate tumor growth. Prior to instituting androgen therapy, a careful breast and digital rectal examination should be performed. Measurement of serum prostate-specific antigen (PSA) may also be useful prior to and during testosterone therapy, especially in older men and those at higher risk for prostate carcinoma (e.g., those with a family history of prostate cancer). Relative contraindications to androgen therapy include patients with untreated obstructive sleep apnea in whom sleep disordered breathing can worsen and patients with significant polycythemia in whom further stimulation of erythrocytosis can result in hyperviscosity and vascular thrombosis (see later discussion). Adequate treatment of these disorders should be instituted prior to starting testosterone therapy.

In general, androgen replacement therapy using either injectable testosterone esters or transdermal testosterone is tolerated very well and serious adverse effects are rare. Mild to moderate weight gain usually occurs as a result of anabolic effects and sodium retention associated with androgens. The latter may cause worsening of edema in men with underlying edematous states, such as congestive heart failure, nephrotic syndrome, or hepatic cirrhosis. Acne and oily skin may also occur during treatment. Excessive stimulation of libido and erections is rare, usually occurring in men with long-standing, severe androgen deficiency and prepubertal boys treated with large dosages of testosterone. These symptoms usually resolve with time or reduction in dosage.

Testosterone may cause excessive stimulation of erythropoiesis, and occasionally, clinically significant erythrocytosis that requires therapeutic phlebotomy.[710] This usually occurs in men with predisposing conditions such as hypoxia due to chronic lung disease or sleep apnea, but may also occur in the absence of underlying disease, especially in elderly men. Excessive increases in hematocrit occur less commonly in hypogonadal men treated with testosterone patches than in those receiving injections of testosterone esters that deliver higher average androgen concentrations.[711] Hematocrit should be monitored yearly in men on androgen therapy. If hematocrit rises above 52 percent during therapy, testosterone should be discontinued temporarily or reduced in dose, and in cases of excessive erythrocytosis, they should undergo phlebotomy. Testosterone therapy may induce or worsen obstructive sleep apnea, and sleep studies should be performed in men who develop clinical manifestations of sleep apnea, such as daytime somnolence, while on therapy.[712,713]

Severe hypogonadism increases and testosterone replacement decreases HDL cholesterol.[714,715] The degree of HDL reduction is small (~10–15 percent) with testosterone administration and much greater with the use of nonaromatizable oral androgens, such as 17 α-alkylated androgens.[709,715,716] The clinical significance and long-term effects of androgen replacement on coronary artery disease risk are unclear. In fact, most epidemiological studies demonstrate higher cardiovascular risk in men with lower testosterone levels.[717] Contrary to popular belief, testosterone therapy improves mood and reduces irritability, and does not increase anger or aggression in hypogonadal men.[718,719]

Testosterone replacement therapy in hypogonadal men increases prostate size to volumes that are similar to those observed in age-matched control men, but does not cause excessive prostatic enlargement.[720] Although there is no evidence that androgen therapy in hypogonadal men worsens bladder outlet obstruction or precipitates urinary retention, caution should be exercised when treating older men with moderate to severe symptoms of BPH.[721,722] Low-dose androgen supplementation and/or therapy for BPH (α-adrenergic antagonists, 5α-reductase inhibitors, or surgery) should be considered in these patients. PSA levels are reduced in hypogonadal men and increased to normal with androgen replacement.[720] There is no evidence that androgen replacement therapy causes prostate carcinoma. However, whether long-term testosterone treatment in older men may stimulate growth of subclinical prostate cancer remains unknown. In men who develop a prostate nodule or progressively rising PSA levels >4 ng/mL on therapy, testosterone should be discontinued, and a urological evaluation that may include a transrectal prostate biopsy should be undertaken.

Although uncommon, potentially serious hepatotoxicity occurs predominantly with the use of oral 17α-alkylated androgens, and does not occur with the use of injectable testosterone esters or transdermal testosterone.[708] Intramuscular injections of testosterone esters may occasionally cause local discomfort or pain. Skin irritation may occur with the use of transdermal testosterone, particularly with the permeation-enhanced nonscrotal testosterone patches.

Other Uses of Androgens

In addition to treatment of hypogonadism, androgens have also been used as stimulation for erythropoiesis in hypoproliferative anemias related to renal and bone marrow failure; as treatment for micropenis and microphallus; as prophylactic treatment for hereditary angioneurotic edema; as adjuvant hormonal therapy for female breast cancer; topically for vulvar lichen sclerosus; and as a stimulant of bone formation in men and women with osteoporosis.[690]

The anabolic effects of testosterone replacement in hypogonadal men and supraphysiological androgen administration in eugonadal men have recently been demonstrated in well controlled clinical trials.[723–725] As described previously, serum testosterone levels are commonly reduced in men with chronic illness (e.g., renal and liver failure), wasting syndromes (e.g., associated with cancer and AIDS), the use of certain medications (e.g., glucocorticoids) and normal aging (see earlier discussion). These clinical conditions are associated with loss of muscle mass and strength, diminished bone mass, sexual dysfunction, and behavioral changes that are also manifestations of androgen deficiency. Although preliminary studies suggest potential beneficial anabolic and behavioral effects of testosterone treatment in many of these conditions,[403–407,726–740] the long-term benefits and risks of therapy are not fully established. The potential for expanded uses of androgens, however, has ignited recent interest in the development of new testosterone delivery systems.

Androgens, mostly testosterone enanthate, either alone or in combination with progestagens or GnRH analogs, have been used to suppress endogenous gonadotropin and sperm production as a male contraceptive strategy.[685–687] Androgen administration is an absolute requirement for hormonal male contraception, both for suppression of gonadotropin secretion and as a replacement for suppressed endogenous testosterone production induced by other agents. Because it plays such a key role in male contraceptive strategies, more practical androgen preparations with zero-order kinetics and longer durations of action are being developed and evaluated.

Abuse of Androgens

Androgens are often used illicitly in extremely high dosages, particularly by athletes and bodybuilders to enhance strength and performance, and by adolescents to "improve" appearance.[741] This has resulted in reclassification of testosterone and anabolic androgenic steroids as Schedule III controlled substances by the Food and Drug Administration (FDA). Androgen preparations (e.g., androstenedione and DHEA) available for purchase over-the-counter as "food supplements" are also being used and abused for their anabolic effects. Physicians should be alert to the significant abuse potential of androgen preparations.

Hepatotoxicity, behavioral disturbances, and impaired spermatogenesis resulting in infertility have been reported in athletes taking large doses of androgenic steroids. The long-term sequelae of taking massive dosages of androgens are not known, and the use of these agents to improve athletic performance or appearance should be strongly discouraged.

Antiandrogens

Broadly defined, antiandrogens are agents that inhibit the synthesis or action of androgens. They are used primarily for hormonal therapy of androgen-dependent malignancies, such as prostatic and breast carcinoma in men. They have also been used to treat male sex offenders and a variety of nonmalignant androgen-dependent conditions, such as acne, hirsutism, hyperandrogenism in women, male pattern baldness, and precocious puberty in boys.

GnRH Agonists

Potent agonist analogs of GnRH effectively suppress endogenous LH and testosterone secretion and induce a "medical castration" in patients.[742] GnRH agonists, such as leuprolide and goserelin, have been used either alone or in combination with androgen receptor antagonists primarily for the treatment of symptomatic stage D_2 metastatic prostate cancer.[743] Although controversial, combined GnRH and androgen receptor antagonist therapy, termed "complete androgen blockade," has the advantage of blocking both testicular and adrenal androgens, and preventing a "flare" in disease activity associated with the transient increase in gonadotropins and testosterone that occurs with initiation of GnRH agonist therapy alone (Fig. 15-33).[742–744] Depot formulations of leuprolide given monthly and goserelin given every three months are available. GnRH agonists have also been used to treat precocious puberty, paraphilia, and occasionally BPH.[745–747]

Megestrol Acetate

Megestrol acetate is a progestational antiandrogen that significantly blocks androgen production and androgen-mediated action. When administered in combination with small doses of estradiol or diethylstilbesterol, it profoundly suppresses serum gonadotropin and testosterone levels. These combinations have been used in the treatment of metastatic prostate cancer.[748] Megestrol acetate has

FIGURE 15-33. Diagrammatic representation of various types of primary and secondary hormonal therapies for prostate cancer. Complete androgen blockade involves measures designed to block the synthesis or action of androgens and androgen precursors made by the testes and adrenals.

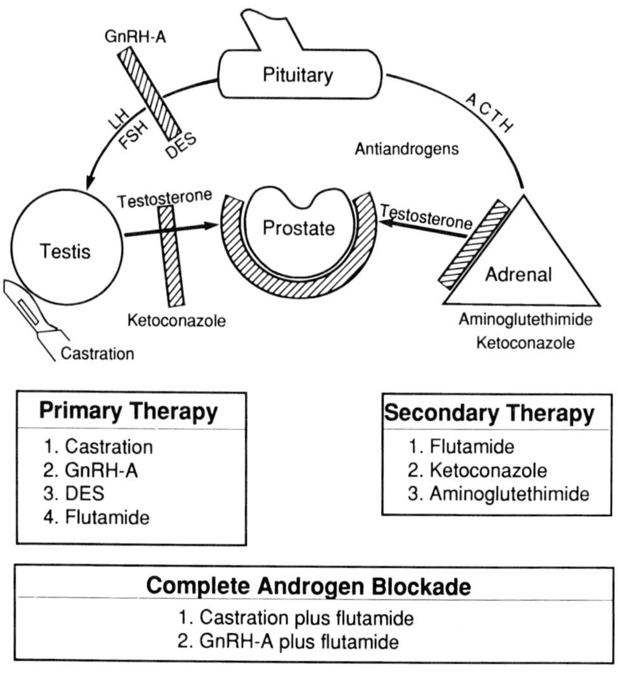

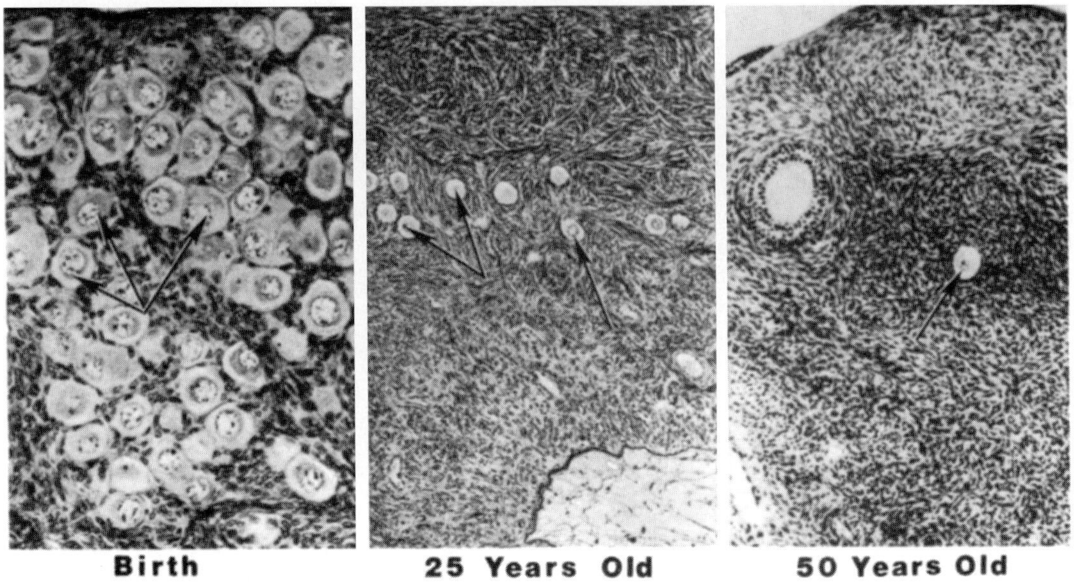

FIGURE 16A-6. Photomicrographs of sections through the cortex of human ovaries at different periods in life, showing the progressive decrease in the number of primordial follicles (arrows).

ing primary follicular growth, both the granulosa and the oocyte undergo striking changes. The first indication of primary follicle development (recruitment) is that individual granulosa cells begin to become round and appear cuboidal rather than squamous in shape; at about this time, the oocyte begins to change, primarily by increasing in size. As oocyte growth progresses, small patches of glycoprotein material begin to form between the granulosa cells juxtaposed to the oolemma; this material eventually covers the entire egg and is termed the *zona pellucida*. At the later primary stage, the oocyte is nearly fully grown (100-μm in diameter) and is completely enveloped by a thin zona pellucida, a single layer of cuboidal granulosa cells, and a basal lamina (Fig. 16A-3).

Secondary Follicle

During the stages of secondary follicle development, the granulosa cells proliferate and the oocyte completes its growth. By the end of the secondary stage, the follicle is organized into a multilayered structure which is strikingly symmetrical. In the center is a full-grown oocyte (120 μm in diameter) covered by a thick zona pellucida, about eight layers of stratified low-columnar granulosa cells, and a basal lamina (Fig. 16A-7).

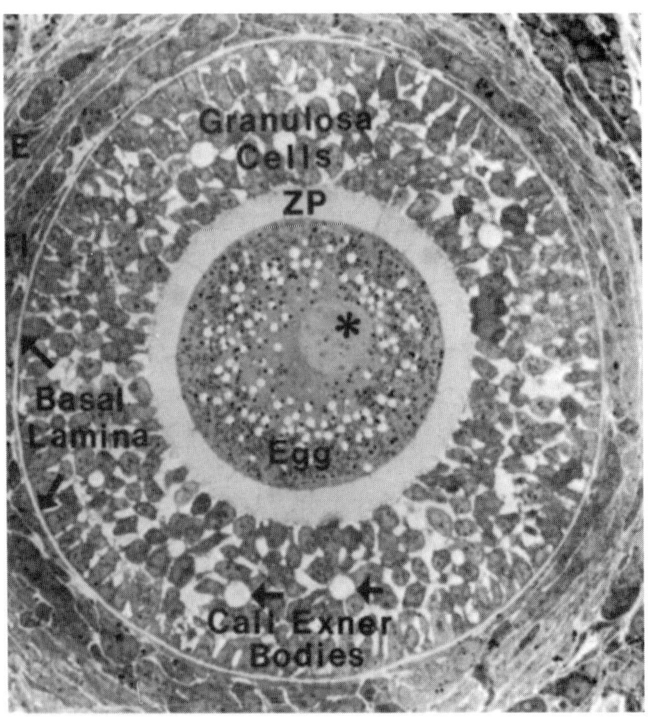

FIGURE 16A-7. Photomicrograph of a section through a preantral secondary follicle. The dictyotene oocyte contains a large germinal vesicle or nucleus (asterisk) and a zona pellucida (ZP). The egg is surrounded by five layers of granulosa cells, which in turn are enclosed by a basal lamina. The presumptive cells of the theca interna (TI) and theca externa (TE) have become associated with the follicle. (*Courtesy of Dr. Everett Anderson, by permission of Saunders.*)

During the course of secondary follicle development, several important morphologic events occur. One critical event involves the acquisition of cells of the prospective theca. When a secondary follicle acquires two to three layers of granulosa cells, a putative signal (yet to be identified) causes a stream of mesenchymal cells to migrate to the outer surface of the follicle.[9] The precise origin of these cells and the pathway they take remain unknown, but there is evidence in the rodent that they arise from stromal fibroblasts outside the immediate vicinity of the secondary follicle.[10] After the mesenchymal cells reach the basal lamina, they align themselves in parallel and form a radial arrangement of highly elongated, fibroblast-like cells around the entire follicle (Fig. 16A-7). This newly acquired tissue layer ultimately gives rise to the theca interna and the theca externa (Fig. 16A-7).

Another critical event which occurs during secondary follicle growth is the acquisition of an independent blood supply. At the secondary stage, a follicle is supplied by one or two arterioles which terminate in a wreathlike network of capillaries.[1] In a broad sense, the investing vessels form two sets of capillaries which are interconnected: an inner wreath of capillaries in the theca interna, which is supplied by branches from an outer wreath of capillaries in the theca externa. Characteristically, the capillaries of the inner wreath become closely associated with the basal lamina; however, they never penetrate beyond this membrane, and thus the granulosa and egg are avascular. The inner capillary wreath is drained by small venules which connect in the theca externa into larger venules, which in turn enter the ovarian veins.[1]

Another interesting morphologic feature which appears in the secondary follicle is the formation of Call-Exner bodies among the granulosa cells (Fig. 16A-7). These bodies have been characterized ultrastructurally (Fig. 16A-8), but nothing is known about the manner in which they form or their physiologic importance. Given the importance of the extracellular matrix in cell division and mitosis,[15] one could speculate that Cell-Exner bodies may play a role in regulating granulosa growth and differentiation by providing novel substrate-to-cell interactions.

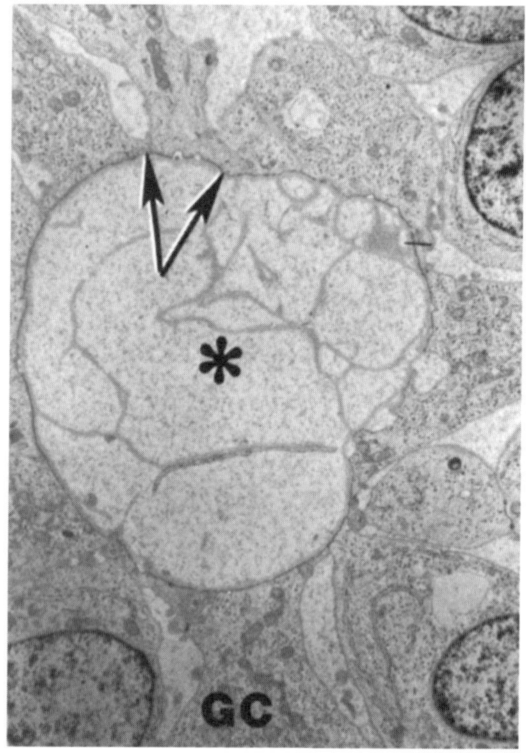

FIGURE 16A-8. Electron micrograph of a Call-Exner body. It consists of a distinct basal lamina (arrow) to which membrana granulosa cells (GC) are attached and a cavity (asterisk) with excess basal lamina material and a flocculant protein-like material. The question of its function remains unanswered.

Tertiary Follicle

The primary characteristic of a tertiary follicle is the presence of a small antrum. Antrum formation occurs when a follicle reaches approximately 400 μm in diameter (Fig. 16A-3). The process of antrum formation in its earliest phase is termed *cavitation*. This event is characterized by the uptake or accumulation of fluid between the granulosa cells and, therefore, the formation of a small internal cavity at one pole of the oocyte. Histologic evidence suggests that the site of initiation of antrum formation is controlled in a highly specific manner, perhaps by the oocyte (Fig. 16A-9). Although the underlying mechanism for cavitation is

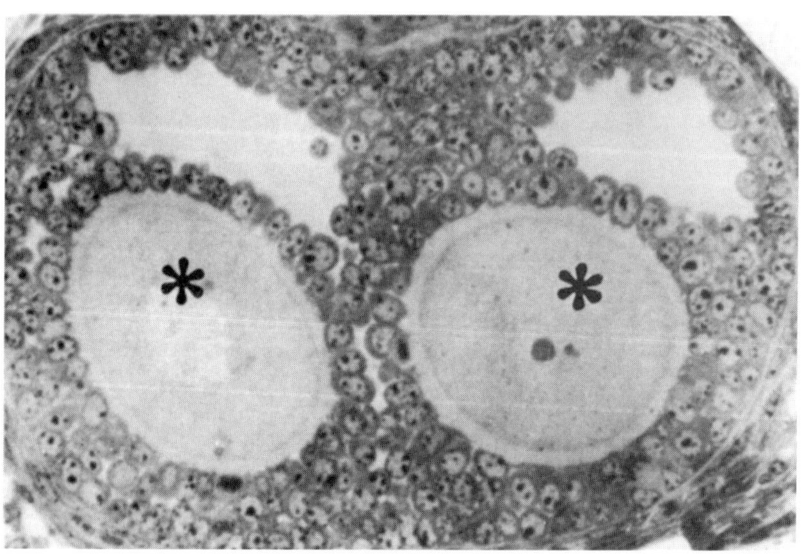

FIGURE 16A-9. Photomicrograph of a polyovular follicle at the early tertiary stage, showing the sites of cavitation or early antrum formation (clear spaces) just above oocytes (asterisk). This event, which is under intraovarian control, seems to arise in a specific synchronized manner and establishes the polarity of the follicle. [*From Zamboni L: Comparative studies on the ultrastructure of mammalian oocytes, in Biggers JD, Schultz AW (eds): Oogenesis. University Park Press, Baltimore, MD, 1972, pp 5–46.*]

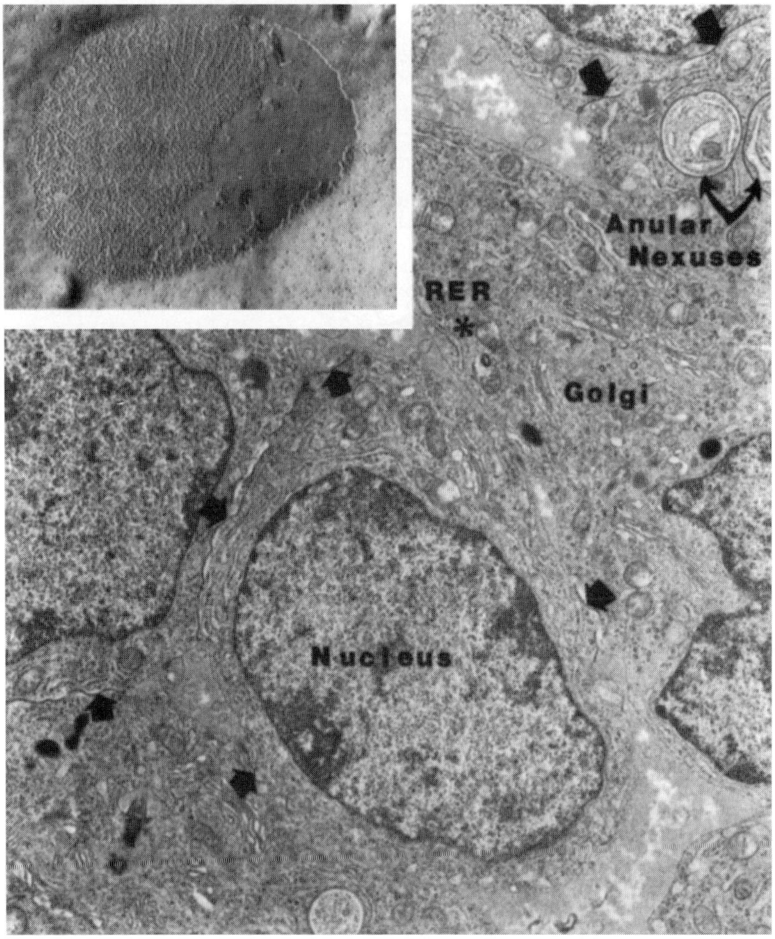

FIGURE 16A-10. Electron micrograph showing extensive gap junctional contacts (arrows) between granulosa cells of a healthy Graafian follicle. (Inset) Replica of a granulosa cell fracture showing the hexagonally ordered connexin proteins which constitute the gap junction. (*Courtesy of Dr. David Albertini.*)

unknown, it occurs in the absence of the pituitary and thus seems to result from a local process intrinsic to the follicle itself. As a result of cavitation, the follicle acquires an inherent polarity and internal organization which remain throughout the rest of folliculogenesis.

Concurrent with the initiation of antrum formation, numerous histologic changes occur in both the theca interna and the granulosa cells. In the case of the theca interna,[10] subpopulations of fibroblasts transform into large epithelial cells termed *theca interstitial cells* (Fig. 16A-3). These cells become highly differentiated steroidogenic cells which synthesize and secrete androgens.[10]

At cavitation, there is an increase in the size and number of gap junctions (Fig. 16A-10) in the follicle.[16] Gap junctions are intracellular channels composed of a family of at least 13 proteins called *connexins* (Cx).[17–19] Studies of the permeability of this cell-to-cell membrane channel have indicated that molecules (including the second messengers calcium and cyclic AMP) with a molecular mass up to 1800 daltons can pass from one cell to another. Gap junctions or Cx43 are present in granulosa cells being detected in primordial and primary follicles.[16] Gap junctions also develop between the oocyte and corona radiata granulosa cells. Cx37 is an oocyte-derived Cx which forms gap junctions between the oocyte and corona cells.[20] Interestingly, evidence from Cx37-deficient mice assigns to Cx37 an obligatory role in Graafian follicle formation, ovulation and fertility.[20] Gap junctions or Cx26 are present between differentiating theca interstitial cells at cavitation.[16] The emerging concept is that gap junctions are obligatory for folliculogenesis and fertility and that by virtue of their presence, the entire follicle has the potential to undergo a synchronized pattern of activities in response to ligand stimulation.

Graafian or Antral Follicles

A Graafian follicle can be defined structurally as a heterogeneous family of relatively large follicles (400 μm to 2 cm at ovulation) characterized by a cavity or antrum containing a fluid termed *follicular fluid* or *liquor folliculi*.[21] The characteristic structural unit of all Graafian follicles is the antrum. Hence, the term antral follicle is used correctly as a synonym for Graafian follicle. In response to FSH brought to the follicle by the inner and outer capillary wreaths, the tertiary follicle increases tremendously in size. If a developing human tertiary follicle is selected to ovulate, it may grow 75-fold, in diameter; the growth of the Graafian follicle is accomplished primarily by follicular fluid accumulation in the antrum and to a lesser extent by granulosa and theca proliferation.[22] Contrary to preantral follicles, this change in size and differentiation in Graafian follicles is not under autonomous control but is dependent on pituitary gonadotropins, most notably FSH.

As seen in Fig. 16A-11, the Graafian follicle is a highly structured mass of precisely positioned cells. Granulosa cells develop as pseudostratified epithelium and are limited peripherally by a basal lamina. By virtue of this architecture, the granulosa cells (and the egg) develop within the microenvironment of the follicular fluid. The follicular fluid is the medium in which regulatory

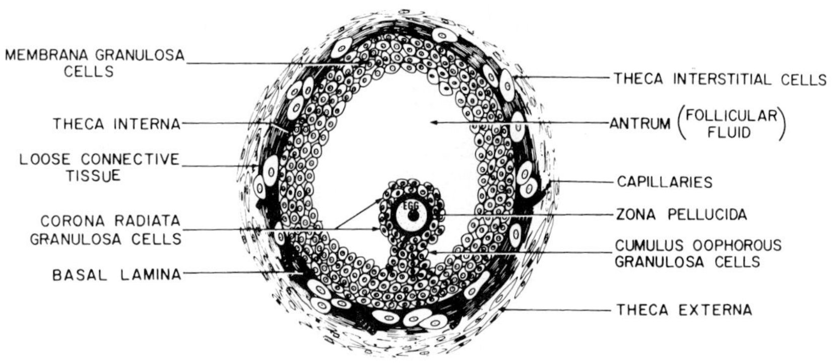

FIGURE 16A-11. Diagrammatic representation of the histology of a section through a healthy Graafian follicle. (*Revised from Erickson,*[66] *by permission of Elsevier Scientific.*)

molecules must pass on their way to and from this microenvironment. In the Graafian follicle, both the number and the size of the gap junctions between the granulosa cells increase,[16] suggesting that the levels of electric and metabolic coupling in this tissue become amplified during folliculogenesis.

During Graafian follicle development the granulosa cells become different from one another with respect to polarity and relative position within the whole follicle (Fig. 16A-11). An important concept is that granulosa cells are a complex tissue containing several subgroups of different cell populations: the corona radiata cells, which make cell-to-cell contact with the egg and the zona pellucida; the cumulus cells, which make cell-to-cell contact with both the corona and the periantral granulosa cells; and the membrana cells, which make direct contact with the basal lamina, Call-Exner bodies and the periantral granulosa cells (Fig. 16A-12). This has led to the concept of heterogeneity in granulosa cell organization and function. An interesting subject (considered below) is how the relative position of a granulosa cell or a group of granulosa cells within the follicle determines the direction in which that cell differentiates.

Throughout Graafian follicle development, the morphologic characteristics of the theca that are established at cavitation remain. Highly differentiated theca interstitial cells progressively accumulate until there are eventually five to eight layers of these

FIGURE 16A-12. Diagram of the structural and functional heterogeneity of the granulosa cells in a healthy Graafian follicle. The granulosa cells express different patterns of proliferation and differentiation as a result of their position or location in the follicle. (*From Erickson GF,*[21] *by permission of Springer-Verlag.*)

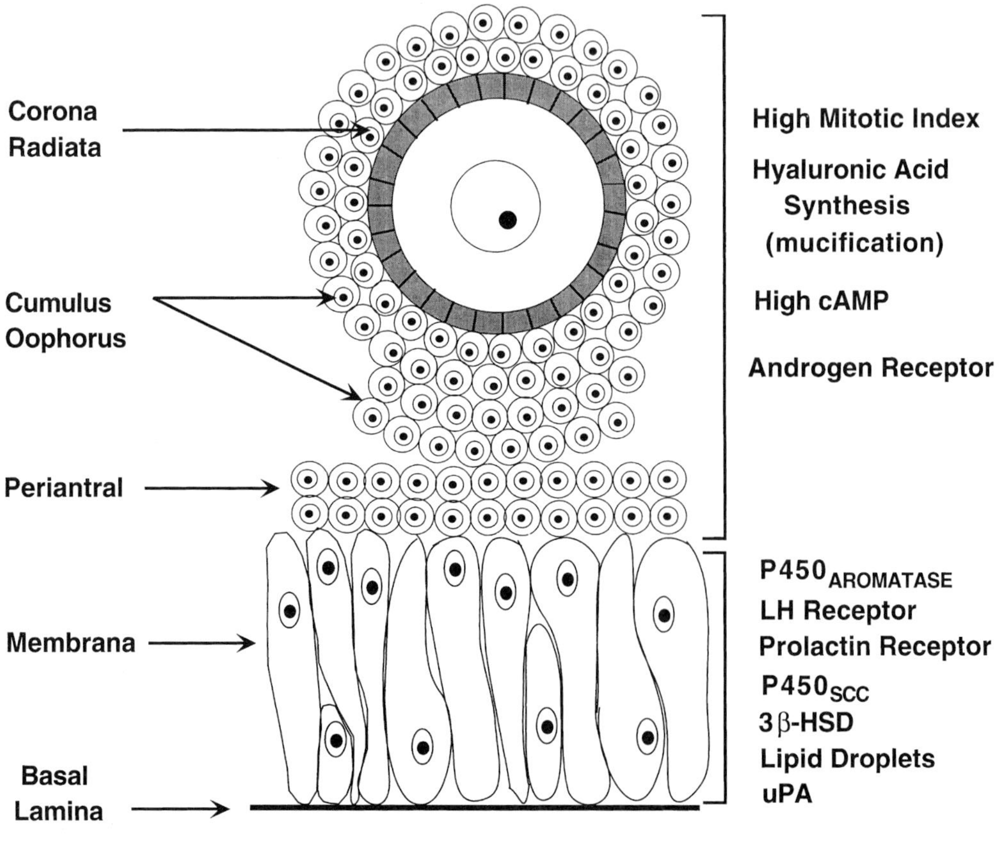

cells in a dominant preovulatory follicle (Fig. 16A-11). The generation of theca interstitial cells results through mitotic division of cells in the theca interna.[10,22]

Electron microscopic studies of the theca externa of Graafian follicles reveal the presence of smooth muscle cells[23] which contain actin and myosin.[24] The contractile cells in the theca externa (Figs. 16A-1 and 16A-11) are innervated by both sympathetic and parasympathetic nerves,[2] and the influence of the associated nerves presumably determines the extent to which the theca externa cells contract. Several lines of evidence point to a role of these cells in ovulation.[21]

Atretic Follicles

Once a primordial follicle is recruited to initiate growth, it either develops into a dominant preovulatory follicle or degenerates by a process termed *atresia*.[21,25] Accordingly, all follicles can be divided broadly into two groups, healthy and atretic. Atresia results in the selective death and clearance of the oocyte and granulosa by a programmed cell death mechanism called apoptosis.[26,27] But the surrounding theca cells appear to undergo hypertrophy[10] and eventually become islands of interstitial gland cells, some of which appear to remain permanently in the ovarian cortex (Fig. 16A-1).[10] In a broad sense, the main difference between healthy and atretic follicle is whether or not apoptosis is occurring in the oocyte and/or granulosa cells.

There seems to be two types of atresia: type A atresia, in which primary changes occur in the oocyte, and type B atresia, in which there are primary changes in granulosa cells. Type A atresia is most common in preantral follicles, whereas type B atresia is most common in Graafian follicles. During the course of both types of atresia, three major successive changes have been identified morphologically: the primary, secondary, and tertiary stages.

In the primary stage of type B atresia (in Graafian follicles), apoptosis first appear in some periantral granulosa cells.[28] In time, the margin of apoptosis expands until all granulosa cells along the antrum are apoptotic. At the secondary stage, apoptosis occurs in the membrana granulosa cells. As atresia continues, large numbers of granulosa cells undergo apoptosis. Directly next to the granulosa cells that are shedding their cytoplasmic and nuclear contents, there can be granulosa cells which appear healthy and show mitotic activity. In this light, cumulus cells appear to show little sign of apoptosis during secondary atresia and thus seem to occupy a privileged position in comparison with membrana granulosa cells in the atretic process.[28] At the tertiary stage, the entire membrana granulosa is apoptotic and large parts of it are often seen lying free in the antrum (Fig. 16A-13). During these late stages of atresia, apoptosis begins appearing in the cumulus cells and the first signs of oocyte degeneration are detected. In some cases, the cumulus breaks up and the oocyte, surrounded only by corona radiata, is set free within the antral cavity. Finally, there is the complete apoptosis and clearance of the granulosa and oocyte; the follicle collapses. With the collapse of the follicle, the theca interstitial cells hypertrophy and eventually become the secondary interstitial gland cells.[10]

The route taken in type A atresia (in preantral follicles) is different from that in the type B pattern. An early morphologic event seen in type A atresia involves the oocyte rather than the granulosa cells.[29] In the early phases of type A atresia the oocyte initiates meiotic maturation and begins to exhibit maturation spindles and polar bodies. In some instances, the activated oocytes in preantral follicles undergo pseudo cleavage or fragmentation into embryoid bodies.[30] Such activated eggs may be the source of ovarian teratomas. Macrophages are often detected within the atretic follicle where they are believed to phagocytize the oocyte and granulosa cells.[29] The basal lamina becomes hyalinized and the theca interna hypertrophies, after which the unit becomes part of the secondary interstitial gland cells.[10]

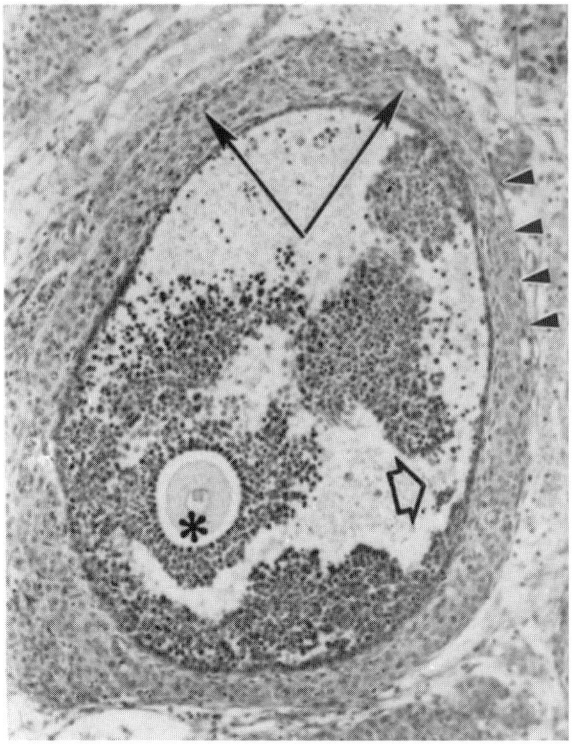

FIGURE 16A-13. Photomicrograph of type B atresia in a Graafian follicle. Note that large numbers of granulosa cells (open arrowhead) have detached from the basal lamina and that many are apoptotic. By contrast, the dictyate egg and cumulus granulosa appear healthy. The theca interstitial cells exhibit hypertrophy (arrows) and are surrounded by a thin theca externa (arrowheads).

Ovarian Interstitial Cells

A characteristic feature of the human ovary is the presence of several different types of interstitial cells which can synthesize and secrete androgens.[10] These cells are found in the stroma of both the cortex and the medulla (Fig. 16A-1). Over the years, considerable attention has been paid to the development of these cells, and as a result, the life cycle of the ovarian interstitial cell type has been worked out. In all cases, the cells which eventually give rise to interstitial cells are derived from mesenchymal cells in the ovarian stroma.[10] In the human, there are four major classes of ovarian interstitial cells: (1) primary, (2) theca interstitial, (3) secondary interstitial, and (4) hilus cells. Because ovarian interstitial cells produce androgens, they are central in regulating a number of fundamental reproductive processes.[10]

Primary Interstitial Cells

The first interstitial cells to develop in the ovary are termed *primary interstitial* cells. In the human, primary interstitial cells are first distinguished at 12 weeks gestation in the fetal ovary where they remain visible until about the 20th week.[31] The

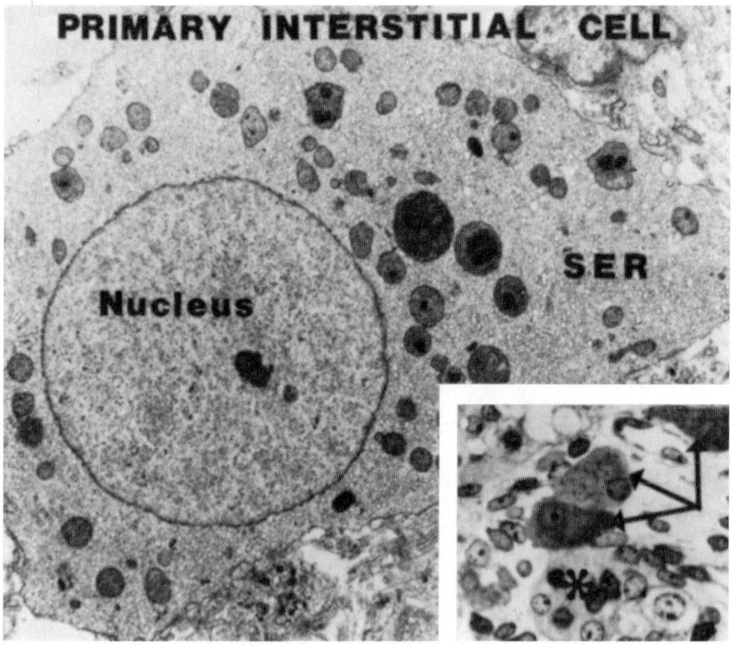

FIGURE 16A-14. Electron micrograph of a primary interstitial cell in the human fetal ovary at 15 weeks gestation. Its ultrastructure strongly resembles that of steroidogenically active testicular Leydig cells. *Inset* shows the intimate relationship between primary interstitial cells (arrows) and oogonia (arrowhead) in the cortical cords (asterisk). (*From Ref. 31, courtesy of Dr. B. Gondos, by permission of Williams & Wilkins.*)

primary interstitial cells are juxtaposed to the basal lamina of the ovarian cortical cords which contain the oogonia and oocytes (Fig. 16A-14).

The ultrastructural properties of primary interstitial cells are consistent with those of active, steroid-secreting cells. It is interesting that these cells bear a striking resemblance to the Leydig cells in the human fetal testis.[31] Based on their ultrastructure one would predict that primary interstitial cells are producing steroids, perhaps androgens, at high rates.

Theca Interstitial Cells

The most widely studied class of ovarian interstitial cells is the theca interstitial cells.[10] Such cells are present in the theca interna of all tertiary follicles (Figs. 16A-3 and 16A-11). In the human, theca interstitial cells are the site of follicular androgen, most notably androstenedione, synthesis.[32]

As was pointed out earlier, presumptive theca interstitial cells first develop when a follicle reaches the end of the secondary stage (Figs. 16A-3 and 16A-7). At this point, some mesenchymal cells undergo significant change and become directed along a path of theca interstitial cell differentiation. This developmental shift involves the acquisition of LH receptors. The stimulus which causes some mesenchymal cells to undergo this change is unknown, but it appears to emanate from the secondary follicle itself and is independent of the pituitary. The remaining mesenchymal cells are thought to be pluripotent stem cells that can divide to produce other theca interstitial cells or differentiate into loose connective tissue as the follicle grows.[10]

The consequence of the transformation from a mesenchymal to a theca interstitial cell is evident. With the acquisition of LH receptors, theca interstitial cells are committed to respond to plasma LH, which is brought to the follicle by the inner capillary wreath. When a follicle reaches the early tertiary stage, the presumptive theca interstitial cells respond to LH by undergoing a major shape change from an elongated fibroblast to an epithelial cell.[10] Once the shape change is initiated (Fig. 16A-3), the cells begin to develop properties that are not found in the precursor stem cells. With increasing periods of time, theca interstitial cells increase markedly in size to 15 to 20 μm in diameter and acquire the fine structure typical of active steroid-synthesizing cells (Fig. 16A-15). This step is particularly striking and is characterized by the increased use of cytoplasmic organelles for de novo androgen biosynthesis. As folliculogenesis proceeds, the number of terminally differentiated theca interstitial cells increases as a result of mitosis.[22] Within the theca interna of developing follicles are transitional cells whose ultrastructure reflects intermediate stages between the ultrastructure of unspecialized mesenchymal cells and that of fully differentiated steroidogenic cells, providing support for the concept of a theca interstitial stem cell.

A characteristic feature of the human theca interna is the presence of what seem to be subpopulations of differentiated theca interstitial cells (Fig. 16A-15). Electron micrographs show that the two main types (dark and light cells) both have the ultrastructure of active steroidogenic cells. Even though data are lacking, the demonstration of cytologic heterogeneity raises the possibility that within a follicle there are theca interstitial cells with differing endocrine capabilities and responsiveness.[10] Whether these cells secrete different classes of regulatory molecules and/or are controlled independently remains to be determined.

Secondary Interstitial Cells

During the process of atresia, the theca interstitial cells survive, becoming cords or clusters of large epithelial cells called *secondary interstitial* cells.[10,33] In this sense, secondary interstitial cells are direct descendants of theca interstitial cells of atretic follicles. Thus, it seems that theca interstitial cells never die but are actually accumulated in the ovary. In humans, secondary interstitial cells can maintain their specialized ultrastructure characteristic of active steroidogenic cells (Fig. 16A-16) and continue responding to LH with increased androstenedione production.[22] This argues that the secondary interstitial cells continue to exhibit properties of their precursors, the theca interstitial cells.

There is, however, one very important property that these two cell types do not have in common: Secondary, but not theca,

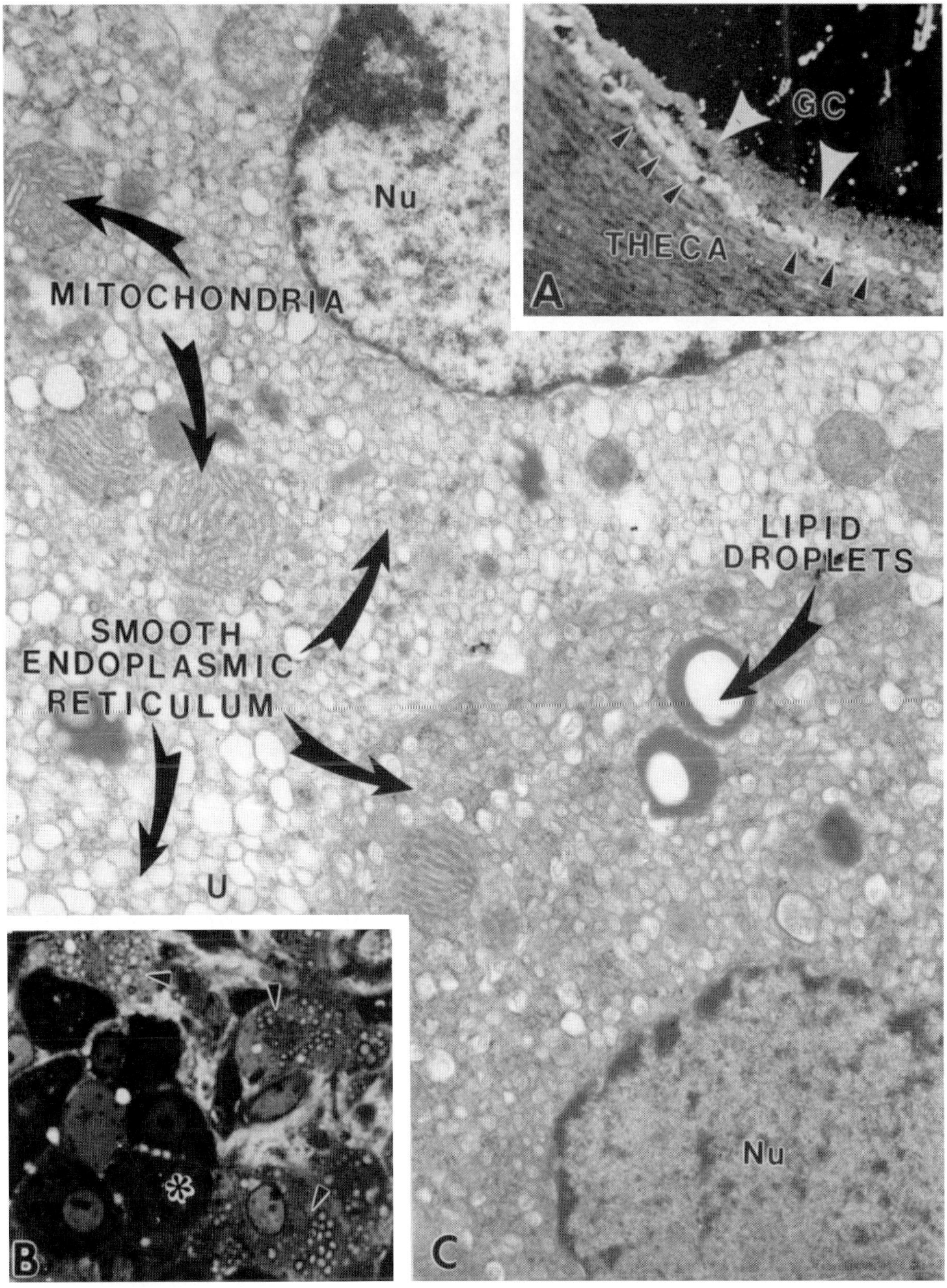

FIGURE 16A-15. Histology of human theca interstitial cells. (*A*) Localization of $P450_{C17}$ in theca cells. $P450_{C17}$ was detected by immunocytochemistry. Note that $P450_{C17}$ is not detected in the granulosa (GC). (*B*) Photomicrograph of theca interna showing the two populations of differentiated theca interstitial cells: dark ones (asterisk) and light ones (arrowheads). (*C*) Electron micrograph of the dark and light cells. Note that both contain mitochondria with tubular cristae (the site of P450ssc), smooth endoplasmic reticulum (the site of $P450_{C17}$), and lipid droplets (site of cholesterol ester storage).

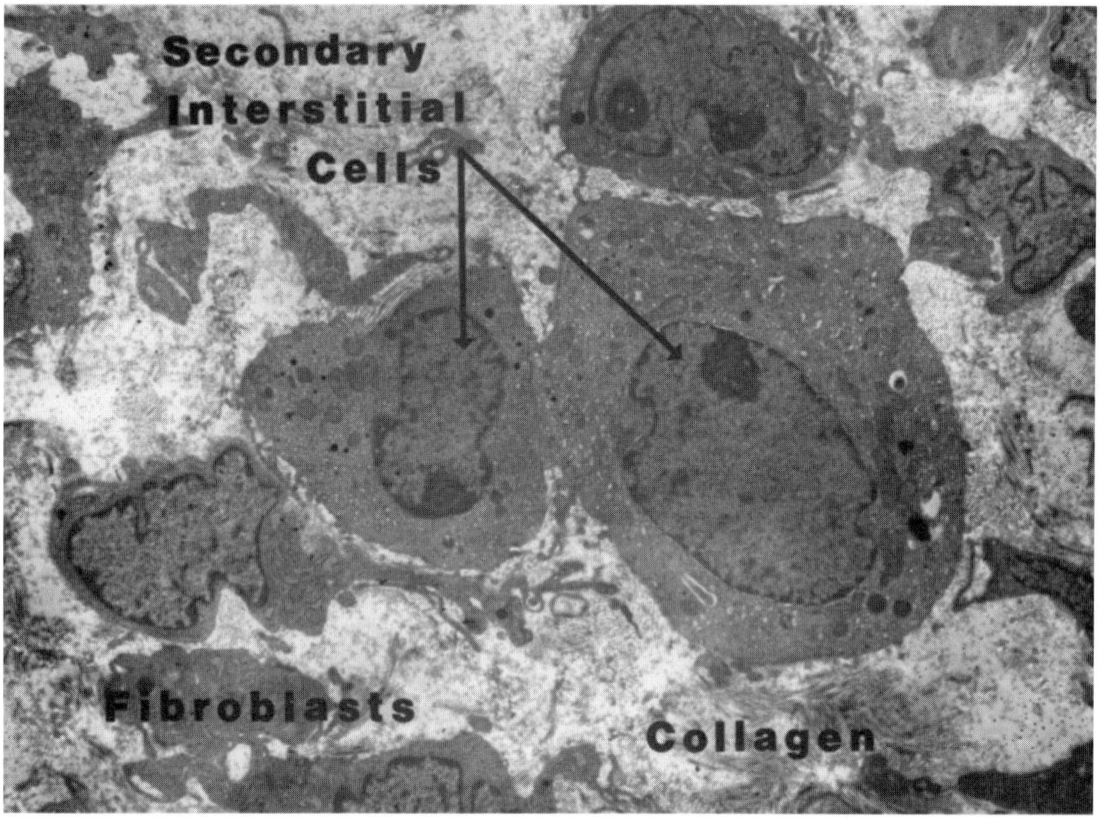

FIGURE 16A-16. Electron micrograph of a cluster of secondary interstitial cells found in the connective tissue of the cortex of a normal human ovary. Their fine structure is typical of active steroidogenic cells in that they have smooth endoplasmic reticulum, lipid droplets, and mitochondria with tubular cristae. During the life of a woman, they can remain as islands of innervated, hormone-responsive androgen-producing cells.

interstitial cells are innervated.[10] As was mentioned earlier, secondary interstitial cells are unique in that they seem to be innervated by sympathetic nerves. Evidence in rodents strongly suggests the existence of point-to-point communication between neurons in the brain and the ovarian steroidogenic cells.[34] Stimulation of selected hypothalamic nuclei in hypophysectomized and adrenalectomized rats stimulates or inhibits estrogen and progesterone synthesis, depending on which nucleus is stimulated.[34] It seems, therefore, that precise information from the brain can be transmitted directly to the ovaries via the secondary interstitial cells. In this regard, direct evidence in the rat that catecholamines can stimulate structural and functional changes in secondary interstitial cells has been reported.[10] Thus, the concept which is emerging is that catecholamines (and perhaps other neuro-transmitters) pass across a synapse bind to receptors and thus regulate androgen activity in the secondary interstitial cell.

Hilus Cells

Along the length of the ovarian hilus are clusters of large (15 to 25 μm in diameter) steroidogenic cells called *hilus cells* (Fig. 16A-1). These are highly unusual cells because all aspects of their structure and function are identical to those of differentiated testicular Leydig cells.[10,35] The hilus and Leydig cells cannot be distinguished on morphologic criteria (Fig. 16A-17): Both contain a unique hexagonal array of crystal lattice termed *crystalloids of Reinke*.[36,37] The nature and importance of these crystalloids remain unknown; however, they may be albumin-like material which provide a reservoir of binding sites for testosterone molecules. It has been established that hilus cells (like Leydig cells) synthesize and secrete testosterone in response to LH stimulation.[38–40] In this context, ovarian tumors of the hilus cell cause virilization. For all intents and purposes, a hilus cell is an ovarian Leydig cell.

What are the endocrine controls and physical importance of ovarian hilus cells? One intriguing feature is the intimate association of hilus cells with nonmyelinated sympathetic nerve fibers (Fig. 16A-1)[35] and the ovarian spiral arteries.[1] Perhaps interactions occur between hilus cells and the nerves and blood vessels which directly or indirectly alter ovarian testosterone production which in turn may have an impact on the decision-making processes in female production. It has been proposed that hilus cells may be a source of testosterone needed for increased striated muscle activities in women during exercise.[41]

Corpora Lutea

After ovulation of the egg-cumulus complex, the follicle wall undergoes a series of histologic changes that result in the formation of a corpus luteum.[42] Cells that make up the corpus luteum are contributed by the membrana and periantral granulosa, and the theca interna and theca externa. Morphologically, a corpus luteum is roughly equivalent to a Graafian follicle (Fig. 16A-18; compare with Fig. 16A-11). In the center, where the antrum and liquor folliculi were once located, is a fibrin clot in which there has been an

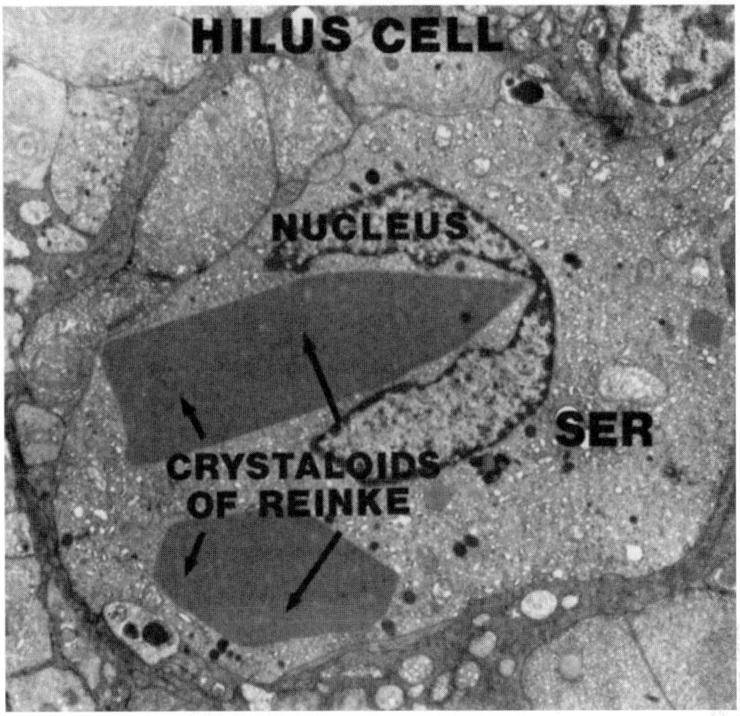

FIGURE 16A-17. Electron micrograph of a hilus cell, showing both abundant smooth endoplasmic reticulum (SER) and numerous large crystalloids of Reinke. (*Courtesy of Dr. Norbert Schnoy, by permission of Springer-Verlag.*)

invasion of loose connective tissue, blood vessels, angiogenesis, and blood cells.

At ovulation, the wall of the Graafian follicle undergoes extensive hypertrophy (Fig. 16A-18). During luteinization, the membrana granulosa cells undergo tremendous changes and attain a large size of 35 to 60 μm in diameter.[43] Such cells are termed *granulosa-lutein* cells. Perhaps the most dramatic event that occurs in the newly forming granulosa-lutein cell is its transformation from a protein secretory-like cell into a highly differentiated steroidogenic cell. In the cytoplasm prominent regions of smooth endoplasmic reticulum develop, the mitochondria develop tubular cristae, and large clusters of lipid droplets containing cholesterol esters accumu-

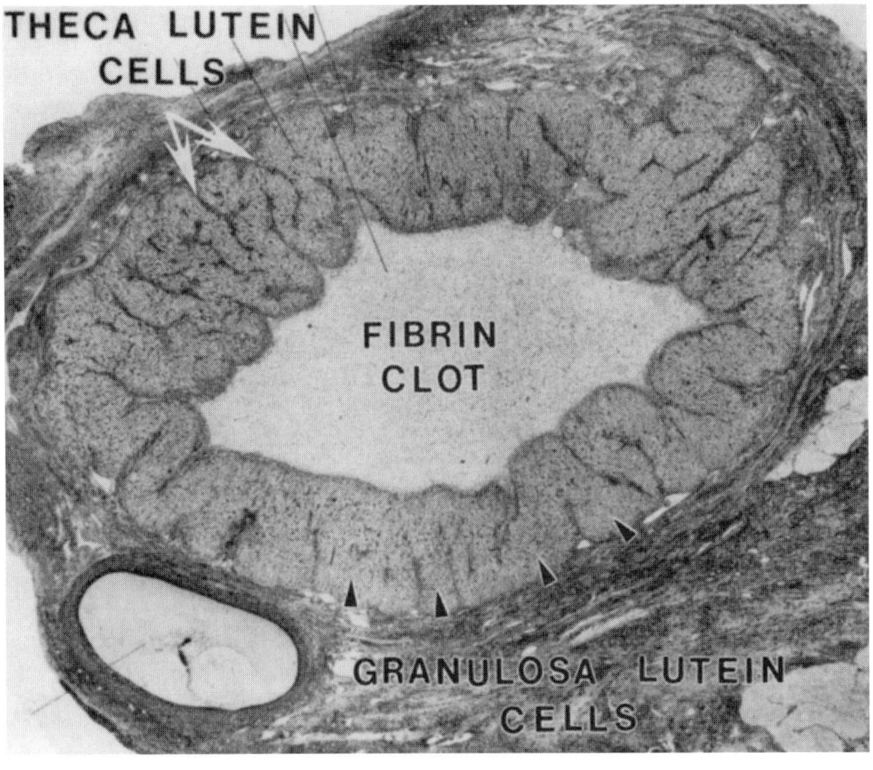

FIGURE 16A-18. Photomicrograph of a section of a human corpus luteum, showing the fibrin clot in the antrum and the hypertrophied follicle wall composed of granulosa and theca lutein cells. (*Revised from Bloom and Fawcett,*[202] *by permission of WB Saunders.*)

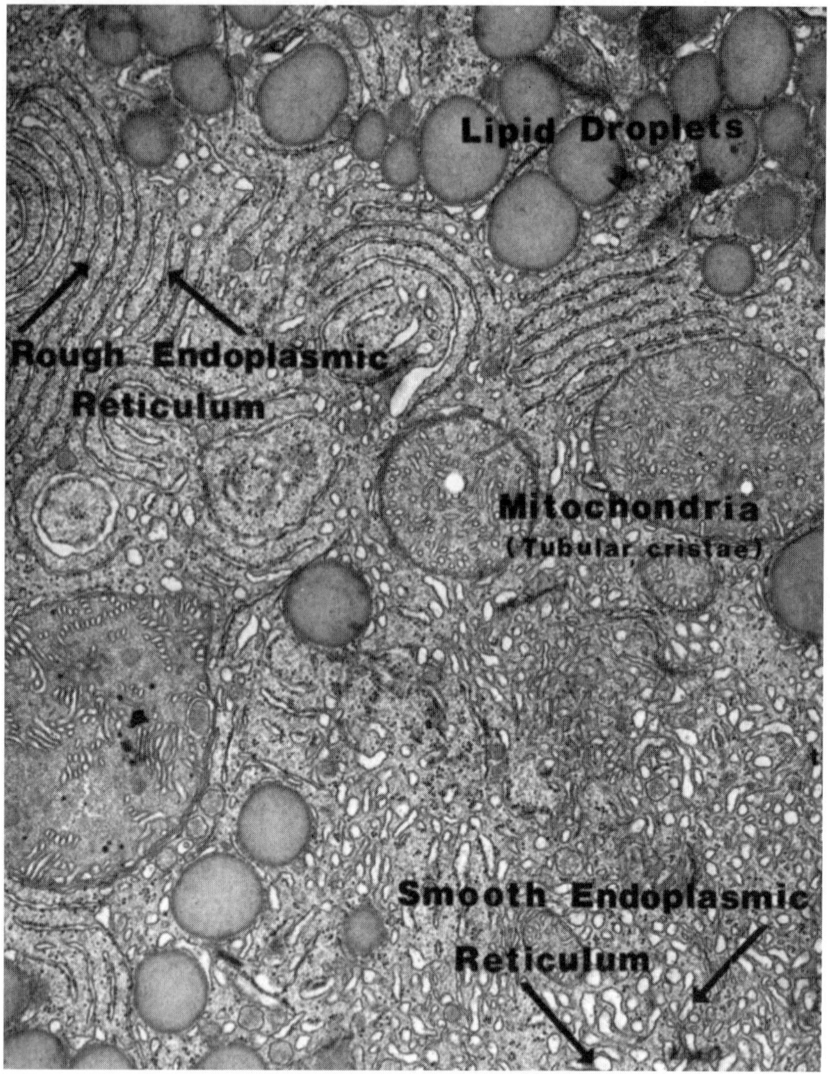

FIGURE 16A-19. Electron micrograph of a section through a human granulosa lutein cell, showing both protein-synthesizing [rough endoplasmic reticulum (ER)] and steroid-synthesizing (smooth ER) potential. The smooth ER is the site of $P450_{AROM}$. Note the prominent tubular cristae (the site of $P450_{scc}$) in the mitochondria and the large number of lipid droplets containing stored cholesterol esters. (*Courtesy of Dr. Tom Crisp, by permission of CV Mosby.*)

late (Fig. 16A-19). Granulosa-lutein cells contain substantial quantities of rough endoplasmic reticulum, indicating that these cells also have protein-synthesizing activity (Fig. 16A-19). These cells have a series of long microvilli which can measure 2 μm or more in length projecting from their apical surface.[43] In rodents, these microvilli have been shown to contain the functional LH receptors.[44]

During luteinization, the theca interstitial cells become incorporated into the periphery of the corpus luteum and are termed *theca lutein* cells. Theca lutein cells can be distinguished from granulosa-lutein cells (Fig. 16A-20) because they are typically smaller (15 μm in diameter) and stain more darkly.[43,45] Ultrastructurally, they appear as active steroid-producing cells, but they also contain stacks of rough endoplasmic reticulum, consistent with the synthesis and secretion of proteins.[43] Like the theca interna, the theca lutein tissue contains cells with differing degrees of density (light, dark, intermediate) (Fig. 16A-20), suggesting that there may be subpopulations of theca lutein cells.[43] Scattered throughout the corpus luteum are many macrophages,[45] the so-called K cells (Fig. 16A-20). Finally, as with the follicle, the entire corpus luteum is surrounded by a theca externa (Fig. 16A-20).

If fertilization and implantation do not occur, the corpus luteum undergoes degeneration by apoptosis.[46] This process, which is termed *luteolysis*, becomes apparent 8 days after ovulation.[47] The first histologic indication of luteolysis is shrinkage of the granulosa-lutein cells. This is characterized by specific decreases in the amount of endoplasmic reticulum and general decreases in the amount of cytoplasmic matrix,[47] followed by the expression of apoptotic bodies.[46] Initially the regression seems to be selective for granulosa-lutein cells as theca lutein cells actually become more prominent.[47] At this time, the theca layer is formed of tightly packed theca-lutein cells which contain profuse amounts of smooth endoplasmic reticulum and large mitochondria with tubular cristae. In this sense, luteolysis seems to be associated with hyperstimulation of the theca lutein cells. This is followed by apoptosis of all lutein cells (granulosa, theca, endothelial). When the glandular corpus luteum disintegrates, all that is left is a nodule of dense connective tissue called the *corpus albicans* (Fig. 16A-1).

BIOGENESIS OF OVARIAN HORMONES

Steroids

In a broad sense, the adult human ovaries secrete three major types of biologically active steroid hormones: progesterone, androstenedione, and estradiol. The ability to produce these steroids

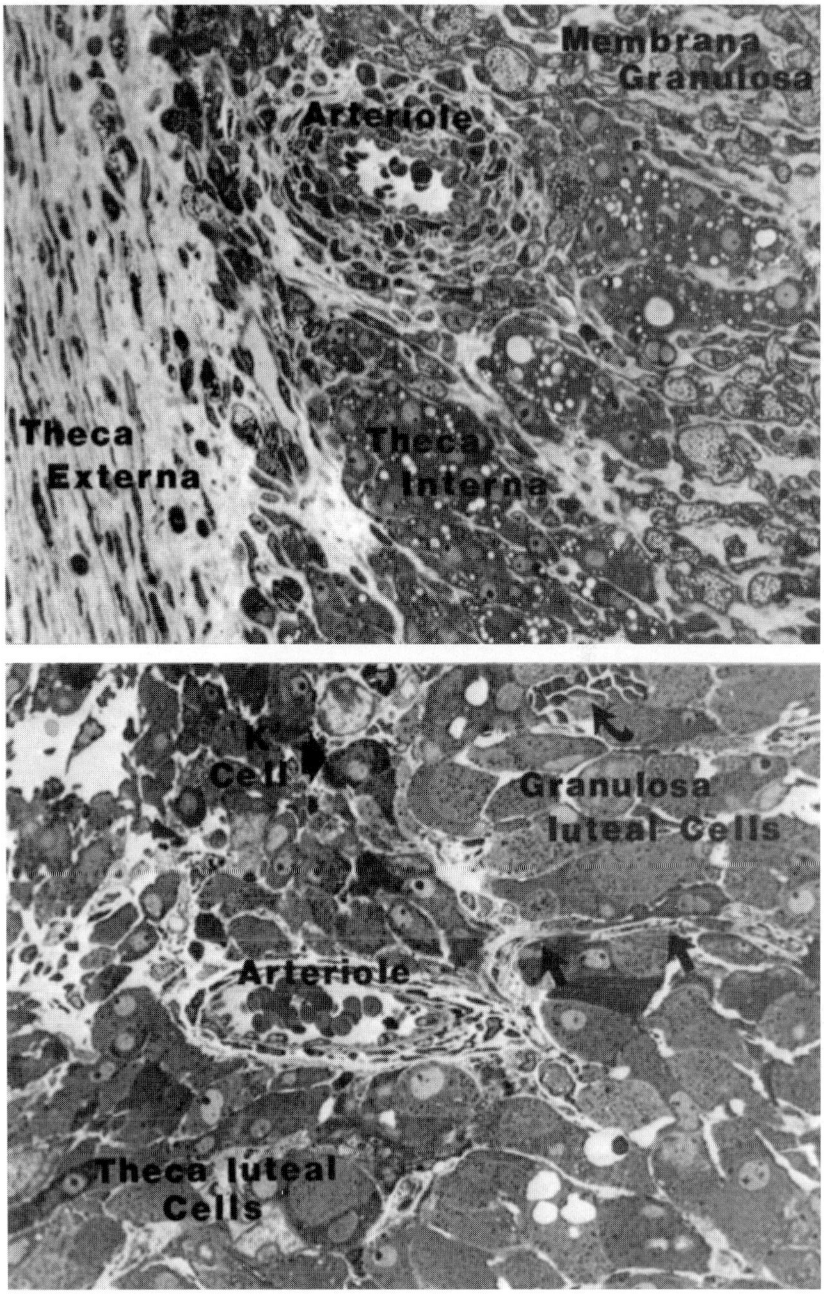

FIGURE 16A-20. Photomicrographs of a section through a human corpus luteum. *(Top)* The three main parts—theca externa, theca lutein, and granulosa lutein—are readily distinguished from one another. *(Bottom)* Larger pale granulosa-lutein cells readily distinguished from smaller (light and dark) theca lutein cells. Note intimate relationship between the K cell (macrophage) and luteal cells. (*Courtesy of Dr. Tom Crisp, by permission of CV Mosby.*)

depends on the presence of a special collection of enzymes termed *mixed-function oxidases*. These enzymes are involved in a variety of oxidation-reduction reactions and require an NADPH-generating system and an oxygen transport system involving cytochrome P450. Recently, researchers have isolated, cloned, and sequenced the genes which encode the human cytochrome P450 enzymes responsible for ovarian steroidogenesis.[48] Therefore, it is now possible to study physiologic and pathologic aspects of their expression at the molecular level.

An important concept in ovarian physiology is that steroidogenic enzymes are distributed throughout the endocrine compartments in a tissue specific manner. The basis for this is the selective transcription of genes which code for specific steroid-metabolizing enzymes. By virtue of differential gene activities, the various steroidogenic cells in the ovary respond to ligands with increases and/or decreases in selective classes of steroid hormones. Consequently, luteal cells secrete primarily C_{21} progestins and interstitial cells preferentially produce C_{19} androgens. Importantly, the capacity to produce C_{18} estrogens de novo does not exist in any one cell type. Rather, ovarian aromatase enzymes are selectively expressed in the granulosa and granulosa-lutein cells.

Cholesterol Substrate

All steroids are derived from cholesterol. Normally, three systems operate to provide a steroidogenic cell with cholesterol: (1) de novo synthesis from acetate, (2) mobilization from intracellular lipid droplets, (3) liberation from low-density lipoprotein (LDL). Under normal physiologic conditions, the de novo synthesis of cholesterol provides little substrate for steroid hormone production by the ovary. Similarly, the storage pool of cholesterol esters

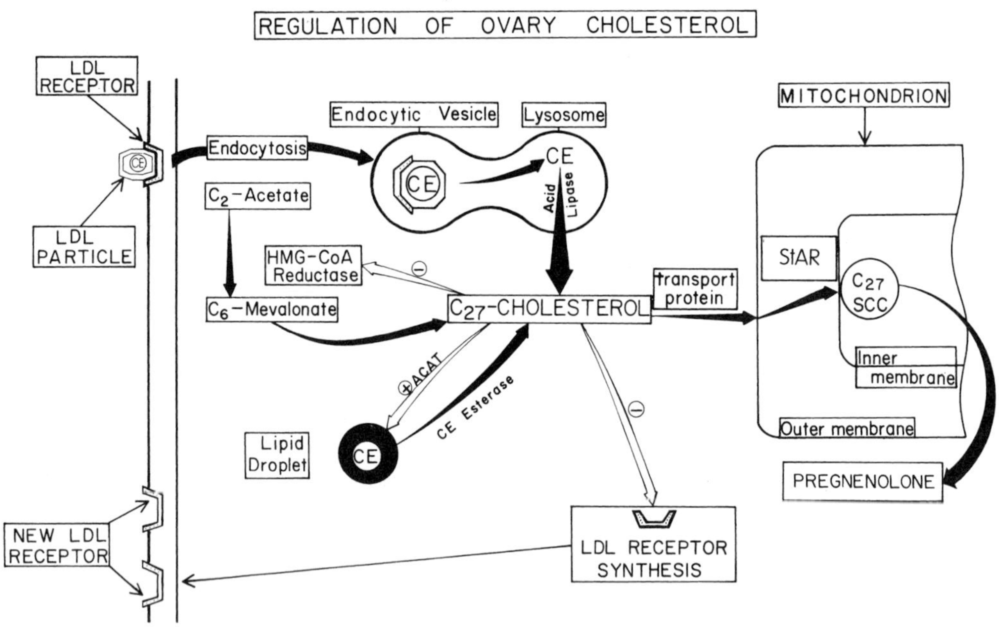

FIGURE 16A-21. Diagram showing the ovarian cellular responses to cholesterol with respect to steroidogenesis.

in the lipid droplets is not a primary source of cholesterol under normal conditions.[49] The most important source of cholesterol used for steroid biosynthesis is the cholesterol liberated from LDL.[49] As can be seen in Fig. 16A-21, the process begins with the binding of LDL to a high-affinity receptor site and the subsequent internalization of the receptor-LDL particle in the form of a coated or endocytic vesicle.[50,51] This is followed by the delivery of the endocytic vesicle to a lysosome, where the LDL particle is hydrolyzed to amino acids by proteinases and the cholesterol esters are cleaved by an acid lipase to generate free cholesterol, which leaves the lysosome for use in cellular reactions.[51]

The cholesterol which is liberated from LDL initiates a set of three feedback control mechanisms within the steroidogenic cell (Fig. 16A-21). First, liberated cholesterol turns off de novo cholesterol synthesis from acetate by inhibiting 3-hydroxy-3-methylglutaryl coenzyme A reductase, which is the rate-controlling enzyme in cholesterol biosynthesis. Second, the LDL-derived cholesterol stimulates the enzyme acyl CoA:cholesterol acyltransferase, which reesterifies excess cholesterol and stores it as cholesterol ester lipid droplets. Third, the incoming cholesterol inhibits the synthesis of new LDL receptors, preventing the entry of LDL and the overaccumulation of cholesterol.

Intracellular Cholesterol Transport

The rate-limiting step in the conversion of cholesterol to steroid hormones is the transfer of the liberated cholesterol into the mitochondrion, where the cholesterol side-chain cleavage enzyme ($P450_{C22}$) is located.[52] It has been proposed that this process involves activation of the cytoskeletal systems (microfilaments and microtubules) by a cyclic AMP (cAMP)-protein A kinase-dependent mechanism.[49] As a consequence of this putative transport system, free cholesterol accumulates in the outer membrane of the mitochondrion (Fig. 16A-21). Here, movement from the outer into the inner mitochondrial membrane, where the cholesterol side-chain cleavage enzyme is located, depends on a labile protein termed *StAR* (steroid acute regulatory protein).[53,54]

Cholesterol Side-Chain Cleavage

The enzyme which is responsible for converting free cholesterol to pregnenolone (the initial step in steroidogenesis) is located at the inner mitochondrial membrane (Figs. 16A-21 and 16A-22). In this enzyme complex, cytochrome $P450_{C22}$ is a terminal oxidase of the mitochondrial electron transport system, which consists of a flavoprotein and an iron-sulfur protein which transports electrons from NADPH to O_2.[52] The consequence of the side-chain cleavage is the transformation of C_{27} cholesterol to C_{21} pregnenolone and a 6-carbon fragment called *isocaproic acid.*

Metabolism of Steroid Hormones

Pregnenolone is the precursor to all steroid hormones. Once formed, pregnenolone is rapidly converted to the biologically active hormone progesterone through the action of Δ^5-3β-ol dehydrogenase-$\Delta^{4,5}$-isomerase.[55] This enzyme is located within the outer mitochondrial membrane and in the smooth endoplasmic reticulum of steroid-secreting cells.[56] The main pathway of steroid synthesis in the human ovary is the Δ^4 pathway, which involves the conversion of progesterone to various C_{19} and C_{18} steroids. The cytochrome $P450_{C22}$, $P450_{C17}$, and P450 aromatase enzymes in the Δ^4 pathway are involved principally with the stepwise removal of carbon atoms from the C_{21} skeleton of progesterone. The formation of C_{19} androgens involves the enzyme $P450_{C17}$, which contains both 17α-hydroxylase and 17,20-lyase activities.[48] The $P450_{C17}$ is located in the smooth endoplasmic reticulum and is responsible for cleavage of the side chain of progesterone to yield Δ^4-androstenedione. In the ovary, the $P450_{C17}$ is selectively expressed in the interstitial cells, including the theca lutein cells (Fig. 16A-15). Importantly, granulosa cells do not contain these enzymes and therefore are unable to convert progesterone to androstenedione (Fig. 16A-15).

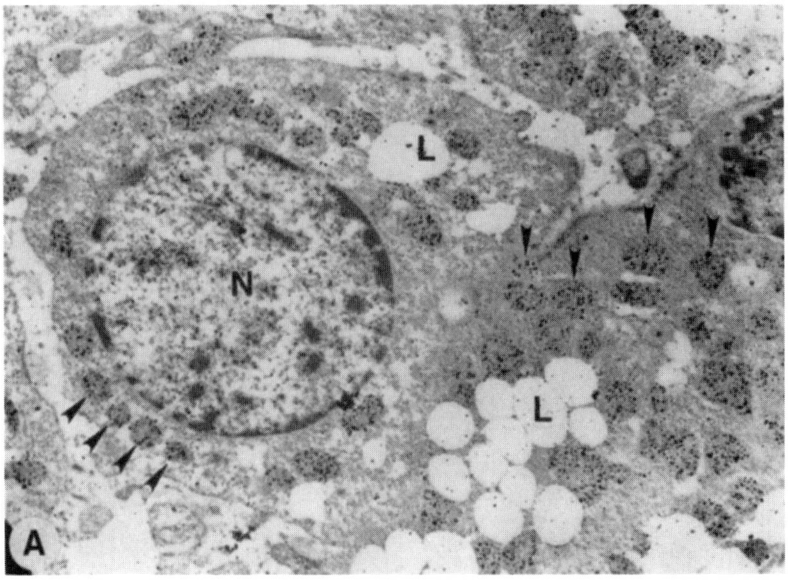

FIGURE 16A-22. Localization of $P450_{scc}$ in mitochondria by staining with immunogold. Colloidal gold particles are specifically located in the mitochondria (arrowheads). N-nucleus; L-lipid droplets. *(Courtesy of Dr. Yosi Orly.)*

The degree to which androstenedione is further metabolized depends on the ovarian cell type. The hilus cells, for example, contain the enzyme 17β-hydroxysteroid dehydrogenase, type I, which converts androstenedione to testosterone.[57] This enzyme is also present in granulosa cells,[58] where it converts androstenedione to testosterone and estrone to estradiol. In the ovary, one of the most important steps in androstenedione metabolism is its conversion to estrogen via a 19-hydroxylase-aromatase enzyme complex, P450 aromatase.[59] This enzyme, which holds the key to much that is characteristic of the female, is found in the granulosa and granulosa lutein cells.[60] The presence of the aromatase leads to the removal of the angular carbon between rings A and B, followed by the aromatization of the A ring of the C_{18} steroid. Finally, the interstitial cells contain a 5α-reductase (NADPH: $\Delta^{4\text{-}3}$-ketosteroid-5α-reductase), which can convert ring A metabolites to 5α-reduced steroids.[61] The 5α-reductase is potentially an important enzyme because (1) the 5α-reduced steroids [such as dihydrotestosterone (DHT)] are potent androgens and because (2) they are competitive inhibitors of the aromatase.[62] Thus, they may play a role in inhibiting estradiol production.

Gonadotropin Control

The control mechanisms governing de novo steroid synthesis in the ovary are almost exclusively regulated by LH and human chorionic gonadotropin (hCG). The ability of LH to stimulate de novo steroidogenesis involves both acute and long-acting mechanisms. The acute effects of LH occur within minutes and involve a G-protein-linked receptor-signaling, A-kinase mechanism followed by phosphorylation of regulatory proteins. The rate-determining step in ovarian steroid biosynthesis is the conversion of cholesterol to pregnenolone by $P450_{C22}$.[52] LH, through its second message, cAMP, causes dramatic and rapid increases in the capacity of $P450_{C22}$ to convert cholesterol to pregnenolone. The underlying control mechanism involves LH-induced increases in the amount of cholesterol which is specifically bound to $P450_{C22}$.[52] The mechanism involves LH-dependent increases in the amount or/and activity of StAR (Fig. 16A-21). Thus, the basis of the immediate effect of LH on steroidogenesis seems to be a rapid delivery of cholesterol to $P450_{C22}$.

The long-term effect of LH on steroidogenesis involves the increased expression of the genes encoding steroid-metabolizing enzymes.[63] Specifically, LH stimulates the synthesis of $P450_{C22}$, 3β-HSD, and $P450_{C17}$. Consequently, the long-term control of steroidogenesis by LH occurs at a rate which is governed by the rate of the synthesis of new enzyme molecules. Although the relation between FSH and de novo steroidogenesis is minimal, FSH plays a central role in regulating ovarian estrogen formation by virtue of its control of the activities of ovarian P450 aromatase and 17β-HSD type I.[64,65] In this sense, FSH is most important in controlling immediate and long-term estrogen responses in the ovary.

OVARIAN CYTODIFFERENTIATION: UNDERLYING CONTROL MECHANISMS

The changing morphologic pattern of the developing follicle and corpus luteum is accompanied by dramatic biochemical changes that reflect continuing processes of cellular differentiation. The underlying basis for this differentiation is the acquisition of specific cell surface and intracellular receptors which provide cells with the ability to respond in a specific way to various ligands, such as the hormones (amino acid derivatives, peptides, and steroid derivatives) and the growth factors. The expression of the receptors occurs in a highly predictable manner and involves both intraovarian and extraovarian mechanisms. In essence, the continued transformation of cells from the undifferentiated state to the fully differentiated state or the activation of the apoptotic pathway is the underlying principle of ovarian physiology.[6,10,63,66]

The Granulosa Cell

Cytodifferentiation

The differentiation of a granulosa cell begins in the primordial follicle when it is recruited to initiate growth. After being committed to the granulosa pathway, these morphologically unspecialized

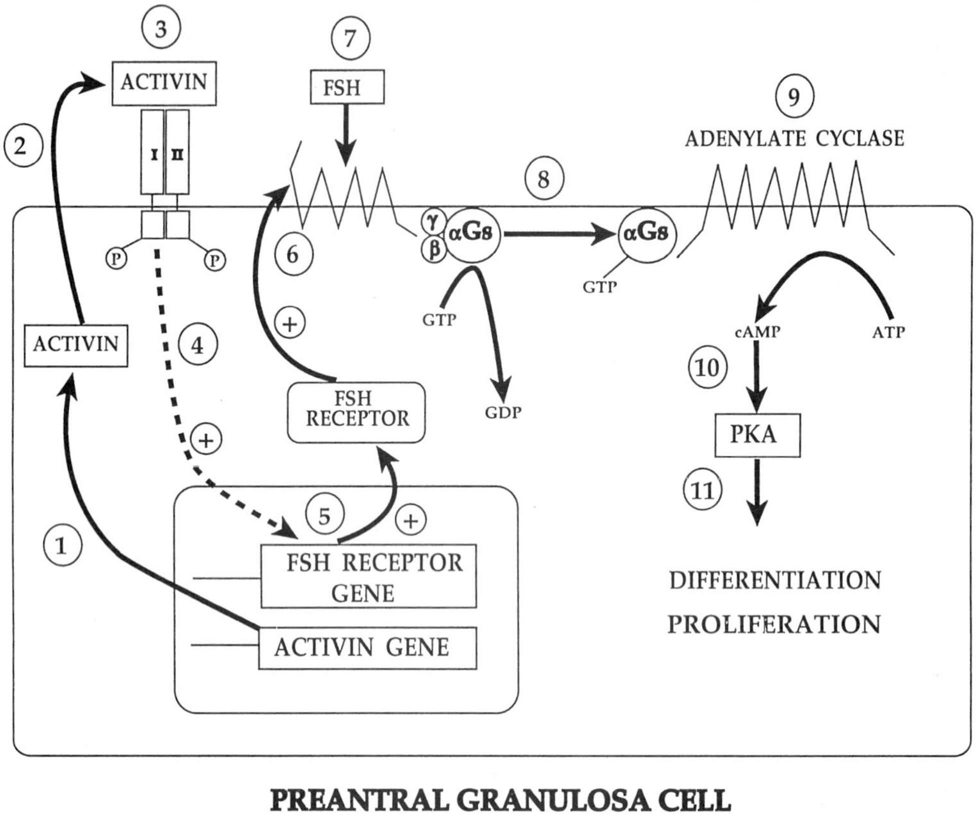

FIGURE 16A-23. The activin autocrine hypothesis for the induction of FSH receptors in the granulosa cells. 1) the activin genes turned on; 2,3) activin ligand binds to cell surface activin receptors; 4,5) activin receptor signaling leads to activation of FSH receptor gene expression; 6,7) FSH receptors integrated into plasma membrane; 8–10) FSH ligand can interreact with FSH receptor to activate signaling pathways that lead to mitosis and differentiation. (*Redrawn from Erickson GF: Dissociation of endocrine and gametogenic ovarian function, in Lobo R (ed): Perimenopause. Serono Symposia Springer-Verlag, New York, 1997, pp 101–118 with permission.*)

cells start to proliferate and produce new cells whose subsequent differentiation is under hormonal control. Granulosa cytodifferentiation can conveniently be divided into four levels which parallel follicular morphology (Fig. 16A-3).

First Level

Only when a primordial follicle is recruited does granulosa cytodifferentiation begin. After changing from a squamous to a cuboidal shape, the granulosa cells are shifted into mitosis.[67] This transition is accompanied by the acquisition of FSH receptors.[68–70] Therefore, one of the first steps in granulosa differentiation occurs in primary follicles and involves the expression of the gene encoding the FSH receptor. There is evidence in rodents to suggest that the basis of FSH receptor induction involves the local production of activin by the granulosa cell[71] (Fig. 16A-23). It can be concluded, therefore, that the first level of granulosa cytodifferentiation involves a shape change from squamous to cuboidal which in turn results in mitosis which in turn results in the induction of FSH receptors. The acquisition of FSH receptors is one of the most important developmental events in folliculogenesis.

Second Level

When a rat follicle reaches the secondary or early tertiary stage, the granulosa cells reach a second level of differentiation. The second transition is accompanied by the acquisition of intracellular receptors for key steroid hormones, most notably the estrogen (estrogen receptor-β)[72] and androgen.[73] Although the factor responsible for inducing these important changes is unknown, it is FSH-independent. In the rat, this differentiative change is fundamental because the granulosa cells (and thus the follicle) are now competent to react in a specific way to a set of very potent determinative stimuli which can modulate folliculogenesis in a positive or negative manner.

The concept of steroid receptors in the human follicle is still in its infancy. There is evidence that human granulosa cells at the second level of differentiation indeed contain receptors for androgen,[74] but not estrogen.[74–77] This supports a local role of androgens in granulosa cell differentiation in humans. The fact that the 17β-HSD type I is expressed constitutively in human granulosa cells beginning as early as the first level of differentiation,[58,78] supports this view of androgen (perhaps testosterone) receptor mediated cytodifferentiation.

Third Level

Up to this point, granulosa cytodifferentiation occurs independently of the pituitary. This is not the case for its subsequent differentiation, which is completely dependent on pituitary FSH. FSH, which is brought to a tertiary follicle by capillaries in the

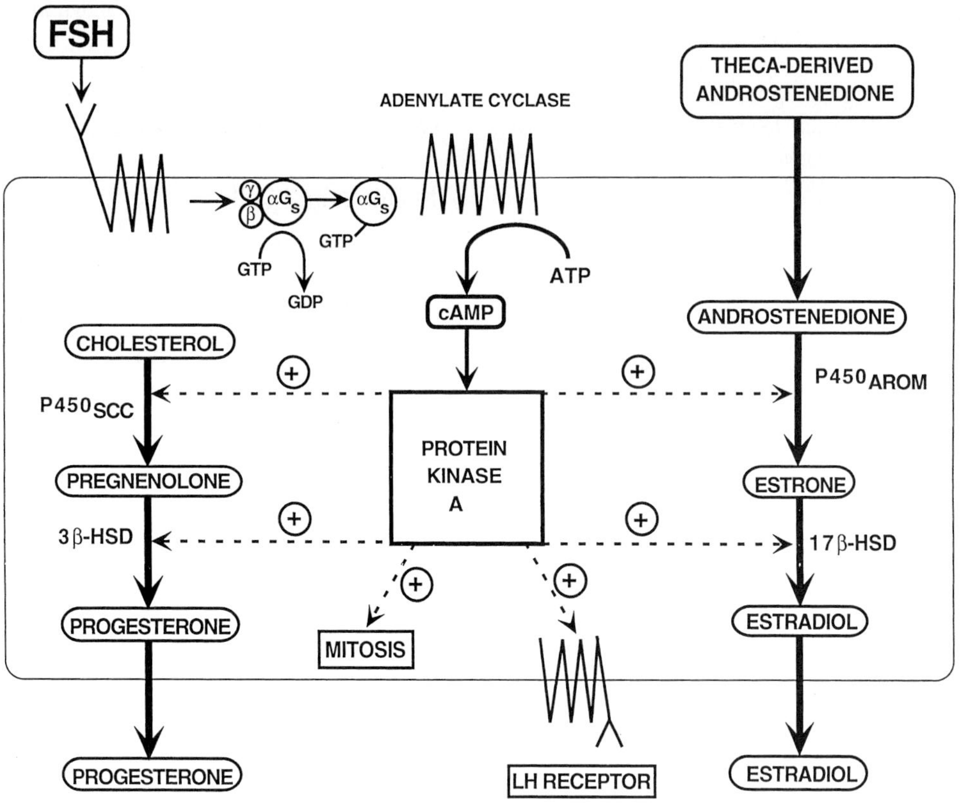

FIGURE 16A-24. Schematic model of FSH signal transduction pathway in granulosa cells of a dominant follicle leading to increased steroidogenic potential, proliferation, and LH receptor expression. (*Redrawn from Erickson GF: Polycystic ovary syndrome: Normal and abnormal steroidogenesis, in Schats R, Schoemaker J (eds): Ovarian Endocrinopathies: Proceedings of the 8th Reinier deGraaf Symposium. Parthenon Publishing, 1994, pp 103–115 with permission.*)

theca interna, crosses the basal lamina, where it binds to the G-protein-linked FSH receptor in the granulosa and stimulates adenylate cyclase (Fig. 16A-24). This causes an increase in cAMP which binds to the cAMP-dependent protein A kinases and causes phosphorylation of regulatory proteins. In this context, estrogen in the rat plays a permissive role in amplifying FSH action by facilitating FSH-stimulated cAMP formation in rat granulosa cells. This action of estrogen is particularly important in the rat because it increases the sensitivity of the granulosa cell to FSH. Because there does not appear to be estrogen receptor in the human granulosa cells at this early stage of folliculogenesis, it would seem that this autocrine concept may not apply to the human. However, the potential role for androgen is the action of FSH in human granulosa cells needs to be explored.

The critical role of FSH in granulosa cytodifferentiation is illustrated by the number of specialized functions which are dependent on FSH stimulation. One of the primary consequences of FSH action is the activation of proliferative cell cycles which lead to increased numbers of granulosa cells. The growth of a tertiary follicle to the ovulatory stage is associated with an increase in the number of granulosa cells from about 1×10^4 to over 50×10^6 cells.[22,67] It is clear that FSH is responsible for the stimulation of mitosis in human granulosa cells.[22,67] Whether this effect is direct or is controlled indirectly by the production of regulatory molecules such as growth factors is unknown. Two growth factors—basic fibroblast growth factor (bFGF) and epidermal growth factor (EGF)—have been shown to stimulate mitosis in human granulosa cells in vitro.[79] Based on such evidence, one explanation for the FSH stimulation of mitosis is that it results from the local production of EGF and/or bFGF. It is clear that further studies are needed to elucidate the regulators that control mitosis in human granulosa cells.

FSH interaction can also cause the granulosa cells to express $P450_{AROM}$. This regulatory process is fundamentally important for the development of the estrogen-synthetic activities of the follicle and thus the homeostatic activities of the female. It appears that FSH stimulation of its G-protein-linked receptor activates the adenylate cyclase-cAMP-A kinase cascade. This results in the phosphorylation of key regulatory peptides, leading to the activation of the transcription of the gene encoding $P450_{AROM}$ (Fig. 16A-24). This positive regulatory effect of FSH on $P450_{AROM}$ activity is time and dose dependent; it increases progressively as a function of both follicle growth and the stage in the follicular phase of the menstrual cycle,[62,65] importantly being restricted to the granulosa cells in the dominant follicle.[60,80]

Fourth Level

During the fourth level, the granulosa cells in the dominant follicle develop LH receptors,[68] estrogen receptor β receptors,[75,77] and receptors for progesterone.[75] In vitro experiments with monkey granulosa cells have shown that FSH regulates the induction of LH receptors.[81] The LH receptors are members of the

G-protein-linked receptor family which can stimulate the effector adenylate cyclase.[82] It is significant that when granulosa cells develop LH receptors, they become competent to respond to the LH that enters the follicular fluid during the late follicular phase.[83] Thus, it is possible that LH in the dominant follicle becomes a regulator of granulosa cell differentiation during the period when FSH levels in the blood are declining.

It is clear from this discussion that FSH plays a crirical role in controlling the differentiation processes that occur in granulosa cells during the growth and development of a primary follicle to the preovulatory stage; however it is clear from animal studies that other ligands, such as estrogen and androgen, can modulate the FSH effect. In this regard, it should be noted that once granulosa cytodifferentiation has been initiated by FSH, the cells become completely dependent on FSH for their survival. In this context, FSH withdrawal results in the loss of all available receptors and aromatase enzymes, followed by cell death by atresia. Therefore, FSH is critical for the life of any granulosa cell that it has activated.

Granulosa Heterogeneity

In developing Graafian follicles, every granulosa cell contains FSH receptors.[68,69] Surprisingly, however, groups of differentiating granulosa cells respond to FSH differently. For example, when challenged by FSH, the LH receptor and aromatase enzymes are selectively induced in the membrana granulosa cells (Fig. 16A-12). These data indicate that the granulosa cells are not a simple equipotent tissue, even though they all have FSH receptors. In this view, the position of the granulosa cell within the follicle determines which way it will differentiate in response to FSH stimulation. Interestingly, it seems that this process is determined by regulatory factors secreted by the oocyte.[84]

The Interstitial Cells

Androgens produced by interstitial cells are involved in both constructive and destructive processes in the ovary.[10] Follicular estradiol formation is causally linked to androgens produced by interstitial cells. This contrasts with other evidence that androgens arising from interstitial cells can induce apoptosis and destruction of granulosa cells and ova through atresia.[10,26] Consequently, changes in interstitial androgen production could affect the direction of folliculogenesis and thus may have important consequences for the reproductive state of the female.

The most important stimulating force in interstitial androgen production is LH.[85] All interstitial cells are competent to react to LH (or hCG) by way of G-protein-linked LH receptors in the plasma membrane (Fig. 16A-25). When LH binds to its receptor, there is an allosteric change which causes the LH-receptor complex to interact with G-proteins. This results in the release of the G-stimulatory protein, which then activates adenylate cyclase, which converts ATP to the second messenger, cAMP; the cAMP binds to the regulatory subunit of A kinase, which then allows the catalytic subunits of protein kinase A to phosphorylate the serine

FIGURE 16A-25. Diagram of a differentiated theca interstitial cell showing the expression of key components in the LH receptor signal transduction pathway leading to androstenedione biosynthesis. (*From Erickson GF,*[85] *from Lippincott-Raven Publishers with permission.*)

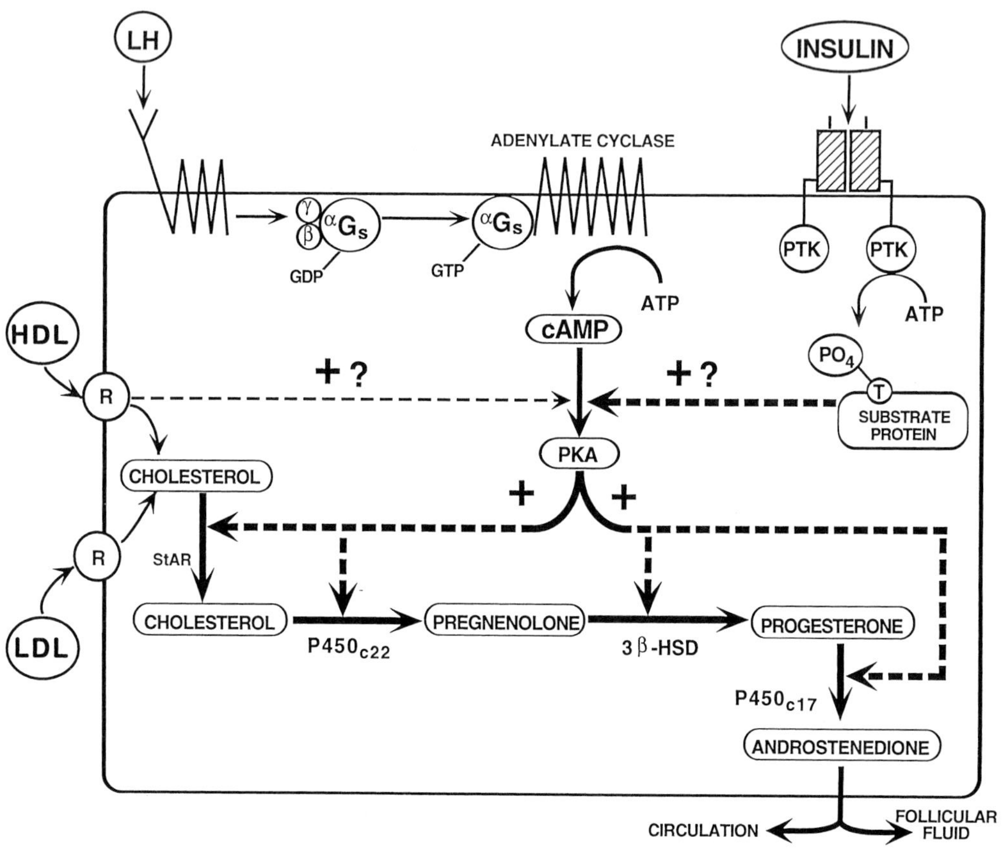

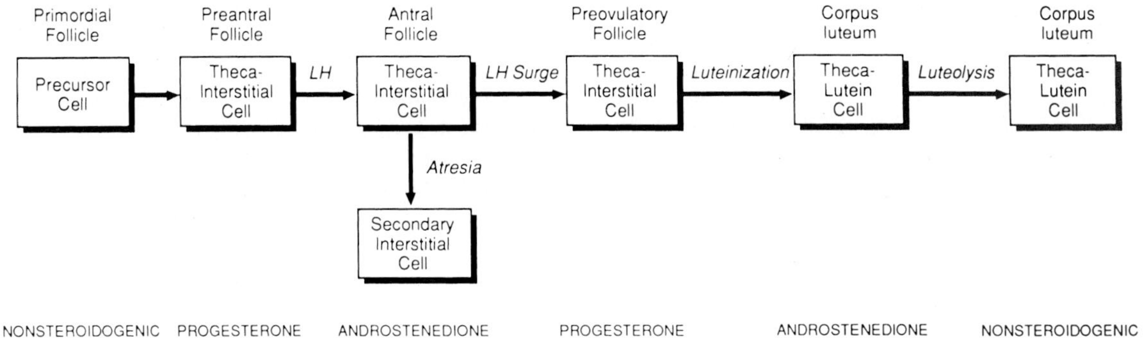

FIGURE 16A-26. Diagram of the steroidogenic changes in the human theca interstitial cells throughout their life cycle.

and threonine residues of regulatory proteins (Fig. 16A-25). This cascade then results in the transcription of genes which encode the genes involved in de novo steroidogenesis including StAR, $P450_{C22}$, 3β-HSD, and $P450_{C17}$.[85] In this regard, theca interstitial cells in preantral follicles express $P450_{C22}$ but not $P450_{C17}$. This indicates that during the first stages of differentiation, the theca cells are primarily progesterone-producing cells (Fig. 16A-26). The failure of theca interstitial cells to produce androgens during early folliculogenesis could ensure that none of the developing preantral follicles dies by atresia. Once antrum formation occurs, an unknown mechanism causes the expression of the $P450_{C17}$ in the theca cells, thus switching them into androgen-producing cell (Fig. 16A-25). The development of $P450_{C17}$ ensures that aromatase substrate is produced by the cohort of Graafian follicles. Interestingly, after the surge of LH at midcycle, the theca cells once again lose $P450_{C17}$ and become primarily a progestin-producing tissue during ovulation (Fig. 16A-25). Then, as the process of luteinization occurs, the theca interstitial cells (now called theca lutein cells) reexpress $P450_{C17}$ activity and once again produce C_{19} androgens (Fig. 16A-25). Thus, the concept that differentiating theca interstitial cells switch back and forth between progesterone- and androgen-producing cells during their life cycle is clearly established.[85] We will return to the physiologic significance of this concept later. It should be noted that other ligands including insulin and lipoproteins (Fig. 16A-25), are potent stimulators of theca progesterone and androgen biosynthesis.[32,85,86]

The Corpus Luteum

Corpus luteum differentiation is typically divided into two periods. It begins in response to the preovulatory surge of gonadotropins by the process called luteinization. After maximal differentiated function is reached at the end of 1 week (day 21 to day 22 of the cycle), the corpus luteum normally undergoes degeneration by the process of luteolysis. What are the primary events leading to luteinization and luteolysis?

Luteinization

Much of what is known about the control of the human corpus luteum has come from studies of hormone levels in peripheral and ovarian venous blood and follicular fluid.[22,87–89] Collectively, the evidence indicates that luteal differentiation is associated with a biphasic secretion of ovarian regulatory steroids, namely, progesterone, 17α-hydroxyprogesterone, androstenedione, and estradiol. This conclusion has been corroborated by in vitro experiments with isolated corpus luteum tissue.[90,91] The concept which emerges is that the biphasic production of a steroid in the corpus luteum is causally connected with biphasic changes of activities of the regulatory steroidogenic enzymes in the Δ^4 pathway, namely, $P450_{C22}$, 3β-SDH, $P450_{C17}$, and $P450_{AROM}$.

What agents are responsible for biphasic changes in corpus luteum steroidogenic enzymes? The fundamental regulator in promoting and maintaining the life of a corpus luteum is LH. LH is the inducer of luteinization, and low levels of LH are critical for maintaining active luteal tissue during the early and midluteal phases.[92] Importantly, hCG produced by the blastocyst can prevent luteolysis and promote further increases in corpus luteum activity; however, this effect is only temporary.[92] The conclusion can therefore be reached that induction and maintenance of the differentiated state of the corpus luteum are controlled directly by LH/hCG, but other regulatory molecules appear to be involved including blood cells and cytokines.[93]

Considering the fact that LH/hCG action is mediated by receptors, the question of the factors involved in changes in the corpus luteum becomes intimately connected with how the LH receptor signaling is controlled in luteal cells. LH receptors in developing human corpora lutea undergo a predictable pattern of activity. As ovulation approaches, a striking decrease in the LH receptor number occurs in granulosa cells, while during the early luteal phase, the LH receptor number increases sharply, reaching a nearly maximal level in the midluteal phase, where it remains until the end of the cycle.[94–97] It thus can be concluded that the LH receptor is first desensitized and down regulated and then reinduced during the process of luteinization.[97–99]

Since reinduction of LH receptor renders the corpus luteum responsive to hCG secreted by the blastocyst, an important question is how the LH receptor is reinduced in luteal cells. In vitro studies with human granulosa luteal cells have shown that the recovery of LH/hCG sensitivity is due to the reinduction of functional LH/hCG receptors in the plasma membrane; significantly, this process is regulated by LH itself.[100] This is an important question clinically because foremost among the characteristics of luteal-phase defects in women is the inability of the corpus luteum to respond appropriately to LH/hCG.[101–103] This defect may be caused by inappropriate formation of new LH/hCG receptors.

The physiologic importance of LH/hCG in regulating progesterone secretion by the human corpus luteum has been clearly established. FSH itself does not appear to stimulate progesterone biosynthesis during luteinization in women. In vitro[104,105] and in vivo[106] studies have demonstrated that progesterone levels are not increased in response to purified FSH during the early, middle, or late luteal phase of the menstrual cycle. This supports the possibility that FSH may not play a physiologic role in controlling progesterone production by the human corpus luteum. Importantly, however, FSH has a high capacity for stimulating estradiol formation by human copora luteal cells in vivo[107] and in vitro.[108] Hence, the physiologic actions of FSH in luteinization seem to promote estradiol rather than progesterone synthesis. It is important that LH/hCG can also stimulate estradiol production.[107] Therefore, by comparison to FSH, the LH/hCG signaling pathway in human granulosa-lutein cells is capable of stimulating both estradiol and progesterone synthesis.

Luteolysis

At the time of luteolysis, a programmed cell death mechanism (apoptosis) is initiated which leads to the destruction of the corpus luteum approximately 5 to 7 days later.[46] Once this mechanism has been initiated, there is a sharp decrease in progesterone production, an event which is unfavorable to pregnancy. What is the mechanism of luteolysis? The answer to this fundamental question is uncertain, but evidence suggests that aromatase activity may be particularly important. Aromatase activity in the corpus luteum increases prior to luteolysis, and the concentration of estrogen in the corpus luteum reaches a peak at that time.[95,104,108] Can the two processes—a decrease in progesterone production and an increase in aromatase activity, be causally linked in luteolysis? In women, injection of estrogen directly into the ovary causes an early onset of menstrual bleeding.[109] Furthermore, treatment with exogenous estrogen inhibits progesterone production by human corpus luteum cells in vitro.[110,111] The site of estrogen action seems to be directly at the level of Δ^4-3β-HDH$\Delta^{4,5}$-isomerase.[112] Consequently, the conclusion may be drawn that estradiol is an important luteolytic agent in humans.

With this concept in mind, a very important question in the differentiation of the corpus luteum concerns the underlying mechanisms for controlling estrogen biosynthesis. The mechanism that controls estrogen formation could act directly at the $P450_{AROM}$ and/or at the level of androgen substrate production. As was noted above, LH/hCG can increase estrogen and progesterone secretion in human corpora lutea while FSH selectively stimulates estrogen but not progesterone production. The picture that emerges is that FSH and LH may be responsible for progressive increases in corpora lutea aromatase activity and progesterone levels, respectively, during the differentiation of the corpus luteum in the early to midluteal phases.

In this context, clomiphene acts directly on the human placenta to decrease progesterone production while increasing 17-hydroxyprogesterone, androstenedione, and estradiol production.[113] How clomiphene exerts this action is unknown, but clomiphene can increase the aromatization of testosterone to estradiol. With respect to luteolysis, the induction of aromatase activity by clomiphene may result in increased concentrations of cellular estrogen, which then enters into the process of luteolysis. This scenario could have important implications for the way in which clomiphene induces luteal defects in women.

To what extent is luteal cytodifferentiation determined by interactions with modulators? It seems clear that LH, FSH, and hCG are the principal positive regulators of corpus luteum differentiation. Several putative hormone modulators of human corpus luteum function have been identified, including prolactin, gonadotropin releasing hormone (GnRH), $PGF_{2\alpha}$, estradiol, and oxytocin.

In human granulosa cells which are undergoing luteinization in vitro, prolactin can inhibit LH/FSH-stimulated progesterone production and prolactin inhibits basal and gonadotropin-stimulated progesterone and estrogen secretion by human ovaries in vitro.[114] By contrast, experiments with human corpus luteum cells have failed to find consistent direct effects of prolactin on hCG-stimulated progesterone production, although prolactin was found to modulate hCG-stimulated estrogen formation.[115] Despite great clinical interest, the consequences of prolactin action on the human corpus luteum remain unsolved.

As with prolactin, a direct effect of GnRH on human ovarian cells is equivocal. Evidence suggests that human corpora lutea do not have high-affinity GnRH receptors[116] and that GnRH does not influence steroidogenesis by human corpus luteum cells in vitro.[117] It was reported that GnRH inhibits granulosa luteinization in culture,[118] but this was not subsequently confirmed.[119] The question of whether GnRH can modulate the differentiation of human corpus luteum cells is still controversial. It is notable that a GnRH-like molecule has been found in the human ovary, raising the possibility that this protein mediates antigonadotropic responses during the luteal phase of the menstrual cycle.[120]

In some animals $PGF_{2\alpha}$ directly inhibits progesterone production by the corpus luteum and therefore has been termed a physiologic luteolysin. In human corpora lutea, $PGF_{2\alpha}$ receptors have been reported[121] and luteal cells have the synthetic capability of producing PGs.[121] Again, despite considerable clinical interest, definitive evidence that $PGF_{2\alpha}$ is a physiologic modulator in human luteal cytodifferentiation is lacking.

As was stated earlier, there is evidence that estradiol and oxytocin act directly on human corpus luteum cells to block LH/hCG activation of progesterone synthesis. Thus, the concept is emerging that the differentiation of the human corpus luteum (like that of the granulosa and interstitial cells) is controlled by positive and negative ligands, some of which are themselves the products of the corpus luteum.

The Oocyte

Primordial Germ Cells

The eggs within the ovary are derived from primordial germ cells (PGCs). These cells, which are set aside very early in embryonic development, arise in the yolk sac endoderm, far from the eventual site of gonad formation. In humans, PGCs can be selectively identified histochemically by virtue of an alkaline phosphatase which is located in their plasma membrane.[122] It is known that from their location in the hindgut they migrate through the dorsal mesentery and into the gonadal ridges; PGCs migrate to the gonad by ameboid movement, presumably via chemotaxis.[123]

When PGCs enter the female genital ridge, they migrate toward the germinal epithelium and are incorporated into cortical cords.[123] Coincident with the colonization of the gonad by PGCs, epithelial cells from mesonephric tubules migrate into the genital area, where they probably become the granulosa and interstitial cells.[124] The conclusion, therefore, is that all the cellular components of the follicle (oocyte, granulosa, theca) originate outside the gonad itself.[123,124]

Oogonia

In the PGCs, only one X chromosome in an XX female is expressed; however, once PGCs enter the presumptive ovary, both X chromosomes are expressed and the germ cells are now called *oogonia*.[125] Subsequently, oogonia initiate an active phase of proliferation, and their number increases tremendously. As the oogonia proliferate, there are dramatic increases in the activity of enzymes which are encoded by genes on the X chromosome. The importance of the expression of twice the gene product in developing female germ cells is emphasized by the fact that XO genetic females exhibit oocyte depletion and sterility.[126] The oogonium is unique in that it is the only cell in which both X chromosomes are active.

As mitosis proceeds and cortical cord growth continues, the dividing oogonia fail to complete cytokinesis. Consequently, subpopulations of oogonia remain joined together by intercellular bridges,[127] and their differentiation then proceeds synchronously in a way resembling germ cell differentiation in the testis.

Oocytes

Beginning at 12 weeks gestation,[11] some of the connected oogonia (those in the deepest regions of the cortical cords nearest the medullary tissue) initiate meiosis (Fig. 16A-4). There is evidence that the mesonephric system is important in triggering the initiation of meiosis in the oocytes and their subsequent incorporation into primordial follicles.[128] In response to the putative meiosis-inducing substance, subgroups of oogonia initiate meiotic DNA synthesis and begin to proceed through leptotene, zygotene, pachytene, and diplotene stages of meiotic prophase (Fig. 16A-4). At the diplotene, the paired homologous chromosomes become less condensed and the oocyte enters a protracted interphase-like stage called the *dictyotene*. It is at this time that the oocytes become incorporated into primordial follicles (Fig. 16A-4).[11] At its shortest, an oocyte will remain in this arrested state for about 12 years (until puberty); at its longest, it can last about 50 years (until the menopause).

Oocyte Growth

To understand oogenesis, two interrelated processes must be considered: oocyte growth and completion of meiosis. Oocyte growth is associated with the accumulation and storage of nutritional and informational materials, some of which are critical to the development of the preimplantation blastocyst. During growth the human oocyte increases in diameter from 20 μm to 120 μm. The basis for growth resides in the active transcription of stable messenger RNA, ribosomal RNA, transfer RNA, and heterogeneous RNA by lampbrush chromosomes of the oocyte.[129,130] A fundamental concept is that the growth of the follicle relative to that of the oocyte can be divided into two distinct phases: Initially, oocyte and follicle diameter are positively and linearly correlated until the follicle reaches the early tertiary stage (cavitation); after that, the oocyte ceases to grow while follicular growth continues (Fig. 16A-27).

The presence of granulosa cells is an absolute requirement for mouse oocyte growth.[131,132] As growth progresses, the oocyte is

FIGURE 16A-27. Regression lines showing the relation between the sizes of the oocyte and follicle in the human ovary. (*From Green and Zuckerman,[203] by permission of Cambridge University Press.*)

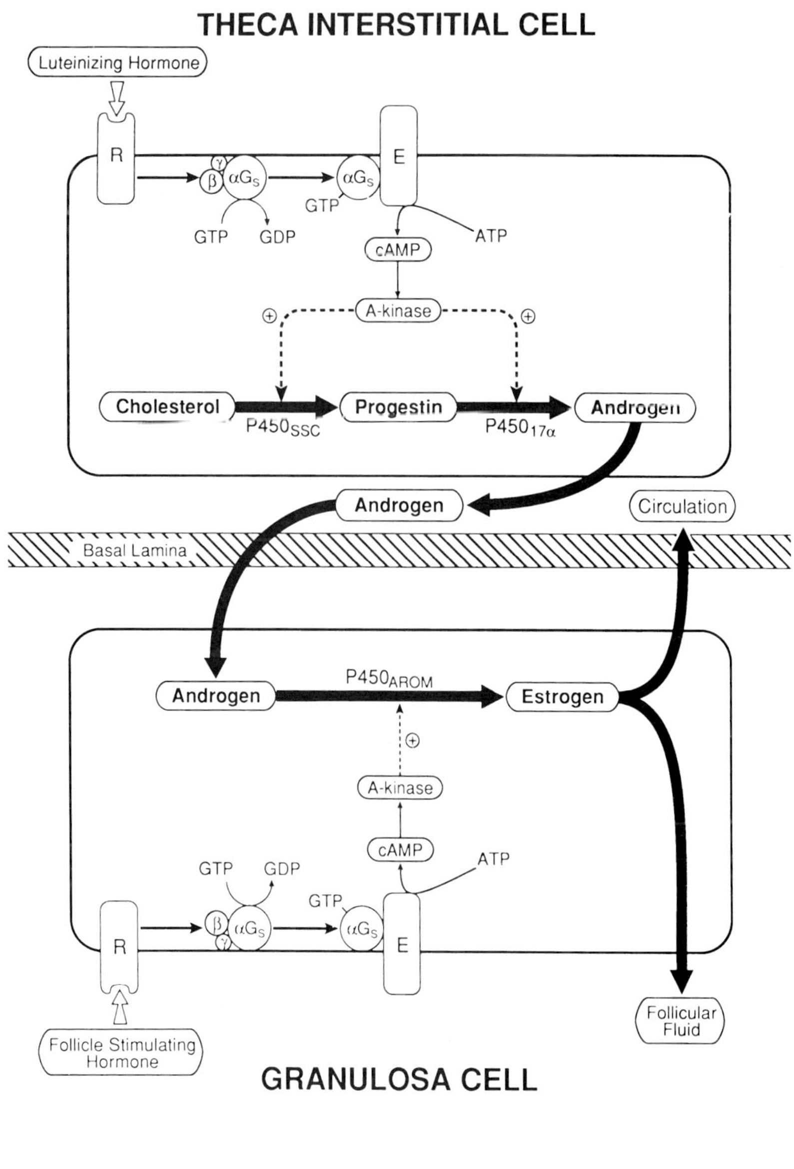

closely surrounded by corona radiata granulosa cells which interact directly with the oocyte via gap junctions and desmosomes. As a result of this metabolic coupling, the oocyte can capitalize on unique nutritional and/or regulatory capacities of granulosa cells. Results obtained with animal species indicate that 85 percent of the metabolites present in follicle-enclosed oocytes are originally taken up by the granulosa cell and then transferred into the oocyte through the gap junctions.[131,132] The concept which emerges is that the obligatory role of granulosa cells in oocyte growth involves special gap junctional contacts which are responsible for the transfer of fundamental nutrients into the oocyte.

During oocyte growth, the zona pellucida is formed. The zona pellucida is a relatively thick, translucent acellular coat which surrounds the oolemma of the fully grown oocyte. The zona pellucida plays an important role in a number of vital biological functions:[133,134] (1) It contains species-specific receptors for capacitated sperm, (2) it provides a block to polyspermy, and (3) it is critical in allowing the embryo to move freely through the fallopian tube into the uterus.

It is apparent that the proteins in the zona pellucida are synthesized and secreted by the growing oocytes.[133,134] The morphologic basis for this event involves multiple replications of the Golgi apparatus and their subsequent migration to the periphery of the oocyte, just beneath the oolemma. The human zona pellucida contains three glycoproteins, designated ZP-1 (molecular mass of ~150 kDa), ZP-2 (molecular mass of ~100 kDa), and ZP-3 (molecular mass of ~55–65 kDa).[135] The physiologic significance of the zona pellucida proteins produced by the egg is emphasized by the fact that they contain the species-specific sperm receptor and initiate the acrosome reaction. The ZP-3 molecule is responsible for these two critical events. Interestingly, however, the sperm receptor for the mouse egg is β-1,4-galactosyltransferase (GalTase) which binds o-linked oligosaccharides on ZP-3.[136] Clinically, there is growing evidence that infertility in some women may be caused by the presence of circulating antibodies to the ZP-3 which block the binding of the sperm to its ZP-3 receptor on the zona pellucida.[137] In this regard, ongoing research is headed toward using ZP-3 as an antigen to develop novel immunologic approaches to contraception.[138–140]

Meiotic Maturation The capacity to resume meiosis is acquired at a specific stage in oocyte growth and differentiation; the ability to complete meiotic maturation is acquired subsequently. Meiotic maturation or resumption of meiosis (Fig. 16A-28) is a process characterized by (1) the dissolution of the nuclear or germinal vesicle membrane, (2) the condensation of dictyotene chromatin into discrete bivalents, (3) the separation of homologous chromosomes, (4) the release of a first polar body, and (5) the arrest of the meiotic process at metaphase II. The completion of meiosis and the release of the second polar body are triggered by fertilization or parthenogenetic activation.

FIGURE 16A-28. Photomicrographs showing the process of meiotic maturation or resumption of meiosis induced by preovulatory surge of LH. (*A*) Germinal vesicle stage of primary (4N) oocyte; (*B*) germinal vesicle breakdown followed by condensation of chromosomes into bivalents; (*C, D*) release of first polar body and arrest of meiotic process at metaphase II of the secondary (2N) oocyte.

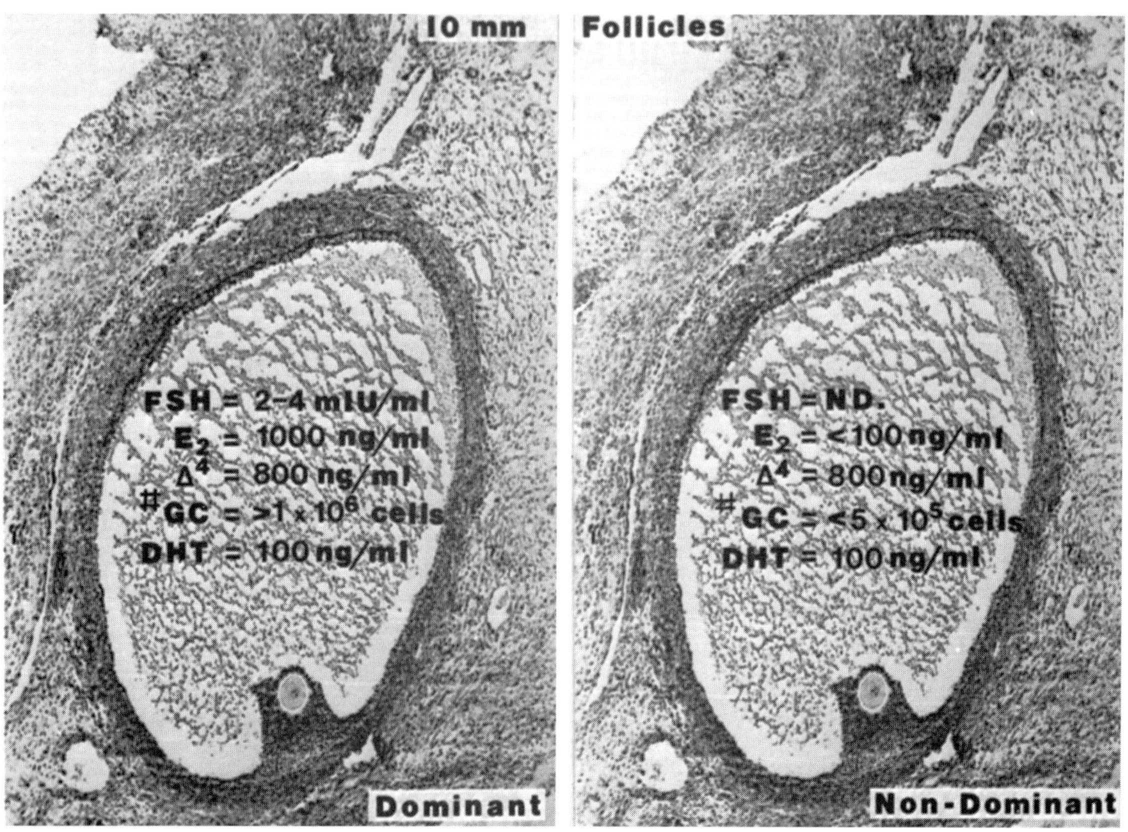

During follicle development, the oocyte acquires the capacity to resume meiosis at or about the time it completes its growth in the preantral follicle. The acquisition of the capacity for meiotic maturation seems to be a two-step process.[141] First, the oocyte acquires the capacity to undergo germinal vesicle breakdown and progress to metaphase I; second, it acquires the capacity to complete the first reductional division and release the first polar body. The mechanisms responsible for the acquisition of meiotic potential are unknown, but they seem to be under intraovarian control. In this connection, it is interesting that isolated mice oocytes which have been allowed to complete their growth in vitro undergo meiotic maturation spontaneously; such eggs can be fertilized in the dish and then give rise to live young when transferred into foster mothers.[142]

Although the oocyte is capable of resuming meiosis early in follicle development, it is kept from doing so by an inhibitory influence. Under normal physiologic conditions, the resumption of meiotic maturation is a highly selective process that occurs only in oocytes which are in dominant preovulatory follicles. There is little doubt that the resumption of meiosis in such oocytes occurs as a result of the preovulatory surge of LH.[143] Interestingly, studies in rodents have demonstrated that EGF[144] and GnRH[145] can induce meiotic maturation. Therefore, the possibility exists that other regulatory molecules play a role in this important process. Based on a large body of data, it is evident that fully grown oocytes from secondary and/or Graafian follicles undergo meiotic maturation spontaneously when the oocyte is placed in tissue culture. Collectively, these observations have led to the hypothesis that there is an inhibiting substance which blocks meiotic maturation in the follicle and that high levels of LH can override the inhibitory influence.

Evidence suggests that granulosa cells supply to the ovum a substance which blocks meiotic maturation.[146] This substance, termed *oocyte meiotic inhibitor* (OMI), is putatively a protein. What is the underlying mechanism by which LH and OMI regulate meiotic maturation? In this concept it is proposed that the membrana granulosa cells secrete OMI into the follicular fluid in response to gonadotropin stimulation. Evidence indicates that OMI does not act directly on the oocyte but exerts its inhibitory influence indirectly through interactions with the cumulus and the corona radiata granulosa cells.[146] It has been proposed that OMI acts as a signal to these cells to stimulate cAMP, which subsequently diffuses through gap junctions into the oocyte, where it suppresses meiotic maturation.[146] When the preovulatory surge of LH occurs, the membrana granulosa becomes desensitized and stops producing OMI. Ultimately, this response leads to decreases in oocyte cAMP levels, followed by a release of intracellular calcium stores and germinal vesicle breakdown (Fig. 16A-29).[147] The nature of the OMI molecule, remains unknown; however, there is evidence that it may be a protein, perhaps müllerian inhibiting substance (MIS)[148] or perhaps the glycoprotein hormone inhibin.[149] However, more work is necessary to prove the nature of physiologic OMI.

An important aspect of this concept concerns the role of steroids in the initiation of meiosis. The best results to date have been obtained in animal species. High concentrations of estradiol are essential for normal cytoplasmic maturation of the oocyte. If there is inadequate estrogen support, meiotic maturation results in abnormalities in fertilization, delayed cleavage, and almost total failure of animal embryos to undergo blastocyst formation.[150] The conclusion is that high levels of estradiol in follicular fluid facilitate the complete differentiation of the egg in vivo and in vitro. The mechanism for this is unknown, but likely involves the estrogen receptor-β in the granulosa cells.

FOLLICLE DEVELOPMENT: CONTROL MECHANISMS

Recruitment

Recruitment is the process in which a primordial follicle is stimulated to leave the pool of nongrowing follicles and initiate development. In humans, recruitment begins in the embryo when primordial follicles are first formed and ends at the menopause when the pool of primordial follicles is depleted.[11,12]

What mechanisms are responsible for recruitment? It is well established that the first transition to the recruited state is accompanied by the transformation of the granulosa cells from a squamous to a cuboidal shape.[151] Thus, a developmental process in the

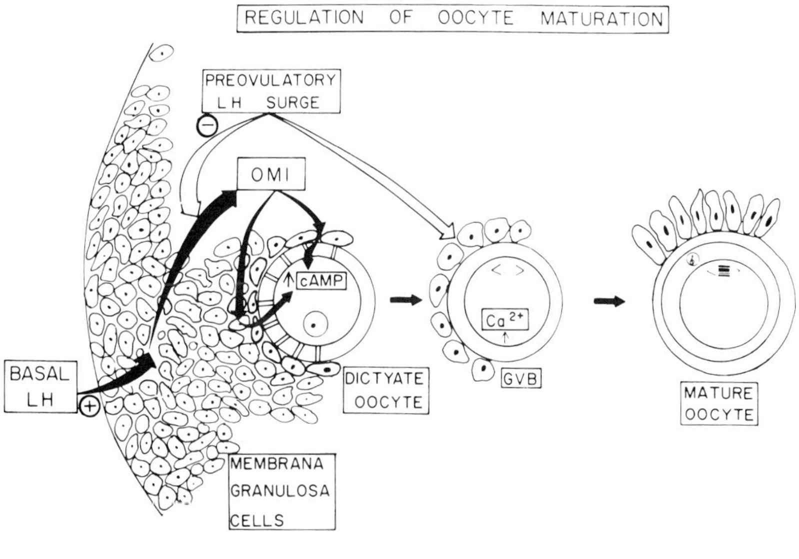

FIGURE 16A-29. Diagram of current concept of control of meiotic maturation.

granulosa must be considered a major event in recruitment. As granulosa cells become round, they acquire the capability to incorporate [^{3}H]thymidine and begin to divide, albeit very slowly.[67] When ≥90 percent of the granulosa cells are cuboidal, there occurs a dramatic activation in rodent oocyte RNA synthesis which results in rapid growth of the cytoplasm and the germinal vesicle.[129,130] Since changes in the synthetic activity of the oocyte appear to arise after prior changes in the granulosa cells, it would seem that the granulosa either responds to or generates a signal that triggers the primordial follicle to follow the pathway of recruitment.

Although the whole process is poorly understood, some information about the nature of the cues for recruitment does exist in animal models. First, the ovaries are endowed with a message capable of initiating recruitment. It has long been recognized that recruitment (including oocyte growth and granulosa proliferation) does not depend on extragonadal hormones such as FSH and LH. The cellular source or chemical nature of recruitment inducers is unknown, but as discussed earlier, it may involve a neurocrine mechanism.

An important concept in laboratory animals is that the process of recruitment can be modulated. Normally, the number of primordial follicles recruited is not constant but varies with age.[152] The greatest growth activity occurs early in life, after which the number of recruited follicles decreases progressively with advancing age.[153] This would indicate that the normal inducers of recruitment are somehow regulated by the actual size of the pool of primordial follicles. In this context, there is a marked reduction (by 30 percent) in the number of follicles recruited during pregnancy compared to the number during the cycle.[154] This suggests that the conditions leading to recruitment may be modulated by hormones. It is clear that the presence of testosterone severely reduces the number of primordial follicles and thus influences the recruitment process.[155] On the basis of these experiments, it has been proposed that recruitment is regulated by intraovarian androgens produced by the interstitial cells. Other experiments of a more complicated nature indicate that recruitment can also be modulated (i.e., attenuated) by the thymus gland,[156] food intake or starvation,[157] and opioid peptides.[158] No modulator has yet been found which can stimulate or amplify the process of recruitment. Finally, next to nothing is known about the recruitment process in humans.

Atresia

Of the estimated 2 million primary oocytes present in the female at birth (Fig. 16A-5), only about 400 are destined to leave the ovary through ovulation. Thus, 99.9 percent of the eggs are destroyed by the process of atresia. There are two classes of atresia (see section on Ovarian Follicles): type A, which occurs in preantral follicles, and type B, which occurs in antral or Graafian follicles. On the basis of recent studies, it is clear that atresia results from the activation of apoptosis or a programmed cell death mechanism in the granulosa and oocyte of growing follicles.[26,27] Despite the fact that atresia embraces so much that is central to ovarian function, almost nothing is known about the nature of the apoptotic signals or the steps in the apoptotic pathway in humans. A possible explanation of the activation of apoptosis in the follicle is a decrease or suppression in FSH action in the granulosa which in turn triggers or activates the program of apoptosis. This could reflect submaximal concentrations of FSH in follicular fluid is the inhibition of FSH action by inhibitory ligands.

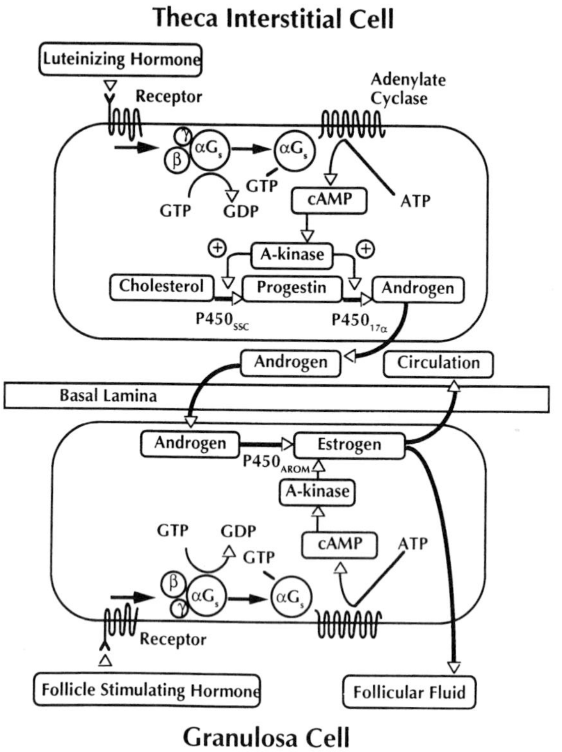

FIGURE 16A-30. Diagram illustrating the two-cell, two-gonadotropin concept of follicle estrogen biosynthesis. (*Reprinted with permission from Kettel M, Erickson GF: Basic and clinical concepts in ovulation induction, in Advances in Obstetrics and Gynecology. St. Louis, Mosby Year Book, Inc., 1994, pp 211–228.*)

Selection

The signaling pathways activated by FSH and LH play a fundamental role in the expression of the differentiated state of a dominant follicle. The primary roles of these signal transduction pathways are to stimulate mitotic and differentiation responses in the granulosa and theca cells. Physiologically, these signaling pathways act in parallel to regulate the expression of a set of genes in a precise quantitative and temporal fashion. One endocrine response associated with the action of FSH and LH is the production of large amounts of estradiol by the dominant follicle. This gonadotropin-dependent mechanism is called the two gonadotrophin-two cell concept (Fig. 16A-30). Because the estradiol response appears to be specific for the dominant follicle, the levels of plasma estradiol can be used as an indicator for follicle differentiation during ovulation induction.

Folliculogenesis in women is a very long process.[159] The dominant follicle that is selected to ovulate originates from a primordial follicle that was recruited to grow about one year earlier (Fig. 16A-31). The early stages of folliculogenesis (class 1, primary and secondary; class 2, early tertiary) proceed slowly, e.g., once recruited, ≥300 days are required for a primordial follicle to complete the preantral period (Fig. 16A-31). The basis for the slow growth is the long doubling time (~250 hrs) of the granulosa cells. When follicular fluid begins to accumulate in class 2 follicles, the size of the Graafian follicle increases relatively rapidly (Fig. 16A-31). During development, the Graafian follicle passes through the small (class 3,4,5), medium (class 6,7), and large (class 8), stages (Fig. 16A-31). Graafian follicle development

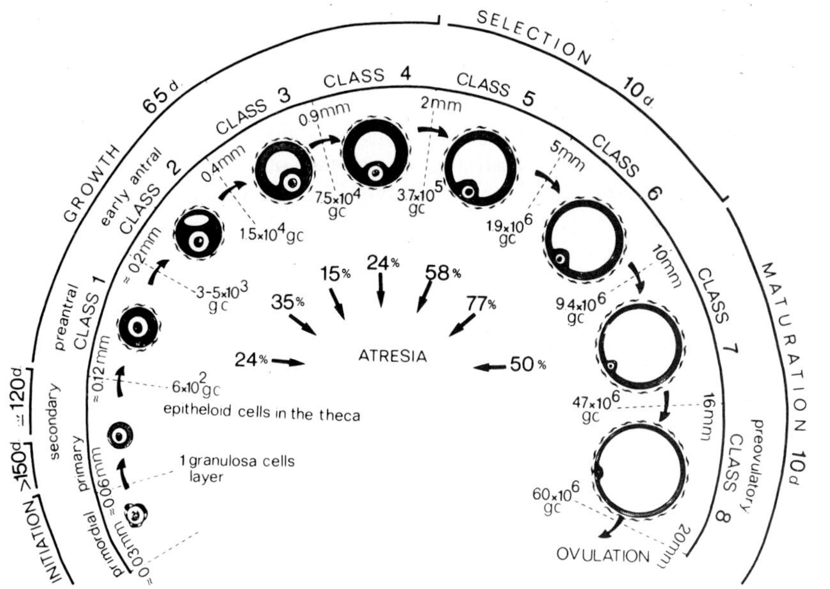

FIGURE 16A-31. The temporal pattern of folliculogenesis in normal human ovaries. The rates (in days) and stages (classes 1 through 8) of folliculogenesis and the levels of atresia (%) in the eight follicle classes are shown. The number of granulosa cells (gc) and the diameters of corresponding follicles are indicated. (*From Gougeon,*[159] *by permission of Oxford University Press.*)

depends critically on the correct level of FSH. Hence it is called the gonadotropin or FSH-dependent period of folliculogenesis.

The dominant follicle appears to be selected from a cohort of healthy class 5 (2–5 mm) follicles.[67,159,160] Once selected, it requires ~20 days for dominant follicles to grow and develop to the ovulatory stage (Fig. 16A-31). Thus, the gonadotropin-dependent pathway is very rapid when compared to the preantral sequence. During the 20-day period, the nondominant cohort follicles undergo atresia with the largest number appearing at the class 6 stage e.g., shortly after selection has occurred. Also note that atresia can take place in the preantral follicles at the class 2, 3, and 4 stages (Fig. 16A-31).

The dominant follicle that will ovulate its egg the next cycle appears to be selected at the end of the luteal phase of the menstrual cycle.[67,159,160] At this time, the ovaries contain a cohort of 4 to 8 follicles (class 5) that measure 4.7 ± 0.7 mm in diameter. Each cohort follicle[22,67] contains a fully grown egg, about 50 μL follicular fluid, about 1 million granulosa cells, a theca interna containing several layers of differentiated theca interstitial cells, and a band of smooth muscle cells in the theca externa (see Fig. 16A-11).

Physiological and morphological studies have shown that selection of a dominant follicle involves a change in the mitotic rate of the granulosa cells. Shortly after the mid luteal phase, the granulosa cells in these follicles exhibit a sharp increase (~2 fold) in the rate of mitosis.[67] The mechanism of stimulation is not clear, but it may be in response to luteolysis. The high rate of mitosis is maintained in the granulosa cells of one follicle while the rate appears to fall in the others. Consequently, the selected follicle becomes the fastest growing follicle in both ovaries. During the follicular phase,[159,161] the dominant follicle grows rapidly reaching 6.9 ± 0.5 mm at days 1 to 5, 13.7 ± 1.2 mm at days 6 to 10, and 18.8 ± 0.5 mm at days 11 to 14. The rapid growth is caused by mitosis and follicular fluid accumulation. In the nondominant cohort follicles, growth and expansion proceed more slowly, and with time, mitosis stops and the granulosa cells undergo apoptosis.[67] Rarely does a nondominant follicle reach >9 mm in diameter.[161]

FSH is obligatory for follicle selection and no other ligand by itself can serve in this regulatory capacity. Furthermore, once selected, the dominant follicle depends on FSH for its survival. Physiologically, the secondary rise in plasma FSH is responsible for follicle selection.[162] This increase in plasma FSH begins a few days before progesterone levels reach basal levels at the end of luteal phase,[163] and continues through the first week of the follicular phase (Fig. 16A-32). The biological importance of the secondary rise in FSH is demonstrated by the fact that the dominant follicle will undergo atresia if plasma FSH levels fall below a critical level during this period. This observation supports the concept that once selected the dominant follicle depends on a threshold level of FSH for its survival.

FIGURE 16A-32. The endocrinology of the luteal-follicular transition in women. Data are mean ±SE of daily serum concentrations of FSH, LH, estradiol (E_2), progesterone (P_4) and immunoreactive inhibin in women with normal cycles. Note the secondary rise in plasma FSH in the late luteal phase (−2 days before menses). (*From Roseff et al,*[163] *with permission.*)

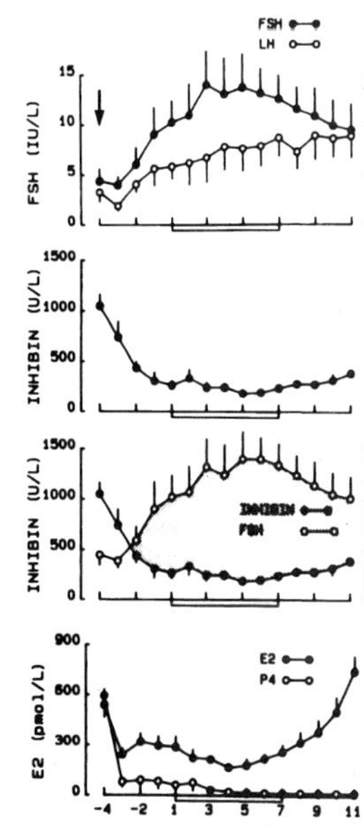

How does the increase in circulating FSH mediate selection? As consequence of the secondary FSH rise, there is a significant increase in the concentration of FSH within the microenvironment of the chosen follicle. The relatively high level of FSH in the microenvironment is critically important for stimulating mitosis and differentiation of the granulosa cells. In follicular fluid of healthy class 5 to 8 follicles, the mean concentration of FSH increases from ~1.3 mIU/mL (~58 ng/ml) to ~3.2 mIU/ml (~143 ng/ml), over the follicular phase.[22] By comparison, FSH levels are low or undetectable in follicular fluid of nondominant or atretic cohort follicles. Thus, a threshold concentration of FSH within the microenvironment is critically important for selection and survival of a dominant follicle, and those follicles that lack it die by atresia. The mechanism that regulates the differential uptake of FSH into the chosen follicle is totally obscure.

One important effect of FSH is the marked, time dependent increase in plasma estradiol during the follicular phase. The rise in estradiol suppresses pituitary FSH secretion (Fig. 16A-32) by a negative feedback mechanism. The fall in plasma FSH is believed to play a key role in the events leading to atresia of the nondominant cohort follicles. Physiologically, this estrogen mediated decrease in FSH is thought to be involved in the mechanism by which the dominant follicle achieves dominance. It is noteworthy that mitosis in nondominant follicles can be stimulated by treatment with hMG in the early follicular phase.[159] This evidence suggests that an immediate consequence of increased FSH levels in a nondominant follicle is a stimulation of mitosis in the granulosa cells. Thus, it is possible that one mechanism by which exogenous FSH or hMG generates multiple preovulatory follicles in women is by rescuing nondominant cohort follicles from atresia. One prediction of this idea is that the effectiveness of FSH or hMG in the rescue process will depend on the level of atresia of the nondominant follicle. One could speculate that this process might contribute to the success or failure of an ovulation induction protocol in a patient.

Ovulation

The expulsion of a mature oocyte from the ovary involves the release of hydrolytic enzymes in selected regions of the preovulatory follicle and a squeezing process in the basal region of the follicle wall (Fig. 16A-33).[164] It follows, therefore, that questions concerning the phenomenon of ovulation center on the generation of proteolytic activity and contractile mechanisms in the theca externa.

There are seven cellular and extracellular components which together serve as a barrier to prevent the escape of the oocyte from the preovulatory follicle. Beginning at the surface of the ovary and moving inward, these components include (1) the surface or germinal epithelium, (2) the basement membrane, (3) the dense connective tissue of the tunica albuginea, (4) the theca externa, (5) the theca interna, (6) the basal lamina of the follicle, and (7) the membrana granulosa cells. It is evident that if an oocyte-cumulus complex is to exit from its follicle, this organized network of cells and extracellular material must be broken down.

One important aspect of the destructive mechanism is that it occurs in a highly localized area called the *stigma* (Figs. 16A-33 and 16A-34). How do the cells in the presumptive stigma become activated to fulfill this fundamental degradative process? Morphologic and biochemical studies have shown that during the ovulatory period surface epithelial cells in the presumptive stigma become filled with large lysosome-like inclusions.[165] With increasing periods of time, the lysosome-like inclusions fuse with the plasma membrane and release their contents toward the tunica albuginea. This is accompanied by the progressive destruction of the basement membrane. This situation continues to progress medially, causing disruptive changes in the theca layers. It appears, therefore, that the steps leading to the formation of the stigma are initiated in a specialized population of surface epithelial cells and involve the formation and subsequent release of large amounts of hydrolytic enzymes. The question that must be analyzed is how this event occurs.

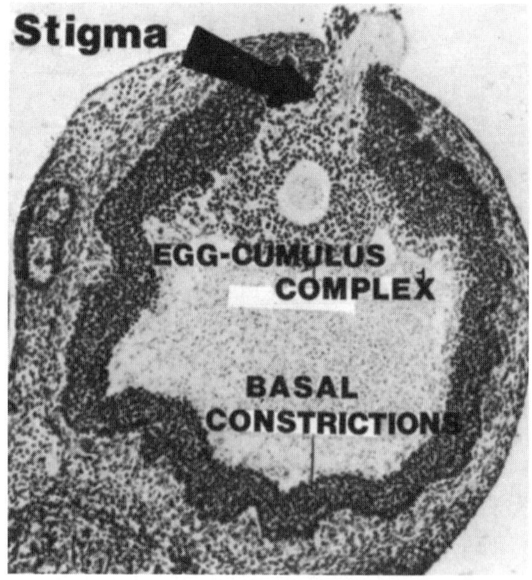

FIGURE 16A-33. Photomicrograph through a preovulatory follicle during ovulation. Note the selective destruction of tissue in the stigma and the constrictions of the basal follicular wall. (*From Hartman and Leathem,*[164] *by permission of Pergamon.*)

It is well established that the most important stimulating force in ovulation is LH. Although the basic mechanisms involved in LH-induced ovulation are unclear, some insights have been generated from studies carried out primarily in laboratory animals. First, the LH surge starts the preovulatory follicle on the path of progesterone production. An important concept is that progesterone is obligatory for ovulation and that the progesterone receptor in the follicle plays an essential role in the process of ovulation.[166] Consequently, LH-stimulated progesterone production and the induction of the expression of its receptor play a fundamental role in the ovulation process.

Results from an extensive variety of animal studies indicate that the mechanisms underlying ovulation involve the generation of PGs by the preovulatory follicle.[167,168] Following the preovulatory surge of LH and the stimulation of progesterone production, marked increases in the synthesis of PGE and PGF occur. If an LH-stimulated preovulatory follicle is injected with indomethacin or antiprostaglandin serum, ovulation is completely blocked.[169]

Prostaglandin G/H synthase is a key rate-limiting enzyme in PG biosynthesis as it catalyzes the conversion of arachidonic acid into PGH_2, a common precursor for the prostanoids.[170] The obligatory role for prostaglandin synthase (PGFH) expression during ovulation is evident from PGHS deficient female mice in which infertility is associated with impaired ovulation.[171] The conclusion

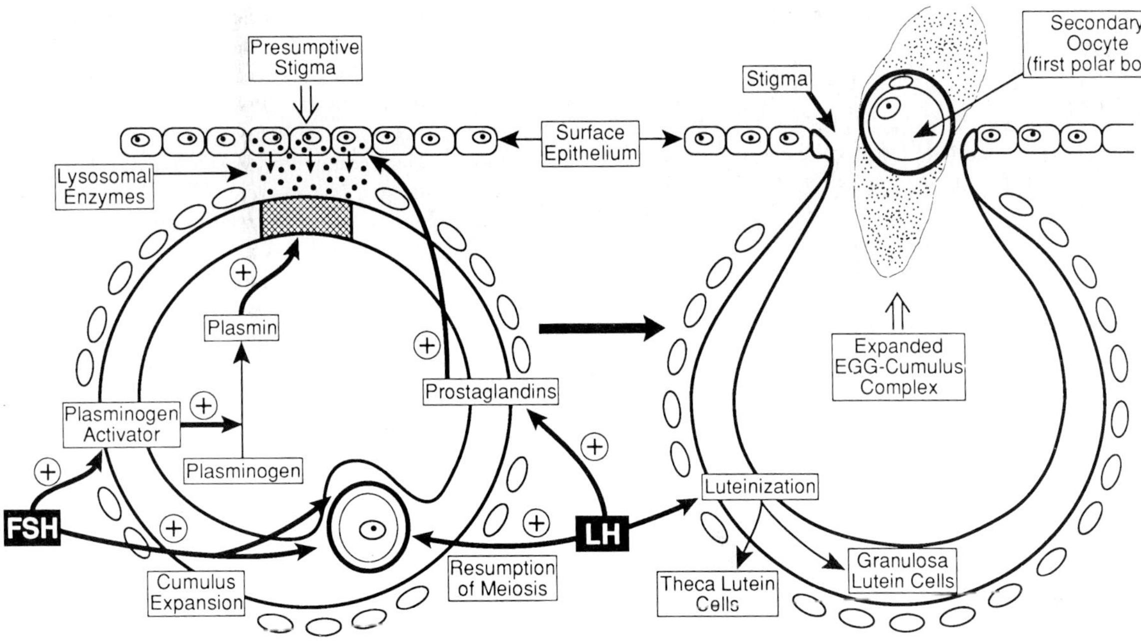

FIGURE 16A-34. Diagram illustrating the mechanisms by which the preovulatory surges of FSH and LH cause the ovulation of a fertilizable egg at midcycle.

that emerges is that LH-stimulated PG production is an obligatory trigger eliciting ovulation. Interestingly, morphologic studies of indomethacin-treated ovaries suggest that the prostaglandins might be involved in the steps by which the stigma is formed.[38] It appears, therefore, that the underlying mechanisms of LH-induced ovulation involve the following scenario: The elevated level of progesterone serves to activate PGHS and PG production, which then promotes the release of hydrolytic enzymes by a subpopulation of surface epithelial cells, which then cause stigma formation (Fig. 16A-34).

Another highly active protease that is involved in ovulation is plasmin.[172] The follicular fluid of a preovulatory follicle contains the plasmin precursor *plasminogen* at the same levels that are found in serum. The granulosa cells in a preovulatory follicle are selectively stimulated by very low levels of FSH to release the protein plasminogen activator.[173] This regulatory molecule then converts plasminogen to the active protease plasmin. Once the process is initiated, holes are formed in the basal lamina and there is a general weakening of the follicular wall, presumably caused by the proteolytic action of plasmin.[174] Questions concerning the physiologic importance of the plasminogen activator in ovulation are unanswered, but the concept is intriguing and raises the possibility that FSH, like LH, plays a basic role in ovulation, perhaps by causing destructive changes in the follicular basal lamina.

As was discussed earlier, the meiotically competent oocyte in the dominant follicle is inhibited from resuming meiosis by an OMI substance. However, under normal physiologic conditions, the high levels of LH at midcycle are capable of overriding the inhibitory influence of OMI. Consequently, meiosis resumes and the oocyte reaches the second meiotic metaphase or first polar body stage (Fig. 16A-34). Meiotic maturation is again arrested, and the egg awaits fertilization. The process of meiotic maturation occurs only in the oocyte of the dominant preovulatory follicle and results from specific stimulation by the high levels of LH reached at midcycle.

During the ovulatory sequence, the cumulus granulosa cells undergo a series of structural and functional changes termed *mucification* or *expansion* (Figs. 16A-33 and 16A-34). In response to the preovulatory surge of gonadotropins, the granulosa cells in the cumulus secrete a hyaluronidase-sensitive mucous substance. This results in the dispersal of the cumulus cells and causes the egg-cumulus complex to expand tremendously.[175] The specific stimulus for mucification is believed to be FSH. The functional significance of mucification is thought to involve the pickup and transport of the egg cumulus complex in the fallopian tube.

To what extent are contractile mechanisms involved in ovulation? It has been established that cells with the ultrastructure of smooth muscle cells are found only in the basal hemisphere of the follicle and that these cells contract before follicle rupture.[176] A number of experiments have been done with human ovarian follicles with regard to the contractile effects of various hormones. The conclusion which emerges is that the smooth muscle cells in the theca externa have beta-adrenergic receptors for norepinephrine and muscarinic receptors for acetylcholine, both of which, when activated by ligand, will stimulate follicle contraction.[177] Since smooth muscle cells in the theca externa are innervated by sympathetic and parasympathetic nerves, it seems certain that autonomic nerves are involved in the contractile mechanisms which occur prior to ovulation. Importantly, direct analysis of intrafollicular pressure during ovulation has ruled out a buildup of intrafollicular pressure in the ovulatory process.[178] These results suggest that contractile mechanisms do not play a direct role in follicular rupture. However, based on morphologic studies, there is little doubt that contractile mechanisms occur prior to ovulation and play an important role in the collapse of the follicle and the actual expulsion of the cumulus-egg complex onto the surface of the ovary.

PHYSIOLOGIC CORRELATES OF OVARIAN ACTIVITY WITH AGING

The Fetal Period

To what extent is the human fetal ovary steroidogenically active? As pointed out earlier, fetal ovaries at 12 to 20 weeks gestation contain a population of differentiated primary interstitial cells (Fig. 16A-13). Analysis of steroid metabolism has led to the concept that the human fetal ovaries do not have the ability to synthesize steroids de novo, presumably because they are unable to metabolize cholesterol to pregnenolone.[179] Furthermore, if human fetal ovaries are incubated with either exogenous pregnenolone or progesterone, there is little or no metabolism to steroid hormones.[179–181]

By contrast, when fetal ovary cells at 12 weeks gestation are incubated with pregnenolone sulfate, it is metabolized to pregnenolone, 17α-hydroxypregnenolone, dehydroepiandrosterone, and androstenedione but not to estrogen or testosterone.[182] This finding suggests that the fetal ovaries at 12 weeks gestation contain a very active sulfatase (three to seven times more active than in the fetal adrenal), as well as key steroidogenic enzymes in the Δ^5 pathway.[182] As development proceeds, there is a progressive decline in the steroidogenic enzymes such that by 17 weeks, the ability of the fetal ovary to metabolize pregnenolone sulfate to C_{19} steroids is very low.[182] It follows from these types of experiments that cells in human fetal ovaries may be able to effectively use pregnenolone sulfate to produce biologically active steroids, including androgens. The physiologic implications of this work lie in the fact that pregnenolone sulfate is present in very high concentrations in the fetal circulation.[183] Taken together, these observations support the idea that during their short existence (between 12 and 20 weeks of gestation), the primary interstitial cells in the ovaries are actively engaged in the production of biologically active androgens, using as substrate the steroid sulfates present in the fetal circulation. The physiologic significance of the androgens produced by the fetal ovaries is unknown. Importantly, LH, FSH, and hCG do not stimulate steroid metabolism by fetal ovarian cells in vitro,[184] suggesting that their activity may be independent of gonadotropin control.

By 26 weeks gestation, the fetal ovaries contain a population of small Graafian follicles that have well-developed thecae internae.[13] During the remainder of gestation, the frequency and size of Graafian follicles increase; the largest diameter reached is about 5 mm at 28 weeks. No follicles progress beyond this size, and all are destroyed by atresia. Nothing is known about the steroidogenic potential of the human fetal ovaries during this latter period, but the presence of well-developed theca interstitial cells could imply they are active in androgen formation.

Premenarche

Typically, the normal ovary in childhood is a dynamic organ which is undergoing constant internal changes associated with recruitment, follicular growth, and atresia.[185–187] A characteristic feature of the human ovary from birth until menarche is the presence of large numbers of Graafian follicles which measure between 1 and 6 mm in diameter (Fig. 16A-35). Generally, these follicles contain three to five layers of granulosa cells, a fully grown oocyte, and a thickened theca interna with apparently highly differentiated theca interstitial cells (Fig. 16A-35). Although evidence is lacking, the premenarcheal ovaries may be actively engaged in steroid biosynthesis. Under normal circumstances, these follicles in the premenarcheal ovary grow to the Graafian state, but all of them undergo atresia.[187] Thus, the regulatory mechanisms of selection are not operative in the prepubertal ovary.

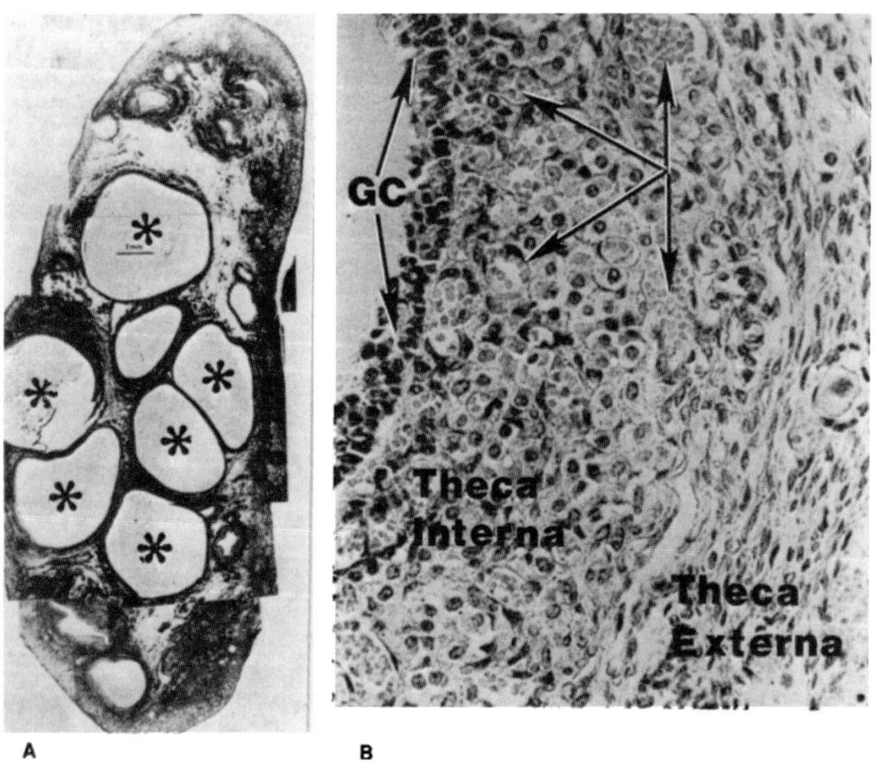

FIGURE 16A-35. Photomicrographs of actively growing human ovary at 7-1/2 years of age. (*A*) Ovaries are polycystic-like with large numbers of Graafian follicles (asterisk) measuring 2 to 6 mm in diameter. (*B*) Higher magnification of follicle shows paucity of granulosa cells (GC) and well-developed theca interna with five to seven layers of highly differentiated theca interstitial cells and numerous large capillaries (arrows). (*From Peters et al,*[186] *by permission.*)

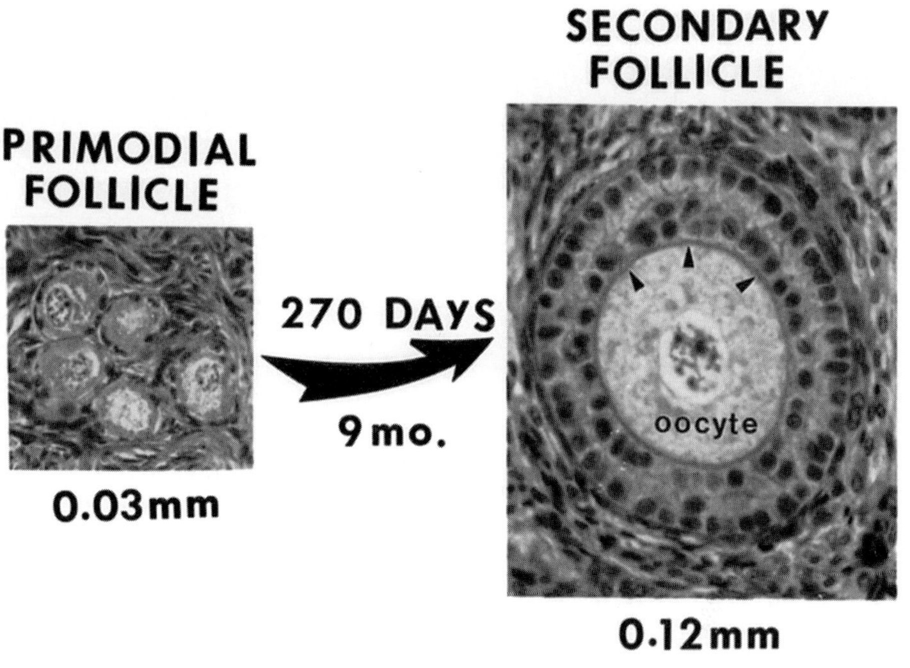

FIGURE 16A-36. Serum concentration of FSH, LH, and estradiol in girls of different ages. (*From Peters,*[204] *by permission of Gauthier Villars.*)

Menarche

When a child reaches 6 years of age, some follicles begin to grow and develop beyond the 5- and 6-mm stage.[188] This situation is accompanied by progressive increases in the levels of estrogen in plasma (Fig. 16A-36).[189] At the same time, steady increases in FSH and LH concentrations in the peripheral plasma occur. Importantly, at about age 10, the concentration of FSH is greater than that of LH, similar to the situation in the early follicular phase of the menstrual cycle.[189] The underlying mechanism that controls the onset of follicular estrogen synthesis certainly involves the stimulatory effect of LH and FSH, in particular the FSH induction of some $P450_{AROM}$ activity in the granulosa cells. As a result of this scenario, the prepubertal ovaries show a progressive increase in the capacity for estrogen production and follicular growth, a process which continues until the events responsible for the initiation of selection occur at menarche. After commitment to a dominant follicle occurs, the ovulatory process is initiated and the follicle becomes a corpus luteum. At this time menarche occurs; the basis for the commitment toward menarche certainly involves a steady increase in the FSH level, which, when high enough in the follicular fluid, drives granulosa cells in ovarian follicles to express their full differentiated state.

Currently, there is interest in the concept that insulin-like growth factor I (IGF-I) acts synergistically with FSH and LH to control the level of androgen and estrogen expression by prepubertal and pubertal ovaries. The basis for this interest is twofold. First, IGF-I levels in the blood of females increase dramatically during normal puberty.[190] Second, specific synergistic interactions between IGF-I and the gonadotropins have been observed in human granulosa and theca cells in vitro.[86,107] Thus, IGF-I is a candidate for amplifying the FSH and LH signaling pathways in the follicle wall. When this occurs there is an increase in ovarian estradiol expression that accompanies menarche in women.

Postmenarche: The Normal Menstrual Cycle

The menstrual cycle is accompanied by the sequence of recruitment, selection, ovulation, luteinization, and luteolysis. The underlying mechanisms responsible for these individual processes have already been described.

Typically, the menstrual cycle is divided into two major periods (Fig. 16A-37): the follicular phase (days 1 to 14) and the luteal phase (days 15 to 28); these major events are divided by ovulation, which occurs early on day 15. If the length of the normal menstrual cycle changes (becoming either shorter or longer), the shift occurs in the length of the follicular phase; normally, the programming of the corpus luteum is highly constant at 14 days.

As discussed earlier, the decision to select the dominant follicle is made at the end of the luteal phase of the preceding cycle. As illustrated in Fig. 16A-37, FSH is the predominant gonadotropin in the peripheral circulation when the dominant follicle is selected. The importance of elevated FSH concentrations in selection is best revealed by studies employing estradiol implants.[191] When the FSH rise is blocked by estradiol, the selected follicle is rendered inactive and the follicular phase is substantially lengthened. In conjunction with the previous discussion, the basis for this process is that the chosen follicle sequesters plasma FSH into its microenvironment which stimulates DNA synthesis and the induction of $P450_{AROM}$ activity in the granulosa cells, followed by dramatic increases in both granulosa cell number and follicular estrogen production. As a result, plasma estradiol levels begin to increase gradually between days 1 and 7, followed by a rapid and sharp increase of estrogen concentration, reaching peak values of about 300 pg/ml on day 12, when the dominant follicle reaches about 20 mm in diameter (Fig. 16A-37).

Unlike FSH, LH levels remain low and uniform during the early to midfollicular phase (Fig. 16A-37). Even though the LH concentration is low, it is evident from the androstenedione levels that LH stimulates theca interstitial cells to secrete large amounts of the aromatase substrate and that the amount formed is the same

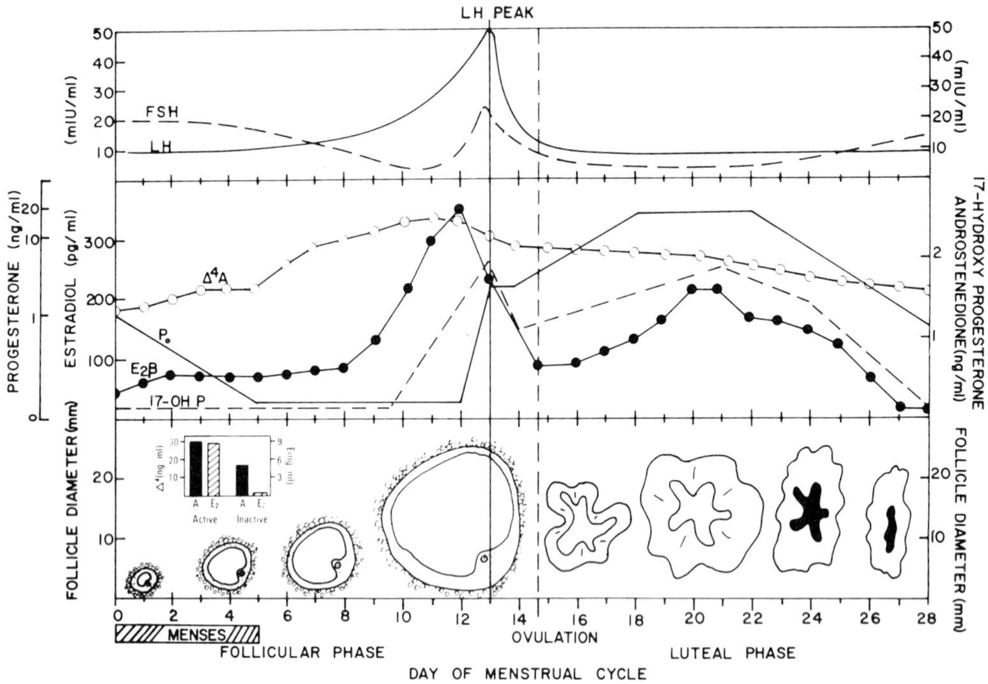

FIGURE 16A-37. Diagrammatic illustration of endocrine events in the human menstrual cycle. The inset (lower left) indicates differences in levels of steroids in ovarian venous effluent between ovaries with (active) and without (inactive) the selected follicle. (*Revised from Erickson and Yen,*[205] *by permission of Thieme-Stratton.*)

in both ovaries (Fig. 16A-37, *inset*). In contrast to estradiol, the concentration of androstenedione (1 to 2 ng/ml) in the peripheral plasma (and ovarian venous effluent) remains relatively constant throughout the menstrual cycle. This is supported by the fact that the concentration of follicular fluid androstenedione is maximal on day 1 of the cycle. Thus, the conclusion can be drawn that LH-stimulated androgen production in the follicular phase is sufficient to ensure that the levels of aromatase substrate are nearly maximal throughout the development of the selected follicle to the preovulatory stage.

Once the estradiol levels rise, the gonadotropins (LH and FSH) undergo a predictable pattern of activity characteristic of negative and positive feedback, respectively (Fig. 16A-37). When LH reaches a concentration of about 30 to 40 mIU/ml on day 12 of the cycle, a signal is triggered in the preovulatory follicle which results in the cessation of estradiol production. The mechanism underlying this change involves a selective inhibition of the $P450_{C17}$ enzyme in the theca interstitial cells.[97] Consequently, the selected follicle stops producing androstenedione (and therefore estradiol) and begins to secrete increased amounts of progestin. The physiologic mechanism by which the $P450_{C17}$ is suppressed might involve a local negative feedback action of estradiol directly on the theca interstitial cells.[10] Altogether, the increases in the plasma progestin (17-hydroxyprogesterone) level during the late follicular phase seem to be a consequence of steroidogenic changes within the affected preovulatory follicle.

In response to the peak levels of LH and FSH which occur on day 13, the process of ovulation is initiated in the dominant follicle and an egg-cumulus complex is released 36 to 38 h later.[192] As a consequence of breaks in the basal lamina caused by plasmin activity, LDL enters the granulosa cell microenvironment for the first time[193] and causes rapid increases in progesterone production by a mechanism that was discussed earlier. Considering the low levels of LH and FSH in the luteal phase (Fig. 16A-37), it is believed that LDL is the principal force stimulating progesterone production in the corpus luteum.[193] Normally, the plasma progesterone concentration reaches maximum levels of 10 to 20 ng/ml on day 19 (the consequence of luteinization) and remains elevated until day 22, when it declines sharply, reaching levels of about 0.8 ng/ml on the first day of menses (the consequence of luteolysis).

It is evident that as the corpus luteum differentiates, estrogen production is reinitiated and the corpus luteum begins progressively increasing estradiol secretion, reaching peak levels on days 21 to 22 of the luteal phase. Afterward, a sharp decline in estradiol concentration occurs, reaching levels of about 40 pg/ml at the end of the luteal phase (Fig. 16A-37). Importantly, as estradiol levels decline in the late luteal phase, the plasma FSH level begins to rise. Undoubtedly, this event is physiologically coupled with the selection of the dominant follicle which will generate the next menstrual cycle.

Menopause

The basis for the menopause is the depletion of the pool of primordial follicles (Fig. 16A-6). Consequently, the processes of recruitment and selection no longer occur, and the ovary loses its ability to synthesize and secrete estradiol and progesterone. Therefore, the menstrual cycle ceases.

Although all the aspects of folliculogenesis cease, the postmenopausal ovaries remain steroidogenically active. As was discussed earlier, the theca interstitial cells of atretic follicles hypertrophy and subsequently accumulate in the ovarian stroma as the secondary interstitial cells. Thus, with increasing age, the number of secondary interstitial cells would appear to increase in human ovaries. It is obvious from the previous discussion that these cells, together with the hilar cells, respond to LH with increased synthesis of androstenedione and testosterone. During the menopause, plasma LH levels are elevated, and therefore the interstitial cells in the postmenopausal ovaries are active secretors of C_{19} androgens, but not of C_{18} estrogens.[194,195]

Altogether, it can be concluded that secondary interstitial and hilar cells in postmenopausal ovaries retain their capacity for androgen biosynthesis and are constantly activated by the high levels of circulating LH in the peripheral plasma. The absence of estradiol production by the postmenopausal ovary certainly is causally connected with the absence of follicular granulosa cells.

THE CONCEPT OF OVARIAN GROWTH FACTORS

It is clear that FSH and LH play an essential role in the physiologic mechanisms of follicle section. However, only a single follicle is selected during each menstrual cycle, despite the fact that the concentrations of LH and FSH are identical in the blood perfusing both ovaries. To explain the variance in behavior between the two ovaries and among the follicles themselves, it is necessary to invoke the existence of local intraovarian/intrafollicular regulatory elements.

Historically, this concept evolved when Gospodarowitz and Bialecki[79] discovered that a number of potent growth factors act directly on human granulosa cells to stimulate mitosis. This finding was of considerable interest because it implied that folliculogenesis may be regulated by factors other than FSH and LH. As researchers began to look more closely at the issue, two significant discoveries were made.[196] First, the oocyte, theca and granulosa cells were found to actually synthesize and secrete a wide variety of potent regulatory proteins, including growth factors, binding proteins and their proteases. Second, these growth factors can act directly on all follicle cells (theca, granulosa, and oocyte) to regulate their activities. Such discoveries have led to the important theory that growth and development of follicles are influenced by interactions with growth factors via autocrine and paracrine mechanisms, which in turn serve to modulate (amplify or attenuate) the signals of endocrine hormones such as FSH and LH. The intellectual excitement of this rapidly progressing field is that gene knockout studies in rodents have demonstrated that some growth factors produced by the follicle are obligatory for folliculogenesis and female fertility i.e., loss of function of IGF-I[197,198] and oocyte-derived growth differentiation factor-9 (GDF-9)[199–201] result in the cessation of folliculogenesis at the preantral stage and the females are infertile. Thus, these studies reveal that ovary growth factors are fundamental in key physiological events in female reproduction.

There can be no doubt that growth factors have significant biological effects on human follicle cells in vitro. However, there are no definitive data as yet to indicate that growth factor actions are physiologically relevant to human reproduction. Certainly, until the in vitro results have been extrapolated to the in vivo situation, the novel idea that growth factors are crucial regulators of human ovarian physiology must remain largely theoretical. Still, the data raise the intriguing possibility that growth factors, acting through autocrine/paracrine mechanisms, may be a fundamental (perhaps obligatory) part of ovarian physiology in women. If this theory is proved true, the clinical question must be raised, To what extent are disorders of ovarian function caused by alterations in ovarian growth factor production and/or mechanism of action? Answering this question is one of the biggest challenges facing researchers in the ovary growth factor field.

CONCLUSION

Finally, it is important to note that our current understanding of ovarian physiology leans heavily on research performed on rodent species. The methods and technology have been adopted by researchers working on the human ovary. The problem that is now evident is that although many physiologic, cellular, and molecular processes found in the rodent are also found in the human, many are not. A difficulty in this situation is the tendency to generalize research findings to all animals. The conclusion is that one must be cautious when attempting to generalize from the laboratory animal to the human. Certainly much more needs to be learned before follicle growth and development can be understood. The more that is understood concerning this process in the human, the more likely we are to understand fertility and alleviate the afflictions of infertility.

REFERENCES

1. Reynolds SRM: The vasculature of the ovary and ovarian function. *Recent Prog Horm Res* 5:65, 1950.
2. Neilson D, Jones GS, Woodruff JD, et al: The innervation of the ovary. *Obstet Gynecol Surv* 25:889, 1970.
3. Owman C, Rosenbren E, Sjöberg NO: Adrenergic innervation of human female reproductive organs: A histochemical and chemical investigation. *Obstet Gynecol* 30:763, 1967.
4. Walles B, Gröschel-Stewart U, Owman C, et al: Fluorescence histochemical demonstration of a relationship between adrenergic nerves and cells containing actin and myosin in the rat ovary, with special reference to the follicle wall. *J Reprod Fertil* 52:174, 1978.
5. Condon WA, Black DL: Catecholamine-induced stimulation of progesterone by the bovine corpus luteum in vitro. *Biol Reprod* 15:573, 1976.
6. Hsueh AJW, Adashi EY, Jones PBC, et al: Hormonal regulation of differentiation of cultured ovarian granulosa cells. *Endocr Rev* 5:76, 1984.
7. Bahr J, Kao L, Nalbandov AV: The role of catecholamines and nerves in ovulation. *Biol Reprod* 10:273, 1974.
8. Schultea TD, Dees WL, Ojeda SR: Postnatal development of sympathetic and sensory innervation of the rhesus monkey ovary. *Biol Reprod* 47:760, 1992.
9. Capps ML, Lawrence LE Jr, Burden HW: Ultrastructure of the cells of the ovarian interstitial gland in hypophysectomized rats. *Cell Tissue Res* 193:433, 1978.
10. Erickson GF, Magoffin DA, Dyer CA, et al: The ovarian androgen producing cells: A review of structure/function relationships. *Endocr Rev* 6:371, 1985.
11. Ohno S, Klinger HP, Atkin NB: Human oogenesis. *Cytogenetics* 1:42, 1962.
12. Baker TG, Sum W: Development of the ovary and oogenesis. *Clin Obstet Gynaecol* 3:3, 1976.
13. Pryse-Davies J, Dewhurst CJ: The development of the ovary and uterus in the foetus, newborn and infant: a morphological and enzyme histochemical study. *J Pathol* 103:5, 1971.
14. Mandl A, Zuckerman A: The relation of age to the number of oocytes. *J Endocrinol* 7:190, 1951.
15. Meredith JE Jr, Winitz S, Lewis JM, et al: The regulation of growth and intracellular signaling by integrins. *Endocr Rev* 17:207, 1996.
16. Grazul-Bilska AT, Reynolds LP, Redmer DA: Gap junctions in the ovaries. *Biol Reprod* 57:947, 1997.
17. Beyer EC: Gap junctions. *Int Rev Cytol* 137C:1, 1993.
18. Bruzzone R, White TW, Paul DL: Connections with connexins: the molecular basis of direct intercellular signaling. *Eur J Biochem* 238:1, 1996.

19. Kumar NM, Gilula NB: The gap junction communication channel. *Cell* 84:381, 1996.
20. Simon AM, Goodenough DA, Li E, et al: Female infertility in mice lacking connexin 37. *Nature* 385:525, 1997.
21. Erickson GF: The graafian follicle: A functional definition., in Adashi EY (ed): *Ovulation: Evolving Scientific and Clinical Concepts*. New York, Springer-Verlaag, 2000.
22. McNatty KP, Moore-Smith D, Osathanondh R, et al: The human antral follicle: Functional correlates of growth and atresia. *Ann Biol Anim Biochim Biophys* 19:1547, 1979.
23. Okamura H, Virutamasen P, Wright KH, et al: Ovarian smooth muscle in the human being, rabbit, and cat. Histochemical and electron microscopic study. *Am J Obstet Gynecol* 112:183, 1972.
24. Amsterdam A, Lindner HR, Groschel-Stewart U: Localization of actin and myosin in the rat oocyte and follicular wall by immunofluorescence. *Anat Rec* 187:311, 1977.
25. Ingram DL: Atresia, in Zuckerman S, Mandl AM, Eckstein P (eds): *The Ovary*. New York, Academic Press, 1962, p 247.
26. Hsueh AJ, Billig H, Tsafriri A: Ovarian follicle atresia: A hormonally controlled apoptotic process. *Endocr Rev* 15:707, 1994.
27. Erickson GF: Defining apoptosis: players and systems. *J Soc Gynecol Investig* 4:219, 1997.
28. Hay MF, Cran DG: Differential response of components of hseep Graafian follicles to atresia. *Ann Biol Anim Biochim Biophys* 18:453, 1978.
29. Byskov AG: Atresia, in Midgley AR, Sadler WA (eds): *Ovarian Follicular Development and Function*. New York, Raven, 1979, p 41.
30. Krafka J: Parthenogenic cleavage in the human ovary. *Anat Rec* 75:19, 1934.
31. Gondos B, Hobel CJ: Interstitial cells in the human fetal ovary. *Endocrinology* 93:736, 1973.
32. Erickson GF: Normal regulation of ovarian androgen production. *Semin Reprod Endocrinol* 11:307, 1993.
33. Mossman HW, Koering MJ, Ferry D Jr: Cyclic changes of interstitial gland tissue of the human ovary. *Am J Anat* 115:235, 1964.
34. Kawakami M, Kubo K, Uemura T, et al: Involvement of ovarian innervation in steroid secretion. *Endocrinology* 109:136, 1981.
35. Sternberg WH: The morphology, androgenic function, hyperplasia, and tumors of the human ovarian hilus cells. *Am J Pathol* 25:493, 1949.
36. Merkow LP, Slifkin M, Acevedo HF, et al: Ultrastructure of an interstitial (Hilar) cell tumor of the ovary. *Obstet Gynecol* 37:845, 1971.
37. Schnoy N: Ultrastructure of a virilizing ovarian Leydig-cell-tumor. *Virchows Arch A Pathol Anat* 397:17, 1982.
38. Downs SM, Longo FJ: An ultrastructural study of preovulatory apical development in mouse ovarian follicles: effects of indomethacin. *Anat Rec* 205:159, 1983.
39. Echt CR, Hadd HE: Androgen excretion patterns in a patient with a metastatic hilus cell tumor of the ovary. *Am J Obstet Gynecol* 100:1055, 1968.
40. Jeffcoate SL, Prunty FTG: Steroid synthesis in vitro by a hilar cell tumor. *Am J Obstet Gynecol* 101:684, 1968.
41. Jezová D, Vigas M: Testosterone response to exercise during blockade and stimulation of adrenergic receptors in man. *Horm Res* 15:141, 1981.
42. Corner JGW: The histological dating of the human corpus luteum of mensturation. *Am J Anat* 98:377, 1956.
43. Crisp TM, Dessouky DA, Denys FR: The fine structure of the human corpus luteum of early pregnancy and during the progestational phase of the mestrual cycle. *Am J Anat* 127:37, 1970.
44. Bramley TA, Ryan RJ: Interations of gonadotropins with corpus luteum membranes. VII. Association of hCG-binding and adenylate cyclase activities with rabbit corpus luteum plasma-membranes. *Mol Cell Endocrinol* 12:319, 1978.
45. Gillim SW, Christensen AK, McLennan CE: Fine structure of the human menstrual corpus luteum at its stage of maximum secretory activity. *Am J Anat* 126:409, 1969.
46. Shikone T, Yamoto M, Kokawa K, et al: Apoptosis of human corpora lutea during cyclic luteal regression and early pregnancy. *J Clin Endocrinol Metab* 81:2376, 1996.
47. van Lennep EW, Madden LM: Electron microscopic observations on the involution of the human corpus luteum of menstruation. *Z Zellforsch Mikrosk Anat* 66:365, 1965.
48. Miller WL: Molecular biology of steroid hormone synthesis. *Endocr Rev* 9:295, 1988.
49. Gwynne JT, Strauss JFd: The role of lipoproteins in steroidogenesis and cholesterol metabolism in steroidogenic glands. *Endocr Rev* 3:299, 1982.
50. Brown MS, Kovanen PT, Goldstein JL: Regulation of plasma cholesterol by lipoprotein receptors. *Science* 212:628, 1981.
51. Brown MS, Goldstein JL: Receptor-mediated endocytosis: insights from the lipoprotein receptor system. *Proc Natl Acad Sci USA* 76:3330, 1979.
52. Simpson ER: Cholesterol side-chain cleavage, cytochrome P450, and the control of steroidogenesis. *Mol Cell Endocrinol* 13:213, 1979.
53. Stocco DM: A StAR search: implications in controlling steroidgenesis. *Biol Reprod* 56:328, 1997.
54. Kiriakidou M, McAllister JM, Sugawara T, et al: Expression of steroidogenic acute regulatory protein StAR in the human ovary. *J Clin Endocrinol Metab* 81:4122, 1996.
55. Penning TM: Molecular endocrinology of hydroxysteroid dehydrogenases. *Endocr Rev* 18:281, 1997.
56. Bara G, Anderson WA: Fine structural localization of 3beta-hydroxysteroid dehydrogenase in rat corpus luteum. *Histochemical Journal* 5:437, 1973.
57. Fauser CJM, Pache TD, Lamberts SWJ, et al: Serum bioactive and immunoreactive luteinizing hormone and follicle-stimulating hormone levels in women with cycle abnormalities, with or without polycystic ovarian disease. *J Clin Endocrinol Metab* 73:811, 1991.
58. Zhang Y, Word RA, Fesmire S, et al: Human ovarian expression of 17 beta-hydroxysteroid dehydrogenase types 1, 2, and 3. *J Clin Endocrinol Metab* 81:3594, 1996.
59. Simpson ER, Mahendroo MS, Means GD, et al: Aromatase cytochrome P450, the enzyme responsible for estrogen biosynthesis. *Endocr Rev* 15:342, 1994.
60. Suzuki T, Sasano H, Tamura M, et al: Temporal and spatial localization of steroidogenic enzymes in premenopausal human ovaries: in situ hybridization and immunohistochemical study. *Mol Cell Endocrinol* 97:135, 1993.
61. Smith OW, Ofner P, Vena RL: In vitro conversion of testosterone-4-14C to androgens of the 5alpha-androstane series by a normal human ovary. *Steroids* 24:311, 1974.
62. Hillier SG: Regulation of follicular oestrogen biosynthesis: a survey of current concepts. *J Endocrinol* 89 Suppl:3P, 1981.
63. Richards JS: Hormonal control of gene expression in the ovary. *Endocr Rev* 15:725, 1994.
64. Steinkampf MP, Mendelson CR, Simpson ER: Regulation by follicle-stimulating hormone of the synthesis of aromatase cytochrome P-450 in human granulosa cells. *Mol Endocrinol* 1:465, 1987.
65. Erickson GF, Hsueh AJW, Quigley ME, et al: Functional studies of aromatase activity in human granulosa cells from normal and polycystic ovaries. *J Clin Endocrinol Metab* 49:514, 1979.
66. Erickson GF: Primary cultures of ovarian cells in serum-free medium as models of hormone-dependent differentiation. *Mol Cell Endocrinol* 29:21, 1983.
67. Gougeon A: Regulation of ovarian follicular development in primates: facts and hypotheses. *Endocr Rev* 17:121, 1996.
68. Yamoto M, Shima K, Nakano R: Gonadotropin receptors in human ovarian follicles and corpora lutea throughout the menstrual cycle. *Horm Res* 37 (Suppl 1):5, 1992.
69. Minegishi T, Tano M, Igarashi M, et al: Expression of follicle-stimulating hormone receptor in human ovary. *Eur J Clin Invest* 27:469, 1997.
70. Oktay K, Briggs D, Gosden RG: Ontogeny of follicle-stimulating hormone receptor gene expression in isolated human ovarian follicles. *J Clin Endocrinol Metab* 82:3748, 1997.
71. Tano M, Minegishi T, Nakamura K, et al: Transcriptional and post-transcriptional regulation of FSH receptor in rat granulosa cells by cyclic AMP and activin. *J Endocrinol* 153:465, 1997.
72. Byers M, Kuiper GG, Gustafsson JA, et al: Estrogen receptor-beta mRNA expression in rat ovary: down-regulation by gonadotropins. *Mol Endocrinol* 11:172, 1997.
73. Tetsuka M, Hillier SG: Androgen receptor gene expression in rat granulosa cells: the role of follicle-stimulating hormone and steroid hormones. *Endocrinology* 137:4392, 1996.
74. Horie K, Takakura K, Fujiwara H, et al: Immunohistochemical localization of androgen receptor in the human ovary throughout the menstrual cycle in relation to oestrogen and progesterone receptor expression. *Hum Reprod* 7:184, 1992.

75. Iwai T, Nanbu Y, Iwai M, et al: Immunohistochemical localization of oestrogen receptors and progesterone receptors in the human ovary throughout the menstrual cycle. *Virchows Arch A Pathol Anat Histopathol* 417:369, 1990.
76. Suzuki T, Sasano H, Kimura N, et al: Immunohistochemical distribution of progesterone, androgen and oestrogen receptors in the human ovary during the menstrual cycle: relationship to expression of steroidogenic enzymes. *Hum Reprod* 9:1589, 1994.
77. Enmark E, Pelto-Huikko M, Grandien K, et al: Human estrogen receptor beta-gene structure, chromosomal localization, and expression pattern. *J Clin Endocrinol Metab* 82:4258, 1997.
78. Sawetawan C, Milewich L, Word RA, et al: Compartmentalization of type I 17 beta-hydroxysteroid oxidoreductase in the human ovary. *Mol Cell Endocrinol* 99:161, 1994.
79. Gospodarowicz D, Bialecki H: Fibroblast and epidermal growth factors are mitogenic agents for cultured granulosa cells of rodent, porcine, and human origin. *Endocrinology* 104:757, 1979.
80. Inkster SE, Brodie AM: Expression of aromatase cytochrome P-450 in premenopausal and postmenopausal human ovaries: an immunocytochemical study. *J Clin Endocrinol Metab* 73:717, 1991.
81. Hillier SG, Harlow CR, Shaw HJ, et al: Cellular aspects of pre-ovulatory folliculogenesis in primate ovaries. *Hum Reprod* 3:507, 1988.
82. McFarland KC, Sprengel R, Phillips HS, et al: Lutropin-choriogonadotropin receptor: An unusual member of the G protein-coupled receptor family. *Science* 245:494, 1989.
83. McNatty KP, Hunter WM, McNeilly AS, et al: Changes in the concentration of pituitary and steroid hormones in the follicular fluid of human graafian follicles throughout the menstrual cycle. *J Endocrinol* 64:555, 1975.
84. Eppig JJ, Chesnel F, Hirao Y, et al: Oocyte control of granulosa cell development: How and why. *Hum Reprod* 12:127, 1997.
85. Erickson GF: Ovarian androgen biosynthesis: endocrine regulation, in Azziz R, Nestler JE, Dewailly D (eds): *Androgen Excess Disorders in Women*, Lippincott-Raven Pub., 1997; p 3.
86. Erickson GF, Magoffin DA, Jones KL: Theca function in polycystic ovaries of a patient with virilizing congenital adrenal hyperplasia. *Fertil Steril* 51:173, 1989.
87. Abraham GE, Odell WD, Swerdloff RS, et al: Simultaneous radioimmunoassay of plasma FSH, LH, progesterone, 17-hydroxyprogesterone, and estradiol-17 beta during the menstrual cycle. *J Clin Endocrinol Metab* 34:312, 1972.
88. Baird DT, Burger PE, Heavon-Jones GD, et al: The site of secretion of androstenedione in non-pregnant women. *J Endocrinol* 63:201, 1974.
89. Baird DT, Fraser IS: Blood production and ovarian secretion rates of estradiol-17 beta and estrone in women throughout the menstrual cycle. *J Clin Endocrinol Metab* 38:1009, 1974.
90. Huang WY, Pearlman WH: The corpus luteum and steroid hormone formation: II. Studies on the human corpus luteum in vitro. *J Biol Chem* 238:1308, 1963.
91. Hammerstein J, Rice RB, Savard K: Steroid hormone formation in the human ovary: I. Identification of steroids formed in vitro from acetate-1-^{14}C in the corpus luteum. *J Clin Endocrinol* 24:597, 1964.
92. Vande Wiele RL, Bogumil J, Dyrenfurth I, et al: Mechanisms regulating the menstrual cycle in women. *Recent Prog Horm Res* 26:63, 1970.
93. Brännström M, Norman RJ: Involvement of leukocytes and cytokines in the ovulatory process and corpus luteum function. *Hum Reprod* 8:1762, 1993.
94. Lee CY, Coulam CB, Jiang NS, et al: Receptors for human luteinizing hormone in human corpora luteal tissue. *J Clin Endocrinol Metab* 36:148, 1973.
95. McNeilly AS, Kerin J, Swanston IA, et al: Changes in the binding of human chorionic gonadotrophin/luteinizing hormone, follicle-stimulating hormone and prolactin to human corpora lutea during the menstrual cycle and pregnancy. *J Endocrinol* 87:315, 1980.
96. Rajaniemi HJ, Rönnberg L, Kauppila A, et al: Luteinizing hormone receptors in human ovarian follicles and corpora lutea during menstrual cycle and pregnancy. *J Clin Endocrinol Metab* 52:307, 1981.
97. Dennefors BL, Hamberger L, Nilsson L: Influence of human chorionic gonadotropin in vivo on steroid formation and gonadotropin responsiveness of isolated human preovulatory follicular cells. *Fertil Steril* 39:56, 1983.
98. Polan ML, Seu D, Tarlatzis B: Human chorionic gonadotropin stimulation of estradiol production and androgen antagonism of gonadotropin-stimulated responses in cultured human granulosa-luteal cells. *J Clin Endocrinol Metab* 62:628, 1986.
99. Vega M, Devoto L, Navarro V, et al: In vitro net progesterone production by human corpora lutea: effects of human chorionic gonadotropin, dibutyryl adenosine 3',5'-monophosphate, cholera toxin, and forskolin. *J Clin Endocrinol Metab* 65:747, 1987.
100. Polan ML, Laufer N, Dlugi AM, et al: Human chorionic gonadotropin and prolactin modulation of early luteal function and luteinizing hormone receptor-binding activity in cultured human granulosa-luteal cells. *J Clin Endocrinol Metab* 59:773, 1984.
101. Jones GS: The luteal phase defect. *Fertil Steril* 27:351, 1976.
102. Wentz AC: Physiologic and clinical considerations in luteal phase defects. *Clin Obstet Gynecol* 22:169, 1979.
103. McNeely MJ, Soules MR: The diagnosis of luteal phase deficiency: a critical review [see comments]. *Fertil Steril* 50:1, 1988.
104. Hunter MG, Baker TG: Effect of hCG, cAMP and FSH on steroidogenesis by human corpora lutea in vitro. *J Reprod Fertil* 63:285, 1981.
105. Ohara A, Mori T, Taii S, et al: Functional differentiation in steroidogenesis of two types of luteal cells isolated from mature human corpora lutea of menstrual cycle. *J Clin Endocrinol Metab* 65:1192, 1987.
106. Ohara A, Taii S, Mori T: Stimulatory effects of purified human follicle-stimulating hormone on estradiol production in the human luteal phase. *J Clin Endocrinol Metab* 68:359, 1989.
107. Erickson GF, Garzo VG, Magoffin DA: Insulin-like growth factor 1 (IGF-1) regulates aromatase activity in human granulosa and granulosa luteal cells. *J Clin Endocrinol Metab* 69:716, 1989.
108. Fujita Y, Mori T, Suzuki A, et al: Functional and structural relationships in steroidogenesis in vitro by human corpora lutea during development and regression. *J Clin Endocrinol Metab* 53:744, 1981.
109. Hoffman F: Unterschungen uber die hormonale beeinflussung der lebensdauer des corpus luteum in zyklus der frau. *Geburtshilfe Frauenheilkd* 20:1153, 1960.
110. Williams MT, Roth MS, Marsh JM, et al: Inhibition of human chorionic gonadotropin-induced progesterone synthesis by estradiol in isolated human luteal cells. *J Clin Endocrinol Metab* 48:437, 1979.
111. Thibier M, el-Hassan N, Clark MR, et al: Inhibition by estradiol of human chorionic gonadotropin-induced progesterone accumulation in isolated human luteal cells: lack of mediation by prostaglandin F. *J Clin Endocrinol Metab* 50:590, 1980.
112. Vega M, Devoto L, Castro O, et al: Progesterone synthesis by human luteal cells: modulation by estradiol. *J Clin Endocrinol Metab* 79:466, 1994.
113. Hagerman DD, Smith OW, Day CF: Mechanism of the stimulatory effect of Clomid on aromatization of steroids by human placenta in vitro. *Acta Endocrinol Copenh* 51:591, 1966.
114. McNatty KP, Sawers RS, McNeilly AS: A possible role for prolactin in control of steroid secretion by the human Graafian follicle. *Nature* 250:653, 1974.
115. Demura R, Ono M, Demura H, et al: Prolactin directly inhibits basal as well as gonadotropin-stimulated secretion of progesterone and 17 beta-estradiol in the human ovary. *J Clin Endocrinol Metab* 54:1246, 1982.
116. Clayton RN, Huhtaniemi IT: Absence of gonadotrp[om-releasing hormone receptors in human gonadal tissue. *Nature* 299:56, 1982.
117. Casper RF, Erickson GF, Yen SSC: Studies on the effect of GnRH and its agonist on human luteal steroidogenesis *in vitro*. *Fertil Steril* 42:39, 1984.
118. Tureck RW, Mastroianni L Jr, Blasco L, et al: Inhibition of human granulosa cell progesterone secretion by a gonadotropin-releasing hormone agonist. *J Clin Endocrinol Metab* 54:1078, 1982.
119. Casper RF, Erickson GF, Rebar RW, et al: The effect of luteinizing hormone-releasing factor and its agonist on cultured human granulosa cells. *Fertil Steril* 37:405, 1982.
120. Aten RF, Polan ML, Bayless R, et al: A gonadotropin-releasing hormone (GnRH)-like protein in human ovaries: Similarity to the GnRH-like ovarian protein of the rat. *J Clin Endocrinol Metab* 64:1288, 1987.
121. Auletta FJ, Flint AP: Mechanisms controlling corpus luteum function in sheep, cows, nonhuman primates, and women especially in relation to the time of luteolysis. *Endocr Rev* 9:88, 1988.
122. McKay DG, Hertig AT, Adams EC, et al: Histochemical observation on the germ cells of human embryos. *Anatomic Record* 117:201, 1953.

123. Eddy EM, Clark JM, Gong D, et al: Origin and migration of primordial germ cells in mammals. *Gamete Res* 4:333, 1981.
124. Wartenberg H: Development of the early human ovary and role of the mesonephros in the differentiation of the cortex. *Ana Embryol* 165:253, 1982.
125. Monk M, McLaren A: X-chromosome activity in foetal germ cells of the mouse. *J Embryol Exp Morphol* 63:75, 1981.
126. Burgoyne PS, Baker TG: Oocyte depletion in XO mice and their XX sibs from 12 to 200 days post partum. *J Reprod Fertil* 61:207, 1981.
127. Ruby JR, Dyer RF, Skalko RG: The occurrence of intercellular bridges during oogenesis. *J Morph* 127:307, 1969.
128. Byskov AG: Regulation of meiosis in mammals. *Annal Biol Animale, Biochim, Biophys (Paris)* 19:1251, 1979.
129. Bachvarova R: Gene expression during oogenesis and oocyte development in mammals, in Browder L (ed): *Developmental Biology: A Comprehensive Synthesis*. New York, Plenum, 1985, p 453.
130. Roller RJ, Kinloch RA, Hiraoka BY, et al: Gene expression during mammalian oogenesis and early embryogenesis: quantification of three messenger RNAs abundant in fully grown mouse oocytes. *Development* 106:251, 1989.
131. Heller DT, Cahill DM, Schultz RM: Biochemical studies of mammalian oogenesis: Metabolic cooperativity between granulosa cells and growing mouse oocytes. *Dev Biol* 84:455, 1981.
132. Brower PT, Schultz RM: Intercellular communication between granulosa cells and mouse oocytes: existence and possible nutritional role during oocyte growth. *Dev Biol* 90:144, 1982.
133. Wassarman PM: Fertilization in mammals. *Sci Am* 259:78, 1988.
134. McLeskey SB, Dowds C, Carballada R, et al: Molecules involved in mammalian sperm-egg interaction. *Int Rev Cytol* 177:57, 1998.
135. Moos J, Faundes D, Kopf GS, et al: Composition of the human zona pellucida and modifications following fertilization. *Hum Reprod* 10:2467, 1995.
136. Gong X, Dubois DH, Miller DJ, et al: Activation of a G protein complex by aggregation of beta-1,4-galactosyltransferase on the surface of sperm. *Science* 269:1718, 1995.
137. Tesarik J: Targeting the zona pellucida for immunocontraception: a minireview. *Hum Reprod* 10 Suppl 2:132, 1995.
138. Jones WR: Gamete immunology. *Hum Reprod* 9 Suppl 2:107, 1994.
139. Skinner SM, Prasad SV, Ndolo TM, et al: Zona pellucida antigens: targets for contraceptive vaccines. *Am J Reprod Immunol* 35:163, 1996.
140. Bagavant H, Fusi FM, Baisch J, et al: Immunogenicity and contraceptive potential of a human zona pellucida 3 peptide vaccine [published erratum appears in Biol Reprod 1997 May;56(5):1361]. *Biol Reprod* 56:764, 1997.
141. Eppig JJ, Downs SM: Chemical signals that regulate mammalian oocyte maturation. *Biol Reprod* 30:1, 1984.
142. Eppig JJ, Schroeder AC: Capacity of mouse oocytes from preantral follicles to undergo embryogenesis and development to live young after growth, maturation, and fertilization *in vitro*. *Biol Reprod* 41:268, 1989.
143. Testart J, Frydman R, De Mouzon J, et al: A study of factors affecting the success of human fertilization in vitro. I. Influence of ovarian stimulation upon the number and condition of oocytes collected. *Biol Reprod* 28:415, 1983.
144. Downs SM, Daniel SA, Eppig JJ: Induction of maturation in cumulus cell-enclosed mouse oocytes by follicle-stimulating hormone and epidermal growth factor: evidence for a positive stimulus of somatic cell origin. *J Exp Zool* 245:86, 1988.
145. Banka CL, Erickson GF: Gonadotropin-releasing hormone induces classical meiotic maturation in subpopulations of atretic preantral follicles. *Endocrinology* 117:1500, 1985.
146. Tsafriri A, Dekel N, Bar-Ami S: The role of oocyte maturation inhibitor in follicular regulation of oocyte maturation. *J Reprod Fertil* 64:541, 1982.
147. Whittingham DG, Siracusa G: The involvement of calcium in the activation of mammalian oocytes. *Exp Cell Res* 113:311, 1978.
148. Dolci S, Eusebi F, Siracusa G: γ-amino butyric-*N*-acid sensitivity of mouse and human oocytes. *Dev Biol* 109:242, 1985.
149. O WS, Robertson DM, de Kretser DM: Inhibin as an oocyte meiotic inhibitor. *Mol Cell Endocrinol* 62:307, 1989.
150. Moor RM: Role of steroids in the maturation of ovine oocytes. *Annal Biol Anim Biochim, Biophys (Paris)* 18:477, 1978.
151. Gougeon A, Chainy GBN: Morphometric studies of small follicles in ovaries of women at different ages. *J Reprod Fertil* 81:433, 1987.
152. Pedersen T: Follicle growth in the immature mouse ovary. *Acta Endocrinol Copenh* 62:117, 1969.
153. Krarup T, Pedersen T, Faber M: Regulation of oocyte growth in the mouse ovary. *Nature* 224:187, 1969.
154. Pedersen T, Peters H: Follicle growth and cell dynamics in the mouse ovary during pregnancy. *Fertil Steril* 22:42, 1971.
155. Peters H, Byskov AGS, Sorensen IN, et al: The development of the mouse ovary after testosterone propionate injection on day 5, in Butt WR, Crooke AC, Ryle E (eds): *Gonadotropins and Ovarian Development*. London, Livingstone, 1979, p 351.
156. Lintern-Moore S: Effect of athymia on the initiation of follicular growth in the rat ovary. *Biol Reprod* 17:155, 1977.
157. Lintern-Moore S, Everitt AV: The effect of restricted food intake on the size and composition of the ovarian follicle population in the Wistar rat. *Biol Reprod* 19:688, 1978.
158. Lintern-Moore S, Supasri Y, Pavasuthipaisit K, et al: Acute and chronic morphine sulfate treatment alters ovarian development in prepuberal rats. *Biol Reprod* 21:379, 1979.
159. Gougeon A: Dynamics of follicular growth in the human: a model from preliminary results. *Hum Reprod* 1:81, 1986.
160. Gougeon A, Lefèvre B: Evolution of the diameters of the largest healthy and atretic follicles during the human menstrual cycle. *J Reprod Fertil* 69:497, 1983.
161. McNatty KP: Hormonal correlates of follicular development in the human ovary. *Australian Journal of Biological Sciences* 34:249, 1981.
162. Erickson GF: Physiologic basis of ovulation induction, in Speroff L (ed): *Seminars in Reproductive Endocrinology*, Thieme Medical Publishers, 1996, p 287.
163. Roseff SJ, Bangah ML, Kettel LM, et al: Dynamic changes in circulating inhibin levels during the luteal-follicular transition of the human menstrual cycle. *J Clin Endocrinol Metab* 69:1033, 1989.
164. Hartman CG, Leathem JH: Oogenesis and ovulation, Conference on Physiological Mechanisms Concerned with Conception: Pergamon, 1963; 205.
165. Cajander S, Bjersing L: Fine structural demonstration of acid phosphatase in rabbit germinal epithelium prior to induced ovulation. *Cell Tissue Res* 164:279, 1975.
166. Graham JD, Clarke CL: Physiological action of progesterone in target tissues. *Endocr Rev* 18:502, 1997.
167. Marsh JM, Yang NS, LeMaire WJ: Prostaglandin synthesis in rabbit graafian follicles in vitro. Effect of luteinizing hormone and cyclic AMP. *Prostaglandins* 7:269, 1974.
168. Armstrong DT: Role of prostaglandins in follicular responses to luteinizing hormone. *Annal Biol Anim, Biochim, Biophys (Paris)* 15:181, 1975.
169. Armstrong DT, Grinwich DL, Moon YS, et al: Inhibition of ovulation in rabbits by intrafollicular injection of indomethacin and prostaglandin F antiserum. *Life Sci* 14:129, 1974.
170. Herschman HR: Prostaglandin synthase 2. *Biochim Biophys Acta* 1299:125, 1996.
171. Dinchuk JE, Car BD, Focht RJ, et al: Renal abnormalities and an altered inflammatory response in mice lacking cyclooxygenase II. *Nature* 378:406, 1995.
172. Beers WH, Strickland S, Reich E: Ovarian plasminogen activator: relationship to ovulation and hormonal regulation. *Cell* 6:387, 1975.
173. Beers WH, Strickland S: A cell culture assay for follicle-stimulating hormone. *J Biol Chem* 253:3877, 1978.
174. Beers WH: Follicular plasminogen and plasminogen activator and the effect of plasmin on ovarian follicle wall. *Cell* 6:379, 1975.
175. Erickson GF: Analysis of follicle development and ovum maturation. *Semin Reprod Endocrinol* 4:233, 1986.
176. Martin GG, Talbot P: The role of follicular smooth muscle cells in hamster ovulation. *J Exp Zool* 216:469, 1981.
177. Walles B, Falck B, Owman C, et al: Characterization of autonomic receptors in the smooth musculature of human Graafian follicle. *Biol Reprod* 17:423, 1977.
178. Bronson RA, Bryant G, Balk MW, et al: Intrafollicular pressure within preovulatory follicles of the pig. *Fertil Steril* 31:205, 1979.
179. Jungmann RA, Schweppe JS: Biosynthesis of sterols and steroids from acetate-14-C by human fetal ovaries. *J Clin Endocrinol Metab* 28:1599, 1968.
180. Bloch E: Metabolism of 4-^{14}C-progesterone by human fetal testis and ovaries. *Endocrinology* 74:833, 1964.

181. Taylor T, Coutts JR, Macnaughton MC: Human foetal synthesis of testosterone from perfused progesterone. *J Endocrinol* 60:321, 1974.
182. Payne AH, Jaffe RB: Androgen formation from pregnenolone sulfate by the human fetal ovary. *J Clin Endocrinol Metab* 39:300, 1974.
183. Huhtaniemi I, Vihko R: Determination of unconjugated and sulfated neutral steroids in human fetal blood of early and mid-pregnancy. *Steroids* 16:197, 1970.
184. Wilson EA, Jawad MJ: The effect of trophic agents on fetal ovarian steroidogenesis in organ culture. *Fertil Steril* 32:73, 1979.
185. Valdes-Dapena MA: The normal ovary of childhood. *Ann NY Acad Sci* 142:597, 1967.
186. Peters H, Himelstein-Braw R, Faber M: The normal development of the ovary in childhood. *Acta Endocrinol Copenh* 82:617, 1976.
187. Himelstein-Braw R, Byskov AG, Peters H, et al: Follicular atresia in the infant human ovary. *J Reprod Fertil* 46:55, 1976.
188. Lintern-Moore S, Peters H, Moore GPM, et al: Follicular development in the infant human ovary. *J Reprod Fertil* 39:53, 1974.
189. Faiman C, Winter JSD: Gonadotropins and sex hormone pattern in puberty, in Grumbach MM, Grave GD, Mayer FE (eds): *The Control of the Onset of Puberty*. London, Wiley, 1974, p 68.
190. Bala RM, Lopatka J, Leung A, et al: Serum immunoreactive somatomedin levels in normal adults, pregnant women at term, children at various ages, and children with constitutionally delayed growth. *J Clin Endocrinol Metab* 52:508, 1981.
191. Zeleznik AJ: Premature elevation of systemic estradiol reduces serum levels of follicle-stimulating hormone and lengthens the follicular phase of the menstrual cycle in Rhesus monkeys. *Endocrinology* 109:352, 1981.
192. Edwards RG: Studies on human conception. *Am J Obstet Gynecol* 117:587, 1973.
193. Carr BR, MacDonald PC, Simpson ER: The role of lipoproteins in the regulation of progesterone secretion by the human corpus luteum. *Fertil Steril* 38:303, 1982.
194. Mattingly RF, Huang WY: Steroidogenesis of the menopausal and postmenopausal ovary. *Am J Obstet Gynecol* 103:679, 1969.
195. Asch RH, Greenblatt RB: Steroidogenesis in the postmenopausal ovary. *Clin Obstet Gynaecol* 4:85, 1977.
196. Adashi E, Leung PCK: *The Ovary: Comprehensive Endocrinology.* 1st ed. New York, Raven Press, Ltd., 1993.
197. Baker J, Hardy MP, Zhou J, et al: Effects of an lgf1 gene null mutation on mouse reproduction. *Mol Endocrinol* 10:903, 1996.
198. Bellvé AR: Differential effects of IGF null mutations in male and female mice, in LeRoith D (ed): *Frontiers in Endocrinology*. Rome, Italy, Ares-Serono Symposia Publications, 1996; p 35.
199. McPherron AC, Lee S-J: GDF-3 and GDF-9: two new members of the transforming growth factor-β superfamily containing a novel pattern of cysteines. *J Biol Chem* 268:3444, 1993.
200. McGrath SA, Esquela AF, Lee S-J: Oocyte-specific expression of growth/differentiation factor-9. *Mol Endocrinol* 9:131, 1995.
201. Dong J, Albertini DF, Nishimori K, et al: Growth differentiation factor-9 is required during early ovarian folliculogenesis. *Nature* 383:531, 1996.
202. Bloom W, Fawcett DW: *A Textbook of Histology*. 10th ed. Philadelphia, W.B. Saunders, 1975.
203. Green SH, Zuckerman S: Quantitative aspects of the growth of the human ovum and follicle. *J Anat* 85:373, 1951.
204. Peters H: The development and maturation of the ovary. *Ann Biol Anim Biochim Biophys* 16:271, 1976.
205. Erickson GF, Yen SSC: New data on follicle cells in polycystic ovaries: A proposed mechanism for the genesis of cystic follicles. *Semin Reprod Endocrinol* 2:231, 1984.

CHAPTER 16

The Ovary: Basic Principles and Concepts B. Clinical

Henry G. Burger
David L. Healy
Beverley J. Vollenhoven

In this section an approach to the management of the clinical disorders of ovarian function is outlined, based on the particular setting in which patients present to the clinician, i.e., in teenagers, young adults, and individuals of middle age.

OVARIAN DISORDERS IN TEENAGERS

Primary Amenorrhea

The time of menarche varies widely among racial groups and families but normally occurs between 9 and 16 years of age. It is preceded by an acceleration of growth and breast development, normally by age 14. These changes reflect the rise in estrogen secretion from the pubertal ovary and the consequent increase in circulating insulin-like growth factor I (IGF1) concentrations. In addition, the development of pubic hair, reflecting a rise in androgen production (adrenarche), precedes menarche by 1 to 3 years. Failure of menses to occur by age 16 years is termed *primary amenorrhea*.

The clinical evaluation of a girl with primary amenorrhea commences with an assessment of her growth and development. The failure of onset of pubertal development (breast development, Fig. 16B-1) to occur by the age of 14, or of menses to occur by 16, should lead to investigation, including karyotype, FSH assay, assessment of bone age, and abdomino-pelvic ultrasound to check for the presence and activity of the ovaries.

A wide variety of disorders of the hypothalamic-pituitary-ovarian axis can result in primary amenorrhea. It is more helpful to classify these conditions clinically according to the girl's stature and the degree, timing, and nature of pubertal change. The more common causes of primary amenorrhea are classified according to clinical presentation in Table 16B-1.

Short Stature and No Pubertal Development

Gonadal Dysgenesis

Turner's Syndrome Short stature, absence of a pubertal growth spurt, and absence of secondary sexual characteristics suggest the syndromes of gonadal dysgenesis which represent an important cause of primary amenorrhea. The most common condition is Turner's syndrome, a sporadic condition which affects approximately 1 in 2,500 girls and results from an abnormality of one X chromosome, leading either to a 45,XO karyotype or some form of X chromosome mosaicism. This may include deletions of the short arm of the X chromosome. Demonstration of X chromosome mosaicism may require the use of microsatellite probes for the X chromosome to show low level mosaicism which may also be tissue specific. The müllerian duct derivatives and genitalia are female; however, the ovaries (in 45,XO patients) are represented by gonads devoid of primordial follicles. The characteristic phenotype includes short stature [>2.5 standard deviations (SD) below the mean for chronologic age, adult mean height <148 cm]. In patients with 45,XO karyotype in particular, infantile female genitalia, and absence of secondary sexual characteristics are found whereas in patients with mosaicism, short stature may be the only phenotypic abnormality and fertility is possible.[1] Somatic abnormalities including short neck are often present in patients with Turner's syndrome, cubitus valgus, short metacarpals, characteristic facies with micrognathia, high arched palate, rotated ears, and otitis media.

Investigation will show low estrogen secretion though this is not particularly diagnostically helpful. Elevation of serum FSH, which may be detectable by age 8–9, is useful in indicating that the patient has primary gonadal failure. Assessment of the karyotype is clearly important as is ovarian ultrasound, as in patients with classic Turner's syndrome, no ovaries are demonstrable. Cardiovascular assessment is indicated in view of a 10- to 20-percent incidence of coarctation of the aorta. Thyroid function should also be measured because of an increased incidence of autoimmune thyroid disease. Routine diagnostic imaging of the kidneys is performed in the initial evaluation because of the increased incidence of renal tract abnormalities, especially horseshoe kidney.

Lifelong estrogen replacement is essential in patients with Turner's syndrome. Significant acceleration of ulnar bone growth has been shown in short-term studies using low-dose estrogen replacement (5 μg ethinyl estradiol), while a dose of 10 μg ethinyl estradiol daily similarly accelerates bone growth but also induces breast budding.[2] Whether this therapy augments eventual adult height is controversial, but it has the clinical advantage of inducing pubertal change, menses, and a growth spurt in line with that of the patient's peers. The maintenance of bone density and normal female lipid profiles (with a likely reduction in the future risk of atherosclerotic vascular disease) are other important advantages

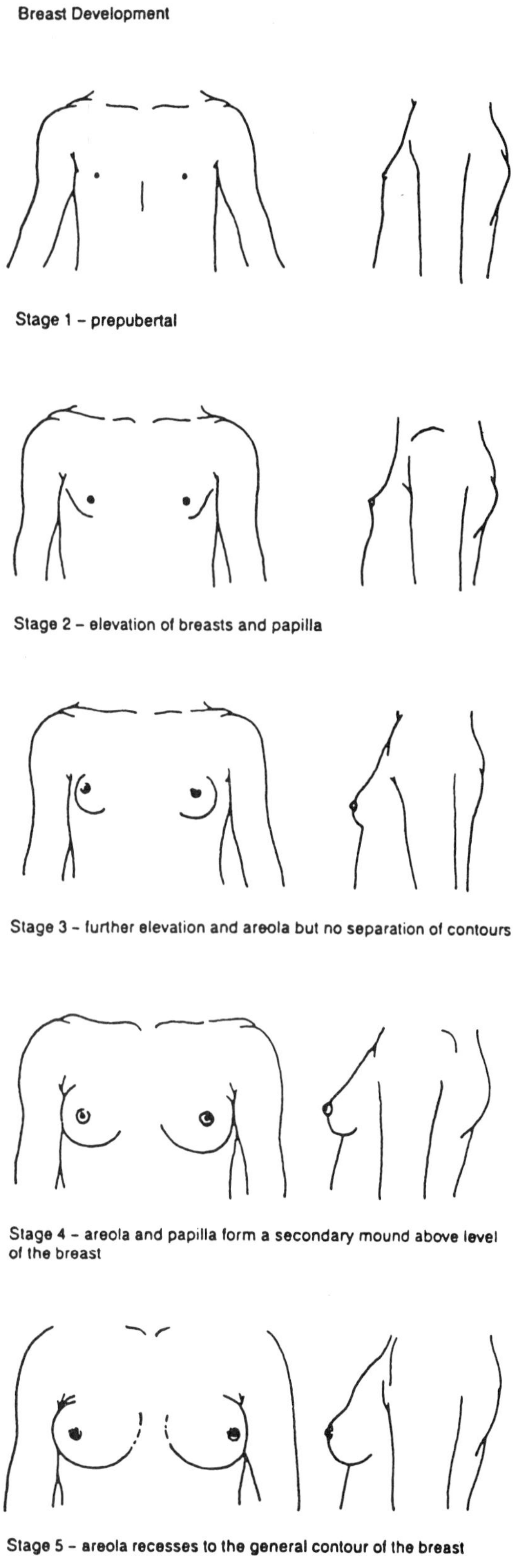

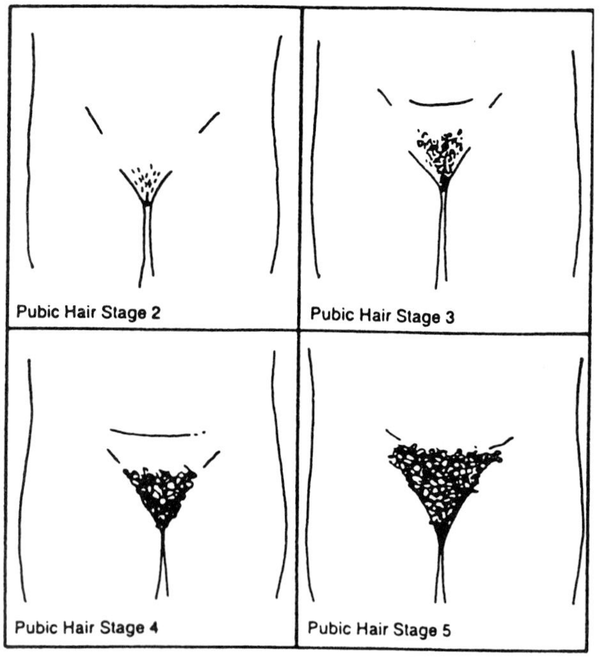

FIGURE 16B-1.
STAGES OF PUBERTY
Pubertal staging is based on the degree of breast and pubic hair development. (*Adapted from Tanner J, Davis PSW: J Paediatrics 107:317, 1985.*)
Breast development: Stages 1–5 as shown.
Pubic hair
Stage 1. Preadolescent. The vellus over the pubes is not further developed than that over the abdominal wall, i.e., no pubic hair.
Stage 2. Sparse growth of long, slightly pigmented downy hair, straight or slightly curled, chiefly along labia.
Stage 3. Considerably darker, coarser, and more curled. The hair spreads sparsely over the junction of the pubes.
Stage 4. Hair now adult in type, but area covered is still considerably smaller than in the adult. No spread to the medial surface of thighs.
Stage 5. Adult in quantity and type with distribution of the horizontal (or classically "feminine") pattern. Spread to medial surface of thighs but not up linea alba or elsewhere above the base of the inverse triangle (spread up linea alba occurs late and is rated stage 6).

of estrogen replacement. Improvement in growth velocity and adult height are the major aims of treatment. Several studies have shown that recombinant human growth hormone (hGH) alone or in combination with androgens or estrogens can accelerate growth velocity and stimulate catch-up growth.[3–5] For example, hGH 1 IU/kg per week is commenced at 4–5 years (if the diagnosis is made early) and continued until completion of growth. If the diagnosis is made later, growth hormone should still be initiated if

TABLE 16B-1. Clinical Classification of Primary Amenorrhea

Short stature, no pubertal development
- Gonadal dysgenesis
  - Turner's syndrome (45,XO)*
  - Turner's mosaicism (e.g., 46,XX, 45,XO)
  - Abnormalities of X chromosome
  - Mosaicism 46,XX, 45,XO + Y variants
  - Pure gonadal dysgenesis
- Hypopituitarism
  - Hypothalamo-pituitary dysfunction: idiopathic or associated with surgery, irradiation, trauma, tumor

Normal stature, no or minimal pubertal development
- Hypogonadotropic hypogonadism (Kallmann's syndrome)
  - Idiopathic*
  - Organic lesions
- Idiopathic delayed puberty*
- Malnutrition, systemic disease, intensive exercise*

Normal stature and pubertal development
- With adrenarche: müllerian (paramesonephric) duct-derivative abnormalities
- Without adrenarche: testicular feminization

Virilization and/or anomalous genitalia
- Miscellaneous rare disorders:
  - Partial testicular feminization
  - Inborn errors of testosterone biosynthesis or conversion to dihydrotestosterone
  - Untreated congenital adrenal hyperplasia

* Most common differential diagnoses.

skeletal age assessed by X-ray of the wrist is <12 years. If the initial response is poor, and in patients presenting at 8–10 years of age, a low dose of an anabolic agent such as oxandrolone may be added. The anabolic agent is ceased when estrogen therapy is begun. Such treatment programs have substantially improved the probability of achieving a more normal adult height. Informed and sensitive medical and psychosocial counselling both for the girl's parents and for her, once old enough to understand her condition, is mandatory—the latter may be from around age 10 in intellectually normal girls.

Although these subjects have no oocytes and have been regarded as sterile, with the advent of donor oocyte in vitro fertilization (IVF) programs, fertility is now possible. Donor oocytes have been used for many years in women with premature ovarian failure, including those with Turner's syndrome. Both mosaic and nonmosaic patients have the same pregnancy rates as others requiring donor eggs, provided that the hormone replacement regimen results in an endometrial thickness ≥6.5 mm, the uterine size is ≥5 cm, and the uterine shape is normal.[6] In the future, ovarian tissue donation may be an option. A possible donor would be the patient's mother, from whom a 1 mm segment of the ovary could be removed and frozen whilst she is of reproductive age (preferably <35 years), and kept until required by her daughter. At that time, the frozen-thawed tissue could be replaced in an easily accessible site in the donor. This is preferable to donation of the tissue to the patient as that would require tissue histocompatibility. The small amount of ovary can be stimulated to produce multiple follicles using controlled ovarian hyperstimulation, with oocyte retrieval, fertilization, and embryo transfer to the patient. During pregnancy, women with Turner's syndrome have a greater risk for hypertension, particularly if they have coarctation of the aorta, and they may also have problems with obstructed labor because of their short stature. In light of the above, a new optimism should permeate the paramedical and lay support groups for Turner's syndrome patients, which are available in many centers for counselling of the patient, her parents, or her husband regarding the nature of the condition. (See also Management of Premature Ovarian Failure, later.)

Mosaicism Compared to the XO karyotype, the XO/XX karyotype is associated with taller stature, fewer somatic abnormalities, and occasionally menstruation and fertility. In fact it has been reported that 8 percent of 45,XO women menstruate spontaneously, the percentage being higher in patients with mosaicism.[7] In patients with Turner's syndrome who become pregnant spontaneously, there is a 29 percent abortion rate and a 22 percent incidence of births with Down's and Turner's syndromes, respectively dictating the need for counseling and amniocentesis. It has been reported that 38 percent of offspring of such patients are normal. There is a 7 percent stillbirth rate and 34 percent have physical or mental abnormalities.[8]

Disorders incorporating XO/XY mosaicism lead to a range of phenotypes from male to female. Predominantly female phenotypes usually present with amenorrhea and a degree of genital virilization. The 30–70 percent frequency of gonadal tumors, especially dysgerminoma, warrants prophylactic removal of the gonads at the time that the diagnosis is made (see Chap. 18).

Hypopituitarism

Conditions that diminish pituitary function are often associated with inadequate growth hormone and gonadotropin secretion, resulting in short stature and failure to enter puberty. Features of thyroid and adrenal deficiency may also be present. Often a history of head trauma, cranial tumor surgery, or irradiation is elicited, although the patient may present with primary amenorrhea reflecting an underlying and often idiopathic hypothalamo-pituitary disorder. Depressed levels of gonadotropins and other pituitary hormones, which may be unresponsive to their normal trophic stimuli, will be found. Computed tomography (CT) or magnetic resonance imaging (MRI) of the pituitary region is essential to exclude a neoplasm, especially a craniopharyngioma. Therapy involves treatment of the underlying cause and replacement of sex steroids and other deficient hormones.

Normal Stature and No or Minimal Pubertal Development

Hypogonadotropic Hypogonadism (Kallmann's Syndrome)

Delayed or absent pubertal change, particularly when associated with hyposmia or anosmia in a subject of normal height, suggests the possibility of idiopathic hypogonadotropic hypogonadism.[9] This congenital, often familial condition results from an isolated deficiency of hypothalamic gonadotropin releasing hormone (GnRH) and therefore of gonadotropins (Fig. 16B-2). This deficiency appears to result from the failure of GnRH neurons to migrate from the olfactory placode into the hypothalamus. Associated somatic abnormalities include cleft lip and palate and congenital deafness. Deletion of the Xp 22.3 region of the X chromosome is associated with Kallmann's syndrome and occasionally with other congenital defects such as ichthyosis and chondromalacia punctata.[10]

Laboratory features include low ovarian steroid production and low to low normal gonadotropin levels. The pituitary, chronically

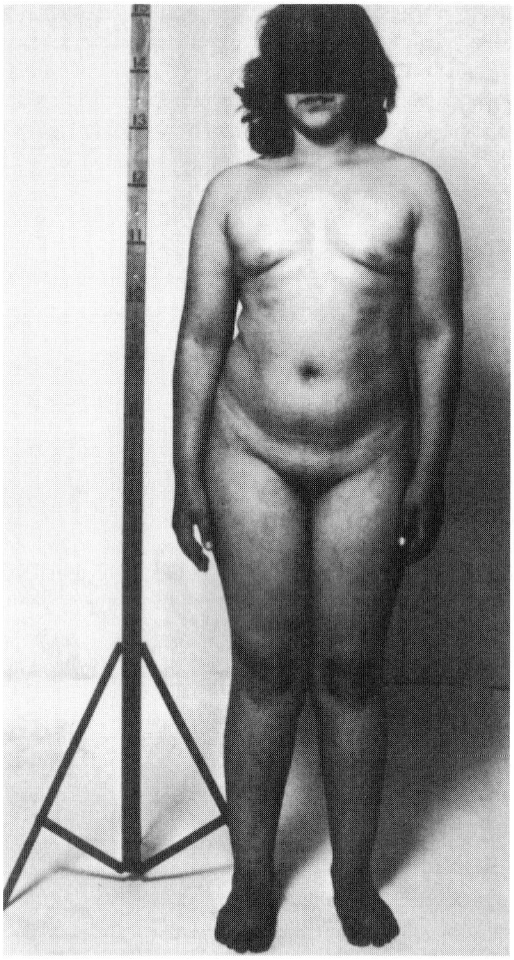

FIGURE 16B-2. Clinical appearance of a 19-year-old female with hypogonadotropic hypogonadism. Note the normal height (152 cm) and absence of a female body habitus. There was no breast development in this patient.

deprived of GnRH stimulation, generally responds poorly to acute GnRH infusion, although normal or exaggerated responses have been described. Basal and stimulated levels of other pituitary hormones are usually normal, although diminished prolactin secretion in response to thyrotropin releasing hormone (TRH) has been described in females. CT or MRI scanning of the hypothalamopituitary region is also indicated in view of the occasional occurrence of tumor, hamartoma, empty sella syndrome, and disorders of the rhinencephalon.

Induction of pubertal changes and menses is achieved with exogenous estrogen and progesterone. Women with this syndrome are characteristically unresponsive to clomiphene. Fertility can be achieved with exogenous gonadotropin ovulation induction (see later) or with pulsatile GnRH infusion therapy. Pulsatile GnRH, either subcutaneous or intravenous, is preferable because of the low rate of multiple pregnancy.

Idiopathic Delayed Puberty

A delay in menarche as a component of delayed puberty is a common cause of presentation with primary amenorrhea. Its differentiation from hypogonadotropic hypogonadism can be very difficult. Features supporting the diagnosis include a family history of delayed puberty, normal development in other respects, and usually some development and progression of pubertal changes by the time of consultation. These subjects are often short (3rd to 10th percentile) with an appropriately delayed bone age. Serum gonadotropin and ovarian steroid secretion either is prepubertal or shows early pubertal changes corresponding to the degree of pubertal development. Neither GnRH infusion nor other tests, such as the prolactin response to TRH or metoclopramide, lead to confident diagnostic discrimination between delayed puberty and hypogonadotropic hypogonadism. Therefore, after other likely causes have been excluded, reassurance and review of these patients should be rewarded by spontaneous menses between ages 17 and 20 years. The pubertal growth spurt is also delayed, but adult height is usually normal. Pubertal development can be hastened, if desired by the patient, by estrogen replacement (as described previously for Turner's syndrome) alone with intermittent withdrawal to observe the underlying state of the pituitary ovarian axis, at which time the possibility of hypogonadotropic hypogonadism can be readdressed.[11] It should be noted that hyperprolactinemia is an occasional cause of primary amenorrhea.

Malnutrition, Systemic Disease, or Intensive Exercise

Normal puberty can be interrupted by intercurrent problems such as the severe weight loss seen in starvation, anorexia nervosa, or severe systemic diseases. Intensive athletic training, particularly ballet and running, can be associated with decreased body weight, particularly fat content, along with menstrual disturbances including amenorrhea. Although more commonly a cause of secondary amenorrhea, such activities, when undertaken and maintained from early puberty, can produce primary amenorrhea. Restoration of good nutrition with weight gain or resolution of underlying illness should restore pubertal progression. In these settings serum gonadotropins show a prepubertal pattern of low levels [particularly of luteinizing hormone (LH)], lack of pulsatile secretion, and blunted response to GnRH.

Normal Stature with Normal Pubertal Development

Müllerian Duct–Derivative Abnormalities

Primary amenorrhea with normal growth and pubertal development to a stage where menses ought to be occurring suggests abnormalities of the müllerian duct–derived structures (uterine tubes, uterus, cervix, and upper vagina).[12] Ovarian function is normal, but menses do not occur because of an absence of normal endometrial tissue or the lack of a conduit for menstrual flow to the exterior. An imperforate vagina (often incorrectly diagnosed as an imperforate hymen) may lead to retention of menstrual fluid behind a membrane (hematocolpos) or cyclic abdominal pain from an accompanying hematometra. The resultant mass may be sufficiently large to produce abdominal distension. Clinical examination, including examination under general anesthesia, will define these anatomic variations. Therapy will depend on the anatomy and may range from simple stellate incision of the vaginal membrane, drainage, and use of prophylactic antibiotics to laparotomy for excision of a noncommunicating uterine horn, to consideration of surrogacy or adoption or an absent uterus.

Testicular Feminization

A normal female phenotype, often with tall stature and breast development but absent or scanty pubic hair, suggests the possibility of testicular feminization, also termed androgen insensitivity

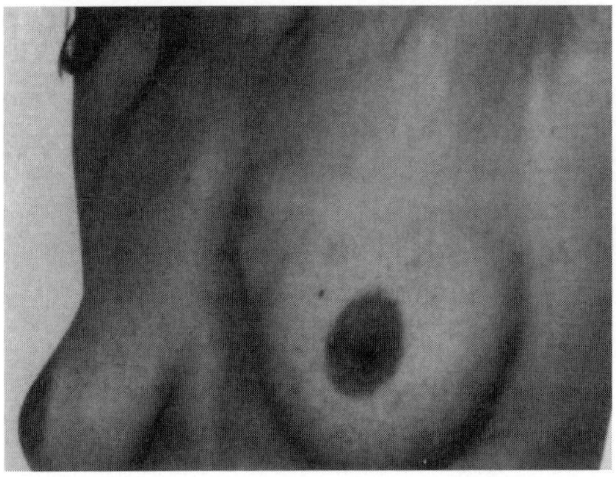

FIGURE 16B-3. Testicular feminization. Note the Tanner stage 5 breast development, resulting from testicular estrogen secretion, and the absence of axillary hair.

syndrome (AIS). This is an X-linked dominant condition in which absent or defective cytosolic testosterone receptors result in androgen insensitivity in genetic males (46,XY). Analysis of the androgen receptor gene reveals a range of mutations (deletions, substitutions) which lead to androgen resistance.[13] Testes are present, but spermatogenesis does not occur and the testes lie in the abdomen, the pelvis, the inguinal canal or labia. This latter key examination feature underlines the importance of a thorough examination of the inguinal and labial region. External genitalia are female; however, the vagina is a short pouch and no müllerian duct derivatives are present. The absence of a uterus can be confirmed by rectal examination and ultrasound. Diagnostic features include the karyotype and a serum testosterone level in the normal male range while serum LH concentration is raised, underlining the insensitivity of the pituitary gonadotrophs to testosterone feedback. Testicular estrogen production and conversion of testosterone to estradiol, in the absence of testosterone effects, lead to pubertal breast development (Fig. 16B-3). Cytosolic androgen receptors are absent or defective. Therapy includes reinforcement of the female gender identity and orchidectomy at any time in the presence of a gonadal hernia or otherwise after puberty in view of an increased incidence of testicular neoplasia. Lifelong estrogen replacement is then required (see Hormonal Replacement Therapy under Postmenopausal Problems, later).

Virilization and/or Anomalous Genitalia

A range of rare disorders may present with amenorrhea and varying degrees of virilization and/or anomalous genitalia in a young girl. Partial testicular feminization occurs when the defect in the androgen receptor is incomplete. Some androgen effect therefore leads to labioscrotal fusion or clitoromegaly. Deficiency of the 5α-reductase enzyme is an autosomal recessive condition of genetic males in which there are normal testosterone levels but inadequate conversion to the more potent androgen dihydrotestosterone (DHT). Ambiguous genitalia (varying degrees of labioscrotal fusion) with a blind-ending vaginal pouch occur. Virilization occurs at puberty, while breast development fails. Finally, a range of inborn errors of the testosterone biosynthetic pathway are other rare causes of female or anomalous genitalia associated with amenorrhea in the genetic male. These conditions are outlined in Chap. 17. They require extensive investigation of steroid metabolism and androgen receptor activity as well as anatomic delineation.

Menarcheal Menorrhagia

The mammalian uterus is a highly specialized fibromuscular and secretory organ in which the myometrium is elastic and contractile properties are responsive to a variety of hormonal regulators secreted both locally and distantly. In contrast, the inner lining of the uterus, the endometrium, is a distinctive tissue in both form and function. Throughout adult reproductive life in humans and other higher primates, the endometrium grows and is shed cyclically as a bloody discharge (i.e., the menstrual cycle) that typically recurs at about 28-day intervals. The temporal nature of this sequence (proliferation, differentiation, and sloughing of the endometrium) is the classic manifestation of an end organ response to the changing steroidal milieu imposed by the ovarian cycle. Until recently little attention was given to the endometrium as a source of hormone secretion. Accordingly, traditional emphasis on clinical disorders of the ovary can now usefully be widened to include endometrial secretion of hormones that may act both locally and distantly. Increasing evidence suggests that endometrial tissue may play a central role in the complement of endocrine signals governing female fertility.[14]

Cyclic ovarian function normally begins in adolescent girls soon after menarche. Before the attainment of gonadotropin secretory capabilities sufficient to support follicular maturation leading to ovulation, a limited degree of intermittent estrogen secretion results in endometrial proliferation and irregular vaginal bleeding; that is, variable degrees and intervals of hypoestrogenism are interspersed with transient elevations of blood estrogen levels. The initial ovulatory cycles in these young women are often characterized by abbreviated intermenstrual intervals and serum progesterone levels below those of the normal adult in the luteal phase. Clinically, these changes can be seen in a young teenager with heavy and irregular menses due to recurrent anovulation. In developed parts of the world menarche normally occurs between 11.5 and 15.5 years (mean 12.8 years, SD 1.0 year). Menstruation occurs regularly; cycles occur between 21 and 35 days apart (28.0 $\pm$ 3.5 days) and persist for 3–7 days. Studies by Baird and associates have proved that dysfunctional uterine bleeding in this age group is often associated with a defect in the positive feedback response to estradiol.[15]

Heavy menarcheal bleeding is not rare. If there is no possibility of pregnancy, the initial therapy should be medical, with progestogen treatment, such as 5–10 mg per day of norethindrone for 10 days (in the absence of cycles). An excellent alternative is the oral contraceptive pill which provides cycle control as well as effective contraception. Tranexamic acid is an antifibrinolytic agent shown to be one of the most effective in decreasing menstrual blood loss in women with heavy, regular periods with no pathological cause. A randomized trial[16] compared the efficacy of mefenamic acid (500 mg 8 hourly), ethamsylate (500 mg 6 hourly) and tranexamic acid (1 g 6 hourly) in 76 women with regular, heavy DUB. The treatment began on cycle day 1 and continued for 5 days. The authors showed that tranexamic acid reduced menstrual blood loss by 50 percent, mefenamic acid by 20 percent, and ethamsylate did not decrease blood loss. The side effects of tranexamic acid include nausea, abdominal pain, diarrhea, dizziness, and headache. The rare but major potential side effect is thrombosis.[17] In young teenagers curettage should be a last resort in attempting to control endometrial hemorrhage as well as in excluding extremely rare diseases such as sarcoma botryoides. A hemorrhagic diathesis should always be excluded in a teenager who presents with catastrophic menarcheal bleeding.

Fifty to 80 percent of patients with hemorrhagic diatheses have excessive menstrual blood loss.

OVARIAN DISORDERS IN YOUNG ADULTS

Secondary Amenorrhea

The cessation of menses for longer than 6 months in a patient who has previously menstruated is termed *secondary amenorrhea*. The most common cause is pregnancy, although a pregnancy beyond 12 weeks gestation should not be missed clinically by any doctor. Early pregnancy findings are minimal, and a pregnancy test therefore is essential in all patients with secondary amenorrhea. Serum gonadotropin assays in pregnancy may reveal a markedly elevated LH level, reflecting cross-reaction of hCG in many LH radioimmunoassays, while follicle stimulating hormone (FSH) concentration is low normal. Another important physiologic cause of amenorrhea is breast-feeding. This is associated with a period of ovarian inactivity, the duration of which depends on the frequency and duration of suckling. It is associated with elevated prolactin levels, failure of positive feedback of estradiol on LH and FSH secretion, and disturbances of pulsatile LH release. With decreased breast-feeding, ovarian function gradually returns, yielding periods of initially increased estradiol production without menses, menses without ovulation or with inadequate luteal function, and, finally, normal ovulatory cycles. Maternal undernutrition prolongs the period of lactational amenorrhea. Finally, the natural menopause generally occurs after age 40. The cessation of menses in the menopause can take the form of oligomenorrhea, menorrhagia, or abrupt cessation. Symptoms of estrogen deficiency (vaginal atrophy, hot flushes) are common, and gonadotropin levels are in the postmenopausal range. A family history in patients with early menopause is common. The most important clinical disorders, after the physiologic causes of secondary amenorrhea, are outlined in Table 16B-2.

TABLE 16B-2. Clinical Classification of Secondary Amenorrhea

Physiologic
Pregnancy
Lactation
Menopause
Premature ovarian failure
Congenital
Acquired
Autoimmune
Idiopathic
Chemotherapy, irradiation
Surgery, trauma
Infection
Hyperprolactinemia and/or galactorrhea
Drug-associated
Prolactinoma
Microadenoma
Macroadenoma
Systemic illness (e.g., hypothyroidism)
Nutrition/exercise-associated
Weight loss
Simple
Anorexia nervosa
Systemic illness
Intensive exercise
Polycystic ovary syndrome
Rare conditions
Uterine synechiae: postcurettage endometritis
Pituitary deficiency
Tumors, especially after surgery or irradiation
Sheehan's syndrome
Ovarian/adrenal neoplasia, empty sella syndrome

Premature Ovarian Failure

Premature ovarian failure (POF) can be defined as the syndrome of amenorrhea, hypoestrogenism, and elevated serum gonadotropin concentrations occurring before age 40 years. It occurs in about 1 percent of women. For practical purposes, 40 years may reasonably be taken as the age after which cessation of menses is most likely to be due to spontaneous cessation of ovarian function. Cessation of ovarian function may occur in the teenage years as a rare cause of primary amenorrhea; most commonly it presents with secondary amenorrhea and accounts for about 5 percent of new cases.[18]

The clinical and hormonal features of POF are similar to those of the normal menopause and commonly develop over a period of several years. Approximately half the subjects present with clinical features of hypoestrogenism (mainly vaginal dryness and hot flushes), while secondary sexual characteristics are usually normal. If the condition develops around the time of menarche, the secondary sexual characteristics may be underdeveloped. The combination of hot flushes and amenorrhea always warrants exclusion of POF. Serum gonadotropin concentrations are elevated and hyperresponsive to GnRH as after the normal menopause. As is also seen in the perimenopausal period, serum FSH levels may fluctuate in and out of the normal range and serum estradiol levels may rise to the midfollicular range. These fluctuations may be seen over a period of several years with a gradual trend toward established hypoestrogenic hypergonadotropic amenorrhea. The variable natural history of this transition was underlined by a study of 67 women suspected of having premature ovarian failure on the basis of an elevated FSH level.[19] More than one-quarter of these women resumed normal ovarian function in 1–5 years; six subjects conceived. Neither clinical features (e.g., age, mode of presentation) nor the degree of FSH concentration elevation predicted which subjects would resume ovarian function. Little is known about the natural history of POF, although spontaneous resumption of menses and fertility may occur in some women.

Etiologies of Premature Ovarian Failure

Genetic In about 50 percent of patients presenting with POF, no cause can be identified. Premature ovarian failure may occur either as a result of ovarian follicular dysfunction or follicular depletion.[18] Follicular dysfunction may arise as a result of autoimmunity, gonadotropin or gonadotropin receptor abnormalities, enzyme deficiencies, chemotherapy, or radiation. Follicular depletion may occur as a result of X chromosome abnormalities, galactosemia, and again as a result of chemotherapy or radiation or of viral illnesses.

Chromosomal abnormalities, particularly variants of gonadal dysgenesis, may present with POF and secondary amenorrhea. The previous pattern of menses and physical findings may be normal and require that karyotyping be performed on all women under the age of 35 years undergoing investigation for POF. Future management may be influenced by an abnormal karyotype, particularly one including a Y chromosome. The majority of subjects, however, have the normal 46,XX karyotype. A family history of POF is found in 10 percent of subjects. The pattern of inheritance is not clear, but reports of vertical transmission of the trait are consistent with autosomal dominant or sex-linked inheritance.[20]

Physical Agents Pelvic surgery and viral (especially mumps) oophoritis are rare causes of POF. Gonadal irradiation and/or chemotherapy (especially with cyclophosphamide or busulfan) for malignant conditions are also known to cause transient (especially with exposure before age 30) or permanent ovarian failure.[21] Finally, cigarette smoking, perhaps via an antiovarian action of polycyclic aromatic hydrocarbons, is associated with menopause 1–3 years earlier than in nonsmokers.

Autoimmunity Evidence for an autoimmune basis for some cases of POF is based on two observations. First, the association of POF with other autoimmune diseases, especially Hashimoto's thyroiditis and Addison's disease, has been reported. In a study of 33 women with POF, 39 percent had an associated autoimmune condition and 18 percent had a family history of such a condition.[22] Another study of 24 patients demonstrated non-organ-specific autoantibodies (e.g., antinuclear) and various organ-specific autoantibodies (adrenal, gastric, pancreatic, ovarian) in 92 percent of subjects, although very few had associated disease states.[23] Second, the presence of anti-ovarian antibodies, including anti–zona pellucida antibodies, in the serum of some of these patients has been reported. The methodology for assessing the presence of antibodies is not universally accepted, and a direct pathogenic role for these antibodies has not been established.[18] Overall, an autoimmune link with POF may be present in 20–50 percent of these patients. Consideration of possible autoimmune thyroid or adrenal disease should be given in initial assessment and intermittently during a review of patients with POF.

Occult Ovarian Failure

Occult ovarian failure is a term for a syndrome of the clinical triad of infertility, regular menses, and hypergonadotropic hypogonadism.[24] Unlike POF, occult ovarian failure is not associated with impaired ovarian steroid synthesis. However, serum FSH and LH concentrations are elevated throughout the spontaneous menstrual cycle in these patients. In addition, autoantibodies to the ovary or the adrenal or thyroid glands are present in 50 percent and anti-ovarian antibodies are detectable in 40 percent. In addition to ovarian estradiol and progesterone secretion equivalent to that seen in the spontaneous ovarian cycle, serum immunoreactive inhibin concentrations are also within the normal range though it seems probable that inhibin B concentration would be reduced (see later discussion). It is believed that occult ovarian failure represents a state of compensated granulosa cell failure where ovarian steroid and glycoprotein secretion is maintained by a compensatory increase in pituitary FSH secretion. Women with occult ovarian failure have an impaired response to ovarian hyperstimulation and may be at increased risk of developing polyglandular autoimmunity. A syndrome of "incipient ovarian failure" in which inhibin levels are below the normal range and FSH is more greatly elevated than in occult ovarian failure has also been described.[25]

Management of Premature Ovarian Failure

The diagnosis of POF is confirmed by the finding of sustained gonadotropin elevation associated with depressed estrogen secretion in a woman less than 40 years of age. Weekly serum gonadotropin determinations and tests of urinary estrogen and progesterone excretion during a 6-week period will establish a true baseline estimate of any ovarian follicular activity. Karyotyping should be performed in all patients under the age of 35 years.

Therapy for POF involves the replacement of estrogen and cyclic progesterone for the maintenance of normal secondary sex characteristics and libido and avoidance of the long-term sequelae of hypoestrogenism. In young women a dose equivalent to 1.25 mg conjugated estrogens daily is recommended together with a progestin for 12–14 days each month to prevent endometrial hyperplasia. Androgen replacement should also be considered in women who are not restored to well-being by estrogen replacement, in particular if they complain of persisting fatigue and low libido.[26] Although achievement of fertility is unlikely, many spontaneous and therapy-associated pregnancies have been reported. Ovarian biopsy has been emphasized by some authors as necessary to differentiate oocyte depletion from the gonadotropin-resistant ovary syndrome, which allegedly is amenable to treatment. However, ovarian biopsy may not provide a representative tissue sample, and patients said to lack primordial follicles may subsequently ovulate. High-dose exogenous gonadotropin therapy has occasionally been associated with pregnancy, but the results of this expensive therapy have generally been disappointing.[18] The majority of POF subjects who subsequently conceive have been exposed to estrogen. In theory, estrogen may act to induce FSH receptors in the remaining follicles, prevent down regulation of ovarian gonadotropin receptors by suppressing circulating gonadotropin levels, or increase the biological activity of the gonadotropins.

None of these therapies for POF has been subjected to a proper prospective trial with due regard to the variable natural history of POF and the spontaneous pregnancy rate.[19,27] In view of these facts, POF patients requesting fertility are not routinely subjected to ovarian biopsy. Review of the underlying ovarian-pituitary axis during sex steroid replacement is undertaken every 3–6 months. The return of a normal serum FSH level may occur spontaneously even years after diagnosis, with the return of menses and fertility. Ovulation induction (see later discussion) may be undertaken during the period of normal circulating FSH levels but is usually not successful. Further studies of the natural history, autoimmunity, and ovarian histology of POF and prospective study of a range of therapies are needed to allow better categorization of POF and particularly to identify subgroups amenable to therapy. Patients with POF desirous of fertility are now managed in a donor oocyte program as described previously for Turner's syndrome.

In these treatments, the oocyte donor has been either anonymous or known to the recipient. The general phenotypic characteristics of the recipient and donor have been matched in a fashion similar to the matching of phenotypic characteristics which occurs in programs of artificial insemination using donor semen. In some countries legislation has established registries of such oocyte donors so that the children born from these procedures may acquire nonidentifying information about the donors upon attaining adulthood.[28]

Hyperprolactinemia and Galactorrhea

Hyperprolactinemia is a common cause of female infertility, accounting for about 20 percent of cases, depending on the referral center. When sustained, hyperprolactinemia is usually associated with oligo- or amenorrhea and infertility. Impairment of reproductive capacity probably occurs at the hypothalamic level with disturbance of the dopaminergic control of pulsatile GnRH release. Defects in the positive feedback of sex steroids on the hypothalamus and a direct anti-ovarian action of prolactin have also been postulated. Galactorrhea is an important and frequent accompaniment of hyperprolactinemia. It is usually defined as any persistent milklike discharge from the nipple or overt lactation occurring in a nulliparous woman or a mother whose offspring has been weaned more than 6 months previously. It may be spontaneous or apparent only on manual expression. The majority of women with galactorrhea and secondary amenorrhea have hyperprolactinemia. Galactorrhea may, however, occur with normal prolactin concentrations and without menstrual disturbance. Such idiopathic galactorrhea was reported as the largest single category (32 percent) in 235 consecutive cases of galactorrhea.[29] The presence of galactorrhea always requires careful exclusion of the causes of hyperprolactinemia, as detailed later. Serial sampling is routinely performed at 20-min intervals for 2 h when a single elevated prolactin value <1,500 mu/ml is detected, as the prolactin may be elevated by the stress of venipuncture or a preceding breast examination.

Etiologies of Hyperprolactinemia

Drug-Related Phenothiazines and other psychotropic agents that act to antagonize hypothalamic dopaminergic pathways are associated with mild to moderate elevations of prolactin concentrations (up to four times normal). Galactorrhea has been reported in one-quarter of female psychiatric patients on high doses of such medications. Amenorrhea in association is less common, occurring in 22 percent of patients with drug-induced galactorrhea. Many other medications are associated with hyperprolactinemia, including metoclopramide, H_2 histamine antagonists, calcium channel blockers, and α-methyldopa.[30] These symptoms generally resolve with the cessation of medication.

Estrogens stimulate prolactin synthesis and mitotic activity in pituitary lactotrophs. Estrogen therapy, particularly the oral contraceptives, may lead to a mild elevation (approximately a doubling) of serum prolactin concentration. Estrogen has been implicated in the development of prolactinoma in cases of postpill amenorrhea syndromes; however, most recent case-control studies have not supported this contention.

Hypothalamic Disorders Pituitary prolactin secretion is under tonic inhibitory control by the hypothalamus via the postulated prolactin inhibitory factor(s) (PIF). Disruption of this system by a hypothalamic tumor, infiltrative disease (e.g., sarcoidosis), or surgical or traumatic stalk section can lead to a moderate elevation of prolactin concentration to four to six times normal. Galactorrhea and amenorrhea may result from the effect of elevated prolactin levels combined with interference with GnRH production in some cases.

Systemic Disease Primary hypothyroidism is associated with elevated hypothalamic TRH secretion, which enhances pituitary thyroid stimulating hormone (TSH) and prolactin secretion. It is therefore an uncommon but important cause of the amenorrhea–galactorrhea syndrome and is easily excluded by clinical assessment and thyroid function tests. Renal failure and hepatic cirrhosis are additional causes of hyperprolactinemia that usually do not present a diagnostic problem.

Local Factors Repetitive nipple stimulation can be associated with hyperprolactinemia and galactorrhea; irritative chest wall diseases (thoracic scarring or herpes zoster) are rare causes.

Polycystic Ovary Syndrome Inappropriately enhanced estrogen feedback leading to increased pituitary lactotroph secretion probably explains the modest (up to fivefold) elevation of prolactin concentration commonly seen in polycystic ovary syndrome (PCOS). Disturbance in the normal dopaminergic control of GnRH release has also been described; this may further explain diminished PIF activity. Clinical features of hirsutism, obesity, and absence of galactorrhea assist in the differentiation from prolactinoma, although occasionally further biochemical and radiologic investigations are needed. The picture is somewhat confused by a purportedly increased risk of prolactinoma in PCOS.

Prolactinoma Pituitary prolactinoma accounts for approximately 50 percent of cases of hyperprolactinemia. Its diagnosis depends on the finding of the following:

1. Sustained hyperprolactinemia, often of marked degree.
2. Normal or suppressed serum gonadotropin levels and estrogen production, as are commonly seen in association with amenorrhea.
3. Radiologic abnormalities of the pituitary. High-resolution CT scanning[31] and MRI scanning (where available) are the essential examinations. The relative merit of the two scanning methods is unclear, but CT may be better at detecting small lesions within a normal or minimally enlarged gland. MRI is superior in visualizing structures adjacent to the pituitary, which is often the most significant issue.[32,33] Conventionally, tumors are classified as microadenomas (<1 cm in diameter) or macroadenomas. Macroadenomas are less common in women; these larger tumors may extend beyond the pituitary fossa superiorly (suprasellar), laterally (parasellar), or antero-inferiorly into the sphenoid sinus.

Clinically, oligo- or amenorrhea may develop in association with prolactinoma at any reproductive age. With the widespread use of oral contraceptives, the problem is frequently recognized when these agents are ceased. As was previously mentioned, an etiologic role for this estrogen therapy in the genesis of prolactinoma has been suggested but not proved. Galactorrhea occurs in approximately 50 percent of cases. Occasionally mild obesity and hirsutism are seen, again with the differential diagnostic problem of PCOS. Estrogen deficiency resulting in frictional dyspareunia and loss of libido may occur. All these symptoms generally resolve upon restoration of normal prolactin levels. Symptoms of tumor enlargement (headache, visual field defects) are uncommon in females but can occur with macroadenomas and are an especially important consideration during pregnancy (see later discussion).

Idiopathic Hyperprolactinemia Idiopathic hyperprolactinemia is differentiated from prolactinoma by the failure to demonstrate a tumor on CT or MRI scanning. This distinction may be somewhat artificial in that the tumor may simply be too small to resolve even on the most sophisticated equipment. Therapeutically, the two conditions can be considered together. Various dynamic tests, such as the prolactin response to TRH or levodopa, have been suggested to differentiate tumorous from idiopathic hyperprolactinemia.

None has been conclusively shown to be superior to the imaging techniques.

Management of Hyperprolactinemia

Therapeutic intervention may be indicated for the following reasons:

1. Tumor-related problems, particularly compressive features such as headache, visual field defects, and cranial nerve palsies.
2. Infertility.
3. Disabling galactorrhea.
4. Short-term symptoms (secondary amenorrhea) and long-term side effects of chronic hypoestrogenemia, which may be avoided by restoration of normal menses and estrogen status. Bone density is reduced in chronic hyperprolactinemic amenorrhea and is improved by correction of hyperprolactinemia.[34,35]

For patients with tumor related problems, infertility and disabling galactorrhea, the management of first choice is generally the use of dopamine agonists. For patients complaining only of secondary amenorrhea, in particular where the hyperprolactinemia is idiopathic or secondary to the presence of a micro prolactinoma, treatment with the oral contraceptive pill is an acceptable option and does not lead to significant tumor growth.[36] In such circumstances, serum prolactin should be checked every 6–12 months to detect the minority of patients in whom tumor growth progresses.

Dopamine Agonists Dopamine agonists are the drugs of choice in the management of hyerprolactinemia. With reduction of prolactin levels, ovulatory menses and fertility are restored and galactorrhea abolished in the majority of patients.[37] Shrinkage of tumors frequently occurs.[31] The dopamine agonist of choice is currently cabergoline in an initial dose of one tablet (0.5 mg) once weekly. Dosage increments should be undertaken at intervals no shorter than one month and control of prolactin secretion is usually achieved within a dose range of 0.5 mg once weekly to 1 mg twice weekly, though occasionally higher doses must be used. Until recently, the most widely used dopamine agonist was bromocriptine. It is initiated at a dose of 1.25 mg at night with food and gradual increase in dosage over two weeks until control of symptoms and hyperprolactinemia is achieved, usually at 5–7.5 mg per day. Side effects of nausea, vomiting, constipation, and postural hypotension are minimized with this gradual introduction. In a direct comparison of cabergoline and bromocriptine in the treatment of hyperprolactinemic amenorrhea it was concluded that cabergoline is more effective and better tolerated,[38] and it has been shown to be capable of successfully reducing serum prolactin and causing tumor shrinkage in patients previously resistant to bromocriptine.[39]

When fertility is desired, it can be achieved in 75–85 percent of patients with dopamine agonists. If they are used to induce pregnancy, tumor enlargement is uncommon in microadenomas or in macroadenomas previously treated with x-ray or surgery.[40] Untreated macroadenoma is associated with a 5–10 percent risk of tumor enlargement. The authors routinely check for symptoms of enlargement and perform two monthly visual field estimates during pregnancy in patients with a macroadenoma. Whereas dopamine agonists are normally withdrawn once pregnancy has been established in patients with idiopathic hyperprolactinemia or a microadenoma, those with a macroadenoma should have dopamine agonist therapy continued. There is no evidence that bromocriptine is teratogenic, while for cabergoline, this has not yet been established with certainty.

There appear to be no adverse long term effects of pregnancy or breast-feeding on the natural history of prolactinoma and in fact serum prolactin has been reported to fall by more than 50 percent in a third of patients 1–9 years post partum.[41]

Surgery Surgical management of prolactinoma has a limited role. Success of transsphenoidal surgery, as judged by short-term normalization of prolactin concentration and resolution of symptoms, has been claimed in 60–90 percent of microadenoma patients, while the cure rate is much lower with larger tumors. Recent studies have indicated a late relapse rate of up to 20 percent at 5 years in previously "cured" subjects.[42,43] In view of the efficacy of dopamine agonists, the role of pituitary surgery is now seen as limited to subjects who are intolerant of or resistant to those drugs and those with tumors causing compressive symptoms, where the drugs have had an inadequate effect.

Nutritional Amenorrhea

Adequate nutrition is essential to the initiation and maintenance of reproductive capacity. Frisch and Revelle showed that the mean weight of normal girls at the time of menarche is 48 kg, independent of their age at sexual maturation.[44] Subsequently, it was postulated that a critical percentage of body weight (17 percent) must be present as fat for menarche to occur and that during puberty this percentage increases, stabilizing at approximately 28 percent in adulthood.[45] The maintenance of normal ovulatory cycles requires about 22 percent body weight as fat. In practical terms weight loss below 10–15 percent of ideal body weight is sufficient to interfere with reproductive capacity. Improved nutrition over the past century may therefore be related to the trend toward an earlier menarche. Undernutrition of any cause can be associated with diminished reproductive capacity, the severity of which is proportional to the degree of weight loss.

The mechanism by which body fat is related to reproductive state has been reviewed recently.[46] Hypothalamic neuropeptide Y appears to be a central link between nutrition and reproductive function. Cell bodies which produce this peptide are functionally and morphologically linked to hypothalamic galanin and opioid networks which in turn have roles in the control of reproduction and eating behavior. The adipose tissue hormone, leptin, has direct feedback effects on neuropeptide Y gene expression. Alterations in neuropeptide Y levels as a result of nutritional deprivation are in turn related to alterations in GnRH pulse frequency and amplitude. This leads to a reversion toward a prepubertal pattern of diminished GnRH responsiveness and a decrease in levels of gonadotropins, particularly LH, which is proportional to the degree of fat loss (Fig. 16B-4).[47] Mediation of these effects by opiate peptide inhibition of GnRH secretion has been suggested; the opiate antagonist naloxone has been successful in restoring LH in weight loss-related amenorrhea.[48] Estrogen production by the ovary and from peripheral conversion of androgen in fat tissue is reduced to prepubertal levels in these women. Overall, these can be considered appropriate adaptive responses to starvation. Other hormonal changes have been described in anorexia nervosa, including diminished serum triiodothyronine (T_3) and prolactin concentrations and increased secretion of cortisol and growth hormone.[49]

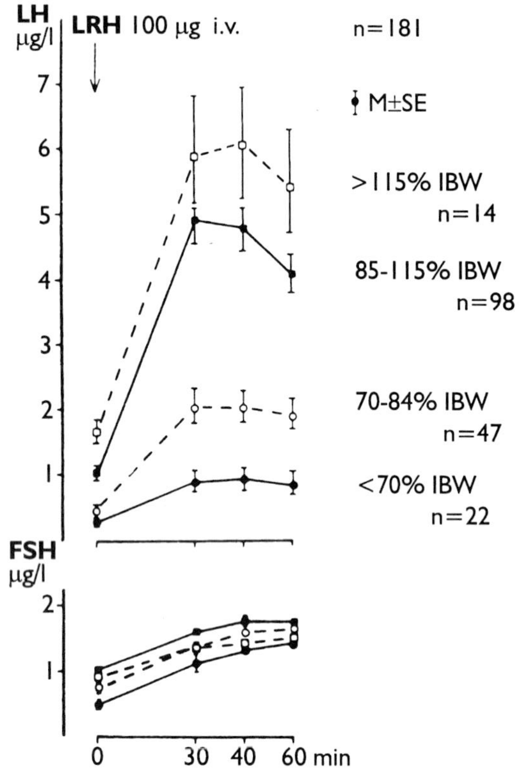

FIGURE 16B-4. As the proportion of body fat decreases, a diminished gonadotropin responsiveness to GnRH occurs. (*Reproduced from Berg et al.,*[47] *with permission.*)

Etiologies of Nutritional Amenorrhea

The common etiologies of nutritional amenorrhea are summarized in the following sections. The endocrine changes outlined previously are essentially common to all these etiologies.

Simple Weight Loss The most common presentation of secondary amenorrhea is that of a girl who complains of absence of menses without obvious cause, occurring either spontaneously or after discontinuation of the oral contraceptive pill. Careful questioning reveals a history of weight loss, often relatively rapid, of about 3–7 kg (7–15 lb), usually because of a conviction that she is somewhat overweight. There may be an accompanying history of fairly intensive exercise. Such weight loss may occur while the contraceptive pill is being taken, in which case the postpill amenorrhea may be falsely ascribed to an effect of the pill rather than the incidental weight loss. There are usually accompanying drops in the levels of LH and estradiol. Regain of weight commonly leads to restoration of the hormone levels to normal and reinitiation of cyclic menses.

Anorexia Nervosa This is a severe psychiatric condition featuring a distortion of body image and perceptions of feelings of hunger and satiety. Such patients are often adolescent girls with extremely manipulative personalities, making treatment difficult. Avoidance of carbohydrate-rich foods in particular is typical; bingeing and self-induced vomiting (bulimia) may occur. Amenorrhea occurs with reduction of body weight and fat; weight may be as low as 25 kg in severe cases. The causes of the psychological changes are unknown, but risk factors that have been suggested include a high-achieving personality, upper socioeconomic class, and careers requiring avoidance of obesity (e.g., ballet dancing). The condition is more subtle in the early stages and should always be considered in underweight amenorrheic subjects. Treatment occasionally involves hospitalization for severe cachexia but primarily involves intensive psychotherapy. Rates of successful treatment vary but are improved by early diagnosis. Mortality rates of up to 19 percent have been reported.[50]

Exercise-Related Amenorrhea Intensive exercise programs require increased caloric intake for the maintenance of body weight. Weight loss, particularly a reduction in the percentage of body weight as fat, may occur if exercise programs are too severe and/or dietary intake is inadequate. In adolescent ballet dancers a delay in the age of menarche compared to normal students matched for career stress has been reported.[51] An increased incidence of secondary amenorrhea in athletes has also been reported.[52] Among 23 runners, the incidence of amenorrhea was highest in those who began running before age 30, those running more than 40 miles per week, and nulliparous compared with multiparous subjects.[53] The occurrence of athletic amenorrhea appears to be the result of chronic low energy availability and not to the effects of the exercise per se.[54]

Management of Nutritional Amenorrhea

Resumption of menstruation and fertility usually accompanies the regain of weight. Improved nutritional status requires treatment of any underlying psychiatric problem and modification of inappropriate diets or exercise programs. Attempts at ovulation induction in the presence of severe weight loss are usually unsuccessful[55] and inadvisable with respect to maternal and fetal health. If weight gain is not practicable, consideration should be given to estrogen replacement therapy to avoid the long-term sequelae of hypoestrogenism, though such patients may be intolerant even of low-dose estrogen therapy. Exercise may not, as previously suspected, protect against the loss of bone density in amenorrheic runners.[56]

Polycystic Ovary Syndrome

The classic description of PCOS is of a syndrome that includes oligo- or amenorrhea, infertility, hirsutism, obesity, and enlarged polycystic ovaries. It is now recognized that PCOS is a heterogeneous group of disorders whose manifestations vary from the classic description to the isolated presence of one or more of the components. Assessment of its prevalence is difficult because of the lack of universally accepted diagnostic criteria. In the past, diagnosis was based on the typical clinical features associated with an elevated plasma LH/FSH ratio and elevated plasma androgen levels. Histologic confirmation of polycystic ovaries has not been widely available. With the advent of high-resolution ovarian ultrasound, ovarian anatomy can be assessed noninvasively. Polycystic ovaries (PCO) defined ultrasonically have been described in nonhirsute, regularly ovulating women.[57] There are generally ten or more subcapsular follicles, 2–10 mm in diameter, with bilateral ovarian enlargement (9 cm in maximal diameter) and increased density and area of stroma.[58] There is a strong familial component to PCOS, with polycystic ovaries on ultrasound being common in asymptomatic first-degree relatives of patients presenting with PCOS.[59] Therefore, this common condition has heterogeneous clinical, anatomic, and biochemical

TABLE 16B-3. Clinical Features of 300 Women with Polycystic Ovary Syndrone Diagnosed by Ultrasound

	Presenting Features, %	Total, %*
Hirsutism	34	64
Acne	9	27
Obesity, BMI >25 kg/m^2	10	35
Infertility	41	42
Amenorrhea	23	28
Oligomenorrhea/irregular cycle	38	52
Dysfunctional bleeding	6	14

*The total in the right-hand column refers to the total number of subjects who on history and/or examination were found to have the clinical abnormalities indicated. Ten women (3%) also had androgen-dependent alopecia, and two (1%) had acanthosis nigricans.

Source: Adapted from Franks.[59]

features. Three minimal criteria have been proposed for the diagnosis: chronic anovulation (leading to menstrual irregularity), hyperandrogenism, and the exclusion of other diseases such as nonclassical congenital adrenal hyperplasia, hyperprolactinemia, Cushing's syndrome, and androgen secreting tumors.[60] When polycystic ovaries are recognized by ultrasonography without other features, the diagnosis of PCOS is inappropriate, though subtle metabolic abnormalities may be found if actively sought.[61]

Clinical Features

A variety of clinical features are associated with PCOS (Table 16B-3). Although patients may present with one or more features, additional ones are often apparent on assessment.[58]

Menstrual Disturbance

Menarche usually occurs normally in PCOS, but there is menstrual irregularity with oligo- or amenorrhea persisting into adulthood. PCOS is probably the most common cause of persistent menstrual disturbance. One study reported a 20 percent incidence of polycystic ovaries on ultrasound in a large group of unselected "normal" women.[57] Three-quarters of these PCO women had a history of menstrual irregularity. Menstrual bleeding may be heavy and painful in view of the continuous unopposed estrogen effect (see later discussion). Cycles are often anovulatory or associated with a deficient luteal phase. Patients may seek help for irregular cycles per se, dysfunctional uterine bleeding, or infertility. The prevalence of PCOS as a cause of infertility varies depending on the referral center but has been reported in up to 50 percent of cases.[62]

Hirsutism

A degree of hirsutism varying from mild to severe (i.e., masculine pattern) is common in PCOS. It may be the primary reason for presentation or may have frustrated cosmetic attempts at management. Frequently acne is a troublesome accompaniment.

Obesity

Weight gain at the time of puberty causing mild to moderate obesity is common in PCOS, although many patients are of normal weight.

Pathophysiology

The complex question of the primary defect in PCOS remains unresolved, but the large body of knowledge available can be considered under the following headings. Figure 16B-5 depicts one schema for the pathogenesis of the PCOS, which may be outlined as follows:

1. Defects in ovarian function
   a. Folliculogenesis
   b. Sex steroid secretion
2. Defects in hypothalamic-pituitary function
3. Abnormal androgen metabolism
4. Insulin resistance

These defects exist concurrently and interact to produce a chronic anovulatory state with or without evidence of hyperandrogenemia. Whatever the primary defect, once these events are established, they are usually self-maintaining.

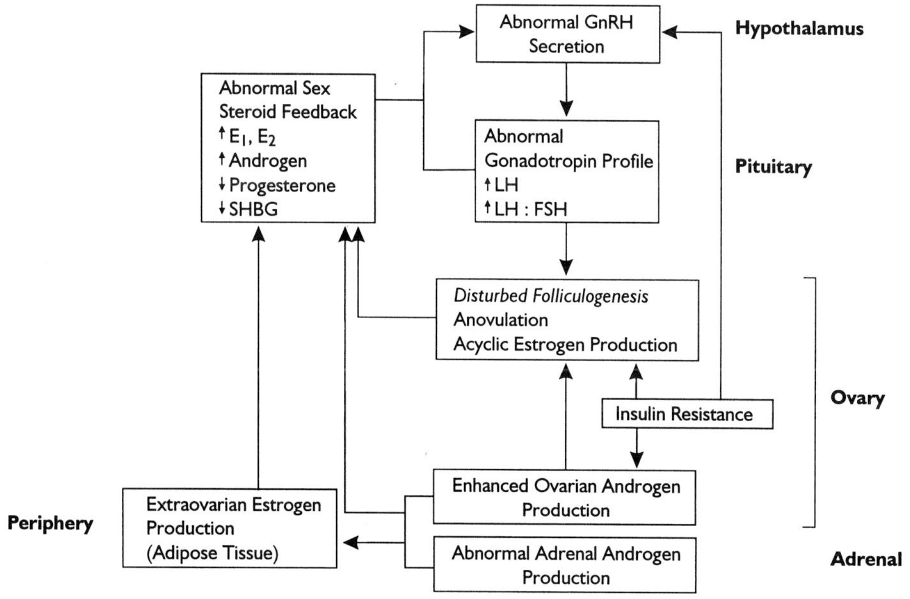

FIGURE 16B-5. Schema for the pathogenesis of the polycystic ovary syndrome.

Defects in Ovarian Function

Folliculogenesis Polycystic ovaries contain numerous small cysts (usually 2–4 mm in diameter) and characteristically increased stromal tissue; the increased stromal tissue is primarily responsible for increased ovarian volume. Granulosa cells from these cysts have a normal appearance and respond to FSH stimulation in vitro.[63] However, there is a failure of one follicle to become dominant and to develop to a preovulatory state with suppression of other follicles. The nature of this defect in intraovarian regulation is unknown. Abnormal regulation of the steroidogenic enzyme cytochrome P450c17 α within ovarian thecal cells may underlie their LH-induced hypersecretion of androgens.[64] Increased intraovarian androgen levels resulting from enhanced thecal cell secretion of androgen may impair FSH action and enhance follicular atresia.

Sex Steroid Secretion Estrogen secretion in the absence of a normal follicular development is acyclic with total estradiol levels in the early to midfollicular range. Increased ovarian and adrenal androgen secretion (see later sections) also bear directly on estrogen levels by acting as a substrate for extraovarian estrogen production (especially of estrone), primarily in fat tissue. Androgens also act to lower sex hormone–binding globulin (SHBG) levels, thereby increasing the free androgen and estrogen levels. Abnormal sex steroid profiles are therefore present to feed back on the hypothalamic-pituitary system.

Defects in Hypothalamic-Pituitary Function

Plasma LH levels are raised approximately twofold, while plasma FSH levels are normal or depressed, leading to the characteristic though not invariable elevation in the LH/FSH ratio.[65] Chronic acyclic elevation of free estrogen levels in PCOS may explain this abnormal profile of gonadotropins. Unopposed estrogen feedback may enhance pituitary LH, but not FSH, release in response to GnRH exposure. Progesterone suppresses LH secretion, and its deficiency in anovulatory PCOS patients may also be important. Coordinated cyclic release of gonadotropins does not occur, and failure of normal folliculogenesis results. Higher LH levels are associated with higher androgen levels, a greater incidence of anovulation, and resistance to ovulation induction therapy. A primary hypothalamic problem independent of abnormal sex steroid feedback has been suggested by the finding of increased LH secretory pulse frequency in adolescent girls and adult PCOS subjects.[66,67] This may suggest alterations in hypothalamic GnRH pulsatility. However, other studies have shown normal LH pulse frequency in PCOS.[68]

Moderate elevation of serum prolactin concentration (one to five times normal) was apparent in 27 percent of 394 PCOS subjects in a review of several published series.[69] Increased LH sensitivity to dopamine inhibition in PCOS compared to the sensitivity in the early follicular phase in normal women has been reported,[70] but this has not been confirmed by others.[71] Whether unopposed estrogen action or abnormal hypothalamic dopamine metabolism is important in producing these elevations is unclear. It seems that most cases are due to a coexisting prolactinoma which occurs with increased frequency in PCOS, warranting careful exclusion of this tumor, particularly in patients with more marked elevations of prolactin concentration.[72]

A possible explanation of the relatively suppressed FSH levels seen in PCOS is a selective elevation in the levels of serum inhibin B, postulated to be secreted by the increased number of small ovarian follicles.[73] Total serum immunoreactive inhibin levels, in contrast, have been reported to be in the normal early follicular phase range.[74]

Abnormal Androgen Secretion

Controversy has existed in regard to whether the ovary or the adrenal is the principal source of hyperandrogenemia in PCOS. Approximately 50 percent of PCOS subjects have elevated levels of total testosterone (generally up to twice the normal level); with the suppression of SHBG seen in this condition, about 75 percent have elevated unbound levels.[75] The specific suppression of gonadotropins using GnRH analogues has been shown to suppress the elevated testosterone and androstenedione levels in PCOS, suggesting that the ovary is the primary source of these androgens. Dehydroepiandrosterone sulfate (DHEA-S) is predominantly an adrenal androgen, and its concentration is elevated in about 50 percent of PCOS subjects.[76]

It is apparent, therefore, that in most subjects both the adrenal and the ovary hypersecrete androgens, while in the remainder either or neither does so. The correlation is poor between total androgen levels and the severity of hirsutism, although free T levels and the 5α reduced urinary T metabolites tend to be higher in more hirsute subjects. It should be emphasized that hyperandrogenemia may be due to other causes (e.g., endocrine tumors or cryptic congenital adrenal hyperplasia), in which the elevation of the 17-hydroxyprogesterone level, especially after ACTH infusion, is characteristic. These diagnoses should therefore be considered.

The interaction of these components is shown in Fig. 16B-5. This self-perpetuating cycle of events can be followed, commencing at the pituitary. In response to elevated and acyclic estrogen exposure and possibly abnormal inhibin levels, pituitary LH release is enhanced, while the FSH/LH ratio is depressed and cyclic release of gonadotropins is abnormal. Orderly folliculogenesis fails to occur because of a relative lack of FSH and therefore of aromatase activity, and ovulation does not occur or occurs infrequently. Enhanced ovarian and/or adrenal androgen secretion provides the substrate for peripheral estrogen production, lowers the SHBG level, and produces hirsutism in some patients. It must be emphasized that not all components of this schema need always be present.

Insulin Resistance

Insulin resistance is common in PCOS[77,78] and has been attributed to defects in both receptor and postreceptor mechanisms. Obesity only partially explains the resistance. The severity of insulin resistance correlates with the degree of hyperandrogenemia.[78] Insulin sensitivity does not consistently improve with a reduction in androgen levels by ovariectomy[79] or GnRH agonist treatment, suggesting that it is one of the primary defects in PCOS. As insulin influences granulosa cell maturation, abnormal insulin action may be involved in the disturbance of folliculogenesis.

An increasing body of evidence suggests that insulin resistance may be the important underlying etiological explanation of PCOS.[80] In at least 50 percent of affected women, it may be due to excessive serine phosphorylation of the insulin receptor.[81] Insulin resistance together with obesity leads to the substantially increased prevalence of impaired glucose tolerance in PCOS, which is in turn an important cause of NIDDM in women. PCOS is associated with an increase in risk factors for cardiovascular disease, including dyslipidemia, with increased LDL cholesterol and decreased HDL cholesterol.[82–85] Whether such increased risk is in fact followed by an actual increase in cardiovascular disease is controversial, though a number of studies are suggestive of the possibility.[80,86–88] Recent publications recommend that an assessment of the fasting glucose : insulin ratio may be a simple way of assessing insulin resistance,[89] which would be actively managed by encouragement of weight loss and exercise together with dietary modification towards a low-fat, high-fiber diet. The use of insulin sensitizing agents is mentioned later.

Management of Polycystic Ovary Syndrome

Indications for therapeutic intervention in PCOS can be summarized as follows:

- Control of menstrual cyclicity and/or bleeding
- Management of infertility
- Management of hirsutism
- Management of insulin resistance

Menstrual Cyclicity

The use of a combined oral contraceptive can control irregular cycles in PCOS. Heavy bleeding may occur in PCOS in view of the anovulatory state, with continuous unopposed estrogen exposure leading to thickening of the endometrial lining. A course of progestogen (norethindrone 5–10 mg daily for 10 days) will usually control this bleeding. A combined oral contraceptive or a regular cyclic progestogen alone can then be used to maintain menstrual control. Induction of regular menses is advisable in patients with anovulatory PCOS in view of the reported increased incidence of endometrial hyperplasia and neoplasia.[90,91]

Infertility

Clomiphene citrate has conventionally been used for the induction of ovulation. Its mechanism of action is presumed to occur by means of the temporary relief of estrogen feedback on gonadotropins, especially FSH. Follicular development is permitted, and the estrogen level increases to stimulate an LH surge. Ovulation can be induced in the majority (80 percent) of PCOS subjects, although the pregnancy rate is often reported as lower (39 percent).[92] In addition, there appears to be a high rate of spontaneous abortion in clomiphene-induced PCOS pregnancy: 40 percent compared with 25 percent in non-PCOS clomiphene-induced pregnancy. Nonetheless, clomiphene offers the most convenient form of ovulation induction for the majority of these subjects. Doses of 50–150 mg daily for 5 days commencing between days 2 and 5 of the cycle are suggested. The response is monitored by charting basal body temperature and with ovarian ultrasound and luteal-phase estimations of progesterone concentration.

For PCOS subjects who fail to ovulate with clomiphene, a range of therapies has been applied,[93] including the addition of hCG or glucocorticoids to clomiphene, although a clear benefit over clomiphene alone has not been shown. Bromocriptine has also been shown to induce ovulation in some PCOS women, especially when hyperprolactinemia is present.[94] Many of these patients require ovulation induction with gonadotropins, although they are generally resistant to therapy with pulsatile GnRH. Treatment using GnRH analogues to suppress endogenous gonadotropin secretion in combination with gonadotropin is an increasingly common approach (see Ovulation Induction, later). Finally, electrocautery of the ovarian surface has been claimed to restore the ovulatory cycle and produce pregnancy rates similar to those with gonadotropin therapy.[95] The mechanism of action of electrocautery is obscure. Because laparoscopy is often undertaken as part of the basic infertility investigation, it has been proposed that electrocautery could be considered prior to gonadotropin therapy.

A recent approach to treatment of infertility in PCOS is the administration of agents that improve insulin sensitivity. Metformin suppresses hepatic glucose production and insulin secretion, and can induce weight loss, which may be its main insulin sensitizing action.[96] It has been reported as leading to ovulation, facilitating the action of clomiphene,[97] and as leading to pregnancy.[98] The thiazolidinedione troglitazone is another insulin sensitizing agent, the role of which in PCOS therapy is under active investigation.[99]

Virilization and Hirsutism

Clinical Assessment and Investigation

The number of advertisements offering the removal of superfluous hair suggests that hirsutism is a common disorder. It may be defined as the excessive growth of terminal hair in a male distribution, and it affects particularly the upper lip, chin, chest, sacral area, lower abdomen, and thighs. It is frequently perceived as being much more severe by the patient than by the doctor to whom she brings her complaint. In contrast, virilization is uncommon. It is manifested by male pattern baldness, clitoral hypertrophy, deepening of the voice, and increased muscularity in addition to hirsutism. The presence of virilization strongly suggests an underlying organic cause.

A variety of methods have been used to measure the degree of hirsutism and the rate of hair growth. From a practical viewpoint, the scoring system of Ferriman and Gallwey has achieved widespread popularity.[100] The degree of hair growth is graded on a scale of 0–4 on the upper lip, chin, chest, upper back, lower back, upper abdomen, lower abdomen, upper arm, forearm, thigh and lower leg, giving a maximal possible score of 44 with an upper limit of normal of 11. A hormonal score omitting the forearm and lower leg is frequently used giving a maximal score of 36 and upper limit of normal of 7. Forty percent of normal white women have a score of 0. More cumbersome objective methods of assessing the velocity of hair growth have been described.[101]

Increased hair growth may occur in otherwise apparently normal subjects, for example, at puberty or in the late teens or early twenties, during pregnancy, or at the time of menopause. It may also occur in response to the administration of certain drugs, including phenytoin, norgestrel, norethindrone, metronidazole, minoxidil, corticosteroids, anabolic steroids, androgens, and cyclosporin. Patients with hypothyroidism, acromegaly, and porphyria may develop increased hair growth, although the classic associations are with increased androgen production of either ovarian or adrenal origin. Ovarian causes include the polycystic ovary syndrome, hyperthecosis, and ovarian tumor; adrenal causes include tumors and congenital adrenal hyperplasia, particularly the late-onset adult type. Patients with Cushing's syndrome usually have some degree of hirsutism.

From a practical clinical viewpoint, by far the most common clinical varieties of hirsutism are the idiopathic form and PCOS. The terminology of the former is somewhat confused, as the majority of patients with idiopathic hirsutism actually have an increase at least in the androgen production rate, though the cause of this remains undefined. An alternative term for this disorder is *functional androgen excess*. The concentration of a peripheral metabolite of DHT, $3\alpha,5\alpha$-androstanediol glucuronide, has been reported to be markedly elevated in hirsute patients and correlates with the degree of hirsutism.[102]

Idiopathic hirsutism is often associated with a family history of excess hair growth in either male or female relatives and tends to come on in the late teens or early twenties. The hirsutism is usually mild to moderate in extent, and menstrual cycles usually remain regular and ovulatory. Nonetheless, many of these women probably have PCOS, as many have ultrasonographic evidence of ovarian enlargement. The PCOS classically has its onset just before or at the time of puberty and is associated with obesity, menstrual irregularity (either oligomenorrhea or amenorrhea, which may be primary or secondary), and infertility. Both idiopathic hirsutism and PCOS may be associated with acne and excessively oily skin. It has become increasingly recognized that a syndrome indistinguishable from PCOS may occur in previously normal women who gain excess weight, often associated with one or more pregnancies, and present in their late twenties or early thirties with obesity, hirsutism, and oligomenorrhea. In these patients, the obesity may be the primary disorder and restoration of menstrual periodicity and some decrease in hirsutism may accompany successful weight loss, though this is difficult to achieve.

Some authors report that between one-third and two-thirds of hirsute women have mild defects in adrenal steroidogenesis that are suggestive of late-onset congenital adrenal hyperplasia, based on measurements of basal and ACTH-stimulated levels of steroids in the androgen pathway.[103,104] The frequency with which this diagnosis is made probably varies with the ethnicity of the patients and the effort applied to studying their steroidogenesis.

The clinical assessment of patients presenting with hirsutism must include taking an appropriate history, including a family history, and paying particular attention to the rapidity of onset of the hirsutism: An abrupt onset suggests the possibility of organic lesions such as an adrenal or ovarian tumor. A careful menstrual history with attention to symptoms suggesting the presence of ovulation should be recorded. It is important to determine whether the patient is also complaining of infertility and whether she requires contraception. Physical examination should include an assessment of the severity of the hirsutism. Using the Ferriman and Gallwey hormonal score with a maximum score of 36, mild hirsutism may be regarded as a score of 8–12, moderate hirsutism as a score of 13–18, and severe hirsutism as a score of over 19.[105] Careful assessment should be made for evidence of accompanying virilization (e.g., clitoral hypertrophy) and for stigmata of rare causes of hirsutism such as Cushing's syndrome and hypothyroidism.

An area of significant concern and controversy is the question of what degree of investigation should be undertaken in patients presenting with apparently uncomplicated hirsutism. Although it is of theoretical interest to establish whether excessive androgen secretion is arising from the ovary or the adrenal, in practice this may not significantly affect the choice of management unless a specific adrenal lesion has been identified and suppressive therapy is contemplated.

Measurements which may be made include the plasma testosterone concentration, or, preferably, the free testosterone level, as total testosterone is occasionally normal despite significant hyperandrogenemia, in part as a result of lower SHBG levels. Salivary testosterone determination is an alternative approach to assessing the unbound steroid level. DHT, DHEA-S, and androstenedione concentrations may be measured, together with that of 17-hydroxyprogesterone. A marked elevation in plasma testosterone to around twice the upper limit of normal is compatible with the PCOS, but if testosterone is substantially above that level, the possibility of an ovarian tumor must be kept in mind and is best evaluated with pelvic examination and vaginal ultrasonography or MRI scanning. A marked elevation in the DHEA-S concentration to more than twice the upper limit of normal suggests the possibility of an adrenal tumor, which should again be excluded by CT scanning. Androstenedione and DHEA-S together with testosterone levels are frequently moderately elevated in PCOS. An elevation in basal levels of 17-hydroxyprogesterone suggests late-onset congenital adrenal hyperplasia; in this disorder a stimulation test with ACTH may establish the diagnosis.[106] We have found late-onset congenital adrenal hyperplasia (CAH) to be most uncommon and screen for it only in severe or atypical cases or in patients with elevated basal levels of 17OH progesterone in addition to DHEA-S. As anti-androgen therapy is effective in most hirsute patients (see later section), the cost-effectiveness of exhaustively investigating all subjects for more subtle abnormalities remains unproven, although this point is controversial.[107] Measurements of FSH, LH, and prolactin levels may also be diagnostically helpful, with an elevation of LH concentration and a high LH/FSH ratio being typical of PCOS. Prolactin-secreting pituitary adenomas may occasionally be associated with excess hair growth.

It is difficult to formulate satisfactory general rules for the degree of investigation that should be undertaken in an individual patient. As a general guide, in mild to moderate hirsutism with normal menses investigations are of extremely doubtful value. In mild to moderate hirsutism with menstrual irregularity, investigations may be directed toward establishing PCOS as the cause with measurements of FSH, LH, and total or, preferably, free testosterone levels. It is well recognized that the free testosterone fraction is much more frequently elevated in hirsutism than is total plasma testosterone, but this observation is of little practical value in terms of management.

In more severe hirsutism, levels of DHEA-S, testosterone, and 17-hydroxyprogesterone, with the latter's response to ACTH, should be assessed, and, where indicated, abdominal CT scanning or vaginal ultrasound should be undertaken to clarify the diagnosis.

When management with anti-androgens, particularly cyproterone acetate, is contemplated, it is also useful to measure baseline cholesterol and triglyceride levels, as cyproterone acetate may cause an increase in plasma lipid levels. In patients in whom spironolactone is to be used, basal renal function should be assessed, with particular reference to serum potassium.

Management

The overall approach to a hirsute patient should be one of empathy and understanding with emphasis on the fact that it is a lifelong disorder for which cosmetic approaches provide the cornerstone of management. The available measures include simple plucking, waxing, and shaving and the use of depilatory creams, all of which require long-term use. Permanent cure may be achieved with properly performed electrolysis, which is, however, tedious, uncomfortable, and expensive. In addition, in obese patients weight loss often has a favorable effect on hirsutism.

Medical measures include regimens of ovarian suppression (with a combination of estrogen and progestogen, e.g., the oral contraceptive pill) and adrenal suppression (with nocturnally administered corticosteroids such as prednisone 7.5 mg daily or dexamethasone 0.5 mg daily) if a defect in adrenal steroid synthesis has been shown. Results with such measures are slow to occur and often disappointing. More successful approaches have involved the use of anti-androgens, such as cyproterone acetate (given in reverse sequential fashion), and spironolactone.

Cyproterone acetate has been extensively tried in Europe and Australia and has been found to be highly effective. It is administered in reverse sequential order with cyclic estrogen (e.g., cyproterone 50–100 mg daily on days 5–15 and ethinyl estradiol 30–50 μg daily on days 5–25 of each calendar month).[108] This treatment also provides effective contraception. An alternative to ethinyl estrodial is to use a combined oral contraceptive. A response is seen within 3–6 months. Both acne and hirsutism respond in about three-quarters of patients. The dose of cyproterone can often be gradually reduced to a maintenance dose of 2 mg daily. Spironolactone in a high dose (100–200 mg daily) is also useful but must be given with contraceptive cover.[109,110] Unfortunately, hirsutism almost always recurs when therapy is discontinued. It is mandatory that pregnancy be avoided during such therapy because of the risks of feminization of a male fetus. In recent years, several new anti-androgens have received limited evaluation for the management of hirsutism, including Flutamide,[111] a pure anti-androgen, and Finasteride,[112] a 5α reductase inhibitor. Both may be effective, but have not come into general use. An alternative approach is the suppression of ovarian androgen production by the use of GnRH agonist.[113] Such an approach of course concomitantly leads to estrogen deficiency, necessitating the addition of an estrogen (plus a progestin) to the regimen. This approach, while effective, is costly and cumbersome.

Female Infertility: Diagnosis of Ovulatory Dysfunction

It has been estimated that 1 couple in 7 will experience difficulty with conception, with male and female factors being equally prevalent. Thus, it is important to see both partners together and to recognize that anxiety and depression are common in both. Eliciting these emotions is an integral part of the initial interview, and the physician must gain the patients' confidence before proceeding with any of the large number of investigations available, particularly in women with possible ovarian dysfunction. The number and outcome of previous pregnancies are also significant, as the prognosis for secondary infertility is better than that for primary infertility.

Previous medical treatments such as cytotoxic or psychopharmacologic agents or irradiation may have caused permanent or temporary damage to folliculogenesis. Surgery, including not only gynecologic procedures such as ovarian cystectomy and abdominal operations such as complicated appendectomy but also tissue handling at laparotomy, may cause adhesions to form in the pelvis and thus affect tubal function. Environmental and occupational factors, for example, frequent night shift work, may disturb ovarian function and also make intercourse in the fertile period less likely.

In a general physical examination, use of a weight index such as the Garrow or body mass index (BMI, weight in kilograms divided by squared height in meters) is recommended. Hair distribution should be scored according to the definitions of Ferriman and Gallwey.[100] Excessive hair growth (bearing in mind the patient's ethnic background) may indicate excessive androgen secretion or action, and this may be associated with anovulation. Hypoestrogenism may be indicated by incomplete breast development and should be recorded by the appropriate Tanner stage (see Fig. 16B-1). Galactorrhea is detected by gentle sustained pressure on the areolae, but the secretion should not be brown or bloodstained, which would indicate organic breast disease, including malignancy. In ideal circumstances, galactorrhea should be confirmed by testing for lactose and by microscopic examination for fat globules.

There are a number of possible tests of ovulation: charting of mucous symptoms and/or basal body temperature, urinary LH monitoring, determination of luteal-phase plasma progesterone concentrations, ultrasonic ovarian follicle assessment, and luteal-phase endometrial biopsy. The emphasis placed on each of these tests will depend on the clinical facilities at hand. The authors use a plasma progesterone assay as a screening test of ovulation, drawing the blood sample on day 21 of an expected 28-day cycle or 7 ± 3 days before the next anticipated menses.

In patients in whom chronic anovulation appears to be the major cause of infertility, a large number of ovulation induction agents are now available for therapy (Table 16B-4 and Fig. 16B-6). Low plasma estradiol concentrations (<100 p*M*) suggest that the response to antiestrogens (e.g., clomiphene citrate) will be inadequate. However, the progestogen withdrawal for estrogen priming of the endometrium does provide useful information, and withdrawal uterine bleeding should be assessed by giving 10 mg

TABLE 16B-4. Ovulation-Inducing Agents

Category	Agents
Anti-estrogens	Clomiphene
Dopamine agonists	Bromocriptine, cabergoline
FSH, LH	hMG
Purified FSH	Metrodin
Recombinant FSH	
Recombinant LH	
Surrogate LH	hCG
GnRH	
GnRH agonists	Buserelin, Nafarelin, Leuprolide, Goserelin

Abbreviations: hMG = human menopausal gonadotropin; hCG = human chorionic gonadotropin.

FIGURE 16B-6. Pulsatile GnRH infuser assembled to allow subcutaneous hormone administration in an ambulatory patient.

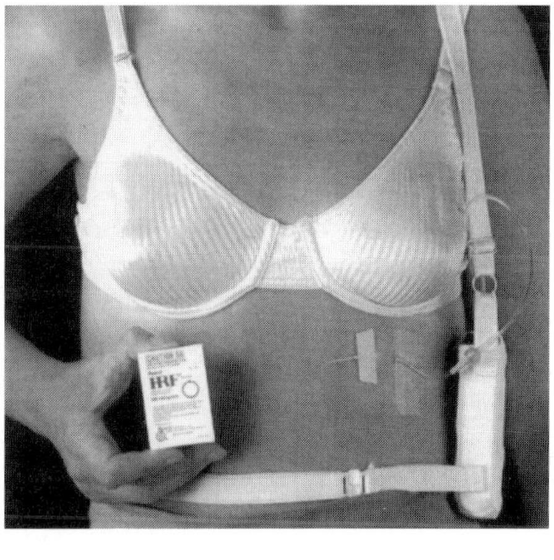

per day of a progestogen such as medroxyprogesterone acetate or 1.25 mg norethindrone orally for 5 days. If no vaginal bleeding occurs, the test is negative; any bleeding up to 1 week after the test is positive and suggests that there is sufficient circulating estrogen present for anti-estrogen therapy to be potentially beneficial.

Anti-estrogen Ovulation Induction

With the anti-estrogen clomiphene citrate, treatment starts at 50 mg per day for 5 days and should be increased by 50-mg increments in each cycle, to a daily maximum of 150 mg or until ovulation occurs. Treatment is begun on day 2–5 of the cycle, and ovulation is assessed by charting basal body temperature as well as measuring serum progesterone concentrations between days 21 and 24. Ovulation may occur anywhere from 5 to 10 days after the last clomiphene tablet. Theoretically, beginning therapy on day 2 or 3 leads to the recruitment of more follicles, while beginning on day 5 augments gonadotropin levels at the time of selection of the dominant follicle and enhances its particular development. The serum progesterone level should be above 30 n*M* per liter in the midluteal phase to support the occurrence of ovulation, but the date of the next menses is of obvious significance in ensuring that the progesterone estimate was made on the appropriate day.

Patients who fail to respond may benefit from the addition of continuous low-dose dexamethasone therapy (0.5 mg decreasing to 0.25 mg after 4–8 weeks) if androgen levels are elevated, or from an hCG bolus to induce ovulation where a leading follicle develops but fails to rupture.

Side effects from clomiphene citrate therapy are infrequent but include hot flushes, mood disturbance, bloating, breast tenderness, and very rarely, visual disturbances. If eyesight is affected, therapy should cease immediately and not be repeated. Low multiple gestations are increased, and on higher doses ovarian enlargement may occur. Repeat cycles should be postponed until this has settled. Efforts are continuing to separate the two stereoisomers of clomiphene citrate for separate clinical use to optimize its efficacy.

Ovulation induction with clomiphene citrate in anovulatory women with no other additional cause for infertility should not usually continue beyond six (approximately a 60 percent prospect of pregnancy) to nine (75 percent prospect) ovulations without considering other options (see later discussion).

Gonadotropin Ovulation Induction

Clinical use of human pituitary FSH resulting in pregnancy was first reported in 1958.[114] Human gonadotropins were initially prepared from cadaver pituitaries or derived from the urine of postmenopausal women. Highly purified FSH/LH preparations from postmenopausal urine were subsequently obtained, and are being replaced worldwide by recombinant gonadotropins. Pituitary gonadotropins have been withdrawn because of the reported transmission of Creutzfeldt-Jakob disease.[115]

Gonadotropins may be given in a fixed dosage regimen in which a predetermined dose of gonadotropin is administered in increasing concentrations in each cycle of treatment until a response occurs. Alternatively, the dose of gonadotropin may be tailored to the patient's response during treatment so that an effective dose is administered during each cycle. This has the advantage of yielding a smaller number of cycles per pregnancy, and in the authors' hands it has produced a pregnancy rate which is equivalent to the natural conception rate in the community, as assessed by life table analysis (Fig. 16B-7).[116]

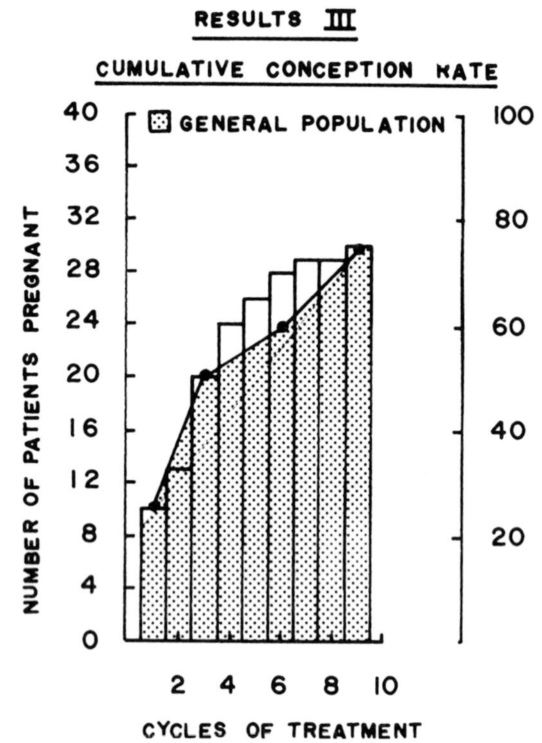

FIGURE 16B-7. Cumulative conception rate in a series of patients receiving human pituitary gonadotropin for ovulation induction. Stippled area shows the conception rate for the general population (*Reproduced from Healy et al.,*[116] *with permission.*)

We use a variable gonadotropin schedule, starting at 75 IU per day human menopausal gonadotropins or recombinant FSH. The dose is increased every 7 days if there is no doubling of serum estradiol values. Monitoring is done by means of serum estradiol and ovarian vaginal ultrasonography, at intervals determined by the individual's responsiveness.

With current human gonadotropin treatments, excessive stimulation of the ovaries is the major complication of therapy. This can be expressed either as the ovarian hyperstimulation syndrome (OHSS), which presents with a spectrum of clinical features varying from palpable ovarian cysts to its most severe form, which includes abdominal distension, nausea, hydrothorax, coagulopathy, and occasionally death,[117] or by multiple ovulation and multiple pregnancy in up to 20–30 percent of patients. To decrease the incidence of these complications, cycles are monitored ultrasonically for follicular development and by serum estradiol levels. Multiple linear regression analysis has shown that the number of follicles greater than 10 mm in diameter at the time of the ovulatory hCG injection is predictive of both pregnancy and the number of fetuses but not of OHSS while the estradiol level at the same point is predictive for OHSS but not of multiple pregnancy.[118]

Mean serum FSH and LH concentrations are markedly elevated during ovulation induction therapy with human gonadotropins.[119] Elevated FSH/LH ratios for more than 8 days provide unrelenting FSH exposure to the cohort of recruited follicles; this appears to be important in inducing the disordered multiple folliculogenesis in these patients. Two or more ovarian follicles develop in approximately 86 percent of gonadotropin-treated cycles, compared with only 23 percent of spontaneous cycles, and at

TABLE 16B-5. Results of Ovulation Induction by Gonadotropin Therapy*

	Percent with Follicles >10 mm	
	2 Follicles	**3 Follicles**
Human gonadotropin-induced cycles (n = 28)	86	50
Spontaneous cycles (n = 13)	23	0

*Percent of cycles with two or three follicles developing to >10 mm in diameter.

least three follicles greater than 12 mm in diameter develop during 50 percent of gonadotropin-stimulated cycles (Table 16B-5).

Various permutations of human gonadotropin or GnRH therapy have been reported for PCOS, where the treatment response is often unpredictable. Pulsatile administration of either human menopausal gonadotropin or FSH has been tried with or without GnRH agonist pituitary down regulation.[120] The results have varied between centers, but one of the larger trials has shown pulsatile FSH to produce a very low incidence of OHSS but also a disappointingly low pregnancy rate, while intramuscular pure FSH has a comparable pregnancy rate with human menopausal gonadotropin and an incidence of OHSS intermediate between the other two regimens.[121] GnRH agonist administration has been used in an attempt to induce pituitary down regulation and convert abnormal secretion of LH and FSH and aberrant LH/FSH ratios to more normal patterns (Fig. 16B-8) prior to gonadotropin therapy. Reports are variable, but the overall complication rate does seem decreased and the ovulation and pregnancy rates are similar to therapy without GnRH agonist suppression.[121] Larger groups of patients must be studied to be confident that these therapies offer a significant advantage over current methods of ovarian stimulation.

An alternative regimen of gonadotrophin administration in which the starting dose is 150 IU per day, with a rapid reduction to 112 and then 75 IU per day, has been proposed,[122] a so-called 'step down' regimen. Results overall have compared favorably with conventional schedules, although further confirmation is required.

Pulsatile GnRH Ovulation Induction

Leyendecker and colleagues were the first to report the pulsatile administration of GnRH in women with hypothalamic amenorrhea.[123] Since then it has been given by both the subcutaneous and intravenous routes (Fig. 16B-6). When endogenous gonadotropins are used, the normal pituitary-ovarian feedback mechanisms remain intact. Therefore, in comparison with gonadotropin therapy it requires less monitoring, both hormonal and ultrasonographic, and the incidences of multiple pregnancy and the ovarian hyperstimulation syndrome are reduced. Its disadvantages include the cost and inconvenience of the GnRH pump and delivery unit and, particularly with the intravenous route, the risk of local and systemic infection. In PCOS the therapy has been disappointing, though pretreatment with a GnRH agonist in a small series has improved the ovulation rates.[124]

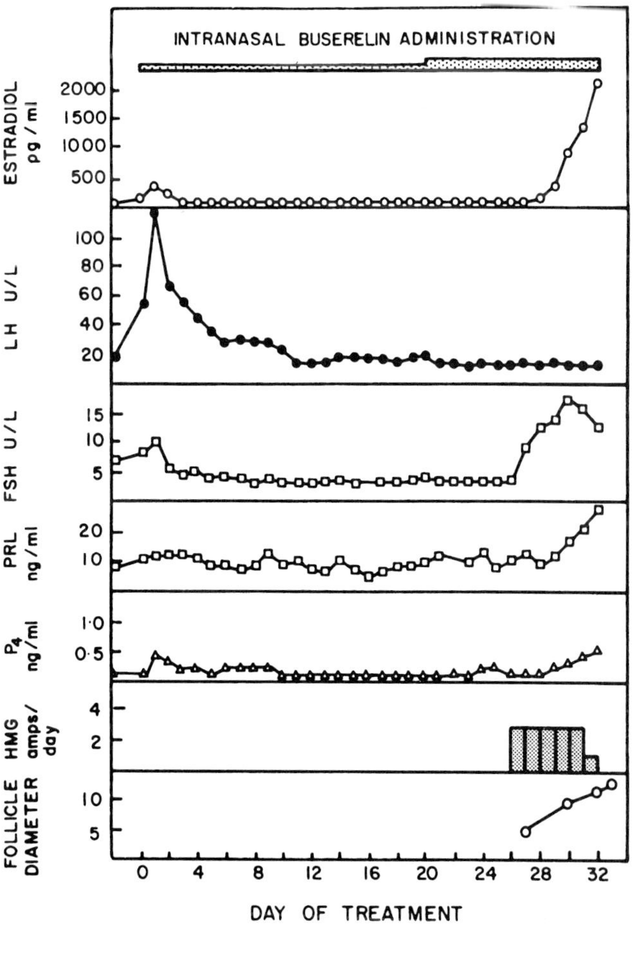

FIGURE 16B-8. Intranasal GnRH agonist (buserelin) administration to an anovulatory patient with polycystic ovary syndrome. Note the initial LH/FSH ratio, the suppression of plasma estradiol levels with buserelin therapy, the exponential increase in estradiol values when hMG treatment has begun, and the rapid increase in follicle growth.

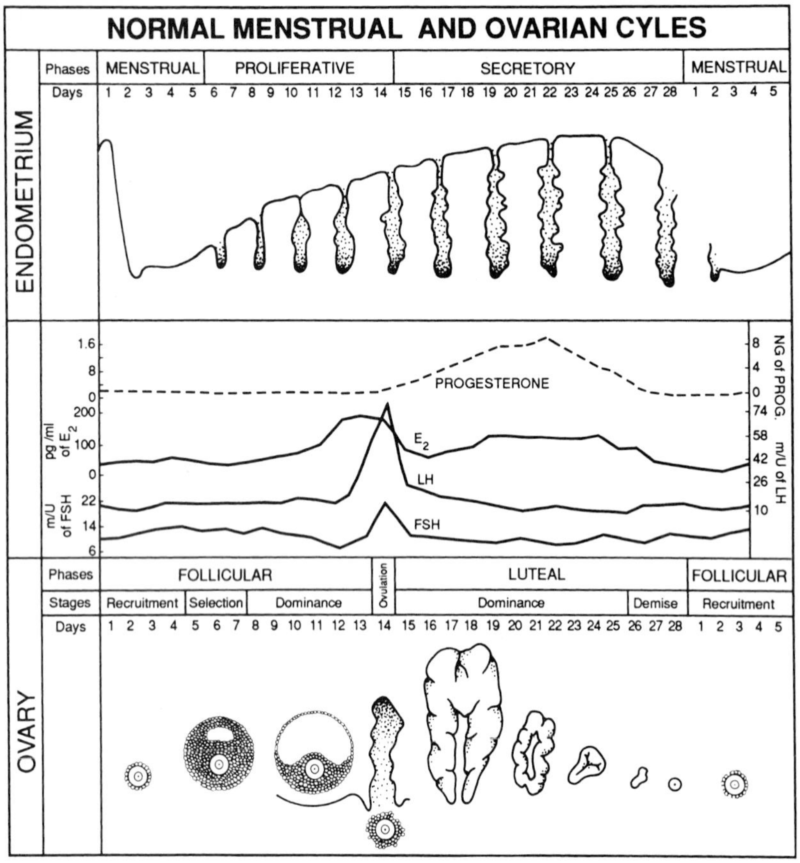

FIGURE 16B-9. Schematic representation of the interactions of the endometrium, pituitary, and ovaries during ovulatory menstrual cycles.

The intravenous route provides a more physiologic profile than does the subcutaneous route and requires less drug. However, although ovulation is increased (90 vs. 75 percent), the conception rate per ovulatory cycle is the same (approximately 30 percent). As the subcutaneous route is more convenient and has a reduced risk of septicemia, it is arguable that the intravenous route should be reserved for patients who fail to respond to the subcutaneous therapy.

In the authors' clinic, we have used 90-min subcutaneous pulses of GnRH, commencing at 5 μg per pulse and increasing by 5 μg every 7–14 days until a progressive rise in the urinary estrone glucuronide level is observed.[125] Twenty-three of the 30 ovulatory cycles with this therapy were induced with 10-μg pulses. There were 13 pregnancies in 14 subjects in our study.

The incidence of multiple pregnancy is lower with GnRH therapy compared with human gonadotropin treatment. In reported series, a multiple pregnancy rate of 8 percent occurred, although it is noteworthy that several cases of triplet pregnancies and one quadruplet pregnancy have been reported, as have other instances of ovarian hyperstimulation. A comprehensive account of ovulation induction and its short- and long-term effects has been published.[126]

Menorrhagia and Dysmenorrhea

The clinical problems of menorrhagia and dysmenorrhea are among the most common which present to a gynecologist. To properly understand the basis of present clinical management of these disorders, a brief review of endometrial anatomy and physiology is necessary.

Endometrial Anatomy and Physiology

Normal endometrium consists of a simple columnar epithelium, which contains estrogen-responsive and progesterone-dependent mucous glands on an underlying stroma. The endometrium is typically classified into a more superficial functional zone, which is supplied by coiled spiral arteries (Fig. 16B-9) and is shed at menstruation, and a deeper basal zone, which is supplied by straight arteries. This remains after menstruation and regenerates the endometrium. Moreover, the functional zone contains a superficial luminal zone (zone 1), an intermediate zone 2 where the glands are straight and widely separated by stroma, and a deeper layer, zone 3, where the glands are coiled and closely packed. These differences are clinically relevant, as the highest mitotic rates are observed in the upper third of human endometrium on days 8 to 10 of the cycle.

In 1950, Noyes, Hertig, and Rock established criteria for dating endometrial biopsies (Fig. 16B-10).[127] They found that the proliferative phase of the menstrual cycle was variable in length and the endometrial changes were too indistinct to permit day-today recognition or "dating" of the endometrium. They recognized early proliferative, midproliferative, and late proliferative endometrium (Fig. 16B-10). Through these phases, the endometrium thickens because of an increase in the number and size of the glands, which become tortuous. Glandular diameter and volume are directly related to plasma estradiol concentrations.

In contrast to the proliferative phase, Noyes and colleagues found that secretory-phase endometrium developed in such a characteristic rate and fashion after ovulation that daily changes were recognizable; the endometrium could therefore be dated. Basal or

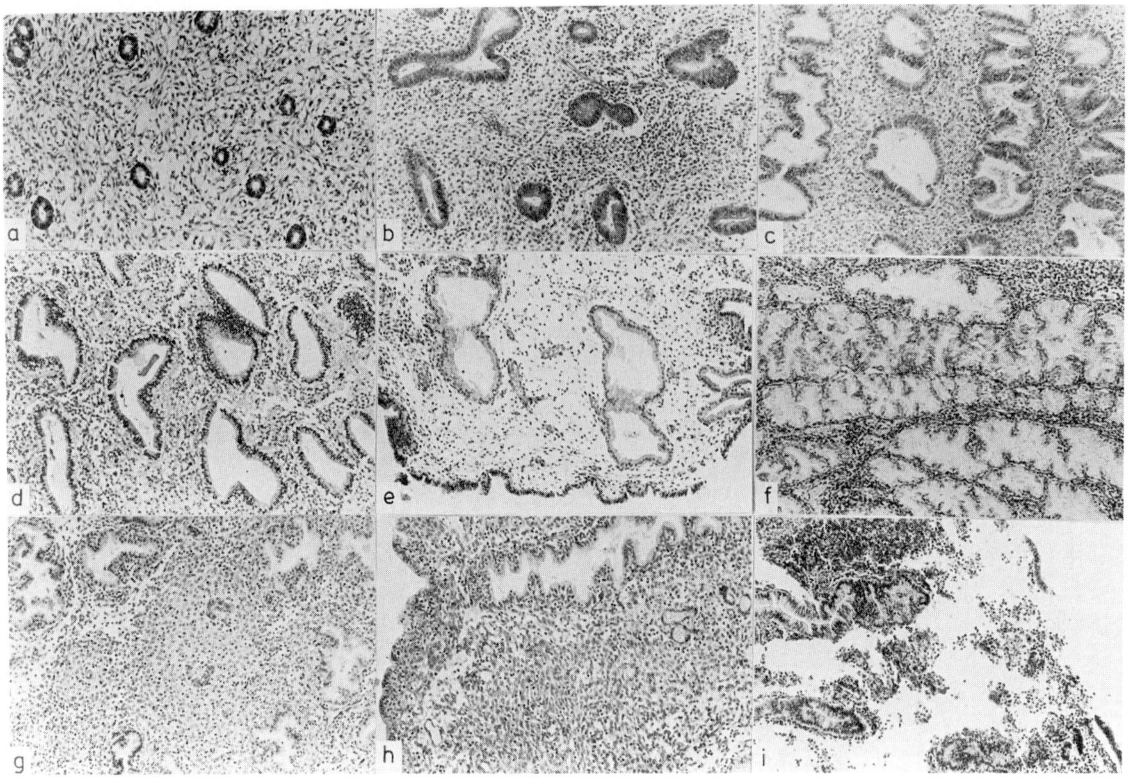

FIGURE 16B-10. Morphologic changes in human endometrium during a normal menstrual cycle: (*A*) early proliferative; (*B*) midproliferative; (*C*) late proliferative. During the follicular phase, the endometrium thickens as a result of an increase in the number and size of the glands. Moderate tortuosity is seen as they become wider and longer. (*D*) Basal vacuolation of the gland epithelium is the earliest morphologic evidence of luteinization. Day 16 endometrium. (*E*) During the secretory stage, basal vacuoles disappear and nuclei are seen at the base of the epithelial cells. Note also stromal edema. Day 20 endometrium. (*F*) During the premenstrual stage, glands may present a pronounced sawtooth appearance. Day 25 endometrium (*G*) Stromal cells first show predecidual change around arterioles. Day 23 endometrium. (*H*) Just before menstruation, a compact layer of predecidual cells is formed. (*I*) During the menstrual phase, the endometrium typically crumbles away and is densely infiltrated with leukocytes.

subnuclear vacuolation of the glandular epithelium was found 36 to 48 h after ovulation and was the first endometrial sign of luteinization. This change was prominent from days 16–19 of a typical menstrual cycle. From day 19, basal vacuoles disappeared as the glycogen-enriched secretion passed by the gland nuclei and into the lumen. The nuclei were thus seen at the base of the epithelial cells. From days 21–23, the spiral arterioles acquired a cuff of stromal cells with enlarged nuclei and cytoplasm. This constituted the earliest predecidual or pseudodecidual change. Predecidua extended to beneath the epithelium by day 25 and at day 27 appeared as solid sheets of decidua-like cells infiltrated by leukocytes. These predecidual cells underwent mitosis as well as hypertrophy. If conception occurs, further enlargement forms polygonal decidual cells in a highly vascular stroma. After implantation, the portion of the decidua between the placenta and myometrium is called the *decidua basalis*. The part covering the blastocyst is the *decidua capsularis*, which fuses with the part lining the remainder of the uterus, the *decidua parietalis*.

In a young adult, menstrual blood loss can be measured by collecting tampons and/or sanitary pads and extracting the iron or hemoglobin. Hallberg and associates found in 476 women that the volume of menstrual blood loss was not normally distributed but rather was skewed in distribution[128]: Median blood loss was 43 ml, and 90 percent of randomly selected women had menstrual blood losses less than 80 ml. Cole and colleagues examined 348 unselected women and confirmed a skewed distribution of menstrual blood loss.[129] In their study, median blood loss was 28 ml; in only 20 percent of these women was the difference in menstrual blood loss in consecutive periods greater than 20 ml. Menstrual blood loss increased with parity, perhaps because of an increased endometrial area or vascularity or both, but did not increase with age. Above 80 ml of menstrual blood loss, most women will develop iron-deficiency anemia.

Approximately 50 to 70 percent of the menstrual discharge is blood. The platelet count found in menstrual fluid is about 10 percent of that in blood. The remainder of the menses consists of fragments of endometrium and mucus. Normal menstrual blood does not readily clot. Although Buller reported that menstrual blood does not contain fibrin and that menstrual clots also contain no fibrin[130] and thus are not true clots, more recent studies by Bonnar and colleagues[131] found fibrin in 85 percent of normal menstrual clots and in 88 percent of patients with dysfunctional uterine bleeding. They found no fibrinogen in menstrual blood but did find large amounts of fibrin degradation products and suggested that thrombin and plasmin generation are central to menstrual hemostasis. This active fibrinolytic system seems to be

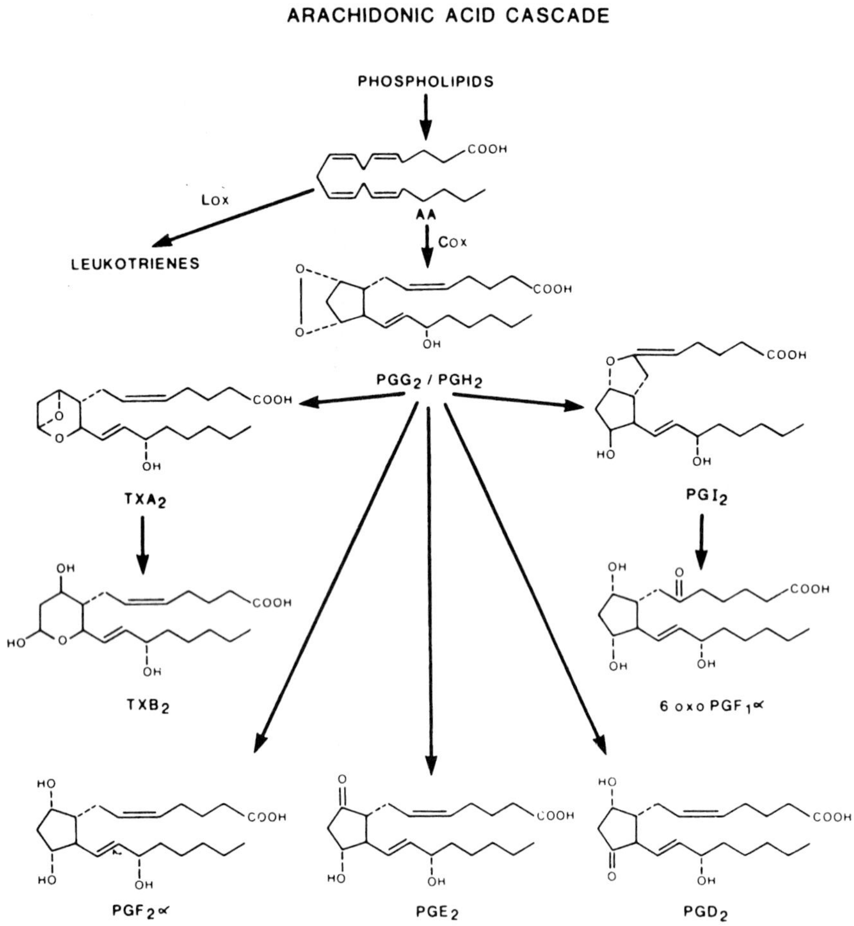

FIGURE 16B-11. The cyclooxygenase (COX) and lipoxygenase (LOX) cascade pathways of arachidonic acid (AA) metabolism. Note the pivotal position of the endoperoxide intermediates PGG_2 and PGH_2 in the production of the three classes of prostanoids, the thromboxanes (TXA_2 and TXB_2), prostacyclin (PGI_2), and the prostaglandins $PGF_{2\alpha}$, PGE_2, and PGD_2.

confined to the endometrial glandular epithelium. Not surprisingly, therefore, antifibrinolytic drugs such as ε-aminocaproic acid and tranexamic acid, 1 g every 6 h for 5 days, have proved effective in decreasing menstrual blood loss.

Endometrial Prostaglandins

Since the discovery of an acidic lipid with oxytocic properties in menstrual fluid,[132] later shown to be $PGF_{2\alpha}$ and PGE_2, these substances have been implicated in normal and abnormal menstruation. Figure 16B-11 presents a scheme of the interrelations of the various prostaglandins (PGs) or prostanoids. Intrauterine PGs derive from arachidonic acid, originating predominantly from the essential fatty acid linoleic acid. Arachidonic acid is a polyunsaturated 20-carbon chain with four double bonds and no nitrogen and is liberated from cell membrane phospholipids by the enzyme phospholipase A_2 in response to many physical and hormonal stimuli. In the best-studied pathway, arachidonic acid is oxygenated rapidly by the enzyme PG synthetase or cyclooxygenase (COX) to form a family of prostaglandins; each contains only two double bonds. Later research discovered a second enzyme, lipoxygenase (LOX); its products, the *leukotrienes*, have a straight-chain conformation. *Eicosanoids* is the generic name for both COX and LOX products. In the COX path, the initial intermediates generated are two endoperoxides: PGG_2 and PGH2. Both substances are pivotal in liberating at least three groups of prostanoids. $PGF_{2\alpha}$ and PGE_2 are among the most studied, in part because of their potency in the induction of myometrial contraction. $PGF_{2\alpha}$ and thromboxane A_2 (TXA_2) are potent vasoconstrictors; conversely, PGE_2 and especially prostacyclin (PGI_2) cause vasodilation. PGI_2 also dissociates platelets, while TXA_2 aggregates platelets. Both PGE_2 and TXA_2 are rapidly converted to more stable products, including 6-oxo-PGF_1 and TXB_2, respectively. Estrogen stimulates COX-mediated synthesis of endometrial $PGF_{2\alpha}$ and PGE_2 in women. In contrast, progesterone inhibits this production from proliferative and secretory-phase endometrium. The precise intracellular mechanisms controlling steroid induction of PG synthesis are unknown.

$PGF_{2\alpha}$ is quantitatively the major endometrial prostanoid liberated during the human menstrual cycle. As estrogen does stimulate COX activity, it is not surprising that prostaglandin production rates are high in the proliferative phase of the menstrual cycle. In early human pregnancy, decidua contains less $PGF_{2\alpha}$ than is found in secretory endometrium. This chronic suppression appears to be due to an inhibitor of COX which is identifiable in amniotic fluid and maternal serum. The origin and nature of this endogenous inhibitor of prostaglandin synthesis by amniochorion are unknown, though suppression by decidual prolactin or a metabolite is possible.[133]

Excessive menstrual blood loss may affect up to 20 percent of women. In the majority of individuals, no organic cause for this menorrhagia is found and the diagnosis of dysfunctional uterine bleeding is made. Clinically, it is important to realize that only approximately one-third of patients presenting with menorrhagia have excessive menstrual blood loss (>80 ml).

It is now evident that excessive menstrual blood loss is associated with changes in PG production by the uterus. Endometrium from women with ovular dysfunctional uterine bleeding, which is common in young adults, synthesizes more PGE_2 than does endometrium from normal women, and the myometrial production of PGI_2 is markedly enhanced.[134] In women with anovular dysfunctional bleeding, excessive menstrual loss is associated with a relative deficiency of PGF_2 synthesis. There is, in fact, a direct relation between the $PGE_2/PGF_{2\alpha}$ ratio and the amount of blood loss; it may be, therefore, that menstrual loss is determined by the relative synthesis of PGs with mainly vasoconstrictive properties on the one hand ($PGF_{2\alpha}$) as opposed to those with vasodilatory properties (PGE_2 and PGI_2) on the other.

The medical treatment of DUB will depend on the patient's age, desire for fertility, amount of blood loss, and if blood loss is acute or chronic in nature. The aims of the treatment are to stop the acute episode and prevent recurrence and long-term complications.

The acute medical treatment of DUB when blood loss is severe but not life-threatening is Premarin 25 mg intravenously (IV) 3 hourly until the bleeding ceases, up to 3 doses may be given. The loss will cease within 4–24 h in 70 percent of patients. If there is no change in the blood flow, a D&C will need to be performed. Premarin acts rapidly and has effects on clotting factor concentrations.[135] Once blood loss has ceased oral Premarin 10 mg is started slowly decreasing to 2.5 mg daily. At this time 10 mg medroxy progesterone acetate (MPA) for 10 days is added to produce an orderly maturation of the endometrium. Norethindrone (NET) at a dose of 2.5 mg for 10 days can be used instead of MPA. Both medications (Premarin and either MPA or NET) are then withdrawn and the endometrium will shed. The patient should be warned that the subsequent withdrawal bleed will be heavy and may be painful. Patients treated with Premarin especially at doses over 1.25 mg will require an antiemetic.

Acute bleeding may also be stopped using 100 μg ethinyl estradiol daily for 5–7 days. A heavy cramping withdrawal bleed will subsequently occur within 5 days of therapy cessation. The oral contraceptive pill (OCP) can then be started on the 5th day after withdrawal bleeding occurs. Oral MPA starting at a dose of 30 mg daily (60 mg if obese) for 3 days, reducing to 20 mg daily for 3 days, then 15 mg daily for 3 days, and finally to 10 mg daily for 5 days, is also effective in stopping bleeding. Alternatively oral NET may also be very effective in causing bleeding cessation. The initial dose is 15 mg daily for 3 days, reducing to 10 mg daily for 3 days, then 7.5 mg daily for 3 days, and finally to 5 mg daily for 5 days.

The chronic medical treatment of DUB may be undertaken using hormonal or nonhormonal medication. The OCP is a valuable drug in the treatment of DUB, especially if contraception is also required. It reduces menstrual flow by at least 60 percent in a normal uterus as well as reducing dysmenorrhoea.[135] An alternative therapy is MPA 10 mg or NET 1.25–2.5 mg both for days 5–25 of the cycle. This treatment may decrease blood loss by 20 percent.[136] Depot MPA (150 mg every 3 months) is an acceptable alternative if the patient is noncompliant with oral medication. The levonorgestrel releasing intrauterine contraceptive device (LNG-IUD) may also be used in women who desire contraception. This device releases 20 μg LNG/day and is effective for 5 years. It has been reported to reduce menstrual blood loss by 50 percent.[17] Progestogens act to diminish the E effects on target cells by decreasing the production of E receptors (ER). Therefore, there is an antiproliferative, antimitotic action which leads to endometrial atrophy. Other hormonal agents which may be used include danocrine 100–200 mg daily. With this dose there are few androgenic side-effects but it is not contraceptive.[137] Gonadotropin releasing hormone agonists are also effective but, in the long-term (greater than 6 months) will produce osteoporosis and therefore will need to be combined with add-back therapy.[138] Of all the hormonal choices the OCP is the better and often cheaper alternative. Nonhormonal therapy for DUB includes cox inhibitors, antifibrinolytic agents, and hemostatic agents, all of which are taken during menstruation. Cyclo-oxygenase inhibitors include mefenamic acid, ibuprofen and naproxen. These will decrease blood loss by 30 percent but only while treatment is continued and, if used for more than 6 months, the therapy loses its effectiveness.[139] The inhibition of cox in the prostaglandin pathway causes a reduction in prostacyclin and thromboxane levels. Because prostacyclin levels are inhibited more effectively, there is blood vessel contraction and platelet aggregation.[140] These drugs are contraindicated in those with peptic ulcer disease, liver, or renal disease and in those who develop bronchospasm with aspirin or who have an aspirin intolerance.[17]

Antifibrinolytic agents include amino caproic acid, and tranexamic acid, and these agents are effective in 50 percent of women with DUB. The minor side effects of these drugs include nausea, abdominal pain, diarrhea, dizziness, and headache, and the major but rare side effect of thrombosis is the potential life-threatening problem.[17]

Hemostatic agents include ethamsylate. Their effectiveness in the treatment of excessive menstrual blood loss is questionable and has been discussed previously (page 756). Iron supplementation may also be required and is often forgotten.

Operative Hysteroscopy

Recent advances in hysteroscopic equipment have allowed new surgical treatments for menorrhagia and dysmenorrhea resistant to medical treatment while avoiding hysterectomy. These techniques aim to destroy not only the full thickness of the endometrium but also the adjoining 1 or 2 mm of myometrium to prevent endometrial regrowth and continuing menstrual ill health.

Endometrial ablation often requires pretreatment using GnRHa for 2–3 months to ensure endometrial atrophy. This medication is more effective than danocrine (800 mg daily) or MPA.[141] Alternatively, the procedure may be carried out in the very early follicular phase of the menstrual cycle. It is effective in 90 percent of women (50 percent will become amenorrheic and 40 percent will have decreased bleeding). The remaining 10 percent will be no better and rarely may be worse.[142] More than 1 procedure may be carried out. O'Connor and Magos[143] followed 525 women for up to 5 years after endometrial resection and reported that 9 percent subsequently underwent hysterectomy. There were no reported long-term complications of the procedure. When the woman reaches menopause and wishes hormone replacement therapy it is important that a progestin is added to the estrogen component.

It is of considerable interest that not only menorrhagia but also previously intractable dysmenorrhea may be effectively treated with operative hysteroscopy. Presumably, endometrial removal reduces the amount of PG production by the uterus, although this has not been proved.

Premenstrual Syndrome

Premenstrual syndrome is diagnosed by the repeated occurrence of behavioral and somatic symptoms severe enough to impair the woman's social and work-related function during the luteal phase of the menstrual cycle. Using strict diagnostic criteria it is estimated that 2.5 percent of women of reproductive age have this condition.[144,145] The range of symptoms commonly includes a disordered mood (irritability, depression), breast tenderness and abdominal bloating, headache, and altered appetite (especially carbohydrate craving) and libido. There have been many unsuccessful attempts to conclusively define clinical, menstrual, or hormonal parameters unique to PMS sufferers, including investigation of the sex steroid profile, the renin-angiotensin system, vitamin deficiency, glucose metabolism, and the opiate neuropeptides.[144,146–147] It has been suggested that ovulation occurs prematurely in PMS patients.[148] Central neurotransmitters are also most likely involved given successful treatment modalities. Social and psychological factors are important in the subjective assessment of PMS severity.[148,149] Effective treatments of PMS proven in randomized placebo-controlled clinical trials include serotonin reuptake inhibitors, alprazolam, and gonadotropin releasing hormone agonists.[144] Unproven therapies include relaxation therapy, pyridoxine hydrochloride, diuretics (including spironolactone), oral contraceptives, bromocriptine, and metronidazole.[150] All may be of some benefit in selected cases.

OVARIAN DISORDERS IN MIDDLE AGE

Endocrinology of the Menopause

The menopause is the permanent cessation of menstruation which results from loss of ovarian follicular activity. The term *perimenopause*, or *climacteric*, signifies the period of months when the endocrine, biological, and clinical features of declining ovarian function commence until the first year after menses have ceased (Fig. 16B-12). The postmenopause dates from the menopause but by convention cannot be determined until spontaneous amenorrhea has persisted for 12 months.[151] Uterine bleeding which recommences after 12 months of amenorrhea in a woman over age 40 years requires investigation to exclude endometrial cancer, although the most likely finding on endometrial sampling is an atrophic endometrium.

The median age at menopause is 51 years for women of European origin in developed countries, but there is no generally agreed on range for this age, making the definition of premature menopause arbitrary. Cessation of ovarian function prior to age 40 years is regarded widely as consistent with the concept of a premature menopause (see Premature Ovarian Failure, earlier).

Cigarette smoking is associated with a slightly reduced age at menopause.[152] The most striking aspect of ovarian morphology as the menopause approaches is the accelerated loss of primordial follicles. Although a gradual decline in follicular numbers is seen from the time of birth, the rate of decline increases markedly from about age 40. In an important study of Richardson et al.[153] the mean number of primordial follicles per ovary was 1392 ± 355 (SEM) in a group of women age 45–50 years who were still experiencing regular cycles. In a group that had entered a phase of cycle irregularity, the mean number fell to 142 ± 72, while in women who were postmenopausal, a single follicle was identified in one of four ovaries subjected to serial section. The overall decline in follicle numbers from both groups is illustrated in Fig. 16B-12.[153]

Endocrinologically, the major features of the loss of ovarian function are a marked fall (by 90–95 percent) in circulating estradiol level (from normal follicular-phase levels of 200–500 pM to 30–50 pM) and in the inhibins, which become undetectable. There are marked elevations of FSH concentration (10- to 15-fold, from normal follicular-phase levels of 3–15 IU/L to 25–100 IU/L

FIGURE 16B-12. Schematic representation of some clinical, biological, and endocrinologic features of the peri- and postmenopausal years.

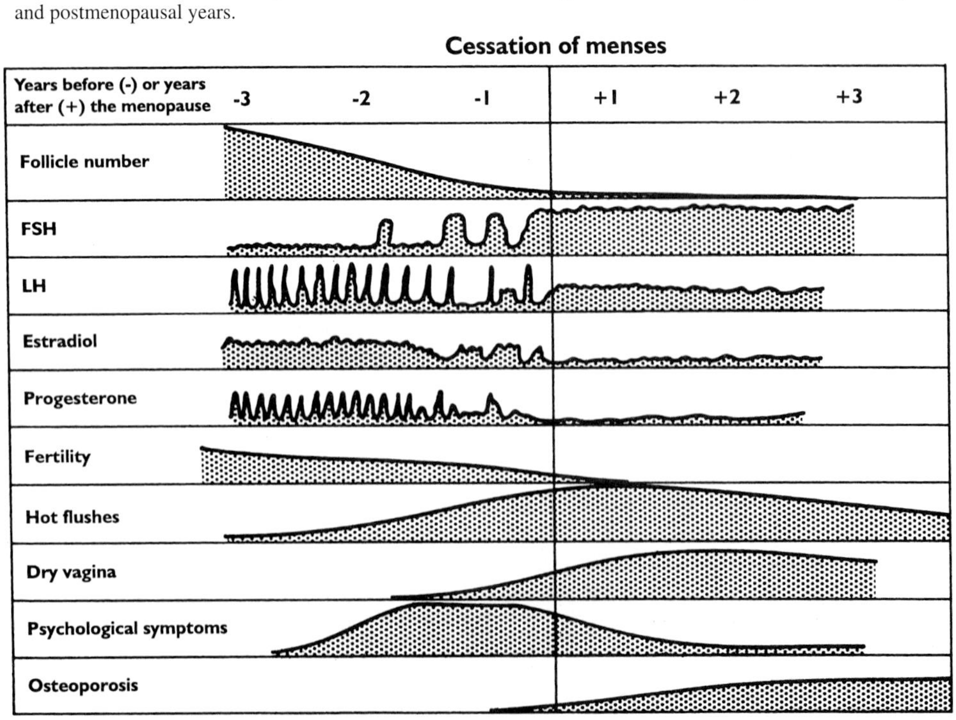

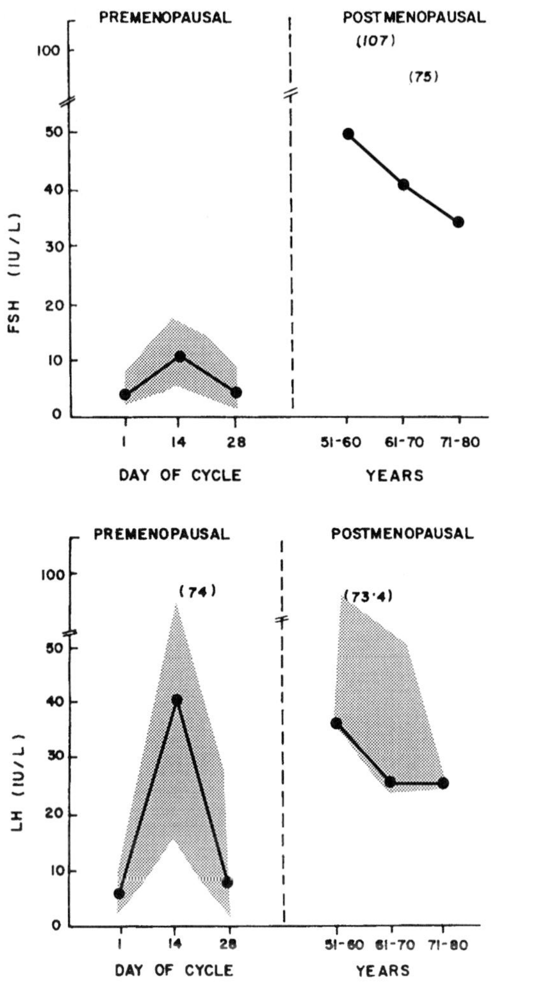

FIGURE 16B-13. Diagrammatic representation of serum FSH and LH concentrations during the follicular, periovulatory, and luteal phases of the normal menstrual cycle and during the postmenopausal period. Note that postmenopausal FSH levels greatly exceed those found during the menstrual cycle.

or more) and LH concentration (threefold, from 3–7 to 15–50 IU/L or more) (Fig. 16B-13). Progesterone secretion virtually ceases. The increase in gonadotropin levels results from loss of ovarian feedback both by estradiol and by the inhibins. During the transition between normal menstrual cyclicity and the postmenopausal period, a variety of hormonal patterns may be encountered. In women over age 40 who continue to have regular cycles, the follicular phase in particular may show moderate to marked elevations in serum FSH and decreases in inhibin, particularly in inhibin B levels,[154–156] with LH, estradiol, and progesterone secretion remaining unchanged. The menopausal transition is marked by considerable variability in menstrual cycle length; during this phase, apparently bizarre hormonal changes are found,[157] including elevation of levels of FSH or LH alone or FSH with LH and high or low levels of estrogens. A critical early event is a decline in circulating inhibin B.[158] In contrast to the decline in ovarian estrogen production, ovarian androgen production persists and there is little change in the circulating testosterone concentration after the menopause.[159] In fact, a 50 percent fall in circulating testosterone levels has been reported between ages 20 and 40.[160] This may be an important consideration when decisions are made regarding removal of the ovaries in peri- and postmenopausal women. Because of the variability in FSH and estradiol levels, the diagnosis of the menopausal state may not be made reliably by means of hormonal measurements alone, especially in women who have experienced lack of menses for only a few months. From a practical viewpoint, the possibility of fertility cannot be excluded until 1 year after the menopause.[161] Estimates of the annual risk of pregnancy are 10–20 percent for women aged 40–44 and 2–3 percent for women aged 45–49.[162] The finding of a clearly elevated serum FSH concentration and a serum estradiol level below 50 pM in a woman with 6 months or more of amenorrhea certainly makes the diagnosis of the postmenopausal state probable, but not certain. The endocrinology of the perimenopausal period has been extensively reviewed.[163]

Climacteric Symptoms

Perimenopausal patients may seek medical advice regarding the desirability of hormone replacement therapy (HRT) when they are asymptomatic because of the widespread prominence given to such therapy in the media. Alternatively, vasomotor symptoms, psychological complaints, and/or loss of sexuality, often in the context of menstrual irregularity, are frequent reasons for presentation.

The most characteristic perimenopausal symptom is the hot flush (or flash), which was found in one study in 17 percent of women in the age range 42–62 years still experiencing regular cycles, 40 percent of those with irregular cycles, 65 percent of those in the 1–2 years after menopause, and 35 percent of those 5–10 years after menopause.[164] The symptom is described as a brief sensation of heat usually involving the face and upper trunk; it is accompanied by a rise in skin temperature (up to 4°C or more), peripheral vasodilation, transient increase in heart rate, and lowering of skin resistance.[165] There may be sweating, chills, nervousness, irritability, and headache. Flushes are thought to be due to a sympathetic discharge [166] and occur more or less simultaneously with pulses of LH secretion, though they are not a result of such pulses.[167] Thus, it is likely that a hypothalamic event in which there is a transient downward resetting of the central thermostat occurs at the same time as the episodic discharge of GnRH.

Flush frequency is variable; occurrence during the night leads to sleep disturbance. Estrogen therapy specifically relieves the symptom, providing strong evidence for the role of estrogen withdrawal in its occurrence. When estradiol was administered transdermally, a dose-related decrease in hot flush frequency occurred with increasing serum estradiol levels.[168] Relief may also be afforded by the central alpha-adrenergic agonist drug clonidine and by progestogens such as medroxyprogesterone. Techniques such as continual recording of such symptoms now allow objective monitoring of flush frequency, permitting proper study of the efficacy of various treatment regimens.[169]

Controversy has surrounded the specificity of psychological symptoms in relation to the menopause; the degree to which symptoms such as fatigue, irritability, depression, and a general sense of feeling unwell are a reflection of "general lack of well-being" or of more specific psychological states such as depression is unclear, but there is substantial evidence that estrogen replacement will alleviate such symptoms, particularly in women who have no prior history of psychological disturbance.[170]

A decline in sexual interest of varying severity may occur after the menopause,[171] although the frequency of this problem has been questioned.[172] There may be associated vaginal dryness and dyspareunia, but correction of the dyspareunia with local or systemic estrogens often fails to restore sexual interest and enjoyment.

Urinary symptoms, such as frequency and urgency of micturition, may be experienced for the first time by peri- and postmenopausal women, but their association with estrogen deficiency has not been established clearly. In the absence of another underlying cause, a trial of vaginal or systemic estrogen therapy may be rewarding.

Alterations in appearance due to declining skin quality are common complaints in perimenopausal women, and the skin has been shown to contain estradiol receptors.[173] The postmenopausal state is associated with a decrease in skin collagen, which can be restored by HRT.[174]

The symptoms of flushes, psychological disturbances, and loss of sexuality are self-limited and respond satisfactorily to HRT. The presence of such symptoms constitutes a strong indication for at least short-term HRT for 6–12 months. During such a limited period the choice of estrogen is not a major issue, and oral therapy with a natural estrogen [e.g., conjugated equine estrogens (Premarin) 0.625–1.25 mg daily or estradiol valerate 1–2 mg daily] is used conventionally. Although not mandatory with short-term therapy, it is prudent to add a cyclic progestogen (e.g., medroxyprogesterone 10 mg or norethindrone 0.7–1.25 mg daily for 12 days per month) in order to avoid unexpected vaginal bleeding. Topical vaginal estrogen creams or tablets are valuable for the specific relief of vaginal dryness or dyspareunia. Conventional contraindications to estrogen therapy include a history of breast cancer or endometrial cancer; recent undiagnosed genital bleeding; active, severe liver disease; or a history of thromboembolism. There is, however, some controversy regarding the seriousness of these contraindications. For example, a patient who has no evidence of recurrence of breast cancer treated more than 5 years previously or who has had a stage 1 or 2 endometrial cancer treated can probably be given HRT without danger, especially if quality of life is taken into consideration.[175,176] Relief of severe flushing or dyspareunia may be an overwhelming indication for HRT despite the theoretical concerns regarding reactivation of a treated malignancy. For patients with mild liver disease or a past history of thromboembolism, parenteral estrogen therapy (e.g., by transdermal patch) is almost certainly safe, as this route is not associated with significant effects on liver function, including levels of clotting factors.[177,178] For patients with loss of libido persisting despite adequate oral estrogen replacement, combined subcutaneous implants of estradiol (40 mg) and testosterone (50 mg) have proved efficacious.[179,180]

Postmenopausal Problems

Osteoporosis

Osteoporosis is defined as a reduction in the mass of bony tissue relative to the volume of anatomic bone. Conventionally, the reference value for normal bones is taken as that derived from a normal young (premenopausal) adult population; a significant reduction is to less than 2.5 SD below that mean. A variety of techniques are available for the measurement of bone mass, including CT, dual x-ray (DEXA), and ultrasonic densitometry of the forearm, the os calcis, the spine, and the neck of the femur. Measurements can be made in the peri- or postmenopausal period in order to identify those at increased risk for the later development of osteoporotic fractures, which especially affect the radius, spine, and femoral neck. Loss of cortical bone in particular predisposes women to radial and femoral fractures, while loss of trabecular bone leads to vertebral crush fractures. Assessment of bone density is the only reliable method for estimating the risk of fracture.[181]

The exact pathogenesis of postmenopausal osteoporosis is not understood; however, there is a clear association between cessation of ovarian function and loss of bone mass, and estradiol receptors have been identified in bone cells.[182] It is hypothesized that estrogens somehow have a protective effect on bone, opposing bony resorption induced by parathormone, vitamin D, or both. Controversy exists regarding the role of calcitonin; there is some evidence that its levels fall after menopause and are stimulated by estrogen. The mean daily calcium requirement to maintain calcium balance was shown to increase after the menopause from about 500–1,500 mg.[183] Despite this, rates of loss of bone after menopause appear to be independent of calcium uptake over a wide range of values.[184] There is a slight rise in serum calcium and phosphate levels after the menopause, as well as in urinary calcium and hydroxyproline levels.[185] Measurement of the fasting urinary calcium/creatinine ratio provides a useful index of the rate of loss of calcium in the urine.

The prevention of postmenopausal osteoporosis is a major reason to consider long-term HRT (further discussed later). Numerous observational studies (summarized in[186,187]) suggest that HRT users are at reduced risk of osteoporotic fracture, though as yet there is no single randomized control trial of HRT in the prevention of the most important of these fractures, that of the hip. Nevertheless fracture prevention is a widely accepted indication for long term HRT. Ensuring an adequate calcium intake (about 1,500 mg daily) and encouragement of physical exercise are useful general measures. A recent study indicated that in men and women 65 years of age or older living in the community, dietary supplementation with calcium (500 mg) plus Vitamin D3 (700 IU) moderately reduced bone loss in the femoral neck, spine, and total body over a 3-year study period and reduced the incidence of nonvertebral fractures.[188]

The treatment of established osteoporosis remains an area of debate, but several approaches have shown promise. These include HRT,[189–191] cyclic or continuous[192,193] bisphosphonates, and calcitonin.[194] The place of sodium fluoride therapy is uncertain, as some studies have failed to show any beneficial effect on fracture prevention despite an increase in radiologic bone density.[195] Supplementary vitamin D in physiologic replacement doses should be given to women whose diet is deficient or who have little exposure to sunlight, but may be of value even in normal community dwellers, as noted earlier.

Atherosclerotic Cardiovascular Disease

Because cardiovascular disease is a leading cause of death, its possible relation to cessation of ovarian function and its possible prevention by HRT assume great importance.[196] It has been shown that the menopause is associated with increases in levels of serum cholesterol and triglycerides, accepted risk factors for atherosclerotic vascular disease.[197–199] Two population studies have examined the relation between carefully defined cardiovascular disease and the menopause. In Goteborg, Sweden, systematic samples from birth cohorts of women were examined and classified on the basis of a past history of myocardial infarction, angina pectoris, and EKG evidence of ischemic heart disease[199] The observed cases were compared to unaffected members of their cohort in three age groups, and those in all three affected groups were found to have undergone earlier menopause. In the Framingham Study, an increase in the incidence of coronary heart disease and in the severity of the presenting syndrome was found to occur after menopause among the 2,873 women who had been followed for up to 24 years after initial assessment.[200] No premenopausal women developed myocardial infarction or died of coronary heart disease, whereas such events were commonly seen among postmenopausal women. Within each of the age groups 40–44, 45–49, and 50–54 years, coronary heart disease was more than twice as common in postmenopausal as in premenopausal women, whether the menopause was spontaneous or surgical. In a study of American nurses, those who had had bilateral oophorectomy before age 35 years had more than seven times the risk of having a nonfatal myocardial infarct compared with premenopausal women of the same age and with the same risk factors.[201] Although there are other data not supportive of these associations,[202,203] it can reasonably be concluded that menopause may be associated with an increase in the risks of morbidity and mortality from atherosclerotic cardiovascular disease.

Estrogen therapy alone given to postmenopausal women has beneficial effects on coronary risk factors, causing a fall in serum cholesterol and low-density lipoprotein levels and an increase in the concentration of high-density lipoprotein,[204,205] with variable effects on levels of plasma triglycerides. Synthetic progestogens tend to nullify these estrogen effects,[206] although their ability to do so varies with the dose and with the precise time during the treatment regimen at which lipid levels are measured. Although an initial report suggested that 17-acetoxyprogestogens are less potent in this regard than are 19-nor-progestogens, the doses of the latter used in that study were relatively much greater than those of medroxyprogesterone.[206] Whether progestogens in the lower doses currently recommended have long-term adverse effects on plasma lipids, in particular on morbidity or mortality from coronary artery disease, remains to be established (see later discussion).[207] Effects of estrogen on blood coagulation factors are variable; dosage, route of administration, and the nature of the estrogen preparation are important. Thus, oral estrogens cause increases in levels of factors VII, IX, X, and X complex[208,209] and lower concentrations of anticoagulation factors such as antithrombin III. Percutaneously administered estradiol has no effect on antithrombin III.[210]

Whether estrogen therapy leads to an alteration in the actual occurrence of cardiovascular disease remains controversial.[211] At least one study of death from ischemic heart disease in a retirement community suggests a strong protective effect of oral estrogen (risk ratio with estrogen therapy 0.43).[212] A report from the Lipid Research Clinics Program follow-up study indicated a marked decrease in all-cause mortality in estrogen users compared with nonusers,[213] mainly as a result of reduced cardiovascular mortality.[214] Confirmatory reports have been published.[215–217] It is now clear that progestogen should be used routinely in patients who have intact uteri to protect against the risk of endometrial cancer arising from unopposed estrogen; the epidemiological data suggest that the effects of combined estrogen/progestogen on coronary risk are equivalent to those of estrogen alone.[218–220] Studies in the cynomolgus monkey suggest that different progestins may have different effects in preventing development of atherosclerosis, independently of their effects on serum lipids.[221,222]

The first well designed double-blind, placebo-controlled randomized study of combined continuous oral HRT in women in whom the presence of coronary artery disease had previously been demonstrated was reported in 1998.[223] It involved 2,763 postmenopausal women of mean age 66.7 and failed to demonstrate any difference in vascular events including myocardial infarction, coronary revascularisation, unstable angina, congestive cardiac

TABLE 16B-6. Types of Estrogen Available for Therapeutic Use

Natural
Estradiol
Estrone and estrone sulfate
Estriol
Conjugated (mixture of sodium estrone sulfate, sodium equilin sulfate, sodium equilenin sulfate, sodium estradiol sulfate and others.
Synthetic
Ethinyl estradiol
Mestranol
Quinestrol
Diethylstilbestrol
Dienestrol

failure, stroke or transient ischaemic attack, or peripheral arterial disease between the active and placebo-treated groups despite changes in their lipid parameters in the expected direction. These results were unexpected and the publications on further trials of secondary prevention are awaited. There are a variety of mechanisms by which estrogens may in principle reduce the vascular processes which lead to atherosclerosis.[224,224a] The major issues in relation to hormone therapy and atherosclerotic vascular disease have been reviewed.[151]

Long-Term Hormone Replacement Therapy

Modes of Administration

From a therapeutic viewpoint, estrogens are arbitrarily classified into those which occur in nature and those which are synthetic (Table 16B-6). Natural estrogens include estradiol and its esters, estrone sulfate (including its piperazine salt), estriol, and conjugated equine estrogens (Premarin, a mixture of several, including estrone sulfate, equilin, and equilenin). The major synthetic estrogen is ethinyl estradiol; mestranol and diethylstilbestrol are additional examples. Estrogens may be given orally or parenterally; approximately equivalent doses of the commonly used preparations are listed in Table 16B-7. Although preparations differ in their relative potencies, depending on the assay end point, the doses listed are approximately equivalent in terms of FSH suppression.[225] The synthetic estrogens are relatively more potent than the natural estrogens in their hepatic effects.

The oral estrogens may be given cyclically (3 weeks on, 1 week off) in the belief that this will minimize the likelihood of development of endometrial hyperplasia, but there is no evidence that continuous oral administration results in a greater risk,[226] and

TABLE 16B-7. Oral Estrogen Preparations and Approximately Equivalent Doses

Preparation	Dose
Oral estrogens	
Conjugated equine estrogens	0.625–1.25 mg daily
Piperazine estrone sulfate	1.25–2.5 mg daily
Estradiol valerate	1–2 mg daily
Micronized estradiol	1–2 mg daily
Ethinyl estradiol	10–20 μg daily
Parenteral estrogens	
Transdermal estradiol	50 μg patch twice weekly
Percutaneous estradiol	3 mg daily
Subcutaneous estradiol implant	50 mg every 6 months

some patients suffer recurrence of hot flushes during the week off therapy on the cyclic regimen.

Oral estrogen administration results in "first-pass" effects on the liver, with maximal opportunity for effects on hepatic protein synthesis. Synthetic estrogens are particularly potent from this standpoint and produce significant increases in the synthesis of renin substrate, SHBG, corticosteroid-binding globulin, thyroxine-binding globulin, and lipoproteins.[227] This has led to the development of various parenteral estrogen preparations (e.g., subcutaneous estradiol implants, estradiol gels for application to the skin, estrogen-containing vaginal creams, and transdermal therapeutic systems).[228] These preparations have little if any effect on hepatic protein synthesis and may thus have at least theoretical advantages for long-term use. In addition, although all natural orally administered estrogens give rise to plasma levels of estrone markedly in excess of that of plasma estradiol, the parenteral preparations produce plasma levels of estradiol greater than those of estrone, mimicking the physiologic situation of the normal follicular phase of the menstrual cycle.[228–230]

In women with an intact uterus, cyclic administration of a progestogen for a minimum of 10 and preferably 12–13 days each month is mandatory in order to avoid the risk of estrogen-induced endometrial hyperplasia, which may progress to endometrial carcinoma.[231] Other possible beneficial effects of the added progestogen (e.g., possible reduction in the risk of occurrence of breast cancer, actual increase in bone mass) remain controversial, and the potential adverse effects (neutralization of the possible beneficial effects of estrogens) have not been well defined. The dose of progestogen required to protect against the development of endometrial hyperplasia and carcinoma varies with the type of progestogen,[232] but the risk of endometrial carcinoma may not be abolished entirely by cyclic progestins.[233] Currently recommended regimens include the use of medroxyprogesterone acetate 5–10 mg daily or norethindrone 0.7–1.25 mg daily, most conveniently given on the first 12 calendar days of the month to facilitate patient compliance. A useful clinical indicator that the dose of progestogen is adequate is that induced menstrual bleeding occurs only after the 10th to 12th day of the month.[232] The occurrence of withdrawal bleeding as a result of cyclic progestogen administration is a major disincentive to some women in considering HRT. An alternative therapeutic regimen that can lead to amenorrhea is the combined continuous administration of a standard dose of estrogen (either orally or parenterally) with a dose of progestogen lower than that required for cyclic therapy (e.g., medroxyprogesterone acetate 2.5 mg, norethindrone 0.35–0.7 mg, or norethisterone acetate 1 mg daily).[234,235] Although breakthrough bleeding in the first 3 to 4 months of such combined continuous therapy may occur in 40–50 percent of patients, amenorrhea is usually induced after 4–6 months. The long-term safety of this type of combined continuous therapy has not yet been established,[235] although the lack of adverse effects on cardiovascular risk factors and the beneficial effects on bone mineral density provide grounds for optimism. The use of progestogens in women who have had a hysterectomy is not regarded as necessary.[236] The development of "nonandrogenic" progestogens gives promise that HRT can be made even safer in the future.

Routine supervision of patients on long-term HRT should include blood pressure measurement, breast examination, and assessment of lipid levels, with endometrial sampling in any patient who develops unexpected uterine bleeding. Whether endometrial biopsy should be undertaken routinely before long-term HRT is instituted is controversial; in a patient previously untreated with estrogen, the procedure may be associated with significant discomfort, and if there is no history of abnormal uterine bleeding and a cyclic progestogen is used, endometrial biopsy is unlikely to yield clinically significant information. Especially in patients with a history of benign breast disease or a family history of breast cancer, routine mammography is desirable prior to initiating therapy and at intervals of 1–2 years thereafter.

Benefits and Risks

The major potential benefits of long-term HRT are the prevention of osteoporosis and hence of lowering the risk of osteoporosis-associated fracture, particularly of the femoral neck, and the theoretical benefit of the prevention of atherosclerotic cardiovascular disease. If the latter is established on the basis of further epidemiologic studies, it will be extremely important to consider using HRT more routinely in the community. In recent years there has been considerable interest in the possibility that HRT may also be protective against the risk of developing dementia of the Alzheimer's type. This remains controversial and the benefit is at present unproven.[237]

It should be noted that there are a number of other potential approaches to the prevention of osteoporosis and to the prevention of atherosclerotic cardiovascular disease. For example, for the former bisphosphonates and Vitamin D therapy are potential alternatives, as are the recently developed selective estrogen modulators (SERMs).[238] For atherosclerotic vascular disease prevention, the use of dietary measures and lipid lowering agents is efficacious.

The major potential risks are of endometrial and breast cancer. Although it has been established that estrogen therapy without accompanying progestogen leads to a substantially increased risk of endometrial hyperplasia and carcinoma, this risk may be largely abolished if regular cyclic progestogen is administered.[233,239] The question of whether HRT causes an increased risk of developing breast cancer is unresolved[151,240]; if a risk does exist, it is relatively small (risk ratio ≤ 2).[241,242] However, because breast cancer is an extremely frightening prospect for the individual patient, the risk must be taken into account in making a decision concerning long-term HRT. It has proved extremely difficult to arrive at an objective resolution of the benefit/risk ratio for HRT,[216] and the situation has become more complex because there are few epidemiologic data on the benefits (and risks) of long-term HRT using both estrogens and progestogens. Further, there are no comprehensive data on regimens of parenteral estrogen administration. The authors have adopted the approach of being ready to administer long-term HRT to any woman who seeks such therapy, provided that no contraindications are present and that she is willing to tolerate the inconvenience of monthly withdrawal bleeding. A regimen commonly used in women who are 1–2 years post-menopausal is oral estradiol valerate 1–2 mg or conjugated equine estrogen 0.625–1.25 mg daily continuously with medroxyprogesterone acetate 10 mg daily or norethindrone 1.25 mg daily for the first 12 calendar days each month. For women who are more than 2 years post-menopausal, combined continuous HRT is commonly given. There is a growing preference for lower dose therapy (e.g. conjugated equine estrogen 0.3 mg plus MPA 2.5 mg daily, or estradiol 1 mg with norethisterone acetate 0.5 mg daily). Patients are reviewed at 6- to 12-month intervals for assessment of blood pressure and breasts and for measurement of serum lipids. Endometrial biopsy is undertaken only when abnormal uterine bleeding is reported.

Use of Androgens

A controversial aspect of menopausal hormone therapy is the use of androgens, particularly for the management of loss of libido in women who have had bilateral oophorectomy. In those circumstances, if libido does not return to normal after adequate estrogen replacement, initiation of testosterone therapy is reasonable. Testosterone can be administered initially on a trial basis, using injections of testosterone esters 50 mg monthly for 3 months. If this therapy is effective a longer acting testosterone implant can be considered.[26,179,180]

Postmenopausal Bleeding

Patients with or without HRT may develop bleeding more than 12 months after the cessation of their spontaneous menstrual cycles. Each patient with unanticipated postmenopausal bleeding must be thoroughly evaluated because of the increased incidence of endometrial adenocarcinoma, which in some series has reached 23 percent.[243]

Outpatient endometrial sampling using a Novak or Randall instrument or a suction device such as the Vabra aspirator has been reported to correlate with formal inpatient cervical dilatation and uterine curettage in approximately 90 percent of subjects.[244] Simpler sampling devices have been developed, such as the Pipelle cannula and Gynoscann,[245] and the use of endometrial sampling in women on HRT has been reviewed.[246] Where available, such outpatient procedures and office diagnostic hysteroscopy are now the diagnostic methods of choice for directed endometrial biopsy in patients with postmenopausal bleeding. In the 10 percent of outpatients in whom the endometrial cavity cannot be sounded or in whom repeated or persistent postmenopausal bleeding occurs, inpatient examination under anesthesia and curettage is mandatory. Gambrell and Greenblatt have emphasized the usefulness of progestogen and estrogen therapy to arrest heavy postmenopausal bleeding and the value of cyclic courses of progestogens such as Provera 20 mg daily to reverse hyperplasia of the endometrium.[247] Patients with any degree of endometrial hyperplasia must have repeat curettage after 3 months of progestogen treatment and hysterectomy if hyperplasia persists.

Endovaginal ultrasound is a noninvasive diagnostic test that may indicate which patients should undergo endometrial sampling. It has been reported that if the endometrial stripe is homogeneously $\leq$5 mm the likelihood of an endometrial abnormality is very small (0.1 percent in users of HRT and 1 percent in nonusers). But if bleeding continues further evaluation should be undertaken.[248,249] If the endometrium is $>$5 mm or irregular or if a mass is suspected sonohysterography is a useful tool. This involves instilling saline into the endometrial cavity during an ultrasound examination. This procedure more clearly delineates the endometrium and helps to differentiate endometrial polyps from submucosal fibroids.[250]

CHEMICAL CONTRACEPTION AND CONTRAGESTION

Oral contraceptives are probably the most studied medicines in the history of therapeutics. Many international conferences, books, and reviews on chemical contraceptives can be found in the literature.[251,252] It is not the aim of this section to provide an exhaustive review of the last 30 years of oral contraceptives, which are now estimated to have been taken at some time by four out of every five western women in their midthirties. Rather, the aim is to briefly review the benefits and risks of oral contraceptives, describe recent advances in progestogen therapy, and review chemical contragestion by progesterone receptor antagonists such as Mifepristone.[253]

During the last three decades there have been major modifications to oral contraceptives. Initially, the amount of progestogen was markedly reduced by the introduction of norgestrel and subsequent isolation of its active isomer, levonorgestrel. This was also associated with a decrease of the estrogen component in 1973 to 30 μg of ethinylestradiol per day. In the 1980s, there were also attempts to further reduce the estrogen content of oral contraceptives with the introduction of the triphasic approach to oral contraception.

Studies during the past 30 years have shown a number of rare but serious adverse effects from chemical contraception, especially in the cardiovascular system. However, it is important to emphasize that current studies on cardiovascular effects, metabolic actions, and the incidence of various tumors tell us about only the previous generation of oral chemical contraceptives, not those in current use. As far as increased cardiovascular risk is concerned, this is mainly concentrated in women who are over 35 years old, smoke cigarettes, or have other risk factors such as obesity, poorly controlled diabetes, or uncontrolled hypertension. The most recent data indicate that healthy nonsmoking women age 35 years to menopause can continue to use oral contraceptives without an increased risk of cardiovascular disease.

A major benefit of the use of chemical contraception has been a clear reduction in the risk of various cancers. At least nine major studies indicate that oral contraceptives have a protective effect against endometrial cancer, the third most common cancer among women in the United States. This protective effect is greatest in women who have no children or only one child, and it is precisely these women who have the greatest risk of acquiring endometrial cancer. Ovarian cancer kills more women than all other genital malignancies combined. There are more than 12 published reports indicating that the use of chemical contraception reduces the risk of ovarian cancer, in particular the most common types of epithelial ovarian cancer. As little as 6 months of oral contraceptive use provides protection, and this protective effect continues for at least 15 years after the use of chemical contraception stops (Table 16B-8).

In terms of possible risks, many studies have looked at the risk of breast cancer among users of chemical contraception. The most extensive report is that of the Collaborative Group on Hormonal Factors in Breast Cancer,[254] which reported their findings on breast cancer in users of the OCP. They obtained data from 54

TABLE 16B-8. Benefits and Risks of Chemical Contraception

Benefits	Risks
Menstrual loss reduced	Hypertension
Iron deficiency anemia decreased	Arterial thromboembolism increased
Dysmenorrhea less	Venous thromboembolism increased
Benign ovarian cysts fewer	Gallbladder disease increased
Endometrial cancer decreased	
Ovarian cancer decreased	
Bone density increased	
Risks of ectopic pregnancy reduced	
Risk of endometriosis reduced	

studies conducted in 25 countries encompassing 53,297 women with breast cancer and 100,239 women without breast cancer. They reported that women who are currently using the OCP or have used it in the past 10 years are at a slightly increased risk of having breast cancer diagnosed (RR 1.24 [1.15–1.33] current users; 1.07 [1.02–1.13] after 10 years). The cancers that have been diagnosed tend to be localized within the breast compared with the cancers diagnosed in never-users. Ten years after cessation of use there is no increase in the risk. They concluded that it was not known if an earlier diagnosis of breast cancer in women on the OCP contributed to the increase in the risk or whether it was a biological effect of the OCP or a combination of reasons.

There have been reports that increased cervical intraepithelial neoplasia may be associated with chemical contraception. It is currently impossible to say whether this is a casual relation because of the confounding difficulties with other risk factors, such as the age of first intercourse, the number of sexual partners, and infection with papilloma or wart virus.

There is a significant trend for the development of invasive cervical cancer with increasing duration of use of the OCP (RR 1.77 after 12 years of use). The risk appears to decline with increasing time after OCP discontinuation. The increased risk may occur because the OCP gives no protection against the human papilloma virus.[255] However, the studies have not been standardized for sexual activity,[256] which is a major risk factor for the development of cervical cancer.

There is a high correlation between oral contraceptive use and benign liver tumors. Such benign hepatocellular adenomas are rare in western countries, and although these tumors may become malignant, the rate of death from this disease has remained unchanged in the United States during the past 25 years, a period when millions of women have used chemical contraception. Furthermore, other tumors, including malignant melanoma and pituitary adenoma, are no more frequent among users of chemical contraception than among nonusers.

New Progestogens

As part of a continuum in the development of chemical contraception, recent research has explored the potential usefulness of a new series of gonane progestogens related to levonorgestrel. The most studied of these newer derivatives are gestodene and desogestrel. Both molecules are derivatives of 19-norprogesterone and, like levonorgestrel, bind with higher affinity to the progesterone receptor than does the natural hormone. There was no affinity for the estrogen receptor and similar affinities with levonorgestrel to the androgen receptor. Gestodene and desogestrel bind three to five times more avidly to the aldosterone receptor than does levonorgestrel. Gestodene and desogestrel inhibit ovulation in doses of approximately 40 μg per day, which is similar to levonorgestrel and compares with an inhibitory action of progesterone at only 300 mg per day. Gestodene and desogestrel cause progestogenic transformation of endometrium at doses of only 2 mg per cycle compared with levonorgestrel (5–6 mg/cycle).[257]

The clinical interest in "third-generation" progestogens arises from data suggesting that the progesterone component of the combined oral contraceptive may contribute to the increased risk of stroke and ischemic heart disease in women taking these medicines. It has been suggested that the progestogen used in combined oral contraceptives modifies the estrogen effect on blood coagulation. It has been reported that these progestogens increase fibrinolytic activity and decrease platelet aggregation; this suggests that these new forms of chemical contraception will have fewer thrombogenic hazards than previous formulations did.

There has been some controversy as to whether the OCPs containing third generation progestogens are associated with an increase in venous thromboembolism. There are several reports of a small increase (doubling) in the incidence of venous thromboembolic disease in women using third generation OCPs compared with those using the second generation OCPs.[258–261] It was not known if this was a true increase or whether selection bias contributed to these results, whereby women at risk of venous thrombosis were prescribed the third rather than the second generation OCPs. Farmer et al[262] have reported that the increase in risk was likely due to residual confounding by age. However, Vanderbroucke and Rosendaal[263] have also reported that the third generation OCPs induce a resistance to the blood's natural anticoagulation system (activated protein C resistance) and that the second generation OCPs show only part of this effect. Winkler[264] has argued that the venous thromboembolism risk is unknown when this is present. It must be remembered that the risk of thromboembolic disease in a pregnant woman is 30 times greater than in a nonpregnant woman.

A second recent advance in chemical regulation of fertility has been the development of progesterone receptor antagonists such as Mifepristone (RU-486).[265] Progesterone receptor antagonists bind avidly to the progesterone receptor and glucocorticoid receptor and have essentially no binding to the mineralocorticoid, estrogen, or androgen receptors. Mifepristone also binds avidly to albumin, resulting in a half-life of approximately 24 h after oral administration.

Progesterone receptor antagonists can induce menstruation by a direct action on the endometrium.[266] This action is produced by the release of PGF_2 and PGE_2 and by a decrease in the metabolism of these eicosanoids.[267]

Baulieu has highlighted the use of progesterone receptor antagonists as contragestives or antigestational agents.[265] Chemical contragestives regulate fertility by preventing or interrupting implantation and act regardless of whether fertilization has occurred. Ulmann[268] has reported that 600 mg of Mifepristone taken on day 27 of the cycle in women who had unprotected intercourse at midcycle resulted in menstruation within 72 h in all patients. However, of the 35 of 102 women who had conceived, 6 of these 35 pregnancies continued and required surgical termination. Further studies are required to establish whether progesterone receptor antagonists alone or in combination with other medicines will be clinically effective for occasional contragestion.

REFERENCES

1. Lippe B: Turner Syndrome. *I Endocrinol Metab Clin North Am* 20: 1, 1991.
2. Ross JL, Cassorla FG, Skerda NC, Valk IM, Loriaux DL, Cutler GB: A preliminary study of the effect of estrogen dose on growth in Turner's syndrome. *N Engl J Med* 309:1104, 1983.
3. Rosenfeld RG, Hintz RL, Johanson AJ, Sherman B, Brasel JA, Burstein S, Chernausek S, Compton P, et al: Three year results of a randomized prospective trial of methionyl human growth hormone and oxandrolone in Turner's syndrome. *J Pediatr* 113:393, 1988.
4. Takano K, Shizume K, Hibi I: Turner's syndrome: Treatment of 203 patients with recombinant human growth hormone for one year: A multicentre study. *Acta Endocrinol (Copenh)* 120:559, 1989.
5. Vanderschueren-Lodeweyckz M, Massa G, Maes M, Craen M, van Vliet G, Heinrichs C, Malvaux P: Growth-promoting effect of

growth hormone and low dose ethinyl estradiol in girls with Turner's syndrome. *J Clin Endocrinol Metab* 70:122, 1990.
6. Khastgir G, Abdalla H, Thomas A, et al: Oocyte donation in Turner's syndrome: An analysis of the factors affecting outcome. *Hum Reprod* 12:279, 1997.
7. Nielsen J, Sillesen I, Hansen KB: Fertility in women with Turner's syndrome: Case report and review of literature. *Brit J Obstet Gynaecol* 86:833, 1979.
8. Tarani L, Lampariello G, Raguso G, et al: Pregnancy in patients with Turner's syndrome: Six new cases and review of literature. Gynecol Endocrinol 12:83, 1993.
9. Seminara SB, Hayes FJ, Crowley WF Jr: Gonadotropin-releasing hormone deficiency in the human (idiopathic hypogonadotropic hypogonadism and Kallman's syndrome): Pathophysiological and genetic considerations. *Endocr Rev* 19:521, 1998.
10. Ballabio A, Bardoni B, Carrozzo R, Andria G, Bick O, Campbell L, Hamel B, Ferguson-Smith MA, et al: Contiguous gene syndromes due to deletions in the distal short arm of the human X chromosome. *Proc Natl Acad Sci USA* 86:10001, 1989.
11. Shalet SM: Treatment of constitutional delay in growth and puberty (CDGP). *Clin Endocrinol (Oxf)* 31:81, 1989.
12. Dewhurst CJ (ed): *Integrated Obstetrics and Gynaecology for Postgraduates*. London, Blackwell, 1981.
13. Quigley CA, De Bellis A, Marschke KB, et al: Androgen receptor defects: Historical clinical and molecular perspectives. *Endocr Rev* 16:271, 1995.
14. Healy DL, Hodgen GD: The endocrinology of human endometrium. *Obstet Gynecol Surv* 38:509, 1983.
15. Fraser IS, Michie EA, Wide L, Baird DT: Pituitary gonadotropins and ovarian function in adolescent dysfunctional uterine bleeding. *J Clin Endocrinol Metab* 37:407, 1973.
16. Bonnar J, Sheppard BL: Treatment of menorrhagia during menstruation: Randomised controlled trial of ethamsylate, mefenamic acid, and tranexamic acid. *Br Med J* 7:579, 1996.
17. Valle RF: Assessing new treatments for dysfunctional bleeding. *Ob Gyn* April: 43, 1994.
18. Kalantaridou SN, Davis SR, Nelson LM. Premature ovarian failure. *Endocrinol Metab Clin North Am* 27:989, 1998.
19. O'Herlihy C, Pepperell RJ, Evans JH: The significance of FSH elevation in young women with disorders of ovulation. *Br Med J* 281:1447, 1980.
20. Keelam CV, Stringfellow S, Frohocfnagel D. Evidence for a genetic factor in the etiology of premature ovarian failure. *Fertil Steril* 40:693, 1983.
21. Warne GL, Fairley KF, Hobbs JH, Martin FIR: Cyclophosphamide-induced ovarian failure. *N Engl J Med* 289:1159, 1973.
22. Alper MM, Garner PR: Premature ovarian failure: Its relationship to autoimmune disease. *Obstet Gynecol* 66:27, 1985.
23. Mignot MH, Shoemaker J, Kleingeld M, Ramanath Rao B, Drexhage HA: Premature ovarian failure: I. The association with autoimmunity. *Eur J Obstet Gynecol Reprod Biol* 30:59, 1989.
24. Cameron IT, O'Shea F, MacLachlan V, Healy DL: Occult ovarian failure: A clinical syndrome of regular menses, infertility and elevated FSH values shows an impaired response to superovulation. *J Clin Endocrinol Metab* 67:1190, 1988.
25. Buckler HM, Evans CA, Mamtora H, Burger HG, Anderson DC: Gonadotropin, steroid, and inhibin levels in women with incipient ovarian failure during anovulatory and ovulatory rebound cycle. *J Clin Endocrinol Metab* 72:116, 1991.
26. Davis SR, Burger HG: Clinical Review: Androgens and the postmenopausal woman. *J Clin Endocrinol Metab* 81:2759, 1996.
27. Kreiner D, Droesch K, Navot D, Scott R, Rosenwaks Z: Spontaneous and pharmacologically induced remissions in patients with premature ovarian failure. Obstet Gynecol 72:926, 1988.
28. Cameron IT, Rogers PAW, Caro C, Harman J, Healy DL, Leeton JF: Oocyte donation: A review. *Br J Obstet Gynaecol* 96:893, 1989.
29. Kleinberg BL, Noel GL, Francz AG: Galactorrhea: A study of 235 cases, including 48 with pituitary tumours. *N Engl J Med* 296:589, 1977.
30. Katz E, Adashi EY: Hyperprolactinemic disorders. *Clin Obstet Gynecol* 33:622, 1990.
31. Bonneville JF, Poulignot D, Cattin F, Couturier M, Mollet E, Dietmann JL: Computed tomographic demonstration of the effects of bromocriptine on pituitary microadenoma size. *Neuroradiology* 143:451, 1982.
32. Davis PC, Hoffman JC Jr, Spencer T, Tindall GT, Braun IF: MR imaging of pituitary adenoma: CT, clinical and surgical correlation. *AJNR* 148:797, 1987.
33. Stein AL, Levenick MN, Kletzky OA: Computed tomography versus magnetic resonance imaging for the evaluation of suspected pituitary adenomas. *Obstet Gynecol* 73:996, 1989.
34. Klibanski A, Neer RM, Beilins JZ, Ridgway EC, Zervas NT, McArthur JW: Decreased bone density in hyperprolactinemic women. *N Engl J Med* 303:1511, 1980.
35. Klibanski A, Greenspan SL: Increase in bone mass after treatment of hyperprolactinemic amenorrhea. *N Engl J Med* 315:542, 1986.
36. Corenblum B, Donovan L: The safety of physiological estrogen plus progestin replacement therapy and of oral contraceptive therapy in women with pathological hyperprolactinemia. *Fertil Steril* 59:671, 1993.
37. Yazigi RA, Quintero CH, Salameh WA: Prolactin disorders. *Fertil Steril* 67:215, 1997.
38. Webster J, Piscitelli G, Polli A, Ferrari CI, Ismail I, Scanlon MF: A comparison of cabergoline and bromocriptine in the treatment of hyperprolactinemic amenorrhea. *N Engl J Med* 331:904, 1994.
39. Colao A, Di Sarno A, Sarnacchiaro F, et al: Prolactinomas resistant to standard dopamine agonists respond to chronic cabergoline treatment. *J Clin Endocrinol Metab* 82:876, 1997.
40. Molitch ME: Pregnancy and the hyperprolactinemic woman. *N Engl J Med* 312:1364, 1985.
41. Rasmussen C, Berg HT, Nillius SJ, Wide L: The return of menstruation and normalization of prolactin in hyperprolactinemic women with bromocriptine-induced pregnancy. *Fertil Steril* 44:31, 1985.
42. Rodman EF, Molitch ME, Post KD, Boller BJ, Reichman S: Long-term followup of transsphenoidal selective adenomectomy for prolactinoma. *JAMA* 252:921, 1984.
43. Serri U, Rasio E, Beauregard H, Hardy J, Sommer AN: Recurrence of hyperprolactinemia after selective transphenoidal adenomectomy in women with prolactinoma. *N Engl J Med* 309:280, 1983.
44. Frisch RE, Revelle ER: Height and weight at menarche and a hypothesis of critical body weight and adolescent events. *Science* 169:397, 1970.
45. Van der Spuy ZM: Nutrition and reproduction. *Clin Obstet Gynecol* 12:579, 1985.
46. Yen SSC. Effects of lifestyle and body composition on the ovary. *Endocrinol Metab Clin North Am* 27:915, 1998.
47. Berg HT, Nillius SJ, Wide L: Serum prolactin and gonadotrophin levels before and after luteinising hormone releasing hormone in the investigation of amenorrhoea. *Br J Obstet Gynaecol* 85:945, 1978.
48. McArthur JW, Bullen BA, Beitins IZ, Pagano M, Badger TM, Klibanski A: Hypothalamic amenorrhea in runners of normal body composition. *Endocr Res Commun* 7:13, 1980.
49. Herd HP, Palumbo PJ, Gharib H: Hypothalamic-endocrine dysfunction in anorexia nervosa. *Mayo Clin Proc* 51:711, 1977.
50. Hsu LKG: Outcome of anorexia nervosa. *Arch Gen Psychiatry* 37:1041, 1980.
51. Warren MP: The effects of exercise on pubertal progression and reproductive function in girls. *J Clin Endocrinol Metab* 51:1150, 1980.
52. Feicht CB, Johnston TS, Martin BJ, Sparkes KE, Wagner WW Jr: Secondary amenorrhoea in athletes. *Lancet* ii:1145, 1978.
53. Baker ER, Mathur RS, Kirk RS, Williamson HO: Female runners and secondary amenorrhea: Correlation with age, parity, mileage, and plasma hormonal and sex-hormone-binding globulin concentrations. *Fertil Steril* 36:183, 1981.
54. Loucks AB, Verdun M, Heath EM: Low energy availability, not stress of exercise, alters LH pulsatility in exercising women. *J Appl Physiol* 84:37, 1998.
55. Marshall JC, Fraser TR: Amenorrhoea and anorexia nervosa: Assessment and treatment with clomiphene citrate. *Br Med J* 4:590, 1971.
56. Drinkwater BL, Nilson K, Chestnut CH, Bremner WJ, Shainholtz S, Southworth MB: Bone mineral content of amenorrheic and eumenorrheic athletes. *N Engl J Med* 311:277, 1984.
57. Polson DW, Adams J, Wadsworth J, Franks S: Polycystic ovaries—a common finding in normal women. *Lancet* 1:870, 1988.
58. Franks S: Polycystic ovary syndrome. *N Engl J Med* 333:853, 1995.
59. Hague W, Adams J, Reeders S, Peto TEA, Jacobs HS: Familial polycystic ovaries: A genetic disease. *Clin Endocrinol (Oxf)* 29:593, 1988.
60. Zawadzki JK, Dunaif A: Diagnostic criteria for polycystic ovary syndrome: Towards a rational approach, in Dunaif A, Haseltine FP,

Merriam GR (eds): *Polycystic Ovary Syndrome.* Oxford, England, Blackwell Scientific, 1992, pp 377–384.

61. Norman RJ, Hague WM, Masters SC, Wang XJ: Subjects with polycystic ovaries without hyperandrogenaemia exhibit similar disturbances in insulin and lipid profiles as those with polycystic ovary syndrome. *Hum Reprod* 10:2258, 1995.
62. Franks S, Adams J, Mason H, Poulson D: Ovulatory disorders in women with polycystic ovary syndrome. *Clin Obstet Gynecol* 12:605, 1985.
63. Erickson GS, Hsueh AJW, Quigley ME, Rebar RW, Yen SSC: Functional studies of aromatase activity in human granulosa cells from normal and polycystic ovaries. *J Clin Endocrinol Metab* 49:514, 1979.
64. Rosenfield RL, Barnes RB, Cara JF, Lucky AW: Dysregulation of cytochrome P450c17α as the cause of polycystic ovarian syndrome. *Fertil Steril* 53:785, 1990.
65. Baird DT, Corker CS, Davidson DW, Hunter WN, Michie EA, Van Look PFA: Pituitary-ovarian relationships in polycystic ovary syndrome. *J Clin Endocrinol Metab* 45:798, 1977.
66. Zumoff B, Freeman R, Coupey S, Saenger P, Markowitz N, Krean J: A chronobiologic abnormality in luteinizing hormone secretion in teenage girls with the polycystic-ovary syndrome. *N Engl J Med* 309:1206, 1983.
67. Waldstreicher J, Santoro NF, Hall JE, Filicori M, Crowley WF Jr: Hyperfunction of the hypothalamo-pituitary axis in women with polycystic ovarian disease: Indirect evidence for partial gonadotroph desensitization. *J Clin Endocrinol Metab* 66:165, 1988.
68. Rebar J, Judd HL, Yen SSC: Characterization of the inappropriate gonadotropin secretion in polycystic ovary syndrome. *J Clin Invest* 57:1320, 1976.
69. Futterweit W: Pathologic anatomy of polycystic ovarian disease, in Futterweit W (ed): *Polycystic Ovarian Disease.* New York, Springer-Verlag, 1984, p 41.
70. Quigley ME, Rakoff JS, Yen SSC: Increased luteinizing hormone sensitivity to dopamine inhibition in polycystic ovary syndrome. *J Clin Endocrinol Metab* 52:231, 1981.
71. Barnes RB, Mileikowsky CN, Cha KY, Spencer CA, Lobo RA: Effects of dopamine and metoclopramide in polycystic ovary syndrome. *J Clin Endocrinol Metab* 65:506, 1986.
72. Futterweit W: Pituitary tumors and polycystic ovarian disease. *Obstet Gynecol* 62:74, 1983.
73. Lockwood GM, Muttukrishna S, Groome NP, Matthews DR, Ledger WL: Mid-follicular phase pulses of inhibin B are absent in polycystic ovarian syndrome and are initiated by successful laparoscopic ovarian diathermy: A possible mechanism regulating emergence of the dominant follicle. *J Clin Endocrinol Metab* 83:1730, 1998.
74. Buckler HM, McLachlan RI, MacLachlan VB, Healy DL, Burger HG: Serum inhibin levels in polycystic ovary syndrome: Basal levels and response to luteinizing hormone-releasing hormone agonist and exogenous gonadotrophin administration. *J Clin Endocrinol Metab* 55:798, 1988.
75. Lobo RA: Disturbances of androgen secretion and metabolism in polycystic ovary syndrome. *Clin Obstet Gynecol* 12:633, 1983.
76. Chang RJ, Loufer LR, Meldrum DR, De Fazio J, Lu JKH, Vale WW, Rivier JE, Hudd HL: Steroid suppression in polycystic ovarian disease after ovarian suppression by a long-acting gonadotropin-releasing hormone agonist. *J Clin Endocrinol Metab* 56:897, 1983.
77. Legro RS, Dunaif A: The role of insulin resistance in polycystic ovary syndrome. *The Endocrinologist* 6: 307, 1996.
78. Burghen GA, Givens JR, Kitabashi AE: Correlation of hyperandrogenism with hyperinsulinism in polycystic ovarian disease. *J Clin Endocrinol Metab* 50:113, 1980.
79. Givens JR, Kerber IJ, Wiser WL, Andersen RN, Coleman SA, Fish SA: Remission of acanthosis nigricans associated with polycystic ovarian disease and a stromal luteoma. *J Clin Endocrinol Metab* 38:347, 1974.
80. Dunaif A: Insulin resistance and the polycystic ovary syndrome: Mechanism and implications for pathogenesis. *Endocr Rev* 18:774, 1997.
81. Dunaif A. Xia J, Book C, et al: Excessive insulin receptor serine phosphorylation in cultured fibroblasts and in skeletal muscle: A potential mechanism for insulin resistance in the polycystic ovary syndrome. *J Clin Invest* 96:801, 1995.
82. Wild RA: Obesity, lipids, cardiovascular risk, and androgen excess. *Am J Med* 98:27S, 1995.
83. Talbott E, Juzick D, Clerici A, et al: Coronary heart disease risk factors in women with polycystic ovary syndrome. *Arter Throm Vas Biol* 15:821, 1995.
84. Conway GS, Agarwall R, Betteridge DJ, et al: Risk factors for coronary artery disease in lean and obese women with the polycystic ovary syndrome. *Clin Endocrinol (Oxf)* 37:119, 1992.
85. Wild RA, Bartholomew MJ: The influence on bodyweight on lipoprotein lipids in patients with polycystic ovary syndrome. *Am J Obstet Gynecol* 159:423, 1988.
86. Dahlgren E, Janson PO, Johansson S, et al: Polycystic ovary syndrome and risk for myocardial infarction. *Acta Obstet Gynecol Scand* 71:599, 1992.
87. Birdsall MA, Farquhar CM, White HD: Association between polycystic ovaries and extent of coronary artery disease in women having cardiac catheritization. *Ann Int Med* 126:32, 1997.
88. Guzick DS, Talbot EO, Sutton-Tyrell K, et al: Carotid atherosclerosis in women with polycystic ovary syndrome: Initial results from a case-control study. *Am J Obstet Gynecol* 174:1224, 1996.
89. Legro RS, Finegood D, Dunaif A: A fasting glucose to insulin ratio is a useful measure of insulin sensitivity in women with polycystic ovary syndrome. *J Clin Endocrinol Metab* 83:2694, 1998.
90. Chamlian DL, Taylor HB: Endometrial hyperplasia in young women. *Obstet Gynecol* 36:659, 1970.
91. Jackson RL, Docherty NB: The Stein-Leventhal syndrome: Analysis of 43 cases with special reference to association with endometrial carcinoma. *Am J Obstet Gynecol* 73:161, 1950.
92. Garcia JE, Jones GS, Wentz AC: The use of clomiphene citrate. *Fertil Steril* 28:707, 1977.
93. Kelly AC, Jewelewicz R: Alternate regimens for ovulation induction in polycystic ovarian disease. *Fertil Steril* 54:195, 1990.
94. Spruce BA, Kendall-Taylor P, Dunlop W, Anderson AJ, Watson MJ, Cook DB, Gray C: The effect of bromocriptine in the polycystic ovary syndrome. *Clin Endocrinol* 20:481, 1984.
95. Gadir AA, Mowafi RS, Alnaser HMI, Alrashid AH, Alonezi DM, Shaw RW: Ovarian electrocautery versus human menopausal gonadotrophins and pure follicle stimulating hormone therapy in the treatment of patients with polycystic ovarian disease. *Clin Endocrinol (Oxf)* 33:585, 1990.
96. DeFronzo RA, Barzilai M, Simonson DC: Mechanism of metformin action in obese and lean non-insulin dependent diabetic subjects. *J Clin Endocrinol Metab* 73:1294, 1991.
97. Nestler J, Jakubowics DJ, Evans WS, Pasquali R: Effects of metformin on spontaneous and clomiphene-induced ovulation in the polycystic ovary syndrome. *N Engl J Med* 338:1876, 1998.
98. Velazquez EM, Mendoza S, Hamer T, et al: Metformin therapy in polycystic ovary syndrome reduces hyperinsulinemia, insulin resistance, hyperandrogenemia, and systolic blood pressure, while facilitating normal menses and pregnancy. *Metabolism* 43:647, 1994.
99. Dunaif A, Scott D, Finegood D, et al: The insulin sensitising agent troglitazone: A novel therapy for the polycystic ovary syndrome. *J Clin Endocrinol Metab* 81:3299, 1996.
100. Ferriman D, Gallwey JD: The clinical assessment of body hair growth in women. *J Clin Endocrinol Metab* 21:1440, 1961.
101. Burgess CA, Edwards CRE: Hirsutography. *Br J Photography* 8:770, 1978.
102. Lobo RA, Groebelsmann U, Horton R: Evidence for the importance of peripheral tissue events in the development of hirsutism in polycystic ovary syndrome. *J Clin Endocrinol Metab* 57:393, 1983.
103. Siegel SF, Finegold DN, Lanes R, Lee PA: ACTH stimulation tests and plasma dehydroepiandrosterone sulfate levels in women with hirsutism. *N Engl J Med* 323:849, 1990.
104. Eldar-Geva T, Hurwitz A, Vecsei P, Pulti Z, Milwidsky A, Rusler A: Secondary biosynthetic defects in women with late-onset congenital adrenal hyperplasia. *N Engl J Med* 323:855, 1990.
105. Holdaway IM, Croxson MS, Frengley PA, Ibbertson HK, Sheehan A, Fraser A, Evans MC, Knox B, et al: Clinical and biochemical evaluation of patients with hirsutism. *Aust NZ J Obstet Gynaecol* 24:23, 1984.
106. Chetkowski RJ, DeFazio J, Shamonki I, Judd HL, Chang RJ: The incidence of late-onset congenital adrenal hyperplasia due to 21-hydroxylase deficiency among hirsute women. *J Clin Endocrinol Metab* 58:595, 1984.
107. Ehrmann DA, Rosenfield RL: Hirsutism—beyond the steroidogenic block. *N Engl J Med* 323:909, 1990.

108. Belisl S, Love EJ: Clinical efficacy and safety of cyproterone acetate in severe hirsutism: Results of a multicentered Canadian study. *Fertil Steril* 46:1015, 1986.
109. Shapiro G, Evron S: A novel use of spironolactone: Treatment of hirsutism. *J Clin Endocrinol Metab* 51:429, 1980.
110. Barth JH, Cherry CA, Wojnarowski F, Dawber RP: Spironolactone is an effective and well tolerated systemic antiandrogen therapy for hirsute women. *J Clin Endocrinol Metab* 68:966, 1989.
111. Ciotta L, Cianci A, Marletta E, et al: Treatment of hirsutism with flutamide and a low-dose oral contraceptive in polycystic ovarian disease patients. *Fertil Steril* 62:1129, 1994.
112. Wong IL, Morris RS, Chang L, et al: A prospective randomised trial comparing finasteride to spironolactone in the treatment of hirsute women. *J Clin Endocrinol Metab* 80:233, 1995.
113. Castelo-Branco C, Martinez de Osaba MJ, Pons F, et al: Gonadotropin-releasing hormone analog plus an oral contraceptive containing desogestrel in women with severe hirsutism: Effects on hair, bone, and hormonal profile after 1-year use. *Metabolism* 46:437, 1997.
114. Gemzell CA, Diczfalusy E, Tillinger KG: Clinical effect of human pituitary follicle stimulating hormone (FSH). *J Clin Endocrinol Metab* 18:1333, 1958.
115. Lazarus L: Suspension of the Australian human pituitary programme. *Med J Aust* 43:57, 1985.
116. Healy DL, Kovacs GT, Pepperell RJ, Burger HG: A normal cumulative conception rate with human pituitary gonadotropin. *Fertil Steril* 34:341, 1980.
117. Schenker JG, Polishuk WZ: Ovarian hyperstimulation syndrome. *Obstet Gynecol* 46:23, 1975.
118. Haning RV Jr, Boehalein LM, Carlson IH, Kuzma DL, Zweibel WJ: Diagnosis-specific serum 17β-estradiol upper limits for treatment with menotropins using a ^{125}I direct E_2 assay. *Fertil Steril* 42:882, 1984.
119. Healy DL, Burger HG: Serum follicle-stimulating hormone, luteinizing hormone and prolactin during the induction of ovulation with exogenous gonadotropin. *J Clin Endocrinol Metab* 56:474, 1983.
120. Fleming R, Haxton MJ, Hamilton MPR, McGune GS, Black WP, MacNaughton MC, Coutts JRT: Successful treatment of infertile women with oligomenorrhea using a combination of an LHRH agonist and exogenous gonadotrophins. *Br J Obstet Gynaecol* 92:369, 1985.
121. McFaul FB, Traub AI, Thompson W: Treatment of clomiphene citrate-resistant polycystic ovarian syndrome with pure follicle-stimulating hormone or human menopausal gonadotropin. *Fertil Steril* 53:792, 1990.
122. Fauser BCJM, van Heusden AM: Manipulation of human ovarian function: Physiological concepts and clinical consequences. *Endocr Rev* 18:71, 1997.
123. Leyendecker G, Struve T, Potz EJ: Induction of ovulation with chronic intermittent (pulsatile) administration of LHRH in women with hypothalamic and hyperprolactinaemic amenorrhea. *Arch Gynecol* 229:177, 1980.
124. Filicori M, Campaniello E, Michelacci L, Pareschi A, Ferrari P, Bolelli G, Flamigni C: Gonadotropin-releasing hormone (GnRH) analog suppression renders polycystic ovarian disease patients more susceptible to ovulation induction with pulsatile GnRH. *J Clin Endocrinol Metab* 66:327, 1988.
125. Hurley DM, Brian RJ, Burger HG: Ovulation induction with subcutaneous pulsatile gonadotropin-releasing hormone: Singleton pregnancies in patients with previous multiple pregnancies after gonadotropin therapy. *Fertil Steril* 40:575, 1983.
126. Vollenhoven BJ, Healy DL: Short and long term effects of ovulation induction. *Endocrinol Metab Clin North Am* 27:903, 1998.
127. Noyes RW, Hertig AT, Rock AJ: Dating the endometrial biopsy. *Fertil Steril* 1:3 1950.
128. Hallberg L, Hogdahl IEM, Nilsson L, Rybog T: Menstrual blood loss—a population study. *Acta Obstet Gynecol Scand* 45:320, 1966.
129. Cole SK, Billewicz WZ, Thomson AM: Sources of variation in menstrual blood loss. *J Obstet Gynaecol Br Cwlth* 78:933, 1971.
130. Buller FJ: Observations on the clotting of menstrual blood and clot formation. *Am J Obstet Gynecol* 111:535, 1971.
131. Bonnar J, Shepherd VL, Dockerey CJ: The haemostatic system and dysfunctional uterine bleeding. *Res Clin Forum* 5:277, 1983.
132. Pickles VR, Hall WS, Best FA, Smith GN: Prostaglandins in endometrium and menstrual fluid from normal and dysmenorrhoeic subjects. *J Obstet Gynaecol Br Cwlth* 72:185, 1965.
133. Healy DL: The clinical significance of endometrial prolactin. *Aust NZ J Obstet Gynaecol* 24:111, 1984.
134. Smith SK, Abel MH, Kelly RW, Baird DT: A role for prostacyclin (PGI_2) in excessive menstrual bleeding. *Lancet* i:522, 1981.
135. Speroff L, Glass RH, Kase NG: Dysfunctional uterine bleeding: Clinical Gynecologic Endocrinology and Infertility, 4th Ed. Baltimore, Williams and Wilkins, 1989, pp 265–283.
136. Shaw RW: Assessment of medical treatments for menorrhagia. *Brit J Obstet Gynaecol* 101:15, 1994.
137. Chimbira TH, Anderson ABM, Naisch C, et al: Reduction of menstrual blood loss by danazol in unexpected menorrhagia: Lack of effect of placebo. *Brit J Obstet Gynaecol* 87:1152, 1980.
138. Thomas EJ, Okuda KJ, Thomas NM: The combination of a depot gonadotrophin-releasing hormone agonist and cyclical hormone replacement therapy for dysfunctional uterine bleeding. *Brit J Obstet Gynaecol* 98:1155, 1991.
139. Fraser IS: Prostaglandin inhibitors in gynaecology. *Aust NZ J Obstet Gynaecol* 25:114, 1985.
140. Owen PR: Prostaglandin synthetase inhibitors in the treatment of primary dysmenorrhoea. *Am J Obstet Gynecol* 148:94, 1984.
141. Brooks PG, Serden SP, Davos I: Hormonal inhibition of the endometrium for resectoscopic endometrial ablation. *Am J Obstet Gynecol* 164:1601, 1991.
142. Hill D, Maher P: Treatment of menorrhagia by endometrial ablation. *Med J Aust* 152:564, 1980.
143. O'Connor H, Magos A: Endometrial resection for the treatment of menorrhagia. *N Engl J Med* 335:151, 1996.
144. Steiner M: Premenstrual syndromes. *Annu Rev Med* 48:447, 1997.
145. Mortola JF: Premenstrual syndrome: Pathophysiologic considerations. *N Engl J Med* 338:256, 1998.
146. Rubinoff DR: The premenstrual syndrome. *JAMA* 268:1908, 1992.
147. Bancroft J, Backstrom T: Premenstrual syndrome. *Clin Endocrinol (Oxf)* 22:247, 1985.
148. Wasp JSF, Butt WR, Edwards RL, Holder G: Hormonal studies in women with premenstrual tension. *Br J Obstet Gynaecol* 92:247, 1985.
149. Steege JF, Stout AL, Rupp SL: Relationships among premenstrual symptoms and menstrual cycle characteristics. *Obstet Gynecol* 65:398, 1985.
150. Muse KN, Cetel NS, Futterman LA, Yen SSC: The premenstrual syndrome: Effects of medical ovariectomy. *N Engl J Med* 311:1345, 1984.
151. World Health Organization. Research on the menopause in the 1990s. Report of a WHO Scientific Group, Geneva, 1996.
152. Kaufman DW, Slone D, Rosenberg L, Miettinen OS, Shapiro S: Cigarette smoking and age of natural menopause. *Am J Public Health* 70:420, 1980.
153. Richardson SJ, Senikas V, Nelson JF: Follicular depletion during the menopausal transition: Evidence for accelerated loss and ultimate exhaustion. *J Clin Endocrinol Metab* 65:1231, 1987.
154. MacNaughton JA, Bangah M, McCloud PI, Hee J, Burger HG: Age related changes in follicle-stimulating hormone luteinising hormone, oestradiol and immunoreactive inhibin in women of reproductive age. *Clin Endocrinol (Oxf)*, 1992, (in press).
155. Klein NA, Illingworth PJ, Groome NP, McNeilly AS, Battaglia DE, Soules, MR: Decreased Inhibin B secretion is associated with the monotrophic rise in older, ovulatory women:A study of serum and follicular fluid levels of dimeric Inhibin A and B in spontaneous menstrual cycles. *J Clin Endocrinol Metab* 81: 2742, 1996.
156. Lee SJ, Lenton EA, Sexton L and Cooke ID: The effect of age on the cyclical patterns of plasma LH, FSH, oestradiol and progesterone in women with regular menstrual cycles. *Hum Reprod* 3:851, 1988.
157. Metcalf MG, Donald RA, Livesey JH: Pituitary-ovarian function in normal women during the menopausal transition. *Clin Endocrinol (Oxf)* 14:245, 1981.
158. Burger HG, Cahir N, Robertson DM, Groome NO, Dudley E, Green A and Dennerstein L: Serum inhibins A and B fall differentially as FSH rises in perimenopausal women. *Clin Endocrinol* 48:809, 1998.
159. Burger HG, Dudley EC, Hopper JL: The endocrinology of the menopausal transition: a cross-sectional study of a population-based sample. *J Clin Endocrinol Metab* 80:3537, 1995.
160. Zumoff B, Strain GW, Miller LK, Rosner W: Twenty-four hour mean plasma testosterone concentration declines with age in normal premenopausal women. *J Clin Endocrinol Metab* 80:1429, 1995.

161. Burger HG: Diagnostic role of follicle-stimulating hormone (FSH) measurements during the menopausal transition—an analysis of FSH, oestradiol and inhibin. *Eur J Endocrinol* 130:38, 1994.
162. Gray RH: Biological and social interactions in the determination of late fertility. *J Biosoc Sci [Suppl]* 6:97, 1979.
163. Prior JC: Perimenopause: The complex endocrinology of the menopausal transition. *Endocr Rev* 19:397, 1998.
164. Jaszmann L, van Lith ND, Zaat JCA: The perimenopausal symptoms. *Med Gynaecol Sociol* 4:268, 1969.
165. Tataryn IV, Lomax P, Bajorek JG, Chesarek W, Meldrum DR, Judd HL: Postmenopausal hot flushes: A disorder of thermoregulation. *Maturitas* 2:101, 1980.
166. Sturdee DW, Wilson KA, Pipili E, Crocker AD: Physiological aspects of menopausal hot flush. *Br Med J* 2:79, 1979.
167. Casper RF, Yen SSC, Wilkes MM: Menopausal flushes: A neuroendocrine link with pulsatile luteinizing hormone secretion. *Science* 205:823, 1979.
168. Chetkowski RJ, Meldrum DR, Steingold KA, Randle D, Lu JK, Eggena P, Hershman JM, Alkjaersig NK, et al: Biological effects of transdermal estradiol. *N Engl J Med* 314:1615, 1986.
169. Meldrum DR, Shamonki IM, Tataryn I, et al: Elevations in skin temperature of the finger as an objective index of postmenopausal hot flushes: Standardization of the technique. *Am J Obstet Gynecol* 135:713, 1979.
170. Dennerstein L, Burrows GD, Hyman GJ, Sharpe K: Hormone therapy and affect. *Maturitas* 1:247, 1979.
171. Hallstrom T: *Mental Disorder and Sexuality in the Climacteric*. Stockholm, Scandinavian University Books, Esselte Studium, 1973.
172. Youngs DD: Some misconceptions concerning the menopause. *Obstet Gynecol* 75:881, 1990.
173. Hasselquist MB, Goldberg N, Schroeter A, Spelsberg TC: Isolation and characterization of the estrogen receptors in human skin. *J Clin Endocrinol Metab* 50:76, 1980.
174. Brincat M, Wong Ten Yuen A, Studd JWW, Montgomery J, Magos AL, Savvas M: Response of skin thickness and metacarpal index to estradiol therapy in postmenopausal women. *Obstet Gynecol* 70:538, 1987.
175. Conference Sponsors: The Hormone Foundation, The Susan G. Komen Breast Cancer Foundation, the Canadian Breast Cancer Research Initiative, the National Cancer Institute of Canada, The Endocrine Society, and the University of Virginia Cancer Center and Woman's place. Treatment of oestrogen deficiency symptoms in women surviving breast cancer. *J Clin Endocrinol Metab* 83:1993, 1998.
176. Vassilopoulou-Sellin R, Theriault R, Klein MJ: Oestrogen replacement therapy in women with prior diagnosis and treatment for breast cancer. *Gynecol Oncol* 65:89, 1997.
177. O'Donohue J, Williams R: Hormone replacement therapy in women with liver disease. *Br J Obstet Gynaecol* 104:1, 1977.
178. Doiuketis JD, Ginsberg JS, Holbrook A, et al: A reevaluation of the risk for venous thromboembolism with the use of oral contraceptives and hormone replacement therapy. *Arch Intern Med* 157:1522, 1997.
179. Burger HG, Hailes J, Menelaus M, Nelson J, Hudson B, Balazs N: The management of persistent symptoms with oestradiol/testosterone implants: Clinical, lipid and hormonal results. *Maturitas* 6:351, 1984.
180. Burger HG, Hailes J, Nelson J, Menelaus M: Effect of combined implants of oestradiol and testosterone on libido in postmenopausal women. *Brit Med J* 294:936, 1987.
181. Conference Report: Consensus Development Conference: Prophylaxis and treatment of osteoporosis. *Am J Med* 90:107, 1991.
182. Eriksen EF, Colvard DS, Berg NJ, Graham ML, Mann KG, Spelsberg TC, Riggs BL: Evidence of estrogen receptors in normal human osteoblast-like cells. *Science* 241:84, 1988.
183. Heaney RP, et al: Calcium balance and calcium requirements in middle-aged women. *Am J Clin Nutr* 30:1603, 1977.
184. Stevenson JC, Whitehead MI, Padwick M, Endacott JA, Sutton C, Banks LM, Freemantle C, Spinks TJ, Hesp R: Dietary intake of calcium and postmenopausal bone loss. *Br Med J* 297:15, 1988.
185. Crilly RG, Francis RM, Nordin BEC: Steroid hormones, ageing and bone. *Clin Endocrinol Metab* 10:115, 1981.
186. Henry D, Robertson J, O'Connell D, Gillespie W: A systematic review of the skeletal effects of oestrogen therapy in postmenopausal women I. An assessment of the quality of randomised trials published between 1977 and 1995. *Climacteric* 1:92, 1998.
187. O'Connell D, Robertson J, Henry D, Gillespie W: A systematic review of the skeletal effects of oestrogen therapy in postmenopausal women II. An assessment of treatment effects. *Climacteric* 1:112, 1998.
188. Dawson-Hughes B, Harris SS, Krall EA, Dallal GE: Effect of calcium and vitamin D supplementation on bone density in men and women 65 years of age or older. *N Engl J Med* 337:670, 1997.
189. Lindsay R, Tohme JF: Estrogen treatment of patients with established postmenopausal osteoporosis. *Obstet Gynecol* 76:290, 1990.
190. Munk-Jensen N, Nielsen SP, Obel EB, Eriksen PB: Reversal of postmenopausal vertebral bone loss by oestrogen and progestogen: A double blind placebo controlled study. *Br Med J* 296:1150, 1988.
191. Christiansen C, Riis BJ: 17β-Estradiol and continuous norethisterone: A unique treatment for established osteoporosis in elderly women. *J Clin Endocrinol Metab* 71:836, 1990.
192. Storm T, Thamsborg G, Steiniche T, Genant HK, Sorensen OH: Effect of intermittent cyclical etidronate therapy on bone mass and fracture rate in women with postmenopausal osteoporosis. *N Engl J Med* 322:1265, 1990.
193 Liberman UA, Weiss SR, Broll J, et al. Effect of oral alendronate on bone mineral density and the incidence of fractures in postmenopausal osteoporosis. The Alendronate Phase III Osteoporosis Treatment Study Group. *N Engl J Med* 30:1437, 1995.
194. Civitelli R, Gonnelli S, Zacchei F, Bigazzi S, Vattimo A, Avioli LV, Gennari C: Bone turnover in postmenopausal osteoporosis: Effect of calcitonin treatment. *J Clin Invest* 82:1268, 1988.
195. Riggs BL, Hodgson SF, O'Fallon WM, Chao EYS, Wahner HW, Muhs JM, Cedel SL, Melton LJ: Effect of fluoride treatment on the fracture rate in postmenopausal women with osteoporosis. *N Engl J Med* 322:802, 1990.
196. Bengtsson C, Lindquist O: Menopausal effects on risk factors for ischaemic heart disease. *Maturitas* 1:165, 1979.
197. Hjortland MC, McNamara PM, Kannel WB: Some atherogenic concomitants of menopause: The Framingham study. *Am J Epidemiol* 103:304, 1976.
198. Shibata H, Matsuzaki T, Hapana S: Relationship of relevant factors of atherosclerosis to menopause in Japanese women. *Am J Epidemiol* 109:420, 1979.
199. Bengtsson C: Ischemic heart disease in women. *Acta Med Scand [Suppl]* 549:75, 1973.
200. Gordon T, Kannell WB, Hjortland MC, McNamara PM: Menopause and coronary heart disease. The Framingham study. *Ann Intern Med* 89:157, 1978.
201. Rosenberg L, Hennekens CH, Rosner B, Belanger C, Rothman KJ, Speizer FE: Early menopause and the risk of myocardial infarction. *Am J Obstet Gynecol* 139:47, 1981.
202. Heller RF, Jacobs RS: Coronary heart disease in relation to age, sex and the menopause. *Br Med Journal* 1:472, 1978.
203. Tunstall-Pedoe H: Myth and paradox of coronary risk and the menopause. *Lancet* 351:1425, 1998.
204. Gustafson A, Svanborg A: Gonadal steroid effects on plasma lipoprotein and individual phospholipids. *J Clin Endocrinol Metab* 35:203, 1972.
205. Wallentin L, Larsson-Cohn V: Metabolic and hormonal effects of post-menopausal estrogen replacement: II. Plasma lipids. *Acta Endocrinol (Copenh)* 86:579, 1977.
206. Hirvonen E, Malkonen M, Manninen V: Effects of different progestogens on lipoproteins during postmenopausal replacement therapy. *N Engl J Med* 304:560, 1981.
207. Hunt K, Vessey M, McPherson K: Mortality in a cohort of long-term users of hormone replacement therapy: An updated analysis. *Br J Obstet Gynaecol* 97:1080, 1990.
208. Von Kaulla E, Droegemuller W, Von Kaulla KN: Conjugated estrogens in hypercoagulability. *Am J Obstet Gynecol* 122:688, 1975.
209. Bonnar J, Haddon M, Hunter DH, Richards D, Thornton C: Coagulation system changes in postmenopausal women receiving oestrogen preparations. *Postgrad Med J* 52(Suppl 6):30, 1976.
210. Elkik F: Potency and hepato-cellular effects of oestrogens after oral, percutaneous, and subcutaneous administration, in van Keep PA, Utian WH, Vermeulen A (eds): *The Controversial Climacteric, Workshop 12*. Lancaster, England, MTP, 1982.
211. Sitruk-Ware R, dePalacios I: Oestrogen replacement therapy and cardiovascular disease in post-menopausal women: A review. *Maturitas* 11:259, 1989.

212. Ross RK, Paganinni-Hill A, Mack TM, Arthur M, Henderson BE: Menopausal estrogen therapy and protection from ischaemic heart disease death. *Lancet* i:858, 1981.
213. Bush TL, Cowan LD, Barrett-Connor E, Criqui MH, Karon JM, Wallace RB, Al Tyroler H, Rifkind BM: Estrogen use and all-cause mortality. *JAMA* 249:903, 1983.
214. Bush TL, Barrett-Connor E, Cowan LD, Criqui MH, Wallace RB, Suchindran CM, Tyroler HA, Rifkind BM: Cardiovascular mortality and noncontraceptive use of estrogen in women. *Circulation* 75:1102, 1987.
215. Henderson BE, Paganini-Hill A, Ross RK: Decreased mortality in users of estrogen replacement therapy. *Arch Intern Med* 151:75, 1991.
216. Grady D, Rubin SM, Petitti DB, et al: Hormone therapy to prevent disease and prolong life in postmenopausal women. *Ann Intern Med* 117:1016, 1992.
217. Grodstein F, Stampfer M: The epidemiology of coronary heart disease and estrogen replacement in postmenopausal women. *Progress in Cardiovascular Disease* 38:199, 1995.
218. Falkeborn M, Persson I, Adami H, et al: The risk of acute myocardial infarction after oestrogen and oestrogen-progestogen replacement. *Br J Obstet Gynaecol* 99:821, 1992.
219. Psaty BM, Heckbert SR, Atkins D, et al: The risk of myocardial infarction associated with the combined use of oestrogens and progestins in postmenopausal women. *Arch Intern Med* 154:1333, 1994.
220. Grodstein F, Stampfer MJ, Manson JE, et al: Postmenopausal oestrogen and progestin use and the risk of cardiovascular disease. *N Engl J Med* 335:453, 1996.
221. Adams MR, Register T, Golden D, Wagner J, Williams K: Medroxyprogesterone acetate antagonises inhibitory effects of conjugated equine oestrogens on coronary artery atherosclerosis. *Arterioscler Thromb Vasc Biol* 17:217, 1997.
222. Adams MR, Kaplan JR, Manuck SB, et al: Inhibition of coronary artery atherosclerosis by 17β oestradiol in ovariectomized monkeys. Lack of an effect of added progesterone. *Arteriosclerosis* 10:1051, 1990.
223. Hulley S, et al: Randomized trial of oestrogen plus progestin for secondary prevention of coronary heart disease in postmenopausal women. Heart and Oestrogen/Progestin Replacement Study (HERS) Research Group. *JAMA* 280:605, 1998.
224. Gerhard M, Ganz P: How do we explain the clinical benefits of estrogen? From bedside to bench. *Circulation* 92:5, 1995.
224a. Mendelsohn ME, Karas RH: The protective effects of estrogen on the cardiovascular system. *N Eng J Med* 340:1801, 1999.
225. Mashchak CA, Lobo RA, Dozono-Takano R, Eggena P, Nakamura RM, Brenner PF, Mishell DR: Comparison of pharmacodynamic properties of various estrogen formulations. *Am J Obstet Gynecol* 144:511, 1982.
226. Schiff I, Seta HK, Cramer D, Tulchinsky D, Ryan KJ: Endometrial hyperplasia in women on cyclic or continuous estrogen regimen. *Fertil Steril* 37:79, 1982.
227. Mandel FP, Geola FL, Lu JKH, Eggena P, Sambhi MP, Hershman JM, Judd HL: Biological effects of various doses of ethinyl estradiol in postmenopausal women. *Obstet Gynecol* 59:673, 1982.
228. Steingold KA, Laufer L, Chetkowski RJ, de Fazio JD, Watt DW, Meldrum DR, Judd HL: Treatment of hot flushes with transdermal estradiol administration. *J Clin Endocrinol Metab* 61:627, 1985.
229. Yen SSC, Martin PL, Burnier AM, Czekala NM, Greaney MD Jr., Callantine MR: Circulating estradiol, estrone and gonadotropin levels following the administration of orally active 17-beta-estradiol in postmenopausal women. *J Clin Endocrinol Metab* 40:518, 1975.
230. Englund DE, Johansson EDB: Pharmacokinetic and pharmacodynamic studies on estradiol valerianate administered orally to postmenopausal women. *Acta Obstet Gynecol Scand* [*Suppl*] 65:27, 1977.
231. Sturdee DW, Wade-Evans T, Paterson MEL, Thom M, Studd JWW: Relations between bleeding pattern, endometrial histology, and oestrogen treatment in menopausal women. *Br Med J* 1:575, 1978.
232. Whitehead MI, Hillard TC, Crook D: The role and use of progestogens. *Obstet Gynecol* 75:595, 1990.
233. Beresford SAA, Weiss NS, Voigt LF, McKnight B: Risk of endometrial cancer in relation to use of estrogen combined with cyclic progestagen therapy in postmenopausal women. *Lancet* 349:458, 1997.
234. Hovik P, Sundsbak HP, Gaasemyr M, Sandvik L: Comparison of continuous and sequential oestrogen-progestogen treatment in women with climacteric symptoms. *Maturitas* 11:75, 1989.
235. Udoff L, Langenberg P, Adashi EY: Combined continuous hormone replacement therapy: A critical review. *Obstet Gynecol* 86:306, 1995.
236. Editorial: Consensus statement on progestin use in postmenopausal women. *Maturitas* 11:175, 1988.
237. Yaffe K, Sawaya G, Lieberburg I, Grady D: Estrogen therapy in postmenopausal women: Effects on cognitive function and dementia. *JAMA* 4:688, 1988.
238. Kearney CE, Purdie DW: Selective estrogen receptor modulators. *Climacteric* 1:143, 1998.
239. Gambrell RD Jr: The prevention of endometrial cancer in postmenopausal women with progestogens. *Maturitas* 1:107, 1978.
240. Hulka BS: When is the evidence for "no association" sufficient? *JAMA* 252:81, 1984.
241. Dupont WD, Page DL: Menopausal estrogen replacement therapy and breast cancer. *Arch Intern Med* 151:67, 1991.
242. Collaborative Group on Hormonal Factors in Breast Cancer. Breast Cancer and Hormone Replacement Therapy: Collaborative reanalysis of data from 51 epidemiological studies of 52,705 women with breast cancer and 108,411 women without breast cancer. *Lancet* 350:1047, 1997.
243. Keirse MJNC: Aetiology of postmenopausal bleeding. *Postgrad Med J* 49:344, 1973.
244. Kahler VL, Creasy RK, Morris JA: Value of the endometrial biopsy. *Obstet Gynecol* 34:91, 1969.
245. Kovacs G, Burger HG, Hailes J, Medley G: A new method of endometrial sampling—the Gynoscann: A comparison with Vabra curettage. *Med J Aust* 148:498, 1988.
246. Kovacs GT, Burger HG: Endometrial sampling for women on perimenopausal hormone replacement therapy. *Maturitas* 10:259, 1988.
247. Gambrell RD, Greenblatt RV: Management of dysfunctional uterine bleeding with norgestrel-ethinyl estradiol. *Curr Med Dialogue* 42:80, 1975.
248. Smith-Bindman R, Kerlikowske K, Feldstein VA, et al: Endovaginal ultrasound to exclude endometrial cancer and other endometrial abnormalities. *JAMA* 280:1510, 1998.
249. Carlson KJ: Vaginal ultrasonography to evaluate post-menopausal bleeding. *JAMA* 280:1529, 1998.
250. Fleischer AC: Optimizing the accuracy of transvaginal ultrasonography of the endometrium. *N Engl J Med* 337:1839, 1997.
251. Shearman RP: Oral contraceptive agents. *Med J Aust* 144:180, 1986.
252. Mishell DR: Contraception. *New Engl J Med* 320:777, 1989.
253. Healy DL, Fraser HM: The antiprogesterones are coming: Menses induction, abortion, labour? *Br Med J* 290:580, 1985.
254. Collaborative Group on Hormonal Factors in Breast Cancer. Breast cancer and hormonal contraceptives: Collaborative reanalysis of individual data on 53,297 women with breast cancer and 100,239 women without breast cancer from 54 epidemiological studies. *Lancet* 347:1713, 1996.
255. Schlesselman JJ: Net effect of oral contraceptive use on the risk of cancer in women in the United States. *Obstet Gynecol* 85:793, 1995.
256. Kaunitz PD, Mishell DR: Progestin only contraceptives: Current perspectives and future direction. *Dialog Contracep* 4: 1, 1994.
257. Elstein M (ed): A New Specific Progestogen for Low Dose Oral Contraception. Parkridge, New Jersey: Parthenon Publishing Group, 1989.
258. Bloemenkamp KWM, Rosendaal FR, Helmerhorst FM, Buller HR, Vandenbroucke JP: Enhancement by factor V Leiden mutation of risk of deep-vein thrombosis associated with oral contraceptives containing a third-generation progestogen. *Lancet* 346:1593 1995.
259. Jick H, Jick SS, Gurewich V, Myers MW, Vasilakis: Risk of idiopathic cardiovascylar death and nonfatal venous thromboembolism in women using oral contraceptives with differing progestogen components. *Lancet* 346:1589, 1995.
260. WHO Collaborative Study of Cardiovascular Disease and Steroid Hormone Contraception. Effect of different progestogens in low oestrogen oral contraceptives on venous thromboembolic disease. *Lancet* 346:1582, 1995.
261. Spitzer WO, Lewis MA, Heinemann LAJ, Thorogood M, Macrae KD: Third-generation oral contraceptives and risk of venous thromboembolic disorders: An international case-control study. *Br Med J* 312:83, 1996.
262. Farmer RDT, Lawrenson RA, Thompson CR, et al: Population-based study of risk of venous thromboembolism associated with various oral contraceptives. *Lancet* 349:83, 1997.

263. Vandenbroucke JP, Rosendaal FR: End of the line for 'third-generation-pill' controversy. *Lancet* 349:1113, 1997.
264. Winkler UH: Effects on hemostatic variables of desogestrel- and gestodene-containing oral contraceptives in comparison with levonorgestrel-containing oral contraceptives: A review. *Am J Obstet Gynecol* 179:S51, 1998.
265. Baulieu EE, Segal S: *The Antiprogestin-Steroid RU486 and Human Fertility Control*. New York, Plenum, 1985.
266. Healy DL, Baulieu EE, Hodgen GD: Induction of menstruation by an antiprogesterone steroid (Mifepristone) in primates: Site of action, dose response relationships and hormonal effects. *Fertil Steril* 40:253, 1983.
267. Kelly RW, Healy DL, Cameron IJ, Cameron IT, Baird DT: The stimulation of prostaglandin production by two antiprogesterone steroids in human endometrial cells. *J Clin Endocrinol Metab* 62:1116, 1986.
268. Ulmann A: Use of RU486 for contragestion: An update. *Contraception* 36(suppl.): 27, 1987.

CHAPTER 17

Sexual Differentiation

Robert M. Couch
Jeremy S. D. Winter

Attempts to explain sexual dimorphism are as old as humankind itself, and countless theories have been promulgated to provide a rational basis for separate patterns of male and female development. Aristotle, with remarkable prescience, suggested that semen determines embryonic sex through its innate ability to impose maleness upon a process which otherwise tends to be female; the role of the female parent was seen to be essentially passive, providing the material and the environment for embryonic development. Two thousand years later light microscopy led to the description of spermatozoa, ova, and the events of fertilization. It was probably Mendel who first perceived that sex might be a genetic character, obeying the laws of inheritance, but, like many of his ideas, the notion remained buried until this century. In 1924, Painter provided direct evidence for the role of the male parent in human sex determination when he showed that human primary spermatocytes contain an unequal pair of chromosomes, termed X and Y, which segregate into different gametes during the first meiotic division,[1] a finding that has since been confirmed by modern techniques of chromosome analysis.

Sexual reproduction requires each parent to contribute equal (*haploid*) amounts of genetic material to the offspring, a mechanism that provides for rapid gene assortment with an increased opportunity for favorable combinations of genes to develop and be selected in a changing environment. In higher organisms the parents are of different sexes, maintained separate and distinct by the actions of unpaired sex chromosomes that contain the genetic information for sex determination. One sex (in mammals XX, or female) is homogametic while the other (XY, or male) is heterogametic. The Y chromosome contains important male-determining factors that direct the embryo away from an otherwise predetermined course of female differentiation. Fisher has pointed out that it is not necessary for all male characters to be under the control of genes on the Y chromosome.[2] Rather, a single Y-linked gene need only cause male differentiation of the gonad; in turn, testicular hormones can activate or repress genes throughout the autosomal complement, a strategy which would allow any gene to become involved in producing sexual dimorphism.

The past quarter century has seen a flood of new information and new insights into both the initial genetic process of sex determination and the endocrine mechanisms that subsequently direct sexual differentiation; indeed, it is probable that no aspect of prenatal development is better understood. Vital clues about these events have been provided by patients with various anatomic abnormalities of sexual differentiation. It is therefore fitting that these insights have led to the development of rapid and exact techniques for diagnosis and specific forms of therapy which, if applied early and properly, can prevent much of the physical and psychological scarring which previously was the lot of these patients.

NORMAL SEX DETERMINATION AND SEXUAL DIFFERENTIATION

The appearance of a fertile adult with congruent secondary sexual characteristics and psychosexual orientation represents the denouement of a logical and ordered sequence which begins at conception with the establishment of *genetic sex*. In turn, the presence or absence of the male-determining portion of the Y chromosome defines *gonadal sex*, causing the indifferent embryonic gonad to become either a testis or an ovary. Subsequent differentiation of the internal genital ducts and the external genitalia follows a similar paradigm in which indifferent common primordia show an innate tendency to feminize unless male patterns of development are imposed by secretions from the fetal testis. At birth the external genitalia provide the basis by which society assigns both gender role and legal sex. Later, during and after puberty, testicular or ovarian hormones induce secondary sexual characteristics, which serve both to reinforce psychosexual identity and to signal adult reproductive capabilities. The six parameters of sexual dimorphism listed in Table 17-1 define the sum of what is meant by the terms *male* and *female*. In clinical situations of disordered sexual differentiation, the physician must be aware that complete diagnosis requires a definitive statement concerning each of these aspects of sexual development. In the absence of such information, the initiation of therapy, or even the assignment of sex of rearing, carries grave risk of a later psychosexual disaster.

Genetic Sex

In some fish and amphibians complete sex reversal can be caused by environmental influences such as hormones, but in mammals sex is solely and decisively determined by chromosomal mechanisms. All physicians are now familiar with the systematized array of metaphase chromosomes known as a *karyotype* (Fig. 17-1). The 22 pairs of autosomes and the unpaired (X and Y) sex chromosomes can each be characterized according to size, centromeric position, and a distinctive pattern of banding. Various techniques are used to demonstrate these bands, including fluorescent staining with quinacrine (Q banding) and several methods of Giemsa staining (G, C, or R banding). The chemical basis for specific

TABLE 17-1. Parameters of Sexual Dimorphism

	Determining Factors		
	Female Development	**Male Development**	**Identified By**
Genetic sex	Homogametic (XX)	Heterogametic (XY)	Karyotype
Gonadal sex	Oocytes	Y-linked testis-determining factor (TDF)	Histology
Genital ducts	Innate tendency	Müllerian inhibiting substance; testosterone	Ultrasound
External genitalia	Innate tendency	Dihydrotestosterone	Examination
Gender role	Psychosocial factors	Psychosocial factors	Observation
Puberty	Estradiol	Testosterone	Hormone assay

bands is not entirely clear, but the bands appear to reflect not only variations in DNA base composition but also the nature and quantity of associated histone and nonhistone proteins. *An International System for Human Cytogenetic Nomenclature*, first developed in 1960 and revised at intervals, provides a standard method for the description of the regions and bands of both normal and structurally altered chromosomes.[3]

Chromosomal Errors

Chromosomal abnormalities include both deviations from the normal number (*aneuploidy*) and various structural changes in individual chromosomes.

Aneuploidy

During cell division a chromosome may be lost; this circumstance, known as *anaphase lag*, is more likely to occur if the chromosome is structurally abnormal. A more common mechanism for losing a chromosome (*monosomy*) or gaining extra chromosomes (*trisomy* or *polysomy*) is primary nondisjunction; in this case a pair of sister chromatids (during mitosis) or homologous chromosomes (during meiosis) fails to separate at metaphase, so that one daughter cell receives both members of the pair while the complementary cell receives none. If nondisjunction occurs during meiotic division, aneuploid gametes will ensue and the resulting embryo will contain a single aneuploid cell line. Nondisjunction occurring after fertilization during an early mitotic division will produce an individual with two or more cell lines. Such mosaicism, particularly for the sex chromosomes, is not uncommon and can be ruled out only by means of karyotype analysis of relatively large numbers of cells from a variety of tissues. *Mosaicism*, in which the different cell lines have the same genetic origin, must be differentiated from the much less common situation of *chimerism*, in which double fertilization of a binucleate ovum or fusion of two zygotes leads to a single embryo having two cell lines of different genetic origin (e.g., 46,XY/46,XX).

Structural Anomalies

Aberrations of chromosome structure arise through breakage, often followed by improper reunion of the fragments; these occurrences can lead to phenotypic abnormalities through a deficiency or duplication of genetic information or through a position effect. A simple *deletion* involves the loss of a portion of the short arm, designated *p* [e.g., 46,X,del(X)(p21), indicating deletion of the short arm of X distal to band Xp21], or of the long arm, designated *q*. *Ring chromosomes* occur after breaks in both the short and long arms, the ends of which then fuse, with loss of the acentric fragments [e.g., 46,X,r(X)]. *Duplications* may involve a portion of a single chromosome or *translocation*, in which genetic material is transferred from one chromosome to another. In translocation, although both chromosomes are structurally abnormal, the translocation may be balanced; however, an offspring receiving one of the translocation chromosomes without the other will be genetically unbalanced and presumably phenotypically abnormal. *Isochromosomes* result from the loss of an entire arm with replication of the remaining one, so that the chromosome comes to have either two identical long arms [e.g., 46,X,iso(Xq)] or two short arms.

The frequency of chromosome abnormalities at conception has been estimated to be between 10 and 50 percent,[4] but most of these abnormalities terminate in early spontaneous abortion. Studies of human spermatozoa show abnormal chromosome complements in about 9 percent (range 0–28 percent in different donors), with aneuploidy and structural anomalies affecting every chromosome.[5] It is of interest that X-bearing sperm normally outnumber Y-bearing sperm by a ratio of 54:46, suggesting selective loss of the latter during gametogenesis. The incidence of significant abnormality involving the sex chromosomes is probably about 17 per 1,000 conceptions[6]; most of these abnormalities, particularly those with a 45,X karyotype, lead to early abortion. Surveys of unselected liveborn infants indicate that sex chromosome abnormalities (mainly 47,XYY, 47,XXY, and 47,XXX) occur in 0.3 percent of males and 0.15 percent of females. The low incidence of 45,X newborns (about 0.01 percent) is in sharp contrast to the high frequency of this karyotype in spontaneous abortions.

The frequency of chromosome abnormalities in adult patients is naturally biased by preselection for reproductive disorders. For example, approximately 25 percent of young women with primary amenorrhea and 4 percent with secondary amenorrhea show an abnormal karyotype, usually 45,X or one of its variants.[7] About 10 percent of males with azoospermia show an abnormality. Similarly, one may expect to find a chromosomal abnormality such as reciprocal autosomal translocation or mosaicism for X chromosome aneuploidy in about 10 percent of couples with a history of recurrent abortion.[8]

The techniques of modern molecular biology, in particular the increasing availability of specific DNA probes for the sex chromosomes and for autosomal loci that regulate pituitary or gonadal hormone production, sex steroid action, and gametogenesis, have made possible the elucidation of point mutations and other minor genetic variants that may underlie reproductive dysfunction.

Properties and Functions of the Sex Chromosomes

It is probable that the X and Y chromosomes evolved from an ancestral pair of autosomes through translocation of sex-specific genes plus a mechanism to discourage crossing-over or gene exchange between the sex chromosomes during meiosis.

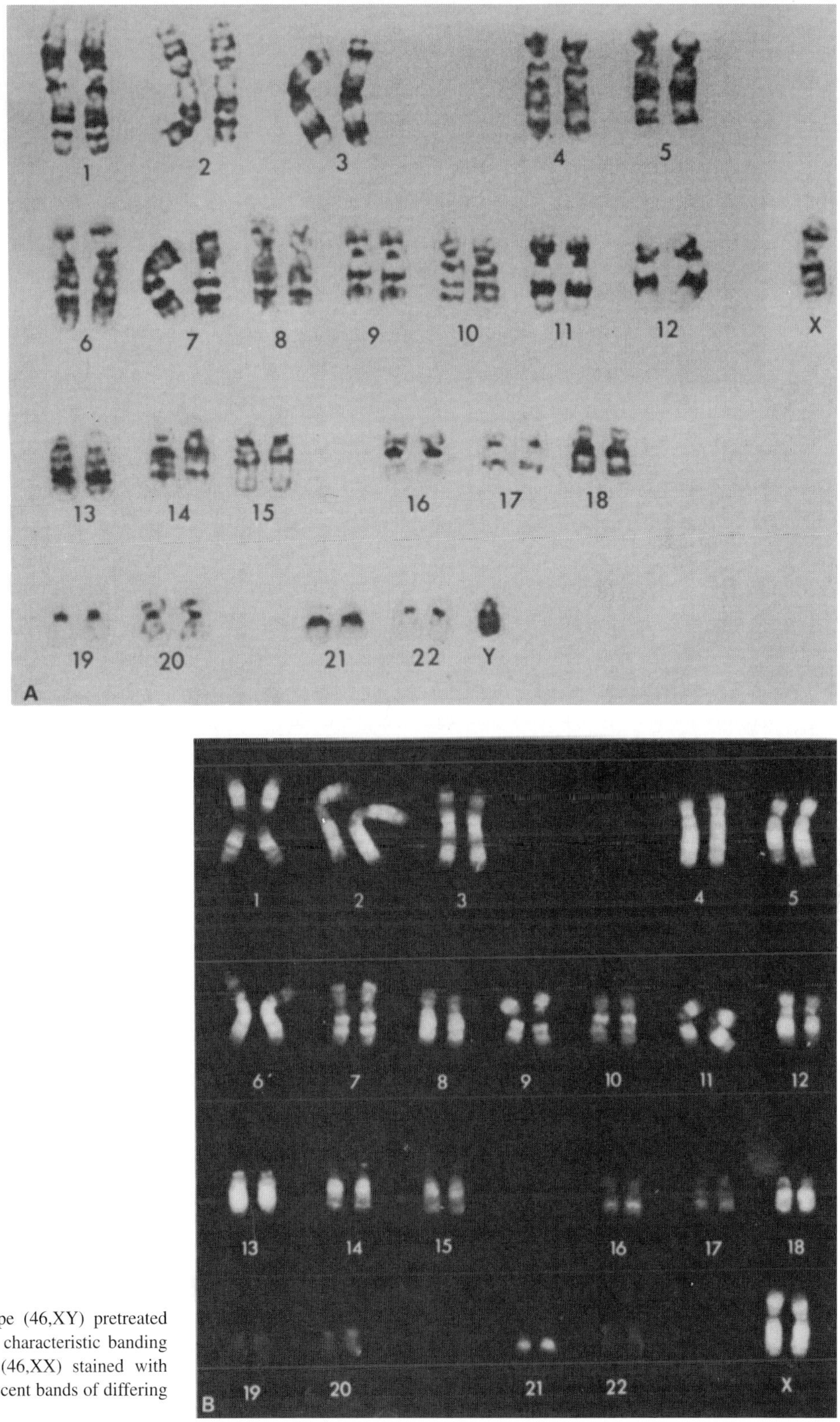

FIGURE 17-1. (*A*) Normal male karyotype (46,XY) pretreated with trypsin and Giemsa-stained to show characteristic banding patterns. (*B*) Normal female karyotype (46,XX) stained with quinacrine dihydrochloride to show fluorescent bands of differing intensity.

The Y Chromosome

The Y chromosome is the most specialized mammalian chromosome, being almost exclusively involved in the control of sex determination and fertility. By conventional cytogenetic methods, it contains a euchromatic portion that includes the entire short arm and the proximal long arm and a quinacrine-positive heterochromatic portion that includes the rest of the long arm and the centromeric region. In quinacrine-stained interphase cells this heterochromatic portion shows up as the fluorescent Y body, which usually is adjacent to the nuclear membrane (Fig. 17-2*A*) and

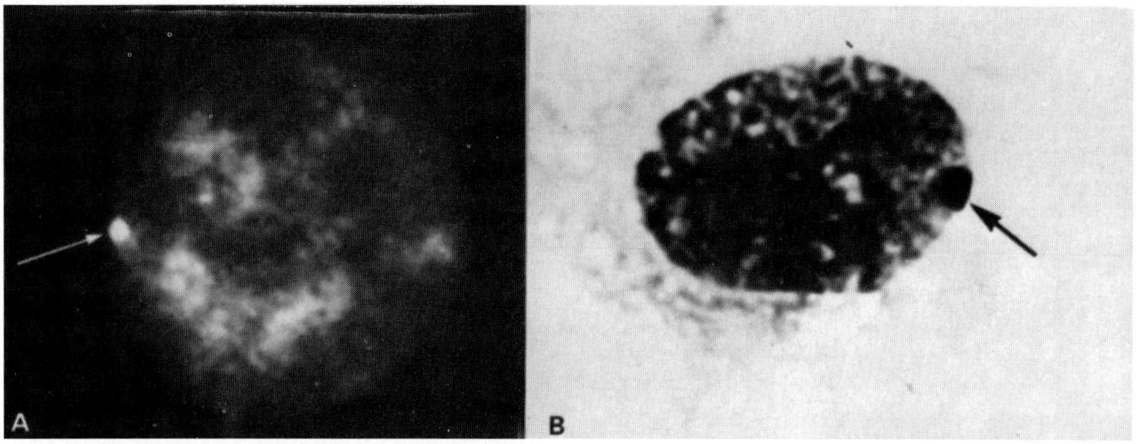

FIGURE 17-2. (*A*) A fluorescent Y chromatin mass (arrow) in an interphase nucleus, indicating the presence of the long arm of the Y chromosome. (*B*) An X chromatin mass in an interphase nucleus. In diploid lines, the number of X chromatin bodies equals the number of X chromosomes minus one.

which provides evidence of the number of Y chromosomes present. The occasional absence of the entire quinacrine-positive region in normal fertile males suggests that this region does not contain functional genes, being composed mainly of tandem DNA repeats.[9]

During male meiosis X/Y genetic exchange normally occurs only within the so-called pseudoautosomal regions at the distal end of both the short and long arms (Fig. 17-3). These regions on the Y are essentially identical to those on the X and the genes encoded on both chromosomes escape inactivation. Several genes have been mapped to the pseudoautosomal regions[10] including one, SHOX (short stature homeobox-containing gene), which is implicated in the short stature of Turner's syndrome.[11]

FIGURE 17-3. Mapping of genes involved in sexual differentiation on the Y chromosome (*top*) and the X chromosome (*bottom*).

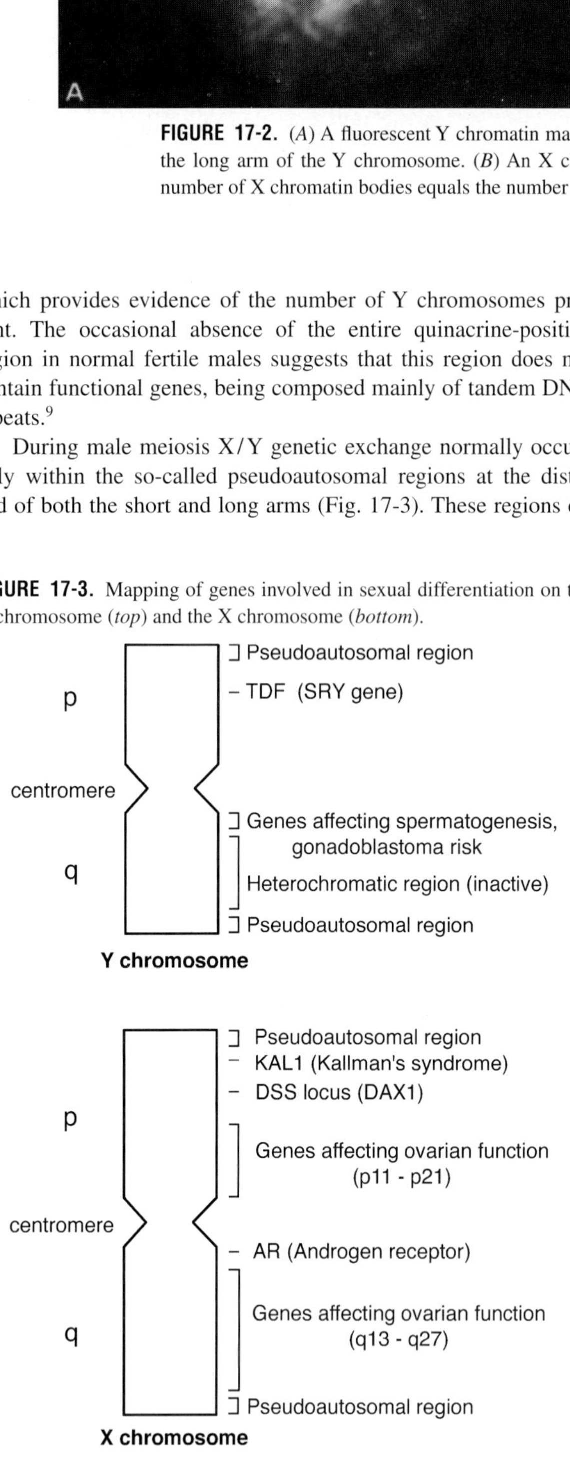

Immediately adjacent to the pseudoautosomal region on the short arm of the Y is the gene for the testis determining factor, SRY (sex-determining region Y). The evidence that this gene is TDF comes from studies of 46,XX males and 46,XY females,[12] and from XX mice in which transgenic SRY induced testis development and sex reversal.[13] SRY encodes a protein with a highly conserved high mobility group (HMG) box DNA-binding domain. This protein likely acts as a type of transcription factor by inducing DNA binding.[14] The target gene(s) remains to be identified, but cell proliferation in the coelomic epithelium is the earliest noted effect.[14a] Several mutations within the HMG box of SRY have been found in sex-reversed XY individuals while SRY translocation to the X chromosome during meiosis results in an XX male.[15]

The large nonrecombining region of the Y containing euchromatin and heterochromatin makes up 95 percent of its length. This region contains at least 9 genes with X homologs and 11 testis-specific genes.[16] The latter include several genes, including DAZ, RBM, and SPGY, which appear necessary for spermatogenesis,[17] as well as a gene associated with development of gonadoblastoma in dysgenetic gonads.[18] This region also contains the gene for H-Y antigen, a male-specific histocompatibility antigen that can lead to rejection of male organ or marrow grafts by female recipients.[19] Other genes not yet identified appear to be involved with stature.[16]

The X Chromosome

The X chromosome (Fig. 17-3) is a large metacentric chromosome that contains about 5 percent of the total DNA in a haploid set (22 autosomes plus the X). In sharp contrast to the Y chromosome, the X chromosome is involved in the function of every system in the body and contains more than 280 mapped genetic loci.[20] These loci include genes that play important roles in the sexual differentiation of both males and females. The gene for the androgen receptor, which is essential in the male for both genital differentiation and secondary sexual characteristics, is located in band Xq11-12.[21] Male carriers of X-autosome translocations, regardless of the position of the break point on the X, usually are azoospermic or severely oligospermic, while ambiguous genitalia have been observed in males carrying a pericentric X inversion. Deletion mapping has shown that genes on the long arm of X (between bands Xq11 and Xq22) are involved in the expression of the stigmata of Klinefelter's syndrome. A region localized to Xp21, dosage sensitive sex reversal locus (DSS), when duplicated in XY individuals causes testicular dysgenesis and sex reversal.[22] Such observations indicate the critical but still incompletely defined role that this chromosome plays in male reproductive function.

Both X chromosomes are necessary for normal ovarian differentiation as evidenced by the gonadal dysgenesis of Turner's syndrome. There is a critical segment on the long arm of the X chromosome, lying between bands Xq13 and Xq27, which is essential for normal ovarian differentiation and function. Females with structural abnormalities or break points in this region present with premature follicular atresia leading to gonadal dysgenesis, primary or secondary amenorrhea, and infertility. Although some deletions of the short arm (Xp) cause only short stature with normal sexual development, more severe abnormalities such as monosomy (45,X) or an isochromosome [46,X,iso(Xq)] give rise to the full Turner's syndrome.[23]

Other genes on the X chromosome are also involved in sexual differentiation. Deletion or mutations of KAL1 at Xp 22.3 result in hypogonadotropic hypogonadism of Kallman's syndrome, of GDXY at Xp22.11 cause some forms of XY gonadal dysgenesis, and of DAX-1 at Xp21 result in congenital adrenal hypoplasia with hypogonadotropic hypogonadism.[20]

The X chromosome also contains a large number of unpaired genes that are not present on the Y chromosome, defects of which cause disease in hemizygous males and females with monosomy X. Examples of these X-linked traits include color blindness, hemophilia A (factor VIII), hemophilia B (factor IX), and glucose-6-phosphate dehydrogenase deficiency, the loci for which are located on the long arm. The steroid sulfatase (STS) locus, which is involved in X-linked ichthyosis and placental sulfatase deficiency, has been assigned to the distal part of the short arm.

Because normal 46,XX females obtain twice as many of these unpaired genes as do normal males, a dosage difference with effects similar to those of aneuploidy might be expected if there were not some mechanism for dosage compensation. This compensation is effected by inactivation of one X chromosome in the female early in development so that the expressed dosage of X-linked genes is equivalent in males and females. This process is random but is fixed thereafter for each cell line; thus the female comes to be a mosaic of active paternal and maternal X chromosomes. Regardless of the number of X chromosomes present in a cell, all but one are inactivated. After inactivation, cell lines in which the active X is structurally abnormal may replicate less efficiently than do their normal counterparts so that selection against this line may occur.

The inactive X chromosome can be identified during cell division in the presence of [^{3}H]thymidine by its asynchronous delayed pattern of DNA synthesis. In interphase cells this late-replicating X can be stained and visualized as an X chromatin, or Barr body, of about 1 m diameter applied to the inner surface of the nuclear membrane (Fig. 17-2*B*). In smears of female buccal mucosa, X chromatin can be found in about 20 percent of cells. Sex chromatin also appears in the form of a drumstick-shaped accessory appendage on 1–15 percent of the nuclei of female polymorphonuclear leukocytes. The number of chromatin bodies in any diploid nucleus is one less than the total number of X chromosomes; thus the buccal smear of a 48,XXXY male will show two chromatin bodies, while that of a 45,X female will show none. Structural anomalies altering the size of the X chromosome may influence the size of the resulting mass of heterochromatin.

In recent years the concept of mammalian X inactivation and dosage compensation has been extended and modified.[24] In the embryo, even though X-linked genes become active in transcription as early as the two-cell stage, X inactivation does not occur until the early blastocyst stage. Thus very early female embryos show levels of X-linked enzyme activity twice those of male embryos. The initiation of X inactivation seems to coincide with the beginning of cell differentiation and is seen first in the trophoderm, then in the primitive endoderm, and finally in the inner cell masses. Both somatic and germ cells appear to be derived from a common pool of X-inactivated cells. However, in females germ cells undergo genetic reactivation before entering meiosis so that both X chromosomes become active again in the primary oocytes of the fetal and postnatal ovary. This pattern is exactly the opposite of what occurs in the normal male during spermatogenesis, when the single active X chromosome undergoes apparent inactivation at the onset of meiosis. These observations may underlie the accelerated oocyte degeneration seen in 45,X females and the azoospermia in 47,XXY males. In Turner's syndrome the lack of two active X chromosomes in the germ cell appears to accelerate follicular atresia; conversely, in Klinefelter's syndrome the extra, presumably active, X chromosome interferes with normal spermatogenesis.

In somatic cells and their descendants X inactivation affects all but a single X chromosome. It has therefore been difficult to explain the somatic abnormalities of 45,X and 47,XXY subjects. Indeed, in polysomy X the severity of the somatic anomalies correlates with the number of X chromosomes, a finding that suggests that dosage compensation as achieved by X inactivation is incomplete. Recent evidence has partially resolved this paradox by demonstrating that several loci clustered around the pseudoautosomal region and Xp11, including those for the Xg^a red blood cell antigen and for microsomal STS, escape complete inactivation and are expressed by both X chromosomes. Therefore, X inactivation does not involve the entire chromosome, and females normally express some gene loci in double dosage. Some inactivated genes may also be reactivated with aging.

The molecular basis of X inactivation is not fully understood but involves underacetylation of histones and methylation of DNA cytosine residues, which both prevent transcription.[24] Initiation of X-inactivation is controlled by an X-inactivation center (Xic), which is postulated to be Xist.[24] This gene is expressed only on the inactivated X and appears to code for a nontranslated RNA. A second locus, the X-controlling element (Xce), is thought to influence the randomness of inactivation.[24]

Gonadal Sex

Although a person's genetic sex is determined at conception, for the first few weeks of fetal life the gonadal anlagen maintain a similar appearance in both sexes. This indifferent gonad forms at about 7–10 days in the mesenchyme at the ventral edge of the cranial medial part of the mesonephros and is invaded in turn by primordial germ cells and cells originating from the mesonephros and the coelomic epithelium. The large spherical germ cells probably arise in or close to the yolk sac endoderm; from there they

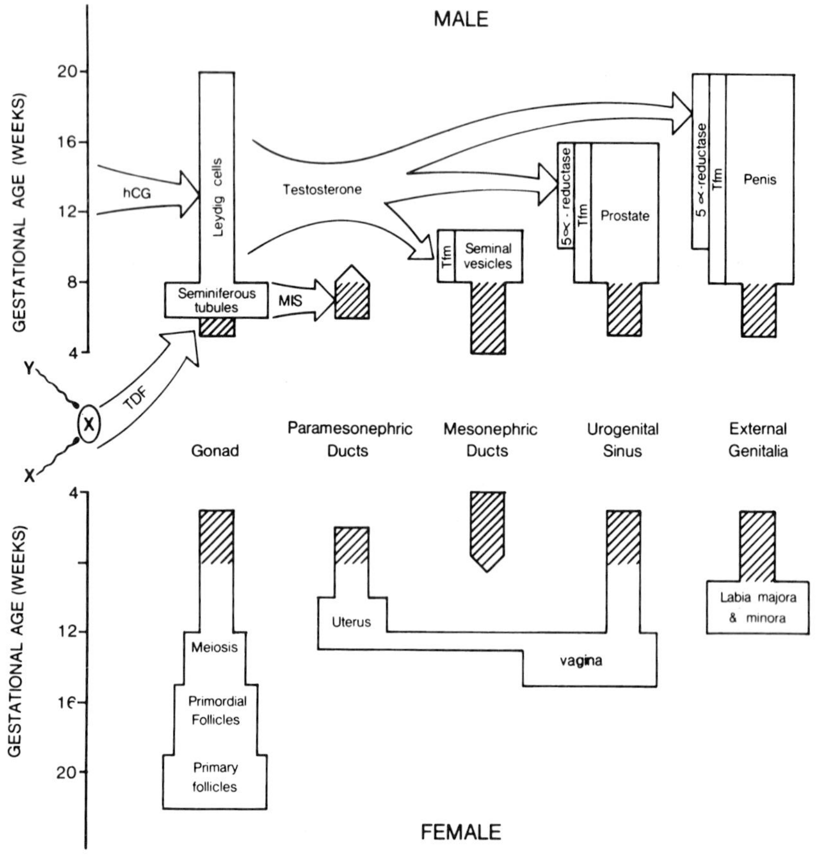

FIGURE 17-4. The major determinants of sexual differentiation, showing the cascade of genetic and endocrine effects and their timing in relation to fetal age in the male (*top*) and the female (*bottom*). The broad arrows show the sequential effects of the Y-linked testis-determining factor (TDF), human chorionic gonadotropin (hCG), müllerian inhibiting substance (MIS), and testosterone in directing male differentiation. Tfm indicates the target cell androgen receptor. The crosshatched segments refer to a sexually undifferentiated structure.

migrate through the hindgut region and the dorsal mesentery to reach the gonadal ridge at around day 35–45, where they proliferate rapidly. The mesonephros itself contributes dense cell cords which in the male will form the rete testis and part of the epididymis and in the female will remain as the rete ovarii. It has been suggested that mesonephric cells within the gonad may give rise to Sertoli and granulosa cells, while Leydig cells, theca, and ovarian stroma arise from mesenchyme.[25] These findings emphasize that although the testis and ovary differentiate into dissimilar organs, they continue throughout life to show numerous homologies in their gametogenic and steroidogenic functions (Fig. 17-4).

Two autosomal genes, WT-1 and SF-1, are necessary for normal development of the primordial bipotential gonad.[26] The Wilm's tumor gene, WT-1, codes for a zinc finger protein required for formation of the primitive kidney and gonadal ridge.[27] Mutations of WT-1 not only can result in Wilms' tumor but also in 3 distinct syndromes (WAGR, Denys-Drash, and Frasier) which all have urogenital anomalies including XY sex reversal.[28] SF-1 codes for an orphan nuclear receptor (steroidogenic factor1) that is essential for formation of both the adrenal cortex and gonad.[29] SF-1 expression is evident in the urogenital ridge at the earliest stage of male and female gonadal organogenesis. Knockout mice which lack SF-1 have female internal and external genitalia regardless of genetic sex and have complete absence of adrenals and gonads. Interstingly, SF-1 appears to play a role in the development of the ventromedial hypothalamus and pituitary gonadotropes as well.[29] Therefore the evidence suggests that both WT-1 and SF-1 function upstream from SRY and influence formation of the indifferent gonad (Fig. 17-5). Another homeobox gene, Lhx9, has recently been found to be essential for somatic cell proliferation in the genital ridge and SF-1 expression.[29a]

Testicular Differentiation

The earliest sign of male differentiation is the appearance within the indifferent gonad of large numbers of Sertoli cells at about 6 to 7 weeks and the subsequent organization of seminiferous tubules containing Sertoli cells and primordial germ cells.[30] Selective destruction of germ cells before they reach the gonad confirms that these cells do not play a role in the initiation of testis differentiation. Rather, it appears that the TDF gene (SRY) product acts autonomously to cause Sertoli cell differentiation and that all subsequent events reflect Sertoli cell activity.[14] Germ cells (gonocytes and spermatogonia) undergo mitotic division within the testicular cords as these structures grow in length, anastomose, and eventually become canalized. In contrast to the female, in the male meiosis does not occur before puberty.

At 8 weeks typical Leydig cells equipped with membrane receptors for human chorionic gonadotropin (hCG) and luteinizing hormone (LH) appear in the interstitium between the testicular cords; by 14 weeks they make up more than half the volume of the testis. These Leydig cells have the typical ultrastructural appearance of steroid-secreting cells and contain abundant amounts of steroidogenic enzymes. After the end of the fourth month the number of fetal Leydig cells decreases, and only a few are visible at term. The appearance and decline of fetal Leydig cells closely parallels the rise and fall of fetal serum hCG levels. Mean testis

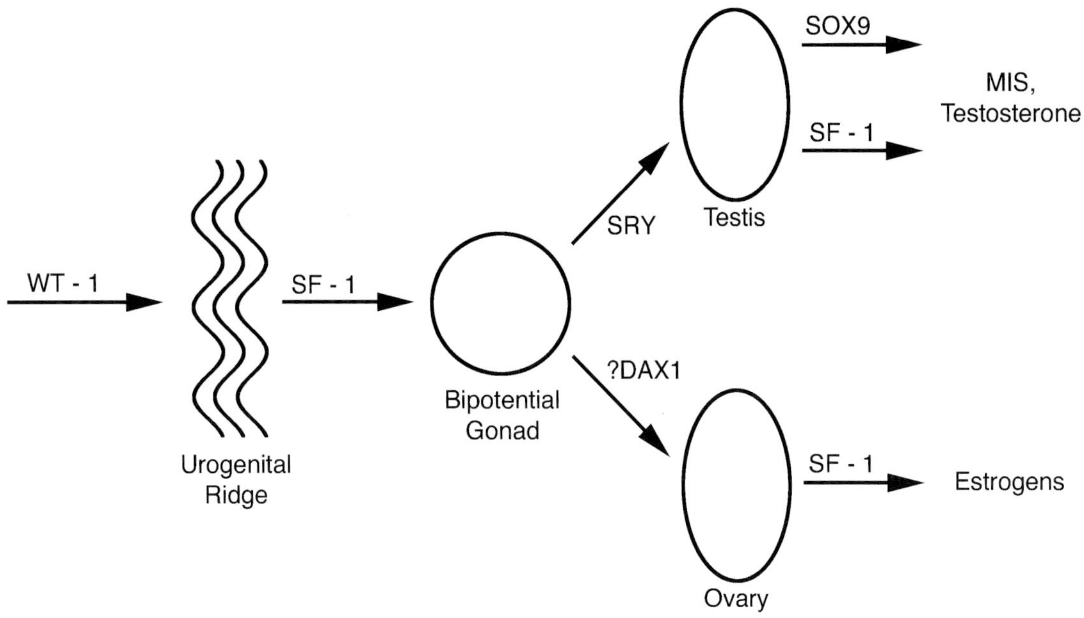

FIGURE 17-5. Genes involved in gonadal differentiation.

weight increases to about 850 mg at term and is greater than ovarian weight at every gestational age. The final stage of testis differentiation is descent through the inguinal canal to reach the scrotum at about 34–35 weeks gestation.

The genetics of testicular differentiation has been further elucidate in recent years, but much remains to be determined. SRY is undoubtedly the TDF gene,[14] but appears not to act alone in testis formation (Fig. 17-5). Deletions of 9p and 10q are associated with XY sex reversal, although the specific genes remain to be identified. In campomelic dysplasia, a congenital syndrome of bone and cartilage malformation, XY sex reversal with failure of testicular differentiation occurs in about 75 percent of genetic males whereas XX females have normal ovarian development.[31] The gene responsible, SOX9, is on chromosome 17q and encodes as HMG-box protein similar to SRY, which likely acts as a transcription factor.[32] A variety of heterozygous mutations have been described suggesting that haploid insufficiency is responsible, but to date there is no correlation between mutation and phenotype.[33] SOX9 expression studies implicate it as a critical factor in Sertoli cell differentiation, likely immediately downstream from SRY.[34] Expression of SF-1 is also dimorphic, persisting in Sertoli and Leydig cells after testicular differentiation but ceasing in ovarian tissue until late gestation.[29] SF-1 is required for induction of Leydig cell steroidogenesis and for regulating synthesis of Müllerian inhibiting substance (MIS) in Sertoli cells. Recent evidence suggests WT-1 synergizes with SF-1 to promote MIS expression whereas DAX-1 antagonizes this synergy.[35]

Ovarian Differentiation

In contrast to testicular development, which is independent of the presence of germ cells, differentiation of the ovary is largely defined in terms of germ cell maturation. At 7 to 9 weeks gestation clumps of oogonia undergoing mitotic division are scattered throughout the ovarian parenchyma. The first definitive sign of ovarian development is the onset of meiotic prophase in primary oocytes at around 10–11 weeks. The first meiotic division is arrested at the diplotene stage shortly before birth and is not completed until ovulation runs its course 12–40 years later. The peak number of germ cells is observed at midpregnancy, when the fetal ovary contains up to 7 million oogonia, oocytes, and degenerating cells. At about 13 weeks gestation, oocytes become surrounded by follicular cells,[36] and by 17 weeks most oocytes are in primordial follicles. After 22–25 weeks, multilayered and even a few antral follicles can be seen; the newborn ovary still contains mainly primary and primordial (single-layer) follicles, although small numbers of more mature and atretic forms occur. Although small amounts of steroid hormones can be produced by theca and interstitial cells, which are homologous with Leydig cells, their nature and local significance for oocyte maturation remain unclear.

The most remarkable phenomenon of ovarian development during the latter half of pregnancy and indeed during postnatal life is a decline in the total germ cell population as a result of atresia. By term, the ovaries contain about 2 million germ cells, but only about 400 of these cells will survive to ovulate during a woman's reproductive life.

Preservation of a viable follicle requires an oocyte equipped with two active X chromosomes. Females with various chromosomal abnormalities show inadequate ovarian development and excessive loss of germ cells. Thus in 45,X Turner's syndrome, germ cells migrate to the gonad and undergo mitosis, but subsequently the rate of loss through degeneration is accelerated, leaving the neonate with only a few follicles.

There is evidence that the genes necessary for normal follicular development are found on both the long and short arms of the X chromosome. One candidate gene is DAX-1, which is located in the DSS region at Xp21.[22] DAX-1 appears to act when present in double dosage by antagonizing the action of SRY.[37] However, recent development of a DAX-1 knockout mouse did not affect ovarian differentiation in females but did prevent spermatogenesis in the males, suggesting that DAX-1 is not critical for ovarian development.[37a] The syndrome of autosomal recessive XX gonadal dysgenesis suggests that other genes are also necessary for normal ovarian differentiation. The presence of XX germ cells in the developing ovary appears to be essential as ovaries depleted of germ cells can develop seminiferous cords.[38]

Differentiation of the Genital Ducts

The mesonephric, or wolffian, ducts appear in the fetus at about 4 weeks gestation; they then grow caudally, become canalized, and open into the cloaca. The mesonophric nephrons, except for those contiguous with the rete system of the gonad, degenerate once the definitive kidney (metanephros) forms, but their ducts become incorporated into the genital system. The paramesonephric (müllerian) ducts originate at about 6 weeks gestation as solid cords of coelomic epithelial cells lateral to the mesonephric ducts, which grow caudally and cross the epithelial cells ventrally to reach the urogenital sinus. These paired cords become canalized; caudally, where they meet in the midline, they fuse to form a single uterovaginal canal. Thus by 7 weeks gestation, each fetus is equipped with the primordia of both male and female genital ducts (Fig. 17-6).

Female Internal Genital Development

In female fetuses the mesonephric ducts degenerate relatively early, leaving only remnants of tubules that can be identified later as the epoöphoron, paraoöphoron, and Gartner's duct. The partially fused paramesonephric ducts provide the paired fallopian tubes, the midline uterine primordium, and, in collaboration with tissue contributed by the urogenital sinus, the vaginal primordium. The development of these structures does not depend on hormonal or other influences from the ovary. However, it is contingent on the prior appearance of the mesonephric ducts; thus renal aplasia is commonly associated with agenesis of the fallopian tube, uterus, and vagina. Although the female internal genitalia differentiate morphologically somewhat later than do those of the male, there is evidence that they are functionally committed to become female by as early as 8 weeks gestation.

Male Internal Genital Development

The development of male internal genitalia involves two separate processes: regression of the paramesonephric ducts and stabilization of the mesonephric ducts. These processes are mediated by two secretions of the fetal testis: müllerian inhibiting substance (MIS), also called antimüllerian hormone, produced by the Sertoli cells; and testosterone from the fetal Leydig cells (Fig. 17-4).

Müllerian Inhibiting Substance

Regression of the paramesonephric ducts begins at about 8 weeks gestation, initially adjacent to the caudal pole of the testis and then extending cranially and caudally. In the normal male only the cranial tip, which becomes the appendix testis, is spared. Close juxtaposition of the paramesonephric duct and the ipsilateral testis is necessary to initiate regression, but even large amounts of testosterone applied locally cannot duplicate the effect. Rather, paramesonephric regression is induced by the local paracrine action of MIS secreted by Sertoli cells of the ipsilateral testis.

FIGURE 17-6. Diagrammatic sagittal sections of the internal genitalia of an 8-week fetus (*A*) and of male (*B*) and female (*C*) fetuses at 13 weeks gestation. [*From Smail P, Reyes FI, Winter JSD, Faiman C, in Kogan SJ, Hafez ESE (eds): Pediatric Andrology. The Hague, Martinus Nijhoff, 1981, p 11.*]

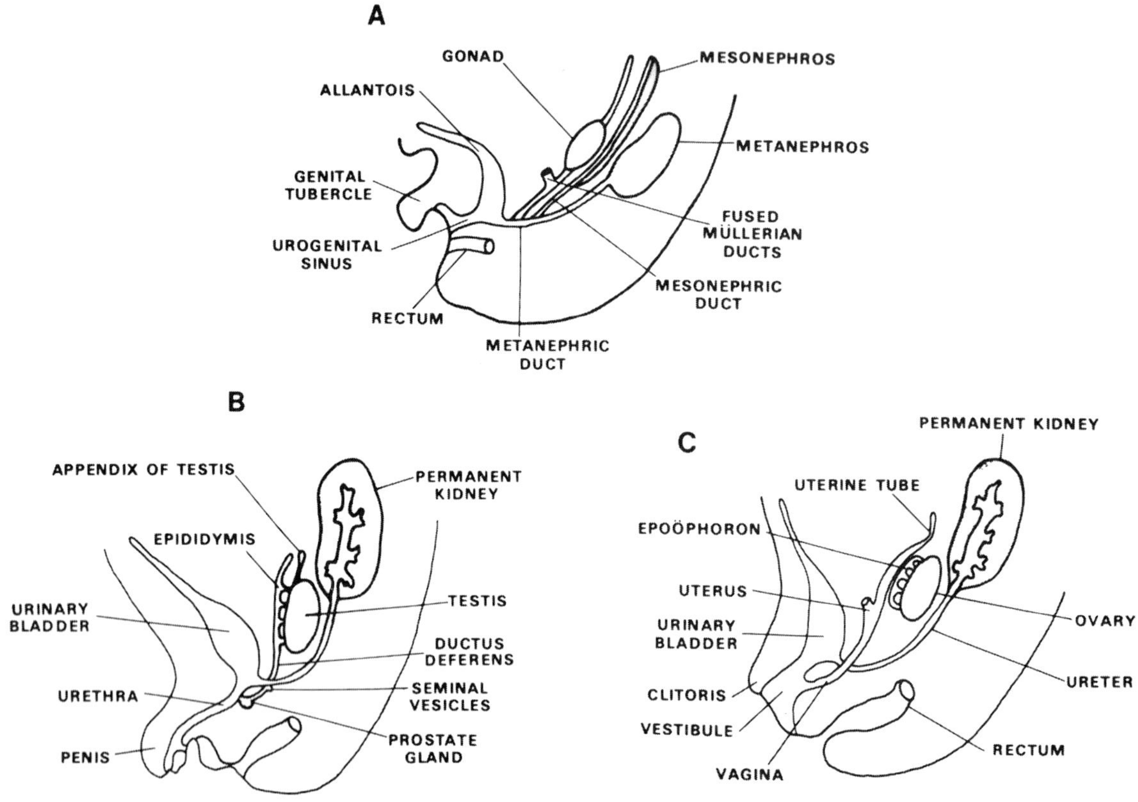

MIS is a dimeric glycoprotein (molecular mass of 140,000 dalton) encoded by a gene in the short arm of chromosome 19.[39,40] It possesses interesting structural homologies with both transforming growth factor b (TGF-b) and the beta chain of inhibin. It is the first secretory product of the testis and appears at around 7 weeks gestation, at the time of Sertoli cell differentiation. Expression of the MIS gene appears to be activated by SF-1.[41] Regression of the paramesonephric ducts occurs in response to the paracrine effect of MIS from the ipsilateral testis. The MIS receptor is a member of the serine-threonine kinase transmembrane receptor superfamily with its gene on chromosome 12.[42] The mechanism of action is not fully understood, but it appears to promote growth of fibroblasts and production of fibronectin while inhibiting the growth of epithelial cells.[43] There is a limited time window during which Müllerian structures will respond to MIS.

MIS is still detectable in males at birth and is secreted postnatally by juvenile and adult Sertoli cells, although levels are lower after the onset of puberty.[43] Circulating MIS is undetectable in females at birth, but some is secreted by postnatal ovarian granulosa cells. The functions of MIS in the male after paramesonephric duct involution is not known; there is some evidence that in the female MIS may act as an inhibitor of oocyte meiosis and of aromatase.[43] Exposure of fetal ovaries to MIS causes inhibition of germ cell replication, suppression of aromatase activity, and the appearance of seminiferous tubulelike structures, suggesting that this factor may also play a role in normal testis development. It is therefore possible to postulate a model of male development in which the TDF gene product triggers Sertoli cell differentiation, perhaps via SF-1 and SOX9, and activates MIS gene expression. MIS could then act in an autocrine fashion to induce further differentiation of the Sertoli cell (which has MIS receptors) and thus could eventually influence Leydig cell differentiation, germ cell proliferation, seminiferous tubule formation, and even testicular descent.[44]

Testosterone

Stabilization and differentiation of the paired mesonephric ducts to form the vasa efferentia, epididymis, vasa deferentia, ejaculatory ducts, and seminal vesicles is dependent on local high concentrations of androgen from the ipsilateral testis. Androgen receptors in the ductal cells bind both testosterone and dihydrotestosterone; however, because only small amounts of the latter are synthesized by the testis and the ductal cells themselves appear to lack 5α-reductase until after differentiation, it is generally assumed that testosterone is the active intracellular mediator that is primarily responsible.[45]

In patients with asymmetric gonadal differentiation, duct development on each side correlates closely with the degree of testicular development on the same side. Patients with enzymatic defects in testosterone biosynthesis or defective androgen receptors show rudimentary mesonephric duct structures, but in genetic 5α-reductase deficiency male genital ducts are normal. That this effect of testosterone is a local paracrine effect rather than a blood-borne endocrine effect is underscored by the failure of adrenal androgens to prevent normal regression of the mesonephric ducts in females with congenital adrenal hyperplasia.

Differentiation of the Urogenital Sinus and External Genitalia

For the first 2 months of prenatal development the external genitalia are identical in both sexes. They consist of a midline genital tubercle (*phallus*) and lateral labioscrotal swellings. Behind these structures lies the urogenital sinus, into which both the ureters and the internal genital ducts open.

Feminization of the External Genitalia

In females the phallus remains small and bends ventrally, the anogenital distance remains short, and the labioscrotal swellings and urethral groove do not fuse in the midline. The labioscrotal swellings become the labia majora, the separate genital folds become the labia minora, and the phallic part of the urogenital sinus becomes the vestibule (Fig. 17-7). The urogenital sinus is divided by downgrowth of a vaginal plate which approaches the perineum to provide separate urethral and uterovaginal access to the exterior. The contribution of paramesonephric duct tissue to the upper vagina is indicated by the abnormally shallow vagina of patients with complete testicular feminization, in whom the paramesonephric ducts regress. It appears that the development of female external genitalia is independent of ovarian influence, although prenatal exposure to diethylstilbestrol can cause persistence of müllerian-derived vaginal epithelium, with vaginal adenosis and a predisposition to malignant transformation.

Masculinization of the External Genitalia

During male differentiation the labioscrotal swellings and urethral folds fuse in the midline to form the scrotum and a penis enclosing the phallic urethra (Fig. 17-7). This process, which is imposed by testicular androgens, begins at 9 weeks and is complete by 14 weeks gestation. The urogenital sinus differentiates into the male urethra and the prostate. During the latter half of pregnancy the penis continues to enlarge, with a rate of growth three to four times that of the female clitoris.[46] During this same period the testes descend into the scrotum, a process that appears to be androgen-dependent, although other testicular factors may play a role.[44] In males with deficient testicular function, the prostatic utricle, which is homologous to the female upper vagina, is commonly larger than normal.

Hormonal Sex: Differentiation of the Hypothalamic-Pituitary-Gonadal Axis

Gonadal Steroid Production

By the time Leydig cells can be recognized at 6 to 7 weeks fetal age, the fetal testis contains the necessary enzymes for the synthesis of testosterone from various substrates, although the preferred substrate is probably circulating low-density lipoprotein cholesterol. Testicular concentrations of testosterone rise to a peak at 12–14 weeks gestation and then decline, a pattern that correlates closely with the growth and involution of fetal Leydig cells and with testicular mRNA levels for certain key steroidogenic enzymes.[47,48] Although the fetal ovaries of some mammalian species contain enzymes for both the synthesis of androgens and their aromatization to estrogen, there is no evidence that the human fetal ovary secretes significant amounts of sex steroids, at least during the first half of pregnancy, when sexual differentiation is taking place.

Sex Steroids in the Fetal Circulation

The initial local or paracrine action of fetal testosterine is to stabilize development of the ipsilateral mesonephric duct and possibly to stimulate growth of the testis itself. Soon, however, male fetal serum testosterone concentrations begin to rise, reaching peak concentrations of 200–600 ng/dl (7–21 nmol/L) at 16–18 weeks

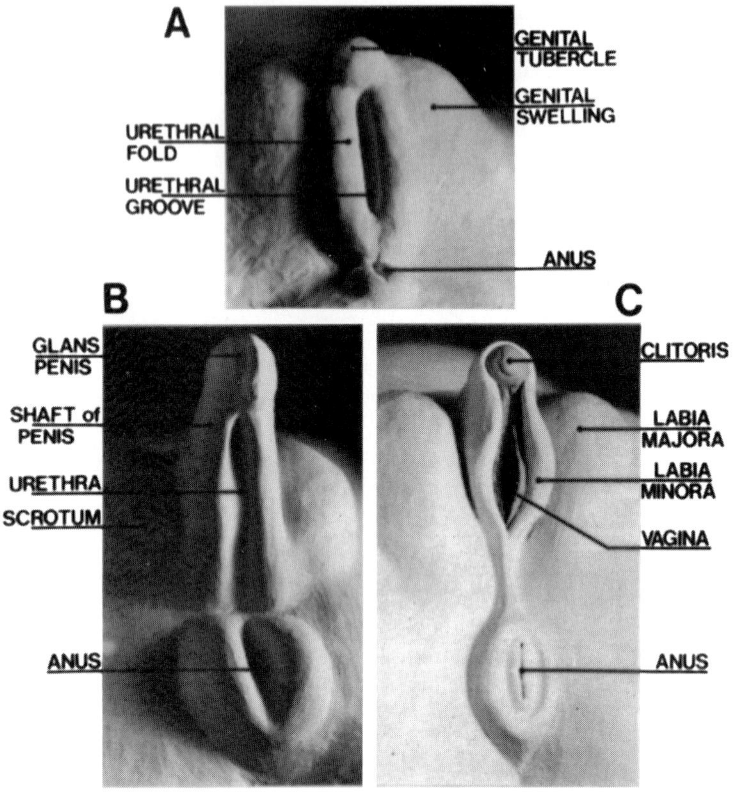

FIGURE 17-7. Models of the external genitalia in an 8-week undifferentiated fetus (*A*) and in male (*B*) and female (*C*) fetuses at 13 weeks gestation. [*From Smail P, Reyes FI, Winter JSD, Faiman C, in Kogan SJ, Hafez ESE (eds): Pediatric Andrology. The Hague, Martinus Nijhoff, 1981, p 12.*]

gestation, values which are in the adult male range.[47] After mid-pregnancy, as Leydig cells involute male serum testosterone levels gradually decline, but they remain higher than female levels until term. At the same time the fetus is exposed to high concentrations of steroids from the placenta, notably estrogens and progesterone, and from the adrenal cortex, in particular dehydroepiandrosterone sulfate. There is no significant sex difference in serum concentrations of these steroids; presumably, therefore, they do not play a direct role in sexual differentiation, but may influence the process through their effects on gonadal steroidogenesis, binding of steroids by serum proteins, and target cell receptor occupancy.

Serum levels of sex steroid-binding globulin (TeBG) are only about one-twentieth of those in maternal serum, and the human fetus does not appear to produce any other high-affinity androgen-binding protein. Although albumin serves as a low-affinity high-capacity carrier of many steroids, its concentration is also low in the fetal circulation. The effect of this low level of sex steroid binding is to increase the fraction of serum testosterone that is free and therefore presumably active.

Actions of Sex Steroids on the Genitalia

The changing patterns of testosterone concentrations in the fetal testis and circulation, in relation to the major events of male genital development, are summarized in Fig. 17-8. Testosterone appears first in high concentrations in the testis itself, where, by a local paracrine effect, it induces masculinization of the ipsilateral mesonephric duct. Subsequently, circulating testosterone levels become sufficiently high to initiate masculinization of the urogenital sinus and external genitalia.

In all these target cells specific high-affinity androgen receptors can be found prior to differentiation. Androgens bind to this nuclear receptor protein, and the steroid-receptor complex binds to specific chromatin acceptor sites to initiate transcription of new messenger RNA[49]; in turn, this RNA is processed and transported to cytoplasmic ribosomes, where it is translated for synthesis of androgen-induced proteins. There is evidence that the actual target for these androgen effects is the mesenchyme of the genital anlagen, which in turn induces specific patterns of morphogenesis, cytodifferentiation, and functional activity in the overlying epithelium.[50]

The androgen receptor protein has a higher binding affinity and a slower rate of dissociation for dihydrotestosterone than for testosterone itself. The enzyme necessary for this intracellular conversion—5α-reductase—does not appear in the mesonephric ducts until development is already well advanced, but high local concentrations of testosterone are sufficient to accomplish masculinization. The urogenital sinus and external genitalia contain active 5α-reductase as soon as testosterone appears in the circulation; it therefore seems likely that masculinization of these structures is accomplished by lower concentrations of the more potent androgen dihydrotestosterone.

The androgen receptor (Tfm) gene has been cloned and localized to band Xq11-12 of the X chromosome.[51,52] The 5α-reductase gene is autosomal. Thus, in normal circumstances both sexes can respond to circulating androgen; the direction of genital differentiation is determined solely by testicular testosterone production. Defects in testosterone synthesis, deficient 5α-reductase activity, and an ineffective androgen receptor will each prevent normal genital masculinization of the genetic male, although in 5α-reductase deficiency mesonephric duct development is normal. Conversely, exposure of a female fetus to high levels of circulating androgen does not induce mesonephric duct development but does inhibit separation of the vagina from the

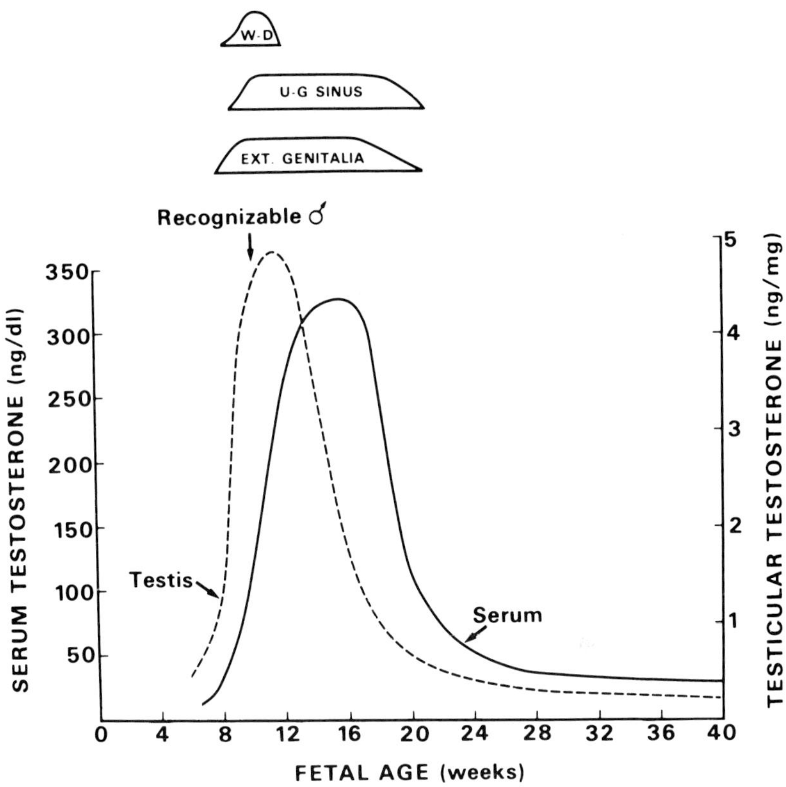

FIGURE 17-8. The relation of changes in mean testicular and serum testosterone concentrations to the time of development of the mesonephric ducts (W.D.) and virilization of the urogenital (U-G) sinus and external genitalia in male fetuses. (*From Winter et al.*[47])

urogenital sinus and promotes labioscrotal fusion and clitoral hypertrophy.

Control of Fetal Gonadal Function

Chorionic Gonadotropin

There is considerable circumstantial evidence that testosterone synthesis by Leydig cells during the period of genital differentiation is dependent on hCG, although one cannot rule out the possibility that steroidogenesis in the very youngest testes may be initiated by other factors.[53] Thus hypopituitary males do not demonstrate genital ambiguity, although micropenis and cryptorchism are often observed. Chorionic gonadotropin appears in the maternal circulation immediately after implantation of the blastocyst; levels rise to a peak at about 10 weeks fetal age and then decline, although significant placental production continues until term. The pattern in the fetal circulation of both sexes is similar, but fetal hCG concentrations are only about one-thirtieth of those in the maternal compartment.[47]

Fetal Leydig cells, but not ovarian cells, have specific membrane receptors for LH and hCG; the number of these receptors increases to a maximum at 15–18 weeks gestation and then declines. Via a mechanism that appears to utilize cyclic AMP as the intracellular second messenger, hCG increases the number of low-density lipoprotein receptors, enhances de novo cholesterol synthesis, and stimulates mitochondrial cholesterol side-chain cleavage, all of which serve to increase the pool of available pregnenolone for androgen biosynthesis.[54]

Pituitary Gonadotropins

Although maternal pituitary gonadotropins do not cross the placental barrier, the fetal pituitary after about 9 weeks gestation produces significant amounts of FSH and LH. By 4–5 weeks, fetal age the pituitary anlage has the ability to synthesize glycoprotein hormone α subunit, but gonadotropin releasing hormone (GnRH)-mediated hypothalamic stimulation is probably necessary for the synthesis of the hormone-specific β subunit and thus of intact FSH and LH.

Both gonadotropins appear in the fetal circulation at about 11–12 weeks and rise to peak concentrations at midpregnancy.[55] Serum FSH concentrations are much higher in female fetuses, in whom adult castrate values occur, than in male fetuses, in whom values are in the normal adult range. This sex difference demonstrates that a negative feedback mechanism mediated by testicular androgens is already operative by midgestation; in experimental animals, castration of the male fetus raises gonadotropin levels to the female range while castration of the female has no effect. After 28 weeks gestation, serum gonadotropin levels decline in both sexes, a phenomenon that probably reflects maturation of placental estrogen-mediated feedback inhibitory mechanisms. The decline in Leydig cell testosterone production in the latter half of pregnancy would appear to result from the combined effects of a decline in circulating levels of hCG, FSH, and LH and direct inhibition of androgen biosynthesis by high levels of circulating placental estrogens.

The pattern of mean serum hCG and pituitary gonadotropin concentrations in the male fetus, in relation to changes in testicular morphology and function, is summarized in Fig. 17-9. Although hCG is the major gonadotropin in the fetal circulation and clearly drives testosterone synthesis during genital differentiation, pituitary gonadotropins become relatively more significant in later gestation and influence such phenomena as phallic growth and testicular descent. The testes of anencephalic and hypogonadotropic fetuses show reduced numbers of Leydig cells. In addition, they may show reduced numbers of spermatogonia, suggesting that FSH- or possi-

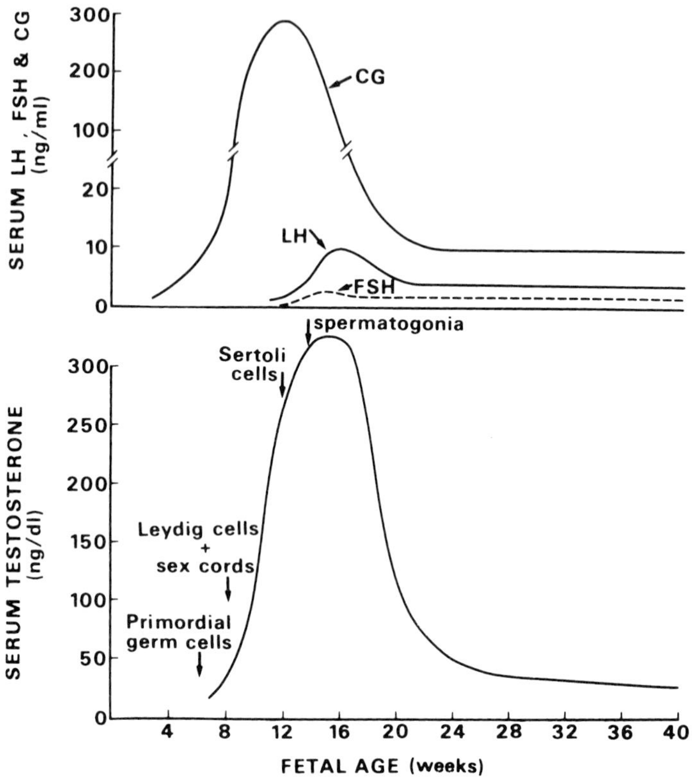

FIGURE 17-9. A schematic summary of the temporal relation between mean serum concentrations of hCG, LH, and FSH; mean serum testosterone concentrations; and morphologic development of the fetal testis. (*From Winter et al.*[47])

bly LH-mediated testosterone secretion plays a role in germ cell maturation.

The relationships between serum gonadotropins and ovarian development are summarized in Fig. 17-10. Ovarian development proceeds normally in anencephalic fetuses until about 32 weeks gestation; after this one observes reduced ovarian size and accelerated atresia with premature loss of germ cells and absence of antral follicles, suggesting inadequate granulosa cell proliferation and differentiation. This coincides with the timing of the appearance of FSH receptors in ovarian granulosa cells.

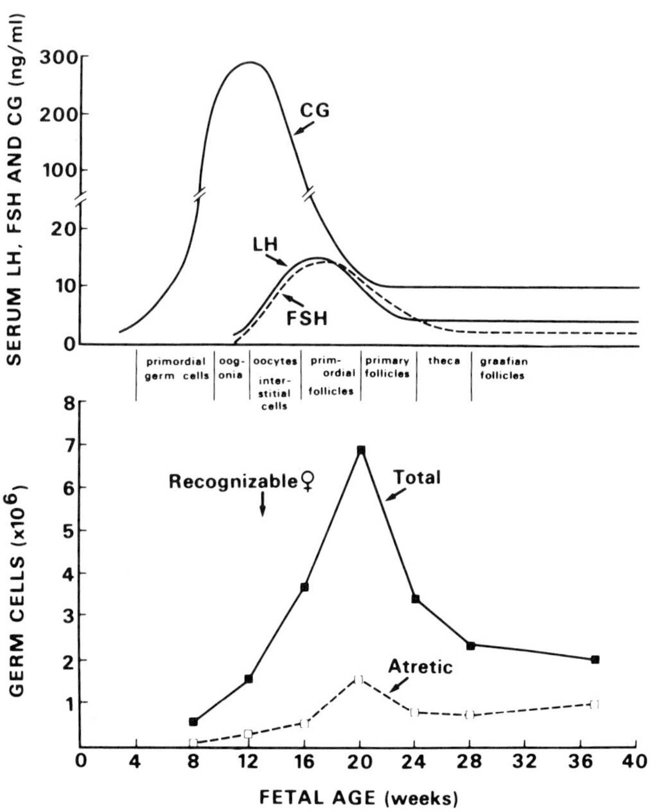

FIGURE 17-10. A schematic summary of the temporal relation between mean serum concentrations of hCG, LH, and FSH; morphologic development of the fetal ovary; and ovarian total content of germ cells. (*From Winter et al.*[47])

There is considerable evidence that fetal pituitary gonadotropin secretion is regulated by hypothalamic GnRH. Neurons expressing pro-GnRH mRNA appear in the nasal area of the brain by 5 weeks fetal age and migrate to the basal hypothalamus.[56] By 9–11 weeks, GnRH-secreting neurons can be demonstrated which have their perikarya in the pericommissural, preoptic, lamina terminalis, and perimamillary regions; their axons end in the median eminence apposed to a capillary plexus that connects to the anterior pituitary, although a clearly defined hypothalamic-hypophyseal portal system develops later. Between 11 and 14 weeks gestation, there is a 14-fold rise in hypothalamic GnRH content, which parallels the increase in pituitary gonadotropin secretion.[55]

By midgestation the fetus demonstrates pulsatile GnRH release; both in vivo and in vitro fetal pituitary gonadotropin secretion is enhanced by GnRH administration[57] and blocked by specific GnRH antagonists.[58] The striking sex difference in circulating FSH and LH levels at midpregnancy suggests that testosterone in the male fetus suppresses gonadotropin release. Thus orchiectomy increases fetal FSH and LH levels, an effect that can be blocked by the administration of testosterone. As one would expect, fetal ovariectomy has no effect on gonadotropin levels. The subsequent decline in gonadotropin secretion in both sexes presumably reflects the appearance of specific estrogen receptors in the hypothalamus and pituitary and maturation of a feedback system mediated by placental estrogens.

Less is known about central nervous system (CNS) regulation of fetal hypothalamic GnRH release. Certainly by midgestation hypothalamic nuclei are developed and can produce significant amounts of potential regulators such as dopamine, norepinephrine, and serotonin. Observations that neurons in the arcuate-median eminence unit of the fetal hypothalamus contain b-endorphin and that fetal hypothalamic GnRH secretion in vitro is responsive to naloxone suggest the possibility that endogenous opiates exert a tonic inhibitory influence on GnRH release at this time.[59] In addition, GnRH and its receptor are produced by the placenta; their relevance for the regulation of fetal pituitary function is unclear, although they do appear to influence placental hCG synthesis.[60,61]

In addition to gonadotropins, other factors of placental or pituitary origin, such as growth hormone, may influence fetal gonadal growth and differentiation. The fetal testis shows significant expression of IGF-II.[62] Other local growth factors, including insulin-like growth factor I (IGF-I), fibroblast growth factor, epidermal growth factor, and (TGFβ), influence the development of other fetal systems and may well play a role in the developing gonad. Inhibin and activin are structurally related dimeric gonadal glycoproteins that may act to modulate both pituitary FSH secretion and various intragonadal processes. Inhibin B levels are much higher in serum from male than female fetuses,[63] which may be a factor in the lower FSH levels in fetal males. Inhibin A is produced by the placenta where it may be involved in the suppression of hCG in late gestation.[64]

Perinatal Adaptations of the Reproductive Endocrine System

By term, the pituitary-gonadal axis of the human infant is structurally complete and capable of relatively mature function.[65] Circulating levels of placental sex steroids such as estrone (900–4,000 ng/dl), estradiol (200–1,600 ng/dl), estriol (1,200–15,000 ng/dl), 17-hydroxyprogesterone (1,000–7,000 ng/dl), and progesterone (12,000–50,000 ng/dl) are extremely high. Surprisingly, the only visible effects of these hormones on the neonate are occasional breast enlargement and some degree of endometrial hyperplasia. However, the feedback effect of these steroids suppresses serum FSH and LH secretion in both sexes. At term, cord serum hCG levels range from 20–9,000 mIU/ml (median 50 mIU/ml). The only hormonal sex difference is in serum testosterone, which is still slightly higher in males than in females. Parturition elicits a transient release of LH in the male, so that at birth circulating LH levels are higher than in the female.[66]

Immediately after birth, placental estrogens, progesterone, and 17-hydroxyprogesterone are cleared from the neonatal circulation. Concentrations of hCG fall more slowly, but by 4 days of age this gonadotropin is no longer detectable, while testosterone levels have become similar in both sexes. During the second week of life, a remarkable phenomenon occurs in all normal infants, which can only be interpreted as an apparent onset of puberty. As the infant is released from the inhibitory influence of placental estrogens, there is brisk pulsatile secretion of pituitary gonadotropins, which is clearly driven by hypothalamic GnRH just as at adolescence.

In male infants serum gonadotropin levels rise until 1 month of age and then decline to prepubertal levels by 4 months. This rise is accompanied by a parallel rise in serum testosterone concentrations to a peak at 1–3 months of age (see Table 17-6). Although levels of sex hormone-binding globulin also increase, values of free testosterone are distinctly raised in normal male infants.[67] This neonatal activation of the pituitary-testicular axis may influence the timing and course of subsequent sexual development, as blockade with a GnRH agonist appears to cause a significant delay in the onset of puberty.[68]

In female or functionally hypogonadal infants, because of a relative lack of gonadal steroid feedback inhibition, serum FSH and LH levels continue to rise until 3–4 months of age and do not decline to their prepubertal nadir until age 3–4 years. The steroidogenic response of the infant ovary to this postnatal gonadotropin surge is neither so immediate nor so dramatic as that of the testis. There is usually an increase in the number of large antral follicles, which can be observed on pelvic ultrasonography, but only a variable, unsustained rise in serum estradiol levels. The major clinical correlate of these events is the common appearance of transient breast enlargement in girls 1–2 years of age, referred to as *benign premature thelarche.*

The most interesting aspect of these neonatal phenomena is the decline in pituitary gonadotropin secretion which occurs in both sexes, even in the absence of gonads. This clearly reflects maturation of a central mechanism for inhibition of pulsatile hypothalamic GnRH secretion. This prepubertal suppression of pituitary gonadotropin secretion is the penultimate stage in sexual differentiation—the final phase is puberty, with the appearance of sexually dimorphic secondary sex characteristics and eventual acquisition of full adult reproductive function.

Gender Role and Psychosexual Differentiation

Gender role encompasses a person's psychosexual self-identity, legal and social gender designation, external manifestations such as dress and social comportment, and erotic responsiveness to one sex or the other. For years a nature-versus-nurture controversy has raged regarding the potential significance of prenatal androgen exposure as an organizer of these postnatal phenomena. At one extreme is the concept that each infant is psychosexually neuter at birth and that gender identity is permanently imposed during the first few years of life by social and environmental influences. Numerous reports of persons raised in a sex discordant with their genetic or gonadal sex certainly testify to the importance of such influences, although it seems simplistic to assume that their effect is limited to infancy. More likely, gender role is continually reinforced through childhood and puberty by both external influences and awareness of one's genital and secondary sexual characteristics. The demonstration of spontaneous and successful gender role reversal in male pseudohermaphrodites after virilization at puberty[69] underscores the important influence of these sex hormone-mediated factors in later life.

The opposite viewpoint holds that postnatal behavior and intellectual function, to the extent that they are dimorphic, are programmed by sex steroids during a critical prenatal phase of neural differentiation. In its most extreme form this theory proposes that subtle deficiencies of androgen in genetic male fetuses can permit female organization of the brain and predispose to homosexuality.[70] Conversely, excess androgen in a genetic female might induce masculine postnatal behavior, homosexuality, and anovulatory infertility. It must be emphasized that this model invokes not just a direct and immediate activational effect of androgens, such as that upon energy expenditure and libido in adults, but also an organizational effect on neuronal growth and synaptogenesis, which is permanent and is expressed for years after the actual hormone exposure. Such organizational effects can be readily demonstrated in female rodents, in which brief exposure to sex steroids at a critical time can permanently impose male-type acyclic gonadotropin secretion and copulatory behavior in later adult life. Gorski has described sexually dimorphic development of the preoptic area of rat brain, which is dependent on the level of circulating androgens during brain differentiation,[71] but it is not clear to what extent these phenomena have a counterpart in human brain development.

The developing fetal brain expresses not only androgen receptor activity but also 5α-reductase and aromatase, suggesting that androgens can be transformed to products that could have greater or lesser biological activity.[72] Prenatal exposure of female primates to testosterone in amounts sufficient to masculinize the genitalia may induce increased postnatal aggressiveness and lead to aberrant adult sexual behavior but does not block normal ovulatory cycles. The human parallel of this situation might be congenital adrenal hyperplasia, but here any permanent organizational effect has been difficult to prove. Early reports of higher IQ scores in androgen-exposed females have not been confirmed. Although some females with this condition may exhibit more aggression and male-type play,[73] no studies of the behavior of children with such endocrine disorders have been able to correct adequately for postnatal variations in sex steroid levels or for the impact that awareness of the disease, its treatment, and its potential implications has on both self-image and parental perceptions of behavior. Prenatal exposure of females to the synthetic estrogen diethylstilbestrol may increase the likelihood of homosexuality,[74] but the observation that the great majority of such women are exclusively heterosexual suggests that other unidentified variables play a more important role in sexual orientation.

A reasonable viewpoint would suggest that prenatal androgen may play a role in the differentiation of human psychosexual behavior but is certainly not the decisive determinant. Successful differentiation of gender role appears to depend primarily on appropriate assignment of the sex of rearing plus continued unambiguous reinforcement by social interaction, concordant genital appearance, and appropriate secondary sexual characteristics. Even in adult life sex steroids continue to interact with psychological and sociocultural factors to maintain patterns of dimorphic behavior we identify as male and female. The implications of this concept for the management of children with disorders of sexual differentiation should be obvious.

ABNORMAL SEXUAL DIFFERENTIATION

Under normal circumstances genetic sex is defined at conception. Subsequently, unambiguous male or female differentiation is effected by the presence or absence of three key determinants: a testis-determining factor (SRY), müllerian inhibiting substance, and testosterone. The synthesis of each is regulated by specific genetic loci, and each requires specific receptor mechanisms that are normally present in the target cells of either sex. Disordered differentiation may occur at any stage in this process and result in inadequate masculinization of a genetic male or inappropriate virilization of a genetic female. Some relatively common situations which should alert the clinician to the possible presence of such a disorder are listed in Table 17-2. In these situations the diagnostic process is not merely an attempt to assign a label but rather a logical stepwise evaluation of the operation of each of the three key determinants until the clinician can define or rationally infer the status of each of the parameters of sexual dimorphism listed in Table 17-1.

Such an approach can also be applied to the classification of disorders of sexual differentiation, as summarized in Table 17-3.

Errors of Primary Sex Determination

Disorders of sex determination involve sex chromosome abnormalities and/or defective gonad formation. For completeness, the relatively common situations of trisomy X and XYY syndrome are included in this category, even though neither produces any consistent abnormality of gonadal structure or function.

Sex Chromosome Anomalies Associated with Functional Testes and Male Phenotype

Klinefelter's Syndrome

In 1942, Klinefelter and associates described in adult males a syndrome of seminiferous tubule dysgenesis characterized by small firm testes, azoospermia, eunuchoid body habitus, and gynecomastia.[75] Subsequent genetic studies disclosed that most of these patients had two X chromosomes; the term *Klinefelter's syndrome* is now usually restricted to persons with a 47,XXY karyo-type, although variant forms with similar clinical features also occur.

TABLE 17-2. Clinical Features Suggestive of a Possible Disorder of Sexual Differentiation

In the neonate or infant
- Ambiguous external genitalia
- Cryptorchidism and/or hypospadias
- Female with mass in the groin or labium majus pudendi
- Lymphedema or other stigmata of Turner's syndrome
- Family history of anomalous sexual development
- Maternal virilization or hormone ingestion

In the child or young adult
- Female with short stature or other stigmata of Turner's syndrome
- Female with sexual infantilism or precocious ovarian failure
- Male with small testes, gynecomastia, or other stigmata of Klinefelter's syndrome
- Unexplained virilization

TABLE 17-3. A Classification of Abnormal Sexual Development

- I. Errors of primary sex determination
  - A. Sex chromosome anomalies
    - 1. With testes and male phenotype
      - *a.* Klinefelter's syndrome (47,XXY and variants)
      - *b.* XYY syndrome
      - *c.* XX males (X-Y interchange)
    - 2. With ovaries and female phenotype
      - *a.* Trisomy X and variants
    - 3. With bisexual gonads
      - *a.* True hermaphroditism (X-Y interchange)
      - *b.* Chimeric (XX/XY) true hermaphroditism
      - *c.* Mosaic (XX/XXY) true hermaphroditism
    - 4. With dysgenetic gonads
      - *a.* Y chromosome anomalies (XYp-)
      - *b.* Mixed gonadal dysgenesis (45,X/46,XY)
      - *c.* Turner's syndrome (45,X and variants)
  - B. Anomalies of gonadogenesis
    - 1. Defective ovary development
      - *a.* XX gonadal dysgenesis
    - 2. Defective testis development
      - *a.* XY gonadal dysgenesis
      - *b.* Dysgenetic male pseudohermaphroditism
      - *c.* Testicular regression syndromes (agonadism, rudimentary testis, anorchia)
- II. Errors of sexual differentiation
  - A. Inadequate masculinization of genetic male
    - 1. Defective paramesonephric duct regression
      - *a.* Persistent paramesonephric ducts
    - 2. Defective genital virilization
      - *a.* Leydig cell hypoplasia (LH/hCG receptor defect)
      - *b.* Inborn errors of corticosteroid and testosterone synthesis
        - (1) Steroidogenic acute regulatory (StAR) protein deficiency
        - (2) 3β-Hydroxysteroid dehydrogenase deficiency
        - (3) 17α-Hydroxylase deficiency
      - *c.* Inborn errors of testosterone synthesis
        - (1) 17,20-Desmolase deficiency
        - (2) 17β-Hydroxysteroid dehydrogenase deficiency
      - *d.* Inborn error of testosterone metabolism
        - (1) 5α-Reductase deficiency
      - *e.* Defective target cell response
        - (1) Complete androgen insensitivity
        - (2) Incomplete androgen insensitivity and variants
      - *f.* Environmental feminization
        - (1) Maternal ingestion of estrogen or progestin
      - *g.* Multigenic/multifactorial
        - (1) Isolated hypospadias and cryptorchism
        - (2) Multiple congenital anomaly syndromes
  - B. Virilization of genetic female
    - 1. Adrenal androgens (congenital adrenal hyperplasia
      - *a.* 21-Hydroxylase deficiency
      - *b.* 11β-Hydroxylase deficiency
      - *c.* 3β-Hydroxysteroid dehydrogenase deficiency
    - 2. Defective estrogen synthesis
      - *a.* Aromatase deficiency
    - 3. Environmental hormones
      - *a.* Maternal virilizing disorders
      - *b.* Iatrogenic virilization
    - 4. Teratologic malformation
      - *a.* Abnormal development of vagina or uterus
      - *b.* Multiple congenital anomaly syndromes

The genetic abnormality arises from nondisjunction during the first or second meiotic division of gametogenesis. In 60 percent of cases, the nondisjunctional error is maternal; therefore, the frequency of this disorder is maternal age-dependent. Testis formation, paramesonephric duct regression, and mesonephric duct development are normal and the external genitalia are male, although micropenis may occur. There does not appear to be any excess prenatal wastage of 47,XXY embryos; the frequency in unselected newborns is approximately 1 per 1,000 males. As a group, 47,XXY infants have a tendency to lower birth weights and minor somatic anomalies such as clinodactyly, but a clinical diagnosis at this time is unusual. There is some evidence that cord serum testosterone concentrations may be lower than those of controls, but no data regarding the neonatal gonadotropin/testosterone surge are available.

During childhood many, but not all, patients with Klinefelter's syndrome show increased stature (above the 50th percentile), with relatively long legs, decreased head circumference, diminished verbal skills, emotional immaturity, and poor neuromuscular coordination. Penile length and testis volume are usually in the low-normal range. Before puberty the testes show reduced numbers of spermatogonia, but tubular hyalinization is not observed. Serum concentrations of FSH, LH, testosterone, and estradiol are in the normal prepubertal range, and responses to stimulation with GnRH and hCG are appropriate for age.[76]

Secondary sex characteristics usually appear at the normal age. Testis size often increases initially, but growth usually ceases before midpuberty at an average volume of 3.5 $\pm$ 1.5 ml.[77] Coincident with the onset of puberty, serum gonadotropin values increase abruptly to abnormal levels (Fig. 17-11). Presumably this hypergonadotropic state reflects diminished testosterone production; in turn, it leads to progressive hyalinization and fibrosis of seminiferous tubules, clumping of Leydig cells, and enhanced testicular secretion of estrogen. Spermatogenesis is rarely present except in a few isolated tubules. Because of tubular shrinkage the Leydig cells appear hyperplastic, but in fact Leydig cell volume is not affected. Serum estradiol concentrations tend to be high-normal, while serum testosterone concentrations fail to rise above the low-normal adult range. In 50–75 percent of unselected patients, clinically apparent gynecomastia develops; in contrast to benign juvenile gynecomastia, this often persists into adult life.

Virtually all adult 47,XXY subjects are azoospermic; the occasional report of paternity may reflect hidden XY/XXY mosaicism or the appearance of a clone of XY spermatocytes through mitotic nondisjunction. Clinical problems possibly related to androgen deficiency include a eunuchoid body habitus, persistent gynecomastia, reduced lean body mass, decreased libido and seminal volume, and a lack of social drive and aggressiveness. It is not clear to what extent these physical and psychosexual handicaps can be prevented or ameliorated by supplementation with exogenous androgens from early puberty.

In addition to consistently elevated values of serum FSH and LH, adults with Klinefelter's syndrome show reduced circulating levels of testosterone (276 $\pm$ 156 ng/dl) and dihydrotestosterone (28 $\pm$ 9.4 ng/dl) and increased levels of estradiol (2.8 $\pm$ 0.9 ng/dl); levels of adrenal androgens are not significantly different from normal. With advancing age, testicular function continues to decline, with a further decrease in serum testosterone levels and testosterone/estradiol ratios.

The prevalence of impaired glucose tolerance, chronic pulmonary disease, and varicose veins appears to be increased in

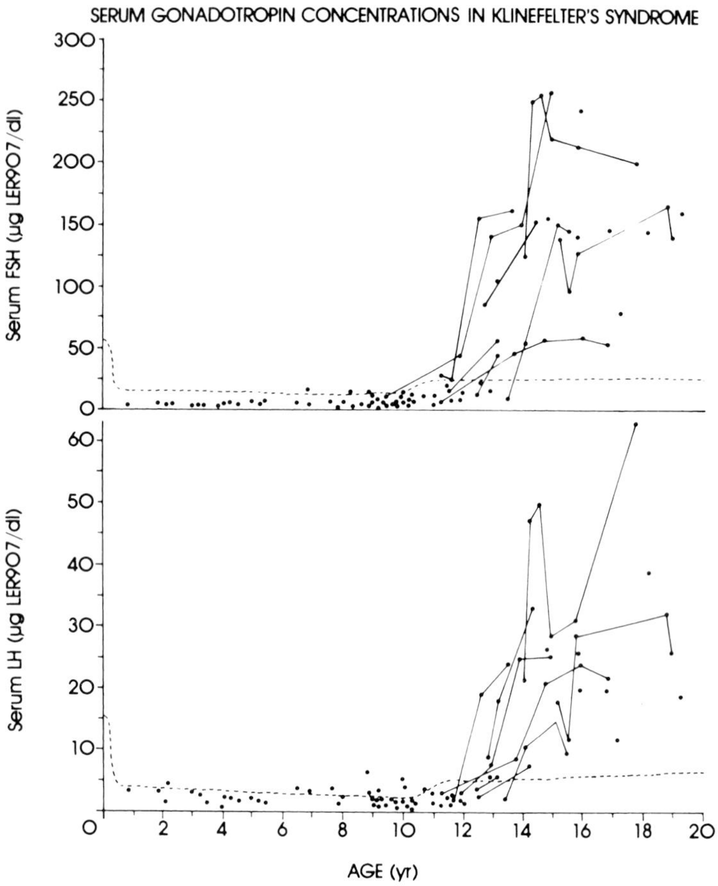

FIGURE 17-11. Basal serum FSH and LH concentrations in boys with Klinefelter's syndrome before and during puberty. The dotted lines show the upper limit of the normal male range. The gonadotropin values may be converted from micrograms of LER907 per deciliter to international units per liter by multiplying FSH by 0.5 and LH by 4.5. (*From Salbenblatt et al.*[76])

adults with Klinefelter's syndrome. In addition, there is a predisposition to various neoplasms, including germ cell tumors, bronchogenic carcinoma, acute lymphocytic leukemia, and carcinoma of the breast. The frequency of breast cancer in Klinefelter's syndrome patients is about 50 times that in normal men.[78]

The diagnosis of Klinefelter's syndrome may be suspected on the basis of the traditional phenotype but should be considered in any male with hypergonadotropic hypogonadism. The diagnosis is confirmed by karyotype analysis.

The most common variant form of Klinefelter's syndrome is 46,XY/47,XXY mosaicism; these patients show lesser degrees of hypogonadism, may be fertile, and may not complain of androgen deficiency until the fourth or fifth decade of life. Patients with more severe sex chromosome anomalies such as 48,XXYY, 48,XXXY, 49,XXXYY, and 49,XXXXY have the typical features of Klinefelter's syndrome but also are mentally retarded and show a wide range of somatic anomalies, particularly radioulnar synostosis, epiphyseal dysplasia, and patent ductus arteriosus. The presence of testes in these syndromes of X polysomy demonstrates the power of the Y chromosome to direct male gonadal differentiation.

The treatment of Klinefelter's syndrome is amelioration of hypergonadotropic hypogonadism and the resulting poor self-image. Most patients benefit psychologically and socially from surgery to reduce gynecomastia and administration of full replacement doses of testosterone esters, coupled with long-term counseling by an informed and sympathetic physician.

XYY Males

Strictly speaking, the 47,XYY karyotype, which occurs in about 1 in every 1,000 males, does not produce a disorder of sexual differentiation, as testicular, internal genital, and external genital development is male. There are no consistent physical anomalies, but hypotonia, delayed speech, and poor neuromuscular coordination appear to be relatively common. Tall stature is often described but is not a consistent finding. Testicular size is usually normal, but up to 10 percent of these individuals may have small testes. Adolescent and adult testicular endocrine function is normal, with no evidence of hypergonadotropic hypogonadism. Although many XYY males are fertile and presumably have normal seminiferous epithelium, biopsy studies of institutionalized adult patients have described variable but often severe abnormalities of spermatogenesis. The XYY disorder initially gained notoriety when it was discovered that its incidence was increased in criminals with persistent violent or aggressive behavior. It is now generally recognized that various sex chromosome anomalies, including but not limited to XYY, may be associated with behavioral difficulties in children and adults, but the suggestion that criminality may be the inevitable result is both naive and simplistic.

XX Males

Although phenotypic males with a 46,XX karyotype occur only once in every 30,000 male infants, this situation provides a useful illustration of the central role played in male sexual differentiation by the testis-determining gene locus found on the Y chromosome. Even though these persons lack a Y chromosome, they have testes which resemble histologically those of XXY males. Recent studies have demonstrated that in 80 percent of XX males X-Y interchange has occurred during paternal gametogenesis, with the testis-determining segment and other DNA sequences normally located on the Y chromosome being translocated to the short arm of the X chromosome; in turn, the paternal X chromosome can be shown to have lost genetic material from its short arm.[79,80] Such X-Y translocation, which presumably occurs during the pairing of the pseudoautosomal regions in meiosis, does not always lead to the development of testes but may result in gonadal dysgenesis with a female phenotype if the testis-determining locus is not involved or is inoperative.[81]

Clinically, XX males resemble those with Klinefelter's syndrome, although they tend to be somewhat shorter (mean height 168 cm). Their internal and external genitalia are usually normal, but hypospadias, cryptorchism, or more severe genital ambiguity occurs in about 10 percent of cases. The testes are small and soft, with uneven hyalinization, peritubular fibrosis, and Leydig cell clumping after the onset of puberty. Spermatogonia are usually absent, possibly because of premature commitment of the XX germ cells to meiosis. It is of interest that although two functioning X chromosomes are essential to the survival of germ cells in the ovary, they are detrimental to survival in a testicular environment. One-third of these patients develop significant gynecomastia. The hormonal profile of adult XX males confirms their hypergonadotropic hypogonadism, with increased serum concentrations of FSH and LH and reduced levels of testosterone. Basal and GnRH-stimulated androgen levels may be normal during childhood, as in Klinefelter's syndrome.

Sex Chromosome Anomalies Associated with Ovaries and Female Phenotype

A 47,XXX karyotype occurs in about 1 per 1,000 female infants, usually as a result of nondisjunction during maternal meiosis; thus, as in Klinefelter's syndrome, there is a maternal age effect. Sexual differentiation is female. No consistent pattern of somatic abnormalities is observed in this condition (trisomy X), but birth weight tends to be low and various minor anomalies have been reported.[82] Although one must be cautious regarding sampling bias due to investigation in institutions, triple-X females do seem to show a greater prevalence of mental retardation, cognitive dysfunction, and schizophreniform psychoses. There is a variable effect on oogenesis: about one-quarter of these patients experience some form of ovarian dysfunction, ranging from delayed menarche to premature ovarian failure, but fertility does occur. Naturally, the hormonal profile is dependent on the degree of ovarian dysfunction. Similar abnormalities, but usually associated with more severe somatic anomalies, have been described in association with 48,XXXX and 49,XXXXX karyotypes.

Sex Chromosome Anomalies Associated with Bisexual Gonadal Development

A person can be classified as a *true hermaphrodite* only if both testicular tissue with distinct tubules and ovarian tissue containing follicles or corpora albicantia are present. The more frequent finding of a dysgenetic gonad containing testicular elements plus fibrous stroma without follicles does not establish true hermaphroditism. About 30 percent of cases are classified as lateral, with a testis on one side and an ovary on the other; 50 percent have one ovotestis; and the rest have bilateral ovotestes containing distinct ovarian and testicular elements.[83,84]

Approximately two-thirds of true hermaphrodites show a 46,XX karyotype. Only in a minority of these individuals can the SRY gene be demonstrated, suggesting X-Y interchange during paternal gametogenesis, as in the XX male.[84,85] Thus interchange between the X and Y chromosomes may result in an XX male (with or without hypospadias), true hermaphroditism, or gonadal dysgenesis, depending presumably on the amount and efficacy of the translocated testis-determining DNA segment. Pedigrees containing both XX males and XX true hermaphrodites are thought to result from familial deletion of an X-linked locus or an autosomal recessive structural gene defect. The cause of testicular development in SRY negative 46,XX true hermophrodites may be unrecognized genetic mosaicism in the gonadal tissue or mutation of an autosomal or X-gene that permits testicular differentiation without SRY. The pathogenesis of the less common 46,XY form of true hermaphroditism is less clear but may involve undetected XX/XY chimerism. Such whole-body chimerism has been documented in several cases and presumably results from double fertilization (by an X and Y sperm) of a binucleate ovum or fusion of XX and XY zygotes. Finally, a few cases of XX/XXY mosaicism have been described as a result of the loss of a Y chromosome from a 47,XXY zygote at an early mitotic division. Thus, a variety of genetic mechanisms may be operative.

The clinical presentation of true hermaphroditism depends on the amount of functioning testicular tissue. In patients with a testis and an ovary, development of the mesonephric and paramesonephric ducts is consistent with the appearance of the ipsilateral gonad. With ovotestes, genital duct development is usually female. According to the level of circulating androgen, the external genitalia may appear female, may be ambiguous, or may be frankly masculine, although hypospadias and cryptorchism are common. Sometimes an inguinal hernia contains an ovotestis. At puberty virilization is variable. Breast development and menstruation are common, reflecting the low serum testosterone/estradiol ratio in most patients. If testicular function is minimal or if all testicular tissue has been removed, cyclical gonadotropin secretion, ovulation, and fertility may be observed. Spermatogenesis is rare, and male fertility has not been documented. Gonadal tumors, usually gonadoblastoma, dysgerminoma, or seminoma, occur in about 4 percent of true hermaphrodites.

The diagnosis of true hermaphroditism can be confirmed only by histologic examination of the gonads. In an infant the sex of rearing should be assigned according to the degree of virilization of the internal and external genitalia. Any discordant or dysgenetic gonadal tissue, together with inappropriate internal genital structures, should be removed, and plastic repair of the external genitalia should be undertaken. In children being raised as males because of the risk of malignancy it is probably wise to retain a testis only if it appears normal and is located in the scrotum. Appropriate sex hormone replacement will usually be required at the age of puberty.

Sex Chromosome Anomalies Associated with Dysgenetic Gonads

Structural Anomalies of the Y Chromosome

Abnormalities of the Y chromosome may include ring formation, deletions, dicentrics, inversions, and isochromosomes. Patients with extensive deletions of the short arm of Y may present with gonadal dysgenesis, a female phenotype, and the somatic stigmata of Turner's syndrome. Conversely, if the short arm is intact, testes and male sexual differentiation may develop. However, the abnormal Y chromosome is frequently lost during an early mitotic division, producing a variable proportion of 45,X cells and some degree of gonadal dysgenesis. The clinical picture then becomes that of mixed gonadal dysgenesis.

Mixed Gonadal Dysgenesis

It is not uncommon for a Y chromosome, particularly one that is structurally abnormal, to be lost from a 46,XY zygote as a result of anaphase lag or mitotic nondisjunction. The karyotype will then show 45,X as well as 46,XY and/or 47,XYY cell lines in varying proportions, and the phenotype will depend on the amount of testicular tissue present. If no testicular development occurs, the clinical presentation will be that of a female with bilateral streak gonads, although short stature and the somatic anomalies of Turner's syndrome (see later discussion) may be less obvious than in the pure 45,X patient.

The term *mixed gonadal dysgenesis* is applied to persons with 45,X/46,XY mosaicism in whom some prenatal virilization has occurred. These patients are SRY-positive and show either one dysgenetic testis (usually intraabdominal) and one streak gonad or bilateral testes, both usually dysgenetic to some degree. Internal genital differentiation depends on the functional integrity of the ipsilateral gonad, but usually one or both paramesonephric ducts fail to regress and a rudimentary uterus is present. Depending on the level of prenatal androgen secretion, the newborn patient may display isolated clitoral hypertrophy, ambiguous external genitalia, or even relatively normal male genitalia, with or without hypospadias.[86] Two-thirds of the reported patients have been raised as females.

The importance of identifying 45,X/46,XY mosaicism, regardless of the phenotype, lies in the potential for significant virilization at puberty and the propensity of the affected gonads to undergo malignant degeneration. In most cases there is fairly good correlation between the degree of genital masculinization and the secretion of testosterone at puberty; this can be assessed directly before puberty by observing the serum testosterone response to several days of hCG stimulation.

The risk of gonadal neoplasm, whether gonadoblastoma, dysgerminoma, or embryonal carcinoma, in patients with 45,X/46,XY mosaicism is approximately 20 percent overall and increases with age.[87] The risk of malignancy is probably highest in dysgenetic testes and lowest in streak gonads. The occurrence of spontaneous breast development nearly always signals the presence of an estrogen-secreting gonadoblastoma. Often a gonadal neoplasm can be detected with pelvic ultrasonography or computed tomography, but regardless of these findings or the clinical phenotype, it is a prudent policy to recommend prophylactic removal of streak gonads and undescended testes during the first decade in all children with 45,X/46,XY mosaicism. Occasionally in a phenotypic male, scrotal testes of normal consistency may be preserved. This requires close and continuing observation which should include annual testicular ultrasounds from the onset of puberty and testicular biopsy in the early adulthood.

Because of the continuum of genital differentiation seen in these patients, decisions regarding the sex of rearing should be based on the potential for normal genital function. In females, clitoroplasty and vaginoplasty should be undertaken in infancy. In males, all paramesonephric duct remnants should be removed, hypospadias repaired, and testicular prostheses placed in the scrotum. In either case, prophylactic gonadectomy is desirable, and appropriate sex steroid replacement will be needed at puberty.

Turner's Syndrome

Classic Turner's syndrome consists of bilateral gonadal dysgenesis with streak gonads, a female phenotype, and sexual infantilism plus short stature and a pattern of distinctive somatic stigmata (Fig. 17-12). The typical syndrome results from monosomy for the X chromosome (45,X), with or without mosaicism, but it may also be seen in patients with two sex chromosomes in which one (X or Y) is structurally defective, producing effective monosomy.

Comparison of the frequency of the 45,X karyotype in spontaneous abortions (approximately 1 in 15) and in live births (1 in 20,000) demonstrates that monosomy X is nearly always lethal in utero; surviving patients often show some degree of mosaicism, indicative of a postfertilization mitotic error. It is of interest that Turner's syndrome is more frequently associated with young maternal age.[88] In 80 percent of 45,X survivors, the single X chromosome is of maternal origin, suggesting preferential loss of the paternal sex chromosome either before or after fertilization. Mosaic forms commonly result from postzygotic loss of a sex chromosome that is structurally abnormal. Monozygotic twinning appears to be more frequent in such mosaicism situations; the twins may be discordant for the Turner's syndrome phenotype because of heterogeneous distribution of the 45,X and other (usually XX, XY, or XXX) cell lines.

The indifferent gonad of the 45,X fetus forms normally and is seeded by germ cells that become incorporated into primordial follicles. However, the rate of follicular atresia and degeneration is greatly increased, so that by birth only a few primary follicles remain. Almost always these, too, disappear before puberty, leaving fibrous streak gonads, the consequence of which is sexual infantilism and primary amenorrhea. As one would expect, the internal and external genitalia are female. Any sign of prenatal or postnatal virilization indicates the presence of a Y-bearing cell line and some testicular tissue (mixed gonadal dysgenesis).

Generalized lymphedema with hygromatous neck masses is characteristic of 45,X fetuses. In newborn infants this same lymphatic hypoplasia can produce the Bonnevie-Ullrich syndrome, with distal lymphedema, loose skin folds at the nape, ascites, and pleural effusion. Birth weight and length are usually low for gestational age.

During childhood, the dominant clinical feature is short stature due to loss of a gene, SHOX, in the pseudoautosomal region of the short arm.[11] Growth in the first 3–5 years may be reasonably normal, but still 75 percent of these girls have a height less than the 5th percentile for age. By 11 years of age, 95 percent have a height less than the 5th percentile due to significant decline in growth velocity after age 5 years. Because of the sexual infantilism, untreated patients show no pubertal growth spurt, and radiologic bone maturation becomes retarded after 11 years of age. The mean adult height is 143 cm, but height can range up to 155 cm, depending on parental stature.[89,90]

Accompanying this short stature is often a characteristic pattern of somatic abnormalities (Fig. 17-12). The skull is brachycephalic, and the facies are distinctive, with a triangular shape, a retruded mandible, epicanthal folds, ptosis, and a narrow high palate. The ears are low-set and often deformed. The nuchal hairline is low and the neck is short in most cases, but frank webbing of the neck (pterygium colli) occurs in only 40 percent. The chest is usually square or shield-shaped, the nipples are relatively wide spaced, and pectus excavatum may be present. There are commonly many pigmented nevi over the face, arms, and chest.

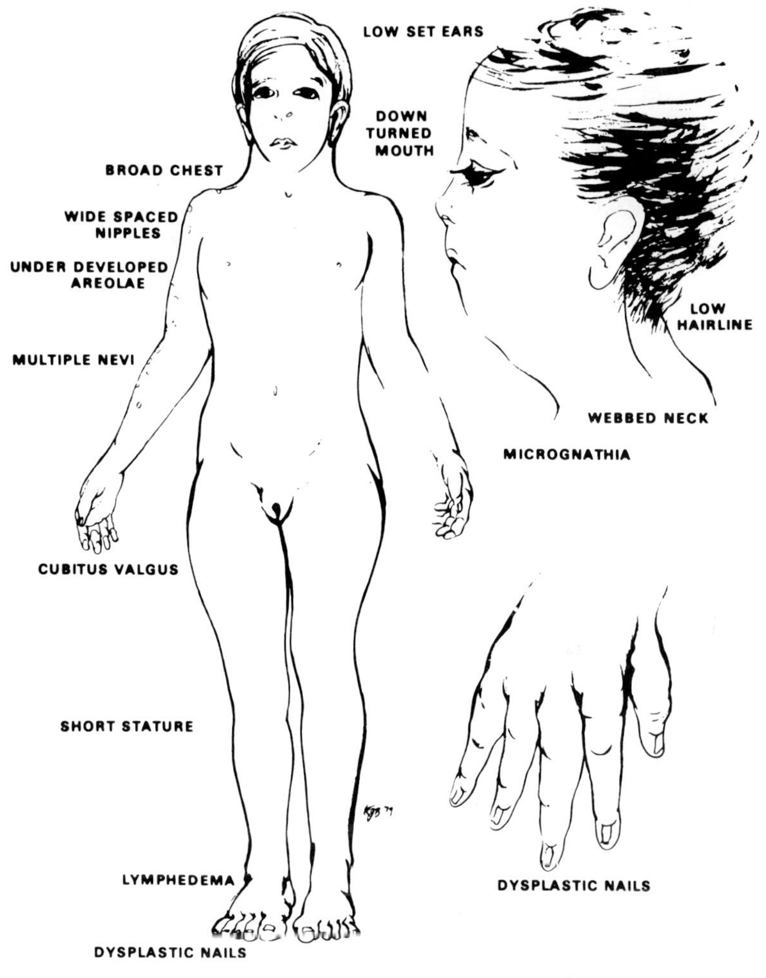

FIGURE 17-12. The major clinical features of a child with Turner's syndrome (45,X gonadal dysgenesis). [*From Dean HJ, Winter JSD, in Collu C, Ducharme JR, Guyda H (eds): Pediatric Endocrinology, 2nd ed. New York, Raven, 1989, p. 345.*]

Anomalies of the extremities include cubitus valgus (in about 50 percent), lymphedema or puffiness of the hands and feet, shortening of the fourth metacarpal, and hypoplastic nails. Kyphoscoliosis is not uncommon. Some of the skeletal abnormalities appear to also be due to the haploinsufficiency of SHOX. Renal anomalies, including unilateral aplasia, horseshoe kidney, and ureteral duplication, are found in 60 percent of cases. Bicuspid aortic valve is the most common cardiovascular anomaly (34–50 percent), but coarctation of the aorta, ventricular septal defect, aortic stenosis, and aortic aneurysm also occur. Occasionally gastrointestinal bleeding may result from congenital intestinal telangiectasia. Strabismus is not uncommon, and there may be hearing loss due to a sensorineural deficit or recurrent otitis media. Although most 45,X patients have normal intelligence and the incidence of severe psychopathology is not increased, they frequently demonstrate social immaturity and problems with visuospatial ability and mathematics.[91] Social adjustment appears to partly depend on whether the retained X is maternally or paternally derived.[92] Individuals with monosomy X from the father have better social cognition than if the X is from the mother.

Radiographic examination often discloses characteristic bony anomalies, including shortening of the fourth metacarpal, the "carpal sign," or a reduced angle in the proximal row of carpals, basilar impression of the skull, hypoplasia of cervical vertebrae, and occasional areas of aseptic necrosis, particularly around the knee. In adults who have not received sex steroids, osteoporosis may become severe. Reactive enlargement of the pituitary fossa has also been described in adult patients with long-standing untreated hypergonadotropic hypogonadism. Excretory urography commonly discloses structural or positional abnormalities of the kidney, occasionally associated with significant ureteropelvic obstruction.

Several other disorders appear to be increased in patients with Turner's syndrome. Hypertension unrelated to aortic coarctation or renal disease occurs in about half of adult patients; although the initial rise in blood pressure occurs during the second decade, there does not seem to be an obvious relation to estrogen therapy. The risk of developing autoimmune endocrine disease, particularly of the thyroid, is considerably increased. Antithyroid antibodies indicative of chronic lymphocytic thyroiditis can be detected in about a third of these patients, and many of them in time develop goiter or become hypothyroid. Impaired carbohydrate tolerance can frequently be demonstrated, but frank diabetes mellitus is less common. Other autoimmune disorders, such as rheumatoid arthritis and inflammatory bowel disease, appear to be more frequent in Turner's syndrome. Keloid formation is also more common.

Phenotype-Karyotype Correlations The key genetic determinants absent in Turner's syndrome appear to be on the short arm of the X or Y chromosome, and the severity of the clinical presentation to some extent correlates with the amount of this loss. Patients with complete monosomy (45,X) or an isochromosome for the long arm [46,X,iso(Xq)] usually show the classic syndrome, with short stature, sexual infantilism, and multiple somatic stigmata. These patients are unlikely to show aortic coarctation or severe lymphedema but appear to be more at risk for developing autoimmune disorders such as Hashimoto's disease and diabetes mellitus. Patients with major deletions of the short arm [46,X(Xp)] or a ring X chromosome [46,X,r(X)] tend to have fewer somatic stigmata, while those with deletions of the long arm [46,X(Xq)] usually present with only sexual infantilism or primary amenorrhea, are of normal stature, and show none of the usual somatic stigmata. However, structurally abnormal sex chromosomes are frequently lost during an early mitotic division, leading to a variable proportion of 45,X cells, which will naturally confute phenotype-karyotype generalizations. For the same reason, the buccal smear may be chromatin-negative or chromatin-positive, depending on the relative proportion of 45,X and 46,XX cells in that tissue. Occasionally a clue to the presence of an isochromosome or major deletion may be provided by a sex chromatin body that is larger or smaller than normal.

There have been many reports of breast development, menses, and even fertility in patients with Turner's syndrome.[93] The incidence of spontaneous puberty with 45,X is 5–15 percent, but the presence of a cell-line with a second X appears to double the incidence. However, if mosaicism cannot be detected in peripheral leukocytes, it may be impossible to determine whether this spontaneous ovarian function represents hidden mosaicism or the rare survival of a 45,X oocyte. To date most reported patients with 45,X/46,XX mosaicism with secondary amenorrhea have also had short stature, but it is not clear to what extent this represents sampling bias.

Several interesting patients have demonstrated either pericentric inversion or balanced X-X or X-autosome translocation; that is, breakage and structural rearrangement of segments of the X chromosome without any detectable loss of genetic material. These studies demonstrate that there is a critical segment on the long arm of X (between bands Xq13 and Xq27) which is essential for normal gonadal development.[94] Females with break points or rearrangements affecting this segment often suffer from primary or secondary amenorrhea; males with the same defect may show disturbed spermatogenesis.

As described previously, patients with 45,X/46,XY or 45,X/47,XYY mosaicism may show varying degrees of virilization, depending on the amount of functional testicular tissue. Not only may their genital development be female, ambiguous, or male, the degree of short stature and the frequency of somatic anomalies are also highly variable. At puberty, they may be virilized because of Leydig cell activity, may remain sexually infantile because of gonadal dysgenesis, or may be feminized because of an estrogen-secreting gonadal neoplasm. Because of the propensity to develop gonadoblastoma or malignant germinoma, the risk of which approaches 20 percent in the second decade, the streak gonads or dysgenetic testes of any patient with 45,X/46,XY mosaicism should be removed. There is not yet sufficient reproducible data to indicate that all Turner's syndrome patients should be screened for Y mosaicism by molecular DNA techniques. Analysis by Southern blotting with Y specific probes or polymerase chain reaction using Y primers suggests a prevalence of undetected Y chromosome DNA in 1–3.5 percent of Turner's syndrome patients.[95] Higher rates of mosaicism may have been found if multiple tissues were studied. However, until more data is available or the gonadoblastoma gene on Yq is identified, molecular studies for Y DNA should be reserved for those with prenatal or pubertal virilization or those with an unidentified chromosome fragment. In classic Turner's syndrome, prophylactic gonadectomy does not appear to be necessary.

Diagnosis and Treatment A definitive diagnosis of Turner's syndrome requires careful karyotype analysis, including banding and study of sufficient cells to confirm or exclude mosaicism. In equivocal situations, particularly when the presence of a Y-bearing or 45,X cell line is critical to patient management, consideration should be given to genetic analysis of additional tissues such as skin fibroblasts. Because of the relatively high proportion of patients with mosaicism, a buccal smear for sex chromatin is an inadequate diagnostic technique.

In the evaluation of females with short stature or late puberty, a clue to the presence of gonadal dysgenesis may be the finding of serum FSH concentrations above the age-specific normal range (Fig. 17-13). In contrast to the situation in Klinefelter's syndrome, children with gonadal dysgenesis will usually show high serum FSH levels[96] and exaggerated responses to stimulation with exogenous GnRH. Even though the absence of gonadal negative feedback leads to increased gonadotropin secretion, the pattern of serum gonadotropin values in agonadal children parallels that in normal girls, with higher values in infancy, a decline in midchildhood, and a rise to the postmenopausal range again at the normal time of puberty.

The short stature of patients with Turner's syndrome is due to a combination of intrauterine growth retardation, subnormal growth velocity during childhood, and lack of a pubertal growth spurt. Spontaneous and stimulated growth hormone levels are normal during childhood but may decline after age 9 years, presumably because of the absence of sex steroid. The current availability of biosynthetic growth hormone has led to numerous studies of its efficacy and safety. Several uncontrolled studies have shown an increase in both short-term growth rate and final height as compared to pretreatment predicted height.[97–99] A randomized controlled trial has demonstrated a mean final height gain of 5 cm from growth hormone therapy (Canadian Growth Hormone Advisory Committee, unpublished data). The variability in response (0–10 cm final height gain) in part seems to relate to age at commencing growth hormone, age at commencing estrogen replacement, and use of oxandrolone with growth hormone. Nevertheless, these results indicate growth hormone should be offered to girls with Turner's syndrome once growth failure is noted.

Patients with Turner's syndrome show normal serum levels of adrenal androgens and a normal adrenarchal rise in these values before the age of puberty; thereafter, because of deficient gonadal contribution, serum testosterone and androstenedione concentrations are slightly lower than in normal females.[100] Several studies have demonstrated improved growth velocity in patients treated with low doses of exogenous androgen (fluoxymesterone or oxandrolone, 0.1–0.3 mg/kg of body weight per day), but it has been difficult to ascertain whether such treatment has a significant effect on eventual adult size.[101] Low doses of ethinyl estradiol (100 ng/kg per day) can also increase short-term growth velocity,[102] but with longer periods of therapy skeletal maturation may be accelerated, with little effect on final height.[103] All patients with gonadal dysgenesis require sex steroid therapy for normal sec-

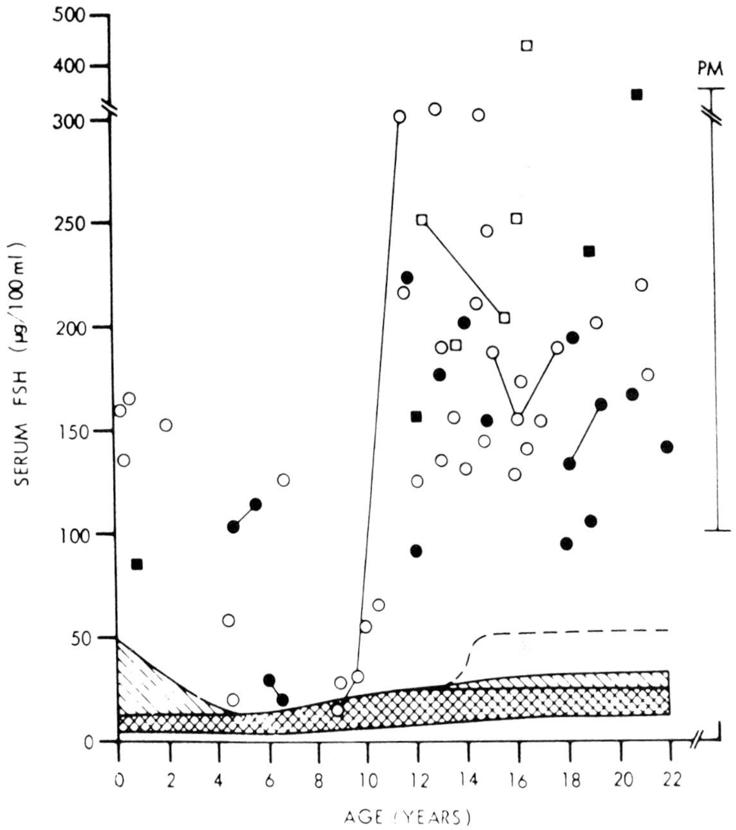

FIGURE 17-13. Serum FSH concentrations in agonadal subjects. The normal male and female ranges are shown by the hatched areas. The dotted line represents the adult female midcycle peak, and the bar (PM) represents the postmenopausal range. Patients with gonadal dysgenesis are shown by open circles. (*From Winter and Faiman.*[96])

ondary sex characteristics. Our approach has been to initiate estrogen replacement in low doses (ethinyl estradiol, 5 µg per day, or 0.3 mg conjugated estrogen) at an age (usually 13–14 years) slightly older than the patient's peers begin puberty. This will elicit gradual development of breasts and pubic hair and appears to induce at least a temporary acceleration of growth.[104] However, the optimal age for introducing estrogen, both for growth and psychosocial adjustment, requires further study. After 6–12 months, the dose of estrogen can be increased (ethinyl estradiol 20 µg or 0.625 mg conjugated estrogen). Because of the significant risk of developing endometrial hyperplasia and carcinoma in patients treated only with estrogen, it is essential that after 6–24 months patients be switched to a combination estrogen-progestin preparation administered in cyclic fashion.

Those who have spontaneous puberty are likely to undergo early menopause. They should, however, be provided with appropriate contraception advise and be referred for genetic counselling as pregnancy is possible, although there is increased risk of fetal anomalies and miscarriage.[105] In vitro fertilization is an option for Turner's syndrome women who have streak gonads.[106] Other general health issues for Turner's syndrome patients need to be followed as outlined in published practice guidelines.[107,108]

Anomalies of Gonadogenesis Without Chromosomal Abnormality

Defective Ovary Formation

Defective ovary formation is exemplified by *XX gonadal dysgenesis*, in which patients have bilateral streak gonads but normal stature, a 46,XX karyotype, and none of the somatic stigmata of Turner's syndrome. Their internal and external genitalia are normal female, and the diagnosis is not suspected until sexual infantilism and hypergonadotropic hypogonadism become apparent at the normal age of puberty. Familial aggregation is common, and siblings may show hypoplastic ovaries and precocious menopause, suggesting variable expression of the basic genetic disorder. In several families gonadal dysgenesis and sensorineural deafness were observed together, but it is not clear whether this represented varied expression of a single mutant gene or coincident occurrence of two genetic disorders. An occasional patient has shown signs of postpubertal virilization, which was thought to reflect hilus cell hyperplasia within the streak gonads in response to high circulating gonadotropin levels. Gonadal neoplasia does not seem to be a feature of XX gonadal dysgenesis.

The common finding of consanguinity in affected families points to the presence of a rare X-linked or autosomal recessive gene that must be present in double dose to prevent normal ovarian development.[109] Genetic heterogeneity seems likely, as occasionally patients show short stature or various neurologic deficits. The pathogenesis remains obscure, but presumably the mutant gene acts to impair oogonial maturation and follicle formation or to accelerate the rate of germ cell attrition, as in Turner's syndrome. Because of the genetic implications of this disorder, it is important to rule out 45,X/46,XX mosaicism with great care. Treatment of the hypergonadotropic hypogonadism is carried out with replacement estrogen and progestin, as in other forms of gonadal dysgenesis.

Defective Testis Formation

XY Gonadal Dysgenesis (Swyer Syndrome) If in spite of normal male genetic sex (46,XY) testes fail to develop, the phenotypic result will be XY gonadal dysgenesis with streak gonads, female internal and external genitalia, and sexual infantilism at the time of puberty. The short stature and somatic stigmata of Turner's syndrome are not features of this syndrome and, if present, probably indicate undetected 45,X/46,XY mosaicism.

XY gonadal dysgenesis is a heterogeneous group clinically and genetically. Some are due to mutations in SRY,[15,110] SF-1,[29] and WT-1.[26,27] In cases with WT-1 deletions or mutations, there are associated renal anomalies, as previously discussed. SOX-9 mutations appear responsible for the XY gonadal dysgenesis associated with campomelic dwarfism.[31,33] Still other cases have been described with deletion or monosomy of 9p24,[111] and others appear due to duplication of the DAX-1 gene.[22] However, to date the majority of cases do not have a known gene mutation or deletion.

Regardless of the etiology, the usual clinical presentation is a phenotypic female with sexual infantilism and primary amenorrhea. Clitoromegaly can occur in untreated adults because of hyperstimulation of androgen-secreting hilus cells in the streak gonads. Spontaneous breast development does not occur unless an estrogen-secreting neoplasm appears.

As in other forms of defective testis development, there is a 20–30 percent risk of gonadal neoplasm, mainly gonadoblastoma or dysgerminoma. Therefore, prophylactic gonadectomy is recommended for all patients with XY gonadal dysgenesis. Sex hormone replacement should be initiated in the same manner as in other forms of gonadal dysgenesis.

Dysgenetic Male Pseudohermaphroditism The term *dysgenetic male pseudohermaphroditism* does not define a distinct clinical entity but rather is a catchall phrase to describe patients with a 46,XY karyotype who present with bilateral dysgenetic testes (usually intraabdominal), incomplete masculinization with ambiguous external genitalia, and variable persistence of paramesonephric duct structures. In most such patients the disorder is not familial. It seems likely that many of these patients have a subtle structural anomaly of the Y chromosome [e.g., 46,X(Yp) or 46,X(Yp)/46,XY mosaicism] or represent unrecognized cases of 45,X/46,XY mosaicism. The latter situation may prove impossible to detect if selective pressures mitigate against survival of the 45,X cell line in peripheral leukocytes or fibroblasts. Other patients may represent a less severe variant of XY gonadal dysgenesis with some testicular differentiation. These cases likely have different mutations of the same genes mentioned above. For example, the Denys-Drash and WAGR syndrome have ambiguous genitalia and renal anomalies due to mutations in WT-1.[28] Most of these patients will show some virilization at puberty if their testes remain, and they are at high risk of developing a gonadoblastoma or germinoma. As in any intersex situation in which sterility is inevitable, sex of rearing should be assigned to provide the greatest opportunity for normal genital function. Because of the high risk of neoplasia, early prophylactic gonadectomy should be performed; appropriate sex steroid replacement will be necessary at the time of puberty.

Testicular Regression Syndromes The general term *testicular regression syndrome* applies to a heterogeneous group of conditions in which, for largely undetermined reasons, there is a cessation of testicular function during fetal life. Obviously, the pathogenesis of these conditions is closely related to that of XY gonadal dysgenesis and dysgenetic male pseudohermaphroditism. As shown in Table 17-4, the clinical phenotype depends on the degree of testicular function and its duration during sexual differentiation. Any of these disorders may be familial.

So-called true agonadism probably is a variant form of dysgenetic male pseudohermaphroditism in which there is some testicular function during early development, after which the testes disappear.[112] The external genitalia are ambiguous, with a phallus the size of an enlarged clitoris, partial labioscrotal fusion, and a persistent urogenital sinus; both paramesonephric and mesonephric ductal structures are absent. Stimulation testing with chorionic gonadotropin in later life may sometimes induce a slight rise in plasma testosterone, even though testes cannot be found. Associated craniofacial or vertebral anomalies have occasionally been observed, suggesting the action of a teratogen or an underlying connective tissue defect.

Complete regression of the testes after 20 weeks gestation leads to congenital anorchia, in which male sexual differentiation is complete but testes are absent. This situation can be distinguished from cryptorchism by the finding of high levels of serum FSH[96] and a failure of serum testosterone to rise after stimulation with hCG.[113] The mechanism underlying this late regression of the testes is unknown but is thought to involve torsion or occulusion of the testicular vascular supply.[114]

Errors of Sexual Differentiation

Once structurally normal gonads have been formed, it is still possible for sexual differentiation to be aberrant if the testes are unable to accomplish normal masculinization of a genetic male (male pseudohermaphroditism) or if an abnormal source of androgen induces inappropriate prenatal virilization of a genetic female (female pseudohermaphroditism).

Persistent Paramesonephric Ducts

A failure of paramesonephric (müllerian) duct regression, ranging from simple enlargement of the prostatic utricle to complete preservation of a uterus and tubes, is expected in disor-

TABLE 17-4. Clinical Features of Testicular Dysgenesis Syndromes

	XY Gonadal Dysgenesis	True Agonadism	Rudimentary Testes	Congenital Anorchia
Genetic sex	46,XY	46,XY	46,XY	46,XY
Time of testis dysfunction (gestational)	Before 8 weeks	8–12 weeks	14–20 weeks	After 20 weeks
External genitalia	Female	Ambiguous	Micropenis	Male
Vagina	Complete	Blind pouch	Absent	Absent
Paramesonephric structures	Present	Rudimentary	Absent	Absent
Mesonephric structures	Absent	Absent	Present	Present
Gonads	Streak	Absent	Rudimentary testis	Absent

Source: Cleary, Caras, Rosenfield, and Young.[112]

ders of testicular dysgenesis, in which case one also sees impaired testosterone-dependent differentiation. However, more than 150 genetic males with normal male external genitalia have been reported in whom were found a cervix, uterus, and fallopian tubes in addition to normal mesonephric duct structures.[115] This situation, referred to as *persistent müllerian duct syndrome* or *hernia uteri inguinalis*, presents most commonly (90 percent) as unilateral cryptorchidism with contralateral inguinal hernia; less common presentation is bilateral cryptorchidism. Testicular endocrine function is normal, spermatogenesis occurs, but development anomalies of the vasa deferentia, epidydidymis, and tunica albuginea may lead to problems with fertility. The disorder is due to either mutations in the MIS gene or in the type II MIS receptor. Serum levels of MIS will distinguish between these 2 possibilities, being low in the former and high in the latter. Both these genes are autosomal. Defects in the MIS gene must be present in both alleles, consistent with autosomal recessive inheritance. Only about half the patients with type II receptor mutations are homozygous, and in these cases the defect is in the ligand-binding domain. The remaining patients have a mutation affecting the intracellular domain that prevents transcriptional responses. These individuals are hetrozygous, indicating the defect produces a dominant negative effect. Females with either MIS or its receptor gene mutations have normal pubertal development and fertility, indicating MIS is not required for reproduction in women. The treatment of affected males requires orchidopexy with proximal salpingectomy and partial hysterectomy in order to preserve fertility.

Defective Genital Virilization (Male Pseudohermaphroditism)

Leydig Cell Hypoplasia

Leydig cell agenesis or hypoplasia is an autosomal recessive condition due to genetic defects in the LH-hCG receptor, resulting in Leydig cell unresponsiveness to gonadotropic stimulation and inadequate testosterone production before and after birth.[116] These are 46,XY patients with female external genitalia, absent paramesonephric duct structures, small intraabdominal testes lacking any Leydig cells, and a lack of serum testosterone response to exogenous hCG. Partial virilization may occur depending on the mutation.[117] Phenotypic females will require gonadectomy and estrogen therapy in adolescence and adulthood. More virilized infants raised as males should receive testosterone for phallic lengthening in infancy and will require testosterone for puberty.

Inborn Errors

Testosterone Biosynthesis Of the five known inborn errors of testosterone synthesis, three also impair adrenal secretion of cortisol and therefore cause variant forms of congenital adrenal hyperplasia (Fig. 17-14). In all cases prenatal androgen deficiency in affected genetic males results in either a female external genetic phenotype or ambiguous genitalia; at puberty there is sexual infantilism in both males and females because of the inability to produce any sex steroids.

Steroidogenic Acute Regulatory (StAR) Protein Deficiency (Congenital Lipoid Adrenal Hyperplasa) Whether in the testis, ovary, or adrenal cortex, the initial and rate-limiting step in steroid hormone biosynthesis is transport of cholesterol across the outer to the inner mitochondrial membrane. This transfer is mediated by a 30-kD protein, *steroidogenic acute regulatory protein (StAR)*, whose gene is on the short arm of chromosome 8.[118,119] StAR is expressed in all steroidogenic tissues except the placenta. SF-1 is required for StAR expression, as it is for all the steroidogenic enzymes. Expression is also induced by ACTH and LH via cyclic AMP and by angiotension II and potassium acting through calcium signalling in the adrenal glomerulosa.[120,121]

Mutations of StAR result in an inability to synthesize sex steroids, glucocorticoids, or mineralocorticoids. Patients with such mutations have the severest form of congenital adrenal hyperplasia. Their adrenals are enlarged and laden with cholesterol esters, hence the term *congenital lipoid adrenal hyperplasia*. Patients usually present with severe salt wasting crisis within a few days to weeks of birth and die without replacement therapy. Affected males have female genitalia, hypoplastic mesonephric duct structures, and a blind vaginal pouch. Affected females have normal internal and external genitalia. Besides having evidence of adrenal crisis with severe dehydration, hyponatremia, hypercalcemia, and hypokalemia, all steroids are usually low, especially for the degree of illness; ACTH and renin are elevated. There is no response to stimulation with synthetic ACTH or hCG. Affected genetic females can be distinguished from congenital adrenal hypoplasia by imaging the adrenals, which reveals enlarged glands engorged with lipid in StAR deficiency. Affected males with female external genitalia should be raised as females and the testes removed. Leydig cell function is severely damaged by the build-up of cholesterol esters early in fetal life. However, ovarian cells remain undamaged until puberty because the fetal ovary is not active in steroidogenesis. Prenatal diagnosis is possible by measuring amniotic fluid steroid levels.[122]

Molecular analysis of the StAR gene in affected individuals has to date revealed mutations confined to the C-terminus of the protein.[123,124] All patients are either homozygotes or compound heterozygotes confirming autosomal recessive inheritance. Carriers for this condition can only be determined by gene analysis because stimulated steroid responses are normal.

This condition was previously thought to be due to a deficiency of the cholesterol side-chain cleavage enzyme, which converts cholesterol to pregnenolone. However, analysis of the P450scc, adrenodoxin, and adrenodoxin reductase genes from individuals with congenial lipoid adrenal hyperplasia failed to reveal any mutations.[125] Because such defects would also affect placental steroidogenesis, it is probable that such a defect is not compatible with life.[126]

3β-Hydroxysteroid Dehydrogenase Deficiency All human biologically active steroid hormones, whether of adrenal or gonadal origin, have in common a Δ^4-3-keto configuration. The enzyme complex responsible for conversion of pregnenolone, 17-hydroxypregnenolone, and dehydroepiandrosterone to their respective Δ^4-3-keto forms (progesterone, 17-hydroxyprogesterone, and androstenedione) is 3β-hydroxysteroid dehydrogenase/isomerase, which utilizes NAD as a cofactor and is located in the smooth endoplasmic reticulum, with lesser amounts in mitochondria. In the human, 2 isozymes (type I and II) have been isolated and the genes cloned.[127,128] Both genes (HSD3B1, HSD3B2) are on the short arm of chromosome 1; there are also 3 known pseudogenes. Type I 3βHSD is expressed in placenta, skin, and adipose tissue, while the type II enzyme is expressed only in the adrenal and gonad. One remarkable characteristic of the type II enzyme is its susceptibility to inhibition by micromolar concentrations of

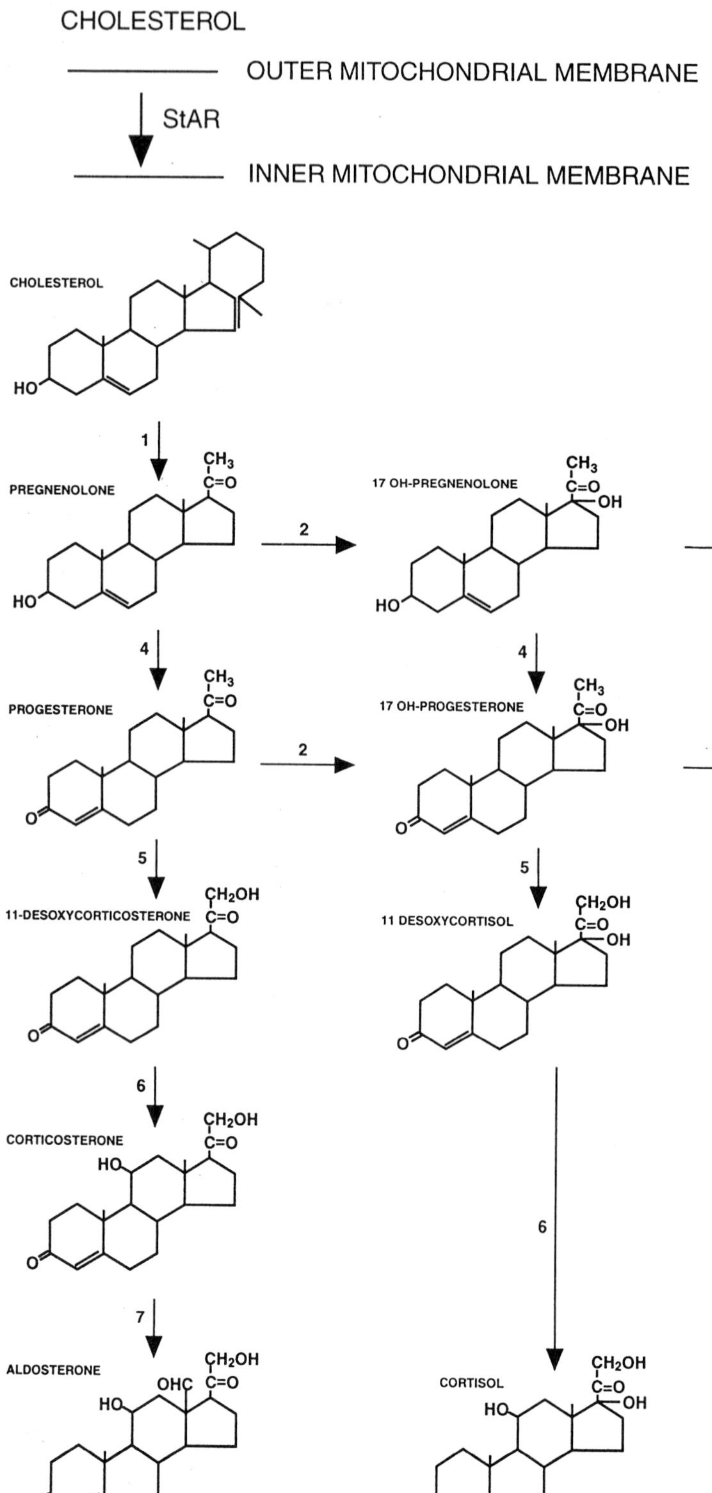

FIGURE 17-14. Pathways of steroidogenesis in the adrenal cortex and gonads. The protein and enzymes involved include steroidogenic acute regulatory protein (StAR); cytochrome $P450_{scc}$ (cholesterol side-chain cleavage) [1]; cytochrome $P450_{C17}$ (responsible for both 17-hydroxylase [2] and 17,20-desmolase [3]); 3β-hydroxysteroid dehydrogenase/isomerase [4]; cytochrome $P450_{C21}$ (21-hydroxylase) [5]; cytochrome $P450_{C11}$ (responsible for 11β-hydroxylase [6], aldosterone synthase [7]); 17β-hydroxysteroid dehydrogenase [8]; and cytochrome $P450_{arom}$ (aromatase) [9].

circulating or intraadrenal steroids. Changes in ambient steroid concentrations appear to account for shifts in adrenal 3β-HSD activity during development[129]; thus in fetal and adult life, 3β-HSD normally becomes a rate-limiting step in cortisol biosynthesis, and large amounts of dehydroepiandrosterone are secreted by the adrenal cortex.

Infants affected with autosomal recessive 3β-HSD deficiency typically present with ambiguous genitalia plus severe adrenal insufficiency. The genitalia of affected females may be normal or show mild clitoromegaly, presumably a result of peripheral transformation of adrenal dehydroepiandrosterone to testosterone. Salt wasting is present in cases with complete enzyme deficiency. At puberty there is no spontaneous breast development. Affected males typically show a small hypospadic phallus, partially fused labioscrotal folds, and a urogenital sinus with a blind vaginal pouch. Paramesonephric duct structures are absent, but surprisingly, mesonephric duct structures are normal, indicating that the prenatal testis was capable of some androgen production. At the time of puberty males show hypergonadotropic hypogonadism, with gynecomastia, inadequate masculinization, and spermatogenic arrest.

The diagnosis of 3β-HSD deficiency requires demonstration of increased concentrations of Δ^5-3β-hydroxysteroids such as pregnenolone, dehydroepiandrosterone, Δ^5-androstenediol, and 17-hydroxypregnenolone in serum or increased urinary excretion of their metabolites (pregnenetriol and 16-pregnenetriol). During the neonatal period attention must be paid to the normally high excretion of Δ^5-3β-hydroxysteroids at this time. Therapy for this disorder requires glucocorticoid and mineralocorticoid replacement from birth and appropriate sex steroid replacement at puberty. Affected males should receive sufficient testosterone in infancy to correct the micropenis and permit satisfactory repair of hypospadias.

All patients with classical 3β-HSD deficiency have to date been found to have a mutation in both alleles of the HSD3B2 gene and a normal HSD3B1 gene. Thus the defect is limited to the adrenal and gonad; placental steroidogenesis is unaffected and peripheral conversion of 17-hydroxyprognenolone by the normal type I enzyme probably accounts for the mildly increased levels of 17-hydroxyprogesterone in these patients. Frameshift or nonsense mutations which destroy all type II enzymatic activity have been found in patients with the salt-wasting form.[130]

Elevated ratios of Δ^5-hydroxysteroids to Δ^4-ketosteroids in the presence of premature pubic hair growth or hirsutism and amenorrhea in postpubertal females has led to the suggestion that a milder, nonclassical form of 3β-HSD deficiency exists.[131,132] However, no mutation of either HSD3B1 or HSD3B2 has been found in these patients.[133,134]

17α-Hydroxylase Deficiency Conversion of pregnenolone to 17-hydroxypregnenolone takes place in the adrenal cortex, testicular Leydig cells, and ovarian theca and granulosa cells. The enzyme complex, which is located in the smooth endoplasmic reticulum, is a typical mixed-function oxidase; NADPH is the preferred electron donor, and the electron transport system involves a flavoprotein which interacts directly with the terminal cytochrome P450. This cytochrome P450 (59,000 dalton) has been purified and shown to have not only 17α-hydroxylase but also 17,20-desmolase activity.[135] A single gene, CYP17, located on chromosome 10q24.3 and expressed in adrenals and gonads, codes for this single enzyme with dual function.[136] Several different molecular defects in the coding sequence of this gene that affected both activities equally have been described.[137]

In males, deficiency of 17α-hydroxylase results in variable genital ambiguity and mesonephric duct differentiation. The phenotype may vary from apparently female external genitalia with a blind vaginal pouch to a hypospadic male with micropenis (Fig. 17-15). The testes are normally formed and may be intraabdominal, inguinal, or in the labioscrotal folds. Affected females have normal internal and external development. Hypertension, with or without hypokalemic alkalosis, due to excessive adrenal secretion of mineralocorticoids such as deoxycorticosterone, becomes evident by 2 years of age.[138] In both sexes there is failure of sexual maturation at puberty, although untreated males usually develop gynecomastia.

The diagnosis of 17α-hydroxylase deficiency can be confirmed by demonstrating increased serum concentrations of pregnenolone, progesterone, corticosterone, and deoxycorticosterone, with increased urinary excretion of their metabolites. Plasma renin activity and serum aldosterone levels are usually suppressed,[139] but plasma ACTH is increased. Occasionally circulating aldosterone levels are increased; such patients may appear to have primary hyperaldosteronism or dexamethasone-suppressible hyperaldosteronism. Affected males show low serum testosterone and cortisol values, with inadequate responses to hCG and ACTH. Serum FSH and LH levels are elevated into the age-specific agonadal range because of the lack of sex steroid-mediated feedback inhibition.

Replacement glucocorticoid therapy (cortisol, 10–20 mg/m^2 daily) suppresses corticosterone and deoxycorticosterone secre-

FIGURE 17-15. External genitalia of a male with 17-hydroxylase deficiency at 10 months of age. Testes were palpable in the labioscrotal folds. (*From Dean et al.*[138])

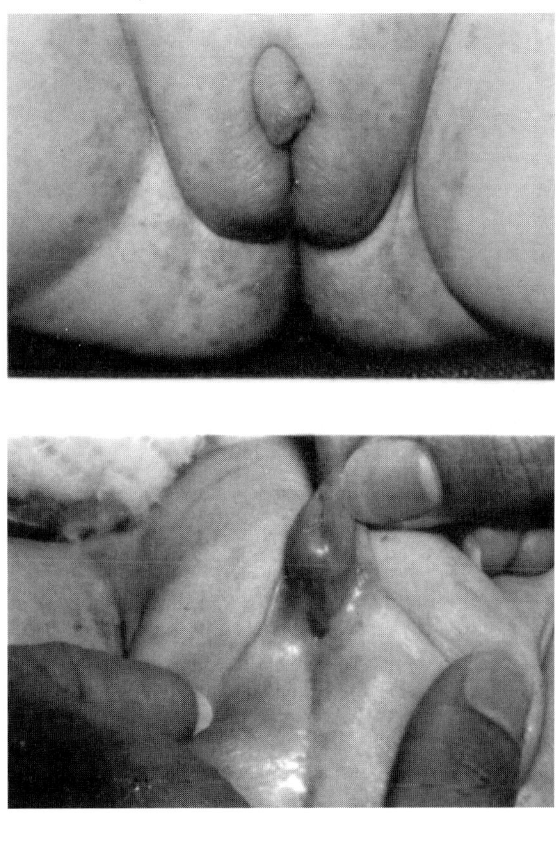

tion and corrects the hypertension and hypokalemic alkalosis. Infant males should receive sufficient testosterone to produce a normal-sized penis, followed by surgical correction of the hypospadias.[138] In both sexes, appropriate sex steroid replacement is required at the time of puberty.

17,20-Desmolase Deficiency Synthesis of testosterone involves two enzymes—17,20-desmolase and 17β-HSD—which are not necessary for biosynthesis of cortisol or aldosterone (Fig. 17-14). Genetic deficiencies of these enzymes cause inadequate virilization of genetic males (male pseudohermaphroditism) without any associated adrenal insufficiency. They are autosomal recessive traits and should also present as sexual infantilism and primary amenorrhea in genetic females, as testosterone is a necessary precursor of estradiol biosynthesis. Few affected females have been described, presumably because of inadequate endocrine investigation of women presenting with hypergonadotropic hypogonadism.

There are at least two clinical variants of this syndrome, which differ in regard to the severity of the block in androgen biosynthesis.[140] Some affected genetic males present with female external genitalia and show little or no spontaneous pubertal development owing to an almost complete inability to secrete testosterone. Others present as undervirilized males with micropenis, perineal hypospadias, and a bifid scrotum; these patients may show some Leydig cell response to hCG and will virilize to some extent at puberty. The testes in either case appear histologically normal, although tubular atrophy and hyalinization have been described after puberty. In most patients mesonephric duct structures are present, but a uterus is uniformly absent. Very few 46,XX females with apparent 17,20-desmolase deficiency have been recognized.[141] They might be expected to present with sexual infantilism, amenorrhea, or possibly just infertility, depending on the capacity for ovarian estrogen production.

In vivo and in vitro studies confirm the inability of the gonad and adrenal cortex to convert pregnenolone or 17-hydroxypregnenolone to C-19 androgens, but secretion of cortisol and aldosterone is normal. Serum concentrations of testosterone, androstenedione, and dehydroepiandrosterone are subnormal, while levels of C-21 precursors such as pregnenolone, 17-hydroxypregnenolone, and 17-hydroxyprogesterone are inappropriately high; this discrepancy is accentuated on stimulation with hCG or ACTH. Patients with ambiguous genitalia excrete significant amounts of pregnanetriolone, a metabolite of 17-hydroxypregnenolone; conversely, patients with a female phenotype do not excrete pregnanetriolone, but some dehydroepiandrosterone is found in serum and urine.

Patients who are identified at birth require plastic repair of the external genitalia and replacement therapy with testosterone. Those who have been raised as females and whose condition is not recognized until adolescence require castration and estrogen replacement therapy.

Because a single enzyme, P450C17, catalyzes both 17-hydroxylation and 17,20 cleavage, it has been difficult to understand isolated 17,20 desmolase deficiency. However, the regulation of these 2 enzyme activities has recently been elucidated.[142] It appears that the ratio of 17,20-desmolase to 17α-hydroxylase activity is increased by increasing the amount of electron-donating redox partners. Mutations in the redox-partner binding site of P450C17 have been found in patients with isolated 17,20-desmolase deficiency.[143,144]

17β-Hydroxysteroid Dehydrogenase Deficiency The final step in the biosynthesis of testosterone is 17-keto reduction of androstenedione (Fig. 17-14). The enzyme that catalyzes this conversion, and also the conversion of estrone to estradiol, is 17β-HSD (also called *17-ketosteroid reductase*). To date, there are 5 human isoenzymes, which bear little homology to each other.[145] The type I enzyme is primarily expressed in the ovary and placenta and converts estrone to estradiol, but has little activity for androgens. The type 3 enzyme is expressed only in testes and converts androstenedione to testosterone. Its gene, HSD17B3, is located on 9q22, and several different mutations have been found to result in undervirilization in affected males.[146]

Genetic males with 17β-HSD deficiency usually present with female external genitalia at birth (although a few show mild clitoromegaly or posterior labioscrotal fusion); thus the sex of rearing has almost always been female. The testes are usually inguinal or in the labioscrotal folds; in infancy such a condition may be misdiagnosed as testicular feminization. There is a blind vagina, and mesonephric duct structures are present.

The diagnosis is usually made at puberty, when, unless castration has already been performed, striking virilization occurs with marked enlargement of the phallus, hirsutism, acne, and deepening of the voice. This pubertal virilization occurs because a different unaffected 17β-HSD isozyme converts androstenedione to testosterone in peripheral tissues. In utero, the placenta likely clears the precursor androgen by aromatization such that testosterone levels do not reach a concentration necessary for masculinization. Some breast enlargement may occur, but primary amenorrhea is constant. In some cases, the degree of virilization has been such that successful transition to a male gender role has been possible.[147]

The diagnostic hallmark of this disorder is a markedly elevated serum concentration of androstenedione after puberty or hCG stimulation, with low-normal levels of testosterone.[147] Serum estradiol values are normal, but estrone levels are increased.

A deficiency of 17β-HSD should be considered in any male pseudohermaphrodite who has normal adrenal glucocorticoid and mineralocorticoid function and an absent uterus, particularly if virilization occurs at puberty. Because these patients have generally already been assigned a female gender, the appropriate therapy is usually castration followed by estrogen replacement at puberty. When a male gender role is assigned or feasible, the patient requires plastic repair of the external genitalia and supplementary testosterone therapy. Spermatogenesis would not be expected because of the lack of testicular testosterone.

Defects in Androgen Target Tissues

The bulk of testosterone in the circulation is bound to either sex hormone-binding globulin or albumin, although levels of both proteins are markedly reduced in the fetus at the time of sexual differentiation. Unbound testosterone enters target cells by passive diffusion and is then converted to the more potent androgen dihydrotestosterone through the action of the enzyme 5α-reductase. Both androgens bind to a specific high-affinity androgen receptor in the nucleus; the hormone-receptor complex binds to chromatin acceptor sites composed of DNA and nonhistone chromosomal protein. This interaction initiates transcription and processing of specific messenger RNAs, which subsequently are translated to initiate ribosomal synthesis of new proteins. The androgen receptor is regulated by a gene on the X chromosome, while the gene for 5α-reductase is autosomal. Thus the cellular mechanisms for androgen action are present in target tissues of both sexes. There is evidence that dihydrotestosterone is the major androgen responsible for virilization of the external genitalia and the later appearance of male secondary sexual characteristics at puberty; testosterone itself appears to mediate differentiation of the mesonephric duct and possibly also spermatogenesis and feedback control of gonadotropin secretion in adult life. In some forms of male pseudohermaphroditism, testosterone synthesis and paramesonephric duct regression are normal, but prenatal masculinization of the external genitalia is inadequate because of target cell resistance to androgen. The molecular basis for such androgen resistance may include a defect in 5α-reductase, in the androgen receptor, or at one or more postreceptor loci.

Defective Androgen Metabolism: 5α-Reductase Deficiency Genetic males with a deficiency of 5α-reductase present with a clinical picture formerly termed *pseudovaginal perineoscrotal hypospadias*. Typical features at birth include a clitoris-sized phallus with a hooded prepuce, a ventral urethral groove, a variable chordee, and a urogenital sinus opening on the perineum.[147] Because paramesonephric duct regression is normal, there is a blind vaginal pouch opening into the urogenital sinus. The testes are normally formed and located in either the inguinal canal or the partially fused labioscrotal folds. Mesonephric duct structures (epididymis, vas deferens, seminal vesicle, and ejaculatory duct) are well differentiated and empty into the blind vagina. Most of these patients have been raised as females.

At puberty, if castration was not accomplished earlier, serum testosterone increases into the adult male range; variable virilization occurs, without gynecomastia. The phallus enlarges to as much as 8 cm in length, the testes enlarge and complete their descent, muscle mass increases, the voice deepens, and spermatogenesis may occur. However, prostatic enlargement, acne, growth of facial and body hair, and temporal hair recession, features which are dihydrotestosterone-dependent, do not occur. Many such patients spontaneously and successfully change to a male gender identity and role, in spite of unambiguous assignment of female gender throughout childhood.[148] Such occurrences demonstrate the powerful influence that self-perceptions of genital and secondary sexual development have on gender identity and cast serious doubts on the previous notion that core psychosexual identity is always permanently imprinted during a critical period in infancy and early childhood. Although most reported patients have chosen this postpubertal gender reassignment, some patients, particularly those with a relatively small phallus, have opted to retain their female psychosexual orientation.[149]

The absence of paramesonephric duct remnants differentiates 5α-reductase deficiency from disorders of gonadogenesis such as 45,X/46,XY mixed gonadal dysgenesis; however, detailed endocrine studies are necessary to rule out a disorder of testosterone biosynthesis or other forms of androgen resistance due to receptor defects. Homozygous postpubertal males show normal or slightly increased levels of circulating FSH and LH. Serum testosterone concentrations are also normal or slightly elevated, but dihydrotestosterone concentrations remain relatively low; thus the testosterone/dihydrotestosterone ratio exceeds 35, in contrast to the normal adult male ratio of 8:16.[150] A similar pattern can be elicited in affected children after Leydig cell stimulation with hCG. Decreased conversion of ^{3}H-labeled testosterone to dihydrotestosterone has been confirmed in vivo. Study of urinary steroids shows diminished ratios of 5α reduced to 5α-reduced C-19 and C-21 steroids (for example, a reduced androsterone/etiocholanolone ratio). Homozygous females show similar urinary steroid patterns but have no clinical manifestations other than decreased body hair; heterozygotes show intermediate 5α/5β steroid ratios. In vitro study of tissue slices or cultured genital skin fibroblasts may confirm the inability to convert [^{3}H]testosterone to 5α-reduced metabolites, but the wide variation observed in normal control preparations can make interpretation of the results problematic.

There are 2 isoenzymes of 5α-reductase. The type 1 enzyme is found primarily in liver and nongenital skin and is coded for by a gene, SRD5A1, located on 5p15. The type 2 enzyme is expressed in genital skin, prostate, and hair follicle and is coded by a gene, SRD5A2, on chromosome 2p23.[147] Mutations in the type 2 gene have been found in undervirilized males with 5α-reductase deficiency, but the type 1 gene is normal.[151,152] Defects is SRD5A2 ranging from point mutations to entire gene deletion have been found, but correlation between phenotype and genotype has not been seen.

If the diagnosis of 5α-reductase deficiency is suspected and confirmed during the neonatal period, the sex of rearing should be male. Therapy with dihydrotestosterone cream can be used to enhance penile growth and facilitate surgical repair of the genitalia.[153] In such patients virilization can be expected at puberty, and fertility is theoretically possible. Those who are diagnosed later and who have an unambiguous female gender identity should undergo orchiectomy and receive estrogen therapy at the time of puberty.

Androgen Insensitivity Syndrome The clinical phenotype in genetic males with various forms of androgen insensitivity may range from female through genital ambiguity to male with hypospadias or infertility, presumably a reflection of the severity of the receptor or postreceptor defect. In all these disorders, regardless of phenotype, the affected males have a 46,XY karyotype and have testes capable of normal testosterone secretion.

The most common form of male pseudohermaphroditism is complete *androgen insensitivty syndrome* (AIS, previously termed testicular feminization), an X-linked recessive disorder due to mutations of the androgen receptor (AR) gene.[154] Phenotypically, the hemizygous male presents with normal female external genitalia; a blind vaginal pouch with absent cervix, uterus, and tubes; and absent or vestigial mesonephric duct structures. The testes may be intraabdominal, inguinal, or labial.

During infancy and childhood, complete androgen resistance should be considered in any girl with an inguinal hernia, particularly if it contains a palpable gonad; 1 in 50 girls with a hernia has this disorder. The diagnosis is almost certain if the karyotype is 46,XY and ultrasonography fails to demonstrate a uterus but should be confirmed by in vitro study of androgen receptors. After puberty the presenting complaint is primary amenorrhea, which in up to 10 percent of cases may be due to AIS. At puberty, these patients acquire a normal female body habitus and well-developed breasts, but the clitoris remains small and pubic and axillary hair is absent or sparse.

The testes are characterized by small seminiferous tubules devoid of spermatogenic elements other than spermatogonia. After puberty varying degrees of Leydig cell hyperplasia, frequently in adenomatous clumps, can be observed. These patients are predisposed to develop germ cell tumors of the testis, of which seminoma is the most common malignant variety. The incidence of malignant degeneration ranges from 5 to 20 percent and is clearly related to the age of the patient. Clinically apparent neoplasm rarely occurs before the third decade, but studies of even prepubertal testes frequently show carcinoma in situ.[155]

The hypothalamus and pituitary of these patients are resistant to the feedback effects of androgen, although gonadotropin suppression by estrogens is normal.[156] After puberty, serum LH concentrations are higher than in normal men, and as a result, levels of testosterone, dihydrotestosterone, and estradiol are also elevated. In spite of defective spermatogenesis, serum FSH concentrations are usually normal or only slightly increased.

Most patients with androgen insensitivity show markedly reduced androgen binding in cultured genital skin fibroblasts.[157] Numerous defects in the AR gene, including total or large section deletions, have been found in patients with complete AIS.[158] However, the majority appear to have a single base mutation that completely inactivates either the ligand-binding or DNA-binding site on the protein.

Therapy for complete androgen-insensitive patients requires positive reinforcement of the female gender identity. The testes should probably be removed as soon as the diagnosis is made, particularly if herniorrhaphy is required. There seems to be little merit in retaining such testes in order to permit spontaneous puberty because later prophylactic orchiectomy to prevent malignancy will be required as a second surgical procedure. Estrogen replacement therapy is required after castration to initiate and maintain secondary sex characters, but as no endometrium is present, there is no need to provide this in cyclic fashion. The blind vagina will usually permit normal sexual intercourse, but occasionally dilatation is required. In adult life the female gender identity remains firm, and marital and maternal attitudes are clearly feminine.

About 10 percent of patients with androgen insensitivity show some evidence of prenatal and adolescent virilization, and their condition is termed *partial androgen insensitivity syndrome* (PAIS). In contrast to typical receptor-negative complete AIS, there is considerable clinical heterogeneity even within the same pedigree. Furthermore, there is little if any correlation between the degree of virilization and the severity of the receptor abnormality demonstrable in vitro. In view of this clinical variability, there seems to be no reason to retain eponymic syndromes based on phenotype, such as those of Reifenstein, Rosewater, Gilbert-Dreyfus, and Lubs. A large number of the more than 300 mutations described to date in the AR gene result in PAIS, but genotype-phenotype correlation has not been possible.[158] A distinct mutation involving elongation of the CAG repeat sequence in exon 1 results in spinal and bulbar muscular atrophy.[159] These patients have small testes and gynecomastia as the only signs of androgen resistance. How this mutation results in neurodegeneration is not understood.

All these patients are 46,XY, have testes, and lack paramesonephric duct structures. In some the genitalia are female, as in complete androgen insensitivity, but distinct mesonephric duct structures can be identified. More commonly the genitalia are ambiguous, with varying degrees of clitoromegaly and labioscrotal fusion and a short blind vagina (pseudovaginal perineoscrotal hypospadias). At puberty such patients show, in addition to gynecomastia and primary amenorrhea, significant virilization with clitoral enlargement, masculine body habitus, and growth of pubic and axillary hair. In most the gender identity is female, and therapy involves immediate orchiectomy, genital reconstruction as necessary, and estrogen replacement.

The term *Reifenstein syndrome* was formerly applied to less severe variants of X-linked partial androgen insensitivity in which affected individuals presented as phenotypic males with hypospadias, inadequate pubertal virilization, gynecomastia, and infertility.[160] Cryptorchism is common; the testes are small, with normal Leydig cells but arrested spermatogenesis. Some patients show defective mesonephric duct development, such as severe hypoplasia of the vas deferens, while other mild cases have normal male genitalia but impotence and infertility.[161,162]

It is obvious that with this wide spectrum of clinical phenotypes, the diagnosis of partial androgen insensitivity is problematic unless there is an obvious family history. Serum concentrations of FSH, LH, testosterone, and estradiol are normal or moderately elevated. The decline in sex hormone binding globulin after administration of androgen in some patients with PAIS is subnormal.[163] However, this test is not useful in the first 6 months of life and has low sensitivity.[157,164] The diagnosis may be suspected because of a poor clinical response to administered androgen but must be confirmed by in vitro assessment of transactivation activity of the receptor in a reporter gene assay.[157] Because of the number of gene mutations found in patients with androgen insensitivity, it is not practical to analyze the gene for diagnosis. However, once a patient's genotype is known, analysis for that specific mutation within the family can be used for carrier detection and prenatal diagnosis.

In patients with male sex of rearing, therapy is even more problematic in view of the limited response to testosterone. Any hypospadias or cryptorchism should be corrected surgically; mastectomy will often be required because of gynecomastia. There is no evidence that the risk of developing a gonadal neoplasm in this situation exceeds that in normal males with undescended testes.

Defective Virilization Due to Exogenous Sex Steroids

Although normal exposure to placental estrogens and progesterone does not disturb fetal sexual differentiation, data derived from studies in experimental animals and some circumstantial epidemiologic evidence have raised the possibility that maternal ingestion of synthetic sex steroids may lead to hypospadias or more severe genital ambiguity.[165] Variable degrees of incomplete masculinization can be induced in rats and rabbits by prenatal exposure to high doses of progestational compounds such as the 19-nor- and 17α-ethinyl derivatives of testosterone. Progesterone and the synthetic progestogen norethindrone have been shown to cause dose-dependent inhibition of 5α-reductase activity in genital skin fibroblasts,[166] but the concentrations required make it seem unlikely that this mechanism could explain any teratogenic effect. However, a recent meta-analysis of studies of progestational agent effects on human genital development failed to show any impact.[167]

A case of male pseudohermaphroditism has been reported in which the mother received large doses of diethylstilbestrol during early pregnancy; in two surveys of boys similarly exposed, no increased incidence of hypospadias was found, although other genital anomalies, such as meatal stenosis, epididymal cyst, testicular hypoplasia, and cryptorchidism were increased.[168] Estrogens are known to be potent inhibitors of the steroidogenic enzyme 3β-HSD, but there is no proof that exogenous estrogens, even in combination with the high levels produced by the placenta, could cause significant inhibition of fetal testosterone biosynthesis.

There is some evidence that the incidences of cryptorchidism[169] and hypospadius[170,171] have increased during the past 20–30 years. The possibility that this is due to increased exposure to environmental pollutants with either estrogenic or antiandrogenic activity has been raised but to date there is no conclusive evidence.[172]

Male Pseudohermaphroditism of Unknown Etiology

Multiple Malformation Syndromes The presence of ambiguous genitalia in a genetic male may alert the physician to the presence of associated somatic anomalies that require immediate therapy.[173] Such situations include the Smith-Lemli-Opitz syndrome, in which hypospadias is associated with mental retardation, short stature, and skeletal defects; the Najjar syndrome of ambiguous genitalia, cardiomyopathy, and mental retardation; and the genito-palato-cardiac (Gardner-Silengo-Wachtel) syndrome[174] of micrognathia, facial asymmetry, cleft palate, cardiac defects, and female external and internal genitalia. These situations probably represent defects in an autosomal gene involved in gonad development but are more readily ascertained in 46,XY individuals because of the discrepancy between genetic and genital sex.

Isolated Hypospadias Failure of fusion of the urethral folds is one of the most common congenital malformations, with an incidence of about 5 per 1,000 live male births. In most cases, there is no obvious underlying endocrine defect; indeed, nonendocrine factors are suggested by the frequent coexistence of associated genitourinary and other anomalies. In about one-quarter of cases, another family member is affected. The overall risk factor for a subsequent male sibling has been estimated as 11 percent[175] but increases with more severe degrees of hypospadias, suggesting a multigenic form of inheritance. The concordance rate in identical twins is about 50 percent. Basal serum gonadotropin and testosterone concentrations are normal in unselected hypospadiac boys, but a slight diminution in mean testosterone levels has been reported in affected young adults.[176,177] More detailed testing, even during childhood, may reveal exaggerated FSH and LH responses to gonadotropin releasing hormone and altered steroid hormone responses to hCG and/or ACTH stimulation suggestive of some degree of testosterone biosynthesis defect.[178,179] Genital skin 5α-reductase activity appears to be normal in hypospadiac boys, but androgen receptor gene mutations may be present in a few.[180] These findings only underscore the heterogeneous nature of simple hypospadias and its multigenic-multifactorial etiology.

Cryptorchism The testes are frequently undescended in various forms of male pseudohermaphroditism and also in association with a number of multiple anomaly syndromes.[181] In some of these latter situations, such as the Prader-Willi syndrome, the cryptorchism reflects hypogonadotropic hypogonadism. Because of the role of pituitary gonadotropins in the regulation of Leydig cell function during the latter half of pregnancy, the occurrence of microphallus and cryptorchism in an infant with otherwise normally formed genitalia should alert the clinician to a possible hypogonadotropic or hypopituitary condition. A high proportion of maldescended testes show abnormalities of germ cells, but it is not clear whether these abnormalities represent a cause or effect of the maldescent.[182]

Virilization of a Genetic Female (Female Pseudohermaphroditism)

Exposure of a female fetus to inappropriate levels of circulating androgen does not affect ovarian or uterine development but results in some virilization of the external genitalia, or so-called female pseudohermaphroditism. The degree of genital ambiguity present at birth, which may be graded according to the classification of Prader,[183] depends mainly on the timing of the androgen exposure. Late exposure, after 12 weeks gestation, causes only clitoral hypertrophy. However, exposure between 4 and 12 weeks gestation results in varying degrees of labioscrotal fusion; the urogenital sinus commonly opens on the perineum but occasionally may reach the tip of the phallus. The most common source of the offending androgens is the adrenal cortex because of an inborn error of cortisol biosynthesis, but occasionally a maternal source of androgen can be identified. In addition, several nonendocrine malformation syndromes affecting the female external genitalia may produce a similar clinical picture.

Congenital Adrenal Hyperplasia

The virilizing syndromes of congenital adrenal hyperplasia (CAH) have in common reduced adrenal capacity to secrete cortisol (and in some forms also aldosterone). This cortisol deficiency, which during fetal life is exacerbated by rapid placental clearance of cortisol, leads to compensatory hypersecretion of ACTH, adrenocortical hyperplasia, and excessive synthesis of steroids proximal to the enzymatic block (Fig. 17-14). These steroids, such as 17-hydroxyprogesterone, may be converted to testosterone and cause virilization. The impact after birth on salt and water handling depends on the specific enzymatic defect: thus in 11β-hydroxylase deficiency there is excessive secretion of steroids that have mineralocorticoid activity, such as 11-deoxycorticosterone, but in 21-hydroxylase deficiency the predominant abnormal steroids, 17-hydroxyprogesterone and progesterone, have an antimineralocorticoid effect through their ability to compete for renal tubular aldosterone receptors.

These CAH syndromes are by far the most common cause of female pseudohermaphroditism and account for the majority of all neonates with ambiguous genitalia. Although it has been customary to consider each disorder, defined in vivo from its steroid secretion patterns, as a genetically distinct and homogeneous entity, recent evidence has demonstrated that there is remarkable phenotypic and genotypic variation.

It may be useful to examine the variables that interact to determine the age of onset and the severity of clinical abnormalities in any patient with CAH. These include both the factors influencing adrenal steroid secretion and those regulating target cell responses. Obviously, the primary variable is the underlying genetic defect. This may be a major deletion rendering the gene incapable of transcription. However, in most cases, varying amounts of gene product are formed that are defective in terms of substrate or cofactor affinity, maximal activity per cell, or susceptibility to intracellular inhibitors. The activities of steroidogenic enzymes are also regulated by hormones such as ACTH and angiotensin, electrolytes such as potassium, and the modulating effects of ambient intracellular steroids.[129]

Because steroids show a significant gradient across the adrenal cortex and these intraadrenal concentrations change with age and adrenal growth,[184] they may influence the relative secretion of mineralocorticoid, glucocorticoid, and androgen in both normal and CAH patients at different stages of development. ACTH and various mitogenic peptides interact to regulate the total mass of adrenal steroidogenic tissue. The interaction of all these variables determines the daily secretion of cortisol, aldosterone, and various other steroids, some of which are metabolically active while others are available for peripheral conversion to active steroids. Finally, the biological effect of secreted cortisol or aldosterone may be altered by the presence of steroids that bind competitively to plasma proteins or target cell receptors. These variables are probably sufficient to explain phenotypic variation in CAH.

Prenatal virilization of a genetic female can result from defects of adrenal 21-hydroxylase, 11β-hydroxylase, or 3β-HSD. The more proximal defects of cortisol biosynthesis, such as steroidogenic acute regulatory protein and 17-hydroxylase, also impair androgen synthesis; thus virilization of the female is not a clinical feature. All these CAH variants demonstrate an autosomal recessive pattern of inheritance.

21-Hydroxylase Deficiency More than 90 percent of CAH patients have a deficiency of 21-hydroxylase. At least two clinical variants have been identified: the classic form, which causes prenatal and continuing postnatal virilization with varying degrees of apparent glucocorticoid and mineralocorticoid insufficiency, and an attenuated, nonclassical or late-onset form expressed as hirsutism, virilism, or infertility during the second or third decade. The usual incidence of homozygous classic 21-hydroxylase deficiency detected by screening is 1 per 14,000 live births with a carrier frequency of 1 in 61; however, in one genetic isolate, the Yupik of Alaska, the incidence may reach 1 in 400 live births.[185]

The 21-hydroxylase complex, which is located in adrenal smooth endoplasmic reticulum, utilizes NADPH as cofactor, atmospheric oxygen, an intermediary flavoprotein, and a terminal substrate-specific cytochrome P450 of about 48,000 dalton. This single enzyme complex catalyzes 21-hydroxylation of both 17-hydroxyprogesterone and progesterone (Fig. 17-14), but the former is the preferred substrate. Extraadrenal 21-hydroxylation does not appear to involve the same enzyme and is not impaired in CAH.

Two 21-hydroxylase genes, termed CYP21 and CYP21P, are located on the short arm of chromosome 6 (6p21.3) between the loci for HLA-B and HLA-DR and adjacent to the two genes for the fourth component of complement (C4A and C4B). The two CYP21 genes are highly homologous (96–98 percent), but only CYP21 encodes an active enzyme. In 90–95 percent of patients with one of the forms of 21-hydroxylase deficiency, mutations converting CYP21 to CYP21P are responsible.[186–188] These mutations result from either unequal crossover during meiosis, which generally produces deletions, or gene conversion from nonreciprocal base change during mitosis. About 20 percent of cases have a large DNA deletion encompassing the 3′ end of CYP21P, all of C4B and several exons at the 5′ end of CYP21, which produces a perfectly spliced CYP21P/CYP21 chimera. Several studies have shown a correlation between the genotype, the expressed enzyme activity and the clinical phenotype (Table 17-5).[188–190a] Because about 10 mutations account for 90–95 percent of cases, allele-specific polymerase chain reaction amplification permits rapid screening for the common mutations.[188]

Close linkage with histocompatibility and complement loci makes it possible to also use extended HLA and complement haplotyping to quickly trace the inheritance of a particular 21-hydroxylase gene (Fig. 17-16). HLA testing combined with careful analysis of basal and ACTH-stimulated 17-hydroxyprogesterone levels can define accurately subjects who are homozygous for classic or late-onset 21-hydroxylase deficiency, genetic compounds carrying both genes, or heterozygous carriers.

This close linkage of 21-hydroxylase with the major histocompatibility locus should not be confused with the phenomenon of genetic linkage disequilibrium, in which the frequency of certain HLA haplotypes differs in affected subjects from that observed in normal persons in the same population. Thus among northern European groups the haplotype Bw47DR7 occurs with increased frequency in association with classic 21-hydroxylase deficiency, while the B8 haplotype frequency is reduced. In the late-onset variant of 21-hydroxylase deficiency the frequency of the B14 haplotype appears to be increased.

The important clinical features of homozygous classic 21-hydroxylase deficiency are virilization and salt wasting. Their pathogenesis is summarized in Fig. 17-17. The primary impairment of cortisol synthesis causes increased pituitary secretion of ACTH, which in turn leads to excessive production of both 17-hydroxyprogesterone and progesterone. Side-chain cleavage of 17-hydroxyprogesterone produces androstenedione, which is then available for adrenal and peripheral conversion to the active androgen testosterone. In untreated patients, plasma ACTH is moderately raised; levels of 17-hydroxyprogesterone, progesterone, androstenedione, testosterone, 21-deoxycortisol, and pregnenolone sulfate are markedly increased, with less striking increases in the levels of dehydroepiandrosterone and its sulfate conjugate. Even if basal serum cortisol levels are in the normal range, stress or ACTH testing may evoke only a blunted rise in spite of a brisk increase in 17-hydroxyprogesterone. Metabolism of these abnormal steroids leads to increased urinary excretion of 17-ketosteroids and pregnanetriol.

Prenatal exposure to adrenal androgens has no effect on male

TABLE 17-5. Common CYP21 Mutations Causing 21-Hydroxylase Deficiency

Mutation	Enzyme Activity*	Phenotype
30kb deletion	0	Salt-wasting
Exon 3, 8 base pair deletion	0	Salt-wasting
Exon 6, 3 clustered mutations	0	Salt-wasting
Exon 7, 1 nucleotide insertion	0	Salt-wasting
Exon 8, nonsense mutation	0	Salt-wasting
Exon 8, missense mutation (Arg356Trp)	0	Salt-wasting
Intron 2 cryptic splice site	0–2	Simple virilizing/Salt-wasting
Exon 4, missense mutation (Ile172Asn)	1–2	Simple virilizing
Exon 1, missense mutation (Pro30Leu)	20–60	Non-classical
Exon 7, missense mutation (Val281Leu)	20–60	Non-classical
Exon 10, missense mutation (Pro453Ser)	20–60	Non-classical

*Percent of normal enzyme activity.

Source: Modified from Speiser and White.[190]

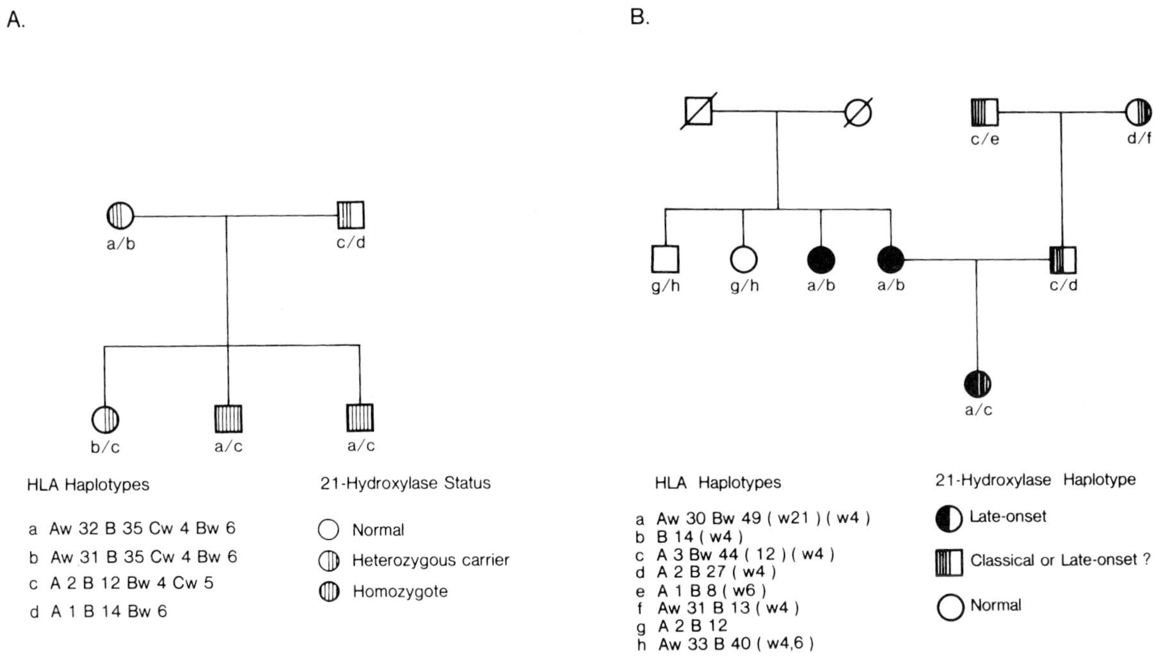

FIGURE 17-16. Application of HLA typing to the genotyping of 21-hydroxylase deficiency. (*A*) Classic 21-hydroxylase deficiency in a family with two affected sons and one heterozygous daughter. (*B*) Pedigree in which the mother is homozygous for late-onset 21-hydroxylase deficiency, the father is heterozygous for 21-hydroxylase deficiency, and the daughter appears to be a genetic compound, showing elevated serum 17-hydroxyprogesterone levels but no virilization.

sexual differentiation. The genitalia of affected males appear normal at birth, but continued androgen exposure becomes apparent by age 2–3 years, with rapid growth and skeletal maturation and precocious appearance of secondary sex characters in the absence of preceding testicular enlargement.

Genetic females who are homozygous for classic 21-hydroxylase deficiency have ambiguous external genitalia at birth (Fig. 17-18). Careful physical examination will demonstrate clitoromegaly, labioscrotal fusion without palpable testes, and a single urogenital sinus, which opens usually on the perineum but occasionally on the phallus. If appropriate therapy to suppress adrenal androgen production is not initiated, this virilism continues during childhood, causing further clitoromegaly, rapid growth, and the appearance of pubic hair, acne, and a masculine body habitus. Even though growth is accelerated, precocious epiphyseal fusion leads to an arrest of growth by about 10 years of age, with marked reduction of adult height. Continued androgen exposure after puberty causes anovular infertility and amenorrhea.

FIGURE 17-17. Pathogenesis of virilization and salt wasting in classic 21-hydroxylase deficiency, showing the close interrelation of these two aspects of the disease and the central importance of serum 17-hydroxyprogesterone (17OH-prog) and plasma renin activity for diagnosis and management. (*From Winter and Couch.*[187])

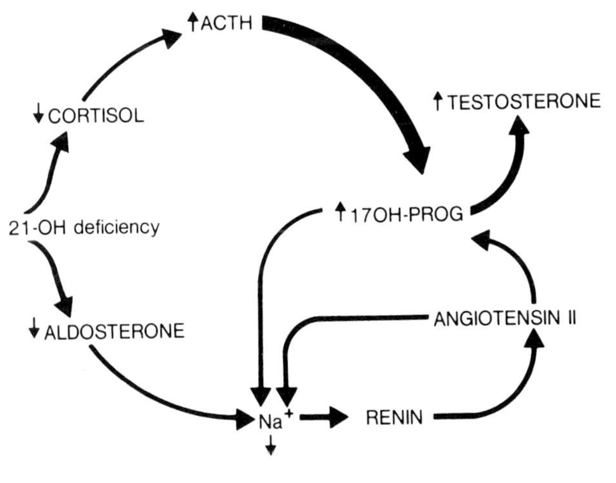

FIGURE 17-18. External genitalia of a newborn female with classic 21-hydroxylase deficiency. No gonads were palpable, and the cervix was felt on rectal examination.

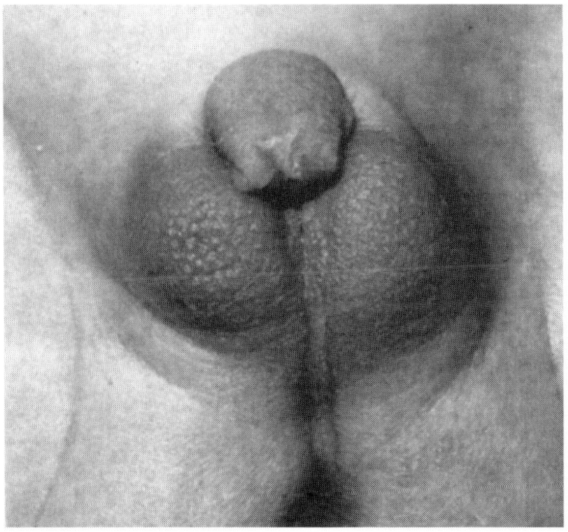

The late-onset or attenuated variant of 21-hydroxylase deficiency is characterized by low-level androgen exposure that does not produce clinically apparent disease until late childhood or adolescence. Affected males are rarely detected unless they present with premature adrenarche. Homozygous females have normal genitalia at birth; the disorder may be suspected in a child with premature adrenarche or a young woman with mild clitoromegaly, hirsutism, or anovular infertility.[191] These patients show moderately increased basal serum concentrations of 17-hydroxyprogesterone and testosterone, with an exaggerated response of 17-hydroxyprogesterone to ACTH stimulation.

Some individuals represent genetic compounds for the classic and late-onset variants of 21-hydroxylase deficiency (Fig. 17-16). The phenotype is most often that of the less severe mutation, such that they have normal genitalia; postnatal signs of androgen excess or infertility may not occur, even though basal serum 17-hydroxyprogesterone levels are persistently increased.[192] Heterozygous carriers for either variant are clinically normal[193] and show normal basal serum concentrations of all adrenal steroids. Examination of basal and ACTH-stimulated 17-hydroxyprogesterone values will usually permit appropriate categorization of individuals within an affected pedigree (Fig. 17-19).

Biochemical evidence of sodium depletion, as evidenced by increased levels of plasma renin activity or concentration, can be observed in virtually all untreated patients with homozygous classic 21-hydroxylase deficiency. However, clinically significant salt wasting develops in only about two-thirds of these patients,[195] usually during early infancy prior to diagnosis. In an affected neonate the first clues to an impending salt-losing crisis are hyperkalemia and rising levels of plasma renin activity, which are usually detectable by 1 week of age. If mineralocorticoid therapy is not initiated, progressive weight loss, vomiting, acidosis, hypoglycemia, and hyponatremic dehydration ensue, leading to peripheral vascular collapse by the third or fourth week. The clinical picture resembles that of hypertrophic pyloric stenosis except that in CAH, because of osmotic diuresis, urinary volume is often maintained in spite of obvious dehydration. The finding of hyponatremia and hyperkalemia in a dehydrated male (or virilized female) infant should lead immediately to investigation of adrenal function, including measurement of serum 17-hydroxyprogesterone levels. The differential diagnosis of a neonatal salt-losing crisis includes other forms of CAH, pyloric stenosis, congenital adrenal hypoplasia, and interstitial pyelonephritis.

Although 21-hydroxylase deficiency is certainly genetically heterogeneous, it is probably simplistic to assume that the presence or absence of a neonatal salt-losing crisis defines two genetically distinct disorders, a salt-losing variant and a simple virilizing variant. In later life most so-called salt losers show a persistent inability to tolerate sodium restriction, but some apparently gain the ability to conserve sodium relatively well.[196] Similarly, one may observe apparent discordance between siblings with the same CYP21 mutation as regards clinically significant salt wasting. It may be useful, therefore, to consider the variables interacting to determine whether and when a salt-losing crisis will occur.

One important determinant is the capacity to secrete aldosterone during sodium deprivation. Although all patients with 21-hydroxylase deficiency show evidence of an aldosterone biosynthetic defect and hypovolemia, those with clinically apparent salt wasting have reduced plasma aldosterone levels and aldosterone secretion rates relative to their plasma renin activities, with little response to sodium restriction; aldosterone levels in those who are not salt losers are typically above normal and may rise further

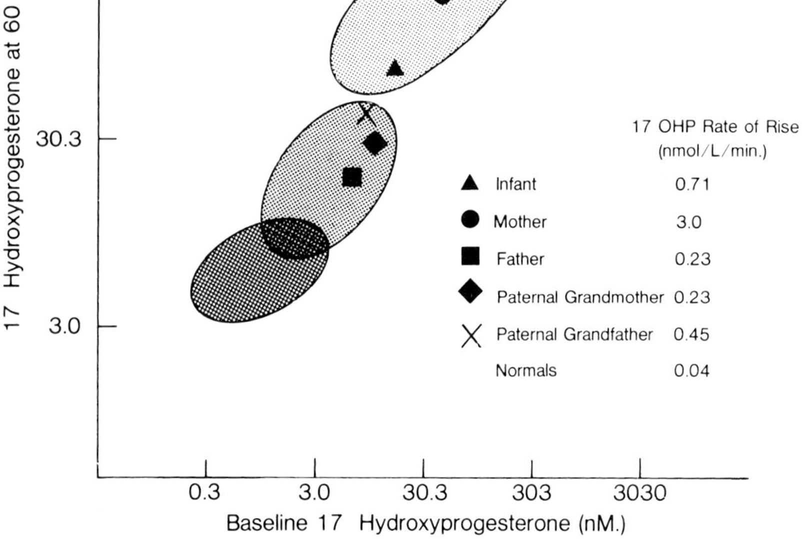

FIGURE 17-19. ACTH stimulation tests (Cortrosyn 0.2 mg/m^2 IV, maximum 0.25 mg). The relation of baseline and 60-min ACTH-stimulated serum 17-hydroxyprogesterone concentrations in normal controls, heterozygous carriers, and patients with homozygous late-onset and homozygous classic forms of 21-hydroxylase deficiency. The application of the nomogram is illustrated, using data from individuals in pedigree B of Fig. 17-16. Data in nanomols per liter may be changed to nanograms per deciliter by multiplying by 33. (*Adapted from New et al.*[194])

with sodium restriction.[197] However, this distinction is not absolute, as clinical salt wasting has been reported in infants with high aldosterone levels. This variability in aldosterone secretory capacity reflects the severity of the defect in 21-hydroxylation. The capacity to secrete aldosterone is also influenced by the total mass of the zona glomerulosa; although this aspect has not been carefully correlated with endocrine and genetic markers, it appears that salt-losing neonates show a deficient zona glomerulosa, while in older children with 21-hydroxylase deficiency this zone is usually hyperplastic.[198]

The second variable is the effect of high circulating levels of steroids such as 17-hydroxyprogesterone and progesterone, which bind to the renal tubular receptor for aldosterone and act as competitive inhibitors of mineralocorticoid action. This phenomenon greatly exacerbates salt wasting unless the patient can compensate with increased secretion of aldosterone. In addition, high intraadenal concentrations of these steroids may act as competitive inhibitors of any residual 21-hydroxylase function and thus exacerbate the defect.[199] A salt-losing crisis tends to be self-accelerating (Fig. 17-17) because both ACTH and angiotensin levels rise and both stimulate increased secretion of these antimineralocorticoid steroids.[200] Thus the glucocorticoid and mineralocorticoid abnormalities interact closely in this disorder: suppression of ACTH with glucocorticoid therapy serves to ameliorate the salt wasting, while suppression of the renin-angiotensin system by salt, fluids, and mineralocorticoid is essential for normalization of 17-hydroxyprogesterone secretion.

The third variable includes various nonendocrine aspects of fluid and electrolyte balance, such as body fluid compartment size, renal function, dietary intake of salt and water, and intercurrent infection, which may predispose a young infant to a salt-losing crisis under circumstances that would be less threatening in later life. The newborn is also relatively mineralocorticoid-resistant as reflected in the normally high levels of aldosterone that decline with age. A distinction between salt losing and simple virilizing forms of homozygous classic 21-hydroxylase deficiency, however, has little impact on therapy, as it is now customary to provide sufficient mineralocorticoid to all patients to ensure normalization of plasma renin activity.

The diagnosis of classic 21-hydroxylase deficiency should be considered in three clinical situations (1) a newborn with ambiguous genitalia (including apparent males with bilateral cryptorchism and hypospadias), (2) a young infant with dehydration, hyponatremia, and hyperkalemia, and (3) a child with precocious virilization. Investigation begins with the immediate determination of serum 17-hydroxyprogesterone levels[201] at the same time that samples are being taken for karyotype analysis and assays of plasma renin activity. Umbilical-cord serum 17-hydroxyprogesterone values are high in normal infants (Table 17-6) but fall to below 200 ng/dl by 48 h (Fig. 17-20). Occasional values above 1,000 ng/dl may be observed in sick or premature infants during the first week.[202] In classic 21-hydroxylase deficiency, serum 17-hydroxyprogesterone levels greatly exceed normal, ranging from 3,000 to 100,000 ng/dl, and rise with age. Similar increases can be observed in levels of androstenedione, testosterone, progesterone, 21-deoxycortisol, and pregnenolone sulfate. Moderate increases in serum 17-hydroxyprogesterone are observed in 11β-hydroxylase deficiency, but in this disorder serum levels of 11-deoxycortisol are raised. Assays of urinary 17-ketosteroids and pregnanetriol were formerly used for the diagnosis of 21-hydroxylase deficiency, but the vagaries of neonatal steroid metabolism and urine collection can create serious errors of interpretation. Plasma renin activity is normal for the first few days of life, but by the fifth day all infants with classic 21-hydroxylase deficiency show elevated and rising values. There seems little merit in waiting to see if this signals a frank salt-losing crisis, and it is now customary to initiate mineralocorticoid therapy at this time.

Deficiency of 21-hydroxylase can be diagnosed prenatally either by DNA analysis for mutant CYP21 or HLA-typing of amniocytes or chorionic villus tissue, or by measurement of amniotic fluid concentrations of 17-hydroxyprogsterone.[203–205] Unfortunately, such a diagnosis by either means does not permit antenatal treatment in time to prevent virilization of affected females. The fetal adrenal cortex can be effectively suppressed during the period of sexual differentiation through the administration to the mother of relatively large doses of dexamethasone (0.5 mg three times a day), provided that the therapy is begun by 4–5 weeks fetal age or as soon as pregnancy can be ascertained.[203–205] This treatment is then continued until the diagnosis of an affected 46,XX fetus can be determined by means of amniocentesis or chorionic villus biopsy; in such a circumstance, therapy is continued to term, but if the fetus is unaffected or male (seven of eight pregnancies), it is discontinued. Provided that dexamethasone therapy was started sufficiently early, affected females at term will have normal genitalia, or at least significantly less virilization. Maternal complications include excessive weight gain, Cushingoid features, and hypertension.[205,206] No teratogenic or other immediate side effects of prenatal treatment have been seen in the newborns but long-term physiological or psychological effects are not yet known; therefore prenatal treatment should likely still be

TABLE 17-6. Normal Values of Hormones Commonly Used for the Diagnosis and Management of Congenital Adrenal Hyperplasia

	Serum					*Plasma*
	17-Hydroxyprogesterone, ng/dl	Androstenedione, ng/dl	Testosterone, ng/dl		Aldosterone, ng/dl	Renin Activity, ng/ml per h
			Male	Female		
Cord	1100–6500	50–200	5–50	5–50	95 ± 10*	8 ± 2*
1–2 days	65–400	20–100	60–400	20–70	7–850	25 ± 8
3–6 days	60–250	10–100	15–25	10–25	35–210	12 ± 2
1–3 weeks	20–220	10–150	50–350	3–25	15–105	6 ± 2
1–12 months	5–150	5–50	5–350	3–20	5–95	6 ± 1
1–3 years	5–90	3–40	3–15	3–15	10–80	5 ± 2
3–6 years	5–90	3–40	3–15	3–15	10–70	3 ± 1
6–15 years	10–160	5–150	10–770	10–60	10–70	2 ± 0.3
Adult	10–285	50–200	260–1000	15–65	5–50	2 ± 0.4

*Mean ± standard error of mean.

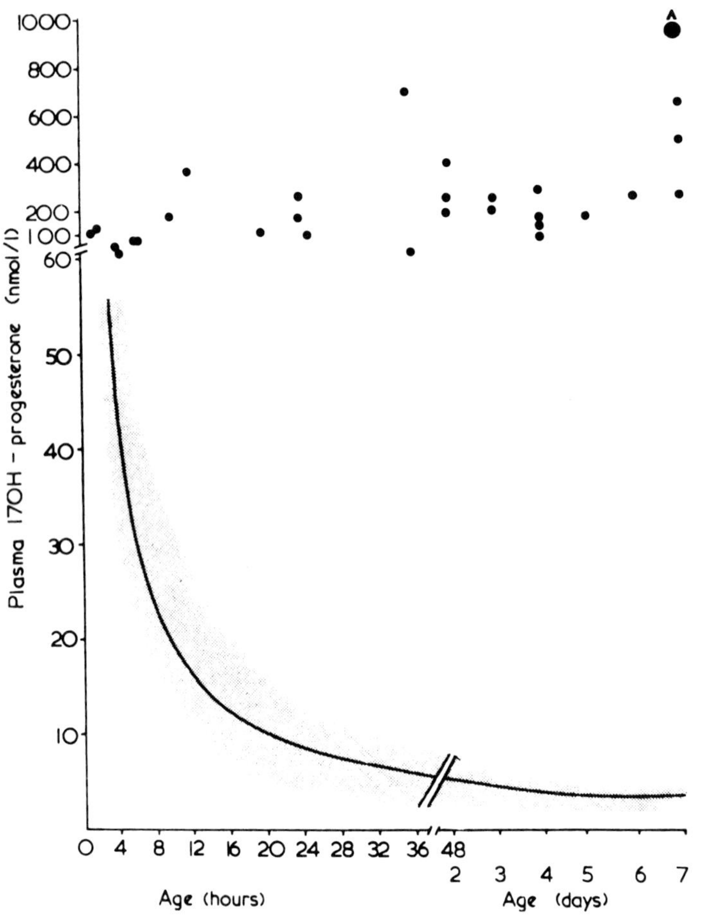

FIGURE 17-20. Plasma 17-hydroxyprogesterone concentrations in normal infants (shaded area indicates mean and range) and in untreated infants with classic 21-hydroxylase deficiency (individual dots) during the first 7 days of life. Values may be changed to nanograms per deciliter by multiplying by 33. (*From Hughes et al.*[201])

considered experimental and be undertaken only after obtaining fully informed consent.[207]

In many jurisdictions neonatal screening for 21-hydroxylase deficiency by means of radioimmunoassay (RIA) of 17-hydroxyprogesterone in blood spots is now routine because studies have demonstrated considerable unrecognized mortality, particularly in male probands with CAH[208]; the disorder has a relatively high incidence; and the screening test is rapid and inexpensive.[185] Neonatal screening demonstrates that many affected male infants show no clinical signs of salt wasting in spite of remarkable hyperkalemia and thus may present as unexpected crib deaths. Unfortunately, because of the relative adrenocortical hyperplasia of normal neonates, even postmortem examination often fails to establish the correct diagnosis. Other benefits of neonatal screening, by comparison with the usual clinical screening,[209] include correct gender assignment in virilized girls and avoidance of significant morbidity resulting from delays in diagnosis.

The diagnosis of the late-onset or attenuated variant of 21-hydroxylase deficiency in patients with premature adrenarche, hirsutism, or infertility requires assessment of serum 17-hydroxyprogesterone concentrations before and after stimulation with ACTH.[210] In postmenarcheal females, this test should be carried out in the early follicular phase to avoid ovarian midcycle and luteal secretion of 17-hydroxyprogesterone. If the morning 17-hydroxyprogesterone level is less than 200 ng/dl (6 nmol/L) the condition is ruled out; similarly if the level is above 500 ng/dl (15.1 nmol/L), the diagnosis is confirmed and ACTH stimulation is not necessary.

Successful treatment of congenital adrenal hyperplasia depends on daily replacement of glucocorticoid and mineralocorticoid in the smallest doses sufficient to reduce pituitary ACTH secretion and the renin-angiotensin system to normal. If this is done correctly, an affected patient can achieve normal growth, healthy psychosexual adjustment, and normal adult reproductive function. Other cornerstones of modern therapy include education of the patient and family to ensure compliance and early perineal repair for affected females to provide normal genital appearance and function.

If the condition is diagnosed during a salt-losing crisis, treatment begins with intravenous fluids, initially with saline (20 ml/kg of body weight in 1 h) to restore intravascular volume and then with a more gradual infusion of 5 percent glucose in saline to replace fluid and electrolyte losses. Hydrocortisone hemisuccinate (50 mg/m^2) is administered as an initial IV bolus, with a similar dose infused over the subsequent 24 h. If available, deoxycorticosterone acetate (1–3 mg IM every 12 h) or aldosterone (0.5 mg IV every 4–6 h) may be added, but mineralocorticoids tend to be relatively ineffective at first because of high levels of circulating 17-hydroxyprogesterone and other inhibitors and the additional mineralocorticoid action of the stress dose of glucocorticoid. In small infants severe hyperkalemia may induce electrocardiographic changes and necessitate the use of rectal cation exchange resins.

Maintenance therapy seeks to provide sufficient glucocorticoid and mineralocorticoid to suppress adrenal 17-hydroxyprogesterone and androgen secretion without causing side effects such as growth failure and hypertension.[187] Irrespective of the presence or absence of a previous frank salt-losing crisis, sufficient mineralocorticoid to reduce plasma renin levels to the age-specific normal range should always be provided. In infancy, 9α-fluorohydrocortisone (fludrocortisone) doses of 0.15–0.2 mg per day are frequently necessary, but in older children and adults the same effect can be achieved with 0.05 to 0.1 mg per day. To avoid hypertension, the dose of 9α-fluorohydrocortisone should always be reduced if the plasma renin activity falls below normal. With such a regimen there appears to be no need for salt supplementation, but patients should not be denied access to salt, particularly during hot weather. Older forms of mineralocorticoid replacement, such as IM injections and subcutaneous pellets of deoxycorticosterone, are ineffective, cumbersome, and potentially dangerous.

If plasma renin activity is normal, adrenal androgen secretion can be suppressed by the use of oral hydrocortisone (cortisol), 10–15 mg/m^2 daily in three divided doses. Cortisone acetate appears to be less effective, with reduced bioavailability; more potent glucocorticoids such as prednisone or dexamethasone are useful in adults but carry too great a risk of growth inhibition for use during childhood.

Therapy should be monitored by measurements of plasma renin activity and serum 17-hydroprogesterone and testosterone at least every 3–6 months. The goal should be to maintain serum 17-hydroxyprogesterone values below 500 ng/dl (15 nmol/L) and renin and testosterone values within the age- and sex-specific normal range (Table 17-6). The sensitivity of serum 17-hydroxyprogesterone to stress-induced fluctuations in ACTH release and its circadian rhythmicity demand careful attention to sampling details such as time of day, time since previous steroid administration, and successful initial venipuncture. Our approach for the past 15 years has been to measure plasma renin activity, serum 17-hydroxyprogesterone, and testosterone at 0900 h, just before the ingestion of medication, and the serum steroid levels again 3 h later. Assays of salivary 17-hydroxyprogesterone and testosterone show excellent correlation with serum levels and provide a noninvasive technique for serial home monitoring.[211] Serum 17-hydroxyprogesterone and testosterone concentrations closely parallel each other in prepubertal children and females (Fig. 17-21), but naturally they deviate in adolescent boys.[212] Serum androstenedione, 17-hydroxypregnenolone, or 21-deoxycortisol determinations also correlate with 17-hydroxyprogesterone and can be used for monitoring therapy; however, levels of dehydroepiandrosterone (and its sulfate conjugate) remain markedly reduced after long-term glucocorticoid therapy and therefore do not provide a sufficiently sensitive index of day-to-day ACTH suppression. Assays of urinary 17-ketosteroids and pregnanetriol were formerly used to monitor therapy in CAH; however, they provide no advantage and are considerably less sensitive and more cumbersome.

In addition, patients should be monitored carefully in regard to growth velocity and skeletal maturation, as there is no biochemical test for overtreatment. At all ages the smallest dose of cortisol that will normalize hormone levels should be used. During major infections the dose of cortisol should be doubled, and extra doses of oral or parenteral glucocorticoid should be provided before surgery requiring general anesthesia. It is our habit to instruct parents to repeat the previous medications any time the child vomits and to give IM hydrocortisone sodium succinate 25–100 mg if there is a second episode of vomiting.

Therapy for late-onset CAH requires only oral hydrocortisone without supplementary mineralocorticoid in the same doses. Once growth is complete, satisfactory control and normal fertility can be achieved more easily with longer-acting agents such as dexamethasone.

Occasionally, if the diagnosis of classic CAH has been delayed or therapy has been inadequate, significant advance of both skeletal maturation and hypothalamic-pituitary maturation may occur, with physical signs and hormonal evidence of true precocious puberty. This complication may require adjunctive use of GnRH analogue therapy, as in other forms of true precocious puberty. From time to time other adjuncts, such as adrenalectomy, have been suggested to treat CAH.[213] However, there is no evidence that such steps are necessary or even beneficial in patients who are compliant with standard glucocorticoid and mineralocorticoid replacement.

In all forms of female pseudohermaphroditism, including 21-hydroxylase deficiency, surgical repair of the external genitalia should be undertaken by 6–12 months of age so that the child is never aware of the deformity. The appropriate procedure includes vaginoplasty to provide labia majora and minora and separate urethral and vaginal communication to the perineum, plus clitoroplasty, in which the separated crura of the clitoris are placed under the symphysis pubis, leaving only the glans visible, with its vascular and nervous supply intact. Occasionally the connection between the upper vagina and the urogenital sinus is proximal to the external sphincter, so far from the perineum that it is necessary to delay creating the appropriate outlet to the perineum until after menarche. However, in all cases the external appearance of the genitalia should be made normal in infancy with no further surgical interference during childhood. Vaginal dilatation may be necessary in young women who underwent vaginoplasty in infancy, but thereafter sexual function is completely normal. It is our custom to recommend cesarean section in women who have undergone this repair, as we have no information regarding the effects of vaginal delivery.

If the diagnosis of 21-hydroxylase deficiency is made soon after birth and appropriate medical care is maintained through childhood, one can expect the majority to have normal growth,[187] bone density,[214] intellectual and psychosexual development.[215] Poor growth is frequently related to overtreatment with glucocorticoid or late diagnosis[216]; some infants with salt-wasting and hypoglycemia at presentation may develop learning difficulties.[217] In young women regular ovulatory menstrual cycles do not occur unless serum testosterone and 17-hydroxyprogesterone levels are reduced to normal. Although apparent well-being and even normal spermatogenesis have been observed in occasional untreated adult males, it seems better to recommend lifelong therapy because infertility due to suppression of gonadotropins is the more likely result of inadequate treatment.[218] Untreated adult males may also develop testicular tumors as a result of chronic ACTH stimulation of adrenal rest cells.

11β-Hydroxylase Deficiency The enzyme complex that catalyzes the conversion of 11-deoxycortisol to cortisol is a mitochondrial oxidase consisting of a flavoprotein, an adrenodoxin, and a substrate-specific cytochrome P450. This enzyme converts 11-deoxycortisol to cortisol and deoxycorticosterone to corticosterone. The gene, CYP11B1, is on 8q22, immediately adjacent to CYP11B2, which codes for the isozyme aldosterone synthase that converts deoxycorticosterone to aldosterone.[219] These genes are 95 percent homologous, but CYP11B1 is expressed in the fasciculata and regulated by ACTH whereas CYP11B2 is expressed in the glomerulosa and regulated by angiotensin II and potassium.

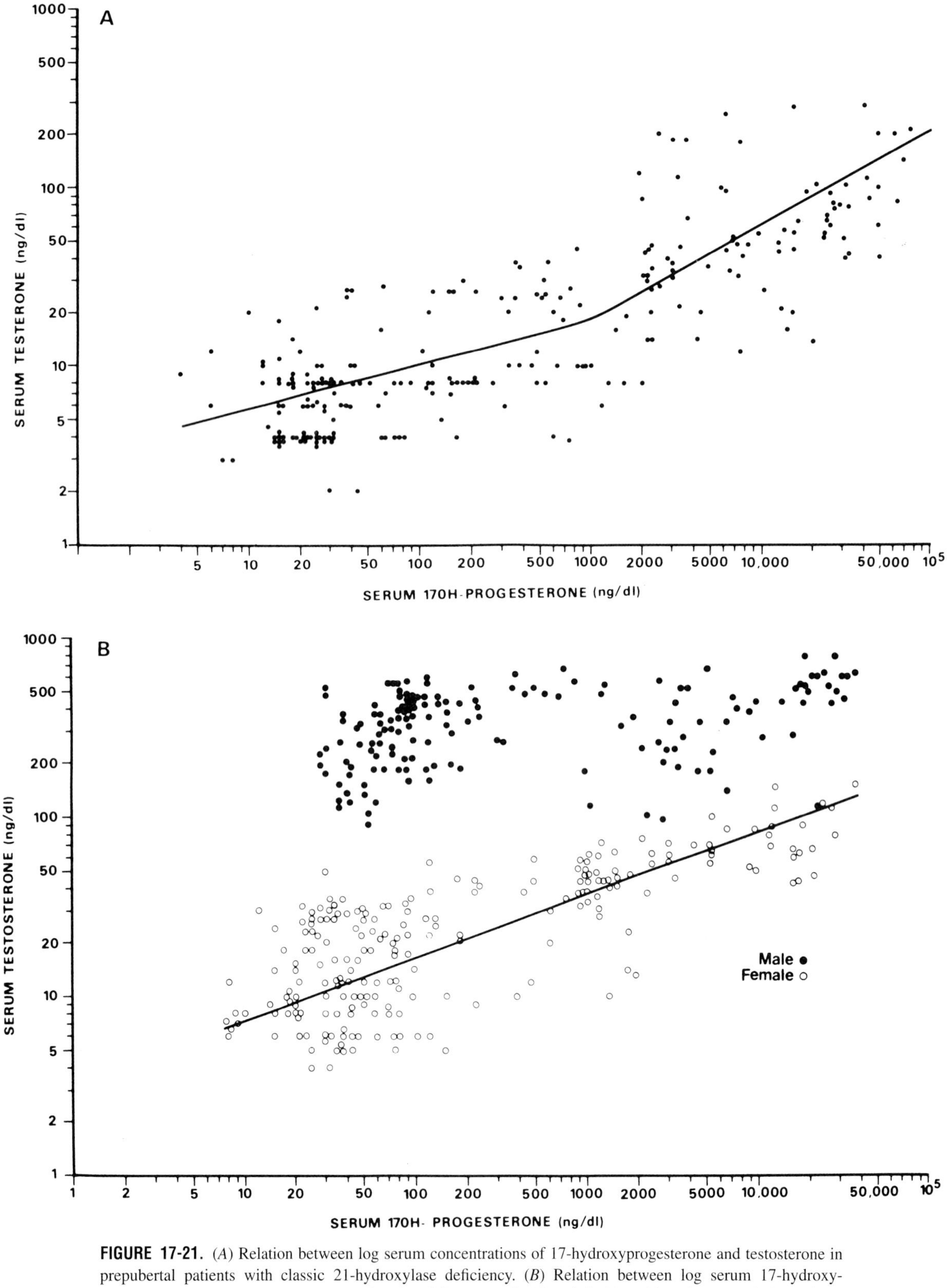

FIGURE 17-21. (*A*) Relation between log serum concentrations of 17-hydroxyprogesterone and testosterone in prepubertal patients with classic 21-hydroxylase deficiency. (*B*) Relation between log serum 17-hydroxyprogesterone and testosterone concentrations in adolescent male (closed circle) and female (open circle) patients with classic 21-hydroxylase deficiency. (*From Hughes and Winter.*[212])

Several different mutations of CYP11B1 that completely inactivate the protein have been found in classical 11-hydroxylase deficiency, but a genotype-phenotype correlation has not been found.[219] Mutations of CYP11B2 produce aldosterone deficiency with resultant salt-wasting, but there is no effect on adrenal androgen production and no abnormality of genital development. Unequal cross-over between the 2 genes with fusion of the 5′ regulatory region of CYP11B1 with the 3′ coding sequence of

CYP11B2 is responsible for glucocorticoid suppressible hyperaldosteronism,[220] but sexual differentiation remains normal.

Deficiency of 11β-hydroxylase is the second most common form of CAH; it accounts, however, for only 5 percent of all CAH cases, although it is relatively more common among Jews of north African origin. It is an autosomal recessive disorder in which the classic signs are virilization plus hypertension. Increased adrenal secretion of 11-deoxycorticosterone (DOC) and 11-deoxycortisol leads to ACTH-dependent hypertension of variable severity. Accumulation of steroids more proximal in the steroidogenic path (such as 17-hydroxyprogesterone) and their subsequent metabolism to androgens lead to prenatal masculinization of the external genitalia in genetic females, as in 21-hydroxylase deficiency.[219] Postnatally, untreated males and females show progressive virilization with rapid skeletal maturation and eventual short stature. Prepubertal gynecomastia of uncertain pathogenesis has been reported in affected males. Severe virilization may occur without hypertension, but the reverse has not been observed. In addition to this classic form of 11-hydroxylase deficiency, milder variants have been described, with onset of hirsutism, acne, amenorrhea, and variable hypertension in adolescence or even latter.[221]

In untreated patients with the classic disorder, hypervolemia suppresses plasma renin activity and aldosterone secretion. After glucocorticoid therapy and suppression of DOC production, plasma renin increases and there is a rise in aldosterone levels. However, the aldosterone response to sodium restriction may be subnormal and salt wasting may occur in a few, but the mechanism is unclear.[219,222]

The hallmark of 11β-hydroxylase deficiency is the presence of elevated serum concentrations of 11-deoxycortisol and DOC and their suppression by exogenous glucocorticoid. Urinary excretion of metabolites such as tetrahydro-11-deoxycortisol (THS) is usually increased but may be normal during early infancy. Prenatal diagnosis can be achieved by determining increased amniotic fluid concentrations of 11-deoxycortisol or increased maternal excretion of THS.[223] Therefore, prenatal therapy with dexamethasone should be feasible to prevent genital virilization in affected females. In obligate heterozygotes, however, basal and ACTH-stimulated 11-deoxysteroid levels cannot be distinguished from normal.[223]

Treatment of 11β-hydroxylase deficiency requires cortisol in doses similar to those used in other forms of CAH. With adequate treatment, virilization ceases and hypertension usually disappears; serum concentrations of DOC and 11-deoxycortisol fall to normal, while plasma renin activity rises to the normal range. Early vaginoplasty and clitoroplasty are required for prenatally virilized females.

3βHSD Deficiency This disorder was discussed in detail earlier under Defective Genital Virilization (Male Pseudohermaphroditism) because it can cause genital ambiguity in both males and females. The originally described classic variant is an autosomal recessive disease that causes a major block in the biosynthesis of mineralocorticoid, glucocorticoid, androgens, and estrogens in both the adrenal cortex and the gonads (Fig. 17-14). Infant girls present with slight to moderate clitoral enlargement plus severe salt wasting; however, a few patients have been described who could maintain normal salt balance and apparently adequate aldosterone production by means of compensatory high renin-angiotensin stimulation. The virilization of affected females is presumably due to peripheral conversion of Δ^5-3β-hydroxysteroid precursors to androgen by the type I isozyme present in adipose tissue and skin.

As in other forms of CAH, phenotypic variation exists. However, in previously described cases of a mild late-onset form presenting with hirsutism and amenorrhea,[131,132] a mutation of HSD3B2 has not ben found.[133,134]

The diagnosis of 3β-HSD deficiency is indicated by the finding of high serum concentrations of dehydroepiandrosterone, pregnenolone, and 17-hydroxypregnenolone with their respective sulfate conjugates. Because of hepatic 3β-HSD activity, one may find increased serum levels of Δ^4-3β-ketosteroids such as 17-hydroxyprogesterone and androstenedione, but these ketosteroids are never as markedly elevated as the Δ^5-3β-hydroxysteroids. There is a similar characteristic Δ^5/Δ^4 imbalance in the urinary excretion of Δ^5-pregnenetriol and pregnanetriol. ACTH and hCG stimulation elicits little rise in circulating levels of cortisol and gonadal sex steroids.

Therapy for 3β-HSD deficiency requires replacement of cortisol, as in other forms of CAH, plus full mineralocorticoid replacement in any patient with elevated plasma renin activity or intolerance to sodium restriction. In addition, patients with the classic variant usually show defective pubertal development[225] and therefore require sex steroid (estrogen and progestin) replacement at the appropriate age. In the less severe variants, normal puberty and regular ovulatory menstrual cycles usually follow suppression of adrenal androgen secretion.

Virilization Due To Defective Estrogen Synthesis
Aromatase Deficiency

Aromatase is a microsomal cytochrome P450 that catalyzes the conversion of testosterone to estradiol and androstenedione to estrone (Fig. 17-14). A single aromatase gene, CYP19, is present on chromosome 15q21 and expressed in several tissues including placenta, gonads, brain, adipose, breast, and liver.[226] During pregnancy, the fetal adrenal produces large amounts of DHEAS and its 16α-hydroxylated metabolite, which are then normally converted to estrogen by sequential action of placental sulfatase and aromatase. Aromatase deficiency is a rare, autosomal recessive condition in which fetal adrenal androgens accumulate and are converted to androstenedione and testosterone by placental 3β-HSD and 17β-HSD. This hyperandrogenism produces virilization of both the mother and female fetus; male infants have normal genital development but maternal virilization again occurs during the pregnancy.[227]

Affected females have clitoromegaly and some degree of labioscrotal fusion. Internal genital structures are normal, but large cystic ovaries may be present.[228] During puberty there is absent breast development and growth spurt, but further virilization may occur. Males have normal masculinization at puberty but prolonged linear growth, tall stature, delayed bone age, and osteoporosis, illustrating the importance of estrogens for normal bone maturation and development.[229]

The diagnosis should be suspected in a virilized female infant after congenital adrenal hyperplasia and a maternal androgen secreting tumour have been excluded. The characteristic laboratory findings are low estradiol; high DHEAS, androstenedione, and testosterone, and elevated LH and FSH. Maternal urinary estriol is low during pregnancy.

Management includes surgical correction of the external genitalia in infancy and lifelong estrogen replacement starting in early adolescence. There is some evidence that very low doses of estrogen during childhood may normalize the multicystic ovaries and bone density.[229]

Prenatal Virilization by Environmental Hormones

Masculinization of the external genitalia of female infants can also occur if the mother ingests androgens or has a virilizing disorder such as an ovarian tumor (usually an arrhenoblastoma or hCG-dependent luteoma of pregnancy), adrenal neoplasm, or inadequately treated CAH. In addition, female pseudohermaphroditism of varying degrees has been observed in the offspring of women treated with synthetic progestins such as norethindrone, ethisterone, norethynodrel, and medroxyprogesterone.[230] Similar virilization may also occur after maternal ingestion of large doses of stilbestrol, perhaps because of inhibition of fetal adrenal 3β-HSD; such offspring would also be at risk for later development of adenocarcinoma of the cervix and vagina.

The only treatment necessary for this form of female pseudohermaphroditism is surgical repair of the external genitalia. There is no need for ongoing hormone replacement therapy, and subsequent physical and psychosexual development should be entirely normal.[231]

Teratologic Malformations of the External Genitalia

Genital abnormalities, occasionally presenting as female pseudohermaphroditism, are frequently observed in association with renal agenesis, imperforate anus, and other malformations of the urinary and intestinal tracts.[232] Usually the internal genitalia are absent or abnormal. Similar apparently nonendocrine masculinization of a female fetus has been observed in association with multiple malformation syndromes, including cryptophthalmos, middle and outer ear maldevelopment, meningoencephalocele, and cardiac malformations; there may be familial recurrence of these anomalies, most of which have been lethal. A familial association of vaginal agenesis, middle ear malformations, and renal hypoplasia has been described.[233] Apparent clitoral enlargement giving the appearance of female pseudohermaphroditism can also occur in neurofibromatosis.

CLINICAL APPROACH TO DISORDERS OF SEXUAL DIFFERENTIATION

The Newborn with Abnormal Genitalia

Genital ambiguity in a neonate presents a psychosocial crisis that demands rapid yet sophisticated investigation before therapy and sex assignment. Such infants should be transferred at once to a center capable of providing within days a definitive diagnosis in terms of genetic sex, gonadal and genital structure, and endocrine function. Although the resources and expertise of a team of physicians are required, a single person, usually the pediatric endocrinologist, should be responsible for communication with the parents in order to explain the problem and proposed investigations and to counsel them regarding the prognosis for health, psychosexual adjustment, and reproductive function. Naming of the child should be delayed until gender assignment is decided; under no circumstances should parents be encouraged to select purposely a sexually ambiguous name. When reassignment of the sex of rearing is necessary because of a previous incorrect diagnosis or ignorance of the principles that govern gender assignment, it becomes doubly important that the reasons for this decision be explained to the parents in simple terms by a physician who is familiar with their cultural, religious, and educational background.

An abnormality of sexual differentiation should be suspected not only in an infant with obviously ambiguous genitalia but also in apparent males with hypospadias, cryptorchidism, or micropenis and in apparent females with partial labial fusion, clitoromegaly, or an inguinal mass. An abbreviated flowchart for the logical application of genetic and endocrine investigations in these circumstances is presented in Fig. 17-22. Only rarely will the genitalia be sufficiently distinctive to diagnose a particular disorder. Rather, examination of the external genitalia serves to document specific points, such as size of the phallus, location of the urethral meatus, number and location of ventral frenula on the phallus, degree of labioscrotal fusion, and presence or absence of palpable gonads. Finally, a careful assessment should be made of any associated congenital malformations, dehydration, or hyperpigmentation. A careful review of both pregnancy history and family history is essential. Maternal virilization during pregnancy may suggest ovarian or adrenal disease with transplacental passage of maternal androgens. Parental consanguinity suggests the possible expression of an autosomal recessive disorder. A family history of genital ambiguity or infertility is often available when an X-linked condition presents.

Initial laboratory investigation in an infant without palpable gonads includes karyotype analysis and assays of serum 17-hydroxyprogesterone levels. The infant's intake, weight, and serum electrolytes should be monitored daily to assess any salt wasting, but assays of plasma renin activity are best delayed until after 4 days of age. Ultrasonography should be performed to confirm the status of the paramesonephric duct structures. Genitography is occasionally necessary. The purpose of this approach is to identify the most common condition, 21-hydroxylase deficiency, before salt-losing complications appear. If, in a genetic female, the serum 17-hydroxyprogesterone concentrations are not significantly raised (over 3,000 ng/dl) and rising by 5 days of age, one should consider other forms of female pseudohermaphroditism and assess serum levels of steroids such as 11-deoxycortisol, dehydroepiandrosterone, and 17-hydroxypregnenolone.

Any gonad felt in the labioscrotal or inguinal area almost certainly contains testicular tissue. If portions of it differ in consistency, one should consider a possible ovotestis or a gonad that has undergone neoplastic transformation. Absence of well-differentiated paramesonephric duct structures on one side provides further evidence that the ipsilateral gonad contains testicular tissue. Complete absence of these structures shown by genitography in a 46,XY infant with ambiguous genitalia suggests one of the several forms of male pseudohermaphroditism; further investigation requires detailed analysis of hCG-stimulated androgen biosynthesis and of target cell receptors and metabolism.

With increasing frequency, a family history of abnormal sexual differentiation raises the question of possible prenatal diagnosis during a subsequent pregnancy. Ultrasonography may permit visualization of the external genitalia after the fifth month of gestation, amniocentesis can often provide a biochemical diagnosis at 15–20 weeks, and chorionic villus biopsy offers an opportunity to assess genetic sex, HLA haplotype and genotype even earlier. These techniques have been used successfully to identify affected fetuses with 21-hydroxylase deficiency and permit prenatal treatment with dexamethasone given to the mother. Such an approach has resulted in the birth of affected females with normal or only minimally virilized genitalia.

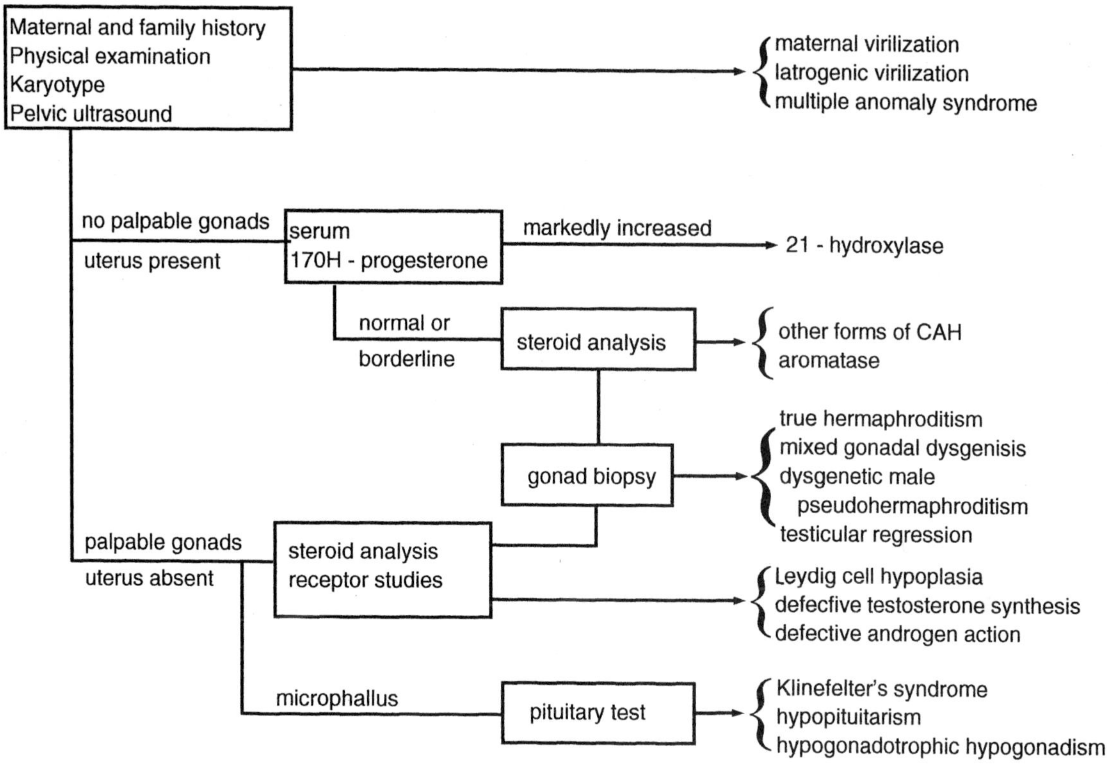

FIGURE 17-22. A simplified flowchart for the investigation and diagnosis of an infant with genital ambiguity.

In a female pseudohermaphrodite capable of normal fertility, it is obvious that the sex of rearing should be female. Similarly, in a male with 5α-reductase deficiency, the potential for dramatic virilization and adult male reproductive function requires that the infant be raised as male regardless of genital appearance. However, in most intersex disorders there is no chance for fertility, and the prime consideration for gender assignment should be the potential to achieve functional and cosmetically acceptable external genitalia with endocrine and surgical therapy. Genetic males with microphallus often benefit from a course of androgen therapy (testosterone cypionate 25 mg IM monthly for three doses) before any surgery. However, if a defect in androgen receptor activity has been demonstrated, such virilization is impossible and assignment of female gender is appropriate.

To ensure family acceptance and normal adjustment of the infant, reconstructive surgery to provide gender-compatible external genitalia should, if possible, be performed before 12 months of age. In females a type of vaginoplasty and clitoroplasty that preserves clitoral innervation and blood supply is most desirable. Thereafter, any further surgery should be delayed until late adolescence. In males the creation of a phallic urethra is more difficult and requires several procedures; if the testes are absent or have been removed, consideration should be given to the insertion of prostheses, usually during adolescence.

Where there is a significant risk of gonadal neoplasia, as in gonadal dysgenesis with a Y-bearing cell line, the gonads should be removed as early as is convenient. It has been customary in complete androgen insensitivity to leave the testes in place until after puberty, but when an infant is already undergoing repair of inguinal hernias, it is probably more reasonable to remove the testes and then to provide estrogen replacement at the time of puberty. If the sex of rearing is female and there is any risk of even partial virilization at puberty (as in incomplete androgen resistance), the gonads should be removed during childhood.

Virilization During Childhood or Adolescence

The precocious appearance of pubic hair and acne or inappropriate hirsutism, clitoral enlargement, or other sign of virilization deserves careful investigation, as outlined in Fig. 17-23. A small but significant fraction of such patients will prove to have a late-onset variant of CAH (21-hydroxylase, 11-hydroxylase, or 3-HSD deficiency). Frequently ACTH stimulation and dexamethasone suppression testing are necessary to demonstrate the defect in steroidogenesis.

Delayed Puberty, Amenorrhea, and Infertility

The initial evaluation of a patient presenting with delayed or unsatisfactory pubertal development, primary or secondary amenorrhea, or unexplained infertility should include assessment of serum gonadotropin concentrations. Those with hypergonadotropic hypogonadism (Fig. 17-24) may turn out to have an unrecognized disorder of sexual differentiations. Females with gonadal dysgenesis may present early with pubertal failure or later with secondary amenorrhea and infertility. If an apparent female shows normal breast development, sparse sex hair, and

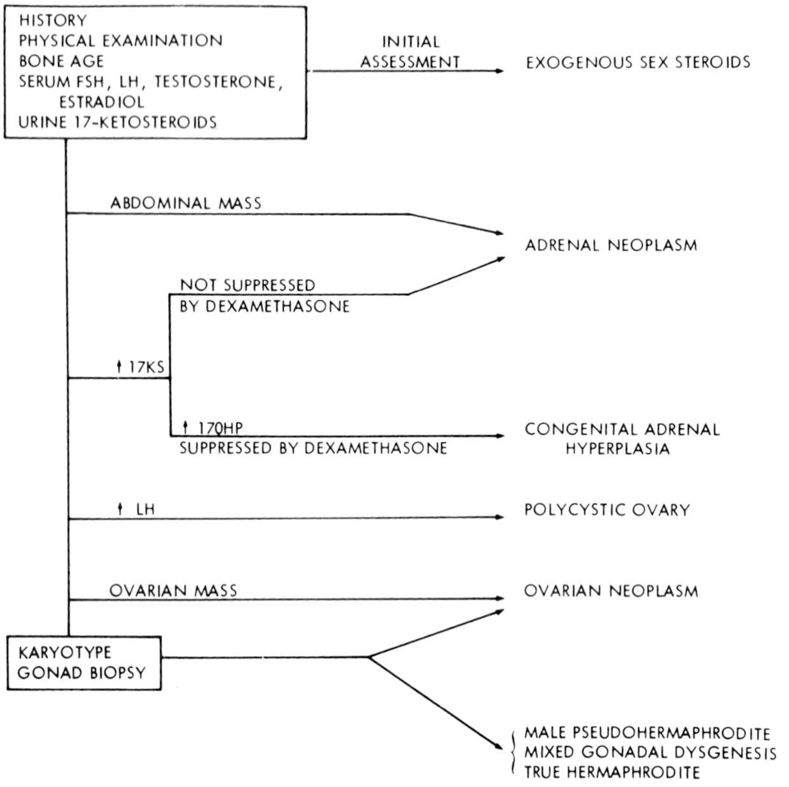

FIGURE 17-23. A flowchart illustrating a practical diagnostic approach to children with inappropriate virilization. [*From Dean HJ, Winter JSD, in Collu R, Ducharme JR, Guyda H (eds): Pediatric Endocrinology. New York, Raven, 1981, p 350.*]

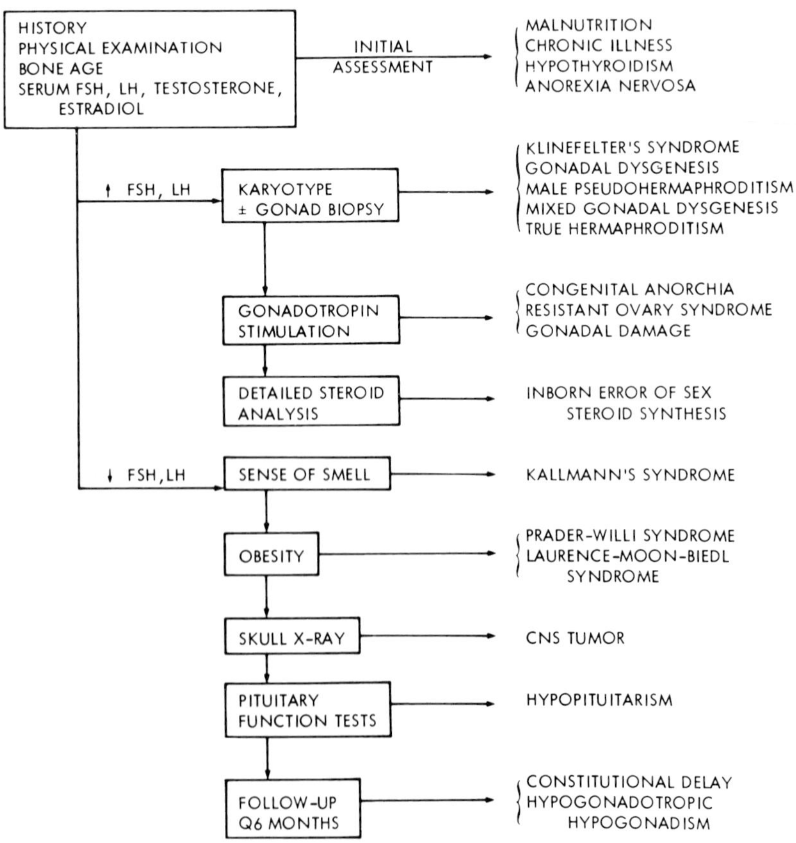

FIGURE 17-24. A flowchart illustrating a practical diagnostic approach to patients with delayed puberty. [*From Dean HJ, Winter JSD, in Collu R, Ducharme JR, Guyda H (eds): Pediatric Endocrinology. New York, Raven, 1981, p 333.*]

primary amenorrhea, the likely diagnosis is testicular feminization.

REFERENCES

1. Painter TS: The sex chromosome of man. *Am Nat* 58:506, 1924.
2. Fisher RA: *The Genetical Theory of Natural Selection*. Oxford, Clarendon, 1930.
3. National Foundation for Birth Defects: *An International System for Human Cytogenic Nomenclature. Birth Defects* 21:1, 1985.
4. Boué J, Boué A, Lazar P: Retrospective and prospective epidemiological studies of 1500 karyotyped spontaneous human abortions. *Teratology* 12:11, 1975.
5. Martin RH, Balkan W, Burns K, Rademaker AW, Lin CC, Rudd NL: The chromosome constitution of 1000 human spermatozoa. *Hum Genet* 63:305, 1983.
6. Jacobs PA: The incidence and etiology of sex chromosome abnormalities in man. New York, The National Foundation, 1979.
7. Opitz O, Zoll B, Hansmann I, Hinney B: Cytogenetic investigation of 103 patients with primary or secondary amenorrhea. *Hum Genet* 65:46, 1983.
8. Diedrich U, Hansmann I, Janke D, Opitz O, Probeck HD: Chromosome abnormalities in 136 couples with a history of recurrent abortions. *Hum Genet* 65:48, 1983.
9. Muller U: Molecular biology of the human Y chromosome, in SS Wachtel (ed): *Evolutionary Mechanisms in Sex Determination*. Boca Raton, FL, CRC Press, 1989, pp 91-98.
10. Vogt PH, Affara N, Davey P, et al: Report of the third international workship on Y chromosome mapping 1997. *Cytogenet Cell Genet* 79:1, 1997.
11. Rao E, Weiss B, Fukami M, et al: Pseudoautosomal deletions encompassing a novel homeobox gene cause growth failure in idiopathic short stature and Turner syndrome. *Nat Genet* 16:54, 1997.
12. Sinclair AH, Berta P, et al: A gene from the human sex-determining region encodes a protein with homology to a conserved DNA-binding motif. *Nature* 346:240, 1990.
13. Koopman P, Gubbay J, Vivian N, Goodfellow P, Lovell-Badge R: Male development of chromosomally female mice transgenic for *Sry*. *Nature* 351:117, 1991.
14. Capel B: Sex in the 90s: SRY and the switch to the male pathway. *Annu Rev Physiol* 60:497, 1998.

14a. Schmahl J, Eicher EM, Washburn LL, Capel B: Sry induces cell proliferation in the mouse gonad. *Development* 127:65, 2000.

15. Haqq CM, Donahoe PK: Regulation of sexual dimorphism in mammals. *Physiol Rev* 78:1, 1998.
16. Lahn BT, Page DC: Functional coherence of the human Y chromosome. *Science* 278:675, 1997.
17. Vogt PH, Affara N, Davey P, et al: Report of the third international workshop on Y chromosome mapping 1997. *Cytogenet Cell Genet* 79:1, 1997.
18. Salo P, Kaariainen H, Petrovic V, et al: Molecular mapping of the putative gonadoblastoma locus on the Y chromsome. *Genes, Chromosomes and Cancer* 14:210, 1995.
19. Wang W, Meadows LR, den Haan JMM, et al: Human H-Y: a male-specific histocompatibility antigen derived from the SMCY protein. *Science* 269:1588, 1995.
20. McKusick VA: *Mendeleian Inheritance in Man. A Catalog of Human Genes and Genetic Disorders*, 12th ed. Baltimore, Johns Hopkins University Press, 1998.
21. Quigley CA, DeBellis A, Marschke KB, et al: Androgen receptor defects: Historical, clinical and molecular perspectives. *Endocrin Rev* 16:271, 1995.
22. Bardoni B, Zanaria E, Guioli S, et al: A dosage sensitive locus at chromosome Xp21 is involved in male to female sex reversal. *Nat Genet* 7:497, 1994.
23. Ogata T, Matsuo N: Turner syndrome and female sex chromosome aberrations: Deduction of the principal factors involved in the development of clinical features. *Hum Genet* 95:607, 1995.
24. Heard E, Clerc P, Avner P: X-chromosome inactivation in mammmals. *Annu Rev Genet* 31:571, 1997.
25. Byskov AG: Gonadal sex and germ cell differentiation, in Austin CR, Edwards RG (eds): *Mechanisms of Sex Differentiation in Animals and Man*. London, Academic, 1981, p 145.
26. Schafer AJ, Goodfellow PN: Sex determination in Humans. *BioEssays* 18:955, 1996.
27. Kreidberg JA, Sariola H, Loring JM, et al: WT-1 is required for early kidney development. *Cell* 74:679, 1993.
28. Little M, Wells C: A clinical overview of WT1 gene mutations. *Hum Mutat* 9:209, 1997.
29. Wong M, Ikeda Y, Luo X, et al: Steroidogenic factor 1 plays multiple roles in endocrine development and function. *Rec Prog Horm Res* 52:167, 1997.

29a. Birk OS, Casiano DE, Wassif CA, et al: The LIM homeobox gene Lhx9 is essential for mouse gonad formation. *Nature* 403:909, 2000.

30. Rabinovici J, Jaffe RB: Development and regulation of growth and differentiated function in human and subhuman primate fetal gonads. *Endocr Rev* 11:532, 1990.
31. Mansour S, Hall CM, Pembrey ME, Young ID: A clinical and genetic study of campomelic dysplasia. *J Med Genet* 32:415, 1995.
32. Foster JW, Dominguez-Steglich A, Guioli S, et al: Campomelic dysplasia and autosomal sex reversal caused by mutations in an SRY related gene. *Nature* 372:525, 1994.
33. Schafter AJ, Foster JW, Kwok C, et al: Campomelic dysplasia with XY sex reversal: Diverse phenotypes resulting from mutations in a single gene. *Ann NY Acad Sci* 785:137, 1996.
34. Morais da Silva S, Hacker A, Harley V, et al: Sox9 expression during gonadal development implies a conserved role for the gene in testis differentiation in mammals and birds. *Nat Genet* 14:62, 1996.
35. Nachtigal MV, Hirokawa Y, Enyeart-VanHouten DL, et al: Wilms' tumour 1 and Dax-1 modulate the orphan nuclear receptor SF-1 in sex-specific gene expression. *Cell* 93:445, 1998.
36. Kurilo LF: Oogenesis in antenatal development in man. *Hum Genet* 57:86, 1981.
37. Swain A, Narvaez V, Burgoyne P, et al: Daxl antagonizes Sry action in mammalian sex determination. *Nature* 391:761, 1998.

37a. Yu RN, Ito M, Saunders TL, et al: Role of Ahch in gonadal development and gametogenesis. *Nat Genet* 20:353, 1998.

38. Whitworth DJ: XX germ cells: The difference between an ovary and a testis. *Trends Endocrinol Metab* 9:2, 1998.
39. Cate RL, Mattalinao RJ, Hesion C, et al: Isolation of the bovine and human genes for Mullerian inhibiting substance and expression of the human genes in animal cells. *Cell* 45:685, 1986.
40. Cohen-Haguenauer O, Picard JY, Mattei MG, et al: Mapping of the gene for antimullerian hormone to the short arm of human chromosome 19. *Cytogenet Cell Genet* 44:2, 1987.
41. Guilli G, Shen W-H, Ingraham HA: The nuclear receptor SF-1 mediates sexually dimorphic expression of Mullerian inhibiting substance, in vivo. *Development* 124:1799, 1997.
42. Imbeaud S, Faure E, Lamarre I, et al: Insensitivity to anti-mullerian hormone due to a mutation in the human anti-mullerian hormone receptor. *Nat Genet* 11:382, 1995.
43. Josso N, Cate RL, Picard JY, et al: Anti-Mullerian hormone: The Jost factor. *Rec Prog Horm Res* 48:1, 1993.
44. Hutson JM, Hasthorpe S, Heyns CF: Anatomical and functional aspects of testicular descent and cryptorchidism. *Endocrine Rev* 18:259, 1997.
45. Siiteri PK, Wilson JD: Testosterone formation and metabolism during male sexual differentiation in the human embryo. *J Clin Endocrinol Metab* 38:113, 1974.
46. Feldman KW, Smith DW: Fetal phallic growth and penile standards for newborn male infants. *J Pediatr* 86:395, 1975.
47. Winter JSD, Faiman C, Reyes FI: Sex steroid production by the human fetus: Its role in morphogenesis and control by gonadotropins, in Blandau RJ, Bergsman D (eds): *Morphogenesis and Malformation of the Genital System*. New York, Liss, 1977, pp 41–58.
48. Voutilainen R, Miller WL: Development expression of genes for the steroidogenic enzymes $P450_{scc}$(20,22-desmolase), $P450_{c17}$(17-alpha-hydroxylase/17,20-lyase) and $P450_{c21}$(21-hydroxylase) in the human fetus. *J Clin Endocrinol Metab* 63:1145, 1986.
49. Rundlett SE, Wu XP, Miesfield RL: Functional characterizations of the androgen receptor confirm the molecular basis of androgen action is transcriptional regulation. *Mol Endocrinol* 4:708, 1990.
50. Cunha GR, Shannon JM, Neubauer BL, et al: Mesenchymal-epithelial interactions in sex differentiation. *Hum Genet* 58:68, 1981.
51. Chang C, Kokontis J, Liao S: Molecular cloning of human and rat

complementary DNA encoding androgen receptors. *Science* 240:324, 1988.
52. Lubahn DB, Joseph Dr, Sullivan PM, Willard HF, French FS, Wilson EM: Cloning of human androgen receptor complementary DNA and localization to the X chromosome. *Science* 240:327, 1988.
53. Word RA, George FW, Wilson JD, Carr BR: Testosterone synthesis and adenylate cyclase activity in the early human fetal testis appear to be independent of human chorionic gonadotropin control. *J Clin Endocrinol Metab* 69:204, 1989.
54. Voutilainen R: Differentiation of the fetal gonad. *Horm Res* 38(suppl 2):66, 1992.
55. Mulchahey JJ, DiBlasio AM, Martin MC, et al: Hormone production and peptide regulation of the human fetal pituitary gland. *Endocrine Rev* 8:406, 1987.
56. Ronnekleiv OK, Resko JA: Ontogeny of gonadotropin-releasing hormone-containing neurons in early fetal development of rhesus macaques. *Endocrinology* 126:498, 1990.
57. Dumesic DA, Pohl H, Kamel F, Terasawa E: Increase in luteinizing hormone content occurs in cultured human fetal pituitary cells exposed to gonadotropin-releasing hormone. *J Clin Endocrinol Metab* 70:606, 1990.
58. Reyes FI, Winter JSD, Faiman C: Endocrinology of the fetal testis, in H. Burger and D. de Kretser (eds): *The Testis*, 2nd ed. New York, Raven Press, 1989, pp 119–142.
59. Rasmussen DD, Liu JH, Wolf PL, Yen SSC: Endogenous opioid regulation of gonadotropin-releasing hormone release from the human fetal hypothalamus in vitro. *J Clin Endocrinol Metab* 57:881, 1983.
60. Petraglia F, Volpe A, Genazzani AR, et al: Neuroendocrinology of human placenta. *Front Neuroendocrinol* 11:6, 1990.
61. Lin LS, Roberts VJ, Yen SS: Expression of human gonadotropin-releasing hormone receptor gene in the placenta and its functional relationship to human chorionic gonadotropin secretion. *J Clin Endocrinol Metab* 80:580, 1995.
62. Voutilainen R, Miller WL: Developmental and hormonal regulation of mRNAs for insulin-like growth factor II and steroidogenic enzymes in human fetal adrenals and gonads. *DNA* 7:9, 1989.
63. Wallace EM, Riley SC, Crossley JA, et al: Dimeric inhibins in amniotic fluid, maternal serum and fetal serum in human pregnancy. *J Clin Endocrinol Metab* 82:218, 1997.
64. Qu J, Thomas K: Inhibin and activin production in human placenta. *Endocrine Rev* 16:485, 1995.
65. Winter JSD, Faiman C, Reyes FI: Sexual endocrinology of fetal and perinatal life, in Austin CR, Edwards RG (eds): *Mechanisms of Sex Differentiation in Animals and Man*. London, Academic, 1981, pp 205–253.
66. Corbier P, Dahennin L, Castanier M, Mebazaa A, Edwards DA, Roffi J: Sex differences in serum luteinizing hormone and testosterone in the human neonate during the first few hours after birth. *J Clin Endocrinol Metab* 7:1344, 1990.
67. Bolton NJ, Tapanainen J, Koivisto M, Vihko R: Circulating sex hormone-binding globulin and testosterone in newborns and infants. *Clin Endocrinol (Oxf)* 31:201, 1989.
68. Mann DR, Gould KG, Collins DC, Wallen K: Blockade of neonatal activation of the pituitary-testicular axis: Effect on peripubertal luteinizing hormone and testosterone secretion and on testicular development in male monkeys. *J Clin Endocrinol Metab* 68:600, 1988.
69. Imperato-McGinley J, Peterson RE, Gautier T, Sturla E: The impact of androgens on the evolution of male gender identity, in Kogan SJ, Hafez ESE (eds): *Pediatric Andrology*. The Hague, Martinus Nijhoff, 1981, pp 99–108.
70. Dorner G: Hormones, brain differentiation and the fundamental process of life. *J Steroid Biochem* 8:531, 1977.
71. Gorski RA: Sexual differentiation of the brain: Possible mechanisms and implications. *Can J Physiol Pharmacol* 63:577, 1985.
72. Sholl SA, Goy RW, Kim KL: 5α-Reductase, aromatase, and androgen receptor levels in the monkey brain during fetal development. *Endocrinology* 124:627, 1989.
73. Berenbaum SA, Duck SC, Bryk K: Behavioral effects of prenatal versus postnatal androgen excess in children with 21-hydroxylase deficient congenital adrenal hyperplasia. *J Clin Endocrinol Metab* 85:727, 2000.
74. Ehrhardt AA, Meyer-Bahlburg HFL, Rosen LR, Feldman JF, Veridiano NP, Zimmerman I, McEwen BS: Sexual orientation after prenatal exposure to exogenous estrogen. *Arch Sex Behav* 14:57, 1985.
75. Klinefelter HF Jr, Reifenstein EC Jr, Albright F: Syndrome characterized by gynecomastia, aspermatogenesis with a-leydigism, and increased excretion of follicle-stimulating hormone. *J Clin Endocrinol Metab* 2:615, 1942.
76. Salbenblatt JA, Bender BG, Puck MH, Robinson A, Faiman C, Winter JSD: Pituitary-gonadal function in Klinefelter syndrome before and during puberty. *Pediatr Res* 19:82, 1985.
77. Topper E, Dickerman Z, Prager-Lewin R, Kaufman H, Maimon Z, Laron Z: Puberty in 24 patients with Klinefelter syndrome. *Eur J Pediatr* 139:8, 1982.
78. Hultborn R, Hanson C, Kopf I, et al: Prevalence of Klinefelter's syndrome in male breast cancer patients. *Anticancer Res* 17:4293, 1997.
79. Page DC, Brown LG, de la Chapelle A: Exchange of terminal portions of X- and Y-chromosomal short arms in human XX males. *Nature* 328:437, 1987.
80. Weil D, Wang I, Deitrich A, et al: Highly homologous loci on the X and Y chromosomes are hot-spots for ectopic recombinations leading to XX maleness. *Nat Genet* 7:414, 1994.
81. Page DC, Fisher EMC, McGillivray B, Brown L: Additional deletion in sex-determining region of human Y chromosome resolves paradox of X,t(Y;22) female. *Nature* 346:279, 1990.
82. Kohn G, Winter JSD, Mellman WJ: Trisomy X in three children. *J Pediatr* 72:248, 1968.
83. Krob G, Braun A, Kuhnle U: True hermephroditism: geographical distribution, clinical findings and gonadal histology. *Eur J Pediatr* 153:2, 1994.
84. Damiani D, Fellous M, McElreavey K, et al: True hermaphroditism: Clinical aspects and molecular studies in 16 cases. *Eur J Endocrinol* 136:201, 1997.
85. Berkovitz GD, Fechner PY, Marcantoni SM: The role of the sex-determining region of the Y chromosome (SRY) in the etiology of 46, XX true hermaphroditism. *Hum Genet* 88:411, 1992.
86. Davidoff F, Federman DD: Mixed gonadal dysgenesis. *Pediatrics* 52:725, 1973.
87. Manuel M, Katayama KP, Jones HW Jr: The age of occurrence of gonadal tumors in intersex patients with a Y chromosome. *Am J Obstet Gynecol* 124:293, 1976.
88. Warburton D, Cline J, Stein Z, Susser M: Monosomy X: A chromosomal anomaly associated with young maternal age. *Lancet* i:167, 1980.
89. Lyon AJ, Preece MA, Grant DB: Growth curve for girls with Turner's syndrome. *Arch Dis Child* 60:932, 1985.
90. Ranke MB: Growth disorder in the Ullrich-Turner Syndrome. *Bailliere's Clin Endocrinol Metab* 6:603, 1992.
91. Kleczkowska A, Kubien E, Dmoch E, et al: Turner syndrome: II. Associated anomalies, mental performance and psychological problems in 218 patients diagnosed in Leuven in the period 1965–1989. *Genet Counselling* 1:241, 1990.
92. Skuse DH, James RS, Bishop DV, et al: Evidence from Turner's syndrome of an imprinted X-linked locus affecting cognitive function. *Nature* 387:705, 1997.
93. Pasquino AM, Passeri F, Pucarelli I, et al: Spontaneous pubertal development in Turner's syndrome. *J Clin Endocrinol Metab* 82:1810, 1997.
94. Krauss CM, Turksoy RN, Atkins L, McLaughlin C, Brown LG, Page DC: Familial premature ovarian failure due to an interstitial deletion of the long arm of the X-chromosome. *N Engl J Med* 317:125, 1987.
95. Chu CE, Donaldson MDC, Smail PJ, et al: Detection of Y mosaicism in patients with Turner's syndrome. *J Med Genet* 32:578, 1995.
96. Winter JSD, Faiman C: Serum gonadotrophin levels in agonadal children and adults. *J Clin Endocrinol Metab* 35:561, 1972.
97. Van den Broeck JV, Massa GG, Attanasio A, et al: Final height after long-term growth hormone treatment in Turner's syndrome. *J Pediatr* 127:729, 1995.
98. Nilsson KO, Albertson-Wikland K, Alm J, et al: Improved final height in girls with Turner's syndrome treated with growth hormone and oxandrolone. *J Clin Endocrinol Metab* 81:635, 1996.
99. Rosenfeld RG, Attie KM, Frane J, et al: Growth hormone therapy of Turner's syndrome: beneficial effect on adult height. *J Pediatr* 132:319, 1998.
100. Apter D, Lenko HL, Perheentupa J, Soderholm A, Vihko R: Subnormal pubertal increases of serum androgens in Turner's syndrome. *Horm Res* 16:164, 1982.
101. Sybert VP: Adult height in Turner syndrome with and without androgen therapy. *J Pediatr* 104:365, 1984.

102. Ross JL, Cassorla FG, Skerda MC, Valk IM, Loriaux DL, Cutler GB Jr: A preliminary study of the effect of estrogen dose on growth in Turner's syndrome. *N Engl J Med* 309:1104, 1983.
103. Martinez A, Heinrich JJ, Domene H, Escobar ME, Jasper H, Moinuori, Bergada C: Growth in Turner's syndrome: Long term treatment with low dose ethinyl estradiol. *J Clin Endocrinol Metab* 65:253, 1987.
104. Demetriou F, Emans SJ, Crigler JF Jr: Final height in estrogen-treated patients with Turner's syndrome. *Obstet Gynecol* 64:459, 1984.
105. Kaneko N, Kawagoe S, Hiroi M: Turner's syndrome—review of the literature with reference to a successful pregnancy outcome. *Gynecol Obstet Invest* 29:81, 1990.
106. Khastgir G, Abdalla H, Thomas A, et al: Oocyte donation in Turner's syndrome: An analysis of the factors affecting the outcome. *Hum Reprod* 12:279, 1997.
107. Committee on Genetics, American Academy of Pediatrics: Health supervision for children with Turner syndrome. *Pediatrics* 96:1166, 1995.
108. Doherty L, Brown DM, Ainslie M, et al: Turner syndrome practice guidelines. *Endocrinologist* 7:443, 1997.
109. Aittomaki K: The genetics of XX gonadal dysgenesis. *Am J Hum Genet* 54:844, 1994.
110. Scherer G, Held M, Erdel M, et al: Three novel SRY mutations in XY gonadal dysgenesis and the enigma of XY gonadal dyspenesis cases without SRY mutations. *Cytogenet and Cell Genet* 80:188, 1998.
111. McDonald MT, Flejter W, Sheldon S, Putzi MJ, Gorski JL: XY sex reversal and gonadal dysgenesis due to 9p24 monosomy. *Am J Med Genet* 73:321, 1997.
112. Cleary RE, Caras J, Rosenfield RL, Young PCM: Endocrine and metabolic studies in a patient with male pseudohermaphroditism and true agonadism. *Am J Obstet Gynecol* 128:862, 1977.
113. Winter JSD, Taraska S, Faiman C: The hormonal response to hCG stimulation in male children and adolescents. *J Clin Endocrinol Metab* 34:348, 1972.
114. Smith NM, Byard RW, Bourne AJ: Testicular regression syndrome—a pathological study of 77 cases. *Histopathol* 19:269, 1991.
115. Josso N, Picard JY, Imbeaud S, et al. Clinical aspects and molecular genetics of the persistent Mullerian duct syndrome. *Clin Endocrinol* 47:137, 1997.
116. Latronico AC, Anasti J, Arnhold IJP: Testicular and ovarian resistance to luteinizing hormone caused by homozygous inactivating mutations of the luteinizing hormone receptor gene. *N Engl J Med* 334:507, 1996.
117. Tsigos C, Latronico C, Chroussos GP: Luteinizing hormone resistance syndromes. *Ann NY Acad Sci* 816:263, 1997.
118. Clark BJ, Wells J, King SR, et al: The purification, cloning, and expression of a novel LH-induced mitochondrial protein in MA-10 mouse Leydig tumor cells: Characterization of the steroidogenic acute regulatory protein (StAR). *J Biol Chem* 269:28314, 1994.
119. Sugarawa T, Holt JA, Driscoll D, et al: Human steroidogenic acute regulatory protein: Functional activity in COS-1 cells, tissue specific expression and mapping of the gene to 8p11.2 and a pseudogene to chromosome 13. *Proc Natl Acad Sci USA* 92:4778, 1995.
120. Stocco DM, Clark BJ: The role of the steroidogenic acute regulatory protein in steroidogenesis. *Steroids* 62:29, 1997.
121. Cheradi N, Capponi AM: The acute regulation of mineralocorticoid biosynthesis: Scenarios for the StAR system. *Trends Endocrinol Metab* 9:412, 1998.
122. Saenger P, Klonari Z, Black SM, et al: Prenatal diagnosis of congenital lipoid adrenal hyperplasia. *J Clin Endocrinol Metab* 80:200, 1995.
123. Bose HS, Sugawara T, Strauss JF, et al: The pathophysiology and genetics of congenital lipoid adrenal hyperplasia. *N Engl J Med* 335:1870, 1996.
124. Nakae J, Tajima T, Sugawara, et al: Analysis of the steroidogenic acute regulatory protein (StAR), gene in Japanese patients with congenital lipoid adrenal hyperplasia. *Hum Mol Genet* 6:571, 1997.
125. Lin D, Gitelman SE, Saenger P, Miller WL: Normal genes for the cholesterol side chain cleavage enzyme, P450scc, in congenital lipoid adrenal hyperplasia. *J Clin Invest* 88:1955, 1991.
126. Miller WL: Why nobody has P450scc (20, 22 desmolase) deficiency. *J Clin Endocrinol Metab* 83:1399, 1998.
127. The VL, Lachance Y, Labrie C, Leblanc G, Thomas JL, Strickler RC, Labrie F: Full-length cDNA structure and predicted amino acid sequence of human placenta 3β-hydroxy-5-ene steroid dehydrogenase. *Mol Endocrinol* 3:1310, 1989.
128. Rheaume E, Lachance Y, Zhao HF, et al: Structure and expression of a new cDNA encoding the almost exclusive 3 beta-hydroxysteroid dehydrogenase/delta 5-delta 4 isomerase in human adrenals and gonads. *Mol Endocrinol* 5:1147, 1991.
129. Byrne GC, Perry YS, Winter JSD: Steroid inhibitory effects upon human adrenal 3β-hydroxysteroid dehydrogenase activity. *J Clin Endocrinol Metab* 62:413, 1986.
130. Morel Y, Mebarki F, Rheaume E, et al: Structure-function relationships of 3β-hydroxysteroid dehydrogenase: Contribution made by the molecular genetics of 3β-hydroxysteroid dehydrogenase deficiency. *Steroids* 62:176, 1997.
131. Pang S, Levine LS, Stoner E, Opitz JM, Pollack MS, Dupont B, New MI: Nonsalt-losing congenital adrenal hyperplasia due to 3β-hydroxysteroid dehydrogenase deficiency with normal glomerulosa function. *J Clin Endocrinol Metab* 56:808, 1983.
132. Pang S, Lerner AJ, Stoner E, Levine LS, Oberfield SE, Engel I, New MI: Late-onset adrenal steroid 3β-hydroxysteroid dehydrogenase deficiency: A cause of hirsutism in pubertal and postpubertal women. *J Clin Endocrinol Metab* 60:428, 1985.
133. Zerah M, Rheaume E, Mani P, et al: No evidence of mutations in the genes for type I and type II 3β-hydroxysteroid dehydrogenase (3β-HSD) in nonclassical 3β-HSD deficiency. *J Clin Endocrinol Metab* 79:1811, 1994.
134. Chang YT, Zhang L, Alkaddour HS, et al: Absence of molecular defect in type II 3β-hydroxysteroid dehydrogenase (3β-HSD) gene in premature pubarche children and hirsute female patients with moderately decreased 3β-HSD activity. *Pediatr Res* 37:820, 1995.
135. Kominami S, Shinzawa K, Takemori S: Purification and some properties of cytochrome P-450 specific for steroid 17α-hydroxylation and C17-C20 bond cleavage from guinea pig adrenal microsomes. *Biochem Biophys Res Commun* 109:916, 1982.
136. Picardo-Leonard J, Miller WL: Cloning and sequence of the human gene encoding P450c17 (steroid 17α-hydroxylase/17,20-lyase): Similarity to the gene for P450c21. *DNA* 6:439, 1987.
137. Yanase T: 17α-hydroxylase/17,20-lyase defects. *J Steroid Biochem Mol Biol* 53:153, 1995.
138. Dean HJ, Shackleton CHL, Winter JSD: Diagnosis and natural history of 17-hydroxylase deficiency in a newborn male. *J Clin Endocrinol Metab* 59:513, 1984.
139. Kater CE, Biglieri EG, Brust N, Change B, Hirai J: The unique patterns of plasma aldosterone and 18-hydroxycorticosterone concentrations in the 17β-hydroxylase deficiency syndrome. *J Clin Endocrinol Metab* 55:295, 1982.
140. Zachmann M, Werder EA, Prader A: Two types of male pseudohermaphroditism due to 17,20-desmolase deficiency. *Acta Endocrinol (Copenh)* 103:400, 1983.
141. Larrea F, Lisker R, Banuelos R, et al: Hypergonadotrophic hypogonadism in an XX female subject due to 17,20-desmolase deficiency. *Acta Endocrinol (Copenh)* 103:400, 1983.
142. Miller WL, Auchus RJ, Geller DH: The regulation of 17,20 lyase activity. *Steroids* 62:133, 1997.
143. Geller DH, Auchus RJ, Mendonca BB, Miller WL: The genetic and functional basis of isolated 17,20-lyase deficiency. *Nat Genet* 17:201, 1997.
144. Biason-Lauber A, Leiberman E, Zachman M: A single amino acid substitution in the putative redox partner-binding site of P450C17 as cause of isolated 17,20-lyase deficiency. *J Clin Endocrinol Metab* 82:3807, 1997.
145. Labrie F, Luu-The V, Lin SX, et al: The key role of 17β-hydroxysteroid dehydrogenases in sex steroid biology. *Steroids* 62:148, 1997.
146. Geissler WM, Davis DL, Wu L, et al: Male pseudohermaphroditism caused by mutations of testicular 17 beta-hydroxysteroid dehydrogenase. *Nat Genet* 7:34, 1994.
147. Zhu YS, Katz MD, Imperato-McGinley J: Natural potent androgens: Lessons from human genetic models. *Bailliere's Clin Endocrinol Metab* 12:83, 1998.
148. Imperato-McGinley J, Peterson RE, Gautier T, Sturla E: Androgens and the evolution of male-gender identity among male pseudohermaphrodites with 5α-reductase deficiency. *N Engl J Med* 300:1233, 1979.
149. Cantu JM, Corona Rivera E, Diaz M, Medina C, Esquinca E, Cortes-Gallegos V, Vaca G, Hernandez A: Post-pubertal female psychosex-

ual orientation in incomplete male pseudohermaphroditism type 2 (5α-reductase deficiency). *Acta Endocrinol (Copenh)* 94:273, 1980.
150. Savage MO, Preece MA, Jeffcoate SL, Ransley PG, Rumsby G, Mansfield MD, Williams DI: Familial male pseudohermaphroditism due to deficiency of 5α-reductase. *Clin Endocrinol (Oxf)* 12:397, 1980.
151. Andersson S, Berman DS, Jenkins EP, Russell DW: Deletion of 5α-reductase 2 gene in male pseudohermaphroditism. *Nature* 354: 159, 1991.
152. Thigpen AE, Davis DL, Milatovich A, et al: Molecular genetics of steroid 5α-reductase 2 deficiency. *J Clin Invest* 90:799, 1992.
153. Imperato-McGinley J: 5α-reductase deficiency, in Bardin CW (ed): *Current Therapy in Endocrinology and Metabolism*, Philadelphia, BC Decker, 1991, p 312.
154. Brinkman A, Jenster G, Ris-Stalpers C, et al: Molecular basis of androgen insensitivity. *Steroids* 61:172, 1996.
155. Müller J, Skakkebaek NE: Testicular carcinoma in situ testis in children with the androgen insensitivity (testicular feminization) syndrome. *Br Med J* 1:1419, 1984.
156. Faiman C, Winter JSD: The control of gonadotropin secretion in complete testicular feminization. *J Clin Endocrinol Metab* 39:631, 1974.
157. Hiort O, Holterhus PM, Nitsche EM: Physiology and pathophysiology of androgen action. *Bailliere's Clin Endocrinol Metab* 12:115, 1998.
158. Quigley CA, DeBellis A, Marschke KB, et al: Androgen receptor defects: Historical, clinical and molecular perspectives. *Endocrine Rev* 16:271, 1995.
159. LaSpada AR, Wilson EM, Lubalm DB, et al: Androgen receptor gene mutations in X-linked spinal and bulbar muscular atrophy. *Nature* 352:77, 1991.
160. Amrhein JA, Klingensmith GJ, Walsh PC, McKusick VA, Migeon CJ: Partial androgen insensitivity: The Reifenstein syndrome revisited. *N Engl J Med* 297:350, 1977.
161. Cundy T, Rees M, Evans B, et al: Mild androgen insensitivity presenting with sexual dysfunction. *Fertil Steril* 46:721, 1986.
162. Hiort O, Sinnecker GHG, Horter T, et al: Minimal androgen receptor gene abnormalities. *Horm Res* 46 suppl 2:96, 1996.
163. Sinnecker GH, Hiort O, Nitsche EM, et al: Functional assessment and clinical classification of androgen sensitivity in patients with mutations of the androgen receptor gene. *Eur J Pediatr* 156:7, 1997.
164. Alberts N, Ulrichs C, Gluer S, et al: Etiologic classification of severe hypospadius: Implications for prognosis and management. *J Pediatr* 131:386, 1997.
165. Aarskog D: Maternal progestins as a possible cause of hypospadias. *N Engl J Med* 300:75, 1979.
166. Dean HJ, Winter JSD: The effect of five synthetic progestational compounds on 5α-reductase activity in genital skin fibroblast monolayers. *Steroids* 43:13, 1985.
167. Raman-Wilms L, Tseng AL, Wighardt S, et al: Fetal genital effects of first-trimester sex hormone exposure: A meta-analysis. *Obstet Gynecol* 85:141, 1995.
168. Gill WB, Schumacher GFB, Bibbo M, et al: Association of diethylstilbestrol exposure in utero with cryptorchidism, testicular hypoplasia and semen abnormalities. *J Urol* 122:36, 1979.
169. John Radcliffe Hospital Cryptorchidism Study: Cryptorchidism: A prospective study of 7500 consecutive male births, 1984-8. *Arch Dis Child* 67:892, 1992.
170. WHO: *Congenital Malformations Worldwide: A Report from the International Clearinghouse for Birth Defects Monitoring Systems*. Oxford, Elsevier, 1991.
171. Paulozzi LJ, Erickson JD, Jackson RJ: Hypospadias trends in two US surveillance systems. *Pediatrics* 100:831, 1997.
172. Toppari J, Skakkebaek NE: Sexual differentiation and environmental disrupters. *Bailliere's Clin Endocrinol Metab* 12:143, 1998.
173. Jones KL: Smith's *Recognizable Patterns of Human Malformation: Genetic, Embryologic and Clinical Aspects*, 5th ed. Philadelphia, Saunders, 1997.
174. Greenberg F, Gresik MW, Carpenter RT, Law SW, Hoffman LP, Ledbetter DH: The Gardner-Silengo-Wachtel or genito-palato-cardiac syndrome: Male pseudohermaphroditism with micrognathia, cleft palate and conotruncal cardiac defects. *Am J Med Genet* 26:59, 1987.
175. Bauer SB, Bull MJ, Retik AB: Hypospadias: A familial study. *J Urol* 121:474, 1979.
176. Svensson J, Eneroth P, Gustafsson JA, Ritzen M, Stenberg A: Metabolism of androstenedione in skin and serum levels of gonadotrophins and androgens in prepubertal boys with hypospadias. *J Endocrinol* 76:399, 1978.
177. Raboch J, Pondelickova J, Starka L: Plasma testosterone values in hypospadias. *Andrologia* 8:255, 1976.
178. Nonomura K, Fujieda K, Sakakibara N, Terasawa K, Matsuno T, Matsuura N, Koyanagi T: Pituitary and gonadal function in prepubertal boys with hypospadias. *J Urol* 132:595, 1984.
179. Aaronson IA, Cakmak MA, Key LL: Defects of the testosterone biosynthetic pathway in boys with hypospadias. *J Urol* 157:1884, 1997.
180. Sutherland RW, Wiener JS, Hicks JP, et al: Androgen receptor gene mutations are rarely associated with isolated penile hypospadias. *J Urol* 156:828, 1996.
181. Hutson JM, Hasthorpe S, Heyns CF: Anatomical and functional aspects of testicular descent and cryptorchidism. *Endocrine Rev* 18:259, 1997.
182. Müller J, Skakkebaek NE: Abnormal germ cells in maldescended testes: A study of cell density, nuclear size and deoxyribonucleic acid content in testicular biopsies from 50 boys. *J Urol* 131:730, 1984.
183. Prader A: Der Genitalbeffund beim Pseudohermaphroditismus feminus des Kongenitalen Adenogenitalen Syndroms. *Helv Paediatr Acta* 9:231, 1954.
184. Dickerman Z, Grant DR, Faiman C, Winter JSD: Intra-adrenal steroid concentrations in man: Zonal differences and developmental changes. *J Clin Endocrinol Metab* 59:1031, 1984.
185. Pang SY, Wallace AM, Hofman L, et al: Worldwide experience in newborn screening for classic congenital adrenal hyperplasia due to 21-hydroxylase deficiency. *Pediatrics* 81:866, 1988.
186. White PC, New MI: Genetic basis of endocrine disease 2: Congenital adrenal hyperplasia due to 21-hydroxylase deficiency. *J Clin Endocrinol Metab* 74:6, 1992.
187. Miller WL: Genetics, diagnosis and management of 21-hydroxylase deficiency. *J Clin Endocrinol Metab* 78:241, 1994.
188. Wedell A: Molecular genetics of congenital adrenal hyperplasia (21-hydroxylase deficiency): Implications for diagnosis, prognosis and treatment. *Acta Paediatrica* 87:159, 1998.
189. Jaaskelainen J, Levo A, Voutilainen R, Partanen J: Population-wide evaluation of disease manifestation in relation to molecular genotype in steroid 21-hydroxylase (CYP21) deficiency: Good correlation in a well-defined population. *J Clin Endocrinol Metab* 82:3293, 1997.
190. Sperser PW, White PC: Congenital adrenal hyperplasia due to steroid 21-hydroxylase deficiency. *Clin Endocrinol* 49:411, 1998.
190a. Krone N, Braun A, Roscher AA, Knorr D, Schwarz HP: Predicting phenotype in steroid 21-hydroxylase deficiency? Comprehensive genotyping in 155 unrelated, well-defined patients from southern Germany. *J Clin Endocrinol Metab* 85:1059, 2000.
191. Blankstein J, Faiman C, Reyes FI, Schroeder M, Winter JSD: Adult-onset familial 21-hydroxylase deficiency. *Am J Med* 68:441, 1980.
192. Speiser PW, Dupont J, Zhu D, et al: Disease specific expression and molecular genotype in congenital adrenal hyperplasia due to 21-hydroxylase deficiency. *J Clin Invest* 90:584, 1992.
193. Knochenhaur ES, Cortet-Rudelli C, Cunningham RD, et al: Carriers of 21-hydroxylase deficiency are not at increased risk for hyperandrogenism. *J Clin Endocrinol Metab* 82:479, 1997.
194. New MI, Lorenzen F, Lerner AJ, et al: Genotyping steroid 21-hydroxylase deficiency: Hormonal reference data. *J Clin Endocrinol Metab* 57:320, 1983.
195. Fife D, Rappaport EB: Prevalence of salt-losing among congenital adrenal hyperplasia patients. *Clin Endocrinol (Oxf)* 18:259, 1983.
196. Speiser PW, Agdere L, Ueshiba H, White PC, New MI: Aldosterone synthesis in salt-wasting congenital adrenal hyperplasia with complete absence of adrenal 21-hydroxylase. *N Engl J Med* 324:145, 1991.
197. Pham-Huu-Trung MT, Raux MC, Gourmelen M, Baron MC, Girard F: Plasma aldosterone concentrations related to 17α-hydroxyprogesterone in congenital adrenal hyperplasia. *Acta Endocrinol (Copenh)* 82:572, 1976.
198. Neville AM, O'Hare MJ: *The Human Adrenal Cortex*. Berlin, Springer-Verlag, 1982.
199. Dickerman Z, Grant DR, Farman C, Winter JS: Intraadrenal steroid concentrations in man: zonal differences and developmental changes. *J Clin Endocrinol Metab* 59:1031, 1984.
200. Schaison G, Couzinet B, Gourmelen M, Elkik F, Bougneres P:

Angiotensin and adrenal steroidogenesis: Study of 21-hydroxylase-deficient congenital adrenal hyperplasia. *J Clin Endocrinol Metab* 51:1390, 1980.

201. Hughes IA, Winter JSD: The application of a serum 17OH-progesterone radioimmunoassay to the diagnosis and management of congenital adrenal hyperplasia. *J Pediatr* 88:766, 1976.
202. Hughes IA, Riad-Fahmy D, Griffiths K: Plasma 17OH-progesterone concentrations in newborn infants. *Arch Dis Child* 54:347, 1979.
203. Forest MG, David M, Morel Y: Prenatal diagnosis and treatment of 21-hydroxylase deficiency. *J Steroid Biochem Molec Biol* 45:75, 1993.
204. Dorr HG, Sippell WG: Prenatal dexamethasone treatment in pregnancies at risk for congenital adrenal hyperplasia due to 21-hydroxylase deficiency: Effect of midgestational amniotic fluid steroid levels. *J Clin Endocrinol Metab* 76:117, 1993.
205. Merado AB, Wilson RC, Cheng KC, et al: Prenatal treatment and diagnosis of congenital adrenal hyperplasia owing to steroid 21-hydroxylase deficiency. *J Clin Endocrinol Metab* 80:2014, 1995.
206. Pang S, Clark AT, Freeman LC, et al: Maternal side effects of prenatal dexamethasone therapy for fetal congenital adrenal hyperplasia. *J Clin Endocrinol Metab* 75:249, 1992.
207. Miller WL: Genetics, diagnosis and management of 21-hydroxylase deficiency. *J Clin Endocrinol Metab* 78:241, 1994.
208. Thompson R, Seargeant L, Winter JSD: Screening for congenital adrenal hyperplasia: Distribution of 17-hydroxyprogesterone concentrations in neonatal blood spot specimens. *J Pediatr* 114:400, 1989.
209. Thilen A, Larsson A: Congenital adrenal hyperplasia in Sweden 1969–1986. *Acta Paediatr Scand* 79:168, 1990.
210. Azziz R, Dewailly D, Owerbach D: Nonclassic adrenal hyperplasia: Current concepts. *J Clin Endocrinol Metab* 78:810, 1994.
211. Hughes IA, Read GF: Simultaneous plasma and saliva steroid measurements as an index of control in congenital adrenal hyperplasia: A longitudinal study. *Horm Res* 16:142, 1982.
212. Hughes IA, Winter JSD: The relationship between serum concentrations of 17OH-progesterone and other serum and urinary steroids in patients with congenital adrenal hyperplasia. *J Clin Endocrinol Metab* 46:98, 1978.
213. Van Wyck JJ, Gunther DF, Ritzen EM, et al: The use of adrenalectomy as a treatment for congenital adrenal hyperplasia. *J Clin Endocrinol Metab* 8:3180, 1996.
214. Girgis R, Winter JSD: The effects of glucocorticoid replacement therapy on growth, bone mineral density, and bone turnover in children with congenital adrenal hyperplasia. *J Clin Endocrinol Metab* 82:3926, 1997.
215. Kuhnle V, Bullinger M, Schwarz HP: The quality of life in adult female patients with congenital adrenal hyperplasia: A comprehensive study of the impact of genital malformations and chronic disease on female patients life. *Eur J Pediatr* 154:708, 1995.
216. Jaaskelainen J, Voutilainen R: Growth of patients with 21-hydroxylase deficiency: An analysis of the factors influencing adult height. *Pediatr Res* 41:30, 1997.
217. Donaldson MDC, Thomas PH, Love JG, et al: Presentation, acute illness, and learning difficulties in salt-wasting 21-hydroxylase deficiency. *Arch Dis Child* 70:214, 1994.
218. Wischusen J, Baker HWG, Hudson B: Reversible male infertility due to congenital adrenal hyperplasia. *Clin Endocrinol (Oxf)* 14:571, 1981.
219. White PC, Curnow KM, Pascoe L: Disorders of 11β-hydroxylase isozymes. *Endocrine Rev* 15:421, 1994.
220. Lifton RP, Dluhy RG, Powers M, et al: A chimaeric 11β-hydroxylase/aldosterone synthase gene causes glucocorticoid-remediable aldosteronism and human hypertension. *Nature* 355:262, 1992.
221. Joehrer K, Geleys, Strasser-Wozack EM, et al: CYP11B1 mutations causing non-classic adrenal hyperplasia due to 11 beta-hydroxylase deficiency. *Hum Molec Genet* 6:1829, 1997.
222. Zadik Z, Kahana L, Kaufman H, Benderli A, Hochberg Z: Salt loss in hypertensive form of congenital adrenal hyperplasia (11β-hydroxylase deficiency). *J Clin Endocrinol Metab* 58:384, 1984.
223. Rosler A, Weshler N, Leiberman E, Hochberg Z, Weidenfeld J, Sack J, Chemke J: 11 β-hydroxylase deficiency congenital adrenal hyperplasia: Update of prenatal diagnosis. *J Clin Endocrinol Metab* 66:830, 1988.
224. Pang S, Levine LS, Lorenzen F, Chow D, Pollack M, Dupont B, Genel M, New MI: Hormonal studies in obligate heterozygotes and siblings of patients with 11β-hydroxylase deficiency congenital adrenal hyperplasia. *J Clin Endocrinol Metab* 50:586, 1980.
225. Zachman M, Forest MG, De Peretti E: 3β-Hydrosteroid dehydrogenase deficiency: Followup study in a girl with pubertal bone age. *Horm Res* 11:292, 1979.
226. Simpson ER, Zhao Y, Argarwal VR, et al: Aromatase expression in health and disease. *Rec Prog Horm Res* 52:185, 1997.
227. Bulun SE: Aromatase deficiency in women and men: Would you have predicted the phenotypes? *J Clin Endocrinol Metab* 81:867, 1996.
228. Mullis PE, Yoshimura N, Kuhlman B, et al: Aromatase deficiency in a female who is compound heterozygote for two point mutations in the P450arom gene: Impact of estrogens on hypergonadotropic hypogonadism, multicystic ovaries and bone densitometry in childhood. *J Clin Endocrinol Metab* 82:1739, 1997.
229. Carani C, Qin K, Simoni M, et al: Effect of testosterone and estradiol in a man with aromatase deficiency. *N Engl J Med* 337:91, 1997.
230. Ishizuka N, Kawashima Y, Nakanishi T, Sugawa T, Nishikawa Y: Statistical observations on genital anomalies of newborns following the administration of progestin to their mothers. *Obstet Gynecol Surv* 19:496, 1964.
231. Lynch A, Mychalkiw W, Hutt SJ: Parental progesterone: I. Its effect on development and on intellectual and academic achievement. *Early Hum Dev* 2:305, 1978.
232. Franks RC, Northcutt R: Female pseudohermaphroditism and renal anomalies. *Am J Dis Child* 105:490, 1963.
233. Winter JSD, Kohn G, Mellman WJ, Wagner S: A familial syndrome of renal, genital, and middle ear anomalies. *J Pediatr* 72:88, 1968.

PART VI

Fuel Metabolism

C H A P T E R 18

Diabetes Mellitus

David M. Nathan
Enrico Cagliero

INTRODUCTION

Diabetes mellitus is probably the most common severe chronic disease in the United States and most of Europe, affecting 8 percent of the adult population and as much as 20 percent of those older than age 65. Diabetes is rapidly reaching pandemic proportions, largely owing to an increase in Type 2 diabetes, as the lifespan is extended and more agricultural and subsistence economies adopt "westernized" life-styles. It is certainly the most common endocrine disease. With its myriad clinical forms, all of which are characterized by hyperglycemia and other perturbations of lipid and protein metabolism, and by long-term complications, including diabetes-specific and nonspecific cardiovascular complications, diabetes is one of the most complex diseases encountered by endocrinologists and other health care providers. Improved understanding of the pathophysiology of diabetes and its complications has resulted in major advances in the treatment of diabetes, and the prevention and treatment of its complications.

Type 1 diabetes, the relatively rare autoimmune form of diabetes that usually arises during childhood and adolescence, has "progressed" from a uniformly fatal disease in the early part of this century to a chronic disorder with a modestly reduced lifespan. Its more common sibling, Type 2 diabetes, continues to increase in frequency and causes enormous morbidity, secondary to the diabetes-specific complications, and mortality from cardiovascular disease. Both of the common forms of diabetes have benefited from advances in therapy. In particular, intensive therapies aimed at achieving and maintaining near-normoglycemia have had a major salutary effect on the development and progression of diabetes-specific long-term complications.

The study and treatment of diabetes inevitably includes attention to obesity, atherosclerotic cardiovascular disease and its risk factors, and the protean long-term manifestations that affect the eye, kidney, and numerous parts of the nervous system. A comprehensive understanding of diabetes mellitus requires near-encyclopedic knowledge. This chapter aims to provide an up-to-date review of the important insights into the epidemiology, pathoetiology, metabolism, and treatment of diabetes mellitus and its complications and associated disorders.

HISTORY

The recorded history of diabetes mellitus is at least 3000 years old.[1-3] Most ancient descriptions are of the clinical form associated with acute metabolic decompensation in children that resulted in death and which we now refer to as Type 1 diabetes. Although there may be older references in Chinese literature to a fatal wasting disease with increased urination, the generally accepted first description of diabetes appears in the Ebers papyrus in 1500 BC. The term "diabetes," coined by Demetrios of Apamaia in 200 BC, is derived from the Greek word diabeinein (διαβεινειν), meaning siphon. It was meant to capture the excessive urination and "melting down of flesh and limbs into urine," noted by Arateus in the first century AD. The Latin appellation "mellitus," meaning honey, was added centuries later with the recognition that the urine of diabetics was sweet tasting.

Despite the prescient naming of diabetes mellitus, a clear distinction between another disease—and an endocrine disease at that—associated with voluminous urination, namely diabetes insipidus, and diabetes mellitus was not clearly made until the eighteenth century. The modern era, characterized by experimentation, followed. Sugar was identified in 1838 as the substance conferring the sweet taste to diabetic urine.[4] Subsequent investigations by Claude Bernard, Paul Langerhans, Minkowski and von Mering,[5] and Eugene Opie,[6] to name a few, provided insights into the roles of the liver and pancreas, and of the islet cells in particular, in the development of diabetes. These observations provided the stage for treating diabetes with various pancreatic extracts by the German physician Georg Zuelzer,[7] a Romanian physician named Paulesco,[8] and finally the successful preparation of an active extract and treatment of dogs and then humans by Frederick Banting, Charles Best, J.J.R. Macleod, and J.B. Collip.[9] (The fascinating story of "The Discovery of Insulin" and the relative roles of the four protagonists is told by Michael Bliss in his book of the same name.[1])

Prior to insulin treatment, first used successfully in 14-year-old Leonard Thompson on January 11, 1922, the relatively acute onset of diabetes during childhood was a death sentence. If children didn't die with the initial episode of diabetic coma, they almost all perished in the next 1–2 years. The only treatments available were a dizzying array of diets, including the starvation diets popularized by Dr. Frederick Allen.[10] In retrospect, many of the diets seem foolish, and even counterintuitive; yet, the desperation of children and their families in the face of this deadly disease made any treatment, no matter how peculiar, worth trying.

The large scale production of insulin so quickly after its discovery may rival the discovery itself as an accomplishment. With insulin therapy, the "juvenile-onset" form of diabetes, as it was often called, was no longer acutely fatal. With longer survival, however, a variety of severe long-term complications were increasingly recognized, belying any notion that diabetes had been cured. Insulin therapy had apparently transformed a uniformly fatal disease to a chronic degenerative one. Beginning in the 1930s, people with juvenile onset diabetes could look forward to a 30–50 percent risk of becoming blind, developing renal failure, requiring an amputation, or suffering a myocardial infarction or stroke during their shortened life-span.[11] Average survival was approximately 40 years after diagnosis, with those developing renal disease dying in their 30s and those without renal disease surviving into their fifth decade, when they often died from cardiovascular disease. Diabetes had been transformed from the disease which was "short, disgusting, and painful," as described by Arateus in the first century AD,[12] to a more chronic condition that was long, disgusting, and, arguably, more painful.

Increased appreciation of the pathophysiology of juvenile-onset diabetes and its complications and the development of improved methods to treat it, including self-monitoring of blood glucose and insulin algorithms that could achieve near-normoglycemia, provided the opportunity to test whether the devastating long-term complications could be prevented or delayed. Studies such as the Diabetes Control and Complications Trial demonstrated that the long-term complications of retinopathy, nephropathy, and neuropathy could all be reduced by more than 50 percent with intensive therapy that reduced glycemic levels, albeit not into the nondiabetic range.[13] This discovery, and the continued evolution of intensive therapies to achieve normal glucose control, have completed an important chapter in the history of diabetes.

Although the juvenile-onset form of diabetes has dominated the interest and attention of clinicians, investigators, and historians alike, it is only a part of the story. Another form of diabetes, with a more insidious onset and which was known to occur in the well-to-do, escaped any clear description or nosologic categorization until relatively recently. In the late ninetheenth century, Lacereaux distinguished two clinical forms of diabetes, "diabete maigre" (thin diabetes) which was resistant to all therapies and was fatal, and "diabete gras" (fat diabetes), which occurred later in life and responded to a change in diet.[14] The "adult-onset" form of diabetes, now known as Type 2 diabetes, was more clearly described as "insulin-resistant," compared with "insulin-sensitive" juvenile-onset diabetes, by Himsworth in 1936.[15] Despite the relative dearth of historical attention to Type 2 diabetes, it represents by far the most prevalent form of diabetes today. An appreciation of its complications has also come rather late. Type 2 diabetes occurs most commonly in the later decades of life. Because the development of complications requires 5–15 years of "exposure" to the disease, many patients with Type 2 diabetes succumbed, usually to cardiovascular disease, before developing the diabetes-specific complications. Now, with the progressive extension of the life-span, more and more persons with Type 2 diabetes are developing the same complications that affect Type 1 diabetes.[16] Intensive therapy aimed at achieving near-normal glycemia has been shown to decrease the long-term complications in Type 2 diabetes, similar to its effect in Type 1 diabetes.[17]

ENDOCRINE PANCREAS

Anatomy

The endocrine portion of the pancreas consists of clusters of endocrine cells (named islets of Langerhans in honor of Paul Langerhans who identified them in 1869) scattered through the exocrine pancreas. In adult humans there are approximately 0.5 to 1 million islets of Langerhans, ranging in size from 40 to 400 μm in diameter. The volume of endocrine tissue relative to that of the entire pancreas decreases from birth to adulthood, going from 20 percent of the pancreatic mass in newborn humans to 1–2 percent in adults. There are four major types of endocrine cells in human islets: alpha or A cells, which produce glucagon; beta or B cells, which produce insulin; delta or D cells, which produce somatostatin; and PP cells, which produce pancreatic polypeptide (see Table 18-1). The different cell types can be identified by ultrastructural characteristics with respect to their secretory granules (Fig. 18-1), as well as by immunostaining. Minor cell types, staining for other hormones such as substance P, gastrin, and vasoactive intestinal polypeptide, have been identified by electron microscopy and immunocytochemical techniques,[18] but their physiologic significance is unclear. Moreover, some of the major endocrine cell types stain for multiple peptides. The islet amyloid polypeptide (IAPP/amylin) has been found to colocalize in the insulin granules of beta cells,[19] and more than 100 proteins have been identified in insulin secretory granule.[20]

The distribution of the endocrine cells in the islets of Langerhans is nonrandom, with beta cells constituting the core of the islets surrounded by a thin layer of cells containing glucagon, somatostatin and PP.[21] Fibroblasts and collagen fibers have been identified in the periphery of islets of Langerhans, forming an often incomplete capsule. The endocrine pancreas is highly vascularized, with approximately 10 percent of the overall pancreatic blood flow directed to serve only 1 percent of the pancreatic tissue.[22] Each islet is perfused by one to five arterioles that enter into the islet and then divide into numerous fenestrated capillaries that form a glomerulous-like structure.[18,22] In large islets, capillaries empty directly in collecting venules, while in smaller islets efferent capillaries extend into exocrine tissue, forming an insuloacinar portal system. Lymphatic vessels have not been observed within the islets. Changes in islet blood flow have been implicated in the regulation of hormonal secretion,[23] with both nitric oxide and angiotensin II playing a potential role in the regulation of islet blood flow and insulin secretion.[24] The pancreas is innervated by sympathetic and parasympathetic fibers; in the islets the nerves follow the blood vessels and terminate within the pericapillary space. Cholinergic and beta-adrenergic stimulation increases insulin, glucagon, and pancreatic polypeptide secretion, while alpha-adrenergic stimulation decreases insulin and somatostatin secretion and has variable effects on glucagon secretion in different species.[25]

Development

The pancreas originates from an evagination of the foregut during early embryonic development. Two outpockets of endoderm form in early gestation (approximately 28 days in humans) on the dor-

TABLE 18-1. Characteristics of Islet-Cell Types

Cell Type	Percentage of Total	Hormone	Secretory Granules
Alpha (α)	15	Glucagon	Dense core, pale periphery
Beta (β)	60	Insulin	Crystalloid, pleomorphic
Delta (δ)	10	Somatostatin	Low density, homogeneous, fill membrane
PP	15	Pancreatic polypeptide	Dense, elongated

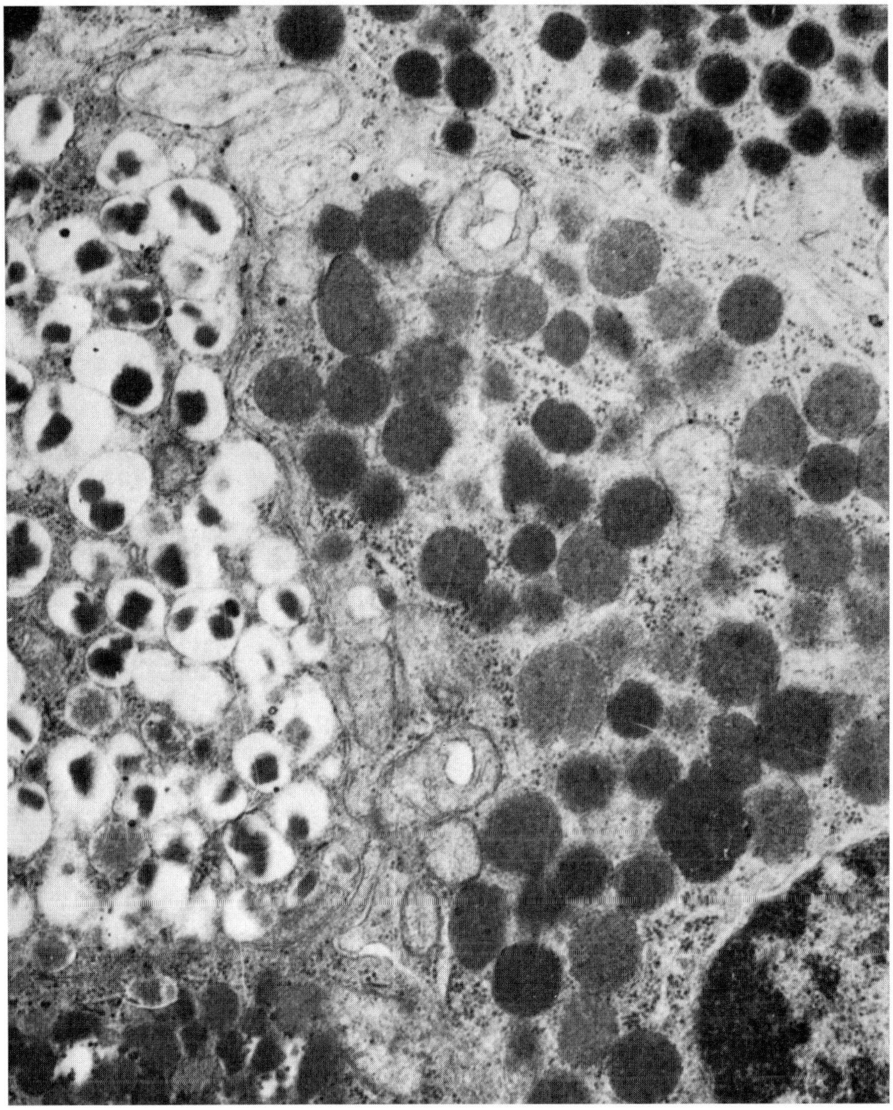

FIGURE 18-1. Electron micrograph of portion of normal human islet showing alpha, beta, and delta cells. In the alpha cell (upper right), the secretory granules show a dense core and a pale periphery. In the beta cells (left), there are pleomorphic granules with a crystalloid matrix. In the delta cell (center), the secetory granules are homogeneous and fill the vesicles.

sal and ventral side of the primitive duodenum. As the stomach and the duodenum rotate, the ventral and dorsal pancreatic buds fuse, with the ventral bud giving origin to the posterior part of the head and the dorsal bud forming the remainder of the organ. This dual origin of the organ is responsible for regional differences in the distribution of islet cells in the adult: the dorsal pancreas is rich in glucagon-containing islets, while the ventral portion contains pancreatic polypeptide rich islets and few glucagon producing cell.[26] Endocrine cells can be visualized in the early stages of pancreatic development, initially associated with the pancreatic ductal epithelium, and then found in islets by the middle of gestation. Initially thought to be of neural crest origin, the endocrine cells have more recently been shown to originate from the endodermal epithelium, with the earliest endocrine cells coexpressing insulin and glucagon, followed by somatostatin and pancreatic polypeptide expressing cells.[26]

Recent studies on transcriptional factors expressed in the pancreas have shed some light on the molecular mechanisms of pancreatic development. The homeodomain protein insulin-promoter-factor 1 or IPF1 (also known as IDX-1, STF-1, and PDX-1) has been proposed as the master regulator of pancreatic development.[27] This protein is selectively expressed in adult beta cells and binds to and transactivates the insulin promoter. Targeted disruption of the gene in mice results in pancreatic agenesis,[28] and a single nucleotide deletion in the human IPF-1 gene was found in a patient with pancreatic agenesis, thus supporting the essential role of this protein in human pancreatic development.[29] In addition to the regulation of the insulin gene, IPF-1 is also implicated in the transcriptional regulation of several important genes, including somatostatin, IAPP, glucose-transporter-2, and glucokinase.

The targeted disruption of genes in experimental animals has provided the opportunity to demonstrate the importance of different proteins in pancreatic development (Table 18-2).[27,30] Mice deficient in the LIM homeodomain protein ISL-1 show deficiency in pancreatic development with complete loss of differentiated islet cells,[31] while disruption of the homeodomain proteins Pax4 and Pax6 result in more targeted abnormalities. Mice deficient in Pax4 show a severe retardation of insulin- and somatostatin-producing cells with resulting hyperplasia of glucagon cells,[32] while deficiency of the Pax6 protein results in animals lacking glucagon-

TABLE 18-2. Gene Knockout Experiments and Pancreatic Development

Protein	Knockout Phenotype
IPF-1	Pancreatic agenesis
ISL-1	Islet agenesis
Pax4	B- and D-cell agenesis A-cell hyperplasia
Pax6	A-cell hypoplasia
Nkx2.2	B-cell agenesis A- and PP-cell hypoplasia
Nkx6.1	B-cell hypoplasia
Beta2/neuroD	B-cell agenesis
Glut-2	Inverted A to B cell ratio
Activin	A- and B-cell hypoplasia

producing cells[33]; mice lacking both Pax4 and Pax6 fail to develop any endocrine cells. Other proteins that have been shown to play a role in the normal endocrine pancreatic development include the homeobox transcriptional factors Nkx2.2 and Nkx6.1,[30] the helix-loop-helix transcriptional factor beta2/neuroD,[30] the glucose transporter Glut-2,[34] and activin.[35]

Pancreatic Hormones

Insulin Chemistry and Biosynthesis

The discovery of insulin in 1921 by Banting and Best[36] opened a new era in diabetes therapy. It also led to an enormous research effort to explore the chemistry, biosynthesis, and cell biology of this hormone. Human insulin was the first human gene to be cloned,[37] and one of the first proteins to be isolated, crystallized, and sequenced. The human insulin molecule consists of two polypeptide chains, named A and B, connected by two disulfide bridges. There is, in addition, a disulfide bridge between the sixth and eleventh amino acid residues of the A chain (Fig. 18-2). The complete molecule contains 51 amino acids and has a molecular weight of 5,800 and an isoelectric pH of 5.35. By definition, 1 mg of pure insulin contains 24.0 international units (IU). Insulin has been found in all vertebrates, and it is highly conserved among different species. The positions of the three disulfide bonds, the N-terminal and C-terminal regions of the A chain, and the hydrophobic residues of the B chain are highly conserved through evolution. Porcine insulin differs from human insulin only in the presence of a terminal alanine rather than threonine in the B chain. There are two additional differences in the A chain between bovine and human insulin, at position 8 (alanine replaces threonine) and 10 (valine replaces isoleucine). In the secretory granules of the beta cells, the presence of zinc ions favors the formation of insulin hexamers made up of three dimers arranged around an axis with two atoms of zinc. The structure of the insulin hexamers is important in the packing of insulin and crystal growth; crystallization of insulin is abnormal in transgenic mice that express mutant insulin.[38] Insulin derived from porcine and bovine pancreases was used until biosynthetic human insulin became available in the 1980s.

The gene for insulin has been cloned from a wide range of animals and has a highly conserved structure consisting of three exons and two introns. Exon 1 is located in the untranslated region of the gene, exon 2 contains sequences coding for the signal peptide, the B chain, and part of the C-peptide, and exon 3 encodes the remainder of the insulin sequence.[37] In humans there is a single copy of the insulin gene located on the short arm of chromosome 11, on band 11p15,[39] and it is flanked on the 5′ side by a polymorphic region of tandem repeats that provides a useful marker for genetic linkage analysis. The human insulin promoter region regulates the transcriptional response to glucose and other nutrients, and limits transcription of the gene to the pancreatic beta cells.[40] These regulatory sequences are located in the −350 basepairs upstream the transcription start, and they are sufficient to provide glucose-responsiveness to a linked reported gene.[41] Of particular importance are the E-boxes (sequences containing the core motif CANNTG) that bind helix-loop-helix transcriptional factors including IEF-1 and USF and A-elements (sequences containing the core motif TAAT) that bind the homeodomain transcriptional factor IPF-1. A cAMP responsive element (CRE) and two SP-1 recognition sequences are also present in the human insulin promoter region.

Insulin, like most secretory proteins, is synthesized as a precursor molecule, called preproinsulin, that carries a leader, or signal peptide. The interaction of the signal recognition peptide (SRP) with the SRP receptor on the ribosome ensures that preproinsulin enters the secretory pathway in the rough endoplastic reticulum (RER).[42] Preproinsulin is a single chain of 110 amino acids with a molecular weight of 11,500. Removal of the 24-amino-acid N-terminal signal peptide by the signal peptidase in

FIGURE 18-2. Amino acid sequence of human insulin. In porcine insulin alanine rather than threonine is the terminal amino acid in the B chain. Bovine insulin differs from human insulin in having an alanine at position 30 in the B chain, alanine (rather than a threonine) at position 8 in the A chain, and valine (rather than isoleucine) at position 10 in the A chain.

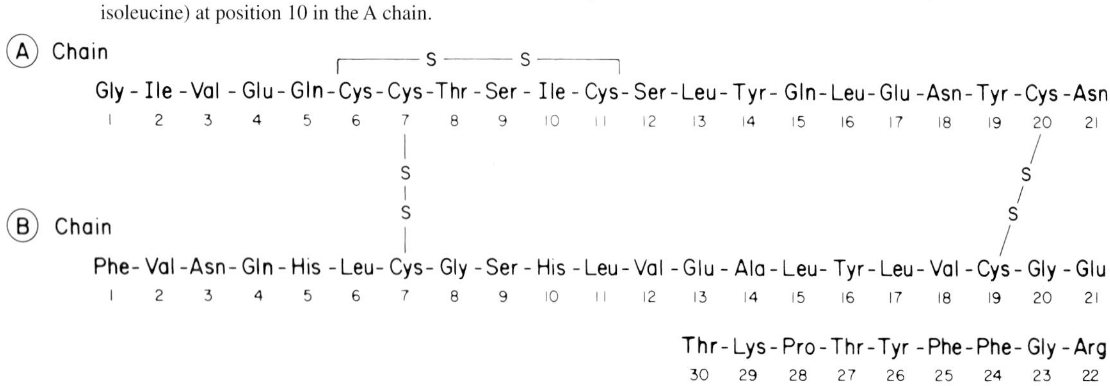

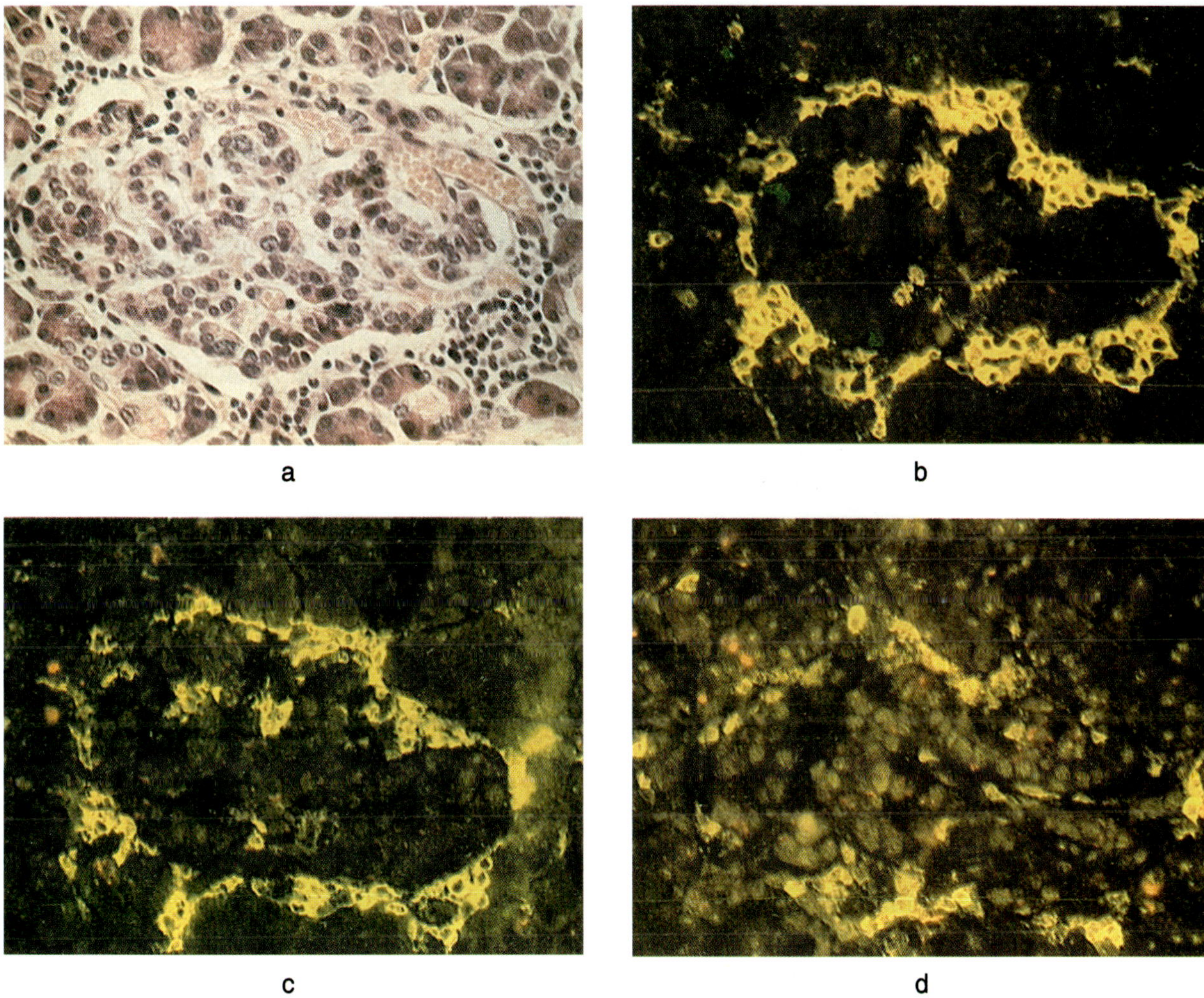

PLATE 1 (FIGURE 18-20). T-lymphocyte invasion of β-cells in a 12-year-old girl with recently diagnosed diabetes. In panel (*a*), hematoxylin and eosin staining shows lymphocyte infiltration. Panel (*b*) shows all types of leukocytes with a monoclonal antibody and fluourescence. Panel (*c*) specifically stains for T8, presumably cytotoxic, lymphocytes while panel (*d*) indicates activated T-cells staining for interleukin-2 receptor lymphocytes. (*From Bottazzo et al.*[184])

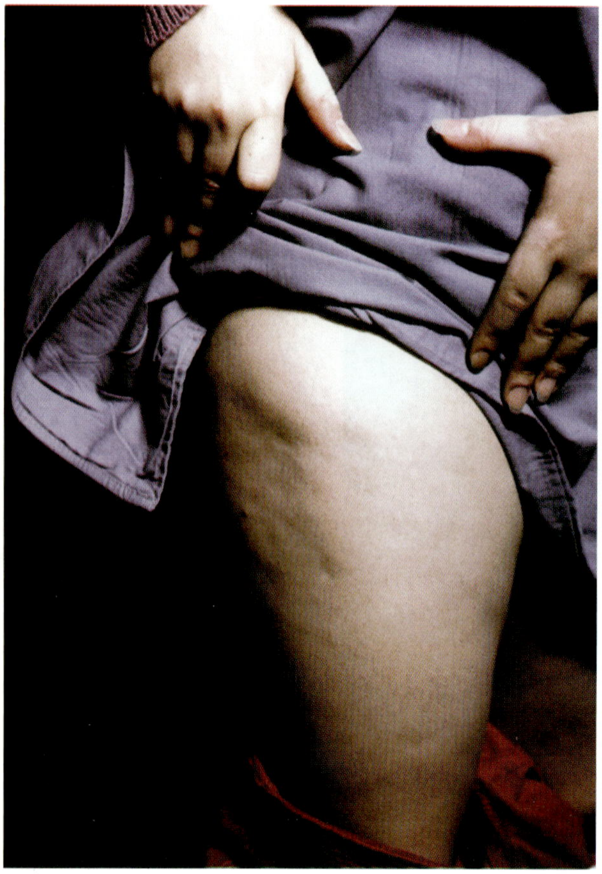

PLATE 3 (FIGURE 18-50). Lipoatrophy represents discrete areas with loss of subcutaneous fat at sites of previous insulin injections and at anatomic sites where insulin has never been injected. An increasingly rare complication of insulin therapy, lipoatrophy appears as "dents" in the skin.

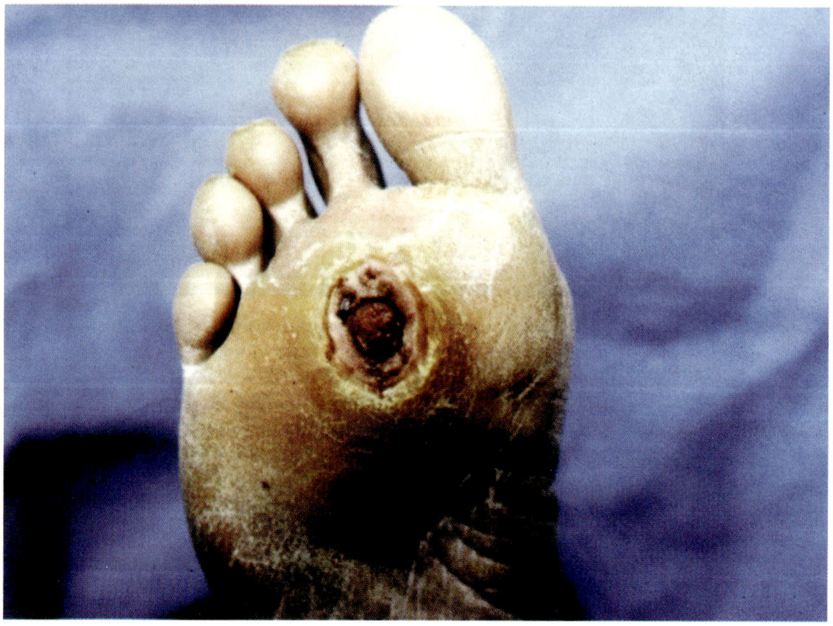

PLATE 4 (FIGURE 18-60). Penetrating pressure ulcer over second metatarsal head in patient with diabetic neuropathy. Changes in innervation of the intrinsic muscles of the foot result in increased flexion with altered weight distribution and increased weight bearing over MT heads. Flexion at the PIP joints of the toes exposes the PIP joints to the risk of abrasion and ulceration. Fitted orthotic devices can spread weight bearing and prevent the ulceration shown here. Extra depth shoes can protect the PIP joints from trauma.

the RER yields the insulin precursor proinsulin. Proinsulin is a stable peptide of ~9,000 molecular weight that is transferred to the Golgi apparatus. The signal peptide is degraded in the RER and is not a secretory product. Proinsulin folds and disulfide bonds form, giving proinsulin its native structure. Proinsulin is then transported to the cis region of the Golgi apparatus where it is cleaved into insulin and the connecting peptide (C-peptide) that links the C-terminus of the B-chain and the N-terminus of the A-chain. The conversion of proinsulin to insulin does not require energy and occurs mostly during maturation of the clathrin-coated secretory granules. Two endoproteases that process proinsulin were initially identified in secretory granules of rat insulinoma and named proinsulin convertase 2 (PC2) and 3 (PC3) (Fig. 18-3).[43] PC2 cleaves proinsulin preferentially at the Lys-Arg-Gly sequence at the junction of the C-peptide and A-chain, while PC3 cleaves the Arg-Arg-Glu sequence at the C-peptide and B-chain junction. These convertases are expressed only in neuroendocrine tissues (islets of Langerhans, pituitary, adrenal medulla) and are responsible for the processing of several prohormones such as proinsulin, proglucagon, and pro-opiomelanocortin. The products of endoproteolytic cleavage are split 32, 33 proinsulin (by action of PC3) or split 65, 66 proinsulin by action of PC2. These intermediates are the substrate of carboxypeptidase-H, an enzyme expressed in many neuroendocrine tissues that removes the carboxy-terminal amino acids of the split proinsulin products so that the more commonly observed intermediary products are des 31, 32 proinsulin and des 64, 65 proinsulin. In human pancreas des 31, 32 proinsulin is present in higher concentrations than des 64, 65 proinsulin, suggesting that the initial cleavage of the proinsulin molecule occurs by action of PC3 at the 31, 32 site (Fig. 18-3). The endopeptidases PC2 and PC3 are calcium- and pH-dependent, and operate maximally at the acidic pH present in secretory granules. In response to high glucose levels, there is a coordinated increase in expression of the PC2 and PC3 genes, occurring both at the transcriptional and translational level, that parallels the changes in proinsulin gene expression.[44,45]

The conversion of proinsulin to insulin is an efficient process that requires 2–4 hours. More than 95 percent of secretory products of the insulin gene are in the form of insulin plus C-peptide in the normal basal state. Small amounts of proinsulin (3–5 percent) are secreted and can be detected in the circulation of normal individuals where they are cleared at a slower rate because of reduced affinity for the insulin receptor (~3 percent of insulin). In cases of progressive beta cell dysfunction such as type 2 diabetes and impaired glucose tolerance, an increased proinsulin/insulin ratio of 25–40 percent has been observed. The increased ratio is thought to be an indicator of reduced beta cell secretory capacity.[43,46] C-peptide is cosecreted in equimolar amounts with insulin; it is not extracted by the liver and it is excreted by the kidneys. For these reasons, it is used to determine endogenous insulin secretion in conditions when direct measurements of insulin levels are technically inaccurate (such as in presence of insulin antibodies) or when surreptitious administration of insulin is suspected. There is considerable variability in C-peptide sequences among different species, and this finding, together with the lack of a specific receptor for C-peptide, has been thought to imply that this molecule has no specific hormonal function. Some recent animal and human data have suggested beneficial role of C-peptide administration in diabetes,[47,48] but these findings are still controversial and there is no consensus for any physiological role for this molecule.[49]

Insulin Secretion

Insulin has an essential role in nutrient disposal and its secretion is regulated in a feedback loop by availability of exogenous nutrients, glucose being most important. Although other anabolic, insulin-like hormones are present in humans, only insulin is

FIGURE 18-3. Conversion of proinsulin to insulin in human β-cells. (*From Rhodes CJ and Alarcon C.*[43])

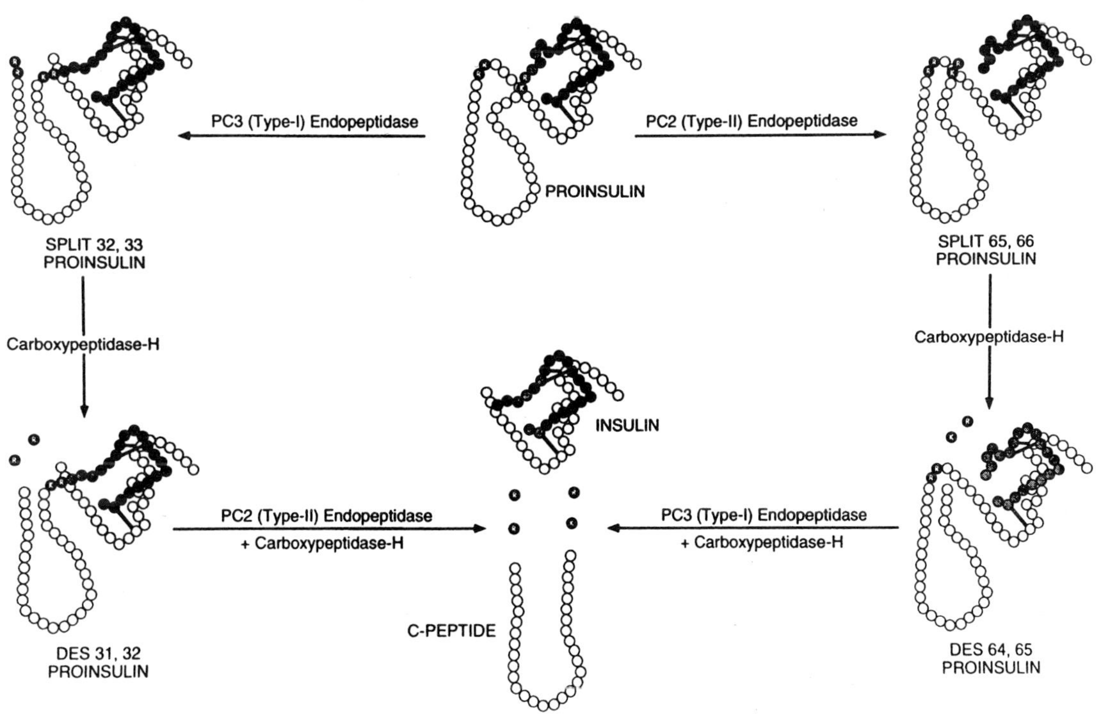

regulated acutely by glucose levels. In the basal fasting state, circulating insulin levels are approximately 10 to 20 μU/ml (0.4 to 0.8 ng/ml), depending on the assay. To maintain these levels, estimated basal insulin secretion rates range from 18 to 32 units/24 hours in normal subjects (0.7 to 1.3 mg).[50] This constitutes approximately 50 percent of total daily insulin secretion, with the remainder being secreted in response to meals.[50,51] Basal insulin secretion is not constant. Like other hormones, secretion is pulsatile. Insulin secretion has major pulses every 1.5 to 2 hours, and more rapid oscillations every 8 to 16 minutes.[50–52] The exact physiological significance of these oscillations is still unclear; however, insulin has a moderately greater hypoglycemic effect when administered in a pulsatile pattern compared with continuous infusion. Because of its crucial role in the regulation of plasma glucose levels and nutrient disposal, insulin secretion is under extremely tight control by a number of compounds including glucose and other nutrients, hormones, and neurotransmitters (Table 18-3).

The regulation of insulin synthesis and secretion occurs at multiple levels, including regulation of insulin gene expression and exocytotic insulin release. Insulin is stored in the secretory granules of the beta cells together with equimolar amounts of C-peptide and small amounts of proinsulin and proinsulin intermediates. These granules form a large cytoplasmatic pool. Exocytotic release of insulin occurs in response to different secretagogues. Although the process of exocytosis is the rate-limiting step in insulin secretion, the renewal of insulin stores in the beta cells is an essential component of the insulin secretory pathway.

Glucose regulates insulin gene expression at several levels: glucose increases gene transcription, stabilizes mRNA, and increases translation. After acute exposure of islets of Langerhans to elevated glucose levels, increased translation of insulin mRNA can be observed within 20 min.[53] This effect is independent of RNA synthesis and occurs at three levels: increased rate of initiation of insulin translation, increased elongation of insulin mRNA, and increased transfer of initiated insulin mRNA from free to membrane-bound ribosomes. The latter process requires the interaction between signal recognition particles (SRP) and docking proteins in the endoplastic reticulum.[53] Increases in insulin gene transcription were initially observed after longer exposure (24 h) of islet cells to high glucose levels,[54] but recent studies using more sensitive techniques have demonstrated short-term (15 minute) glucose regulation of insulin gene transcription.[55] Insulin pre-RNA splicing is also stimulated by elevated glucose levels.[56] Another level of regulation of insulin gene expression by glucose is at the level of mRNA stability, with the half-life of insulin mRNA being threefold longer in cells cultured in high glucose levels.[57] The physiological role of changes in insulin gene expression are still debated; interestingly, transgenic mice expressing the human insulin gene under the control of its promoter showed doubling of total insulin mRNA, but normal content of immunoreactive insulin and normal glucose homeostasis,[58] emphasizing the importance of posttranscriptional regulation of the insulin gene.

TABLE 18-3. Regulation of Insulin Secretion in Vivo

Secretagogues	Inhibitors
Nutrients	Hormones
Glucose	Somatostatin
Amino acids	Leptin
Ketone bodies	Neural factors
Fatty acids	α-adrenergic activity
Hormones	
GIP	
CCK	
GLP-1	
VIP	
Secretin	
Gastrin	
Glucagon	
Growth hormone	
Prolactin	
Glucocorticoids	
Placental lactogen	
Sex steroids	
Neural factors	
Acetylcholine	
β-adrenergic activity	

Mature insulin is stored in secretory granules in the cytoplasm of pancreatic beta cells; these granules serve as a storage pool of hormone as well as transport vesicles. Under maximal stimulation only a small fraction of stored insulin is released. The regulation of circulating insulin levels occurs primarily at the level of secretion itself. Exocytosis includes recruitment of secretory granules, docking to the plasma membrane, vesicle priming in an ATP-dependent reaction, and finally fusion with the plasma membrane and insulin release.[59] This process is dependent on cytosolic Ca^{++} concentrations, and the Ca^{++}/calmodulin-dependent protein kinase CaM kinase II has recently been proposed to play an important role in insulin secretion by controlling the interaction of secretory granules with the cell cytoskeleton, thus facilitating the transport of mature granules from the intracellular synthesis sites to the plasma membrane.[60]

Under physiological conditions, insulin stores are maintained constant by coordinated regulation of insulin secretion and biosynthesis. Unique among hormones, insulin release is dependent on the metabolism of glucose, its major secretagogue, and not on the interaction between an agonist and a receptor. Substrate-induced insulin secretion and synthesis, however, can be modified by other hormones and neurotransmitters. Glucose analogs that are not metabolized do not stimulate insulin secretion; conversely, glycolytic intermediates are able to induce insulin release. Glucose is transported into pancreatic beta cells by the high-capacity, low-affinity glucose transporter GLUT-2.[61,62] Once inside the cell, glucose is phosphorylated by glucokinase to generate glucose-6-phosphate, the rate limiting step for glucose metabolism in pancreatic beta cells.[63] Glucokinase effectively serves as the pancreatic glucose sensor. Its role in insulin secretion has been emphasized by transgenic knockout experiments showing that underexpression of pancreatic beta cell glucokinase is associated with reduced insulin secretion and glucose intolerance,[64] and by the finding that glucokinase mutations are the cause of maturity onset diabetes of the young type 2 (MODY-2), a familiar cause of mild diabetes associated with abnormalities in insulin secretion.[65,66]

The metabolism of glucose through the glycolytic pathway results in an increase in the intracellular ATP/ADP ratio that leads to closure of the ATP-sensitive potassium channels (K^+-ATP) in the plasma membrane (Fig. 18-4). K^+-ATP channels are found in a variety of cells, are inhibited by increased ATP concentrations, and are responsible for setting cell resting membrane potential. In the beta cells, ATP-induced closure of the K^+-ATP channels leads to reduction in K^+ outflow, depolarization, activation of L-type

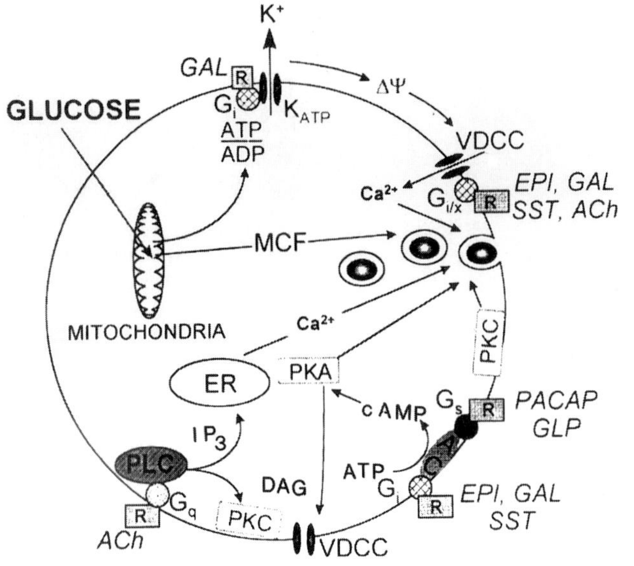

FIGURE 18-4. Proximal events in insulin secretion. (*Modified from Lang J.*[59])

calcium channels with calcium influx, and insulin exocytosis.[67] Beta cell K^+-ATP channels consist of a complex of two subunits, the sulfonylurea receptor (a member of the ATP-binding cassette superfamily to which sulfonylureas bind) and a small inward rectifier K^+ channel subunit named Kir6.2.[68,69] Both subunits have been cloned, and mutations in these genes have been observed in patients with hyperinsulinemic hypoglycemia of infancy, an autosomal recessive disorder.[70]

More recently, another glucose signaling pathway, independent of the K^+-ATP channels, has been shown to play an important role in insulin secretion.[71] The K^+-ATP channel-independent pathway does not cause an increase in cytoplasmic Ca^{++} concentration, but potentiates the response to increased Ca^{++} levels. This effect is dependent on glucose metabolism and is thought to be secondary to increased malonyl-CoA levels, which inhibit fatty acid beta-oxidation, which in turn results in an increase in long-chain fatty acid acyl-CoA.[71,72] Increased glycolysis leads to increased levels of malonyl-CoA which, by inhibiting carnitine palmitoyl-transferase I (CPT-I), the rate limiting step in fatty acid oxidation, decreases fatty acid oxidation. The resulting increase in long-chain fatty acids is currently thought to play a potentiating role in insulin secretion, although not in insulin biosynthesis, through still undetermined cellular mechanisms.[73]

Other mechanisms that potentiate insulin secretion involve the activation of protein kinase A (PKA) and protein kinase C (PKC) pathways. In the presence of forskolin and the phorbol ester TPA, agents that activate PKA and PKC respectively, glucose can strongly augment insulin secretion under Ca^{++} free conditions.[71] A number of receptor-mediated insulin secretagogues, such as glucagon and glucagon-like peptide-1 (GLP-1), potentiate insulin secretion via PKA-dependent mechanisms. Under basal conditions, PKA is an inactive tetramer with two regulatory and two catalytic subunits. Binding of agonists such as glucagon to cell surface receptors that are linked to the heterotrimeric G protein Gs activates adenylate cyclase with consequent generation of cAMP. The cAMP then binds to the PKA regulatory subunits causing activation of PKA, phosphorylation of protein substrates, and potentiation of insulin secretion. Activation of the PKA pathway probably cannot initiate insulin secretion at low glucose concentrations, thus making it a potentiatior rather than an initiator of insulin secretion.[74] Although the PKA-dependent potentiation of insulin secretion has usually been thought to be distinct from the traditional ATP-dependent pathway, recent data suggest that ATP can be a source of cAMP and donate phosphate for PKA-mediated phosphorylation of substrates important for insulin exocytosis, thus playing a more central role in insulin secretion.[75]

Insulin secretagogues such as acetylcholine and cholecystokinin bind to surface receptors that are coupled to phospholipase C (PLC) via the G protein G_q. Binding to the receptor activates PLC, with resulting hydrolysis of phosphatidylinositol bisphosphate (PIP_2) and generation of diacylglycerol (DAG) and inositol trisphospate (IP_3). DAG and IP_3 can in turn activate PKC either directly or, in the case of IP_3, through Ca^{++} release from the endoplasmic reticulum. PKC activation can in turn potentiate insulin secretion.[74]

Inhibition of insulin secretion (as modulated by hormones and peptides such as somatostatin and norepinephrine) appears to be mediated through activation of G proteins, and involves different mechanisms such as inhibition of PKA, increased permeability to K^+, reduction of Ca^{++} entry through the Ca^{++} channels, and inhibition of late stages in the process of exocytosis.[76] Insulin itself plays an important role in its secretion via interaction with the insulin receptor. Overexpression of insulin receptors in betacells results in increased biosynthesis and secretion of insulin,[77] and knockout mice lacking insulin receptors only in pancreatic beta cells exhibit a selective decrease in glucose induced insulin secretion.[78]

Insulin is secreted in vivo under the positive and negative regulation of many substances that can be categorized as nutrients, hormones, and neural factors (Table 18-3). Among the various factors capable of stimulating insulin secretion, glucose is physiologically the most important. The coordinated secretion of insulin and glucagon, one of the central counterregulatory hormones (see section later), to glucose levels maintains glucose in a tight physiological range. The major role of glucose in controlling insulin levels is reflected by the moment-to-moment fluctuations in plasma insulin concentration, which accompany fluctuations in plasma glucose (Fig. 18-5). A characteristic kinetic feature of the insulin response to glucose is its biphasic nature, with an early insulin peak followed by a slower, more sustained increment (Fig. 18-6). The initial rapid secretory burst begins within 1 minute of the intravenous (IV) glucose stimulus, reaches a peak within 2 minutes, and declines during the following 3 to 5 minutes. A second phase, characterized by a more gradual increase in insulin levels, commences 5 to 10 min after the initiation of the glucose infusion and continues through the next hour. In the perfused pancreas, inhibitors of protein synthesis do not alter the first phase of insulin secretion, although such agents attenuate the second phase. These observations have led to the concept that insulin exists within the beta cells in a two-pool system[79]: an immediately releasable pool consisting of preformed insulin is discharged rapidly during the early secretory phase, while newly synthesized insulin in addition to stored insulin is discharged during the second phase. The characteristic two-phase insulin response to an IV glucose challenge is generally not detectable with oral glucose, probably owing to the attenuated absorption and presentation of secretagogues to the β-cell. Other sugars, sugar derivatives, and sugar alcohols have been shown to induced insulin secretion in vitro; in vivo sorbitol and xylitol have been shown to potentiate insulin secretion.[80]

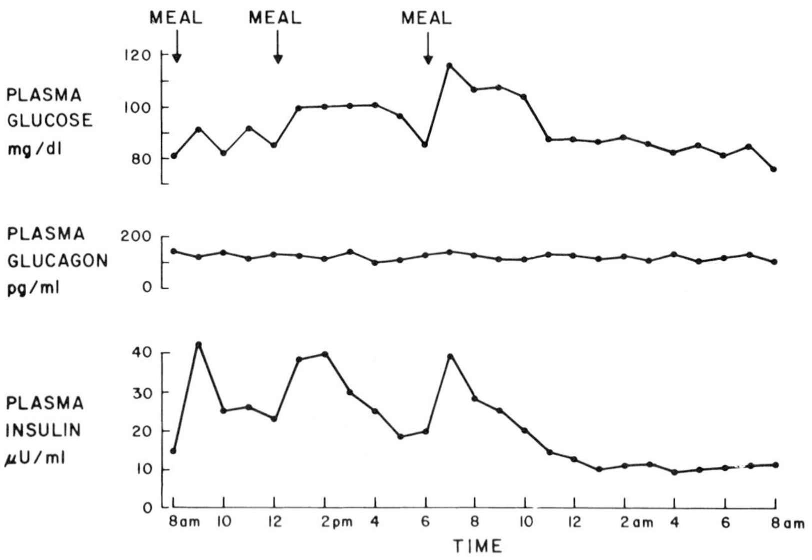

FIGURE 18-5. Fluctuations in plasma glucose, glucagon, and insulin concentrations over 24-h period in normal healthy subjects ingesting mixed meals. The maximal excursion in plasma glucose concentration over 24 h is generally less than 30 mg/dl. The minimal degree of fluctuation of plasma glucose level is a consequence of the feedback relationship to insulin secretion and the enhancement of insulin secretion by gastrointestinal hormones in response to meal ingestion. In contrast to the changes in plasma insulin concentration, there is virtually no change in plasma glucagon level when mixed meals are fed. (*Modified from Tasaka et al. Horm Metab Res 7:205, 1975.*)

The plasma insulin response to an oral glucose load is two or more times greater than after an IV load despite lower or equal plasma glucose levels (Fig. 18-7). This observation lead to the concept of "incretin," factor(s) produced by the gastrointestinal tract that stimulate insulin secretion.[81] Glucose-dependent insulin-releasing polypeptide (previously named gastric inhibitory polypeptide) (GIP), and glucagon-like peptide 1 (GLP-1) are thought to be the "legitimate" incretins.[82,83] GIP is a polypeptide secreted by endocrine cells of the duodenum and jejunum after carbohydrate ingestion, which stimulates insulin secretion.[84] GIP receptors are present on beta cells and are functionally coupled to the PKA/adenylate cyclase transduction system. GLP-1 was originally predicted from the nucleotide sequence of the preproglucagon gene.[85] It is one of the multiple gene products of the proglucagon gene, and is highly conserved among different species. GLP-1 is posttranslationally modified with cleavage after position 6 resulting in the bioactive molecule GLP-1(7-37) and further modified by C-terminal truncation and amidation to GLP1(7-36)amide. In humans, the majority of GLP-1 in the circulation occurs in the GLP1(7-36)amide form. This molecule is a potent stimulator of insulin release both in perfused pancreas[86] and in vivo,[87] and it is thought to contribute the major incretin effect in humans.[88] Its exact physiological importance is still debated,[89] but studies in transgenic mice with a null mutation in the GLP-1 receptor gene show abnormal glucose tolerance to oral glucose,[90] supporting the role of GLP-1 in glucose homeostasis.

FIGURE 18-6. Plasma insulin concentrations in portal and peripheral venous blood and after IV administration of glucose. The portal concentration of insulin is 3 times the peripheral level in the fasting state and may increase to 10 times the peripheral level immediately after glucose is infused. The changes in portal insulin concentration indicate the presence of a biphasic secretory response by the beta cell in which an acute rise in insulin release is followed by a slower, more sustained increment. (*From Blackard WG, Nelson NC. Diabetes 19:302, 1970.*)

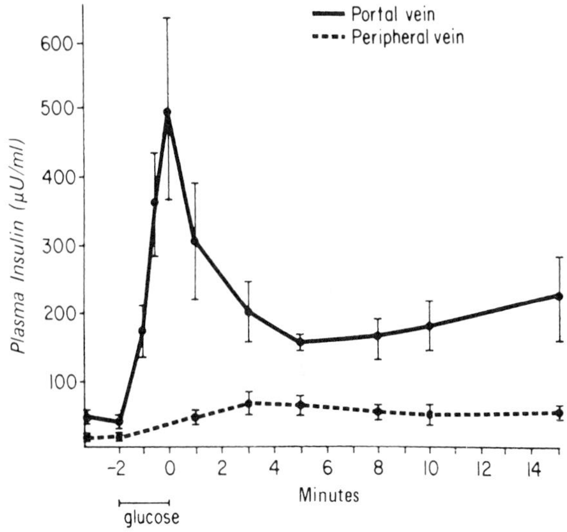

Ingestion of protein or infusion of single or multiple amino acids stimulates insulin secretion, with the most potent secretagogues being leucine, arginine, and lysine. A pure protein meal induces an increase in insulin levels of a lesser magnitude than a pure carbohydrate meal, with the concomitant secretion of glucagon to counteract the hypoglycemic effect of insulin. In contrast to amino acids, triglycerides, fatty acids, and ketones have only minimal effects on insulin secretion in humans.

The hormones secreted by the alpha and delta cells of the endocrine pancreas modulate insulin secretion. Glucagon stimulates insulin secretion while somatostatin inhibits it. Whether the effects of these hormones are paracrine or endocrine is not clear, and the physiological importance of glucagon and somatostatin in the regulation of insulin secretion is also debated.[80] Other hormones that are associated with hyperinsulinemia include growth hormone, glucocorticoids, prolactin, placental lactogen, estrogen, and progestins.[80] Because glucose levels are not reduced and sometimes are even raised in the presence of these hormones, it may be inferred that induction of insulin resistance is their major effect. However, the possibility of a direct action at the level of the beta cells has not been excluded. Gastrointestinal hormones such as gastrin, secretin, and vasoactive intestinal polypeptide (VIP) may influence insulin secretion in response to oral stimuli, but their physiological role remains to be elucidated. Recently, leptin has been found to inhibit insulin secretion and biosynthesis by activating (opening) the ATP-sensitive K^+ channels on beta cells.[91]

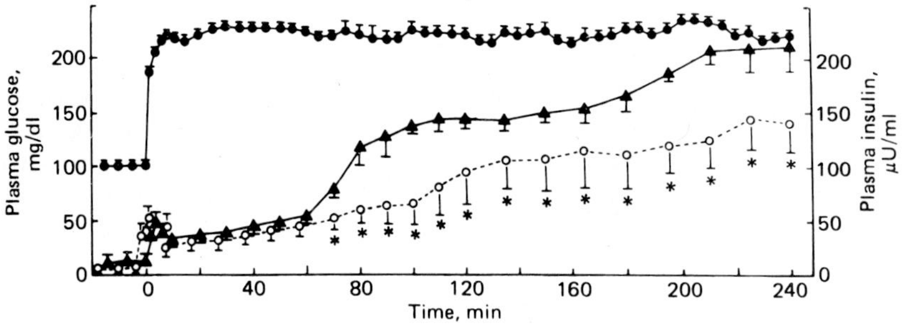

FIGURE 18-7. Enhancing effect of the oral route of glucose administration on the plasma insulin response to hyperglycemia. Hyperglycemia was induced and maintained constant (•) by a variable IV infusion of glucose. After 60 min, additional glucose was ingested by mouth while the plasma glucose level was maintained at the same hyperglycemic plateau. Despite the constancy of the plasma glucose level, there was a significantly greater rise in plasma insulin concentration after oral glucose (▲) than when hyperglycemia was maintained solely via the IV administration of glucose (○). (*From Defronzo et al. Proc Natl Acad Sci USA 75:5173, 1978.*)

Both the cholinergic and adrenergic arms of the autonomic nervous system innervate the islets. Adrenergic stimulation inhibits insulin secretion through the alpha-adrenergic receptors, while beta-adrenergic stimulation with isoproterenol results in increased insulin secretion. However, the inhibitory alpha-adrenergic action predominates, with the net effect of epinephrine being inhibition of glucose-stimulated insulin release, with minimal changes in basal insulin secretion.[80] The alpha-adrenergic receptors in the beta cells appear to alter insulin secretion via alterations in intracellular cAMP concentrations. In contrast to the action of epinephrine, stimulation of the parasympathetic nervous system (e.g., the vagus nerves) increases insulin secretion. This effect of acetylcholine is glucose-dependent, but its effect in human subjects is modest. Other neurotransmitters, such as neuropeptide Y (NPY) and galanin, have been found in human pancreas, but their effects on insulin release are still unclear, and likely to be minor at most.[92,93]

The regulatory role of the autonomic nervous system and circulating catecholamines in the control of insulin secretion is manifested both in the physiologic hypoinsulinemia that accompanies exercise and in pathologic circumstances such as stress hyperglycemia. During moderate or severe exercise, plasma insulin levels decline in association with a rise in plasma catecholamine concentrations. In stress hyperglycemia (e.g., with severe body burns), the failure of basal insulin levels to rise in association with increases in blood glucose concentration is probably a consequence of catecholamine action. By contrast, the very modest (two- to threefold) increment in plasma epinephrine concentrations that occurs with mild viral illness results in glucose intolerance by interfering with insulin action rather than by inhibiting secretion. The role of vagal control of insulin secretion is thought to be exemplified by the "cephalic" phase of insulin release, i.e., the insulin release that occurs at the sight and smell of food.[94] The physiological importance of neural regulation of insulin secretion is underscored by the decrease in glucose-stimulated early insulin secretion rates observed in pancreas transplant recipients[95]; however, despite these changes, the majority of such patients maintain normal glucose levels following transplantation without hypoglycemic therapy.

Insulin Action

Insulin is the primary hormone that controls the storage and metabolism of ingested metabolic fuels. After a meal, secretion of insulin facilitates the uptake, utilization, and storage of glucose, fat, and amino acids. Conversely, a reduction in the circulating insulin concentration leads to mobilization of endogenous fuels and reduced uptake of ingested nutrients. The action of insulin involves all three major metabolic fuels—carbohydrate, protein and fat—and occurs in three principal tissues: liver, muscle, and adipose tissue. In each of these tissues there are anticatabolic as well as anabolic effects of insulin that act to reinforce each other (Table 18-4). All these actions of insulin are initiated by insulin receptors binding the ligand at the plasma membrane.

The insulin receptor is a heterotetramer consisting of two 723 amino acid α-subunits and two 620 amino acid β-subunits that are linked to each other by disulfide bonds (Fig. 18-8). The two extracellular α-subunits contain the insulin binding site, while the transcellular β-subunits contain the insulin-regulated tyrosine kinase domain.[96] The insulin receptor derives from a single 150 kilobases (kb) gene located on the short arm of chromosome 19 near the low-density lipoprotein (LDL) receptor gene and contains 22 exons, with the first 11 coding for the α-subunits. Alternative splicing of exon 11 yields two distinct mRNA species coding for different α-subunits, termed HIR-A (human insulin receptor variant A) and HIR-B, differing for 12 amino acids at the carboxyl terminal. Although small biochemical differences between the

TABLE 18-4. Insulin Action on Liver, Adipose Tissue, and Muscle

	Liver	Adipose Tissue	Muscle
Anticatabolic effects	↓ Glycogenolysis	↓ Lipolysis	↓ Proteolysis
	↓ Gluconeogenesis		↓ Amino acid output
	↓ Ketogenesis		
Anabolic effects	↑ Glycogen synthesis	↑ Fatty acid uptake, synthesis, and esterification	↑ Amino acid uptake
	↑ Fatty acid synthesis		↑ Protein synthesis
			↑ Glycogen synthesis

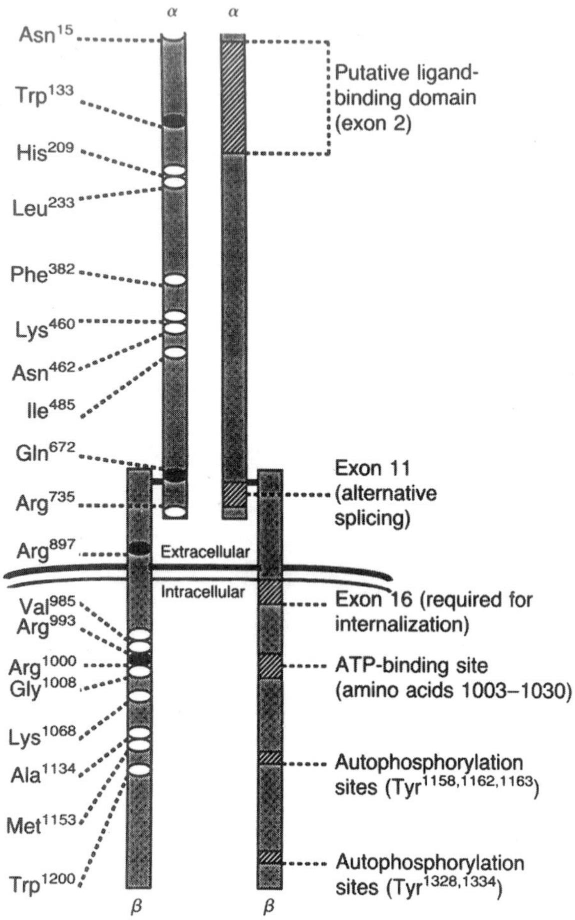

FIGURE 18-8. Structure of the human insulin receptor. (*From Moller and Flier, N Engl J Med 325:938, 1991.*)

variant subunits have been reported,[97] they do not appear to play a major role in diabetes.[98] Mutations in the insulin receptor gene have been described in patients with rare diseases associated with severe insulin resistance, including leprechaunism, type A severe insulin resistance, and lipoatrophic diabetes,[99] but are not associated with type 2 diabetes. These mutations fall in two groups: those that affect ligand binding and those that interfere with tyrosine kinase activity.

Insulin action begins when the insulin molecule binds to the α-subunits of the insulin receptor, followed by autophosphorylation of the β-subunits on tyrosine residues. As a tyrosine kinase, the insulin receptor belongs to a large family of tyrosine kinases that includes the receptors for insulin-like growth factor 1 (IGF-1), platelet-derived growth factor (PDGF), nerve growth factor (NGF), fibroblast growth factor (FGF), and the src-like oncogene. Insulin binding to the α-subunit releases an inhibitory constraint on the tyrosine kinase activity and triggers the autophosphorylation cascade on multiple tyrosine residues that has been shown in mutagenesis experiments to be essential for signal transduction.[100] Serine and threonine residues of the β-subunits are also phosphorylated after insulin binding, as a result of protein kinase C activation, and this constitutes another layer of regulation. In addition to autophosphorylation of the β-subunit, several endogenous molecules have been identified as substrates for further phosphorylation. This expanding family now has nine members, including insulin receptor substrate (IRS) 1, IRS-2, IRS-3, IRS-4, Gab-1, Shc, which has three isoforms, and p62^{dok}.[101]

The different members of the IRS family contain a PH (pleckstrin homology) domain near the amino terminus, involved in the targeting of the IRS proteins to the plasma membrane adjacent to the insulin receptor, and a PTB (phosphotyrosine binding) domain that recognizes the NPXpY motif present in the β-subunit of the insulin receptor. The tyrosine phosphorylation sites present in IRS molecules lie within motifs that bind proteins possessing Src homology-2 (SH2) domains. This relates to homology with pp60$^{v\text{-}src}$, the sarc oncogene with protein kinase activity. Many signaling molecules have SH2 domains, which allow IRS proteins to function as docking proteins and ultimately provide fine regulation of insulin-signal transmission. The role of individual IRS proteins is still not completely clear, and they are likely to represent multiple pathways for insulin signal transduction. Experiments in knockout mice have given very interesting results; IRS-1 homologous knockout mice show reduced size (suggesting a role of IRS-1 in the growth promoting effects of insulin) but only mild insulin resistance and no diabetes,[102,103] while a polygenic model of mice heterozygous for null alleles in the IRS-1 and insulin receptor genes develop age-dependent diabetes.[104] More recently the potential role of IRS-2 in the pathogenesis of type 2 diabetes has been suggested by the IRS-2 knockout mice model in which both insulin resistance at the liver and skeletal muscle sites and lack of compensatory beta cell hyperplasia are present, thus exhibiting a phenotype similar to human type 2 diabetes.[105]

Divergence of the insulin-signaling pathway into metabolic, growth promoting, and other biological effects probably occurs downstream from the IRS proteins, at the level of SH2 adaptor proteins, molecules that recognize and bind to tyrosine-phosphorylated proteins through their SH2 domains (Fig. 18-9).[101] Grb-2 is one of the best characterized adaptor proteins. It docks with IRS upon insulin stimulation and through an SH3 binding domain associates with SOS (mammalian homologue of the Drosophila son-of-sevenless protein). This prepares SOS for activation of the Ras (rat sarcoma protein) signaling pathway, including activation of Raf-1 kinase, activation of MAP (mitogen activated protein) kinase kinase, MAP kinase, and pp90 S6 kinase (Fig. 18-9). This cascade mediates the mitogenic effects of insulin and activates glycogen synthase through pp90 S6 kinase activation of the glycogen-associated protein 1. However, the key element of the pathway leading to insulin's metabolic effects is activation of the PI-3 kinase (phosphatidylinositol 3 kinase). PI-3 kinase is a heterodimer protein consisting of a regulatory subunit that associates with IRS and a catalytic subunit that phosphorylates phosphatidylinositols in cellular membranes. There are at least eight different isoforms of the regulatory subunit, and it is easy to envision specific functions being associated with different isoforms dependent on specific affinity to IRS proteins. The critical role of this pathway in transducing the metabolic effects of insulin has been demonstrated in experiments using either inhibitors of PI-3 activation[106] or expression of dominant-negative regulatory subunit lacking the binding site for the catalytic subunit.[107] In either case, inhibition of PI-3 kinase is associated with lack of insulin-stimulated glucose uptake and inhibition of GLUT4 translocation to the plasma membrane, as well as inhibition of other cellular effects of insulin. Activation of PI-3 kinase is also seen with other hormones and growth factors such as PDGF, but glucose transport is not stimulated in these cases. The precise mechanism(s) by which activation of the insulin receptor results in a specific pattern

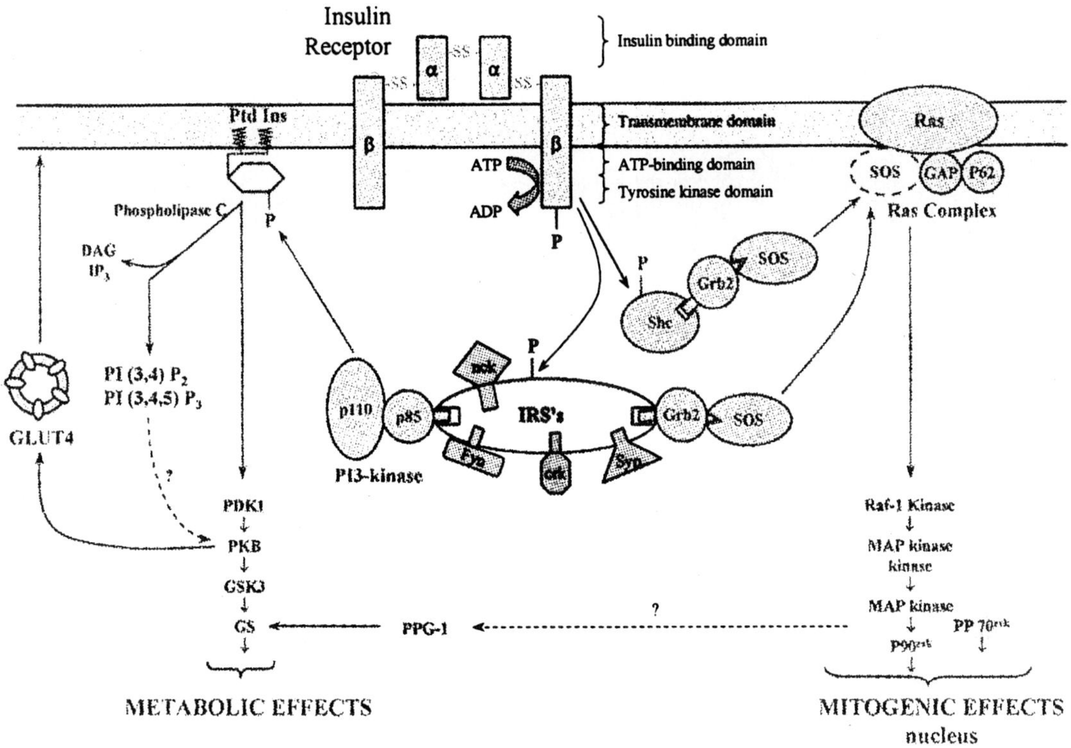

FIGURE 18-9. Metabolic and mitogenic signaling pathways in insulin action. (*From Hunter SJ, Garvey T. Am J Med 105:331, 1998.*)

of PI-3 dependent metabolic effects is still unclear, but activation through IRS docking and possibly subcellular localization of PI 3 kinase activity could play an important role.[101] Activation of PI-3 leads to phosphorylation of the inositol ring at the D-3 position, thus increasing the levels of several phosphoinositides. The downstream sequence of events includes activation of protein kinase B and certain isoforms of protein kinase C; activation of protein kinase B leads to stimulation of glucose transport and translocation of GLUT4.[101]

One of the most important actions of insulin is to facilitate glucose transport into muscle and fat cells. Glucose transport across cell membranes occurs via glucose transporters, energy-independent proteins that facilitate the transport of glucose down a concentration gradient in almost all cells. The mammalian glucose transporter family is involved not only in the action of insulin on glucose metabolism, but also in the entry of glucose in cells and tissues that are insulin-independent. Several genes have been cloned that encode for different isoforms of glucose transporters. The proteins they code for have structural homologies and tissue-specific distribution (Table 18-5).[109] Five glucose transporters are involved in the sodium-independent transport of glucose and other hexoses into cells, and they all share a 12-membrane–spanning α-helical domain, amino and carboxyl terminals extending into the cytoplasm, a large exoplasmic loop between helices 1 and 2, and a long cytoplasmic hydrophilic segment between helices 6 and 7 (Fig. 18-10). With regard to insulin action, the most important glucose transporter is GLUT-4, which is expressed in tissues where glucose transport is regulated by insulin such as skeletal muscle, adipocytes, and cardiac muscle. Insulin activates glucose transport in these tissues predominantly by recruiting intracellular glucose transport protein and translocating it to the plasma membrane. The increased number of glucose transporters on cell membranes facilitates diffusion of glucose into cells. In insulin-sensitive cells, glucose transport is rate limiting for glucose metabolism.

The exact mechanism by which activation of the insulin receptor leads to translocation of glucose transporters is still unclear. In the basal state, GLUT-4 is located mostly in vesicular compartments within the cell interior, and slowly cycles between these intracellular compartments and the plasma membrane.[110] Insulin action stimulates a large increase in the rate of GLUT-4 exocytosis and a small decrease in endocytosis. GLUT-4 appears to be localized in separate subpopulation of vesicles, with some in the constitutively recycling endosomal proteins, but most in a unique storage compartment comprising vesicles and tubulovesicular elements. This may account for the different magnitude of the effects of insulin on different recycling proteins: insulin stimulates a 2–4 fold increment in plasma membrane levels of GLUT-1 or transferrin receptors, but a 10–40 fold increase in GLUT-4.[11] The movement of GLUT-4 molecules within cells is determined by targeting motifs intrinsic to the GLUT-4 protein and by multiple proteins

TABLE 18-5. Human Glucose Transporters

Isoforms	Tissue Distribution	Function
GLUT-1	Erythrocytes, brain microvessels	Basal glucose transport
GLUT-2	Liver, β-cells, kidney	High-capacity, low-affinity transport
GLUT-3	Brain, fibroblasts	Basal glucose transport
GLUT-4	Skeletal muscle, fat, heart	Insulin-stimulated glucose transport
GLUT-5	Small intestine, testes	Intestinal absorption of fructose

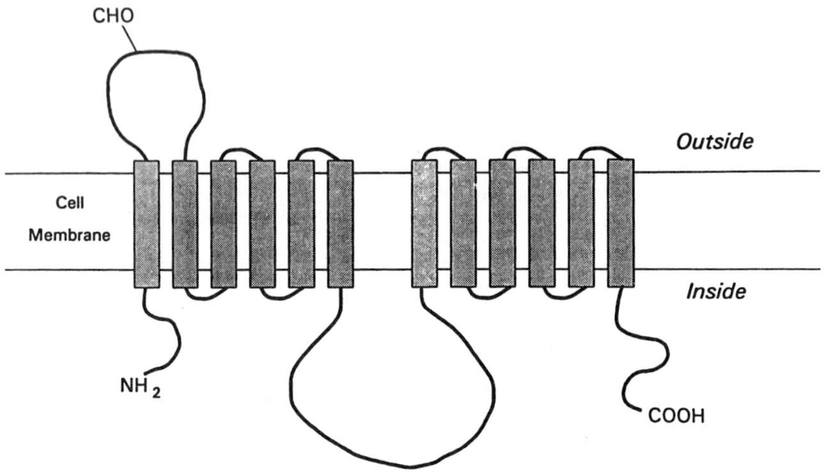

FIGURE 18-10. Schematic model of glucose transporters. (*From White MF, Kahn CR.*[100])

that are known to regulate the flow of cellular vesicles and the proteins they contain. Different motifs have been identified in GLUT-4 molecules that are likely to contribute to trafficking of this molecule. Among these, a di-leucine motif in the cytosolic C-terminus has been associated with intracellular retention and/or internalization signals.[111] Moreover, multiple proteins involved in the synaptic vesicle movements according to the v-SNARE/t-SNARE (vesicle associated and target membrane soluble N-ethylmaleimide-sensitive attachment protein receptors) model [110] regulate GLUT-4 vesicular traffic. According to this model, docking and fusion to the plasma membrane occurs via high affinity interactions between a ligand on the transport vesicle (v-SNARE) and a receptor on the target membrane (t-SNARE). Several proteins have been proposed as facilitating this interaction in the case of GLUT-4 vesicle translocation.[110,111]

The essential role of insulin in glucose transport at the level of skeletal muscle and adipose tissue has led to numerous studies of abnormalities of GLUT-4 in experimental diabetes. GLUT-4 knockout mice have been developed and the heterozygous animals exhibits a decrease in GLUT-4 expression, reduced glucose uptake in skeletal muscle and adipose tissue, hypertension, and increased glucose and insulin levels, thus providing a reasonable model of type 2 diabetes.[112] Interestingly, homozygous mice do not express GLUT-4 at all and yet do not develop diabetes. In human type 2 diabetes, decreased glucose transport in adipocytes is associated with decreased expression of GLUT-4 transporters,[113] but normal levels of GLUT-4 mRNA and protein have been found in patients with insulin resistance associated with obesity or type 2 diabetes.[114] Recent evidence suggests that in skeletal muscles of type 2 diabetic patients there is a defect in insulin-induced GLUT-4 translocation, and this defect correlates with maximal in vivo glucose disposal rates, suggesting that an abnormality in GLUT-4 translocation could cause insulin resistance.[115]

Termination of the insulin signal is mainly due to insulin degradation. The biological half-life of insulin is in the range of 6 to 10 minutes. There are three major sites of insulin degradation. After secretion, 40 to 60 percent of insulin undergoes first-pass elimination by the liver. In addition, insulin binds to its peripheral receptors where it is internalized, translocated to lysosomes, and then degraded. Two insulin-degrading enzymes have been identified: glutathione-insulin transhydrogenase cleaves the disulfide bonds of insulin, releasing intact A and B chains, and proteases inactivate insulin by peptide bond cleavage. The kidney accounts for 15 to 20 percent of insulin degradation. The renal clearance of insulin is larger than the GFR, indicating that the hormone is removed by the tubules as well as by filtration. In patients with renal insufficiency, insulin uptake by the kidney may fall by ~9 percent.[116] This accounts in part for the diminished insulin requirements often seen in diabetic patients with end stage renal disease. The kidney assumes increased importance in the degradation of exogenous insulin because subcutaneously injected insulin is absorbed via the systemic circulation while endogenous insulin is released into the portal vein.

Glucagon Chemistry and Biosynthesis

Glucagon is a polypeptide consisting of a single chain of 29 amino acids with a molecular mass of 3,485 daltons. Recent studies of structure-activity relations indicate that the terminal amino group is active in both receptor binding and cellular action of the hormone. However, the terminal carboxyl group confers high affinity of the hormone for its receptor, which permits hormone binding and action at physiologic concentrations. Unlike insulin, the amino acid sequence of glucagon is identical in all mammalian species examined. The alpha cells of the islets of Langerhans are the site of glucagon biosynthesis: these cells are situated on the outer rim of the islets and constitute ~15 percent of the islet-cell population. A single gene located on the long arm of chromosome 2 has been found to code for preproglucagon in humans,[85,117] and this gene gives rise to "true" glucagon in the pancreas and glucagon-like immunoreactivity in the intestinal tract and in the hypothalamus.[118,119] The processing of the large proglucagon molecule differs in the pancreas, the intestine, and the brain (Fig. 18-11). The preproglucagon gene codes for a signal peptide, glicentin-related polypeptide (GRPP); glucagon; a hexapeptide, GLP-1 (glucagon-like peptide-1); and GLP-2 (glucagon-like peptide-2). The segment that contains GRPP, glucagon, and the hexapeptide has been named glicentin, and cleavage at the Lys-Arg site located between GRPP and glucagon releases oxyntomodulin in the intestine (Fig. 18-11). Both glicentin and oxyntomodulin are thought to affect gastrointestinal function, potentially by inhibiting gastric emptying and HCl production, as well as decreasing exocrine pancreatic secretion.[119] GLP-1 and GLP-2 form part of a large proglucagon fragment in the pancreas, while in the intestine

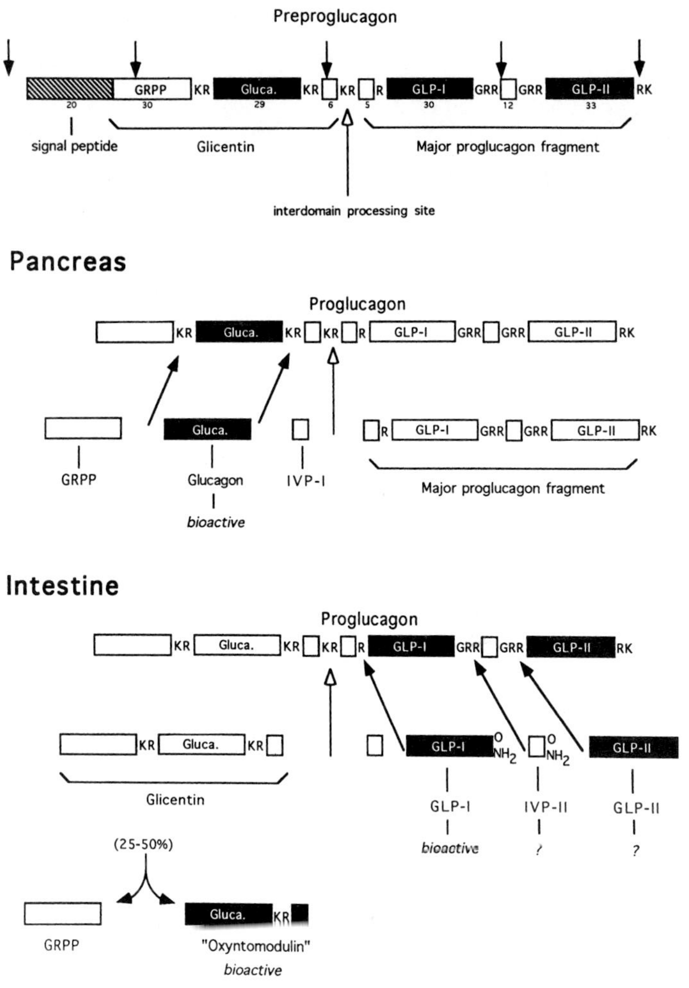

FIGURE 18-11. Tissue specific processing of preproglucagon. (*From Steiner et al.*[137])

they exist as independent molecules. GLP-1, glicentin, oxyntomodulin, and very small amounts of glucagon have been identified in the brain; whether they function as neurotransmitters is not known.[120]

Glucagon Secretion

Glucagon secretion does not markedly fluctuate throughout the day in normal subjects receiving mixed meals (Fig. 18-5). The relative constancy of glucagon concentration contrasts with the frequent daily fluctuations of insulin concentration, which accompany mixed-meal ingestion or even minor changes (10 to 20 mg/dl), in blood glucose concentration. Plasma glucose level has an overriding effect on glucagon secretion, which is the inverse of its effect on insulin. Hypoglycemia causes a twofold to fourfold increase in plasma glucagon levels, while hyperglycemia lowers them by approximately 50 percent. Other major physiologic stimuli of glucagon secretion in normal humans are protein ingestion, infusion of amino acids, and exercise, particularly if it is strenuous or prolonged.[119,121] Increases in glucagon secretion are also seen after the infusion of large doses of epinephrine (mediated through alpha 2A and beta 2 adrenergic receptors), and in association with hypercortisolism.[119] After 5–10 years of disease duration, the stimulating effect of hypoglycemia on glucagon secretion is markedly reduced in patients with Type 1 diabetes. Glucagon secretion with hypoglycemia is restored with successful pancreatic transplantation.[122] The hyperglucagonemia observed with starvation is largely due to decreased catabolism rather than augmented secretion (see later discussion).

Suppression of glucagon secretion occurs after the ingestion or infusion of glucose. The hypoglucagonemic effects of glucose may depend on insulin-mediated uptake of glucose by the alpha cells and/or the absence of marked hyperglycemia, as well as by the concomitant rise in other hormones that suppress glucagon secretion,[123] such as GLP-1. Somatostatin is also a potent inhibitor of glucagon as well as insulin and GH secretion.

Glucagon Action

Although glucagon was discovered in the 1930s in crude insulin preparations as a "hyperglycemic-glycogenolytic factor," its physiologic role and mechanism of action have been elucidated only recently. Early studies were hampered by the inability to produce a pure glucagon-deficient state without concomitant insulin deficiency and the lack of data on circulating levels and secretory rates of glucagon.

It is now apparent that physiologic increments in glucagon concentration produce a rise in blood glucose concentration by stimulating hepatic glycogenolysis and gluconeogenesis (Fig. 18-12). In contrast, a fall in glucagon concentration to below basal levels results in a decrease in hepatic glucose production.[124] However, when an increment in glucagon concentration is accompanied by a small (50 to 150 percent) rise in the circulating insulin concentration, hepatic glucose production remains unchanged.

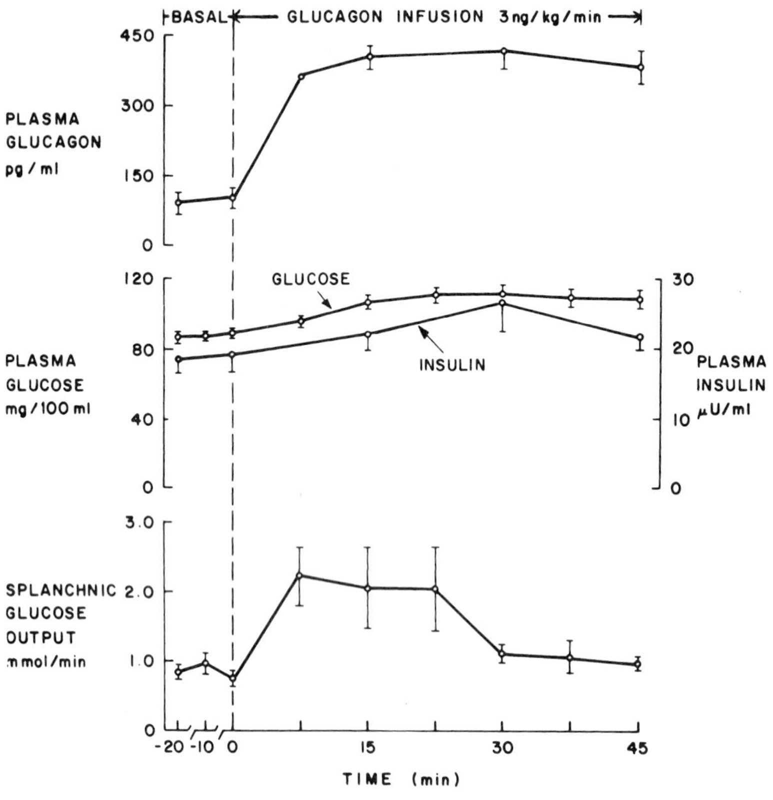

FIGURE 18-12. Stimulation by glucagon of hepatic (splanchnic) glucose production in normal humans. Physiologic hyperglucagonemia causes a prompt rise in hepatic glucose production. The effect is transient, however, lasting less than 45 min. The stimulatory action of glucagon on glucose production thus results from changes in concentrations of glucagon rather than absolute concentrations themselves. (*From Felig et al.*[127])

The latter phenomenon accounts for the importance of the bihormonal response (i.e., rise in glucagon concentration as well as insulin concentration) to the ingestion of a protein meal (Fig. 18-13). Glucagon has been shown to play a critical role in vivo in the disposition of amino acids by increasing their transport and conversion to glucose.[125] The insulin response engendered by the protein meal ensures the cellular uptake and utilization of amino acids contained in the meal. However, the rise in insulin concentration alone would inhibit hepatic glucose output, resulting in hypoglycemia. The simultaneous increase in glucagon concentration mitigates such an effect by ensuring that glucose production is maintained (Fig. 18-12).

Because of the opposing actions of insulin and glucagon on the liver, and inasmuch as glucose suppresses glucagon secretion while stimulating insulin secretion, Unger has suggested that the insulin/glucagon molar ratio (I/G), rather than the concentration of either hormone alone, governs overall carbohydrate homeostasis.[126] The applicability of this bihormonal hypothesis to the intact organism has been challenged in studies involving infusions of glucagon in physiologic doses.[127,128] High plasma glucagon levels of 300 to 400 pg/ml (comparable to those observed in a variety of hyperglucagonemic states) fail to alter glucose tolerance in normal subjects. Moreover, despite a marked fall in I/G (from 34:1 to 6:1) when glucagon is infused, no change in glucose tolerance occurs.[119] Glucagon-induced changes in glucose tolerance thus require insulin deficiency or pharmacologic doses of glucagon.

Glucagon is the primary hormone that restores glucose levels in the setting of hyperinsulinemia. Glucagon's dominant counterregulatory effect in hypoglycemia is confirmed by the inability of increased epinephrine secretion to compensate entirely when glucagon is missing.[129]

In addition to its action on carbohydrate and protein metabolism, glucagon is involved in the regulation of ketogenesis. Livers obtained from rats given physiologic doses of glucagon display augmented ketone production from FFA.[130] In vivo, ketonemia may occur in the absence of glucagon, as in pancreatectomized patients.[131] However, in insulin-deficient diabetic patients, hyperglucagonemia increases the ketogenic capacity. It should be emphasized that glucagon's effects in raising blood glucose concentration and enhancing ketosis are entirely a consequence of its actions on the liver. Increases in FFA oxidation and ketogenesis result from glucagon's inhibitory effect on hepatic lipogenesis decreasing malonyl CoA availability, rather than from stimulation of peripheral lipolysis.

The first step in the action of glucagon on the liver is interaction with a specific receptor on the cell membrane. The glucagon receptor has homologies to the calcitonin and parathyroid hormone receptors, and transduces signals via accumulation of two second messengers, cAMP and calcium.[132] Hormone binding causes signaling through the GTP-binding proteins, with subsequent activation of adenylate cyclase with resulting increases in intracellular cAMP levels. The rise in cAMP concentration, through activation of cAMP-dependent protein kinase, triggers several phosphorylation reactions, resulting in activation of glycogen phosphorylase and simultaneous inhibition of glycogen synthase. Insulin antagonizes this action by reducing the activity of cAMP-dependent protein kinase[133] and/or augmenting the activity of phosphodiesterase responsible for cAMP degradation.[134] There is also evidence suggesting that elevation of intracellular calcium, independent of cAMP accumulation, may play a role in the action of glucagon.[119] It appears that influx of calcium, possibly secondary to activation of a calcium pump by the GTP-binding proteins, is essential for the metabolic actions of glucagon, because

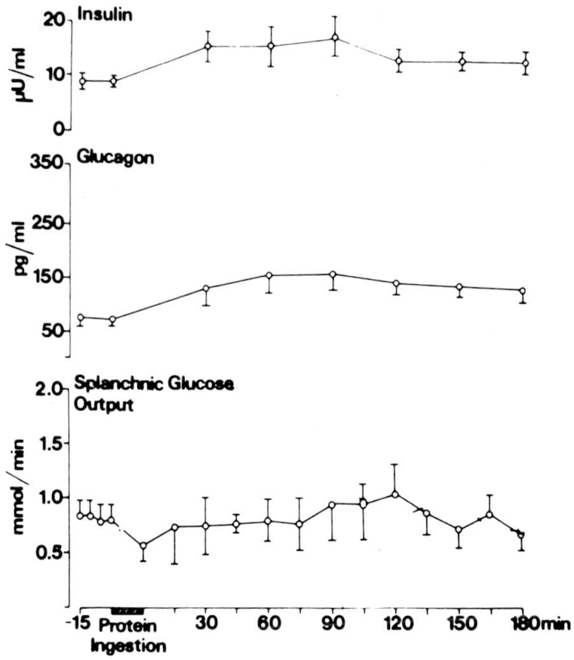

FIGURE 18-13. Influence of protein feeding on plasma insulin and glucagon concentrations and on splanchnic (hepatic) glucose production in normal humans. The rise in glucagon concentration induced by protein feeding is necessary for the uptake and anabolic utilization of the amino acids contained in the protein meal. (*Based on data of Wahren et al. J Clin Inv 58:761,1976.*)

blocking calcium influx inhibits glycogenolysis and gluconeogenesis in hepatocytes.[135] Glucagon also lowers serum potassium and calcium concentrations, decreases gastric acid and pancreatic enzyme secretion, raises serum GH secretion, and increases myocardial contractility. However, each of these effects requires pharmacologic doses of the hormone.

In contrast to insulin, glucagon degradation is carried out primarily in the kidney rather than liver. As a result, plasma glucagon concentration is elevated in uremia despite the absence of hypersecretion. Glucagon removal by the kidney normally exceeds the filtered load, suggesting that peritubular uptake contributes to renal clearance. A reduction in glucagon catabolism is also the major factor responsible for the hyperglucagonemia observed in short-term (3-day) starvation. Although hyperglucagonemia is observed in cirrhosis patients, particularly when accompanied by portal hypertension, augmented secretion rather than diminished degradation is the major mechanism of the elevated plasma glucagon concentration in such patients.[136]

Somatostatin

Somatostatin is a tetradecapeptide hormone, initially isolated from hypothalamic extracts and defined by its role in inhibiting growth hormone secretion. Further studies quickly led to the discovery that this peptide is present in many tissues, including other regions of the CNS, pancreas, stomach, and intestine. Somatostatin can suppress the secretion of several hormones including growth hormone, thyrotropin, insulin, and glucagon, and inhibits gastric acid and pepsin secretion and intestinal smooth muscle contractility.[137] The human somatostatin gene has been cloned,[138] and processing of prosomatostatin is known to produce two bioactive forms of somatostatin: the larger somatostatin-28, found predominantly in the intestine, and somatostatin-14.[137] In pancreatic islets somatostatin-14 is secreted by D-cells, and it is thought to have paracrine effects on adjacent A, B, and PP cells.[139] The biological actions of somatostatin are mediated by binding to a family of high-affinity receptors coupled to GTP-binding proteins.[140] The physiological role of pancreatic somatostatin secretion is still unclear, and the initial enthusiasm for a potential role of somatostatin in the therapy of type 1 diabetic patients has now faded.[141] The amount of somatostatin-14 secreted by pancreatic D cells is very small compared to the amount released by the intestine.[139]

Pancreatic Polypeptide

Pancreatic polypeptide (PP) is a 36-amino-acid peptide produced by the PP cells of the pancreas (Table 18-1). PP belongs to a family of biologically active peptides that include peptide YY and neuropeptide Y, peptides that are present in many neurons of the central and peripheral nervous systems. The human PP gene has been cloned,[142] is located on chromosome 17, and is expressed almost exclusively in the duodenal pancreas. Secretion of PP is mainly regulated by food intake and vagal cholinergic mechanisms. PP does not appear to alter carbohydrate metabolism, but is thought to inhibit exocrine pancreatic secretions and biliary tract motility.[143] PP secretion decreases in chronic pancreatitis and has been proposed to contribute to the increased hepatic glucose production and impaired glucose tolerance observed in these patients.[144]

Islet Amyloid Polypeptide

Islet amyloid polypeptide (IAPP), or "amylin," is a 37-amino-acids peptide that is cosecreted with insulin in pancreatic beta cells. IAPP was initially described as the main component of amyloid deposits that had long been observed in the islets of elderly type 2 diabetic patients. IAPP has major homology with the calcitonin-gene related peptide (CGRP).[145] The human IAPP gene is located on the short arm of chromosome 12, and structure analysis suggests that IAPP, CGRP, and calcitonin all derive from a common ancestral gene.[146] IAPP is colocalized with insulin to the secretory granules of human beta cells and is cosecreted in a molar ratio of ~1–2 percent with insulin.[147] The physiological role of IAPP is still debated. Effects of IAPP on insulin resistance (inhibition of peripheral glucose uptake and stimulation of hepatic glucose production) and on the regulation of insulin secretion have been described.[148] However, most experiments were performed with pharmacological doses of IAPP, and the physiological significance of these observations is debatable. A role of IAPP on gastric motility and food intake has also been proposed and is thought to be the basis of the small effects of a synthetic analog of human amylin on glucose control in type 2 diabetic patients.[149]

An open issue is the role of IAPP and amyloid deposits in the pathogenesis of type 2 diabetes. At autopsy, as many as 90 percent of patients with type 2 diabetes have amyloid deposits in their islets,[150] although they are rarely observed in individuals with normal glucose tolerance. Whether islet amyloid formation plays a pathogenetic role in type 2 diabetes or is an epiphenomenon is still debated. Human IAPP has been shown to have an amino acid sequence that confers amyloidogenic properties that are essential for fibril formation in pancreatic islets. However, because nondiabetic individuals do not develop islet amyloid, other unrecognized factors are probably necessary for development of amyloid deposits in type 2 diabetes. There is no evidence of an abnormal IAPP gene in type 2 diabetes,[151] and transgenic mice for human IAPP did not develop amyloid deposits or glucose intolerance unless exposed to a high fat diet.[152] A potential role of increased dietary fat consumption in inducing abnormal beta cell IAPP production, processing, and secretion, with consequent amyloid fibril deposition and eventual development of beta cell failure and type 2 diabetes, has been recently proposed.[153]

FUEL HOMEOSTASIS

Regulatory and Counterregulatory Hormones

The large number of hormones that influence fuel metabolism may be categorized as favoring either the storage or the dissipation of energy. In this regard, insulin is unique because it favors the storage of each of the major body fuels (glucose, fat, and protein). In contrast, five hormones (epinephrine, glucagon, cortisol, GH, and thyroid hormone) promote the dissipation of body fat, glycogen, and/or protein. These hormones may also be classified with respect to the feedback effect of plasma glucose concentration on their secretion and in terms of their action on blood glucose concentration. Insulin is the only hormone whose secretion is influenced on a moment-to-moment basis by physiologic fluctuations in blood glucose concentration (Fig. 18-5) and which brings about a fall in the blood glucose concentration. In contrast, each of the energy-dissipating hormones (except for thyroxine) causes a rise in the blood glucose concentration. Furthermore, an increase in their secretion requires either the development of frank hypoglycemia or the interposition of signals other than a change in blood glucose concentration (e.g., protein feeding, exercise, and stress). Consequently, with respect to blood glucose control, insulin is generally considered the major regulatory hormone, while glucagon, catecholamines, cortisol, and GH are collectively referred to as *counterregulatory* hormones. The actions of the counterregulatory hormones in raising blood glucose concentration may result from coordinate effects on glycogen metabolism and/or gluconeogenesis or antagonism of insulin-mediated glucose uptake.

Metabolism and Energy Stores

The homeostasis of body fuels is dependent not only on the availability of enzymatically regulated pathways and a variety of hormonal signals, but also on finely coordinated substrate-hormone interactions. These interactions are best understood by considering the changes that occur in conditions of fuel availability (the fed state), fuel need (starvation, exercise), or fuel imbalance ("stress" hyperglycemia). These perturbations, however, require an understanding of normal body composition (e.g., fuel stores) and the conditions existing in the basal state.

The caloric composition of a typical American or western European diet consists of 40 to 45 percent carbohydrate, 40 percent fat, and 15 to 20 percent protein. The composition of the fuels stored in the human body is far different from that of fuels ingested in the diet (Table 18-6). Carbohydrate represents a calorically insignificant fuel store. The combined caloric value of liver glycogen (70 g), muscle glycogen (200 g), and circulating blood glucose (20 g) amounts to ~ 1,200 kcal, well below the average caloric expenditure of a single day. Nevertheless, liver glycogen represents an important source of carbohydrate for the ongoing supply to the brain and the needs of muscle during exercise (see later discussion). The teleologic basis for limiting carbohydrate as a major source of stored energy includes not only its low caloric density (4 kcal/g, compared with 9 kcal/g in fat), but the large amount of tissue water obligatory for the storage of glycogen (4 ml/g).

By far the largest reservoir of body fuel is fat, which is stored as triglyceride. In a nonobese subject, body fat amounts to ~ 20 percent of total body weight, representing 130,000 to 140,000 kcal and accounting for 80 percent of total body fuel depots. The compact nature of this large fuel depot is due to its caloric density and anhydrous nature. To store an equivalent amount of energy as carbohydrate would require more than eight times the weight of fat. The fat depot is sufficient to meet the caloric requirements for ~ 2 months. In obese subjects, fat tissue may store more than 500,000 kcal. Regardless of the degree of adiposity, fat clearly represents the most expendable, as well as the most plentiful, fuel available to humans.

The major reservoir of body protein is in muscle tissue, amounting to 10 kg (exclusive of tissue water) or 40,000 kcal. Because of protein's indispensable role in body structure, muscle function, and as a catalytic agent (e.g., enzymes), loss of >50 percent of body protein is incompatible with survival despite residual mobilizable fat tissue. Death from starvation generally results not from hypoglycemia but from dissolution of protein stores. Loss of respiratory muscle function leads to terminal pneumonia.

Of particular importance in considering the homeostatic response to the need for fuel is an understanding of the relationships among body fuels. Protein (by virtue of its constituent amino acids other than leucine or valine) is readily converted to glucose (gluconeogenesis). Carbohydrate availability for glucose-dependent tissues (e.g., brain) thus does not cease with depletion of liver glycogen. In contrast, fatty acids cannot generally be converted to

TABLE 18-6. Body Composition and Fuel Reserves in a Normal 70-kg Human

Fuel	Tissue	Weight (kg)	Body Weight (%)	Energy Value (kcal)
Fat	Adipose tissue	11–17	15–25	100,000–150,000
Protein	Muscle (primarily)	8–12	12–17	32,000–48,000
Carbohydrate	Liver (glycogen)	0.070	<1	280
	Muscle (glycogen)	0.200	<1	800
	Blood (glucose)	0.020	<1	80

glucose because mammalian tissue lacks the enzymatic capacity for net gluconeogenesis from substrates with less than three carbons, e.g., acetyl CoA. Thus, to the extent that glucose is terminally oxidized (by brain) and must be replenished by gluconeogenesis, there is an obligate dissolution of body protein stores in total starvation.

The Basal State

The basal or postabsorptive state, the condition that exists 6 to 12 h after food ingestion, represents the transition from feeding to fasting. Although this interval represents a nonsteady state, it is nevertheless a readily identifiable reference point with which various perturbations may be compared. In the postabsorptive condition, adipose tissue releases FFA to meet the fuel requirements of muscle and heart as well as parenchymal tissues (liver, kidney). The respiratory quotient of most muscles is close to 0.7, reflecting virtual dependence on fat oxidation. Carbohydrate utilization occurs primarily in the brain, which terminally oxidizes glucose at a rate of 50 to 100 g per day. Smaller amounts of glucose are utilized by resting muscle, by adipose tissue, and by obligate anaerobic tissues such as the formed elements of the blood and the renal medulla (Fig. 18-14).[154]

Although several tissues utilize glucose, the production of glucose is limited largely to the liver. Maintenance of euglycemia depends on the release of glucose from the liver at a rate equal to the combined utilization in brain and peripheral tissues (100 to 200 g per day or 2 to 2.5 mg/min per kilogram of body weight). Approximately 75 percent of the glucose produced during an overnight fast is derived from glycogen, and the remainder is formed by gluconeogenesis from lactate, alanine, and, to a lesser extent, pyruvate and glycerol.[155] In the complete absence of hepatic glucose production, the blood glucose level would be halved in 40 to 60 min. The increased delivery of FFA to the liver results in the formation of ketone bodies. However, the rate of ketogenesis in the basal state is such that it maintains the concentration of circulating ketone acids at < 0.5 m*M* only.

The hormonal signal that permits the initiation of glycogenolysis, gluconeogenesis, and ketogenesis in the basal state is the fall in plasma insulin concentration from the level observed in the fed state (30 to 100 μU/ml) to values of 10 to 20 μU/ml. Glucose utilization in the basal state is largely ($\sim$70 percent) non-insulin–dependent, occurring primarily in the brain. In contrast, the presence of basal insulin levels (and basal secretory rates of 0.25 to 1.5 U/h) ensures maximal efficiency in fuel economy by preventing excessive gluconeogenesis and unrestrained FFA mobilization and ketogenesis. There is an apparent "redundant regulation" of insulin secretion at low glucose levels, probably mediated by FFA levels or the products of their oxidation. Thus, the rates of glucose and ketone production do not exceed the rates of glucose and ketone utilization, precluding the development of hyperglycemia and hyperketonemia. When there is no basal insulin secretion (as in type 1 diabetes) or if hormonal perturbations that occur interfere with basal insulin action (see Stress Hyperglycemia, later) occur, the blood glucose and ketone concentrations rise.

Fuel Availability: The Fed State

The hormonal response to the fed state is determined in part by the nature of the ingested substrate (Table 18-7). If pure glucose is ingested, a multihormonal response involving a rise in insulin concentration and decreases in glucagon and GH concentrations ensues. If pure protein is ingested, the multihormonal response consists of a rise in insulin as well as glucagon and GH

FIGURE 18-14. Glucose turnover in the postabsorptive and postprandial states. In the postabsorptive state (overnight fast, basal state), the liver is the sole site of the production of glucose by glycogenolysis (75 percent) and gluconeogenesis (25 percent). The brain is the major site of glucose utilization which is not insulin-dependent. Muscle provides gluconeogenic precursors in the form of lactate, alanine, and glutamine, while fat cells are a source of glycerol. In the postprandial state, glucose uptake is insulin-dependent and occurs in liver, muscle, and fat cells. Some of the glycogen stored in the liver is synthesized via the indirect (gluconeogenic) pathway. (*From Dineen et al.*[154])

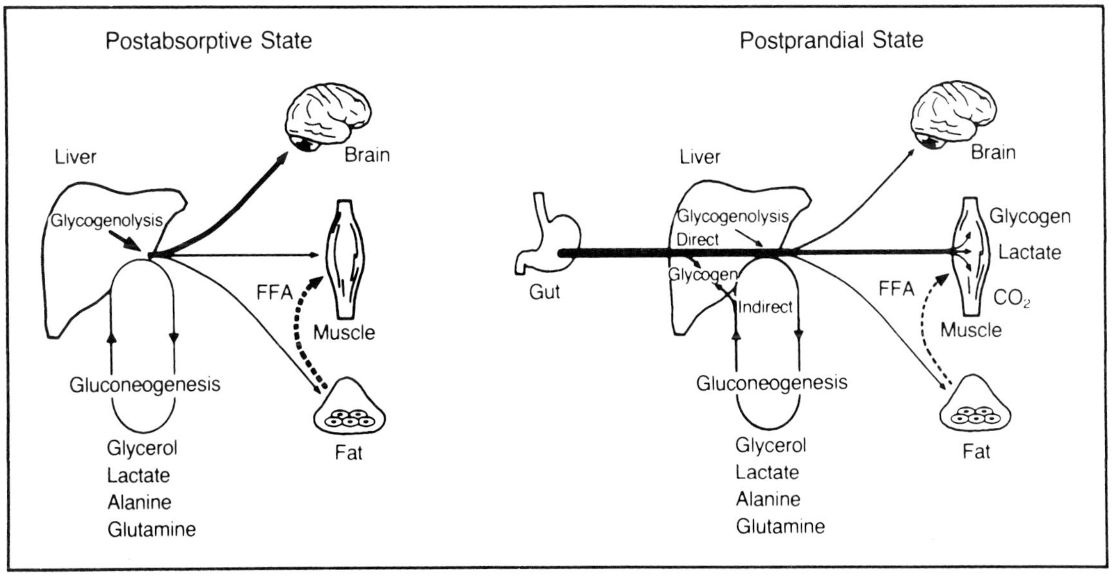

TABLE 18-7. Hormonal Response to Altered Fuel Availability or Need

Condition	Insulin	Glucagon	Growth Hormone	Epinephrine	Cortisol
Fuel availability					
Glucose ingestion	↑	↓	↓	±	±
Protein ingestion	↑	↑	↑	±	±
Mixed-meal ingestion	↑	±	±	±	±
Fuel need					
Starvation	↓	↑	↑ or ±	↑ or ±	↓
Acute hypoglycemia	↓	↑	↑	↑	↑
Exercise	↓	↑	↑	↑	↑

Abbreviations: ↑ = increased secretion; ↓ = decreased secretion; ± = unchanged.

concentrations. In contrast, when mixed meals are eaten (the usual dietary intake), a rise only in insulin level is observed. Regardless of the substrate ingested, the rise in insulin concentration is the key signal that shifts metabolism to the fed state by stimulating cellular uptake of glucose and amino acids and inhibiting lipolysis. When the rise in insulin concentration is not accompanied by a rise in glucagon concentration (e.g., with glucose or mixed-meal ingestion), glucose output from the liver is inhibited and net hepatic uptake of glucose occurs. Some hepatic gluconeogenesis may continue even during periods of net hepatic glucose storage by virtue of glycogen formation via the "indirect" (gluconeogenic) pathway (Fig. 18-14).[156] The fall in GH concentration that accompanies glucose ingestion may enhance insulin's antilipolytic effects. When both insulin and glucagon levels rise (e.g., with protein feeding), glucose output from the liver is maintained at basal rates. The importance of the latter derives from the fact that ingested protein cannot by itself supply the fuel requirements of the brain. Note that feeding fails to alter abruptly the secretion of catecholamines or cortisol (Table 18-7).

Fuel Need: Starvation

If the basal state is not interrupted by the ingestion of food, the metabolic response progresses to one that characterizes starvation. The major hormonal signals governing the fasting state are a fall in insulin concentration and, to a lesser extent, a rise in glucagon concentration. The progressive decline in insulin concentration is triggered by a small decline in blood glucose concentration but may be initiated by caloric lack per se. Hypoinsulinemia leads to increased lipolysis and hepatic fatty acid oxidation, resulting in a gradual increase in ketogenesis. The outflow of amino acids (particularly alanine) from muscle and the key rate-limiting enzymes involved in hepatic gluconeogenesis are stimulated. In this manner, hepatic glucose production is sustained despite the fact that liver glycogen stores are depleted within 24 h.

When starvation is prolonged for >3 weeks, the kidney, in addition to the liver, contributes to glucose production. Nevertheless, the total rate of gluconeogenesis as well as glucose utilization is markedly reduced. In this circumstance, ketones become an increasingly important substrate for the brain (replacing some glucose) and may provide the signal to muscle by which protein catabolism and alanine outflow are diminished.[157] Although growth hormone levels rise with starvation, the increment is transient and is not essential for the lipolytic or ketogenic response.

Exercise

A marked increase in fuel requirements occurs in either fed or fasted humans during muscular exercise. The major fuel consumed (carbohydrate or fat) depends on the duration as well as the intensity of the exercise performed (Fig. 18-15).[158] With very brief exercise (a run lasting only a few minutes), the major fuel consumed is muscle glycogen. With longer periods of exercise, extending to 1 to 2 h, blood glucose levels account for ~40 percent of the increased fuel consumption, with the rest being provided by FFA. The rate of glucose uptake by muscle is stimulated up to 40 times the resting level, while total body glucose turnover may increase three- to fourfold. With very prolonged exercise, there is progressively less dependence on glucose and increased utilization of fat. The stimulatory effect of exercise on glucose utilization occurs in the face of a declining insulin concentration. The multihormonal response to exercise (Table 18-7) is thus largely directed at providing a milieu that favors hepatic glycogenolysis and gluconeogenesis as well as lipolysis.

Fuel-Hormone Imbalance

Hypoglycemia

When the blood glucose level is suddenly lowered by the administration of insulin, there is an immediate need to restore circulating glucose levels so that brain function will not be irreversibly disturbed. The homeostatic response consists of a marked increase in the secretion of each of the counterregulatory hormones and inhibition of endogenous insulin secretion (Table 18-7). As a result, within 15 to 30 min of bolus administration of insulin, a reversal of its inhibitory effects on hepatic glucose production is observed. The redundant nature of the counterregulatory hormone response to hypoglycemia is particularly important in diabetic patients. In such patients, the glucagon response to hypoglycemia may be blunted, increasing their dependency on catecholamines (see section on Complications of Insulin Therapy).[159]

Stress Hyperglycemia

The hormonal response characteristic of acute fuel need (low insulin concentration and increased glucagon, catecholamine, cortisol, and GH concentrations) is occasionally observed in the absence of starvation, exercise, or hypoglycemia. In patients with various types of stress (extensive body burns, compound fractures, sepsis, etc.), high levels of counterregulatory hormones and a low plasma insulin concentration are often noted. In the absence of a

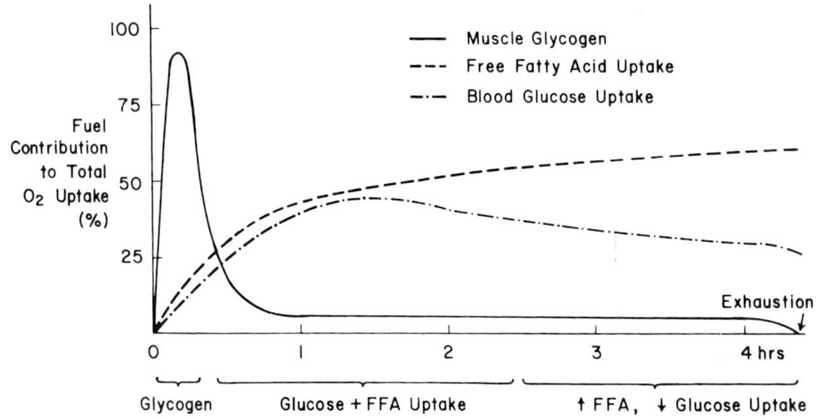

FIGURE 18-15. Pattern of fuel utilization by muscle during exercise of varying duration. During the initial few minutes of exercise, muscle glycogen is a major fuel for the production of ATP. Between 10 and 40 min of exercise, blood-borne glucose and FFA each account for 40 percent of total fuel oxidation. Thereafter (i.e., with very prolonged exercise), there is a progressive rise in the utilization of FFA and lessened uptake of blood glucose. Although muscle glycogen makes only a small contribution to fuel utilization in prolonged exercise, its total depletion is associated with the development of fatigue.

stimulus for glucose utilization (e.g., exercise), such a hormonal pattern results in a rise in blood glucose concentration (*stress hyperglycemia*). This phenomenon involves overproduction as well as underutilization of glucose. It is due to synergistic interaction among the various counterregulatory hormones.[160,161] Thus, although glucagon, epinephrine, or cortisol causes only minor rises in the blood glucose concentration when elevated individually, the effect of a multihormonal response is more than additive (Fig. 18-16). The synergism derives from the fact that while cortisol itself has little effect on glucose production, it converts the transient hepatic effect of glucagon or epinephrine to one of sustained glucose overproduction. In addition, epinephrine, by virtue of its suppressive effects on insulin secretion as well as its antagonism of insulin action, exaggerates the hyperglycemic response by decreasing glucose utilization. If insulin levels are already reduced, as in a diabetic patient, the effect of such a multihormonal response is to intensify the diabetic state.

CLINICAL DIABETES

Definition, Classification, and Diagnosis

Definition Diabetes mellitus is a heterogeneous set of disorders characterized by two shared features—disordered metabolism, most notably hyperglycemia, and the propensity to develop specific long-term complications including retinopathy, nephropathy, and neuropathy. The underlying cause of all forms of diabetes is relative or absolute insulin deficiency.

Classification The modern classification of diabetes mellitus continues to evolve with increasing understanding of its epidemiology, pathophysiology, and genetics. The similar classifications promulgated by the National Diabetes Data Group (NDDG)[162] and World Health Organization[163] in 1979 and 1985, respectively, have recently been updated by an Expert Committee of the American Diabetes Association (ADA).[164] All three classifications are remarkably similar except for modest changes in nomenclature, a recent decrease in the diagnostic level for fasting glucose level, and changes in the recommendations for screening.

The major forms of diabetes, the conditions that precede diabetes, and the most recent nomenclature are shown in Table 18-8. The major forms of diabetes include Type 1 (previously called juvenile-onset or insulin-dependent) diabetes mellitus, Type 2

FIGURE 18-16. The synergistic effects of cortisol (C), glucagon (G), and epinephrine (E) in raising plasma glucose concentration, stimulating glucose production, and reducing glucose clearance. The hyperglycemic response to the triple hormone infusion (C + G + E) is far greater than the additive response to all three hormones given singly or the response to any combination of two hormones given together plus one hormone given singly. The development of "stress" hyperglycemia is a consequence of this hormone synergism, which also includes GH. (*From Eigler et al.*[160])

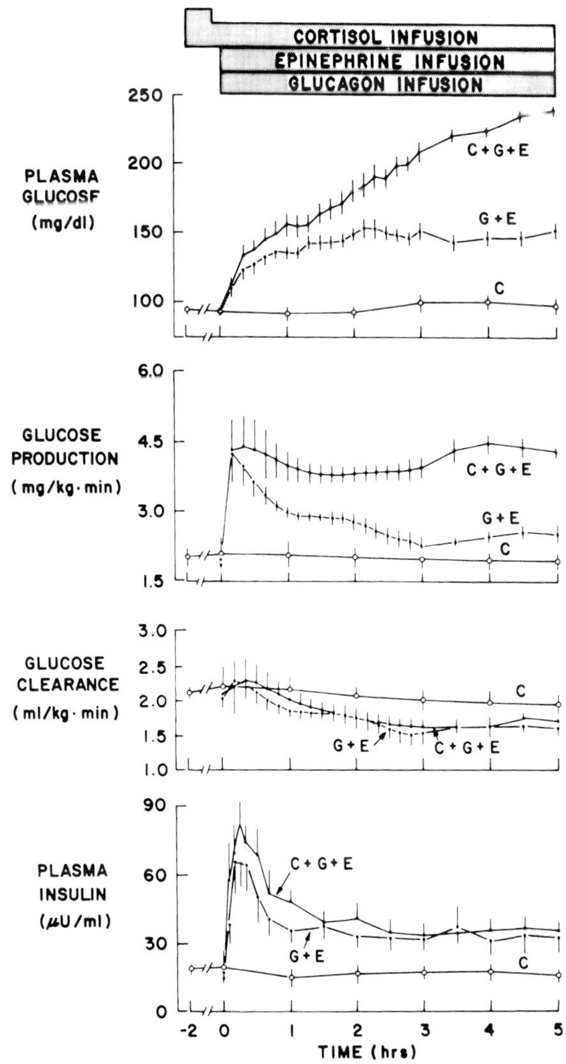

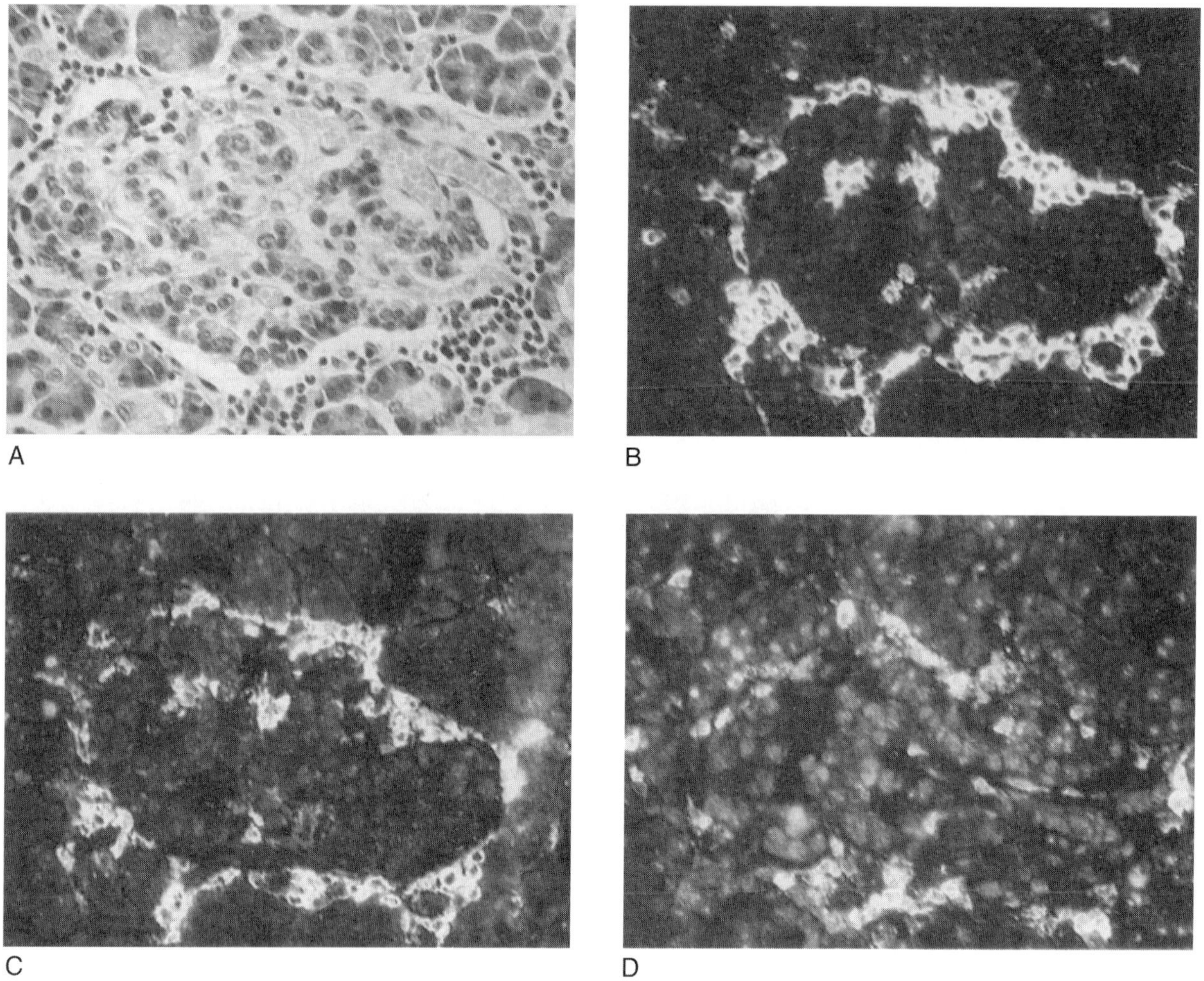

FIGURE 18-20. T-lymphocyte invasion of β-cells in a 12-year-old girl with recently diagnosed diabetes. In panel (*a*), hematoxylin and eosin staining shows lymphocyte infiltration. Panel (*b*) shows all types of leukocytes with a monoclonal antibody and fluourescence. Panel (*c*) specifically stains for T8, presumably cytotoxic, lymphocytes while panel (*d*) indicates activated T-cells staining for interleukin-2 receptor lymphocytes. (*From Bottazzo et al.*[184])

more specific antigens, such as ICA 512 (IA2), which is a tyrosine phosphatase, or glutamic acid decarboxylase (GAD), and/or insulin is generally considered to be an epiphenomenon, rather than the cause of beta cell destruction. Although some antibodies have been suggested to impair β-cell function,[185] anti-islet cell antibodies generally don't fix complement and passive transfer of diabetes has not been accomplished. The presence of these markers is useful in identifying siblings or children of Type 1 diabetics, and even persons in the general population, who are at heightened risk for developing diabetes.[170,186]

In addition to the autoimmune destruction of the beta cell, roles for oxidation, apoptosis, decreased β-cell regeneration, and other factors that may make the beta cell population more vulnerable to destruction have been proposed in the pathogenesis of Type 1 diabetes.

Clinical Presentation

Characteristically, Type 1 diabetes has a clinically acute onset with symptoms secondary to hyperglycemia and the attendant osmotic diuresis, including polyuria, nocturia, increased thirst, and polydipsia. Unregulated metabolism results in weight loss, initially from dehydration with osmotic diuresis, then from fat loss, and eventually from protein loss with loss of muscle mass. Although appetite is often increased in the early stages, development of ketosis results in nausea and vomiting. Other presenting symptoms of diabetes include the consequences of acute fluctuations in glucose level, such as blurred vision secondary to osmotic swelling of the lens with changes in its refractive properties. Other less specific symptoms, such as vaginitis or balanitis with recurrent or intractable yeast infections, occur owing to high tissue glucose levels, which provide a hospitable environment for yeast overgrowth.[187] With the onset of ketosis, acute gastrointestinal symptoms including abdominal pain, anorexia, nausea, and vomiting supervene. As many as 20 percent of patients with Type 1 diabetes present in diabetic ketoacidosis.[188] Indigent or underserved populations may have a higher rate of ketoacidosis as the presenting sign of Type 1 diabetes.

The absolute insulin deficiency that characterizes established Type 1 diabetes results in labile glucose levels unless physiologic levels of insulin are restored by frequent administration of exogenous insulin (Fig. 18-21a).[189] Because β-cells can no longer respond to physiologic stimuli, such as eating or exercise, glucose

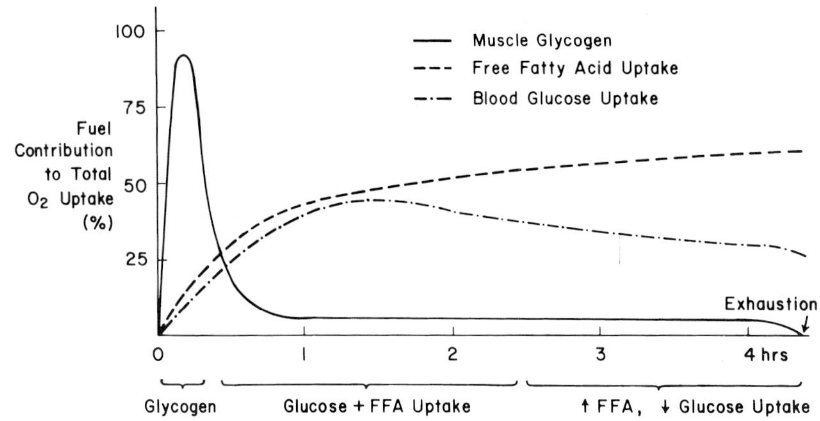

FIGURE 18-15. Pattern of fuel utilization by muscle during exercise of varying duration. During the initial few minutes of exercise, muscle glycogen is a major fuel for the production of ATP. Between 10 and 40 min of exercise, blood-borne glucose and FFA each account for 40 percent of total fuel oxidation. Thereafter (i.e., with very prolonged exercise), there is a progressive rise in the utilization of FFA and lessened uptake of blood glucose. Although muscle glycogen makes only a small contribution to fuel utilization in prolonged exercise, its total depletion is associated with the development of fatigue.

stimulus for glucose utilization (e.g., exercise), such a hormonal pattern results in a rise in blood glucose concentration (*stress hyperglycemia*). This phenomenon involves overproduction as well as underutilization of glucose. It is due to synergistic interaction among the various counterregulatory hormones.[160,161] Thus, although glucagon, epinephrine, or cortisol causes only minor rises in the blood glucose concentration when elevated individually, the effect of a multihormonal response is more than additive (Fig. 18-16). The synergism derives from the fact that while cortisol itself has little effect on glucose production, it converts the transient hepatic effect of glucagon or epinephrine to one of sustained glucose overproduction. In addition, epinephrine, by virtue of its suppressive effects on insulin secretion as well as its antagonism of insulin action, exaggerates the hyperglycemic response by decreasing glucose utilization. If insulin levels are already reduced, as in a diabetic patient, the effect of such a multihormonal response is to intensify the diabetic state.

FIGURE 18-16. The synergistic effects of cortisol (C), glucagon (G), and epinephrine (E) in raising plasma glucose concentration, stimulating glucose production, and reducing glucose clearance. The hyperglycemic response to the triple hormone infusion (C + G + E) is far greater than the additive response to all three hormones given singly or the response to any combination of two hormones given together plus one hormone given singly. The development of "stress" hyperglycemia is a consequence of this hormone synergism, which also includes GH. (*From Eigler et al.*[160])

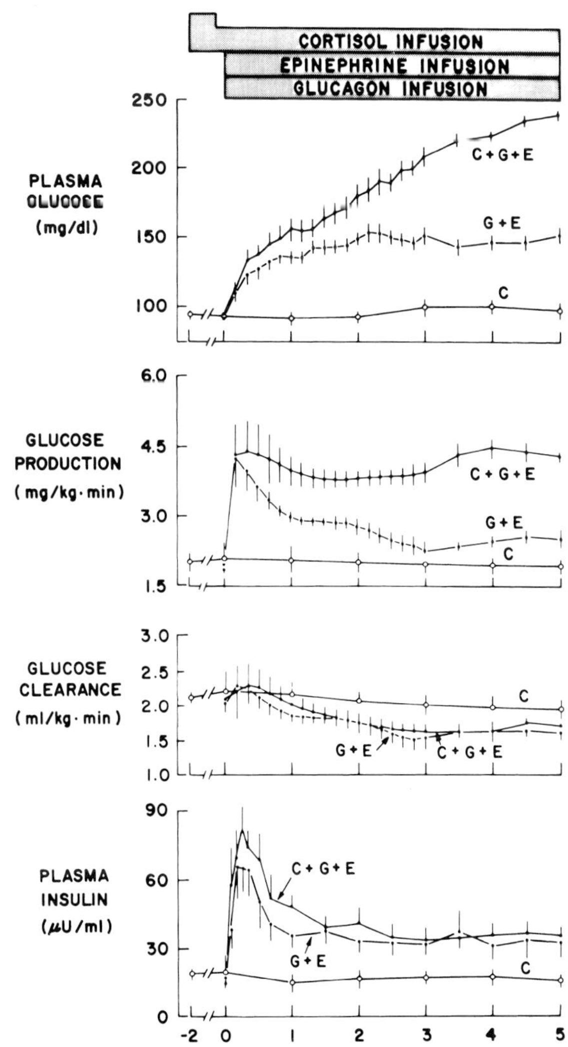

CLINICAL DIABETES

Definition, Classification, and Diagnosis

Definition Diabetes mellitus is a heterogeneous set of disorders characterized by two shared features—disordered metabolism, most notably hyperglycemia, and the propensity to develop specific long-term complications including retinopathy, nephropathy, and neuropathy. The underlying cause of all forms of diabetes is relative or absolute insulin deficiency.

Classification The modern classification of diabetes mellitus continues to evolve with increasing understanding of its epidemiology, pathophysiology, and genetics. The similar classifications promulgated by the National Diabetes Data Group (NDDG)[162] and World Health Organization[163] in 1979 and 1985, respectively, have recently been updated by an Expert Committee of the American Diabetes Association (ADA).[164] All three classifications are remarkably similar except for modest changes in nomenclature, a recent decrease in the diagnostic level for fasting glucose level, and changes in the recommendations for screening.

The major forms of diabetes, the conditions that precede diabetes, and the most recent nomenclature are shown in Table 18-8. The major forms of diabetes include Type 1 (previously called juvenile-onset or insulin-dependent) diabetes mellitus, Type 2

TABLE 18-8. Classification of Diabetes Mellitus*

- **Type 1** diabetes (formerly "insulin-dependent" or "ketosis prone," owing to absolute insulin deficiency with β-cell destruction)
  - Immune-mediated
  - Idiopathic
- **Type 2** diabetes (formerly "noninsulin-dependent," reflecting the presence of endogenous insulin secretion, although as many as 50 percent of Type 2 diabetics will likely require insulin to correct hyperglycemia. Caused by combination of insulin resistance and relative insulin deficiency, insufficient to meet increased demands imposed by resistance. Spectrum of mild to severe resistance and secretory deficits.)
- **Other types**
  - Genetic defects of β-cell function
    - **M**aturity **O**nset **D**iabetes of the **Y**oung (autosomal dominant—relative insulin deficiency)
      - Type 1-Hepatic nuclear transcription factor-4α, chr 20
      - Type 2-Glucokinase mutations, chr 7
      - Type 3-Hepatic nuclear transcription factor-1α, chr 12
      - Type 4-Mutation in Islet promoter factor-1, chr 13
      - Type 5-Hepatic nuclear transcription factor 1β, chr 17
    - Mitochondrial DNA—associated with sensorineural hearing loss, predominantly in Japanese
    - Others
  - Genetic defects in insulin action—mediated by insulin receptor abnormalities
    - Type A insulin resistance—associated with acanthosis nigricans, PCO
    - Leprechaunism—severe growth retardation, death soon after birth
    - Rabson-Mendenhall syndrome
    - Lipoatrophic diabetes—numerous forms with different anatomic patterns of subcutaneous fat atrophy
    - Others
  - Diseases of exocrine pancreas—result in relative or absolute B-cell dysfunction
    - Pancreatectomy
    - Pancreatitis—usually chronic/recurrent
    - Neoplasia
    - Cystic fibrosis
    - Hemochromatosis
    - Fibrocalculous pancreatitis
    - Other infiltrative/inflammatory disorders
  - Endocrinopathies—increase insulin resistance, decrease insulin secretion, or both
    - Predominantly worsen resistance
      - Acromegaly
      - Cushing's syndrome
      - Glucagonoma
      - Hyperthyroidism
    - Predominantly decrease secretion
      - Somatostatinoma—decreased insulin secretion
      - Aldosteronoma—decreased insulin secretion probably mediated by hypokalemia
    - Effects resistance and secretion
      - Pheochromocytoma
  - Drug- or chemical-induced
    - Predominantly increase resistance
      - Glucocorticoids
      - Thyroid hormone
    - Predominantly decrease secretion
      - Vacor—rodenticide toxic to islets
      - Pentamidine
      - Cyclosporin
      - Nicotinic acid
      - Diazoxide
      - B-adrenergic blockers
      - Thiazides—may be mediated by hypokalemia
      - Dilantin
      - α-interferon
      - Others
  - Infections—β-cell inflammation/destruction
    - Congenital rubella
    - Mumps
    - CMV
    - Coxsackie
  - Other autoimmune forms
    - "Stiff man" syndrome
    - Anti-insulin receptor antibodies (Type B insulin resistance)
    - Other
- **Gestational diabetes**—defined as diabetes with onset during pregnancy. Usually remits after delivery, only to return usually as Type 2 diabetes in approximately 50 percent of women who had GDM

* Adapted from Expert Committee report.[164]

(previously known as adult-onset or non-insulin–dependent) diabetes mellitus, gestational diabetes mellitus (GDM), and other types. Other types include diabetes secondary to other well-recognized diseases that affect pancreatic function and inherited and other diseases associated with the development of diabetes. The conditions that most often precede Type 2 diabetes and screening recommendations have been classified based on glucose levels and include impaired glucose tolerance (IGT) and impaired fasting glucose (IFG), with the latter group first defined in the 1997 classification (Tables 18-9 and 18-10).[164]

The separation of the clinical forms of diabetes is based predominantly on differences in clinical presentation and pathophysiology. The most recent classification also incorporates new genetic insights. To date, only a small fraction (<5 percent) of all cases of diabetes have had a clear genetic basis identified. As the genetic basis for more forms of diabetes is elucidated, the classification of diabetes will inevitably change.

Type 1 Diabetes

The major phenotypic characteristic of Type 1 diabetes is absolute insulin deficiency, leading to unregulated carbohydrate and fat metabolism with hyperglycemia and ketoacidosis in the untreated state. The most common cause of Type 1 diabetes is autoimmune destruction of the insulin-producing beta cells. Evidence supporting the autoimmune pathogenesis of Type 1 diabetes includes: the association with HLA-haplotypes related to immune function; the presence of lymphocytic (T-cell) "insulitis" in pancreatic specimens; the presence of a variety of autoantibodies against the islet cell and islet cell constituents prior to the development of clinical diabetes; and the common cooccurrence of other diseases of autoimmune etiology. Other causes of beta cell destruction, such as viral infections, have been identified, but are not likely causes of most cases of Type 1 diabetes. Although absolute insulin deficiency and its clinical and metabolic consequences are the sine qua non of established Type 1 diabetes, its preclinical and early clinical course often includes a period of variable duration when a small fraction of beta cells continues to function. This period, commonly termed the "honeymoon" after diagnosis, is characterized by metabolic stability with little or no requirement for exogenous insulin. Insulin is not necessary to prevent ketoacidosis and sustain life during this period. However, virtually all patients with Type 1 diabetes eventually develop absolute insulin defi-

TABLE 18-9. Recommendations for Screening for Diabetes Mellitus*

Nonpregnant, asymptomatic adults
Fasting (after 8 hr fast) plasma glucose preferred to oral glucose tolerance test
Screen all adults 45 years and older at least every three years
Nonpregnant, asymptomatic adults with any of the following to be tested at earlier age and/or more frequently:
Obesity (BMI $\geq$ 27 kg/m^2)
First-degree family history of diabetes
High-risk ethnic/racial group
Previous baby > 9 lb
Previous history of GDM
Hypertensive
HDL $\leq$ 35 or triglyceride $\geq$ 250 mg/dL
IGT or IFG on previous testing
Pregnant women†
50 gram OGTT (fasting unnecessary) with 1 hr result at 24–28 weeks of gestation (if prior GDM, test earlier in pregnancy)
If preliminary screen positive, 100 gm, 3 hr OGTT

*Adapted from Expert Committee Report.[164]

†May not be necessary in women at low risk, i.e., age < 25, nonobese, no prior history of GDM, negative first-degree family history, and not a member of a high-risk group.

TABLE 18-10. Diagnostic Criteria

	Test	Plasma Glucose Value (mg/dL)
Diabetes	Fasting glucose*	≥126
	2 h after 75 gm OGTT* or	≥200
	Casual glucose in setting of symptoms of diabetes	
Gestational Diabetes Mellitus (GDM)		
Screening (1 hour after 50 gm OGTT)		≥140
Diagnostic† (100 gm OGTT)		
Fasting		≥105
1-hour		≥190
2-hour		≥165
3-hour		≥145
Impaired Glucose Tolerance (IGT)		
Fasting		<126
and 2 h after 75 gm OGTT*		140–200
Impaired Fasting Glucose (IFG)		
Fasting*		110–125

*Must be confirmed with repeat testing.

†At least two abnormal results required.

ciency and, if not treated with insulin, develop hyperglycemia with the attendant consequences of osmotic diuresis, loss of body mass owing to a catabolic state, and ketoacidosis secondary to unrestrained lipolysis and ketogenesis.

Epidemiology

Although the classifications of the last 20 years have avoided the age criteria formerly imputed by the juvenile-onset vs. adult or maturity-onset terminology, Type 1 diabetes is generally a disease with onset during childhood or adolescence with the majority of cases appearing before age 20 (peak onset is around time of puberty). A relatively small percentage (< 10 percent) of Type 1 diabetes may have its onset after age 50. Such patients are thin, ketosis-prone, and share genetic and immunologic markers with more typical Type 1 diabetes patients who have onset in youth.[165] Patients who develop Type 1 diabetes in the setting of autoimmune polyendocrinopathy (polyglandular autoimmune syndrome Type II) typically have an older age onset.[166] Finally, a group of diabetics who have been called Type 1 & 1/2 or latent autoimmune diabetes in adults (LADA)[167] may represent slowly progressive autoimmune disease. Despite their older age at onset, such patients are usually thin—or at least thinner than Type 2 diabetics—and have serologic markers of autoimmunity, and ultimately require insulin to manage their hyperglycemia.

Type 1 diabetes has its highest prevalence in Northern Europe and in populations of Northern European descent[168] (Fig. 18-17). Several "hot spots" for Type 1 diabetes, for example in Finland and Sardinia, have been investigated. The prevalence in Asian and African populations has been said to be lower, although there is a dearth of good epidemiologic data. The overall prevalence of Type 1 diabetes in the US is approximately 0.5 percent, with a total population of 750,000 to 1 million.[169]

Pathoetiology

The autoimmune, inherited basis of Type 1 diabetes has been advanced by studies in human diabetes and in animal models, especially in the non-obese Diabetic (NOD) mouse.[165,170] Identical twin studies have demonstrated a concordance rate of approximately 50 percent, strongly supporting a genetic basis of Type 1 diabetes with superimposed environmental factors that affect its occurrence (Table 18-11).[171] Children of a father with Type 1 diabetes have a 10- to 12-fold risk (5–6 percent lifetime risk) of developing Type 1 diabetes compared with children of nondiabetic parents. Children of a mother with Type 1 diabetes have a lower risk compared with children of Type 1 diabetic fathers (6- to 8-fold risk compared with children of nondiabetic parents or 2–4 percent lifetime risk), for unclear reasons, but probably not related to fetal loss in utero.[172] The role of environmental factors has been strongly implicated on the basis of the 50 percent concordance rate in identical twins; however, specific environmental factors have not been clearly identified. The role of breast-feeding and exposure to cows milk,[173] effect of immunizations, such as with BCG,[174] viral infections,[175] and a variety of other factors have been vigorously debated; however, no single or combination of environmental factors has been firmly established in the development of Type 1 diabetes. Viral infections with Coxsackie B strains have been shown to cause diabetes in several well documented cases.[176] However, they have been very atypical, with onset during infancy and death related to overwhelming viremia. Viruses may play a precipitating, or triggering, role in the pathogenesis of Type 1 diabetes, perhaps by initiating an autoimmune reaction in genetically susceptible individuals, but are an unlikely primary cause.

Genes Although specific genes have not been identified, several loci have been shown to be associated with Type 1 diabetes. The earliest observations noted an association of Type 1 diabetes with histocompatability genes on the short arm of chromosome 6.[177] The histocompatability genes closest to the centromere encode the MHC class II molecules, DR, DQ, and DP, while those farther away encode Class I molecules A, B, and C (Fig. 18-18). Although the first associations between genetic markers and Type 1 diabetes were between allelic Class I molecules B8 and B15, sub-

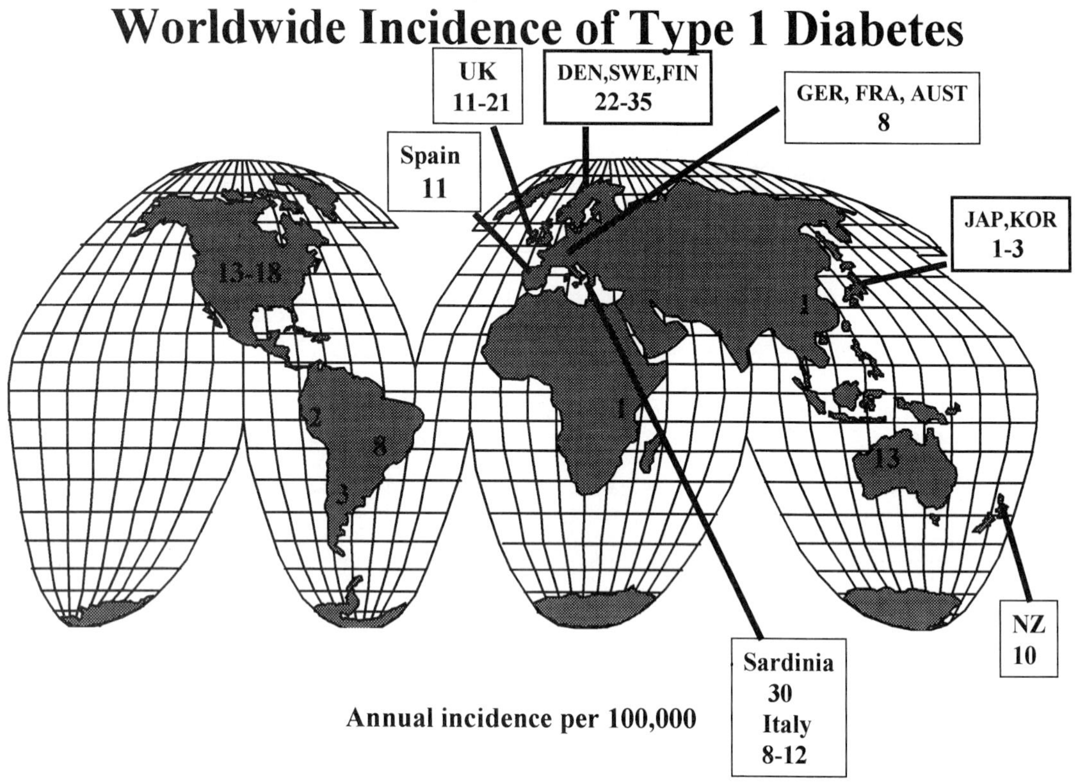

FIGURE 18-17. Incidence of Type 1 diabetes in different parts of the world. Annual incidence per 100,000. By comparison, incidence of Type 2 diabetes in the U.S. is 250 per 100,000 per year. (*Data from Kitigawa et al.*[168] *and LaPorte R et al.*[169])

sequent studies have established Class II molecules (in linkage dysequilibrium with the Class I alleles) as more reliable predictors of Type 1 diabetes. The presence of HLA DR3 and/or DR4 was noted in > 90 percent of Type 1 diabetics, compared to 40 percent of controls.[178] The relative risk for developing Type 1 diabetes associated with some combinations of DR3/DR4 was 10- to 20-fold. More specific serotyping revealed an even stronger association with the DQβ-chain. The presence of a noncharged amino acid, such as valine or serine, at position 57 increased the risk of Type 1 diabetes by as much as 50-fold, while the presence of aspartate appeared to be protective.[179] Analogous associations with histocompatability genes in the NOD mouse reinforced the importance of these associations.[180]

The appeal of these observations rested on the recognized function of the MHC Class II molecules in the immune system, the demonstration of similar associations in other autoimmune diseases, and analogous findings in the NOD animal model of autoimmune diabetes. Although associations with MHC Class I molecules (which appear to be more involved with recognition and processing of endogenous antigens, compared with MHC Class II, which are involved in processing exogenous antigens) have been postulated,[181] the majority of the observations support MHC Class II as being involved in the pathogenesis of Type 1 diabetes. How these alleles specifically affect the autoimmune process is not clear.

Other genetic loci have been identified through genomic screening to be associated with Type 1 diabetes. In addition to the locus on chromosome 6 associated with MHC class II ("IDDM1"), loci on chromosome 11p15 (the insulin coding region, "IDDM2"), 11q, and others have been identified.[182] Many of

TABLE 18-11. Risk of Developing Type 1 and Type 2 Diabetes Based on Family History*

	Monozygotic Twin†	*Family Member Affected*					General Population
		Sibling	Mother	Father	Both Parents	Any 1° Relative	
Risk of developing (percent):							
Type 1@	50	5	2–4	6	10–12	5	0.5
Type 2‡	95	15–20	10–12	8–10	18–20	8–12	6–7

* Risk is an estimate of life-time occurrence for the U.S. population.

† From ref. 171.

† Based on data from ref. 171 and 172.

‡ Based predominantly on national survey calculations (*National Health Interview Survey, 1989, and National Health and Nutrition Examination Survey, 1976–80*).

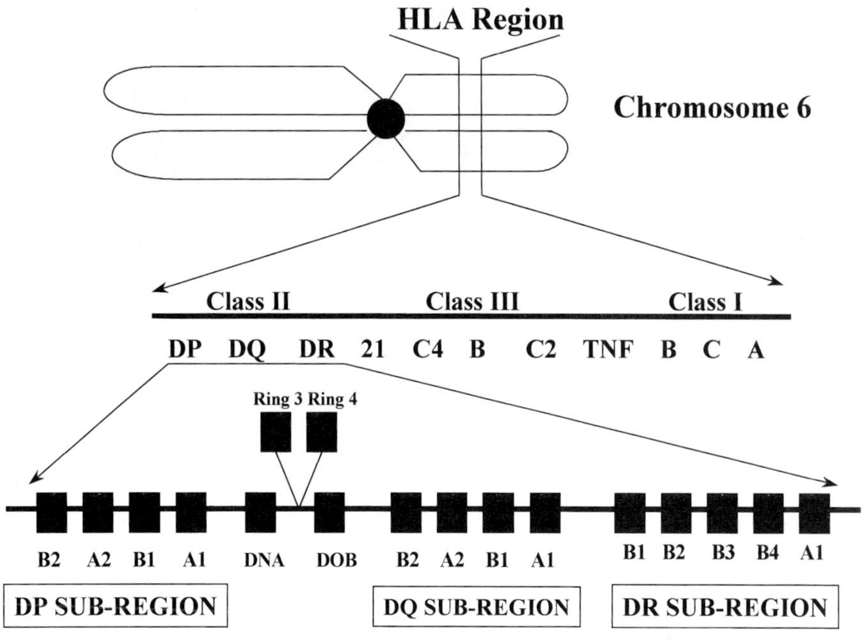

FIGURE 18-18. Human histocompatability loci on chromosome 6. The areas most closely associated with risk for developing Type 1 diabetes include DR3, DR4, and DQβ. (*From Trucco.*[179])

these are weakly linked and their protein products have not been identified. To date, no genetic loci have been identified that have as large an association with Type 1 diabetes as IDDM1. Polygenic inheritance is most likely.

Autoimmunity The autoimmune process that leads to the development of Type 1 diabetes appears to occur over many years prior to demonstrable abnormalities in insulin secretion or the clinical appearance of glucose abnormalities and diabetes. The timeline proposed by Eisenbarth has been popularly accepted (Fig. 18-19).[170] Those children who develop Type 1 diabetes early in life presumably have a more aggressive destruction of their beta cells, while those who develop their diabetes in later life either have a more attenuated destruction of the beta cells and/or the process is initiated later. Markers of autoimmune destruction have been observed for as long as 10–15 years prior to the development of diabetes.[170]

Current understanding of the pathogenesis suggests that some as yet to be identified constituent of the beta cell is identified by the immune system as foreign and is destroyed through a T-cell–mediated attack. "Insulitis" with T-cell infiltration of the beta cells has been observed in most of the cases of recent onset diabetes where pancreatic tissue was available for examination (Fig. 18-20, [Color Plate 1]).[183,184] A shift of T lymphocytes from TH1 to TH2 accompanies the development of Type 1, autoimmune diabetes. The development of antibodies to the islet cell or

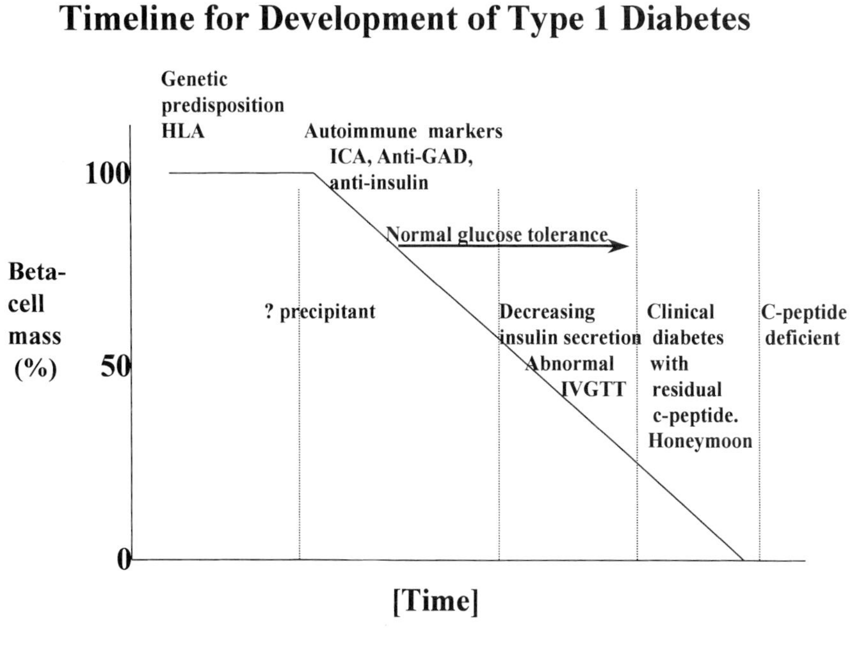

FIGURE 18-19. Timeline for development of Type 2 diabetes. A preclinical phase during which autoimmune destruction of the insulin secreting β-cells occurs may precede the development of clinical diabetes by as much as 10 years. Increased glycemia doesn't occur until more than 80 percent of the β-cells have been destroyed. (*Adapted from Eisenbarth.*[170])

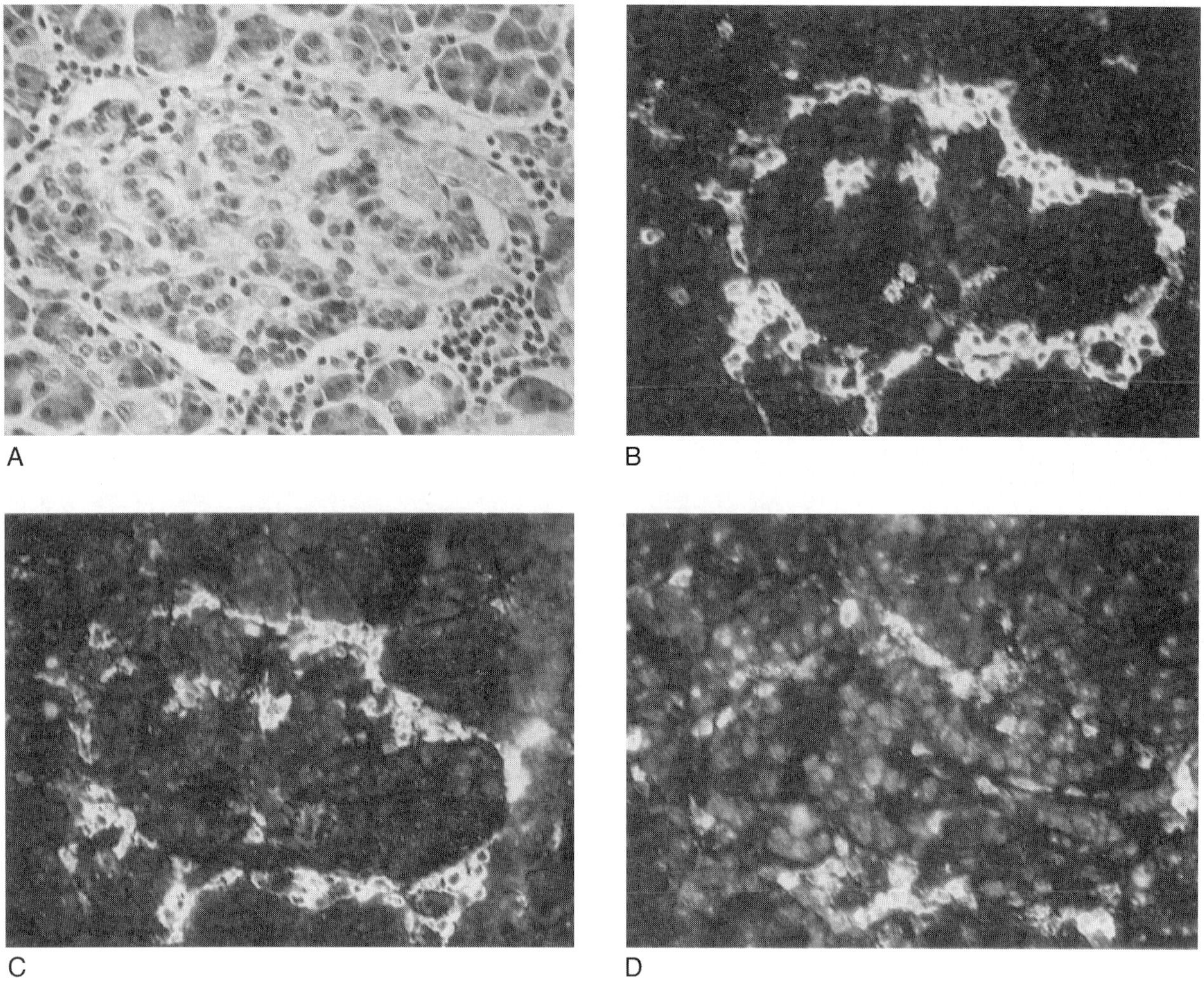

FIGURE 18-20. T-lymphocyte invasion of β-cells in a 12-year-old girl with recently diagnosed diabetes. In panel (*a*), hematoxylin and eosin staining shows lymphocyte infiltration. Panel (*b*) shows all types of leukocytes with a monoclonal antibody and fluourescence. Panel (*c*) specifically stains for T8, presumably cytotoxic, lymphocytes while panel (*d*) indicates activated T-cells staining for interleukin-2 receptor lymphocytes. (*From Bottazzo et al.*[184])

more specific antigens, such as ICA 512 (IA2), which is a tyrosine phosphatase, or glutamic acid decarboxylase (GAD), and/or insulin is generally considered to be an epiphenomenon, rather than the cause of beta cell destruction. Although some antibodies have been suggested to impair β-cell function,[185] anti-islet cell antibodies generally don't fix complement and passive transfer of diabetes has not been accomplished. The presence of these markers is useful in identifying siblings or children of Type 1 diabetics, and even persons in the general population, who are at heightened risk for developing diabetes.[170,186]

In addition to the autoimmune destruction of the beta cell, roles for oxidation, apoptosis, decreased β-cell regeneration, and other factors that may make the beta cell population more vulnerable to destruction have been proposed in the pathogenesis of Type 1 diabetes.

Clinical Presentation

Characteristically, Type 1 diabetes has a clinically acute onset with symptoms secondary to hyperglycemia and the attendant osmotic diuresis, including polyuria, nocturia, increased thirst, and polydipsia. Unregulated metabolism results in weight loss, initially from dehydration with osmotic diuresis, then from fat loss, and eventually from protein loss with loss of muscle mass. Although appetite is often increased in the early stages, development of ketosis results in nausea and vomiting. Other presenting symptoms of diabetes include the consequences of acute fluctuations in glucose level, such as blurred vision secondary to osmotic swelling of the lens with changes in its refractive properties. Other less specific symptoms, such as vaginitis or balanitis with recurrent or intractable yeast infections, occur owing to high tissue glucose levels, which provide a hospitable environment for yeast overgrowth.[187] With the onset of ketosis, acute gastrointestinal symptoms including abdominal pain, anorexia, nausea, and vomiting supervene. As many as 20 percent of patients with Type 1 diabetes present in diabetic ketoacidosis.[188] Indigent or underserved populations may have a higher rate of ketoacidosis as the presenting sign of Type 1 diabetes.

The absolute insulin deficiency that characterizes established Type 1 diabetes results in labile glucose levels unless physiologic levels of insulin are restored by frequent administration of exogenous insulin (Fig. 18-21a).[189] Because β-cells can no longer respond to physiologic stimuli, such as eating or exercise, glucose

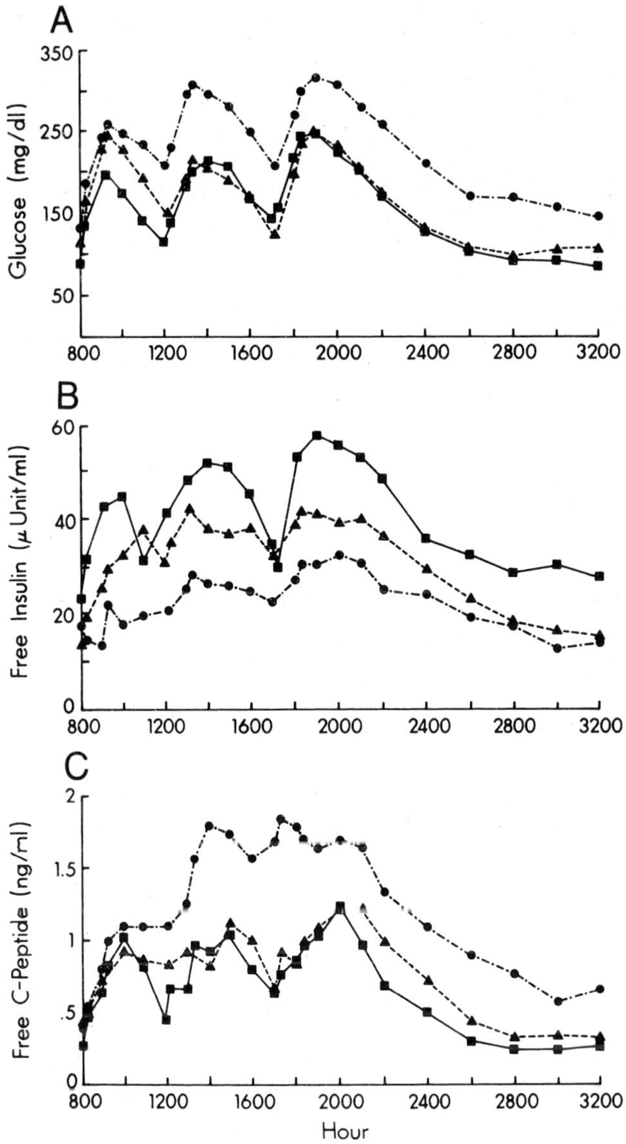

FIGURE 18-21. Blood glucose profiles obtained with frequent monitoring in a regimented inpatient setting for (*a*) Type 1 diabetes (*From Molnar et al. Diabetes 14:279–88, 1965*) and (*b*) Type 2 diabetes (5 Type 2 diabetic patients treated with ultralente or lente insulin Δ once per day, or with an implantable pump and continuous intravenous regular insulin □. (*From Blackshear et al.*[384]) Glucose levels with nonphysiologic insulin delivery (twice per-day intermediate-acting insulin) are chaotic in Type 1 diabetes. In Type 2 diabetes, the endogenous secretion of insulin, measured as c-peptide in panel (*c*), prevents the labile glucose excursions commonly seen in Type 1 diabetes.

levels are totally dependent on administered insulin and are subject to the vicissitudes of erratic absorption of insulin, changing meal content and absorption of carbohydrate, variable activity levels, and numerous other factors. The end result is a frequent mismatch of insulin requirements and insulin delivery and labile glucose levels. Glucose levels are not as labile in Type 2 diabetes (Fig. 18-21b) where endogenous insulin levels suppress post-prandial glucose levels (Fig. 18-21c).

The poor wound healing popularly ascribed to diabetes is rarely seen as a presenting sign or symptom in modern times. This historic feature of diabetes was probably related to delayed diagnosis and the profound cachexia that often occurred in the pre-insulin era. Complications of diabetes, such as retinopathy, neuropathy, and nephropathy, are a consequence of long-term (>5 years) exposure to diabetes and hyperglycemia and are rarely seen at the time of diagnosis of Type 1 diabetes.[190]

Type 2 Diabetes Mellitus

Type 2 diabetes is by far the most common form of diabetes in all parts of the world. Although classification according to age of onset is no longer used because of the considerable overlap between Type 1 and Type 2 diabetes, most persons developing Type 2 diabetes are adults, and usually beyond their fourth decade of life. The major characteristic that differentiates Type 2 from Type 1 diabetes is relative vs. absolute insulin deficiency. In Type 2 diabetes, a functional β-cell defect results in relative insulin deficiency, which is incapable of meeting the heightened demand for insulin imposed by insulin resistance. Several studies have suggested a relative deficiency of β-cells in Type 2 diabetes.[191,192] The hierarchy of tissue and enzyme sensitivity to insulin effects results in hyperglycemia (with identical clinical consequences as in Type 1 diabetes), but generally an absence of unrestrained lipolysis and ketogenesis. The preserved insulin secretion in Type 2 diabetes, albeit decreased, is sufficient to suppress ketogenesis in most circumstances. Although the majority of Type 2 diabetics will eventually require insulin therapy to control glucose levels acceptably, they don't require exogenous insulin to prevent ketoacidosis and death, as is the case for Type 1 diabetes.

Type 2 diabetes has a strong genetic basis, which is probably polygenic; however, it is not associated with the same genetic loci as Type 1 diabetes. No associations with specific HLA haplotypes have been identified. Moreover, the strong evidence for autoimmunity in Type 1 diabetes is absent in Type 2 diabetes. Whereas more than 90 percent of Type 1 diabetic patients have one or a combination of autoantibodies present at the time of diagnosis,[170] less than 5 percent of the Type 2 population has such antibodies. Several studies have shown a higher (10 percent) prevalence of autoantibodies present in patients with phenotypic Type 2 diabetes, but these studies have generally been in Northern European populations with a higher prevalence of Type 1 diabetes.[193] Presumably these populations contain an admixture of Type 1 diabetic patients or may have serologic markers of autoimmunity coincident with, but unrelated to, the development of Type 2 diabetes. Of note, the presence of more than one autoantibody, which is most predictive of Type 1 diabetes, is very unusual in phenotypic Type 2 diabetic populations. In addition, the percent of patients with phenotypic Type 2 diabetes who are ICA- or GAD-positive decreases with the age of the population.

Epidemiology

The majority of Type 2 diabetes occurs after age 40, with more than 50 percent of cases developing in patients older than age 55.[194] From an epidemiologic point of view, Type 2 diabetes is more problematic than Type 1 because it has a more insidious onset than Type 1 diabetes, often going undetected either because symptoms are unrecognized or are ignored. In addition, early in the course of Type 2 diabetes increasing blood glucose levels are often in a range not associated with osmotic diuresis. In the aggregate, this results in diagnosis of Type 2 diabetes being delayed for an estimated 4–7 years after it actually develops.[195] A relatively small percentage of Type 2 diabetic patients develop diabetes in

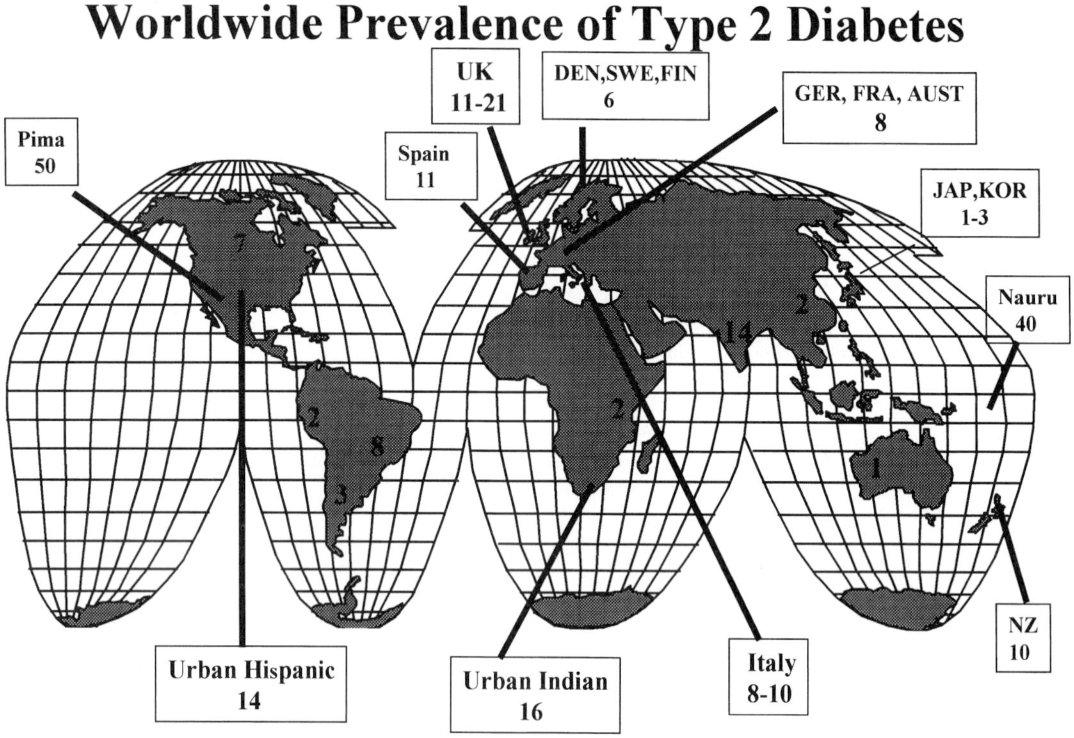

FIGURE 18-22. Prevalence of Type 2 diabetes in different parts of the world in populations aged 30–64. (*Based on data from King et al.* [194])

their twenties and thirties. Such patients are often very obese, the offspring of two parents with Type 2 diabetes, or members of an ethnic or racial group with a particularly high prevalence of Type 2 diabetes. The highest prevalence of Type 2 diabetes has been found in the Pima Indians of the Gila River reservation in Arizona (Fig. 18-22).[196] Similarly high rates of diabetes have developed in the micronesian island population of Nauru.[197] Of note, Pima Indians who live in Mexico, farming and living at a subsistence level, have not developed obesity or diabetes. Similarly, the development of diabetes in the native Nauruan population didn't occur until the mining of guano changed their life-style from subsistence fishing and farming to a more sedentary westernized life-style with motorbikes, a high-fat diet, and the development of obesity. These same factors (obesity, high-fat diets, sedentary life-style) have played a role in the development of Type 2 diabetes worldwide, although not with the exaggerated effect seen in these very high-risk populations. Other populations in the US that have been documented to have a particularly high risk for developing Type 2 diabetes include Hispanic Americans, African Americans, and Asian Americans.[198] These populations are at 1.5- to 2.2-fold risk to develop diabetes compared to the general population (Fig. 18-23). The study of Japanese who have emigrated to Hawaii or the US has been particularly instructive[199]and reflects the same phenomenon as seen in the American Indians and Nauruans.

In addition to ethnic and racial factors, the following risk factors for the development of Type 2 diabetes have been identified. Age is a major determinant, with more than 50 percent of the Type 2 population diagnosed in their fifth decade and risk increasing with every decade (Fig. 18-23).[194,200] Overweight and obesity have been recognized for centuries as risk factors.[201–203] Risk for developing Type 2 diabetes begins to increase at almost any level above ideal body weight, but escalates most rapidly with body mass levels considered to be obese (i.e., > 20 percent over ideal) (Fig. 18-24). More recently, the distribution of body fat has been shown to be an important risk factor.[204–206] Body habitus described as "android"—as opposed to "gynoid" [204]—with a waist-to-hip ratio greater than 0.8 in men and 0.9 in women, has been associated with an increased risk for developing diabetes at all levels of obesity. Most[207–209] studies utilizing CT or MRI scanning that directly measure intraabdominal—also called visceral or mesenteric—fat, compared with subcutaneous fat, have documented that intra-abdominal fat, rather than abdominal subcutaneous fat, appears to be the mediator of hyperinsulinemia, and an increased risk for developing Type 2 diabetes and cardiovascular disease. The role that visceral fat may play in the pathogenesis of Type 2 diabetes may be mediated by its predisposition to catecholamine-induced lipolysis[210,211] with direct delivery of fatty acids to the liver and pancreas.[212] Expensive measurements of intra-abdominal fat are not necessary for epidemiologic studies or assessment of clinical risk, as simple measurements of waist-to-hip ratio or waist circumference provide comparable information for calculating risk.[213] Epidemiologic studies have also suggested that weight status early in life may contribute to the risk of developing Type 2 diabetes.[214]

Other established risk factors include sedentary life-style [215,216] and poor cardiorespiratory fitness[217] independent of body mass, history of gestational diabetes[218] (see later discussion), and maternal nutritional status, including that leading to low birth weight.[219,220] Type 2 diabetes is also a heritable disease and positive family history is a well-recognized risk factor.[221,222] The concordance rate among identical-monozygotic twins approaches 100 percent.[171] Having one diabetic parent results in a 1.5- to 2-fold

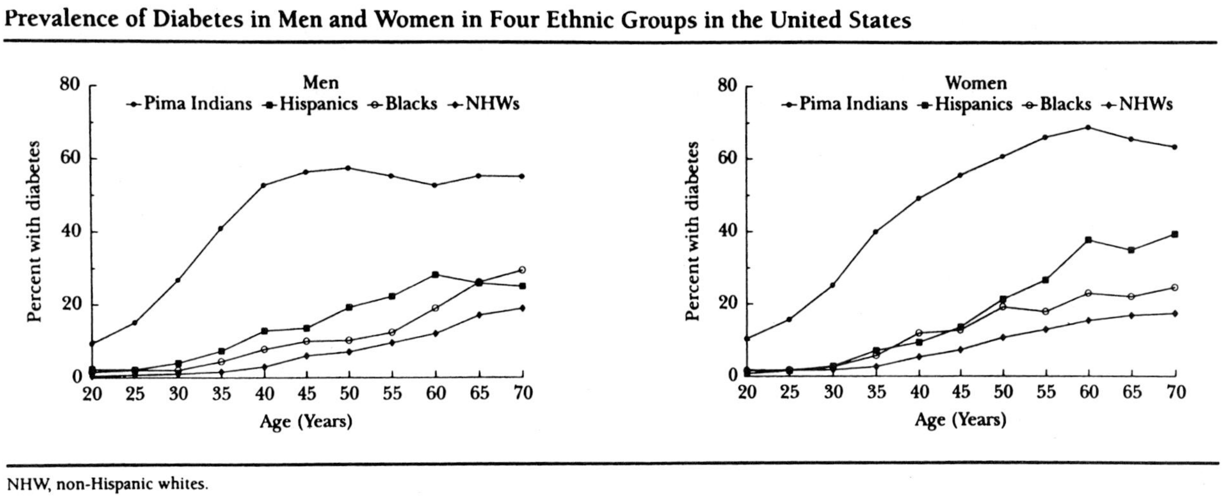

FIGURE 18-23. Risk of developing Type 2 diabetes in different ethnic/racial groups in the U.S. according to age and gender. (*From King et al.*[194])

risk; two parents with Type 2 diabetes results in a 4-fold increased risk compared with persons without diabetic parents (Table 18-11). The risk imparted by a positive family history of diabetes may be genetic in origin, a function of shared environment, or both.

Screening

Current recommendations to screen the adult population with fasting glucose levels on a regular basis[164] (Table 18-9) are predicated on the observation that almost one-half of Type 2 diabetes goes undiagnosed. To the extent that screening programs are routinely implemented, the proportion of Type 2 diabetes that goes undiagnosed will decrease. The performance of the oral glucose tolerance test (OGTT) compared with fasting glucose level and glycosylated hemoglobin level for screening purposes has been analyzed extensively.[223,224] Although the OGTT remains more sensitive than fasting glucose, the greater ease of performing repeated fasting glucose tests has been suggested to outweigh the increased sensitivity of repeated OGTTs. HbA1c testing performs well if appropriate cut-offs are selected[223,224]; moreover, a measure of chronic glycemia is probably more biologically relevant with regard to glycemic exposure and risk of long-term complications. Unfortunately, the absence of standardization of the assay has prevented it from being recommended as a routine screening tool. The current efforts to standardize glycohemoglobin assays to a DCCT standard may make it more feasible to use glycohemoglobin testing for screening and diagnosis in the future.

FIGURE 18-24. Incidence of Type 2 diabetes (per 1,000 person-years) for different racial/ethnic groups based on body mass index. (*From Edelstein et al.*[198])

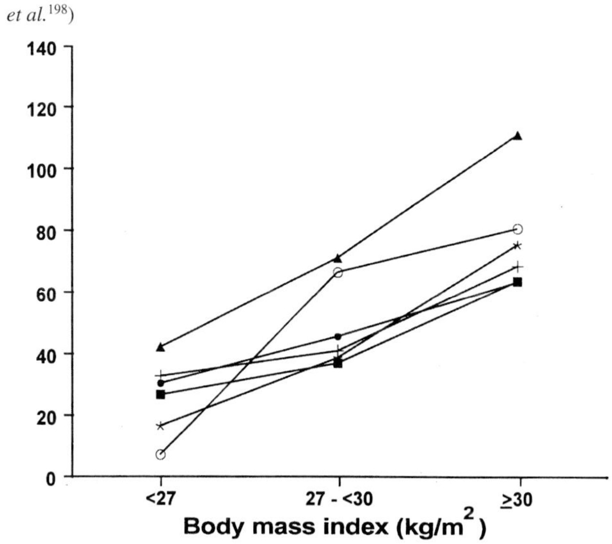

Pathoetiology

Type 2 diabetes has an inherited basis, but is not associated with the HLA markers or markers of autoimmunity that are present in Type 1 diabetes. The most widely accepted theory of the pathogenesis for Type 2 diabetes includes a combination of insulin resistance compounded by deficient insulin secretion (Fig. 18-25).[225,226] Insulin resistance, simply expressed as reduced sensitivity to the effects of insulin, is the most common underlying abnormality in Type 2 diabetes. Insulin resistance may be inherited or acquired as a result of obesity, aging, medications, or specific endocrinopathies such as acromegaly or Cushing's syndrome. Although hyperinsulinemic euglycemic clamps were originally used to establish insulin resistance,[227] simpler tests, or even the level of fasting or postchallenge insulin, have been used to establish insulin resistance.[228] In hyperinsulinemic euglycemic clamp studies, insulin is infused to achieve high physiologic or supraphysiologic levels and sufficient glucose is simultaneously infused to "clamp" the glucose concentration at normal levels. The amount of glucose infused (the M value) is an index of the sensitivity to insulin (Fig. 18-26).

Insulin resistance is a ubiquitous condition, affecting as much as 30 percent of the adult U.S. population.[229] It is associated with a constellation of other cardiovascular risk factors including obesity, hypertension, dyslipidemia (most commonly elevated triglycerides and reduced HDL concentrations), hyperuricemia, and other factors (increased plasminogen activator inhibitor, fibrinogen, and inflammatory factors or markers such as C-reactive

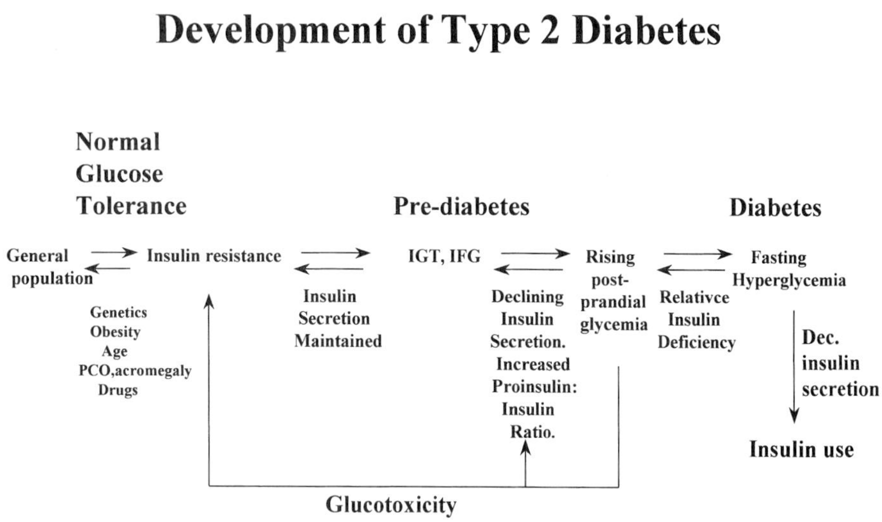

FIGURE 18-25. Pathophysiology of Type 2 diabetes.

protein) that increase thrombosis, decrease fibrinolysis, and may worsen cardiovascular risk.[229–232] The original concept of insulin resistance and its coexistent conditions—termed syndrome X by Reaven and including obesity, hypertension, increased triglycerides and decreased HDL cholesterol concentration, and glucose intolerance—visualized insulin resistance at the center of the complex.[230] More recent studies have suggested that there may be several distinct domains that overlap. These domains include: a "central metabolic syndrome" including hyperinsulinemia, increased body mass, central obesity, increased triglyceride and decreased HDL-cholesterol levels; an impaired glucose tolerance domain including glucose intolerance and hyperinsulinemia; and a hypertension domain with systolic and diastolic hypertension and increased body mass (Fig. 18-27).[229]

FIGURE 18-26. Hyperinsulinemic-euglycemic clamp. Insulin is infused to maintain a steady state level (100 uU/ml in this study) and glucose is infused at a rate sufficient to maintain glucose levels in the normal range (here 90 mg/dL). The amount of glucose infused to maintain a normal glucose level (the "M" value) is an index of insulin sensitivity. All values are mean ± SE. (*From DeFronzo RA, Tobin JD, and Andres R.*[227])

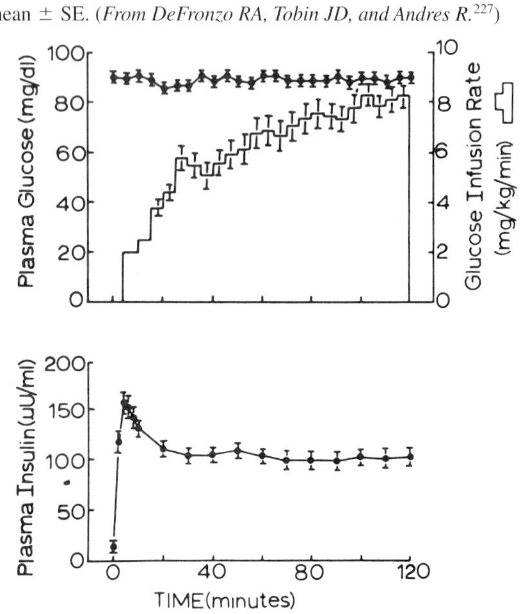

The majority of patients with obesity and insulin resistance do not develop Type 2 diabetes. The critical factor that appears to determine which at-risk patients go on to develop diabetes (estimated at 20–80 percent, depending on the underlying prevalence of Type 2 diabetes in the population) is whether increased insulin secretion, which is necessary to maintain normal metabolism in the face of insulin resistance, is sustained.[191,233,234] During the development of glucose intolerance, insulin secretion and levels increase progressively. Those persons who go on to develop Type 2 diabetes are unable to maintain the high rate of insulin secretion (Fig. 18-28a). Moreover, their ratio of proinsulin to insulin increases, presumably secondary to the release of immature insulin granules coincident with increased demand on the beta cell, resulting in decreased insulin bioactivity (Fig. 18-28b).[235] Glucose intolerance worsens progressively until frank diabetes develops. The abnormal insulin secretory capacity continues to worsen over the course of diabetes.[236] The abnormality in beta cell function is quite specific to glucose, as responsiveness to other insulin secretagogues is often preserved.[237] In addition, increased glucose levels can further worsen beta cell responsiveness to glucose, so called glucotoxicity.[191] Decreased insulin secretion in the setting of hyperglycemia may be secondary to glucose-induced changes in transcription factors or glucose transport.[238] This generic effect of hyperglycemia is partially reversible. Reduction of glucose levels results in restoration of insulin secretion, although not to normal levels.[239–242]

Genetics

The origin of this double defect (insulin resistance and insulin secretory failure) is not well understood. Insulin resistance appears to segregate in families and is probably heritable.[243] Family studies of nondiabetic children of two parents with Type 2 diabetes have demonstrated the occurrence of insulin resistance in the children years before any defects in glucose metabolism are demonstrable.[244] To date, despite an ever-increasing number of candidate genes related to insulin resistance, insulin secretion, and insulin action, and genomic approaches,[222,245,246] only a small fraction of the phenotypic Type 2 diabetic population has been

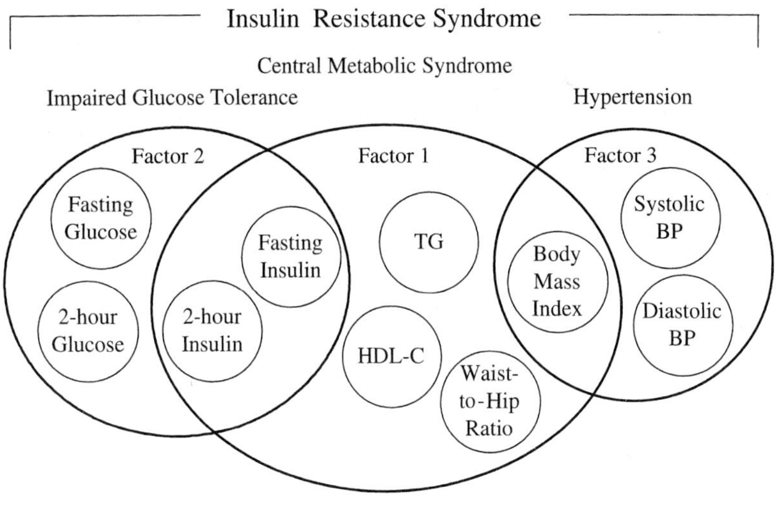

FIGURE 18-27. Three overlapping domains of insulin resistance. (*From Meigs, et al.*[229])

successfully genotyped. Although polymorphisms in the flanking region of the insulin gene, mutations in the insulin receptor gene, polymorphisms in glycogen synthase, sequence variations in the sulfonylurea receptor, and a host of other potential genetic causes of Type 2 diabetes have been identified, none of them appears to explain Type 2 diabetes.[247–252] A recent study has identified a relatively common polymorphism in PPAR-α as contributing to risk for Type 2 diabetes.[253] Animal models utilizing genetic manipulation have not uniformly provided support for simple genetic explanations of Type 2 diabetes. For example, knockout models of insulin receptor substrate 1 (IRS-1) or the glucokinase gene do not result in diabetes.[102,103] On the other hand, a knockout of IRS-2 [105] and a double knockout that resulted in disruption of IRS-1 and the β-cell glucokinase genes in mice caused metabolic abnormalities similar to those found in human Type 2 diabetes.[104]

Not surprisingly, the autosomal dominant form of diabetes known as maturity onset diabetes of youth (MODY) was the first form of Type 2 diabetes to surrender its genetic secret.[254–258] The genes that give rise to this rare form of diabetes are related to insulin secretion. Mutations in the gene that encodes glucokinase, which serves as the glucose sensor of the β-cell, results in one form of MODY, MODY 2, while abnormalities in hepatic nuclear transcription factors 4α, 1α, and 1β cause MODY 1, 3, and 5, respectively. MODY 4 is linked to a mutation in Islet promoter factor-1. Insulin secretory abnormalities in non-MODY Type 2 diabetes may also be inherited. Normoglycemic first degree relatives of patients with Type 2 diabetes have been shown to have abnormalities in phasic insulin secretion.[259,260]

It is highly likely that Type 2 diabetes is heterogeneous and polygenic in origin with a large contribution from acquired, envi-

FIGURE 18-28. Association of (*a*) decreasing insulin secretory capacity with rising glycemia (*From Brunzell et al.*[233]) and (*b*) increasing proinsulin:insulin ratio in the setting of evolving Type 2 diabetes (*From Yoshioka et al.*[235]). In the cross-sectional study in (*a*), subjects were given an intravenous glucose challenge. The incremental insulin responses were compared with fasting blood glucose levels, arbitrarily divided as shown. Rising glucose levels are associated with rising insulin levels; however, fasting blood glucose levels in excess of 100 mg/dL are associated with falling insulin secretion. In addition, in (*b*) the fraction of total insulin secreted as proinsulin, which has less than 10 percent of the bioactivity of insulin, is increased at blood glucose levels >100 mg/dL.

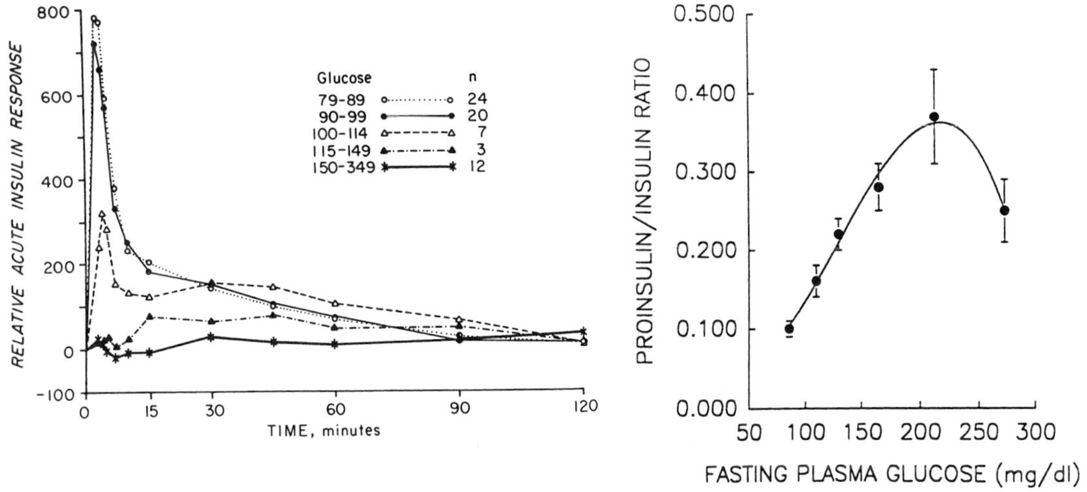

ronmental factors. Environmental factors that contribute to insulin resistance include obesity, medications, and aging. Insulin secretion may be adversely affected by medications, glucotoxicity, and other factors (Table 18-8).

Clinical Presentation

The development of glucose intolerance in Type 2 diabetes is much less acute than in Type 1 diabetes. The majority of persons with Type 2 diabetes probably go through a preclinical period of hyperinsulinemia associated with underlying insulin resistance, slowly develop increasing glucose intolerance with increases in postprandial glycemia more prominent than postabsorptive (fasting) levels, and then develop diabetic levels of glycemia as insulin secretion fails to keep up with the heightened demand imposed by insulin resistance (Figs. 18-25 and 18-28).

The gradual increase in glycemic levels over time, which is characteristic of Type 2 diabetes, and the absence of ketoacidosis, result in a different clinical presentation than in Type 1 diabetes. Although some patients may report symptoms consistent with the osmotic diuresis of hyperglycemia, many do not. The absence of symptoms may be secondary to the gradual rise in glucose levels with patients becoming inured to subtle changes in urination or thirst. Alternatively, the decreased glomerular filtration rate associated with aging may protect patients who are developing diabetes from symptomatic hyperglycemia. With decreased delivery of glucose to the tubules, patients may tolerate higher plasma glucose levels without glycosuria. Finally, the diagnostic levels of glycemia may be too low to cause sufficient glycosuria to elicit symptoms. Regardless of the mechanism, a substantial fraction of Type 2 diabetic patients deny symptoms at the time of presentation.

In IGT and early Type 2 diabetes, glucose levels initially rise in the postprandial period owing to decreased disposal of carbohydrate into muscle as a function of insulin resistance.[261] With progressively worse hyperglycemia, fasting glucose levels rise substantially, secondary to unrestrained hepatic glucose output.[262] Regardless of the stage or severity of Type 2 diabetes, the pattern of glucose levels is less chaotic than in Type 1 diabetes (Fig. 18-21b). Glucose levels usually are lowest before meals and rise to a peak approximately 2 h after the meal, paralleling the profile in nondiabetics. The glucose pattern remains stable from day to day; endogenous insulin secretion prevents blood glucose levels from being as chaotic as they are in Type 1 diabetes.

A small number of patients with Type 2 diabetes may have ketoacidosis at the time of diagnosis. This usually occurs in patients with more profound abnormalities in insulin secretion. They have often lost substantial weight or are thin at the time of diagnosis. Alternatively, patients with previously undiagnosed Type 2 diabetes who suffer an extremely stressful clinical event, such as a myocardial infarction or sepsis, with elevated levels of counterregulatory hormones, may present in ketoacidosis. Another group of Type 2 diabetic patients who develop ketoacidosis are obese African-Americans, usually of Caribbean origin, who have a form of Type 2 diabetes that has been called "Flatbush" diabetes.[263] These patients have no specific genetic or serologic markers of Type 1 diabetes, but appear to have relatively severe insulin deficiency. After initial therapy, these patients often have prolonged remissions with no requirement for exogenous insulin.

The more common presentation of Type 2 diabetes is either through routine blood or urine screening when hyperglycemia or glycosuria is detected, or with symptoms referable to hyperglycemia, similar to those in type 1 diabetes. Because Type 2 diabetes may go unrecognized for long periods of time, complications are present in 20–30 percent of patients at the time of diagnosis.[195,264] Retinopathy and neuropathy, including sensorimotor and autonomic neuropathy such as erectile dysfunction, are often present at the time of diagnosis.

Gestational Diabetes

Gestational diabetes is defined as diabetes that develops during pregnancy. Women who develop this form of diabetes may have had it during previous pregnancies. Gestational diabetes (GDM) most commonly develops during the third trimester of pregnancy and affects 3–5 percent of all pregnant women.[265] The clinical appearance is most often asymptomatic, owing to the modestly increased glycemia, and virtually all cases are detected through widely promulgated screening programs (Table 18-9).[164,266] GDM is generally considered to be most similar to Type 2 diabetes with regard to pathophysiology. Insulin resistance is heightened by placental hormones, especially human placental lactogen (sommatomammotropin), which increases most prominently beginning at weeks 20–24 of gestation.[267] More than 95 percent of women with GDM revert to normal glucose metabolism within 6 weeks of delivery; however, at least 50 percent of them will develop Type 2 diabetes later in life, with a large fraction developing it within 10 years of the index GDM pregnancy.[268]

The major risk factors for developing GDM include history of GDM with previous pregnancies, large for gestational age birthweights (>4.5 kg) with previous pregnancies, family history of Type 2 diabetes, GDM with previous pregnancies, and obesity.[269] Progression to Type 2 diabetes is more likely in women who have had GDM during more than one pregnancy or required insulin to treat their GDM. In addition, obesity and family history of diabetes increases the risk of developing Type 2 diabetes after GDM.[270] Although most diabetes that develops during pregnancy is GDM, a small number of women develop their Type 1 diabetes during pregnancy, either by chance or owing in part to the superimposed stress of the pregnancy. In addition, some women, especially in populations with a high prevalence of Type 2 diabetes, develop Type 2 diabetes at a young age and become pregnant in the setting of pregestational Type 2 diabetes.

Other Types of Diabetes

Other types of diabetes occur for a variety of reasons, some of which are well understood. For example, well-defined insults to the pancreas, such as pancreatitis, pancreatectomy, cystic fibrosis, or hemochromatosis may result in decreased insulin secretion. Some medications and endocrine conditions may precipitate diabetes by increasing insulin resistance and/or decreasing insulin secretion. A list of these forms of diabetes and their presumptive or established cause is included in Table 18-1.

Genetic forms: As noted above, although both Type 1 and Type 2 diabetes have a strong genetic basis, as demonstrated in identical twin studies, the specific genetic cause of diabetes has been demonstrated for only a small fraction of cases.

Maturity onset diabetes of youth (MODY). First described by Tattersall, MODY resembles a noninsulin dependent form of diabetes that characteristically has its onset in relatively young persons and affects multiple generations, consistent with autosomal dominant inheritance.[271] Subtle differences among families regarding age of onset and severity of the metabolic abnormalities have been identified.[272] Initially using a candidate gene approach, a variety of mutations were identified in the gene for glucokinase,[254] long suspected to be the functional glucose receptor for the islet β-cells.[273] Deficient insulin secretion was documented in the families with these glucokinase mutations, completing the understanding of this form of diabetes, thought to account for <1 percent of all Type 2 diabetes. Other families with autosomal Type 2 diabetes have been demonstrated to have mutations in transcription factors suspected to play a role in beta cell function. Five distinct genetic forms of MODY have now been identified: MODY 1 is linked to mutations in hepatic nuclear factor (HNF) 4α[255] on chromosome 20; MODY 2 is secondary to glucokinase mutations on chromosome 7[254]; MODY 3 is associated with HNF 1α mutations on chromosome 12[256]; MODY 4 is related to Islet promoter factor-1 on chromosome 13[257]; and MODY 5 is associated with HNF1β on chromosome 17.[258] Mutations in the transcription factors may cause glucose intolerance owing to their effect(s) on glucose signaling in the islet (GLUT 2, glucokinase, and glycolysis) or on islet development and function (PDX 1).

Another relatively rare form of diabetes that occurs predominantly in Japan includes nerve deafness and diabetes; it most closely resembles Type 2 diabetes.[274] A mutation in mitochondrial DNA has been demonstrated.

Diagnosis

The clinical presentation of Type 1 diabetes mellitus, with the relatively acute development of gross hyperglycemia resulting in an osmotic diuresis of calorie rich urine and polyuria, polydipsia, and weight loss, and occasional ketoacidosis, is sufficiently characteristic that it doesn't usually require more than a history and random blood glucose test for diagnosis. However, Type 2 diabetes mellitus occurs in the setting of a continuum of glucose levels that increase with increasing age (fasting glucose levels increase by 1–2 mg/dl per decade and levels of plasma glucose 2 hours after an oral glucose tolerance test increase by 10 mg/dL per decade after age 40).[275] Moreover, glucose levels in Type 2 diabetes usually increase progressively and slowly over time, with postprandial levels increasing from normal to impaired glucose tolerance to diabetic levels over 5–10 years. The insidious rise of glycemia in Type 2 diabetes may inure patients to the symptoms of hyperglycemia.

In order to distinguish abnormal glucose tolerance from age-related worsening of glucose tolerance, nonphysiologic testing such as the glucose tolerance test has been employed. Defining diagnostic glucose levels required long-term epidemiologic studies that established the glucose threshold at which the characteristic complications of diabetes developed (Fig. 18-29).[276–278] These studies were reviewed by the ADA Expert Committee that updated the diagnostic glucose levels for diabetes in 1997.[164]

The relative attributes of different measures of glycemia have been discussed and debated,[223,224] and the accepted measure of glycemia for the diagnosis of diabetes is plasma glucose (whole blood or capillary glucose levels are usually 12–15 percent lower than plasma or serum levels when measured by the same method). The choice of plasma glucose, over a variety of glycosylated proteins, urine glucose, or other intermediate metabolites that are abnormal in diabetes, is predicated on the widespread ability to measure its level accurately with uniform methods, and the large number of long-term studies relating glucose levels to the risk of developing retinopathy. Depending on the setting, either a fasting or random plasma glucose level or the level after an oral glucose tolerance test is acceptable (Table 18-2). If obvious symptoms of hyperglycemia are present, a random plasma glucose level greater than 200 mg/dL is sufficient to diagnose diabetes. In the absence of symptoms, a fasting plasma glucose level ≥140 mg/dL or a level ≥200 mg/dL two hours after a 75 gm oral glucose tolerance test was advised in the WHO recommendations in 1979. These results were to be confirmed by repeat testing. In 1997, based on new epidemiologic studies, the diagnostic level of fasting plasma glucose was adjusted to ≥126 mg/dL (7 mmol/L).[164]

FIGURE 18-29. Association between different measures of glycemia (fasting and 2 h plasma glucose levels after a 75 gm oral glucose tolerance test and HbA1c levels) and risk of developing retinopathy. These epidemiologic studies provided the rationale for changing the diagnostic level of fasting plasma glucose from 140 to 126 mg/dL. (*From the ADA Expert Committee Report.*[164])

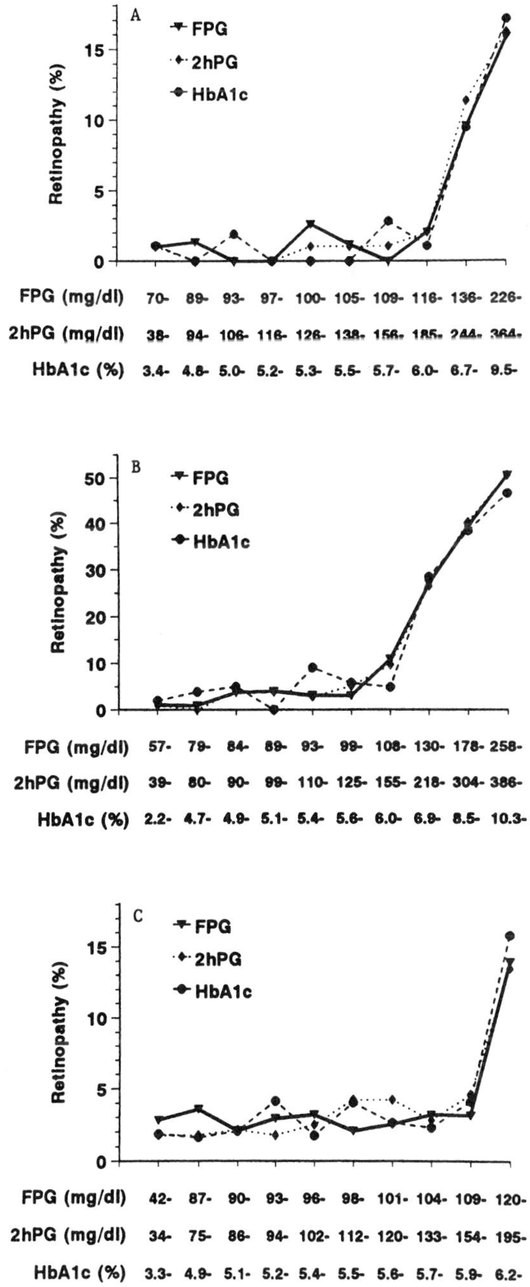

TABLE 18-14. DCCT Intensive Therapy

Metabolic Goals	
Premeal	70–120 mg/dL
90–120 min postmeal	<180
3 A.M.	>65
HbA1c	<6.05 percent
Monitoring	
Self-glucose	Premeals (more as necessary) and at bed 3 A.M. once per week
HbA1c	monthly
Insulin	≥ 3 injections per day or CSII with external pump Premeal regular doses adjusted based on glucose levels, meal size, and anticipated exercise
Dietary	Frequent counseling
Education	Intensive therapy initiated in hospital
Supervision	Monthly visits Frequent phone calls

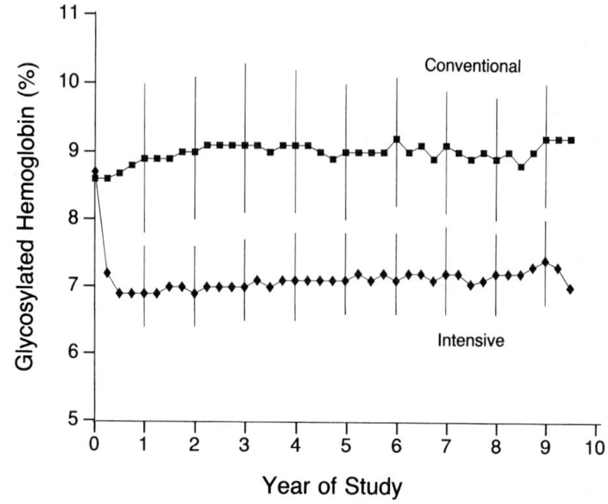

FIGURE 18-31. Median HbA1c levels in the DCCT conventional and intensive treatment groups. The bars represent the interquartile distribution of values. The difference between the treatment groups was highly significant ($p < .0001$) from 3 months to study end. The difference in HbA1c between the groups was approximately 2 percent during the study. HbA1c was measured centrally with an ion exchange HPLC method every three months in all subjects. The nondiabetic mean was 5.05 ± 0.5 percent (1 SD). (*From DCCT Research Group.*[13])

association among glycemia, long-term complications, and other risk factors were also described.[301,323] A long-term followup study of the DCCT cohort, the Epidemiology of Diabetes Interventions and Complications study is underway[324] and is providing further insight into the long-term consequences of intensive therapy.[325]

During the 6.5-year mean follow-up of the study (range 3–9 years), compliance was excellent, with 99 percent of the cohort completing the trial. In addition, there was virtually no crossover between assigned treatments. Subjects adhered to their assigned treatment more than 97 percent of study time. Intensive therapy decreased HbA1c to a nadir of approximately 6.9 percent by 6 months and maintained mean HbA1c levels during the remainder of the trial that were approximately 2 percent lower than with conventional treatment (7 percent versus 9 percent) (Fig. 18-31). Of note, intensive therapy did not lower mean HbA1c to the nondiabetic range.

Retinopathy was evaluated every 6 months by 7-field stereoscopic fundus photography. Although many analytic levels[307] of retinopathy were assessed, the principal outcome in the primary prevention study was the development of a sustained (seen on two consecutive exams) three-step or greater progression on a retinopathy severity scale adopted from the Early Treatment of Diabetic Retinopathy Study (ETDRS).[326] Similarly, the principal outcome in the secondary intervention study was a sustained progression of three or more steps from the baseline level. Intensive therapy reduced the development of these end points by 76 percent in the primary prevention study and by 54 percent in the secondary intervention study compared with conventional therapy (Figs. 18-32a and 18-33b). Other retinopathy outcomes and the effects of intensive therapy are shown in Table 18-15.

The overall effect of intensive therapy was to decrease all stages of retinopathy included in the DCCT. However, intensive therapy was relatively more effective when initiated early in the course of diabetes (shorter versus longer duration) and when retinopathy was less severe at baseline.[307,308] Although intensive therapy reduced the risk somewhat less for more advanced stages of retinopathy than for earlier stages, patients with more advanced retinopathy still benefited from intensive therapy. Their retinal status was much more likely to stabilize or even to improve with intensive compared with conventional therapy. The beneficial effects of intensive therapy were not seen for the first 3 years of therapy, presumably because of the natural "momentum" of diabetic complications. In addition, intensive therapy was associated with a transient worsening of retinopathy during the first year of therapy.[309] Both of these factors conspired to delay the beneficial effects of intensive therapy on retinopathy, which were similar in almost all subgroups of patients defined by age, gender, and other baseline characteristics.

The long-term followup of the DCCT cohort in the EDIC study has shown further improvement in retinal status in the previous intensive treatment group compared with the previous conventional treatment group (Table 18-16).[327] The difference between the two treatment groups persists 4.5 years after DCCT end, even though the majority of the previous conventional treatment cohort has changed to intensive therapy and the mean HbA1c levels have drifted closer between the two treatment groups. The persistent benefit of 6.5 years of intensive therapy during the DCCT further supports the concept of "momentum" with regard to diabetic complications.

The study of families of DCCT volunteers, in which there are more than one person with diabetes, has revealed clustering of retinopathy within families.[328] The tendency for some families with diabetes to develop retinopathy, while other families do not, may be mediated by genetic factors or by some as yet to be identified shared environmental factor. Interestingly, regardless of the cause of clustering, intensive therapy decreased the development and progression of retinopathy in DCCT volunteers who were members of "high risk" families as well as in DCCT volunteers in "low risk" families.

Nephropathy was assessed by measurements of albumin excretion and standard creatinine clearance, based on an annual standardized 4-hour collection and by periodically measured iothalamate clearance. As with retinopathy, the risk for progression of nephropathy was reduced by intensive therapy (Fig.

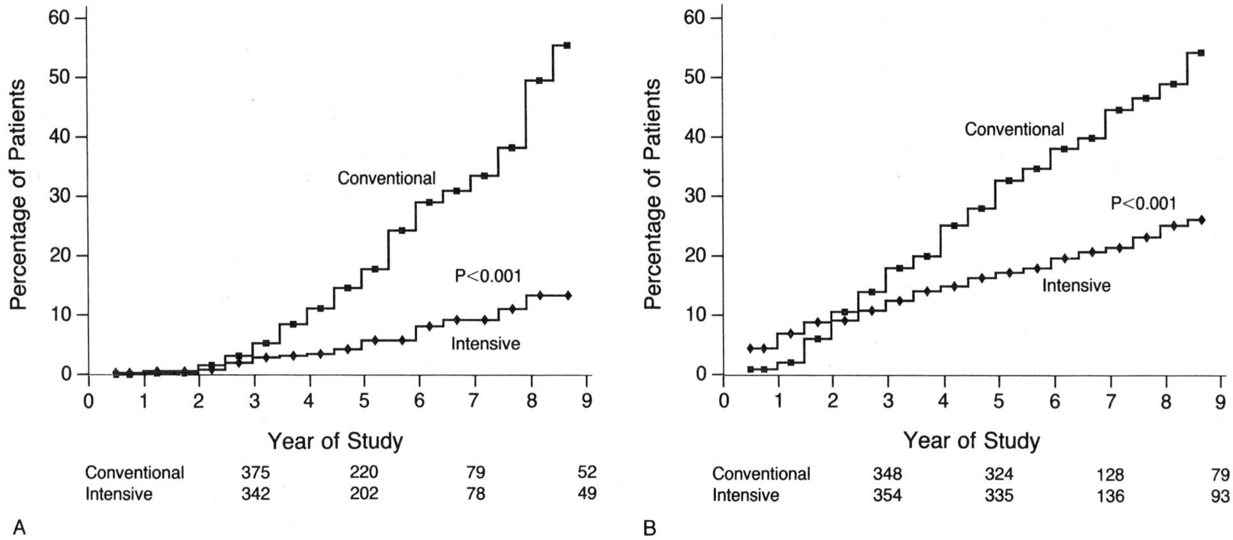

FIGURE 18-32. Retinopathy results in the DCCT for conventional and intensive treatment groups for the (*a*) primary prevention cohort (no retinopathy at baseline and 1–5 years diabetes duration) and (*b*) secondary intervention cohort (at least 1 microaneurysm in either eye). The primary outcome was a 3-step change in retinopathy according to the ETDRS scales that was sustained for at least 6 months. Centrally graded stereoscopic seven-field fundus photography was performed every 6 months in all subjects. Note that no beneficial effect was detected in the primary prevention cohort for the first 3 years of intensive therapy; in the secondary intervention cohort, intensive therapy was associated with worse retinopathy, so called "transient worsening,"[309] with improved results compared with conventional therapy first noted at 3 years. The difference between therapy groups appears to widen over time. (*From DCCT Research Group.*[13])

18-33). This included reduction in the development of microalbuminuria (≥40 mg/24 h) and clinical grade albuminuria (>300 mg/24 h). The small number of patients developing clinical nephropathy, defined as a creatinine clearance <70 mL/min/1.73^2 with albumin excretion >300 mg/24 hours, precluded a statistically valid analysis of any difference between treatment groups. However, the number of conventional treatment patients who developed this level of renal dysfunction (n = 5) was more than twice the number of intensive treatment patients (n = 2). The relatively small number of secondary intervention patients who had microalbuminuria at baseline (n = 70) made it difficult to demonstrate a benefit of intensive therapy with regard

FIGURE 18-33. Nephropathy results of intensive therapy vs. conventional therapy in the DCCT in the (*a*) primary prevention cohort and (*b*) secondary intervention cohort. The cumulative incidence of urinary albumin excretion ≥300 mg/24 h (dashed lines) and ≥40 mg/24 h (solid lines) was measured annually. Intensive therapy reduced the development of microalbuminuria by 34 percent and 43 percent in the primary prevention and secondary intervention cohorts, respectively, and reduced clinical grade albuminuria by 56 percent in the secondary intervention cohort. (*From DCCT Research Group.*[13])

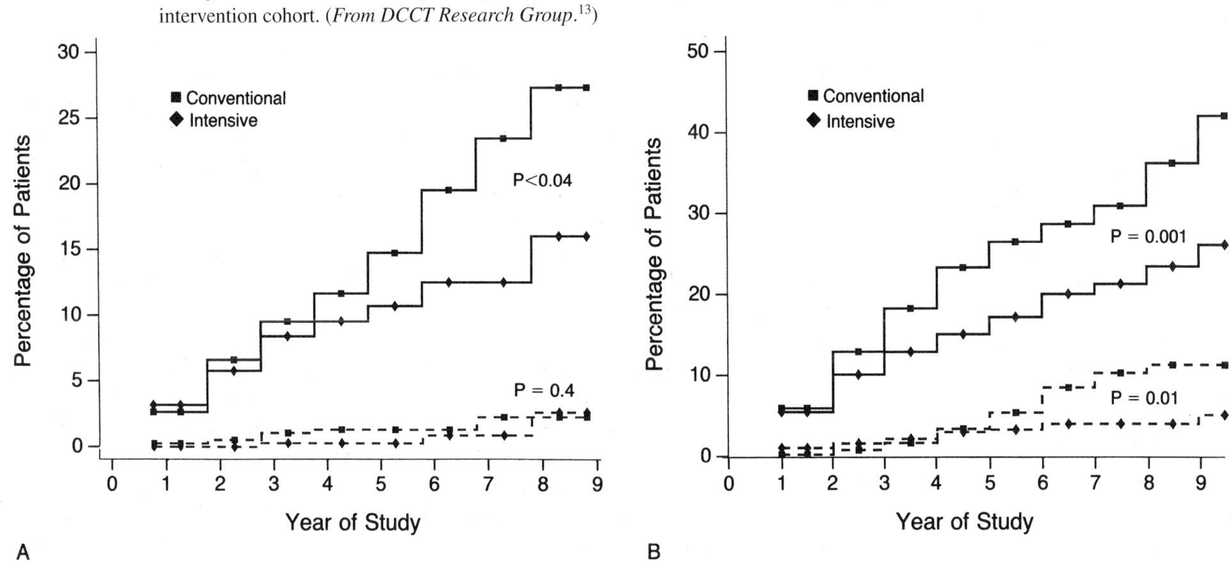

TABLE 18-15. Effects of Intensive Therapy in DCCT

	Percent Risk Reduction		
Complications	**Primary Prevention**	**Secondary Intervention**	**Both Cohorts**
Retinopathy			
≥ 3-step sustained	76†	54†	63†
Macular edema		23	26
Severe NPDR or PDR		47‡	47‡
Laser therapy		56†	51‡
Nephropathy			
≥ 40 mg/24 h	34‡	43†	39†
≥ 300 mg/24 h	44	56‡	54‡
Clinical neuropathy*	69‡	57†	60†

NPDR—Non-proliferative diabetic retinopathy; PDR—Proliferative diabetic retinopathy

*Defined as occurrence at 5 yr of symptoms or signs of peripheral neuropathy confirmed by either abnormal nerve conduction or autonomic neuropathy testing in patients without clinical neuropathy at baseline.

†P ≤ .002.

‡P ≤ .04.

to slowing progression to clinical grade albuminuria once microalbuminuria had occurred.[310] The long-term followup of the DCCT cohort has reinforced the role of intensive therapy in delaying and perhaps preventing diabetic nephropathy (Table 18-16).[327]

Confirmed clinical *neuropathy* was defined as the presence of signs or symptoms of peripheral neuropathy plus either abnormal nerve conduction in at least two peripheral nerves or unequivocally abnormal autonomic nerve testing. Intensive therapy reduced the risk of developing clinical neuropathy by 60 percent in the combined cohorts (Table 18-15).[13,311–313] In addition to the decreased development of confirmed clinical neuropathy, the most stringent of the neurologic outcomes, intensive therapy reduced the risk of deterioration of nerve function, as measured with electrophysiologic methods, that occurred with conventional therapy.[313] The decline in autonomic nerve function, assessed with measures of cardiovascular autonomic function, that occurred with conventional therapy was significantly reduced with intensive therapy in the primary prevention, but not in the secondary intervention cohort.[312]

The DCCT did not demonstrate a significant difference in major *macrovascular outcomes* (death from cardiovascular disease, myocardial infarction, and major peripheral vascular events) between treatment groups.[314] Although the risk for these combined events was reduced by 41 percent with intensive therapy, the difference between groups failed to achieve conventional levels of statistical significance ($p = 0.06$). However, several risk factors for cardiovascular disease were improved with intensive therapy, including a 34 percent reduction in low-density lipoprotein cholesterol ($p = 0.02$).

Accompanying the salutary effects of intensive therapy on long-term complications was an approximately threefold increase in severe hypoglycemia, defined as an episode that required assistance to treat.[13,319,320] Although the majority of these episodes were clinically benign, the incidence of hypoglycemia resulting in coma or seizures or requiring emergency room treatment was also increased by approximately two- to threefold. The more severe hypoglycemic reactions, such as those resulting in seizure or coma, were relatively rare (16 vs. 5 episodes per 100 patient-years

TABLE 18-16. Follow-up of DCCT Cohort After End of DCCT*

	Risk Reduction (percent) Intensive vs. Conventional Therapy	
Complication	**After DCCT†**	**Between End of DCCT and After 4 Years Additional Follow-up‡**
Retinopathy		
> 3-step change	76	77
≥ Severe NPDR	68	76
Macular edema	26	77
Laser Treatment	51	77
Nephropathy		
Albumin excretion		
≥ 40 mg/24 h	39	53
≥ 300 mg/24 h	54	86

*Adapted from ref. 327.

†Mean follow-up 6.5 years with HbA1c 9.1 vs 7.2 percent in intensive vs. conventional therapy, respectively.

‡Adjusted for level at DCCT closeout. Mean A1c approximately 8.2 percent in both treatment groups over 4 years follow-up after end of DCCT. The continued difference in outcomes between the two treatment groups, even with similar HbA1c levels during the 4 years after the end of the DCCT, is probably attributable to the "momentum" of complications in the conventional group, the time necessary to see a beneficial effect of intensive therapy, and the persistent benefit of intensive therapy in the former intensive treatment group.

in the intensive and conventional treatment groups, respectively). Other adverse events that accompanied intensive therapy included an increased risk for weight gain, secondary in part to the decrease in caloric wasting with decreased glycosuria, and catheter-related infections in patients using insulin pumps. Taken together, none of these adverse events caused significant morbidity or mortality. There were no patient deaths or macrovascular events ascribed to hypoglycemia. Moreover, the increased frequency of hypoglycemia had no adverse effects on neurocognitive function as judged by frequent testing in both treatment groups.[316] Finally, despite the demands of intensive therapy, quality of life, measured yearly by self-report,[315] did not differ between the two treatment groups.

Several secondary analyses of DCCT data have clearly established the association between chronic glycemic levels and complications.[301,323] These analyses have revealed a continuous relationship between mean HbA1c levels during the DCCT and the risk of developing retinopathy (Fig. 18-35) and nephropathy, with no obvious breakpoint. Every 10 percent reduction in HbA1c is associated with a 43 percent reduction in development of a 3-step change in retinopathy, and a similar decrease in the risk of retinopathy progression. There is no level of HbA1c in the diabetic range below which further lowering in risk does not occur.

DCCT Treatment Recommendations The DCCT Research Group, the American Diabetes Association, and other groups have concluded that the significant and consistent effects of intensive therapy in reducing the risk of development and progression of long-term complications of diabetes outweigh its costs, the considerable effort to implement it, and the increased patient risk for hypoglycemia.[13,303] Intensive therapy has been endorsed as the treatment of choice for most patients with Type 1 diabetes. This conclusion is further supported on the basis of the projected economic impact of intensive therapy.[321] Although the annual cost of intensive therapy exceeds the cost of conventional therapy and must be incurred for at least 3 years before a benefit is seen, the long-term benefits of intensive therapy—in the form of reducing loss of vision and the need for laser therapy, reducing the incidence of end-stage renal disease and the need for dialysis and transplantation, and reducing the number of amputations—and the costs associated with all these problems make intensive therapy an economically viable therapy. The long-term followup in EDIC, demonstrating further benefits of intensive therapy even 4.5 years after the end of the DCCT, supports this conclusion.[327]

Realistically, not all Type 1 diabetic patients are able to implement intensive therapy; however, the goal for all patients should be to lower glycemia as close to the normal range as safety and lifestyle allow. For patients who cannot implement intensive treatment, therapies of variable intensity are available (Table 18-17). All patients should be evaluated and advised to increase the intensity of their therapy as needed. Lower HbA1c levels should translate into appreciably lower risk for complications (Fig. 18-34).

Elements of Metabolic Therapy of Type 1 Diabetes

Monitoring metabolic status in Type 1 diabetes includes monitoring acute and chronic glycemic levels and measuring the presence of ketones when ketosis or ketoacidosis is suspected.[329–331] Much of the monitoring is performed by the patient.

Acute Glycemia Considering the labile nature of glucose profiles in Type 1 diabetes, the potentially severe consequences of hypoglycemia, and the inability of urine glucose tests to provide accurate information regarding contemporaneous blood glucose levels,[329] an accurate, user-friendly method for measuring blood glucose on a frequent outpatient basis is necessary. Reagent strips impregnated with glucose oxidase and coupled to colorimetric indicators have been available for more than thirty years; however, convenient and accurate methods, including meters that store data, did not become available until the 1980s. A large variety of meters and strips using dry methodology (i.e., not requiring washing the strips) and requiring very small volumes of capillary blood are now available.[331]

The frequency of monitoring in Type 1 diabetes is predicated on decreasing the risk of hypoglycemia and the need to guide therapy, specifically the size of preprandial doses of rapid- or very-rapid-acting insulin. Few studies have directly studied the role of monitoring, or the specific frequency required, in intensive regimens. However, most clinical trials of intensive therapy have required premeal and prebed monitoring in order to adjust each dose of rapid- or very-rapid-acting insulin. Intensive regimens that don't use insulin at lunch may be able to eliminate the prelunch glucose test, which is sometimes difficult to perform at work or school. The DCCT also required a 3 A.M. test once per week to safeguard against nocturnal hypoglycemia. The difficulty in maintaining a high frequency of testing has been demonstrated in the DCCT and subsequent followup in EDIC. During the 6.5 years of the DCCT, 80–90 percent of intensive therapy patients tested blood glucose at least 4 times per day.[318] During the 4 years of followup after the end of the DCCT, when intensive therapy patients were returned to their own health care providers, only 45 percent tested 4 or more times per day.[324]

Not all patients will be able to perform or maintain intensive therapy. In general, the frequency of monitoring should parallel the intensiveness of the treatment program (Table 18-17). At a minimum, Type 1 diabetic patients should be capable of SMBG when insulin doses, diet, or activity change, or when hypoglycemia would be particularly dangerous, e.g., before a car trip. In addition, SMBG during intercurrent illnesses can help patients adjust insulin.

The role of office-based testing of acute glucose levels has become more limited with the widespread implementation of SMBG. Single, infrequent measures of glucose are not usually useful with regard to clinical management. Office-based measurements can be used to assess the accuracy of simultaneously measured results with the patient's meter or to identify and treat hypoglycemia that occurs during a visit. In rare patients who are unwilling or unable to perform any SMBG, office-based measurements of glucose, performed with an office-meter or in a chemistry laboratory, may be helpful in adjusting doses.

Urine glucose monitoring is generally considered an outmoded method. It provides semiquantitative data at best, is an indirect measure of blood glucose concentration with a temporal delay, and cannot help distinguish between normal and hypoglycemic blood glucose levels. Urine glucose monitoring should not be encouraged in Type 1 diabetes.

Chronic Glycemia The lability of glucose levels, especially in Type 1 diabetes, makes the assessment of chronic glycemia, even with repeated measures of acute glycemia, problematic. An accurate, objective measure of chronic glycemia was necessary for epidemiologic studies, clinical trials of the effect of intensive intervention on long-term complications, and for clinical management.

TABLE 18-17. Treatment Regimens for Type 1 Diabetes Mellitus

Level of Therapy	SMBG* per Day	Insulin Regimen Injections per Day (Type†)	Diet	Exercise	Risks‡	Expected HbArc (%)[@]
Minimal	0–1	1 or 2 Generally stable doses without frequent adjustments (I ± R)	45–60 percent carbohydrate, limited sucrose <300 mg cholesterol, protein 0.8 g/kg Consistent meal time and content	Patient preference Snack to prevent hypoglycemia	Increased risk for all microvascular and neurologic complications	>9
Average	1–3 (fasting and pre supper or prebed)	2 (I and R) Adjust regular dose based on premeal blood glucose & meal size	As above with exchange list	As above	Increased risk for all microvascular and neurologic complications	7.5–10
Intensive#	4–7 (premeals and prebed; 3 A.M. once per week; postprandial as needed).	≥ 3 injections (I or UL and R) or CSII. Match insulin delivery to insulin requirements	More accurate carbohydrate exchange—use glycemic indices when appropriate	Adjust insulin and/or meals to prevent hypoglycemia	Hypoglycemia** weight gain, catheter inflammation and infection, transient worsening of retinopathy	<7.5

*SMBG = self-monitoring of blood glucose levels.

†I = intermediate-acting (NPH or Lente); R = rapid-acting or very rapid-acting; UL = ultralente; CSII = continuous subcutaneous insulin infusion.

‡Risks relative to other therapy regimens.

**Intensive therapy may decrease threshold for counterregulation.

#Recommended for most patients with Type 1 diabetes.

@ Normal range 4.8–6.1.

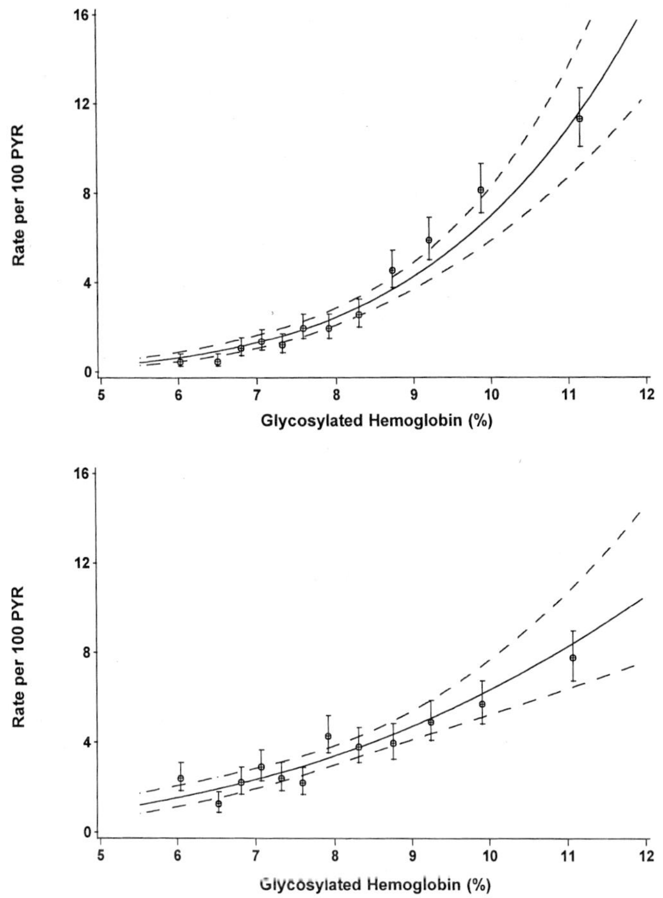

FIGURE 18-34. Association of chronic glycemia as measured by mean HbA1c with (*a*) risk of developing a 3-step progression of retinopathy and (*b*) risk of developing microalbuminuria in the DCCT. This secondary analysis of DCCT results demonstrates a continuous risk for developing retinopathy and nephropathy (hazard rate per 100 patient-years) based on mean HbA1c with no apparent level of glycemia at which lower HbA1c does not provide a benefit. For every 10 percent (relative, not absolute) reduction in HbA1c (for example, reducing HbA1c from 9 to 8.1 percent), there is a 43 percent reduction in risk of developing retinopathy. (*From DCCT Research Group Diabetes 45:1289, 1996.*)

The recent recognition of the importance of chronic glycemia in the development of long-term complications has made such measures indispensable in clinical management. The assay for glycosylated hemoglobin revolutionized diabetes management and has become one of the most commonly performed assays in medical practice.

Prior to the recognition that the concentration of glycated (glycosylated) proteins reflected circulating blood glucose concentrations integrated over time,[332,333] there was no reliable, accurate index of chronic glycemia. The utility of measuring the concentration of glycated (glycosylated) proteins (the nonenzymatic product of glucose and amino groups of circulating and membrane proteins), as an index of chronic glucose levels has now been well established.[332,334] The concentration of a glycated protein reflects the mean blood glucose concentration integrated over the half-life of the protein (Fig. 18-35). Thus, the concentration of glycosylated hemoglobin (HbA1 or HbA1c depending on the specific method used) reflects mean glucose levels over approximately 60 days (average erythrocyte life span is 120 days); glycated albumin or serum protein (e.g., fructosamine) reflects mean blood glucose levels over a 20-day period.[335] Two studies have demonstrated the correlation between mean glucose levels and HbA1c levels.[332,333] These measures provide an objective means of assessing long-term glycemia and judging the efficacy of therapeutic interventions. At least one study has demonstrated that performing HbA1c measurements leads to better health status with lower glycemia and fewer hospitalizations than in a randomly selected group that did not have HbA1c measured.[334] In Type 1 diabetes, three to four

FIGURE 18-35. Relationship between glycosylated hemoglobin level and mean blood glucose. Blood glucose levels were measured pre- and 90–120 min postmeals in 21 patients with diabetes mellitus during an eight-week period. Accuracy of self-monitored results was confirmed with laboratory-based plasma glucose assays. At the end of the eight-week period, HbA1c was measured with an ion exchange HPLC method. The arithmetic mean of the blood glucose levels are plotted against the HbA1c level. The calculated regression equation [Mean blood glucose = 33.3 × HbA1c-86] has been used to provide a mean blood glucose equivalent for HbA1c values. (*From Nathan.*[284])

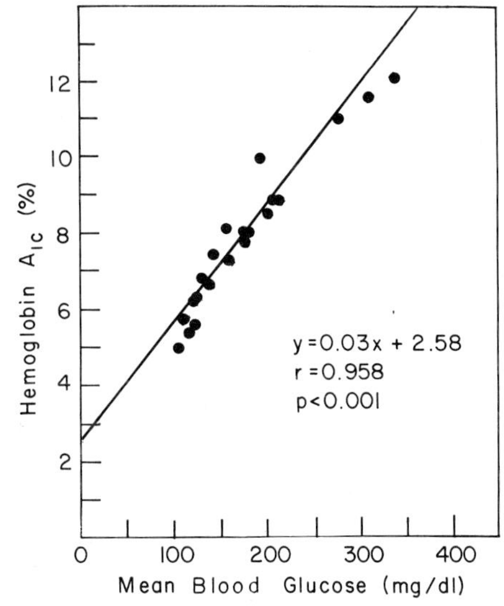

TABLE 18-18. Routine Laboratory Tests and Examinations in the Management of Diabetes

	Frequency (per year)	
Assay	**Type 1**	**Type 2**
Glycohemoglobin	4	2–4
Ketones	PRN	PRN
Fasting lipids	1	1
Microalbuminuria*	1	1
Serum creatinine†	<1	1
Electrolytes (Na, K)	1	1
Thyroid function tests (TSH)	<1	—
Adrenal	<1	—
B12	<1	—
Retinopathy		
Dilated exam‡	1	1
Neuropathy and foot examinations		
Foot exam	each visit	each visit
Sensory exam	each visit	each visit
Cardiovascular		
Blood pressure	each visit	each visit
EKG**	<1	1
Peripheral pulses	each visit	each visit

*Can screen patients with a spot urine, corrected for urine creatinine. To establish presence of microalbuminuria definitively, a 12- or 24-h urine collection should be performed and the result confirmed.

†Frequent (annual) serum creatinine not necessary in otherwise healthy Type 1 diabetic patients if albuminuria not present. In older patients, use of antihypertensives and more common occurrence of other conditions and use of specific drugs (metformin) that may affect, or be affected by, renal function require more frequent measurement of serum creatinine levels. Other tests, such as liver function monitoring, may be required depending on medications (thiazolidinediones, HMG CoA reductase inhibitors) used.

‡In Type 1 diabetes, examinations should commence after 5 years of diabetes duration. In Type 2 diabetes, patients should be examined from the time of diagnosis.

**EKGs need not be performed routinely in patients with Type 1 diabetes until they reach an age when they are at increased risk, e.g., older than 30. However, Type 1 diabetic patients at particularly high risk for cardiac disease (cardiac autonomic neuropathy, micro- or macroalbuminuria, renal failure) require routine surveillance. Other cardiac evaluation, such as exercise tolerance testing, should be performed when patients with Type 2 diabetes or older Type 1 diabetic patients plan a change in activity level or exercise, or if patients have any exercise related symptoms, even if atypical for angina.

HbA1c measurements per year are sufficient for clinical management (Table 18-18).

Many assay methods are available to measure glycosylated hemoglobin.[331] These include chromatographic and electroendosmotic methods that separate glycated hemoglobin from nonglycosylated hemoglobin on the basis of differences in charge distribution, affinity assays and radioimmunoassays that bind specifically to the glycated species, and other colorimetric assays. Some of these assays measure "total" glycohemoglobin, while others can separate different glycated moieties, i.e., different sugars attached to hemoglobin (Table 18-19). Of note, virtually all of these assays have very tight interassay correlations. However, confusion has occurred owing to differences in nomenclature and nondiabetic ranges for these assays, the wide variety of assays, and frequent switching between assay methods in commercial laboratories. Efforts are underway to standardize the diverse assays to the DCCT method,[336,337] a very precise high-performance liquid chromatography assay which has stable high and low standards and a nondiabetic value of 5.05 ± 0.5 percent (mean ± 1 SD). Many laboratories report a calculated mean blood glucose concentration along with the percent of glycated hemoglobin using the regression equation calculated from the data in Fig. 18-35.

Depending on which glycohemoglobin assay is used, specific factors may interfere with the accuracy of the result (Table 18-19). All of the assays can be affected by a change in the turnover of the red cell mass. For example, acute blood loss with a resultant increase in erythrocyte turnover will spuriously lower glycated hemoglobin levels. The large influx of young erythrocytes alters the usual age distribution of the red cell population with a predominance of nonglycated cells. In addition to acute blood loss, pregnancy represents another common state in which the usual relationship between glycemia and glycohemoglobin levels may be perturbed. Other factors that can affect the assay results include hemoglobinopathies such as sickle cell trait or disease (lowers HbA1c measured by chromatography because glycated sickle cell hemoglobin elutes with nonglycated hemoglobin), persistent fetal hemoglobinopathy (raises HbA1c since HbF elutes with glycated hemoblobin), and uremia (minor effect).

Other measures of chronic glycemia have been proposed, but none has achieved the popular use of the glycohemoglobin assay. Assays that reflect a shorter period of glycemia, such as fructosamine, which measures glycemia over 20 days, would need to be repeated more frequently. Their role in diabetes therapy has not been established, and glycohemoglobin measurements are usually preferred.

Ketones The risk of ketoacidosis in the setting of a superimposed illness or inadequate insulin, reflected by unusually high blood glucose levels, should prompt testing for urine ketones. Urine ketones can be conveniently measured with semiquantitative reagent strips that rely on an enzymatic assay coupled to colorimetric reaction. Most assays rely on a nitroprusside reaction which detects acetoacetate and acetone but not hydroxybutyrate. Patients should be instructed to call their health care provider if more than trace or minimal urine ketones are present. Ketone testing should be performed whenever a patient is nauseated or vomiting, as these may represent the early symptoms of ketoacidosis. Office-based testing with a reagent strip can be performed when a patient has an intercurrent illness with gastrointestinal symptoms or when blood glucose levels are extremely elevated. Monitoring of serum ketones should be reserved for the management of ketoacidosis (see section on ketoacidosis).

Other In addition to monitoring acute and chronic glycemia, other routine monitoring of Type 1 diabetes takes into account associated metabolic abnormalities and the need for surveillance for and treatment of long-term complications (Table 18-18). The presence of microalbuminuria (>30 mg albumin per 24 h) is a highly predictive marker for the development of later "clinical" albuminuria (>300 mg albumin per 24 h).[338] The demonstrated efficacy of blood pressure management, and angiotensin converting enzyme inhibitors in particular, in delaying progression of diabetic nephropathy supports regular surveillance.[339] Although most guidelines suggest confirmation of microalbuminuria with repeated 24-h urines, screening can be performed with a spot urine, corrected for creatinine excretion (>15–20 μg/mg creatinine) which should be followed by a timed (12 or 24 h) collection.[340] Clinical albuminuria, which can be detected as a positive dipstick test, results in end-stage renal disease in more than 90 percent of cases. Routine surveillance of creatinine, in the absence of

TABLE 18-19. Assays for Glycosylated Hemoglobin

Assay	Glycated Species Measured*	Typical Non-diabetic Range (mean ± 2 SD)	Interfering Factors† Falsely Lower	Interfering Factors† Falsely Raise
Ion exchange chromatography (HPLC, microcolumn separates on the basis of charge changes)	HbA_{1c} or HbA_1	5.0 ± 1	HbS,C,D, E,A_2†	HbF, uremia, labile‡**, lipids#
Radioimmunoassay (recognizes HbA_{1c})	HbA_{1c}	4.7 ± 0.6		HbF (>30 percent)
Affinity (Boronate binds to cis-diol of glucose)	Total glycohemoglobin	6.0 ± 1.0		Lipids#
Colorimetric (based on chemical reactivity of glucose)	Total glycohemoglobin	5.5 ± 1.2		High (>200) plasma glucose
Electroendosmotic (separates on basis of charge)	HbA_1	6.7 ± 1.0		HbF, labile**
Isoelectric focusing (separates on basis of charge)	HbA_{1c}	5.85 ± 0.3		Labile**, HbF (>30 percent)

Ion exchange, radioimmunoassay-based, and affinity assays are most commonly used.

*The classification of different glycated and nonglycated hemoglobin fractions is based on the elution pattern originally described with ion exchange (liquid) chromatography. HbA (normal adult hemoglobin) includes nonglycated HbA_0 (no glucose at the N-terminal β-chain valine, although glucose adducts may be located on internal lysines), and the minor glycated fractions that elute before HbA_0. The minor glycated fractions include HbA_{1c}, which is the largest component and measures glucose bound to the N-terminal valine, and HbA_{1a} and HbA_{1b}, each of which has subfractions that represent other sugars binding to hemoglobin. Combined, HbA_{1c}, HbA_{1a}, and HbA_{1b} are called HbA_1. The ion exchange assays can provide either HbA_1 or HbA_{1c} results, with the former usually 1.5 percent higher than HbA_{1c}. The correlation between the two measures exceeds r of 0.99.

†Any condition that increases the influx of new, young erythrocytes into the circulation (e.g., hemolytic anemia, recent acute blood loss) will spuriously lower HbA1c levels, regardless of assay method.

‡Several automated HPLC assays are capable of removing the labile glycated hemoglobin and separating some of the hemoglobinopathies (HbS, HbF) so that a corrected HbA_{1c} can be reported.

**The labile, intermediate aldimine, which forms before final rearrangement to the stable ketoamine, will artifically raise HbA_{1c} levels, reflecting ambient glucose levels at the time of blood sampling. A variety of strategies remove this interfering substance during sample preparation or assay.

#Very high triglyceride levels cause lactescence and can interfere with any chromatographic method.

albuminuria, is probably not merited because proteinuria virtually always precedes falling glomerular filtration rate in diabetic nephropathy; however, this inexpensive test may detect nondiabetic renal disease and should be performed regularly. Periodic measurement of electrolytes (Na^+ and K^+) should be performed, especially in any patient with renal dysfunction or treated with antihypertensive medications, to detect the hyperkalemia associated with hyporeninemic hypoaldosteronism or other electrolyte abnormalities secondary to diuretic use.

Type 1 diabetes is less commonly affected by lipid abnormalities than Type 2 diabetes; nevertheless, the increased cardiovascular risk associated with Type 1 diabetes and abnormalities in lipids that accompany poor glycemic control (especially increased triglyceride levels) and nephrotic syndrome (increased total and LDL cholesterol) dictate regular monitoring and aggressive therapy.[341]

Other commonly associated conditions, such as Grave's disease and Hashimoto's thyroiditis, require regular monitoring of TSH levels. Similarly, in patients with anemia or features suggestive of polyglandular autoimmune syndrome, monitoring for adrenal dysfunction and pernicious anemia may be required.

Insulin Therapy

Insulin is available in various formulations, species and degrees of purification (Table 18-11).[342] The development of highly purified human insulin, either synthesized by modifying pork insulin or with recombinant methods in *E. coli* or yeast, has largely supplanted animal species insulin in most of Europe and North America. As of 1998, the major supplier of insulin in the U.S., Eli Lilly and Co., stopped producing animal species insulins, largely for financial reasons. European manufacturers will probably follow, but currently continue to make animal species insulin that are highly purified. Purity of insulin has traditionally been measured as parts per million of proinsulin. Almost all of the insulins currently marketed have < 50 ppm proinsulin, and often < 10 ppm.

Pork and beef insulins differ from human insulin by one and three amino acids, respectively (Fig. 18-2). Despite the differences in amino acid sequence and the increased generation of anti-insulin antibodies when beef, pork, or beef/pork insulin is administered,[343] these insulins retain similar potency to human insulin and rarely cause clinical problems. The increased use of highly purified human insulin has largely eliminated the local pruritus at injection sites, representing a cellular mediated delayed hypersensitivity that was commonly seen with the initiation of insulin therapy with less pure animal species insulin in the past. It has also decreased the occurrence of the very rare episodes of IgE mediated allergic reactions and severe insulin resistance secondary to high titers of IgG insulin binding antibodies.[344] The latter conditions have been reported, albeit rarely, even with the use of highly purified human insulin. When the rare cases of antibody-mediated insulin resistance or local or systemic insulin allergy occur, either a change in insulin (to highly purified pork or human insulin) or desensitization is effective.[345] With the increasing use of highly purified human insulin, cases of insulin allergy have become even more rare; however, patients with intermittent insulin use (e.g., gestational diabetes) are at greater risk for developing immune mediated complications and should be treated with pure pork or human insulin.

Table 18-11 shows the different formulations available and their profiles of action. Variability in insulin absorption from person to person, and even in a single individual, renders these profiles only crude estimates.[346] Human insulins generally have a slightly faster onset and shorter duration than corresponding animal species insulins. Several fixed combination formulations (e.g., 70 percent NPH and 30 percent regular) are available. These are only rarely useful in Type 1 diabetes because they obligate

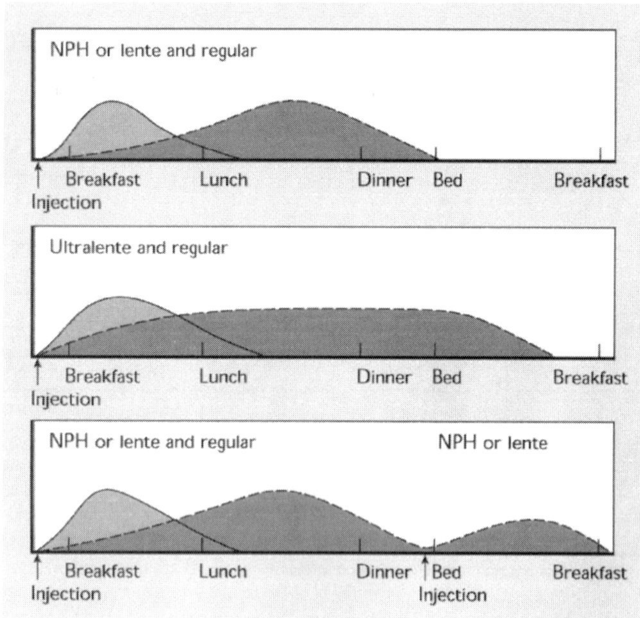

A

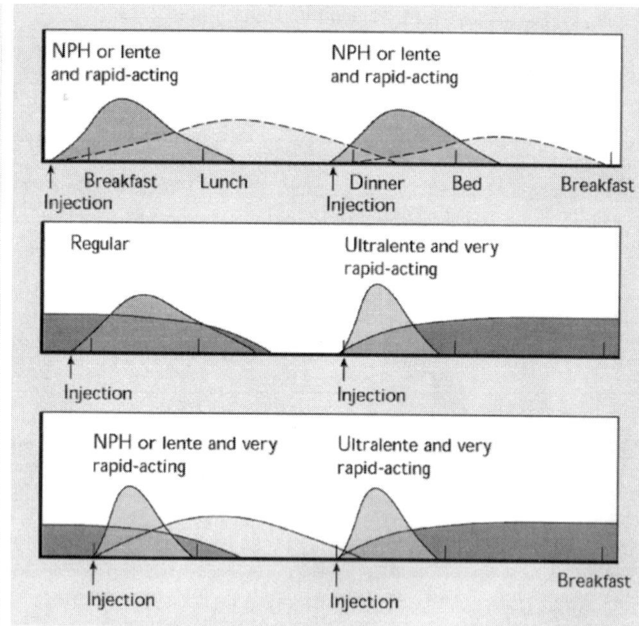

B

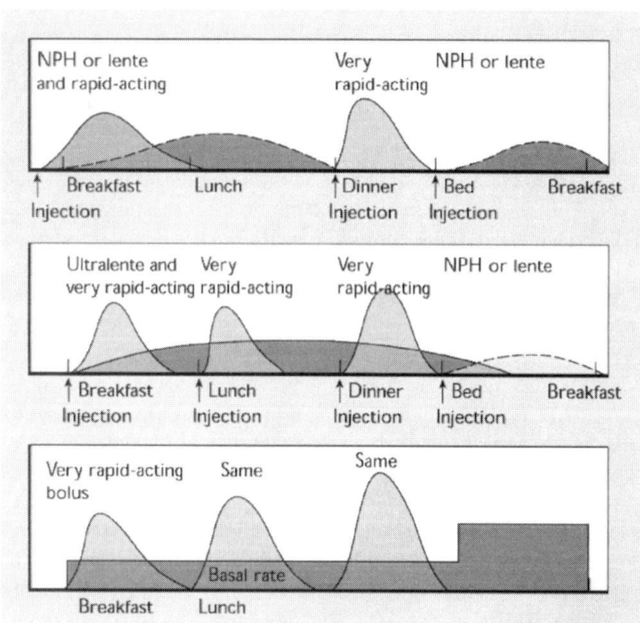

C

FIGURE 18-36. Insulin regimens to treat Type 1 diabetes. Ideally, combinations of insulin formulations are designed to provide basal insulin delivery plus sufficient insulin around meals to suppress postprandial glucose excursions. In (*a*), intermediate or long-acting insulins are combined with rapid-acting (regular) insulin and given once or twice per day. This minimal therapy may be adequate to avoid ketosis, but acceptable glycemic control is highly unlikely with these regimens. In (*b*), twice-per-day injections of intermediate and rapid-acting or very-rapid-acting insulin and ultralente (long-acting) and rapid- or very-rapid-acting insulins are adequate to lower glucose levels compared with the minimal regimen in 37 (*a*). Only rarely will these intermediate intensity regimens achieve a goal of HbA1c <7 percent. In (*c*), more physiologic patterns of insulin delivery are achieved with ≥ 3 injections or with delivery of rapid- or very-rapid-acting insulin with an insulin pump. These "intensive" regimens achieved HbA1c levels of approximately 7 percent in the DCCT. The long-term benefits of intensive therapy are accompanied by a threefold increase in hypoglycemia. (*From Nathan DM in Atlas of Endocrinology, 1999.*)

patients to use the same fixed ratio of NPH to regular insulin. Different formulations can be combined to provide insulin delivery that approximates normal physiology (Fig. 18-36).

The key elements of physiological insulin delivery include the provision of "basal" insulin to suppress unrestrained hepatic glucose output and inhibit ketogenesis in the postabsorptive (fasting) and interprandial periods, and administration of preprandial boluses of rapid- or very-rapid-acting insulin in doses sufficient to limit glucose excursions immediately after meals. The more complex regimens require more frequent injections and glucose tests to guide the choice of dose. Patients treated with intensive regimens have individual algorithms to help them select the correct dose of regular (rapid-acting) or very-rapid-acting insulin for a given blood glucose level, meal, and anticipated exercise.

The delayed onset of action of subcutaneous regular insulin obligates patients to administer preprandial insulin 30 to 60 min before the meal. The interval between injection and eating can be decreased to 10–15 min when lispro (very-rapid-acting) insulin is used.

In addition to basal and bolus insulin delivery, the insulin regimen must address the rise in insulin requirements that occurs in nondiabetics and diabetic patients between 4 and 6 A.M., the so-called dawn phenomenon. A nocturnal increase in growth hormone secretion appears to cause the dawn phenomenon. Intermediate-acting insulin given at bedtime, or an increase in the pump basal rate of regular insulin at 2–3 A.M. or of very-rapid-acting insulin at 3 to 4 A.M. is usually effective in suppressing the rise in blood glucose overnight.

Insulin delivery devices have been developed to facilitate the frequent administration of regular insulin that is part of intensive treatment regimens. Mechanical syringes, air jet injectors, battery-powered external pumps, and implantable pumps have all been shown to be effective in intensive regimens and can result in near normal glycemia.[347,348] Similar metabolic results can be obtained with multiple (≥ 3) daily injections or continuous subcutaneous insulin infusion with an external pump.[318] The major risk shared by all intensive regimens, with the exception of implantable pump therapy,[348,349] is a two- to three-fold increase in severe hypoglycemia (see section on complications of insulin therapy later).[320] In addition, the devices that use subcutaneous catheters can result in inflammation or infections at the catheter insertion sites.[319] Finally, weight gain occurs commonly with intensive therapies, owing to decreased caloric loss with reduced glycosuria, treatment of hypoglycemia, and a decrease in basal metabolic rate as glycemia is normalized.[319]

Diet Therapy

Diet therapy is a crucial component of diabetes care. As with monitoring and insulin therapy, different levels of therapeutic intensity should be chosen based on the patient's lifestyle, motivation, and overall goals of diabetes care (Table 18-17). Moreover, the amount of attention focused on diet should be integrated into a consistent approach. Intensive treatment strategies generally require a different level of attention than a therapeutic program with less intensive metabolic goals.[350]

The fundamental aspects of a diet for Type 1 diabetes include consistent, regular meals (to facilitate matching insulin doses to meals and to avoid hypoglycemia) with high carbohydrate (45–50 percent of calories), low-fat (<30 percent of calories), and low-cholesterol (<300 mg) content.[351] In addition, limiting concentrated sweets prevents frequent, exuberant increases in blood glucose levels that are difficult to control. However, the opportunity to inject rapid- or very-rapid-acting insulin frequently and easily, using insulin pumps or pen-devices, can loosen these restrictions, allowing patients to have sweet snacks without paying the penalty of high glucose excursions.[352] When intensive metabolic goals are not achieved, the problem can often be tracked back to inconsistent meal times and content, and the failure of the patient to accommodate specific meals with the appropriate amount of insulin.

A variety of exchange lists help patients maintain similar carbohydrate content from meal to meal and facilitate the choice of insulin doses.[353] Alternatively, "carbohydrate counting" approaches provide the patient treated intensively with a guideline to the amount of carbohydrate in a particular food and meal and help guide the choice of the preprandial dose.[354] Appreciation that different carbohydrates have different rates of digestion and impact on glucose levels[355] has led to the use of glycemic indices, which take into account the differential effect of different carbohydrate containing foods on glucose levels. Although the glycemic index applies when single foods are eaten, its relevance in the setting of complex meals when different food types with variable fat, carbohydrate, and protein mix in the stomach, has been questioned.[356,357] Given the importance of diet in management of Type 1 diabetes, a dietitian should be incorporated as part of the health care team.

In addition to the important role of diet, integrated with the insulin and exercise regimen, in achieving glucose goals, therapeutic diets should include attention to fat content. Although persons with Type 1 diabetes don't have the same constellation of cardiovascular disease (CVD) risk factors as found in Type 2 diabetes, they are also at heightened risk for CVD, especially in the setting of renal dysfunction. A prudent low-fat diet, as recommended by the American Diabetes Association and the American Heart Association, is appropriate for all patients with Type 1 diabetes.[351,358] For patients with hypercholesterolemia or other CVD risk factors, the National Cholesterol Education Program (NCEP) guidelines [359] have been adapted for the diabetic population (Table 18-20).[341] The primary goal of limiting dietary fat and cholesterol is to decrease cardiovascular risk; however, an additional goal is limiting calorically dense, i.e., fat-rich, foods in order to prevent or control the excess weight gain that occurs with intensive therapies.[319] Other aspects of nutritional therapy for patients with Type 1 diabetes include limited salt diets for patients with hypertension, congestive heart failure, or renal failure; low-potassium diets for patients with hyporeninemic hypoaldosteronism or renal failure; and low-protein diets for patients with renal dysfunction.[360]

TABLE 18-20. Lipid Goals for Diabetic Patients

	LDL-Cholesterol Goals			
	Medical Nutrition Therapy		*Drug Therapy*	
	Initiation Level	**Goal**	**Initiation Level**	**Goal**
With CVD	>100 mg/dL	≤100	>100	≤100
Without CVD	>100	≤100	≥130*	≤100

*Therapy with medications is recommended by many experts for LDL 100–130 in the setting of multiple risk factors, such as low HDL (<35 mg/dL), hypertension, smoking, positive family history of CVD, or proteinuria. Medical nutrition therapy should always by instituted prior to any drug therapy. For elevated triglyceride levels, improved glycemic control (in addition to low—<10 percent—fat diet, increased exercise and elimination of alcohol) will often ameliorate triglyceride levels. Drug therapy with a fibric acid should be instituted for triglyceride levels >1,000 mg/dL to decrease the risk of pancreatitis. Levels that remain greater than 400 mg/dL after dietary and life-style modification should also usually be treated with drugs. No evidence supports more rigorous therapy.

From American Diabetes Association. *Diabetes Care* 22:S56, 1999.

Exercise

Exercise is another component of diabetes care that must be integrated into the treatment program.[361] In addition to its cardiovascular benefits, aerobic exercise, if performed on a frequent basis,[362] can reduce insulin resistance. Patients must be instructed to adjust meals and/or insulin to prevent hypoglycemia during, immediately after, or even 6–12 hours after exercise. In nondiabetics, the balance between increased glucose utilization by exercising muscle and increased hepatic glucose output, which maintains stable blood glucose levels, is mediated by a decrease in insulin levels and an increase in catecholamines (Fig. 18-37a). In the diabetic patient, any imbalance in these levels can lead to hypoglycemia or hyperglycemia. If insulin levels are too low, as occurs in inadequately replaced, hypoinsulinemic Type 1 diabetics, the catecholamine surge associated with exercise and low insulin levels lead to excessive hepatic glucose production. In addition, the low insulin levels decrease glucose transport into muscle and liver and increase the likelihood of ketogenesis. In this setting, exercise may not lower glucose levels but, paradoxically, can lead to worse hyperglycemia and ketosis (Fig. 18-37b). Conversely, if insulin levels are inappropriately high at the time of exercise, glucose uptake by the recovering muscle is heightened and hepatic glucose production is suppressed, leading to hypoglycemia (Fig. 18-37c). Hypoglycemia that occurs 4–8 hours or more after exercise is a result of continued glucose uptake by recovering muscle.[363]

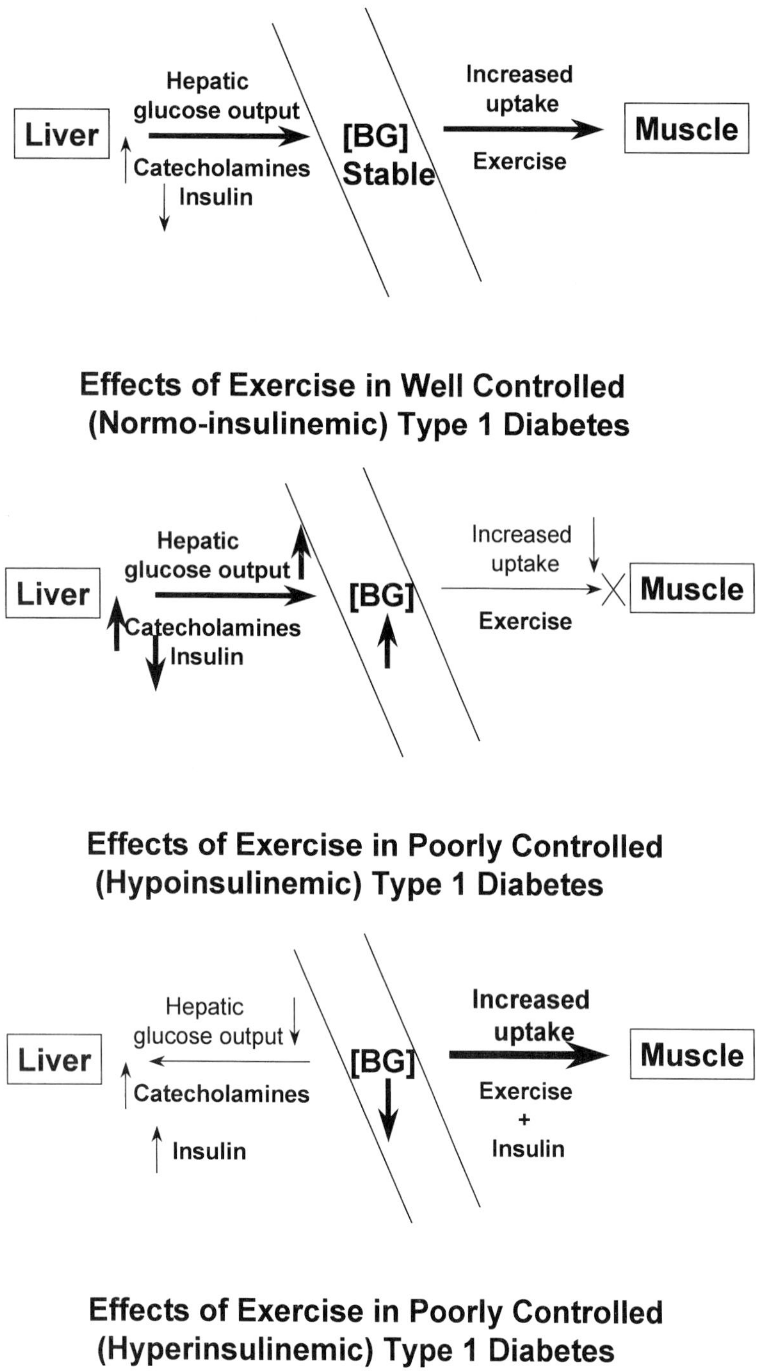

FIGURE 18-37. Physiology of glucose homeostasis during and after exercise in (*a*) well controlled diabetic patients with physiologic supply of insulin; (*b*) in the presence of inadequate insulin; and (*c*) in the presence of excessive insulin.

Intensive therapy regimens that aim to replace insulin physiologically can be adjusted to accommodate exercise.[364,365] Depending on the timing of exercise, preprandial doses of rapid- or very-rapid-acting insulin, or the longer-acting insulins can be adjusted. With continuous subcutaneous insulin infusion, pump infusion can often be suspended during 1–2 hours of moderate or intensive exercise and then restarted.

Particular care must be taken to ensure that patients don't have cardiovascular disease, especially in view of the masked or atypical symptoms that may occur in the setting of autonomic neuropathy. Exercise tolerance tests are highly recommended prior to instituting a more vigorous exercise program in any diabetic patient who may be at higher risk for CVD. In addition, high-impact sports can be particularly hazardous in patients with advanced retinopathy or in patients with peripheral neuropathy who are at risk for foot trauma.

Whole Organ Pancreas Transplantation

First attempted in 1966, whole organ pancreas transplantation has increasingly become an effective and relatively safe procedure.[366,367] The use of enteric or urinary bladder drainage of the exocrine drainage has surmounted, to a great extent, the obstacle of pancreatic inflammation and destruction that affected the early trials of pancreatic transplantation (Fig. 18-38). The immunologic

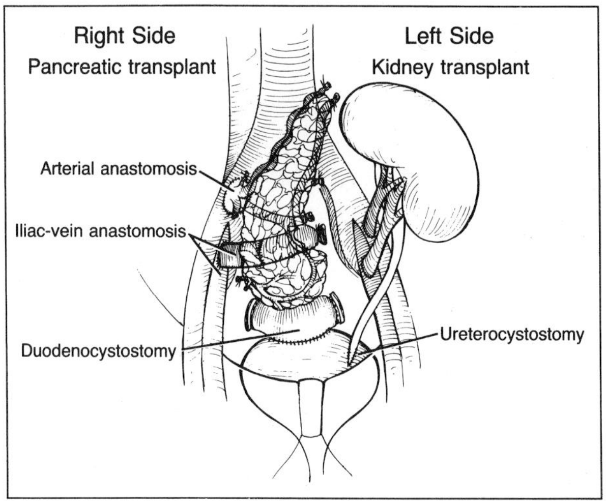

FIGURE 18-38. Whole organ pancreas transplantation with simultaneous renal transplantation. The donor pancreas is harvested with a duodenal cuff, the ends of which are oversewn. The duodenal cuff is attached to the dome of the bladder and exocrine secretion drains into the bladder, often requiring bicarbonate repletion. The endocrine pancreas is anastamosed to the peripheral circulation through the iliac artery and vein. The donor kidney is anastamosed to the peripheral circulation with attachment of the ureter to the bladder. (*From Robertson P. N Engl J Med 327:1861, 1992.*)

barriers of whole organ allotransplantation require life-long immunosuppression; however, improvements in immunosuppression have benefited pancreas transplantation similar to other organ transplantation. The requirement for general anesthesia, major surgery, and life-long immunosuppression has relegated most pancreas transplantation to be performed concurrent with cadaver kidney transplantation for patients with end-stage renal disease, because such patients assume the risk of surgery and immunosuppression for the kidney. Most centers performing pancreas transplantation consider the balance between the risk added when pancreas transplantation is combined with kidney transplantation and the benefit of eliminating the need for exogenous insulin acceptable. Only a minority of centers perform solitary cadaver pancreas transplantation or partial transplants from living related donors. Solitary pancreas transplantation has generally been reserved for patients with severe diabetic instability that causes major disruption in their schooling or employment. The hesitancy to perform solitary pancreas transplants on a more regular basis is based on the risk–benefit analysis above and the observation that the success rate (measured by achievement of normal glycemia without the need for exogenous hypoglycemic medications) is lower in solitary transplantation than with combined kidney-pancreas transplantation. The difference has widely been ascribed to the kidney transplant serving as a "sentinel" organ, alerting clinicians to impending rejection. With solitary pancreas transplantation, monitoring blood glucose levels or urinary amylase excretion is the only way to monitor the status of the transplant and is often not satisfactory.

The most successful programs have demonstrated greater than 90 percent patient and graft survival at 1–3 years.[366,367] In addition to eliminating the need for exogenous insulin and restoring true normoglycemia, pancreas transplantation has been shown to improve quality of life and reduce the development of diabetic nephropathic changes in the transplanted kidney and improve indices of neuropathy.[366,368–371] Because most programs have included only patients with advanced complications, the clinical significance of these changes remains arguable. In addition, no randomized, controlled trials have been done to compare the benefits and risks of combined kidney pancreas transplantation and kidney transplantation alone. As kidney transplantation has beneficial effects on long-term complications, well-matched control groups, i.e., diabetic kidney transplant recipients, are necessary to test any additional impact of the pancreas transplantation.

In addition to perioperative morbidity and mortality and rejection episodes, a variety of other complications including peripancreatic collections and effusions, sterile and bacterial peritonitis, and non-anion gap acidosis secondary to bicarbonate loss in the urine have required more frequent hospital admissions and care compared with kidney-only transplantation.[366] Availability of cadaver organs remains a significant barrier, especially because they must be harvested with extreme care. Several long-term pancreas transplants have lost function apparently secondary to recurrent autoimmune destruction of the islets, rather than to immune rejection.

Future Therapies

Experimental approaches to treatment include the development of new modified insulins, including insulin analogs, that provide more convenient and more physiologic insulin delivery; the development and refinement of insulin delivery devices, such as new automatic syringes and implantable pumps; alternative routes of insulin delivery such as nasal or inhaled insulin; the development of noninvasive or minimally invasive glucose monitors capable of providing frequent feedback to insulin delivery devices, effectively creating an artificial pancreas; and "biological" solutions to the challenge of restoring normal metabolism such as islet transplantation and engineered beta cells. Some of these new methods have already been advanced and ushered into clinical practice, while others have defied long-term intensive study and remain tantalizing opportunities.

The first approved insulin analog, lispro insulin, was designed to provide a more rapid acting and shorter duration insulin than regular (clear zinc) insulin.[372] Regular insulin tends to self-aggregate, forming hexamers that must dissociate to monomers and dimers before they can be absorbed. Reversing the order of the proline and lysine located at positions 28 and 29, respectively, on the beta chain reduces the tendency of insulin to self-aggregate and results in an insulin that is predominantly monomeric and has an onset of action within 10–15 minutes of injection and an offset of action by four hours. Lispro insulin has been used in MDI and external pump regimens,[373] proving to be more convenient[374] than regular insulin because it can be injected shortly before the meal, and resulting in a modest decrease in hypoglycemia because of its shorter duration of action.[375] Its shorter duration requires adjustments to intermediate- and long-acting insulins.[376] Other insulin analogs under development are designed to provide a wide spectrum of action.[377] Previous clinical studies with proinsulin, initiated because of the putative liver specificity of proinsulin's bioactivity, were suspended owing to an apparent increase in cardiovascular morbidity and mortality.[378]

Alternative routes of insulin administration, prompted by the desire to avoid the inconvenience and discomfort of injections and to decrease the delay in absorption and inconsistent profiles associated with subcutaneous injection, have been explored for more than 30 years. Insulin has been administered by nasal insufflation

TABLE 18-21. Whole Organ vs. Islet Transplantation

	Transplantation	
	Whole Organ	*Islet*
Procedure	Major surgery Exocrine drainage necessary	Infusion No exocrine drainage
Immunosuppression	Major immunosuppression	Potential for limited or no immunosuppression—masking epitopes
Donor	Human source Single donor	Animal sources possible Potential multiple donors
Success (normoglycemia without hypoglycemic agents 1 year posttransplant)	>90 percent	<10 percent

with transmucosal absorption enhanced with the use of detergents,[379] rectally, transdermally using ultrasound,[380] and by inhalation.[381] Inhaled insulin appears to be well absorbed, but consistency of absorption and long-term safety need to be established.

Insulin delivery with implantable pumps has the theoretical advantage of eliminating the need for insulin injections and providing more physiologic profiles and delivery.[382] Implantable pumps, placed in subcutaneous pockets like a pacemaker, deliver insulin intravenously or intraperitoneally and can be controlled by telemetry. They have been tested in long-term (>3 year) studies and found to be safe, well tolerated, and capable of achieving near-normal glycemia in Type 1[348,383] and Type 2[384] diabetic patients. Although the level of glycemia achieved in long-term studies is similar to that achieved by conventional intensive regimens, the frequency of hypoglycemia is substantially less.[348,349] Quality of life has been improved in patients treated with implantable pumps.[348] The ultimate goal of such pumps is to connect them to continuous glucose monitoring with dosing adjusted automatically, thus creating a true artificial pancreas. The absence of reliable continuous monitoring has precluded "closing the loop" and made implantable pumps less appealing.

One of the holy grails in clinical diabetes research has been the development of noninvasive monitors capable of providing continuous feedback of ambient glucose levels.[385] The results of such monitoring could be connected with an external or implantable pump, which could be programmed to maintain glucose in the near normal range. Reliable implantable and external pumps have already been developed (see previous discussion) and the algorithms to control glycemia have been tested with indwelling sensors.[386,387] The critical link, continuous noninvasive monitoring, has proved elusive. Recent advances include microdialysis and iontophoresis as means of sampling interstitial fluid[388]; however, technical barriers, including assay drift, continue to impede the development of reliable long-term monitors using enzymatic, e.g., hexokinase, or noble metal sensors.[385] Difficulty in detecting a clear and unique signal for glucose using infrared spectroscopy has been one of the barriers to the development of reliable noninvasive monitoring. Signal drift and the need to calibrate frequently have also been major obstacles. The form of continuous monitoring that is most likely to be available in the near future will use implanted catheters and interstitial sampling.

Other metabolic therapies of Type 1 diabetes have been studied. Administration of C-peptide, which has no intrinsic metabolic activity, has been suggested as a means to decrease complications, specifically neuropathy.[47,48] Insulin-like growth factor-1 (IGF-1) has metabolic activity mediated by binding to its own receptor, or, with large enough doses, to the insulin receptor. It has been studied in both Type 1 and Type 2 diabetes and shown to lower glycemia.[389,390] In addition, the frequency of hypoglycemia may be decreased compared to treatment with insulin alone. Enthusiasm for IGF therapy, which was envisioned as an adjunct with, and not a replacement for, insulin, has waned owing to concern regarding the potential role of IGF in the pathogenesis of retinopathy and oncogenesis.

Finally, recognition of the major barriers to widespread whole organ transplantation, including the need for major surgery and lifelong immunosuppression, limited organ supply, and early and late perioperative complications, has spurred investigation into isolated islet transplantation as a potential cure for Type 1 diabetes (Table 18-21).[391] Islet isolation, purification, and transplantation have been intensively investigated for almost 30 years. Animal and human source islets have been studied and allografts and autografts have been successfully performed in humans.[392–394] In animal models of diabetes, cross-species (xenografts) islet transplantation has been accomplished[395] by masking immunogenic sites on the donor islets, giving rise to the prospect of using animal source islets for human transplantation in the future. In humans, isolation and purification of large numbers of islets with infusion into the liver (either through the umbilical vein or portal vein) has been effective in preventing diabetes in patients undergoing pancreatectomy because of chronic pancreatitis (autografting) or because of widespread malignancy (allografting with multiple other organs, so called "cluster" transplants).[392,393] However, results in human autoimmune diabetes have been far less successful, with less than 10 percent of islet recipients having normal glycemia restored without the need for exogenous insulin. The poor results have occurred even with large numbers (>5,000 islets per kg body weight) of highly purified, viable islets being transplanted with immunosuppression capable of abrogating whole organ rejection. One likely explanation for the failure of these programs is that the autoimmune process that caused diabetes in the first place is interfering with successful engraftment. The success of islet transplantation in nonimmune diabetes, e.g., after pancreatectomy, reinforces this explanation. Other possible explanations for the lack of success of these programs include: vulnerability of transplanted islets to either endogenous or exogenous toxins, or to immune destruction, especially given their lack of vascularization immediately after transplantation; the inhospitable environment of the liver, into which most islets have been transplanted; or the toxic effects of immunosuppressive agents, such as cyclosporin or pred-

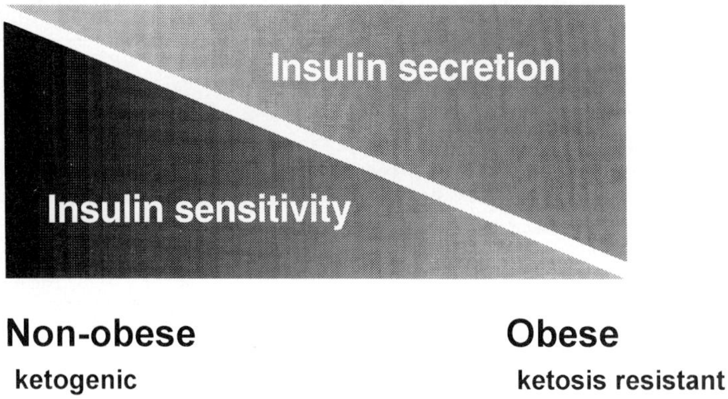

FIGURE 18-39. Pathophysiology of Type 2 diabetes. Type 2 diabetes may occur with any combination of abnormal insulin sensitivity (insulin resistance) and/or insulin deficiency. Some patients may develop Type 2 diabetes with normal insulin sensitivity but deficient secretion, while others may have relatively high secretory rates with very decreased sensitivity. The heterogeneous pathophysiology suggests more than one cause of Type 2 diabetes.

nisone on islets (cyclosporin has direct effects on islets while prednisone adversely affects islets by causing hyperglycemia). Unfortunately, all studies of human islet transplantation have failed to examine the islets after they fail, making it difficult to understand the source of islet failure. One recent study, using repeated transplantation of uncultured islets and avoiding prednisone in the immuno-suppression regimen, has demonstrated a high degree of success in restoring normoglycemia to Type 1 diabetic patients without prior kidney transplantation.[395a] This approach must be confirmed.

Innovative programs that mask immunogenic sites on the islets,[395] block specific effectors of islet rejection such as anti-CD 154 antibodies,[396] immunoprotect islets by sequestering them in capsules,[397] or try to induce immune tolerance to transplanted tissues are underway. Most of these programs are examining new means of specific immunosuppression and are not focusing on alternative sites for transplantation.

The source of insulin producing cells is of great interest, especially because availability of human organs would likely be a limiting factor. Masking programs that have allowed xenografting in animals make transplantation of pig islets into humans, for example, a possibility. Other studies have concentrated on "bioengineering" cells to behave like beta cells.[398] Although genetic manipulation can insert the gene for human insulin into fibroblasts and convert them into insulin secreting cells, the transformation of such cells into glucose sensing cells with regulated insulin secretion is a far greater challenge.

Prevention of Type 1 Diabetes

Previous attempts to prevent the development of Type 1 diabetes have relied on identification of persons at high risk and the use of immunosuppressants or immunomodulating agents.[398a–398e] "High-risk" patients were originally identified after the clinical onset of diabetes, usually with the first episode of ketoacidosis, but with residual functioning β-cells present. Treatment with prednisone, azathioprine, or cyclosporin A appeared to prolong β-cell function in these poorly controlled studies, albeit variably. As soon as the immunosuppressant agent was stopped, any evidence of a prolonged "honeymoon" period rapidly disappeared. More recent studies have tried to identify at-risk individuals prior to the autoimmune destruction of most of their β-cells. First degree relatives of Type 1 diabetic patients with high titers of anti-islet cell antibodies and/or evidence of early β-cell dysfunction have been selected for these studies. In addition to studies with immunosuppressants, trials using insulin therapy with the goal of sparing β-cell function, and perhaps immunomodulating the autoimmune destruction, have been initiated. To date, no interventions have been shown to have a convincing lasting effect in delaying the onset of Type 1 diabetes.

Therapy of Type 2 Diabetes

Pathophysiology Relevant to Therapy

Although the principal or initial metabolic abnormality that underlies Type 2 diabetes remains controversial, everyone agrees that Type 2 diabetes is the result of both insulin resistance (decreased sensitivity to insulin action) and deficient insulin secretion.[399] Most patients who develop Type 2 diabetes progress through a stage of worsening postprandial hyperglycemia (impaired glucose tolerance), probably genetically mediated and caused by insulin resistance, and then subsequently develop even higher postprandial glycemia and ultimately fasting hyperglycemia when insulin secretion fails to keep up with the increased demand (Figs. 18-25 and 18-28).[226,234] Because only a minority of patients with insulin resistance, for example obese patients, develop Type 2 diabetes, the rate-limiting step in the development of Type 2 diabetes is probably the capacity to achieve and maintain high levels of insulin secretion in the face of insulin resistance. Those persons who can't maintain insulin secretion develop Type 2 diabetes. Increased proinsulin secretion in this setting probably reflects the release of immature insulin secretory granules and is a function of a beta cell mass struggling to maintain normoglycemia.[235]

Patients with Type 2 diabetes do not suffer from the same autoimmune destruction of islet cell mass as patients with Type 1 diabetes; their insulin secretory failure appears to be predominantly functional, rather than anatomic. It is important to recognize that Type 2 diabetes may be caused by any combination of defective insulin secretion and increased resistance where the insulin sensitivity is so low that even high levels of secretion cannot compensate or where sensitivity is relatively normal but secretion is severely impaired (Fig. 18-39). Understanding the pathophysiologic feature that predominates in the individual patient with Type 2 diabetes may help to select more effective, directed therapy. Whether the relatively expensive attempts to characterize patients with Type 2 diabetes on the basis of degree of insulin resistance or C-peptide secretion provide more useful information than demographic or clinical features, such as body mass, remains to be shown.

The other important variable in the pathogenesis of Type 2 diabetes with regard to therapy is the toxic effect of hyperglycemia

TABLE 18-22. UKPDS Patient Characteristics at Baseline*

Age (yr)	53	Blood pressure (mm Hg)	135/82
Female (percent)	39	HbA1c (percent)	7.08
Race		Triglycerides (mg/dL)	208
Caucasian (percent)	81	Cholesterol (mg/dL)	209
Indian-Asian (percent)	10	LDL (mg/dL)	135
Afro-Caribbean (percent)	8	HDL (mg/dL)	41
Duration (yr)	<1	Retinopathy (percent)	36
Hypertension (percent)	27	Proteinuria >300 mg/dL (percent)	2
		Neuropathy (percent)	12

*Diagnosed within 1 year of enrollment in UKPDS. The presence of complications at baseline strongly suggests that diagnosis was made >1 year after the actual development of diabetes in a substantial fraction of the population.

on insulin resistance and insulin secretion, so called "glucotoxicity."[191] Regardless of the pathoetiology of Type 2 diabetes, any elevation in glycemic levels will secondarily result in increased resistance and decreased secretion. (This is also true in evolving Type 1 diabetes.) Animal models of Type 2 diabetes and human studies have demonstrated that the glucotoxic effect, especially on the beta cell, is reversible to a limited degree. Lowering fasting glycemia to the normal or near-normal range by almost any means, including diet, sulfonylurea, or insulin, will improve insulin secretion.[239-242]

The relevance of these observations to treatment of Type 2 diabetes is the following: (1) therapy can be directed at reducing resistance, improving secretion, or altering the rate of delivery of glucose from the gut; (2) any treatment that decreases glycemic levels will be effectively amplified through improved endogenous insulin secretion (improved glycemia begets further improvement in glycemia); and (3) conversely, worsening glycemia further hampers insulin secretion, resulting in a vicious cycle of higher and higher glucose levels with progressively lower insulin secretion.

Metabolic Goals of Therapy—UKPDS

The DCCT demonstrated the role of intensive therapy in decreasing the risk of development and progression of all diabetes-specific complications in Type 1 diabetes, and in doing so, established justifiable metabolic goals of therapy.[13] Whether the lessons learned in the DCCT applied to patients with Type 2 diabetes was unclear until recently, as almost no comparable data existed for Type 2 diabetes.[400] However, a recent study in Japanese patients virtually duplicated the results of the DCCT in insulin-treated patients with Type 2 diabetes.[302] Retinopathy and neuropathy were reduced by intensive therapy that decreased HbA1c to a mean of 7.1 percent, compared with 9.4 percent in the conventional treatment group, over 6 years. Intensive therapy decreased the average risk of worsening retinopathy and nephropathy by 69 percent and 70 percent, respectively, compared with conventional diabetes management. The results of this study would have been more compelling if the Japanese Type 2 diabetes patients had resembled non-Asian Type 2 diabetes patients more than they did. Typical for most Japanese Type 2 diabetics, they were relatively thin and required extremely small doses of insulin.

If there was any residual doubt regarding the role of intensive therapy in Type 2 diabetes, the United Kingdom Prospective Diabetes Study (UKPDS) finally settled the issue.[17,286] Originally planned and initiated in 1977 in order to address the confusion left by the University Group Diabetes Program (UGDP) results,[401] the UKPDS results were published in 1998. The UGDP had failed to establish a benefit of intensive therapy (sulfonylurea, phenformin, standard dose insulin based on body mass, or variable dose insulin adjusted for glucose results), compared with diet therapy, on long-term complications. Unfortunately, the means of measuring the complications were insensitive and the study may have been underpowered. After more than 9 years of therapy, there were no significant differences in outcomes among the therapies, despite significantly lower mean fasting glucose levels achieved in the variable dose insulin group. An unexpected finding, which captured the headlines at the time, was a higher rate (1 percent per year) of cardiovascular mortality in the sulfonylurea-treated group.

UKPDS Design The UKPDS was originally designed to answer two questions: (1) Is an "intensive strategy" aimed at achieving fasting glucose levels <6 mmol (108 mg/dL) superior to conventional therapy with diet in preventing the complications of diabetes in patients with relatively recent onset Type 2 diabetes (Table 18-22)[402] and (2) Are any glucose lowering therapies particularly advantageous or disadvantageous with regard to preventing or delaying diabetic complications? The outcomes were aggregated into diabetes-specific complications (combining retinopathy, nephropathy, cataracts, and cardiovascular outcomes), all-cause mortality, and diabetes-related mortality.

The study design included stepwise addition of therapies in the conventional and intensive treatment groups if glucose goals were not met. The intensive therapies were numerous including three types of sulfonylureas and insulin (Fig. 18-40). The obese subset of patients were also randomly assigned to metformin. Metabolic control in the UKPDS worsened over time (Fig. 18-41a), regardless of treatment assignment, and required the addition of alternative therapies to the originally assigned therapy.[17,236,286] Over the course of the study, the majority of conventional treatment subjects had one or more of the intensive therapies added, and a substantial fraction (often ≥ 20 percent) of the intensive treatment subjects had the alternative intensive therapies added or substituted for their originally assigned intensive therapy. This design feature, which was intended to keep glycemia as low as possible in the intensive treatment group, severely undercut the comparison of the specific intensive therapy modalities.[305] Finally, other randomized interventions (early addition of metformin or insulin to sulfonylurea therapy if fasting plasma glucose was greater than 6 mmol, use of acarbose, and intensive vs. conventional hypertension treatment) made the UKPDS protocol byzantine in its complexity.

UKPDS Results The UKPDS results, analyzed by intention to treat, revealed a benefit of intensive therapy, which lowered

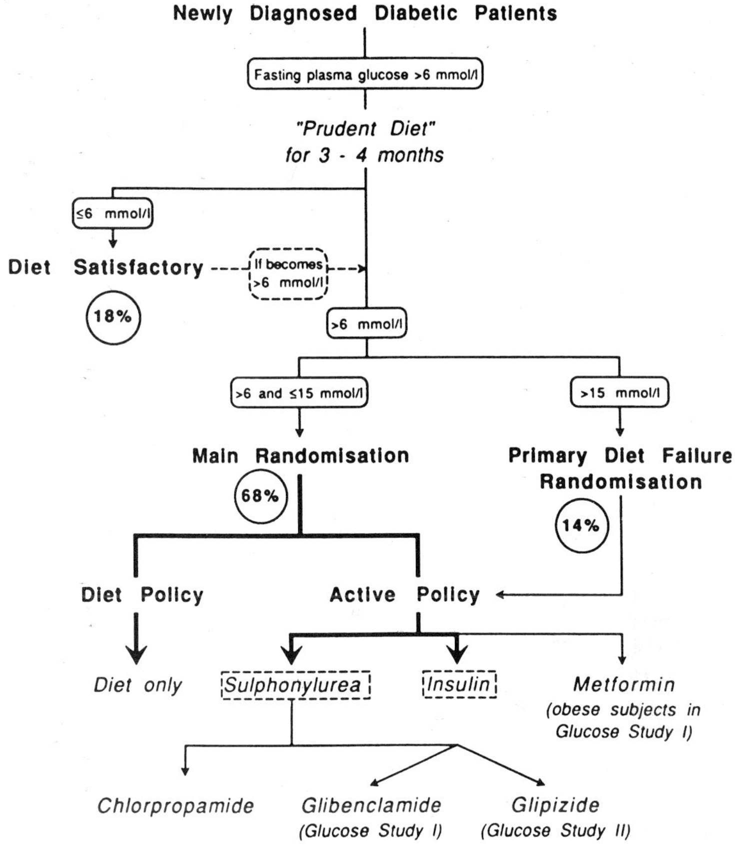

FIGURE 18-40. Design of United Kingdom Prospective Diabetes Study (UKPDS). After randomized assignment to treatment groups, conventional ("diet policy") and intensive ("active policy") subjects could have other therapies added if glycemic goals were not being met. In practice, more than one-half of the subjects assigned to conventional therapy had one or more medications added and variable fractions of the specific drug therapy groups had other medications added, or were changed to other medications (e.g., metformin added to sulfonylurea, or sufonylurea-treated subjects changed to insulin) over the course of the study. This stepped intervention strategy made comparison between the different medication groups problematic. (*From the UKPDS Research Group.*[402])

HbA1c by 1 percent absolute (11 percent relative reduction), on the development of the aggregate diabetes outcomes, decreasing risk by 12 percent.[17] This benefit was predicated to a great extent on a beneficial effect on retinopathy and cataracts. There was no significant benefit with regard to cardiovascular disease (Table 18-23). Of interest, glycemic control was not appreciably different in patients randomly assigned to insulin therapy compared with those assigned to sulfonylurea or metformin. The failure to achieve, or maintain, lower glycemia in the insulin-treated subjects may have been due to the reluctance to use the large doses of insulin necessary to control glycemia. The mean daily insulin dose was 0.42 units/kg (median daily dose of 24 units in the subjects with BMI < 25 and 60 units in the obese subjects with BMI > 35) at 12 years. The investigators ascribed the relatively low doses of insulin to concern, on the part of clinicians and patients, regarding hypoglycemia and weight gain.

The results with metformin in the overweight subjects were analyzed separately as diet therapy vs. metformin therapy, excluding the sulfonylurea- and insulin-treated overweight subjects from the primary analysis.[286] (The validity of this analytic strategy has been called into question.[305]) Metformin therapy resulted in less weight gain and hypoglycemia than other intensive therapies. In addition, aggregate diabetes mortality, but not diabetes-related outcomes, was significantly reduced by metformin.[286] Conversely, early addition of metformin to sulfonylurea resulted in a large and statistically significant increase in cardiovascular mortality. The complex design, numerous crossovers, and controversial analytic strategy of the UKPDS cast some of its results into question. However, the fundamental observation that intensive diabetes management improves outcome, specifically microvascular outcomes, is unquestionable. Secondary, epidemiologic analyses of the UKPDS data have shown that there is a continuum of decreased risk for the development of complications with lower levels of glycosylated hemoglobin (35 percent reduction in microvascular complications for every 1 percent decrease in HbA1c), with no apparent threshold.[403] These results mirror those of the DCCT in Type 1 diabetes.[323]

The results of the UKPDS and Kumamoto study have established intensive therapy with the goal of normoglycemia as the most appropriate therapy to decrease long-term complications in Type 2 diabetes, similar to Type 1 diabetes. These goals have been widely endorsed.[404] As with Type 1 diabetes, the balance between risks/costs and benefits may vary for specific groups of patients, and metabolic goals may need to be modified.[405] For example, older persons with Type 2 diabetes may not experience the same benefit from intensive therapy with regard to long-term complications by virtue of having a shorter projected life-span.

Therapeutic options

While intensive therapy goals were clearly established by the UKPDS, the best means of achieving those goals remain less clear. Moreover, the balance among benefits, risks, and cost is not well understood. Although the UKPDS did not provide a clear answer with regard to the most advantageous choice of therapies, it was reassuring with regard to the safety of insulin, metformin, and sulfonylurea monotherapy. The UGDP findings of excessive cardiovascular disease with tolbutamide and phenformin[401] were not confirmed by the UKPDS; moreover, concern regarding potential

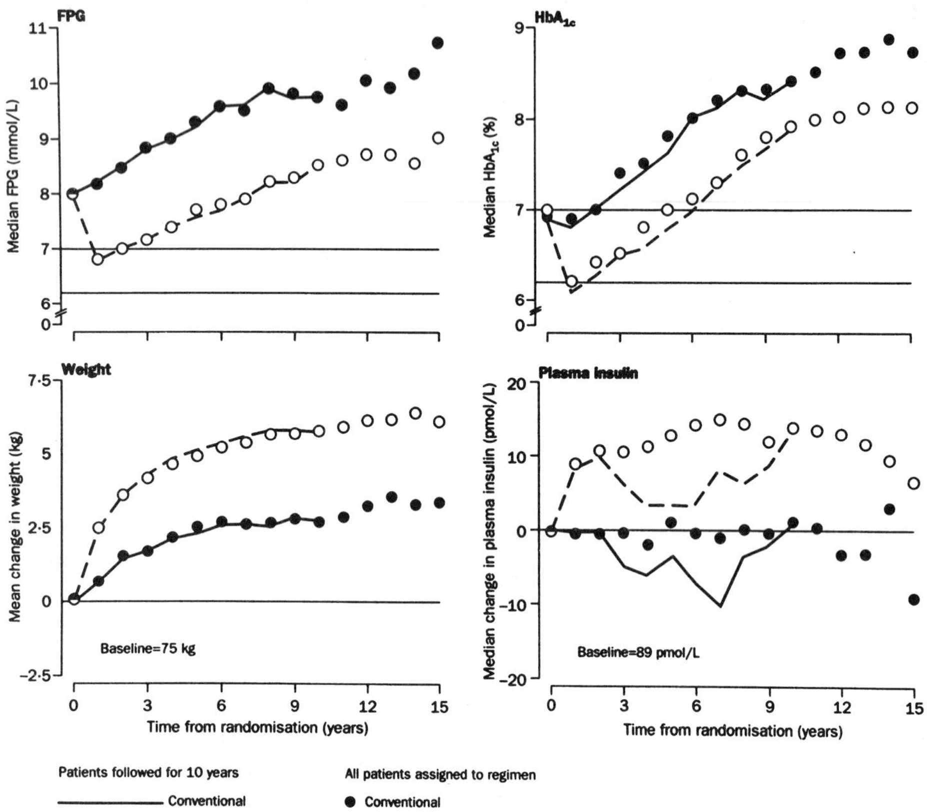

FIGURE 18-41. Results of United Kingdom Prospective Diabetes Study for nonobese and obese subjects randomly assigned to conventional treatment with "diet policy" or to intensive therapy with sulfonylureas or insulin. (*From UKPDS Research Group.*[17])

cardiovascular toxicity of exogenous insulin therapy[406] was also assuaged. None of the active monotherapies in the UKPDS was associated with excessive cardiovascular disease compared with the dietary intervention. Other, generally short-term, studies have contributed to understanding the benefits and risks of specific therapies and combinations of therapies.

The number and combinations of therapies, available for the treatment of Type 2 diabetes expanded in the 1990s, providing flexibility for practitioners and patients.[285] Whether the expanded number of therapies will achieve better (lower) glycemia than past regimens is not known. Many patients sequentially fail diet and oral agent therapy over time and are eventually treated with insulin. However, physicians and patients appear to be reluctant to use the relatively high doses of insulin necessary to achieve acceptable glucose control. Moreover, physicians have historically been unwilling to use insulin early in the clinical history, although recent studies demonstrate that patients can often achieve a remission of sorts with this strategy.[407] The usual pattern of therapy has included diet followed by the sequential addition of oral agents and finally insulin, either alone or in combination with oral agents. The transition from one therapy to the next has usually been slow. By the time patients are treated with insulin, they have many years of diabetes, and long-term complications are often present.

Diet and Exercise Because obesity[201] and a sedentary lifestyle[215,216] are well-recognized risk factors for the development of Type 2 diabetes, it should not be surprising that manipulation of these two environmental factors would be used as first-line

TABLE 18-23. Major UKPDS Findings

Nonobese + Obese	Obese Only
Intensive therapy **reduced***	Metformin **reduced***
Aggregate diabetes outcomes by 12 percent, P = .029	Aggregated diabetes outcomes by 32 percent, P = .003
Laser therapy by 29 percent, P = .003	Diabetes related death by 42 percent, P = .02
Cataract extraction by 24 percent, P = .046	All cause death by 36 percent, P = .011
Sudden death by 46 percent, P = .047	Metformin **did not reduce**
Intensive therapy **did not** reduce	Laser therapy—31 percent, P = .17
Diabetes-related deaths—10 percent, P = .34	
All cause mortality—6 percent, P = .44	
Fatal MI—6 percent, P = .63	
Nonfatal MI—21 percent, P = .057	
Renal failure—27 percent, P = .45	

*Compared with conventional therapy.

TABLE 18-24. Dietary Recommendations for Diabetes Mellitus

	Type 1	Type 2
Overall goals	Maintenance of near-normal glucose levels including prevention of hypoglycemia. Normal growth and development. Maintenance of "reasonable" weight. Maintenance of optimal lipid levels.	
Calories	Adequate for growth & development.* Meals should be consistent in timing and caloric content to facilitate matching insulin to caloric intake.	For the 90 percent of patients who are obese, realistic hypocaloric diet to achieve weight loss. Frequent small (vs. infrequent large) meals preferable.*
Carbohydrate (percent of daily calories)	≈ 50 percent	≈ 50 percent
Fat (percent of daily calories)		
Total	<30 percent	<30 percent
Saturated	<10 percent†	<10 percent†
Monounsaturated	≥10 percent	≥10 percent
Cholesterol	<300 mg/d†	<300 mg/d†
Protein	0.8 g/kg*	0.8 g/kg*
Renal failure	0.6 g/kg	0.6 g/kg
Fiber (dietary)	20–35 g/d	20–35 g/d

* Adjusted for children for growth, and for women during pregnancy and breast feeding.

† Saturated fat and daily cholesterol reduced to <7 percent and <200 mg/d, respectively (NCEP step 2 diet), if LDL levels elevated, CAD present, or ≥2 CVD risk factors present.

Source: Adapted from American Diabetes Association "Nutrition Recommendations and Principles for People with Diabetes Mellitus." *Diabetes Care* 22:S42, 1999.

therapy. Numerous studies, almost all short-term, have demonstrated the beneficial effect of diet (predominantly hypocaloric diets to achieve weight loss), with or without exercise, on hyperglycemia.[408–411] Only a modest degree of weight loss is often required to ameliorate hyperglycemia.[408,411] The major feature of medical nutrition therapy (MNT) necessary to ameliorate hyperglycemia is a hypocaloric diet, which improves glycemia, insulin secretion, insulin resistance, and dyslipidemia acutely, even before significant weight loss has occurred.[412] Other features of MNT, such as limitation of fat content, substituting complex for simple carbohydrates, substitution of monounsaturated for saturated fat, and the use of high fiber diets have been used to effect weight loss, decrease glycemic levels, and decrease cardiovascular risk.[413–415,415a] Although a high carbohydrate, high fiber diet has been recommended (Table 18-24), a prolonged debate regarding the relative benefits of high (> 50 percent) complex carbohydrate vs. relatively higher-fat diets, with polyunsaturated and monounsaturated fats, has been waged without a consensus.[416,417]

Despite the demonstrated benefit of dietary intervention, long-term results have been abysmal. The rate of recidivism, defined as patients returning to their previous weight and hyperglycemia, or redeveloping hyperglycemia even if they maintain a lower weight, is very high, even within a year of the original MNT. The United Kingdom Prospective Diabetes Study provides the largest prospective trial that examines the impact of diet on Type 2 diabetes, albeit in a group of patients with relatively brief duration (within 1 year of diagnosis), only modest hyperglycemia, and only moderately intensive diet intervention (Fig. 18-41).[17,286] The poor results of dietary therapy were recognized almost 30 years ago by Kelly West in "Diet therapy of diabetes: an analysis of failure."[418] Relatively little has changed in the ensuing three decades, although behavioral strategies have modestly improved results of MNT.[419] In addition, therapies other than MNT that promote or achieve weight loss, including pharmacotherapy[420] and bariatric surgery,[421] have successfully ameliorated glucose intolerance and virtually all other metabolic sequelae of diabetes and obesity.

Exercise has been employed as an adjunct to MNT to increase caloric expenditure, promote weight loss, and improve aerobic conditioning. In addition, regularly performed exercise decreases insulin resistance.[362] The high prevalence of cardiovascular disease, including relatively asymptomatic CVD, in the Type 2 diabetic population dictates careful clinical assessment, often with exercise tolerance testing, prior to beginning a new exercise regimen. In addition, patients with sensory neuropathy and/or peripheral vascular disease must be instructed to avoid foot trauma. Patients with active proliferative retinopathy should also be instructed to avoid high-impact exercise, which might precipitate bleeding.

Medications The eventual failure of MNT in the vast majority of overweight Type 2 diabetic patients means that the majority of Type 2 diabetes patients will require hypoglycemic medication(s) (Table 18-25) in addition to diet and exercise if normoglycemia is the goal.

Sulfonylureas are a relatively old class of drugs, developed almost fifty years ago (Fig. 18-42).[422] The first generation drugs (chlorpropamide, tolbutamide, acetohexamide, and tolazamide) have largely been supplanted by a "second generation" (glyburide and glibenclamide, and more recently glimepiride) which has been available for more than a decade. The second generation sulfonylureas are more potent on a mg-per-mg basis and have fewer drug interactions and side effects, but generally have the same mechanism of action and limitations as the first generation drugs (Table 18-26). At maximal doses, the second generation sulfonylureas are no more potent than most of the first generation agents.[423].

Sulfonylureas act almost entirely by stimulating insulin secretion through binding to a specific beta cell receptor, the sulphonylurea receptor (SUR1).[68] The receptor is part of the ATP sensitive K^+ channel (KIR) complex that maintains intracellular potassium concentrations and depolarization. Binding of sulfonylurea to the receptor results in closure of the ATP-sensitive potassium channels with depolarization of the cell and consequent opening of the

TABLE 18-25. Comparison of Type 2 Diabetes Therapies

	Diet	Sulfonylurea*	Biguanides	Acarbose	TZD@	Insulin
Metabolic effects						
Improves						
Resistance	++	+	+	+	+++	+
Secretion	+	++	−	+	−	−
Overnight HGO	+	+	++	−	+	++
Postprandial bg excursions	+	+	+	++	+	++
Atherogenic† lipid profiles	++	+	+	+	+	++
Lowers						
Insulin levels	++	−	+	+	++	−
Free fatty acids	+	+	+	+	+	+
Weight gain∞	−	+	−	−	+	++
Hypoglycemia∞	−	+	−	−	−	+
Allergies	−	+	+	+	+	+
Other side effects						
Antabuse effect	−	+‡	−	−	−	−
Hyponatremia	−	+‡	−	−	−	−
Lactic acidosis	−	−	+#	−	−	−
Gastrointestinal	−	−	+	++	−	−
Liver function abnl.	−	−	−	−	+$^{\alpha}$	−

*Repaglinide probably has similar characteristics, except for possibly less hypoglycemia.

†Lowers triglycerides and VLDL-cholesterol. Insulin raises HDL-cholesterol. Troglitazone raises LDL- and HDL-cholesterol levels to a similar degree.

‡Uncommon with second generation sulfonylureas.

#Frequency <3/100,000 patient-years of use with metformin.

∞ When used in combination, most agents take on the adverse event profile of the more toxic drug. For example, weight gain is minimal with metformin as monotherapy, but is more prominent when it is used in combination with insulin or sulfonylurea.

$^{\alpha}$Elevated transaminase levels in ≈2 percent of patients treated with troglitazone; less frequent with other TZDs.

@TZD = thiazolidinediones include troglitazone, rosiglitazone, and pioglitazone. Although troglitazone was removed from the U.S. market, most published clinical data with TZDs are with troglitazone.

voltage-dependent calcium channel. Influx of calcium is the first step in stimulus-secretion coupling which ultimately leads to insulin secretion (Fig. 18-4). Sulfonylureas are ineffective in Type 1 diabetes patients and relatively impotent in thin Type 2 diabetes patients, who are usually insulin deficient. Because they stimulate insulin secretion, they can cause hypoglycemia. The longer acting agents (especially chlorpropamide) can cause severe, prolonged hypoglycemia.[424]

The sulfonylureas succeed in lowering glycemia in 85–90 percent of newly treated Type 2 diabetes patients (1° failure rate of 10–15 percent), lowering fasting plasma glucose and HbA1c levels by 50–70 mg/dL and 1–1.5 percent, respectively, in most monotherapy studies.[422] The secondary failure rate (patients redevelop hyperglycemia after an initial response) is approximately 10 percent per year.[425] Therefore, for a majority of Type 2 diabetic patients sulfonylurea therapy is only a temporizing measure; a second drug will need to be added (e.g., metformin or insulin) or substituted (insulin), usually within 5 years of starting a sulfonylurea, if achieving near-normal glycemia is the goal. The two longest interventional studies with sulfonylureas, the UGDP and UKPDS, both of which included patients with relatively mild hyperglycemia, demonstrated the transient efficacy of sulfonylureas.[17,401] After an initial response to sulfonylureas, glycemic control worsened such that glycemia had returned to baseline levels, or higher, within several years of beginning therapy.

In addition to chemical substitutions creating sulfonylureas with different durations of activity, protein binding characteristics, and slightly different side-effect profiles, long-acting formulations based on gastrointestinal therapeutic system (gits) have been developed.[426] The most common potentially severe side effect of sulfonylureas is hypoglycemia. Long-acting agents such as chlorpropamide, which is largely excreted unchanged by the kidneys and can accumulate with renal dysfunction, pose the greatest risk for hypoglycemia, which may be prolonged. Shorter-acting agents are less likely to cause frequent or prolonged hypoglycemia.

Other than the risk of hypoglycemia, which is relatively rare at <2 percent per year,[424] sulfonylureas, and especially the second generation drugs, are well-tolerated with few side-effects. Weight gain secondary to poor regulation of caloric intake in the setting of decreased glycosuria typically results in 1–3 kg gain over the first year of therapy. The UGDP suggested that the first-generation sulfonylurea tolbutamide was associated with excess cardiovascular mortality of approximately 1 percent per year.[401] The UGDP results were highly contentious, and the UKPDS did not substantiate its results with regard to sulfonylurea.[17] Allergies to sulfonylureas are more likely to occur in patients with allergies to other sulfa drugs. Other side effects such as alcohol intolerance and hyponatremia are very rare with the second-generation oral agents.

Sulfonylureas are approved for combination therapy with insulin, metformin, thiazolidinediones, and the alpha-glycosidase inhibitors (see later discussion). Generic second generation sulphonylureas are available and are relatively inexpensive.

Repaglinide is the first approved drug in the meglitinide family (Fig. 18-43). It is unique in structure from the sulfonylureas

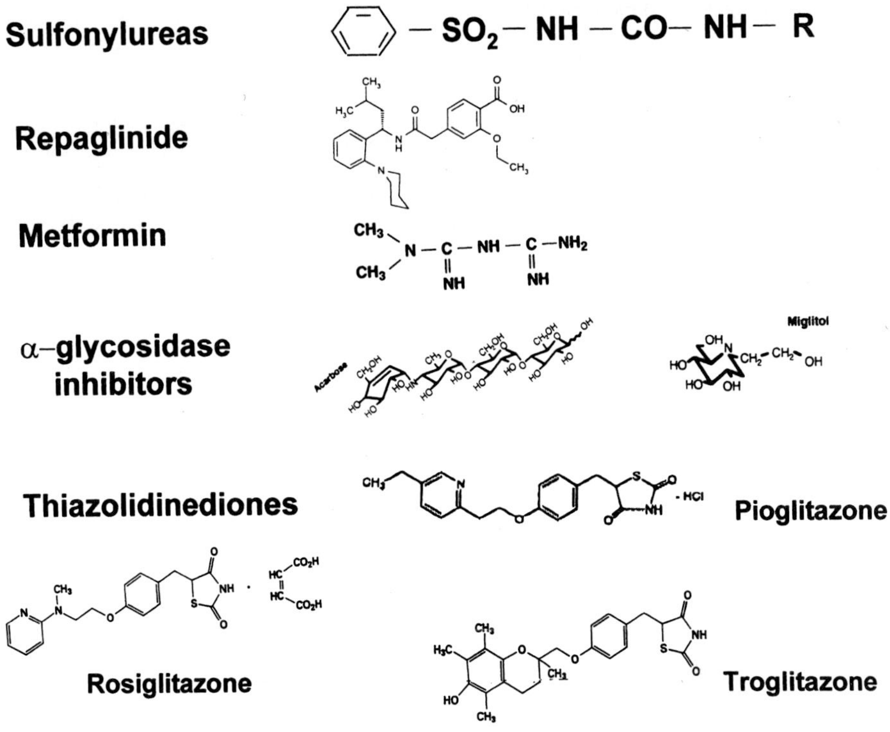

FIGURE 18-42. The structure of commonly available oral antidiabetic agents. Sulfonylureas all share the structure shown. Repaglinide stimulates insulin secretion similar to the sulfonylureas, although it binds to a distinct site on the β-cell and has a shorter duration of action. Metformin is the only biguanide currently available in the U.S. Two α-glycosidase inhibitors are available and three thiazolidinediones have been approved, although troglitazone was withdrawn from the U.S. market in 1999.

and binds to a different site on the ATP-sensitive potassium channel; however, it causes insulin secretion in the presence of glucose similar to the sulfonylureas.[427] It differs from the sulfonylureas in being more rapidly active with a very brief (1-hour) metabolic half-life. The short half-life requires administration before each meal in order to achieve a mean decrease in HbA1c level of 1–1.5 percent, similar in magnitude to the sulfonylureas.[428] With a more rapid on-and-off effect, the expectation was that this oral agent would be safer than sulfonylureas with regard to hypoglycemia, especially in the elderly. This putative benefit of repaglinide has yet to be clearly demonstrated, and considering the relative rarity of severe hypoglycemia with oral agents, it's not clear that this benefit will ever be a major clinical advantage. Because repaglinide has a rapid clearance that is not affected by renal failure, it is the only oral hypoglycemic agent other than acarbose that can be used, albeit cautiously, in the setting of renal failure.

Hypoglycemia and weight gain similar to the sulfonylureas are the major complications experienced with repaglinide. Repaglinide is approved for combination therapy with metformin[429] (see later discussion). Repaglinide is not available as a generic medication and is relatively expensive compared with generic sulfonylureas.

The *biguanide metformin*, although only recently approved (in 1993) in the U.S. has been in use for 40 years, having been developed in 1959 (Fig. 18-43).[430] Extensive use in Canada and Europe, and more recent clinical trials in the US have helped characterize its activity, safety profile, and role in combination therapy (Table 18-27).[430–436] The biguanides, including phenformin, metformin, and buformin, have a mechanism of action that is unique from the other oral medications. Although the cellular mechanism of action is unknown, biguanides act predominantly by suppressing hepatic glucose output.[436] The presence of insulin is necessary, but insulin

TABLE 18-26. Properties of Sulfonylurea Agents

Characteristic	Tolbutamide	Tolazamide	Chlorpropamide	Glipizide	Glyburide
Relative Potency	1	5	6	100	150
Duration of action (h)	6–10	16–24	24–72	16–24	18–24
Protein binding*	Ionic/nonionic	Ionic/nonionic	Ionic/nonionic	Nonionic	Nonionic
Activity of hepatic metabolites	Weak	One active, others nonactive	Weak	Weak	One active, others nonactive
Dose range (mg)	500–3000	100–1000	100–500	2.5–40	1.25–20
Dose frequency (/day)	2–3	1–2	1	1–2	1–2
Usual initial daily dose (mg)	500	100	100	5	2.5
Dosage forms available (mg)	250, 500	100, 250, 500	100, 250	5, 10	1.25, 2.5, 5
Diuretic effect	Yes	Yes	No	No	No
Antidiuretic (hyponatremia)	Yes	No	Yes	No	No
"Disulfiram effect"	No	No	Yes	No	No
Frequency of hypoglycemia (percent)	1	1	4–6	2–4	4–6
Overall frequency of side effects (percent)	3	4	9	6	7

*Greater than 95 percent binding for all drugs.

TABLE 18-27. Metformin Characteristics

- Suppresses hepatic glucose output
- Effective in obese and nonobese Type 2 diabetes
- Lowers HbA1c by 1–1.5 percent
- Usual effective dose is 850 mg taken with breakfast and dinner
- Maximum dose 3,000 mg/day
- Antihyperglycemic—doesn't cause hypoglycemia as single agent
- Not associated with weight gain with monotherapy
- Without benefit if substituted for sulfonylurea in sulfonylurea failures
- May be beneficial in combination with sulfonylurea in sulfonylurea failures
- Most common side effects are gastrointestinal with sense of bloating, abdominal distention and, more rarely, diarrhea. Frequency of these side effects may be reduced if dose is escalated slowly.
- Lactic acidosis extremely rare if patients with decreased GFR, binge drinkers, liver disease, hypovolemia excluded
- Discontinue drug in patients about to have dye studies or general anesthesia to limit cases of lactic acidosis should dye induced renal failure or shock occur

secretion is not stimulated; rather, insulin levels may be modestly decreased with metformin therapy. In addition to suppressing hepatic glucose output, metformin increases anaerobic glycolysis in the intestinal wall.

Monotherapy with metformin decreases glycosylated hemoglobin levels by 1–1.5 percent, comparable to sulfonylurea therapy (Fig. 18-43a). Patients who have failed sulfonylurea are not likely to respond to substitution with metformin, and vice versa.[434] Because metformin does not stimulate insulin secretion, it is generally not associated with hypoglycemia when used as monotherapy. It also does not appear to cause weight gain,[286,430] which is unique to the biguanides and may be secondary to its gastrointestinal side effects. Although phenformin use was largely discontinued in the 1960s owing to cases of lactic acidosis, 25–40 percent of which were fatal, metformin is much less likely to cause lactic acidosis. Compared with phenformin, metformin does not accumulate in mitochondria, is less bound to proteins, and has a shorter half-life. The best estimate of the risk for lactic acidosis with metformin is 0.05 cases of lactic acidosis per 1,000 patient-years.[437] The rate can be decreased further by screening carefully for patients who are at higher risk. Eliminating patients with reduced glomerular filtration or who are at risk for decreased renal function or renal perfusion (e.g., patients with congestive heart failure or who are undergoing radiographic studies with intravenous dye), or who have liver dysfunction, is projected to reduce the frequency of lactic acidosis cases even more. Similar to sulfonylureas, phenformin was associated with excess cardiovascular mortality in the UGDP.[401] However, phenformin was also associated with increased blood pressure and tachycardia, a characteristic not shared by metformin. Moreover, the UKPDS did not demonstrate increased risk for cardiovascular disease with metformin monotherapy.[286] In fact, metformin may have resulted in a decreased risk for all cause and diabetes related mortality in the UKPDS, although the validity of the analyses has been challenged.[305]

In addition to extremely rare, but potentially fatal, lactic acidosis, metformin decreases vitamin B12 absorption, but rarely causes anemia. Gastrointestinal intolerance with abdominal discomfort may lead to discontinuation of metformin in 5–10 percent of treated patients. Increasing metformin doses slowly, beginning with 500 mg with breakfast, and adding 500 mg at dinner before changing to 850 mg two to three times per day, increases patients' acceptance of metformin. Combination therapy with sulfonylureas (Fig. 18-43b), insulin and rosiglitazone has been approved in the U.S. (see later discussion). Generic metformin is relatively inexpensive.

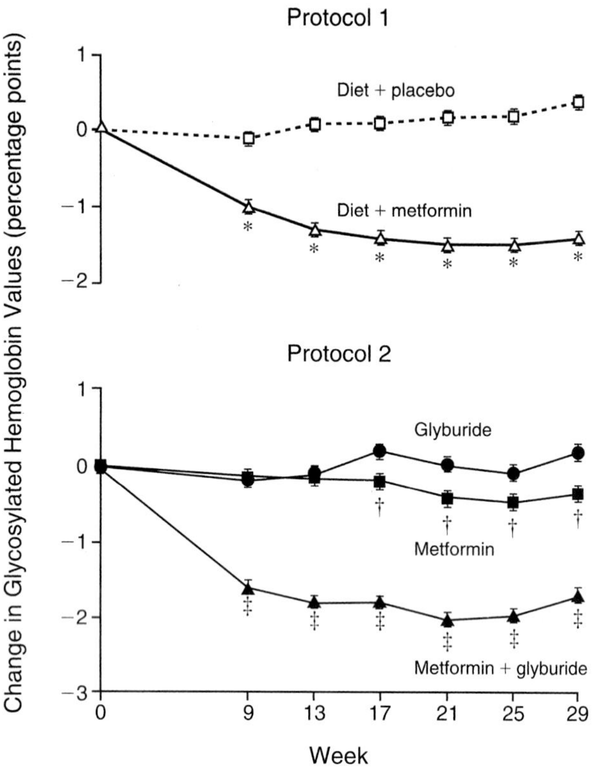

FIGURE 18-43. Hemoglobin A1c change from baseline with metformin therapy when (*a*) used as monotherapy in patients with Type 2 diabetes who "failed" dietary therapy and (*b*) used in combination with sulfonylurea in patients who "failed" sulfonylurea therapy. In (*a*), mean baseline HbA1c was 8.3 percent and patients were randomly assigned to continue diet with placebo or with metformin. In fig. (*b*) mean baseline HbA1c was 8.8 percent and patients were randomly assigned to continue their sulfonylurea, to change to metformin, or to continue sulfonylurea and add metformin. (*From DeFronzo et al.*[434])

α-glucosidase inhibitors, acarbose and miglitol, have been developed and approved for therapy of Type 1 and Type 2 diabetes (Fig. 18-42).[438] These synthetic oligosaccharides have an entirely different principle of action than sulfonylureas or metformin. By binding competitively to intestinal luminal polysaccharidases, they inhibit enzymatic hydrolysis and absorption of carbohydrate in the small intestine. Miglitol may be even more potent than acarbose. The unabsorbed carbohydrate is delivered to the large intestine where bacterial fermentation results in increased methane formation with predictable gastrointestinal side effects of flatulence and discomfort. Although the α-glucosidase inhibitors may be associated with a small degree of malabsorption, alpha glucosidase activity is apparently induced in the large intestine so that the absorption of carbohydrate is delayed rather than decreased. Significant malabsorption of vitamins or other nutrients and weight loss does not occur.

The predominant metabolic effect of α-glucosidase inhibitors is a reduction in postprandial glucose excursions. When used as

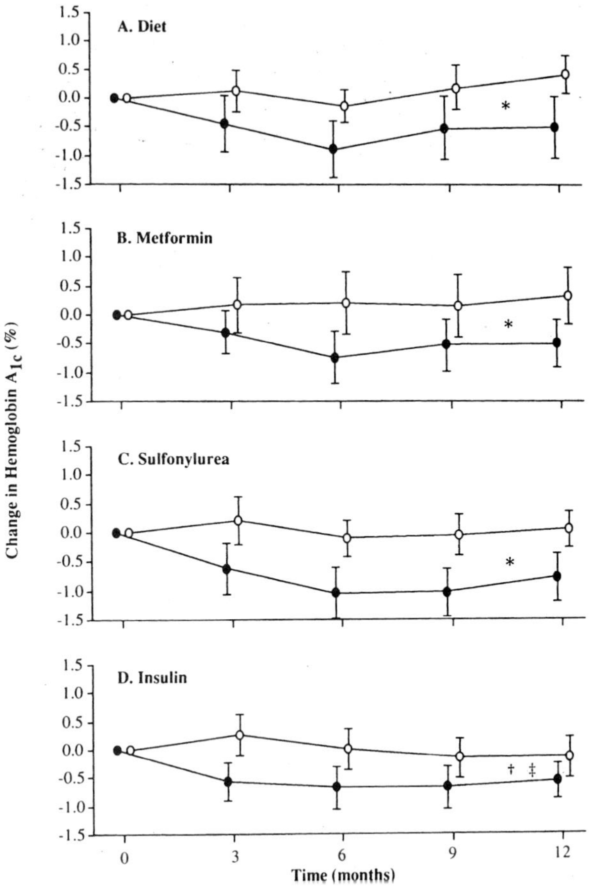

FIGURE 18-44. Hemoglobin A1c change from baseline with acarbose added to diet, sulfonylurea, metformin, or insulin therapy of Type 2 diabetes. At baseline, mean HbA1c was 6.7 percent in the diet treatment group, 7.8 percent in the metformin group, 8.0 percent in the sulfonylurea group, and 7.7 percent in the insulin treatment group. (*From Chiasson et al.*[439])

monotherapy, it is particularly useful in patients with mild glucose intolerance associated with postprandial hyperglycemia. In general, however, it is usually a weaker hypoglycemic agent than sulfonylurea or metformin, lowering HbA1c by 0.5–1.0 percent (Fig. 18-44).[439] The α-glucosidase inhibitors are generally not absorbed and have few, if any, systemic effects. Assuming that patients can tolerate the gastrointestinal side effects, which occur in at least 30 percent of patients and are more common and severe with higher dietary carbohydrate content, the α-glucosidase inhibitors may be used as a single agent in patients with mild Type 2 diabetes, or in combination therapy with other oral agents, insulin, and even in Type 1 diabetes to decrease postprandial glycemic excursions.[440] Titration of dose may limit the gastrointestinal side effects. No generic formulations exist, and acarbose and miglitol remain relatively expensive compared with other oral hypoglycemic agents that are available in generic formulations.

Thiazolidinediones (troglitazone, pioglitazone, and rosiglitazone) were originally identified while screening for potential hypolipidemic agents (Fig. 18-42).[441,442] Their direct mechanism of action is different than that of the other hypoglycemic agents. The thiazolidinediones primarily decrease insulin resistance, i.e., lower glycemia with lower insulin levels. (In fact, both metformin and acarbose therapy also promote lower glucose levels in the setting of lower insulin levels.) Thiazolidinediones act as insulinomimetic agents, or insulin "sensitizers." They bind to a family of nuclear receptors known as the peroxisome proliferator-activator receptors (PPAR-γ). Activation of the receptor through binding to a variety of ligands, including the fibric acids, promotes the differentiation of preadipocytes to adipocytes, amongst other effects. How the thiazolidinediones lower glycemia is unknown, but it may be a function of increased metabolic flux into differentiated fat stores and small adipocytes. The decrease in free fatty acids may improve insulin resistance. Binding to PPAR-γ parallels the hypoglycemic potency of thiazolidinediones.

Thiazolidinediones lower glucose levels modestly when used as monotherapy, with HbA1c levels decreased by less than 1 percent (Fig. 18-45a).[443,444] They are not associated with hypoglycemia, but are accompanied by modest weight gain. Troglitazone was initially approved for use as combination therapy in the setting of insulin-treated Type 2 diabetes, in which it was particularly effective.[445] HbA1c was lowered by 1–1.5 percent (Fig. 18-45b). Modest weight gain and hypoglycemia can occur with combination therapy. Troglitazone was subsequently approved for use as monotherapy in Type 2 diabetes in 1997. Thiazolidinediones have also been used in combination with sulfonylureas[446] and metformin.[443]

In general, troglitazone was well tolerated. The original preapproval clinical trials of troglitazone, the first thiazolidinedione approved, demonstrated a low incidence of liver function test abnormalities (approximately 2 percent vs. 0.6 percent in controls). The greater than threefold elevations in transaminase levels returned to normal with or without discontinuation of troglitazone. In the first year after FDA and Japanese approval of troglitazone, almost 1 million patients were treated. During postmarketing surveillance, relatively rare episodes of severe liver dysfunction (approximately 20–30 cases) attributed to troglitazone were reported.[447] These severe, idiosyncratic reactions resulted in liver failure, liver transplantation, and death, with an estimated rate of occurrence of 1 episode for every 30–50,000 treated patients. The occurrence of severe cases of liver dysfunction with troglitazone prompted the FDA to require monthly monitoring of liver function tests for the first year of use, and every three months thereafter. With the recognition that frequent monitoring did not effectively prevent cases of severe liver dysfunction, troglitazone was withdrawn from the market in 1999.

Two new thiazolidinediones, rosiglitazone and pioglitazone, were approved for use in 1999. During clinical testing, treated patients did not develop an increased frequency of liver function test abnormalities compared with placebo-treated patients. Based on these preliminary results, rosiglitazone and pioglitazone have been suggested to be less likely to cause idiosyncratic liver toxicity compared with troglitazone. Mindful that severe liver disease with troglitazone did not appear until large numbers of patients were treated, the FDA is requiring monitoring of liver test function every other month during the first year of therapy and "periodically" thereafter.

Rosiglitazone is approved for use as monotherapy or use with metformin, and pioglitazone is approved for use as monotherapy or in combination with insulin, sulfonylurea, or metformin. Troglitazone has also been used to lower glycemic levels, albeit modestly, in patients with impaired glucose tolerance and insulin resistance.[448] It has also been used to treat women with polycystic ovarian syndrome, in whom it lowers insulin resistance and insulin levels and can restore fertility.[449]

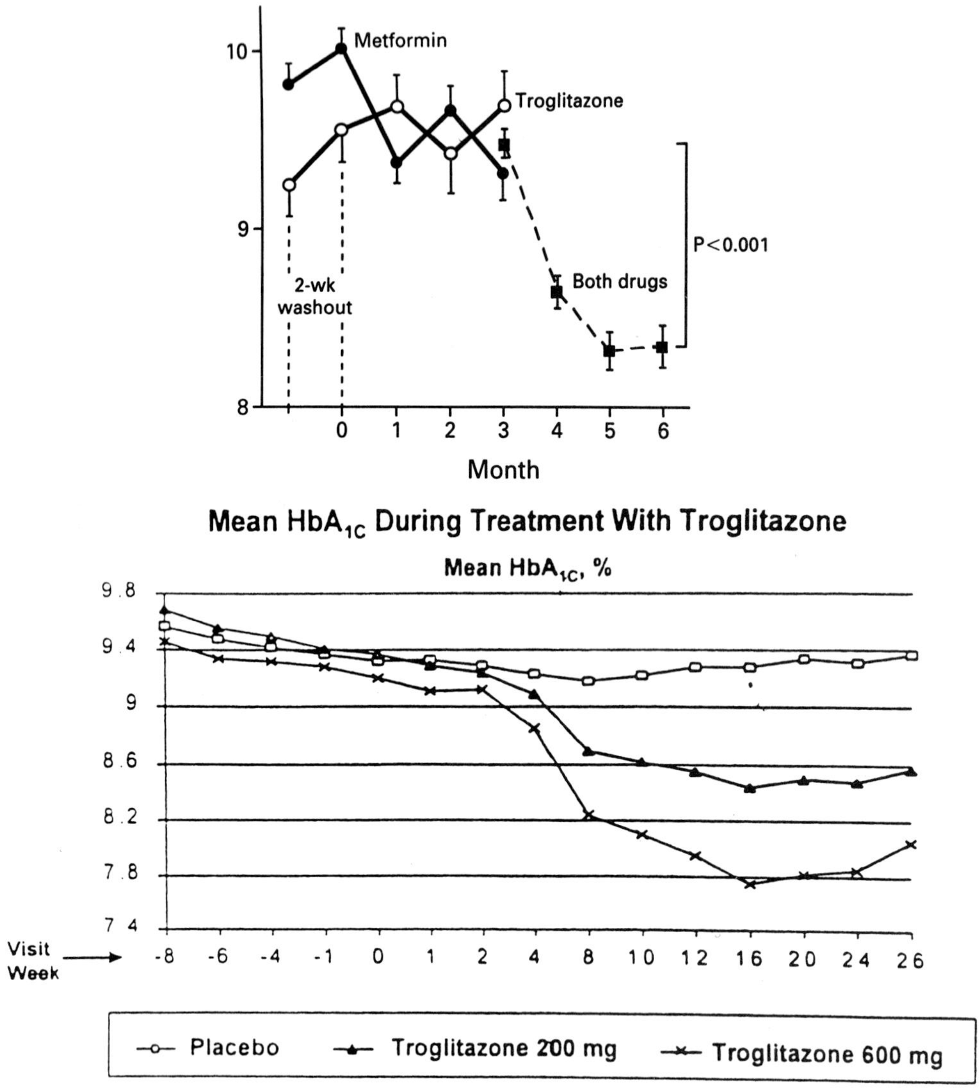

FIGURE 18-45. Hemoglobin A1c levels achieved with troglitazone (*a*) monotherapy, (*b*) in combination with metformin, and (*c*) in combination with insulin. (*From Inzucchi et al.*[443] *and Schwartz et al.*[445])

Insulin is the oldest of all hypoglycemic agents and the only naturally occurring substance.[450] Insulin remains the most effective drug to treat Type 2 diabetes, assuming that patients and care providers are willing to use the large doses that are necessary to achieve near normoglycemia. All of the oral agents have maximal doses beyond which no additional effect occurs. In contrast, insulin has no maximal dose and increasing doses result in increased biological effects. Virtually all studies attempting to normalize glucose levels in overweight Type 2 diabetes with insulin have documented insulin requirements of at least 55 units per day (Fig. 18-46). The goal of insulin therapy in Type 2 diabetes is to supplement endogenous insulin with quantities sufficient to normalize glycemia. From a physiologic point of view, it would be advantageous to correct fasting glycemia with exogenous insulin and allow endogenous insulin secretion to control postprandial glycemic excursions. Decreasing overnight glycemia or 24-hour glycemia with exogenous insulin decreases glucotoxicity and improves beta cell function.[239,241,242]

Unfortunately, most studies of insulin therapy in Type 2 diabetes have been relatively short-term. The four longest-term studies have been the Kumamoto study (6 years mean followup in relatively thin Japanese patients),[302] the Veterans Administration Cooperative study (28 months),[451] the UGDP (9 years),[401] and the UKPDS (10 years).[17] Of note, all of the studies, with the exception of the UKPDS, demonstrated near-normal glycemia that was stable over time with insulin therapy. In the UKPDS, after an initial decrease in HbA1c with insulin, a steady increase occurred over the course of the study. Although mean insulin doses were increased over time, they peaked at 24 and 60 units per day in the nonobese and obese subjects, respectively. When calculated as units per kg per day, the insulin dose used in the UKPDS was substantially less than that used in DCCT intensive therapy (0.42 vs. 0.67). On the basis of an unpublished survey of UKPDS investigators and patients, the UKPDS investigators attributed the failure to raise insulin doses further to fear of hypoglycemia on the part of investigators and patients and concern regarding weight gain on the part of the participants.

As noted earlier, the usual pattern of therapy in Type 2 diabetes is a stepwise introduction of diet and exercise followed by one or more oral agents, and finally the introduction of insulin

FIGURE 18-46. Decrease in Hemoglobin A1c levels achieved with intensive insulin therapy regimens in Type 2 diabetes. The hemoglobin A1c level before and after institution of intensive therapy are shown in the left and right columns, respectively. The upper-limit-of-normal for the HbA1c assay for each study is represented by the white horizontal line, and the mean dose of insulin (units per day) used with intensive therapy is indicated on the intensive therapy column. The insulin regimen for the individual studies was the following: Veterans Administration Cooperative Study (VA), twice per day intermediate-acting insulin[451]; United Kingdom Prospective Diabetes Study (UKPDS), long-acting insulin supplemented with rapid-acting insulin[17]; Kumamoto study, premeal rapid acting insulin and bedtime intermediate-acting insulin[302]; Nathan et al., morning intermediate-acting insulin adjusted according to self-glucose monitoring results[457]; Cusi et al., bedtime intermediate-acting insulin adjusted based on fasting glucose level.[458]

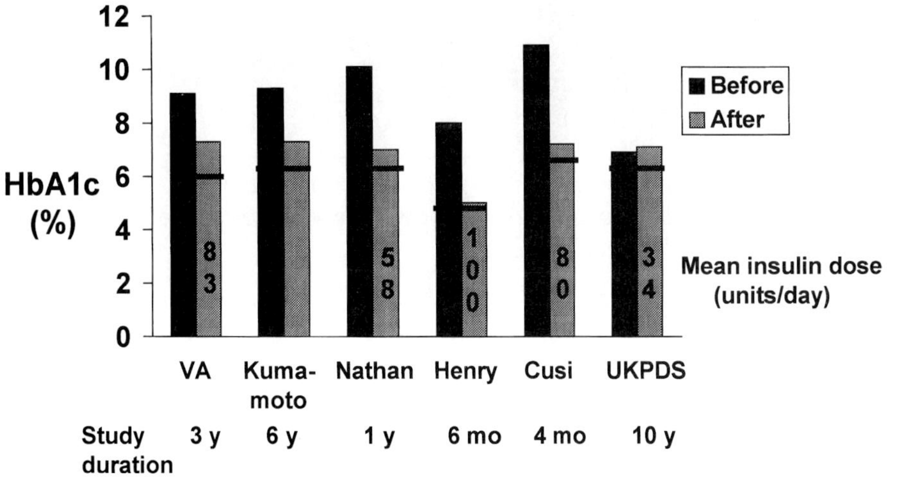

therapy, either alone or in combination with oral agents. Insulin is usually not added until late in the clinical course. More aggressive, i.e., earlier, therapy with insulin has been suggested as a means of putting Type 2 diabetes into "remission."[407]

Insulin can be administered with a variety of regimens (Table 18-28).[452–459] Although nocturnal insulin has been recommended as the most efficient way to normalize fasting glycemia, decrease glucotoxicity, and potentiate endogenous insulin secretion,[459] relatively few studies have compared nocturnal and daily insulin. Many studies of "intensive insulin therapy" in Type 2 diabetes have achieved glycosylated hemoglobin levels comparable to those achieved in the DCCT, regardless of the specific insulin regimen used (Fig. 18-47). The mean daily insulin dose, while considerably higher than those required with intensive therapy of Type 1 diabetes, are usually only modestly higher than the doses used in the DCCT when expressed on a unit/kg/day basis.

The major side effects of insulin therapy are hypoglycemia and weight gain. Although hypoglycemia has not been studied as

TABLE 18-28. Insulin Regimens Used to Treat Type 2 Diabetes

Intermediate-acting insulin (NPH or Lente)
Prebreakfast
Prebed
Twice per day
Prebreakfast and dinner
With rapid- or very rapid-acting
Prebreakfast and bed
With rapid- or very rapid-acting prebreakfast and/or predinner (3 injections)
Long-acting insulin (ultralente)
Prebreakfast
Prebed
Premixed insulin (70/30)
Prebreakfast
Predinner
Prebreakfast and predinner

extensively during intensive therapy of Type 2 diabetes as in intensive therapy of Type 1 diabetes, the relatively low frequency of severe hypoglycemia with intensive therapy is striking (Fig. 18-47). Weight gain, on the other hand, is almost universal with insulin therapy aimed at achieving normoglycemia. The cause of weight gain is probably the same as with sulfonylurea therapy—elimination of glycosuria and decreased basal metabolic rate associated with improved glycemia.

The reluctance to use insulin may be secondary to patient or physician concerns and resistance to using an injectable medication. Interestingly, once Type 2 diabetes patients are treated with insulin, compliance with injections is at least as good as compliance with oral diabetic medications.[460]

Combination Therapies Virtually every combination of therapies has been used to treat Type 2 diabetes. The UKPDS demonstrated a seemingly inexorable increase in glycemia, despite adding medications sequentially. These data can be interpreted to mean that combinations of therapies are necessary to maintain glycemia as low as possible, or that the strategy of stepwise additions of therapies fails to maintain glycemia in the near-normal range.

The most common, and probably most important combination therapy is diet, exercise, and pharmacologic therapy. Continued application of dietary therapy and exercise when medications are begun makes therapy more effective, at least in part by limiting weight gain. The combination of insulin and sulfonylurea has been espoused as a means of achieving lower glycemia with less insulin.[461–470] The use of this combination decreases insulin doses by approximately 10 percent at almost twice the cost of insulin therapy alone (Fig. 18-48). Similar metabolic results can usually be achieved with insulin alone, assuming that sufficient doses are used.[468–470] A recent study suggests an advantage of combining metformin and insulin, compared with once-per-day or twice-per-day insulin, although the dose of insulin wasn't "forced" in the insulin alone groups.[471] In this study, insulin combined with metformin resulted in modestly lower glycemia with less weight gain; compared with insulin alone.

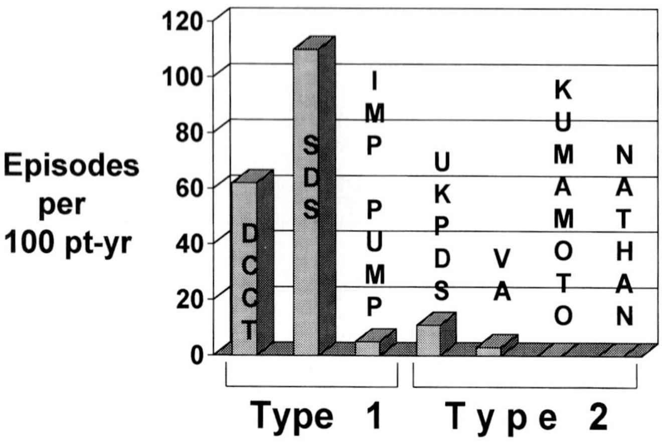

FIGURE 18-47. Frequency of severe hypoglycemia in intensive insulin therapy studies in Type 1 [Diabetes Control and Complications Trial (DCCT) and Stockholm Diabetes Intervention Study (SDIS)] and in Type 2 diabetes. The definition of severe hypoglycemia is the DCCT definition of any clinical episode of hypoglycemia that requires assistance to treat. The subset of episodes with coma or seizure represented approximately 25 percent of the total number of episodes in the DCCT.

Combining acarbose with insulin, sulfonylurea or diet lowers HbA1c by 0.5–1.0 percent (Fig. 18-45).[439] Combining metformin and sulfonylurea also lowers HbA1c results in patients who have failed to normalize glycemia with either agent alone (Fig. 18-44b).[434] Thiazolidinediones have been approved for use with insulin, sulfonylureas, or metformin. Short-term studies have suggested that combination therapy is effective in lowering HbA1c with stable or lower insulin doses (Figs. 18-45b and 18-45c).[445]

The costs of combining oral agent therapies or adding oral agents to insulin include increasing the risk of hypoglycemia, the risk of side effects associated with the individual drugs, and a large increase in economic costs (Fig. 18-48). Whether such combination therapy is preferable to initiating or increasing insulin has not been examined carefully.

Other Components of Therapy of Type 2 Diabetes

Monitoring of glycemia and other biochemical analytes is similar as in Type 1 diabetes with several differences (Table 18-14). Because glycemic levels are generally more stable in Type 2 diabetes, and many patients (treated with diet alone or with oral agents not asociated with hypoglycemia) are not at risk for hypoglycemia, SMBG may not be necessary. Even in insulin-treated patients with Type 2 diabetes, SMBG may not need to be performed as frequently as in Type 1 diabetes. In addition, because ketosis is rare in Type 2 diabetes, urine ketone testing is usually unnecessary.

On the other hand, lipid abnormalities are more common in Type 2 than Type 1 diabetes and require more frequent surveillance. Elevated triglyceride and VLDL cholesterol levels (secondary to increased hepatic production and decreased clearance associated with reduced insulin sensitive lipase activity) and decreased HDL cholesterol levels are the most common abnormal lipid patterns. Owing to their increased age, and the constellation of CVD risk factors that commonly accompany Type 2 diabetes, patients with Type 2 diabetes require assiduous attention to all CVD risk factors. (See section on CVD and Tables 18-18 and 18-20.)

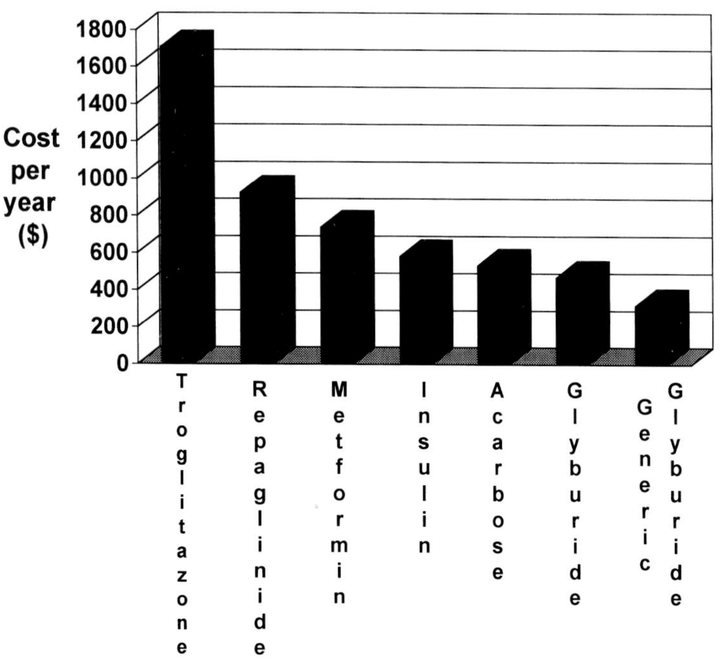

FIGURE 18-48. Relative costs of medications for diabetes therapy. The costs are the Redbook costs (to the pharmacist) for a one-month supply of the specific agent. For medications with available generic substitutes, the lower cost generic medications are included. The doses of medications were the following: Troglitazone 400 mg per day, Repaglinide 2 mg three times per day, Metformin 850 mg twice per day, Insulin 60 units per day (cost of syringes and alcohol wipes included), Acarbose 50 mg three times per day, Glyburide 5 mg twice per day.

Alternative Therapies A large number of herbal therapies have been advocated to treat Type 2 diabetes. Few, if any, have been studied rigorously in controlled trials. Chromium and other trace minerals such as vanadium have been suggested as effective therapies for Type 2 diabetes for more than 30 years. A recent study in a Chinese population that may have been chromium deficient demonstrated a significant decrease in HbA1c after 4 months treatment with 1,000 μg of chromium as the picolinate salt.[472]

The Future The medications currently under development include glucagon-like peptide 1,7-36amide (GLP), several weight loss medicines, glucagon antagonists, and other insulinomimetic medications and insulin secretagogues. GLP is a naturally occurring gut peptide that stimulates insulin secretion, inhibits glucagon secretion, and slows gastric motility.[87,473] Currently, it is administered intravenously or subcutaneously, although oral formulations are under development. Weight loss medications currently approved include sibutramine, an appetite suppressant, which can raise blood pressure,[474] and orlistat, a pancreatic lipase inhibitor that causes fat malabsorption.[475] Other potential therapies include d-chiroinositol, proposed as an insulomimetic agent.[476]

Gestational Diabetes

The documented benefit of therapy of gestational diabetes on fetal outcomes[477] is the rationale for identifying and treating gestational diabetes. On the other hand, there is a paucity of data regarding the most appropriate therapy for GDM. The goals of therapy are shown in Table 18-29. The most common therapy for GDM is diet and exercise, which is satisfactory to achieve target glucose goals in the majority of patients.[478] The recognition that a standard amount of weight gain is not necessary for overweight pregnant women has resulted in diet therapy that provides sufficient nutrition to maintain fetal growth but does not result in excess maternal weight gain. The original ADA recommendation of 35 kcal/kg with 50–60 percent carbohydrate resulted in unnecessary weight gain and postprandial hyperglycemia. A moderately restricted diet (approximately 1,800 kcal for women who are 120–150 percent of ideal body weight) resulted in reduced glycemia and no ketonemia. (Concern regarding ketonemia stems from a study that reported decreased IQ scores associated with the development of ketonemia during pregnancy. This finding has been confirmed by some, but not other, studies.) Exercise has also been used successfully to control glycemia during GDM.[479]

TABLE 18-29. Goals of Therapy of Gestational Diabetes Mellitus and Women with Pregestational Diabetes Mellitus

	Blood Glucose Levels mg/dL (mmol/L)
Before breakfast	60–90 (3.3–4.9)
Before lunch & dinner	60–105 (3.3–5.8)
1 h after meals	70–140 (3.9–7.8)
2 h after meals	60–120 (3.3–6.7)
Caloric prescription	35–38 kcal/kg prepregnancy body weight*

*A hypocaloric diet of 1,200–1,500 kcal/d, instead of an isocaloric diet, has been recommended for overweight women with GDM. In GDM, if diet therapy does not maintain glucose goals of fbg ≤105 mg/dL and/or 2-h postprandial levels ≤120 mg/dL, on two occasions at 1–2 week intervals, insulin therapy should be instituted. Intermediate acting insulin combined with rapid-acting insulin given prebreakfast and predinner (usually 2/3 in A.M. and 1/3 in P.M.) is usually sufficient. Fasting hyperglycemia without postprandial hyperglycemia can be treated effectively with prebed intermediate-acting insulin.

None of the oral hypoglycemic agents are approved for use during pregnancy; however, experience during pregnancy with metformin and the α-glycosidase inhibitors has suggested that they may be safe and do not increase congenital malformations.[480]

The first choice of pharmacologic therapy when diet and exercise fail to lower glucose levels adequately is insulin. Therapy can be initiated with either intermediate- or a combination of intermediate- and rapid-acting insulins before breakfast and dinner. Approximately two-thirds of the dose can be given in the morning and the remainder before dinner. Glucose monitoring, usually performed by the patient, is most effective if 90–120 min postprandial levels are tested and controlled.[481] Although HbA1c levels can be followed, the large normal range, into which most GDM patients fall, and the changes in HbA1c that occur during nondiabetic pregnancies, make HbA1c less useful than glucose monitoring.

Metabolic Emergencies—Diabetic Ketoacidosis (DKA), Hyperosmolar Hyperglycemic Nonketotic Coma (HHNKC), Hypoglycemia

A spectrum of acute metabolic emergencies can occur in Type 1 or Type 2 diabetes. Gross increases in plasma glucose or ketone levels, or both, with dehydration, and either alone or in combination with lactic acidosis can occur with insulin deficiency. An abnormally low blood glucose level, secondary to a mismatch of insulin supply and requirements, that results in neurologic manifestations characterizes hypoglycemia. The major clinical syndromes encountered are DKA (hyperglycemia plus ketone accumulation), alcoholic ketoacidosis (ketone accumulation with modest hyperglycemia), hyperosmolar hyperglycemic nonketotic coma (profound hyperglycemia without ketonemia), any of these disorders plus lactic acidosis, and hypoglycemia. These severe acute metabolic abnormalities require special attention because of the need for prompt, accurate diagnosis and treatment so that the condition does not progress to death.

Diabetic Ketoacidosis (DKA)

The most severe clinical manifestation of insulin deficiency is the development of DKA. Since the advent of insulin therapy >75 years ago, the importance of DKA as a cause of death in the diabetic population has progressively declined. The incidence of DKA is approximately 30–50 cases per 1,000 patient-years in Type 1 diabetes, and probably 100-fold less in Type 2 diabetes.[188] In the DCCT population, followed between 1983 and 1993 and composed predominantly of adults with only 15 percent adolescents, the rate of DKA was approximately 20 cases per 1,000 patient-years, with no significant difference between intensive and conventional therapy.[319] DKA may be a recurrent disorder, particularly in patients who have not been taught, or who have not followed, specific management strategies for "sick days." Behavioral problems, especially during adolescence, may manifest as recurrent DKA. Only a minority of all DKA cases occur at the time of diagnosis of Type 1 diabetes; the majority occur in the setting of an intercurrent illness when patients did not, or could not, adjust insulin appropriately.[482] The most common mistake is stopping insulin administration when oral intake is decreased, for example owing to a gastroenteritis. With the availability of self-monitoring of blood glucose and urine ketones, most patients should be able to prevent or recognize evolving DKA and prevent worsening to

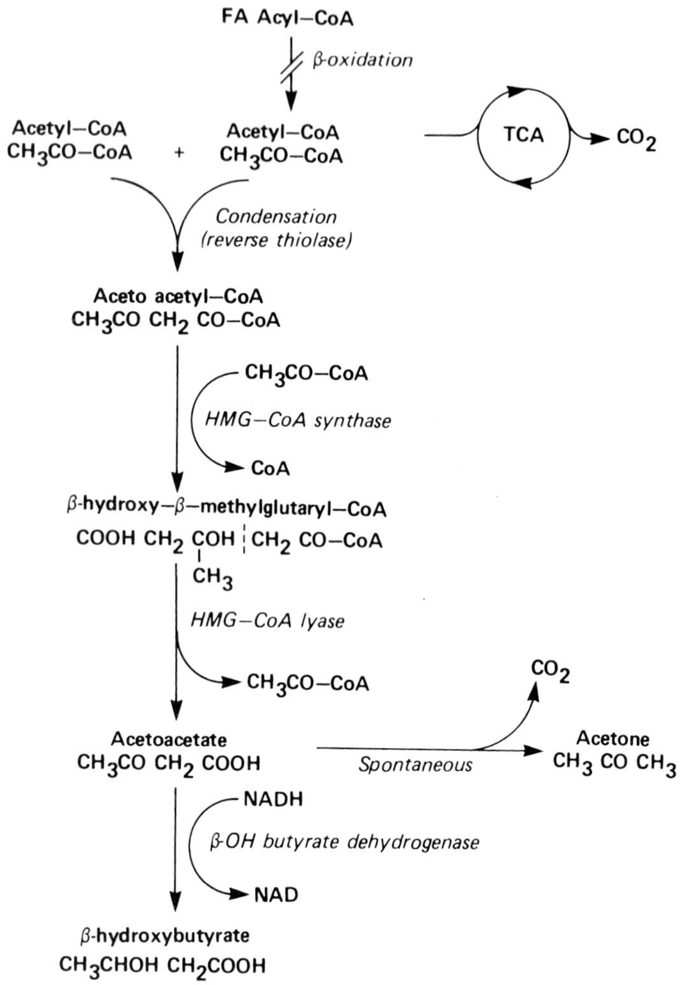

FIGURE 18-49. Biochemical pathway of ketogenesis. In the presence of large amounts of acetyl CoA derived from excessive FFA oxidation, condensation into acetoacetyl CoA takes place in liver mitochondria. Earlier it was thought that during enhanced ketogenesis acetoacetate may be directly formed by deacylation of acetoacetyl CoA, an intermediate in the last stage of β oxidation. It is known today that the main pathway requires an additional condensation with acetyl CoA to form β-hydroxy-β-methylglutaryl CoA (HMG-CoA) catalyzed by *HMG-CoA synthase.* Acetoacetate is formed and released from the mitochondria after cleavage of HMG-CoA by *HMG-CoA lyase,* which also results in the recovery of acetyl CoA. Acetoacetate may be converted to β-hydroxybutyrate, which is quantitatively the predominant ketone body in the circulation, or decarboxylated to acetone. Neither of the above reactions is rate-limiting; FFA supply is the major determinant of ketogenesis.

full-blown DKA. Early and aggressive treatment with extra insulin and fluids can often forestall the development of DKA. DKA often represents a failure of patient education or inability to comply with prescribed regimen.

Although the treatment of DKA in Type 1 diabetes is usually straightforward, lending itself to treatment algorithms, DKA remains a potentially lethal disorder, with a mortality rate that may be as high as 5 percent, especially in the elderly.[188,483] In most circumstances death is due not to DKA per se, but to some intercurrent catastrophic event (e.g., sepsis, myocardial infarction, pancreatitis) that may have precipitated or complicated the course of DKA. In children, cerebral edema may complicate recovery from DKA and result in severe morbidity or mortality.[484]

Only a tiny minority of cases of DKA occur in the setting of Type 2 diabetes, owing to preserved insulin secretion, which inhibits ketogenesis. When DKA does occur in the setting of Type 2 diabetes it is usually associated with major stress, such as sepsis or an acute myocardial infarction. In this setting, the case fatality may be higher than 40 percent, secondary to the severe underlying precipitant, rather than the DKA itself.

Pathogenesis

From a metabolic standpoint, the major findings in DKA are the accumulation of the organic acids ("ketone bodies") acetoacetate and β-hydroxybutyrate, elevation in serum acetone concentration, a marked increase in blood glucose concentration, and cation loss in urine (Fig. 18-49). Clinically, the major life-threatening abnormalities are metabolic acidosis (owing to hyperketonemia), hyperosmolarity (owing to hyperglycemia and water loss), and dehydration (owing to the osmotic diuresis accompanying hyperglycemia and the vomiting that generally accompanies ketoacidosis) (Table 18-30). The hyperosmolarity is more important than acidosis in causing obtundation and coma.[485] All of these abnormalities may be traced directly to an absolute or relative lack of insulin, which may develop over a period of several hours or days. Relative or absolute insulin deficiency may result from failure of endogenous insulin secretion (as in an individual with newly discovered diabetes); inadequate administration of exogenous insulin (in a patient with known Type 1 diabetes); increased requirements for insulin engendered by the stress associated with intercurrent infections, or inflammatory, traumatic, or endocrinologic disorders; or, as is often the case, a combination of these factors. The increased insulin requirements in such disorders may be attributed to the augmented secretion of hormones with an action antagonistic to insulin (e.g., epinephrine, cortisol, glucagon, and GH) (Figs. 18-12 and 18-16).[486] In the setting of decreased counterregulatory hormones such as hypopituitarism or glucagon deficiency, the development of DKA may be attenuated.[487]

TABLE 18-30. Clinical and Laboratory Findings in Diabetic Ketoacidosis

Clinical Signs and Symptoms	Laboratory Values
Dehydration	Hyperglycemia
Tachycardia	(usually 350–700 mg/dL)
Abnormal skin turgor	Bun, Cr increased*
Dry mucous membranes	Hyperosmolar
Hypotension	Hypokalemia†
Nausea and vomiting	Hypophosphatemia
Abdominal pain	Anion gap acidosis
Ileus	Low bicarbonate
Kussmaul respiration	(<15 meq/l)
Ketotic (fruity) breath	Serum and urine ketones
Altered mental status	Arterial pH <7.3
Somnolence to coma	Leukocytosis
(coma unusual)	

*Creatinine increased secondary to dehydration and because of interference by ketones with standard creatinine assay.

†Serum levels may initially be high or normal in setting of acidosis; however, total K^+ deficit is usually profound.

Severely decreased tissue utilization of glucose and glucose overproduction by the liver and kidney characterize the insulin-deficient state.[399] Whereas glucose is released by the liver at a rate of 150–200 mg/min (2 to 3 mg per kilogram of body weight per min) in normal postabsorptive subjects, in DKA the rate of glucose production may rise to 600 mg/min. The kidney contributes to the hyperglycemia by acidosis-stimulated gluconeogenesis. Hyperglycemia arises predominantly from excessive production of glucose from endogenous precursors, rather than a failure to metabolize ingested carbohydrate. Consequently, a diabetic patient may have had no intake of carbohydrate or other food for 12 to 24 h yet manifest hyperglycemia of 500 mg/dl (28 m*M*). In addition, the dehydration that occurs with osmotic diuresis leads to hypovolemia, which in turn concentrates glucose levels to even higher levels. Finally, as GFR falls, the filtered load of glucose decreases and urinary glucose excretion decreases. Typically, plasma glucose levels are in the 350–700 mg/dL (approximately 20–40 mmol/L) range.

Because protein-derived amino acids are the major precursors for de novo glucose synthesis, implicit in this increase in gluconeogenesis are dissolution of body protein stores and the development of negative nitrogen balance. Massive mobilization of adipose tissue in the form of free fatty acids (FFA), which are ketone precursors and glycerol (a gluconeogenic substrate), causes an additional loss of body weight, which is superimposed on the osmotic diuresis that accompanies severe hyperglycemia. In a Type 1 diabetic patient, repeated episodes of DKA or chronically poor metabolic control may interfere with normal growth (Mauriac syndrome) owing to protein loss and decreased somatostatin levels.

Osmotic diuresis leads to dehydration as a result of urinary losses of water and to the development of hyperosmolarity. The osmotic diuresis also results in large urinary electrolyte losses (compared with plasma, the urine in osmotic diuresis is always hypotonic with respect to sodium concentration). Cation losses are aggravated by the need to neutralize the organic acids before excreting them in urine. Insulin deficiency may of itself (independent of the osmotic diuresis) also contribute to renal sodium losses. Insulin administration has been shown to have an antinatriuretic effect, whereas an acute reduction in insulin concentration results in natriuresis.[488] If fluid intake is reduced, often because of nausea and vomiting, which are harbingers of DKA, dehydration proceeds rapidly, blood volume drops, peripheral resistance is reduced, blood pressure falls, and renal function is impaired. Loss of water in vomitus dehydrates the intracellular space further. Loss of gastric acid may modify the development of acidosis.

In fully developed DKA, all body compartments are dehydrated, and there are absolute deficiencies of water, sodium, potassium, magnesium, chloride, and bicarbonate. The hypovolemia may in turn aggravate the ketosis, perhaps by acting as a stimulus for the secretion of epinephrine. On the other hand, if fluids and electrolytes are given to diabetic patients in whom insulin treatment has been withdrawn, hyperketonemia is delayed or reduced even in the absence of insulin administration.

Coincident with the increase in blood glucose concentration, acetoacetate, β-hydroxybutyrate, and acetone progressively accumulate in blood, reaching levels of 8 to 15 m*M*. Insulin deficiency is responsible for the unrestrained FFA outflow from adipose tissue. Increased hepatic ketogenesis is the outcome of the sheer mass of FFA and regulatory adjustments within the liver. The entry of fatty acyl CoA into the mitochondria, with consequent β-oxidation, is preferred over esterification of fatty acyl CoA with glycerol 3-phosphate because of the decrease in malonyl CoA concentration coincident with cessation of de novo lipogenesis. The reduction in malonyl CoA concentration removes the inhibition of CAT 1, the enzyme responsible for intramitochondrial transfer of long-chain fatty acyl CoA,[489] resulting in excessive acetyl CoA production. The increasing concentrations of acetyl CoA exceed the capacity for its oxidation to CO_2 via the Krebs cycle, resulting in condensation of acetyl CoA to ketone acids. (Fig. 18-49). Hyperglucagonemia conditions the liver to be ketogenic by increasing the level of carnitine, decreasing the concentration of malonyl CoA, and increasing the activity of CAT in excess of that attributable to insulin deficiency alone.

In addition to increased ketone production, hyperketonemia in diabetes is a consequence of decreased utilization of the ketoacids by muscle tissue. Even in patients with mild insulin deficiency, a diminution in the ability to dispose of the ketones is demonstrable; this diminished disposal becomes increasingly important as serum ketone levels reach 10 m*M*.[490]

The ketone acids are generally present in plasma in a ratio of 3 to 1, β-hydroxybutyrate to acetoacetate, dictated in part by the redox state (NADH to NAD ratio). Changes in the redox state with treatment may alter the ratio of the ketoacids.[491] Acetone is also formed (by the spontaneous decarboxylation of acetoacetate) and circulates in a concentration which may reach 10 to 15 m*M*. Because of its low vapor pressure, acetone is excreted by the lungs, causing the characteristic fruity odor. The presence of acetone may be detected on the patient's breath and may serve as a useful diagnostic clue. The presence of large amounts of ketone bodies, which are moderately strong acids, causes an increase in the hydrogen ion concentration of the body fluids. As a result, there is a fall in the concentration or serum bicarbonate and an increase in the anion gap (i.e., the difference between the serum sodium concentration and the sum of chloride plus bicarbonate exceeds the normal range of 10 to 12 mEq/liter).

Clinical Characteristics

The typical clinical presentation of DKA (Table 18-30) includes signs and symptoms of dehydration (2° to osmotic diuresis and vomiting), rapid, deep (Kussmaul) respirations (to increase expiration of volatile acids), nausea and vomiting (perhaps 2° to altered prostaglandin metabolism and resultant gastroparesis and decreased gastrointestinal motility), and depressed mentation, depending on the degree of hyperosmolarity. Abdominal pain often accompanies the nausea and vomiting and may mimic an acute abdomen.

Plasma glucose is elevated, usually from 350–700 mg/dL, and an anion gap acidosis is typically present with elevated ketone bodies (acetoacetate, β-hydroxybutyrate, and acetone) detectable in urine and serum. Although potassium and phosphate may initially be normal or even high, hydration and correction of the acidosis invariably lowers serum levels, unmasking a profound total body depletion. Other factors can alter the usual laboratory values of DKA. Preliminary insulin treatment by the patient, profound inanition, or DKA during pregnancy can result in "euglycemic" DKA with glucose levels < 250 mg/dL.[492] Because specific enzymatic techniques are cumbersome, reliance is placed on the semiquantitative reagent strip or tablet (nitroprusside) test for urinary ketone determinations. Unfortunately, the test measures only acetoacetate and acetone, but not β-hydroxybutyrate concentration. Consequently, when acetoacetate accounts for < 25 percent of the total ketone acids (as in combined DKA and lactic acidosis or in alcoholic ketoacidosis), the test may give a spuriously low value. Conversely, a spuriously high value is seen with the nitroprusside test after insulin treatment has been instituted because the unmeasured β-hydroxybutyrate component falls, owing to a fall in the NADH to NAD ratio, with an increase in measured acetoacetate concentration.

Elevations in serum amylase concentration and in the amylase/creatinine clearance ratio are not uncommon in DKA. Although in some patients hyperamylasemia may signify accompanying pancreatitis, in most circumstances there is no clinical evidence of pancreatitis. The data suggest that the elevated amylase concentrations in DKA are of salivary rather than pancreatic origin.[493]

In addition to the increased blood urea nitrogen concentration, consistent with dehydration and the prerenal state, serum creatinine levels are often elevated. Although the creatinine level may indicate compromised renal function (consider outflow obstruction with necrotizing papillitis if pyelonephritis present), more often than not the elevated serum creatinine is spurious, owing to the interference of high ketone levels in the commonly used assay for creatinine based on picric acid.[494] An elevated hematocrit is also a common manifestation of the dehydration accompanying DKA. Leukocytosis, frequently with increased numbers of young polymorphonuclear leukocytes, may be present and must be interpreted with care. Sometimes this finding reflects the precipitating cause of acidosis, such as infection, but even in the absence of such a complication, leukocytosis may be present, probably reflecting the stress state with demargination of polymorphonuclear leukocytes from the bone marrow.

Diagnosis

Prompt diagnosis of DKA requires a high index of suspicion in patients with obtundation, dehydration, hyperpnea, vomiting, and abdominal pain or with an acetone odor on the breath. In the era of self-monitoring, the diagnosis of early DKA, or diabetes "out-of-control" prior to the development of DKA, can—and should—be made by the patient. Early detection of severe hyperglycemia and the presence of urine ketones should lead to aggressive efforts to provide adequate insulin, replete volume losses, and treat the underlying cause of the problem (e.g., start antibiotics for a urinary tract infection, give antiemetics to decrease vomiting and fluid loss). Such therapy may be initiated at home, in the office, or in an emergency care facility, depending on the degree of hyperglycemia and ketosis and the clinical state of the patient. The earlier that the abnormal metabolic state is identified and addressed, the more likely that DKA can be prevented, or, if it develops, the more likely that hospital treatment will be rapidly effective.

The diagnosis of DKA is established in the presence of hyperglycemia and an anion gap acidosis with ketonuria or ketonemia. Specifically, (1) blood glucose concentration > 200 mg/dl, (2) presence of moderate or greater ketones in urine or serum, and (3) arterial pH below 7.3 or serum bicarbonate < 20 meq/L will diagnose DKA. The differential diagnosis includes other types of metabolic acidosis and coma. An accumulation of ketone acids sufficient to cause metabolic acidosis may be seen in the absence of diabetes in poorly nourished alcoholic patients with repeated bouts of vomiting.[495] In such cases of *alcoholic ketoacidosis,* blood glucose levels are < 200 mg/dl (in 30 percent of cases frank hypoglycemia is present), and urine tests do not show a 4+ reaction for glucose. In addition, the plasma ketone reaction is generally only mildly or moderately positive because the ratio of β-hydroxybutyrate to acetoacetate is increased. The change in this ratio reflects the ability of alcohol to increase cellular levels of NADH. Treatment consists of glucose infusion, which will increase endogenous insulin secretion; exogenous insulin is usually not required. Often, it is not possible to separate the effects of ingested alcohol from those of diabetes, and Type 1 diabetic patients may have combined diabetic and alcoholic ketoacidoses.

Acidosis associated with uremia or various types of poisoning may present diagnostic problems, especially because patients with diabetic acidosis may also have impaired renal function owing to diabetic nephropathy as well as prerenal azotemia as a consequence of dehydration. Ketosis, however, is not present in uncomplicated uremic acidosis or methanol toxicity.

Hypoglycemia may also cause coma, but differentiation from DKA with coma is usually not difficult. In DKA, the onset is gradual and signs of acidosis are present, including hyperventilation, dehydration, hypotension, and tachycardia. In contrast, hypoglycemia occurs relatively rapidly, and the patient is not dehydrated or hyperventilating. The availability of near instantaneous fingerstick glucose results will clarify whether DKA or hypoglycemia is the cause of coma. If glucose results are not immediately available and uncertainty remains, health care personnel should draw a blood sample for determination of glucose and electrolyte concentrations and administer IV glucose (25 g) while awaiting the laboratory report. Coma may also occur with severe hyperglycemia without ketoacidosis: this syndrome—*hyperglycemic hyperosmolar nonketotic coma*—is discussed later. Severe metabolic acidosis and coma may be present in the absence of ketosis in patients with lactic acidosis. The latter condition is characterized by a reduction in arterial pH and serum bicarbonate concentration in the absence of a positive plasma ketone determination. However, a mildly positive reaction for ketones in a hyperglycemic patient with anion gap acidosis may signify the coexistence of DKA and lactic acidosis or combined alcoholic and diabetic acidoses.

Treatment Treatment of DKA has been relatively stable since the introduction of "low dose" intravenous insulin therapy in

TABLE 18-31. Treatment of DKA

1. Protect airway if mental status and/or gag reflex depressed.
2. Establish adequate IV access.
3. Assess volume state—clinical exam, calculate volume, and electrolyte deficit.
4. Replete volume with normal saline—usually 5–10 ml/kg/h for first 2 h; then 5 ml/kg/h. If hypernatremic or in congestive heart failure, may need to use 1/2 normal saline and consider central venous pressure monitoring.
5. Replete potassium—document urine output and infuse 0.3 to 0.5 meq/kg/hr.
6. Insulin—suggest 10 unit IV bolus, followed immediately by 5–10 u/h (regular insulin only). If improvement in anion gap and decrease in plasma glucose do not begin within 1–2 h, check access, rebolus and double intravenous insulin rate.
7. Monitor glucose levels and anion gap and or arterial pH regularly (hourly glucose monitoring recommended initially). On flow sheet record plasma glucose and electrolyte values and IV fluids, insulin, and urine output. Plasma glucose should decline by 40–100 mg/dl/h, more rapid decline may be dangerous, especially in children.
8. If serum phosphate is < 2.0 meq/l, replace 1/2 of potassium as KCl and 1/2 as K phosphate (not to exceed 1.5 meq/kg/h).
9. NPO until bowel sounds normal and acidosis resolved.
10. Test urine ketones twice per day.
11. Treat infection, myocardial infarction, other identified precipitants.
12. As plasma glucose levels fall to 250–300 mg/dl, add 5 percent dextrose to intravenous fluids.
13. When patient stable and acidosis resolved (anion gap resolved), make transition to subcutaneous insulin therapy. Overlap subcutaneous intermediate (or long-acting) *and* rapid- or very rapid-acting insulin with intravenous insulin. Recommend giving subcutaneous insulin at least 90 minutes (30–60 min if very rapid-acting insulin used) before discontinuing IV insulin.
14. Identify cause of DKA and re-educate patient to prevent future cases

1974.[496] The fundamental principles of treatment include replacement of lost volume and electrolytes including potassium, insulin administration, and diagnosis and treatment of underlying medical conditions (Table 18-31). Depending on the degree of obtundation and the presence or absence of a gag reflex, intubation may be necessary to protect the patient from aspiration. Although treatment in an intensive care unit is not mandatory, the clinical setting should permit frequent monitoring of vital signs, glucose and electrolytes, and administration of insulin. A large caliber intravenous line is required for the administration of large volumes of intravenous fluid. Critical features of intravenous replacement are the inclusion of adequate volume (mean volume and NaCl deficits in a 70 kg patient in DKA are 5–8 liters and 350–600 meq, respectively) and potassium repletion (mean deficit 200–400 meq). As the anion gap is corrected, a hyperchloremic metabolic acidosis often supervenes.[497]

Although DKA can be satisfactorily managed with insulin given intramuscularly or even subcutaneously, intravenous administration is far more predictable and results in less hypoglycemia and hypokalemia.[498,499] In addition, it is advantageous to give all insulin intravenously in the initial phases of treatment, as hypovolemia and impaired circulation may slow the absorption of subcutaneously or intramuscularly administered hormone. All insulin should be rapid-acting. With intravenous therapy, an initial loading dose of 6 to 10 U by bolus administration, immediately followed by a continuous infusion of 5–10 U/h until the plasma glucose concentration falls to 250 mg/dl, is recommended in adults. At that point, the intravenous insulin rate can be titrated and dextrose is added to the intravenous fluid. In children, a dose of 0.1 U per kilogram of body weight is usually appropriate. If glucose levels and acidosis don't begin to correct with the therapy above, patency of the intravenous lines and correct function of the intravenous pumps should be ascertained. In addition, IV lines should be checked to make certain that filters that may bind insulin have not been placed. The patient should be rebolused and a fresh insulin solution prepared from a different bottle of rapid-acting insulin. The insulin rate should be doubled. In very rare instances, the patient may still not respond, and insulin rates will need to be increased further. In such instances, antibody-mediated insulin resistance may be present and the insulin species may need to be changed. Alternatively, U-500 insulin, a highly concentrated regular insulin, or IGF therapy has been used successfully in such cases.[500,501]

One of the major challenges in treating DKA is the successful transition to subcutaneous therapy. Because discontinuation of intravenous insulin results in a precipitous fall in insulin levels within 30 minutes, administration of subcutaneous regular insulin, with or without an intermediate or long-acting insulin, should precede discontinuation of IV insulin by at least 60 minutes. The transition from IV to SC insulin should occur when glucose levels have been stabilized to less than 200 mg/dL and the anion gap acidosis has cleared with no ketonuria. (The hyperchloremic non-anion gap acidosis that often occurs after treatment of DKA should not prevent transition to a subcutaneous insulin regimen.) Usually, subcutaneous therapy should be reinstituted when the patient is ready to eat with resolution of any gastroparesis and resumption of normal bowel sounds.

Major controversies regarding treatment of DKA have focused on the role of bicarbonate and phosphate repletion. No studies have provided support for the use of bicarbonate,[502] although most textbooks continue to advise bicarbonate when the acidosis is "severe" (arterial pH < 7.05). Severe phosphate depletion (< 2.0 meq/L) can result in rhabdomyolysis, diaphragmatic abnormalities, and abnormal hemoglobin/oxygen dissociation secondary to depletion of 2,3-DPG. Although all of these abnormalities can be reversed by phosphate administration, their clinical import is questionable because controlled clinical trials have not demonstrated a significant difference in outcome of DKA whether phosphate is repleted or not.[503] Phosphate repletion has been associated with the development of tetany.

Despite the many advances in our understanding of diabetic ketoacidosis and its treatment, it is still a potentially fatal disorder. The major reasons for mortality include delayed recognition and treatment, aspiration associated with decreased mentation, cardiac arrhythmias, especially those associated with inadequate potassium repletion, and from the underlying clinical event (e.g., myocardial infarction or sepsis) that may have precipitated the DKA. In children, the development of cerebral edema after treatment is initiated is also a cause of mortality.[484] The usual clinical course of cerebral edema, which virtually never occurs in adults, includes apparently successful treatment of DKA with the development of worsening mental status as glucose levels fall. Children lapse into a coma with evidence of cerebral edema. Emergency treatment includes administration of decadron and mannitol and intubation with hyperventilation. The most likely explanation for cerebral edema in this setting is the rapid shift of fluid into the central nervous system as glucose levels fall too rapidly. The accumulation of "idiogenic osmoles", presumably to protect the brain from dehydration in the setting of hyperglycemia and hypertonicity, attracts solute into the brain and causes swelling as serum glucose levels fall.[504] In order to decrease the risk of developing cerebral edema, pediatric guidelines emphasize lowering glucose by no more than 50–150 mg/dL/hr, although there is little evidence to suggest that it is effective in preventing cerebral edema.

Hyperosmolar Hyperglycemic Nonketotic Coma (HHNKC)

Impaired consciousness may occur in a diabetic patient as a consequence of severe hyperglycemia, hyperosmolarity, and dehydration in the absence of ketoacidosis.[505] Hyperosmolar nonketotic coma, by definition, has blood ketone acid concentrations that are normal or only mildly elevated. Typically, this syndrome develops in middle-aged or elderly patients, often in the setting of previously mild type 2 diabetes. Symptoms of polydipsia and polyuria generally develop over a period of several days, culminating in disturbances of consciousness which cause the patient to come to medical attention. As in DKA, mental obtundation varying from lethargy to coma occurs. However, in contrast to DKA, patients with hyperosmolar coma often have focal or generalized seizures. In many instances the syndrome is temporally related to the prior administration of drugs such as diuretics, glucocorticoids, immunosuppressive agents, or phenytoin, or to the institution of tube feedings or total parenteral alimentation that can increase glucose levels acutely. Patients who develop HHNKC are often unable to replete their volume losses owing to impaired level of consciousness or thirst sensation, or because they are in a setting, such as a nursing home or intensive care unit, where they don't have free access to water.

The laboratory findings consist of marked hyperglycemia (>600 mg/dl or 33 mM), hyperosmolarity (generally >310 mOsm), azotemia, and, by definition, the absence of hyperketonemia. The degree of azotemia is on average greater than that observed in DKA, (BUN 70 to 90 mg/dl, compared with 40 mg/dl in DKA).[485] The serum sodium concentration may be normal, elevated, or even reduced. The failure to observe a consistent elevation of serum sodium concentration in the face of marked dehydration is a consequence of redistribution of body fluids from the intracellular to the extracellular compartment engendered by hyperglycemia. The expected reduction in serum sodium concentration brought about by hyperglycemia may be calculated as 1.6 mEq/liter for each 100-mg/dl increment in serum glucose concentration above normal.[506] Thus, in a patient with a markedly elevated blood glucose level and a normal or elevated serum sodium concentration, a severe state of dehydration is likely to be present.

The pathogenesis of the syndrome of nonketotic hyperosmolar coma remains somewhat unclear. Two factors require explanation: the presence of hyperglycemia, which exceeds that generally observed in DKA, and the absence of ketoacidosis. With respect to the former, the diminution in renal function may limit the extent to which glucose can be excreted in urine, thus resulting in the progressive accumulation of glucose in the blood. Supporting this possibility is the observation that alloxan-treated animals develop nonketotic hyperosmolar coma if the ureters are tied and glucocorticoids are administered.[507] The presence of small amounts of insulin sufficient to inhibit lipolysis (but not gluconeogenesis) has been postulated to account for the failure to develop ketoacidosis. C-peptide levels tend to be higher and plasma FFA levels tend to be lower in hyperosmolar nonketotic coma than in DKA.[508,509]

Treatment consists of continuous IV infusion of insulin in low doses (6 to 10 U/h), together with large amounts of fluids as hypotonic saline (unless the patient is in shock, in which case isotonic saline is infused) and repletion of body potassium.[510,511]

The mortality rate has been reported to vary from 5 to 40 percent. Many of the fatal cases have accompanying lactic acidosis, as reflected by reduced arterial pH, absent or low ketone concentrations, and a large anion gap. In many instances, death is due to an underlying disease process such as pancreatitis or sepsis.

Complications of Insulin Therapy (Hypoglycemia, Allergy, Lipodystrophy)

Hypoglycemia is more common than DKA, and potentially as dangerous a metabolic emergency. Clinical hypoglycemia can range from an annoying set of symptoms accompanying a biochemically low (<65 mg/dL) glucose level to the occurrence of confusion, seizures, and/or loss of consciousness. The "warning" symptoms that most commonly constitute nonsevere hypoglycemia are adrenergic in character and include tremulousness, diaphoresis, and tachycardia. The central nervous system manifestations that occur with severe hypoglycemia result in cognitive dysfunction ranging from lethargy, confusion, and difficulty in concentrating to loss of consciousness and seizures. When hypoglycemia occurs during sleep, the only symptoms may be nightmares, sweating, and a headache on awakening in the morning.

The functional definition of "severe" hypoglycemia established by the DCCT[13,320] is now commonly employed in epidemiologic studies and clinical trials and provides a useful clinical definition. Severe hypoglycemia is defined as any episode of chemical hypoglycemia (with blood glucose level <65 mg/dL, and usually lower) and with symptoms or neurologic findings consistent with clinical hypoglycemia (see later discussion) that could not be treated by the patient without assistance. These severe episodes most commonly include modest confusion or lethargy with the patient requiring assistance from a family member to "get the juice" so that the patient can treat the "reaction" with oral carbohydrate. Only a small fraction (≈25 percent) of severe episodes include more profound disruption in central nervous system function such as loss of consciousness or seizures. The reasoning behind the conservative DCCT definition of severe hypoglycemia is the concern that if a family member had not been available to help treat, the hypoglycemia might have progressed to more severe sequelae. Obviously, severe hypoglycemia can have disastrous acute consequences depending on the setting (e.g., driving a car or operating potentially dangerous equipment).

Glucagon and epinephrine are the major counterregulatory hormones that restore glucose levels as insulin levels dissipate.[159] Cortisol, growth hormone, and thyroxine play a less acute role in maintaining glucose levels. Elevated catecholamine levels provide an "alert" signal that should prompt the affected person to treat the episode. In addition, glucagon and epinephrine stimulate hepatic glucose output. After 5–10 years of Type 1 diabetes, the glucagon response to hypoglycemia may decrease, leaving catecholamines as the only defense against hypoglycemia.[512] If the catecholamine response is also hampered, as may occur in the setting of autonomic neuropathy, patients will be at heightened risk for severe hypoglycemia.[513]

Hypoglycemic unawareness is a relatively new phenomenon that came to light in the wake of intensive therapy. Within weeks

TABLE 18-32. Treatment of Hypoglycemia

Oral*	Parenteral
Orange juice—6 oz	25 cc 50 percent dextrose
Coca-cola—4 oz	1 mg glucagon†
Table sugar—4 teaspoons	
Glucotabs—3	
Lifesavers—5	

*Common sources of 12–15 gram of rapidly absorbable carbohydrate.

†0.25–0.5 mg for children < 5 y. Can be given IM or IV. May cause nausea and vomiting.

to months of initiating intensive therapy, patients with Type 1 diabetes would often note that they no longer perceived hypoglycemia at the same blood glucose level as they had in the past. The lower glucose level necessary to activate adrenergic responses was welcomed as evidence that normoglycemia was being restored. With time, however, it became clear that the lessening or disappearance of adrenergic warning symptoms, either until very low glucose levels occurred or no matter how low glucose levels fell, robbed patients of a protective barrier against very severe clinical hypoglycemia. The frequency of coma and seizure increase by threefold or more in patients treated intensively compared with conventional therapy.[13,300] Subsequent studies revealed that the occurrence of one episode of hypoglycemia decreased the blood glucose threshold at which adrenergic activation occurred with subsequent episodes and increased the risk for recurrent severe hypoglycemia.[514,515] The mechanism by which antecedent hypoglycemia affects adrenergic discharge may involve upregulated glucose transport in the central nervous system, which protects the brain from subsequent hypoglycemia but paradoxically makes repeated episodes of severe hypoglycemia more likely.[516] Avoidance of hypoglycemia can restore adrenergic response at higher glucose levels.[517]

Most episodes of hypoglycemia will be rapidly recognized by the patient and effectively treated with a rapidly absorbed oral carbohydrate. Approximately 15 grams of carbohydrate are sufficient to restore blood glucose levels to normal. Common sources of 15 gm of carbohydrate are listed in Table 18-32. Use of complex carbohydrates and foods with high fat content, such as chocolate, may delay digestion/absorption of saccharides and is not appropriate for hypoglycemia treatment. In addition, treatment with one of the glycosidase inhibitors may decrease digestion and absorption of sugars.

If a patient is unable to swallow or cooperate, either intravenous dextrose or IM or SC, glucagon should be given. Twenty five cc (1/2 ampule) of 50 percent dextrose (12.5 grams) given IV push is generally sufficient to reverse clinical hypoglycemia. Even less may be required in infants and children. Glucagon injection kits contain 1 mg of glucagon, which increases glucose levels in 15 to 30 min. Glucagon can cause nausea, vomiting, and headache, especially in children.

Patients with severe hypoglycemia usually respond rapidly to treatment, although patients with prolonged coma or who are postictal may require days to regain normal mental status and cognitive function. Amnesia for the events preceding and immediately following a seizure or loss of consciousness hypoglycemic episode is not uncommon. Rarely, neurological deficits can be permanent after hypoglycemia.[518,519] On the other hand, the intensively treated patients in the DCCT, studied after a mean of 6.5 years of intensive therapy with a threefold increase in severe hypoglycemia, did not have any measurable difference in cognitive function compared with the conventional therapy patients.[316] Whether longer-term therapy or follow-up will result in or reveal cognitive deficits is unknown. Nevertheless, considering the potential consequences of any severe episode of hypoglycemia, therapy should always be provided on an emergent basis. When in doubt as to the cause of altered mental status (e.g., a confused patient with no immediately available glocuse results) treat as if hypoglycemia is the cause.

Although all patients taking hypoglycemic medications including sulfonylureas, some of which can cause prolonged, severe hypoglycemia should be instructed in how to recognize and treat hypoglycemia, and need to have ready access to a source of rapidly absorbable carbohydrate (glucose tablets, hard candy, icing), the major focus should be on prevention. Understanding the time course of different insulin formulations, the need for consistent timing and size of meals, the impact of exercise, and the need to adjust insulin to accomodate meal size and content, exercise, and ambient glucose levels should help prevent hypoglycemia. In addition, frequent glucose monitoring, especially when activity or dietary regimens change and before beginning any activity that hypoglycemia would make particularly hazardous (e.g., driving), is highly recommended.

A "rebound" in glycemia, often termed the Somogyi phenomenon, may be seen after an episode of hypoglycemia. The phenomenon of posthypoglycemia hyperglycemia was first investigated more than 40 years ago. Increased urine glucose excretion was noted in the 24–48 hours after a severe reaction.[520] The hyperglycemia was secondary to the increased counterregulatory hormones after hypoglycemia. Unfortunately, the Somogyi phenomenon has been misinterpreted, and fasting hyperglycemia is often ascribed to undetected nocturnal hypoglycemia. More recent studies have demonstrated that nocturnal hypoglycemia is usually associated with relatively low fasting glucose levels in the morning, unless the patient has overetreated the hypoglycemic reaction.[521]

Other Complications of Insulin Treatment

Insulin Lipodystrophy

Insulin lipodystrophy is a distressing, although generally benign, complication of insulin treatment that may take the form of hypertrophy or atrophy of subcutaneous tissues. Lipohypertrophy is a direct effect of high local concentrations of insulin stimulating lipid synthesis and storage. The hypertrophied lipid mass that can develop after repeated injections in a single anatomic site is hypoesthetic; the problem is therefore often perpetuated, as these sites are favored for injection. Unfortunately, the absorption of insulin from these sites is often erratic and incomplete and may lead to a deterioration in the control of diabetes. Avoidance of hypertrophied injection sites and rotation of injection sites may ameliorate lipohypertrophy, but it may take years for an appreciable decrease in the size of the mass to occur.

Lipoatrophy represents the loss of subcutaneous fat at the site of previous injections or even at distant sites (Fig. 18-50, [Color Plate 3]). Patients often describe lipoatrophic areas as "dents," or "craters," and they may be disfiguring. The mechanism is thought to be immune in nature.[344] Injection into the center of these lipoat-

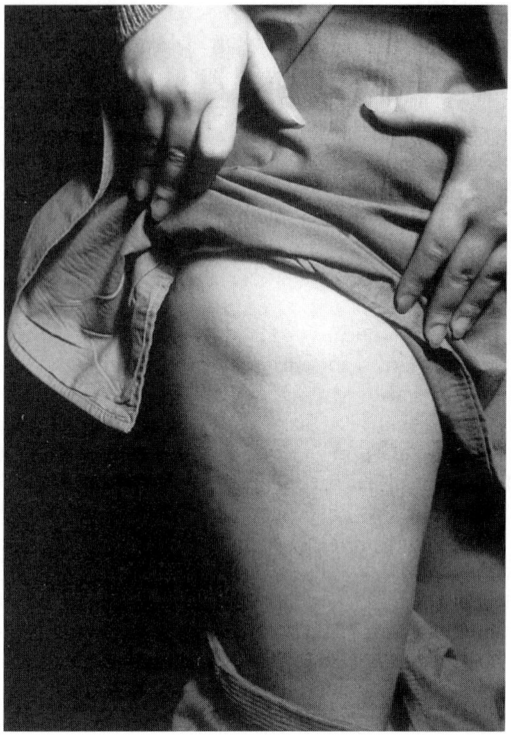

FIGURE 18-50. Lipoatrophy (color photograph). Lipoatrophy represents discrete areas with loss of subcutaneous fat at sites of previous insulin injections and at anatomic sites where insulin has never been injected. An increasingly rare complication of insulin therapy, lipoatrophy appears as "dents" in the skin.

rophic areas is essentially intramuscular, may be painful, and should be avoided. Treatment with highly purified insulin preparations has reduced the incidence of this complication. The use of human insulin may also be advantageous in this circumstance. Lipoatrophic areas should be injected gradually from the periphery toward the center of the "crater" until they are filled in.

Insulin Allergy

Insulin allergy has become an extremely uncommon problem since highly purified animal and human insulins have been introduced. The delayed hypersensitivity reaction, characterized by pruritus, erythema, or pain at the injection site, that commonly occurred when insulin therapy was initiated is rarely seen with modern day insulin preparations. In most patients, the reactions disappeared spontaneously after several weeks. These local skin reactions could be treated by switching to monospecies insulin (e.g., pure pork), to human insulin, or to the local use of small doses of glucocorticoids. Antibody-mediated resistance (usually IgGs mediated) or IgE-mediated systemic allergy has also become vanishingly rare.[344] Intermittent administration of insulin, particularly with beef-pork or beef insulins, has been documented as a risk factor for these phenomena in the past. Although human insulin of recombinant DNA origin is less immunogenic than pork or beef insulin, low-titer antibody formation may still occur, resulting in insulin allergy in rare patients.

Systemic allergy may be manifested as a generalized pruritus and urticaria, angioedema, or acute anaphylaxis; such anaphylaxis, fortunately, is extremely rare. Cutaneous testing to determine the insulin species and formulation that is least immunogenic may be helpful in selecting the insulin to use. Treatment consists of desensitization with human or porcine insulin at an initial dose of 0.001 U.[345]

Although there are few, if any, demonstrated advantages of human insulin compared with comparably pure animal species insulins, most insulin manufacturers are phasing out animal species insulins for economic reasons. One of the disadvantages of the change to human insulin is the generally shorter duration of the intermediate-acting formulations, compared with animal species insulin, perhaps owing to decreased binding to antibodies.

LONG-TERM COMPLICATIONS

Overview

The long-term complications of diabetes mellitus cause most of the morbidity and mortality associated with the disease and make it a chronic, degenerative disease. The complications can be divided into two general categories: diabetes-specific, which are relatively unique to diabetes, and nonspecific, which occur in patients without diabetes, but affect persons with diabetes disproportionately. The diabetes-specific complications occur with generally similar frequencies in all types of diabetes.[523,524]

The *diabetes-specific* complications include retinopathy, nephropathy, and neuropathy. Although these complications share certain features, they also differ in many respects. No obvious common pathophysiological feature or underlying cellular or tissue abnormality, except for their association with hyperglycemia, unites all three diabetes-specific complications.[525] The development of all of the diabetes-specific complications appears to have a glycemic threshold. Nephropathy, retinopathy, and neuropathy do not develop in the setting of subdiabetic glucose levels. (This is to some extent a circular observation since the glucose threshold for diagnosing diabetes is based on the level at which retinopathy occurs.) Moreover, the risk for developing any of the complications is associated with the level of glycemia over time, that is, glycemic exposure.[323] The specific organs affected by diabetic complications appear to be relatively permeable to glucose even in the absence of insulin. Thus, tissue glucose levels are likely to reflect ambient plasma glucose. Finally, studies in animal models of diabetes[291,526,527] and clinical trials in Type 1[13,300] and Type 2 diabetes[17,302] have demonstrated a profound salutary effect of lowering blood glucose on the diabetes-specific complications. The observations above have established the primacy of hyperglycemia in the development and progression of diabetic complications. Of note, not all patients with diabetes develop these complications over time, and glycemia, although a relatively potent factor in the development of complications, only explains a modest fraction of the risk of developing diabetic complications.[323] Other environmental and clinical factors have been identified that influence the risk for developing complications,[528–531] and genetic factors[328,532] may also influence their development and progression.

Differences in the development and progression of the different complications are notable. First, prior to the widespread implementation of intensive therapies aimed at normalizing glycemia, the majority of patients with long-term diabetes developed some degree of retinopathy and/or neuropathy[11,16,533,534]; however, only 30–40 percent of Type 1 patients[11,535,536] and only 10 percent of patients with Type 2 diabetes developed nephropathy.[537,538] Second, the risk for developing retinopathy and neuropathy appears to persist over the entire duration of diabetes[533,534,539]; conversely, the risk of developing nephropathy reaches a peak at 15–20 years duration of diabetes and then plummets.[540] These observations suggest that some complications appear to follow a continuous risk curve over time, while others show a threshold effect. Third, the underlying pathology of the specific complications differ, with microvascular disease apparent in retinopathy and nephropathy, but other, nonvascular factors underlying the most common forms of neuropathy. Finally, even within specific complications, different stages may have different risk factors and causes. For example, the development of nonproliferative retinopathy, the most common form of retinopathy, appears to be most closely associated with glycemic levels X duration; however, the further development of vascular occlusion, ischemia, and proliferative retinopathy, which is less common, is associated with other factors, including angiogenic growth factors,[541] that are not obviously related to glycemia.

The *nonspecific* complications associated with diabetes mellitus are secondary to atherosclerotic macrovascular disease. The risk for coronary artery and cerebral and peripheral vascular disease is increased 2- to 10-fold, compared with that in nondiabetic persons.[542] The clinical manifestations of macrovascular disease in diabetes including myocardial infarctions, stroke, and amputations cause 75 percent of all mortality and result in a significantly reduced life-span.[543] In contrast to the diabetes-specific complications, the development of macrovascular disease is not related to diabetes duration, but is more closely associated with attained age. Diabetes has a disproportionate effect on women, effectively erasing their gender-mediated protection from CVD.[542] In addition, the prevalence of macrovascular disease in diabetes, although increased in all diabetic populations, reflects the underlying risk in the specific racial and ethnic population. For example, in populations with a relatively low frequency of coronary artery disease, diabetes increases the frequency, but in a range that parallels the nondiabetic population's risk.[544,545]

In diabetes mellitus, and especially in Type 2 diabetes, an increased prevalence of risk factors for CVD accounts for a significant fraction of the increased risk for CVD; however, even when the increased prevalence of risk factors for CVD established in the nondiabetic population is taken into account, an excess risk for CVD in the diabetic population remains.[546,547] Whether the remaining risk is secondary to glycemia per se, or to other diabetes-specific risk factors is not known. Epidemiologic studies suggest that glycemia is associated with CVD.[548,549] Moreover, CVD risk factors increase across the entire spectrum of glycemia, from subdiabetic to IGT to diabetic levels,[550] in contrast to the diabetes-specific complications where a definite threshold has been identified. An excess of "classical" cardiac risk factors not specific to diabetes, such as renal failure, combined with changes in lipoproteins, endothelial function, thrombogenesis, and fibrinolysis, that may be specific to the diabetic state, may play a role in the excess macrovascular disease.

Pathophysiology

Glycemia has been demonstrated to play a major role in the pathogenesis of the diabetes-specific complications.[13,17,286,291,300,323] Its role in the nonspecific macrovascular complications is, not surprisingly, less certain. The mechanism by which glycemia influences the development and progression of complications is controversial. Whether a unitary mechanism explains all complications, or the different clinical stages of any given complication, is unknown.[525] It seems increasingly clear that some complications may have one mechanism that initiates the complications (e.g., the development of nonproliferative retinopathy) and another mechanism that results in progression (to proliferative retinopathy). The diverse neurologic complications are probably caused by different mechanisms (a metabolic cause of peripheral sensorimotor neuropathy, but a vascular cause of mononeuropathies).

The most common mechanisms invoked to explain the development of microvascular complications include glycation (and glycooxidation)[551,552]; the accumulation of sorbitol and other sugar alcohols[553]; alterations in intermediate metabolites such as protein kinase C (PKC)[554]; an increased tendency for oxidative damage in diabetes[555]; alteration in growth factors or cytokines[556]; and changes in endothelium that may lead to leakage from and obstruction of small vessels in the eye and glomerulus and the vasa nervorum.[557,558] None of these putative mechanisms is exclusive; some combination of them is likely.

Nonenzymatic glycation of proteins is a universal phenomenon that occurs on N-terminal valines and internal lysines.[329] Higher concentrations of glucose and longer exposure of proteins to glucose result in higher levels of glycated proteins. The turnover of specific proteins also affects the period over which the concentration of glycated proteins reaches an equilibrium. For proteins with a relatively rapid turnover and short life-span, such as albumin with a circulating life-span of 20–30 days, the concentration of glycated albumin reflects the integrated level of glycemia over the half-life of the protein. This property of nonenzymatic glycation has been harnessed to create clinical assays reflecting the average level of glycemia.[332] Glycated serum protein levels measure short-term glycemia, while glycated levels of hemoglobin measure integrated mean glucose levels over approximately 2–3 months.[332] Longer-lived proteins such as Type IV collagen and other glomerular basement membranes proteins remain glycated for longer periods because they turnover more slowly.[559]

Glycation is an attractive pathophysiologic mechanism for long-term complications because glycated protein concentrations reflect average glycemia. Moreover, many of the tissues that suffer diabetic complications have been demonstrated to contain glycated structural proteins or glycated enzymes that might affect function.[551] This includes glycated myelin sheath protein, lens protein, and glomerular basement proteins. After initial glycation, subsequent rearrangements result in advanced glycation endproducts (AGE) that cause structural and functional changes that may explain the development of some or many of the complications (Fig. 18-51). In addition to the structural changes, receptors for AGE have been demonstrated.[551] Binding to the receptors may initiate other processes, such as fibroblast proliferation and intimal hyperplasia, that may contribute to the development of complications. In addition, glycation promotes oxidation that may further increase the atherogenic potency of lipids.[560] Glycation has also been demonstrated to affect the binding of LDL and HDL to their respective receptors, providing a possible mechanism for atherogenesis.[561,562] The role of glycation in the development and progression of diabetic complications has been supported by studies with drugs, such as aminoguanidine, that inhibit the formation of AGE. The early glycosylation (Amadori) products bind preferentially to aminoguanidine, preventing AGE formation and collagen crosslinking. In animal models of diabetes, the development of histologic changes consistent with diabetic complications,

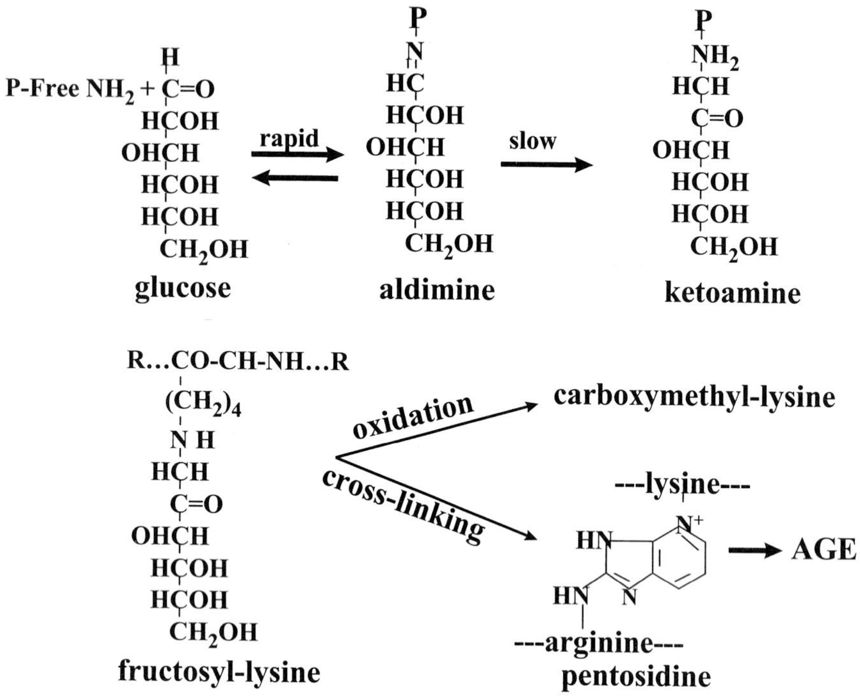

FIGURE 18-51 Glycation and formation of advanced glycation end products.

including retinopathy, nephropathy, and neuropathy, has been reduced with aminoguanidine.[563-565] The interpretation of these studies is somewhat unclear, as the drugs that inhibit AGE formation have other effects, including antioxidation.[566] Studies with drugs that inhibit glycation in human diabetes are ongoing.

An even older proposal for the pathophysiologic mechanism of diabetic complications is the accumulation of sorbitol and other sugar alcohols in specific tissues.[567] The accumulation of sorbitol is secondary to the transport of glucose and its subsequent metabolism by aldose reductase to sorbitol. Sorbitol is subsequently metabolized to fructose by sorbitol dehydrogenase. Aldose reductase and increased sorbitol levels have been demonstrated to be present in many tissues, including those affected by diabetic complications.[568] In some tissues, such as the lens, sorbitol accumulation results in an osmotic gradient that causes swelling and potential disruption in structure and function. In other tissues, such as peripheral nerve, sorbitol accumulation has been implicated as a cause of altered function. However, whether sorbitol accumulation or some other associated change, such as myoinositol depletion or decreased sodium-potassium activated ATPase activity, is responsible for the functional or histologic changes is unclear.[568] The potential role of aldose reductase and sorbitol in the pathogenesis of diabetic complications has been advanced by studies in animal models of diabetes with aldose reductase inhibitors (ARIs). ARIs reduce the levels of sorbitol, increase nerve conduction, and decrease the development of diabetic cataracts in experimental diabetes.[569,570] Unfortunately, numerous clinical studies with a variety of aldose reductase inhibitors have failed to demonstrate any convincing or clinically significant effects on complications in human diabetes.[571-573] Although the failure of aldose reductase inhibitors to have a salutary effect in human diabetes may be secondary to poor bioavailability of the available drugs in the affected tissues, or to some other factors, clinical trial results have weakened support for the sorbitol hypothesis of diabetic complications.

Vascular abnormalities including endothelial dysfunction,[574] abnormalities in supporting cells such as pericytes in the retina[575] and mesangial cells in the glomerulus,[576] and hyperfiltration and intrarenal hypertension in the kidney[577] may be secondary to glycation, oxidation, sorbitol accumulation, or other factors. Some of the advanced vascular changes may not be diabetes specific, i.e., after hyperglycemia initiates cellular abnormalities, the late vascular changes, such as neovascularization in the retina in response to ischemia and progressive glomerular dropout in the kidney, may be nonspecific responses. Finally, other mechanisms including abnormalities in platelet function[578] and growth factors[556,579,580] and genetic factors[328,532] may play a contributory role in the genesis of complications.

Retinopathy

Clinical Characteristics

Retinopathy occurs in all forms of diabetes. The natural history of retinopathy in Type 1 and Type 2 diabetes has been well-described in several long-term studies using stereoscopic fundus photography, a relatively sensitive and objective means of detailing changes in the fundus.[533,539,581,582] Depending on the number of fields in the fundus photography, as much as 160° of the fundus may be encompassed. Other methods of assessing retinal changes include nondilated (nonmydriatic) photography; fluorescein angiography that utilizes a small (300 dalton) molecular weight dye, which fluoresces to visualize the vessels and detect leakage through abnormal endothelial cell junctions in the microvasculature[583]; electroretinograms that measure electrophysiological changes that may precede detectable structural microvascular changes[584]; and direct and indirect ophthalmoscopy and slit lamp biomicroscopy, which are the most common clinical tools to assess retinopathy.

The development of retinopathy is duration dependent, similar to all diabetes-specific complications.[16,533-535] With the use of

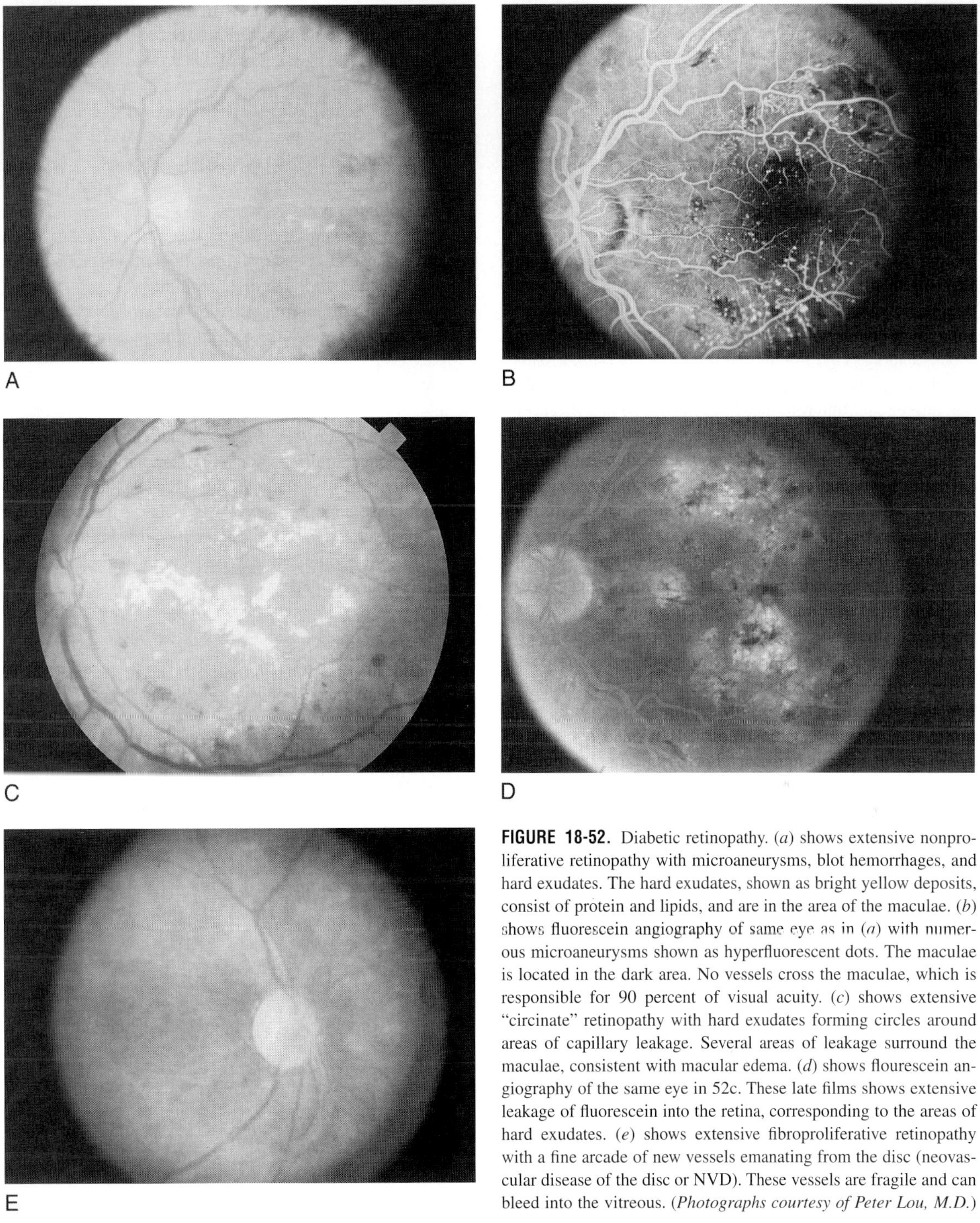

FIGURE 18-52. Diabetic retinopathy. (*a*) shows extensive nonproliferative retinopathy with microaneurysms, blot hemorrhages, and hard exudates. The hard exudates, shown as bright yellow deposits, consist of protein and lipids, and are in the area of the maculae. (*b*) shows fluorescein angiography of same eye as in (*a*) with numerous microaneurysms shown as hyperfluorescent dots. The maculae is located in the dark area. No vessels cross the maculae, which is responsible for 90 percent of visual acuity. (*c*) shows extensive "circinate" retinopathy with hard exudates forming circles around areas of capillary leakage. Several areas of leakage surround the maculae, consistent with macular edema. (*d*) shows flourescein angiography of the same eye in 52c. These late films shows extensive leakage of fluorescein into the retina, corresponding to the areas of hard exudates. (*e*) shows extensive fibroproliferative retinopathy with a fine arcade of new vessels emanating from the disc (neovascular disease of the disc or NVD). These vessels are fragile and can bleed into the vitreous. (*Photographs courtesy of Peter Lou, M.D.*)

flourescein angiography and histologic studies of trypsin digested eyes from diabetic humans and animals with experimental diabetes, the earliest abnormalities in the diabetic eye appear to be loss of pericytes, the supporting cells that provide integrity and perhaps nutrition to the endothelial cells that make up the retinal capillaries.[585] The first visible lesions are small (10–100 micron diameter) microaneurysms arising from the terminal capillaries of the retina, perhaps secondary to the loss of the supporting pericytes (Fig. 18-52a, [Color Plate2]). Dot and blot hemorrhages appear when erythrocytes occupy or escape from the microaneurysms. The most common location for these microaneurysms is in the midperiphery, often one to one and one-half disc diameters (500 to 1,000 microns) from the disc. The retinal vessels are abnormally permeable and leak protein and lipid rich serous fluid leading to the formation of hard exudates.

Microaneurysms, dot and blot hemorrhages, and hard exudates are commonly referred to as "background" (because of their common occurrence in diabetes) or, preferably, as nonproliferative diabetic retinopathy (NPDR). Unless NPDR occurs near the maculae and causes macular edema, it does not lead to vision loss. Macular edema occurs when leakage of fluid from abnormal vessels near the maculae causes thickening and disrupts the light path to the maculae, resulting in loss of visual acuity.[586] With increasing severity, the abnormal vessels can become occluded, leading

TABLE 18-33. High Risk Characteristics for Proliferative Retinopathy

New vessel proliferation within one disk diameter of the optic disk and exceeding 1/4 the disk area in size
Any proliferation within one disk diameter of optic disk and associated with vitreous or preretinal hemorrhage
Proliferation elsewhere at least 1/2 the disk area in size and associated with hemorrhage

to retinal ischemia with infarctions in the nerve layer of the retina, seen as soft (cotton wool) exudates ("pre-proliferative retinopathy," Fig. 18-52b, [Color Plate 2]). Increased tortuosity, dilated veins "venous beading," and intraretinal microvascular abnormalities (IRMA) develop during the preproliferative phase. In response to ischemia, angiogenic humoral factors are released and promote the development of new vessels (neovascularization).[541] The new vessels proliferate out of the retinal surface and into the vitreous cavity ("proliferative diabetic retinopathy," or PDR, Fig. 18-52c, [Color Plate 2]). They are attenuated, fragile, and tend to bleed into the vitreous. The vitreous hemorrhages can obscure vision, but are usually reabsorbed in 1 to 3 months. Subsequent fibroproliferative changes can cause retinal traction and detachment and loss of vision. Proliferative retinopathy is clinically divided into neovascularization of the disc (NVD), i.e., within one disc diameter of the disc, or neovascularization elsewhere (NVE), based on the differential risks for vision loss associated with these lesions.[587] Retinal lesions that are considered "high risk characteristics" with regard to loss of vision are described in Table 18-33.

Although nonproliferative and proliferative retinopathy are the characteristic lesions of diabetic retinopathy, patients with diabetes are also at higher risk for nonspecific ophthalmic disease, such as cataracts.[588] Whether the increased risk for the development of cataracts is predicated on sorbitol accumulation in the lens,[589] glycation of lens crystallin protein,[590] or both, is unknown. Cataracts are more likely than retinopathy to be the cause of loss of vision in patients with late-onset diabetes.[591] Finally, increased intraocular pressure and glaucoma may occur as a consequence of neovascularization that blocks the aqueous outflow (rubeosis).

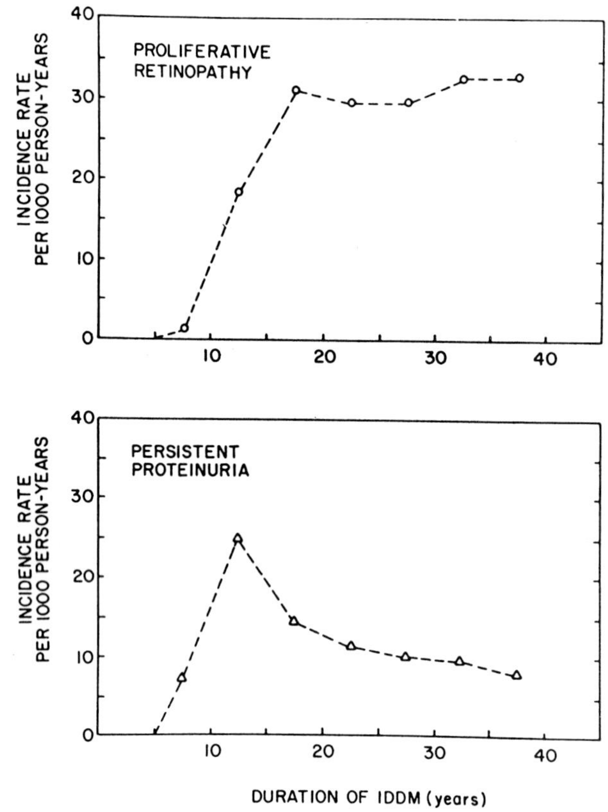

FIGURE 18-53. Epidemiology of diabetic retinopathy and nephropathy in Type 1 diabetes. For 40 years 292 patients with Type 1 diabetes were followed. The risk of proliferative retinopathy continued unabated over the entire followup period. On the other hand, the risk of persistent proteinuria, which results in end-stage renal disease in more than 90 percent of affected subjects, peaked after approximately 15 years. Patients who have not developed proteinuria after 25 years of diabetes duration are unlikely to develop clinically significant renal disease. (*From Krolewski et al. Diabetes Care 9:443–52, 1986.*)

Prevalence and Incidence

The natural history and occurrence of diabetic retinopathy has been defined best in Type 1 diabetes where the date of onset of clinical diabetes can be ascertained accurately. Most of the available epidemiologic data reflect the development of retinopathy during an era when glycemic control was suboptimal (Fig. 18-53). Taking into account the now demonstrated beneficial effect of intensive diabetes therapy and decreased glycemia on the development of retinopathy[13,17,307,308] and the increased efforts to attain improved glycemia, it is likely that the prevalence and incidence of retinopathy demonstrated in the past will be largely reduced in the future. The estimated long-term benefit of intensive therapy suggests a >75 percent decrease in the development and progression of retinopathy.[327]

In general, nonproliferative retinopathy doesn't appear until after 3 to 5 years duration. It may not appear at all prior to puberty, regardless of duration.[592] After 7 years duration, approximately 50 percent of Type 1 diabetic patients have some degree of retinopathy detectable by stereoscopic fundus photography.[533] (Direct ophthalmoscopy is less sensitive, especially for the presence of a small number of lesions).[593] In past studies, prevalence of any retinopathy reached more than 90 percent after 20 years duration.[533] The development of macular edema and proliferative retinopathy is also duration-dependent, albeit at a lower frequency than nonproliferative retinopathy. The natural history of retinopathy in Type 2 diabetes is more difficult to delineate because Type 2 diabetes may be present for many years before it is diagnosed, precluding accurate assessment of duration.[195] As a result, approximately 20 percent of Type 2 diabetic patients have retinopathy and, more rarely, even advanced retinopathy at the time of diagnosis.[195,594] Nevertheless, the development of retinopathy is generally duration-dependent in Type 2 diabetes as in Type 1 diabetes.

Whereas >90 percent of Type 1 diabetic patients and 60 percent of Type 2 diabetic patients develop some degree of retinopathy over 20 years of diabetes duration, only 50 percent and 10 percent, respectively, develop proliferative retinopathy.[539,582] Diabetes remains the most common cause of vision loss in adults in the U.S.

Pathogenesis and Risk Factors

Risk factors identified for the development and progression of retinopathy include the level of chronic glycemia and glycemia X duration,[292,293,294,323] hypertension,[531] smoking in some studies[595] but not others,[596] and pregnancy in Type 1 diabetes.[528,597] The risk imparted by pregnancy is usually transient, with the major impact in the third trimester and up to six months after delivery. Elevated lipid, and especially triglyceride, levels have a minor effect.[598] A positive family history of retinopathy in the setting of multiplex families (with more than one member with diabetes) is also associated with a higher risk of retinopathy.[328] Whether this is secondary to a genetic effect on the development of complications, or some other shared environmental influence, is not known. Finally, intensive therapy is a recognized risk factor for transient worsening of established retinopathy during the first 6 to 12 months of therapy.[309] Major risk factors for transient worsening are the HbA1c level at the time of initiation of intensive therapy and the magnitude of the reduction of this level in the first 6 months. Overall, the benefit of intensive therapy becomes manifest, even taking transient worsening into consideration, after 2–3 years of therapy.

Screening

Screening for complications is supportable if treatment applied in the presymptomatic phase improves outcome when compared with treatment initiated only after symptoms develop. The preclinical phases of retinopathy represent appropriate targets for screening. Intensive glycemic control has been demonstrated to decrease development and progression of retinopathy.[13,17,307,308] The demonstration of early lesions may motivate patients who have not initiated intensive therapy previously. Laser therapy has been demonstrated to decrease subsequent vision loss associated with macular edema[586] and proliferative retinopathy, both of which are usually asymptomatic.[587] Screening recommendations have been formulated based on the natural history of diabetic retinopathy, the risk of vision loss associated with certain high-risk characteristics, and the demonstrated benefit of laser therapy, taking into account the sensitivity, specificity, and cost of specific screening modalities. The American Diabetes Association, American College of Ophthalmology, and American College of Physicians have promoted the screening recommendations shown in Table 18-18.[599] More frequent screening may be necessary after the initiation of intensive therapy and during pregnancy and shortly after delivery because of the recognized risk of progression in these settings.[309,528,597] The level of increased risk imposed by these conditions is usually related to the underlying level of retinopathy. Patients with no retinopathy at baseline are unlikely to develop severe retinopathy; conversely, patients with more advanced retinopathy must be followed carefully because they may develop advanced retinopathy requiring laser therapy.

Therapy

Several high quality clinical trials have unequivocally demonstrated a salutary effect of intensive diabetes therapy on retinopathy. The DCCT (Fig. 18-32) and Stockholm Diabetes Study in Type 1 and Kumamoto and UKPDS in Type 2 diabetes have shown a beneficial effect of intensive therapy.[13,17,300,302] The beneficial effect can be demonstrated before retinopathy develops (primary prevention), and in slowing progression after minimal to moderate retinopathy has developed (secondary intervention). Intensive therapy after the development of proliferative retinopathy has not been demonstrated to be effective, although relatively few studies have been performed.[600] In Type 1 diabetes, transient worsening of pre-existent retinopathy during the first 6–12 months of intensive diabetes treatment has been well-described.[309]

Two major clinical trials have demonstrated a substantial beneficial effect of laser (xenon arc or argon) therapy on proliferative retinopathy[587] and macular edema.[586] Both studies have demonstrated a preventative role for laser therapy, i.e., it reduces the development of new vision loss. With proliferative retinopathy, laser therapy generally doesn't reverse vision loss already present; however, if macular edema is present, visual acuity may improve as the maculae "dries out."

The Diabetic Retinopathy Study (DRS) randomized diabetic patients' eyes with proliferative retinopathy to either deferred therapy or panretinal laser photocoagulation (Fig. 18-54).[587] Laser therapy reduced severe central vision loss by approximately 50 percent for all levels of proliferative retinopathy. The decision to recommend laser therapy for patients with high risk characteristics (Table 18-33) was predicated on balancing the expected benefits with the risk of decreased peripheral and night vision resulting from panretinal photocoagulation. The Early Treatment Diabetic Retinopathy Study (ETDRS) utilized a similar study design but examined treatment of early proliferative and mild to severe nonproliferative retinopathy and macular edema.[586] ETDRS results

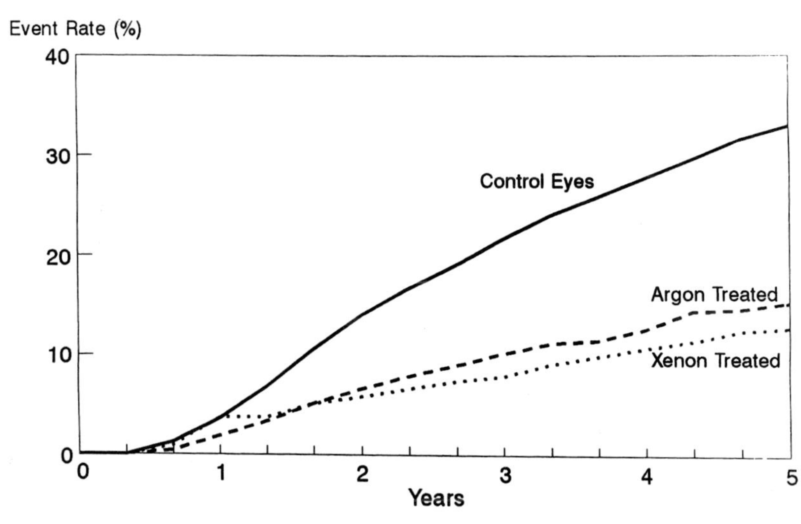

FIGURE 18-54. The effect of laser photocoagulation on proliferative diabetic retinopathy. In this study, eyes with proliferative retinopathy were randomly assigned to laser therapy or no therapy. Over the 5 years of the study, panretinal laser therapy decreased severe visual loss by approximately 50 percent. The benefit–risk ratio (panretinal photocoagulation results in decreased night vision and peripheral vision) was judged to be best for patients with high risk characteristics (see Table 18-33). (*From the DRS Research Group.*[587])

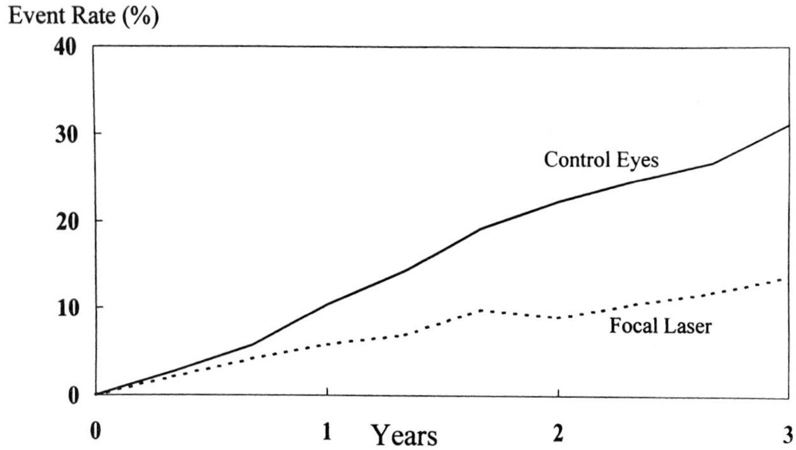

FIGURE 18-55. The effect of focal laser photocoagulation on visual acuity in patients with macular edema. As in the Diabetic Retinopathy Study, eyes were randomly assigned to either laser therapy or no treatment. Focal laser therapy reduced the rate of moderate visual loss by 50 percent. "Clinically significant" macular edema (see Table 18-34) was judged to be the most appropriate target for focal laser therapy. (*From the ETDRS Research Group.*[586])

showed that focal laser therapy of macular edema (Fig. 18-55) produced a 50 percent reduction in subsequent vision loss. Subgroup analyses established patients with "clinically significant macular edema" (Table 18-34) as benefiting most from laser therapy. Early treatment of mild to moderate nonproliferative retinopathy with scatter therapy was of little net benefit.

Other treatments of retinopathy that have proved beneficial include vitrectomy for far advanced retinopathy.[601] Patients with significant vitreous hemorrhage, scarring, and retinal detachment or imminent detachment that results in legal blindness (5/200 or worse) are appropriate candidates for vitrectomy. Using microsurgical techniques, the scarred, fibrotic vitreous content is removed and vitreoretinal adhesions released. Early vitrectomy has been shown to be advantageous in restoring vision with 25 percent of eyes achieving 10/20 or better visual acuity at 1 year, compared with 5 percent of untreated eyes.

Aspirin therapy, directed at a putative platelet or vascular pathogenesis of retinopathy, neither helped nor harmed patients with mild to moderate nonproliferative retinopathy in the ETDRS.[586] Another randomized study of aspirin therapy in Type 1 and Type 2 diabetic patients with early retinopathy (usually microaneurysms only) demonstrated a modest decrease in the rate of microaneurysm development over 3 years.[602] Other experimental approaches are being studied, including attempts to interfere with the underlying pathogenesis of retinopathy with drugs that inhibit glycation or the angiogenic factors that promote proliferation.

When vision loss occurs, either owing to severe retinopathy or as a consequence of laser therapy, low vision aids, including "talking" glucose meters, are available. Vision loss associated with macular edema most often results in loss of central acuity, while proliferative retinopathy can result in complete loss of vision.

TABLE 18-34. Characteristics of Clinically Significant Macular Edema*

Thickening of the retina within 500 microns of the center of the macula
Hard exudates within 500 microns of the center of the macula, in association with thickening of the adjacent retina
Zones of retinal thickening at least one disk diameter in size, any part of which is within one disk diameter of the center of the macula

* In general, macular thickening and edema cannot be detected with two-dimensional direct ophthalmoscopy. However, the presence of microaneurysms and/or hard exudates near the macula, or decreased visual acuity not correctable with pinhole or refraction, should suggest possible macular edema prompt referral to an ophthalmologist.

Nephropathy

Clinical Characteristics

Nephropathy is the diabetes-specific complication associated with the most mortality. Clinically detectable, albeit asymptomatic, diabetic nephropathy in Type 1 diabetes begins with the development of microalbuminuria (30 to 300 mg/24 h) which may occur as early as 5 years after diabetes onset (Fig. 18-56).[538,603–608] This stage of "incipient" nephropathy may be more likely to occur in patients who had hyperfiltration, i.e., glomerular filtration rate (GFR) > 150 ml/min, earlier.[607] After another 5 to 10 years of diabetes, patients destined to develop end-stage renal disease (ESRD) develop clinical or "dipstick positive" proteinuria (> 500 mg protein per liter, equivalent to > 300 mg albuminuria per 24 hours).[538,608] Hypertension almost always occurs during this time period. In the next 5 to 10 years, nephrotic syndrome develops and GFR falls, resulting in ESRD. Prior to the current period of intense attention to glucose and blood pressure control, the mean durations of Type 1 diabetes prior to development of clinical proteinuria and ESRD were 17 years and 23 years, respectively.[608] Considering the widespread availability of renal replacement therapy in the US, either with dialysis or preferably transplantation, only a small fraction of Type 1 diabetic patients who develop nephropathy succumb to uremia. The majority die from concurrent cardiovascular disease, the risk of which increases 30- to 40-fold compared with cardiovascular disease prevalence in Type 1 diabetic patients without nephropathy.[609] Microalbuminuria has been associated with the occurrence of CVD, giving rise to the suggestion that it is a marker—or cause—of abnormal endothelial function.[610]

Unlike retinopathy, the prevalence of nephropathy does not rise continuously with increasing diabetes duration (Fig. 18-54).[538,608] If dip-stick proteinuria, the most reliable indicator of diabetic nephropathy, has not developed after 25 years of diabetes duration, the risk of developing nephropathy begins to decrease. Other causes of nephropathy can occur in patients with Type 1 diabetes, and should be suspected in patients who don't have coexistent diabetic complications, especially retinopathy.

Our understanding of nephropathy in Type 2 diabetes is complicated by the uncertain duration of Type 2 diabetes and the

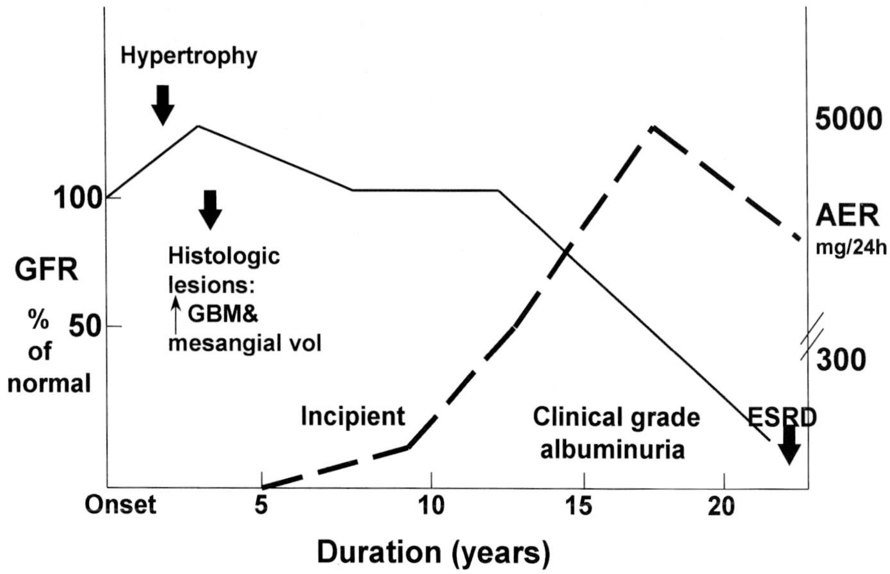

FIGURE 18-56. The course of diabetic nephropathy. No more than 40 percent of patients with Type 1 diabetes and 15 percent of patients with Type 2 diabetes develop clincal nephropathy. The natural history of nephropathy is best understood in Type 1 diabetes. Several studies have demonstrated increased glomerular filtration rate (GFR, solid line) in patients who are at risk for nephropathy. Renal hypertrophy has been documented early in the course. Microalbuminuria, defined as >20 μg/min or >30 mg/24 hr, occurs after approximately 4–7 years of diabetes, and 70–80 percent of patients with so called "incipient" nephropathy proceed to clinical grade albuminuria (>300 mg/24 h). Of those patients who develop clinical grade albuminuria, >90 percent will develop decreasing GFR and end-stage renal disease (ESRD). Protein excretion begins to fall as GFR decreases. The rate of progression of almost all stages of nephropathy can be attenuated by antihypertensive therapy. Intensive diabetes therapy has been demonstrated to have a salutary effect on the early stages of nephropathy.

high prevalence of coexistent hypertension, which may cause nephrosclerosis. Microalbuminuria appears to precede nephropathy in Type 2 diabetes as in Type 1 diabetes.[610]

Although histopathological changes do not always mirror clinical severity, they too follow a stereotypical course.[612–614] Initially, renal hypertrophy occurs with expansion of the glomeruli, including the mesangium and glomerular basement membrane (GBM), and an increase in kidney size.[576,612] Glomerular composition changes more slowly over time leading to characteristic mesangial expansion and GBM thickening (Fig. 18-57).[613] Afferent and efferent arteriosclerosis are also characteristic. With more advanced nephropathy (progressive proteinuria), glomerular closure occurs. Compensatory hypertrophy of the nonoccluded functioning glomeruli occurs during this stage.[614] Classic Kimmelstein-Wilson nodular glomerulosclerosis is a relatively late phenomenon and occurs in only a minority of diabetic kidneys (Fig. 18-58).[615] End-stage renal disease is characterized by small, atrophic kidneys with diffuse glomerulosclerosis.[616]

In addition to the afferent and efferent atherosclerosis of the glomeruli, renal artery stenosis (RAS) is a common occurrence, especially in Type 2 diabetes. Hypertension that is difficult to manage and increasing creatinine with the use of angiotensin converting enzyme inhibitors suggest underlying RAS. Angiography, with its attendant risk of contrast induced renal failure, radionuclide scanning, and magnetic resonance angiography can be used to diagnose RAS.[617]

Another kidney complication that usually occurs in the setting of mild to moderate nephropathy, but can occur even in the setting of a normal glomerular filtration rate, is hyporeninemic, hypoaldosteronemic hyperkalemia. This abnormality in the juxtaglomerular apparatus can affect as many as 10 percent of diabetic patients and causes a Type IV renal tubular acidosis.[618] Finally, bladder infections, ascending infections with pyelonephritis, and emphysematous pyelonephritis and necrotizing papillitis (papillary necrosis) are more common in diabetes.

Prevalence and Incidence

As with retinopathy, the widespread implementation of intensive therapy with improved glycemic levels is likely to change the incidence and prevalence of nephropathy. Moreover, intensive blood pressure control and the use of angiotensin converting enzyme inhibitors should decrease the occurrence or rate of development of nephropathy. Unlike retinopathy, the development of nephropathy appears to occur in only a small fraction of persons with Type 1 diabetes and an even smaller fraction of patients with Type 2 diabetes. Over a lifetime, no more than 35 percent of persons with Type 1 diabetes and only 10 percent of persons with Type 2 diabetes develop end-stage renal disease.[535,537,538] Some,[619] but not all[536] recent studies have suggested that the prevalence of nephropathy in Type 1 diabetes has already begun to decrease.

Even though a smaller fraction of Type 2 diabetics develop nephropathy compared with persons with Type 1 diabetes, the enormously larger size of the Type 2 diabetic population has resulted in more patients having Type 2 than Type 1 diabetes developing renal failure. Diabetes is the most common cause of renal failure in adults in the US and more patients in dialysis progams have had Type 2 than Type 1 diabetes since the 1980s.[620]

Pathogenesis and Risk Factors

The same evidence that has established chronic glycemia as a risk factor for retinopathy has been applied to nephropathy. Intervention studies have demonstrated a remarkable decrease in development and progression of nephropathy with intensive therapy[13,17,300,302,310] and have established glycemia as a prime factor in the pathogenesis of nephropathy. Whether glycation of basement membrane,[551] stimulation of mesangial proliferation by advanced glycated end-products binding to their receptors,[621] or some other factor is ultimately responsible for nephropathy is not known. Once glomerular attrition begins, further glomerular dropout resulting in renal failure may be inevitable,[577] although blood pressure control,[529,622,623] low protein diets,[624] and use of

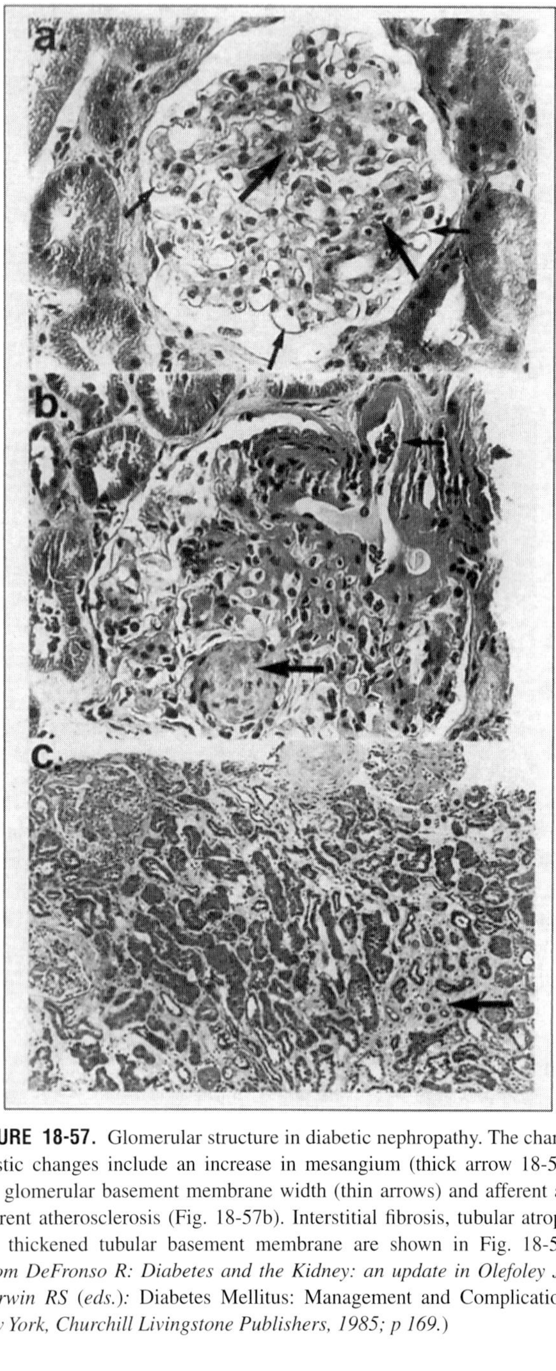

FIGURE 18-57. Glomerular structure in diabetic nephropathy. The characteristic changes include an increase in mesangium (thick arrow 18-57a) and glomerular basement membrane width (thin arrows) and afferent and efferent atherosclerosis (Fig. 18-57b). Interstitial fibrosis, tubular atrophy and thickened tubular basement membrane are shown in Fig. 18-57c. (*From DeFronso R: Diabetes and the Kidney: an update in Olefoley JM, Sherwin RS (eds.):* Diabetes Mellitus: Management and Complications. *New York, Churchill Livingstone Publishers, 1985; p 169.*)

ACE inhibitors[625-632] may attenuate the rate of glomerular decline. (A similar effect of angiotensin receptor blockers, although predicted, has not yet been demonstrated.) Whether glycemic control has an impact at advanced stages of nephropathy is unknown.

The risk factors for the development and progression of nephropathy are similar to those for retinopathy. Higher glycemic levels over time,[323] hypertension, and pregnancy[633] have an adverse effect on nephropathy. As with retinopathy, the impact of pregnancy is usually transient.[597] A positive family history of hypertension[634] and of nephropathy in other diabetic family members[328] are also risk factors.

The susceptibility of diabetic patients to bladder infections and pyelonephritis may result from decreased leukocyte bactericidal activity and/or bladder dysfunction[635] (see europathy section). The increased frequency of severe renal complications, such as emphysematous pyelonephritis and papillary necrosis, may be related to microvascular disease predisposing to more invasive infections.[636]

Screening

Although treatment of nephropathy in its preclinical phase, e.g., microalbuminuria or macroproteinuria, has been shown to decrease the rate of progression of nephropathy,[13,625-627,628,629] controlled clinical studies have been of short duration relative to the long "gestation" period for end-stage renal disease (ESRD). Whether the ultimate development of ESRD is decreased or delayed has not been well established. At least one relatively long-term study in Type 2 diabetes has suggested progressive decrease in GFR despite a salutary effect of ACE inhibitors on protein excretion. Nevertheless, several of the interventions that appear to have a short-term salutary effect (see later disussion) are relatively innocuous, and screening for macroproteinuria and microalbuminuria on a regular basis has been recommended (Table 18-18).

Treatment

Intensive diabetes therapy aimed at normalizing glycemia decreases the development and progression of nephropathy in Type 1[13,300,310] and Type 2 diabetes (Fig. 18-33).[17] A beneficial effect on the rate of progression from microalbuminuria to macroproteinuria has been demonstrated most clearly; the impact of intensive diabetes therapy during the later stages of glomerular dysfunction, while not as clear, is probably less.[637] Several other interventions have been effective in decreasing the rate of development of nephropathy in diabetes. Treatment with antihypertensive agents (especially angiotensin converting enzyme inhibitors), even in normotensive patients with Type 1 diabetes, can decrease microalbuminuria,[625-627] postpone the evolution from micro- to macroproteinuria,[628,629] decrease protein excretion in patients with macroproteinuria,[631,632] and slow the anticipated decline in GFR (Fig. 18-59).[622,623] Whether angiotensin II receptor antagonists provide the same effects has not been clearly demonstrated, although ongoing studies are examining the issue. Several studies have demostrated decreased microalbuminuria,[638] macroproteinuria,[639] and the anticipated rate of fall in GFR[640] with dietary protein restriction; however, the effects are small and have not been uniform across studies.[641] The majority of intervention studies have been of short duration and included small numbers of Type 1, and almost no Type 2, diabetic patients.

No intervention has been demonstrated to halt progression of nephropathy. Moreover, except for the studies of antihypertensive treatment in patients with progressively falling GFR,[622] none of the studies has been long enough in duration to examine whether development of ESRD is delayed.

For patients who develop ESRD, dialysis or transplantation are viable options for treatment. Although diabetic patients often have a remarkable acceleration of cardiovascular disease in the setting of dialysis,[642] many patients can be treated with either continuous ambulatory peritoneal dialysis (CAPD) or hemodialysis (HD), with the following caveats. Heparinization, albeit "regional," and the blood pressure changes that occur with HD may further threaten unstable retinopathy, causing bleeding and vision loss. In Type 2 diabetes, the altered metabolism of sulfonylureas and metformin with renal failure, predisposing patients to hypo-

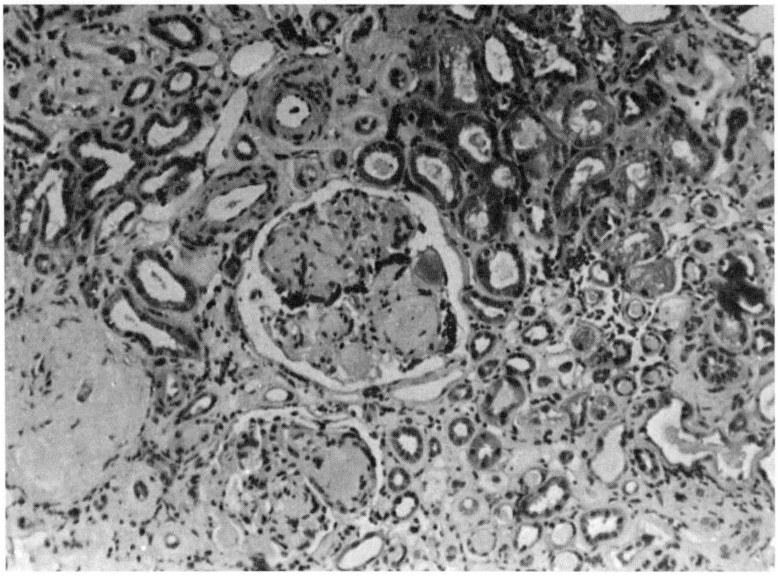

FIGURE 18-58. Section of kidney from a patient with Type I (insulin-dependent) diabetes demonstrating the nodular intercapillary glomerulosclerosis (Kimmelstiel-Wilson lesions) characteristic of diabetic nephropathy. (*Courtesy of M Kashgarian.*)

glycemia and lactic acidosis, respectively, mitigates against the use of these agents in the setting of renal failure. Repaglinide, which stimulates insulin release as do sulfonylureas but has a very brief duration of action, is not affected by renal failure and may be used in this setting. Insulin requirements often decrease dramatically with progressive glomerular failure. Effective treatment with dialysis or transplantation reverses this phenomenon and increased insulin requirements must be anticipated. The large concentrations of dextrose in CAPD fluid may increase glucose levels dramatically and often require adjustments in insulin dose. Insulin can be administered in the dialysate because it is well absorbed across the peritoneum. Depending on the concentration of glucose (e.g., 2.5 vs. 4.25 percent), variable quantities of regular insulin may be added to each bag of dialysate to supplement subcutaneous insulin. The general care of patients with ESRD, including assiduous attention to calcium and phosphate levels, Vitamin D replacement, multivitamins, and aggressive treatment of cardiovascular risk factors, does not differ substantially from the treatment of nondiabetics.

For many young patients with Type 1 diabetes and ESRD, renal replacement therapy with a kidney transplant, either from a living-related or cadaver donor, represents the best way to restore them to health and full function. Unfortunately, the limited number of available donors often means that patients must wait for long periods before having their transplant. During this waiting period, when dialysis is often necessary, patients may suffer an acceleration of retinopathy and macrovascular disease, resulting in further loss of vision, foot ulcers and amputations, and coronary artery disease. Renal transplantation is performed with a high degree of success, with 1-year patient and kidney survival currently approaching 95 and 90 percent, respectively, in most programs.[643] The five-year results are 75 percent and 70 percent, respectively, with most mortality secondary to cardiovascular disease. In the past, there was a distinct advantage with living related donors (LRD). Although closer matching of major histocompatability loci with LRD kidney often translates into lower immunosuppressive requirements, the patient and kidney survival from LRD and cadaver donor kidneys have become similar in recent years in the setting of new, more effective immunosuppressants.[643] The risks of immunosuppression in diabetic patients generally parallel those in nondiabetics.

Though acute or chronic transplant rejection remains the major risk for renal failure in the transplant kidney during the first 10 years posttransplant, patients with long-term transplants face the risk of recurrent diabetic nephropathy. Intensive diabetes therapy can probably slow, if not prevent, the redevelopment of nephropathy in the transplanted kidney, but carefully controlled studies have not been carried out.

Concurrent whole organ pancreas transplantation, usually from the same cadaver donor, but sometimes with a segmental pancreas from a LRD, has become increasingly popular and successful in recent years.[366,367] Pancreas transplants performed concurrently with a kidney transplant have a 1-year survival (no exogenous insulin and normal glycemia) that approaches 90 percent in the best programs.[366,367] In addition to being freed from the need for exogenous insulin, patients with successful pancreas transplants appear to be protected from the redevelopment of the microscopic diabetic changes that are seen in transplanted kidneys when insulin therapy is given conventionally.[371,644] This result is presumably a result of the normoglycemia achieved with the pancreas transplant compared with the frequent occurrence of poor glycemic control after a kidney transplant—in part owing to steroid therapy—in the absence of a pancreas transplant. Pancreas transplantation also improves peripheral nerve function,[369,645] but not retinopathy.[646] Interestingly, the longevity of pancreas transplants performed after a kidney transplant, or as an isolated pancreas transplant, are not as good as when performed concurrent with a kidney transplant.[647]

The treatment of other, nonspecific, renal complications of diabetes such as pyelonephritis is similar to treatment in the nondiabetic, keeping in mind the greater risk for emphysematous pyeleonephritis and necrotizing papilitis in the setting of diabetes. Hyporeninemic hypoaldosteronism can be effectively treated with a loop diuretic or low doses of a mineralocorticoid such as florinef, when electrolyte abnormalities call for it.

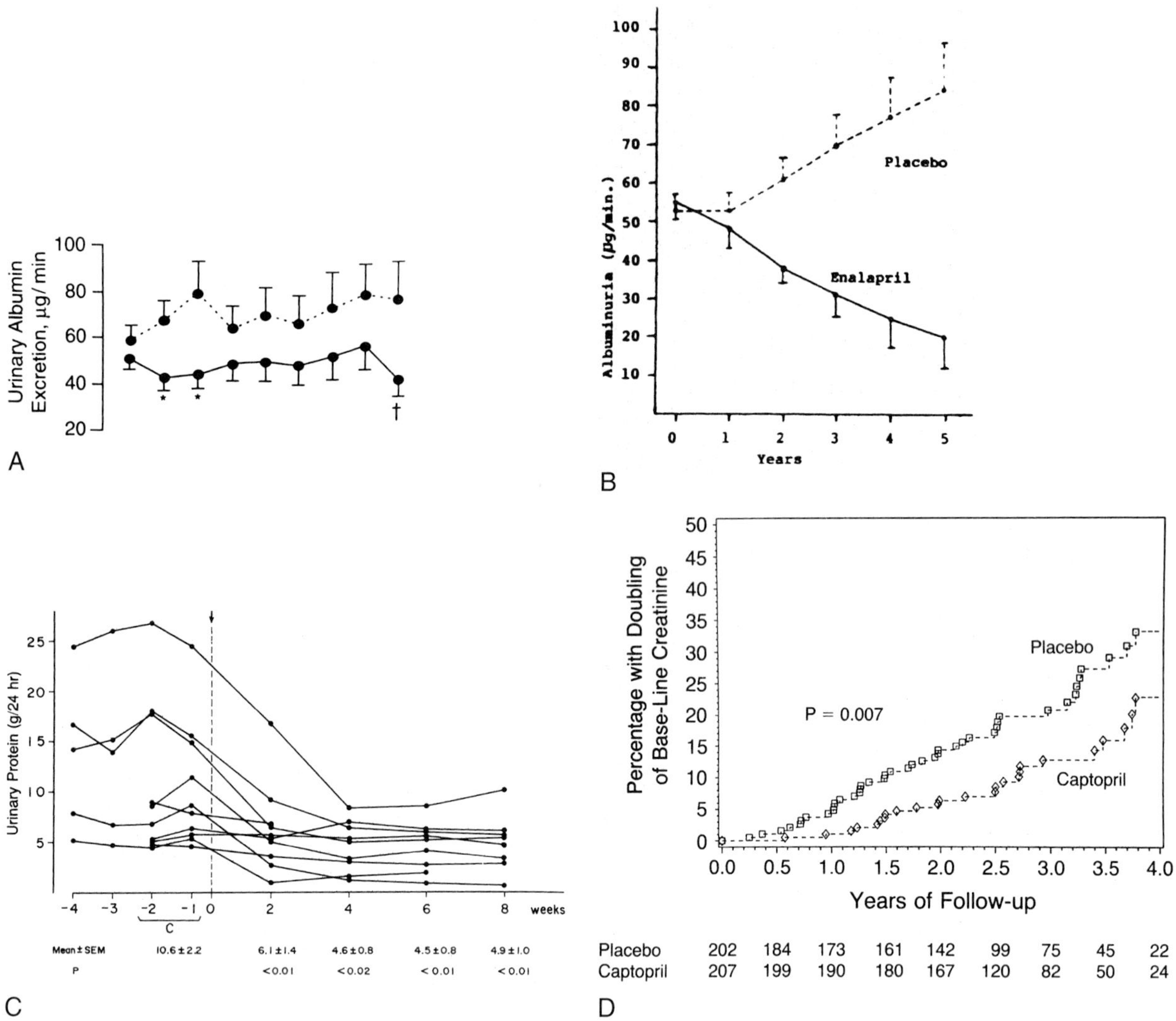

FIGURE 18-59. Improvement in (*a*) microalbuminuria in normotensive Type 1 diabetic patients with captopril therapy compared with placebo (*From Viberti et al. JAMA 271:275–79, 1994*); (*b*) microalbuminuria in Type 2 diabetic patients treated with enalapril compared with placebo (*From Ahmad et al. Diabetes Care 20:1576–1581, 1997*); (*c*) heavy proteinuria in diabetic patients treated with captopril (*From Taguma et al. N Engl J Med 313:1617–20, 1985*); and (*d*) loss of glomerular filtration rate with captopril compared with placebo in Type 1 diabetic patients who had protein excretion >500 mg/24 h and serum creatinine <2.5 mg/dL at baseline. (*From Lewis et al. N Engl J Med 329:1456–62,1993*).

Neuropathy

Neuropathy has protean clinical manifestations in Type 1 and Type 2 diabetes including the most common peripheral, symmetric sensorimotor neuropathy, cranial and peripheral motor neuropathies, and autonomic neuropathy (Table 18-35).[648] Other neurologic complications occur in diabetes including an increased risk for cerebrovascular disease[542] with an attendant increase in strokes, transient ischemic attacks (TIA), and multi-infarct dementia (see macrovascular disease later).

The myriad forms of diabetes-specific neuropathy share several characteristics with the other diabetes-specific long-term complications. First, the neurologic complications are duration-dependent.[16] In Type 1 diabetes, where the onset of disease can be more accurately ascertained, neuropathic complications increase with duration and don't usually occur before 5–10 years of duration. (In Type 2 diabetes, where the true duration of diabetes is usually underestimated, as many as 20 percent of patients will have demonstrable neuropathy at the time of diagnosis.[594]) Second, abnormalities in biochemical, histologic, and functional (electrophysiologic) measurements precede clinical manifestations.[648] Therefore, the prevalence of neuropathy is highly dependent on the methods used to detect it. Third, chronic levels of glycemia play a role in the pathogenesis of neuropathy as demonstrated by epidemiologic associations and by the results of controlled clinical trials.[13,300,311] Finally, neuropathy causes profound clinical complications that have a major effect on the health and quality of life in the diabetic population. For example, diabetes is the most common cause of amputations and of impotence in men in the U.S. population.[649]

Although diabetic neuropathy is often considered as a single entity, it has several distinct components that are sufficiently different to merit individual attention, including peripheral sensorimotor, mononeuropathies, and autonomic neuropathies.

TABLE 18-35. Classification of Diabetic Clinical Neuropathy

Distal symmetrical, sensorimotor polyneuropathy
Most common. Affects longest peripheral nerves first, resulting in "stocking and glove" paraesthesias and eventually hypoesthesia. More rarely results in dysesthesias including lancinating or formicating pain. Also affects intrinsic musculature of foot and alters foot architecture and weight bearing. Sensory function compromised secondary to large and small fiber dysfunction and includes decreased vibratory, light touch, and two-point discrimination. Proprioception may also be adversely affected and may result in unstable, ataxic gait ("pseudotabes").
Focal and multifocal mononeuropathies
Cranial mononeuropathies—oculomotor ophthalmoplegia. Usually resolves spontaneously in weeks to months.
Entrapment neuropathies—e.g., carpal tunnel, peroneal nerve
Mononeuropathy multiplex—asymmetric proximal motor neuropathy "amyotrophy," usually affects pelvic girdle with weakness in hips and thighs. Resolves spontaneously.
Intercostal mononeuropathies—truncal and abdominal sensory neuropathy
Autonomic neuropathy (manifestations of parasympathetic failure generally precede sympathetic failure)
Gastrointestinal
Gastroparesis diabeticorum—delayed gastric emptying with abdominal pain, fullness, reflux, and retained gastric contents, which can affect glucose control.
Diabetic diarrhea—intermittent diarrhea with or without incontinence; may alternate with constipation.
Genitourinary
Erectile dysfunction—decreased frequency and inadequate degree of tumescence (parasympathetic failure)
Retrograde ejaculation—manifestation of sympathetic failure with decreased contraction of trigone and poor closure of bladder outlet during ejaculation. Bladder—urinary retention with distention, predisposes to ascending infections
Cardiovascular
Postural hypotension, resting tachycardia, increased perioperative and anesthesia-related sudden death. Decreased R-R variation with respiration.
Other
Gustatatory sweating
Dyshidrosis secondary to altered sweating and abnormal vasodilatation
Decreased catecholamine secretion in response to hypoglycemia

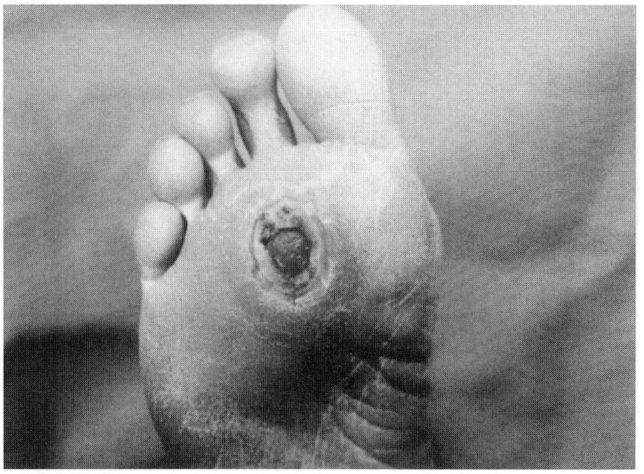

FIGURE 18-60. Penetrating pressure ulcer over second metatarsal head in patient with diabetic neuropathy. Changes in innervation of the intrinsic muscles of the foot result in increased flexion with altered weight distribution and increased weight bearing over MT heads. Flexion at the PIP joints of the toes exposes the PIP joints to the risk of abrasion and ulceration. Fitted orthotic devices can spread weight bearing and prevent the ulceration shown here. Extra depth shoes can protect the PIP joints from trauma. See Color Plate 4.

Distal Sensorimotor Neuropathy

Clinical Characteristics

Although neuropathy is more common with longer duration of diabetes, a relatively severe early-onset polyneuropathy has been described in rare cases.[650] Distal symmetric sensorimotor neuropathy detectable on physical examination is only minimally bothersome for most patients. When questioned, Type 1 diabetic patients will often note numbness or "pins and needles" paraesthesias of their toes or forefoot after 5–10 years duration; however, patients often will not complain spontaneously of these minor symptoms. Considering the 7-years average duration of Type 2 diabetes that precedes its diagnosis, it is not surprising that approximately 20 percent of patients may have neuropathy at the time of diagnosis.[594] The longest peripheral nerves are affected most commonly, with the toes affected first and the foot and distal leg affected over time. Peripheral neuropathy rarely progresses above the knee. Although the upper extremities can be affected by the clinical manifestations of distal sensorimotor neuropathy, only the fingers are usually involved.

Paraesthesias are characteristically worse at night and symptoms often wax and wane. With time, paraesthesias often abate, replaced by decreased sensitivity. This clinical phenomenon may reflect modestly abnormal nerve function progressing to more severely affected function. The clinical manifestations of advancing peripheral neuropathy include alterations in the innervation of the small muscles or intrinsic musculature of the foot. Extensor tone is disproportionately affected, resulting in flexion of the distal joints. The flexed posture of the foot results in the PIP joints projecting above their usual plane on the dorsal surface of the foot (Fig. 18-60, [Color Plate 4]). On the plantar surface, weight distribution changes, with increased weight distributed over the MTP joints. The combination of loss of sensation and altered foot architecture and weight distribution poses a major risk for foot trauma from weight bearing and foot wear that can lead to diabetic ulcers. When decreased peripheral circulation and changes in the integument, including dry skin (dyshidrosis) caused by autonomic nerve dysfunction with altered sweating and vasomotor function, are added to the clinical manifestations of peripheral neuropathy, as is often the case, the end result may be penetrating bacterial infections, osteomyelitis, nonhealing foot ulcers, and amputations. Loss of sensation, position sense, and motor innervation to the intrinsic musculature of the foot can also lead to a Charcot foot.

The usual signs of peripheral neuropathy reflect the different sized fibers that are usually affected.[648] Sensitivity to light touch and vibration are often lost early (small unmyelinated fibers), followed by a decrease and then loss of deep tendon reflexes, specifically the Achilles tendon reflex. Loss of position sense is a relatively late finding. Quantitative means of assessing vibratory, temperature, and light touch sensation have been developed and have revealed deficits in all three.[651] From a clinical point of view, assessment of reflexes, light touch with a 10-gram monofilament, and vibratory sensation with a middle C tuning fork is adequate to detect clinical neuropathy and to identify patients who are at particular risk for foot trauma.

A minority of patients develop painful peripheral neuropathy with lancinating or burning dysesthesias, and, paradoxically, pain to light touch—so severe that even the weight of a sheet is unbearable. The symptoms may be associated with depression, anorexia, and insomnia.[652] Why this rare subset of diabetic patients develops painful manifestations is not understood. Moreover, no specific electrophysiologic abnormality has been identified in patients with painful neuropathy.[653] Acutely elevated glucose levels can decrease pain tolerance.[654] Although small in number, patients who develop painful neuropathy present major treatment problems for the clinician. Although their symptoms wax and wane, they remain symptomatic over long periods.[654]

The differential diagnosis of peripheral neuropathy includes several fairly common conditions such as uremia and alcohol, and other conditions such as syphilis, leprosy, porphyria, sarcoidosis, vasculitis, paraneoplastic syndromes, heavy metal poisoning, and the side effects of medications (vinca alkaloids, cisplatin). B_{12} deficiency must be considered because of the heightened risk for pernicious anemia in the setting of Type 1 diabetes. In general, history, physical examination, and a simple battery of tests (serum creatinine, B_{12} levels, and VDRL) will eliminate other causes of neuropathy.

Prevalence and Incidence

Assessment of the prevalence and incidence of peripheral neuropathy is highly dependent on the means with which it is measured.[655] Electrophysiological studies demonstrate subclinical abnormalities including slowed motor and sensory nerve conduction in more than 50 percent of patients by 5 to 10 year's duration.[648] On the other hand, abnormalities detected on usual clinical exam are less common, affecting only 50 percent of patients. Development of an insensate foot is even less common. The increasing application of intensive therapy will decrease the occurrence of neuropathy. In the DCCT, intensive therapy decreased the development of peripheral neuropathy by 60 percent.[13]

Pathogenesis and Risk Factors

Peripheral neuropathy has been linked to hyperglycemia on the basis of studies in animal models, epidemiologic studies, and interventional studies. Although some investigators have suggested that microvascular abnormalities of the small vessels supplying the peripheral nerves, the vasa nervorum, underly peripheral neuropathy,[558] the consensus is that metabolic abnormalities related to hyperglycemia are pathogenetic. This conclusion is predicated on the diffuse and symmetric occurrence of peripheral sensorimotor neuropathy in the absence of demonstrably diffuse vascular obstruction and the demonstration of diffuse histologic abnormalities of the axons. Finally, a large volume of data supports metabolic abnormalities associated with hyperglycemia affecting peripheral nerve function.[648,656]

Electrophysiologic studies reveal slowing of nerve conduction that occurs in parallel with myoinositol depletion and decreased Na^+-K^+ ATPase activity. The resultant sodium accumulation in the nodes of Ranvier is postulated to cause the axoglial dysjunction and slowed nerve conduction characteristic of diabetes. Studies that replete myoinositol have reversed neuropathy.[657] Although abnormalities in sorbitol metabolism have been championed as the most likely cause of diabetic neuropathy, the generally supportive results of studies with aldose reductase inhibitors in experimental models of diabetes have not been replicated in human diabetes.[658,659]

Risk factors for the development of peripheral neuropathy, in addition to duration of diabetes and hyperglycemia, include smoking.[660]

Screening

As noted earlier, peripheral neuropathy can be detected with increasing sensitivity depending on the method used.[655] Electrophysiologic studies examining sensory and motor nerve conduction can detect subclinical neuropathy, while quantitative sensory testing can often determine the presence of peripheral neuropathy prior to the development of changes on usual physical examination.[651,655] All of these changes usually precede symptomatic neuropathy. From a practical point of view, intensive therapy is indicated for most patients with diabetes to decrease the development of all complications; therefore, specific measures to screen for subclinical neuropathy would not change therapy and would not appear to be warranted. On the other hand, the very nature of peripheral sensory neuropathy may rob patients of the ability to feel anything. Considering the major clinical problems that can develop in the setting of an insensate foot and the demonstrated ability of screening coupled with education programs to lessen the risk of foot ulcers and hospitalizations,[661] some level of screening is recommended. A program of education regarding foot care and routine examination of feet, screening for abnormal anatomy and loss of sensation to light touch, is appropriate.[662]

Therapy

The most effective form of prevention of peripheral neuropathy is intensive glycemic control. The DCCT and Stockholm Study demonstrated that intensive therapy decreases the development and progression of peripheral neuropathy by as much as 60 percent.[13,300] The DCCT data suggest that intensive therapy may even reverse peripheral neuropathy,[313] an observation that is supported by studies with pancreas transplantation.[645] Data in Type 2 diabetes are sparse. For patients who escape the benefits of intensive therapy, careful foot care, including the use of appropriately fitted shoes (extra depth to prevent abrasions and trauma to the dorsal surface of the toes) and orthotics to help protect feet from barotrauma, are critical in preventing calluses and foot ulcers. Patients who are identified through screening as having insensate feet require the attention of specialists, while persons without severe neuropathy can usually be taught appropriate self-care.

Much attention has been focused on the treatment of the relatively small fraction of patients with painful neuropathy. Although several pharmacological therapies have been identified, none are more than partially effective.[663-668] Patients can often be treated with nonaddictive analgesics such as acetaminophen or a nonsteroidal anti-inflammatory agent. Because the symptoms wax and wane, these agents are often effective in the short term. Narcotics and other addictive drugs should be avoided because there is a high risk for dependence. For patients who don't respond, the best experimental data from controlled trials—keeping in mind that a powerful placebo effect must be considered—support the use of tricyclic antidepressants, which both improve neuropathic symptoms compared with placebo and address the insomnia that often accompanies painful neuropathy.[663] The cardiac and bladder complications and other side effects that can occur with tricyclic antidepressants such as dry mouth, can be reduced by using drugs with a lower anticholinergic profile, such as nortriptyline. Carbemazepine, diphenylhydantoin, mexilitene, and intravenous lidocaine have all been used with variable success, but should be reserved as second-line agents.[664–667] If the affected area is relatively small, a topical agent such as capsaicin, a derivative of hot peppers which works by releasing substance P from local nerve endings, is moderately effective.[666] The most recent medication demonstrated to be effective in the treatment of painful neuropathy is gabapentin, a drug that may act through the gamma aminobutyric acid (GABA) receptor.[668]

Motor (Cranial and Peripheral) and Compression Neuropathies, and Mononeuritis Multiplex

The compression and focal motor diabetic neuropathies most commonly affect the median or ulnar nerve (usually on the dominant side), the peroneal nerve (affecting either side similarly), or cranial nerves with the third, fourth, or sixth nerve most commonly involved. The characteristic clinical changes include the motor and sensory changes associated with carpal tunnel syndrome and ulnar compression in the upper extremity, foot drop (peroneal nerve) in the lower extremity, and ophthalmoplegia, depending on which of the cranial nerves is affected. The time course of the motor deficit is predicated, to some extent, on the underlying cause. If the neuropathy is caused by compression, the symptoms and signs may not improve until the compression is relieved. On the other hand, if the focal nerve damage is caused by a nerve infarct, which is the suspected cause for the cranial neuropathies and some of the focal peripheral neuropathies,[669,670] supportive therapy is all that is required as they improve spontaneously in several weeks to months. Recurrent episodes affecting the same nerve can occur. Ischemic focal neuropathies have a sudden clinical onset and are usually painless. Differentiating compression neuropathies from focal neuropathies of ischemic origin relies on physical examination and electrophysiologic studies that can localize the area of compression.

Another form of mononeuropathy is mononeuropathy multiplex, inaccurately named diabetic amyotrophy in the past.[671] This rare condition, which appears to affect men with diabetes more than women, also has a sudden onset and tends to affect the girdle muscles with lancinating pain and asymmetric weakness. Strength of flexion, abduction, and adduction at the hip may be decreased, resulting in difficulty in walking. Nerve conduction studies may reveal abnormalities in multiple nerve roots without any evidence electrophysiologically or on physical exam of a primary myopathy. Paraneoplastic and multiple-level disc disease, and spinal stenosis must be ruled out. As with the mononeuropathies, diabetic "amyotrophy" resolves spontaneously, usually in 6 weeks to 6 months. Some patients have recurrent episodes.

Finally, relatively rare radiculopathies that can cause truncal paraesthesias and dysaesthesias have been described.[672] These conditions mimic postherpetic radiculopathy and usually affect only one side of the trunk. No specific therapy is known and they resolve spontaneously.

The focal neuropathies are much less common than the sensorimotor neuropathies. No screening is appropriate or required for these relatively rare conditions. Patients usually complain spontaneously of the functional changes they note with the acute onset of mononeuropathies. The compression neuropathies, such as carpal tunnel syndrome, may require surgical decompression. The use of splints to decrease repeated flexion trauma at the wrist, or decrease flexion during sleep, is often effective in ameliorating symptoms. The other focal motor neuropathies usually resolve spontaneously in 6 weeks to 6 months. No data exist on the ability of intensive diabetes management to prevent or ameliorate these forms of neuropathy.

Autonomic Neuropathy

Clinical Characteristics

Autonomic neuropathies can affect any part of the autonomic nervous system including gastric or intestinal motility, erectile function, bladder function, and/or cardiac function and vascular tone. The most common clinical manifestations include gastroparesis,[673] impotence,[674] abnormal bladder function with loss of bladder tone, distension, and overflow incontinence, "diabetic diarrhea,"[675] and postural hypotension (Table 18-35).[676] Although subclinical changes (e.g., loss of R-R variation with respiratory phase or altered gastrointestinal contractions) can be detected frequently within 5 to 10 years of the onset of Type 1 diabetes, clinical autonomic neuropathy is more rare.

Gastroparesis Gastroparesis causes discomforting symptoms with meals including abdominal bloating and a sense of fullness and satiety after even small meals, gastric esophageal reflux, and postprandial vomiting. The gastric stasis results in undigested food remaining in the stomach for many hours after a meal. The slowed digestion of meals slows absorption of nutrients, including carbohydrate, and may manifest as erratic glycemic control. The differential diagnosis must consider the use of drugs that slow gastric motility, such as the tricyclic antidepressants.

Diabetic Diarrhea and Incontinence These are rare but can be disabling. A pattern of alternating constipation and diarrhea is often described. Although symptoms wax and wane, the diarrhea is often resistant to all therapies and can be associated with fecal incontinence. The differential diagnosis of diarrhea in a diabetic patient should specifically include celiac disease, which is more common in Type 1 diabetes,[677] and bacterial overgrowth with steatorrhea.

Genitourinary Impotence may be the most common clinical autonomic neuropathy, affecting as many as 50 percent of men with diabetes over their lifetime. The impotence usually has the characteristics of an organic form of erectile dysfunction—as opposed to psychogenic forms—with the progressive loss of erectile function with all forms of stimulation and decreased nocturnal tumescence. During the period of worsening erectile function, psychogenic impotence may be superimposed, making a causal diagnosis more problematic. Another consequence of smooth muscle dysfunction is retrograde ejaculation. Whether autonomic neuropathy in diabetic women is associated with anorgasmia is not clear.

Bladder dysfunction often manifests itself initially as a decreased sense of urgency and frequency of urination, presumably concurrent with decreased stretch receptor sensation. As the bladder becomes increasingly distended, overflow incontinence supervenes. The distended bladder may be more likely to predispose patients, and especially women, to develop cystitis and ascending infections.

Cardiac Autonomic Neuropathy (CAN) CAN most commonly results in resting tachycardia and postural hypotension. The latter complaint is relatively rare, but can be disabling. Cardiac autonomic neuropathy has been described as a serious risk factor for sudden death and complications during anesthesia.[678]

Finally, the loss of counterregulation that is associated with an increased risk of severe hypoglycemia is secondary, in part, to sympathoadrenal failure, a manifestation of autonomic neuropathy.

Prevalence and Incidence

As with the other diabetes-specific complications, the means of detecting autonomic neuropathy has a major effect on its prevalence. The most common clinical manifestations of autonomic neuropathy are probably impotence and the gastrointestinal manifestations, which have been reported in as many as 50 percent of diabetic men and as much as 40 percent of the diabetic population, respectively. However, the high prevalence of these disorders, especially impotence, diarrhea, and constipation, in the nondiabetic population, makes an interpretation of the impact of diabetes difficult. In the DCCT, intensive therapy reduced the development and progression of abnormal autonomic cardiovascular testing results, but did not affect any of the clinical manifestations of autonomic neuropathy.[312] This probably reflects the relatively low prevalence of clinical autonomic disease in the relatively healthy DCCT population with brief diabetes duration. It is reasonable to expect that the prevalence of clinical manifestations of autonomic neruopathy will decrease over time with intensive therapy.

Pathogenesis

The origin of autonomic neuropathy is not known. However, the myriad, diffuse manifestations suggest a metabolic rather than a vascular cause. Parasympathetic dysfunction usually precedes sympathetic abnormalities.

Screening and Diagnosis

Although electrophysiologic and other functional testing will detect abnormalities in a relatively large fraction of the diabetic population, screening for subclinical disease is generally not warranted. Moreover, the methods for detecting subclinical disease are not widely available. Whether screening for cardiac autonomic neuropathy prior to anesthesia should be performed is arguable. All diabetic patients undergoing general anesthesia should be appropriately hydrated, and those with long duration of diabetes and with documented or suspected coronary artery disease should have careful cardiac monitoring. It is by no means clear that demonstration of cardiac autonomic neruopathy will provide added benefit.

Methods to document abnormal gastrointestinal and genitourinary function have been developed.[679] Unfortunately, the results of expensive gastric emptying studies often don't correlate with symptoms or clinical response to therapy. The diagnosis of erectile dysfunction in the diabetic man is often straightforward on historical grounds. After eliminating other, relatively rare, organic causes of impotence (testing for testosterone and prolactin levels), formal sleep testing of nocturnal erections and tumesence probably adds little useful information.

Therapy

Gastroparesis can be treated effectively with several medications that increase propulsion in the upper GI tract.[680–682] After eliminating medications that slow gastrointestinal motility, such as tricyclic antidepressants and narcotics, metoclopropamide or cisapride can be used with excellent clinical relief of symptoms. These medications are often needed in postoperative diabetic patients where gastric motility is especially slow to return after general anesthesia and surgery. In very rare patients with intractable vomiting secondary to gastroparesis, hospitalization, prolonged periods of parenteral nutrition, and intravenous reglan plus oral cisapride may be required. Owing to severe cardiac arrhythmias, metoclopropamide is no longer widely available. The macrolide antibiotics, including erythromycin, bind to the motilin receptor and increase gastric motility. They can be given intravenously or by mouth and are moderately effective.[682]

Diabetic diarrhea and constipation and incontinence can be improved by providing a reasonable "bowel regimen" that includes high dietary fiber. Training can improve sensitivity to the presence of feces in the distal colon and frequent attempts to defecate, independent of urgency, can reduce episodes of incontinence. Severe diabetic diarrhea, with or without incontinence, needs to be evaluated to rule out infectious causes and cases of malabsorption such as blind loop syndrome with bacterial overgrowth and celiac disease. If other causes of diarrhea are excluded, the alpha adrenergic agent clonidine, which inhibits enterocyte secretion, has been used to treat intractable cases.[683] Drugs that slow motility, such as loperamide, are often helpful. Rarely, chronic incapacatating diarrhea with incontinence has required colostomies to improve quality-of-life.

Bladder neuropathy is often asymptomatic until overflow incontinence or recurrent ascending urinary tract infections occur. Patients should be instructed to urinate frequently, independent of any sense of urgency, and perform the credet maneuver, trying to empty the bladder as completely as possible and restore tone to the bladder wall. Routine surveillance for asymptomatic bacteruria is warranted.

Impotence can be treated with pharmacologic agents that cause vasodilatation. Local application of vasodilators by injection[684] or intraurethral application[685] is effective in more than 50 percent of impotent diabetic men. The use of systemic medications is limited by systemic hypotension; however, systemically administered drugs that have relatively restricted activity on the penile vasculature, such as the phosphodiesterase inhibitor sidenafil, have recently been demonstrated to be effective.[686] Other naturally occurring herbs and drugs, such as yohimbine, have not been carefully studied. Although the availability of several effective medications has reduced surgical treatment, penile implants have been used effectively with minimal complications.[687] Microvascular surgery has also been used in a few centers.

Postural hypotension is the manifestation of cardiovascular autonomic neuropathy that may require therapy. Because postural hypotension in diabetic patients frequently coexists with supine hypertension, careful adjustment of antihypertensive drugs is required. If postural symptoms persist, improved glycemic control to decrease osmotic diuresis and hypovolemia and salt repletion are important first steps. In addition, hypoadrenalism and hypothyroidism, both of which are more common in Type 1 diabetes, must be ruled out. If postural symptoms still persist, therapy with a salt-retaining drug, such as florinef, and use of compression stockings may ameliorate the symptoms. Finally, a relatively new alpha agonist, midodrene, has been helpful in treating resistant cases.[688]

Cardiovascular Disease

Cardiovascular disease (CVD), including coronary artery (CAD), cerebral, and peripheral vascular disease (PVD) secondary to atherosclerosis, is arguably the most important of all diabetic

TABLE 18-36. Relative Impact of Diabetes on Cardiovascular Disease

	*Relative Risk**	
Cardiovascular Disease Outcome	**Men**	**Women**
Coronary artery disease (CAD)	1.9	3.6
Congestive heart failure	2.8	7.7
CAD death	2.6	7.2
Intermittent claudication	4.7	8.9
Stroke	3.3	5.6

*Relative risk for specified outcomes is for diabetic men (virtually all with Type 2 diabetes) compared with nondiabetic men, and diabetic women compared with nondiabetic women during 20-year followup (1948–68). Diabetes was defined as treatment with oral agents or insulin or casual blood glucose >150 mg/dL.

Source: From Framingham Heart Study.[542]

TABLE 18-37. Risk Factors for Cardiovascular Disease Associated with Type 2 Diabetes

Nonspecific*	Specific†
Hypertension	Microalbuminuria
Lipids	Glycated LDL
Decreased HDL	Glycated HDL
Obesity	Hypertriglyceridemia
Renal failure	Small dense LDL
	Cardiac autonomic neuropathy
	Endothelial dysfunction
	Altered fibrinolysis and thrombosis

*Risk factors for cardiovascular disease that have been identified in nondiabetic populations but which are more prevalent in Type 2 diabetes.

†These risk factors are specific to diabetes. Glycated LDL and HDL bind to their respective receptors and are metabolized differently than nonglycated LDL and HDL. They may contribute to CVD in diabetes. Small dense LDL is more vulnerable to oxidation and may be more atherogenic than larger, more bouyant LDL particles.

complications because it contributes most to the premature mortality that shortens the life-span of patients with Type 1 and Type 2 diabetes mellitus. Although CVD is generally similar in character to its occurrence in nondiabetics, and therefore a nonspecific long-term complication, its clinical impact is far greater in the setting of diabetes than in the nondiabetic population. The greater impact of CVD in diabetes is predicated on the following: 1) The risk of developing CVD is 2- to 10-fold greater in the diabetic population than in the nondiabetic population, with a disproportionate effect in women with diabetes.[542,543,689] The most common manifestation is CAD, which is increased 2- to 5-fold compared with similarly aged nondiabetics (Table 18-36).[542] Less common manifestations such as PVD are increased 10-fold compared with nondiabetic populations. 2) The outcome of clinical CVD events, such as a myocardial infarction (MI), is worse than in the nondiabetic population.[690,691] For example, mortality and morbidity, especially the development of congestive heart failure, after an MI is at least 150 percent of the rate in nondiabetics. 3) The difference in the occurrence and outcomes of CVD between diabetic and nondiabetic patients has not been substantially altered by the widespread availability of numerous treatments, suggesting that CVD and its risk factors may be resistant to improvement with conventional medications. 4) Diabetes-specific risk factors amplify the risk for and worsen the outcome of CVD. For example, the dyslipidemia and coagulopathy associated with diabetes probably contribute to the excess development of atherosclerosis and the cardiac autonomic neuropathy, coagulopathy, diastolic dysfunction, and hypertension that commonly accompany diabetes probably worsen outcome. Small vessel disease in the foot and peripheral neuropathy, when combined with PVD, result in a 25- to 40-fold increased risk of foot ulcers requiring amputations in the diabetic population.[692]

Prevalence and Incidence

Most of the epidemiologic data have been collected in populations with Type 2 diabetes. The major difference in cardiovascular disease in diabetic patients compared with the nondiabetic population is its increased frequency, especially in diabetic women compared with nondiabetic women (Table 18-36).[542,543,689] The usual protective effect of female gender with regard to coronary artery disease is eliminated by diabetes. Although asymptomatic, "silent" coronary artery disease and myocardial infarction are probably not much more common in diabetic patients than nondiabetic patients,[690,693] atypical anginal symptoms, including congestive heart failure symptoms, are a more common clinical presentation of coronary artery disease in the diabetic population.[690] Mortality from first and repeat myocardial infarctions is higher in diabetic than nondiabetic patients.[690,691]

Relatively few studies have examined the epidemiology of CVD in Type 1 diabetes. Though the prevalence and incidence of CVD is lower in Type 1 than in Type 2 diabetes, owing largely to their younger age, the incidence of CVD is considerably higher in patients with Type 1 diabetes than in age matched nondiabetic populations.

Pathogenesis

Not surprisingly, the increased prevalence of coronary artery disease in diabetes is preceded by a constellation of risk factors for coronary artery disease (Table 18-37).[229,547,694-696] Type 2 diabetic (and IGT) patients are commonly obese, hypertensive, and dyslipidemic (increased triglycerides, decreased HDL-C). However, independent of these variables, diabetes remains a major risk factor for coronary artery disease. Its effect may be mediated in part through the increased occurrence of renal disease. Level of chronic glycemia, measured by HbA1c, may also be an independent risk factor for coronary artery disease, particularly in women.[548,549] A large number of abnormalities, some of which are associated with glycemia or glycation, and which may cause increased risk of CVD, are more prevalent in diabetes. The most common lipid abnormalities in Type 2 diabetes are increased triglyceride and VLDL cholesterol levels and decreased HDL cholesterol levels. The triglyceride and VLDL cholesterol levels are a function of increased hepatic production and decreased clearance associated with decreased insulin-sensitive lipase activity. Both of these abnormalities can be at least partially corrected with improved insulin availability or insulin therapy. Other factors associated with atherosclerosis and present in Type 2 diabetes include glycated LDL[561] and HDL[562]; small dense LDL particles that are more prone to oxidation[553] and, therefore, are more atherogenic; increased plasminogen activator inhibitor-1 (PAI-1), which effectively decreases fibrinolysis[698]; increased fibrinogen[697] and endothelin levels[699]; increased platelet reactivity and aggregation[700]; and increased insulin levels (in Type 2 diabetes) that have been associated with increased risk of CVD in the nondiabetic population.[701,702] Similar changes in established and putative risk factors

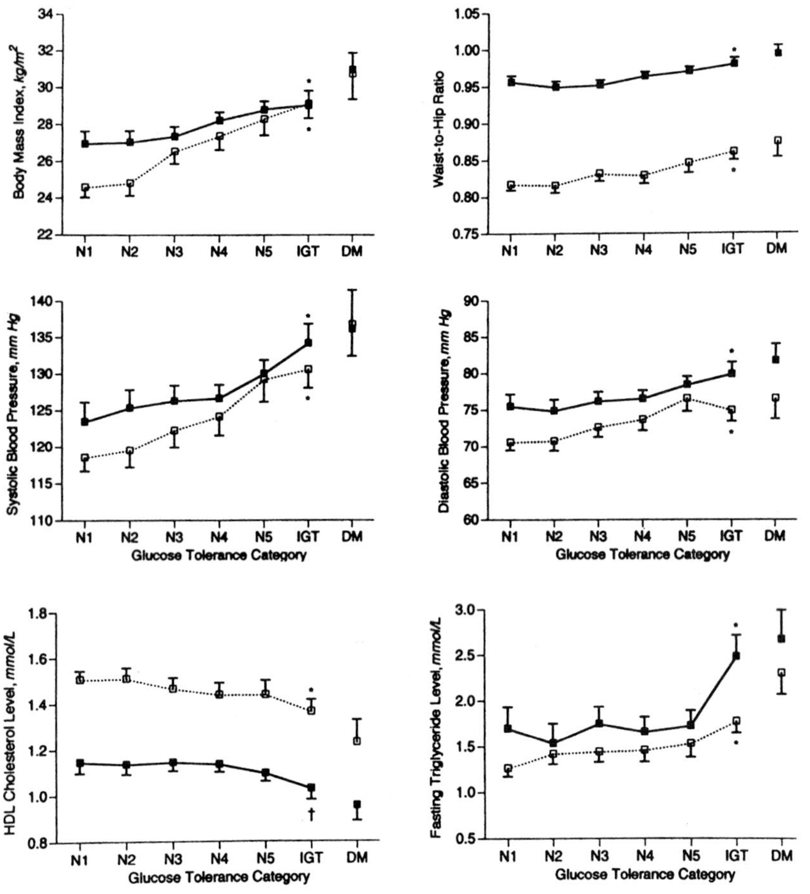

FIGURE 18-61. Risk factors for cardiovascular disease increase over the entire spectrum of glucose intolerance. More than 2,500 volunteers in the Framingham Offspring Study without previously diagnosed diabetes were classified according to their fasting glucose. The quintiles of fasting plasma glucose for the non-IGT and nondiabetic volunteers are shown as N1, N2 . . . N5. In general, previously identified CVD risk factors worsen continuously in the nondiabetic range. (*From Meigs et al.*[550])

for CVD have been demonstrated to increase progressively across the entire range of glycemia in the nondiabetic and IGT population (Fig. 18-61).[550]

The major factor predisposing patients with Type 1 diabetes to early CVD is the development of renal disease, which can increase the risk for CVD by as much as 25- to 40-fold. Type 1 diabetes does not have the same constellation of CVD risk factors (e.g., dyslipidemia, hypertension, obesity) as found commonly in Type 2 diabetes.

Screening and Diagnosis

All health care providers should be aware of the increased risk of CVD in the diabetic population, and the propensity of diabetic patients to have subtle or atypical symptoms of CVD. More frequent surveillance of CVD and its risk factors has been recommended including frequent assessment of peripheral pulses on physical examination and looking for decreased peripheral perfusion and the presence of femoral and carotid bruits (Table 18-18).[703] Periodic electrocardiograms should be performed in patients with Type 2 diabetes as often as annually in patients with established risk factors. Exercise tolerance testing, with or without radionuclide scanning or echocardiography, should be performed in patients at risk prior to a significant change in physical activity level. In addition, most diabetic patients undergoing peripheral revascularization (bypass or angioplasty) will fall into the high-risk category and should have coronary assessments.[704]

Therapy

Treatment of macrovascular complications in patients with diabetes parallels treatment of nondiabetics with several prominent differences. Diabetic patients have largely been excluded from primary prevention and secondary intervention studies of cardiovascular disease, making necessary extrapolation of results from studies in nondiabetic populations. However, several recent studies have included a sufficient number of diabetic subjects to compare results with specific interventions with the nondiabetic population.[705-709]

The role of intensive diabetes treatment to achieve near-normal glucose control with regard to CVD prevention or intervention is debatable. Although intensive treatment regimens may ameliorate the atherogenic lipid profile in Type 1 and Type 2 diabetes,[314,457] randomized controlled clinical trials of intensive glycemia therapy have not demonstrated a significant decrease in cardiovascular disease.[13,17,314] The University Group Diabetes Program observed an excess cardiovascular mortality of approximately 1 percent per year with sulfonylurea and biguanide therapy compared with diet or insulin,[401] which was not confirmed in the UKPDS.[17,286] The UKPDS showed an improvement in diabetes related mortality in the overweight patients assigned to metformin therapy, compared with those treated with diet alone, but paradoxically noted a large increase in cardiovasacular mortality in patients assigned to sulfonylurea plus early addition of metformin.[286] The validity of these findings has been challenged.[305]

Conventional treatments of coronary, peripheral, and cerebral vascular disease including use of beta-adrenergic blockers,

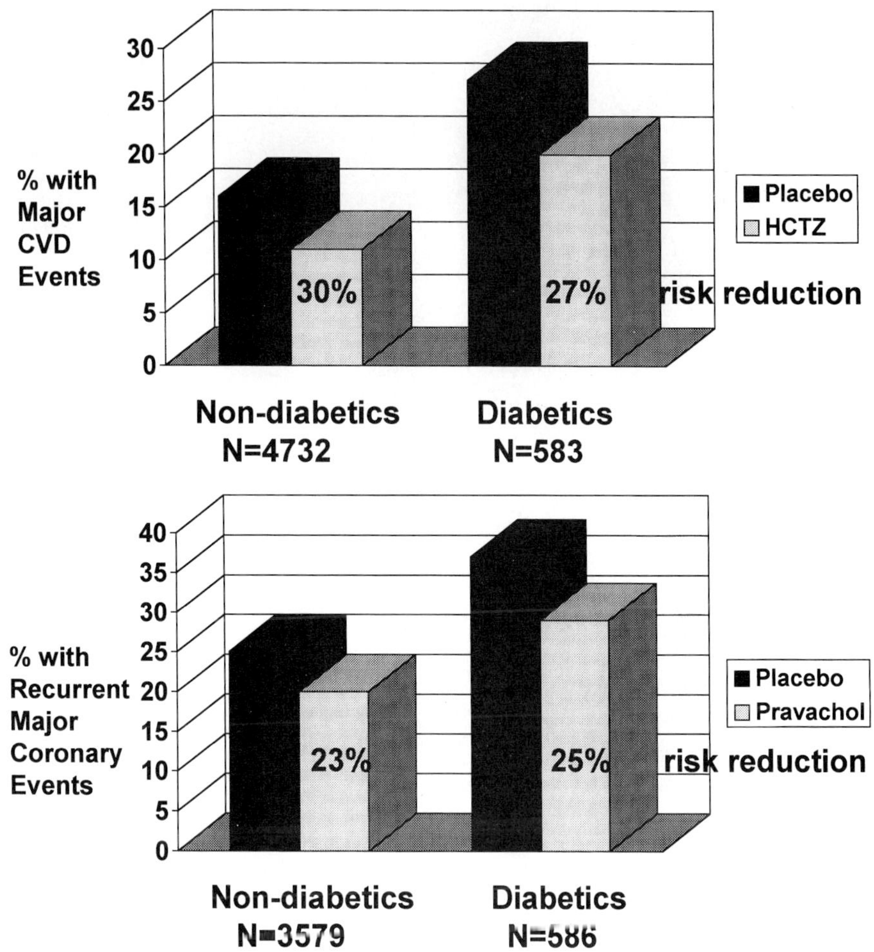

FIGURE 18-62. Treatment of identified cardiovascular disease risk factors in diabetes (predominantly Type 2) and effect on CVD outcomes. In (*a*) treatment of systolic hypertension with hydrochlorthiazide reduced major CVD events by 27 percent in the diabetic particpants, compared with 30 percent reduction in the nondiabetics. In (*b*), treatment of hypercholesterolemia with the HMG CoA-reductase inhibitor simvistatin reduced recurrent major coronary events by 25 percent compared with 23 percent reduction in the nondiabetics. Note that the diabetic participants randomly assigned to active therapy still had higher event rates than the placebo treated nondiabetics. (*From Curb et al.*[708] *and Goldberg et al.*[706])

calcium channel blockers, thrombolytic agents, aspirin, angioplasty, and bypass surgery can all be applied in patients with diabetes and vascular disease with several caveats (Fig. 18-62). Beta-adrenergic blockade may subject insulin-treated patients to more severe hypoglycemia[159] and should be implemented with care, although a recent study has suggested the risk may be more apparent than real.[710] On the other hand, a Norwegian study demonstrated a major decrease in mortality with timolol treatment in diabetic patients after an acute myocardial infarction.[711] When hypertension and/or hyperlipidemia occur in the setting of diabetes, selection of therapeutic agents must be guided by both their efficacy and the risk for exacerbation of glucose intolerance or other coexistent risk factors.[712] Thiazide and beta-adrenergic blocker treatment of hypertension and nicotinic acid treatment of hyperlipidemia may worsen glucose control.

Several recent secondary intervention clinical trials have demonstrated similar or greater[705,706] benefit in diabetic patients treated with HMG CoA-reductase inhibitors compared with nondiabetic patients. Although the reduction in risk was comparable for the diabetic patients as for the nondiabetic patients, the absolute rate of CVD events continued to be higher in the diabetics so that the diabetic patients treated with active agents had higher cardiovascular disease event rates than the placebo-treated nondiabetics. A primary prevention trial treating systolic hypertension with thiazide diuretics demonstrated a beneficial effect in diabetes.[708] In addition, the United Kingdom Prospective Diabetes Study included a study of hypertension therapy with either beta-adrenergic blockers or ACE inhibitors. Intensive hypertension therapy reduced blood pressure to 144/82 mm Hg, compared with 154/87 in the conventional therapy group, and resulted in a potent (24 percent reduction compared with less tight control) effect on aggregate diabetes outcomes, a 32 percent reduction in diabetes related deaths, a 44 percent reduction in strokes, and a 34 percent reduction in microvascular end points. There was no effect on myocardial infarctions.[713] Aspirin therapy has also been shown to decrease CVD mortality in diabetes, similar to the results in nondiabetics.[705,709] Although diabetic patients benefit from revascularization procedures, at least one study has suggested that bypass grafting is preferable to angioplasty in diabetic patients.[714] Finally, a clinical trial has demonstrated a significant improvement in outcome from acute myocardial infarctions in predominantly Type 2 diabetic patients when intensive insulin therapy (intravenous insulin-glucose infusion during the acute period followed by four-times-per-day subcutaneous insulin therapy for ≥ 3 mo) was used.[715]

On the basis of accumulating data in nondiabetic and predominantly Type 2 diabetic populations, regular surveillance of CAD risk factors and aggressive therapy are recommended (Tables 18-18 and 18-20).[341,703] The relatively atypical presentation of CAD, including painless ischemia, in the setting of diabetes should sensitize clinicians to possible CAD in patients with risk factors. Screening such patients is recommended, although false positive

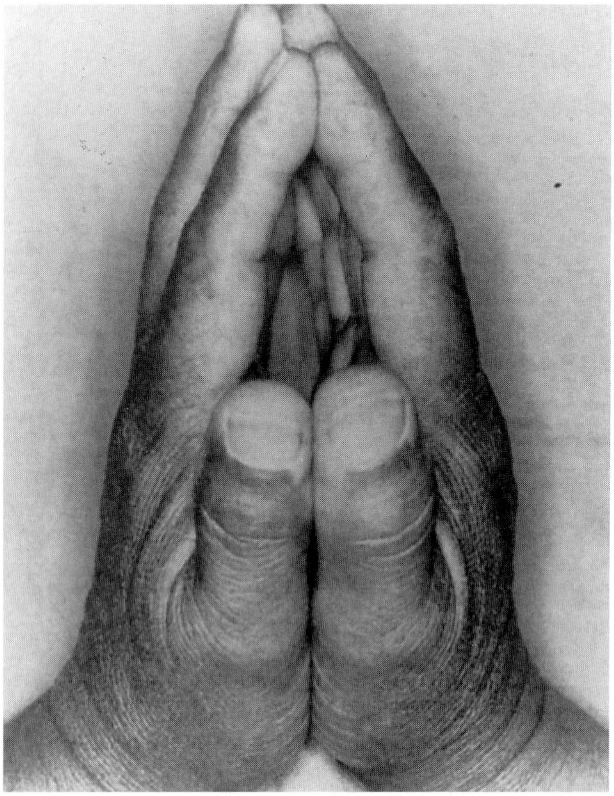

FIGURE 18-63. The "prayer" sign represents periarticular stiffening with inability to extend fingers completely. More severe degrees of flexion can affect dexterity. A similar phenomenon, probably a function of abnormal, glycated collagen, may account for adhesive capsulitis resulting in "diabetic frozen shoulder." (*From Lundbaek.*[718])

exercise and exercise scintographic studies are not uncommon.[716] Data are much more scarce regarding the effects of therapy in the prevention or treatment of peripheral and cerebrovascular disease in diabetes. The UKPDS demonstrated a significant effect of intensive blood pressure control on prevention of stroke and mortality from stroke.[713]

Other Complications

Other long-term complications including a predilection for certain infections (e.g., pseudomonas "malignant" external otitis, monilial skin infections, and rhinocerebral mucormycosis)[636] and cognitive impairment have been identified.[717] An increased prevalence of Dupuytren's contractures and periarticular thickening of the skin leading to decreased mobility of fingers also occurs in diabetic patients.[718] The "prayer sign" can be detected in a substantial fractrion of patients with long-term diabetes and a history of poor glycemic control (Fig. 18-63).[719] Adhesive capsulitis, resulting in "frozen" shoulders, and palmar fascial thickening causing triggering are also seen more frequently in patients with long-term diabetes.

REFERENCES

1. Bliss M: *The Discovery of Insulin*. Chicago, IL, University of Chicago Press, 1982.
2. Schadewalt H: The history of diabetes, in von Engelhardt D (ed): *Diabetes Mellitus: Its Medical and Cultural History*. New York, Springer-Verlag, 1989, pp 3–12.
3. Krall LP, Levine R, Barnett DM: The history of diabetes, in Kahn CR, Weir GC (ed): *Joslin's Diabetes Mellitus*, 13th ed. Lea & Febiger, Phil., 1994, pp 1–14.
4. Hoffman JPH: Die Geschichte des diabetes mellitus. Med Dis Dusseldorf, 1960.
5. von Mering J, Minkowski O: Diabetes Mellitus after the Extirpation of the Pancreas. 1889.
6. Opie EL: *Disease of the Pancreas*. Philadelphia, 1910.
7. Zuelzer GL: Experimetell Untersuchungen Uber dern diabetes. *Berliner Klinische Wochenschrift* 44:475, 1907.
8. Paulesco NC: Action de l'extrait pancreatique. *Comptes rendus des seances de la Societe de Biologie*. 27:555, 1921.
9. Banting FG, Best CH, Collip JB, Campbell WR, Fletcher AA: Pancreatic extracts in the treatment of diabetes mellitus. Preliminary Report. *Can Med Assoc J* 141:141, 1922.
10. Allen FM, Stillman E, Fitz R: *Total Dietary Regulation in the Treatment of Diabetes*. New York, 1919.
11. Deckert T, Poulsen JE, Larsen M: Prognosis of diabetics with diabetes onset before the age of thirty-one. I. Survival, causes of death, and complications. *Diabetologia* 14:363, 1978.
12. Arateus, The Capadocian, The Extant Works, ed and trans by Francis Adams, London, 1856.
13. DCCT Research Group: The effect of intensive treatment of diabetes on the development and progression of long-term complications in insulin-dependent diabetes mellitus. *N Engl J Med* 329:977, 1993.
14. Poulet J: Le diabete avant la decouverture de l'insuline. *Vie med.* Nr spec 52:5, 1971.
15. Himsworth HP: Diabetes mellitus: Its differentiation into insulin-sensitive and insulin-insensitive types. *Lancet*: 127-30, 1936.
16. Pirart J: Diabetes mellitus and its degenerative complications: A prospective study of 4,400 patients observed between 1947 and 1973. *Diabetes Care* 1:168, 1978.
17. UK Prospective Diabetes Study Group: Intensive blood-glucose control with sulfonylureas or insulin compared with conventional treatment and risk complications in patients with type 2 diabetes (UKPDS 33). *Lancet* 352:837, 1998.
18. Bonner-Weir S, Smith FE: Islets of Langerhans: Morphology and its implications, in Kahn CR, Weir GC (eds): *Joslin's Diabetes Mellitus*. Philadelphia, Lea & Febiger, 1994, pp 15–28.
19. Lukinius A, Wilander E, Westermark GT, Engstrom U, Westermark P: Co-localization of islet amyloid polypeptide and insulin in the B cell secretory granules of the human pancreatic islets. *Diabetologia* 32:240, 1989.
20. Guest PC, Bailyes EM, Rutherford NG, Hutton JC: Insulin secretory granule biogenesis. *Biochem J* 274:73, 1991.
21. Brelje TC, Scharp DW, Sorenson RL: Three-dimensional imaging of intact isolated islets of langerhans with confocal microscopy. *Diabetes* 38:808, 1989.
22. Lifson N, Lassa CV, Dixit PK: Relation between blood flow and morphology in islet organ of rat pancreas. *Am J Physiol* 248:E43, 1985.
23. Jansson L: The regulation of pancreatic islet blood flow. *Diab Metab Rev* 10:407, 1994.
24. Carlsson PO, Berne C, Jansson L: Angiotensin II and the endocrine pancreas: Effects on islet blood flow and insulin secretion in rats. *Diabetologia* 41:127, 1998.
25. Ahren B, Taborsky GJ, Porte D, Jr: Neuropeptidergic versus cholinergic and adrenergic regulation of islet hormone secretion. *Diabetologia* 29:827, 1986.
26. Slack JMW: Developmental biology of the pancreas. *Development* 121:1569, 1995.
27. Habener JF, Stoffers DA: A newly discovered role of transcription factors involved in pancreas development and the pathogenesis of diabetes mellitus. *Proc Assoc Am Phys* 110:12, 1998.
28. Jonsson J, Carlsson L, Edlund T, Edlund H: Insulin-promotor-factor 1 is required for pancreas development in mice. *Nature* 371:606, 1994.
29. Stoffers DA, Zinkin NT, Stanojevic V, Clarke WL, Habener JF: Pancreatic agenesis attributable to a single nucleotide deletion in the human IPF1 gene coding sequence. *Nat Genet* 15:106, 1997.
30. Edlund H: Transcribing pancreas. *Diabetes* 47:1817, 1998.
31. Ahigren U, Pfaff SL, Jessell TM, Edlund T, Edlund H: Independent requirement for ISL 1 in formation of pancreatic mesenchyme and islet cells. *Nature* 385:257, 1997.
32. Sosa-Pineda B, Chowdhury K, Torres M, Oliver G, Gruss P: The Pax4 gene is essential for differentiation of insulin-producing β-cells in the mammalian pancreas. *Nature* 386:399, 1997.

33. St-Onge L, Sosa-Pineda B, Chowdhury K, Mansouri A, Gruss P: Pax6 is required for differentiation of glucagon-producing α-cells in mouse pancreas. *Nature* 387:406, 1997.
34. Guillam MT, Hummler E, Schaerer E, Wu JY, Birnbaum MJ, Beermann F, et al: Early diabetes and abnormal postnatal pancreatic islet development in mice lacking Glut-2. *Nat Genet* 17:327, 1997.
35. Yamaoka T, Idehara C, Yano M, Matsushita T, Yamada T, Li S, Moritani M, et al: Hypoplasia of pancreatic islets in transgenic mice expressing activin receptor mutants. *J Clin Invest* 102:294, 1998.
36. Banting FG, Best CH: The internal secretion of the pancreas. *J Lab Clin Med* 7:251, 1922.
37. Bell GI, Pictet RL, Rutter WJ, Cordell B, Tischer E, Goodman HM: Sequence of the human insulin gene. *Nature* 284:26, 1980.
38. Dodson G, Steiner D: The role of assembly in insulin's biosynthesis. *Curr Opin Struct Bio* 8:189, 1998.
39. Harper ME, Ullrich A, Saunders GF: Localization of the human insulin gene to the distal end of the short arm of chromosome 11. *Proc Natl Acad Sci USA* 78:4458, 1981.
40. Docherty K, Macfarlane WM, Read ML, Smith SB, Wilson ME, Bujalska I, Gilligan M: Regulation of insulin gene transcription by nutrients. *Biochem Soc Trans* 24:368, 1996.
41. Sander M, Griffen SC, Huang J, German MS: A novel glucose-responsive element in the human insulin gene functions uniquely in primary cultured islets. *Proc Natl Acad Sci USA* 95:11572, 1998.
42. Halban PAA, Irminger JC: Sorting and processing of secretory proteins. *Biochem J* 299:1, 1994.
43. Rhodes CJ, Alarcon C: What β-cell defect could lead to hyperproinsulinemia in NIDDM? *Diabetes* 43:511, 1994.
44. Skelly RH, Schuppin GT, Ishihara H, Oka Y, Rhodes CJ: Glucose-regulated translational control of proinsulin biosynthesis with that of the proinsulin endopeptidases PC2 and PC3 in the insulin-producing MIN6 cell line. *Diabetes* 45:37, 1996.
45. Schuppin GT, Rhodes CJ: Specific co-ordinated regulation of PC3 and PC2 gene expression with that of preproinsulin in insulin-producing βTC3 cells. *Biochem J* 313:259, 1996.
46. Roder ME, Porte D Jr, Schwartz RS, Kahn SE: Disproportionately elevated proinsulin levels reflect the degree of impaired B cell secretory capacity in patients with noninsulin-dependent diabetes mellitus. *J Clin Endocrinol Metab* 83:604, 1998.
47. Wahren J, Johansson BL, Wallberg-Henriksson H, Linde B, Fernqvist-Forbes E, Zerath Jr: C-peptide revisited—new physiological effects and therapeutic implications. *J Intern Med* 240:115, 1996.
48. Ido Y, Vindigni A, Chang K, Stramm L, Chance R, Heath WF, Dimarchi RD, DiCera E, Williamson JR: Prevention of vascular and neural dysfunction in diabetic rats by C-peptide. *Science* 277:563, 1997.
49. Steiner DF, Rubenstein AH: Proinsulin C-peptide biological activity? *Science* 277:531, 1997.
50. Kruszynska YT, Home PD, Hanning I, Alberti KGMM: Basal and 24-h C-peptide and insulin secretion rate in normal man. *Diabetologia* 30:16, 1987.
51. Polonsky KS, Given BD, VanCauter E: Twenty-four-hour profiles and pulsatile patterns of insulin secretion in normal and obese subjects. *J Clin Invest* 81:442, 1988.
52. Lefebvre PJ, Paolisso G, Scheen AJ, Henquin JC: Pulsatility of insulin and glucagon release: Physiological significance and pharmacological implications. *Diabetologia* 30:443, 1987.
53. Welsh M, Scherberg N, Gilmore R, Steiner DF: Translational control of insulin biosynthesis. *Biochem J* 235:459, 1986.
54. Nielsen DA, Welsh M, Casadaban MJ, Steiner DF: Control of insulin gene expression in pancreatic B-cells and in an insulin-producing cell line, RIN-5F Cells. *J Biol Chem* 260:13585, 1985.
55. Leibiger B, Moede T, Schwarz T, Brown GR, Kohler M, Leibiger IB, Berggren PO: Short-term regulation of insulin gene transcription by glucose. *Proc Natl Acad Sci USA* 95:9307, 1998.
56. Wang J, Shen L, Najafi H, Kolberg J, Matschinsky FM, Urdea M, German M: Regulation of insulin preRNA splicing by glucose. *Proc Natl Acad Sci USA* 94:4360, 1997.
57. Welsh M, Nielsen DA, MacKrell AJ, Steiner DF: Control of insulin gene expression in pancreatic B-cells and in an insulin-producing cell line, RIN-5F cells. *J Biol Chem* 260:13590, 1985.
58. Schnetzler B, Murakawa G, Abalos D, Halban P, Selden R: Adaptation to supraphysiologic levels of insulin gene expression in transgenic mice: Evidence for the importance of posttranscriptional regulation. *J Clin Invest* 92:272, 1993.
59. Lang J: Molecular mechanisms and regulation of insulin exocytosis as a paradigm of endocrine secretion. *Eur J Biochem* 259:3, 1999.
60. Easom RA: CaM kinase II: A protein kinase with extraordinary talents germane to insulin exocytosis. *Diabetes* 48:675, 1999.
61. Thorens B, Sarkar HK, Kaback HR, Lodish HF: Cloning and functional expression in bacteria of a novel glucose transporter present in liver, intestine, kidney, and B-pancreatic islet cells. *Cell* 55:281, 1988.
62. Johnson JH, Newgard CB, Milburn JL, Lodish HF, Thorens B: The high K_m transporter of islets of langerhans is functionally similar to the low affinity transporter of liver and has an identical primary sequence. *J Biol Chem* 265:6548, 1990.
63. Matschinsky FM, Glaser B, Magnuson MA: Pancreatic β-cell glucokinase. Closing the gap between theoretical concepts and experimental realities. *Diabetes* 47:307, 1998.
64. Grupe A, Hultgren B, Ryan A, MA YH, Bauer M, Stewart TA: Transgenic knockouts reveal a critical requirement for pancreatic β cell glucokinase in maintaining glucose homeostasis. *Cell* 83:69, 1995.
65. Froguel P, Zouali H, Vionnet N, Velho G, Vaxillaire M, Sun F, Lesage S, Stoffel M, et al: Familial hyperglycemia due to mutations in glucokinase. *N Engl J Med* 328:697, 1993.
66. Byrne MM, Sturis J, Clement K, Vionnet N, Pueyo M, Stoffel M, et al: Insulin secretory abnormalities in subjects with hyperglycemia due to glucokinase mutations. *J Clin Invest* 93:1120, 1994.
67. Rorsman P: The pancreatic beta-cell as a fuel sensor: An electrophysiologist's viewpoint. *Diabetologia* 40:487, 1997.
68. Aguilar-Bryan L, Nichols CG, Wechsler SW, Clement JP, Boyd AE, Gonzalez G, Herrera-Sosa H, et al: Cloning of the β cell high-affinity sulfonylurea receptor: A regulator of insulin secretion. *Science* 268:423, 1995.
69. Sakura H, Ammala C, Smith PA, Gribble FM: Ashcroft FM. Cloning and functional expression of the cDNA encoding a novel ATP-sensitive potassium channel subunit expressed in pancreatic β-cells, brain, heart and skeletal muscle. *FEBS Lett* 377:338, 1995.
70. Thomas PM, Cote GJ, Wohllk N, Haddad B, Mathew PM, Rabl W, et al: Mutations in the sulfonylurea receptor gene in familial persistent hyperinsulinemic hypoglycemia of infancy. *Science* 268:426, 1995.
71. Komatsu M, Schermerhorn T, Noda M, Straub SG, Aizawa T, Sharp GWG: Augmentation of insulin release by glucose in the absence of extracellular Ca^{2+}. *Diabetes* 46:1928, 1997.
72. Prentki M, Tornheim K, Corkey BE. Signal transduction mechanisms in nutrient-induced insulin secretion. *Diabetologia* 40:S32, 1997.
73. Skelly RH, Bollheimer LC, Wicksteed BL, Corkey BE, Rhodes CJ: A distinct difference in the metabolic stimulus–response coupling pathways for regulating proinsulin biosynthesis and insulin secretion that lies at the level of a requirement for fatty acyl moieties. *Biochem J* 331:553, 1998.
74. Jones PM, Persaud SJ: Protein kinases, protein phosphorylation, and the regulation of insulin secretion from pancreatic β-cells. *Endocrine Rev* 19:429, 1996.
75. Takahashi N, Kadowaki T, Yazaki Y, Ellis-Davies GCR, Miyashita Y, Kasai H: Post-priming actions of ATP on Ca^{2+}-dependent exocytosis in pancreatic beta cells. *Proc Natl Acad Sci USA* 96:760, 1999.
76. Sharp GWG: Mechanisms of inhibition of insulin release. *Am J Physiol* 271: C1781, 1996.
77. Xu GG, Rothenberg PL: Insulin receptor signaling in the β-cell influences insulin gene expression and insulin content. *Diabetes* 47:1243, 1998.
78. Kulkarni RN, Bruning JC, Winnay JN, Postic C, Magnuson MA, Kahn CR: Tissue-specific knockout of the insulin receptor in pancreatic β cells creates an insulin secretory defect similar to that in Type 2 diabetes. *Cell* 96:329, 1999.
79. Porte D, Pupo AA: Insulin responses to glucose: Evidence for a two pool system in man. *J Clin Invest* 48:2309, 1969.
80. O'Meara NM, Polonsky KS: Insulin secretion in vivo, in Kahn CR, Weir GC (eds): *Joslin's Diabetes Mellitus*, 13th Edition. Philadelphia, Lea & Febiger, 1994, pp 81–96.
81. Creutzfeldt W, Ebert R: New developments in the incretin concept. *Diabetologia* 28:565, 1985.
82. Ensinck JW, D'Alessio DA: The enteroinsular axis revisited. *N Engl J Med* 326:1352, 1992.
83. Fehmann HC, Goke R, Goke B: Cell and molecular biology of the incretin hormones glucagon-like peptide-I and glucose-dependent insulin releasing polypeptide. *Endocrine Rev* 16:390 1995.

84. Andersen DK, Elahi D, Brown JC, Tobin JD, Andres R: Oral glucose augmentation of insulin secretion. *J Clin Invest* 62:152, 1978.
85. Bell GI, Sanchez-Pescador R, Laybourn PJ, Najarian C: Exon duplication and divergence in the human preproglucagon gene. *Nature* 304:368, 1983.
86. Mojsov S, Weir GC, Habener JF: Insulinotropin: Glucagon-like peptide I (7-37) co-encoded in the glucagon gene is a potent stimulator of insulin release in the perfused rat pancreas. *J Clin Invest* 79:616, 1987.
87. Gutniak M, Orskov C, Holst JJ, Ahren B, Efendic S: Antidiabetogenic effect of glucagon-like peptide-1 (7-36)amide in normal subjects and patients with diabetes mellitus. *N Engl J Med* 326:1316, 1992.
88. Drucker DJ: Glucagon-like peptides. *Diabetes* 47:159, 1998.
89. Nauck MA: Is glucagon-like peptide 1 an incretin hormone? *Diabetologia* 42:373, 1999.
90. Scrocchi LA, Brown TJ, MacLusky N, Brubaker PL, Auerbach AB, Joyner AL, Drucker DJ: Glucose intolerance but normal satiety in mice with a null mutation in the glucagon-like peptide 1 receptor gene. *Nature Med* 2:1254, 1996.
91. Seufert J, Kieffer TJ, Leech CA, Holz GG, Moritz W, Ricordi C, Habener JF: Leptin suppression of insulin secretion and gene expression in human pancreatic islets: Implications for the development of adipogenic diabetes mellitus. *J Clin Endocrinol Metab* 84:670, 1999.
92. Holst JJ, Bersani M, Hvidberg A, Knigge U, Christiansen E, Madsbad S, Harling H, Kofod H: On the effects of human galanin in man. *Diabetologia* 36:653, 1993.
93. Bennet WM, Wang ZL, Jones PM, Wang RM, James RF, London NJ, Ghatei MA, Bloom SR: Presence of neuropeptide Y and its messenger ribonucleic acid in human islets: Evidence for a possible petacrine role. *J Clin Endocrinol Metab* 81:2117, 1996.
94. Bruce DG, Storlien LH, Furler SM, Chisholm DJ: Cephalic phase metabolic responses in normal weight adults. *Metabolism* 36:721, 1987.
95. Christiansen E, Tibell A, Volund AA, Holst JJ, Rasmussen K, Schaffer L, Madsbad S: Metabolism of oral glucose in pancreas transplant recipients with normal and impaired glucose tolerance. *J Clin Endocrinol Metab* 82:2299, 1997.
96. Lee J, Pilch PF: The insulin receptor: Structure, function, and signaling. *Am J Physiol* 266:C319, 1994.
97. McClain DA: Different ligand affinities of the two human insulin receptor splice variants are reflected in parallel changes in sensitivity for insulin action. *Mol Endocrinol* 5:734, 1991.
98. Benecke H, Flier JS, Moller DE: Alternatively spliced variants of the insulin receptor protein. *J Clin Invest* 89:2066, 1992.
99. Hunter SJ, Garvey WT: Insulin action and insulin resistance: Diseases involving defects in insulin receptors, signal transduction, and the glucose transport effector system. *Am J Med* 105:331, 1998.
100. White MF, Kahn CR: Molecular aspects of insulin action, in Kahn CR, Weir GC (eds.): *Joslin's Diabetes Mellitus*. Philadelphia: Lea & Febiger, 1994, pp 139–62.
101. Virkamaki A, Ueki K, Kahn CR: Protein-protein interaction in insulin signaling and the molecular mechanisms of insulin resistance. *J Clin Invest* 103:931, 1999.
102. Tamemoto H, Kadowaki T, Tobe K, Yagl T, Sakura H, Hayakawa T, Terauchi Y, et al: Insulin resistance and growth retardation in mice lacking insulin receptor substrate-1. *Nature* 372:182, 1994.
103. Araki E, Lipes MA, Patti ME, Bruning JC, Haag, B, Johnson RS, Kahn CR: Alternative pathway of insulin signaling in mice with targeted disruption of the IRS-1 gene. *Nature* 372:186, 1994.
104. Bruning JC, Winnay J, Bonner-Weir S, Taylor SI, Accili D, Kahn CR: Development of a novel polygenic model of NIDDM in mice heterozygous for IR and IRS-1 null alleles. *Cell* 88:561, 1997.
105. Withers DJ, Gutierrez JS, Towery H, Burks DJ, Ren JM, Previst S, et al: Disruption of IRS-2 causes type 2 diabetes in mice. *Nature* 391:900, 1998.
106. Okada T, Kawano Y, Sakakibara T, Hazeki O, Ui M: Essential role of phosphatidylinositol 3-kinase in insulin-induced glucose transport and antilipolysis in rat adipocytes: Studies with a selective inhibitor wortmannin. *J Biol Chem* 269:3568, 1994.
107. Hara K, Yonezawa K, Sakaue H, Ando A, Kotani K, Kitamura T, Kitamura Y, et al: 1-phosphatidylinositol 3-kinase activity is required for insulin-stimulated glucose transport but not for RAS activation in CHO cells. *PNAS* 91:7415, 1994.
108. Calera MR, Martinez C, Liu H, El Jack AK, Birnbaum MJ, Pilch PF: Insulin increases the association of Akt-2 with Glut4-containing vesicles. *J Biol Chem* 273:7201, 1998.
109. Mueckler M: Facilitative glucose transporters. *Eur J Biochem* 219:713, 1994.
110. Pessin JE, Thurmond DC, Elmendorf JS, Coker KJ, Okada S: Molecular basis of insulin-stimulated GLUT4 vesicle trafficking. *J Biol Chem* 274:2593, 1999.
111. Rea S, James DE: Moving GLUT4. The biogenesis and trafficking of GLUT4 storage vesicles. *Diabetes* 46:1667, 1997.
112. Stenbit AE, Tsao TS, Li S, Burcelin R, Geenen DL, Factor SM, Houseknecht K, et al: GLUT4 heterozygous knockout mice develop muscle insulin resistance and diabetes. *Nature Med* 3:1096, 1997.
113. Sinha MK, Raineri-Maldonado C, Buchanan C, Pories WJ, et al: Adipose tissue glucose transporters in NIDDM. *Diabetes* 40:472, 1991.
114. Pedersen O, Bak JF, Andersen PH, Lund S, Moller DE, et al: Evidence against altered expression of GLUT1 or GLUT4 in skeletal muscle of patients with obesity or NIDDM. *Diabetes* 39:865, 1990.
115. Garvey WT, Malanu L, Zhu JH, Brechtel-Hook G, Wallace P, Baron AD: Evidence for defects in the trafficking and translocation of GLUT4 glucose transporters in skeletal muscle as a cause of human insulin resistance. *J Clin Invest* 101:2377, 1998.
116. Rabkin R, Simon N, Steiner S, Colwell JA: Effect of renal disease on renal uptake and excretion of insulin in man. *N Engl J Med* 282:182, 1970.
117. Tricoli JV, Bell GI, Shows TB: The human glucagon gene is located on chromosome 2. *Diabetes* 33:200, 1984.
118. Mojsov S, Heinrich G, Wilson IB, Ravazzola M, Orci L, Habener JF: Preproglucagon gene expression in pancreas and intestine diversifies at the level of post-translational processing. *J Biol Chem* 261:11880, 1986.
119. Unger RH, Orci L: Glucagon, in Porte D, Sherwin RS (eds): *Ellenberg & Rifkin's Diabetes Mellitus*. Stamford, Appleton & Lange, 1997, pp 115–139.
120. Blache P, Kervran A, Bataille D: Oxyntomodulin and glicentin: Brain-gut peptides in the rat. *Endocrinology* 123:2782, 1988.
121. Sherwin RS, Felig P: Glucagon physiology in health and disease, in McCann SM (ed): *International Review of Physiology*, vol. 16: Endocrine Physiology. Baltimore, University Park, 1977, p 151.
122. Diem P, Redmon B, Abid M, Moran A, Sutherland DER, et al: Glucagon, catecholamine and pancreatic polypeptide secretion in Type 1 diabetic recipients of pancreas allografts. *J Clin Invest* 86:2008, 1990.
123. Komatsu R, Matsuyama T, Namba M, Watanabe N, et al: Glucagonostatic and insulinotropic action of glucagonlike peptide I-(7-36)-amide. *Diabetes* 38:902, 1989.
124. Cherrington AD, Chiasson JL, Liljenquist JE, et al: The role of insulin and glucagon in the regulation of basal glucose production in the postabsorptive dog. *J Clin Invest* 58:1407, 1976.
125. Boden G, Tappy L, Jadali F, Hoeldtke RD, Rezvani I, Owen OS: Role of glucagon in disposal of an amino acid load. *Am J Physiol* 259:E225, 1990.
126. Unger RH: Glucagon physiology and pathophysiology in the light of new advances. *Diabetologia* 28:574, 1985.
127. Felig P, Wahren J, Sherwin RS, Hendler R: Insulin, glucagon and somatostatin in normal physiology and diabetes mellitus. *Diabetes* 25:1091, 1976.
128. Sherwin RS, Fisher M, Hendler R, Felig P: Hyperglucagonemia and blood glucose regulation in normal, obese and diabetic subjects. *N Engl J Med* 294:455, 1976.
129. DeFeo P, Perriello G, Torlone E, Fanelli C, Ventura MM, et al: Evidence against important catecholamine compensation for absent glucagon counterregulation. *Am J Physiol* 260:E203, 1991.
130. McGarry JD, Foster DW: Regulation of hepatic fatty acid oxidation and ketone body production. *Annu Rev Biochem* 49:395, 1980.
131. Barnes AJ, Bloom SR, Alberti KGMM, et al: Ketoacidosis in pancreatectomized man. *N Engl J Med* 296:1250, 1977.
132. Jelinek LJ, Lok S, Rosenberg GB, Smith RA, Grant FJ, Biggs S, Bensch PA, Kuijper JL, et al: Expression cloning and signaling properties of the rat glucagon receptor. *Science* 259:1614, 1993.
133. Gabbay RA, Lardy HA: Site of insulin inhibition of cAMP-stimulated glycogenolysis: cAMP-dependent protein kinase is affected independent of cAMP changes. *J Biol Chem* 259:6052, 1984.

134. Denton RM, Brownsey RW, Belsham GJ, et al: A partial view of the mechanism of insulin action. *Diabetologia* 21:347, 1981.
135. Mine T, Kojima I, Ogata E: Role of calcium fluxes in the action of glucagon on glucose metabolism in rat hepatocytes. *Am J Physiol* 265:G35, 1993.
136. Sherwin RS, Fisher M, Bessoff J, et al: Hyperglucagonemia in cirrhosis. Altered secretion and sensitivity to glucagon. *Gastroenterology* 74:1224, 1978.
137. Steiner DF, Bell GI, Tager HS, Rubenstein AH: Chemistry and biosynthesis of the islet hormones: Insulin, islet amyloid polypeptide (amylin), glucagon, somatostatin, and pancreatic polypeptide, in DeGroot LJ (ed): *Endocrinology*. Philadelphia, W.B. Saunders Company, 1995, pp 1296–1328.
138. Shen LP, Rutter WJ: Sequence of the human somatostatin I gene. *Science* 224:168, 1984.
139. Weir GC, Bonner-Weir S: Islets of Langerhans: The puzzle of intraislet interactions and their relevance to diabetes. *J Clin Invest* 85:983, 1990.
140. Yamada Y, Post SR, Wang K, Tager HS, Bell GI, Seino S: Cloning and functional characterization of a family of human and mouse somatostatin receptors expressed in brain, gastrointestinal tract, and kidney. *PNAS* 89:251, 1992.
141. Reichlin S: Somatostatin. *N Engl J Med* 309:1556, 1983.
142. Boel E, Schwartz TW, Norris KE, Fiil NP: A cDNA encoding a small common precursor for human pancreatic polypeptide and pancreatic icosapeptide. *EMBO* 3:909, 1984.
143. Schwartz TW: Pancreatic polypeptide: A hormone under vagal control. *Gastroenterology* 85:1411, 1983.
144. Brunicardi FC, Chaiken RL, Ryan AS, Seymour NE, Hoffmann JA, et al: Pancreatic polypeptide administration improves abnormal glucose metabolism in patients with chronic pancreatitis. *J Clin Endocrinol Metab* 81:3566, 1996.
145. Clark A, Lewis CE, Willis AC, Cooper GJS, Morris JF, Rein KBM, Turner RC: Islet amyloid formed from diabetes-associated peptide may be pathogenic in Type 2 diabetes. *Lancet* 231, 1987.
146. Nishi M, Sanke T, Seino S, Eddy RL, et al: Human islet amyloid polypeptide gene: Complete nucleotide sequence, chromosomal localization, and evolutionary history. *Mol Endocrinol* 3:1775, 1989.
147. Kahn SE, D'Alessio DA, Schwartz MW, Fujimoto WY, et al: Evidence of cosecretion of islet amyloid polypeptide and insulin by β-cells. *Diabetes* 39:634, 1990.
148. Cooper GJS: Amylin compared with calcitonin gene-related peptide: Structure, biology, and relevance to metabolic disease. *Endocrine Rev* 15:163, 1994.
149. Thompson RG, Pearson L, Schoenfeld SL, Kolterman OG, et al: Pramlintide, a synthetic analog of human amylin, improves the metabolic profile of patients with type 2 diabetes using insulin. *Diabetes Care* 21.987, 1998.
150. Clark A, Saad MF, Nezzer T, Urn C, Knowler WC, Bennett PH, Turner RC: Islet amyloid polypeptide in diabetic and non-diabetic Pima Indians. *Diabetologia* 33:285, 1990.
151. Nishi M, Bell GI, Steiner DF: Islet amyloid polypeptide (amylin): No evidence of an abnormal precursor sequence in 25 Type 2 (non-insulin-dependent) diabetic patients. *Diabetologia* 33:628, 1990.
152. Verchere CB, D'Alessio DA, Palmiter RD, Weir GC, Bonner-Weir S, et al: Islet amyloid formation associated with hyperglycemia in transgenic mice with pancreatic beta cell expression of human islet amyloid polypeptide. *PNAS* 93:3492, 1996.
153. Kahn SE, Andrikopoulos S, Verchere CB: Islet amyloid. A long-recognized but underappreciated pathological feature of type 2 diabetes. *Diabetes* 48:241, 1999.
154. Dineen S, Gerich J, Rizza R: Carbohydrate metabolism in non-insulin dependent diabetes mellitus. *N Engl J Med* 327:707, 1992.
155. Felig P: The glucose-alanine cycle. *Metabolism* 22:179, 1973.
156. Magnusson I, Shulman GI: Pathways of hepatic glycogen synthesis in humans. *Med Sci Sports Exerc* 23:939, 1991.
157. Felig P: The metabolic events of starvation. *Am J Med* 60:117, 1976.
158. Felig P, Wahren J: Fuel homeostasis in exercise. *N Engl J Med* 293:1078, 1975.
159. Cryer PE, Gerich JE: Glucose counterregulation, hypoglycemia and intensive insulin therapy of diabetes mellitus. *N Engl J Med* 313:232, 1985.
160. Eigler N, Sacca L, Sherwin RS: Synergistic interactions of physiologic increments of glucagon, epinephrine, and cortisol in the dog: A model for stress-induced hyperglycemia. *J Clin Invest* 63:114, 1979.
161. Felig P, Sherwin RS, et al: Hormonal interactions in the regulation of blood glucose. *Recent Prog Horm Res* 35:501, 1979.
162. National Diabetes Data Group: Classification and diagnosis of diabetes mellitus and other categories of glucose intolerance. *Diabetes* 28:1039, 1979.
163. World Health Organization: Diabetes mellitus: Report of a WHO study group. Geneva. World Health Org. (Tech Report Series no 727), 1985.
164. The Expert Committee on the Diagnosis and Classification of Diabetes Mellitus: Report of the Expert Committee on the Diagnosis and Classification of diabetes mellitus. *Diabetes Care* 20:1183, 1997.
165. Krolewski AS, Warram JH, Rand LI, Kahn CR: Epidemiologic approach to the etiology of type I diabetes mellitus and its complications. *N Engl J Med* 317:1390, 1987.
166. Leshnin M: Polyglandular autoimmune syndromes. *Am J Med Sci* 290:77, 1985.
167. Zimmet PZ, Tuomi T, Mackay IR, Rowley MJ, Knowles W, Cohen M, Lang DA: Latent autoimmune diabetes mellitus in adults (LADA): The role of antibodies to glutamic acid decarboxylase in diagnosis and prediction of insulin dependency. *Diabet Med* 11:299, 1994.
168. Kitagawa T, Fujita H, Hibi I, Aagenaes O, Laron Z, LaPorte RE, Tajima N, Drash AL: A comparative study on the epidemiology of IDDM between Japan, Norway, Israel and the United States. *Acta Paediatr Jpn* 26:275, 1984.
169. LaPorte R, Matsushima M, Chang YF: Prevalence and Incidence of Insulin-Dependent diabetes, in Harris, M (ed) *Diabetes in America*, 2nd ed. National Institutes of Health, NIH Publication No. 95-1468, 1995, pp 37–46.
170. Eisenbarth GS: Type 1 diabetes mellitus. A chronic autoimmune disease. *N Engl J Med* 314:1360, 1986.
171. Barnett AH, Eff C, Leslie RDG, Pyke DA: Diabetes in identical twins. *Diabetologia* 20:87, 1981.
172. Warram JH, Krolewski AJ, Gottlieb MS, et al: Differences in risk of insulin-dependent diabetes in offspring of diabetic mothers and diabetic fathers. *N Engl J Med* 311:149, 1984.
173. Mayer EJ, Hamman RF, Gay EC, Lezotte DC, et al: Reduced risk of IDDM among breast-fed children. *Diabetes* 37:1625, 1988.
174. Parent ME, Simiatycki J, Menzies R, Fritschi L, Colle E. Bacille Calmette-Guerin vaccination and incidence of IDDM in Montreal, Canada. *Diabetes Care* 20:767, 1997.
175. Maclaren N, Atkinson M: Is insulin-dependent diabetes mellitus environmentally induced? *N Engl J Med* 327:348, 1992.
176. Yoon JW, Austin M, Onodera T, Notkins AL: Virus induced diabetes mellitus: Isolation of a virus from the pancreas of a child with diabetic ketoacidosis. *N Engl J Med* 300:1173, 1979.
177. Nerup J, Platz P, Anderson O, Christy M, Lyngsoe J, Poulsen J, Ryder L, Staub R, Nielsen L, Thomsen M, Svejgaard A: HLA antigens and diabetes mellitus. *Lancet* 2:864, 1974.
178. Thompson G: HLA-DR antigens and susceptibility to insulin-dependent diabetes mellitus. *Am J Hum Genet* 36:1309, 1984.
179. Trucco M: To be or not to be ASP 57, that is the question. *Diabetes Care* 15:705, 1992.
180. Acha-Orbea H, McDevitt HO: The first external domain of the nonobese diabetic mouse class II, I-A beta chain is unique. *PNAS* 84:2435, 1987.
181. Faustman D, Li X, Lin HY, Fu Y, Eisenbarth G, Avruch J, Guo J: Linkage of faulty major histocompatibility complex class I to autoimmune diabetes. *Science* 254:1756, 1991.
182. Davies JL, Kawaguchi Y, Bennett ST, Copeman JB, Cordell HJ: A genome-wide search for human type 1 diabetes susceptibility genes. *Nature* 371:130, 1994.
183. Foulis AK, Liddle CN, Farquharson MA, Richmond JA, Weir RS: The histopathology of the pancreas in type 1 (insulin-dependent) diabetes mellitus: A 25-year review of deaths in patients under 20 years of age in the United Kingdom. *Diabetologia* 29:267, 1986.
184. Bottazzo GF, Dean BM, McNally JM, MacKay EH, Swift PGF, Gamble DR: In situ characterization of autoimmune phenomena and expression of HLA molecules in the pancreas in diabetic insulitis. *N Engl J Med* 313:353, 1985.
185. Johnson JH, Crider BP, McCorkle K, Alford M, Unger RH: Inhibition of glucose transport into rat islet cells by immunoglobulins from patients with new-onset insulin-dependent diabetes. *N Engl J Med* 323:1167, 1990.

186. Ziegler AG, Herskowitz RD, Jackson RA: Predicting type I diabetes. *Diabetes Care* 13:762, 1990.
187. Bohannon NJ: Treatment of vulvovaginal candidiasis in patients with diabetes. *Diabetes Care* 21:451, 1998.
188. Faich GA, Fishbein HA, Ellis SE: Epidemiology of diabetic acidosis: A population based study. *Am J Epidemiol* 117: 551, 1983.
189. Molnar GD, Gastineau CF, Rosevear JW, Moxness KE: Quantitative aspects of labile diabetes. *Diabetes* 14: 279, 1965.
190. Palmberg P, Smith M, Waltman S, et al: The natural history of retinopathy in insulin-dependent juvenile-onset diabetes. *Ophthalmology* 88:613, 1981.
191. Leahy JL: Natural history of β-cell dysfunction in NIDDM. *Diabetes Care* 13:992, 1990.
192. Clark A, Wells CA, Buley ID, Cruickshank JK, Vanhagen RI, Matthews DR, Cooper GJS, Holman RR, Turner RC: Islet amyloid, increased A-cells, reduced B-cells and exocrine fibrosis: Quantitative changes in the pancreas in type 2 diabetes. *Diabetes Res* 9:151, 1988.
193. Turner R, Stratton I, Horton V, Manley S, Zimmet P, Mackay IR, Shattock M, Bottazzo GF, Holman R, for UKPDS: UKPDS 25: Autoantibodies to islet-cell cytoplasm and glutamic acid decarboxylase for prediction of insulin requirement in type 2. *Lancet* 350:1288, 1997.
194. King H, Rewers M: WHO Ad Hoc Diabetes Reporting Group: Global estimates for prevalence of diabetes mellitus and impaired glucose tolerance in adults. *Diabetes Care* 16:157, 1993.
195. Harris MI, Klein R, Welborn TA, Knuiman WM: Onset of NIDDM occurs at least 4–7 yr before clinical diagnosis. *Diabetes Care* 15:815, 1992.
196. Knowler WC, Bennett PH, Hamman RF, Miller M: Diabetes incidence and prevalence in Pima Indians: A 19-fold greater incidence than in Rochester, Minnesota. *Am J Epidemiol* 108:497, 1978.
197. Zimmet P, King H, Taylor R, et al: The high prevalence of diabetes mellitus, impaired glucose tolerance and diabetic retinopathy in Nauru—The 1982 Survey. *Diabetes Research* 1:13, 1984.
198. Edelstein SL, Knowler WC, Bain RP, Andres R, Barrett-Connor EL, Dowse GK, Haffner SM, Pettitt DJ, Sorkin JD, Muller DC, Collins VR, Hamman RF: Predictors of progression from impaired glucose tolerance to NIDDM: An analysis of six prospective studies. *Diabetes* 46:791, 1997.
199. Burchfiel CM, Curb D, Rodriguez BL, Yano K, Hwang LJ, Fong KO, Marcus EB: Incidence and predictors of diabetes in Japanese-American men. The Honolulu Heart Program. *Ann Epidemiol* 5:33, 1995
200. Harris MI, Hadden WC, Knowler WC, Bennett PH: Prevalence of diabetes impaired glucose tolerance and plasma glucose levels in U.S. population aged 20–74 yr. *Diabetes* 36:523, 1987.
201. Barrett-Connor E: Epidemiology of obesity and non-insulin-dependent diabetes mellitus. *Epidemiol Rev* 11:172, 1989.
202. Ford ES, Williamson DF, Liu S: Weight changes and diabetes incidence: Findings from a national cohort of US adults. *Am J Epidemiol* 146:214, 1997.
203. Colditz GA, Willett WC, Rotnizky A, Manson JE: Weight gain as a risk factor for clinical diabetes mellitus in woman. *Ann Intern Med* 122:481, 1995.
204. Vague J: The degree of masculine differentiation of obesities: A factor determining predisposition to diabetes, atherosclerosis, gout and uric calculous disease. *Am J Clin Nutr* 4:20, 1956.
205. Hartz AJ, Rupley DC, Rimm AA: The association of girth measurements with disease in 32,856 women. *Am J Epidemiol* 119:71, 1984.
206. Bjorntorp PA: Abdominal obesity and the development of non-insulin-dependent diabetes mellitus. *Diabetes Metab Rev* 4:615, 1988.
207. Kissebah AH: Central obesity: Measurements and metabolic effects. *Diabetes Rev* 5:8, 1997.
208. Sparrow D, Borkan GA, Gerzof SG, Wisniewski C, Silbert CK: Relationship of fat distribution to glucose intolerance: Results of computed tomography in male participants of the Normative Aging Study. *Diabetes* 35:411, 1986.
209. Cassano PA, Rosner B, Vokonas PS, Weiss ST: Obesity and body fat distribution in relation to incidence of non-insulin dependent diabetes mellitus: A prospective cohort study of men in a normative aging study. *Am J Epidemiol* 136:1474, 1992.
210. Abate N, Garg A, Peshock RM, Stray-Gundersen J, Grundy SM: Relationships of generalized and regional adiposity to insulin sensitivity in men. *J Clin Inv* 96:88, 1995.
211. Richelson B, Pedersen SB, Moller-Pedersen T, Bak JF: Regional differences in triglyceride breakdown in human adipose tissue: Effects of catecholamines, insulin, and prostaglandin E2. *Metab Clin Exp* 40:990, 1991.
212. Boden G: Role of fatty acids in the pathogenesis of insulin resistance and NIDDM. *Diabetes* 46:3, 1997.
213. Peiris AN, Hennes MI, Evans DJ, Wilson CR, Lee MB, Kissebah AH: Relationship of anthropometric measurements of body fat distribution to metabolic profile in premenopausal women. *Acta Med Scand Suppl* 723:179, 1988.
214. Colditz G, Willett W, Rotnitzky A, Manson JE: Weight gain as a risk factor for clinical diabetes mellitus in women. *Ann Intern Med* 122;481, 1995.
215. Helmrich SP, Ragland DR, Leung RW, Paffenbarger RS: Physical activity and reduced occurrence of non-insulin-dependent diabetes mellitus. *N Engl J Med* 325:147, 1991.
216. Manson JE, Nathan DM, Krolewski AS, Stampfer MJ, Willett WC, Hennekens CH: A prospective study of exercise and incidence of diabetes among US male physicians. *JAMA* 268:63, 1992.
217. Wei M, Gibbons LW, Mitchell TL, Kampert JB, Lee CD, Blair SN: The association between cardiorespiratory fitness and impaired fasting glucose and type 2 diabetes mellitus in men. *Ann Intern Med* 130:89, 1999.
218. O'Sullivan JB, Mahan CM: Prospective study of 352 young patients with chemical diabetes. *N Engl J Med* 278:1038, 1968.
219. Hales CN, Barker DJ, Clark PM, Cox LI, Fall C, Osmond C, et al: Fetal and infant growth and impaired glucose tolerance at age 64. *Br Med J* 303:1019, 1991.
220. Rich-Edwards JW, Colditz GA, Stampfer MJ, Willett WC, et al: Birthweight and the risk for Type 2 diabetes mellitus in adult women. *Ann Intern Med* 130:278, 1999.
221. Simpson NE: Diabetes in the families of diabetics. *Can Med Assoc J* 98:427, 1968.
222. Rewers M, Hamman R: Risk factors for non-insulin-dependent diabetes, in Harris M (ed): *Diabetes in America*, edition 2. NIH Publication No 95-1468, 1995, pp 79–230.
223. Singer DE, Coley CM, Samet JM, Nathan DM: Screening for diabetes mellitus. *Ann Intern Med* 109:639, 1988.
224. Peters AL, Davidson MB, Schriger DL, Hasselblad V: A clinical approach for the diagnosis of diabetes mellitus. *JAMA* 276:1246, 1996.
225. Saad MF, Knowler WC, Pettitt DJ, Nelson RG, Charles MA, Bennett PA: A two-step model for development of non-insulin-dependent diabetes. *Am J Med* 90:229, 1991.
226. Polonsky KS, Sturis J, Bell IG: Non-insulin-dependent diabetes mellitus—A genetically programmed failure of the beta cell to compensate for insulin resistance. *N Engl J Med* 334:777, 1996.
227. DeFronzo RA, Tobin JD, Andres R: Glucose clamp technique: a method for quantifying insulin secretion and resistance. *Am J Physiol* 237:E214, 1979.
228. Anderson RL, Hamman RF, Savage PJ, Saad MF, Laws A, Kades WW: Exploration of simple insulin sensitivity measures derived from the frequently sampled intravenous glucose tolerance (FSIGT) tests. The Insulin Resistance Atherosclerosis Study. *Am J Epidemiol* 142:724, 1995.
229. Meigs JB, D'Agostino RB, Wilson PWF, Cupples LA, Nathan DM, Singer DE: Risk variable clustering in the insulin resistance syndrome: The Framingham Offspring Study. *Diabetes* 46:1594, 1997.
230. Reaven GM: Role of insulin resistance in human disease. *Diabetes* 37:1595, 1988.
231. Haffner SM, Valdez RA, Hazuda HP, Mitchell BD, Morales PA, Stern MP: Prospective analysis of the insulin resistance syndrome (syndrome X). *Diabetes* 41:215, 1992.
232. Meigs JB, Mittleman MA, Sutherland P, Lipinska I, Muller JE, Nathan DM, Wilson PWF, Singer DE: Hemostatic function and fasting insulin across the spectrum of glucose tolerance: The Framingham Offspring Study. *Diabetes* 45:193A, 1996.
233. Brunzell JD, Robertson RP, Lerner RL, Hazzard WR, et al: Relationships between fasting plasma glucose levels and insulin secretion during intravenous glucose tolerance tests. *J Clin Endocrinol Metab* 42:222, 1976.
234. Ward WK, Bolgiano DC, McKnight B, Halter JB, Porte D Jr: Diminished B cell secretory capacity in patients with noninsulin-dependent diabetes mellitus. *J Clin Invest* 74:318, 1984.

235. Yoshioka N, Kuzuya T, Matsuda A, Taniguchi M, Iwamoto Y: Serum proinsulin levels at fasting and after oral glucose load in patients with Type 2 diabetes mellitus. *Diabetologia* 31:355, 1988.
236. UK Prospective Diabetes Study Group: U.K. Prospective Diabetes Study 16. Overview of 6 years' therapy of type II diabetes: A progressive disease. *Diabetes* 44:1249, 1995.
237. Ward WK, Beard JC, Halter JB, Pfeiffer MA, Porte D: Pathophysiology of insulin secretion in non-insulin-dependent diabetes mellitus. *Diabetes Care* 7:491, 1984.
238. Zangen DH, Bonner-Weir S, Lee CH, Latimer JB, Miller CP, Habener JF, Weir GC: Reduced insulin, GLUT2 and IDX-1 in β-cells after partial pancreatectomy. *Diabetes* 46:258, 1997.
239. Andrews WJ, Vasquez B, Nagulesparan M, et al: Insulin therapy in obese, non-insulin-dependent diabetes induces improvements in insulin action and secretion that are maintained for two weeks after insulin withdrawal. *Diabetes* 33:634, 1984.
240. Kosaka K, Kuzuya T, Akanuma Y, Hagura R: Increase in insulin response after treatment of overt maturity onset diabetes is independent of mode of treatment. *Diabetologia* 18:23, 1980.
241. Glaser B, Leibovich G, Nesher R, Hartling S, et al: Improved β-cell function after intensive insulin treatment in severe non-insulin-dependent diabetes. *Acta Endocrinologica* 118:365, 1988.
242. Garvey WT, Olefsky JM, Griffin J, Hamman RF, Kolterman OG: The effect of insulin treatment on insulin secretion and insulin action in Type II diabetes mellitus. *Diabetes* 34:222, 1985.
243. Lillioja S, Mott DM, Zawadzki JK, Young AA, Abbott WG, Knowler WC, Bennett PH, Moll P, Bogardus C: In vivo insulin action is a familial characteristic in nondiabetic Pima Indians. *Diabetes* 36:1329, 1987.
244. Warram JH, Martin BC, Krolewski AJ, Soeldner JS, Kahn CR: Slow glucose removal rate and hyperinsulinemia precede the development of type II diabetes in the offspring of diabetic parents. *Ann Intern Med* 113:909, 1990.
245. Rich SS: Mapping genes in diabetes. *Diabetes* 39:1315, 1990.
246. Thomson G: Strategies involved in mapping diabetes genes: An overview. *Diabetes Rev* 5:106, 1997.
247. Rotwein PS, Chirgwin J, Province M, Knowler WC, Pettitt DJ, Cordell B, Goodman HM, Permutt A: Polymorphism in the 5' flanking region of the human insulin gene: A genetic marker for non-insulin-dependent diabetes. *N Engl J Med* 308:65, 1983.
248. O'Rahilly S, Choi WH, Patel P, Turner RC, Flier JS, Moller DE: Detection of mutations in insulin-receptor gene in NIDDM patients by analysis of single-stranded conformation polymorphisms. *Diabetes* 40:777, 1991.
249. Inoue H, Ferrer J, Welling CM, Elbein SC, Hoffman M, Mayorga R, Warren-Perry M, Zhang Y, Millns H, Turner R, Province M, Bryan J, Permutt MA, Aguilar-Bryan L: Sequence variants in the sulfonylurea receptor (SUR) gene are associated with NIDDM in caucasians. *Diabetes* 45:825, 1996.
250. Murakami K, Wilk J, Nishida K, Sussman KE, Draznin B: Hep-G2 glucose transporter gene polymorphism in Caucasian, black, Hispanic and Japanese patients with NIDDM. *Diabetes Res Clin Pract* 9:115, 1990.
251. Baroni MG, Oelbaum RS, Pozzilli P, Stocks J, Li SR, Fiore V, Galton DJ: Polymorphisms at the GLUT1 (HepG2) and GLUT4 (muscle/adipocyte) glucose transporter genes and non-insulin-dependent diabetes mellitus (NIDDM). *Hum Genet* 88:557, 1992.
252. Bjorbaek C, Vestergaard H, Heding LG, Cohen P, Pedersen O: Analysis of genes encoding 3 key proteins in insulin resistant glucose utilization of skeletal muscle from type 2 diabetics. *Diabetologia* 35(Suppl 1):A72, 1992.
253. Altshuler D, Hirschhorn JN, Klannemark M, Lindgren CM, Vohl MC, Nernesh J, Lane CR, Schaffner SF, Bolk S, Brewer C, Tourni T, Gaudet D, Hudson TJ, Daly M, Groop L, Lander ES: The common PPAR α Pro 12 Ala polymorphism is associated with decreased risk of type 2 diabetes. *Nat Genet* 26:76, 2000.
254. Stoffel M, Froguel P, Takeda J, Zouali H, Viionnet N, Nishi S, Weber IT, et al: Human glucokinase gene: isolation, characterization, and identification of two missense mutations liked to early-onset non-insulin-dependent (type 2) diabetes mellitus. *PNAS* 89:7698, 1992.
255. Yamagata K, Furuta H, Oda N, Kaisaki PJ, Menzel S, Cox NJ, Fajans SS, Signorini S, Stoffel B, Bell GI: Mutations in the hepatocyte nuclear factor-4 α gene in maturity-onset diabetes of the young (MODY 1). *Nature* 384:458, 1996.
256. Yamagata K, Oda N, Kaisaki PJ, Menzel S, Furuta H, Vaxillarie M, Southman L, Cox RD, et al: Mutations in the hepatocyte nuclear factor-1 α gene in maturity-onset diabetes of the young (MODY 3). *Nature* 384:455, 1996.
257. Stoffers DA, Ferrer J, Clarke WL, Habener JL: Early onset type 2 diabetes mellitus (MODY 4) linked to IPF-1. *Nat Genet* 17:138, 1997.
258. Horikawa Y, Iwasaki N, Hara M, Furuta H, Hinikio Y, Cockburn BN, Linder T, Yamagata K, Ogata M, Tomonaga O, Kuroki H, Kasahara T, Iwamoto Y, Bell GI: Mutation in hepatocyte nuclear factor 1-β gene (TCF2) associated with MODY. *Nat Genet* 17:384, 1997.
259. O'Rahilly S, Turner RC, Matthews DR: Impaired pulsatile secretion of insulin in relatives of patients with non-insulin-dependent diabetes mellitus. *N Engl J Med* 318:1225, 1988.
260. Pimenta W, Korytkowski M, Mitrakou A, Jenssen T, Yki-Jarvinen H, Evron W, Dailey G, Gerich J: Pancreatic beta-cell dysfunction as the primary genetic lesion in NIDDM. *JAMA* 273:1855, 1995.
261. Campbell P, Mandarino L, Gerich J: Quantification of the relative impairment in actions of insulin on hepatic glucose production and peripheral glucose uptake in non-insulin dependent diabetes mellitus. *Metabolism* 37:15, 1988.
262. Perriello G, Pampanelli S, DelSindaco P, Lalli C, Ciofetta M, Volpi E, Santeusanio F, Brunetti P, Bolli GB: Evidence of increased systemic glucose production and gluconeogenesis in an early stage of NIDDM. *Diabetes* 46:1010, 1997.
263. Banerji MA, Chaiken RL, Huey H, Tuomi T, Norin AJ, Mackay IR, Rowley MR, Zimmet PZ, Lebovitz H: GAD antibody negative NIDDM in adult black subjects with diabetic ketoacidosis and increased frequency of human leukocyte antigen DR3 and DR4. *Diabetes* 43:741, 1994.
264. UKPDS Group: Complications in newly diagnosed type 2 diabetic patients and their association with different clinical and biochemical risk factors. *Diabetes* Res 13:1, 1990.
265. Magee MS, Walden CE, Benedetti TJ, Knopp RH: Influence of diagnostic criteria on the incidence of gestational diabetes and perinatal morbidity. *JAMA* 269:609, 1993.
266. Diabetes and pregnancy. In *ACOG Technical Bulletin* 200, 1994.
267. Kuhl C: Etiology and pathogenesis of gestational diabetes. *Diabetes Care* 21:B19, 1998.
268. Kjos SL, Peters RK, Xiang A, Henry OA, Montoro M, Buchanan TA: Predicting future diabetes in Latino women with gestational diabetes: Utility of early postpartum glucose tolerance testing. *Diabetes* 44:586, 1995.
269. Solomon CG, Willett WC, Carey VJ, Rich-Edwards J, Hunter DJ: A prospective study of pregravid determinants of gestational diabetes mellitus. *JAMA* 278:1078, 1997.
270. Coustan D, Carpenter M, O'Sullivan P, Carr S: Gestational diabetes: predictors of subsequent disordered glucose metabolism. *Am J Obstet Gynecol* 1139, 1993.
271. Tattersall RB: Mild familial diabetes with dominant inheritance. *Q J Med* New Series XLIII:339, 1974.
272. Fajans SS: Scope and heterogeneous nature of MODY. *Diabetes Care* 13:49, 1990.
273. Matchinsky FM: Glucokinase as glucose sensor and metabolic signal generator in pancreatic beta-cells and hepatocytes. *Diabetes* 39:647, 1990.
274. Kadowaki T, Kadowaki H, Mori Y, et al: A subtype of diabetes mellitus associated with a mutation of mitochondrial DNA. *N Engl J Med* 330:962, 1994.
275. Davidson MD: The effect of aging on carbohydrate metabolism. A review of the English literature and practical approach to the diagnosis of diabetes mellitus in the elderly. *Metabolism* 28:688, 1979.
276. McCance DR, Hanson RL, Charles MA, Jacobsson LTH, Pettit DH, Bennett PH, Knowler WC: Comparison of tests for glycated hemoglobin and fasting and two hour plasma glucose concentrations as diagnostic methods for diabetes. *Br Med J* 308:1323, 1994.
277. Engelgau MM, Thompson TJ, Herman WH, Boyle JP, Aubert RE, Kenny SJ, Badran A, Sous ES, Ali MA: Comparison of fasting and 2-hour glucose and HbA1c levels for diagnosing diabetes: Diagnostic criteria and performance revisited. *Diabetes Care* 20:785, 1997.
278. Bennett PH, et al: Epidemiologic studies of diabetes in the Pima Indians. *Recent Prog Horm Res* 32:333, 1976.
279. Nathan DM: To screen or not to screen, in Alberti KGGM, Mazze R (eds.): *Frontiers of Diabetes Research: Current Trends in Non-Insulin-Dependent Diabetes Mellitus*. Amsterdam, Elsevier Science Publishers, 1990.

280. O'Sullivan JB, Mahan CM: Criteria for the oral glucose tolerance test in pregnancy. *Diabetes* 13:278, 1964.
281. Kitzmiller J, Buchanan T, Kjos S, Combs A, Ratner R: Pre-conception care of diabetes, congenital malformations, and spontaneous abortions. *Diabetes Care* 19:514, 1996.
282. DCCT Research Group: Pregnancy outcomes in the Diabetes Control and Complications Trial. *Am J Obstet Gynecol* 174:1343, 1996.
283. Drexel H, Bichler A, Sailer S, Breier C, Lisch H, Braunsteiner H, Patsch JR: Prevention of perinatal morbidity by tight metabolic control in gestational diabetes mellitus. *Diabetes Care* 11:761, 1988.
284. Nathan DM: Modern management of insulin-dependent diabetes mellitus. *Med Clin North Am* 72:1365, 1988.
285. Dagogo-Jack S, Santiago JV: Pathophysiology of type 2 diabetes and modes of action of therapeutic interventions. *Arch Intern Med* 157:1802, 1997.
286. UK Prospective Diabetes Study (UKPDS) Group: Effect of intensive blood-glucose control with metformin on complications in overweight patients with type 2 diabetes (UKPDS 34). *Lancet* 352:854, 1999.
287. Boyd JD, Jackson RL, Allen JH: Avoidance of degenerative lesions in diabetes mellitus. *JAMA* 118:694, 1942.
288. Dolger H: Clinical evaluation of vascular damage in diabetes mellitus. *JAMA* 134:1289, 1947.
289. Lawrence RD: Insulin Therapy: Successes and problems. *Lancet* 2:401, 1949.
290. Knowles HC Jr: The problem of the relation of the control of diabetes to the development of vascular disease. *Transactions of the American Clinical and Climatological Association* 76:142, 1964.
291. Engerman R, Bloodworth JM, Neslon S: Relationship of microvascular disease in diabetes to metabolic control. *Diabetes* 26:760, 1977.
292. Klein R, Klein BE, Moss SE, Davis MD, DeMets DL: Glycosylated hemoglobin predicts the incidence and progression of diabetic retinopathy. *JAMA* 260:2864, 1988.
293. Chase HP, Jackson WE, Hoops LS, Cockerham RS, Archer PG, O'Brien D: Glucose control and the renal and retinal complications of insulin-dependent diabetes. *JAMA* 261:1155, 1989.
294. Nathan DM, Singer DE, Godine JE, Harrington CH, Perlmuter LC: Retinopathy in older type II diabetics: Association with glucose control. *Diabetes* 35:797, 1986.
295. Kroc Collaborative Study Group: Blood glucose control and the evolution of diabetic retinopathy and albuminuria. *N Engl J Med* 311:365, 1984.
296. Feldt-Rasmussen B, Mathiesen ER, Deckert T: Effect of two years of strict metabolic control on progression of incipient nephropathy in insulin-dependent diabetes. *Lancet* 2:1300, 1986.
297. Holman RR, Mayon-White V, Orde-Peckar C, Steemson J, Smith B, McPherson K, Rizza C, Knight AH, Dornan TL, Howard-Williams J, Jenkins L, Rolfe R, Barbour D, Poon Pyw, Mann JI, Bron AJ, Turner RC: Prevention of deterioration of renal and sensory-nerve function by more intensive management of insulin-dependent diabetic patients. *Lancet* 1:204 1993.
298. Dahl-Jorgensen K, Brinchmann-Hansen O, Hanssen KF, Sandvik L, Aagenaes O, Aker Diabetes Group: Rapid tightening of blood glucose control leads to transient deterioration of retinopathy in insulin dependent diabetes mellitus: The Oslo study. *Br Med J* 290:811, 1985.
299. Lauritzen T, Frost-Larsen K, Larsen HW, Deckert T, and the Steno Study Group: Two year experience with continuous subcutaneous insulin infusion in relation to retinopathy and neuropathy. *Diabetes 34* (Suppl. 3):74, 1985.
300. Reichard P, Nilsson BY, Rosenqvist U: The effect of long-term intensified insulin treatment on the development of microvascular complications of diabetes mellitus. *N Engl J Med* 329:304, 1993.
301. DCCT Research Group: The absence of a glycemic threshold for the development of long-term complications: The perspective of the Diabetes Control and Complications Trial. *Diabetes* 45:1289, 1996.
302. Ohkubo Y, Kishikawa H, Araki E, et al: Intensive insulin therapy prevents the progression of diabetic microvascular complications in Japanese patients with non-insulin-dependent mellitus: A randomized prospective 6-year study. *Diab Res Clin Prac* 28:103, 1995.
303. American Diabetes Association: Position statement: Implications of the Diabetes Control and Complications Trial. *Diabetes Care* 16:1517, 1993.
304. St. Vincents Declaration: Diabetes care and research in Europe. *Diabetic Med* 7:360, 1990.
305. Nathan DM: Some answers, more controversy, from UKPDS. *Lancet* 352:832, 1998.
306. DCCT Research Group: The Diabetes Control and Complications Trial: Design and methodologic considerations for the feasibility phase. *Diabetes* 35:530, 1986.
307. DCCT Research Group: The effect of intensive diabetes treatment on the progression of diabetic retinopathy in insulin-dependent diabetes mellitus: The Diabetes Control and Complications Trial. *Arch Ophthalmol* 113:36, 1995.
308. DCCT Research Group: Progression of retinopathy with intensive vs conventional therapy in the Diabetes Control and Complications Trial. *Ophthalmology* 102:647, 1995.
309. DCCT Research Group: Early worsening of diabetic retinopathy in the Diabetes Control and Complications Trial. *Arch Ophthalmol* 116:874, 1998.
310. DCCT Research Group: The effect of intensive therapy on the development and progression of diabetic nephropathy in the Diabetes Control and Complications Trial. *Kidney Int* 47:1703, 1995.
311. DCCT Research Group: The effect of intensive diabetes therapy on the development and progression of neuropathy. *Ann Intern Med* 122:561, 1995.
312. DCCT Research Group: The effect of intensive diabetes therapy on measures of autonomic nervous system function in the Diabetes Control and Complications Trial (DCCT). *Diabetologia* 41:416, 1998.
313. DCCT Research Group: The effect of intensive treatment of diabetes on nerve conduction measures in the Diabetes Control and Complications Trial. *Ann Neurol* 38:869, 1995.
314. DCCT Research Group: The effect of intensive diabetes therapy on macrovascular disease and its risk factors in the Diabetes Control and Complications Trial. *Am J Cardiol* 75:894, 1995.
315. DCCT Research Group: The effect of intensive therapy on quality of life outcome in the Diabetes Control and Complications Trial. *Diabetes Care* 19:195, 1996.
316. DCCT Research Group: The effects of intensive diabetes therapy on neuropsychological function in adults in the Diabetes Control and Complications Trial. *Ann Intern Med* 124:379, 1996.
317. DCCT Research Group: Effect of intensive therapy on residual B-cell function in patients with type 1 diabetes in the Diabetes Control and Complications Trial. *Ann Intern Med* 128:517, 1998.
318. DCCT Research Group: Implementation of treatment protocols in the Diabetes Control and Complications Trial. *Diabetes Care* 18:361, 1995.
319. DCCT Research Group: Treatment related adverse events in the Diabetes Control and Complications Trial. *Diabetes Care* 18:1415, 1995.
320. DCCT Research Group: Hypoglycemia in the Diabetes Control and Complications Trial. *Diabetes* 46:271, 1997.
321. DCCT Research Group: Lifetime benefits of intensive therapy as practiced in the Diabetes Control and Complications Trial: An economic evaluation. *JAMA* 276:1409, 1996.
322. DCCT Research Group: Pregnancy outcomes in the Diabetes Control and Complications Trial. *Am J Obstet Gynecol* 174:1343, 1996.
323. DCCT Research Group: The relationship of glycemic exposure to the risk of developing retinopathy in the Diabetes Control and Complications Trial. *Diabetes* 44:968, 1995.
324. EDIC Research Group: Epidemiology of Diabetes Interventions and Complications (EDIC): Design and implementation of a long-term followup of the Diabetes Control and Complications Trial Cohort. *Diabetes Care* 22:99, 1999.
325. EDIC Study Group: The effect of intensive diabetes treatment on carotid artery wall thickness in the Epidemiology of Diabetes Interventions and Complications (EDIC). *Diabetes* 48:383, 1999.
326. Early Treatment Diabetic Retinopathy Study Research Group: Fundus photographic risk factors for progression of diabetic retinopathy. *Ophthalmology* 98:823, 1991.
327. EDIC Research Group: Retinopathy and nephropathy in patients with Type 1 diabetes four years after a trial of intensive therapy. *N Engl J Med* 342:381, 2000.
328. DCCT Research Group: Clustering of long-term complications in families with diabetes in the Diabetes Control and Complications Trial. *Diabetes* 46:1829, 1997.

329. Singer DE, Samet JM, Coley CM, Nathan DM: Tests of glycemia in diabetes mellitus. *Ann Intern Med* 110:125, 1989.
330. Weir GC, Nathan DM, Singer DE: American Diabetes Association technical review on standards of care for diabetes. *Diabetes Care* 17:1514, 1994.
331. Goldstein DE, Little RR, Lorenz RA, Malone JI, Nathan DM, Peterson CM: Technical review on tests of metabolic status to monitor diabetes mellitus. *Diabetes Care* 18:896, 1995.
332. Nathan DM, Singer DE, Hurxthal K, Goodson JD: The clinical information value of the glycosylated hemoglobin assay. *N Engl J Med* 310:341, 1984.
333. Svendsen PA, Lauritzen T, Soegaard U, Nerup J: Glycosylated haemoglobin and steady-state mean blood glucose concentration in Type 1 (insulin-dependent) diabetes. *Diabetologia* 23:403, 1982.
334. Larsen MG, Horder M, Mogensen EF: Effect of long-term monitoring of glycosylated hemoglobin levels in insulin-dependent diabetes mellitus. *N Eng J Med* 323:1021, 1990.
335. Armbruster DA: Fructosamine: Structure, analysis, and clinical usefulness. *Clin Chem* 33:2153, 1987.
336. Goldstein DE, Soeldner S, Cleary PA, Nathan DM: Feasibility of centralized measurements of glycated hemoglobin in the Diabetes Control and Complications Trial (DCCT): A multicenter trial. *Clin Chem* 33:2267, 1987.
337. Goldstein DE, Little RR, Wiedmeyer H, Eckfeldt J, Myers GL, Nathan DM, Parker M, Reed RG, Messenger LJ, Steffes MW, Gunter EW, Robbins DC: The National glycohemoglobin standardization program (NGSP): A progress report. *Diabetes* 48: LB-34, 1999.
338. Mogensen CE, Christensen CK: Predicting diabetic nephropathy in insulin-dependent patients. *N Engl J Med* 311:89, 1984.
339. Mogensen CE: Microalbuminuria, blood pressure and diabetic renal disease: Origin and development of ideas. *Diabetologia* 42:263, 1999.
340. Nathan DM, Rosenbaum C, Protasowicki VD: Single void urine samples can be used to estimate quantitative microalbuminuria. *Diabetes Care* 10:414, 1987.
341. ADA Clinical Practice Recommendations: Management of dyslipidemia in adults with diabetes. *Diabetes Care* 22:S56, 1999.
342. Zinman B: The physiological replacement of insulin. *N Engl J Med* 321:363, 1989.
343. Fineberg SE, Galloway JA, Fineberg NS, Goldman J: Effects of species of origin, purification levels and formulation on insulin immunogenicity. *Diabetes* 32:585, 1983.
344. Schernthaner G: Immunogenicity and allergenic potential of animal and human insulins. *Diabetes Care* 16(Suppl 3):155, 1993.
345. Kahn CR, Rosenthal AS: Immunologic reactions to insulin: Insulin allergy, insulin resistance, and the autoimmune insulin syndrome. *Diabetes Care* 2:283, 1979.
346. Galloway JA, Spradlin CT, Howey DC, Dupre J: Intrasubject differences in pharmokinetic responses: The immutable problem of present-day treatment? in Serrano-Rios M, Lefebvre PJ (eds): *Diabetes 1985*, New York, NY, Elsevier Scientific Publishing, pp 877–886.
347. Malone JI, Lowitt S, Grove NP, Shah SC: Comparison of insulin levels after injection by jet stream and disposable insulin syringes. *Diabetes Care* 9:637, 1986.
348. Dunn FL, Nathan DM, Scavini M, Selam JL: Long-term therapy of IDDM with an implantable insulin pump. *Diabetes Care* 20:59, 1997.
349. Nathan DM, Dunn FL, Bruch J, McKitrick C, Larkin M, Haggan C, Lavin-Tompkins J, Norman D, Rogers D, Simon D: Post-prandial insulin profiles with implantable pump therapy may explain decreased frequency of severe hypoglycemia, compared with subcutaneous intensive regimens, in IDDM. *Am J Med* 100:412, 1996.
350. Grinvalsky MA, Nathan DM: Diets for insulin pump and multiple daily injection therapy. *Diabetes Care* 6:241, 1983.
351. American Diabetes Association: Nutrition recommendations and principles for people with diabetes mellitus. *Diabetes Care* 22(Suppl 1):S42, 1999.
352. Nathan DM, Godine JE, Gauthier-Kelley C, Kawahara D, Grinvalsky M: Ice cream in the diet of insulin-dependent diabetic patients. *JAMA* 251:2825, 1984.
353. American Diabetes Association, American Dietetic Association: *Exchange Lists for Meal Planning*. Alexandria, VA: The American Diabetes Association, Chicago, IL, 1986.
354. DCCT Research Group: Nutrition interventions for intensive therapy in the Diabetes Control and Complications Trial. *J Am Diet Assoc* 93:768, 1993.
355. Jenkins DJA, Wolever TMS, Jenkins AL. Josse RG, Wong GS: The glycemic response to carbohydrate foods. *Lancet* 2:388, 1984.
356. Hermansen K, Rasmussen O, Arnfred J, Winther E, Schmitz O: Glycemic effects of spaghetti and potato consumed as part of mixed meal on IDDM patients. *Diabetes Care* 10:401, 1987.
357. Nathan DM: The glycemic index: Meat and potatoes or just gravy? *Diabetes Care* 10:524, 1987.
358. Fletcher G, Greenland P, Hiratzka LF, Houston-Miller N, Kris-Etherton P, Krumholz HM, LaRosa J, Ockene IS, Pearson TA, Reen J, Smith SC, Washington R: When to start cholesterol-lowering therapy in patients with coronary heart disease: A statement for healthcare professionals from the American Heart Association task force on risk reduction. *Circulation* 95:1683, 1997.
359. National Cholesterol Education Program (NCEP) Expert Panel: Summary of the Second Report (Adult Panel II). *JAMA* 209:3015, 1993.
360. Pedrini MT, Levey AS, Lau J, Chalmers TC, Wang PH: The effect of dietary protein restriction on the progression of diabetic and nondiabetic renal diseases: A meta-analysis. *Ann Intern Med* 124:627, 1996.
361. ADA Clinical Practice Recommendations: Diabetes and Exercise. *Diabetes Care* 22(Suppl 1):S49, 1999.
362. Schneider SH, Ruderman NB: Exercise and Type 2 diabetes *Diabetes Care* 13:785, 1990.
363. Wahren J, Felig P, Hendler R, Ahlborg G: Glucose and amino acid metabolism during recovery after exercise. *J Appl Physiol* 34:838, 1973.
364. Schiffrin A, Parikh S: Accommodating planned exercise in Type 1 diabetic patients on intensive treatment. *Diabetes Care* 8:337, 1985.
365. Nathan DM, Madnek SF, Delahanty L: Programming pre-exercise snacks to prevent post-exercise hypoglycemia in intensively treated insulin-dependent diabetes. *Ann Intern Med* 102:483, 1985.
366. Nathan DM, Fogel HA, Norman D, Russell PS, Tolkoff Rubin N, Delmonico FL, Auchincloss H, Camuso J, Cosimi AB: Long-term metabolic and quality of life results with pancreatic/renal transplantation in IDDM. *Transplantation* 52:85, 1991.
367. Sutherland DER: Pancreas transplantation as a treatment for diabetes: Indications and outcome, in Bardin CW (ed): *Current Therapy in Endocrinology and Metabolism*, 6th edition. St Louis, Mosby, 1997, pp 496–99.
368. Kendall DM, Rooney DP, Smets YFC, Bolding LS, Robertson RP: Pancreas transplantation restores epinephrine response and symptom recognition during hypoglycemia in patients with long-standing type 1 diabetes and autonomic neuropathy. *Diabetes* 46:249, 1997.
369. Navarro X, Kennedy WR, Loewenson RB, Sutherland DER: Influence of pancreas transplantation on cardiorespiratory reflexes, nerve conduction, and mortality in diabetes mellitus. *Diabetes* 39:802, 1990.
370. Landgraf R: Impact of pancreas transplantation on diabetic secondary complications and quality of life. *Diabetologia* 39:1415, 1996.
371. Bilous RW, Mauer SM, Sutherland DER, Najarian JS, Goetz FC, Steffes MW: The effects of pancreas transplantation on the glomerular structure of renal allografts in patients with insulin-dependent diabetes. *N Engl J Med* 321:80, 1989.
372. Howey DC, Bowher RR, Brunelle RL, Woodworth JR: [Lys(B28), Pro(B29)]-human insulin. A rapidly absorbed analogue of human insulin. *Diabetes* 43:396, 1994.
373. Zinman B, Tildesley H, Chiasson JL, Tsui E, Strack T: Insulin Lispro in CSII. *Diabetes* 46:440, 1997.
374. Kotsanos JG, Vignati L, Huster W, Andrejasich C, Boggs MB, et al: Health-related quality-of-life results from multinational clinical trials of insulin lispro. *Diabetes Care* 20:948, 1997.
375. Heinemann L: Hypoglycemia and insulin analogues: Is there a reduction in the incidence? *J Diabetes Complications* 13:105, 1999.
376. Ebeling P, Jansson PA, Smith U, Lalli C, Bolli G, Koivisto V: Strategies toward improved control during insulin lispro therapy in IDDM. *Diabetes Care* 20:1287, 1997.
377. Lee WL, Zinman B: From insulin to insulin analogs: Progress in the treatment of type 1 diabetes. *Diabetes Rev* 6:73, 1998.
378. Galloway JA, Hooper SA, Spradlin CT, Howey DC, Frank BH, Bowsher RR, Anderson JH: Biosynthetic human proinsulin: Review of

chemistry, in vitro and in vivo receptor binding, animal and human pharmacology studies, and clinical trial experience. *Diabetes Care* 15:666, 1992.

379. Moses AC, Gordon, GS, Carey MC, Flier JS: Insulin administered intranasally as an insulin-bile salt aerosol. *Diabetes* 32:1040, 1983.
380. Mitragotri S, Blankschtein D, Langer R: Ultrasound-mediated transdermal protein delivery. *Science* 269:850, 1995.
381. Kipnes M, Otulana B, Clauson P, Fischer J, Farr SJ, Hatorp V, Schwartz S: A comparison of the pharmacodynamic effects of inhaled insulin versus subcutaneous insulin in Type 1 diabetic patients. *Diabetes* 48:A95, 1999.
382. Jaremko J, Rorstad O: Advances toward the implantable artificial pancreas for treatment of diabetes. *Diabetes Care* 21:444, 1998.
383. Saudek CD, Selam JL, Pitt HA, Waxman K, Rubio M, Turner D, Jeandidier N, Charles MA, Fischell RE: A preliminary trial with the programmable implantable medication system for insulin delivery. *N Engl J Med* 321:575, 1989.
384. Blackshear PJ, Roussell AM, Cohen AM, Nathan DM: Basal rate intravenous insulin infusion compared to conventional insulin treatment in patients with type II diabetes. *Diabetes Care* 12:455, 1989.
385. Klonoff D: Noninvasive blood glucose monitoring. *Diabetes Care* 20:433, 1997.
386. Bremer T, Gough DA: Is blood glucose predictable from previous values? *Diabetes* 48:445, 1999.
387. Schichiri M, Asakawa N, Yamasaki Y, Kawamori R, Abe H: Telemetry glucose monitoring device with needle-type glucose sensor: A useful tool for blood glucose monitoring in diabetic individuals. *Diabetes Care* 9:298, 1986.
388. Service FJ, O'Brien PC, Wise SD, Ness S, LeBlanc SM: Dermal interstitial glucose as an indicator of ambient glycemia. *Diabetes Care* 20:1426, 1997.
389. Acerini C, Patton C, Savage M, Kernell A, Westphal O, Dunger D: Randomised placebo-controlled trial of human recombinant insulin-like growth factor I plus intensive insulin therapy in adolescents with insulin-dependent diabetes mellitus. *Lancet* 350:1199, 1997.
390. Moses A, Young S, Morrow L, O'Brien M, Clemmons D: Recombinant human insulin-like growth factor I increases insulin sensitivity and improves glycemic control in type II diabetes. *Diabetes* 45:91, 1996.
391. Kenyon NS, Ranuncoli A, Masetti M, Chatzipetrou M, Ricordi C: Islet transplantation: Present and future perspectives. *Diabetes Metab Rev* 14:303, 1998.
392. Pyzdrowski KL, Kendall DM, Halter JB, Nakhleh RE, Sutherland DE, Robertson RP: Preserved insulin secretion and insulin independence in recipients of islet autografts. *N Engl J Med* 327:220, 1992.
393. Tzakis AG, Ricordi C, Alejandro R, Zeng Y, Fung JJ, Todo S, Demetris AJ, Mintz DH, Starzl TE: Pancreatic islet transplantation after upper abdominal exenteration and liver replacement. *Lancet* 336:402, 1990.
394. Scharp DW, Lacy PE, Santiago JV, McCullough CS, Weide LG, Boyle PJ, Falqui L, Marchetti P, Ricordi C, Gingerich RL, Jaffee AS, Cryer PE, Hanto DW, Anderson CB, Flye MW: Results of our first nine intraportal islet allografts in type 1, insulin-dependent diabetic patients. *Transplantation* 51:76, 1991.
395. Faustman D, Coe C: Prevention of xenograft rejection by masking donor HLA class I antigens. *Science* 252:1700, 1991.
395a. Shapiro AM, Lakey JR, Ryan EA, et al: Islet transplantation in screen patients with Type 1 diabetes mellitus using a glucocorticoid-free immunosuppressive regimen. *N Engl J Med* 343:230, 2000.
396. Kenyon NS, Fernandez LA, Lehman R, Masetti M, Chatzipetrou M, Ranuncoli A, Iaria G, Han D, Wagner JL, Ruiz P, Berho M, Inverardi L, Alejandro R, Mintz DH, Kirk AD, Harlan DM, Burkly LC, Ricordi C: Long-term survival and function of intrahepatic islet allografts in baboons treated with humanized anti-CD154. *Diabetes* 48:1473, 1999.
397. Juang JH, Bonner-Weir S, Ogawa Y, Vacanti JP, Weir GC: Outcome of subcutaneous islet transplantation improved by polymer device. *Transplantation* 61:1557, 1996.
398. Hohmeier HE, BeltrandelRio H, Clark SA, Henkel-Rieger R, Normington K, Newgard CB: Regulation of insulin secretion from novel engineered insulinoma cell lines. *Diabetes* 46:968, 1997.
398a. Cook JJ, Hudson I, Harrison LC, et al: Double-blind controlled trial of azathioprine in children with newly diagnosed Type 1 diabetes. *Diabetes* 38:779, 1989.
398b. Mistura L, Beccaria L, Meschi F, et al: Prednisone treatment in newly diagnosed Type 1 diabetic children: 1 year followup. *Diabetes Care* 10:39, 1987.
398c. De Filippo G, Carel J-L, Boitard C, Bougheres PF: Long-term results of early cyclosporin therapy in juvenile IDDM. *Diabetes* 45:101, 1996.
398d. Canadian-European Randomized Control Trial Group: Cyclosporin-induced remission of IDDM after early intervention. *Diabetes* 37:1574, 1988.
398e. Eliot RB, Chase HP: Prevention or delay of Type 1 diabetes mellitus in children using nicotinamide. *Diabetologia* 34:362, 1991.
399. DeFronzo RA: Lilly Lecture. The Triumvirate: beta cell, muscle, liver. A collusion responsible for NIDDM. *Diabetes* 37:667, 1988.
400. Nathan DM: Inferences and implications: Do the DCCT results apply in NIDDM? *Diabetes Care* 18:251, 1995.
401. University Group Diabetes Program: A study of the effects of hypoglycemic agents on vascular complications in patients with adult onset diabetes. II. Mortality results. *Diabetes* 19:787, 1970.
402. UKPDS Group: UK Prospective Diabetes Study VIII: Study design, progress and performance. *Diabetologia* 34:877, 1991.
403. UKPDS Group: Epidemiological association of glycaemia with macrovascular and microvascular complications of Type 2 diabetes (UKPDS 35). *Br Med J* In press, 1999.
404. Genuth S, Eastman R, Kahn R, Klein R, Lachin J, Lebowitz H, Nathan DM, Vinicor F: Implications of the United Kingdom Diabetes Prospective Study. *Diabetes Care* 21:2180, 1998.
405. Vijan S, Hofer TP, Hayward RA: Estimated benefits of glycemic control in microvascular complications in Type 2 diabetes. *Ann Intern Med* 127:788, 1997.
406. Stout, RW: Insulin and Atheroma. *Diabetes Care* 13:631, 1990.
407. Ilkova H, Glaser B, Tunckale A, Bagriacik N, Cerasi E: Induction of long-term glycemic control in newly diagnosed type 2 diabetic patients by transient intensive insulin treatment. *Diabetes Care* 20:1353, 1997.
408. Hadden DR, Blair ALT, Wilson EA, et al: Natural history of diabetes presenting age 40–69 years: A prospective study of the influence of intensive dietary therapy. *Q J Med* 59:579, 1986.
409. Heilbronn LK, Noakes M, Clifton PM: Effect of energy restriction, weight loss, and diet composition on plasma lipids and glucose in patients with type 2 diabetes. *Diabetes Care* 22:889, 1999.
410. Henry RR, Scheaffer L, Olefsky JM: Glycemic effects of intensive caloric restriction and isocaloric refeeding in noninsulin dependent diabetes mellitus. *J Clin Endocrinol Metab* 61:917, 1985.
411. Wing RR, Koeske R, Epstein LH, Nowlak MP, Gooding W, Becker D: Long-term effects of modest weight loss in type 2 diabetic patients. *Arch Intern Med* 147:1749, 1987.
412. Gannon MC, Nuttall FQ, Lane JT, Fang S, Gupta V, Sandhoffer CR: Effect of twenty-four hours of starvation on plasma glucose and insulin concentrations in people with untreated non-insulin dependent diabetes mellitus. *Metabolism* 45:492, 1996.
413. Howard BV, Abbott WGH, Swinburn BA: Evaluation of metabolic effects of substitution of complex carbohydrates for saturated fat in individuals with obesity and NIDDM. *Diabetes Care* 14:786, 1991.
414. Garg A, Bonanome A, Grundy SM, Zhang ZJ, Unger RH: Comparison of a high carbohydrate diet with a high-monunsaturated-fat diet in patients with non-insulin-dependent diabetes mellitus. *N Engl J Med* 319:829, 1988.
415. Abbott WGH, Boyce VL, Grundy SM, Howard BV: Effects of replacing saturated fat with complex carbohydrate in diets of subjects with NIDDM. *Diabetes Care* 12:10207, 1989.
415a. Chandalia M, Garg A, Lutjohann D, et al: Beneficial effects of high dietary fiber intake in patients with Type 2 diabetes mellitus. *N Engl J Med* 342:1392, 2000.
416. Coulston AM, Hollenbeck CB, Swislocki ALM, Reaven GM: Persistence of hypertriglyceridemic effect of low-fat high-carbohydrate diets in NIDDM patients. *Diabetes Care* 12:94, 1989.
417. Howard BV, Abbott WGH, Swinburn BA: Evaluation of metabolic effects of substitution of complex carbohydrates for saturated fat in individuals with obesity and NIDDM. *Diabetes Care* 14:786, 1991.
418. West KM: Diet therapy of diabetes: An analysis of failure. *Ann Intern Med* 79:425, 1973.
419. Wing RR: Behavioral strategies for weight reduction in obese type II diabetic patients. *Diabetes Care* 12:139, 1989.

420. Redmon JB, Raatz SK, Kwong CA, Swanson JE, Thomas W, Bantle JP: Pharmacologic induction of weight loss to treat Type 2 diabetes. *Diabetes Care* 22:896, 1999.
421. Pories WJ, MacDonald KG, Morgan EJ, Sinha MK, Dohm GL, Swanson MS, Barakat HA, Khazanie PG, Leggett-Frazier N, Long SD: Surgical treatment of obesity and its effect on diabetes: 10-year followup. *Am J Clin Nutr* 55:582S, 1992.
422. Groop L: Sulfonylureas in NIDDM. *Diabetes Care* 15:737, 1992.
423. Lev JD, Zeidler A, Kumar D: Glyburide and glipizide in treatment of diabetic patients with secondary failures to tolazamide or chlorpropamide. *Diabetes Care* 10:679, 1987.
424. van Staa T, Abenhaim L, Monette J: Rates of hypoglycemia in users of sulfonylureas. *J Clin Epidemiol* 50:735, 1997.
425. Haupt E, Laube F, Loy H, Schoffling K: Secondary failures in modern therapy of diabetes mellitus with blood glucose lowering sulfonamides. *Med Klin* 72:1529, 1977.
426. Simonson DC, Kourides IA, Feinglos M, Shamoon H, Fischette CT: Efficacy, safety, and dose-response characteristics of glipizide gastrointestinal therapeutic system on glycemic control and insulin secretion in NIDDM. *Diabetes Care* 20:597, 1997.
427. Fuhlendorff J, Rorsman P, Kofod H, Brand CL, Rolin B, MacKay P, Shymko R, Carr RD: Stimulation of insulin release by repaglinide and glibenclamide involves both common and distinct processes. *Diabetes* 47:345, 1998.
428. Goldberg R, Einhorn D, Lucas CP, Rendell MS, Damsbo P, Huang W, Strange P, Brodows R: A randomized placebo-controlled trial of repaglinide in the treatment of type 2 diabetes. *Diabetes Care* 21:1897, 1998.
429. Moses R, Slobodniuk R, Boyages S, Colagiuri S, Kidson W, Carter J, Donnelly T, Moffitt P, Hopkins H: Effect of repaglinide addition to metformin monotherapy on glycemic control in patients with type 2 diabetes. *Diabetes Care* 22:119, 1999.
430. Bailey CJ, Path MRC, Turner RC: Metformin. *N Engl J Med* 334:574, 1996.
431. Cusi K, DeFronzo RA: Metformin: A review of its metabolic effects. *Diabetes Rev* 6: 89, 1998.
432. Lee AJ: Metformin in non-insulin-dependent diabetes mellitus. *Pharmacotherapy* 16:327, 1996.
433. Campbell IW, Howlett HCS: Worldwide experience of metformin as an effective glucose lowering agent: A meta-analysis. *Diabetes Metab Rev* 11:S57, 1995.
434. DeFronzo RA, Goodman AM: The Multicenter Metformin Study Group. Efficacy of metformin in patients with non-insulin-dependent diabetes mellitus. *N Engl J Med* 333:541, 1995.
435. Hermann LS, Schersten B, Bitzen PO, Kjellstrom T, Lindgarde F, Melander A: Therapeutic comparison of metformin and sulfonylurea, alone and in various combinations: A double blind controlled study. *Diabetes Care* 17:1100, 1994.
436. Strumvoll N, Nurjhan N, Perriello G, Dailey G, Gerich JE: Metabolic effects of metformin in non-insulin-dependent diabetes mellitus. *N Engl J Med* 333:550, 1995.
437. Misbin RI, Green L, Stadel BV, Gueriguian JL, Gubbi A, Fleming GA: Lactic acidosis in patients with diabetes treated with metformin. *N Engl J Med* 338: 265, 1998.
438. Lebovitz HE: α-Glucosidase inhibitors as agents in the treatment of diabetes. *Diabetes Rev* 6:132, 1998.
439. Chiasson JL, Josse RG, Hunt JA, Palmason C, Rodger NW, Ross SA, Ryan EA, Tan MH, Wolever TMS: The effectiveness of acarbose in the treatment of patients with NIDDM. *Ann Intern Med* 121:928, 1994.
440. Hollander P, Pi-Sunyer X, Coniff RF: Acarbose in the treatment of Type 1 diabetes. *Diabetes Care* 20:248, 1997.
441. Saltiel A, Olefsky JM: Thiazolidinediones in the treatment of insulin resistance and type 2 diabetes. *Diabetes* 45:1661, 1996.
442. Saleh Y, Mudaliar SR, Henry RR: Metabolic and vascular effects of the thiazolidinedione troglitazone. *Diabetes Rev* 7:55, 1999.
443. Inzucchi SE, Maggs DG, Spollet GR, Page SL, Rife FS, Walton V, Shulman GI: Efficacy and metabolic effects of metformin and troglitazone in type II diabetes mellitus. *N Engl J Med* 338:867, 1998.
444. Kumar S, Boulton AJM, Beck-Nielsen H, Berthezene F, Muggeo M, Persson B, Spinas GA, Donoghue S, Lettis S, Stewart-Long P: Troglitazone an insulin action enhancer improves metabolic control in NIDDM patients. *Diabetologia* 39:701, 1996.
445. Schwartz S, Raskin P, Fonseca V, Graveline JF: Effect of troglitazone in insulin-treated patients with Type II diabetic mellitus. Troglitazone and Exogenous Insulin Study Group. *N Engl J Med* 338:861, 1998.
446. Iwamoto Y, Kosaka K, Kuzuya T, Akanuma Y, Shigeta Y, Kaneko T: Effect of combination therapy of troglitazone and sulphonylureas in patients with Type 2 diabetes who were poorly controlled by sulphonylurea therapy alone. *Diabetic Med* 13:365, 1996.
447. Gitlin N, Julie NL, Spurr CL, Lim KN, Juarbe HM: Two cases of severe clinical and histologic hepatotoxicity associated with troglitazone. *Ann Intern Med* 129:36, 1998.
448. Nolan JJ, Ludvik B, Beerdsen P, Joyce M, Olefsky J: Improvement in glucose tolerance and insulin resistance in obese subjects treated with troglitazone. *N Engl J Med* 331:1188, 1994.
449. Hasegawa I, Murakawa H, Suzuki M, Yamamoto Y, Kurabayashi T, Tanaka K: Effect of troglitazone on endocrine and ovulatory performance in women with insulin-resistance related polycystic ovary syndrome. *Fertil Steril* 71:323, 1999.
450. Genuth S: Insulin use in NIDDM. *Diabetes Care* 13:1240, 1990.
451. Abraira C, Johnson N, Colwell J, VA CSDM Group: VA Cooperative study on glycemic control and complications in Type II diabetes. *Diabetes Care* 18:1113, 1995.
452. Henry RR, Gumbiner B, Ditzler T, Wallace P, et al: Intensive conventional insulin therapy for Type II diabetes. *Diabetes Care* 16:21, 1993.
453. Jennings AM, Lewis KS, Murdoch S, Talbot JF, et al: Randomized trial comparing continuous insulin infusion and conventional insulin therapy in type II diabetic patients poorly controlled with sulfonylureas. *Diabetes Care* 14:738, 1991.
454. Lindstrom T, Eriksson P, Olsson AG, Amqvist HJ: Long-term improvement of glycemic control by insulin treatment in NIDDM patients with secondary failure. *Diabetes Care* 17:719, 1994.
455. Lindstrom TH, Arnqvist HJ, von Schenk HH: Effect of conventional and intensified insulin therapy on free-insulin profiles and glycemic control in NIDDM. *Diabetes Care* 15:27, 1992.
456. Wolffenbuttel BHR, Sels JP, Rondas-Colbers GJ, Menheere P, Kruseman AC: Comparison of different insulin regimens in elderly patients with NIDDM. *Diabetes Care* 19:1326, 1996.
457. Nathan DM, Roussell A, Godine JE: Glyburide or insulin for metabolic control in non-insulin-dependent diabetes mellitus in the elderly. *Am J Med* 81:837, 1986.
458. Cusi K, Cunningham G, Comstock J: Safety and efficacy of normalizing fasting glucose with bedtime NPH insulin alone in NIDDM. *Diabetes Care* 18:843, 1995.
459. Riddle MC: New tactics for type 2 diabetes: Regimens based on intermediate-acting insulin taken at bedtime. *Lancet* 1:192, 1985.
460. Diehl AK, Sugarek NJ, Bauer RL: Medication compliance in non-insulin-dependent diabetes: A randomized comparison of chlorpropamide and insulin. *Diabetes Care* 8:219, 1985.
461. Genuth SM: Treating diabetes with both insulin and sulfonylurea drugs: What is the value? *Clin Diabetes* 5:74, 1987.
462. Longnecker M, Elsenhans V, Leiman S, Owen E, Boden G: Insulin and sulfonylurea agent in non-insulin-dependent diabetes mellitus. *Arch Intern Med* 146:673, 1986.
463. Schade D, Mitchell W, Griego G: Addition of sulfonylurea to insulin treatment in poorly controlled type II diabetes. *JAMA* 257:2441, 1987.
464. Riddle M, Hart J, Bouma D, Phillipson Y: Efficacy of bedtime NPH insulin with daytime sulfonylurea for subpopulation of type II diabetic subjects. *Diabetes Care* 12:623, 1989.
465. Groop L, Harno K, Tolppanen E: The combination of insulin and sulphonylurea in the treatment of secondary drug failure in patients with type II diabetes. *Acta Endocrinol* 106:97, 1984.
466. Karlander S, Gutniak M, Efendic S: Effects of combination therapy with glyburide and insulin on serum lipid levels in NIDDM patients with secondary sulfonylurea failure. *Diabetes Care* 14:963, 1991.
467. Lewitt M, Yu, Vincent K, Rennie G, Carter J, Marel G, Yue D, Hooper M: Effects of combined insulin-sulfonylurea therapy in type II patients. *Diabetes Care* 12:379, 1989.
468. Chow C, Sorensen J, Tsang L, Cockram C: Comparison of insulin with or without continuation of oral hypoglycemic agents in the treatment of secondary failure in NIDDM patients. *Diabetes Care* 18:307, 1995.
469. Pugh J, Wagner M, Sawyer J, Ramirez G, Tuley M, Friedberg S: Is combination sulfonylurea and insulin therapy useful in NIDDM patients? *Diabetes Care* 15:953, 1992.

470. Peters AL, Davidson MB: Insulin plus a sulfonylurea agent for treating Type 2 diabetes. *Ann Intern Med* 115:45, 1991.
471. Yki-Jarvinen H, Ryysy L, Tulokas T, Venamo R, Heikkila M: Comparison of bedtime insulin regimens in patients with type 2 diabetes mellitus. *Ann Intern Med* 130:389, 1999.
472. Anderson RA, Cheng N, Bryden NA, Polansky MM, Cheng N, Chi J, Feng J: Elevated intakes of supplemental chromium improve glucose and insulin variables in individuals with type 2 diabetes. *Diabetes* 46:1786, 1997.
473. Nathan DM, Schreiber E, Fogel HA, Mojsov S, Habener JF: Preliminary studies of insulinotropic action of glucagon-like peptide-1 (7-37) in diabetic and nondiabetic human subjects. *Diabetes Care* 15:270, 1992.
474. FDA Pink Sheet: Endocrinologic and Metabolic Drugs Advisory Committee Review of New Drug Application for Sibutramine. Washington, DC, US Govt, Printing Office, Sept 26, 1996.
475. Hollander PA, Elbein SC, Hirsch IB, Kelley D, McGill J, Taylor T, Weiss SR, Crockett SE, Kaplan RA, Comstock J, Lucas CP, Lodewick PA, Canovatchel W, Chung J, Hauptman J: Role of orlistat in the treatment of obese patients with type 2 diabetes: A 1 year randomized double-blind study. *Diabetes Care* 21:1288, 1998.
476. Nestler JE, Jakubowicz DJ, Reamer P, Gunn RD, Allan G: Ovulatory and metabolic effects of D-chiro-inositol in the polycystic ovary syndrome. *N Engl J Med* 340:1314, 1999.
477. Langer O, Mazze R: The relationship between large-for-gestational age infants and glycemic control in women with gestational diabetes. *Am J Obstet Gynecol* 159:1478, 1988.
478. Coustan D: Gestational diabetes. *Diabetes Care* 16:8, 1993.
479. Mulford MI, Jovanovic-Peterson L, Peterson CM: Alternative therapies for the management of gestational diabetes. *Clin Perinatol* 20:619, 1993.
480. Coetzee EJ, Jackson WPU: Oral hypoglycemic agents in treatment of gestational diabetes, in Jovanovic-Peterson L (ed): *Controversies in Diabetes and Pregnancy*. New York, Springer-Verlag, 1988, pp 71–73.
481. DeVecian M, Major CA, Morgan MA, et al: Postprandial versus preprandial blood glucose monitoring in women with gestational diabetes mellitus requiring insulin therapy. *N Engl J Med* 333:1237, 1995.
482. Rosenbloom AL, Schatz DA: Diabetic ketoacidosis in childhood. *Pedatric Ann* 23:284, 1994.
483. Elleman K, Soerensen JN, Pedersen L, et al: Epidemiology and treatment of diabetic ketoacidosis in a community. *Diabetes Care* 7:528, 1984.
484. Bello FA, Sotos JF: Cerebral edema in diabetic ketoacidosis in children. *Lancet* 2:64, 1990.
485. Siperstein MD: Diabetic ketoacidosis and hyperosmolar coma. *Endocrinol Metab Clinic North Am* 21:415, 1992.
486. Cryer P, Gerich J: Glucose counterregulation, hypoglycemia, and intensive insulin therapy in diabetes mellitus. *N Engl J Med* 313:232, 1985.
487. Barnes AJ, Bloom SR, Alberti KGMM, et al: Ketoacidosis in pancreatectomized man. *N Engl J Med* 296:1250, 1977.
488. DeFronzo RA, Sherwin RS, Dillingham M, et al: Influence of basal insulin and glucagon secretion on potassium and sodium metabolism. *J Clin Invest* 61:426, 1978.
489. McGarry JD, Foster DW: Regulation of hepatic fatty acid oxidation and ketone body production. *Annu Rev Biochem* 49:395, 1980.
490. Fery F, Ballasse EO: Ketone body production and disposal in diabetic ketosis: A comparison with fasting ketosis. *Diabetes* 34:326, 1985.
491. Marliss EB, Ohman JL, Aoki TT, Kozak GP: Altered redox state obscuring ketoacidosis in diabetic patients with lactic acidosis. *N Engl J Med* 283:978, 1970.
492. Munro JF, Campbell IW, McCuish AC, Duncan LJP: Euglycemic diabetic ketoacidosis. *Br Med J* 2:578, 1973.
493. Vinicor F, Lehrner LM, Karn RG, Merritt AD: Hyperamylasemia in diabetic ketoacidosis: Sources and significance. *Ann Intern Med* 91:200, 1979.
494. Molitch ME, Rodman E, Hirsch CA, Dubinsky E: Spurious serum creatinine elevations in ketoacidosis. *Ann Intern Med* 93:280, 1980.
495. Wrenn KD, Slovis CM, Minion GE, Rutkowski R: The syndrome of alcoholic ketoacidosis. *Am K Med* 91:119, 1991.
496. Page MM, Alberti KGMM, Greenwood R, Gumaa KA, Hockaday TDR, Lowy C, Nabarro JDN, Pyke DA, Sonsen PH, Watkins PJ, West TET: Treatment of diabetic coma with continuous low dose infusion of insulin. *Br Med J* 2:687, 1974.
497. Androgue HJ, Wilson H, Boyd AE, Suki WN, Eknoyan G: Plasma acid-base patterns in diabetic ketoacidosis. *N Engl J Med* 307:1603, 1982.
498. Carol P, Matz R: Uncontrolled diabetes mellitus in adults: Experience in treating diabetic ketoacidosis and hyperosmolar nonketotic coma with low-dose insulin and a uniform treatment regimen. *Diabetes Care* 6:579, 1983.
499. Fisher J, Shahshahani M, Kitabchi A: Diabetic ketoacidosis: Low dose insulin therapy by various routes. *N Engl J Med* 297:238, 1977.
500. Nathan DM, Axelrod L, Flier JS, Carr D: U-500 insulin in the treatment of antibody mediated insulin resistance. *Ann Intern Med* 94:653, 1981.
501. Cusi K, DeFronzo RA: Treatment of Type 2 diabetes, IDDM and other insulin resistant states with IGF-I. *Diabetes Rev* 3:206, 1995.
502. Carol P, Matz R: Uncontrolled diabetes mellitus in adults: Experience in treating diabetic ketoacidosis and hyperosmolar nonketotic coma with low-dose insulin and a uniform treatment regimen. *Diabetes Care* 6:579, 1983.
503. Fisher JN, Ketabchi AE: A randomized study of phosphate therapy in the treatment of diabetic ketoacidosis. *J Clin Endocrinol Metab* 57:177, 1983.
504. Arieff AL, Kleeman CR: Cerebral edema in diabetic comas: II. Effects of hyperosmolarity, hyperglycemia and insulin in diabetic rabbits. *J Clin Endocrinol Metab* 38:1057, 1974.
505. Arieff AL, Carrol JH: Non-ketotic hyperosmolar coma with hyperglycemia: Clinical features, pathophysiology, renal function, acid-base balance, plasma-cerebrospinal fluid equilibria and the effects of therapy. *Medicine (Baltimore)* 51:73, 1972.
506. Katz JA: Hyperglycemia-induced hyponatremia: Calculation of expected serum sodium depression. *N Engl J Med* 289:843, 1973.
507. Bavli S, Gordon EE: Experimental diabetic hyperosmolar coma in rats. *Diabetes* 20:92, 1971.
508. Malchoff CD, Pohl SL, Kaiser DL, Carey RM: Determinants of glucose and ketoacid concentrations in acutely hyperlgycemic diabetic patients. *Am J Med* 77:275, 1984.
509. Turpin P, Duckworth WC, Solomon SS: Simulated hyperglycemic hyperosmolar syndrome: Impaired insulin and D-epinephrine effects upon lipolysis in the isolated rat fat cell. *J Clin Invest* 63:403, 1979.
510. Podolsky S: Hyperosmolar nonketotic coma in the elderly diabetic. *Med Clin North Am* 62:815, 1978.
511. Kitabchi AE, Fisher JN, Murphy MB, Rumbak MJ: Diabetic ketoacidosis and the hyperglycemic, hyperosmolar nonketotic state, in Kahn CR, Weir GC (eds): *Joslin's Diabetes Mellitus*. Philadelphia, Lea & Febiger, 1994, pp 738–770.
512. Gerich J, Langlois M, Noacco C, Karam J, Forsham P: Lack of a glucagon response to hypoglycemia in diabetes: Evidence for an intrinsic pancreatic alpha-cell defect. *Science* 182:171, 1993.
513. DeFeo P, Bolli G, Perriello G, DeCosmo S, Compagnucci P, Santeusanio F, Brunetti P, Gerich J, Motolese J, Brunelti P: The adrenergic contribution to glucose counterregulation in type I diabetes mellitus. *Diabetes* 32:887, 1983.
514. Amiel SA, Pottinger RC, Archibald HR, Chusney G, Cunnah DTF, Prior PF, Gale EAM: Effect of antecedent glucose control on cerebral function during hypoglycemia. *Diabetes Care* 14:109, 1991.
515. Fanelli C, Pampanelli S, Lalli C, DelSindaco P, Ciofetta M, Lepore M: Long-term intensive therapy of IDDM patients with clinically overt autonomic neuropathy. *Diabetes* 46:1172, 1997.
516. Boyle P, Kempers SF, O'Connor AM, Nagy RJ: Brain glucose uptake and unawareness of hypoglycemia in patients with insulin-dependent diabetes mellitus. *N Engl J Med* 333:1726, 1995.
517. Lingenfelser T, Buettner U, Martin J, Tobis M, Renn W, et al: Improvement of impaired counterregulatory hormone reponse and symptom perception by short-term avoidance of hypoglycemia in IDDM. *Diabetes Care* 18:321, 1995.
518. Wredling R, Levander S, Adamson U, Lins PE: Permanent neuropsychological impairment after recurrent episodes of severe hypoglycaemia in man. *Diabetologia* 33:152, 1990.
519. Chalmers J, Risk MT, Kean DM, Grant R, Ashworth B, Campbell IW: Severe amnesia after hypoglycemia. Clinical, psychometric, and magnetic resonance imaging correlations. *Diabetes Care* 14:922, 1991.
520. Somogyi M: Insulin as a cause of extreme hyperglycemia and instability. *Bull St Louis Med Soc* 32:498, 1938.

521. Hirsch IB, Smith LJH, Havlin CE, Shah SD, Clutter WE, Cryer PE: Failure of nocturnal hypoglycemia to cause daytime hyperglycemia in patients with IDDM. *Diabetes Care* 13:133, 1990.
522. No reference.
523. Nathan DM: Long-term complications of diabetes mellitus. *N Engl J Med* 328:1676, 1993.
524. Clark CM, Lee DA: Prevention and treatment of the complications of diabetes mellitus. *N Engl J Med* 332:1210, 1995.
525. Nathan DM: The pathophysiology of diabetic complications: How much does the glucose hypothesis explain? *Ann Intern Med* 124:86, 1996.
526. Steffes MW, Brown DM, Bosgen JM, Mouer SM: Amelioration of mesangial volume and surface alterations following islet transplantation in diabetic rats. *Diabetes* 29:509, 1980.
527. Engerman RL, Kern TS: Progression of incipient diabetic retinopathy during good glycemic control. *Diabetes* 36:808, 1987.
528. Klein BEK, Moss SE, Klein R: Effect of pregnancy on progression of diabetic retinopathy. *Diabetes Care* 13:34, 1990.
529. Parving HH, Smidt UM, Friisberg B, et al: A prospective study of glomerular filtration rate and arterial blood pressure in insulin-dependent diabetics with diabetic nephropathy. *Diabetologia* 20:457, 1981.
530. Krolewski AS, Canessa M, Warram JH, et al: Predisposition to hypertension and susceptibility to renal disease in insulin-dependent diabetes mellitus. *N Engl J Med* 318:140, 1988.
531. Chase PH, Garg SK, Jackson WE, et al: Blood pressure and retinopathy in Type I diabetes. *Ophthalmology* 97:155, 1990.
532. Quinn M, Angelico MC, Warram JH, et al: Familial factors determine the development of diabetic nephropathy in patients with IDDM. *Diabetologia* 39:940, 1996.
533. Palmberg P, Smith M, Waltman S, Krupin T, et al: The natural history of retinopathy in insulin-dependent juvenile-onset diabetes. *Ophthalmology* 88:613, 1981.
534. Krolewski AS, Warram JH, Rand LI, et al: Risk of proliferative diabetic retinopathy in juvenile onset type I diabetes; A 40-yr follow-up study. *Diabetes Care* 9:443, 1986.
535. Andersen AR, Christiansen JS, Andersen JK, et al: Diabetic nephropathy in Type I (insulin-dependent) diabetes: An epidemiological study. *Diabetologia* 25:496, 1983.
536. Rossing P, Rossing K, Jacobsen P, Parving HH: Unchanged incidence of diabetic nephropathy in IDDM patients. *Diabetes* 44:739, 1995.
537. Ballard DJ, Humphrey LL, Melton J III, et al: Epidemiology of persistent proteinuria in type II diabetes mellitus. *Diabetes* 37:405, 1988.
538. Selby JV, FitzSimmons SC, Newman JM, Katz PP, et al: The natural history and epidemiology of diabetic nephropathy. *JAMA* 263:1954, 1990.
539. Klein R, Klein BEK, Moss SE, et al: The Wisconsin Epidemiologic Study of Diabetic Retinopathy: II. Prevalence and risk of diabetic retinopathy when age at diagnosis is less than 30 years. *Arch Ophthalmol* 102:520, 1984.
540. Krolewski AS, Warram JH, Christlieb R, et al. The changing natural history of nephropathy in Type I diabetes. *Am J Med* 78:785, 1985.
541. Aiello LP, Avery RL, Arrigg PG, et al: Vascular endothelial growth factor in ocular fluid of patients with diabetic retinopathy and other retinal disorders. *N Engl J Med* 331:1480, 1994.
542. Kannel WB, McGee DL: Diabetes and cardiovascular disease. The Framingham Study. *JAMA* 241:2036, 1979.
543. Geiss LS, Herman WH, Smith PJ: Mortality in non-insulin-dependent diabetes, in Harris M (ed.): *Diabetes in America*, 2nd ed. Bethesda, MD, National Institutes of Health, 1995.
544. Howard BV, Lee ET, Fabsitz RR, et al: Diabetes and coronary heart disease in American Indians: The Strong Heart Study. *Diabetes* 45:6, 1996.
545. WHO Multinational study of vascular disease in diabetics. Prevalence of small vessel and large vessel disease in diabetic patients from 14 centers. *Diabetologia*, 28:615, 1985.
546. Kannel WB, McGee DL: Diabetes and glucose tolerance as risk factors for cardiovascular disease: The Framingham study. *Diabetes Care* 2:120, 1979.
547. Stammler J, Vaccaro O, Neaton JD, et al: Diabetes, other risk factors, and 12-year cardiovascular mortality for men screened in the Multiple Risk Factor Intervention Trial. *Diabetes Care* 16:434, 1993.
548. Singer DE, Nathan DM, Anderson KM, et al: Association of HbA1c with prevalent cardiovascular disease in the original cohort of the Framingham Heart Study. *Diabetes* 41:202, 1992.
549. Coutinino M, Wang Y, Gerstein HC, et al: Continuous relationship of glucose with cardiovascular events in non-diabetic subjects: A metaregression analysis in 18 studies in 88,000 individuals. *Circulation* 94:I-214, 1996.
550. Meigs JB, Nathan DM, Wislon PWF, et al: Metabolic risk factors worsen continuously across the spectrum of nondiabetic glucose tolerance. *Ann Intern Med* 128:524, 1998.
551. Vlassara H: Recent progress in advanced glycation endproducts and diabetic complications. *Diabetes* 46:S19, 1997.
552. Lyons TJ, Jemkins AJ: Glycation, oxidation, and lipoxidation in the development of the complications of diabetes: A carbonyl stress hypothesis. *Diabetes Rev* 5:365, 1997.
553. Frank RN: The aldose reductase controversy. *Diabetes* 43:169, 1994.
554. Ishii H, Daisuke K, King GL: Protein kinase C activation and its role in the development of vascular complications in diabetes mellitus. *J Mol Med* 76:21, 1998.
555. Baynes JW, Thorpe SR: Role of oxidative stress in diabetic complications. *Diabetes* 48:1, 1999.
556. Pfeiffer A, Schatz H: Diabetic microvascular complications and growth factors. *Exp Clin Endocrinol Diabetes* 103:7, 1995.
557. Williamson JR, Chang K, Frangos M, et al: Hyperglycemic pseudohypoxia and diabetic complications. *Diabetes* 42:801, 1993.
558. Tesfaye S, Malik R, Ward JD: Vascular factors in diabetic neuropathy. *Diabetologia* 37:847, 1994.
559. Brownlee M, Spiro RG: Glomerular basement membrane metabolism in the diabetic rat. *Diabetes* 28:121, 1979.
560. Reaven GM, Chen IYD, Jeppensen J, et al: Insulin resistance and hyperinsulinemia in individuals with small dense low density lipoprotein particles. *J Clin Invest* 92:141, 1993.
561. Gonen B, Baenziger J, Schonfeld G, et al: Nonenzymatic glycosylation of low density lipoproteins in vitro. *Diabetes* 30:875, 1981.
562. Duell PB, Oram JF, Bierman EL: Nonenzymatic glycosylation of HDL resulting in inhibition of high-affinity binding to cultured human fibroblasts. *Diabetes* 39:1257, 1990.
563. Hammes HP, Martin S, Federlin K, et al: Aminoguanidine treatment inhibits the development of experimental diabetic retinopathy. *PNAS* 88:11555, 1991.
564. Ellis EN, Good BH: Prevention of glomerular basement membrane thickening by aminoguanidine in experimental diabetes mellitus. *Metabolism* 40:1016, 1991.
565. Kihara M, Schmelzer JD, Poduslo JF, et al: Aminoguanidine effects on nerve blood flow, vascular permeability, electrophysiology and oxygen free radicals. *PNAS* 88:5107, 1991.
566. Picard S, Parthasarathy S, Fruebis J, et al: Aminoguanidine inhibits oxidative modification of LDL protein and the subsequent increase in uptake by macrophage scavenger receptors. *J Clin Invest* 92:1407, 1993.
567. Gabbay KH: The sorbitol pathway and the complications of diabetes. *N Engl J Med* 288:831, 1973.
568. Greene DA, Lattimer SA, Sima AAF: Sorbitol, phosphoinositides, and sodium-potassium-ATPase in the pathogenesis of diabetic complications. *N Engl J Med* 316:599, 1987.
569. Engerman RL, Kern TS, Larson ME: Nerve conduction and aldose reductase inhibition during 5 years of diabetes or galactosemia in dogs. *Diabetologia* 37:141, 1994.
570. Beyer-Mears A, Cruz E: Reversal of diabetic cataract by sorbinil, an aldose reductase inhibitor. *Diabetes* 34:15, 1985.
571. Fagius J, Brattber A, Jameson S, et al: Limited benefit of treatment of diabetic polyneuropathy with an aldose reductase inhibitor: A 24 week controlled trial. *Diabetologia* 28:323, 1985.
572. Lewin IG, O'Brien IAD, Morgan MH, et al: Clinical and neurophysiological studies with the aldose reductase inhibitor, sorbinil, in symptomatic diabetic neuropathy. *Diabetologia* 26:445, 1984.
573. Krentz AJ, Honigsberger L, Ellis SH, et al: A 12-month randomized controlled study of the aldose reductase inhibitor ponalrestat in patients with chronic symptomatic diabetic neuropathy. *Diabetic Med* 9:463, 1992.
574. Lorenzi M, Cagliero E: Pathobiology of endothelial and other vascular cells in diabetes mellitus. *Diabetes* 40:653, 1991.
575. Engerman RL: Pathogenesis of diabetic retinopathy. *Diabetes* 38:1203, 1989.

576. Steffes MW, Osterby R, Chavers B: Mesangial expansion as a central mechanism for loss of kidney function in diabetic patients. *Diabetes* 38:1077, 1989.
577. Hostetter TH, Rennke HG, Brenner BM: The case of intrarenal hypertension in the initiation and progression of diabetic and other glomerulopathies. *Am J Med* 72:375, 1982.
578. Colwell JA, Winocour PD, Halushka PV: Do platelets have anything to do with diabetic microvascular disease? *Diabetes* 32:14, 1983.
579. Merimee TJ, Zapf J, Froesch ER: Insulin-like growth factors. *N Engl J Med* 309:527, 1983.
580. Dills DG, Moss SE, Klein R, et al: Is insulinlike growth factor I associated with diabetic retinopathy? *Diabetes* 39:191, 1990.
581. Frank RN, Hoffman WH, Podgor MJ, et al: Retinopathy in juvenile-onset type I diabetes of short duration. *Diabetes* 31:874, 1982.
582. Klein R, Klein BEK, Moss SE, et al: The Wisconsin Epidemiologic Study of Diabetic Retinopathy: Prevalence and risk of diabetic retinopathy when age at diagnosis is 30 or more years. *Arch Ophthalmol* 102:527, 1984.
583. Novotny HR, Alvis DL: A method of photographing fluorescence in circulating blood in the retina. *Circulation* 24:82, 1961.
584. Uccioli L, Parisi V, Monicone G, et al: Electrophysiological assessment of visual function in newly-diagnosed IDDM patients. *Diabetologia* 38:804, 1995.
585. Cogan DG, Toussaint D, Kuwabara T: Retinal vascular patterns. *Arch Ophthalmol* 66:366, 1961.
586. ETDRS Research Group: Photocoagulation for diabetic macular edema. *Arch Ophthalmol* 103:1796, 1985.
587. Diabetic Retinopathy Study Group: Photocoagulation treatment of proliferative diabetic retinopathy: The second report of Diabetic Retinopathy Study findings. *Ophthalmology* 85:82, 1978.
588. Nathan DM, Singer DE, Godine JE, Perlmuter LC: Non-insulin-dependent diabetes in older patients. Complications and risk factors. *Am J Med* 81:837, 1986.
589. Kador PF, Akagi Y, Kinoshita JH: The effect of aldose reductase and its inhibition on sugar cataract formation. *Metabolism* 35:15, 1986.
590. Lyons TJ, Silvestri G, Dunn JA, et al: Role of glycation in modification of lens crystallins in diabetic and nondiabetic senile cataracts. *Diabetes* 40:1010, 1991.
591. Klein R, Klein BEK, Moss SE: Visual impairment in diabetes. *Ophthalmolgy* 91:1, 1984.
592. Klein BEK, Moss SE, Klein R: Is menarche associated with diabetic retinopathy. *Diabetes Care* 13:1034, 1990.
593. Singer DE, Nathan DM, Fogel HA, et al: Screening for diabetic retinopathy. *Ann Intern Med* 116:660, 1992.
594. UKPDS Group: UK Prospective Diabetes Study 6. Complications in newly diagnosed Type 2 diabetic patients and their association with different clinical and biochemical risk factors. *Diabetes Research* 13:1, 1990.
595. Muhlhauser I, Sawicki P, Berger M: Cigarette-smoking as a risk factor for macroproteinuria and proliferative retinopathy in type 1 (insulin-dependent) diabetes. *Diabetologia* 29:500, 1986.
596. Moss RP, SE, Klein R, Klein BEK: Association of cigarette smoking with diabetic retinopathy. *Diabetes Care* 14:119, 1991.
597. DCCT Research Group: Pregnancy increases the risk of complications in the DCCT. *Diabetes* 47:A50, 1998.
598. Chew EY, Klein ML, Ferris FL, et al: Association of elevated serum lipid levels with retinal hard exudates in diabetic retinopathy. *Arch Ophthalmol* 114:1079, 1996.
599. Singer DE, Schachat AP, Nathan DM, Patz A, et al: Screening guidelines for diabetic retinopathy. *Ann Intern Med* 116:684, 1992.
600. Tamborlane WV, Puklin JE, Bergman M, et al: Long-term improvement of metabolic control with the insulin pump does not reverse diabetic microangiopathy. *Diabetes Care* 5:58, 1982.
601. The Diabetic Retinopathy Vitrectomy Study Research Group: Early vitrectomy for severe vitreous hemorrhage in diabetic retinopathy. *Arch Ophthalmol* 103:1644, 1985.
602. The DAMAD Study Group: Effect of aspirin alone and aspirin plus dipyridamole in early diabetic retinopathy. *Diabetes* 38:491, 1989.
603. Viberti G, Keen H: The patterns of proteinuria in diabetes mellitus. *Diabetes* 33:686, 1984.
604. Viberti GC, Hill RD, Jarrett RJ, Argyropoulos A: Microalbuminuria as a predictor of clinical nephropathy in insulin-dependent diabetes mellitus. *Lancet* 1:1430, 1982.
605. Mathiesen ER, Oxenboll B, Johansen K, et al: Incipient nephropathy in type I (insulin-dependent) diabetes. *Diabetologia* 26:406, 1984.
606. Mogensen CE, Christensen CK: Predicting diabetic nephropathy in insulin-dependent patients. *N Engl J Med* 311:89, 1984.
607. Mogensen CE: Early glomerular hyperfiltration in insulin-dependent diabetics and late nephropathy. *Scand J Clin Lab Invest* 46:201, 1986.
608. Kussman MJ, Goldstein H, Gleason RE: The clinical course of diabetic nephropathy. *JAMA* 236:1861, 1976.
609. Borch-Johnsen K, Kreiner S: Proteinuria: Value as predictor of cardiovascular mortality in insulin dependent diabetes mellitus. *Br Med J* 294:1651, 1987.
610. Mogensen CE: Microalbuminuria predicts clinical proteinuria and early mortality in maturity-onset diabetes. *N Engl J Med* 310:356, 1984.
611. Stehouwer CDA, Navta JJP, Zeldenrust GC, et al: Urinary albumin excretion, cardiovascular disease and endothelial dysfunction in non-insulin-dependent diabetes mellitus. *Lancet* 340:319, 1992.
612. Osterby R: Early phases in the development of diabetic glomerulopathy: A quantitative electron microscopic study. *Acta Med Scand* 574:1, 1985.
613. Mauer SM, Steffes MW, Sutherland DER, et al: Structural-functional relationships in diabetic nephropathy. *J Clin Invest* 74:1143, 1984.
614. Osterby R: Advanced diabetic glomerulopathy. *Diabetes* 36:612, 1987.
615. Kimmelstiel P, Wilson C: Intercapillary lesions in the glomeruli of the kidney. *Am J Pathol* 12:83, 1936.
616. Bilous RW, Mauer SM, Sutherland DER, Steffes MW: Mean glomerular volume and rate of development of diabetic nephropathy. *Diabetes* 38:1142, 1989.
617. Sawicki PT, Kaiser S, Heinemann L, Frenzel H, Berger M: Prevalence of renal artery stenosis in diabetes mellitus—an autopsy study. *J Intern Med* 229:489, 1991.
618. Perez GO, Lespier L, Jacobi J, et al: Hyporeninemia and hypoaldosteronism in diabetes mellitus. *Arch Intern Med* 137:852, 1977.
619. Kofoed-Enevoldsen A, Borch-Johnsen K, Kveiner S, et al: Declining incidence of persistent proteinuria in type 1 diabetic patients in Denmark. *Diabetes* 36:205, 1982.
620. U.S. Renal Data System: USRDS 1994 Annual Data Report. Bethesda, MD, National Institutes of Health, NIDDK, July, 1994.
621. Schmidt AM: Advanced glycation endproducts interacting with their endothelial receptor induce expression of vascular cell adhesion molecules (VCAM-1): A potential mechanism for the accelerated vasculopathy of diabetes. *J Clin Invest* 96:1395, 1995.
622. Mogensen CE: Long-term antihypertensive treatment inhibiting progression of diabetic nephropathy. *Br Med J* 285:685, 1982.
623. Kasiske BL, Kalil RSN, Ma JZ, et al: Effect of antihypertensive therapy on the kidney in patients with diabetes: A meta-regression analysis. *Ann Intern Med* 118:129, 1993.
624. Pedrini MT, Levey AS, Lau J, et al: The effect of dietary protein restriction on the progression of diabetic and nondiabetic renal diseases: A meta-analysis. *Ann Intern Med* 124:627, 1996.
625. Marre M, LeBlanc H, Suarez L, et al: Converting enzyme inhibition and kidney function in normotensive diabetic patients with persistent microalbuminuria. *Br Med J* 294:1448, 1987.
626. Cook J, Daneman D, Spino M, et al: Angiotensin converting enzyme inhibitor therapy to decrease microalbuminuria in normotensive children with insulin-dependent diabetes mellitus. *J Pediatr* 117:39, 1990.
627. Wiegmann TB, Herron KG, Chonko AM, MacDougall ML, et al: Effect of angiotensin-converting enzyme inhibition on renal function and albuminuria in normotensive type I diabetic patients. *Diabetes* 41:62, 1992.
628. Marre M, Chatellier G, Leblanc H, Guyene TT, et al: Prevention of diabetic nephropathy with enalapril in normotensive diabetics with microalbuminuria. *Br Med J* 296:1092, 1989.
629. Mathiesen ER, Hommel E, Giese J, Parving HH: Efficacy of captopril in postponing nephropathy in normotensive insulin dependent diabetic patients with microalbuminuria. *Br Med J* 303:81, 1991.
630. Parving HH, Hommel E, Nielsen MD, Giese J: Effect of captopril on blood pressure and kidney function in normotensive insulin dependent diabetics with nephropathy. *Br Med J* 299:533, 1989.
631. Hommel E, Mathiesen E, Edsberg B, Bahnsen M, et al: Effect of captopril on kidney function in insulin dependent diabetic patients with nephropathy. *Br Med J* 293:467, 1986.

632. Taguma Y, Yasunori K, Futaki G, Ueda H, et al: Effect of captopril on heavy proteinuria in azotemic diabetics. *N Eng J Med* 313:1617, 1985.
633. Kitzmiller JL, Coombs CA: Diabetic nephropathy and pregnancy. *Obstet Gynecol Clin North Am* 23:173, 1996.
634. Viberti GC, Keen H, Wiseman MJ: Raised arterial pressure in parents of proteinuric insulin-dependent diabetics. *Br Med J* 295:515, 1987.
635. Hostetter MK: Handicaps to host defense. Effects of hyperglycemia on C3 and *Candida albicans*. *Diabetes* 39:271, 1990.
636. Wheat LJ: Infection and diabetes mellitus. *Diabetes Care* 3:187, 1980.
637. Viberti GC, Bilous RW, MacKintosh D, et al: Long term correction of hyperglycaemia and progression of renal failure in insulin dependent diabetes. *Br Med J* 286:598, 1983.
638. Cohen D, Dodds R, Viberti G: Effect of protein restriction in insulin dependent diabetics at risk of nephropathy. *Br Med J* 294:795, 1987.
639. Ciavarella A, DiMizio G, Stefoni S, et al: Reduced albuminuria after dietary protein restriction in insulin-dependent diabetic patients with clinical nephropathy. *Diabetes Care* 10:407, 1987.
640. Zeller K, Whittaker E, Sullivan L, et al: Effect of restricting dietary protein on the progression of renal failure in patients with insulin-dependent diabetes mellitus. *N Engl J Med* 324:78, 1991.
641. Pedrini MT, Levey AS, Lau J, Chalmers TC: The effect of dietary protein restriction on progression of diabetic and nondiabetic renal diseases: A meta-analysis. *Ann Intern Med* 124:627, 1996.
642. Port FK, Wolf RA, Mauger EA, Berling DP, Jiang K: Comparison of survival probabilities for dialysis patients cadaveric renal transplant recipients. *JAMA* 270:1339, 1993.
643. Shaffer D, Simpson MA, Madras PN, Sahyoun AI, Conway PA, Davis CP, Monaco AP: Kidney transplantation in diabetic patients using cyclosporine: Five year followup. *Arch Surg* 130:283, 1995.
644. Fioreto P, Steffes MW, Sutherland DER, et al: Reversal of lesions of diabetic nephropathy after pancreas transplantation. *N Engl J Med* 339:69, 1998.
645. Kennedy WR, Navarro X, Goetz F, et al: Effects of pancreatic transplantation on diabetic neuropathy. *N Engl J Med* 322:1031, 1990.
646. Ramsay RC, Goetz FC, Sutherland DER, Mauer SM, et al: Progression of diabetic retinopathy after pancreas transplantation for insulin-dependent diabetes mellitus. *N Engl J Med* 318:208, 1988.
647. Pirsch JD, Andrews C, Hricik DE, Josephson MA et al. Pancreas transplantation for diabetes mellitus. *Am J Kid Dis* 3:444, 1996.
648. Thomas PK, Eliasson SG: Diabetic neuropathy, in Dyck PJ (ed.): *Peripheral neuropathy*. Philadelphia, PA, W.B. Saunders, 1984.
649. Eastman RC: Neuropathy in diabetes, in Harris, M (ed.): *Diabetes in America*, 2nd ed. National Institute of Diabetes and Digestive and Kidney Diseases, NIH. NIH Publication No 95-1468, 1995.
650. Said G, Goulon Goeau C, Slama G: Tchobroutsky G. Severe early-onset polyneuropathy in insulin-dependent diabetes mellitus. *N Engl J Med* 326:1257, 1992.
651. Maser RE, Nielsen VK, Bass EB, et al: Measuring diabetic neuropathy: Assessment and comparison of clinical examination and quantitative sensory testing. *Diabetes* 12:270, 1989.
652. Ellenberg M: Diabetic neuropathic cachexia. *Diabetes* 23:418, 1974.
653. Young RJ, Ewing DJ, Clarke BF: Chronic and remitting painful diabetic polyneuropathy. *Diabetes Care* 11:34, 1988.
654. Morley GK, Mooradian AD, Levine AS, Morley JE: Mechanism of pain in diabetic peripheral neuropathy. *Am J Med* 77:79, 1984.
655. Lehtinen JM, Uusitupa M, Siitonen O, Pyorala K: Prevalence of neuropathy in newly diagnosed Type 2 diabetes and nondiabetic control subjects. *Diabetes* 38:1307, 1989.
656. Greene DA, Lattimer SA, Sima AAF: Sorbitol, phophoinositides, and sodium-potassium-ATPase in the pathogenesis of diabetic complications. *N Engl J Med* 316:599, 1987.
657. Gregensen G, Borsting H, Theil P, et al: Myoinositol and function of peripheral nerve in human diabetics: A controlled clinical trial. *Acta Neurol Scand* 58:241, 1978.
658. Lewin IG, O'Brien IAD, Morgan MH, Corrall RJM: Clinical and neurophysiological studies with the aldose reductase inhibitor, sorbinil, in symptomatic diabetic neuropathy. *Diabetologia* 26:445, 1984.
659. Sundkvist G, Armstrong FM, Bradbury JE, Chaplin JE, et al: Peripheral and autonomic nerve function in 259 diabetic patients with peripheral neuropathy treated with ponalrestat (an aldose reductase inhibitor) or placebo for 18 months. *J Diab Comp* 6:123, 1992.
660. The DCCT Research Group: Factors in development of diabetic neuropathy. *Diabetes* 37:476, 1988.
661. Litzelman DK, Slemenda CW, Langefeld CD: Lower extremity amputation risk reduction in persons with diabetes. *Clin Res* 39:581A, 1991.
662. American Diabetes Association: Preventive foot care in people with diabetes. *Diabetes Care* 22:S54, 1999.
663. Max MB, Lynch SA, Muir J, Shoaf SE, et al: Effects of desipramine, amitriptyline, and fluoxetine on pain in diabetic neuropathy. *N Engl J Med* 326:1250, 1992.
664. Ellenberg M: Treatment of diabetic neuropathy with diphenylhydantoin. *NY State J Med* 68:2653, 1968.
665. Rull JA, Quibrera R, Gonzalez-Millan H, et al: Symptomatic treatment of peripheral diabetic neuropathy with carbamazepine (Tegretol): Double blind crossover trial. *Diabetologia* 5:215, 1969.
666. Capsaicin Study Group: Treatment of painful diabetic neuropathy with topical Capsaicin. *Arch Intern Med* 151:2225, 1990.
667. Oskarsson P, Ljunggren JG, Lins PE: Efficacy and safety of mexiletine in the treatment of painful diabetic neuropathy. *Diabetes Care* 20:1594, 1997.
668. Backonja M, Beydoun A, Edwards KR, et al: Gabapentin for the symptomatic treatment of painful neuropathy in patients with diabetes mellitus. *JAMA* 280:1831, 1998.
669. Raff MC, Asbury AK: Ischemic mononeuropathy and mononeuropathy multiplex in diabetes mellitus. *N Engl J Med* 279:17, 1968.
670. Asbury AK, et al: Oclolmotor palsy in diabetes: A clinicopathologic study. *Brain* 93:555, 1970.
671. Garland, H: Diabetic amyotrophy. *Br Med J* 1287, 1955.
672. Longstreth G, Newcomer A: Abdominal pain caused by diabetic radiulopathy. *Ann Intern Med* 86:166, 1977.
673. Horowitz M, Fraser R: Disordered gastric motor function in diabetes mellitus. *Diabetologia* 37:543, 1994.
674. Kaiser FE, Korenman SG: Impotence in diabetic men. *Am J Med* 85:147, 1988.
675. Valdovinos MA, Camilleri M, Zimmerman BR: Chronic diarrhea in diabetes mellitus: Mechanism and an approach to diagnosis and treatment. *Mayo Clin Proc* 68:691, 1993.
676 Ziegler D, Gries FA, Spuler M, Lessman F, DiaCAN Multicenter Study Group: The epidemiology of diabetic neuropathy. *Diabetic Med* 10:82S, 1993.
677. Rensch MJ, Merenich JA, Lieberman M, et al: Gluten-sensitive enteropathy in patients with insulin-dependent diabetes mellitus. *Ann Intern Med* 124.564, 1996.
678. Ewing DJ, Campbell IW, Clarke BF: The natural history of diabetic autonomic neuropathy. *Q J Med* 193:95, 1980.
679. McLeod J, Tuck R: Disorders of the autonomic nervous system: II Investigations and treatment. *Ann Neurol* 22:519, 1987.
680. Snape WJ, Battle WM, Schwartz SS, Braunstein SN, Goldstein HA, et al: Metoclopramide to treat gastroparesis due to diabetes mellitus. *Ann Intern Med* 96:444, 1982.
681. Chen HT, Goh MH, Pan S: The effect and mechanism of the prokinetic action of cisapride on gastrointestinal smooth muscle. *Gastroent Jap* 28:218, 1993.
682. Janssens J, Peeters TL, Vantrappen G, et al: Improvement of gastric emptying in diabetic gastroparesis by erythromycin. *N Engl J Med* 322:1028, 1990.
683. Fedorak RN, Field M, Chang EB: Treatment of diabetic diarrhea with clonidine. *Ann Intern Med* 102:197, 1985.
684. Gasser TC: Intracavernous injections for impotence. *J Urol* 137:678, 1987.
685. Harin PN, Hellstrom WJG, Kaiser FE, et al: Treatment of men with erectile dysfunction with transurethral alprostadil. *N Engl J Med* 336:1, 1997.
686. Rendell MS, Rajfer J, Wicker PA, Smith MD, for the Sildenafil Diabetes Study Group: Sidenafil for treatment of erectile dysfunction in men with diabetes: A randomized controlled trial. *JAMA* 281:421, 1999.
687. Scott FB, Fishman IJ, Light JK: An inflatable penile prosthesis for treatment of diabetic impotence. *Ann Intern Med* 92:340, 1980.
688. Low PA, Gilden JL, Freeman R, Sheng KN, McElligott MA: Efficacy of midodrine vs placebo in neurogenic hypotension. A randomized, double-blind multicenter study. Midodrine Study Group. *JAMA* 277:1046, 1997.
689. Gordon T, Castelli WP, Hjortland MC, et al: Diabetes, blood lipids, and the role of obesity in coronary heart disease risk for women. The Framingham Study. *Ann Intern Med* 87:393, 1977.

690. Singer DE, Moulton AW, Nathan DM: Diabetic myocardial infarction. Interaction of diabetes with other preinfarction risk factors. *Diabetes* 38:350, 1989.
691. Rytter L, Troelsen S, Beck-Nielsen H: Prevalence and mortality of acute myocardial infarction in patients with diabetes. *Diabetes Care* 8:230, 1985.
692. Palumbo PJ, Melton J: Peripheral vascular disease and diabetes, in Harris M (ed): *Diabetes in America*, 2nd edition. National Institute of Diabetes Digestive and Kidney Diseases, NIH. NIH Publication 95-1468, 1995.
693. Margolis JR, Kannel WB, Feinfeib M, Dawber TR, McNamara PM: Clinical features of unrecognized myocardial infarction—silent and symptomatic: Eighteen year follow-up: The Framingham study. *Am J Cardiol* 32:1, 1973.
694. Wingard DL, Barrett-Connors E, Criqui MH, Suarez L: Clustering of heart disease risk factors in diabetic compared to nondiabetic adults. *Am J Epidemiol* 117:19, 1983.
695. Jarret RJ, McCarntey P, Keen H: The Bedford Survey: Ten year mortality rates in newly diagnosed diabetics, borderline diabetics and normoglycaemic controls and risk indices for coronary heart disease in borderline diabetics. *Diabetologia* 22:79, 1982.
696. Haffner SM, Stern MP, Hazuda HP, Mitchell BD, Patterson JK: Cardiovascular risk factors in confirmed prediabetic individuals: Does the clock for coronary heart disease start ticking before the onset of diabetes? *JAMA* 1990:2893, 1990.
697. Gray RP, Patterson DLH, Yudkin JS: Plasminogen activator inhibitor activity in diabetic and non-diabetic survivors of myocardial infarction. *Arteriosclerosis and Thrombosis* 13:415, 1993.
698. Kannel WB, D'Agostino RB, Wilson PW, Belanger AJ, Gagnon DR: Diabetes, fibrinogen, and risk of cardiovascular disease: The Framingham experience. *Am Heart J* 120:672, 1990.
699. Collier A, Leach PJ, McLellan A, Jardine A: Plasma endothelinlike immunoreactivity levels in IDDM patients with microalbuminuria. *Diabetes Care* 15:1038, 1992.
700. Colwell JA, Sagel J, Crook L, Chambus A, Laimins M: Correlation of platelet aggregation, "plasma factor activity," and megathrombocytes in diabetic subjects with and without vascular disease. *Metabolism* 26:279, 1977.
701. Ducimetiere P, Eschwege E, Papoz, et al: Relationship of plasma insulin levels to the incidence of myocardial infarction and coronary heart disease mortality in a middle aged population. *Diabetologia* 19:205, 1980.
702. Pyorala K, Savolainen E, Kaukola S, et al: Plasma insulin as coronary heart disease factor: Relationship to other risk factors and predictive value during 91/2 year followup of the Helsinki policemen study population. *Acta Med Scand* (suppl) 38, 1985.
703. American Diabetes Association: Standards of medical care for patients with diabetes mellitus. *Diabetes Care* 21:523, 1999.
704. Eagle K, Coley C, Newell J, Brewster D, Darling R, Strauss H, Guiney T, Boucher C: Combining clinical and thallium data optimizes preoperative assessment of cardiac risk before major vascular surgery. *Ann Intern Med* 110:859, 1989.
705. ETDRS Investigators: Aspirin effects on mortality and morbidity in patients with diabetes mellitus. *JAMA* 268:1292, 1992.
706. Goldberg R, et al: Cardiovasacular events and their reduction with pravastatin in diabetic and glucose intolerant myocardial infarction survivors with average cholesterol levels. *Circulation* 98:2513, 1998.
707. Pyorala K, et al: Cholesterol lowering with simvistatin improves prognosis of diabetic patients with coronary heart disease. *Diabetes Care* 20:614, 1997.
708. Curb JD, et al: Effect of diuretic based antihypertensive treatment on cardiovascular disease risk in older patients with isolated systolic hypertension. *JAMA* 276:1886, 1996.
709. Physicians' Health Study Research Group: Final report of the aspirin component of the ongoing Physicians' Health Study. *N Engl J Med* 321:129, 1989.
710. Shorr RI, Ray WA, Daugherty JR, Griffin MR: Antihypertensives and the risk of serious hypoglycemia in older persons using insulin or sulfonylureas. *JAMA* 278:40, 1997.
711. Gundersen T, Kjekshus J: Timolol treatment after myocardial infarction in diabetic patients. *Diabetes Care* 6:285, 1983.
712. Kaplan NM, Rosenstock J, Raskin P: A differing view of treatment of hypertension in patients with diabetes mellitus. *Arch Intern Med* 147:1160, 1987.
713. UK Prospective Diabetes Study Group: Tight blood pressure control and risk of macrovascular and microvascular complications in type 2 diabetes. *Br Med J* 317:703, 1998.
714. BARI investigators: Comparison of coronary bypass surgery with angioplasty in patients with multivessel disease. The Bypass Angioplasty Revascularization Investigation. *N Engl J Med* 336:147, 1997.
715. Malmberg K, for the DIGAMI Study Group: Prospective randomized study of intensive insulin treatment on long term survival after acute myocardial infarction in patients with diabetes mellitus. *Br Med J* 314:1512, 1997.
716. Janand-Delenne B, Savin B, Habib G, Bory M, Vague P, Lassmann-Vague V: Silent myocardial ischemia in patients with diabetes. Who to screen. *Diabetes Care* 22:1396, 1999.
717. Perlmuter LC, Hakami MK, Hodgson-Harrington C, et al: Decreased cognitive function in aging non-insulin-dependent diabetic patients. *Am J Med* 77:1043, 1984.
718. Kapoor A, Sibbitt WL: Contractures in diabetes mellitus: The syndrome of limited joint mobility. *Semin Arthritis Rheum* 18:168, 1989.
719. Lundbaek K: Stiff hands in long-term diabetes. *Acta Med Scand* 158: 447, 1957.

CHAPTER 19

Hypoglycemia

Harry Shamoon

The concentration of blood glucose normally is regulated within exceedingly narrow limits, reflecting the virtually complete dependence of the brain on glucose for energy metabolism. In healthy individuals the venous plasma glucose concentration remains between 60 and 90 mg/dl (3.3 and 5.0 mmol/L) after overnight fasting and only transiently increases to 120–130 mg/dl (6.7–7.2 mmol/L) after a mixed meal. Because the total amount of intracellular (free) glucose in humans is relatively small and the largest pool is confined to the extracellular space, a variety of mechanisms exist to ensure precise homeostasis. Disruption of this system may lead to hypoglycemia severe enough to be catastrophic or mild enough to escape clinical attention. This wide range of nonspecific manifestations leads to difficulties in diagnosis. Nevertheless, recent advances in the understanding of glucose regulation at a physiologic and molecular level have provided powerful tools that enable the clinician to arrive at the underlying causes of hypoglycemic states.

DEFINITION

Much of the difficulty in the diagnosis of hypoglycemia stems from the confusion of biochemical abnormalities and clinical symptoms. Both factors must be taken into consideration as the apparent severity of symptoms and their episodic nature do not always correlate with plasma glucose values. Although the symptoms of hypoglycemia are usually relieved by ingestion of carbohydrate, the diagnosis should never be made on the basis of this observation alone. Although it is generally agreed that a venous plasma glucose concentration below 50 mg/dl (2.8 mmol/L) in adults is significant, no absolute level can be reliably established because women who are otherwise healthy may have a plasma glucose nadir as low as 25–30 mg/dl (1.4–1.7 mmol/L) after a 72-h fast.[1,2] In children, the diagnosis is complicated by difficulty in appreciating hypoglycemic symptoms, and plasma glucose levels as low as 30 mg/dl (1.7 mmol/L) in newborns once were considered normal.[3] Most authorities, however, agree that a child or infant who has a plasma glucose level below 50 mg/dl (2.8 mmol/L) should be observed carefully and that diagnostic evaluation and therapeutic intervention should begin at concentrations below 40 mg/dl (2.24 mmol/L).[4]

Whether symptoms result from a given reduction in the plasma glucose concentration and the severity of those symptoms depend on other factors, including (1) the age of the patient, (2) the glucose threshold at which counterregulatory responses are triggered, (3) prior glucose concentrations in the individual, and (4) the availability of ketones for brain metabolism. Older persons and those with underlying central nervous system (CNS) disorders may exhibit focal neurologic deficits, an altered mental state, or seizures at plasma glucose concentrations seemingly well tolerated by others.[5]

The physiological changes that produce, defend against, and prevent hypoglycemia have been extensively studied. Because the brain can neither store a large supply of glucose nor synthesize glucose de novo, it derives most of its metabolic fuels from the blood. The rate of GLUT1 facilitated glucose transport across the blood-brain barrier is higher than the rate of brain glucose metabolism under normal conditions. As blood glucose concentrations fall below a critical level, glucose transport now becomes rate-limiting. Hypoglycemia sensed in the brain (and probably also the liver and/or the portal vein)[6] activates a cascade of counterregulatory mechanisms. The plasma glucose threshold for release of counterregulatory hormones in healthy persons ranges between 60 and 70 mg/dl (3.3–3.9 mmol/L), although in some patients with diabetes or a chronic hypoglycemic state (e.g., insulinoma) these thresholds may be reduced.[7–9]

The perception of hypoglycemia and counterregulatory hormone responses appear to occur at plasma glucose levels below 50 mg/dl (2.8 mmol/L) in intensively treated patients with type 1 diabetes.[8] Conversely, poorly controlled subjects with type 1 diabetes appear to exhibit both symptoms and counterregulatory hormone release at higher than normal thresholds,[10] suggesting that hyperglycemia may influence the response to subsequent reduction of the plasma glucose level. It has also been observed that persons who have fasted for several weeks are better able to tolerate the effects of hypoglycemia. This has been attributed to the increased circulating concentrations of ketones, and perhaps to augmented brain capacity to utilize other metabolic fuels, particularly ketones.[11]

SIGNS AND SYMPTOMS

The extensive symptomatology of hypoglycemia was not fully appreciated until the advent of insulin treatment for patients with diabetes. Because insulin-induced hypoglycemia is the only experimental model which can be studied in humans, it remains uncertain whether patients with hypoglycemia not due to hyperinsulinemia suffer from the same clinical symptoms and signs. Nevertheless, it is apparent that the CNS and the sympathetic nervous system give rise to most of the symptoms and signs of hypoglycemia. Because many of these manifestations are nonspecific, confusion with various functional complaints may lead to overdiagnosis of hypoglycemia.

Neuroglycopenia

Changes in cerebral function probably accompany all levels of hypoglycemia, although subtle degrees of dysfunction may not be apparent at plasma glucose concentrations above 50 mg/dl. Experiments using sensory evoked potentials have indicated that some neurologic parameters, such as reaction time and cognitive function, may be slowed in healthy subjects at arterial plasma glucose levels of 60 mg/dl (3.3 mmol/L) and that recovery of function may lag 30–60 min after the restoration of euglycemia.[12,13] Overall brain energy metabolism and glucose utilization appear to be normal at this level of hypoglycemia, in keeping with the known kinetic characteristics of the glucose transport system.[14,15] A critical level of plasma glucose for the development of overt neurologic signs in most mammalian species appears to be 2 mmol/L (36 mg/dl).[14] This is also the threshold at which changes in behavior and slowing of alpha waves and increased delta waves in the electroencephalogram (EEG) can be discerned in humans.[16,17] Finally, this glucose concentration is also approximately that at which brain glucose transport becomes limiting; intracellular glucose concentrations approach zero when arterial plasma glucose falls below 2 mmol/L.[16]

The mechanisms underlying neural dysfunction, including the possibility that regional brain metabolism may make certain areas of the brain more vulnerable to hypoglycemia, have not been clarified. However, most of the neurologic signs and symptoms that accompany severe hypoglycemia can be reversed within a few minutes after restoration of euglycemia. Thus, the term neuroglycopenia has been used to denote manifestations of cellular glucose deficiency in the brain including inability to concentrate, fatigue, headache, irrational behavior, amnesia, and confusion. In infants and children, irritability, feeding difficulties, lethargy, cyanosis, and tachypnea may be the only findings. At the most severe extreme, grand mal or focal seizures, hemiparesis (in older adults), and coma may occur.

It should be emphasized that the associated behavioral and cognitive dysfunction may be extremely subtle, particularly in insulin-treated diabetics with hypoglycemia unawareness. Such patients may exhibit no obvious sign of hypoglycemia except the denial of the symptoms or refusal of assistance from others. Because these patients may be combative or abusive or display inappropriate responses, hypoglycemia may be mistaken for drug or ethanol intoxication, on occasion with devastating medical or legal consequences as a result of a delay in diagnosis.

A catastrophic result of severe and/or prolonged hypoglycemia is the development of irreversible coma. Experiments in nonhuman primates indicate that the plasma glucose concentration must fall to 1.1 mmol/L (20 mg/dl) for hypoglycemia to produce brain damage.[18] However, coexisting hypotension or hypoxemia can provoke the same changes at higher plasma glucose levels. Because most of the neuropathologic changes associated with severe hypoglycemia resemble those induced by cellular ischemia, differentiation from other causes may be difficult. Cerebral edema may also play a role in the development of irreversible coma. In patients who have survived hypoglycemic coma for more than a few months, cortical atrophy and enlargement of the ventricular system may be seen. In some patients with repeated hypoglycemic episodes, a distal, symmetric peripheral neuropathy may develop.[13] This entity is most often reported in patients with islet-cell tumors who have experienced prolonged periods of hypoglycemia.[20] Motor neuron involvement is somewhat more common than sensory findings.

Long-term sequelae of hypoglycemic coma in type 1 diabetes have been suggested to occur as a result of recurrent bouts of hypoglycemia. The results from large clinical trials in which intensive therapy was used with attendent increases in the frequency of severe hypoglycemia have not reported irreversible defects in cognitive function when measured by neuropsychological tests.[21,22] These data have been confirmed in cross-sectional studies in adults with well-controlled type 1 diabetes.[23] However, data in children is lacking and neuropsychological and neurophysiological tests may not be sensitive enough to detect subtle cognitive deficits, particularly as type 1 diabetes may of itself be associated with mild deficits in patients with longer disease duration. Certainly, prolonged hypoglycemic coma in type 1 diabetes can cause permanent cognitive damage, especially in children.[24]

Sympathoadrenal Symptoms

The symptoms resulting from stimulation of the sympathoadrenal system consist of anxiety, tremulousness, perspiration, palpitations, and hunger. These symptoms often constitute the warning signs of hypoglycemia as they are likely to precede overt impairment of cortical function. The patient can therefore usually prevent a further deepening of hypoglycemia by ingesting carbohydrate. However, this should not be assumed to be an automatic response and must be taught to patients who are at the highest risk of suffering hypoglycemia.

Other Symptoms and Signs

Apart from its effects on the CNS and on the secretion of counter-regulatory hormones, acute hypoglycemia has a number of other physiologic sequelae. Hemodynamic changes include tachycardia, a widened pulse pressure, and a dramatic increase in cardiac output. Changes in the electrocardiogram are common and include ST segment depression, T wave flattening, and prolongation of the Q-T interval.[25] Dysrythmias are also common, especially ectopic atrial or ventricular beats. These hemodynamic changes are responsible for the rare occurrence of angina or myocardial infarction in susceptible persons.[26]

Thermogenesis is increased during hypoglycemia[27] but is not usually accompanied by a rise in body temperature. In fact, comatose or severely obtunded patients with hypoglycemia may present with hypothermia. This is especially true in patients with alcohol-induced hypoglycemia. As with many of the signs of this entity, hypothermia is not specific for hypoglycemia because it can be encountered in all forms of shock, in sepsis, after cold exposure, and in severe myxedema.

Biochemical changes during hypoglycemia are multitudinous but depend somewhat on the inciting cause. These changes include decreases in plasma potassium, inorganic phosphate, free fatty acids (FFA), and ketones. All these changes may be due to the prevailing hyperinsulinemia rather than to hypoglycemia per se; within 60 to 90 min of acute hypoglycemia, plasma FFA and blood ketone concentrations increase severalfold. Abnormalities of platelet function have been noted during insulin-induced and spontaneous hypoglycemia.[28] Plasma cAMP levels and urinary cAMP excretion also rise during acute hypoglycemia.[29] Finally, lymphocytosis followed by neutrophilia has also been reported.[30]

Two features of hypoglycemia may complicate the diagnosis. The first is the episodic nature of hypoglycemic symptoms.

Although these symptoms may recur, they usually last for periods of minutes to hours. The reason for this relatively brief duration is that endogenous glucose counterregulatory mechanisms or the ingestion of carbohydrate will restore the plasma glucose concentration to normal. Without these responses, the plasma glucose concentration will continue to decline to levels resulting in loss of consciousness, seizures, or coma. Thus, when patients complain of prolonged fatigue, lassitude, or inability to concentrate lasting for several hours or days, hypoglycemia is not likely to be the cause of these symptoms.

The second feature of hypoglycemia which may lead to an incorrect diagnosis is the misconception that reversal of symptoms after the ingestion of carbohydrate denotes underlying hypoglycemia. Symptomatic relief associated with glucose ingestion as such does not constitute a specific sign of hypoglycemia. A variety of symptoms associated with anxiety states may be relieved by eating. Thus, a low plasma glucose concentration must be documented *before* the administration of glucose to establish the presence of hypoglycemia. When such documentation is not available but the patient is suffering from neuroglycopenia, prompt reversal of the symptoms with glucose or glucagon is advisable.

TESTS FOR EVALUATION OF HYPOGLYCEMIA

Plasma Glucose

It is imperative that a low plasma or serum glucose be documented, particularly in the setting of symptoms attributed to hypoglycemia. A normal or elevated plasma glucose at the time of the occurrence of symptoms usually excludes hypoglycemia as a cause, and no further evaluation for such disorders is indicated. Reflectance meters should not be employed in the diagnostic evaluation, either by the patient at home or by hospital staff during supervised fasting. In the first case, patients without diabetes are not sufficiently experienced with the technique, and may not provide reliable information. In the second case, most reflectance systems do not have the requisite precision to allow for an unequivocal diagnosis. Thus, a laboratory glucose determination is always preferable. Self monitoring of blood glucose may be helpful for *management* of patients once the diagnosis has been established.

Plasma Insulin

Accurate determination of plasma insulin by means of radioimmunoassay (RIA) is easily obtainable and should be included in the initial evaluation of all patients with fasting hypoglycemia. After an overnight fast plasma insulin concentrations are generally below 10 μU/ml, but higher values may be seen in simple obesity or after glucose infusion. In certain RIAs, unheparinized serum should be employed because the heparin anticoagulant may affect the test adversely. In the conventional radioimmunassay used by the author, plasma insulin levels in healthy individuals fall below 5 μU/ml during prolonged fasting. New immunochemiluminometric (ICMA) assays specific for the insulin peptide and no cross-reactivity with proinsulin have been developed. In such assays with sensitivities lower than 1 μU/ml, values above 2–3 μU/ml may be sufficiently diagnostic of hyperinsulinism. It is imperative that the physician be familiar with the insulin assay employed, particularly as specimens may be sent to a variety of laboratories with differing methodologies in place.

Insulin antibodies can variably interfere with the RIA, spuriously raising or lowering the measured insulin value. In assays which employ a second ("double") antibody to separate the bound fraction, insulin values are falsely high. Most commercially available RIAs are of the double-antibody type. Maneuvers to detect insulin antibodies in the patient's plasma include measurement of precipitable insulin tracer in a tube to which no antibody is added, the pretreatment of plasma with polyethylene glycol to precipitate insulin antibody before the RIA, and the use of high-performance liquid chromatography (HPLC) to resolve insulin-antibody complexes from free insulin. An important clue to the presence of interfering antibodies is the apparent monotony of elevated plasma insulin values when determined over time in the patient.

Of greater importance than the isolated plasma insulin concentration is the relation between plasma insulin and plasma glucose determined simultaneously, preferably in the same sample of blood. Because the plasma glucose concentration normally exerts the major negative feedback on insulin secretion, a low plasma glucose should be associated with a relatively suppressed plasma insulin concentration. In the past, an elevated insulin–glucose ratio was considered highly suggestive of hyperinsulinism.[31] However, the utility of this ratio as a diagnostic test is seriously limited,[32] and it should only be considered suggestive. In particular, newer assays for plasma insulin have rendered published ratios misleading. When both plasma insulin and glucose are determined repetitively during supervised fasting (see later discussion), the likelihood of documenting inappropriate hyperinsulinemia is considerably enhanced.

In addition to the concentration of insulin in plasma, it may be useful to determine the species of insulin in order to distinguish endogenous insulin from surreptitious (animal species) insulin administration. Bovine or porcine insulin can be distinguished from human insulin by means of HPLC[33] or species-specific insulin antisera.[34] The gradual disappearance of insulin preparations derived from animal species have made this testing less useful.

C Peptide

C peptide determinations are readily available by means of RIA and are essential in differentiating endogenous from exogenous hyperinsulinism. In as much as, (1) insulin and the C peptide fragment are secreted in equimolar amounts from the beta cell, (2) the peptides are immunologically distinct, and (3) the metabolic clearance rate of C peptide is slower than that of insulin, elevated C peptide values in the fasting state almost always indicate increased endogenous beta cell activity.[34,35] C peptide determinations at the time of hypoglycemia (e.g., during a prolonged supervised fast) should be performed to corroborate the finding of hyperinsulinism. When combined with exogenous insulin infusion to induce hypoglycemia (C peptide suppression test), the presence of C peptide concentrations above 0.5 ng/ml suggests the presence of an unregulated islet-cell tumor. This test is best reserved for difficult diagnostic problems and should not precede the use of fasting plasma insulin and glucose measurements. Because of the lack of published data regarding the sensitivity and specificity of this test, it should only be performed in centers with substantial experience with the method.[32]

Proinsulin

Normally, proinsulin represents less than 20 percent of total insulin immunoreactivity in plasma.[34,35] In certain conditions, including islet-cell tumors, proinsulin makes up as much as 70 percent of the circulating insulin.[35] This measurement cannot be relied on as the sole means of distinguishing these patients. Proinsulin levels are significantly elevated in patients with renal failure and in members of families with benign hyperproinsulinemia.[36] It should be noted that proinsulin cross-reacts with C peptide in most RIAs for C peptide and that proinsulin determination with HPLC or newer ICMA assays is more specific. Using an ICMA assay, proinsulin levels have been shown to be generally reflective of plasma C peptide.[37]

Supervised Prolonged Fasting

The most reliable test for a diagnostic evaluation of fasting hypoglycemia is a prolonged fast (up to 72 h) in the supervised, controlled setting of a hospital. The onset of the fast and the sampling intervals should be timed carefully to coincide with the most likely time of occurrence of hypoglycemia. For example, in a patient with spontaneous episodes occurring after fasting for more than 8 h, the fast should be initiated in the early morning and samples should be obtained every 2 h. As noted below, rarely will patients require a full 72 h of fasting to provoke hypoglycemia. A practical sampling interval in the first 24–48 h may be every 4 h and whenever symptoms appear. The patient should be permitted to drink water, and sampling from an indwelling catheter is convenient and provides ready intravenous access for glucose infusion, if necessary. Blood should be drawn for glucose, insulin, and C peptide determinations, but only plasma glucose should be determined immediately. Urinary ketones, if present, are helpful in documenting that the patient is fasting and will be suppressed in the face of persistent insulin secretion. The blood samples should be carefully labeled with the time and day to allow subsequent assays in the proper sequence. This is especially important when frank symptomatic hypoglycemia does not develop during the fast; under these circumstances, a pattern of unchanging (or rising) plasma insulin concentrations in the face of declining plasma glucose levels may be diagnostic. Generally, however, the fast should be considered diagnostic when symptoms occur simultaneously with low plasma glucose (see later discussion). An additional sample should be drawn at that moment for determinations of cortisol and growth hormone to exclude hypopituitarism, and the patient should then be fed. Repeated plasma glucose values below 45–50 mg/dl (2.5–2.8 mmol/L) with strongly suggestive symptoms of hypoglycemia will increase the diagnostic yield. However, if neuroglycopenic symptoms develop, blood sampling at that time should be followed immediately by intravenous glucose infusion and feeding.

A common occurrence in the hospital setting is for a patient suspected of having a hypoglycemic disorder to receive parenteral glucose infusion. One can obtain semiquantitative information from the effect of this glucose infusion and the prevailing plasma glucose values. Thus, in an adult in whom euglycemia is maintained only at the expense of glucose infusion rates exceeding 2 mg/kg per minute, one can infer that there may be abnormal glucose homeostasis (i.e., an increase in glucose consumption, an impairment in glucose production, or both). However, in the face of unmonitored glucose administration in a hospital setting, an elevated plasma insulin concentration may not reflect abnormal insulin secretion. Only after several hours' withdrawal from parenteral glucose should the diagnostic fast be initiated.

Oral Glucose Tolerance Test

Unfortunately, this is probably the most overused test in the diagnostic evaluation of hypoglycemia and the one with the lowest degree of specificity. The oral glucose tolerance test (OGTT) is rarely helpful in the diagnosis of fasting hypoglycemia, yet it is likely to have been performed at an early stage of the patient's evaluation. In the diagnosis of reactive hypoglycemia, a 5- to 6-h test is advised. The patient should be fasted overnight and should refrain from ethanol, smoking, and severe exertion before the test. The test should not be performed if the patient is ill (even with a mild upper respiratory infection), but prior preparation with adequate carbohydrate intake as necessary for the diagnosis of diabetes is not required. An indwelling catheter for blood sampling will markedly reduce the likelihood of artifactual symptoms. After a sample for glucose and insulin determinations has been obtained, an oral load of 75 g glucose is administered. Blood samples should be withdrawn at 30-min intervals during the entire test, and a competent observer should be present to record the patient's reported symptoms and perform a repeat determination when severe symptoms occur. The pattern of plasma glucose values during OGTT can vary a great deal, though in the typical case of reactive hypoglycemia the nadir values tend to occur in the third to fifth hour following glucose ingestion. Frequently, the earlier symptoms reported will be due to nausea after the ingestion of glucose or vasovagal complaints associated with frequent venipuncture.

Other Tests

Provocative tests involving the administration of oral arginine or leucine[38,39] or IV tolbutamide,[38,39] glucagon,[40] or calcium[41] generally have limited utility in the usual differential diagnosis. In the case of islet-cell tumors, false-negative tests occur in 25 percent or more of cases. Intravenous tolbutamide appears to yield the greatest sensitivity, but the risk of hypoglycemia as a result of the persistent hyperinsulinemia induced by this agent has rendered the test obsolete. Oral leucine (150 mg/kg) in patients with insulin-producing tumors increases insulin secretion and produces hypoglycemia that is generally milder than that induced by tolbutamide. In the rare leucine-sensitive child, ingestion of leucine also provokes hyperinsulinemia and severe hypoglycemia, but the amino acid produces small changes in plasma insulin concentrations (5–10 μU/ml) and plasma glucose (5–10 mg/dl) in normal subjects.[39]

Glucagon is a direct insulin secretagogue only in high concentrations (as a paracrine factor); physiologic concentrations induce insulin secretion secondary to hyperglycemia. Islet-cell tumors are especially responsive to glucagon (in contrast to glucose) in vitro, and some workers have exploited this aberrant response to design a rapid outpatient test.[38,40] Patients with an insulinoma may display an exaggerated plasma insulin response (with or without subsequent hypoglycemia) after IV injection of 1 mg glucagon. The maximal plasma insulin concentration 5 min after injection is normally below 150 μU/ml and may be severalfold greater in some patients with islet-cell tumors. Similarly, calcium infusion (5 mg/kg per hour infused over 2 h) induces hyperinsulinemia in such patients.[38,41] Neither test, however, has the required sensitivity or reproducibility to be recommended for inclusion in the routine diagnostic battery. Finally, it is possible to measure both first- and second-generation sulfonylureas in plasma or urine when there is suspicion of surreptitious use or erroneous administration of such drugs. These drugs increase plasma insulin, C peptide, and proinsulin in a manner similar to that seen with insulinoma. The presence of first-generation agents (tolbutamide, tolazamide, and chlorpropamide) in urine and plasma can be ascertained by gas chromatography. Less widely available methods can detect the second-generation sulfonylureas.

CLASSIFICATION

Hypoglycemia is not a diagnosis per se; rather, it is a marker for an underlying disorder of glucose homeostasis. Once it has been established as the cause of a patient's symptoms, the etiology of hypoglycemia should be established. The most useful diagnostic classification is one that divides hypoglycemia into the three major categories in which this marker presents: fasting hypoglycemia, reactive hypoglycemia, and induced hypoglycemia (Table 19-1).

Although patients with fasting hypoglycemia may also have postprandial symptoms, individuals with reactive hypoglycemia should never have symptoms in the fasting state. Another useful clinical distinction is the fact that fasting hypoglycemic episodes almost never reverse without intervention whereas individuals with reactive symptoms always recover spontaneously without further food ingestion.

TABLE 19-1. Classification of Hypoglycemias

- I. Fasting hypoglycemia
  - A. Endocrine
    - 1. Excess insulin or insulin-like factors
      - *a.* Insulin-producing islet-cell tumors
      - *b.* Islet hyperplasia (adenomatosis, nesidioblastosis, etc.)
      - *c.* Extrapancreatic tumors
    - 2. Deficiency of anti-insulin hormones
      - *a.* Hypopituitarism
      - *b.* Isolated ACTH or growth hormone deficiency
      - *c.* Addison's disease
  - B. Hepatic
    - *a.* Glycogen storage diseases
    - *b.* Congenital deficiencies of gluconeogenic enzymes
    - *c.* Acute hepatic necrosis
      - (1) Toxins
      - (2) Viral hepatitis
      - (3) Reye's syndrome
    - *d.* Congestive heart failure
  - C. Gluconeogenic substrate defects
    - *a.* Pregnancy and lactation
    - *b.* Ketotic hypoglycemia of infancy
    - *c.* Chronic renal failure
    - *d.* Severe malnutrition
    - *e.* Maple syrup urine disease
  - D. Miscellaneous
    - *a.* Insulin autoimmune syndromes
    - *b.* Systemic carnitine deficiency
    - *c.* Hyperinsulinemia hypoglycemia in childhood
- II. Reactive hypoglycemia
  - A. Reactive "functional"
  - B. Alimentary
- III. Induced hypoglycemia
  - A. Insulin and sulfonylureas
    - *a.* Diabetes mellitus
    - *b.* Factitious
  - B. Alcohol-induced
  - C. Drug-induced

Fasting Hypoglycemia

These entities are characterized by unbalanced glucose homeostasis resulting in hypoglycemia when food is withheld. Although some reactive and induced hypoglycemias may present with hypoglycemia in the fasting state, the following disorders have in common the absence of factors inciting hypoglycemia such as food, drugs, and toxins. *Fasting hypoglycemia is always pathologic.* The response to prolonged fasting in normal humans can provide a framework for understanding the pathophysiology of these diseases.

Glucose Homeostasis during Fasting and Exercise

The remarkable degree of glucose control in humans occurs despite glucose input and outflow from a relatively small glucose pool of 15–20 g (80–110 mmol), a fasting glucose turnover rate in adults of 150 mg/min, and the addition of a glucose load up to 10 times larger than this pool during a meal. Humans, like most large mammals, feed intermittently. Between meals, a constant supply of glucose is maintained by hepatic production of glucose *via* combined glycogenolysis and gluconeogenesis. The more prolonged the period of fasting, the more dramatic the adaptive changes required and the greater the stress on the organism. Thus, brief periods of fasting which occur routinely (e.g., during sleep) are not accompanied by a detectable fall in plasma glucose in healthy humans. Longer-term fasting (12–72 h), by contrast, does produce a gradual decline in circulating glucose and tissue adaptation to the utilization of alternative fuels.

The dynamics of glucose metabolism after overnight fasting are well-documented. In healthy subjects, glucose production is almost entirely derived from hepatic glycogenolysis (75 percent) and gluconeogenesis (25 percent). Of the total glucose flux averaging 2 mg/kg of body weight per minute, 70 to 80 percent is taken up by noninsulin-requiring uptake processes, predominantly in the brain. Other insulin-requiring tissues, such as resting muscle and adipose tissue, mainly consume FFA as an energy source. The major substrates for gluconeogenesis by the liver include lactate, pyruvate, amino acids (mainly alanine), and glycerol. The balanced rates of glucose production and uptake under normal conditions result in no net change in the plasma glucose concentration (Fig. 19-1).

The major hormonal signals that regulate these processes are insulin (acting on hepatic and extrahepatic tissues) and glucagon (acting on the liver). The decline in peripheral circulating insulin concentrations from peak values (50–100 μU/ml) 1–3 h after meal ingestion to basal values of 10–20 μU/ml removes the restraint on hepatic glucose production, which is supported primarily by glucagon. The decline in peripheral plasma insulin serves to limit glucose uptake in extrahepatic insulin-sensitive tissues and promotes the flux of gluconeogenic substrates such as lactate, amino acids, and glycerol from these sites.

More prolonged fasting begins to deplete hepatic glycogen stores (within 24 h), and glucose production shifts progressively to gluconeogensis. A gradual decline in plasma glucose concentration (by 25 percent after 3 days) invariably accompanies a 72-h fast under controlled conditions. Peripherally-derived substrate availability becomes more critical and is enhanced by a further

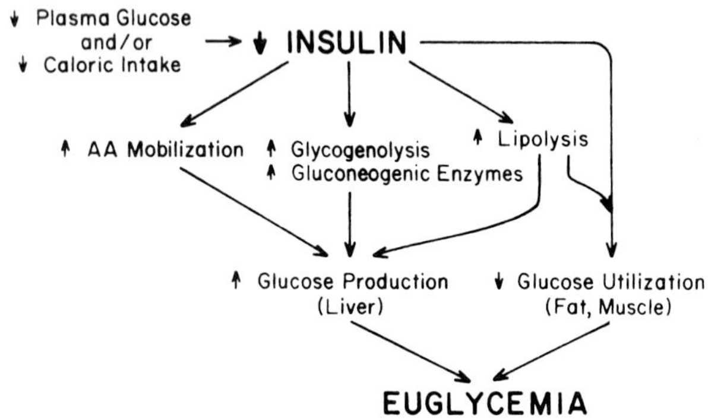

FIGURE 19-1. The hormonal and substrate changes by which euglycemia is maintained (and hypoglycemia is prevented) in normal subjects during a fast. The fall in plasma insulin concentration is the key hormonal change resulting in increased glucose production and decreased glucose utilization. The decline in plasma insulin level is, in turn, a result of a small decrease in plasma glucose concentration (5–10 mg/dl) and/or a decrease in caloric intake per se.

decline in plasma insulin concentrations from basal values to levels below 5–10 μU/ml. This relative hypoinsulinemia leads to increased mobilization of alanine from muscle and FFA from adipose tissue as lipolysis is stimulated. This process allows for sparing of glucose for the brain as increased fatty acid uptake provides a greater proportion of energy for muscle. The liver is another important site for fatty acid metabolism because conversion to glucose in the liver occurs pari passu with enhanced oxidation of fatty acids to ketone bodies. Under prolonged fasting conditions, the renal medulla may contribute a small proportion of endogenous glucose production *via* gluconeogenesis.

Plasma glucagon levels also begin to increase as fasting is extended, in part because of the small decline in plasma glucose concentration and perhaps as a result of direct neural sympathetic stimulation and/or the effect of decreased insulin secretion. Hyperglucagonemia further enhances the gluconeogenic and ketogenic effects of hypoinsulinemia. Other counterregulatory factors appear to be increased during prolonged fasting, including growth hormone, cortisol, and sympathoadrenal hormones. It is unlikely that all these effects are mediated by the small decrease in plasma glucose, but experimental and clinical data suggest that these hormonal and metabolic changes prevent the development of severe hypoglycemia. For example, the persistence of basal insulin infusion in fasting persons with type 1 diabetes will eventually produce hypoglycemia.

Exercise has been used as another modality for inducing hypoglycemia during evaluation for islet-cell tumors. In 72-h fasted subjects who have not developed clear-cut hypoglycemia, a 30-min bout of exercise frequently produces a further, and diagnostic, decline in plasma glucose concentrations. Glucose homeostasis during even brief exercise bears some resemblance to that in the fasting state; both a decline in portal venous insulin levels and an increase in glucagon secretion seem to be necessary signals for hepatic glucose output to increase sufficiently to match the augmented demands of exercising muscle. Exercise in the face of fixed basal insulin concentrations will result in hypoglycemia.

Glucose Counterregulation

Experimental data in animals and humans suggest that glucose counterregulatory hormone secretion is triggered at plasma glucose concentrations higher than the level that produces symptoms of hypoglycemia. This observation highlights the clinical concern that symptoms of "hypoglycemia" may not be accompanied by the presence of a low plasma glucose level and establishes the relative importance of glucose counterregulatory mechanisms in preventing a dangerous decline in blood glucose to levels that threaten the brain. Impaired glucose counterregulation may be defined as the failure to restore plasma glucose concentrations to normal or to prevent further decline.[42]

Counterregulatory hormone secretion during hypoglycemia has been studied extensively in humans during experimental insulin-induced reduction of the plasma glucose concentration.[42,43] It should be emphasized that dissipation of insulin action is an essential component of the recovery of plasma glucose. The suppression of hepatic glucose release and the increased peripheral utilization of glucose induced by insulin—the inciting factors leading to hypoglycemia—are reversed in part by declining plasma insulin concentrations. This mechanism is critical to the restoration of the plasma glucose concentration after hypoglycemia in patients with insulin-treated diabetes.[43,44] The suppression of insulin secretion in the normal beta cell at an arterial plasma glucose threshold ~83 mg/dl (4.6 mmol/L) can be defined as the earliest detectable defense against hypoglycemia.[45] Counterregulatory hormones can overcome the effects of insulin even under conditions in which the plasma insulin concentration does not decrease.[46] Among the counterregulatory hormones, epinephrine (released from the adrenal medullae) and glucagon (secreted by the alpha cells of the islets of Langerhans) appear to be the most potent insulin antagonists. These hormones are secreted promptly after plasma glucose levels fall, and both induce a rapid increase in hepatic glucose production.[47] The glycemic thresholds for secretion of these hormones is normally ~68 mg/dl (3.8 mmol/L), considerably higher than the threshold for symptoms of hypoglycemia (~54 mg/dl [3.0 mmol/L]) or that for cognitive dysfunction (~49 mg/dl [2.7 mmol/L]).[48–50] The independent contribution of each of these hormones to hepatic glucose production appears to be quantitatively similar; hence, a deficient response of either hormone alone does not impair glucose counterregulation. This is best demonstrated in patients with type 1 diabetes, most of whom have a marked reduction in glucagon secretion during hypoglycemia[44] but counterregulate appropriately if epinephrine is not deficient. Conversely, glucose counterregulation appears to be normal in patients after adrenalectomy who are given adequate glucocorticoid replacement and in subjects receiving combined alpha- and beta-adrenergic blockade.[42,51] Finally, in many patients with type 1 diabetes of greater than a few years' duration, failure of epinephrine secretion in response to hypoglycemia develops; the combined deficiencies of glucagon and epinephrine are most likely responsible for the greater propensity to severe and/or prolonged hypoglycemia in such patients (Fig. 19-2).[42–45,52]

The contributions of the other major counterregulatory hormones seem to be less critical in the initial glycemic recovery (30 to 60 min) but are nonetheless important in the latter stage of glucose stabilization. Cortisol and growth hormone both have significant late effects on the ability of the liver to sustain glucose output in the face of hyperinsulinemia.[53,54] In addition, these hormones reduce peripheral glucose utilization during recovery from hypoglycemia, an action shared by epinephrine.[55] These effects are both direct[56] and indirect, e.g., by stimulation of FFA release. In patients with type 1 diabetes and impaired hepatic glucose release, the reduction in peripheral glucose uptake is vital in glycemic

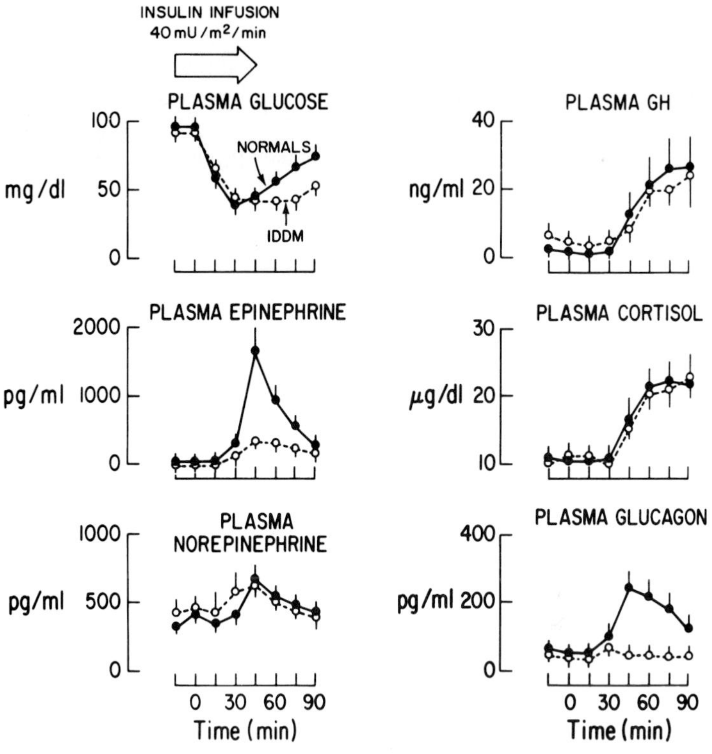

FIGURE 19-2. Hormonal responses to insulin-induced hypoglycemia in normal subjects (solid circles) compared with patients with insulin-dependent diabetes mellitus (IDDM) (open circles). The subjects received a 40 mU/m^2 per minute insulin infusion to induce equivalent hypoglycemia, yet the recovery of plasma glucose was significantly retarded in the patients with IDDM. With a mean duration of 10 years of diabetes, the IDDM patients displayed blunted secretion of epinephrine as well as glucagon. (*From Hirsch BR, Shamoon H, Diabetes 36:20, 1987, by permission of American Diabetes Association, Inc.*)

recovery from hypoglycemia.[52] Finally, chronic glucocorticoid and growth hormone deficiency can cause severe hypoglycemia. In particular, patients with hypopituitarism who suffer from these combined hormonal deficiencies may present with profound hypoglycemia despite the absence of hyperinsulinemia or known abnormalities in glucagon or epinephrine secretion.[57,58]

Other counterregulatory factors are known to exist, but their contribution is of uncertain importance. For example, it is likely that glucose per se exerts feedback control on its own production by the liver either directly (so-called autoregulation) or *via* neural pathways originating in the CNS.[6,59] Also, norepinephrine is known to activate glucose production and impair glucose utilization, but its concentrations in plasma during hypoglycemia do not achieve the levels required to affect glucose metabolism.[60] The secretion of a variety of other hormones and neurotransmitters is induced by hypoglycemia (e.g., vasopressin, angiotensin, prolactin, and pancreatic polypeptide), but none of these substances seem to possess major glucoregulatory actions.

Counterregulation in Diabetes

Impaired glucose counterregulation has emerged as a clinical syndrome of considerable importance in patients who are the most likely to suffer hypoglycemia: those with type 1 diabetes.[61] As noted above, combined defects in the secretion of glucagon and epinephrine lead to inadequate hepatic glucose production during recovery from insulin-induced hypoglycemia. The etiology of these hormonal defects is uncertain. Although some affected patients clearly suffer from autonomic neuropathy (which has been implicated in defective adrenergic responses to hypoglycemia), most patients with impaired glucose counterregulation do not exhibit other clinical symptoms of autonomic neuropathy.[52,62,63] There is evidence that the defect in both glucagon and epinephrine release in diabetics may be specific to the hypoglycemic stimulus per se and that these hormones can be secreted in response to other stimuli.[63,64] The observation that intensive insulin therapy in diabetic patients further impairs epinephrine secretion (as well as the secretory responses of cortisol and growth hormone) suggests that "functional" defects in hormonal responses to hypoglycemia may be common.[8,65] Indeed, other syndromes of hypoglycemia may share such defects in glucose counterregulation. Some patients with islet-cell tumors have been shown to have reduced secretion of the major counterregulatory hormones,[7,9,66] and in one such patient reversal of this phenomenon occurred after surgical cure.[9] A clinical hallmark of impaired glucose counterregulation is "hypoglycemic unawareness."[43,44] As a result of the deficient epinephrine response in such patients, lack of adrenergic warning symptoms and impaired glucose production exacerbate the risk of developing prolonged and/or more severe hypoglycemia. It is of interest that not all the adrenergic symptoms of hypoglycemia can be attributed to epinephrine secretion,[67,68] suggesting that there may be defects other than reduced adrenomedullary epinephrine secretion.

Recent clinical trials have provided better quantification of the risk of hypoglycemia—in particular, severe hypoglycemia—in both type 1 and type 2 diabetes. The landmark Diabetes Control and Complications Trial (DCCT) in type 1 diabetes reported severe hypoglycemic event rates of 19/100 patient-years in conventionally-treated patients and 62/100 patient-years in intensively-treated patients.[69,70] The risk of severe hypoglycemia was inversely related to the mean HbA1c achieved, but it was clear that glycemic control, prior history of severe hypoglycemic events, and duration of type 1 diabetes did not completely account for the frequency of severe hypoglycemia. In type 2 diabetes, the reported frequency of severe hypoglycemia is lower, such that 1–5 percent of patients experienced at least one severe hypoglycemic episode per year when treated with insulin in the United Kingdom Prospective Diabetes Study.[71] The proportions of patients per year with any type of hypoglycemic event were 4.2 percent (metformin), 12.1 percent (chlorpropamide), 17.5 percent (glibenclamide), and 34 percent (insulin). The duration of insulin treatment may be a factor in the apparent greater frequency of severe hypoglycemia in type 1 diabetes,[61] and the underlying presence of peripheral insulin resistance may be a critical factor in preventing hypoglycemia in poorly-controlled type 2 diabetes.[72]

From this discussion it is apparent that the maintenance of euglycemia in the fasting state is dependent on three factors: (1) a hormonal milieu characterized by basal or reduced insulin secretion and increased secretion of glucagon, growth hormone, and cortisol; (2) intact glycogenolytic and gluconeogenic process in the liver; and (3) substrate availability for hepatic gluconeogenesis as well as sparing of glucose utilization in the periphery. Severe impairment of any of these defenses (or, usually, generalized partial defects in more than one) will result in fasting hypoglycemias (Table 19-1). In addition, impairment of glucose counterregulatory mechanisms may exacerbate and prolong hypoglycemia.

Insulin-Producing Islet-Cell Tumors

Clinical Characteristics

Insulin-producing tumors of the islet are rare, with an estimated annual incidence of 1–2 per million persons.[43,73] Although the majority of these tumors are benign, 10–15 percent are malignant as defined by the presence of metastases. Malignant insulinomas may secrete human chorionic gonadotropin (hCG), a sensitive test for which is measurement of the subunit of hCG.[74] Multiple benign tumors occur in about 10 percent of cases, usually in association with type 1 multiple endocrine neoplasia (MEN 1).[75] In such families the incidence of multiple adenomas may be as high as 50 percent. The average age at diagnosis of an insulinoma is 42 years, though patients have been reported from birth to the ninth decade. In prepubertal children with this diagnosis, a careful search for endocrine neoplasia in the patient and family members is necessary to uncover MEN 1. Malignant insulinoma has been reported in a 9-year-old child.[76]

Most insulinomas are small (2 cm) and evenly distributed throughout the pancreas. They are usually, but not invariably, vascular and palpable at the time of surgery. The histologic appearance is usually that of clusters of normal beta cells, although secretory granules may not be demonstrable with traditional staining methods. Immunohistochemical stains or electron microscopy generally reveals insulin-containing granules, though some tumors are associated with other secretory products, such as adrenocorticotropic hormone (ACTH) and calcitonin. Coexisting islet-cell adenomatosis has been reported,[32,76,77] and normal islet tissue is usually not atrophic. Differentiation between benign and malignant tumors cannot be made on the basis of histologic criteria but rather on the finding of regional lymph node or hepatic metastases. Ectopic insulin-secreting tumors are extremely rare but can occur at sites in which pancreatic rests occur, including the wall of the duodenum, the porta hepatis, and the pancreatic bed.

The clinical presentation of patients with insulinomas includes psychiatric symptomatology, organic brain syndrome, suspected brain tumor, epilepsy, and intoxication. The duration of symptoms may be as short as a few weeks to as long as 30 years, although in some series most patients had symptoms of less than 12 months' duration.[32,76] The history suggests episodes of neuroglycopenia of increasing frequency provoked by abstinence from food, therapeutic dieting, or exercise. In rare cases, preexisting diabetes mellitus may gradually "improve" and insulin requirement may disappear. Between episodes, patients are likely to feel well; only about 30 percent of these patients develop obesity. Many patients are not aware of the connection between their symptoms and fasting or of the relief experienced after eating.

The mechanism underlying hypoglycemia in such patients is absolute or relative hyperinsulinemia. The normal suppression of insulin secretion as plasma glucose levels decline ensures that hepatic glucose production will increase as hypoglycemia develops. Beta cell tumors lack this negative feedback control on insulin secretion. Thus, earlier in the course of the disease glucose homeostatic mechanisms which tend to fail reflect failure of a decrease in fasting plasma insulin (e.g., during exercise or after prolonged fasting), whereas absolute hyperinsulinemia tends to characterize long-standing disease.

Increased glucose utilization in insulin-sensitive tissues has not been a prominent feature in carefully studied patients. Indeed, patients with insulinoma may be insulin-resistant, presumably as a result of the down regulation of insulin action mediated by peripheral hyperinsulinemia. Insulin resistance, especially when combined with the reduced responsiveness of insulinoma tissue to glucose, may result in carbohydrate intolerance in some patients.

Diagnosis

A history suggestive of the recent onset of episodic confusion, bizarre behavior, or neurologic symptoms relieved by eating should prompt evaluation with fasting plasma glucose and insulin measurements. If hypoglycemia is present in the face of unequivocal hyperinsulinemia in an adult, the diagnosis of islet-cell tumor is almost certain. A repeat evaluation, however, may be necessary to confirm the biochemical diagnosis before one proceeds to localizing procedures. Because insulinomas may secrete insulin only intermittently, patients with suspicious symptoms may also require periodic reevaluation.

Various series have reported on the duration of the supervised fast required to detect the presence of hypoglycemia. Almost half of all patients with islet-cell tumors have a fasting plasma glucose concentration below 60 mg/dl (3.4 mmol/L) and a plasma insulin level above 20 μU/ml after overnight fasting.[78] The simple maneuver of prolonging the fast to a total period of 14–18 h will result in the development of diagnostic hypoglycemia in more than 90 percent of patients.[78] Only a minority of patients will need to undergo the full 72-h fast, and an even smaller number will require the addition of exercise after the 3-day fast to provoke hypoglycemia. Under these extreme conditions, less than 2 percent of reported patients fail to exhibit hypoglycemia or neuroglycopenia.[79]

It is important to note the pattern of plasma insulin concentrations and the concomitant plasma glucose values obtained during fasting, particularly in patients who do not exhibit absolute hyperinsulinemia or clear-cut evidence of neuroglycopenia (Fig. 19-3). The lack of a decline in plasma insulin concentrations over time, if associated with decreasing plasma glucose levels, may be diagnostic. Supporting evidence for the presence of unrestrained beta cell secretion is provided by C peptide measurements. In a few patients the diagnosis of abnormal insulin secretion has required additional tests (see previous discussion). Although data on the specificity of such ancillary tests is not available, the C peptide suppression test may be the most likely to yield unequivocal results.

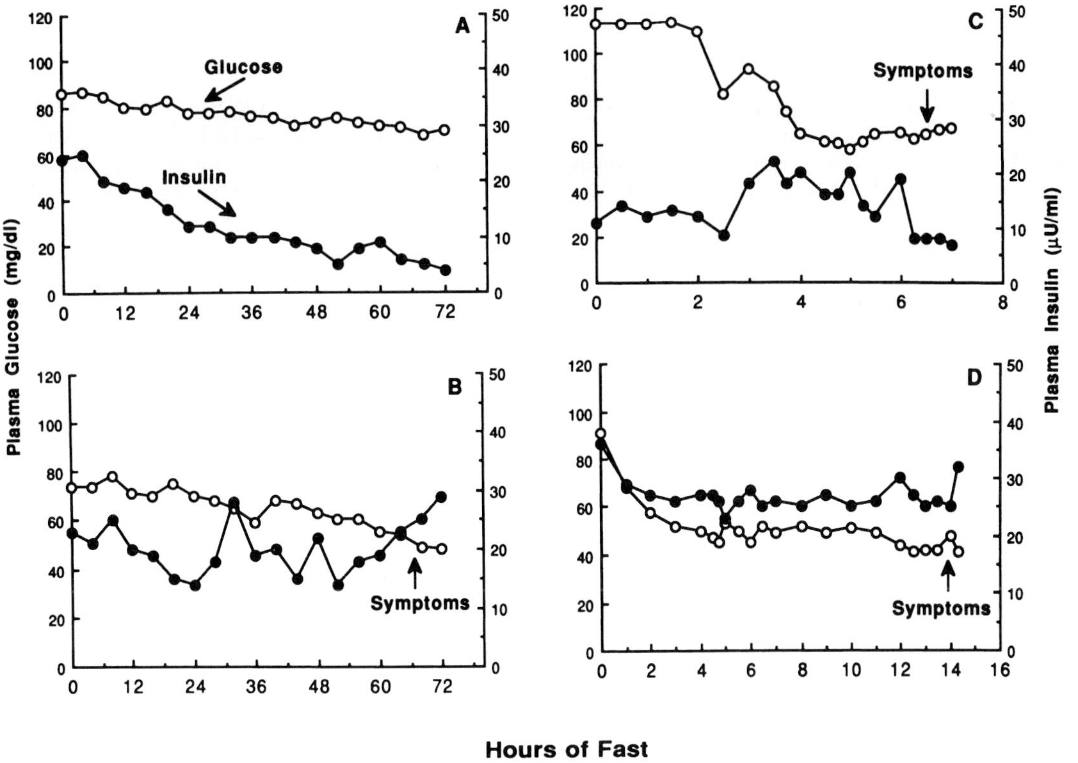

FIGURE 19-3. Examples of the response of plasma glucose and insulin to fasting in a normal patient and in three patients with islet-cell tumors and mild hyperinsulinemia. (*A*) A 72-h fast in a normal man results in a progressive decline in plasma insulin to the limits of detection together with a roughly parallel decrease in plasma glucose without symptoms of neuroglycopenia. (*B*) In a patient found to have a benign insulinoma and mild hyperinsulinemia, symptoms did not appear until late in the 3-day fast. (*C*) A patient with a malignant islet-cell tumor requiring intravenous glucose infusion to maintain plasma glucose levels. Only after a lag of several hours after discontinuation of the glucose infusion did plasma glucose fall to symptomatic levels. Sequential insulin values taken during hours 2–4 of the fast suggested unregulated insulin secretion. (*D*) Despite the initial decline in plasma glucose, this patient experienced symptoms coinciding with rising plasma insulin and falling glucose after 15 h of fasting. A benign islet-cell tumor was resected. Note the shorter time frames in (*C*) and (*D*) compared with (*A*) and (*B*).

Establishing the biochemical diagnosis is important in view of the current limitations of localizing procedures. Imaging studies should not be performed in lieu of diagnostic tests, but should be reserved for the management stage of the work-up. Because of the unavoidability of false-negative findings with many of the procedures noted below, these tests should generally be undertaken after a decision to operate has been made (or when evidence of malignant metastases is sought).

Computerized tomography (CT) and transabdominal ultrasonography are generally safe but, because of the small size of tumors, yield localizing information in less than half the cases. Magnetic resonance imaging (MRI) has not altered this yield dramatically.[80] In the hands of a skilled radiologist, selective arteriography is often helpful. Most tumors located with this technique have been vascular, yet many avascular lesions have been reported using other localizing methods. Nonselective celiac angiography is less sensitive and probably no better than CT.[81] Intraoperative and endoscopic sonography have yielded helpful localizing information (see later discussion).

Selective percutaneous transhepatic venous sampling combined with plasma insulin determinations to detect a gradient in insulin levels has been employed to definitively localize hyperinsulinism to the head, body, or tail of the pancreas.[82] However, several factors make this test problematic. First, considerable experience in selective venous catheterization is required on the part of the radiologist. Second, morbidity from the procedure includes intraperitoneal hemorrhage, infection, and bile leakage. Third, it is probable that adequate surgical exploration will suffice in the majority of first operations, and it is uncertain whether unusual cases (e.g., multiple adenomas and concomitant hyperplasia) are readily localizable with this technique. Because sampling takes place along the splenic and portal venous systems, where blood flow rates are relatively high, dilution of samples may yield falsely low plasma insulin values. Fourth, agents that inhibit insulin secretion generally must be discontinued for at least 24 h before sampling and can expose the patient to recurrent hypoglycemia. Consequently, this procedure should probably be reserved as a test to reevaluate patients in whom initial surgery was unsuccessful.

Recently, endoscopic ultrasonography has been utilized to localize islet cell tumors of the pancreas,[83,84] and the method is useful for detecting tumors <3 cm in size. The technique is more sensitive than CT scanning, and has been combined with angiography to detect vascular invasion.[85] Intraoperative ultrasound may add a significant benefit during surgical exploration. This approach involves the application of an ultrasound probe directly to the pancreas during laparotomy to differentiate tumors from normal tissue.[86] Because surgery is the treatment of choice for most patients, the utility of this technique generally exceeds any small risks associated with prolongation of surgical exploration.

The use of a [^{111}indium]-labeled OCTREOTIDE as a scanning agent is useful in localizing islet-cell tumors and their metastases that possess specific somatostatin receptors.[87,88] Whether such procedures will become helpful in preoperative tumor localization (particularly of insulinomas, which respond clinically to octreotide) remains to be elucidated. The methodology appears to be comparable in specificity and sensitivity to CT.

Treatment

Initial medical management with dietary measures may be entirely effective in alleviating symptoms in some patients; certainly, all patients should be instructed to increase the frequency of feedings, particularly at night. Carbohydrates should not be restricted, and more slowly absorbed complex forms (e.g., bread, potatoes, and rice) are preferable. During hypoglycemic episodes, more rapidly absorbed carbohydrates (e.g., fruit juices and sucrose) should be used. [Patients with diabetes who take medications with the potential of causing hypoglycemia should be instructed to have readily-absorbable sucrose or glucose tablets on hand.]

In patients with severe, refractory hypoglycemia, a continuous IV glucose infusion may be required to supplement oral feeding. At glucose infusion rates above 10 g/h (which would roughly approximate hepatic glucose delivery rates in a resting normal-weight adult), concentrations of 10 percent or higher of dextrose infusate will be needed, preferably delivered *via* a large-caliber vein.

In the hands of an experienced surgeon, cure of insulinomas is likely in the majority of benign cases. In the Mayo Clinic series, 154 patients underwent surgery, with 5.4 percent mortality.[89] Surgery was successful in removing a tumor in 85 percent of all patients and in 93 percent of patients with adenomas. In some patients in whom no definite tumor was found a blind resection of the body and tail of the pancreas was performed. The success rate in patients with carcinomas was much lower, with only 50 percent found at surgery. The remainder manifested as metastases from a primary tumor that was too small to be identified at the time of the original surgery. It is often possible to detect an abrupt, intraoperative rise in plasma glucose after successful surgery. Although the response to surgical resection may vary and other factors can alter blood glucose levels in this setting, determinations of plasma glucose after presumed surgical resection can provide reassurance with relatively little risk.

Nonsurgical treatment of insulinomas plays a limited but important role. The oral drug with the greatest clinical utility—diazoxide—is a potent inhibitor of insulin secretion and can thus ameliorate the symptoms of hyperinsulinism. The dose needed ranges from 100 to 200 mg two to three times per day (12 mg/kg of body weight in children), with maintenance doses generally being lower than initial requirements. Diazoxide frequently causes sodium and water retention, resulting in edema, and so the drug should be used cautiously in persons with impaired cardiovascular function or should be combined with diuretic treatment. Occasional side effects include anorexia, tachycardia, and hirsutism (after prolonged use). In general, however, this agent is safe enough to be considered in the interim management of patients awaiting localizing tests or surgery and patients who are not candidates for surgery or have functional malignant metastases. Other drugs that may provide adjunctive treatment of hyperinsulinism include phenytoin (diphenylhydantoin), adrenocorticosteroids, and calcium-channel antagonists, including verapamil and diltiazem.[78]

Somatostatin is a potent inhibitor of insulin secretion, but its short half-life has made it impractical as a clinically useful agent. The long-acting somatostatin analog octreotide provides an alternative in the medical management of insulinomas. Because this octapeptide has a half-life of 90–120 min, subcutaneous injections given several times daily have sustained effects on the secretion of some hormones. Unfortunately, most patients do not appear to experience adequate or long-term suppression of insulin secretion that would justify the use of this agent alone.[90] There have been reports of successful use of OCTREOTIDE administered by continuous subcutaneous infusion.[91] It may also act synergistically with diazoxide treatment or be employed as a second agent in patients with unremitting side effects of higher doses of diazoxide.

In patients with inoperable or malignant insulinoma, streptozocin (streptozotocin; STZ) has been employed because of its relative affinity for neuroendocrine cells and its beta-cytolytic properties in animals. This drug, however, has significant toxicity when given systemically, including transient nausea and vomiting, renal tubular damage, and hepatotoxicity. Although it has been reported to have some benefit in metastatic islet-cell carcinomas in general, STZ has relatively disappointing potency in the treatment of insulin-producing tumors. This is true both for reduction of the frequency of hypoglycemia and for tumor size and the survival of patients. Regimens for the palliative treatment of malignant insulinomas include combined STZ and 5-fluorouracil, mithramycin, doxorubicin, and interferon-alpha, all of which have been used with dismal results.[92]

Non-Islet–Cell Tumor Hypoglycemia

The relative frequency of non-islet–cell tumors that cause hypoglycemia is difficult to ascertain because nutritional hypoglycemia may accompany the late stages of malignancy and because such patients may not be referred for evaluation unless their hypoglycemia is severe and unremitting. However, it has become increasingly clear that a variety of nonpancreatic tumors are associated with hypoglycemia and suppressed plasma insulin concentrations. These tumors include retroperitoneal fibrosarcomas, hepatomas, gastrointestinal tumors, mesotheliomas, adrenal cortical carcinomas, and hypernephromas. As many of these tumors are large (some mesenchymal tumors weighing several kilograms have been reported), the clinical presentation is usually obvious with tumor in the abdominal or thoracic areas. However, some fairly common malignancies have on rare occasions been associated with hypoglycemia (e.g., breast carcinoma, prostate carcinoma, and lymphoma).

Based on occasional reports of substantial glucose uptake as measured across the tumor bed, excess tumor consumption of glucose has been one postulated mechanism for the hypoglycemia of extrapancreatic tumors.[93] The increased uptake of glucose by the tumor may be mediated by activated oncogenes that enhance the activity of the glucose transporter system within the tumor mass.[94] Other studies have suggested that in more than 50 percent of such patients there are elevated plasma concentrations of an insulin-like peptide.[95] Classical RIAs for insulin-like growth factor I (IGF-I) or IGF-II have been less helpful than radioreceptor assays in establishing the presence of these peptides. A number of technical considerations cloud the interpretation of the conflicting data.[95,96] Results from independent laboratories, however, have shown the presence of IGF-II mRNA in tumors associated with clinical hypoglycemia.[97,98] These observations cannot be considered conclusive because the relatively modest IGF-II elevations in the plasma of most reported patients cannot account for the hypoglycemia. It is unclear whether IGF-I– or IGF-II–mediated tumor hypoglycemia results from the activation of the insulin receptor by the peptide, whether the IGF receptor mediates these hypoglycemic effects, or whether high local concentrations of the IGF in the tumor itself may be responsible for the increased rates of glucose removal. Recent studies suggest a role of an IGF binding protein (BP) 3 on the bioavailability of tumor-secreted IGF-II.[99] The ability of IGFBP3 to form a ternary complex with IGF-II and a liver-derived glycoprotein, ALS (acid-labile subunit), appears to be critical because in some patients with tumor hypoglycemia the IGF-II and IGFBP3 are present in a binary complex with a resultant excess of free IGF-II capable of causing hypoglycemia.[100,101] The reversal of this binding pattern occurs with surgical removal of the tumor; GH treatment may also serve to reduce hypoglycemia by increasing IGFBP3.[99] An interesting associated finding in some patients is the concomitant absence of a growth hormone (GH) response to hypoglycemia.[98] The return of the GH response after successful tumor resection is taken to indicate that the tumor caused IGF-II–mediated feedback inhibition of pituitary GH secretion. Thus, some impairment in glucose counterregulatory hormones may also play a role in the pathogenesis of tumor-associated hypoglycemia. Finally, it should be pointed out that various cytokines released by tumors or macrophages activated by tumors can affect glucose metabolism, including interleukin-1, interferon-alpha, and tumor necrosis factor, although the role of such factors in hypoglycemia is far from settled.[95]

Diagnostic evaluation in such patients is limited by the lack of understanding of the cause of hypoglycemia and the absence of clinically available assays for the putative hormonal mediators of hypoglycemia. Certainly, hypoglycemia associated with low plasma insulin levels in a patient with a mesenchymal tumor is highly suggestive of the diagnosis. Treatment of hypoglycemia associated with non-islet–cell tumors is directed at the tumor itself (e.g., surgery or chemotherapy). As hypoglycemia in such patients is accompanied by hypoinsulinemia, therapy directed at reducing insulin secretion (e.g., diazoxide) is not indicated. Anecdotal reports also fail to suggest a prominent role for octreotide in treating such patients.

Hypoglycemia in Endocrine Deficiency States

As was discussed above, the prevention and reversal of hypoglycemia involve both attenuation of insulin secretion and secretion of cortisol, GH, glucagon, and catecholamines. Hypoglycemia may be the presenting symptom in patients with hypopituitarism with multiple deficiencies (e.g., in Sheehan's syndrome with combined ACTH and GH deficiency) or isolated deficiencies (e.g., in isolated GH deficiency). Hypoglycemia may also occur in Addison's disease. The occurrence of hypoglycemia may be more common in children, perhaps because the relatively greater rate of glucose turnover places a greater demand on the liver for glucose production.[102] In all these clinical conditions hypoglycemia is accompanied by an appropriate reduction in plasma insulin concentration and an increase in urinary ketones. The diagnostic evaluation depends on tests of pituitary and/or adrenal function (discussed in Chaps. 7 and 11). Although glucagon is clearly important in the maintenance of glucose production and its absence contributes to insulin-induced hypoglycemia in patients with diabetes, a clinical syndrome of hypoglycemia due to glucagon deficiency per se in nondiabetic individuals has not been convincingly documented.

Hepatic Disease

Fasting hypoglycemia occurs only when there is widespread damage to hepatic parenchyma, but the level of the fasting plasma glucose does not correlate with the degree of liver dysfunction reflected in standard laboratory tests.[103] Patients with cirrhosis, hepatitis, or metastatic liver disease rarely display hypoglycemia (though portacaval shunting may increase the likelihood of developing hypoglycemia). Fulminant hepatitis due to infectious or toxic agents, however, may be associated with severe hypoglycemia. In infectious hepatitis, about 10 percent of individuals progress to a stage of fulminant hepatic failure and account for most of the hypoglycemia observed in these disorders. A variety of drugs causing hepatic failure [acetaminophen, isoniazid, valproic acid (sodium valproate), methyldopa, tetracycline, halothane] as well as chemical toxins (carbon tetrachloride, phosphorus, urethan) may be associated with hypoglycemia. Parenteral glucose infusions must be used in the acute stages of such disorders, and if the clinical condition improves, a gradual transition to frequent oral feedings is indicated. Intravenous glucagon is usually not useful in counteracting acute hypoglycemia in such cases.

Severe right-sided congestive heart failure with hepatomegaly in both children and adults can be associated with hypoglycemia. Because most of these patients exhibit signs of cardiac cachexia and there is little evidence of hepatic parenchymal necrosis, the mechanism underlying hypoglycemia may be nutritional.[104] Once heart failure has been treated, however, hypoglycemia usually remits.

Infiltrative diseases such as amyloidosis, sarcoidosis, and hemochromatosis rarely produce sufficient parenchymal loss to cause hypoglycemia. However, hypoglycemia is a frequent concomitant of the rare acute fatty liver that occurs in late pregnancy.[105] A brief illness characterized by nausea, vomiting, epigastric pain, and jaundice precedes the development of hypoglycemia. Hemolysis, thrombocytopenia, and renal failure may ensue as terminal events. Appropriate treatment of hypoglycemia may reduce the incidence of encephalopathy and permit continued supportive management.

Hypoglycemia Due to Substrate Deficiency

A diverse group of clinical entities is characterized by deficiency in gluconeogenic precursors with consequent hypoglycemia upon prolonged fasting. In childhood, the demands on glucose production by the liver may be outstripped because of the relatively larger brain weight (glucose uptake) and smaller muscle mass (source for gluconeogenic precursors). Glucose-6-phosphatase deficiency [glycogen storage disease (GSD), type 1] is due to a defect in the final common pathway for hepatic glucose release resulting from both glycogenolysis and gluconeogenesis. As such, it is one of the forms of GSD associated with hypoglycemia. As in the fructose-1,6-diphosphatase deficiency syndrome, plasma insulin concentrations are low and the child consequently presents with ketosis. Other, even rarer inborn errors resulting in hypoglycemia may present with a similar picture.[102] In children with defective gluconeogenesis, continuous nocturnal gastric infusions of glucose supplementing frequent feeding during the waking hours have been employed successfully.

Defects in gluconeogenic amino acid metabolism also cause hypoglycemia, as one would predict. In patients with maple syrup urine disease, an enzymatic defect in the decarboxylation of the alpha-ketoacids of leucine, isoleucine, and valine associated with profound hypoglycemia is due to decreased alanine production by muscle. In ketotic hypoglycemia of infancy and childhood, alanine deficiency has also been implicated in the pathogenesis of hypoglycemia.[106,107] Although these children are frequently small for age, the mechanism of the hypoalaninemia is unknown. Clinical hypoglycemia tends to become exaggerated during periods of stress or caloric deprivation and responds to feeding. The disorder remits by 8–9 years of age and has become increasingly uncommon.[107]

In adults, alanine deficiency has been the postulated mechanism to explain spontaneous hypoglycemia associated with renal failure. As in other patients with defective gluconeogenesis, these patients are generally calorie-deprived, but the precise pathogenesis of the disorder remains uncertain.

Systemic carnitine deficiency is associated with hypoglycemia. As a result of the generalized carnitine-dependent defect in the transport of long-chain fatty acid into mitochondria, this disorder results in skeletal muscle weakness, hepatic dysfunction, and cardiomyopathy as well. Hypoglycemia is due to decreased hepatic synthesis coupled with greater muscle dependence on glucose for oxidative energy. Because ketogenesis is also impaired in these patients, this syndrome presents with hypoinsulinemic hypoglycemia without ketosis.[108] Treatment consists of frequent high-carbohydrate feeding and dietary administration of medium-chain triglycerides that do not depend on carnitine for oxidation. Finally, hypoglycemia may be associated with disordered fatty acid β-oxidation. Medium chain acyl-coenzyme A dehydrogenase (MCAD) deficiency is an autosomal recessively inherited disease that occurs in one in 23,000 live births.[109]

Insulin Autoimmune Hypoglycemia

Several rare syndromes in which autoimmunity is associated with fasting hypoglycemia have been identified. These syndromes are caused by the presence of autoantibodies to the insulin receptor or to insulin itself.

Antibodies to the insulin receptor were first discovered in patients with extreme insulin resistance and hyperglycemia.[110] However, fasting hypoglycemia developed in some patients whose diabetes resolved. In addition, several patients with anti-insulin receptor antibodies have been reported in whom severe fasting hypoglycemia was not preceded by a history of diabetes.[111] Potential mechanisms include the insulinomimetic effect of the antibody and reduced insulin clearance from plasma. The latter explanation is consistent with the fact that the major mechanism for the removal of insulin from plasma is receptor-mediated endocytosis, which is reduced in patients with antireceptor antibodies. Diagnosis in these patients is a challenge because plasma insulin concentrations are usually elevated disproportionately to plasma C peptide levels[111] and because determinations of antireceptor antibody are not reliable unless performed in a research laboratory. Treatment of these patients has involved the use of corticosteroids, immunosuppressive drugs, and plasmapheresis while the disease is active; in most reported patients, antireceptor antibody titers declined over time.

Another form of autoimmune hypoglycemia is that associated with insulin autoantibodies. This syndrome must be distinguished from the more commonly occurring surreptitious use of exogenous insulin by the patient. The majority of cases of the so-called autoimmune insulin syndrome have been reported from Japan, and most of these patients have had associated autoimmune diseases [e.g., Graves' disease, systemic lupus erythematosus (SLE), or rheumatoid arthritis]. Both fasting and reactive patterns of hypoglycemia have been reported.[112] The presence of insulin autoantibodies will interfere with insulin RIAs (see previous discussion), although the "total" insulin concentration in the plasma in such patients is clearly elevated. The hypoglycemia in most of these patients has been mild and self-limited, with symptoms resolving within a year. Supportive therapy with frequent small feedings usually suffices; a few patients have required glucocorticoids.

The pathophysiology of hypoglycemia in these patients is obscure. Because of the large pool of antibody-bound insulin (which is in equilibrium with free insulin in plasma), inappropriate hyperinsulinism may occur at unpredictable times of the day. It is also hypothesized that insulin antibodies per se mimic insulin at the receptor (anti-idiotypic antibody) or that the antibodies may potentiate insulin action.

Hyperinsulinemic Hypoglycemia in Childhood

Recent studies have elucidated the pathogenesis of several forms of hyperinsulinism presenting in infancy with hypoglycemia.[113] The usual clinical presentation is that of hypoglycemia that does not respond to diazoxide or octreotide and requires near total (99 percent) pancreatectomy. The term persistent hyperinsulinemic hypoglycemia of infancy (PHHI) has been used to describe this cluster of disease phenotypes characterized by uncoupling of β-cell stimulus-secretion. It has been suggested that PHHI should be subdivided on the basis of the severity of the β-cell dysfunction. In the Type I variant, the disorder is familial with truncation of the SUR1 (sufonylurea receptor) gene and an absence of K^+_{ATP} channels.[113] These patients have a severe form of the disease and do not respond to diazoxide or octreotide. In the Type II (nonfamilial) variant of PHHI, patients lack functional of K^+_{ATP} channels, but retain some diazoxide responsiveness due to presumed compensation by a novel nucleotide-regulated K^+ channel in the β-cell membrane, which has not been fully characterized. In patients with Type III PHHI, there is a later onset of disease (>6 months), which is usually milder with diazoxide-sensitive K^+ channels.[114,115]

Reactive Hypoglycemias

A great deal of controversy surrounds the subject of reactive or "functional" hypoglycemia. The debate centers not on whether reactive symptoms associated with low blood glucose can be produced under the appropriate conditions but on whether spontaneous reactive hypoglycemia represents a common clinical entity. The recognition that fasting hypoglycemia, as discussed earlier, may be associated with disastrous sequelae has unfortunately resulted in more attention being paid to its poor cousins, the reactive hypoglycemias. Indeed, it is not uncommon to find that an evaluation for the symptoms of fasting hypoglycemia was initiated incorrectly with an OGTT.

Definition

It is well known that the ingestion of large amounts of glucose is often followed by a transient decline in plasma glucose below the fasting concentration.[116] The decline in plasma glucose during the later (3–5 h) stage of a 75-g OGTT is also associated with a small but detectable increase in the secretion of counterregulatory hormones.[116] Thus, reactive hypoglycemia has probably been overdiagnosed as a result of indiscriminate use of the OGTT. In fact, an international group has defined reactive hypoglycemia as a clinical disorder in which the patient has postprandial symptoms accompanied by a plasma or serum glucose below 45–50 mg/dl (2.5–2.8 mmol/L) in an arterialized specimen.[117] This definition requiring that symptoms be associated with documented chemical evidence of hypoglycemia under normal feeding conditions has rarely been met in various series reporting reactive hypoglycemia; thus, many patients with hypoglycemic-type symptoms in fact have "nonhypoglycemia."[118] Indeed, in a study of 28 patients with suspected postprandial hypoglycemia in whom capillary blood was collected at the time of symptoms, it was found that almost 50 percent of patients experienced symptoms at glucose levels >3.3 mmol/L (60 mg/dl). There was no correlation found between the plasma glucose values during oral glucose administration and the levels measured during symptoms.[119]

Symptoms

In contrast to fasting hypoglycemia, severe neuroglycopenia is rarely observed in patients who experience only postprandial symptoms. Glucose concentrations generally do not decline below 40 mg/dl (2.2 mmol/L), and the hypoglycemic period is also usually brief. Adrenergic symptoms accompany the transient decrease in blood glucose in the late stage of the OGTT, though a wide array of nonspecific symptomatology may be reported in patients allegedly suffering from this syndrome (Fig. 19-4).

Alimentary Hypoglycemia

Alimentary hypoglycemia represents one of the diverse pathologic causes of reactive hypoglycemia. Some patients who have undergone gastric surgery display an exaggerated early increase in both plasma glucose and insulin after oral glucose administration, followed by a rapid decline to hypoglycemic levels by 3 h. The symptoms accompanying this hypoglycemia tend to be predominantly of the adrenergic type, though loss of consciousness and seizures have been reported. These reactive symptoms can usually be distinguished from those due to the "dumping" syndrome as those symptoms tend to occur within 1 h of feeding and are generally associated with nausea and epigastric fullness induced by the rapid transit of a large osmotic and fluid load.

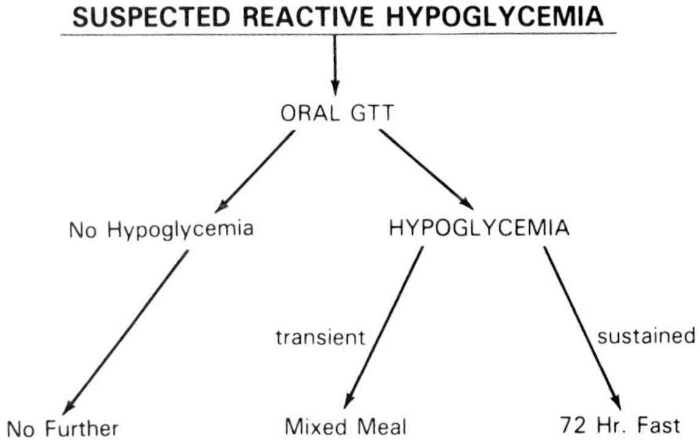

FIGURE 19-4. Flow sheet for the evaluation of a patient with suspected reactive (postprandial) hypoglycemia. "Mixed meal test" refers to the determination of the response of the plasma glucose concentration to mixed meals.

The mechanism underlying alimentary hypoglycemia has not been established with certainty. Rapid gastric emptying resulting from a reduced gastric pouch size (e.g., partial gastrectomy) or caused by vagal interruption has been postulated to result in rapid, early glucose absorption, which in turn leads to excessive hyperglycemia and hyperinsulinemia. Augmentation of insulin secretion as a result of increased gastric inhibitory peptide (GIP) and other gut hormones may also play a role.

Reactive Hypoglycemia in Diabetes

A reactive pattern of hypoglycemia is occassionally observed in patients who have subsequently developed diabetes.[120] It is unclear whether this is a true association or simply a coincidence in which a common disease (diabetes) is combined with the overdiagnosed "idiopathic" hypoglycemia. Postprandial hypoglycemia has also been reported in patients with obesity, renal glycosuria, hypothyroidism, and congenital adrenal hyperplasia.

Treatment

Carbohydrate restriction, especially limitation of simple sugars in the diet, has been the empirical approach to the treatment of most of these patients. Although controlled studies of such dietary changes are not available, most patients experience relief and only rare patients require other modalities (e.g., drugs, reoperation on the gastric stoma). Patients with milder symptoms may need only minimal dietary interventions (such as the avoidance of simple sugars), whereas certain patients will require a carefully designed diet containing only 120–150 g per day of total carbohydrate and supervised by a qualified nutritionist. Meal size should be reduced, and the frequency of feedings should be increased as needed.

In patients who fail to respond to dietary manipulations, the physician should be concerned about the possibility of the patient having fasting hypoglycemia or alternatively that hypoglycemia is not responsible for the symptoms. Pharmacologic interventions that may be attempted include anticholinergics, especially in patients with alimentary hypoglycemia.[121] Long-acting somatostatin analogues have been successful in a few patients.

Induced Hypoglycemias

Drug-induced hypoglycemias (Table 19-2) are the most common forms of hypoglycemia because of the frequency of insulin and sulfonylurea use in patients with diabetes. However, a wide variety of other drugs have been reported to cause severe hypoglycemia, and more than 50 individual agents have been implicated in published reports.[122] Treatment must include discontinuation of the agent when possible and supportive therapy for the hypoglycemia. The counterregulatory responses triggered by insulin-induced hypoglycemia and the syndrome of hypoglycemia unawareness are discussed earlier in glucose counterregulation and counterregulation in diabetes.

Sulfonylureas

These drugs account for a substantial proportion of drug-induced hypoglycemia. Because of their widespread clinical use, it is difficult to assess the true incidence of sulfonylurea hypoglycemia in patients with diabetes. The majority of reported cases of severe hypoglycemia have occurred in patients given chlorpropamide or glyburide. However, severe episodes characterized by coma have been reported with all the agents in common use

TABLE 19-2. Causes of Induced Hypoglycemia

1. Hypoglycemic drugs
   a. Insulin
   b. Sulfonylureas
   c. Biguanides
   d. Benzoic acid derivatives
   e. Thiazolidinediones
2. Nonhypoglycemic therapeutic agents
   a. Salicylates
   b. Propranolol
   c. Phenylbutazone
   d. Sulfonamides
   e. Dicumarol (bishydroxycoumarin)
   f. Quinine
   g. Pentamidine isethionate
   h. Ritodrine and β_2 agonists
   i. Disopyramide
3. Ethanol
4. Toxins
   a. Hypoglycine A (akee fruit)
   b. Pyriminil (Vacor)

(Table 19-2). In part, the hypoglycemic potential of an agent is related to its potency, its plasma and biological half-lives, and the use of concomitant substances. For example, liver disease prolongs the hypoglycemic actions of tolbutamide, acetohexamide, glyburide, and glipizide as these drugs are normally metabolized in the liver. The effects of chlorpropamide and acetohexamide are accentuated in patients with renal insuffiency, though even older patients without overt renal disease may suffer severe and prolonged hypoglycemia. Chlorpropamide may also cause hypoglycemia in patiens treated for diabetes insipidus or when it has been mistakenly prescribed or dispensed.

In addition to the inherent potential of these drugs to lower plasma glucose, they may interact with other agents to produce severe hypoglycemia. The additive (or possibly synergistic) effects during combined insulin and sulfonylurea therapy account for an increasing number of such episodes. Drugs that interfere with sulfonylurea metabolism or compete for circulating plasma protein binding with sulfonylureas can also potentiate these effects (Table 19-2). Important among these agents is coumarin, heparin, warfarin, and phenindione do not possess these effects. The increasing use of sulfonylurea drugs together with metformin and/or trogletazone (see later section) has also increased the incidence of sulfonylurea-induced hypoglycemia.

Pentamidine Isethionate

The earliest report of hypoglycemia associated with the use of this drug appeared in 1977.[123] Since then, the widespread use of this agent in the treatment of *Pneumocystis carinii* infection in immunocompromised hosts has resulted in many reported cases of severe hypoglycemia in patients with the acquired immunodeficiency syndrome (AIDS).[122] Although pentamidine is a biguanide derivative, the mechanism of the hypoglycemia is not clear. It is most likely that this agent causes beta cell injury with leakage of insulin, as plasma insulin concentrations during hypoglycemia may be increased and diabetes has ultimately developed in a few patients.

Ethanol

Ethanol ingestion is a recognized cause of hypoglycemia among all age groups. Most of these patients have a history of chronic alcoholism and/or poor nutrition, but accidental ingestion in healthy children and binge drinking among adults also have been reported in association with hypoglycemia. The diagnosis may be obscured by the absence of signs of acute inebriation, although blood alcohol levels are usually detectable. Ketonuria is often present, in keeping with the reduction in insulin secretion; liver function tests and amylase and phosphate levels are usually normal. Although plasma glucagon concentrations are appropriately increased, a hallmark of the disease is that exogenous glucagon administration has little effect on blood glucose.

The mechanism underlying this disorder most likely involves disruption of gluconeogenesis at the liver. This is suggested by the observation that hypoglycemia occurs when healthy volunteers are given ethanol after fasting for 36–72 h (at which time liver glycogen is depleted) but not after overnight fasting. During the hepatic oxidation of ethanol to acetaldehyde and acetate, nicotinamide-adenine dinucleotide (NAD) is reduced to NADH. The increased NADH/NAD ratio results in a redox state that does not promote the oxidation of substrates for gluconeogenesis such as lactate.[124] The levels of pyruvate fall, oxaloacetate, and phosphoenolpyruvate are not formed, and gluconeogenesis is hampered. Hypoglycemia results when hepatic glycogen stores are also depleted, hence the relation to the nutritional state of the patient. Alcohol consequently also potentiates the hypoglycemic actions of insulin and sulfonylurea agents. It is particularly important to emphasize this risk for type 1 diabetes patients because death and irreversible brain damage have been attributed to hypoglycemia induced by the combination.[125]

Other Drugs

Recently, several new classes of oral antidiabetic agents have been introduced in the United States for the treatment of type 2 diabetes. There is limited experience regarding the effect of most of these agents on the risk of hypoglycemia. Metformin has been available worldwide for 40 years, though its association with hypoglycemia has only recently been quantified.[71] The absence of severe hypoglycemia with metformin use as monotherapy in the United Kingdom Prospective Diabetes Study suggests that when hypoglycemia occurs in patients taking this agent that it may be due to other factors such as concomitant treatment with a sulfonylurea. The benzoic acid derivatives, which act as insulin secretagogues, have the potential to cause hypoglycemia by inducing insulin secretion; among these, repaglinide has been approved for use in the United States.[126] The thiazolidinedione troglitazone acts to sensitize peripheral tissues to insulin, and hence may cause hypoglycemia when insulin is used concomitantly.[127] Hypoglycemia can also be observed with monotherapy or when the drug is used in combination with other oral agents, particularly sulfonylureas. Finally, use of the α-glucosidase inhibitor acarbose is not of itself associated with hypoglycemia. However, in theory its use in a patient with hypoglycemia (e.g., due to concomitant sulfonylurea) may prevent orally-administered carbohydrate from being metabolized to glucose in the gut.

Diagnostic and Therapeutic Approach to Fasting Hypoglycemia

In the majority of patients historical clues (symptoms arising from neuroglycopenia) will point to the presence of fasting hypoglycemia. In some circumstances a diagnostic evaluation will be required not because of the patient's symptoms but by reason of

TABLE 19-3. Laboratory Findings in Fasting Hypoglycemia

	Sulfonylurea Ingestion*	Non-Islet–Cell Tumor Hypoglycemia	Insulinoma	Insulin Antibodies†	Insulin Receptor Antibodies	Factitious Hypoglycemia (Insulin)
Plasma Insulin‡	↑	↓	↑	↑↑↑	↑	↑
Plasma C peptide‡	↑	↓	↑	↓	↓	↓
Plasma proinsulin‡	↑	↓	↑	↓	↑	↓
Urine or plasma sulfonylurea	+	−	−	−	−	−
Insulin antibodies	−	−	−	+	−	−
Insulin receptor antibody	−	−	−	−	+	−

*(−) negative; (+) positive.

†In double-antibody radioimmunoassays of insulin, insulin antibodies will be elevated.

‡Measurement coinciding with the time of hypoglycemia.

laboratory (e.g., plasma glucose) or radiologic tests performed for other reasons (e.g., abdominal CT). Thus, in this latter instance, establishing the presence of fasting hypoglycemia is critical.

If postprandial hypoglycemia is considered on clinical grounds, only a 5-h OGTT is required (Fig. 19-4). The reactive hypoglycemias may be excluded if hypoglycemia fails to develop or if symptoms do not occur despite a fall in plasma glucose concentrations to a level <50 mg/dl (2.8 mmol/L). If biochemical hypoglycemia or symptomatic hypoglycemia is observed, it is usually not necessary to test for fasting hypoglycemia unless the hypoglycemia is sustained. It is important, however, to determine whether the hypoglycemia is also provoked by the usual mixed meal before embarking on a therapeutic regimen.

In patients suspected of having fasting hypoglycemia, a supervised fast is mandatory. Of course, patients with hypoglycemia after brief periods of fasting (12–18 h) should not be subjected to a full 72-h fast. Conversely, it may be sufficient for the patient to undergo an 18-h fast as an outpatient by merely skipping breakfast and giving a blood sample for plasma glucose and insulin before lunch. If plasma glucose remains above 70 mg/dl (3.9 mmol/L), further studies may not be warranted. If plasma glucose falls below 50–60 mg/dl (2.8–3.4 mmol/L), insulin and C peptide levels should be obtained. Self-testing of blood glucose with a reflectance meter should not substitute for a diagnostic evaluation to establish that laboratory glucose values confirm hypoglycemia coinciding with symptoms and the simultaneous measurement of plasma hormones.

The development of hypoglycemia during a brief or prolonged fast is the sine qua non of diagnosis (Table 19-3). In contrast, hyperinsulinemia without concomitant hypoglycemia indicates neither the presence of an islet-cell tumor nor that of another hypoglycemic disorder. The most common form of nonhypoglycemic hyperinsulinemia is obesity. The concurrence of symptomatic hypoglycemia with relative or absolute hyperinsulinemia provides the highest degree of confidence in the clinical diagnosis of islet-cell pathology. No further tests are warranted in a patient who does not develop hypoglycemia after a prolonged fast. Long-term observation may, however, be necessary to reevaluate a patient with suspicious symptoms. A repeated fast with the addition of a bout of exercise in the last hour may be helpful in eliciting symptomatic hypoglycemia.

In a patient with both hypoglycemia and hyperinsulinemia, plasma C peptide determinations should help distinguish factitious or iatrogenic hypoglycemia caused by exogenous insulin. However, hypoglycemia due to sulfonylurea drugs cannot be excluded by the C peptide assay; detection of these agents in plasma or urine may be necessary.

When hypoglycemia is found in the presence of low plasma insulin concentratioins, underlying hepatic or renal dysfunction is the most probable cause. However, these conditions are not likely to escape detection in a routine clinical evaluation. In other cases a careful search for an undetected endocrine deficiency or occult extrapancreatic malignancy is warranted.

If the plasma insulin concentration is equivocal, additional examinations such as a C peptide suppression test or proinsulin determinations should be considered. If these examinations are abnormal, the diagnosis of an islet-cell lesion should be pursued (Table 19-3).

Only after unequivocal demonstration of fasting hypoglycemia and relative or absolute hyperinsulinemia should one consider tests to localize an islet-cell tumor. Because the frequency of false-negative imaging studies is substantial and reliance on the operative findings will be critical, a surgical consultation should be obtained. A trial of medical therapy with dietary and pharmacologic intervention (diazoxide and/or octreotide) should be considered at this stage. This is especially important if a tumor cannot be found at the time of laparotomy (estimated to occur in 10 percent of patients with biochemical evidence of autonomous insulin secretion). Before subjecting the patient to the risk of a partial or subtotal blind resection of the distal pancreas, one can utilize the preoperative response to medical therapy to direct the appropriate course of action. In addition, one may choose to defer definitive surgery until more invasive tests (i.e., pancreatic venous sampling) allow better localization of pancreatic pathology. Such testing should only be performed in specialized centers.

REFERENCES

1. Merimee TJ, Tyson JE: Stabilization of plasma glucose during fasting. Normal variations in two separate studies. *N Engl J Med* 291:1275, 1979.
2. Field JB: Hypoglycemia, definition, clinical presentations, classification, and laboratory tests. *Endocrinol Clin North Am* 18:27, 1989.
3. Cornblath M, Schwartz R: *Disorders of Carbohydrate Metabolism in Infancy*, 2nd ed. Philadelphia, Saunders, 1976.
4. Haymond MW, Karl E, Clark WL, Pagliara AS, Santiago JV: Differences in circulating gluconeogenic substrates during short-term fasting in men, women, and children. *Metabolism* 31:34, 1982.
5. Marks V, Rose FC: *Hypoglycaemia*, 2nd ed. Oxford, Blackwell, 1981.
6. Moore MC, Connnolly CC, Cherrington AD: Autoregulation of hepatic glucose production. *Eur J Endocrinol* 138:240, 1998.
7. Marks V, Greenwood FC, Howorth PJN, Samols E: Plasma growth hormone levels in spontaneous hypoglycemia. *J Clin Endocrinol Metab* 27:523, 1967.

8. Amiel SA, Sherwin RS, Simonson DC, Tamborlane WV: Effect of intensive insulin therapy on glycemic thresholds for counterregulatory hormone release. *Diabetes* 37:901, 1988.
9. Davis MR, Shamoon H: Deficient counterregulatory hormone responses during hypoglycemia in a patient with insulinoma. *J Clin Endocrinol Metab* 72:788, 1991.
10. Boyle P, Schwartz NS, Shah, Clutter WE, Cryer PE: Plasma glucose concentrations at the onset of hypoglycemic symptoms in patients with poorly controlled diabetes and in nondiabetics. *N Engl J Med* 318:1487, 1988.
11. Owen OE, Morgan AO, Kemp HG, Sullivan JM, Herrera MG, Cahill GF Jr: Brain metabolism during fasting. *J Clin Invest* 46:1589, 1967.
12. Holmes CS, Hayford JT, Gonzalez JL, Weydert JA: A survey of cognitive functioning at different glucose levels in diabetic persons. *Diabetes Care* 6:180, 1983.
13. Herold KC, Polonsky KS, Cohen RM, Levy J, Douglas F: Variable deterioration in cortical function during insulin-induced hypoglycemia. *Diabetes* 34:677, 1985.
14. Siejo BK: Hypoglycemia, brain metabolism, and brain damage. *Diabetes Metab Rev* 4:113, 1988.
15. Bryan RM Jr, Keefer KA, MacNeill C: Regional cerebral glucose utilization during insulin-induced hypoglycemia in unanesthetized rats. *J Neurochem* 46:1904, 1986.
16. Ferrendelli JA: Hypoglycemia and the: Then CNS, in Ingrar DH, Lassen NA (eds): *Brain Work Coupling of Function, Metabolism and Blood Flow in the Brain.* Copenhagen, Munksgaard, 1975, p 298.
17. Horton RW, Meldrum BS, Bachelard HS: Enzymic and cerebral metabolic effects of 2-deory-D-glucose. *J Neurochem* 21:507, 1973.
18. Myers RE, Kahn KJ: Insulin-induced hypoglycemia in the nonhuman primate: II. Long-term neuropathological consequences, in Brierley JB, Meldrum BS (eds): *Brain Hypoxia. Clinics in Developmental Medicine 39/40.* London, Heinemann, 1971, p 195.
19. Danta G: Hypoglycemic peripheral neuropathy. *Arch Neurol* 21:121, 1969.
20. Bertoye A, Bourrat C, Bolot JF, Robert D: Neuropathie amyotrophique quadridistale par hyperinsulinisme. *Rev Neurol (Paris)* 126:220, 1972.
21. Reichard P, Berglund A, Britz A, Levander S, Rosenquist: Hypoglycaemic episodes during intensified insulin treatment: Increased frequency but no effect on cognitive function. *J Intern Med* 229:9, 1991.
22. The Diabetes Control and Complications Trial Research Group: Effects of intensive diabetes therapy on neuropsychological function in adults in the Diabetes Control and Complications Trial. *Ann Intern Med* 124:379, 1996.
23. Kramer L, Fasching P, Madl C, Schneider B, Damjancic P, Waldhäusl W, Irsigler K, Grimm G: Previous episodes of hypoglycemic coma are not associated with permanent cognitive brain dysfunction in IDDM patients on intensive insulin treatment. *Diabetes* 47:1909, 1998.
24. Northam EA, Anderson PJ, Werther GA, Warne GL, Adler RG, Andrewes D: Neuropsychological complications of IDDM in children 2 years after disease onset. *Diabetes Care* 21:379, 1998.
25. Lloyd-Mostyn RH, Oram S: Modification by propranolol of cardiovascular effects of induced hypoglycemia. *Lancet* i:1213, 1975.
26. Pladziewicz DS, Nesto RW: Hypoglycemia-induced silent myocardial ischemia. *Am J Cardiol* 63:1531, 1989.
27. Bennett T, Gale EAM, Green JH, MacDonald IA, Walford S: The influence of beta-adrenoceptor antagonists on thermoregulation during insulin induced hypoglycemia. *J Physiol* 308:26, 1980.
28. Hutton RA, Mikhailidis D, Dormandy KM, Ginsburg J: Platelet aggregation studies during transient hypoglycemia. *J Clin Pathol* 32:434, 1979.
29. Brodows RG, Ensinck JW, Campbell RG: Mechanism of plasma cyclic AMP response to hypoglycemia in man. *Metabolism* 6:659, 1976.
30. Frier BM, Corrall RJM, Davidson NM, Webber RG, Dewar A, French EB: Peripheral blood cell changes in response to acute hypoglycemia in man. *J Clin Invest* 13:33, 1983.
31. Fajans S, Floyd JC: Fasting hypoglycemia in adults. *N Engl J Med* 294:766, 1976.
32. Service FJ: Hypoglycemia. *Endocinol Metab Clin North Am* 26:937, 1997.
33. Shoelson SE, Polonsky KS, Zeidler A, Rubenstein AH, Tager HS: Human insulin B24(PHE—SER): Secretion and metabolic clearance of the abnormal insulin in man and in a dog model. *J Clin Invest* 73:1351, 1984.
34. Rubenstein AH, Steiner DF, Horwitz DL, Mako ME, Block MB, Starr JI, Kuzaya H, Melani F: Clinical significance of circulating proinsulin and C-peptide. *Recent Prog Horm Res* 33:435, 1977.
35. Gorden P, Sherman B, Roth J: Proinsulin-like component of circulating insulin in the basal state and in patients and hamsters with islet cell tumors. *J Clin Invest* 50:2113, 1971.
36. Gabbay KH, De Luca K, Fisher JN Jr, Mako ME, Rubenstein AH: Familial hyperproinsulinemia: An autosomal dominant defect. *N Engl J Med* 294:911, 1976.
37. Kao PC, Taylor RL, Service FJ: Proinsulin by immunochemiluminometric assay for the diagnosis of insulinoma. *J Clin Endocrinol Metab* 78:1046, 1994.
38. Johansen K: Insulinoma: Clinical manifestation, diagnosis and treatment. *J Endocrinol Invest* 2:285, 1979.
39. Floyd JC, Fajans SS, Knopf RF, Conn JW: Plasma insulin in organic hyperinsulinism: Comparative effects of tolbutamide, leucine and glucose. *J Clin Endocrinol Metab* 24:747, 1964.
40. Marks V, Samols E: Glucagon test for insulinoma: A chemical study in 25 cases. *J Clin Pathol* 21:346, 1968.
41. Roy BK, Abuid J, Wendorff H, Nitiyanant W: Insulin release in response to calcium in the diagnosis of insulinoma. *Metabolism* 28:1029, 1975.
42. Cryer PE: Glucose counterregulation in man. *Diabetes* 30:261, 1981.
43. Gerich JE, Campbell PJ: Overview of counterregulation and its abnormalities in diabetes mellitus and other conditions. *Diabetes Metab Rev* 4:93, 1988.
44. Cryer PE, Gerich JE: Glucose counterregulation, hypoglycemia and intensive insulin therapy in diabetes mellitus. *N Engl J Med* 313:232, 1985.
45. Cryer PE: Glucose counterregulation: The prevention and correction of hypoglycemia in humans. *Am J Physiol* 264:E149, 1993.
46. Bolli G, De Feo P, Compagnucci P, Cartechini MG, Angeletti G, Santeusanio F, Brunetti P, Gerich JE: Abnormal glucose counterregulation in insulin-dependent diabetes mellitus: Interaction of anti-insulin antibodies and impaired glucagon and epinephrine secretion. *Diabetes* 32:134, 1983.
47. Shamoon H, Hendler R, Sherwin R: Synergistic interactions among anti-insulin hormones in the pathogenesis of stress hyperglycemia in hormones. *J Clin Endocrinol Metab* 52:1235, 1981.
48. Schwartz NS, Clutter WE, Shah SD, Cryer PE: The glycemic thresholds for activation of glucose counterregulatory systems are higher than the thresholds for symptoms. *J Clin Invest* 79:777, 1987.
49. Mitrakou A, Ryan C, Veneman T, Evron W, Jensen T, Cryer P, Gerich J: Hierarchy of glycemic thresholds for activation of counterregulatory hormone secretion, initiation of symptoms and onset of cerebral dysfunction in normal humans. *Am J Physiol* 260:E67, 1991.
50. Davis M, Mellman M, Friedman S, Chang CJ, Shamoon H: Recovery of epinephrine response but not hypoglycemic symptom threshold after intensive therapy in type 1 diabetes. *Am J Med* 97:1, 1994.
51. Gerich JE, Rizza R, Haymond M, Cryer PE: Hormone mechanisms in acute glucose counterregulation: The relative roles of glucagon, epinephrine, nonepinephrine growth hormones and cortisol. *Metabolism* 29:1164, 1980.
52. Kleinbaum J, Shamoon H: Impaired counterregulation of hypoglycemia in insulin-dependent diabetes mellitus. *Diabetes* 32:493, 1983.
53. De Feo P, Perriello G, Torlone E, Ventura MM, Fanelli C, Santeusanio F, Burnetti P, Gerich JE, Bolli GB: Contribution of cortisol to glucose counterregulation in humans. *Am J Physiol* 20:E35, 1989.
54. De Feo P, Perriello G, Torlone E, Ventura MM, Santeusanio F, Brunetti P, Gerich JE, Bolli GB: Demonstration of a role for growth hormone in glucose counterregulation. *Am J Physiol* 19:E835, 1989.
55. Rizza R, Cryer P, Haymond M, Gerich JE: Adrenergic mechanisms for the effects of epinephrine on glucose production and clearance in man. *J Clin Invest* 65:682, 1980.
56. Cohen N, Rossetti L, Shlimovich P, Halberstam M, Hu M, Shamoon H: Counterregulation of Hypoglycemia: Skeletal muscle glycogen metabolism during physiologic hyperinsulinemia in humans. *Diabetes* 44:423, 1995.
57. Hopwood NJ, Forsham PJ, Kenny FM, Drash AL: Hypolycemia in hypopituitary children. *Am J Dis Child* 129:918, 1975.

58. Smallright RC, Corrigan DF, Thomason AM, Blue PW: Hypoglycemia in pregnancy: Occurrence due to adrenocorticotropic hormone and growth hormone deficiency. *Arch Intern Med* 140:564, 1980.
59. Sacca L, Sherwin RS, Hendler R, Felig P: Influence of continuous physiologic hyperinsulinemia on glucose kinetics and counterregulatory hormones in normal and diabetic humans. *J Clin Invest* 63:849, 1979.
60. Silverberg AB, Shah SD, Haymond MW, Cryer PE: Norepinephrine: Hormone and neurotransmitter. *Am J Physiol* 234:E252, 1978.
61. Cryer PE, Fisher JN Jr, Shamoon H: Hypoglycemia. *Diabetes Care* 17:734, 1994.
62. Polonsky K, Bergenstal R, Pons G, Schneider M, Jaspan J, Rubenstein AH: Relation of counterregulatory response to hypoglycemia in type I diabetics. *N Eng J Med* 307:1106, 1982.
63. Hirsch BR, Shamoon H: Defective epinephrine and growth hormone responses in IDDM are stimulus-specific. *Diabetes* 36:20, 1987.
64. Gerich JE, Langlois M, Noacco C, Karam JH, Forsham PH: Lack of glucagon response to hypoglycemia in diabetes: Evidence for an intrinsic pancreatic alpha-cell defect. *Science* 182:171, 1973.
65. Simonson DC, Tamborlane WV, DeFronzo RA, Sherwin RS: Intensive insulin therapy reduces counterregulatory hormone responses to hypoglycemia in patients with type I diabetes. *Ann Intern Med* 103:184, 1985.
66. Cloutier MG, Pek S, Crowther RL, Floyd JC Jr, Fajans SS: Glucagon-insulin interactions in patients with insulin producing pancreatic islet lesions. *J Clin Endocrinol Metab* 48:201, 1979.
67. French EB, Kilpatric R: Role of adrenaline in hypoglycaemic reactions in man. *Clin Sci* 14:639, 1955.
68. Ginsburg J, Paton A: Effects of insulin after adrenalectomy. *Lancet* ii:491, 1965.
69. The Diabetes Control and Complications Trial Research Group: The effect of intensive treatment of diabetes on the development and progression of long-term complications in insulin-dependent diabetes mellitus. *N Engl J Med* 329:977, 1993.
70. The Diabetes Control and Complications Trial Research Group: Hypoglycemia in the DCCT. *Diabetes* 46:271, 1997.
71. UK Prospective Diabetes Study Group: Effect of intensive blood-glucose control with metformin on complications in overweight patients with type 2 diabetes (UKPDS 34). *Lancet* 352:854, 1998.
72. Shamoon H, Friedman S, Canton C, Zacharowicz L, Hu M, Rossetti L: Increased epinephrine and skeletal muscle responses to hypoglycemia in noninsulin-dependent diabetes mellitus. *J Clin Invest* 93:2562, 1994.
73. Marks V, Samols E: Insulinoma: Natural history and diagnosis. *Clin Gastroenterol* 3:559, 1974.
74. Kahn CR, Rosen SW, Weintraub BD, Fajans SS, Gorden P: Ectopic production of chorionic gonadotropin and its subunits by islet-cell tumors. *N Engl J Med* 297:565, 1977.
75. Anderson A, Bergdahl L: Insulinomas and multiple endocrine neoplasia. *Acta Chir Scand* 142:297, 1976.
76. Stefanini P, Carboni M, Patrassi N, Basoli A: Beta-islet cell tumors of the pancreas: Results of a study on 1,067 cases. *Surgery* 75:597, 1974.
77. Tibaldi JM, Lorber D, Shamoon H, Lomasky S, Steinberg JJ, Reisman R: Postprandial hypoglycemia in islet beta cell hyperplasia with adenomatosis of the pancreas. *J Surg Onc* 50:532, 1992.
78. Fajans SS: Insulin-producing islet cell tumors. *Endocrinol Metab Clin North Am* 18:45, 1989.
79. Merimee TJ, Tyson JE: Hypoglycemia in man: Pathologic and physiologic variants. *Diabetes* 24:161, 1977.
80. Stark D, Moss AA, Goldberg HI, Deveney CW, Way L: Computed tomography and nuclear magnetic resonance imaging of pancreatic islet cell tumors. *Surgery* 94:1024, 1983.
81. Fulton RE, Sheedy PF, McIlrath DC, Ferris DO: Preoperative angiographic localization of insulin-producing tumors of the pancreas. *Am J Radiol* 123:367, 1975.
82. Roche A, Raissonnier A, Gillon-Savouret MC: Pancreatic venous sampling and arteriography in localizing insulinomas and gastrinomas: Procedure and results in 55 cases. *Radiology* 145:621, 1982.
83. Ueno N, Tomiyama T, Tano S, Wada S, Aizawa T, Kimura K: Utility of endoscopic ultrasonography with color doppler function for the diagnosis of islet cell tumor. *Am J Gastroenterol* 91:772, 1996.
84. Pitre J, Soubrana O, Palazzo L, Chapuis Y: Endoscopic ultrasonography for the preoperative localization of insulinomas. *Pancreas* 13:55, 1996.
85. Kato T, Tsukamoto Y, Naitoh Y, Hirooka Y, Furukawa T, Hayakawa T: Ultrasonographic and endoscopic untrasonographic angiography in pancreatic mass lesions. *Acta Radiol* 36:381, 1995.
86. Grant CS, Van Heerden J, Charboneau JW, James EM, Reading CC: Insulinoma: The value of intraoperative ultrasonography. *Arch Surg* 123:843, 1988.
87. Modlin IM, Cornelius E, Lawton GP: Use of an isotopic somatostatin receptor probe to image endocrine tumors. *Arch Surg* 130:367, 1995.
88. Breeman WAP, van Hagen PM, Kwekkeboom DJ, Visser TJ, Krenning EP: Somatostatin receptor scintigraphy using [^{111}In-DTPA0]RC-160 in humans: a comparison with [^{111}In-DTPA0]octreotide. *Eur J Nuc Med* 25:182, 1998.
89. Laroche GP, Ferris DO, Priestly JT, Scholz DA, Dockerty MB: Hyperinsulinism: Surgical results and management of occult functioning islet cell tumors: Review of 154 cases. *Arch Surg* 96:763, 1968.
90. Laron Z: Somatostatin analogues in the management of benign insulinomas. *Isr J Med Sci* 26:1, 1990.
91. Glaser B, Rosler A, Halperin Y: Chronic treatment of a benign insulinoma using the long-acting somatostatin analogue SMS 201-995. *Isr J Med Sci* 26:16, 1990.
92. Comi RJ, Gorden P, Doppman J, Norton J: Insulinoma, in Go VLW (ed): *The Exocrine Pancreas: Biology, Pathobiology and Diseases*. New York, Raven Press, 1986, p 745.
93. Chowdhury F, Bleicha JJ: Studies of tumor hypoglycemia. *Metabolism* 22:663, 1973.
94. Flier JS, Mueckler MM, Usher P, Lodish HF: Elevated levels of glucose transport and transporter messenger RNA are induced by ras or src oncogenes. *Science* 235:1492, 1987.
95. Daughaday WH: Hypoglycemia in patients with non-islet cell tumors. *Endocrinol Metab Clin North Am* 18:91, 1989.
96. Merimee TJ: Insulin-like growth factors in patients with non-islet cell tumors and hypoglycemia. *Metabolism* 35:360, 1986.
97. Daughaday WH, Emanuele MA, Brooks MH, Barbato AL, Kapadia M, Rotwein P: Synthesis and secretion of insulin-like growth factor II by a leiomyosarcoma with associated hypoglycemia. *N Engl J Med* 319:1434, 1988.
98. Axelrod L, Ron D: Insulin-like growth factor II and the riddle of tumor-induced hypoglycemia. *N Engl J Med* 319:1477, 1988.
99. Baxter RC: Insulin-like growth factor binding proteins as glucoregulators. *Metabolism* 44:12, 1995.
100. Daughaday WH, Trivedi B, Baxter RC: Serum "big" insulin-like growth factor-II from patients with tumor hypoglycemia lacks normal E-domain *O*-linked glycosylation, a possible determinant of normal propeptide processing. *Proc Natl Acad Sci USA* 90:5823, 1993.
101. Baxter RC, Daughaday WH: Impaired formation of the ternary insulin-like growth factor binding protein complex in patients with hypoglycemia due to non-islet cell tumors. *J Clin Endocrinol Metab* 73:696, 1991.
102. Bier D, Rosemary DL, Haymond MW, Arnold KJ, Gruenke LD, Sperling MA, Kipnis DM: Measurement of "true" glucose production rates in infancy and childhood with 6,6-dideuteroglucose. *Diabetes* 26:1016, 1977.
103. Comi RJ, Gorden P: Approach to hypoglycemia in adults. *Compr Ther* 13:38, 1987.
104. Block MB, Gambetta M, Resnekov L, Rubenstein AH: Spontaneous hypoglycemia and congestive heart-failure. *Lancet* ii:736, 1972.
105. Breen KJ, Penkins KW, Mistilis SP, Shearman R: Idiopathic acute fatty liver of pregnancy. *Gut* 11:82, 1970.
106. Haymond MW: Hypoglycemia in infants and children. *Endocrinol Metab Clin* 18:211, 1989.
107. Haymond MW, Pagliara AS: Ketotic hypoglycemia. *Clin Endocrinol Metab* 12:447, 1983.
108. Rebouche CJ, Engel AG: Carnitine metabolism and deficiency. *Mayo Clin Proc* 58:533, 1983.
109. Verrotti A, Fusilli P, Pallotta R, Morgese G, Chiarelli F: Hypoglycemia in childhood. A clinical approach. *J Ped Endocrinol Metab* 11:147, 1998.
110. Kahn CR, Flier JS, Bar RS, Archer JA, Gorden P, Martin MM, Roth J: The syndromes of insulin resistance and acanthosis nigricans: Insulin-receptor disorders in man. *N Engl J Med* 294:739, 1976.

111. Taylor SI, Grunberger G, Marcus-Samuel B, Underhill LH, Dons RF, Ryan J, Roddam RF, Rupe CE, Gorden P: Hypoglycemia associated with antibodies to the insulin receptor. *N Engl J Med* 307:1422, 1982.
112. Hirata Y: Autoimmune insulin syndrome, in Andreani D, Marks V, Lefebvre PJ (eds): *Hypoglycemia*. New York, Raven Press, 1987, p 105.
113. Aynsley-Green A, Dunne MJ, James RFL, Lindley KJ: Ions and genes in persistent hyperinsulinaemic hypoglycaemia in infancy: A commentary on the implications for tailoring treatment to disease pathogenesis. *J Ped Endocrinol Metab* 11:121, 1998.
114. Dunne MJ, Kane C, Shepherd RM, Sanchez JA, James RFL, Johnson PRV, Aynsley-Green A, Lu S, Clement JP IV, Lindley KJ, Seino S, Aguilar-Bryan L: Familial persistent hyperinsulinemic hypoglycemia of infancy and mutations in the sulfonylurea receptor. *N Engl J Med* 336:703, 1997.
115. Nichols CG, Shyng SL, Nestorowicz A, Glaser B, Clement JP IV, Gonzalez G, Aguilar-Bryan L, Permutt MA, Bryan J: Adenosine diphosphate as an intracellular regulator of insulin secretion. *Science* 272:1785, 1996.
116. Kleinbaum J, Shamoon H: Selective counterregulatory hormone responses after oral glucose in man. *J Clin Endocrinol Metab* 55:787, 1982.
117. Lefebvre PJ, Andreani D, Marks V: Statement on "postprandial" or reactive hypoglycemia, in Andreani D, Marks V, Lefebvre PJ (eds): *Hypoglycemia*. New York, Raven Press, 1987, p 79.
118. Cahill GF, Soeldner JS: A non-editorial on non-hypoglycemia. *N Engl J Med* 291:905, 1974.
119. Palardy J, Havrankova J, Lepage R, Matte R, Bélanger R, D'Amour P, Ste Marie LG: Blood glucose measurements during symptomatic episodes in patients with suspected postprandial hypoglycemia. *N Engl J Med* 321:1421, 1989.
120. Seltzer HS, Fajans SS, Conn JW: Spontaneous hypoglycemia as an early manifestation of diabetes mellitus. *Diabetes* 5:437, 1956.
121. Permutt MA: Postprandial hypoglycemia. *Diabetes* 25:719, 1976.
122. Seltzer HS: Drug-induced hypoglycemia: A review of 1418 cases. *Endocrinol Metab Clin* 18:163, 1989.
123. Grant AM, Sandler RM, Carrell RW: Hypoglycaemic effect of pentamidine detected by glucose screen. *Lancet* ii:510, 1977.
124. Krebs HA, Freedland RA, Hems R, Stubbs M: Inhibition of hepatic gluconeogenesis by ethanol. *Biochem J* 112:117, 1969.
125. Arky R, Veverbrants E, Abramson EA: Irreversible hypoglycemia: A complication of alcohol and insulin. *JAMA* 206:575, 1968.
126. Goldberg RB, Einhorn D, Lucas CP, Rendell MS, Damaso P, Huang WC, Strange P, Brodows, RG: A randomized placebo-controlled trial of repaglinide in the treatment of type 2 diabetes. *Diabetes Care* 21:1897, 1998.
127. Buse JB, Gumbiner B, Mathias NP, Nelson DM, Faja BW, Whitcomb RW: Troglitazone use in insulin-treated type 2 diabetic patients. *Diabetes Care* 21:1455, 1998.

CHAPTER 20

Obesity

John M. Amatruda
David L. Linemeyer

DEFINITION AND DIAGNOSIS OF OBESITY

Obesity is a chronic metabolic disorder characterized by an excess of body fat. This distinguishes obesity from *overweight*, which is defined as excess weight in reference to an arbitrary standard, usually a "desirable weight" from height–weight tables. A bodybuilder will probably be overweight for his or her height but will be very lean and therefore not obese. Generally, normal females have 18–30 percent body fat and normal males have less than 25 percent body fat.

There are currently several methods of assessing fatness, all of which have certain advantages and disadvantages (Table 20-1). These techniques were extensively reviewed by Forbes[1] and Amatruda.[2]

Underwater weighing to determine body density is considered the gold standard and requires few assumptions. This method, however, requires a specialized tank and the ability to measure residual lung volumes accurately. Furthermore, it requires substantial cooperation because in most cases the patient must be completely submerged. For these reasons, it is largely a research tool. Total body water and other ion dilution measurements require the administration of radioactive or stable isotopes of hydrogen, oxygen, or other elements and assume that a constant percentage of lean body mass is composed of water. This percentage can vary, potentially introducing error. This method is also expensive and is currently used primarily as a research tool. A third method is potassium 40 (^{40}K) measurement. Because potassium is distributed in fat-free mass, measuring total body potassium allows one to estimate lean body mass. This is another research tool requiring expensive and not widely available equipment, and it depends on assumptions about the potassium content of lean tissue. A simpler and far less expensive method of estimating lean body mass (and, by subtraction, fat) is to measure the 24-h excretion of creatinine (Cr). Forbes and Bruining[3] found that on an ad lib diet, lean body mass in kilograms = 0.0291 Cr (mg/day) + 7.38, with an r value of 0.97. This technique gives different results depending on the amount of meat in the diet and varies with day-to-day variation in creatinine excretion. Recently, electrical impedance has shown promise in measuring lean body mass, with correlation coefficients from 0.9 to 0.97 between fat-free mass by densitometry and by impedance.[4] This technique is easy to perform and relatively inexpensive, although one must be cautious if weight is changing[4–6] as changes in bioelectrical impedance may reflect changes in total body water rather than lean body mass. Two measurement techniques used to measure bone mass are now being applied successfully to measure body composition. These dual-energy absorption techniques are dual x-ray absorptiometry (DXA), which uses x-rays as an energy source, and dual photon absorptiometry (DPA), which uses a radionucleotide as a source of energy. DXA is now the standard for measuring bone density and equipment is usually readily available.[7,8] Recent studies indicate that even morbidly obese patients can be scanned by doing half-body scans.[8]

Another measure of fatness is skin fold measurements, or anthropometry.[1] Skin fold measurements measure mostly subcutaneous fat and are usually made over the triceps at the tip of the scapula. Because the thickness of fat varies in different depots and because subcutaneous fat may not reflect total body fat, these measurements are not accurate.

Although it is not a true measure of fatness, the most commonly used indirect measure of obesity is body mass index [BMI = weight (kg)/height^2 (m)]. Although normal ranges for this index from Metropolitan Life Insurance Tables correlate with percentile values from height-weight tables from the National Health and Nutrition Survey in 1982 and body fat in some studies, they do not necessarily reflect body fat. BMIs for the midpoint of medium-frame men of all heights from the Metropolitan Life Insurance Tables, after adjusting for shoes and clothes, are 22 kg/m^2, which equals a Metropolitan relative weight of 100. The 85th percentile values are a BMI of 27.8 for males and 27.3 for females, which correspond to 124 percent of ideal body weight for a male of average height and 120 percent of ideal body weight for a female of average height based on the 1983 Metropolitan Life Insurance Tables. The range of the midpoint for all heights and frames is 19.8–25.7 kg/m^2. The midpoint for medium-frame females of all heights is 21.5 kg/m^2, and the range of midpoint values for females of all heights and frames is 19 to 26 kg/m^2.[3,9] From the NHANES III data[10] (1988 to 1994) the mean BMI for all men and women ≥20 years old is 26.5 while the median BMI is 25.5 for men and 25.1 for women.

An expert committee convened by the World Health Organization recommended a classification of obesity based on low, moderate, and high risk that was modified in 1997 by the International Obesity Task force and defined as pre-obese (BMI 25–29.9), class 1 obesity (BMI 30–34.9), class II obesity (BMI 35–39.9), and class III obesity (BMI ≥ 40).[11,12] A recent report from the National Institutes of Health defined overweight as a BMI from 25 to 29.9 kg/m^2 and obesity as a BMI ≥ 30 kg/m[11] with class I, II, and III as defined above and as used in NHANES. These classifications are associated with disease risk and modified by waist circumference (Table 20-2).

TABLE 20-1. Body Composition Measurement Techniques: Advantages and Disadvantages

	Advantages	Disadvantages
Density	Apparatus inexpensive Estimates lean body mass and fat simultaneously Nonhazardous Can be repeated frequently	Subject cooperation necessary for underwater weighing Unsuitable for young children and the elderly Error from intestinal gas
Total body water and ion dilution	Estimate body fluid volumes Inexpensive Great variety: NA, K, Cl (Br), H_2O	Radiation exposure (some materials) Blood samples needed for some materials (some require several samples) Incomplete equilibration Na, K; overestimation by D_2O, $3H_2O$; value for extracellular fluid depends on method used; ^{18}O assay requires elaborate equipment
Dual-energy X-ray absorptivity (DXA)	Equipment readily available, inexpensive, quick, noninvasive, not affected by tissue dimensions and level of hydration	Limited dimensions of table (overcome with half-body scans) Variations in equipment calibration and algorithms
^{40}K counting	No hazard Minimal subject cooperation Can be repeated frequently	Instrument expensive Proper calibration necessary Problem in interpretation in subjects with K deficiency
Creatinine excretion	No hazard Estimate of muscle mass	Meticulous subject cooperation Influenced by diet; collection time critical Day-to-day variation (5–10 percent)
Electrical impedance	Noninvasive Easy to perform Minimal patient cooperation Quick	Inaccurate when weight or body H_2O is changing
Anthropometry (skin fold)	Cheap Indirect estimate of body fat and muscle mass	Poor precision in obese subjects and those with firm subcutaneous fat tissue Regional variation in subcutaneous fat layer; uncertainty about the ratio of subcutaneous fat to total fat
Metabolic balance	No hazard Suitable for many elements Can detect small changes in body content (<1 percent) Many laboratory analyses needed	Measures only the change in body composition Meticulous subject cooperation Metabolic ward expensive Error from unmeasured skin losses
Neutron activation	Minimal subject cooperation Body content Ca, P, N, Na, Cl	Apparatus very expensive Calibration very difficult Radiation exposure
Fat-soluble gases	Direct estimate of body fat	Cyclopropane, xenon, 85Kr Apparatus expensive Long equilibration time
Ultrasound	Organ size No hazard	Poor definition of subcutaneous fat layer
3-Methylhistidine excretion	Estimate of muscle mass	Meat-free diet 2 days before collection Subject cooperation Variable contribution from gastrointestinal tissue (?) Magnitude of day-to-day variations (?)
Functions of height and weight (BMI)	Easy Quick Cheap	Not an accurate measure of body composition

Source: Modified from Forbes,[1] with permission.

Height–weight tables are based on the levels of overweight associated with excess mortality.[13] The most commonly used tables are the Metropolitan Life Insurance Tables (Table 20-2), which are based on the 1979 Build Study published by the Society of Actuaries and the Association of Life Insurance Medical Directors. These tables give relative body weights, which do not necessarily reflect adiposity. The Build Study was flawed in many ways in its attempt to relate relative weight to mortality. It disproportionately included men, whites, people under 60 years old, and the middle and upper classes. Furthermore, the unit of analysis was the insurance policy, not the person. Thus, a person who had more than one policy was included more than once. A person with more than one policy would obviously disproportionately affect the mortality data whether that person lived or died. The length of time a person was followed depended on how long that person was insured. The average length of follow-up was only 6.6 years, which minimizes the ability to see the effect of weight on mortality. Smoking and other variables were not considered. Also, frame size

TABLE 20-2. Classification of Overweight and Obesity by BMI, Waist Circumference, and Associated Disease Risks

	BMI (kg/m^2)	Obesity Class	*Disease Risk* Relative to Normal Weight and Waist Circumference* Men ≤102 cm (≤40 in.) Women ≤88 cm (≤35 in.)	>102 cm (>40 in.) >88 cm (>35 in.)
Underweight	<18.5		—	—
Normal†	18.5–24.9		—	—
Overweight	25.0–29.9		Increased	High
Obesity	30.0–34.9	I	High	Very high
	35.0–39.9	II	Very high	Very high
Extreme obesity	≥40	III	Extremely high	Extremely high

*Disease risk for type 2 diabetes, hypertension, and CVD.

†Increase waist circumference can also be a marker for increased risk even in persons of normal weight.

Source: From Ref. 11.

was not actually measured, and patients were weighed with their shoes and clothes. Among approximately 4.2 million subjects, only 100,000 (2.5 percent) died during the course of the study. Finally, 10 percent of the heights and weights were self-reported. Other studies relating mortality to weight, including the Framingham, American Cancer Society, and National Health and Nutrition Examination Survey (NHANES) studies, all suffer from one or more of these problems, limiting the usefulness of height–weight tables. Of great importance is the fact that none of these studies considered the distribution of the body fat by measuring the waist circumference or waist-to-hip ratio, which has recently been shown to be predictive of multiple complications of obesity.

In summary, the usual methods to assess the fatness of patients in clinical practice—height–weight tables and BMI—do not measure fatness, and the databases on which risk is assessed are either inadequate or flawed. Nevertheless, these measurements are easy to acquire, and most evidence indicates that assigning a patient as obese on the basis of these data, while not quantitatively accurate, is usually qualitatively correct. Furthermore, there are ample data relating obesity based on height–weight tables and

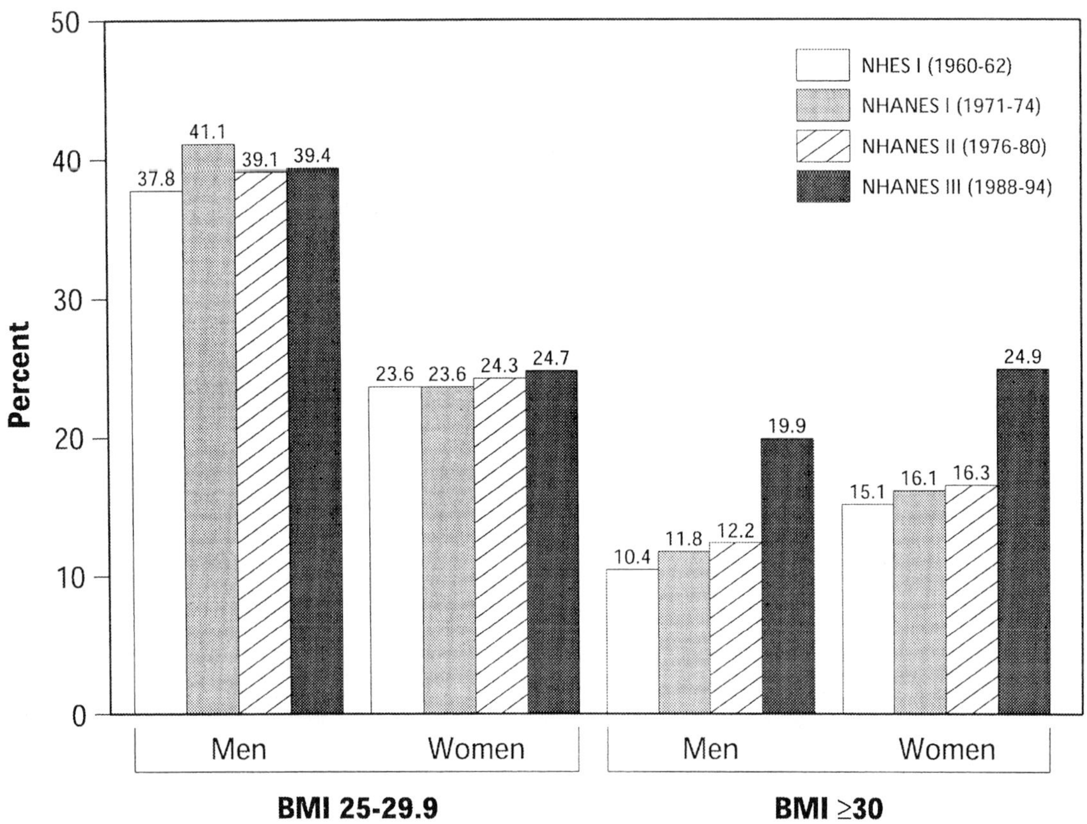

FIGURE 20-1. Age adjusted prevalence of overweight (BMI 25–29.9) and obesity (BMI ≥ 30) from 1960 to 1994. (*From ref.* 11 *with permission.*)

BMI to morbidity and mortality and demonstrating that weight loss lessens risk by reducing concomitant risk factors such as hypertension. Furthermore, supplementing BMI with waist/hip ratios or waist circumference may be extremely useful. Until inexpensive, easy to use, precise, and accurate methods for measuring adiposity become available, the current height–weight measurements or BMI, supplemented with waist measurements, are useful if not ideal. The waist-to-hip ratio and waist circumference are discussed below under Body Fat Distribution. The NIH Expert Panel[11] has recommended that in clinical practice, the abdominal fat content should be assessed and followed by measuring the waist circumference, as waist circumference has been found to be a better marker of abdominal fat content than the waist-to-hip ratio.[14] The recommended method to measure waist circumference is to mark the uppermost lateral border of the right iliac crest at the midaxillary line and place a measuring tape in a horizontal plane around the abdomen at the level of this mark parallel to the floor. The tape should be snug but not compress the skin and the measurement made during a normal minimal inspiration.[7]

PREVALENCE AND ECONOMIC COSTS OF OBESITY

Based on the NIH definitions of overweight and obesity using BMI as cited previously (Table 20-2), the prevalence of obesity in the United States is not only high but is rising rapidly.[12] As reviewed in the NIH document, 97 million adults in the United States are overweight or obese. According to NAHNES III[11] (Fig. 20-1), during the period from 1960 to 1994, the prevalence of overweight increased from 30.5 to 32 percent and obesity from 12.8 to 22.5 percent. In 1994, 39.4 percent of men and 24.7 percent of women were overweight and 19.9 percent of men and 24.9 percent of women were obese. For adults over the age of 20, 32.6 percent are overweight and 22.3 percent obese. The prevalence is also increasing among children and adolescents, an effect attributed to a more sedentary lifestyle. The prevalence of overweight and obesity is especially alarming among minority populations. For example, among Mexican-American and non-Hispanic black women, 66 percent are overweight and 33.3 to 37.7 percent are obese, respectively. Other minorities such as Puerto Ricans, Cuban-Americans, and Pacific Islanders have similar high prevalences. The prevalence of overweight and obesity (BMI > 27.8 for men and > 27.3 for women) among American Indians from New Mexico, Arizona, and North Dakota ranges from 54 to 67 percent for men and 66–80 percent for women.

The economic costs of obesity are staggering. In 1995,[15] the total costs attributed to obesity in the U.S. were \$99.2 billion. Of that, \$51.6 billion are direct costs associated with diseases attributed to obesity and \$47.6 billion are indirect costs (i.e., the costs of lost output due to the morbidity and mortality of obesity) that are comparable to the costs of cigarette smoking. The direct costs of obesity are 5.7 percent of our national health care expenditures.

MEDICAL COMPLICATIONS OF OBESITY (TABLE 20-3)

Obesity is associated with increased mortality and documented increased morbidity due to hypertension; type 2 diabetes; coronary artery disease; stroke; gallbladder disease; osteoarthritis; sleep apnea and respiratory problems; some types of cancer including endometrial, breast, prostate, and colon; complications of pregnancy; menstrual irregularities; hirsutism; stress incontinence, and depression.

TABLE 20-3. Medical Complications of Obesity

Cardiovascular
Coronary artery disease
Myocardial infarction
Congestive heart failure
Sudden death
Cerebrovascular accidents
Hypertension
Left ventricular hypertrophy
Metabolic
Hyperlipidemia
Insulin resistance
Noninsulin-dependent diabetes mellitus
Cholesterol gallstones
Cancer
Males: colon, rectum, prostate
Females: breast, ovary, endometrium, cervix, gallbladder, bile ducts
Hormonal
Menstrual abnormalities
Hyperandrogenism
Hirsutism
Acanthosis nigricans
Polycystic ovaries
Decreased sex hormone-binding globulin
Increased estrogens
Decreased testosterone in males
Decreased growth hormone
Decreased prolactin responsiveness
Enhanced cortisol production
Rheumatic
Osteoarthritis
Pulmonary
Decreased functional residual capacity, expiratory reserve volume, total lung capacity
Increased residual volume and diffusing capacity
Decreased maximum expiratory flow rate in males
Sleep apnea and obesity hypoventilation syndrome

Mortality

The relation between body weight and mortality has been reviewed.[11,16] Data from the Framingham study[17] evaluated mortality in men followed for 30 years from the date of entry. These data and those from the 1979 Build Study[9,18] indicate that the effects of obesity on mortality are delayed by approximately 10 years (Fig. 20-2). Framingham data (Fig. 20-2) also indicate that in both nonsmokers and smokers the effects of obesity on mortality are demonstrable in each age decade, with the lowest mortality in men who are 100–109 percent of ideal body weight (IBW). In smokers, mortality curves are J-shaped, with those below IBW having a higher mortality than do those at IBW. In nonsmokers the mortality curves are also J-shaped, but there are an inadequate number of men who are underweight to evaluate mortality risk in this group. Overweight nonsmoking men age 30–39 at entry have mortality rates before age 70 that are 3.9 times those of nonsmoking men who are 100 to 109 percent of IBW. The relative risk is 8.8 for smoking men and 9.8 for overweight smoking men, indicating that the risk of smoking far exceeds that of obesity.[19] The 1979 Build

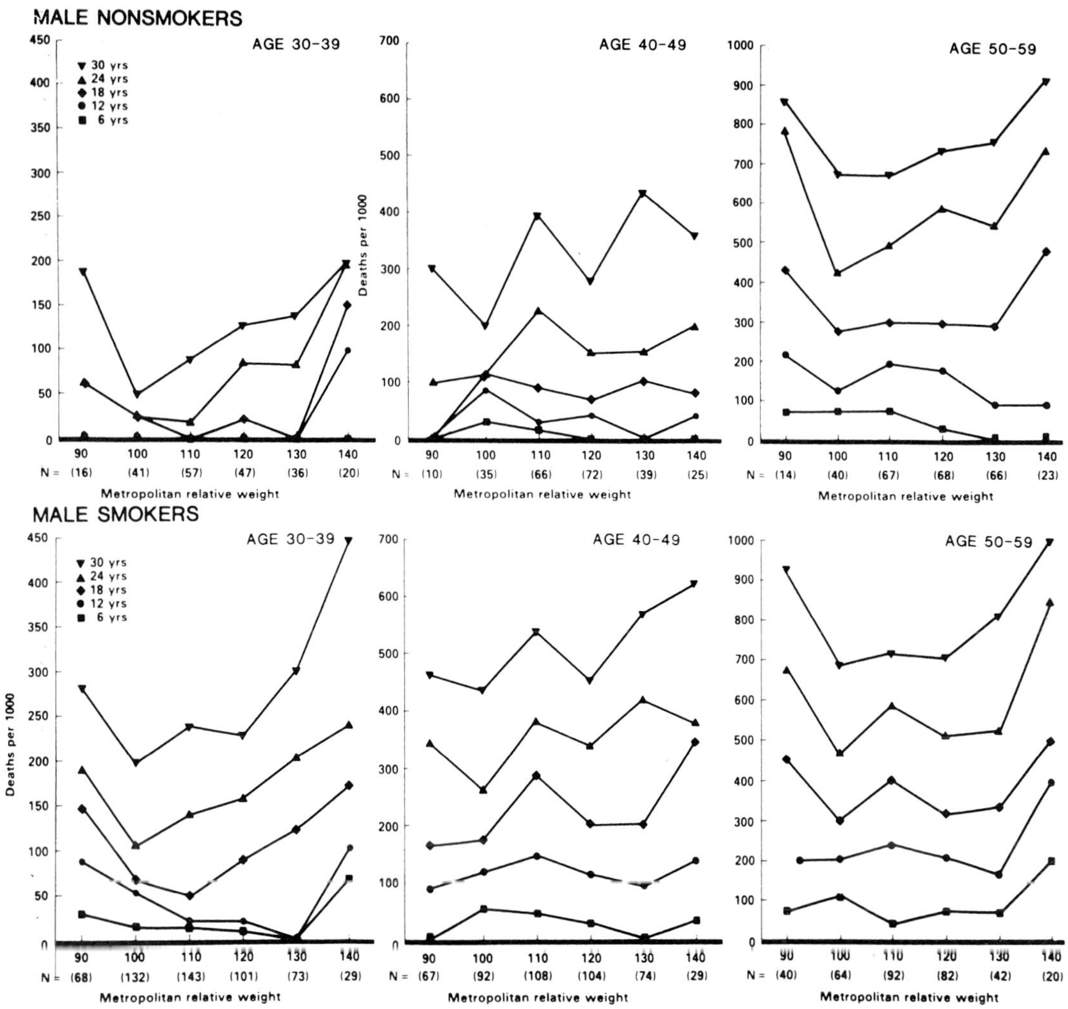

FIGURE 20-2. Cumulative death rates per 1,000 male nonsmokers (top graphs) and smokers (bottom graphs) according to age group and duration of follow-up in 6-year intervals (6, 12, 18, 24, and 30 years). (*From Feinleib,*[17] *with permission.*)

Study[9,18] was conducted from 1950 to 1972 and included approximately 4 million people. The lowest mortality in men, adjusted for length of follow-up, was at 25 percent below to 5 percent above average weight, and in females it was from 15 percent below to 5 percent above average weight. Similar data were obtained in the American Cancer Society study[9,20] and the Harvard Alumni[21] study, with the lowest mortality occurring in nonsmoking persons 80 to 89 percent of average weight adjusted for height. When cigarette smoking and duration of obesity are taken into consideration, obesity is clearly a risk factor for early death. Studies of insured persons show that underweight people have a high initial mortality that decreases with time, while obese individuals have a low initial mortality that increases with time. Thus, most epidemiologic studies show that the lowest mortality occurs at slightly below average weight for both sexes and that mortality increases both above and below the "optimal" weight. Troiano et al[22] in a meta-analysis of 19 studies points out the limitations of insurance studies including the relatively affluent populations they represent. This attenuates the risk of a low BMI. These authors found a U-shaped curve for mortality with increased mortality at a BMI <23 and >28. In a review of 25 major prospective studies evaluating the association of body weight and longevity, Manson et al.[16] noted that separating obesity from other risk factors such as cholesterol, systolic blood pressure, left ventricular hypertrophy, and glucose intolerance can be difficult. In the Framingham Study, only 8 percent of males and 18 percent of females in the highest weight class were free of risk factors. These conditions are effects of obesity with complex interrelationships, not confounding variables.[16,22,23] If obesity is directly causal for these factors, then obesity may exert its influence on longevity through them, and controlling for them will produce an independent but not a true effect of obesity on longevity. Manson et al[24] recently published the results of the prospective Nurses' Health Study in which prospective data were collected by questionnaire during 16 years of follow-up. The data indicated that the J-shaped curvilinear relationship between BMI and total mortality existed only when smokers were included in the analysis. The relative risk of death from all causes (Fig. 20-3), death from cardiovascular disease (Fig. 20-4), and

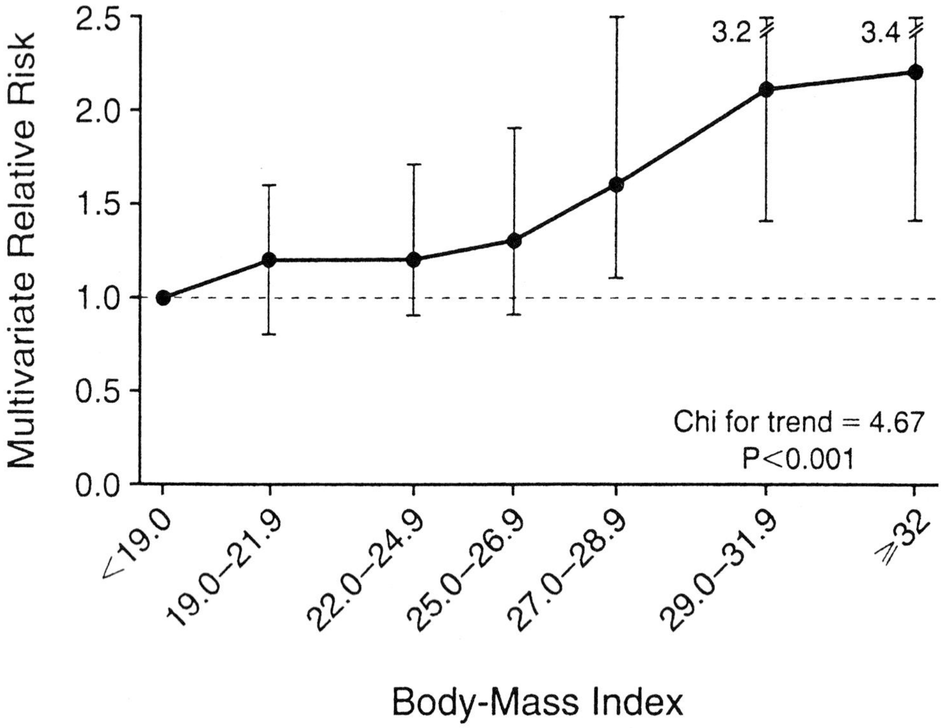

FIGURE 20-3. The relationship between body mass index and the relative risk of death from all causes in 531 deaths when the analysis (1980–1992) is restricted to women who never smoked and who had a stable weight for the previous four years. (*From Manson et al.,*[24] *with permission.*)

death from cancer was lowest at a BMI of <19 and rose to 2.1, 4.1, and 2.1, respectively, for a BMI ≥32. Weight gain was associated with increased mortality, especially from coronary heart disease. Subjects who gained 10–19 kg and ≥20 kg had a relative risk of death from coronary heart disease of 2.6 and 7.4, respectively. Women who lost ≥10 kg had a relative risk of 0.3. Obesity in adolescents is also associated with an increased risk of mortality and morbidity and, with the exception of diabetes, the risk is independent of adult weight.[25] Other reviews and studies showing that weight loss and weight cycling has an adverse effect on mortality[26–28] have been criticized.[29,30] These studies are all subject to significant potential problems such as failure to consider smoking, to exclude people with health problems at entry, to consider cultural and socioeconomic variability and numerous other problems.[30] Sorkin et al.,[31] however, recently concluded that hypothesized errors such as these do not significantly distort the analyses.

The ratio of the waist circumference to hip circumference was recently shown to be positively associated with all-cause mortality in primarily white women aged 55–69 years old (Table 20-4).[29] The relationship did not show the usual J-shaped curve (Fig. 20-4).[24] In this study, every 0.15-unit increase in the waist to hip ratio was associated with a 1.6-fold increase in the relative risk of death after adjusting for other factors including BMI. The women at most risk for death had a low BMI and a high waist-to-hip ratio.

The association of BMI with mortality is applicable to African Americans but weakens in older individuals, especially those aged 75 and above.[11,32]

Cardiovascular Disease

There has been substantial controversy about the relation between obesity and coronary artery disease.[32] Autopsy studies in general do not show an association between coronary artery disease and obesity, whereas epidemiologic studies do. Most notable is the Framingham Study,[34] which showed a positive relation between obesity as an independent risk factor for the 26-year incidence of cardiovascular disease, particularly among women (Fig. 20-5). The percentage of desirable weight on initial examination predicted the 26-year incidence of coronary disease, coronary death, and congestive heart failure in men independent of other risk factors. In women, relative weight was positively and independently associated with coronary disease, stroke, congestive heart failure, and death from coronary and cardiovascular disease. For example, in men below 50, the 26-year incidence of coronary heart disease per 1,000 subjects was 177 for a Metropolitan relative weight less

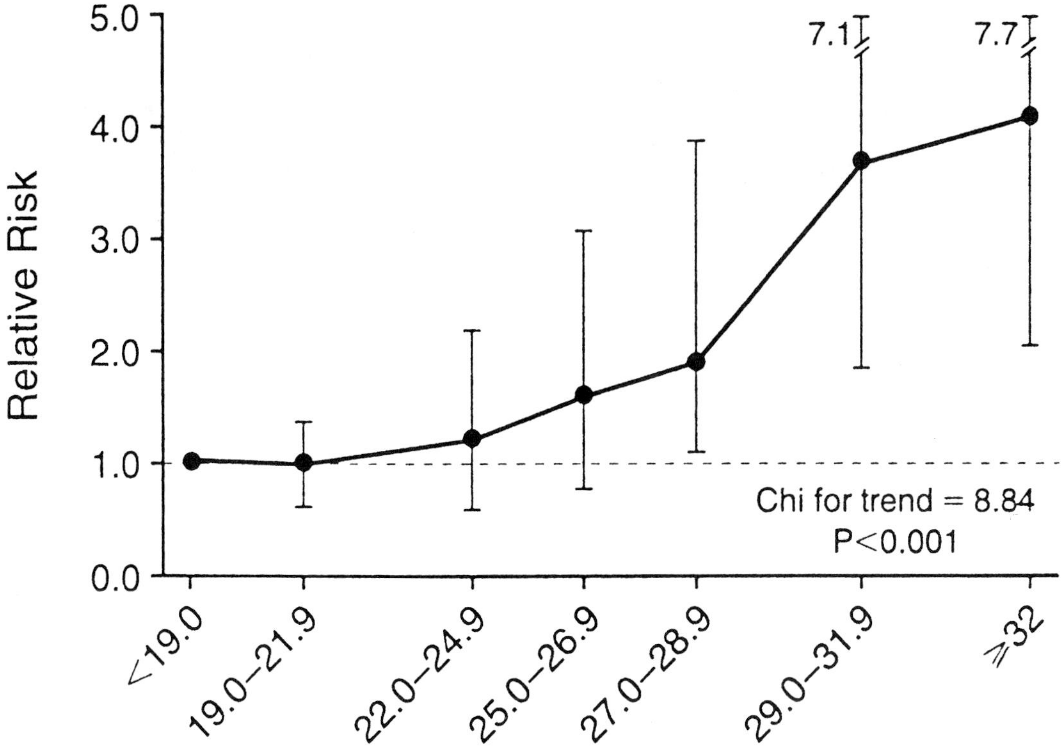

FIGURE 20-4. Relative risk of death from cardiovascular disease in 184 deaths according to body mass index among women who never smoked. (*From Manson et al.,*[24] *with permission.*)

than 110 percent and 350 for a Metropolitan relative weight greater than 130 percent. In women below 50 years old, the 26-year incidence was 76 per 1,000 for women less than 110 percent and 179 per 1,000 for women greater than 130 percent. For myocardial infarction in men below 50, the 26-year incidence was 110 per 1,000 for men less than 110 percent of Metropolitan relative weight and 187 per 1,000 for men greater than 130 percent of Metropolitan relative weight. In women who were below 50 years

TABLE 20-4. Multivariate Adjusted Relative Risk of Death Within a 5-Year Follow-Up Period, According to Quintiles of Body Mass Index or Waist–Hip Circumference Ratio (WHR), in Women Aged 55–69 Years

Model No.	Subjects	No. of Deaths	Variable*	Relative Risk for Quintile 1	2	3	4	5	Trend, *P*
1	All	1469	BMI	1.00	0.75	0.68	0.64	0.74	<.001
			WHR	1.00	1.51	1.63	2.09	2.56	<.001
2	Never smokers	720	BMI	1.00	0.83	0.64	0.65	0.80	.02
			WHR	1.00	1.44	1.56	2.11	2.39	<.001
3	Never smokers, excluding those who lost >5 kg since age 50 yr or died in first 2 follow-up years	410	BMI	1.00	1.09	0.75	0.93	1.13	.85
			WHR	1.00	1.16	1.20	1.68	2.05	<.001
4	Ever smokers	725	BMI	1.00	0.68	0.74	0.66	0.69	.008
			WHR	1.00	1.50	1.60	1.87	2.42	<.001

*Dummy variables for BMI quintiles and WHR quintiles were included in each model along with the following covariates: model 1, age, education level, marital status, alcohol use, estrogen use, and smoking status; models 2 and 3, age, education level, marital status, alcohol use, and estrogen use; and model 4, age, education level, marital status, alcohol intake, estrogen use, smoking status (current/past), and pack-years of cigarettes.

Source: From Folsom et al.[29]

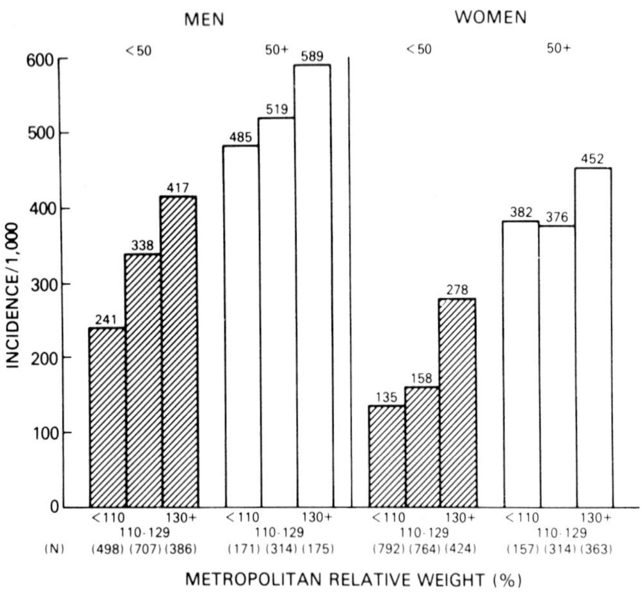

FIGURE 20-5. Twenty-six-year incidence of coronary heart disease from the Framingham Heart Study by Metropolitan Relative Weight at entry among men and women less than or more than 50 years old. N = number at risk. The numbers over the bars indicate incidence rate per 1,000. (*From Hubert et al.,*[34] *with permission.*)

old upon entering the study, the 26-year incidence was 24 per 1,000 if less than 110 percent of IBW and 59 per 1,000 if greater than 130 percent of IBW. Similar differences were observed for sudden death, congestive heart failure, and cerebrovascular accidents. Perhaps of greatest interest is the fact that the relative odds of developing cardiovascular disease were related to the degree of change of Metropolitan relative weight before age 25 years and entry into the Framingham Study. The men and women who lost weight decreased their relative odds, while those who gained weight increased their relative odds (Fig. 20-6).[34] Similarly, the American Cancer Society[20] and Manitoba studies[34] showed positive relations between the percent overweight or BMI and mortality from or incidence of coronary heart disease. The Nurses' Health Study[24,36] showed that higher levels of BMI even within the "normal range" and weight gain after 18 years old were associated with an increased risk of coronary heart disease as well as a positive relationship between BMI and death due to cardiovascular disease (Fig. 20-4). Several other studies, however, have shown no such relation.[33,37]

Recent data from the Nurses' Health Study[37] has shown that both obesity and weight gain are risk factors for ischemic but not hemorrhagic stroke.

As mentioned above, overweight and obesity as well as duration of obesity are important risk factors for congestive heart failure (CHF).[11,34,38,39] Duration of obesity is a predictor of CHF.[11] These associations may be related to the association of obesity with hypertension, left ventricular hypertrophy, and sleep apnea. [38,40,41] The cardiomyopathy associated with obesity is manifest as ventricular dilation and eccentric hypertrophy, is associated with both systolic and diastolic dysfunction, and may result from elevated blood volume and high cardiac output.[40,41]As mentioned later, CHF is also associated with the obesity hypoventilation syndrome or sleep apnea.

Body Fat Distribution

Of great importance and of considerable recent interest and attention has been the issue of body fat distribution and the metabolic

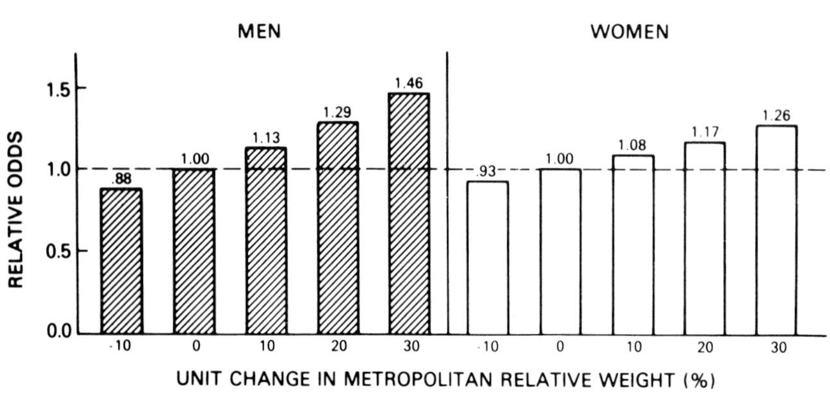

FIGURE 20-6. The relative odds of developing cardiovascular disease corresponding to the percent change in Metropolitan Relative Weight between age 25 and entry into the Framingham Heart Study. (*From Hubert et al.,*[34] *with permission.*)

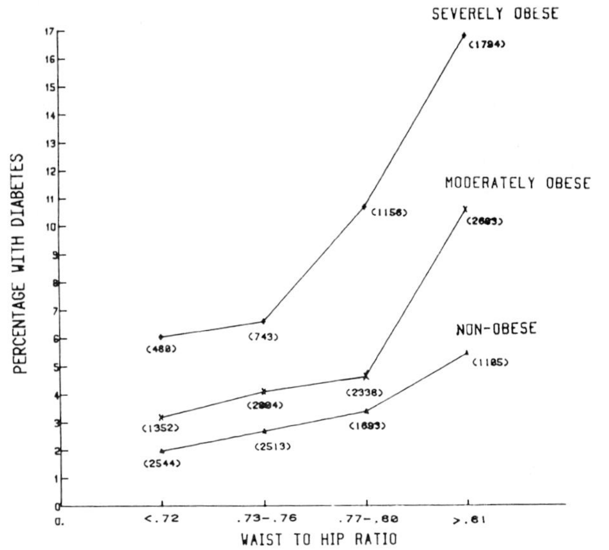

FIGURE 20-7. The prevalence of diabetes according to relative weight and body fat distribution in 20,325 women. (*From Hartz et al.,*[44] *with permission.*)

complications of obesity.[42] Jean Vague drew attention to "android" (waist-predominant) and "gynoid" (hip-predominant) obesity and the association of android obesity with diabetes and atherosclerosis.[43] The relation between the metabolic complications of obesity and the distribution of body fat was greater than the relation with weight alone.

Subsequent studies have confirmed and extended these observations. Hartz et al. evaluated data on 2,165 women 40–59 years of age and 11,791 women 20–39 years of age who were enrolled in a weight-reduction program.[44] They found that the ratio of waist girth to hip girth was significantly associated with diabetes (Fig. 20-7), hypertension (Fig. 20-8), and gallbladder disease in women age 40–59 and with menstrual abnormalities in women age 20–39. The distribution of fat was associated with higher disease prevalence even among women with comparable total body fat. In the study of Kissebah et al., plasma glucose and insulin levels during oral glucose loading as well as fasting plasma triglycerides were significantly higher in women with predominately upper body obesity.[45] Krotkiewski et al. studied 930 obese men and women and found similar relations.[46] Peiris et al. demonstrated in a group of 33 healthy but modestly obese women that visceral fat distribution assessed by computed tomography accounts for a greater degree of variance than does total body fat mass in regard to cumulative insulin levels during a glucose tolerance test, triglyceride levels, and systolic and diastolic blood pressure.[47] Evans et al. demonstrated that an increase in the percentage of free testosterone in women was associated with an increasing waist–hip ratio, increased plasma glucose and insulin levels, and diminished insulin sensitivity.[48] This group also showed insulin resistance in muscle in subjects with higher waist–hip ratios as well as a decreased hepatic extraction of insulin.[49,50] Interestingly, in women receiving testosterone, increases in intraabdominal fat have been observed consistent with associations in women between high androgen levels and increased intraabdominal fat.[51] Glucocorticoids have also been postulated to play a role.[52] Others[53–56] have shown similar relations between abdominal obesity and insulin, triglycerides, hypertension, low-density lipoprotein (LDL), and plasminogen activator inhibitor-1 as well as low high-density lipoprotein (HDL) cholesterol levels. Among epidemiologic studies, the Gothenberg study[55] followed 792 men born in 1913 for 13 years and found statistically significant associations between the ratio of waist to hip circumference and the occurrence of stroke and ischemic heart disease. Among 1,452 women in Gothenberg followed for 12 years,[57] there was a significant positive association between the ratio of waist-to-hip circumference and the 12-year incidence of myocardial infarction, angina, stroke, and death. In a multivariate analysis, the association of the waist–hip ratio with myocardial infarction remained.

The mechanism of the relation between the waist–hip ratio and the metabolic complications of obesity is unknown. Obese individuals with high waist–hip ratios have decreased hepatic extraction of insulin, higher posthepatic insulin levels, and more insulin resistance.[49] The increased insulin resistance has led to the suggestion that enhanced free fatty acid delivery to the liver from intraabdominal stores may decrease insulin uptake by the liver and lead to peripheral hyperinsulinemia. This might explain the association of increased intra-abdominal fat with conditions associated with hyperinsulinemia, such as noninsulin-dependent diabetes (NIDDM), hypertension, hyperlipidemia, and atherosclerosis.[58] The combination of obesity, hyperinsulinemia, insulin resistance, hypertension, and a predisposition to NIDDM has been postulated to be part of a common metabolic abnormality caused by a combination of hyperinsulinemia and insulin resistance.[59] Interestingly, when obese women reduce to ideal body weight, intra-abdominal and hip subcutaneous fat depots are reduced to normal. The waist-to-hip ratio and subcutaneous fat, however, remain significantly increased compared to a never-obese control group.[60] Finally, cigarette smoking, an important risk factor for cardiovascular disease, is associated with an in-

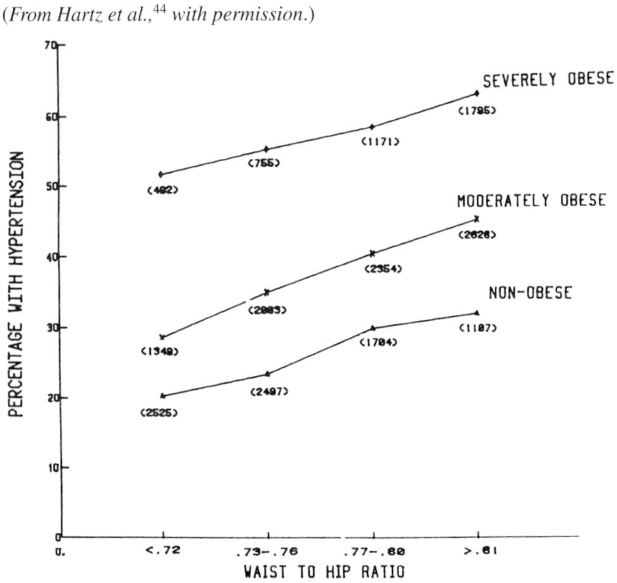

FIGURE 20-8. The prevalence of hypertension according to relative weight and body fat distribution in 20,380 women from 40 to 59 years old. (*From Hartz et al.,*[44] *with permission.*)

creased waist–hip ratio in a dose-dependent manner.[61] This is independent of BMI, and while it was seen in both sexes, the association was stronger in women. This stronger association has been postulated to be due to the enhanced adrenal androgen levels associated with cigarette smoking.

Metabolic Disorders

Diabetes

The well-established association between obesity, duration of obesity and weight gain,[62–66] and insulin resistance and type 2 diabetes is discussed in Chap. 19. Table 20-5 illustrates the relative risk for type 2 diabetes from the Nurses' Health Study.[62] Even women with an average body mass index of 24–24.9 had an age adjusted relative risk of type 2 diabetes of 5.0 compared to women with a BMI of <22. A BMI of ≥35 increases the age-adjusted relative risk to 93.2. Weight loss decreases and weight gain increases the age-adjusted risk of type 2 diabetes (Table 20-5). This relationship is further modified by the BMI at age 18, that is, the higher the BMI at age 18, the greater the relative risk of developing diabetes with any given weight gain. As expected, a family history of type 2 diabetes also increases risk with weight gain.

Insulin resistance and hyperinsulinemia are characteristic features of human obesity.[67–76] This resistance is especially pronounced at physiologic concentrations of insulin in patients with normal glucose tolerance,[71] is closely related to plasma insulin levels,[73] and involves glucose storage and oxidation.[69,77] Both glucose storage and glucose oxidation are directly related to glucose uptake during euglycemic hyperinsulinemia, but glucose storage makes a progressively greater contribution to glucose uptake from the most to the least insulin-resistant subjects with normal glucose tolerance. The degree of insulin resistance associated with obesity and whether resistance occurs at both maximal and submaximal insulin concentrations vary from study to study.[68,70,71,73,75] The reasons for such variability could include the use of height–weight tables or BMI[68–71,74,78] rather than true measures of the percentage of fat,[72,73,76,77] the lumping together of upper and lower body obese patients,[67–73,75–78] and the inclusion of obese patients with impaired glucose tolerance.[68,70,75,78,79] Peiris et al. performed multiple-dose euglycemic clamp studies on 10 females with lower and upper body obesity and found significant reductions in glucose utilization with the 300 $mU/m^2/min$ clamp only in the group with upper body obesity (waist–hip ratio >0.85).[74] These authors did not measure the percentage of body fat directly, and their obese subjects did not have glucose tolerance tests. Some studies have included only patients with normal glucose tolerance,[69,71–73,77] and some have included patients with impaired glucose tolerance.[67,69,75,78,79] Only a few have studied patients with both normal glucose tolerance and measured the percentage of fat,[72,73,77,80] and several have done neither.[40,67,69,78] In the Pima Indian population, the degree of obesity does not account for the distribution of insulin action, which is a mixture of three normal distributions. However, a greater proportion of the more obese Pimas are in the more insulin-resistant groups.[76] Pima Indians who are insulin resistant are more likely to become obese. This is consistent with the strong association between obesity and type 2 diabetes and the paucity of studies of obese subjects with normal glucose tolerance. To our knowledge, a study of obese Caucasians prior to weight gain or after weight loss to IBW to evaluate the hypothesis that insulin resistance predisposes individuals to obesity has never been conducted. One could postulate that a defect in glucose uptake in muscle would lead to hyperinsulinemia, which could lead to increased storage of calories as fat or lean body mass as a result of normal or enhanced insulin action in areas such as lipoprotein lipase or protein synthesis and insulin resistance in other areas (i.e., glucose uptake and apolipoprotein B secretion).[81] Indeed, there are many examples of differential insulin resistance in the same and different tissues.[81–84] Insulin resistance has been implicated in the etiology of type 2 diabetes, hypertension, and hypertriglyceridemia.[59,81,85–89] It is possible that insulin resistance is also etiologic in the development of obesity. In recent studies of Pima Indians, however, most insulin resistance was associated with lower rates of weight gain.[90]

The primary mechanism of insulin resistance in human obesity is unknown, although several potential contributing factors have been identified including elevated free fatty acids,[91–93] leptin,[94] TNF alpha,[95,96] variants of PPAR gamma[97,98] polymorphisms of the Beta 3 adrenergic receptor,[99–101] dietary fat and muscle triglyceride,[102] and others including cortisol.[52] The roles of

TABLE 20-5. Attained Body Mass Index and Relative Risk for Noninsulin-Dependent Diabetes Mellitus in U.S. Women Aged 30–55 Years in 1976 and Followed for 14 Years

Body Mass Index (kg/m^2)	Cases (*n*)	Person-Years of Follow-Up	Age-Standardized Incidence Rate* (%)	Age-Adjusted Relative Risk (95 percent CI)
>22.0	55	466,052	13.0	1.0 (reference)
22.0–22.9	71	194,433	37.4	2.9 (2.0–4.1)
23.0–23.9	88	156,770	54.9	4.3 (3.1–5.8)
24.0–24.9	94	142,392	62.9	5.0 (3.6–6.6)
25.0–26.9	227	198,484	103.5	8.1 (6.2–10.5)
27.0–28.9	267	119,662	200.4	15.8 (12.7–19.8)
29.0–30.9	329	84,880	354.5	27.6 (22.7–33.5)
31.0–32.9	263	47,119	521.2	40.3 (33.7–48.3)
33.0–34.9	224	29,885	703.6	54.0 (45.6–64.0)
≥35.0	579	46,636	1190.5	93.2 (81.4–106.6)

*Rate per 100,000 persons standardized to the age distribution of length of follow-up in the cohort.

Source: From Colditz et al.[62]

leptin,[94] TNF alpha,[97] and the Beta 3 receptor[103,104] are controversial. Other proposed mechanisms of insulin resistance are decreased capillary density,[89] a decreased ability of insulin to increase blood flow,[105] and decreased physical fitness as reflected in a decreased V_{O2max}.[75,106] Whatever the underlying cause, the insulin resistance in the periphery is manifested as a decrease in insulin stimulated glucose transport/phosphorylation.[80] In preliminary studies in our laboratory, this defect is ameliorated with weight loss.

Lipid Abnormalities

Obesity is frequently associated with hypertriglyceridemia, and plasma triglyceride levels and the very low density lipoprotein (VLDL) production rate are related to insulin levels[107–114] and the percentage of body weight that is fat.[114,115] It has been postulated that this hypertriglyceridemia is due to hyperinsulinemia.[115,116] However, in studies in humans[111,112,117,118] and in human[119] and rat hepatocytes,[120,121] insulin acutely inhibited both apolipoprotein B and VLDL triglyceride secretion from the liver. This is due to both direct mechanisms at the level of the liver cell and the ability of insulin to decrease free fatty acids released from adipose tissue, which decreases the substrate supply for VLDL triglyceride synthesis.[81,111,112,115] It is possible that an inability of insulin to elicit these effects—i.e., insulin resistance—combined with enhanced triglyceride synthesis, increases the production of VLDL and causes the hypertriglyceridemia of obesity.[81,111,112,118,119,122,123] There is also substantial variability in lipoprotein lipase levels in obese subjects, and it is likely that the balance between VLDL triglyceride production and triglyceride clearance determines whether an obese subject will have hypertriglyceridemia.[111,112,116] In fact, patients with hypertriglyceridemia have been shown to be insulin-resistant,[59,113,122–124] and subjects with high insulin levels have higher blood pressure and serum triglycerides. HDL cholesterol levels are also lower in obese individuals,[110,113,125] consistent with their hypertriglyceridemia.[110] Obese subjects, especially those with predominately abdominal obesity, also have a higher prevalence of increased total and LDL cholesterol.[113,126–128] Weight loss generally leads to favorable changes in plasma lipids and lipoproteins.[129,130]

Hypertension

The relationship between obesity and hypertension has been reviewed recently.[131,132] In the Framingham study,[133] 70 percent of hypertension in men and 61 percent in women was directly attributable to excess adiposity. For every 10 lb of excess weight, systolic blood pressure increases 4.5 mmHg. Changes in insulin secretion and/or action have been implicated in the pathogenesis of hypertension associated with obesity.[123,124,131,132,134–136] Hypertension is related to insulin resistance[48,123,124,136,137] and central obesity.[138,139] In young, healthy, nonobese, nondiabetic, hypertensive subjects, stimulation of nonoxidative glucose disposal is impaired, and the severity of insulin resistance is closely related to the increase in blood pressure.[48,132] Normotensive, nonobese offspring of hypertensive parents are also insulin resistant.[132]

There are several possible mechanisms by which insulin might produce hypertension.[123,131,132] Insulin increases sodium reabsorption in both the proximal and distal tubules.[140–143] Indeed, obese individuals have normal responsiveness to the sodium-retaining effects of insulin.[144] Obese patients have increased total body sodium,[145–147] and weight loss leads to a natriuresis and dramatic decreases in blood pressure and insulin levels.[148–150] A second postulated mechanism of hypertension in obesity involves activation of the sympathetic nervous system.[110,123,151–153] In this regard, both hyperinsulinemia[154,155] and dietary intake[132] increase the activity of the sympathetic nervous system. As expected, weight reduction leads to sodium losses and decreases in sympathetic nervous system activity.[144,149,156–158] Rocchini et al. studied 60 obese adolescents and found an increased sensitivity of blood pressure to sodium restriction compared with nonobese adolescents.[159] This sensitivity to sodium disappeared with weight reduction and was not closely associated with decreases in insulin, norepinephrine, and aldosterone levels. These authors postulated that the sodium sensitivity of hypertensive obese individuals might be due to a combination of hyperinsulinemia, hyperaldosteronism, and increased activity of the sympathetic nervous system. Obese individuals also have increased plasma volume[123,144,145] and increased thickness of the left ventricular wall.[160] Weight loss leads to reduction in both parameters. Visceral obesity, which is associated with hyperinsulinemia and insulin resistance, is also associated with a higher incidence of hypertension,[44,55,161,162] increasing the association between hyperinsulinemia, activation of the sympathetic nervous system, obesity, and hypertension. Although insulin normally induces vasodilatation, this effect of insulin is impaired in insulin-resistant states including obesity.[163,164] It is not known, however, what effect, if any, obesity has on the ability of insulin to activate the sympathetic nervous system.

Thus, obesity is associated with an expanded plasma volume, hyperinsulinemia that increases sodium resorption by the kidney and activates the sympathetic nervous system, increased sensitivity of blood pressure to changes in body sodium, and resistance to the vasodilating effects of insulin. Variable sensitivities to any of these factors could explain why some obese subjects are hypertensive and others are normotensive. Additionally, it should be kept in mind that not all obese subjects become normotensive with weight reduction and that not all hyperlipidemic obese subjects become normolipidemic with weight loss. Thus, some obese subjects have other underlying causes of hypertension.

Gallstones

There is a strong association between obesity and cholesterol gallstones. In a recent study the risk was linearly related to weight and increased with age. A person approximately 50 percent above IBW has an approximately six-fold increase in the incidence of symptomatic gallstones.[165,166] These data have recently been confirmed.[167,168] Obesity and overnutrition both increase biliary secretion of cholesterol.[169,170] Total body cholesterol synthesis is increased in obesity,[171–173] and hepatic cholesterol synthesis is increased in patients with gallstones[174] and is enhanced by insulin.[175] The Pima Indians have an extremely high incidence of cholesterol gallstones, affecting approximately 80 percent of Pima women.[176] In addition to enhanced cholesterol secretion in bile as a result of obesity, Pima Indians also have decreased bile acid pool sizes.[177] Together, these factors lead to supersaturation of bile. Such a defect has not been demonstrated in Caucasians. Thus, obesity is associated with increased hepatic cholesterol synthesis, increased biliary cholesterol secretion, and gallbladder bile supersaturation with cholesterol. As discussed later, the risk of gallstone formation rises during weight loss in an exponential fashion, with the risk increasing dramatically at rates of weight loss above 1.5 kg per week.

Cancer

Obesity is also associated with a higher incidence of cancer. Obese males have higher mortality from cancer of the colon, rectum, and prostate, and obese females have higher mortality from cancer of the gallbladder, bile ducts, breast, endometrium, cervix, and ovaries.[110,178–183] The mechanism of the enhanced risk of cancer in obese patients is unknown. Studies have cast doubt on the relation between dietary fat and breast and colon cancer.[184–186] As reviewed, however, the role of diet has not been excluded.[110,186] Because androgens are converted to estrogens in adipose tissue, a role for increased estrogen levels in the development of breast and uterine cancer is a possibility.[187] It is well known that adipose tissue aromatizes androgens to estrogens.[188–192] Furthermore, body weight and the percentage of conversion of androstenedione to estrone are highly correlated in women.[193] In obese postmenopausal women, estrogen levels are also increased.[194]

Endocrine Disorders

Obesity,[195] especially abdominal obesity,[44] is associated with menstrual abnormalities. Rogers and Mitchell reported that among 100 patients with menstrual disorders, 43 were 20 percent or more above IBW.[196] In the control group of women of similar age with normal menstrual periods, the overall incidence of obesity was 13 percent. In a subsequent study these authors reported that 13 of 15 patients who lost weight had a return of menstrual function.[197] Hartz et al. also reported a higher incidence of menstrual abnormalities as well as hirsutism in obese women.[198] Hyperandrogenism is also associated with menstrual abnormalities in obese women and frequently with acanthosis nigricans.[199,200] Flier et al. reported that acanthosis nigricans occurred in 5 percent of patients being evaluated for hyperandrogenism and that all these patients were obese and insulin-resistant.[201] Compared with hyperandrogenized women of similar body weight, patients with acanthosis nigricans were more hyperinsulinemic and insulin-resistant. With weight loss, acanthosis nigricans remitted as insulin resistance improved.

The polycystic ovary syndrome consists of anovulation and hyperandrogenemia.[202] Data from the Nurses Health Study[203] indicated that the greater the BMI at age 18, even at levels lower than those considered to be obese, the greater the risk of ovulatory infertility. This was true both with and without the diagnosis of polycystic ovarian disease. Obesity is present in 40 percent of patients with polycystic ovaries.[204] As reviewed by Barnes and Rosenfield, obesity may contribute to the insulin resistance in the polycystic ovary syndrome; however, nonobese women with polycystic ovaries are also insulin-resistant.[204] The insulin resistance in the polycystic ovary syndrome correlates with the degree of hyperandrogenemia and in some, but not all studies, decreases with a reduction of androgen levels. It is likely that the hyperinsulinemia associated with insulin resistance is the cause of polycystic ovarian syndrome rather than the result of it. In obese women with this syndrome, weight loss reduces estrone levels and returns gonadotropin secretion to normal with resumption of regular menstrual cycles.[205,206] Also, because there is little or no improvement in insulin resistance with ovariectomy[207] or medical reduction of androgens,[208,209] it is possible that hyperinsulinemia is at least in part causal for hyperandrogenism. Evidence for this hypothesis includes the fact that there are insulin and IGF-I receptors on granulosa cells and other cells in the ovary; the fact that insulin and IGF-I stimulate steroidogenesis in granulosa, thecal, and stromal cells; the fact that insulin and IGF-I act synergistically with luteinizing hsormone (LH) or follicle stimulating hormone (FSH) to increase steroidogenesis in vitro; and the fact that insulin increases LH receptors and IGF-I enhances FSH induction of LH receptors in granulosa cells.[210,211] Further supporting a role for insulin in the hyperandrogenism of obese women with polycystic ovaries, Nestler et al. reduced serum insulin levels with diazoxide for 10 days and observed significant reductions in serum total testosterone and unbound testosterone.[212] Other studies have generally confirmed that lowering insulin improves ovulatory function and lowers androgen levels.[202,213,214] It has been proposed that the development of the polycystic ovary syndrome in obese patients may be caused by abnormal gonadotropin secretion induced by increased levels of estrone and by amplification of the action of LH on the ovary in the presence of insulin.[206,211]

Hirsute women with the polycystic ovary syndrome have higher insulin levels than do women with this syndrome alone, and there is a significant correlation between plasma insulin and plasma testosterone or androstenedione. The hyperandrogenism can be due to the effects of insulin on granulosa cells or possibly to the effect of insulin to increase gonadotropin secretion or enhance gonadotropin action.[208,209,214–216] Adipose tissue can also convert preandrogens to testosterone, and obesity is associated with the reduced sex hormone-binding globulin concentrations characteristic of hyperandrogen states.[215] Finally, it has been proposed that hyperandrogenemia may be responsible for the upper body fat localization in women with high waist–hip ratios (android obesity)[48] and decreased hepatic extraction of insulin.[217] In obese women with PCO the first line treatment is weight reduction.[204]

Decreased plasma testosterone and decreased sex hormone-binding globulin levels have been reported in men more than 160 percent of IBW.[218–220] Free testosterone levels are decreased in only some morbidly obese men who are more than 200 percent of IBW. The normal free testosterone level in most obese males is reflected in their normal masculinization, libido, potency, and spermatogenesis.[218,219] In morbidly obese men, the hypothalamic-hypophyseal-gonadal axis is normal as determined by the testicular response to human chorionic gonadotropin (hCG), the pituitary response to gonadotropin releasing hormone (GnRH), and the hypothalamic pituitary testicular response to clomiphene.[219,220] However, LH levels and LH pulse amplitude are decreased in morbidly obese men with decreased free testosterone levels.[219] As in women, estrogen levels rise with increasing obesity in men and decrease after weight reduction.[219]

Despite enhanced growth, growth hormone levels are reduced in obesity, especially abdominal obesity. Growth hormone responses to GnRH, sleep, exercise, fasting, protein, and pharmacologic stimuli such as L-dopa, L-dopa plus propranolol, glucagon plus propranolol, insulin, arginine GHRH, GHRH and pyriidostigmine, growth hormone releasing peptides, and other drugs are blunted.[219,221,222] Weight loss improves the growth hormone response. Despite decreased growth hormone levels, IGF-1 levels tend to be normal.[221] It has been proposed that hyperinsulinemia or increased nutrition may enhance IGF-1 production. Recent data indicate that reducing free fatty acid levels restores growth hormone responsiveness in obese subjects[222] but not obese patients with hypopituitarism.[223] Naltrexone also restores the growth hormone response to GHRH.[224] Prolactin levels are normal in obesity, but the response to pharmacologic stimuli such as thyrotropin releasing hormone (TRH) and chlorpromazine is blunted.[219,220] The significance of this is currently unknown.

Other endocrine abnormalities in obesity include enhanced cortisol production and clearance rates with normal cortisol levels, a normal pituitary response to corticotrophin releasing factor (CRF), and a normal adrenal responsiveness to ACTH.[219,225] The overnight 1-mg dexamethasone suppression is usually normal in obese subjects, although 13 percent of obese control subjects have false-positive tests.[225] Although urinary 17-hydroxycorticosteroids are increased in 27 percent of obese subjects, urinary free cortisol levels and diurnal cortisol rhythms are normal.[219,225,226] Interesting recent data evaluating cortisol metabolism suggest increased metabolism of cortisone to cortisol via 11-beta-HSD1, perhaps leading to local tissue hypercortisolism.[227,228]

Skeletal Disorders

Osteoarthritis has been associated with obesity in several cross-sectional studies. Felson et al., in reviewing Framingham data, found a strong association between being obese in 1948–1952 and having either symptomatic or asymptomatic knee osteoarthritis approximately 36 years later.[229] The association was stronger for women and persisted after controlling for other risk factors. More recent studies have confirmed these observations[230–233] and demonstrated a 9–13 percent risk of developing osteoarthritis for every kg increase in weight[230] and a reduction in knee osteoarthritis of 50 percent over 10 years with a decrease in BMI of 2 units.[234] Similarly, other studies have shown an improvement in symptoms with weight loss.[235–237] The cause in obese subjects may be related to the increased force on cartilage and increased subchondral bony stiffness. The association of osteoarthritis with obesity in nonweight-bearing joints suggests that obesity-related metabolic abnormalities may also be responsible.[230,232]

Obesity is protective for osteoporosis.[238–240] In a recent study, weight was positively correlated with midshaft radius, lumbar spine, and femoral neck bone densities, yet risk factors alone were poor predictors of bone mass.[240] Other studies have shown normal[241] and increased[242] bone mass in obese individuals. Both increased estrogens and increased weight bearing in obese women have been postulated as etiologic in protecting against osteoporosis.[110,241]

In addition, obese subjects have elevated PTH, 1,25-dihydroxyvitamin D, osteocalcin, and urinary cyclic AMP with lower 25-hydroxyvitamin D and urinary calcium, consistent with secondary hyperparathyroidism.[243] Parathyroid hormone levels fall with weight loss.[244] This is consistent with the postulate that increased bone mass results because increased muscle mass diminishes the skeletal response to PTH.[243,245]

Pulmonary Disorders

Obesity is also associated with abnormalities in pulmonary function. These abnormalities were recently studied by Rubenstein et al. in 103 obese nonsmokers without cardiopulmonary disease compared with 190 healthy, nonobese nonsmokers.[246] These authors found that obese patients had lower functional residual capacity, expiratory reserve volume, and total lung capacity than did nonobese controls. In addition, residual volume and diffusing capacity were higher in obese patients. Obese men, but not women, had a reduced maximum expiratory flow rate at 15–75 percent of exhaled vital capacity. As reviewed by Rubenstein et al., obesity adversely affects chest wall mechanics and causes a decrease in total respiratory compliance, perhaps as a result of deposition of subcutaneous adipose tissue.[246] In addition, respiratory muscle function may also be impaired as a result of the mechanical disadvantage of the chest wall configuration, fat deposition, and the increased energy expenditure needed to expand the lungs. Decreased peripheral airway size may be due to increased pulmonary blood volume, congestion of bronchial vessels in the submucosa, and narrowing of the airway wall.[246] The decrease in peripheral airway dimensions in morbidly obese men can predispose them to chronic airflow limitation or to rapid deterioration in airway function if they are exposed to cigarette smoke or respiratory infections that could contribute to airway narrowing.

Severe obesity is associated with obstructive sleep apnea and the obesity hypoventilation syndrome. Sleep apnea syndrome[247,248] is associated with loud snoring, frequent nocturnal awakening, daytime somnolence, and nocturnal oxyhemoglobin desaturation. Sleep apnea can be obstructive, central, or mixed. The obstructive type is the most common. Frequently, patients fall asleep during the day, as in the Pickwickian syndrome. Other associated problems include morning headaches, loss of libido, intellectual deterioration, systemic and pulmonary hypertension, congestive heart failure, and cardiac arrhythmias.[247,248] Patients with severe sleep apnea have a higher rate of automobile accidents.[249] The etiology of obstruction of the upper airway during sleep in obese patients is not completely understood,[247,248] but a recent study found a correlation between the severity of obstructive sleep apnea and the volume of pharyngeal adipose tissue as determined by MRI.[250] The arrhythmias associated with sleep apnea may be related to increased plasma catecholamines, which are directly related to oxygen saturation.[251] Sleep apnea may also be an independent risk factor for myocardial infarction.[252]

In obese subjects with obstructive sleep apnea syndrome, weight loss is the treatment of choice. Relatively small amounts of weight loss can lead to significant improvement.[253,254] The relation between apneic episodes per hour and body weight was shown to be a logarithmic function in one study.[255] Changes in weight of 10–20 kg can lead to marked changes in sleep apnea.[253–256] Other treatments for sleep apnea include sleeping in a lateral position and avoiding sedatives and alcohol. Various pharmacologic approaches have been tried with mixed results,[247,248,254] including protriptyline, progesterone, and acetazolamide. These and other pharmacologic agents are reviewed by Hugel.[254] Nonsedating antidepressants such as protriptyline decrease REM sleep when apneas are most common. Selective serotonin reuptake inhibitors and serotonin agonists may also be useful.[254] There is conflicting data on the usefulness of medroxyprogesterone and acetazolamide, which may be more useful in patients with central apnea.[254] Nasal continuous positive airway pressure is frequently effective and improves survival[254] but often is not well tolerated. Surgical procedures include tracheostomy, removal of a discrete obstruction, uvulopalatopharyngoplasty, mandibular and maxillary advancement, midline glossectomy, sectioning of the hyoid, and laser uvulopalatoplasty.[247,248,254] Dental appliances are also being evaluated.[254] In morbidly obese patients, gastric bypass should be considered.[257] In one study comparing conservative treatment-weight loss to tracheostomy, the conservatively treated group had more extreme daytime somnolence and greater vascular morbidity after 7 years of follow-up.[258]

Miscellaneous Disorders

Obesity is also associated with an increased history of pregnancy-associated hypertension and a previous stillborn infant as well as increased frequencies of hypertension, gestational diabetes, multiple gestation, inadequate weight gain, and anemia during current pregnancies.[259] In addition, morbid obesity can be associated with the nephrotic syndrome.[260] Even overweight (BMI 25–29.9) is a significant risk factor for obstetrical complications.[261] Anecdotally, morbid obesity has been associated with esophageal reflux, but this is difficult to document experimentally.[262]

ETIOLOGY OF OBESITY

Obesity results from positive energy balance (i.e., energy intake exceeding energy expenditure). All people are in a state of positive energy balance as growing children. As adults, lean individuals maintain energy balance close to zero over the long run, but even lean adults often go through periods of positive or negative energy balance. Obese adults also maintain their energy balance close to zero for prolonged periods, although at a higher level of energy stores. Because obesity may develop over many years, only small differences in energy intake and expenditure are required, and these differences may be impossible to detect with current methods. The cause of the excessive positive energy balance in obesity has not been clearly defined. It is likely that there are numerous causes of obesity, including metabolic, psychological, hormonal, and socioeconomic factors. It may never be possible to point to a single factor as being the predominant cause of obesity. Thus, the following discussion covers a variety of potential influences on the development of obesity, any of which may have a role in a particular obese patient.

Genetic Factors

There is no question that obesity tends to run in families. However, this observation does not indicate whether this familial clustering is genetic or is related to the similarity of environmental influences on members of the same family. The strongest evidence for a significant genetic influence comes from studies of adoptees in Denmark[263] and twins who were reared in separate families in Sweden.[264] The BMI of adoptees was closely related to that of their biological parents but not that of their adoptive parents (Fig. 20-9). An overweight adoptee was more than twice as likely to have an overweight biological mother than was a thin adoptee and 40 percent more likely to have an overweight biological father. In 93 pairs of identical twins who were reared apart, the intrapair correlation coefficient for BMI was 0.70 for men and 0.66 for women. Identical twins reared together had very similar intrapair correlations for BMI (0.74 in men and 0.66 in women). Dizygotic twins reared apart or together had intrapair correlations that were less than half the values observed in monozygotic twins. There was no evidence that sharing the same childhood environment contributed to the similarity in BMI later in life.

Most studies of the genetic transmission of obesity have used indirect indexes of obesity, such as BMI or percentage of IBW. However, in one study of Canadian subjects, fat mass and percentage of body fat were measured directly using the underwater weighing method.[265] Based on consideration of nine different types of family relationships in these subjects, it was concluded that about half the variance in fatness was transmissible, with 25 percent being genetic transmission and 30 percent being cultural transmission.

First-degree relatives of obese patients whose obesity first became evident in childhood are more likely to be obese than are relatives of obese patients whose obesity began later in life.[266] After controlling for gender, degree of obesity, and family size, the relatives of those with childhood-onset obesity are about twice as likely to be obese as are relatives of those with adult-onset obesity.

The results that genetic factors may correlate with obesity have initiated studies to identify human genes linked to this condition; however, there is little information on specific genes being linked to obesity in humans. Linkage studies and positional cloning of genes involved in complex diseases, like obesity, are difficult due to complications resulting from confusion of genetic and environmental factors, and the need for complete genome searches with large family pedigrees. A number of reports have appeared in the literature regarding gene linkage studies in humans with correlation to obesity. Many of these studies were reviewed recently by Perusse et al.[267] and include genetic markers linked to BMI[268] and to fat mass.[269] Most studies indicate that the strongest genetic linkages are associated with morbid obesity

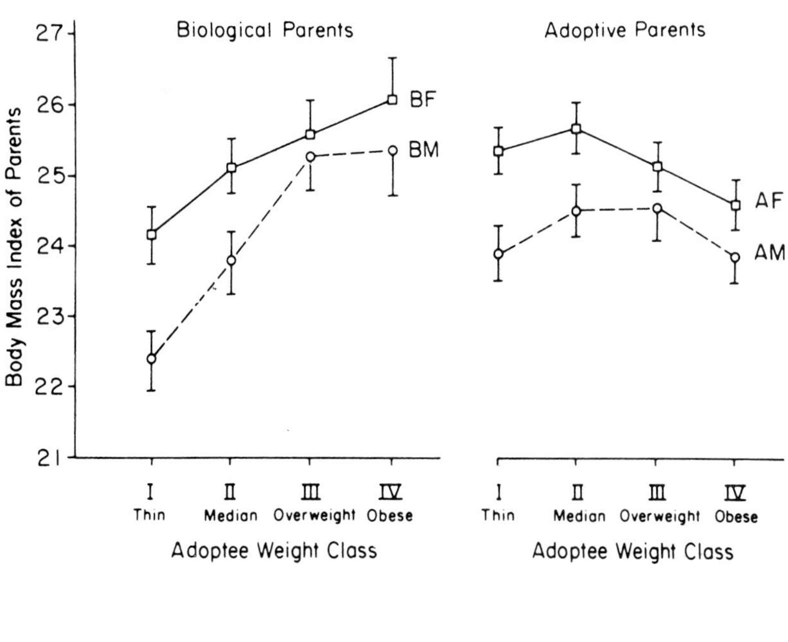

FIGURE 20-9. Mean body mass index (BMI) (±SEM) of biological fathers (BF), biological mothers (BM), adoptive fathers (AF), and adoptive mothers (AM) as a function of the weight class of adoptees (class I = thin with BMI in lowest 25 percent; class II = medium with BMI in the 26th through 91st percentile; class III = overweight with BMI in the 92nd to 96th percentile; class IV = obese with BMI above the 96th percentile). (*From Stunkard et al.,*[263] *with permission.*)

(BMI > 40)[270] and that most of these are rare mutations which would not explain the high prevalence of the disease. The linkage of morbid obesity to mutations in the genes encoding leptin and its receptor have been described and will be discussed later.[271,272] More recently, mutations have been described in the melanocortin-4 receptor gene that are associated with morbid obesity in humans.[273] In addition, in a woman with a history of early-onset obesity, mutations were found in the gene that encodes the endopeptidase prohormone convertase 1 (PC1), an enzyme that processes many precursors to hormones such as insulin, corticotropin, and leutenizing hormone releasing hormone.[274] Lastly, there is much controversy about the relevance of a common missense mutation in the gene that encodes the beta-3 adrenergic receptor. Some studies show a linkage of this mutation to obesity and insulin resistance while others find no association.[275–278] Further investigation will be needed to determine the importance of this mutation in the disease or whether other genes that are close to this gene on the chromosome are involved in the disease.

Animal models have provided potential useful information in gaining an understanding of the control of body mass and adiposity. Five monogenetic animal models that lead to obesity have been described and the genes for each of these mutations have been isolated, providing evidence of different pathways involved in the control of body weight and fat mass. Mice homozygous for the *obese* mutation (ob/ob) exhibit obesity, hyperphagia, decreased energy expenditure and impaired reproduction.[279–281] Parabiosis studies indicated that this gene encodes a circulating factor which regulates food intake by interaction with a second gene which is mutated in the *diabetes* (db/db) mouse strain.[281] The *diabetes* mutation also results in animals that display the major traits of obesity and diabetes.[282] As discussed later, the *obese* gene has been isolated and its product has been named leptin,[283] while the isolated diabetes gene has been shown to produce the receptor through which leptin signals.[282] The *yellow* or *agouti* (A^y) mouse strain imparts a maturity onset obesity where an increase in adipose tissue occurs gradually during the adult life of the mice. The defective gene codes for a 133-amino acid secreted peptide that acts as a competitive antagonist for melanocortin receptors. In wild-type mice this peptide is expressed in the skin and regulates hair color, however, in the *agouti* mouse the gene is expressed in many other tissues leading to increased food intake and decreased energy expenditure.[284,285] As stated earlier, mutations in one of these melanocortin receptors (MC-4) are associated with morbid obesity in humans.[273] Most recently, the mahogany (mg) locus has been shown to act as a suppressor of the *agouti* mutation and, in mice homozygous for mg, the yellow coat color and obesity resulting from the *agouti* mutation are blocked and diet-induced obesity is suppressed.[286,287] The fourth mouse obesity gene is embodied in the *fat* mutation. *Fat* mice also display a late-onset obesity phenotype and hyperproinsulinemia found to be caused by mutation of the carboxypeptidase E (CPE) gene. CPE is required for processing many prohormones and proneuropeptides including the precursors of insulin, peptides known to act at melanocortin receptors, neurotensin, and melanin concentrating hormone.[288–290] This defect in hormone processing is analogous to the PC1 mutations described previously that led to obesity in a female patient. Lastly, the *tubby* mutation has been described by a phenotype of late-onset obesity, hyperinsulinemia, and progressive retinal degeneration.[291] However, unlike other models of obesity, these mice remain mildly hypoglycemic and, thus, do not demonstrate insulin resistance. Although the gene mutated in *tubby* mice has been cloned,[292,293] the mechanism of the resulting obesity is unknown, and it remains the most poorly understood of the monogenetic mouse models of obesity.

The predisposition to human obesity could result from inheritance of a metabolic efficiency or of a tendency to eat more food than lean individuals eat. The resting metabolic rate, which accounts for more than half of total energy expenditure, appears to have a significant genetic component (Fig. 20-10).[294,295] For example, it has been estimated that after the resting metabolic rate is adjusted for fat-free mass, age, and gender, 40 percent of the remaining variance is explained by genetic factors. Similar heritability estimates were made for the increase in energy expenditure associated with meals and low-intensity exercise.[295] A low resting metabolic rate and a low 24-h energy expenditure in a respiration chamber were associated with an increased risk of gaining a significant amount of weight in a prospective study of a group of southwestern American Indians.[296] However, it seems unlikely that inheritance of a low energy expenditure explains most cases of obesity because obese individuals usually do not have a low metabolic rate. This issue will be discussed further.

Although there is familial resemblance in food intake, it is controversial whether this is entirely environmental or whether genetic influences play a role.[297,298] If the children of obese parents inherit a gene (or set of genes) that causes them to consume too much food, the nature of this genetic factor is unknown. As will

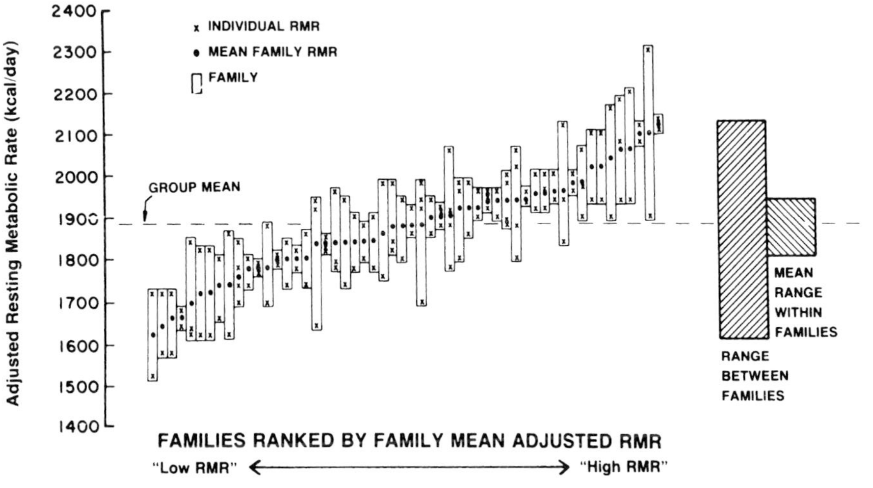

FIGURE 20-10. Mean family and individual resting metabolic rates in Pima Indians adjusted for the covariances of fat-free mass, age, and sex. (*From Bogardus et al.,*[294] *with permission.*)

be discussed later, the regulation of energy intake is extremely complex, and numerous metabolic and/or psychological factors may be involved.

In considering the genetics of obesity, it should be noted that throughout most of human evolution famine was very common. Those who were able to store energy efficiently as body fat when food was available would have been more likely to survive periods of famine and pass along their genes to offspring. Thus, obesity should not necessarily be viewed as a genetic abnormality but rather, a predictable consequence of natural selection. Only when the obese genotype is placed in a situation of a constant supply of food that does not require much physical effort to obtain is the obese phenotype expressed.

Environmental Factors

Genetic makeup only determines the tendency to become obese. The interactions between genes and the environment determine whether obesity actually develops. For example, if food is scarce because of poverty or regional famine, even those who are highly predisposed toward obesity will not become obese.

Cultural factors may play a significant role in determining the prevalence of obesity. In developed societies there is an inverse relation between socioeconomic status and obesity in women; i.e., women with a low socioeconomic status are much more likely to be obese.[299] However, in underdeveloped countries women with a high socioeconomic status are more likely to be obese.[299] The most likely explanation for this discrepancy is that obesity signifies the desirable traits of wealth and sexual attractiveness in poorer societies with limited access to food. In contrast, obesity often is looked upon as a sign of low intelligence or lack of self-control in wealthy nations.

Among children, the prevalence of obesity is related to the amount of time spent watching television.[300,301] This relation may be explained by a lower rate of energy expenditure during television viewing than during alternative activities or by snacking during television viewing. Moreover, the large amount of food advertising may lead children to eat more even when not watching television.

Among children there are regional and seasonal influences on the prevalence of obesity. In the United States (data from 1963 to 1965), obesity was much more common in the northeast than in the western part of the country and was more prevalent in the winter than in the summer in all regions.[302]

Exposure to a high-fat diet may increase one's probability of becoming obese. Results from multiple clinical trials shows that a reduction of 10 percent in the proportion of energy from fat was associated with a reduction in weight of 16 g/d.[303] A high percentage of fat in the diet is associated with adiposity, probably because a high-fat diet is associated with an increase in energy intake (Table 20-6)[304] and an increase in body fat storage.[305] Thus, a person who would not become obese on a high-carbohydrate diet, as is consumed by most of the world's population, may become obese when exposed to the typical high-fat western diet.

Although it has been difficult to assign any psychological disorder to the etiology of obesity, it has been a common observation that many obese patients have been abused as children or have a history of dysfunctional families. This was confirmed in a study by Filitti,[306] who interviewed 100 obese patients applying to a VLCD program at Kaiser Permanente and compared them to 100 always slender adults. The author found that the obese patients had a significantly higher incidence of sexual and nonsexual abuse in infancy, childhood, and adolescence; chronic depression and anxiety; rage reactions; and alcohol and drug abuse. The onset of obesity frequently coincided with identifiable events. Thirty-three percent of applicants stated that obesity defended them against the threat of sexual proposals or helped marital stability by reducing spousal jealousy. These factors are important in the treatment of obesity because they may play an important role in patients dropping out of programs after some weight loss and their regain of lost weight. Becoming sexually attractive is a frequent reason given for these events.

TABLE 20-6. Effect of a High- or Low-Fat Diet on Spontaneous Food Intake of Normal-Weight Young Men

	Low-Fat Diet	High-Fat Diet
Energy intake (kcal/day)	2987 ± 421	4135 ± 484*
Protein (g)	111 ± 13	122 ± 14
Fat (g)	73 ± 8	245 ± 28*
Carbohydrate (g)	488 ± 86	358 ± 59*

*$p < .01$. Values are mean ± SD of measured intake over 2 days.

Source: From Tremblay et al.[184]

Energy Expenditure

One popular theory[307] of obesity is that preobese individuals have a low rate of energy expenditure. According to this theory, preobese persons with low energy expenditure eat the same amount of food as do individuals with normal energy expenditure. Total energy expenditure then increases as weight is gained because of the increased energy cost of maintaining and moving a larger body. Eventually energy expenditure matches energy intake, and body weight stabilizes at an obese level, with both energy intake and energy expenditure being "normal." This theory is attractive because many studies have indicated that obese subjects do not consume more energy than lean subjects consume.[308–311]

The major problem with this theory is that numerous studies have demonstrated that the average total energy expenditure is higher in obese subjects than in lean subjects (Fig. 20-11). Increased energy expenditure in obesity has been demonstrated using precise calorimetry chambers,[312–317] has been inferred from the increased weight-maintenance energy requirements of obese patients living in metabolic wards[318,319] and from measurements of the energy costs of various activities in lean and obese subjects,[320] and has been demonstrated under free-living conditions using the doubly labeled water method.[321–323] These studies indicate that the normal or low self-reported intake of groups of obese subjects results from underreporting of food intake. Nevertheless, there were a few obese individuals in these studies whose energy expenditure was in the range of values observed in lean subjects. Such individuals probably had a subnormal energy expenditure before they became obese, as energy expenditure increases as weight is gained. Of course, the finding that energy expenditure generally is increased in obesity only demonstrates that increased energy intake is usually needed to maintain the obese state. It does not prove that energy expenditure was not subnormal before obesity developed.

The doubly labeled water method has been used to study the free-living energy expenditure of infants born to lean and obese mothers.[324] Among six infants of lean mothers, none became

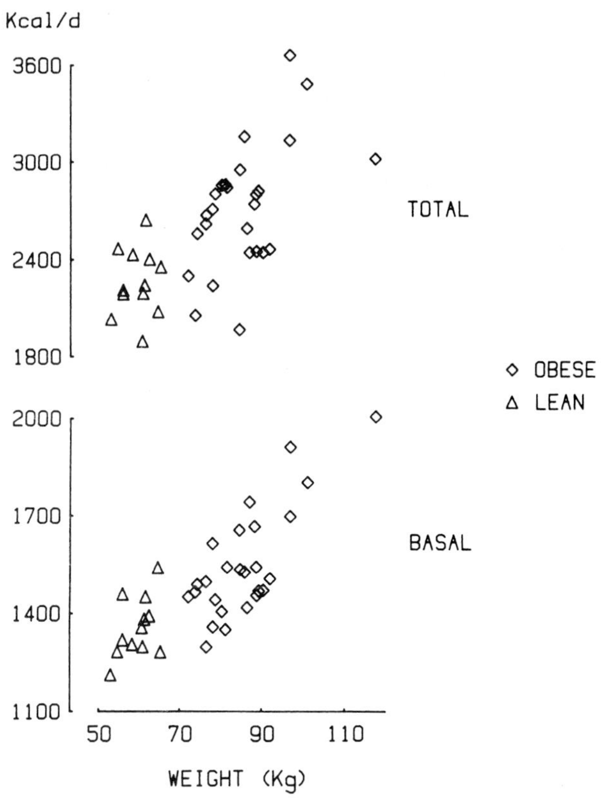

FIGURE 20-11. Total (top) and basal (bottom) energy expenditure in obese and lean subjects as a function of body weight. Total energy expenditure was measured by the doubly labeled water method. (*From Welle et al.,*[321] *with permission.*)

obese in the first year of life, whereas six of 12 infants of overweight mothers became obese within the first year. The energy expenditure of the infants was measured when they were 3 months old, a time when the mean body weights and energy intakes of the different groups were similar. The mean total energy expenditure of the six infants who later became obese was 20 percent lower than that of the other groups. However, their mean resting metabolic rate was not low, indicating that their low energy expenditure was related to reduced physical activity. Only three of these six infants were considered to be obese when the follow-up period ended at 1 year, and so the question remains whether infants with a low energy expenditure will be plagued with obesity throughout life. Among normal-weight children 4–5 years old it was found that the average resting metabolic rate of those with an obese parent was 16 percent lower than that of children whose parents had always been of normal weight.[325] The total daily energy expenditure of the group with obese parents was 22 percent lower than the energy expenditure in the group with lean parents. Although total expenditure was estimated with the imprecise heart rate method, these data suggest that those predisposed to obesity may have a reduced energy expenditure early in life. Unfortunately, no long-term follow-up was done to determine whether these children had an increased incidence of obesity later in life.

One approach to defining the energy expenditure of preobese people is to study reduced-obese subjects, assuming that their metabolic state reverts to its preobese condition when weight is normalized (although this assumption could be incorrect). Numerous studies have documented the fact that energy expenditure declines during weight loss in obese patients.[326–329] However, these subjects have an elevated metabolic rate before weight loss, and so a reduction in energy expenditure does not demonstrate that reduced-obese subjects are hypometabolic relative to normal-weight subjects. There is extremely little information regarding the energy expenditure of obese subjects who were reduced and stabilized at a normal body weight. The most convincing evidence for reduced energy expenditure in reduced-obese subjects comes from a study of 16 reduced-obese women and 16 normal-weight controls whose 24-h energy expenditure was measured in a respiration chamber at three different levels of activity.[330] At all activity levels, the reduced-obese women had metabolic rates about 15 percent lower than those of the normal-weight women. A similar study with fewer subjects did not confirm this finding, although total energy expenditure did tend to be lower (mean 6.5 percent) in reduced-obese subjects.[331]

Other investigations of the energy expenditure of reduced-obese subjects have involved subjects who were still overweight after their weight loss. Twenty-nine women who had lost some weight but who claimed that they could not lose any more on a low-energy diet (1,000–1,500 kcal/day) were isolated in a country house and fed 1,500 kcal/day for 3 weeks.[332] One of them gained more than 1 kg, and nine maintained their weight within 1 kg. Their expected weight-maintenance requirement would be in excess of 2,000 kcal/day, suggesting that a low metabolic rate contributed to their obesity. Unfortunately, body composition was determined by the imprecise skin fold thickness method, and so changes in energy stores during the study could not be calculated accurately. A change in body weight of 1 kg in 3 weeks could represent a change in energy stores of several hundred kilocalories per day. In another study, the weight-maintenance energy intake of 26 reduced-obese patients who were given a liquid formula diet in a metabolic ward was compared with that of age- and sex-matched controls who had never been obese.[318] The reduced-obese subjects had a mean energy requirement that was slightly less than that of the normal-weight subjects even though they were still 60 percent heavier. When energy requirements were expressed per square meter of surface area, the reduced-obese subjects had an energy requirement that was 25 percent below normal. Because the lean body mass was not determined, it is impossible to know if the difference could be explained by a lower active cell mass in the reduced-obese subjects. Body cell mass is the primary determinant of the resting metabolic rate, which is the primary determinant of total energy expenditure under sedentary conditions. In a similar experiment, the energy requirements of 10 reduced-obese patients were 18 percent below those of weight-matched subjects who had never dieted.[333] Both the reduced-obese and the control subjects were obese, suggesting that the weight loss itself rather than the predisposition to obesity was the main factor associated with reduced expenditure. The resting metabolic rate was normal when adjusted for lean body mass, suggesting that reduced physical activity could explain the lower energy requirement of the reduced-obese subjects. In contrast to these studies, other investigators have failed to find subnormal resting metabolic rates or total energy expenditure in obese subjects who had lost a substantial amount of weight.[326,334,335]

In one study, 24-h total, resting, and nonresting energy expenditures were measured in nonobese and obese subjects at their usual body weight and after losing 10 or 20 percent of their body weight by underfeeding and after gaining 10 percent of their body weight by overfeeding.[329] In all cases, measurements were made after body weights had stabilized for 14 days. Energy expenditures were higher in obese than in nonobese subjects and a 10-percent increase or decrease in initial body weight was associated with a 16-percent increase or 15-percent decrease in 24-h total energy expenditure, respectively. Unfortunately, total energy expenditure was not measured in these subjects but was estimated from caloric intake during short-term weight stability. The fat mass of the subjects was significantly related to energy expenditure and the preceding values were corrected for body composition. There were no significant differences in energy expenditure as measured by caloric intake at weights 10 and 20 percent below the initial body weight, which indicates that the maximal compensatory change was reached at the 10 percent decreased body weight level. In addition, there was no difference in the decrease in energy expenditure seen in nonobese versus obese subjects. Because of the methods used, these results would need to be reproduced using a precise method to measure total energy expenditure before any conclusions can be drawn.

The *thermic effect* of food is the increase in metabolic rate that follows meals. The increase persists for several hours, and in an average person the thermic effect of food accounts for about 8 percent of total energy expenditure. Several studies have indicated that the thermic effect of food is reduced in obese subjects.[336–341] However, others have failed to find a reduced thermic effect in obesity.[342–346] A reduction in the thermic effect of food (or at least carbohydrate) may be related more to impaired glucose tolerance[346–348] or to the degree of insulin resistance[349] than to obesity per se. This suggests that a reduced thermic response may be a result rather than a cause of obesity, but it has been reported that the thermic response to a glucose meal or a mixed meal remains low after weight loss.[334, 350] The argument is often put forth that even though the decrease in the thermic effect of food amounts to only a few percent of total energy requirements, it can lead to obesity because even a positive energy balance of only 50 kcal/day will cause a weight gain of 5 pounds in a year. This argument is flawed because the basal metabolic rate and the energy cost of activity increase as weight is gained, so that the initial weight gain associated with a reduced thermic effect of food would quickly be offset by the increase in total energy expenditure. In one study even a decreased thermic effect of 50–150 kcal/day was unable to explain a significant role in increased body weight.[351] Hence, it is unlikely that a low thermic effect of food has more than a minor role in the development of obesity.

Inactivity has been described in obese children and adults.[352–356] However, the energy required to perform all types of activities is elevated in obese subjects, so that the actual amount of energy used for physical activity is slightly higher in obese than in lean individuals.[321–323] It is likely that the increased effort needed to perform activities causes obese people to limit their activity, and this could help perpetuate obesity. Reduced physical activity in preobese or reduced-obese subjects could contribute to lower total energy expenditure. An increase in the basal metabolic rate and an increase in the energy cost of activity would eventually offset this decrease as weight is gained, but only after the subjects had become overweight. The extent of inactivity in preobese or reduced-obese individuals is not clear. A study of total energy expenditure of preobese infants,[324] which was discussed earlier, indicated that their lower energy expenditure was related to inactivity. In obese adults who had lost an average 21.5 percent of their body weight, the nonresting energy expenditure (estimated as the difference between weight-maintenance intake and resting metabolic rate) was several hundred kilocalories per day below the level observed in moderately obese patients who had not lost weight.[333] These results suggest that inactivity may contribute to the rebound in body weight usually seen after weight loss in obese patients.

A study of 18 obese women before and after attaining and maintaining ideal body weight for at least 2 months and 14 nonobese women showed that obese women had a higher total energy expenditure, which was reduced upon weight loss.[357] However, the reduced-obese subjects did not show hypometabolism when compared to the nonobese women. After one year, 10 of the reduced-obese women had regained weight, but there was no low energy expenditure seen in these women to explain the increase in weight. In yet another study, 24 normal-weight women were compared to 24 moderately obese women with a familial history towards obesity after weight loss (average 12.9 kg) to near-normal levels.[358] Mean resting energy expenditure, thermic effect of food, and fasting and postprandial fuel utilization were similar between the nonobese and reduced-obese women. Following four years, the reduced-obese women regained weight (average 10.9 kg) and the nonobese women gain little weight (average 1.7 kg). There were no significant differences in metabolic parameters between the reduced-obese and nonobese women to explain the increase in weight seen in the reduced-obese group. Instead, the data suggest that decreased physical activity and/or increased energy intake were responsible for the gain of weight.

Patients with the Prader-Willi syndrome are obese. It has been reported that such patients have a total energy expenditure, estimated with the doubly labeled water method, 47 percent lower than that of weight-matched controls.[359] When the data are normalized for their lower lean body mass, the difference is only 14 percent and the basal metabolic rate is normal.

Some obese patients claim that they cannot lose weight in spite of consuming only a very low energy diet, often less than 1,000 kcal/day. We have measured the basal metabolic rates of many such patients and have not found one with an abnormally low basal metabolism. Usually the basal metabolic rate is higher than the self-reported total energy intake. Hence, the accuracy of self-reported very low energy requirements in obese patients should be viewed with suspicion. Treatment based on the assumption of hypometabolism should be undertaken with caution in the absence of direct evidence of low energy expenditure.

Regardless of whether energy expenditure is below normal in preobese individuals, it is clear that energy intake must exceed energy expenditure for obesity to develop. It has been pointed out that when subjects voluntarily overeat, there is considerable variability in the ease with which weight is gained.[360,361] The variability in weight gained observed in the famous Vermont overfeeding study[360] resurrected the notion of "luxuskonsumption," or the wastage of excess energy as heat during periods of overeating. If some subjects increase their thermogenesis more than others do when they overeat, they should be less susceptible to becoming obese. Unfortunately, this hypothesis was not tested by direct measurements of energy expenditure in the Vermont study. More recently, a correlation was found within twin pairs for weight gain during prolonged experimental overfeeding, suggesting a genetic component to the susceptibility to weight gain.[361] Although increased metabolic rates have been documented in overfeeding studies,[362–364] they are never great enough to prevent weight gain completely during periods of overeating. Thus individual differences in overfeeding-induced thermogenesis can explain only differences in the degree of obesity and are not sufficient to explain why some individuals become obese and others remain lean.

Food Intake

Because energy expenditure tends to be higher in weight-stable obese subjects, obese subjects generally must eat more food to maintain the obese state. In most cases it is likely that this increased food intake is the primary cause of obesity. Body weight then stabilizes at a high level of food intake because energy expenditure increases as weight is gained. These statements contradict the many studies indicating that the self-reported food intake of obese subjects is not increased.[308–311] However, the consistency with which increased energy expenditure is observed in obese patients necessitates acceptance of the fact that many obese patients underreport their intake.[312–324,357] This fact, along with the poor accuracy of self-reported intake even in normal-weight subjects, makes studies of food intake under free-living conditions extremely difficult. Many investigations have been done of food intake in the laboratory or in metabolic wards, but the extent to which these studies reflect the regulation of food intake under actual living conditions is uncertain. Thus, it is very difficult to compare the regulation of food intake in lean and obese subjects.

It is often stated that obese individuals have a higher "set point" for body weight than do lean individuals. This concept suggests that some comparator exists in the central nervous system (CNS) that causes a person to eat more when weight is below the set point and eat less when weight is above the set point. The comparator presumably senses either body weight or body fat (the lipostatic theory), and would appear to be located in the hypothalamus, according to studies done in rats and other animals. When lesions are made in the lateral hypothalamus (LH), a rat will become hypophagic but will usually survive (if postoperative care is intense enough) and maintain its weight at a subnormal level. However, if the rat is reduced to a weight below this reduced set point level before the LH lesion is made, it will actually become hyperphagic and gain weight after the lesion to reach the new set point.[365] In contrast, rats with lesions of the ventromedial hypothalamus (VMH) become obese and appear to defend an elevated body weight.[366] In addition, animals defend this set point only when fed a normal chow containing nutrients low in fat. On a high fat "cafeteria" diet, the set point is not maintained and the animals become obese.[367]

Two mutant strains of mice, *obese* (ob/ob) and *diabetes* (db/db), have been described that are phenotypically similar with major traits of obesity and diabetes.[280] Parabiosis studies with *obese*, *diabetes,* and normal mice suggested that a peripheral signal exists which senses body weight or body fat.[281] Recently, the gene that is responsible for the *obese* phenotype has been cloned.[283] It codes for a peptide produced in adipose tissue that has been called leptin. Also, the gene responsible for the *diabetes* mutant mouse strain has been identified as the receptor for the leptin peptide.[282] This receptor is located in peripheral tissues[368] and in various regions of the brain[369] including the choroid plexus and the hypothalamus. Together this peptide sensor and receptor signal could explain the possible mechanism of the lipostatic theory.

Leptin production increases with the increase in fat mass, thus sensing body fat. In human subjects, plasma leptin concentrations are strongly associated with body fat mass, waist girth, and cross-sectional areas of abdominal subcutaneous and visceral fat tissue.[370] Men exhibit 2–3 times lower levels of plasma leptin than females.[370,371] Because some variation could be explained by peripheral fat distribution, this may have implications relating to differences in body composition between men and women.[370–372] In animals, injections of leptin by intraperitoneal, intravenous, or intracranial routes cause a decrease in appetite and an increase in energy expenditure and weight loss.[279,373,374] Leptin expression in adipocytes is regulated by nutrients being increased after food intake and decreased after fasting.[375] In mice, there is a saturable system located in the choroid plexus of the brain that allows leptin penetration across the blood-brain barrier.[376] A form of the leptin receptor that is upregulated by a high-fat diet is located in the choroid plexus and believed to be responsible for this transport of leptin.[377] Thus, leptin is secreted from adipose tissue into the blood and transferred to the brain through leptin receptors in the choroid plexus. It then travels to the hypothalamus, where interaction with other leptin receptors produces a negative signal to suppress appetite.[375] Leptin also acts to increase energy expenditure, possibly via the sympathetic nervous system. However, in humans, a relationship between leptin and energy expenditure has not been seen.[372]

Leptin has been shown to interact with other neuronal systems known to affect food intake and energy metabolism. Leptin has been reported to inhibit the synthesis and release of NPY,[375,378] a neuropeptide known to induce feeding in animals.[379] Thus, lowered NPY levels may be responsible for the decreased food intake seen after leptin treatment. Also, leptin has been shown to stimulate pro-opiomelanocortin gene expression, which would lead to an increase in MSH production,[380] and an antagonist of MSH action can block the anorexic activity of leptin.[381] This suggests that the melanocortin system is important for the activity of leptin. Leptin has been reported to increase the expression of uncoupling protein genes, UCP-1, -2, and -3, which are involved in energy homeostatsis.[382] Furthermore, mice that lack brown adipose tissue, a tissue that has uncoupling activity and that regulates energy expenditure in rodents, are resistant to the effects of leptin.[383] Thus, multiple mechanisms are involved in the actions of leptin on satiety and energy expenditure.

Because leptin decreases appetite and body weight, the increased leptin concentrations seen in obese humans suggests a decreased sensitivity to leptin. Although plasma levels of leptin in humans are closely correlated with adipose mass as in rodents, obese patients do not respond to this increased leptin by suppressing food intake or increasing energy expenditure. This ineffective action of leptin has been called *leptin resistance*, but the nature of this resistance is not well understood. Obesity caused by hypothalamic damage is very rare in humans, and there is no evidence for any subtle anatomic or neurochemical abnormality in the hypothalamus of most obese patients. However, a homozygous leptin gene mutation has been found in two obese children who are members of the same pedigree[271] and a homozygous mutation in the leptin receptor gene has been found in obese patients from another family.[272] These mutations, which are associated with early-onset obesity, indicate the importance of leptin in energy balance in humans. However, they do not explain the causes of obesity in most human subjects.

Other studies done in human patients indicate a possible mechanism for leptin resistance. Schwartz et al.[384] and Caro et al.[385] have reported that although there is a positive correlation between the levels of leptin in the CSF and BMI, the ratio of CSF to serum leptin levels is negatively correlated with BMI. In other words, the efficiency by which leptin is taken up in the brain from the plasma is lower in obese than in lean subjects. This reduced transport of leptin into the brain in obese individuals with high plasma leptin levels could explain the apparent resistance to leptin. In support of this theory, Ramsey et al.[386] have reported that inefficient transport of leptin could be responsible for the limitation of leptin action in primates. They demonstrated that while IV injections of leptin in rhesus monkeys led to a 10-fold increase in serum leptin, there was no affect on food intake. However, when leptin was administered directly into the brain via intracerebroventricular injection, leptin caused a dose-dependent decrease in food intake.

In further discussing the set point theory, it should be noted that neither normal nor VMH-lesioned rats defend their body weight very avidly. If normal animals are given a highly palatable diet, they become hyperphagic and obese,[387] and if VMH-lesioned rats are given an unpalatable diet, they lose weight.[388] Likewise, obese humans do not maintain their body weight when placed on a monotonous liquid diet even though they are allowed to eat ad libitum.[389] Obese subjects also fail to maintain a constant food intake when the energy density of the diet is covertly reduced with sugar or fat substitutes[390,391] and fail to increase energy intake when expenditure is increased by additional exercise.[392] These studies suggest that if leptin or some other factors contribute to the control of food intake and energy expenditure, and if a hypothalamic set point for weight or fat does exist in humans, obese patients generally are above this set point and will go into negative energy balance under a variety of conditions.

The nature of leptin resistance and whether there are other set point comparators that are altered in human obesity and/or whether there are other signals emanating from adipose tissue that influence food intake are questions that will continue to be explored. The fact that obese patients almost always regain weight after losing weight and that lean subjects who are experimentally overfed return to their original weight by reducing food intake[393] makes the set point concept attractive. However, explanations other than a set point can account for these observations. Lean subjects who are overfed may consciously reduce their intake to lose weight. If reduced-obese subjects return to their former eating habits they also will return to their former weight simply because a certain level of food intake will support a certain amount of body weight.

If there is no physiologic set point that is avidly defended, it follows that short-term hunger and satiety cues are the primary determinants of food intake. There does not appear to be a single overriding signal that determines meal onset or termination. Thus, the probability of starting or ending a meal can be influenced by numerous neural, hormonal, metabolic, psychological, and environmental factors.

Since the early work on LH and VMH lesions, a vast amount of research has been done to elucidate the finer details of the anatomic and neurochemical regulation of feeding in the CNS of animals, mostly rodents. Not only the hypothalamus but many nuclei in the hindbrain and forebrain are involved in regulating food intake, as are ascending and descending pathways that traverse the hypothalamus. Because no anatomic or biochemical CNS lesion is apparent in human obesity, such research has not succeeded in elucidating the specific etiology of obesity in humans. However, in the future the use of positron emission tomography (PET) scans may uncover changes in human obesity in areas of the brain that regulate food intake. To date PET studies on patients with eating disorders have shown that underweight anorectic patients show global and regional hypometabolism of glucose in the brain as compared to control subjects, especially in the parietal cortex, and that this hypometabolism is normalized with weight gain.[394,395] Similar findings have been reported in studies of bulimic patients indicating common parietal cortex dysfunction in patients with eating disorders or a sensitivity of this region to consequences of eating disorders.[396]

Because glucose ordinarily provides all the brain's energy, the role of glucose in the regulation of feeding has been an important area of investigation. The glucostatic theory holds that hunger is related to the circulating glucose concentration, or the rate of glucose metabolism in some critical area of the CNS.[397] Glucoreceptors also exist in the liver, which may relay information regarding hepatic glucose metabolism to the brain through vagal afferents.[398] Hypoglycemia induced by insulin or the inhibition of glucose metabolism with 2-deoxy-D-glucose can induce an intense craving for food. However, the degree of glucoprivation with these stimuli is much greater than that which ordinarily occurs between meals. Obese subjects tend to have higher rather than lower glucose levels, and this, according to the glucostatic theory, would tend to suppress food intake rather than stimulate it. Even though obese subjects tend to have glucose intolerance as a result of insulin resistance, the brain does not require insulin for glucose uptake and metabolism. Thus, it is unlikely that the hyperphagia of obesity is related to altered CNS glucose metabolism.

It is worth noting that animal studies have demonstrated a key role for monoaminergic neurons (containing norepinephrine, dopamine, or serotonin) in regulating food intake. This may explain the fact that previous and some current appetite suppressants used to treat obesity are sympathomimetics that cause the release of or inhibit the deactivation of catecholamines and serotonin (e.g., amphetamines, phentermine, Mazindol, fenfluramine, dexfenfluramine, sibutramine, phendimetrazine, diethylpropion, and phenylpropanolamine hydrochloride). The anorexic effects of norepinephrine are most likely mediated by alpha-1 and beta-adrenergic receptors,[399,400] while serotonin is thought to reduce feeding by acting at 5-HT_{1B} and 5-HT_{2C} receptors.[401,402]

It has been proposed that the rate of tryptophan or tyrosine uptake into the brain is a determinant of appetite. These amino acids are precursors of dopamine and norepinephrine (tyrosine) and serotonin (tryptophan). The large neutral amino acids (LNAAs) compete with one another for uptake into the brain via a competitive transport system. Hence, the ratio of a particular LNAA to the others, not their absolute concentrations, can determine the availability of the precursors for monoamine synthesis, which apparently can influence concentrations of these neurotransmitters in the brain.[403,404] The ratio of tryptophan to total LNAA concentrations was reported to be lower than normal in obese subjects after a carbohydrate meal.[405] The obese subjects were classified as carbohydrate cravers, and it was suggested that the reduced Trp/LNAA ratio caused reduced appetite suppression because of reduced CNS serotonin synthesis.[406] The reduced Trp/LNAA ratio probably resulted from the insulin resistance of obesity, which led to hyperinsulinemia and subsequently to an altered amino acid pattern. Thus, the proposed mechanism may explain why obese carbohydrate cravers have an increased food intake after they become hyperinsulinemic, but there is no evidence that preobese individuals have abnormal patterns of LNAAs that can explain the hyperphagia that eventually causes obesity. Nevertheless, the idea that a subgroup of obese subjects may overeat carbohydrates because of a need to increase serotonergic transmission in the CNS deserves further study.[407]

The fact that a high-fat diet tends to promote obesity raises the question of whether fat is less satiating than are other macronutrients. Fat has been reported to be as effective in reducing subsequent food intake and hunger ratings as other nutrients in single-meal studies.[408,409] When subjects were allowed to eat ad lib for 2 days in a laboratory setting, their energy intake was 38 percent greater with a high-fat diet (54 percent of energy as fat) than with a low-fat diet (22 percent of energy as fat) (Table 20-6).[304] Moreover, self-reported energy intake was greater in men with high-fat diets (45 ± 4 percent of energy) than in men with low-fat diets (30 ± 5 percent of energy), and the body fat content of the men on high-fat diets was 5 kg greater.[304] Obese subjects consume a greater percentage of their calories from fat, according to self-reports, but in these same studies there was no relation between obesity and self-reported energy intake.[410,411] Because a high-fat diet can promote obesity only by increasing energy intake or reducing energy expenditure, these studies are difficult to interpret. There is no good evidence that a high-fat diet increases energy efficiency in humans[412] apart from the slightly lower thermic effect of fat than of carbohydrate or protein.[413] Moreover, as was discussed earlier, there is ample evidence that obese subjects expend more energy than lean subjects do. Thus, if obese subjects underreport their energy intake, the accuracy of their self-reported diet composition must be questioned. The available evidence suggests that the high-fat diet consumed in western societies increases the prevalence of obesity, but there are many individuals who remain lean in spite of a high-fat diet and many who become obese with a dietary fat composition similar to that of lean individuals.

Adipose tissue lipoprotein lipase (LPL) activity is greater in obese subjects than in lean subjects.[414–419] This enzyme is responsible for hydrolyzing triglycerides in chylomicrons and circulating VLDLs to free fatty acids for uptake into adipocytes. The finding of higher activity of an enzyme that promotes the filling of adipocytes with fat is of obvious interest. However, as has been emphasized throughout this discussion, obesity can be understood only in terms of factors that increase energy intake or reduce energy expenditure. Because there is no reason to suspect that increased LPL activity reduces energy expenditure, this increased activity must increase energy intake to cause obesity. Because increased LPL activity enhances the storage of fat in adipocytes, less fat may be available to "feed" other tissues and increased food intake could result. The most attractive aspect of the theory that increased LPL activity is involved in the etiology of obesity is that adipose tissue LPL activity is unchanged or even increased after weight loss,[414–416,420,421] although a few studies have shown a decrease after weight loss.[417,422,423] Thus, increased adipose tissue LPL activity may be an inherent characteristic of obese subjects rather than a secondary consequence of obesity.

The role of insulin in regulating food intake is of obvious interest, given the hyperinsulinemia of obesity. It is known that insulin levels in the CSF are proportional to peripheral circulating insulin levels and that there are insulin receptors in certain areas of the brain.[424,425] In baboons, intracerebroventricular infusion of insulin suppresses food intake and body weight, suggesting that insulin is a satiety hormone.[424] There are some reports that plasma leptin levels correlate with plasma insulin levels and that insulin may upregulate leptin secretion, which could explain the effects of insulin on food intake.[370,371] Other studies indicate that increased serum insulin does not increase serum leptin levels in humans.[426] However, it is well known that animals become hyperphagic if they receive sufficiently large doses of insulin peripherally. This effect often is assumed to be caused by the hypoglycemia induced by insulin. However, human subjects report increased hunger and increased palatability of sweet solutions and consume more of a liquid meal during peripheral hyperinsulinemia even when euglycemia is maintained by means of intravenous glucose infusion.[427] This finding suggests that hyperinsulinemia can contribute to hyperphagia. If this is true, the hyperinsulinemia of obesity could contribute to the maintenance of the obese state. However, there is no evidence that hyperinsulinemia precedes obesity, and it is therefore unknown whether it is a primary cause of the overeating that initially leads to obesity. Additionally, in a study of 31 obese, nondiabetic women, it has been shown that neither insulin resistance nor hyperinsulinemia affect the ability of obese patients to lose weight during a short time when placed on a calorie-restricted diet.[428] Thus, the relationship between the incidence of obesity and insulin resistance or hyperinsulinemia remain controversial.

Endogenous opioids have been implicated in the control of food intake. It has long been known that opiate agonists stimulate hunger, and more recently it has been shown that opioid antagonists can inhibit food intake in certain situations.[429–431] Concentrations of the endogenous opioid agonist β-endorphin have been reported to be increased in the blood and CSF of obese humans.[430] However, it was reported that elevated plasma β-endorphin levels occur in obese women but not in obese men.[432] In studies of normal weight relatives of obese families, low rates of β-endorphin infusion leading to physiological increases of plasma opioid levels cause increases in plasma insulin and glucagon concentrations, but only in relatives of obese families.[433] This suggests a primary role of opioid peptides in metabolic events of obesity and increased islet hormone release in early phases of human obesity. Several trials of the effects of opioid antagonists on the food intake and body weight of obese subjects have been published.[429,430] Although some inhibitory effects of naloxone on food intake have been observed in short-term studies, long-term controlled studies of naltrexone have demonstrated little or no inhibitory effects on food intake or body weight. (Naloxone must be given intravenously and therefore is not useful for long term studies in humans.) Hence, it appears that even if opioids are involved in regulating short-term food intake, during longer periods other factors predominate in determining body weight in obese humans. However, this area of research must be reevaluated periodically as newer antagonists that act on specific opiate receptor subtypes are developed. A newer opioid-like receptor has been described with homology to other opioid receptors but which does not bind traditional opioid peptides.[434] The natural ligand for this receptor was isolated[435] and, like other opioid peptides, it stimulates food intake, which is reversible by naloxone treatment.[436] Further studies will be required to determine if antagonists of this receptor act to reduce feeding and body weight in humans.

Many neuropeptide hormones that affect hunger or satiety have been identified and recently reviewed.[437] These include neuropeptide Y (NPY), galanin, melanin-concentrating hormone (MCH), the orexins, neurotensin, melanocortin (alpha-MSH), agouti peptide, cocaine and amphetamine-regulated transcript peptide (CART), glucagon-like peptide-1 (GLP-1) and, of course, leptin. Some of these peptides increase appetite while others decrease appetite to reduce food intake by acting in the brain. Identification of agonists and antagonists of the receptors through which these neuropeptides act is an intense area of research for the discovery of new pharmacological agents which could be used in the treatment of obesity.

Satiety is mediated by numerous factors, including gastric distension, gut peptides (cholecystokinin, bombesin), and receptors that relay information from the large intestine and liver to the brain through the vagus nerve. These factors are important in terminating meals but probably are not very important in regulating food intake during long periods. It is not known whether obese humans respond differently than lean subjects to these signals. These short-term satiety cues could be involved in the etiology of obesity only if long-term food intake or body weight itself were poorly regulated.

Sensory, cognitive, and psychological factors may override the physiologic regulation of food intake and contribute to obesity in some individuals. Although both lean and obese people tend to eat more food when it is very palatable, this effect appears to be exaggerated among obese subjects.[438] Obese people also may be more likely to prefer food with a higher fat content,[439] which tends to cause increased food intake. Obese subjects have been shown to be unusually responsive to nonphysiologic stimuli, such as time of day and level of anxiety, and less responsive to internal physiologic cues in determining their food intake.[438,440,441] However, many studies of the nonphysiologic factors that influence food intake in lean and obese subjects must be interpreted cautiously because they used contrived laboratory settings, did not carefully define obesity, and studied intake at only a single meal.[441]

Although many obese individuals suffer from psychological problems, it is difficult to evaluate the extent to which such problems are the result rather than the cause of obesity. At this point there is no evidence for a common underlying psychological disturbance or personality trait that is typical of obese individuals.[438] However, it is possible that a significant proportion (30 percent) of obese subjects engage in binge eating, a form of compulsive behavior.[442]

Lastly, it has been shown that obesity is correlated with an increase in energy expenditure. An increase in food intake leads to an increase in total energy expenditure in both obese subjects and in subjects who have never been obese. In contrast, a decreased food intake leads to decreased energy expenditure in these patients.[329] Thus, the maintenance of a reduced or increased body weight by change in the diet is coupled with an opposing change in energy expenditure that counteracts the maintenance of a different body weight.

Endocrine Systems and the Autonomic Nervous System

The thyroid hormones are the most important regulators of energy expenditure. Untreated hypothyroid individuals may have basal metabolic rates that are only 50 percent of normal, yet weight gain is not always present with this condition and obesity very rarely is caused by hypothyroidism.[443] Thyroid hormone levels are almost always within normal ranges in obese subjects, although it has been reported that the nuclear binding capacity for T_4 and T_3 is reduced in the monocytes of obese subjects.[444] As was discussed earlier, there is no strong evidence that low energy expenditure is a common cause of obesity, and so it is unlikely that obese subjects have a generalized thyroid hormone receptor defect that leads to low energy expenditure in spite of normal thyroid hormone levels. Recently it has been reported that increased leptin levels are reversibly associated with hypothyroidism.[445] The implications of leptin concentrations and the association with thyroid hormone levels on metabolic rates and obesity will require further study.

Over the years there has been interest in the possible role of adrenal steroids in the etiology of obesity. Experimental obesity in animals is reversed or attenuated by adrenalectomy, an effect that appears to be mediated by the removal of the adrenal cortex.[446] Adrenalectomy normalizes body weight in obese animals by both reducing food intake and increasing energy expenditure.[446] However, the relevance of these animal models to human obesity is tenuous. Although the cortisol excess seen in Cushing's syndrome leads to a characteristic deposition of excess fat in the face, interscapular area, and mesenteric bed, there is no good evidence that the excess body fat in primary obesity is caused by high cortisol levels. Some early studies suggested that obese subjects hypersecrete cortisol, but other studies have not supported these results.[447] A more recent report indicates that although urinary cortisol excretion is elevated in obese subjects, the plasma levels of cortisol are not elevated and suggests that the clearance of cortisol may be altered in obesity.[448] Even if some obese patients have slightly elevated cortisol production, this does not prove that high cortisol levels are the cause rather than the result of obesity.

Dehydroepiandrosterone (DHEA) is an adrenal steroid that in high doses has an antiobesity effect in animals.[449,450] A negative correlation between the percentage of excess body weight and DHEA excretion has been observed.[451] However, circulating levels of DHEA and DHEA sulfate are normal in obese subjects in spite of increased DHEA production.[452,453] Large doses of DHEA given to obese men for 28 days had no effect on body weight,[454] however, longer-acting analogs of DHEA may be required to allow further progress in this area.

Insulin and β-endorphin were discussed earlier in this chapter in the context of the regulation of food intake. It also is possible that these hormones influence energy balance through effects on energy expenditure. Although insulin appears to have no thermogenic effect per se, it indirectly increases energy expenditure through its stimulatory effect on glycogen synthesis and lipogenesis. Opiates may increase energy expenditure.[430] However, it should be noted that the high levels of insulin and β-endorphin in obese subjects would tend to increase rather than reduce energy expenditure and therefore would tend to attenuate rather than promote weight gain. Thus, these hormones could contribute to obesity only through their effects, if any, on food intake.

As discussed earlier in this chapter, obesity is associated with a number of changes in endocrine systems. From the standpoint of the etiology of obesity, only changes that are present before the onset of obesity (which may be reflected by their persistence after weight loss) can be causative. Endocrine abnormalities that disappear when weight is normalized are unlikely to be involved in the development of obesity. In the vast majority of cases there is no evidence for any endocrine abnormality that is the cause of obesity.

Catecholamines (epinephrine and norepinephrine) are thermogenic hormones, and reduced sympathetic nervous system activity therefore could lead to reduced energy expenditure. Epinephrine and norepinephrine are secreted from the adrenal medulla, and norepinephrine is released from sympathetic nerves. (Most of the circulating norepinephrine comes from sympathetic nerves and reflects spillover from the synapses; thus, norepinephrine should be regarded more as a neurotransmitter than as a hormone.) Genetic obesity in *ob/ob* mice has been related to reduced sympathetic nervous system activity due to lack of leptin activity, especially in the nerves innervating brown adipose tissue,[455,456] but the relevance of this animal model to human obesity is questionable, as discussed previously.

It has been reported that plasma norepinephrine and epinephrine levels were inversely related to body fat in a select group of healthy men with body fat ranging from 5 to 50 percent.[457] Other measures of sympathetic and parasympathetic activity also were inversely related to the percentage of body fat.[457] However, other data do not support the concept that obese or postobese subjects have impaired autonomic activity.[458] There is a tendency for higher rather than lower norepinephrine levels in obese subjects.[459] In view of the lack of data supporting the notion that impaired thermogenesis is an important causal factor in obesity (as discussed earlier), it seems unlikely that abnormal sympathetic nervous system activity plays a significant role in the pathogenesis of this condition.

Summary

The predisposition to become obese is inherited, but genetic factors apparently interact with environmental influences in complex ways to determine the body weight phenotype. Most obese subjects consume more energy than lean subjects do to maintain their obese condition, and it seems likely that this hyperphagia also is the primary cause of obesity. Although some obese individuals do not consume more energy than does the average lean person, they are hyperphagic in the sense that they consume more energy than they require to maintain a healthy body weight. Numerous factors that can influence food intake have been identified, but there is no evidence that an abnormality in any of these factors is a common cause of obesity. The mechanism by which energy intake is linked to either energy expenditure or body energy stores has not been elucidated. Thus, while it can be said that obesity definitely results from positive energy balance, it is not understood why some individuals are much more likely than others to go through periods of positive energy balance. Obesity is probably a multifactorial process with complex interactions among genetic, metabolic, hormonal, and psychological factors. It may be unrealistic to think that a single overriding cause is operative.

Other Causes of Obesity

In the evaluation of an obese patient, secondary causes such as hypothyroidism, glucocorticoid excess, hypopituitarism, hypogonadism, and insulinoma should be considered. The signs and symptoms as well as the evaluation of these conditions are discussed in other chapters. Drugs such as phenothiazines and tricyclic antidepressants should also be considered.

Trauma, granulomatous disease, tumors, aneurysms, acute leukemia, and pseudotumor cerebri can cause hypothalamic obesity. This type of obesity is usually mild (5–15 kg overweight), although more severe obesity can occur with a sudden onset and can be associated with other symptoms of a space-occupying lesion, such as headache, impaired vision, hypogonadism, diabetes insipidus, impaired growth, seizures, and behavioral changes.[460,461]

Genetic syndromes associated with obesity include Prader-Willi syndrome, the Laurence-Moon-Biedl and Bardet-Biedl syndromes,[462] Cohen syndrome,[463] and Blount disease.[464] Prader-Willi syndrome is characterized by infantile hypotonia, mental deficiency, obesity, hypogonadism, hypopigmentation, behavioral abnormalities, and dysmorphic features.[465–467] Approximately 60 percent of these patients have a partial deletion of chromosome 15, 37 percent have normal chromosomes, and 3.6 percent have other abnormalities of chromosome 15.[468] Inheritance of both chromosome 15s from the mother may be causal in patients with normal chromosomes.[469] Some studies show that chromosome 15 changes associated with Prader-Willi syndrome occur in the gene encoding the small nuclear ribonucleoprotein N (SNRPN)[470,471]; however, there is no known mechanism to explain the occurrence of this disease. Treatment of Prader-Willi syndrome with both fluoxetine[472] and fenfluramine[473] has been reported.

TREATMENT OF OBESITY

Despite the numerous health and social problems associated with obesity as well as the physical limitations it imposes, the treatment of obesity is frustrating and usually unsuccessful. In a classic study, Stunkard and McLaren-Hume reviewed the literature on the treatment of obesity in 1959[474] and reported that less than 5 percent of patients were successful in losing 18 kg or more. The results of this study, as well as the experience of physicians in treating obese patients, have led to numerous strategies to treat obesity, including hypocaloric-balanced diets, "fad" diets, drugs, surgery, total starvation, jaw wiring, behavioral modification, exercise programs, very low calorie diets, and combinations of these treatments. Many of these treatments used alone are ineffective, and some are associated with significant side effects, are only transiently effective, or are dangerous.

Because of the frustrating nature of the treatment of obesity and the lack of a simple cure, misinformation and misinterpretation of information are rampant. Also, in a quest for a "cure," patients are susceptible to gimmicks and fad diets. The medically acceptable treatments for obesity are prevention, some diets, exercise, behavioral modification, surgery, and some drugs. There are several reviews on the treatment of obesity in adults.[11,182,475]

The NHLBI Expert Panel on the Identification, Evaluation, and Treatment of Overweight and Obesity in adults has formulated guidelines for the treatment of overweight and obesity.[11] The approach recommended is to measure weight and height in undergarments without shoes, measure waist circumference, and calculate BMI. For overweight and obese patients, a nutritional and physical activity assessment is also recommended. For those with a history of overweight or obesity, counseling concerning weight maintenance, evaluation of other risk factors, and periodic evaluation are advised. For those with a BMI $\geq$25 *or* a waist circumference of >88 cm in women and 103 cm in men, assessment of risk factors (CVD risk factors and obesity-associated diseases) is recommended. If the BMI is $\geq$30 *or* [BMI is 25–29.9 or the waist circumference is $\geq$88 cm (F) $\geq$102 cm (M) *and* $\geq$2 risk factors exist] weight loss is recommended. For those with a BMI between 25 and 29.9 who have one or no risk factors, maintaining weight is advised. It is recommended that the decision to lose weight should be a joint one between the physician and patient. If the patient does not want to lose weight, weight maintenance and treatment of other risk factors is recommended.

Prevention

Prevention of obesity is obviously the best treatment. Unfortunately, as reviewed earlier, the prevalence of obesity in children, adolescents, and adults in the United States is increasing.[11,12,476] Williamson et al. estimated the 10-year incidence of weight gain and concluded that obesity prevention should begin among adults in their early twenties, with special emphasis on young women who are already overweight.[477] Risk factors for weight gain include development periods (i.e., early childhood, adolescence, ages 25–35 years, and life events such as pregnancy, menopause, and the period after weight loss). In addition, a mother with gestational diabetes, overweight family members, and a history of depression, substance abuse, or sexual abuse, increase the risk of obesity.[182]

Although the 1988 Surgeon General's Report on Nutrition and Health, the NIH Consensus Conference on the Health Implications of Obesity,[478] and the recent NHLBI[11] and AACE[182] position statements recommend that obesity be treated because of increased morbidity and mortality, it is important that health professionals not promote an excessive preoccupation with weight and dieting, which might provoke eating disorders in susceptible individuals.[479] Some longitudinal studies have shown that obese babies do not necessarily become obese children.[480] This is in contrast to the generally accepted concept that fat children grow into fat adults.[481,482] The most important risk factor for obesity in children is parental obesity,[483] with both genetic[484] and environmental[485,486] factors. Because of the importance of parental modeling and supportive behaviors, Epstein and Cluss evaluated a program incorporating behavioral change reinforced by child and parent groups for the treatment of childhood obesity.[486] The 10-year follow-up of this program indicated that the techniques used were effective in achieving and maintaining long-term weight loss during a 10-year period.[487,488] This program involved several behavioral procedures, including contracting, self-monitoring, social reinforcement and modeling, and contingency management. If confirmed in other studies, this approach may be extremely useful in limiting obesity in adulthood. It should be mentioned that this treatment limited but did not prevent obesity. Patients in the child and parent treatment group were still approximately 35 percent overweight 10 years after intervention. This is in contrast to the nonspecific group, which was heavier 10 years later and was approximately 60 percent overweight.[488] In children, it is important that interventions not interfere with normal growth or promote the development of eating disorders.[489] It is recommended by the American Dietetic Association that intervention programs (1) be adaptable to individual needs, (2) include nutritionally sound and sensible eating patterns, (3) use psychologically sound family-oriented approaches and bring about positive behavioral modification, (4) be supportive of social needs, (5) include physical activity components, (6) be coordinated with medical care, (7) continue long enough to establish attitudinal and behavioral changes, (8) promote a positive attitude toward life and self, and (9) recognize that there is a wide range of acceptable body sizes and shapes.

Work site programs are often the most effective community approaches to weight control. As reviewed by Stunkard, weight-loss competitions are often extremely effective and attractive to groups that often ignore health promotion programs, such as men and blue-collar workers.[490] The effective elements of weight-loss competitions appear to be a combination of competition and cooperation because neither cooperation nor individual competition alone is effective. The advantage of such cooperative competition against natural competitors such as business rivals is its very low cost. As outlined by Stunkard, the cost of work site competition is less than a dollar per 1 percent reduction in percentage overweight as opposed to \$6.30 for commercial programs and \$89.20 for a university clinic.[490]

A primary objective for health care professionals should be the prevention of obesity in children and adults through nutrition and health education. Optimal weight should be determined by considering health risks, heredity, age, sex, percentage of body fat, and realistic goal setting. Primary prevention should include strategies that address social issues related to calorie overconsumption and inadequate physical exercise.[491] Children should not be placed on restricted-calorie diets but should be encouraged to be physically active and eat a well-balanced diet. Parents should be included in programs for children. Finally, weight-control programs should include behavioral management techniques for food intake, exercise, stress, and improved self-esteem. These programs should focus on the avoidance of repeated diet failures.[489] For adults, the inclusion of partners in weight-loss programs may facilitate weight loss and improve long-term maintenance of weight reduction for the patient while also promoting weight loss in the partner. Patients with normal-weight partners tend to lose more weight than do those with overweight partners; however, the body weight of overweight partners significantly decreases over time.[492,493] Commercial groups such as Weight Watchers and Tops can be extremely effective, but the attrition rates in these programs are very high.[494] Community programs for weight reduction and prevention have with few exceptions generally been ineffective.[495–497]

Exercise

Based on epidemiologic evidence and randomized trials supporting the association between exercise and weight control,[498] the report for the U.S. Preventive Services Task Force[499] has stated that the efficacy of exercising in the prevention of obesity warrants a category A recommendation; that is, there is good evidence to support the recommendation that the conditions be specifically considered in a periodic health examination. Based on a careful review of the literature, this report recommends the guidelines for physician action counseling outlined in Table 20-7. The NHLBI[11] has issued the following statements based on a review of the literature:

1. Physical activity (i.e. aerobic exercise) in overweight and obese adults results in modest weight loss independent of the effect of caloric reduction through diet.
2. Physical activity in overweight and obese adults modestly reduces abdominal fat.
3. Physical activity in overweight and obese adults increases cardiorespiratory fitness independent of weight loss.

They conclude that exercise is recommended as part of a comprehensive weight loss and maintenance program. Even small amounts of exercise may be beneficial, including weight training.[499] As reviewed by Wanger and Bell,[500] improvement in cardiovascular fitness can be achieved at relatively low levels of exercise intensity and is graded from intensities of 50–100 percent V_{O_2max}, frequencies of two to four times per week, and a duration of 15–45 min. Low-intensity exercise can be especially efficacious in the elderly and in persons with poor baseline fitness.[499] Also, low-intensity exercise (50–70 percent V_{O_2max}) during a longer period (35–45 min) can have an effect equal to or greater than that of higher-intensity (90–100 percent V_{O_2max}) exercise during a shorter period (25–35 min).[500]

An exercise prescription should take into account the patient's cardiopulmonary status, illnesses, exercise tolerance, and current life-style. As with most life-style changes, including diet, the smaller the increment in the change and the less radical the

TABLE 20-7. Guidelines for Physical Activity Counseling

1. Incorporate questions regarding the physical activity level of patients into history taking during routine health care visits.
2. Identify inactive patients who do not appear to meet the minimal level of physical activity associated with gains in cardiorespiratory fitness: intensity of >50 percent V_{O_2max},* duration of 15–45 min, and frequency of 2–4 times per week.
3. Attempt to interest patients in adopting a program of regular physical activity by discussing the role of physical activity disease prevention and addressing each patient's individual risk of conditions associated with inactivity and perceived health status.
4. Guide patients in choosing an appropriate type of physical activity that will be efficacious for health—such as an activity that is predominantly weight-bearing, results in energy expenditure, contributes to cardiorespiratory fitness, and has a low potential for adverse effects—and effective for adherence—such as an activity with moderate intensity; low perceived exertion; low cost; convenience; proximity to home; flexible time and location; lack of need for specialized facilities, equipment, skills, or formal programs; opportunity for simultaneous social interaction; and the potential to be incorporated into the patient's usual daily activities. Walking is the optimal activity in most cases.
5. Guide the patient to choose an appropriate level of participation in terms of intensity, duration, and frequency. The initial level should be only a small increment above baseline status. Gradual progression should be made over a period of several months, with a goal of reaching the minimum level outlined above. Familiarize the patient with measuring the pulse rate during exercise and set appropriate goals for intensity based on estimating the V_{O_2max} on the basis of the heart rate. (An intensity of 50–85 percent of the V_{O_2max} corresponds to 65–90 percent of the maximal heart rate. The maximal heart rate can be crudely estimated by subtracting one's age in years from 220.) Encourage patients at each visit to set at least one specific goal in terms of intensity, duration, and frequency that can be built on in the future. An exercise diary may be useful for this purpose.
6. Monitor compliance with physical activity and provide positive reinforcement during future health care visits.
7. Large increments in the physical activity level should be discouraged because of increased risk of injury and adverse effects as well as increased noncompliance. Patients should be told to consult a physician if they encounter persistent injury or adverse effects.
8. Encourage the social support of significant others.
9. Identify barriers that arise to optimal adherence and discuss strategies for overcoming them.
10. Encourage adherence to activity, particularly after major lifestyle transitions such as graduation from high school or college, marriage, job change, residence change, and recovery from illness or injury.
11. An exercise ECG is not necessary for asymptomatic, generally healthy persons planning to increase their level of physical activity. Patients needing specific medical attention and those in whom exercise is contraindicated should be identified.

* V_{O_2max} indicates maximal uptake.

Source: Modified from Harris et al.[499]

change, the more likely it is to be accepted by the patient. Intervention should be achieved in small increments. Although the initial motivation for exercise is health-related, the motivation for continuing includes enjoyment, convenience, cost, and social support of the exercise. Low-intensity exercise has a greater compliance rate,[501] although King et al. have found that higher intensity home-based exercise has better long-term adherence.[502] Few people over age 35 who are not currently exercising are likely to take on a program of vigorous exercise.[501] Physicians can have a significant impact on whether a patient exercises[499] and should focus on the reasons for recommending exercise and encouraging social support. Brisk walking is an excellent additional recommendation because it is weight-bearing; improves cardiovascular fitness; is convenient; has little perceived discomfort; can be done at flexible times and locations; has the potential for social interactions; can be incorporated into usual daily activities, making it less disruptive; and requires no special facilities, equipment, or skills.

Exercise could theoretically improve weight loss and help maintain a reduced weight by increasing caloric expenditure, decreasing energy intake, or making changes in life-style that promote better adherence to a diet. The effect of exercise on weight loss is modest. In a review of 12 articles by the NHLBI, the average weight loss was 5.3 pounds compared to controls.[11] In a meta-analysis of 28 studies, aerobic exercise alone produced a weight loss of 6.6 lbs in men and 3.1 pounds in women.[503] Woo et al. have presented evidence that obese individuals do not increase intake to compensate for increased energy expenditure, though lean individuals do.[504,505] The obese individuals did not, however, lose a significant amount of weight.[504] In a review of 10 studies that contained a diet-only and an exercise-only group, the exercise-only groups did not lose as much weight as the diet-only groups with one exception.[11] Obviously, the effects of exercise on weight loss and body composition depend on the intensity, duration, and type of exercise. The greater the intensity and duration, the more calories are used, and the more resistance training is done, the more lean body mass (LBM) is preserved.[506] The greatest effect of exercise, however, is on the ability to maintain weight loss.[507] The more lean body mass can be preserved, the less the decrease is in resting energy expenditure, and the more total energy that is expended in exercise, the greater the weight loss will be. It is likely, however, that an exercise program in most middle-aged obese individuals represents a substantial life-style change.

As mentioned earlier, the major effect of exercise is in the maintenance of weight reduction. Pronk and Wing[508] have reviewed this. Studies show with remarkable consistency that exercise is an important determinant of long-term maintenance of weight loss. In one study subjects who exercised during weight reduction and continued to exercise afterward maintained their weight loss during an 18-month follow-up, whereas those who never exercised or stopped exercising regained most or all of their weight.[507] As shown in Fig. 20-12, among 52 subjects who lost an average of approximately 10 kg without exercise and were followed for 18 months after the diet, 47 who continued to abstain from exercise regained all their weight, while 5 subjects who began exercising after weight gain lost weight to approximately their original weight loss. Among the subjects who exercised during weight loss, all 36 who continued to exercise maintained their weight loss for 18 months. Those who stopped exercising regained most or all of their weight loss (Fig. 20-9). The authors concluded that treatment programs must be multidisciplinary and include a supervised exercise component, that exercise instruction alone is insufficient, that maintenance of weight loss requires a continuation of exercise at a level of at least three times weekly for a total of approximately 1,500 calories per week, and that maintenance exercise need not be supervised if the treatment phase is conducted properly.

It can be concluded that exercise is a critical component of any weight-loss program and that emphasis should be placed on life-style changes that will lead to continued exercise after weight has been lost. Patients should exercise three to four times per

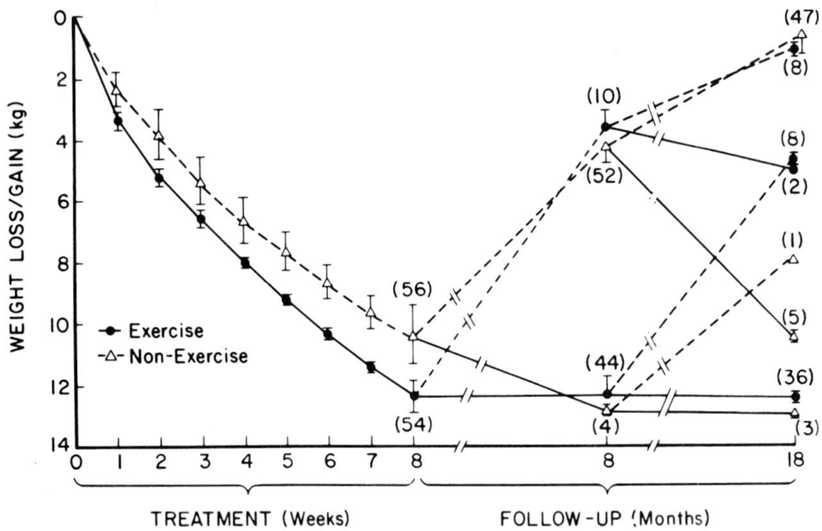

FIGURE 20-12. Weight loss or gain in exercise and nonexercise groups during an 8-week diet period and 18 months of follow-up. There was a small increase in weight loss in the exercise group during the first 8 weeks; however, the main difference was in weight maintenance. Subjects who continued to exercise (solid lines) maintained weight loss; those who discontinued exercise (dashed lines) gained weight. Subjects who never exercised regained their weight, whereas the poststudy introduction of exercise had a positive effect. (*From Pavlou et al.,*[341] *with permission.*)

week at activities they enjoy in order to avoid burnout. They should plan ahead and develop realistic exercise patterns that can be sustained in the future. The physician should provide reinforcement and encouragement and emphasize life-style changes. Exercise focuses patients on leading a healthy life-style, which includes attention to diet and body image. This may be more important in sustaining weight loss than is the increase in caloric expenditure induced by exercise. Other potential actions of exercise, such as effects on resting energy expenditure, modifying the thermic effect of food, and sustaining increased energy expenditure, along with the possible benefits of exercise before or after a meal, are of minor significance.[338,340,509–516]

Behavioral Modification

An organized behavioral modification program is critical to successful weight reduction and maintenance.[11,182] Without significant changes in life-style and eating habits, along with group support, a weight-reduction program is likely to fail. A successful behavioral modification program will describe the behavior to be changed, set goals for behavioral change and outcomes, modify the stimuli that precede eating, and modify the consequences of eating inappropriate foods. Such a program involves (1) setting goals for caloric intake, weight loss, and exercise, and (2) keeping a diary to help recognize the cues that trigger eating behavior and develop appropriate responses to these cues. Patients should record the feelings that lead to eating behavior and list alternative behaviors related to what they are feeling at the time. Eventually, eating responses will be replaced by more productive behavior. This process of deconditioning old behavior and reconditioning new behavior does not occur rapidly and requires patience and repeated reinforcement. It is important to help patients realize that eating is often not done out of physical need. One should emphasize the importance of eating only three meals per day, as snacking behavior can lead to large increases in caloric intake, and to be aware of the potential caloric intake from beverages. Patients are instructed in how to slow down eating to prolong a meal and how to have only one place in the house where they eat to avoid eating while engaging in activities such as watching television and driving.

Diet

Any treatment for obesity will require a diet. As was mentioned earlier, exercise alone is usually not effective unless it involves extreme exertion, which is unlikely for the vast majority of obese patients. The standard or conventional hypocaloric diets (1,000–1,500 cal/day), when used alone, are usually ineffective primarily because patients are hungry, their weight loss is slow, and they have difficulty controlling their energy intake. For example, a 5-foot, 2-inch woman who does not exercise would be expected to utilize a minimum of 1,500 to 1,700 kcal/day. On a 1,000-calorie diet, with each 500 kcal/day caloric deficit resulting in a 1 lb/week weight loss, she would lose approximately 1 to 1.3 lb/week. If she weighed 180 lb and wanted to achieve a weight of 130 lbs, this would require from 37 to 48 weeks of dieting without ever exceeding 1,000 cal/day, a nearly impossible task. Recently, more modest goals for weight reduction have been proposed with goals of 10 percent weight loss over 6 months[11] using a diet deficient in 300–500 kcal per day for a BMI of 27–35 and 500–1,000 kcal per day for a BMI of >35. The AACE[182] has recommended goals of 10 percent to no more than 30 percent weight loss with a goal of 1 lb per week for the first month. This group recommends a daily caloric deficit of 500 kcal with total energy expenditure based on the formula REE = 9.99 wt(kg) + 6.25 ht(cm) − 4.92 age(yr) + 166 × sex (males = 1, females = 0) − 161. Multiply REE × 1.5 for women and 1.6 for men to get TEE. A simpler method for average levels of activity is to calculate 30 kcal per kg body weight or 35 kcal per kg for moderate activity. In our studies using $^{2}H^{18}0$, TEE (kcal/24 h) in women equaled 1,056 + 19.6 wt(kg).[357]

The AACE has recently affirmed that all programs for the treatment of obesity require five essential components: (1) Attainable weight loss goals, (2) at least monthly contact for the first year with group sessions, (3) emphasis on weight-loss maintenance, (4) informed consent, and (5) physician involvement.[182] For modest weight reduction, such an approach through an inexpensive, organized, reputable program such as Weight Watchers, Diet Workshop, or TOPS is reasonable. These programs all have organized behavioral modification programs and long-term follow-up. To be successful, however, patients must stay in the program, and this is often not the case. Volkmar et al. found that 50 percent of the members of commercial weight-reduction programs dropped out in 6 weeks and 70 percent in 12 weeks.[494] Diets containing less than 1,200 kcal per day require vitamin and mineral supplementation.[182] For patients with large amounts of weight to lose (more than 30 percent above IBW), a low-energy diet (<800 to 1,000 cal/day) should be considered, but only after failure of the methods listed above. Patients should be given a chance with a commercial diet program first, with encouragement and a scientific explanation of expected weight loss on such a diet.

Patients should also be instructed in the importance of weighing and measuring food. Most patients underestimate their caloric consumption by an average of 23 percent.[310] In a more recent study,[518] 24-h energy expenditure, resting energy expenditure, body composition, thermic effect of food, oxygen consumption in response to exercise, and food intake were measured in diet-resistant and control obese subjects. Total and resting energy expenditure were within 5 percent of predicted and the thermic effect of food and response to exercise were the same in the diet-resistant and control groups. The diet-resistant group, however, underreported their actual food intake by 47 ± 16 percent and overreported their physical activity by 51 ± 75 percent. This confirms what all those who care for obese patients have experienced, that patients who report an inability to lose weight on a restricted diet are not accurately reporting their energy intake or expenditure. With refractory patients, I routinely measure their resting metabolic rate. This almost always convinces them that they are underreporting their energy intake. I also emphasize weighing and measuring all food and recording all exercise.

Patients not enrolled in commercial programs should see a dietician. Diets should be individualized based on life-style, ethnicity, coexisting medical conditions, and current drug therapy. I also emphasize eating only three meals per day, eliminating all snacks and desserts, and drinking only noncaloric beverages unless incorporated into the diet plan.

A multidisciplinary team including a physician, a mental health professional who specializes in the psychological treatment of eating disorders, and a dietician[519] should treat patients who meet the criteria of binge eaters. The criteria for diagnosis, psychiatric comorbidity, and treatment are discussed in a recent article.[519]

Maintenance of long-term weight loss is a critical problem for obese patients who are successful at losing weight. A recent descriptive study[520] of individuals who were successful at keeping off a minimum of 13.6 kg for 5 years indicated that only 55 percent used a formal program or professional assistance and 77 percent reported a triggering event that preceded successful weight loss. The triggering event appears to be critical in the motivation for increased exercise and a stricter dietary approach than previous weight loss attempts. Many different strategies were employed for weight loss and maintenance including limiting intake of certain foods, limiting quantities, limiting fat, counting calories, etc. Exercise was also widely used. More than 90 percent reported improved quality of life, energy, mood, mobility, and self-confidence. Although this study was not controlled, used self-reported data, and was conducted on a primarily white, highly-educated group, it does point out that weight loss can be maintained using individual strategies.

Very-low-energy diets (400–800 cal/day, 1,760–3,350 kJ) have recently been reviewed[521] and the National Institutes of Health National Task Force on the Prevention and Treatment of Obesity has issued a review and position statement.[522] The conclusion of the National Task Force[522] was that "Current VLCDs are generally safe when used under proper medical supervision in moderately and severely obese patients" but that "long-term maintenance of weight lost . . . is no better than with other forms of obesity treatment. Incorporation of behavioral therapy and physical therapy . . . seems to improve maintenance." Similarly, as discussed below, the AACE has concluded that ". . . long-term success of VLCDs does not seem any better than that with LCDs."[182] New data suggests that treating patients with sibutramine after losing weight on a VLCD is beneficial (see later discussion). The criteria for LCDs, VLCDs, and surgical treatment are outlined in Table 20-8.

The liquid protein diets popularized in the 1970s proved to be unsafe. Based on research observations that 55 g of protein per day is accompanied by minimal negative nitrogen balance during the first week of a fast with subsequent return to equilibrium,[523] numerous investigators added protein to a total fast to reduce the protein loss associated with total fasting. Although these research diets contained high-quality protein with some mineral and vitamin supplementation,[521,524] many commercial very-low-calorie or liquid protein diets consisted of collagen hydrolysates and lacked necessary minerals and micronutrients. In 1977, based on the book *The Last Chance Diet*,[525] it was estimated that more than

TABLE 20-8. General Criteria for Selecting a Weight-Management Strategy*

Basic Treatment with LCD	Basic Treatment with LCD or VLCD†	Basic Treatment with LCD or VLCD† and Pharmacotherapy	Surgical Treatment
BMI ≥ 25	BMI ≥ 35	BMI ≥ 35	BMI > 40
Good diet history	BMI ≥ 30 with comorbid conditions	BMI ≥ 30†	BMI ≥ 35 with life-threatening or disabling comorbid condition(s)
		BMI 27–29 with comorbid conditions‡	
	Poor diet history	Poor diet history	Obesity history ≥5 yr No history of alcoholism or major psychiatric disorders ≥18 yr old

*BMI = body mass index; LCD = low-calorie diet; VLCD = very-low-calorie diet.

† VLCDs are reserved for nonelderly adults with high health risk due solely to BMI or BMI with serious comorbid condition(s).

‡ In combination with LCD only.

Source: From Ref. 182.

100,000 people used this 300-cal hydrolyzed collagen diet exclusively for at least 1 month. In the same year, at least 60 deaths were reported among persons who used these formulations. Among the 60 deaths between July 1977 and January 1978, Isner and colleagues[526] reported on 17 patients who were healthy prior to initiation of the diet and had detailed clinical information, autopsy data, or both at the time of death. All 17 patients had serious cardiac arrhythmias prior to death, including ventricular tachycardia, and autopsy findings showed significant cardiac muscle wasting compatible with cachexia.

A 6-week study of patients in a controlled clinical research setting ingesting a very-low-energy diet similar to those that were commercially available[527] demonstrated potentially life-threatening arrhythmias in 50 percent of the patients. The arrhythmias were observed as early as 10 days after the start of the diet and increased in frequency and complexity as the diet continued. These arrhythmias were not seen on routine electrocardiograms but were detectable only by 24-h ambulatory ECG monitoring. Despite numerous balance studies, we could not find an association between the cardiac arrhythmias and imbalances of nitrogen or minerals. A follow-up report in which obese subjects were given a highly supplemented 420-kcal diet under the same controlled conditions[528] indicated that with this highly supplemented diet, no cardiac arrhythmias or significant mineral depletions were detected. We concluded that a vigorously supplemented, very-low-energy diet under proper medical supervision could be used safely. In a subsequent study we evaluated patients with obesity and NIDDM, again using a highly supplemented very-low-energy diet.[149] This study demonstrated that in a controlled clinical research center environment such a diet is both safe and efficacious in patients with complicated obesity and is highly effective in reducing blood glucose, cholesterol, triglycerides, and blood pressure in patients with type 2 diabetes. Cholesterol declined from a mean of 6.38 ± 0.51 mmol/L (247 ± 55 mg/dl) to 4.49 ± 0.32 mmol/L (174 ± 12.5 mg/dl), triglycerides declined from 3.01 ± 0.62 mmol/L (267 ± 55 mg/dl) to 1.58 ± 0.16 mmol/L (150 ± 15 mg/dl), and blood pressure declined from a mean of $136 \pm 9/81 \pm 2$ to $116 \pm 8/71 \pm 2$. We concluded that such diets under proper medical supervision are the initial treatment of choice for patients with type 2 diabetes who are 30 percent or more above IBW.

Very-low-energy diets, as they are used today, provide 420–800 kcal/day (1,760–3,350 kJ) in the form of dietary protein alone or in combination with carbohydrate and fat. They contain 45–100 g of protein, 30 to 100 g of carbohydrate, and approximately 2 g of fat per day. VLCDs should provide at least 1g of protein per kg of desirable body weight. Most diets use a milk- or egg-based protein formula served as a liquid diet. These diets contain the minimum daily requirements of vitamins, minerals, and trace elements. For some trace elements minimum daily requirements have not been established, and in such cases supplements are usually based on average daily intake. Because of the significant potassium losses that can occur with the 420 calorie formulations, potassium supplements are frequently necessary, especially if patients are losing weight very rapidly, were on diuretics before starting the diet, or have low or low-normal serum potassium. Some diets use animal protein in food form (i.e., meat, fish, or fowl). Proponents of these diets argue that patients learn to successfully handle conventional foods and can make the transition from a very-low-energy diet to a weight-maintenance diet more easily. Those who favor liquid formula diets argue that they promote better dietary adherence by simplifying the diet and removing food choices. Both diets produce similar weight loss, but there have been no controlled studies comparing the merits of the two diets for long-term maintenance. Over-the-counter supplements should be used only for replacement of one or two meals per day and their use as the sole source of nutrition could be dangerous.

Since the advent of commercially available very-low-energy diets that contain high-quality protein, daily minimum requirements of vitamins, minerals, and trace elements, and 45–100 g of protein per day, there have been no reports of sudden death attributable to these diets when used under medical supervision. Based on this information and studies in the literature directly demonstrating safety,[149,528] it is reasonable to conclude that these diets are safe when medically supervised and used for a short period in a properly selected group of patients. Because studies indicate that there is no significant difference in weight loss on formula diets less than 800 calories compared to 800 calories,[528] it is recommended that the 800-calorie diet be used.

The major advantages of very-low-energy diets compared with standard hypocaloric diets (from 800 to 1,000 cal/day) are the more rapid rate of weight loss and the suppression of hunger.

Weight loss on a very-low-energy diet varies substantially depending primarily on the initial weight of the patient, complicating medical illnesses and medications, and the sex of the patient. During the first week of a very-low-energy diet, the majority of the weight loss is related to fluid loss. Thus, a patient who is fluid-depleted as a result of diuretic use or hyperglycemia secondary to poorly regulated diabetes mellitus may lose less weight in the first 1 or 2 weeks. For example, the correlation coefficient between the percentage weight loss over 6 weeks and initial fasting plasma glucose level was $r = -0.98$.[149] The initial fluid loss is related to decreasing insulin levels that lead to decreased sodium resorption by the kidney, increased ketone body production resulting in sodium and water loss, and the utilization of carbohydrate stores, which, unlike lipid, must be stored in hydrated form. Obese patients without diabetes lose approximately 13 percent of their initial weight in the first 6 weeks of a very-low-energy diet,[528,529] while patients with hyperglycemia and type II diabetes lose approximately 10 percent of their initial body weight in the first 6 weeks.[149] The average weight loss on very-low-energy diets during the active dieting phase is 1.5–2.0 kg/week in women and 2.0–2.5 kg/week in men.[523] Conventional low-calorie diets produce average weight losses during the active dieting phase of 0.4–0.5 kg/week.[523]

Obese women expend an average of approximately 32 calories per kilogram of total body weight.[321] Thus, the expected weight loss in subsequent weeks can be easily calculated, taking into account the fact that the metabolic rate decreases approximately 15 percent on restrictive diets. A 5-foot, 2-inch, 180-lb woman would be expected to lose approximately 38 lb in 12 weeks: 13 percent in the first 6 weeks and 2 to 3 lb/week thereafter depending on her exercise level. Because of increased lean body mass in males, the metabolic rate is higher than it is in females of comparable height. Thus, males on average will lose more weight than females. Finally, obese individuals have more lean body mass than do normal individuals of comparable height, and consequently, the resting metabolic rate in obese individuals is increased because the resting metabolic rate is closely related to lean body mass.[321,357] As total energy expenditure is best correlated with body weight, obese individuals have greater total energy expenditure than do lean individuals. Thus, the more a patient weighs, the greater that patient's resting and total energy expenditure and the faster that patient would be expected to lose weight.

The metabolic changes that occur with very-low-energy diets include decreases in blood pressure, plasma glucose, cholesterol, triglycerides, and edema, and dramatic improvements in pulmonary function.[149,527–530] Sleep apnea syndrome frequently resolves within a few weeks.[253] In most patients plasma glucose declines very rapidly in the first week and subsequently declines more slowly.[149] Cardiac performance and exercise tolerance also improve.[149] Other benefits of weight reduction frequently include changes in body image and sense of well-being as well as improvements in joint and low back pain and, frequently, regulation of menses and enhanced fertility.

Unfortunately, there have been few long-term follow-up studies of these metabolic and clinical parameters in patients who have been treated with very-low-energy diets for the standard period of 12–16 weeks. Studies evaluating long-term follow-up of glucose, blood pressure, pulmonary function, lipids, and other parameters are necessary to evaluate the long-term benefit of very-low-energy diets in complicated obesity. The few long-term studies evaluating success at maintaining a reduced weight indicate that patients on a VLCD plus behavioral modification lose and maintain greater weight loss than patients on conventional diets for periods up to one year, but at 5 years of follow-up sustained weight loss is poor and there is no difference between the diet groups.[531–534] However, several published reports have demonstrated the importance of behavioral modification in long-term success[522,531,533,535] as well as the importance of exercise.[507,522] Clinical trials have not demonstrated that VLCDs lead to greater weight loss after one year than do conventional hypocaloric diets.[532] There have been no publications of controlled trials evaluating weight maintenance several years later. A recent descriptive study of self-reported weights followed 621 patients who had completed a 26-week weight loss program that included 12 weeks of a very-low-calorie diet.[534] Of these patients, 281 participated in all follow-up assessments for 5 years. Men lost a mean of 25.5 percent and women 22.6 percent of their weight. At follow-up at 2, 3, 4, and 5 years, the percent of weight loss that was maintained for men and women followed for all 5 years was 36.1 and 44, 28 and 42.2, 25.9 and 27.9, and 22.7 and 30.5, respectively. At 5 years, 47.8 percent maintained a reduction in weight of ≥5 percent. Participation in additional weight loss programs did not significantly affect treatment outcome. Though these results are encouraging, it is critical that new methods be developed to help patients maintain weight loss. A recent study evaluating sibutramine for the long-term maintenance of weight loss after a VLCD has suggested that this approach may be effective (see later discussion). Additional controlled long-term studies of drug treatment after weight loss, the intermittent use of very-low-energy diets, and the use of a combination of supplements and food are important areas for future research.

As with weight loss on conventional diets, the people with diabetes who remain euglycemic will probably be those with diabetes of shorter duration (i.e., <5–10 years).[530,536] Those who are hypertensive secondary to obesity will have permanent resolution of blood pressure with persistent weight reduction. Those whose hypertension is only exacerbated by obesity will not have normalization of blood pressure. Similarly, secondary hyperlipidemias due to diet and obesity are corrected, whereas patients with primary hyperlipidemia will still have lipid abnormalities after weight reduction.

The complications of very-low-energy diets are generally minor and include fatigue, orthostatic dizziness, inability to concentrate, feelings of euphoria, constipation or diarrhea, dry skin, hair loss, cold intolerance, menstrual irregularities, and, rarely, muscle cramps. Rarely, patients complain of loss of libido, and a few patients have complained of worsening of migraine or the appearance of ocular migraine.[537] On carefully controlled refeeding, cholelithiasis and pancreatitis are rare. However, they can be a complication of binge eating on a very-low-energy diet. Hyperuricemia is common, but gout is rare. Some patients also experience problems with self-identity and body image, but serious psychiatric problems are rarely encountered. The two most frequent problems—constipation and orthostatic hypotension—are usually easily treated with fiber and bouillon, respectively.

Of recent interest and some concern has been the appearance of gallstones while patients are ingesting a very-low-energy diet.[538,539] It has been known for some time that weight-reducing diets are associated with decreased bile acid output, decreased cholesterol saturation of bile, decreased contraction of the gallbladder, increased biliary glycoproteins, and increased bile prostaglandin E_2 concentrations. In the study of Mok et al., bile acid pools in obese subjects decreased on caloric restriction to 1,000 kcal/day.[540] In patients on a 520-cal/day diet,[539] bile saturation increased after 4 weeks and this was associated with an increase in percent cholesterol, a decrease in percent bile acids, and a decrease in percent phospholipids. In addition, prostaglandin E_2 increased significantly. Total parenteral nutrition and gastric and ileal bypass surgery are also associated with an increased incidence of gallstones,[511–513] although the relationship between bariatric surgery and gallstone formation has recently been challenged.[544] It has been proposed that decreased bile acid flow and gallbladder stasis may be important etiologic events. On very-low-energy diets, 5 of 19 patients developed gallstones in one study[539] and 13 of 51 subjects did so in another study.[538] In patients with gallstones who do not require surgery, 33–40 percent still have gallstones 6–36 months after completion of the diet. In one study, ursodeoxycholic acid was used to prevent the supersaturation of bile during weight reduction and aspirin was used to decrease prostaglandin-dependent glycoprotein formation.[539,545–548] Two of 21 subjects on aspirin developed gallstones, but both patients had low salicylate levels. In the ursodeoxycholate-treated groups[539] only one patient developed cholesterol crystals. Some have proposed that increasing the fat content of the diet will prevent gallstones.[549] A recent review of the literature, however, indicates that the rate of weight loss is most important (Fig. 20-13) and that the incidence of gallstones increases dramatically above an average weight loss of 1.5 kg per week.[550] A recent publication compared a 900-calorie liquid diet with 30 g of fat, including one 10 g fat meal to stimulate maximal gallbladder emptying, to a 520-calorie diet with less than 2 g of fat.[551] Both diets produced comparable weight loss, but gallstones developed in 4 of 6 patients on the 520-calorie diet and none of nine on the 900-calorie diet plus the added fat. The 10 g fat meal maximally stimulated gallbladder emptying. Though these data need to be confirmed, adding a small amount of fat to the diet during rapid weight loss may prevent gallstone formation.[551] Approximately one-third of gallstones formed during a VLCD disappear during the first 6 months after refeeding.[552]

The safety and efficacy of very-low-energy diets depend on proper patient selection, careful medical supervision, and the availability of an organized program that includes the participation of physicians, behaviorists, and nutritionists. It is mandatory to include

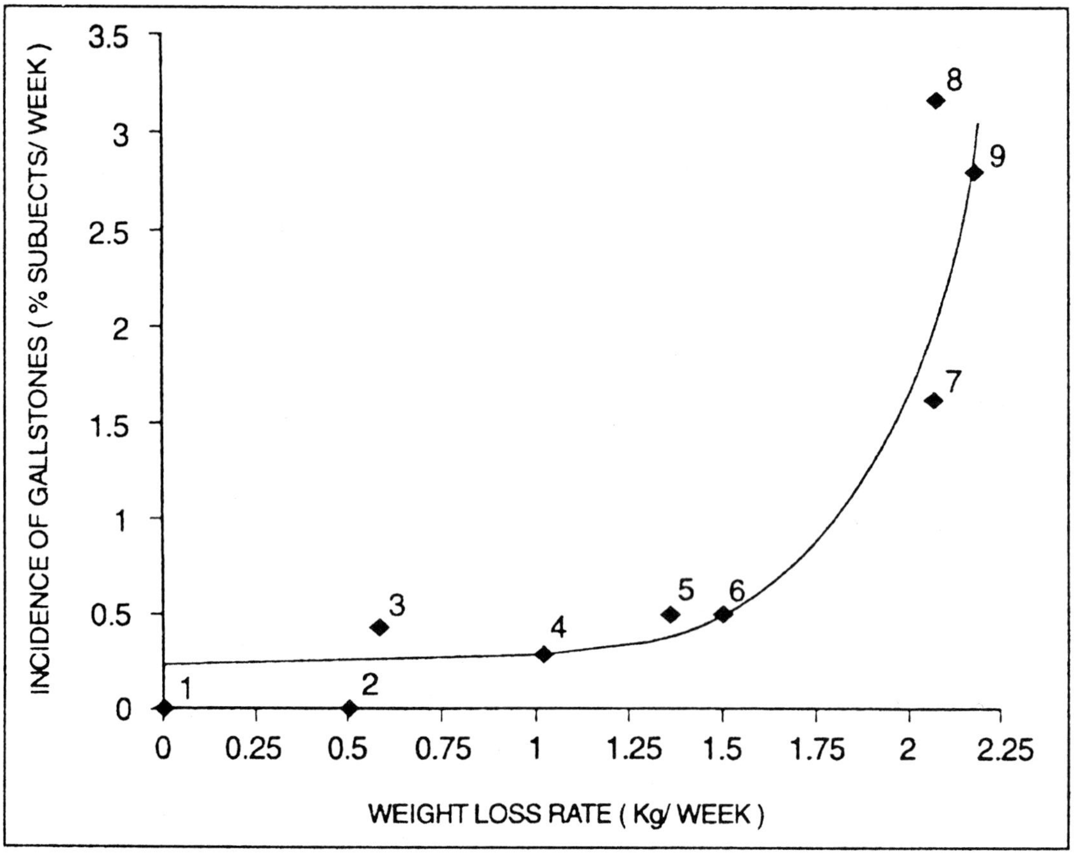

FIGURE 20-13. The relationship of incidence of gallstone formation to rate of weight loss in obese patients based upon published studies. (*From Weisner et al.,*[550] *with permission.*)

an organized long-term maintenance program. Because exercise tolerance and exercise preferences vary substantially among individuals, it is difficult to include an exercise program as part of a weight-loss program. Nevertheless, to facilitate maintenance of weight loss, all patients should be required to enter into an exercise program of their choosing. The exercise should be something they enjoy and something that can be sustained for long periods. Patients should be encouraged to exercise 3–4 days per week and should be discouraged from developing unrealistic expectations about exercise. They should not plan on exercising vigorously only while losing weight and should expect to continue exercising after weight loss has been achieved.

Proper patient selection is critical. Patients must be at least 30 percent above IBW ($BMI > 30$) with comorbid conditions or have a BMI of $\geq$35 with obesity alone, be less than 60 years old, and have failed at more conservative approaches to weight loss. As patients approach IBW, the proportion of weight loss which is lean body mass increases.[553] This is accelerated even more by a very-low-energy diet. It is therefore critical that patients who are below 120 percent of IBW not be maintained on a very-low-energy diet. Normal body composition can be achieved at IBW if caloric intake is increased to 800 calories when body weight has fallen to 120 percent above and gradually increased to maintenance calories when IBW has been achieved.[357]

Generally, although most programs do not accept patients with serious underlying illnesses, the patients who have the most serious complications of obesity are the ones most likely to benefit from weight reduction. It is critical, however, that if such patients are accepted, a physician who is skilled in caring for patients on very-low-energy diets monitor them. Definite contraindications include cancer, cerebrovascular disease, a recent myocardial infarction, unstable angina, malignant dysrhythmias, prolonged QT syndromes, cardiac syncope, hepatic disease, a serious untreated psychiatric disease, and pregnancy. Any patient with psychiatric disease who is accepted into a program should have clearance from the psychiatrist or psychologist who is treating the illness, and medications known to prolong the QT interval such as phenothiazines and tricyclic antidepressants should be avoided. A history of bulimia nervosa or anorexia is a contraindication. Although diets below 800 calories per day are no longer recommended, patients over 60, less than 30 percent above IBW, or with significant cardiopulmonary disease or renal disease should be treated with a minimum of 800 cal/day under close supervision with appropriate subspecialty consultations. Patients with type 1 diabetes can be treated with very-low-energy diets if great care is given to the decreased insulin requirements. It should be required that all patients with insulin-treated diabetes use home glucose monitoring. Oral agents are discontinued upon initiation of the VLCD. Obese patients with renal failure can be treated, but it must be recognized that these patients usually have other serious medical problems and should not be treated with less than an 800-cal formula diet or a 1,000-cal food diet. The National Task Force on the Prevention and Treatment of Obesity[554] reviewed recommendations for the use of VLCDs.

During the initial evaluation for treatment with very-low-energy diets the physician should explain to the patient the physiologic basis for recommending the diet program and emphasize possible side effects and the importance of behavioral modification, exercise, and a long-term maintenance group in sustaining the reduced weight. Consistent attendance and tracking or records keeping are essential. These points should be reinforced by a lecture or tape dealing with the history and theory of low-energy diets as well as the issues mentioned earlier. Weekly visits include a physician visit and a behavioral modification class. Support sessions should be conducted in closed groups of 10–20 patients since it has been shown that open-group programs have a higher attrition rate.[555] Helpful information is included in the AACE/ACE Obesity statement.[182] For patients in whom exercise may constitute a risk, referral to a cardiac rehabilitation program may be indicated.

During the first visit prior to starting a very-low-energy diet, the physician and patient set a weight goal that is achievable and realistic for the time the patient is to be in the program. Long-term weight goals can also be established. Patients should sign a contract that includes the goal weight and very specific program rules. The criteria for expulsion from the program are specified, as is the warning system for expulsion. It is important that patients abide by these rules both to ensure the safety of the program and to maximize the chances of long-term success. The points to be emphasized include (1) eating the diet and supplement as three meals per day to extinguish snacking behavior and (2) the importance of the avoidance of eating food.[521] Most patients who eat food while on a very-low-energy diet are not successful in achieving their weight-loss goal. Patients are encouraged to keep a diary and take the behavioral modification seriously.

Patients with potassium below 4 mEq/dl and those who have been taking diuretics are started on a potassium supplement. For patients with type 2 diabetes, oral antidiabetic agents are discontinued. If a patient with type 2 diabetes is on less than 40 U/day of insulin, it is discontinued. If the patient is on more than 40 U/day of insulin, the insulin is decreased by 50 percent, blood sugars are followed by home glucose monitoring, and insulin is decreased appropriately. In most patients with type II diabetes insulin can be discontinued at the onset of the program. Antihypertensives are usually either discontinued or tapered at the first visit, depending on the level of hypertension and the number of antihypertensive agents. With rare exceptions, diuretics are discontinued. Because the vast majority of the weight loss in the first 1–2 weeks of a very-low-energy diet is fluid loss, except in unusual cases, diuretics are unnecessary and will exacerbate potassium wasting and lead to postural hypotension. Patients are informed that the weight loss during the first 1–2 weeks will be substantially greater than the subsequent weight loss.

In some programs patients are given a 1,200-kcal balanced food diet for the initial week to 2 weeks. This introductory phase is optional. Most programs involve three phases. Phase I is the reduced-energy diet phase using the formula diet of 800 cal. This phase usually lasts up to 12 weeks. Phase II is a refeeding phase, and phase III is a maintenance phase. We now recommend that all patients be placed on the 800-calorie formula because there is no known advantage to the 420-calorie formulation.

Once the diet is begun, the physician sees the patient each week and reviews the patient's weight loss, compliance, blood pressure, blood sugars if appropriate, medication lists, and any problems or complications the patient is having. Adjustments are made as necessary. Electrolytes, glucose, and blood urea nitrogen (BUN) are obtained on weeks 2 and 4 and every 4 weeks thereafter in phase I. The use of excessive laboratory testing is discouraged. For example, cholesterol and triglyceride levels will fall on a very-low-energy diet. There is generally no need to repeat cholesterol and triglyceride levels until after the patient is on a maintenance diet. At that time, if additional intervention other than weight loss is indicated (e.g., hypolipidemia drugs), appropriate measures can be taken. We have not detected significant changes in liver function studies or other routine tests,[149,528,529] and repetitive routine screening panels are also discouraged. Uric acid levels may rise on a very-low-energy diet because of the competition between ketones and uric acid for renal excretory mechanisms. In patients who do not have elevated uric acid before entering the program or a history of gout, complications related to the increase in uric acid observed during the program are extremely rare. It is important, however, to obtain electrolytes and a BUN, with special attention paid to serum potassium as patients may become potassium-depleted. Routine ECGs are also recommended in many programs. In our studies evaluating the cardiac effects of incomplete, unsupplemented very-low-energy diets, we detected arrhythmias only on 24-h avionics. Even in patients with abnormal 24-h avionics, the routine ECG was always within normal limits. Though many programs require routine ECGs, in noncomplicated obesity repeated routine ECGs should be considered optional.

During the second phase the supplement is gradually decreased as food is increased. Patients continue in the weekly behavioral modification classes during this period and meet regularly with the dietitian on an individual basis and less frequently with the physician. Food is introduced slowly to prevent the complications of rapid refeeding, allow for continued weight reduction, and give patients time to apply behavioral modification techniques to their eating. The reintroduction of food usually makes patients apprehensive and considerable encouragement is needed during this phase. It is again reemphasized that patients should continue the exercise program.

The maintenance phase consists of group support sessions. The behaviorist and a dietician lead the group sessions. After 3 months, blood studies, including a lipid profile, are repeated.

Patients who still have substantial weight to lose after successful completion of 3 months of maintenance may reenter phase I. Despite patients' firm conviction that they can do this, however, it is very difficult for patients to go back on a very-low-energy diet, and a longer period of weight maintenance may be indicated. Long-term maintenance is encouraged, and it often takes several years before patients feel comfortable and in control of their eating. If patients regain weight, they can be allowed to reenter phase I only if they have regained less than 50 lb and are 30 percent above IBW.

For patients who have known gallstones or have symptoms of gallstones, ultrasonography is performed before the diet is started. If gallstones are confirmed, patients should not be enrolled in the program or should be on a minimum 800-calorie diet with 30 g of fat and should take ursodeoxycholic acid (8–10 mg/kg per day) during the weight-loss phase. Follow-up ultrasonography should be performed on the eighth week of the low-energy diet or any time the patient develops symptoms. Routine ultrasonography or treatment with ursodeoxycholic acid is not recommended at this time for patients who have neither symptoms nor a history of gallbladder disease. Aspirin use is still considered experimental.

Weight-reduction programs and behavioral modification classes are not intended to be psychotherapy sessions and cannot address an individual's specific problems. When a patient shows signs of psychological difficulty, the issue should be addressed immediately. This usually involves referral for proper help.

Four issues frequently arise with regard to weight loss: caloric utilization, plateaus in weight loss, whether the decrease in energy expenditure with dieting hinders weight loss, and the possible danger of repeated weight fluctuations, weight cycling, or "yo-yo" dieting. The first issue relates to patients who state that they eat very little food and yet either gain weight or cannot lose weight. Studies using metabolic chambers and studies measuring the ambulatory metabolic rate in adolescents and in women with postpartum obesity, as well as our own studies,[321] indicate that obesity is generally associated with increased caloric utilization. Though there is some overlap between obese and lean individuals in ambulatory metabolic rate, there are no obese individuals who utilize fewer calories than lean individuals do. Reports by obese individuals that they gain or maintain weight on a reduced caloric intake must be considered suspect. We have noted that in a clinical research center setting, when obese patients are fed three meals a day at isocaloric levels, they routinely claim that they are getting too much food to eat. We believe that this is related to their usual eating habits, which include frequent snacking which never gives them the sense of fullness that comes with eating three meals a day. For this reason, modifying behavior to eat only three meals a day is important.

The second issue concerns the commonly held belief that plateaus in weight loss are due to a decreased metabolic rate secondary to the diet. The resting metabolic rate does decrease with severe caloric restriction and also decreases with weight loss as a result of decreases in lean body mass.[326,357,556] For patients who follow the diet, this decrease can be factored into a reliable prediction of expected weight loss. Upon refeeding, the resting metabolic rate rises, as one would expect, based on body composition and is not altered in a pathologic way. Patients lose substantially more weight during the first week or two of any diet as a result of fluid loss. Thereafter, weight loss continues at a predictable level, with some variations from week to week that are primarily dependent on the patient's fluid status. It is possible that a premenstrual patient could retain enough fluid to offset a week's weight loss, but if energy expenditure and energy intake remain constant, the body is using fat stores for energy and the patient will be losing fat and lean tissue at a predictable rate. Problems arise when patients weigh themselves too often as the weight loss from day to day may not be apparent on home scales or may be obliterated by fluid shifts. We encourage patients to weigh themselves only once a week.

Finally, repeated cycles of weight loss and regain have been reported to lead to more rapid weight gain and a lower metabolic rate.[557,558] Unfortunately, most of these studies in animals and people have failed to measure body composition adequately, did not have proper controls, did not control for effects of gender and aging, and were generally not based on strong experimental evidence.[559] In studies of people[558,559] and animals,[560] when properly controlled, repeated weight loss and regain do not lead to excessive fatness or fat redistribution, a decreased rate of weight loss, an increased rate of weight gain, or a decrease in the metabolic rate.[558,561] Fluctuations in body weight have been reported to increase the risk for coronary heart disease and death comparable to the risk of being obese.[558,562] Additional studies will be necessary to confirm these observations, especially in the absence of a clear hypothesis as to why this should be true. The National Task Force on the Prevention and Treatment of Obesity has concluded that "The currently available evidence regarding increased morbidity and mortality with variation in body weight is not sufficiently compelling to override the potential benefits of moderate weight loss in significantly obese patients . . . obese individuals should not allow concerns about hazards of weight cycling to deter them from efforts to control their body weight." In addition it concluded that "There is no convincing evidence that weight cycling in humans has adverse effects on body composition, energy expenditure, risk factors for cardiovascular disease, or the effectiveness of future efforts at weight loss."[558]

Fad Diets

Fad diets, such as the grapefruit diet, should be discouraged because they frequently do not provide adequate nutrition, have severe side effects, and are not based on sound scientific principles.[563] Patients with a disease understandably are looking for a cure, and most of these subjects, frustrated with numerous past attempts, are vulnerable to so-called experts who promote fad diets that are "nutritional nonsense." Many fads come and go including rice diets, high protein–low carbohydrate diets, and numerous other examples. It is important for the health professional to review the scientific basis of these diets as published in peer-reviewed journals and not be misled by so called experts' books. Basically, if caloric intake is less than caloric expenditure, patients will lose weight. This can occur safely on any diet that is nutritionally complete. However, for weight maintenance I believe it is best for patients to learn good dietary habits. Dieting on the same foods that the patient will be ingesting at maintenance best does this. A good example of promoting a diet by inappropriately quoting the literature is the book *The Last Chance Diet*,[525] which promoted a collagen hydrolysate diet on the basis of research done with other sources of nutrients. The result was sudden death in more than 60 people.[527] It is important to instruct patients in the scientific basis of weight reduction and the importance of weight maintenance.

Pharmacological Treatment

Drugs to treat obesity have had a history of failure, weight regain, drug abuse, adverse side effects, and inappropriate use. Nevertheless, several agents have limited or no potential for abuse and have been shown to be effective in enhancing weight reduction during short periods. In more than 200 studies using amphetamine-like drugs which included almost 10,000 patients, active drugs produced more weight loss than did placebo in more than 90 percent of the studies.[564] However, in 160 trials comparing placebo and active drugs, patients receiving active drug lost significantly more weight than patients receiving placebo in only 40 percent of the studies. The dropout rate at the end of the studies was 49 percent for placebo-treated patients and 47.9 percent for patients receiving active drug. Anorexic drugs enhanced weight loss by an average of 0.56 lb per week more than placebo. On the basis of these data, the FDA has approved several amphetamine-like drugs for marketing on the basis of their short-term efficacy. Amphetamine-like drugs led to a weight loss of at least 1 lb/week in 44 percent of subjects taking active drugs, compared with 26 percent of subjects taking placebo.[564] There was no significant difference between any of the active drugs. As reviewed by Weintraub and Bray,[565] weight loss occurs at a decelerating rate, stabilizing while patients are on active drug and increasing with discontinuation of drug.

Phentermine, an amphetamine-like drug with low addictive potential, is effective in inducing weight loss.[566] With dropouts included, average weight loss during 24 weeks (16 weeks of drug use) was 10.0 kg in the phentermine group and 4.4 kg in the placebo group. The group treated with fenfluramine, which both stimulates serotonin release from nerve endings and prevents its reuptake, lost 7.5 kg in 24 weeks. Combining the drugs to take advantage of the stimulatory effects of phentermine by giving one-half the usual dose in the morning and the sedative effects of fenfluramine by giving one-half the usual dose before supper led to a weight loss of 8.4 kg. All active treatment groups lost significantly more weight than the placebo group did. Adverse effects were less common with the combination group than with either phentermine or fenfluramine alone. The difference in weight loss between placebo and active drug was small: 3.1 vs. 5.6 kg with a plateau in weight loss. The FDA never approved the combination of phentermine and fenfluramine (Phen-Fen) yet this combination was extensively used.

Because the *d*-isomer of fenfluramine is the active isomer, studies have evaluated the effects of dexfenfluramine in obese subjects. A European cooperative study[567] of 822 obese patients evaluated dexfenfluramine in a placebo-controlled, double-blind fashion for 1 year. At 12 months, mean weight loss was 9.82 kg in the dexfenfluramine group and 7.15 kg in the placebo group. This represented 10.76 percent and 7.18 percent of initial weight, respectively. Again, 1 year of medication for a 2.7-kg differential in weight loss does not appear to be a cost-effective option. It is of interest that weight loss in the placebo and drug-treatment groups reached a plateau between the fourth and sixth months and increased slightly thereafter. An over-the-counter drug, phenylpropanolamine hydrochloride, leads to a weight loss of approximately 0.25 kg/week more than with placebo in short-term studies, not different from prescription appetite suppressants.[566] Dexfenfluramine (*d*-fenfluramine) and fenfluramine were pulled from the market in 1997 due to the occurrence of pulmonary hypertension and heart valve abnormalities similar to that seen with carcinoid syndrome.[568–575]

A class of atypical β-adrenergic receptor agonist (β_3 agonist) that stimulates thermogenesis in brown adipose tissue and muscle[576,577] has been described. One of these drugs, BRL 26830A, has been studied in obese humans for 18 weeks.[578] Mean weight loss was 15.4 kg in obese subjects and 10.0 kg in subjects who were given placebo. This was significant at week 18 only and represents a difference of 0.3 kg/week, not unlike all the other drugs tested. No adverse effects were detected on blood pressure, lipids, glucose, or other parameters. The only side effect regularly observed was tremulousness. Tremors should be less common with the newer β_3 agonists that are currently being tested and are reported to be more specific. Of interest is that BRL 26830A did increase energy expenditure 2 h after an oral dose but did not affect the resting metabolic rate. The effect on 24-h energy expenditure is not known.

Sibutramine was approved for chronic use in the U.S. and became available for use in the beginning of 1998. Sibutramine is a serotonin and norepinephrine reuptake inhibitor which, in animals, also leads to increased metabolic rate thought to be related to central stimulation of brown adipose tissue.[579] Studies provided by Knoll Pharmaceutical Company demonstrate that after 1 year of treatment, patients on placebo and 10 and 15 mg/day of sibutramine lost an average of 3.5, 9.8, and 14 pounds, respectively. For patients who completed the 1-yr study the weight loss was 4.8, 13.6, and 15.2 pounds, respectively, and for patients who lost at least 4 lbs. in the first 4 weeks, weight loss was 10.7, 18.2, and 18.8 lbs, respectively. In a study in which patients were treated with a VLCD for 4 weeks, those who lost at least 6 kg on the VLCD were treated for 1 yr with 10 mg/day sibutramine or placebo.[580] Placebo and sibutramine treated patients lost 15.2 and 28.4 lbs, respectively. For patients who completed the study, weight loss was 16.7 and 29.7 lbs, respectively, and for patients who lost at least 4 lbs in the first 4 weeks weight loss was 21.5 and 33 lbs, respectively. Thus, in all groups, patients treated with sibutramine weighed 8.1 to 13.4 lbs less than placebo treated patients after 1 yr. From the time of completion of the VLCD to the end of the study, placebo-treated patients gained a mean of 1.1 lbs, while the sibutramine-treated patients lost an additional 11.4 pounds.[580] Thus, sibutramine may be especially useful in patients who have lost weight to maintain the weight loss. Sibutramine can be used in patients with a BMI $\geq$ 30 or a BMI $\geq$ 27 in the presence of other risk factors (i.e., hypertension, dyslipidemia, and diabetes). In some patients, sibutramine raises blood pressure, so monitoring of blood pressure is required. Sibutramine should not be used in patients with uncontrolled hypertension. Patients on sibutramine have decreases in cholesterol and triglycerides consistent with their weight loss. In studies with mean treatment duration of 7.6 months, there was no excess occurrence of cardiac valvular disease in patients treated with sibutramine. Sibutramine is contraindicated in patients taking MAO inhibitors and other centrally-acting appetite suppressant drugs.

Tetrahydrolipstatin, a pancreatic lipase inhibitor, has been approved for use in the United States and recently became available. In a recent study,[581] the difference in weight loss between placebo and Orlistat (120 mg tid) treated patients after 1 yr of treatment was 8.6 lbs. After 2 years of treatment, patients on Orlistat lost 5.3 lbs more than placebo-treated patients. Patients on Orlistat had small but statistically significant decreases in glucose and blood pressure. Total and LDL cholesterol fell more after 1 year in Orlistat-treated patients, while HDL cholesterol and triglycerides were the same in Orlistat and placebo-treated patients. The major side effects were GI, with 31 percent of patients having fatty or oily stool, 20 percent increased defecation, 18 percent oily spotting, 7 percent flatus with discharge and fecal incontinence, and 6 percent oily evacuation. Small changes were seen in fat-soluble vitamins but few patients required supplementation. In a second similar study, the difference in weight loss between placebo and Orlistat (120 mg tid) at one year was 6.5 lbs. During the second year of the study, patients on placebo regained 63.4 percent of the weight lost. Patients who continued to take Orlistat at 120 mg tid regained 35.2 percent of the weight lost while those who took 60 mg tid during the second year regained 51.3 percent of the weight lost.[582] Side effects were frequent and included flatus with discharge (40.1 percent), oily spotting (32.7 percent), fecal urgency (29.7 percent), fatty/oily stool (19.8 percent), oily evacuation (14.3 percent), fecal incontinence (11.8 percent), and increased defecation (11.1 percent). Because of the side effects related to steatorrhea, many believe that the effectiveness of Orlistat lies primarily in the lower fat intake required to avoid embarrassing side effects.

Other drugs used to treat obesity, such as hCG,[583] opioid antagonists, and phenytoin, are ineffective and have no place in current therapy.[565] Thyroid hormone has been used, but it enhances the loss of lean body mass, and its use is subject to all the complications associated with hyperthyroidism. It also has no place in the treatment of obesity. Bile acid resins are ineffective. α-glucosidase inhibitors[584] have been shown to lower postprandial glucose levels, are approved for the treatment of type 2 diabetes, and will prevent the weight gain frequently associated with treatment with sulfonylureas. Weight loss is not observed at approved doses because carbohydrate absorption is delayed but not inhibited. The data on sucrose polyester (Olestra) indicate that it reduces serum cholesterol but has minimal or no effects on body weight beyond that caused by diet alone.[585,586] Fiber added to a weight-reducing diet has been shown to lead to small increases in weight loss (mean = 1.8 kg over 12 weeks).[587]

Growth hormone has been used in conjunction with diets of 24 cal/kg[588] and 18 cal/kg.[589] These studies have demonstrated that short-term growth hormone administration is effective in decreasing loss of LBM. However, loss of LBM is a normal accompaniment of weight reduction because lean individuals have less LBM than do obese individuals. Body composition at reduced weight is normal in subjects treated with low-energy diets. Thus, growth hormone would be an expensive method to alter body composition, a situation that will probably change when growth hormone is discontinued. The more cost-effective and physiologic approach would be exercise with a resistance component.

Endogenous cholecystokinin has been postulated to be a mediator of postprandial satiety. Animals treated with a potent agonist to the CCK_1 receptor have decreased food intake.[590] The usefulness of cholecystokinin or potential cholecystokinin agonists in the treatment of human obesity is unknown.

In patients with obesity and type 2 diabetes, the biguanide metformin decreases blood glucose and body weight, probably by inhibiting glucose absorption from the GI tract. Selective serotonin reuptake inhibitors, especially fluoxetine, have been studied extensively for weight reduction in obese patients with mixed results.[591] The only controlled, randomized clinical trial lasting one year demonstrated a significantly greater weight loss in fluoxetine-treated patients at 28 weeks, but there was no difference in weight loss between fluoxetine and placebo-treated patients at 52 weeks.[592] Doses of fluoxetine used in obesity trials were 60 mg per day, three times the dose used to treat depression. Though fluoxetine is approved for the treatment of bulimia nervosa, it is not approved for the treatment of obesity.

There are numerous other potential therapies that are under investigation including leptin, GLP-1, GLP-1 agonists, and GLP-1-like proteins; motilin; and other early principles.

Surgery for Morbid Obesity

Clinically severe obesity, formerly called morbid obesity, is defined as either 100 percent or 100 lbs above IBW or a BMI > 40 kg/m^2.[593] The excess mortality associated with morbid obesity comes largely from extrapolated data.[594] However, Drenick et al. compared a group of 200 morbidly obese men followed for a mean of 7.5 years with mortality statistics for men in the general population.[595] Complete follow-up data were available on 185 men. Fifty of the 200 morbidly obese men died during the course of the study, which was a 12-fold excess in the age group from 25 to 34 years of age and a sixfold excess in the age group from 35 to 45 years of age. Excess frequencies of cardiovascular disease, diabetes, and accidents as the cause of death were found in the morbidly obese men. It is of interest that the excess mortality of morbidly obese men over 65 years old diminished to approximately twofold.

Because of the marked excess mortality associated with morbid obesity as well as the other conditions associated with obesity and because of the failure of morbidly obese patients to respond to conventional modalities for the treatment of obesity,[11,182,594] various surgical techniques to induce weight reduction have been developed.[11,182,593,596–600] Both the NIH consensus conference[593] and the AACE[182] recommend surgery as an option in patients with a BMI > 40 or with a BMI between 35 and 40 with life-threatening or disabling comorbid conditions and acceptable surgical risk. In 1991 a NIH consensus conference[593] developed guidelines for selection, counseling, and follow-up of patients for the surgical treatment of obesity. These guidelines are as follows: The surgeon should be knowledgeable in the fields of obesity surgery, gastroenterology, and nutrition and should regularly perform such operations with a commitment to postoperative care and long-term follow-up. Patients should have failed a multidisciplinary nonsurgical program and comorbidities should be treated. A multidisciplinary team with medical, surgical, psychiatric, and nutritional expertise should evaluate the patient. All treatment options, the need for lifelong medical surveillance, and possible risks and benefits as well as the effects on everyday life should be discussed. Pregnancy should be avoided until weight has stabilized and all potential micronutrient deficiencies corrected.

With this in mind, several operations have been used to treat morbid obesity.[596–602] The two procedures recommended are gastric bypass and vertical banded gastroplasty.[11,182,593] Jejunoileal bypass is no longer performed because of the multiple complications including liver failure.[603,604] The two procedures, advantages and disadvantages, efficacy, complications, and indications have been reviewed.[11,182,593] Pories et al.[598] reviewed their experience with gastric bypass in 608 patients during 14 years of follow-up. Mean excess weight loss was 68.9 percent, 57.7 percent, 54.7 percent, and 49.2 percent at 1, 5, 10, and 14 yr, respectively. The perioperative mortality was 1.5 percent. Postoperative complications occurred in from 2.5 to 8.7 percent of patients. The most frequent late complications included vitamin B_{12} deficiency in 40 percent, anemia in 39 percent, hospital readmission in 38.1 percent, incisional hernia in 23.9 percent, depression in 23.4 percent, staple line failure in 15.1 percent, gastritis in 13.2 percent, cholelithiasis in 11.4 percent, and bile acid reflux in 8.7 percent. Dumping syndrome developed in 70.6 percent of the patients, but the authors state that this is controlled by avoiding sweets.

Benotti et al. compared the results of gastric bypass and vertical banded gastroplasty.[597] Weight tends to plateau at 30–40 percent above ideal body weight after gastric bypass and 60–70 percent above ideal body weight after vertical banded gastroplasty. Sugerman et al. compared the Roux-en-Y gastric bypass with the vertical banded gastroplasty and demonstrated that after 3 years of follow-up the gastric bypass led to significantly greater weight loss.[605] These authors also showed that vertical banded gastroplasty patients who were "sweet eaters" tended to lose less weight than did those who were not, whereas there was no difference in patients who had the gastric bypass procedure.[596,606] It is suggested that "superobese" (>150 kg) patients show poorer results with gastroplasty and should have a gastric bypass.[596] Comorbid conditions usually show dramatic improvement.[182,593,597,598] In a comparison of gastroplasty vs. gastric bypass, the failure rate for gastroplasty patients at 2 years of follow-up was approximately 45 percent, whereas for gastric bypass patients it was only approximately 10 percent.[607] The complications of the two procedures are similar,[182] with stomal obstruction being more common earlier in the vertical banded gastroplastic group and vitamin B_{12} deficiency, dumping syndrome, and transient neuropathy being more common as late complications in the gastric bypass group.[182, 608] The neurologic syndromes following gastric surgery for morbid obesity include polyneuropathy.[597,609,610]

In summary, in severely obese patients the only treatment that leads to consistent weight loss is surgery. The surgical procedures of choice are the vertical banded gastroplasty and the Roux-en-Y gastric bypass procedure. These procedures should be performed in accordance with the guidelines outlined of the NIH consensus conference.[593]

Summary

The treatment of obesity begins with prevention and good diet and exercise habits. A well-balanced hypocaloric diet should be combined with an established behavioral modification program and long-term maintenance. In more refractory cases and especially in patients with complications of obesity, very-low-energy diets should be considered, but only in conjunction with an established program, behavioral modification, and a long-term maintenance group. To ensure safety and maximize long-term success, the program should conform to the standards discussed previously. There is no cost-effective pharmacologic approach to obesity at the present time, although many drugs can enhance weight loss a small amount and, if continued, help sustain the loss. They may be especially useful for weight maintenance after weight loss is achieved by a diet approach. Surgery is recommended only for severe or morbid obesity, and the program should conform to the guidelines of the NIH consensus conference.[593]

REFERENCES

1. Forbes GB: Techniques for estimating body composition, in *Human Body Composition*. New York, Springer-Verlag, 1987, pp 5–100.
2. Amatruda JM: Assessment of body composition, in Mogensen CE, Standl E (eds): *Research Methodologies in Human Diabetes–Part 2*. Walter de Gruyter, Berlin, New York, 1995, pp 85–96.
3. Forbes GB, Bruining GJ: Urinary creatinine excretion and lean body mass. *Am J Clin Nutr* 29:1359, 1976.
4. Gray DS, Bray GA, Gemayel N, Kaplan K: Effect of obesity on bioelectrical impedance. *Am J Clin Nutr* 50:255, 1989.
5. Gray DS: Changes in bioelectrical impedance during fasting. *Am J Clin Nutr* 48:1184, 1988.
6. Kushner RF, Kunigk A, Alspaugh M, Andronis PT, Leitch CA, Schoeller DA: Validation of bioelectrical-impedance analysis as a measurement of change in body composition in obesity. *Am J Clin Nutr* 52:219, 1990.
7. Wellens R, Chumlea WC, Guo S, Roche AF, Reo NV, Siervogel RM: Body composition in white adults by dual-energy X-ray absorptiometry, densitometry, and total body water. *Am J Clin Nutr* 59:547, 1994.
8. Tataranni PA, Ravussin E: Use of dual-energy X-ray absorptiometry in obese individuals. *Am J Clin Nutr* 62:730, 1995.
9. Simopoulos AP, VanItallie TB: Body weight, health, and longevity. *Ann Intern Med* 100:285, 1984.
10. Kuczmarski RJ, Carroll MD, Flegal KM, Troiano RP: Varying body mass index cutoff points to describe overweight prevalence among U.S. Adults: NHANES III (1988 to 1994). *Obes Res* 5:542, 1997.
11. NHLBI Expert Panel on The Identification, Evaluation, and Treatment of Overweight and Obesity in Adults: Clinical Guidelines on The Identification, Evaluation, and Treatment of Overweight and Obesity in Adults. *Obes Res* 6:515, 1998.
12. Flegal KM, Caroll MD, Kuczmarski RJ, Johnson CL: Overweight and obesity in the United States: Prevalence and trends, 1960–1994. *Int J Obes* 22:39, 1998.
13. Harrison GG: Height-weight tables. *Ann Intern Med* 103:989, 1985.
14. Despres JP, Nadeau A, Tremblay A, et al: Role of deep abdominal fat in the association between regioal adipose tissue distribution and glucose tolerance in obese women. *Diabetes* 38:304, 1989.
15. Wolf AM, Colditz GA: Current estimates of the economic costs of obesity in the United States: *Obes Res* 6:97, 1998.
16. Manson JE, Stampfer MJ, Hennekens CH, Willett WC: Body weight and longevity: A reassessment. *JAMA* 257:353, 1987.
17. Feinleib M: Epidemiology of obesity in relation to health hazards. *Ann Intern Med* 103:1019, 1985.
18. Build study, 1979. Chicago, Society of Actuaries and Association of Life Insurance Medical Directors, 1980.
19. Garrison RJ, Castelli WP: Weight and thirty-year mortality of men in the Framingham Study. *Ann Intern Med* 103:1006, 1985.
20. Lew EA: Mortality and weight: Insured lives and the American Cancer Society Studies. *Ann Intern Med* 103:1024, 1985.
21. Lee IM, Manson JE, Hennekens CH, Paffenbarger RS: Body weight and mortality: A 27-year follow-up of middle-aged men. *JAMA* 270:2823, 1993.
22. Troiano RP, Frongillo EA, Sobal J, Levitsky DA: The relationship between body weight and mortality: A quantitative analysis of combined information from existing studies. *Int J Obes* 20:63, 1996.
23. Stallones RA: Epidemiologic studies of obesity. *Ann Intern Med* 103:1003, 1985.
24. Manson JE, Willett WC, Stampfer MJ, Colditz GA, Hunter DJ, Hankinson SE, Hennekens CH, Speizer FE: Body weight and mortality among women. *N Engl J Med* 333:677, 1995.
25. Must A, Jacques PF, Dallal GE, Bajema CJ, Dietz WH: Long-term morbidity and mortality of overweight adolescents. *N Engl J Med* 327:1350, 1992.
26. Andres R, Muller DC, Sorkin JD: Long-term effects of change in body weight on all-cause mortality. *Ann Intern Med* 119:737, 1993.
27. Pamuk ER, Williamson DE, Serdula MK, Madans J, Byers TE: Weight loss and subsequent death in a cohort of U.S. adults. *Ann Intern Med* 119:744, 1993.
28. Blair SN, Shaten J, Brownell L, Collins G, Lissner L: Body weight change, all-cause mortality, and cause-specific mortality in the Multiple Risk Factor Intervention Trial. *Ann Intern Med* 119:749, 1993.
29. Folsom AR, Kaye SA, Sellers TA, Hong CP, Cerhan JR, Potter JD, Prineas RJ: Body fat distribution and 5-year risk for death in older women. *JAMA* 269:483, 1993.
30. Kuller L, Wing R: Weight loss and mortality. *Ann Intern Med* 117:630, 1993.
31. Sorkin JD, Zonderman AB, Costa PT, Andres R: Twenty year follow-up of the NHANES I cohort: Tests of metholodologic hypotheses. *Obes Res* 4:12S, 1996.
32. Stevens J, Jianwen C, Pamuk ER, Williamson DF, Thun MJ, Woods JL: The effect of age on the association between body mass index and mortality. *N Engl J Med* 338:1, 1998.
33. Barrett-Conner EL: Obesity, atherosclerosis, and coronary artery disease. *Ann Intern Med* 103:1010, 1985.
34. Hubert HB, Feinleib M, McNamara PM, Castelli WP: Obesity as an independent risk factor for cardiovascular disease: A 26-year follow-up of participants in the Framingham Heart Study. *Circulation* 67:968, 1983.
35. Rabkin SW, Mathewson FAL, Hsu PH: Relation of body weight to development of ischemic heart disease in a cohort of young North American men after a 26 year observation: The Manitoba Study. *Am J Cardiol* 39:452, 1977.
36. Willett WC, Manson JE, Stampfer MJ, Colditz GA, Rosner B, Speizer FE, Hennekens CH: Weight, weight change, and coronary heart disease in women. *JAMA* 273:461, 1995.
37. Rexrode KM, Hennekens CH, Willett WC, Colditz GA, Stampfer MJ, Rich-Edwards JW, Speizer FE, Manson JE: A prospective study of body mass index, weight change, and risk of stroke in women. *JAMA* 277:1539, 1997.

38. Urbina EM, Gidding SS, Bao W, Pickoff AS, Berdusis K, Berenson GS: Effect of body size, ponderosity, and blood pressure on left ventricular growth in children and young adults in the Bogalusa Heart Study. *Circulation* 91:2400, 1995.
39. Hoffmann RM, Psaty BM, Kromal RA: Modifiable risk factors for incident heart failure in the coronary artery surgery study. *Arch Intern Med* 154:417,1994
40. Alpert MA, Hashimi MW: Obesity and the heart. *Am J Med Sci* 306:117, 1993.
41. Garavaglia GE, Messerli FH, Nunez BD, Schmieder RE, Grossman E: Myocardial contractility and left ventricular function in obese patients with essential hypertension. *Am J Cardiol* 62:594, 1988.
42. Yamashita S, Nakamura T, Shimomura I, Nishida M, Yoshida S, Kotani K, Kameda-Takemuara K, Tokunaga K, Matsuzawa Y: Insulin resistance and body fat distribution: Contribution of visceral fat accumulation to the development of insulin resistance and atherosclerosis. *Diabetes Care* 19:287, 1996.
43. Vague J: The degree of masculine differentiation of obesities: A factor determining predisposition to diabetes, atherosclerosis, gout and uric calculous disease. *Am J Clin Nutr* 4:20, 1956.
44. Hartz AJ, Rupley DC, Rimm AA: The association of girth measurements with disease in 32,856 women. *Am J Epidemiol* 119:71, 1984.
45. Kissebah AH, Vydelingum N, Murray R, Evans DJ, Hartz AJ, Kalkhoff RK, Adams PW: Relation of body fat distribution to metabolic complications of obesity. *J Clin Endocrinol Metab* 54:254, 1982.
46. Krotkiewski M, Bjöntorp P, Sjöström L, Smith U: Impact of obesity on metabolism in men and women: Importance of regional adipose tissue distribution. *J Clin Invest* 72:1150, 1983.
47. Peiris AN, Sothmann MS, Hoffmann RG, Hennes MI, Wilson CR, Gustafson AB, Kissebah AH: Adiposity, fat distribution, and cardiovascular risk. *Ann Intern Med* 110:867, 1989.
48. Evans DJ, Hoffman RG, Kalkhoff RK, Kissebah AH: Relationship of androgenic activity to body fat topography, fat cell morphology, and metabolic aberrations in premenopausal women. *J Clin Endocrinol Metab* 57:304, 1983.
49. Evans DJ, Murray R, Kissebah AH: Relationship between skeletal muscle insulin resistance, insulin-mediated glucose disposal, and insulin binding: Effects of obesity and body fat topography. *J Clin Invest* 74:1515, 1984.
50. Peiris AN, Mueller RA, Smith GA, Struve MF, Kissebah AH: Splanchnic insulin metabolism in obesity. *J Clin Invest* 78:1648, 1986.
51. Elbers JM, Asscheman H, Seidell JC, Megens JA, Gooren LJ: Long-term teatosterone administration increases intraabdominal fat in female to male transsexuals. *J Clin Endocrinol Metab* 82:2044, 1997.
52. Peeke PM, Chrousos GP: Hypercortisolism and obesity. *Ann NY Acad Sci* 771:665, 1995.
53. Haffner SN, Fong D, Hazuda HP, Pugh JA, Patterson JK: Hyperinsulinemia, upper body adiposity, and cardiovascular risk factors in non-diabetics. *Metabolism* 37:338, 1988.
54. Anderson AJ, Sobocinski KA, Freedman DS, Barboriak JJ, Rimm AA, Gruchow HW: Body fat distribution, plasma lipids, and lipoproteins. *Arteriosclerosis* 8:88, 1988.
55. Larsson B, Svardsudd K, Welin L, Wilhelmsen L, Björntorp P, Tibblin G: Abdominal adipose tissue distribution, obesity, and risk of cardiovascular disease and death: 13 year follow-up of participants in the study of men born in 1913. *Br Med J* 288:1401, 1984.
56. Landin K, Stigendal L, Eriksson E, Krotkiewski M, Risberg B, Tengborn L, Smith U: Abdominal obesity is associated with an impaired fibrinolytic activity and elevated plasminogen activator inhibitor-1. *Metabolism* 39:1044, 1990.
57. Lapidus L, Bengtsson C, Larsson B, Pennert K, Rybo E, Sjöström L: Distribution of adipose tissue and risk of cardiovascular disease and death: A 12 year follow-up of participants in the population study of women in Gothenburg, Sweden. *Br Med J* 289:1257, 1984.
58. Kissebah AH: Intra-abdominal fat: is it a major factor in developing diabetes and coronary artery disease. *Diabetes Res Clin Pract* 30:25, 1996.
59. Reaven GM: Role of insulin resistance in human disease. *Diabetes* 37:1595, 1988.
60. Hendler RG, Welle SL, Statt MC, Barnard R, Amatruda JM: The effects of weight reduction to ideal body weight on body fat distribution. *Metabolism* 44:1413, 1995.
61. Barrett-Connor E, Khaw KT: Cigarette smoking and increased central adiposity. *Ann Intern Med* 111:783, 1989.
62. Colditz GA, Willett WC, Rotnitsky A, Manson JE: Weight gain as a risk factor for clinical diabetes in women. *Ann Intern Med* 122:481, 1995.
63. Chan JM, Rimm EB, Colditz GA, Stamfer MJ, Willett WC: Obesity, fat distribution, and weight gain as risk factors for clinical diabetes in men. *Diabetes Care* 17:961, 1994.
64. Ford ES, Williamson DF, Liu S: Weight change and diabetes incidence: Findings from a national cohort of US adults. *Am J Epidemiol* 146:214, 1997.
65. Ferrannini E, Camastre S: Relationship between impaired glucose tolerance, non-insulin dependent diabetes mellitus and obesity. *Eur J Clin Invest* 28:3, 1998.
66. Everson SA, Goldberg DE, Helmrich SP, Lakka TA, Lynch JW, Kaplan GA, Salonen JT: Weight gain and the risk of developing insulin resistance syndrome. *Diabetes Care* 21:1637, 1998.
67. Rabinowitz D, Zierler KL: Forearm metabolism in obesity and its response to intraarterial insulin: Characterization of insulin resistance and evidence for adaptive hyperinsulinism. *J Clin Invest* 41:2173, 1962.
68. Kolterman OG, Insel J, Saekow M, Olefsky JM: Mechanisms of insulin resistance in human obesity: Evidence for receptor and postreceptor defects. *J Clin Invest* 65:1272, 1980.
69. Felber JP, Ferrannini E, Golay A, Meyer HU, Theibaud D, Curchod B, Maeder E, Jequier E, et al: Role of lipid oxidation in pathogenesis of insulin resistance of obesity and Type II diabetes. *Diabetes* 36:1341, 1987.
70. Prager R, Wallace P, Olefsky JM: Hyperinsulinemia does not compensate for peripheral insulin resistance in obesity. *Diabetes* 36:327, 1987.
71. Bonadonna RC, Groop L, Kraemer N, Ferrannini E, DelPrato S, DeFronzo RA: Obesity and insulin resistance in humans: A dose-response study. *Metabolism* 39:452, 1990.
72. Lillioja S, Bogardus C, Mott DM, Kennedy AL, Knowler WC, Howard BV: Relationship between insulin-mediated glucose disposal and lipid metabolism in man. *J Clin Invest* 75:106, 1985.
73. Bogardus C, Lillioja S, Mott D, Reaven GM, Kashiwagi A, Foley JE: Relationship between obesity and maximal insulin-stimulated glucose uptake in vivo and in vitro in Pima Indians. *J Clin Invest* 73:800, 1984.
74. Peiris A, Struve MF, Mueller RA, Lee MB, Kissebah AH: Glucose metabolism in obesity: Influence of body fat distribution. *J Clin Endocrinol Metab* 67:760, 1988.
75. Devlin JT, Horton ES: Effects of prior high-intensity exercise on glucose metabolism in normal and insulin-resistant men. *Diabetes* 34:973, 1985.
76. Bogardus C, Lillioja S, Nyomba BL, Zurlo F, Swinburn B, Esposito-Del Puente A, Knowler WC, Ravussin E, et al: Distribution of in vivo insulin action in Pima Indians as mixture of three normal distributions. *Diabetes* 38:1423, 1989.
77. Lillioja S, Mott DM, Zawadzki JK, Young AA, Abbott WG, Bogardus C: Glucose storage is a major determinant of in vivo "insulin resistance" in subjects with normal glucose tolerance. *J Clin Endocrinol Metab* 62:922, 1986.
78. Laasko M, Edelman SV, Brechtel G, Baron AD: Decreased effect of insulin to stimulate skeletal muscle blood flow in obese man. *J Clin Invest* 85:1844, 1990.
79. Kida Y, Esposito-Del Puente A, Bogardus C, Mott DM: Insulin resistance is associated with reduced fasting and insulin-stimulated glycogen synthase phosphatase activity in human skeletal muscle. *J Clin Invest* 85:476, 1990.
80. Petersen KF, Hendler R, Price T, Perseghin G, Rothman DL, Held N, Amatruda JM, Shulman GI: $^{13}C/^{31}P$ NMR studies on the mechanism of insulin resistance in obesity. *Diabetes* 47:381, 1998.
81. Amatruda JM, Salhanick AI: Insulin and steatonecrosis: Are they related? *Hepatology* 10:1024, 1989.
82. Cech JM, Freeman RB, Caro JF, Amatruda JM: Insulin action and binding in isolated hepatocytes from fasted, streptozotocin-diabetic, and older, spontaneously obese rats. *Biochem J* 188:839, 1980.
83. Amatruda JM, Salhanick AI, Chang CL: Hepatic insulin resistance in non-insulin-dependent diabetes mellitus and the effects of a sulfonylurea in potentiating insulin action. *Diabetes Care* 7:47, 1984.
84. Amatruda JM, Livingston JN, Lockwood DH: Cellular mechanisms in selected states of insulin resistance: Human obesity, glucocorticoid excess, and chronic fetal failure. *Diabetes Metab Rev* 1:293, 1985.

85. Ferrannini E, Buzzigoli G, Bonadonna R, Giorico MA, Oleggini M, Graziadei L, Pedrinelli R, Brandi L, et al: Insulin resistance in essential hypertension. *N Engl J Med* 317:350, 1987.
86. Zavaroni I, Bonora E, Pagliara M, Dall'Aglio E, Luchetti L, Buonanno G, Bonati PA, Bergonzani M, et al: Risk factors for coronary artery disease in healthy persons with hyperinsulinemia and normal glucose tolerance. *N Engl J Med* 320:702, 1989.
87. Haffner SM, Stern MP, Hazuda HP, Mitchell BD, Patterson JK: Increased insulin concentrations in nondiabetic offspring of diabetic parents. *N Engl J Med* 319:1297, 1988.
88. Laakso M, Sarlund H, Mykkänen L: Insulin resistance is associated with lipid and degrees of glucose tolerance. *Arteriosclerosis* 10:223, 1990.
89. Lillioja S, Bogardus C: Insulin resistance in Pima Indians. *Acta Med Scand* 723:103, 1990.
90. Swinburn BA, Nyomba BL, Saad MF, Zurlo F, Raz I, Knowlder WC, Lillioja S, Bogardus C, et al: Insulin resistance associated with lower rates of weight gain in Pima Indians. *J Clin Invest* 88:168, 1991.
91. Boden G: Role of fatty acids in the pathogenesis of insulin resistance and NIDDM. *Diabetes* 46:3, 1996.
92. McGarry JD: Glucose-fatty acid interactions in health and disease. *Am J Clin Nutr* 67:500S, 1998.
93. Roden M, Price TB, Perseghin G, Petersen KF, Rothman DL, Cline GW, Shulman GI: Mechanism of free fatty acid-induced insulin resistance in humans. *J Clin Invest* 97:2859, 1996
94. Pi-Sunyer FX, Laferrere B, Aronne LJ, Bray GA: Obesity—A modern day epidemic. *J Clin Endocrinol Metab* 84:3, 1999.
95. Peraldi P, Spiegelman B: TNF-alpha and insulin resistance: Summary and future prospects. *Mol Cell Biochem* 182:169, 1998.
96. Uysal KT, Wiebrock SM, Marino MW, Hotamisligil GS: Protection from obesity-induced insulin resistance in mice lacking TNF-alpha function. *Nature* 389:610, 1997.
97. Spiegelman BM: PPAR gamma: Adipogenic regulator and thiazolidinedione receptor. *Diabetes* 47:507, 1998.
98. Ristow M, Muler-Wieland D, Pfeiffer A, Krone W, Kahn CR: Obesity associated with a mutation in a genetic refulator of adipocyte differentiation. *N Engl J Med* 339:953, 1998.
99. Walston J, Silver K, Bogardus C, Knowler WC, Celi FS, Austin S, Manning B, Strosbers AD, Stern MP, Raben N, Sorkin JD, Roth J, Schuldiner AR: Time of onset of non-insulin-dependent diabetes mellitus and genetic variation in the Beta 3 adrenergic receptor gene. *N Engl J Med* 333:343, 1995.
100. Widen E, Lehto M, Kanninen T, Walston J, Schuldiner AR, Groop LC: Asociation of polymorphism in the Beta 3 adrenergic receptor gene with features of the insulin resistance syndrome in finns. *N Engl J Med* 333:348, 1995.
101. Clement K, Vaisse CV, Manning BSJ, Basdevant A, Guy-Grand B, Ruiz J, Silver KD, Shuldiner AR, Froguel P, Strosberg AD: Genetic variation in the Beta 3 adrenergic receptor and an increased capacity to gain weight in patients with morbid obesity. *N Engl J Med* 333:352, 1995.
102. Storlien LH, Baur LA, Kriketos AD, Pan DA, Cooney GJ, Jenkins AB, Calvert GD, Campbell LV: Dietary fats and insulin action: *Diabetologia* 39:621, 1996.
103. Buettner R, Schaffler A, Arndt H, Rogler G, Nusser J, Zietz B, Enger I, Hugl S, Cuk A, Scholmerich J, Palitzsch KD: The Trp64Arg polymorphism of the beta 3-adrenergic receptor geneis not associated with obesity or type 2 diabetes mellitus in a large population-based cohort. *J Clin Endocrinol Metab* 83:2892, 1998.
104. Mitchell BD, Biangero J, Comuzzie AG, Almasy LA, Shuldiner AR, Silver K, Stern MP, MacCluer JW, Hixson JE: A paired sibling analysis of the beta-3 adrenergic receptor and obesity in Mexican Americans. *J Clin Invest* 101:584, 1998.
105. Baron AD: Hemodynamic actions of insulin. *Am J Physiol* 267:E187, 1994.
106. Rosenthal M, Haskell WL, Solomon R, Widstromo A, Reaven GM: Demonstration of a relationship between level of physical training and insulin-stimulated glucose utilization in normal humans. *Diabetes* 32:408, 1983.
107. Olefsky JM, Farquhar JW, Reaven GM: Reappraisal of the role of insulin in hypertriglyceridemia. *Am J Med* 57:551, 1974.
108. Grundy SM, Mok HYI, Zech L, Steinberg D, Berman M: Transport of very low density lipoprotein triglycerides in varying degrees of obesity and hypertriglyceridemia. *J Clin Invest* 63:1274, 1979.
109. Olefsky J, Reaven GM, Farquhar JM: Effects of weight reduction and obesity on lipid and carbohydrate metabolism in normal and hyperlipoproteinemic subjects. *J Clin Invest* 53:64, 1974.
110. Grundy SM, Barnett JP: Metabolic and health complications of obesity. *Dis Mon* 36:645, 1990.
111. Steiner G, Lewis GF: Hyperinsulinemia and triglyceride-rich lipoproteins. *Diabetes* 45:S24, 1996.
112. Lewis GF, Steiner G: Acute effects of insulin in the control of VLDL production in humans. *Diabetes Care* 19:390, 1996.
113. Garg A: Insulin resistance in the pathogenesis of dyslipedemia. *Diabetes Care* 19:387, 1996.
114. Ginsberg HN: Diabetic dyslipedemia: Mechanisms underlying the common hypertriglyceridemia and low HDL cholesterol levels. *Diabetes* 45:S27, 1996.
115. Equsa G, Beltz WF, Grundy SM, Howard BV: Influence of obesity on metabolism of apolipoprotein B in humans. *J Clin Invest* 76:596, 1985.
116. Kazumi T, Vranic M, Steiner G: Changes in very low density lipoprotein particle size and production in response to sucrose feeding and hyperinsulinemia. *Endocrinology* 117:1145, 1985.
117. Dunn FL, Carroll PB, Beltz WF: Treatment with artificial β-cell decreases very-low-density lipoprotein triglyceride synthesis in Type I diabetes. *Diabetes* 36:661, 1987.
118. Rosenstock J, Vega GL, Raskin P: Effect of intensive diabetes treatment on low-density lipoprotein apolipoprotein B kinetics in Type I diabetes. *Diabetes* 37:393, 1988.
119. Salhanick AI, Schwartz SI, Amatruda JM: Insulin inhibits apolipoprotein B secretion in isolated human hepatocytes. *Metabolism* 40:275, 1991.
120. Sparks CE, Sparks JD, Bolognino M, Salhanick AI, Strumph PS, Amatruda JM: Insulin effects on apolipoprotein B lipoprotein synthesis and secretion by primary cultures of rat hepatocytes. *Metabolism* 35:1128, 1986.
121. Jackson TK, Salhanick AI, Elovson J, Deichman ML, Amatruda JM: Insulin regulates apolipoprotein B turnover and phosphorylation in rat hepatocytes. *J Clin Invest* 86:1746, 1990.
122. Yki-Järvinen H, Taskinen MR: Interrelationships among insulin's antilipolytic and glucoregulatory effects and plasma triglycerides in nondiabetic and diabetic patients with endogeneous hypertriglyceridemia. *Diabetes* 37:1271, 1988.
123. DeFronzo RA, Ferrannini E: Insulin resistance: A multifaceted syndrome responsible for NIDDM, obesity, hypertension, dyslipidemia, and atherosclerotic cardiovascular disease. *Diabetes Care* 14:173, 1991.
124. Reaven GM: Insulin resistance, hyperinsulinemia, hypertriglyceridemia and hypertension: Parallels between human disease and rodent models. *Diabetes Care* 14:195, 1991.
125. Garrison RJ, Wilson PW, Castelli WP, Feinleib M, Kannel WB, McNamara PM: Obesity and lipoprotein cholesterol in the Framingham offspring study. *Metabolism* 29:1053, 1980.
126. Denke MA, Sempos CT, Grundy SM: Excess body weight. An unrecognized contributor to high blood cholesterol levels in white American men. *Arch Intern Med* 153:1093, 1993.
127. Denke MA, Sempos CT, Grundy SM: Excess body weight: An unrecognized contributor to dyslipedemia in white American women. *Arch Intern Med* 154:401, 1994.
128. Reeder BA, Angel A, Ledoux M, Rabkin SW, Young TK, Sweet LE: Obesity and its relation to cardiovascular disease risk factors in Canadian adults. Canadian Heart Health Surveys Research Group. *Can Med Assoc J* 146:2009, 1992.
129. Follick MJ, Abrams DB, Smith TW, Henderson LO, Herbert PN: Contrasting short- and long-term effects of weight loss on lipoprotein levels. *Arch Intern Med* 144:1571, 1984.
130. Wood PD, Stefanick ML, Dreon DM, Frey-Hewitt B, Garay SC, Williams PT, Superko HR, Fortmann SP, et al: Changes in plasma lipids and lipoproteins in overweight men during weight loss through dieting as compared with exercise. *N Engl J Med* 319:1173, 1988.
131. Kaplan NM: Obesity in hypertension: Effects on prognosis and treatment. *J Hypertens* 16:S35, 1998.
132. Reaven GM, Lithell H, Landsberg L: Hypertension and associated metabolic abnormalities—the role of insulin resistance and the sympathoadrenal system. *N Engl J Med* 334:374, 1996.
133. Kannel WB, Garrison RJ, Dannenberg AL: Secular blood pressure trends in normotensive persons: The Framingham study. *Am Heart J* 125:1154, 1993.

134. Dustan HP: Obesity and hypertension. *Ann Intern Med* 103:1047, 1985.
135. Stamler R, Stamler J, Riedlinger W, Algera G, Roberts RH: Weight and blood pressure findings in hypertension screening of 1 million Americans. *JAMA* 240:1607, 1978.
136. Modan M, Halkin H, Almog S, Lusky A, Eskol A, Shefi M, Shitrit A, Fuchs Z: Hyperinsulinemia: A link between hypertension, obesity and glucose intolerance. *J Clin Invest* 75:809, 1985.
137. Pollare T, Lithell H, Berne C: Insulin resistance is a characteristic feature of primary hypertension independent of obesity. *Metabolism* 39:167, 1990.
138. Pouliot MC, Despres JP, Lemieux S, Moorjani S, Bouchard C, Tremblay A, Nadeau A, Lupien PJ: Waist circumference and abdominal sagittal diameter: Best simple anthropometric indexes of abdominal visceral adipose tissue accumulation and related cardiovascular risk in men and women. *Am J Cardiology* 73:460, 1994.
139. deVisser DC, van Hooft IMS, van Doornen LJP, Hofman A, Orlebeke JF, Grobbee DE: Anthropometric measures, fitness and habitual physical activity in offspring of hypertensive parents: Dutch hypertension and offspring study. *Am J Hypertens* 7:242, 1994.
140. DeFronzo RA, Cooke CR, Andres R, Faloona GR, Davis PJ: The effect of insulin on renal handling of sodium, potassium, calcium and phosphate in man. *J Clin Invest* 55:845, 1975.
141. DeFronzo RA, Goldberg M, Agus ZS: The effects of glucose and insulin on renal electrolyte transport. *J Clin Invest* 58:83, 1976.
142. Skott P, Hother-Nielsen O, Bruun NE, Giese J, Nielsen MD, Beck-Nielsen H, Parving HH: Effects of insulin on kidney function and sodium excretion in healthy subjects. *Diabetologia* 32:694, 1989.
143. Baum M: Insulin stimulates volume absorption in the rabbit proximal convoluted tubule. *J Clin Invest* 79:1104, 1987.
144. Rocchini AP, Katch V, Kveselis D, Moorehead C, Martin MN, Lampman R, Gregory M: Insulin and renal sodium retention in obese adolescents. *Hypertension* 14:367, 1989.
145. Dustan HP: Mechanisms of hypertension associated with obesity. *Ann Intern Med* 98:860, 1983.
146. Mujais SK, Tarazi RC, Dustan HP, Fouad FM, Bravo EL: Hypertension in obese patients: Hemodynamic and volume studies. *Hypertension* 4:84, 1982.
147. Frohlich ED: Mechanisms contributing to high blood pressure. *Ann Intern Med* 98:709, 1983.
148. Singler MH: The mechanism of natriuresis of fasting. *J Clin Invest* 55:377, 1975.
149. Amatruda JM, Richeson JF, Welle SL, Brodows RG, Lockwood DH: The safety and efficacy of a controlled low-energy ('very-low-calorie') diet in the treatment of non-insulin-dependent diabetes and obesity. *Arch Intern Med* 148:873, 1988.
150. Tuck ML, Sowers J, Dornfeld L, Kledzik G, Maxwell M: The effect of weight reduction on blood pressure, plasma renin activity and plasma aldosterone levels in obese patients. *N Engl J Med* 304:930, 1981.
151. Landsberg L, Krieger DR: Obesity, metabolism, and the sympathetic nervous system. *Am J Hypertens* 2:1255, 1989.
152. Grassi G, Cattaneo BM, Seravalle G, Colombo M, Cavagnini F, Mancia G: Obesity and the sympathetic nervous system. *Blood Pressure* 5:43, 1996.
153. Gudbjornsdottir S, Lonnroth P, Sverrisdottir YB, Wallin BG, Elam M: Sympathetic nerve activity and insulin in obese normotensive and hypertensive men. *Hypertension* 27:276, 1996.
154. Rowe JW, Young JB, Minaker KL, Stevens AL, Pallotta J, Landsberg L: Effect of insulin and glucose infusions on sympathetic nervous system activity in normal man. *Diabetes* 30:219, 1981.
155. Liang CS, Doherty JU, Faillace R, Maekawa K, Arnold S, Gavras H, Hood WB Jr: Insulin infusion in conscious dogs: Effects on systemic and coronary hemodynamics, regional blood flows, and plasma catecholamines. *J Clin Invest* 69:1321, 1982.
156. DeHaven J, Sherwin R, Hendler R, Felig P: Nitrogen and sodium balance and sympathetic-nervous-system activity in obese subjects treated with a low-calorie protein or mixed diet. *N Engl J Med* 302:477, 1980.
157. Jung RT, Shetty PS, Barrand M, Callingham BA, James WPT: Role of catecholamines in hypotensive response to dieting. *Br Med J* 1:12, 1979.
158. Sowers JR, Whitfield LA, Catania RA, Stern N, Tuck ML, Dornfeld L, Maxwell M: Role of sympathetic nervous system in blood pressure maintenance in obesity. *J Clin Endocrinol Metab* 54:1181, 1982.
159. Rocchini AP, Key J, Bondie D, Chico R, Moorehead C, Katch V, Martin M: The effect of weight loss on the sensitivity of blood pressure to sodium in obese adolescents. *N Engl J Med* 321:580, 1989.
160. MacMahon SW, Wilcken DEL, MacDonald GH: The effect of weight reduction on left ventricular mass. *N Engl J Med* 314:334, 1986.
161. Krotkiewski M, Bjödorntorp P, Sjöström L, Smith U: Impact of obesity on metabolism in men and women: Importance of regional adipose tissue distribution. *J Clin Invest* 72:1150, 1983.
162. Blair D, Habicht JP, Sims EAH, Sylwester D, Abraham S: Evidence for an increased risk for hypertension with centrally located body fat and the effect of race and sex on the risk. *Am J Epidemiol* 119:526, 1984.
163. Baron AD: Hemodynamic actions of insulin. *Am J Physiol* 267: E187, 1994.
164. Vollenweider P, Randin D, Tappy L, Jequier E, Nicod P, Scherrer U: Impaired insulin-induced sympathetic activation and vasodilation in skeletal muscle in obese humans. *J Clin Invest* 93:2365, 1994.
165. Maclure KM, Hayes KC, Colditz GA, Stampfer M, Speizer FE, Willett WC: Weight, diet, and the risk of symptomatic gallstones in middle-aged women. *N Engl J Med* 321:563, 1989.
166. Bennion LJ, Grundy SM: Risk factors in the development of cholelithiasis in man. *N Engl J Med* 299:1161, 1978.
167. Stampfer MJ, Maclure KM, Colditz GA, Manson JE, Willett WC: Risk of symptomatic gallstones in women with severe obesity. *Am J Clin Nutr* 55:652, 1992.
168. Khare M, Everhart JE, Maurer KR, Hill MC: Association of ethnicity and body mass index (BMI) with gallstone disease in the United States. *Am J Epidemiol* 141:569, 1995.
169. Bennion LJ, Grundy SM: Effects of obesity and caloric intake on biliary lipid metabolism in man. *J Clin Invest* 56:996, 1975.
170. Mabee TM, Meyer P, DenBesten L, Mason EE: The mechanism of increased gallstone formation in obese human subjects. *Surgery* 79:460, 1976.
171. Shaffer EA, Small DM: Biliary lipid secretion in cholesterol gallstone disease: The effect of cholecystectomy and obesity. *J Clin Invest* 59:828, 1977.
172. Miettinen TA: Cholesterol production in obesity. *Circulation* 44:842, 1971.
173. Nestel PJ, Schreibman PH, Ahrens EH Jr: Cholesterol metabolism in human obesity. *J Clin Invest* 52:2389, 1973.
174. Salen G, Nicholan G, Shefer S, Mosbach EH: Hepatic cholesterol metabolism in patients with gallstones. *Gastroenterology* 69:676, 1975.
175. Nepokroeff CM, Lakshmanan MR, Ness GC, Dugan RE, Porter JW: Regulation of diurnal rhythm of rat liver β-hydroxy-β-methylglutaryl coenzyme A reductase activity by insulin, glucagon, cyclic AMP and hydrocortisone. *Arch Biochem Biophys* 160:387, 1974.
176. Sampliner RE, Bennett PH, Comess LJ, Rose FA, Burch TA: Gallbladder disease in Pima Indians: Demonstration of high prevalence and early onset by cholecystography. *N Engl J Med* 283:1358, 1970.
177. Grundy SM, Metzger AL, Alder RD: Mechanisms of lithogenic bile formation in American Indian women with cholesterol gallstones. *J Clin Invest* 51:3026, 1972.
178. Willett WC, Browne ML, Bain C, Lipnick RJ, Stampfer MJ, Rosner B, Colditz GA, Hennekens CH, et al: Relative weight and risk of breast cancer among premenopausal women. *Am J Epidemiol* 122:731, 1985.
179. London SJ, Colditz GA, Stampfer MJ, Willett WC, Rosner B, Speizer FE: Prospective study of relative weight, height, and risk of breast cancer. *JAMA* 262:2853, 1989.
180. Wolff GL: Body weight and cancer. *Am J Clin Nutr* 45:168, 1987.
181. Snowdon DA, Phillips RL, Choi W: Diet, obesity, and risk of fatal prostate cancer. *Am J Epidemiol* 120:244, 1984.
182. AACE/ACE Obesity Task Force: AACE/ACE position statement on the prevention, diagnosis and treatment of obesity. *Endo Practice* 3:162, 1997.
183. Willett WC: Implications of total energy intake for epidemiological studies of breast and large-bowel cancer. *Am J Clin Nutr* 45:354, 1987.
184. Willett WC, Stampfer MJ, Colditz GA, Rosner BA, Hennekens CH, Speizer FE: Dietary fat and the risk of breast cancer. *N Engl J Med* 316:22, 1987.
185. Kolonel LN: Fat and colon cancer: How firm is the epidemiologic evidence? *Am J Clin Nutr* 45:336, 1987.

186. Hunter DJ, Willett WC: Diet, body size and breast cancer. *Epidemiol Rev* 15:110, 1993.
187. Simopoulos AP: Obesity and carcinogenesis: Historical perspective. *Am J Clin Nutr* 45:271, 1987.
188. Nimrod A, Ryan KJ: Aromatization of androgens by human abdominal and breast fat tissue. *J Clin Endocrinol Metab* 40:367, 1975.
189. Edman CD, MacDonald PC: Effect of obesity on conversion of plasma androstenedione to estrone in ovulatory and anovulatory young women. *Am J Obstet Gynecol* 130:456, 1978.
190. Loncope C, Pratt JH, Schneider SH, Fineberg SE: Aromatization of androgens by muscle and adipose tissue in vivo. *J Clin Endocrinol Metab* 46:146, 1978.
191. Cleland WH, Mendelson CR, Simpson ER: Aromatase activity of membrane fractions of human adipose tissue stromal cells and adipocytes. *Endocrinology* 113:2155, 1983.
192. Schindler AE, Ebert A, Friedrich E: Conversion of androstenedione to estrone by human tissue. *J Clin Endocrinol Metab* 35:627, 1972.
193. Sitteri PK, MacDonald PC: Role of extraglandular estrogen in human endocrinology, in Greep RO (ed): *Handbook of Physiology*. Washington, D.C., American Physiological Society, 1973, p 615.
194. Klinga K, VonHolst T, Runnebaum B: Influence of severe obesity on peripheral hormone concentrations in pre-menopausal and postmenopausal women. *Eur J Obstet Gynecol Reprod Biol* 15:103, 1983.
195. Bray G: Complications of obesity. *Ann Intern Med* 103:1052, 1985.
196. Rogers J, Mitchell GW: The relation of obesity to menstrual disturbances. *N Engl J Med* 247:53, 1952.
197. Mitchell GW, Rogers J: The influence of weight reduction on amenorrhea in obese women. *N Engl J Med* 249:835, 1953.
198. Hartz AJ, Barboriak PN, Wong A, Katayama KP, Rimm AA: The association of obesity with infertility and related menstrual abnormalities in women. *Int J Obes* 3:57, 1979.
199. Glass AR, Dahms WT, Abraham G, Atkinson RL, Bray GA, Swerdloff RS: Secondary amenorrhea in obesity: Etiologic role of weight-related androgen excess. *Fertil Steril* 30:243, 1978.
200. Barbieri RL, Ryan KJ: Hyperandrogenism, insulin resistance, and acanthosis nigricans syndrome: A common endocrinopathy with distinct pathophysiologic features. *Am J Obstet Gynecol* 147:90, 1983.
201. Flier JS, Eastman RC, Minaker KL, Matteson D, Rowe JW: Acanthosis nigricans in obese women with hyperandrogenism: Characterization of an insulin-resistant state distinct from the Type A and B syndromes. *Diabetes* 34:101, 1985.
202. Legro RS: Polycystic ovary syndrome: Current and future treatment paradigms. *Am J Obstet Gynecol* 179:S101, 1998.
203. Rich-Edwards JW, Goldman MB, Willett WC, Hunter DJ, Stampfer MJ, Colditz GA, Manson JE: Adolescent body mass index and infertility caused by ovulatory disorder. *Am J Obstet Gynecol* 171:171, 1994.
204. Barnes R, Rosenfield RL: The polycystic ovary syndrome: Pathogenesis and treatment. *Ann Intern Med* 110:386, 1989.
205. Harlass FE, Plymate SR, Fariss BL, Belts RP: Weight loss is associated with correction of gonadotropin and sex steroid abnormalities in the obese anovulatory female. *Fertil Steril* 42:649, 1984.
206. McKenna TJ: Pathogenesis and treatment of polycystic ovary syndrome. *N Engl J Med* 318:558, 1988.
207. Annos T, Taymor ML: Ovarian pathology associated with insulin resistance and acanthosis nigricans. *Obstet Gynecol* 58:662, 1981.
208. Geffner ME, Kaplan SA, Bersch N, Golden DW, Landaw EM, Chang R: Persistance of insulin resistance in polycystic ovarian disease after inhibition of ovarian steroid secretion. *Fertil Steril* 45:327, 1986.
209. Taylor AE: Understanding the underlying metabolic abnormalities of polycystic ovary syndrome and their implications. *Am J Obstet Gynecol* 179:S94, 1998.
210. Poretsky L, Kalin MF: The gonadotropic function of insulin. *Endocr Rev* 8:132, 1987.
211. Dunaif A: Insulin resistance and the polycystic ovary syndrome: Mechanism and implications for pathogenesis. *Endo Rev* 18:774, 1997.
212. Nestler JE, Barlascini CO, Matt DW, Steingold KA, Plymate SR, Clore JM, Blackard WG: Suppression of serum insulin by diazoxide reduces serum testosterone levels in obese women with polycystic ovary syndrome. *J Clin Endocrinol Metab* 68:1027, 1989.
213. Nestler JE, Jakubowicz DJ, Evans WS, Pasquali R: Effects of metformin on spontaneous and clomiphene-induced ovulation in the polycystic ovary syndrome. *N Engl J Med* 338:1876, 1998.
214. Nestler JE, Jakubowicz DJ: Decreases in ovarian cytochrome P250c17a activity and serum free testosterone after reduction of insulin secretion in polycystic ovary syndrome. *N Engl J Med* 335:617, 1996.
215. Rittmaster RS, Loriaux DL: Hirsutism. *Ann Intern Med* 106:95, 1987.
216. Adashi EY, Hsueh HW, Yen SSC: Insulin enhancement of luteinizing hormone and follicle stimulating hormone release by cultured pituitary cells. *Endocrinology* 108:1441, 1981.
217. Peiris AN, Mueller RA, Struve MF, Smith GA, Kissebah AH: Relationship of androgenic activity to splanchnic insulin metabolism and peripheral glucose utilization in premenopausal women. *J Clin Endocrinol Metab* 64:162, 1987.
218. Amatruda JM, Harman SM, Pourmotabbed G, Lockwood DH: Depressed plasma testosterone and fractional binding of testosterone in obese males. *J Clin Endocrinol Metab* 47:268, 1978.
219. Glass AR: Endocrine aspects of obesity. *Med Clin North Am* 73:139, 1989.
220. Amatruda JM, Hochstein M, Hsu TH, Lockwood DH: Hypothalamic and pituitary dysfunction in obese males. *Int J Obes* 6:183, 1981.
221. Shalet SM, Toogood A, Rahim A, Brennan B: The diagnosis of growth hormone deficiency in children and adults. *Endo Rev* 19:203, 1998.
222. Pontirolo AE, Manzoni MF, Malighetti ME, Lanzi R: Restoration of growth hormone (GH) response to GH-releasing hormone in elderly and obese subjects by acute pharmacological reduction of plasma free fatty acids. *J Clin Endocrinol Metab* 81:3998, 1996.
223. Cordido F, Fernandez T, Martinez T, Penalva A, Peino R, Casanueva FF, Dieguez C: Effect of acute pharmacological reduction of plasma free fatty acids on growth hormone (GH) releasing hormone-induced GH secretion in obese adults with and without hypopituitarism. *J Clin Endocrinol Metab* 83:4350, 1998.
224. Villa P, Fulghesu AM, DeMarinis L, Valle D, Mancini A, Pavone V, Caruso A, Lanzone A: Impact of long-term naltrexone on growth hormone and insulin secretion in hyperandrogenic and normal obese patients. *Metabolism* 46:538, 1997.
225. Crapo L: Cushing's syndrome: A review of diagnostic tests. *Metabolism* 28:955, 1979.
226. Pasquali R, Biscotti D, Spinucci G, Vicennati V, Genazzani AD, Sgarbi L, Casimirri F: Pulsatile secretion of ACTH and cortisol in premenopausal women: Effect of obesity and body fat distribution. *Clin Endocrinol* 48:603, 1998.
227. Andrew R, Phillips DI, Walker BR: Obesity and gender influence cortisol secretion and metabolism in man. *J Clin Endocrinol Metab* 83:1806, 1998.
228. Bujalska IJ, Kumar S, Stewart PM: Does central obesity reflect "Cushing's disease of the omentum." *Lancet* 349:1210, 1997.
229. Felson DT, Anderson JJ, Naimark A, Walker AM, Meenan RF: Obesity and knee osteoarthritis: The Farmington Study. *Ann Intern Med* 109.18, 1988.
230. Cicuttini FM, Baker JR, Spector TD: The association of obesity with osterarthritis of the hand and knee in women: A twin study. *J Rheumatol* 23:1221, 1996.
231. Hart DJ, Spector TD: The relationship of obesity, fat distribution, and osteoarthritis in women in the general population: The Chingford Study. *J Rheumatol* 20:331, 1993.
232. Hochberg MC, Lethbridge-Cejku M, Scott WW Jr, Reichle R, Plato CC, Tobin JD: The assoiation of body weight, body fatness and body fat distribution with osteoarthritis of the knee: Data from the Baltimore Longitudinal Study of Aging. *J Rheumatol* 22:488, 1995.
233. Carmen WJ, Sowers M, Hawthorne VM, Weissfeld LA: Obesity as a risk factor for osteoarthritis of the hand and wrist: A prospective study. *Am J Epidemiol* 139:119, 1994.
234. Felson DT, Zhang Y, Anthony JM, Naimark A, Anderson JJ: Weight loss reduces the risk for symptomatic knee osteoarthritis in women. The Framingham study. *Ann Intern Med* 116:535, 1992.
235. Felson DT: Weight reduction and osteoarthritis. *J Rheumatol* 43:7, 1995.
236. McGoey BV, Deitel M, Saplys RJ, Kliman ME: Effect of weight loss on musculoskeletal pain in the morbidly obese. *J Bone Surg* [*Br*] 72-B:322, 1990.
237. Williams RA, Foulsham BM: Weight reduction in osteoarthritis using phentermine. *Practitioner* 335:231, 1981.
238. Kreiger N, Kelsey JL, Holford TR, O'Connor T: An epidemiologic study of hip fracture in postmenopausal women. *Am J Epidemiol* 116:141, 1982.

239. Kelsey JL, Hoffman S: Risk factors for hip fracture. *N Engl J Med* 316:404, 1987.
240. Slemenda CW, Hui SL, Longcope C, Wellman H, Johnston CC: Predictors of bone mass in premenopausal women: A prospective study of clinical data using photo absorptiometry. *Ann Intern Med* 112:96, 1990.
241. Teitelbaum SL, Halverson JD, Bates M, Wise L, Haddad WG: Abnormalities of circulating 25-OH vitamin D after jejunal bypass for obesity: Evidence of an adaptive response. *Ann Intern Med* 86:289, 1977.
242. Dalen N, Hallberd D, Lamke B: Bone mass in obese subjects. *Acta Med Scand* 197:353, 1975.
243. Bell NH, Epstein S, Greene A, Shary J, Oexmann MH, Shaw S: Evidence for alteration of the vitamin D-endocrine system in obese subjects. *J Clin Invest* 76:370, 1985.
244. Atkinson RL, Dahms WT, Bray GA, Schwartz AA: Parathyroid hormone levels in obesity: Effects of intestinal bypass surgery. *Miner Electrolyte Metab* 1:315, 1978.
245. Cohen SH, Abesamis C, Yasamura S, Aloia JF, Zanzi I, Ellis KJ: Comparative skeletal mass and radial bone mineral content in black and white women. *Metab Clin Exp* 26:171, 1977.
246. Rubinstein I, Zamel N, DuBarry L, Hoffstein V: Airflow limitation in morbidly obese, nonsmoking men. *Ann Intern Med* 112:828, 1990.
247. Kaplan J, Staats BA: Obstructive sleep apnea syndrome. *Mayo Clin Proc* 65:1087, 1990.
248. Prowse K, Allen MB: Sleep apnoea. *Br J Dis Chest* 82:329, 1989.
249. Findley LJ, Fabrizio M, Thommi M, Suratt PM: Severity of sleep apnea and automobile crashes. *N Engl J Med* 320:868, 1989.
250. Shelton KE, Woodson H, Gay S, et al: Pharyngeal fat in obstructive sleep apnea: *Am Rev Respir Dis* 148:462, 1993.
251. Eisenberg E, Zimlichman R, Lavie P: Plasma norepinephrine levels in patients with sleep apnea syndrome. *N Engl J Med* 322:932, 1990.
252. Hung J, Whitford EG, Parsons RW, Hillman DR: Association of sleep apnoea with myocardial infarction in men. *Lancet* 336:261, 1990.
253. Smith PL, Gold AR, Meyers DA, Haponik EF, Bleecker ER: Weight loss in mildly to moderately obese patients with obstructive sleep apnea. *Ann Intern Med* 103:850, 1985.
254. Hudgel DW: Treatment of obstructive sleep apnea. *Chest* 109:1346, 1996.
255. Browman CP, Sampson MG, Yolles SF, Gujavarty KS, Weiler SJ, Walsleben JA, Hahn PM, Mitler MM: Obstructive sleep apnea and body weight. *Chest* 85:434, 1984.
256. Suratt PM, McTier RF, Findley LJ, Pohl SL, Wilhit SC: Effect of very-low-calorie diets with weight loss on obstructive sleep apnea. *Am J Clin Nutr* 56:183S, 1992.
257. Charuzi I, Ovnat A, Peiser J, Saltz H, Weitzman S, Lavie P: The effect of surgical weight reduction on sleep quality in obesity-related sleep apnea syndrome. *Surgery* 97:535, 1985.
258. Partinen M, Guilleminault G: Daytime sleepiness and vascular morbidity at seven-year follow-up in obstructive sleep apnea patients. *Chest* 97:27, 1990.
259. Gross T, Sokol RJ, King KC: Obesity in pregnancy: Risks and outcome. *Obstet Gynecol* 56:446, 1980.
260. Weisinger JR, Kempson RL, Eldridge FL, Swenson RS: The nephrotic syndrome: A complication of massive obesity. *Ann Intern Med* 81:440, 1974.
261. Galtier-Dereure F, Montpeyroux F, Boulot P, Bringer J, Jaffiol C: Weight excess before pregnancy: Complications and cost. *Int J Obesity* 19:443, 1995.
262. O'Brien TF, Stroop EM: Lower esophageal sphincter pressure (LESP) and esophageal function in obese humans. *J Clin Gastroenterol* 2:145, 1980.
263. Stunkard AJ, Sorensen TIA, Hanis C, Teasdale TW, Chakraborty R, Schull WJ, Schulsinger F: An adoption study of human obesity. *N Engl J Med* 314:193, 1986.
264. Stunkard AJ, Harris JR, Pedersen NL, McClearn GE: The body-mass index of twins who have been reared apart. *N Engl J Med* 322:1483, 1990.
265. Bouchard C: Current understanding of the etiology of obesity: Genetic and nongenetic factors. *Am J Clin Nutr* 53:1561S, 1991.
266. Price RA, Stunkard AJ, Ness R, Wadden TH, Heshka S, Kanders B, Cormillot A: Childhood onset (age <10) obesity has high familial risk. *Int J Obesity* 14:185, 1989.
267. Perusse L, Chagnon YC, Weisnagel J, Bouchard C: The human obesity gene map: The 1998 update. *Obes Res* 7:111, 1999.
268. Lee JH, Reed DR, Li WD, Xu W, Joo EJ, Kilker RL, Nanthakumar E, North M, Sakul H, Bell C, Price RA: Genome scan for human obesity and linkage to markers in 20q13. *Am J Hum Genet* 64:196, 1999.
269. Borecki IB, Blangero J, Rice T, Perusse L, Bouchard C, Rao DC: Evidence for at least two major loci influencing human fatness. *Am J Hum Genet* 63:831, 1998.
270. Perusse L, Chagnon YC, Bouchard C: Etiology of massive obesity: Role of genetic factors. *World J Surg* 22:907, 1998.
271. Montague CT, Farooqi IS, Whitehead JP, Soos MA, Rau H, Wareham NJ, Sewter CP, Digb, JE, Mohammed SN, Hurst JA, Cheetham CH, Earley AR, Barnett AH, Prins JB, O'Rahilly S: Congenital leptin deficiency is associated with severe early-onset obesity in humans. *Nature* 387:903, 1997.
272. Clement K, Vaisse C, Lahlou N, Cabrol S, Pelloux V, Cassuto D, Gourmelen M, Dina C, Chambaz J, Lacorte JM, Basdevant A, Bougneres P, Lebouc Y, Froguel P, Guy-Grand B: A mutation in the human leptin receptor gene causes obesity and pituitary dysfunction. *Nature* 392:398, 1998.
273. Hinney A, Schmidt A, Nottebom K, Heibult O, Becker I, Ziegler A, Gerber G, Sina M, Gorg T, Mayer H, Siegfried W, Fichter M, Remschmidt H, Hebebrand J: Several mutations in the melanocortin-4 receptor gene including a nonsense and a frameshift mutation associated with dominantly inherited obesity in humans. *J Clin Endocrinol Metab* 84:1483, 1999.
274. Jackson RS, Creemers JW, Ohagi S, Raffin-Sanson ML, Sanders L, Montague CT, Hutton JC, O'Rahilly S: Obesity and impaired prohormone processing associated with mutations in the human prohormone convertase 1 gene. *Nat Genet* 16:303, 1997.
275. Clement K, Vaisse C, Manning BS, Basdevant A, Guy-Grand B, Ruiz J, Silver KD, Shuldiner AR, Froguel P, Strosberg AD: Genetic variation in the beta 3-adrenergic receptor and an increased capacity to gain weight in patients with morbid obesity. *N Engl J Med* 333:352, 1995.
276. Mitchell BD, Blangero J, Comuzzie AG, Almasy LA, Shuldiner AR, Silver K, Stern MP, MacCluer JW, Hixson JE: A paired sibling analysis of the beta-3 adrenergic receptor and obesity in Mexican Americans. *J Clin Invest* 101:584, 1998.
277. Buettner R, Schaffler A, Arndt H, Rogler G, Nusser J, Zietz B, Enger I, Hugl S, Cuk A, Scholmerich J, Palitzsch KD: The Trp64Arg polymorphism of the beta 3-adrenergic receptor gene is not associated with obesity or type 2 diabetes mellitus in a large population-based Caucasian cohort. *J Clin Endocrinol Metab* 83:2892, 1998.
278. Ghosh S, Langefeld CD, Ally D, Watanabe RM, Hauser ER, Magnuson VL, Nylund SJ, Valle T, Eriksson J, Bergman RN, Tuomilehto J, Collins FS, Boehnke M: The W64R variant of the beta 3-adrenergic receptor is not associated with type II diabetes or obesity in a large Finnish sample. *Diabetologia* 42:238, 1999.
279. Pelleymounter MA, Cullen MJ, Baker MB, Hecht R, Winters D, Boone T, Collins F: Effects of the obese gene product on body weight regulation in ob/ob mice. *Science* 269:540, 1995.
280. Coleman DL: Obese and diabetes: Two mutant genes causing diabetes-obesity syndromes in mice. *Diabetologia* 14:141, 1978.
281. Coleman DL: Effects of parabiosis of obese with diabetes and normal mice. *Diabetologia* 9:294, 1973.
282. Tartaglia LA, Dembski M, Weng X, Deng N, Culpepper J, Devos R, Richards GJ, Campfield LA, Clark FT, Deeds J, Muir C, Sanker S, Moriarty A, Moore KJ, Smutko JS, Mays GG, Woolf EA, Monroe CA, Tepper RI: Identification and expression cloning of a leptin receptor, OB-R. *Cell* 83:1263, 1995.
283. Zhang Y, Proenca R, Maffei M, Barone M, Leopold L, Friedman JM: Positional cloning of the mouse obese gene and its human homologue. *Nature* 372:425, 1994.
284. Bultman SJ, Michaud EJ, Woychik RP: Molecular characterization of the mouse agouti locus. *Cell* 71:1195, 1992.
285. Yen TT, Gill AM, Frigeri LG, Barsh GS, Wolff GL: Obesity, diabetes, and neoplasia in yellow A(vy)/-mice: Ectopic expression of the agouti gene. *FASEB J* 8:479, 1994.
286. Dinulescu DM, Fan W, Boston BA, McCall K, Lamoreux ML, Moore KJ, Montagno J, Cone RD: Mahogany (mg) stimulates feeding and increases basal metabolic rate independent of its suppression of agouti. *Proc Natl Acad Sci USA* 95:12707, 1998.

287. Nagle DL, McGrail SH, Vitale J, Woolf EA, Dussault BJ Jr, DiRocco L, Holmgren L, Montagno J, Bork P, Huszar D, Fairchild-Huntress V, Ge P, Keilty J, Ebeling C, Baldini L, Gilchrist J, Burn P, Carlson GA, Moore KJ: The mahogany protein is a receptor involved in suppression of obesity. *Nature* 398:148, 1999.
288. Naggert JK, Fricker LD, Varlamov O, Nishina PM, Rouille Y, Steiner DF, Carroll RJ, Paigen BJ, Leiter EH: Hyperproinsulinaemia in obese fat/fat mice associated with a carboxypeptidase E mutation which reduces enzyme activity. *Nat Genet* 10:135, 1995.
289. Rovere C, Viale A, Nahon J, Kitabgi P: Impaired processing of brain proneurotensin and promelanin-concentrating hormone in obese fat/fat mice. *Endocrinology* 37:2954, 1996.
290. Cool DR, Normant E, Shen F, Chen HC, Pannell L, Zhang Y, Loh YP: Carboxypeptidase E is a regulated secretory pathway sorting receptor: Genetic obliteration leads to endocrine disorders in Cpe(fat) mice. *Cell* 88:73, 1997.
291. Coleman DL, Eicher EM: Fat (fat) and tubby (tub): Two autosomal recessive mutations causing obesity syndromes in the mouse. *J Hered* 81:424, 1990.
292. Noben-Trauth K, Naggert JK, North MA, Nishina PM: A candidate gene for the mouse mutation tubby. *Nature* 380:534, 1996.
293. Kleyn PW, Fan W, Kovats SG, Lee JJ, Pulido JC, Wu Y, Berkemeier LR, Misumi DJ, Holmgren L, Charlat O, Woolf EA, Tayber O, Brody T, Shu P, Hawkins F, Kennedy B, Baldini L, Ebeling C, Alperin GD, Deeds J, Lakey ND, Culpepper J, Chen H, Glucksmann-Kuis MA, Carlson GA, Duyk GM, Moore KJ: Identification and characterization of the mouse obesity gene tubby: A member of a novel gene family. *Cell* 85:281, 1996.
294. Bogardus C, Lillioja S, Ravussin E, Abbott W, Zawadzki JK, Young A, Knowler WC, Jacobowitz R, et al: Familial dependence of the resting metabolic rate. *N Engl J Med* 315:96, 1986.
295. Bouchard C, Tremblay A, Nadeau A, Despres JP, Theriault G, Boulay MR, Lortie G, Leblanc C, Fournier G: Genetic effect in resting and exercise metabolic rates. *Metabolism* 38:364, 1989.
296. Ravussin E, Lillioja S, Knowler WC, Christin L, Freymond D, Abbott WGH, Boyce V, Howard BV, et al: Reduced rate of energy expenditure as a risk factor for body-weight gain. *N Engl J Med* 318:467, 1988.
297. Wade J, Milner J, Krondl M: Evidence for a physiological regulation of food selection and nutrient intake in twins. *Am J Clin Nutr* 34:143, 1981.
298. Perusse L, Tremblay A, Leblanc C, Cloninger CR, Reich T, Rice J, Bouchard C: Familial resemblance in energy intake: Contribution of genetic and environmental factors. *Am J Clin Nutr* 47:629, 1988.
299. Sobal J, Stunkard AJ: Socioeconomic status and obesity: A review of the literature. *Psychol Bull* 105:260, 1989.
300. Dietz WH, Gortmaker SL: Do we fatten our children at the television set? Obesity and television viewing in children and adolescents. *Pediatrics* 75:807, 1985.
301. Gortmaker SL, Must A, Sobol AM, Peterson K, Colditz GA, Dietz WH: Television viewing as a cause of increasing obesity among children in the United States, 1986-1990. *Arch Pediatr Adolesc Med* 150:356, 1996.
302. Dietz WH, Gortmaker SL: Factors within the physical environment associated with childhood obesity. *Am J Clin Nutr* 39:619, 1984.
303. Bray GA, Popkin BMN: Dietary fat intake does affect obesity. *Am J Clin Nutr* 68:1157, 1998.
304. Tremblay A, Plourde G, Despres JP, Bouchard C: Impact of dietary fat content and fat oxidation on energy intake in humans. *Am J Clin Nutr* 49:799, 1989.
305. Proserpi C, Sparti A, Schutz Y, DiVetta V, Milon H, Jequier E: Ad libitum intake of a high-carbohydrate or high-fat diet in young men: Effects on nutrient balances. *Am J Clin Nutr* 66:539, 1997.
306. Felitti VJ: Childhood sexual abuse, depression, and family dysfunction in adult obese patients. *South Med J* 86:732, 1993.
307. James WPT, Trayhurn P: An integrated view of the metabolic and genetic basis for obesity. *Lancet* 2:770, 1976.
308. McCarron DA, Morris CD, Henry HJ, Stanton JL: Blood pressure and nutrient in the United States. *Science* 224:1391, 1984.
309. Myers RG, Klesges RC, Eck LH, Hanson CL, Klem ML: Accuracy of self-reports of food intake in obese and normal-weight individuals: Effects of obesity on self-reports of dietary intake in adult females. *Am J Clin Nutr* 48:1248, 1988.
310. Romieu I, Willett WC, Stampfer MJ, Colditz GA, Sampson L, Rosner B, Hennekens CH, Speizer FE: Energy intake and other determinants of relative weight. *Am J Clin Nutr* 47:406, 1988.
311. Lissner L, Habicht J-P, Strupp BJ, Levitsky DA, Haas JD, Roe DA: Body composition and energy intake: Do overweight women overeat and underreport? *Am J Clin Nutr* 49:320, 1989.
312. Irsigler K, Veitl V, Sigmund A, Tschegg E, Kunz K: Calorimetric results in man: Energy output in normal and overweight subjects. *Metabolism* 28:1127, 1979.
313. Ravussin E, Burnard B, Schutz Y, Jequier E: Twenty-four-hour energy expenditure and resting metabolic rate in obese, moderately obese, and control subjects. *Am J Clin Nutr* 35:566, 1982.
314. Bessard T, Schutz Y, Jequier E: Energy expenditure and postprandial thermogenesis in obese women before and after weight loss. *Am J Clin Nutr* 38:680, 1983.
315. Ravussin E, Lillioja S, Anderson TE, Christin L, Bogardus C: Determinants of 24-hour energy expenditure in man. *J Clin Invest* 78:1568, 1986.
316. DeBoer JO, VanEs AJH, VanRaaij JMA, Hautvast JGAJ: Energy requirements and energy expenditure of lean and overweight women, measured by indirect calorimetry. *Am J Clin Nutr* 46:13, 1987.
317. Lean MEJ, James WPT: Metabolic effects of isoenergetic nutrient exchange over 24 hours in relation to obesity in women. *Int J Obes* 12:15, 1988.
318. Leibel RL, Hirsch J: Diminished energy requirements in reduced-obese patients. *Metabolism* 33:164, 1984.
319. Forbes GB, Brown MR: Energy need for weight maintenance in human beings: Effects of body size and composition. *J Am Diet Assoc* 89:499, 1989.
320. Blair D, Burkirk ER: Habitual daily energy expenditure and activity levels of lean and adult-onset and child-onset obese women. *Am J Clin Nutr* 45:540, 1987.
321. Welle S, Forbes GB, Statt M, Barnard RR, Amatruda JM: Energy expenditure under free-living conditions in normal-weight and overweight women. *Am J Clin Nutr* 55:14, 1992.
322. Prentice AM, Black AE, Coward WA, Davies HL, Goldberg GR, Murgatroyd PR, Ashford J, Sawyer M, Whitehead RG: High levels of energy expenditure in obese women. *Br Med J* 292:983, 1986.
323. Bandini LG, Schoeller DA, Dietz WH: Energy expenditure in obese and nonobese adolescents. *Pediatr Res* 27:198, 1990.
324. Roberts SV, Savage J, Coward WA, Chew B, Lucas A: Energy expenditure and intake in infants born to lean and overweight mothers. *N Engl J Med* 318:461, 1988.
325. Griffiths M, Payne PR: Energy expenditure in small children of obese and non-obese parents. *Nature* 260:698, 1976.
326. Welle SL, Amatruda JM, Forbes GB, Lockwood DH: Resting metabolic rates of obese women after rapid weight loss. *J Clin Endocrinol Metab* 59:41, 1984.
327. Weigle DA: Contribution of decreased body mass to diminished thermic effect of exercise in reduced-obese men. *Int J Obes* 12:567, 1988.
328. Elliot DL, Goldberg L, Kuehl KS, Bennett WM: Sustained depression of the resting metabolic rate after massive weight loss. *Am J Clin Nutr* 49:93, 1989.
329. Leibel RL, Rosenbaum M, Hirsch J: Changes in energy-expenditure resulting from altered body-weight. *N Engl J Med* 332:621, 1995.
330. Geissler CA, Miller DS, Shah M: The daily metabolic rate of the post-obese and the lean. *Am J Clin Nutr* 45:914, 1987.
331. McNeill G, Bukkens SGF, Morrison DC, Smith JS: Energy intake and energy expenditure in post-obese women and weight-matched controls. *Proc Nutr Soc* 49:1190, 1990.
332. Miller DS, Parsonage S: Resistance to slimming adaptation or illusion? *Lancet* 1:773, 1975.
333. Weigle DA, Sande KJ, Iverius PH, Monsen ER, Brunzell JD: Weight loss leads to a marked decrease in nonresting energy expenditure in ambulatory human subjects. *Metabolism* 37:930, 1988.
334. Bessard T, Schutz Y, Jequier E: Energy expenditure and postprandial thermogenesis in obese women before and after weight loss. *Am J Clin Nutr* 38:680, 1983.
335. Dore C, Hesp R, Wilkins D, Garrow JS: Prediction of energy requirements of obese patients after massive weight loss. *Hum Nutr Clin Nutr* 36C:41, 1982.
336. Kaplan ML, Leveille GA: Calorigenic response in obese and nonobese women. *Am J Clin Nutr* 29:1108, 1976.
337. Shetty PS, Jung RT, James WPT, Barrand MA, Callingham BA: Postprandial thermogenesis in obesity. *Clin Sci* 60:519, 1981.
338. Segal KR, Gutin B: Thermic effects of food and exercise in lean and obese women. *Metabolism* 32:581, 1983.

339. Schutz Y, Bessard T, Jequier E: Diet-induced thermogenesis measured over a whole day in obese and nonobese women. *Am J Clin Nutr* 40:542, 1984.
340. Segal KR, Gutin B, Nyman AM, Pi-Sunyer X: Thermic effect of food at rest, during exercise, and after exercise in lean and obese men of similar body weight. *J Clin Invest* 76:1107, 1985.
341. Segal KR, Gutin B, Albu J, Pi-Sunyer X: Thermic effects of food and exercise in lean and obese men of similar lean body mass. *Am J Physiol* 252:E110, 1987.
342. Nair KS, Halliday D, Garrow JS: Thermic response to isoenergetic protein, carbohydrate or fat meals in lean and obese subjects. *Clin Sci* 65:307, 1983.
343. Felig P, Cunningham J, Levitt M, Hendler R, Nadel E: Energy expenditure in obesity in fasting and postprandial state. *Am J Physiol* 244:E45, 1983.
344. D'Alessio DA, Kavle EC, Mozzoli MA, Smalley KJ, Polansky M, Kendrick ZV, Owen LR, Bushman MC, et al: Thermic effect of food in lean and obese men. *J Clin Invest* 81:1781, 1988.
345. Bronstein MN, Mak RP, King JC: The thermic effect of food in normal-weight and overweight pregnant women. *Br J Nutr* 74:261, 1995.
346. Tataranni PA, Larson DE, Snitker S, Ravussin E: Thermic effect of food in humans: Methods and results from use of a respiratory chamber. *Am J Clin Nutr* 61:1013, 1995.
347. Ravussin E, Acheson KJ, Vernet O, Danforth E, Jequier E: Evidence that insulin resistance is responsible for the decreased thermic effect of glucose in human obesity. *J Clin Invest* 76:1268, 1985.
348. Nair KS, Webster J, Garrow JS: Effect of impaired glucose tolerance and type II diabetes on resting metabolic rate and thermic response to glucose meal in obese women. *Metabolism* 35:640, 1986.
349. de Jonge L, Bray GA: The thermic effect of food and obesity: A critical review. *Obes Res* 5:622, 1997.
350. Schutz Y, Golay A, Felber JP, Jequier E: Decreased glucose-induced thermogenesis after weight loss in obese subjects: A predisposing factor for relapse of obesity? *Am J Clin Nutr* 39:380, 1984.
351. Tappy L: Thermic effect of food and sympathetic nervous system activity in humans. *Reprod Nutr Dev* 36:391, 1996.
352. Chirico AM, Stunkard AJ: Physical activity and human obesity. *N Engl J Med* 263:935, 1960.
353. Hutson EM, Cohen NL, Kunkel ND, Steinkamp RC, Rourke MH, Walsh HE: Measures of body fat and related factors in normal adults. *J Am Diet Assoc* 47:179, 1965.
354. Bloom WL, Eidex MF: Inactivity as a major factor in adult obesity. *Metabolism* 16:679, 1967.
355. Stefanik PA, Heald FP, Mayer J: Caloric intake in relation to energy output of obese and non-obese adolescent boys. *Am J Clin Nutr* 7:55, 1959.
356. Bullen BA, Reed RB, Mayer J: Physical activity of obese and nonobese adolescent girls appraised by motion picture sampling. *Am J Clin Nutr* 14:211, 1964.
357. Amatruda JM, Statt MC, Welle SL: Total and resting energy expenditure in obese women reduced to ideal body weight. *J Clin Invest* 92:1236, 1993.
358. Weinsier RL, Nelson KM, Hensrud DD, Darnell BE, Hunter GR, Schutz Y: Metabolic predictors of obesity. Contribution of resting energy expenditure, thermic effect of food, and fuel utilization to four-year weight gain of post-obese and never-obese women. *J Clin Invest* 95:980, 1995.
359. Schoeller DA, Levitsky LL, Bandini LG, Dietz WW, Walczak A: Energy expenditure and body composition in Prader-Willi syndrome. *Metabolism* 37:115, 1988.
360. Sims EAH: Experimental obesity, dietary-induced thermogenesis, and their clinical implications. *J Clin Endocrinol Metab* 5:377, 1976.
361. Bouchard C, Tremblay A, Despres JP, Nadeau A, Lupien PS, Theriault G, Dussault J, Moorjan S, et al: The response to long-term overfeeding in identical twins. *N Engl J Med* 322:1477, 1990.
362. Welle S, Campbell RG: Stimulation of thermogenesis by carbohydrate overfeeding. *J Clin Invest* 71:916, 1983.
363. Norgan NG, Durnin VGA: The effect of 6 weeks of overfeeding on the body weight, body composition, and energy metabolism of young men. *Am J Clin Nutr* 33:978, 1980.
364. Ravussin E, Schutz Y, Acheson KJ, Dusmt M, Bourquin L, Jequier E: Short-term, mixed-diet overfeeding in man: No evidence for "luxuskonsumption." *Am J Physiol* 249:E470, 1985.
365. Powley RL, Keesey RE: Relationship of body weight to the lateral hypothalamic feeding syndrome. *J Comp Physiol Psychol* 70:25, 1970.
366. Hoebel BG, Teitelbaum P: Weight regulation in normal and hypothalamic hyperphagic rats. *J Comp Physiol Psychol* 61:189, 1966.
367. Frederich RC, Hamann A, Anderson S, Lollmann B, Lowell BB, Flier JS: Leptin levels reflect body lipid-content in mice—evidence for diet-induced resistance to leptin action. *Nat Med* 1:1311, 1995.
368. Kielar D, Clark JS, Ciechanowicz A, Kurzawski G, Sulikowski T, Naruszewicz M: Leptin receptor isoforms expressed in human adipose tissue. *Metabolism* 47:844, 1998.
369. Elmquist JK, Bjorbaek C, Ahima RS, Flier JS, Saper CB: Distributions of leptin receptor mRNA isoforms in the rat brain. *J Comp Neurol* 395:535, 1998.
370. Couillard C, Mauriege P, Prud'homme D, Nadeau A, Tremblay, Bouchard C, Despres JP: Plasma leptin concentrations: Gender differences and associations with metabolic risk factors for cardiovascular disease. *Diabetologia* 40:1178, 1997.
371. Lonnqvist F, Wennlund A, Arner P: Relationship between circulating leptin and peripheral fat distribution in obese subjects. *Int J Obes Relat Metab Disord* 21:255, 1997.
372. Kennedy A, Gettys TW, Watson P, Wallace P, Ganaway E, Pan Q, Garvey WT: The metabolic significance of leptin in humans: Gender-based differences in relationship to adiposity, insulin sensitivity, and energy expenditure. *J Clin Endocrinol Metab* 82:1293, 1997.
373. Halaas JL, Gajiwala KS, Maffei M, Cohen SL, Chait BT, Rabinowitz D, Lallone RL, Burley SK, Friedman JM: Weight-reducing effects of the plasma protein encoded by the obese gene. *Science* 269:543, 1995.
374. Campfield LA, Smith FJ, Guisez Y, Devos R, Burn P: Recombinant mouse OB protein: evidence for a peripheral signal linking adiposity and central neural networks. *Science* 269:546, 1995.
375. Girard J: Is leptin the link between obesity and insulin resistance? *Diabetes Metab* 23:16, 1997.
376. Banks WA, Kastin AJ, Huang W, Jaspan JB, Maness LM: Leptin enters the brain by a saturable system independent of insulin. *Peptides* 17:305, 1996.
377. Boado RJ, Golden PL, Levin N, Pardridge WM: Up-regulation of blood-brain barrier short-form leptin receptor gene products in rats fed a high fat diet. *J Neurochem* 71:1761, 1998.
378. Stephens TW, Basinski M, Bristow PK, Bue-Valleskey JM, Burgett SG, Craft L, Hale J, Hoffmann J, Hsiung HM, Kriauciunas A, Mackellar W, Rosteck PR, Schoner B, Smith D, Tinsley FC, Shang XY, Heiman M: The role of neuropeptide Y in the antiobesity action of the obese gene product. *Nature* 377:530, 1995.
379. Levine AS, Morley J: Neuropeptide Y: A potent inducer of consummatory behavior in rats. *Peptides* 5:1025, 1984.
380. Mizuno TM, Kleopoulos SP, Bergen HT, Roberts JL, Priest CA, Mobbs CV: Hypothalamic pro-opiomelanocortin mRNA is reduced by fasting and in ob/ob and db/db mice, but is stimulated by leptin. *Diabetes* 47:294, 1998.
381. Kask A, Rago L, Wikberg JE, Schioth HB: Evidence for involvement of the melanocortin MC4 receptor in the effects of leptin on food intake and body weight. *Eur J Pharmacol* 360:15, 1998.
382. Scarpace PJ, Nicolson M, Matheny M: UCP2, UCP3 and leptin gene expression: Modulation by food restriction and leptin. *J Endocrinol* 159:349, 1998.
383. Mantzoros CS, Frederich RC, Qu D, Lowell BB, Maratos-Flier E, Flier JS: Severe leptin resistance in brown fat-deficient uncoupling protein promoter-driven diphtheria toxin A mice despite suppression of hypothalamic neuropeptide Y and circulating corticosterone concentrations. *Diabetes* 47:2308, 1998.
384. Schwartz MW, Peskind E, Raskind M, Boyko EJ, Porte D Jr: Cerebrospinal fluid leptin levels: Relationship to plasma levels and to adiposity in humans. *Nat Med* 2:589, 1996.
385. Caro JF, Kolaczynski JW, Nyce MR, Ohannesian JP, Opentanova I, Goldman WH, Lynn RB, Zhang PL, Sinha MK, Considine RV: Decreased cerebrospinal-fluid/serum leptin ratio in obesity: A possible mechanism for leptin resistance. *Lancet* 348:159, 1996.
386. Ramsey JJ, Kemnitz JW, Colman RJ, Cunningham D, Swick AG: Different central and peripheral responses to leptin in rhesus monkeys: Brain transport may be limited. *J Clin Endocrinol Metab* 83:3230, 1998.
387. Sclafani A, Springer D: Dietary obesity in adult rats: Similarities to hypothalamic and human obesity syndromes. *Physiol Behav* 17:461, 1976.

388. Sclafani A, Springer D, Kluge V: Effects of quinine adulterated diets on the food intake and body weight of obese and non-obese hypothalamic hyperphagic rats. *Physiol Behav* 16:631, 1976.
389. Campbell RG, Hashim SA, VanItallie TB: Studies of food-intake regulation in man. *N Engl J Med* 285:1402, 1971.
390. Porikos KP, Booth G, VanItallie TB: Effect of covert nutritive dilution on the spontaneous food intake of obese individuals: A pilot study. *Am J Clin Nutr* 30:1638, 1977.
391. Glueck CJ, Hastings MM, Allen C, Hogg E, Baehler L, Gartside PS, Phillips D, Jones M, et al: Sucrose polyester and covert caloric dilution. *Am J Clin Nutr* 35:1352, 1982.
392. Pi-Sunyer FX: Exercise effects on calorie intake. *Ann NY Acad Sci* 499:94, 1987.
393. Roberts SB, Young VR, Fuss P, Fiatarone MA, Richard B, Rasmussen H, Wagner D, Joseph L: Energy expenditure and subsequent nutrient intakes in overfed young men. *Am J Physiol* 259:R461, 1990.
394. Delvenne V, Goldman S, De Maertelaer V, Simon Y, Luxen A, Lotstra F: Brain hypometabolism of glucose in anorexia nervosa: Normalization after weight gain. *Biol Psychiatry* 40:761, 1996.
395. Delvenne V, Goldman S, De Maertelaer V, Wikler D, Damhaut P, Lotstra F: Brain glucose metabolism in anorexia nervosa and affective disorders: Influence of weight loss or depressive symptomatology. *Psychiatry Res* 74:83, 1997.
396. Delvenne V, Goldman S, De Maertelaer V, Lotstra F: Brain glucose metabolism in eating disorders assessed by positron emission tomography. *Int J Eat Disord* 25:29, 1999.
397. Mayer J: Regulation of energy intake and body weight: The glucostatic theory and the lipostatic hypothesis. *Ann NY Acad Sci* 63:15, 1955.
398. Novin D, VanderWeele DA: Visceral involvement in feeding: There is more to regulation than the hypothalamus, in Sprague JM, Epstein AN (eds): *Progress in Psychobiology and Physiological Psychology*. New York, Academic, 1977, p 193.
399. Morien A, McMahon L, Wellman PJ: Effects on food and water intake of the alpha 1-adrenoceptor agonists amidephrine and SK&F-89748. *Life Sci* 53:169, 1996.
400. Leibowitz SF: Reciprocal hunger-regulating circuits involving alpha- and beta-adrenergic receptors located, respectively, in the ventromedial and lateral hypothalamus. *Proc Natl Acad Sci USA* 67:1063, 1970.
401. Kennett GA: 5-HT drugs and eating disorders. *Drugs* 1:456, 1998.
402. Tecott LH, Sun LM, Akana SF, Strack AM, Lowenstein DH, Dallman MF, Julius D: Eating disorder and epilepsy in mice lacking 5-HT2c serotonin receptors. *Nature* 374:542, 1995.
403. Fernstrom JD: Effects of tryptophan and the diet on brain serotonin formation and brain function, in Beers RF, Bassett EG (eds): *Nutritional Factors: Modulating Effects on Metabolic Processes*. New York, Raven, 1981, p 217.
404. Gibson CJ: Nutritional control of catecholamine synthesis, in Beers RF, Bassett EG (eds): *Nutritional Factors: Modulating Effects on Metabolic Processes*. New York, Raven, 1981, p 217.
405. Caballero B, Finer N, Wurtman RJ: Plasma amino acids and insulin levels in obesity: Response to carbohydrate intake and tryptophan supplements. *Metabolism* 37:672, 1988.
406. Wurtman R, Wurtman J: Serotoninergic mechanisms and obesity. *J Nutr Biochem* 9:511, 1998.
407. Wurtman JJ: The involvement of brain serotonin in excessive carbohydrate snacking by obese carbohydrate cravers. *J Am Diet Assoc* 84:1004, 1984.
408. Geliebter AA: Effects of equicaloric loads of protein, fat, and carbohydrate on food intake in the rat and man. *Physiol Behav* 22:267, 1979.
409. Rolls BJ, Kim S, McNelis AL, Fischman MW, Foltin RW, Moran TH: Time course of effects of preloads high in fat or carbohydrate on food intake and hunger ratings in humans. *Am J Physiol* 260:R756, 1991.
410. Miller WC, Lindeman AK, Wallace J, Niederpruem M: Diet composition, energy intake, and exercise in relation to body fat in men and women. *Am J Clin Nutr* 52:426, 1990.
411. Dreon DM, Frey-Hewitt B, Ellsworth N, Williams PT, Terry RB, Wood PD: Dietary fat: Carbohydrate ratio and obesity in middle-aged men. *Am J Clin Nutr* 47:995, 1988.
412. Hill JO, Peters JC, Reed GW, Schlundt DG, Sharp T, Greene HL: Nutrient balance in humans: Effects of diet composition. *Am J Clin Nutr* 54:10, 1991.
413. Schwartz RS, Ravussin E, Massari M, O'Connell M, Robbins DC: The thermic effect of carbohydrate versus fat feeding in man. *Metabolism* 34:285, 1985.
414. Smolin LA, Grosvenor MB, Handelsman DJ, Brasel JA: Diet composition and lipoprotein lipase (EC 3.1.1.34) activity in human obesity. *Br J Nutr* 58:13, 1987.
415. Schwartz RS, Brunzell JD: Increased adipose-tissue lipoprotein-lipase activity in moderately obese men after weight reduction. *Lancet* 1:1230, 1978.
416. Schwartz RS, Brunzell JD: Increase of adipose tissue lipoprotein lipase activity with weight loss. *J Clin Invest* 67:1425, 1981.
417. Reitman JS, Kosmakos FC, Howard BV, Taskinen MR, Kuusi T, Nikkila EA: Characterization of lipase activities in obese Pima Indians. *J Clin Invest* 70:791, 1982.
418. Ong JM, Kern PA: Effect of feeding and obesity on lipoprotein lipase activity, immunoreactive protein, and messenger RNA levels in human adipose tissue. *J Clin Invest* 84:305, 1989.
419. Berman DM, Rogus EM, Busby-Whitehead MJ, Katzel LI, Goldberg AP: Predictors of adipose tissue lipoprotein lipase in middle-aged and older men: Relationship to leptin and obesity, but not cardiovascular fitness. *Metabolism* 48:183, 1999.
420. Eckel RH, Yost TJ: Weight reduction increases adipose tissue lipoprotein lipase responsiveness in obese women. *J Clin Invest* 80:992, 1987.
421. Kern PA, Ong JM, Saffari B, Carty J: The effects of weight loss on the activity and expression of adipose tissue lipoprotein lipase in very obese humans. *N Engl J Med* 322:1053, 1990.
422. Taskinen MR, Nikkila EA: Basal and postprandial lipoprotein lipase activity in adipose tissue during caloric restriction and refeeding. *Metabolism* 36:625, 1987.
423. Rebuffe-Scrive M, Basdevant A, Guy-Grand B: Nutritional induction of adipose tissue lipoprotein lipase in obese subjects. *Am J Clin Nutr* 37:974, 1983.
424. Woods SC, Lotter EC, McKay LD, Porte D Jr: Chronic intracerebroventricular infusion of insulin reduces food intake and body weight of baboons. *Nature* 282:503, 1979.
425. Ciaraldi T, Robbins R, Leidy JW, Thamm P, Berhanu P: Insulin receptors on cultured hypothalamic cells: Functional and structural differences from receptors on peripheral target cells. *Endocrinology* 116:2179, 1985.
426. Kolaczynski JW, Nyce MR, Considine RV, Boden G, Nolan JJ, Henry R, Mudaliar SR, Olefsky J, Caro JF: Acute and chronic effects of insulin on leptin production in humans: Studies in vivo and in vitro. *Diabetes* 45:699, 1996.
427. Rodin J, Wack J, Ferrannini E, DeFronzo RA: Effect of insulin and glucose on feeding behavior. *Metabolism* 34:826, 1985.
428. McLaughlin T, Abbasi F, Carantoni M, Schaaf P, Reaven G: Differences in insulin resistance do not predict weight loss in response to hypocaloric diets in healthy obese women. *J Clin Endocrinol Metab* 84:578, 1999.
429. Alger SA, Schwalberg MD, Bigaouette JM, Michalek AV, Howard LJ: Effect of a tricyclic antidepressant and opiate antagonist on binge-eating behavior in normoweight bulimic and obese, binge-eating subjects. *Am J Clin Nutr* 53:865, 1991.
430. Atkinson RL: Opioid regulation of food intake and body weight in humans. *Fed Proc* 46:178, 1987.
431. Fantino M, Hosotte J, Apfelbaum M: An opioid antagonist, naltrexone, reduces preference for sucrose in humans. *Am J Physiol* 251:R91, 1986.
432. Ritter MM, Sönnichsen AC, Mohrle W, Richter WO, Schwandt P: β-endorphin plasma levels and their dependence on gender during an enteral glucose load in lean subjects as well as in obese patients before and after weight reduction. *Int J Obes* 15:421, 1991.
433. Cozzolino D, Sessa G, Salvatore T, Sasso FC, Giugliano D, Lefebvre PJ, Torella R: The involvement of the opioid system in human obesity: A study in normal weight relatives of obese people. *J Clin Endocrinol Metab* 81:713, 1996.
434. Mollereau C, Parmentier M, Mailleux P, Butour JL, Moisand, Chalon P, Caput D, Vassart G, Meunier JC: ORL1, a novel member of the opioid receptor family. Cloning, functional expression and localization. *FEBS Lett* 341:33, 1994.
435. Reinscheid RK, Nothacker HP, Bourson A, Ardati A, Henningsen RA, Bunzow JR, Grandy DK, Langen H, Monsma FJ Jr, Civelli O: Orphanin FQ: A neuropeptide that activates an opioidlike G protein-coupled receptor. *Science* 270:792, 1995.

436. Pomonis JD, Billington CJ, Levine AS: Orphanin FQ, agonist of orphan opioid receptor ORL1, stimulates feeding in rats. *Neuroreport* 8:369, 1996.
437. Kalra SP, Dube MG, Pu S, Xu B, Horvath TL, Kalra PS: Interacting appetite-regulating pathways in the hypothalamic regulation of body weight. *Endocr Rev* 20:68, 1999.
438. Rodin J, Schank D, Striegel-Moore R: Psychological features of obesity. *Med Clin North Am* 73:47, 1989.
439. Drewnowiski A, Brunzell JD, Sande K, Iverisu PH, Greenwood MRC: Sweet tooth reconsidered: Taste responsiveness in human obesity. *Physiol Behav* 35:617, 1985.
440. Schachter S: Obesity and eating. *Science* 161:751, 1968.
441. Leon GR, Roth L: Obesity: Psychological causes, correlations, and speculations. *Psychol Bull* 84:117, 1977.
442. Loro A, Orleans C: Binge eating in obesity: Preliminary findings and guidelines for behavioral analysis and treatment. *Addict Behav* 6:155, 1981.
443. Werner SC: Hypothyroidism: Introduction, in Werner SC, Ingbar SH (eds): *The Thyroid*, 3rd ed. New York, Harper & Row, 1971, p 715.
444. Burman KD, Latham KR, Djuh YY, Smallridge RC, Tseng YCL, Lukes YG, Maunder R, Wartofsky L: Solubilized nuclear thyroid hormone receptors in circulating human mononuclear cells. *J Clin Endocrinol Metab* 51:106, 1980.
445. Pinkney J, Goodrick S: Leptin and the pituitary-thyroid axis: A comparative study in lean, obese, hypothyroid and hyperthyroid subjects. *Clin Endocrinol* 49:583, 1998.
446. Bray GA: Obesity—a disease of nutrient or energy balance? *Nutr Rev* 45:33, 1987.
447. Rivera MP, Svec F: Is cortisol involved in upper-body obesity? *Med Hypotheses* 30:95, 1989.
448. Andrew R, Phillips DI, Walker B: Obesity and gender influence cortisol secretion and metabolism in man. *J Clin Endocrinol Metab* 83:1806, 1998.
449. Clearly MP: Antiobesity effect of dehydroepiandrosterone in the Zucker rat, in Lardy H, Stratman F (eds): *Hormones, Thermogenesis, and Obesity*. New York, Elsevier, 1989, p 365.
450. MacEwen EG, Kurzman ID, Haffa ALM: Antiobesity and hypocholesterolemic activity of dehydroepiandrosterone (DHEA) in the dog, in Lardy H, Stratman F (eds): *Hormones, Thermogenesis, and Obesity*. New York, Elsevier, 1989, p 399.
451. Lopez SA, Krehl WA: A possible interrelation between glucose-6-phosphate dehydrogenase and dehydroepiandrosterone in obesity. *Lancet* 2:485, 1967.
452. Barrett-Connor E, Khaw KT, Yen SSC: A prospective study of dehydroepiandrosterone sulfate, mortality, and cardiovascular disease. *N Engl J Med* 315:1519, 1986.
453. Kurtz BR, Givens JR, Komindr S, Stevens MD, Karas JG, Bittle JB, Judge D, Kitabchi AE: Maintenance of normal circulating levels of Δ4-androstenedione and dehydroepiandrosterone in simple obesity despite increased metabolic clearance rates: Evidence for a servo-control mechanism. *J Clin Endocrinol Metab* 64:1261, 1987.
454. Usiskin KS, Butterworth S, Clore JN, Arad Y, Ginsberg HN, Blackard WG, Nestler JE: Lack of effect of dehydroepiandrosterone in obese men. *Int J Obes* 14:457, 1990.
455. Knehans AW, Romsos DE: Reduced norepinephrine turnover in brown adipose tissue of ob/ob mice. *Am J Physiol* 242:E253, 1982.
456. Young JB, Landsberg L: Diminished sympathetic nervous system activity in genetically obese (ob/ob) mouse. *Am J Physiol* 245:E148, 1983.
457. Peterson HR, Rothschild M, Weinberg CR, Fell RD, McLeish KR, Pfeifer MA: Body fat and the activity of the autonomic nervous system. *N Engl J Med* 318:1077, 1988.
458. Jung RT, Shetty PS, James WPT, Barrand MA, Callingham BA: Plasma catecholamines and autonomic responsiveness in obesity. *Int J Obes* 6:131, 1982.
459. Welle SL, Campbell RG: Normal thermic effect of glucose in obese women. *Am J Clin Nutr* 37:87, 1983.
460. Bray GA, Gallagher TF Jr: Manifestations of hypothalamic obesity in man: A comprehensive investigation of eight patients and a review of the literature. *Medicine (Baltimore)* 54:301, 1975.
461. Bray GA: Syndromes of hypothalamic obesity in man. *Pediatr Ann* 13:525, 1984.
462. Green JS, Parfrey PS, Harnett JD, Farid NR, Cramer BC, Johnson G, Heath O, McManamon PJ, et al: The cardinal manifestations of Bardet-Biedl syndrome, a form of Laurence-Moon-Biedl syndrome. *N Engl J Med* 321:1002, 1989.
463. Goecke T, Majewski F, Kauther KD, Sterzel U: Mental retardation, hypotonia, obesity, ocular, facial, dental, and limb abnormalities (Cohen Syndrome). *Eur J Pediatr* 138:338, 1982.
464. Dietz WH, Gross WL, Kirkpatrick JA: Blount disease (tibia vara): Another skeletal disorder associated with childhood obesity. *J Pediatr* 101:735, 1982.
465. Cassidy SB, Ledbetter DH: Prader-Willi Syndrome. *Neurol Clin* 7:37, 1989.
466. Aughton DJ, Cassidy SB: Physical features of Prader-Willi syndrome in neonates. *Am J Dis Child* 144:1251, 1990.
467. Butler MG, Moore J, Morawiecki A, Nicolson M: Comparison of leptin protein levels in Prader-Willi syndrome and control individuals. *Am J Med Genet* 75:7, 1998.
468. Ledbetter DH, Greenberg F, Holm VA, Cassidy SB: Conference report: Second annual Prader-Willi syndrome scientific conference. *Am J Med Genet* 28:779, 1987.
469. Nicholls RD, Knoll JHM, Butler MG, Karam S, Lalande M: Genetic imprinting suggested by maternal heterodisomy in non-deletion Prader-Willi syndrome. *Nature* 342:281, 1989.
470. Kuslich CD, Kobori JA, Mohapatra G, Gregorio-King C, Donlon TA: Prader-Willi syndrome is caused by disruption of the SNRPN gene. *Am J Hum Genet* 64:70, 1999.
471. Farber C, Dittrich B, Buiting K, Horsthemke B: The chromosome 15 imprinting centre (IC) region has undergone multiple duplication events and contains an upstream exon of SNRPN that is deleted in all Angelman syndrome patients with an IC microdeletion. *Hum Molec Genet* 8:337, 1999.
472. Dech B, Budow L: The use of fluoxetine in an adolescent with Prader-Willi syndrome. *J Am Acad Child Adolesc Psychiatry* 30:298, 1991.
473. Selikowitz M, Sunman J, Pendergast A, Wright S: Fenfluramine in Prader-Willi syndrome: A double blind, placebo controlled trial. *Arch Dis Child* 65:112, 1990.
474. Stunkard A, McLaren-Hume H: The results of treatment for obesity: A review of the literature and report of a series. *Arch Intern Med* 103:79, 1959.
475. AMA Council on Scientific Affairs: Treatment of obesity in adults. *Conn Med* 53:21, 1989.
476. Gortmaker SL, Dietz WH, Sobol AM, Wehler CA: Increasing pediatric obesity in the United States. *Am J Dis Child* 141:535, 1987.
477. Williamson DF, Kahn HS, Remington PL, Anda RF: The 10-year incidence of overweight and major weight gain in U.S. adults. *Arch Intern Med* 150:665, 1990.
478. National Institutes of Health Consensus Development Conference Statement: Health implications of obesity. *Ann Intern Med* 103:1073, 1985.
479. Health and Public Policy Committee, American College of Physicians: Eating disorders: Anorexia nervosa and bulimia. *Ann Intern Med* 105:790, 1986.
480. Shapiro LR, Crawford PB, Clark MJ, Pearson DL, Raz J, Huenemann RL: Obesity prognosis: A longitudinal study of children from the age of 6 months to 9 years. *Am J Public Health* 74:968, 1984.
481. Sorensen TIA, Sonne-Holm S: Risk in childhood of development of severe adult obesity: Retrospective population-based care-cohort study. *Am J Epidemiol* 127:104, 1988.
482. Stark O, Atkins E, Wolff OH, Douglas JWB: Longitudinal study of obesity in the National Survey of Health and Development. *Br Med J* 283:13, 1981.
483. Garn SM, Clark DC: Trends in fatness and the origins of obesity. *Pediatrics* 57:433, 1976.
484. Stunkard AJ, Foch TT, Hrubel Z: A twin study of human obesity. *JAMA* 256:51, 1986.
485. Epstein LH, Wing RR: Behavioral treatment of childhood obesity. *Psychol Bull* 101:331, 1987.
486. Epstein LH, Cluss PA: Behavioral genetics of childhood obesity. *Behav Ther* 17:324, 1986.
487. Epstein LH, Valoski A, Wing RR, McCurley J: Ten-year follow-up of behavioral, family-based treatment for obese children. *JAMA* 264:2519, 1990.
488. Stunkard AJ, Berkowitz RI: Treatment of obesity in children. *JAMA* 264:2550, 1990.
489. Position of the American Dietetic Association: Optimal weight as a health promotion strategy: ADA Reports. *J Am Diet Assoc* 89:1814, 1989.

490. Stunkard AJ: Some perspectives on human obesity: Treatment. *Bull NY Acad Med* 64:924, 1988.
491. James WP: A public health approach to the problem of obesity. *Int J Obes Relat Metab Disord* 19:S37, 1995.
492. Black DR, Threfall WE: Partner weight status and subject weight loss: Implications for cost-effective programs and public health. *Addict Behav* 14:279, 1989.
493. Brownell KD, Stunkard AJ: Couples training pharmacotherapy and behavior in the treatment of obesity. *Arch Gen Psychiatry* 38:1224, 1981.
494. Volkmar FR, Stunkard AJ, Woolston J, Bailey RA: High attrition rates in commercial weight reduction programs. *Arch Intern Med* 141:426, 1981.
495. Brownell KD: Public health approaches to obesity and its management. *Annu Rev Public Health* 7:521, 1986.
496. Winkleby MA, Feldman HA, Murray DM: Joint analysis of three U.S. community intervention trials for reduction of cardiovascular disease risk. *J Clin Epidemiol* 50:645, 1997.
497. Carleton RA, Lasater TM, Assaf AR, Feldman HA, McKinlay S: The Pawtucket heart health program: Community changes in cardiovascular risk factors and projected disease risk. *Am J Public Health* 85:777, 1995.
498. Epstein LH, Wing RR: Aerobic exercise and weight. *Addict Behav* 5:371, 1980.
499. Harris SS, Caspersen CJ, DeFriese GH, Estes FH: Physical activity counseling for healthy adults as a primary preventive intervention in the clinical setting: Report for the US Preventive Services Task Force. *JAMA* 262:2094, 1989.
500. Wanger HA, Bell GJ: The interactions of intensity, frequency and duration of exercise training in altering cardiovascular fitness. *Sports Med* 3:346, 1986.
501. Sallis JF, Haskell WL, Fortmann SP, Vraiult KM, Taylor CB, Solomon DS: Predictors of adaption and maintenance of physical activity in a community sample. *Prev Med* 15:331, 1986.
502. King AC, Haskell WL, Young DR, Oka RK, Stefanick ML: Long-term effects of varying intensities and formats of physical activity on participation rates, fitness, and lipoproteins in men and women. *Circulation* 91:2596, 1995.
503. Garrow JS, Summerbell CD: Meta-analysis: Effect of exercise with or without dieting, on the body composition of overweight subjects. *Eur J Clin Nutr* 49:1, 1995.
504. Woo R, Garrow JS, Pi-Sunyer FX: Effect of exercise on spontaneous calorie intake in obesity. *Am J Clin Nutr* 36:470, 1982.
505. Woo R, Pi-Sunyer FX: Effect of increased physical activity on voluntary intake in lean women. *Metabolism* 34:836, 1985.
506. Ballor DL, Katch VL, Becque MD, Marks CR: Resistance weight training during caloric restriction enhances lean body weight maintenance. *Am J Clin Nutr* 47:19, 1988.
507. Pavlou KN, Krey S, Steffee WP: Exercise as an adjunct to weight loss and maintenance in moderately obese subjects. *Am J Clin Nutr* 49:1115, 1989.
508. Pronk NP, Wing RR: Physical activity and long-term maintenance of weight loss. *Obes Res* 2:587, 1994.
509. Henson LC, Poole DC, Donahoe CP, Heber D: Effects of exercise training on resting energy expenditure during caloric restriction. *Am J Clin Nutr* 46:893, 1987.
510. Freedman-Akabas S, Colt E, Kissileff HR, Pi-Sunyer FX: Lack of sustained increase in VO_2 following exercise in fit and unfit subjects. *Am J Clin Nutr* 41:545, 1985.
511. Bielinski R, Schutz Y, Jequier E: Energy metabolism during the post-exercise recovery in man. *Am J Clin Nutr* 42:69, 1985.
512. Segal KR, Presta E, Gutin B: Thermic effect of food during graded exercise in normal weight and obese men. *Am J Clin Nutr* 40:995, 1984.
513. Dallosso HM, James WPT: Whole-body calorimetry studies in adult men. *Br J Nutr* 52:65, 1984.
514. Brehm BA, Gutlin B: Recovery energy expenditure for steady state exercise in runners and nonexercisers. *Med Sci Sports Exerc* 18:205, 1986.
515. Segal KR, Pi-Sunyer FX: Exercise and obesity. *Med Clin North Am* 73:217, 1989.
516. Welle S: Metabolic responses to a meal during rest and low-intensity exercise. *Am J Clin Nutr* 40:990, 1984.
517. Romieu I, Willett WC, Stampfer MJ, Colditz GA, Sampson L, Rosner B, Hennekens CH, Speizer FE: Energy intake and other determinants of relative weight. *Am J Clin Nutr* 47:406, 1988.
518. Lichtman SW, Pisarka MS, Berman ER, Pestone M, Dowling H, Offenbacher E, Weisel H, Heshka S, Matthews DE, Heymsfield SB: Discrepancy between self-reported and actual caloric intake and exercise in obese individuals. *N Engl J Med* 327:1893, 1992.
519. Bruce B, Wilfley D: Binge eating among the overweight population: A serious and prevalent problem. *J Am Diet Asoc* 96:58, 1996.
520. Klem ML, Wing RR, McGuire MT, Seagle HM, Hill JO: A descriptive study of individuals successful at long-term maintenance of substantial weight loss. *Am J Clin Nutr* 66:239, 1997.
521. Amatruda JM: Very low energy diets for the treatment of simple and complicated obesity. *Endocrinologist* 1:171, 1991.
522. National Task Force on the Prevention and Treatment of Obesity: Very low-calorie diets. *JAMA* 270:967, 1993.
523. Apfelbaum M: The effects of very restrictive high protein diets. *J Clin Endocrinol Metab* 5:417, 1976.
524. Bistrian BR, Blackburn GL, Flatt JP, Sizer J, Scrimshaw NS, Sherman M: Nitrogen metabolism and insulin requirements in obese diabetic adults on a protein-sparing modified fast. *Diabetes* 25:494, 1976.
525. Linn R, Stuart SL: *The Last Chance Diet*. Secaucus, NJ, Lyle Stuart, 1976.
526. Isner JM, Sours HH, Paris AL, Ferraus VJ: Sudden unexpected death in avid dieters using the liquid-protein-modified-fast diet: Observations in 17 patients and the role of the prolonged QT interval. *Circulation* 60:1401, 1979.
527. Lantigua RA, Amatruda JM, Biddle TL, Forbes GB, Lockwood DH: Cardiac arrhythmias associated with a liquid protein diet for the treatment of obesity. *N Engl J Med* 303:735, 1980.
528. Amatruda JM, Biddle TL, Patton ML, Lockwood DH: Vigorous supplementation of a hypocaloric diet prevents cardiac arrhythmias and mineral depletion. *Am J Med* 74:1016, 1983.
529. Amatruda JM, Brodows RG, Lockwood DH: Very low calorie diets: Efficacy, cardiac arrhythmias, nitrogen sparing mineral depletion, and hormone and substrate levels. *J Obes Weight Regul* 3:3, 1984.
530. Henry RR, Schaeffer L, Olefsky JM: Glycemic effects of intensive caloric restriction and isocaloric feeding in noninsulin-dependent diabetes mellitus. *J Clin Endocrinol Metab* 61:917, 1985.
531. Wadden TA: Treatment of obesity by moderate and severe caloric restriction. *Ann Intern Med* 119:688, 1993.
532. Ryttig KR, Flaten H, Rossner S: Long-term effects of a very low calorie diet (Nutrilett) in obesity treatment. A prospective, randomized, comparison between VLCD and a hypocaloric diet + behavior modification and their combination. *Int J Obes* 21:574, 1997.
533. Wadden TA, Foster GD, Letizia, KA: One-year behavioral treatment of obesity: Comparison of moderate and severe caloric restriction and the effects of weight maintenance therapy. *J Consult Clin Psychol* 62:165, 1994.
534. Wadden TA, Frey DL: A multicenter evaluation of a proprietary weight loss program for the treatment of marked obesity: A five-year follow-up. *Int J Eat Disord* 22:203, 1997.
535. Wadden TA, Stunkard AJ: Controlled trial of very low calorie diet, behavioral therapy, and their combination in the treatment of obesity. *J Consult Clin Psychol* 54:482, 1986.
536. Nagulesparan M, Savage PJ, Bennion LJ, Unger RH, Bennett PH: Diminished effect of caloric restriction on control of hyperglycemia with increasing known duration of type II diabetes mellitus. *J Clin Endocrinol Metab* 53:560, 1981.
537. Lockwood DH, Amatruda JM: Very low calorie diets in the management of obesity. *Annu Rev Med* 35:373, 1984.
538. Liddle RA, Goldstein RB, Saxton J: Gallstone formation during weight-reduction dieting. *Arch Intern Med* 149:1750, 1989.
539. Broomfield PH, Chopra R, Sheinbaum RC, Bonorris GG, Silverman A, Schoenfield LJ, Marks JW: Effects of ursodeoxycholic acid and aspirin on the formation of lithogenic bile and gallstones during loss of weight. *N Engl J Med* 319:1567, 1988.
540. Mok HY, Von Bergmann K, Crouse JR, Grundy SM: Biliary lipid metabolism in obesity: Effects of bile acid feeding before and during weight reduction. *Gastroenterology* 76:556, 1978.
541. Roslyn JJ, Pitt HA, Mann LL, Ament ME, DenBesten L: Gallbladder disease in patients on long term parenteral nutrition. *Gastroenterology* 84:148, 1983.
542. Wattchow DA, Hall JC, Whiting MJ, Bradley B, Iannos J, Watts JM: Prevalence and treatment of gallstones after gastric bypass surgery for morbid obesity. *Br Med J* 286:763, 1983.

543. Hocking MP, Duerson MC, O'Leary P, Woodward ER: Jejunoileal bypass for morbid obesity: Late follow-up in 100 cases. *N Engl J Med* 308:995, 1983.
544. Shiffman ML, Sugarman HJ, Kellum JH, Brewer WH, Moore EW: Gallstones in patients with morbid obesity. Relationship to body weight, weight loss, and gallbladder bile cholesterol solubility. *Int J Obesity* 17:153, 1993.
545. Carey MC, Cahalane J: Whither biliary sludge? *Gastroenterology* 95:508, 1988.
546. Gallinger S, Tayler RD, Harvey PR, Petrunka CN, Strasberg SM: Effect of mucous glycoprotein on nucleation time of human bile. *Gastroenterology* 89:648, 1985.
547. Lee SP, LaMont JT, Carey MC: Role of gall bladder mucus hypersecretion in the evolution of cholesterol gallstones: Studies in the prairie dog. *J Clin Invest* 67:1712, 1981.
548. Lee SP, Carey MC, LaMont JT: Aspirin prevention of cholesterol gallstone formation in prairie dogs. *Science* 211:1429, 1981.
549. Klawansky S, Chalmers TC: Fat content of very low-calorie diets and gallstone formation. *JAMA* 268:873, 1992.
550. Weisner RL, Wilson LJ, Lee J: Medically safe rate of weight loss for the treatment of obesity: A guideline based on risk of gallstone formation. *Am J Med* 98:115, 1995.
551. Gebhard RL, Prigge WF, Ansel HJ, Schlasner L, Ketover SR, Sande D, Holtmeier K, Peterson FJ: The roll of gallbladder emptying in gallstone formation during diet-induced rapid weight loss. *Hepatology* 24:544, 1996.
552. Little RA, Goldstein RB, Saxton J: Gallstone formation during weight-reduction dieting. *Arch Intern Med* 149:1750, 1989.
553. Forbes GB: Lean body mass-body fat interrelationships in humans. *Nutr Rev* 45:225, 1987.
553. National Task Force on the Prevention and Treatment of Obesity: Very low-calorie diets. *JAMA* 270:967, 1993.
555. Institute of Medicine Food and Nutrition Board Committee to Develop Criteria for Evaluating the Outcomes of Approaches to Prevent and Treat Obesity: Weighing the options: Criteria for evaluating weight-management programs. Thomas PR (ed), Washington, DC, National Academy Press, 1995.
556. Wadden TA, Foster GD, Leitzia KA, Mullen JL: Long-term effects of dieting on resting metabolic rate in obese outpatients. *JAMA* 264:707, 1990.
557. Steen SN, Oppliger RA, Brownell KD: Metabolic effects of repeated weight loss and regain in adolescent wrestlers. *JAMA* 260:47, 1988.
558. National Task Force on the Prevention and Treatment of Obesity: Weight cycling. *JAMA* 272:1196, 1994.
559. vanDale D, Saris WHM: Repetitive weight loss and weight regain: Effects on weight reduction, resting metabolic rate, and lipolytic activity before and after exercise and/or diet treatment. *Am J Clin Nutr* 49:409, 1989.
560. Gray DS, Fisler JS, Bray GA: Effects of repeated weight loss and regain on body composition in obese rats. *Am J Clin Nutr* 47:393, 1988.
561. Bouchard C: Is weight fluctuation a risk factor? *N Engl J Med* 324:1887, 1991.
562. Lissner L, Odell PM, D'Agostino RB, Stokes J, Kreger BE, Belanger A, Brownell KD: Variability of body weight and health outcomes in the Framingham population. *N Engl J Med* 324:1839, 1991.
563. Mirkin GB, Shore RN: The Beverly Hills diet. *JAMA* 246:2235, 1981.
564. Scoville BA: Review of amphetamine-like drugs by the Food and Drug Administration: Clinical data and value judgments, in Bray GA (ed): *Obesity in Perspective*. DHEW (NIH) 75-708. Bethesda, MD, National Institutes of Health, 1975, p 441.
565. Weintraub M, Bray GA: Drug treatment of obesity. *Med Clin North Am* 73:237, 1989.
566. Weintraub M, Hasday JD, Mushlin AI, Lockwood DH: A double-blind clinical trial in weight control: Use of fenfluramine and phentermine alone and in combination. *Arch Intern Med* 144:1143, 1984.
567. Guy-grand B, Apfelbaum M, Crepaldi G, Gries A, Lefebvre P, Turner P: International trial of long-term dexfenfluramine in obesity. *Lancet* 2:1142, 1989.
568. Abenhaim L, Moride Y, Brenot F, Rich S, Benichou J, Kurz X, Higenbottam T, Oakley C, Wouters E, Aubier M, Simonneau G, Begaud B: Appetite-suppressant drugs and the risk of primary pulmonary hypertension. International Primary Pulmonary Hypertension Study Group. *N Engl J Med* 335:609, 1996.
569. Mark EJ, Patalas ED, Chang HT, Evans RJ, Kessler SC: Fatal pulmonary hypertension associated with short-term use of fenfluramine and phentermine. *N Engl J Med* 337:602, 1997.
570. Connolly HM, Crary JL, McGoon MD, Hensrud DD, Edwards BS, Edwards WD, Schaff HV: Valvular heart disease associated with fenfluramine-phentermine. *N Engl J Med* 337:581, 1997.
571. Cannistra LB, Cannistra AJ: Regression of multivavular regurgitation after cessation of fenfluramine and phentermine treatment. *N Engl J Med* 339:771, 1998.
572. Curfman GD: Diet pills redux. *N Engl J Med* 337:629, 1997.
573. Jick H, Vasilakis C, Weinrauch LA, Meier CR, Jick SS, Derby LE: A population-based study of appetite-suppressant drugs and the risk of cardiac-valve regurgitation. *N Engl J Med* 339:719, 1998.
574. Kahn MA, Herzog CA, St. Peter JV, Hartley GG, Madlon-Kay R, Dick CD, Asinger RW, Vessey JT: The prevalence of cardiac vavular insufficiency assessed by transthoracic echocardiography in obese patients treated with appetite-suppressant drugs. *N Engl J Med* 339:713, 1998.
575. Wee CC, Phillips RS, Aurigemma G, Erban S, Kriegel G, Riley M, Douglas PS: Risk for valvular heart disease among users of fenfluramine and dexfenfluramine who underwent echocardiography before use of medication. *Ann Intern Med* 129:870, 1998.
576. Thurlby PL, Ellis RDM: Differences between the effects of noradrenaline and the β-adrenoceptor agonist BRL 28410 in brown adipose tissue and hind limb of the anaesthetized rat. *Can J Physiol Pharmacol* 64:1111, 1986.
577. Cunningham S, Leslie P, Hopwood D, Illingworth P, Jung RT, Nicholls DG, Peden N, Rafael J, et al: The characterization and energetic potential of brown adipose tissue in man. *Clin Sci* 69:343, 1985.
578. Connacher AA, Jung RT, Mitchell PEG: Weight loss in obese subjects on a restricted diet given BRL 26830A, a new atypical β adrenoceptor agonist. *Br Med J* 296:1217, 1988.
579. Stock MJ: Sibutramine: A review of the pharmacology of a novel anti-obesity agent. *Int J Obesity* 21:S25, 1997.
580. Apfelbaum M, Vgue P, Ziegler O, Hanotin C, Thomas F, Leutenegger E: Long-term maintenance of weight loss after a very-low calorie diet: A randomized blinded trial of the efficacy and tolerability of sibutramine. *Am J Med* 106:179, 1999.
581. Sjostrom L, Rissanen A, Andersen T, Boldrin M, Golay A, Koppeschaar HPF, Krempf M: Randomized placebo-controlled trial of Orlistat for weight loss and prevention of weight regain in obese patients. *Lancet* 352:167, 1998.
582. Davidson MH, Hauptman J, DiGirolamo M, Foreyt JP, Halsted CH, Huber D, Heimburger DC, Lucas CP, Robbins DC, Chung J, Heymsfield SB: Weight control and risk factor reduction in obese subject treated for 2 years with Orlistat. *JAMA* 281:235, 1999.
583. Greenway FL, Bray GA: Human chorionic gonadotropin (HCG) in the treatment of obesity. *West J Med* 127:461, 1977.
584. Coniff RF, Shapiro J, Seaton TB, Bray GA: Multicenter, placebo-controlled trial comparing acarbose (Bay g5421) with placebo, tolbutamide, and tolbutamide-plus-acarbose in non-insulin-dependent diabetes mellitus. *Am J Med* 98:443, 1995.
585. Glueck CJ, Jandacek R, Hogg E, Allen C, Baehler L, Tewksbury M: Sucrose polyester: Substitution for dietary fats in hypocaloric diets in the treatment of familial hypercholesterolemia. *Am J Clin Nutr* 37:347, 1983.
586. Mellies MJ, Vitale C, Jandacek RJ, Lamkin GE, Clueck CJ: The substitution of sucrose polyester for dietary fat in obese, hypercholesterolemic outpatients. *Am J Clin Nutr* 41:1, 1985.
587. Solum TT, Ryttig KR, Solum E, Larsen S: The influence of a high-fibre diet on body weight, serum lipids and blood pressure in slightly overweight persons. *Int J Obes* 11:67, 1987.
588. Clemmons DR, Snyder DK, Williams R, Underwood LE: Growth hormone administration conserves lean body mass during dietary restriction in obese subjects. *J Clin Endocrinol Metab* 64:878, 1987.
589. Snyder DK, Clemmons DR, Underwood LE: Treatment of obese, diet-restricted subjects with growth hormone for 11 weeks: Effects on anabolism, lipolysis, and body composition. *J Clin Endocrinol Metab* 67:54, 1988.
590. Bignon E, Alonso R, Arnone M, Boigegrain R, Brodin R, Gueudet C, Heaulme M, Keane P, Landi M, Molimard JC, Olliero D, Poncelet M, Seban E, Simiand J, Soubrie P, Pascal M, Maffrand JP, Le Fur G: SR146131: A new potent, orally active, and selective nonpeptide cholecystokinin subtype 1 receptor agonist. II: In vivo pharmacological characterization. *J Pharmcol Exp Ther* 289:752, 1999.

591. Mayer LES, Walsh BT: The use of selective serotonin reuptake inhibitors in eating disorders. *J Clin Psychiatry* 59:28, 1998.
592. Goldstein DJ, Rampey AH, Enas GG, Potvin JH, Fludzinski LA, Levine LR: Fluoxetine: A randomized clinical trial in the treatment of obesity. *Int J Obesity* 18:129, 1994.
593. National Institutes of Health: Gastrointestinal surgery for severe obesity: National Institutes of Health consensus development conference statement. *Am J Clin Nutr* 55:615S, 1992.
594. VanItallie TB: "Morbid" obesity: A hazardous disorder that resists conservative treatment. *Am J Clin Nutr* 33:358, 1980.
595. Drenick EJ, Gurunanjappa SB, Seltzer F, Johnson GA: Excessive mortality and causes of death in morbidly obese men. *JAMA* 243:443, 1980.
596. Sugerman HJ, Kellum JM, Engle KM, Wolfe L, Starkey JV, Birkenhauer R, Fletcher P, Sawyer MJ: Gastric bypass for treating severe obesity. *Am J Clin Nutr* 55:560S, 1992.
597. Benotti PN, Forse A: The role of gastric surgery in the multidisciplinary management of severe obesity. *Am J Surg* 169:361, 1995.
598. Pories WJ, Swanson MS, MacDonald KG, Long SB, Morris PG, Brown BM, Barakat HA, deRamon RA, Israel G, Dolezal JM, Dohm L: Who would have thought it? An operation proves to be the most effective therapy for adult-onset diabetes mellitus. *Ann Surg* 222:339, 1995.
599. Brolin RE, Kenler HA, Gorman JH, Cody RP: Long limb gastric bypass in the superobese. *Ann Surg* 215:387, 1992.
600. Azagra JS, Goergen M, Ansay J, DeSimone P, Vanhaverbeek M, Devuyst L, Squelaert J: Laparoscopic gastric reduction surgery. Preliminary results of a randomized prospective trial of laparoscopic vs open vertical banded gastroplasty. *Surg Endosc* 13:555, 1999.
601. Kral JG: Malabsorptive procedures in surgical treatment of morbid obesity. *Gastroenterol Clin North Am* 16:293, 1987.
602. Linner JH: Overview of surgical techniques for the treatment of morbid obesity. *Gastroenterol Clin North Am* 16:253, 1987.
603. Zollinger RW, Coccia MR, Zollinger RW II: Critical analysis of jejunoileal bypass. *Am J Surg* 146:626, 1983.
604. Hocking MP, Duerson MC, O'Leary JP, Woodward ER: Jejunoileal bypass for morbid obesity. *N Engl J Med* 308:995, 1983.
605. Sugerman JH, Starkey JV, Birkenhauer R: A randomized prospective trial of gastric bypass versus vertical banded gastroplasty for morbid obesity and their effects on sweets versus non-sweets eaters. *Ann Surg* 205:613, 1987.
606. Sugerman HJ, Londrey GL, Kellum JM, Wolf L, Liszka T, Engle KM, Birkenhauer R, Starkey JV: Weight loss with vertical banded gastroplasty and roux-Y gastric bypass for morbid obesity with selective versus random assignment. *Am J Surg* 157:93, 1989.
607. Linner JH: Treatment of morbid obesity. *Arch Surg* 117:697, 1982.
608. Fobi MAL, Fleming AW: Vertical banded gastroplasty vs gastric bypass in the treatment of obesity. *J Natl Med Assoc* 78:1091, 1986.
609. Pasulka PS, Bistrian BR, Benotti PN, Blackburn GL: The risks of surgery in obese patients. *Ann Intern Med* 104:540, 1986.
610. Abarbanel JM, Berginer VM, Osimani A, Solomon H, Charuzi I: Neurologic complications after gastric restriction surgery for morbid obesity. *Neurology* 37:196, 1987.

CHAPTER 21

Disorders of Lipid Metabolism

P. Barton Duell
D. Roger Illingworth
William E. Connor

Hyperlipidemia warrants special concern and interest because it is found with exceptional frequency in the American population. Ten percent of children and at least 25 percent of adults in the United States, Canada, and western Europe have lipid values that put them at increased risk of developing premature cardiovascular disease. Although most affected individuals have hyperlipidemia secondary to dietary factors or other metabolic disorders, some have genetic causes of hyperlipidemia. These are estimated to be among the most common hereditary disorders seen in adult medical practice. Thus, asymptomatic hyperlipidemia may be detected both in so-called healthy people and in patients seeking medical attention for a variety of other problems. Hyperlipidemia is especially noted today because plasma cholesterol and triglyceride concentrations are so frequently determined in the course of routine chemical screening.

Hyperlipidemia involves an elevation of plasma lipid levels, cholesterol, and triglyceride, singly or in combination. Because these lipids are transported in the plasma as components of lipoprotein molecules, hyperlipidemia implies an associated lipoprotein abnormality as well.

There are four important clinical reasons for concern about the correct diagnosis and treatment of hyperlipidemia. The first reason is the strong causative relation between hyperlipidemia and atherosclerotic vascular disease: coronary heart disease, stroke, visceral atherosclerosis, and peripheral vascular disease. The second is the direct correlation of hyperlipidemia with the occurrence in the skin and tendons of xanthomas, which should be regarded as external manifestations of lipid deposits in tissues that are analogous to similar deposits occurring internally in the arteries. Xanthomas present cosmetic problems and because of their unique characteristics may be of value in the differential diagnosis of the exact type of hyperlipidemia. Both atherosclerosis and xanthomas will be the subject of more extensive discussion in subsequent sections of this chapter.

The third reason relates to the diagnosis of obscure abdominal distress and even acute abdominal pain. In some patients, the episode of abdominal pain may progress to acute pancreatitis. Many hyperlipidemic patients with abdominal pain on the basis of a lipemic state have even been surgically explored for the presence of an acute abdomen. Thus, hyperlipidemia should be considered as a possible cause of both acute pancreatitis and obscure abdominal pain.

The fourth reason for clinical concern is that the occurrence of hyperlipidemia may point to another disease to which the hyperlipidemia is secondary. In many cases the primary condition may be obvious, but in others the hyperlipidemia may alert one to the possibility of hypothyroidism, for example.

THE PLASMA LIPOPROTEINS

The plasma of all vertebrates, including human beings, contains lipids transported as soluble complexes called *lipoproteins*. Individually such lipids have very limited solubility in aqueous environments, whereas as lipoprotein complexes they are readily held in solution. It is the lipid moieties with hydrated densities of 0.8 to 0.9 g/ml that give lipoproteins a unique density range that is lighter than that of the other plasma proteins. Notable landmarks in the separation of lipoproteins have been the development of ultracentrifugal flotation by Gofman and coworkers[1] and the development of electrophoretic separation techniques by Lees and Hatch.[2]

Lipoprotein Classification

The separation of different lipoproteins has been achieved by means of two principal techniques—electrophoresis and ultracentrifugation in salt solutions—and their classification is most commonly expressed in operational terms. On the basis of ultracentrifugal separation of plasma, four lipoprotein classes are recognized: chylomicrons, very low density lipoproteins (VLDL), low-density lipoproteins (LDL), and high-density lipoproteins (HDL). The relation between this ultracentrifugal classification and the size and electrophoretic mobility of lipoproteins is shown in Fig. 21-1. Further refinements in these density classes have been made and are a topic of considerable current interest. Low-density lipoproteins may be separated into two or more fractions: LDL_1 [also commonly referred to as intermediate-density lipoprotein, IDL; density (*d*) 1.006 to 1.019] and LDL_2 (*d* 1.019 to 1.063). High-density lipoproteins may be similarly divided into HDL_2 (*d* 1.063 to 1.125) and HDL_3 (*d* 1.125 to 1.21). A fifth lipoprotein, lipoprotein (a), is present in plasma and has a hydrated density between 1.06 and 1.08 g/ml.[3] Lp(a) is usually a minor constituent of lipoproteins isolated by ultracentrifugation. Lp(a) consists of an LDL particle to which an additional protein termed apo (a) is covalently bound.[3]

In addition to this operational classification, Alaupovic has proposed a concept of lipoprotein families, each of which is

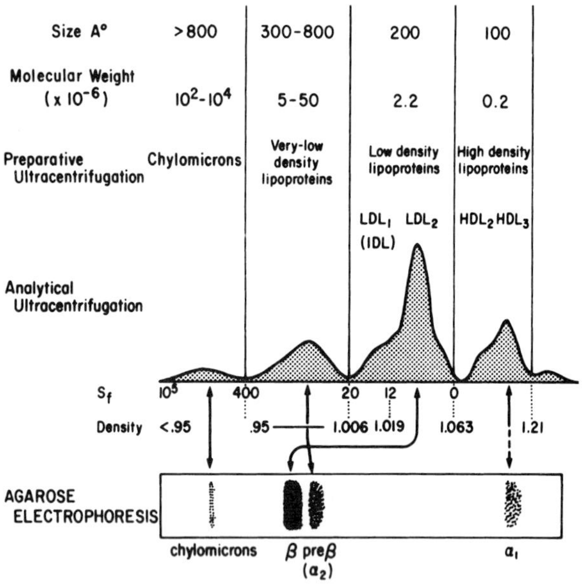

FIGURE 21-1. Diagrammatic representation of the major classes and properties of human lipoproteins separated by electrophoresis and ultracentrifugation.

distinguished by its apoprotein moiety.[4] These moieties are designated alphabetically as apo-A, apo-B, apo-C, apo-D, and apo-E. The apo-A family in turn contains three separate apoproteins designated A-I, A-II, and A-IV, and the C family also has three: C-I, C-II, and C-III. The distribution of these apoproteins within the four operational density classes is shown in Table 21-1. It is evident that when lipoproteins are classified according to their density, each class represents a polydisperse system of particles that differ in size, hydrated density, and constituent apoproteins. In contrast, the lipoprotein family classification[5,6] defines five families, each of which consists of a polydisperse system of lipid-apoprotein associations characterized by the presence of a single distinct apoprotein or its constituent polypeptides. We shall rely on the operational definition in this review.

Lipoprotein Composition

Chylomicrons

Chylomicrons are the largest of the lipoprotein particles whose primary role in the transport of exogenously derived fat from the intestine is well defined. Their size varies from 800 to 10,000 Å, with larger particles being produced under conditions of high dietary fat intake. The larger particles contain relatively more triglycerides and less polar phospholipids and free cholesterol than do their smaller counterparts. Typical values for the composition of plasma chylomicrons are shown in Table 21-2. After a lipid-rich meal, the fatty acid composition of chylomicron triglycerides generally resembles that of consumed dietary fat, although with lower fat intakes the proportions of linoleic acid, which is derived from biliary lecithin, are higher. The large size and high triglyceride content of chylomicrons are responsible for the lactescent appearance of plasma with a high content of these particles. When present, a chylomicron layer will float to the surface of plasma stored overnight at 4°C. Despite their low content of protein, the A, B, and C apoproteins all appear to be integral components of chylomicrons. Human chylomicrons contain a unique form of apoprotein B (B-48), which is synthesized in the intestinal mucosal cells. Recent studies have demonstrated that B-48 represents a unique intestine-derived form of apoprotein B that consists of the amino-terminal 2,152 amino acids of the normal hepatic apo-B-100, which is 4,536 amino acids in length.[7,8] Apo-B-48 is produced from the apo-B-100 gene by a novel mechanism involving the editing of message RNA in the intestine that results in insertion of a stop codon (UAA) in place of the normal CAA, with a resultant termination of protein synthesis at amino acid number 2,152. Why the intestinal mucosal cells have evolved to synthesize this unique form of apoprotein B is not clear; possibilities include a more rapid adaptation to increase fat intake with a greater and more rapid synthetic capacity than would be observed for a longer protein (B-100) or the possibility that apo-B-48 containing chylomicrons can accommodate more apo-E molecules per particle than can apo-B-100 containing lipoproteins, which in turn may enhance their subsequent uptake by the liver. Because of apoprotein transfer reactions, the C-apoprotein content of chylomicrons isolated from plasma is higher than that of similar particles isolated from thoracic duct lymph. The reverse

TABLE 21-1. Apoprotein Content of Human Plasma Lipoproteins

Chylomicrons	VLDL	LDL	Lp(a)	HDL
Major apoproteins				
Apo-B-48	Apo-B-100	Apo-B-100	Apo-B-100	Apo-A-I
Apo-C-I	Apo-C-I		Apo(a)	Apo-A-II
Apo-C-II	Apo-C-II			
Apo-C-III	Apo-C-III			
Apo-E	Apo-E			
Minor apoproteins				
Apo-A-I	Apo-D			Apo-C-I
Apo-A-II				Apo-C-II
Apo-A-IV				Apo-C-III
Apo-D				Apo-D
				Apo-E

Note: Apoproteins A-I, A-II, and A-IV each constitute 5 to 10 percent of the apoproteins in lymph chylomicrons but are minor components of the chylomicron particles present in plasma.

TABLE 21-2. Composition of Human Plasma Lipoproteins

	Chylomicrons	VLDL	LDL	HDL
Protein	2	8	21	50
Phospholipid	7	19	22	23
Cholesterol-free	2	7	8	4
Cholesterol ester	5	13	37	18
Triglyceride	84	51	11	4
Nonesterified fatty acid		2	1	1

Note: Values are expressed as percent total dry weight of the lipoprotein.

situation is true for apoproteins A-I, A-II, and A-IV, whose concentrations are higher in chylomicron particles isolated from lymph compared with their plasma counterparts. As will be discussed later, such a transfer is physiologically important in the activation of lipoprotein lipase and the subsequent hydrolysis of chylomicron triglycerides.

Very Low Density Lipoproteins

Very low density lipoproteins, which are the major transport vehicle for endogenous triglycerides in plasma, are smaller than chylomicrons and constitute a heterogeneous series of particles ranging in diameter from 300 to 800 Å. Typical values for VLDL composition are shown in Tables 21-1 and 21-2. The size of VLDL particles is sufficient to scatter transmitted light and gives plasma containing these particles a turbid appearance. However, in contrast to lipemia due to chylomicrons, the turbidity due to VLDL does not separate after storage of plasma for 12 to 18 h at 4°C. Various methods have been used to show that the size heterogeneity of VLDL particles is paralleled by variations in both their lipid composition and their protein composition. Larger particles contain relatively more of the nonpolar triglycerides and less phospholipid and cholesterol than do their smaller counterparts. Thus, as a VLDL particle gets smaller, its relative content of both free and esterified cholesterol is increased. The proportion of apo-C present is also directly related to the size and triglyceride content of the VLDL particle, whereas the apo-B content shows an inverse relation with these parameters. VLDL particles contain the higher-molecular-weight form of apoprotein B termed *B-100*, which is the same apoprotein B present in LDL but is different from the B-48 protein present in chylomicrons.[8]

Low-Density Lipoproteins

Low-density lipoproteins (α-lipoproteins) are the major carrier of cholesterol, cholesteryl ester, and phospholipid in human plasma. A typical LDL molecule has a molecular weight of 2.2×10^6 and is composed of 20 to 25 percent protein and 75 to 80 percent lipid (Tables 21-1 and 21-2). A single molecule of apo-B-100 constitutes more than 95 percent of the protein content of LDL, with trace quantities of A, C, and E apoproteins also being present. Lower-density fractions of LDL do, however, contain higher proportions of apo-E and C, but apo-B-100 still contributes more than 90 percent of the total protein.

High-Density Lipoproteins

High-density lipoproteins (α-lipoproteins) are the heaviest (*d* 1.063 to 1.21) and smallest (diameter 90 to 120 Å) of the human lipoproteins and contain about equal proportions of lipid and protein (Table 21-2). Apo-A-I (55 percent) and apo-A-II (30 percent) constitute the major apoproteins in HDL, with smaller quantities of apo-C, apo-D, and apo-E also being present. A number of other plasma proteins also are associated with HDL particles, such as paraoxonase, an enzyme that hydrolyzes lipid peroxides and is believed to help protect LDL against oxidative modification. Some polymorphisms of paraoxonase are associated with increased risk of atherosclerosis.

The lipoproteins isolated in the HDL density range have frequently been further separated into HDL_2 (*d* 1.063 to 1.125) and HDL_3 (*d* 1.125 to 1.21). The latter are smaller and contain relatively more apo-A-I and apo-A-II and less apo-C and apo-E. Although the significance of HDL_2 and HDL_3 in physiologic terms remains unclear, the concentration of HDL_2 is some three times higher in premenopausal women than in men. Perturbations in HDL levels caused by factors such as increased exercise also seem to specifically increase the concentrations of HDL_2 in plasma. Based on the apoprotein content, HDL may also be separated into particles containing only apo A-I (Lp:A-I) or both apo A-I and A-II (Lp:A-I/A-II). It has been hypothesized that Lp:A-I and Lp:A-I/A-II particles are functionally distinct. Lp:A-I particles may protect against atherosclerosis whereas Lp:A-I/A-II particles may counteract the anti-atherogenic effects of Lp:A-I.

Lipoprotein (a)

Lipoprotein (a) [Lp(a)] is an LDL-like particle that contains cholesterol, phospholipid, triglycerides, and apo-B-100, which is linked via a single disulfide bond to a second large protein termed apolipoprotein (a) [apo(a)].[9] Each Lp(a) particle contains one molecule each of apo(a) and apo B. Apo(a) is extensively glycosylated, which causes Lp(a) to have a carbohydrate content that is approximately four-fold higher than that of LDL. Removal of the apo(a) moiety from Lp(a) by reducing the disulfide linkage yields an LDL particle. Lp(a) can be isolated by ultracentrifugation between the densities of 1.06 and 1.08 g/ml, but unlike HDL, Lp(a) is precipitated by heparin manganese, and in this respect it resembles LDL. Because Lp(a) has pre-ß migration on agarose gel electrophoresis, and is more dense than VLDL (the predominant pre-β lipoprotein), Lp(a) has sometimes been referred to as sinking pre-β lipoprotein. The structure of apo(a) is very similar to that of plasminogen and contains a number of pretzel-like structures that have been termed "kringles." The number of copies of the 114 amino acid kringle IV that are present in apo(a) varies substantially among different patients. This variability is one of the factors responsible for considerable interindividual heterogeneity in the molecular weight of apo(a) and plasma concentrations of Lp(a). The size of apo(a) ranges between 450,000 and 750,000 daltons, and the relation between molecular mass and plasma concentrations is an inverse one, with the highest plasma concentrations being observed in patients with the lowest-molecular-weight forms of apo(a).[10] The frequency distribution of Lp(a) concentrations in the general population is highly skewed toward zero, such that the prevalence of a given concentration of Lp(a) is inversely related to the plasma concentration (ranging from <0.1 mg/dl to >100 mg/dl).

The species distribution of Lp(a) is unusual and fascinating. Other than in humans, Lp(a) is found only in old world monkeys, great apes, and hedgehogs, but not in new world monkeys, which diverged from old world monkeys about 40 million years ago. The occurrence of Lp(a) in hedgehogs and primates is probably a consequence of convergent evolution resulting from the origin of 2 distinct apo(a) genes from the plasminogen gene at two different times in evolutionary history.

It is estimated that about 80–90 percent of interindividual heterogeneity in plasma concentrations of Lp(a) is attributable to inheritance, primarily related to sequence differences in the apo(a) gene locus. Plasma concentrations of Lp(a) greater than 20 to 30 mg/dl are associated with an increased risk of atherosclerosis, but the precise physiologic function of Lp(a) remains unknown.[11] Although Lp(a) may have a role in repair mechanisms at sites of endothelial injury, no deficiency syndrome has been identified in the large number of patients who have low (or even undetectable) levels of Lp(a).

Abnormal Lipoproteins

Certain pathologic conditions may be associated with the presence of abnormal lipoprotein particles in plasma. This is most commonly seen in patients with cholestasis in which an abnormal cholesterol-rich lipoprotein termed lipoprotein X (LPX) is present in plasma.[12] Lipoprotein X appears as bilamellar discoidal structures measuring 40 to 60 nm in diameter and 10 nm in thickness when studied under electron microscopy. Lipoprotein X contains phospholipid and free cholesterol in a 1:1 molar ratio and albumin and apoproteins C-I, C-II, and C-III as the protein moieties. The cholesteryl ester content is low. The lecithin contained in LPX contains fatty acid moieties of similar composition to those of biliary lecithin, and this lipoprotein is believed to contain phospholipid and cholesterol which are transported into plasma when their normal route of excretion in bile is impaired. Similar lipoprotein particles also occur in the plasma of patients with lecithin cholesterol acyltransferase deficiency (LCAT).[13]

The Apoproteins

Structure

The apoprotein moieties of plasma lipoproteins have in common the requirement that they bind and transport lipid in the bloodstream. During the past decade, major advances have occurred that have delineated the synthesis, structure, and function of these unique proteins. Eleven major apoproteins—A-I, A-II, A-IV, B-48, B-100, C-I, C-II, C-III, D, E, and apo(a)—have been sequenced, and the genes responsible for their synthesis have been mapped in the human genome.[14,15] With the exception of apo(a), these apoproteins have one common structural feature: a domain containing an amphipathic helix.[16] The amino acid sequences of these regions of the protein are such that hydrophobic amino acids are arranged on one side of the helix and hydrophilic polar amino acids form the other side. The hydrophobic face of the helix is thought to interact with the acyl chains of phospholipids, whereas the hydrophilic region faces the polar region of phospholipid head groups. With the exception of apo-B-48, apo-B-100, and apo(a), all of the other apoproteins appear to be capable of dissociating from one lipoprotein particle and moving to another. This movement of apoproteins between lipoproteins not only serves to enhance metabolic processing of given lipoprotein particles but also prolongs the residence time of the apoproteins in plasma.

Studies of the biosynthesis of several apoproteins have indicated that the apoproteins are initially synthesized as preapolipoproteins or preproapolipoproteins, with pre- and pro-segments of the apolipoprotein being cleaved posttranslationally within the cell or after secretion of the proapolipoprotein into plasma.[17,18] The gene locations of the major apoproteins have been delineated; examples include apo-B on chromosome 2; apo(a) on chromosome 6; apo-A-I, A-IV, and C-III on chromosome 11; and apo-C-II, apo-E, and the LDL receptor gene on chromosome 19.[15] Application of the techniques of modern molecular biology to plasma apolipoproteins has resulted in the identification of regulatory and structural mutations in the genes for these apoproteins, several of which appear to predispose individuals to dyslipoproteinemias and the premature development of atherosclerosis. Different allelic forms of apoprotein E resulting from amino acid substitutions in the receptor-binding region of this apoprotein have been described and underlie susceptibility to type III hyperlipoproteinemia. Mutations in apo-B have been identified that result in hypercholesterolemia in the case of familial defective apo-B-100, or hypocholesterolemia in the case of mutations resulting in truncated forms of apo-B.[8,14,15] A variety of apolipoprotein A-I isoproteins resulting from amino acid substitutions have also been described, and it is likely that many more variations will be identified in the future. In addition to alterations in apoprotein composition caused by amino acid substitutions resulting from structural gene mutations, differences in the sialic acid content of apoproteins also contribute to the apparent variations detected on isoelectric focusing. For example, three forms of apoprotein C-III can be resolved by means of isoelectric focusing; apoprotein C-III_0 contains no sialic acid, apoprotein C-III_1 has 1 mol of sialic acid per mole of protein, and apoprotein C-III_2 has 2 mol.[19] Various dietary and hormonal manipulations have been shown to alter the degree of sialation of apo-C-III.[20]

The major sites of biosynthesis of apolipoproteins are the liver and the intestinal mucosal cells; both organs appear to contribute to the plasma pool of apoproteins of the A and C families as well as apoprotein E.[21] Current data[8] indicate that the biosynthesis of human apoprotein B-48 occurs exclusively in the intestine, whereas apoprotein B-100 appears to be almost exclusively of hepatic origin. The biosynthesis of apoprotein E occurs in many nonhepatic tissues,[22] including muscle and macrophages; muscle tissue also appears capable of synthesizing apolipoprotein A-I.[21]

Function

In addition to their structural role in maintaining lipoprotein stability, several apolipoproteins are known to play distinct roles in the intravascular metabolism and cellular uptake of lipoproteins (Table 21-3). Apolipoprotein C-II serves as a cofactor for lipoprotein lipase, the enzyme that hydrolyzes the triglycerides in plasma chylomicrons and VLDL,[23] and a deficiency of apo-C-II is associated with severe hypertriglyceridemia.[24] The infusion of normal plasma or isolated apo-C-II fractions dramatically reduces the hypertriglyceridemia seen in patients with apo-C-II deficiency.[24,25] Apolipoprotein A-I, the major apoprotein in HDL, is a cofactor for lecithin cholesterol acyltransferase (LCAT), a plasma enzyme that catalyzes the conversion of cholesterol and phosphatidylcholine to cholesteryl esters and lysophosphatidylcholine.[14,26] Apo-C-I may also serve as an activator of LCAT. Apoproteins A-I, A-II, and A-IV are ligands for the ATP binding cassette-1 (ABC-1), the recently identified peripheral tissue HDL receptor, and apo A-I is also a ligand for cubulin, a primarily renal HDL receptor, and scavenger receptor B-1 (SR-B1), which mediates hepatic, gonadal, and adrenal uptake of HDL cholesteryl esters.

Distinct roles for apoprotein E and apoprotein B-100 in the cellular uptake of lipoprotein particles have been well established. The uptake of chylomicron and VLDL remnant particles is dependent on a specific hepatic receptor that has been termed the LDL receptor–related protein (LRP), which recognizes the apoprotein E moieties contained in these lipoprotein particles and facilitates their uptake from plasma.[27,28] A single amino acid substitution between residues 140 and 160 of the 299-amino acid sequence of apoprotein E can profoundly affect receptor binding, and a substitution of cysteine for arginine at residue 158 is primarily responsible for the decreased receptor binding of apoprotein E-2, which is believed to underlie the clinical development of type III hyperlipoproteinemia.[29] The synthesis of apoprotein B-48 within intestinal mucosal cells and of apoprotein B-100 within the liver appears to be necessary for the normal formation of chylomicron and VLDL-LDL particles, respectively.[8] Although the hepatic uptake of chylomicron remnants does not require the interaction of apo-B-48 with hepatic receptors, the removal of LDL particles from plasma is facilitated by binding domains present in the C-terminal portion of apo-B-100 that are recognized by specific high-affinity LDL receptors.[8] Monoclonal antibodies directed against epitopes on apo-B-100 located between amino acids 2,980 and 3,780 completely block the specific binding of LDL particles to the LDL receptor and indicate that this region of apoprotein B contains the receptor-binding domain. These studies are also consistent with the observation that patients with familial defective apo-B-100, in which the amino acid glutamine is substituted for the normal arginine at position 3,500, exhibit increased plasma concentrations of LDL particles that bind poorly to the LDL-receptor.[8] Chemical modification of LDL with agents that block the charge on lysine or arginine residues inhibits the recognition of LDL by specific high-affinity LDL receptors and blocks this receptor-mediated pathway of cellular LDL uptake without having an apparent effect on receptor-independent pathways.[30]

Lipoprotein Structure

When viewed under the electron microscope, all normal mature lipoproteins appear as spherical particles without any discernible subunit structure.[26] The nonpolar triglycerides and cholesteryl esters are found in the central core of the lipoprotein particle, and the more polar phospholipids and free cholesterol are found at the surface. The apoproteins are also thought to be primarily located in an alpha-helical arrangement at the surface, although apolar regions of the protein chain may extend into the milieu of the lipid core. This lipid core model is consistent with the greater exchange of phospholipids and free cholesterol compared with the exchange of triglyceride and cholesteryl esters between lipoproteins.[26] A diagrammatic representation of the structure of LDL is shown in Fig. 21-2.[31]

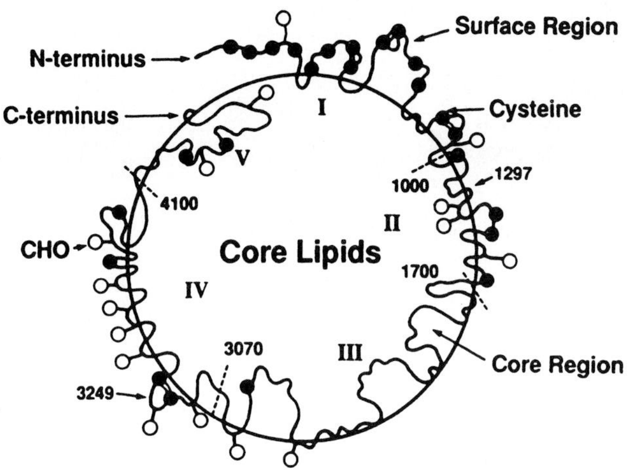

FIGURE 21-2. Schematic structure of low-density lipoprotein indicating the location of apoprotein B-100. The locations of two sites where thrombin cleaves apoprotein B (residues 1297 and 3249) are indicated. The locations of the sixteen *N*-linked carbohydrates (CHO ○), cysteine residues (●), and disulfide bridges (-) are also shown. The five hypothetical domains of apo-B are indicated by roman numerals and separated by dashed lines. (*Reproduced from Yang et al.*[31] *with permission.*)

SYNTHESIS AND CATABOLISM OF LIPIDS AND LIPOPROTEINS

Lipids

Cholesterol

In the schemata for the cholesterol balance of the body (Table 21-4), cholesterol is synthesized from acetate by the liver and intestinal mucosa and released into the plasma in lipoproteins.

TABLE 21-3. Metabolic Functions of the Major Plasma Apoproteins

Apoprotein	Molecular Weight	Metabolic Role
A-I	28,000	Activates LCAT, ligand for HDL receptor
A-II	17,500	Activated hepatic lipase; may inhibit LCAT
A-IV	46,000	Unknown; has been tentatively linked to satiety in rats
B-48	210,000	Transport of lipids from the gut as chylomicrons
B-100	350,000	Transport of lipids from the liver as VLDL and LDL; recognized by cellular LDL receptors
C-I	7,000	Activates LCAT
C-II	9,000	Activates lipoprotein lipase
C-III	9,000	May inhibit activation of lipoprotein lipase by apo-C-II
D	22,000	May be involved in lipid transfer between lipoproteins
E	34,000	Recognized by hepatic apo-E receptors and cellular LDL receptors; recognition facilitates hepatic uptake of chylomicron and VLDL remnants
Transfer proteins	Variable	Facilitate the transfer of triglycerides, phospholipids, and cholesteryl esters between lipoproteins

TABLE 21-4. The Cholesterol Balance of the Body

	Milligrams per day
Input	
From synthesis	500–1000
Absorbed from the diet	0–400
	500–1400
Output	
Excretion in the bile (cholesterol and bile acids) and subsequently in the feces	400–1300
Skin excretion	80–100
Synthesis of steroid hormones	Variable
Losses during pregnancy and lactation	Variable
Storage in the tissues	Variable
	500–1400

Cholesterol biosynthesis is regulated in the liver by the enzyme 3-hydroxy-3-methylglutaryl coenzyme A reductase (HMG CoA reductase). This enzyme catalyzes the production of mevalonic acid, which is converted to cholesterol. Cholesterol absorbed from the diet also enters the body pool of cholesterol and thus provides a second major source of cholesterol which circulates in the plasma. Only about 40 percent of dietary cholesterol is absorbed by the intestine. Although cells in the body have the capacity to synthesize cholesterol, in most cells the locally synthesized cholesterol is utilized for membrane formation within the cell and does not contribute en masse to the plasma cholesterol concentration.

A variety of circumstances favor cholesterol biosynthesis, including excessive calories in the diet, saturated fat in the diet, and perhaps the total fat content of the diet. Cholesterol synthesis is depressed with hypocaloric and starvation diets. As will be indicated in the section on Pharmaceutical Agents, some of the lipid-lowering drugs act by altering cholesterol biosynthesis, although in general earlier agents such as triparanol, which inhibited a late stage in cholesterol biosynthesis, were too toxic for therapeutic use.

Cholesterol synthesis may also be inhibited by the presence of cholesterol in the liver cells; this is known as *feedback inhibition*. Likewise, the presence of bile acids through feedback inhibition tends to inhibit the synthesis of additional bile acids from cholesterol. In humans, however, the inhibition of cholesterol biosynthesis is insufficient to prevent a rise in plasma cholesterol concentrations when a large quantity of cholesterol is present in the diet.

Besides the efflux of cholesterol from the plasma as carried by LDL to supply cholesterol for membranes in growing cells, cholesterol from the plasma may be utilized for the synthesis of the steroid hormones and bile acids.

The primary route of excretion of cholesterol from the body begins in the liver, where cholesterol and bile acids synthesized from cholesterol are secreted in the bile. Thus, the chief pathway of excretion of cholesterol from the body ultimately occurs via the feces, where this steroid nucleus appears either as cholesterol or as its bacterially altered products coprosterol (coprostanol) and coprostanone and as bile acids. The bile acids in the stool represent the small fraction excreted in the bile and not absorbed by the enterohepatic circulation. The usual output of cholesterol from the body is approximately 600 to 1,000 mg per day. About 60 percent of the output is as cholesterol (or coprostanol), and the other 40 percent is as the secondary bile acids.

Cholesteryl ester is the predominant circulating form of cholesterol, with some 70 to 80 percent of the total plasma cholesterol being esterified through the action of the LCAT enzyme, as will be discussed subsequently. The predominant cholesteryl ester is cholesteryl linoleate, followed by cholesteryl oleate, cholesteryl palmitate, and cholesteryl stearate. Some arachidonic acid is also transported as a cholesteryl ester. The cholesterol of the bodily tissues is largely in the free form, except for the storage of cholesteryl ester in the adrenal glands and other steroid-synthesizing endocrine glands, where it becomes readily available for the synthesis of steroid hormones under conditions of rapid need. Some cholesteryl ester is also present in the liver, but in general normal tissues contain only free cholesterol, which is present primarily in cell membranes; of course, cholesteryl ester predominates in atheroma and xanthoma. Finally, it must be appreciated that cholesterol is unique in that once it is present in the body, it remains until it is excreted. The steroid nucleus cannot be broken down by the tissues, unlike lipids such as triglyceride.

Triglyceride

Like cholesterol, the triglyceride of the plasma lipoproteins is synthesized either by the intestinal tract (from absorbed fatty acids) or by the liver from both acetate and fatty acids and enters the plasma in the form of one of the four major lipoprotein classes: chylomicrons, VLDL, LDL, and HDL. Plasma triglyceride constitutes a readily available source of energy for the body, again through the action of lipoprotein lipase at the cellular level. The free fatty acid produced from the hydrolysis of triglyceride is then taken up by the cells of the body either for storage, as in adipose tissue, or for oxidation by muscle cells. Thus, hypertriglyceridemia can result from oversynthesis, impaired catabolism, or a combination of both circumstances. Caloric excess and adiposity apparently favor both increased synthesis of triglycerides in liver and gut and impaired removal by the peripheral tissue.

Phospholipids

The plasma phospholipids are derived almost entirely from synthesis in the liver and intestinal mucosa but can be synthesized by most body tissues. Dietary phospholipids are not absorbed as such and undergo hydrolysis by phospholipases in the intestinal juices with formation of both lysophosphatides and the basic constituent phosphorus-containing amine, 2 mol of fatty acids, and glycerol. Phospholipids are catabolized as components of their respective lipoproteins and also readily exchange between lipoproteins and cell membranes. Catabolism of individual phospholipids may proceed to their basic constituents or may undergo deacylation-reacylation reactions during which the fatty acid composition is altered. Lysolecithin may be formed by tissue phospholipases or may be formed in plasma by LCAT, and this somewhat toxic molecule is rapidly metabolized.

Enzymes and Transfer Proteins Active in Lipoprotein Metabolism

Four enzymes—lipoprotein lipase (LPL), hepatic lipase (HL), LCAT, and endothelial lipase—the activities of which can all be measured in plasma, are of physiologic importance in lipoprotein metabolism. In addition, a specific transfer protein, cholesteryl ester transfer protein (CETP), facilitates the interchange of cholesteryl esters between HDL and triglyceride-rich lipoproteins. Phospholipid transfer protein (PLTP) facilitates the interchange of phospholipid between lipoproteins. These enzymes and transfer proteins collectively play a major role in modulating the size and

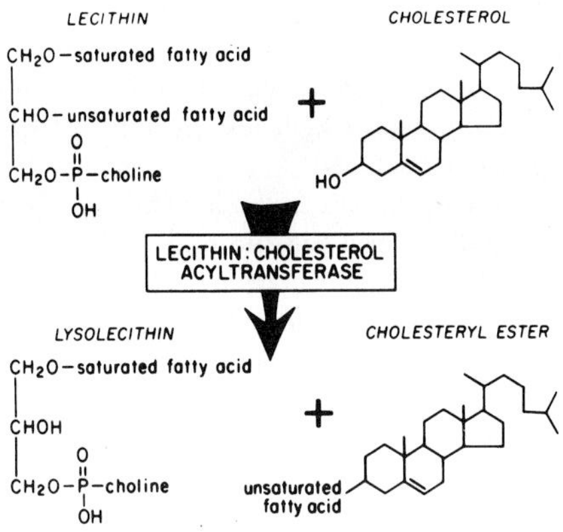

FIGURE 21-3. Lipid reactants in the plasma lecithin cholesterol acyltransferase reaction. (*Reproduced from Glomset et al.*[35] *with permission.*)

composition of plasma HDL particles. Microsomal triglyceride transfer protein (MTP) is involved in the formation of chylomicrons in the gut and VLDL in the liver. Mutations in MTP can be associated with abetalipoproteinemia.[32–34]

Lecithin Cholesterol Acyltransferase (LCAT)

The enzyme LCAT catalyzes the transfer of fatty acid from the 2 position of phosphatidylcholine to cholesterol with the formation of cholesteryl ester and lysophosphatidyl choline[35,36] (Fig. 21-3). Current evidence suggests that this enzyme is responsible for the formation of most of the esterified cholesterol present in plasma, although lesser amounts of cholesteryl ester also enter plasma as native constituents of VLDL and probably as chylomicrons. Phosphatidylcholine and free cholesterol present on HDL are the preferred substrate for LCAT, for which apo-A-I, the major apoprotein of HDL, and apo-C-I act as specific activators. The enzyme itself is secreted by the liver and is present in plasma, lymph, and cerebrospinal fluid. LCAT shows fatty acid specificity, which results in the preferential formation of cholesteryl linoleate. The absence of LCAT has been described in a rare disease which will be discussed later. LCAT deficiency alone is associated with low HDL cholesterol concentrations, but may not cause atherosclerosis unless LDL cholesterol concentrations also are increased. Overall, LCAT appears to have favorable effects on lipoprotein metabolism, which include enhanced clearance of proatherogenic apo B-containing lipoproteins and increased HDL cholesterol concentrations as well as enhanced reverse cholesterol transport.[37] Overexpression of LCAT in transgenic mice, however, does not protect against atherosclerosis unless CETP and apo A-I also are expressed. In the absence of this triad, overexpression of LCAT alone produces dysfunctional HDL particles and impaired reverse cholesterol transport. Thus, the presumed antiatherosclerotic properties of LCAT require the presence of functional apo A-I, CETP, and other key components of the reverse cholesterol transport pathway.

Lipoprotein Lipase (LPL)

Lipoprotein lipase is an important enzyme consisting of 448 amino acids that is present in a number of tissues, including muscle, adipose tissue, lung, brain, and breast tissue.[38] This enzyme is present primarily on endothelial cells in tissue capillary beds, where it is bound to heparan sulfate proteoglycans present as components of the glycocalyx on the plasma membrane. The enzyme is present in very low concentrations in plasma but may be released by the injection of heparin. Physiologically, LPL acts in capillary beds to hydrolyze triglycerides present in chylomicrons and VLDL particles, with subsequent liberation of free fatty acids and monoglycerides. Apoprotein C-II functions as a specific activator for LPL, and defects in the synthesis or activity of either LPL or apo-C-II result in impaired triglyceride catabolism and severe hypertriglyceridemia. Classically, deficiency of LPL is associated with familial type I hyperlipidemia that is detected early in life, often due to the development of pancreatitis. Patients with heterozygous LDL deficiency have a variable lipoprotein phenotype (increased triglyceride, decreased HDL cholesterol, possibly increased LDL cholesterol) that in some cases may be a subgroup of familial combined hyperlipidemia. The activity of LPL in adipose tissue is increased in response to insulin and is reduced by fasting.[38] The activity of LPL increases in breast tissue during lactation, and this enzyme facilitates the provision of free fatty acids to this tissue. Lipoprotein lipase deficiency has been associated with a reduced content of essential fatty acids in breast milk.[39] LPL has an LRP binding site that facilitates LPL-mediated delivery of lipolytically modified triglyceride-rich lipoproteins to LRP for cellular uptake and catabolism. Binding of LPL to extracellular proteoglycans is also involved in this process.

Hepatic Lipase (HL)

Hepatic lipase is a distinct lipolytic enzyme consisting of 477 amino acids that is synthesized in hepatocytes and can be released into plasma by intravenous injection of heparin.[40] HL does not require an apoprotein activator, in contrast to LPL, and appears to function in the hydrolysis of triglycerides and phospholipids present in VLDL and VLDL remnant particles, possibly enhancing their conversion to LDL. HL also facilitates uptake of remnant particles in a process that probably involves binding of HL to cell surface proteoglycans. HL also hydrolyzes triglyceride and phospholipid in HDL particles, and in concert with transfer proteins modulates the size and level of HDL particles in plasma.[41] Deficiency of HL has been associated with the accumulation of small triglyceride-rich VLDL particles in plasma as well as an increase in the concentration of HDL_2.[42] Kinetic studies of VLDL metabolism in a patient with hepatic lipase deficiency have indicated that the deficiency results in impaired conversion of small VLDL particles into LDL but that the initial delipidation of VLDL is normal.[43] These studies indicate that LPL and HL play complementary roles in the intravascular catabolism of triglyceride-rich lipoproteins and modulation of HDL particle composition and metabolic fate. The results of recent studies indicate that HL facilitates SR-B1 mediated uptake of cholesteryl esters from HDL particles in a process that requires both the proteoglycan binding capacity and lipolytic activity of HL.[44]

Endothelial Lipase (EL)

Endothelial lipase is a recently discovered member of the triglyceride lipase family.[44B] The other members of this family are pancreatic lipase, LPL, and HL. As its name implies, EL is synthesized by endothelial cells, but it also is synthesized by macrophages, hepatocytes, and other cell types. EL is predominantly a phospholipase, in contrast to LPL which is predominantly a triglyceride lipase, and HL which has both phospholipase and triglyceride lipase activity. EL enzymatic activity is not dependent on apo-C-II or any other serum factor for activity. EL may be involved in HDL metabolism, placental lipid metabolism, and the generation of fatty acids from lipoprotein phospholipids for energy utilization.

Cholesteryl Ester Transfer Protein (CETP)

Cholesteryl ester transfer protein mediates the transfer of cholesteryl esters from HDL particles to VLDL, with a reciprocal transfer of triglycerides from VLDL to HDL.[45] Deficiency of CETP has been associated with marked increases in the plasma concentrations of HDL cholesterol, and this deficiency supports the view that CETP is important in the normal physiology of lipid transport.[46] CETP activity has been shown to be increased in hypertriglyceridemia and in patients with diabetes or hypothyroidism but is decreased in response to alcohol consumption.[45] Whether reductions in CETP activity, which may lead to increases in HDL cholesterol, should be viewed as beneficial is unclear, as patients with CETP deficiency appear to have an increased risk of CHD.[46B]

Phospholipid Transfer Protein (PLTP)

Phospholipid transfer protein is a member of the lipopolysaccharide binding/lipid transfer protein family that includes CETP, lipopolysaccharide-binding protein (LBP), and bacteriocidal/permeability-increasing protein (BPI). This hydrophobic glycoprotein is partially associated with HDL particles in plasma,[47] where it is a major modulator of HDL metabolism. Two lipid-binding pockets in PLTP participate in the transfer of phospholipid between lipoproteins in a process that is still not well understood. During lipolysis of triglyceride-rich lipoproteins by LPL, PLTP may mediate the transfer of phospholipids to the surface of nascent HDL particles. PLTP may also facilitate the recycling of HDL_3 back to discoidal HDL (which are the best acceptors of cholesterol in the initial steps of reverse cholesterol transport) in a process that may involve transfer of phospholipids from one HDL particle to another. It has been suggested that PLTP has antiatherogenic properties.[48]

Lipoprotein Metabolism

Chylomicrons

Chylomicrons are synthesized by the small intestine, principally the jejunum, in response to the absorption of dietary fat. After a fat-rich meal, lipids are hydrolyzed in the intestinal lumen; the digestive products are then absorbed and utilized in the synthesis of triglycerides, cholesteryl esters, and phospholipids within the mucosal cell. Synthesis of apoproteins A-I, A-II, A-IV, and B-48 and possibly some C and E apoproteins occurs concurrently, and the resultant chylomicron particle is subsequently released from the mucosal cell into the lacteals, from where it progresses to enter the systemic circulation via the thoracic duct. Fatty acids with a chain length less than 12 carbon atoms are transported in the portal blood.

Upon entry into the systemic circulation, chylomicrons are metabolized rapidly with a half-life of 5 to 15 min. Transfer of apo-A-I and A-II to HDL and reciprocal transfers of C and E apoproteins from HDL serve to enhance the hydrolysis of chylomicron triglycerides by LPL and provide a source of chylomicron surface components that act as a precursor of nascent HDL particles. Hydrolysis of chylomicron triglycerides by this enzyme occurs at the endothelial cell surface and results in chylomicron remnants that are relatively enriched in cholesterol. These particles are taken up by the liver via a specific apo-E receptor, probably LRP,[27] but this uptake may also involve the apo-B or LDL receptor. As was previously discussed, apo-E is the apoprotein responsible for receptor-mediated clearance of chylomicron (and VLDL) remnants by the liver. Such uptake results in an increased hepatic cholesterol content and is associated with a decrease in de novo cholesterol synthesis.

Very Low Density Lipoproteins

The liver is the major site of synthesis of VLDL, with a minor contribution being derived from the intestine. Transport of endogenous triglyceride from the liver to peripheral tissues is probably the principal function of VLDL, but it also serves as the major precursor of LDL (Fig. 21-4). Many factors, including thc basal diet; time of day; levels of insulin, glucagon, and epinephrine in plasma; and degree of adiposity, appear to modulate the rate of secretion of hepatic VLDL. Apo-B-100 appears to be essential for VLDL synthesis. Like chylomicrons, newly secreted VLDL rapidly acquire some C and possibly E apoproteins from HDL in plasma. The acquisition of apo-C-II by VLDL particles facilitates their subsequent hydrolysis by LPL. Clearance of VLDL is slower than that of chylomicrons, and their half-life in plasma is normally 6 to 12 h. Hydrolysis of VLDL triglycerides and phospholipids by LPL and HL results in a progressively smaller particle with lower S_f but with a constant content of one apoprotein B-100 molecule per VLDL particle. The content of C and E apoproteins in VLDL, however, decreases as the particle is metabolized, as a consequence of transfer of these apoproteins back to HDL. The catabolism of VLDL remnant particles by the liver is facilitated by their binding to high-affinity LDL receptors, as well as to proteoglycans and the LDL receptor–related protein (LRP),[27,28] as shown in

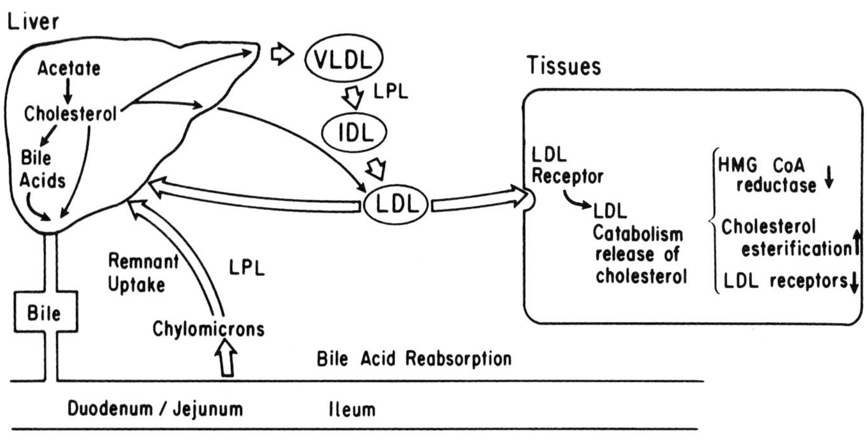

FIGURE 21-4. Metabolism and transport of lipoproteins in humans and the cellular changes that result from receptor-mediated uptake of low-density lipoproteins.

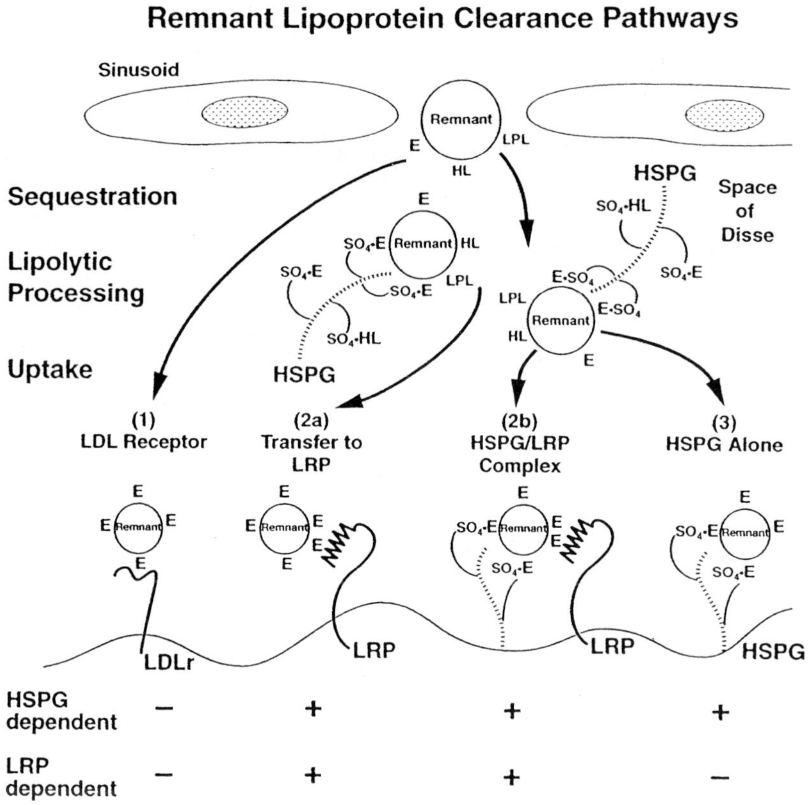

FIGURE 21-5. Three major pathways for hepatic uptake of VLDL remnant particles via the LDL receptor, LRP, and heparan sulfate proteoglycans. (*Reproduced from Mahley et al.*[28])

Fig. 21-5. In this model, there are 3 major catabolic pathways for partially lipolyzed VLDL (and chylomicron) remnant particles. Some particles may bind via apo E to the LDL receptor or LRP for subsequent hepatic uptake. Apo B-100 in VLDL, but not chylomicrons (which contain apo B-48), may also serve as a ligand for binding to the LDL receptor. The 2 other catabolic pathways involve binding of remnant particles to heparan sulfate proteoglycans, which may lead directly to receptor-independent uptake of remnant particles or their subsequent delivery to LRP for LRP-mediated uptake.

The importance of apo E in the catabolism of VLDL particles is apparent in patients with apo-E variants, such as apo E-2, that have reduced affinity for receptor binding. Such patients have a defect in VLDL clearance that can produce type III hyperlipidemia in the setting of overproduction of triglyceride-rich lipoproteins. HDL functions as a reservoir for C apoproteins, which are transferred between VLDL and HDL in a process that economizes the use of C apoproteins and prolongs their half-life in plasma. In normolipidemic humans, virtually all the apoprotein B that enters plasma as a constituent of VLDL is preserved as the particle is metabolized to intermediate-density lipoproteins (IDL) and eventually to LDL. In contrast, in patients with severe hypertriglyceridemia, most of the VLDL particles are removed before conversion to LDL, and LDL concentrations are low. In addition to apo-B, a considerable proportion of the phospholipid, free cholesterol, and some of the cholesteryl esters of the plasma VLDL are retained during metabolism of VLDL to LDL. This precursor-product relation between VLDL and LDL may be seen clinically in patients with type IV hyperlipidemia who are treated with either diet or drugs. In such cases, initial falls in VLDL are not uncommonly accompanied by reciprocal rises in LDL.

Low-Density Lipoproteins

In humans, most of the LDL in plasma are derived from the intravascular catabolism of VLDL; LDL may therefore be regarded as the end product of VLDL metabolism (Fig. 21-4). Catabolism of LDL occurs in both peripheral cells and the liver (the liver is the major site of removal) and is facilitated by both receptor-mediated and non-receptor–mediated pathways.[49,50] The turnover of LDL is considerably slower than that of VLDL; the half-life in normal humans is from 3 to 4 days and is prolonged in patients with familial hypercholesterolemia. Based largely on the elegant studies of Goldstein and Brown, a variety of cells have been shown to contain specific receptors for LDL.[49,50] The uptake of LDL by cells results in suppression of endogenous cholesterol biosynthesis, an enhanced rate of intracellular cholesterol esterification, and a reduction in the number of high-affinity LDL receptors expressed on the cell surface (Fig. 21-6). Functional high-affinity LDL receptors are absent from the cells of most patients with homozygous familial hypercholesterolemia. Although the liver is quantitatively the most important organ for the removal of LDL from plasma, the *relative* rate of uptake is greatest in certain endocrine tissues (e.g., adrenal cortex and corpus luteum of the ovary) that have a high capacity for the synthesis of steroid hormones for which cholesterol contained in LDL serves as an important precursor.[51,52] Clinical and epidemiologic studies have shown a strong positive relation between elevated levels of LDL cholesterol and an increased risk of cardiovascular morbidity and mortality.

High-Density Lipoproteins

The synthesis and secretion of HDL from the liver are well documented.[53] In addition, some HDL particles are also derived from the surface components of chylomicrons and VLDL particles during lipolysis (Fig. 21-7). This dual etiology for HDL explains

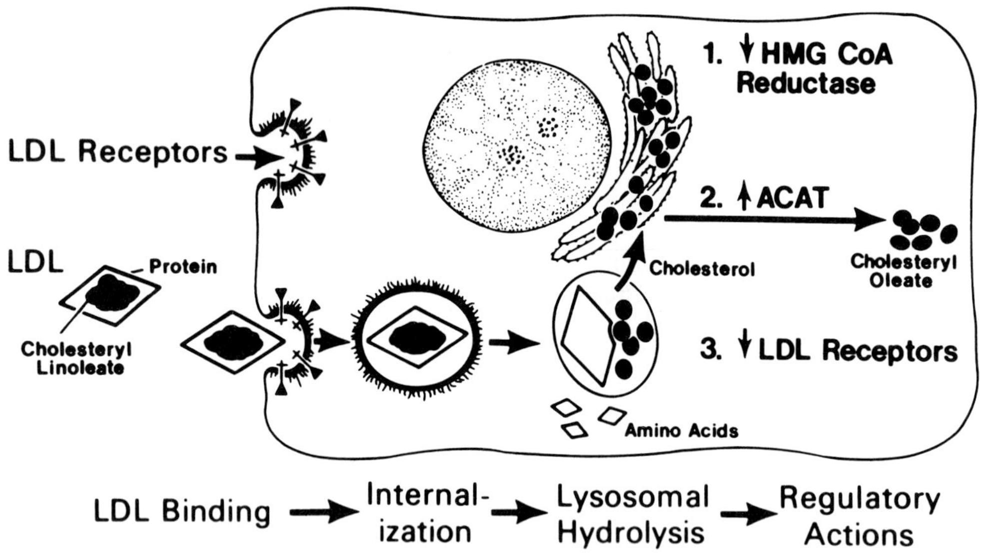

FIGURE 21-6. Sequential steps in the pathway of LDL metabolism in cultured human fibroblasts. The central role of the LDL receptor in controlling the binding, uptake, lysosomal hydrolysis, and regulation of cholesterol synthesis and cholesteryl ester formation is illustrated. (*Reproduced from Goldstein and Brown*[67] *with permission.*)

the inverse correlation between plasma triglycerides and HDL as well as the known presence of HDL in patients with abetalipoproteinemia (who do not form chylomicrons and VLDL). Newly secreted HDL appears as flat, disk-shaped structures containing predominantly protein, phospholipid, and free cholesterol. Discoidal HDL particles are believed to acquire cholesterol from peripheral cells via binding of apo A-I to the ABC-1 receptor. ABC-1-mediated efflux of cholesterol from peripheral tissues may be a major source of plasma HDL cholesterol. When cholesterol-loaded nascent HDL particles are exposed to the action of LCAT, these particles are converted to spherical particles that are enriched in cholesteryl esters. Indeed, the formation of cholesteryl esters in plasma catalyzed by LCAT appears to be an important function of HDL, which may help to create a concentration gradient that favors removal of cholesterol from peripheral tissues in the process of reverse cholesterol transport. HDL also provides a reservoir for C apoproteins, which transfer to chylomicrons and VLDL during alimentary lipemia and subsequently move back to HDL during hydrolysis of triglycerides in larger triglyceride-rich particles in plasma. The half-life of HDL, as assessed by that of apo-A-I and A-II, is from 4 to 6 days and is influenced by both diet and drugs. Thus, diets high in carbohydrate that raise VLDL cause a lowering of HDL and an enhanced HDL turnover. Thus, the modest drop in HDL cholesterol after low-fat feeding may be an indication of a beneficial increase in the flux of HDL cholesterol from peripheral tissues to the liver. Nicotinic acid depresses VLDL synthesis, raises HDL cholesterol concentrations, and prolongs the half-life of HDL. Both effects on HDL metabolism probably are a consequence of changes in both the synthesis of VLDL and the catabolic rate of HDL[54] and support the general view that VLDL (and triglyceride) and HDL levels change reciprocally. The major sites of HDL catabolism are the liver and kidney. Hepatic catabolism of HDL is mediated by selective uptake of HDL cholesteryl esters via the SR-B1 receptor in the liver and steroidogenic organs. Renal catabolism of HDL may be mediated by cubulin, as described later. Glomset and Norum[13] have proposed that a major function of HDL is to transport cholesterol from peripheral tissues back to the liver.[13] Thus, high levels of HDL, with normal delivery of

FIGURE 21-7. Diagrammatic representation of the origin and intravascular metabolism of high-density lipoproteins.

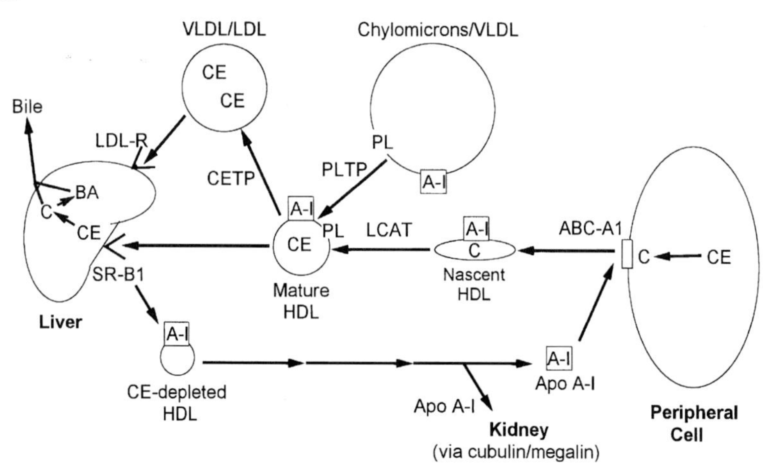

HDL lipids to the liver (and kidney), may enhance removal of cholesterol from tissues, including the arterial wall, and protect against the development of atherosclerosis. Several factors have been shown to increase the concentrations of HDL in plasma,[55,56] and fluctuations in total HDL concentrations are sometimes due to alterations in the levels of the predominant HDL_2 subfraction. Variations in the concentration of HDL_2 also show the strongest inverse correlation with cardiovascular risk. Thus, increased concentrations of HDL_2 are viewed as protective, whereas low concentrations may be detrimental,[57] but the results of other studies indicate that the total HDL and HDL_3 concentrations also correlate with cardiovascular risk. Factors that have been shown to increase the concentrations of HDL include moderate ethanol consumption,[56] sustained regular exercise, correction of hypertriglyceridemia, and certain drugs, such as phenobarbital, phenytoin, clofibrate, estrogens, nicotinic acid, and gemfibrozil.[55,57,58] Statin drugs also have a modest HDL-raising effect. Decreases in the plasma concentrations of HDL may be seen in association with weight gain, cigarette smoking, hypertriglyceridemia, and the use of probucol.

Lipoprotein(a)

The precise steps involved in production of Lp(a) are still uncertain, but several lines of evidence suggest that Lp(a) is formed in plasma as a consequence of a two-step process involving the association of circulating free apo(a) with LDL. Apo(a) may initially bind noncovalently to an LDL particle, but subsequently forms a covalent disulfide linkage between a free cysteine residue in kringle 4-36 of apo(a) and a cysteine residue in the C-terminal region of the apo B-100 molecule on LDL. The resulting disulfide bond is subsequently stable unless it is cleaved by chemical reduction.

The almost exclusive site of apo(a) synthesis is the liver,[59] which secretes apo(a) into plasma. In the absence of acceptor LDL particles, apo(a) circulates free of lipoproteins, but under normal circumstances more than 95 percent of apo(a) in plasma becomes bound to circulating LDL particles to form Lp(a). The rate of synthesis of Lp(a) appears to be the predominant determinant of plasma Lp(a) concentrations.[60]

The pathways for clearance of Lp(a) from plasma remain unclear. Although Lp(a) binds to and is internalized by the LDL receptor, the LDL receptor pathway probably does not contribute to a great extent to catabolism of plasma Lp(a). This conclusion is supported by the observation that factors that increase LDL receptor activity (e.g., treatment with HMG-CoA reductase inhibitors) or decrease LDL receptor activity (e.g., the genetic disorder familial hypercholesterolemia or hypothyroidism) do not appreciably influence plasma concentrations of Lp(a), in contrast to the association of these conditions with marked changes in LDL cholesterol concentrations.

Plasma Lp(a) concentrations are not significantly influenced by body mass index, weight loss, exercise, age (in adults), or diet-composition, except for the Lp(a)-raising effects of trans fatty acids.[61,62] Plasma Lp(a) concentrations may increase 15 to 50 percent after menopause,[63] but may be reduced by administration of estrogen replacement therapy. Chronic renal failure and proteinuria are associated with markedly increased plasma Lp(a) concentrations, which are one of many atherogenic changes associated with renal disease. In addition to treatment with estrogen, plasma Lp(a) concentrations can be lowered by treatment with niacin, anabolic steroids, and plasma exchange or LDL apheresis. Although niacin can be used in many patients to achieve modest lowering of Lp(a) concentrations, treatment to reduce plasma LDL cholesterol concentrations may be a more important endeavor in patients with elevated Lp(a) and high risk of atherosclerosis. This suggestion is supported by several lines of evidence. First, elevated plasma Lp(a) concentrations may not be associated with atherogenesis if the LDL cholesterol concentration is low (<80–100 mg/dl). Second, aggressive lowering of plasma LDL cholesterol concentrations in the Familial Atherosclerosis Treatment Study eliminated the association between Lp(a) concentrations and cardiac events and disease progression.[64] Third, lowering LDL cholesterol and Lp(a) concentrations with LDL apheresis had no added benefit in prevention of coronary artery lesion progression compared to treatment with an HMG-CoA reductase alone or in combination with a bile acid sequestrant, which lowered plasma concentrations of LDL cholesterol, but not Lp(a).[65,66] Thus, the primary therapeutic goal in patients with high concentrations of Lp(a) may be to aggressively lower plasma LDL cholesterol concentrations.

Free Fatty Acids

Free fatty acids (FFA) constitute the fifth class of lipoproteins. They consist of long-chain fatty acids bound to albumin, occupying up to two high-affinity binding sites on the albumin molecule; if FFA levels are elevated, additional lower affinity binding sites are then occupied. FFA constitute a major metabolic fuel of the body. They are derived in part from lipolysis of triglycerides stored in the adipose tissue cell. The tissue lipase in these cells is under neuroendocrine control and operates through the adenyl cyclase system. A second origin of FFA is through the hydrolysis of plasma triglyceride present in chylomicrons and VLDL through the action of LPL.

FFA have a very short half-life of 4 to 8 min and are readily taken up from plasma by the muscle cells of the body. A second pathway for their catabolism is uptake by the liver and resynthesis into triglyceride, which then may be transported from the liver in VLDL, or oxidation to acetyl CoA. Physiologically, FFA levels may rise and fall in the blood with great rapidity in order to meet the body's needs for this form of energy. Levels tend to be low after the absorption of carbohydrate associated with increased insulin secretion but rise postprandially as blood glucose falls. In the fasting state, levels of 400 to 600 μEq/L are common; with a prolonged fast of 24 to 72 h, the levels of FFA may range from 1,000 to 1,500 μEq/L. Glucagon, epinephrine, growth hormone, and adrenocorticotropic hormone (ACTH) may also increase FFA levels. The major physiologic regulators of the plasma FFA are insulin and epinephrine.

The chief fatty acids of the plasma FFA fraction are oleic, palmitic, linoleic, and stearic acids, which reflect in most instances the composition of the adipose tissue triglyceride. Three of these four fatty acids (oleic, palmitic, and stearic acids) may be synthesized by the body from acetate. Linoleic acid is unique in being an essential fatty acid that cannot be synthesized in humans but is necessary for the body's growth and for membrane formation. The syndrome of essential fatty acid deficiency results when linoleic acid accounts for less than 1 percent of the total calories in the diet, as occurs after prolonged total parenteral nutrition. Linoleic acid is of special importance as the precursor substance for arachidonic acid, which in turn has multitudinous functions, of which a most important one is as a precursor for prostaglandin formation. Linolenic (18:3) and other omega-3 fatty acids are also components of adipose tissue and the plasma FFA. Deficiency states of omega-3 fatty acids occur with fat-free diets. Linolenic

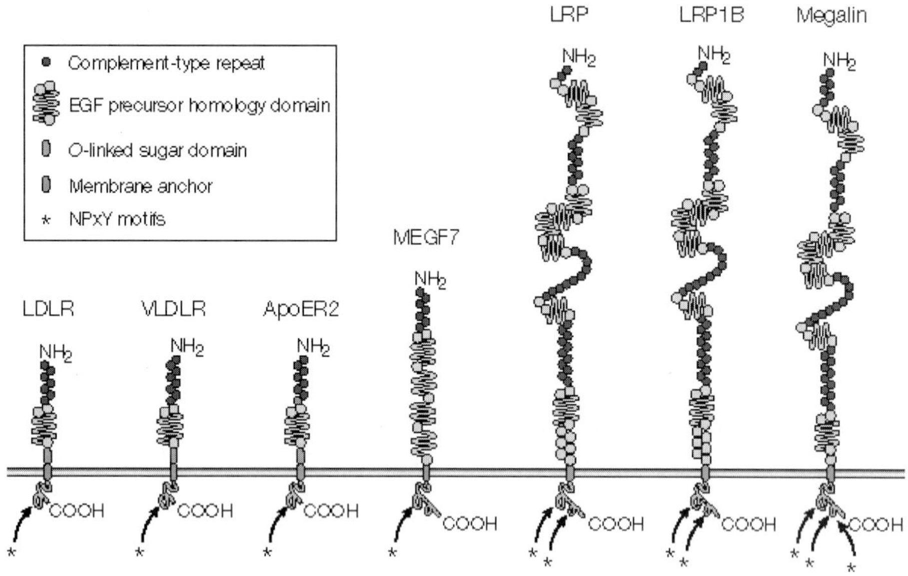

FIGURE 21-8. Members of the LDL receptor family that are expressed in mammals. (*Adapted from Herz and Beffert.*[68])

acid is the substrate for the synthesis of eicosapentaenoic acid and docosahexaenoic acid of this series, which are important in membrane formation, especially for the brain and retina, and in eicosanoid metabolism.

Lipoprotein Receptors

Our understanding of lipoprotein physiology has been greatly expanded as a consequence of the identification and sequencing of a multitude of lipoprotein receptors during the last decade. The traditional LDL-receptor,[67] previously thought to be a unique receptor, is now regarded as a member of the growing LDL-receptor gene family (Fig. 21-8). Members of this receptor family that are expressed in mammals include the LDL receptor, VLDL receptor, apo E receptor 2(Apo ER 2; also known as LR8B and neuro apo E receptor), MEGF7, LDL receptor-related protein (LRP), (LRPIB), and megalin/gp330.[68] Vitellogenin is another member of the family that is expressed in a smaller form in birds and in a larger form with an additional EGF-precursor domain in insects. LRP is a multifunctional receptor that binds a variety of ligands. Although its primary role in lipoprotein metabolism may be the apo E-mediated binding and uptake of remnant lipoproteins, LRP also mediates uptake of LPL, α_2-macroglobulin-endoproteinase complexes, plasminogen activator inhibitor (PAI) complexes, tissue-type plasminogen activator (tPA), lactoferrin, and other substrates. All members of the LDL receptor family bind apo E, as well as other receptor-specific ligands. Binding of remnant lipoproteins to LRP is facilitated by binding to adjacent proteoglycans, which is followed by coated pit-mediated endocytosis of LRP-remnant lipoprotein complexes (Fig. 21-5). LRP, the VLDL receptor, Apo ER2, and megalin also are expressed in the central nervous system (CNS), where they appear to serve essential roles brain development and neuronal signaling. In the CNS, the VLDL-receptor and apo ER2 also bind Roelin, a large extracellular matrix protein that controls neuronal migration and positioning. Polymorphisms in LRP and α_2-macroglobulin, a ligand for LRP, may be associated with late onset Alzheimer's disease. Apo E4, another ligand for members of the LDL receptor family, is associated with early onset Alzheimer's disease. Megalin mediates endocytic uptake of retinolds and steroids. LR11, which was named for the presence of 11 ligand-binding repeats. LR11 appears to be a new 250 kDa LDL receptor that is expressed in brain, where it may mediate uptake of apo E-containing lipoproteins,[69–71] but also is expressed by smooth muscle cells in atheromatous lesions. LR11 is not a core member of the LDL receptor family.

As the name implies, members of the scavenger receptor family generally facilitate the uptake and degradation of modified lipoproteins, a variety of other biomolecules, and apoptotic and senescent cells. Class A scavenger receptors consist of a trimeric

FIGURE 21-9. The predicted structures of macrophage class A scavenger receptors, types I and II. Roman numerals indicate domains I–VI. Numbers in parentheses indicate number of amino acids in each domain. SRCR = scavenger receptor cysteine-rich domain (absent in type II receptor); TM = transmembrane domain. (*Reproduced from Krieger.*[72])

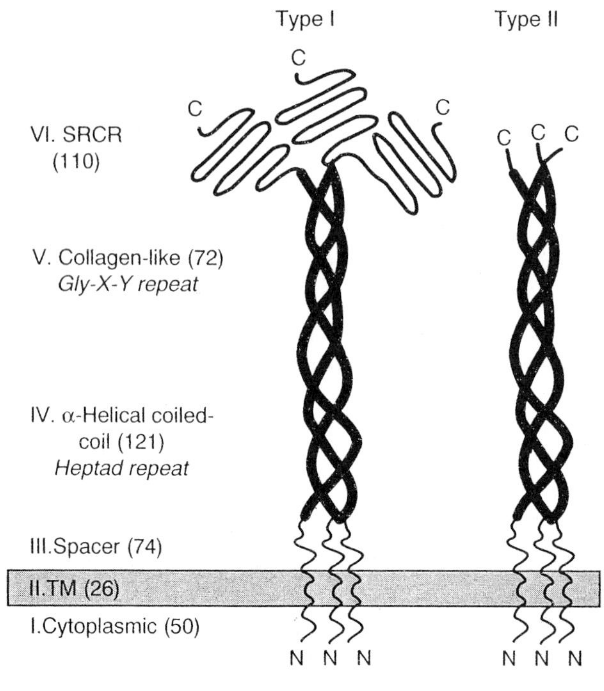

complex composed of 6 domains. On the basis of the extracellular C-terminal structure, Class A scavenger receptors have been classified into types I (SR-AI) and II (SR-AII)[72] (Fig. 21-9). The major site of expression of SR-AI and SR-AII in vivo appears to be tissue macrophages. These receptors bind both acetylated LDL and oxidized LDL, as well as a wide variety of other polyanionic molecules and molecular complexes.

Class B scavenger receptors include CD36, an 88 kDa glycoprotein that may play a major role in macrophage receptor-mediated uptake of oxidized LDL. Additional members of this class include scavenger receptor class B, type I (SR-BI), which was recently cloned by Krieger and colleagues,[73] and an SR-BI splicing variant, SR-BII. Both CD36 and SR-BI bind acetylated LDL and oxidized LDL, but not the broad spectrum of polyanionic molecules that bind to class A receptors. In contrast to CD36, SR-BI is expressed primarily in the liver, gonads, and adrenals. SR-BI also binds native LDL and HDL, and is believed to serve in the important role of a key HDL receptor that mediates selective uptake of HDL-derived cholesteryl ester by the liver and steroidogenic tissues.[74] The human cutaneous lymphocyte antigen-1 (CLA-1) is the human analogue of the rodent SR-B1.

Class C macrophage scavenger receptors (SR-CI) also have been recently described in *Drosophila melanogaster*, but their possible role in humans is unknown. A variety of other candidate macrophage receptors for oxidized LDL have been described, such as FcγRII-B2 (an Fc receptor), macrosialin (CD68), and lectin-like oxidized LDL receptor-1 (LOX-1).

There are currently 3 main members of the HDL receptor family (Fig. 21-10), which are structurally and genetically unrelated proteins. These receptors are SR-BI, cubulin, and ABC-1. The newest member of the family is ATP-binding cassette transporter-1 (ABC-1), a 2,201-amino acid protein that appears to be the major receptor responsible for removal of cholesterol from peripheral tissues by nascent HDL particles.[75–77] ABC-1 also is referred to as ABC subfamily A, member 1 (ABCA-1). Because deficiency of ABC-1 is associated with markedly reduced plasma concentrations of HDL cholesterol,[78] ABC-1 may also be a major mediator of the formation of new HDL particles from circulating apo A-I and peripheral tissue-derived cholesterol. In this role, ABC-1 appears to be the starting point of the process of reverse cholesterol transport. ABC-1 is a member of the large ABC family of more than 30 transporter proteins that share the characteristic of utilizing ATP hydrolysis as a source of energy to facilitate transmembrane transport of various substances. Examples of other diseases that are caused by ABC mutations include cystic fibrosis, some forms of retinitis pigmentosa, multidrug resistance syndrome, inherited immune deficiencies, macular degeneration, adrenoleukodystrophy, intrahepatic cholestasis, peroxisomal dysfunction, and persistent hyperinsulinemic hypoglycemia of infancy. The ABC-1 receptor was initially cloned in 1994 in relation to studies of apoptosis, but its role as an HDL receptor and the defective Tangier disease gene was unrecognized until recently.[79–81] Mutations in the ABC-1 gene are the cause of the rare autosomal recessive HDL deficiency syndrome, Tangier disease,[75,76] as well as more common autosomal dominant familial hypoalphalipoproteinemia syndromes.[78] Thirty-six mutations in the ABC-1 gene have been reported to date.

The results of recent studies have indicated that ABC-1 also is involved in modulation of cholesterol absorption from the gut,[81B] which may facilitate disposal of excess cholesterol that is delivered to the liver during reverse cholesterol transport. Upregulation of ABC-1 in the gut appears to allow enterocytes to export absorbed cholesterol back into the intestinal lumen, thereby reducing net absorption of cholesterol. Accumulation of cholesterol in the liver, as a result of reverse cholesterol transport, also increases CYP7A1-mediated bile acid synthesis and concurrently increases excretion of hepatic cholesterol into the intestinal lumen. The expression of ABC-1 in the gut and in peripheral cells (e.g., macrophages) is under the regulatory influence of heterodimers of two nuclear hormone receptors, retinoid X receptors (RXR) and liver X (oxysterol) receptors (LXR).[81B] Expression of the rate limiting enzyme for bile acid synthesis in the liver, CYP7A1, is modulated by heterodimers of RXR and farnesoid X (bile acid) receptors (FXR).[81B]

SR-BI, which is described earlier, is believed to mediate the selective uptake of HDL cholesteryl ester (and other lipids) by the liver (and to a lessor extent by the gonads and adrenals) at the hypothetical terminus of the reverse cholesterol transport pathway.

Cubulin (also historically designated as gp280) is the established receptor that mediates uptake of intrinsic factor-vitamin B12 complexes in the gut.[82] Cubulin is a 460,000 Mr protein consisting of 27 C-terminal C1r/C1s Uegf Bmp1 (CUB) domains, 8 epidermal growth factor (EGF) repeats, and a short amino terminal region with a putative amphipathic helix structure (Fig. 21-10). It is coexpressed with megalin, a 600,000 Mr member of the LDL receptor family, and is localized in coated pits, endosomes, and recycling vesicles.

FIGURE 21-10. Members of the HDL receptor "family," which are genetically and structurally distinct proteins.

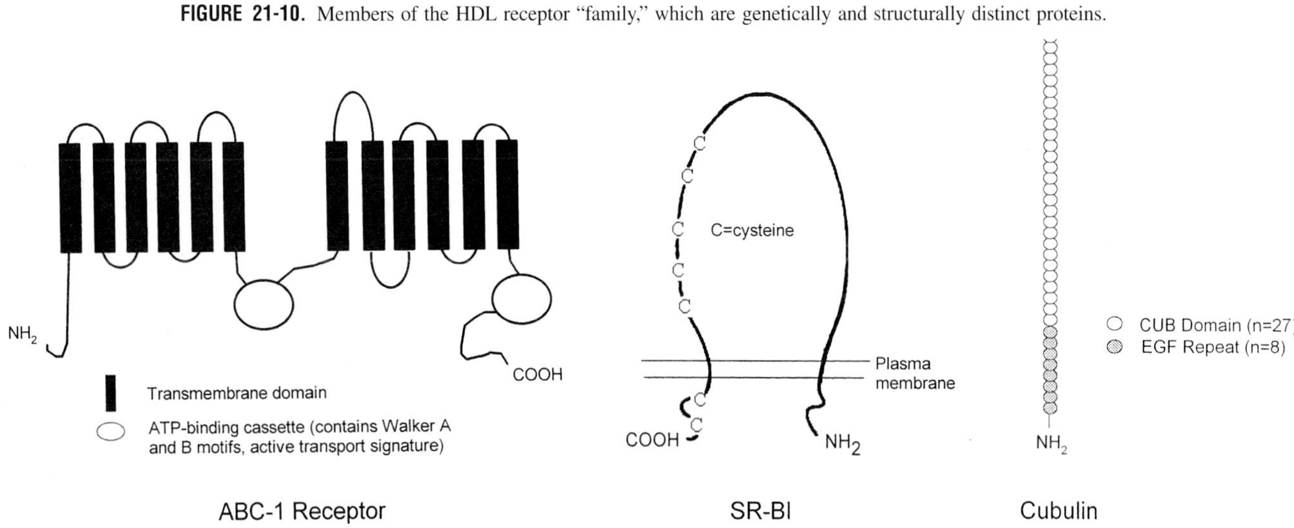

TABLE 21-5. Relative Atherogenicity of Individual Lipoprotein Particles

Lipoprotein	Atherogenicity	Typical Associated Dyslipoproteinemia
Chylomicrons (lipoprotein lipase deficiency)	0	Type I
VLDL	+	Type IV (familial hypertriglyceridemia)
Chylomicron and VLDL remnants	+++	Type III (dysbetalipoproteinemia)
LDL	++++	Type II (familial hypercholesterolemia)
Lp(a)	++++	Various
HDL	Negatively correlated with atherosclerosis	Familial hyperalphalipoproteinemia

The results of recent studies have indicated that cubulin also is a novel receptor for endocytosis of HDL and apo A-I.[83,84] Although cubulin is expressed in a variety of epithelial cells, the major site of cubulin-mediated HDL and apo A-I catabolism appears to be in the kidney, primarily in the proximal tubule. Because only filtered proteins and particles would have access to cubulin in this site, cubulin may primarily mediate uptake of free apo A-I and small filterable HDL particles. Cubulin is also expressed in syncytiotrophoblasts in the early human placenta, where it might mediate uptake of HDL.

A novel apo B-48 receptor (apoB48R), which appears to mediate uptake of chylomicrons and/or chylomicron remnants was recently cloned.[85] The expression of this receptor in foam cells in human atherosclerotic lesions suggests that the apoB48R may play a role in the putative atherogenic effects of postprandial lipemia.

Atherogenicity of Individual Lipoprotein Particles

The lipoprotein particles in human plasma all contain cholesterol, but the extent to which elevated levels of each of these particles may contribute to the development of atherosclerosis differs widely (Table 21-5). Increased plasma concentrations of LDL, Lp(a), and cholesterol-rich remnant particles, the latter of which accumulate in the plasma of patients with type III hyperlipidemia, are all highly atherogenic,[8,9,11,29] whereas increased levels of HDL cholesterol appear to afford protection from atherosclerosis.[57]

Plasma concentrations of the major LDL apoprotein (apoprotein B) may provide a better prediction of the risk of coronary artery disease than does measurement of LDL cholesterol.[86] Similarly, plasma concentrations of the major HDL apoproteins (A-I and A-II) may be better discriminators for cardiovascular risk associated with low concentrations of HDL particles than are measurements of HDL cholesterol.[86,87] Hyperchylomicronemia as an isolated entity (e.g., that seen in patients with LPL deficiency) does not appear to be associated with an increased risk of atherosclerosis,[88] but concurrent or isolated elevations of VLDL do appear to be moderately atherogenic, as do lipoprotein particles produced from the intravascular hydrolysis of triglycerides from VLDL and chylomicrons.[89]

Modifications in lipoproteins, particularly oxidation of LDL, markedly enhance the uptake of these lipoproteins by macrophages when studied under in vitro conditions[90–92] and lead to foam cell development. It is believed that oxidation of LDL particles occurs in atherosclerotic plaques, but local oxidation of LDL may occur under conditions of endothelial cell injury and potentially under other circumstances in which plasma concentrations of natural antioxidants are reduced. The potential role of modified lipoproteins in the pathogenesis of atherosclerosis in humans is currently a subject of intense research, as is the potential role of antioxidants in the prevention of atherosclerosis.

THE HYPERLIPIDEMIAS

Classification of Hyperlipidemias

Classification of hyperlipidemias on the basis of plasma lipoprotein patterns, as originally proposed by Fredrickson, Levy, and Lees[93] and modified by the WHO,[94] is the most widely used system of nomenclature. As shown in Table 21-6, the six types are classified with respect to increased levels of chylomicrons, VLDL, IDL, and LDL. Although this classification provides a simple way in which to categorize increases in the concentrations of given lipoproteins, it does not provide any information about the etiology of the abnormality. Thus, a given phenotype may occur as a primary genetic disorder or may be secondary to a variety of associated conditions. Similarly, this classification system does not consider variations in HDL concentrations as an independent variable. Despite these limitations, the Fredrickson classification provides a useful basis for describing most hyperlipoproteinemias.

Determination of the plasma concentrations of cholesterol and triglycerides, with a concurrent determination of the concentrations

TABLE 21-6. Classification of Hyperlipidemias Based on Lipoprotein Concentrations

Type	Lipoprotein Abnormality	Lipid Profiles	Typical Values, mg/dl
I	Chylomicrons markedly ↑, VLDL and LDL both normal or low	Chol ↑ Tg ↑↑	320 4000
IIa	LDL ↑, VLDL normal	Chol ↑ Tg N	370 90
IIb	LDL ↑, VLDL ↑	Chol ↑ Tg ↑	350 400
III	Abnormal cholesterol-enriched VLDL remnants (IDL) present in excess	Chol ↑ Tg ↑	500 700
IV	VLDL ↑, LDL normal	Chol N Tg ↑	220 400
V	Chylomicrons markedly ↑, VLDL ↑, LDL normal or low	Chol ↑ Tg ↑↑	700 5000

Source: Based on Fredrickson, Levy, and Lees[93] and the WHO committee.[94]

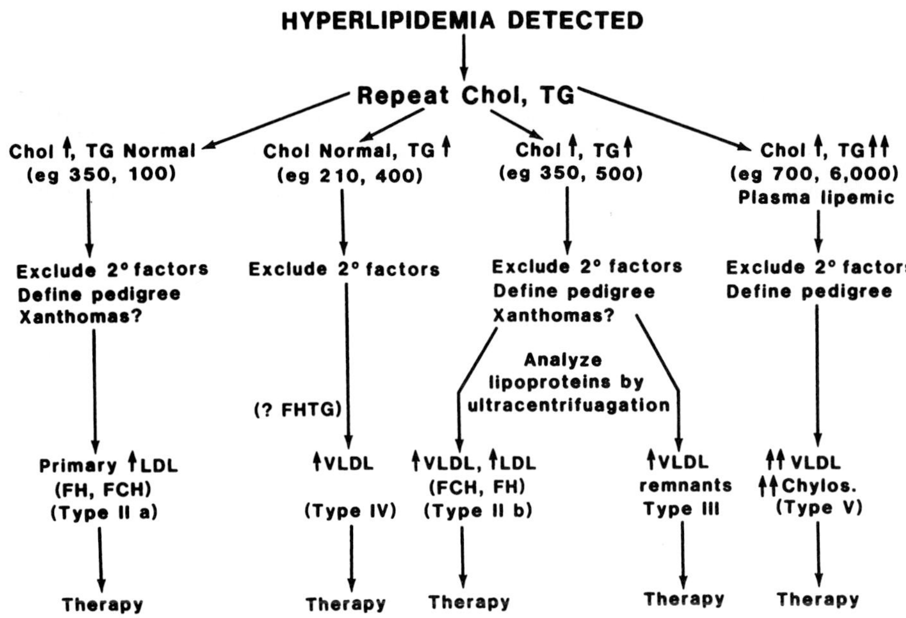

FIGURE 21-11. Algorithm for the progressive characterization and delineation of hyperlipidemia after its initial detection.

of HDL cholesterol, remains the basic lipid profile necessary for the diagnosis of most hyperlipidemias. Despite the fact that a number of dyslipidemias are now characterized on the basis of apoprotein abnormalities, apoprotein measurements are not in routine clinical use and are available only in specialized centers with a major interest in lipoprotein disorders. To avoid the postprandial increase in plasma triglycerides, it is advisable to request that patients fast for 12 to 15 h before venipuncture. In contrast, plasma cholesterol concentrations are minimally affected by eating, and nonfasting blood samples are adequate for the determination of total plasma cholesterol concentrations. The importance of determining plasma lipid and lipoprotein concentrations under steady-state conditions cannot be overemphasized; concentrations of cholesterol and triglyceride both decrease during periods of weight loss and commonly fall for 2 to 3 months after a myocardial infarction.

Hyperlipidemia can be divided into four basic patterns (Fig. 21-11) based on the initial determination of total plasma (or serum), cholesterol, and triglyceride concentrations: (1) hypercholesterolemia with normal concentrations of triglycerides (type IIa phenotype), (2) combined elevation of cholesterol and triglyceride in which the plasma triglyceride concentrations are one to three times higher than the cholesterol concentration (phenotypes IIb and III), (3) a primary elevation of triglycerides in which cholesterol concentrations are normal or only slightly increased (type IV phenotype), and (4) moderately to markedly elevated levels of cholesterol (>300 mg/dl) with a simultaneous marked increase in plasma triglycerides (>1,000 mg/dl) in which the plasma appears lipemic (type I and type V phenotypes). In adult patients, such severe hypertriglyceridemia is invariably associated with increased plasma concentrations of both chylomicrons and VLDL particles. A fifth category of patients with dyslipidemia, who would not be identified on the basis of measurements of cholesterol and triglycerides alone, are patients with very low concentrations of HDL cholesterol who may also be at increased risk for developing coronary artery disease.[95] Disorders associated with variations in the plasma concentrations of HDL will be discussed later in this chapter.

Criteria for the Diagnosis of Hyperlipoproteinemia

In assessing the concentrations of lipids and lipoproteins in a given patient, it is important to consider the age of the patient and be familiar with the average concentrations of lipids and lipoproteins for that age and sex, in addition to the cutpoints recommended by expert panels for potential therapeutic intervention (Table 21-7).[61] Criteria for the diagnosis of hypercholesterolemia, with a particular emphasis on increased concentrations of LDL cholesterol, have been established, but these cutpoints are somewhat arbitrary and take into account the curvilinear relation between increased plasma concentrations of total and LDL cholesterol and the risk of coronary artery disease, which increases substantially when plasma cholesterol concentrations exceed 240 mg/dl or when LDL cholesterol concentrations exceed 160 mg/dl. The relation between serum cholesterol concentrations and the 6-year risk of coronary artery disease in 362,000 men studied in the MRFIT Study is illustrated in Fig. 21-12.[97]

The Consensus Conference on Lowering Blood Cholesterol to Prevent Heart Disease recommended that dietary modifications and potential drug therapy should be considered in adult patients in whom plasma concentrations of total cholesterol exceed the 90th percentile.[98] In this report, moderate hypercholesterolemia was defined as plasma cholesterol concentrations between the 75th and 90th percentiles. More recently, several expert panels in the United States,[99] Europe,[100] the United Kingdom,[101] and Canada[102] have defined more specific cutpoints for the diagnosis of hypercholesterolemia in adults and have made recommendations concerning concentrations of LDL cholesterol above which diet and drug therapy should be considered. The expert panels have concluded that desirable levels of total cholesterol for adults in western societies are under 200 mg/dl, and for most patients in this category further characterization of lipoproteins is not generally advocated. With the caveat that these recommendations will fail to detect patients with atypically low concentrations of HDL cholesterol in whom total cholesterol concentrations remain below

TABLE 21-7. Average Values for Lipids and Lipoproteins in American Men and Women*

Age, years	Total Plasma Cholesterol	LDL Cholesterol	HDL Cholesterol	Total Plasma Triglyceride
		Men		
20–24	162 (212)†	103 (147)	45 (63)	89 (165)
25–29	179 (234)	117 (165)	45 (63)	104 (204)
30–34	193 (258)	126 (185)	46 (63)	122 (253)
35–39	201 (267)	133 (189)	43 (62)	141 (316)
40–44	205 (260)	136 (186)	44 (67)	152 (318)
45–49	213 (275)	144 (202)	45 (64)	143 (279)
50–54	213 (274)	142 (197)	44 (63)	154 (313)
		Women		
20–24	162	98	52	68
25–29	174 (22)	106 (151)	56 (81)	71 (128)
30–34	174 (220)	109 (148)	55 (75)	74 (138)
35–39	186 (251)	119 (173)	56 (82)	89 (174)
40–44	196 (253)	125 (174)	57 (87)	92 (179)
45–49	205 (167)	130 (188)	58 (86)	105 (192)
50–54	222 (292)	145 (214)	60 (89)	112 (214)
55–59	231 (296)	150 (212)	60 (86)	132 (280)

*Data obtained from 11 communities across the United States.[96]

† Values given in milligrams per deciliter are means and 95th percentiles (in parentheses) for white men and women.

200 mg/dl, the latter value is an appropriate goal of therapy for patients who do not have evidence of coronary or peripheral vascular disease and who do not have a family history of premature atherosclerosis.

The Expert Panel of the National Cholesterol Education Program recommended determination of total cholesterol concentrations in serum or plasma for all adult patients in the United States.[99] Further decisions are based on the initial total plasma cholesterol concentrations and take into account the presence or absence of atherosclerosis and other cardiovascular risk factors in determining the recommendations for specific therapy. Measurement of lipoprotein concentrations (LDL and HDL cholesterol) were advocated in patients with known cardiovascular disease or in those with two or more established cardiovascular risk factors in whom total cholesterol levels ranged between 200 and 239 mg/dl and were recommended in all patients in whom initial concentrations of total cholesterol exceeded 240 mg/dl. The NCEP Panel considered desirable concentrations of LDL cholesterol to be <130 mg/dl, borderline elevations to be between 130 and 159 mg/dl, and high-risk concentrations of LDL cholesterol to be greater than 160 mg/dl.[99] Some authorities have recommended an additional classification of "severe hypercholesterolemia" to identify patients in need of the most aggressive intervention.[103] This is illustrated in Table 21-8. The second revision of the NCEP Guidelines was published in 1994.[99]

FIGURE 21-12. Relation between serum cholesterol concentrations and death from coronary artery disease in 361,662 men age 35 to 57 during an average follow-up of 6 years in MRFIT screens. Each point represents a medium value for 5 percent of the population. (*From Ref. 97.*)

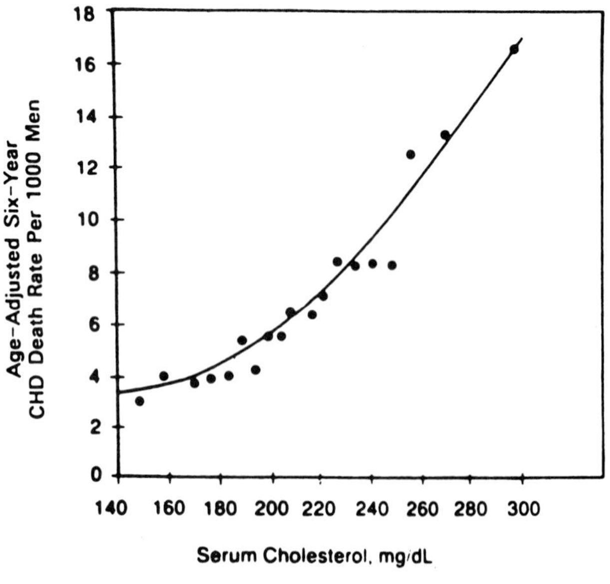

The NCEP Expert Panel has provided recommended thresholds for initiation of diet and drug therapy for elevated concentrations of total and LDL cholesterol (Table 21-9). These recommendations should be considered as guidelines, and in specific patients a more or less aggressive approach may be justified depending on the age, the family history, and the potential benefit to be derived from diet and drug therapy. A particularly aggressive approach is indicated in patients with known coronary atherosclerosis in whom concentrations of LDL cholesterol less than 100 mg/dl may be necessary if no further progression of atherosclerosis and, potentially, some regression are to occur.[104,105] Updated NCEP guidelines are anticipated in 2001.

Despite a broad consensus on the criteria for the diagnosis and potential treatment of hypercholesterolemia, the significance and treatment of isolated hypertriglyceridemia remains controversial.[106,107] Two consensus conferences on hypertriglyceridemia[108,109] have concluded that borderline hypertriglyceridemia occurs in patients with plasma triglyceride concentrations between 250 and 500 mg/dl and that distinct (overt) hypertriglyceridemia occurs in patients in whom triglyceride concentrations exceed 500 mg/dl. Severe hypertriglyceridemia can be considered to be present when plasma triglyceride concentrations exceed 1,000 mg/dl. A significant relation has been observed between hypertriglyceridemia and increased risk for coronary artery disease in some, but not all, stud-

TABLE 21-8. Classification of Plasma Total and LDL Cholesterol

	Total Cholesterol, mg/dl	LDL Cholesterol, mg/dl	Relative CHD Risk
Desirable serum cholesterol	<200	<130	<1.0
Borderline-high serum cholesterol	200–239	130–159	1.0–2.0
High serum cholesterol	>240	>160	
Moderate hypercholesterolemia	240–289	160–209	2.0–4.0
Severe hypercholesterolemia	>290	>210	>4.0

LDL = low density lipoprotein; CHD = coronary heart disease.

Source: Adapted from Grundy.[103]

ies in which multivariate statistical analysis have been performed and in which concentrations of total and LDL cholesterol have been controlled. However, in studies that have also controlled for HDL cholesterol concentrations, this association has often disappeared, particularly in studies involving men. In contrast, studies in women and in patients with diabetes have demonstrated significant positive univariate relations between plasma triglyceride concentrations and the risk for premature development of atherosclerosis.[110] Treatment guidelines for the institution of diet and drug therapy in patients with hypertriglyceridemia have not been precisely formulated, but in the opinion of the authors, dietary therapy is appropriate for patients with triglyceride concentrations that exceed 250 to 300 mg/dl and drug therapy should be considered in patients without cardiovascular disease or diabetes in whom the levels of triglycerides exceed 800 to 1,000 mg/dl, with a goal of therapy being to reduce the increased risk of hepatic steatosis and, potentially, pancreatitis. Drug therapy may also be appropriate in individual patients with more modest degrees of hypertriglyceridemia in the setting of familial combined hyperlipidemia or in patients with known cardiovascular disease who concurrently have low levels of HDL cholesterol. An aggressive approach to the treatment of hypertriglyceridemia in patients with diabetes also appears to be justified, although clinical trials to document benefit from such therapy have not been conducted.

The recent report of the expert panel on blood cholesterol levels in children and adolescents has defined concentrations of total and LDL cholesterol that should be considered as acceptable, borderline, and high.[111] Acceptable concentrations of total and LDL cholesterol were defined as less than 170 and 110 mg/dl, respectively, and borderline elevations were considered to be present when the total cholesterol ranged between 170 and 199 mg/dl, with LDL values between 110 and 129 mg/dl, whereas hypercholesterolemia was considered to be present in children whose total plasma cholesterol concentrations exceeded 200 mg/dl and in whom LDL exceeded 130 mg/dl. The panel did not establish guidelines for the diagnosis of hypertriglyceridemia. The pediatric panel recommended that dietary therapy be the mainstay of treatment in children but that drug therapy be considered in children age 10 years or older in whom, after adequate trials of dietary therapy, LDL cholesterol concentrations remained greater than 190 mg/dl in children with fewer than two cardiovascular risk factors or greater than 160 mg/dl in those with a strongly positive family history of coronary artery disease or two or more risk factors. In the opinion of the authors, these guidelines for drug therapy are too aggressive and, if widely instituted, would lead to the excessive use of lipid-lowering drugs in this population. We believe that additional factors, including the sex of the child (treat boys more aggressively than girls) and plasma concentrations of Lp(a), should be taken into consideration before the institution of drug therapy in children whose LDL cholesterol concentrations remain less than 220 to 250 mg/dl on dietary therapy.

In addition to criteria for the diagnosis of hyperlipidemia in children and adults, the NCEP panel and the recent Consensus Conference on Hypertriglyceridemia have both recommended that concentrations of HDL cholesterol, below 35 mg/dl should be considered abnormally low. Hygienic measures are the cornerstone of therapy for patients with low concentrations of HDL cholesterol, which frequently coexists with hypertriglyceridemia. Current data do not support the use of drugs aimed solely at increasing plasma concentrations of HDL cholesterol in the absence of concurrent elevated levels of LDL cholesterol or, in selected patients, hypertriglyceridemia.

Secondary Hyperlipidemias

Dietary

The majority of hyperlipidemias in western societies are secondary to predisposing conditions. Among the secondary

TABLE 21-9. Treatment Decisions Based on LDL Cholesterol

	Initiation Level, mg/dl	Minimal Goal, mg/dl
Dietary treatment		
Without CHD and <2 other risk factors	>160	<160
Without CHD but with >2 other risk factors	>130	<130
With CHD	>100	<100
Drug therapy		
Without CHD and <2 other risk factors after diet	>190	<160
Without CHD but with ≥2 other risk factors after diet	>160	<130
With CHD after diet	>130	<100

Source: Adapted from The Second Report of the National Cholesterol Education Program Expert Panel on Detection, Evaluation, and Treatment of High Blood Cholesterol in Adults.[99]

TABLE 21-10. Examples of Primary Versus Secondary Hyperlipidemia

Primary (genetic)
Familial combined hyperlipidemia (incidence 1/100)
Familial hypercholesterolemia (incidence 1/500 heterozygous)
Familial defective apo B (incidence 1/1000)
Type III hyperlipidemia (incidence 1/10,000)
Familial hypertriglyceridemia
Apo C-II deficiency (incidence 1/1,000,000)
Lipoprotein lipase deficiency (incidence 1/1,000,000)
Secondary
Diet
Excess saturated fat, cholesterol, or calories
Endocrine/Metabolic
Diabetes
Insulin resistance/impaired glucose tolerance
Hypothyroidism
Obesity
Cushing syndrome
Acromegaly
Anorexia nervosa
Lipodystrophy
Acute intermittent porphyria
Glycogen storage disease
Werner syndrome
Drugs
Alcohol
Glucocorticoids
Oral estrogen
Tamoxifen
Thiazides
Beta-adrenergic blockers
Cyclosporin
Retinoic acid derivatives (e.g. isotretinoin, Accutane)
Protease inhibitors/Antiretroviral agents
Other
Nephrotic syndrome
Chronic renal failure
Cholestatic liver disease/biliary obstruction
Monoclonal gammopathy (e.g., multiple myeloma)
Autoimmune disease (e.g., systemic lupus erythematosis)
Hepatitis

hyperlipidemias (Table 21-10), the most common cause in Americans is excess dietary intake of saturated fat and cholesterol. American children, who typically consume a relatively high-fat diet, have a mean plasma cholesterol level of 168 mg/dl, compared with the Mexican Tarahumara Indian children, who consume a low-fat diet and have cholesterol levels of 118 mg/dl.[112] Tarahumara adults have values that are only a little higher than the levels in children (136 mg/dl). In contrast, among Americans, there is a much greater rise with age—a mean value of about 250 mg/dl among adults (Fig. 21-13) which continues to at least age 55 to 60 years.[113] The rise of plasma cholesterol with age is believed to be caused by functional impairment of the LDL receptor.[114] As a group, American children and adults have much higher levels of blood cholesterol compared to many nonwestern societies. A major cause of this difference is the increased amount of fat, cholesterol, and excess calories in the American diet. Accordingly, blood cholesterol concentrations are rising in many nonwestern populations around the world as their diets become more affluent with increased amounts of saturated fat, total fat, and cholesterol. This relation in adults is illustrated in Fig. 21-14.[96,99]

Factors that contribute to dietary hyperlipidemia include the intake of total fat, saturated fat, dietary cholesterol, and excessive calories. Among these dietary factors, the intake of total fat and saturated fat appears to exert the greatest influence on the serum cholesterol level. Dietary cholesterol is the next most important factor, which causes maximal increases in cholesterol concentrations when the daily intake reaches 300 to 400 mg per day, as shown in Fig. 21-15. Excessive caloric intake is typically manifested as obesity and hypertriglyceridemia. Dietary deficiency of fiber is a minor contributor to hyperlipidemia. These factors are discussed further in the section on the dietary treatment of hyperlipidemia.

Diabetes

The next most common cause of secondary hyperlipidemia is diabetes mellitus. The hyperlipidemia associated with diabetes appears to be due in part to insulin deficiency (relative or absolute) and/or insulin resistance. Consequently, individuals with impaired glucose tolerance who have hyperinsulinemia without significant hyperglycemia may exhibit a pattern of hyperlipidemia that is typical for diabetic patients.

Patients with diabetes mellitus have a two- to sixfold increase in the risk of developing atherosclerosis. Part of this risk is attributable to the associated hyperlipidemia, but other aspects of diabetes and insulin resistance syndrome are also contributory. Thus, diabetic patients deserve careful monitoring and treatment of other risk factors for atherosclerosis, including hypertension, smoking, obesity, and dietary excesses of saturated fat, cholesterol, and calories. The risk of atherosclerosis is severely accelerated in patients with proteinuria and possibly in those with microalbuminuria. The risk of atherosclerosis in women with diabetes appears to be nearly identical to the risk in diabetic men despite the relative resistance to atherosclerosis that is observed in nondiabetic women.

Because the abnormalities in lipid metabolism in diabetes include both qualitative (i.e., functional) and quantitative (e.g., hypertriglyceridemia) changes, the term *dyslipidemia* is often applied to this syndrome. The severity of dyslipidemia in diabetic patients is influenced by the type of diabetes, [non-insulin-dependent/type 2 (NIDDM) or insulin-dependent/type 1 diabetes mellitus (IDDM)], the severity of hyperglycemia, the degree of insulin deficiency, and the underlying genetic predisposition to hyperlipidemia.

Diabetic patients with dyslipidemia may be divided into the five following groups.

IDDM (Type 1 Diabetes) with Ketoacidosis

Diabetic ketoacidosis (DKA) is associated with an overproduction of VLDL and impaired clearance of VLDL and chylomicrons from plasma. In some patients, this may lead to a type IV or V pattern of hyperlipidemia. The overproduction of triglyceride and VLDL is primarily the result of an increased flux of FFA from insulin-deficient adipocytes to the liver. The extremely high circulating levels of FFA (800 to 1,600 mEq/L) are derived from lipolysis of adipose tissue triglyceride and correlate directly with the blood glucose levels. When glucose cannot enter the cells because of absolute or relative insulin deficiency, the endocrine and biochemical effects are those of starvation. In this setting, increased plasma FFA levels provide an alternative source of energy for the working cells of the body. FFA elevations may also promote vascular damage and platelet aggregation, although the clinical significance of this tendency to thrombosis has not been elucidated.

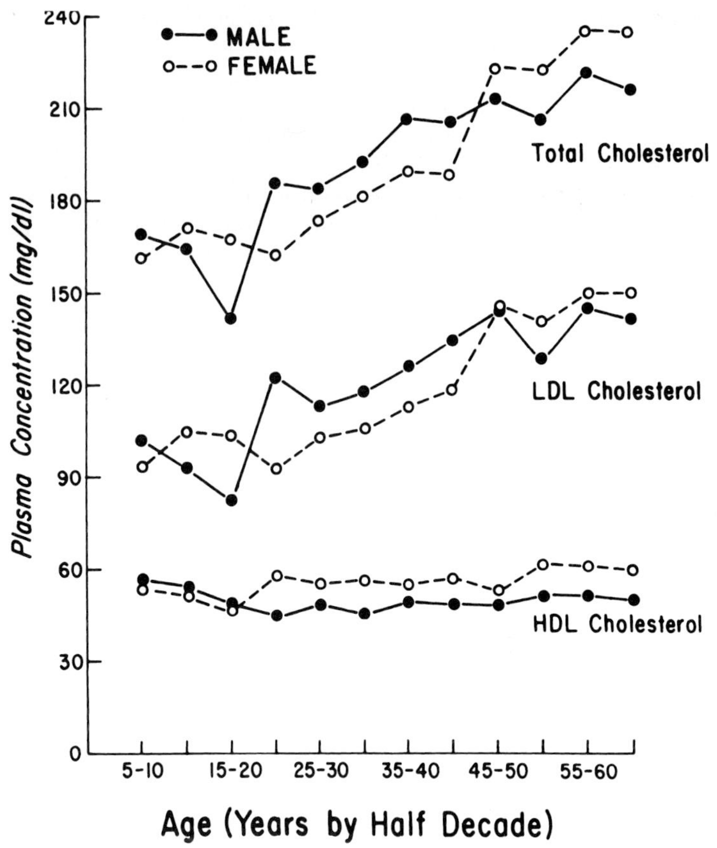

FIGURE 21-13. Age-related changes in the plasma concentrations of total, high-density, and low-density lipoprotein cholesterol in men and women age 6 to 65 years. Data derived from lipid analyses on 619 subjects residing in Portland, Oregon. (*Reproduced from Connor et al.*[113] *with permission.*)

The decrease in clearance of VLDL and chylomicrons in DKA occurs primarily because the activity of the enzyme LPL, which is responsible for the clearance of triglyceride from VLDL and chylomicrons, is diminished in insulin-deficient states. Triglyceride clearance is also impeded by saturation of catabolic pathways when the triglyceride concentration exceeds about 1,000 mg/dl (11.29 mmol/L). When DKA occurs in a patient with baseline hypertriglyceridemia greater than 400 to 500 mg/dl (4.52 to 5.65 mmol/L), the triglyceride level may increase to more than 5,000 to 10,000 mg/dl (56.5 to 112.9 mmol/L) and lead to pancreatitis.

Correction of the ketoacidotic state by administering insulin will promptly ameliorate the hyperlipidemia. Even when plasma triglyceride concentrations are as high as 10,000 to 15,000 mg/dl

FIGURE 21-14. Estimated effect of conversion to a phase I diet. Curve A represents the typical distribution of cholesterol levels among middle-aged (40 to 44 years) American men.[96] Curve B represents the hypothetical effects of conversion of all individuals from a typical American diet (about 37% fat, 400 mg cholesterol) to a phase I American Heart Association diet (>30% fat, >300 mg cholesterol).[99] For women in the same age group, curves A and B are shifted to the left by about 10 mg/dl.

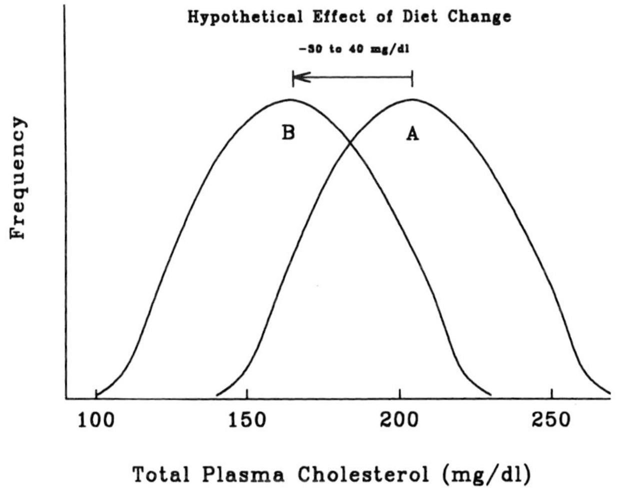

FIGURE 21-15. The effects of gradually increasing amounts of dietary cholesterol on the plasma cholesterol levels of human subjects whose background diet is very low in cholesterol content. (See text for a discussion of threshold and ceiling concepts.)

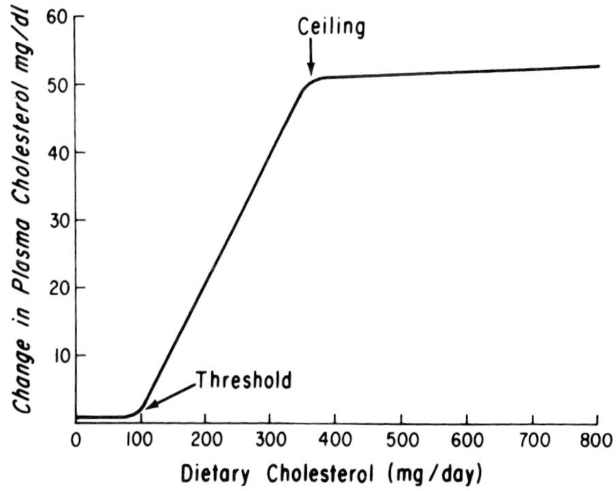

(112.9 to 169.4 mmol/L), administration of insulin in combination with a very low-fat diet will reduce plasma triglyceride levels by more than 1,000 mg/dl per day (see Fig. 21-32, which shows data for type 2 diabetes). Because DKA is a temporary state, it does not present a long-term management problem.

Poorly Controlled Diabetes without Ketoacidosis

Poorly controlled IDDM or NIDDM is an insulin-deficient state that can be associated with persistent combined hyperlipidemia that is similar to the type observed in DKA. The predominant lipoprotein abnormality is hypertriglyceridemia, which reflects the increased levels in plasma of VLDL, VLDL remnants, and chylomicron remnants. Triglyceride concentrations greater than 1,000 mg/dl also are commonly associated with increased plasma levels of chylomicrons due to delayed clearance of dietary fat from the blood. The hyperlipidemia is primarily a consequence of relative insulin deficiency and is associated with increased production of VLDL and diminished clearance of triglyceride-rich lipoproteins. As a consequence of insulin deficiency at the cellular level, the mass and activity of LPL are reduced, resulting in attenuated clearance of VLDL and chylomicron triglyceride. As a consequence of diminished insulin-mediated inhibition of lipolysis of adipocyte triglyceride stores, plasma concentrations of FFA rise, resulting in increased flux of FFA to the liver. Increased uptake of FFA and glucose by the liver stimulates increased synthesis and secretion of triglyceride and VLDL. Increased synthesis of cholesterol and its accumulation in LDL also may occur in such patients.[115] The qualitative abnormalities in these patients, particularly those with NIDDM, may include the presence of small dense VLDL, increased IDL (including remnants of VLDL and chylomicrons), small dense LDL (with or without an increase in the level of LDL cholesterol), decreased levels of HDL_2, and increased glycation of various apoproteins. These atherogenic abnormalities collectively comprise diabetic dyslipidemia. Increased formation of advanced glycosylation end products (AGEs), which are formed in proportion to the magnitude of hyperglycemia, may contribute to accelerated development of atherosclerosis in diabetes.

Well-Controlled Diabetes

Patients with well-controlled IDDM tend to be normolipidemic or may have slightly increased levels of HDL cholesterol. Nonetheless, recent results from the diabetes control and complications trial (DCCT) have demonstrated beneficial effects of intensive glycemic control on the lipoprotein profile in patients with type 1 diabetes.[116] In this study, intensive insulin therapy reduced the mean HgbA1c level from 9.2 to 7.3 percent and was associated with decreased plasma concentrations of VLDL cholesterol and total apo B, slightly lower concentrations of LDL cholesterol and Lp(a), a shift in LDL density and size toward more buoyant larger (less atherogenic) particles, and increased HDL cholesterol. The results of other studies have indicated that such a change in the HgbA1c level also will be associated with decreased levels of glycated apoproteins, which may improve normal pathways of lipoprotein catabolism and reduce the atherogenicity lipoprotein particles. Thus, intensive glycemic control in type 1 diabetes produces several positive qualitative and quantitative changes in the lipoprotein profile in type 1 diabetes.

In contrast, patients with well-controlled NIDDM tend to have persistent qualitative and quantitative lipoprotein abnormalities, although the hyperlipidemia is improved compared with the uncontrolled diabetic state. The activity of LPL tends to be normal and the production of VLDL is only mildly elevated, but the stigmata of diabetes-associated dyslipidemia may be present. These abnormalities may include the presence of small dense VLDL, increased IDL, small dense LDL, and decreased total HDL and subfraction HDL_2 concentrations.

Several other abnormalities in lipoprotein metabolism may be present. Nonenzymatic glycation of apoproteins in LDL and HDL occurs in the hyperglycemic state[117] and may be associated with potentially atherogenic functional abnormalities in these lipoproteins.[118,119] The results of other preliminary studies have suggested that the diabetic state may also be associated with the following conditions: abnormalities in CETP and PLTP activity and reverse cholesterol transport, abnormalities in the balance of activities of LPL and HL, an increased tendency for oxidative modification of LDL, increased trapping of LDL in the subendothelial space, adverse effects of AGEs in the artery wall, and enhanced accumulation of cholesteryl ester from LDL by macrophages in the artery wall.

Diet-Induced Hyperlipidemia in Diabetes

During recent years there has been a resurgence of the promotion of diets for diabetic patients that are high protein, high fat, high saturated fat, high cholesterol, and relatively low carbohydrate. Although such diets may have the beneficial effect of promoting modest weight loss, they also can have a variety of adverse effects that may include worsening hyperlipidemia, increased urinary protein excretion and accelerated decline in renal function, gout, and other sequella. Moreover, such diets also lack the spectrum of antiatherosclerotic and anticancer compounds found in fruits, vegetables, legumes, and grains. Although there has been general moderation of this dietary approach in the medical community, there still is a tendency among some physicians to shun carbohydrate in the diet and to recommend a diet high in animal protein and fat. The rationale behind such recommendations is often based on an incomplete understanding of the pathophysiology of type 2 diabetes and the profound atherosclerotic complications of diabetes. Thus, despite the ongoing popularity of high protein, high fat diets among the general public, such diets are not advisable as a long-term approach to treatment of dyslipidemia and excess body weight in patients with type 2 diabetes, as well as nondiabetic patients.

Coexisting Genetic Hyperlipidemia in Diabetes

A further cause of hyperlipidemia in diabetic patients is the coexistence with diabetes of primary genetic hyperlipidemias, the most common of which are familial hypertriglyceridemia and familial combined hyperlipidemia. As a consequence, the severity of dyslipidemia in diabetic patients varies widely in terms of both qualitative and quantitative abnormalities. Increases in chylomicrons, VLDL, remnants and IDL, small dense LDL, Lp(a), and FFA may occur, and HDL levels are frequently decreased. The characteristics of dyslipidemia in diabetes are influenced by the type of diabetes, the severity of insulin deficiency and hyperglycemia, and underlying genetic and environmental factors. Diabetic patients with a coexisting genetic cause of hyperlipidemia usually have the most severe hyperlipidemia. Patients with well-controlled diabetes and persistent hypertriglyceridemia greater than 400 to 600 mg/dl commonly have an underlying genetic or additional acquired cause of hypertriglyceridemia. For similar reasons, patients with uncontrolled diabetes and plasma triglyceride concentrations greater than 1,000 to 2,000 mg/dl are also very likely to have an additional underlying cause of hypertriglyceridemia.

Hypothyroidism

Apart from diabetes, hypothyroidism is the second most common endocrine cause of secondary hyperlipidemia. The results of several studies, including a review of patients in the Lipid Disorders Clinic at the Oregon Health Sciences University, have suggested that 2 to 4 percent of patients with hyperlipidemia have hypothyroidism.[120,121] The majority of these patients were not suspected to have hypothyroidism on the basis of clinical findings, despite thyroid stimulating hormone (TSH) concentrations in some cases greater than 20 μU/ml. Among other patients with previously stable lipid concentrations, a marked increase in the plasma cholesterol (and LDL cholesterol) concentration is a strong indication that the patient has acquired secondary hyperlipidemia, possibly due to hypothyroidism. Thus, routine screening of hyperlipidemic patients is likely to identify a few percent of patients with unsuspected hypothyroidism.

Any of the lipoprotein phenotypes may occur in hypothyroidism, but elevations of plasma cholesterol in the range of 250 to 600 mg/dl (6.5 to 15.5 mmol/L) with or without associated triglyceride elevation occur most commonly (i.e., type IIa or IIb pattern). The increased total plasma cholesterol concentration is usually a reflection of increased levels of LDL cholesterol resulting from decreased catabolism of LDL particles. The degree of hyperlipidemia shows a positive correlation with the severity of hypothyroidism. If hypothyroidism occurs concurrently with familial hyperlipidemia, the plasma lipid elevations are more extreme. Indeed, young patients with the heterozygous form of familial hypercholesterolemia and hypothyroidism may present with xanthomas and plasma lipid concentrations resembling those seen in homozygous familial hypercholesterolemia.[122]

The mechanisms responsible for hyperlipidemia in the setting of hypothyroidism include reduced high-affinity receptor-mediated catabolism of LDL[123] (due to decreased hepatic expression of LDL receptors), lower biliary excretion of cholesterol and bile acids, and decreased LPL activity. These factors more than counteract a concomitant decrease in cholesterol biosynthesis.

The dramatic lipid-lowering response that accompanies thyroid hormone replacement is particularly gratifying. Plasma cholesterol values as high as 350 mg/dl (9.05 mmol/L) frequently return to normal within 4 to 6 weeks of full-replacement doses of thyroxine and may begin to decline within days after the initiation of therapy. The results of recent studies have indicated that even mild hypothyroidism (subclinical hypothyroidism) is a risk factor for coronary artery disease, possibly because of the association with hypercholesterolemia. The results of other studies have indicated that treatment of subclinical hypothyroidism with thyroid hormone is associated with modest reductions in total and LDL cholesterol concentrations. Thus, it is reasonable to screen most, if not all, hyperlipidemic patients for hypothyroidism in order to identify this important but easily missed diagnosis.

Renal Disease

Hyperlipidemia is common in renal disease and may be manifested by a variety of lipid and lipoprotein abnormalities.[124] Three categories of hyperlipidemic renal patients may be observed: uremic patients undergoing dialysis; renal-transplant patients receiving immunosuppressive therapy with corticosteroids, azathioprine, and/or cyclosporine; and nephrotic patients.

The characteristic abnormality in patients undergoing dialysis is hypertriglyceridemia with an increase in VLDL resulting in a type IV pattern. These patients have reduced clearance of triglyceride from the plasma, presumably because LPL activity is reduced. Transplant patients most frequently have an elevation of LDL cholesterol with a type IIa pattern but commonly also show elevated levels of VLDL cholesterol and triglycerides with a type IV or IIb phenotype. Rarely, patients with type V hyperlipidemia have been observed after transplantation. Although the mechanism for transplant hyperlipidemia is multifactorial, it presumably is related in part to increased appetite, weight gain, and the use of corticosteroids. Cyclosporine is an additional cause of increased levels of LDL and total cholesterol. This effect may be mediated in part by cyclosporine-induced selective activation of sterol regulatory element binding protein-2 (SREBP-2).[125] Prednisone therapy, given for posttransplant immunosuppression, commonly causes insulin resistance and exacerbation of hypertriglyceridemia.

Patients with the nephrotic syndrome frequently have a mixed form of hyperlipidemia with elevation of both plasma cholesterol and triglyceride levels (type IIb is the most common). The hyperlipidemia is roughly related to the severity of hypoalbuminemia associated with this syndrome. Remission of the nephrotic state invariably brings about correction of the hyperlipidemia.

The numbers of patients with hyperlipidemia attributable to renal disease have dramatically increased in the last few decades as a consequence of the development of dialysis and transplantation programs, which have resulted in prolonged survival of patients with end-stage kidney disease. The major cause of death in these patients is atherosclerotic coronary heart disease. Carotid and aortoileofemoral atherosclerosis are also common, which emphasizes the importance of aggressive management of hyperlipidemia in patients with renal disease. The same principles of dietary management should be applied to patients with hyperlipidemia secondary to renal disease, especially among those with renal transplants. In those in whom satisfactory control of hyperlipidemia has not been achieved, the use of lipid-lowering drugs is appropriate. The HMG CoA reductase inhibitors[126] or niacin may be efficacious in these patients.

An additional potential contributor to accelerated atherosclerosis in patients with renal failure is increased plasma concentrations of Lp(a), an atherogenic lipoprotein particle. The mechanism responsible for the increase is unclear, but it may be related to decreased clearance. Levels of Lp(a) greater than 20 to 30 mg/dl are associated with an increased risk of stroke, myocardial infarction, and peripheral vascular disease. Niacin and postmenopausal estrogen, as well as less commonly prescribed anabolic steroids, are medications that may reduce the level of Lp(a), but the benefits of a reduced level of Lp(a) remain unproven.

Human Immunodeficiency Virus (HIV) and Acquired Immunodeficiency Syndrome (AIDS)

AIDS has been reported to be associated with hypertriglyceridemia, presumably as a consequence of increased levels of interferon alpha,[127] resulting in decreased clearance of triglyceride-rich lipoproteins and increased hepatic production of VLDL. The prevalence of small dense LDL (pattern B) also is increased in patients with AIDS and hypertriglyceridemia.

With the recent advent of highly active antiretroviral therapy (HAART), survival of patients with AIDS has improved dramatically, but a new endocrine disorder has emerged that is characterized by lipodystrophy, insulin resistance with or without diabetes, and hypertriglyceridemia with reduced HDL cholesterol concentrations.[128] The prevalence of lipodystrophy among patients receiving HAART may be greater than 80 percent after prolonged therapy. The prevalence of overt diabetes in lipodystrophic patients may be relatively low, but abnormalities in glucose homeostasis have been reported in about 25 percent of patients.

HAART regimens typically include at least one HIV-1 protease inhibitor or a nonnucleoside reverse transcriptase inhibitor in combination with two nucleoside analog HIV-1 reverse transcriptase inhibitors. Both protease inhibitors and nucleoside analog HIV-1 reverse transcriptase inhibitors appear to play a role in the development of HAART-related lipodystrophy, but they may contribute to this disorder through separate mechanisms. The lipodystrophy typically involves loss of peripheral adipose tissue and development of central adiposity, but also may involve fat deposition over the dorsocervical spine ("buffalo hump") and in the breasts of women. The severity of lipodystrophy has been correlated with the duration of HAART, body weight before therapy (increased risk with lower pretreatment weight), fasting triglyceride and C-peptide concentrations, and inversely with HDL cholesterol concentrations.[129] Protease inhibitor-induced hypertriglyceridemia may be mediated by reduced lipoprotein lipase activity and increased hepatic synthesis of apo B. The prevalence of dyslipidemia among users of protease inhibitors may approximate 75 percent, and may be most prevalent among users of the protease inhibitor ritonavir.

The pathogenesis of HAART-associated lipodystrophy and dyslipidemia is believed to be related to inhibition of LRP, which mediates uptake of triglyceride-rich remnant lipoproteins, and cytoplasmic retinoic acid binding protein type I (CRABP-1), which indirectly activates peroxisome-proliferator activated receptor type γ (PPARγ) to stimulate adipocyte differentiation and inhibit apoptosis. The catalytic site of HIV protease, to which protease inhibitors bind, may be 70 percent homologous with regions of LRP and CRABP-1, which might allow protease inhibitors to block the activity of LRP and CRABP-1.

The optimal treatment for hypertriglyceridemia related to HAART-associated lipodystrophy is uncertain, but attentiveness to the identification and treatment of hyperglycemia is essential. Drugs that alter the severity of insulin resistance, such as thiazolidinediones or metformin, may have utility in this disorder, but there are concerns about the risk of hepatotoxicity (and lactic acidosis with metformin) in patients already taking a variety of potentially hepatotoxic medications. The same concerns apply to the use of gemfibrozil or fenofibrate for treatment of hypertriglyceridemia, or statin drugs for treatment of elevated concentrations of LDL cholesterol. Niacin may have beneficial triglyceride-lowering efficacy, but may exacerbate insulin resistance and also can be hepatotoxic. Fish oil appears to be a reasonably nontoxic agent that has the capability of lowering plasma triglyceride concentrations when administered in sufficient doses. Studies are required to define the proper role of these agents in patients with HAART-associated lipodystrophy.

Biliary Obstruction and Alpha$_1$ Antitrypsin Deficiency

Hyperlipidemia invariably occurs in the setting of cholestatic liver disease. This type of secondary hyperlipidemia is commonly seen in various forms of biliary cirrhosis and biliary atresia. Plasma cholesterol values over 1,500 mg/dl are not unusual. Planar xanthomas frequently occur as a result of the severe hyperlipidemia. Less severe hyperlipidemia is also seen in biliary obstruction arising from reversible conditions, such as obstruction of the common bile duct by a stone (or tumor) or drug-induced obstructive liver disease. In such conditions, the hypercholesterolemia resolves when the biliary obstruction is ameliorated. In the setting of chronic biliary obstruction, the severity of hyperlipidemia may diminish over time as hepatocellular function becomes progressively impaired, resulting in diminished capacity for hepatic lipoprotein synthesis. Hyperlipidemia has also occurred in a child with severe liver disease present at birth caused by alpha$_1$ antitrypsin deficiency.[130] Lipoprotein X was present, but the bilirubin was only mildly elevated. Thus, liver disease in the absence of biliary obstruction may be a rare cause of the same lipoprotein abnormality seen with biliary obstruction.

The unique lipoprotein particle that is elevated in cholestatic liver disease is termed *lipoprotein X.* This lipoprotein has beta-electrophoretic mobility but has an unusual lipid composition consisting of predominantly free cholesterol and phospholipid, greatly reduced amounts of cholesteryl esters, complexed with a protein moiety consisting primarily of apo C and albumin. Although it is not routinely determined, the total plasma phospholipid concentration is also greatly increased, whereas plasma triglyceride is only moderately elevated. Lipoprotein X can be characterized by immunologic techniques and is often diagnostic of biliary obstruction, but it may also be associated with rare forms of LCAT deficiency.

The etiology of this hyperlipidemia is related to impaired excretion of bile acids (and probably cholesterol) into bile. The level of serum bile acids becomes elevated, and the conversion of cholesterol to bile acids in the liver is decreased. The activity of the enzyme LCAT is also reduced and probably contributes to the reduced level of cholesteryl ester in plasma. Abnormal discoidal HDL particles are present, which may be a consequence of decreased LCAT activity and the reduced content of cholesteryl ester. Cholestyramine may be used to control the itching these patients invariably have and may also reduce plasma lipid levels, but therapy is aimed primarily at correcting the underlying hepatic disease of biliary obstruction. Plasmapheresis may be useful to remove cholesterol in patients with xanthomatous neuropathy. Liver transplantation corrects the hyperlipidemia associated with cholestatic liver disease.

Alcohol

A common cause of hypertriglyceridemia in western societies is excessive alcohol intake.[124] Considerable variation exists in the plasma lipid response of a given individual to alcohol, as is discussed later, and only about 10 percent of patients who habitually abuse alcohol develop hyperlipidemia, usually with a type IV phenotype. Combined elevations of cholesterol and triglycerides (type IIb) also occur, as do cases with more severe hypertriglyceridemia and a type V phenotype. The latter pattern is most apt to occur in chronic alcohol abusers during periods of high fat intake and may lead to pancreatitis. Alternatively, patients with baseline plasma triglyceride levels of 600 to 1,000 mg/dl (6.8 to 11.2 mmol/L) may develop severe chylomicronemia (type V) and pancreatitis after a brief period of high-level alcohol consumption. Such individuals also may experience worsening of hypertriglyceridemia as a consequence of consuming as little as one alcoholic drink per day.

The mechanisms responsible for alcohol-induced hyperlipidemia are complex and are related in part to the high caloric content of alcoholic beverages. In addition, alcohol increases the magnitude and duration of food-related postprandial lipemia. This increase appears to be due to enhanced secretion of VLDL, which occurs concomitantly with postprandial hyperchylomicronemia, and results in a prolonged clearance of both particles. In the fasting state, alcohol also enhances hepatic synthesis and secretion of VLDL and is the main factor responsible for the development of the type IV phenotype. This occurs because increased levels of nicotinamide adenine dinucleotide (NADH), which are produced during the metabolism of ethanol by alcohol dehydrogenase, inhibit oxidation of FFA and thereby enhance synthesis of triglycerides and VLDL. Alcohol may also promote the induction of hepatic microsomal enzymes with additional stimulatory effects on lipoprotein synthesis.

Anorexia Nervosa

Anorexia nervosa was previously reported more than 35 years ago as a cause of secondary hypercholesterolemia, presumably related to decreased biliary excretion of bile acids and cholesterol. In contrast to these historical reports, however, the results of a recent small study in 23 women with anorexia nervosa demonstrated normal plasma concentrations of total and LDL cholesterol.[131] The presence or absence of hypercholesterolemia in various studies of patients with anorexia nervosa may be a function of underlying genetically-mediated forms of hyperlipidemia, diet composition, and whether the patient is in the process of refeeding, starvation, or is weight stable.

Drug-Induced Hyperlipoproteinemia

A number of drugs and hormones have been reported to have an adverse effect on plasma lipoprotein concentrations in humans (Table 21-11). In the case of glucocorticoids,[132,133] estrogen,[134] and 13-*cis*-retinoic acid (isotretinoin, Accutane),[135,136] the primary effect appears to be stimulation of VLDL production and an increase in the concentrations of triglyceride-rich lipoproteins. Progestins and Danazol may have variable effects.[137,138] In patients with underlying familial hypertriglyceridemia, familial combined hyperlipidemia, or diabetes-associated hypertriglyceridemia, the use of these agents may result in a profound elevation in the concentration of serum triglyceride. In some patients, the triglyceride level may increase from a baseline of 600 to 800 mg/dl (6.8 to 9.0 mmol/L) to more than 5,000 mg/dl (56.5 mmol/L), resulting in clinical symptoms of abdominal pain, pancreatitis, and the development of eruptive xanthomas. The thiazide diuretics have also been reported to increase the concentrations of cholesterol and triglyceride, an effect that is attributable to increased concentrations of VLDL and LDL particles in plasma.[139,140] Beta-adrenergic blocking agents such as propranolol may also cause plasma triglyceride concentrations to increase and may concurrently reduce HDL cholesterol levels.[139,140] Beta-adrenergic blocking agents with intrinsic sympathomimetic activity (e.g., pindolol and labetalol) do not cause hyperlipidemia. Therapy with thiazide diuretics and beta-adrenergic blockers should be avoided in patients with known hyperlipidemia if other avenues of therapy are available. The immunosuppressant drug, cyclosporine, is commonly used in transplant patients and is a cause of drug-induced increases in plasma concentrations of total and LDL cholesterol. This effect may be mediated in part by cyclosporine-induced selective activation of sterol regulatory element binding protein-2 (SREBP-2).[125]

TABLE 21-11. The Influence of Drugs on Plasma Lipids and Lipoproteins

	Lipid/Lipoprotein				
Drug	**Total Chol**	**TG**	**LDL Chol**	**HDL Chol**	**Reference**
Corticosteroids	↑	↑↑	± ↑	± ↑	132, 133
Estrogens	↑	↑	↓	↑	134
Progestins	± ↑	± ↑	± ↑	↓	137
Androgens	↓	—	± ↑	↓	138
Beta blockers			± ↑	↓	139, 140
(without ISI)	↑	↑			
Thiazide			± ↑	↓	139, 140
diuretics	↑	↑			
Vitamin A	± ↑	↑↑	↓	↓	135, 136
derivatives					
Cimetidine	± ↑	↑	↓	↓	141
Cyclosporin	↑	—	↑	—	125, 142
Phenytoin	↑	—	—	↑	143
Barbiturates		—	—	↑	143

TG = triglycerides; chol = cholesterol; ISI = intrinsic sympathomimetic activity.

HYPERCHOLESTEROLEMIA

Elevated levels of plasma cholesterol in the setting of normal triglyceride concentrations are usually attributable to an increased number of LDL particles in plasma. Less commonly, hypercholesterolemia reflects cholestasis in which an abnormal lipoprotein (LPX) accumulates or is seen in the occasional patient with an atypically high level of HDL cholesterol; in this case, no treatment is indicated (see Familial Hyperalphalipoproteinemia under Disorders of High-Density Lipoproteins). The causes of hypercholesterolemia may be divided into primary (genetic) etiologies, secondary causes, and a combination of the two. Evaluation of a patient with hypercholesterolemia should therefore include satisfactory exclusion of secondary factors and a detailed family history. The potential value of identifying asymptomatic children and young adults with primary hypercholesterolemia cannot be overemphasized if preventive therapeutic measures to minimize the future development of atherosclerosis are to be successful. Increased concentrations of LDL cholesterol with normal triglycerides can be seen in patients with familial hypercholesterolemia, familial combined hyperlipidemia, familial defective apolipoprotein B-100, and so-called polygenic hypercholesterolemia. Polygenic hypercholesterolemia is a poorly characterized disorder of unknown etiology in which affected adults display moderate hypercholesterolemia (220 to 280 mg/dl) without evidence of tendon xanthomas. Whether it is a distinct disorder has not been established.

Familial Hypercholesterolemia

Definition

This condition (synonyms: familial xanthomatous hypercholesterolemia, type IIa and IIb hyperlipoproteinemia, hyperbetalipoproteinemia) is characterized by increased LDL, or β-lipoproteins, which are the chief carriers of cholesterol and cholesteryl ester in the plasma. Consequently, the plasma cholesterol concentration is always moderately to profoundly elevated, with plasma triglyceride levels usually normal or low (type IIa) but at times elevated (type IIb). The etiology of hypercholesterolemia is related to a deficiency of hepatic LDL receptor numbers and/or function, which diminishes hepatic removal of LDL from the plasma. Of all the hyperlipidemias, familial hypercholesterolemia especially is characterized clinically by premature atherosclerosis and coronary heart disease as well as by the occurrence of tuberous and tendon xanthomas.[67]

Clinical Characteristics

The heterozygous form of familial hypercholesterolemia occurs in approximately 1 in 500 individuals and is one of the most common genetic causes of moderate to severe hypercholesterolemia in North America.[67] The disorder may be found at any age in either sex and may be diagnosed in the homozygous state during intrauterine life.[144] The chief clinical manifestations of this disease are the occurrence of xanthomatous deposits in the skin and tendons and greatly accelerated rates of atherosclerosis. The homozygous form of familial hypercholesterolemia is usually detected in childhood. Affected patients develop planar, tuberous, and tendon xanthomas during the first 5 years of life and in some cases may even be born with these skin manifestations. Plasma cholesterol concentrations in these patients are generally in excess of 600 to 700 mg/dl. Because of their inherently lower levels of total (240 to 450 mg/dl) and LDL cholesterol (160 to 400 mg/dl), children and young adults with heterozygous familial hypercholesterolemia frequently have no physical abnormalities.[145] Small planar xanthomas (slightly raised yellow lesions) may occasionally be seen in the digital webs or behind the knees. Recurrent episodes of Achilles tendonitis, usually exercise-related, occur in 50 to 75 percent of heterozygotes and frequently have their onset in the patient's late teens or early twenties.[146] These episodes are a reflection of the insidious deposition of LDL cholesterol in the tendons of patients with familial hypercholesterolemia and often precede clinical evidence of thickening or xanthomatous deposits in the Achilles tendons. These nodular lipid-rich lesions have a mild inflammatory tissue reaction and an associated collagen accumulation. Tendon xanthomas, which are the hallmark of familial hypercholesterolemia, become more prominent as the patient gets older, and their development is often accelerated by local trauma. In the experience of the authors, tendon xanthomas are also more prominent in patients with heterozygous familial hypercholesterolemia who concurrently have increased plasma concentrations of Lp(a). In adult patients with heterozygous familial hypercholesterolemia who are over age 30 to 35, tendon xanthomas are usually detectable by means of clinical examination. Tendon xanthomas characteristically involve the extensor tendons of the hands (Figs. 21-16 and 21-17), the olecranon tendon, the patellar tendon, and the Achilles tendon (Fig. 21-18). An increased thickening and nodularity of the Achilles tendon is often noted on palpation. Xanthelasmas (Fig. 21-19) are present in less than 20 percent of older patients[147] but are not specific for familial hypercholesterolemia, occurring frequently in patients with normal lipid values.[145] The presence of a corneal arcus (Fig. 21-20) in patients under age 35 years constitutes another external hallmark of familial hypercholesterolemia[145] but is surprisingly absent in some patients with severe hypercholesterolemia. In many patients, however, a long latent period with only hypercholesterolemia precedes the clinical manifestations of cholesterol accumulation in the tendons, skin, and arterial walls. Lipid accumulation in these tissues, however, tends to proceed in parallel, and manifestations of cardiovascular disease are more likely to be present in patients with prominent tendon xanthomas than in patients in whom such lesions are less conspicuous.[148]

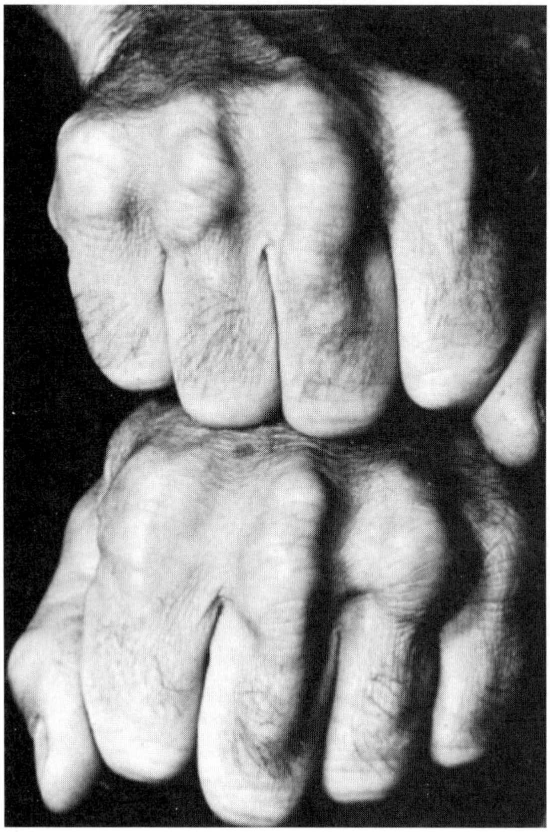

FIGURE 21-16. Tendon xanthomas in a patient with heterozygous familial hypercholesterolemia.

The high incidence of premature coronary artery disease in patients with familial hypercholesterolemia has been well documented.[145,148–152] Homozygotes are the most severely affected individuals and develop symptoms of coronary atherosclerosis by 10 to 15 years of age.[67] Myocardial infarction has been reported at $^1/_2$ and 3 years of age.[153,154] In addition to precocious coronary artery disease, patients with homozygous familial hypercholesterolemia are also predisposed to both valvular and supravalvular aortic stenosis[155,156] and to atherosclerosis of the carotid and femoral arteries. Premature coronary artery disease is also characteristic of

FIGURE 21-17. The appearance of tendon xanthomas before surgical removal in a patient with heterozygous familial hypercholesterolemia.

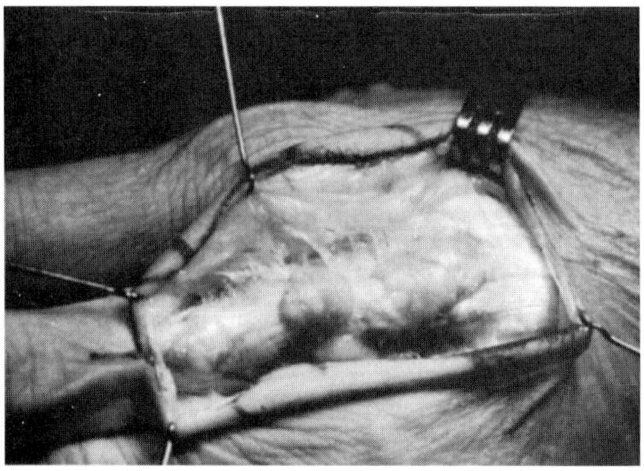

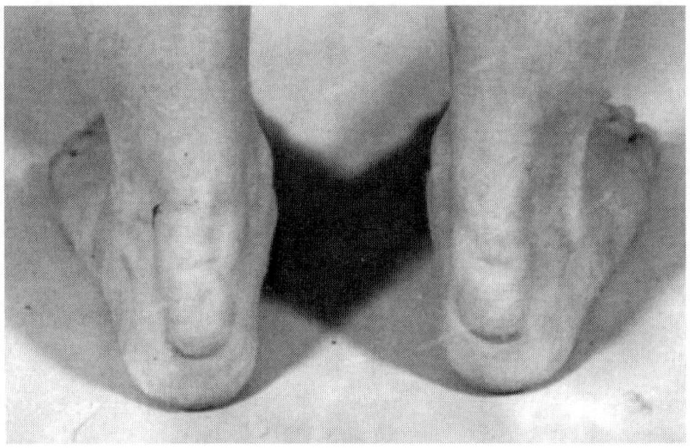

FIGURE 21-18. Xanthomas of the Achilles tendons in a patient with heterozygous familial hypercholesterolemia.

patients with heterozygous familial hypercholesterolemia; it is influenced by the magnitude of hypercholesterolemia, family history, and other cardiovascular risk factors and is also higher in patients who concurrently have increased plasma concentrations of Lp(a).[157,158] Unlike the situation in homozygotes, among whom vascular complications appear to be similar in men and women, the predilection for atherosclerosis is greater in men. The average age of onset for symptomatic coronary artery disease is 40 to 45 years in men and 50 to 60 years in women with heterozygous familial hypercholesterolemia (Table 21-12). Angiographic studies have also disclosed a higher than expected incidence of proximal lesions of the coronary arteries, including left main coronary artery disease, in patients with familial hypercholesterolemia.[159,160]

Diagnostic Laboratory Features

It must be stressed that many individuals with hypercholesterolemia resulting from elevated plasma levels of LDL will not have a distinctly definable genetic disorder and will have hypercholesterolemia on the basis of dietary or other secondary factors. These patients in general have plasma cholesterol concentrations that are lower than those of the genetically affected individuals, although severe hypercholesterolemia may be seen in association with both hypothyroidism and renal disease. Patients with familial hypercholesterolemia in the heterozygous form usually present with elevated levels of total and LDL cholesterol and normal levels of plasma triglycerides. Concentrations of HDL cholesterol are infrequently reduced by 5 to 10 mg/dl in heterozygotes and are even lower in homozygotes.[161] Plasma cholesterol levels in heterozygous patients generally range from 280 to 550 mg/dl in adults, and in homozygous patients they generally exceed 600 mg/dl during childhood. These increases correlate with increased concentrations of LDL cholesterol. Although not associated with other metabolic disorders, the concurrent presence of familial hypercholesterolemia with obesity, diabetes, or renal disease often results in increased triglyceride levels and the expression of a type IIb phenotype. Similarly, the coexistence of heterozygous familial hypercholesterolemia and another primary disorder of lipid metabolism (e.g., familial combined hyperlipidemia),[162] type III hyperlipoproteinemia,[163] or a secondary disorder such as hypothyroidism or the nephrotic syndrome may lead to more profound elevations of total cholesterol (often exceeding 500 to 600 mg/dl) than are usually seen in patients with heterozygous familial hypercholesterolemia alone.

FIGURE 21-19. Xanthelasma in a patient with heterozygous familial hypercholesterolemia.

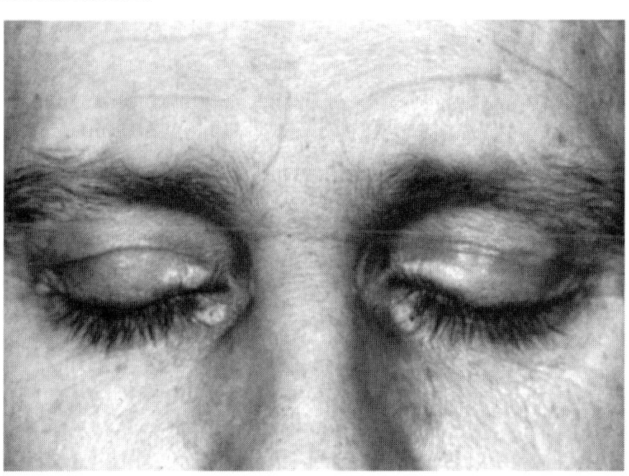

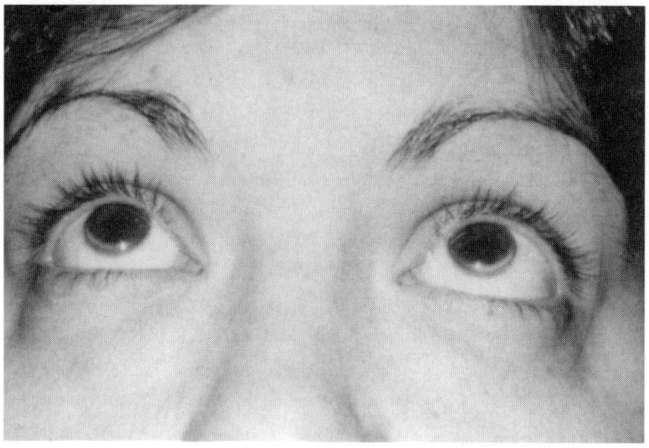

FIGURE 21-20. Corneal arcus in a young woman with heterozygous familial hypercholesterolemia.

Pathophysiology

Major insights into the biochemical basis of familial hypercholesterolemia have been provided by the elegant studies of Goldstein and Brown. These investigators have proceeded from the initial demonstration of specific membrane receptors for LDL on normal cultured fibroblasts and their absence in cells cultured from patients with homozygous familial hypercholesterolemia to delineation of the molecular heterogeneity of the cellular abnormalities in familial hypercholesterolemia[164] and, most recently, delineation of the precise gene defects in cells from different

TABLE 21-12. Coronary Artery Disease in Familial Hypercholesterolemia

	Mean Age for Onset of Coronary Artery Disease	*Chance of Myocardial Infarction Before*		
		Age 30, percent	Age 50, percent	Age 60, percent
Men	40	5	50	85
Women	55	<1	15	50

Source: Data from Refs. 145, 148–152.

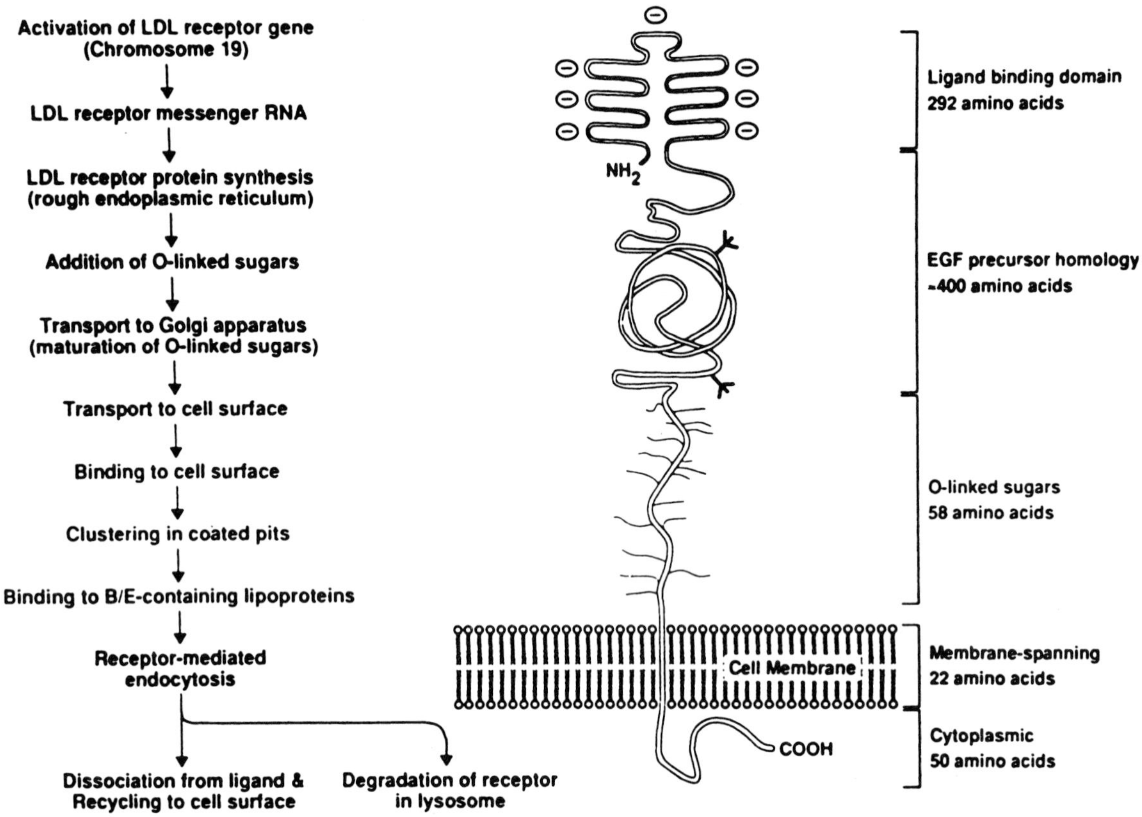

FIGURE 21-21. Structure of the mature human LDL receptor, a single protein with five domains. The pathway of synthesis, intracellular transport, and degradation of the LDL receptor is shown on the left, and the five different domains of the LDL receptor structure are shown on the right. (*Reproduced from Grundy and Vega*[473] *with permission.*)

patients with homozygous familial hypercholesterolemia.[165] The structure and functional domains of the human LDL-receptor are illustrated in Fig. 21-21. Specific mutations that have been identified in the LDL-receptor gene and result in impaired LDL-receptor function with a concurrent clinical phenotype of familial hypercholesterolemia are illustrated in Fig. 21-22. To date, several hundred mutations in the LDL receptor that cause familial hypercholesterolemia have been identified. Various classes of mutations may cause a variety of defects that may involve impaired synthesis or secretion of the LDL receptor, defective LDL binding, impaired transport to clathrin-coated pits, or defective internalization and degradation of LDL receptor-LDL complexes. As previously discussed, specific high-affinity LDL receptors appear to be present on virtually all cells, including hepatocytes and mononuclear leukocytes. From the pathophysiologic point of view, the inability of cells in the body to incorporate LDL via the specific receptor pathway has a number of consequences, including an elevation in the concentration of LDL in plasma and an inappropriately higher rate of cellular cholesterol biosynthesis and LDL production from the liver. Patients with familial hypercholesterolemia show a decrease in the fractional rate of catabolism of LDL, which is most marked in the homozygous state.[166] The biosynthesis of LDL, however, is normal or only modestly increased in heterozygotes but is two to three times greater than normal in homozygous patients.[166] Although genetic defects that reduce the number or functional capacity of LDL receptors explain the marked hypercholesterolemia in patients with familial hypercholesterolemia, the high rate of atherosclerosis that occurs in these patients is mediated by other receptor-mediated pathways for uptake LDL and modified LDL particles into cells. Such non-LDL-receptor-mediated pathways (e.g., scavenger receptors) for LDL uptake into certain cells (including macrophages)[167] contribute to accelerated deposition of lipid in the arterial wall in the setting of severely elevated plasma concentrations of LDL.

A new form of inherited hypercholesterolemia, termed "familial recessive hypercholesterolemia," was recently described in 2 Sardinian families as an autosomal recessive condition with a phenotype that mimics familial hypercholesterolemia.[168] In contrast to familial hypercholesterolemia, subjects with this presumably rare disorder appear to have normal LDL receptor activity, as measured in cultured fibroblasts ex vivo, but a 50 percent reduction in the LDL fractional catabolic rate in vivo. The condition is not caused by the common familial defective apoprotein B mutation, but other mutations in apo B that affect receptor binding of LDL could be contributory.

Genetics

Familial hypercholesterolemia is transmitted by an autosomal dominant mode of inheritance. Because of the large number of possible mutations, routine genetic screening of individual patients is unfeasible. Genetic testing can, however, be useful for genotypic identification of cases within families with a known mutation. Because this disorder is seldom lethal in the heterozygous form until after or during the childbearing period, the

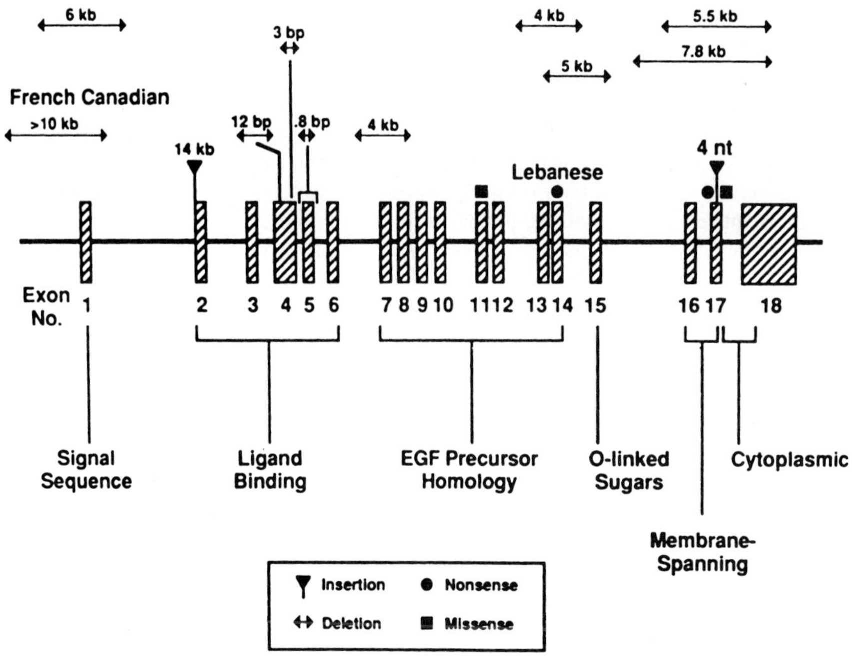

FIGURE 21-22. Location of mutations in the LDL receptor gene that cause familial hypercholesterolemia. Exons are represented by hatched boxes, and introns by lines between boxes. The sites of 16 mutations are indicated, and the key for the symbols is given in the box. (*Reproduced from Russell et al.*[468] *with permission.*)

passage of the disorder from one generation to the next readily explains the large pedigrees of the disorder that have been described. The homozygous form may be diagnosed in utero by tissue culture studies of the LDL receptor in cells derived from the amniotic fluid[144] as well as in children or adults by means of skin biopsies with subsequent studies of the LDL-receptor mechanism in cultured skin fibroblasts or in patients in whom the precise gene defect is known by amplification of DNA obtained from white blood cells by the polymerase chain reaction and subsequent hybridization studies.[165] However, in most patients, this technique is not necessary; the diagnosis can be made on the basis of clinical and usual laboratory features. Only in the homozygote is such precise characterization desirable from the point of view of the demonstration of deficient LDL receptors.

To facilitate the detection of couples at risk for having a child with homozygous familial hypercholesterolemia, it is advisable to check lipid values in the spouses or future spouses of all young patients with known familial hypercholesterolemia. The incidence of heterozygous familial hypercholesterolemia is about 1 in 500 in Europe and North America but appears to be higher in certain populations, most notably in the Afrikaans (Dutch) population of South Africa,[169] in Quebec, and in Lebanon.[170]

Treatment

The increased predilection for premature coronary artery disease that occurs in patients with both heterozygous and homozygous familial hypercholesterolemia justifies the use of intensive treatment regimens to lower plasma LDL cholesterol concentrations with a view to preventing the premature development of atherosclerosis. Treatment in all patients should initially consist of the low-cholesterol, low-fat diet described in Dietary Treatment of Hyperlipidemia. In patients in whom plasma concentrations of total cholesterol are greater than 250 to 300 mg/dl, the response to dietary treatment may be most gratifying. However, in the vast majority of adult patients with heterozygous familial hypercholesterolemia, drug therapy in addition to intensive dietary treatment is almost always necessary. In the opinion of the authors, the goal of such therapy is to reduce the concentrations of LDL cholesterol to less than 130 to 160 mg/dl in adult patients with heterozygous familial hypercholesterolemia who do not have evidence of coronary artery disease and to less than 100 mg/dl in patients with evidence of atherosclerosis.

The development of specific competitive inhibitors of the rate-limiting enzyme in cholesterol biosynthesis, HMG CoA reductase, has provided an important and effective new avenue of therapy for adult patients with heterozygous familial hypercholesterolemia. At the present time, six of these drugs—lovastatin, simvastatin, pravastatin, fluvastatin, atorvastatin, and cerivastatin—have been approved in North America, and one or more of these drugs is available in other countries throughout the world. As a class, the HMG CoA reductase inhibitors are the most effective agents available for the treatment of patients with elevated levels of LDL cholesterol. In patients with heterozygous familial hypercholesterolemia, lovastatin has been shown to reduce concentrations of LDL cholesterol by 17 to 40 percent at doses of 10 to 80 mg per day.[171,172] At the maximum dose of 40 mg per day, simvastatin has been shown to reduce LDL cholesterol concentrations by 37 to 44 percent,[173,174] whereas the same dose of pravastatin resulted in a mean decrease of 28 percent in the concentrations of LDL cholesterol in 40 patients with heterozygous familial hypercholesterolemia.[175] Considerable individual variability exists, however, in the magnitude of the LDL reduction attained in individual patients treated with HMG CoA reductase inhibitors.[171,173] To address the question "How effective is lovastatin as monotherapy in the treatment of adult patients with heterozygous familial hypercholesterolemia?" the efficacy of this drug at doses of 40 and 80 mg per day has been evaluated in patients attending our Lipid Disorders Clinic. In 69 men, mean concentrations of LDL cholesterol decreased from 301 mg/dl to 212 mg/dl during treatment, with 40 mg per day of lovastatin. However, the concentrations of LDL cholesterol remained above 200 mg/dl in 50.7 percent of the patients and fell to less than 160 mg/dl in only 11.6 percent and to less than 130 mg/dl in only 4.3 percent. Similar data from 83 women treated with the same dose of lovastatin indicated that mean concentrations of LDL cholesterol decreased from 294 mg/dl on diet to 196 mg/dl on lovastatin; 41 percent of the female patients had LDL concentrations exceeding 200 mg/dl, while the LDL values fell to under 160 mg/dl in 19.3 percent of the patients and to under 130 mg/dl in 7.2 percent. Similar analyses in patients treated with 80 mg per day of lovastatin indicated that as a group, female patients with heterozygous familial hypercholesterolemia responded better than their male counterparts but that in both groups more than one-third maintained LDL cholesterol concentrations above 250 mg/dl during treatment with the maximum approved dose of lovastatin. These results indicate that single-drug therapy with maximal doses of lovastatin fails to achieve optimal control of hypercholesterolemia in the majority of adult patients with heterozygous familial hypercholesterolemia. However, these are the most effective agents available for the treatment of this disorder and, in the opinion of the authors, are an appropriate first-choice therapy to use in adult patients with heterozygous familial hypercholesterolemia; however, they should not be used in women who plan to have children in the near future or during pregnancy and lactation. The use of this class of drugs in pediatric patients with heterozygous familial hypercholesterolemia is investigational, and the drugs cannot be recommended for general use in the pediatric age group.

The bile acid–binding resins cholestyramine and colestipol are also drugs of first choice for the treatment of patients with heterozygous familial hypercholesterolemia. Notable exceptions include patients with a concurrent elevation in plasma triglyceride levels and patients with a history of severe constipation. Cholestyramine and colestipol are not absorbed and, in the opinion of the authors, are the drugs of first choice (if drug therapy is warranted) for pediatric patients with heterozygous familial hypercholesterolemia; such therapy should not be begun before 5 to 6 years of age and is most appropriate for patients with LDL concentrations exceeding 220 mg/dl on maximum dietary therapy. The dose response curves for both cholestyramine and colestipol are nonlinear, but in compliant patients these drugs reduce concentrations of LDL cholesterol by 23 to 36 percent when given at doses of 16 and 24 g per day in the case of cholestyramine or 20 to 30 g per day in the case of colestipol. An analysis of the lipid-lowering effect of colestipol as monotherapy (mean dose 21 g per day) in 38 patients with heterozygous familial hypercholesterolemia treated in our Lipid Disorders Clinic indicated that mean concentrations of LDL were reduced by 30 percent but that LDL concentrations remained greater than 190 mg/dl in 25 of the 38 patients and decreased to less than 160 mg/dl in only 3. These results indicate that in adult patients with heterozygous familial hypercholesterolemia, single-drug therapy with a bile acid sequestrant fails to achieve optimal concentrations of LDL cholesterol in the vast majority of cases.

Nicotinic acid (niacin) at doses of 3 to 6 g per day, taken in divided doses, is also an effective drug for adult patients with heterozygous familial hypercholesterolemia and is most appropriate to use as monotherapy in patients with concurrent hypertriglyceridemia. In the opinion of the authors, nicotinic acid should not be used in pediatric patients with heterozygous familial hypercholesterolemia. When used as monotherapy, nicotonic acid in doses of 3 to 8 g per day results in 15 to 40 percent decreases in the plasma concentrations of LDL cholesterol, with a modest increase in HDL concentrations. In 12 adult patients with heterozygous familial hypercholesterolemia treated in our Lipid Disorders Clinic who received a mean dose of 4.5 g per day (range: 3 to 6 g per day), concentrations of LDL cholesterol decreased from 318 mg/dl to 220 mg/dl (−30.8 percent), but in the group as a whole, they remained above 190 mg/dl in 9 of the 12 patients and decreased to under 160 mg/dl in only 1.[173]

Probucol is no longer available in the USA, but was a modestly effective drug in the treatment of adult patients with heterozygous familial hypercholesterolemia and, at the recommended dose of 500 mg bid, reduces LDL cholesterol concentrations by 8 to 15 percent.[176] Individual patient response to probucol is, however, quite variable, and the use of this drug appears to be more effective in patients with homozygous familial hypercholesterolemia than it is in heterozygotes.[177] Despite a modest ability to lower LDL concentrations, however, probucol has been shown to cause regression of tendon xanthomas in patients with both homozygous and heterozygous familial hypercholesterolemia.[178]

Gemfibrozil and clofibrate have been shown to reduce concentrations of LDL cholesterol by less than 10 percent in patients with heterozygous familial hypercholesterolemia and cannot be recommended for general use in this disorder. Newer fibrate drugs, including fenofibrate, bezafibrate, and ciprofibrate, are, however, more effective, and with these three drugs, decreases in LDL cholesterol concentrations ranging from 18 to 30 percent have been observed.[173]

The effectiveness of a variety of combined drug regimens that take advantage of the different mechanisms of action of the most effective LDL-lowering drugs have been evaluated in a number of clinical trials in adult patients with heterozygous familial hypercholesterolemia.[179–185] The majority of these studies have utilized combinations that include one of the bile acid sequestrants (which act to increase sterol excretion) in combination with drugs that act to reduce the synthesis of VLDL and/or LDL (e.g., nicotinic acid) or agents that inhibit hepatic cholesterol biosynthesis (e.g., lovastatin, simvastatin, and pravastatin). Referral to a lipid specialist is appropriate for the optimal management of patients with severe heterozygous familial hypercholesterolemia in whom combination drug therapy is required. The efficacy of the combined drug regimens in the treatment of adult patients with heterozygous familial hypercholesterolemia is summarized in Table 21-13.

A number of surgical techniques have been used to treat patients with both heterozygous and homozygous familial hypercholesterolemia, but none can be generally recommended. In patients with heterozygous familial hypercholesterolemia, distal ileal bypass surgery, with surgical resection of the distal 200 cm of the ileum, has been reported to reduce concentrations of LDL cholesterol by 30 to 40 percent,[186] but this operation is ineffective in patients with homozygous familial hypercholesterolemia.[187] Distal ileal bypass surgery may be an appropriate treatment option for selected patients with heterozygous familial hypercholesterolemia who are intolerant to bile acid sequestrant therapy and in whom additional drug therapy with lovastatin may lead to overall reductions in LDL cholesterol greater than 50 percent.[188] Recent data have indicated that ileal bypass surgery leads to a reduction in cardiovascular morbidity and mortality,[189] but the individual lipid-lowering response to this surgical procedure is variable, and in the opinion of the authors, it cannot be generally recommended. LDL-apheresis may be appropriate for selected patients with severe heterozygous familial hypercholesterolemia in whom optimal drug therapy fails to reduce LDL cholesterol concentrations to less than 160 mg/dl.[190]

TABLE 21-13. Efficacy of Combined Drug Regimens in Heterozygous Familial Hypercholesterolemia

Drug Combination	Percent Decrease in LDL Cholesterol	No. Patients Studied	References
Cholestyramine + NA	−48	6	Packard et al., 1980[179]
Cholestipol + NA	−47	11	Illingworth et al., 1981[180]
Colestipol + lovastatin	−54	10	Illingworth, 1984[181]
Cholestyramine + simvastatin	−54	13	Lintott et al., 1989[182]
Cholestyramine + pravastatin	−45	30	Hoogerbrugge et al., 1990[183]
Cholestyramine + bezafibrate	−31	18	Curtis et al., 1988[184]
Lovastatin + NA	−49	8	Illingworth and Bacon, 1989[173]
Lovastatin + Colestipol + NA	67	21	Malloy et al., 1987[185]

NA = Nicotinic acid (niacin).

Intensive therapeutic intervention is necessary to reduce the severely elevated plasma concentrations of total and LDL cholesterol in patients with homozygous familial hypercholesterolemia. However, these patients, particularly those who are true homozygotes with no functional LDL receptors, respond poorly to single-drug therapy or combination drug therapy and invariably require other adjunctive measures to optimally reduce their LDL cholesterol concentrations. At the present time, LDL-apheresis is the treatment of choice for patients with homozygous familial hypercholesterolemia, and this technique affords an opportunity to reduce plasma concentrations of LDL cholesterol by 80 to 90 percent in the immediate postapheresis period, with average reductions of 50 to 60 percent between treatments when the procedure is performed at weekly intervals.[190] The rate of increase in the plasma concentrations of LDL cholesterol can be reduced by concurrent therapy with lipid-lowering drugs, particularly HMG CoA reductase inhibitors or nicotinic acid.[191,192] Treatment of patients with homozygous familial hypercholesterolemia by plasmapheresis has been shown to favorably affect the natural history of the premature coronary artery disease which occurs in these patients.[193] Liver transplantation has been the most effective of the surgical procedures used in the treatment of homozygous familial hypercholesterolemia but is associated with all the complications of long-term immunosuppressive therapy. Liver transplantation, however, offers the advantage of providing functional LDL receptors in the transplanted liver; this procedure reduced concentrations of LDL cholesterol by 81 and 83 percent, respectively, in two children with homozygous familial hypercholesterolemia.[194,195] The National Institutes of Health recently approved gene replacement therapy for the treatment of homozygous familial hypercholesterolemia, and this technique may afford the potential to provide functional LDL receptors to the liver without the complications associated with liver transplantation.

Familial Defective Apolipoprotein B-100

Definition

Familial defective apolipoprotein B-100 (FDB) is an autosomal dominant disorder in which substitution of the amino acid glutamine for arginine at residue 3,500 in apoprotein B-100 results in LDL particles which have defective binding to the LDL receptor. This results in hypercholesterolemia; all patients identified to date have been heterozygous for FDB, and their plasma contains both normal and defective binding LDL particles. The diagnosis of FDB is based on an analysis of DNA and the demonstration of the G to A substitution at nucleotide 10,699 by polymerase chain reaction techniques.

Clinical Characteristics

Initial studies in which FDB was identified in patients with moderate hypercholesterolemia suggested that this disorder is not associated with any ocular, cutaneous, or tendon manifestations of hypercholesterolemia.[196] However, more recent studies in which patients with hypercholesterolemia attending specialty lipid clinics have been screened for FDB have indicated that the clinical phenotype mirrors that seen in patients with heterozygous familial hypercholesterolemia and that patients with FDB may have a premature corneal arcus and frequently have tendon xanthomas.[196–198] The development of tendon xanthomas in patients with FDB appears to increase with increasing age and may be higher in patients with more severe degrees of hypercholesterolemia. Figure 21-23 illustrates the frequency of tendon xanthomas in male and female patients with FDB identified in the Lipid Disorders Clinic at Oregon Health Sciences University when stratified according to the age of individual patients and plasma concentrations of LDL cholesterol obtained on diet only. Deposition of LDL-derived cholesterol in the tendons of patients with FDB also appears to be paralleled by an increased risk of coronary and, potentially, carotid artery disease. The incidence of coronary atherosclerosis is clearly increased and, on the basis of data from patients identified in Oregon and Europe, parallels that seen in patients with heterozygous familial hypercholesterolemia.[197–199]

Genetics

FDB is inherited as an autosomal dominant trait that shows complete penetration in children and young adults. The gene frequency of FDB varies among different populations but has an estimated frequency of 1 in 700 in the United Kingdom, Germany, and North America.[197,198,200] FDB was present in 3 percent of patients with a clinical phenotype consistent with heterozygous familial hypercholesterolemia attending a lipid clinic in Munich, Germany, and represents 8 percent of this patient population attending our Lipid Disorders Clinic in Portland, Oregon.[197,199]

Diagnostic Laboratory Features

The diagnosis of FDB is based on demonstration of the G → A mutation at nucleotide 10,699 in the apolipoprotein B gene by means of amplification of genomic DNA and subsequent hybridization with allele-specific oligonucleotide probes.[197,201] The presence of defective binding LDL particles isolated from the

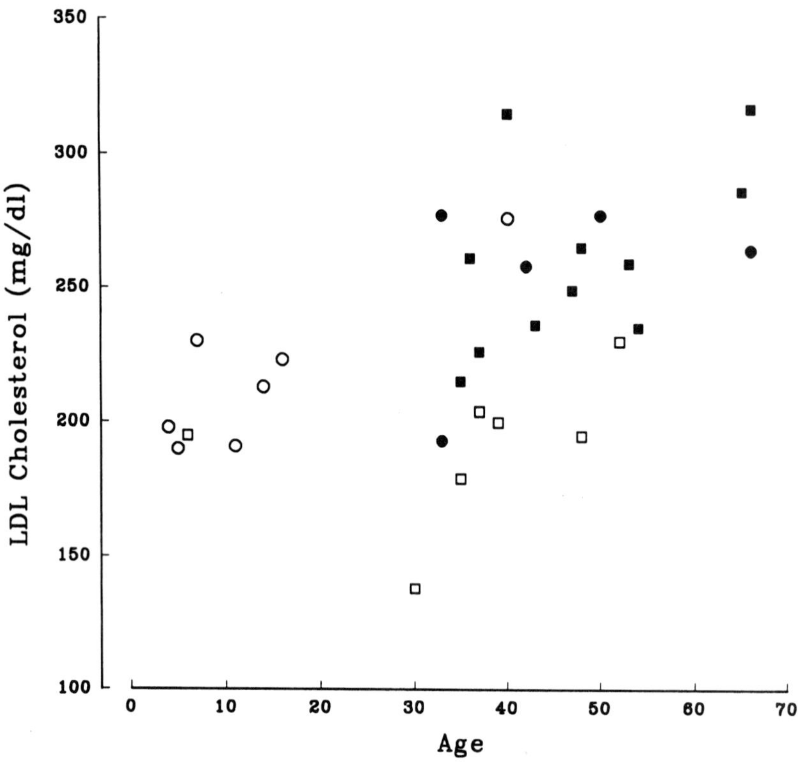

FIGURE 21-23. Plasma LDL concentrations in patients with familial defective apolipoprotein B-100 plotted as a function of age. The data are from patients identified to have this disorder attending the Lipid Disorders Clinic at Oregon Health Sciences University. Note that with increasing age, the number of patients who have tendon xanthomas increases. Male, no xanthoma; female, no xanthoma; male, with xanthoma; female, with xanthoma.

plasma of patients with FDB can also be demonstrated by competitive binding studies with ^{125}I-labeled LDL and cultured human fibroblasts, but the latter technique is more labor-intensive and less specific. It is likely that other amino acid substitutions in the apolipoprotein B molecule exist, and the latter technique would serve to identify these before precise delineation of the molecular defect in the apo-B gene. To date, all patients with FDB have been heterozygous for this disorder, and their plasma contains both defective binding and normal LDL particles in a ratio of approximately 7:3.[200] Despite a specific genetic etiology for FDB, the magnitude of LDL elevation observed in patients with this disorder is quite variable (Fig. 21-23), although in the majority of patients, LDL cholesterol concentrations exceed 190 mg/dl. Plasma triglyceride concentrations are generally normal, and in contrast to the situation in patients with heterozygous familial hypercholesterolemia, in whom concentrations of HDL cholesterol are reduced, HDL cholesterol concentrations appear to be normal in patients with FDB.[197,200]

Pathophysiology

The initial identification of a patient with defective binding of LDL was made during kinetic studies of homologous and autologous LDL metabolism in patients with primary hypercholesterolemia in which it was observed that the fractional catabolic rate of ^{125}I LDL isolated from one patient was impaired irrespective of whether the LDL was injected into the patient himself or into another patient with primary hypercholesterolemia. Subsequent studies have indicated that LDL particles isolated from the plasma of patients with FDB exhibit extremely poor binding to the LDL receptor on cultured human fibroblasts.[202] Thus, the hypercholesterolemia in patients with FDB results from an impairment in high-affinity receptor-mediated catabolism of the abnormal LDL particles present in the plasma of these patients. Predictably, patients with FDB show abnormalities only in the concentrations of LDL and do not have hypertriglyceridemia or accumulate increased plasma concentrations of remnant lipoproteins. On theoretical grounds, we predict that the magnitude of hypercholesterolemia in patients with FDB will be exacerbated by factors known to increase the production of VLDL apoprotein B and that double heterozygotes for FDB and heterozygous familial hypercholesterolemia will exhibit more severe hypercholesterolemia and be more refractory to lipid-lowering therapy.

Treatment

The goals of therapy in patients with FDB are to reduce the plasma concentrations of LDL cholesterol and, in patients with concurrent increased levels of Lp(a), to reduce the plasma concentrations of this lipoprotein as well. Data on the response to specific dietary interventions in patients with FDB are unavailable, but it may be predicted that factors which would either decrease hepatic VLDL and LDL synthesis or enhance LDL receptor expression would promote reductions in the synthesis of LDL particles in the plasma of these patients and concurrently enhance the catabolism of the normal LDL particles. Although an initial report[203] in two patients with FDB suggested that they were hyporesponders to simvastatin, studies in a larger number of patients[199] have indicated that the overall response to lovastatin in patients with FDB is similar to that seen in patients with other primary causes of hypercholesterolemia, but the individual magnitude of LDL reduction is heterogeneous. Surprisingly, patients with FDB appear to be as responsive to treatment with bile acid sequestrants as are patients with heterozygous familial hypercholesterolemia[204] (and unpublished observations). The ability of these drugs to reduce LDL concentrations in patients with FDB seems unlikely to be due to an enhanced metabolism of LDL particles in the plasma of these patients but may reflect an increase in hepatic catabolism of VLDL remnants, thereby reducing the ultimate production of LDL particles with defective binding present in the plasma of FDB patients. Recent studies have demonstrated a 24 percent decrease in LDL cholesterol concentrations in patients with FDB treated with 3 g per day of niacin compared with a mean reduction of 14 percent in patients with heterozygous familial hypercholesterolemia treated with the same dose.[205] These results suggest that nicotinic acid may be a particularly effective drug in the treatment of patients with FDB.

Combined Hypercholesterolemia and Hypertriglyceridemia

Combined elevations of cholesterol and triglyceride can be due to the presence of an increased number of VLDL and LDL particles of normal composition (type IIb phenotype) or may reflect the presence of abnormal chylomicron and VLDL remnant particles that are typical of dysbetalipoproteinemia (type III hyperlipoproteinemia). It is in this group of patients with total plasma cholesterol values ranging between 280 and 700 mg/dl and concurrent triglyceride values ranging between 300 and 1,500 mg/dl that more detailed studies should always be undertaken to precisely define the lipoprotein phenotype. Differentiation between patients with increased concentrations of VLDL and LDL (type IIb phenotype) and patients with type III hyperlipoproteinemia requires ultracentrifugal separation of VLDL in order to document the abnormal cholesterol-rich particles which are present in the plasma of patients with type III hyperlipoproteinemia. The detection of beta-VLDL by agarose gel electrophoresis and the identification of the abnormal apoprotein E-2/E-2 phenotype can help confirm the diagnosis of type III hypolipoproteinemia.

Increased concentrations of LDL in the presence of concurrent hypertriglyceridemia (phenotypic type IIb) may be secondary to other disorders (Table 21–10) or may be attributable to familial hypercholesterolemia, familial combined hyperlipidemia, or other genotypically less well defined causes. The elevated levels of VLDL present in the plasma of these patients are commonly accompanied by reduced levels of HDL cholesterol.[161] In many patients with phenotypic type IIb hyperlipidemia, the presence of a primary genetic disorder may be exacerbated by concurrent secondary disorders such as non-insulin–dependent diabetes mellitus, obesity, excessive alcohol intake, and medications. Thus, attainment of ideal weight, restricted use of alcohol, and control of other causes of secondary hyperlipidemia should be strongly encouraged in these patients. Because weight gain can cause a marked exacerbation of hypertriglyceridemia, patients should be cautioned to strive for modest levels of maintainable weight loss. More extreme weight loss is frequently associated with subsequent weight gain, potentially leading to chylomicronemia and pancreatitis.

The presence of tendon xanthomas and/or primary hypercholesterolemia in children within a given family indicates an underlying genotypic diagnosis of familial hypercholesterolemia, whereas in a family with multiple different phenotypes and an autosomal dominant pattern of inheritance, the genotypic diagnosis is most likely to be familial combined hyperlipidemia. The risk of premature cardiovascular disease is increased in patients with these hereditary disorders (type IIa or IIb phenotype).

Familial Combined Hyperlipidemia

Definition

Familial combined hyperlipidemia is an autosomal dominant inherited disorder in which affected family members may display different phenotypic forms of hyperlipidemia. The disorder appears to be due to an inherent overproduction of apoprotein B and the apoprotein B–containing lipoproteins, VLDL and LDL, by the liver. This defect may result in the expression of increased levels of LDL cholesterol (type IIa phenotype), combined elevations of VLDL and LDL cholesterol (type IIb phenotype), or singular elevation in the concentration of VLDL (type IV phenotype).

Clinical Characteristics

There are no typical physical findings associated with the underlying presence of familial combined hyperlipidemia. Tendon xanthomas are usually absent in patients with this disorder, but have been reported in rare patients.[206] The absence of tendon xanthomas in patients with primary hypercholesterolemia cannot be used to exclude the diagnosis of familial hypercholesterolemia, as not all patients with familial hypercholesterolemia have tendon xanthomas, especially among younger patients. Severe hypertriglyceridemia with the development of eruptive xanthomas may occur in patients with familial combined hyperlipidemia who concurrently develop diabetes or other secondary disorders, whereas patients who are homozygous for apoprotein E-2 may present clinically with tuberous xanthomas and a type III phenotype. In patients with familial combined hyperlipidemia who have elevated levels of only LDL cholesterol, the total plasma cholesterol concentration usually ranges from 250 to 350 mg/dl (6.47 to 9.05 mmol/L), with LDL cholesterol ranging from 180 to 300 mg/dl (4.65 to 7.76 mmol/L).

Because familial combined hyperlipidemia shows incomplete penetration in children and young adults, lipid values in affected patients often do not increase substantially until the third or fourth decade of life. This, together with the lower absolute lipid values usually seen in familial combined hyperlipidemias compared with familial hypercholesterolemia, may explain the lower incidence of premature coronary artery disease in patients with familial combined hyperlipidemia. The typical age of onset for symptomatic coronary artery disease in men with familial combined hyperlipidemia is approximately 50; it occurs 10 to 15 years later in women patients.[207]

Genetics

Familial combined hyperlipidemia is a genetically and clinically heterogeneous disorder that is inherited as an autosomal dominant trait with incomplete penetration in children and young adults. It is a common genetic disease, with an estimated frequency of 1 or 2 in 200 in North America. Because no specific marker for familial combined hyperlipidemia exists, it is likely that many patients with moderate inherited hypercholesterolemia who do not have tendon xanthomas have familial combined hyperlipidemia. Heterozygous deficiency of LPL may constitute one subtype of this disorder.[208] In another recent study, familial combined hyperlipidemia was linked to the apoprotein A-I-C-III-A-IV gene cluster on chromosome 11q23-q24 in 16 unrelated probands of northern European origin.[209] Further studies are required to better delineate the genetic determinants of this heterogeneous disorder.

Diagnostic Laboratory Features

Patients with familial combined hyperlipidemia may present with primary hypercholesterolemia, primary hypertriglyceridemia, or combined elevations of cholesterol and triglyceride. Because the expression of this disorder appears to be exacerbated by factors such as weight gain and increasing age, the diagnosis of familial combined hyperlipidemia rests on a demonstration of multiple different lipoprotein phenotypes in different family members with an autosomal dominant pattern of inheritance. The detection of an elevated level of apoprotein B is consistent with this disorder but is not diagnostic. Some patients with familial combined hyperlipidemia appear to have proportionally higher levels of LDL apoprotein B than would be expected from their LDL cholesterol concentrations.[210] Studies by Sniderman and colleagues[211] suggest that these patients with high levels of apoprotein B also have an increased incidence of premature cardiovascular disease even when the LDL cholesterol level is not elevated.

Pathophysiology

Lack of a specific marker for familial combined hyperlipidemia has hindered investigations of the biochemical causes of this disorder(s). Kinetic studies in which radioiodinated lipoproteins have been injected into patients with familial combined hyperlipidemia have shown an inherently high production rate of apoprotein B, VLDL, and LDL in these patients. In contrast to the low fractional catabolic rate of LDL seen in patients with familial hypercholesterolemia, the rate of catabolism of LDL is normal in patients with familial combined hyperlipidemia, and the expression of LDL receptors in cells from these patients is also normal.[212] By current diagnostic criteria, familial combined hyperlipidemia undoubtedly represents a heterogeneous group of disorders in which the hepatic production of apoprotein B-100 is increased. Further insights into the causes of this defect should be rapidly forthcoming now that the gene for apoprotein B has been cloned.[213,214]

Treatment

The primary goal of therapy for patients with familial combined hyperlipidemia is to reduce the levels of LDL cholesterol and apoprotein B in plasma. Because hepatic production of VLDL and LDL may be increased by secondary factors such as obesity, type II diabetes, and excessive alcohol intake, correction of secondary predisposing factors should be attempted in all patients with this disorder. Knowledge about the pathophysiology of familial combined hyperlipidemia suggests that lipid-lowering agents which primarily inhibit the synthesis of apoprotein B, VLDL, and LDL may be the most effective therapy in patients with this disorder. Based on these criteria, nicotinic acid is the drug of choice for patients with familial combined hyperlipidemia. The bile acid–binding resins cholestyramine and colestipol are second-choice agents but can be useful in combination with niacin or HMG CoA reductase inhibitors. The use of bile acid–binding resins as single-drug therapy can exacerbate preexisting hypertriglyceridemia and should be avoided.[215] Gemfibrozil and probucol are third-choice drugs that are variably effective in this disorder. The results of a recent angiographic study of men with presumed familial combined hyperlipidemia showed that net regression of established coronary artery disease could be detected after $21\frac{1}{2}$ years of aggressive treatment [LDL cholesterol reduced to less than 100 mg/dl (2.59 mmol/L)] with diet and colestipol combined with niacin or lovastatin.[104]

Primary Type III Hyperlipoproteinemia

Definition

Type III hyperlipoproteinemia, also referred to as broad-beta disease, floating beta disease, and dysbetalipoproteinemia, is a rare disorder characterized by the accumulation in plasma of abnormal chylomicron and VLDL remnant particles. Such particles have a density in the range of intermediate-density lipoproteins (*d* 1.006 to 1.019), have an abnormally high ratio of cholesterol to triglyceride, and exhibit beta mobility on agarose gel electrophoresis. Patients with this disorder are usually homozygous for the abnormal apoprotein E-2. Plasma lipid values vary widely but generally reveal cholesterol levels in the range of 300 to 600 mg/dl with triglyceride levels of 400 to 800 mg/dl.

Clinically, patients with type III hyperlipidemia sometimes have palmar and tuberous xanthomas and display an increased incidence of premature coronary and peripheral vascular disease.

Clinical Characteristics

The initial recognition of type III hyperlipidemia as "xanthoma tuberosum" was made by Goffman and colleagues[216] more than 40 years ago. Although the physical findings in patients with type III vary widely, certain features are strongly suggestive of this diagnosis.[217] The most characteristic and common[218] xanthomas seen in type III, termed xanthoma striatum palmare or palmar xanthomas, are present on the hands. These lesions, which may be the only skin manifestation of the disorder, vary from a yellow-orange discoloration of the palmar creases of both hands to more advanced lesions with planar elevation of the skin and eventually, in the most severe form, to raised tuberous xanthomas on the palms and fingers (Fig. 21-24). Palmar xanthomas occur in less than 50 percent of patients with this disorder, but usually are considered diagnostic of type III hyperlipidemia when present.

Tuberoeruptive xanthomas (Fig. 21-25), which consist of raised erythematous nodular lesions 0.5 cm or greater in diameter that commonly coalesce into larger lesions, are also typical of type III. They have a tendency to occur in areas of pressure, most notably the extensor surface of the elbows and knees and on the buttocks. Tuberous xanthomas were present in 51 percent of the patients studied by Morganroth and associates,[218] whereas in other series their incidence has varied from 35 to 100 percent. Xanthelasmas and corneal arcus are uncommon, but tendon xanthomas are present in

FIGURE 21-24. Tuberous palmar xanthomas in a patient with type III hyperlipoproteinemia.

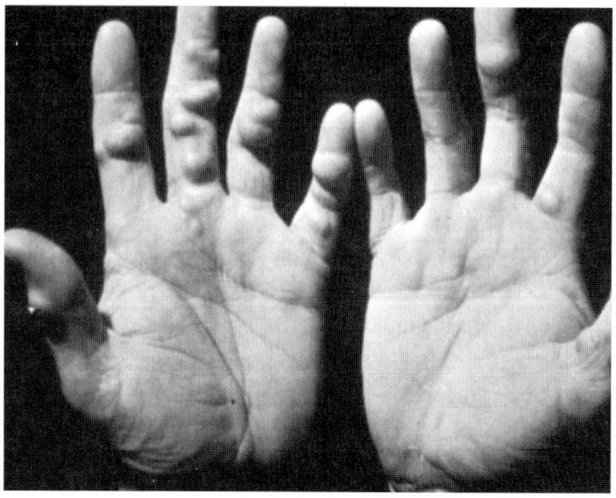

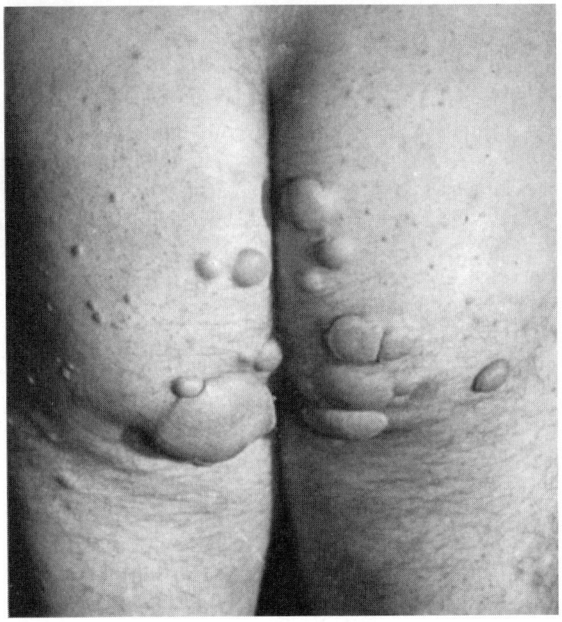

FIGURE 21-25. Tuberoeruptive xanthomas on the buttocks of a patient with type III hyperlipoproteinemia. The lesions regressed with hypolipidemic therapy.

about 10 percent of patients with type III. Patients with type III have an increased incidence of premature coronary and peripheral vascular disease, both of which have been present in 20 to 40 percent of the patients studied in most reports.[219] The likelihood of both complications is higher in patients who present with advanced tuberous xanthomas than in those with less severe skin lesions.

Few cases of phenotypic type III have been described in patients under 20 years of age, and these have frequently been associated with coexisting hypothyroidism. Phenotypic expression of the type III disorder in older patients is also commonly associated with obesity, hypothyroidism, diabetes mellitus, high fat diet, or a coexistent familial hyperlipidemia. By far the most common of these factors is obesity, which is present in up to 75 percent of cases. Screening of the family members of a patient with type III hyperlipidemia is indicated to allow detection of other coexistent familial lipid disorders or rare cases of autosomal dominant type III hyperlipidemia. Because the pattern of inheritance is nearly always autosomal recessive, heterozygous family members have no manifestations of the disorder. Phenotypic expression of type III hyperlipidemia is more common in men than in premenopausal women, but menopause is a common cause of the development of type III hyperlipidemia in apo E2 heterozygotes.

The autosomal recessive pattern of inheritance of type III hyperlipoproteinemia has been clarified by the recognition that apoprotein E exists in three common allelic forms—apoproteins E-2, E-3, and E-4—and that the vast majority of patients with this disorder are homozygous for apoprotein E-2.[220] The different allelic forms of apoprotein E can be identified by isoelectric focusing or can be confirmed by analysis of DNA samples obtained from peripheral white blood cells. The frequency of homozygosity for apoprotein E-2 has been estimated at 1 percent of the population,[219] whereas heterozygosity occurs in approximately 15 percent of the population. As discussed later, however, only about 1 percent of patients who are homozygous for apoprotein E-2 actually develop hyperlipidemia. Thus, the prevalence of the type III phenotype has been estimated at 1 or 2 in 10,000. The majority of patients who are homozygous for the apoprotein E-2 phenotype are actually mildly hypolipidemic, but many of these individuals have an abnormal ratio of VLDL cholesterol to triglyceride and may accumulate abnormal beta-VLDL in plasma. The absence of functional apo E3 or E4 causes a defect in clearance of triglyceride-rich lipoproteins, but type III hyperlipidemia ensues only when a second disorder associated with overproduction of VLDL (e.g., hypothyroidism, menopause, diabetes, familial combined hyperlipidemia) is present. Rare forms of type III hyperlipidemia may be inherited in an autosomal dominant mode.

Diagnostic Laboratory Features

Lipid concentrations in patients with type III hyperlipidemia vary widely, but plasma cholesterol levels commonly are 300 to 600 mg/dl and triglyceride levels are 400 to 800 mg/dl. These parameters alone, however, are not diagnostic, as similar values may occur in patients with forms of hyperlipidemia. Determination of the ratio of VLDL cholesterol to the total plasma triglyceride concentration is the most readily available method for the diagnosis of type III hyperlipoproteinemia,[221] but this determination requires ultracentrifugation. A ratio greater than 0.30 is diagnostic, whereas values of 0.25 to 0.30 should be considered suggestive. This method is reliable at triglyceride values of 150 to 1,000 mg/dl, above which spuriously low ratios may be obtained because of the contribution of chylomicrons to the calculated ratio. An older and less optimal criterion for the diagnosis of type III hyperlipidemia is based on the identification of a beta-migrating band, sometimes referred to as β-VLDL, on agarose gel electrophoresis of plasma lipoproteins. The presence of β-VLDL on agarose gel electrophoresis is, however, not specific and may be seen in some patients with the type IV phenotype.

Although still available primarily in research laboratories, separation of the apoprotein E isoproteins by isoelectric focusing is a reliable method for the diagnosis of most patients with type III hyperlipoproteinemia.[219,220] These studies have disclosed that the vast majority of patients with type III hyperlipoproteinemia are homozygotes for apoprotein E-2 and lack apoproteins E-3 and E-4. This disorder may also occur in patients with a complete deficiency of apoprotein E[222] and is likely to be found in patients with aberrant hepatic receptors for apoprotein E[223] and patients with other amino acid substitutions in the apoprotein E receptor-binding domain that do not affect the isoelectric point of the variant. Analysis of the apoprotein E genotype using DNA isolated from anticoagulated blood can be accomplished using the polymerase chain reaction and specific probes. This sophisticated method of analysis is available for clinical use at only a limited number of research laboratories.

Pathophysiology

Type III hyperlipoproteinemia is an inherited disorder in which the phenotypic expression requires the absence of functional apo E-3 or E-4 (which causes a defect in clearance of triglyceride-rich lipoproteins) in association with overproduction of chylomicrons and VLDL. Homozygosity for the dysfunctional apo E2 alone is usually insufficient to cause hyperlipidemia. Factors that may contribute to increased production of triglyceride-rich lipoproteins include obesity, hypothyroidism, diabetes, and concomitant familial hyperlipidemia. Thus, apo E-2 homozygosity often is "silent" unless the defect in triglyceride clearance is unmasked by overproduction of lipoproteins.

Studies of the binding of apoprotein E–containing lipoproteins to receptors of various cells have shown that apoprotein E-2 has a markedly reduced binding affinity for the LDL-receptor and VLDL-receptor. The normal interaction of apoprotein E with its receptor depends on the presence of specific lysine and arginine residues situated between amino acids 140 and 160 in the apoprotein E molecule. The decrease in binding affinity of apoprotein E-2 is commonly due to a substitution of cysteine for the positively charged amino acid arginine at residue 158 in the apoprotein E molecule. The difference in isoelectric point between apoproteins E-3 and E-4 reflects a substitution of cysteine for arginine at residue 112. Because this does not affect receptor binding, the affinities for binding of apoproteins E-3 and E-4 to the LDL and VLDL receptors are comparable. In patients with type III hyperlipoproteinemia, defective receptor binding of apoprotein E-2 results in delayed clearance of these particles from plasma, leading to accumulation in plasma of remnant lipoproteins (e.g., beta-VLDL). Small amounts of remnant lipoproteins may accumulate in the plasma of patients who are homozygous for apoprotein E-2, but the development of hyperlipidemia requires the concurrent presence of a second disorder leading to overproduction of chylimicrons and/or VLDL (Fig. 21–26). Homozygosity for apo E-2 in the absence of overproduction of chylomicrons and/or VLDL tends to be associated with slightly reduced plasma concentrations of total and LDL cholesterol, presumably due to impaired conversion of VLDL to LDL.[220,223] Although LDL cholesterol concentrations often are low in type III hyperlipidemia, high plasma concentrations of atherogenic remnant lipoproteins substantially increase the risk of myocardial infarction, stroke, and peripheral vascular disease. The accelerated atherosclerosis that develops in patients with type III hyperlipoproteinemia is believed to be due to the uptake of cholesterol-rich beta-VLDL particles by macrophages and smooth muscle cells in the arterial wall.

Treatment

Patients with type III hyperlipidemia often respond very well to therapy with a regimen of lifestyle modification and drug therapy. Diet modification is especially important in this endeavor because these patients often are very sensitive to the adverse effects of dietary cholesterol and saturated fat on hyperlidemia. As will be discussed later, we favor a unified approach to dietary treatment of hyperlipidemias and encourage a low-fat (20 percent), 100-mg-cholesterol diet together with caloric restriction to achieve ideal body weight. Identification and treatment of reversible secondary causes of hyperlipidemia is essential. Thus, appropriate studies to exclude hypothyroidism, excessive alcohol consumption, diabetes mellitus, and a concomitant second familial hyperlipidemia should be undertaken in all patients. Treatment of hyperglycemia in diabetic patients is a critical part of management of type III hyperlipidemia. Reduction of caloric intake to achieve ideal body weight in obese patients is extremely beneficial and by itself was successful in achieving normal lipid values in 25 of 29 patients treated by Morganroth and associates.[218] In the absence of a contraindication such as breast cancer, estrogen replacement therapy should be given to women who are postmenopausal or are otherwise estrogen-deficient. Although estrogen replacement often elevates plasma triglyceride concentrations in ordinary patients, such therapy can ameliorate type III hyperlipidemia in some patients. Women who are postmenopausal or perimenopausal may respond well to treatment with ethinyl estradiol (1 μg per kilogram per day),[224] but will require coadministration of a progestational agent to help minimize the risk of endometrial carcinoma.

In patients whose response to diet treatment is less than adequate, drug therapy may still be highly effective. Fibric acid derivatives usually are the first choice for drug therapy. Gemfibrozil can be given at a dose of 600 mg orally twice daily, clofibrate at a dose of 1 g orally twice daily, and fenofibrate can be given as a single daily dose of 200 mg. Despite reservations about the use of clofibrate as therapy for other disorders of lipid metabolism, this drug is extremely effective in patients with type III hyperlipoproteinemia. Therapy with 1 g twice daily usually results in rapid decreases in the concentrations of cholesterol and triglyceride (Fig. 21–27), and in some cases patients can be maintained on lower doses (e.g., 500 mg twice daily) with equal efficacy. Nicotinic acid 3 to 6 g per day and statin drugs may also be effective as monotherapy. Although statins are only modestly efficacious in the treatment of ordinary hypertriglyceridemia, patients with type III may respond well to statins because these drugs enhance clearance of remnant lipoproteins from plasma as a consequence of upregulation of hepatic expression of LDL receptors. Fish oil (in adequate doses, e.g., more than 5 to 6 grams daily) also may be efficacious in the treatment of type III hyperlipidemia, and can be used safely with other lipid-lowering drugs. Refractory patients, particularly those in whom the expression of type III hyperlipoproteinemia occurs as a consequence of underlying familial combined hyperlipidemia, may be treated with a combination of nicotinic acid and a fibrate or a statin. Patients receiving combination drug therapy should be monitored closely because of the increased risk of hepatic dysfunction and rhabdomyolysis. The bile acid–binding resins

FIGURE 21-26. Diagrammatic representation of the factors contributing to clinical expression of type III hyperlipoproteinemia.

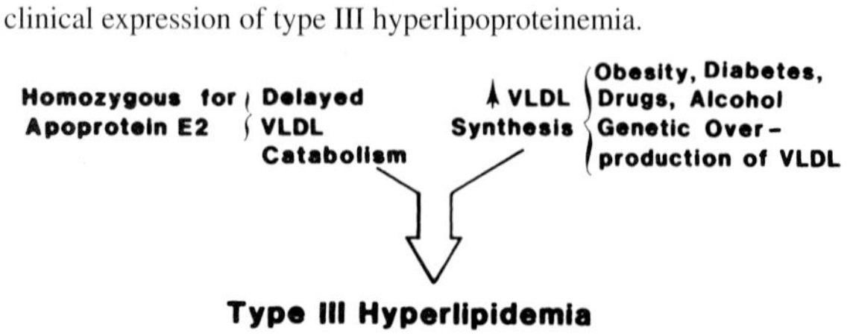

FIGURE 21-27. The effects of an isocaloric >300 mg cholesterol diet plus clofibrate (2 g per day) on the plasma cholesterol, triglyceride, and peak reactive hyperemic blood flow (RHBF) in six patients with type III hyperlipoproteinemia. (*Adapted from Zelis et al.*[225])

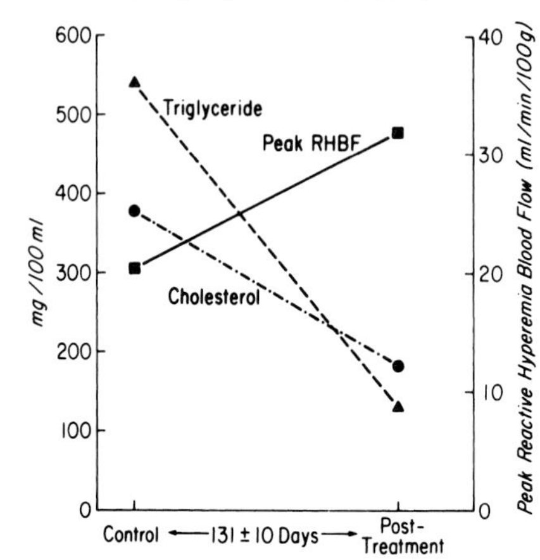

are contraindicated in patients with type III hyperlipidemia. The use of bile acid–binding resins will exacerbate this disorder, as will distal ileal bypass surgery.

The response to diet and drug therapy is usually dramatic, and, as occurred with the patient shown in Figs. 21-24 and 21-25, regression of xanthomas frequently occurs in less than 1 year. Marked improvement in the symptoms of angina pectoris and intermittent claudication have also been noted and suggest that regression of xanthomas may be paralleled by similar changes in lesions of the arterial wall. Objective evidence of such changes was obtained by Zelis and associates[225] (Fig. 21-27), who noted a 55 percent improvement in maximal blood flow in patients with type III treated with diet plus clofibrate. The excellent therapeutic response found in patients with type III hyperlipidemia justifies an aggressive approach to both the diagnosis and the treatment of this interesting disorder.

Hepatic Lipase Deficiency

Combined hyperlipidemia with elevated plasma concentrations of cholesterol (260 to 1,500 mg/dl) and triglyceride (395 to 8,200 mg/dl) has been ascribed to a deficiency of hepatic lipase in two Canadian patients.[226] Clinically, the index patient had palmar and tuberoeruptive xanthomas and was noted to have a corneal arcus at age 38. Lipoprotein studies demonstrated the accumulation of small VLDL particles with beta mobility, but no abnormality in apoprotein E could be demonstrated. After intravenous injection of heparin, concentrations of HL in plasma were less than 5 percent of normal whereas LPL activity was not reduced. The ratio of VLDL cholesterol to total plasma cholesterol (which is generally greater than 0.3 in patients with type III hyperlipoproteinemia) ranged between 0.16 and 0.22 in patients with HL deficiency, whereas analysis of the composition of LDL disclosed a characteristic enrichment of these particles with triglyceride (28 percent of LDL by weight; normal, 6 percent). Dietary restriction of calories, total fat, and cholesterol was effective in reducing plasma lipid values in this disorder, but clofibrate appeared to be ineffective.

Hypertriglyceridemia

Hyperchylomicronemia: Types I and V Hyperlipoproteinemia, Familial Apoprotein C-II Deficiency

Definition

An abnormal accumulation of chylomicrons in plasma is characteristic of both type I and type V hyperlipidemia and justifies discussing them together. In type I hyperlipidemia, chylomicronemia is detectable in plasma obtained after an overnight (12 to 16 h) fast, and levels of VLDL are normal; in the type V phenotype, chylomicronemia is accompanied by a concomitant increase in concentrations of VLDL. Both phenotypes may occur as primary familial disorders or secondary to a variety of associated conditions. The biochemical defect in type I is due to a functional deficiency or absence of the enzyme LPL; in type V, impaired clearance of chylomicrons has not been correlated with lipolytic activity, and the nature of the deficit or deficits is not known. In familial apoprotein C-II deficiency, the clearances of both chylomicrons and VLDL are impaired because C-II is a cofactor for LPL activation. The clinical aspects of this rare apoprotein disorder are identical to those of type I hyperlipidemia due to LPL deficiency.[227]

Clinical Features

Both the type I and type V phenotypes may occur as primary familial disorders or may be secondary to a number of associated underlying conditions (Table 21-10). In children the disorder is most likely to be familial, whereas in adults secondary causes constitute the most common etiology. In many cases, however, secondary factors are the provoking stimulus that exacerbates the expression of an underlying familial hyperlipidemia and brings it to clinical attention. The clinical features of both type I and type V are similar and are attributable to the presence of hyperchylomicronemia.[227–230] The age of presentation, however, is different, and in most cases type I is detected in childhood. In a review of 32 cases, Fredrickson and Levy noted that the diagnosis was made before age 10 in 22 patients and prior to age 1 in 7.[228] In contrast, patients with type V usually, although not invariably,[231] are detected after age 20 and generally do not have severe hyperchylomicronemia in childhood.

Abdominal pain is the most frequent symptom that brings the patient to medical attention. The pain may be mild to severe and may mimic an "acute abdomen." The pain may be generalized or localized to the upper abdomen and frequently radiates to the back. Associated tenderness of the liver or spleen is common and is accompanied by hepatomegaly, splenomegaly, or both in more than 50 percent of cases. The abdominal pain may proceed to acute pancreatitis. In the series of 32 patients with type I reported by Fredrickson and Levy, 24 reported abdominal pain and 12 had episodes of pancreatitis, with the latter being responsible for four fatalities.[228] Similarly, in reports of patients with type V hyperlipidemia, abdominal pain has been noted in up to 70 percent, with pancreatitis seen in 50 percent.[232,233] Because chylomicrons may interfere with the chemical determination of amylase and result in falsely low readings, such assays should be performed on diluted or chylomicron-free plasma, or alternatively, the serum lipase level or the amylase creatinine clearance ratios should be determined on urine samples.[234] Values greater than 0.04 are suggestive of pancreatitis. The mechanism by which hyperchylomicronemia produces abdominal pain and pancreatitis remains an enigma. Stretching of the hepatic and splenic capsule secondary to enlargement of these organs from the infiltration of fat seems a likely cause of the pain and tenderness of these organs, especially the liver. It has been postulated that the chylomicronemic state leads to occlusion of the microvasculature of the pancreas; with the resultant ischemia and necrosis, pancreatic enzymes are released locally to induce pancreatitis.

Two physical findings—lipemia retinalis and eruptive xanthomas—are diagnostic of severe hyperchylomicronemia. Eruptive xanthomas appear as 1- to 5-mm yellow papules on an erythematous base. The lesions are nonpruritic and characteristically appear on the trunk and the extensor surfaces of the arms, buttocks, and thighs (Figs. 21-28 and 21-29) during a period of several weeks. Their presence implies severe hyperchylomicronemia (triglycerides usually greater than 4,000 mg/dl). After therapeutic reduction of the hyperchylomicronemia, eruptive xanthomas gradually disappear during a 4- to 12-week period. In lipemia retinalis, the other hallmark of hyperchylomicronemia, the retinal arteries and veins have a salmon-pink color on funduscopic examination. This also disappears with treatment.

The type I phenotype is rarely associated with hyperglycemia or abnormal glucose tolerance, and affected patients are usually of normal body weight. In contrast, patients with the type V phenotype have a high incidence of hyperglycemia with hyperinsulinism

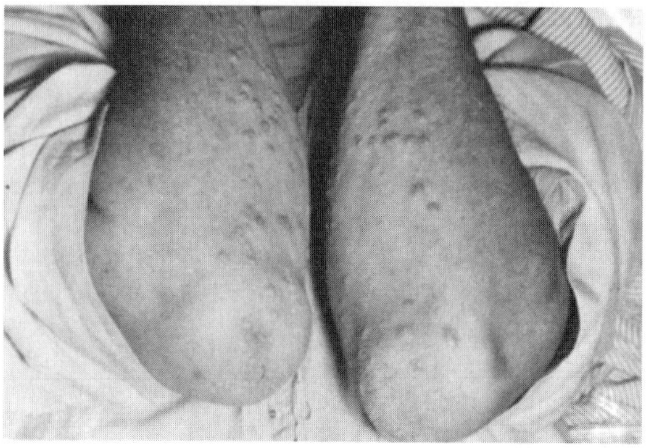

FIGURE 21-28. Eruptive xanthomas on the arms of a patient with severe hypertriglyceridemia and phenotypic type V hyperlipoproteinemia.

TABLE 21-14. Incidence of Atherosclerosis in Patients with Type V Hyperlipidemia and in Familial Hypercholesterolemia (Type IIa) (Percent of the Total Number)

	Type V (n = 83)*	Type IIa (n = 83)*
Coronary heart disease	32.5	38.6
Peripheral atherosclerosis	15.7	18.2
Cerebral vascular disease	7.2	6.8
Any atherosclerotic disease	43.4	44.6

*There were 44 men and 39 women in both groupings

and are frequently above ideal body weight. Although the relation between these abnormalities is complex, a positive correlation has been documented between the degree of hypertriglyceridemia and both body weight and hyperglycemia.[232] Type I hyperlipidemia does not appear to be associated with an increased incidence of atherosclerotic vascular disease.[227,228,230]

In patients with type V hyperlipidemia, by contrast, there is a high incidence of atherosclerotic disorders, including coronary, cerebral, and peripheral atherosclerosis (Table 21-14). A comparison of the incidence of atherosclerotic disorders in type V patients and in patients with familial hypercholesterolemia (type IIa) reveals a remarkable similarity. The numbers of type V and type IIa patients were 83 men and women in both groups, age- and sex-matched from our lipid clinic patients. Forty-three percent of the type V patients seen in our lipid clinic had clinical atherosclerotic disease, compared with 44.6 percent in patients with type IIa hyperlipidemia. As will be stressed subsequently, type V patients have particularly low LDL concentrations as well as low HDL. The predominant lipoproteins are chylomicrons, VLDL, and the remnant particles, which are particularly atherogenic. This is in contrast to the predominant lipoprotein LDL in the type IIa patients.

Genetics

Familial lipoprotein lipase deficiency (type I hyperlipoproteinemia) is inherited as an autosomal recessive trait. Obligate heterozygotes may have combined hyperlipidemia but have reduced levels of adipose tissue lipoprotein lipase.[25,208,235] Many different molecular defects result in a deficiency of lipoprotein lipase. The identification of the lipoprotein lipase gene has offered the possibility of determining the different mutations of this condition.[236]

The genetics of type V hyperlipoproteinemias are not well characterized, in part because of the heterogenous etiologies of these disorders. Family members of an index patient with phenotypic type V hyperlipoproteinemia show a high incidence of both the type IV and type V phenotypes, the frequencies of which both increase with age. In the largest study to date,[232] the distribution of lipoprotein phenotypes in 181 first-degree relatives from 32 patients with familial type V revealed 57 percent to be normal, 11 percent with type II phenotype, 15 percent with type IV, and 16 percent with type V. Fallat and Glueck noted an even higher incidence of type IV and type V phenotypes in first-degree relatives and concluded that the inheritance was consistent with an autosomal dominant mode of transmission.[233] These studies are consistent with the view that patients with the type V phenotype represent a heterogeneous population in which most appear to have familial hypertriglyceridemia or familial combined hyperlipidemia as the underlying genetic disorder.[230] Familial apoprotein C-II deficiency is inherited as an autosomal recessive trait.[24,227]

FIGURE 21-29. Eruptive xanthomas on the buttocks of a patient with severe hypertriglyceridemia and phenotypic type V hyperlipoproteinemia.

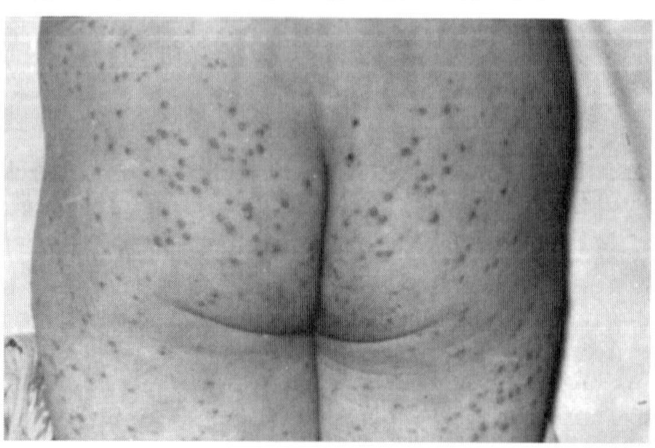

Diagnostic Laboratory Features

The determinations of cholesterol and triglyceride in plasma obtained after a 12- to 14-h fast, together with the visual inspection of a plasma sample that has been allowed to stand for 12 to 18 h at 4°C for the presence of chylomicronemia, will permit diagnosis of the type I or type V phenotype in most cases. In type I hyperlipidemia, increases in triglyceride are paralleled by a much smaller rise in cholesterol such that the triglyceride/cholesterol ratio is usually greater than 10:1 (e.g., triglyceride 4,200 mg/dl, cholesterol 320 mg/dl). Upon refrigeration, the chylomicron layer is seen to overlay a clear subnatant that does not contain increased concentrations of VLDL. The levels of both LDL and HDL in type I hyperlipidemia are low, typically averaging 50 percent of normal. Lipid values in the type V phenotype reflect the combined increase in both VLDL and chylomicrons; the triglyceride/cholesterol ratio is therefore lower than in type I and usually ranges from 5:1 to 8:1 (e.g., triglyceride 4,800 mg/dl, cholesterol 730 mg/dl). Concentrations of LDL and HDL in type V are 50 percent or more lower than normal and reflect the impaired catabolism of both VLDL and chylomicrons to smaller particles in this disorder. As previously discussed, hyperglycemia frequently coexists in patients with the type V phenotype but does not occur at increased frequency in patients with the type I disorder. Documentation of very low or absent levels of lipoprotein lipase mass and/or activity either in adipose tissue or in plasma after the intravenous injection of heparin remains the sine qua non for the diagnosis of type I hyperlipidemia. In contrast, the activity of both HL and LPL is usually normal in patients with type V hyperlipidemia.

Pathophysiology

The biochemical defect in type I hyperlipidemia involves an abnormality in the synthesis, storage, or, less likely, release of lipoprotein lipase. Abnormalities in chylomicrons obtained from patients with type I have not been demonstrated, and such particles are metabolized at a normal rate when infused into control subjects or used as a substrate for LPL in vitro. The profound impairment in chylomicron metabolism that occurs in patients with type I clearly illustrates the key role of LPL in normal chylomicron metabolism. It is also not clear why only chylomicrons accumulate in patients with type I, when in fact both chylomicrons and VLDL are thought to require LPL for hydrolysis of their triglycerides. The etiologic factors responsible for the development of phenotypic type V hyperlipidemia remain poorly understood. Most patients have an underlying hereditary disorder associated with enhanced VLDL production (familial hypertriglyceridemia or familial combined hyperlipidemia) plus a secondary factor which concurrently stimulates triglyceride synthesis (e.g., diabetes or estrogen therapy).[230] The activities of both LPL and HL are normal in most patients with type V[237] and do not explain the impaired triglyceride clearance found in this disorder. Enhanced production of VLDL has been demonstrated in some patients with type V and may, in the presence of a high fat intake, lead to overload of the normal lipolytic pathway, with resultant elevation of both VLDL and chylomicrons. Impaired chylomicron and VLDL catabolism occurs concomitantly and is responsible for the low levels of LDL and HDL that typically occur. A deficiency of apo-C-II, the apoprotein activator of lipoprotein lipase, has been reported in several families, with one family member being originally diagnosed as type V.[24,42]

Treatment

In both the type I and the type V phenotypes, elimination of secondary factors is important if a readily treatable etiology is not to be overlooked (Tables 21-10 and 21-11). Lipid values in first-degree relatives should also be determined and are valuable both for verification of a familial pattern and to detect other hyperlipidemic family members. Therapy for both type I and type V hyperlipidemia is primarily aimed at reduction or elimination of hyperchylomicronemia so that episodes of abdominal pain and pancreatitis can be prevented. Correction of hyperchylomicronemia is accomplished by means of a reduction in dietary fat and total calories, as described in Dietary Treatment. Alcohol is contraindicated. Fish oils and fatty fish may be useful in the type V disorder and possibly also in type I, as will be amplified later. Hypolipidemic drugs have no place in therapy for type I. In the authors' experience, gemfibrozil (Lopid) is especially helpful in patients with type V hyperlipidemia.[238] Niacin is of some value; other drugs have not been useful. Infusions of normal plasma containing apoprotein C-II will temporarily correct the defect in familial apoprotein C-II deficiency.[24,42] This may be helpful during episodes of acute pancreatitis.

The response to the appropriate treatment in type V patients is dramatic. Triglyceride values of 4,000 to 8,000 mg/dl may decrease to 300 to 400 mg/dl within 2 weeks with a 10 percent fat diet, weight loss, and gemfibrozil. Frequently, type V patients develop a lipoprotein pattern characteristic of type IV patients. Unfortunately, relapse is common as the patients regain weight and consume a high-fat diet again.

Hypertriglyceridemia in Pregnancy

As is well known, there are pronounced increases in plasma triglyceride and cholesterol concentrations during pregnancy, presumably because of the hormonal effects along with weight gain.[239] The hyperlipidemia reaches a peak during the third trimester of pregnancy. In some women who have prepregnancy hypertriglyceridemia, the pregnant state may bring on severe hypertriglyceridemia with the occurrence of the chylomicronemia syndrome. There is both increased production of triglyceride and VLDL and decreased removal because of lower LPL activity. Acute pancreatitis may develop as a most severe complication in hypertriglyceridemic pregnant women.

There are two aspects to the management of this condition. The very low fat diet can be employed; dietary fat is restricted to less than 10 percent of total calories. If this first step is not successful, omega-3 fatty acids in a dose of 10 to 15 g per day can be utilized. Such administration decreases the synthesis of triglyceride in the liver and also promotes clearance. This has been successfully employed in one pregnant woman to avoid acute pancreatitis (Farquhar J, personal communication). The second method of management utilized in a recent clinical report is the hospitalization of the patient and the provision of intravenous glucose feeding.[240] Calories can be administered via this modality without stimulating triglyceride synthesis, whereas carbohydrate taken orally may in some instances further aggravate the problem.[241] Successful conclusion of the pregnancy resulted with this treatment.[240] Also, the relative reduction of caloric intake will reduce triglyceride synthesis.

Type IV Hyperlipoproteinemia

Definition

Type IV hyperlipidemia, also called hyperprebetalipoproteinemia, is characterized by an increased concentration of VLDL in plasma without the concomitant presence of chylomicrons or increased levels of LDL. The disorder may be secondary to a number of associated conditions or may result from primary familial disorders, most notably familial hypertriglyceridemia and familial combined hyperlipidemia. Lipid values obtained after a 12- to 14-h fast characteristically reveal elevated triglyceride levels greater than 140 mg/dl, usually above 200 mg/dl and under 1,000 mg/dl, without chylomicronemia. Cholesterol levels are average or only mildly elevated. HDL is usually decreased.

Clinical Characteristics

The clinical presentation of type IV hyperlipidemia varies markedly. The disorder may be primary or, more commonly, secondary.[242] Most patients are asymptomatic, and the abnormality is frequently detected on a routine multichannel chemistry screen. Xanthomas are seldom seen. Xanthelasmas are likewise uncommon; their presence in patients with increased triglycerides is more suggestive of the type IIb phenotype. Vascular disease, particularly coronary heart disease, is a frequent complication in patients over age 45 with type IV hyperlipidemia, particularly those with genotypic familial combined hyperlipidemia. Peripheral vascular disease is less common. The importance of type IV hyperlipidemia as a risk factor in coronary heart disease was illustrated in a study of 500 survivors of myocardial infarction,[243] among whom this phenotype was present in 15 percent. Secondary causes should be sought in all patients who present with a type IV phenotype. Obesity, chronic renal failure or nephrotic syndrome, diabetes mellitus, and hypothyroidism together with excessive consumption of alcohol are the most commonly associated conditions. It must be stressed that the vast majority of patients with type IV are overweight. Only in families with endogenous familial hypertriglyceridemia or familial combined hyperlipidemia is obesity not common. Included in this group are children and slender individuals with type IV. A variety of medications, most notably estrogen-containing oral contraceptives, β-adrenergic blocking agents, and thiazide diuretics, have also been implicated.

Genetics

In addition to secondary causes, the type IV phenotype may occur in patients with endogenous familial hypertriglyceridemia and in familial combined hyperlipidemia. The distinction between the two is dependent on the lipid values in first-degree family members. In the former, the proband comes from a family in which all affected relatives have isolated hypertriglyceridemia with increased levels of VLDL. In familial combined hyperlipidemia, the affected relatives are heterogeneous and may have isolated hypercholesterolemia (IIa), hypertriglyceridemia (IV or V), or both (IIb).[207] Both disorders appear to be inherited as an autosomal dominant trait that frequently shows penetrance only after the first two decades of life.

Diagnostic Laboratory Features

The hallmark of type IV hyperlipidemia is an elevation of endogenously synthesized VLDL. The criteria for the diagnosis of this disorder are not absolute and are influenced by the race, age, sex, and diet of the patient and by the reliability of the available lipid determinations. For North American adults over age 45, the combination of a plasma cholesterol level lower than 240 mg/dl with a triglyceride level higher than 200 mg/dl without chylomicrons present may be considered diagnostic. Visualization of turbid plasma without chylomicrons together with an increased triglyceride level and a slightly elevated cholesterol level is all that is required in the diagnosis of type IV (see Laboratory Tests). Frequently, HDL will be low; this is probably partly responsible for the vascular disease in these patients. Associated laboratory abnormalities commonly seen in patients with type IV include hyperuricemia, hyperglycemia, and an abnormal glucose tolerance test.

Pathophysiology

The accumulation of endogenously synthesized VLDL may result from enhanced synthesis of this lipoprotein with overload of the normal removal mechanism or, alternatively, from impaired removal in the presence of normal rates of synthesis. In some cases, both mechanisms may be operative together. The secondary forms of hypertriglyceridemia, particularly those associated with obesity and hyperinsulinism, excessive alcohol intake, and the use of oral contraceptives, are associated with enhanced synthesis of VLDL; this seems to be the primary factor responsible for the type IV phenotype. In contrast, both increased synthesis and decreased catabolism may occur in obese patients and in poorly controlled insulin-dependent diabetics. The primary mechanism underlying VLDL accumulation in the familial hypertriglyceridemias has not been clearly established but may involve increased synthesis of VLDL. Enhanced hepatic VLDL and triglyceride synthesis, possibly mediated by an increased responsiveness to insulin, has been proposed to explain the lipid abnormalities in patients with endogenous familial hypertriglyceridemia.[244]

Treatment

Because of the common association of the type IV phenotype with obesity, adult-onset diabetes mellitus, and excessive alcohol intake, correction of secondary predisposing factors should be attempted in all patients. Thus, the attainment of ideal weight and restricted use of alcohol should be strongly encouraged; caloric restriction is essential if the patient is overweight. Estrogens, unless prescribed for a compelling medical reason, should be withdrawn or changed to a transdermal preparation in patients with type IV. As discussed elsewhere, we favor a single dietary approach to the treatment of hyperlipidemias and recommend a low-cholesterol (100-mg) diet in which the fat content is reduced to 20 percent of total calories, with an emphasis on restriction of saturated fat.

Drug therapy for type IV should be reserved for patients in whom an adequate trial of dietary therapy (6 to 8 months) and correction of secondary factors have failed to reduce the elevated VLDL levels. Drug therapy should be regarded as an adjunct to, rather than a substitute for, dietary therapy. Gemfibrozil 600 mg twice daily is the most widely accepted and most tolerated drug for therapy for type IV (see Pharmaceutical Agents). Gemfibrozil is successful in reducing triglyceride and VLDL levels in most patients. In some cases, however, decreases in VLDL are not paralleled by reductions in total cholesterol, which may actually increase.[215] This paradox is attributable to enhanced conversion of VLDL to LDL and to mild increases in HDL and may on occasion convert a type IV phenotype to a mild type IIa pattern. Strict control of dietary cholesterol and saturated fat will frequently correct the increase in LDL cholesterol, but if this does not occur, serious thought should be given to the discontinuation of gemfibrozil or the addition of a second drug effective in type IIa. Nicotinic acid is probably more effective than gemfibrozil in reducing VLDL triglyceride and apoprotein B levels and rarely produces a paradoxic increase in LDL. As discussed in Pharmaceutical Agents, side effects are much more common with this medication and result in much poorer patient compliance. Bile acid sequestrants (cholestyramine and colestipol), HMG CoA reductase inhibitors (e.g., lovastatin), and probucol (Lorelco) have no place in the treatment of type IV hyperlipidemia.

DISORDERS OF HIGH-DENSITY LIPOPROTEINS

A number of epidemiologic studies conducted during the last three decades have established a strong inverse relation between the concentrations of HDL cholesterol in plasma and the incidence of coronary heart disease observed in western populations.[245–247] Although these studies support the view that HDL may facilitate the transport of cholesterol from peripheral tissues back to the liver, the precise role of HDL in the pathogenesis of the atherosclerotic process has not been clarified. Thus, it is not clear whether high levels of HDL are themselves protective or whether they are simply a marker for other, more fundamental differences in lipoprotein metabolism (for example, more efficient lipolysis and hepatic uptake of triglyceride-rich lipoproteins) that occur in patients with high levels of HDL cholesterol. Concentrations of HDL cholesterol are low (25 to 30 mg/dl) in some societies habituated to a very low fat, low-cholesterol diet in which the incidence of coronary heart disease is also very low.[113] Notably, concentrations of LDL are also low in these populations, suggesting that the inverse correlations noted between low concentrations of HDL cholesterol and high rates of coronary heart disease in western societies may require the concurrent presence of a permissive level of LDL cholesterol (e.g., >120 mg/dl) that is not normally present in more "primitive" societies.

Despite strong epidemiologic associations between low levels of HDL cholesterol and an increased incidence of coronary heart disease, it is not clear whether therapeutic measures intended to increase HDL cholesterol levels in individuals in whom these are low are of therapeutic benefit.[109] Although the results of the recent VA HIT trial showed reduced risk of cardiovascular events in men treated with gemfibrozil who had CAD and low HDL cholesterol concentrations,[400] it is uncertain whether treatment intended to increase HDL cholesterol is the optimal intervention for such patients. In contrast, the use of other measures (e.g., diet, weight loss, increase in exercise, and cessation of cigarette smoking) that may raise HDL cholesterol levels as a secondary phenomenon should be encouraged. Because a low-fat diet can sometimes lower plasma HDL cholesterol concentrations, some investigators have recommended consumption of a diet enriched in monounsaturated fatty acids to avoid reducing the HDL cholesterol concentration. However, there is little to no evidence to suggest that diet-induced reductions in the concentration of HDL cholesterol are proatherogenic.

Reduced levels of HDL cholesterol may occur in association with several secondary factors (Table 21-15), including hypertriglyceridemia, obesity, cigarette smoking, and physical inactivity, and are 10 mg/dl lower in men than in premenopausal women.[96] The plasma levels of HDL cholesterol are identical in prepubertal boys and girls, but the levels decrease during puberty in boys,[248] and remain depressed throughout life. This effect is mediated by testosterone. Reductions in plasma concentrations of HDL cholesterol may also be seen in patients receiving probucol[249] and during the administration of anabolic steroids.

A number of secondary factors have been shown to increase concentrations of HDL cholesterol in human plasma (Table 21-15). These include exercise, moderate consumption of alcohol, cessation of cigarette smoking, and correction of hypertriglyceridemia. Several medications, including estrogens, phenytoin, and barbiturates, also are known to increase plasma concentrations of HDL cholesterol. The consumption of a high-fat diet is associated with an increase in the HDL cholesterol level, but any potential benefit from the increased HDL is overshadowed by a disproportionate increase in the level of LDL cholesterol.

TABLE 21-15. Secondary Factors That Influence HDL Cholesterol Concentrations

Decrease	Increase
Hypertriglyceridemia	Exercise
Obesity	Ethanol consumption
Cigarette smoking	Weight loss
Androgens	Cessation of cigarette smoking
Puberty in boys	Estrogens
NIDDM (type II diabetes mellitus)	Lipid-lowering drugs
Physical inactivity	Niacin (most potent)
Probucol	Fibric acid derivatives
Low-fat diet	HMG CoA reductase inhibitors
	Bile acid–binding resins
	Phenytoin
	Barbiturates
	High-fat diet

A number of familial syndromes in which HDL cholesterol levels are reduced below the 10th percentile in the absence of severe hypertriglyceridemia have been described. These disorders include familial apo-A-I and -C-III deficiency,[250–252] familial apo-A-I, C-III, A-IV deficiency,[250,253] Tangier disease,[254,255] HDL deficiency with planar xanthomas,[256,257] LCAT deficiency,[258,259] fish eye disease,[260,261] apo-A-I variants (Milano, Glessen, Marburg, Munster 1-3),[262–265] familial hypoalphalipoproteinemia,[266,267] and some individuals with familial hypertriglyceridemia.[207] In addition to these disorders of HDL deficiency, increased plasma concentrations of HDL cholesterol and a low risk of atherosclerosis have been described in familial hyperalphalipoproteinemia.[268] In the following section, the salient features of these disorders will be briefly reviewed. Distinguishing clinical and biochemical features of the familial HDL deficiency disorders are outlined in Table 21-16.

Familial Apolipoprotein A-I and C-III Deficiency

Three patients from two separate kindreds have been described with a marked reduction in the concentrations of HDL cholesterol (1 to 6 mg/dl) and a virtual absence of apoproteins A-I and C-III from plasma.[250,251] Corneal opacification was noted in all three patients, and prominent planar xanthomas were present on the trunk, neck, and eyelids of the two sisters from the second family. Coronary atherosclerosis was present in one patient by age 40 and was present in the other two by their late twenties. Reduced concentrations of HDL cholesterol (25 to 35 mg/dl) were found in obligate heterozygotes from both kindreds, but of 17 heterozygotes in one kindred, none developed premature coronary artery disease before age 40 and only 2 did so before age 60. Thus, the heterozygous form of this disorder does not appear to be associated with a marked increase in premature coronary artery disease. The defect in this disease appears to be an inability to synthesize apoproteins A-I and C-III because of a DNA insertion in the coding region of the apo-A-I gene.[252] Although it is of unproven efficacy in this rare disorder, it would seem prudent to attempt to reduce the LDL cholesterol concentrations with a view to reversing the tendency for accelerated atherosclerosis and possibly causing regression of the cutaneous xanthomas.

Familial Apo-A-I, C-III, A-IV Deficiency

This rare disorder was first described in 1982 in a 45-year-old woman who had mild corneal opacifications, severe coronary artery disease, normal tonsils, and no xanthomas.[250,253] The level of LDL cholesterol was normal, but the levels of VLDL cholesterol and apoprotein C-II were reduced and the HDL cholesterol concentration was severely diminished. Apolipoproteins A-I and C-III were undetectable, and the apoprotein A-II level was decreased 90 percent. The activity and mass of the LCAT enzyme were 40 percent of normal. Seventeen heterozygotes were identified in the kindred and had levels of HDL cholesterol and apoproteins A-I, C-III, and A-IV that were 50 percent of normal. The

TABLE 21-16. Clinical and Biochemical Findings in Familial HDL Deficiency Disorders

	Familial Apo-A-I, C-III Deficiency	Familial Apo-A-I, C-III, A-IV Deficiency	Tangier Disease	HDL Deficiency with Planar Xanthomas	Apo-A-I Variants (e.g., Milano)	LCAT Deficiency	Fish Eye Disease	Familial Alphalipo-proteinemia
Corneal opacities	+	+	+	+	—	+++	+++	—
Planar xanthomas	+	—	—	+	—	—	—	—
Abnormal tonsils	—	—	+	—	—	—	—	—
Neuropathy	—	—	+	—	—	—	—	—
Hepatosplenomegaly	—	—	+	+	—	—	—	—
Premature CAD	+++	+++	+	++	—	—	—	+++
Plasma cholesterol (mg/dl)								
Total	138	111	65	260	182	170–500	207	165
LDL	120	106	42	134	137	225	199	115
HDL	6	1	2	3	18	5–15	7	26
Plasma triglycerides (mg/dl)	62	62	200	290	188	105–1800	424	113
Apo-A-I	ND	ND	1.3	2	74	51	38	65

CAD = coronary artery disease; ND not detectable.

For premature CAD, +++ indicates onset before age 40, ++ before age 50, and + before age 60. Patients with apo-A-I Milano and familial hypoalphalipoproteinemia are heterozygous, whereas for the other disorders, the description refers to homozygotes.

Source: Modified from Schaefer[269] and Breslow.[270]

frequency of coronary artery disease was increased among the heterozygotes. The molecular defect in this disorder may be due to a major deletion in the apoprotein A-I, C-III, A-IV gene complex.

HDL Deficiency with Planar Xanthomas

This disorder of unknown etiology[256,257] has been described in one Swedish woman who presented with an HDL cholesterol of 3 mg/dl and extensive cutaneous planar xanthomas. The patient developed coronary artery disease in her late forties, and apoprotein analyses disclosed a marked decrease in the concentrations of apo-A-I, with concentrations of apo-C-III that were slightly above normal. Corneal opacification was also observed, but the patient's tonsils were normal. The molecular defect responsible for this disorder has not been determined.

Lecithin Cholesterol Acyltransferase Deficiency

This disorder is discussed in further detail in Other Lipoprotein Disorders.

Fish Eye Disease

Severe corneal opacification and low concentrations of HDL cholesterol (7 mg/dl) have been reported in two Swedish kindreds, and this abnormality has been termed *fish eye disease* because of the ocular findings.[260,261] Despite modest elevations in the concentrations of LDL cholesterol and modest hypertriglyceridemia, the reported patients did not develop coronary artery disease before the sixth decade of life. Concentrations of apo-A-I and A-II were reduced in the homozygous patients, and concentrations of HDL cholesterol were approximately 50 percent of normal in heterozygotes. The metabolic defect in this disorder has not been determined, but it appears to be related to a selective deficiency in LCAT-mediated esterification of cholesterol in HDL.[258]

Familial Apo-A-I Variants

Eleven distinct structural variants of the apoprotein A-I molecule have been identified, primarily by isoelectric focusing. Each of these variants is associated with a point mutation in the apoprotein A-I gene, resulting in a single amino acid substitution. Apoprotein A-I Milano was initially reported in an Italian man who had low levels of HDL cholesterol (11 mg/dl) with no clinical evidence of coronary artery disease. The low concentrations of HDL cholesterol were due to heterozygosity for a substitution of cysteine for arginine at residue 173 in apo-A-I; this resulted in an enhanced rate of catabolism of these lipoprotein particles from plasma.[262,271] Corneal opacification, xanthomas, and hepatosplenomegaly were not reported in this patient, and there was no family history of premature coronary artery disease. The other variants include apoproteins Gleesen, Marburg, and Munster 1-3.[263–265] All of these were identified as heterozygous defects. None of these apoprotein A-I variants have been associated with coronary artery disease or other clinical abnormalities despite the exceptionally low levels of HDL cholesterol.

Familial Hypoalphalipoproteinemia

Familial hypoalphalipoproteinemia is a relatively common autosomal dominant inherited trait that is associated with concentrations of HDL cholesterol below the 10th percentile (less than 30 mg/dl in men; less than 35 mg/dl in women) and an accelerated rate of premature coronary artery disease.[266,267] There are no specific clinical findings, and corneal opacities are not characteristic of this disorder. Recent studies suggest that familial hypoalphalipoproteinemia may have a gene frequency as common as 1 in 400 in the United States. Although the cause of this disorder is not known, patients with familial hypoalphalipoproteinemia appear to have a 15-fold increase in the frequency of a restriction enzyme polymorphism after DNA digestion with the restriction enzyme PstI.[270] Familial hypoalphalipoproteinemia has also been associated with an increased incidence of stroke in children.[272] Therapy for patients with familial hypoalphalipoproteinemia should aim to minimize other potential risk factors for cardiovascular disease and maintain the level of LDL cholesterol below 100 mg/dl. Whether pharmaceutical measures that raise HDL cholesterol levels have any benefit in this disorder is not known, but therapy with nicotinic acid would be an attractive strategy to reduce LDL and increase HDL cholesterol levels. The results of recent studies have indicated that mutations in the ABC-1 protein may be a common cause of familial hypoalphalipoproteinemia.

Tangier Disease

Definition

Tangier disease is a rare disorder characterized by severe deficiency of normal HDL in plasma and the accumulation of cholesteryl esters in many tissues throughout the body, including the characteristic deposition in the tonsils. The disorder takes its name from Tangier Island, Virginia, where the first cases were reported. To date, fewer than 50 cases have been reported in North America, Japan, Europe, and Australia.[254,255]

Clinical Features

Suspicion of Tangier disease is most commonly aroused by the unique appearance of the tonsils. Oral pharyngeal examination reveals large lobulated tonsils that have a distinctive orange or yellow color that is attributable to deposits of cholesteryl esters within the tissue. Deposition of this lipid in other tissues frequently results in splenomegaly (80 percent), hepatomegaly (30 percent), and lymphadenopathy (20 percent) and may provoke suspicion of a malignancy. Cholesteryl esters are also deposited in the rectal mucosa, which shows 1- to 2-mm orange and brown spots on proctosigmoidoscopic examination. Rectal biopsy reveals foamy cholesteryl ester–laden histiocytes in the mucosa and submucosa. Corneal infiltration is usually detectable by means of slit-lamp examination in patients over age 40 years but does not impair vision. A variety of neurologic symptoms occur in patients with Tangier disease, and these symptoms may constitute the initial reason for seeking medical attention. Symptoms include weakness, paresthesias, diplopia, and increased sweating. Objectively, reduced muscle strength with wasting, decreased tendon reflexes, ocular palsies, and selective loss of pain and temperature sensation have been described. Electromyography (EMG) reveals signs of denervation in affected muscles, but nerve conduction is normal. No episodes of premature coronary artery disease or cerebral vascular disease have been noted in homozygous or heterozygous patients with Tangier disease before age 40. However, among eight homozygotes over age 40, five had evidence of coronary artery disease or cerebral vascular disease,[273] whereas the other three are alive and well in their fifth and sixth decades. Thus, patients homozygous for Tangier disease have increased risk for the premature development of atherosclerosis, which is a consequence of severely impaired reverse cholesterol transport.

Genetics

Full expression of Tangier disease occurs in patients homozygous for this disorder and is consistent with an autosomal dominant mode of transmission.[254,255] Heterozygous patients frequently have reduced levels of HDL cholesterol (25 to 30 mg/dl) and reduced concentrations of apoprotein A-I but do not have any of the tonsillar or neuropathic findings noted in the homozygous form and remain asymptomatic. Because of their reduced concentration of HDL cholesterol, heterozygous patients may be at increased risk for the premature development of coronary artery disease.[274] Tangier disease is caused by a variety of mutations in the ABC-1 gene on chromosome 9_q31, which encodes the peripheral tissue HDL receptor. A total of 14 mutations have been reported to date.

Diagnostic Laboratory Features

The plasma lipid profile of patients who are homozygous for Tangier disease is characterized by a low concentration of cholesterol (60 to 100 mg/dl) with moderately increased triglyceride levels (100 to 300 mg/dl). Lipoprotein fractionation discloses a marked reduction in the concentration of HDL cholesterol (1 to 3 mg/dl). Plasma concentrations of apoprotein A-I and A-II are reduced to 1 percent and 9 percent of normal, respectively, and concentrations of other major apoproteins are 50 to 80 percent of normal. Patients who are heterozygous for Tangier disease have plasma concentrations of HDL cholesterol, apo-A-I, and apo-A-II that are approximately 50 percent of normal. Although familial hypoalphalipoproteinemia also is caused by heterozygous mutations in ABC-1, HDL cholesterol concentrations in Tangier disease heterozygotes are higher than HDL cholesterol concentrations in patients with familial hypoalphalipoproteinemia.[275] The laboratory findings taken in conjunction with the usual clinical picture permit a definitive diagnosis of Tangier disease to be made in virtually all cases.

Pathophysiology

The biochemical defects underlying the lipoprotein abnormalities and presumed secondary storage of cholesteryl esters in Tangier disease are a consequence of mutations in the ABC-1 gene, which severely impair the capacity of nascent HDL particles to acquire cholesterol from peripheral tissues. Studies utilizing apoprotein A-I isolated from the plasma of patients with Tangier disease have demonstrated an increased content of proapo-A-I,[276] which has a reduced affinity to associate with HDL particles.[274] The amino acid composition of apo-A-I Tangier may also differ slightly from that of normal apoprotein A-I.[277] Kinetic studies have indicated an enhanced fractional catabolic rate for proapoprotein A-I in patients with Tangier disease, but the activity of the converting enzyme responsible for the formation of apo-A-I from proapo A-I is normal. The accelerated catabolism of apoprotein A-I in this disorder appears to be a consequence of the failure of apo A-I to form HDL particles by acquiring lipid from peripheral cells. The increased catabolism of apoprotein A-I and blockage of revers cholesterol transport presumably are responsible for increased uptake of cholesteryl ester–rich chylomicron remnants by macrophages of the reticuloendothelial system, which results in the selective storage of this lipid in these tissues from homozygous patients with Tangier disease.

Treatment

There is no treatment for Tangier disease. Dietary restriction of fat to minimize the formation of chylomicron remnants has been advocated by some authors; although of unproven benefit, such a regimen would seem prudent until further evidence becomes available. Gene therapy to replace or modify the defective ABC-1 gene may become feasible at some point in the distant future.

Familial Hyperalphalipoproteinemia

Familial hyperalphalipoproteinemia is characterized by distinct elevations in the concentrations of HDL cholesterol in association with normal levels of LDL and VLDL cholesterol and normal plasma triglyceride concentrations.[268] When adjusted for age and sex, total cholesterol concentrations are mildly elevated and typically lie in the range of 230 to 280 mg/dl. The condition is of interest largely because it is the only known hyperlipidemia that actually appears to be beneficial to the patient. As with familial hypobetalipoproteinemia, patients with this disorder have a low incidence of cardiovascular disease and show increased longevity. Familial hyperalphalipoproteinemia should be suspected when the HDL cholesterol level is in excess of 70 mg/dl in male patients and in excess of 85 to 90 mg/dl in female patients in whom secondary causes of HDL elevation have been excluded. Genetic studies by Glueck and associates have indicated that familial hyperalphalipoproteinemia is inherited as an autosomal dominant trait with full penetrance in neonates and children.[278] The incidence of this condition in the general population is not known but is probably greater than 1 in 3,000. The condition may be benign, and treatment may not be indicated. Marked familial hyperalphalipoproteinemia (HDL cholesterol above 150 mg/dl) has been identified in Japanese patients with cholesteryl ester transfer protein deficiency.[279,280] Although CETP deficiency is associated with very high very plasma concentrations of HDL cholesterol, the disorder may be associated with increased risk of CHD as a consequence of impaired reverse cholesterol transport, particularly when the plasma concentration of LDL cholesterol is increased.

OTHER LIPOPROTEIN DISORDERS

Abetalipoproteinemia

Definition

The term *abetalipoproteinemia* refers to a group of disorders characterized by a complete absence of apoprotein B-100, the protein essential for the formation of LDL and VLDL, from plasma.[281] To date, three distinct genetic conditions have been described in which there is a complete absence of VLDL and LDL from plasma. In classic abetalipoproteinemia and homozygous hypobetalipoproteinemia there is a concurrent absence of apoprotein B-48–containing chylomicron particles from plasma, whereas in normotriglyceridemic abetalipoproteinemia the intestinal production of apoprotein B-48–containing chylomicron particles is normal and hepatic production of apoprotein B-100 in VLDL and LDL is impaired.[240,241] Patients with these disorders have profound hypocholesterolemia (20 to 40 mg/dl), which in classic abetalipoproteinemia and homozygous hypobetalipoproteinemia is accompanied by marked hypotriglyceridemia (5 to 10 mg/dl).

Clinical Characteristics

Patients with phenotypic abetalipoproteinemia due to the classic form of this disorder or to homozygous hypobetalipoproteinemia show similar clinical features. Such patients manifest steatorrhea from birth that is attributable to the block in mucosal formation of chylomicron particles, with a resulting impairment of fat absorption. There is concomitantly an impairment of the absorption of the fat-soluble vitamins (A, D, E, and K) and of essential fatty acids and cholesterol. Biopsies of intestinal mucosal cells show intense engorgement of fat within the enterocytes. Because of the malabsorption of fat-soluble vitamins, patients with abetalipoproteinemia may manifest vitamin A and vitamin K deficiency at a young age[284] and clearly develop profound vitamin E deficiency.[285,286] This results from two factors. First, absorption of vitamin E is impaired, as is absorption of all other fat-soluble vitamins, because of the blockade of chylomicron formation. Second, plasma transport of vitamin E is greatly disturbed because the chief transport form—LDL—is not present at all. Thus, vitamin E deficiency in humans may be most clearly seen in patients with abetalipoproteinemia. Steatorrhea and, in patients who remain undiagnosed, a general failure to thrive may be the only manifestations of the disease for the first 5 to 7 years of life. Subsequent to this, in untreated patients there is progressive development of neurologic and retinal dysfunction, which if unrecognized ultimately will prove profoundly disabling. Initially, deep tendon reflexes disappear and there is mild impairment of sensation. Signs of abnormal cerebellar, posterior column, and peripheral nerve function together with muscle weakness progress if the disease is not recognized, and in untreated patients severe ataxia is present by the second decade of life. Retinal dysfunction is manifested by the insidious development of retinitis pigmentosa with loss of night vision and progressive visual impairment. Although some of the visual loss may reflect vitamin A deficiency, treatment with vitamin A alone does not halt further progression of disease, suggesting that vitamin E deficiency may be the primary insult responsible for these retinal abnormalities.

The abnormal lipoprotein environment also affects the erythrocytes, and the peripheral smear reveals large numbers of acanthocytes, which form because of the abnormal cholesterol and phospholipid composition of the erythrocyte membranes. These patients do not, however, generally develop anemia as a result of the abnormal red cell membranes.

Because of the important role of LDL in delivering cholesterol to steroid hormone–producing tissues, the question of whether corticosteroid or progesterone production may be impaired in abetalipoproteinemia has been addressed. Studies of the adrenal response to prolonged ACTH infusion have documented a modest impairment in corticosteroid production, which is probably not of clinical significance.[287,288] Reduced progesterone levels were reported in one patient with homozygous hypobetalipoproteinemia[289] who was followed through pregnancy. Although pregnancy proceeded normally without the need for exogenous progesterone in this patient, such a supplement may be necessary in other patients.

Recognition of the key role of vitamin E deficiency in the pathogenesis of the neurologic abnormalities in abetalipoproteinemia has radically changed the prognosis for patients with this disorder. Current data strongly suggest that with appropriate therapy, the disabling neurologic and visual deterioration can be totally prevented.[290–292]

Reported findings in normotriglyceridemic abetalipoproteinemia have included hypocholesterolemia (25 mg/dl) with plasma triglyceride concentrations of 25 to 35 mg/dl, a lack of significant steatorrhea, and the presence of acanthocytes on peripheral blood smears.[282,283] In one patient[282] neurologic symptoms of ataxia were present at 8 years of age, suggesting that even in the presence of normal chylomicron formation, and therefore normal absorption of vitamin E, transport of this vitamin in plasma and its subsequent delivery to tissues are severely compromised when apoprotein B-100–containing lipoproteins are absent.

Genetics

The inherited pattern of phenotypic abetalipoproteinemia takes two forms. The most common disorder (classic abetalipoproteinemia) is inherited as an autosomal recessive trait for which affected patients are homozygotes. Obligate heterozygous parents have normal concentrations of plasma lipids and lipoproteins, and the carrier state cannot be identified. In the second form, phenotypic abetalipoproteinemia represents the homozygous form of hypobetalipoproteinemia, which is inherited as an autosomal dominant trait. Fewer than 10 cases of homozygous hypobetalipoproteinemia have been reported, and obligate heterozygotes show LDL cholesterol concentrations ranging from 15 to 40 mg/dl.[293] Normotriglyceridemic abetalipoproteinemia appears to be inherited as an autosomal recessive trait, and obligate heterozygous parents have normal plasma lipid values.[283] Defects in the MTP gene are an additional cause of abetalipoproteinemia.[32–34]

Laboratory Findings

Patients with phenotypic abetalipoproteinemia show extremely low levels of plasma cholesterol (20 to 30 mg/dl), and their levels of triglycerides are generally lower than 10 mg/dl. Lipoprotein fractionation studies disclose a total absence of chylomicrons, VLDL, and LDL, and plasma concentrations of HDL are reduced approximately 50 percent. A fatty meal does not result in the appearance of chylomicrons in the blood or elevation of the plasma triglyceride concentrations. In untreated patients, plasma concentrations of carotene and vitamin A are very low whereas vitamin E levels are usually undetectable. Because of vitamin K deficiency, the vitamin K–dependent coagulation factors may be reduced, resulting in a prolonged prothrombin time; hemorrhagic bleeding has been the initial presentation in several cases.[284] The synthesis of vitamin D in the skin appears to be adequate to compensate for the presumed decrease in the absorption of vitamin D, and rickets is not described as a complication of abetalipoproteinemia. The content of linoleic acid and linolenic acid as well as the long-chain polyunsaturated fatty acids derived from these two essential fatty acids is reduced in the plasma lipids of patients with abetalipoproteinemia, and this reduction is also reflected in reduced levels in adipose tissue, erythrocytes, and breast milk.[294] Mild elevations in alkaline phosphatase, lactic acid dehydrogenase (LDH), and serum glutamic oxaloacetic transaminase (SGOT) have been observed in some patients and are presumed to reflect hepatic steatosis.

Pathophysiology

Considerable progress in elucidating the biochemical defects responsible for abetalipoproteinemia have occurred since the cloning and characterization of apoprotein B. Studies in patients with classic abetalipoproteinemia have failed to detect any abnormalities in the apo-B gene,[295] and in two patients, concentrations of mRNA in liver biopsies were increased fivefold to sixfold, suggesting that apo-B-100 is inducible and that the defect in this disorder does not involve a transcriptional abnormality. Immunofluorescence for apoprotein B-100–like material has also been detected in liver biopsies, suggesting that in these particular patients, the disorder resulted from a posttranslational defect in the assembly or secretion of apoprotein B–containing lipoprotein from hepatocytes. It seems likely that multiple molecular defects result in the clinical phenotype in abetalipoproteinemia. In contrast to abetalipoproteinemia, studies in patients with hypobeta-lipoproteinemia have indicated that this disorder results from a series of mutations in the apo-B gene that result in premature termination of apo-B synthesis and lead to the synthesis of truncated species of apoprotein B which are unable to associate adequately with lipids and are rapidly catabolized.[281,296,297] In a series of elegant experiments, Hardman and associates demonstrated that the molecular defect in normotriglyceridemic abetalipoproteinemia results from the synthesis of a truncated form of apo-B-100 (B-50), which is secreted into plasma as a VLDL-like particle but is rapidly catabolized without any subsequent production of LDL particles.[298] Current data[290–292] strongly support the view that the acquired neurologic and retinal degeneration that occurs in untreated patients with abetalipoproteinemia represents a manifestation of vitamin E deficiency. A current hypothesis suggests that the formation of peroxides in the face of low levels of vitamin E may create damage to certain tissues (the retina and the posterior columns of the spinal cord) which are rich in long-chain polyunsaturated fatty acids. Symptoms of deficiency of essential fatty acids have not been reported in patients with abetalipoproteinemia despite profound fat malabsorption and low concentrations of linoleic acid in plasma and adipose tissues.

Treatment

Steatorrhea in patients with phenotypic abetalipoproteinemia can be readily controlled with a very low fat diet (5 to 10 percent of total calories as fat). The degree of fat restriction necessary to prevent steatorrhea is greater in infants and children than in adults, in whom a diet with 15 to 20 percent of calories derived from fat is usually well tolerated. Deficiencies of fat-soluble vitamins can be completely corrected by the administration of water-soluble forms of vitamin A (Aquasol A) 10,000 to 25,000 U daily and vitamin K (Synkayvite) 5 mg weekly. Plasma levels of vitamin E can never be restored to normal, but high-dose vitamin E therapy has been shown to result in normal tissue concentrations of vitamin E in both adults and children[299,300] and clinical improvement and lack of further deterioration in newly diagnosed patients. We recommend that vitamin E be administered at 200 mg per kilogram of body weight per day in single or divided doses.[286] Treatment of patients with normotriglyceridemic abetalipoproteinemia is aimed at providing adequate intake of the fat-soluble vitamins, particularly vitamin E, but the ability of these patients to form chylomicrons allows the use of lower doses (400 U per day). The use of medium-chain triglycerides should be regarded as contraindicated in all patients with abetalipoproteinemia.[301] In the face of defective hepatic triglyceride secretion, medium-chain triglycerides may result in the accumulation of two-carbon fragments in the liver and may lead to the development of cirrhosis.

Hypobetalipoproteinemia

Reduced plasma concentrations of LDL cholesterol in the absence of hypertriglyceridemia (less than 40 mg/dl) can be seen in association with hyperthyroidism, malabsorption, and resection of the ileum and can also be seen in patients with autoantibodies directed against apoprotein B.[302] Low plasma concentrations of LDL may also occur in patients with heterozygous familial hypobetalipoproteinemia, which represents a heterogenous group of disorders characterized by the synthesis of abnormal truncated forms of apoprotein B, which undergo rapid catabolism in plasma.[281,296,297] These disorders are inherited as autosomal dominant traits and show full phenotypic expression in childhood.[303,304] Heterozygous familial hypobetalipoproteinemia has an estimated gene frequency of 1 in 1,000 to 1 in 2,000,[305] and because of the low risk of coronary heart disease, it is associated with an overall increase in longevity.[306] Patients with heterozygous familial hypobetalipoproteinemia usually have no clinical abnormalities but occasionally may develop neuromuscular symptoms suggestive of vitamin E deficiency; in these cases, supplemental treatment with vitamin E is advisable. Additional supplementation with vitamin A and vitamin K should be dictated based on serum concentrations of vitamin A and the prothrombin time. In a family in which two patients with heterozygous hypobetalipoproteinemia are to marry, the risk of having a child homozygous for this disorder will be one of four, and such a child will have the clinical features of abetalipoproteinemia.

Chylomicron Retention Disease

Several patients have been reported in whom fat malabsorption and lipid storage in enterocytes appear to be due to an inability to synthesize or secrete chylomicrons in response to oral intake of fat.[281] These patients have all presented with severe diarrhea in childhood and have concurrently had low levels of total and LDL cholesterol but a total absence of chylomicrons and lack of a rise in plasma triglycerides after an oral fat challenge. Apoprotein B was detectable immunologically in the enterocytes obtained from patients with chylomicron retention disease, suggesting that the disorder is due to an undefined abnormality in the formation or secretion of chylomicrons. Chylomicron retention disease appears to be inherited as an autosomal recessive trait. Absorption of other fat-soluble vitamins is impaired, and these patients should concurrently receive supplemental vitamin E and, potentially, vitamins A and K. In addition to fat-soluble vitamin supplementation, treatment is directed at maintaining adequate caloric intake in the setting of a low-fat diet to prevent steatorrhea.

Familial Lecithin Cholesterol Acyltransferase Deficiency

Absence of the enzyme LCAT is a rare disorder characterized by moderately increased total cholesterol and triglyceride levels with markedly reduced levels of cholesteryl ester and lysolecithin and an increased level of free cholesterol in plasma. Clinically, these patients have corneal opacities and normochromic anemia and develop progressive renal insufficiency.[36]

Clinical Features

Corneal opacities develop in early childhood and consist of numerous gray dots in the corneal stroma, especially in the periphery, resembling an arcus senilis. They are the most consistent and sometimes the only abnormal physical findings in patients with LCAT deficiency. The disorder is associated with premature atherosclerosis and progressive renal dysfunction, both of which are commonly present in the third and fourth decades.[36]

Genetics

Familial LCAT deficiency appears to be an autosomal recessive disorder, the clinical expression of which occurs only in homozygotes. Obligate heterozygotes typically have normal levels of both plasma LCAT and esterified cholesterol and do not develop corneal opacities. However, in one kindred the heterozygotes had low levels of plasma LCAT activity, HDL cholesteryl ester, and apoprotein A-I and higher levels of triglyceride and apoprotein B, but without a detectable increased risk of developing atherosclerosis.[307]

Diagnostic Laboratory Features

The plasma lipid profile in patients with LCAT deficiency is variable but generally reveals total cholesterol of 250 to 400 mg/dl and triglycerides of 250 to 800 mg/dl. Chromatographic separation of plasma lipids reveals 85 to 90 percent of the cholesterol to be in the free form, with only 10 to 15 percent esterified. Various lipoprotein abnormalities can be demonstrated; paper electrophoresis reveals a prominent beta band with faint or absent pre-beta and alpha bands, whereas ultracentrifugal separation shows reduced HDL levels. Documentation of the absence of LCAT remains the key to diagnosis. Some other disorders, notably obstructive jaundice, primary biliary cirrhosis, and $alpha_1$ antitrypsin deficiency, may be associated with marked elevations in free cholesterol and the presence of an abnormal low-density lipoprotein, termed LPX, similar to that seen in LCAT deficiency. Such conditions, however, are usually evident clinically and are not associated with a total deficiency of LCAT. Laboratory findings in patients with LCAT deficiency frequently include a normochromic anemia with hemoglobin concentrations of 10 g/dl and target cells visible on peripheral smear. Proteinuria of 1 to 2 g/24 h is also commonly seen and increases as renal function deteriorates. Bone marrow aspiration has revealed foam cells that stain as sea-blue histiocytes on Giemsa stain.

Pathophysiology

The primary defect in this disease is a failure in the hepatic synthesis or secretion of the enzyme LCAT. This in turn leads to above-normal concentrations of free cholesterol and phosphatidylcholine in plasma and is manifested by a variety of abnormal lipoproteins. Although the precise pathophysiologic mechanisms by which these lipids affect blood vessels and the renal glomerulus and are responsible for the pathologic features of LCAT deficiency are not known, these may be mediated by an enhanced transfer of free cholesterol from plasma lipoproteins to cell plasma membranes or, alternatively, by a reduction in the normal egress of this lipid from the cells to the plasma. Patients with LCAT deficiency and those with Tangier disease both have a block in reverse cholesterol transport, but the defect in LCAT deficiency is less severe because the initial steps of reverse cholesterol transport (i.e., removal of cholesterol from peripheral cells by nascent HDL particles) proceed normally.

Treatment

At present, there is no specific therapy for patients with LCAT deficiency. Restriction of fat and cholesterol has been advocated and seems efficacious in lowering both cholesterol and triglyceride levels. Progressive renal disease has been managed with hemodialysis and transplantation, but both maneuvers must be regarded as palliative rather than curative.

Smith-Lemli-Opitz Syndrome

Smith-Lemli-Opitz Syndrome (SLOS) is an autosomal recessive disorder that is associated with physical malformations, metal retardation, and growth failure. The cause of SLOS was recently shown to be related to reduced activity of 7-dehydrocholesterol 7-reductase,[308] the final enzyme in cholesterol biosynthesis. Decreased activity of 7-dehydrocholesterol 7-reductase is a consequence of mutations in the human sterol 7-reductase gene at 11q12-13.[309,310] Characteristic biochemical abnormalities in SLOS include reduced tissue and plasma concentrations of cholesterol and increased accumulation of cholesterol precursors such as 7-dehydrocholesterol. It is unknown whether the lack of cholesterol or excess of potentially toxic cholesterol precursors, or both, contribute to the pathology in this disorder. The results of recent studies in 4 patients with SLOS have indicated that supplementation of the diet with cholesterol in egg yolk for 35 to 90 weeks increased the mean plasma cholesterol concentration 116 percent from 53 to 114 mg/dl and decreased the plasma 7-dehydrocholesterol concentration 67 percent from 11.3 mg/dl to 3.5 mg/dl.[311] If such therapy may help prevent complications associated with SLOS, it would most likely need to be initiated early in gestation because severe irreversible abnormalities are typically present at birth.

STEROL STORAGE DISEASES

Atherosclerosis

The common atherosclerotic lesions of the coronary arteries, the extracranial arteries of the head, and the distal aorta and arteries of the lower extremities represent fundamentally a biochemical storage disease with a tremendous accumulation of cholesterol, particularly cholesteryl ester.[312] This great storage of sterol initially occurs intracellularly but later occurs mainly extracellularly. There is associated proliferation of smooth muscle cells and macrophages that become foam cells as a result of the storage of cholesteryl ester. A second biochemical event is the synthesis of collagen, which occurs as a reaction to the presence of cholesterol in the arterial intima. Thrombosis and platelet aggregation are important late events that occur after the endothelial surface of the growing atheromatous plaque has been disrupted.

This storage of cholesteryl ester and free cholesterol in the intima of the arteries has its counterpart in only a few other conditions. A similar storage occurs in xanthomatous lesions, whose chemistry will be discussed later in this chapter. An accumulation of free cholesterol clearly occurs in cholesterol gallstones, with the cholesterol content being 60 to 80 percent by weight. Large quantities of cholesteryl ester under physiologic circumstances are stored in the steroid-secreting endocrine glands as precursors for hormonal synthesis. Cholesteryl ester, of course, circulates physiologically in the blood as a vital constituent of lipoproteins. In only the latter two circumstances is the presence of cholesteryl ester other than pathologic.

The majority of the cholesterol in atherosclerotic plaques originates from the circulating plasma. Although the arterial wall has a small capacity to synthesize cholesterol, its synthetic rate is insufficient to account for the tremendous mass of cholesterol present. Cholesterol enters the arterial wall as a part of the LDL molecule or other atherogenic lipoproteins. The mechanisms by which LDL induces cholesterol uptake in macrophages leading to foam cell formation remain unclear. Native LDL cannot stimulate foam cell formation in vitro, but LDL modified by malondialdehyde, acetylation, or oxidation is avidly taken up by macrophages. Thus, it is hypothesized that LDL must be modified first possibly by oxidation in the artery wall to "activate" its atherogenic potential. There is mounting evidence to support this feasible hypothesis.

With hypercholesterolemia and concomitant increases in LDL cholesterol, the arterial wall picks up the modified LDL molecule and its cholesterol load at an accelerated rate that is greater than the amount of cholesterol exchanged back into the plasma and picked up by the HDL molecule for transport to the liver. Thus, the physiologic disposal system for excess cholesterol in any tissue, but particularly in the arterial intima, becomes overloaded when the plasma LDL cholesterol concentration is high.

This concept of cholesterol transport and storage in the artery has been greatly clarified by tissue culture experiments in which a variety of cells from animals and humans have been incubated with both LDL and HDL. When modified LDL is in high concentration, there is a tremendous uptake of cholesterol, particularly cholesteryl ester. The resultant mass accumulation within the cell may be reversed by incubation of the cells in a medium containing HDL.

After the uptake of LDL and modified LDL by cultured cells, there is intracellular digestion of the LDL molecule, and its load of cholesterol, especially cholesteryl ester, is left within the cell in a storage form which the cell is unable to excrete as long as the medium contains a high content of LDL (Fig. 21-6). Some internal rearrangement with further esterification of free cholesterol taken up by the cell may also be occurring.[41] Note that the cholesterol molecule cannot be broken down by the cells of the arterial intima; hence, storage and excretion are the only possible metabolic pathways. It has been suggested that there is a relative enzymatic deficiency of cholesteryl ester hydrolase in the arterial wall that would tend to promote the accumulation of cholesteryl ester that has come into the wall carried by LDL. This cellular uptake of cholesteryl ester from the medium may be considered as a model system for the uptake of cholesterol and cholesteryl ester by the arterial wall in atherosclerosis and by the skin and tendons in xanthomatosis. Thus, the lifetime accumulation of cholesterol in countless numbers of smooth muscle cells and macrophages and in the extracellular milieu brings about the atherosclerotic process.

The pathogenicity of other lipoproteins for the development of atherosclerosis varies greatly (see Table 21-5). Epidemiologically, many studies reveal an association between VLDL and triglyceride levels and the development of coronary heart disease, especially in older women.[313] Clinically, premature coronary heart disease has been observed in families with type IV hyperlipidemia. The VLDL molecule, unlike HDL, can be picked up by tissue-culture cells and does contain apoprotein B. Furthermore, it carries a considerable amount of cholesterol, albeit less than does LDL. Thus, a moderate view would acknowledge that VLDL in excess may be associated with an increased risk for developing coronary heart disease in some patients. IDL, which is found in type III hyperlipoproteinemia, has an undisputed relation with both atherosclerosis and xanthomatosis. Both coronary heart disease and peripheral atherosclerosis occur at an accelerated rate with IDL elevation.

Chylomicrons would appear to have a minimum of atherogenicity because of the large size of the particle. Atherosclerosis is reportedly rare in type I hyperlipoproteinemia with an absence or deficiency of lipoprotein lipase. However, there is considerable evidence that the chylomicron remnant, which is produced during the action of the tissue enzyme lipoprotein lipase on chylomicron triglycerides, is very atherogenic. The chylomicron remnant is less rich in triglyceride and richer in cholesterol and cholesteryl ester than is the original chylomicron. In type V hyperlipidemia, with poor clearing of chylomicrons, a great accumulation of remnants and VLDL, and low HDL, atherosclerosis and coronary heart disease certainly do occur. The remnant of chylomicron metabolism may be analogous to the remnant—IDL—from VLDL metabolism. However, HDL has a negative relation to atherosclerosis.[314] The data from all sources place HDL as having a protective role against the development of atherosclerosis. This applies particularly to American women before menopause, who have an attack rate for coronary heart disease much lower than that for similarly aged men and in whom HDL levels are 10 to 15 mg/dl higher. As has already been stressed,[55] the current thinking about HDL in this connection is that HDL may be a transport mechanism to carry cholesterol from the tissues back to the liver. Animals, for example, that have high HDL levels are relatively resistant to atherosclerosis, e.g., the rat and the dog. In tissue-culture systems, HDL does not induce the deposition of cholesteryl ester. Instead, its presence in the medium seems to prevent this occurrence and actually produce regression of cholesteryl esters in cells previously incubated in LDL. Both autopsy and, more recently, coronary angiographic evidence afford further confirmation of these concepts about the atherogenicity of various lipoproteins and plasma lipids.

Xanthomas

In this discussion of the various types of hyperlipidemia, considerable emphasis has been placed on xanthomas as one of the chief and cardinal clinical manifestations. In this section, emphasis will be placed on their collective characteristics, particularly as representing another disorder of lipid storage. Tendon and tuberous xanthomas represent sterol (ester) storage,[312] but in eruptive xanthomas of the skin, triglyceride (from chylomicrons) is the chief constituent.

Ordinarily xanthomas represent a clinical manifestation of severe hyperlipidemia, but xanthelasmas may be seen in patients with normal plasma lipid concentrations, particularly among patients who are homozygous for apo E-2. The vast majority of patients with tendon xanthomas have familial hypercholesterolemia, but rarely have cerebrotendinous xanthomatosis or sitosterolemia. The more severe the hyperlipidemia, the earlier in life the xanthomas appear. This concept is expressed most fully in the homozygote of familial hypercholesterolemia when the xanthomas appear in the first decade of life or at birth.

Although the appearance of xanthomas is usually related to the duration and level of hypercholesterolemia, important exceptions occur. These include several other sterol storage diseases: cerebrotendinous xanthomatosis (the CTX syndrome) and "sitosterolemia and xanthomatosis." The presence of other sterols in the blood and in the tissues, cholestanol (CTX syndrome) and the plant sterols (sitosterolemia and xanthomatosis), potentiates greatly the development of xanthomas, particularly tendon xanthomas, as will be discussed subsequently.

Xanthomas may be regarded as the outward manifestation of sterol and lipid storage, analogous to the internal sterol storage occurring in developing atherosclerotic lesions or in other tissues; xanthomas have been found in the lung and the soft tissues of the buttocks.[315] These two manifestations generally can be correlated, and when xanthomas are present, suspicion of underlying latent atherosclerosis must always be entertained. Xanthomas may also provide a clue to the diagnosis of a particular hyperlipidemia. Eruptive xanthomas indicate the presence of type I or type V hyperlipidemia with chylomicronemia. Tuberous xanthomas may indicate type II familial hypercholesterolemia or type III. Tendon xanthomas are also found in these two conditions. Xanthelasmas have no absolute predilection for a given form of hyperlipidemia, although they are most commonly seen in association with hypercholesterolemia and patients homozygous for apoprotein E-2 without hyperlipidemia. The fact that many patients with severe familial hypercholesterolemia may not have xanthelasmas at all is also puzzling. The appearance of corneal arcus, another lipid storage entity, is certainly not predictable on the basis of hyperlipidemia: it may or may not be present. However, when it is found early in life without there having been injury to the eye, the presence of a profound corneal arcus is highly suggestive of severe hypercholesterolemia.

As is the case with early atherosclerotic plaques, xanthomas are composed principally of foam cells laden with cholesteryl esters, a mild inflammatory reaction with the presence of Touton giant cells, and some increased collagen. Cholesteryl ester is the chemical constituent most characteristically increased.[312,316] It is presumed that LDL [or Lp(a) or IDL] is taken up by the cells of the tendons and skin, much in the same way that these lipoproteins are taken up from the plasma into the atherosclerotic plaque.

It is worth emphasizing the potential reversibility of all xanthomas in response to decreases in plasma lipid concentrations because xanthoma cholesterol exchanges with plasma cholesterol.[316] Reversibility has occurred most dramatically with regard to the eruptive xanthomas of types I and V hyperlipidemia. These lesions may disappear completely in a month. Xanthelasmas and tuberous xanthomas have been observed to disappear during a period of 1 to 2 years with pronounced plasma lipid lowering. Tendon xanthomas are slower to regress, and significant changes take 2 or more years of effective therapy to become evident. The surgical removal of xanthomatous lesions, usually for cosmetic reasons, is almost invariably succeeded by their recurrence unless attention is paid to concomitant lowering of plasma lipids. This has occurred especially in regard to xanthelasmas but also for surgically removed tendon and tuberous xanthomas.

Acid Cholesteryl Ester Hydrolase Deficiency

Two other sterol storage diseases—Wolman disease and cholesteryl ester storage disease—in which cholesteryl esters and triglycerides accumulate in lysosomes have been described[317] and appear to be allelic. In both inherited disorders, the biochemical defect involves the deficiency of a lysosomal esterase, which at optimal acidic pH is capable of the hydrolysis of both cholesteryl esters and triglycerides. Etiologically, both diseases appear to be similar to other lysosomal storage diseases associated with catabolic enzyme deficiencies, such as the sphingolipidoses and gangliosidoses.

Wolman Disease

Wolman disease is usually detected within the first few weeks of life. Symptoms include vomiting, abdominal distension, steatorrhea, and a general failure to thrive.[317] Examination reveals hepatosplenomegaly with normal tonsils. Calcification of the adrenal glands is usually apparent on x-ray, and the plasma lipids are normal or low. Bone marrow aspiration reveals foam cells laden with cholesteryl esters and triglycerides; at autopsy, increased concentrations of these lipids are found throughout the body, most notably in the liver, spleen, and lymph nodes. A definitive diagnosis is based on the clinical picture together with a demonstrable absence of acid cholesteryl esterase in cultured fibroblasts or peripheral leukocytes. Studies of the known cases suggest that the disorder is inherited as an autosomal recessive trait; obligate heterozygotes may have reduced acid esterase activity but are clinically normal. Treatment is supportive, and the disease is fatal within the first year of life.

Cholesteryl Ester Storage Disease

Clinically less severe than Wolman disease, cholesteryl ester storage disease is usually but not invariably detected in childhood.[317] Affected infants are usually asymptomatic, and the only consistent finding on physical examination has been hepatomegaly, which may be associated with splenomegaly in older subjects. Adrenal calcification is unusual in children but may occur in older subjects. Portal hypertension and esophageal varices have been reported secondary to hepatic fibrosis and cirrhosis in some of the reported cases. Plasma lipid values have shown moderate hypercholesterolemia (250 to 400 mg/dl) with increased levels of VLDL and LDL and low levels of HDL. Xanthomas have not been reported, but there is autopsy evidence for premature atherosclerosis in two subjects.

The diagnosis of this autosomal recessive disorder is based on clinical findings together with enzyme studies similar to those in Wolman disease, which reveal a virtual absence of lysosomal cholesteryl esterase. In addition to dietary restriction of fat and cholesterol, recent studies have suggested that treatment of patients with cholesteryl ester hydrolase deficiency with lovastatin or simvastatin reduces plasma concentrations of total and LDL cholesterol and also leads to a diminution in liver size;[318,319] the latter observation suggests that this treatment reduces the storage of cholesteryl esters within the liver. Favorable effects were not, however, observed in response to lovastatin treatment in three patients with cholesteryl ester hydrolase deficiency evaluated at the NIH.[320] Use of lovastatin or simvastatin in patients with cholesteryl ester hydrolase deficiency must be regarded as investigational, and long-term follow-up of the patients currently being treated will be necessary to objectively assess whether such therapy is beneficial.

Lp(a) Hyperlipidemia

Increased plasma concentrations of Lp(a) have been associated with an increased risk of premature atherosclerosis in western societies.[9,11] The plasma concentrations of Lp(a) do not show a normal distribution, and the majority of the population exhibits Lp(a) concentrations between 5 and 20 mg/dl. Although the definition is arbitrary, plasma concentrations of Lp(a) that exceed 30 mg/dl should be considered abnormally high. As previously discussed in the section on familial hypercholesterolemia, the incidence of coronary artery disease in patients with that disorder appears to be higher in individuals who concurrently have increased plasma concentrations of Lp(a).[157,158] Tendon xanthomas may be particularly prominent in patients with heterozygous familial hypercholesterolemia who concurrently have high plasma concentrations of Lp(a).

Data on proof of benefit from reducing plasma concentrations of Lp(a) in individuals in whom the levels are increased are incomplete, but in view of the evidence linking high plasma concentrations of Lp(a) with an increased risk of atherosclerosis and, potentially, thrombosis, strategies to reduce elevated plasma concentrations of this lipoprotein seem to be appropriate in selected patients. Plasma concentrations of Lp(a) do not appear to change appreciably in response to different dietary perturbations[321]; treatment with a number of lipid-lowering drugs, including bile acid sequestrants,[322] fibrates,[215] and lovastatin or simvastatin,[323,324] also fails to alter concentrations of Lp(a). In contrast, treatment with nicotinic acid has been shown to reduce plasma Lp(a) concentrations.[325] Estrogen replacement therapy in postmenopausal women has also been shown to reduce plasma concentrations of Lp(a).[326]

FAMILIAL DISEASES WITH STORAGE OF STEROLS OTHER THAN CHOLESTEROL

This section describes two lipid storage diseases characterized by the accumulation of unusual sterols in the blood and tissue. In cerebrotendinous xanthomatosis (CTX syndrome), cholestanol (dihydrocholesterol) accumulates in the blood and tissues. The second disease, sitosterolemia and xanthomatosis, involves the accumulation of plant sterols, particularly sitosterol, in the blood and tissues, notably in the tendons. Xanthomas can occur in the absence of hypercholesterolemia in both disorders.[327,328] In both conditions, premature coronary heart disease also occurs.

Cerebrotendinous Xanthomatosis (CTX)

Cerebrotendinous xanthomatosis (CTX) is a rare autosomal recessive disease characterized by the development of xanthomas of the tendons, lungs, and brain in the setting of normal or low plasma cholesterol levels.[327,328] Other clinical manifestations include cataracts, subnormal intelligence, progressive cerebellar ataxia, dementia, and spinal cord paresis. Cholestanol accumulates in the white matter of the cerebrum and cerebellum and in xanthomas as a consequence of increased plasma concentrations of cholestanol. The disease appears to be caused by homozygous mutations that result in deficiency of 27-hydroxylase, a key hepatic enzyme that is involved in cholesterol oxidation and bile acid synthesis. The resulting block in bile acid synthesis causes the accumulation of cholestanol and other precursors.[329] It is estimated that more than 150 CTX homozygotes have been reported around the world.

Clinical Manifestations

The onset of CTX is insidious and unpredictable. Dementia has been observed at age 10 years, cataracts by age 15, tendon xanthomas at age 15, and ataxia by age 18 years.

The course may be divided into several time phases. The initial stage usually begins in childhood, when borderline intelligence, mental retardation, mental deterioration, or even dementia may be found. This is not invariable, however, and in some patients mentation has been found to be normal even in the third and fourth decades of life.

During adolescence and young adulthood, spasticity and at times ataxia develop and become progressively more severe. Juvenile cataracts and tendon xanthomas are frequently observed in this second stage of disease and are usually well developed by young adulthood. The Achilles tendon is the most common site of xanthoma formation, but xanthomas also may occur in the triceps, the tibial tuberosities, and the extensor tendons of the fingers. These lesions are similar in appearance to those seen in familial hypercholesterolemia. Tuberous xanthomas and xanthelasmas (palpebral xanthomas) may also be present.

In the third stage of CTX, enlargement of xanthomas and neurologic deterioration with spasticity, ataxia, difficulties of speech, tremors, and atrophy of the distal musculature become prominent. There may be bilateral Babinski signs and loss of pain and vibratory sensation. The disease follows a deteriorating course characterized by cerebellar ataxia, systemic spinal cord involvement, and finally a phase of pseudobulbar paresis leading to death. Four of the ten deaths reported so far, however, resulted from acute myocardial infarction. In the others, death presumably resulted from neurologic dysfunction. Death has usually occurred between the fourth and sixth decades.

Laboratory and Pathologic Findings

In most patients, the plasma cholesterol and triglyceride levels have been within the normal range, e.g., 117 to 220 mg/dl. The plasma cholestanol (5 -cholestan-3 -ol) concentration may be elevated nearly 10-fold compared to normal (e.g., 4 mg/dl vs. <0.6 mg/dl). Cholestanol is a saturated sterol that differs from cholesterol by the absence of the 5,6 double bond. Cholestanol is normally present in small amounts in tissues and plasma and occurs in both the free and the ester forms.

Cholestanol is normally excreted in trace amounts in the bile, but in the CTX syndrome its excretion is greatly increased (4 to 11 percent of total sterols). Abnormalities of the secretion of bile acid occur concomitantly and reveal decreased concentrations of chenodeoxycholic acid, with an increase in cholic acid to about 80 percent of the total bile acids. Allocholic acid, which is formed from cholestanol, is also increased and represents the other bile acid abnormality.

In the CTX syndrome, large quantities of cholestanol are found in the tissues throughout the body. This phenomenon is particularly manifest in the nervous system, where cholestanol may constitute up to 25 percent of the total sterols. Although in the tendon xanthomas cholestanol may constitute up to 11 percent of the total sterols, cholesterol is still the predominant steroid present. Considerable amounts of cholestanol may be found in any tissue examined, including that of the skin, lung, liver, spleen, adipose tissue, and muscle. Large ectopic xanthomas that are particularly rich in cholestanol may be found internally, particularly in the lung and brain.

Pathophysiology

The origin of the great increase of tissue cholestanol hypothetically includes increased local synthesis, influx from the blood after synthesis elsewhere, absorption from the diet, or a block in catabolism or excretion from the tissues. The underlying biochemical defect in the CTX syndrome is a lack of the liver enzyme 27-hydroxylase, which is necessary for the normal synthesis of bile acids, especially chenodeoxycholic acid.[282,283] In this disorder, as already indicated, there is decreased synthesis of chenodeoxycholic acid. Thus, many intermediate metabolites that occur in bile acid synthesis are excreted in the bile, the feces, and the urine. At least part of the excess cholestanol in CTX patients may be formed from these accumulated intermediates in bile acid synthesis. There is also increased synthesis of both cholestanol and cholesterol.

Treatment

Because cholestanol is present in certain foods of animal origin, mainly eggs and dairy products, reduction in or elimination of their consumption in a very low cholesterol diet has led to a lowering of plasma cholestanol levels. The logical drug treatment has been chenodeoxycholic acid administered orally.[330] This treatment can increase the size of the bile acid pool, produce normal concentrations of chenodeoxycholic acid in bile, reduce the levels of abnormal bile acid precursors in bile, and diminish levels of cholestanol in the plasma. Adjunctive administration of HMG CoA reductase inhibitors may augment the biochemical improvement and possibly improve the clinical outcome.[330B,330C] Whether these treatments will ultimately change the course of this progressively deteriorating disorder is not yet certain because the disease seems to continue to progress in some patients despite treatment.

Sitosterolemia and Xanthomatosis

This rare autosomal recessive disease was initially described 25 years ago by Bhattacharyya and Connor in two sisters[331] and has now been reported in more than 40 patients worldwide.[328] It is characterized by tendon and tuberous xanthomas, premature atherosclerosis, and the accumulation of plant sterols, particularly sitosterol, in the blood and tissues.[332] Xanthomas may appear in childhood despite normal or only slightly elevated plasma cholesterol concentrations, presumably as a consequence of foam cell formation resulting from greatly increased plasma concentrations of sitosterol and other phytosterols.

The metabolic defects that cause the disease are twofold: greatly increased intestinal absorption of all dietary sterols, including sitosterol and other plant sterols that are normally absorbed only in minute amounts, and impaired excretion of sitosterol from the body. The exact nature of these metabolic defects is not known. The mutation responsible for sitosterolemia was recently mapped to a 15 cM interval at chromosome 2p21 between microsatellite markers D2S1788 and D2S1352.[333]

The disorder now appears to be caused by mutations in two new members of the adenosine triphosphate (ATP)-binding cassette (ABC) transporter family, ABCG5 and ABCG8. ABCG5 and ABCG8 are believed to attenuate intestinal absorption of dietary sterols and facilitate biliary excretion of endogenous sterols. This process seems to promote selective absorption of cholesterol and excretion of sitosterol. The mechanism responsible for normal discrimination between these sterols is currently unknown.

Clinical Features

In the patients in the initial report, xanthomas were first noted in childhood in the extensor tendons of both hands; in later years, they subsequently developed in the patellar, plantar, and Achilles tendons. The plant sterols—sitosterol, campesterol, and stigmasterol—are present in high concentrations in the blood and tissues. Cholestanol levels are also increased.

As might be expected from the extensive tendon xanthomas found in this disease, severe atherosclerosis also occurs at an early age. Indeed, the severity of the atherosclerotic disease mirrors that found in familial hypercholesterolemia. Altogether, three males have died of coronary atherosclerosis at ages 13, 18, and 42 years and one female has died at age 39.[328] Three living patients have sustained myocardial infarction; one had coronary bypass surgery, and two other patients had severe coronary atherosclerosis demonstrated by angiography. The postmortem examination of the 18-year-old male, who died suddenly of acute myocardial infarction, revealed diffuse and extensive coronary atherosclerosis in the proximal left main and proximal right coronary arteries as well as in the right and left anterior descending and circumflex arteries.[334]

The thoracic and abdominal aorta and iliac vessels also had severe atherosclerosis.

Because most of these patients have average plasma cholesterol levels for western populations, the cause of the severe atherosclerosis cannot be just cholesterol carried in the LDL molecule. The presence of the plant sterols in the lipoproteins somehow increases the propensity to foam cell formation both in the tendons as xanthoma and in the medium- and large-size arteries as atherosclerosis. Biochemical examination of the tendon xanthomas has revealed a higher cholesterol/plant sterol ratio than is found in the blood. A uterine artery removed at the time of elective surgery in one of the sitosterolemic patients revealed the presence of plant sterols as well as cholesterol in the arterial wall.[335] Sitosterolemia should be considered in the differential diagnosis of any patient with myocardial infarction before age 40.

Although the red cell membranes contain the characteristic plant sterols of sitosterolemia, anemia has not been a problem in the majority of these patients. However, in four patients hemolysis and chronic hemolytic anemia have been described, along with hypersplenism and platelet abnormalities.[328] These findings of an autoimmune state may be accompanied by arthritis and a positive ANA test. It may well be that sitosterolemia does not represent a single gene defect and may express itself in several clinical entities, one of which leads to hemolytic anemia.

Chemistry, Absorption, and Metabolism of Plant Sterols in Humans

The three plant sterols—sitosterol, campesterol, and stigmasterol—are usually found only in the lipids of plants and thus are particularly plentiful in vegetable oils, nuts, and fat-rich vegetables and fruits. In chemical structure, the three plant sterols resemble cholesterol except for minor differences in their side chains.

Plant sterols are habitually consumed by human beings in the usual diet. A typical American diet may contain up to 250 mg of these sterols per day, of which sitosterol makes up to 75 percent of the total, with lesser proportions of campesterol and stigmasterol.

Intestinal absorption of plant sterols in humans is normally less than 5 percent of the amount in the diet and is responsible for their low plasma concentration (0.3 to 1.73 mg/dl). However, during infancy, considerable amounts of sitosterol can be found in the blood (up to 9 mg/dl) and also in the aortas of infants fed vegetable oil–rich formulas. Twenty percent of the absorbed dietary sitosterol is converted to bile acids, and the remainder is excreted in the bile as free sterol.

Laboratory Abnormalities

High concentrations of sitosterol and the other two plant sterols in the plasma are the chief characteristic of sitosterolemia and xanthomatosis. Sitosterol predominates in concentrations ranging between 12 and 27 mg/dl. The campesterol concentration is 6 to 10 mg/dl, with less than 1 mg/dl of stigmasterol present. About 60 percent of the plasma sitosterol and campesterol is esterified. The plasma plant sterols are distributed between the low-density (about 70 percent of the total) and high-density lipoproteins. The very low density lipoproteins carry only trace amounts. Hypercholesterolemia is a variable feature that is most prominent in children with sitosterolemia who are also consuming and hyperabsorbing a high-cholesterol diet. Cholestanol may also be increased.

Erythrocytes also contain unesterified plant sterols. The ratio of cholesterol to sitosterol in these cells is similar to that in the plasma and suggests that free exchange of both sterols occurs.

Considerable accumulation of plant sterols, mainly unesterified sitosterol, occurs in the tendon xanthomas. However, despite the high content of plant sterols, cholesterol is still the predominant sterol, constituting 73 to 88 percent of the total. Histologically, these xanthomatous lesions are indistinguishable from the tendon xanthomas found in hyperlipoproteinemia and CTX.

The subcutaneous adipose tissue and the skin of patients also have been found to contain plant sterols. Other tissues of the body also probably contain them in abnormal amounts.

Pathophysiology

The principal metabolic defect in sitosterolemia and xanthomatosis appears to be the greatly increased intestinal absorption of dietary sitosterol and other sterols including cholesterol, but the exact mechanism is not known. One hypothesis is that the esterification of plant sterols is abnormally enhanced and that this in turn promotes absorption. The biliary excretion of sitosterol as neutral sterol or as bile acid is critically limited, resulting in slow turnover of sitosterol.

The accumulation of sitosterol and the other two plant sterols in smaller amounts in the tendons implies that the plant sterols probably produce the major manifestations of the disease and initiate xanthoma formation. Analogous to the situation in CTX, it is noteworthy that despite high concentrations of sitosterol in the xanthomas, the increase in the xanthoma cholesterol is quantitatively more important. It has been hypothesized that the incorporation of the plant sterols into the plasma lipoproteins affects the stability of the lipoprotein complexes, favoring deposition of sterols generally into the tissues.

In this context, a role of plant sterols in the development of atherosclerotic vascular disease should also be considered. Plant sterols favor deposition of cholesterol in the arterial wall and lead to premature atherosclerotic lesions. The development of overt coronary disease in patients with sitosterolemia and xanthomatosis provides evidence in support of this view.

Diagnosis

Sitosterolemia and xanthomatosis should be considered in every patient who has developed xanthomas in childhood and does not have either familial hypercholesterolemia or the CTX syndrome. The diagnosis of this disease can be established by analyzing the sterols of the plasma by means of gas-liquid chromatography. The variable hypercholesterolemia that some of these patients manifest is noteworthy. There should be a high index of suspicion that sitosterolemia may be the underlying diagnosis in any young person with xanthomas whose cholesterol level is normal or elevated to the range of 300 to 500 mg/dl. Some of these hypercholesterolemic sitosterolemia patients have been termed pseudohomozygotes of familial hypercholesterolemia because their parents were completely normal. When plasma sterols were determined, they were found to have sitosterolemia.[328] Some patients with sitosterolemia will be identified because of reversible marked diet-induced hypercholesterolemia that is a consequence of hyperabsorption of dietary cholesterol.

Treatment

The logical treatment for this sterol storage disease is a diet low in or devoid of plant sterols, as the excessive plant sterols in the body originate from the diet. The results of such treatment in two patients revealed a 29 percent decrease in the level of plasma sitosterol. Presumably the great stores of plant sterols in the tissues are in equilibration with the plant sterols of plasma, and prolonged dietary treatment is required to reduce the plasma sitosterol level to normal.

The guiding principles in the formulation of a diet with a low content of plant sterol are to (1) eliminate all sources of vegetable fats such as vegetable oil, shortenings, and margarines, (2) eliminate all plant foods with a high fat content such as nuts, seeds, chocolate, olives, and avocado, and (3) use only refined cereal products that have the germ (rich in fat and plant sterols) removed. In general, foods that have a high content of vegetable fat will also have a high content of plant sterols. The detailed composition of such a diet has been published elsewhere.[327] The diet also should be low in cholesterol and shellfish sterols because all sterols are hyperabsorbed. Margarines containing sitosterol or sitostanol, which are marketed as cholesterol-lowering foods, should be avoided by patients with sitosterolemia.

Theoretically, drugs that may interfere with the intestinal absorption of plant sterols may prevent the expression of sitosterolemia and xanthomatosis. No such drug trial has been conducted. However, two drugs have been found to be useful in greatly reducing the plasma levels of all sterols, including the plant sterols as well as cholestanol and cholesterol. These agents are the bile acid–binding resins such as cholestyramine and the HMG CoA reductase inhibitors of cholesterol biosynthesis. These include lovastatin, which has an effective sterol-lowering action in some patients with sitosterolemia.

TABLE 21-17. Dietary Effects on Plasma Lipids and Lipoproteins in Humans

Hyperlipidemic dietary factors
1. Dietary cholesterol
2. Saturated fat
3. *Trans* fatty acids
4. Total fat
5. Total calories with adiposity
6. Alcohol (in some individuals)
Lipid-lowering dietary factors
7. Polyunsaturated fat: omega-6-rich vegetable oils* and omega-3-rich fish and fish oils
8. Monounsaturated fat*
9. Soluble fibers (pectin, guar gum)
10. Carbohydrate as starches replacing fat
11. Possibly vegetable protein or other substances from vegetables
Dietary factors with no discrete long-term effects
12. Protein generally
13. Vitamins and minerals
14. Lecithin

*Very high amounts of polyunsaturated or monounsaturated vegetable fat, while resulting in a hypocholesterolemic effect overall, would produce postprandial hypertriglyceridemia and increased remnant formation.

DIETARY TREATMENT OF HYPERLIPIDEMIA

The cornerstone in the treatment of hyperlipidemia is dietary alteration. This is true regardless of the degree to which primary genetic abnormalities are partly or completely responsible for the development of the hyperlipidemia. Dietary factors in the American population inevitably exacerbate any genetic abnormality when this is largely responsible for the hyperlipidemic state. Dietary treatment will almost always result in some improvement of the condition. Therapy has been simplified by the concept that a single basic diet may be used initially in the treatment of all forms of hyperlipidemia.[336] This single diet is low in cholesterol and low in total and saturated fat; it is high in complex carbohydrate. It is of low caloric density and provides only enough calories to achieve and maintain ideal body weight.

The aim of the dietary treatment of hyperlipidemia is straightforward: the achievement of "normal" plasma cholesterol and triglyceride concentrations. Dietary treatment should be initiated when the plasma cholesterol concentration is above 200 mg/dl in older adults and 180 mg/dl in young adults and children; the upper limit for plasma triglyceride concentration is 140 mg/dl.

The recommended dietary treatment is appropriate and safe for both adults and children. Such treatment must clearly answer all the nutritional needs of the body and at the same time have beneficial effects on the elevated plasma lipid and lipoprotein concentrations. These criteria have been satisfied both theoretically and practically.[336]

The Effects of Specific Nutrients on the Plasma Lipids and Lipoproteins

Historically and to the present time, a vast amount of evidence in both humans and animals has pointed to certain dietary factors that have hyperlipidemic effects (Table 21-17). Some have a hypolipidemic action. Many other factors have no or minimal effects. These nutritional factors will be discussed briefly to provide a theoretical and practical basis for dietary prescription in the treatment of hyperlipidemia. It must also be appreciated that certain dietary factors can affect thrombosis, an event that adds greatly to the organ ischemia produced by atherosclerotic blockage of blood flow.

Cholesterol

Cholesterol in the diet has important effects on lipid metabolism.[337] Cholesterol-rich diets have regularly caused hypercholesterolemia, atherosclerosis, and even at times myocardial infarction in a large number of species of experimental animals, including primates.[338,339] Dietary cholesterol enters the body by way of the chylomicron pathway and is removed from the plasma by the liver as a component of chylomicron remnants. Only about 40 percent of ingested cholesterol is absorbed; the remaining 60 percent passes out in the stool. Dietary cholesterol is thus added to the cholesterol synthesized by the body, as feedback inhibition of cholesterol biosynthesis in the body only partially occurs in humans, even when a large amount of dietary cholesterol is ingested.[340] Because the ring structure of the sterol nucleus cannot be broken down by the tissues of the body, as occurs with fat, protein, and carbohydrate, cholesterol must be either excreted or stored. Thus, it is easy to see how the body or a particular tissue (i.e., a coronary artery) can become overloaded with cholesterol if there are limitations in cholesterol excretion from the body. Cholesterol is excreted in the bile and ultimately in the stool, either as cholesterol or as bile acids, synthesized in the liver from cholesterol. Both pathways of excretion are limited, and furthermore, much of what is excreted in the bile is returned to the body by the very efficient enterohepatic reabsorption.

Dietary cholesterol does not directly enter into the formation of the very low density lipoproteins and low-density lipoproteins synthesized in the liver because it is removed by the liver as a component of the chylomicron remnants. It can, however, profoundly affect the catabolism of LDL as mediated through the

LDL receptor. Because dietary cholesterol ultimately contributes to the total amount of hepatic cell cholesterol, it can affect the biosynthesis of both cholesterol and LDL receptors in the liver. In particular, an increase in hepatic cell cholesterol will decrease the synthesis of mRNA for the LDL receptor, which decreases the number of LDL receptors and subsequently, as in other conditions that decrease LDL receptors, will cause an *increase* in the plasma level of LDL cholesterol.[341–344] Conversely, a drastic decrease in dietary cholesterol will increase the number of LDL receptors in the liver, enhance LDL removal, and hence lower plasma LDL levels. The effects of dietary cholesterol follow.

1. Increased chylomicrons and remnants
2. Increased hepatic cell cholesterol, which has the following consequences:
   a. Decreased cholesterol biosynthesis
   b. Partial compensation in excretion of biliary cholesterol and bile acids to lessen hepatic cholesterol
   c. Decreased synthesis of LDL receptors
   d. Increased plasma LDL
3. Increased plasma LDL and deposition of cholesterol into the arterial wall

During the past 30 years, 26 separate metabolic experiments involving 196 human subjects have demonstrated that dietary cholesterol exerts decisive effects on plasma cholesterol and LDL levels.[345–347] However, as was pointed out years ago, the doubling or tripling of the amount of dietary cholesterol will not necessarily increase the plasma levels if the initial amount of dietary cholesterol is already substantial (e.g., an increase in intake from 475 mg per day to 950 mg per day).[346] This phenomenon is restudied from time to time and mistakenly interpreted as showing that dietary cholesterol has no effect on the plasma levels, as will be explained later. For those who wish to explore the subject more fully, the results of various cholesterol feeding studies have been reviewed.[348]

The effects on the plasma cholesterol levels as the amount of dietary cholesterol is gradually increased are depicted in Fig. 21-15. These data are supported by both animal and human experiments. With a baseline cholesterol-free diet, the amount of dietary cholesterol necessary to produce an increase in the plasma cholesterol concentration is referred to as the *threshold amount*. Then, as the amount of dietary cholesterol is increased, the plasma cholesterol increases until the second important point on this curve—the *ceiling amount*—is reached. Further increases in dietary cholesterol do not lead to higher levels of plasma cholesterol even though phenomenally high amounts may be ingested. Each animal or human being probably has its own distinctive threshold and ceiling amounts. Generally speaking, however, and again based on the experimental literature, we suggest that an average threshold amount for human beings is 100 mg per day; an average ceiling amount of dietary cholesterol is in the neighborhood of 300 to 400 mg per day. Further experiments are necessary to provide more precise information about the ceiling. Thus, a baseline dietary cholesterol intake of 500 mg per day from two eggs would already exceed the ceiling for most individuals. The addition of two more egg yolks, for a total dietary cholesterol intake of 1,000 mg per day, would not then further increase the plasma cholesterol concentration. Yet beginning with a baseline very low cholesterol diet under 100 mg per day and adding the equivalent of two egg yolks, or 500 mg, to this baseline amount would produce a striking increase in plasma cholesterol concentrations, perhaps, as shown in many experiments, by up to 60 mg/dl.

Dietary surveys indicate that the average American intake of dietary cholesterol is about 400 mg per day for women and 500 mg per day for men.[349] Decreasing these amounts of dietary cholesterol to 100 mg per day, as would take place in the therapeutic and preventive diets, would then have a profound effect on plasma cholesterol concentrations, because, as shown in Fig. 21-15, operationally one would be on the descending limb of the curve.

Dietary Fat, Amount and Saturation, Kinds of Polyunsaturation

The amount and kind of fat in the diet have a well-documented effect on plasma lipid concentrations. The *total* amount of dietary fat is important because the formation of chylomicrons in the intestinal mucosa and their subsequent circulation in the blood are directly proportional to the amount of fat that has been consumed in the diet. A fatty meal will result in the production of large numbers of chylomicrons and will impart the characteristic lactescent appearance to postprandial plasma that is observed some 3 to 5 h after meal consumption. A typical American diet containing 110 g of fat will produce 110 g of chylomicron triglyceride per day. *Remnant* production from chylomicrons is proportional to the number of chylomicrons synthesized. Chylomicron remnants resulting from the action of lipoprotein lipase are cholesterol-rich and are atherogenic particles.[89]

Postprandial lipemia is, of course, intense after the usual American diet and may be present for many hours before being cleared. Not only is this lipemia (the composite of chylomicrons and remnants) suspected to be atherogenic, it may also promote thrombosis. Postprandial lipemia is lessened by physical activity and by a diet low in fat and/or containing omega-3 fatty acids from fish. It is worse and very prolonged in patients with fasting hypertriglyceridemia whose clearance mechanisms are already impaired.

Different types of fat have different effects on plasma lipids and lipoproteins. Fats may be divided into three major classes identified by saturation and unsaturation characteristics. Long-chain saturated fatty acids have no double bonds, are not essential nutrients, and may be readily synthesized in the body from acetate. Dietary saturated fatty acids typically have a profound hypercholesterolemic effect, increase the concentrations of LDL, and are thrombogenic. All animal fats are highly saturated (30 percent or more of the fat is saturated) and contains little polyunsaturated fatty acid. The molecular basis for the effects of dietary saturated fat on the plasma cholesterol level is now well understood. It rests on the influence of saturated fat on the LDL receptor activity of liver cells as described by Brown and Goldstein.[341] Dietary saturated fat suppresses mRNA synthesis for the LDL receptor, which decreases hepatic LDL receptor activity, decreases the removal of LDL from the blood, and thus increases the concentration of LDL cholesterol in the blood.[342–344] Cholesterol in this diet augments the effect of saturated fat by further suppressing hepatic LDL receptor activity and raising the plasma LDL cholesterol level. Conversely, a decrease in dietary cholesterol and saturated fat increases the LDL receptor activity of the liver cells, enhances the hepatic pickup of LDL cholesterol, and lowers the concentration of LDL cholesterol in the blood.[342] Some saturated fats, such as coconut oil, increase the synthesis of cholesterol and LDL in the liver. Metabolic studies suggest that one can expect an average plasma cholesterol decrease of 20 percent by maximally decreasing dietary cholesterol and saturated fat.

Besides natural sources of saturated fats, the hydrogenation of liquid vegetable oils can saturate the unsaturated fatty acids. Soft margarines and shortenings are lightly hydrogenated. The softer a margarine is at room temperature, the less hydrogenated it is. Peanut butter is so lightly hydrogenated that its fatty acid composition is little affected. Large quantities of highly hydrogenated fat should be avoided to keep the total saturated fat low. The daily use of small quantities of soft margarines is acceptable in the context of a low-fat diet. Monounsaturated *trans* fatty acids, isomers of the *cis* oleic acid, are important byproducts of this process. *Trans* fatty acids are oxidized for energy, as are other fatty acids. In a recent study in which large amounts of *trans* fatty acids were consumed, the plasma LDL cholesterol level was significantly elevated.[350] However, the presence of small amounts of *trans* fatty acids in lightly hydrogenated margarines (those in which a liquid vegetable oil is listed as the first ingredient) does not appear to constitute a problem in the diet for the treatment of hyperlipidemia.

Attention has been called to the fact that some saturated fats do not seem to cause hypercholesterolemia. Medium-chain triglycerides (C8 and C10 saturated fatty acids) are water-soluble and are handled metabolically more like carbohydrate than like fat. They are transported to the liver in portal vein blood rather than as chylomicrons. These fatty acids do not elevate the plasma cholesterol concentration.

Stearic acid, an 18-carbon saturated fatty acid, also has a limited effect on the plasma cholesterol concentration. Excessive stearic acid from the diet is converted into oleic acid, a monounsaturated fatty acid, by a desaturase enzyme. Feeding animals large quantities of stearic acid does not result in the deposition of stearic acid in the adipose tissue, as would occur with mono- and polyunsaturated fat feeding. This is due to the action of the desaturase enzyme. The practical importance of these observations about stearic acid is limited because stearic acid is present in foods that also contain appreciable amounts of other fatty acids that cause hypercholesterolemia. Palmitic acid is the most common saturated fat found in our food supply. It has 16 carbons and is intensely hypercholesterolemic. Myristic acid and lauric acid, with 14 and 12 carbons, respectively, also are intensely hypercholesterolemic. It is these fatty acids present in "saturated" dietary fats that cause their untoward effects. Amounts of stearic acid in the American diet are not great compared with amounts of palmitic acid.

The second class of dietary fats consists of the characteristic monounsaturated fatty acids that are present in all animal and vegetable fats. For practical purposes, oleic acid, which has one double bond at the omega-9 position, is the only significant dietary monounsaturated fatty acid. In general, the effects of dietary monounsaturated fatty acids on the plasma lipids are neutral, neither raising nor lowering their concentrations. They are, however, cholesterol-lowering compared to saturated fat. Reports that Mediterranean basin populations that consume olive oil in large quantities have fewer heart attacks than do people in the United States have led to further investigations of the antiatherogenic properties of the monounsaturates. Studies have shown that large amounts of monounsaturated fat, like polyunsaturated oils, lower plasma total and LDL cholesterol levels compared with saturated fat.[351] Furthermore, unlike polyunsaturated oils, monounsaturated fat did not lower the plasma HDL cholesterol level.

There are several additional points to be made in regard to these recent studies:

1. The "Mediterranean diet" is also rich in fish, beans, fruits, and vegetables and is *low* in both saturated fat and cholesterol. These could be the decisive factors that influence the lessened incidence of coronary disease and lower plasma cholesterol levels.
2. Olive oil is low in saturated fatty acids, which raise plasma cholesterol levels; this is why recent metabolic experiments have shown some cholesterol lowering as a result of large amounts of monounsaturated fat in the diet.
3. Large amounts of any kind of fat should be avoided to lower the risk of other diseases, such as colon or breast cancer and obesity. In addition, all fats, after absorption as chylomicrons, are acted on by LPL to form remnant particles that circulate in the blood. These are atherogenic.

Based on these considerations, it is prudent to include monounsaturated fat as part of a general lower-fat eating style but not to consider them as particularly antiatherogenic or hypolipidemic.

The third class of fatty acids—the polyunsaturated fatty acids—are vital constituents of cellular membranes and serve as prostaglandin precursors. Because they cannot be synthesized by the body and can be obtained only from the diet, they are "essential" fatty acids.[352] The two classes of essential fatty acids are the omega-6 and omega-3 fatty acids (Fig. 21-30). The most common examples of omega-6 fatty acids are arachidonic acid, 20 carbons in length with four double bonds, and its dietary precursor, linoleic acid. Linoleic acid is converted to arachidonic acid in the liver. Because the basic structure of omega-6 fatty acids cannot be synthesized by the body, 2 to 3 percent of the total energy in the diet must consist of linoleic acid to meet the metabolic requirements for the omega-6 structure.

Omega-3 fatty acids differ in the position of the first double bond. Counting from the methyl end of the molecule, this double

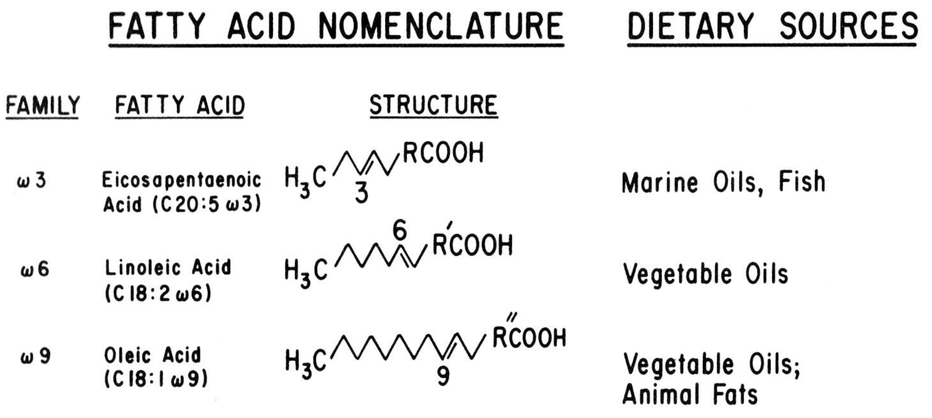

FIGURE 21-30. The structure and sources of dietary fatty acids. Fatty acids can be organized into families according to the position of the first double bond from the terminal methyl group. The omega-3 fatty acids all have three carbons between the methyl end and the first double bond. Fatty acids in this family include eicosapentaenoic acid (C20:5), linolenic acid (C18:3), and docosahexaenoic acid (C22:6). Linoleic acid (C18:2) and arachidonic acid (C20:4) are the most important omega-6 fatty acids, while oleic acid (C18:1) is the most common fatty acid in the omega-9 family.

bond is at the third rather than the sixth carbon. Omega-3 fatty acids are also "essential." They constitute important membrane components of the brain, retina, and sperm.[352,353] Omega-6 and omega-3 fatty acids are not interconvertible. The dietary sources of omega-6 fatty acids are plant foods, some but not all vegetable oils, and leafy vegetables. Fish and shellfish are especially rich in omega-3 fatty acids. Linolenic acid, C18:3, is obtained from vegetable products. Eicosapentaenoic acid (EPA), C20:5, and docosahexaenoic acid (DHA), C22:6, are derived from fish, shellfish, and phytoplankton. They are highly concentrated in fish oils. Like omega-6 fatty acids, omega-3 fatty acids are viewed as essential nutrients, and a safe intake would be 0.4 to 0.6 percent of total calories. Once either the omega-3 or omega-6 structure comes into the body as the 18-carbon linoleic or linolenic acid, the body can synthesize the longer-chain and more highly polyunsaturated omega-6 or omega-3 fatty acids (20 and 22 carbons, respectively).

EPA and DHA are present in the diet in two forms: as triglyceride in the adipose tissue of fish, usually present between muscle fibers, and as membrane phospholipids of the muscle of fish. These highly polyunsaturated fatty acids occupy the middle position of the glycerol skeleton for both triglycerides and phospholipids. In either of these dietary forms, EPA and DHA are efficiently absorbed from the intestinal tract. After absorption, EPA and DHA readily associate with membranes and are found in all four lipid classes: triglycerides, FFA, cholesteryl esters, and phospholipids. Ultimately, they are stored in the adipose tissue, and in experimental animals they even reach the brain and the retina.

Polyunsaturated fatty acids in large amounts, either the omega-6 or omega-3 structure, reduce plasma total and LDL cholesterol concentrations in normal and hypercholesterolemic individuals.[354,355] The situation is somewhat different in hypertriglyceridemic individuals or in those with combined hyperlipidemia. Only the omega-3 fatty acids from fish and fish oil have a decided triglyceride-lowering effect. VLDL in particular is decreased by the omega-3 fatty acids[356] (Fig. 21-31). Isotopic studies have shown that the triglyceride-lowering effect of omega-3 fatty acids occurs as a result of the depression of triglyceride and VLDL synthesis in the liver and from the accelerated catabolism of VLDL from the plasma. In some patients with type IV hypertriglyceridemia and in some patients with combined hyperlipidemia, there have been reports of an increase in LDL as the plasma triglycerides fall. This also occurs when gemfibrozil is given to these patients. In severely hypertriglyceridemic type V patients, however, large doses of fish oil (10 to 15 g/day) produce a dramatic clearing of chylomicronemia and lower both triglyceride and cholesterol concentrations. Fish oil also seems to promote the clearing of chylomicrons after the administration of a fatty meal. This would be of particular benefit in type V patients in whom there is great difficulty in clearing chylomicrons. Most experiments have not shown plasma triglyceride lowering from the omega-6 vegetable oils.

It is not known exactly how the intake of dietary omega-3 fatty acids should be altered to achieve the optimum effect. One study from The Netherlands indicated that men who included fish in their diet twice a week had fewer deaths from heart disease. A similar protective effect from eating fish was demonstrated in Japan. In a prospective trial in Wales, the prescription of two fish meals per week led to a reduction in both total mortality and the number of coronary events.[357] Even very low fat seafood contains an appreciable amount of omega-3 fatty acids, up to 40 or more percent of total fatty acids. Eating a total of 12 oz of a variety of

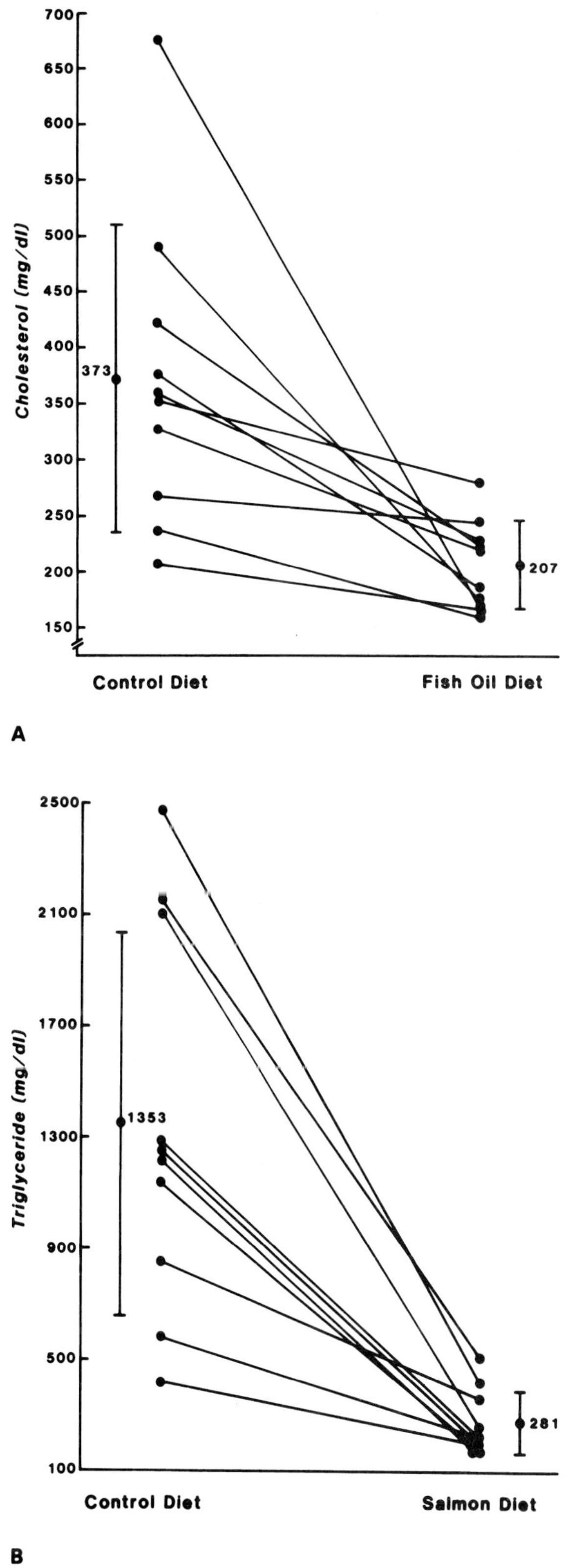

FIGURE 21-31. The hypocholesterolemic and hypotriglyceridemic effects of fish oils rich in omega-3 fatty acids in patients with phenotypic type V hyperlipoproteinemia. Changes in the plasma concentrations of total cholesterol = −166 mg/dl ($p > 0.01$), and triglyceride = −1072 mg/dl ($p > 0.001$), from 10 patients fed a fish oil–supplemented diet containing 20 to 30 g of omega-3 fatty acids. (*Reproduced from Phillipson et al.*[356] *with permission.*)

fish and shellfish each week would provide 3 to 5 g of omega-3 fatty acids as well as protein, vitamins, and minerals. The fish can be fresh, frozen, or canned without affecting the quantity of omega-3 fatty acids. The beneficial effects from following this dietary advice are especially evident if the fish replaces meat in the diet, meat being a major source of saturated fat. Also to be considered are the antithrombotic actions of fish oil, which seem to be mediated through the inhibition of the thromboxane A_2 in platelets,[353] and the enhanced clearance of chylomicrons.[358,359] Other effects of fish oil include inhibition of platelet-derived growth factor, alteration of leukocyte function, reduction of blood viscosity, increased fibrinolysis, and the inhibition of intimal hyperplasia in vein grafts used for arterial bypass. Thus, fish oils not only influence plasma lipids and lipoproteins, they also affect the thrombotic process.

The results of several recent studies have demonstrated beneficial effects of fish oil consumption on cardiovascular risk. In the GISSI study, 11,324 subjects with previous coronary artery disease were randomized to receive placebo or 1 gram daily of concentrated fish oil (Omacor) containing about 85–88 percent ethyl esters of EPA and DHA.[360] Compared to subjects who received placebo treatment, those who received fish oil had a 14 percent lower risk of events (death, nonfatal myocardial infarction, and nonfatal stroke). Other results from this study have been interpreted to indicate a possible reduction in fatal cardiac arrhythmias by omega-3 fatty acids in the setting of myocardial infarction. Additional recent results from the Health Professionals Study and the Physicians Health Study indicated that consumption of fish and fish oil products conferred protection against cardiovascular disease.[361,362]

Calories and Obesity

Excessive caloric intake from any source (fat, carbohydrate, protein, or alcohol) promotes hyperlipidemia (especially hypertriglyceridemia) in some individuals. Plasma triglyceride levels rise, and levels of high-density lipoprotein fall. The immediate metabolic consequence of excessive calories is an increased substrate for triglyceride synthesis in the liver, with subsequent elevated plasma VLDL triglyceride.[363] Furthermore, overproduction of VLDL triglyceride combined with reduced clearance of VLDL triglyceride from the blood may be responsible in part for the hypertriglyceridemia of obesity. The enlarged adipose tissue cells, because of their lessened sensitivity to the circulating insulin that stimulates lipoprotein lipase, the "clearing factor" enzyme, may have a reduced capacity to remove circulating triglyceride from the plasma.

In hypertriglyceridemic overweight patients, there is usually an associated hypercholesterolemia, partly because of the increased intake of dietary cholesterol and saturated fat that occurs in the obese but also because the VLDL that carries the increased triglyceride content transports cholesterol as well. The lower HDL concentrations apparently reflect the shunting of HDL apoproteins into the VLDL molecule. Moderate reduction of caloric intake in hypertriglyceridemic overweight patients and the subsequent loss of adiposity invariably lead to lower plasma triglyceride levels, often to a normal range. Plasma cholesterol levels concomitantly fall; HDL levels reciprocally rise.[363,364]

Although caloric control is the most important consideration for these hypertriglyceridemic patients, the source of the calories in weight-loss diets is of some importance in the establishment of patterns of food consumption that will be useful when a more ideal weight has been achieved. Many patients have combined hyperlipidemia (i.e., type IIb), and whatever hypercholesterolemia remains after both body weight and plasma triglyceride stabilize at lower levels will require attention in regard to the reduction of dietary cholesterol and saturated fat. Furthermore, the pattern of food intake should then be such that future weight gain will be avoided. The low-fat, high-complex-carbohydrate diet concept can be useful for both the period of weight reduction and the subsequent period of stabilization of body weight.

When excessive dietary cholesterol and fat are combined with excessive calories, a particularly potent hyperlipidemic effect occurs. Such a "holiday" diet occurs in the United States between Thanksgiving and New Year's day. The effects of such dietary excesses were studied in the Tarahumara Indians of Mexico, a people habitually accustomed to a very low fat diet.[365] After a suitable baseline period in which they consumed their typical diet, Tarahumara Indians were given a diet high in cholesterol, fat, and calories. Within 2 weeks, their plasma lipids had increased tremendously: total cholesterol 31 percent, LDL 39 percent, HDL 31 percent, and a plasma triglyceride 18 percent. Body weight gain averaged 7 to 8 lb for each individual. The composite effect of these potent dietary hyperlipidemic factors (fat, cholesterol, calories) was greater than that of any one of them alone.

Carbohydrate

If the total fat content of a hypolipidemic diet is reduced from the current American fat intake of 40 percent of total calories to only 20 percent and if the protein in the diet is kept constant, the difference in caloric intake between a high-fat diet and a low-fat diet must be made up by increasing the carbohydrate content of the diet. Epidemiologic evidence buttresses this basic concept, as populations ingesting a high-carbohydrate diet from complex carbohydrates have low plasma cholesterol levels and a low incidence of coronary disease. Are there harmful effects from a high-carbohydrate diet? It was demonstrated more than 25 years ago that a sudden increase in the amount of dietary carbohydrate in Americans accustomed to a high-fat diet can dramatically increase the plasma triglyceride concentration. After many weeks of the new diet, however, adaptation occurs and the hypertriglyceridemia subsides. If the dietary carbohydrate is gradually increased as fat is reduced, hypertriglyceridemia does not occur. Thus, high dietary carbohydrate need not be regarded as a problem but rather as a caloric replacement for the saturated fat removed from the diet. For example, we recently increased the dietary carbohydrate intake gradually from 45 percent kcal to 65 percent kcal during a 28-day period in eight mildly hypertriglyceridemic subjects. There was a significant fall in the mean plasma cholesterol level, from 232 to 198 mg/dl. The mean plasma triglyceride level remained constant, at 213 to 230 mg/dl.[366]

In the low-fat, high-carbohydrate diet described earlier, the majority of the carbohydrate is in the form of cereals and legumes, not in the form of sucrose or other simple sugars. Americans commonly consume about 20 percent of their total calories, half of their carbohydrate intake, as sucrose or other simple sugars. In the dietary changes being suggested, simple sugars fall to about 10 percent of the total. Sucrose, in large quantities, is hypertriglyceridemic. The primary point is that all simple sugars, including sucrose, are potent promoters of obesity; they are extremely low in bulk and have a high caloric density. Thus, in substituting carbohydrate for fat, a hypolipidemic effect can be expected only to the extent that total caloric intake is not increased and simple sugars are restricted.

Fiber, Saponins, and Antioxidants

Dietary fiber is a broad and nondescript term that includes several carbohydrates thought to be indigestible by the human gut. These include cellulose, hemicellulose, lignin, pectin, and beta glucans. Dietary fiber is found only in plants and is commonly present in unprocessed cereals, legumes, vegetables, and fruits. In ruminant animals, dietary fiber is completely digested by the microbial flora of the rumen; in these animals, fiber provides a major source of energy. In humans, however, dietary fiber contributes little to the caloric content of the diet but promotes satiety through its bulk. The bulk also greatly affects colonic function. A high-fiber diet produces larger stools and a more rapid intestinal transit, factors that may prevent certain diseases of the colon (i.e., diverticulitis, colon cancer).

Interest in the hypolipidemic effects of fiber dates back at least 30 years. Fiber added to semisynthetic diets fed to rats usually has a plasma cholesterol–lowering effect. Feeding fiber, predominantly in an insoluble form such as wheat bran, does not have a cholesterol-lowering effect in humans. Soluble fiber may be different. Large amounts of soluble fiber (17 g/2,000 kcal), such as that contained in oat bran or beans, produced a 20 percent reduction of the plasma total and LDL cholesterol levels.[367] These decreases were, at least in part, a result of concurrent weight loss. Rich sources of soluble fiber include fruits, oats and some other cereals, legumes, and vegetables. One way in which soluble fiber acts to lower cholesterol is by binding bile acids in the gut and preventing their reabsorption. This is the same mechanism used by bile acid–binding resins such as cholestyramine. Soluble fibers also may reduce cholesterol absorption.

A high-fiber diet is certainly an integral part of the dietary concept for the treatment of hyperlipidemia. The consumption of more foods from vegetable sources will automatically mean a higher consumption of both total and soluble fiber. Such foods are bulky and have a lower caloric density, which is helpful for overweight patients. A feeling of satiety occurs from the consumption of high-fiber foods that also are low in calories. If oat bran is consumed in place of bacon and eggs for breakfast, this high-fiber food will also have a beneficial effect indirectly because it has replaced foods high in cholesterol and saturated fat. Finally, plant foods rich in fiber also may contain other cholesterol-lowering substances. One of these substances is a group of compounds called saponins, which in monkeys have a cholesterol-lowering action.[368] Saponins bind cholesterol in the gut lumen and prevent its absorption.

Other dietary factors contained in fruits, vegetables, grains, and beans that may be important in the prevention of the atherogenic process are the antioxidants. The antioxidants may block the oxidation of LDL, which is believed to be central to the atherosclerotic process.[369,370] The antioxidant factors in plant foods include beta carotene, ascorbic acid (vitamin C), and alpha tocopherol (vitamin E). There is little evidence that consuming these vitamins in the form of vitamin supplements has an antiatherogenic effect. The important point is that when dietary fat is reduced, the consumption of fruits, vegetables, and beans is enhanced, which will increase the intake of the desirable antioxidants in a more natural and physiologic fashion.

Plant Sterols (Sitosterol and Sitostanol)

Two margarines containing esterified plant sterols (sitosterol and sitostanol) have recently become commercially available for general use. These products, which can be purchased in most grocery stores, may be useful as adjunctive therapy for hypercholesterolemia, particularly when these margarines are substituted for dietary butter. Consumption of the equivalent of 1 pat of sitosterol or sitostanol margarine three times daily can lower plasma LDL cholesterol concentrations by 10 to 14 percent.[371] The same magnitude of LDL cholesterol-lowering may also be achieved among patients who merely add these margarines to their diet and also in patients who already are being treated with a "statin" drug. The 2 commercially available margarines are Take Control, which contains sitosterol-esters, and Benecol, which contains sitostanol-esters. The mechanism of action involves the inhibition of cholesterol absorption by sitosterol and sitostanol, which are normally poorly absorbed sterols. These margarines, particularly the sitosterol ester margarine, may exacerbate hypercholesterolemia in the rare patient who hyperabsorbs plant sterols as a consequence of the genetic disorder, β-sitosterolemia.

Alcohol

In the past few years, there has been confusion about the relation between alcohol consumption and factors related to coronary heart disease. Alcohol consumption correlates well with higher values of HDL in the blood and reduced mortality from coronary heart disease.[372–375] Because HDL plays a role in "reverse" cholesterol transport, this finding has encouraged some researchers to conclude that drinking ethanol is "good for the heart." From a clinical point of view, the typical patient attending a lipid clinic who is overweight and consumes two or more drinks a day could have a problem directly related to alcohol consumption. Many of these patients are hypertriglyceridemic and have low HDL concentrations.[376] A key aspect of the treatment for hypertriglyceridemia is to reduce alcohol consumption or even stop it completely, as alcohol increases hypertriglyceridemia. Alcohol also has a high caloric content of 140 kcal per drink. Two to three drinks a day can contribute 300 to 400 kcal to an already hypercaloric state, stimulating further the synthesis of triglyceride and VLDL by the liver. We therefore generally suggest that alcohol consumption in hyperlipidemic patients be restricted to no more than two to four drinks per week in order to avoid adverse effects on the plasma lipids and lipoproteins. However, if this amount of alcohol produces hyperlipidemia, the use of alcohol should be completely discontinued. The use of alcohol is clearly precluded in type I and type V patients who have had pancreatitis. If liver disease and hyperlipidemia occur together, alcohol should not be used in any circumstances. Consumption of more than 1–2 alcoholic drinks daily can contribute to hypertension, cardiac arrhythmias (e.g., atrial fibrillation), cardiomyopathy, and other adverse cardiovascular complications.

Although consumption of alcohol in small amounts can be an effective tool for elevating HDL concentrations in some patients, the decision to recommend such treatment must be carefully weighed against the possible risk of excessive alcohol intake. For example, patients who are prone to alcohol abuse may be adversely affected by the suggestion that alcohol promotes good health. Thus, although regular consumption of alcoholic beverages (<1–2 drinks daily) may reduce the risk of atherosclerosis, practitioners must not lose sight of the high prevalence of alcohol abuse and its associated morbidity and mortality. In addition, some patients may also develop the impression that drinking wine or beer every day will somehow alleviate the need for other health promoting behaviors, such as regular exercise and a cholesterol-lowering diet, both of which are much less enticing than alcohol consumption. Hence, it may not be advisable for health care professionals to promote consumption of alcohol as a therapeutic agent.

Protein

Dietary protein has been studied extensively for possible effects on plasma lipid concentrations. These studies have utilized both single protein sources and mixtures of different proteins with range of protein intake from 25 to 150 g per day. No changes in the plasma cholesterol and triglyceride concentrations have resulted from these different amounts of protein, provided that at least the minimum amounts of essential amino acids were ingested. It has been suggested on the basis of animal studies that animal protein (such as casein from milk) is hypercholesterolemic and that vegetable protein (such as soybean protein) has a cholesterol-lowering effect. Well-designed experiments in humans to test the differential effects of casein and soy protein have not been conclusive. However, the rabbit experiments are not completely translatable to humans. Many human studies used formula diets with casein as the sole protein source. Because these diets were also free of cholesterol, plasma lipid levels fell greatly; this suggests that casein is probably not hypercholesterolemic. Although the single-diet concept makes extensive use of proteins from vegetable sources, it does contain casein and is not a vegetarian diet. Thus, the inclusion of more protein from vegetable sources may confer some benefit to hyperlipidemic patients.

Lecithin

This phospholipid derived from soybeans is commonly sold in health food stores and is widely publicized as a popular remedy for hypercholesterolemia. Aside from its high content of linoleic acid, the consumption of lecithin is irrational because this lipid is not absorbed as such from the digestive tract but is hydrolyzed into its constituent fatty acids, glycerol and choline. A higher content of linoleic acid in the diet can therefore be obtained much more inexpensively from a liquid polyunsaturated vegetable oil. There are no practical or theoretical reasons for the discrete use of lecithin, but no harm occurs.

Minerals and Other Vitamins

Assuming that the minimum daily requirements for minerals and vitamins have been met in the diet, there is no information to indicate that additional vitamins and minerals will have any effect on the plasma lipid concentrations. Recent information suggests that the antioxidant vitamins such as vitamin E and vitamin C may be antiatherogenic,[370] but the current evidence showing benefit from administration of these vitamins is limited.[377,377B] Moreover, in 2 studies, ingestion of beta-carotene appeared to increase the risk of lung cancer among smokers and did not reduce the risk of CHD, despite ample epidemiologic evidence that suggested protection against CHD and cancer by carotenoids. These findings underscore the uncertainties about the safety and efficacy of high dose vitamin supplements in disease prevention. The consumption of fruits, vegetables, grains, and beans would enhance the consumption of all vitamins and minerals, as well as flavonoids and other beneficial compounds, and has been shown to reduce the risk of CHD. There is little evidence that adding vitamins as supplements to a low-fat, high-complex-carbohydrate, fruit and vegetable-rich diet would have an additional benefit. One exception is niacin (vitamin B_3), which, when given as a drug in a dose 50 times its requirement as a vitamin, does have a lipid-lowering effect. In this instance, niacin is used as a pharmaceutical preparation, not as a nutrient. Daily ingestion of vitamin E 400 to 800 IU and vitamin C 500 mg is a common practice that is not likely to cause harm and might have cardioprotective benefit, but definitive proof of benefit is currently unavailable.

Coffee and Tea

Because of the enjoyment people derive from drinking coffee, there is great interest in the conflicting reports on the relation between coffee and coronary heart disease. Most of the reports are contradictory. One study from Europe does make some sense in that boiled coffee, in which most of the ingredients that might have an effect on health are extracted into the beverage, is positively associated with increased cholesterol levels and higher incidence of coronary heart disease.[378] Other methods of coffee preparation (instant coffee, percolated coffee, filtered coffee) do not appear to raise cholesterol levels. In a recent U.S. study, only the consumption of 720 ml of filtered caffeinated coffee raised the plasma cholesterol slightly (both LDL and HDL alike), in contrast to no effect from the same amount of decaffeinated coffee.[379] A theoretical reason why larger quantities of coffee may be harmful relates to the caffeine content. Caffeine stimulates the release of epinephrine, which increases FFA concentrations. The production of VLDL and triglyceride would be expected to increase as a consequence. No one has defined precisely what constitutes an excessive intake of coffee. When patients ask, we generally suggest no more than two to four cups per day. Other adverse effects that may be associated with consumption of more than this amount of caffeinated coffee (or other caffeinated beverages) include increased urinary calcium excretion, which might contribute to decreased bone mass and osteoporosis. Whether a patient chooses to drink small amounts of decaffeinated or regular coffee or tea is a matter of personal choice. Tea, by contrast, has not been associated with heart disease. In fact, tea consumption may reduce the risk of coronary heart disease, possibly as a consequence of flavonoids present in black and green teas.

Implementation of the Single-Diet Concept for the Treatment of Hyperlipidemia

Instead of multiple diets, each for a different form of hyperlipidemia, we favor a "single-diet" concept for the treatment of hyperlipidemia. The chemical formulation of the single diet, low in total and saturated fat and cholesterol and high in complex carbohydrates and fiber, is presented in terms of major components, as follows. Of course, the ultimate and optimal objectives in terms of a diet to produce maximal plasma lipid lowering will be achieved in a series of phases that have been fully described in detail, with appropriate menu planning and recipes, in recent publications.[380–382]

Dietary cholesterol is reduced from the usual American intake of 500 mg per day to 100 mg per day. This change will lower LDL cholesterol, which is elevated in types IIa and IIb hyperlipidemia, and also both VLDL and intermediate-density lipoproteins in types IV and III hyperlipidemias, respectively (Table 21-18). In many patients with "diet-induced" IIa or IIb hypercholesterolemia, a reduction of dietary cholesterol to 100 mg per day will lower the plasma lipids to "normal" values (plasma cholesterol level below 220 mg/dl). Frequently, hyperlipidemic patients are also overweight. For overweight patients, the same diet at a hypocaloric level should be prescribed initially until the patient

TABLE 21-18. Dietary Factors in the Causation and Correction of Lipoprotein Abnormalities

Lipoprotein Abnormality	Cause	Dietary Factor Increasing Lipoprotein Synthesis	Dietary Correction
Increased Chylomicrons (types I and V)	Impaired removal	Fat, except for omega-3 fatty acids from fish	Reduction of dietary fat to 5–10 percent of total calories*
Increased VLDL (types IV and IIb) and IDL (type III)	Impaired removal (obesity) and/or increased synthesis	Excessive calories from any source Dietary cholesterol and saturated fat	A hypocaloric 20% fat diet to induce loss of excess adiposity; reduction of dietary cholesterol and saturated fat
Increased LDL (types IIa and IIb)	Increased synthesis and impaired removal	Dietary cholesterol, saturated fat, and total fat	Reduction of dietary cholesterol to 100 mg, saturated fat to 5 percent of total calories, and total fat to 20 percent
Decreased HDL	Utilization of HDL apoproteins in triglyceride-carrying lipoproteins in types I, V, IV, IIb, and III hyperlipidemias	Excessive calories with adiposity	Correction of obesity as noted above

*All overweight hyperlipidemic patients should have the appropriate dietary factor modified as above and should be provided with a hypocaloric diet to help in the attainment of normal body weight. For an insulin-dependent diabetic, appropriate use of insulin may also aid in the correction of the hyperlipidemia. The omega-3 fatty acids from fish may help reduce plasma VLDL and triglyceride levels.

attains optimum weight. At that time, the low-fat, high-complex-carbohydrate diet at a eucaloric level is prescribed.

In patients with genetically determined severe hypercholesterolemia, normal plasma cholesterol levels cannot be achieved by means of diet alone; combined diet plus drug therapy is needed. Restrictions on dietary cholesterol and saturated fat are nevertheless critically important in severe type IIa patients.

Dietary fat content is lowered to 20 percent of total calories compared with the usual American fat intake of 40 percent of total calories. Most of this decrease is in saturated fat, which is reduced to no more than 5 percent of total calories. This change in total fat content and composition has a beneficial effect in all forms of hyperlipidemia for reasons already discussed but especially in type II and types I and V hyperlipidemia (Table 21-18). In the latter two cases, when dietary fat is reduced to a minimum, the chylomicrons present in the blood gradually clear and the plasma triglycerides fall. Plasma cholesterol levels also decline, and HDL and LDL, both very low, rise. This "minimum" of dietary fat varies from patient to patient with hyperchylomicronemia; the exact level necessary for chylomicron clearance can be ascertained only by means of a trial of several diets with a fat content varying from 5 to 20 percent.[383]

In some patients with extreme chylomicronemia who are in danger of acute pancreatitis, a 1 percent fat or fat-free formula diet (protein, glucose, minerals, and vitamins) can be employed to promote maximal chylomicron lowering. Another simple but effective approach is the use of fruit juices for a few days of initial therapy. In both cases, triglyceride levels fall rapidly (Fig. 21-32).

Although the basic problem in types I and V hyperlipidemia is not an excess of dietary cholesterol and the suggested diets need not restrict cholesterol per se, they are lower in cholesterol content because most foods that contain cholesterol are also high in fat. However, shellfish, which are relatively high in cholesterol content, are low in fat content and in saturated fat. Consequently, shellfish and fish can be freely used by patients with types I and V hyperlipidemia.

Omega-3 fatty acids derived from fish may be added to the low-fat diet to achieve a specific hypolipidemic effect beyond what can be obtained from the dietary measures suggested in the single-diet concept. The omega-3 fatty acids from fatty fish, or even fish oil used experimentally, will have a pronounced plasma triglyceride (VLDL)–lowering action in hypertriglyceridemic patients with an exaggerated synthesis of VLDL. The result of giving omega-3 fatty acids to type V patients is illustrated in Fig. 21-31.[356] Polyunsaturated vegetable oil, as is well known, raises triglyceride levels in type V patients, and its use is therefore contraindicated. Fatty fish such as salmon, mackerel, and sardines

FIGURE 21-32. Reduction in chylomicronemia by means of a 1 percent fat formula diet plus insulin replacement in a patient with adult-onset diabetes mellitus and phenotypic type V hyperlipoproteinemia. Note that the fall in chylomicron and VLDL levels is associated with a reciprocal rise in LDL cholesterol. Concentrations of HDL cholesterol also rose (not shown).

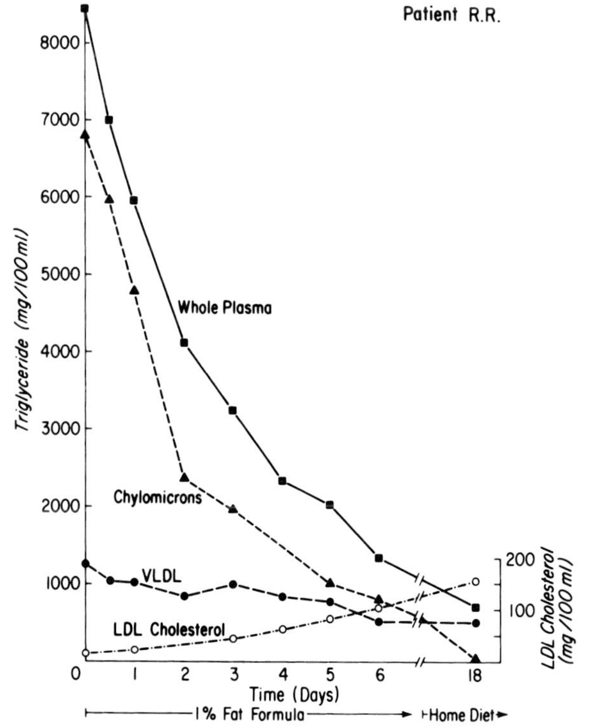

may be particularly effective. Fish oil in doses of 15 g per day or more may also be used in type V patients.

Saturated fat in the diet is reduced greatly to maximize the lowering of LDL in types IIa and IIb. The polyunsaturated fat content remains little changed from the usual American intake of 6 to 8 percent of total calories. Most of the reduction of the total fat from 40 percent of total calories to 20 percent is accomplished by cutting down on foods that are rich in saturated fatty acids.

Of particular importance is the decrease in the HDL cholesterol level that occurs with a low-fat, low cholesterol diet. Populations that eat low-fat diets have been observed to have low HDL cholesterol levels.[384,385] Because these populations have low LDL cholesterol levels and little coronary heart disease, the low HDL cholesterol level is not a risk factor. The physiologic response to a low-fat diet is a 10 to 20 percent decrease in the HDL cholesterol level.[383] Because LDL cholesterol is lowered even more, the LDL to HDL ratio is little changed or even improved. Also, a lower HDL cholesterol level resulting from a low fat, high-complex-carbohydrate diet is different from a genetically low HDL cholesterol level in that the coronary risk is not enhanced.[386]

The Cholesterol–Saturated Fat Index of Foods

The major plasma cholesterol–elevating effects of a given food reside in its content of cholesterol and saturated fat. To understand the contribution of these two factors in a single food item and to compare one food with another, we have computed a cholesterol–saturated fat index (CSI) for selected foods.[387,388] The formula for the CSI is CSI $= (1.01 \times$ g saturated fat$) + (0.05 \times$ mg cholesterol), where the amounts of saturated fat and cholesterol in a given amount of a food item are entered into this equation. The higher the CSI of a food, the greater the hypercholesterolemic and atherogenic effect. This index is a representation of how much a given food will decrease the activity of the LDL receptor and hence raise the level of LDL cholesterol in plasma.

In this context, it is particularly instructive to compare the CSI of fish with that of moderately fatty beef. An 85-g portion of cooked fish contains 51 mg of cholesterol and 0.14 g of saturated fat. This contrasts to 80 mg of cholesterol and 11.3 g of saturated fat in 30 percent fat beef. The CSI for 85 g (3 oz) of fish is 3; that of 85 g of beef is 15. The caloric value of these two portions also differs greatly (71 for fish and 323 for beef). The CSI of cooked chicken and turkey (without the skin) is also lower than that of beef and other red meats. The total fat content is considerably lower. The saturated fat in an 85-g serving is 1.6 g, and the cholesterol is 71 mg. The CSI of poultry is 5. Table 21-19 lists the CSI for various foods. Shellfish have a low CSI because their saturated fat content is extremely low despite the fact that their cholesterol content is 2.5 to 3 times higher than that of fish, poultry, or red meat. Shellfish have a CSI of 3. This means that when one is considering both cholesterol and saturated fat, shellfish, like poultry, is a better choice than even the leanest red meats. Salmon also has a low CSI and is preferred to meat. The CSI of 1,000 foods, as well as information about selection for categories of foods and more than 300 recipes with low CSIs, can be found in *The New American Diet System*.[382]

The *protein* intake is kept at an amount similar to what Americans commonly eat: about 15 percent of total calories. The decrease in fat content is thus offset by a reciprocal increase in dietary *carbohydrate*, ultimately to 65 percent of total calories. This is provided primarily in terms of complex carbohydrate ordinarily associated with protein. Other constituents of the diet are not reduced or are enhanced in terms of nutritional adequacy.

Caloric control is vitally important in overweight patients for decreasing the VLDL of types IIb and IV and the IDL of type III hyperlipidemia and in improving the chylomicron clearance in type V hyperlipidemia (Table 21-18). These overweight patients have elevated plasma triglyceride levels, often with concomitant adult-onset diabetes. Such hyperlipidemias are particularly sensitive to the state of caloric balance. Dietary factors operate indirectly but crucially in supplying the substrate for triglyceride synthesis. Type III hyperlipidemia is rare, and because its dietary treatment is similar to that for type IV, it will not be referred to specifically in the subsequent comments other than to emphasize the extreme importance of weight control.

Reduction of excess body weight is the most important measure for the correction of type IV hyperlipidemia. We stress gradual rather than sudden weight loss so that the weight-loss diet will be balanced in nutrients and will not have untoward effects. For overweight patients, the caloric content of the diet can be reduced to one-third or two-fifths of the patient's caloric requirements. We then expect a gentle weight loss of about 2 lb per week.

The plasma triglyceride and cholesterol response to caloric restriction and weight loss is prompt and dramatic. Within 1 to 2 weeks, the plasma triglyceride and cholesterol levels decrease, and they remain lower as long as weight loss continues. With the achievement of normal weight, the plasma triglyceride level usually is in the normal range. Glucose intolerance and the associated diabetic state may also disappear with the hypertriglyceridemia.

The special case of overweight type IIb patients warrants further comment. After the excessive plasma triglyceride levels are corrected by means of weight loss, such patients will be left with some hypercholesterolemia carried by LDL. Particular attention will have to be directed toward the restriction of dietary cholesterol and fat when the eucaloric diet to maintain weight is initiated.

It should be noted that in some hypertriglyceridemic patients, caloric control and a reduction in serum triglycerides will not be achieved unless dietary carbohydrate is restricted. This reduction in dietary carbohydrate should be accompanied by a decrease in dietary fat.

A Phased Approach to the Dietary Treatment of Hyperlipidemia

A realistic view is that even highly motivated patients have difficulty making abrupt changes in their dietary habits. It may take many months and even years to change patterns of food consumption. Therefore, the changes recommended from the current American diet of most hyperlipidemic patients should be approached in a gradual manner, with each of three phases introducing more changes toward the eating pattern ultimately required for maximal therapy.

The goal of phase I is to modify the customary consumption of foods very high in cholesterol and saturated fat (Table 21-20). This can be accomplished by deleting egg yolk, butterfat, lard, and organ meats from the diet and by using substitute products when possible: soft margarine for butter, vegetable oils and shortening for lard, skim milk for whole milk, and egg whites for whole eggs.

In phase II, a reduction in meat consumption is the goal, with a gradual transition from the presumed American ideal of up to a pound of meat a day to no more than 6 to 8 oz per day (Table 21-

TABLE 21-19. The Cholesterol-Saturated Fat Index (CSI) and Kilocalorie Content of Selected Foods

	CSI*	Calorie, kcal*
Fish, poultry, red meat [3 oz (85 g) cooked]		
Shellfish (oysters, scallops, clams)	3	100
Whitefish (snapper, perch, sole, cod, halibut, etc.)	3	100
Salmon	5	168
Shellfish (shrimp, crab, lobster)	5	85
Poultry, no skin	5	154
Beef, pork and lamb		
10 percent fat (ground sirloin, flank steak)	7	170
15 percent fat (ground extra lean, round steak, pork chop)	9	215
25 percent fat (ground lean, rump roasts)	12	278
30 percent fat (typical ground beef, ground lamb, steaks, ribs, lamb chops, pork sausage, roasts)	15	323
Cheese [1 oz (28 g)]		
Low-fat ricotta, tofu (bean curd), Dorman's Light†, Alpine Lace Free N Lean, Kraft Free Singles	<1	53
Imitation mozzarella†, Hickory Farms Lyte†, Heart Beat Sharp Cheddar†	1	74
Lite-line, part-skim ricotta, Reduced Calories Laughing Cow, lite part-skim mozzarella, Mini Chol (Swedish low fat)†	2	62
Lite n'Lively, Olympia's Low Fat, Green River Part-Skim, Kraft Light Naturals, Light cream cheese, Heidi Ann Low Fat Ched-Style, Lappi, String, part-skim mozzarella	4	73
Cheese spreads (jars), Neufchatel (lower-fat cream cheese), Velveeta, Brie, Swiss, gruyere	6	93
Cheddar, roquefort, jack, American, cream cheese, havarti, feta	8	111
Eggs		
Whites (two)	0	32
Egg substitute (equivalent to two eggs)	0	98
Whole (two)	25	158
Fats (1/4 cup or 4 tablespoons)		
Peanut butter	6	380
Mayonnaise, fat free, cholesterol free	trace	40
Mayonnaise, Light	3	200
Mayonnaise, regular	8	404
Most vegetable oils	7	491
Olive oil	8	486
Soft vegetable margarines	8	405
Soft shortenings	13	464
Bacon grease	20	464
Butter	36	432
Coconut oil, palm oil	37	491
Frozen desserts (1 cup)		
Fruit ices, sorbets	0	255
Nonfat frozen yogurt	trace	224
Sherbet or frozen yogurt (low-fat)	3	249
Ice milk	4	224
Ice cream, 10 percent fat	15	329
Rich ice cream, 12 percent fat	19	480
Specialty ice cream, 18 percent fat	30	580
Milk products (1 cup)		
Skim milk or powdered nonfat	1	85
1 percent milk, buttermilk	2	100
2 percent milk	4	122
Whole milk (3.5 percent fat)	7	149
Cottage cheese, low-fat (2 percent)	4	204
Cottage cheese, regular	8	222
Liquid nondairy creamers: soybean oil	4	326
Liquid nondairy creamers: coconut oil	23	326
Sour cream	36	468
Imitation sour cream (IMO)	40	480

*Averages.

†Cheeses made with skim milk and vegetable oils.

TABLE 21-20. Summary of the Suggested Dietary Changes in the Different Phases of the Diet

Phase I
Avoid foods very high in cholesterol and saturated fat
Delete egg yolk, butterfat, lard, and organ meats
Substitute soft margarine for butter, vegetable oils and shortening for lard, skim milk for whole milk, egg whites for whole eggs
Phase II
Gradually use less meat and more fish, chicken, and turkey
No more than 6–8 oz a day
Use less fat and cheese
Acquire new recipes
Phase III
Eat mainly cereals, legumes, fruits, and vegetables
Use meat as a condiment
Use low-cholesterol cheeses
Save these foods for use only on special occasions:
extra meats, regular cheese, chocolate, candy, and coconut

20). Meat can no longer be the center of the meal, particularly for two or three meals a day. Some ideas for lunch with and without sandwiches have been detailed in sample menus and recipes.[380–382] In addition, in phase II we propose the use of less fat and cheese.

Substitute recipes have been developed to replace recipes that are centered on meat or high-fat dairy products (cream cheese, butter, sour cream, cheese) as the principal ingredients. Because these foods are to be eaten in smaller amounts or even omitted (butterfat), the patient needs to find recipes that use larger amounts of grains, legumes, vegetables, and fruits. Examples of such recipes are included in Refs. 380 through 382.

In phase III, the maximal diet for the treatment of hyperlipidemia is attained (Table 21-20). The cholesterol content of the diet is reduced to 100 mg per day, and saturated fat is lowered to 5 to 6 percent of total calories. Because cholesterol is contained only in foods of animal origin, these changes mean that meat consumption in particular must be further reduced. Meat, fish, and poultry should be used as "condiments" rather than "aliments." With this philosophy, the meat dish will no longer occupy the center of the table. Instead, meat in smaller quantities will spice up dishes based on vegetables, rice, cereal, and legumes, much as Asian, Indian, and Mediterranean cookery has been doing for eons. The total of meat and poultry should average 3 to 4 oz per day, but the use of poultry should be stressed because of its lower content of saturated fat. The use of fish is also preferred. Note the low CSI of fish in Table 21-19, shared also by shellfish, as alluded to subsequently. Because of a low CSI, up to 6 oz of fish can be used in place of meat during phase III of the diet. All fish contain omega-3 fatty acids.

Shellfish are divided into two groups: high-cholesterol shellfish (shrimp, crab, and lobster) and low cholesterol shellfish (oysters, clams, and scallops). Both groups contain omega-3 fatty acids and have a low fat content. Because of these differences, high-cholesterol shellfish are more restricted in the daily diet than are low-cholesterol shellfish, i.e., 3 oz vs. 6 oz per day. The low-cholesterol shellfish contain other sterols (e.g., brassicasterol) that are more analogous to plant sterols. These are poorly absorbed by humans. The use of special low-cholesterol cheeses is an important component of phase III (Table 21-19). The sample menus in Refs. 380 through 382 give some idea about the eating pattern in phase III.

A new eating habit questionnaire, the Diet Habit Survey, can be used to classify the diet into the typical U.S. diet and into phases I, II, and III of the low-fat, high-complex-carbohydrate diet.[389] The Diet Habit Survey is related to plasma cholesterol change, measures eating habits directly, reflects nutrient composition indirectly, is quick to administer, and is inexpensive to analyze. Thus, it is useful as a research questionnaire and helpful in the dietary management of patients with hyperlipidemia and coronary heart disease.

The Chemical Composition of the Low-Fat, High-Complex-Carbohydrate Diet

The American diet contains approximately 400 to 500 mg of cholesterol per day. This is decreased in phase I to 300 mg, in phase II to 200 mg, and in phase III to 100 mg. The fat content decreases from 34 percent of calories in the typical American diet to 30 percent in phase I, 25 percent in phase II, and 20 percent in phase III, with special consideration given to the decrease in saturated fat. To provide sufficient calories to meet body needs, the carbohydrate content should be increased as the fat content is decreased, with emphasis on the use of the fiber-containing complex carbohydrates contained in whole grains, cereal products, and legumes. The carbohydrate content increases from 45 percent of the calories in the American diet to 55 percent in phase I, 60 percent in phase II, and 65 percent in phase III. The bulk or fiber in the diet is enhanced considerably, a feature that induces satiety sooner per unit of calories and helps promote weight loss. The dietary fiber content increases from 18 to 45 g per day.

Predicted Plasma Cholesterol Lowering from the Three Phases of the Low-Fat, High-Complex-Carbohydrate Diet

As has been emphasized, both dietary cholesterol and saturated fat elevate plasma cholesterol levels, whereas monounsaturated and polyunsaturated fats have a mild depressing effect. In stepwise fashion, the cholesterol and saturated fat of each phase of the diet are successively reduced, with phase III providing for the lowest intakes. According to calculations derived from Hegsted and coworkers,[390] phase III of the diet would provide for maximal plasma cholesterol lowering, an estimated average change of 20 percent. Phase II would produce a lowering of 14 percent; and phase I, 7 percent. These plasma cholesterol changes for all phases offer the possibility of improved plasma lipids, depending on the amount of dietary modifications, with phase III as the ultimate goal.

The Use of the Low-Fat, High-Complex-Carbohydrate Diet in Diabetic Patients, Pregnant Patients, Children, and Hypertensive Patients

The approach to diabetic patients who are also hyperlipidemic involves the same dietary considerations for the treatment of the hyperlipidemia. Phase III of the diet has been used successfully in both juvenile-onset and maturity-onset and insulin-dependent and non-insulin-dependent diabetic patients. Clearly involved in this treatment is the appropriate control of carbohydrate as well as lipid metabolism by means of adequate amounts of insulin and weight reduction when the patient is overweight. The great propensity of diabetic patients to atherosclerotic vascular disease makes control of their hyperlipidemia of particular importance. The principles we have outlined can be utilized fully with benefit to the patient.

Pregnancy constitutes a particularly difficult situation, because in most pregnant women there will be a 40 to 50 percent increase in plasma lipids and lipoproteins (chiefly LDL) in physiologic circumstances. A hyperlipidemic patient who becomes pregnant should continue on the same diet recommended previously for the treatment of her hyperlipidemia, supplemented by vitamins and minerals as is usual in pregnancy. In patients with familial hypercholesterolemia, the phase III diet is utilized as before, with some increase in calories to permit the desired weight gain. In type I or V hypertriglyceridemic pregnant patients, there is apt to be a profound augmentation of the usual hyperchylomicronemia, and strict adherence to the 5 to 10 percent fat diet is often necessary to avoid pancreatitis.

The single-diet concept for the treatment of hyperlipidemic children can be applied as for adults, with the exception that a child up to 4 years of age is allowed less cholesterol than an older child. Above age 4 years, no more than 3 oz of meat per day is the goal. Egg yolk, organ meat, and butterfat are eliminated from the diet, even for infants. Dietary iron is supplemented from fortified cereals. Human breast milk or whole cow's milk is recommended before weaning or until the infant eats enough table food to provide adequate calories for growth. This is usually from 1 to 2 years. From that time on, the child should drink skim milk.

For the rare infant with type I hyperlipidemia, the fat content of the usual human breast or cow's milk is much too high. A basic skim milk formula will have to be used to avoid the abdominal pain and episodes of pancreatitis to which these patients are so prone. The main objective of such therapy is the provision of sufficient amounts of essential fatty acids, which can be prescribed separately as canola or soybean oil, to yield at least 2 to 4 percent of the total calories. Such oils will provide both omega-6 and omega-3 fatty acids. In this way much of the fat intake will be from linoleic and linolenic acids, and very little other fat will be taken in. Success in several infants with the type I disorder has been achieved using this dietary approach, resulting in the abolition of episodes of abdominal pain.

Special attention must be given to hypertensive, hyperlipidemic patients for several reasons. First, coronary heart disease and atherosclerotic brain disease are common causes of death in hypertensive patients. Second, some diuretic agents (thiazides) and -adrenergic blocking agents are hyperlipidemic in themselves so that the usual hypertensive patient will have an increase in plasma lipids from the use of these agents alone. Thus, hypertensive individuals who are given thiazides or adrenergic blocking agents should have additional dietary therapy in the form of the single-diet approach. Furthermore, the genetic syndrome of both hypertension and hypertriglyceridemia requires simultaneous treatment of both conditions. Finally, a salt-restriction program can readily be incorporated to provide for the additional treatment of the essential hypertension as this is desired by the physician. The correction of obesity and lessening of alcohol intake may also have blood-pressure-lowering effects. To combine the dietary treatment of hypertension and that of hyperlipidemia in a single diet, a stepwise reduction in salt use is also advocated and incorporated into the different phases.[381]

Interrelations Between Dietary and Pharmaceutical Therapy of Hyperlipidemic States

Although dietary therapy remains the cornerstone in the treatment of hyperlipidemia, many patients require pharmaceutical treatment to attain the therapeutic objectives. In this connection, some patients may believe that once they are started on drug therapy, they no longer need to pay as much attention to their diet. Nothing could be farther from the truth. The two modes of therapy are not mutually exclusive but are complementary. Maximum dietary treatment may lower plasma LDL and total cholesterol as much as 15 to 20 percent. This will continue to be the case when pharmaceutical treatment is added.

The complementary nature of diet and drugs is easily noted during the holiday period from Thanksgiving to New Year's day, when weight gain and additional intake of cholesterol and saturated fat from holiday foods occur. When patients were given a diet high in cholesterol and saturated fat while still maintaining the usual dose of lovastatin, the plasma cholesterol level increased from 246 to 289 mg/dl, a 17.5 percent increase. LDL cholesterol increased 20 percent. When it is considered that dietary cholesterol and saturated fat decrease LDL receptor activity[242] and that lovastatin increases LDL receptor activity,[241] it becomes apparent that a diet high in cholesterol and saturated fat may nullify some of the beneficial effects of lovastatin. Similar responses may occur in patients with type IV or type V hyperlipidemia. Weight gain and a high-fat diet or an increase in carbohydrate intake can nullify the effects of gemfibrozil in maintaining lower plasma triglyceride concentrations. When a patient whose lipid values have previously been under good control with diet and medication has a deterioration in lipid values, it is reasonable to question whether the previous dietary lifestyle changes have been disregarded. In diabetic hypertriglyceridemic patients, the dietary deviations will upset glycemic control as well. When this matter is explained to the patient, he or she is then able to return to the previous excellent dietary lifestyle, with a concomitant decrease in the plasma triglyceride levels and, if the patient is diabetic, better glucose control.

PHARMACEUTICAL AGENTS FOR THE TREATMENT OF HYPERLIPOPROTEINEMIA

The rationale for the treatment of hyperlipoproteinemia is based on the premise that a successful reduction in lipid levels will lead to slowing of the rate of progression of atherosclerosis or, potentially, a reversal of this process with a subsequent reduction in cardiovascular morbidity and mortality. A substantial body of evidence now supports the view that reductions in the plasma concentrations of LDL cholesterol and, possibly, concurrent decreases in Lp(a) and increases in HDL cholesterol, are associated with a reduction in coronary morbidity and mortality. The results of older studies using drugs with modest cholesterol-lowering efficacy demonstrated small decreases in the risk of CHD.[391,392] In other studies of patients with pre-existing CHD, changes in the severity of coronary artery stenosis (quantified angiographically) were used as a surrogate endpoint. Such studies showed that small, but significant, differences in rates of progression or regression of lesions could be achieved by markedly lowering LDL cholesterol concentrations.[104,105,393,394] Although the measured changes in lumen diameter in these studies were unlikely to have direct hemodynamic significance, these small differences corresponded to marked reductions in the risk of clinical events. This paradox has been attributed to other important consequences of cholesterol-lowering, such as improved endothelial function and increased plaque stability.

The most valuable data have come from several large clinical

TABLE 21-21. Characteristics of the 5 Recent Randomized, Placebo-Controlled Primary and Secondary Prevention "Megatrials" Using Statin Drugs

Trial	Statin	Number of Subjects
4S	Simvastatin	4444
WOSCOPS	Pravastatin	6595
CARE	Pravastatin	4159
LIPID	Pravastatin	9014
AFCAPS	Lovastatin	6605
	TOTAL	30,817

4S = Scandinavian Simvastatin Survival Study,[395] WOSCOPS = West of Scotland Coronary Prevention Study,[398] CARE = Cholesterol and Recurrent Events Trial,[396] LIPID = Long Term Intervention with Pravastatin in Ischemic Heart Disease,[397] AFCAPS = Air Force/Texas Coronary Atherosclerosis Prevention Study.[399]

trials that have been completed during the last 6 to 7 years, all of which used statin drugs. The collective results from these studies have demonstrated consistent reductions in the risk of fatal and nonfatal myocardial infarction, revascularization procedures, stroke, and (in most of the studies) total mortality (Table 21-21).[395–399] The cardioprotective benefit from cholesterol-lowering in these studies has been verified in both men and women, younger and older subjects, and in the setting of primary (prior to diagnosis of CHD) or secondary (after diagnosis of CHD) prevention. The relationship between CHD risk and LDL cholesterol-lowering suggests that the risk of CHD is reduced proportionately to the LDL cholesterol concentration down to a level at least as low as 90 mg/dl (Fig. 21-33), without convincing evidence of a threshold effect above this level. The results of these clinical trials provide a solid foundation for current recommendations for aggressive treatment of hypercholesterolemia, especially in patients with multiple CHD risk factors, diabetes, or known CHD.

The results from the recent VA HIT trial suggested that raising low HDL cholesterol concentrations by 6 percent (without affecting LDL cholesterol levels) with gemfibrozil in men with CAD could reduce the risk of CHD events (CHD death, nonfatal myocardial infarction, and stroke) by 24 percent.[400] These results are confounded, however, by a concurrent 31 percent decrease in the mean plasma triglyceride concentration. Thus, although the results of statistical analyses have suggested that HDL-raising in this study was the best predictor of event reduction, the intricate physiological intertwining of HDL and triglyceride metabolism prevents solid conclusions about the efficacy of HDL-raising in this study. Another outstanding question about this study is whether treatment with statins, niacin, or other fibrates instead of gemfibrozil may have improved the clinical outcome.

Treatment of patients with severe hypertriglyceridemia is aimed at the prevention of abdominal pain and pancreatitis (associated with plasma triglyceride concentrations greater than 1,000 to 2,000 mg/dl), as well as the long-term risk of atherosclerosis. Unfortunately, data from clinical intervention trials are still too limited to define and verify the utility of treatment guidelines.

Because hyperlipoproteinemia is a lifelong disorder, the decision to begin drug therapy should be made only after satisfactory exclusion of secondary factors and after an adequate trial of diet has failed to achieve satisfactory lipid levels. When drugs are prescribed to treat hyperlipoproteinemia, it is worthwhile to emphasize to patients the need for continued dietary therapy. The overall success of treatment will be maximized when this twofold approach is employed, and also will allow the use of minimum dosages of cholesterol-lowering drugs. A limited number of drugs are available, and their clinical indications will be reviewed in this section. Several reviews have been published recently.[401]

Bile Acid Sequestrants

Three products are currently available: cholestyramine (Questran, Questran Light, and Lo-Cholest) and colestipol (Colestid), and colesevelam (WelChol). They are high-molecular-weight polymers to which anionic bile acids are ionically bound in exchange for chloride ions. Colesevelam is poly(allylamine hydrochloride) cross-linked with epichlorohydrin and alkylated with 1-bromodecane and (6-bromohexyl)-trimethyl-ammonium bromide. These agents are not absorbed, and their activities are based entirely on sequestration of bile acids in the intestinal lumen. The bile acid–resin complex is excreted in the stools.

Mechanism of Action

The primary action of cholestyramine, colesevelam and colestipol is to bind bile acids in the intestinal lumen. This, in turn, results in an interruption of the enterohepatic circulation of bile acids and a markedly increased excretion of these steroids in the feces. The size of the bile acid pool is decreased, and this reduction stimulates increased hepatic synthesis of bile acids from cholesterol. Depletion of the hepatic pool of cholesterol results in two compensatory changes: an increase in cholesterol biosynthesis and an increase in the number of specific high-affinity receptors for LDL on the hepatocyte membrane.[402,403] The increased number of hepatic LDL receptors stimulates the rate of LDL catabolism from plasma and thus lowers the concentration of this

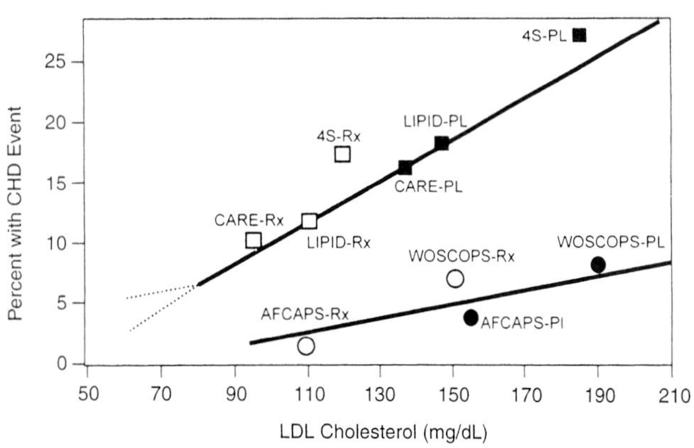

FIGURE 21-33. The relationship between reductions in plasma LDL cholesterol concentrations and 5-year risk of CHD events in 5 large clinical trials. Primary prevention trials (circles): WOSCOPS = West of Scotland Coronary Prevention Study,[398] AFCAPS = Air Force/Texas Coronary Atherosclerosis Prevention Study.[399] Secondary prevention trials: 4S = Scandinavian Simvastatin Survival Study,[395] LIPID = Long Term Intervention with Pravastatin in Ischemic Heart Disease,[397] CARE = Cholesterol and Recurrent Events Trial.[396] PL = placebo treatment; Rx = statin treatment. (*Reproduced from Illingworth.*[401])

lipoprotein. The selective stimulation of hepatic LDL receptors explains why concentrations of LDL are selectively reduced during therapy with a bile acid sequestrant. Bile acid sequestrants are ineffective in patients with homozygous familial hypercholesterolemia who lack the ability to make more high-affinity LDL receptors. The increase in hepatic cholesterol biosynthesis that occurs during therapy with a bile acid sequestrant may be paralleled by an increase in hepatic VLDL production and often results in a slight increase in plasma concentrations of triglyceride and VLDL.

Side Effects

The most common side effects of cholestyramine, colesevelam and colestipol consist of changes in bowel function, including constipation, bloating, epigastric fullness, nausea, and flatulence. Colesevelam may be less likely to cause these side effects. Constipation, which is the most frequent side effect, may be relieved with stool softeners, but the gritty nature of these medications may exacerbate hemorrhoids. Patients frequently complain that these medications are bulky, and some find the sandy or gritty texture of cholestyramine and colestipol unpleasant. Rare side effects have included intestinal obstruction and the development of hyperchloremic acidosis. Decreased absorption of fat-soluble vitamins and folic acid may occur with prolonged high doses of these medications, and oral supplementation with these vitamins may be advisable in children. Because of their avidity for anionic molecules, cholestyramine and colestipol may interfere with the absorption of other drugs, and it is advisable to take other medications 1 h before or 4 h after taking the resin. Colesevelam may cause fewer drug interactions than cholestyramine and colestipol. Such effects have been reported with digoxin, thyroxine, warfarin, pravastatin, and thiazides and may occur with any anionic drug. Biochemical side effects include a modest increase in plasma triglyceride concentrations in many patients; mild increases in alkaline phosphatase and transaminases have also been reported.

Indications and Dosage

Cholestyramine is available in 9-g packets (Questran), which contain 4 g of cholestyramine and 5 g of orange flavoring, and in cans that contain 378 g. Two other preparations of this drug (Questran Lite and Lo-Cholest) contain the same 4 g of cholestyramine but 1 g of orange or strawberry flavoring, which is sweetened with Nutrasweet. The formulation of the latter 2 products seems to be associated with improved tolerability for many patients. Cholestyramine is available in 5-g packets and 210-g cans. Colestipol is available in 5-g packets and 500-g bottles; this formulation contains no additives. The cholesterol-lowering effects of 4 g of cholestyramine appear to be equivalent to those obtained with 5 g of colestipol. Both medications must be mixed with water or juice and are taken in two (or occasionally three) divided doses with or just after meals. Colesevelam is available as 625 mg tablets usually given at a dosage of 2 tablets three times daily or 3 tablets twice daily with meals. It can be given at a dosage of 6 tablets once daily with a meal. Colestipol also is available as one gram tablets that may improve the ease of use for some patients, but still cause the same gastrointestinal side-effects and require the patient to ingest plenty of water. The total daily dose of cholestyramine is 8 to 24 g a day, and the daily dose of colestipol is 10 to 30 g; however, the benefits of increasing the dose above 16 g of cholestyramine or 20 g of colestipol per day must be balanced against the high incidence of gastrointestinal side effects and poorer patient compliance at these higher doses.

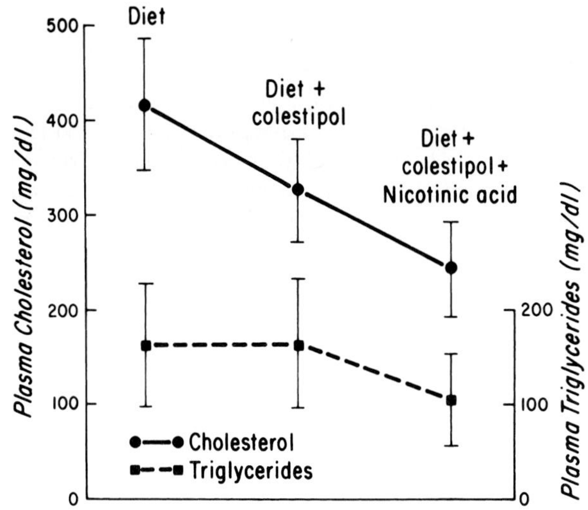

FIGURE 21-34. The effects of sequential therapy with diet, colestipol, and colestipol plus nicotinic acid on the plasma concentrations of cholesterol and triglycerides in 13 patients with heterozygous familial hypercholesterolemia. (*Redrawn from Illingworth et al.*[180])

As was discussed in the section on Hypercholesterolemia, bile acid sequestrants are among the drugs of choice for patients with primary elevations in the concentrations of LDL cholesterol who do not have concurrent hypertriglyceridemia. These agents have no place in the treatment of other hyperlipidemias and may in fact aggravate the hypertriglyceridemia seen in patients with type III hyperlipoproteinemia and patients with chylomicronemia. The response to therapy in patients with primary hypercholesterolemia is variable, but 15 to 25 percent reductions in concentrations of LDL cholesterol may be achieved with 16 g a day of cholestyramine, or 20 g of colestipol or 3.8 g of colesevelam.[173] The addition of nicotinic acid to this regimen may result in further decrements of 20 to 25 percent, and this combination remains one of the most effective for patients with severe type IIa hypercholesterolemia (Table 21-13). This is illustrated in Fig. 21-34. Combined drug therapy with a bile acid sequestrant and probucol[404] or gemfibrozil is sometimes effective in patients who are unable to take nicotinic acid. Combined drug therapy with an inhibitor of HMG CoA reductase plus a bile acid sequestrant is the most consistently effective regimen available, resulting in a greater than 50 percent reduction in the concentrations of LDL cholesterol in patients with familial hypercholesterolemia (Table 21-13).

Cholestyramine was the drug used in the Lipid Research Clinic's Primary Prevention Trial.[391] The results from this large clinical trial have established the long-term safety and efficacy of bile acid sequestrants and have provided conclusive proof that reduction of LDL cholesterol reduces morbidity and mortality from cardiovascular disease. Because they are not absorbed, bile acid sequestrants are the only drugs safe for use in the treatment of children with heterozygous familial hypercholesterolemia; if clinically indicated, these drugs can also be used for the treatment of patients with severe type II hypercholesterolemia during pregnancy.

Nicotinic Acid

The lipid-lowering action of nicotinic acid, or niacin, has been recognized for 30 years[405] and appears to be unrelated to its action as a vitamin coenzyme in intermediary metabolism. It is well absorbed from the gastrointestinal tract and is excreted in the urine.

Mechanism of Action

The precise mechanism of action of nicotinic acid at the cellular level that is responsible for reducing plasma concentrations of VLDL and LDL is not known. Considerable evidence, however, points to an effect in reducing the hepatic synthesis of VLDL,[406] which in turn leads to a reduction in LDL synthesis. Factors responsible for the decreased hepatic production of VLDL include inhibition of lipolysis with a concomitant decrease in FFA levels in plasma, decreased hepatic esterification of triglycerides, and possible effects on the hepatic production of apoprotein B.

Side Effects

The main side effects of nicotinic acid involve the skin and gastrointestinal tract. Cutaneous flushing occurs 15 min to 2 h after a patient takes the medication, but the duration and magnitude usually diminish with prolonged therapy and can be minimized by starting at a low dose and always taking the medication after the ingestion of food. The flushing appears to be mediated by prostaglandins and can be reduced by means of the concurrent administration of 150 to 325 mg of aspirin.[407] Nausea, abdominal discomfort, and diarrhea constitute the most common gastrointestinal side effects, and the drug is contraindicated in patients with active liver disease, peptic ulcer disease, or hyperuricemia. Less common side effects include itching, development of rash, hyperpigmentation of the skin with development of acanthosis nigricans, and blurred vision due to macular edema; blurred vision is not common but will necessitate the discontinuation of therapy. Other side effects have included activation of peptic ulcer disease and exacerbation of both hyperuricemia and diabetes. Laboratory disturbances noted in patients on nicotinic acid are more common with higher doses (>3 g per day) and include increases in alkaline phosphatase and transaminases and elevation of uric acid and glucose. The incidence of elevated transaminases and alkaline phosphatase is higher in patients receiving time-release formulations of niacin,[408] and patients should be advised not to change from regular to sustained-release formulations of this drug because of the increased risk of hepatotoxicity at the same daily dose.[409] Liver function tests and uric acid should be monitored during the initiation of nicotinic acid and should be checked periodically once an appropriate dosage regimen has been established.

Indications and Dosage

Nicotinic acid is available in tablets containing 100, 250, or 500 mg and in time-release preparations containing 125, 250, or 500 mg. The authors do not recommend the older time-release forms of nicotinic acid, which increase the risk of abnormal liver function. An intermediate-release preparation of niacin, that is marketed as Niaspan, appears to be well tolerated and efficacious in doses ranging from 500 to 2,000 mg taken once daily in the evening. Niacinamide, which is widely available in health food stores, has no effect on lipid or lipoprotein concentrations. Therapy with nicotinic acid is best initiated with a low-dose regimen (e.g., 100 to 250 mg once to three times daily with or just after meals), with the dose then being gradually increased at 7- to 14-day intervals to a total dose of 3 g per day. Lipid values as well as tests of liver function, blood glucose, and uric acid should be assessed at this point; if a satisfactory reduction in plasma lipids has not been achieved, the dose should be increased a further 1.5 g per day. Periodic increases in the dose up to a maximum of 7.5 to 8 g per day may be administered, but the increased hypolipidemic effect of such higher doses must be balanced against the higher incidence of side effects noted at doses above 4.5 g per day. Nicotinic acid is useful in the treatment of all hyperlipoproteinemias except those due to familial LPL deficiency. The drug is used chiefly in the treatment of primary hypercholesterolemia; when used by itself, it results in 15 to 30 percent decreases in concentrations of LDL cholesterol with a concurrent 10 to 20 percent rise in HDL levels.[173] In addition to reducing LDL concentrations, nicotinic acid at a dose of 4 g per day has been reported to reduce Lp(a) concentrations by 30 percent.[325] Forty to eighty percent reductions in the concentrations of plasma triglycerides may be obtained with nicotinic acid, and this drug is effective in reducing both VLDL and LDL levels in patients with phenotypic type IIb hyperlipidemia. Nicotinic acid is a second-choice drug for patients with type III hyperlipoproteinemia (clofibrate is the drug of choice) and is a good second choice drug for patients with severe hypertriglyceridemia (type V phenotype), in whom gemfibrozil is currently the drug of choice. As was discussed previously, combined treatment with nicotinic acid and a bile acid sequestrant is an effective therapy for patients with severe hypercholesterolemia and LDL concentrations greater than 300 mg/dl. Although combination therapy with nicotinic acid and an HMG CoA reductase inhibitor (e.g., lovastatin) may also be an effective regimen, the use of these two drugs together cannot be generally recommended because of an increased risk of myopathy.[410]

HMG CoA Reductase Inhibitors

The recent development of specific competitive inhibitors of HMG CoA reductase, the rate-limiting enzyme in cholesterol biosynthesis, has provided an important therapeutic approach to the treatment of hypercholesterolemia and combined hyperlipidemia.[411] Lovastatin, the first agent in this class to become available, was approved for prescription use in the United States in 1987, and five other agents in this class, simvastatin, pravastatin, fluvastatin, atorvastatin, and cerivastatin have become available during the last decade. In addition, Colestin, which is a partially purified fungal preparation containing low doses of lovastatin, is available over-the-counter without a prescription.

Mechanism of Action

The structures of the currently available HMG CoA reductase inhibitors, which are also known as "statins," are shown in Fig. 21-35. Lovastatin is made by a soil fungus (*Aspergillus terrius*), and simvastatin is a methylated derivative of this drug. Pravastatin is produced by microbial transformation of mevastatin. Lovastatin and simvastatin are administered as prodrugs (lactones), and conversion to the open acid occurs after gastrointestinal absorption. In contrast, pravastatin is administered orally as the open acid formulation. Fluvastatin, atorvastatin, and cerivastatin are synthetic drugs, as shown in Fig. 21-35. Studies in animals and in tissue culture on the relative rates of uptake of these drugs by the liver and by peripheral tissues are contradictory,[411B,412,413] and further work is needed to assess whether the greater hydrophilicity of pravastatin compared with other statins results in lower rates of uptake of this drug in peripheral tissues. At the present time, no definitive clinical advantage of pravastatin resulting from potential hydrophilic "tissue selectivity" activity has been demonstrated.[414] At clinically effective doses, all statins are primarily taken up by the liver, where they exert their lipid-lowering effects by inhibiting hepatic HMG CoA reductase. Lovastatin and simvastatin reduce the 24-h rates of excretion of mevalonic acid (the product of HMG CoA reductase) by 30 to 40 percent at doses of 40 mg per day in patients with heterozygous familial hypercholesterolemia.[415,416]

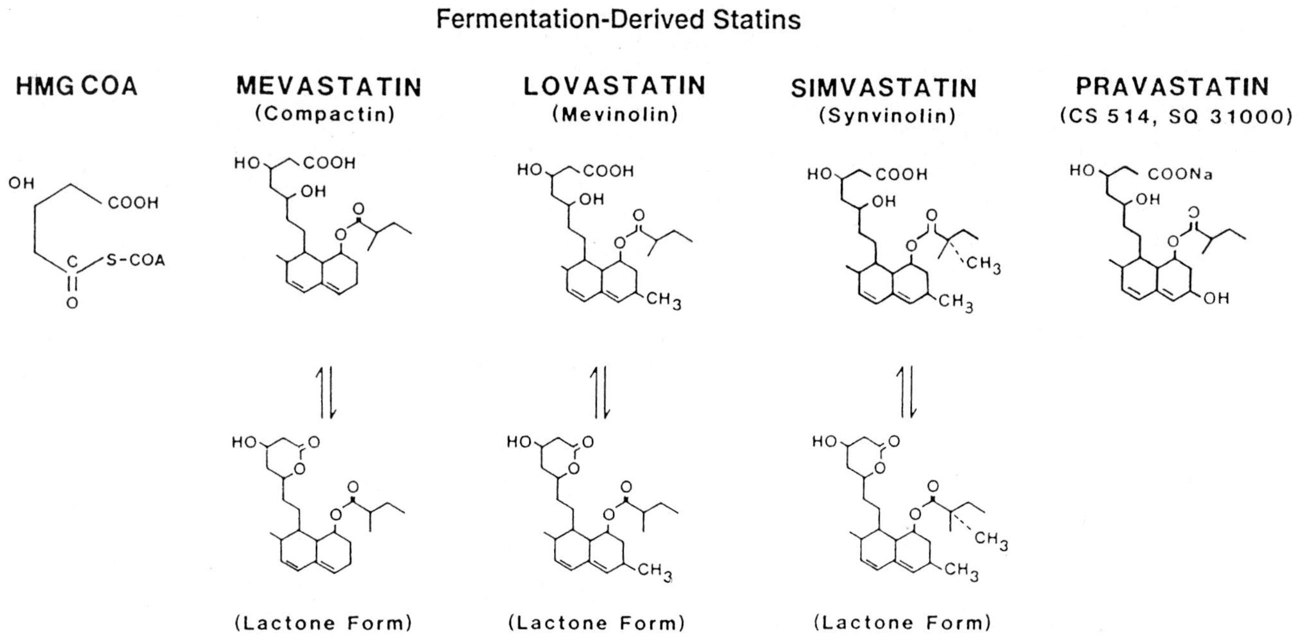

FIGURE 21-35. Structure of HMG CoA and the HMG CoA reductase inhibitors ("statins") that are available for prescription use. Mevastatin is not used as a therapeutic agent, but is a precursor for pravastatin. The 3 newest statins are synthetic, whereas the older drugs are purified or modified fungal metabolites.

Other statins have similar effects when given at therapeutically equivalent doses. Reduced formation of mevalonic acid leads to a corresponding decrease in hepatic cholesterol biosynthesis and a reduction in the cellular pool of cholesterol. This leads to a compensatory increase in the number of high-affinity LDL receptors expressed on the cell surface, and this in turn stimulates an increase in receptor-mediated catabolism of VLDL remnant particles and LDL.[411] Hepatic synthesis of VLDL and LDL may be concurrently reduced in response to drug therapy with HMG CoA reductase inhibitors,[417] which contributes to modest triglyceride-lowering efficacy that is associated with all available drugs in this class.

Side Effects

HMG CoA reductase inhibitors have been well tolerated, and side effects in both short-term and more extended (up to 14 years) use have been fairly uncommon.[418–420] The reported side effects include changes in bowel function, headache, nausea, fatigue, insomnia, and skin rashes. Less common but more severe side effects include myopathy and hepatitis, with elevated liver enzymes. The development of myopathy does not appear to be due to an unusual susceptibility to the inhibition of mevalonic acid production by lovastatin,[421] and the etiologic factors responsible for this remain to be better defined. Fortunately, myopathy is uncommon in patients treated with statins as monotherapy and the risk appears to be dose-dependent and may be somewhat proportional to the amount of LDL lowering. The incidence of myopathy is, however, increased in patients treated with statins who also receive cyclosporine, nicotinic acid, gemfibrozil, antifungal agents (e.g., ketoconazole), or erythromycin.[410] Until proved otherwise, these drug interactions should be regarded as a class effect, but recently released data suggest the cerivastatin may have an increased proclivity to cause rhabdomyolysis when it is given in combination with fibric acid derivatives. Pravastatin, which is not metabolized by the cytochrome P450 isoform 3A4, may be associated with a slightly lower risk of rhabdomyolysis in patients taking cyclosporine. All of the HMG CoA reductase inhibitors should be used very cautiously in combination with these other drugs; combined therapy with gemfibrozil or niacin cannot be recommended for general use,[422] despite the popularity of such combinations among some physicians. HMG CoA reductase inhibitors do not exert any adverse effects on steroid hormone biosynthesis.[423] Biochemical tests to monitor the safety of these drugs should be assessed at 6- to 8-week intervals for the first 9 or 12 months of therapy, and at 3- to 6-month intervals thereafter. These should include assessment of liver function in addition to cholesterol-lowering efficacy. Measurements of serum creatine kinase concentrations are not routinely indicated, but should be done in patients who experience symptoms of muscle discomfort or weakness. Although initial studies in dogs indicated that HMG CoA reductase inhibitors occasionally cause cataracts when administered at doses 30 to 60 times the maximal human dose, subsequent studies in patients treated with these drugs for periods of 3 to 9 years have failed to document any increased frequency of lenticular opacities. Accordingly, the FDA does not currently require slit lamp examinations during the treatment of patients with this class of drugs. Lovastatin, simvastatin, and their metabolites are excreted primarily in bile, and toxic levels can easily be reached if these drugs are given to patients with cholestasis or other disorders in which hepatic excretion and metabolism are significantly compromised. Renal excretion and hepatic metabolism appear to be important mechanisms for the elimination of pravastatin.[424]

Indications and Dosage

Lovastatin is available in 10-, 20-, and 40-mg tablets (maximum dose 80 mg daily), whereas simvastatin (maximum dose 80 mg daily) and pravastatin (maximum dose 40 mg daily) are available in 10-, 20-, and 40-mg tablets. Fluvastatin is available as 20 and 40 mg capsules (maximum dose 80 mg daily), atorvastatin is available as 10, 20, and 40 mg tablets (maximal dose 80 mg daily), and cerivastatin is available as 0.2, 0.3, and 0.4 mg tablets. The cholesterol-lowering effects of lovastatin, pravastatin, simvastatin, fluvastatin, atorvastatin, and cerivastatin have been extensively investigated, and all six drugs have been found to be effective in

TABLE 21-22. Relationship Between Various Dosages of HMG CoA Reductase Inhibitors and Percent Reduction in Plasma LDL Cholesterol Concentrations

	LDL-C Percent Change					
Dose (mg/d)	Lovastatin (Mevacor)	Simvastatin (Zocor)	Pravastatin (Pravachol)	Fluvastatin (Lescol)	Atorvastatin (Lipitor)	Cerivastatin (Baycol)
0.3	—	—	—	—	—	−29
0.4	—	—	—	—	—	−34
0.8	—	—	—	—	—	−42
10	−18	−28	−19		−35	
20	−26	−34	−26	−18	−44	
40	−33	−41	−32	−27	−50	
80	−39	−48		−34	−56	

patients with heterozygous familial hypercholesterolemia, familial combined hyperlipidemia, and moderate primary hypercholesterolemia.[171,148,425] The comparative efficacy of these drugs is presented in Table 21-22. Based on these data, it appears that on a milligram basis, lovastatin and pravastatin are equipotent, whereas simvastatin is twice as potent, fluvastatin is about half as potent, atorvastatin is 4 times as potent, and cerivastatin is about 100 times more potent. Single-drug therapy with statins has been associated with a 10 to 55 percent dose-dependent decrease in plasma triglycerides and an overall tendency for HDL cholesterol to increase by 2 to 15 percent.[171,411] The results of several recent studies of the comparative efficacy of higher doses of simvastatin and atorvastatin have demonstrated that simvastatin may raise HDL and apo A-I levels significantly more than equivalent doses of atorvastatin. Although statin-induced increases in HDL cholesterol and apo A-I may contribute to reduction of clinical events, the significance of this difference between the two drugs is unknown.

In light of the current safety and efficacy data, HMG CoA reductase inhibitors are often the drugs of first choice for the treatment of adult patients with primary hypercholesterolemia and are also effective in the treatment of many patients with combined hyperlipidemia and type III hyperlipidemia. They may also be preferable in selected patients with secondary causes of hyperlipidemia, such as nephrotic syndrome, and in many patients with diabetes, particularly those who do not have marked hypertriglyceridemia. The usual starting dose of lovastatin is 20 mg once daily in the evening, but at doses above this level, the drug is more effective in a twice-daily regimen. In contrast, the other statins appear to be equally effective when given as single doses in the evening. It is usually recommended that simvastatin be taken with dinner, whereas the other statins may be taken at bedtime. In humans, cholesterol biosynthesis increases at night, and this may explain the greater efficacy of HMG CoA reductase inhibitors when given as a single dose in the evening, compared with the same dose given in the morning.[426,427] HMG CoA reductase inhibitors do not influence plasma concentrations of Lp(a)[323,324] and should not be used for the treatment of severe hypertriglyceridemia.[428]

The cholesterol-lowering effects of HMG CoA reductase inhibitors can be enhanced by using these drugs in combination with bile acid sequestrants. The use of low doses of both drugs may be a particularly efficacious and cost-effective means of treating moderately severe hypercholesterolemia[429] (Fig. 21-36). As illustrated in Table 21-13, the combination of lovastatin, colestipol, and nicotinic acid has been shown to reduce LDL concentrations by 60 to 70 percent in patients with heterozygous familial hypercholesterolemia. Certain drug combinations cannot be recommended because of a lack of efficacy or the potential for increased toxicity. These include therapy with an HMG CoA reductase inhibitor and gemfibrozil.[430,431] Although the latter combination may have potential therapeutic appeal in patients with combined hyperlipidemia, it does not exert a significant further LDL-lowering effect compared with lovastatin alone in patients with heterozygous familial hypercholesterolemia and is associated with an increased risk of myopathy.[422,430,431] Treatment with statins plus fish oil is an excellent option for treatment of combined hyperlipidemia.

FIGURE 21-36. Changes in concentrations of low-density lipoprotein cholesterol in 10 patients with heterozygous familial hypercholesterolemia during sequential therapy with diet, lovastatin (80 mg per day), and lovastatin plus colestipol (15 to 20 g per day). (*Reproduced from Illingworth*[181] *with permission.*)

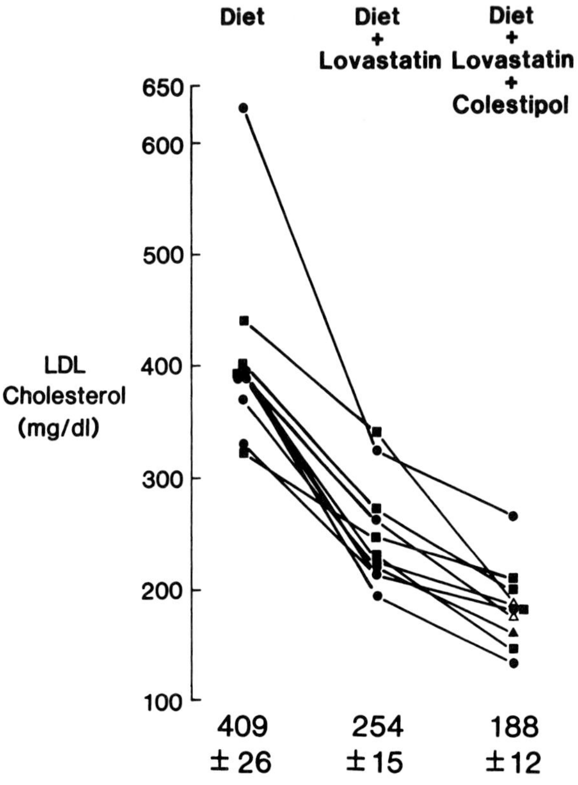

Probucol

Probucol (Lorelco) is no longer available in the USA, but was a second-line drug for the treatment of primary hypercholesterolemia. Less than 10 percent of probucol is absorbed in the intestinal tract, and the hydrophobic nature of this drug contributes to its prolonged storage in adipose tissue. When used as a single agent, probucol has been shown to reduce plasma LDL cholesterol concentrations 8 to 15 percent and concurrently to lower HDL levels up to 25 percent.[176]

Mechanism of Action

The mechanism by which probucol influences plasma lipoprotein levels has not been completely defined.[176] The drug has been shown to increase the fractional rate of clearance of LDL[432] and to increase biliary secretion of cholesterol. The increased removal of LDL may be due to an increase in nonreceptor-mediated pathways, and this would explain the modest efficacy of probucol in patients with homozygous familial hypercholesterolemia who lack LDL receptors. The decrease in HDL levels seen with probucol is due to a decrease in apoprotein A-I synthesis, a decrease in lipoprotein lipase, and an increase in cholesterol ester transfer protein activity.[433,434]

Side Effects

Probucol is well tolerated and appears to have minimal side effects; in order of decreasing frequency, these include diarrhea (10 percent of patients), flatulence, abdominal pain, and nausea and vomiting.[176] Less common side effects have included hyperhidrosis, fetid sweat, and angioneurotic edema. With the possible exception of mild eosinophilia, no consistent biochemical abnormalities have been reported. Probucol causes prolongation of the QT interval, and although no arrhythmias have been attributed to its use in humans, the drug should probably be regarded as contraindicated in patients with electrocardiographic (ECG) findings suggestive of ventricular irritability.[176] Probucol is stored in adipose tissue, and blood levels fall slowly after therapy is discontinued. For this reason, the drug should not be given to women who plan to have children in the near future or to children.

Indications and Dosage

Probucol is available in 500-mg tablets. The recommended dose is 500 mg twice daily with the morning and evening meals. Probucol should be regarded as a second-line drug for the treatment of primary hypercholesterolemia, and 8 to 15 percent reductions in plasma concentrations of LDL can be expected. The drug concurrently lowers HDL levels up to 25 percent and may adversely affect the ratio of LDL to HDL. Probucol has been shown to cause regression of tendon xanthomas in patients with familial hypercholesterolemia[178] and may exert other potentially beneficial effects on lipoproteins, including inhibition of LDL oxidation[91] and an increase in reverse cholesterol transfer.[434] Probucol was used in one placebo-controlled secondary prevention trial, but no benefit was seen in prevention of progression of femoral atherosclerosis. Probucol is ineffective in the treatment of hypertriglyceridemia.

Clofibrate

Clofibrate (Atromid-S) is the ethyl ester of *p*-chlorophenoxyisobutyrate and is well absorbed from the gastrointestinal tract. In plasma, the ester bond is hydrolyzed and the free acid is transported bound to albumin. The plasma half-life is 12 to 15 h. The drug is excreted in the urine, and its clearance is decreased in patients with chronic renal failure.

Mechanism of Action

The mechanism of action of clofibrate at the molecular level is not known. The most important effect, however, is to increase the rate of metabolism of triglyceride-rich lipoproteins as a result of increases in the activity of lipoprotein lipase.[215] Small and variable reductions in the synthesis and/or secretion of hepatic VLDL into plasma may also occur; these may be mediated by a number of mechanisms, including decreases in the hepatic synthesis of cholesterol and fatty acids and enhanced biliary excretion of cholesterol.

Side Effects

Clofibrate is generally well tolerated and has a low incidence of side effects. Nausea, abdominal discomfort, and in men decreased libido and breast tenderness are the most commonly reported. Less common side effects include dry skin, alopecia, and the development of a myositis-like syndrome with muscle tenderness and increased creatine phosphokinase (CPK/CK).[215] The latter syndrome is more likely to occur in patients with hypoalbuminemia or impaired renal function. Rarely, ventricular arrhythmias and a lupus-like syndrome have been associated with clofibrate therapy. Biochemical abnormalities have included a decrease in alkaline phosphatase and transient increases in transaminases. Two long-term clinical trials, The Coronary Drug Research Project[435] and the WHO Primary Prevention Trial,[436] have provided data concerning the long-term safety and efficacy of clofibrate. In both studies there was an increased incidence of gallstones, whereas in the WHO study clofibrate-treated patients had a higher noncardiac mortality rate than did control subjects. This was mainly attributable to an increased incidence of malignant neoplasms and complications resulting from cholecystectomy. The increased incidence of noncardiac deaths did not persist after discontinuation of clofibrate therapy.[437] The increased incidence of noncardiac deaths in the WHO trial has led to a marked reduction in the use of clofibrate in the treatment of hyperlipidemia. Drug interactions may occur between clofibrate and other albumin-bound drugs, most notably warfarin (Coumadin).

Indications and Dosage

Clofibrate is available in 500-mg capsules; the usual dose is 1 g twice daily. Clofibrate is one of the drugs of choice for patients with type III hyperlipoproteinemia and should be regarded as a second choice drug for patients with severe hypertriglyceridemia (type V phenotype) who are unable to take gemfibrozil or nicotinic acid. In patients with type III hyperlipoproteinemia, clofibrate therapy frequently reduces cholesterol and triglyceride concentrations 50 to 80 percent and leads to the regression of xanthomas. When given to patients with primary hypertriglyceridemia, clofibrate lowers VLDL cholesterol and plasma triglyceride concentrations up to 50 percent but frequently results in increased concentrations of LDL cholesterol. The drug is generally ineffective in patients with primary hypercholesterolemia and has no role in the treatment of disorders associated with increased plasma concentrations of LDL cholesterol. The drug is contraindicated in patients with chronic renal disease or the nephrotic syndrome; use in this population frequently results in the development of muscle tenderness and a myositis-like syndrome.

Gemfibrozil

Gemfibrozil (Lopid) is a fibric acid derivative that is structurally related to clofibrate. The drug is well absorbed from the intestinal tract and is transported, in part, bound to albumin. Although gemfibrozil undergoes enterohepatic circulation, the primary route of excretion is in urine.[215]

Mechanism of Action

The triglyceride-lowering effect of gemfibrozil results primarily from a reduction in VLDL triglyceride and, to a lesser extent, apoprotein B synthesis with a concurrent increase in the rate of removal of triglyceride-rich lipoproteins from plasma.[215] The latter effect is believed to result from an increased activity of lipoprotein lipase, but the ability of gemfibrozil to inhibit VLDL triglyceride production appears to be much greater than that seen with clofibrate. Although gemfibrozil has also been shown to reduce the rate of synthesis of LDL apoprotein B,[438] this may simply be a reflection of a reduced rate of synthesis of VLDL, the precursor for LDL, in plasma.

Side Effects

Gemfibrozil is well tolerated in most patients; the most frequent side effects are changes in bowel function, abdominal pain, diarrhea, and occasionally nausea. These effects occur in 3 to 5 percent of patients and may necessitate the discontinuation of gemfibrozil. Less common side effects include muscle tenderness and skin rash. Biochemical changes are uncommon; they include eosinophilia, decreases in the plasma concentration of alkaline phosphatase, and occasionally rises in transaminases. Like clofibrate, gemfibrozil potentiates the effects of oral anticoagulants and may increase biliary lithogenicity, with a predicted long-term increase in the incidence of gallstones.

Indications and Dosage

Gemfibrozil is available in 600-mg tablets; the usual dose is 600 mg twice daily. Gemfibrozil has been shown to reduce the incidence of coronary artery disease in middle-aged men with primary hyperlipidemia,[392] and in this study, the greatest benefit was noted in patients with combined hyperlipidemia. In these patients, gemfibrozil reduced concentrations of total cholesterol and triglycerides as well as the level of LDL cholesterol and resulted in an increase in the levels of HDL cholesterol.[392] Debate continues on which factor was most influential in reducing coronary artery disease in this study, although it is noteworthy that the beneficial effects of gemfibrozil were limited to patients without coronary artery disease at the outset and that no benefit was observed in patients with preexistent coronary artery disease. In contrast, the results of the VA HIT trial demonstrated reduced risk of CHD events in men with low plasma HDL cholesterol concentrations who were treated with gemfibrozil, as discussed earlier. Gemfibrozil and fenofibrate (and alternatively niacin) are the drugs of choice for patients with severe hypertriglyceridemia (type V phenotype), when given in combination with a very low fat diet. In the authors' experience, gemfibrozil and fenofibrate are superior to clofibrate in treating this disorder. Reductions of 75 to 90 percent in plasma concentrations of triglycerides may be achieved in patients with severe hypertriglyceridemia, which can be effective in reducing the risk of pancreatitis, and possibly the risk of atherosclerosis. Gemfibrozil and fenofibrate should be regarded as the potential first choice drugs for patients with type III hyperlipoproteinemia, but are second choice agents for treatment of elevated concentrations of LDL cholesterol.[215] In patients with combined elevations of LDL cholesterol and triglycerides, particularly those unable to take nicotinic acid, combined drug therapy with gemfibrozil or fenofibrate and a bile acid sequestrant is often quite effective. In the authors' experience, 25 to 45 percent reductions in concentrations of LDL cholesterol can be achieved in some patients on this regimen, whereas in other patients no additional LDL-lowering effect is seen with the addition of gemfibrozil. Fenofibrate appears to have greater LDL cholesterol-lowering efficacy compared to gemfibrozil. Concentrations of HDL cholesterol increase 10 to 20 percent during therapy with gemfibrozil and fenofibrate, and even greater increases may be seen in patients with severe hypertriglyceridemia. As was discussed previously, combination drug therapy with fibric acid derivatives and HMG CoA reductase inhibitors may be associated with an increased risk of myopathy and therefore is not recommended or approved by the Food and Drug Administration.

Fenofibrate

Fenofibrate (Tricor) is another useful fibric acid derivative that has the same mechanisms of action as gemfibrozil, but seems to have somewhat better LDL cholesterol-lowering efficacy. The usual dosage is 200 mg taken once daily, but lower dosages (e.g., 67 mg tablets) may be indicated in some patients with increased risk of drug toxicity or adverse side-effects.

Miscellaneous Agents

A number of other drugs have been used in the past for treatment of hyperlipidemia, but now are only of historical interest and are not recommended for general use. Such agents include neomycin, which increased fecal excretion of cholesterol and neutral steroids[439,440]; dextrothyroxine (the optical isomer of L-thyroxine), which lowered LDL cholesterol concentrations by 10 to 15 percent at the expense of causing mild hyperthyroidism[441]; anabolic steroids (e.g., oxandrolone) for treatment of hypertriglyceridemia[442]; and progestational agents (e.g., norethindrone acetate) for treatment of severe hypertriglyceridemia.[443] The drug appears to increase postheparin lipolytic activity and results in an enhanced clearance of triglyceride-rich lipoproteins from plasma. Norethindrone acetate may be useful in women patients with severe hypertriglyceridemia who fail to respond to other therapeutic regimens.

Estrogens

Concentrations of LDL cholesterol are known to increase in women after menopause; the magnitude of this increase is greatest in women with preexistent hypercholesterolemia (e.g., heterozygous familial hypercholesterolemia). Estrogen deficiency has also been associated with the phenotypic expression of type III hyperlipidemia in women homozygous for apoprotein E-2. In both of these situations, estrogen therapy significantly reduces the magnitude of hyperlipidemia and may minimize the need for concurrent hypolipidemic drug therapy. Although estrogens increase concentrations of HDL cholesterol, they also stimulate VLDL synthesis and may lead to severe hypertriglyceridemia in patients with preexisting hypertriglyceridemia. The use of transdermal preparations of estradiol minimizes the tendency to exacerbate hypertriglyceridemia and can be effective in women in whom hormone replacement therapy is advocated for other reasons (e.g., prevention of osteoporosis). Estrogens have no role as lipid-modifying agents in men for a variety of reasons, including the risk of feminization. Moreover, the results of the Coronary Drug Project showed that administration of 2.5-mg and 5-mg doses of conjugated estrogens (Premarin) to men was associated with increased cardiovascular morbidity, which led to premature termination of this arm of the study.[444] Although the results of epidemiologic studies have suggested that postmenopausal estrogen replacement may reduce the risk of CHD by 50 percent, recent results from the heart and estrogen/progesterone replacement study (HERS) showed an increased risk of CHD during the first 1 to 2 years and no net benefit after 4.1 years of treatment among women with preexisting CAD.[445] Moreover, the results from a recent angiographic regression trial indicate no protective benefit of estrogen replacement compared to placebo.[446]

Orlistat

Orlistat (Xenical) is an intestinal lipase inhibitor that causes malabsorption of about 30 percent of ingested fat and has recently been marketed as a drug to promote weight loss. The high cost of the drug (greater than $100 per month) and lack of coverage by most insurance plans have limited the use of this drug in clinical practice. Although the average net weight loss after 6 to 12 months of treatment compared to placebo was only about 4 percent of initial body weight, the results of a recent report suggest that orlistat may have some utility as an adjunctive lipid lowering agent in selected patients.[447] Among subjects who lost more than 10 percent of their initial body weight, LDL cholesterol concentrations decreased by an additional 9 to 10 percent compared to placebo treatment with comparable weight loss. Thus, orlistat may have modest LDL lowering benefit that may be attributable to the malabsorptive properties of the drug.

Future Advances

Fibric Acid Derivatives

Three fibric acid derivatives—clofibrate, gemfibrozil, and fenofibrate—have been approved for clinical use in the United States, and several other derivatives are currently undergoing clinical trials or have been approved for general use in Europe. These drugs, which include bezafibrate and ciprofibrate, are more effective than either clofibrate or gemfibrozil in reducing LDL concentrations in patients with primary hypercholesterolemia.[215] Fenofibrate and ciprofibrate may be the most effective, and both may reduce LDL cholesterol concentrations by 20 to 25 percent in patients with heterozygous familial hypercholesterolemia (Table 21-23). The cholesterol-lowering effects of these drugs appear to be mediated by an enhanced rate of receptor-mediated clearance of LDL from plasma.[215]

Nicotinic Acid Derivatives

Several derivatives of nicotinic acid have been developed in an attempt to maintain the lipid-modifying effects of nicotinic acid with a concurrent reduction in the side effect profile, particularly cutaneous flushing. Several esters of nicotinic acid, including xanthinol nicotinate and niceritrol, have been evaluated, and both preparations show a hypolipidemic profile similar to that of the parent compound, but with fewer side effects.[448] Etofibrate is an interesting derivative of nicotinic acid in which the nicotinic acid moiety is esterified to clofibrate. Etofibrate has been shown to reduce plasma triglyceride and cholesterol concentrations in patients with hypercholesterolemia and enhance catabolism of LDL via the LDL-receptor pathway.[449] Perhaps the most interesting of the nicotinic acid derivatives is acipimox, which at a dose of 250 mg three times daily has been shown to reduce LDL cholesterol concentrations by 11 percent, with a concurrent 20 percent increase in concentrations of HDL cholesterol.[450] In contrast to nicotinic acid, which exacerbates hyperglycemia, acipimox may exert a glucose-lowering effect, making this agent potentially useful for the treatment of lipid disorders in diabetics.

Agents that Reduce Cholesterol Biosynthesis

The clinical utility and safety of HMG CoA reductase inhibitors in the treatment of hypercholesterolemia has been well demonstrated, as described previously. Six drugs in this class—lovastatin, simvastatin, pravastatin, fluvastatin, atorvastatin, and cerivastatin—have been approved by regulatory authorities for use in different countries. These drugs are effective in doses ranging from 0.2 to 80 mg per day. In view of the availablity of six efficacious and well-tolerated drugs in this class, newer agents may be unlikely to provide any additional benefit beyond those provided by the available drugs.

The clinical efficacy of the HMG CoA reductase inhibitors indicates that inhibition of other enzymes in the cholesterol biosynthetic pathway may have clinical utility in the treatment of

TABLE 21-23. Comparative Efficacy of Fibric Acid Derivatives in Decreasing LDL Cholesterol Concentrations in Patients with Heterozygous Familial Hypercholesterolemia

Drug	Dose, g/day	Initial LDL Cholesterol, mg/dl	No. Patients Studied	Percent Decrease in LDL Cholesterol	References
Clofibrate	2.0	286	10	4.6	Levy et al., 1972[475]
Gemfibrozil	1.2	309	9	9.6	Meinertz, 1987[476]
Bezafibrate	0.6	313	12	28.0	Eisenberg et al., 1987[477]
Bezafibrate	0.6	262	18	18.3	Curtis et al., 1988[184]
Ciprofibrate	0.1	293	10	24.0	Illingworth et al., 1982[478]
Ciprofibrate	0.1	336	20	19.5	Rouffy et al., 1985[479]
Ciprofibrate	0.2	336	20	27.0	Rouffy et al., 1985[479]
Fenofibrate	0.3	309	9	24.0	Weisweiler et al., 1984[480]
Fenofibrate	0.3	309	21	25.0	Rouffy et al., 1985[479]
Fenofibrate	0.4	309	21	31.0	Rouffy et al., 1985[479]

hypercholesterolemia. Inhibition of late steps in sterol biosynthesis has resulted in the accumulation of lipid-soluble precursors in tissues and has been associated with the development of cataracts and icthyosis. Inhibition of squalene synthase is a particularly attractive therapeutic target, as this enzyme represents the first committed step in cholesterol biosynthesis, and the substrate for this enzyme—farnesyl pyrophosphate—can be metabolized to other water-soluble products which would not be expected to accumulate and lead to toxicity. Three structurally related fungal metabolites that are potent inhibitors of squalene synthase have been identified, and the structure of these compounds resembles that of presqualene pyrophosphate. The compounds identified have been named either "Zaragozic Acids"[451] or "Squalestatin,"[452] which have similar chemical structures. They are effective in inhibiting squalene synthase in nanomolar concentrations. These agents are a new class of fungal metabolites that inhibit cholesterol biosynthesis, but their toxicity may limit their utility as cholesterol-lowering agents in humans.

Inhibitors of Acyl Coenzyme A Cholesterol Acyltransferase

The enzyme acyl coenzyme A cholesterol acyltransferase (ACAT) catalyzes the esterification of cholesterol and is present in intestinal mucosal cells, liver, and monocytes and macrophages. A number of inhibitors of this enzyme have been synthesized,[453] and these agents exert cholesterol-lowering effects in cholesterol-fed animals. Their potential as lipid-lowering agents in humans is based on their ability to reduce cholesterol esterification in the small intestine, reducing cholesterol absorption, and potentially to influence cholesterol esterification in the liver, with a concurrent reduction in VLDL production. At the present time, ACAT inhibitors remain investigational and may not be effective as cholesterol-lowering agents in humans.[454] The potential adverse effects of ACAT inhibitors, including impairment of cholesterol esterification in steroid hormone–producing tissues, remain to be better defined. Thus, the therapeutic potential of ACAT inhibitors in humans may be limited.

MTP Inhibitors

Inhibitors of MTP have the potential to block the absorption of dietary fat and cholesterol, and have been tested in animal models, but their utility and safety as lipid-lowering agents in humans remains to be demonstrated.

Inhibitors of Cholesterol Absorption

Ezetimibe (SCH-58235) is a 2-azetidinone member of a new class of inhibitors of cholesterol absorption. It blocks absorption of cholesterol, but not bile acids, by unknown mechanisms. The results of phase II studies indicated that ezetimibe reduces LDL cholesterol concentrations by 15 to 18 percent at doses of 5 and 10 mg once daily compared to placebo. Phase III studies of ezetimibe as monotherapy and in combination with statins are underway.

THE SURGICAL TREATMENT OF HYPERLIPOPROTEINEMIA

Although surgery is rarely, if ever, indicated at the present time for the treatment of hyperlipidemia, a variety of surgical procedures have been performed in the past on patients with familial hypercholesterolemia in an attempt to reduce plasma concentrations of total and LDL cholesterol. The distal ileal bypass operation was the most widely used surgical procedure for the treatment of severe hypercholesterolemia but is less effective than combined drug therapy in lowering LDL cholesterol concentrations, and may cause serious late complications such as renal failure and hepatic failure. Thus, this surgical procedure is not recommended. Gastric bypass surgery is an effective tool for inducing permanent dramatic weight loss in patients with a BMI greater than 40 kg/m^2. Patients with severe hypercholesterolemia who undergo this procedure for treatment of obesity are likely to experience marked decreases in LDL cholesterol concentrations in addition to substantial weight loss.

A variety of surgical procedures have been performed in patients with homozygous familial hypercholesterolemia in an attempt to reduce their markedly elevated LDL cholesterol concentrations. Distal ileal bypass surgery and total biliary diversion do not work in these patients because of compensatory increases in cholesterol biosynthesis that nullify the increased excretion of bile acid.[187] Portacaval shunt surgery has been shown to be effective in some patients,[455] but the 25 to 40 percent decrease in LDL cholesterol concentrations achieved after this procedure still leaves these patients markedly hypercholesterolemic. Liver transplantation has been successful in two patients.[194,195] By providing a transplanted liver that normally expresses LDL receptors, this procedure is physiologically attractive, but suffers from the significant adverse sequella associated with chronic immunosuppression.

TREATMENT OF SPECIAL PATIENT POPULATIONS

The criteria for the diagnosis of hyperlipoproteinemia in both adults and children were discussed earlier in this chapter. In the year 2000, there is very little controversy about the benefits of lipid-lowering drug therapy in a variety of patient populations such as men versus women and younger versus older subjects. The safety of the statin drugs, in particular, has been excellent. The benefits of treatment have included decreased risk of fatal and nonfatal myocardial infarction, decreased risk of revascularization procedures, reduced risk of stroke, and decreased risk of total mortality in some studies. This section describes treatment of some special patient populations.

Hyperlipidemia in Women

Because most earlier primary and secondary intervention trials of diet or drug treatment of hyperlipidemia focused on middle-aged men, proof of benefit from treatment of hyperlipidemia in women was not clearly documented until the last 8 years. With the exception of patients with major genetic lipid disorders such as familial hypercholesterolemia, men typically develop coronary artery disease in their fifties and sixties, whereas women are more often affected in their late sixties and seventies, when they are postmenopausal.[456] In women who do not receive estrogen replacement therapy, the postmenopausal period is associated with a decrease in LDL-receptor activity and a rise in the plasma concentrations of LDL cholesterol.[457] Although some investigators have questioned whether high concentrations of LDL cholesterol represent risk factors in women,[458] data from the Honolulu Heart Study and several other epidemiologic studies have indicated that women have the same risk factors for coronary artery disease that men have, including elevated plasma concentrations of total and LDL cholesterol, reduced concentrations of HDL cholesterol, and hypertriglyceridemia.[459,460] Despite the fact that women develop coronary artery disease at a later age than do men, the absolute number of men and women who die from coronary heart disease (CHD) is quite similar, and CHD represents the number one cause of death among American women.[459] Thus, female gender appears to only delay the onset of CHD rather than conferring absolute protection against CHD. Indeed, aggressive lipid lowering with combination drug treatment in patients with heterozygous familial hypercholesterolemia was associated with greater degrees of angiographic regression in women than was observed in men.[393] The results from multiple clinical trials (4S, CARE, AFCAPS/TexCaps, LIPID) have demonstrated that women and men achieve the same cardioprotective benefit from lipid-lowering.[395–397,399]

The decision to use lipid-lowering drugs aimed at the primary prevention of coronary artery disease in women must take into account a number of factors, of which a family history of atherosclerosis and the presence of other risk factors [e.g., low concentrations of HDL, increased levels of Lp(a), concurrent presence of diabetes] are the most important. With the exception of women with heterozygous familial hypercholesterolemia, it may be reasonable to postpone drug therapy until the postreproductive years. Even in women with heterozygous familial hypercholesterolemia who have LDL cholesterol values below 220 mg/dl, there is usually little urgency to commence drug therapy during adolescence or in the early twenties, but there also is no reason to delay treatment in young adults, unless pregnancy is being attempted. Among women who are planning to become pregnant, the use of systemically acting drugs should be avoided. Aggressive measures to reduce concentrations of atherogenic lipoproteins are indicated in women who have developed premature coronary artery disease, in whom the goal of therapy should be to reduce LDL concentrations to under 100 mg/dl.

Hyperlipidemia in Older Patients

Coronary artery disease remains the leading cause of mortality in men and women over age 65; the prevalence of hypercholesterolemia and coronary artery disease is also highest in this age group.[461] In the Honolulu Heart Program, the incidence of coronary artery disease was twofold higher in subjects age 65 to 75 years old whose total cholesterol concentrations exceeded 240 mg/dl compared with participants whose values were under 190 mg/dl, but the risk of CHD in both groups was substantially greater than the risk in younger subjects at any level of cholesterol.[462] The results from recent clinical trials have shown comparable cardioprotective benefit in subjects up to age 70 years at entry into the study compared to younger subjects. Thus, older patients who are in relatively good health should not be excluded from testing and possible therapy for hyperlipidemia. If moderate dietary changes fail to produce the desired goals of LDL reduction, the risk of drug therapy must be weighed carefully against the expected benefits. Drug therapy should be reserved for patients in whom the expected potential benefit outweighs the potential side effects and increased medical costs.[461] In our Lipid Disorders Clinic, we rely heavily on family history and the personal wishes of the patient in deciding which patients should be treated with lipid-lowering medications. The NCEP guidelines provide a broad framework for cutpoints above which medications could be considered after satisfactory exclusion of potentially exacerbating secondary factors. Side effects associated with bile acid sequestrant therapy and nicotinic acid may be more commonly observed in older patients, and for this reason, the HMG CoA reductase inhibitors are preferred as the initial therapeutic agents. In many older patients, 10 or 20 mg per day of lovastatin, or equivalent doses of other statins, will achieve the desired result. It has been the policy of the authors not to discontinue hypolipidemic drug therapy in patients with genetic lipid disorders on the basis of increasing age unless another life-limiting illness is diagnosed. For older patients who have evidence of coronary or peripheral vascular disease and who concurrently have hypercholesterolemia, clinical benefits from lipid-lowering drug therapy can be seen in as short a time as 3 to 6 months, related in part to improved endothelial function and decreased myocardial ischemia, which can be manifested as decreased angina and possibly improved functional status. Hence, an aggressive approach to treatment of older patients with increased risk of CHD can be justified, particularly if it can be accomplished without adversely affecting the quality of life.[105]

Hyperlipidemia in Children

Criteria for the diagnosis of hypercholesterolemia in children have been formulated by the Pediatric Expert Panel of the National Cholesterol Education Program,[111] and there is uniform agreement that once the secondary causes of hyperlipidemia have been excluded, dietary therapy is the cornerstone of treatment in this patient population. As discussed previously, the cutpoints for drug therapy in children with heterozygous familial hypercholesterolemia may be too aggressive. In deciding which children should be treated with lipid-lowering medications, the familial occurrence of CAD prior to age 30 years is a strong indication for initiating drug therapy before the age of 18 to 20 years. At the present time, the bile acid sequestrants (cholestyramine and colestipol) are recommended for initial treatment, based on their proven efficacy and safety.[463] Depending on the age of the child and the magnitude of hypercholesterolemia, one or two (rarely, up to four) packets or scoops daily of a bile acid sequestrant may be used. Supplements of folic acid and fat-soluble vitamins are advisable in children who are maintained on long-term therapy with these drugs. Insufficient data are available concerning the efficacy and long-term safety of HMG CoA reductase inhibitors or fibrates to recommend their widespread use in children with heterozygous familial hypercholesterolemia, but safety and efficacy of lovastatin at doses of 10 to 40 mg daily for 48 weeks.[464] Referral to a medical center specializing in lipid disorders is recommended for pediatric patients in whom drug therapy is being considered and is mandatory for the effective management of the rare child with homozygous familial hypercholesterolemia.

Hyperlipidemia in Patients with Diabetes

It has been recommended that patients with type 2 diabetes or longstanding type 1 diabetes be treated as if they have coronary artery disease within the NCEP guidelines. This recommendation is based on the observation that 20 percent or more of type 2 diabetic patients may have occult CAD at the time of diagnosis of diabetes. Moreover, the risk of CAD events in diabetic patients who are not known to have CHD is increased two- to four-fold to a level that equals the risk of events in nondiabetic subjects who are known to have CAD. Thus, it has been recommended to lower

101. Betteridge DJ, Dodson PM, Durrington PN: Management of hyperlipidemia. Guidelines of the British Hyperlipidemia Association. *Postgrad Med J* 69:359, 1993.
102. Basinki A, Frank JW, Naylor CC, Rachlas MM: Detection and management of asymptomatic hypercholesterolemia: A policy document by the Toronto Working Group on Cholesterol Policy. Toronto, Ontario Ministry of Health, 1989.
103. Grundy SM: Multifactorial etiology of hypercholesterolemia: Implications for prevention of coronary heart disease. *Arterioscler Thromb* 11:1619, 1991.
104. Brown G, Albers JJ, Fisher LD, Schaefer SM, Lin JT, et al: Regression of coronary artery disease as a result of intensive lipid-lowering therapy in men with high levels of apolipoprotein B. *N Engl J Med* 323:1289, 1990.
105. Cashin-Hemphill L, Mack WJ, Pagoda JM, SanMarco ME, Azen SP, Blankenhorn DH: Beneficial effects of colestipol niacin on coronary atherosclerosis: A four-year follow-up. *JAMA* 264:3013, 1990.
106. Grundy SM, Vega GL: Two different views of the relationship of hypertriglyceridemia to coronary artery disease: Implications for treatment. *Arch Intern Med* 152:28, 1992.
107. Hulley SB, Avins AL: Asymptomatic hypertriglyceridemia: Insufficient evidence to treat. *Br Med J* 304:395, 1992.
108. National Institutes of Health Consensus Conference: Treatment of hypertriglyceridemia. *JAMA* 251:1196, 1984.
109. National Institutes of Health Consensus Conference: Triglycerides, high density lipoprotein and coronary artery disease. *JAMA* 269:505, 1993.
110. Austin MA: Plasma triglyceride and coronary heart disease. *Arterioscler Thromb* 11:2, 1991.
111. The Expert Panel: Report of the Expert Panel on blood cholesterol levels in children and adolescents. *Pediatrics* 89(Suppl 2):525, 1992.
112. Connor WE, Cerquiera MT, Connor RW, Wallace RB, Malinow MR, Casdorph HR: The plasma lipids, lipoproteins and diet of the Tarahumara Indians of Mexico. *Am J Clin Nutr* 31:1131, 1978.
113. Connor SL, Connor WE, Sexton G, Calvin L, Bacon S: The effects of age, body weight and family relationships on plasma lipoproteins and lipids in men, women and children of randomly selected families. *Circulation* 65:1290, 1982.
114. Grundy SM, Vega GL, Bilheimer DW: Kinetic mechanism determining variability in low density lipoprotein levels and rise with age. *Arteriosclerosis* 5:623, 1985.
115. Brunzell JB, Chait A: Lipoprotein pathophysiology and treatment, in Rifkin H, Porte D Jr (eds): *Diabetes Mellitus: Theory and Practice*, 4th ed. New York, Elsevier, 1990, pp 756–767.
116. Purnell JQ, Marcovina SM, Hokansen JE, et al: Levels of lipoprotein(a), apoprotein B, and lipoprotein cholesterol distribution in IDDM: Results from follow-up in the diabetes control and complications trial. Diabetes 44:1218, 1995.
117. Curtiss LK, Witztum JL: Plasma apolipoproteins AI, AII, B, CI and E are glucosylated in hyperglycemic diabetic subjects. *Diabetes* 34:452, 1985.
118. Duell PB, Oram JF, Bierman EL: Nonenzymatic glycosylation of HDL resulting in inhibition of high-affinity binding to cultured human fibroblasts. *Diabetes* 39:1257, 1990.
119. Duell PB, Oram JF, Bierman EL: Nonenzymatic glycosylation of HDL and impaired HDL-receptor-mediated cholesterol efflux. *Diabetes* 40:377, 1991.
120. Glueck C, Lang J, Tracy T, Spers J: High prevalence of hypothyroidism in patients with hyperlipoproteinemia. *Clin Chim Acta* 201:113, 1991.
121. Ball MJ, Griffiths D, Thorogood M: Asymptomatic hypothyroidism in hypercholesterolemic patients. *J R Soc Med* 84:527, 1991.
122. Illingworth DR, McClung MR, Connor WE, Alaupovic P: Familial hypercholesterolemia and primary hypothyroidism: Coexistence of both disorders in a young woman with severe hypercholesterolemia. *Clin Endocrinol (Oxf)* 14:145, 1981.
123. Chait A, Bierman EL, Albers JJ: Regulatory role of triiodothyronine in the degradation of low density lipoprotein by cultured human skin fibroblasts. *J Clin Endocrinol Metab* 48:887, 1979.
124. Lewis B: *The Hyperlipidemias: Clinical and Laboratory Practise*. Oxford, Blackwell, 1976, p 292.
125. Wu J, Zhu YH, Patel SB: Cyclosporin-induced dyslipoproteinemia is associated with selective activation of SREBP-2. *Am J Physiol* 277(6 Pt 1):E1087, 1999.
126. Golper TA, Illingworth DR, Morris CD, Bennett WM: Lovastatin in the treatment of multifactorial hyperlipidemia associated with proteinuria. *Am J Kidney Dis* 13:312, 1989.
127. Grunfeld C, Pang M, Doerrler W, Shigenaga JK, Jensen P, Feingold KR: Lipids, lipoproteins, triglyceride clearance, and cytokines in human immunodeficiency virus infection and the acquired immunodeficiency syndrome. *J Clin Endocrinol Metab* 74:1045, 1992.
128. Pett SL, Milliken S: Current review of the metabolic and endocrine disturbances in human immunodeficiency virus infection. *Curr Opin Endocrinol Diabetes* 7:96, 2000.
129. Carr A, Samaras K, Thorisdottir A, Kaufmann GR, Chisholm DJ, Cooper DA: Diagnosis, prediction, and natural course of HIV-1 protease-inhibitor-associated lipodystrophy, hyperlipidemia, and diabetes mellitus: A cohort study. *Lancet* 353:2093, 1999.
130. DeLiberti JH, McMurry MP, Connor WE, Alaupovic P: Hypercholesterolemia associated with alpha-I antitrypsin deficiency and hepatitis: Lipoprotein and apoprotein determinations, sterol balance and treatment. *Am J Med Sci* 288:81, 1984.
131. Mehler PS, Lezotte D, Eckel R: Lipid levels in anorexia nervosa. *Int J Eating Disorders* 24:217, 1998.
132. Ettinger WH, Hazzard WR: Prednisone increases very low density lipoprotein and high density lipoprotein in healthy men. *Metabolism* 36:1055, 1988.
133. Shaboury AM, Hayes TM: Hyperlipidemia in asthmatic patients receiving long term steroid therapy. *Br Med J* 1:85, 1973.
134. Molitch ME, Oill P, Odell WD: Massive hyperlipidemia during estrogen therapy. *JAMA* 227:522, 1974.
135. Bershad S, Rubenstein A, Paterniti JR Jr, et al: Changes in plasma lipids and lipoproteins during isotretinoin therapy for acne. *N Engl J Med* 313:981, 1985.
136. Katz RA, Jorgensen H, Nigra TP: Elevation of serum triglyceride levels from oral isotretinoin in disorders of keratinization. *Arch Dermatol* 116:1369, 1980.
137. Crook D, Godsland I, Winn V: Oral contraceptives and coronary heart disease: Modulation of glucose tolerance and plasma lipids by progestins. *Am J Obstet Gynecol* 158:1612, 1988.
138. Burry KA, Patton PE, Illingworth DR: Metabolic changes during medical treatment of endometriosis: Nafarelin acetate *vs.* Danazol. *Am J Obstet Gynecol* 160:1454, 1989.
139. Lardinois CK, Newman SL: The effects of antihypertensive agents on serum lipids and lipoproteins. *Arch Intern Med* 148:1280, 1988.
140. Krone W, Nagele H: Effects of antihypertensives on plasma lipids and lipoprotein metabolism. *Am Heart J* 116:1729, 1988.
141. Iverius PH, Brunzell JD: Chylomicronemia induced by cimetidine. *Gastroenterology* 89:664, 1985.
142. Ballantyne CM, Podet EJ, Patsch WP, et al: Effects of cyclosporine therapy on plasma lipoprotein levels. *JAMA* 262:53, 1989.
143. Wallace RB, Hunninghake DB, Reiland S, et al: Alterations of plasma high density lipoprotein cholesterol levels associated with consumption of selected medications. *Circulation* 62(Suppl 4):77, 1980.
144. Brown MS, Kovanen PT, Goldstein JL, Eeckles R, Vandenberg K, et al: Prenatal diagnosis of homozygous familial hypercholesterolemia. *Lancet* 1:526, 1978.
145. Gagne C, Moorjani S, Grun D, Doussaint M, Lupen PJ: Heterozygous familial hypercholesterolemia: The relationship between plasma lipids, lipoproteins, clinical manifestations, and ischemic heart disease in men and women. *Atherosclerosis* 34:13, 1979.
146. Shapiro JR, Fallet RW, Tsang RC, Glueck CJ: Achilles tendonitis and tenosinovitis: A diagnostic manifestation of familial Type II hyperlipoproteinemia in children. *Am J Dis Child* 128:486, 1974.
147. Watanabe A, Yoshimura A, Wacasugi T, Tatami R, Takada R: Serum lipids, lipoproteins and coronary heart disease in patients with xanthelasma palpebrarum. *Atherosclerosis* 38:283, 1981.
148. Mabuchi M, Ito S, Haba T: Achilles tendon thickness and ischemic heart disease in familial hypercholesterolemia. *Metabolism* 27:1672, 1978.
149. Jensen D, Blankenhorn DH, Kornerup V: Coronary disease in familial hypercholesterolemia. *Circulation* 36:77, 1967.
150. Stone NY, Levy RI, Fredrickson DS, Vetter J: Coronary artery disease in 116 kindred with familial Type II hypercholesterolemia. *Circulation* 49:476, 1974.
151. Slack J: Risks of ischemic heart disease in familial hypercholesterolemia. *Lancet* 2:1380, 1969.
152. Hale JS, Hayden NR, Frohlich J, Pritchard PH: Genetic and environmental factors affecting the incidence of coronary artery disease in

heterozygous familial hypercholesterolemia. *Arterioscler Thromb* 11:290, 1991.

153. Coetze GA, VanderWesthuyzen DR, Berger JMB, Henderson HE, Gevers W: Low density lipoprotein metabolism in cultured fibroblasts from a new group of patients presenting clinically with homozygous familial hypercholesterolemia. *Arteriosclerosis* 2:303, 1982.
154. Rose V, Wilson G, Steiner G: Familial hypercholesterolemia: Report of coronary death at age 3 in a homozygous child and prenatal diagnosis in a heterozygous sibling. *J Pediatr* 100:757, 1982.
155. Allen JM, Thompson GR, Myant MB, Steiner R, Oakley MC: Cardiovascular complications of homozygous familial hypercholesterolemia. *Br Heart J* 44:361, 1980.
156. Forman MB, Kinsley RH, Duplessis JP, Danskey R, Milner S, Levine SE: Surgical correction of combined supravalvular and valvular aortic stenosis in homozygous familial hypercholesterolemia. *S Afr Med J* 61:579, 1982.
157. Seed M, Hoppichler F, Reaveley D, Thompson GR: Relation of serum lipoprotein(a) concentration and apolipoprotein(a) phenotype to coronary heart disease in patients with familial hypercholesterolemia. *N Engl J Med* 322:1494, 1990.
158. Wiklund O, Angelian B, Olofsson SO, Eriksson M, Fajer G, et al: Apolipoprotein(a) and ischemic heart disease in familial hypercholesterolemia. *Lancet* 335:1360, 1990.
159. Bloch A, Dinsmore RE, Lees RS: Coronary angiographic findings in Type II and Type IV hyperlipoproteinemia. *Lancet* 1:928, 1976.
160. Sugrue DD, Thompson GR, Oakley CM, Trainer IM, Steiner RE: Contrasting patterns of coronary atherosclerosis in normocholesterolemic smokers and patients with familial hypercholesterolemia. *Br Med J* 283:1358, 1981.
161. Streja D, Steiner G, Kwiterovich PO: Plasma high density lipoproteins in ischemic heart disease: Studies in a large kindred with familial hypercholesterolemia. *Ann Intern Med* 89:871, 1978.
162. Ginsberg H, Davidson N, Le NA, Gibson J, Ahrens EH, Brown WV: Marked overproduction of low density lipoprotein apoprotein B in a subject with heterozygous familial hypercholesterolemia. *Biochim Biophys Acta* 712.250, 1982.
163. Hazzard WR, Albers JJ, Caron P, Lewis B: Association of isoapolipoprotein EIII deficiency with heterozygous familial hypercholesterolemia: Implications for lipoprotein physiology. *Lancet* 1:298, 1981.
164. Tolleshaug H, Hopgood KK, Brown MS, Goldstein JL: The LDL receptor locus in familial hypercholesterolemia: Multiple mutations disrupt transport and processing of a membrane receptor. *Cell* 32:941, 1983.
165. Hobbs HH, Russell DW, Brown MS, Goldstein JL: The LDL receptor locus in familial hypercholesterolemia: Mutational analysis of a membrane protein. *Annu Rev Genet* 24:133, 1990.
166. Bilheimer DW, Stone NJ, Grundy SM: Metabolic studies in familial hypercholesterolemia: Evidence for a gene dosage effect *in vivo*. *J Clin Invest* 64:524, 1979.
167. Fogelman AM, Hokam MM, Haberland ME, Tanaka RD, Edwards PA: Lipoprotein regulation of cholesterol metabolism in macrophages derived from human monocytes. *J Biol Chem* 258:14081, 1982.
168. Zuliani G, Arca M, Signore A, Bader G, Fazio S, et al: Characterization of a new form of inherited hypercholesterolemia: familial recessive hypercholesterolemia. *Arterioscler Thromb Vasc Biol* 19:802, 1999.
169. Seftel HC, Baker CG, Sundler MP: A host of hypercholesterolemic homozygotes in South Africa. *Br Med J* 281:633, 1980.
170. Khachadurian AK, Uthman SM: Experiences with homozygous cases of hypercholesterolemia: A report of 52 patients. *Nutr Metab* 15:132, 1973.
171. Illingworth DR, Sexton GJ: Hypocholesterolemic effects of mevinolin in patients with heterozygous familial hypercholesterolemia. *J Clin Invest* 74:1972, 1984.
172. Havel RG, Hunninghake DB, Illingworth DR, Stein EA: Lovastatin (mevinolin) in the treatment of heterozygous familial hypercholesterolemia: A multicenter study. *Ann Intern Med* 107:609, 1987.
173. Illingworth DR, Bacon S: Treatment of heterozygous familial hypercholesterolemia with lipid-lowering drugs. *Arteriosclerosis* 9(Suppl 1):1, 1989.
174. Mol MJTM, Erkelens DW, Gevers-Leuven JA: Effects of synvinolin (MK 733) on plasma lipids in familial hypercholesterolemia. *Lancet* 2:936, 1986.
175. Wiklund O, Angelin B, Fager G: Treatment of familial hypercholesterolemia: A controlled trial of the effects of pravastatin or Cholestyramine therapy on lipoprotein and apoprotein levels. *J Intern Med* 228:241, 1990.
176. Buckley MMT, Goa KL, Price AH, Brogden RN: Probucol: A reappraisal of its pharmacological properties and therapeutic use in hypercholesterolemia. *Drugs* 37:761, 1989.
177. Baker SG, Joffe BI, Mendelsohn D, Seftel HC: Treatment of homozygous familial hypercholesterolemia with Probucol. *S Afr Med J* 62:7, 1982.
178. Yamamota A, Matsuzawa Y, Yokoyama S: Effects of Probucol on xanthoma regression in familial hypercholesterolemia. *Am J Cardiol* 57:29H, 1986.
179. Packard CJ, Stewart JM, Morgan HG, Shepherd J: Combined drug therapy for familial hypercholesterolemia. *Artery* 7:281, 1980.
180. Illingworth DR, Phillipson BE, Rapp JH, Connor WE: Colestipol plus nicotinic acid in treatment of heterozygous familial hypercholesterolemia. *Lancet* 1:296, 1981.
181. Illingworth DR: Mevinolin plus Colestipol in therapy for severe heterozygous familial hypercholesterolemia. *Ann Intern Med* 101:598, 1984.
182. Lintott CJ, Scott RS, Nye ER, Sutherland EW: Simvastatin (MK 733): An effective treatment for hypercholesterolemia. *Aust N Z J Med* 19:317, 1989.
183. Hoogerbrugge N, Mol NJTM, van Dormaal JJ: The efficacy and safety of pravastatin compared to and in combination with bile acid-binding resins in familial hypercholesterolemia. *J Intern Med* 228:261, 1990.
184. Curtis LD, Dixon AC, Ling KLE, Betteridge J: Combination treatment with Cholestyramine and Bezafibrate for heterozygous familial hypercholesterolemia. *Br Med J* 297:173, 1988.
185. Malloy MJ, Kane JP, Kunitake ST, Havel RJ: Complimentarity of Colestipol, niacin and lovastatin in treatment of severe familial hypercholesterolemia. *Ann Intern Med* 107:616, 1987.
186. Spengel FA, Jadhav A, Duffield RGM, Wood CB, Thompson GR: Superiority of partial illeal bypass over Cholestyramine in reducing cholesterol in familial hypercholesterolemia. *Lancet* 2:768, 1981.
187. Buchwald H, Moore RB, Varco RL: Surgical treatment of hyperlipidemia. *Circulation* 49(Suppl 1):1, 1974.
188. Illingworth DR, Connor WE: Hypercholesterolemia persisting after distal ileal bypass: Response to mevinolin. *Ann Intern Med* 100:850, 1984.
189. Buchwald H, Varco RL, Matts JP, et al: Effect of partial ileal bypass surgery on mortality and morbidity from coronary heart disease in patients with hypercholesterolemia: Report of the Program on the Surgical Control of the Hyperlipidemias. *N Engl J Med* 323:946, 1990.
190. Keller C: LDL apheresis: Results of long-term treatment and vascular outcome. *Atherosclerosis* 86:1, 1991.
191. Thompson GR, Barbir M, Okabayashi K: Plasmapheresis in familial hypercholesterolemia. *Arteriosclerosis* 9(Suppl 1):152, 1989.
192. Eisenhauer T, Armstrong VW, Wieland H, Fuchs C, Scheler F, Seidel D: Selective removal of low density lipoprotein by precipitation at low pH: First clinical application of the HELP System. *Klin Wochenschr* 65:1, 1987.
193. Thompson GR, Miller JP, Breslow JL: Improved survival of patients with homozygous familial hypercholesterolemia treated by plasma exchange. *Br Med J* 291:1671, 1985.
194. Bilheimer DW, Goldstein JL, Grundy SM, Starzle TE, Brown MS: Liver transplantation to provide low density lipoprotein receptors and lower plasma cholesterol in a child with homozygous familial hypercholesterolemia. *N Engl J Med* 311:1658, 1984.
195. Hoeg JM, Starzle TE, Brewer HP Jr: Liver transplantation for treatment of cardiovascular disease: Comparison of medication and plasma exchange in homozygous familial hypercholesterolemia. *Am J Cardiol* 59:705, 1987.
196. Innerarity TL, Weisgraber KH, Arnold KS, Grundy SM, Mahley RW: Familial defective apolipoprotein B-100: Low density lipoproteins with abnormal receptor binding. *Proc Natl Acad Sci USA* 84:6919, 1987.
197. Schuster H, Rauh G, Kormann B, Hepp T, Humphries S, et al: Familial defective apolipoprotein B-100: Comparison with familial hypercholesterolemia in eighteen cases detected in Munich. *Arteriosclerosis* 10:577, 1990.
198. Myant MB, Gallagher JJ, Knight BL, McCarthy SN, Frostegard J, et al: Clinical signs of familial hypercholesterolemia in patients with

familial defective apoprotein B-100 and normal low density lipoprotein receptor function. *Arterioscler Thromb* 11:691, 1991.
199. Illingworth DR, Vakar F, Mahley RW, Weisgraber KH: Hypocholesterolemic effects of lovastatin in familial defective apolipoprotein B-100. *Lancet* 339:598, 1992.
200. Innerarity TL, Mahley RW, Weisgraber KH, Bersot TP, Krauss RM, et al: Familial defective apolipoprotein B-100: A mutation of apolipoprotein B that causes hypercholesterolemia. *J Lipid Res* 31:1337, 1990.
201. Hansen PS, Rudigen N, Tybjærg-Hansen A: Detection of the apo B 3,500 mutation (glutamine arginine) by gene amplification and cleavage with Mspl. *J Lipid Res* 32:1229, 1991.
202. Vega GL, Grundy SM: *In vivo* evidence for reduced binding of low density lipoproteins to receptors as a cause of primary moderate hypercholesterolemia. *J Clin Invest* 78:1410, 1986.
203. Corsini A, Mazzotti M, Fumagalli R, Catapano AL, Romano L, Romano C: Poor response to simvastatin in familial defective apolipoprotein B-100. *Lancet* 337:305, 1991.
204. Maher VMG, Gallagher JJ, Thompson GR, Myant NB: Response to cholesterol-lowering drugs in familial defective apolipoprotein B-100. *Atherosclerosis* 91:73, 1991.
205. Schmidt EB, Illingworth DR, Bacon S, Mahley RW, Weisgraber KH: Hypocholesterolemic effects of nicotinic acid in patients with familial defective apoprotein B-100. *Metabolism* 42:137, 1993.
206. Vega GL, Illingworth DR, Grundy SM, Lindgren FT, Connor WE: Normocholesterolemic tendon xanthomas with overproduction of apolipoprotein B. *Metabolism* 32:118, 1983.
207. Goldstein JL, Schrott HG, Hazzard WR: Hyperlipidemia in coronary heart disease: Genetic analysis of lipid levels in 176 families and delineation of a new inherited disorder, combined hyperlipidemia. *J Clin Invest* 52:1544, 1973.
208. Babirak SP, Inverius PH, Fujimoto WY, Brunzell JD: Detection and characterization of the heterozygote state for lipoprotein lipase deficiency. *Arteriosclerosis* 9:326, 1989.
209. Wojciechowski AP, Farrall M, Cullen P, Wilson TME, Bayliss JD, et al: Familial combined hyperlipidemia linked to the apolipoprotein AI-CIII-AIV gene cluster on chromosome 11q23-q24. *Nature* 349:161, 1991.
210. Sniderman AD, Shapiro S, Marpole D, Skinner B, Tang G, Kwiterovich PO Jr: Association of coronary atherosclerosis with hyperapobetalipoproteinemia. *Proc Natl Acad Sci USA* 77:604, 1980.
211. Sniderman AD, Wolfson C, Tang B, Franklin FA, Bachorik PS, Kwiterovich PO Jr: Association of hyperapobetalipoproteinemia with endogenous hypertriglyceridemia and atherosclerosis. *Ann Intern Med* 97:833, 1982.
212. Janus ED, Nicoll AM, Turner PL, Lewis B: Kinetic basis of the primary hyperlipoproteinemias: Studies of apolipoprotein B turnover in genetically defined subjects. *Eur J Clin Invest* 10:161, 1980.
213. Deeb SS, Motulsky AG, Albers JJ: A partial cDNA clone for human apolipoprotein B. *Proc Natl Acad Sci USA* 82:4983, 1985.
214. Knott TJ, Rall SC, Innerarity TL, Jacobson SF, Urdea MS, et al: Human apolipoprotein B: Structure of carboxyterminal domains, cytogenic expression and chromosomal localization. *Science* 230:37, 1985.
215. Illingworth DR: Fibric acid derivatives, in Rifkind BM (ed): *Drug Treatment of Hyperlipidemia*. New York, Marcel Dekker, 1991, p 103.
216. Goffman JW, Dipalla O, Glazier F, Freeman NK, Linguen FT, et al: The serum lipoprotein transport system and health, metabolic disorders, atherosclerosis and coronary heart disease. *Plasma* 2:413, 1954.
217. Brewer HB, Zech LA, Gregg RE, et al: Type III hyperlipoproteinemia: Diagnosis, molecular defects, pathology and treatment. *Ann Intern Med* 98:623, 1983.
218. Morganroth J, Levy RI, Fredrickson DS: The biochemical, clinical and genetic features of Type III hyperlipidemia. *Ann Intern Med* 82:158, 1975.
219. Davignon J, Gregg RE, Sing CF: Apoprotein E polymorphism and atherosclerosis. *Arteriosclerosis* 8:1, 1988.
220. Mahley RW, Angelin B: Type III hyperlipoproteinemia: Recent insights into the genetic defects of familial dysbetalipoproteinemia. *Adv Intern Med* 29:395, 1984.
221. Fredrickson DS, Morganroth J, Levy RI: Type III hyperlipidemia: An analysis of two contemporary definitions. *Ann Intern Med* 82:150, 1975.
222. Ghiselli G, Schaffer EJ, Gascon P, Brewer HB Jr: Type III hyperlipoproteinemia associated with apolipoprotein E deficiency. *Science* 214:1239, 1981.
223. Havel RJ: Familial dysbetalipoproteinemia: New aspects of pathogenesis and diagnosis. *Med Clin North Am* 66:441, 1982.
224. Kushwaha RS, Hazzard WR, Gagne C, Chait A, Albers JJ: Type III hyperlipoproteinemia: Paradoxical hypolipidemic response to estrogen. *Ann Intern Med* 87:517, 1977.
225. Zelis R, Mason DT, Braunwald E, Levy RI: Effects of hyperlipoproteinemias and their treatment on the peripheral circulation. *J Clin Invest* 49:1007, 1970.
226. Breckenridge WC, Little JA, Alaupovic P, Wang CS, Kuksis A, et al: Lipoprotein abnormalities associated with a familial deficiency of hepatic lipase. *Atherosclerosis* 45:161, 1982.
227. Brunzell JD: Familial lipoprotein lipase deficiency and other causes of the chylomicronemia syndrome, in Scriver CR, Beaudet AL, Sly WS, Valler D (eds): *The Metabolic Basis of Inherited Disease*, 6th ed. New York, McGraw-Hill, 1989, pp 1165–1180.
228. Fredrickson DS, Levy RI: Familial hyperlipoproteinemia, in Stanbury JB, Wyngaarden JB, Fredrickson DS (eds): *The Metabolic Basis of Inherited Disease*, 3rd ed. New York, McGraw-Hill, 1972, p 545.
229. Brown WV, Baginsky ML, Ehnholm C: Primary type I and V hyperlipoproteinemia, in Rifkind BM, Levy RI (eds): *Hyperlipidemia: Diagnosis and Therapy*. New York, Grune & Stratton, 1977, p 93.
230. Brunzell JD, Bierman EL: Chylomicronemia syndrome: Interaction of genetic and acquired hypertriglyceridemia. *Med Clin North Am* 66:455, 1982.
231. Kwiterovich PO, Farah JR, Brown WV, Bachorik PS, Baylin SB, Neill CA: The clinical, biochemical, and familial presentation of type V hyperlipoproteinemia in childhood. *Pediatrics* 59:513, 1977.
232. Greenberg BM, Blackwelder WC, Levy RI: Primary type V hyperlipoproteinemia. *Ann Intern Med* 87:526, 1977.
233. Fallat RW, Glueck CJ: Familial and acquired type V hyperlipoproteinemia. *Atherosclerosis* 23:41, 1976.
234. Lesser PB, Warshaw AL: Diagnosis of pancreatitis masked by hyperlipidemia. *Ann Intern Med* 82:795, 1975.
235. Harlan WR, Winesett PS, Wasserman AJ: Tissue lipoprotein lipase in normal individuals and in individuals with exogenous hypertriglyceridemia and the relation of this enzyme to the assimilation of fat. *J Clin Invest* 46:239, 1967.
236. Santamarina-Fojo S, Brewer HB Jr: The familial hyperchylomicronemia syndrome. *JAMA* 265:904, 1991.
237. Sigurdson G, Nicoll A, Lewis B: Metabolism of very low density lipoproteins in hyperlipidemia: Studies of apoprotein B kinetics in man. *Eur J Clin Invest* 6:167, 1976.
238. Leaf DA, Connor WE, Illingworth DR, Bacon SP, Sexton G: The hypolipidemic effects of gemfibrozil in type V hyperlipidemia: A double blind crossover study. *JAMA* 262:3154, 1989.
239. McMurry MP, Connor WE, Goplerud CP: Effects of dietary cholesterol upon the hypercholesterolemia of pregnancy. *Metabolism* 30:869, 1981.
240. Sanderson SL, Iverius PH, Wilson DE: Successful hyperlipidemic pregnancy. *JAMA* 265:1858, 1991.
241. DenBesten L, Reyna RH, Connor WE, Stegink LD: The different effects on the serum lipids and fecal steroids of high carbohydrate diets given orally or intravenously. *J Clin Invest* 52:1384, 1973.
242. Mishkel MA, Stein EA: Primary type IV hyperlipoproteinemia, in Rifkind BM, Levy RI (eds): *Hyperlipidemia: Diagnosis and Therapy*. New York, Grune & Stratton, 1977, p 177.
243. Goldstein JL, Hazzard WR, Schrott HG, Bierman EL, Motulsky AG, et al: Hyperlipidemia in coronary heart disease: I. Lipid levels in 500 survivors of myocardial infarction. *J Clin Invest* 52:1533, 1973.
244. Brunzell JD, Bierman EL: Plasma triglyceride and insulin levels in familial hypertriglyceridemia. *Ann Intern Med* 87:198, 1977.
245. Kannel WB: Lipids, diabetes, and coronary heart disease: Insights from the Framingham study. *Am Heart J* 110:1100, 1985.
246. Kannel WB, McGee DL: Diabetes and cardiovascular disease—the Framingham study. *JAMA* 241:2035, 1979.
247. Garcia MJ, McNamara PM, Gordon T, Kannel WB: Morbidity and mortality in diabetics in the Framingham population: Sixteen year follow-up study. *Diabetes* 23:105, 1974.
248. Kirkland RT, Keenan BS, Probstfield JL, et al: Decrease in plasma high density lipoprotein cholesterol levels at puberty in boys with delayed adolescence. *JAMA* 257:502, 1987.

249. Mellies MJ, Gartside PS, Galtfelter L, Blueck CJ: Effect of probucol on plasma cholesterol high and low density lipoprotein cholesterol and apolipoprotein AI and AII in adults with primary familial hypercholesterolemia. *Metabolism* 29:956, 1980.
250. Schaefer EJ, Heaton WH, Wetzel MG, Brewer HG Jr: Plasma apolipoprotein AI absence associated with a marked reduction of high density lipoproteins and premature coronary artery disease. *Arteriosclerosis* 2:16, 1982.
251. Norum RA, Lakier JB, Goldstein S, Angel A, Goldberg RB, et al: Familial deficiency of apolipoproteins AI and CIII and precocious coronary artery disease. *N Engl J Med* 306:1513, 1982.
252. Karathanasis SK, Norum RA, Zannis VI, Breslow JL: An inherited polymorphism in the human apolipoprotein AI gene locus related to the development of atherosclerosis. *Nature* 301:718, 1983.
253. Schaefer EJ, Ordovas JM, Law S, et al: Familial lipolipoprotein AI and CIII deficiency, variant II. *J Lipid Res* 26:1089, 1985.
254. Assman G, Schmitz G, Brewer HB Jr: Familial high density lipoprotein deficiency: Tangier disease, in Scriver CR, Beaudet AL, Sly WS, Valle D (eds): *The Metabolic Basis of Inherited Disease*, 6th ed. New York, McGraw-Hill, 1989, p 1267.
255. Frederickson DA: The inheritance of high density lipoprotein deficiency (Tangier disease). *J Clin Invest* 43:228, 1964.
256. Lindeskog GR, Gustafson A, Enerback L: Serum lipoprotein deficiency and diffuse planar xanthoma. *Arch Dermatol* 106:529, 1972.
257. Gustafson A, McCounathy W, Alaupovic P, Curry MD, Persson B: Identification of apoprotein families in a variant of human plasma apolipoprotein A deficiency. *Scand J Clin Lab Invest* 39:377, 1979.
258. Norum KR, Gjone E, Glomset JA: Familial lecithin: Cholesterol acyltransferase deficiency, including fish eye disease, in Scriver CR, Beaudet AL, Sly WS, Valle D (eds): *The Metabolic Basis of Inherited Disease*, 6th ed. New York, McGraw-Hill, 1989, p 1181.
259. Gjone E, Norum KR: Familial serum cholesterol ester deficiency: Clinical study of a patient with a new syndrome. *Acta Med Scand* 183:107, 1968.
260. Carlson LA, Phillipson B: Fish eye disease: A new familial condition associated with massive corneal opacities and dyslipoproteinemia. *Lancet* 2:921, 1979.
261. Carlson LA: Fish eye disease: A new familial condition with massive corneal opacities and dyslipoproteinemia. *Eur J Clin Invest* 12:41, 1982.
262. Weisgraber KH, Rall SC Jr, Bersot TP, et al: Apolipoprotein AI Milano: Detection of normal AI in affected subjects and evidence for a cysteine for arginine substitution in the variant AI. *J Biol Chem* 258:2508, 1983.
263. Rall SC, Menzel HG, Assmann G, et al: Identification of amino acid substitutions in five human apolipoproteins AI variants. *Arteriosclerosis* 3:515a, 1983
264. Utermann G, Feussner G, Franceschini G, et al: Genetic variants of group A apolipoproteins, lipid methods for screening and characterization without ultracentrifugation. *J Biol Chem* 257:501, 1982.
265. Menzel HJ, Kladetzky RG, Assmann G: One step screening method for the polymorphisms of apolipoprotein AI, AII, and AIV. *J Lipid Res* 23:9156, 1982.
266. Vergani C, Bettale A: Familial hypoalphalipoproteinemia. *Clin Chim Acta* 114:45, 1981.
267. Third JHLC, Montag J, Freidel J, et al: Primary and familial hypoalphalipoproteinemia. *Metabolism* 33:136, 1984.
268. Glueck DJ, Fallet RW, Millet F, Gottside P, Elston RC, Go RCP: Familial hyperalphalipoproteinemia: Studies in 28 kindreds. *Metabolism* 24:1243, 1975.
269. Schaefer EJ: Clinical, biochemical and genetic features in familial disorders of high density lipoprotein deficiency. *Arteriosclerosis* 4:303, 1984.
270. Breslow JL: Familial disorders of high density lipoprotein metabolism, in Scriver CR, Beaudet AL, Sly WS, Valle D (eds): *The Metabolic Basis of Inherited Disease*, 6th ed. New York, McGraw-Hill, 1989, p 1251.
271. Franceschini G, Sirtori CR, Capurso A, Weisgraber KH, Mahley RW: AI Milano apoprotein: Decreased high density lipoprotein cholesterol levels with significant lipoprotein modifications and with clinical atherosclerosis in an Italian family. *J Clin Invest* 66:892, 1980.
272. Daniels SR, Bates S, Lutkin RR, Benton C, Third JLHC, Glueck CJ: Cerebral vascular arteriopathy (arteriosclerosis) and ischemic childhood stroke. *Stroke* 13:360, 1982.
273. Schaefer EJ, Zech LA, Schwartz DS, Brewer HP Jr: Coronary heart disease prevalence and other clinical features in familial high density lipoprotein deficiency (Tangiers disease). *Ann Intern Med* 93:261, 1980.
274. Schmitz G, Assmann G, Rall SE Jr, Mahley RW: Tangier disease: Defective recombination of a specific Tangier apolipoprotein AI isoform (proapo AI) with high density lipoproteins. *Proc Natl Acad Sci USA* 80:6081, 1983.
275. Hayden MR, Clee SM, Brooks-Wilson A, Genest J, Attie A, Kastelein JJP: Cholesterol efflux regulatory protein, Tangier disease and familial high-density lipoprotein deficiency. *Curr Opin Lipidol* 11:117, 2000.
276. Zannis VI, Lees AM, Lees RS, Breslow JL: Abnormal apo AI isoprotein composition in patients with Tangier disease. *J Biochem* 257:4978, 1982.
277. Kay L, Ronan R, Schaefer EJ, Brewer HG Jr: Tangier disease: A structural defect in apolipoprotein AI. *Proc Natl Acad Sci USA* 79:2485, 1982.
278. Glueck CJ, Kostis PM, Tsang RC, Mellies MJ, Steiner PM: Neonatal familial hyperalphalipoproteinemia. *Metabolism* 26:469, 1977.
279. Koizumi J, Mabuchi H, Yoshimura A, Michishita I, Takeda M, et al: Deficiency of serum cholesterol-ester transfer activity in patients with familial hyperalphalipoproteinemia. *Atherosclerosis* 58:175, 1985.
280. Kurasawa T, Yokoyama S, Miyake Y, Yamamura T, Yamamoto A: Rate of cholesterol-ester transfer between high and low density lipoproteins in human serum and a case with decreased transfer rate in association with hyperalphalipoproteinemia. *J Biochem* 98:1499, 1985.
281. Kane JP, Havel RJ: Disorders of the biogenesis and secretion of lipoproteins containing the B apoproteins, in Scriver CR, Beaudet AL, Sly WS, Valle D (eds): *The Metabolic Basis of Inherited Disease*, 6th ed. New York, McGraw-Hill, 1989, p 1139.
282. Malloy MJ, Kane JP, Hardman DA, Hamilton RL, Dalal KB: Normotriglyceridemic abetalipoproteinemia: Absence of the B100 apolipoprotein. *J Clin Invest* 67:1441, 1981.
283. Takashimo Y, Kodama T, Lida H, Kawamura M, Aburatani H, et al: Normotriglyceridemic abetalipoproteinemia in infancy: An isolated apolipoprotein B100 deficiency. *Pediatrics* 75:541, 1985.
284. Caballero FM, Buchanan GR: Abetalipoproteinemia presenting as severe vitamin K deficiency. *Pediatrics* 65:161, 1980
285. Muller DPR, Lloyd JK, Bird AC: Long term management of abetalipoproteinemia: Possible role for vitamin E. *Arch Dis Child* 52:209, 1977.
286. Illingworth DR, Connor WE, Miller RG: Abetalipoproteinemia: Report of two cases and review of therapy. *Arch Neurol* 37:659, 1980.
287. Illingworth DR, Kenny TA, Orwolll ES: Adrenal function in heterozygous and homozygous hypobetalipoproteinemia. *J Clin Endocrinol Metab* 54:27, 1982.
288. Illingworth DR, Kenny TA, Connor WE, Orwoll ES: Corticosteroid production in abetalipoproteinemia: Evidence for an impaired response to ACTH. *J Lab Clin Med* 100:115, 1982.
289. Parker CR Jr, Illingworth DR, Bissonnette J, Carr BR: Endocrinology of pregnancy in abetalipoproteinemia: Studies in a patient with heterozygous familial hypobetalipoproteinemia. *N Engl J Med* 314:557, 1986.
290. Muller DPR, Lloyd JK: Effect of large oral doses of vitamin E on the neurological sequelae of patients with abetalipoproteinemia. *Ann NY Acad Sci* 393:133, 1982.
291. Hegele RA, Angel A: Arrest of neuropathy and myopathy in abetalipoproteinemia with high dose vitamin E therapy. *Can Med Assoc J* 132:41, 1985.
292. Runge P, Muller DPR, McCallister J, Calver D, Lloyd JK, Taylor D: Oral vitamin E supplements can prevent the retinopathy of abetalipoproteinemia. *Br J Ophthalmol* 70:166, 1986.
293. Illingworth DR, Connor WE, Buist NRM, Jhaveri DJ, Lin DS, McMurray MP: Sterol balance in abetalipoproteinemia: Studies in a patient with homozygous familial hypobetalipoproteinemia. *Metabolism* 28:1152, 1979.
294. Wang CS, Illingworth DR: Lipid composition and lipolytic activities in milk from a patient with homozygous familial hypobetalipoproteinemia. *Am J Clin Nutr* 45:730, 1987.
295. Lackner KJ, Monge JC, Greg RE, Hoeg JM, Triche TJ, et al: Analysis of the apoprotein B gene and messenger ribonucleic acid in abetalipoproteinemia. *J Clin Invest* 78:1707, 1986.

296. Young SG, Hubi ST, Smith RS, Snyder SM, Terdiman JF: Familial hypobetalipoproteinemia caused by a mutation in the apolipoprotein gene that results in a truncated species of apolipoprotein B (B31). *J Clin Invest* 85:933, 1990.
297. Talmud P, King-Underwood L, Krul E, Schonfeld G, Humphries SE: The molecular basis of truncated forms of apolipoprotein B in a kindred with compound heterozygous hypobetalipoproteinemia. *J Lipid Res* 30:1773, 1989.
298. Hardman DA, Pulinger CR, Hamilton RL, Kane JP, Malloy MJ: Molecular and metabolic basis for the metabolic disorder normotriglyceridemic abetalipoproteinemia. *J Clin Invest* 88:1722, 1991.
299. Bieri JG, Hoeg JM, Schaefer EJ, Zech LA, Brewer HB Jr: Vitamin A and vitamin E replacement in abetalipoproteinemia. *Ann Intern Med* 100:238, 1984.
300. Kayden HJ, Hatem LJ, Traber MG: The measurement of nanograms of tocopherol from needle aspiration biopsies of adipose tissue: Normal and abetalipoproteinemic subjects. *J Lipid Res* 24:652, 1983.
301. Partin JS, Partin JC, Schubert WK, McAdams AJ: Liver ultrastructure in abetalipoproteinemia: Evolution of micronodular cirrhosis. *Gastroenterology* 67:107, 1974.
302. Noseda G, Riesen W, Schlumph E, Morrell A: Hypobetalipoproteinemia associated with autoantibodies against betalipoproteins. *Eur J Clin Invest* 2:342, 1972.
303. Cottrill C, Glueck CJ, Leuba V, Millett F, Puppinone D, Brown WV: Familial homozygous hypobetalipoproteinemia. *Metabolism* 23:779, 1974.
304. Salt HB, Wolff OH, Lloyd JK, Fosbrooke AS, Cameron AH, Hubble DV: On having no betalipoprotein: A syndrome comprising abetalipoproteinemia, acanthocytosis, and steatorrhea. *Lancet* 2:325, 1960.
305. Andersen GE, Brokhatting NK, Lous P: Familial hypobetalipoproteinemia in nine children diagnosed as the result of cord blood screening for hypolipoproteinemia in 10,000 Danish newborns. *Arch Dis Child* 54:691, 1979.
306. Glueck CJ, Gartside PS, Steiner PM, Miller M, Todd-Hunter T, et al: Hyperalpha and hypobetalipoproteinemia in octogenarian kindreds. *Atherosclerosis* 27:387, 1977.
307. Frohlich J, McLeod R, Pritchard PH, Fesmire J, McConathy W: Plasma lipoprotein abnormalities in heterozygotes for familial lecithin: Cholesterol acyltransferase deficiency. *Metabolism* 37:3, 1988.
308. Salen G, Shefer S, Batta AK, et al: Abnormal cholesterol biosynthesis in the Smith-Lemli-Opitz syndrome *J Lipid Res* 37:1169, 1996.
309. Wassif CA, Maslen C, Kachilele-Linjewile S, et al: Mutations in the Human Sterol ^{7}-Reductase Gene at 11q12-13 Cause Smith-Lemli-Opitz Syndrome. *Am J Hum Genet* 63:55, 1998.
310. Yu H, Tint GS, Salen G, Patel SB: Detection of a common mutation in the RSH or Smith-Lemli-Opitz syndrome by a PCR-RFLP assay: IVS8-G—>C is found in over sixty percent of US propositi. *Am J Med Genet* 90:347, 2000.
311. Linck LM, Lin DS, Flavell D, Connor WE, Steiner RD: Cholesterol supplementation with egg yolk increases plasma cholesterol and decreases plasma 7-dehydrocholesterol in Smith-Lemli-Opitz Syndrome. *Am J Med Genet* 93:360, 2000.
312. Rapp JH, Connor WE, Lin DS, Inahara T, Porter JM: The lipids of human atherosclerotic plaques and xanthomas: Clues to the mechanism of plaque progression. *J Lipid Res* 24:1329, 1983.
313. Austin MA: Plasma triglyceride as a risk factor for coronary heart disease: The epidemiologic evidence and beyond. *Am J Epidemiol* 129:249, 1989.
314. Gordon T, Castelli WP, Hjortland MC, Kannel WM: High density lipoprotein as a protective factor against coronary heart disease: The Framingham study. *Am J Med* 62:707, 1977.
315. Bhattacharyya AK, Preacher AB, Connor WE: Ectopic xanthomas in familial (Type II) hypercholesterolemia. *Atherosclerosis* 37:319, 1980.
316. Bhattacharyya AK, Connor WE, Mausolf FA, Flatt AE: Turnover of xanthoma cholesterol in hyperlipoproteinemic patients. *J Lab Clin Med* 87:503, 1976.
317. Schmidtz G, Assmann G: Acid lipase deficiency, Wolman disease and cholesterol ester storage disease, in Scriver CR, Beaudet AL, Sly WS, Valle D (eds): *The Metabolic Basis of Inherited Disease*, 6th ed. New York, McGraw-Hill, 1989, p 1623.
318. Tarrantino MD, McNamarra DJ, Granstrom P, Ellefson RD, Unger EC, Udall JM Jr: Lovastatin therapy for cholesterol ester storage disease in two sisters. *J Pediatr* 118:131, 1991.
319. Leone L, Ippoliti PF: Use of simvastatin plus Cholestyramine in the treatment of lysosomal acid lipase deficiency. *J Pediatr* 119:1008, 1991.
320. Bisceglie AND, Ishak KG, Rabin L, Hoeg JN: Cholesterol ester storage disease: Hepatopathology and effects of therapy with lovastatin. *Hepatology* 11:764, 1990.
321. Mbewu AD, Durrington PN: Lipoprotein (a): Structure, properties and possible involvement in thrombogenesis and atherogenesis. *Atherosclerosis* 85:1, 1990.
322. Vessby B, Kostner G, Lithell J, Thomas J: Diverging effects of Cholestyramine on apolipoprotein B and lipoprotein Lp(a): A dose response study of the effects of Cholestyramine in hypercholesterolemia. *Atherosclerosis* 44:61, 1982.
323. Berg K, Laren TP: Unchanged serum lipoprotein (a) concentrations with lovastatin. *Lancet* 2:812, 1989.
324. Kostner GM, Gavish O, Leopold B, Bolzano K, Weintraub MS, Breslow JL: HMG CoA reductase inhibitors lower LDL cholesterol without reducing Lp(a) levels. *Circulation* 80:1313, 1989.
325. Carlson LA, Hamsten A, Asplund A: Pronounced lowering of serum levels of lipoprotein Lp(a) in hyperlipidemic subjects treated with nicotinic acid. *J Intern Med* 226:271, 1989.
326. Soma M, Fumagalli R, Paolett R, Meschia M, Maini MC, et al: Plasma Lp(a) concentration after estrogen and progesterone in post menopausal women. *Lancet* 337:612, 1991.
327. Bhattacharyya AK, Connor WE: Familial diseases with storage of sterols other than cholesterol (cerebrotendinous xanthomatosis and sitosterolemia and xanthomatosis), in Stanbury JB, Wyngaarden JB, Fredrickson DS (eds): *The Metabolic Basis of Inherited Disease*, 4th ed. New York, McGraw-Hill, 1978, p 656.
328. Bjorkem I, Boberg KM: Inborn errors in bile acid biosynthesis and storage of sterols other than cholesterol, in Scriver CR, Beaudet AL, Sly WS, Valle D (eds): *The Metabolic Basis of Inherited Disease*, 7th ed. New York, McGraw-Hill, 1995, pp 2073–2102.
329. Salen G, Shefer S, Cheng FW, Dayal B, Batta AK, Tint GS: Cholic acid biosynthesis: The enzymatic defect in cerebrotendinous xanthomatosis. *J Clin Invest* 63:38, 1979.
330. Berginer VN, Salen G, Shefer S: Long-term treatment of cerebrotendinous xanthomatosis with chenodeoxycholic acid. *N Engl J Med* 311:1649, 1984.
330B. Nakamura T, Matsuzawa Y, Takemura K, et al: Combined treatment with chenodeoxycholic acid and pravastatin improves plasma cholestanol levels associated with marked regression of tendon xanthomas in cerebrotendinous xanthomatosis. *Metabolism* 40:741, 1991.
330C. Peynet J, Laurent A, De Liege P, et al: Cerebrotendinous xanthomatosis: treatments with simvastatin, lovastatin, and chenodeoxycholic acid in 3 siblings. *Neurology* 41:434, 1991.
331. Bhattacharyya AK, Connor WE: Sitosterolemia and xanthomatosis: A newly described lipid storage disease in two sisters. *J Clin Invest* 53:1033, 1974.
332. Salen G, Shefer S, Nguyen L, Ness GC, Tint GS, Shore V: Sitosterolemia. *J Lipid Res* 33:945, 1992.
333. Patel SB, Salen G, Hidaka H, Kwiterovich PO, Stalenhoef AF, et al: Mapping a gene involved in regulating dietary cholesterol absorption. The sitosterolemia locus is found at chromosome 2p21. *J Clin Invest* 102:1041, 1998.
334. Salen G, Horak I, Rothkopf M, Cohen JL, Speck J, et al: Lethal atherosclerosis associated with abnormal plasma and tissue sterol composition in sitosterolemia with xanthomatosis. *J Lipid Res* 26:1126, 1985.
335. Gregg RA, Connor WE, Lin DS, Brewer H Jr: Abnormal metabolism of shellfish sterols in a patient with sitosterolemia and xanthomatosis. *J Clin Invest* 77:1864, 1986.
336. Connor WE, Connor SL: The key role of nutritional factors in the prevention of coronary heart disease. *Prev Med* 1:49, 1972.
337. Lin DS, Connor WE: The long-term effects of dietary cholesterol upon the plasma lipids, lipoproteins, cholesterol absorption, and the sterol balance in man: The demonstration of feedback inhibition of cholesterol biosynthesis and increased bile acid excretion. *J Lipid Res* 21:1042, 1981.
338. Taylor CB, Patton DE, Cox GE: Atherosclerosis in rhesus monkeys: VI. Fatal myocardial infarction in a monkey fed fat and cholesterol. *Arch Pathol* 76:404, 1963.

339. Armstrong ML, Warner ED, Connor WE: Regression of coronary atheromatosis in rhesus monkeys. *Circ Res* 27:59, 1970.
340. Connor WE, Connor SL: The dietary treatment of hyperlipidemia: Rationale, technique and efficacy, in Havel RJ (ed): Lipid disorders. *Med Clin North Am* 66:485, 1982.
341. Brown MS, Goldstein FL: A receptor-mediated pathway for cholesterol homeostasis. *Science* 232:34, 1986.
342. Spady DK, Dietschy JM: Interaction of dietary cholesterol and triglycerides in the regulation of hepatic low density lipoprotein transport in the hamster. *J Clin Invest* 81:300, 1988.
343. Sorci-Thomas M, Wilson MD, Johnson FL, Williams DL, Rudel LL: Studies on the expression of genes encoding apolipoproteins B100 and B48 and the low density lipoprotein receptor in nonhuman primates. *J Biol Chem* 264:9039, 1989.
344. Fox JC, Mcgill HC Jr, Carey KD, Getz GS: In vivo regulation of hepatic LDL receptor mRNA in the baboon—differential effects of saturated and unsaturated fat. *J Biol Chem* 262:7014, 1987.
345. Hopkins PN: Effects of dietary cholesterol on serum cholesterol: A meta-analysis and review. *Am J Clin Nutr* 55:1060, 1992.
346. Connor WE, Hodges RE, Bleiler RE: The serum lipids in men receiving high cholesterol and cholesterol-free diets. *J Clin Invest* 40:894, 1961.
347. Connor WE, Stone DB, Hodges RE: The interrelated effects of dietary cholesterol and fat upon the human serum lipid levels. *J Clin Invest* 43:1691, 1964.
348. Roberts SL, McMurry M, Connor WE: Does egg feeding (i.e. dietary cholesterol) affect plasma cholesterol levels in humans? The results of a double-blind study. *Am J Clin Nutr* 34:2092, 1981.
349. Gordon T, Fisher M, Ernst M, et al: Relation of diet to LDL cholesterol, VLDL cholesterol and plasma total cholesterol and triglycerides in white adults. *Atherosclerosis* 2:502, 1982.
350. Mensink RP, Katan MB: Effect of dietary trans fatty acids on high-density and low-density lipoprotein cholesterol levels in healthy subjects. *N Engl J Med* 323:439, 1990.
351. Mattson FH, Grundy SM: Comparison of effects of dietary saturated, monounsaturated and polyunsaturated fatty acids on plasma lipids and lipoproteins in men. *J Lipid Res* 26:194, 1985.
352. Neuringer MD, Connor WE: Omega-3 fatty acids in the brain and retina: Evidence for their essentiality. *Nutr Rev* 44:285, 1986.
353. Goodnight SH Jr, Harris WS, Connor WE, Illingworth DR: Polyun saturated fatty acids, hyperlipidemia and thrombosis. *Arteriosclerosis* 2:87, 1982.
354. Connor WE, Connor SL: Diet, atherosclerosis and fish oil, in Stollerman H, Siperstein MD (eds): *Advances in Internal Medicine*. Chicago, Year Book, 1989, p 139.
355. Harris WS, Connor WE, McMurry MP: The comparative reductions of the plasma lipids and lipoproteins by dietary polyunsaturated fats: Salmon oil versus vegetable oils. *Metabolism* 32:179, 1983.
356. Phillipson BE, Rothrock DW, Connor WE, Harris WS, Illingworth DR: The reduction of plasma lipids, lipoproteins, and apoproteins in hypertriglyceridemic patients by dietary fish oils. *N Engl J Med* 312:1210, 1985.
357. Burr ML, Gilbert JF, Holliday RM, Elwood PC, Fehly AM, et al: Effects of changes in fat, fish, and fibre intakes on death and myocardial infarction: Diet and reinfarction trial (DART). *Lancet* 2:757, 1989.
358. Harris WS, Connor WE, Alam N, Illingworth DR: The reduction of postprandial triglyceridemia in humans by dietary n-3 fatty acids. *J Lipid Res* 29:1451, 1988.
359. Weintraub MS, Zechner R, Brown A, Eisenberg S, Breslow JL: Dietary polyunsaturated fats of the w-6 and w-3 series reduce postprandial lipoprotein levels: Chronic and acute effects of fat saturation on postprandial lipoprotein metabolism. *J Clin Invest* 82:1884, 1988.
360. GISSI-Prevenzione Investigators: Dietary supplementation with n-3 polyunsaturated fatty acids and vitamin E after myocardial infarction: Results of the GISSI-Prevenzione trial. *Lancet* 354:447, 1999.
361. Ascherio A, Rimm EB, Stampfer MJ, Giovannucci EL, Willett WC: Dietary intake of marine n-3 fatty acids, fish intake and the risk of coronary artery disease among men. *N Engl J Med* 332:977, 1995.
362. Albert CM, Hennekens CH, O'Donnell CJ, et al: Fish consumption and risk of sudden death. *JAMA* 279:23, 1998.
363. Olefsky J, Reaven GM, Farquhar JW: Effects of weight reduction on obesity. *J Clin Invest* 53:64, 1974.
364. Schwartz RS, Brunzell JD: Increase of adipose tissue lipoprotein lipase activity with weight loss. *J Clin Invest* 67:1425, 1981.
365. McMurry MP, Cerqueira MT, Connor SL, Connor WE: Changes in lipid and lipoprotein levels and body weight in Tarahumara Indians after consumption of an affluent diet. *N Engl J Med* 325:1704, 1991.
366. Ullmann D, Connor WE, Hatcher LF, Connor SL, Flavell DP: Will a high carbohydrate, low-fat diet lower plasma lipids and lipoproteins without producing hypertriglyceridemia? *Arterioscler Thromb* 11:1059, 1991.
367. Anderson JW, Story L, Sieling B, Chen WJL, Petro MS, Story J: Hypocholesterolemic effects of oat-bran or bean intake for hypercholesterolemic men. *Am J Clin Nutr* 40:1146, 1984.
368. Malinow MR, Connor WE, McLaughlin P, Stafford C, Lin DS, et al: Sterol balance in Macaca fascicularis: Effects of alfalfa saponins. *J Clin Invest* 67:156, 1981.
369. Witzam JL, Steinbert D: Role of oxidized low density lipoprotein in atherogenesis. *J Lipid Res* 26:194, 1985.
370. Princen HMG, van Poppel G, Vogelezang C, Buytenhek R, Kok FJ: Supplementation with vitamin E but not B-carotene in vivo protects low density lipoprotein from lipid peroxidation in vitro: Effect of ciagarette smoking. *Arterioscler Thromb* 12:554, 1992.
371. Miettinen TA, Puska P, Gylling H, Vanhanen H, Vartianen E: Reduction of serum cholesterol with sitostanol-ester margarine in a mildly hypercholesterolemic population. *N Engl J Med* 333:1308, 1995.
372. Marmot M, Brunner E: Alcohol and cardiovascular disease—the status of the U shaped curve. *Br Med J* 303:565, 1991.
373. Hennekens CH, Rosner B, Cole DS: Daily alcohol consumption and coronary heart disease. *Am J Epidemiol* 107:196, 1978.
374. Hegsted DM, Ausman LM: Diet, alcohol and coronary heart disease in men. *J Nutr* 118:1184, 1988.
375. Suh IL, Shaten BJ, Cutler JA, Kuller LH: Alcohol use and mortality from coronary heart disease: The role of high-density lipoprotein cholesterol. *Ann Intern Med* 116:881, 1992.
376. Fry MM, Spector AA, Connor SL, et al: Intensification of hypertriglyceridemia by either alcohol or carbohydrate. *Am J Clin Nutr* 26:798, 1973.
377 Gaziano JM: Do antioxidants protect against cardiovascular disease? *Prev Cardiol* 1:59, 1999.
377B. Rimm EB, Stampfer MJ: Antioxidants for vascular disease. *Med Clin North Am* 84:239, 2000.
378. Zock PL, Katan MB, Merkus MP, van Dusseldorp M, Harryvan JL: Effect of a lipid-rich fraction from boiled coffee on serum cholesterol. *Lancet* 335:1235, 1990.
379. Fried RE, Levine DM, Kwiterovich PO, Diamond EL, Wilder LB, et al: The effect of filtered-coffee consumption on plasma lipid levels. *JAMA* 267:811, 1992.
380. Connor WE, Connor SL: The dietary prevention and treatment of coronary heart disease, in Connor WE, Bristow JD (eds): *Coronary Heart Disease: Prevention, Complications, and Treatment*. Philadelphia, Lippincott, 1985, pp 43–64.
381. Connor SL, Connor WE: *The New American Diet*. New York, Simon & Schuster, 1986.
382. Connor SL, Connor WE: *The New American Diet System*. New York, Simon & Schuster, 1991.
383. Connor WE, Connor SL: Dietary treatment of hyperlipidemia: Rationale and benefit. *Endocrinologist* 1:33, 1991.
384. Knuiman JT, Hermus RJJ, Hautvast JGAJ: Serum total and high density lipoprotein (HDL) cholesterol concentrations in rural and urban boys from 16 countries. *Atherosclerosis* 36:529, 1980.
385. Miller GJ, Miller NE: Dietary fat, HDL cholesterol, and coronary disease: One interpretation. *Lancet* 2:1270, 1982.
386. Brinton EA, Eisenberg S, Breslow JL: A low-fat diet decreases high density lipoprotein (HDL) cholesterol levels by decreasing HDL apolipoprotein transport rates. *J Clin Invest* 85:144, 1990.
387. Connor SL, Artand-Wild SM, Classick-Kohn CJ, Gustafson JR, Flavell DP, et al: The cholesterol/ç saturated fat index: An indication of the hypercholesterolemic and atherogenic potential of food. *Lancet* 1:1229, 1986.
388. Connor SL, Gustafson JR, Artand-Wild SM, Classick-Kohn CJ: The cholesterol-saturated fat index for coronary prevention: Background, use, and a comprehensive table of foods. *J Am Diet Assoc* 89:807, 1989.
389. Connor SL, Gustafson JR, Sexton G, Becker N, Artand-Wild SM, Connor WE: The Diet Habit Survey: A new method of dietary as-

sessment that relates to plasma cholesterol changes. *J Am Diet Assoc* 92:41, 1992.
390. Hegsted DM, McGandy RB, Myers ML, Stare FJ: Quantitative effects of dietary fat on serum cholesterol in man. *Am J Clin Nutr* 17:281, 1965.
391. The Lipid Research Clinics Program: The Lipid Research Clinic's Coronary Prevention Trial Results. *JAMA* 251:365, 1984.
392. Frick MH, Elo O, Haapa K, et al: Helsinki Heart Study: Primary Prevention Trial with gemfibrozil in middle-aged men with dyslipidemia: Safety and treatment, changes in risk factors and instance of coronary heart disease. *N Engl J Med* 317:1237, 1987.
393. Kane JP, Malloy MJ, Ports TA, Philips NR, Diehl JC, Havel RJ: Regression of coronary atherosclerosis during treatment of familial hypercholesterolemia with combined drug regimens. *JAMA* 264:3007, 1990.
394. Watts GF, Lewis B, Brunt JNH, Lewis ES, Coltart DJ, et al: Effects on coronary artery disease of lipid-lowering diet or diet plus Cholestyramine in the St. Thomas' Atherosclerosis Regression Study. *Lancet* 339:563, 1992.
395. Scandinavian Simvastatin Survival Study Group: Randomised trial of cholesterol lowering in 4444 patients with coronary heart disease; the Scandinavian Survival Study. *Lancet* 344:1383, 1994.
396. Sacks FM, Pfeffer MA, Moye LA, et al: The effect of pravastatin on coronary events after myocardial infarction in patients with average cholesterol levels. *N Engl J Med* 335:1001, 1996.
397. The Long-Term Intervention with Pravastatin in Ischaemic Disease (LIPID) Study Group: Prevention of cardiovascular events and death with pravastatin in patients with coronary heart disease and broad range of initial cholesterol levels. *N Engl J Med* 339:1349, 1998.
398. Shepherd J, Cobbe SM, Ford I, et al: For the West of Scotland Coronary Prevention Study Group. Prevention of coronary heart disease with pravastatin in men with hypercholesterolaemia. *N Engl J Med* 333:1301, 1995.
399. Downs GR, Clearfield M, Weiss S, et al: Primary prevention of acute coronary events with lovastatin in men and women with average cholesterol levels: Results of the AFCAPS/TexCAPS (Air Force/Texas Coronary Atherosclerosis Prevention Study). *JAMA* 279:1615, 1998.
400. Rubins H, Robins SJ, Collins D, et al: Gemfibrozil for the secondary prevention of coronary heart disease in men with low levels of high-density lipoprotein cholesterol. *N Engl J Med* 341:410, 1999.
401. Illingworth DR: Management of hypercholesterolemia. *Med Clin North Am* 84:23, 2000.
402. Shepherd J, Packard CJ, Bicker S, Laurie TDV, Morgan HG: Cholestyramine promotes receptor mediated low density lipoprotein catabolism. *N Engl J Med* 302:1029, 1980.
403. Kovanen PT, Bilheimer DW, Goldstein JL, Jaramillow JJ, Brown MS: Regulatory role for hepatic low density lipoprotein receptors *in vivo* in the dog. *Proc Natl Acad Sci USA* 78:194, 1981.
404. Dujovne CA, Krehbiel P, DeCoursey S, Jackson B, Chernoff SB, Pitteman A, Garty M: Probucol with Colestipol in the treatment of hypercholesterolemia. *Ann Intern Med* 100: 477, 1984.
405. Altschul R, Hoeffer A, Stephen JD: Influence of nicotinic acid on serum cholesterol in man. *Arch Biochem Biophys* 54:558, 1955.
406. Grundy SM, Mok HYI, Zack L, Berman M: The influence of nicotinic acid on metabolism of cholesterol and triglycerides in man. *J Lipid Res* 22:24, 1981.
407. Olsson AG, Carlson LA, Anggard E, Ciabattoni G: Prostacyclin production augmented in the short term by nicotinic acid. *Lancet* 2:565, 1983.
408. Knopp RH, Ginsberg J, Albers JJ, Hoff C, Ogilvie JT, et al: Contrasting effects of unmodified and time released forms of niacin on lipoproteins in hyperlipidemic subjects: Clues to mechanism of action of niacin. *Metabolism* 34:642, 1985.
409. Mullin GE, Greenson JK, Mitchell MC: Fulminant hepatic failure after ingestion of sustained release nicotinic acid. *Ann Intern Med* 111:253, 1989.
410. Tobert JA: Efficacy and long-term adverse effect pattern of lovastatin. *Am J Cardiol* 62:28J, 1988.
411. Grundy SM: HMG CoA reductase inhibitors for treatment of hypercholesterolemia. *N Engl J Med* 319:24, 1988.
411B. Tsugita Y, Kuroda M, Shimada Y: CS 514, a competitive inhibitor of 3-hydroxy-3-methylglutaryl-coenzyme reductase: Tissue selective inhibition of sterol synthesis and hypolipidemic effect in various animal species. *Biochim Biophys Acta* 877:50, 1986.
412. Alberts AW: Discovery, biochemistry and biology of lovastatin. *Am J Cardiol* 62:10J, 1988.
413. Koga T, Shimada Y, Kuroda M, Tsujita Y, Hasegawa K, Yamazaki M: Tissue selective inhibition of ch synthesis *in vivo* by pravastatin sodium: A 3-hydroxy-3-methylglutaryl-coenzyme reductase inhibitor. *Biochim Biophys Acta* 1045:115, 1990.
414. Raasch RH: Pravastatin sodium: A new HMG CoA reductase inhibitor. *DICP* 25:388, 1991.
415. Pappu AS, Illingworth DR, Bacon S: Reduction in plasma low density lipoprotein cholesterol in urine and mevalonic acid by lovastatin in patients with heterozygous familial hypercholesterolemia. *Metabolism* 38:542, 1989.
416. Hagemenas FC, Pappu AS, Illingworth DR: The effects of simvastatin on plasma lipoproteins and cholesterol homeostasis in patients with heterozygous familial hypercholesterolemia. *Eur J Clin Invest* 20:150, 1990.
417. Ginsberg HN, Le NA, Short MP, Ramakrishnan R, Desnick RJ: Suppression of apolipoprotein B production during treatment of cholesterol ester storage disease with lovastatin: Implication for regulation of apolipoprotein synthesis. *J Clin Invest* 80:1692, 1987.
418. Bradford RH, Shear CL, Chremos AN: Expanded clinical evaluation of lovastatin (EXCEL): Study results: I. Efficacy in modifying plasma lipoproteins and adverse event profile in 8,245 patients with moderate hypercholesterolemia. *Arch Intern Med* 151:43, 1991.
419. Stalenhoef AF, Mol MGT, Stuyt PM: Efficacy and tolerability of simvastatin. *Am J Med* 87:39S, 1989.
420. Illingworth DR, Bacon S, Larson KK: Long-term experience with HMG CoA reductase inhibitors in the therapy of hypercholesterolemia. *Atherosclerosis Revs* 18:161, 1988.
421. Maher VM, Pappu AS, Illingworth DR, Thompson GR: Plasma mevalonate response in lovastatin-related myopathy. *Lancet* 2:1098, 1989.
422. Pierce LR, Wysowski DK, Gross TP: Myopathy and rhabdomyolysis associated with lovastatin/gemfibrozil combination therapy. *JAMA* 264:71, 1990.
423. Prihoda JS, Pappu AS, Smith FE, Illingworth DR: The influence of simvastatin on adrenal corticosteroid production and urine mevalonate during adrenal corticotropin stimulation in patients with heterozygous familial hypercholesterolemia. *J Clin Endocrinol Metab* 72:567, 1991.
424. Everett DW, Chando TJ, Didonato GC, Signhvi SM, Pan HY, Weinstein SH: Biotransformation of pravastatin sodium in humans. *Drug Metab Dispos* 19:740, 1991.
425. Malini PL, Ambrosioni E, Rosiello G, Trimarco B: Simvastatin *versus* pravastatin: Efficacy and tolerability in patients with primary hypercholesterolemia. *Clin Ther* 13:500, 1991.
426. McTavish D, Sorkin EM: Pravastatin: A review of its pharmacological properties and therapeutic potential in hypercholesterolemia. *Drugs* 42:65, 1991.
427. Todd PA, Goa KL: Simvastatin: A review of its pharmacological properties and therapeutic potential in hypercholesterolemia. *Drugs* 40:583, 1990.
428. Illingworth DR: Use and abuse of lovastatin. *Endocrinologist* 1:323, 1991.
429. Illingworth DR: New horizons in combination drug therapy for hypercholesterolemia. *Cardiology* 76(Suppl 1):83, 1989.
430. Duell PB, Illingworth DR: Combination therapy with HMG CoA reductase inhibitors and gemfibrozil: Practical or perilous? *Heart Disease Stroke* 2:260, 1993.
431. Illingworth DR, Bacon S: Influence of lovastatin plus gemfibrozil on plasma lipids and lipoproteins in patients with heterozygous familial hypercholesterolemia. *Circulation* 79:590, 1989.
432. Nestel PJ, Billington T: Effects of probucol on low density lipoprotein removal and high density lipoprotein synthesis. *Atherosclerosis* 38:203, 1981.
433. Miettinen TA, Huttenen LK, Kusi T: Effect of probucol on the activity of post heparin plasma lipoprotein lipase and hepatic lipase. *Clin Chim Acta* 113:59, 1981.
434. Franceschini G, Sirtori M, Vaccarino V, Sirtori C: Mechanisms of LDL reduction after probucol: Changes in HDL subfractions and increased reverse cholesterol ester transfer. *Arteriosclerosis* 9:462, 1989.
435. Coronary Drug Project Research Group: Clofibrate and niacin in coronary artery disease. *JAMA* 231:360, 1975.

436. Committee of Principal Investigators: A cooperative trial in the primary prevention of eschemic heart disease using clofibrate. *Br Heart J* 40:1069, 1978.
437. Committee of Principal Investigators, WHO: A cooperative trial on primary prevention of eschemic heart disease using clofibrate to lower cholesterol: Final mortality follow-up. *Lancet* 2:600, 1984.
438. Vega GL, Grundy SM: Gemfibrozil therapy in primary hypertriglyceridemia associated with coronary artery disease: Effects on metabolism of low density lipoproteins. *JAMA* 253:2398, 1985.
439. Samuel P: Treatment of hypercholesterolemia with neomycin: A time for reappraisal. *N Engl J Med* 301:595, 1979.
440. Hoeg JM, Maher MB, Bou E, Zeck LA, Bailey KR, et al: Normalization of plasma lipoprotein concentrations in patients with Type II hyperlipoproteinemia by combined use of neomycin and niacin. *Circulation* 70:1004, 1984.
441. Bantle JP, Oppenheimer JH, Schwartz HL, Hunninghake DB, Probstielz JL, Hansom RL: TSH response to TRH in euthyroid hypercholesterolemic patients treated with graded doses of dextrothyroxin. *Metabolism* 30:63, 1981.
442. Glueck CJ: Effects of oxandrolone on plasma triglycerides and postheparin lipolytic activity in patients with Types III, IV and V familial hyperlipoproteinemia. *Metabolism* 20:691, 1971.
443. Glueck CJ, Levy RI, Fredrickson DS: Norethindrone acetate, postheparin lipolytic activity and plasma triglycerides in familial Type I, III, IV and V hyperlipoproteinemia: Studies in twenty-six patients and five normal patients. *Ann Intern Med* 75:343, 1971.
444. Coronary Drug Project: Findings leading to discontinuation of the 2.5 mg per day estrogen group. *JAMA* 226:652, 1973.
445. Hulley S, Grady D, Bush T, et al: Randomized trial of estrogen plus progestin for secondary prevention of coronary heart disease in postmenopausal women. *JAMA* 280:605, 1988.
446. Herrington DM, Reboussin DM, Brosnihan KB, et al: Effects of estrogen replacement on the progression of coronary-artery atherosclerosis. *N Engl J Med* 343:522, 2000.
447. Hollander PA, Elbein SC, Hirsch IB, et al: Role of orlistat in the treatment of obese patients with type 2 diabetes. *Diabetes Care* 21:1288, 1998.
448. Fattore PC, Sirtori CR: Nicotinic acid and derivatives. *Curr Opin Lipidol* 2:43, 1991.
449. Series JJ, Caslake MJ, Kilday C, Crookshank A, Demant T, et al: Influence of etofibrate on low density lipoprotein metabolism. *Atherosclerosis* 69:233, 1988.
450. Sirtori CR, Gianfranceschi G, Sirtori M, Bernini F, Descovich GC, Montaguti V, Fuccella L, Musatti M: Reduced triglyceridemia and increased high density lipoprotein cholesterol levels after treatment with acipimox, a new inhibitor of lipolysis. *Atherosclerosis* 38:267, 1981.
451. Bergstrom JD: The Zaragozic acids: Pontent natural product derived inhibitors of squalene synthesis and cholesterol synthesis. *Proc XIth Int Symp on Drugs Affecting Lipid Metabolism*, Florence, Italy, 120, 1992.
452. McCarthy AD, Fitzgerald BJ, Hutson JL, Motteram JM, Sappora M, Snowden MA, Watson NS, Williams RJ, Wright C: Squalene synthesis inhibition: Effects of a novel natural product on cholesterol metabolism. *Proc XIth Int Symp on Drugs Affecting Lipid Metabolism*, Florence, Italy, 120, 1992.
453. Suckling KE: Drugs working on the intestine. *Curr Opin Lipidol* 2:31, 1991.
454. Harris WS, Dujovne CA, vonBergman K, Neal J, Akester J, Windsor SL, Greene D, Look Z: Effects of the ACAT inhibitor CL277082 on cholesterol metabolism in humans. *Clin Pharmacol Ther* 48:189, 1990.
455. Forman MB, Baker SG, Many CJ: Treatment of homozygous familial hypercholesterolemia with portacaval shunt. *Atherosclerosis* 41:349, 1982.
456. Lerner DJ, Kannel WB: Patterns of coronary heart disease morbidity and mortality in the sexes: A 26-year follow-up of the Framingham population. *Am Heart J* 111:383, 1986.
457. Erikson M, Bergman L, Rudling M, Henriksson T, Angelin B: Effect of estrogen on low density lipoprotein metabolism in males: Short-term and long-term studies during hormonal treatment of prostatic carcinoma. *J Clin Invest* 84:802, 1989.
458. Crouse JR III: Gender lipoproteins, diet and cardiovascular risk: Sauce for the goose may not be sauce for the gander. *Lancet* 1:318, 1989.
459. Castelli WP: Cardiovascular disease in women. *Am J Obstet Gynecol* 158:1553, 1988.
460. Castelli WP: The triglycerides issue: A view from Framingham. *Am Heart J* 112:432, 1986.
461. Denke MA, Grundy SM: Hypercholesterolemia in elderly persons: Resolving the treatment dilema. *Ann Intern Med* 112:780, 1990.
462. Bilheimer DW: Clinical considerations regarding treatment of hypercholesterolemia in the elderly. *Atherosclerosis* 91:S35, 1991.
463. West RJ, Lloyd JK, Leonard JV: Long-term follow-up of children with familial hypercholesterolemia treated with cholestyramine. *Lancet* 2:873, 1980.
464. Stein EA, Illingworth DR, Kwiterovich PO, et al: Efficacy and safety of lovastatin in adolescent males with heterozygous familial hypercholesterolemia. *JAMA* 281:137, 1999.
465. Bachorik PS, Wood PDS: Laboratory considerations in diagnosis and management of hyperlipidemia, in Rifkind BM, Levy RI (eds): *Hyperlipidemia: Diagnosis and Therapy*. New York, Grune & Stratton, 1977, p 41.
466. Lipid Research Clinics Program: *Manual of Laboratory Operations: vol 1: Lipid and Lipoprotein Analysis*. Bethesda, Md., NIH, DHEW Publication (NIH) 75-628, 1974.
467. Brown MS, Kovanen PT, Goldstein JL, Eeckles R, Vandenberg K, et al: Prenatal diagnosis of homozygous familial hypercholesterolemia. *Lancet* 1:526, 1978.
468. Russell DW, Esser V, Hobbs HH: Molecular basis of familial hypercholesterolemia. *Arteriosclerosis* 9:8, 1989.
469. Ridker PM, Glynn RJ, Hennekens CH: C-reactive protein adds to the predictive value of total and HDL cholesterol in determining the risk of first myocardial infarction. *Circulation*, 97:2007, 1998.
470. Ridker PM, Buring JE, Shih J, Matias M, Hennekens CH: Prospective study of C-reactive protein and the risk of future cardiovascular events among apparently healthy women. *Circulation* 98:731, 1998.
471. Gerhard GT, Duell PB: Homocysteine and atherosclerosis. *Curr Opin Lipidol* 10:417, 1999.
472. Duell PB, Malinow MR: Homocysteine as a risk factor for coronary artery disease, in Robinson K (ed): *Homocysteine and vascular disease*. Kluwer Academic Publishers, Dordecht,The Netherlands 2000, pp 173–202.
473. Grundy SM, Vega GL: Causes of high blood cholesterol. *Circulation* 81:412, 1990.
474. Betteridge DJ, Illingworth DR, Shepherd J (eds): *Lipoproteins in Health and Disease*. Arnold, London, Great Britain, 1999.
475. Levy RI, Fredrickson DS, Shulman R: Dietary and drug treatment of primary hyperlipoproteinemia. *Ann Intern Med* 77:267, 1972.
476. Meinertz H: Effects of gemfibrozil on plasma lipoproteins in patients with Type II hyperlipoproteinemia and familial hypercholesterolemia, in *Royal Soc Med Int Congress and Symposium Series: Further Progress with Gemfibrozil*. London, Royal Soceity of Medicine, 1987, vol 15.
477. Eisenberg S, Gavish D, Oschry Y, Fainaru M, Deckelbaum RJ: Abnormalilites in very low, low and high density lipoproteins in hypertriglyceridemia: Reversal toward normal with bezafribrate treatment. *J Clin Invest* 74:470, 1984.
478. Illingworth DR, Olson DG, Cook SF, Wendell H, Connor WE: Ciprofibrate in the therapy of Type II hypercholesterolemia: A double-blind trial. *Atherosclerosis* 44:211, 1982.
479. Rouffy J, Chanu B, Bakir R: Comparative evalution of the effects of Ciprofibrate and fenofibrate on lipids, lipoproteins and apoproteins A and B. *Atherosclerosis* 54:273, 1985.
480. Weisweiler P, Merck W, Janetschek P, Schwandt P: Effect of fenofibrate on serum lipoproteins in subjects with familial hypercholesterolemia and combined hyperlipidemia. *Atherosclerosis* 53:321, 1984.

PART VII

Calcium and Bone Metabolism

CHAPTER 22

Mineral Metabolism

Jan M. Bruder

Theresa A. Guise

Gregory R. Mundy

CELLULAR AND EXTRACELLULAR CALCIUM METABOLISM

The divalent calcium cation (Ca^{2+}; ionized calcium) serves an important role in the physiology and metabolism of virtually all living things from unicellular organisms to mammals. Extracellular levels of calcium in humans and other mammals are tightly regulated within a narrow physiologic range to ensure appropriate excitation-contraction of the heart, expression of bioactivity for a number of hormones, and normal functioning of muscles, nerves, platelets, neutrophils, and several coagulation factors. The central physiologic role of calcium derives mechanistically from its actions as a cofactor for certain enzymes and as an electrochemical agent involved in membrane activation, permeability, or stabilization and from its ability to serve as an intracellular second messenger. Calcium also plays a role in cell growth and division and in cellular secretion for exocrine function, endocrine function, and neurotransmitter release, when the ion bonds to the membrane of preformed secretory vesicles and promotes fusion with the plasma membrane or stimulates the intracellular microtubule/microfilament system.

Within the cell, calcium concentrations are integrated as a result of a number of complex and interacting component calcium fluxes created by the activity of several plasma membrane "pumps" or "exchangers" (Fig. 22-1).

Furthermore, the activity of these transmembrane macromolecules that transport calcium can be modulated by extracellular calcium levels, membrane electric activity or potential gradient, physical distension ("stretch"), or hormonal activity.

When cells are bathed in extracellular fluid (ECF) containing calcium ion at a concentration of 10^{-6} *M*, the concentration of calcium ions in cytosol is 10^{-6} *M*.[1] Most (90 to 99 percent) of the intracellular calcium is stored within mitochondria or in microsomes, where it is largely complexed to phosphate. From these locales, it leaks into the cytosol. The low intracellular calcium level is preserved by calcium pumps (analogous to those present on the plasma membrane) that return calcium to the intramitochondrial or intramicrosomal space in an energy-dependent fashion or transport calcium out of the cell (Fig. 22-1). However, the levels of intracellular calcium can be self-modulating. Because calcium can serve as an intracellular signal, or "second messenger,"[1] calcium is directly linked to calmodulin function and the inositol polyphosphate–protein kinase C pathway. In many cases, several second messengers interact to produce an integrated intracellular calcium response.

It is the ionized or "free" calcium that is metabolically active and critical for normal physiologic function; hence, it is the form of calcium that is regulated. In the ECF, calcium is present in a free form, which accounts for 50 percent of ECF calcium, while 40 percent is bound reversibly to proteins and 10 percent is complexed with citrate and phosphate.[2,3] About 90 percent of the protein-bound calcium is associated with albumin, bound to its carboxyl groups in a pH-dependent manner. Because the amount of calcium present in the blood and ECF represents 1 percent of the total calcium in the body,[4–6] only 0.5 percent of total body calcium is ionized and plays the critical role in physiologic functions described previously (Fig. 22-2). The picture is complicated by the fact that calcium normally circulates at a concentration approaching its saturation point—the solubility product constant for calcium phosphate [$K_{sp} = (Ca^{2+})(PO_4^{-})$]—and this accounts for some of the major clinical problems encountered in patients with hypercalcemia, such as soft tissue calcification and kidney stones.

The maintenance of blood calcium levels within the narrow range dictated by normal physiology requires the action of at least two hormones acting on three organs. Parathyroid hormone (PTH, a polypeptide hormone) and vitamin D (a steroid hormone) act on bone, kidney, and gut to ensure calcium homeostasis and close regulation of extracellular calcium levels. In humans and other mammals, this hormonal system is designed to defend the organism against the major metabolic threat of hypocalcemia. In fish, calcitonin acts to lower blood calcium levels and protects against hypercalcemia. Therefore, it follows logically that this regulatory system did not appear in evolution until the time when animals left the calcium-rich sea.

Although the absolute quantity of ionized calcium that is tightly regulated is small, calcium flux at various organs over time is extremely large in comparison (Fig. 22-3). The kidney filters 5 to 7 g of calcium per day, a quantity in large excess over the total amount present at any time in the circulation and ECF. Although the kidney reabsorbs 96 to 98 percent of the calcium it filters, it cannot recover 100 percent of this calcium even when it is maximally stimulated. In addition, there is an obligatory loss of calcium from sweat and from the gut as a result of gastrointestinal secretions and the sloughing of lining cells of the gastrointestinal tract into its lumen.

Bone, which contains 99 percent of the calcium present in the body, not only plays a structural role for the organism, but also acts as an internal reservoir for calcium. Calcium stored in the skeleton can be used as a defense against hypocalcemia if the dietary intake

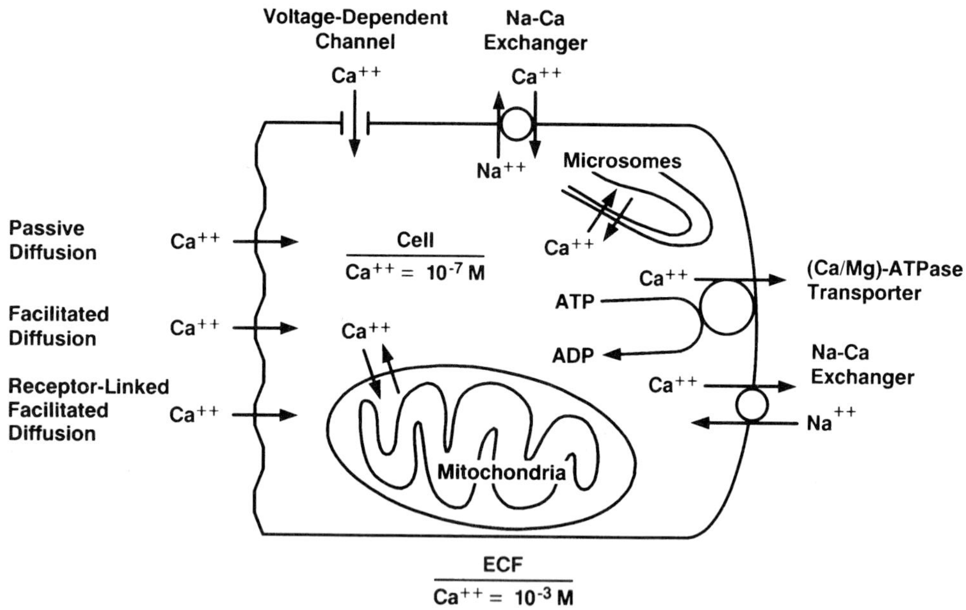

FIGURE 22-1. Schematic representation of calcium flux across the plasma membrane of cells and between the cytoplasm and organelles.

of calcium is deficient for a short period or chronically. A substantial amount of calcium can be rapidly mobilized from bone. In fact, quantities of calcium comparable to the total amount present in the ECF can be released within hours. The reservoir is also large enough to sustain normal physiologic function without the development of hypocalcemia for months to years.

Hormonal regulation of calcium by PTH and vitamin D plays two roles: tight regulation of calcium levels in the ECF and maintenance of long-term calcium balance. PTH is responsible for the minute-to-minute regulation of ECF calcium levels. It acts on the kidney to stimulate calcium reabsorption and on bone to stimulate bone resorption and the release of calcium stores into the ECF. However, reliance of the organism on PTH alone for the maintenance of normocalcemia without adequate calcium intake can lead in the long term only to negative calcium balance (particularly from bone) because of the obligatory calcium losses. This loss of bone mineral ultimately compromises the biomechanical strength of bone.

Therefore, the struggle for calcium homeostasis ultimately is won or lost at the level of the gut, which is the point of entry for

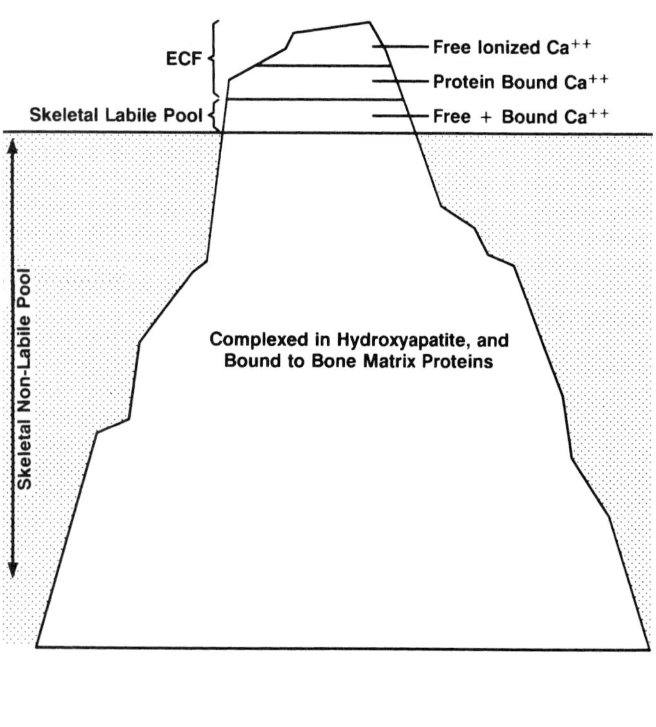

FIGURE 22-2. Illustration of relative amounts of calcium within the total body calcium pool.

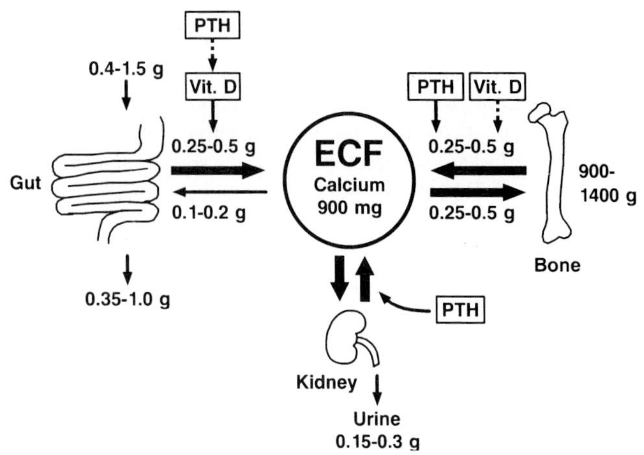

FIGURE 22-3. Schematic representation of calcium flux and balance in a normal human. Arrows indicate direction of movement of calcium between the gut, bone, kidneys, and extracellular fluid (ECF). Modulation of flux by vitamin D (Vit. D) or parathyroid hormone (PTH) is shown. Solid arrows depict a direct effect; dashed arrows depict an indirect effect. The numeric values indicate quantities of elemental calcium stored or transferred in a 24-h period. Thickness of arrows indicates relative magnitude of flux.

calcium to replace the obligatory losses described. The principal hormone responsible for enhancing the absorption of dietary calcium is vitamin D.[7–9] Its effects on the absorption of dietary calcium from the gut are discussed in the Vitamin D section. Vitamin D levels are determined in part by the circulating levels of PTH, which act on an enzyme in the kidney, 1α-hydroxylase, to convert 25-hydroxyvitamin D_3 into the active form of the hormone, 1α,25-$(OH)_2D_3$. The average American diet contains 0.4 to 1.5 g of calcium per day (1 quart of milk contains approximately 1 g of calcium). However, the dietary intake of many individuals, particularly the elderly, falls well below this amount (Fig. 22-3). In some countries, such as Japan, the majority of elderly people have diets frankly deficient in calcium. Under these circumstances, even maximally stimulated and efficient calcium absorption cannot offset the cumulative obligatory losses.

PARATHYROID HORMONE

Anatomy and Embryology of the Parathyroid Glands Anatomy

Anatomy

The four parathyroid glands weigh an average of 40 mg each. Although they are usually found in two symmetric pairs in proximity to the thyroid, their adult location is variable. The two superior glands are usually found near the posterior aspect of the thyroid capsule; the inferior glands are most often located near the inferior thyroid margin. The position of the inferior glands is more variable than that of the superior glands, and they are sometimes found within or near the thymus in the anterior superior mediastinum. Interthyroidal and retroesophageal glands also occur. Five percent of the population has only three parathyroid glands. A supernumerary fifth gland is found in 12 to 15 percent of individuals, and six or more parathyroids are occasionally present. The variability of parathyroid number and position are important features of their surgical anatomy.[10]

The parathyroids are composed of epithelial cells and stromal fat. The predominant epithelial element is the chief cell, with clear cytoplasm and a slightly hyperchromatic nucleus. The other epithelial component is the oxyphil cell, which is slightly larger than the chief cell, with eosinophilic granular cytoplasm and a small, extremely hyperchromatic nucleus. Both cell types contain PTH, and it is not known whether they have separate secretory regulation.

Embryology

The two pairs of parathyroid glands arise from the dorsal endoderm of the branchial pouches at the end of the sixth week of gestation. The superior parathyroid glands (parathyroids 4) are derived from the fourth, and the inferior glands (parathyroids 3) from the third branchial pouch. The parathyroids 4 migrate a short distance caudad to assume their superior position; the inferior glands migrate farther caudad with the thymus, ordinarily separating from the thymus at the inferior thyroid margin. If they do not separate, they may be found in association with the thymus or its fat pad in the upper anterior mediastinum.

Biosynthesis, Processing, and Secretion of Parathyroid Hormone Physiology of Parathyroid Hormone Secretion

Physiology of Parathyroid Hormone Secretion

Consistent with the function of PTH as an acute regulator of extracellular calcium homeostasis, the secretion of the hormone is under negative feedback regulation by the concentration of ionized calcium in the extracellular fluid. The dynamics of PTH secretion in normal humans are shown in Fig. 22-4.[11] To maintain the serum concentration of calcium within the very narrow normal range, the secretion of PTH must be exquisitely sensitive to the calcium concentration. Thus, the relation of serum ionized calcium to serum PTH levels (Fig. 22-4) is steeply sigmoidal. The steep portion of the curve corresponds precisely to the normal range of ionized calcium, so that the level of PTH is maximal at the lower limit and minimal at the upper limit of the normal range—precisely the desirable relation to maximize the sensitivity of these glands to small changes in ionized calcium and ensure maintenance of the normal calcium level by PTH. Small changes in ionized calcium produce large changes in PTH secretion. The midpoint or set point of this parathyroid function curve determines the concentration at which extracellular calcium is set in vivo. The calcium "sensor" responsible for detecting extracellular levels of calcium and transmitting an intracellular signal to parathyroid cells is a G protein-coupled seven-transmembrane spanning receptor. Its role in the physiology and pathophysiology of PTH secretion is discussed later.[12]

Note that the PTH level is still detectable in the face of markedly elevated ionized calcium concentrations. The nonsuppressible secretion of PTH from suppressed glands may play a role in the development of primary hyperparathyroidism and in secondary hyperparathyroidism in chronic renal failure and after renal transplantation. The regulation of PTH secretion by calcium

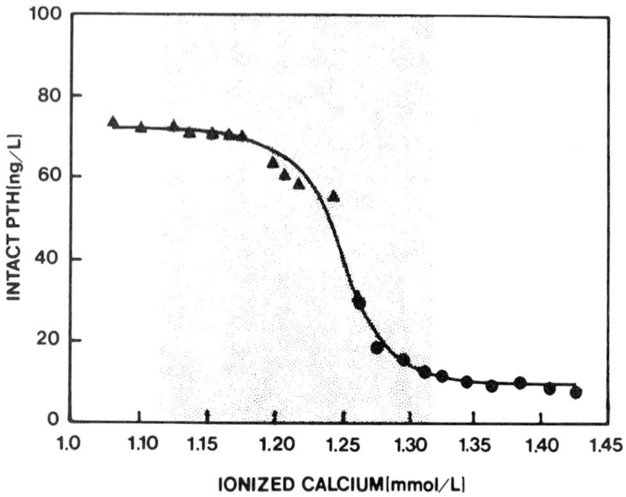

FIGURE 22-4. The relation between the serum ionized calcium level and the simultaneous serum concentration of intact PTH in normal humans. The serum calcium concentration was altered by the infusion of calcium (closed circles) or citrate (closed triangles). Parathyroid sensitivity to changes in serum calcium is maximal within the normal range (the shaded area). Low concentrations of PTH persist in the face of hypercalcemia. *(Modified from Conlin PR, Fajtova VT, Mortensen RM, Brown EM,[11] by permission of Journal of Clinical Endocrinology and Metabolism.)*

has also been studied in vitro, using dispersed human parathyroid cells, and similar results have been obtained.[13] As will be discussed in detail later, other factors also influence the secretion of PTH. However, the only physiologically significant regulator of minute-to-minute changes in PTH secretion is the ionized calcium concentration.

Like many other hormones, PTH is secreted episodically, and PTH levels in blood display both a circadian rhythm with a peak at midnight, and episodic pulses with a mean interpulse interval of 60 min.[14] The episodic nature of PTH secretion is preserved in primary hyperparathyroidism. In postmenopausal females, PTH is secreted in a fashion similar to young adults with significant tonic secretion and PTH pulse occurrence averaging every 18–19 minutes. Pulsatile PTH accounted for 25 percent of the total and no differences in such secretion were noted in women with low bone mineral density or with estrogen deficiency compared with young normals.[15]

Chemistry, Biosynthesis, and Processing of Parathyroid Hormone

Parathyroid hormone is an 84-amino acid linear peptide with a molecular weight of 9,300 (Fig. 22-5). Its sequence is strongly conserved among mammalian species. Although most of the recognized biological actions of the intact hormone are encoded by the amino-terminal amino acids 1-34, there is accumulating evidence that the mid- and carboxyl-terminal regions may have distinct biologic properties.[16–19]

The human PTH gene is located on the short arm of chromosome 11. It contains three exons: The first encodes a short 5′ untranslated domain, the second a prepro region consisting of a 29-amino acid precursor sequence, and the third the last two amino acids of pro-PTH, the mature 84-amino acid peptide, and the 3′ untranslated domain.[18] After nuclear processing of primary transcripts to remove introns, PTH mRNA is transported into the cytoplasm, where the coding sequence is translated by the ribosomal machinery into the 115-amino acid precursor prepro-PTH.[20] Nascent peptide chains emerging from the ribosome are guided through the membrane of the rough endoplasmic reticulum by a

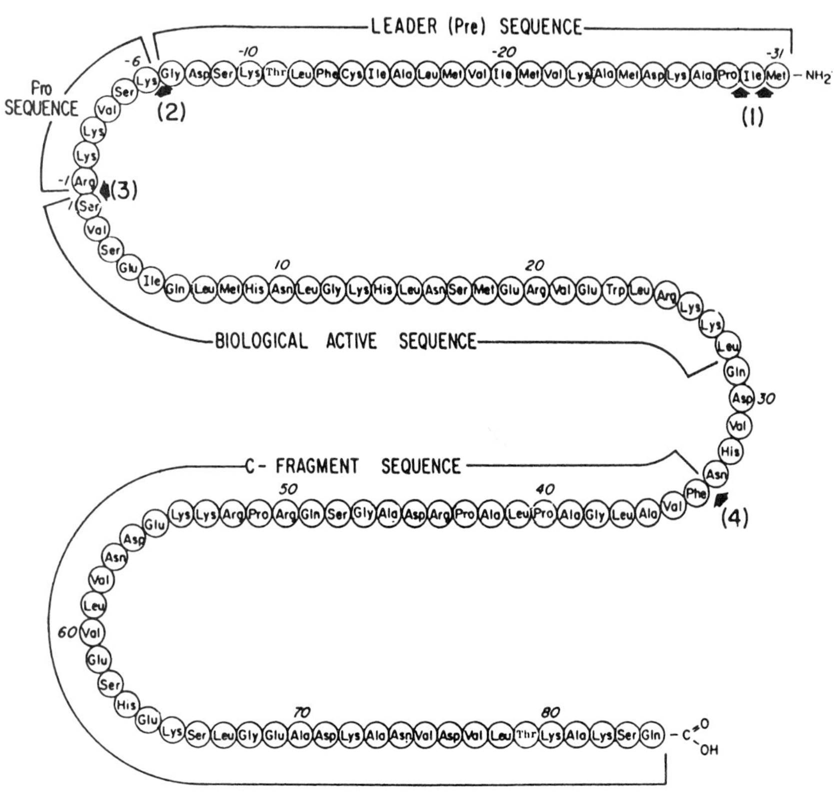

FIGURE 22-5. Primary structure of human preparathyroid hormone. The arrows indicate sites of specific cleavages which occur in the sequence of biosynthesis and peripheral metabolism of the hormone. The biologically active sequence is enclosed in the center of the molecule.

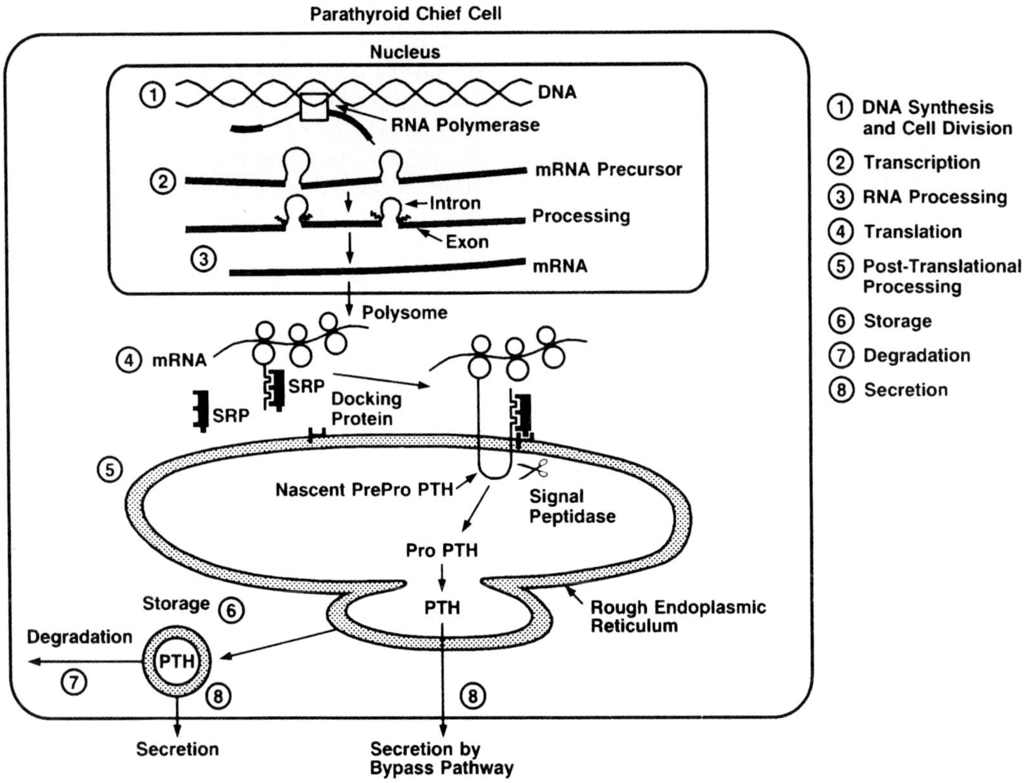

FIGURE 22-6. Schematic representation of major points at which the level of PTH biosynthesis and secretion appears to be regulated. Each point represents a potential site of dysfunction in hyperparathyroid disorders. *(Reprinted with permission from Lynn H. Caporale and Michael Rosenblatt, Parathyroid hormone secretion: Molecular events and regulation, Contributions to Nephrology 50:73–95, 1986.)*

signal recognition particle that recognizes the "signal" sequence in the prepro region of the hormone precursor and guides it to a docking protein on the outer surface of the endoplasmic reticulum. As the signal peptide sequence emerges into the lumen of the endoplasmic reticulum, it is cleaved at position −6/−7, leaving the 90-amino acid pro-PTH (Fig. 22-6). The process of binding of nascent chains by the signal recognition particle, docking, insertion, and cleavage of the prepro sequence occurs cotranslationally and so rapidly that nascent chains containing the prepro sequence of PTH are barely detectable unless translation is carried out in vitro in the absence of endoplasmic reticulum.[20,21]

The sequence of prepro-PTH has many of the general features of signal sequences that direct secretory proteins into the lumen of the endoplasmic reticulum[22]: at least one positively charged residue near the amino terminus, an uninterrupted segment of hydrophobic or neutral amino acids, and small amino acids just proximal to and two residues removed from the cleavage site (i.e., positions −7 and −9). A synthetic fragment of the prepro sequence from PTH can block the processing of secretion illustrating the relative interchangeability of signal sequences and suggesting that many, if not all, secreted proteins utilize the same processing apparatus for intracellular transport. The sequence features of prepro-PTH required for efficient processing have been studied by expressing mutants of the prepro region in cell-free systems or in intact cells. Deletion of the first six amino acids result in translation initiation at *met*,[25] but the truncated peptide is processed normally. In contrast, the deletion of 10 or more residues, including portions of the hydrophobic core, results in peptides that do not enter the secretory pathway and are degraded rapidly.[23,24] Thus, the first six residues of prepro-PTH are relatively dispensable, the hydrophobic core is required for entry into the endoplasmic reticulum, and cleavage of the signal sequence is required for secretion. Along these lines, the signal peptidase—the enzyme that cleaves the signal region from the nascent protein—has an unusually large recognition sequence, requiring 11 amino acids of the PTH signal sequence for recognition as substrate. Another unusual feature of the enzyme is that conformation (secondary structure) appears more critical for recognition than does the primary amino acid sequence per se. A spontaneous mutation that disrupts the hydrophobic core of the signal sequence and blocks translocation is associated with familial hypoparathyroidism,[25] as discussed later.

In contrast to the evanescent existence of prepro-PTH, pro-PTH has a life span of about 15 min in pulse-chase studies and is converted to mature PTH coincidentally with arrival in the Golgi apparatus.[20,26] The Golgi cleavage enzyme presumably recognizes the dibasic sequence lys^{-2}-arg^{-1}; similar dibasic sequences are present at the cleavage sites of other prohormones, e.g., insulin. However, the processing of pro-PTH is more efficient than insulin processing because pro-PTH, unlike proinsulin, is not secreted.[27] The functional significance of the two-step cleavage of prepro-PTH is not fully understood, but mutational analysis suggests that the hexapeptide pro-PTH sequence is necessary for the correct transport and cleavage of prepro-PTH. Mutants in which the hydrophobic core is intact but the pro sequence is deleted are translocated and cleaved inefficiently. In such mutants, both the correct cleavage site and an incorrect one in the signal sequence are utilized[26]; only the cleaved forms are secreted. Because a normal amino terminus of mature PTH is critical for its biological activity, the pro sequence may have evolved as an "adaptor," first assuring correct cleavage of prepro-PTH and then being cleaved off itself.

After its biogenesis in the Golgi apparatus, mature PTH is packaged in dense secretory granules like those of other endocrine cells and stored to await secretion. It has been estimated that glandular stores of PTH are sufficient to maintain maximal rates of secretion for about 1.5 h.[21] PTH is stored and cosecreted with the peptide chromogranin A (parathyroid secretory protein-1).[29] The significance of the presence of chromogranin A as a passenger in secretory granules of parathyroid and other endocrine cells is unknown. It appears that 10 to 20 percent of PTH is postranslationally modified by phosphorylation on serine residues near the amino terminus before secretion[30]; this is also of unknown significance.

Regulation of PTH Synthesis

Acutely, extracellular calcium regulates the secretion of preformed PTH rather than the synthesis of PTH. However, over a period of hours to days, increases in extracellular calcium inhibit the transcription of the PTH gene.[31] The converse is also true: hypocalcemia also increases the transcription of the PTH gene.[32] The increase in the synthesis of PTH is appropriate in the face of relatively small glandular stores of the hormone, serving to maintain high secretory rates during sustained hypocalcemia.

The synthesis of PTH is also regulated by vitamin D. Metabolites of vitamin D, most notably 1,25-dihydroxyvitamin D3, play an important role in the long-term regulation of parathyroid function by affecting PTH secretion, gene expression as by controlling expression of the calcium-sensing receptor and the vitamin D receptor. High levels of 1α,25-dihydroxyvitamin D inhibit transcription of the PTH gene,[33] providing yet another short loop of negative feedback in the remarkably complex interrelations of PTH and vitamin D in the control of calcium homeostasis. This effect occurs within 2 h and involves a vitamin D response element within the first 690 base pairs upstream of the cap site of the PTH gene.[34] The inhibition of PTH gene expression by 1α,25-dihydroxyvitamin D has been observed both in dispersed parathyroid cells in vitro and with the administration of vitamin D analogs in vivo under conditions in which the serum calcium does not perceptibly change.[33] Whether or not vitamin D plays a physiologic role in the minute-to-minute regulation of PTH secretion, the effect of 1α,25-dihydroxyvitamin D is relevant therapeutically in the treatment of secondary hyperparathyroidism in chronic renal failure.

Phosphate stimulates PTH secretion and proliferation of parathyroid cells, likely through its effects on calcium.[35,36] This action of hyperphosphatemia could potentially contribute to the secondary hyperparathyroidism of end stage renal failure.[37] Hypo- and hyperphosphatemia decrease and increase, respectively, mRNA for PTH through a mechanism independent of changes in extracellular calcium or 1,25-dihydroxyvitamin D3.

Cellular Regulation of PTH Secretion by Calcium

The parathyroid cell is unique in its ability to sense and respond to changes in the ambient calcium concentration. For PTH to be secreted in response to hypocalcemia, it must function differently from other secretory cells, which require calcium for stimulus-secretion coupling and are paralyzed by exposure to low calcium concentrations. The regulation of PTH secretion by extracellular calcium has been studied in collagenase-dispersed parathyroid cells from bovine and human glands.[12,13] Like other mammalian cells, the parathyroid cell maintains a large [Ca^{2+}] gradient between the extracellular fluid (free [Ca^{2+}] about 10^{-3} *M*) and its cytosol (free [Ca^{+}] about 10^{-7} *M*) Unlike most other cells, in which the cytosolic calcium concentration is well buffered against changes in extracellular calcium, the parathyroid cell responds to acute increases in extracellular calcium with a transient rise in cytoplasmic free calcium[13,38]; this transient rise is followed by a sustained plateau. Most of the calcium entering the cytosolic compartment in response to increased extracellular calcium appears to originate from intracellular stores. However, the sustained increase in intracellular calcium that follows is dependent on the presence of extracellular calcium. Experiments using the calcium ionophore ionomycin suggest that the regulation of cytoplasmic free calcium is important in the regulation of PTH secretion by extracellular calcium. Intracellular calcium transients induced by ionomycin treatment are associated with inhibition of PTH secretion.[38] It is possible that other potential cellular second messengers (cAMP, protein kinase C) also play a role in the inhibition of PTH secretion by calcium.[12,13,39]

A major advance in the field of calcium metabolism has been the discovery of an extracellular calcium-sensing receptor on the surface of parathyroid cells.[12] The receptor contains seven transmembrane-spanning domains and belongs to the superfamily of G protein-coupled receptors (Fig. 22-7). It has a molecular mass of approximately 120 kDa and shares limited homology with metabotropic glutamate receptors. It possesses a large extracellular domain containing clusters of amino acids known to play a role in sensing extracellular calcium. The receptor is expressed on the surface of all tissues involved in calcium homeostasis: parathyroid cells, calcitonin-secreting parafollicular C-cells of the thyroid, proximal renal tubular and distal collecting tubule cells, bone (osteoblasts and cells of the monocyte macrophage lineage), and intestinal cells where calcium is absorbed. In addition, the receptor is also expressed in cells of the kidney, intestine, and bone that are not involved in calcium homeostasis. For example, the calcium-sensing receptor is expressed in the squamous epithelial cells of the esophagus, the surface cells of the gastric mucosa, and enteric nervous system. Its expression in the apical membrane of the inner medullary collecting duct of the kidney suggests that the calcium-sensing receptor contributes to the known inhibitory effect of hypercalcemia on vasopressin-stimulated water reabsorption. In the bone marrow, the calcium-sensing receptor is expressed in red blood cell precursors, megakaryocytes and monocytes. Other tissues that express this receptor include epithelial cells of breast ducts, keratinocytes, the central nervous system, and lens epithelial cells.[40] The role of the calcium-sensing receptor in these tissues remains to be determined. It has a relatively low (millimolar) affinity for calcium, consistent with its role in regulating PTH secretion.[40,41]

The intracellular domains of the calcium-sensing receptor couple the activated receptor to stimulation of guanine nucleotide regulatory or G proteins. The receptor activates phospholipase C and inhibits adenylate cyclase via $G_{9/11}$ and G_1 families of G proteins, respectively.[40] It also activates phospholipases A_2 and D[42] as well as the mitogen-activated protein (MAP) kinase pathway.[43]

The evidence that convincingly supports the role of the calcium-sensing receptor in regulating PTH secretion is the alterations in extracellular calcium-regulated PTH release observed in

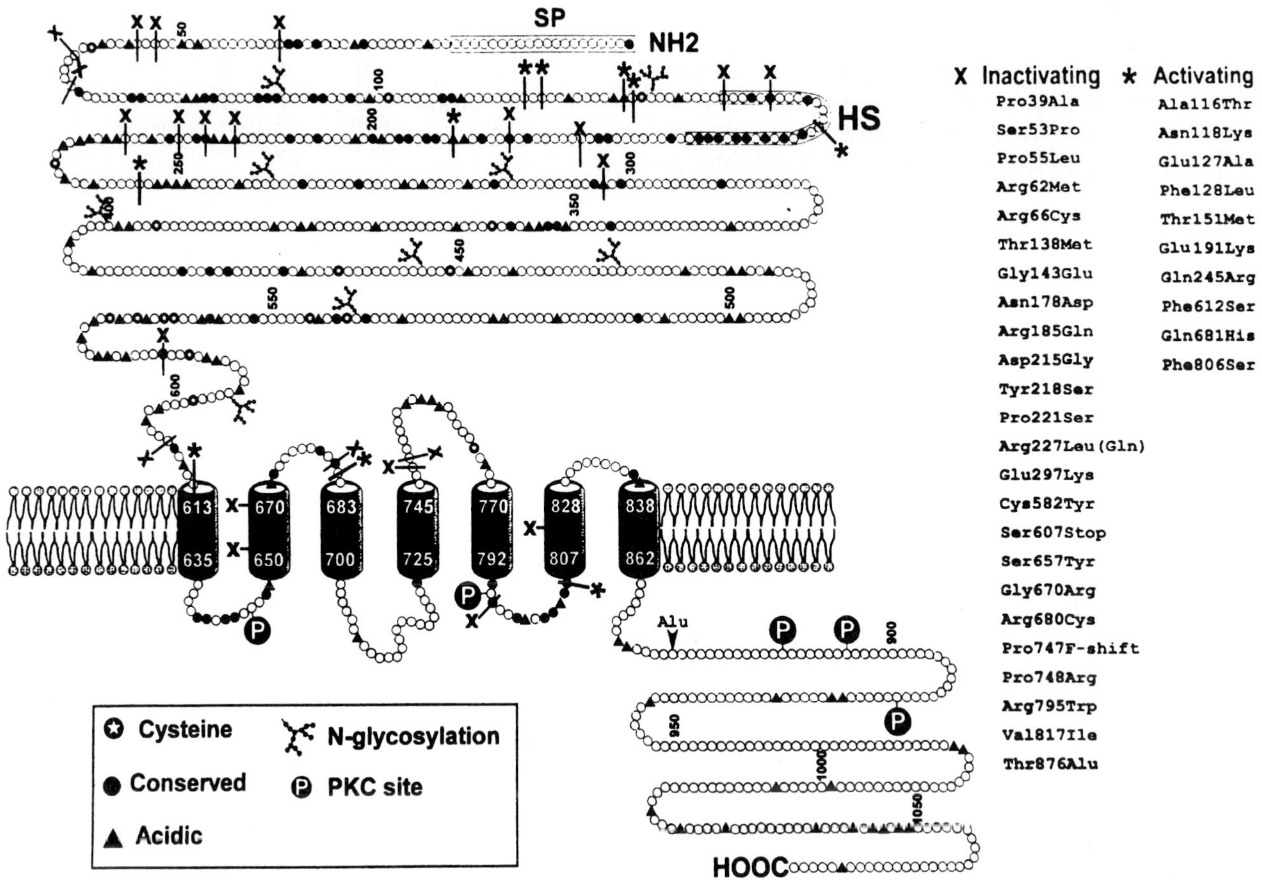

FIGURE 22-7. Predicted topology of the calcium-sensing receptor cloned from human parathyroid. SP = signal peptide; HS = hydrophobic segment. Indicated are missense and nonsense mutations that cause either familial hypocalciuric hypercalcemia or autosomal dominant hypocalcemia. These are represented using the three-letter amino acid code. The normal amino acid is shown before and the mutated amino acid is indicated after the numbers of the relevant codons. (Reprinted with permission from Brown ER, Bai M, Pollak M, Familial benign hypocalciuric hypercalcemia and other syndromes of altered responsiveness to extracellular calcium, in Krane SM, Avioli LV (eds): *Metabolic Bone Diseases*, 3rd ed. San Diego, Academic Press, 1997, pp. 479–499.)

inherited human diseases or mouse models where the CaR functions abnormally.[41] As discussed later, the calcium-sensing receptor is mutated in disorders of familial hypocalciuric hypercalcemia,[44] neonatal severe hyperparathyroidism, and autosomal dominant hypocalcemia.[45] Furthermore, mice with targeted disruption of the calcium-sensing receptor gene[46] have reduced suppression of PTH secretion at any given extracellular calcium concentration, similar to humans with familial hypocalciuric hypercalcemia and neonatal severe hyperparathyroidism.

Other Parathyroid Hormone Secretagogues

Magnesium

Like its sister divalent cation, magnesium inhibits the secretion of PTH at high concentrations and stimulates it at low concentrations.[47] On a molar basis, magnesium is severalfold less potent than calcium as a modulator of PTH secretion, making it unlikely that changes in the physiologic range have an important influence on the gland. The effects of hypermagnesemia to decrease PTH secretion are also mediated by the calcium-sensing receptor, which senses other divalent cations besides calcium.[40] The high serum magnesium concentrations attained during treatment of premature labor have been shown to inhibit PTH secretion and occasionally to produce hypocalcemia.[48] In contrast to the stimulatory effects of mild hypomagnesemia, profound chronic magnesium deficiency, as seen with chronic gastrointestinal or renal magnesium wasting, can produce a state of functional hypoparathyroidism. This is discussed further in the section on hypoparathyroidism. However, from the perspective of control of PTH secretion, it is likely that in the parathyroid gland magnesium is required for the release of parathyroid hormone from secretory granules, fulfilling the essential role in stimulus-secretion coupling that calcium subserves in most other secretory tissues, and that depletion of glandular stores of magnesium interferes with the secretory mechanism.

Catecholamines

Acting through beta-adrenergic receptors, catecholamines acutely stimulate the secretion of PTH from parathyroid cells in vitro. This effect is mediated by cAMP. Stimulation of alpha-adrenergic receptors inhibits cAMP accumulation and PTH release. Although early studies showed a small effect of the beta-adrenergic antagonist propranolol in reducing basal levels of

PTH,[49] evidence for a tonic role of catecholamines in the parathyroid gland is rather sparse.[50] Hypercalcemia is rarely seen in the state of catecholamine excess produced by a pheochromocytoma, but this phenomenon is probably caused by secretion of the homologous peptide parathyroid hormone–related protein (PTHrP) by some pheochromocytomas (discussed in the malignancy-associated hypercalcemia section).

Other Secretagogues

Acute administration of phosphate is a powerful stimulus to the secretion of PTH, but this effect is indirect and is entirely attributable to the fall in ionized calcium produced by a phosphate bolus. Exposure of parathyroid cells in vitro to lithium induces a shift to the right in the set point for the secretion of PTH, i.e., decreased sensitivity to suppression by extracellular calcium.[51] The administration of lithium in therapy for bipolar affective disorders is associated with increased PTH secretion and sometimes with hypercalcemia (see the section on hypercalcemia). Ingestion of alcohol acutely inhibits the secretion of PTH.[52]

Metabolism of Parathyroid Hormone

Heterogeneity of Circulating PTH

In Berson and Yalow's pioneering studies, it was recognized that circulating PTH differs immunochemically from glandular PTH, and it soon became clear that PTH circulates in several distinct forms.[53] These forms have different tissue origins, plasma half-lives, and metabolic fates and are affected differentially by disease states such as chronic renal failure. An understanding of the heterogeneous forms of circulating PTH has been crucial to the interpretation of clinical assay data using region-specific assays, and considerable effort has been expended in this quest.

It is now clear that there are two major forms of circulating PTH. One is the intact, biologically active hormone PTH(1-84); the other is a family of closely related fragments that constitute the midportion and carboxyl terminus of PTH and are biologically inactive in calcium homeostasis, as they do not contain the biologically active 1-34 domain. These will be referred to as carboxyl-terminal fragments.

Clearance of PTH from Plasma

The clearance of intact PTH(1-84) from plasma is very rapid, with a half-life of 2 to 3 min. The principal sites of clearance are the liver and kidney, with the liver accounting for up to two-thirds of the total (Fig. 22-8).[54,55] The major route of clearance is into a degradative pathway. In the liver, this pathway is located primarily in the Kupffer's cells.[56] In the kidney, degradation of PTH(1-84) takes place mainly in tubule cells after uptake either directly from the peritubular circulation or from the tubule lumen after filtration of PTH(1-84) at the glomerulus.[54,55,57]

PTH is also taken up by its target tissues, including osteoblasts in bone, renal tubule cells, and hepatocytes.[20] This is a receptor-mediated process that has a low capacity (probably less than 1 percent of the overall clearance rate) and a high affinity for PTH, in contrast to the high-capacity, nonsaturable uptake of PTH(1-84) by bulk degradative sites in the liver and kidney.[58]

Origins of Circulating Fragments of PTH

In vivo, both of the main circulating forms of PTH are probably secreted directly from the gland. Secretion of carboxyl-terminal fragments of PTH is detectable in careful gel filtration studies

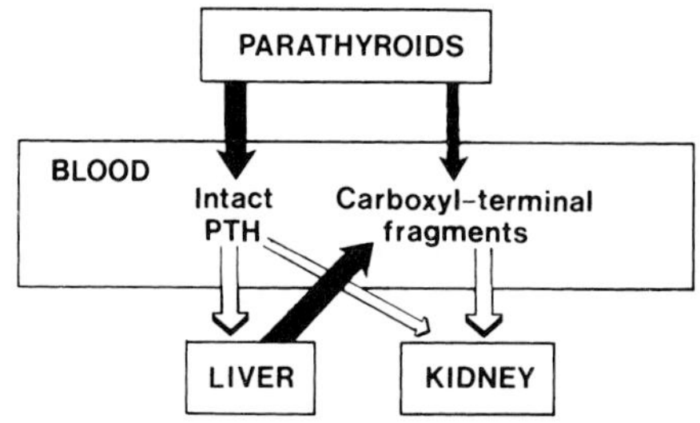

FIGURE 22-8. Secretion and metabolism of intact PTH and carboxyl-terminal fragments. Secretion is indicated by solid arrows, and major directions of metabolism by open arrows.

of parathyroid venous effluent sera.[59] However, parathyroid venous effluents do not appear to contain fragments that possess the amino-terminal domain of PTH or are bioactive. The principal enzyme thought to be responsible for the intraglandular cleavage of PTH is the lysosomal proteinase cathepsin B, which cleaves PTH between residues 36 and 37.[60] Intraglandular degradation of PTH appears to be calcium-dependent[61] and could be a mechanism for diminishing glandular stores of PTH under conditions of chronic suppression of the glands. Pro-PTH, the storage form of PTH, does not appear to be secreted. During hypocalcemia, the bulk of the hormone that is released from the parathyroid cell is intact PTH(1-84). As calcium increases, more intracellular PTH is degraded, and with hypercalcemia, the majority of secreted PTH consists of carboxyl-terminal fragments.[37]

Carboxyl-terminal fragments of PTH are cleared in the kidney (Fig. 22-8). Although intact PTH is cleared by a combination of peritubular uptake from blood and glomerular filtration, carboxyl-terminal fragments are cleared mainly by glomerular filtration.[57] Hormone that is filtered at the glomerulus is efficiently reabsorbed along the nephron, and very little reaches the final urine. The half-life of circulating carboxyl-terminal fragments is much longer than the half-life of intact PTH. Their clearance half-time has been estimated at 20 to 30 min with normal renal function and is greatly prolonged in the presence of renal failure, reflective of the importance of glomerular filtration in this process. Clinically, the accumulation of carboxyl-terminal fragments has complicated the use of PTH radioimmunoassays that are specific for the midregion and carboxyl terminus to quantitate the degree of secondary hyperparathyroidism present in patients with renal insufficiency. Although true secondary hyperparathyroidism is present in most such patients, its effect on circulating levels of PTH is greatly magnified by the reduced clearance of carboxyl-terminal fragments.

Assay of Parathyroid Hormone

Historically, the interpretation of assays for PTH has been complicated greatly by the immunoheterogeneity of the circulating hormone. A variety of different radioimmunoassays have been developed, mostly using antisera to the intact hormone. With the availability of synthetic and natural fragments of the hormone, it became clear that one major class of radioimmunoassays for PTH was directed toward amino-terminal determinants, and another toward determinants in the carboxyl-terminal domain, often to a "midregion" consisting of amino acids 43-68. The predominant species of PTH recognized by "midregion" assays are carboxyl-terminal fragments, which, by virtue of their long half-life, are the major circulating forms of PTH. Surprisingly, antisera to the biologically inactive midregion provided assays that were both sensitive and highly reliable in the diagnosis of primary hyperparathyroidism.[62] For the past 20 years, such assays have been in wide use.

Despite their utility in the diagnosis of hyperparathyroidism, to varying degrees all first and second-generation radioimmunoassays for PTH shared certain problems. None were sensitive or specific enough to detect the suppression of PTH consistently, for example, in patients with nonparathyroid hypercalcemia. Quantitative comparison of results from different assays was rendered nearly impossible by the immunoheterogeneity of circulating PTH, coupled with limited information about the relevant epitopes for different polyclonal antisera and by the use of different standard PTH preparations in different laboratories. None of the assays clearly measured biologically active hormone, and the potential for excess accumulation of biologically inactive fragments in renal failure complicated the interpretation of assay results in that setting.

The development of two-site assays for PTH in the mid-1980s was a great step forward. Several different assays have been developed and are available commercially.[63,64] They have in common the use of two antibodies, one directed toward an amino-terminal determinant and the other directed toward a carboxyl-terminal determinant. One is immobilized and used as a capture antibody; the other is labeled and used for the detection of bound hormone. The antibody used for detection is labeled either with radioactive iodine (immunoradiometric assays, IRMA) or with a luminescent tag (immunochemiluminescent assays) (Fig. 22-9). Because the only major circulating form of PTH that possesses both amino- and carboxyl-terminal determinants is PTH(1-84), such assays should theoretically be specific for the intact hormone.

The normal range for immunoreactive PTH(1-84) in serum determined using two-site techniques is about 10 to 60 pg/ml (Fig. 22-10). It is likely that this corresponds closely to the concentration of biologically active PTH. The normal range in two-site assays is in good agreement with bioassay results, and the ability of such assays to detect dynamic changes in the secretion of PTH suggests that a labile species such as authentic PTH(1-84) is being measured. In practical terms, two-site assays for PTH have two distinct advantages over previous techniques: They are more sensitive, and they are less subject to nonspecific effects of serum. Together, these characteristics provide for the ability to quantitate PTH throughout the normal range and detect the suppression of PTH when present as illustrated by the results in sera from patients with malignancy-associated hypercalcemia (Fig. 22-10). Wide experience with assays performed in commercial laboratories or using commercially available kits indicates that the level of performance shown in Fig. 22-10 is maintained.

With the advantages of two-site assays for intact PTH, is there a compelling reason to use a region-specific PTH assay in specific clinical circumstances? Midregion assays and amino-terminal assays remain excellent for the detection of primary hyperparathyroidism. They have been widely used for the management of secondary hyperparathyroidism in renal osteodystrophy, and clinicians are accustomed to using results in region-specific PTH assays to adjust treatment. However, aside from familiarity, no clear advantage is gained by the use of region-specific assays. Levels of intact PTH correlate well with midregion PTH levels in chronic renal failure, and although the sensitivity of assays for intact PTH for the detection of primary hyperparathyroidism is no better than

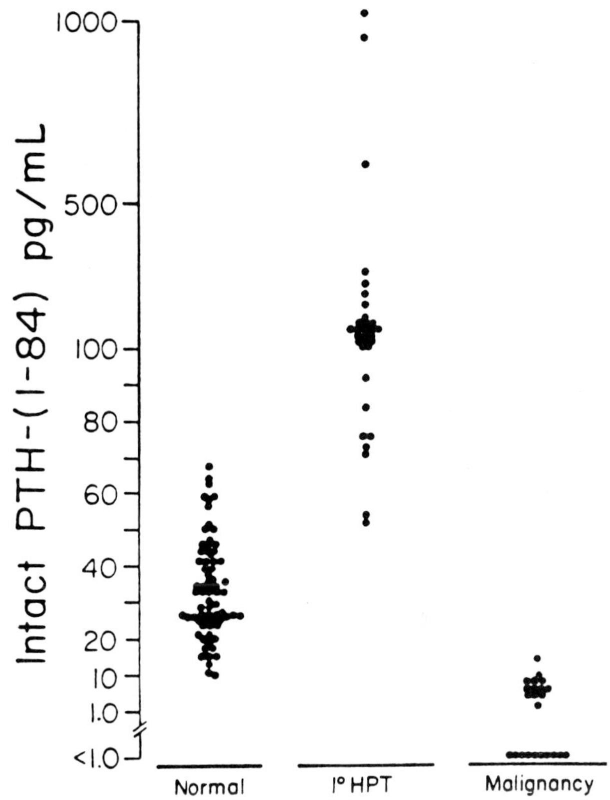

FIGURE 22-10. Levels of intact PTH in primary hyperparathyroidism and malignancy using the two-site technique. The serum level of PTH is typically elevated in hypercalcemic subjects with hyperparathyroidism but is uniformly suppressed in hypercalcemic patients with malignancy. (*From Nussbaum SR, Zahradnik RJ, Lavigne JR, et al[54] by permission of Clinical Chemistry.*)

FIGURE 22-9. Two-site immunoradiometric assay for intact PTH. The hormone is captured by anti-carboxyl-terminal antibodies (anti-PTH 39–84) coupled to a bead. Captured PTH is detected by binding of radioactively labeled anti-amino-terminal antibodies (anti-PTH 1–34). (*After SR Nussbaum.*)

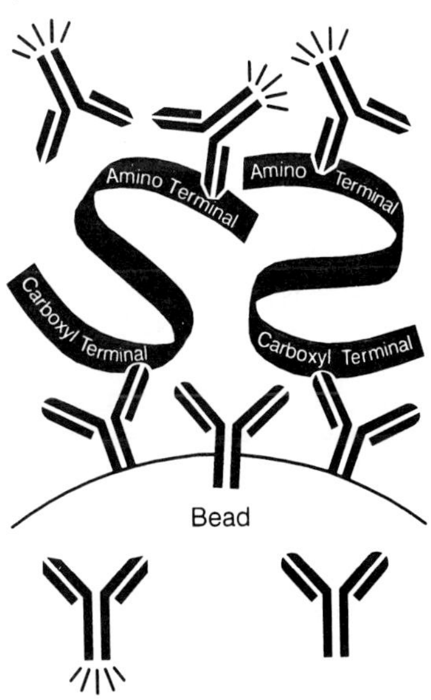

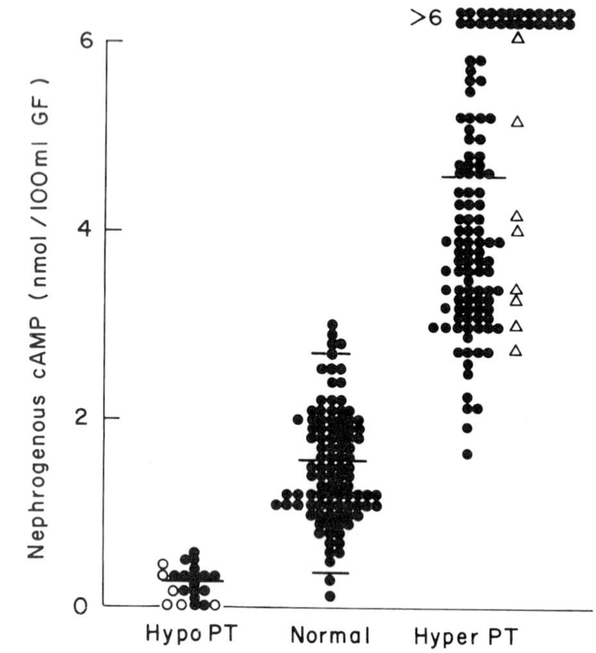

FIGURE 22-11. Values for nephrogenous cAMP in normal subjects and patients with hypoparathyroidism (HypoPT), nonparathyroid hypercalcemia (0), primary hyperparathyroidism (HyperPT), and nonazotemic secondary hyperparathyroidism (Δ). The marginated bars represent mean ± 2 SD in the normal subjects and mean values in the patients with hypoparathyroidism and hyperparathyroidism. (*By permission of Broadus AE, Nephron 23:136, 1978.*)

that of region-specific assays, their enhanced specificity, in particular their ability to detect the suppression of PTH in nonparathyroid hypercalcemia, makes them superior instruments for the differential diagnosis of hypercalcemia.

Bioactive PTH can also be determined using bioassay techniques. A cytochemical technique is based on quantitating the effect of PTH on glucose-6-phosphate dehydrogenase activity measured microspectrophotometrically in distal tubules of guinea pig renal cortex.[65,66] This is a remarkably sensitive assay but is rather cumbersome and not suited to routine use.

Because the renal PTH receptor is coupled to adenylyl cyclase and a fraction of the cAMP produced in the proximal tubule in response to PTH is secreted into the urine, determination of urinary cAMP can be used as a bioassay for PTH. In research studies, the excretion of the secreted component, called *nephrogenous* cAMP, can be determined specifically by subtracting the filtered load of cAMP [plasma (cAMP) × glomerular filtration rate (GFR)] from the total urinary excretion. When measured carefully, nephrogenous cAMP is a reliable test of parathyroid function (Fig. 22-11), and determination of total urinary cAMP, which is technically easier, is also useful.[67] Bioassays have the advantage of detecting other molecules that mimic PTH, and determination of urinary cAMP was critical in the detection of a PTH-like peptide in malignancy-associated hypercalcemia. However, this same property makes them unable to distinguish PTH from PTHrP. At present, the principal use of urinary cAMP assays is in the differential diagnosis of hypocalcemic disorders, where the unresponsiveness of urinary cAMP to PTH is the hallmark of pseudohypoparathyroidism.

Biological Effects and Mechanism of Action of Parathyroid Hormone

Parathyroid hormone plays a critical role in the acute regulation of calcium levels in the ECF, while vitamin D plays an important long-term role in overall calcium balance by modulating the efficiency of the absorption of dietary calcium from the gut. PTH "fine-tunes" the blood levels of calcium, which otherwise would be subject to peaks and troughs related to intermittent dietary intake. PTH acts directly on bone to stimulate its resorption and the release of calcium salts into the ECF. Similarly, PTH acts directly on the kidney to promote phosphate excretion and increase calcium reabsorption. The response to PTH at the level of the kidney is rapid, but the response in bone typically occurs much more slowly, probably reflecting a more complex cascade of events which must be put in motion to effect bone resorption. The action of PTH in promoting increased dietary absorption of calcium is indirect: The hormone acts at the level of the kidney to stimulate 25-hydroxyvitamin D 1α-hydroxylase. This enzyme acts on the weakly active precursor form of vitamin D, 25-hydroxyvitamin D_3, to generate the fully active form, $1\alpha,25\text{-}(OH)_2D_3$. The active hormone then acts on the gut to stimulate increased activity of calcium-binding protein and facilitated transport of calcium from the gut lumen into the bloodstream (Fig. 22-3). The activity of the 1α-hydroxylase enzyme is in part regulated by PTH, as discussed later.

It is the action of PTH in concert on bone, kidney, and gut that increases the inflow of calcium into the ECF and defends the organism against hypocalcemia (Fig. 22-3).[20] The relative contribution of each of these three principal target organs to calcium homeostasis as a result of PTH action has not been definitively delineated and almost certainly varies with the nature of the stress to homeostasis. However, the contribution of PTH is clear: Surgical removal of the parathyroid glands in animals or humans without replacement of the hormone or other maneuvers designed to increase calcium influx (such as the administration of vitamin D and a high-calcium diet) leads to hypocalcemia, tetany, and even death within hours.

Parathyroid Hormone Action

Receptors for PTH

Parathyroid hormone, like other peptide hormones, produces its biological actions by interacting with a hormone-specific receptor on the cell surface of target tissue cells. This interaction results in the production of intracellular second messengers which initiate a series of metabolic events. The PTH signal transduction cascade consists of 1) receptors that detect ligand, 2) signal-generating enzymes, and 3) heterotrimeric (α,β,γ) G proteins. PTH mediates its effects of mineral ion homeostasis via the PTH/parathyroid hormone-related protein (PTHrP) receptor, which is coupled to adenylyl cyclase and phospholipase C.[68,69] This classical PTH receptor, also known as the type 1 PTH receptor, binds both PTH and PTHrP, a factor identified initially (Fig. 22-12) as that responsible for malignancy-associated hypercalcemia.[70–72] The receptor belongs to the family of seven-transmembrane–spanning G protein-coupled receptors and mediates the biological actions of PTH and PTHrP with similar efficacy. The PTH/PTHrP receptor is most abundantly expressed in the target tissues for PTH, such as kidney and bone, as well as in growth plate chondrocytes.[37] In the tissues other than bone and kidney, the receptor mediates the autocrine and paracrine actions of PTHrP,[73] rather than the endocrine

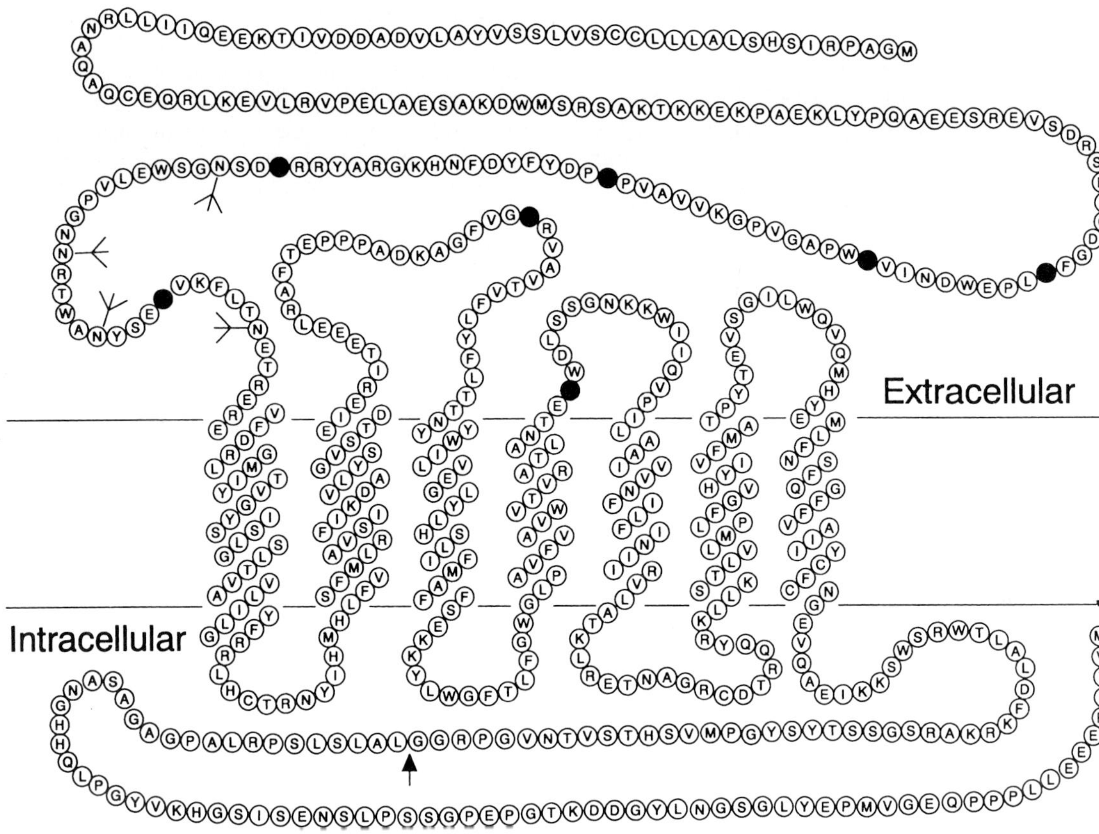

FIGURE 22-12. Schematic representation of the PTH/PTHrP receptor (NH_2 terminus at top) from opossum kidney cells, potential N-glycosylation sites (⋏), and cysteine residues that are conserved in the calcitonin receptor (●). In OK-H, residues 508 to 515 (to the left of the arrow) are WPCSALD. The peptide ends eight residues after the arrow. (*Reprinted with permission from Jüppner et al.*[68])

effects of PTH. The receptor has a major role in bone growth as it mediates the effects of PTHrP on chondrocyte proliferation and differentiation. The functional domains of the PTH molecule are shown in Fig. 22-13.

A second PTH receptor (PTH-2) is activated by PTH and not PTHrP.[74] The highest expression of this PTH-2 receptor is in the brain, where PTH itself is undetectable. Recently, a potent and selective agonist of the PTH-2 receptor was purified from bovine hypothalamus and named tubuloinfundibular peptide of 39 residues (TIP39).[75] TIP39 does not bind the PTH/PTHrP receptor. The biological effects of the TIP39 activation of the PTH-2 receptor are currently unknown.

The seven-transmembrane–spanning receptors are coupled by G proteins[76] to signal effectors localized to the inner surface of the cell membrane. Specific associations among at least 20α, 6β, and 12γ chains generate a diversity of heterotrimeric G proteins that

FIGURE 22-13. A functional map of the parathyroid hormone molecule. All the structural determinants required for full biological activity reside within the N-terminal 1–34 sequence. Contained within this region is a domain critical for activation of the receptor, positions 1–6. The sequence 7–34 forms the core for most PTH antagonists. Within this inhibitory domain lies the principal binding domain of the hormone, positions 25–34. (*Modified and reprinted with permission from Rosenblatt.*[99])

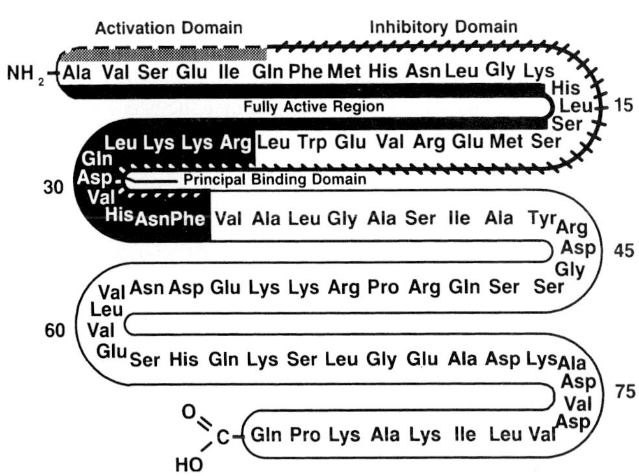

have the capacity to discriminate among a multitude of receptor and effector molecules.[77] Hormone binding to a receptor facilitates activation of the G protein. In this process the α chain exchanges bound GDP for GTP and dissociates from the $\beta\gamma$ dimer and the receptor. The free GTP-bound form of the α chain is the primary modulator of relevant effector molecules. An intrinsic GTPase associated with the α chain hydrolyzes GTP to GDP after a predetermined interval. The inactive GDP-bound α then reassociates with the $\beta\gamma$ dimer, and the heterotrimeric G protein is ready for another cycle of hormone activation.[77]

PTH binding to its receptor activates intracellular signal effector systems that generate the second messengers cAMP,[78,79] inositol 1,4,5-triphosphate and diacylglycerol,[80,81] and cytosolic calcium.[82–85] The most completely characterized second messenger for PTH is cAMP, which activates protein kinase A.[86]

Receptors thus far characterized that are linked to adenylyl cyclase activation[87,88] and other G-linked second messenger systems contain a number of common structural features. These include the receptors for rhodopsin,[87] the beta-adrenergic receptor agonists,[89] acetylcholine (muscarinic),[90,91] luteinizing hormone (LH),[92] thyrotropin stimulating hormone,[93] and others.[94] They possess seven membrane-spanning domains, although they may vary in the size of the extracellular N-terminal domain, which in many cases interacts with hormone, the size of the cytoplasmically oriented C-terminal domain and intracellular loops (which may be involved in signal transduction or regulation of receptor number) varies from receptor to receptor. Of interest is the fact that despite their common interaction with G proteins, the specific transmembrane domains involved in G protein interaction display considerable sequence heterogeneity across receptors.

PTH receptors from rat osteoblast-like bone [ROS 17(2.8)] and opossum kidney (OK) cell lines[68] encode for 591- and 585-amino acid proteins, respectively, which are 78 percent identical despite differences in species and organ of origin. The receptor, as expected, appears to contain seven membrane-spanning regions (Fig. 22-12). However, the receptor contains little homology to other guanyl nucleotide regulatory protein–linked receptors. There is striking homology to the sequence of the calcitonin receptor,[95] as well as the receptors for glucagon, secretin, and VIP, indicating that these receptors form a new subgroup in the family of G protein-linked receptors. For example, transmembrane domain number VII is nearly identical (17 of 18 amino acid identity) to the corresponding domain in the calcitonin receptor. The overall similarity between the PTH and calcitonin receptors is approximately 50 percent; there is 32 percent identity in amino acid sequence. The structural determinants of PTH required for full biological activity reside within the N-terminal 1-34 sequence (Fig. 22-13).

The PTH/PTHrP receptor, like the CT receptor and the receptor for large glycoprotein hormones but unlike the beta-adrenergic receptor, contains a signal sequence at the N terminus. In the exoplasmic domain, there are four potential sites for N-linked glycosylation and six cysteines in each of the first two extracellular loops that are thought to be important in maintaining a bioactive conformation for the receptor (two additional cysteines in the signal sequence). The third intracellular loop and the carboxyl-terminal intracellular tail contain potential phosphorylation sites. The gene encoding the receptor contains 4 introns and 4 exons.

PTH Effects on the Kidney

PTH has three effects on the kidney. It stimulates reabsorption of calcium, inhibits reabsorption of phosphate, and stimulates synthesis of $1\alpha,25\text{-}(OH)_2D_3$. PTH acts on the distal tubule to promote the reabsorption of calcium although the majority of calcium reabsorption occurs in the proximal tubule and is PTH-independent.[37] Because large quantities of calcium (7 to 10 g/day) are filtered, even a small increase in an already efficient process, such as going from 95 to 98 percent efficacy, can have a dramatic salutary effect when calcium homeostasis and balance are stressed. PTH action on the distal tubule stimulates transport against both a calcium concentration and an electric potential gradient.[96–100] The calcium-sensing receptor directly regulates renal calcium reabsorption by inhibiting tubular reabsorption of calcium when the peritubular calcium concentration increases. This effect is independent of PTH.

PTH inhibits phosphate reabsorption at the proximal and distal tubules.[101] In the proximal tubular cells, phosphate is transported into the cell via the membrane-anchored sodium-phosphate contransporter, Npt2.[102,103] PTH reduces cell surface Npt2 by several mechanisms.[103,104] Targeted disruption of the Npt2 gene in mice causes severe renal phosphate wasting. PTH also inhibits phosphate reabsorption in the distal tubules, by mechanisms yet unknown.[105]

PTH also stimulates the formation of the active form of vitamin D, $1\alpha,25\text{-}(OH)_2D$, in the nephron. PTH stimulates the activity of the renal 25-hydroxy-vitamin D 1α-hydroxylase present in proximal tubular cells.[106] The mechanism of regulation of this enzyme by PTH has not been clearly established but appears to be linked to PTH-dependent production of cAMP; however, low phosphate levels intracellularly, which occur secondarily as a result of PTH action, can also stimulate the enzyme.[107,108] Hypercalcemia suppresses the 1α-hydroxylase activity and limits the production of $1\alpha,25\text{-}(OH)_2D$.[109] PTH decreases renal vitamin D 24 hydroxylase, which enhances the effect on $1\alpha,25\text{-}(OH)_2D$ synthesis.[110,111]

Actions on Bone

To understand the actions of parathyroid hormone on bone and appreciate the contribution of PTH to mineral metabolism, it is necessary to provide some general information regarding bone biology. Bone is a complex organ. It is not metabolically static, but is in dynamic balance. Throughout life, bone is actively involved in remodeling. The continuous resorption of discrete quanta of the skeleton followed by stepwise "programmed" replacement (formation) is termed *bone turnover* (Fig. 22-14). Throughout bone, there are thousands of sites involved in the asynchronous process of first removing and then replacing bone along its surfaces. The discussion that follows is not intended to be comprehensive. Rather, it provides a background oriented toward a discussion of the participation of bone in mineral ion homeostasis.

Bone is composed of cells and extracellular matrix. Cells account for 2 percent of the total volume of bone. The extracellular matrix is rich in collagen and glycosaminoglycans. A unique feature of the extracellular matrix in this connective tissue is that it can be calcified. Bone can be subdivided into cortical (compact) bone and trabecular (cancellous) bone. Approximately 80 to 90 percent of the volume of compact bone is calcified, while 15 to 25 percent of trabecular bone is calcified; the rest is occupied by marrow. Therefore, much of the biomechanical strength of bone is derived from the cortical component, while trabecular bone participates more fully in the metabolic function of mineral ion homeostasis. However, it is important to emphasize that both categories of bone participate in structural and metabolic functions.

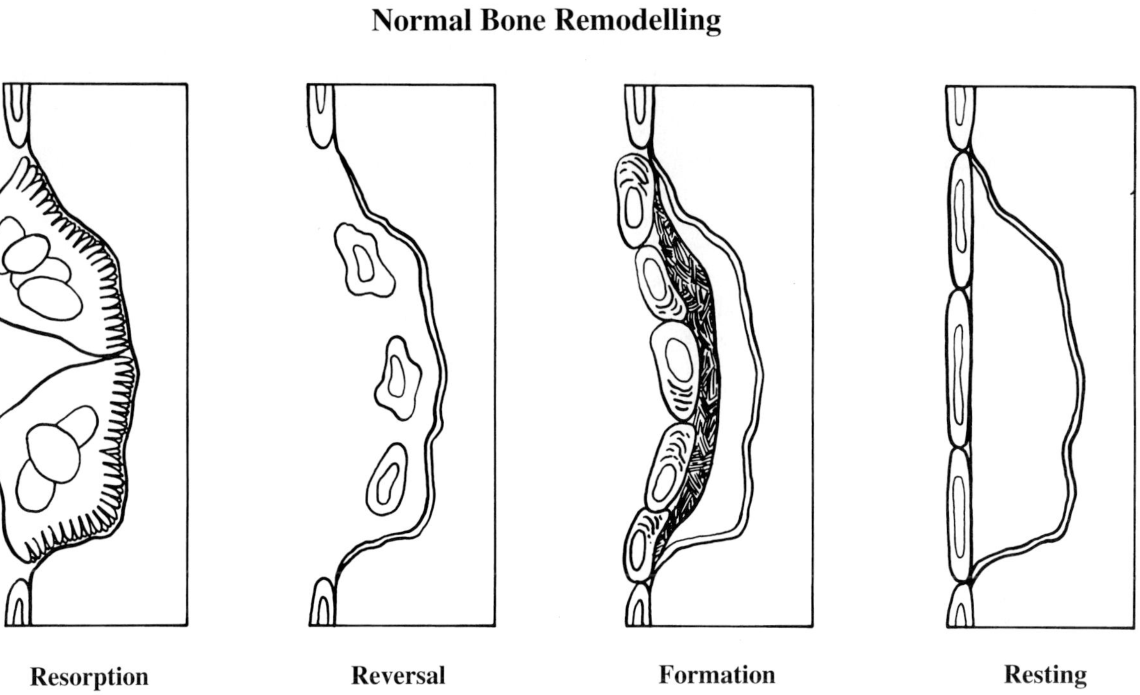

FIGURE 22-14. Schematic representation of the cycle of bone resorption by osteoclasts followed by bone formation by osteoblasts.

Cortical bone is largely found in the appendicular regions and accounts for 80 percent of the adult skeleton, whereas the vertebrae and axial skeleton are rich in trabecular bone.

In mature bone, collagen fibers are arranged in layers, termed *lamellae*, that are concentrically deposited around a central channel based on a blood vessel (haversian system). These lamellae become calcified. The combination of hydroxyapatite $[Ca_{10}(PO_4)_6(OH)_2]$ and matrix proteins (especially collagen) gives bone its strength. Given the correct ionic milieu in ECF, the organic matrix of bone will mineralize spontaneously. In humans, the calcification process is complete within 10 to 20 days after the biosynthesis of organic matrix. If an appropriate ionic environment is not present, mineralization will be delayed. A prolonged lag between matrix formation and mineralization is the hallmark of certain diseases, such as osteomalacia and rickets.

When bone is formed rapidly, the organization of collagen fibers is sacrificed: fiber bundles are oriented randomly. Such bone is found in healing fractures and in certain metabolic bone diseases; it is termed "woven" bone. Although there are at least 13 types of collagen, type 1 collagen is the only form found in bone. Several noncollagenous proteins constitute the 10 to 15 percent of bone protein that is not type 1 collagen. The most abundant of these proteins is osteonectin, a phosphorylated glycoprotein. This protein binds ionic calcium and hydroxyapatite. Other proteins synthesized in bone that bind calcium are osteocalcin, bone sialoprotein (BSP), thrombospondin (TSP), and osteopontin (OP). Osteocalcin contains residues of γ-carboxyl glutamic acid (gla), an amino acid that is biosynthesized posttranslationally by a vitamin K–dependent process. Chondroitin sulfate and heparin sulfate are also present.

A separate process for the mineralization of cartilage (endochondral calcification) involves exocytosis of matrix vesicles from the plasma membrane of osteoblasts. Mineralization occurs at specific gap regions in the matrix fibers. These gaps provide space for inorganic ions within the fibril structure.

The *osteoblast* is the principal bone-forming cell. It is responsible for the biosynthesis of the components of the matrix, collagen and ground substance. The enzyme alkaline phosphatase is displayed on the plasma membrane of osteoblasts and plays a critical role in matrix calcification. In fact, genetic alkaline phosphatase deficiency (hypophosphatasia) leads to osteomalacia. Hence, the osteoblast not only synthesizes the organic matrix of bone but also plays a role in its subsequent mineralization. Thus, serum alkaline phosphatase is a marker for bone formation. Osteoblasts arise from stem cells within the bone marrow, different from those that give rise to hematopoietic cells. Under appropriate stimulation, these cells proliferate and differentiate into osteoblast precursors and then mature osteoblasts. The osteoblast is always found adjacent to the lining layer of bone matrix that these cells are synthesizing, the osteoid seam, which is not yet calcified. Osteoblasts possess receptors for parathyroid hormone but not for calcitonin. In addition, they contain intracellular estrogen receptors.

Eventually osteoblasts trap themselves within the calcified matrix they have formed. Now embedded within the bone, they are termed *osteocytes*. They remain bathed in ECF via a network of canaliculi, which are the remnants of a network of thin cellular processes extending from the osteoblast along the bone surface during its formation. Whether an osteocyte is capable of resorbing calcified matrix around its perimeter is a subject of controversy. For the most part, osteocytes are considerably less active metabolically than are osteoblasts and osteoclasts.

The *osteoclast* is the bone cell responsible for resorption of matrix and release of calcium salts from the large reservoir of mineralized matrix into the ECF. Like the osteoblast, the osteoclast lines the calcified bone surface. The osteoclast etches a pit, or *Howship lacuna*, also termed a resorption bay. The progenitor of the osteoclast appears to be a member of the monocyte/macrophage family. Differentiation occurs from the promonocyte stage; promonocyte precursor cells fuse to generate osteoclasts. The osteoclast is a giant multinucleated cell that contains 4 to 20 nuclei. It contains receptors for calcitonin but not for parathyroid hormone. The osteoclast adheres to the bony surface through a receptor-mediated attachment process.

When activated, osteoclasts mediate bone resorption by attaching to mineralized matrix of bone that has had surface collagen removed by collagenase, which is latent in bone and is activated by osteoclasts or secreted by the osteoclast itself. It has also been suggested that osteoblasts or bone lining cells may produce collagenase, which is activated by the acid and lysosomal enzymes released by osteoclasts. Thus, the osteoblasts "prepare" the bone surface for osteoclastic resorption. Other studies using electron microscopy, however, indicate that osteoclasts can resorb bone without a need for other supporting cells. Heterodimeric plasma membrane receptors on the surface of the osteoclast, termed *integrins*, interact with macromolecules present in the matrix of bone, such as osteocalcin, osteopontin, and other proteins.[112,113] These macromolecules share a common sequence of arginine-glycine-aspartic acid (R-G-D). When enough integrins on the cell surface of an osteoclast bind to bone matrix, the osteoclast is anchored and a microscopic sealed environment termed the *ruffled border* is created[114]; in reality, this is a series of folds and invaginations of the plasma membrane. Contractile proteins within the cytoplasm of an activated osteoclast help the osteoclast form and maintain this sealed environment as well as move along the surface of bone, resulting in the excavation of a trough.

The space between the ruffled border and the mineralized bone matrix becomes the functional equivalent of an extracellular lysosome. The osteoclast releases numerous enzymes and acid via the hydrogen-potassium-ATPase (proton) pump[115–118] into this sequestered space. The enzyme carbonic anhydrase (type II) also contributes to the creation of an acid microenvironment.[119,120] The coordinated action of these enzymes and acid results in catabolism of bone by breakdown of bone proteins and release of calcium salts into the ECF. Cysteine proteinases such as cathepsin B are also released and/or activated.[121] The importance of each of these individual components to the process of osteolysis is demonstrated by the fact that blockade of the cysteine proteases, carbonic anhydrase, or the proton pump can independently block bone resorption in vitro and in vivo in animal models and in human genetic disorders such as one type of osteopetrosis in which there is a deficiency of carbonic anhydrase type II and vastly diminished bone resorption.[122,123]

These processes of resorption and formation are closely coupled, resulting in the maintenance of bone volume and structural integrity as well as mineral ion homeostasis. The sequence of events is a cycle of activation-resorption-formation (Fig. 22-14). Once osteoclasts have been activated and have formed a pit, they depart. Osteoblasts are then able to move into the resorption bay and fill it with new bone matrix.

The local regulation or coupling of bone resorption and formation is not well understood. There is intensive research under way to identify a coupling factor or factors. It is clear that osteoclastic activity can be influenced by cytokines such as interleukin 1, tumor necrosis factor (TNF), interferons, prostaglandins, and growth factors. These substances may be produced by bone cells and act in an autocrine or paracrine fashion or enter through the circulation. There is speculation that osteoblasts may "seed" their own anabolic activity for bone. It is known that osteoblasts secrete insulin-like growth factor-I (IGF-I), transforming growth factor β (TGF-β), or other growth factors. These proteins may be encased within the bone matrix during formation. Later, during resorption by osteoclasts, they may be released and recruit osteoblasts to the resorption pit and stimulate their biosynthetic activity. TGF-β may also inhibit osteoclastic activity at the same resorption site, setting the stage for osteoblastic activity. Hence, sequestered growth factors within the bone matrix may be the actual coupling factors. Their diffusion locally may result in the proliferation and differentiation of osteoblast precursors.

The actions of PTH on bone are expressed through an unusual cascade. An increase in the number and activity of osteoclasts is the hallmark of PTH action. Yet when examined in vitro, osteoclasts appear to have few if any PTH receptors.[124] Rather, the hormonally responsive cell is the osteoblast, the cell normally associated with bone formation.[125] Presumably, when exposed to PTH, osteoblasts secrete a cytokine(s) that acts locally and directly on osteoclasts to recruit them to sites ready for bone resorption and increase the resorptive activity of osteoclasts.[126,127] Alternatively, PTH-stimulated osteoblasts may secrete factors that act through an intermediate cell, such as a monocyte, which in turn secretes a factor that stimulates or recruits osteoclasts. Candidate molecules that are secreted locally in bone and are known to stimulate bone resorption include interleukin 1 (IL-1), tumor necrosis factor (TNF-α, interleukin 6 (IL-6), prostaglandin E_2 (PGE_2), granulocyte-macrophage colony-stimulating factor (GM-CSF), and leukemia inhibitory factor (LIF or DIF),[128–136] as discussed earlier.

A recently discovered family of molecules have been identified as mediators of the effect of PTH to stimulate osteoclastic bone resorption. The stromal cell-derived RANK (receptor activator of NF kappa B) Ligand, also known as osteoclast differentiation factor (ODF), osteoprotegerin ligand (OPGL), and TRANCE, has been identified, and a soluble form of the molecule in combination with M-CSF can generate osteoclasts from hematopoietic cells in the absence of osteoblastic stromal cells.[137–140] PTH, as well as IL-11, prostaglandin E_2, and $1\alpha,25\text{-}(OH)_2D_3$, promotes osteoclast differentiation and function by stimulating osteoblast production of RANKL (Fig. 22-15). RANKL was also identified by its ability to induce NFkB and apoptosis of T-cells as RANKL and TRANCE, respectively.[141–143] For simplicity, the nomenclature of RANK Ligand as indicated by a recent review and consensus[144] will be used. RANK Ligand is a member of the TNF family and is a membrane-bound molecule. Two receptors for RANK Ligand exist. The first, which aided the identification of RANK Ligand, was osteoprotegerin (OPG), also reported as osteoclastogenesis inhibitory factor (OCIF).[145,146] OPG is a secreted TNF receptor family member and has a relatively wide distribution. Overexpression of OPG in mice resulted in osteopetrosis.[145] Conversely, mice deficient in OPG demonstrate osteoporosis and calcification of the aorta. In agreement with the phenotypes of mice with altered OPG production, recombinant OPG inhibited osteoclast formation in cocultures of mouse osteoblastic cells and hematopoietic cells.[138,139] The ability of OPG to bind to RANK Ligand and limit the biological actions of RANK Ligand suggested that OPG may function as a decoy receptor.[138,139,146] The putative receptor responsible for signaling RANK Ligand biological actions appears to be receptor activator of NF-κB (RANK),[141] although other unrecognized receptors of the TNF-receptor family may have similar

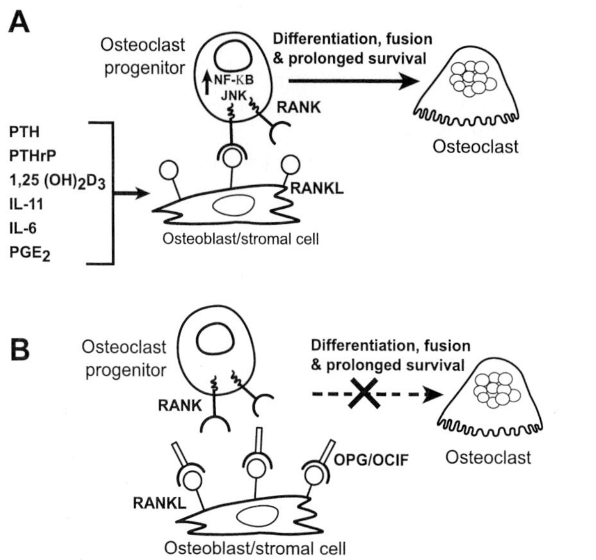

FIGURE 22-15. Mechanisms of osteoclast differentiation, fusion, and survival induced by RANK ligand. *A*. Factors, such as PTH, PTHrP, 1,25 dihydroxyvitamin D3, IL-11, IL-6, and PGE2 stimulate the production of the membrane-bound RANK ligand by osteoblasts and stromal cells in the bone microenvironment. RANK ligand, in the absence of osteoprotegerin (OPG), also known as osteoclast inhibitory factor (OCIF), binds to RANK on osteoclast progenitors to stimulate the differentiation, fusion, and survival of osteoclasts via JNK and NF kappa B signaling pathways. *B*. In the presence of the decoy receptor, Opg, Osteoclast formation is blocked.

capabilities. Fig. 22-15 demonstrates the role of RANKL and OPG in PTH-mediated osteoclastic bone resorption.

Through its action on osteoblasts, PTH can have effects that stimulate bone formation and result in an overall anabolic rather than catabolic effect on the skeleton.[147–153] It seems likely that bone formation mediated by PTH results from an osteoblast autocrine mechanism. Exposure of osteoblasts to PTH leads to increased secretion or activity of certain growth factors, such as insulin-like growth factors I and II, TGF-β, and fibroblast growth factor (FGF). These factors may then, in an autocrine manner, stimulate osteoblastic activity and bone formation,[154–156] as discussed earlier.

Although the discussion has focused on osteoblasts as the PTH target cell, it is fair to say that the true target cell has not been definitively identified. Osteoblast progenitor cells may represent the actual target cell, as has been proposed.[157–159]

Disorders Resulting from Molecular Defects in the PTH/PTHrP Receptors

PTH/PTHrP receptor mutations have been identified in two rare genetic disorders, Jansen's metaphyseal chodrodysplasia and Blomstrand's lethal chondrodysplasia. Jansen's metaphyseal chondrodysplasia is characterized by short-limbed dwarfism and severe hypercalcemia and hypophosphatemia despite normal or undetectable concentrations of PTH or PTHrP in the circulation. This autosomal dominant disease is the result of an activating mutation of the PTH/PTHrP receptor that leads to ligand-independent accumulation of cAMP.[160] Conversely, inactivating PTH/PTHrP receptor mutations were identified in patients with Blomstrand disease. These patients are born prematurely and die at birth, and have advanced bone maturation, accelerated chondrocyte differentiation, and likely abnormalities in mineral ion homeostasis.[161–163] Consistent with the clinical condition of Blomstrand chondrodysplasia, targeted disruption of the PTH/PTHrP receptor gene resulted in fetal death during middle or late gestation and severe skeletal abnormalities in mice that inherit both alleles of the defective gene.[164] Mice that are heterozygous for the abnormal gene have no apparent defects in calcium or bone metabolism.

CALCITONIN

Introduction and Historical Notes

Although calcitonin has potent effects on mineral ion flux through its actions on kidney and bone, its role in the normal physiology of humans is not known. The hormone was discovered by Copp and coworkers in the early 1960s.[165,166] It is a 32-amino acid peptide whose amino terminus contains a cyclic structure involving seven amino acids bridged by a disulfide bond (Fig. 22-16). The hormone decreases blood calcium levels by inhibiting bone resorption and promoting renal excretion of calcium.[167–169] Phosphaturia is also stimulated by calcitonin.

The existence of the hormone was postulated after Copp and colleagues found that perfusion of the parathyroid and thyroid glands with a hypercalcemic perfusate produced a more rapid fall in systemic blood calcium than that produced by surgical removal of the parathyroid glands.[170] Although there was initial confusion regarding the glandular and cellular origin of calcitonin and although for a period of time the parathyroid glands were thought to be the source,[170] the hormone has been documented to be

FIGURE 22-16. The sequence of human calcitonin. The molecule contains a seven-membered ring linked by a disulfide bridge at the N terminus.

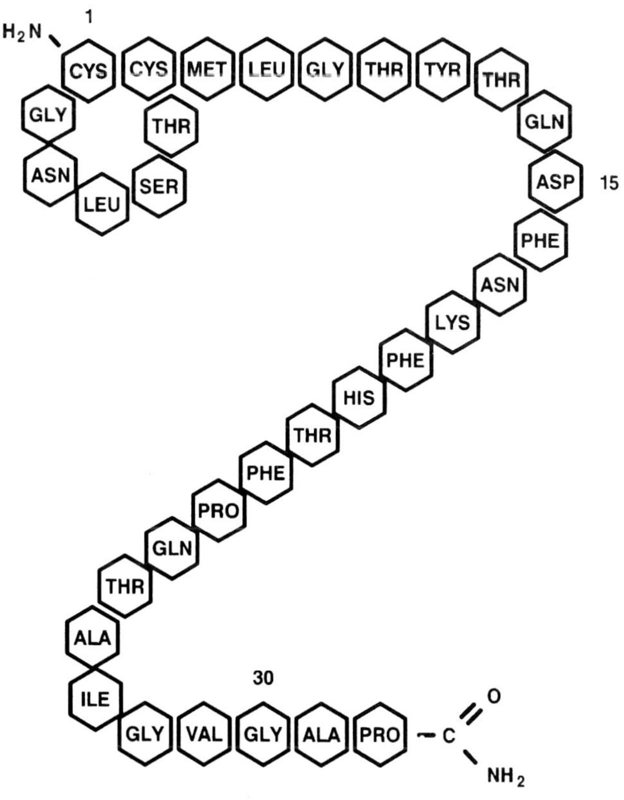

biosynthesized by the parafollicular or C cells of the thyroid gland, which have a different embryologic origin than the rest of the gland, arising from neural crest cells.[171] Calcitonin clearly plays an important role in calcium regulation in lower species such as fish, in which the major homeostatic challenge is maintenance of blood calcium levels when the organism is literally bathed in an external environment (the sea) containing a high concentration of calcium. The evolutionary precursor of the thyroid C cell in fish is the ultimobranchial gland, an older structure (phylogenetically) than the parathyroid gland.

In humans and other terrestrial animals, it is unlikely that calcitonin plays an essential physiological role. Evidence supporting this notion includes the finding that the hormone circulates at very low levels in humans and that surgical removal of the thyroid gland (normally the only source of the hormone) has no appreciable effect on calcium metabolism. Furthermore, the high levels of circulating calcitonin that occur with medullary carcinoma of the thyroid are not accompanied by hypocalcemia. In humans, calcitonin remains "a hormone in search of a function."[169]

Therefore, much of the medical interest in calcitonin arises because this hormone serves as a tumor marker: Calcitonin is secreted by medullary carcinoma of the thyroid (one of the neoplasms which occur as part of the hereditary disorders of multiple endocrine neoplasia type II and type III.[169,172] Removal of the tumor is accompanied by the return of calcitonin to normal or undetectable levels; recurrence of tumor is often heralded by renewed elevation of blood calcitonin levels. Thus, the CT radioimmunoassay can be used to monitor the status of the malignancy and the efficacy of surgical treatment. In addition to basal secretion of calcitonin by such tumors, secretagogues of calcitonin such as calcium and gastrin can be used in stimulatory tests to reveal the presence of early and otherwise undetectable or premalignant lesions[167–169] in subjects with a hereditary predisposition to developing the disease.

Clinical interest in calcitonin also stems from its use as therapeutic agent for the treatment of hypercalcemia, Paget disease of bone, and osteoporosis (discussed later). The hormone is available in several homologues from different species,[167,168] and there is a 10- to 40-fold range in potency between human calcitonin and the highly potent salmon form of the hormone. It was first chemically synthesized in 1968.[173,174]

At the basic level, the biosynthesis and intracellular processing of calcitonin (discussed later) are complex and make a fascinating story, serving as one of the paradigms for hormonal biosynthesis in modern molecular biology.

Biological Effects and Mechanism of Action

When administered intravenously, calcitonin produces a rapid and dramatic decline in levels of serum calcium and phosphorus. These fluxes in mineral ions result from the action of the hormone directly on bone and kidney. At the level of bone, calcitonin directly inhibits bone resorption by inhibiting osteoclast activity. Calcitonin receptors have been documented to be present on mammalian osteoclasts, the principal bone-resorbing cell.[175,176] Calcitonin appears to have no influence on the inhibition of bone formation or mineralization.[177] The magnitude of its action is increased in conditions that increase bone turnover and therefore the number of active osteoclasts recruited to mineralized surfaces of bone, such as skeletal growth in young animals, immobilization, Paget disease, disorders of increased parathyroid hormone levels, or Graves' disease (of the thyroid).

After exposure to calcitonin, the morphology of the active osteoclast changes rapidly.[178] The multinucleated cell shrinks in size, and its ruffled border, which is presumed to be the essential morphologic feature for the conduct of bone resorption, retracts from the resorptive surface.

At the level of the kidney, calcitonin, like PTH, decreases the threshold for urinary reabsorption of phosphorus, thus promoting increased urinary phosphorus excretion.[167,168] In addition, calcitonin promotes an increase in the renal fractional excretion of calcium. These effects are thought to result from the action of the hormone on the proximal tubule. However, these renal actions are unlikely to be of physiologic or even pathophysiologic consequence, as demonstrated by the presence of normal mineral metabolism in patients with medullary carcinoma of the thyroid who exhibit extraordinarily high levels of calcitonin in the blood.

Calcitonin utilizes cAMP as the second messenger for expression of bioactivity on bone and on the renal tubule. Although calcitonin works through cAMP, it is not a contributor to nephrogenous cAMP and therefore does not complicate the evaluation of patients with hyperparathyroidism or hypercalcemia of malignancy. Calcitonin is related in sequence to several other bioactive peptides, calcitonin gene-related peptide (CGRP), adrenomedullin, and amylin. Except for CT and CGRP1, each of these peptides are derived from a separate gene and exert characteristic actions in specific target.[179,180] CGRP1 and 2 are vasodilators and immunomodulators, with effects on the CNS and other targets. Adrenomedullin is also a vasodilator and has CNS actions. In addition to having effects on carbohydrate metabolism, gastric emptying and CNS function, amylin has been shown to increase trabecular bone mass in rats[181] and stimulate osteoblast activity.[182]

The newest insights into the CT system come from the recent cloning of the porcine CT receptor.[66] The deduced nucleotide sequence of the receptor cDNA encodes a 482-amino acid protein. Like other receptors that stimulate adenylyl cyclase activity, the CT receptor interacts with a guanyl nucleotide regulatory protein and therefore possesses the characteristic scaffold of seven membrane-spanning domains (Fig. 22-17). In one of the transmembrane domains (domain VII, discussed previously), the CT receptor shares great homology (17 of 18 amino acids) with the PTH/PTHrP receptor (Fig. 22-12) and approximately 32 percent homology and 56 percent similarity across four of the seven (IV, V, VI, VII) transmembrane domains. Except for the secretion receptor, the homology of the CT receptor and the PTH/PTHrP receptor with other G protein–linked receptors is low (<12 percent). Therefore, these three receptors, together with the glucagon, VIP, and secretin receptors, may represent a newly identified subgroup of the family of G protein–linked rhodopsin-like receptors. Like the PTH/PTHrP receptor, but unlike the beta-adrenergic receptor, the CT receptor contains a signal sequence at the N terminus. The N-terminal exoplasmic domain contains three potential N-linked glycosylation sites and conserved extracellular cysteine residues (Fig. 22-17). As predicted, the CT receptor has a moderate- to large-sized N-terminal extracellular domain 147 amino acids long, intermediate in size between that of the beta-adrenergic receptor and the luteinizing hormone receptor, which is thought to bind the hormone, and a unique long C-terminal intracellular region that contains several potential phosphorylation sites. Like the PTH receptor,[68] the CT receptor appears to be able to interact not only with $G_s\alpha$ but also with the G protein involved in the activation of protein kinase C.[183] The structural domain(s) within the receptor

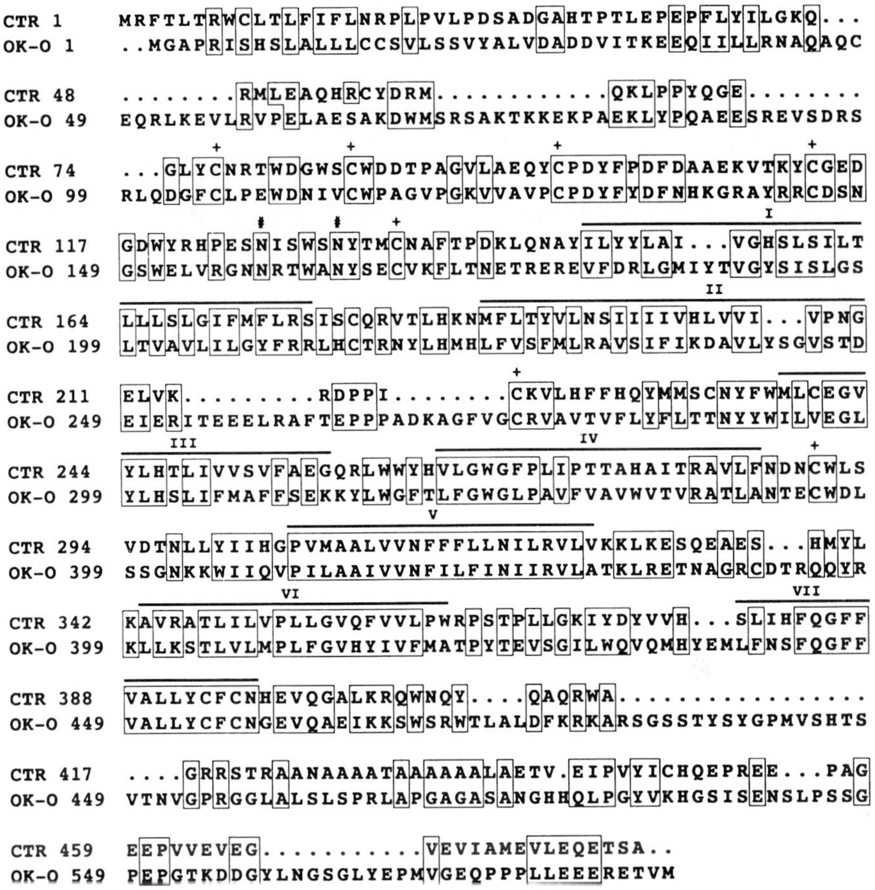

FIGURE 22-17. An alignment of the calcitonin receptor vs. the PTH/PTHrP receptor (OK-O) from opossum kidney cells. Shaded boxes represent identity or similarity. The bars above the sequences represent the transmembrane domains. The symbol # indicates N-linked glycosylation sites, and + indicates conserved cysteins. The Gen-Bank accession number is M74420 for the calcitonin receptor and M74445 for the PTH/PTHrP receptor. *(Reprinted with permission from Lin et al.*[87]*)*

responsible for this biological property has not been identified. The cloned expressed receptor binds CT with 6 nM affinity and also binds calcitonin gene–related peptide (CGRP) (see later discussion), but less avidly than CT (as predicted), and displays down regulation. It is found in osteoclasts and human giant cell tumors of bone but not in osteoblasts. Preliminary Southern blot analysis indicates the presence of only one gene encoding the CT receptor.

Each of the calcitonin family of peptides binds to a specific receptor, all of which are members of the seven-transmembrane-spanning G protein-coupled receptor family.[179] There is some cross reactivity between the peptides and respective receptors. Interactions of these ligands with the receptors is influenced by newly identified receptor modulating proteins, which expand the biological actions mediated by the receptors and their respective ligands alone.[184–186] The CGRP receptor component protein (CGRP-RCP) modulates a CGRP-unresponsive receptor to a responsive state and is a hydrophilic protein that is highly conserved and expressed in all tissues.[184] The receptor-activity-modifying proteins (RAMPs) are membrane proteins with one transmembrane domain and are comprised of 3 family members: RAMP1–3.[185] RAMPs interact with a separate calcitonin receptor-like receptor (CRLR), which has >50 percent homology with the CT receptor to transport it to the cell surface. RAMP1 transport of CRLR results in a receptor that recognizes CGRP, while RAMP2 and 3 transport of CRLR results in a receptor that recognizes adrenomedullin.[179]

Biochemistry and Molecular Biology

Although many questions remain regarding the role of calcitonin in normal physiology and its contribution to pathophysiology, considerable information has emerged from basic investigations regarding its interaction with receptors and its molecular biology.

The 32-amino acid size of the hormone is invariant across species.[167,168] In addition, all the homologs contain a 7-amino acid cyclic structure at the N terminus and a proline amide at the carboxyl terminus. Although homology within the ring structure is largely conserved across various species, the central linear portion of the hormone displays great diversity (Fig. 22-18). Only 9 of the 32 amino acid residues across the 10 species that have been structurally elucidated are constant. Interestingly, the nonmammalian calcitonins have higher potency than do mammalian calcitonins even when used in mammalian-based systems or in vivo in humans. Salmon CT, for instance, appears to be approximately 10- to 40-fold more active than human calcitonin in humans.[187] In fact, the interaction of salmon CT with receptors is so avid that almost no dissociation is observed; the interaction with receptor is functionally irreversible.[188–190] This is a very unusual feature of the calcitonin hormone–receptor system.

Beyond the information regarding structure-function relations for the hormone provided by the great sequence diversity present in nature, numerous structure-activity studies have been performed with synthetic analogs of the hormone.[187,191,192]

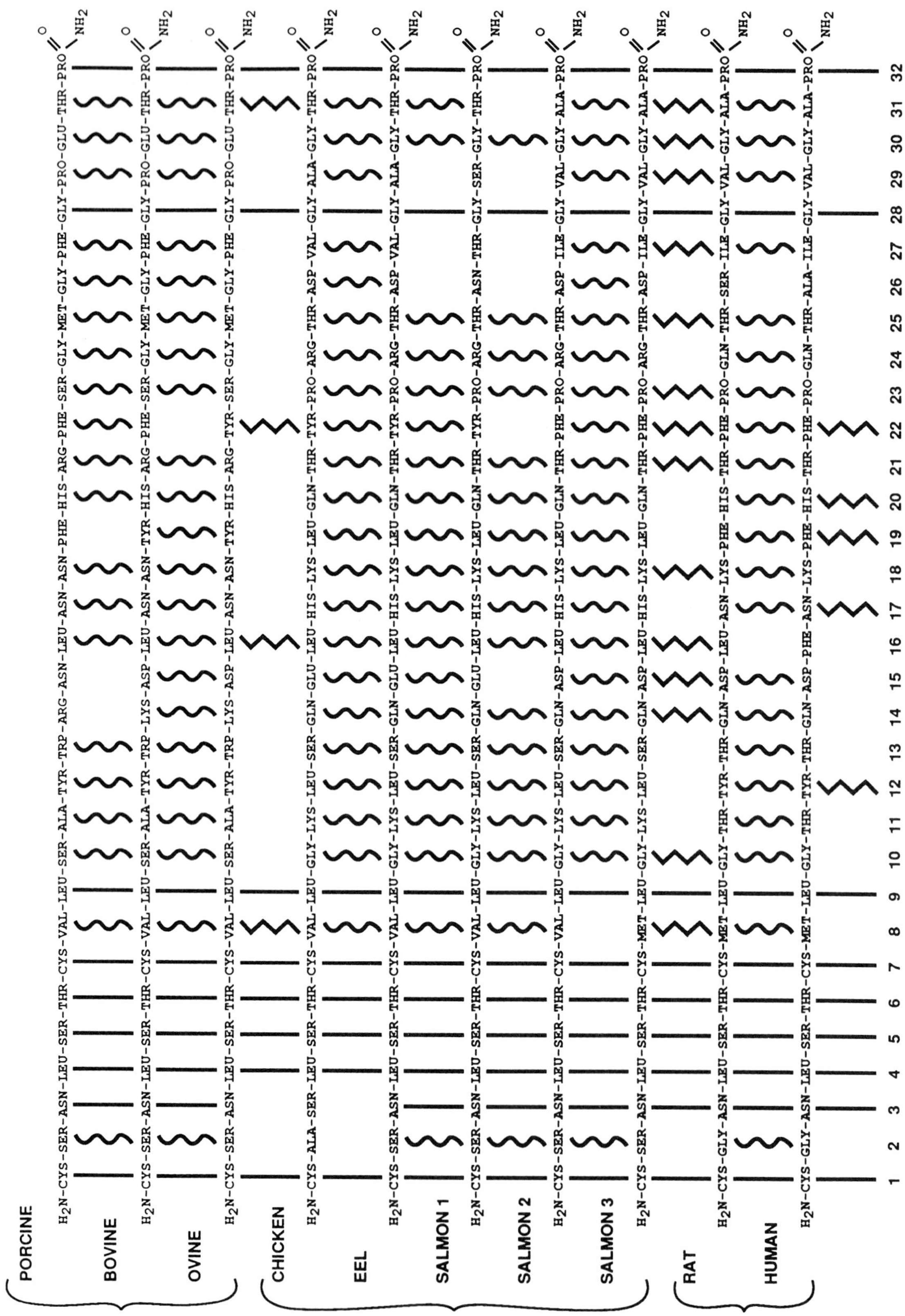

FIGURE 22-18. Comparison of the sequence of homologues of calcitonin from various species. Straight lines indicate conservation across all species. Wavy lines indicate conservation within groups only. (*Modified and reprinted with permission from Leonard J. Deftos, Calcitonin, in Primer on the Metabolic Bone Diseases and Disorders of Mineral Metabolism, Murray J. Favus, ed., Am. Soc. Bone and Mineral Research, Kelseyville, California, p. 53, 1990.*)

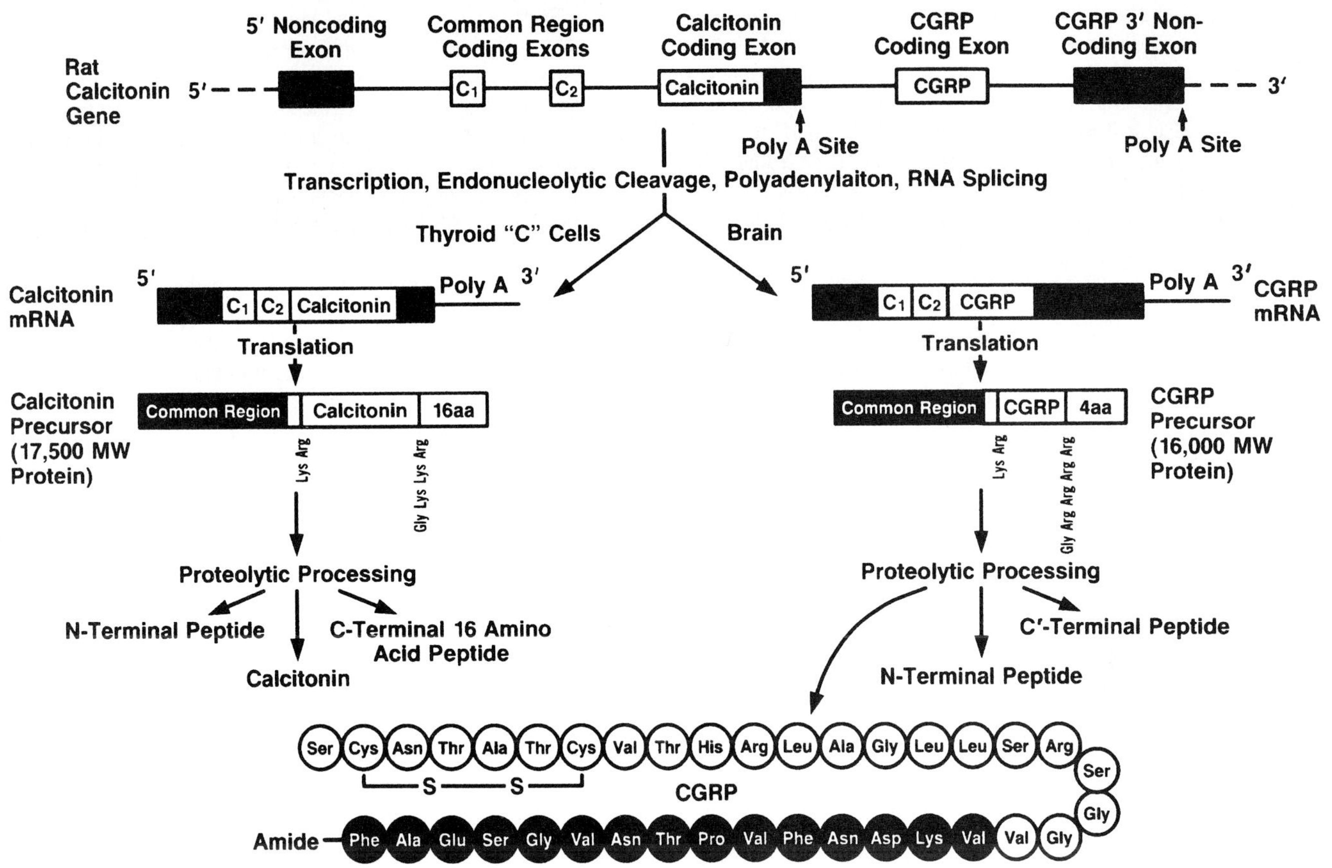

FIGURE 22-19. Alternative RNA processing pathways in the expression of the calcitonin gene. Calcitonin is biosynthesized in thyroid C cells; CGRP mRNA is produced in the brain. In addition to calcitonin and CGRP, N-terminal and C-terminal peptides are encoded in both the precursor of calcitonin and the precursor of CGRP. (*Reprinted with permission from Rosenfeld et al.*[279])

Shortening of the peptide at either end of the molecule results in nearly complete loss of biological activity,[187,193] although there is at least one exception to this general observation.[194] In the central portion of the molecule, many of the amino acids appear to serve a spacer role and can be substituted without having much of an impact on bioactivity. The 7-amino acid disulfide-linked ring is important for bioactivity but is not essential. The sulfur atoms can be replaced with methylenes,[195] and there is one example of opening of the ring with preservation of bioactivity.[196]

The biosynthesis of calcitonin from its gene occurs by a complex and intriguing process (Fig. 22-19).[197,198] The calcitonin gene is composed of six exons. The gene has the potential to generate at least two different mature mRNAs and the peptides each of them encodes. By one set of splicing routes, the calcitonin precursor of 141 amino acids is generated. Calcitonin is encoded at the C terminus of the precursor molecule and is the major processed peptide. The thyroid C cell follows this pattern of splicing to produce calcitonin. In other tissues, such as neurons, a 128-amino acid precursor is generated that contains a peptide termed calcitonin gene–related peptide (CGRP) but no calcitonin.[198] CGRP is a 37-amino acid peptide with considerable homology to calcitonin. Like calcitonin, it contains a cyclic disulfide bridge region and an amidated C terminus. CGRP biosynthesis has been localized to the dorsal spinal cord and the pituitary.[199] Like calcitonin, it is located at the C terminus of its precursor protein and is encoded by the fourth exon in the series of five that are spliced together to generate the mature mRNA. The calcitonin-coding exon is excised in this splicing arrangement and therefore is not present in the mature mRNA encoding CGRP.

Through interaction with its own receptor, CGRP possesses striking vasodilatory activity: It is one of the most potent vasodilators known.[200] It causes vascular dilatation whether administered intravenously or into the cerebrospinal fluid,[201] leading to the speculation that the hormone may play a role in cerebral vascular regulation. Arterial dilatation stimulated by CGRP appears to involve the activation of K^+ channels,[202] particularly a K^+/ATPase channel. In this regard, CGRP appears to act through a mechanism shared by that of vasoactive intestinal peptide (VIP) and endothelium-derived relaxant factor (EDRF). CGRP probably can also act as a neurotransmitter.[203] It has been shown to have effects on food intake in laboratory rats when administered into the central nervous system, decreasing food intake and spontaneous nocturnal eating[204] and inhibiting gastric acid secretion.[205] CGRP is also able to interact with and activate the calcitonin receptor.[206,207] The calcitonin-like biological properties of CGRP on osteoclasts and elsewhere are therefore directly traceable to the hormone's interaction with calcitonin receptors.[208–210] This ability of both CT and CGRP to interact with the other hormone's receptor has provided the impetus for the synthesis of new "hybrid" analogs that combine structural elements of each hormone in a new molecule.[211]

Interestingly, both calcitonin and CGRP precursor mRNAs also code for additional peptides that are presumed to be translated, termed "cryptic" peptides.[212–215] For the calcitonin precursor, which contains a signal sequence and a pro region, there is also a 16-amino acid carboxyl-terminal adjacent peptide (C-CAP) and an N-terminal adjacent peptide (N-CAP). C-CAP is known to be cosecreted with calcitonin by medullary carcinomas.[216] Such cryptic peptides have now been found in the precursors of many other peptide hormones. Their physiologic role in the CT/CGRP precursor is still uncertain, although some calcium-regulating actions have been reported.[214,217] However, the discovery of new and potentially biologically active peptides within the genes for established hormones indicates that there is a capacity for diversity of biological active peptides not previously envisioned in the endocrine system.

Calcitonin as a Therapeutic Agent

Calcitonin is effective in the acute treatment of hypercalcemia of malignancy.[218–225] Both humoral hypercalcemia of malignancy and hypercalcemia associated with extensive metastases to bone are associated with recruitment of the normal cellular apparatus for bone resorption, osteoclasts, by the tumor. Therefore, calcitonin, which acts on osteoclasts, is effective in blocking further bone resorption and produces a rapid lowering of serum calcium levels. Although the effects of administered calcitonin on mineral ion flux are prompt and large in magnitude, in many instances they are limited to the acute period. Chronic administration of calcitonin leads to a classic picture of tachyphylaxis within days.[218] It seems most likely that this tachyphylaxis is due to down regulation of receptors.[226] In some patients, tachyphylaxis of the response to calcitonin may be delayed for a few days by the coadministration of glucocorticoids.[227] Similarly, although acute hypercalcemia is a documented stimulus for calcitonin secretion, chronic hypercalcemia has not been consistently associated with increased levels of calcitonin.

In Paget's disease of bone, there are many localized regions throughout bone where bone turnover (both formation and resorption) is highly accelerated. Although the linkage of formation and resorption in Paget's disease is close enough to prevent the development of hypercalcemia, calcitonin is nevertheless able to reduce the metabolic activity and associated pain resulting from increased bone turnover.[225] Symptomatic relief occurs within weeks in approximately two-thirds of patients. Biochemical indexes of improvement such as reduction in serum alkaline phosphatase usually follow within 3 to 6 months. The usual starting dose is 100 units per day subcutaneously. After biochemical efficacy is evident, the dose can be reduced, but usually not below 50 units three times per week. Unfortunately, "escape" from calcitonin's effects occurs commonly, perhaps acutely as a result of down regulation of receptors or long-term via the development of anticalcitonin (salmon) antibodies.[228]

At this time, calcitonin is available in the United States as both parenteral and intranasal formulations. Salmon calcitonin is used more widely in the United States because of its enhanced potency and for historical reasons, while human calcitonin is used more widely in Europe. The clinical use of salmon calcitonin generates antibodies in most patients. However, despite the differences in amino acid sequence between the isoforms (Fig. 22-18), the antibodies generated usually are not neutralizing, and their presence does not seem to correlate with resistance to the hormone.[229,230] In cases where resistance to salmon calcitonin develops after long-term administration and is presumed to be antibody-mediated, switching to the human form is indicated.[225]

The use of calcitonin as a therapeutic agent for the treatment of osteoporosis varies in different regions of the world. In Europe, calcitonin is used to prevent loss of bone mineral and ameliorate the pain associated with osteoporosis-related vertebral fractures and sometimes with metabolic bone disease. How calcitonin produces analgesia is uncertain; this may be due to a central, perhaps endorphin-mediated, effect. Calcitonin treatment may increase bone mineral density for 1 or 2 years. However, the positive effects of calcitonin or bone mineral density in postmenopausal osteoporosis are modest and may begin to plateau or even reverse within 12 to 24 months despite continued treatment.[231] Furthermore, there is no convincing evidence that calcitonin treatment reduces fractures.[232,233] Therefore, in the United States, calcitonin is used less frequently than in Europe for the treatment of osteoporosis, although it does have Food and Drug Administration approval for this indication.

VITAMIN D

Historical Introduction

Rickets became endemic in European cities during their explosive growth in the industrial revolution. By the late nineteenth century epidemiologic investigations in several European countries had found that environmental factors having to do with crowding rather than poor nutrition made city dwellers prone to rickets, which was virtually unheard of among impoverished children in the countryside. As early as 1822, the Polish physician Sniadecki wrote that "if the parents' financial status permits, it is best to take the children [with rickets] out into the country and keep them as much as possible in the dry, open and pure air. If not, at least they should be carried out in the open air, especially in the sun, direct action of which on our bodies must be regarded as one of the most efficient methods for the prevention and cure of the disease."[234] In the British Isles, "systematic use of sunbaths . . . and the education of the public to the appreciation of sunshine as a means of health" was proposed by Palm in 1890. However, this simple notion never caught on. In 1919 Huldschinsky cured rickets with phototherapy[235]; by then, the nutritional and photochemical approaches to rickets were about to merge.

Cod liver oil had been used for treatment of rickets in the nineteenth century. In 1922, McCollum and colleagues identified a specific antirachitic activity in cod liver oil by showing that destruction of vitamin A activity by oxidation did not abolish antirachitic activity.[236] Shortly thereafter, two groups showed that UV irradiation of food substances could also produce the antirachitic activity that by then was called vitamin D.[237,238] By the 1930s milk in the United States was fortified with vitamin D by irradiation, leading to the virtual abolition of rickets. The form of vitamin D produced by the irradiation of yeast extract was shown to be ergocalciferol (vitamin D_2); that produced in skin was cholecalciferol (vitamin D_3). What was referred to as vitamin D_1 turned out to be a mixture of two forms, and the term is now obsolete.

Knowledge of the chemistry of vitamin D did not advance until the late 1960s, when work in the laboratories of DeLuca, Fraser, Norman, and others established that vitamin D is a prohormone which is converted to highly active forms by successive hydroxylation at the 25- and 1-positions.[239] This work emphasized what was clear from their forerunners: Vitamin D is both a vitamin when ingested from nutritional sources and a hormone, which they showed is produced in the skin and activated sequentially in the liver and kidney.

Biosynthesis and Chemistry

Cholecalciferol (vitamin D_3) is produced nonenzymatically in the skin from 7-dehydrocholesterol (provitamin D_3) upon exposure to ultraviolet (UV) light of 290 to 310 nm. Upon absorption of photons of this wavelength by the 5,7-diene, the B ring is split and an unstable intermediate (previtamin D_3) is formed. Previtamin D is then slowly converted to cholecalciferol by a temperature-dependent nonenzymatic process.[240] The concentration of 7-dehydrocholesterol in skin is not limiting; the amount of cholecalciferol produced is a function of the dose of UV light and the solar zenith angle. At northern latitudes, where the incident angle of the sun's rays is low, little vitamin D is produced, particularly during the winter months. This probably accounts for the appearance of nutritional rickets in late winter. Total-body sun exposure can provide 250 ug (10,000 IU) of vitamin D per day.[241] A person older than 70 years produces approximately 30 percent less than that.[242] Ultraviolet light of 290 to 310 nm is efficiently absorbed by sunscreens and by the endogenous pigment melanin, so that for a given exposure blacks produce considerably smaller amounts of vitamin D than do whites.[243]

Cholecalciferol (vitamin D_3) is the form of vitamin D in fish liver oils and other animal sources, whereas the other major calciferol, ergocalciferol (vitamin D_2), is similarly produced from its precursor ergosterol by irradiation in plants and irradiated yeast. Cholecalciferol differs from ergocalciferol only in the side chain (Fig. 22-20), and the two compounds have equivalent biological activity in humans (40,000 IU/mg) and undergo identical metabolic conversion to active forms. Thus, both the endogenous form of vitamin D, cholecalciferol, and the plant form, ergocalciferol,

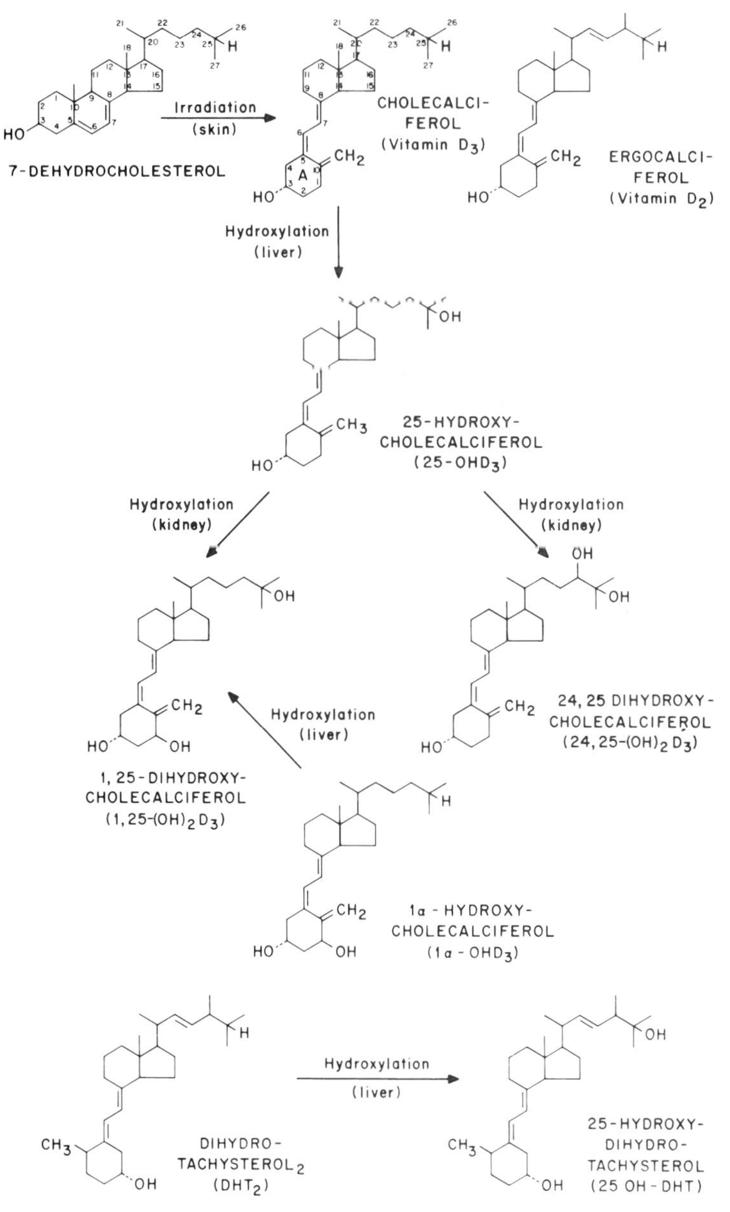

FIGURE 22-20. Chemical structures of the major vitamin D metabolites and analogues. The numbering system is based on that of cholesterol, and the A ring of cholecalciferol is so designated.

can be ingested in foodstuffs. In this chapter, the term *vitamin D* without a subscript will be used generically to apply to both forms.

As will be discussed in detail later, vitamin D is activated by sequential hydroxylations in the 25- and 1α-positions (Fig. 22-20). The structures of two therapeutically useful analogs are also shown there. 1α-hydroxycholecalciferol can be synthesized from cholesterol and is useful as an analog of 1α,25-dihydroxycholecalciferol. Dihydrotachysterol (DHT) is a synthetic analog in which the A ring is rotated 180° so that the position of the 3-hydroxyl sterically resembles that of the 1α-hydroxyl in active vitamin D metabolites. Although its potency is only threefold higher than that of vitamin D, it has a rapid onset of action. Both 1α-hydroxycholecalciferol and DHT appear to require 25-hydroxylation for full activity in vivo. However, because these analogs do not require 1α-hydroxylation in vivo, they are useful in vitamin D–resistant states where 1α-hydroxylation is impaired, such as chronic renal failure and hypoparathyroidism.

Absorption, Activation, and Transport of Vitamin D

Absorption

Vitamin D_3 produced in the skin by exposure to ultraviolet light enters the circulation by a process that is not well understood but which may involve a serum binding protein for vitamin D.[240] Vitamin D has a circulating half-life of approximately 48 h and is stored in adipose tissue and muscle. Dietary forms of vitamin D are fat-soluble substances that are primarily absorbed from the proximal small bowel and transported through the lymphatic system bound to chylomicrons. Absorption may fail in individuals with generalized or fat malabsorption disorders (Whipple's disease, celiac disease, pancreatic insufficiency).

Activation

Vitamin D is transported from the skin and body stores to the liver bound to a specific protein, vitamin D–binding protein, whose role is discussed in detail later. In the liver, vitamin D undergoes hydroxylation at the 25-position by enzymes in the microsomes and mitochondria of parenchymal cells (Fig. 22-21). The enzyme system is a mixed-function oxidase that utilizes reduced NADP and molecular oxygen.[244] 25-hydroxylation of vitamin D is not a closely regulated process. The effect of 1α,25-dihydroxyvitamin D [1α-25-$(OH)_2D$] in reducing circulating levels of 25-hydroxyvitamin D in vivo[245] is attributable primarily to an increase in the metabolic clearance rate of 25-hydroxyvitamin D[246] (see discussion on metabolism of vitamin D). Whether 1α,25-$(OH)_2D$ affects hepatic synthesis of 25-hydroxyvitamin D directly is controversial.[247]

FIGURE 22-21. Transport and metabolic sequence of activation of vitamin D in humans.

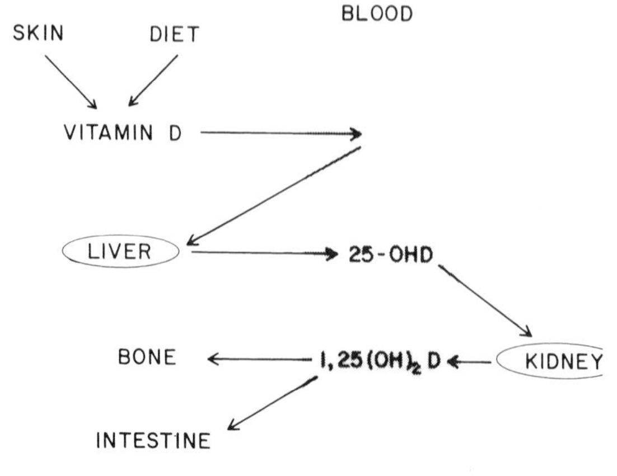

25-hydroxyvitamin D is the principal circulating form of the vitamin. Its concentration in serum is 10 to 50 ng/ml (25 to 125 nmol/liter). The circulating pool is presumed to be in equilibrium with body stores in muscle and fat, and the half-life of 25-hydroxyvitamin D has been estimated at 15 to 20 days. As 25-hydroxyvitamin D is produced in a relatively unregulated fashion from either endogenous or exogenous sources of the hormone and enters a large stable circulating pool, the serum concentration of 25-hydroxyvitamin D is the best clinical measure of nutritional vitamin D status, and chronic vitamin D deficiency is reflected in low serum 25-hydroxyvitamin D levels. Note that in vitamin D–replete individuals, acute increases in serum levels of vitamin D induced by brief exposure to sunlight have little impact on the much larger circulating pool of 25-hydroxyvitamin D (Fig. 22-22). Assay of the serum concentration of 25-hydroxyvitamin D is thus a key part of the evaluation of certain disorders of mineral metabolism (see section on assay of vitamin D metabolites).

The liver has a large excess capacity to 25-hydroxylate vitamin D, and in the United States chronic liver disease is not generally associated with a clinically significant deficiency of this metabolite. Although circulating levels of 25-hydroxyvitamin D are reduced in liver disease, this is largely a consequence of reduced hepatic synthesis of the carrier protein, vitamin D–binding protein, as discussed in transport of vitamin D metabolites. Treatment with anticonvulsants (phenytoin, phenobarbital) can also reduce 25-hydroxyvitamin D levels, presumably by inducing hepatic microsomal enzymes that inactivate vitamin D and its metabolites. In addition, 25-hydroxyvitamin D undergoes accelerated clearance, together with its binding protein, in the nephrotic syndrome, leading to lower circulating levels of this metabolite.

With the discovery of 25-hydroxyvitamin D, it was briefly thought that the most active metabolite of the vitamin had been identified, but within a few years it became clear that a further hydroxylation would produce a thousandfold increase in biological activity. 25-hydroxyvitamin D is further hydroxylated in the kidney to 1α,25-dihydroxyvitamin D [1α,25-$(OH)_2D$] or 24,25-dihydroxyvitamin D [24,25-$(OH)_2D$ (Fig. 22-21). In contrast to 25-hydroxylation in the liver, 1α-hydroxylation is under exquisite metabolic control (Table 22-1), providing for integration of vitamin D activation into the overall schema for the regulation of mineral homeostasis.[248,249] Although 1α,25-$(OH)_2D$ is clearly the most active metabolite, 24-hydroxyvitamin D can also exert calcium absorptive activity although its potency is 1/100th that of 1α,25-$(OH)_2D$.[250]

The renal 1α-hydroxylase is a mitochondrial cytochrome P450 mixed-function oxidase that requires reduced NADP and molecular oxygen. The cytochrome P450 probably participates directly in the hydroxylation of 25-hydroxyvitamin D, transferring electrons from reduced NADP via a reductase and renal renodoxin.[7,251] The enzyme has been localized to the proximal convoluted tubule and the pars recta of the rat nephron. At the former site, it is regulated by parathyroid hormone but not calcitonin; at the latter, it is regulated by calcitonin exclusively.[108] The 1α-hydroxylase cDNA was cloned from rodents and humans in 1997.[252] 25-hydroxyvitamin D 24-hydroxylase (24-OHase) is a separate

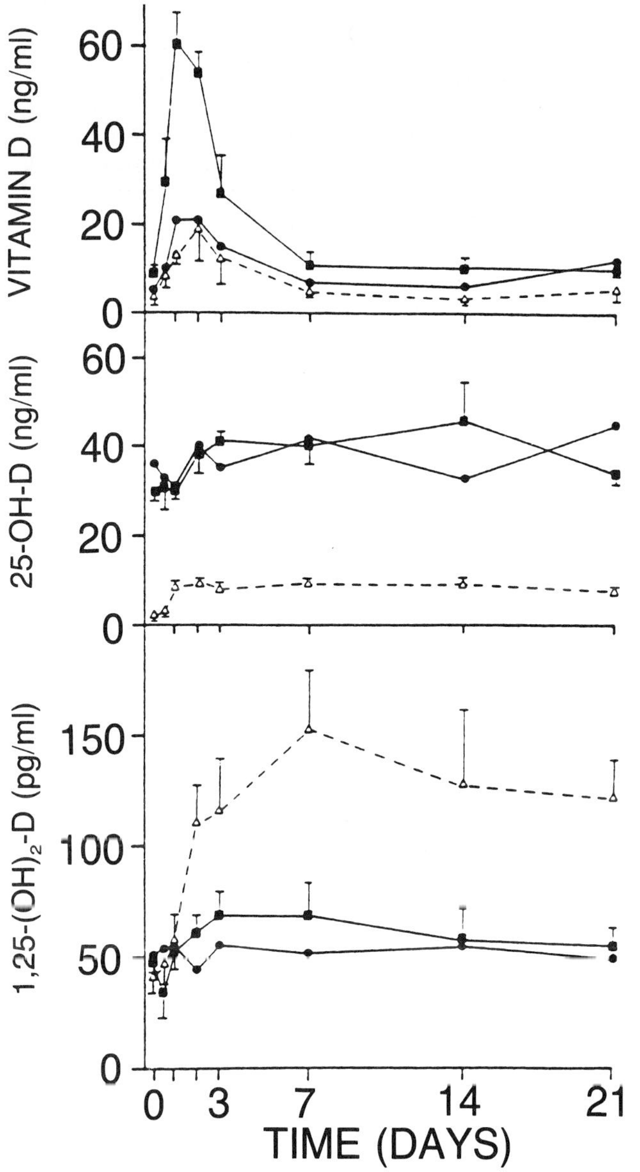

FIGURE 22-22. Changes in serum concentrations of vitamin D and its metabolites after exposure to ultraviolet radiation (UVR). Normal subjects (solid circle, solid square) were exposed to one (solid circle) or three (solid square) minimal erythemal doses of UVR. Vitamin D-deficient subjects (open triangles) were exposed to one minimal erythemal dose of UVR. The transient increase in serum vitamin D levels does not affect the serum level of 25-OH-D or 1α,25-$(OH)_2D$ in normal subjects but markedly increases the serum level of both metabolites in patients with vitamin D deficiency. (*From Adams JS, Clemens TL, Parrish JA, Holick MF, N Engl J Med 306:722, 1982, by permission of the New England Journal of Medicine.*)

P450 mixed-function oxidase that is also located in the proximal renal tubule and under many circumstances is regulated inversely to the 1α-hydroxylase, as discussed later. The cloned enzyme has less than 30 percent homology to other cytochrome P450s and thus represents a new family.[253] To prevent sustained production of 1α,25-$(OH)_2D$ that would lead to hypercalcemia, 1α,25-$(OH)_2D$ hormone induces the expression of 24-OHase. This enzymes catalyzes the addition of an hydroxyl group on carbon 24. When the substrate is 1α,25-$(OH)_2D$, the product is 1,24,25-trihydroxy vitamin D, which is inactive. Animals homogeneous for 24-OHase inactivating mutation cannot clear 1α,25-$(OH)_2D$, resulting in increased circulating concentrations. This leads to hypercalcemia and perinatal lethality.[254] 24-OHase also catalyzes 25-$(OH)_2D$ to 24,25-$(OH)_2D$. Literature also suggests that 24,25-$(OH)_2D$ is important in cartilage development[255,256] and fracture repair.[257,258]

Parathyroid Hormone

Parathyroid hormone stimulates renal 1α-hydroxylase activity and reciprocally decreases the activity of 24-hydroxylase.[248,249,259] Based on the ability of cAMP analogues and the nonhormonal activator of adenylyl cyclase forskolin to mimic the effect of PTH, the second messenger for this effect appears to be cAMP.[260,261] PTH exerts its effects within hours, a time course consistent with the induction of new enzyme protein, but a direct effect of phosphorylating a regulatory component of the complex has not been excluded. The effect of PTH on 24-hydroxylase activity appears to be transcriptional.[262] It is also conceivable that part of the effect of PTH on the enzyme in vivo could result from PTH action to change intrarenal handling of phosphate and ultimately serum phosphorus levels (see later discussion).

In hyperparathyroidism, the serum level of 1α,25-$(OH)_2D$ tends to be increased, although many patients have levels in the high-normal range, presumably because of the countervailing influence of hypercalcemia.[263] PTH is the primary mediator of the marked increases in renal 1α-hydroxylase activity in hypocalcemic states. The response to hypocalcemia is blunted in hypoparathyroid states, so that the serum level of 1α,25-$(OH)_2D$ is low or low-normal in hypocalcemic patients with hypoparathyroidism and pseudohypoparathyroidism.[264] However, hypocalcemia per se probably can increase 1α-hydroxylase activity in the absence of PTH[248] (see later discussion).

The plasma level of 1α,25-$(OH)_2D$ is regulated by changes in calcium intake within the normal range,[265] and increased 1α,25-$(OH)_2D$ levels in response to a low calcium intake play a role in the adaptation of intestinal calcium absorption. Diet-induced changes in 1α,25-$(OH)_2D$ are highly correlated with changes in the level of PTH, suggesting that the system is sufficiently sensitive for PTH to play a role in homeostatic adjustments to changing calcium intake within the usual dietary range.

Phosphorus

Although early studies suggested that only extreme changes in phosphate intake might affect the production of 1α,25-$(OH)_2D$, it is now clear that the production of this metabolite can be regulated by alterations in phosphate intake within the range of normal

TABLE 22-1. Factors That Influence Renal 1α-Hydroxylase Activity

Parathyroid hormone
Phosphate
1,25-$(OH)_2D$
Serum calcium
Growth hormone
Glucocorticoids
Prolactin
pH
Calcitonin
Estrogen

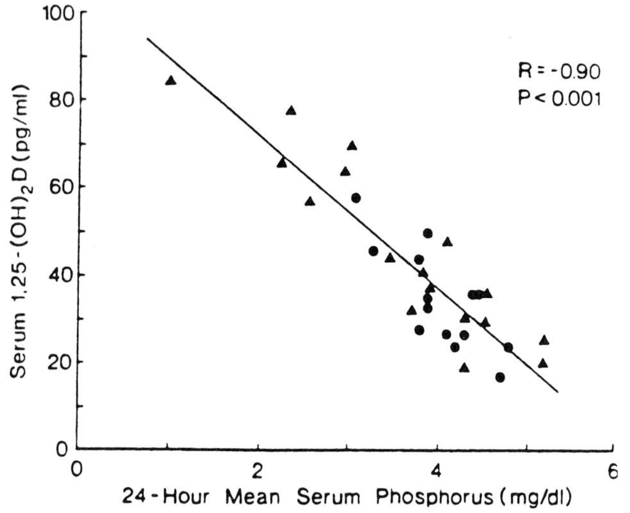

FIGURE 22-23. The relation between serum levels of phosphorus and serum levels of 1α,25-$(OH)_2D$ in normal men in whom serum phosphorus was manipulated by varying phosphate intake. Data are combined from two studies in which dietary phosphorus was maintained at <50, 1500, or >3000 mg/day (closed triangles) or at 625 or 2300 mg/day (closed circles). Changes in dietary phosphorus within the normal range (closed circles) regulate 1α,25-$(OH)_2D$ levels similarly to extreme changes (closed triangles). (*From Portale, Halloran, and Morris*[337] *by copyright permission of the American Society for Clinical Investigation.*)

(Fig. 22-23) and that this occurs independently of changes in PTH.[266] It is also clear that dietary phosphate intake can override the effect of PTH on the production of 1α,25-$(OH)_2D$ in several circumstances. Oral phosphate therapy for primary hyperparathyroidism or idiopathic hypercalciuria decreases the serum 1α,25-$(OH)_2D$ level in the face of a rise in the PTH level[267]; conversely, phosphate restriction in children with moderate chronic renal insufficiency increases the serum concentration of 1α,25-$(OH)_2D$ as PTH levels fall.[268] The changes in the production of 1α,25-$(OH)_2D$ induced by alterations in dietary phosphate are correlated with changes in the serum phosphorus level, but it is not clear how changes in phosphorus intake are sensed and transmitted to the enzymes of vitamin D metabolism. Altered dietary phosphate intake produces adaptive changes in phosphate transport, but the effect of altered phosphate transport on phosphate levels in intracellular compartments relevant to vitamin D metabolism cannot be predicted. This process may also be under hormonal control. The adaptation of 1α-hydroxylase activity to a low phosphate intake requires the presence of growth hormone, acting through IGF-I.[269] There is evidence for humoral factors that simultaneously produce increased renal phosphate clearance and decreased 1α,25-$(OH)_2D$ levels in tumor-induced osteomalacia.[270] Renal 24-hydroxylase activity is regulated inversely to 1α-hydroxylase activity at the extremes of phosphate intake (Fig. 22-24), but it is not known whether the 24-hydroxylase is subject to fine control by smaller changes.

Vitamin D Status

Renal 1α-hydroxylase activity is markedly increased (Fig. 22-22) and 24-hydroxylase activity is negligible in vitamin D deficiency.[249,271] Both are rapidly restored to normal by the administration of 1α,25-$(OH)_2D$. These effects are blocked by inhibitors of RNA and protein synthesis, suggesting that they occur at the transcriptional level. The reduction in 24-hydroxylase activity has been shown directly to involve a reduction in the level of mRNA.[262] Conversely, vitamin D excess is associated with a reduction in renal 1α-hydroxylase activity, protecting against vitamin D intoxication.

Serum and Intracellular Calcium

Studies in animals and in normal humans indicate that sustained hypercalcemia produces a reduction in the serum concentration of 1α,25-$(OH)_2D$, which can override the stimulatory effect of PTH in experimental hyperparathyroidism.[109] This effect of hypercalcemia may explain the finding of normal serum levels of 1α,25-$(OH)_2D$ in some patients with primary hyperparathyroidism[263] and could contribute to the finding of low serum concentrations of 1α,25-$(OH)_2D$ in malignancy-associated hypercalcemia.

It appears (as discussed previously) that the stimulation of 1α-hydroxylase activity in hypocalcemic states is primarily attributable to secondary hyperparathyroidism, with a minor direct effect of hypocalcemia.[7] However, the normal levels sometimes observed in hypoparathyroidism despite the combined effects of PTH deficiency and hyperphosphatemia are compatible with an independent effect of hypocalcemia to stimulate 1α-hydroxylase activity. This has been shown directly in the rat.[272]

In isolated mitochondria, normal metabolism of vitamin D appears to require a fixed range of ionized calcium.[273] However, it is not clear whether acute changes in cytoplasmic $[Ca^{2+}]$ in the intact cell are involved in the physiologic regulation of enzyme activity.

Other Regulators

Estrogen treatment increases serum levels of 1α,25-$(OH)_2D$. This is attributable partly to increased synthesis of the vitamin D–binding protein, but free 1α,25-$(OH)_2D$ concentrations are also elevated.[274,275] The level of 1α,25-$(OH)_2D$ is markedly elevated in the third trimester of pregnancy,[278] a situation to which estrogen-dependent increases in renal synthesis, placental production of 1α,25-$(OH)_2D$ (see later discussion), and other hormones such as prolactin may all contribute. The plasma level of 1α,25-$(OH)_2D$ may be increased in markedly hypercalcitonemic

FIGURE 22-24. Relation between serum phosphorus and accumulation of radioactive vitamin D metabolites in the serum of thyroparathyroidectomized rats in which serum phosphorus was manipulated by variations in phosphate intake. The high level of serum phosphorus in these studies reflects both the effects of parathyroidectomy and the fact that serum phosphorus is normally higher in rats than it is in humans. (*By permission of Tanaka Y, DeLuca HF, Arch Biochem Biophys 154:566, 1973.*)

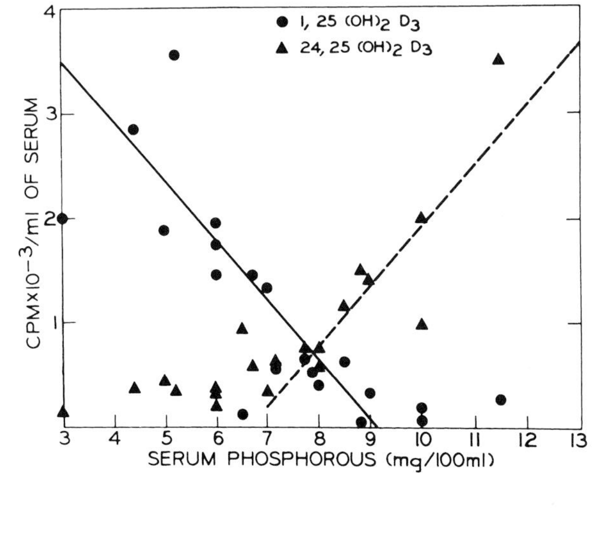

states,[277] but there is no evidence for physiologic regulation of renal production by calcitonin. A number of other factors, including growth hormone, prolactin, glucocorticoids, thyroid hormone, and systemic metabolic acidosis have been shown to affect the activity of renal 1α-hydroxylase in animal studies, but data supporting significant effects of any of these agents on the activity of the human enzyme are lacking or conflicting.[249]

Integrated Control

The fine control of its synthesis in the kidney serves to integrate 1α,25-$(OH)_2$D into the regulatory scheme for calcium homeostasis. The most important regulators of vitamin D metabolism in the kidney are PTH and phosphate. The parathyroids can respond to minute-to-minute changes in serum calcium and can sense changes induced by altered calcium intake within the normal dietary range. In pathologic states, the various regulators interact in complex ways. In nutritional vitamin D deficiency hypophosphatemia, secondary hyperparathyroidism and the reduced supply of vitamin D act in concert to increase enzyme activity. Their combined effect may maintain normal serum levels of 1α,25-$(OH)_2$D in the face of reduced substrate levels (Fig. 22-22). Note that in vitamin D–deficient individuals, exposure to sunlight produces a small increase in 25-(OH)D pool but an exaggerated rise in serum levels of 1α,25-$(OH)_2$D up to high levels, reflecting the high activity state of 1α-hydroxylase. In vitamin D excess, the combined effects of substrate, product, hypercalcemia, and hyperphosphatemia act to inhibit 1α-hydroxylase activity strongly, maintaining relatively normal levels of 1α,25-$(OH)_2$D. Thus, the integrated control of renal 1α-hydroxylase activity is remarkably successful in protecting the circulating level of the most important vitamin D metabolite against changes in intake or production. In other circumstances, individual factors work in opposition, with a hierarchy of dominance that is not fully predictable. For example, a large increase in phosphate intake suppresses 1α-hydroxylase activity even though it induces secondary hyperparathyroidism. The contrary effects of hypercalcemia, hypophosphatemia, and PTH excess produce variable increases in 1α,25-$(OH)_2$D in primary hyperparathyroidism.

Circulating and Extrarenal 1α,25-$(OH)_2$D

The circulating concentration of 1α,25-$(OH)_2$D is 20 to 60 pg/ml (50 to 150 pmol/liter), and its plasma half-life is 12 to 15 h. The relatively rapid turnover of 1α,25-$(OH)_2$D is a factor in its physiologic role as a day-to-day regulator of calcium homeostasis. The most important extrarenal source of 1α,25-$(OH)_2$D in humans is the placenta.[278] Production of 1α,25-$(OH)_2$D at that site probably contributes to high circulating 1α,25-$(OH)_2$D levels in the third trimester of pregnancy,[276] which in turn probably contribute to physiologic calcium hyperabsorption in pregnancy and lactation.[279] The plasma concentration of 1α,25-$(OH)_2$D is greatly reduced in anephric individuals, suggesting that in nonpregnant humans there is no major extrarenal source of circulating 1α,25-$(OH)_2$D, although 1α-hydroxylase activity is clearly present at other extrarenal sites. Low levels of 1α-hydroxylase activity are detectable in dermal keratinocytes in vitro,[280] in bone,[281] and in other target tissues. It is not known whether there is a paracrine tissue role of 1α,25-$(OH)_2$D produced at extrarenal sites. However, extrarenal production can be pathophysiologically critical. 1α-hydroxylase is present in activated macrophages,[282] and excessive production of 1α,25-$(OH)_2$D can lead to hypercalcemia in sarcoidosis and other granulomatous diseases, as discussed later.

Role of 24,25-$(OH)_2$D

24,25-$(OH)_2$D is the principal circulating metabolite of 25-hydroxyvitamin D. Its serum concentration of 2 to 4 ng/ml (5 to 10 nmol/liter) is 100-fold higher than the concentration of 1α,25-$(OH)_2$D and, in contrast to 1α,25-$(OH)_2$D, is a function of the 25-hydroxy-vitamin D concentration. In most circumstances, the renal production of 1α,25-$(OH)_2$D and 24,25-$(OH)_2$D is regulated reciprocally. However, the actual biological role of 24,25-$(OH)_2$D is obscure. There is a large body of literature suggesting that 24,25-$(OH)_2$D is important in cartilage development[255,256] and fracture repair.[257,258] There have been reports that 24,25-$(OH)_2$D has several biological actions that are not fully mimicked by 1α,25-$(OH)_2$D. These include increased bone formation in vitro in the presence of PTH and 1α,25-$(OH)_2$D, increased proteoglycan synthesis in chondrocytes, and improved mineralization of bone when it is added to 1α,25-$(OH)_2$D in therapy for vitamin D-deficient osteomalacia.[283] However, studies in intact animals are complicated by renal conversion of 24,25-$(OH)_2$D to the biologically active trihydroxylated 1α,24,25-trihydroxyvitamin D. Difluoro analogs in which C-24 is incapable of hydroxylation have the same biological activity as 25-hydroxyvitamin D with regard to intestinal calcium transport and healing of rickets in rats. This has been taken as evidence that hydroxylation at the 24-position is not essential for the actions of vitamin D.[283] However, 24-(OH)ase null mutants have a mineralization defect at the growth plate that is reversed by treatment with 24,25$(OH)_2$D,[254] suggesting that 24,25$(OH)_2$D does in fact have a physiological role.

Transport of Vitamin D Metabolites

All forms of vitamin D are transported in blood predominantly bound to a specific carrier protein, vitamin D–binding protein (also called Gc-globulin). This is an alpha globulin with a molecular weight of 58,000 that is a member of the same gene family as albumin and α-fetoprotein, and it binds actin in addition to vitamin D.[284] The protein has a single binding site for vitamin D metabolites. Its affinity for 25-hydroxyvitamin D and 24,25-$(OH)_2$D is equivalent and is higher than its affinity for 1α,25-$(OH)_2$D. In addition to the fraction bound to the specific vitamin D–binding protein, a small fraction of vitamin D metabolites circulates bound to albumin. Vitamin D–binding protein is produced in the liver. Its levels are increased by estrogen therapy[274,275] and reduced in severe liver disease and in the nephrotic syndrome.[284] The latter two states are not generally associated with the development of osteomalacia, and free levels of 25-hydroxyvitamin D are normal.[285]

It is uncertain whether the physiologic actions of vitamin D in vivo occur in conformity with the "free hormone hypothesis," that is, whether only the free fraction is biologically active. However, it is clear that the presence of vitamin D–binding protein limits the availability of 1α,25-$(OH)_2$D to its receptor and that when levels of vitamin D–binding protein are varied in vitro, the cellular effects of 1α,25-$(OH)_2$D are tightly correlated with the free concentration of the hormone.[286]

Further Metabolism of 1α,25-$(OH)_2$D

1α,25-$(OH)_2$D is metabolized by several pathways (Fig. 22-25).[249] A monoglucuronide and sulfates are produced in the liver, and 1α,25-$(OH)_2$D undergoes enterohepatic recirculation. Side-chain oxidation gives rise to the biologically inert metabolite calcitroic acid (1α-hydroxy-23-carboxy-tetranor vitamin D). 1α,25-$(OH)_2$D is also hydroxylated in the 24-position to 1α,24,25-$(OH)_3$D, which

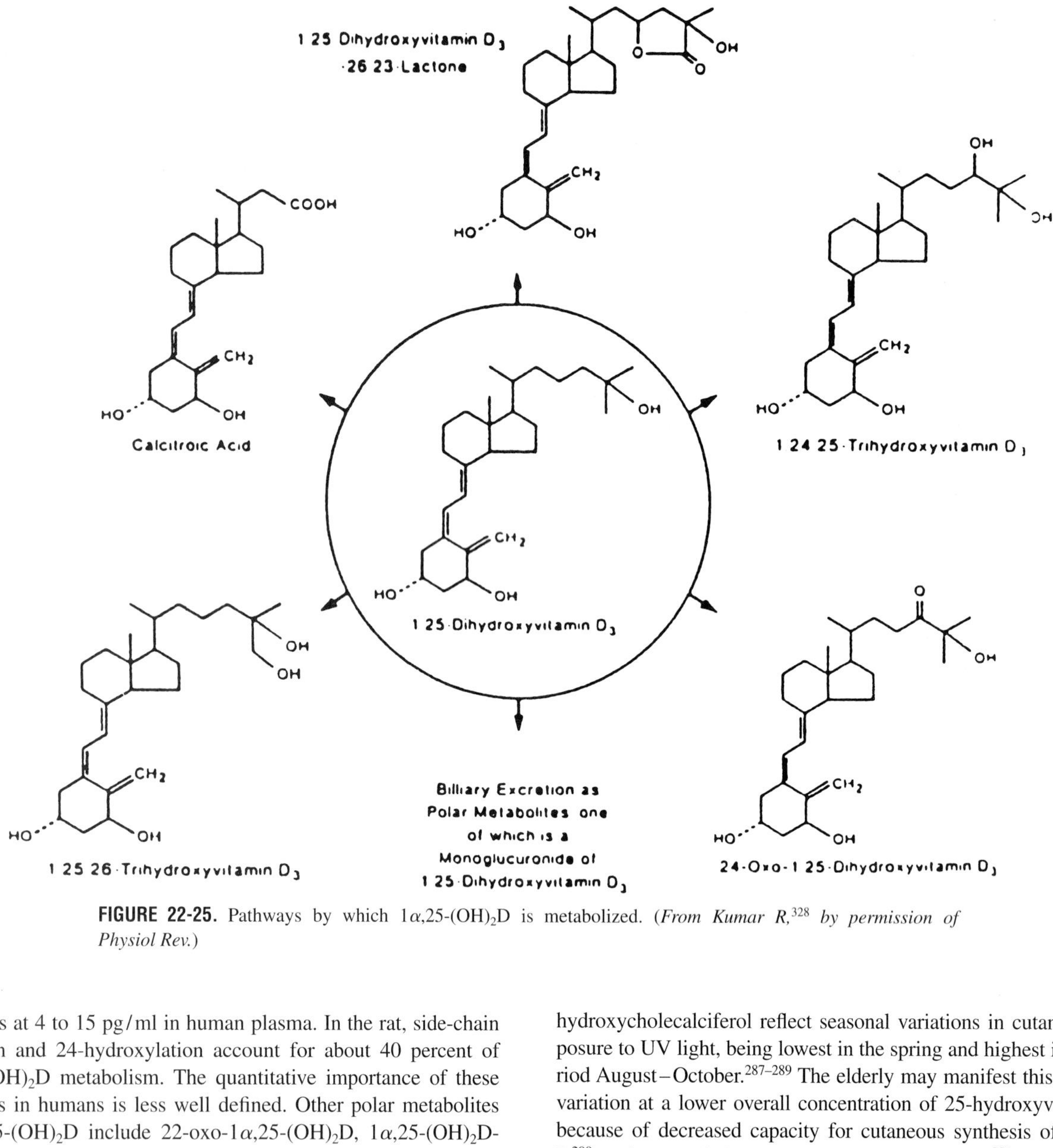

FIGURE 22-25. Pathways by which 1α,25-$(OH)_2$D is metabolized. (*From Kumar R,*[328] *by permission of Physiol Rev.*)

circulates at 4 to 15 pg/ml in human plasma. In the rat, side-chain oxidation and 24-hydroxylation account for about 40 percent of 1α,25-$(OH)_2$D metabolism. The quantitative importance of these pathways in humans is less well defined. Other polar metabolites of 1α,25-$(OH)_2$D include 22-oxo-1α,25-$(OH)_2$D, 1α,25-$(OH)_2$D-26,23-lactone, and 1α,25,26-$(OH)_3$D. All these metabolites have reduced biological activity relative to 1α,25-$(OH)_2$D. In all, some 30 metabolites of vitamin D have been identified to date.

The clearance of vitamin D metabolites is regulated by 1α,25-$(OH)_2$D.[246] In the rat, the administration of 1α,25-$(OH)_2$D lowers the serum concentrations of 25-(OH)D and 24,25-$(OH)_2$D by 50 percent and 70 percent, respectively, by increasing their metabolic clearance rate. The administration of 1α,25-$(OH)_2$D also increases its own metabolic clearance rate. Part of these effects is probably attributable to the sevenfold increase in renal 24-hydroxylase activity induced by 1α,25-$(OH)_2$D administration. It is likely that a human counterpart to this phenomenon exists, as the administration of 1α,25-$(OH)_2$D has also been shown to decrease the serum concentration of 25-(OH)D in humans.[245]

Vitamin D Nutrition

In much of the world, the requirement for vitamin D is satisfied by endogenous synthesis. In temperate zones, serum levels of 25-hydroxycholecalciferol reflect seasonal variations in cutaneous exposure to UV light, being lowest in the spring and highest in the period August–October.[287–289] The elderly may manifest this seasonal variation at a lower overall concentration of 25-hydroxyvitamin D because of decreased capacity for cutaneous synthesis of vitamin D[290] or decreased absorption of dietary vitamin D.[291] A substantial fraction of healthy individuals in the northen United States have 25-hydroxyvitamin D levels at the lower limit of normal in the spring.[288]

The recommended daily allowance of vitamin D for adults is 200 IU. Vitamin D is rarely found naturally in food but in the United States, food is supplemented with vitamin D. Both ergocalciferol and cholecalciferol are used as additives in milk and, in some locales, in cereals and bread products. Milk is usually supplemented with 400 IU per quart, but most milk sampled contain $<$50 percent of the amount stated on the label.[292] Presumably as a consequence of these practices, Americans have higher 25-hydroxy-vitamin D levels than do the residents of European countries in which dietary supplementation is not practiced (for example, Great Britain), and many researchers believe that this accounts for a decreased incidence of vitamin D insufficiency in the United States, particularly in those in whom the system is additionally stressed by illness that compromises the absorption or metabolism of the vitamin (e.g., liver disease, anticonvulsant therapy, nephrotic syndrome). Natural sources of dietary vitamin D are fatty fish, such as salmon and mackerel, and fatty fish oils such as cod liver oil.

The recommended daily allowance (RDA) of vitamin D is 400 IU per day. Some researchers believe that the elderly should receive more than the current RDA, as vitamin D deficiency has been detected frequently in the elderly, especially in the winter months. Among postmenopausal women in New England, seasonal variations in 25-hydroxyvitamin D levels are correlated inversely with the level of PTH.[289] This relation is accounted for by seasonal increases in PTH in women whose intake of vitamin D is <220 IU per day. This suggests that in the late winter and spring, when body stores of vitamin D are at their nadir, secondary hyperparathyroidism may develop to compensate for a relative state of vitamin D deficiency. In keeping with this interpretation, supplementation of this group with vitamins lessens hyperparathyroidism and increases bone density.[293] In 1997 the Institute of Medicine recommended 600 IU/d for adults >71 years.[242]

Vitamin D deficiency among patient hospitalized on a general medical service was recently reported to be as high as 57 percent. Some patients were considered to have severe vitamin D deficiency. It is unclear why the prevalence is so high, but supports the argument that the recommended amount may still not be sufficient.[294]

Cellular Basis of Vitamin D Action

The vitamin D receptor is a member of the steroid hormone receptor supergene family. It is a 50,000-molecular-weight protein with a DNA-binding domain whose sequence is 39 to 55 percent homologous to other members of the family.[295] Evidence that the cloned receptor is physiologically relevant comes from studies of patients with hereditary $1\alpha,25\text{-(OH)}_2\text{D}$–resistant rickets. These individuals have receptor mutations that interfere with the binding of hormone or association of the occupied receptor with DNA.[296] The vitamin D receptor binds $1\alpha,25\text{-(OH)}_2\text{D}$ with an affinity of 50 pmol/liter, consistent with the binding of $1\alpha,25\text{-(OH)}_2\text{D}$ from a cellular pool that is in diffusion equilibrium with circulating $1\alpha,25\text{-(OH)}_2\text{D}$. The relative affinities of other vitamin D metabolites for the receptor are 1:3 for $1\alpha,24,25\text{-(OH)}_3\text{D}$, 1:1,000 for 25-(OH)D, and 1:1,500 for $24,25\text{-(OH)}_2\text{D}$. Binding of hormone activates the receptor, and the hormone-receptor complex binds to nuclear chromatin. The means by which binding of its ligand activates the vitamin D receptor are relatively less well understood than for other members of the superfamily.[297,298]

The number of receptors is controlled at the transcriptional level, as $1\alpha,25\text{-(OH)}_2\text{D}$ is known to induce the synthesis of receptor mRNA and protein in several target tissues, including the intestine, kidney, and parathyroid glands.[299,300] This increase in available receptor is potentially important in the adaptation to states such as a low calcium intake, amplifying the effects of increased $1\alpha,25\text{-(OH)}_2\text{D}$ concentrations on intestinal calcium transport. The vitamin D receptor is a phosphoprotein, and phosphorylation may be important for its function.[301]

Direct evidence that the vitamin D receptor is a transcriptional activator has come from studies of the gene for osteocalcin, a bone matrix–specific protein.[298] Other VDR regulated proteins include osteopontin, bone-specific alkaline phosphatase, and calcium-binding protein. A vitamin D response element about 500 base pairs upstream of the transcriptional start site of the osteocalcin gene has been shown to confer vitamin D responsivity to this and heterologous promoters. The vitamin D response element in the osteocalcin gene consists of three copies of the half palindrome GGGTGA and an overlapping site for the transcription factor AP-1.[302] It appears that the vitamin D receptor has options of binding to its response elements as a homodimer, or as a heterodimer with a member of the retinoic acid receptor family, RXRβ.[303,304] The complex structure of the response element provides for complex regulatory interactions between vitamin A, vitamin D, and AP-1 binding factors such as the products of the proto-oncogenes *jun* and *fos*, which are responsive to serum, to activation of the protein kinase C pathway, or to interleukin 1. Thus, steroid hormones that bind to soluble receptors and hormones and growth factors that activate cell surface receptors may induce coordinated responses at key target genes.

It is likely that not all the effects of vitamin D are genomic. In fibroblasts and liver, exposure to $1\alpha,25\text{-(OH)}_2\text{D}$ produces rapid increases in cGMP[305] or in the intracellular calcium concentration.[306] Although these effects are likely to be nongenomic, those in fibroblasts require the presence of the vitamin D receptor. As we shall see, there is also evidence for a nongenomic effect of vitamin D on intestinal calcium transport, and this probably involves the vitamin D receptor as well. Thus, the same receptor may mediate the genomic and nongenomic actions of vitamin D.

Actions of Vitamin D in Intestine, Bone, and Kidney

Intestinal Transport of Calcium

The primary effect of vitamin D on mineral metabolism is the induction of increased calcium absorption across the intestinal epithelium. This conclusion is strongly supported by observations in individuals with hereditary $1\alpha,25\text{-(OH)}_2\text{D}$–resistant rickets, in whom active vitamin D receptors are lacking. Their severe bone disease can be healed by supplying calcium in the form of chronic intravenous infusions.[307]

The average diet contains 400 to 1,500 mg of calcium. From this dietary load, the net absorption of calcium averages 100 to 250 mg, or about 20 percent of dietary calcium (Fig. 22-3); the remainder is excreted as fecal calcium. Calcium is absorbed throughout the small bowel and specific nuclear receptors for $1\alpha,25\text{-(OH)}_2\text{D}$ are found throughout the small intestine. The highest concentration is in the duodenum. In animal studies, the efficiency of absorption per unit length of bowel is duodenum > jejunum ≥ ileum. In humans, the absolute rates of transport are similar in the jejunum and the ileum. However, because of the prolonged transit through the lengthy ileum, the bulk of calcium is absorbed at this site. Net absorption of calcium varies with the dietary load of calcium, the ambient serum concentration of $1\alpha,25\text{-(OH)}_2\text{D}$, and the bioavailability of dietary calcium. In cow's milk, 40 percent of calcium is in solution. Acidification of food in the stomach tends to solubilize calcium, and absorption of calcium may be reduced in achlorhydric states,[308,309] but the fraction that is available for absorption varies with dietary composition. Less calcium may be available in foods, such as leafy vegetables, which are high in oxalate, or in cereals, which may be high in nondigestible organic phosphates such as phytate. Finally, the ability of the intestine to absorb calcium probably decreases with age,[310] an important consideration in the pathogenesis of osteoporosis.

The jejunum and ileum are relatively leaky to calcium such that there is net diffusion of calcium passively from the intestinal lumen to the plasma through a paracellular pathway when the

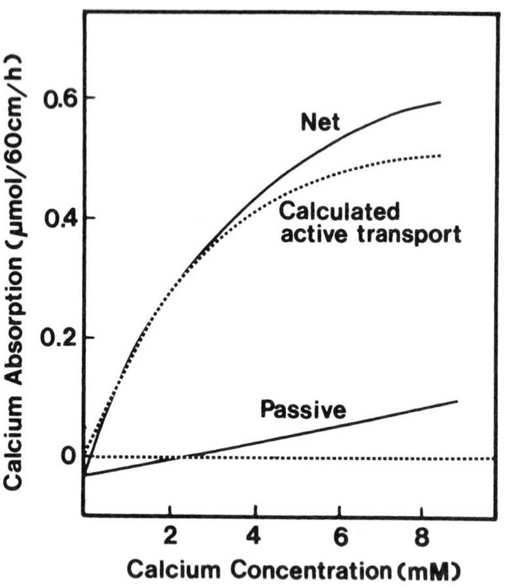

FIGURE 22-26. The active and passive components of intestinal calcium absorption in normal humans. The data were obtained by perfusion of jejunal segments. (*Modified from Ireland P, Fordtran JS, J Clin Invest 52:2672, 1973, by copyright permission of the American Society for Clinical Investigation.*)

luminal concentration of calcium is high, but net diffusion is in the opposite direction when the luminal concentration is low. The intestinal calcium transport system that is induced by vitamin D is superimposed on this passive process (Fig. 22-26). The hormonally sensitive transport process is transcellular, unidirectional, and saturable. Thus, at a given calcium intake and a given ambient concentration of vitamin D, the rate of intestinal transport is the sum of an inwardly directed, saturable active component and a linear diffusive component.[311,312]

The vitamin D–sensitive cellular transport of calcium through the intestinal epithelial cell can be viewed as occurring in three steps (Fig. 22-27). Vitamin D increases the uptake of calcium through the brush border membrane of intestinal microvilli. This is presumably the rate-limiting step in the hormone-sensitive transport of calcium. Subsequently, calcium crosses the cell, probably bound to specific carrier proteins that are induced by vitamin D. Finally, calcium is actively extruded from the cell by an energy-requiring process whose activity is stimulated by vitamin D.

Uptake of calcium across the brush border is a passive process driven by the large electrochemical gradient of calcium (luminal concentration >1 mM, cytoplasmic concentration approximately 100 nM). Several lines of evidence support the view that the induction of this process is a nongenomic action of vitamin D: Uptake is rapid, occurring within 4 min after exposure to the hormone; it is not blocked by inhibitors of RNA synthesis; and it is also not blocked by inhibitors of de novo protein synthesis.[313,314] However, it presumably requires either the binding of vitamin D to its receptor or cellular components induced by vitamin D–receptor complexes, as intestinal calcium transport is drastically reduced in the absence of a functional receptor in patients with 1α,25-$(OH)_2$D–resistant rickets. Both increased calmodulin binding to a specific brush border membrane–associated protein[315] and increased membrane fluidity[316] have been found after exposure to vitamin D.

Intestinal epithelial cells possess two specific cytosolic calcium-binding proteins called calbindins, with molecular mass of 9 and 28 kDA.[317,318] The calbindins are members of the troponin-C superfamily of calcium-binding proteins. The 9-kDa and 28-kDa forms bind two and four moles of calcium per mole, respectively, to approximately 29-amino acid domains known as EF hands. With an affinity for calcium of about 1×10^{-6} *M*, these proteins are suited to buffer intracellular calcium and potentially to shuttle calcium from the lumen of the microvillus to the basolateral surface of the intestinal epithelial cell, from which calcium can be extruded. The synthesis of both forms of calbindin is induced by vitamin D with a time course that lags behind the onset of calcium transport but parallels the achievement of maximal rates of transepithelial calcium flux after exposure to 1α,25-$(OH)_2$D. However, the evidence for a direct role in calcium absorption is still circumstantial.

FIGURE 22-27. Proposed mechanism of action of 1α,25-$(OH)_2$D in the intestine. Binding of 1α,25-$(OH)_2$D to the vitamin D receptor (VDR) affects the transcription of genes including calbindin and may also permit calcium entry through channels in the luminal (brush border) membrane by a nongenomic mechanism. Calbindin is proposed to ferry calcium through the cell. The exit step through the basolateral membrane may involve a calcium pump (Ca-ATPase) and/or Na/Ca exchange.

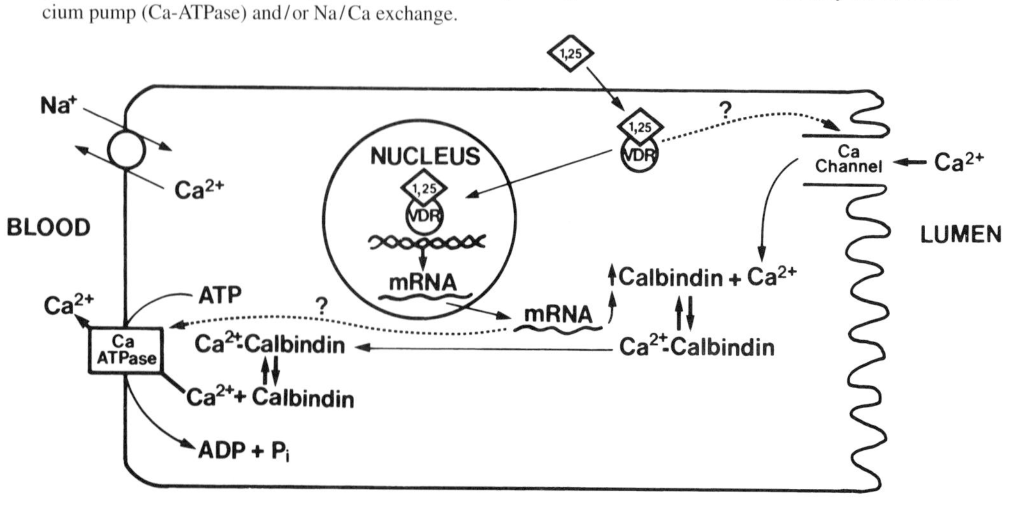

An ATP-driven calcium pump present in the basolateral membrane of the intestinal epithelial cell is capable of active extrusion of calcium into the blood against the existing electrochemical gradient. Calcium transport across the basolateral membrane is stimulated by the exposure of cells to $1\alpha,25\text{-}(OH)_2D$, and it is thought that this could be a third site at which vitamin D acts to stimulate transepithelial transport of calcium.[311,319] Calcium exit could also be driven by a basolateral Na/Ca exchanger driven by the sodium gradient. The overall schema presented in Fig. 22-27—that the transport of calcium across the intestinal epithelium is composed of a passive vitamin D–sensitive entry step, transcellular shuttling of calcium via the vitamin D–inducible calbindins, and active extrusion via a vitamin D–sensitive ATP-driven calcium pump—is attractive and consistent with a mass of data but remains to be proved in detail.

Adaptation to Calcium Intake

The regulation of calcium absorption in response to a changing intake[312] illustrates the way metabolism is integrated. Adaptation to a low calcium intake is thought to begin with an imperceptible fall in the serum calcium concentration, which is a stimulus to secondary hyperparathyroidism. The resultant increment in PTH is the primary driver for accelerated renal synthesis of $1\alpha,25\text{-}(OH)_2D$,[265] and the ensuing increase in serum $1\alpha,25\text{-}(OH)_2D$ concentration has several compensatory actions: Intestinal $1\alpha,25\text{-}(OH)_2D$ receptors are induced,[299] the active component of intestinal calcium absorption is increased by the direct action of $1\alpha,25\text{-}(OH)_2D$ on these receptors, and bone resorption is increased by a direct action of $1\alpha,25\text{-}(OH)_2D$.[267] Of course, PTH participates directly in the response to a low calcium intake, decreasing urinary calcium excretion and increasing bone resorption. Adaptation to a high calcium intake has the opposite effects, with suppression of $1\alpha,25\text{-}(OH)_2D$ and reduced active calcium transport.[312] The total absorption of calcium increases progressively with intake, however, because the passive influx pathway is not saturable (Fig. 22-26). Thus, adequate levels of calcium absorption can be achieved at high levels of intake even in individuals with impaired metabolism of vitamin D (hypoparathyroidism, chronic renal failure). Very high intakes of calcium (greater than 10 g per day) can produce hypercalcemia despite activation of all the compensatory mechanisms discussed.

Intestinal Absorption of Phosphate

Phosphate is principally absorbed passively, with a smaller component of active transport; the details are discussed in the section on disorders of phosphate metabolism. It is likely that vitamin D stimulates cellular uptake of phosphate by a sodium-coupled phosphate transporter by increasing the V_{max}, most likely by increasing the number of carriers.[320] However, because the vitamin D–dependent component of phosphate absorption is small, the impact of vitamin D deficiency on phosphate absorption is much smaller than it is on calcium absorption. The hypophosphatemia that accompanies osteomalacia results not from this but primarily from resetting of the renal phosphate threshold by associated hyperparathyroidism.

Actions of Vitamin D in Bone

The most prominent clinical effect of vitamin D deficiency is *osteomalacia*, or defective mineralization of bone matrix. Whether this form of bone disease is a direct consequence of defective vitamin D action on bone cells or an indirect effect of impaired absorption of calcium and phosphates, with a reduction in the concentrations of calcium and phosphate available for mineralization of the organic matrix of bone, has been debated for many years. Several lines of evidence support the view that the development of osteomalacia is a secondary result of the systemic effects of vitamin D deficiency. Rachitic cartilage will mineralize in vitro in the presence of adequate concentrations of calcium and phosphate. Experimental vitamin D–deficient osteomalacia will heal after the provision of calcium and phosphorus. Most impressively, the severe form of rickets seen in patients with hereditary resistance to $1\alpha,25\text{-}(OH)_2D$ can be healed by a chronic intravenous infusion of calcium that bypasses the defect in intestinal calcium absorption. Healing of osteomalacia is apparent by both radiologic and histomorphometric examination in individuals who lack functional vitamin D receptors.[307]

Despite the evidence that the clinically most apparent osseous effects of vitamin D deficiency may be indirect, vitamin D has a number of direct effects on bone cells.[321] The primary target cell is the osteoblast. Vitamin D receptors are demonstrable by autoradiographic effects in mature rat osteoblasts and in osteoprogenitor cells. Receptors have also been identified in the direct binding studies of a variety of cultured osteoblast-like cells and osteosarcoma cells from humans and rodents. Most osteoblast functions that have been carefully studied are affected by vitamin D. Transcription of type I collagen genes and collagen synthesis are inhibited by the administration of $1\alpha,25\text{-}(OH)_2D$ in vivo,[322] and collagen synthesis is also inhibited by vitamin D in isolated rat and mouse calvaria in organ culture and cultured bone cells. However, collagen synthesis is stimulated by vitamin D in other bone cell lines.[321] Exposure to vitamin D also has bidirectional effects on the activity of alkaline phosphatase in different bone-derived cell lines. Transcription of the gene encoding the bone matrix protein osteocalcin is stimulated by vitamin D in vivo and in vitro. Exposure to $1\alpha,25\text{-}(OH)_2D$ also affects the synthesis of bone growth factors such as TGF-β.

Vitamin D also stimulates bone resorption in organ culture[321] and in vivo.[323] The hypercalcemia that accompanies vitamin D intoxication is sustained by increased resorption of bone. Mature osteoclasts are reportedly lacking in vitamin D receptors, and coculture experiments suggest that activation of the osteoclast by vitamin D requires the release of a trophic factor from the osteoblast.[324] Besides its effects on the mature osteoclast, $1\alpha,25\text{-}(OH)_2D$ accelerates the maturation of osteoclast precursors in bone organ culture,[325,326] an effect that may be related to its ability to induce the differentiation of circulating mononuclear cells, which is discussed later.

Administration of pharamacologic doses of $1\alpha,25\text{-}(OH)_2D$ in excess of the replacement dose results in the appearance of large amounts of undermineralized osteoid on bone surfaces.[327] There is a certain irony in these observations, considering the origins of vitamin D as an antirachitic agent. However, it is not clear whether a primary defect in the mineralization of osteoid is indeed present in this circumstance.

It is not possible at present to create a coherent picture of the physiology of vitamin D action in bone. In individual cells, the hormone can act as a differentiation factor, as a regulator of various differentiated functions, and to modulate cell-cell interactions. This may account for some of the complexity of its effects in various bone-derived systems. In any case, it is difficult to reconcile the remarkably diverse direct effects of vitamin D on bone cells with the view that only its systemic actions (i.e., providing an adequate supply of calcium and phosphate) are required for the health of bone.

Actions of Vitamin D in the Kidney

Because of the complex interrelations among vitamin D, PTH, and phosphate intake, the nature of the direct renal effects of vitamin D has been controversial. However, there is an emerging consensus that $1\alpha,25\text{-}(OH)_2D$ acutely stimulates phosphate reabsorption in the proximal tubule.[328] It is unlikely that vitamin D is a primary regulator of renal phosphate handling under physiologic circumstances. Indeed, in the chronic state, the direct tubular effect of $1\alpha,25\text{-}(OH)_2D$ administration is counterbalanced by a fall in proximal tubule phosphate reabsorption induced by the simultaneous increase in intestinal phosphate absorption that results from the administration of $1\alpha,25\text{-}(OH)_2D$, as discussed in the phosphate homeostasis section. Thus, although the systemic effects of $1\alpha,25\text{-}(OH)_2D$ on phosphate transport can be conceptualized as serving to maintain the availability of phosphate for mineralization of bone by enhancing intestinal absorption and diminishing renal excretion, the superimposed homeostatic effects of increased phosphate absorption by the intestine and of PTH tend to minimize the physiologic importance of the direct renal effects of $1\alpha,25\text{-}(OH)_2D$.

The same complexities that have confused the interpretation of the role of vitamin D in renal phosphate transport apply to the renal handling of calcium. The most convincing interpretation is that vitamin D deficiency impairs renal calcium reabsorption and that the administration of vitamin D restores a normal threshold for renal calcium reabsorption and also sensitizes the tubule to PTH.[329] The tubule site of this action of vitamin D is not known, although calbindins induced by vitamin D are present in the distal tubule segments where PTH-regulated reabsorption of calcium occurs and preliminary data suggest that the effects of vitamin D on calcium transport occur in these cells.[317,318]

Actions of Vitamin D in Other Tissues

Outside the classic target tissues, vitamin D receptors are widely distributed in fibroblasts, skin, brain, pituitary, parotid, stomach, testis, ovary, placenta, breast, and other tissues. In several tissues $1\alpha,25\text{-}(OH)_2D$ has been shown to regulate physiologic functions. The role of vitamin D as a regulator of PTH synthesis in the parathyroids was discussed earlier.

The Immune System

The finding that exposure to $1\alpha,25\text{-}(OH)_2D$ induced the maturation of M-1 and HL-60 myeloblastic leukemia cells to a macrophage phenotype led to demonstrations that $1\alpha,25\text{-}(OH)_2D$ at physiologic concentrations induces the maturation of human peripheral monocytes.[330] Activated T lymphocytes also express vitamin D receptors, and exposure to $1\alpha,25\text{-}(OH)_2D$ inhibits their proliferation and the production of interleukin 2. The physiologic significance of these observations in vitro is unclear.[330] Vitamin D–deficient individuals may have recurrent infections, but rachitic individuals lacking vitamin D receptors do not, even though the receptor deficiency is expressed in their peripheral monocytes. However, the effect of $1\alpha,25\text{-}(OH)_2D$ on monocyte maturation may be related to its ability to influence the maturation of osteoclast precursors in bone.[325,326]

Skin

Keratinocytes can metabolize 25-(OH)D to $\alpha,25\text{-}(OH)_2D352$, and $1\alpha,25\text{-}(OH)_2D$ is a potent inducer of the differentiation of keratinocytes.[331] The antiproliferative effects of $1\alpha,25\text{-}(OH)_2D$ have led to its use as an experimental treatment for psoriasis. Although abnormalities of the epidermis are not prominent in vitamin D–deficient individuals, alopecia totalis is present in many kindreds with $1\alpha,25\text{-}(OH)_2D$–resistant rickets. This suggests a possible role of $1\alpha,25\text{-}(OH)_2D$ in the differentiation of the hair follicle.

Tissue-Specific Analogs

Several vitamin D analogs are reported to have tissue-specific effects.[332] The best studied is 22-oxa-$1\alpha,25\text{-}(OH)_2D$, which is a potent activator of the differentiation of myeloid leukemia cells[333] and inhibits the secretion of PTH but is not a potent bone-resorbing agent in vitro and does not readily produce hypercalcemia in vivo.[333,334] It thus may be of use in treating secondary hyperparathyroidism. Preferential activity in myeloid differentiation over systemic calcemic effects has also been reported for 24-homo-$1\alpha,25\text{-}(OH)_2D$ and an analog with a cyclopropyl group at the end of the side chain.[321,332,335]

Summary

In cells of the osteoclast lineage, leukocytes, and keratinocytes, $1\alpha,25\text{-}(OH)_2D$ is a differentiation factor with antiproliferative effects. The absence of prominent defects in these systems in vitamin D–deficient or receptor-deficient humans suggests that the effects of the hormone are not essential but modulatory.

Assay of Vitamin D Metabolites

The two metabolites whose assay is clinically vital are 25-(OH)D and $1\alpha,25\text{-}(OH)_2D$. Assay of 25-(OH)D gives the best available measure of body stores of vitamin D and is the assay of choice for the diagnosis of suspected vitamin D deficiency and vitamin D intoxication. The 25-hydroxyvitamin D level can be used to follow therapy in patients treated with vitamin D or 25-hydroxycholecalciferol (calcifediol). In patients with liver disease, the nephrotic syndrome, or hyperestrogenemic states, the results must be interpreted in light of possible changes in levels of the vitamin D–binding protein. Direct assays of the vitamin D–binding protein or free 25-(OH)D are not commercially available.

Prior to 1985, assays of 25-hydroxyvitamin D employed competitive protein binding assays. Radioimmunoassays for assessing the serum concentration of 25-hydroxyvitamin D were introduced using ^{1,25}I-labeled tracer in 1993 and have become the method of choice.[242]

Despite its central role in calcium homeostasis, there are only a few clinical indications for assay of $1\alpha,25\text{-}(OH)_2D$ in serum. Because the production of $1\alpha,25\text{-}(OH)_2D$ is so closely regulated, assay of this metabolite is not a good measure of body stores of vitamin D in suspected states of deficiency or excess. Specific indications for assay of $1\alpha,25\text{-}(OH)_2D$ involve states in which the activity of 25-(OH)D-1α-hydroxylase is thought to be reduced (heritable defects in vitamin D metabolism, renal failure) or increased (hypercalcemic patients with sarcoidosis, other granulomatous disorders, idiopathic hypercalcemia of infancy, or lymphoma) and suspected intoxication with exogenous $1\alpha\text{-}(OH)D_3$ or $1\alpha,25\text{-}(OH)_2D_3$.

Of all the steroid hormones $1\alpha,25\text{-}(OH)_2D$ is the most difficult to measure because it circulates at low picogram per milliliter concentrations.[242] Nearly all methods for determinations of $1\alpha,25\text{-}(OH)_2D$ prior to 1996 utilized the vitamin D receptor as a binding protein in a competitive binding assay or utilized extracts of calf thymus, which binds $1\alpha,25\text{-}(OH)_2D_2$ and $1\alpha,25\text{-}(OH)_2D_3$ with

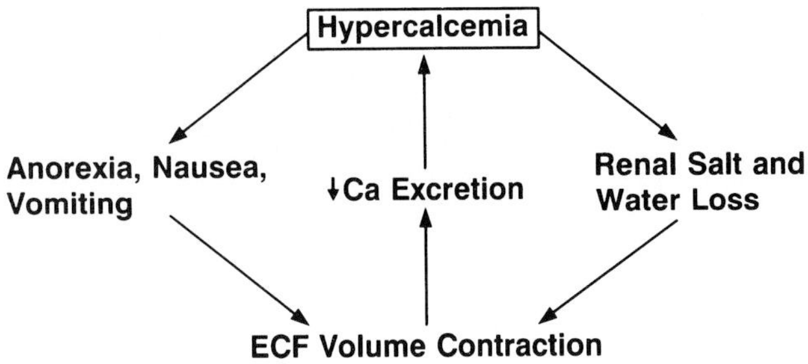

FIGURE 22-28. Once established, hypercalcemia can be maintained or aggravated as depicted. (*Courtesy of Dr. Maurice Attie, University of Pennsylvania School of Medicine.*)

equivalent affinity.[336] Other vitamin D metabolites that bind to the receptor, of which there are many, must be separated before the assay. In 1996 a radioimmunoassay was designed using ^{125}I based tracer. To date, however, no method used in the determination of circulating 1α,25-$(OH)_2$D has received FDA approval.

HYPERCALCEMIA

Introduction

Although many diseases are associated with hypercalcemia, they each produce hypercalcemia through only a limited number of mechanisms: (1) increasing bone resorption (either generalized or localized, such as at the site of malignant metastases) and release of calcium into the systemic circulation, (2) decreasing urinary calcium excretion, and (3) increasing gastrointestinal absorption of calcium. In essentially all instances, at least two of these mechanisms act in concert. For example, in primary hyperparathyroidism, hypercalcemia occurs as a consequence of increased bone resorption, increased renal tubular calcium reabsorption (probably the major mechanism), and increased gut calcium absorption. In malignancy-associated hypercalcemia, there is almost always increased bone resorption and increased renal tubular calcium reabsorption. Once established, hypercalcemia can become self-perpetuating or can be aggravated by dehydration (Fig. 22-28). Table 22-2 summarizes the differential diagnosis of hypercalcemia. A number of symptoms and signs accompany the hypercalcemic state including central nervous system effects such as lethargy, depression, stupor or coma, ataxia, and psychosis; neuromuscular effects such as weakness, proximal myopathy, and hypertonia; cardiovascular effects such as hypertension, bradycardia, and eventually asystole, and a shortened QT interval on electrocardiogram; renal effects such as renal stones, decreased glomerular filtration, polyuria, hyperchloremic acidosis, and nephrocalcinosis; gastrointestinal effects such as nausea, vomiting, constipation and anorexia; eye findings such as band keratopathy; and systemic metastatic calcification (Fig. 22-29 and Table 22-3).

The Defense Against Hypercalcemia

Hypercalcemia is defined as a total serum calcium, adjusted for protein concentration, above 10.2 mg/dl (2.55 mmol/liter) in adults.[337] Ionized calcium is a more precise measure of calcium concentration, the normal plasma concentrations ranging from 1.12–1.23 mmol/liter.[337] With the advent of automated biochemical testing, hypercalcemia is now recognized to be more common than once realized. By far, the commonest causes of hypercalcemia are primary hyperparathyroidism and malignancy.

The clinical features of hypercalcemia are listed in Table 22-3. Symptoms may vary in individual patients and are related both to the absolute concentration of serum calcium and to the rate of rise in serum calcium. Symptoms also reflect the underlying cause of the hypercalcemia as well as intercurrent medical conditions. In older or critically ill patients, symptoms of hypercalcemia may be more prominent with relatively small increases in serum calcium concentration. Hypercalcemia most often results in neuromuscular, gastrointestinal, and renal manifestations. Severe hypercalcemia is likely the result of a vicious cycle. The hypercalcemic effects of anorexia, nausea, vomiting, and impaired renal concentrating ability lead to dehydration and, subsequently, altered mental status. This, in turn, may promote immobilization and lead to worsening hypercalcemia. In addition to the symptoms of hypercalcemia, clinical features of hypercalcemia of malignancy include signs and symptoms of the underlying cancer. Generally, the cancer is well advanced when hypercalcemia occurs, and the prognosis is poor. Survival beyond 6 months is uncommon.[338–340]

Malignancy is the most common cause of hypercalcemia in the hospitalized patient, and malignancy-associated hypercalcemia is one of the more common paraneoplastic syndromes. The relative frequencies of malignancies associated with hypercalcemia are listed in Table 22-4.[341] Hypercalcemia occurring in the setting of malignancy may be due to (1) humoral factors secreted by tumors that act systemically on target organs of bone, kidney, and

TABLE 22-2. Causes of Hypercalcemia

Hyperparathyroidism
Idiopathic
Associated with multiple endocrine neoplasia type 1 or type 2a
Familial
After renal transplantation
Malignancies
Humoral hypercalcemia of malignancy
Solid tumors with local osteolysis (breast, lung, kidney, etc.)
Hematologic malignancies (multiple myeloma, lymphoma, leukemia, etc.)
Sarcoidosis or other granulomatous disease
Endocrinopathies
Thyrotoxicosis
Adrenal insufficiency
Pheochromocytoma
Acromegaly
VIPoma
Drug-induced
Vitamin D excess
Vitamin A excess
Thiazide diuretics
Lithium
Milk-alkali syndrome
Estrogens, androgens, tamoxifen (in breast carcinoma)
Miscellaneous
Familial hypocalciuric hypercalcemia (FHH)
Dehydration
Immobilization (in growing children or adults with increased bone turnover, ie, Pagets)
Acute renal failure
Idiopathic hypercalcemia of infancy
ICU hypercalcemia
Serum protein disorders
Jansen's metaphyseal chondrodysplasia

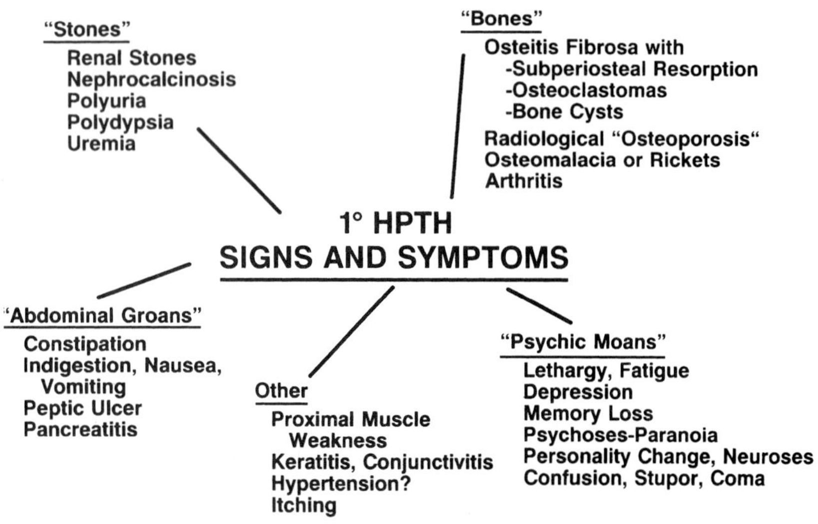

FIGURE 22-29. Mnemonic used for categorizing the signs and symptoms of hyperparathyroidism.

intestine to disrupt normal calcium homeostasis; (2) local factors secreted by tumors in bone, either metastatic or hematological, which directly stimulate osteoclastic bone resorption; and (3) coexisting primary hyperparathyroidism.

It is probably more accurate to think of the first two situations as a continuing spectrum rather than as discrete groups. The pathophysiology of hypercalcemia is very different in patients with solid tumors and without bone metastases at one end of the spectrum, and myeloma associated with extensive local bone destruction adjacent to the tumor cells at the other. However, in between these two extremes are hypercalcemic patients with squamous cell carcinomas in which hypercalcemia may occur with some, but not extensive, osteolytic bone metastases and hypercalcemic patients with advanced breast carcinoma in which hypercalcemia almost never occurs in the absence of extensive osteolytic bone destruction. Separating hypercalcemia into subcategories based on the assumption that the underlying mechanisms are distinct is not entirely satisfactory because the mediators may be identical except that in one situation the mediator may be locally produced while in another the same mediator may be responsible, but produced at a distant site. Additionally, if the tumor burden in bone is great, local tumor-produced mediators of bone resorption may be produced in sufficient quantities to have systemic effects. Although this review will discuss the effects of cancer on bone organized into such subcategories, it is important that the reader understand that a significant portion of cancer patients will fall into the middle of this spectrum, having both humoral and local effects of tumor on bone.

Because of the efficiency of the renal response to a calcium load, hypercalciuria is more common than hypercalcemia in most situations where a calcium load is imposed; the exceptions are primary hyperparathyroidism, hypercalcemia associated with PTHrP excess, where the hypocalciuric effect of PTH or PTHrP persists and the ability of the kidney to respond is thus impaired (Fig. 22-30). However, profoundly hypercalciuric patients are in precarious balance because several factors conspire against the renal adaptation to hypercalcemia (Fig. 22-28). Glomerular filtration is impaired by hypercalcemia. The urinary concentrating ability is diminished, poor mentation may interfere with access to fluids, and nausea or vomiting may occur such that the patient is subject to dehydration and prerenal azotemia. Renal insufficiency in turn compromises calcium clearance, potentially leading to a downward spiral that can culminate in severe hypercalcemia and renal failure.

TABLE 22-3. Clinical Features of Hypercalcemia

Neurologic and psychiatric	Lethargy, drowsiness Confusion, disorientation Disturbed sleep, nightmares Irritability, depression Hypotonia, decreased deep tendon reflexes Stupor, coma
Gastrointestinal	Anorexia, vomiting Constipation Peptic ulceration Acute pancreatitis
Cardiovascular	Arrhythmias Synergism with digoxin ? Hypertension
Renal	Polyuria, polydipsia Hypercalciuria Nephrocalcinosis Impaired glomerular filtration

TABLE 22-4. Malignancies Associated with Hypercalcemia

Malignancy	Frequency (%)
Lung	35
Breast	25
Hematologic	14
Head and neck	6
Renal	3
Prostate	3
Unknown primary	7
Others	7

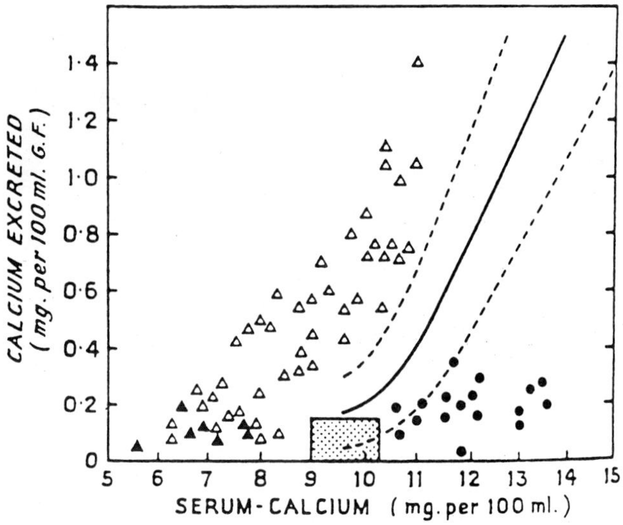

FIGURE 22-30. The effect of hyperparathyroidism and hypoparathyroidism on the relation between serum and urinary calcium. At any level of serum calcium, the urinary calcium is increased in hypoparathyroidism (open and closed triangles) and decreased in hyperparathyroidism (closed circles) compared with normal subjects. Normal subjects were studied in the basal state (shaded area) or during the infusion of calcium, where the response is shown as the mean (—) plus or minus 2 standard deviations (- - - -). *(By permission of BEC Nordin and M Peacock, Lancet 2:1280, 1969.)*

Approach to the Hypercalcemic Patient

The approach to the hypercalcemic patient takes account of the demographics and pathophysiology of hypercalcemia. Thus, the causes of hypercalcemia can be divided into three categories: primary hyperparathyroidism, malignancy, and other causes. Primary hyperparathyroidism and malignancy comprise 90 percent of all other causes of hypercalcemia. To differentiate nonparathyroid hypercalcemia from primary hyperparathyroidism, the clinician relies on shared clinical features of nonparathyroid hypercalcemia, the consequences of suppression of PTH secretion. Once nonparathyroid hypercalcemia has been diagnosed, its cause can usually be found by using other features of its presentation to identify the underlying disorder.

In ambulatory patients with asymptomatic or mildly symptomatic hypercalcemia, primary hyperparathyroidism is the likely diagnosis. The prevalence of primary hyperparathyroidism is much higher than that of all other causes of hypercalcemia combined. A high level of intact PTH in a hypercalcemic patient is virtually diagnostic of primary hyperparathyroidism, as in assays for the intact hormone, the PTH level in nonparathyroid hypercalcemia is suppressed. It is these considerations of the prevalence of primary hyperparathyroidism and the relative ease of diagnosis which led to the recommendation (presented later) for an abbreviated work-up of hypercalcemia in asymptomatic ambulatory patients. Other laboratory features, such as hypophosphatemia and hyperchloremia, are often present in primary hyperparathyroidism, reflecting the renal actions of excess PTH, but need not be relied on to make the diagnosis.

Although the *incidence* of malignancy-associated hypercalcemia is about half the incidence of primary hyperparathyroidism, the *prevalence* of malignancy-associated hypercalcemia is much lower owing to the short survival in malignancy-associated hypercalcemia (mean life expectancy, 30 days). However, malignancy is the most common etiology of hypercalcemia in hospitalized patients. If the underlying malignancy is not already recognized, it is usually readily apparent by physical examination or laboratory screening of the hypercalcemic patient. Because PTHrP is the etiologic agent that produces hypercalcemia in most patients with malignant tumors, other features reminiscent of hyperparathyroidism are also often present. The serum phosphorus level is often low, and the tubular maximum for phosphate/glomerular filtration rate (TmP/GFR) is correspondingly decreased. (Of note is the fact that, unlike patients with primary hyperparathyroidism who have a hyperchloremic acidosis, most patients with malignancy have a metabolic alkalosis.)

The other causes of hypercalcemia are diverse but have some common features. A key feature is suppression of PTH secretion. The intact PTH level is suppressed below 2 pmol/liter (20 pg/ml). Thus, a determination of the intact PTH level using a two-site assay readily distinguishes all other entities from primary hyperparathyroidism (Fig. 22-10). The suppression of PTH also has several consequences that are useful in making the diagnosis of nonparathyroid, non-PTHrP–related hypercalcemia. The urinary excretion of calcium is significantly increased (Fig. 22-30). The TmP/GFR is generally normal or increased, setting the serum phosphorus concentration in the midnormal range or higher (the occasional finding of a low-normal serum phosphorus in hypercalcemic patients without increased plasma PTH or PTH-rP is probably attributable to a direct effect of hypercalcemia in decreasing renal phosphate reabsorption).

A patient with hypercalcemia in the setting of chronic renal failure presents the physician with a special challenge. Because secondary hyperparathyroidism is common in such patients and phosphorus excretion is impaired, the interpretation of the intact PTH and serum phosphorus levels must be tempered with caution.

Hypercalcemia is usually caused by increased bone resorption. Bone resorption involves destruction of the collagen-rich bone matrix as well as the release of mineral. This often leads to increased urinary excretion of the metabolites of type I collagen, such as the collagen-specific amino acid hydroxyproline and pyridinium cross-links. Measurement of urinary hydroxyproline is the traditional test for bone resorption, but it is insensitive because hydroxyproline is also released from dietary collagen in meats and gelatin and from collagen-rich tissues other than bone. The pyridinium compounds are the cross-links between collagen chains that remain after extensive hydrolysis, and they are more sensitive and specific than hydroxyproline as measures of bone resorption.[342,343] One (hydroxylysylpyridinoline, or simply pyridinoline) is derived mainly from the degradation of type I collagen in bone and type II collagen in cartilage. The other (lysylpyridinoline or deoxypyridinoline) has been found only in type I collagen of bone. Urinary excretion of the pyridinoline cross-links involving the N- or C-terminals of type I collagen are more sensitive measures of bone resorption. They are coming into use as the preferred clinical assay marker reflecting increased rates of bone resorption, although their ability in this clinical situation remains unclear.[343a] These assays of collagen degradation products are undergoing rapid development as their potential uses have become apparent. Serum assays are under development.

Because bone formation usually follows bone resorption, most states of increased bone resorption are also characterized by high rates of bone formation. This is usually manifested as an increase in serum alkaline phosphatase levels. However, because alkaline phosphatase has multiple sources, determination of bone specific serum alkaline phosphatase is more sensitive and specific as a measure of bone formation. Assays for the bone matrix–specific protein osteocalcin (bone gla protein) are now generally available and provide a highly specific measure of bone formation.[342] The osteocalcin level is elevated in many hypercalcemic states.[342,344] Although bone formation is usually coupled to bone resorption in primary hyperparathyroidism, bone formation rates are often impaired in patients with malignancy, and particularly in myeloma. The reasons are unknown. Additional markers of bone formation include procollagen C- or N- terminal peptides that are cleaved in the process of type I collagen formation.[343a]

Intestinal absorption of calcium is increased in primary hyperparathyroidism, granulomatous disorders, vitamin D intoxication, and the milk-alkali syndrome. The milk-alkali syndrome may be the only disorder in which increased intestinal absorption of calcium is the primary cause of hypercalcemia, as excessive bone resorption plays a role in all the other states, including vitamin D intoxication. Intestinal absorption of calcium can be estimated from metabolic balance studies or from a variety of tests that measure the unidirectional or bidirectional flux of isotopic calcium. These are all research procedures, and which is best is disputed.[312] However, there is no reliable and readily available clinical measure of intestinal calcium absorption.

Primary Hyperparathyroidism

The most common cause of hypercalcemia is primary hyperparathyroidism. The prevalence is as high as 1 in 500 to 1 in 1,000. It occurs in approximately 0.2 percent of women over 65 years old and 0.1 percent of men over 65 years old. The frequency of diagnosis has dramatically increased since 1970 due to widespread use of auto-analyzers for routine serum calcium determinations. The disease occurs more commonly in women (3:1 ratio) than in men, and the incidence increases markedly with age, particularly over age 60. Although the majority of these cases occur sporadically in postmenopausal women, hyperparathyroidism also has an hereditary association. If it is found in children it is likely to be genetic. It is a component of two of the three autosomal dominant multiple endocrine neoplasia syndromes (discussed later). Although any or all of the symptoms and signs described earlier can be produced by primary hyperparathyroidism, the majority of cases arise without symptoms (discussed in the section on diagnosis and management of asymptomatic primary hyperparathyroidism).

History

The history of hyperparathyroidism is recounted in a review by Schwartz.[345] The first description of a parathyroid gland was made by Sandstrom in 1880.[346] Although von Recklinghausen described osteitis fibrosis cystica in 1891, the connection between bone disease and parathyroid tumors was not made until more than a decade later by Askanazy.[345] The link between the hormone secreted by the parathyroid gland and calcium mobilization from bone was later established by Erdheim in Vienna. Until that time, the causes of excessive levels of calcium in the blood were not known. In fact, one school of thought held that inadequate parathyroid hormone was the etiology of hypercalcemia and that the parathyroid enlargement observed with hypercalcemia resulted secondarily as a response to elevated blood calcium levels. Therefore, some physicians advocated transplantation with parathyroid glands as a treatment for the disorder.[345] The causal link between the increased activity of one or more parathyroid glands and hyperparathyroidism and hypercalcemia became most clearly established in American medicine by the pioneering efforts of Fuller Albright in his famous studies of the patient (and coinvestigator!) Captain Martell[347] (Fig. 22-31). Linking the abnormal gland to the disease hyperparathyroidism would require an exceptional effort because it was a novel concept: "This gland is so small that few doctors have ever seen one on the dissecting table. . . . This little gland is so powerful, however, that its over- or underfunction can be fatal."[348]

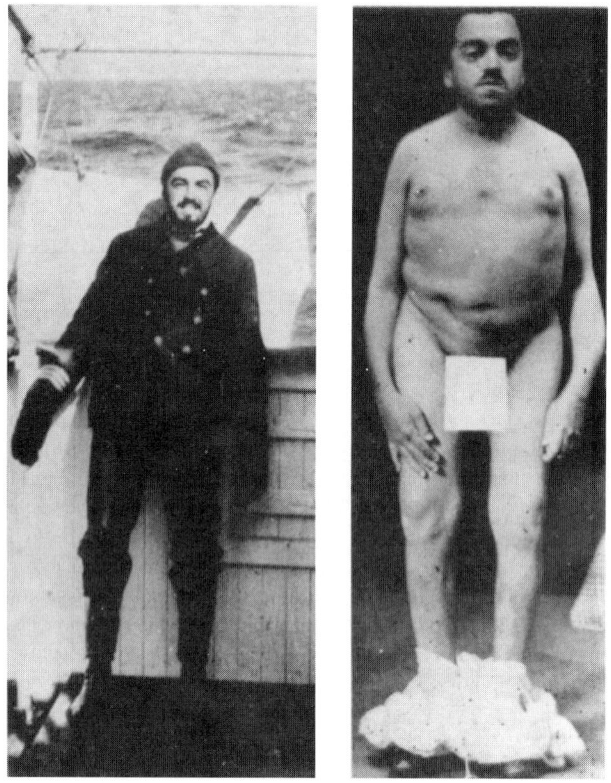

FIGURE 22-31. Captain Charles Martell. The picture on the left shows him a few months before his first symptom. On the right, he is pictured 8 years later at the time of entry to the hospital in 1926. (*Reprinted with permission from W. Bauer and D. D. Federman, Hyperparathyroidism epitomized: The case of Captain Charles Martell, Metabolism 11:22, 1962.*)

The remarkable story of Captain Martell and the intensive clinical investigation for which he served as the subject is one of the most dramatic accounts of biomedical research in the history of American medicine. Martell's disease was severe; skeletal involvement was dramatic. His habitus was altered remarkably by years of excess secretion of parathyroid hormone. Albright described the situation as follows: "The Captain . . . lay in a ward slowly excreting his skeleton into his urine."[348] Captain Martell's case exemplified the course of others severely incapacitated with the disease, which was fatal at the time because there was no medical or surgical treatment: "The patients [became] more and more skeletonless, more and more plant-like, until finally they were jellyfish incapable of locomotion, in some cases dying of suffocation, unable to move the chest in respiration."[348] Martell underwent six unsuccessful surgical neck explorations in an attempt to identify and remove the abnormally functioning parathyroid gland before an adenoma finally was found ectopically located in the mediastinum.[348]

Albright's efforts to elucidate the pathophysiology of hyperparathyroidism represent a brilliant chapter in endocrine research. While Albright championed the concept that PTH acts principally on kidney to produce its systemic effects on calcium metabolism, the Canadian physician James Bertram Collip argued that the hormone acts principally on bone to mobilize calcium; he thought that the renal effects were secondary. The controversy sparked experimentation for more than a decade before the researchers finally realized that both hypotheses were actually correct.[345] The hormone acts directly on both bone and kidney. Using nephrectomized animals, Collip and coworkers showed a direct effect of PTH on bone.[349] The decisive proof that the hormone acts on bone came from later experiments by Barnicot, who transplanted parathyroid glands into a position adjacent to cranial bone, producing local bony resorption.[345,350]

Primary hyperparathyroidism affects women more commonly than men (ratio 3:1) and increases in prevalence progressively after age 30. Postmenopausal women have the highest risk of having not only hyperparathyroidism but also osteoporosis.[351] Hence, a postmenopausal woman who has hyperparathyroidism is at risk for compromise of bone strength because of the combined accelerated bone loss which accompanies both disorders.

The incidence of primary hyperparathyroidism appears to have increased by an order of magnitude since the advent of multiphasic screening of blood on a routine basis some three decades ago.[351] This vast increase in the detection of the syndrome in the general population has raised controversy regarding the natural history and management of the disease. It now seems likely that many, perhaps most, patients with this disorder have normal life expectancy and do not suffer from the dramatic bone, renal, and other disorders associated with the disease in an earlier era. In fact, it is likely that many patients suffer no symptoms or adverse sequelae from the disorder. Therefore, the important issues regarding the management of "asymptomatic" hyperparathyroidism will be discussed later in a separate section.

Etiology

The "anatomic" etiology of hyperparathyroidism can be divided into several categories. The pathology in 80 to 85 percent of cases of primary hyperparathyroidism is caused by a single adenoma of one of the four parathyroid glands. These adenomas are monoclonal in origin, as recently documented using recombinat DNA techniques,[352,353] lending strong support to the surgical approach of removing only the single abnormal gland. It is not known why adenomas arise spontaneously, but in at least one (minor) subgroup of patients there was previous exposure to neck irradiation.[346,354,355]

Most parathyroid adenomas are clonal in origin suggesting a defect in the gene controlling growth of the parathyroid cell or expression of PTH. An intriguing mechanism accounting for at least 4 percent of adenomas examined is a DNA rearrangement in the region of the PTH gene.[356–358] This genetic alteration is present in all the cells of the adenoma but not in the same patient's normal tissue. In these cases, one PTH gene has been severed between its coding region and the upstream regulatory domain. The chromosome then inverts and is ligated together, resulting in a new linkage of the PTH gene regulatory domain to an unrelated gene. The alteration is termed a pericentromeric inversion. It brings the proto-oncogene PRAD1 (for *para*thyroid *ad*enoma) located in chromosome band 11q13 (Fig. 22-32) under the influence of the putative tissue-specific PTH regulatory domain. PRAD1 (also known as cyclin D1) is markedly overexpressed in this arrangement and appears to be an oncogene. This realignment places a growth factor under control of the regulatory element that controls PTH. Overexpression of PRAD1 (cyclin D1) has been demonstrated in 18 percent of parathyroid adenomas.[359] The same oncogene may be involved in lymphoma and breast cancer.[360,361] The PTH produced by the adenoma presumably arises from the unaffected remaining PTH allele, although this does not explain the "set point" error that may be present in some adenomas.

The role of PRAD1 in normal physiology is not known. PRAD1 is not known to be calcium-regulated. The proto-oncogene's product has structural homology to the cyclin families of proteins involved in the cell division cycle,[362] and PRAD1 may regulate the crucial cell cycle checkpoint between the G_1 and S phases.[362] Whether overexpression of PRAD1 or other cell cycle regulators is involved more generally in parathyroid adenomas without detectable PTH rearrangement is not known.

Another molecular mechanism that may explain the clonal expansion of a parathyroid cell into an adenoma is the loss of a

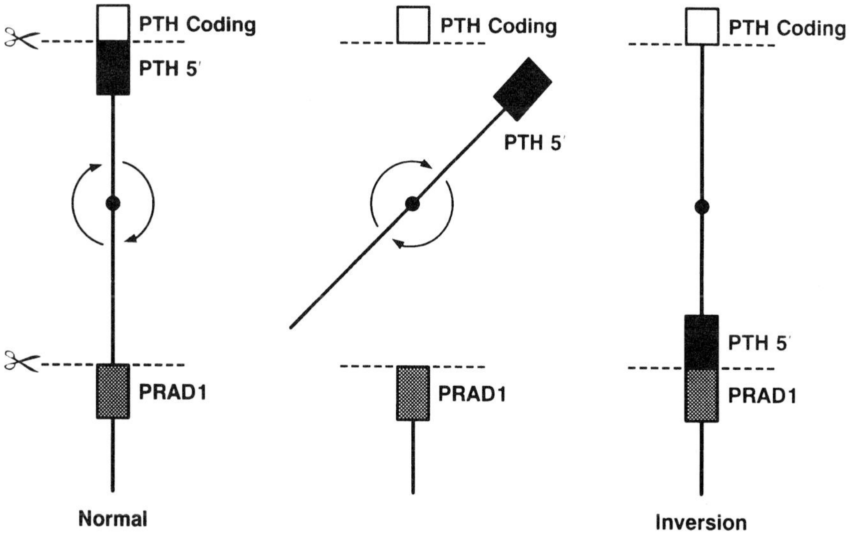

FIGURE 22-32. The genetic abnormality present in a subset of parathyroid adenomas has been structurally elucidated. The abnormality appears to arise from a gene rearrangement (inversion) in which the 5′ regulatory region of PTH is separated from the coding region of the hormone. Instead, the PRAD1 gene occupies the position adjacent to the 5′ regulatory region of PTH. (*Courtesy of Dr. Andrew Arnold. Massachusetts General Hospital.*)

tumor suppressor gene. This mechanism is suggested by the finding of deletions in chromosome 11 that have been mapped to 11q13. This region of chromosome 11 also is often deleted in parathyroid tumors from patients with multiple endocrine neoplasia syndrome type 1 (discussed later) who have four-gland disease.[363,364] It is known as the MEN I gene and has been recently cloned. Mutations have also been identified. The MEN I gene codes for a novel 610-amino acid protein referred to as MENIN.[365] The precise function of MENIN, which is not homologous to other proteins involved in cell proliferation, remains to be elucidated.[366] Mutations in the MENIN gene has been identified in association with MEN type I and has been demonstrated to be abnormal in 17 percent of patients with parathyroid adenoma.[367] This model for adenoma development may parallel the paradigm described for oncogenesis in retinoblastoma by loss of a tumor suppressor gene product or antioncogene,[368–370] although parathyroid adenomas are benign. Another candidate gene is also a tumor suppressor gene found on chromosome 1p.[371] The autosomal dominant hyperparathyroidism-jaw syndrome was recently localized to 1q21-q31. Isolated hyperparathyroidism in some families have been isolated to this region.[372] No mutations in the calcium receptor gene have been identified in parathyroid tumors.[373]

The pathology of an adenoma may differ only subtly from that of a normal gland. The balance between parenchymal hormone-secreting chief cells or oxyphil cells and fat cells is shifted toward the former group. Because the proportion of fat cells in the gland increases normally with age, an adenomatous gland may simply resemble the "normal" gland of a younger patient. Sometimes the pathologic diagnosis is facilitated by the presence of a rim of normal or "compressed" parathyroid tissue at the edge of the adenoma. The noninvolved glands, which are "suppressed" and hence are synthetically inactive, are not usually distinctive in appearance and appear "normal."

The observed pathology in 10 to 15 percent of patients with primary hyperparathyroidism is four-gland hyperplasia, which typically is polyclonal in origin in the nonfamilial forms but involves a genomic mutation when associated with the multiple endocrine neoplasia (MEN) syndromes (discussed later).[352,374,375] It presents in two pathologic variants. Primary chief cell hyperplasia is the more common form and predominates (or is the only form that occurs) in the hereditarily associated disorders such as the MEN syndromes and familial hyperparathyroidism. Clear cell hyperplasia is much more rare; the cell type of origin is not known. Both kinds of pathology can arise sporadically. Although four-gland hyperplasia can arise spontaneously, its presence should always raise the possibility of a MEN syndrome in the patient and should therefore alert the physician to perform a diagnostic evaluation for the related hereditary disorders as well as the relevant endocrine evaluation of relatives.

The pathology in the remaining small proportion (<1 percent) of patients is a parathyroid carcinoma that secretes parathyroid hormone autonomously. The role PRAD1/cyclin D1 overexpression in parathyroid carcinoma may be greater than parathyroid adenomas.[359] Calcium levels typically are markedly elevated in these patients, as are PTH levels; both are considerably higher than usual in typical hyperparathyroidism. Patients with parathyroid carcinoma more often have nephrolithiasis (56 percent), renal insufficiency (84 percent), and bone involvement (91 percent).[375] The morphology of the gland reveals extensive mitosis, vascular invasion, and fibrous trabeculae. Local invasion or distant metastasis confirms the diagnosis. The course of the disease usually is rapid, in contrast to the indolent course of primary hyperparathyroidism.

The pathophysiologic mechanism responsible for inappropriately elevated secretion of parathyroid hormone by adenomas and hyperplastic tissue appears to be complex. Much of the increased secretion appears to result from an inappropriate "set point" for hormonal secretion by the abnormal cells.[21,377,378] In other words, the dose-response curve for PTH secretion as regulated by extracellular calcium levels is inappropriately shifted to the right so that higher calcium levels are required to suppress PTH secretion (Fig. 22-33). Once higher levels of calcium are achieved, normal "suppression" of secretion occurs. This "thermostat-like" error appears to be present in both adenomatous and hyperplastic parathyroid tissue. However, for both normal and abnormal parathyroid tissue, total suppression of hormonal secretion cannot be achieved.[21,377] There is always a small but obligatory secretion of hormone that persists even at extremely high levels of extracellular calcium. Therefore, it is reasonable to suppose that when the absolute quantity of parathyroid tissue increases, the obligatory secretion or "nonsuppressible" component of PTH secretion increases and becomes sufficiently high to produce hyperparathyroidism and hypercalcemia (Fig. 22-33). In fact, hyperparathyroidism can be created experimentally in rats by transplanting multiple isologous glands into a single animal.[379] In parathyroid carcinomas, secretion is autonomous and is not affected by extracellular calcium concentrations; continuously high levels of hormone are released by carcinomatous cells.

The particular step(s) in hormonal biosynthesis and secretion that fails to be appropriately regulated and is therefore responsible for excess secretion of PTH is unknown. All the steps in the biosynthesis, processing, and secretion of the hormone are potential sites of malfunction, including transcription, translation, posttranslational modification, packaging, and release of secretory granules (Fig. 22-6). Thus far, efficiency of transcription and translation, conversion of precursor mRNA to mature mRNA, and the intracellular metabolism of preproparathyroid homone to proparathyroid hormone and then to native parathyroid hormone appears to be normal. Only the actual regulation of release of hormone into the circulation appears to be defective in primary hyperparathyroidism.[374]

Clinical Presentation and Pathophysiology

The presentation of primary hyperparathyroidism has evolved considerably since the early days of identification of the syndrome.[351,380] As was mentioned previously, the hallmark of the disease used to be severe bone changes associated with osteitis fibrosa cystica. During the next several decades, the association with kidney stones was recognized and became the most common presenting sign of hyperparathyroidism, approximately 3 to 10 times more common than bone complications. The routine screening of blood chemistry values in large portions of the population has led to the current clinical profile in which "asymptomatic" hyperparathyroidism predominates (Fig. 22-34).

It is difficult to specifically attribute signs and symptoms other than renal stones and bone disease to primary hyperparathyroidism for several reasons (Fig. 22-29). First, there can be a concurrence of common disorders such as hyperparathyroidism and hypertension or hyperparathyroidism and peptic ulcer disease.[351,380–383] These illnesses previously were thought to be associated with hyperparathyroidism. With the exception of the linkage that occurs between hyperparathyroidism and peptic ulcers

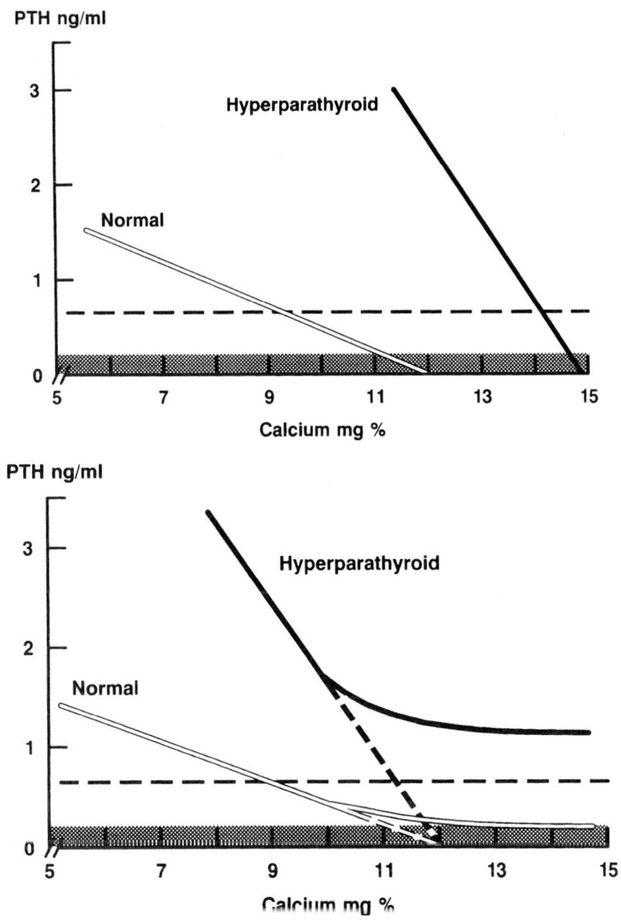

FIGURE 22-33. Possible mechanism for parathyroid hormone oversecretion in various disorders. In instances such as lithium-induced hyperparathyroidism, familial hypercalciuric hypercalcemia, and many parathyroid adenomas, a "set point" error appears to account for the abnormality *(top)*. Glands from such hyperparathyroid individuals show steeper slopes of response than normal, and a higher level of calcium is required to suppress hormone secretion. When the total mass of parathyroid hormone (PTH) is increased, the amount of hormone secreted as a result of the "nonsuppressed" component of PTH secretion is sufficient to produce hypercalcemia without evoking any other abnormality in stimulus-secretion coupling owing to a larger mass of tissue *(bottom)*. The hypothesis requires that a small amount of hormone secretion persists despite elevated calcium. In the normal parathyroid gland, this secretion is small and insignificant. In hyperparathyroidism, greatly increased tissue mass leads to persistent secretion of the hormone above the normal range (dashed line). The slopes of both normal and hyperparathyroid states extrapolate to the same calcium subpoint (12 mg/100 ml). PTH values within the shaded area are below the limits of assay detection. *(Reprinted with permission from Lynn H. Caporale and Michael Rosenblatt, Parathyroid Hormone Secretion: Molecular Events and Regulation, Contributions to Nephrology 50:73–95, 1986.)*

caused by the Zollinger-Ellison syndrome as part of multiple endocrine neoplasia syndrome type I (discussed later), there does not appear to be an increased incidence of hypertension or peptide ulcer disease with hyperparathyroidism. Similarly, pancreatitis appears to be associated by chance with primary hyperparathyroidism.[384] Other findings, such as fatigue, weakness, and depression, are common in the general population and therefore are not specific or readily quantified. Although physicians who care for patients with primary hyperparathyroidism believe that many of these patients have subtle complaints either originating from the metabolic consequences of hyperparathyroidism or exacerbated by the disease,[385] these disturbances often cannot be reversed by surgical intervention.

A variety of articular manifestations are observed in patients with primary hyperparathyroidism. The most common is chronic chondrocalcinosis, with or without acute attacks of pseudogout. Chondrocalcinosis may affect as many as 5 percent of patients with primary hyperparathyroidism and is seen radiologically as calcification of articular cartilage, most often in the knee. Pseudogout occurs less frequently. It is usually an acute arthritis of the large joints, most commonly the knee, induced by deposition of calcium pyrophosphate crystals. The diagnosis of pseudogout can be made by demonstrating rhomboidal calcium phosphate crystals in joint fluid. Attacks of acute gouty arthritis also occur in a few percent of patients. Both pseudogout and urate gout may occur after parathyroidectomy.

Distinguishing hyperparathyroidism from malignancy (the second most common cause of hypercalcemia) was once the most challenging diagnostic problem facing the clinician. Measuring serum intact PTH concentrations readily distinguishes the two.

Hyperparathyroid Bone Disease

Increased bone turnover is characteristic of primary hyperparathyroidism. However, in most cases, bone formation and bone resorption remain nearly balanced and there are no short-term clinical sequelae of the increased metabolic bone turnover other than hypercalcemia. In severe cases, osteitis fibrosa is present and is associated with bone pain, which can be the presenting complaint. An x-ray is shown in Fig. 22-35. The disorder is characterized by distorted and disorganized remodeling of bone, accelerated bone resorption leading to pathologic fractures, and fibrotic infiltrates. The cortical surfaces of bone are thinned, and much of the bone is demineralized (Fig. 22-36). The fibrotic bulging lesions within bone are histologically termed "brown tumors" (Fig. 22-37). Often, fluid-filled cysts also occur, termed osteitis fibrosa cystica (Fig. 22-38). Present in the hands is a characteristic subperiosteal resorption on the medial aspects of the middle phalanges

FIGURE 22-34. Clinical presentation of primary hyperparathyroidism in the current era. *(Courtesy of Maurice Attie, University of Pennsylvania School of Medicine.)*

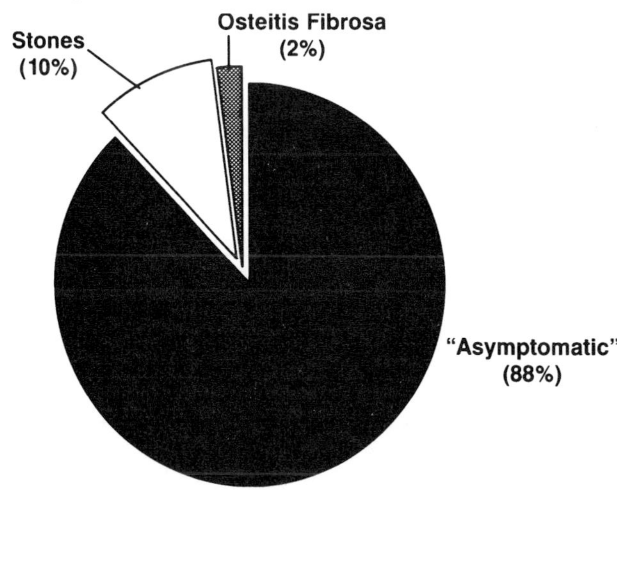

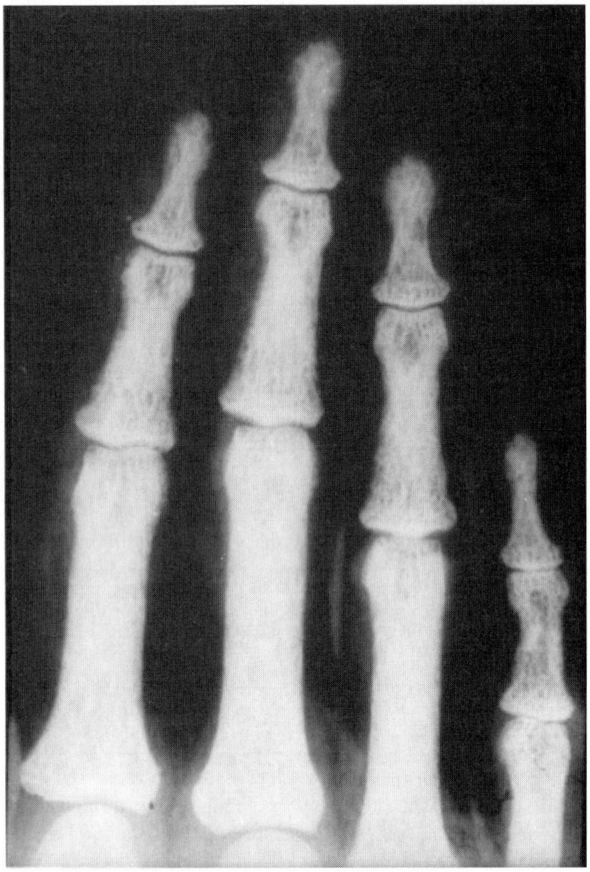

FIGURE 22-35. Radiograph of osteitis fibrosa in primary hyperparathyroidism. Subperiosteal resorption of the medial aspects of the middle phalanges is present. This finding is thought to be pathognomonic for hyperparathyroidism. (*Courtesy of Dr. Maurice Attie, University of Pennsylvania School of Medicine.*)

of the third and fourth fingers (Fig. 22-35); this is also present in the toes and ribs. Subperiosteal resorption in the hand is pathognomonic of hyperparathyroidism. A similar process in the skull leads to a so-called salt and pepper appearance (Fig. 22-39). Disappearance of the lamina dura of the teeth is also seen, but this is a nonspecific finding that occurs commonly in periodontal disease.

During the period 1925–1950, as many 50 percent of patients presented with skeletal complications. Today, this number has fallen sharply to below 10 percent (Fig. 22-34).[351,380] Of greater concern now is osteopenia and its potential aggravation of underlying osteoporosis. Loss of bone mineral density is known to be accompanied by a loss of the biomechanical strength of bone. Such a loss of bone mineral density is clinically silent until the appearance of the first fracture. In most surveys of patients with documented hyperparathyroidism, it is clear that the levels of bone mineral density are below those found in age-, sex-, and race-matched normal cohorts (Figs. 22-40 and 22-41).[386–389] Measuring bone mineral density by bone densitometry has become very important in the routine evaluation of patients with primary hyperparathyroidism. Bone loss has been predominately demonstrated in cortical bone such as the proximal third of the distal radius. The cancellous bone of the spine is relatively preserved. This is in contrast to postmenopausal bone loss which involves cancellous sites first. Such a local shift of calcium within bone might actually strengthen vertebral bone and prevent crush fractures, although the risk for hip fracture might be increased. Although there is paucity of information related to the mechanism of cancellous bone preservation, histomorphometric examination of patients with hyperparathyroidism has demonstrated elevated indexes of bone turnover. Eroded surfaces, osteoid surfaces, mineralization surface, bone formation rate, and activation frequently are increased. Higher values of adjusted mineral apposition rates and active bone formation rates have also been demonstrated.[390] Indices of bone formation such as serum osteocalcin and bone specific alkaline phosphatase are mildly elevated. Similarly, the markers of bone resorption such as the type I collogen crosslinks are also elevated.[391]

The precise risk of fractures in patients with primary hyperparathyroidism is unknown. In a retrospective population-based study, the risk of vertebral, wrist, rib, and pelvic fractures were increased in patients with asymptomatic primary hyperparathyroidism.[392] In another 10-year prospective study, bone mineral density increased after parathyroidectomy in the femoral neck by 6.1 percent after 1 year and 14 percent after 10 years.[393]

Hyperparathyroid Kidney Disease

The occurrence of calcium-containing kidney stones is clearly associated with hyperparathyroidism and can lead to renal compromise.[351,380] Hence, nephrolithiasis is generally considered an indication for surgery.[394] However, currently less than 15 percent of these patients have kidney stones at the time of presentation. In addition to the increased calcium clearance, the decreased acid content of the urine may contribute as a risk factor for the development of kidney stones. Although there have been reports indicating an increased incidence of kidney stones in patients whose vitamin D levels are higher than average for hyperparathyroidism,[262] increased vitamin D levels do not predict the future occurrence of kidney stones and certainly should not be used as an indication for surgery.[395] Nephrocalcinosis occurs even less commonly, is mostly associated with more severe disease, and is rare in the modern era. Typically, calcium deposits ectopically in the kidney in an anatomic distribution corresponding to locales where the solute-concentrating function of the kidney is greatest. Nephrocalcinosis can lead to renal failure. However, more subtle renal disturbances occur commonly, such as increased urinary calcium excretion and mild electrolyte disorders. In general, these disturbances are correctable surgically.[389] Renal concentrating ability also may be compromised by long-standing hyperparathyroidism, as occurs with hypercalcemia of other causes but does not necessarily reverse with surgical treatment.

Nonspecific Features of Primary Hyperparathyroidism

Although many symptoms have been commonly ascribed to primary hyperparathyroidism, it has been difficult to establish a true causal relation between primary hyperparathyroidism and many of these symptoms. This is especially true for central nervous system symptoms,[396] for extremes of hypercalcemia, lethargy, stupor and even coma occur and clearly are attributable to hypercalcemia. However, more subtle or often nonspecific symptoms such as fatigue, difficulty concentrating, and a decline in one's general sense of well-being occur in certain individuals in association with hyperparathyroidism.[385] Along the same lines, constipation, mild nausea, polyuria, polydipsia, and nocturia are difficult to link to hyperparathyroidism. These symptoms can be vague, are difficult to quantify, and are prevalent in the general population. There are undoubtedly many patients with hyperparathyroidism who report an improvement in symptoms as a

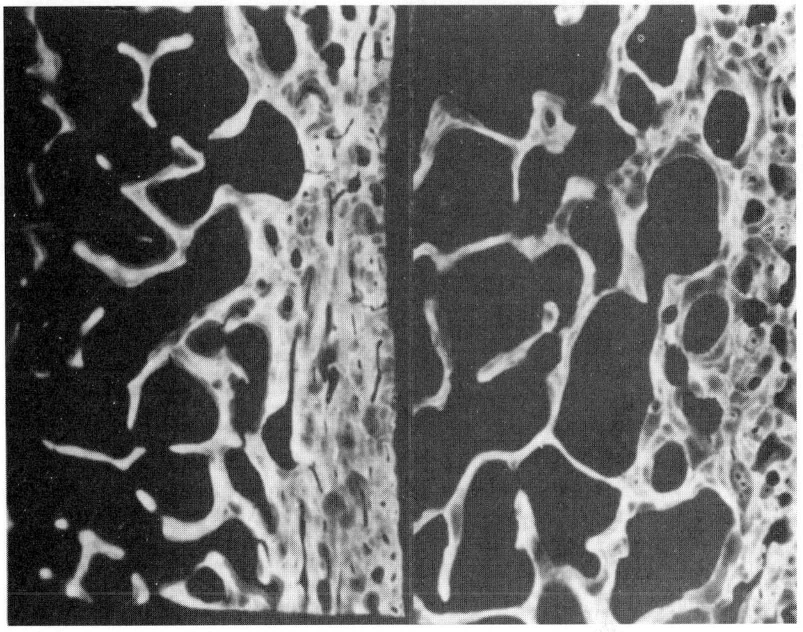

FIGURE 22-36. Normal bone (*left*) vs. bone from a patient with chronic hyperparathyroidism (*right*). The cortex and the trabecular meshwork are thinned in hyperparathyroidism, compromising biomechanical strength and predisposing to fracture. (*Reprinted with permission from Jenifer Jowsey, Bone histology and hyperparathyroidism, Clinics in Endocrinology and Metabolism, vol. 3, p. 268, 1974.*)

result of surgery. For example, baseline scores of a health survey indicated substantial disability that improved 6 months after parathyroidectomy.[397] Some patients report not realizing that they were not feeling well until the contrast they experienced after parathyroidectomy. However, in many cases, surgery does not reverse mild or nonspecific symptoms. Furthermore, surgery is known to have a large placebo effect, complicating the evaluation of its benefit in hyperparathyroidism. In any case, it can be said

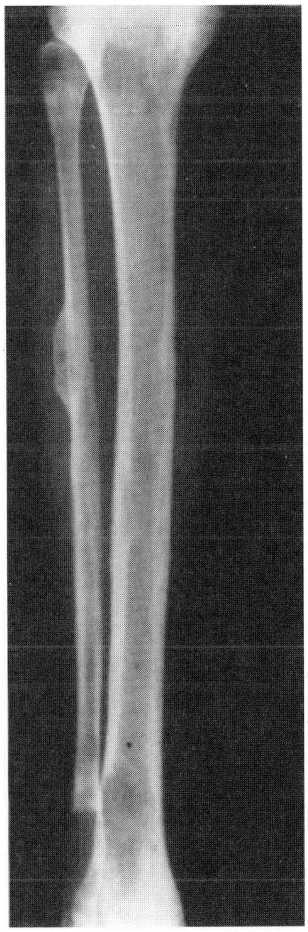

FIGURE 22-37. Radiograph of a "brown tumor," actually fibrous tissue, replacing resorbed bone. (*Courtesy of Dr. Maurice Attie, University of Pennsylvania School of Medicine.*)

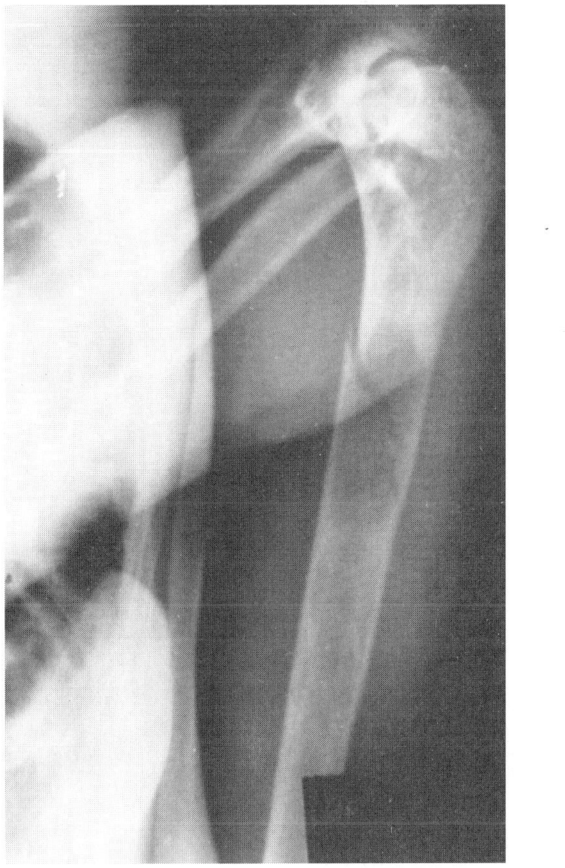

FIGURE 22-38. Osteitis fibrosa cystica. "Brown tumors" can appear "cystic" on a radiograph. The fibrous infiltrate is weaker than normal bone, predisposing to fracture, as seen in this case. (*Courtesy of Dr. Maurice Attie, University of Pennsylvania School of Medicine.*)

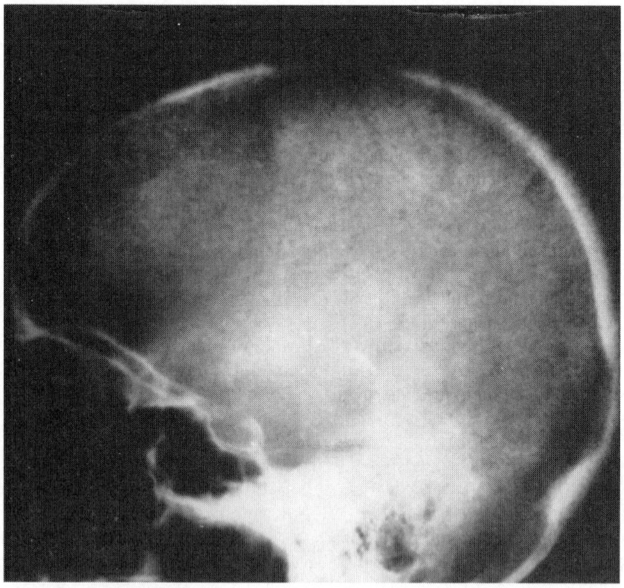

FIGURE 22-39. Radiograph of a "salt and pepper" skull reflecting resorption and demineralization. (*Courtesy of Dr. Maurice Attie, University of Pennsylvania School of Medicine.*)

with certainty that it is difficult to predict which patients will respond symptomatically to surgical intervention.

For some disorders, such as the muscle weakness that accompanies hyperparathyroidism, a neuromuscular deficit has been defined which appears to be specific to primary hyperparathyroidism. Characteristic electromyographic (EMG) changes have been observed.[398,399] Some clinicians contend that these abnormalities are neurogenic. Although the muscle weakness and EMG changes seem to be less common now than in earlier times,[399] when present, they may be reversed by parathyroid surgery.[398]

Therefore, in considering a recommendation for surgery in patients with mild elevations of calcium, the physician should be careful to avoid advocating surgery in hopes of reversing nonspecific symptoms. Rather, the recommendation for surgery should be based on biochemical indexes of the disease, evidence of end organ compromise or deterioration, or the presence of fairly clear changes in mental status (such as confusion or altered psyche and mood, which generally occur at moderate to severe elevations of calcium and PTH). A more specific set of guidelines for surgical intervention is provided later in the section on diagnosis and management of asymptomatic primary hyperparathyroidism.

Multiple Endocrine Neoplasia

Although hyperparathyroidism occurs most often sporadically, in a minority of cases there is a link to a familial syndrome. Familial hyperparathyroidism without other associated endocrine abnormalities has been reported in a few kindreds.[400] In general, it is inherited as an autosomal dominant pattern, and the pathology is four-gland chief cell hyperplasia. An even more rare form has single-gland parathyroid adenoma as the underlying pathology and is inherited in an autosomal recessive pattern.[401] Clinically, there appear to be no particular features that distinguish these forms of hyperparathyroidism from sporadic primary hyperparathyroidism.

The multiple endocrine neoplasia (MEN) syndromes constitute a well-defined set of hereditary endocrine disorders, some of which include hyperparathyroidism as a component. For the purpose of this chapter, some aspects of the MEN syndromes as they relate to hyperparathyroidism are highlighted. Hyperparathyroidism is a prominent component in two of the three MEN syndromes (type 1 and type 2a) and is rare in or absent from the third (type 2b). In these syndromes, hyperparathyroidism occurs as a result of four-gland hyperplasia. Table 22-5 lists the components of MEN type 1 (Wermer's syndrome, the three P's),[402] in which hyperparathyroidism is almost always present (penetrance approaches 100 percent by age 50) and is associated with tumors of the pituitary gland (usually chromophobe prolactin-secreting adenomas) and pancreatic adenomas (which typically secrete gastrin, insulin, or glucagon). The age of onset of hyperparathyroidisim tends to be younger (between age 15 and 35) than in primary hyperparathyroidism, and the ratio of afflicted men to women is approximately equal, as opposed to a ratio of 3:1 for women to men in sporadic primary hyperparathyroidism.

The pattern of inheritance is that of an autosomal dominant trait. Using restriction fragment length polymorphism (RFLP) analysis, the genetic defect has been mapped to the long arm of chromosome 11, 11q12-13, in all kindreds with MEN 1 that have

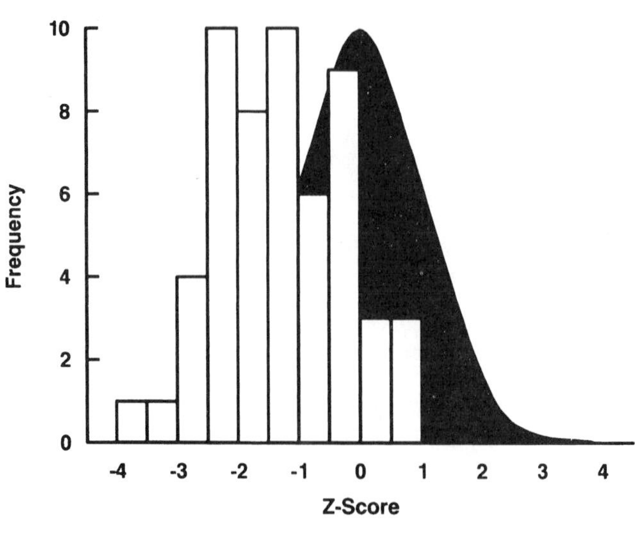

FIGURE 22-40. The Z-score, an index of bone mineral density in the distal radius in asymptomatic primary hyperparathyroidism (open bars) compared to that in normal subjects (darkened arrow). Diminished bone mineral density is evident for the population with this disorder. [*Reprinted with permission from B.H. Mitlak, et al, Asymptomatic Primary Hyperparathyroidism, J Bone Mineral Res 6(Suppl 2):S103–S110, 1991.*]

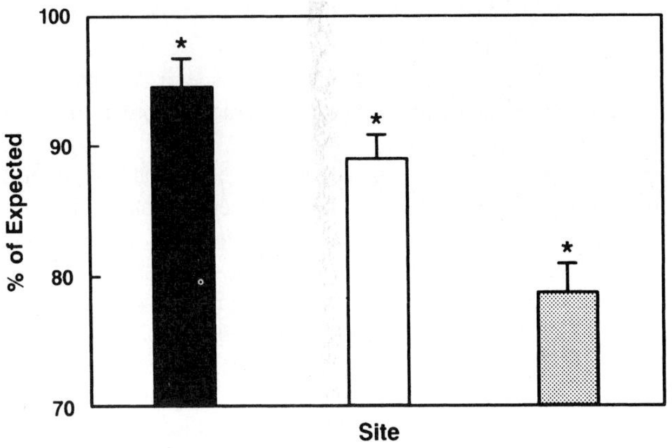

FIGURE 22-41. Decreased bone mineral density in primary hyperparathyroidism at several skeletal sites. ■, Lumbar, □, femoral; ■, radius. (*Reprinted with permission from Silverberg et al.*[449])

been examined.[403] The mutation is thought to result in inactivation of a tumor suppressor gene or antioncogene, as occurs with retinoblastoma, and is thought to be the cause of some parathyroid adenomas. The MEN 1 gene has been cloned and mutations have been identified. The gene on chromosome 11 codes for a novel 610-amino acid protein referred to as MENIN.[366,367] Because both alleles for the tumor suppressor are inactivated or altered, the disease must represent a "two-hit" phenomenon. The germ line may contain a point mutation with no clinical consequences. However, on this background, a second event, such as somatic mutation, will lead to tumorigenesis. Hence, the glandular abnormality is "monoclonal" even though all four glands become hyperplastic (the hyperplasia can be asymmetric across the glands). The markedly increased gland mass per se can account for the excess PTH secretion without a set point abnormality based on the nonsuppressible component of PTH secretion by parathyroid cells.

By producing hypercalcemia, the primary hyperparathyroidism of MEN 1 can exacerbate gastrin and acid secretion in patients who also harbor a gastrinoma (Zollinger-Ellison syndrome). Hence, parathyroidectomy is often indicated when the two disorders coexist and some improvement in peptic ulcer disease can be expected after parathyroidectomy.

Primary hyperparathyroidism occurs in approximately 10 percent of cases (although it may be present histologically in 50 percent) of the MEN type 2a syndrome (Sipple's syndrome).[404,405] The other components of the disorder are pheochromocytomas and medullary carcinoma of the thyroid gland, the latter of which dominates the syndrome (Table 22-5). The different endocrine tumors share a common developmental origin from the neuroectoderm. Any of the tumor types can present first, not all the types in each syndrome arise in each individual, and there is no set pattern of appearance. The allelic mutations responsible for both MEN type 2a and MEN type 2b (3) map to different chromosome than do the abnormalities in MEN type 1; both are found on the same locus of chromosome 10 as opposed to chromosome 11.[406]

It is always important to obtain a family history regarding the presence of any of the other components of the MEN type 1 or 2a syndromes in a patient suspected of having primary hyperparathyroidism. Certainly in patients who are discovered to have four-gland hyperplasia at the time of surgery, it is important to undertake diagnostic evaluation not only of the patient but also of close relatives for the potential relevant endocrine abnormalities.

TABLE 22-5. Multiple Endocrine Neoplasia Syndromes

Type 1
>95% hyperparathyroidism (four-gland hyperplasia)
~50% pancreatic tumors (gastrinoma, insulinoma, glucagonoma, etc.)
15–50% pituitary adenomas (prolactinoma, growth hormone-secreting, etc.)
Type 2 (2a)
100% medullary carcinoma of the thyroid
<50% pheochromocytoma or adrenal medullary hyperplasia
10–50% hyperparathyroidism (four-gland hyperplasia)
Type 3 (2b)
100% medullary carcinoma of the thyroid
<50% pheochromocytoma or adrenal medullary hyperplasia
100% mucosal neuromas

Familial Hypocalciuric Hypercalcemia

Familial hypocalciuric hypercalcemia (FHH), although rare, has fascinated clinical investigators. It is also referred to as familial benign hypercalcemia (FBH).[407–409] This disorder is characterized by chronically elevated serum calcium, somewhat depressed phosphorus, and PTH values that are usually detectable and normal or slightly elevated in some cases. Even normal levels of PTH are "inappropriate" in the setting of hypercalcemia and imply that PTH may play an etiologic role in maintenance of the hypercalcemia. Along the same line, the parathyroid glands are usually normal in size or slightly enlarged. On microscopic examination, they are normal or somewhat hyperplastic.

Patients with this disorder tend to excrete low quantities of calcium in the urine, typically one-third of the value observed in patients with primary hyperparathyroidism and below a value of 0.10 for the ratio of calcium to creatinine clearance. This appears to reflect a renal defect, as the increased tubular reabsorption of calcium persists even after parathyroidectomy. These patients also display somewhat elevated blood magnesium levels. Although these biochemical parameters are true of the population with the disorder, they cannot be used to make the diagnosis in any given individual because the values overlap with those present in classical primary hyperparathyroidism (Fig. 22-42). The disorder is lifelong and is inherited as an autosomal dominant trait with virtually 100 percent penetrance. The age of onset is much earlier than in hyperparathyroidism; hypercalcemia can be demonstrated from birth and is usually detected by age 20. However, because FHH is asymptomatic, the disorder may not be detected until much later in life.

Although the low urine calcium excretion, presentation early in life, and positive family history are findings that strongly suggest the diagnosis of FHH, none of these features alone can distinguish the disorder from primary hyperparathyroidism. Fortunately, however, as far as can be determined at this point, these patients develop no long-term sequelae of the disease other than rare instances of relapsing pancreatitis. Although bone mass is normal in these patients, markers of bone turnover may be increased.[410] If they mistakenly undergo neck exploration, an adenoma is not found. Normal or somewhat hyperplastic-appearing glands may be found. If one or more of these glands are removed, the hypercalcemia remains unchanged; therefore, it is important not to send such patients for unnecessary surgery. Attempts to regulate serum calcium concentrations with medications have not been successful so far.

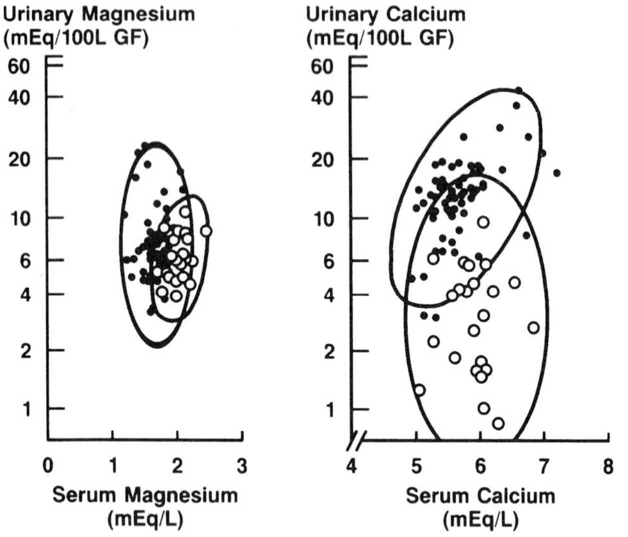

FIGURE 22-42. Biochemical abnormalities in familial hypocalciuric hypercalcemia (FHH). As shown, there is considerable overlap between patients with primary hyperparathyroidism and patients with FHH. ○, FHH; ●, 1° PTH. (*Modified from Marx et al.*[464])

The etiology of FHH has been elucidated recently.[44,411,412] The pathophysiology seems to derive from a set point error in the response of parathyroid tissue to calcium that is directly related to a mutation in the calcium-sensing receptor (Fig. 22-7).[12] Several distinct mutations have been elucidated which render the calcium sensor's responsiveness markedly diminished. This error accounts for the normal levels of PTH accompanying hypercalcemia. However, the tissues that are exposed to elevated PTH and calcium levels also may respond less than normally; hence, adverse effects do not seem to develop. Because the disorder is inherited as an autosomal dominant trait with high penetrance, it is important to identify family members with the disorder in order to avoid unnecessary surgery.

Although the disease is usually benign, occasionally it presents in the neonate as severe life-threatening hypercalcemia. Individuals with this disorder are homozygous for a defective calcium-sensing receptor gene.[44,411,412] The double dose cases represent one of the few instances where surgical total parathyroidectomy is recommended. Some of the affected offspring can also have severe hypercalcemia because of secondary hyperparathyroidism, but usually this evolves into asymptomatic hypercalcemia. In constrast, the unaffected offspring of a mother with FHH may show symptomatic hypocalcemia from fetal parathyroid suppression.[413]

Physical Findings

There are a limited number of physical findings associated with hyperparathyroidism. Band keratopathy is seen at the outer edge of the cornea at the upper and lower poles (Fig. 22-43). This finding must be distinguished from age-related nonspecific or inflammatory calcification in the limbic girdle by slitlamp examination. Weakness may be apparent on physical examination, particularly of the proximal muscles of the lower extremities. Confusion or altered mental status may also be present. Only rarely can an abnormal parathyroid gland (sometimes a parathyroid carcinoma) be palpated. In fact, according to "Albright's dictum," if a mass is detected in the neck, it usually is in the thyroid gland or may represent a parathyroid carcinoma. Bone involvement can sometimes be detected by finding tenderness in the region of the distal tibia. Collapse of the terminal phalanges may occur, giving rise to "pseudo clubbing."

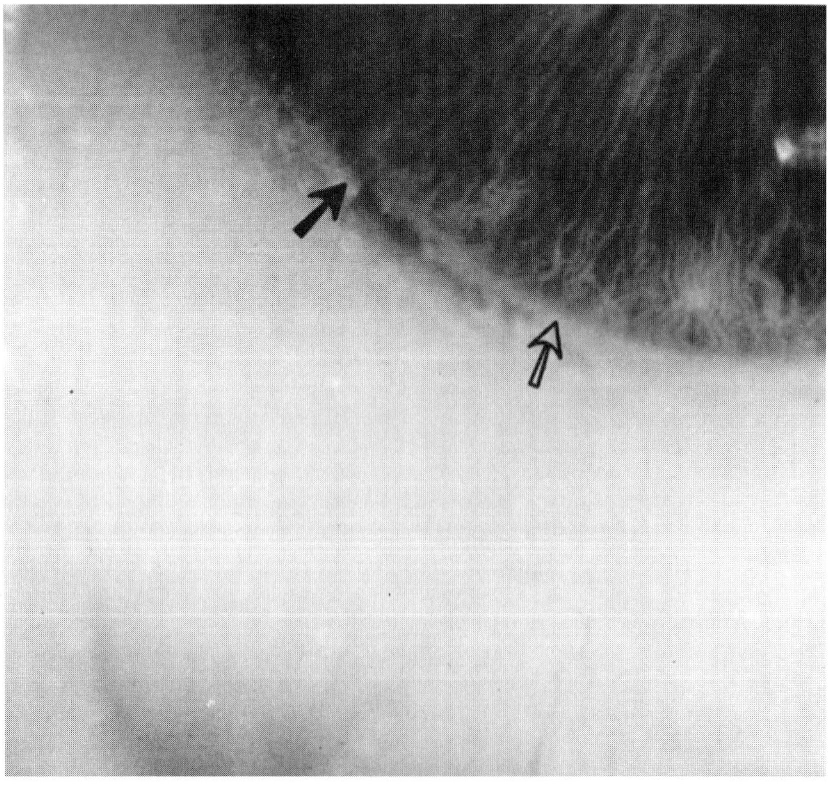

FIGURE 22-43. Band keratopathy. The open arrow identifies the limbic girdle, a region of linear calcium salt deposition associated with aging. Band keratopathy (solid arrow) is a moth-eaten and irregular region of calcium deposition, usually at the medial and lateral limbic margins. These locations are thought to result from diffusion of carbon dioxide from air-exposed regions of the cornea, with local precipitation of calcium phosphate crystals.

Laboratory Findings and Definitive Diagnosis

Consistent elevations in serum calcium above the normal level are the sine qua non of hyperparathyroidism. The measurement of serum calcium is accurate in clinical laboratories nearly universally now that multiphasic automated screening devices are employed. Detection of a calcium level above 10.4 mg/dl (2.6 mmol/liter) should always raise the suspicion of hypercalcemia. This is true regardless of the normal range listed by the laboratory, as some laboratories failed to change the normal range indicated on their lab reports after switching to automated analyzers. Although the entity of "normocalcemic hyperparathyroidism" or "intermittent hypercalcemia" has received some attention in the literature,[414] when truly hyperparathyroid patients with borderline or occasional elevations in calcium are monitored and serial calcium determinations are obtained, a clear pattern of repeatedly frank hypercalcemia generally becomes evident. Chronicity of calcium elevation is also a hallmark of hyperparathyroidism. As the disease is usually asymptomatic in the early stages, it is often possible to review a medical record and discover that a patient had documented mild elevations of calcium during a period of years. Hyperparathyroidism and its associated familial disorders are the only clinical disorders that produce hypercalcemia without other signs or symptoms for a period of years. It is also important to avoid misinterpretation of the calcium determination reported by the clinical laboratory. Because calcium circulates bound principally to albumin, abnormalities in the albumin level can alter the total serum calcium value without having a true physiologic consequence. In general, deviation in serum albumin of 1.0 mg/dl results in a change of 0.8 mg/dl in the same direction for calcium; this shift needs to be taken into account when one is assessing a potential calcium abnormality. If the significance of a total calcium determination is in question, ionized calcium should be measured.

In recent years, definitive establishment of the diagnosis of hyperparathyroidism has been greatly facilitated by the development of reliable, sensitive, and accurate radioimmunoassays for PTH (discussed elsewhere in this chapter). In particular, the two-site IRMA[63] and immunochemiluminescent (ICMA) can accurately determine the quantity of biologically active full-length PTH present in the circulation and is considered to be the gold standard. In almost all cases of hyperparathyroidism, PTH levels are found to be clearly elevated using such assays (Fig. 22-10), obviating the need for provocative testing or calcium-PTH histograms or other devices for assigning a diagnosis based on a combination of laboratory values. For the most part, it is no longer necessary to invoke previously employed diagnostic principles in which an "inappropriately" normal PTH level at the time of hypercalcemia was used to establish the diagnosis of hyperparathyroidism. Using the IRMA, PTH levels are usually elevated in 85–90 percent of patients with hyperparathyroidism. There is no crossreactivity with parathyroid-related peptide, PTH-rP. Furthermore, there is a general correlation between the level of PTH detected, the degree of hypercalcemia, and the mass of abnormal parathyroid tissue. When this assay method is employed in complex clinical situations, many previously confusing diagnostic issues are clarified. Hypercalcemia caused by hyperparathyroidism as opposed to that caused by malignancy can be readily distinguished using the newer assays; PTH levels are depressed or undetectable in patients with hypercalcemia due to malignancy. Even in renal failure, where earlier radioimmunoassay (RIA) systems indicated increased levels of PTH (as a result of accumulation of carboxyl-terminal inactive fragments detected by the RIA system), the IRMA reveals elevated levels of PTH only when biologically active hormone and true secondary hyperparathyroidism are present. Though not essential for determining the status of PTH secretion, use of the PTH IRMA can be advantageous compared to previous RIAs for detecting PTH levels in blood. A modified two-site immunochemiluminometric assay has been developed with results available in only 10 minutes. It is now being utilized intraoperatively to monitor the success of the surgery.[415]

Other indicators of increased PTH activity such as low fasting serum phosphorus and bicarbonate levels and elevated chloride levels can be helpful in an ancillary manner in supporting the diagnosis. The action of PTH on the proximal tubule inhibits the reabsorption of bicarbonate, resulting in bicarbonate wasting. Consequently, in chronic states of parathyroid excess such as hyperparathyroidism, renal tubular acidosis develops. The resulting retention of hydrogen ions obligates chloride, resulting in a hyperchloremic acidosis. X-ray changes in bone can also corroborate the diagnosis. A determination of bone mineral density, though not helpful in establishing the diagnosis, will provide a useful baseline measurement of bone status by which to later monitor the course of the disease. Once the diagnosis of hyperparathyroidism has been made, an abdominal radiograph should be obtained to assist in the search for calcified renal stones. Elevations in alkaline phosphatase serve as a biochemical indicator of bone involvement before x-ray changes are apparent. The QT interval on the electrocardiogram may be shortened, reflecting hypercalcemia, not hyperparathyroidism specifically. Measurement of 24-h urine calcium should be performed once the diagnosis of hyperparathyroidism has been confirmed to investigate the possibility of FHH syndrome, to evaluate the need for surgery in asymptomatic patients, and as a baseline for future monitoring. However, measurements of vitamin D levels or 24-h urine phosphorus excretion are not necessary in establishing the diagnosis. Therefore, it is emphasized that in the current era the diagnosis of hyperparathyroidism can be established definitively and exclusively or disproven by the biochemical determinations of blood calcium and PTH levels.

Preoperative Localization Studies

Until recently the techniques available for localizing abnormal parathyroid glands before surgery had problems yielding false negative and false positive results. These included venous catheterization with determination of PTH levels, angiography, ultrasound, and radio-thallium/technetium imaging.[416–418] In fact, the skilled surgeon had a much better chance of identification of the abnormal gland or glands than did any of the preoperative localization techniques. During the last 5 years, technetium-99m sestamibi has become established as the best and most convenient localization test. It is a 2-phase test that includes readings initially and at 2 hours. Sestamibi is taken up by the parathyroid and thyroid tissue but is rapidly washed out by the thyroid. Uptake persists in the abnormal parathyroid tissue at 2 hours. False positive and negative results remain an issue[419] and its routine use remains controversial.

Preoperative localization studies are particularly useful in patients in whom there has been previous surgery and failure to identify the abnormal gland in the neck.[420] In such cases, technitium 99m Sestamibi, computed tomography of the mediastinum or angiography may be used to search for the rare abnormal parathyroid gland within the mediastinum (intrathymic or otherwise); CT is noninvasive and less expensive than angiography. If a mediastinal mass is not discovered, selective venous catheterization with measurement of PTH values should be considered to identify secretion from an abnormal gland in the neck. Because the success of invasive techniques depends in part on the skill of the practitioner, patients should be referred to one of the small number of institutions with substantial experience in these procedures. Localization techniques, particularly selective venous catheterization, should also be considered when there has been previous neck surgery which has altered the local anatomy, complicating the anticipated parathyroid surgery, whether or not the previous neck surgery was for hyperparathyroidism. In some cases, localization can be coupled with an ablation technique, such as destructive infusion of angiographic contrast medium, to effectively treat the disease.[421] Ablative methods should be considered when previous surgery has been unsuccessful and the patient is at high risk for complications of neck exploration and no longer amenable to surgery or when the abnormal gland has been localized to the mediastinum and an attempt is being made to avoid sternotomy. Looking back on all the effort undertaken thus far to develop localization techniques for the parathyroids, one is reminded of Albright's quip, "There is no time like the initial operation to find and remove the tumor."

Parathyroid Surgery

Parathyroid surgery can be technically difficult. The adjacent vital structures in the neck require that surgery be performed with considerable skill. Complications from surgery in this area include hypoparathyroidism and vocal cord paralysis from damage to the recurrent laryngeal nerve, causing pemanent hoarseness. If the laryngeal nerves are damaged bilaterally, respiratory compromise or death can result. The variation in the anatomic location of abnormal glands in ectopic sites such as the lateral neck, retroesophageal region, intrathyroidal position, and mediastinum may complicate surgery. Furthermore, the differences in pathology between single-gland adenoma, four-gland hyperplasia, and parathyroid carcinoma dictate different operative treatments. Hence, the need for engaging a surgeon experienced in parathyroid surgery cannot be overemphasized. As was mentioned previously, the surgeon can expect to find a single abnormal parathyroid gland in approximately 85 percent of cases. The extent of the operative dissection is controversial but four-gland exploration with frozen section confirmation is the approach most recommended. Preoperative technetium-99m sestamibi imaging and the measurement of parathyroid hormone concentrations intraoperatively allows for a more streamlined approach with a reduced operative time and number of complications. In addition, there are cost savings from the reduced number of frozen sections required for histopathology. The technetium-99m sestamibi scan localizes the adenoma and allows for a unilateral exploration. An intraoperative drop in PTH assures the surgeon that no more hyperfunctioning tissue is present.[422] Larger clinical trials using this approach are needed before it becomes universally accepted.

In the 10 to 15 percent of cases where four-gland hyperplasia is found, the surgeon should remove three glands and a portion of the fourth. Such surgery can be extremely difficult and runs the risk of inadequately treating the condition, thus leaving residual persistent hyperparathyroidism, or removing too much parathyroid tissue, thus producing hypoparathyroidism.[423,424] Even when normocalcemia is achieved postoperatively, within months some patients with hyperplasia develop recurrent hyperparathyroidism, especially those patients whose hyperplasia results from an MEN syndrome. Within 12 years, 50 percent of MEN patients who underwent successful subtotal parathyroidectomy for hyperplasia developed recurrent hyperparathyroidism.[423] For these reasons, some surgeons have resorted to removing all the abnormal parathyroid glands and then autotransplanting a portion of the abnormal parathyroid tissue into an antecubital position in the brachioradialus muscle in the forearm, where it is more accessible if hyperparathyroidism recurs and the tissue has to be removed.[425–427] Unfortunately, this approach runs the risk of transplanting too much parathyroid tissue or losing all the parathyroid tissue if the transplant fails, producing hypoparathyroidism. Furthermore, although the transplanted tissue is theoretically located in a more accessible site than the neck, it often cannot be found after transplantation. Finally, the autotransplant approach does not preclude possible recurrent disease from remaining and growing parathyroid tissue in the neck or mediastinum. The best surgical approach toward four-gland hyperplasia therefore remains controversial, with most surgeons preferring to remove three glands and a portion of the fourth. Some also cryopreserve the extracted parathyroid tissue for possible future transplantation.

For parathyroid carcinoma, the surgeon must be careful to excise around a margin of the gland. Parathyroid carcinomas are notorious for seeding locally and recurring. Therefore, the capsule of the carcinoma should not be disrupted.[375,428,429] Unusually high calcium or PTH levels should alert the surgeon to the possible presence of a parathyroid carcinoma preoperatively. Metastases occur frequently, however, with parathyroid carcinoma. Because PTH secretion appears to correlate with the size of the tumor, periodic surgical removal of one or a few parathyroid carcinoma metastases should be used to manage the patient. As the tumors are usually slow-growing and hypercalcemia is often the worst or only complication of the malignancy, such patients can often be maintained in this manner for years. Nevertheless, the level of serum calcium increases progressively and at a rate more rapid than is typical of hyperparathyroidism. The tumors become truly inoperable when the location or number of metastases precludes this surgical approach.

In the immediate postoperative period, some patients become mildly or even severely hypoparathyroid until the remaining suppressed glands, which have been "dormant" for months or years, resume normal function. This situation can last for several days. It is typified by low serum calcium and elevated serum phosphorous. Hence, calcium should be monitored every 12 h until a stable plateau has been reached or the levels have returned to normal. Postoperative transient hypoparathyroidism usually can be managed with dietary calcium supplementation (1 to 2 g/day) alone. Some patients even develop symptoms of hypocalcemia with tingling in the fingertips and around the mouth or even a positive Chvostek's sign on physical examination despite absolute values of calcium level within the normal range. It appears that the rapid relative decline in calcium alone can produce "hypocalcemic" symptoms. Permanent hypoparathyroidism can also develop either in the immediate postoperative period or rarely after a long delay. Treatment with vitamin D analogs and calcium along the lines described elsewhere in this chapter is required in such cases.

Patients with extensive bone disease characterized by changes apparent on x-ray and elevated serum alkaline phosphatase levels are at risk for developing a severe and life-threatening hypocalcemic syndrome postoperatively. It is important to distinguish this syndrome, termed "hungry bones," from transient postoperative hypoparathyroidism.[430] It arises because bone has been under a tremendous resorptive stimulus chronically, which is then abruptly interrupted by removal of the overactive parathyroid tissue. Bone formation is now unopposed and is able to catch up with resorption. As a result, a large calcium influx into bone ensues, depleting the ECF of calcium and sometimes resulting in marked hypocalcemia. This hypocalcemia is distinguished from transient hypoparathyroidism by the serum phosphorus levels, which, instead of being elevated, are below normal because both calcium and phosphate move into bone as part of the remineralization process. This condition usually persists for days to weeks and requires large amounts of calcium supplementation, often administered intravenously, as well as large doses of vitamin D, preferably a relatively short-acting analog (see previous discussion of vitamin D). Once normocalcemia is established after subtotal parathyroidectomy, calcium should be tested at 1-, 3- to 6-, and 12-month intervals and annually thereafter.

Diagnosis and Management of Asymptomatic Primary Hyperparathyroidism

The diagnosis and management of asymptomatic primary hyperparathyroidism remain one of the most controversial areas in endocrinology and internal medicine. The majority of patients who present with hypercalcemia in an ambulatory setting have primary hyperparathyroidism. The vast majority of these patients are asymptomatic (Fig. 22-34). It appears likely that this management problem will confront internists with increasing frequency as the population ages and more patients are detected by multiphasic screening.

In 1990, the NIH convened a Consensus Development Conference on the diagnosis and management of this disorder.[420] The panel reaffirmed the common practice of recommending surgery as the treatment of choice for primary hyperparathyroidism. However, although control of serum calcium, recurrent kidney stones, and osteitis fibrosa cystica clearly can be managed effectively with surgery, complications and symptoms such as muscle weakness, neuropsychiatric effects, and hypertension do not necessarily respond to surgical treatment, as was discussed earlier.

Although all these patients should be considered candidates for surgery because it is relatively safe and is the only proven treatment for primary hyperparathyroidism, some patients are truly asymptomatic and can be considered for medical management under rigorous conditions of selection and monitoring. These patients have neither symptoms nor signs commonly attributable to primary hyperparathyroidism. Because the natural history of the disease is uncertain, there are no signs or absolute laboratory criteria that can be used to predict the future development of long-term complications in any given patient. However, in a recent 10-year follow-up study of 52 asymptomatic patients with primary hyperparathyroidism who did not undergo surgery, 14 (27 percent) had progression of disease as defined by the development of at least one indication for parathyroid resection. Marked hypercalcemia developed in 2 patients, marked hypercalcuria in 8, and low cortical bone density in 6. The patients who progressed were younger at base-line than those with no disease progression, and 6 became menopausal during follow-up.[393] No symptomatic complications such as kidney stones or fractures developed. This study, although observational in design, suggests that asymptomatic patients with confirmed primary hyperparathyroidism should undergo surgery.

Although controversy continues regarding the surgical treatment of the asymptomatic patient,[431] surgery is definitely indicated in the asymptomatic patient if any of the following are present: markedly elevated serum calcium levels [above 11.4 to 12 mg/dl or 1 to 1.6 mg/dl above normal (above 2.8 to 3 mmol/liter or 2.5 to 2.7 mmol/liter above normal)], a previous episode of life-threatening hypercalcemia, reduced creatinine clearance (30 percent below normal), presence of a kidney stone on radiography, markedly elevated 24-h urine calcium excretion (>400 mg), or substantially reduced bone mass (approximately 2 standard deviations below normal for age, sex, and race). Hence, medical monitoring can be undertaken in selected patients who are defined by not meeting the criteria for surgery listed.

In addition, medical surveillance is not considered desirable or suitable for patients who (1) requested surgery, (2) are unlikely to be monitored regularly because of issues of patient compliance or because of the physician's circumstances, (3) have a coexisting illness complicating their management, or (4) are young (less than 50 years old, particularly premenopausal women). Finally, physician judgment in consultation with the patient should be applied instead of rigorous adherence to these guidelines.

Not enough is known to predict the occurrence of fractures in primary hyperparathyroidism on the basis of determinations of bone mass or bone mineral density. No subgroup at risk for future fractures can be clearly identified. However, it is assumed that the same paradigm that is operative for osteoporosis—that decreased bone mineral density is associated with increased fractures—is applicable to primary hyperparathyroidism. This would be of special importance when there is a combination of postmenopausal status and primary hyperparathyroidism. At this time, however, there have been no controlled studies with the requisite power (in terms of numbers of patients or duration of follow-up) to resolve the fracture issue for asymptomatic primary hyperparathyroidism. In an observational study of 407 patients, 10 asymptomatic patients with hyperparathyroidism had an increase in vertebral distal forearm and pelvic fractures. Increasing age and female gender was associated with a great risk.[392] Certainly, in established hyperparathyroidism, bone mineral density is known to be below normal (Figs. 22-40 and 22-41) and fracture rates are increased (Fig. 22-44). Furthermore, successful surgery leads to sustained increase in bone mineral density that is persistent 4 years after

FIGURE 22-44. Increased incidence of fractures at multiple skeletal sites in patients with primary hyperparathyroidism. □, Observed; ■, expected; $P < 0.001$. *(Reprinted with permission from M. Peacock, Osteoporosis 1:463, 1984.)*

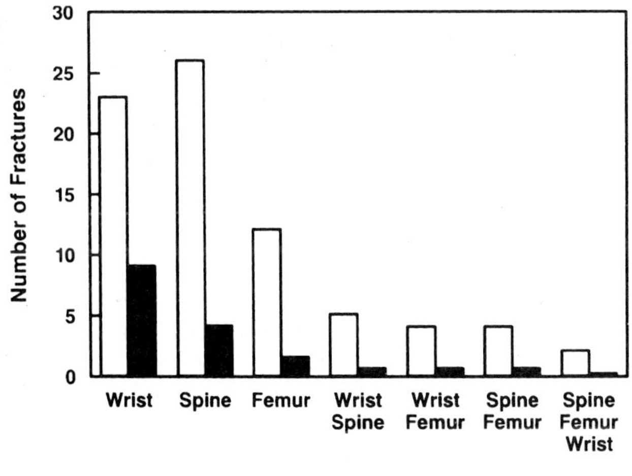

surgery. The greatest increases in bone mineral density are seen in the lumbar spine and femoral neck.[391,432]

A somewhat related issue is the question of hyperparathyroidism contributing to the etiology of postmenopausal osteoporosis. There has been speculation that subtle hyperparathyroidism or increased sensitivity to normal circulating levels of PTH may cause or exacerbate osteoporosis. This hypothesis has not been proved conclusively even for a subset of osteoporotic patients. Therefore, osteoporosis per se is not an indication for subtotal parathyroidectomy.

Once a decision has been made to follow a patient with medical surveillance, subsequent deterioration in organ status should be considered an indication for surgery. Although definite numbers cannot be recommended and individual physician judgment is paramount, deterioration of renal or bone parameters or elevation of serum calcium to the values previously listed as initial criteria for surgery or the development of kidney stones would seem to warrant surgical intervention. Many physicians will intervene in the presence of a less marked abnormality for any of the parameters cited.

After an initial determination to ascertain a baseline, monitoring of bone mineral density should be performed on a semiannual basis until lack of progression is confirmed. Thereafter, if a patient is stable, monitoring should be performed at 1- to 3-year intervals, depending on the status of the patient and the particular techniques available for determinations of bone mineral density. It remains unclear whether patients with asymptomatic hyperparathyroidism, once diagnosed, actually continue to lose bone at a more rapid rate than do their peers.

Concerns about the long-term complications of the disease on other organs have not been specifically addressed. For instance, one pathologic survey found that chronic hypercalcemia was associated with accelerated deposition of calcium in cardiac annuli and valvular cusps and in the media and intima of coronary arteries.[433] The coronary intimal calcification might be accelerated in the presence of hypercholesterolemia and thus contribute as a risk factor for atherosclerosis.

Medical Management of Primary Hyperparathyroidism and Asymptomatic Hyperparathyroidism

A limited number of general mechanistic approaches can be used to treat hypercalcemia.[434] Urinary calcium excretion should be increased first by expanding intravascular volume and then by prescribing loop diuretics, if needed and tolerated. Several medical agents inhibit bone resorption; plicamycin, bisphosphonates, calcitonin, and gallium nitrate all diminish osteoclastic bone resorption by different biochemical mechanisms.

The treatment of hypercalcemia depends on the severity of the abnormality. For "asymptomatic" hyperparathyroidism and in the absence of factors that would make the patient no longer suitable for medical monitoring, as described previously, no specific treatment is recommended except avoidance of dehydration, immobilization, and thiazide diuretics. Estrogens provide the theoretical advantage of lowering calcium, perhaps by reducing the action of PTH on bone and simultaneously providing known beneficial effects on the cardiovascular system and bone (osteoporosis) in postmenopausal women.[435–437] Weighing against the use of estrogen, however, is its potential for promoting malignancies of the uterus and breast and the associated side effects, including uterine bleeding, all of which limit the practical use of estrogens for many patients. Furthermore, estrogen administration results in raised levels of PTH. Although estrogen appears promising, we feel that if a patient requires treatment to control calcium levels, it is more appropriate to recommend surgery. For calcium levels of 12 mg/dl (3 mmol/liter) or less, promotion of urinary excretion of calcium is the best approach. This can usually be accomplished by increasing the oral intake of salt and fluids. Patients with even mild hypercalcemia tend to be relatively dehydrated as a result of the obligatory loss of water that accompanies hypercalciuria. Correction of the fluid derangement alone will usually substantially correct the blood calcium level.

Although diuretics such as furosemide may promote calciuria, they should be used with caution as they can dehydrate the patient further, leading to decreased glomerular filtration and thus exacerbating the hypercalcemia. Thiazide diuretics should be avoided because they may worsen hypercalcemia. Dietary restriction of calcium is controversial; if the pathophysiology of the disease is a set point error in calcium regulation of PTH secretion by the parathyroid gland, dietary restriction will have the adverse effect of raising PTH levels and promoting bone resorption to maintain elevated levels of calcium. Therefore, we favor a moderate calcium intake.

Though some clinicians have advocated the use of oral phosphate salts in treating mild cases of hypercalcemia under carefully controlled conditions,[438] it is our feeling that this merely treats the biochemical abnormality of elevated serum calcium. Furthermore, diminishing calcium levels by administering phosphate salts is not without risk. First, such treatment has the undesirable effect of elevating PTH levels.[438] Second, if the solubility product constant for calcium and phosphate is exceeded, ectopic precipitation of calcium phosphate can occur in the soft tissues, including the kidney, where it can lead to renal compromise or failure. Finally, the dose of oral phosphate required to reduce calcium levels into the normal range regularly produces diarrhea. Phosphate appears to act by three mechanisms. It interferes with intestinal calcium absorption, inhibits bone resorption, and inhibits renal production of $1\alpha,25\text{-}(OH)_2D$ vitamin D.

In the past, several other agents appeared promising for the management of mild hypercalcemia due to primary hyperparathyroidism. Preliminary reports indicated that propranolol[439] or cimetidine[440] might be useful, but ultimately their efficacy was not observed consistently. Bisphosphonates have been used but thus far they do no appear to lead to a sustained reduction in serum calcium concentrations. It appears that serum calcium concentrations decrease transiently and PTH levels increase.[441–443] A new class of agents called calcimimetics can reduce PTH levels and serum calcium in patients with primary hyperparathyroidism. These agents activate the calcium-sensing receptors on the parathyroid cells. When activated they signal the G protein transducing pathways to increase intracellular calcium concentration. This in turn inhibits PTH secretion. Larger clinical trials will establish their clinical potential.[444] Finding an effective medical therapy not only provides an option for asymptomatic patients, it also would be invaluable for those in whom surgery is contraindicated or in situations when surgical resection is not possible, such as parathyroid carcinoma.

Hypercalcemic Crisis

Patients with calcium levels of 12.5 mg/dl (3.1 mmol/liter) or greater, who are often said to have a "parathyroid storm" or "crisis," require aggressive or emergency treatment as these levels can be life-threatening. Although surgery is definitely required, it should not be undertaken when calcium levels are higher than 12.5 mg/dl because of a substantially increased risk of mortality. Only after reduction of calcium levels to below 12.5 mg/dl should surgery be performed. If it is not known whether the patient's calcium level has been stably but markedly elevated, hospitalization should be considered because of the seriousness of the metabolic disturbance. Again, saline rehydration is the first line of treatment. One to 4 liters of saline should be administered intravenously during a 2- to 6-h period if the patient's cardiovascular status will tolerate such an infusion. Only after complete rehydration should intravenous loop diuretics such as furosemide be administered to promote calcium along with sodium excretion. Calcitonin (100 to 400 units/day) parenterally alone or in conjunction with corticosteroids can effectively decrease calcium levels.[227] Calcium levels will generally fall within 24 to 48 h. However, tachyphylaxis to calcitonin usually occurs within days, thus limiting its utility to acute treatment.[218,226] This loss of responsiveness can be reversed by conconcitant corticosteroid therapy.[218] Once calcium has been restored to normal or nearly normal levels by any of these maneuvers, parathyroidectomy should be performed before hypercalcemia recurs.

For patients with parathyroid carcinoma who are inoperable (described earlier), it is necessary to eventually achieve a maintenance regimen. The physician should consider the addition of other therapeutic modalities early in the treatment of acute hypercalcemia, especially because these other agents are effective only after a lag period of several days. If orchestrated properly, their beneficial effects can begin just as calcitonin's effectiveness is declining and attempts are being made to discontinue intravenous fluid infusions. These drugs are discussed in more detail in the section on the treatment of hypercalcemia of malignancy.

FIGURE 22-45. Serum calcium and excretion of nephrogenous cAMP (NcAMP) in hyperparathyroidism and malignancy. Patient groups are normocalcemic patients with cancer ("cancer controls"), patients with primary hyperparathyroidism (HPT), patients with humoral hypercalcemia of malignancy (HHM), and patients with local osteolytic hypercalcemia (LOH). The HHM group includes patients with squamous carcinomas, renal carcinoma, bladder carcinomas, and miscellaneous tumors; the LOH group includes patients with breast carcinoma, multiple myeloma, lymphoma, and pulmonary adenocarcinoma. *(From Stewart, Horst, Deftos, Cadman, Lang, and Broadus,[499] by permission of the New England Journal of Medicine.)*

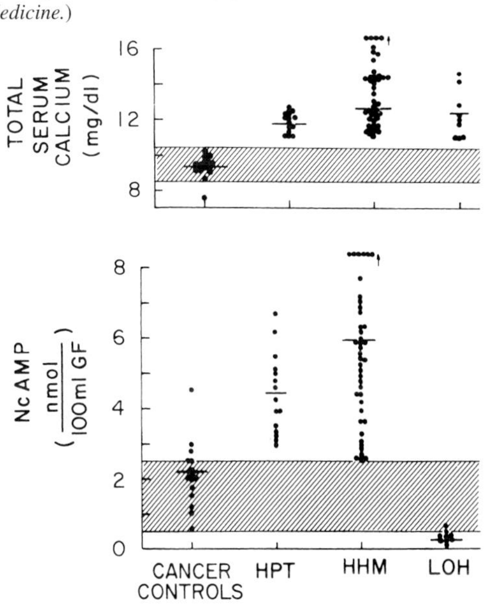

Plicamycin (mithramycin) (25 μg/kg for 3 to 4 days) is quite effective in treating the hypercalcemia of malignancy as well as primary hyperparathyroidism or parathyroid carcinoma because it blocks bone resorption, probably through a toxic effect on the osteoclast.

Bisphosphonates are effective in short-term treatment of hypercalcemia due to primary hyperparathyroidism survival.[441] Clondronate, which unlike etidronate does not inhibit bone mineralization or produce osteomalacia, has been shown to be effective in short-term studies.[445] The drug of first choice in the treatment of hypercalcemia presently is Pamidroniate, with which there has been large experience over many years.[446] Zoledronate will likely be approved soon and may replace Pamidroniate. The drug is not available in the United States, although it is used commonly in Europe. It will be useful in both acute and maintenance regimens for the treatment of parathyroid carcinoma or hyperparathyroidism in cases where medical control of hypercalcemia is required.[446–448]

Gallium nitrate has recently been approved in the United States for the treatment of hypercalcemia of malignancy.[449] Experience with this agent in treating severe hypercalcemia due to hyperparathyroidism has not been reported, although the agent has been used effectively on a short-term basis in treating parathyroid carcinoma.[450]

Malignancy-Associated Hypercalcemia and Osteolysis

Parathyroid Hormone-Related Protein (PTHrP)

Malignancy is the most frequent cause of hypercalcemia in hospitalized patients. It usually occurs in the setting of advanced disease, and is a poor prognostic factor. The majority of patients have associated osteolytic bone metastases, but in a few, the humoral hypercalcemia syndrome occurs in the absence of tumor cells in bone. The mechanisms responsible have been clarified in the last 15 years.

Biochemical features of malignancy-associated hypercalcemia share some similarities to those seen in primary hyperparathyroidism (1°HPT). Specifically, in addition to the hypercalcemia, hypophosphatemia can occur (depending on the patient's renal function) as well as hypercalciuria, hyperphosphaturia, and increased excretion of nephrogenous cyclic AMP (Fig. 22-45).[451] Plasma intact PTH concentrations are suppressed in this syndrome except in rare cases of ectopic PTH production or concomitant primary hyperparathyroidism. Plasma $1,25(OH)_2D_3$ concentrations are generally low except in certain hematologic malignancies when the humoral mediator is $1,25(OH)_2D_3$ (Fig. 22-46). Serum PTHrP concentrations are increased (Fig. 22-47).

In 1941 Fuller Albright proposed that hypercalcemia in a patient with renal carcinoma was due to ectopic secretion of PTH.[452] As the patient had normal parathyroid glands at the time of the neck operation, Albright postulated that the tumor produced PTH but when assayed for PTH, it was not detected. When more sensitive PTH assays became available, it was clear that the mediator was not PTH, but rather an immunologically distinct factor that had PTH-like biological activity.[451]

Almost 50 years after Albright's observations, this parathyroid hormone-related protein was purified from human lung cancer,[453]

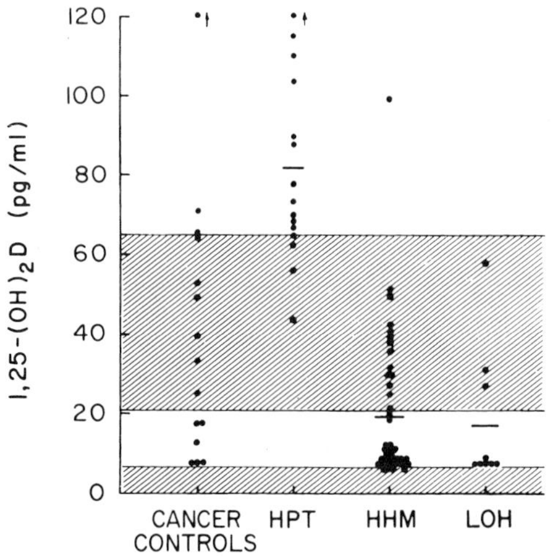

FIGURE 22-46. Values for plasma 1α,25-$(OH)_2D$ in the patients described in Fig. 23-60. Plasma 1α,25-$(OH)_2D$ values are elevated in patients with hyperparathyroidism (HPT) but are normal or reduced in patients with humoral hypercalcemia of malignancy (HHM) or local osteolytic hypercalcemia (LOH). (*From Stewart, Horst, Deftos, Cadman, Lang, and Broadus,*[499] *by permission of the New England Journal of Medicine.*)

breast cancer,[454] and renal cell carcinoma[455] simultaneously by several independent groups and was cloned shortly thereafter.[456] PTHrP and not PTH, is the major mediator of humoral hypercalcemia of malignancy,[457,458] although 7 cases of authentic tumor-produced PTH have been reported.[459–465] PTHrP has 70 percent homology to the first 13 amino acids of the N-terminal portion of PTH,[456] (Fig. 22-48) binds to PTH receptors[69] and shares similar biologic activity to PTH.[466] PTHrP stimulates adenylate cyclase in renal and bone cells,[454,455,466–468] increases renal tubular reabsorption of calcium and osteoclastic bone resorption,[467,468] decreases renal phosphate uptake,[466,467,469] and stimulates 1-hydroxylase.[466] PTHrP has been found in a variety of tumor types associated with hypercalcemia including squamous, breast, and renal carcinoma.[470,471] Although the majority of squamous cell carcinomas produce PTHrP,[472] the capacity to cause hypercalcemia may depend on the level of PTHrP gene expression, which in turn may be determined by differential transcription of the PTHrP gene promoters.[473] The regulation of PTHrP is complex. Factors such as prolactin,[474] epidermal growth factor (EGF),[475–478] insulin,[476] insulin-like growth factor (IGF) I[476,479] and II,[478] transforming growth factor (TGF)-α,[480] TGF-β,[478,481–483] angiotensin II,[484] stretch,[485] and the src proto-oncogene[486] increase expression, while glucocorticoids[476,479,487,488] and 1,25$(OH)_2D_3$[475,476] decrease it. Estrogen increases PTHrP expression in uterine tissue and in vitro studies suggest that an estrogen response element is present in the PTHrP gene.[489,490] Mutations in codons 248 and 273 of the p53 tumor suppressor gene repress PTHrP gene expression in some squamous cell carcinomas.[491]

The human PTHrP gene is larger and more complex than the human PTH gene. It spans approximately 15 kilobases of genomic DNA and has 9 exons and 3 promoters. Three PTHrP isoforms of 139, 141, or 173 amino acids as well as multiple PTHrP messenger RNA species exist.[478] There is considerable sequence homology across species up to amino acid 111.[492] Cell line-specific utilization of the promoters and of the 3′ alternative splicing pathways among bone, breast, kidney, and lung cell lines have been demonstrated.[478]

Like PTH, PTHrP undergoes endoproteolytic posttranslational processing that results in several secretory forms: (1) an amino-terminal PTHrP-(1–36), (2) a mid-region species that begins at amino acid 38 that has an undefined carboxyl terminus,[493,494] and (3) a carboxyl-terminal species that is recognized by an antibody directed against the 109–138 region.[494–496] The arrangement of basic residues suggest that members of the subtilisin family of endoproteases such as furin,[497] PC 1/3, PC-2, PACE-4, and PC8[498] are responsible for such processing.[493,499,500] Posttranslational modification of PTHrP also occurs as glycosylation of an amino-terminal PTHrP species produced by keratinocytes has been reported.[501] The subject of posttranslational processing of PTHrP as well as the receptor and signal transduction pathways employed by the mature secretory forms of PTHrP has been extensively reviewed by Orloff et al.[499] Although PTHrP mediates its calcemic effects through the classical PTH/PTHrP receptor, there is evidence for a separate PTHrP receptor.[502] However, the function of such a receptor remains unclear.

PTHrP has been detected in a variety of tumor types as well as in normal tissue.[470,471] The widespread expression of PTHrP in normal tissue was the first evidence that the hormone had a role in normal physiology. PTHrP appears to be important in (1) the regulation of cartilage differentiation and bone formation

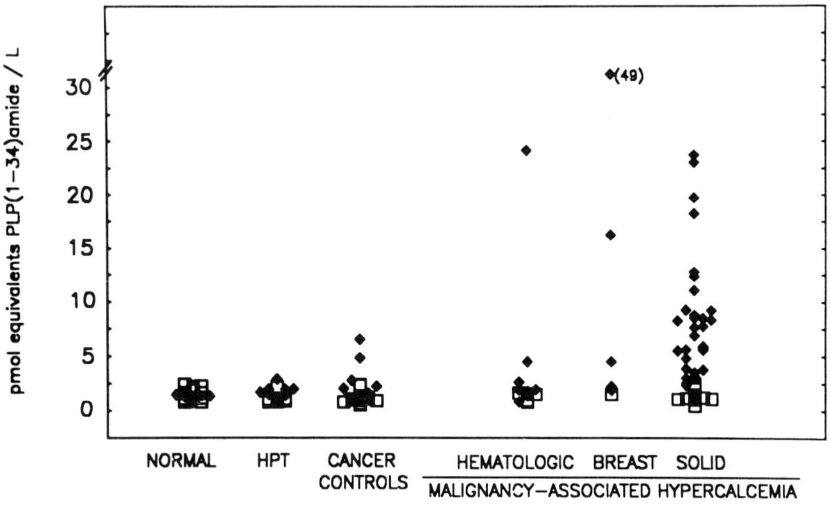

FIGURE 22-47. Serum levels of PTHrP in normal subjects, hyperparathyroidism (HPT), and malignancy. "Cancer controls" are normocalcemic patients with cancer. (*From Budayr, Nissenson, Klein, Pun, Clark, Diep, Arnaud, Strewler,*[510] *permission of the Annals of Internal Medicine.*)

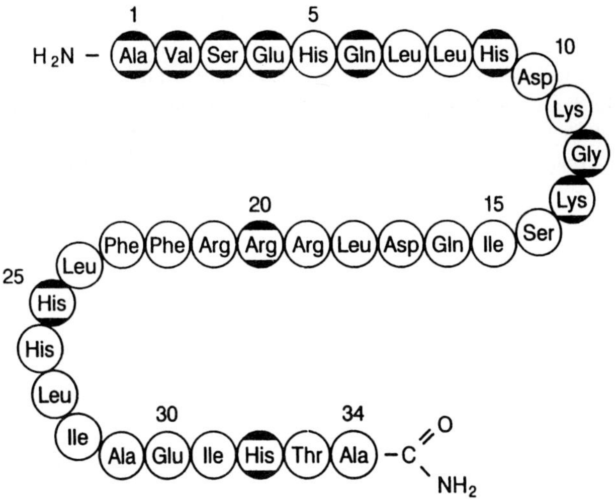

FIGURE 22-48. The sequence of PTHrP(1–34). Amino acids that are identical to those in PTH are partly shaded.

through endochondral ossification[164,503,504], (2) growth and differentiation of skin,[505] mammary gland,[506,507] and pancreatic islets[508]; (3) cardiovascular function[509]; (4) transepithelial calcium transport in the distal nephron, mammary epithelia, and the placenta[507,510]; (5) relaxation of smooth muscle in uterus, bladder, arteries, stomach, and ileum[484,511–513]; and (6) host immune function.[514–516] Bone perichondrial cell production of PTHrP regulates cartilage cell differentiation and has been linked to expression of Indian Hedgehog gene.[517] Indian Hedgehog protein expressed by prehypertrophic cartilage cells inhibited cartilage differentiation and this inhibitory effect was mediated by PTHrP. The normal physiologic functions of PTHrP have been extensively reviewed elsewhere.[518,519]

PTHrP likely plays a role in normal breast physiology,[520,521] which is discussed in later portions of this review. PTHrP is expressed in lactating mammary tissue[522] and secreted into milk at concentrations 10,000–100,000 times greater than plasma concentrations of humans with malignancy-associated hypercalcemia.[523–527] Increased plasma PTHrP concentrations have been documented in at least 2 patients with the rare syndrome of lactational hypercalcemia[528–530] in addition to some breast-feeding mothers.[531] Thus, PTHrP may be responsible for mobilizing calcium from maternal bone for use in milk production, and it may mediate lactation-associated bone loss.

The hypercalcemia of malignancy syndrome was the first identified consequence of increased PTHrP production. In this syndrome, tumor-produced PTHrP interacts with PTH receptors in bone and kidney to cause hypercalcemia, osteoclast-mediated bone resorption, increased nephrogenous cAMP, and phosphate excretion. The PTH-like properties of PTHrP, and specifically increasing osteoclastic bone resorption and renal tubular calcium reabsorption, appear to be responsible for the hypercalcemia. Approximately 80 percent of hypercalcemic patients with solid tumors have detectable or increased plasma PTHrP concentrations.[495] Plasma PTHrP concentrations, as measured by a sensitive 2-site immunoradiometric assay, are low or undetectable in the plasma of normals,[532] but the C-terminal fragment is increased in patients with chronic renal failure,[495] and the plasma C-terminal PTHrP concentration increases as the glomerular filtration rate decreases.[496]

Humoral Hypercalcemia of Malignancy (HHM) vs. 1°HPT

Despite similarities between HHM and 1°HPT and the similar biologic actions of PTHrP and PTH, respectively, unexplained differences between these syndromes exist. First, patients with PTHrP-mediated HHM have low serum concentrations of $1,25(OH)_2D_3$ compared with patients with 1°HPT,[533] even though both proteins stimulate renal 1α-hydroxylase activity. Clinical studies in which normal humans received short-term infusions of PTHrP-(1-34)[534] or PTHrP-(1-36)[535] revealed increased serum 1,25-dihydroxyvitamin D concentrations comparable to those that had received a similar infusion of PTH-(1-34). Animal studies have revealed similar findings.[536,537] Female nude mice infused with synthetic PTHrP-(1-40) for 7 days developed hypercalcemia, hypophosphatemia, and increased serum 1,25-dihydroxyvitamin D concentrations.[537] Likewise, male nude mice bearing Chinese hamster ovarian (CHO) cell tumors transfected with the cDNA for human preproPTHrP or preproPTH developed similar hypercalcemia and increased plasma concentrations of 1,25-dihydroxyvitamin D when compared with control animals bearing untransfected CHO tumors.[538] Additionally, similar increases in blood ionized calcium and 1,25-dihydroxyvitamin D concentrations were observed in nude mice bearing CHO tumors that were engineered to secrete PTHrP mutants truncated at the carboxyl terminus.[536]

Second, human studies using either quantitative bone histomorphometry[539] or biochemical markers of bone turnover[540] have demonstrated that although patients with either HHM or 1°HPT have increased osteoclastic bone resorption, many patients with HHM do not have the coupled increase in osteoblastic bone formation that those with 1°HPT have. Serum osteocalcin concentrations, a marker for bone formation, were significantly increased in patients with 1°HPT compared with normals.[541] In the same study, serum osteocalcin concentrations in hypercalcemic patients with bone metastasis were significantly lower compared with those of normal controls, while normocalcemic patients with bone metastases had values similar to normals. These osteocalcin concentrations correlated with histomorphometric parameters of bone formation, but not bone resorption.[541] In the studies by Fraher and Everhart-Caye, in which normal humans have received infusions of PTH or PTHrP,[534,535] bone histomorphometry or biochemical markers of bone turnover were not measured. Such studies done with PTHrP infusions in rodents have revealed increased osteoclastic bone resorption as well as increased bone formation as assessed by dynamic bone histomorphometry.[537] In contrast, nude mice bearing a PTHrP-secreting human squamous cell carcinoma demonstrated increased bone resorption and decreased bone formation as assessed by dynamic bone histomorphometry.[542] Thus, whether PTHrP alone is responsible for the uncoupling of bone formation from bone resorption is an issue that remains controversial.

Unlike the metabolic acidosis seen in patients with primary hyperparathyroidism, patients with malignancy-associated hypercalcemia often have a metabolic alkalosis with a low plasma chloride and high plasma bicarbonate concentration. Although many explanations have been postulated for the discrepancies between HHM and 1°HPT, such as differences between the pulsatile secretion of PTH and the presumed continuous secretion of PTHrP, suppression of bone formation and 1-hydroxylase activity by other tumor-associated factors, biologically active PTHrP fragments, or hypercalcemia per se,[109] the reasons for these differences have not been identified.

Modulation of PTHrP Effects by Other Tumor-Associated Factors

Regardless of the reasons for the clinical differences between HHM and 1°HPT, there is clear evidence that other tumor-produced factors can modulate the end-organ effects of PTHrP as well as its secretion from tumors. Excess production of PTH and PTHrP in vivo by tumors in which the corresponding genes were transfected and then inoculated into nude mice caused similar hypercalcemia as well as increases in osteoclastic bone resorption, more committed marrow mononuclear osteoclast precursors, and mature osteoclasts.[543] No stimulatory effects were seen on the multipotent osteoclast precursors, the granulocyte/macrophage colony-forming unit. In a similar model system, IL-6 potentiated the hypercalcemia and bone resorption mediated by PTHrP in vivo by stimulating production of early osteoclast precursors.[544] Likewise, TGFα has been shown to enhance the hypercalcemic effects of PTHrP in an animal model of malignancy-associated hypercalcemia[545] as well as to modulate the renal and bone effects of PTHrP.[546,547] Sato demonstrated that IL-1 and PTHrP may have synergistic effects in vivo[548] and others have shown that IL-1 may modulate the renal effects of PTHrP.[549] Finally, TNFα has been shown to enhance the hypercalcemic effect of PTHrP by increasing the pool of committed osteoclast progenitors with a subsequent increase in osteoclastic bone resorption. Bone formation parameters in these nude mice indicate that TNFα did not inhibit the new bone formation stimulated by PTHrP.[550]

Such tumor-associated factors also appear to be important regulators of PTHrP expression and secretion by tumors. EGF has been shown to stimulate PTHrP expression in a keratinocyte cell line[551] as well as a mammary epithelial line[476] while TGFα enhanced PTHrP expression in a human squamous cell carcinoma of the lung.[552] Interleukin-6 (IL-6), tumor necrosis factor (TNF), IGF-I, and IGF-II increased the production of PTHrP in vitro by a human squamous cell carcinoma.[479] TGFβ, which is abundant in bone, released in active form by resorbing bone and expressed by some breast cancers[553,554] and cancer-associated stromal cells,[555] has been shown to enhance secretion of and stabilize the message for PTHrP in a renal cell carcinoma[481] as well as in a squamous cell carcinoma.[482,483] Other data[556,557] demonstrate that this relationship also exists in a human breast adenocarcinoma cell line, MDA-MB-231.

PTHrP in Hypercalcemia Associated with Breast Cancer

Hypercalcemia in breast cancer represents one end of a spectrum of hypercalcemia associated with solid tumors. Hypercalcemia is associated with breast cancer in at least 10% of afflicted women during the course of their disease,[558] and is more common in those with advanced breast cancer. Osteoclast-mediated skeletal destruction by metastatic tumor is a major mechanism responsible for hypercalcemia, as increased osteoclastic bone resorption has been documented histologically in areas surrounding breast cancer metastases.[559–562] Humoral mechanisms contribute in 10–60 percent of cases of breast cancer-associated hypercalcemia as evidenced by increased nephrogenous cAMP and plasma PTHrP.[562–566]

PTHrP plays a major role in mediating hypercalcemia in breast cancer.[567] Because PTHrP is expressed in normal breast tissue and appears to play an important role in normal breast physiology, its overproduction in breast cancer is not surprising. One of the three tumors from which PTHrP was originally purified was a breast cancer from a patient with humoral hypercalcemia of malignancy.[453] PTHrP was detected by immunohistochemical staining in 60 percent of 102 invasive breast tumors removed from normocalcemic women, but not in normal breast tissue.[568] At least four other studies have confirmed these percentages[569–572] and one of these has demonstrated immunoreactive PTHrP within the cytoplasm of lobular and ductal epithelial cells in normal and fibrocystic breast tissues.[569] Furthermore, 65–92 percent of hypercalcemic breast cancer patients (with and without bone metastasis) had detectable plasma PTHrP concentrations by radioimmunoassay (RIA) similar to those documented in patients with humoral hypercalcemia of malignancy due to nonbreast tumors.[571,573] Not only is PTHrP an important mediator of hypercalcemia in breast cancer, it also has a significant role in the pathophysiology of breast cancer metastasis to bone as evidenced by the clinical studies which indicate that PTHrP expression by the primary breast cancer is more commonly associated with the development of bone metastasis and hypercalcemia.[571] This topic will be discussed in a later section.

PTHrP in Hypercalcemia Associated with Hematologic Malignancies

The mechanisms responsible for hypercalcemia associated with hematologic malignancies are multifactorial and include secretion of local bone-active cytokines, such as IL-6, IL-1, and lymphotoxin or TNFα, from tumor in bone or from systemic effects of tumor-produced factors such as $1,25(OH)_2D_3$ (discussed later). Recent data from a clinical study of 76 patients with various hematologic malignancies demonstrate that PTHrP also may be an important pathogenetic factor in the development of hypercalcemia in some patients.[574] In this study, 8 of the 14 hypercalcemic patients had non-Hodgkin's lymphoma and, of these, 62 percent had significant increases in plasma PTHrP concentrations. The serum $1,25(OH)_2D_3$ concentrations, when measured, were low in the hypercalcemic non-Hodgkin's lymphoma patients who had increased plasma PTHrP concentrations.[574] Additionally, 1 of 2 hypercalcemic patients with Hodgkin's disease and 1 of 4 hypercalcemic patients with multiple myeloma had increased plasma PTHrP concentrations. Also of interest in this study is the fact that several normocalcemic patients with non-Hodgkin's lymphoma, Hodgkin's lymphoma, multiple myeloma, and Waldenstrom's macroglobulinemia had increased plasma PTHrP concentrations as measured by an amino-terminal PTHrP assay.[574] Using a sensitive 2-site immunoradiometric assay, other investigators have noted increased plasma PTHrP concentrations in patients with adult T-cell leukemia and B-cell lymphoma.[575] Finally, circulating concentrations of PTHrP, comparable to those in humoral hypercalcemia of malignancy, were present in 2 of 4 hypercalcemic patients with non-Hodgkin's lymphoma, in 3 of 9 with myeloma[576] and in a patient with myeloid blast crisis of chronic myeloid leukemia.[577] Thus, the humoral mediators in the hypercalcemia associated with hematologic malignancies include both $1,25(OH)_2D_3$ and PTHrP.

$1,25(OH)_2D_3$

In the setting of hypercalcemia, serum concentrations of $1,25(OH)_2D_3$ are normally suppressed unless an autonomous source of PTH is the cause, such as a parathyroid adenoma. Lack of $1,25(OH)_2D_3$ suppression in this situation is evidence of disordered regulation of $1,25(OH)_2D_3$ synthesis and indicates extrarenal production such as that observed in the hypercalcemia associated with granulomatous disease. Less commonly, tumors may secrete other humoral factors responsible for hypercalcemia. A major mediator of hypercalcemia in Hodgkin's disease, non-Hodgkin's lymphoma, and other hematologic malignancies appears to be extrarenal production of $1,25(OH)_2D_3$.[578] The mechanism is similar to that observed in hypercalcemia associated with granulomatous disease in which activated macrophages within the granuloma synthesize $1,25(OH)_2D_3$.[579–581] These patients usually have increased plasma $1,25(OH)_2D_3$ concentrations in addition to low or normal plasma PTH and urinary cAMP concentrations[582] in the absence of bone involvement. Affected patients have also been shown to have increased fasting urinary calcium excretion[582] as well as increased intestinal calcium (^{47}Ca) absorption.[583] Increased $1,25(OH)_2D_3$ concentrations were noted in 12 of 22 hypercalcemic patients with non-Hodgkin's lymphoma. In addition, 71 percent of 22 normocalcemic patients with non-Hodgkin's lymphoma were hypercalciuric and 18 percent had increased serum $1,25(OH)_2D_3$ concentrations. These findings led the investigators to conclude that dysregulated $1,25(OH)_2D_3$ production is common in patients with diffuse large cell lymphoma.[578]

Thus, the mechanisms responsible for hypercalcemia in these lymphomas appear to be multifactorial and include increased intestinal calcium absorption as well as increased osteoclastic bone resorption. Additionally, many of the reported patients had altered renal function, a finding which suggests that impaired renal calcium clearance may also be contributing to the hypercalcemia in certain patients. The low serum PTH and urinary cAMP concentrations indicate that neither PTH nor PTHrP mediates the hypercalcemia. Prostaglandins, when measured, have been low and selected patients had no calcium-lowering effect from indomethacin therapy.[576] It is likely that the lymphoma tissue itself hydroxylates 25-hydroxyvitamin D to the active $1,25(OH)_2D_3$ similar to the situation in hypercalcemia associated with granulomatous disease.[579,581] One alpha hydroxylase activity has been demonstrated in human T-cell lymphotrophic virus type I transformed lymphocytes.[584] None of the reported patients with $1,25(OH)_2D_3$-mediated hypercalcemia had concomitant granulomatous disease and hypercalcemia often improved with medical or surgical therapy that resulted in a decrease in serum $1,25(OH)_2D_3$ concentrations. Recurrence of hypercalcemia and increased plasma $1,25(OH)_2D_3$ concentrations has been documented with recurrence of disease.[585]

PTH

Following Fuller Albright's observations in 1941, it was postulated that malignancy-associated hypercalcemia was due to tumor production of PTH. This notion was strengthened by the early PTH radioimmunoassay data in hypercalcemic patients with malignancy, which suggested that tumors produced factors recognized in these PTH radioimmunoassays.[586–589] Although for many years malignancy-associated hypercalcemia was attributed to ectopic tumor-produced PTH, it is now clear that PTHrP is responsible for most cases. Analysis of 13 human and 3 animal nonparathyroid tumors of diverse origin associated with hypercalcemia did not detect PTH RNA transcripts.[590] Since that time, 7 cases of authentic tumor-produced PTH have been convincingly demonstrated in 2 cases a small cell carcinoma of the lung,[461,465] an ovarian cancer,[460] a widely-metastatic primitive neuroectodermal tumor,[459] thymoma,[462] papillary thyroid cancer,[463] and a squamous cell lung cancer.[464] Molecular analysis of the ovarian carcinoma revealed both DNA amplification and rearrangement in the upstream regulatory region of the PTH gene.[460] Interestingly, the primitive neuroectodermal tumor produced both PTH and PTHrP that resulted in severe hypercalcemia.[459] These reported patients did not have coexisting primary hyperparathyroidism because the parathyroid glands were normal at the time of neck exploration or at autopsy in all cases. However, the fact remains that ectopic production of PTH is a rare event and it is clearly documented that most patients with malignancy-associated hypercalcemia have suppressed plasma PTH concentrations.[451] It should be emphasized that the most likely cause of hypercalcemia in the setting of malignancy that is associated with a normal or increased serum PTH concentration is coexisting primary hyperparathyroidism.

Other Tumor-Associated Factors

There is abundant evidence that solid tumors may produce other factors, alone or in combination with PTHrP, which have the capacity to stimulate osteoclastic bone resorption and cause hypercalcemia.[591] These factors include interleukin-1 (IL-1), IL-6, transforming growth factor-α (TGF-α), and tumor necrosis factor (TNF). Administration of IL-1 injections to mice caused mild hypercalcemia,[592,593] and this IL-1-induced hypercalcemia has been effectively blocked by the IL-1 receptor antagonist.[594] Mice bearing Chinese hamster ovarian (CHO) tumors transfected with the cDNA for IL-6 developed mild hypercalcemia[595] as did mice bearing a renal carcinoma which cosecreted IL-6 and PTHrP.[596] Human TGF-β and TNF-α have been demonstrated to stimulate osteoclastic bone resorption in vitro and cause hypercalcemia in vivo.[597–602] TNF-α also caused hypercalciuria, without an increase in nephrogenous cAMP, and increased osteoclastic bone resorption in vivo in a mouse model.[603] Some of these factors have been shown to modulate the end organ effects of PTHrP on bone and kidney, and TGF-β, IL-1, IL-6, and TNF have been shown to enhance the hypercalcemic effects of PTHrP. The ability of IL-6 to enhance PTHrP-mediated hypercalcemia appears to be due to increased production of the early osteoclast precursor, CFU-GM, by IL-6 in combination with increased production of the more committed osteoclast precursors stimulated by PTHrP.[544]

Prostaglandins of the E series are powerful stimulators of bone resorption[604] although their role in bone destruction associated with malignancy remains unclear.[605] Some of the effects of cytokines on bone may be mediated in part through prostaglandins as indomethacin, a prostaglandin synthesis inhibitor, has been shown to block part of the osteoclast-stimulatory effects of interleukin-1 in vivo.[592,593] Although prostaglandins have been demonstrated to be produced by cultured tumor cells in vitro, indomethacin treatment of malignancy-associated hypercalcemia is only occasionally effective.[606] Thus, it is unlikely that prostaglandins have a major causal role in hypercalcemia associated with malignancy.

Treatment of Hypercalcemia Associated with Malignancy

Treatment of hypercalcemia due to malignancy should always involve treating the underlying tumor. Unfortunately, because this is often not effective or cannot be accomplished with the rapidity needed when the patient is faced with life-threatening hypercalcemia, therapy should also be directed against the mechanisms responsible for the hypercalcemia. In essentially all patients with hypercalcemia of malignancy, there is an increase in osteoclastic bone resorption, and in many there is also an increase in renal tubular calcium reabsorption, even in malignancies that are not associated with PTHrP production.[607] Medical therapy is therefore aimed at inhibiting bone resorption and promoting renal calcium excretion. Because hypercalcemia associated with cancer is often accompanied by dehydration, volume expansion with isotonic saline is essential. This serves to increase the glomerular filtration rate and reduces the fractional reabsorption of both sodium and calcium. Because hydration alone will normalize serum calcium concentrations only transiently,[608] inhibitors of bone resorption such as the bisphosphonates or calcitonin should be administered as well. When possible, mechanism-specific treatment should be attempted.[609] Glucocorticoids, for example, are more effective in reducing the serum calcium concentration in hematologic malignancies and $1,25(OH)_2D_3$-mediated hypercalcemia than in solid tumors. Dietary calcium restriction is ineffective in reducing serum calcium concentrations except in cases of vitamin D-mediated hypercalcemia. In these cases, dietary calcium should be restricted to 400 mg daily until the underlying disorder is corrected. It is not desirable or advantageous to reduce calcium intake in hypercalcemia due to malignancy.

Bisphosphonates, analogs of pyrophosphate, have become the most useful antiresorptive agents among the currently available armamentarium for the treatment of hypercalcemia. They have a high affinity for hydroxyapatite in bone and concentrate in areas of high bone turnover. The mechanisms by which bisphosphonates inhibit bone resorption are not clearly understood, but potentially include induction of osteoclast apoptosis, inhibition of osteoclast formation and recruitment, or stimulation of osteoblasts to produce an inhibitor of osteoclast formation.[610,611] Another mechanism by which bisphosphonates might affect bone resorption is by decreasing the function of the osteoclast with respect to attachment and ruffled border formation.[610]

Bisphosphonates vary in potency but, in general, are poorly absorbed and are most effective in treating hypercalcemia when given intravenously. Bisphosphonates are concentrated in bone and remain there until the bone is resorbed. Etidronate, the first available bisphosphonate in the United States, is the least potent. Intravenous etidronate, given in doses of 7.5 mg/kg intravenously over 3 consecutive days normalized calcium concentration in 30 percent to 40 percent of patients.[612–614] Oral etidronate is generally ineffective in treating hypercalcemia[606] and at sustained dosages of 25 mg/kg per day for more than 6 months, it can cause bone mineralization defects.[611] Etidronate can also cause hyperphosphatemia which, in addition to hypercalcemia, may lead to a high calcium-phosphate solubility product.

Pamidronate is a potent aminobisphosphonate available for the treatment of hypercalcemia of malignancy. The drug combines high efficacy with a low toxicity profile, and thus has become the current bisphosphonate of choice for the treatment of hypercalcemia of malignancy. It is highly effective in normalizing serum calcium concentrations and, when used in dosages recommended for hypercalcemia of malignancy, is not associated with bone mineralization defects. Pamidronate, administered as a single 24-hour infusion normalized serum calcium concentrations in 30 percent of patients who received 30 mg, 61 percent of patients who received 60 mg, 100 percent of patients who received 90 mg.[340] Successful therapy with bisphosphonates is associated with an increase in the plasma PTH and $1,25(OH)_2D_3$ concentrations as well as a decrease in the biochemical markers of bone resorption.[340,533,566] Clinical studies of pamidronate treatment in patients with hypercalcemia of malignancy indicate that the calcium-lowering response to bisphosphonates positively correlates with the presence of bone metastases[615–617] and negatively correlates with plasma PTHrP concentrations.[339,615,616] Such a relationship has also been demonstrated with clodronate, an oral bisphosphonate.[618] This is presumably due to the effects of PTHrP to increase renal tubular reabsorption of calcium, which are not blocked by bisphosphonates. Nonetheless, pamidronate compares favorably to other inhibitors of bone resorption such as plicamycin, calcitonin, and gallium nitrate, and is well-tolerated. Pamidronate should be delivered as an intravenous infusion over 4–24 hours. Clinical studies using 90 mg infusion of pamidronate over 4 hours, indicate that the mean time to achieve normocalcemia is approximately 4 days while the mean duration of normocalcemia is 28 days.[619] Similarly, intravenous pamidronate, given as 60 mg every 2 weeks maintained normocalcemia in a majority of patients with malignancy-associated hypercalcemia.[620] An effective method for achieving more rapid reduction of the serum calcium is to use the combination of calcitonin and pamidronate.[621] Calcitonin acts rapidly to lower the serum calcium although usually its effects are only transient. Although escape from calcitonin therapy may occur within 48 hours, by that time pamidronate is beginning to exert its maximal effects. Calcitonin can be administered either intramuscularly or subcutaneously every 12 hours in doses of 200–400 MRC units. Reported side effects of pamidronate include transient low-grade fever and asymptomatic mild hypocalcemia.[340] Bone mineralization defects have been reported only in patients receiving high-dose pamidronate at weekly intervals for the treatment of Paget's disease.[622] It is possible that other bisphosphonates such as alendronate, risedronate, and tiludronate will be effective oral therapy for hypercalcemia of malignancy. Due to its propensity to cause mouth ulcers, oral pamidronate, although effective, is not likely to be approved for such use in the United States.

Calcitonin inhibits osteoclastic bone resorption and renal tubular reabsorption of calcium. The main advantages of calcitonin are its rapid onset of action and its relative lack of serious side effects. Unfortunately, calcitonin alone only transiently normalizes the calcium concentration in patients with hypercalcemia of malignancy. Tachyphylaxis, probably due to down regulation of calcitonin receptors, frequently develops with calcitonin administration, although this can be delayed with concomitant glucocorticoid treatment.[623] However, calcitonin use can be particularly effective in the setting of severe hypercalcemia while waiting for the more sustained hypocalcemic effect of administered bisphosphonates to occur. Calcitonin use with bisphosphonates lowers calcium concentrations more quickly and effectively than either alone.[624] Although human calcitonin is available, salmon calcitonin is generally used. If salmon calcitonin is used, a test dose of 1 MRC unit should be administered first, as rare anaphylactic reactions have been reported.[625]

Plicamycin, or mithramycin, an antineoplastic agent used in the treatment of certain embryonal cancers,[626] is also a potent inhibitor of bone resorption. Plicamycin inhibits DNA-dependent RNA synthesis[627] in tumor cells by binding to the promoter regions on DNA, thus preventing transcription.[628] Presumably, osteoclastic bone resorption is inhibited by this mechanism as well. The dosage used to treat hypercalcemia (25 $\mu g/kg$) is one tenth of the usual chemotherapeutic dose and should be infused over 4 hours. Although plicamycin is almost invariably effective in lowering serum calcium concentrations, its considerable toxicity has limited its use in more recent years as more potent bisphosphonates have become available. Plicamycin has serious hepato- and nephrotoxicity in addition to local irritation and thrombocytopenic effects, which can limit its use in cancer patients as well as in those with renal impairment.

Gallium nitrate is another antineoplastic agent that, like plicamycin, was found to induce hypocalcemia in normocalcemic cancer patients receiving it.[629] It inhibits osteoclastic bone resorption and appears to be more effective in lowering serum calcium concentration than calcitonin[449] and etidronate. Gallium is administered as a continuous infusion over 5 days, making it somewhat less convenient than some other antihypercalcemic agents. Gallium is excreted unchanged by the kidneys and has significant nephrotoxicity. Thus, it should not be administered to patients with renal impairment or to those receiving other nephrotoxic drugs.[630]

About 30 percent of patients treated with glucocorticoids for hypercalcemia associated with nonparathyroid malignancy respond with a fall in calcium concentration.[608] However, the response is often not complete and the responsiveness to glucocorticoids is unpredictable.[606] Glucocorticoids are most effective in hypercalcemic patients with hematologic malignancies, multiple myeloma in particular, as well as in vitamin D-associated disorders such as lymphomas. In hematologic malignancies, glucocorticoids inhibit osteoclastic bone resorption by decreasing tumor production of locally active cytokines, in addition to having direct tumorolytic effects.[631] Glucocorticoids in dosage equivalents of prednisone 40 to 60 mg daily should be given for 10 days. If the calcium has not decreased in this period, glucocorticoids should be discontinued. Long-term adverse effects of glucocorticoids, such as osteopenia and Cushing's syndrome, occur with continued administration over several months. This is usually not a consideration in patients with widespread malignancy, who have a very limited prognosis.

Localized Osteolysis (with or without Hypercalcemia)

It is clear that hypercalcemia associated with cancer conveys a poor prognosis, with survival of less than 3 months.[338,339] However, the majority of patients with metastatic bone disease are not hypercalcemic and, in the case of breast cancer, patients may survive up to 90 months after the detection of the first bone metastases.[632,633] Autopsy studies reveal bone metastasis in 70 percent of women that died of breast cancer.[634–636] Thus, it behooves us to understand the mechanisms responsible for this complication of cancer in order to effectively decrease the associated morbidity or to prevent it altogether.

Clinical Manifestations

Both solid tumors and hematologic malignancies frequently affect the most vascular areas of the skeleton, specifically in the red bone marrow of the axial skeleton, the proximal ends of the long bones, ribs and the vertebral bodies. The most common way cancer affects the skeleton is directly through local tumor-mediated stimulation of osteoclastic bone resorption. Such osteolytic bone lesions are typical of breast and lung carcinoma as well as hematologic malignancies such as multiple myeloma. Although breast cancer cells have been shown to resorb bone directly in vitro,[637] most evidence (scanning electron microscopic examination of adjacent bone surfaces[560] and response to osteoclast inhibitors) is consistent with the notion that factors secreted by cancer cells can activate osteoclasts locally. Thus, local and systemic effects of cancer on bone are mediated through one common final pathway, the osteoclast. The resulting osteolytic bone destruction can lead to pain, pathologic fractures, nerve compression syndromes, and hypercalcemia.

Hypercalcemia associated with metastatic bone disease or hematologic malignancies has been referred to as local osteolytic hypercalcemia, as clinical studies have demonstrated that many patients with bone involvement and hypercalcemia did not have the increase in plasma PTHrP or nephrogeneous cAMP concentration observed in patients with humoral hypercalcemia of malignancy.[451,495] The mechanism of hypercalcemia in this situation was postulated to be local tumor production of factors that stimulate osteoclastic bone resorption, such as TNF-α, IL-6, and IL-1 as in the case of myeloma. However, it is now clear that humoral mediators of hypercalcemia, such as PTHrP, may mediate local osteolysis, even in the absence of hypercalcemia and increased plasma PTHrP concentrations.[638] Additionally, if tumor burden in bone is great enough, tumor-produced factors in bone may be produced in enough quantity locally to reach the systemic circulation and have effects on sites distant from affected bone.

Pathophysiology of Osteolytic Metastases

Cancer metastatic to bone often causes bone destruction or osteolysis. Although several tumor types, such as prostate, lung, renal cell, and thyroid, are associated with osteolytic lesions, breast cancer is the most common. A comprehensive review of more than 500 patients dying of breast cancer revealed that 69 percent had bone metastasis and bone was the most common site of first distant relapse.[558] In those patients with disease confined to the skeleton, the median survival was 24 months compared with three months in those patients whose first relapse occurred in the liver.

A variety of common characteristics are necessary for tumor cells to possess the metastatic phenotype. Such properties include (1) the production of proteolytic enzymes necessary for detachment from the primary site, invasion into surrounding soft tissues, intravasation, extravasation, and bone matrix degradation; (2) expression or loss of cell adhesion molecules essential for detachment from the primary site and arrest at a metastatic site; (3) migratory activity to travel in the circulation; (4) escape from the host immune surveillance to survive; and (5) capacity to respond to a chemoattractant. Although these properties are common to tumor cells metastasizing to any organ, they are insufficient to explain the propensity of breast cancer to metastasize to bone. Therefore, it is likely that breast cancer cells have additional characteristics that are specifically required for causing metastases in bone.

Because bone is mainly composed of a hard mineralized tissue, it is more resistant to destruction than other soft tissues. Thus, in order for cancer cells to grow in bone, they must possess the capacity to cause bone destruction. Histologic review of breast cancer metastatic to bone reveals that tumor cells are adjacent to osteoclasts resorbing bones[560–562] and indicate that breast cancer cells posses the capacity to stimulate osteoclastic bone resorption. Breast cancer cells may either induce osteoclastic differentiation of hematopoietic stem cells, activate mature osteoclasts already present in bone, or do both, through releasing soluble mediators or via cell-to-cell contact. Clinical and experimental evidence indicates that tumor-produced PTHrP is a major candidate factor responsible for the osteoclastic bone resorption present at sites of breast cancer metastatic to bone.[639–641] PTHrP has been detected by immunohistochemistry[639] and in situ hybridization[640] in 92 percent of breast cancer metastases in bone compared with only 17 percent of similar metastases to nonbone sites, an observation that prompted speculation that production of PTHrP as a bone-resorbing agent may contribute to the ability of breast cancers to grow as bone metastases. Bundred and colleagues found positive immunohistochemical staining for PTHrP in 56 percent of 155 primary breast tumors from normocalcemic women, and PTHrP expression was positively correlated to the development of bone metastases and hypercalcemic episodes.[571] PTHrP expression was detected by reverse transcriptase PCR in 37 of 38 primary breast cancers, and subsequent development of bone metastases was associated with a higher PTHrP expression.[641] Finally, PTHrP was detected by immunohistochemistry in 83 percent of patients who developed bone metastases compared with 38 percent in those who developed lung metastases and 38 percent in those without recurrence.[572] There have been no consistent correlations between PTHrP expression in the primary breast tumor and standard prognostic factors, recurrence, or survival. The only significant and consistent correlations have been between PTHrP positivity and the development of bone metastases and hypercalcemia.

These clinical observations have been extended by using a mouse model of bone metastases[642,643] in which inoculation of a human breast cancer cell line, MDA-MB-231,[643a] into the left cardiac ventricle reliably cause osteolytic metastases. MDA-MB-231 cells produce low amounts of PTHrP in vitro and when the cells were engineered to overexpress PTHrP, by transfection with the cDNA for human preproPTHrP, an increase in the number of osteolytic metastases was observed.[557] In contrast, when mice were treated with monoclonal antibodies directed against the 1-34 region of PTHrP/ prior to inoculation with parental MDA-MB-231 cells, the number and size of observed osteolytic lesions were dramatically less than similar animals treated with control. Mice with established osteolytic metastases due to MDA-MB-231, treated with the antibody, had a decrease in the rate of progression of metastases when compared with mice that received a control injection.[638,643b] Similar findings have been demonstrated in this model using a human lung squamous cell carcinoma.[644] Taken together, these data strongly suggest that PTHrP expression by breast cancer cells is important for the development and progression of breast cancer metastases in bone. It stands to reason, then, that production of other osteoclast-stimulating factors should potentiate the development of bone metastases as well.

Just as production of bone-resorbing factors by breast cancer cells enhance bone metastases, production of other factors may render the breast cancer cell ineffective as a seed and result in fewer metastases in bone or other sites. Using the same mouse model of breast cancer metastases to bone, MDA-MB-231 cells transfected to overexpress either the cell adhesion molecule, E-cadherin, or tissue inhibitor of metalloproteinase-2 (TIMP-2) inoculated into nude mice resulted in a decrease in osteolytic metastases compared with nontransfected MDA-MB-231 cells.[645,646]

The Role of the Bone Microenvironment as the "Soil"

Bone is unique among metastatic target tissues as it undergoes continual remodeling under the influence of systemic hormones and local bone-derived growth factors. Mineralized bone matrix is a repository for growth factors, of which TGF-β and IGF-II comprise the majority. As described earlier, these growth factors are released from the bone matrix as a result of normal osteoclastic bone resorption, a part of the normal remodeling process necessary for maintenance of the structural integrity of bone. The hematopoietic stem cells in the bone marrow can differentiate into bone-resorbing osteoclasts. Other cells in the bone marrow, stromal and immune cells in particular, produce cytokines and growth factors that may potentiate tumor cell growth or expression of osteolytic factors. Thus, once breast cancer cells arrest in bone, the high concentrations of growth factors and cytokines in the bone microenvironment provide a fertile soil on which the cells can grow. Such host cytokines may also enhance osteoclastic bone resorption stimulated by tumor-produced factors such as PTHrP. Furthermore, when the tumor cells stimulate osteoclastic bone resorption, this bone microenvironment is even more enriched with bone-derived growth factors that enhance survival of the cancer. Finally, bone-derived TGF-β may have an important role as a chemoattractant for breast cancer cells.

A large body of indirect evidence to support the concept that bone is a fertile soil, further enriched by the process of osteoclastic bone resorption, has accumulated in studies using bisphosphonates in the treatment of bone metastases. It is already clear from clinical studies that the use of bisphosphonates, potent inhibitors of bone resorption, significantly reduces skeletal morbidity in advanced breast cancer.[647–658] In a recent multicenter trial consisting of more than 700 patients with stage IV breast cancer with 2 or more predominantly lytic lesions, with at least one lesion that was one centimeter or greater in diameter, treatment with pamidronate 90 mg intravenously every 3 to 4 weeks for 12 months in conjunction with chemotherapy or hormonal therapy resulted in a significant reduction in skeletal complications and bone pain compared with the control group.[656] Bisphosphonates have also been shown to decrease the number of bone metastases as well as tumor burden in animal models.[643,659,660] Thus, by decreasing osteoclastic bone resorption, the bone microenvironment is a less fertile soil for the growth of tumor.

TGF-β, which is present in high concentrations in the bone microenvironment and expressed by some breast cancers[556,557] and cancer-associated stromal cells,[555] has been shown to enhance secretion of and stabilize the mRNA for PTHrP in a renal cell carcinoma,[481] a squamous cell carcinoma,[482,483] and a human breast adenocarcinoma, MDA-MB-231.[556,557] Of the known growth factors present in the mineralized bone matrix other than TGF-β, such as IGF-I and -II, FGF 1 and 2, BMPs and PDGF, only TGF-β has been shown to significantly stimulate PTHrP secretion from the human breast cancer cell line, MDA-MB-231.[557] The fact that TGF-β is abundant in bone[3] and can enhance PTHrP expression by cancer cells makes it an important candidate factor in the establishment and progression of breast cancer metastases to bone.

TGF-β is a member of a large superfamily of proteins that are important regulators of bone cell activity.[661] Multiple isoforms of TGF-β exist in mammals and appear to control cell proliferation and differentiation in many human cell types.[662] The prototype of these isoforms, TGF-β1, is highly expressed by differentiated osteoblasts and osteoclasts, is stored in bone matrix and released in active form during osteoclastic bone resorption.[5] The effects of TGF-β include stimulation of cell proliferation of mesenchymal cells, growth inhibition of epithelial cells, synthesis of extracellular matrix proteins, and enhancing cell adhesion. These effects of TGF-β are mediated through complex receptor interactions.[663] TGF-β binds to the type II receptor and this complex recruits and phosphorylates the type I receptor, which in turn initiates signal transduction mediated by the recently identified Smad protein family.[663] The effects of TGF-β on cancer cells are complex and variable.[664] In some cancer cells, TGF-β inhibits growth, while in others growth is stimulated.[665] It likely has effects on apoptosis as well.

Further evidence for the role of bone-derived TGF-β in the development and progression of breast cancer metastasis to bone has been demonstrated in the same in vivo animal model of osteolysis described previously. Because TGF-β increases PTHrP expression by MDA-MB-231 cells in vitro, this cell line was transfected with a cDNA encoding a TGF-β type II receptor lacking a cytoplasmic domain (TβRIIΔ*cyt*).[666] This receptor binds TGF-β, but as it cannot phosphorylate the type I receptor, signal transduction is not initiated and it acts in a dominant-negative fashion to block the biologic effects of TGF-β.[667] Stable clones expressing TβRIIΔ*cyt* did not increase PTHrP secretion in response to TGF-β stimulation compared with controls of untransfected MDA-MB-231 cells or those transfected with the empty vector. Mice inoculated into the left cardiac ventricle with MDA-MB-231 cells expressing TβRIIΔ*cyt* had fewer osteolytic lesions as well as a smaller area of osteolytic lesions by radiography and histomorphometry compared with the controls of parental cells or those transfected with the empty vector.[668] These data indicate that TGF-β responsiveness of this human breast cancer cell line is important for the expression of PTHrP in bone and the development of osteolytic bone metastasis in vivo.

The Role of PTHrP in Breast Cancer-Mediated Osteolysis

These findings have important implications for breast cancer effects on the skeleton. First, breast cancers expressing PTHrP may affect the skeleton through humoral and osteolytic mechanisms. Second, the effects of PTHrP on bone may be enhanced if the breast cancer expresses other bone-active factors, such as TGF-β or IL-6, in addition to PTHrP. Finally, growth of breast cancer cells in bone may be enhanced if the tumor cells express PTHrP or other bone-resorbing factors. TGF-β, as well as other bone derived growth factors, increase PTHrP expression by breast cancer cells in bone, so that TGF-β-responsive tumors may preferentially grow in bone. Thus, enhanced osteoclastic bone resorption causes increased release of TGF-β and other growth factors into the bone microenvironment. The result is (1) greater PTHrP expression by the breast cancer cells, (2) enhanced growth of the cancer cells, and (3) chemoattraction of more tumor cells by bone-derived factors. Thus, a cycle is established that ends in bone destruction and the other consequences of lytic bone metastases. The clinical finding of increased PTHrP expression in bone compared with other sites supports the notion that production of PTHrP as a bone-resorbing agent may contribute to the ability of breast cancers to grow as bone metastases and/or that the bone microenvironment enhances production of PTHrP. These and other reasons may, in part, explain the propensity of breast cancers to metastasize to bone and the alacrity with which breast cancer grows in bone.

If PTHrP expression in the primary breast tumor indicates a propensity to metastasize and destroy bone due to its potent bone resorbing capability, early treatment with inhibitors of bone resorption or agents that inhibit the production of or biologic effects of PTHrP are likely to prevent or delay the development of bone metastases as well as reduce the catastrophic complications of pain, hypercalcemia, fracture, and nerve compression syndromes.

Hematologic Malignancy (with or without Hypercalcemia)

Multiple myeloma is a plasma cell malignancy that is almost invariably associated with destructive bone lesions, either in the form of diffuse osteopenia or localized osteolysis throughout the skeleton.[669] Eighty percent of patients with myeloma first present with pain that can be related to the bone disease, and bone complications are the most obvious clinical feature in most patients.[669] The bone lesions of myeloma may be diffuse or localized, and are comprised of three types. In the majority of patients (more than 95 percent), they are osteolytic. These lesions occur predominantly in those bones that are rich in red marrow such as the axial skeleton, and are associated with increased osteoclast activity adjacent to sites of myeloma cell accumulation. This suggests that myeloma cells produce locally active soluble factors that stimulate the remaining osteoclasts to resorb bone.[670] In some patients, the bone loss is more generalized and the appearances more closely resemble those of osteoporosis. In these patients the myeloma cells tend to be more diffusely spread throughout the axial skeleton. Some patients may have a combination of these two pictures, osteopenia of vertebral bodies but discrete osteolytic bone lesions of the skull. Myeloma bone disease is always an important differential diagnosis in the patient who presents with apparent osteoporosis. The bone disease of myeloma tends to be steadily progressive in most patients, and can be used as one of the parameters to monitor the course of the disease. For example, obvious progression of the bone lesions or the appearance of new discrete lesions indicates that the disease is active. On the other hand, vertebral body collapse can occur in patients in remission because of the weakened state of the skeleton, and bone pain itself is not a reliable indicator of the state of the disease activity.

The type of osteolytic disease that occurs in myeloma may be quite different from the bone disease associated with other types of malignancy, such as carcinoma of the breast. In myeloma bone disease there is often no increase in bone formation or osteoblast activity. The reason for this complete uncoupling of bone formation and bone resorption is unknown. It is paralleled clinically by the absence of an increase in the markers of bone formation, which are frequently present in other types of osteolytic bone disease due to malignancy, such as serum osteocalcin and alkaline phosphatase.[541] In addition, the radionuclide bone scan shows no evidence of increased isotope uptake at the site of bone lesions.

A small number of patients with myeloma bone disease present with an entirely different picture of diffuse osteosclerosis.[671,672] Osteosclerotic myeloma often occurs as a part of a syndrome of polyneuropathy and is associated with the cutaneous and endocrine features that comprise POEM's syndrome (polyneuropathy, organomegaly, endocrinopathy, M-protein, and skin changes).[673]

Thus, the majority of patients with myeloma have a crippling form of bone disease associated with intractable pain, susceptibility to fracture upon trivial injury, and nerve compression syndromes (most frequently spinal cord compression) associated with vertebral body collapse. About 30 percent of patients develop hypercalcemia at some stage during the course of the disease, usually in association with impaired renal function.[669] The pathophysiology of bone destruction that is so characteristic of myeloma bone disease remains unclear. Cultures of myeloma cells in vitro produce several osteoclast activating factors such as interleukin-6, interleukin-1α, and tumor necrosis factor α or lymphotoxin,[674–676] which have been implicated. Lymphotoxin (or TNFβ) is a powerful bone-resorbing cytokine that is produced by lymphoid cell lines in vivo. It is expressed by many B-cell lines in culture, including cell lines derived from patients with myeloma.[676] It is capable of causing hypercalcemia in vivo and has effects on bone resorption that are indistinguishable from those of tumor necrosis factor-α, namely an increase in osteoclast formation and activity, associated with impaired osteoblast differentiation and increased osteoblast precursor proliferation.[602] Although produced by many cell lines derived from patients with myeloma, it has not been detected in freshly isolated marrow cells from these patients.

The second cytokine that has been implicated in the bone lesions in myeloma is interleukin-1α.[674,675] Interleukin-1α is also a powerful stimulator of osteoclastic bone resorption, which increases osteoclast formation, increases osteoblast proliferation, and can cause hypercalcemia in vivo. Freshly isolated marrow cells from patients with myeloma that contain myeloma cells plus other marrow cells, have been shown to contain interleukin-1α in the conditioned medium harvested from these cells. Moreover, bone resorbing activity present in these conditioned media can be neutralized by antibodies to interleukin-1α.

Finally, interleukin-6 is a cytokine that has an important growth regulatory role in many patients with myeloma.[677] IL-6 concentrations in bone marrow and in plasma correlate with the stage of disease.[678–680] It may be produced by the myeloma cells or other stromal cells in the marrow microenvironment. Endogenous IL-6 production is 2–30 times greater in patients with myeloma than in normals.[679] Administration of a murine-human chimeric anti IL-6 antibody to patients with multiple myeloma resistant to second-line chemotherapy suppressed this IL-6 production, but did not prevent infection-induced IL-6 production.[679] Such results suggest that this IL-6 antibody inhibited a positive feed-back IL-6-dependent loop.

IL-6 is not a powerful bone resorbing factor in its own right, but is capable of enhancing the effects of other factors on bone resorption, presumably by increasing generation of precursors for cells in the osteoclast lineage.[544] Myeloma cells occasionally produce PTHrP and because IL-6 may potentiate the osteoclastic bone resorption mediated by PTHrP, such cytokine interactions have important implications in the genesis of the bone destruction associated with myeloma.

Just as there may be a vicious cycle in the bone microenvironment between the tumor cells and bone-derived growth factors in breast cancer, there may be a similar relationship between the process of bone resorption and myeloma cell behavior. In this latter case, the responsible mediator may be interleukin-6, which is the major growth factor for myeloma cells. In myeloma, stimulation of bone resorption may lead to interleukin-6 generation,[681] which in turn may be responsible for maintaining aggressive growth of the malignant cells. Primary tumor cells from myeloma patients induced IL-6 secretion by adherent cells from long-term bone marrow cultures.[680] Interestingly, this IL-6 production did not occur when tissue-culture inserts, which prevented direct contact between the adherent cells from bone marrow and the myeloma cells, were used in the wells. Such findings imply an important role for cell-cell contact in mediating the bone marrow cell induction of IL-6 by myeloma cells. Binding of myeloma cells to adherent cells from long-term bone marrow cultures was partly inhibited by antibodies against the adhesion molecules, very late antigen-4 (VLA-4), CD44, and lymphocyte function-associated antigen 1 (LFA-1), as was IL-6 production.[680] These data indicate that one source of IL-6 may be the normal cells in the bone marrow and that adhesion molecules expressed on myeloma cells may mediate the induction of IL-6.

Other properties of myeloma cells contribute to its predilection to grow in the bone microenvironment. Cell surface adhesion molecules expressed by myeloma cells may bind to bone marrow stromal or endothelial cells. A variety of adhesion molecules, such as the VLAs, intercellular adhesion molecules (ICAM), and LFAs[682–687] are expressed on myeloma cells. VLA-5 and MPC-1 were reported to be involved in the adhesion of mature myeloma cells to bone marrow stromal cells.[688] Additionally, expression of the cell surface adhesion molecule, CD21, was demonstrated on both mature and immature myeloma cells. CD23 present on bone marrow stromal cells bind CD21 and, thus, may mediate myeloma cell adhesion in the bone microenvironment.[689] VLA-4 is the principal integrin present on the U266, ARH-77, IM-9, and HS-Sultan human myeloma cell lines and work by Uchiyama et al. reveal that such cells bind fibronectin through VLA-4 as well as through RGD-dependent mechanisms.[683] This binding was downregulated by IL-6. Studies from human subjects with myeloma and monoclonal gammopathy of unknown significance indicate that expression of plasma cell adhesion molecules LFA-1, VLA-4, and CD44 was highest in myeloma patients and was associated with increased evidence of angiogenesis.[690] Finally, CD44 expression by myeloma cells may mediate colonization in bone by binding osteopontin.[691]

At this point in time, it is not possible to say which is the most important cytokine involved in myeloma. The bone disease may be due to the combination and interaction of a number of cytokines and other molecules working in parallel, derived from both myeloma as well as from the normal host cells. Several animal models of myeloma bone disease have been developed recently that should provide significant insight into the pathophysiology of this disease.[692,693]

Until recently, the management of myeloma bone disease comprised treatment of the underlying malignancy, management of bone pain with analgesics, radiation therapy if the bone disease was localized, and treatment of hypercalcemia when it occurred with caution, because it is likely accompanied by impaired glomerular filtration. Recently, this has changed with the availability of more potent bisphosphonates. The Food and Drug Administration approved the use of pamidronate for myeloma bone disease in 1995. Pamidronate has been shown to reduce skeletal events associated with myeloma, including the need for radiation therapy and pathologic fractures. It also probably reduces the number of episodes of hypercalcemia. When given in doses of 90 mg by intravenous infusion over 4 hours monthly for 9 months, it has been shown to be very effective in patients with advanced disease, and the number of skeletal events is almost halved in patients taking pamidronate. Moreover, an objective assessment of quality of life in treated patients has shown a beneficial effect of pamidronate.[694] Similar studies in Europe have also suggested that potent bisphosphonates such as clodronate are effective in improving performance status and in reducing bone pain, vertebral fractures, and progression of osteolytic bone lesions as well as preventing hypercalcemic episodes. Animal studies using a mouse model of myeloma with the bisphosphonate, risedronate, reveal similar findings.[695] Previous clinical studies with less potent bisphosphonates in patients with myeloma have been less successful as oral etidronate was ineffective[696] and oral clodronate inhibited the progression of osteolytic bone lesions but did not reduce bone pain or fracture rate.[697] Clinical studies in patients with myeloma indicate that adjuvant treatment with low-dose gallium nitrate attenuates the rate of bone loss as well as the associated bone pain.[698] There is no definitive evidence as yet for a beneficial effect of inhibition of bone resorption on tumor burden.

Bisphosphonates seem to be most effective in patients with minimal disease, but are appropriate for almost all patients.

As with solid tumors that cause destructive bone lesions and hypercalcemia, hypercalcemia is also frequent in myeloma, occurring in about 30 percent of all patients sometime during the course of the disease. Hypercalcemia is always associated with bone destruction and often with impaired renal function. When hypercalcemia occurs in patients with myeloma, it is usually accompanied by impaired renal function, which limits the availability of specific therapies for treatment of the hypercalcemia. Under these circumstances, the most appropriate medical agent to use is a new generation bisphosphonate, although experience with these drugs is limited in patients with markedly impaired glomerular filtration. An alternative is the use of a combination of calcitonin and glucocorticoids, which has been shown to be very effective in reducing hypercalcemia in patients with myeloma.[341,623] However, because calcitonin must be given by injection, this combination is not as convenient as the new generation bisphosphonates.

In myeloma, bone destruction occurs as a consequence of osteoclastic bone resorption as osteoclasts accumulate on bone-resorbing surfaces adjacent to myeloma cells. In an early clinical study of patients with myeloma, biopsy samples indicate that active osteoclastic bone resorption correlated with the presence of greater than 20 percent myeloma cells in the adjacent marrow cell population.[670,699] The striking feature in myeloma is that there is a marked increase in osteoclastic bone resorption, usually without manifestations of increased bone formation.[699] These abnormalities in bone formation were confirmed by transiliac bone biopsies from 118 patients with myeloma in which quantitative bone histomorphometry demonstrated that osteoid seams were reduced in thickness and had a lowered calcification rate.[700] This is in contrast to breast cancer, where although the bone lesions are mainly destructive, there is usually a slight increase in bone formation and an increase in serum alkaline phosphatase and radionuclide uptake at sites of osteolytic deposits associated with increased osteoblast activity. The mechanism of this uncoupling of bone formation from bone resorption is not known, but is the subject of intense study.

Therapy of Osteolytic Lesions Due to Malignancy

Most patients with bone metastasis are normocalcemic. In a majority of breast cancer patients with bone metastases, local osteolysis occurs without hypercalcemia,[633] increases in nephrogenous cyclic AMP,[451] or PTHrP.[495] Osteolytic bone lesions are most frequent in patients with carcinoma of the breast, carcinoma of the lung, and myeloma, the same malignancies that are associated with hypercalcemia. However, there are also other solid tumors where hypercalcemia is rare but osteolytic bone lesions are relatively frequent. These include patients with carcinoma of the thyroid. These patients suffer considerably because their bone lesions cause intractable pain, pathological fracture after trivial injury, nerve compression syndrome such as spinal cord compression, and propensity to develop hypercalcemia. Until recently, therapy of tumor in bone was directed against tumor cells for breast and prostate cancer as well as myeloma and other malignancies. This usually involved chemo- or hormonal therapy, local field irradiation, radionuclide therapy, or surgery.[632,701,702] The advent of bisphosphonates has changed this perspective somewhat in that it has added therapy directed against the osteoclast to our current armamentarium of anticancer drugs.

As metastatic bone disease is mediated by osteoclastic bone resorption, and factors that stimulate osteoclastic bone resorption, such as PTHrP, enhance bone destruction by tumor, it is logical to consider therapy with inhibitors of bone resorption to prevent the development of bone metastasis or to delay their progression. Other mechanisms by which bisphosphonates exert their effects to decrease bone metastases may involve tumor cell adhesion to bone. In vitro studies demonstrate that a number of bisphosphonates decrease attachment of MDA-MB-231 breast cancer cells to extracellular bone matrix. Of interest is the fact that the effect of these bisphosphonates to decrease tumor adhesion positively correlated to the antiresorptive potency.[703]

Several prospective, double-blind, placebo-controlled trials have been published documenting the efficacy of the bisphophonate pamidronate in decreasing the skeletal complications associated with breast cancer[656] and myeloma.[694] For patients with myeloma, the FDA has recently approved pamidronate for use in patients with osteolytic lesions who are not hypercalcemic. This is based on a recent study,[694] showing that intravenous pamidronate given every 4 weeks for 9 cycles in almost 400 patients with myeloma caused a significant reduction in skeletal complications (defined as pathologic fracture, requirement for radiation to bone or surgery, or spinal cord compression), decreased the occurrence of new pathologic fractures, and prevented development of hypercalcemia. In addition, this treatment alleviated bone pain and improved quality of life. There was a suggestion in these patients that there may have also been a beneficial effect on overall survival. Pamidronate is therefore now being widely used early in the course of myeloma because it is a relatively nontoxic drug and may have a beneficial effect on more than bone complications. There is no definitive evidence as yet for a beneficial effect on tumor burden or survival and this will require careful controlled studies in more extended numbers of patients.

Clinical studies have been ongoing for 20 years in normocalcemic patients with solid tumors and osteolytic bone metastases. All of the available evidence from these studies suggests that drugs which decrease bone resorption such as the potent bisphosphonates have a beneficial effect on skeletal complications, including pain and pathologic fracture, prevention of hypercalcemia, and improved quality of life. In a recent multicenter trial which consisted of more than 700 patients with stage IV breast cancer with 2 or more predominantly lytic lesions, with at least one lesion that was one centimeter or greater in diameter, treatment with pamidronate 90 mg intravenously every 3 to 4 weeks for 12 months in conjunction with chemotherapy or hormonal therapy resulted in a significant reduction in skeletal complications and bone pain compared with the control group.[656] However, there may be an added beneficial effect of the bisphosphonates that is even more important. In experimental studies in which human breast cancer cells are inoculated into the left ventricle of the nude mouse, Sasaki et al.[643] have shown that bisphosphonates such as risedronate and ibandronate not only prevent the development of skeletal complications and bone metastases, but also reduce tumor burden in bone. This likely occurs because the bisphosphonates make bone a less favorable environment for the growth of tumor cells by reducing bone turnover and decreasing the supply of local bone-derived growth factors which also act as tumor growth factors in the bone microenvironment. It is apparent from clinical studies that the use of bisphosphonates reduces significant skeletal morbidity in advanced breast cancer.[647–658] These data suggest that drugs which inhibit bone resorption may be useful adjuvant therapy in patients with malignant disease by preventing the growth of tumor cells in the skeleton.

Studies using bisphosphonates in the treatment of prostate cancer metastatic to bone are fewer and less impressive. Clodronate treatment of men with advanced prostate cancer not only resulted in decreased osteoclastic bone resorption, as assessed histomorphometrically, but also in osteomalacia. The authors explained the transient relief of bone pain in the clodronate group to this resultant osteomalacia.[704] In a small study of breast and prostate cancer patients with osteosclerotic lesions, treatment with pamidronate resulted in a decrease in bone pain. This response was mostly predicted by a decrease in the urinary marker of bone resorption, deoxypyridinoline.[705]

Despite the encouraging results presented in these and other studies, several important questions remain regarding the use of bisphosphonates for treatment of tumor in bone. They include (1) Will bisphosphonates be useful as adjuvant therapy in tumor types other than breast cancer and myeloma? (2) Will bisphosphonate treatment in cancer improve survival? (3) Will bisphosphonates be beneficial in prevention of bone metastasis if therapy is initiated prior to the development of bone metastasis in patients with limited disease? (4) Will bisphosphonate therapy in cancer prove to be cost-effective? (5) Is there a role for bisphosphonate therapy in osteoblastic metastasis? Although animal studies suggest that the answers to these questions may already be obvious, only prospective trials in humans will provide us with the definitive answers.

Other Hypercalcemic Disorders

Sarcoidosis and other Granulomatous Disorders

Hypercalcemia occurs in about 10 percent of patients with sarcoidosis, and hypercalciuria is considerably more common, although precise figures are not available. It was originally thought that hypercalcemia reflects direct bone involvement, but in the 1950s it was found that patients with sarcoidosis had findings suggestive of unusual sensitivity to vitamin D[706] and 25 years later the serum concentration of 1α,25-$(OH)_2D$ was found to be increased in hypercalcemic patients.[707] A remarkable case report subsequently documented that 1α,25-$(OH)_2D$ levels were high in an anephric patient with sarcoidosis, establishing unexpectedly that the source of 1α,25-$(OH)_2D$ was extrarenal.[708] More recently, it has been shown that sarcoid tissue and macrophages lavaged from the lungs in pulmonary sarcoidosis are capable of 1α-hydroxylation of 25-(OH)D to produce 1α,25-$(OH)_2D$.[581]

As macrophages from normocalcemic sarcoidosis patients[581] and even normal macrophages[282] metabolize vitamin D to its active form, factors other than intrinsic enzyme activity may be responsible for hypercalciuria and hypercalcemia. Thus, one determinant of hypercalcemia is the mass and activity of sarcoid tissue. A second is the availability of substrate. In contrast to the kidney, macrophages from sarcoid granulomas synthesize 1α,25-$(OH)_2D$ in an unregulated fashion. When challenged with vitamin D, normal individuals regulate the 1α,25-$(OH)_2D$ concentration tightly,[709] but in sarcoidosis patients serum levels of 1α,25-$(OH)_2D$ increase concomitantly with the increase in serum 25-(OH)D levels. This occurs even in normocalcemic patients, suggesting that the development of hypercalcemia may be substrate-limited. Similarly, exposure to UV light increases cutaneous vitamin D synthesis but does not affect the serum concentration of 1α,25-$(OH)_2D$ in normal humans (Fig. 22-22). In sarcoidosis, hypercalcemia has long been recognized as occurring in the summer months, and episodes of hypercalcemia with increased 1α,25-$(OH)_2D$ levels have been reported in English patients after vacations on the Costa del Sol. Most hypercalcemic patients are azotemic, consistent with the notion that impairment of renal function by compromising renal calcium excretion is probably a key element in tipping chronically hypercalciuric patients over into hypercalcemia, although this scenario is not well documented in longitudinal studies.

Hypercalcemia generally presents in patients with active and obvious disease, manifesting high serum levels of angiotensin converting enzyme.[710] The serum 25-(OH)D level is normal, and the serum level of 1α,25-$(OH)_2D$ is increased. Urinary calcium excretion is increased, and calcium-containing renal stones may occur. Serum phosphorus is usually normal. When present, increased levels of alkaline phosphatase most commonly reflect the presence of liver disease. When assayed with immunoradiometric techniques capable of detecting suppression, the serum concentration of intact PTH is in the suppressed range. Hypercalcemia responds to corticosteroid therapy over a few days, and the serum 1α,25-$(OH)_2D$ level falls pari passu with the serum calcium. Doses of 40 mg prednisone daily can be used initially; most patients can be titrated to a lower maintenance dose. Chloroquine has also been used to treat hypercalcemia.[711] The differential diagnosis of hypercalcemia in suspected sarcoidosis has historically been vexing, and short-term suppression tests with hydrocortisone (40 mg tid for 10 days) have been used to rule out hyperparathyroidism, in which hypercalcemia does not respond to corticosteroid therapy. With the advent of assays for 1α,25-$(OH)_2D$ and intact PTH, the hydrocortisone suppression test is often formally unnecessary, but the effect of corticosteroid therapy can be observed during a therapeutic trial of prednisone.

Hypercalcemia is also seen in a variety of other granulomatous disorders. Mild hypercalcemia may be relatively common in untreated pulmonary tuberculosis (up to 28 percent of patients).[712–714] Hypercalcemia also occurs in berylliosis, disseminated candidiasis, disseminated coccidiomycosis, pulmonary eosinophilic granuloma, histoplasmosis, leprosy, and with silicone granulomas. The role of 1α,25-$(OH)_2D$ in these disorders is controversial.[715–719]

Endocrinopathies

Hyperthyroidism

Mild hypercalcemia is observed in about one-fourth of patients with thyrotoxicosis,[720] and the ionized calcium may be high in up to one-half. The serum phosphorus is in the high-normal range or slightly elevated, and the TmP/GFR is correspondingly high. The serum calcium and serum phosphorus levels are correlated with the level of thyroid hormone, and patients with significant hypercalcemia usually have clinically obvious thyrotoxicosis. The serum alkaline phosphatase and urinary hydroxyproline may also be mildly increased. The urinary excretion of calcium is high. Both PTH and 1α,25-$(OH)_2D$ levels are reduced.[721,722] Severe hypercalcemia occurs rarely, usually in patients with high levels of thyroid hormone who have coexisting hyperparathyroidism or are further compromised by immobilization or impaired renal function. Hypercalcemia is best understood as a manifestation of hyperthyroid bone disease. Thyrotoxicosis is a state of increased bone turnover resulting from a direct ability of thyroid hormone to stimulate bone resorption.[722] Despite compensatory increases in bone formation, losses of bone mineral may be substantial, as reflected in persistent hypercalciuria in the face of reduced 1α,25-$(OH)_2D$ levels. Osteopenia is now recognized as common even in mild hyperthyroidism, although symptomatic osteoporosis is found mainly in postmenopausal women. Even hypothyroid patients who are overreplaced with thyroid hormone, as indicated by suppression of thyroid stimulating hormone (TSH), may have significant reductions in bone density. The manifestations of hypercalcemia in hyperthyroid patients thus reflect accelerated bone resorption with suppression of PTH and 1α,25-$(OH)_2D$. Hypercalcemia responds to antithyroid therapy and may respond to beta-adrenergic blocking agents.

Adrenal Insufficiency

Hypercalcemia can be a feature of acute adrenal crisis and responds to corticosteroid replacement therapy. Animal studies suggest that hemoconcentration is a critical factor in elevating total serum calcium; in experimental adrenal insufficiency, plasma ionized calcium is normal.[723] However, the ionized calcium is reported to be elevated in some patients,[724] and the pathogenesis of hypercalcemia is not fully understood.

Pheochromocytoma

Hypercalcemia occurring in a patient with pheochromocytoma is generally due to concomitant hyperparathyroidism, most often as part of MEN type 2A. However, hypercalcemia is also found occasionally in uncomplicated pheochromocytoma. Recent evidence favors production of PTHrP by the pheochromocytoma as the cause of hypercalcemia in such patients.[725,726]

Pheochromocytoma is the only benign neoplasm for which there is evidence that PTHrP is secreted, although the PTHrP gene is also expressed in certain parathyroid adenomas.[727]

Vipoma

Hypercalcemia has been recorded in about 40 percent of patients with the watery diarrhea, hypokalemia, achlorhydria syndrome (WDHA syndrome, Verner-Morrison syndrome). Some patients may have intercurrent primary hyperparathyroidism, but reversal of hypercalcemia has occurred with resection of the VIP-producing tumor. VIP is known to increase bone resorption. In view of the role of PTHrP in pheochromocytoma and the association of ganglioneuromas and pheochromocytomas with the WDHA syndrome, PTHrP may also be involved.

Drug-Induced Hypercalcemia

Thiazide Diuretics

The administration of thiazides and related diuretics such as chlorthalidone, metolazone, and indapamide can produce an increase in the total serum calcium. This results in part from hemoconcentration, but ionized calcium is also increased.[728] Hypercalcemia is usually transient, lasting for days or weeks, but occasionally persists. Thiazide administration can also exacerbate the effects of mild primary hyperparathyroidism; in fact, a several-week course of thiazides has been employed as a provocative test in patients with borderline hypercalcemia. It appears that most cases of thiazide-associated hypercalcemia involve underlying hyperparathyroidism. In a large cross-sectional screening study in Sweden, the prevalence of hypercalcemia was increased threefold in thiazide users. In one-fourth of patients, hypercalcemia remitted after the thiazide medication was stopped; most thiazide users with persistent hypercalcemia when the drug was stopped proved to have primary hyperparathyroidism.[729]

The mechanism by which thiazide diuretics cause hypercalcemia is controversial. The hypocalciuric effect of thiazides is well known and is used therapeutically in the treatment of renal stone disease and hypoparathyroidism.[730] Urinary calcium excretion is reduced by about 40 percent with chronic thiazide use. Thiazides inhibit calcium reabsorption in the early distal convoluted tubule; the cellular basis for this effect is incompletely understood but may be secondary to the effects of the drugs on sodium chloride or sodium entry.[731] In addition, extracellular volume depletion will increase proximal sodium reabsorption and thus reduce delivery to distal sites. Increased sodium intake blunts the hypocalciuric effect of thiazides. However, in the presence of intact calcium homeostasis, a simple reduction in urinary calcium excretion should be compensated. Indeed, thiazide administration has extrarenal effects, increasing the serum calcium concentration in end stage renal failure.[732] Thus, there may be effects of thiazides on bone either directly or by potentiating the effect of PTH on bone resorption. Theoretically, thiazides could also stimulate the secretion of PTH or intestinal calcium absorption, but there is no compelling evidence for such actions.

Vitamin D

Hypercalcemia occurs in patients taking large doses of vitamin D (usually greater than 50,000 units daily).[733] It is seen in hypoparathyroid patients treated with vitamin D and in patients who selfadminister large amounts as an anodyne. In the latter instance, the history of drug use may not be readily obtainable. The presenting symptoms and signs are those of hypercalcemia. The glomerular filtration rate is reduced, and calcium urolithiasis may also occur. Hypercalcemia persists in fasting patients, indicating a contribution of bone resorption as well as increased intestinal calcium absorption. In patients taking ergocalciferol, cholecalciferol, or calcifediol [25-$(OH)D_3$], the diagnosis may be established by measurement of the serum 25-(OH)D level, which is often 5 to 10 times normal. The level of 1α,25-$(OH)_2D$ may be normal or slightly raised, a tribute to the tight control of its synthetic rate.[733–735] Thus, much of the toxicity of vitamin D probably results from the action of 25-(OH)D, which has an appreciable affinity for the receptor [one-thousandth that of 1α,25-$(OH)_2D$]. Hypercalcemia in vitamin D intoxication is treated with withdrawal of vitamin D and calcium, increased intake of fluids, and high-dose corticosteroid therapy; it responds to corticosteroids within a few days. In contrast to the effects of corticosteroids on the production of 1α,25-$(OH)_2D$ in sarcoidosis, the effect of steroids seen here appears to be attributable to blockade of vitamin D action. Intoxication with calcitriol [1α,25-$(OH)_2D_3$] can be diagnosed by determining its serum level; the other available short-acting agent, dihydrotachysterol, produces a metabolite that cross-reacts in some assays for 1α,25-$(OH)_2D$ but not in assays that use the calf thymus receptor.

Vitamin A

Large doses of vitamin A (50,000 to 200,000 units daily) produce a syndrome of lassitude, headache, anorexia, cheilitis, glossitis, a scaly pruritic rash, alopecia, hepatomegaly, and bone pain and tenderness. This syndrome is sometimes complicated by hypercalcemia. In hypercalcemic patients, the serum phosphorus is normal and the alkaline phosphase and other hepatic enzymes may be increased. Bone radiographs may show characteristic periosteal calcifications.[736] The vitamin A level in serum is elevated. Food faddism and self-medication with high-dose vitamin preparations are the most common causes of this rare disorder, and a history of excessive vitamin A intake may be difficult to obtain. It appears that dialysis patients are sensitive to smaller doses of vitamin A.[737] Hypercalcemia has also been reported as a complication of treatment with the retinoic acid derivative isotretinoin. The occurrence of hypercalcemia is probably attributable to a direct effect of vitamin A on bone resorption. Hypercalcemia responds to corticosteroids.

Lithium

Hypercalcemia is one of several endocrine complications in lithium-treated patients. As with lithium-induced hypothyroidism and nephrogenic diabetes insipidus, hypercalcemia occurs in patients with therapeutic serum levels of lithium. The serum calcium level is increased in populations of lithium-treated patients, and about 10 percent have frank hypercalcemia.[44,738] PTH levels tend to be increased in hypercalcemic patients, and studies in vitro indicate that lithium increases the set point for calcium suppression of PTH secretion.[51] Lithium therapy also decreases urinary calcium excretion and increases the serum magnesium.[738] Overall, the constellation of hypercalcemia with detectable PTH levels, hypocalciuria, and hypermagnesemia is reminiscent of familial benign hypercalcemia (familial hypocalciuric hypercalcemia), discussed earlier, and it is conceivable that lithium therapy induces abnormalities of calcium sensing that closely resemble those in the familial disorder. Lithium may also increase parathyroid gland growth.[739,740] It also appears that like other drugs that predispose to hypercalcemia, lithium can exacerbate the hypercalcemia of primary hyperparathyroidism. The diagnosis of "true" primary hyperparathyroidism in the face of lithium therapy may be difficult, particularly because withdrawal of lithium from a well-controlled patient may be unacceptable.[741] Some patients with good evidence for a parathyroid tumor have been operated on, partly in the hope that the psychiatric disturbance would be ameliorated, but in this regard the results of surgery have been disappointing. Expectant management of mild hypercalcemia is often indicated.

The Milk-Alkali Syndrome

The ingestion of large quantities of calcium together with an absorbable alkali can produce hypercalcemia with alkalosis, renal impairment, and often nephrocalcinosis.[742] The serum phosphorus is normal. Hypercalciuria is classically absent despite the high filtered load of calcium. The syndrome was commonplace when the Sippy diet consisting of a milk-cream mixture and either sodium bicarbonate or bismuth subcarbonate was a standard peptic ulcer regimen. It is seen much less frequently now that nonabsorbable antacids are in common use but still occurs, as witnessed by a recent epidemic of 65 cases in cardiac transplant patients treated prophylactically for peptic ulcer disease with large doses of calcium carbonate (8 to 12 g daily).[743] The pathophysiology of the syndrome is incompletely known. Clearly, large amounts of calcium can be absorbed passively from the intestine even if 1α,25-$(OH)_2D$ is suppressed; presumably hypercalcemia occurs when renal calcium excretion is impaired.

Miscellaneous Conditions

Immobilization

From the perspective of bone, immobilization is an example of a pure resorptive state. Histomorphometric studies indicate that immobilization produces an uncoupling of bone remodeling, with a decreased rate of bone formation and less pronounced increases in bone resorption.[744] The net effect is a loss of mineral from bone, and the consequences are predictable: osteoporosis, marked hypercalciuria, suppression of PTH, decreased 1α,25-$(OH)_2D$ levels, and an increased renal phosphate threshold.[745]

Hypercalcemia is seen predominantly in immobilized individuals with a preexisting state of high bone turnover: the young, in whom physiologic remodeling is active; the pagetic patient, with extensive osteolysis from a bony neoplasm (e.g., multiple myeloma); and in thyrotoxicosis. After a spinal cord injury, peak levels of hypercalciuria occur between 1 and 4 months, and the incidence of hypercalcemia is also highest during this period. Overall, 24 percent of children under age 16 experience hypercalcemia after a spinal cord injury, usually in conjunction with a decreased GFR.

The treatment of immobilization hypercalcemia consists of early resumption of weight bearing. Passive range-of-motion exercises are not helpful. In situations such as spinal cord injury in which weight bearing is not possible, a variety of pharmacologic approaches have been tried. Glucocorticoids, calcitonin, and oral phosphate have been used with minimal success. Several cases have been reported in which bisphosphonate treatment promptly returned serum calcium levels to normal.[746]

Acute Renal Failure

Hypercalcemia is occasionally seen in acute renal failure, usually in the early diuretic phase. It has most commonly been reported in renal failure induced by rhabdomyolysis, which is characterized by severe hyperphosphatemia and hypocalcemia in the oliguric phase. Hypercalcemia appears in the early diuretic phase, at a time when the serum phosphorus level is falling but often still above normal, and resolves over a few weeks.[747] It is not certain what leads to transient hypercalcemia. Substantial amounts of calcium and phosphate are deposited in the injured muscle and are released during recovery. This occurs at a time when levels of PTH and 1α,25-$(OH)_2D$ are reported to be high. Treatment consists of low-calcium dialysis, phosphate binders, and hydration.

ICU Hypercalcemia

An apparently new form of hypercalcemia has been reported over the past decade in critically ill patients. The etiology is unclear but may be multifactorial. At least two of the following factors are commonly present: immobilization, parenteral nutrition, and renal insufficiency.[748] The underlying illnesses are diverse, but the disorder is prevalent in patients with end stage liver disease.[749] Hypoalbuminemia is often present, serum phosphorus concentrations are normal, and marked hypercalciuria is sometimes observed. The serum level of 25-(OH)D is normal, and intact PTH and 1α,25-$(OH)_2D$ are usually suppressed. In a few patients, serum PTHrP levels have been normal. Fluctuating hypercalcemia may persist for weeks but is reversible in patients who survive the ICU. Parenteral nutrition may be a key factor in some patients, as hypercalcemia has also been reported in patients maintained on chronic parenteral nutrition, often in association with low-turnover bone disease. However, hypercalcemia generally does not respond to the removal of calcium or vitamin D from the total parenteral nutrition (TPN) solution. No satisfactory therapy is available.

Idiopathic Hypercalcemia of Infancy

There are at least three forms of hypercalcemia in the newborn. Severe neonatal hypercalcemia is seen in families with familial benign hypercalcemia (familial hypocalciuric hypercalcemia), and some cases may be homozygotes for this autosomal dominant trait.[411] Hypercalcemia responds to subtotal parathyroidectomy. A second form occurs in Williams syndrome, which includes supravalvular aortic stenosis, other cardiac anomalies, mental retardation, and a characteristic elfin facies. High plasma concentrations of 1α,25-$(OH)_2D$ have been found in some patients with this disorder,[750] but vitamin D metabolite levels are normal in other patients and the role of 1α,25-$(OH)_2D$ is disputed. A third form of neonatal hypercalcemia occurs transiently in patients who lack the somatic features of Williams syndrome.

Serum Protein Disorders

Hemoconcentration leads to hyperalbuminemia and a consequent increase in the total serum calcium; ionized calcium levels are normal. Binding of calcium by myeloma paraproteins has also been reported.[751] These patients present with chronic hypercalcemia and a normal ionized calcium level. Measurement of ionized calcium is unnecessary in patients with symptomatic hypercalcemia but should be performed in asymptomatic myeloma patients.

Familial Hypocalciuric Hypercalcemia

This important hereditary form of hypercalcemia is considered in the section on primary hyperparathyroidism.

Jansen's Metaphyseal Chondrodysplasia

Jansen's metaphyseal chondrodysplasia is characterized by short-limbed dwarfism and severe hypercalcemia and hypophosphatemia, despite normal or undetectable concentrations of PTH or PTHrP in the circulation. This autosomal dominant disease is the result of an activating mutation of the PTH/PTHrP receptor which leads to ligand-independent accumulation of cAMP.[160]

HYPOCALCEMIA

Hypocalcemia is defined as a total serum calcium concentration, corrected for protein, of <8.4 mg/dl (2.1 mmol/L) or an ionized calcium concentration of <4.48 mg/dl (1.12 mmol/L).[732] Total calcium concentration should be corrected for protein concentration using the formula cited in the beginning of this chapter. A reduction in the serum albumin will result in a low total calcium concentration while the ionized calcium concentration remains normal. Many chronic illnesses are associated with reductions in the albumin concentration, but not necessarily true hypocalcemia. The most common causes of hypocalcemia are hypoparathyroidism, abnormalities in vitamin D, hypomagnesemia, and chronic renal failure. The causes of hypocalcemia are listed in Table 22-6.

TABLE 22-6. Causes of Hypocalcemia

Hypoparathyroidism
Idiopathic
Branchial dysembryogenesis (DiGeorge's syndrome)
Congenital absence of parathyroids
Associated with polyglandular autoimmune disorders
Isolated late-onset
Postsurgical
Transient suppression
Infiltrative diseases
Irradiation
Hypomagnesemia
Autosomal dominant hypocalcemia
PTH resistance
Pseudohypoparathyroidism
Hypomagnesemia
Vitamin D deficiency
Nutritional
Renal failure
Malabsorption
Anticonvulsant therapy
Liver disease
α-hydroxylase deficiency (vitamin D-dependant rickets, type 1)
Vitamin D resistance (vitamin D-dependant rickets, type II)
Medications
Plicamycin, calcitonin, bisphosphonates, phosphate
Phenobarbital, dilantin
Citrated blood, radiographic contrast dyes
Fluoride
Foscarnet, pentamidine
Malignancy
Osteoblastic metastases
Tumor-lysis syndrome
Acute pancreatitis
Toxic shock syndrome
Neonatal

FIGURE 22-49. The sequence of adjustments initiated in response to hypocalcemia.

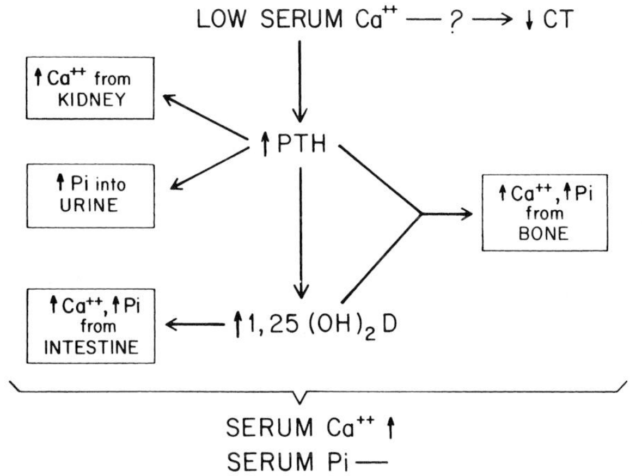

Defenses against hypocalcemia are very effective and are illustrated in Fig. 22-49. Serum calcium does not drop below 4.5 mg/dl. Calcium deficiency that is caused, for example, by dietary deficiency or hormonal deficiency is compensated for by

1. Glomerular filtration—as the ionized serum calcium falls, the filtered load of calcium decreases.
2. Compensatory mechanisms in the skeleton and kidney—as the ionized serum calcium level falls, PTH synthesis and secretion is enhanced, and this will tend to increase plasma calcium by the effects of PTH on the renal tubules to enhance renal tubular calcium reabsorption, and by effects of PTH on osteoclasts to stimulate bone resorption.
3. Gut adaptation—as the serum calcium levels fall, PTH will be increased and stimulate the production of 1,25 dihydroxyvitamin D3, which enhances dietary absorption of calcium. The fractional absorption of dietary calcium will subsequently increase.

TABLE 22-7. Clinical Features of Hypocalcemia

Neurologic/neuromuscular
Peripheral
Parasthesias
Tetany
Laryngospasm
Bronchospasm
Muscle cramps
Chvostek sign
Trousseau sign
Central
Irritability
Seizures
Intracranial calcification
Papilledema
Mental status changes
Cataracts
Abnormal dentition
Dry skin, coarse hair, brittle nails
Cardiovascular
Abnormal EKG (prolonged QT interval)
Congestive heart failure
Arrhythmias
Hypotension
Bradycardia

Clinical Features of Hypocalcemia

The clinical features of hypocalcemia are listed in Table 22-7. Most of the signs and symptoms of hypocalcemia result from either increased neuromuscular excitability (tetany, parasthesia, seizures) or calcium deposition (cataract, calcification of basal ganglia). Symptoms of hypocalcemia are characterized by abnormal neurologic sensations and neuromuscular excitability and reflect both the absolute calcium concentration as well as the rate of fall in calcium concentration. The threshold for development of symptoms also depends on the serum pH, severity of concomitant hypomagnesemia, hypokalemia and hyponatremia, and administered sedatives. Sensations of numbness and tingling involving the fingers, toes, and circumoral region are early symptoms. Spontaneous tonic muscle contractions, referred to as tetany in the hypocalcemic patient, are due to increased neural excitability that occurs as a consequence of the low extracellular fluid calcium concentration reducing the threshold for excitation of the neural tissue. The clinical manifestations of tetany occur as a result of spontaneous discharges of both sensory and motor fibers in peripheral nerves. The result is carpopedal spasm and despite the appellation, it more often involves the hands than the feet (Fig. 22-50). Electromyographically, tetany is typified by repetitive motor-unit action potentials, usually grouped as doublets. These changes are characteristic of tetany but not of hypocalcemia per se. Extracellular calcium and magnesium are thought to affect the local electric field of the membrane near ion channels in such a fashion that hypocalcemia or hypomagnesemia reduces the amount of depolarization necessary to induce an increase in sodium conductance and depolarize nerve cells.[753] In milder forms, or latent tetany, a tetanic attack will occur if provoked, as seen when a physician elicits a Chvostek's or Trousseau's sign. Chvostek's sign is elicited by tapping the facial nerve about 2 cm anterior to the earlobe just below the zygoma. The reaction can be graded semiquantitatively: grade 1, twitching of the angle of the mouth; grade 2, additional twitching of the alae nasi; grade 3, contraction of the orbicularis oculi; grade 4, hemifacial contractions. A grade 1 Chvostek's sign is present in 25 percent of normal individuals. Trousseau's sign, a typical carpal spasm, is provoked by placing a sphygmomanometer cuff on the upper arm and inflating it to 10 mmHg above the systolic blood pressure for 3 minutes. The response depends on the induction of regional ischemia in the ulnar nerve, not generalized ischemia of the forearm. This can be shown by deflating the cuff after placing a second cuff distally. The carpal spasm will recede and then reoccur after several minutes, a response that can be used to outwit the occasional malingerer. Trousseau's sign is more specific than Chvostek's sign, but a positive Trousseau's sign may occur in 1 to 4 percent of normal subjects. It should be noted that significant hypocalcemia may be present in the absence of Chvostek's and Trousseau's sign. Variations in expression of tetany may manifest as muscle cramping, laryngeal stridor, or bronchospasm.

The most important cause of normocalcemic tetany is hyperventilation. Although respiratory alkalosis lowers the ionized calcium by increasing protein binding, alkalosis causes tetany primarily by an independent effect on neuromuscular excitability.[754] However, latent tetany in hypocalcemic persons may become overt during hyperventilation. Other causes of tetany include metabolic alkalosis and hypomagnesemia. Regardless of its cause, tetany worsens during pregnancy and lactation. Tetany in hypocalcemic individuals may be masked by uremia, hypokalemia, or hypermagnesemia.

Central nervous system manifestations of hypocalcemia include seizures, mental status changes, and irritability. The seizures may be focal, jacksonian, petit mal, or grand mal. Long standing hypocalcemia may be associated with papilledema and basal ganglia calcifications. Other manifestations of chronic hypocalcemia include cataracts, dry skin, coarse hair, and brittle nails.

FIGURE 22-50. Carpal spasm in tetany. The wrist is flexed, the thumb is adducted, the metacarpophalangeal joints are flexed, and the interphalangeal joints are extended. [*By permission of Arnaud CD, The calcitropic hormones and metabolic bone disease in FS Greenspan (ed): Basic and Clinical Endocrinology, 3d ed. Norwalk, CT Appleton and Lange, p. 264, 1991.*]

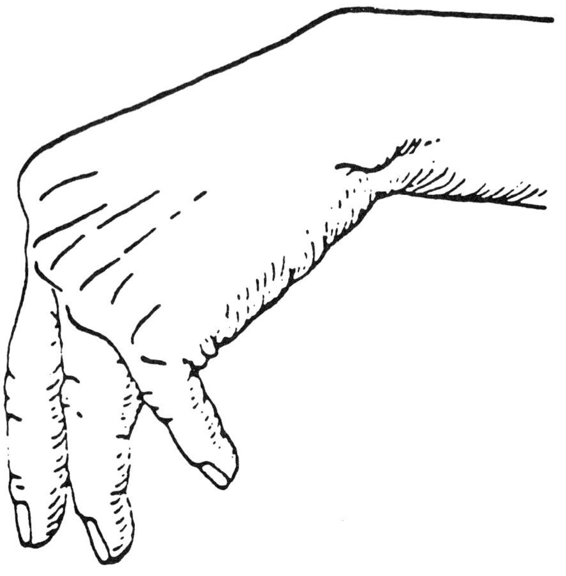

Hypocalcemia may be associated with an exacerbation of pustular psoriasis.[755] Defective dentition may date the onset of hypocalcemia to childhood. If hypocalcemia is a result of a vitamin D deficiency state, signs of osteomalacia or rickets may be present.

Cardiovascular manifestations of hypocalcemia include arrhythmias, bradycardia, hypotension, and impaired cardiac contractility.[756] Hypotension results from diminished smooth muscle tone and usually occurs when the hypocalcemia has developed rapidly. The hypotension is unresponsive to fluids and pressors until calcium is administered. Likewise, the impaired cardiac contractility responds poorly to inotropic agents until the hypocalcemia is corrected. The electrocardiogram may have a prolonged QT interval, ST-segment prolongation, and T wave abnormalities. The prolonged QT interval, in the absence of drugs, indicates significant hypocalcemia.

Hypoparathyroidism

Hypoparathyroidism may be due to a wide variety of inherited or acquired diseases of the parathyroid gland that cause impaired synthesis and secretion of PTH. Pseudohypoparathyroidism refers to a state of PTH resistance that renders affected patients functionally hypoparathyroid and will be discussed separately. Functional hypoparathyroidism may also result from magnesium deficiency. The signs and symptoms of hypoparathyroidism are those of hypocalcemia. Biochemically, the serum level of phosphorus is high or high-normal as a result of a high renal phosphate threshold. This results primarily from absence of the phosphaturic effect of PTH. However, hypocalcemia per se may independently increase the renal phosphate threshold, accounting for the variable improvement in hyperphosphatemia when hypoparathyroid patients are treated with vitamin D.[757]

Idiopathic hypoparathyroidism refers to diseases of the parathyroid gland associated with insufficient PTH secretion that are not secondary or acquired. Rare individuals born without parathyroid glands will manifest the hypocalcemia in the neonatal period. Hypoparathyroidism due to branchial dysembryogenesis will also be evident in the neonatal period and may be associated with other branchial cleft abnormalities. DiGeorge Syndrome is a sporadic developmental disorder involving the third and fourth branchial clefts that results in dysgenesis of the thymus and the parathyroids.[758] Hypoparathyroidism presents as tetany in infancy, but defective T-cell function dominates the subsequent course unless thymic tissue is transplanted. Associated cardiac abnormalities and craniofacial anomalies are also common.[758,759] It was recently reported that deletion of both copies of the homeobox gene hox 1.5 in the mouse produces a similar development defect.[760]

Hypoparathyroidism associated with the polyglandular autoimmune syndrome, type I, is the most common variety of idiopathic hypoparathyroidism.[761] The syndrome is usually sporadic but can be familial, although the pattern of inheritance is not known. Hypoparathyroidism in this syndrome is most associated with chronic mucocutaneous candidiasis and primary adrenal insufficiency although primary hypogonadism, diabetes mellitus, pernicious anemia, vitiligo, and autoimmune thyroid disease can occur as well. Typically, the condition begins, usually by age 4, with candidiasis, and hypoparathyroidism follows several years later. Primary adrenal insufficiency presents next, usually during adolescence. The combination of hypoparathyroidism, primary adrenal insufficiency, and mucocutaneous candidiasis is known as HAM syndrome. Although these patients demonstrate autoantibodies to parathyroid tissue, the significance of this remains unclear. Recently, antibodies to the calcium-sensing receptor were detected in a significant number of patients with idiopathic hypoparathyroidism.[762] Isolated late-onset hypoparathyroidism occurs in adulthood and although patients may have parathyroid antibodies, it is not usually associated with the polyglandular autoimmune syndrome.

Postsurgical hypoparathyroidism is associated with extensive thyroid surgery such as that performed as treatment of thyroid cancer or of Graves' hyperthyroidism. Because radioactive iodine ablation has become the mainstay of therapy for Graves' disease, postsurgical hypoparathyroidism is usually seen in patients who have had a near-total thyroidectomy for thyroid cancer or in patients who have had recurrent parathyroid surgery for parathyroi hyperplasia or a persistent parathyroid adenoma. Hypoparathyroidism may occur following head and neck surgery for malignancy, particularly when radical removal of tumor tissue en bloc requires removal of the thyroid and adjacent structures. The frequency of hypoparathyroidism varies with the amount of cervical dissection; it is highest after cancer surgery, it is more common after total than after subtotal thyroidectomy, and with skilled hands it occurs in less than 1 percent of parathyroidectomies.[763] The skill and experience of the surgeon are probably as important a variable as the nature of the procedure. The mechanism of injury to the parathyroid glands is obscure, but ischemia due to excessive use of ligatures in the vicinity of the glands is the most likely cause; rarely are all the parathyroid glands identified in the surgical specimen.

Postsurgical hypoparathyroidism can be transient or permanent. Patients whose parathyroid glands are inadvertently removed during surgery are clearly hypocalcemic within 24 hours and remain hypoparathyroid for the remainder of their lives. Occasionally, the parathyroids may undergo ischemic vascular damage or trauma that causes transient hypoparathyroidism. Typically, these patients are hypocalcemic in the immediate postoperative period but recover parathyroid function anywhere from 2 weeks to 6 months after the offending operation. Such patients may have impaired parathyroid reserve and experience periodic hypocalcemia during periods of stress. Transient hypoparathyroidism may also occur following removal of a single parathyroid adenoma as a result of transient suppression of the remaining parathyroid tissue by the adenoma.

Most patients experience a fall of about 1 mg/dl in the serum calcium during the 24 to 48 h after neck exploration as a nonspecific response to surgery. Patients who develop severe hypocalcemia with overt symptoms of tetany are suspect for the development of postsurgical hypoparathyroidism. Tetany usually appears during the first two postoperative days. About half of patients with postoperative tetany will recover sufficiently to require no chronic therapy, but most of them will have a decreased parathyroid reserve. Some patients with transient tetany and some patients who were asymptomatic in the immediate postoperative period will go on to develop late hypoparathyroidism months or years after neck surgery. Thus, surgical hypoparathyroidism must always be suspected in a hypocalcemic individual with a scar on the neck.[764]

"Hungry bone" syndrome is another cause of postsurgical hypocalcemia that may occur in patients with severe hyperparathyroidism and osteitis fibrosa cystica that undergo parathyroidectomy. In this situation, the relative hypoparathyroidism induced by the surgical procedure is complicated by deposition of available calcium into the healing bone lesions.

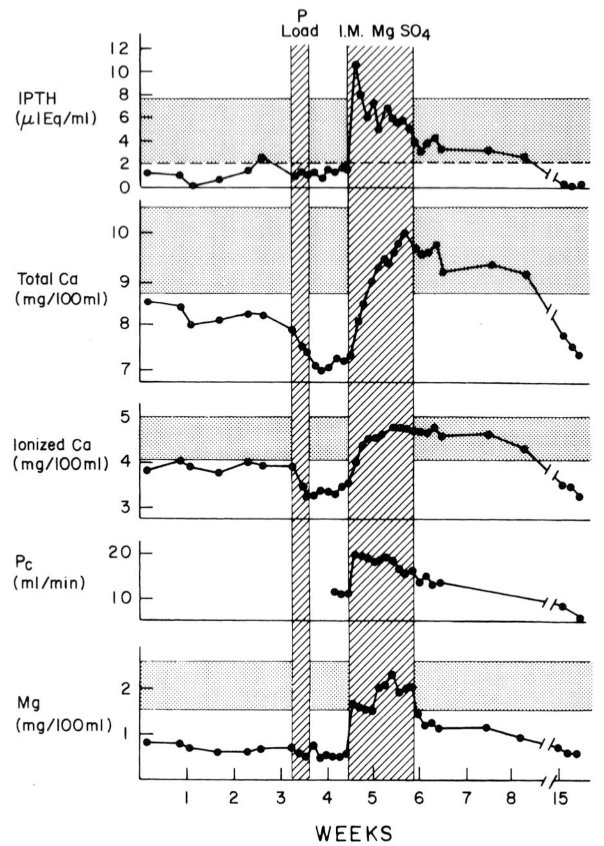

FIGURE 22-51. Response of serum calcium, parathyroid hormone, and phosphorus clearance (P_c) to magnesium replacement in a patient with severe hypomagnesemia. The hypocalcemia produced by an oral phosphate challenge before magnesium replacement did not result in an increase in PTH secretion. The shaded areas represent the normal ranges, and the dotted line represents the detection limit of the PTH assay. (*Adapted from and by permission of Anast CS, Mohs JM, Kaplan SL, Burns TW, Science 177:606, 1972.*)

Severe magnesium deficiency is a common cause of functional hypoparathyroidism. Hypomagnesemia results in impaired secretion of PTH as well as resistance to the action of PTH on the end organs of bone and kidney.[48,765–767] Patients with hypocalcemia due to hypomagnesemia are also resistant to parenteral calcium and vitamin D therapy. The response of calcium PTH and phosphorous clearance to magnesium replacement in a patient with severe hypomagnesium is shown in Fig. 22-51. Hypocalcemic patients are often significantly hypomagnesemic (serum magnesium concentration <1.5 mEq/L), although occasionally, the serum magnesium concentration is normal.[768] Magnesium deficiency may occur because of internal electrolyte shifts, decreased absorption of magnesium from the gut, or renal losses due to intrinsic tubular disorders or drug effects. Renal magnesium wasting can occur with loop diuretics, aminoglycosides, pentamidine[769] cisplatinum, cyclosporin, and amphotericin B.[770] A common scenario in which magnesium deficiency occurs is in the poorly nourished alcoholic patient who has recently been binge-drinking. Chronic diarrhea can also lead to magnesium deficiency.

Hypoparathyroidism may result from external radiation to the neck, and it has also been reported following low-dose radioactive iodine therapy for Graves' disease.[771,772] Infiltrative diseases, such as hemochromatosis, amyloidosis and granulomatous, and Wilson's disease can cause hypoparathyroidism as can metastatic carcinoma. Hypoparathyroidism is sometimes seen in congenitally transfusion-dependent patients with thalassemia or pure red cell aplasia who survive until the third decade of life.[773] Pathologically, abundant iron and a fibrous reaction are present in the glands. Hypoparathyroidism is rare in hemochromatosis. Frank hypoparathyroidism and decreased parathyroid reserve can occur in Wilson's disease, presumably because of copper deposition.[774] Aluminum deposition may impair the parathyroid reserve in renal osteodystrophy.

Familial Hypoparathyroidism

This rare disorder can be inherited in autosomal dominant, autosomal recessive, and X-linked patterns. It presents in infancy and can thus be considered a subcategory of persistent neonatal hypoparathyroidism. Linkage analysis of multiple kindreds has excluded a parathyroid gene mutation in about half the families examined; in these families, a developmental syndrome may lead to congenital aplasia.[775] In two kindreds the prepro-PTH gene was abnormal. In a family with autosomal dominant inheritance of hypoparathyroidism, a missense mutation (Cys^{17} Arg) disrupts the hydrophobic core of the signal sequence; expression of this trait results in inefficient uptake of prepro-PTH into the endoplasmic reticulum.[25] A family with an autosomal recessive disorder carries a splicing mutation that deletes the prepro sequence in exon 2.[776]

The most obvious clinical manifestation of hypoparathyroidism is hypocalcemia. Patients with hypocalcemia, hyperphosphatemia, and normal renal function are most likely to have either idiopathic or acquired hypoparathyroidism, or pseudohypoparathyroidism. The presence of cataracts or basal ganglia calcification indicate that the hypocalcemia has been longstanding. Coexisting endocrine disorders suggest the polyglandular autoimmune syndromes as an etiology. Infiltrative diseases should also be excluded before classifying the hypoparathyroidism as idiopathic. Magnesium deficiency should obviously be ruled out. Laboratory features of hypoparathyroidism (Table 22-9) include hypocalcemia and hyperphosphatemia concomitant with a low serum concentration of PTH and $1,25(OH)_2D_3$. The Ellsworth-Howard test (described later), formerly used to differentiate hypoparathyroidism from pseudohypoparathyroidism and to subclassify the types of pseudohypoparathyroidism, is probably not necessary to make the diagnosis of hypoparathyroidism now that sensitive PTH assays are available.[63]

Treatment of hypoparathyroidism is difficult as PTH is not available for therapeutic purposes. The serum calcium is increased through the administration of oral calcium and vitamin D supplements, the use of which is described in more detail in the later section on treatment of hypocalcemia. Vitamin D increases intestinal absorption of calcium. However, in the absence of PTH, which increases renal tubular reabsorption of calcium, vitamin D administration to bring the serum calcium into the normal range causes hypercalciuria, nephrolithiasis, and nephrocalcinosis. Therefore, when vitamin D or an active metabolite is used to increase the serum calcium concentration of patients with PTH deficiency, the goal is to maintain the calcium concentration in the low-normal range without causing hypercalciuria. When the corrected serum calcium concentration is in the target range (i.e., 8.0–9.0 mg/dL) and the patient is taking a stable dose of calcium and vitamin D, the 24-hour excretion of urinary calcium should be measured. In this situation, 24-hour urinary excretion of calcium should be less than 250 mg. The dosage of vitamin D should be decreased if urinary calcium excretion is greater. Alternatively, thiazide diuretics may be a useful adjunct to decrease the urinary calcium excretion. The choice of vitamin D and calcium preparations are discussed under therapy of hypocalcemia. When hypoparathyroidism is due to magnesium deficiency, supplemental magnesium must be given to maintain the serum magnesium concentration within the normal range, as calcium therapy alone will not correct the hypocalcemia.

Pseudohypoparathyroidism

The term pseudohypoparathyroidism describes a heterogeneous syndrome characterized by functional hypoparathyroidism, increased serum PTH concentrations, and peripheral resistance to the biological actions of PTH.[777] Fuller Albright first recognized that end-organ resistance to PTH can produce a syndrome that resembles true hypoparathyroidism. His classic paper in 1942 defining the syndrome reported three hypocalcemic patients with hyperphosphatemia who shared some unusual somatic features (Fig. 22-52). Unlike patients with idiopathic hypoparathyroidism, these individuals had no response to the infusion of parathyroid extract, and one had normal parathyroid glands. Albright proposed that their hypocalcemia had resulted from unresponsiveness to PTH and titled the paper "Pseudo-hypoparathyrodism—an example of Seabright-Bantam syndrome"[778] after a strain of domestic fowl in which the roosters have female feathering. Albright's report was the first clear description of end-organ resistance to a hormone, as the Seabright bantam syndrome, ironically, has now been shown to be caused by abnormal aromatization of androgen rather than resistance to the tissue effects of androgens.[779] In 1969, shortly after the discovery of cAMP, it was found that the normally brisk increase in urinary cAMP in response to PTH was markedly blunted in pseudohypoparathyroidism (Fig. 22-53), providing a clue that the molecular defect lay in the PTH receptor–adenylyl cyclase complex.[780] The rare opportunity to study renal tissue from a pseudohypoparathyroid patient subsequently led to the discovery of abnormalities in guanosine triphosphate (GTP) stimulation of renal adenylyl cyclase, focusing attention directly on the coupling

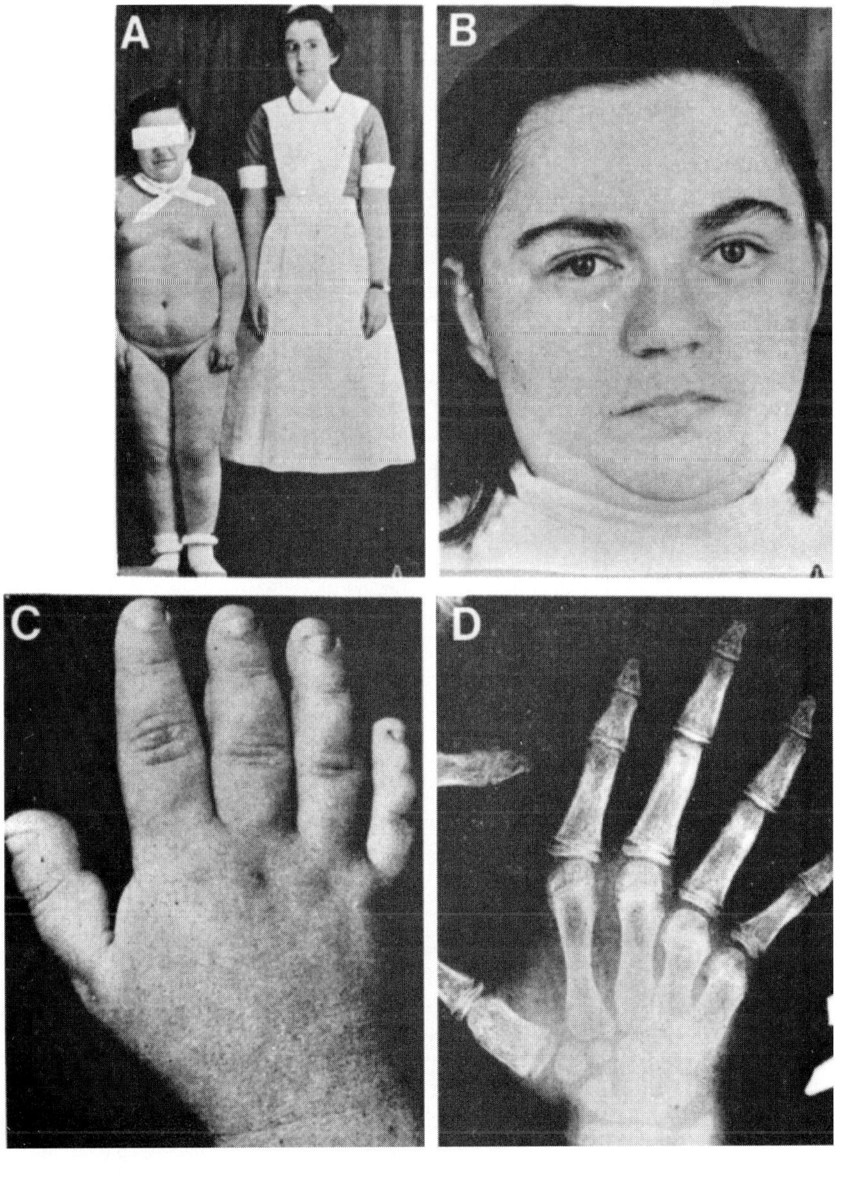

FIGURE 22-52. Phenotypic abnormalities in pseudohypoparathyroidism: (*A*) short, stocky habitus; (*B*) round face; (*C* and *D*) short metacarpals. (*A, B, and C by permission of Albright F, Burnett CH, Smith PH, Parson W, Endocrinology 30:922, 1942. D by permission of Kolb FO, Steinbach HJ, J Clin Endocrinol Metab 22:59, 1962.*)

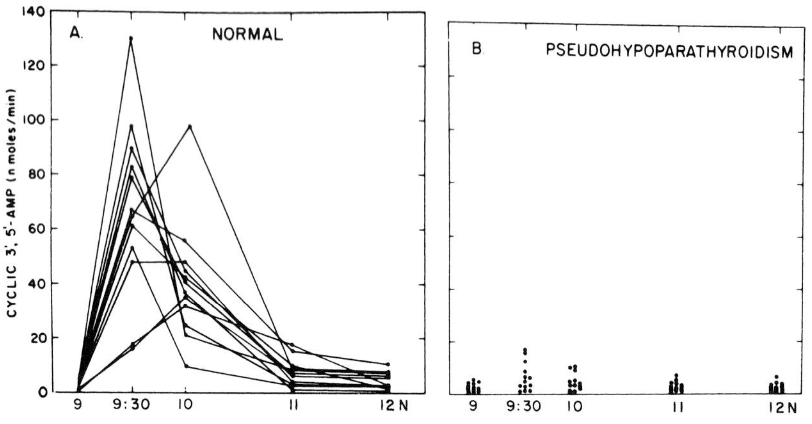

FIGURE 22-53. Urinary cAMP response to parathyroid hormone administration in normal subjects and patients with pseudohypoparathyroidism. (*From Chase, Melson, and Aurbach,*[614] *by permission of the Journal of Clinical Investigation.*)

of the PTH receptor–adenylyl cyclase complex, which is known to be GTP-dependent.[781] Subsequently, it was shown that many patients with pseudohypoparathyroidism display a 50 percent reduction in the content of the stimulatory G protein subunit of adenylyl cyclase, G_s, as described in detail later, providing a presumptive molecular basis for one form of the disorder.[782,783]

Many patients also have a number of somatic abnormalities, which are referred to collectively as the phenotype of Albright's hereditary osteodystrophy. Other hormone resistance syndromes may be present as well.

Clinical and Biochemical Features

The symptoms and signs of hypocalcemia develop in childhood. The average age at the onset of symptoms is 8 years, although the diagnosis is not made until adulthood in some relatively asymptomatic persons. As in other hypocalcemic disorders, the presenting symptoms are tetany and seizures.[784] Subsequently, pseudohypoparathyroid patients are prone to the complications of chronic hypocalcemia including calcification of the basal ganglia, which occurs in 50 percent; cognitive defects; cataracts; and dental abnormalities, including hypoplasia of dentin or enamel and delay or absence of eruption (Table 22-8).

TABLE 22-8. Symptoms and Signs in Pseudohypoparathyroidism

Symptom or Sign	Incidence, %
Somatotype	
Short stature	80
Round face	92
Stocky or obese habitus	50
Mental retardation	75
Dystrophic changes in bone	
Short metacarpals	68
Short metatarsals	43
Calvarial thickening	62
Ecotopic ossification	56
Symptoms or signs of hypocalcemia	
Tetany	86
Seizures	59
Cataracts	44
Calcification of the basal ganglia	45
Dental abnormalities	55

Many patients present with the somatic features described in the original report. The combination of short stature, brachydactyly (short digits), and soft tissue calcification is distinctive and is known as Albright's hereditary osteodystrophy (AHO). Patients are short (usually less than 150 cm) and obese and have round faces and short necks (Fig. 22-52). Brachydactyly most commonly affects the fourth and fifth metacarpal bones (brachymetacarpia), but shortened metatarsals (brachymetatarsia) are seen in 43 percent and brachyphalangia in 68 percent of patients (Table 22-8). Brachydactyly may be asymmetrical, and short thumbs are the most common abnormality in the digits. Brachydactyly may be diagnosed on physical examination or radiographs. On examination of the clenched fists, knuckles that would represent the ends of normal metacarpals are absent; instead, dimples overlie the shortened metacarpals. A straight edge laid over the fourth and fifth metacarpal heads in a clenched fist will normally miss the third metacarpal head but may touch it if the fourth is short. Similarly, on hand films, a line tangential to the fourth and fifth metacarpal heads should not intersect the third. Subcutaneous calcifications that histologically represent ectopic ossification are seen in more than half of these patients. These forms of soft tissue ossifications are not seen in hypoparathyroidism or other chronic hypocalcemic states and may be observed prior to the development of hypocalcemia in patients with AHO. Numerous other syndromes involving brachydactyly are recognized, but the complete picture of AHO is virtually pathognomic of pseudohypoparathyroidism or the related disorder pseudopseudohypoparathyroidism (see later discussion).

In addition to their disorder of mineral metabolism, patients with AHO may have clinical or biochemical evidence of other hormone resistance syndromes, most prominently hypothyroidism and ovarian failure. These problems are discussed in the section on pathogenesis.

Pseudohypoparathyroidism presents with hypocalcemia, hyperphosphatemia, and secondary hyperparathyroidism. The urinary excretion of calcium may be lower than in hypoparathyroid patients with a similar serum calcium level, and it is not clear whether the renal defect in responsiveness to PTH extends to the distal site of calcium reabsorption.[785] However, the serum 1α,25-$(OH)_2D$ level is in the low-normal range in the face of hyperparathyroidism and hypocalcemia and does not respond normally to the infusion of PTH.[786] The serum level of alkaline phosphatase is normal. The bones may appear to be dense radiographically. However, in contrast to patients with hypoparathyroidism, pseudohypoparathyroid patients have evidence of increased bone turnover, with increased urinary excretion of hydroxyproline and reduced bone density, and some actually have hyperparathyroid bone disease (see later discussion).[787]

Pathogenesis

The finding of Chase, Melson, and Aurbach that the urinary cAMP response to PTH was markedly blunted (but not abolished) in pseudohypoparathyroidism (Fig. 22-53) provides strong evidence that the molecular defect has to do with the synthesis or metabolism of cAMP.[780] In confirmation of this conclusion, infusion of dibutyryl cAMP has a normal has a normal effect on urinary phosphorus excretion and serum levels of 1α,25-$(OH)_2D$.[788,789] Theoretical possibilities for the underlying defect include defective function of the PTH receptor, reduced coupling of the occupied receptor to the catalytic subunit of adenylyl cyclase, abnormal synthesis of cAMP by the catalytic subunit, and rapid degradation of cAMP. Subsequent work has shown that the disorder is heterogeneous. Some patients have a reduced level of the coupling protein component of adenylyl cyclase, G_s; this disorder has been termed pseudohypoparathyroidism type IA. The exact etiology in the remaining patients (pseudohypoparathyroidism type IB) is unknown, but may also involve yet undefined abnormalities in $Gs\alpha$.

Pseudohypoparathyroidism Type IA

In this disorder, pseudohypoparathyroidism is associated with a deficiency of functional G_s resulting from mutations in the subunit $G_s\alpha$. The PTH receptor occupied by hormone is coupled inefficiently by G_s, to the catalytic subunit of adenylyl cyclase, with defective production of cAMP in response to PTH and a consequent defect in PTH action. The level of the coupling protein G_s in erythrocytes[782,783] or other tissues (fibroblasts, lymphocytes, platelets)[790] was reduced to 50 percent of normal in a group of pseudohypoparathyroid patients First citation (Fig. 22-54), as measured either by a functional assay or by labeling its α-subunit with cholera toxin. As discussed in the section on biochemical events in parathyroid hormone action, the G proteins are heterotrimeric GTP-binding proteins that couple occupied receptors to effector molecules, including catalytic adenylyl cyclase. The G proteins share common β and γ subunits. The specificity of a G protein for a receptor and for its cognate effector moiety are properties of the GTP-binding α subunit, and $G_s\alpha$ specifically couples stimulatory receptors to catalytic adenylyl cyclase. Thus, a generalized reduction in functional $G_s\alpha$ to one-half of normal levels would be expected to uncouple a fraction of occupied PTH receptors from the catalytic subunit of adenylyl cyclase and also to uncouple from adenylyl cyclase other receptors that normally stimulate the enzyme, engendering a generalized disorder of unresponsiveness of the hormones that utilize this signaling system.

The reduction in $G_s\alpha$ levels is not uniformly associated with unresponsiveness to PTH, as some members of families with pseudohypoparathyroidism have normal mineral metabolism despite a 50 percent reduction in $G_s\alpha$ levels (pseudopseudohypoparathyroidism). However, most patients with reduced levels of $Gs\alpha$ have AHO (Fig. 22-54). Thus, the defect in adenylyl cyclase function, independently of abnormal mineral metabolism, must directly produce the complex developmental abnormalities that eventuate in AHO.

A number of mutations in the gene that encodes $Gs\alpha$ (GNAS1)[791] can produce the phenotype of pseudohypoparathyroidism type IA. Cell membranes from most of these patients have an approximately 50 percent reduction in levels of expression or activity of $G_s\alpha$[792] $Gs\alpha$ deficiency in patients with AHO results from heterozygous inactivating mutations in the GNAS1 gene, which maps to chromosome 20q13.2.[793] The human GNAS1 gene is complex and comprised of at least 17 exons, including three alternative first exons.[794,795] Alternative splicing of transcripts derived from exons 1–13 generates four mRNAs that encode two $Gs\alpha$ proteins with apparent molecular weights of 45 kDa and two with molecular weights of 52 kDa[791] that exhibit specific patterns of tissues expression.[796] These forms of $Gs\alpha$ stimulate adenylyl cyclase but have subtle differences in the binding constant for GDP, the rate at which the forms are activated by agonist binding, efficiency of adenylyl cyclase stimulation, and the rate of GTP hydrolysis.[797–800] The biological significance of these differences are unknown. The processing of the GNAS1 gene is complicated by use of alternative first exons that generate novel transcripts. It is unlikely that alternate forms which lack amino acids encoded by exon 1 interact with $G\beta\gamma$ or attach to the plasma membrane.[77] Molecular analysis of DNA from patients with pseudohypoparathyroidism type Ia and AHO have revealed inactivating mutations in the GNAS1 gene that account for the 50 percent reduction in expression or function of the $Gs\alpha$ protein.[801–813] All patients are heterozygous and have one normal GNAS1 allele and one defective allele. Novel mutations have been discovered in

FIGURE 22-54. Activity of G_s in erythrocyte membranes from control subjects and from patients with pseudohypoparathyroidism, with or without Albright's hereditary osteodystrophy (AHO). The activity of G_s was assayed as the ability to reconstitute the adenylyl cyclase activity of turkey erythrocyte membranes containing the catalytic subunit of adenylyl cyclase. (*From Levine, Downs, and Moses,[635] by permission of the American Journal of Medicine.*)

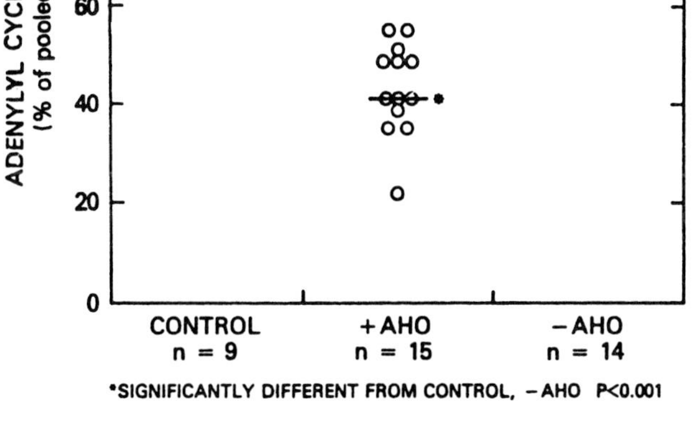

•SIGNIFICANTLY DIFFERENT FROM CONTROL, –AHO P<0.001

nearly all kindreds studied with the exception of a 4-base pair deletion in exon 7 detected in several families[814–816] and a missense mutation in exon 13 identified in two unrelated young boys.[802] The described mutations in GNAS1 include missense mutations, point mutations in sequences required for efficient splicing, and small deletions.

The association of peripheral resistance to PTH with an abnormality of the protein that is responsible for coupling the PTH receptor provides a very powerful inference of causality, yet these findings raise as many questions as they answer. What is the basis for hypocalcemia in these individuals? Why do some individuals in families with pseudohypoparathyroidism inherit an abnormal G_s, protein and AHO but respond normally to PTH? Because the abnormality in G_s, is expressed in many tissues, it would be expected to affect the action of many hormones coupled to adenylyl cyclase. This appears to be the case, but it is not clear why the clinical syndrome is often limited to abnormal PTH action.

Although renal unresponsiveness to PTH, with consequent hyperphosphatemia and possibly increased renal calcium excretion, would predispose a patient to hypocalcemia, it is likely that the genesis of hypocalcemia is multifactorial and involves bone and the gut as well as the kidney. In pseudohypoparathyroid patients, PTH does not mobilize calcium normally from bone, yet there is evidence of increased bone remodeling, with increased urinary hyroxyproline and decreased bone density,[787] and some patients actually manifest the skeletal changes of osteitis fibrosa cystica that occur in other forms of hyperparathyroidism.[790,817] Thus, in patients with pseudohypoparathyroidism, the remodeling function of PTH in bone seems to be dissociated from its function in calcium homeostasis. One theoretical explanation involves the use of multiple cellular second messengers by the PTH receptor (or receptors) in bone cells. Thus, cAMP may be the intracellular second messenger for the regulation of calcium homeostasis by bone cells, which would thus be abnormal in pseudohypoparathyroidism, whereas a different effector for the bone remodeling effects of PTH (e.g., phospholipase C, which is probably coupled to the PTH receptor by a G protein other than G_s.) is unaffected in the disorder.

It is also likely that reduced $1\alpha,25\text{-}(OH)_2D$ levels are important in the pathogenesis of hypocalcemia. Evidence from several circumstances suggests that $1\alpha,25\text{-}(OH)_2D$ may be required for PTH to mobilize calcium from bone,[818] and normalization of plasma $1\alpha,25\text{-}(OH)_2D$ concentrations in patients with pseudohypoparathyroidism may normalize plasma calcium.[819] In addition, intestinal calcium absorption is reduced in patients with pseudohypoparathyroidism.

Albright recognized that in families with pseudohypoparathyroidism there are individuals who inherit AHO without a clinical disorder of mineral metabolism and called this state pseudopseudohypoparathyroidism.[820] These individuals have the same inherited abnormality of G_s as do their kin with pseudohypoparathyroidism but have a normal urinary cAMP response to the infusion of PTH.[780] Thus, the inheritance of abnormal G_s is closely linked to the inheritance of AHO. Analysis of pedigrees has implicated genomic imprinting of the GNAS1 gene as a possible regulatory mechanism. In most cases, maternal transmission of the $Gs\alpha$ deficiency is associated with pseudohypoparathyroidism type Ia while paternal transmission is associated with pseudopseudohypoparathyroidism.[812,821–823]

As expected in view of the defect in $G_s\alpha$, resistance to the action of other hormones whose receptors are coupled to adenylyl cyclase is common in patients with pseudohypoparathyroidism type IA, although this resistance does not usually cause clinically apparent disorders.[824] Most of these patients have compensated primary hypothyroidism, in which thyroid hormone levels are slightly low and TSH is increased, but some present with frank hypothyroidism. Most women patients are oligomenorrheic, and some have increased gonadotropins and an exaggerated LH and FSH response to gonadotropin releasing hormone (GnRH). The cAMP response to glucagon and isoproterenol may be blunted, but resistance to the action of these hormones is not otherwise evident. These patients show no resistance to ACTH or ADH. The spectrum of impaired hormone action observed in pseudohypoparathyroidism type IA parallels the spectrum of impairment in PTH action in individuals with deficient $G_s\alpha$. The modifying factors that account for the differences in hormone responsiveness among tissues and among individuals are unidentified.

Two different animal models of pseudohypoparathyroidism type Ia have been generated by targeted disruption of the GNAS1 gene at exon 1 and exon 2 respectively.[825,826] Homozygosity for the mutant GNAS1 allele results in embryonic lethality. These mice have reduced expression of $G_s\alpha$ protein, but lack some of the features of the human disease. Heterozygous mice are smaller and fatter than wild-type mice. Unlike mice with pseudohypoparathyroidism la, affected mice have no heterotopic ossifications, no brachypodia, and bone histology is normal. Biochemical analysis of these heterozygous knockout mice suggest that $G_s\alpha$ expression may derive from only the maternal allele in some tissues, such as the renal cortex, and from both alleles in other tissues, such as the renal medulla.[825,826]

Pseudohypoparathyroidism Type IB

This is a syndrome of peripheral resistance to PTH, including a severely blunted nephrogenous cAMP response to the infusion of PTH, without either AHO or a deficiency of G_s. However, patients with pseudohypoparathyroidism Ib who have increased circulating concentrations of PTH often manifest skeletal lesions similar to those observed in patients with hyperparathyroidism. Thus, the PTH resistance appears to be limited to the kidney. The responsiveness to other hormones is normal.[824] Until recently, it was thought that the pathogenesis of this disorder resulted in decreased expression or function of the PTH/PTHrP receptor because there was renal resistance to PTH and normal activity of $G_s\alpha$. Extensive molecular studies have failed to disclose mutations in the coding exons and promoter regions of the PTH/PTHrP receptor gene or its mRNA.[827–829] Furthermore, mice and humans that are heterozygous for inactivation of the gene encoding the PTH/PTHrP receptor do not manifest PTH resistance or hypocalcemia.[161,164] Finally, inheritance of two inactive PTH/PTHrP receptor genes results in the letal disorder of Blomstraad chondrodysplasia, which is characterized by advanced endochondral bone formation.[161]

Pseudohypoparathyroidism type Ib has been described as a sporadic disorder. However, a recent study of four unrelated New England kindreds demonstrate an autosomal dominant pattern of transmission for this disorder.[830] These investigators mapped the molecular defect to a small region of chromosome 20q13.3, which is near the GNAS1 gene. Similar to pseudohypoparathyroidism type Ia, the genetic transmission appears to involve imprinting. Specifically, the gene appears to be paternally transmitted.

Pseudohypoparathyroidism Type II

This disorder was originally described as consisting of resistance to the phosphaturic effect of PTH despite a normal increase in urinary cAMP. It is rare and is likely to be heterogeneous.[831,832] Some cases may result from a defect in renal cAMP action leading to impairment of its second messenger function. Others may actually represent forms of vitamin D resistance. Syndromes of vitamin D resistance characterized by hyperphosphatemia have been recognized.[819] In them, osteomalacia may be mild or inapparent. In some cases of vitamin D resistance, the urinary cAMP responses to PTH are normal while the phosphaturic response may be impaired. Finally, the phosphaturic response to PTH is variable in normal subjects, and one must be cautious in ascribing a blunted response to a primary defect in the action of PTH.[833]

Diagnosis

The biochemical findings associated with hypocalcemia states are shown in Table 22-9. Pseudohypoparathyroidism should be considered in the differential diagnosis of hypocalcemia with hyperphosphatemia and normal renal function regardless of somatic features, as pseudohypoparathyroidism in the absence of AHO is not unusual. The elevated serum concentration of PTH in a patient with chronic hypocalcemia, hyperphosphatemia, and normal renal function excludes hypoparathyroidism and is suggestive of pseudohypoparathyroidism. The diagnosis of pseudohypoparathyroidism type I can be confirmed by a short infusion of PTH (the Ellsworth-Howard test; see the section on testing for pseudohypoparathyroidism, later). The primary responses to PTH that are of value in a short infusion protocol are the increase in urinary phosphorus and the increase in urinary cAMP excretion. Although the former is the classic index of renal responsiveness, the phosphaturic effect of PTH is variable, and marked blunting of the robust normal urinary cAMP response to PTH is the most reliable diagnostic maneuver. The response of serum 1α,25-$(OH)_2D$ levels and of serum calcium levels to the Ellsworth-Howard protocol is too small to use these as diagnostic criteria; a more prolonged infusion of PTH is necessary for this purpose.

Clinical features of pseudohypoparathyroidism include those of hypocalcemia from other causes. The phenotype of Albright's hereditary osteodystrophy suggests type Ia, although it may be present in other types. Osteitis fibrosa cystica or osteomalacia suggests pseudohypoparathyroidism type II. Other hormone resistance syndromes may be present as well. Laboratory abnormalities (Table 22-9), as in hypoparathyroidism, include hypocalcemia, hyperphosphatemia, and a decreased serum 1,25$(OH)_2D_3$ concentration. The biochemical feature that distinguishes pseudohypoparathyroidism from hypoparathyroidism is an increased serum PTH concentration. The alkaline phosphatase may be increased in cases of type II pseudohypoparathyroidism when osteitis fibrosa cystica or osteomalacia is present. The Ellsworth-Howard test or its modifications[834] can be used to classify the type of pseudohypoparathyroidism. In this test, PTH is administered to the fasting patient after control serum and urine samples are obtained. Serum and urine are then collected during the first and second half-hours followed by the second and third hours after the PTH infusion. Samples are analyzed for cAMP, phosphorous, and creatinine. Normal and hypoparathyroid patients display a 10 to 20-fold increase in urinary cAMP excretion, while patients with pseudohypoparathyroidism, type I (a and b), have a markedly blunted response. Patients with pseudohypoparathyroidism, type II, have a normal cAMP response, but an abnormal phosphaturic response to PTH. This test has previously used bovine PTH or parathyroid extract, which is no longer available. Synthetic human PTH-(1-34), now approved, can be used, and protocols for its use have been developed.[835] Classification of the type of pseudohypoparathyroidism has no impact on the choice of therapy, however. Therapy for the hypocalcemic pseudohypoparathyroid patient is similar to that of the hypoparathyroid patient and involves the administration of calcium and vitamin D.

Autosomal Dominant Hypocalcemia

This disorder, which is the mirror image of familial hypocalciuric hypocalcemia, is characterized by mild to moderate and occasionally severe hypocalcemia with hyperphosphatemia, low normal plasma PTH concentrations, and a tendency toward hypomagnesemia.[40] The hypocalcemia is the result of activating mutations of the calcium-sensing receptor and can be viewed as a form of hypoparathyroidism in that the hypocalcemia is the result of insufficient circulating concentrations of PTH to maintain normocalcemia. Unlike hypoparathyroidism, there is a shift of the set point for PTH secretion downward such that it defends a stable, albeit lower than normal concentration of calcium.[836] In this

TABLE 22-9. Biochemical Findings in Hypocalcemic States

Diagnosis	Phosphate	PTH	25(OH)D	1,25$(OH)_2D_3$
Hypoparathyroidism	↑	↓	N	↓
Pseudohypoparathyroidism	↑	↑	N	↓
Vitamin D deficiency	↓	↑	↓	↓,N, ↑
Renal failure	↑	↑	N	↓
Severe liver disease	↓	↑	↓	↑,N
Nephrotic syndrome	↓	↑	↓	↓,N
Hypomagnesemia	N, ↑	↓	N	↓,N
Vitamin D dependent rickets, type I	↓	↑	N, ↑	↓
Vitamin D dependent rickets, type II	↓	↑	N, ↑	↑

setting, if EDTA is infused to lower the calcium even further, PTH will increase.[40] This demonstrates that there is not a deficiency of PTH per se, but rather a reset calciostat in the parathyroid glands.

A number of activating mutations have been described in affected kindreds (Fig. 22-7).[45,837,838] The disorder follows an autosomal dominant pattern of inheritance, although some cases report de novo activating mutations of the calcium-sensing receptor as a cause of sporadic hypocalcemia.[838,839] Most of the mutations are located in the extracellular domain of the calcium-sensing receptor.

Most patients with autsomal dominant hypocalcemia are aymptomatic, but occasionally they experience hypocalcemic symptoms such as carpopedal spasm and seizures. It is recommended that patients with this disorder be treated only if they are symptomatic because the usual therapy of hypocalcemia with vitamin D and calcium will result in excretion of twice the daily amount of urinary calcium compared with other forms of hypoparathyroidism,[837,838] even when the serum calcium is normal or subnormal. This could eventually result in the complications of nephrocalcinosis, nephrolithiasis, and reduced renal function. This hypercalciuria is a consequence of activated calcium-sensing receptors in the kidney that reduce renal tubular calcium reabsorption, a phenotype which is the mirror-image of familial hypocalciuric hypercalcemia.

As recommended by Brown, the diagnosis should be considered when the patient has a constellation of the following: (1) low-normal concentrations of serum PTH under treated conditions, (2) hypomagnesemia, (3) the occurrence of hypocalcemia in other family members with an autosomal dominant pattern of inheritance, and (4) a tendency to marked hypercalciuria that is accompanied by impaired renal function, nephrolithiasis, or nephrocalcinosis during treatment ith vitamin D and calcium.[40]

Vitamin D Abnormalities

Vitamin D deficiency as a cause of hypocalcemia may be due to an absolute deficiency of vitamin D or an abnormality in metabolism of vitamin D to the biologically active form, $1,25(OH)_2D_3$. Nutritional deficiency as a cause of vitamin D deficiency is rare in the United States because of supplementation of milk and food with vitamin D. Generally, it occurs in the elderly and poorly nourished alcoholics, particularly when combined with poor exposure to sunlight. Because vitamin D is a fat-soluble vitamin, vitamin D deficiency can also occur with fat malabsorptive states such as celiac disease, cystic fibrosis, chronic pancreatitis, primary biliary cirrhosis, and in short bowel syndromes and patients who have undergone gastrectomy. Anticonvulsant use is associated with vitamin D deficiency, although the mechanism is not entirely clear.[195] Phenobarbital is a potent inducer of hepatic microsomal enzymes and enhances the catabolism of vitamin D and 25(OH)D in the liver. Phenytoin does not have a direct effect on vitamin D catabolism but can lead to hypocalcemia through impaired calcium release from bone and reduced intestinal calcium absorption. In any event, anticonvulsant use increases the requirement for vitamin D. Hypocalcemia due to chronic renal disease is associated with decreased production of 1,25-dihydroxyvitamin D by the proximal renal tubule. There appears to be a correlation between the amount of functioning renal parenchyma and α-hydroxylase activity.[840] Hepatocellular disease may lead to vitamin D deficiency if it is severe enough to impair hydroxylation of 25-vitamin D to 25-hydroxyvitamin D.

Vitamin D-dependent rickets or osteomalacia refers to a group of syndromes associated with either abnormalities in the conversion of 25-hydroxyvitamin D to 1,25-dihydroxyvitamin D or resistance of target organs to active vitamin D metabolites. These are rare inborn errors of vitamin D metabolism that are characterized by all the clinical features of vitamin D deficiency despite adequate vitamin D intake and without a therapeutic response to the usual vitamin D replacement therapy. Patients with these disorders usually present early in life with hypocalcemia and rickets. Vitamin D-dependent rickets type I is due to defective activity of the renal 1-hydroxylase and is an autosomal recessive disorder. Patients with this disorder have low serum concentrations of $1,25(OH)_2D_3$, but respond to treatment with physiologic doses of $1,25(OH)_2D_3$ (calcitriol) with healing of rickets and normalization of hypocalcemia. Conversely, patients with vitamin D-dependent rickets, type II, have dramatically increased circulating concentrations of $1,25(OH)_2D_3$ and respond poorly to doses of calcitriol used to treat patients with vitamin D-dependent rickets, type I. These patients are resistant to the effects of $1,25(OH)_2D_3$ due to mutations in the vitamin D receptor.[296,841,842] In these patients, a series of point mutations in the vitamin D receptor have been described,[296] some in the DNA binding domain (leucine zipper) and some in the hormone binding domain. The site of these mutations determines the nature of impaired vitamin D receptor function, which may be represented by decreased hormone binding to the receptor, decreased affinity of the hormone for the receptor, deficient nuclear localization of the receptor, or decreased activation of target genes by hormone-receptor complexes. The type of receptor defect appears to predict whether the patient will respond to treatment with pharmacologic doses of active vitamin D metabolites, which is the treatment of choice. The presence of alopecia seems to be associated with a more severe form of the disease, but its relationship to the vitamin D resistance is unclear. Parenteral high dose calcium has been effective in healing rickets in the few patients that do not respond to active vitamin D metabolites.[843,844]

Clinical features of vitamin D deficiency include those due to hypocalcemia as well as bone mineralization defects. These defects, rickets in children and osteomalacia in adults, are characterized by bone pain, susceptibility to fracture, and subsequent deformity. Vitamin D deficiency is also accompanied by muscle weakness and tenderness, particularly in the proximal muscles of the lower extremities. The bone disease is characterized by impaired mineralization of newly formed bone that results in excess unmineralized bone matrix. In children, weight-bearing produces a bowing deformity of the long bones. The rachitic rosary, due to prominence of the costochondral junctions, is a characteristic feature. Diffuse bone pain is the most common manifestation of osteomalacia, although there is a tendency for localization of pain in the hip area.

Vitamin D deficiency with normal renal function is characterized by hypocalcemia and severe hypophosphatemia. The severe hypophosphatemia is a result of both decreased phosphate absorption from the gut and increased urinary phosphate excretion due to the development of secondary hyperparathyroidism. Serum PTH concentrations are increased due to hypocalcemia, and the serum alkaline phosphatase is also increased. When the vitamin D deficiency is due to nutritional causes, anticonvulsants or liver disease, the 25-hydroxyvitamin D (25(OH)D) concentration is low. Serum $1,25(OH)_2D_3$ concentrations may be low, normal, or increased, depending on the amount of substrate, 25(OH)D, available. If the vitamin D abnormality is due to chronic renal disease or deficiency of renal 1-hydroxylase, the 25(OH)D concentration will be normal

TABLE 22-10. Pharmacology of Vitamin D and Its Analogs

Characteristic	Calciferol (Ergocalciferol, Vitamin D_2)	Calcifediol (25-OH-D_3)	Dihydrotachysterol (DHT)	Calcitriol [1α25-$(OH)_2D_3$]	1α-Hydroxy-cholecalciferol*
Need for 25-hydroxylation	+	−	+	−	−
Need for 1-hydroxylation	+	+	−	−	−
Time for normocalcemia (weeks)†	4–8	2–4	1–2	0.5–1	1–2
Persistence after cessation (weeks)	6–18	4–12	1–3	0.5–1	1–2
Approximate daily dose (μg)	1,000–3,000 (40,000–20,000 U)‡	75–225	300–1,000	0.75–2.25	1–3
Dosage forms	50,000‡	20, 50 μg	0.125, 0.2, 0.4 mg	0.25, 0.5 μg	*

*Not available in United States.

†Can be decreased by use of loading dose.

‡40,000 U = 1 mg.

Source: Parfitt AM: Surgical, idiopathic, and other varieties of parathyroid hormone-deficient hypoparathyroidism, DeGroot LJ (ed): *Endocrinology*, Philadelphia, Saunders, 1989, pp 1049–1064.

and the $1,25(OH)_2D_3$ will be decreased. In cases of resistance to $1,25(OH)_2D_3$, serum 25(OH)D concentrations are normal and $1,25(OH)_2D_3$ concentrations are markedly increased.

Roentgenographically, vitamin D deficiency may show the characteristic features of osteomalacia including pseudofractures and osteopenia. Pseudofractures are lines of rarefaction that occur at sites where arteries cross bone and are often seen in the scapula, the pubic rami, and the ribs. Thin cortical radiolucent lines (stress fractures) at right angles to the bone shaft may be seen in osteomalacia. In children, rickets is characterized by irregular expansion of the growth plates. The growth plate is widened, cupped, and has an irregular appearance at the end of the metaphysis.

Vitamin D deficiency is corrected with administration of oral calcium and vitamin D. The form of vitamin D that is beneficial depends on the nature of the vitamin D abnormality and is discussed in the later section on treatment. Vitamin D preparations are listed in Table 22-10.

Medications

Hypocalcemia may result from a variety of medications, including those used to treat hypercalcemia and states of increased bone resorption such as bisphosphonates, plicamycin, calcitonin, gallium nitrate, and phosphates. As discussed earlier, anticonvulsants, phenobarbital, and phenytoin can cause hypocalcemia due to alterations in vitamin D metabolism. Blood, given as transfusion, and radiographic contrast dyes that contain EDTA and/or citrate may cause hypocalcemia by chelating calcium.[845,846] Fluoride may cause hypocalcemia, particularly when taken in excess, as illustrated recently when a town in Alaska experienced an outbreak of fluorosis due to excessive fluoride addition to the drinking water. Foscarnet, a pyrophosphate analog used to treat cytomegalovirus infections in patients with AIDS, can cause significant hypocalcemia by chelating calcium in the extracellular fluid as well as through induction of hypomagnesemia.[847] Other drugs used in the treatment of AIDS-related disorders, such as ketoconazole[848] and pentamidine, have been shown to induce hypocalcemia. Pentamidine causes renal magnesium wasting, leading to hypomagnesemia and subsequent hypocalcemia.[769] Finally, any other medication that causes hypomagnesemia can induce a functional hypoparathyroidism and subsequent hypocalcemia.

Biochemical abnormalities in medication-induced hypocalcemia depend on the mechanism involved. Those drugs that decrease bone resorption or complex calcium will be associated with an increased serum PTH concentration and normal vitamin D metabolites. The drugs that cause hypomagnesemia will be associated with an inappropriate decreased plasma PTH concentration. Finally, drugs that alter vitamin D metabolism will be associated with an increased serum PTH concentration and a decrease in the serum 25(OH)D concentration. Treatment of medication-associated hypocalcemia is to stop the offending agent when possible and/or supplement with calcium and vitamin D when appropriate. Magnesium should be replaced to maintain the magnesium concentration within the normal range when the offending drug causes magnesium wasting. This may be necessary after discontinuation of the drug as magnesium wasting may continue if the drug half-life is particularly long.

Hypocalcemia Associated with Malignant Disease

Osteoblastic metastases, most commonly associated with prostate and breast cancer, can cause profound hypocalcemia as a consequence of accelerated bone formation.[849] Tumor cells in bone may produce growth factors that stimulate osteoblastic bone formation and, as a result, there is enhanced calcium entry into the skeleton. Affected patients have widespread osteoblastic metastases or osteosclerosis evident on plain radiography and marked increases in the serum alkaline phosphatase.

Another potential cause of hypocalcemia associated with malignancy is tumor lysis, which may occur as a consequence of successful therapy of neoplastic disease.[850] This is often seen during therapy of hematologic malignancies, particularly high-grade lymphomas, in which a large amount of tumor cells are lysed in a short period of time. This leads to the release of intracellular ions such as phosphate and potassium into the extracellular fluid. The resultant hyperphosphatemia leads to hypocalcemia. Patients may also develop renal failure and hyperuricemia.

The majority of patients with cancer and apparent hypocalcemia are not hypocalcemic at all, but rather have hypoalbuminemia and a normal ionized calcium concentration. True hypocalcemia associated with malignancy is usually of rapid onset and may be associated with profound symptoms of hypocalcemia. In the absence of other medications that may cause hypocalcemia in a cancer patient, such as bisphosphonates, plicamycin, or gallium nitrate, the diagnosis is usually obvious. The serum PTH concentration is increased and vitamin D metabolites should be normal. Magnesium deficiency should also be excluded as cancer patients often receive drugs that cause renal magnesium wasting, such as amphotericin B. In this case, serum PTH concentration should be inappropriately decreased, indicating the functional hypoparathyroidism associated with hypomagnesemia. Treatment of malignancy-associated hypocalcemia involves supplemental calcium and vitamin D. If the hypocalcemia is severe, symptomatic and potentially life-threatening parenteral calcium should be administered as discussed later.

Other Diseases Associated with Hypocalcemia

Chronic renal insufficiency is almost always associated with hypocalcemia, which occurs by several mechanisms. As kidney function declines, 1-hydroxylase activity decreases proportionately. Thus, there is decreased hydroxylation of 25-hydroxyvitamin D to 1,25-dihydroxyvitamin D, the biologically active metabolite. Serum $1,25(OH)_2D_3$ concentrations decline below normal when the glomerular filtration rate reaches 30 to 50 mL/minute and are approximately 20 percent of normal in those patients with glomerular filtration rate <1 mL/minute.[840] Anephric patients usually have undetectable serum concentrations of $1,25(OH)_2D_3$.[851] This leads to decreased calcium absorption from the gastrointestinal tract. Additionally, as renal function declines, phosphate excretion decreases and affected patients develop hyperphosphatemia. The serum calcium concentration is further decreased by calcium binding to phosphate. Patients with chronic renal failure who have intact parathyroid function will respond to this hypocalcemia by increasing PTH secretion. The calcium concentration will then increase, mostly at the expense of the increased bone resorption stimulated by PTH. When this is longstanding, patients will develop parathyroid hyperplasia and parathyroid bone disease. This secondary hyperparathyroidism, which is a significant cause of morbidity in chronic renal failure patients, can be prevented by adequate calcium and vitamin D supplementation early in the course of renal insufficiency.

Hypocalcemia is occasionally associated with pancreatitis. The mechanisms may be multifactorial and related to the association of acute pancreatitis with acute renal failure, or increased circulating concentrations of calcitonin that lower the serum calcium, or possibly the release of pancreatic enzymes that cause calcium deposition at sites of fat necrosis to form insoluble calcium soaps.[852] However, the amount of calcium deposited in areas of fat necrosis is unlikely to be sufficient to account for the hypocalcemia. Glucagon release has also been implicated as a potential mechanism. Whenever patients with acute pancreatitis are normocalcemic or hypercalcemic, then primary hyperparathyroidism should be considered, because occasionally primary hyperparathyroidism can present as acute pancreatitis. Toxic shock syndrome and bacteremic septic shock can be associated with hypocalcemia through mechanisms that remain unclear. It is possible that mediators of septic shock, such as tumor necrosis factor and interleukin-1, may be responsible for the hypocalcemia. Hypocalcemia in these situations should be treated symptomatically.

Neonatal hypocalcemia may be the result of congenital hypoparathyroidism, or transient hypoparathyroidism caused by a hypercalcemic state in the mother such as hyperparathyroidism or FHH. Hypocalcemia appears to be more common in premature infants, particularly those of diabetic mothers and those with the respiratory distress syndrome. The mechanisms that cause hypocalcemia in this situation are unclear, but the hypocalcemic state is usually temporary and should be treated symptomatically.

Approach to the Hypocalcemic Patient

Together with knowledge of the clinical circumstances, the serum levels of calcium, magnesium, and phosphorus and a confirmatory determination of the serum PTH level will often suffice for the differential diagnosis of hypocalcemia. Unless there is a history of recent neck surgery, acute development of hypocalcemia suggests that one of the acute antecedent conditions listed has overwhelmed the homeostatic system. When one is armed with this idea, the cause of hypocalcemia (Table 22-6) is usually obvious. In addition to measuring serum phosphorus, creatinine, and PTH, it is important to exclude hypomagnesemia as a cause of functional hypoparathyroidism.

In a chronically hypocalcemic patient, the presence of *hyper*phospatemia suggests a failure of secretion of PTH (hypoparathyroidism) or of the response to PTH (pseudohypoparathyroidism) unless renal insufficiency is present. The genesis of hypocalcemia in renal failure is a complex issue. Renal failure rarely causes hypocalcemia unless it is profound (creatinine clearance less than 15 ml/min). Conversely, *hypo*phosphatemia will often be present in a chronically hypocalcemic patient if the parathyroid glands can respond. The combination of hypocalcemia and hypophosphatemia is seen in states of excessive skeletal mineralization (hungry bones syndrome) and in disorders of the vitamin D endocrine system. In both instances, the presence of secondary hyperparathyroidism can be confirmed by direct assay of PTH.

Diagnostic Evaluation of Hypocalcemia

The diagnosis of hypocalcemia should be based on the corrected calcium concentration and, if in doubt, an ionized calcium should be measured. Ionized calcium measurements may be more useful than total calcium in the critically ill patient. Etiology of the hypocalcemia should be sought as it will impact on the ultimate therapy. As with hypercalcemia, the cause of the hypocalcemia is often evident from the history, physical examination, and routine laboratory evaluation that includes phosphate, protein, BUN, creatinine, and liver function tests. Most hypocalcemic patients with hyperphosphatemia and normal renal function will have idiopathic or acquired hypoparathyroidism or pseudohypoparathyroidism. Because medications are also a significant cause of hypocalcemia, careful attention should be paid to exactly what drugs the patient has been receiving. The nutritional status of the hypocalcemic patient should be considered, particularly in the elderly or alcoholic patient, as vitamin D deficiency as a cause of hypocalcemia is not uncommon. The clinical situation should also alert one to the cause of the hypocalcemia. A hypocalcemic patient seen in the period following a neck operation should suggest hypoparathyroidism, while severe symptomatic hypocalcemia in a cancer patient should suggest osteoblastic metastases or tumor lysis as the cause for hypocalcemia. The presence of other endocrine abnormalities should suggest either hypoparathyroidism in association with the polyglandular autoimmune syndrome or pseudohypoparathyroidism in association with other hormone resistance syndromes. Magnesium deficiency should always be considered as the hypocalcemic patient will remain resistant to therapy until magnesium is replete. Clinical settings for severe hypomagnesemia include ethanol abuse, chronic diarrhea, diuretics, hyperalimentation, posttreatment for diabetic ketoacidosis and after administration of gentamicin, cisplatinum, amphotericin, and cyclosporin. Initial diagnostic testing should include serum concentrations of PTH, magnesium, and vitamin D metabolites, 25(OH)D, and $1,25(OH)_2D_3$. Biochemical abnormalities for various hypocalcemic states are illustrated in Table 22-9. Additional tests that may be helpful when considering vitamin D deficiency and osteomalacia include serum alkaline phosphatase (bone-specific when possible) and radiographs of particular bones that may be painful to the patient. Bone biopsy may be indicated if osteomalacia is suspected. The renal responsiveness to PTH may be tested using the modification of the Ellsworth-Howard test.[853]

Treatment of Hypocalcemia

The objectives of treatment of the hypocalcemic patient are (1) to increase the serum calcium concentration into the range in which symptoms and complications directly related to hypocalcemia do not occur; (2) to prevent skeletal deformity due to secondary hyperparathyroidism, in those situations where chronic hypocalcemia is present; (3) to avoid hypercalciuria and hypercalcemia and their consequences; and (4) in children, to promote normal growth and development.

Indications for Treatment

In general, all patients with signs or symptoms of hypocalcemia should be treated. The absolute concentration of the serum calcium as well as the rate of the fall in the calcium concentration are important points to consider in determining how quickly the hypocalcemia should be reversed. Total calcium concentration, corrected for albumin, of <7.5 mg/dL in a patient with or without symptoms is an indication for treatment.

Urgent Treatment

Hypocalcemia may be associated with severe and life-threatening symptoms, in which case urgent treatment with parenteral calcium is indicated. Patients that require immediate attention may exhibit a positive Chvostek's or Trousseau's sign, seizures, papilledema, hypotension, and prolonged ST segment and QT intervals on EKG, with or without arrhythmia. This is most likely to occur in the postsurgical setting when the parathyroids are damaged and onset of hypoparathyroidism is abrupt. It may also occur in the patient with widespread osteoblastic metastases, tumor lysis, acute pancreatitis, or hungry bone syndrome. In any of these situations, the hypocalcemia is usually of abrupt onset and associated with significant symptoms. Thus, the calcium concentration should be corrected rapidly. For frank tetany, 10 to 20 mL of calcium gluconate (90 mg elemental calcium in 10 mL), diluted in 50–100 mL of 5 percent dextrose, should be infused intravenously over 10 minutes.[854] During infusion, continuous cardiac monitoring should be instituted, particularly if the patient is digitalized, as serious cardiac arrhythmias may occur. This procedure should be repeated as necessary to control symptomatic hypocalcemia. When there is an ongoing process leading to recurrent and symptomatic hypocalcemia, a continuous infusion of calcium gluconate should be instituted to provide 10–15 mg/kg of elemental calcium over approximately 6–8 hours. Calcium chloride can also be used but is more irritating at the site of venous access. Likewise, infusions containing >200 mg/100 mL of elemental calcium should be avoided because of propensity for irritation of veins and soft tissues, if extravasation at the site of the venous catheter should occur. If hypocalcemia is likely to persist, therapy should be initiated early with oral calcium supplements (1–2 g elemental calcium) and calcitriol (0.5–1.0 μg) daily.

The magnesium deficient patient that is hypocalcemic will require treatment of the hypomagnesemia before the hypocalcemia will resolve. Magnesium sulfate can be administered intramuscularly or intravenously. A dose of 16 mEq magnesium intramuscularly three times daily is usually effective in normalizing the calcium concentration.[855] Intramuscular injections may be painful, in which case a continuous infusion of 48 mEq magnesium/24 hr may be administered. Magnesium therapy should continue for several days in order to restore intracellular magnesium. If magnesium losses are ongoing, therapy should be appropriately continued. The dose of magnesium should be reduced by 50 percent in patients with renal insufficiency, and the serum magnesium concentration should be followed closely.

Chronic Treatment

Once it has been determined that the patient will need long-term treatment for hypocalcemia, oral supplementation with calcium and vitamin D should be started. Most patients with chronic hypocalcemia will require both calcium (1–2 g elemental) and vitamin D to maintain a serum calcium concentration in the low normal range.

A variety of vitamin D preparations are available, and the choice will depend on biological activity, cost, and duration of effect. The particular vitamin D abnormality involved should also be considered when determining the appropriate preparation. Simplistically, $1,25(OH)_2D_3$ (calcitriol) could be used for treatment of all chronic hypocalcemic states as it is the biologically active form of vitamin D, but its cost may preclude this. The principal advantages of calcitriol are its rapid onset and short duration of action. This minimizes the duration of hypercalcemia should overdosage occur. Theoretically, it is advantageous for use in hypoparathyroidism, pseudohypoparathyroidism, and renal failure as these states are characterized by a deficiency of $1,25(OH)_2D_3$. However, treatment with high doses of cholecalciferol, ergocalciferol, or calcifediol will increase serum concentrations of 25-hydroxyvitamin D enough to act directly on the vitamin D receptor. 25-hydroxyvitamin D binds to the vitamin D receptor, but with an affinity that is three orders of magnitude lower than that of $1,25(OH)_2D_3$. These preparations also have a longer duration of action than calcitriol and could result in prolonged toxicity due to hypercalcemia should overdosage occur. The major advantage of these preparations over calcitriol is cost. In malabsorption, there is a deficiency of vitamin D itself so that it would be appropriate to treat with the parent vitamin D compound, ergocalciferol. In severe liver disease, because the formation of 25-hydroxyvitamin D is impaired, calcifediol may be used as the form of vitamin D replacement. Dihydrotachysterol (DHT), a synthetic analog of $1,25(OH)_2D_3$ that was once more popular than it is today, has similar biologic activity to calcitriol. DHT is hydroxylated in the liver to 25-hydroxydihydrotachysterol, which is the major circulating active form of the drug.

Changes in vitamin D requirements may occur as a consequence of concomitant administration of drugs such as anticonvulsants, thiazide diuretics, oral contraceptives, and antacids, or the development of electrolyte disturbances such as hypomagnesemia or hyperphosphatemia. Requirements may also change during pregnancy due to changes in estrogen[856] and production of $1,25(OH)_2D_3$ by the placenta.[207] It is advisable to choose the most appropriate vitamin D preparation and stick with it in most patients. If a new preparation must be instituted, then a useful rule is to use one-third less to decrease the risks of toxicity.

Given along with vitamin D, 1–2 g of elemental calcium should be sufficient to satisfy the objectives of therapy. The dose of calcium should be adjusted to maintain the total serum calcium concentration in the low normal range (8.0–9.0 mg/dl) with the 24-hour urinary calcium excretion not exceeding 250 mg. Higher serum calcium concentrations are associated with hypercalciuria which, if longstanding, may result in nephrolithiasis, nephrocalcinosis, or impaired renal function. Calcium carbonate has the greatest amount of elemental calcium (40 percent) and is relatively inexpensive. However, it may not be absorbed by achlorhydric patients unless given with food.[857] Calcium citrate is better absorbed in the achlorhydric state. Calcium gluconate is more palatable than the other preparations, but is also more expensive. Addition of a thiazide diuretic may decrease vitamin D requirements by decreasing urinary excretion of calcium when used in combination with moderate salt restriction.[730]

Foods that are high in phosphate content (milk and dairy products) should be limited to avoid hyperphosphatemia. The presence of hyperphosphatemia may cause soft tissue calcification and make the achievement of eucalcemia difficult. Although the use of phosphate-binding antacids may be used in this situation it will not be necessary in the majority of patients as restoration of serum calcium concentration decreases renal threshold of phosphorus excretion and lowers serum phosphorus concentration.

DISORDERS OF PHOSPHATE METABOLISM

Phosphate Homeostasis

Intracellular and Extracellular Phosphate

The total body content of phosphate is about 1 percent of body weight. About 85 percent is contained in the skeleton, and most extraskeletal phosphate is intracellular. Phosphate is the principal intracellular anion, with a total cellular concentration of 100 mmol/liter, most of which is present as metabolically crucial organic phosphates (ATP, other nucleotides, sugar phosphates, etc). Organic phosphate in cells plays a number of roles. When linked to the purines or pyrimidines of DNA, it has a structural role; in membranes, phosphate-containing phospholipids help create the physicochemical features of membrane bilayers with hydrophobic interiors and hydrophilic (charged) layers to interface with the cytoplasm on one side and ECF on the other side. Phosphate is covalently attached to or removed from ATP and ADP via high-energy bonds for the generation, storage, or utilization of energy. It has been estimated that the intracellular concentration of *free* inorganic phosphate is only about 1 mmol/liter,[858] and because of metabolic demands, this small pool must turn over rapidly. It is not understood how intracellular free phosphate levels are regulated, although they appear to be,[858] but the rapid entry of phosphate into cells that occurs together with the entry and metabolism of carbohydrates can be viewed as a mechanism for maintaining this pool.

Phosphate in plasma and extracellular fluid is in dynamic equilibrium not only with the exterior and with bone (Fig. 22-55)

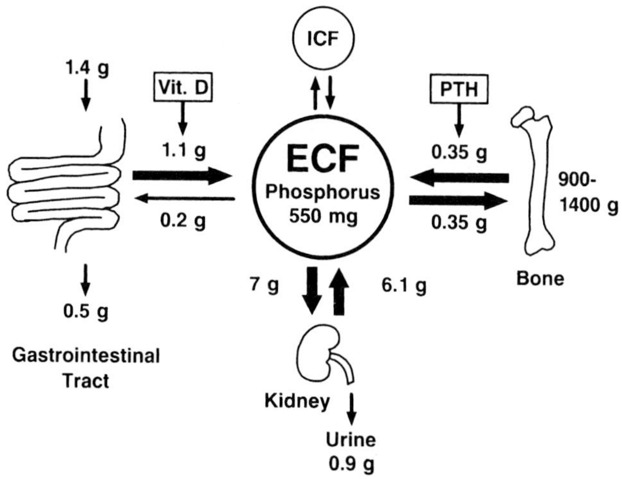

FIGURE 22-55. Schematic representation of phosphorus flux and balance in a normal human. Arrows indicate the direction of movement of phosphorus between the gut, kidneys, and extracellular fluid (ECF). Modulation of flux by vitamin D (Vit. D) or parathyroid hormone (PTH) is shown; the direction of hormonal influence on flux is indicated by the positioning of each hormone directly over the effect which that hormone increases. The numeric values indicate quantities of elemental phosphorus stored or transferred in a 24-h period. The intensities of the arrows indicate relative magnitude of flux.

but also with the larger intracellular pool. In adults, the serum concentration of inorganic phosphorus is 0.8 to 1.5 mmol/liter (2.5 to 4.5 mg/dl). In growing children, the serum concentration is higher, averaging 1.5 to 1.6 mmol/liter (4.5 to 5.0 mg/dl) during the first 15 years of life. Because the buffer pair HPO_4^{-2}/H_2PO_4- has a pK_a of 6.8, both monovalent and divalent phosphate ions are present in blood at a ratio dependent on the blood pH. For clinical purposes, the level in serum or urine is expressed as the concentration of phosphorus, because precise conversion to a molar concentration of phosphate would require knowledge of the blood pH. Thus, we refer clinically to measurements of serum phosphorus, recognizing that the ion in question is actually phosphate. About 25 percent of inorganic phosphate in serum is protein-bound, but 90 percent is filterable because of the Gibbs-Donnan equilibrium.

The serum concentration of phosphorus is not as closely regulated as is the concentration of calcium. The fasting concentration is set primarily by the renal phosphate threshold. This contrasts markedly with the complex regulation of the serum calcium concentration, which occurs at the boundaries of the extracellular fluid with bone, the gut, and the kidney. Serum phosphorus levels may fall after meals as phosphate enters cells together with carbohydrates. This postcibal change is superimposed on a marked diurnal variation, with the nadir at 11 A.M. and a peak at about 4 A.M.[859]

Intestinal Absorption of Phosphate

The normal diet contains 800 to 2,000 mg of phosphorus per day. Throughout this range, approximately 60 percent of dietary phosphate is absorbed (Fig. 22-55). This is higher than the 20 percent of calcium normally absorbed and is relatively independent of the intake of phosphate. The linearity of phosphate absorption is consistent with absorption primarily by a diffusional process without a large saturable component.

Most foods contain phosphates, but the most important dietary sources are dairy products, grains, and meats. In the American diet, food additives present in baked goods, cheeses, and carbonated beverages can contribute as much as 30 percent of the dietary phosphate intake. Organic phosphate is released during the digestive process. Phosphate is absorbed most efficiently in the duodenum and jejunum, but as with calcium, the greatest net absorption may be from the ileum. Phosphate absorption can be reduced by a high intake of calcium or by aluminum hydroxide–containing compounds, because both calcium and aluminum bind phosphate to form relatively insoluble salts in the intestinal lumen.

Little is understood about the cellular basis of phosphate absorption.[320] The absorption can be passive or active. With a transepithelial potential difference of 3 mV (lumen negative), the Ussing equation predicts passive phosphate reabsorption of phosphate anion by the paracellular route when the luminal concentration exceeds 1.5 mmol/liter, as probably occurs postprandially. This is probably the quantitatively most significant process. A separate cellular pathway for phosphate uptake involves sodium-coupled phosphate entry by a carrier in the brush border membrane. Energy for this electrochemically uphill process is provided by the sodium gradient, which is maintained by sodium-potassium ATPase. The exit of phosphate across the basolateral membrane into the blood may be passive. It is thought that vitamin D primarily regulates sodium-coupled phosphate entry (see earlier discussion).[320] Vitamin D deficiency can reduce intestinal phosphate absorption, but this has little impact on the adaptation to changing dietary intake.

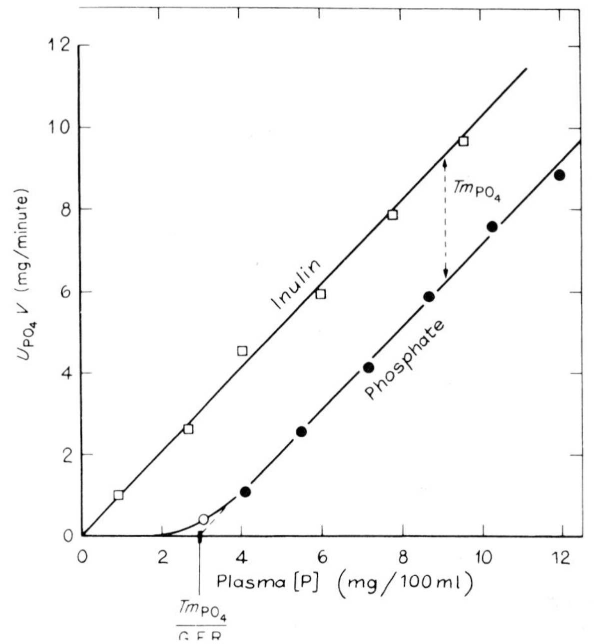

FIGURE 22-56. The relation between the plasma phosphorus concentration (mg/dl) and the urinary excretion rate of phosphate (mg/min) in a normal individual while fasting (○) and during an intravenous infusion of phosphate (●). Also shown is the relation between the urinary excretion rate and the plasma concentration of inulin when inulin was simultaneously infused. The slopes of the lines through the inulin and phosphate data are identical and are numerically equal to the glomerular filtration. The vertical distance between the two lines is the maximum rate of tubular reabsorption of phosphate (TmP/GFR) in mg/dl. (*By permission of Bijvoet OLM, Clin Sci 37:23, 1969.*)

Renal Phosphate Handling

Of the filtered load of phosphate, 80 to 97 percent is normally reabsorbed. The level of renal phosphate reabsorption defines the concentration of phosphate in serum and is thus an important contributor to extracellular mineral homeostasis. Renal phosphate reabsorption can be quantified as the fractional excretion (C_p/C_{creat}) or as tubular resorption of phosphorus ($1\text{-}C_p/C_{creat}$) but is best expressed as the theoretical renal phosphate threshold (TmP/GFR).[860] Because the renal phosphate threshold sets the serum phosphorus concentration, the normal range of TmP/GFR (2.5 to 4.2 mg/dl) closely mirrors the normal range of serum phosphorus. Although the TmP/GFR can be measured by infusion of phosphate (Fig. 22-56), this is impractical clinically, and so it is usually estimated from measurements of serum and urinary phosphorus and creatinine using a nomogram (Fig. 22-57), (see also testing, later). Renal phosphate handling is deranged in renal insufficiency, and the TmP/GFR is not readily interpretable with a GFR less than 30 ml/min.

Under normal circumstances, phosphate reabsorption is essentially limited to the proximal tubule.[861,862] The proximal convoluted tubule reabsorbs about 75 percent of filtered phosphate, and most of the remainder is reabsorbed in the proximal straight tubule. Although distal tubule segments may have a limited capacity for reabsorption of phosphate (5 percent of filtered load), this is evident experimentally mainly after acute parathyroidectomy and is probably not of physiologic importance.

The rate-limiting step for phosphate reabsorption in the proximal tubule is sodium-coupled phosphate entry through the apical membrane via a carrier.[102,862,863] Entry is thus driven by the energy of the sodium gradient, which is maintained by Na-K ATPase. This process is largely electroneutral, involving carriage of divalent phosphate with two equivalents of sodium, but a small component is electrogenic, probably involving the transport of monovalent phosphate together with two equivalents of sodium. Phosphate exit across the basolateral membrane is primarily diffusive and is driven by the electrochemical potential difference (interior negative) maintained by Na-K ATPase. An anion exchange mechanism also may contribute to the exit of phosphorus, but the counterion has not been identified.[862–864]

The most important factors regulating proximal phosphate reabsorption are PTH and the dietary phosphate intake. The cellular basis for the effect of PTH was discussed earlier. It is dependent on cAMP as an intracellular mediator, requires a cAMP-dependent protein kinase,[865] and probably involves phosphorylation of the apical sodium-phosphate transporter or a regulatory component, although this has not been demonstrated directly. By resetting the renal phosphate threshold, PTH allows the kidney to compensate for changes in bone resorption. Teleologically, the phosphaturic effect of PTH tends to prevent increases in serum phosphate, which would result from release of phosphate from bone together with calcium in hyperparathyroid states, from dampening the homeostatic increase in the serum calcium concentration by complexing calcium. This protective mechanism is inoperative in renal failure, where the hypocalcemic effect of phosphate released from bone in patients with secondary hyperparathyroidism is an important contributor to progressive hyperparathyroidism as part of a positive feedback loop. PTHrP mimics the action of PTH on the renal reabsorption of phosphate.

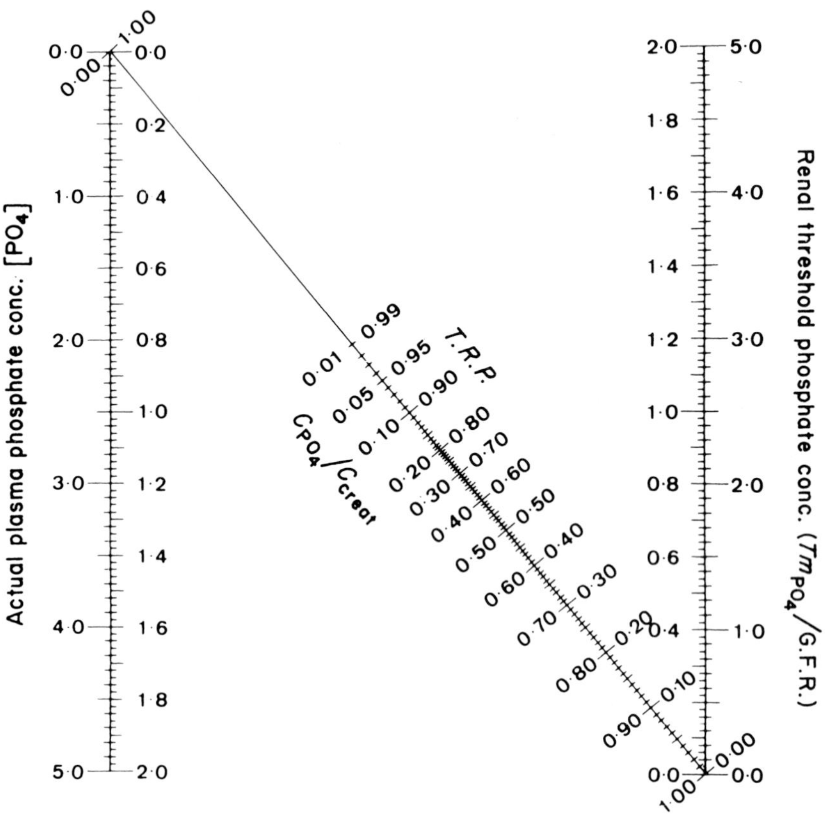

FIGURE 22-57. Nomogram for deriving TmP/GFR from known values for serum phosphorus and the fractional excretion of phosphorus (C_{Pi}/C_{creat}) or TRP. The estimation of (C_{Pi}/C_{creat}) and TRP is described in the section on testing. The outer scale on each ordinate represents units as mg/dl, and the inner scale on each ordinate represents units as mmol/liter. The diagonal connecting the two ordinates has a scale for values for TRP to the right and a scale for values for (C_{Pi}/C_{creat}) to the left. A straight line through the appropriate values for serum phosphorus concentrations and (C_{Pi}/C_{creat}) (or TRP) intersects the TmP scale at the appropriate value for TmP/GFR. The scale used (mg/dl or mmol/liter) must be the same. All data in the text are presented as mg/dl. For example, at a serum phosphorus concentration of 2.5 mg/dl and a C_{Pi}/C_{creat} of 0.14, the TmP/GFR is 2.3 mg/dl. *(By permission of Walton RJ, Bijvoet OLM, Lancet, i:309, 1975.)*

The effect of phosphate intake on urinary phosphate handling is independent of PTH. Under conditions of phosphate deprivation, the TmP is increased until phosphate reabsorption is virtually quantitative.[866] The adaptation involves an increase in the V_{max} for phosphate without a change in K_m and probably reflects the insertion of additional transporters into the apical membrane.[861,862,867] This process occurs over days and probably involves both genomic and nongenomic mechanisms. It cannot be overridden by infusion of phosphaturic agents such as PTH. With continual phosphate deprivation, the serum phosphorus concentration eventually falls. In this circumstance, homeostatic mechanisms have been overridden and the renal tubule is no longer able to regulate the serum phosphorus levels.

Other clinically relevant factors that regulate phosphate reabsorption include other hormones, acid-base status, and the level of serum calcium.[861,862] *Growth hormone* increases renal phosphate reabsorption,[868] largely accounting for the finding of hyperphosphatemia in acromegaly. *Insulin* also appears to have a direct ability to increase proximal phosphate reabsorption, independent of its effects on glucose entry. *Glucocorticoids* directly inhibit phosphate reabsorption, and this may be evident clinically as hypophosphatemia in Cushing's syndrome.[869] *Calcitonin* in high concentrations has a phosphaturic effect; it is not clear that this is physiologically significant.[167,168] The ability of *vitamin D* to increase proximal reabsorption of phosphate was discussed earlier. The bisphosphonate etidronate disodium also increases renal phosphate reabsorption.

Acidosis both acute and chronic, causes phosphaturia. This is at least partly due to titration of phosphate as tubule fluid is acidified, as monovalent phosphate is transported less well than is the divalent form. Chronically, the number of transporters may also be increased.[870] The increased phosphate excretion provides a urinary buffer for the excretion of acid and also provides for the excretion of phosphate liberated as part of the buffering of metabolic acidosis by bone. In this way, the kidney and bone cooperate in the response to acidosis. Although acute *hypercalcemia* has complex effects on renal phosphate handling, chronic hypercalcemia appears uniformly to decrease renal phosphate reabsorption.[757] This may account for the fall in serum phosphate often observed with treatment of hypoparathyroidism and in some cases for the hypophosphatemia associated with hypercalcemia in malignancy.

Disorders Causing Hypophosphatemia

Hypophosphatemia and phosphate depletion can result from decreased intake or dietary absorption, increased renal losses, or shifts of phosphate into the intracellular space (Table 22-11). The elements of the defense against hypophosphatemia are shown in Fig. 22-58. The primary lines of defense are adaptive increases in the intrinsic phosphate-reabsorbing capacity of the renal tubule, increased renal synthesis of $1\alpha,25\text{-}(OH)_2D$ (which increases intestinal phosphorus and calcium absorption), and increases resorption of bone. The net effect is to protect the serum phosphorus concentration and body phosphate stores, with secondary increases in calcium influx from bone and gut, which, together with suppression of PTH, may give rise to hypercalciuria. Hypophosphatemia can be a manifestation of depleted body phosphate stores, but the correlation is imperfect. With acute shifts of phosphate induced by glucose and insulin or by respiratory alkalosis, transient severe hypophosphatemia may occur in the face of unchanged stores of total body phosphate. A reduction in the renal phosphate threshold (e.g., in hyperparathyroidism) will also

TABLE 22-11. Causes of Hypophosphatemia

Disorders of phosphorus intake and absorption
- Starvation
- Malabsorption, diarrhea
- Continuous nasogastric suction
- Phosphorus-binding antacids*

Renal phosphorus losses
- Diuresis (saline infusion, loop and thiazide diuretics, acetazolamide, osmotic diuresis)
- First-, second-, or third-degree hyperparathyroidism
- Humoral hypercalcemia of malignancy
- Oncogenic osteomalacia
- X-linked hypophosphatemia
- Chronic metabolic acidosis
- Bicarbonate therapy
- Hypercalcemia
- Calcitonin therapy
- Cushing's syndrome
- After renal transplant

Extracellular-intracellular shifts
- Respiratory alkalosis*
- Diabetic ketoacidosis*
- Glucose and insulin therapy*
- Nutritional recovery*

Shifts into bone
- Osteoblastic metastases
- Hungry bones syndrome

Miscellaneous conditions
- Alcoholism*
- Burns
- Sepsis
- Dialysis against phosphorus-poor dialysate

*Causes severe hypophosphatemia.

induce mild hypophosphatemia without by itself influencing body stores of phosphate. Conversely, in states of chronically diminished phosphate intake, renal adaptation will essentially eliminate urinary excretion and thus maintain a relatively normal serum phosphorus level in the face of reduced stores until body stores have been markedly depleted.

Hypophosphatemia with levels below 0.3 mmol/liter (1 mg/dl) is thought of as severe.[871,872] As indicated in Table 22-11, profound hypophosphatemia is primarily associated with chronic antacid abuse, alcohol abuse, diabetic ketoacidosis, respiratory alkalosis, hyperalimentation, and the nutritional recovery syndrome. There are many clinical consequences of severe hypophosphatemia with phosphate deficiency. Metabolic encephalopathy may occur. Erythrocyte glycolysis is impeded by dysfunction of glyceraldehyde-3-phosphate dehydrogenase, limiting the formation of ATP and 2,3-DPG.[873] Reduced levels of erythrocyte 2,3-DPG and ATP shift the oxyhemoglobin dissociation curve to the left, reducing oxygen release in the periphery, and can rarely produce hemolytic anemia, which is generally not life-threatening. Depletion of muscle phosphocreatine can induce clinically significant weakness or even rhabdomyolysis. Rhabdomyolysis occurs in profoundly phosphate-depleted patients with alcoholism or during nutritional recovery.[874] Myocardial dysfunction has been reported.[875] Phosphate is required for the mineralization of bone, and chronic hypophosphatemia can produce osteomalacia.[876,877] Profound hypophosphatemia with phosphate deficiency may also produce metabolic acidosis. It is plausible that many of these complications result from a reduction in tissue ATP stores, but this has rarely been shown directly.

FIGURE 22-58. The sequence of adjustments initiated in response to hypophosphatemia.

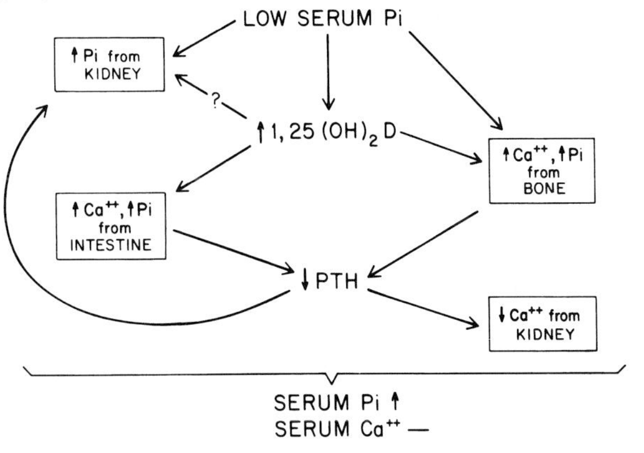

Increased Renal Excretion

A variety of systemic states and renal disorders can result in a fall in the renal phosphate threshold and hypophosphatemia (Table 22-11). In general, these disorders produce only moderate hypophosphatemia that is rarely symptomatic and do not by themselves lead to phosphate depletion. Primary hyperparathyroidism and malignancy-associated hypercalcemia are among the systemic disorders that give rise to hypophosphatemia. Renal tubule disorders include heritable diseases such as X-linked hypophosphatemic rickets and acquired tubule disorders such as oncogenic osteomalacia,[270] Fanconi syndrome, osmotic diuresis, diuretic therapy, bicarbonate administration, and glucocorticoid therapy. Patients with X-linked hypophosphatemia have a reduced sodium–phosphate transport in the proximal tubule. The gene for X-linked hypophosphatemia has been mapped to chromosome Xp22-1. The gene is termed PEX, and has been shown to be mutated in X-linked hypophosphatemia.[878] PEX codes for a yet unidentified neutral endopeptidase hypothesized to be responsible for the degradation of a phosphaturic hormone known as "phosphatonin."[879] Oncogenic osteomalacia is hypophosphatemia associated with a malignant tumor that generates the substance "phosphatonin" that inhibits the renal tubular reabsorption of phosphate.[880]

Decreased Absorption

Phosphate is ubiquitous in foodstuffs, and dietary deficiency short of starvation does not by itself produce profound hypophosphatemia. Chronic diarrheal states do not by themselves induce severe phosphate wasting, but intestinal malabsorption syndrome can result in a decreased phosphate and vitamin D absorption. Vitamin D deficiency can also lead to hypophosphatemia. Another common cause of hypophosphatemia is alcohol abuse due to poor intake, vomiting, and use of antacids. Chronic abuse or rigorous use of phosphate-binding antacids can produce osteomalacia with bone pain, increased alkaline phosphatase, marked hypercalciuria, and increased levels of 1α,25-$(OH)_2D$.[876,877]

Respiratory Alkalosis

Acute respiratory alkalosis from hyperventilation may produce transient severe hypophosphatemia.[881] It is thought that the resulting intracellular alkalosis markedly activates glycolysis with a rapid flux of free phosphate into sugar phosphates, leading to a dramatic shift of phosphate into the intracellular space. The finding of severe hypophosphatemia in a patient presenting with tetany sometimes leads to an extensive evaluation of calcium and phosphate metabolism when the only real disorder is hyperventilation. In recent years, it has become evident that moderate hypophosphatemia often results from treatment of respiratory failure.[882,883] The acute shifts with mechanical hyperventilation may be superimposed on previous renal losses of phosphate occasioned by respiratory acidosis or by therapy with glucocorticoids, diuretics, or xanthines. Hypophosphatemia produces reversible respiratory muscle dysfunction[884] and sometimes acute respiratory failure.[885] Respiratory muscle weakness is associated with depleted stores of phosphocreatine in muscle.[886] Treatment of moderate hypophosphatemia may markedly improve respiratory muscle function.[884,885]

Diabetic Ketoacidosis

Both metabolic acidosis and osmotic diuresis produce urinary phosphate wasting, but the resultant phosphate deficit is obscured by shifts of phosphate into the extracellular space because of acidosis and insulin deficiency, and ketoacidotic patients present with normal or elevated serum phosphorus levels. Treatment with insulin and glucose produces rapid shifts into the intracellular space and a fall in the serum phosphorus (Fig. 22-59). The serum phosphorus rarely falls below 0.3 mmol/liter (1 mg/dl) unless there was a long prodrome of polyuria with chronic phosphate wasting. Controlled studies indicate that routine treatment of hypophosphatemia in diabetic ketoacidosis is not beneficial.[887] However, severely hypophosphatemic patients could benefit from phosphate replacement. Precise guidelines for phosphate replacement in diabetic ketoacidosis have not been agreed on.

Nutritional Recovery

Severe hypophosphatemia is precipitated by refeeding after chronic protein-calorie malnutrition. Originally seen as a fatal complication of refeeding survivors of concentration camps after World War II, hypophosphatemia also occurs during the first 2 to 5 days of enteral and parenteral hyperalimentation (Fig. 22-59) as large quantities of phosphate enter cells. Central nervous system manifestations, peripheral neuropathy, and respiratory muscle failure dominate the clinical picture when hyperalimentation is instituted.[871,888] It is important that hyperalimentation solutions contain phosphate and that serum phosphorus levels be monitored and phosphate be replaced as necessary.

Alcoholism

The pathogenesis of hypophosphatemia in alcoholism is complex and not fully understood.[871,889] Contributory factors are poor intake, vomiting, antacid use, and urinary wasting due to magnesium depletion. Hospitalization and alcohol withdrawal may precipitate severe hypophosphatemia with rhabdomyolysis, respiratory failure, or CNS manifestations. Respiratory alkalososis occurring with alcohol withdrawal and glucose feeding probably contributes to the rapid appearance of hypophosphatemia.

Miscellaneous

Hypophosphatemia also occurs in thermal burns, where hyperventilation may be the proximate cause; in leukemia during

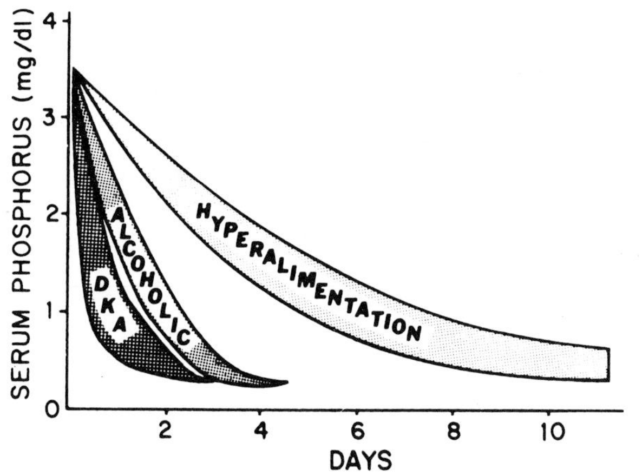

FIGURE 22-59. Approximate time course of the development of severe hypophosphatemia in patients with diabetic ketoacidosis, chronic alcoholics, and patients receiving intravenous hyperalimentation without phosphorus supplementation. (*From Knochel,[667] by permission of the Archives of Internal Medicine.*)

blast crisis; and after renal transplantation in which persistent hyperparathyroidism, glucocorticoid therapy, and poor graft function are probably involved.

Treatment

The decision to treat is based on the evidence for a phosphate depletion state, the level of hypophosphatemia, and the presence of symptoms. Hypophosphatemia does not always require treatment. The syndrome associated with acute respiratory alkalosis or with nutritional recovery may be self-limited and may not require specific therapy. Symptomatic phosphate depletion can usually be treated orally with 1 g per day of elemental phosphorus provided as milk (contains about 1 g per liter) or as a phosphate supplement (Table 22-12). Intravenous therapy should be approached cautiously and only in patients with severe, symptomatic hypophosphatemia [0.3 mmol/liter (1.0 mg/dl)] because of the risk of overshooting and producing hypocalcemia with tetany or soft tissue calcification. Great caution must be exercised in treating renal insufficiency. A dose of 2.5 mg phosphorus/kg body weight as a slow infusion is recommended.[890] This can be administered as sodium phosphate or potassium phosphate (Table 22-12). Close monitoring of serum levels of calcium, phosphorus, and creatinine is necessary.

Disorders Causing Hyperphosphatemia

Chronic hyperphosphatemia with normal renal function reflects an increased renal phosphate threshold. This occurs in hypoparathyroidism and pseudohypoparathyroidism, in acromegaly, and in some patients treated with the bisphosphonate drug etidronate disodium. Chronic hyperphosphatemia is also part of the tumoral calcinosis syndrome characterized by massive ectopic calcification around large joints. Renal insufficiency is the most common cause of hyperphosphatemia. The ability to excrete phosphate falls off sharply when the GFR is reduced below 30 ml/min, and the TmP/GFR and serum phosphorus levels rise. The hyperphosphatemia of chronic renal failure is a major clinical problem because it leads to soft tissue calcification and contributes

TABLE 22-12. Oral and Intravenous Preparations of Phosphate

Preparation	Phosphorus, Mg	Na, MEq	K, mEq
Oral			
Cow's milk	1,000 mg/liter	25	35
Fleet Phospho-Soda	645 mg/5 ml	24	0
K-Phos Neutral	250 mg/capsule	13	1.1
Neutra-Phos	250 mg/capsule	7.1	7.1
Neutra-Phos K	250 mg/capsule		14.2
Parenteral			
K phosphate	93 mg/ml	0	4.4
Na phosphate	93 mg/ml	4	0

significantly to the progression of secondary hyperparathyroidism and renal osteodystrophy. It is treated with dietary phosphate restriction and phosphate-binding antacids. Aluminum containing phosphate-binding antacids have been replaced with calcium acetate as a phosphate-binder.

Acute hyperphosphatemia occurs with rhabdomyolysis in crush and compartment syndromes[747] and in the tumor lysis syndrome[850] and may produce hypocalcemia and tetany. Administration of pharmocologic doses of vitamin D, overzealous use of oral phosphate, or phosphate-containing enemas may result in hyperphosphatemia. It is also seen because of cellular shifts in acute respiratory acidosis and in metabolic acidosis (both ketoacidosis and lactic acidosis). A decreased GFR probably contributes to all these conditions by decreasing phosphate excretion.

The most important short-term consequence of hyperphosphatemia is hypocalcemia and tetany. Soft tissue calcification and secondary hyperparathyroidism are the long-term consequences. Treatment consists of limiting dietary intake of phosphorous and adding a phosphate-binding agent such as aluminum hydroxide, aluminum carbonate, calcium citrate, or calcium carbonate.

DISORDERS OF MAGNESIUM METABOLISM

Although the intracellular environment is relatively poor in calcium, it is rich in magnesium. The ratio of magnesium to calcium is critically important for maintenance of an electrochemical gradient across the plasma membrane and for transmembrane excitation. Therefore, magnesium is maintained within a tight physiologic concentration range both intracellularly and extracellularly. Magnesium is often handled by the same transporters that act on calcium, and so it may often share the same pattern of flux. Nevertheless, there appears to be no direct hormonal regulation of magnesium levels in blood, in ECF, or within the cell[891–894]; no classical feedback loops for magnesium regulation are known. Rather, maintenance of magnesium levels is achieved by modifying the efficiency of dietary absorption or urinary excretion of the mineral (Figs. 22-60, 22-61). Magnesium, however, influences PTH secretion. An acute drop in magnesium will stimulate PTH secretion, but chronic and severe magnesium depletion impairs PTH secretion.[898]

Within cells, magnesium is the most abundant divalent cation and is second only to potassium as a cation. The actions of magnesium are similar to those of calcium in some cases, but because magnesium is present in lower concentrations, it has little or no effect unless extremes of magnesium concentration are present. However, magnesium is a cofactor for many enzymes, especially those involved in phosphorylation and dephosphorylation. These include enzymes that catalyze energy production and storage, such as those involved in making and breaking high-energy bonds in ATP, in intracellular metabolism, and in the polymerization reactions involved in the biosynthesis of DNA and RNA.

The normal adult has approximately 25 g (2,000 mEq) of magnesium present in total throughout the body.[895] Approximately two-thirds of this magnesium is found in the skeleton; the remaining one-third is present in soft tissues.[895] Within the skeleton, magnesium is not part of the crystalline lattice; rather, it is present on the crystalline surface of mineralized bone, from which location it is not freely exchangeable with magnesium in the ECF.

Although the stores of total body magnesium are large and the role of magnesium is vital, only 1 percent of magnesium is found in the ECF. Furthermore, total body magnesium and the levels present intracellularly or in soft tissue do not necessarily correspond with the ECF level. The normal plasma range for magnesium is 1.5 to 2.2 mEq/liter (1.8 to 2.6 mg/dl). Of the magnesium present in the ECF, 55 percent is ionized. Of the remaining 45 percent, two-thirds is bound to proteins such as albumin and one-third is complexed to counterions. Intracellularly, 60 percent of magnesium is found in the mitochondria (concentration $= 1 \times 10^{-3}$ *M*); the remaining intracellular magnesium is in the cytosol (concentration $= 5 \times 10^{-4}$ *M*). Only 5 to 10 percent of intracellular magnesium is present in a free ionic form.

FIGURE 22-60. Schematic representation of magnesium flux and balance in a normal human. Arrows indicate direction of movement of magnesium between the gut, kidneys, and extracellular fluid (ECF). The numeric values indicate quantities of elemental magnesium stored or transferred in a 24-h period. The thickness of arrows indicates the relative magnitude of flux.

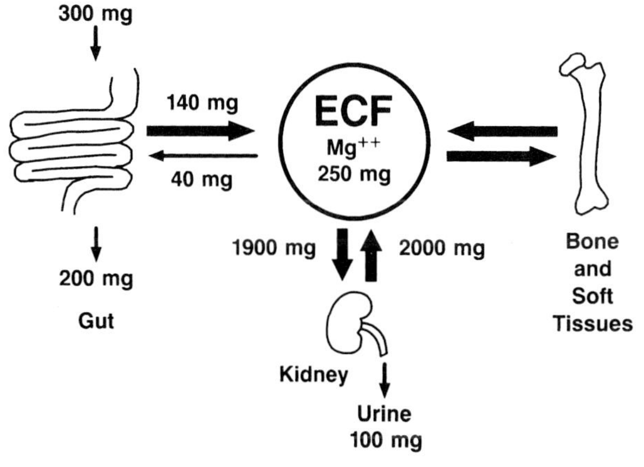

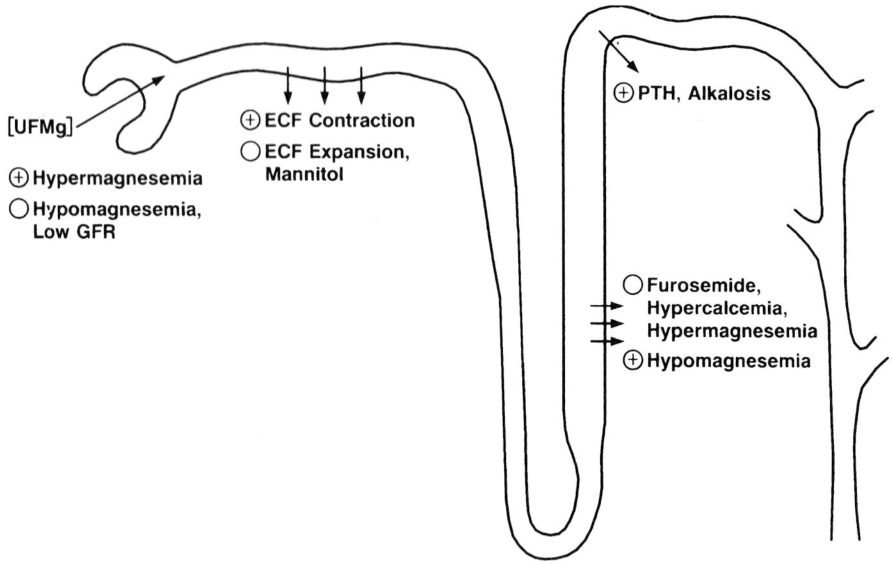

FIGURE 22-61. Handling of magnesium by the nephron. (*Reprinted with permission from Lemann.*[689])

Magnesium Balance

It is possible to construct a diet that is calorically sufficient yet deficient in calcium. However, this is very difficult to do with magnesium. Magnesium is present in all cells; therefore, all normal diets have magnesium present in approximate proportion to caloric intake. The normal adult needs 0.3 to 0.35 mEq/kg of magnesium per day (Fig. 22-60). The average diet exceeds this amount, containing 20 to 40 mEq per day, found principally in green vegetables and meat. The amount of magnesium absorbed from the diet varies linearly with the intake and on average is approximately 30 to 40 percent of the total ingested.[896]

Therefore, the principal homeostatic challenge for the maintenance of normal magnesium levels rests with excretion of the excess magnesium that enters through the diet.[897] This is accomplished by the kidney. The kidney filters an enormous quantity of magnesium. Seventy percent of the magnesium in blood is ultrafilterable, but 95 percent of this filtered magnesium is reabsorbed and only 5 to 10 percent of the filtered load is excreted. Reabsorption within the nephron occurs in the thick limb of the ascending loop of Henle. Hence, renal efficiency of reabsorption is very high and can be most impressive under conditions of dietary deficiency. Under such conditions, magnesium excretion can fall to less than 1 mEq/day in the urine. The excretion of magnesium by the kidney appears to be regulated by the mechanism of a tubular maximum for reabsorption of the ion. Levels in the tubule which exceed a predetermined threshold spill into the urine. The Tm-limited renal process is the principal determinant of ambient serum magnesium. Therefore, in conditions of renal failure, magnesium excretion is inadequate and the mineral accumulates systemically (Fig. 22-61).

Parathyroid hormone, calcitonin, and vitamin D do not play a regulatory role for magnesium but can influence magnesium flux because magnesium tends to be handled similarly to calcium by many cellular transport apparatuses. In fact, the tubular mechanism for the reabsorption of magnesium may be shared with calcium and appears to be sodium-linked. In contrast, vitamin D does not influence magnesium intestinal absorption; the calcium-binding protein responsible for the absorption of dietary calcium does not transport magnesium.

Hypomagnesemia

For hypomagnesemia to develop, increased losses or inadequate intake of magnesium must occur for a prolonged period.[898] Diffuse intestinal disease can lead to failure to absorb magnesium adequately from the diet. However, inadequate intake is more often the cause. Alcoholism is the leading cause of hypomagnesemia, which occurs in 50 percent of alcoholics because of decreased dietary intake, vomiting or diarrhea, secondary aldosteronism, or a direct effect of alcohol on promoting renal magnesium excretion. Certain drugs, such as loop diuretics, cyclosporin, gentamicin, cisplatin, pentamidine, and amphoterrin B can also cause renal magnesium wasting and hypomagnesemia. Magnesium can be depleted in total body stores even in the presence of a normal plasma level (Table 22-13). Metabolic acidosis such as diabetic ketoacidosis, starvation, or alcoholism may also result in magnesium wasting. Treatment of diabetic ketoacidosis with fluid replacement can lead to decreased serum magnesium and unmask the preexisting total body magnesium depletion; therefore, magnesium supplementation is often required along with other components of the treatment regimen. The hungry bones syndrome, in which calcium influx into bone can be extraordinary, is often accompanied by hypomagnesemia. In such instances, calcium replacement alone is not adequate; magnesium needs to be replaced as well in order to relieve tetany. In addition, hypomagnesium per se can produce hypocalcemia and its complications by causing functional hypoparathyroidism. In intensive care units, 65 percent of patients have hypomagnesemia.[898]

The symptoms of hypomagnesemia are similar to those of hypocalcemia, but the electrocardiogram changes differ.[898] The ST segments are depressed, and T waves are inverted in the precordial leads in hypomagnesemia. PR & QT intervals are prolonged. Arrhythmias such as premature atrial contractions, atrial tachycardia, and atrial fibrillation can occur. Such findings usually do not occur until magnesium levels are substantially decreased in the blood, usually below 1 mg/dl. Seizures, arrhythmias, coarse tremors, and carpal pedal spasm may occur; muscle fasciculations and a positive Chvostek's or Trousseau's sign are also part of the syndrome. Once plasma levels of magnesium fall below normal, repletion may take a long time as a result of the large total body deficit that has occurred. A magnesium value <1.5 meq/L indicates magnesium

TABLE 22-13. Causes of Hypomagnesemia and Magnesium Depletion

Decreased intake or absorption
- Dietary deficiency: protein-calorie malnutrition
- Vomiting, diarrhea, nasogastric suction
- Malabsorption syndromes: pancreatic and intestinal
- Parenteral hyperalimentation without adequate magnesium
- Primary hypomagnesemia

Renal disorders
- Osmotic diuresis: mannitol, glucose, urea
- After relief of obstructive uropathy or resolution of acute tubular necrosis
- After renal transplantation
- Drug-induced: loop diuretics, cisplatin, amphotericin, digoxin, aminoglycoside antibiotics, cyclosporine, pentamidine
- ECF expansion, hyperaldosteronism, Bartter's syndrome
- Congenital, hereditary renal magnesium wasting

Miscellaneous disorders
- Alcoholism
- Diabetes mellitus/diabetic ketoacidosis
- Primary hyperparathyroidism
- After parathyroidectomy with hungry-bone syndrome
- Thyrotoxicosis
- Syndrome of inappropriate ADH
- Chronic hypoparathyroidism
- Hypoalbuminemia
- Dialysis against a magnesium-deficiency dialysate
- Excessive lactation
- Pancreatitis

Combinations of the above

depletion. Suspect magnesium deficiency when vitamin D and calcium therapy are ineffective in correcting hypocalcemia. Parenteral administration of up to 200 to 400 mEq of magnesium for several days may be required. This can be administered as $MgSO_47H_2O$ given intravenously during emergent situations, such as seizures. Five hundred mg (40 mEq) can be given under such circumstances, but the administration rate should not exceed 15 mg/min. Thereafter, 600 mg of magnesium sulfate can be given in the first 3 to 4 h; subsequently, another 900 mg can be given over the next 24 h.[899] Although painful, 2 gm of $MgSO_47H_2O$ (16.2 mEq magnesium) can also be given as a 50 percent solution every 8 hours intramuscularly. Magnesium acetate and other magnesium salts can also be used. Maintenance dosing can be achieved with oral formulations of magnesium salts such as magnesium oxide or magnesium chloride. A total of 300 mg elemental magnesium in divided doses should be administered. In our experience, magnesium oxide appears to cause less diarrhea than do other forms of magnesium supplementation. When diarrhea limits oral treatment, intramuscular administration may be required. Hypokalemia is a common finding with magnesium deficiency and may contribute to the cardiac findings. Hypocalcemia is also a common manifestation of hypomagnesemia and may contribute to the neuromuscular hyperexcitability. PTH secretion increases within minutes after beginning magnesium administration.

Caution must be taken to avoid producing hypermagnesemia as a result of treatment in patients with renal impairment.

Hypermagnesemia

Hypermagnesemia most often occurs when there is normal or increased intake of magnesium in the setting of renal failure. Both patients and physicians often fail to recognize that antacids, enemas, and laxatives commonly contain quantities of magnesium sufficient to aggravate hypermagnesemia in the setting of renal compromise (Fig. 22-61). Magnesium-containing enemas and treatment with hemiacidrin can produce hypermagnesia in the absence of renal compromise. $MgSO_4$ administration is the conventional treatment for preeclampsia and eclampsia and can readily produce hypermagnesemia and hypocalcemia. Levels of magnesium above 5 mEq/liter can actually block the action of PTH at its target organs or inhibit its secretion by the gland and can cause hypotension and somnolence. Hence, like hypomagnesemia, hypermagnesemia can produce hypocalcemia. Electrocardiogram changes include a prolonged PR interval and a widened QRS wave. Extremely high magnesium levels—above 15 mEq/liter—lead to muscular flaccidity, respiratory paralysis, and cardiac asystole. Disappearance of the deep tendon reflexes is one of the early signs of hypermagnesemia. Treatment usually is effected simply by stopping the source of magnesium intake. The kidney will usually clear the excess magnesium over time. In emergent situations, dialysis against a low magnesium bath can be performed. Calcium administration can antagonize the toxic effect of hypermagnesemia.

Acknowledgments

The authors have taken or modified for this chapter portions of the corresponding section of the third edition of this textbook written by Gordon J. Strewler and Michael Rosenblatt. We gratefully acknowledge their contributions to our chapter.

The authors also wish to thank Lee Ann Trafton and Christa Martinez for their secretarial assistance during the preparation.

REFERENCES

1. Rasmussen H: The calcium messenger system: Parts 1 and 2. *N Engl J Med* 314:1094, 1986.
2. McLean FC, Hastings AB: A biological method for the estimation of calcium ion concentration. *J Biol Chem* 107:337, 1934.
3. Marshall RW: Plasma fractions, in Nordin BEC (ed): *Calcium, Phosphate and Magnesium Metabolism.* London, Churchill Livingstone, 1976, p 162.
4. Krane SM: Calcium, phosphate and magnesium, in Rasmussen H (ed): *International Encyclopedia of Pharmacology and Therapeutics.* Oxford, Pergamon, 1970, p 19.
5. Bronner F: Dynamics in function of calcium, in Comar LC, Bronner F (eds): *Mineral Metabolism.* New York, Academic Press, 1964, p 342.
6. Neer R, Berman M, Fisher L, et al: Multicompartmental analysis of calcium kinetics in normal adult males. *J Clin Invest* 46: 1364, 1967.
7. DeLuca HF, Schnoes HK: Vitamin D: Recent advances. *Annu Rev Biochem* 52:411, 1983.
8. Norman AW, Roth J, Orci L: The vitamin D endocrine system: Steroid metabolism, hormone receptors, and biological response. *Endocr Rev* 3:331, 1982.
9. Haussler MR, McCain TA: Basic and clinical concepts related to vitamin D metabolism and action. *N Engl J Med* 297:974, 1977.
10. Akerstöm G, Malmaeus J, Bergstrom R: Surgical anatomy of human parathyroid glands. *Surgery* 95:14, 1983.
11. Conlin PR, Fajtova VT, Mortensen RM, et al: Hysteresis in the relationship between serum ionized calcium and intact parathyroid hormone during recovery from induced hyper- and hypocalcemia in normal humans. *J Clin Endocrinol Metab* 69:593, 1989.
12. Brown EM, Gamba G, Riccardi D, et al: Cloning and characterization of an extracellular Ca^{2+} -sensing receptor from bovine parathyroid. *Nature* 366:575, 1993.
13. Brown EM, LeBoff MS, Oetting M, et al: Secretory control in normal and abnormal parathyroid tissue, in Clark JH (ed): *Recent Prog Horm Res.* New York, Harcourt Brace Jovanovich, 1987, p 337.

14. Kitamura N, Shigeno C, Shiomi K, et al: Episodic fluctuation in serum intact parathyroid hormone concentration in men. *J Clin Endocrinol Metab* 70:252, 1990.
15. Samuels MH, Veldhuis JD, Kramer P, et al: Episodic secretion of parathyroid hormone in postmenopausal women: Assessment by deconvolution analysis and approximate entropy. *J Bone Miner Res* 12:616, 1997.
16. Kaji H, Sugimoto T, Kanatani M, et al: Carboxyl-terminal PTH stimulate osteoclast-like cell formation and osteoclastic activity. *Endocrinology* 134:1897, 1994.
17. Inomata N, Akiyama M, Kubota N, et al: Characterization of a novel PTH-receptor with specificity for the carboxyl-terminal region of PTH(1-84). *Endocrinology* 136:4732, 1995.
18. Erdmann S, Muller W, Bahrami S, et al: Differential effects of parathyroid hormone fragments on collagen gene expression in chondrocytes. *J Cell Biol* 135:1179, 1996.
19. Vasicek TJ, McDevitt BE, Freeman MW, et al: Nucleotide sequence of the human parathyroid hormone gene. *Proc Natl Acad Sci USA* 80:2127, 1983.
20. Rosenblatt M, Kronenberg M, Potts JT Jr: Parathyroid hormone: Physiology, chemistry, biosynthesis, secretion, metabolism, and mechanism of action, in DeGroot LJ (ed): *Endocrinology.* Philadelphia, Saunders, 1989, p 848.
21. Habener JF, Rosenblatt M, Potts JT Jr: Parathyroid hormone: Biochemical aspects of biosynthesis, secretion, action, and metabolism. *Physiol Rev* 64:985, 1984.
22. Von Heijne G: Patterns of amino acids near signal-sequence cleavage sites. *Eur J Biochem* 133:17, 1983.
23. Szczesna-Skorupa E, Mead DA, Kemper B: Mutations of the NH2-terminal domain of the surgical peptide of preproparathyroid hormone inhibit translocation without affecting interaction with signal recognition particle. *J Biol Chem* 262:8896, 1987.
24. Freeman M, Wiren K, Rapoport A, et al: Consequences of amino-terminal deletions of preproparathyroid hormone signal sequence. *Mol Endocrinol* 1:628, 1987.
25. Arnold A, Horst SA, Gardella TJ, et al: Mutation of the signal peptide-encoding region of the preproparathyroid hormone gene in familial isolated hypoparathyroidism. *J Clin Invest* 86:1084, 1990.
26. Habener JF, Amherdt M, Ravazzola M, et al: Parathyroid hormone biosynthesis: Correlation of conversion biosynthetic precursors with intracellular protein migration as determined by electron microscope autoradiography. *J Cell Biol* 80:715, 1979.
27. Habener JF, Stevens TD, Tregear GW, et al: Radioimmunoassay of human proparathyroid hormone: Analysis of hormone content in tissue extracts and in plasma. *J Clin Endocrinol Metab* 42:520, 1976.
28. Wiren KM, Potts JT Jr, Kronenberg HM: Importance of the propeptide sequence of human preproparathyroid hormone for signal sequence function. *J Biol Chem* 263:19771, 1988.
29. Cohn DV, Zangerle R, Fischer-Colbrie R, et al: Similarity of secretory protein-I from parathyroid gland to chromogranin-A from adrenal medulla. *Proc Natl Acad Sci USA* 79:6056, 1982.
30. Rabbani SA, Kremer R, Bennett HPJ, et al: Phosphorylation of parathyroid hormone by human and bovine parathyroid glands. *J Biol Chem* 259:2949, 1984.
31. Russell J, Sherwood LM: The effects of 1,25-dihyroxyvitamin D_3 and high calcium on transcription of the pre-proparathyroid hormone gene are direct. *Trans Assoc Am Physicians* 100:256, 1987.
32. Naveh-Many T, Silver J: Regulation of parathyroid hormone gene expression by hypocalcemia, hypercalcemia, and vitamin D in the rat. *J Clin Invest* 86: 1313, 1990.
33. Silver J, Naveh-Many T, Mayer H, et al: Regulation of vitamin D_3 metabolites of parathyroid hormone gene transcription in vivo in the rat. *J Clin Invest* 78:1296, 1986.
34. Okazaki I, Igarashi T, Kronenberg HM: 5'-Flanking region of the parathyroid hormone gene mediates negative regulation by 1,25-$(OH)_2D_3$. *J Biol Chem* 263:2203, 1988.
35. Naveh-Many T, Rahaminov R, Livini N, et al: Parathyroid cell proliferation in normal and chronic renal failure in rats: The effects of calcium, phosphate, and vitamin D. *J Clin Invest* 96:1786, 1995.
36. Slatopolsky E, Finch J, Denda M, et al: Phosphous restriction prevents parathyroid growth: High phosphorus directly stimulates PTH secretion in vitro. *J Clin Invest* 97:2534, 1996.
37. Jüppner H, Brown EM, Kronenberg HM: *Parathyroid Hormone. Primer on metabolic bone diseases and disorders of mineral metabolism,* 4th ed. 1999, p 84.
38. Brown EM, Chen CJ, Kifor O, et al: Ca^{2+}-sensing, second messengers, and the control of parathyroid hormone secretion. *Cell Calcium* 11:333, 1990.
39. Brown EM, Enyedi P, LeBoff MS, et al: High extracellular Ca^{2+} and Mg^{2+} stimulate accumulation of inositol phosphates in bovine parathyroid cells. *FEBS Lett* 218:113, 1987.
40. Brown EM: Physiology and pathophysiology of the extracellular calcium-sensing receptor. *Am J Med* 106:238, 1999.
41. Brown EM, Pollack M, Seidman CE, et al: Calcium-ion-sensing cell-surface receptors. *N Engl J Med* 333:234, 1995.
42. Kifor O, Diaz R, Butters R, et al: The Ca^{2+}-sinsing receptor activates phopholipases C, A2 and D by high extracellular Ca^{2+} in bovine parathyroid and Car-transfected, human embryonic kidney cells. *J Bone Miner Res* 1997, 12:715, 1997.
43. McNeill SE, Hobson SA, Nipper KD, et al: Functional calcium-sensing receptors in rat fibroblasts are required for activation of SRC kinase and mitogen-activated protein kinase in response to extracellular calcium. *J Biol Chem* 273:1114, 1998.
44. Pollack M, Brown EM, Chou YH, et al: Mutations in the human Ca2+-sensing receptor gene cause familial hypocalciuric hypercalcemia and neonatal sever hyperparathyroidsim. *Cell* 75:1297, 1993.
45. Pollack M, Brown E, Estep H, et al: Autosomal dominant hypocalcaemia caused by Ca^{2+}-sensing receptor gene mutation. *Nat Genet* 8:303, 1994.
46. Ho C, Conner DA, Pollak M, et al: A mouse model for familial hypocalciuric hypercalcemia and neonatal severe hyperparathyroidism. *Nat Genet* 11:389, 1995.
47. Brown EM, Thatcher JG, Watson EJ, et al: Extracellular calcium potentiates the inhibitory effects of magnesium on parathyroid function in dispersed bovine parathyroid cells. *Metabolism* 33:171, 1984.
48. Cholst IN, Steinberg SF, Tropper PJ, et al: The influence of hypermagnesemia on serum calcium and parathyroid hormone levels in human subjects. *N Engl J Med* 310:1221, 1984.
49. Broadus AE, Mangin M, Ikeda K, et al: Humoral hypercalcemia of cancer: Identification of a novel parathyroid hormone-like peptide. *N Engl J Med* 319:556, 1988.
50. Heath H: Biogenic amines and the secretion of parathyroid hormone and calcitonin. *Endocr Rev* 1:319, 1980.
51. Brown EM: Lithium induces abnormal calcium-regulated PTH release in dispersed bovine parathyroid cells. *J Clin Endocrinol Metab* 52:1046, 1981.
52. Laitinen K, Lamberg-Allardt C, Tunninen R, et al: Transient hypoparathyroidism during acute alcohol intoxication. *N Engl J Med* 324:721, 1991.
53. Berson SA, Yalow RS: Immunochemical heterogenity of parathyroid hormone in plasma. *J Clin Endocrinol Metab* 28:1037, 1968.
54. Martin KJ, Hruska KA, Greenwalt A: Selective uptake of intact parathyroid hormone by the liver: Differences between hepatic and renal uptake. *J Clin Invest* 60:808, 1977.
55. Segre GV, D'Amour P, Hultman A, et al: Effects of hepatectomy, nephrectomy, and nephrectomy/uremia on the metabolism of parathyroid hormone in the rat. *J Clin Invest* 67:438, 1981.
56. Segre GV, Perkins AS, Witters LA, et al: Metabolism of parathyroid hormone by isolated rat Kupffer cells and hepatocytes. *J Clin Invest* 67:449, 1981.
57. Martin KJ, Hruska KA, Lewis J, et al: The renal handling of parathyroid hormone: Role of peritubular uptake and glomerular filtration. *J Clin Invest* 60:808, 1977.
58. Rouleau MF, Warshawsky H, Goltzman D: Parathyroid hormone binding in vivo to renal, hepatic, and skeletal tissues of the rat using a radioautographic approach. *Endocrinology* 118:919, 1986.
59. Flueck JA, Dibella FB, Edis AJ, et al: Immunoheterogeneity of parathyroid hormone in venous effluent serum from hyperfunctioning parathyroid glands. *J Clin Invest* 60:1367, 1977.
60. MacGregor RR, Hamilton JW, Shofstall RE, et al: Isolation and characterization of porcine parathyroid cathepsin B. *J Biol Chem* 254:4423, 1979.
61. Habener JF, Kemper B, Potts JT Jr: Calcium-dependent intracellular degradation of parathyroid hormone: A possible mechanism for the regulation of hormone stores. *Endocrinology* 97:431, 1975.
62. Arnaud CD, Tsao HS, Littledike T: Radioimmunoassay of human parathyroid hormone in serum. *J Clin Invest* 50:21, 1971.
63. Nussbaum SR, Zahradnik RJ, Lavigne JR, et al: Highly sensitive two-site immunoradiometric assay of parathyrin and its clinical utility in evaluating patients with hypercalcemia. *Clin Chem* 33:1364, 1987.

64. Brown RC, Aston JP, Weeks I, et al: Circulating intact parathyroid hormone measured by a two-site immunochemiluminometric assay. *J Clin Endocrinol Metab* 6:407, 1987.
65. Goltzman D, Henderson B, Loveridge N: Cytochemical bioassay of parathyroid hormone. *J Clin Invest* 65:1309, 1980.
66. Chambers DJ, Dunham J, Zanelii JM, et al: A sensitive bioassay of parathyroid hormone in plasma. *Clin Endocrinol (Oxf)* 9:375, 1978.
67. Broadus AE: Nephrogenous cyclic AMP. *Recent Prog Horm Res* 37:667, 1981.
68. Jüppner H, Abou-Samra AB, Freeman MW, et al: A G protein-linked receptor for parathyroid hormone and parathyroid hormone-related peptide. *Science* 254:1024, 1991.
69. Abou-Samra AB, Jüppner H, Force T, et al: Expression cloning of a common receptor for parathyroid horone and parathyroid hormone-related peptide from rat osteoblast-like cells: A single receptor stimulates intracellular accumulation of both cAMP and inositol triphosphates and increases intracellular free calcium. *Proc Natl Acad Sci USA* 89:2732, 1992.
70. Moseley JM, Kubota M, Diefenbach-Jagger J: Parathyroid hormone-related protein purified from a human lung cancer cell line. *Proc Natl Acad Sci USA* 84:5048, 1987.
71. Stewart AF, Wu T, Goumas D, et al: N-Terminal amino acid sequence of two novel tumor-derived adenylate cyclase-stimulating proteins: Identification of parathyroid hormone-like and parathyroid hormone-unlike domains. *Biochem Biophys Res Commun* 146:672, 1987.
72. Strewler GJ, Stern PH, Jacobs JW, et al: Parathyroid hormone-like protein from human renal carcinoma cells: Structural and functional homology with parathyroid hormone. *J Clin Invest* 80:1803, 1987.
73. Strewler GJ: The physiology of parathyroid hormone-related protein. *N Engl J Med* 342:177, 2000.
74. Usdin TB, Gruber C, Bonner TI: Identification and functional expression of a receptor selectively recognizing parathyroid hormone, the PTH2 receptor. *J Biol Chem* 270:15455, 1995.
75. Usdin TB, Hoare SRJ, Wang T, et al: TIP39: a new neuropeptide and PTH2-receptor agonist from hypothalamus. *Nat Neurosci* 2:941, 1999.
76. Neer EJ: Heterotrimeric G proteins: Organizers of transmembrane signals. *Cell* 80:249, 1995.
77. Levine MA: Pseudohypoparathyroidism: From bedside to bench and back. *J Bone Miner Res* 14:1255, 1999.
78. Melson GL, Chase LR, Aurach GD: Parathyroid hormone-sensitive adenyl cyclase in isolated renal tubules. *Endocrinology* 84:511, 1970.
79. Chase LR, Fedak SA, Aurbach GD: Activation of skeletal adenyl cyclase by parathyroid hormone in vitro. *Endocrinology* 84:761, 1969.
80. Civatelli R, Reid IR, Westbrook S, et al: PTH elevates inositol polyphosphates and diacylglycerol in a rat osteoblast-like cell line. *Am J Physiol* 255:E660, 1988.
81. Dunlay R, Hruska K: PTH receptor coupling to phospholipase C is an alternate pathway of signal transduction in bone and kidney. *Am J Physiol* 258:F223, 1990.
82. Gupta A, Martin KJ, Miyauchi A, et al: Regulation of cytosolic calcium by parathyroid hormone and oscillations of cytosolic calcium in fibroblasts from normal and pseudohypoparathyroid patients. *Endocrinology* 128:2825, 1991.
83. Civatelli R, Martin TJ, Fausto A, et al: Parathyroid hormone-related peptide transiently increases cytosolic calcium in osteoblast-like cells: Comparison with parathyroid hormone. *Endocrinology* 125:1204, 1989.
84. Reid IR, Civitelli R, Halstead LR, et al: Parathyroid hormone acutely elevates intracellular calcium in osteoblast-like cells. *Am J Physiol* 253:E45, 1987.
85. Yamaguchi DT, Hahn TJ, Iida-Klein A, et al: Parathyroid hormone-activated calcium channels in an osteoblast-like clonal osteosarcoma cell line. *J Biol Chem* 262:7711, 1987.
86. Bringhurst FR, Zajac JD, Daggett AS, et al: Inhibition of parathyroid hormone responsiveness in clonal osteoblastic cells expressing a mutant form of 3',5'-cyclic adenosine monophosphate-dependent protein kinase. *Mol Endocrinol* 3:60, 1989.
87. Nathans J, Hogness DS: Isolation and nucleotide sequence of the gene encoding human rhodopsin. *Proc Natl Acad Sci USA* 81:4851, 1984.
88. Lefkowitz RJ: Variations on a theme. *Nature* 351:353, 1991.
89. Dixon RAF, Kobilka BK, Strader DJ, et al: Cloning of the gene and cDNA for mammalian β-adrenergic receptor and homology with rhodopsin. *Nature* 321:75, 1986.
90. Kubo T, Fukuda K, Mikami A, et al: Cloning, sequencing and expression of complementary DNA encoding the muscarinic acetylcholine receptor. *Nature* 323:411, 1986.
91. Colquhoun D: Structure and function of acetylcholine-receptor ion channels. *Nature* 321:382, 1986.
92. McFarland KC, Sprengel R, Phillips HS, et al: Lutropin-choriogonadotropin receptor: An unusual member of the G protein-coupled receptor family. *Science* 245:494, 1989.
93. Parmentier M, Libert F, Maenhaut C, et al: Molecular cloning of the thyrotropin receptor. *Science* 246:1620, 1989.
94. Hanley MR, Jackson T: Return of the magnificent seven. *Nature* 329:766, 1987.
95. Lin HY, Harris TL, Flannery MS, et al: Expression cloning of an adenylate cyclase-coupled calcitonin receptor. *Science* 254:1022, 1991.
96. Pullman TN, Lavender AR, Aho I, et al: Direct renal action of a purified parathyroid extract. *Endocrinology* 67:570, 1960.
97. Widrow SH, Levinsky NG: Effect of parathyroid extract on renal tubular calcium reabsorption in the dog. *J Clin Invest* 41:2151, 1962.
98. Agus ZS, Gardner LB, Beck LH, et al: Effects of parathyroid hormone on renal tubular reabsorption of calcium, sodium, and phosphate. *Am J Physiol* 224:1143, 1973.
99. Scoble JE, Mills S, Hruska KA: Calcium transport in canine renal basolateral membrane vesicles: Effects of parathyroid hormone. *J Clin Invest* 75:1096, 1985.
100. Bouhtiauy D, Lajeunesse D, Brunette MG: The mechanism of parathyroid hormone action on calcium reabsorption by the distal tubule. *Endocrinology* 128:251, 1991.
101. Bringhurst FR: Calciuma and phophate distribution, turnover and metabolic actions, in DeGroot LJ (ed): *Endocrinology,* 2nd ed. Vol 2. Philadelphia, WB Saunders, 1989, p 805.
102. Cheng L, Sacktor B: Sodium gradient-dependent phophate transport in renal brush border vesicles. *J Biol Chem* 256:1556, 1981.
103. Pfister MF, Ruf I, Strange G, et al: Parathyroid hormone leads to the lysosomal degradation of the renal type II Na/Pi cotransporter. *Proc Natl Acad Sci USA* 95:1909, 1998.
104. Pfister PNAS, Malmstom K, Murer H: Parathyroid hormone regulates phosphate transport in OK cells via an irreversible inactivation of a membrane protein. *FEBS Lett* 216:257, 1997.
105. Beck L, Karaplis AC, Amizuka N, et al: Targeted inactivation of Ntp2 in mice leads to sever renal phosphate wasting, hypercalciuria, and skeletal abormalities. *Proc Natl Acad Sci USA* 95:5372, 1998.
106. Kurokawa K, Kawashima H, Torikai S: Parathyroid hormone (PTH)-sensitive and calcitonin (CT)-sensitive 25-(OH)-D_3-1-alpha-hydroxylase along the nephron—distinct distribution and mechanisms of action. *Clin Res* 29:541, 1981.
107. Horiuchi N, Suda T, Takahashi H: In vivo evidence for the intermediary role of 3',5'-cyclic AMP in parathyroid hormone-induced stimulation of 1α,25-dihydroxyvitamin D_3 synthesis in rats. *Endocrinology* 101:969, 1977.
108. Kawashima H, Torikai S, Kurokawa K: Localization of 25-hydroxyvitamin D_3-1α-and -24-dihydroxylase along the rat nephron. *Proc Natl Acad Sci USA* 78:1199, 1981.
109. Hulter HN, Halloran BP, Toto RD, et al: Long-term control of plasma calcitriol concentration in dogs and humans. Dominant role of plasma calcium concentration in experimental hyperparathyroidism. *J Clin Invest* 76:695, 1985.
110. Shigematsu T, Horiuchi N, Ogura Y: Human parathyroid hormone inhibitis renal 24-hydroxylase activity of 25-hydroxyvitamin D3 by a mechanism involving adenosine 3',5'-monophosphate in rats. *Endocrinology* 118:1583, 1986.
111. Brenza HL, Kimmel-Jehan C, Jehan F, et al: Parathyroid hormone activation of the 25-hydroxyvitamin D3-1α hydroxylase gene promoter. *Proc Natl Acad Sci USA* 95:1387, 1998.
112. Sato M, Sardana MK, Grasser WA, et al: Echistatin is a potent inhibitor of bone resorption in culture. *J Cell Biol* 111:1713, 1990.
113. Horton MA, Davies J: Perspectives: Adhesion receptors in bone. *J Bone Miner Res* 4:803, 1989.
114. Blair HC, Ghandur-Mnaymneh L: Macrophase-mediated bone resorption occurs in an acidic environment. *Calcif Tissue Int* 37:547, 1985.
115. Vaes G: The role of lysosomes and of their enzyme in the development of bone resorption induced by parathyroid hormone, in Talmage RV, Belanger LF, Clerk I (eds): *Proceedings of the 3rd Parathyroid Conference.* Amsterdam, Excerpta Medica, 1968, p 318.
116. Walker DG, Lapier CM, Gross J: A collagenolytic factor in rat bone promoted by parathyroid extract. *Biochem Biophys Res Commun* 15:397, 1964.

117. Tuukkanen J, Vaananen HK: Omeprazole, a specific inhibitor of H^+-K^+ ATPase, inhibits bone resorption in vitro. *Calcif Tissue Int* 38:123, 1986.
118. Blair HC, Teitelbaum SL, Ghiselli R, et al: Osteoclastic bone resorption by a polarized vacuolar proton pump. *Science* 245:855, 1989.
119. Waite LC: Carbonic anhydrase inhibitors, parathyroid hormone and calcium metabolism. *Endocrinology* 91:1160, 1972.
120. Mahgoub A, Stern PH: Carbon dioxide and the effect of parathyroid hormone on bone in vitro. *Am J Physiol* 226:1272, 1974.
121. Delaisse JM, Eeckhout Y, Vaes G: In vivo and in vitro evidence for the involvement of cysteine proteinases in bone resorption. *Biochem Biophys Res Commun* 125:441, 1984.
122. Sly WS, Whyte MP, Sundaram V: Carbonic anhydrase II deficiency in 12 families with the autosomal recessive syndrome of osteopetrosis with renal tubular acidosis and cerebral calcification. *N Engl J Med* 313:139, 1985.
123. Sly WS, Hewett-Emmett D, Whyte MP: Carbonic anhydrase II deficiency identified as the primary defect in the autosomal recessive syndrome of osteopetrosis with renal tubular acidosis and cerebral calcification. *Proc Natl Acad Sci USA* 80:2752, 1983.
124. Barling PM, Bibby NJ: Study of the localization of [^{3}H] bovine parathyroid hormone in bone by light microscope autoradiography. *Calcif Tissue Int* 37:441, 1985.
125. Silve CM, Hradek GT, Jones AL, et al: Parathyroid hormone receptor in intact embryonic chicken bone: Characterization and cellular localization. *J Cell Biol* 94:379, 1982.
126. Rodan GA, Martin TJ: Role of osteoblasts in hormonal control of bone resorption—a hypothesis. *Calcif Tissue Int* 33:349, 1982.
127. McSheehy PMJ, Chambers TJ: Osteoblastic cells mediate osteoclastic responsiveness to parathyroid hormone. *Endocrinology* 118:824, 1986.
128. Raisz LG, Martin TJ: Prostaglandins in bone and mineral metabolism, in Peck WA (ed): *Bone and Mineral Research.* Amsterdam, Excerpta Medica, 1984, p 286.
129. Rodan GA, Heath JK, Yoon K, Noda M, Rodan SB: Diversity of the osteoblastic phenotype, in Evered D, Harnett S (eds): *CIBA Symposium on Cell and Molecular Biology of Vertebrate Hard Tissues.* Chichester, UK, Wiley, 1988, p 79.
130. Ralston SH, Russell RGG, Gowen M: Estrogen inhibits release of tumor necrosis factor from peripheral blood mononuclear cells in postmenopausal women. *J Bone Miner Res* 5:983, 1990.
131. Pacifici R, Rifas L, McCracken R, et al: Ovarian steroid treatment blocks a postmenopausal increase in blood monocyte interleukin 1 release. *Proc Natl Acad Sci USA* 86:2398, 1989.
132. Girasole G, Sakagami Y, Hustmyer FG, et al: 17β-Estradiol inhibits cytokine induced IL-6 production by bone marrow stromal cells and osteoblasts. *J Bone Miner Res* 5:S273, 1990.
133. Tabibzadeh SS, Santhanam U, May L, et al: Cytokine-induced production of IL-6 by freshly explanted human endometrial stromal cells: Modulation by estradiol-17β. *Ann NY Acad Sci* 557:543, 1989.
134. Ishimi Y, Miyaura C, Jin CH, et al: IL-6 is produced by osteoblasts and induces bone resorption. *J Immunol* 145:3297, 1990.
135. Gearing DP, Gough NM, King JA, et al: Molecular cloning and expression of cDNA encoding a murine myeloid leukemia inhibitory factor (LIF). *EMBO J* 6:3995, 1987.
136. Weir EC, Insogna KL, Horowitz MC: Osteoblast-like cells secrete granulocyte-macrophage colony-stimulating factor in response to parathyroid hormone and lipopolysaccharide. *Endocrinology* 124:899, 1989.
137. Quinn JM, Elliott J, Gillespie MT, et al: A combination of osteoclast differentiation factor and macrophage-colony stimulating factor is sufficient for both human and mouse osteoclast formation in vitro. *Endocrinology* 139:4424, 1998.
138. Lacey DL, Timms E, Tan HL, et al: Osteoprotegerin ligand is a cytokine that regulates osteoclast differentiation and activation. *Cell* 93:165, 1998.
139. Yasuda H, Shima N, Nakagawa N, et al: Osteoclast differentiation factor is a ligand for osteoprotegerin/osteoclastogenesis-inhibitory factor and is identical to TRANCE/RANKL. *Proc Natl Acad Sci USA* 95:3597, 1998.
140. Fuller K, Wong B, Fox S, et al: TRANCE is necessary and sufficient for osteoblast-mediated activation of bone resorption in osteoclasts. *J Exp Med* 188:997, 1998.
141. Anderson DM, Maraskovsky E, Billingsley WL, et al: A homologue of the TNF receptor and its ligand enhance T-cell growth and dendritic-cell function. *Nature* 390:175, 1997.
142. Wong BR, Josien R, Lee SY, et al: TRANCE (tumor necrosis factor [TNF]-related activation-induced cytokine), a new TNF family member predominantly expressed in T cells, is a dendritic cell-specific survival factor. *J Exp Med* 186:2075, 1997.
143. Wong BR, Rho J, Arron J, et al: TRANCE is a novel ligand of the tumor necrosis factor receptor family that activates c-Jun N-terminal kinase in T cells. *J Biol Chem* 272:25190, 1997.
144. Suda T, Takahashi N, Udagawa N, et al: Modulation of osteoclast differentiation and function by the new members of the tumor necrosis factor receptor and ligand families. *Endocr Rev* 20:345, 1999.
145. Simonet WS, Lacey DL, Dunstan CR, et al: Osteoprotegerin: A novel secreted protein involved in the regulation of bone density. *Cell* 89:309, 1997.
146. Yasuda H, Shima N, Nakagawa N, et al: Identity of osteoclastogenesis inhibitory factor (OCIF) and osteoprotegerin (OPG): A mechanism by which OPG/OCIF inhibits osteoclastogenesis in vitro. *Endocrinology* 139:1329, 1998.
147. Slovik DM, Neer RM, Potts JT Jr: Short term effects of synthetic human parathyroid hormone-(1-34) administration on bone mineral metabolism in osteoporotic patients. *J Clin Invest* 68:1261, 1981.
148. Howard GA, Bottemiller BL, Turner RT, et al: Parathyroid hormone stimulates bone formation and resorption in organ culture: Evidence for a coupling mechanism. *Proc Natl Sci USA* 78:3204, 1981.
149. Tam CS, Heersche JNM, Murray TM, et al: Parathyroid hormone stimulates the bone apposition rate independently of its resorptive action: Differential effects of intermittent and continual administration. *Endocrinology* 110:506, 1982.
150. Reeve J, Davies UM, Hesp R, et al: Treatment of osteoporosis with human parathyroid peptide and observations on effect of sodium fluoride. *Br Med J* 301:314, 1990.
151. Reeve J, Williams D, Hesp R, et al: Anabolic effect of low doses of a fragment of human parathyroid hormone on the skeleton in postmenopausal osteoporosis. *Lancet* 1:1035, 1976.
152. Tada K, Yamamuro T, Okumura H, et al: Restoration of axial and appendicular bone volumes by h-PTH(1-34) in parathyroidectomized and osteopenic rats. *Bone* 11:163, 1990.
153. Hock JM, Gera I, Fonseca J, et al: Human parathyroid hormone-(1-34) increases bone mass in ovariectomized and orchidectomized rats. *Endocrinology* 122:2899, 1988.
154. McCarthy TL, Centrella M, Canalis E: Parathyroid hormone enhances the transcript and polypeptide levels of insulin-like growth factor I in osteoblast-enriched cultures from fetal rat bone. *Endocrinology* 124:1247, 1989.
155. Linkhart TA, Keffer MJ: Differential regulation of insulin-like growth factor-I (IGF-I) and IGF-II release from cultured neonatal mouse calvaria by parathyroid hormone, transforming growth factor-$\beta\beta$, and 1,25-dihydroxyvitamin D_3. *Endocrinology* 128:1511, 1991.
156. Centrella M, McCarthy TL, Canalis E: Parathyroid hormone modulates transforming growth factor β activity and binding in osteoblast-enriched cell cultures from fetal rat parietal bone. *Proc Natl Acad Sci USA* 85:5889, 1988.
157. Rouleau MF, Mitchell J, Goltzman D: In vivo distribution of parathyroid hormone receptors in bone: Evidence that a predominant osseous target cell is not the mature osteoblast. *Endocrinology* 123:187, 1988.
158. Bellows CG, Ishida H, Aubin JE, et al: Parathyroid hormone reversibly suppresses the differentiation of osteoprogenitor cells into functional osteoblasts. *Endocrinology* 127:3111, 1990.
159. Rouleau MF, Mitchell J, Goltzman D: Characterization of the major parathyroid hormone target cell in the endosteal metaphysis of rat long bones. *J Bone Miner Res* 5:1043, 1990.
160. Schipani E, Langman CB, Parfitt AM, et al: Constitutively activated receptors of parathyroid hormone and parathyroid hormone-related peptide in Jansen's metaphyseal chondrodysplasia. *N Engl J Med* 335:708, 1996.
161. Jobert AS, Zhang P, Couvineau A, et al: Absence of functional receptors for parathyroid hormone and parathyroid hormone-related peptide in Blomstrand chondrodysplasia. *J Clin Invest* 102:34, 1998.
162. Zhang P, Jobert AS, Couvineau A, et al: A homozygous inactivating mutation in the parathyroid hormone/parathyroid hormone-related peptide receptor causing Blomstrand chondrodysplasia. *J Clin Endocrinol Metab* 83:3373, 1998.
163. Karaplis AC, Bin He MT, Nguyen A, et al: Inactivating mutation in the human parathyroid hormone receptor type I gene in Blomstrand chondrodysplasia. *Endocrinology* 139:5255, 1998.

164. Lanske B, Karaplis AC, Luz A, et al: PTH/PTHrP receptor in early development and Indian hedgehog-regulated bone growth. *Science* 273:663, 1996.
165. Copp DH: Parathyroids, calcitonin and control of plasma calcium. *Recent Prog Horm Res* 20:59, 1964.
166. Copp DH, Cameron EC, Cheney BA, et al: Evidence for calcitonin—a new hormone from the parathyroid that lowers blood calcium. *Endocrinology* 70:638, 1962.
167. Foster GV, Byfield PGH, Gudmundsson TV: Calcitonin. *Clin Endocrinol Metab* 1:93, 1972.
168. Munson PL: Physiology and pharmacology of thyrocalcitonin, in Aurbach GD (eds): *Handbook of Physiology, Section 7: Endocrinology.* Washington, DC, American Physiological Society, 1976, p 443.
169. Austin LA, Heath H: Calcitonin physiology and pathophysiology. *N Engl J Med* 304:269, 1981.
170. MacIntyre I: Calcitonin: Physiology, biosynthesis, secretion, metabolism, and mode of action, in DeGroot LJ (ed): *Endocrinology.* Philadelphia, Saunders, 1989, p 892.
171. Pearse AGE, Carvalheira AF: Cytochemical evidence for an ultimobranchial origin of rodent thyroid C cells. *Nature* 214:929, 1967.
172. Goltzman D, Tischler AS: Characterization of the immunochemical forms of calcitonin released by a medullary thyroid carcinoma in tissue culture. *J Clin Invest* 61:449, 1978.
173. Seiber P, Brugger M, Kamber B: Menschliches calcitonin: IV. Die synthese von calcitonin M. *Helv Chir Acta* 51:2057, 1968.
174. Guttmann S, Pless J, Sandrin E: Synthese des thyrocalcitonins. *Helv Chir Acta* 51:1155, 1968.
175. Nicholson GC, Moseley JM, Sexton PM, et al: Abundant calcitonin receptors in isolated rat osteoclasts: Biochemical and autoradiographic characterization. *J Clin Invest* 78:355, 1986.
176. Warshawsky H, Goltzman D, Rouleau MF, et al: Direct in vivo demonstration by radioautography of specific binding sites for calcitonin in skeletal and renal tissues of the rat. *J Cell Biol* 85:682, 1980.
177. Raisz LG, Kream BE: Regulation of bone formation. *N Engl J Med* 309:29, 1983.
178. Kallio DM, Garant PR, Minkin C: Ultrastructural effects of calcitonin on osteoclasts in tissue culture. *J Ultrastruct Res* 39:205, 1972.
179. Deftos LJ, Roos BA, Oates EL: *Calcitonin. Primer on metabolic bone diseases and disorders of mineral metabolism.* 4th ed, 1999, p 99.
180. Muff R, Born W, Fischer JA: Calcitonin, calcitonin gene related peptide, adrenomedullin and amylin: Homologous peptides, separate receptors and overlapping biological actions. *Eur J Endocrinol* 133:17, 1995.
181. Cornish J, Callon KE, King AR, et al: Systemic administration of amylin increases bone mass, linear growth, and adiposity in adult male mice. *Am J Physiol* 275(4 Pt 1):E694, 1998.
182. Cornish J, Callon KE, Lin CQ, et al: Comparison of the effects of calcitonin gene-related peptide and amylin on osteoblasts. *J Bone Miner Res* 14:1302, 1999.
183. Chakraborty M, Chatterjee D, Kellokumpu S, et al: Cell cycle-dependent coupling of the calcitonin receptor to different G proteins. *Science* 251:1078, 1991.
184. Luebke AE, Dahl GP, Roos BA, et al: Identification of a protein that confers calcitonin gene-related peptide responsiveness to oocytes by using a cystic fibrosis transmembrane conductance regulator assay. *Proc Natl Acad Sci USA* 93:3455, 1996.
185. McLatchie LM, Fraser NJ, Main MJ, et al: RAMPs regulate the transport and ligand specificity of the calcitonin-receptor-like receptor. *Nature* 393:333, 1998.
186. Balkan W, Oates L, Howard GA, et al: Testes exhibit elevated expression of calcitonin gene-related peptide receptor component protein. *Endocrinology* 140:1459, 1999.
187. Potts JT Jr, Niall HD, Keutmann HT, et al: Chemistry of the calcitonins: Species variation plus structure-activity relations, and pharmacologic implications, in Talmage RV, Munson PL (eds): *Calcium, Parathyroid Hormone, and the Calcitonins: Proceedings of the Fourth Parathyroid Conference.* Amsterdam, Excerpta Medica, 1972, p 121.
188. Tashjian AH, Wright DR, Ivey JL, et al: Calcitonin binding sites in bone: Relationships to biological response and "escape." *Recent Prog Horm Res* 34:285, 1977.
189. Lamp SJ, Findlay DM, Moseley JM, et al: *J Biol Chem* 256:12269, 1981.
190. Michelangeli VP, Findlay DM, Moseley JM, et al: *J Cyclic Nucleotide Protein Phosphor Res* 9:129, 1983.
191. D'Santos CS, Nicholson GC, Moseley JM, et al: Biologically active, derivatizable salmon calcitonin analog: Design, synthesis, and applications. *Endocrinology* 123:1483, 1988.
192. Findlay DM, Michelangeli VP, Martin TJ, et al: Conformational requirements for activity of salmon calcitonin. *Endocrinology* 117:801, 1985.
193. Rittel W, Maier R, Brugger M, et al: Structure-activity relationships of human calcitonin III: The biologic activity of systemic analogues with the shortened or terminally modified peptide chains. *Experientia* 32:246, 1976.
194. Schwartz K, Orlowski R, Marcus R: Des-Ser^{2} salmon calcitonin: A biologically potent synthetic analog. *Endocrinology* 108:831, 1981.
195. Morikawa T, Munekata E, Sakakibara S, et al: Synthesis of ERI calcitonin and (Asu$^{1-7}$)-eel calcitonin: Contribution of the disulphide bond to hormonal activity. *Experientia* 32:1104, 1979.
196. Yates AJ, Gutierrez GE, Garrett IR, et al: A noncyclical analog of salmon calcitonin (N alpha-PropionylDi-Ala^{1,7},des-Leu^{19}sCT) retains full potency without inducing anorexia in rats. *Endocrinology* 126:2845, 1990.
197. Amara SG, Jonas V, Rosenfeld MG, et al: Alternative RNA processing in calcitonin gene expression generates mRNAs encoding different polypeptide products. *Nature* 298:240, 1982.
198. Rosenfeld MG, Mermond JJ, Amara SG, et al: Production of a novel neuropeptide encoded by the calcitonin gene via tissue-specific RNA processing. *Nature* 304:129, 1983.
199. Petermann JB, Born W, Chang JY, et al: Identification in the human central nervous system, pituitary, and thyroid of a novel calcitonin gene-related peptide, and partial amino acid sequence in the spinal cord. *J Biol Chem* 262:542, 1987.
200. Brain SD, Williams TJ, Tippins JR, et al: Calcitonin gene-related peptide is a potent vasodilator. *Nature* 313:54, 1985.
201. McCulloch J, Uddman R, Kingman TA, et al: Calcitonin gene-related peptide: Functional role in cerebrovascular regulation. *Proc Natl Acad Sci USA* 83:5731, 1986.
202. Nelson MT, Huang Y, Brayden JE, et al: Arterial dilations in response to calcitonin gene-related peptide involve activation of K^{+} channels. *Nature* 344:770, 1990.
203. Goodman EC, Iversen LL: Calcitonin gene-related peptide: Novel neuropeptide. *Life Sci* 38:2169, 1986.
204. Krahn DD, Gosnell BA, Levine AS, et al: Effects of calcitonin gene-related peptide on food intake. *Peptides* 5:861, 1984.
205. Hughes JJ, Levine AS, Morley JE, et al: Intraventricular calcitonin gene-related peptide inhibits gastric acid secretion. *Peptides* 5:665, 1984.
206. Goltzman D, Mitchell J: Interaction of calcitonin and calcitonin gene-related peptide at receptor sites in target tissues. *Science* 227:1343, 1985.
207. Seitz PK, Thomas ML, Cooper CW: Binding of calcitonin and calcitonin gene-related peptide to calvarial cells and renal cortical membranes. *J Bone Miner Res* 1:51, 1986.
208. Zaidi M, Chambers TJ, Gaines Das RE, et al: A direct action of human calcitonin gene-related peptide on isolated osteoclasts. *J Endocrinol* 115:511, 1987.
209. D'Souza SM, MacIntyre I, Girgis SI, et al: Human synthetic calcitonin gene-related peptide inhibits bone resorption in vitro. *Endocrinology* 119:58, 1986.
210. Tannenbaum GS, Goltzman D: Calcitonin gene-related peptide mimics calcitonin actions in brain on growth hormone release and feeding. *Endocrinology* 116:2685, 1985.
211. Zaidi M, Brain SD, Tippins JR, et al: Structure-activity relationship of human calcitonin-gene-related peptide. *Biochem J* 269:775, 1990.
212. Craig RK, Hall L, Edbrooke MR, et al: Partial nucleotide sequence of human calcitonin precursor mRNA identifies flanking cryptic peptides. *Nature* 295:345, 1982.
213. Jacobs JW, Goodman RH, Chin WW, et al: Calcitonin messenger RNA encodes multiple polypeptides in a single precursor. *Science* 213:457, 1981.
214. MacIntyre I, Hillyard CJ, Murphy PK, et al: A second plasma calcium-lowering peptide from the human calcitonin precursors. *Nature* 300:460, 1982.
215. Birnbaum RS, Mahoney W, Roos BA: Purification and amino acid sequence of a noncalcitonin secretory peptide derived from preprocalcitonin. *J Biol Chem* 258:5463, 1983.
216. Roos BA, Huber MB, Birnbaum RS, et al: Medullary thyroid carcinomas secrete a noncalcitonin peptide corresponding to the carboxyl-terminal region of preprocalcitonin. *J Clin Endocrinol Metab* 56:802, 1983.

217. Roos BA, Fischer JA, Pignat W, et al: Evaluation of the in vivo and in vitro calcium-regulating actions of noncalcitonin peptides produced via calcitonin gene expression. *Endocrinology* 118:46, 1986.
218. Martin TJ: The therapeutic uses of calcitonin. *Scott Med J* 23:161, 1978.
219. Nilsson O, Almqvist S, Karlberg B: Salmon calcitonin in the acute treatment of moderate and severe hypercalcemia in man. *Acta Med Scand* 204:249, 1978.
220. Silva O, Becker K: Salmon calcitonin in the treatment of hypercalcemia. *Arch Intern Med* 132:337, 1973.
221. Sjöberg H, Hjern B: Acute treatment with calcitonin in primary hyperparathyroidism and severe hypercalcemia of other origin. *Acta Chir Scand* 141:90, 1975.
222. Vaughn C, Vitkevicium K: The effects of calcitonin in hypercalcemia in patients with malignancy. *Cancer* 34:1268, 1974.
223. Deftos L, Neer R: Medical management of the hypercalcemia of malignancy. *Annu Rev Med* 23:323, 1974.
224. Wisneski L, Croom W, Silva O, et al: Salmon calcitonin in hypercalcemia. *Clin Pharmacol Ther* 24:219, 1978.
225. Deftos LJ, First BP: Calcitonin as a drug. *Ann Intern Med* 95:192, 1981.
226. Deftos LJ: Calcitonin, in Gray CH, James VHT (eds): *Hormones and Blood.* London, Academic Press, 1979, p 97.
227. Au WYW: Calcitonin treatment of hypercalcemia due to parathyroid carcinoma: Synergistic effect of prednisone on long-term treatment of hypercalcemia. *Arch Intern Med* 135:1594, 1975.
228. Singer F, Ginger K: Resistance of calcitonin, in Singer F, Wallach S (eds): *Paget's Disease of Bone: Clinical Assessment, Present and Future Therapy, Procedings of the Symposium on Treatment of Paget's Disease of Bone, 1989.* New York, Elsevier, 1991, p 75.
229. Staehelin A: Possible therapeutic value of calcitonin in disorders of arterial circulation. *Schweiz Med Wochenshcr* 107:1865, 1977.
230. Carman JS, Wyatt RJ: Use of calcitonin in psychotic agitation or mania. *Arch Gen Psychiatry* 35:72, 1979.
231. McDermott MT, Kidd GS: The role of calcitonin in the development and treatment of osteoporosis. *Endocr Rev* 8:377, 1987.
232. Synthetic calcitonin for postmenopausal osteoporosis. *Med Lett Drug Ther* 27:53, 1985.
233. Fatourechi V, Heath H III: Salmon calcitonin in the treatment of postmenopausal osteoporosis. *Ann Intern Med* 107:923, 1987.
234. Mozolowski W: Jedrzej Sniadecki (1768–1838) on the cure of rickets. *Nature* 143:121, 1939.
235. Huldschinsky K: Heilung von rachitis durch kunstlicht hohensonne. *Dtsch Med Wochenschr* 45:712, 1919.
236. McCollum EV, Simmonds N, Becker JE, et al: Studies on experimental rickets: An experimental demonstration of the existence of a vitamin which promotes calcium deposition. *J Biol Chem* 53:293, 1922.
237. Steenbock H, Black A: The induction of growth promoting and calcifying properties in a ration by exposure to ultraviolet lights. *J Biol Chem* 61:408, 1924.
238. Hess AF, Weinstock M: Antirachitic properties imparted to inert fluids and green vegetables by ultraviolet irradiation. *J Biol Chem* 62:301, 1924.
239. DeLuca HF: Remembrance: Discovery of the vitamin D endocrine system. *Endocrinology* 130:1763, 1992.
240. Holick MF, MacLaughlin JA, Clark MB, et al: Photosynthesis of previtamin D3 in human skin and the physiologic consequences. *Science* 210:203, 1980.
241. Vieth R: Vitamin D supplementation, 25-hydroxyvitamin D concentrations, and safety. *Am J Clin Nutr* 69:842, 1999.
242. Holick MF, Vitamin D: Photobiology, metabolism, mechanism of action, and clinical applications, in Favus MJ (ed): *Primer on the Bone Metabolic Bone Diseases and Disorders of Mineral Metabolism,* 4th ed. Pennsylvania, Lippincott Williams & Wilkins, 1999, p 92.
243. Clemens TL, Adams JS, Henderson SL, et al: Increased skin pigment reduces the capacity of the skin to synthesize vitamin D. *Lancet* 1:74, 1982.
244. Yoon PS, DeLuca HF: Resolution and reconstitution of soluble components of rat liver microsomal vitamin D_3-25 hydroxylase. *Arch Biochem Biophys* 203:529, 1980.
245. Bell NH, Shaw S, Turner RT: Evidence that 1,25-dihydroxyvitamin D_3 inhibits the hepatic production of 25-hydroxyvitamin D in man. *J Clin Invest* 74:1540, 1984.
246. Halloran BP, Bikle DD, Levens MJ, et al: Chronic 1,25-dihydroxyvitamin D_3 administration in the rat reduces the serum concentration of 25-hydroxyvitamin D by increasing metabolic clearance rate. *J Clin Invest* 78:622, 1986.
247. Haddad P, Gascon-Barre M, Brault G, et al: Influence of calcium or 1,25-dihydroxyvitamin D_3 supplementation on the hepatic microsomal and in vivo metabolism of vitamin D_3 in vitamin D-depleted rats. *J Clin Invest* 78:1529, 1986.
248. Breslau NA: Normal and abnormal regulation of 1,25-$(OH)_2D$ synthesis. *Am J Med Sci* 296:417, 1988.
249. Kumar R: Metabolism of 1,25-dihydroxyvitamin D_3. *Physiol Rev* 64:478, 1984.
250. Heany RP, Barger-Lux MJ, Dowell MS, et al: Calcium absorptive effects of vitamin D and its major metabolites. *J Clin Endocrinol Metab* 82:4111, 1997.
251. Mandel ML, Moorthy B, Ghazarian JG: Reciprocal post-translational regulation of renal 1 alpha- and 24-hydroxylases of 25-hydroxyvitamin D_3 by phosphorylation of ferredoxin: mRNA-directed cell-free synthesis and immunoisolation of ferredoxin. *Biochem J* 266:385, 1990.
252. Miller WL, Portale AA: Genetic disorders of vitamin D biosynthesis. *Endocrinol Metab Clin North Am* 28:825, 1999.
253. Ohyama Y, Noshiro M, Okuda K: Cloning and expression of cDNA encoding 25-hydroxyvitamin D_3 24-hydroxylase. *FEBS Lett* 278: 195, 1991.
254. St. Arnaud R, Glorieux FH: (editorial) 24, 25-Dihydroxyvitamin D-Active metabolite or inactive catabolite? *Endocrinology* 139:3371, 1998.
255. Boyan BK, Dean DD, Sylvia VL, et al: Cartilage and vitamin D: Genomic and nongenomic regulation by 1.25$(OH)_2D_3$ and 24,25$(OH)_2D_3$, in Feldman D, Glorieux FH, Pike JW (eds): *Vitamin D.* San Diego, Academic Press, 1997, p 395.
256. Schwartz Z, Dean DD, Walton JK, et al: Treatment of resting zone chondrocytes with 24,25-dihydroxyvitamin D_3 [24,25-$(OH)_2D_3$] induces differentiation into a 1.25-$(OH)_2D_3$-responsive phenotype characteristic of growth zone chondrocytes. *Endocrinology* 136:402, 1995.
257. Seo EG, Norman AW: Three-fold induction of renal 25-hydroxyvitamin D_3-24-hydroxylase activity and increased serum 24,25-dihydroxyvitamin D_3 levels are correlated with the healing process after chick tibial fracture. *J Bone Miner Res* 12:598, 1997.
258. Seo EG, Einhorn TA, Norman AW: 24R,25-dihydroxyvitamin D3: An essential vitamin D_3 metabolite for both normal bone integrity and healing of tibial fracture in chicks. *Endocrinology* 138:3864, 1997.
259. Henry HL: Regulation of the hydroxylation of 25-hydroxyvitamin D_3 in vivo and in primary cultures of chick kidney cells. *J Biol Chem* 254:2722, 1979.
260. Henry HL: Parathyroid hormone modulation of 25-hydroxyvitamin D_3 metabolism by cultured chick kidney cells is mimicked and enhanced by forskolin. *Endocrinology* 116:503, 1985.
261. Korkor AB, Gray RW, Henry HL, et al: Evidence that stimulation of 1,25$(OH)_2D_3$ production in primary cultures of mouse kidney cells by cyclic AMP requires new protein synthesis. *J Bone Miner Res* 2:517, 1987.
262. Shinki T, Jin CH, Nishimura A, et al: Parathyroid hormone inhibits 25-hydroxyvitamin D_3-24-hydroxylase mRNA expression stimulated by 1 α, 25-dihydroxyvitamin D_3 in rate kidney but not in intestine. *J Biol Chem* 267:13757, 1992.
263. Broadus AE, Horst RL, Lang R, et al: The importance of circulating 1,25-dihydroxyvitamin D in the pathogenesis of hypercalciuria and renal-stone formation in primary hyperparathyroidism. *N Engl J Med* 302:421, 1980.
264. Lund B, Srenson OH, Lund B, et al: Vitamin D metabolism in hypoparathyroidism. *J Clin Endocrinol Metab* 51:606, 1980.
265. Adams ND, Gray RW, Lemann J: The effects of oral $CaCO_3$ loading and dietary calcium deprivation on plasma 1,25-dihydroxyvitamin D concentrations in healthy adults. *J Clin Endocrinol Metab* 48:1008, 1979.
266. Portale AA, Halloran BP, Morris RC Jr: Physiologic regulation of the serum concentration of 1,25-dihydroxyvitamin D by phosphorus in normal men. *J Clin Invest* 83:1494, 1989.
267. Van den Berg CJ, Kumar R, Wilson DM, et al: Orthophosphate therapy decreases urinary calcium excetion and serum 1,25-dihydroxyvitamin D concentrations in idiopathic hypercalciuria. *J Clin Endocrinol Metab* 51:998, 1980.

268. Portale AA, Booth BE, Halloran BP, et al: Effect of dietary phosphorus on circulating concentrations of 1,25-dihydroxyvitamin D and immunoreactive parathyroid hormone in children with moderate renal insufficiency. *J Clin Invest* 73:1580, 1984.
269. Halloran PB, Spencer EM: Dietary phosphorus and 1,25-dihydroxyvitamin D metabolism: Influence of insulin-like growth factor I. *Endocrinology* 123:1225, 1988.
270. Ryan EA, Reiss E: Oncogenous osteomalacia: Review of the world literature of 42 cases and report of two new cases. *Am J Med* 77:501, 1984.
271. Colston KW, Evans IMA, Spelsberg TC, et al: Feedback of regulation of vitamin D metabolism by 1,25-dihydroxycholecalciferol. *Biochem J* 164:83, 1977.
272. Trechsel U, Eisman JA, Fischer JA, et al: Calcium-dependent, parathyroid hormone-independent regulation of 1,25-dihydroxyvitamin D. *Am J Physiol* 239:E119, 1980.
273. Bikle DD, Rasmussen H: The ionic control of 1,25-dihydroxyvitamin D_3 production in isolated chick renal tubules. *J Clin Invest* 55:292, 1975.
274. Bikle DD, Gee E, Halloran BP, et al: Free 1,25-dihydroxyvitamin D levels in serum from normal subjects, pregnant subjects, and subjects with liver disease. *J Clin Invest* 74:1966, 1984.
275. Cheema C, Grant BF, Marcus R: Effects of estrogen on circulating "free" and total 1,25-dihydroxyvitamin D and on the parathyroid-vitamin D axis in postmenopausal women. *J Clin Invest* 83:537, 1989.
276. Kumar R, Cohen WR, Silva P, et al: Elevated 1,25-dihydroxyvitamin D plasma levels in normal human pregnancy and lactation. *J Clin Invest* 63:342, 1979.
277. Emmersten K, Melsen F, Mosekilde L, et al: Altered vitamin D metabolism and bone remodelling in patients with medullary thyroid carcinoma and hypercalcitoninemia. *Metab Bone Dis Rel Res* 4:17, 1981.
278. Gray TK, Lester GE, Lorenc RS: Evidence for extrarenal 1α-hydroxylation of 25-dihydroxyvitamin D_3 in pregnancy. *Science* 204:1311, 1979.
279. Gertner JM, Coustan DR, Kliger AS, et al: Pregnancy is a state of physiological absorptive hypercalciuria. *Am J Med* 81:451, 1986.
280. Bikle DD, Nemanic MK, Whitney JO, et al: Neonatal human foreskin keratinocytes produce 1,25-dihydroxyvitamin D_3. *Biochemistry* 25:1545, 1986.
281. Howard GA, Turner RT, Sherrard DJ, et al: Human bone cells in culture metabolize 25-hydroxyvitamin D_3, and 24,25-dihydroxyvitamin D_3. *J Biol Chem* 256:7738, 1981.
282. Reichel H, Koeffler HP, Bishop JE, et al: 25-hydroxyvitamin D_3 metabolism by lipopolysaccaride-stimulated normal human macrophages. *J Clin Endocrinol Metab* 64:519, 1987.
283. Brommage R, DeLuca HF: Evidence that 1,25-dihydroxyvitamin D_3 is the physiologically active metabolite of vitamin D_3. *Endocr Rev* 6:491, 1985.
284. Cooke NE, Haddad JG: Vitamin D binding protein (Gc-globulin). *Endocr Rev* 10:294, 1989.
285. Bikle DD, Halloran BP, Gee E, et al: Free 25-hydroxyvitamin D levels are normal in subjects with liver disease and reduced total 25-hydroxyvitamin D levels. *J Clin Invest* 78:748, 1986.
286. Bikle DD, Gee E: Free, and not total, 1,25-dihydroxyvitamin D regulates 25-hydroxyvitamin D metabolism by keratinocytes. *Endocrinology* 124:649, 1989.
287. McLaughlin M, Raggatt PR, Fairney A, et al: Seasonal variation in serum 25-hydroxycholecalciferol in healthy people. *Lancet* 1:536, 1974.
288. Arnaud SB, Matthusen M, Gilkinson JB, et al: Components of 25-hydroxyvitamin D in serum of young children in upper midwestern United States. *Am J Clin Nutr* 30:1082, 1977.
289. Krall EA, Sahyoun N, Tannenbaum S, et al: Effect of vitamin D intake on seasonal variations in parathyroid hormone secretion in postmenopausal women. *N Engl J Med* 321:1777, 1989.
290. MacLaughlin J, Holick MF: Aging decreases the capacity of human skin to produce vitamin D_3. *J Clin Invest* 76:1536, 1985.
291. Barragry JM, France MW, Corless D, et al: Intestinal cholecalciferol absorption in the elderly and in younger adults. *Clin Sci Mol Med* 55:213, 1978.
292. Holick MF, Shao Q, Liu WW, et al: The vitamin D content of fortified milk and infant formula. *N Engl J Med* 326:1178, 1992.
293. Dawson-Hughes B, Dallal GE, Krall EA, et al: Effect of vitamin D supplementation on wintertime and overall bone loss in healthy postmenopausal women. *Ann Intern Med* 115:505, 1991.
294. Thomas MK, Lloyd-Jones DM, Thadhani RI, et al: Hypovitaminosis D in medical inpatients. *N Engl J Med* 338:777, 1998.
295. Baker AR, McDonnell DP, Jughes M, et al: Cloning and expression of full-length cDNA encoding human vitamin D receptor. *Proc Natl Acad Sci USA* 85:3294, 1988.
296. Hughes MR, Malloy PJ, Kieback DK, et al: Point mutation in the human vitamin D receptor gene associated with hypocalcemic rickets. *Science* 242:1702, 1988.
297. Liao J, Ozono K, Sone T, et al: Vitamin D receptor interaction with specific DNA requires a nuclear protein and 1,25-dihydroxyvitamin D_3. *Proc Natl Acad Sci USA* 87:9751, 1990.
298. Ozono K, Sone T, Pike JW: The genomic mechanism of action of 1,25-dihydroxyvitamin D_3. *J Bone Miner Res* 6:1021, 1991.
299. Strom M, Sandgren ME, Brown TA, DeLuca HF: 1,25-dihydroxyvitamin D_3 up-regulates the 1,25-dihydroxyvitamin D_3 receptor in vivo. *Proc Natl Acad Sci USA* 86:9770, 1989.
300. Naveh-Many T, Marx R, Keshet E, Pike JW, Silver J: Regulation of 1,25-dihydroxyvitamin D_3 receptor gene expression by 1,25-dihydroxyvitamin D_3 in the parathyroid in vivo. *J Clin Invest* 86:1968, 1990.
301. Hsieh JC, Jurutka PW, Galligan MA, Terpening CM, Haussler CA, Shimizu YK, Shimizu N, Haussler MR: Human vitamin D receptor is selectively phosphorylated by protein kinase C on serine 51, a residue crucial to its trans-activation function. *J Bone Miner Res* 6:S118, 1991.
302. Schüle R, Umesono K, Pike JW, Evans RM: Jun-Fos and receptors for vitamins A and D recognize a common response element in the human osteocalcin gene. *Cell* 61:497, 1990.
303. Yu VC, Delsert C, Andersen B, et al: RXR beta: a coregulator that enhances binding of retinoic acid, thyroid hormone, and vitamin D receptors to their cognate response elements. *Cell* 67:251, 1991.
304. Carlberg C, Bendik I, Wyss A, et al: Two nuclear signalling pathways for vitamin D. *Nature* 361:657, 1993.
305. Barsony J, Marx SJ: Receptor-mediated rapid action of 1 alpha, 25-dihydroxycholecalciferol: Increase of intracellular cGMP in human skin fibroblasts. *Proc Natl Acad Sci USA* 85:1223, 1988.
306. Baran DT, Milne ML: 1,25 dihydroxyvitamin D increases hepatocyte cytosolic calcium levels: A potential regulator of vitamin D-25-hydroxylase. *J Clin Invest* 77:1622, 1986.
307. Balsan S, Garabédian M, Larchet M, et al: Long-term nocturnal calcium infusions can cure rickets and promote normal mineralization in hereditary resistance to 1,25-dihydroxyvitamin D. *J Clin Invest* 77:1661, 1986.
308. Recker RR: Calcium absorption and achlorhydria. *N Engl J Med* 313:70, 1985.
309. Sheikh MS, Santa Ana CA, Nicar MJ, et al: Gastrointestinal absorption of calcium from milk and calcium salts. *N Engl J Med* 317:532, 1987.
310. Heaney RP, Gallagher JC, Johnston CC, et al: Calcium nutrition and bone health in the elderly. *Am J Clin Nutr* 36:986, 1982.
311. Favus MJ: Factors that influence absorption and secretion of calcium in the small intestine and colon. *Am J Physiol* 248:G147, 1985.
312. Sheikh MS, Schille LR, Fordtran JS: In vivo intestinal absorption of calcium in humans. *Miner Electrolyte Metab* 16:130, 1990.
313. Bikle DD, Zolock DT, Morrissey RL, et al: Independence of 1,25-dihydroxyvitamin D_3-mediated calcium transport from de novo RNA and protein synthesis. *J Biol Chem* 253:484, 1978.
314. Norman AW: Intestinal calcium absorption: A vitamin D-hormone-mediated adaptive response. *Am J Clin Nutr* 51:290, 1990.
315. Bikle DD, Munson S: 1,25-dihydroxyvitamin D increases calmodulin binding to specific proteins in the chick duodenal brush border membrane. *J Clin Invest* 76:2312, 1985.
316. Rasmussen H, Matsumoto T, Fontaine O, et al: Role of changes in membrane lipid structure in the action of 1,25-dihydroxyvitamin D_3. *Fed Proc* 41:72, 1982.
317. Christakos S, Gabrielides C, Rhoten WB: Vitamin D-dependent calcium binding proteins: Chemistry, distribution, functional considerations, and molecular biology. *Endocr Rev* 10:3, 1989.
318. Gross M, Kumar R: Physiology and biochemistry of vitamin D-dependent calcium binding proteins. *Am J Physiol* 259:F195, 1990.
319. Ghijsen WEJM, Van Os CH: 1,25-dihydroxyvitamin D_3 regulates ATP-dependent calcium transport in basolateral plasma membranes of rat enterocytes. *Biochim Biophys Acta* 689:170, 1982.
320. Cross HS, Debiec H, Peterlik M: Mechanism and regulation of intestinal phosphate absorption. *Miner Electrolyte Metab* 16:115, 1990.

321. Tern PH: Vitamin D and bone. *Kidney Int* 38:S17, 1990.
322. Rowe DW, Kream BE: Regulation of collagen synthesis in fetal rat calvaria by 1,25-dihydroxyvitamin D_3. *J Biol Chem* 257:8009, 1982.
323. Maierhofer WJ, Lemann J Jr, Gray RW, et al: Dietary calcium and serum 1,25-$(OH)_2$-vitamin D concentrations as determinants of calcium balance in healthy men. *Kidney Int* 26:752, 1984.
324. McSheehy PMJ, Chambers TJ: 1,25-dihydroxyvitamin D_3 stimulates rat osteoblastic cells to release a soluble factor that increases osteoclastic bone resorption. *J Clin Invest* 80:425, 1987.
325. Abe E, Miyaura C, Tanaka H, et al: 1α, 25-dihydroxyvitamin D_3 promotes fusion of mouse alveolar macrophages both by a direct mechanism and by a spleen cell-mediated indirect mechanism. *Proc Natl Acad Sci USA* 80:5583, 1983.
326. Udagawa N, Takahashi N, Akatsu T, et al: Origin of osteoclasts: Mature monocytes and macrophages are capable of differentiating into osteoclasts under a suitable microenvironment prepared by bone marrow-derived stromal cells. *Proc Natl Acad Sci USA* 87:7260, 1990.
327. Bikle DD, Halloran BP, McGalliard-Cone C, et al: Different responses of trabecular and cortical bone to 1,25$(OH)_2D_3$ infusion. *Am J Physiol* 259:E715, 1990.
328. Hruska KA, Kurnik BRC: Regulation of renal phosphate transport, in Avioli LV, Krane SM (eds): *Metabolic Bone Disease*. Philadelphia, Saunders, 1990, p 222.
329. Yamamoto M, Kawanobe Y, Takahashi H, et al: Vitamin D deficiency and renal calcium transport in the rat. *J Clin Invest* 74:507, 1984.
330. Manolages SC, Hystmyer FG, Yu XP: 1,25-dihydroxyvitamin D_3 and the immune system. *Proc Soc Exp Biol Med* 191:238, 1989.
331. Hosomi J, Hosoi J, Abe E, et al: Regulation of terminal differentiation of cultured mouse epidermal cells by 1α,25-dihydroxyvitamin D_3. *Endocrinology* 113:1950, 1983.
332. Bikle DD: Clinical counterpoint: Vitamin D: new actions, new analogs, new therapeutic potential. *Endocr Rev* 13:765, 1992.
333. Abe J, Takita Y, Nakano T, et al: A synthetic analog of vitamin D3, 22-oxa-1α,25-dihydroxyvitamin D_3, is a potent modulator of in vivo immunoregulating activity without inducing hypercalcemia in mice. *Endocrinology* 124:2654, 1989.
334. Brown AJ, Ritter CR, Finch JL, et al: The noncalcemic analogue of vitamin D, 22-oxacalcitriol, suppresses parathyroid hormone synthesis and secretion. *J Clin Invest* 84:728, 1989.
335. Zhou JY, Norman AW, Lubbert M, et al: Novel vitamin D analogs that modulate leukemic cell growth and differentiation with little effect on either intestinal calcium absorption or bone calcium mobilization. *Blood* 74:82, 1989.
336. Shepard RM, Horst RL, Hamstra AJ, et al: Determination of vitamin D and its metabolites in plasma from normal and anephric man. *Biochem J* 182:55, 1979.
337. Murray J, Favus: Laboratory values of importance for calcium metabolism and metabolic bone disease, in Lippincott-Raven Publishers (ed): *Primer on the Metabolic Bone Diseases and Disorders of Mineral Metabolism*, 3rd ed. Philadelphia, New York, 1996, p 451.
338. Ralston SH, Gallacher SJ, Patel U, et al: Cancer-associated hypercalcemia: Morbidity and mortality. Clinical experience in 126 treated patients. *Ann Intern Med* 112:499, 1990.
339. Wimalawansa SJ: Significance of plasma PTH-rP in patients with hypercalcemia of malignancy treated with bisphosphonate. *Cancer* 73:2223, 1994.
340. Nussbaum SR, Younger J, Vandepol CJ, et al: Single-dose intravenous therapy with pamidronate for the treatment of hypercalcemia of malignancy: Comparison of 30-, 60-, and 90-mg dosages. *Am J Med* 95:297, 1993.
341. Mundy GR, Martin TJ: The hypercalcemia of malignancy: Pathogenesis and management. *Metabolism* 31:1247, 1982.
342. Delmas PD: Biochemical markers of bone turnover for the clinical assessment of metabolic disease. *Endocrinol Metab Clin North Am* 19:1, 1990.
343. Eyre D: New biomarkers of bone resorption (editorial). *J Clin Endocrinol Metab* 74:470, 1992.
343a. Miller PD, Baran DT, Bilezikian JP: Practical clinical application of biochemical markers of bone turnover. *J Clin Bone Densitometry* 2:323, 1999.
344. Delmas PD, Demiaux B, Malaval L, Chapuy MC, Edouard C, Meunier PJ: Serum bone gamma carboxyglutamic acid-containing protein in primary hyperparathyroidism and in malignant hypercalcemia. *J Clin Invest* 77:985, 1986.
345. Schwartz TB: Giants with tunnel vision: The Albright-Collip controversy. *Perspec Biol Med* 34:327, 1991.
346. Schachner SH, Hall A: Parathyroid adenoma and previous head-and-neck irradiation. *Ann Intern Med* 88:804, 1978.
347. Albright F: A page out of the history of hyperparathyroidism. *J Clin Endocrinol Metab* 8:637, 1948.
348. Albright F, Ellsworth R: *Unchartered Seas*. Portland OR, Kalmia Press, 1990.
349. Collip JB, Pugsley LI, Selye H, et al: Observations concerning the mechanism of action of parathyroid hormone. *Br J Exp Pathol* 15:335, 1934.
350. Barnicot NA: The local action of the parathyroid and other tissues on bone in intracerebral grafts. *J Anat* 82:233, 1948.
351. Heath H, Hodgson SF, Kennedy MA: Primary hyperparathyroidism: Incidence, morbidity and potential economic impact in a community. *N Engl J Med* 302:189, 1980.
352. Arnold A, Staunton CE, Hyung Goo Kim BS, et al: Monoclonality and abnormal parathyroid hormone genes in parathyroid adenomas. *N Engl J Med* 318:658, 1988.
353. Marx SJ: Genetic defects in primary hyperparathyroidism. *N Engl J Med* 318:699, 1988.
354. Tissell LE, Carlsson S, Lindberg S, et al: Autonomous hyperparathyroidism—a possible late complication of neck radiotherapy. *Acta Chir Scand* 142:367, 1976.
355. Paloyan E, Lawrence AM, Prinz RA, et al: Radiation-associated hyperparathyroidism (letter). *Lancet* 1:949, 1977.
356. Rosenberg CL, Kim HG, Shows TB, et al: Rearrangment and overexpression of D11S287E, a candidate oncogene, on chromosome 11q13 in benign parathyroid tumors. *Oncogene* 6:449, 1991.
357. Friedman E, Bale AE, Marx SJ, et al: Genetic abnormalities in sporadic parathyroid adenomas. *J Clin Endocrinol Metab* 71:293, 1990.
358. Arnold A, Kim HG, Gaz RD, et al: Molecular cloning and chromosomal mapping of DNA rearranged with the parathyroid hormone gene in a parathyroid adenoma. *J Clin Invest* 83:2034, 1989.
359. Hsi ED, Zukerberg LR, Yang WI, et al: Cyclin D1/PRAD1 expression in parathyroid adenomas: An immunohistochemical study. *J Clin Endocrinol Metab* 81:1736, 1996.
360. Lammie GA, Fantl V, Smith R, et al: D11S287, a putative oncogene on chromosome 11q13, is amplified and expressed in squamous cell and mammary carcinomas, and linked to BCL-1. *Oncogene* 6:439, 1991.
361. Rosenberg CL, Wong E, Petty EM, et al: PRAD1, a candidate BCL1 oncongene: Mapping and expression in centrocytic lymphoma. *Proc Natl Acad Sci USA* 88:9638, 1991.
362. Motokura T, Bloom T, Kim HG, et al: A novel cyclin encoded by a BCL1-linked candidate oncogene. *Nature* 350:512, 1991.
363. Bystrom C, Larsson C, Blomberg C, et al: Localization of the MEN1 gene to a small region within chromosome 11q13 by deletion mapping in tumors. *Proc Natl Acad Sci USA* 87:1968, 1990.
364. Friedman E, Sakaguchi K, Bale AE, et al: Clonality of parathyroid tumors in familial multiple endocrine neoplasia type 1. *N Engl J Med* 321:213, 1989.
365. Chandrasekharappa SC, Guru SC, Manickam P, et al: Positional cloning of the gene for multiple endocrine neoplasia type I. *Science* 276:404, 1997.
366. Bassett JHD, Forbes SA, Pannett AAJ, et al: Characterization of mutations in patients with multiple endocrine neoplasia type I. *Am J Hum Genet* 62:232, 1998.
367. Heppner C, Kester MB, Agarwal SK, et al: Somatic mutation of the MEN I gene in parathyroid tumors. *Nat Genet* 16:375, 1997.
368. Bishop JM: The molecular genetics of cancer. *Science* 235:305, 1987.
369. Bishop JM: Molecular themes in oncogenesis. *Cell* 64:235, 1991.
370. Friend SH, Horowitz JM, Gerber MR: Deletions of a DNA sequence in retinoblastomas and mesenchymal tumors: Organization of the sequence and its encoded protein. *Proc Natl Acad Sci USA* 84:9059, 1987.
371. Cryns VL, Yi SM, Tahara H, et al: Frequent loss of chromosome arm 1p DNA in parathyroid adenomas. *Genes Chromosomes Cancer* 13:9, 1995.
372. Szabo J, Heath B, Hill VM, et al: Hereditary hyperparathyroidism—jaw tumor syndrome: The endocrine tumor gene HRPT2 maps to chromosome Iq21-q31. *Am J Hum Genet* 56:944, 1995.
373. Hosokawa Y, Pollak MR, Brown EM, et al: Mutational analysis of the extracellular Ca^{2+}-sensing receptor gene in human parathyroid tumors. *J Clin Endocrinol Metab* 80:3107, 1995.

374. Habener JF, Potts JT Jr: Parathyroid physiology and primary hyperparathyroidism, in Avioli LV, Krane SM (eds): *Metabolic Bone Disease*. New York, Academic Press, 1978, p 1.
375. Roth SI: Recent advances in parathyroid gland pathology. *Am J Med* 50:612, 1971.
376. Wynne AG, Van Heerden J, Carney JA, et al: Parathyroid carcinoma: Clinical and pathological features in 43 patients. *Medicine* 71:197, 1992.
377. Brown EM: Four-parameter model of the sigmoidal relationship between parathyroid hormone release and extracellular calcium concentration in normal and abnormal parathyroid tissue. *J Clin Endocrinol Metab* 56:572, 1983.
378. Brown EM, Garner DG, Brennan MF, et al: Calcium-regulated parathyroid hormone release in primary hyperparathyroidism. *Am J Med* 66:923, 1979.
379. Gittes RR, Radde IC: Experimental hyperparathyroidism from multiple isologous parathyroid transplants: Homostatic effect of simultaneous thyroid transplants. *Endocrinology* 78:1015, 1966.
380. Mundy GR, Cove DH, Fisken R: Primary hyperparathyroidism: Changes in the pattern of clinical presentation. *Lancet* 1:1317, 1980.
381. Barreras RF: Calcium and gastric secretion. *Gastroenterology* 64:1168, 1973.
382. Ostrow JD, Blandshard G, Gray SJ: Peptic ulcer in primary hyperparathyroidism. *Am J Med* 24:769, 1960.
383. Wilson SD, Singh RB, Kalkhoff RK, et al: Does hyperparathyroidism cause hypergastrinemia? *Surgery* 80:231, 1976.
384. Bess MA, Edis AJ, van Heerden JA: Hyperparathyroidism and pancreatitis. *JAMA* 243:246, 1980.
385. Joborn C, Hetta J, Lind L, et al: Self-rated psychiatric symptoms in patients operated on because of primary hyperparathyroidism and in patients with long-standing mild hypercalcemia. *Surgery* 105:72, 1989.
386. Wishart J, Horowitz M, Need A, et al: Relationship between forearm and vertebral mineral density in postmenopausal women with primary hyperparathyroidism. *Arch Intern Med* 150:1329, 1990.
387. Mautalen C, Reyes HR, Ghiringhelli G, et al: Cortical bone mineral content in primary hyperparathyroidism: Changes after parathyroidectomy. *Acta Endocrinol (Copenh)* 111:494, 1986.
388. Christiansen P, Steiniche T, Mosekilde L, et al: Primary hyperparathyroidism: Changes in trabecular bone remodeling following surgical treatment—evaluated by histomorphometric methods. *Bone* 11:75, 1990.
389. Potts JT Jr: Management of asymptomatic hyperparathyroidism. *J Clin Endocrinol Metab* 70:1489, 1990.
390. Dempster DW, Parisien M, Silverberg SJ, et al: On the mechanism of cancellous bone preservation in postmenopausal women with mild primary hyperparathyroidism. *J Clin Endocrinol Metab* 84:1562, 1999.
391. Silverberg SJ, Gartenberg F, Jacobs TP, et al: Longitudinal measurements of bone density and biochemical indices in untreated primary hyperparathyroidism. *J Clin Endocrinol Metab* 80:723, 1995.
392. Khosla S, Melton LJ III, Wermers RA, et al: Primary hyperparathyroidism and the risk of fracture: a population–based study. *J Bone Miner Res* 14:1700, 1999.
393. Silverberg SJ, Shane E, Jacobs TP, et al: A 10-year prospective study of primary hyperparathyroidism with or without parathyroid surgery. *N Engl J Med* 341:1249, 1999.
394. Bilezikian JP: Surgery or no surgery for primary hyperparathyroidism. *Ann Intern Med* 102:402, 1985.
395. Silverberg SJ, Shane E, Jacobs TP, et al: Nephrolithiasis and bone involvement in primary hyperparathyroidism. *Am J Med* 89:327, 1990.
396. Cogan MG, Covey CM, Arieff AI, et al: Central nervous system manifestations of hyperparathyroidism. *Am J Med* 65:963, 1978.
397. Burney RE, Jones KR, Christy B, et al: Health status improvement after surgical correction of primary hyperparathyroidism in patients with high and low preoperative calcium levels. *Surgery* 125:608, 1999.
398. Patten BM, Bilezikian JP, Mallette LE, et al: Neuromuscular disease in primary hyperparathyroidism. *Ann Intern Med* 80:182, 1974.
399. Turken SA, Cafferty M, Silverberg SJ, et al: Neuromuscular involvement in mild, asymptomatic primary hyperparathyroidism. *Am J Med* 87:553, 1989.
400. Goldsmith RE, Sizemore GW, Chen IW, et al: Familial hyperparathyroidism. *Ann Intern Med* 84:36, 1976.
401. Law WM, Hodgson SF, Heath H: Autosomal recessive inheritance of familial hyperparathyroidism. *N Engl J Med* 309:650, 1983.
402. Wermer P: Genetic aspects of adenomatosis of endocrine glands. *Am J Med* 16:363, 1954.
403. Larsson C, Skogseid B, Oberg K, et al: Multiple endocrine neoplasia type 1 maps to chromosome 11 and is lost in insulinoma. *Nature* 332:85, 1988.
404. Keiser HR, Beaven MA, Doppman J, et al: Sipple's syndrome: Medullary thyroid carcinoma, pheochromocytoma, and parathyroid disease. *Ann Intern Med* 78:1973.
405. Sizemore GW, Health H, Carney JA: Multiple endocrine neoplasia type 2. *Clin Endocrinol Metab* 9:299, 1980.
406. Norum RA, Lafreniere RG, O'Neal LW: Linkage of the multiple endocrine neoplasia type 2B gene (MEN2B) to chromosome 10 markers linked to MEN2A. *Genomics* 8:313, 1990.
407. Marx SJ, Spiegel AM, Levine MA, et al: Familial hypocalciuric hypercalcemia. *N Engl J Med* 307:416, 1982.
408. Marx SJ, Attie MF, Levine MA, et al: The hypocalciuric or benign variant of familial hypercalcemia: Clinical and biochemical features in fifteen kindreds. *Medicine (Baltimore)* 60:397, 1981.
409. Law WM, Heath H: Familial benign hypercalcemia (hypocalciuric hypercalcemia). *Ann Intern Med* 102:511, 1985.
410. Kristiansen JH, Rodbro P, Christiansen C, et al: Familial hypocalciuric hypercalcemia III: Bone mineral metabolism. *Clin Endocrinol* 26:713, 1987.
411. Pollak MR, Chou YHW, Marx SJ, et al: Familial hypocalciuric hypercalcemia and neonatal severe hyperparathyroidism: Effects of mutant gene dosage on phenotype. *J Clin Invest* 93:1108, 1994.
412. Clapham DE: Mutations in G protein-linked receptors: Novel insights on disease. *Cell* 75:1237, 1993.
413. Marx SJ: Familial hypocalciuric hypercalcemia, in Favus MJ (ed): *Primer on the Bone Metabolic Bone Diseases and Disorders of Mineral Metabolism*, 4th ed. Pennsylvania, Lippincott Williams & Wilkins, 1999, p 195.
414. Broadus AE, Horst RL, Littledike ET, et al: Primary hyperparathyroidism with intermittent hypercalcemia: Serial observations and simple diagnosis by means of an oral calcium tolerance test. *Clin Endocrinol (Oxf)* 12:225, 1980.
415. Boggs JE, Irvin GL III, Molinari AS, et al: Intraoperative parathyroid hormone monitoring as an adjunct to parathyroidectomy. *Surgery* 120:954, 1996.
416. Winzelberg GG: Parathyroid imaging. *Ann Intern Med* 107:64, 1989.
417. Mallette LE, Gomez L, Fisher RG: Parathyroid angiography: A review of current knowledge and guidelines for clinical application. *Endocr Rev* 2:124, 1981.
418. Eisenberg H, Pallotta J, Sacks B, et al: Parathyroid localization, three-dimensional modeling, and percutaneous ablation techniques. *Endocrinol Metab Clin North Am* 18:659, 1989.
419. Johnston LB, Carroll MJ, Britton KE, et al: The accuracy of parathyroid gland localization in primary hyperparathyroidism using sestamibi radionuclide imaging. *J Clin Endocrinol Metab* 81:346, 1996.
420. CDC Panel: Diagnosis and management of asymptomatic primary hyperparathyroidism: Consensus development conference statement. *Ann Intern Med* 114:593, 1991.
421. Pallotta JA, Sacks BA, Moller DE, et al: Arteriographic ablation of cervical parathyroid adenomas. *J Clin Endocrinol Metab* 69:1249, 1989.
422. Garner SC, Leight GS Jr: Initial experience with intraoperative PTH determinations in the surgical management of 130 consecutive cases of primary hyperparathyroidism. *Surgery* 126:1132, 1999.
423. Rizzoli R, Green J III, Marx SJ: Primary hyperparathyroidism in familial multiple endocrine neoplasia type 1: Long term follow-up of serum calcium levels after parathyroidectomy. *Am J Med* 78:467, 1985.
424. Wang C: Parathyroid re-exploration: A clinical and pathological study of 112 cases. *Ann Surg* 186:140, 1977.
425. Niederle B, Roka R, Brennan MF: The transplantation of parathyroid tissue in man: Development, indications, techniques, and results. *Endocr Rev* 3:245, 1982.
426. Wells SA, Ellis GJ, Gunnells JC, et al: Parathyroid autotransplantation in primary parathyroid hyperplasia. *N Engl J Med* 295:57, 1976.
427. Cope O: Hyperparathyroidism—too little, too much surgery? *N Engl J Med* 295:100, 1976.
428. Schantz A, Castleman B: Parathyroid carcinoma. *Cancer* 31:600, 1973.
429. Shane E, Bilezikian JP: Parathyroid carcinoma: A review of 62 patients. *Endocr Rev* 3:218, 1982.

430. Brasier AR, Nussbaum SR: Hungry bone syndrome: Clinical and biochemical predicators of its occurrence after parathyroid surgery. *Am J Med* 84:654, 1988.
431. Silverberg SJ, Bilezikian JP, Bone HG, et al: Therapeutic controversy: Therapeutic controversies in primary hyperparathyroidism. *J Clin Endocrinol Metab* 84:2275, 1999.
432. Abdelhadi M, Nordenstrom J: Bone mineral recovery after parathyroidectomy in patients with primary and renal hyperparathyroidism. *J Clin Endocrinol Metabol* 83:3845, 1998.
433. Roberts WC, Waller BF: Effect of chronic hypercalcemia on the heart: An analysis of 18 necropsy patients. *Am J Med* 71:371, 1981.
434. Bilezikian JP: The medical management of primary hyperparathyroidism. *Ann Intern Med* 96:198, 1982.
435. Selby PL, Peacock M: Ethinyl estradiol and norethindrone in the treatment of primary hyperparathyroidism in postmenopausal women. *N Engl J Med* 314:1481, 1986.
436. Coe FL, Favus MJ, Parks JH: Is estrogen preferable to surgery for postmenopausal women with primary hyperparathyroidism? *N Engl J Med* 314:1508, 1986.
437. Horowitz M, Wishart J, Need AG, et al: Treatment of postmenopausal hyperparathyroidism with norethindrone. *Arch Intern Med* 147:681, 1987.
438. Broadus AE, Magee JS, Mallette LE, et al: A detailed evaluation of oral phosphate therapy in selected patients with primary hyperparathyroidism. *J Clin Endocrinol Metab* 56:953, 1983.
439. Caro JF, Castro JC, Glennon JA: Effect of long-term propanolol administration on parathyroid hormone and calcium concentration in primary hyperparathyroidism. *Ann Intern Med* 91:740, 1979.
440. Glaser B, Kraiem Z, Rotem M, et al: Effect of acute cimetidine administration on indices of parathyroid hormone action in healthy subjects and patients with primary and secondary hyperparathyroidism. *J Clin Endocrinol Metab* 59:993, 1984.
441. Reasner CA, Stone MD, Hosking DJ, et al: Acute changes in calcium homeostasis during treatment of primary hyperparathyroidism with risedronate. *J Clin Endocrinol Metab* 4:1067, 1993.
442. Jansson S, Tisell LE, Lindstedt G, et al: Disodium pamidronate in the preoperative treatment of hypercalcemia in patients with primary hyperparathyroidism. *Surgery* 3:480, 1991.
443. Adami S, Zamberlan N, Mian M, et al: Duration of the effects of intravenous alendronate in postmenopausal women and in patients with primary hyperparathyroidism and Paget's disease of bone. *Bone Miner* 2:75, 1994.
444. Silverberg SJ, Bone HG, Marriott TB, et al: Short-term inhibition of parathyroid hormone secretion by a calcium receptor agonist in patients with primary hyperparathyroidism. *N Engl J Med* 337:1506, 1997.
445. Shane E, Baquiran DC, Bilezikian JP: Effects of dichloromethylene diphosphate on serum and urinary calcium in primary hyperparathyroidism. *Ann Intern Med* 95:23, 1981.
446. Fleisch H: Osteoporosis: *Bisphosphonates in Bone Disease: from the Laboratory to the Patient.* New York, The Parthenon Publishing Group, 1995, p 115.
447. Pedrazzoni M, Palummeri E, Ciotti G, et al: Short-term effects on bone and mineral metabolism of 4-amino-1-hydroxybutylidene-1, 1-diphosphonate (ABDP) in Paget's disease of bone. *Bone Min* 7:301, 1989.
448. Thompson DD, Seedor JG, Weinreb M, et al: Aminohydroxybutane bisphosphonate inhibits bone loss due to immobilization in rats. *J Bone Miner Res* 5:279, 1990.
449. Warrell RP Jr, Israel R, Frisone M, et al: Gallium nitrate for acute treatment of cancer-related hypercalcemia: A randomized, double-blind comparison to calcitonin. *Ann Intern Med* 108:669, 1988.
450. Warrell RP Jr, Issacs M, Alcock NW, et al: Gallium nitrate for treatment of refractory hypercalcemia from parathyroid carcinoma. *Ann Intern Med* 107:683, 1987.
451. Stewart AF, Horst R, Deftos LJ, et al: Biochemical evaluation of patients with cancer-associated hypercalcemia: Evidence for humoral and nonhumoral groups. *N Engl J Med* 303:1377, 1980.
452. Case Records of the Massachusetts General Hospital (case 27461). *N Engl J Med* 22:789, 1941.
453. Moseley JM, Kubota M, Diefenbach-Jagger H, et al: Parathyroid hormone-related protein purified from a human lung cancer cell line. *Proc Natl Acad Sci USA* 84:5048, 1987.
454. Burtis WJ, Wu T, Bunch C, et al: Identification of a novel 17,000-dalton parathyroid hormone-like adenylate cyclase-stimulating protein from a tumor associated with humoral hypercalcemia of malignancy. *J Biol Chem* 262:7151, 1987.
455. Strewler GJ, Stern PH, Jacobs JW, et al: Parathyroid hormone-like protein from human renal carcinoma cells. Structural and functional homology with parathyroid hormone. *J Clin Invest* 80:1803, 1987.
456. Suva LJ, Winslow GA, Wettenhall REH, et al: A parathyroid hormone-related protein implicated in malignant hypercalcemia: Cloning and expression. *Science* 237:893, 1987.
457. Wysolmerski JJ, Broadus AE: Hypercalcemia of malignancy: The central role of parathyroid hormone-related protein. *Annu Rev Med* 45:189, 1994.
458. Strewler GJ, Nissenson RA: Hypercalcemia in malignancy. *West J Med* 153:635, 1990.
459. Strewler GJ, Budayr AA, Clark OH, et al: Production of parathyroid hormone by a malignant nonparathyroid tumor in a hypercalcemic patient. *J Clin Endocrinol Metab* 76:1373, 1993.
460. Nussbaum SR, Gaz RD, Arnold A: Hypercalcemia and ectopic secretion of parathyroid hormone by an ovarian carcinoma with rearrangement of the gene for parathyroid hormone. *N Engl J Med* 323:1324, 1990.
461. Yoshimoto K, Yamasaki R, Sakai H, et al: Ectopic production of parathyroid hormone by small cell lung cancer in a patient with hypercalcemia. *J Clin Endocrinol Metab* 68:976, 1989.
462. Rizzoli R, Pache JC, Didierjean L, et al: A thymoma as a cause of true ectopic hyperparathyroidism. *J Clin Endocrinol Metab* 79:912, 1994.
463. Iguchi H, Miyagi C, Tomita K, et al: Hypercalcemia caused by ectopic production of parathyroid hormone in a patient with papillary adenocarcinoma of the thyroid gland. *J Clin Endocrinol Metab* 83:2653, 1998.
464. Nielsen P, Rasmussen A, Feldt-Rasmussen U, et al: Ectopic production of intact parathyroid hormone by a squamous cell lung carcinoma in vivo and in vitro. *J Clin Endocrinol Metab* 81:3793, 1996.
465. Schmelzer HJ, Hesch RD, Mayer H: Parathyroid hormone and PTH mRNA in human small cell lung cancer. *Recent Results Cancer Res* 909:88, 1985.
466. Horiuchi N, Caulfield MP, Fisher JE, et al: Similarity of synthetic peptide from human tumor to parathyroid hormone *in vivo* and *in vitro*. *Science* 238:1566, 1987. [Published erratum appears in *Science* 239:128, 1988]
467. Kemp BE, Moseley JM, Rodda CP, et al: Parathyroid hormone-related protein of malignancy: Active synthetic fragments. *Science* 238:1568, 1987.
468. Yates AJP, Gutierrez GE, Smolens P, et al: Effects of a synthetic peptide of a parathyroid hormone-related protein on calcium homeostasis, renal tubular calcium reabsorption, and bone metabolism *in vivo* and *in vitro* in rodents. *J Clin Invest* 81:932, 1988.
469. Sartori L, Weir EC, Stewart AF, et al: Synthetic and partially-purified adenylate cyclase-stimulating proteins from tumors associated with humoral hypercalcemia of malignancy inhibit phosphate transport in a PTH-responsive renal cell line. *J Clin Endocrinol Metab* 66:459, 1988.
470. Asa SL, Henderson J, Goltzman D, et al: Parathyroid hormone-like peptide in normal and neoplastic human endocrine tissues. *J Clin Endocrinol Metab* 71:1112, 1990.
471. Danks JA, Ebeling PR, Hayman J, et al: Parathyroid hormone-related protein: Immunohistochemical localization in cancers and in normal skin. *J Bone Miner Res* 4:273, 1989.
472. Dunne FP, Lee S, Ratcliffe WA, et al: Parathyroid hormone-related protein (PTHrP) gene expression in solid tumors associated with normocalcemia and hypercalcemia. *J Pathol* 171:215, 1993.
473. Wysolmerski JJ, Vasavada R, Foley J, et al: Transactivation of the PTHrP gene in squamous carcinomas predicts the occurrence of hypercalcemia in athymic mice. *Cancer Res* 56:1043, 1996.
474. Thiede MA: The mRNA encoding a parathyroid hormone-like peptide is produced in mammary tissue in response to elevations in serum prolactin. *Mol Endocrinol* 3:1443, 1989.
475. Kremer R, Karaplis AC, Henderson J, et al: Regulation of parathyroid hormone-like peptide in cultured normal human keratinocytes. Effect of growth factors and 1,25 dihydroxyvitamin D_3 on gene expression and secretion. *J Clin Invest* 87:884, 1991.
476. Sebag M, Henderson J, Goltzman D, et al: Regulation of parathyroid hormone-related peptide production in normal human mammary epithelial cells *in vitro*. *Am J Physiol* 267:C723, 1994.
477. Ferrari SL, Rizzoli R, Bonjour JP: Effects of epidermal growth factor on parathyroid hormone-related protein production by mammary epithelial cells. *J Bone Miner Res* 9:639, 1994.

478. Southby J, Murphy LM, Martin TJ, et al: Cell-specific and regulator-induced promoter usage and messenger ribonucleic acid splicing for parathyroid hormone-related protein. *Endocrinology* 137:1349, 1996.
479. Rizzoli R, Feyen JHM, Grau G, et al: Regulation of parathyroid hormone-related protein production in a human lung squamous cell carcinoma line. *J Endocrinol* 143:333, 1994.
480. Burton PBJ, Knight DE: Parathyroid hormone-related peptide can regulate growth of human lung cancer cells. *FEBS Lett* 305:228, 1992.
481. Zakalik D, Diep D, Hooks MA, et al: Transforming growth factor increases stability of parathyroid hormone-related protein messenger RNA. *J Bone Miner Res* 7(Suppl 1):104A, S118, 1992.
482. Merryman JI, DeWille JW, Werkmeister JR, et al: Effects of transforming growth factor on parathyroid hormone-related protein production and ribonucleic acid expression by a squamous carcinoma cell line *in vitro*. *Endocrinology* 134:2424, 1994.
483. Kiriyama T, Gillespie MT, Glatz JA, et al: 1993 Transforming growth factor stimulation of parathyroid hormone-related protein (PTHrP): A paracrine regulator? *Mol Cell Endocrinol* 92:55, 1993. [Published erratum appears in *Mol Cell Endocrinol* 94:145, 1993].
484. Pirola CJ, Wang HM, Kamyar A, et al: Angiotensin II regulates parathyroid hormone-related protein expression in cultured rat aortic smooth muscle cells through both transcriptional and posttranscriptional mechanisms. *J Biol Chem* 268:1987, 1993.
485. Daifotis AG, Weir EC, Dreyer BE, et al: Stretch-induced parathyroid hormone-related protein gene expression in the rat uterus. *J Biol Chem* 267:23455, 1992.
486. Li X, Drucker DJ: Parathyroid hormone-related peptide is a downstream target for ras and src activation. *J Biol Chem* 269:6263, 1994.
487. Glatz JA, Heath JK, Southby J, et al: Dexamethasone regulation of parathyroid hormone-related protein (PTHrP) expression in a squamous cancer cell line. *Mol Cell Endocrinol* 101:295, 1994.
488. Lu C, Ikeda K, Deftos LJ, et al: Glucocorticoid regulation of parathyroid hormone-related peptide gene transcription in a human neuroendocrine cell line. *Mol Endocrinol* 3:2034, 1989.
489. Thiede MA, Harm SC, Hasson DM, et al: *In vivo* regulation of parathyroid hormone-related peptide messenger ribonucleic acid in the rat uterus by 17-estradiol. *Endocrinology* 128:2317, 1991.
490. Paspaliaris V, Petersen DN, Thiede MA: Steroid regulation of parathyroid hormone-related protein expression and action in the rat uterus. *J Steroid Biochem Mol Biol* 53:259, 1995.
491. Foley J, Wysolmerski JJ, Broadus AE, et al: Parathyroid hormone-related protein gene expression in human squamous carcinoma cells is repressed by mutant isoforms of p53. *Cancer Res* 56:4056, 1996.
492. Martin TJ, Moseley JM, Gillespie MT: Parathyroid hormone-related protein: Biochemistry and molecular biology. *Crit Rev Biochem Mol Biol* 26:377, 1991.
493. Soifer NE, Dee KE, Insogna KL, et al: Parathyroid hormone-related protein. Evidence for secretion of a novel mid-region fragment by three different cell types. *J Biol Chem* 267:18236, 1992.
494. Burtis WJ, Fodero JP, Gaich G, et al: Preliminary characterization of circulating amino- and carboxyl-terminal fragments of parathyroid hormone-related peptide in humoral hypercalcemia of malignancy. *J Clin Endocrinol Metab* 75:1110, 1992.
495. Burtis WJ, Brady TG, Orloff JJ, et al: Immunochemical characterization of circulating parathyroid hormone-related protein in patients with humoral hypercalcemia of cancer. *N Engl J Med* 322:1106, 1990.
496. Orloff JJ, Soifer NE, Fodero JP, et al: Accumulation of carboxyl-terminal fragments of parathyroid hormone-related protein in renal failure. *Kidney Int* 43:1371, 1993.
497. Liu B, Amizuka N, Goltzman D, et al: Inhibition of processing of parathyroid hormone-related peptide by antisense furin: Effect *in vitro* and *in vivo* on rat leydig (H-500) tumor cells. *Int J Cancer* 63:276, 1995.
498. Bruzzaniti A, Goodge K, Jay P, et al: 1996 PC8, a new member of the convertase family. *Biochem J* 314:727, 1996. [Published erratum appears in *Biochem J* 316:1007, 1996].
499. Orloff JJ, Reddy D, de Papp AE, et al: Parathyroid hormone-related protein as a prohormone: posttranslational processing and receptor interactions. *Endocr Rev* 15:40, 1994.
500. Plawner LL, Philbrick WM, Burtis WJ, et al: Cell type-specific secretion of parathyroid hormone-related protein via the regulated versus the constitutive secretory pathway. *J Biol Chem* 270:14078, 1995.
501. Wu TL, Soifer NE, Burtis WJ, et al: Glycosylation of parathyroid hormone-related peptide secreted by human epidermal keratinocytes. *J Clin Endocrinol Metab* 73:1002, 1991.
502. Orloff JJ, Kats Y, Urena P, et al: Further evidence for a novel receptor for amino-terminal parathyroid hormone-related protein on keratinocytes and squamous carcinoma cell lines. *Endocrinology* 136:3016, 1995.
503. Karaplis AC, Luz A, Glowacki J, et al: Lethal skeletal dysplasia from targeted disruption of the parathyroid hormone-related peptide gene. *Genes Dev* 8:277, 1994.
504. Weir EC, Philbrick WM, Amling M, et al: Targeted overexpression of parathyroid hormone-related peptide in chondrocytes causes chondrodysplasia and delayed endochondral bone formation. *Proc Natl Acad Sci USA* 93:10240, 1996.
505. Wysolmerski JJ, Broadus AE, Zhou J, et al: Overexpression of parathyroid hormone-related protein in the skin of transgenic mice interferes with hair follicle development. *Proc Natl Acad Sci USA* 91:1133, 1994.
506. Wysolmerski JJ, McCaughern-Carucci JF, Daifotis AG, et al: Overexpression of parathyroid hormone-related protein or parathyroid hormone in transgenic mice impairs branching morphogenesis during mammary gland development. *Development* 121:3539, 1995.
507. Wysolmerski JJ, Carucci JM, Broadus AE, et al: PTH and PTHrP antagonize mammary gland growth and development in transgenic mice. *J Bone Miner Res* 9(Suppl 1):S121, 1994. (abstract)
508. Vasavada RC, Cavaliere C, D'Ercole AJ, et al: Overexpression of parathyroid hormone-related protein in the pancreatic islets of transgenic mice causes islet hyperplasia, hyperinsulinemia, and hypoglycemia. *J Biol Chem* 271:1200, 1996.
509. Massfelder T, Helwig JJ, Stewart AF: Parathyroid hormone-related protein as a cardiovascular regulatory peptide. *Endocrinology* 137:3151, 1996.
510. Kovacs CS, Lanske B, Hunzelman JL, et al: Parathyroid hormone-related peptide (PTHrP) regulates fetal-placental calcium transport through a receptor distinct from the PTH/PTHrP receptor. *Proc Natl Acad Sci USA* 93:15233, 1996.
511. Nakayama T, Ohtsuru A, Enomoto H, et al: Coronary atherosclerotic smooth muscle cells overexpress human parathyroid hormone-related peptides. *Biochem Biophys Res Commun* 200:1028, 1994.
512. Hongo T, Kupfer J, Enomoto H, et al: Abundant expression of parathyroid hormone-related protein in primary rat aortic smooth muscle cells accompanies serum-induced proliferation. *J Clin Invest* 88:1841, 1991.
513. Pirola CJ, Wang HM, Strgacich MI, et al: Mechanical stimuli induce vascular parathyroid hormone-related protein gene expression *in vivo* and *in vitro*. *Endocrinology* 134:2230, 1994.
514. Funk JL, Lausier J, Moser AH, et al: Endotoxin induces parathyroid hormone-related protein gene expression in splenic stromal and smooth muscle cells, not in splenic lymphocytes. *Endocrinology* 136:3412, 1995.
515. Funk JL, Shigenaga JK, Moser AH, et al: Cytokine regulation of parathyroid hormone-related protein messenger ribonucleic acid levels in mouse spleen: Paradoxical effects of interferon- and interleukin-4. *Endocrinology* 135:351, 1994.
516. Funk JL, Krul EJ, Moser AH, et al: Endotoxin increases PTHrP mRNA levels in mouse spleen: Mediation by tumor necrosis factor. *J Clin Invest* 92:2546, 1992.
517. Vortkamp A, Lee K, Lanske B, et al: Regulation of rate of cartilage differentiation by Indian hedgehog and PTH-related protein. *Science* 273:613, 1996.
518. Philbrick WM, Wysolmerski JJ, Galbraith S, et al: Defining the roles of parathyroid hormone-related protein in normal physiology. *Physiol Rev* 76:127, 1996.
519. Guise TA, Mundy GR: Physiological and pathological roles of parathyroid hormone-related peptide. *Curr Opin Nephrol Hypertens* 5:307, 1996.
520. Strewler GJ, Nissenson RA: The parathyroid hormone-related protein as a regulator of normal tissue functions. *Curr Opin Endocrinol Diabetes* 1:286, 1994.
521. Ratcliffe WA: Role of parathyroid hormone-related protein in lactation. *Clin Endocrinol (Oxf)* 37:402, 1992.
522. Thiede MA, Rodan GA: Expression of a calcium-mobilizing parathyroid hormone-like peptide in lactating mammary tissue. *Science* 242:278, 1988.
523. Budayr AA, Halloran BP, King JC, et al: High levels of parathyroid hormone-like protein in milk. *Proc Natl Acad Sci USA* 86:7183, 1989.
524. Yamamoto M, Fisher JE, Thiede MA, et al: Concentrations of parathyroid hormone-related protein in rat milk change with duration

of lactation and interval from previous suckling, but not with milk calcium. *Endocrinology* 130:741, 1992.
525. Khosla S, Johansen KL, Ory SJ, et al: Parathyroid hormone-related peptide in lactation and in umbilical cord blood. *Mayo Clin Proc* 65:1408, 1990.
526. Stewart AF, Wu TL, Insogna KL, et al: Immunoaffinity purification of parathyroid hormone-related protein from bovine milk and human keratinocyte-conditioned medium. *J Bone Miner Res* 6:305, 1991.
527. Ratcliffe WA, Thompson GE, Care AD, et al: Production of parathyroid hormone-related protein by the mammary gland of the goat. *J Endocrinol* 133:87, 1992.
528. Lepre F, Grill V, Danks JA: Hypercalcemia in pregnancy and lactation due to parathyroid hormone-related protein production. *Bone Miner* 10:s317, 1990.
529. Khosla S, van Heerden JA, Garib H, et al: Parathyroid hormone-related protein and hypercalcemia secondary to massive mammary hyperplasia [letter]. *N Engl J Med* 322:1157, 1990.
530. Lepre F, Grill V, Ho PWM, et al: Hypercalcemia in pregnancy and lactation associated with parathyroid hormone-related protein. *N Engl J Med* 328:666, 1993.
531. Grill V, Hillary J, Ho PM, et al: Parathyroid hormone-related protein: A possible endocrine function in lactation. *Clin Endocrinol (Oxf)* 37:405, 1992.
532. Pandian MR, Morgan CH, Carlton E, et al: Modified immunoradiometric assay of parathyroid hormone-related protein: Clinical application in the differential diagnosis of hypercalcemia. *Clin Chem* 38:282, 1992.
533. Schilling T, Pecherstorfer M, Blind E, et al: Parathyroid hormone-related protein (PTHrP) does not regulate 1,25-dihydroxyvitamin D serum levels in hypercalcemia of malignancy. *J Clin Endocrinol Metab* 76:801, 1993.
534. Fraher LJ, Hodsman AB, Jonas K, et al: A comparison of the *in vivo* biochemical responses to exogenous parathyroid hormone-(1-34)[PTH-(1-34)] and PTH-related peptide-(1-34) in man. *J Clin Endocrinol Metab* 75:417, 1992.
535. Everhart-Caye M, Inzucchi SE, Guinness-Henry J, et al: Parathyroid hormone (PTH)-related protein(1-36) is equipotent to PTH(1-34) in humans. *J Clin Endocrinol Metab* 81:199, 1996.
536. Guise TA, Chirgwin JM, Taylor S, et al: Deletions of C-terminal end of parathyroid hormone-related protein (PTHrP) have equivalent effects on bone and calcium homeostasis *in vivo. J Bone Miner Res* 8(Suppl 1):229A, 1993. (abstract)
537. Rosol TJ, Capen CC, Horst RL: Effects of infusion of human parathyroid hormone-related protein-(1-40) in nude mice: Histomorphometric and biochemical investigations. *J Bone Miner Res* 3:699, 1988.
538. Guise TA, Chirgwin JM, Boyce B, et al: Comparison of similar models of parathyroid hormone (PTH) and parathyroid hormone-related protein (PTHrP) excess in nude mice. *J Bone Miner Res* 7(Suppl 1):S241, 593, 1992. (abstract)
539. Stewart AF, Vignery A, Silverglate A, et al: Quantitative bone histomorphometry in humoral hypercalcemia of malignancy: Uncoupling of bone cell activity. *J Clin Endocrinol Metab* 55:219, 1982.
540. Nakayama K, Fukumoto S, Takeda S, et al: Differences in bone and vitamin D metabolism between primary hyperparathyroidism and malignancy-associated hypercalcemia. *J Clin Endocrinol Metab* 81:607, 1996.
541. Delmas PD, Demiaux B, Malaval L, et al: Serum bone gamma carboxyglutamic acid-containing protein in primary hyperparathyroidism and in malignant hypercalcemia. Comparison with bone histomorphometry. *J Clin Invest* 77:985, 1986.
542. Kukreja SC, Rosol TJ, Shevrin DH, et al: Quantitative bone histomorphometry in nude mice bearing a human squamous cell lung cancer. *J Bone Miner Res* 3:341, 1988.
543. Uy HL, Guise TA, De La Mata J, et al: Effects of parathyroid hormone (PTH)-related protein and PTH on osteoclasts and osteoclast precursors *in vivo. Endocrinology* 136:3207, 1995.
544. de la Mata J, Uy HL, Guise TA, et al: IL-6 enhances hypercalcemia and bone resorption mediated by PTHrP *in vivo. J Clin Invest* 95:2846, 1995.
545. Guise TA, Yoneda T, Yates AJP, et al: The combined effect of tumor-produced parathyroid hormone-related peptide and transforming growth factor- enhance hypercalcemia *in vivo* and bone resorption *in vitro. J Clin Endocrinol Metab* 77:40, 1993.
546. Pizurki L, Rizzoli R, Caverzasio J, et al: Effect of transforming growth factor and parathyroid hormone-related protein on phosphate transport in renal cells. *Am J Physiol* 259:F929, 1990.
547. Pizurki L, Rizzoli R, Caverzasio J, et al: Stimulation by parathyroid hormone-related protein and transforming growth factor of phosphate transport in osteoblast-like cells. *J Bone Miner Res* 6:1235, 1991.
548. Sato K, Fujii Y, Kasono K, et al: Parathyroid hormone-related protein and interleukin-1 alpha synergistically stimulate bone resorption *in vitro* and increase the serum calcium concentration in mice *in vivo. Endocrinology* 124:2172, 1989.
549. Torring O, Turner RT, Carter WB, et al: Inhibition by human interleukin-1 of parathyroid hormone-related peptide effects on renal calcium and phosphorous metabolism in the rat. *Endocrinology* 131:5, 1992.
550. Uy HL, Mundy GR, Boyce BF, et al: Tumor necrosis factor enhances parathyroid hormone-related protein (PTHrP)-induced hypercalcemia and bone resorption without inhibiting bone formation in vivo. *Cancer Res* 57:3194, 1997.
551. Allinson ET, Drucker DJ: Parathyroid hormone-like peptide shares features with members of early response gene family: Rapid induction by serum growth factors and cyclohexamide. *Cancer Res* 52:3103, 1992.
552. Burton PB, Moniz C, Knight DE: Parathyroid hormone-related peptide can function as an autocrine growth factor in human renal cell carcinoma. *Biochem Biophys Res Commun* 167:1134, 1990.
553. Dublin EA, Barnes DM, Wang DY, et al: TGF alpha and TGF beta expression in mammary carcinoma. *J Pathol* 170:15, 1993.
554. Herman ME, Katzenellenbogen BS: Alterations in transforming growth factor-alpha and -beta production and cell responsiveness during the progression of MCF-7 human breast cancer cells to estrogen-autonomous growth. *Cancer Res* 54:5867, 1994.
555. van Roozendaal CEP, Klijn JGM, van Ooijen B, et al: Transforming growth factor beta secretion from primary breast cancer fibroblasts. *Mol Cell Endocrinol* 111:1, 1995.
556. Firek A, Jennings J, Tabuenca A, et al: TGF- stimulates PTHrP release from human mammary cancer. *Program and Abstracts Endocrine Society Meeting* 769A, 395, 1994.
557. Guise TA, Taylor SD, Yoneda T, et al: PTHrP expression by breast cancer cells enhance osteolytic bone metastases *in vivo. J Bone Miner Res* 9(Suppl 1):33, S128, 1994.
558. Coleman RE, Rubens RD: The clinical course of bone metastases from breast cancer. *Br J Cancer* 55:61, 1987.
559. Galasko CSB: Mechanisms of bone destruction in the development of skeletal metastasis. *Nature* 263:517, 1976.
560. Boyde A, Maconnachie E, Reid SA, et al: Scanning electron microscopy in bone pathology: Review of methods. Potential and applications. *Scanning Electron Microscopy* IV:1537, 1986.
561. Taube T, Elomaa I, Blomqvist C, et al: Histomorphometric evidence for osteoclast-mediated bone resorption in metastatic breast cancer. *Bone* 15:161, 1994.
562. Francini G, Petrioloi R, Maioli E, et al: Hypercalcemia in breast cancer. *Clin Exp Metastasis* 11:359, 1993.
563. Kimura S, Adachi I, Yamaguchi K, et al: Stimulation of calcium reabsorption observed in advanced breast cancer patients with hypercalcemia and multiple bone metastasis. *Jpn J Cancer Res* 76:308, 1985.
564. Gallacher SJ, Fraser WD, Patel U, et al: Breast cancer-associated hypercalcemia: A reassessment of renal calcium and phosphate handling. *Ann Clin Biochem* 27:551, 1990.
565. Coleman RE, Fogelman I, Rubens RD: Hypercalcemia and breast cancer—an increased humoral component in patients with liver metastases. *Eur J Surg Oncol* 14:423, 1988.
566. Budayr AA, Zysset E, Jenzer A, et al: Effects of treatment of malignancy-associated hypercalcemia on serum parathyroid hormone-related protein. *J Bone Miner Res* 9:521, 1994.
567. Heath DA: Parathyroid hormone related protein. *Clin Endocrinol (Oxf)* 38:135, 1993.
568. Southby J, Kissin MW, Danks JA, et al: 1990 Immunohistochemical localization of parathyroid hormone-related protein in breast cancer. *Cancer Res* 51:7710, 1990.
569. Liapis H, Crouch EC, Grosso LE, et al: Expression of parathyroid like protein in normal, proliferative, and neoplastic human breast tissues. *Am J Pathol* 143:1169, 1993.

570. Bundred NJ, Walker RA, Ratcliffe WA, et al: Parathyroid hormone related protein and skeletal morbidity in breast cancer. *Eur J Cancer* 28:690, 1992.
571. Bundred NJ, Ratcliffe WA, Walker RA, et al: Parathyroid hormone related protein and hypercalcaemia in breast cancer. *Br Med J* 303:1506, 1991.
572. Kohno N, Kitazawa S, Fukase M, et al: The expression of parathyroid hormone-related protein in human breast cancer with skeletal metastases. *Surg Today* 24:215, 1994.
573. Grill V, Ho P, Body JJ, et al: Parathyroid hormone-related protein: Elevated levels in both humoral hypercalcemia and hypercalcemia complicating metastatic breast cancer. *J Clin Endocrinol Metab* 73:1309, 1991.
574. Kremer R, Shustik C, Tabak T, et al: Parathyroid hormone-related peptide in hematologic malignancies. *Am J Med* 100:406, 1996.
575. Ikeda K, Ohno H, Hane M, et al: Development of a sensitive two-site immunoradiometric assay for parathyroid hormone-related peptide: Evidence for elevated levels in plasma from patients with adult T-cell leukemia/lymphoma and B-cell lymphoma. *J Clin Endocrinol Metab* 79:1322, 1994.
576. Firkin F, Seymour JF, Watson AM, et al: Parathyroid hormone-related protein in hypercalcaemia associated with haematological malignancy. *Br J Haematol* 94:486, 1996.
577. Seymour JF, Grill V, Martin TJ, et al: Hypercalcemia in the blastic phase of chronic myeloid leukemia associated with elevated parathyroid hormone-related protein. *Leukemia* 7:1672, 1993.
578. Seymour JF, Gagel RF, Hagemeister FB, et al: Calcitriol production in hypercalcemic and normocalcemic patients with non-Hodgkin lymphoma. *Ann Intern Med* 121:633, 1994.
579. Schwartz Z, Dean DD, Walton JK, et al: Treatment of resting zone chondrocytes with 24,25-dihydroxyvitamin D_3 [24,25-$(OH)_2D_3$] induces differentiation into a 1.25-$(OH)_2D_3$-responsive phenotype characteristic of growth zone chondrocytes. *Endocrinology* 136:402, 1995.
580. Mason RS, Frankel T, Chan YL, et al: Vitamin D conversion by sarcoid lymph node homogenate. *Ann Intern Med* 100:59, 1984.
581. Adams JS, Sharma OP, Gacad MA, et al: Metabolism of 25-hydroxyvitamin D3 by cultured pulmonary alveolar macrophages in sarcoidosis. *J Clin Invest* 72:1856, 1983.
582. Rosenthal N, Insogna KL, Godsall JW, et al: Elevations in circulating 1,25-dihydroxyvitamin D in three patients with lymphoma-associated hypercalcemia. *J Clin Endocrinol Metab* 60:29, 1985.
583. Breslau NA, McGuire JL, Zerwekh JE, et al: Hypercalcemia associated with increased serum calcitriol levels in three patients with lymphoma. *Ann Int Med* 100:1, 1984.
584. Fetchik DA, Bertolini DR, Sarin PS, et al: Production of 1,25-dihydroxyvitamin D_3 by human T-cell lymphotrophic virus-1 transformed lymphocytes. *J Clin Invest* 78:592, 1986.
585. Mercier RJ, Thompson JM, Harman GS, et al: Recurrent hypercalcemia and elevated 1,25-dihydroxyvitamin D levels in Hodgkin's disease. *Am J Med* 84:165, 1988.
586. Munson PL, Tashjian Jr AH, Levine L: Evidence for parathyroid hormone in nonparathyroid tumors associated with hypercalcemia. *Cancer Res* 25:1062, 1965.
587. Benson Jr RC, Riggs BL, Pickard BM, et al: Radioimmunoassay of parathyroid hormone in hypercalcemic patients with malignant disease. *Am J Med* 56:821, 1974.
588. Benson Jr RC, Riggs BL, Pickard BM, et al: Immunoreactive forms of circulating parathyroid hormone in primary and ectopic hyperparathyroidism. *J Clin Invest* 54:175, 1974.
589. Sherwood LM, O'Riordan JL, Aurbach GD, et al: Production of parathyroid hormone by nonparathyroid tumors. *J Clin Endocrinol Metab* 27:140, 1967.
590. Simpson EL, Mundy GR, D'Souza SM, et al: Absence of parathyroid hormone messenger RNA in nonparathyroid tumors associated with hypercalcemia. *N Engl J Med* 309:325, 1983.
591. Mori H, Aoki K, Katayama I, et al: Humoral hypercalcemia with elevated plasma PTHrP, TNF alpha and IL-6 in cutaneous squamous cell carcinoma. *J Dermatol* 23:460, 1996.
592. Sabatini M, Boyce B, Aufdemorte T, et al: Infusions of recombinant human interleukins 1 and 1 cause hypercalcemia in normal mice. *Proc Natl Acad Sci USA* 85:5235, 1988.
593. Boyce BF, Aufdemorte TB, Garrett IR, et al: Effects of interleukin-1 on bone turnover in normal mice. *Endocrinology* 125:1142, 1989.
594. Guise TA, Garrett IR, Bonewald LF, et al: The interleukin-1 receptor antagonist inhibits hypercalcemia mediated by interleukin-1. *J Bone Miner Res* 8:583, 1993.
595. Black K, Garrett IR, Mundy GR: Chinese hamster ovarian cells transfected with the murine interleukin-6 gene cause hypercalcemia as well as cachexia, leukocytosis and thrombocytosis in tumor-bearing mice. *Endocrinology* 128:2657, 1991.
596. Weissglas M, Schamhart D, Lowik C, et al: Hypercalcemia and cosecretion of interleukin-6 and parathyroid hormone related peptide by a human renal cell carcinoma implanted into nude mice. *J Urol* 153:854, 1995.
597. Stern PH, Krieger NS, Nissenson RA, et al: Human transforming growth factor-alpha stimulates bone resorption *in vitro*. *J Clin Invest* 76:2016, 1985.
598. Ibbotson KJ, Harrod J, Gowen M, et al: Human recombinant transforming growth factor stimulates bone resorption and inhibits formation *in vitro*. *Proc Natl Acad Sci USA* 83:2228, 1986.
599. Ibbotson KJ, Twardzik DR, D'Souza SM, et al: Stimulation of bone resorption *in vitro* by synthetic transforming growth factor-alpha. *Science* 228:1007, 1985.
600. Tashjian Jr. AH, Voelkel EF, Lloyd W, et al: Actions of growth factors on plasma calcium. Epidermal growth factor and human transforming growth factor-alpha cause elevation of plasma calcium in mice. *J Clin Invest* 78:1405, 1986.
601. Yates AJ, Boyce BF, Favarato G, et al: Expression of human transforming growth factor alpha by Chinese hamster ovarian tumors in nude mice causes hypercalcemia and increased osteoclastic bone resorption. *J Bone Miner Res* 7:847, 1992.
602. Bertolini DR, Nedwin GE, Bringman TS, et al: Stimulation of bone resorption and inhibition of bone formation *in vitro* by human tumour necrosis factors. *Nature* 319:516, 1986.
603. Johnson RA, Boyce B, Mundy GR, et al: Tumors producing human tumor necrosis factor induce hypercalcemia and osteoclastic bone resorption in nude mice. *Endocrinology* 124:1424, 1989.
604. Klein DC, Raisz LG. Prostaglandins: Stimulation of bone resorption in tissue culture. *Endocrinology* 86:1436, 1970.
605. Mundy GR: Hypercalcemia, in Mundy GR (ed) *Bone Remodeling and Its Disorders*. Martin Dunitz, London, 1995, p 88.
606. Mundy GR, Wilkinson RB, Heath DA: Comparative study of available medical therapy for hypercalcemia of malignancy. *Am J Med* 74:421, 1983.
607. Tuttle KR, Kunau RT, Loveridge N, et al: Altered renal calcium handling in hypercalcemia of malignancy. *J Am Soc Nephrol* 2:191, 1991.
608. Hosking DJ, Cowley A, Bucknall CA: Rehydration in the treatment of severe hypercalcemia. *Q J Med* 51:473, 1981.
609. Nussbaum SR: Pathophysiology and management of severe hypercalcemia. *Endocrinol Metab Clin North Am* 22:343, 1993.
610. Rodan GA, Fleisch HA: Bisphosphonates: Mechanisms of action. *J Clin Invest* 97:2692, 1996.
611. Fleisch H: Bisphosphonates: Pharmacology and use in the treatment of tumor-induced hypercalcemia and metastatic bone disease. *Drugs* 42:919, 1991.
612. Singer FR, Ritch PS, Lad TE, et al: Treatment of hypercalcemia of malignancy with intravenous etidronate-a controlled, multicenter study. *Arch Intern Med* 151:471, 1991.
613. Gucalp R, Ritch P, Wiernik PH, et al: Comparative study of pamidronate disodium and etidronate disodium in the treatment of cancer-related hypercalcemia. *J Clin Oncol* 10:134, 1992.
614. Kanis JA, Urwin GH, Gray RE, et al: Effects of intravenous etidronate disodium on skeletal and calcium metabolism. *Am J Med* 82(suppl 2A):55, 1987.
615. Walls J, Ratcliffe WA, Howell A, et al: Response to intravenous bisphosphonate therapy in hypercalcaemic patients with and without bone metastases: The role of parathyroid hormone-related protein. *Br J Cancer* 70:169, 1994.
616. Pecherstorfer M, Schilling T, Blind E, et al: Parathyroid hormone-related protein and life expectancy in hypercalcemic cancer patients. *J Clin Endocrinol Metab* 78:1268, 1994.
617. Dodwell DJ, Abbas SK, Morton AR, et al: Parathyroid hormone-related protein[(50–69)] and response to pamidronate therapy for tumour-induced hypercalcaemia. *Eur J Cancer* 27:1629, 1991.
618. Kanis JA: Bone and cancer: Pathophysiology and treatment of metastases. *Bone* 17:101S, 1995.

619. Purohit OP, Radstone CR, Anthony C, et al: A Randomised double-blind comparison of intravenous pamidronate and clodronate in the hypercalcaemia of malignancy. *Br J Cancer* 72:1289, 1995.
620. Wimalawansa SJ: Optimal frequency of administration of pamidronate in patients with hypercalcaemia of malignancy. *Clin Endocrinol (Oxf)* 41:591, 1994.
621. Ralston SH, Alzaid AA, Gardner MD, et al: Treatment of cancer associated hypercalcemia with combined aminohydroxypropylidene diphosphonate and calcitonin. *Br Med J* 292:1549, 1986.
622. Adamson BB, Gallacher SJ, Byars J, et al: Mineralisation defects with pamidronate therapy for Paget's disease. *Lancet* 342:1459, 1993.
623. Binstock MD, Mundy GR: Effect of calcitonin and glucocorticoids in combination of the hypercalcemia of malignancy. *Ann Intern Med* 93:269, 1980.
624. Thiebaud D, Jacquet AF, Burckhardt P: Fast and effective treatment of malignant hypercalcemia. *Arch Intern Med* 151:2125, 1990.
625. *Physicians Desk Reference*. 51st ed. Montvale NJ, Medical Economics Data, 1997, pp 2176–2178.
626. Brown JH, Kennedy BJ: Mithramycin in the treatment of disseminated testicular neoplasms. *N Engl J Med* 272:111, 1965.
627. Yarbro JW, Kennedy BJ, Barnum CP: Mithramycin inhibition of ribonucleic acid synthesis. *Cancer Res* 26:36, 1966.
628. Ray R, Snyder RC, Thomas S, et al: Mithramycin blocks protein binding and function of the SV40 early promoter. *J Clin Invest* 83:2003, 1989.
629. Warrell RP Jr, Bockman RS, Coonley CJ, et al: Gallium nitrate inhibits calcium resorption from bone and is effective treatment for cancer-related hypercalcemia. *J Clin Invest* 73:1487, 1984.
630. *Physicians Desk Reference*, 51st ed. Montvale NJ, Medical Economics Data, 1997, pp 2711–2712.
631. Mundy GR, Rick ME, Turcotte R, et al: Pathogenesis of hypercalcemia in lymphosarcoma cell leukemia. Role of an osteoclast activating factor-like substance and a mechanism of action for glucocorticoid therapy. *Am J Med* 65:600, 1978.
632. Aaron AD: The management of cancer metastatic to bone. *JAMA* 272:1206, 1994.
633. Miyauchi A, Fukase M, Tsutsumi M, et al: Hemangiopericytoma-induced osteomalacia: tumor transplantation in nude mice causes hypophosphatemia and tumor extracts inhibit renal 25-hydroxyvitamin D1-hydroxylase activity. *J Clin Endocrinol Metab* 67:46, 1988.
634. Walther HE: Krebsmetastasen. Bens Schwabe Verlag, Basel, Switzerland, 1948.
635. Weiss L: Comments on hematogenous metastastic patterns in humans as revealed by autopsy. *Clin Exp Met* 10:191, 1992.
636. Cifuentes N, Pickren JW: Metastases from carcinoma of mammary gland: An autopsy study. *J Surg Oncol* 11:193, 1979.
637. Eilon G, Mundy GR: Direct resorption of bone by human breast cancer cells *in vitro*. *Nature* 276:726, 1978.
638. Guise TA, Yin JJ, Taylor SD, et al: Evidence for a causal role of parathyroid hormone-related protein in breast cancer-mediated osteolysis. *J Clin Invest* 98:1544, 1996.
639. Powell GJ, Southby J, Danks JA, et al: Localization of parathyroid hormone-related protein in breast cancer metastases: Increased incidence in bone compared with other sites. *Cancer Res* 51:3059, 1991.
640. Vargas SJ, Gillespie MT, Powell GJ, et al: Localization of parathyroid hormone-related protein mRNA expression and metastatic lesions by in situ hybridization. *J Bone Miner Res* 7:971, 1992.
641. Bouizar Z, Spyratos F, Deytieux S, et al: Polymerase chain reaction analysis of parathyroid hormone-related protein gene expression in breast cancer patients and occurrence of bone metastases. *Cancer Res* 53:5076, 1993.
642. Arguello F, Baggs RB, Frantz CN: A murine model of experimental metastasis to bone and bone marrow. *Cancer Res* 48:6876, 1988.
643. Sasaki A, Boyce BF, Story B, et al: The bisphosphonate risedronate reduces metastatic human breast cancer burden in bone in nude mice. *Cancer Res* 55:3551, 1995.
643a. Cailleau R, Yong R, Olive M, et al: Breast tumor cell lines from pleural effusions. *J Natl Cancer Inst* 53:661, 1974.
643b. Yin JJ, Taylor SD, Yoneda T, et al: Evidence that parathyroid hormone-related protein (PTHrP) causes osteolytic metastases without hypercalcemia. *J Bone Miner Res* 10:S169, 122 (abstract), 1995.
644. Iguchi H, Tanaka S, Ozawa Y, et al: An experimental model of bone metastasis by human lung cancer cells: The role of parathyroid hormone-related protein in bone metastasis. *Cancer Res* 56:4040, 1996.
645. Mbalaviele G, Dunstan CR, Sasaki A, et al: E-cadherin expression in human breast cancer cells suppresses the development of osteolytic bone metastases in an experimental metastasis model. *Cancer Res* 56:4063, 1996.
646. Williams P, Mbalaviele G, Sasaki A, et al: Multi-step inhibition of breast cancer metastasis to bone. *J Bone Miner Res* 10:S169 121 (abstract), 1995.
647. Thurlimann B, Morant R, Jungi WF, et al: Pamidronate for pain control in patients with malignant osteolytic bone disease: A prospective dose-effect study. *Support Care Cancer* 2:61, 1994.
648. Glover D, Lipton A, Keller A, Miller AA, et al: Intravenous pamidronate disodium treatment of bone metastases in patients with breast cancer. A dose-seeking study. *Cancer* 74:2949, 1994.
649. van Holten-Verzantvoort AT, Bijvoet OL, Cleton FJ, et al: Reduced morbidity from skeletal metastases in breast cancer patients during long-term bisphosphonate (APD) treatment. *Lancet* 2:983, 1987.
650. Cleton FJ, van Holten-Verzantvoort AT, Bijvoet OL: Effect of long-term bisphosphonate treatment on morbidity due to bone metastases in breast cancer patients. *Recent Results Cancer Res* 116:73, 1989.
651. Burckhardt P, Thiebaud D, Peres L, von Fliedner V: Treatment of tumor-induced osteolysis by APD. *Recent Results Cancer Res* 116:54, 1989.
652. Grutters JC, Hermus AR, de Mulder PH, Beex LV: Long-term follow up of breast cancer patients treated for hypercalcaemia with aminohydroxypropylidene bisphosphonate (APD). *Breast Cancer Res Treat* 25:277, 1993.
653. Paterson AHG, Ernst DS, Powles TJ, et al: Treatment of skeletal disease in breast cancer with clodronate. *Bone* 2:S25, 1991.
654. Morton AR, Cantrill JA, Pillai GV, McMahon A, Anderson DC, Howell A: Sclerosis of lytic bone metastases after disodium aminohydroxypropylidene bisphosphonate (APD) in patients with breast carcinoma. *Br Med J* 297:772, 1988.
655. Paterson AH, Powles TJ, Kanis JA, McCloskey E, Hanson J, Ashley S: Double-blind controlled trial of oral clodronate in patients with bone metastases from breast cancer. *J Clin Oncol* 11:59, 1993.
656. Hortobagyi GN, Theriault RL, Porter L, et al: Efficacy of pamidronate in reducing skeletal complications in patients with breast cancer and lytic bone metastases. Protocol 19 Aredia Breast Cancer Study Group. *N Engl J Med* 335:1785, 1996.
657. Delmas PD: Bisphosphonates in the treatment of bone diseases. *N Engl J Med* 335:1836, 1996.
658. Delmas PD, Balena R, Confravreaux E, Hardouin C, Hardy P, Bremond A: Bisphosphonate risedronate prevents bone loss in women with artificial menopause due to chemotherapy of breast cancer: A double blind placebo-controlled trial. *J Clin Oncol* 15:955, 1997.
659. Bassani D, Sabatini M, Scanziani E, et al: Bone invasion by Walker 256 carcinoma, line A in young and adult rats: Effects of etidronate. *Oncology* 47:160, 1990.
660. Sasaki A, Boyce BF, Story B, et al: Bisphosphonate risedronate reduces metastatic human breast cancer burden in bone in nude mice. *Cancer Res* 55:3551, 1995.
661. Massague J, Blain SW, Lo RS: TGFβ signalling in growth control, cancer, and heritable disorders. *Cell* 103:295, 2000.
662. Derynck R: TGFβ—receptor-mediated signaling. *Trends Biochem Sci* 19:548, 1994.
663. Massagué J, Hata A, Liu F: TGF-β signaling through the Smad pathway. *Trends Cell Biol* 7:187, 1997.
664. Arteaga CL, Dugger TC, Hurd SD: The multifunctional role of transforming growth factor (TGF) 3 on mammary epithelial cell biology. *Breast Cancer Res Treat* 38:49, 1996.
665. Nørgaard P, Hougaard S, Poulsen HS, et al: Transforming growth factor and cancer. *Cancer Treat Rev* 21:367, 1995.
666. Wieser R, Attisano L, Wrana JL, et al: Signaling activity of transforming growth factor type II receptors lacking specific domains in the cytoplasmic region. *Mol Cell Biol* 13:7239, 1993.
667. Wrana JL, Attisano L, Wieser R, et al: 4 Mechanism of activation of the TGF-receptor. *Nature* 370:341, 1994.
668. Yin JJ, Taylor SD, Dallas M, et al: Dominant negative blockade of the transforming growth factor type II receptor decreases breast cancer-mediated osteolysis (abstract). *J Bone Miner Res* 11:S139, 1996.
669. Mundy GR, Bertolini DR: Bone destruction and hypercalcemia in plasma cell myeloma. *Seminars in Oncology* 13:291, 1986. [Published erratum appears in Semin Oncol 1986; 13:Ixiii]

670. Mundy GR, Raisz LG, Cooper RA, et al: Evidence for the secretion of an osteoclast stimulating factor in myeloma. *N Engl J Med* 291:1041, 1974.
671. Case Records of the Massachusetts General Hospital (case 29-1972). *N Engl J Med* 287:138, 1972.
672. Bardwick PA, Zvaifler NJ, Gill GN, et al: Plasma cell dyscrasia with polyneuropathy, organomegaly, endocrinopathy, M protein, and skin changes: The POEMS syndrome. Report on two cases and a review of the literature. *Medicine* 59:311, 1980.
673. Farhangi M, Merlini G: The clinical implications of monoclonal immunoglobulins. *Sem Oncol* 13:366, 1986.
674. Cozzolino F, Torcia M, Aldinucci D, et al: 1989 Production of interleukin-1 by bone marrow myeloma cells. *Blood* 74:380, 1989.
675. Kawano M, Tanaka H, Ishikawa H, et al: Interleukin-1 accelerates autocrine growth of myeloma cells through interleukin-6 in human myeloma. *Blood* 73:2145, 1989.
676. Garrett IR, Durie BG, Nedwin GE, et al: Production of lymphotoxin, a bone-resorbing cytokine, by cultured human myeloma cells. *N Engl J Med* 317:526, 1987.
677. Bataille R, Chappard D, Klein B: The critical role of interleukin-6, interleukin-1 and macrophage colony-stimulating factor in the pathogenesis of bone lesions in multiple myeloma. *Int J Clin Lab Res* 21:283, 1992.
678. Bataille R, Jourdan M, Zhang XG: Serum levels of interleukin-6, a potent myeloma cell growth factor, as a reflect of dyscrasias. *J Clin Invest* 84:2008, 1989.
679. van Zaanen HCT, Koopmans RP, Aarden LA, et al: Endogenous interleukin 6 production in multiple myeloma patients treated with chimeric monoclonal anti-IL6 antibodies indicates the existence of a positive feed-back loop. *J Clin Invest* 98:1441, 1996.
680. Lokhorst HM, Lamme Tanja, de Smet M, Klein S, et al: Primary tumor cells of myeloma patients induce interleukin-6 secretion in long-term bone marrow cultures. *Blood* 84:2269, 1994.
681. Feyen JH, Elford P, Di Padova FE, Trechsel U: Interleukin-6 is produced by bone and modulated by parathyroid hormone. *J Bone Miner Res* 4:633, 1989.
682. Harada H, Kawano MM, Huang N, Harada Y, et al: Phenotypic difference of normal plasma cells from mature myeloma cells. *Blood* 81:2658, 1993.
683. Uchiyama H, Barut BA, Chuhan D, Cannistra SA, Anderson KC: Characterization of adhesion molecules on human myeloma cell lines. *Blood* 80:2306, 1992.
684. Hamilton MS, Ball J, Bromidge E, Franklin IM: Surface antigen expression of human neoplastic plasma cells includes molecules associated with lymphocyte recirculation and adhesion. *Br J Haematol* 78:60, 1991.
685. Barker HF, Hamilton MS, Ball J, Drew M, Franlkin IM: Expression of adhesion molecules LFA-3 and N-CAM on normal and malignant human plasma cells. *Br J Haematol* 81:331, 1992.
686. Van Reit I, De Waele M, Remels L, et al: Expression of cytoadhesion molecules (CD56, CD54, CD18 and CD29) by myeloma plasma cells. *Br J Haematol* 79:421, 1991.
687. Kawano MM, Huang N, Tanaka H, Ishikawa H, et al: Homotypic cell aggregations of human myeloma cells with ICAM-1 and LFA-1 molecules. *Br J Haematol* 79:583, 1991.
688. Huang N, Kawano MM, Harada H, Harada Y, Sakai A, Kuramoto A, Niwa O: Heterogeneous expression of a novel MPC-1 antigen on myeloma cells: Possible involvement of the MPC-1 antigen in the adhesion of mature myeloma cells to bone marrow stromal cells. *Blood* 82:3721, 1993.
689. Huang N, Kawano MM, Mahmoud MS, Mihara K, et al: Expression of CD21 antigen on myeloma cells and its involvement in their adhesion to bone marrow stromal cells. *Blood* 85:3704, 1995.
690. Vacca A, Di Loreto M, Ribatti D, Di Stefano R, et al: Bone marrow of patients with active multiple myeloma: angiogenesis and plasma cell adhesion molecules LFA-1, VLA-4, LAM-1 and CD44. *Am J Hematol* 50:9, 1995.
691. Weber GF, Ashkar S, Glimcher MJ, Cantor H: Receptor-ligand interaction between CD44 and osteopontin (Eta-1). *Science* 271:509, 1996.
692. Alsina M, Boyce B, Devlin RD, Anderson JL, et al: Development of an in vivo model of human multiple myeloma bone disease. *Blood* 87:1495, 1995.
693. Garrett IR, Dallas S, Radl J, Mundy GR: A murine model of myeloma bone disease. *Bone* 20:515, 1997.
694. Berenson JR, Lichtenstein A, Porter L, Dimopoulos MA, et al: Efficacy of pamidronate in reducing skeletal events in patients with advanced multiple myeloma. *N Engl J Med* 334:488, 1996.
695. Garrett IR, Dallas SL, Bonewald LF, Boyce BF, Radl J, Mundy GR: Evidence for bidirectional interactions between osteoclasts and myeloma cells. *J Bone Miner Res* 10:S195 P267 (abstract), 1995.
696. Belch AR, Bergsagel DE, Wilson K, O'Reilly S, et al: Effect of daily etidronate on the osteolysis of multiple myeloma. *J Clin Oncol* 9:1397, 1991.
697. Lahtinen R, Laakso M, Palva I, Virkkuned P, Elomaa I: Randomised, placebo-controlled multicentre trial of clodronate in multiple myeloma. Finnish Leukaemia Group. *Lancet* 340:1049, 1992. [Published erratum appears in *Lancet* 1992; 340:1420]
698. Warrell Jr RP, Lovett D, Dilmanian FA, Schneider R, Heelan RT: Low-dose gallium nitrate for prevention of osteolysis in myeloma: Results of a pilot randomized study. *J Clin Oncol* 11:2443, 1993.
699. Mundy GR, Luben RA, Raisz LG, et al: Bone-resorbing activity in supernatants from lymphoid cell lines. *N Engl J Med* 290:867, 1974.
700. Valentin-Opran A, Charhon SA, Meunier PJ, Edouard CM, Arlot ME: Quantitative histology of myeloma-induced bone changes. *Br J Haematol* 52:601, 1982.
701. Ackery D, Yardley J: Radionuclide-targeted therapy for the management of metastatic bone pain. Seminars in oncology 20:27, 1993. [Published erratum appears in *Semin Oncol* 20:551; 1993]
702. Robinson RG, Preston DF, Schiefelbein M, Baxter KG: Strontium 89 therapy for the palliation of pain due to osseous metastases. *JAMA* 274:420, 1995.
703. van der Pluijm G, Vloedgraven H, van Beek E, van der Wee-Pals L, Löwik C, Papapoulos S: Bisphosphonates inhibit the adhesion of breast cancer cells to bone matrices in vitro. *J Clin Invest* 98:698, 1996.
704. Taube T, Kylmala T, Lamberg-Allardt C, Tammela TL, Elomaa I: The effect of clodronate on bone in metastatic prostate cancer. Histomorphometric report of a double-blind randomised placebo-controlled study. *Eur J Cancer* 30A:751, 1994.
705. Vinholes J, Guo CY, Purohit OP, Eastell R, Coleman RE: Metabolic effects of pamidronate in patients with metastatic bone disease. *Br J Cancer* 73:1089, 1996.
706. Henneman PH, Dempsey EF, Carroll EL, Albright F: The cause of hypercalciuria in sarcoid and its treatment with cortisone and sodium phytate. *J Clin Invest* 35:1229, 1956.
707. Bell NH, Stern PH, Pantzer E, Sinha TK, DeLuca HF: Evidence that increased circulating 1α,25-dihydroxyvitamin D is the probable cause for abnormal calcium metabolism in sarcoidosis. *J Clin Invest* 64:218, 1979.
708. Barbour GL, Coburn JW, Slatopolsky E, Norman AW, Horts RL: Hypercalcemia in an anephric patient with sarcoidosis: Evidence for extrarenal generation of 1,25-dihydroxyvitamin D. *N Engl J Med* 305:440, 1981.
709. Stern PH, De Olazabal J, Bell NH: Evidence for abnormal regulation of circulating 1α,25-dihydroxyvitamin D in patients with sarcoidosis and normal calcium metabolism. *J Clin Invest* 66:852, 1980.
710. DeRemee RA, Lufkin EG, Rohrbach MS: Serum angiotensin-converting enzyme activity. *Arch Intern Med* 145:677, 1985.
711. Adams JS, Diz MM, Sharma OP: Effective reduction in the serum 1,25-dihydroxyvitamin D and calcium concentration in sarcoidosis-associated hypercalcemia with short-course chloroquine therapy. *Ann Intern Med* 111:437, 1989.
712. Abbasi AA, Chemplavil JK, Farah S, Muller BF, Arnstein AR: Hypercalcemia in active pulmonary tuberculosis. *Ann Intern Med* 90:324, 1979.
713. Gkonos PJ, London R, Hendler ED: Hypercalcemia and elevated 1,25-dihydroxyvitamin D levels in a patient with end-stage renal disease and active tuberculosis. *N Engl J Med* 311:1683, 1984.
714. Epstein S, Stern PH, Bell NH, Dowdeswell I, Turner RT: Evidence for abnormal regulation of circulating 1α,25-dihydroxyvitamin D in patients with pulmonary tuberculosis and normal calcium metabolism. *Calcif Tissue Int* 36:541, 1984.
715. Kantarjian HM, Saad MF, Estey EH, Sellin RV, Samaan NA: Hypercalcemia in disseminated candidiasis. *Am J Med* 74:721, 1983.
716. Parker MS, Dokoh S, Woolfenden JM, Buchsbaum HW: Hypercalcemia in coccidioidomycosis. *Am J Med* 76:341, 1984.
717. Murray JJ, Heim CR: Hypercalcemia in disseminated histoplasmosis. *Am J Med* 78:881, 1985.
718. Ryzen E, Rea TH, Singer FR: Hypercalcemia and abnormal 1,25-dihydroxyvitamin D concentrations in leprosy. *Am J Med* 84:325, 1988.

719. Kozeny GA, Barbato AL, Bansal VK, Vertuno LL, Hano JE: Hypercalcemia associated with silicone-induced granulomas. *N Engl J Med* 311:1103, 1984.
720. Mosekilde L, Christensen MS: Decreased parathyroid function in hyperthyroidism: Interrelationships between serum parathyroid hormone, calcium-phosphorus metabolism and thyroid function. *Acta Endocrinol (Copenh)* 84:566, 1977.
721. Bouillon R, Muls E, DeMoor P: Influence of thyroid function on the serum concentration of 1,25-dihydroxyvitamin D. *J Clin Endocrinol Metab* 51:793, 1980.
722. Mosekilde L, Melsen F, Bagger JP, Myhre-Jensen O, Sorensen NS: Bone changes in hyperthyroidism: Interrelationships between bone morphometry, thyroid function and calcium-phosphorus metabolism. *Acta Endocrinol (Copenh)* 85:515, 1977.
723. Walser M, Robinson BHB, Duckett JW Jr: The hypercalcemia of adrenal insufficiency. *J Clin Invest* 42:456, 1963.
724. Muls E, Bouillon R, Boelaert J, Lamberigts G, et al: Etiology of hypercalcemia in a patient with Addison's disease. *Calcif Tissue Int* 34:523, 1982.
725. Stewart AF, Hoecker JL, Mallette LE, Segre GV, Amatruda TT: Hypercalcemia in pheochromocytoma. *Ann Intern Med* 102:776, 1985.
726. Kimura S, Nishimura Y, Yamaguchi K, Nagasaki K, Shimada K, Uchida H: A case of pheochromocytoma producing parathyroid hormone-related protein and presenting with hypercalcemia. *J Clin Endocrinol Metab* 70:1559, 1990.
727. Ikeda K, Arnold A, Mangin M, Kinder B, et al: Expression of transcripts encoding a parathyroid hormone-related peptide in abnormal human parathyroid tissues. *J Clin Endocrinol Metab* 69:1240, 1989.
728. Stote RM, Smith LH, Wilson DM, Dube WJ, Goldsmith RS, Arnaud CD: Hydrochlorothiazide effects on serum calcium and immunoreactive parathyroid hormone concentrations. *Ann Intern Med* 77:587, 1972.
729. Christensson T, Hellström K, Wengle B: Hypercalcemia and primary hyperparathyroidism. *Arch Intern Med* 137:1138, 1977.
730. Porter RH, Cox BG, Heaney D, Hostetter TH, Stinbaugh BJ, Suki WN: Treatment of hypoparathyroid patients with chlorthalidone. *N Engl J Med* 298:577, 1978.
731. Kelepouris E, Agus ZS: Effects of diuretics on calcium and phosphate transport. *Semin Nephrol* 8:273, 1988.
732. Koppel MH, Massry SG, Shinaberger JH, Hartenbower DL, Coburn JW: Thiazide-induced rise in serum calcium and magnesium in patients on maintenance hemodialysis. *Ann Intern Med* 72:895, 1970.
733. Jacobus CH, Holick MF, Shao Q, Chen TC, et al: Hypervitaminosis D associated with drinking milk. *N Engl J Med* 326:1173, 1992.
734. Mawer EB, Hann JT, Berry JL, Davies M: Vitamin D metabolism in patients intoxicated with ergocalciferol. *Clin Sci* 68:135, 1985.
735. Mason RS, Lissner D, Grunstein HS, Posen S: A simplified assay for dihydroxylated vitamin D metabolites in human serum: Application to hyper- and hypovitaminosis D. *Clin Chem* 26:444, 1980.
736. Frame B, Jackson CE, Reynolds WA, Umphrey JE: Hypercalcemia and skeletal effects in chronic hypervitaminosis A. *Ann Intern Med* 80:44, 1974.
737. Farrington K, Miller P, Varghese Z, Baillod RA, Moorhead JF: Vitamin A toxicity and hypercalcaemia in chronic renal failure. *Br Med J* 282:1999, 1981.
738. Christiansen C, Baastrup PC, Lindgreen P, Transbol I: Endocrine effects of lithium: II. "Primary" hyperparathyroidism. *Acta Endocrinol (Copenh)* 88:528, 1978.
739. Saxe AW, Gibson G: Lithium increases tritated thymidine uptake by abnormal human parathyroid tissue. *Surgery* 110:1067, 1991.
740. Mellette LE, Khouri K, Zengotita H, Hollis BW, Malini S: Lithium treatment increases intact and midregion parathyroid hormone and parathyroid volume. *J Clin Endocrinol Metab* 68:654, 1989.
741. Mallette LE, Eichhorn E: Effects of lithium carbonate on human calcium metabolism. *Arch Intern Med* 146:770, 1986.
742. Orwoll ES: The milk-alkali syndrome: Current concepts. *Ann Intern Med* 97:242, 1982.
743. Kapsner P, Langsdorf L, Marcus R, Kraemer FB, Hoffman AR: Milk-alkali syndrome in patients treated with calcium carbonate after cardiac transplantation. *Arch Intern Med* 146:1965, 1986.
744. Minaire P, Meunier P, Edouard C, Bernard J, Courpron P, Bourret J: Quantitative histological data on disuse osteoporosis—comparison with biological data. *Calcif Tissue Res* 17:57, 1974.
745. Stewart AF, Adler M, Byers CM, Segre GV, Broadus AE: Calcium homeostasis in immobilization: An example of resorptive hypercalciuria. *N Engl J Med* 306:1136, 1982.
746. Merli GJ, McElwain GE, Adler AG, Martin JH, et al: Immobilization hypercalcemia in acture spinal cord injury treated with etidronate. *Arch Intern Med* 144:1286, 1984.
747. Llach F, Felsenfeld AJ, Haussler MR: The pathophysiology of altered calcium metabolism in rhabdomyolysis-induced acute renal failure. *N Engl J Med* 305:117, 1981.
748. Forster J, Querusio L, Burchard KW, Gann DS: Hypercalcemia in critically ill surgical patients. *Ann Surg* 202:512, 1985.
749. Gerhardt A, Greenberg A, Reilly JJ Jr, Van Thiel DH: Hypercalcemia: A complication of advanced chronic liver disease. *Arch Intern Med* 147:274, 1987.
750. Garabédian M, Jacqz E, Guillozo H, Grimberg R, Guillot M, Gagnadoux MF, BroyerMenoir G, et al: Elevated plasma 1,25-dihydroxyvitamin D concentrations in infants with hypercalcemia and an elfin facies. *N Engl J Med* 312:948, 1985.
751. Lingärde F, Zettervall O: Hypercalcemia and normal ionized serum calcium in a case of myelomatosis. *Ann Intern Med* 37:396, 1973.
752. Gagel RF: Laboratory values of importance for calcium metabolism and metabolic bone disease, in Favus MJ (ed): *Primer on the Metabolic Bone Diseases and Disorders of Mineral Metabolism.* New York, Raven Press, 1993, pp 411-412.
753. Layzer RB: *Neuromuscular Manifestations of Systemic Disease.* Philadelphia, Davis, 1985.
754. Edmondson JW, Brashear RE, Li TK: Tetany: Quantitative interrelationships between calcium and alkalosis. *Am J Physiol* 228:1082, 1975.
755. Stewart AF, Battaglini-Sabetta J, Millstone L: Hypocalcemia-induced pustular psoriasis of Von Zumbusch, new experience with an old syndrome. *Ann Intern Med* 100:677, 1984.
756. Rimailho A, Bouchard P, Schaison G: Improvement of hypocalcemic cardiomyopathy by correction of serum calcium level. *Am Heart J* 109:611, 1985.
757. Eisenberg E: Effect of serum calcium level and parathyroid extracts on phosphate and calcium excretion in hypoparathyroid patients. *J Clin Invest* 44:942, 1965.
758. Conley ME, Beckwith JB, Mancer JFK, Tenckhoff L: The spectrum of the DiGeorge syndrome. *J Pediatr* 94:883, 1979.
759. Mallette LE, Cooper JB, Kirkland JL: Transient congenital hypoparathyroidism: Possible association with anomalies of the pulmonary valve. *J Pediatr* 101:928, 1982.
760. Chisaka O, Capecchi MR: Regionally restricted developmental defects resulting from targeted disruption of the mouse homeobox gene hox-1.5. *Nature* 350:473, 1991.
761. Nuefeld M, Maclaren NK, Blizzard RM: Two types of autoimmune Addison's disease associated with different polyglandular autoimmune (PGA) syndromes. *Medicine* 60:355, 1981.
762. Li Y, Song YH, Rais N, et al: Autoantibodies to the extracellular domain of the calcium sensing receptor in patients with acquired hypoparathyroidism. *J Clin Invest* 97:910, 1996.
763. Parfitt AM: The incidence of hypoparathyroid tetany after thyroid operations: Relationship to age, extent of resection and surgical experience. *Med J Aust* 1:1103, 1971.
764. Parfitt AM: Surgical, idiopathic, and other varieties of parathyroid hormone-deficient hypoparathyroidism, in DeGroot LJ (ed): *Endocrinology.* Philadelphia, Saunders, 1989, p 1049.
765. Anast CS, Mohs JM, Kaplan SI, Burns TW: Evidence of parathyroid failure in magnesium deficiency. *Science* 177:606, 1972.
766. Anast CS, Winnacker JL, Forte LF, Burns TW: Impaired release of parathyroid hormone in magnesium deficiency. *J Clin Endocrinol Metab* 42:707, 1976.
767. Rude RK, Oldham SB, Singer FR: Functional hypoparathyroidism and parathyroid hormone end-organ resistance in human magnesium deficiency. *Clin Endocrinol* 5:209, 1976.
768. Rude RK: Magnesium metabolism and deficiency. *Endocrinol Metab Clin North Am* 22:377, 1993.
769. Shah GM, Alvarado P, Kirschenbaum MA: Symptomatic hypocalcemia and hypomagnesemia with renal magnesium wasting associated with pentamidine therapy in a patient with AIDS. *Am J Med* 89:380, 1990.
770. Barton CH, Pahl M, Vaziri ND, Cesario T: Renal magnesium wasting associated with amphotericin B therapy. *Am J Med* 77:471, 1984.

771. Burch WM, Posillico JT: Hypoparathyroidism after I-131 therapy with subsequent return of parathyroid function. *J Clin Endocrinol Metab* 57:398, 1983.
772. Richards GE, Brewer ED, Conley SB, Saldana LR: Combined hypothyroidism and hypoparathyroidism in an infant after maternal 131-Iodine administration. *J Pediat* 99:141, 1981.
773. Brezis M, Shalev O, Leibel B, Bernheim J, Ben-Ishay D: Phosphorus retention and hypoparathyroidism associated with transfusional iron overload in thalassaemia. *Min Elect Metab* 4:57, 1980.
774. Carpenter TO, Carnes DL Jr, Anast CS: Hypoparathyroidism in Wilson's disease. *N Engl J Med* 309:873, 1983.
775. Ahn TG, Antonarakis SE, Kronenberg HM, Igarashi T, Levie MA: Familial isolated hypoparathyroidism: A molecular genetic analysis of 8 families with 23 affected persons. *Medicine (Baltimore)* 65:73, 1986.
776. Parkinson DB, Thakker RV: Hypoparathyroidism due to a donor splice site mutation in the parathyroid hormone gene. *J Bone Miner Res* 6:S300, 1991.
777. Caulfield MP, McKee RL, Goldman ME, Duong LT, Fisher JE, Gay CT, DeHaven PA, Levy JJ, et al: The bovine renal parathyroid hormone (PTH) receptor has equal affinity for two different amino acid sequences: The receptor binding domains of PTH and PTH-related protein are located within the 14-34 region. *Endocrinology* 127:83, 1990.
778. Albright F, Burnett CH, Smith PH, Parson W: Pseudohypoparathyroidism—an example of "Seabright-Bantam syndrome." *Endocrinology* 30:922, 1942.
779. Wilson JD, George FW, Leshin M: Genetic control of extraglandular aromatase activity in the chicken. *Steroids* 50:235, 1987.
780. Chase LR, Melson GL, Aurbach GD: Pseudohypoparathyroidism: Defective excretion of 3′,5′-AMP in response to parathyroid hormone. *J Clin Invest* 48:1832, 1969.
781. Drezner MK, Burch WM JR: Altered activity of the nucleotide regulatory site in the parathyroid hormone-sensitive adenylate cyclase from the renal cortex of a patient with pseudohypoparathyroidism. *J Clin Invest* 62:1222, 1978.
782. Farfel Z, Brickman AS, Kaslow HR, Brothers VM, Bourne HR: Deficiency of receptor cyclase coupling protein in pseudohypoparathyroidism. *N Engl J Med* 303:237, 1980.
783. Levine MA, Downs RW, Singer MJ, Marx SJ, Aurbach GD, Spiegel AM: Deficient activity of guanine nucleotide regulatory protein in erythrocytes from patients with pseudohypoparathyroidism. *Biochem Biophys Res Commun* 94:1319, 1980.
784. Nagant de Deuxchaisnes C, Kane SM: Hypoparathyroidism, in Avioli LV, Krane SM (eds): *Metabolic Bone Disease*. New York, Academic Press, 1978, p 217.
785. Yamamoto M, Takuwa Y, Masuko S, Ogata E: Effects of endogenous and exogenous parathyroid hormone on tubular reabsorption of calcium in pseudohypoparathyroidism. *J Clin Endocrinol Metab* 66:618, 1988.
786. Drezner MK, Neelon FA, Haussler M, McPherson HT, Lebovitz HE: 1,25-dihydroxycholecalciferol deficiency: The probable cause of hypocalcemia and metabolic bone disease in pseudohypoparathyroidism. *J Clin Endocrinol Metab* 42:621, 1976.
787. Breslau NA, Moses AM, Pak CYC: Evidence for bone remodeling but lack of calcium mobilization response to parathyroid hormone in pseudohypoparathyroidism. *J Clin Endocrinol Metab* 57:638, 1983.
788. Bell NH, Avery S, Sinha T, Clark CM Jr, Allen DO, Johnston C Jr: Effects of dibutyryl cyclic adenosine 3′,5′-monophosphate and parathyroid extract on calcium and phosphorus metabolism in hypoparathyroidism and pseudohypoparathyroidism. *J Clin Invest* 51:816, 1972.
789. Yamaoka K, Seino Y, Ishida M, Ishii T, Shimotsuji T, Tanaka Y, Kurose H, Matsuda S, et al: Effect of dibutyryl adenosine 3′,3′-monophosphate administration on plasma concentrations of 1,25-dihydroxyvitamin D in pseudohypoparathyroidism type I. *J Clin Endocrinol Metab* 53:1096, 1981.
790. Spiegel AM: Pseudohypoparathyroidism, in Scriver CR, Beaudet AL, Sly WS, Valle D (eds): *The Metabolic Basis of Inherited Disease*. New York, McGraw-Hill, 1989, p 2013.
791. Kozasa T, Itoh H, Tsukamoto T, Kaziro Y: Isolation and characterization of the human $G_s\alpha$ gene. *Proc Natl Acad Sci USA* 85:2081, 1988.
792. Levine MA, Ahn TG, Klupt SF, Kaufman KD, et al: Genetic deficiency of the alpha subunit of the guanine nucleotide-binding protein G_s as the molecular basis for Albright's hereditary osteodystrophy. *Proc Natl Acad Sci USA* 85:617, 1988.
793. Levine MA, Modi WS, O'Brien SJ: Mapping of the gene encoding the alpha subunit of the stimulatory G protein of adenylyl cyclase (GNAS1) to 20q13.2-q13.3 in human by in situ hybridization. *Genomics* 11:478, 1991.
794. Hayward BE, Moran V, Strain L, Bonthron DT: Bidirectional imprinting of a single gene: GNAS1 encodes maternally, paternally and biallelically derived proteins. *Proc Natl Acad Sci USA* 95:15475, 1998.
795. Hayward BE, Kamiya M, Strain L, Moran V, et al: The human GNAS1 gene is imprinted and encodes a distict paternally and biallelically expressed G proteins. *Proc Natl Acad Sci USA* 95:10038, 1998.
796. Bhatt B, Burns J, Flanner D, Mcgee: Direct visualization of a single copy genes on banded metaphase chromosomes by nonisotopic in situ hybridization. *Nucleic Acids Res* 16:3951, 1988.
797. Mattera R, Graziano MP, Yatani A, Zhou Z, et al: Splice variants of the alpha subunit of the G protein Gs Activate both adenylyl cyclase and calcium channels. *Science* 243:804, 1989.
798. Jones DT, Masters SB, Bourne HR, Reed RR: Biochemical characterization of three stimulatory GTP-binding proteins. *J Biol Chem* 265:2671, 1990.
799. Graziano MP, Freissmuth M, Gilman AG: Expression of Gs alpha in *Escherichia coli*: Purification and properties of two forms of the protein. *J Biol Chem* 264:409, 1989.
800. Novotny J, Svoboda P: The long Gs(alpha)—L and short Gs(alpha)-S variants of the stimulatory guanine nucleotide-binding protein. Do they behave in an identical way? *J Mol Endocrinol* 20:163, 1998.
801. Lin CK, Hakakha MJ, Nakamoto JM, Englund AT, et al: Prevalence of three mutations in the $Gs\alpha$ gene among 24 families with pseudohypoparathyroidism type Ia. *Biochem Biophys Res Commun* 189:343, 1992.
802. Iiri T, Herzmark P, Nakamoto JM, Van Dop C, Bourne HR: Rapid GDP release from $Gs\alpha$ in patients with gain and loss of function. *Nature* 371:164, 1994.
803. Luttikhuis ME, Wilson LC, Leonard JV, Trembath RC: Characterization of a de novo 43-bp deletion of the $Gs\alpha$ gene (GNAS1) in Albright hereditary osteodystrophy. *Genomics* 21:455, 1994.
804. Patten JL, Johans DR, Valle D, Eil C, et al: Mutation in the gene encoding the stimulatory G protein of adenylate cyclase in Albright's hereditary osteodystrophy. *N Engl J Med* 322:1412, 1990.
805. Weinstein LS, Gejman PV, Friedman E, Kadowaki T, et al: Mutations of the $Gs\alpha$ subunit gene in Albright hereditary osteodystrophy detected by denaturing gell electrophoresis. *Proc Natl Acad Sci USA* 87:8287, 1990.
806. Miric A, Vechio JD, Levine MA: Heterogeneous mutations in the gene encoding the alpha ubunit of the stimulatory G protein of adenylyl cyclase in Albright hereditary osteodystrophy. *J Clin Endocrinol Metab* 76:1560, 1993.
807. Schwindinger WF, Miric A, Zimmerman D, Levine MA: A novel $Gs\alpha$ mutant in a patient with Albright hereditary osteodystrophy uncouples cell surface receptors from adenylyl cyclase. *J Biol Chem* 269:25387, 1994.
808. Farfel Z, Iiri T, Shapira H, Roitman A, Mouallem M, Bourne HR: Pseudohypoparathyroidism, a novel mutation in the $\beta\gamma$-contact region of $Gs\alpha$ impairs receptor stimulation. *J Biol Chem* 271:19653, 1996.
809. Shapira H, Mouallem M, Shapiro MS, Weisman Y, Farfel Z: Pseudohypoparathyroidism type Ia: Two new heterozygous frameshift mutations in exons 5 and 10 of the $Gs\alpha$ gene. *Hum Genet* 97:73, 1996.
810. Fischer JA, Egert F, Werder E, Born W: An inherited mutation associated with functional deficiency of the alpha-subunit of the guanine nucleotide-binding protein Gs in pseudo- and pseudopseudohypoparathyroidism. *J Clin Endocrinol Metab* 83:935, 1998.
811. Jan de Beur SM, Deng Z, Ding CL, Levine MA: Amplification of the GC-rich exon 1 of GNAS1 and identification of three novel nonsense mutations in Albright's hereditary osteodystrophy. Endocrine Society 80th annual meeting, p. 62 (Abstract), 1998.
812. Nakamoto JM, Sandstrom AT, Brickman AS, Christenson RA, Van Dop C: Pseudohypoparathyroidism type Ia from maternal but not paternal transmission of a $Gs\alpha$ gene mutation. *Am J Med Genet* 77:261, 1998.
813. Warner DR, Weng G, Yu S, Matalon R, Weinstein LS: A novel mutation in the switch 3 region of $Gs\alpha$ in a patient with Albright heredi-

tary osteodystrophy impairs GDP binding and receptor activation. *J Biol Chem* 273:23976, 1998.
814. Ahmed SF, Dixon PH, Bonthron DT, Stirling HF, et al: GNAS1 mutational analysis in pseudohypoparathyroidism. *Clin Endocrinol* 49:525, 1998.
815. Weinstein LS, Gejman PV, de Mazancourt P, American N, Spiegel AM: A heterozygous 4-bp deletion mutation in the Gsα gene (GNAS1) in a patient with Albright hereditary osteodystrophy. *Genomics* 13:1319, 1992.
816. Yu S, Yu D, Hainline BE, Brener JL, et al: A deletion hot-spot in exon 7 of the Gsα (GNAS1) in patients with Albright hereditary osteodystrophy. *Hum Mol Genet* 4:2001, 1995.
817. Kolb FO, Steinbach HL: Pseudohypoparathyroidism with secondary hyperparathyroidism and osteitis fibrosa. *J Clin Endocrinol Metab* 22:59, 1962.
818. Stogmann W, Fischer JA: Pseudohypoparathyroidism: Disappearance of the resistance to parathyroid extract during treatment with vitamin D. *Am J Med* 59:140, 1975.
819. Metz SA, Baylink DJ, Hughes MR, Haussler MR, Robertson RP: Selective deficiency of 1,25-dihydroxycholecalciferol: A cause of isolated skeletal resistance to parathyroid hormone. *N Engl J Med* 292:1084, 1977.
820. Albright F, Forbes AP, Henneman PH: Pseudo-pseudohypoparathyroidism. *Trans Assoc Am Physicians* 65:337, 1952.
821. Levine MA, Jap TS, Mauseth RS, Downs RW, Spiegel AM: Activity of the stimulatory guanine nucleotide-binding protein is reduced in erthrocytes from patients with pseudohypoparathyroidism and pseudopseudohypoparathyroidism: Biochemical, endocrine, and genetic analysis of Albright's hereditary osteodystrophy in six kindreds. *J Clin Endocrino Metab* 62:497, 1986.
822. Wilson LC, Oude Luttikhuis ME, Clayton PT, Fraser WD, Trembath RC: Parental origin of Gsα gene mutations in Albrights hereditary osteodystrophy. *J Med Genet* 31:835, 1994.
823. Davies SJ, Hughes HE: Imprinting in Albrights hereditary osteodystrophy. *J Med Genet* 30:101, 1993.
824. Levine MA, Downs RW Jr, Moses AM: Resistance to multiple hormones in patients with pseudohypoparathyroidism: Association with deficient activity of the guanine nucleotide regulatory protein. *Am J Med* 74:919, 1983.
825. Yu S, Yu D, Lee E, Eckhaus M, et al: Variable and tissue-specific hormone resistance in heterotrimeric Gs protein alpha (Gsα-subunit knockout mice is due to tissue-specific imprinting of the Gsα gene. *Proc Natl Acad Sci USA* 95:8715, 1998.
826. Schwindinger WF, Lawler AM, Gearhart JD, Levine MA: A murine model of Albright hereditary osteodystrophy. Endocrine Society, 80th annual meeting, p. 480 (abstract), 1998.
827. Schipani E, Weinstein LS, Bergwitz C, Iida-klein A, et al: Pseudohypoparathyroidism Ib is not caused by mutations in the coding exons of the human parathyroid hormone (PTH)/PTH-related peptide receptor gene. *J Clin Endocrinol Metab* 80:1611, 1995.
828. Ettoun JD, Minagawa M, Kwan MY, Lee HS, et al: Cloning and characterization of the promoter regions of the human parathyroid hormone (PTH)/PTHrP receptor gene: Analysis of deoxyribonucleic acid from normal subjects and patients with pseudohypoparathyroidism type Ib. *J Clin Endocrinol Metab* 82:1031, 1997.
829. Fukumoto S, Suzawa M, Takeuchi Y, Kodama Y, et al: Absence of mutations in parathyroid hormone (PTH)/PTH-related protein receptor complementary deoxyribonucleic acid in patients with pseudohypoparathyroidism type Ib. *J Clin Endocrinol Metab* 81:2554, 1996.
830. Jüppner H, Schipani E, Astepe M, Cole DE, et al: The gene responsible for pseudohypoparathyroidism type Ib is paternally imprinted and maps in four unrelated kindreds to chromosome 20q13.3. *Proc Natl Acad Sci USA* 95:11798, 1998.
831. Drezner M, Neelon FA, Lebovitz HE: Pseudohypoparathyroidism type II: A possible defect in the reception of the cyclic AMP signal. *N Engl J Med* 289:1056, 1973.
832. Rodriguez HJ, Villarreal H Jr, Klahr S, Slatopolsky E: Pseudohypoparathyroidism type II: Restoration of normal renal responsiveness to parathyroid hormone by calcium administration. *J Clin Endocrinol Metab* 39:693, 1974.
833. Aurbach GD, Marcus R, Winickoff RN, Epstein EH Jr, Nigra TP: Urinary excretion of 3′,5′-AMP in syndromes considered refractory to parathyroid hormones. *Metabolism* 19:799, 1970.
834. Chase LR, Melson GL, Aurbach GD: Pseudohypoparathyroidism: Defective excretion of 3′,5′-AMP in response to parathyroid hormone. *J Clin Invest* 48:1832, 1969.
835. Mallette LE, Kirkland JL, Gagel RF, Law WM Jr, Heath H III: Synthetic human parathyroid hormone-(1-34) for the study of pseudohypoparathyroidism. *J Clin Endocrinol Metab* 67:964, 1988.
836. Chattopadhyay N, Mithal A, Brown EM: The calcium-sensing receptor: A window into the physiology and pathophysiology of mineral ion metabolism. *Endocr Rev* 17:289, 1996.
837. Pearce SHS, Williamson C, Kifor O, et al: A familial syndrome of hypocalcemia with hypercalciuria due to mutations in the calcium-sensing receptor. *N Engl J Med* 335:1115, 1996.
838. Baron J, Winer KK, Yanovski JA, et al: Mutations in the Ca^{2+}-sensing receptor gene cause autosomal dominant and sporadic hypoarathyroidism. *Human Mol Genet* 5:601, 1996.
839. DeLuca F, Ray K, Mancilla EE, et al: Sporadic hypoparathyroidism caused by de novo gain-of-function mutations in the Ca^{2+}-sensing receptor. *J Clin Endocrinol Metab* 82:2710, 1997.
840. McCarthy JT, Kumar R: Renal osteodystrophy. *Endocrinol Metab Clin North Am* 19:65-93, 1990.
841. Ritchie HH, Hughes MR, Thompson ET, et al: An ochre mutation in the vitamin D receptor gene causes hereditary 1,25-dihydroxyvitamin-D3 resistant rickets in three families. *Proc Natl Acad Sci* 86:9783, 1989.
842. Sone T, Marx SJ, Liberman UA, Pike JW: A unique point mutation in the human vitamin D receptor chromosomal gene confers hereditary resistance to 1,25-dihydroxyvitamin D_3. *Mol Endocrinol* 4:623, 1990.
843. Balsan S, Garabedian M, Larchet M, et al: Long-term nocturnal calcium infusions can cure rickets and promote normal mineralization in hereditary resistance to 1,25-dihydroxyvitamin D. *J Clin Invest* 77:1661, 1986.
844. Weisman Y, Bab I, Gazit D, Spirer Z, Jaffe M, Hochberg Z: Long-term intracaval calcium infusion therapy in end-organ resistance to 1,25-dihydroxyvitamin D. *Am J Med* 83:984, 1987.
845. Mallette LE, Gomez LS: Systemic hypocalcemia after clinical injection of radiographic contrast media: Amelioration by omission of calcium chelating agents. *Radiology* 147:677, 1982.
846. Tofalletti J, Nissenson RA, Endres D, McGarry E, Mogollon G: Influence of continuous infusion of citrate on responses of immuno-reactive PTH, calcium, magnesium components, and other electrolytes in normal adults during plasmapheresis. *J Clin Endocrinol Metab* 60:874, 1985.
847. Jacobson MA, Gambertoglio JG, Aweeka FT, Causey DM, Portale AA: Foscarnet-induced hypocalcemia and effects of foscarnet on calcium metabolism. *J Clin Endocrinol Metab* 72:1130, 1991.
848. Grinspoon SK, Bilezikian JP: HIV disease and the endocrine system. *N Engl J Med* 327:1360, 1992.
849. Raskin P, McClain CJ, Medsger TA Jr: Hypocalcemia associated with metastatic bone disease. *Arch Intern Med* 132:539, 1973.
850. Zusman J, Brown DM, Nesbit ME: Hyperphosphatemia, hyperphosphaturia and hypocalcemia in acute lymphoblastic leukemia. *N Engl J Med* 289:1335, 1973.
851. Kumar R: The metabolism and mechanism of action of 1,25-dihydroxyvitamin D. *Kidney Int* 30:793, 1986.
852. Stewart AF, Longo W, Kreutter D, Jacob R, Burtis WJ: Hypocalcemia due to calcium soap formation in a patient with a pancreatic fistula. *N Engl J Med* 315:496, 1986.
853. Rall TW, Sutherland EW: Formation of a cyclic adenine ribonucleotide by tissue particles. *J Biol Chem* 232:1065, 1958.
854. Tohme JF, Bilezikian JP: Hypocalcemic emergencies. *Endocrinol Metab Clinics North Am* 22:363, 1993.
855. Rude RK: Magnesium depletion and hypermagnesemia, in Favus MJ (ed): *Primer on the Metabolic Bone Diseases and Disorders of Mineral Metabolism*. New York, Raven Press, 1996, pp 234–238.
856. Breslau NA, Zerwekh JE: Relationship of estrogen and pregnancy to calcium homeostasis in pseudohypoparathyroidism. *J Clin Endocrinol Metab* 62:45, 1986.
857. Recker R: Calcium absorption and achlorhydria. *N Engl J Med* 313:70, 1985.
858. Freeman D, Bartlett S, Radda G, Ross B: Energetics of sodium transport in the kidney: Saturation transfer 31P-NMR. *Biochem Biophys Acta* 762:325, 1983.
859. Markowitz M, Rotkin L, Rosen JF: Circadian rhythms of blood minerals in humans. *Science* 213:672, 1981.

860. Bijvoet OLM: Relation of plasma phosphate concentration to renal tubular reabsorption of phosphate. *Clin Sci* 37:23, 1969.
861. Suki WN, Rouse D: Renal transport of calcium, magnesium, and phosphorus, in Brenner BM, Rector FC Jr (eds): *The Kidney*. Philadelphia, Saunders, 1991, p 380.
862. Murer H, Werner A, Reshkin S, Wuarin F, Biber J: Cellular mechanisms in proximal tubular reabsorption of inorganic phosphate. *Am J Physiol* 260:C885, 1991.
863. Hammerman MR: Phosphate transport across renal proximal tubular cell membranes. *Am J Physiol* 251:F385, 1986.
864. Low I, Friedrich T, Burckhardt G: Properties of an anion exchanger in rat renal basolateral membrane vesicles. *Am J Physiol* 246:F334, 1984.
865. Segal JH, Pollock AS: Transfection-mediated expression of a dominant cAMP-resistant phenotype in the opposum kidney (OK) cell line prevents parathyroid hormone-induced inhibition of Na-phosphate cotransport: A protein kinase-A mediated event. *J Clin Invest* 86:1442, 1990.
866. Trohler V, Bonjour JP, Fleisch J: Inorganic phosphate homeostasis: Renal adaptation to the dietary intake in intact and thyroparathyroidectomized rats. *J Clin Invest* 57:264, 1976.
867. Stoll R, Kinne R, Murer H: Effect of dietary phosphate intake in phosphate transport by isolated rat renal brush border vesicles. *Biochem J* 180:465, 1978.
868. Corvilain J, Abramow M: Effect of growth hormone on tubular transport of phosphate in normal and parathyroidectomized dogs. *J Clin Invest* 43:1608, 1964.
869. Anderson J, Forster JB: Effect of cortisone on urinary phosphate excretion in man. *Clin Sci* 18:437, 1959.
870. Kempson SA: Effect of metabolic acidosis on renal brush border membrane adaptation to low phosphorus diet. *Kidney Int* 22:225, 1982.
871. Knochel JP: The pathophysiology and clinical characteristics of severe hypophosphatemia. *Arch Intern Med* 137:203, 1977.
872. Rubin MF, Narins RG: Hypophosphatemia: Pathophysiological and practical aspects of its therapy. *Semin Nephrol* 10:536, 1990.
873. Travis SF, Sugarman HJ, Ruberg RL: Alterations of red cell glycolytic intermediates and oxygen transport as a consequence of hypophosphatemia in patients receiving intravenous hyperalimentation. *N Engl J Med* 285:763, 1971.
874. Knochel JP, Barcenas C, Cotton JR, Fuller TJ, Haller R, Carter NW: Hypophosphatemia and rhabdomyolysis. *J Clin Invest* 62:1240, 1978.
875. O'Connor LR, Wheeler WS, Bethune JG: Effect of hypophosphatemia on myocardial performance in man. *N Engl J Med* 297:901, 1978.
876. Lotz M, Zisman E, Bartter FC: Evidence for a phosphorus-depletion syndrome in man. *N Engl J Med* 278:409, 1968.
877. Godsall JW, Baron R, Insogna KL: Vitamin D metabolism and bone histomorphometry in a patient with antacid-induced osteomalacia. *Am J Med* 77:747, 1984.
878. The HYP Consortium: A gene (PEX) with homologies to endopeptidases is mutated in patients with x-linked hypophosphatemic rickets. *Nat Genet* 11:130, 1995.
879. Kumar R: Phosphatonin—a new phosphaturetic hormone? (Lessons from tumour-induced osteomalacia and X-linked hypophosphataemia). *Nephrol Dial Transplant* 12:11, 1997.
880. Cai Q, Hodgson SF, Kao PC, Lennon VA, Klee GG, Zinsmiester AR, Kumar R: Brief report: inhibition of renal phosphate transport by a tumor product in a patient with oncogenic osteomalacia. *N Engl J Med* 330:1645, 1994.
881. Mostellar ME, Tuttle EP: The effects of akalosis on plasma concentrations and urinary excretion of inorganic phosphate in man. *J Clin Invest* 43:138, 1964.
882. Laaban JP, Waked M, Laromiguiere M, Vuong TK, Rochemaure J: Hypophosphatemia complicating management of acute severe asthma. *Ann Intern Med* 112:68, 1990.
883. Fiaccadori E, Coffrini E, Ronda N, Vezzani A, et al: Hypophosphatemia in course of chronic obstructive pulmonary disease. *Chest* 97:857, 1990.
884. Aubier M, Murciano D, Lecocguic Y, Viires N, et al: Effect of hypophosphatemia on diaphragmatic contractility in patients with acute respiratory failure. *N Engl J Med* 313:420, 1985.
885. Newman JH, Neff RA, Ziporin P: Acute respiratory failure associated with hypophosphatemia. *N Engl J Med* 296:1101, 1977.
886. Lewis JF, Hodsman AB, Driedger AA, Thompson RT, McFadden RG: Hypophosphatemia and respiratory failure: Prolonged abnormal energy metabolism demonstrated by nuclear magnetic resonance spectroscopy. *Am J Med* 83:1139, 1987.
887. Fisher JN, Kitabchi AE: A randomized study of phosphate therapy in the treatment of diabetic ketoacidosis. *J Clin Endocrinol Metab* 57:177, 1983.
888. Hayek ME, Eisenberg PG: Severe hypophosphatemia following the institution of enteral feedings. *Arch Surg* 124:1325, 1989.
889. Angeli P, Gatta A, Caregaro L, Luisetto G, et al: Hypophosphatemia and renal tubular dysfunction in alcoholics. *Gastroenterology* 100:502, 1991.
890. Lentz RD, Brown DM, Kjellstrand CM: Treatment of severe hypophosphatemia. *Ann Intern Med* 89:941, 1978.
891. Wacker WEC, Parisi AF: Magnesium metabolism. *N Engl J Med* 278:658, 1968.
892. Agus ZS, Wasserstein A, Goldfarb S: Disorders of calcium and magnesium homeostasis. *Am J Med* 72:473, 1982.
893. Dirks JH: The kidney and magnesium regulation. *Kidney Int* 23:771, 1983.
894 Broadus AE: Physiological functions of calcium, magnesium, and phosphorus, in Favus MJ (ed): *Primer on the Metabolic Bone Diseases and Disorders of Mineral Metabolism*. Richmond VA, American Society for Bone and Mineral Research, William Byrd Press, 1990, p 29.
895 Silverberg SJ: The distribution and balance of calcium, magnesium and phosphorus, in Favus MJ (ed): *Primer on the Metabolic Bone Diseases and Disorders of Mineral Metabolism*. Richmond VA, American Society for Bone and Mineral Research, William Byrd Press, 1990, p 30.
896. Lemann J Jr: Intestinal absorption of calcium, magnesium, and phosphorus, in Favus MJ (ed): *Primer on the Metabolic Bone Diseases and Disorders of Mineral Metabolism*. Richmond VA, William Byrd Press, 1990, p 32.
897. Lemann J Jr: The urinary excretion of calcium, magnesium, and phosphorus, in Favus MJ (ed): *Primer on the Metabolic Bone Diseases and Disorders of Mineral Metabolism*. Richmond VA, William Byrd Press, 1990, p 36.
898. Rude RK: Magnesium depletion and hypermagnesemia, in Favus MJ (ed): *Primer on the Bone Metabolic Bone Diseases and Disorders of Mineral Metabolism*, 4th ed. Pennsylvania, Lippincott Williams & Wilkins, 1999, p 241.
899. Flink EF: Therapy of magnesium deficiency. *Ann NY Acad Sci* 162:901, 1969.

CHAPTER 23

Metabolic Bone Disease

Frederick R. Singer

A *metabolic bone disease* can best be defined as a skeletal disorder that is generalized in extent.[1] This may not always be clinically apparent, as in patients with osteoporosis, in whom the vertebral lesions are often the clinical focus of attention. However, more subtle abnormalities of a generalized nature can be demonstrated in these patients with bone biopsy or bone densitometry.

Metabolic bone diseases, particularly osteoporosis, constitute a growing public health problem that to a great extent is a consequence of the longer life span of the population. These disorders often have a complex pathogenesis that includes abnormal hormone secretion rates, deficiency of vitamin D, impaired metabolic activation of vitamin D or resistance to its actions, other nutritional deficiencies, immobilization, genetic abnormalities of connective tissue matrix and enzyme synthesis, and failure of normal bone stem cell differentiation. In addition, osteoporosis is associated with a number of unrelated primary disorders, such as rheumatoid arthritis, in which the pathogenetic relation between bone loss and the primary disorder is ill defined. Finally, there are instances of "idiopathic" bone disease in which no clues to the pathogenesis are apparent.

CLINICAL EVALUATION OF METABOLIC BONE DISEASE

History and Physical Examination

Patients with a metabolic bone disease may have a prolonged asymptomatic course during which only the appropriate laboratory tests will reveal an abnormality. Such a situation is typical of postmenopausal osteoporosis before bone mass has decreased enough to allow a compression fracture of a vertebral body to occur.

The most common symptoms that occur in adult patients with bone disease are pain and deformity. Pathologic fractures of the vertebral bodies or femoral neck are sometimes the first indication of underlying disease. In children, failure of normal growth is a common feature. Rarely, neurologic deficits may develop as a consequence of abnormal remodeling of bone; for example, optic and auditory nerve compression may complicate osteopetrosis. In patients with hypocalcemia, tetany and seizures may be present. In vitamin D-deficient and phosphate-deficient states, muscle weakness and tenderness may be striking features of the physical examination.

It is particularly important to ascertain the dietary history and the family history and to find out whether there was a period of prolonged immobilization in the past, as these are important determinants of normal skeletal development.

Routine Clinical Chemistry

Important information concerning the type and underlying etiology of metabolic bone disease can be obtained from several routine blood and urine analyses. These are discussed in detail in Chap. 22 and will be only briefly reviewed here.

The fasting serum calcium, phosphorus, and alkaline phosphatase concentrations, usually a part of screening chemistry panels, are simple but valuable parameters in assessing metabolic bone disease.

The serum calcium concentration may be normal, high, or low in patients with bone disease. An elevated concentration suggests that bone resorption is increased, and a low concentration may indicate a failure of adequate release of bone mineral to maintain a normocalcemic state. The presence of a normal serum calcium concentration should not be taken as evidence of normal bone metabolism, as crippling bone disease may be present in normocalcemic patients with osteoporosis, osteomalacia, and renal osteodystrophy.

The serum phosphorus concentration is almost always reduced in osteomalacia and rickets, excluding patients with chronic renal failure. Patients with osteoporosis usually have a normal serum phosphorus concentration. It should be stressed that the serum phosphorus is best measured after an overnight fast to avoid dietary influences and diurnal variation.

The serum alkaline phosphatase activity can be used as an index of osteoblastic activity in the absence of a concomitant disorder which raises extraskeletal enzyme activity. As is stressed in Chap. 22, this parameter is a rather insensitive measure of osteoblastic activity, and mild degrees of bone disease in which increased osteoblasts are found on bone biopsy may be associated with normal circulating alkaline phosphatase activity.

Acid-base status, renal function, and liver function tests may be useful in the differential diagnosis of bone disease but are secondary tests.

Twenty-four-hour urinary calcium and phosphorus excretion have commonly been measured in the evaluation of patients with disturbed mineral homeostasis. These measurements, particularly phosphorus excretion, are often of little use when obtained under uncontrolled conditions, because urinary excretion of these substances is influenced by a variety of factors. More relevant information can be obtained by spot urine collections after an overnight fast. The fasting calcium excretion (expressed as milligrams Ca per 100 ml glomerular filtrate) provides an indirect index of bone mineral resorption. Occasionally, fasting calcium excretion may be increased as a result of impaired renal tubular reabsorption of calcium. The best index of phosphorus excretion is the maximum tubular reabsorption of phosphate (TmP) expressed as a function of the glomerular filtration rate (GFR), or TmP/GFR

(Chap. 22). The TmP/GFR is decreased in hyperparathyroidism; however, a markedly reduced TmP/GFR is typical of various states of primary renal phosphorus wasting unrelated to parathyroid hormone secretion.

Radioimmunoassays for parathyroid hormone provide a more specific test for parathyroid function. Measurements of circulating parathyroid hormone are helpful in determining the pathogenesis of bone disease in patients with primary and secondary hyperparathyroidism. Assays for intact parathyroid hormone in the circulation are excellent.[2] Unlike previous assays, the best of the present two-site immunometric assays exhibit little overlap between hormone levels in normal individuals and those in hyperparathyroid patients.

Urinary cAMP or nephrogenous cAMP measurements are sensitive indexes of parathyroid hormone activity. They are particularly useful in patients in whom parathyroid hormone resistance is suspected. These patients fail to exhibit a normal increase in cAMP production after the administration of parathyroid extract.

Biochemical Markers of Bone Turnover

More sophisticated tests of the metabolic activity of bone formation and bone resorption have been in development during the past 20 years.[3] In Table 23-1 some of the most widely applied and/or clinically useful tests are listed. Other assays have been developed to assess bone formation (serum type I procollagen peptides) or bone resorption (urinary galactosyl hydroxylysine, urinary free pyridinoline crosslinks, serum tartrate-resistant acid phosphatase) but are either not commercially available or are less useful in clinical practice.

The assay of bone specific alkaline phosphatase utilizing reasonably specific antibodies is particularly useful in patients with significant hepatic disease although there is some cross-reactivity between bone and liver alkaline phosphatase.[3]

A second index of osteoblast activity, serum osteocalcin (also termed bone GLA protein), is nearly specific for osteoblast activity.[3] Increased concentrations of osteocalcin are often found in patients with postmenopausal osteoporosis, primary hyperparathyroidism, hyperthyroidism, and acromegaly. Low levels are present in patients with glucocorticoid excess and hypoparathyroidism. In Paget's disease the alkaline phosphatase activity appears to be a better reflection of disease activity than osteocalcin, possibly due to differences in the state of differentiation of osteoblasts in pagetic bone than in other skeletal disorders.

In the past urinary hydroxyproline excretion was the main index used to estimate the rate of bone resorption in patients with metabolic bone disease.[3] Because this amino acid is nearly unique to the collagen molecule, it reflects the rate of metabolic activity in bone, particularly in disorders with high levels of bone resorption such as Paget's disease. Subsequently it has been appreciated that assays which measure various forms of collagen crosslinks are more specific and somewhat more sensitive in estimating the rate of bone resorption. The collagen crosslinks initially were measured in spot or 24-h urine specimens and more recently in serum. The latter assays may become the more standard assays because of ease of collection and avoidance of creatinine assay required for the urine tests.

TABLE 23-1. Biochemical Markers of Bone Metabolism

1. Biochemical markers of bone formation
   - A. Serum bone specific alkaline phosphatase
   - B. Serum osteocalcin
2. Biochemical markers of bone resorption
   - A. Urinary hydroxyproline
   - B. Urinary cross-linked N-telopeptides
   - C. Urinary cross-linked C-telopeptides
   - D. Urinary total deoxypyridinoline crosslinks

Calcium balance studies, as devised by Albright and Reifenstein, have been extensively used as a research tool in the investigation of bone disease, but can be carried out only in a research ward. Various isotopic studies of intestinal calcium absorption have been devised but also have not been widely applied to patients outside research centers.

Radiology and Nuclear Medicine

Radiologic evaluation of the skeleton is a valuable noninvasive means of determining the extent, severity, and nature of bone disease. The "metabolic bone survey" usually consists of a lateral skull x-ray, hand x-rays, lateral thoracic and lumbar x-rays, and a pelvic x-ray. In most patients with a severe generalized bone disease, an abnormal radiologic finding will be apparent in one or more of these sites. If hyperparathyroidism is in the differential diagnosis, films of the clavicles or lamina dura may prove revealing. If osteomalacia is suspected, a search for pseudofractures in the long bones and scapulae is worthwhile if they are not discovered in other areas.

The types of radiologic abnormality that should be sought are a reduction in bone density, unusual bone texture, widening of the epiphyseal cartilage growth plate, thinning or thickening of the cortex, periosteal new bone formation, endosteal scalloping, fractures, pseudofractures, and abnormalities in the size and shape of a bone. These types of abnormality are illustrated in subsequent sections.

Quantitative assessment of bone mineral is of particular importance in view of the high incidence of osteoporosis. Utilization of standard radiographs of bone has long been known to be inadequate to detect as much as 20–40 percent of bone loss in the spine and in following longitudinal changes in bone density. Standard radiographs are useful to detect spinal compression fractures and other fractures. Presently dual x-ray absorptiometry (DXA) is the most widely used method to measure bone density.[4] The technique, introduced in 1987, utilizes two energy level beams to measure spine and hip density as well as peripheral and whole body density, if desired. Reproducibility is good and a low radiation dose has contributed to the broad acceptability of this technique. One disadvantage is found in measurement of spine density in the presence of sclerotic changes produced by arthritis and intervertebral disc disease. In this setting a better estimate of density is obtained from the hip measurement.

Quantitative computerized tomography (QCT) of the lumbar spine has considerable advantages over DXA for spine measurements. It provides a true density measurement and measures the spongy bone density, which is more sensitive to metabolic influences than the surrounding cortical bone. The disadvantage of QCT is that CT scanners are seldom dedicated to bone density measurements. There is a higher radiation exposure than with DXA measurements, but the amount is much less than that received from spinal radiography. The development of 3-dimensional QCT technology has improved the reproducibility to a similar level as DXA measurements.

There has been considerable interest in reducing the cost of assessing bone mineral measurements and in developing portable instruments. This has led to the development of peripheral DXA and QCT instruments, as well as quantitative ultrasound devices to measure speed of sound and broadband ultrasound attenuation in the calcaneous and tibia. A comparison of a number of these techniques indicated considerable differences in distinguishing normal from osteoporotic individuals.[5] With time the role of the peripheral measurements in diagnosis and follow-up should be clarified.

The development of high-resolution bone scanners and the use of technetium-labeled bisphosphonates have brought about major improvements in the quality of bone scans. The bone scan provides a visual display of the metabolic activity in different regions of the skeleton. Scans are used primarily to detect occult bone metastases in patients with cancer. Approximately 4 h after receiving an intravenous injection of the radiolabeled bone-seeking agent, the patient is scanned in the supine position. An example of the scan of a patient initially thought to have metastatic cancer is shown in Fig. 23-1. Further evaluation revealed severe osteoporosis and that the increased tracer uptake reflected pelvic insufficiency fractures and rib fractures. The areas of increased uptake are believed to represent both increased osteoblastic activity and increased blood flow in the involved regions.

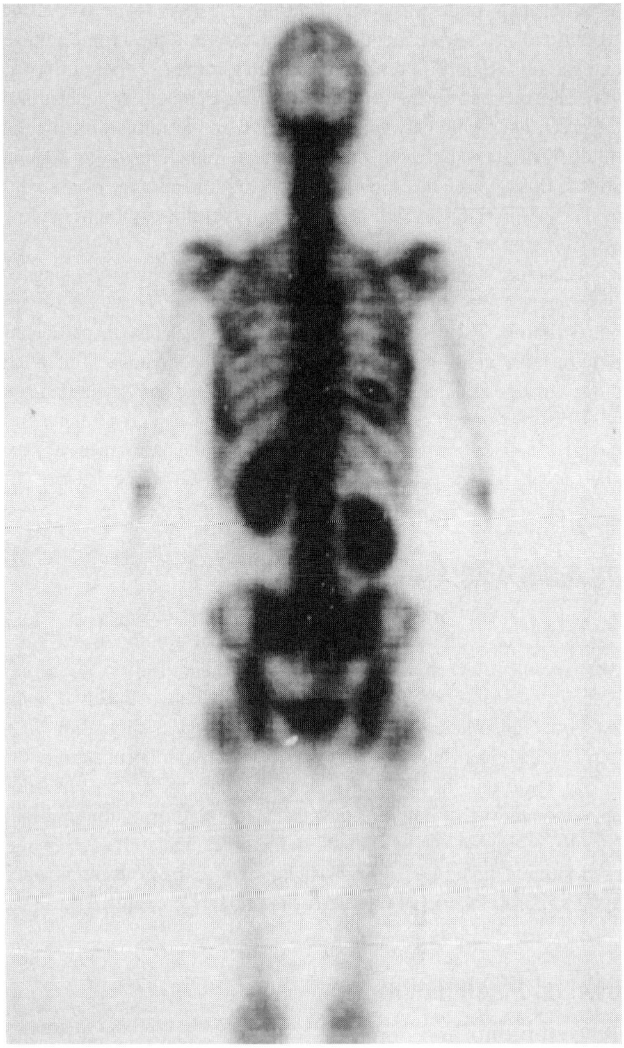

FIGURE 23-1. Technetium-labeled bisphosphonate bone scan of an osteoporotic patient with rib fractures and pelvic insufficiency fractures originally thought to represent metastatic cancer.

Bone Biopsy

A bone biopsy may provide valuable information that is not supplied by other techniques. This is particularly true in patients with milder forms of metabolic bone disease, in whom the radiologic and biochemical parameters are nearly normal or are not specific for a particular disease entity. Unfortunately, the application of bone biopsies and appropriate histologic techniques to clinical problems in the United States has been quite limited. The lack of a sufficient number of physicians trained in obtaining bone biopsies and the limited number of routine pathology laboratories that have experience in the proper processing of bone specimens account for the underutilization of this important technique.

In the past, bone biopsy material was obtained by resecting part of a rib and required the services of a surgeon. The design of a trocar by Bordier and colleagues[6] has made it possible to obtain an iliac crest biopsy specimen in an outpatient setting. After infiltration of the skin, soft tissues, and marrow cavity with lidocaine (Xylocaine) a biopsy can be obtained from the iliac crest adjacent to the anterior superior spine with minimal discomfort in most cases. A repeat biopsy after therapeutic intervention can be carried out on the opposite iliac crest.

In most pathology departments, the bone biopsy is fixed in formalin, decalcified, and embedded in paraffin prior to staining with hematoxylin and eosin (H&E). Examination of a bone specimen prepared in this manner allows identification of the number and types of bone cells present and of the overall structure of the bone. Unfortunately, the H&E stain of decalcified bone sections does not allow consistent identification of the unmineralized osteoid, which may be present in increased amounts in a variety of disorders. This requires the preparation of undecalcified bone sections. The bone specimen is fixed and then embedded in plastic before sectioning with a special microtome. Several stains can be used to delineate the amount of unmineralized osteoid in the sections.

Quantitative histomorphometry of bone biopsies is the most sophisticated approach to analyzing histologic sections.[7] With a variety of specialized microscopes as well as computerized instrumentation, precise quantitation of many parameters can be achieved, including assessment of the bone volume, the percentage of bone surface covered by osteoid, the average thickness of osteoid, the surface of bone undergoing resorption and formation, and the number of osteoclasts.

The discovery that the antibiotic tetracycline localizes at the sites of mineralization in bone led to the development of a dynamic test of bone metabolic activity.[8] A patient receives 500 mg of tetracycline on 2 consecutive days, nothing for 10 days, and 500 mg daily for 3 days; a bone biopsy is done the next day. The iliac crest bone specimen is processed, and the sections are evaluated by fluorescent microscopy. Two types of tetracycline which fluoresce differently can be used. In a normal subject, two bands of tetracycline fluorescence will be found on the surfaces of bone at which new bone was formed during the period of tetracycline labeling. The inner tetracycline band represents the initial course, and the outer band represents the second course of the antibiotic. The rate of bone formation can then be calculated by measuring the average width between the bands and dividing this by the number of days between tetracycline administration. In normal adults, this approaches 1 μg per day.[9] In patients with osteomalacia, in whom the principal defect is in mineralization, tetracycline uptake by bone is impaired.

A biopsy is indicated when there is a need to establish a diagnosis in patients in whom noninvasive parameters of bone disease are not definitive. Patients with subclinical osteomalacia, in particular, require bone biopsies for confirmation of the diagnosis. The bone biopsy may also be used to monitor the results of therapy in patients with disorders such as osteoporosis and renal osteodystrophy. Sequential biopsies are particularly important in the assessment of new pharmacologic agents used in treating patients with bone disease.

OSTEOMALACIA AND RICKETS

Osteomalacia is characterized by an excess of unmineralized bone which results from an impairment of bone mineralization. It is a disorder of diverse etiology which can be subdivided into two main categories: disorders associated with a reduction in circulating vitamin D metabolites and those associated with hypophosphatemia.

In children, the term *rickets* is used to indicate a disorder characterized by epiphyseal dysplasia, retardation of longitudinal growth, and a variety of skeletal deformities. Osteomalacia is the predominant histologic lesion. Rickets arises from etiologic factors similar to those that produce osteomalacia in adults.

Clinical Presentation

Symptoms and Signs

The manifestations of rickets depend not only on the severity and duration of the underlying disorder but to a great extent on the patient's age, because rickets affects the areas of bone that are growing most rapidly, and these vary at different ages.[10] Short stature reflects the epiphyseal dysplasia at the ends of the long bones of the lower extremities. The types of skeletal deformity associated with rickets include areas of thinning and softening of the cranium, protuberance of the frontal bone, thickening of the rib ends (rachitic rosary), lateral indentation of the chest wall (Harrison's groove), bowing of long bones, and knock-knee (Fig. 23-2).

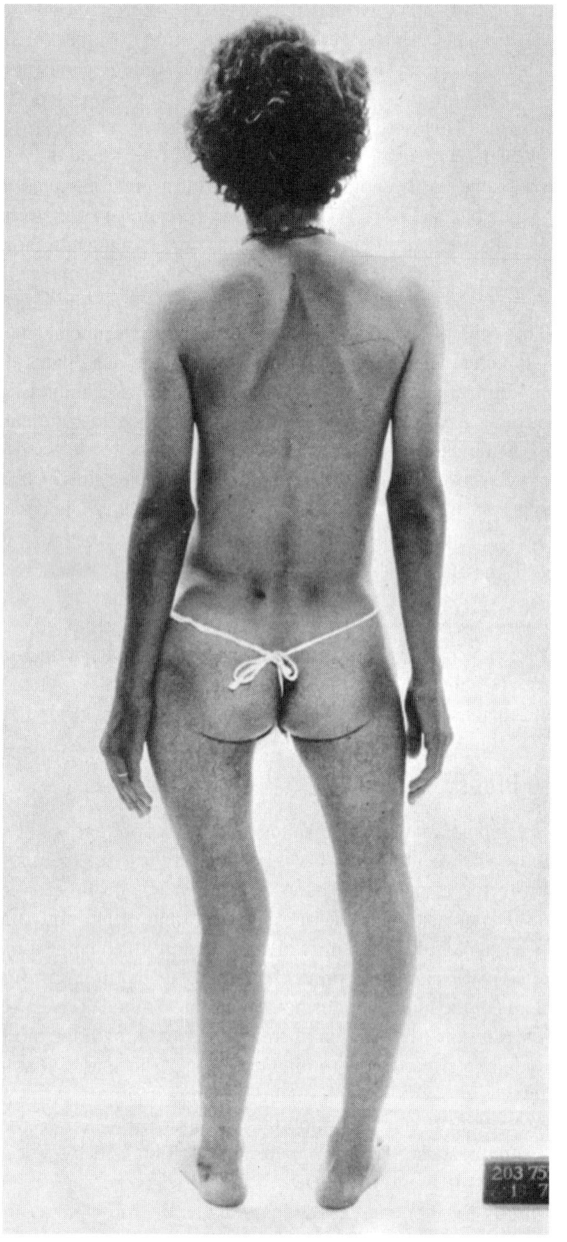

FIGURE 23-2. Bowing and knock-knee deformities in a 19-year-old male with familial X-linked hypophosphatemic rickets.

In adult-onset disease, skeletal deformities are seldom encountered except in the most severe cases. Abnormal spinal curvature, a bell-shaped thorax, or pelvic deformity may develop.

Bone pain is common in both children and adults. It is often experienced in the pelvis, lower extremities, spine, and ribs. The pain is worsened by activity in weight-bearing regions. In severe cases, bone tenderness is present on palpation. This is best elicited by thumb pressure on the distal tibia.

Muscle weakness and tenderness, particularly of the proximal musculature of the lower extremities, may be the dominant features in some patients. This is much more likely to occur in vitamin D-deficient patients than in hypophosphatemic patients.

In vitamin D-deficient patients, hypocalcemia may be reflected by the presence of paresthesias, tetany, seizures, and impaired mentation.

Radiologic Features

Radiologic examination of the skeleton can provide information of a highly specific nature with regard to the diagnosis of rickets or osteomalacia.[11] The radiologic signs of advanced rickets include widening of the epiphyseal growth plates, a frayed appearance of the metaphyses, and cupping and widening of the metaphyses (Fig. 23-3). These abnormalities are most readily detected at the metaphyseal sites that are growing most rapidly. Up to the age of 1 year, both the upper and lower extremities are likely to exhibit these findings. After 1 year, the lower extremities are more likely to reveal the abnormalities of rickets. Within several weeks of the initiation of appropriate therapy, mineralization of the epiphyseal cartilage can be discerned as a radiodense line adjacent to the metaphyses. In subsequent years, Harris lines, which are

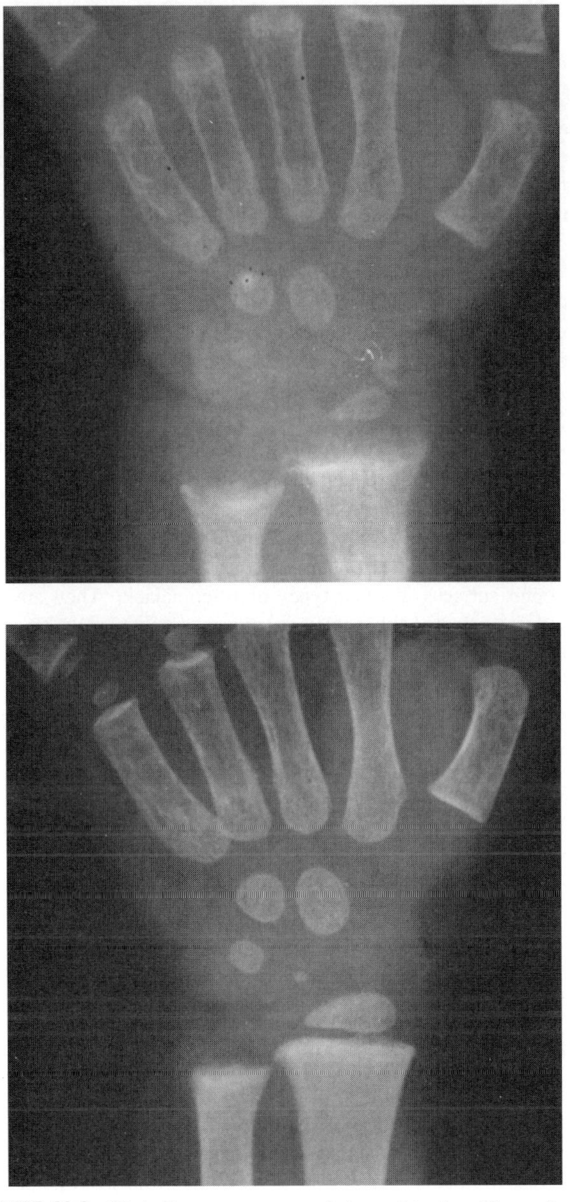

FIGURE 23-3. (*Top*) Roentgenograms of the wrist of a 13-month-old child with rickets due to vitamin D deficiency. Note the frayed appearance associated with widening and cupping of the metaphyses. A pseudofracture is present at the distal radius. (*Bottom*) Nearly total healing of the rickets after 5 months of treatment with vitamin D_2.

transverse radiodense lines across the shafts of long bones, may be noted in patients who have had a fluctuating degree of activity of the disease.

Gross deformity of the skeleton is more likely to occur in children than in adults. Kyphoscoliosis, a bell-shaped thorax, a triangular configuration of the pelvic lumen, and bowing of the upper and lower extremities are abnormalities that may be encountered in patients with severe long-standing disease.

In the adult, the radiologic findings in patients with osteomalacia often mimic those found in osteoporosis. A generalized loss of bone density with thinning of the cortex may be impossible to distinguish from that found in patients with osteoporosis. Expansion of intervertebral disk spaces and pathologic compression fractures of the vertebral bodies may be observed. Occasionally the trabecular pattern of bone is thickened, and mottled radiolucencies may be discerned. Osteosclerosis may rarely occur in isolated bones, most often affecting vertebral bodies. This unexpected finding remains unexplained. It is much more likely to be seen in the healing phase of the disease, when the mineralization defect is corrected.

In osteomalacic patients who have vitamin D deficiency, secondary hyperparathyroidism may be reflected by subperiosteal resorption of the phalanges, loss of the lamina dura, widening of the spaces at the symphysis pubis and sacroiliac joints, and the presence of brown tumors or bone cysts. These abnormalities rarely if ever occur in hypophosphatemic patients.

The pathognomonic radiologic feature of osteomalacia is the presence of pseudofractures, also known as Looser zones or Milkman fractures (Fig. 23-4). These narrow zones of rarefaction are often bilateral and symmetric. Common sites at which they may be found include the femoral neck and shaft, ulna and radius, pubic and ischial rami, clavicles, ribs, scapulae, and metacarpals, metatarsals, and phalanges. The origin of these lesions is not known with certainty. There is an underlying excess of unmineralized osteoid, which may reflect healing of a microfracture. In severe long-standing cases, the borders of a pseudofracture may appear sclerotic.

Laboratory Findings

Biochemical abnormalities in patients with rickets and osteomalacia can be classified into two categories. In patients whose disorder develops as a consequence of vitamin D lack, abnormal vitamin D metabolism, or vitamin D resistance, the concentrations

FIGURE 23-4. Pseudofractures of the medial border of the scapula and acromion in a 52-year-old man with malabsorption syndrome.

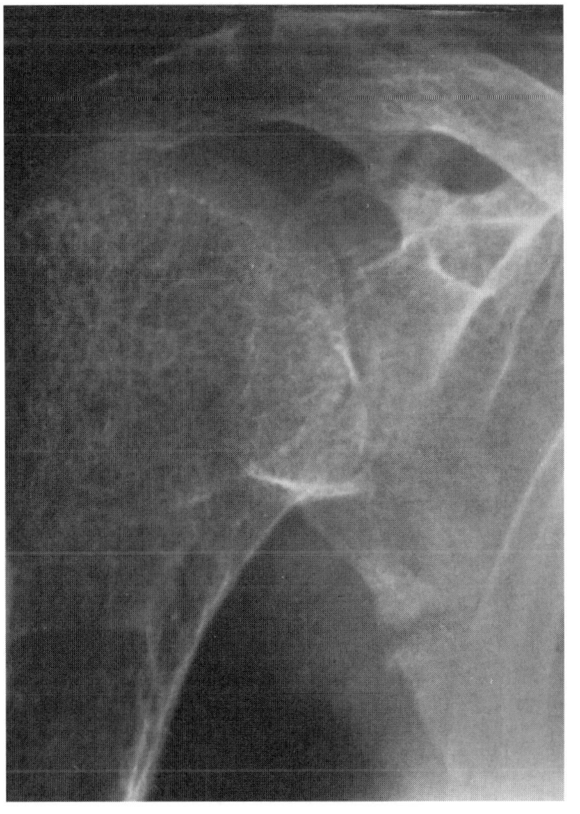

of serum calcium and phosphorus are usually reduced and the serum alkaline phosphatase activity is elevated.[12–14] Patients who develop bone disease on the basis of chronic hypophosphatemia also have elevated serum alkaline phosphatase activity but have a normal serum calcium concentration.[10] Serum total or bone specific alkaline phosphatase measurements appear to be more sensitive to the osteomalacic state than other indices of bone formation. The hypocalcemic state of vitamin D deficient patients is associated with elevated serum parathyroid hormone levels.[15] The state of secondary hyperparathyroidism is further manifested by a decreased renal phosphate threshold,[12] elevated urinary cAMP excretion,[16] and generalized aminoaciduria,[12] including hydroxyprolinuria. The hypophosphatemic group has seldom been reported to have elevated serum parathyroid hormone levels,[10] but a lowered renal phosphate threshold is usually present, and generalized aminoaciduria is not found.[10] Urinary calcium excretion is markedly reduced in hypocalcemic patients but may be less so in hypophosphatemic patients.[10] Urinary collagen crosslink excretion is elevated in osteomalacic patients.[17]

Assays of vitamin D metabolites have also been applied to the assessment of patients with rickets and osteomalacia.[18] The best measure of vitamin D status is the serum 25-hydroxyvitamin D concentration, as it is the major vitamin D metabolite in the circulation (Chap. 22). As expected, 25-hydroxyvitamin D and 24,25-dihydroxyvitamin D are found in low concentrations in the circulation of patients with classical vitamin D deficiency. Levels of serum 1α,25-dihydroxyvitamin D may be within the normal range in such patients,[19] but in the context of hypocalcemia these "normal" levels reflect inadequate synthesis of the renal vitamin D metabolite. Other quantitative abnormalities of circulating vitamin D metabolites have been described and are discussed under Classification and Pathogenesis.

Bone Pathology

To allow for a better understanding of the pathologic features of rickets, the histology of endochondral ossification at the epiphyseal growth plate is briefly described here.

Longitudinal bone growth occurs at the epiphyseal growth plate, a cartilaginous band separating the epiphysis from the metaphyseal region of the shaft.[11] In the proliferative zone of the growth plate, hypertrophic cartilage cells form orderly columns extending toward the shaft. These cell columns are then penetrated by blood vessels extending from the marrow and subsequently are destroyed by chondroclasts. Simultaneously, calcification of the cartilage matrix occurs, and osteoblasts arise around the blood vessels. They synthesize the bone matrix adjacent to the calcified cartilage, and this is rapidly mineralized.

In rickets, replication of cartilage cells in the proliferative zone proceeds in a normal fashion. However, the proliferating cells fail to form orderly columns advancing toward the shaft.[11] The marrow vessels also fail to penetrate the cartilage, and the cartilage cells are only partially removed. Thus, the zone of proliferating cartilage widens. Inadequate mineralization of cartilage and osteoid is noted, along with penetration of this zone by vessels from the perichondrium and adjacent resting cartilage. The weakened structure at the cartilage shaft junction and the proliferation of cartilage account for the deformities, which become apparent on radiologic and clinical examination.

Biopsy of the growth plate of a long bone is not recommended because future bone growth may be impaired. Biopsy of the iliac apophysis can be carried out with less likelihood of skeletal distortion.

The hallmark of osteomalacia is the accumulation of unmineralized osteoid.[20] This occurs as a result of impairment of matrix mineralization and despite a reduction in the rate of bone matrix formation. The increase in osteoid volume is reflected by a greater extent of osteoid seams covering both cortical and trabecular bone surfaces and by an increased width of the osteoid seams. Because excess osteoid may also be a feature of disorders such as thyrotoxicosis, primary hyperparathyroidism, and Paget disease, it may be necessary to label the bone with tetracycline to establish definitively whether an osteomalacic state is present. In osteomalacic patients, the percentage of osteoid seams labeled with tetracycline is reduced; tetracycline uptake, when present, may be diffuse rather than concentrated at the calcification front; bone matrix formation is reduced; and there is an increased mineralization lag time.[20] In states of high bone turnover, tetracycline labels most osteoid seams, and bone matrix formation and mineralization rates are increased. The width of the osteoid seams is usually normal.

Numerous active osteoblasts are usually found lining trabecular bone surfaces in most types of osteomalacia. They are not found in patients with adult hypophosphatasia, in patients with bone disease associated with total parenteral nutrition, and in a small minority of patients with renal osteodystrophy.

Patients with vitamin D deficiency exhibit features of secondary hyperparathyroidism, including increased numbers of osteoclasts and a fibrovascular marrow. Evidence of secondary hyperparathyroidism is generally not found in patients with osteomalacia associated with hypophosphatemic states. The latter patients exhibit increased osteoid volume and a mineralization defect indistinguishable from that found in simple vitamin D deficiency. A partially reversible decrease in mineral surrounding osteocyte lacunae has been reported in hypophosphatemic patients. This may reflect abnormal osteocyte function.[21]

Classification and Pathogenesis

Osteomalacia or rickets may develop as an isolated pathologic state or as a complication of another disorder. Table 23-2 shows a classification of osteomalacia and rickets. In the majority of patients, the pathogenesis can be ascribed to an abnormality of vitamin D supply, metabolic activation or action, or chronic hypophosphatemia. Patients who have an abnormality of vitamin D metabolism are unable to absorb sufficient calcium and phosphorus from their diets to allow normal mineralization of osteoid. A direct effect of vitamin D metabolites on bone mineralization is possible but not definitively proven.[20] Patients who develop osteomalacia or rickets as a result of hypophosphatemia probably do so in part because phosphorus is an essential constituent of hydroxyapatite.

Vitamin D Abnormalities

Vitamin D Deficiency

Classic vitamin D deficiency can develop only in a subject whose skin exposure to ultraviolet light is inadequate *and* whose diet contains insufficient vitamin D.[22] Vitamin D–deficiency rickets has been considered an extremely uncommon disorder since vitamin D supplementation of dairy products and other foods in the United States became a national policy. However, it has been noted that there is an increased susceptibility to rickets in infants

TABLE 23-2. Classification of Causes of Osteomalacia and Rickets

1. Reduction of circulating vitamin D metabolites
   - A. Inadequate ultraviolet light exposure and inadequate dietary vitamin D
   - B. Vitamin D malabsorption
     1. Small intestine disease or surgical bypass
     2. Pancreatic insufficiency
     3. Insufficient bile salts
   - C. Abnormal vitamin D metabolism
     1. Liver disease
     2. Chronic renal failure
     3. Drugs (anticonvulsants, glutethimide)
     4. Mesenchymal tumors, prostatic cancer
     5. Vitamin D-dependent rickets type I or pseudovitamin D deficiency 25-hydroxyvitamin D-1α-hydroxylase
   - D. Renal loss
     1. Nephrotic syndrome
2. Peripheral resistance to vitamin D
   - A. Vitamin D-dependent rickets, type II
   - B. Chronic renal failure
3. Hypophosphatemia
   - A. Renal phosphate wasting
     1. Hypophosphatemic rickets
        - a. Familial X-linked
        - b. Autosomal recessive
        - c. Autosomal dominant
        - d. Sporadic
     2. Hypophosphatemic osteomalacia
        - a. Autosomal dominant
        - b. Sporadic
     3. Familial renal phosphate leak with hypercalciuria, nephrolithiasis, and osteomalacia and rickets
     4. Fanconi's syndrome
     5. Mesenchymal tumors, fibrous dysplasia, epidermal nevus syndrome, prostatic cancer
     6. Primary hyperparathyroidism
   - B. Malnutrition
   - C. Malabsorption due to gastrointestinal disease or phosphate-binding antacids
   - D. Chronic dialysis
4. Miscellaneous
   - A. Inhibitors of calcification
     1. Sodium fluoride
     2. Etidronate disodium
   - B. Calcium deficiency
   - C. Hypoparathyroidism
   - D. Hypophosphatasia
   - E. Fibrogenesis imperfecta ossium
   - F. Systemic acidosis
   - G. Total parenteral nutrition

of mothers who follow certain dietary practices. Children who are breast-fed but not given vitamin D supplements and those on vegetarian diets without vitamin D supplementation are susceptible to rickets.[23,24] These "outbreaks" of rickets have occurred in northern cities where air pollution may reduce ultraviolet exposure. Dressing in long garments and the use of hoods and veils were contributing factors in one group.[23]

There are three stages in the pathogenesis of human rickets.[10] In stage I, hypocalcemia is the only significant biochemical abnormality. In stage II, the calcium concentration returns to the normal range and hypophosphatemia is apparent, presumably because of secondary hyperparathyroidism. Stage III is associated with severe clinical manifestations of rickets and the return of hypocalcemia.

Vitamin D Malabsorption

Malabsorption of vitamin D may occur in patients with small intestine disease, pancreatic insufficiency, and/or inadequate bile salts.[25] Because osteomalacia may develop in malabsorption states despite adequate ultraviolet light exposure, it is possible that malabsorption of 25-hydroxyvitamin D also occurs after the latter is excreted into the small intestine as a constituent of bile.[26] Biliary excretion of vitamin D metabolites may also be increased by calcium malabsorption and secondary hyperparathyroidism.[20] The pathogenesis of bone disease in malabsorption syndromes may be more complex than simply malabsorption of dietary vitamin D and its liver metabolite because other important nutrients, such as trace elements, may be poorly absorbed. The heterogeneity of bone disease was striking in a study of 21 patients after intestinal bypass surgery for obesity.[27] Only six patients had clear evidence of osteomalacia by rigorous histomorphometric criteria. The majority had evidence of bone loss without osteomalacia.

Abnormal Vitamin D Metabolism

Osteomalacia appears to be a very uncommon complication of severe parenchymal liver disease.[28] In some patients, poor nutrition and lack of exposure to ultraviolet light may produce low levels of circulating vitamin D metabolites and osteomalacia. In others, reduced serum vitamin D-binding protein levels account for low serum total 25-hydroxyvitamin D levels.[29] The latter patients have normal free 25-hydroxyvitamin D levels.

In patients with chronic renal failure, there is a reduction in both 1α,25-dihydroxyvitamin D and 24,25-dihydroxyvitamin D in the circulation.[18,30] The pathogenesis of renal osteodystrophy will be discussed later.

Patients on long-term anticonvulsant drugs have developed rickets and/or osteomalacia,[31] which has been interpreted to be a consequence of inactivation of 25-hydroxyvitamin D by cytochrome P-450 enzymes. However, the bulk of the evidence suggests that the majority of such patients reside in institutions where sunshine exposure and dietary vitamin D is inadequate.[20] In the outpatient setting rickets and/or osteomalacia in anticonvulsant-treated patients is quite unusual. In some patients a syndrome of low plasma 25-hydroxyvitamin D levels; intestinal malabsorption of calcium, mild hypocalcemia, secondary hyperparathyroidism, and low density of cortical bone may occur.[32] Although these patients have lost bone, they do not have the histological criteria of osteomalacia. Increased exposure to sunshine and/or an intake of 3,000 units of vitamin D weekly should help prevent this problem.

The association of osteomalacia with a variety of vascular and mesenchymal tumors has been observed in numerous patients.[33] An identical syndrome has also been observed in patients with prostatic cancer[34] and other carcinomas. The patients are usually adults and often present with bone pain and generalized muscle weakness. In most patients, a marked reduction in circulating 1α,25-dihydroxyvitamin D levels has been found. The patients were normocalcemic and often markedly hypophosphatemic because of renal phosphate wasting. Complete excision of the neoplasm generally produces resolution of the biochemical abnormalities and osteomalacia, whereas treatment with phosphate and 1α,25-dihydroxyvitamin D_3 has been less effective. No tumor factor has been identified that could account for the syndrome although tumor extracts do impair phosphate reabsorption and 1α hydroxylation.[20]

Vitamin D-dependent rickets type I is a rare autosomal recessive disorder that is due to mutations in the vitamin D hydroxylase gene, which encodes a mitochondrial P450c enzyme.[35] These patients have the same clinical course as vitamin D-deficient patients but do not respond to vitamin D therapy.[13] Administration of physiologic amounts of 1α,25-dihydroxyvitamin D_3 does produce healing of the bone lesions.[13]

Renal Loss

Subtle degrees of osteomalacia and secondary hyperparathyroidism may develop in patients with the nephrotic syndrome, presumably on the basis of renal losses of vitamin D-binding protein and 25-hydroxyvitamin D.[36,37] Radiological abnormalities are usually not observed but osteomalacia is common in bone biopsies and correlates with duration of nephrotic syndrome and degree of proteinuria.[38]

Peripheral Resistance to Vitamin D

Since 1978 it has been recognized that a subset of patients with early-onset rickets, termed *vitamin D-dependent rickets type II*, develop this disorder as a consequence of tissue insensitivity to 1α,25-dihydroxyvitamin D.[14] These patients characteristically have hypocalcemia, secondary hyperparathyroidism, elevation of circulating 1α,25-dihydroxyvitamin D_3, and a normal intake of vitamin D as well as adequate exposure to sunshine. In some patients, alopecia is a striking clinical feature.[39] A poor response to high doses of 1α,25-dihydroxyvitamin D_3 has also been reported.[40] The syndrome is characterized by autosomal recessive transmission and results from a variety of mutations of the vitamin D receptor.[41] The mutations produce abnormalities of DNA binding/nuclear localization, hormone binding, or heterodimerization with retinoid X receptors. Defective induction of 25-hydroxyvitamin D_3-24-hydroxylase by 1α,25-dihydroxyvitamin D_3 in cultured skin fibroblasts has been shown to predict the in vivo response to calciferol therapy.[40] Profound resistance to 1α,25-dihydroxyvitamin D appears to be present in alopecic patients.[40]

Patients with chronic renal failure require supraphysiologic doses of 1α,25-dihydroxyvitamin D_3 to increase intestinal calcium absorption.[42] This suggests that peripheral resistance to vitamin D is a factor in the impaired calcium absorption found in patients with chronic renal failure.

Hypophosphatemia

Chronic hypophosphatemia produces metabolic bone disease as a consequence of impaired mineralization of osteoid. A chronic hypophosphatemic state may arise from inadequate dietary phosphorus, reduced intestinal absorption of dietary phosphorus, or renal wasting of phosphorus. Renal wasting is the mechanism most commonly encountered clinically.

Renal Phosphate Wasting

The most common cause of rickets in the United States is the dominantly inherited genetic disorder termed *familial X-linked hypophosphatemic* or *vitamin D-resistant rickets*. This entity was first recognized by Albright in 1937.[43] The phenotypic trait of hypophosphatemia is transmitted on the X chromosome by a gene now termed PHEX (phosphate-regulating gene with homologies to endopeptideases on the x-chromosome).[44,45] Mutational analysis of the PHEX gene from numerous families indicates many mutations are present scattered throughout the putative extracellular domain of the encoded 749-amino acid protein.[45] It remains to be demonstrated how this genetic abnormality induces renal phosphate wasting. Bone disease and short stature are usually more severe in males who carry the abnormal genotype, whereas heterozygous females exhibit a more variable penetrance of these somatic traits.[46] Spinal stenosis and cord compression that are produced by new bone formation in the ligamentum flavum are late complications of the disorder.[47]

Hypophosphatemia develops as a consequence of a reduction in TmP/GFR. The exact nature of the abnormality in renal transepithelial phosphorus transport is not known and how this relates to the PHEX gene mutations has not been established. Renal phosphate wasting cannot be attributed to excessive secretion of parathyroid hormone, as hormone levels in blood are usually normal or only modestly elevated.[48] In one study, an increased phosphaturic response to exogenous parathyroid hormone was found, and led the investigators to speculate that an increased responsiveness to normal levels of the hormone might be a factor.[49] However, in a careful study of one patient with idiopathic hypoparathyroidism and familial X-linked hypophosphatemic rickets, a marked renal tubular phosphorus leak was present when the serum calcium was restored to normal by calcium and 1α,25-dihydroxy vitamin D_3 therapy.[50] A few patients have been reported to have reduced intestinal phosphorus absorption,[51] but this is not an invariable finding.

Studies of vitamin D metabolites in the circulation of patients with hypophosphatemic rickets have raised questions concerning the pathogenesis of the bone disease in these patients. It would be expected that chronic hypophosphatemia would raise the level of circulating 1α,25-dihydroxyvitamin D. Instead, normal or frankly reduced levels of this metabolite have been reported by several laboratories.[52–54] Low levels of the metabolite are usually found in patients treated with vitamin D.[52,54] Further evidence of an abnormality in renal hydroxylation of vitamin D was provided by a study that demonstrated a subnormal rise in serum 1α,25-dihydroxyvitamin D levels in untreated patients in response to an infusion of parathyroid hormone.[55] Impaired synthesis of 1α,25-dihydroxyvitamin D might explain the diminished rate of intestinal calcium absorption found in some patients,[43] but the normocalcemic state which is typical of the disorder suggests that significant 1α,25-dihydroxyvitamin D deficiency is not present. The low levels of 1α,25-dihydroxyvitamin D do not account for the hypophosphatemic state, as physiologic doses of the metabolite do not correct the abnormality.[56]

At least three inherited forms of hypophosphatemic rickets other than the X-linked type have been described. In two families evaluated with autosomal recessive inheritance patterns,[57,58] an unusual clinical aspect was gross osteosclerosis. A Bedouin tribe with a probable autosomal recessive inheritance pattern in which striking hypercalciuria appeared to develop as a consequence of marked elevation of 1α,25-dihydroxyvitamin D levels has been described.[59] Members of the tribe with milder degrees of hypophosphatemia and slight elevations of 1α,25-dihydroxyvitamin D exhibited hypercalciuria only. Hypophosphatemic rickets has been observed to be transmitted as an autosomal dominant trait in which, surprisingly, some of the affected may lose the renal phosphate-wasting defect after puberty.[60] A gene linkage study has placed the locus on chromosome 12p13.[61]

Sporadic hypophosphatemic rickets may occur in the absence of hypophosphatemia and/or bone disease in any other family member. This form of rickets is clinically indistinguishable from familial X-linked hypophosphatemic rickets and presumably arises from the same mutation responsible for that disorder.

Hypophosphatemic osteomalacia in adults may occur as a sporadic condition,[62] but a familial X-linked syndrome has been described in a single large kindred.[63,64] The biochemical findings in this syndrome are similar to those of familial X-linked hypophosphatemic rickets, but great phenotypic variability in the kindred suggested a different genetic abnormality than in X-linked hypophosphatemic rickets.[63] However, the family has been demonstrated to have a PHEX gene mutation, signifying that adult-onset vitamin D-resistant hypophosphatemic osteomalacia is not distinct from X-linked hypophosphatemic rickets.[64]

Autosomal dominant hypophosphatemic osteomalacia is a syndrome in which patients present with renal phosphate wasting as adolescents or adults but no lower extremity deformities.[60] Bone pain, fractures, and weakness may be present. Some members of the kindreds do present with rickets and deformities. Genetic analysis of one large kindred has indicated the genetic abnormality is on chromosome 12p13, as previously indicated.[61]

Osteomalacia and rickets may develop as a complication of a variety of generalized renal tubular disorders.[10,20] These disorders have been classified under the general term *Fanconi's syndrome*. Not only renal phosphate wasting but also excessive renal loss of bicarbonate, glucose, uric acid, and amino acids may be detected in affected patients. The bone disease may then be a manifestation of chronic hypophosphatemia and/or systemic acidosis. Acquired renal tubular disorders of phosphate transport differ in one major respect from X-linked hypophosphatemia. Muscle pain and weakness often are prominent features of the acquired disorders, but are seldom a problem in X-linked hypophosphatemia. Distal renal tubular acidosis also may cause bone disease in the absence of hypophosphatemia. Rarely, hypophosphatemic rickets may be associated with reversible renal tubular acidosis.[65]

Patients with a variety of benign or malignant mesenchymal tumors,[33] fibrous dysplasia,[66,67] epidermal nevus syndrome,[68] and prostatic cancer[34] may develop rickets and/or osteomalacia in association with hypophosphatemia. In most of these patients there is renal phosphate wasting, normal or slightly low serum calcium concentrations, normal serum parathyroid hormone concentrations, and reversal of the syndrome after removal of the pathologic lesions. Tumor cells have been demonstrated to produce an unidentified factor which inhibits renal tubular phosphate transport in vitro.[69] It has been suggested that the term phosphatonin be applied to describe what is probably a sodium-dependent phosphate cotransporter found in a variety of tissues.[70] As discussed previously, the significance of low levels of 1α,25-dihydroxyvitamin D in these patients is uncertain, although therapy with 1α,25-dihydroxyvitamin D_3 is often ineffective.[33]

Primary hyperparathyroidism is associated with hypophosphatemia in approximately 70 percent of cases. It is conceivable that osteomalacia could develop in certain patients with severe hypophosphatemia. In one study, quantitative histomorphometry of bone biopsies revealed a reduction of the calcification rate in some patients, but there was no increase in the width of osteoid seams.[71] At present, it does not appear that uncomplicated primary hyperparathyroidism produces significant osteomalacia. However, a patient with primary hyperparathyroidism may more readily develop osteomalacia in the presence of risk factors such as inadequate exposure to sunshine and anticonvulsant therapy. Also, during the postoperative period after parathyroid surgery, osteomalacia may develop as a consequence of the increased need for phosphorus and calcium in the process of healing of osteitis fibrosa.

Malnutrition and Malabsorption

An isolated deficiency of phosphorus due to malnutrition or malabsorption is distinctly uncommon.[20] It is more likely that a combination of vitamin D deficiency and inadequate supplies of calcium and phosphorus would be responsible for osteomalacia or rickets. Persistent use of phosphate-binding antacids is rarely associated with clinical osteomalacia.[72]

Chronic Dialysis

Hypophosphatemia may occur during the course of chronic dialysis in patients with chronic renal failure.[73] Presumably, this occurs as a consequence of excessive loss of phosphorus from the extracellular fluid into the dialysate. The use of phosphate-binding antacids to control hyperphosphatemia may also contribute. Osteomalacia may be severe in a hypophosphatemic patient on dialysis, but is promptly reversible with appropriate therapy. The involvement of aluminum in the production of osteomalacia in certain patients with renal failure is described in a later section.

Miscellaneous

Inhibitors of Calcification

Fluoride is a potent inhibitor of bone mineralization and may cause severe rickets and osteomalacia in areas of endemic fluorosis[74] and osteomalacia in patients treated with pharmacologic doses of sodium fluoride.[75] The latter patients usually receive sodium fluoride, 50 mg or more daily, for the treatment of osteoporosis. Osteomalacia is much less likely to develop if an intermittent slow release form of sodium fluoride is administered.

Etidronate disodium, a bisphosphonate used to treat Paget's disease and osteoporosis and to prevent heterotopic ossification, is an inhibitor of mineralization at doses of 10–20 mg per kilogram per body weight.[76] Fortunately, at a dose of 5 mg/kg, Paget's disease can be suppressed without diffuse impairment of mineralization. However, focal osteomalacia has been found in bone biopsies of patients treated with low doses of etidronate disodium.[77] Mineralization defects of uncertain clinical significance have also been reported in patients treated with intravenous pamidronate.[78]

Calcium Deficiency

Radiologic evidence of rickets has been observed in a child with severe dietary calcium restriction in the presence of normal vitamin D intake and normal circulating 25-hydroxyvitamin D levels.[79] Hypocalcemia, hypophosphatemia, secondary hyperparathyroidism, and elevated alkaline phosphatase were biochemical features in this patient. A group of South African children with poor calcium intake were also found to have a similar rickets-like syndrome, which was corrected by increasing dietary calcium intake.[80] However, these children inexplicably had normal serum calcium and phosphorus levels. Histologic evidence of osteomalacia in three South African children on calcium-deficient diets has been reported.[81] Each of these patients was hypocalcemic. Three Belgian infants who were given soy milk developed severe rickets but had a rapid reversal of bone disease when placed on regular diets.[82] It is not known whether isolated calcium deficiency can produce osteomalacia in adults.

Hypoparathyroidism

Rickets and/or osteomalacia have been reported in a few patients with hypoparathyroidism.[83,84] The pathogenesis is unclear, but successful treatment of the hypocalcemia produced healing of the bone disease. Rickets has also been thought to be present in an infant with hypoparathyroidism whose mother had hyperparathyroidism[85] and in two infants whose mothers had received long-term intravenous $MgSO_4$ therapy.[86] At least one patient with pseudohypoparathyroidism has been reported with convincing features of rickets and osteomalacia.[87]

Hypophosphatasia

Hypophosphatasia is a rare cause of rickets and osteomalacia that is usually inherited as an autosomal recessive trait.[88] A milder adult form of the disorder may be inherited as an autosomal dominant trait. The recessive form is due to various mutations in the bone/liver/kidney isoenzyme of alkaline phosphatase. In infancy the disease may be lethal, whereas in adults early loss of permanent teeth, calcium pyrophosphate arthropathy, and fractures may occur. The biochemical abnormalities characteristic of this disorder are (1) low serum alkaline phosphatase activity, (2) elevated serum and urine inorganic pyrophosphate and phosphoryl-ethanolamine levels, and (3) elevated serum pyridoxal-5′-phosphate levels. The high levels of these substances probably reflect decreased alkaline phosphatase activity in bone and perhaps other organs. Inorganic pyrophosphate may be an important intermediary in the initiation of bone mineralization by extracellular matrix vesicles and failure of alkaline phosphatase to hydrolyze this substrate may account for the impaired mineralization in the patients. The pathogenesis of hypercalcemia sometimes seen in children with hypophosphatasia is unknown.

A study of bone histology in a kindred of patients with adult hypophosphatasia demonstrated a paucity of osteoblasts despite the excess of osteoid.[89] The authors proposed that osteoblast dysfunction might be manifested first by mineralization defects and later by a reduction in the numbers of osteoblasts.

Fibrogenesis Imperfecta Ossium

Fibrogenesis imperfecta ossium is a rare disorder that affects previously healthy males over age 50.[90] Skeletal pain and tenderness may be so severe as to cause total incapacitation. Pseudofractures may be seen on roentgenograms, but, unexpectedly, there is a generalized increase in bone density with a lack of trabeculation and a mottled appearance. Bone histology reveals an increased amount of osteoid, impaired uptake of tetracycline, and absence of a normal lamellar pattern of the collagen fibers. The latter finding suggests an underlying defect in collagen synthesis. Consistent with this hypothesis are the findings of normal plasma calcium and phosphorus concentrations. Plasma alkaline phosphatase activity is increased. Monoclonal IgG paraproteins may be found in plasma and in some patients melphalan and corticosteroids may produce clinical and histological improvement.[91]

Systemic Acidosis

Systemic acidosis due to isolated renal tubular acidosis, Fanconi's syndrome, ureterosigmoidoscopy, or chronic renal failure may be an important factor in the pathogenesis of osteomalacia associated with these disorders.[20] Normal levels of vitamin D metabolites have been found in the circulation of patients with renal tubular acidosis[92] and in volunteers with induced metabolic acidosis.[93] The mineralization defect associated with chronic acidosis probably arises as a direct consequence of acidemia.[94]

Total Parenteral Nutrition

Long-term use of total parenteral nutrition has been associated with bone pain, patchy osteomalacia, low serum levels of parathyroid hormone and 1α,25-dihydroxyvitamin D, hypercalciuria, and intermittent hypercalcemia.[95,96] In patients receiving casein hydrolysate, inadvertent infusion of aluminum has been implicated as the factor responsible for the syndrome. Such patients have been demonstrated to have aluminum localized to the surface of mineralized bone from which tetracycline uptake was absent.[97] However, the syndrome has also been found in patients infused with free amino acids, which are relatively devoid of aluminum.[95]

Treatment

The treatment of osteomalacia and rickets is as heterogeneous as are the underlying causes. Knowledge of the pathogenesis of the disease is critical in assuring an optimum result of therapy, particularly in infants.

Classic vitamin D deficiency can be prevented by the ingestion of 400 IU (10 μg) of vitamin D_2 daily by children and 100 IU daily by adults. These amounts of vitamin D_2 may be used to treat patients with established bone disease, but doses as much as two- to tenfold greater have been used to produce a more rapid clinical recovery.[20] Patients also must receive adequate calcium and phosphorus from their diets or, if necessary, from supplementation. In most patients, the recommended normal daily intake is adequate.

The earliest biochemical response to vitamin D therapy is a rise in serum 1α,25-dihydroxyvitamin D levels.[20] Serum phosphorus concentrations usually increase to normal within 4–8 days. Initially, serum calcium may actually decline and alkaline phosphatase may rise, but both move toward normal levels within weeks. Vitamin D intoxication can be avoided or minimized by measuring the plasma calcium concentration every 2–4 weeks. The dose should be reduced, if pharmacologic, when the biochemical parameters approach the normal range and when radiologic healing of rickets is apparent.

Patients with vitamin D malabsorption require only short-term vitamin D therapy if the underlying disorder can be treated effectively. This is particularly true in patients with celiac disease, in whom a gluten-free diet will produce a complete remission of the malabsorptive state and concomitant vitamin D deficiency. If the disorder is irreversible, pharmacologic doses of vitamin D are required. The dose of vitamin D varies widely, but up to 100,000 IU per day by the oral route may be necessary. In some patients, parenteral administration of smaller doses is required. Greater than usual amounts of calcium and phosphorus also may be needed to overcome the inefficiency of intestinal absorption.

In patients with impaired vitamin D metabolism, vitamin D_2 therapy in pharmacologic amounts is usually effective in preventing or reversing rickets and osteomalacia. Up to 15,000 IU daily has been used to induce healing of established bone disease. Lower doses of 25-hydroxyvitamin D_3 have been effective in these patients.[98] In patients with low circulating levels of 1α,25-dihydroxyvitamin D, near-physiologic doses of this metabolite can produce healing of bone lesions. This has been demonstrated in patients with vitamin D–dependent rickets type I[13] and in some patients with chronic renal failure. In children with vitamin D-dependent rickets type II, pharmacologic doses of vitamin D_2 or its metabolites may be effective. In resistant patients, intravenous or oral calcium (one patient) has been demonstrated to heal rickets.[99,100] The role of 1α,25-dihydroxyvitamin D_3 in the treatment of renal osteodystrophy is discussed further under Renal Osteodystrophy.

The main principle in the treatment of hypophosphatemic bone disease is restoration of the serum phosphorus concentration to the normal range. This may prove difficult if administration of vitamin D_2 or a vitamin D analog is the sole therapy given to patients with renal phosphate wasting. Pharmacologic doses of vitamin D_2 or dihydrotachysterol were the earliest forms of treatment for patients with familial X-linked hypophosphatemic rickets. These drugs often were administered at toxic levels and caused hypercalciuria and hypercalcemia. Despite this high dosage, the rickets was not uniformly healed and there was seldom a significant reversal of short stature.

In 1972, Glorieux and colleagues reported a major improvement in the clinical course of children with X-linked hypophosphatemic rickets who received oral phosphate supplementation.[101] The phosphate was administered every 4 h throughout a 24-h period to maintain the serum phosphorus concentration within the normal range. The children experienced a marked increase in linear growth velocity. Because phosphate therapy alone usually induces hypocalcemia and secondary hyperparathyroidism because of an increased rate of bone mineralization, it has become customary to simultaneously administer vitamin D_2[101,102] or, more recently, 1α,25-dihydroxyvitamin D_3.[103–105] The latter agent is preferable because it has a more rapid onset of action, has a shorter half-life, and has been observed to correct the mineralization defect in trabecular bone more fully than does vitamin D_2.[104,105] Careful observation of the patients is mandatory to avoid hypercalcemia, particularly as bone mineralization nears normalization,[104] and to prevent chronic hypocalcemia, which may result in parathyroid hyperplasia and hypercalcemia after many years of therapy.[106] The occurrence of hypercalcemia associated with increased serum parathyroid hormone levels may require parathyroidectomy to prevent bone and renal complications. A promising means of avoiding this outcome may be through the addition of 24,25-dihydroxyvitamin D_3 to the standard regimen.[107] In one study this reduced parathyroid hormone levels by 50 percent and appeared to improve radiologic and histologic findings. At this time this vitamin D metabolite remains experimental. Urinary calcium excretion should be monitored as a high percentage of patients treated with vitamin D or its renal metabolite have evidence of medullary nephrocalcinosis determined by renal ultrasonography.[108]

If optimum treatment is begun early in the course of hypophosphatemic bone disease in children, dwarfism and rachitic deformities should be reversible or prevented. However, there is some controversy as to whether the achieved adult height is actually increased in treated individuals. After a retrospective analysis of patients at the Mayo Clinic, it was concluded that there was no evidence that any form of treatment had any effect on adult height, symptoms, or alkaline phosphatase levels.[109] Unfortunately, documentation of the serum phosphorus concentrations maintained in these patients was not available. In three studies in which metabolic control was emphasized, combined phosphate and 1α,25-dihydroxyvitamin D_3 or 1α-hydroxyvitamin D_3 did appear to enhance the mature height level.[110–112] The doses of these agents that are needed to achieve maximal benefit are empiric. Phosphate is used in divided doses approximately every 4 h, providing from 1 g of elemental phosphorus daily in infants to 3 to 5 g daily in children or adults, depending on the achievement of normal serum phosphorus concentrations. Diarrhea may limit the dose in some patients. From 0.25 to 1 μg of 1α,25-dihydroxyvitamin D_3 daily is needed to prevent hypocalcemia and stimulate healing of rickets and osteomalacia. Because the phosphorus-vitamin D metabolite regimen does not always produce optimum results, particularly in males, some investigators have added recombinant growth hormone to the regimen. In one three-year study growth hormone appeared to have increased growth velocity, phosphate retention, and bone density without side effects.[113]

It is uncertain whether treatment should be continued in adults if metabolic parameters are normal and bone pain is absent. Bone biopsies in untreated adults have revealed persistent osteomalacia in a similar degree in asymptomatic and symptomatic individuals,[114] although mineralized bone volume was normal in all specimens. Controlled trials of combined therapy are needed in both children and adults to settle the uncertainties regarding medical management.

Surgical intervention to correct skeletal deformities may be needed in patients who have not received appropriate medical therapy. Procedures such as osteotomy and epiphyseal stapling may increase the mobility of the patient and prevent the long-term complication of degenerative joint disease. Preoperative and postoperative metabolic control have been found to be important in avoiding the recurrence of lower extremity deformity.[115]

Patients with autosomal recessive hypophosphatemic rickets, sporadic hypophosphatemic rickets or osteomalacia, and Fanconi's syndrome with hypophosphatemia all respond well to phosphate-vitamin D regimens.[20]

In patients with hypophosphatemia due to mesenchymal tumors, treatment with 1α,25-dihydroxy vitamin D_3 and phosphate is generally effective if the tumor is not resectable.[33]

No effective treatment program for hypophosphatasia has been developed. The infusion of alkaline phosphatase-rich plasma in several patients failed to produce any clinical benefit despite increasing the circulating alkaline phosphatase activity into the normal range during a 2-month period.[116]

Correction of systemic acidosis with oral alkali therapy can fully heal the osteomalacic lesions. Vitamin D therapy is not necessary.[20]

OSTEOPOROSIS

Osteoporosis is the most common metabolic bone disease and is responsible for significant morbidity in elderly men and women and in patients who are treated chronically with glucocorticosteroids in pharmacologic doses.

The disorder is not a single entity but rather a pathologic state which can arise from a variety of disturbances of skeletal homeostasis. It is characterized in all instances by a decreased mass of bone which is normally mineralized.

Clinical Presentation

Symptoms and Signs

In the clinical evolution of osteoporosis, there is a long subclinical phase that occurs in most patients before recognition of the disorder. During this time no symptoms or signs may be detected, but radiologic and histologic abnormalities would be noted if sought. The term *osteopenia* is sometimes used to describe the existence of a reduced bone mass in the absence of symptoms or signs of osteoporosis.[117]

The initial complaint often experienced by these patients is back pain. This may occur suddenly without warning and may be of great intensity. It frequently results from lifting a heavy object. The pain is sharp or burning in quality, is aggravated by movement or weight bearing, and reflects an underlying compression fracture of a vertebral body. The twelfth thoracic and first lumbar vertebrae are most often affected. After healing of the bone, back pain may resolve completely. More commonly, residual pain reflects spasm of the paravertebral muscles.

Spinal deformity may develop after repeated acute episodes of compression fracture or may slowly evolve in the absence of severe back pain. A progressive loss in stature occurs as a result of reduction in the height of multiple vertebral bodies. Dorsal kyphosis is typical of long-standing spinal osteoporosis. In the most severely affected persons the spinal curvature may be so great as to cause the lower ribs to touch the iliac crests.

Osteoporosis does not produce deformities of the extremities unless fractures occur. The common sites of extremity fractures are the femoral neck and the distal radius.

Radiologic Features

The radiologic feature most characteristic of osteoporosis is a decreased density of bone. This is best visualized with routine films of the spine. Cortical thinning and loss of transverse trabeculation are common findings. If the latter feature dominates, a paradoxic accentuation of cortical density and vertical trabeculation may result. The weakened vertebral bodies allow ballooning of the nuclei pulposi into the classical biconcave "codfish" deformities of the intervertebral disk spaces (Fig. 23-5). A localized herniation of a nucleus pulposus into a vertebral body, a *Schmorl's node*, may occasionally occur. Anterior wedging of vertebral bodies is usually a sign of a marked decrease in bone density, but may arise at an earlier stage as a complication of trauma.

FIGURE 23-5. "Codfish" deformities of the lower thoracic and lumbar spine in a 13-year-old male with juvenile osteoporosis.

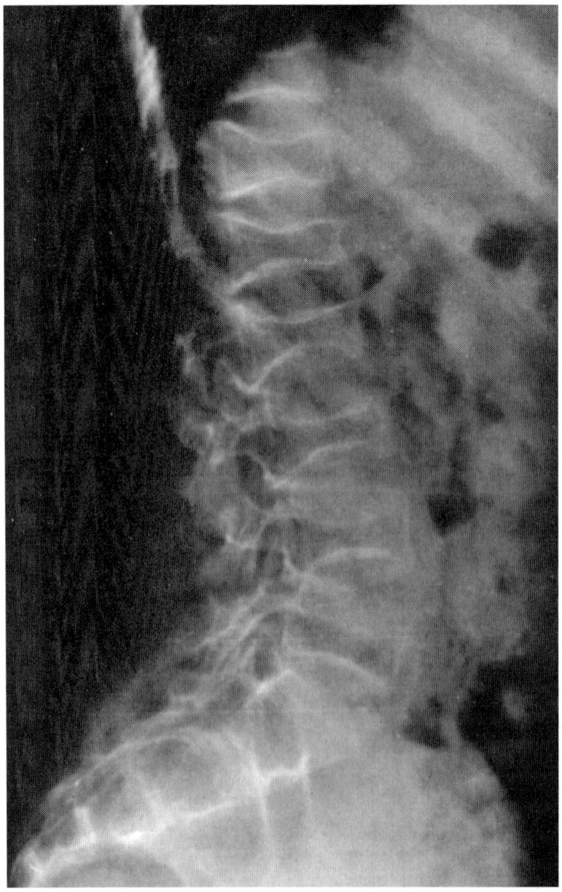

Radiologic manifestations of osteoporosis at sites other than the spine include a patchy loss of density of the calvarium, decreased cortical density of phalanges and long bones, and vertical striation of long bones. Bowing of the bones of the lower extremity is not typical of osteoporosis but does occur in patients with osteogenesis imperfecta.

Bone densitometry has become the standard means of defining the existence of osteoporosis, although bone density measurements are low in disorders of impaired mineralization also. Therefore serum chemistries and, if necessary, a bone biopsy are required to exclude the more unusual problem of osteomalacia.

The most widely accepted classification of densitometry measurements was proposed by the World Health Organization in 1993. A bone mass measurement more than 2.5 SD below peak bone mass (T-scores below -2.5) defines osteoporosis whereas measurement 1–2.5 SD below peak bone mass (T scores -1 to -2.5) define osteopenia. Treatment decisions should not be rigidly based on such a classification as it is believed that there is a continuous gradient of increasing fracture risk as bone mass decreases.[4]

The indications for ordering a bone density include (1) the evaluation of early postmenopausal women who refuse estrogen replacement, (2) the evaluation of patients suspected to have osteoporosis on x-rays, (3) the evaluation of patients whose medical history suggests osteoporosis may be present (hormone disorders, drug therapy, alcoholism), and (4) the monitoring of the effect of treatment or the clinical course. The latter indication is less clearly defined in individual patients than in large clinical trials. In the latter statistical evaluation of bone density effects of treatment has been very successful in defining drug effects in groups of patients. In an individual the changes in density, either spontaneous or related to therapy, may not be much greater than the precision of the measurements. In clinical practice it is not unusual to observe increases in bone density at one site and simultaneous decreases at another. In such circumstances, measurements of a biochemical marker of bone turnover may be useful.

Laboratory Findings

In the great majority of patients, there are no significant abnormalities of the calcium, phosphorus, or alkaline phosphatase concentrations in the circulation. A subset of patients who have thyrotoxicosis may have elevated concentrations of all three parameters,[118] and patients with primary hyperparathyroidism may be hypercalcemic, hypophosphatemic, and hyperphosphatasemic (Chap. 22). Although not in routine use at this time, biochemical markers of bone turnover can provide useful information concerning overall metabolic activity in the skeleton. For example, serum bone alkaline phosphatase activity and urinary N-telopeptide excretion, indices of bone formation and bone resorption, respectively, are more than twice as high in postmenopausal women than in premenopausal women.[119]

Occult vitamin D deficiency and associated secondary hyperparathyroidism appear to be significant factors in postmenopausal women in Northern regions. Fifty percent of women with acute hip fractures had serum 25-hydroxyvitamin D levels below 12 ng/ml and 37 percent had elevated serum intact PTH levels in one study.[120] Secondary hyperparathyroidism could also be a consequence of the reduced intestinal calcium absorption that occurs with aging.[121,122] This may occur because of reduced renal synthesis of 1α,25-dihydroxyvitamin D in the aging kidney. It is also possible that reduced numbers of vitamin D receptors or a change in receptor affinity could impair calcium absorption in the aging intestine because calcium absorption relative to serum 1α,25-dihydroxyvitamin D levels is lower in osteoporotic women than in normal women.[123]

In patients with evolving osteoporosis, urinary calcium excretion may be significantly elevated, a reflection of an increased rate of bone resorption.[124] This is most likely to be found in patients with hyperthyroidism or in a completely immobilized patient. It has also been proposed that in severe postmenopausal osteoporosis there is a defect in renal calcium conservation independent of parathyroid hormone.[125] This could account for a greater increase in urinary calcium excretion than that accounted for by bone resorption alone.

Calcitonin is measurable in low concentrations in the circulation of men and women. Women have a lower concentration than men[126] and hormone concentration fell with age in women in one study.[127] It is unknown whether calcitonin is a significant factor in determining the greater bone mass of men. It is also uncertain whether calcitonin levels are lower in postmenopausal women with osteoporosis[128–133] or whether it is stimulated by estrogen[134–139] because of conflicting data in publications examining these issues.

Bone Pathology

The histologic features of osteoporosis are quite heterogeneous, but in all instances bone volume is decreased, and in the absence of accompanying osteomalacia, bone is normally mineralized.

In postmenopausal osteoporosis bone turnover assessed by bone histomorphometry could be high, low, or normal.[140] In high-turnover specimens osteoclasts and osteoblasts are numerous and in low-turnover specimens they are sparse. In cancellous bone there may be thinning of individual trabeculae and/or trabecular perforation. A decrease in the mean wall thickness coupled with a decrease in the duration of formation periods of cancellous bone in women with postmenopausal osteoporosis has been stressed as indicative of impaired osteoblast function.[141] In general, histologic parameters measured in the iliac crest do not correlate closely with biochemical markers of bone turnover that reflect overall skeletal metabolism. This should not be surprising because the skeleton does not respond in a homogeneous manner to the influences of hormones[142] and perhaps other influences.

The heterogeneity of the bone pathology of osteoporosis is further reflected by studies of patients with adrenal glucocorticosteroid excess and hyperthyroidism. Cushing's syndrome, spontaneous or iatrogenic, is associated with a marked reduction in bone volume. Studies utilizing either quantitative microradiography or quantitative histomorphometry have demonstrated evidence of increased bone resorption and decreased bone formation in these patients.[142–146] In steroid-induced osteoporosis, a decrease in trabecular width associated with decreased bone formation has been suggested to be a characteristic feature.[146]

The histology of hyperthyroidism is characterized by a marked increase in bone remodeling.[118] Numerous osteoclasts and osteoblasts are present, as well as a fibrous bone marrow. The percentage of trabecular bone covered with osteoid is increased, but there is no widening of the osteoid seams, and the mineralization rate is normal. Decreased cortical and trabecular bone volume must ensue if the rate of bone resorption exceeds that of bone formation. Bone disease induced by hyperthyroidism may be difficult to distinguish from that produced by hyperparathyroidism. It has been reported that the two disorders can be distinguished by measuring the size of the periosteocytic lacunae.[118] There is no increase in this parameter in hyperthyroidism, unlike hyperparathyroidism.

Osteoporosis associated with prolonged immobilization has not been studied extensively. In one study, osteoclastic bone resorption was increased and osteoblastic activity was decreased.[147]

Few studies of bone histology in patients with idiopathic juvenile osteoporosis have been reported.[148–150] In a study utilizing quantitative microradiography, there was an increase in bone resorption surfaces and bone formation surfaces were normal.[148] Quantitative histomorphometry revealed normal osteoclast numbers and a reduced osteoblast surface.[149] In the most recent study of 9 patients, tetracycline labeling indicated a reduced bone formation rate per bone surface associated with decreased wall thickness but no evidence of increased bone resorption.[150]

The histologic findings in patients with osteogenesis imperfecta are unique.[151] There is persistence of primitive woven bone and an absence of well-organized haversian systems. Osteoclasts are not present in excessive numbers, and the osteoblasts that are present are spindle-shaped and flattened, suggesting they are inactive cells.

Classification and Pathogenesis

Osteoporosis and osteopenia are associated with genetic polymorphisms, aging, hormonal deficiencies and excesses, nutritional deficiencies, genetic disorders, hematologic malignancy, immobilization, and a variety of other unrelated disorders (Table 23-3). The pathogenesis of bone disease in many of these states is not completely understood, but modern biochemical and histologic techniques have increased our knowledge to a great extent in the past three decades.

Genetic Polymorphisms

Numerous studies indicate that genetic factors are an important determinant of peak bone mineral density.[152–154] Daughters of women with osteoporosis [153] and first-degree relatives of males with idiopathic osteoporosis[154] have lower bone densities than control populations.

A variety of candidate genes have been studied to determine which may have significant influence on bone mineral density. Studies of the vitamin D receptor gene, collagen type 1α1 gene, estrogen receptor gene, interleukin-6 gene, and transforming growth factor-beta 1 gene have shown that polymorphisms of these genes, at least in some studies, may predict bone density and even fractures.[155] Segregation analysis indicates that bone density is a polygenic trait.[156] Therefore many more studies of genetic influences on bone will be needed for a more complete understanding of the determinants of peak bone density. As yet little evidence has accumulated addressing genetic influences on bone loss.

Aging

The incidence of osteoporosis and fractures rises with advancing age in women and men. It has been suggested that two distinct syndromes of osteoporosis may occur in the aging population.[157] Type I osteoporosis is defined as affecting women

TABLE 23-3. Classification of Causes of Osteoporosis and Osteopenia

1. Genetic polymorphisms
2. Aging
3. Endocrine abnormality
   A. Estrogen deficiency
   B. Testosterone deficiency
   C. Cushing's syndrome
   D. Thyrotoxicosis
   E. Primary hyperparathyroidism
   F. Diabetes mellitus
4. Immobilization or weightlessness
5. Genetic
   A. Osteogenesis imperfecta
   B. Ehlers-Danlos syndrome
   C. Homocystinuria
   D. Marfan syndrome
   E. Menkes' syndrome
   F. Lysinuric protein intolerance
6. Juvenile osteoporosis
7. Chronic hypophosphatemia
8. Idiopathic hypercalciuria
9. Chronic alcholism
10. Immunosuppressive therapy post-organ–transplantation
11. Intestinal disease
    A. Celiac sprue
    B. Inflammatory
12. Cigarettes
13. Nutritional abnormality
    A. Calcium deficiency
    B. Vitamin C deficiency
    C. Protein deficiency
14. Anticonvulsant therapy
15. Heparin therapy
16. Methotrexate therapy
17. Rheumatoid arthritis
18. Chronic liver disease
19. Systemic mastocytosis
20. Hematologic malignancy
    A. Multiple myeloma
    B. Leukemia
    C. Lymphoma
21. Pregnancy-associated
22. Idiopathic

during the first 15–20 years after menopause. During this time there is a dominance of cancellous bone loss, which results in vertebral compression fractures and distal forearm fractures. In type II osteoporosis in both women and men there is a slower rate of loss of cancellous and cortical bone, which in women is present after about age 70 years and in men at an earlier age. In type II osteoporosis, fractures of the proximal femur and vertebrae are common. Estrogen deficiency plays a dominant role in type I osteoporosis, but as there is no major difference in estrogen levels between women with and without fractures, it is proposed that another factor linked to estrogen deficiency may account for greater bone loss in some individuals.[157] This could be linked to genetic polymorphisms. In type II osteoporosis, it is proposed that the slow phase of bone loss also is a consequence of estrogen deficiency but is manifested through an effect on extraskeletal calcium homeostasis. Secondary hyperparathyroidism may contribute to bone loss as a consequence of impaired intestinal calcium absorption and a defect in renal calcium conservation due to estrogen deficiency.[157] Although controversial, it is also possible that estrogen deficiency decreases bone formation over time. Recent evidence suggests that declining estrogen levels with aging as well as declining testosterone levels may help explain type II osteoporosis in men.

Clearly a variety of other factors also contribute to the end result of fractures in elderly women and men. As discussed, genetic determinants of peak bone mineral density must be a major factor. Cigarette smoking and alcohol use are established risk factors.[158–160] Decreased exercise as a consequence of arthritis in weight-bearing joints, poor nutrition, impaired intestinal calcium absorption, reduced renal function, and pharmacologic doses of thyroid hormone or glucocorticoids are additional factors that may contribute to abnormal skeletal homeostasis in the elderly. Obesity and black ancestry seem to confer some protection against osteoporosis.[159–161]

Estrogen Deficiency

The incidence of osteoporosis is highest in postmenopausal females. As has been discussed in the aging section, evidence has accumulated that implicates estrogen deficiency as a major factor in the pathogenesis of the disorder in these persons. There is evidence that elderly women with serum estradiol levels from 10 to 25 pg/ml have greater bone density and less vertebral deformity than those with levels less than 5 pg/ml.[162]

Estrogen probably acts directly and indirectly to inhibit bone resorption. Estrogen receptors have been identified on osteoblasts[163] and osteoclasts.[164] Estrogen deficiency also increases the sensitivity of bone to parathyroid hormone[165] and possibly to other factors which induce bone resorption. Cytokines such as interleukin-1, interleukin-6, tumor necrosis factor, and prostaglandin E_2 may be local mediators of the effects of estrogen on bone cells.[166,167] Further insights into the mechanisms of action of estrogen on bone will evolve from studies of the newly discovered members of the tumor necrosis factor receptor and ligand families.[168]

Indirect effects of estrogen on skeletal homeostasis may come from estrogen influencing renal calcium conservation[125] and intestinal calcium absorption.[122] It is not certain whether estrogen deficiency produces low levels of 1α,25-dihydroxyvitamin D in the circulation[122,137,169,170] or whether there is a direct effect on intestinal function. Renal wasting of calcium and impaired intestinal calcium absorption may produce an increase in bone resorption through stimulation of parathyroid hormone secretion. An increase in parathyroid hormone secretion is blunted in the early postmenopausal years, perhaps as a consequence of the marked increase in bone resorption typical of the initial years of estrogen deficiency.[157]

Because the ovary is a source of both estrogens and androgens, several investigators have examined blood androgen levels as a factor in normal and osteoporotic postmenopausal women. Both androstenedione and testosterone blood production rates were reduced in osteoporotic subjects in one study.[171] Serum dehydroepiandrosterone was somewhat reduced in osteoporotic women in another study.[172] In postmenopausal women with Addison's disease, bone mineral density of the wrist is much lower than expected and may have been related to low concentrations of adrenal androgens in the circulation.[173]

The role of the osteoblast in the pathogenesis of postmenopausal osteoporosis is still somewhat unsettled, although bone histomorphometry studies imply diminished osteoblast function,[141] as was proposed to be the dominant mechanism by Albright.[174] However, biochemical evidence of increased bone resorption in the postmenopausal woman is extremely convincing[119,175] and biochemical markers of bone formation are also increased but not to the same degree as bone resorption markers.[119,175] It would appear that estrogen deficiency can blunt a compensatory increase in bone formation that normally would be expected in response to increased bone resorption.

Reversible estrogen deficiency with associated reduced bone density is now well-documented in premenopausal women with athletic oligomenorrhea-amenorrhea,[176] anorexia nervosa,[177,178] hyperprolactinemia,[179] and endometriosis treated with gonadotropin-releasing hormone agonists.[180] It is generally felt that decreased bone density can be attributed to estrogen deficiency in these individuals, although the cortisol excess found in anorexia nervosa may also contribute.[177] The complexity of the reduced bone density in patients with anorexia nervosa is further underscored by the observation that oral contraceptive therapy is only partially effective in preventing bone loss.[178] It does appear that nutritional factors are of great importance in the pathogenesis of bone loss and that lean body mass, independent of estrogen deficiency, is an important determinant of bone loss in these patients.[181]

The role of phytoestrogens in bone health and disease is receiving increasing attention but definitive studies are lacking.[182]

It has been proposed that progesterone deficiency may be a factor in the pathogenesis of osteoporosis but this concept has not been established.[183]

Testosterone Deficiency

Severe hypogonadism in males is associated with loss of bone but much less is known about the biochemical and histologic consequences of testosterone deficiency than of estrogen deficiency. Men treated by orchiectomy for prostate cancer have more fractures than control patients.[184] Prospective studies of patients treated with gonadotropin-releasing hormone agonists with or without an androgen antagonist indicate that lumbar spine density and femoral neck density can decrease by 6.5–7.1 percent within 6–18 months.[185,186] This is associated with an increase in bone turnover documented by elevations of serum osteocalcin concentrations and urinary deoxypyridinoline excretion.[185,186] There are relatively few studies of bone histomorphometry in hypogonadal males.[187,188] No consistent features have been observed. In one study a history of constitutionally delayed puberty was associated with decreased bone density in the radius and the spine.[189] It is likely that these individuals will be at risk for osteoporotic fractures in later years. Androgen receptors have been identified in human osteoblast-like cells[190] and androgens can inhibit bone resorption activity of isolated osteoclasts in vitro.[191] Therefore it is likely that androgens can have a direct influence on skeletal metabolism.

Despite the clear evidence that hypogonadism can cause bone loss in men, in most series of male osteoporosis frank hypogonadism accounts for less than half of the cases.[192,193] Glucocorticoid therapy and alcoholism are other common etiologies, and a significant proportion of patients have no discernible cause.

Cancellous bone loss in the spine decreases slowly and continuously in normal males after peak bone density is reached.[194] In a population-based study of 23–90 year old men it was found that serum bioavailable testosterone and estrogen levels decreased by 64 and 47 percent respectively, and serum parathyroid hormone increased by 84 percent over the life-span.[195] Both sex steroids correlated positively with bone density by univariate analyses, but bioavailable estrogen was the consistent independent predictor of bone density in the men as it is in women. Urinary N-telopeptide excretion increased 77 percent between ages 50 and 85 years in the men and was negatively associated with bone density. It is proposed that age-related bone loss may be the result of estrogen deficiency in males as well as in females. This hypothesis does not explain why iliac crest bone histomorphometry in normal males aged 20–80 years provides evidence of decreased bone formation but no increased bone resorption in elderly males.[196] It has also been reported in other studies of elderly males that urinary N-telopeptide excretion does not increase with age.[197] The concept of the essential role of estrogen in male skeletal physiology is intriguing, particularly in view of the report of an estrogen-induced increase in bone mass in a male with aromatase deficiency.[198] Further studies are needed to validate the concept that estrogen is more essential than testosterone in the male skeleton and to determine if testosterone has any role other than as a precursor of estrogen.

Cushing's Syndrome

Chronic therapy for disorders such as rheumatoid arthritis, systemic lupus erythematosus, and asthma with glucocorticosteroids often produces a virulent form of osteoporosis. The morbidity resulting from the bone disease may approach or even surpass that of the primary disease being treated. Spontaneous Cushing's syndrome may also cause a severe form of osteoporosis, but spontaneous Cushing's syndrome is a rare finding in the osteoporotic population.

The pathogenesis of glucocorticosteroid-induced osteoporosis is complex and probably involves both direct and indirect effects of glucocorticoids on bone.[199] Bone loss is probably mainly induced through a direct inhibition of bone matrix synthesis by osteoblasts, by reduction in calcium absorption in the intestine, and by reduction of renal tubular calcium reabsorption. Steroid-induced hypogonadism, particularly in men, may be another important factor.

Recent biopsy studies indicate that glucocorticoids promote apoptosis of osteoblasts and osteocytes in patients with glucocorticoid-induced osteoporosis.[200] Parallel studies in mice also demonstrated inhibition of osteoblastogenesis. These observations fit with the impressive reduction in bone formation markers found with glucocorticoid therapy.[201] Less certain is whether secondary hyperparathyroidism is a major contributor to the bone loss, particularly in view of the fact that elevated serum parathyroid hormone levels are not a consistent finding in all studies[202–205] and that urinary collagen crosslink excretion may be normal in patients with glucocorticoid-induced osteoporosis.[201]

Pharmacologic doses of glucocorticoids have long been known to inhibit intestinal calcium absorption.[206] No consistent effect of these drugs on vitamin D metabolite levels in animals or humans has been reported. It has been suggested that end-organ resistance is a major factor in the impairment of intestinal calcium absorption, but near-physiologic doses of 1α,25-dihydroxyvitamin D_3 significantly increased calcium absorption in five patients receiving high-dose prednisone therapy for rheumatologic disorders.[207]

Urinary calcium excretion rises considerably in response to glucocorticoid therapy. It has been presumed to be a consequence of a direct effect of the steroids on renal tubular calcium reabsorption, but it is unknown how this might be mediated. It is conceivable that part of the hypercalciuric response could be accounted for by increased bone resorption.

Thyrotoxicosis

Spontaneous thyrotoxicosis is a relatively uncommon cause of osteoporosis, but with the increasing use of bone densitometry, it has become apparent that excessive thyroid hormone replacement therapy in women may have a deleterious impact on bone density.[208] Thyroid hormone has been shown to stimulate bone resorption in vitro.[209] Radioactive calcium turnover studies[210] and bone histology[118] indicate that the rates of both bone resorption and bone formation are increased in thyrotoxicosis. The loss of bone in patients with this "high-turnover" type of osteoporosis must reflect a dominance of bone resorption, but the factors that account for a relative uncoupling of resorption from formation are not known. The role of reduced intestinal calcium absorption, probably due to low levels of 1α,25-dihydroxyvitamin D in the circulation, is uncertain, but this may also contribute to the reduced bone mass found in thyrotoxicosis.[211,212]

Primary Hyperparathyroidism

Severe long-standing primary hyperparathyroidism is known to produce major skeletal abnormalities. More commonly, patients are now discovered in an asymptomatic state. Bone densitometry may detect some patients with significant vertebral bone loss who experience a considerable increase in density after parathyroidectomy.[213] It is still not well-defined to what degree mild hyperparathyroidism is a risk factor for osteoporotic fractures.[214] This problem is discussed in Chap. 22.

Diabetes Mellitus

Decreased bone density has been found in association with diabetes mellitus,[215] particularly in young insulin-dependent patients. Despite this, the incidence of fractures in diabetic subjects does not appear to be high.[216] Because insulin promotes amino acid uptake by bone cells and stimulates bone collagen synthesis, it is possible that insulin deficiency or resistance reduces bone formation directly. Alternatively, the hypercalciuria associated with poor diabetic control or impaired vitamin D metabolism may be an important factor.[215,217,218] In rats, experimental diabetes mellitus produces a reduction in serum 1α,25-dihydroxyvitamin D levels,[218] but this has not been found in humans[219] except in young insulin-dependent diabetic patients[220] and patients with severe diabetic ketoacidosis.[221]

Immobilization and Weightlessness

Osteoporosis is a serious complication in patients confined to bed for prolonged periods as a consequence of spinal trauma or neuromuscular disorders. Bone loss appears to arise from a combination of increased osteoclastic activity and diminished osteoblastic activity.[148] Patients under 30 years of age may become hypercalcemic and hypercalciuric. The absence of weight bearing and of muscular activity, rather than hormonal abnormalities, is responsible for the derangement in skeletal homeostasis. A related loss of bone density occurs during space flight and is not influenced by exercise in the weightless state.

Genetic Disorders

A variety of rare genetic disorders are associated with osteoporosis. Osteogenesis imperfecta, Ehlers-Danlos syndrome, homocystinuria, Menkes' syndrome, and Marfan syndrome all appear to evolve as a consequence of specific gene defects resulting in abnormal bone matrix synthesis.[222,223]

Juvenile Osteoporosis

Juvenile osteoporosis is a rare disorder that is characterized by a rapid loss of bone in prepubertal children of both sexes.[224] Multiple fractures of long bones, ribs, and vertebral bodies may occur in the absence of any apparent abnormality of skin, sclera, joints, or endocrine function. With the onset of puberty, most patients go into remission.[225] The reason for the remarkable spontaneous improvement in bone density is not known, but low serum 1α,25-dihydroxyvitamin D levels were found in four children in one study.[226] Three of the four received replacement 1α,25-dihydroxyvitamin D_3 therapy and exhibited major improvement in bone mineral density.

Chronic Hypophosphatemia

Osteoporosis has been demonstrated in the bone biopsies of 19 adults with chronic hypophosphatemia due to renal tubular wasting of phosphate.[227] This was associated with hypercalciuria, increased urinary hydroxyproline excretion, and low levels of serum immunoreactive parathyroid hormone. How this syndrome relates to the more common problems of hypophosphatemic rickets and osteomalacia is unclear.

Idiopathic Hypercalciuria

Relatively few studies have been done to evaluate the status of bone mineral content in hypercalciuric renal stone patients. Conceivably, patients who have a renal leak of calcium and secondary hyperparathyroidism could become osteopenic. This was the case in a group of patients with renal hypercalciuria in whom single energy photon absorptiometry of the radius was done.[228] The mean density in these subjects was about 10 percent below that of age- and sex-matched controlled subjects, whereas the mean density in patients with absorptive hypercalciuria was normal. In another study patients with fasting hypercalciuria and nephrolithiasis had low bone density measured by quantitative computerized tomography, normal serum parathyroid hormone levels, and elevated monocyte interleukin-1 levels.[229]

Chronic Alcoholism

Bone density and histomorphometric measurements in eight middle-aged males with a history of high alcohol intake for at least 10 years revealed a significant degree of osteoporosis.[230] The patients were otherwise generally in good health and had no evidence of cirrhosis of the liver. Impaired osteoblast function leading to reduced bone formation has been proposed as the mechanism by which osteoporosis emerges in alcoholism.[231] In vitro studies indicate that ethanol and its main metabolite, acetaldehyde, inhibit the formation of early osteoblast progenitors in murine and human bone marrows.[232]

Immunosuppressive Therapy Postorgan Transplantation

The growing use of organ transplantation to treat patients with end-stage renal, cardiac, pulmonary, and hepatic disease has extended the life-span of numerous patients at the cost of increased incidence of fractures, particularly during the first year after transplantation.[233] The incidence of fractures during the first year may be as high as 65 percent. Fractures are most likely to occur in liver transplant patients with biliary cirrhosis and least likely in renal transplant patients. A combination of high doses of glucocorticoids and cyclosporines can produce major decreases in bone density, probably by suppressing bone formation and stimulating bone resorption. After allogeneic bone marrow transplants patients are also highly susceptible to bone loss.[234]

Intestinal Disease

Bone loss is commonly found in patients with celiac disease even after treatment with a gluten-free diet.[235] Bone density deficits have been attributed to secondary hyperparathyroidism since a negative relationship between bone density in the forearm and serum parathyroid hormone concentration has been observed.[235] Osteoporosis has also been reported to be common in patients with inflammatory bowel disease even in the absence of glucocorticoid therapy.[236] It is likely that nutritional deficiencies and possibly circulating cytokines are factors producing bone loss.

Miscellaneous

There is an association of osteoporosis with cigarette smoking.[237] The pathogenesis of bone loss in smokers has not been well-defined but in part may be related to the reduction in weight found in heavy smokers. Reduced intestinal calcium absorption has also been found in smokers[238] as well as relative estrogen deficiency in women.[239]

Nutritional abnormalities, particularly during growth and development, may produce a reduced skeletal mass. Low calcium intake, which is a common feature of the American diet, probably contributes significantly to the pathogenesis of osteoporosis.[240] There is some evidence of osteoporosis in patients treated with heparin,[241] anticonvulsants,[242] and methotrexate.[243,244] Associations of osteoporosis with rheumatoid arthritis,[245] chronic liver disease,[246] systemic mastocytosis[247] and hematologic malignancies[248] also have been reported. Rarely osteoporosis has been reported in association with pregnancy.[249] In the absence of a definable underlying disease or known risk factors, osteoporosis is termed idiopathic.

Prevention of Osteoporosis

If the present body of knowledge pertaining to the prevention of osteoporosis were applied to the population, it is likely that in the future the incidence of osteoporosis would be reduced dramatically. This would begin with an attempt to optimize nutrition and exercise in children and deal with the gonadal dysfunction that may arise through anorexia and overexercise. Young adults would be encouraged to maintain an adequate intake of calcium, approximately 1,000 mg daily, and avoid harmful habits such as cigarette smoking and excessive alcohol.

There are now a large variety of antiresorptive agents that can prevent postmenopausal bone loss with varying degrees of effectiveness. These are listed in Table 23-4.

Estrogen replacement has the longest record of use and is known to provide very long-term protection in women with spontaneous or surgically induced menopause.[250–253] This can be achieved with average replacement doses of the various estrogens, although the majority of the data has been obtained in studies utilizing conjugated equine estrogens.[254] A dose of 0.625 mg daily can increase bone density by 3.5–5 percent after three years in the spine, with the greater increase occurring in patients also receiving continuous progestin therapy. Transdermal estradiol (0.05 mg twice a week)[255] and low-dose esterified estrogen (0.3 mg daily) with 1,000 mg calcium daily[256] can also increase bone density but

TABLE 23-4. Prevention of Postmenopausal Osteoporosis

Antiresorptive Therapy
Estrogen
Tamoxifen (breast cancer patients)
Raloxifene
Alendronate
Risedronate
Etidronate*
Pamidronate*
Salmon calcitonin
Calcium compounds

* = Not FDA-approved

to a lesser degree. Although the increase in bone density is modest, estrogen/progestin therapy produces large reductions in biochemical markers of bone resorption. Urinary N-telopeptide excretion decreased by 52 percent at 12 months in women treated with 0.625 mg conjugated equine estrogens, a progestin daily or cyclically, and a 500 mg calcium supplement.[257] There is a growing consensus that reduction in bone resorption, with presumed preservation of the microarchitecture of cancellous bone, is an important determinant of vertebral fracture prevention. As most of the studies indicating that estrogen replacement prevents fractures are retrospective,[258] it will require prospective studies to verify this hypothesis. It should also be noted that in numerous estrogen intervention trials an average calcium intake of 1,200 mg daily produced significantly greater increments in bone density than with hormone therapy alone.[259] The addition of 400 units of vitamin D daily to a prevention regimen should help assure adequacy of vitamin D stores. A small dose of methyltestosterone in combination with conjugated estrogens produces a greater increase in bone density than estrogen alone.[260]

Despite the proven benefits of estrogen in protecting the skeleton, the majority of postmenopausal women do not receive long-term estrogen replacement therapy. This is a consequence of unacceptable side effects in some individuals, but the main reason for this is the fear of estrogen-induced cancers in the breast and uterus. This situation has stimulated the development of numerous alternative therapies for the protection of the postmenopausal skeleton.

A class of agents termed selective estrogen receptor modulators (SERM) has proven beneficial in preventing postmenopausal bone loss. The first of these, tamoxifen, was actually developed to treat breast cancer. Tamoxifen at a 20-mg daily dose has been demonstrated to prevent lumbar spine and femoral neck bone loss in early postmenopausal women with breast cancer.[261] Because tamoxifen also is known to stimulate the endometrium of the uterus and induce uterine cancers, the search for safer SERMs led to development of raloxifene for prevention of postmenopausal osteoporosis. Raloxifene is a nonsteroidal benzothiophene that has antiestrogenic effects on breast and endometrial tissue and estrogenic effects on bone, lipid metabolism, and blood clotting.[262] During a two-year period 60 mg raloxifene daily increased lumbar spine and total hip density by 1.6 percent and reduced urinary C-telopeptide excretion and serum osteocalcin levels by 34 and 23 percent, respectively, in postmenopausal women.[263] These results indicate that raloxifene is less potent than estrogen in inhibiting bone resorption. Raloxifene is an alternative to estrogen in postmenopausal women but does not relieve hot flashes. It reduces LDL cholesterol but does not increase HDL cholesterol, as does estrogen.[263] Clinical effects on cardiovascular disease are under study.

The bisphosphonates are synthetic analogs of inorganic pyrophosphate that bind to the internal surfaces of bone and inhibit bone resorption. Bisphosphonates that are more similar in structure to pyrophosphate (etidronate) may be metabolized into nonhydrolyzable metabolites of ATP and inhibit osteoclast function after intracellular accumulation.[264] The more potent nitrogen-containing bisphosphonates (pamidronate, alendronate) appear to inhibit enzymes of the mevalonate pathway and impair protein prenylation.[264] Part of the inhibitory effect on bone resorption may be mediated by osteoclast apoptosis.

Etidronate, the first available bisphosphonate, has been shown to prevent early postmenopausal bone loss when administered on a cyclical schedule of 400 mg/day for 14 days followed by 500 mg/day elemental calcium for 11 weeks, repeated over a total of two years.[265] The drug was used cyclically to try to avoid producing a mineralization defect in bone.[76] After two years bone density of the lumbar spine and femoral neck were not reduced, whereas in subjects on placebo and calcium bone density had decreased about 2 percent. Biochemical markers of bone turnover were decreased by 15–20 percent at two years in the etidronate-treated subjects. Etidronate has not been FDA approved for prevention or treatment of osteoporosis although it is widely used, particularly in patients who do not tolerate other drugs.

Alendronate is a potent aminobisphosphonate that is highly effective in preventing postmenopausal bone loss. In women under 60 years of age a daily dose of 5 mg alendronate produced a 3.5 percent increase in lumbar spine density and a 1.9 percent increase in hip density during a two-year period.[266] In comparison an estrogen/progestin regimen produced a 1–2 percent greater increment in density.

Risedronate is the most recent aminobisphosphonate to be approved for prevention of bone loss in post-menopausal women. A 5 mg per day dose over a two year period increased lumbar spine bone density by 4 percent in women who were less than five years postmenopausal.[267]

Salmon calcitonin is an antiresorptive agent that has been used for 25 years to inhibit bone resorption in patients with Paget's disease and osteoporosis. Parenteral administration has been shown to produce a small increase in total body calcium[268] and to stabilize or slightly increase regional bone density measurements.[269] At this time a nasal spray form of salmon calcitonin is most widely used in patients with osteoporosis, but it is not approved for use in early postmenopausal women (up to 5 years postmenopausal) because of low potency.

Attempts have been made to prevent early postmenopausal bone loss by increasing calcium intake. In women whose intake was increased to greater than 1,300 mg/day, bone density still decreased by nearly 2 percent after two years.[270] If calcium supplementation is applied to women 65 years of age or greater, considerable benefit has been demonstrated. In a three-year, double-blind, placebo-controlled study of 213 women the administration of 500 mg calcium (calcium citrate malate) and 700 units of vitamin D resulted in significantly higher bone densities in the calcium-vitamin D-treated patients than in placebo-treated patients.[271] At the end of three years the placebo-treated patients had more than twice the number of nonvertebral fractures (26 versus 11). The largest biochemical changes were increases in urinary calcium excretion and serum 25-hydroxyvitamin D levels and decreases in serum osteocalcin and parathyroid hormone levels. Similar results were found in another study of normal postmenopausal women (mean age $\pm$ SE, 66.3 $\pm$ 0.2 years) given 1,600 mg calcium (calcium citrate) with an average dietary intake of 700 mg calcium.[272] In this study serum parathyroid hormone fell by 18.9 percent and urinary free pyridinoline by 32.2 percent. There is no convincing evidence that dietary calcium is better absorbed than supplemental calcium.

Intestinal calcium absorption can be increased with daily 0.25–0.75 μg doses of 1α,25-dihydroxyvitamin D_3.[273,274] In one study of early postmenopausal women 0.25 μg 1α,25-dihydroxyvitamin D_3 failed to prevent forearm bone loss.[275] Possible complications of hypercalciuria and hypercalcemia limit the appeal of this type of therapy.

Studies of the prevention of bone loss in men are far fewer than in women. Androgen replacement therapy in hypogonadal males is highly effective.[276] A monthly total of 400 mg of testosterone by intramuscular injection can increase lumbar spine density by 14 percent in 18 months as measured by QCT.[277] A three-year trial of testosterone by scrotal patch delivery produced a 7.5 percent increase in density of the lumbar spine and a lessor increase in hip density measured by DXA.[278] Alendronate therapy at a dose of 10 mg daily for a year increased lumbar spine density by 7 percent (DXA) in men with osteoporosis of variable etiologies.[279] Cyclicetidronate increased lumbar spine density by 7.8 percent (QCT) in six months in men given a gonadotropin agonist for the previous six months.[185] Calcium supplements of 500 mg/day with 700 units of vitamin D in elderly males was as effective in men as in women in preventing bone loss.[271]

There is a growing literature documenting the efficacy of the bisphosphonates in preventing glucocorticoid-induced osteoporosis. Etidronate,[280] alendronate,[281] pamidronate,[282] and risedronate[283] are all effective in maintaining or increasing bone density in patients requiring pharmacologic doses of glucocorticoids. This is somewhat surprising in view of the general belief that the main factor in the pathogenesis of glucocorticoid-induced osteoporosis is a reduction in bone formation. Because the greatest bone loss occurs in the first six months of steroid therapy the maximum protection would come from early treatment with a bisphosphonate and calcium supplementation.

Prior to the use of bisphosphonates high doses of vitamin D were used to prevent bone loss in glucocorticoid-treated patients, but objective evidence of efficacy was sparse. Both 25-hydroxyvitamin D_3[284] and 1α,25-dihydroxyvitamin D_3[285] have been reported to prevent bone loss, but these agents have not received FDA approval for this use. Postmenopausal women receiving chronic glucocorticoid therapy should receive partial protection from estrogen therapy.[286] Testosterone therapy has been shown to increase bone density in men who were receiving long-term glucocorticoid therapy,[287] and presumably would aid in preventing bone loss if given at the beginning of treatment. Salmon calcitonin has been used to prevent steroid-induced bone loss[288] but is not FDA-approved.

Intermittent infusions of pamidronate have been reported to prevent vertebral fractures in liver transplant patients treated with immunosuppressive agents,[289] but this bisphosphonate is not FDA-approved for osteoporosis prevention.

Treatment of Established Osteoporosis

Patients with moderate to severe osteoporosis often have spinal deformities that are associated with intermittent or persistent back pain. The recurrence of back pain may indicate a new compression fracture, perivertebral muscle spasm, or, rarely, spinal cord or nerve root irritation. Chronic back pain may also be related to degenerative arthritis in the area of deformed vertebrae as manifested by osteophyte formation and facet joint sclerosis.

The following program has been proposed as an excellent means of managing patients after acute compression fractures:[290] (1) During the initial three weeks, bed rest for 4–8 days until the patient is able to turn easily from side to side, and then with a back brace the patient can arise for frequent but brief periods. (2) For about the next 10 weeks the ambulatory patient should lie down for 20 min every two hours and gradually reduce the use of the back support, and (3) If afternoon or evening low back pain then occurs continue 20 min rest every two hours for another 10 weeks. If pain persists seek other causes.

After recovering from an acute compression fracture patients should be encouraged to walk regularly or ride an exercise bicycle to maintain muscle strength in the lower extremities in order to prevent falls.

Anecdotal evidence and small randomized trials of salmon calcitonin therapy[291] suggest that the hormone may reduce pain in patients with compression fractures. There is no harm in a short trial of this medication but much larger studies are needed to determine the efficacy of analgesic agents. Potent analgesic agents such as narcotics should be used with great caution to avoid the possibility of falls and severe constipation.

In patients with severe osteoporosis the ideal treatment would be an effective anabolic agent which stimulates bone formation to such a degree that bone mass would be restored to an amount which would markedly reduce fracture risk. Drugs such as sodium fluoride[292,293] and human parathyroid hormone 1-34[294] or 1-84[295] can produce considerable increases in bone mass, but as yet have not had FDA approval.

The administration of antiresorptive drugs to patients with established osteoporosis has surprisingly produced considerable benefit with respect to fracture prevention. This has most convincingly been demonstrated in clinical trials with alendronate and risedronate. A daily 10-mg dose of alendronate for two years increased lumbar spine density 7.21 percent and total hip density 5.27 percent in postmenopausal women with low bone density.[296] Urinary deoxypyridinoline excretion fell by 47.3 percent after three months. A three-year alendronate study of daily 5 mg, 10 mg, and 20 mg for two years and 5 mg for one-year doses demonstrated an overall 48 percent reduction in the number of women with new vertebral fractures as compared to a control group receiving 500 mg calcium.[297] Alendronate therapy has also been shown to lower the risk of hip fractures by 51 percent and wrist fractures by 48 percent in a three-year randomized trial of 2,027 postmenopausal women who had previously experienced at least one vertebral fracture[298] (Fig. 23-6). The approximately 50 percent reduction in fracture risk is associated with 7–8 percent increases in lumbar spine density (DXA) and 3–5 percent increases in total hip density (Fig. 23-7) and as much as a 60 percent decrease in urinary N-telopeptide excretion.[299] The relative contribution of increasing bone density and suppressing bone resorption to the reduced fracture risk is uncertain. Alendronate is generally well tolerated. During the formal clinical trials there was little difference in gastrointestinal side effects between treatment and placebo groups.[296–299] The drug should be used with great caution or withheld from patients with esophageal dysfunction as esophageal irritation or even ulceration may be a complication of alendronate therapy,[300] particularly if it is not taken with a full glass of water and if the patient does not avoid a recumbent position for at least 30 minutes after taking the pill. At present it is uncertain how long a patient should remain on daily alendronate therapy as a gain in bone density and suppression of bone resorption may be maintained one to two years after stopping treatment of one or two years' duration.[301] Vertebral fracture incidence was decreased by 41 percent in patients treated with 5 mg risedronate daily over three years and nonvertebral fractures by 39 percent.[302] Bone density of the lumbar spine increased by 5.2 percent (DXA). The drug was well tolerated.

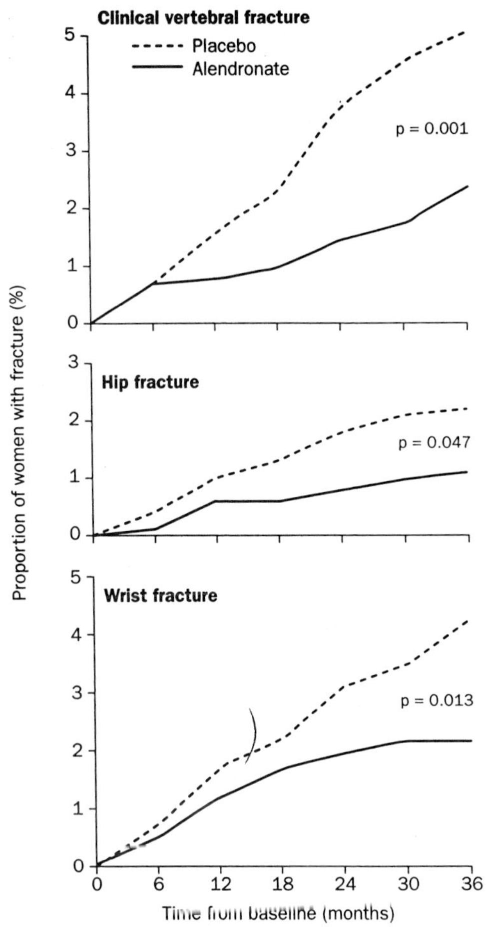

Number of women

Placebo	1005	1004	1000	999	998	993	742
Alendronate	1022	1022	1021	1020	1015	1010	753

FIGURE 23-6. Cumulative proportions of postmenopausal osteoporotic women who developed vertebral, hip or wrist fractures while taking alendronate for 36 months. The dose of alendronate was 5 mg daily for 24 months and then 10 mg daily for 12 months. All subjects had a calcium intake of at least 1,000 mg/day. (*From Black DM et al: Lancet 348:1535, 1996.*)

Etidronate has been used cyclically (400 mg daily for two weeks, 2½ months off) to treat postmenopausal bone loss for up to seven years.[303] Lumbar spine density (DXA) has been observed to increase up to 8.6 percent after five years of treatment and bone density appears to be maintained for at least two years after stopping treatment.[303] Vertebral fracture incidence appears to decrease particularly during long-term treatment, but an adequate-sized study to provide more definitive data on fracture prevention has not been done. A combination of cyclical etidronate and estrogen

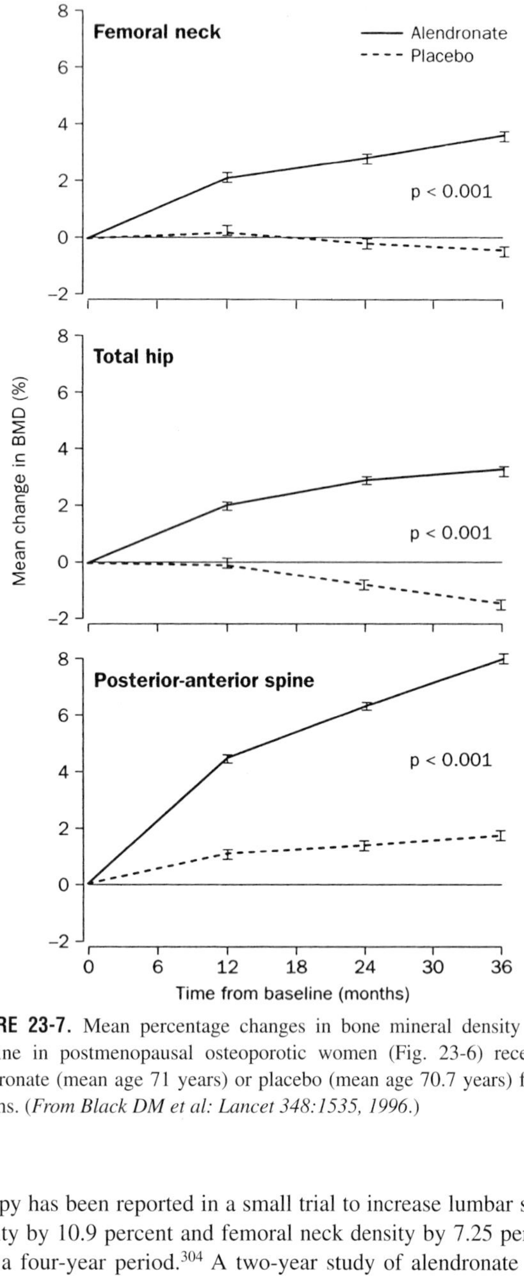

FIGURE 23-7. Mean percentage changes in bone mineral density from baseline in postmenopausal osteoporotic women (Fig. 23-6) receiving alendronate (mean age 71 years) or placebo (mean age 70.7 years) for 36 months. (*From Black DM et al: Lancet 348:1535, 1996.*)

therapy has been reported in a small trial to increase lumbar spine density by 10.9 percent and femoral neck density by 7.25 percent over a four-year period.[304] A two-year study of alendronate with conjugated estrogens produced an 8.3 percent increase in lumbar spine density (DXA)[305].

Ongoing studies with more potent aminobisphosphonates than pamidronate, alendronate, and risedronate will increase the choice of therapeutic agents for treatment of osteoporosis. Ibandronate by intravenous injection[305] appears to be effective therapy[306] in postmenopausal women. It is likely that a once weekly dose of 70 mg alendronate will be used in the future as it produces equivalent results as the 10 mg daily dose.[307]

Parenteral and nasal spray salmon calcitonin have been approved for treatment of postmenopausal osteoporosis for years, but evidence of a reduction in fracture incidence has been lacking. A preliminary report of the results of a multicenter 5-year trial indicates that 200 units daily nasal spray calcitonin reduced vertebral fracture incidence by 36 percent as compared to a placebo group.[308] The 100- and 400-unit doses reduced fracture incidence, but these data were not statistically significant.

There has been interest in using growth hormone as a possible anabolic therapy of osteoporosis. Theoretically this might prove effective because of the temporal relationships of decreased function of the growth hormone/IGF-1 axis and age-related bone loss.[309] The results of clinical trials with growth hormone have proven disappointing thus far.[310]

In patients receiving statins for hyperlipidemia, it has been noted in several studies that the incidence of hip fractures is reduced by about 50 percent.[311] Prospective trials are needed to verify this finding and define the mechanism by which these drugs may produce such a response.

Human parathyroid hormone[1-34] produced a 35 percent increase in lumbar spine density (QCT) in postmenopausal women on glucocorticoid therapy and estrogen.[312]

Recognition that thiazide diuretics reduce urinary calcium excretion has led to retrospective and prospective studies of the potential value of these agents in the management of osteoporosis. A meta-analysis evaluating epidemiological studies relating thiazide use to fracture incidence led to the conclusion that there may be a 20 percent reduction of fracture risk with long-term use.[313]

In patients with other endocrine abnormalities that produce osteoporosis, treatment of the underlying abnormality is of greatest value. Resolution of thyrotoxicosis results in an increase in bone mass, although this is less evident in postmenopausal women.[314] Insulin therapy in juvenile-onset diabetes mellitus appears to exert a protective effect on the skeleton.

The osteoporosis of immobilization is best managed by early mobilization of the patient, if this is possible. Bisphosphonate therapy should prevent bone loss but no large trials have been reported.

The treatment of the osteoporosis associated with genetic disorders has been disappointing until recently. Intravenous pamidronate administered at four-to six-month intervals for up to five years produced remarkable clinical, radiologic, and biochemical improvement in an uncontrolled study in 3–16-year-old children.[315] A mean annualized increase in bone density of 41.9 ± 29 percent was noted as well as sustained reductions in serum alkaline phosphatase concentrations and urinary excretion of calcium and N-telopeptide. The mean incidence of radiologically confirmed fractures decreased by 1.7 per year. Pain relief was reported in all and mobility improved in more than half of the children.

A study of a boy with juvenile osteoporosis demonstrated a dramatic effect of the bisphosphonate pamidronate on the clinical course of the disease.[316] A rapid reduction in bone resorption followed by signs of sclerosis near the growth plates of affected metaphyses and at the end plates of the vertebrae was observed during a period of 3 months of treatment with this drug. The improvement of bone density in three children treated with 1α,25-dihydroxyvitamin D_3 has already been discussed.[226]

OSTEOPETROSIS

Osteopetrosis (*Albers-Schönberg disease, marble bone disease, osteosclerosis fragilis generalisata*) is a rare heritable disorder of bone characterized by increased skeletal density.[317] The pattern of inheritance is either autosomal recessive or autosomal dominant. Patients with recessive inheritance usually have a more severe form of clinical involvement. Common abnormalities include an enlarged skull, hearing loss, optic atrophy, pathologic fractures, osteomyelitis, retarded growth, leukoerythroblastosis, anemia, thrombocytopenia, lymphadenopathy, and hepatosplenomegaly.

Patients often do not survive past age 20 and usually die as a consequence of infection, anemia, or hemorrhage. This type of osteopetrosis is often termed malignant osteopetrosis. There are several other very rare types of autosomal recessive osteopetrosis. These include a syndrome of osteopetrosis, type I renal tubular acidosis and basal ganglia calcification associated with carbonic anhydrase II deficiency,[317,318] and malignant osteopetrosis associated with neuronal storage disease.[319] Mutations of the carbonic anhydrase II gene[317] and the osteoclast-specific 116-Kd subunit gene of the vacuolar proton pump[320] have been described in autosomal recessive osteopetrosis patients. In approximately 50 percent of patients with an autosomal dominant pattern of inheritance, osteopetrosis is asymptomatic. Fractures, osteomyelitis, and cranial nerve palsies may occur in some patients. Studies in Denmark suggest that there are two types of benign osteopetrosis.[321] In one family with benign (autosomal dominant) osteopetrosis linkage studies have implicated a locus in 1p21.[322] Serum calcium, phosphorus, and alkaline phosphatase concentrations are generally normal in the recessive and dominant types of osteopetrosis. Serum acid phosphatase is often increased. Occasionally a patient with infantile osteopetrosis will be found to have hypocalcemia, hypophosphatemia, and elevated alkaline phosphatase.

The radiologic features of osteopetrosis are often quite striking. A generalized increase in skeletal density may be associated with a diminution in or absence of marrow cavities, clublike deformities of the long bones, and a "bone within a bone" appearance of the vertebral bodies (Fig. 23-8).

Bone biopsies in patients with osteopetrosis may be difficult to obtain because of increased bone density. Histologic examination of the bone reveals an increased density of bone, often with obliteration of the marrow cavities. The bone may be woven in character in an adult, and remnants of fetal calcified cartilage are a characteristic feature. Numerous osteoclasts may be present, but there is an absence of Howship lacunae, a finding indicative of inactivity of the osteoclasts. This is probably explained by the poorly developed ruffled borders of the osteoclasts observed by electron microscopy.[323] In some patients, few or no osteoclasts may be found in bone specimens. In children, features of rickets may be apparent.[324]

The studies of Walker in osteopetrotic mice dramatically increased our understanding of the pathogenesis of osteopetrosis.[325] He demonstrated that impaired bone resorption in osteopetrotic mice could be restored by transplanting normal bone marrow or splenic cells and that infusions of splenic cells from osteopetrotic mice to lethally irradiated normal littermates could produce osteopetrosis. These elegant studies provided strong evidence for the hematopoietic origin of osteoclasts and stimulated clinical studies of a similar nature. Bone marrow transplantation has been successful in children with the lethal form of osteopetrosis. Remarkable radiologic and histologic improvement in bone and amelioration of hematologic abnormalities have been reported.[326,327] The data obtained from these patients are consistent with the hypothesis that a normal hematopoietic stem cell is not present in some osteopetrotic subjects and that transplantation of normal marrow provides normal osteoclast precursors, which, when fully differentiated, restore normal osteoclast function.

Large oral doses of 1α,25-hydroxyvitamin D_3 and a low calcium diet may bring about changes in children with malignant osteopetrosis equivalent to those provided by bone marrow transplantation.[328] Interferon gamma-1b treatment may also produce clinical improvement.[329]

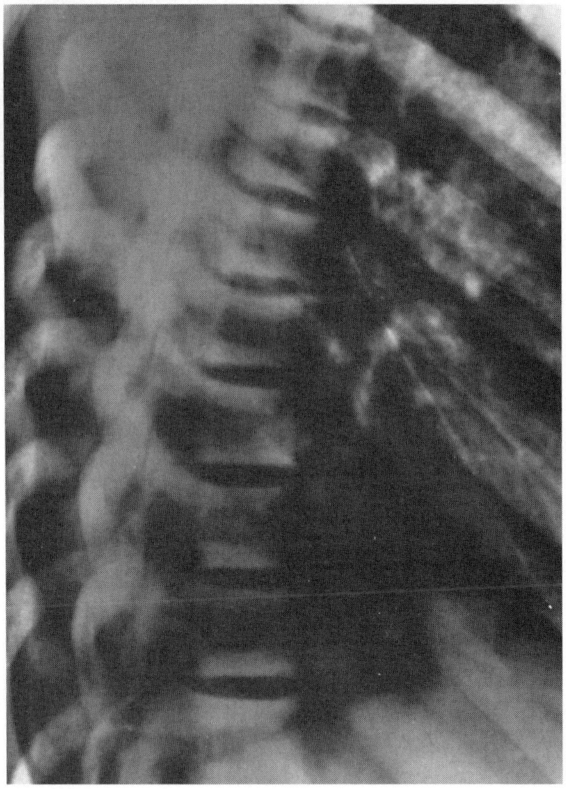

FIGURE 23-8. Roentgenogram of the thoracic spine of a 54-year-old patient with osteopetrosis. Note the marked density of the vertebral end plates, the "bone within a bone" appearance of two vertebral bodies, and the great density of the ribs

RENAL OSTEODYSTROPHY

Renal osteodystrophy is the general term used in connection with the variety of skeletal abnormalities that may complicate the clinical course of patients with chronic renal failure. Osteomalacia, secondary hyperparathyroidism, osteoporosis, and osteosclerosis may be encountered in a given patient either as isolated abnormalities or in combination.

Clinical Presentation

Symptoms and Signs

Bone pain, muscle weakness and tenderness and, rarely, gangrene of the fingers or toes are dramatic complications in patients with renal osteodystrophy.[330] In children, short stature and rachitic deformities are additional features.

Soft tissue calcification often can be detected in the corneas and conjunctivas and gives rise to "red eye." Calcinosis cutis may be associated with generalized pruritus. Calcium deposits may occur around large joints and in muscle. Cardiac and pulmonary calcification may cause congestive heart failure and pulmonary insufficiency.

Radiologic Features

The radiologic findings in patients with renal osteodystrophy are highly variable and reflect the presence of osteomalacia, secondary hyperparathyroidism, osteoporosis, or osteosclerosis in adults and rickets in children. Pseudofractures and rachitic deformities, subperiosteal bone resorption and other lesions of hyperparathyroidism, and, uncommonly, generalized osteopenia may be observed. Osteosclerosis is a common finding, primarily in the spine. A "rugger jersey spine" is characterized by sclerosis of the inferior and superior borders of the vertebral bodies. Sclerosis of the skull and long bones is less common.

Laboratory Findings

Serum calcium concentrations may be low, normal, or even elevated. Serum magnesium is normal or moderately elevated. Serum phosphorus is usually elevated but may fall within the normal range. Serum total and bone specific alkaline phosphatase activity are often elevated, as is serum osteocalcin.[330] Part of the increase in osteocalcin is due to impaired renal clearance. Serum intact parathyroid hormone increases with moderately impaired renal function and may be markedly elevated in dialysis patients. An exception to this is found in patients with aluminum excess.[331] Serum 1α,25-dihydroxyvitamin D and 24,25-dihydroxyvitamin D levels are low,[18,30] but 25-dihydroxyvitamin D is normal if vitamin D intake or sun exposure is adequate.[332] Impaired intestinal calcium absorption is a common finding in severe renal failure.[330] Urinary calcium excretion is low as a consequence of a decreased filtered load of calcium. In patients with elevated serum parathyroid hormone, urinary cAMP excretion is increased and the renal TmP/GFR is reduced. However, the measurement of urinary cAMP and TmP/GFR may not provide a reliable measure of parathyroid function if the GFR is less than 20 to 30 ml/min.

Bone Pathology

The two main types of histologic abnormalities in renal osteodystrophy are those of osteomalacia and hyperparathyroidism.[333] Patients who develop osteomalacia as the dominant lesion exhibit all the characteristic features of osteomalacia, including widened osteoid seams, which cover an increased percentage of the trabecular bone surface, and impaired uptake of tetracycline. Osteomalacia may be present in the near absence of evidence of secondary hyperparathyroidism in dialysis patients. This is usually associated with aluminum accumulation.[331]

When hyperparathyroidism is dominant, a marked increase in osteoclastic bone resorption, severe marrow fibrosis, and osteocytic osteolysis are present.[334] The rate of bone formation in these patients may be increased, in contrast to the osteomalacic type of renal osteodystrophy. A mixed type of renal osteodystrophy exhibiting features of osteomalacia and secondary hyperparathyroidism may represent patients with previously established hyperparathyroid bone disease who experienced aluminum excess.[330]

A more recently recognized form of osteodystrophy is termed "aplastic" or "adynamic." This form is characterized by normal osteoid, no marrow fibrosis, reduced number of bone cells, and low rates of bone formation. This may or may not be associated with aluminum excess, but has also been attributed to reduction of parathyroid hormone levels.[335]

Osteosclerosis is characterized by increased bone density. Widened osteoid seams may be seen, but the amount of mineralized bone is greater than normal.

Decreased bone volume is most likely to be observed with evidence of secondary hyperparathyroidism.

Pathogenesis

The pathogenesis of osteomalacia in patients with renal osteodystrophy is multifactorial. Although circulating levels of 1α,25-dihydroxyvitamin D decrease as the functional renal mass decreases,[336,337] this may not be the critical determinant of osteomalacia, as it is a very common finding but only a relatively small proportion of patients with end-stage renal failure develop full-blown osteomalacia. Vitamin D deficiency, aluminum content of bone, prior parathyroidectomy, metabolic acidosis, and dialysis-induced hypophosphatemia are other important risk factors in producing clinically relevant defects in bone mineralization.[73,338–340]

The syndrome of aluminum-induced osteomalacia in hemodialysis patients has received considerable attention because of the severity of the symptoms and the potential for reversal of the problem. As was previously discussed, these patients exhibit osteomalacia without evidence of secondary hyperparathyroidism. They may develop hypercalcemia despite modest parathyroid hormone levels,[341] probably as a consequence of the failure of bone to take up calcium from the extracellular fluid. If vitamin D of any type is administered in even small doses to treat the osteomalacic state, severe hypercalcemia may ensue because of increased intestinal calcium absorption[331] together with the defective mineralization. This problem is presently much less common due to the widespread use of dialysate with low aluminum concentration and the avoidance of aluminum-containing antacids to control hyperphosphatemia.

Secondary hyperparathyroidism is the most common abnormality in chronic renal failure. A complex series of metabolic interactions leads to the development of parathyroid hyperplasia and high levels of parathyroid hormone in the circulation.[330] A decrease in serum 1α,25-dihydroxyvitamin D levels may contribute to hypocalcemia through impairing intestinal calcium absorption and thereby indirectly stimulate parathyroid hormone secretion. A direct effect on parathyroid secretion is also likely because there is evidence that 1α,25-dihydroxyvitamin D modulates parathyroid cell proliferation; low levels may allow parathyroid cells to proliferate. Alterations in the vitamin D receptor may also be involved, as it has been shown that parathyroid glands from patients with renal failure have reduced numbers of receptors as compared to parathyroid adenomas.[330] A nonsuppressible component of the parathyroid secretory system could also be a factor in perpetuating high parathyroid hormone levels in patients with severe parathyroid hyperplasia. Another factor in parathyroid function in renal failure is the insensitivity to the suppressive effect of calcium on parathyroid hormone secretion. There is an increase in the set point for calcium-regulated parathyroid hormone secretion. This may be related to low 1α,25-dihydroxyvitamin D levels, decreased numbers of vitamin D and calcium receptors in uremic parathyroid glands, and monoclonal transformation of previously hyperplastic parathyroids.[330] Phosphate retention also is felt to be an important contributor to the pathogenesis of secondary hyperparathyroidism. Reducing dietary phosphorus intake can produce a significant reduction in serum parathyroid hormone levels. In some patients this could be modulated by a rise in serum 1α,25-dihydroxyvitamin D levels, but not in patients with advanced renal failure. New laboratory studies suggest that phosphate may directly influence parathyroid hormone synthesis.[330] Finally, skeletal resistance to the calcemic action of parathyroid hormone may contribute to hypocalcemia and secondary hyperparathyroidism. The mechanism of skeletal resistance remains uncertain.

TABLE 23-5. Prevention of Renal Osteodystrophy

1. Maintenance of normal serum phosphate
2. Provide adequate calcium intake
3. Avoid aluminum-containing antacids if possible
4. Oral or intravenous calcitriol, or intravenous paricalcitriol
5. Consider subtotal parathyroidectomy for severe secondary hyperparathyroidism unresponsive to medical therapy.

The pathogenesis of osteosclerosis in patients with chronic renal failure is unknown. It has been suggested that osteosclerosis is more likely to occur in patients with severe secondary hyperparathyroidism.

Treatment

Successful renal transplantation restores vitamin D metabolism to normal and usually produces healing of osteomalacia within 1 year.[341] Resolution of secondary hyperparathyroidism may take longer because the glomerular filtration rate frequently remains slightly reduced. Persistence of elevated parathyroid hormone levels and long-term posttransplant hypercalcemia are well documented.[342] Other complications of renal transplantation affecting the skeleton include steroid-induced osteoporosis, growth retardation in children, and aseptic necrosis of bone.[342] Measures that are likely to be helpful in the prevention of renal osteodystrophy are outlined in Table 23-5. Maintenance of a normal serum phosphate may require limiting dietary phosphorus intake to 600–800 mg/day and providing 1–4 g of calcium carbonate or 0.5–3 g of calcium acetate to reduce phosphate absorption with each meal.[330] Avoidance of aluminum containing antacids is desirable, but if the serum phosphorus is greater than 8 mg/dl short-term use may be acceptable to bind phosphate. It may be helpful to give oral calcium supplements at night (1–2 g) when the serum phosphorous is normal. In dialysis patients the dialysate calcium concentration should not exceed 5–5.5 mg/dl in order to minimize the chance of hypercalcemia.[330] Careful use of alkali will correct systemic acidosis. Hypocalcemia can be corrected with 1α,25-dihydroxyvitamin D_3 in early renal failure and can reverse resistance to parathyroid hormone and other metabolic abnormalities.[343] The institution of a prophylactic regimen to prevent renal osteodystrophy requires close follow-up to avoid hyperphosphatemia, hypercalcemia, and extraskeletal calcification.

The treatment of renal osteodystrophy with 25-hydroxyvitamin D_3, 1α,25-dihydroxyvitamin D_3, and 1α-hydroxyvitamin D_3 has received intensive scrutiny because of the greater potency and shorter half-life of these agents. The 1α derivatives of vitamin D have been demonstrated to be particularly effective in hypocalcemic patients with secondary hyperparathyroidism. Chronic therapy with 2 μg or less daily of 1α,25-dihydroxyvitamin D_3 produces normocalcemia, suppression of the parathyroid hormone concentration, and a decrease in alkaline phosphatase activity as well as reversal of the histologic lesions of secondary hyperparathyroidism.[344] Relief of bone pain and muscle weakness and an increased growth rate in children have been documented in numerous clinical trials. Less consistent results have been reported in respect to improvement of bone mineralization. In some studies, 1α,25-dihydroxyvitamin D_3 has been reported to produce healing of histologic lesions of osteomalacia,[345] but other investigators have reported incomplete healing with this metabolite.[346] It has been claimed that 25-hydroxyvitamin D_3 is a more effective agent in healing osteomalacia.[347] It is not known at present whether 25-hydroxyvitamin D_3 or the induction of 24,25-dihydroxyvitamin D_3 synthesis is responsible for superior healing or whether inadequate doses of 1α,25-dihydroxyvitamin D_3 in some trials account for the preceding observations.

If these potent agents are used, the physician must be aware of the danger of hypercalcemia as a complication. A previously normocalcemic patient often becomes hypercalcemic shortly after a significant fall in alkaline phosphatase activity is observed. Hypercalcemia is also likely to occur early in the course of treatment in patients with severe secondary hyperparathyroidism who are normocalcemic or have borderline hypercalcemia before therapy. These patients may require subtotal parathyroidectomy because of massive parathyroid hyperplasia.[330] Symptomatic hypercalcemia, intractable pruritus, bone pain, fractures, extraskeletal calcifications, and cutaneous gangrene are indications for parathyroid surgery. The studies of Wells suggest that total parathyroidectomy with transplantation of parathyroid tissue in a forearm is the surgery of choice.[348]

In hemodialysis patients with secondary hyperparathyroidism, it may prove difficult to control bone disease with oral vitamin D metabolites because small doses may induce hypercalcemia. Another approach is to infuse 1α,25-dihydroxyvitamin D_3 three times weekly (1–2.5 μg) in the dialysis tubing. This has been reported to markedly improve osteitis fibrosa in bone biopsies and lower serum parathyroid hormone concentrations in dialysis patients who are refractory to oral 1α,25-dihydroxyvitamin D_3.[349] The goal is to maintain serum intact parathyroid hormone levels at 150–250 pg/ml. The efficacy of this form of therapy is probably related to the direct inhibition of parathyroid hormone gene transcription by the vitamin D metabolite. An effective alternative to intravenous therapy with 1α,25-dihydroxyvitamin D is to give 2–4 μg orally two or three times a week.[350] Paricalcitol, a recently approved vitamin D analog, is an effective alternative to 1α,25-dihydroxyvitamin D_3.[351] Intravenous doses administered three times a week have lowered serum parathyroid hormone levels by 60 percent in dialysis patients while hypercalcemia was rarely observed.

A particularly difficult group of patients to treat is the subset of dialysis patients with aluminum excess who have severe osteomalacia in the absence of biochemical or histologic evidence of secondary hyperparathyroidism.[331,338] These patients often do not respond adequately to treatment with 1α,25-dihydroxyvitamin D_3. Deferoxamine infusions may remove aluminum from bone and reverse the osteomalacic lesion.[352] Fortunately, aluminum-induced renal osteodystrophy has become much less common because of a reduced aluminum content in the dialysate and reduced use of aluminum hydroxide.

HEREDITARY HYPERPHOSPHATASIA

Hereditary hyperphosphatasia is a rare autosomal recessive disorder that usually presents during infancy.[353] This condition has been described by a variety of eponyms, including chronic idiopathic hyperphosphatasia, hyperostosis corticalis deformans juvenilis, osteochalasia desmalis familiaris, familial osteoectasia, chronic progressive osteopathy with hyperphosphatasia, hereditary bone dysplasia with hyperphosphatasemia, and juvenile Paget disease. Enlargement of the skull and facial bones and bowing of the extremities are common features of the disease. Skin temperature may be increased over affected bones. Bone pain and pathologic fractures are common.

The radiologic features of hereditary hyperphosphatasia include loss of the normal cortical architecture, disruption of the corticomedullary border, expansion of the diaphysis, and strikingly increased density of the calvarium with a patchy "cotton-wool" pattern. The latter abnormality is quite similar to the radiologic appearance of the skull in patients with advanced Paget disease of bone.

The laboratory characteristics of this disorder are identical to those of polyostotic Paget disease of bone. Serum calcium and phosphorus concentrations are normal. Serum alkaline phosphatase activity and urinary hydroxyproline excretion may be markedly elevated.

The reported histologic findings in patients with hereditary hyperphosphatasia have been heterogeneous, an indication that the classification of patients may be imperfect. There is agreement that the bone is laid down in a chaotic manner indistinguishable from the mosaic pattern of bone characteristic of Paget disease. Numerous osteoblasts and a fibrovascular bone marrow are present. There is disagreement about whether woven or lamellar bone is the dominant type of bone formed. Another point of controversy concerns which bone cells are responsible for the increased rate of bone resorption. In one study of several patients,[353] numerous osteoclasts were present in bone biopsies, but in another study, osteoclasts were rarely observed.[354] Instead, the investigators found a marked degree of osteocytic osteolysis and concluded that the osteocytes were responsible for the accelerated rate of bone resorption. They also described ultrastructural abnormalities in both the osteocytes and the osteoblasts of their patients.[355] Intramitochondrial microcrystalline bodies that were thought to represent calcium deposits were observed. The significance of these intracellular deposits is unknown, but they have been reported to disappear after calcitonin therapy.

The pathogenesis of hereditary hyperphosphatasia is unknown. The disease is clearly not a childhood form of Paget disease, as it is generalized in its distribution and the characteristic nuclear and cytoplasmic inclusions found in the osteoclasts of Paget disease are not present.

Despite the lack of understanding of the pathogenesis of hereditary hyperphosphatasia, remarkable progress has been made in treating this disorder. Chronic treatment with calcitonin is associated with dramatic clinical improvement of both subjective and objective parameters.[356–358] Reduction in bone pain and in the incidence of pathologic fractures has been reported. The rate of bone turnover is decreased, as manifested by a reduction of alkaline phosphatase activity and urinary hydroxyproline excretion. Improvement of radiologic abnormalities has been observed, as well as improvement of the histologic abnormalities in bone biopsies. These improvements in skeletal structure and metabolism appear to be maintained during years of therapy. An impressive biochemical and radiologic response also has been reported in a child treated with intravenous then oral pamidronate.[359]

FIBROUS DYSPLASIA

Fibrous dysplasia of bone (Albright's syndrome, Albright-McCune-Sternberg syndrome) is a rare disorder that may be monostotic or polyostotic in distribution. It is clearly not a metabolic bone disease, but because of numerous associated endocrinopathies it seems appropriate to include this entity in a discussion of metabolic bone disease.

The disorder was lucidly described by Albright and colleagues in 1937,[360] but Albright subsequently pointed out that the first cases in the medical literature were reported by von Recklinghausen in 1891.[361] Cases 5 and 6 of von Recklinghausen's monograph were mistakenly believed to be examples of osteitis fibrosa generalisata.[362]

Fibrous dysplasia is usually recognized between the ages of 3 and 10. There is no evidence of genetic transmission. A triad of abnormalities is often present: bone lesions, sexual precocity (primarily in girls), and café-au-lait skin lesions that have serrated edges.[360] The bone lesions most often affect the femur, tibia, pelvis, hand, rib, humerus, and skull.[363] In patients with polyostotic fibrous dysplasia, there is a tendency to unilateral distribution of the disease. Skeletal deformity, pain, and pathologic fractures are the main manifestations of the bone lesions. Sarcomas may rarely arise in a lesion of fibrous dysplasia.[364] Intramuscular myxomas are a rare associated condition.[365] A great variety of endocrinopathies have been described in patients with fibrous dysplasia since the initial reports of sexual precocity. These include acromegaly, gigantism, hyperprolactinemia, hyperthyroidism, hyperparathyroidism, Cushing's syndrome, hypothalamic hypogonadism, and hypophosphatemic rickets.[366–369] The skin pigmentation occurs most frequently over the sacrum, buttocks, and cervical spine. Cardiovascular and hepatic disease are more recently recognized features of fibrous dysplasia.[370]

The characteristic radiologic feature of fibrous dysplasia is a ground-glass appearance of the lesions. Focal cortical thinning, expansion of the diaphysis, and a multilocular configuration of the lesions are also features (Fig. 23-9). Gross deformities of the skeleton are often apparent. Shepherd's-crook deformity of the femur, coxa vara, tibial bowing, protrusio acetabuli, and enlarged facial bones are common abnormalities. Increased radiodensity of the base of the skull and thickening of the occiput may be observed. Computerized tomography is particularly helpful in defining the extent of craniofascial disease.

Serum calcium and phosphorus determinations are usually normal, except in the few patients who have associated hyperparathyroidism or hypophosphatemic rickets. Serum alkaline phosphatase activity and urinary hydroxyproline excretion may be increased, a reflection of accelerated bone turnover. The turnover of fibrous connective tissue in bone lesions may also contribute to the level of hydroxyproline excretion.

Pathologically, fibrous dysplasia is characterized by highly cellular marrow in which there is dense fibrous connective tissue encircling fragments of trabecular bone[363] (Fig. 23-10). The bone is woven in character and resembles letters of the alphabet. The randomly oriented collagen fibers appear to extend into the adjacent fibrous tissue. Osteoblasts are not abundant, but recent studies indicate that the fibrotic areas consist of an excess of preosteogenic cells producing a disorganized collagenous matrix.[371,372] Widened osteoid seams occasionally are noted at sites where there are few osteoblasts. Osteoclasts may be present in areas adjacent to those in which there is increased osteoblastic activity. Islands of cartilage may represent remnants of the epiphysis or abortive callus formation. Callus formation after trauma may be inadequate. Fluid-filled cysts sometimes develop in areas of previous trauma or surgery. Pathologic examination of the endocrine glands in patients with endocrine disease has revealed hy-

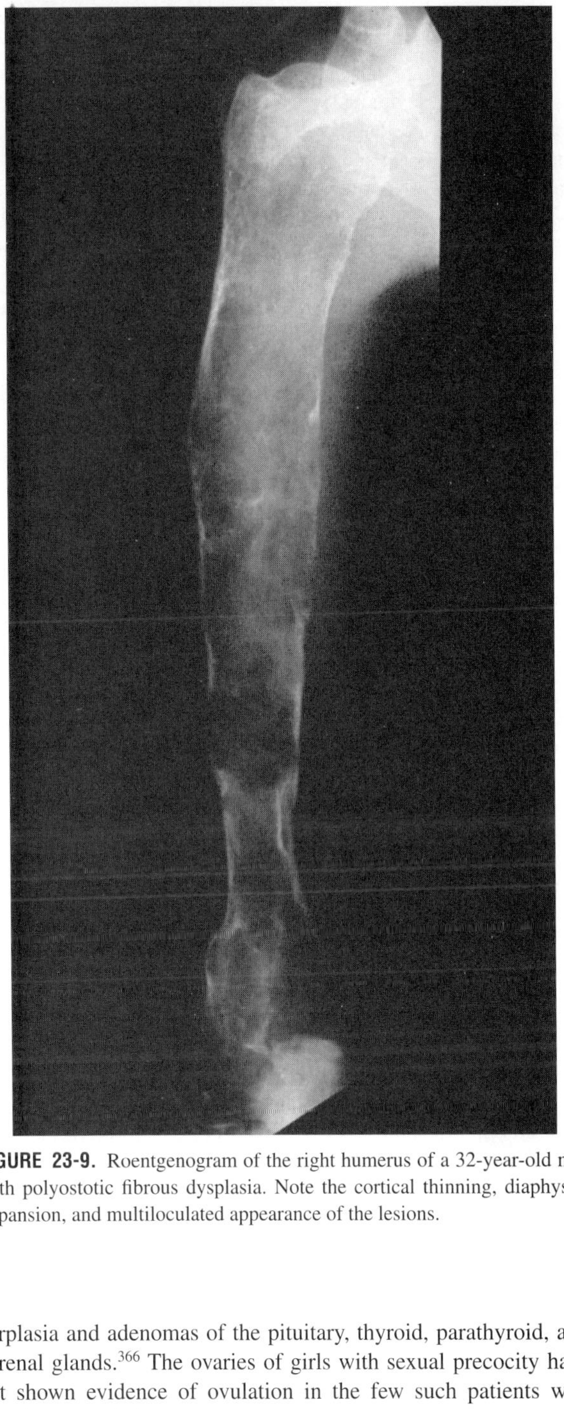

FIGURE 23-9. Roentgenogram of the right humerus of a 32-year-old man with polyostotic fibrous dysplasia. Note the cortical thinning, diaphyseal expansion, and multiloculated appearance of the lesions.

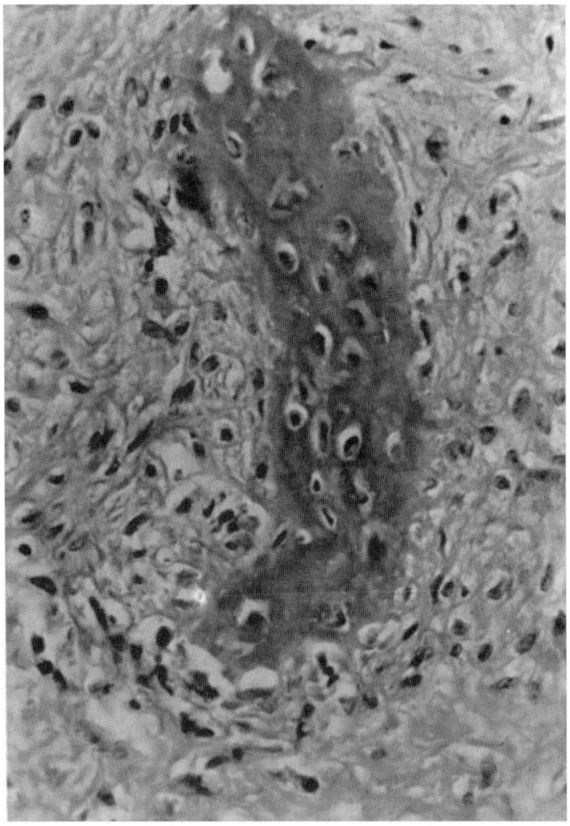

FIGURE 23-10. A trabecula of bone surrounded by dense fibrous connective tissue from a patient with fibrous dysplasia. Decalcified, H&E.

perplasia and adenomas of the pituitary, thyroid, parathyroid, and adrenal glands.[366] The ovaries of girls with sexual precocity have not shown evidence of ovulation in the few such patients who have been studied.

There is now abundant evidence that fibrous dysplasia and its associated endocrine and nonendocrine pathology is linked to somatic mutations in the gene that codes for the α subunit of the stimulatory guanine nucleotide-binding protein.[373] This leads to a cascade of biochemical consequences that include increased cyclic AMP and interleukin-6 production by affected cells.[374] The former appears to account for the proliferation of cells in the skeleton and other organs, and the latter may increase osteoclast differentiation in the bone.[375] The resolution of associated hypophosphatemic bone disease after resection of the lesions of fibrous dysplasia in one patient does suggest that a phosphaturic factor may be secreted by the bone lesions.[66]

In the past, medical treatment of fibrous dysplasia proved unsatisfactory. Recent studies indicate that pamidronate, a potent bisphosphonate, can decrease bone pain, increase the density of the skeletal lesions, and apparently slow the progress of the disease into normal adjacent bone.[376–378] Presumably these effects are mediated through inhibition of osteoclasts. Radiation therapy of the skeletal lesions may lead to sarcomatous degeneration. Testolactone, an inhibitor of estrogen synthesis, has been demonstrated to reduce estradiol levels, ovarian volume, and growth rates in young girls with precocious puberty.[379] Standard treatments of the other endocrinopathies are usually successful.

Various orthopedic procedures on the upper extremities, spine, pelvis, and lower extremities are necessary to treat pain, deformity, and fractures.[380]

PAGET'S DISEASE OF BONE

Paget's disease of bone is a common localized disorder of bone that is often included in a consideration of metabolic bone diseases because in its polyostotic form the level of metabolic activity of the skeleton is as great as that in any bone disease.

Sir James Paget provided a brilliant description in 1876 of a crippling bone disorder he termed *osteitis deformans*.[381] Although he thought that it was a rare disorder, the advent of roentgenograms revealed it to be a common albeit often asymptomatic affliction. An incidence of 3 percent or more in persons over age 50 has been found in regions of the world where there are large concentrations of people of Anglo-Saxon origin.[382] The disease is rare in the Orient, India, and Scandinavia. Males and females are almost equally affected. A positive family history of Paget's disease has been reported in up to 40 percent of patients.[383] The disease is transmitted as an autosomal dominant trait. In some families genetic markers indicate linkage of the disease to a locus on 18q.[383] Patients with familial expansile osteolysis, a purely osteolytic disorder with some features shared with Paget's disease, have mutations in the 18q gene encoding the receptor activator of nuclear factor-kappa B (RANK).[384]

Clinical Presentation

Symptoms and Signs

A significant proportion of patients with Paget's disease do not have symptoms of the disease. In these patients, the disease is discovered by screening blood chemistry or chance findings on radiologic examinations.

Pain and skeletal deformity are the most common presenting complaints in patients with symptomatic Paget's disease. The pain may arise in bone or joints or from spinal cord or nerve impingement.[385] Bone pain is usually not severe and is only slightly worsened by weight bearing if present in the spine, pelvis, or lower extremities. There is a puzzling lack of correlation between the degree of pain and the severity of skeletal deformity. Patients with polyostotic disease, which is associated with marked deformity, may never experience bone pain, whereas moderate pain may arise in a lesion that is demonstrable only by radiologic examination. Joint pain due to degenerative arthritis is usually more severe than bone pain. The most common sites are the hip and knee joints. Weight bearing typically increases the severity of the joint pain. The most excruciating pain occurs as a consequence of impingement by deformed vertebrae on the spinal cord or nerve roots. This pain is often felt in the back and/or lower extremities. Some patients experience pain as a result of a combination of Paget's involvement, degenerative changes, and nerve impingement, and it may be difficult to judge the relative contributions of each type of pain in these patients.

The deformities that may appear in patients with long-standing Paget's disease are most readily appreciated by examining the skull, clavicles, and long bones. The involved bones are generally both increased in size and of an abnormal contour. An increase in skin temperature over affected long bones is a typical finding and is explained by soft tissue vascularity surrounding the bones.[386]

Loss of auditory acuity occurs in approximately 50 percent of patients with skull involvement.

In about 15 percent of patients, disruptions of Bruch's membrane produce cracks in the retina that are termed *angioid streaks*. They rarely produce visual impairment.

A variety of other complications may occur in patients with Paget's disease. Pathologic fractures of the femur, tibia, and vertebral bodies are not uncommon.[387] Nonunion of femoral fractures is relatively common. Bone tumors present with an increase in pain and/or a rapidly growing mass at sites of Paget's disease. Sarcomas are most common, but fortunately occur in less than 1 percent of patients.[387] Benign giant-cell tumors may arise in skull and facial lesions. Multiple myeloma and metastatic carcinoma appear to be chance associations. Gout has been reported to affect males with great frequency, but this has not been a uniform finding.[385] An increase in cardiac output may be found in patients whose disease involves 20 percent or more of the skeleton,[388] but intractable high-output cardiac failure is seldom encountered.

Radiologic Features

The earliest lesions of Paget's disease that can be detected radiologically are osteolytic in nature. In the skull, these early lesions have been termed *osteoporosis circumscripta* (Fig. 23-11). Osteolytic lesions in the extremities are usually found at either end of the affected bone and advance as a V-shaped osteolytic front at an average rate of 1 cm per year.

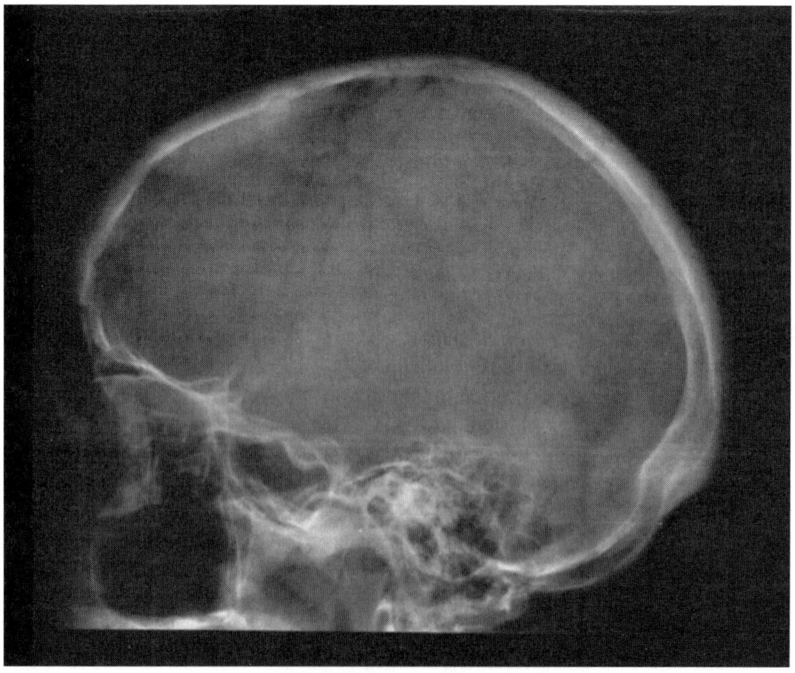

FIGURE 23-11. Roentgenogram of the skull of a 48-year-old patient with osteoporosis circumsripta due to Paget's disease.

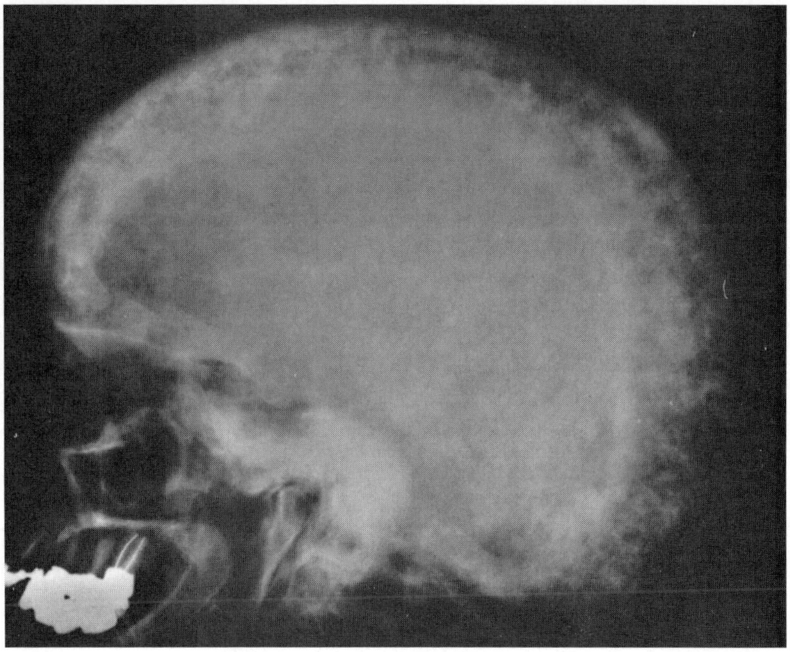

FIGURE 23-12. Roentgenogram of the skull of a 63-year-old patient with the osteoblastic phase of Paget's disease.

The evolution of osteolytic lesions into an osteoblastic phase may require years or even decades. In the skull, there is thickening of the calvarium with a loss of definition of the inner and outer tables. A "cotton wool" appearance due to a patchy increase in bone density is common (Fig. 23-12). Platybasia or basilar invagination may occur in far advanced disease. In the long bones, the osteolytic lesions are replaced by thickened trabeculae that obscure the corticomedullary border. Anterior and lateral bowing of the femur and tibia may develop. Incomplete fissure fractures can be seen on the convex surface of the femur. Pathologic fractures of the lower extremity produce a "chalk stick" rather than a spiral disruption of the bone. Osteoblastic lesions of the vertebrae may produce a "picture frame" appearance because of sclerosis of the vertebral borders, or they may produce a homogeneous increase in density.

Narrowing of the joint spaces of the hip and knee is observed in patients with Paget's disease and degenerative arthritis.[385] Osteophyte formation may be present at these sites and in the spine. Protrusio acetabuli may occur with extensive pagetic involvement of the pelvis.

The radiologic features of a sarcoma include cortical destruction and a soft tissue mass which may exhibit patchy calcification.

Computed tomography and magnetic resonance imaging of the spine are valuable techniques for demonstrating lesions such as spinal stenosis and are quite useful in the evaluation of patients with severe back pain.[382]

The metabolic activity of the lesions of Paget's disease is most easily assessed by nuclear medicine techniques (Fig. 23-13). The administration of bone-seeking radioisotopes such as technetium-labeled bisphosphonates to patients with localized disease may be the only noninvasive means of demonstrating disease activity, since biochemical parameters may be normal in monostotic cases.[389] Bone scans also can detect early lesions of Paget's disease before there is a discernible radiologic abnormality.[390] During treatment of Paget's disease with a variety of agents, bone scans can reflect suppression of disease activity. In one study,[391] gallium scans were found to correlate better with suppression of biochemical parameters than did technetium bisphosphonate bone scans.

Laboratory Findings

The serum calcium and phosphorus concentrations are usually normal in ambulatory patients with Paget's disease. Immobilization because of neurologic complications or after a fracture may cause serious hypercalcemia.[392] Hypercalcemia also may reflect the presence of associated primary hyperparathyroidism, and it has been suggested that there is an increased incidence of hyperparathyroidism in patients with Paget's disease.[393] Control studies of an age-matched population have not been adequate to establish this association convincingly.

Radiocalcium kinetic studies have revealed a markedly increased rate of bone turnover in patients with polyostotic Paget's disease.[392] This is more easily demonstrated by the elevated serum alkaline phosphatase activity and increased urinary hydroxyproline excretion found in these patients. In patients with monostotic disease involving a small bone such as a vertebra, all the above studies may be normal. Serum osteocalcin and urinary collagen crosslink levels may be abnormal in Paget's disease, but do not clearly provide a better index of bone formation and bone resorption in most patients than do alkaline phosphatase and hydroxyproline measurements, respectively.

Urinary calcium excretion is usually normal, although hypercalciuria may be present if the rate of bone resorption exceeds that of bone formation.[392] This occurs primarily in immobilized patients. In ambulatory patients, even with extensive active Paget's disease, the resorption and formation rates are usually closely coupled.

Bone Pathology

The earliest lesion of Paget's disease is a localized area of osteolysis which is produced by an increased number of osteoclasts.[382]

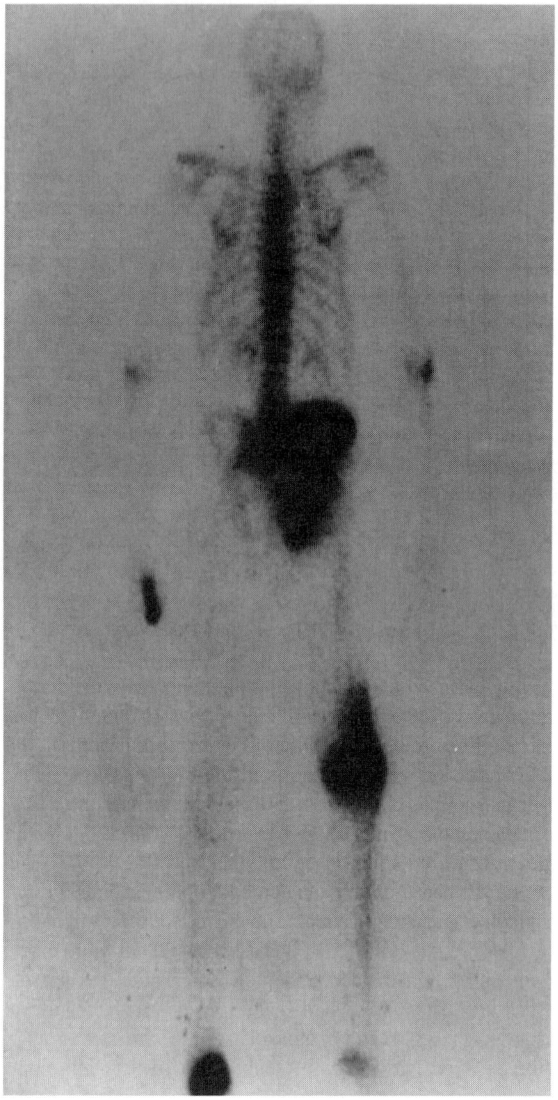

FIGURE 23-13. Bone scan of a 73-year-old patient with Paget's disease involving the left hemipelvis, the distal left femur, the right hand, and the right foot.

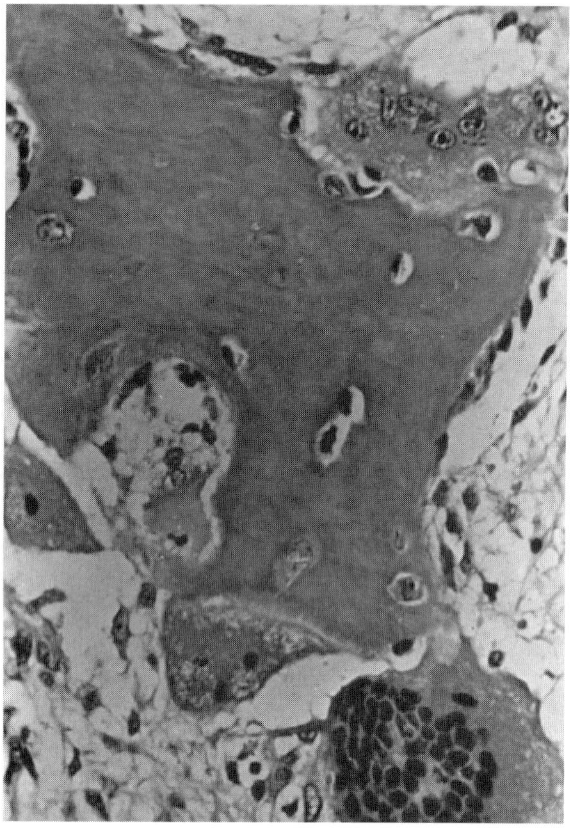

FIGURE 23-14. Several large multinucleated osteoclasts in Howship lacunae. More than 50 nuclei are present in the osteoclast at the bottom. Note the numerous osteoblasts at the bone surface on the right. Decalcified, H&E.

The osteoclasts of Paget's disease are heterogeneous in size; some may have up to 100 nuclei in a single cross section (Fig. 23-14). Giant osteoclasts of this size are rarely found in metabolic bone disease.

Most bone biopsies or surgical specimens show a combination of intensive osteoclastic bone resorption and large numbers of active osteoblasts which are forming bone at sites of previous osteoclastic resorption (Fig. 23-14). The marrow is also found to contain dense fibrovascular tissue containing numerous fibroblasts and osteoprogenitor cells.

In the quiescent, or "burned-out," phase of Paget's disease, the number of bone cells is markedly reduced and the bone marrow consists mainly of fat cells. A single bone may harbor an advancing osteolytic front, a trailing mixed osteoclastic-osteoblastic pattern, and a burned-out stage of the disease.

The intense cellular activity of Paget's disease produces a characteristic chaotic pattern of bone matrix termed the *mosaic pattern*. The bone is partly lamellar in character, with woven bone interspersed between incomplete osteons. A high percentage of bone surface is covered by osteoid, but mineralization is usually normal. The rate of bone formation as determined by double labeling with tetracycline is often increased.

Studies of the ultrastructure of bone cells in Paget's disease have demonstrated characteristic nuclear and cytoplasmic inclusions in the osteoclasts of all patients whose cells have been examined.[394,395] These inclusions consist of numerous microfibrillar structures that are similar in appearance to the viral nucleocapsids of paramyxoviruses and pneumoviruses (Fig. 23-15). The inclusions have not been found in the osteoblasts or osteocytes of Paget's disease or in bone cells from normal subjects. In variable degree, they have also been observed in the osteoclasts of some patients with pycnodysostosis, giant cell tumor of bone, and osteopetrosis.[396]

Pathogenesis

Sir James Paget believed that Paget's disease is inflammatory in nature—hence the term *osteitis deformans*.[381] Because no infectious agent could be recovered from pathologic specimens, this hypothesis was discarded early in this century. The uniform finding of nuclear and cytoplasmic inclusions in the osteoclasts of Paget's disease has revived the search for an infectious cause of the disorder. It is now appreciated that viruses may produce chronic indolent disorders of the nervous system, termed *slow*

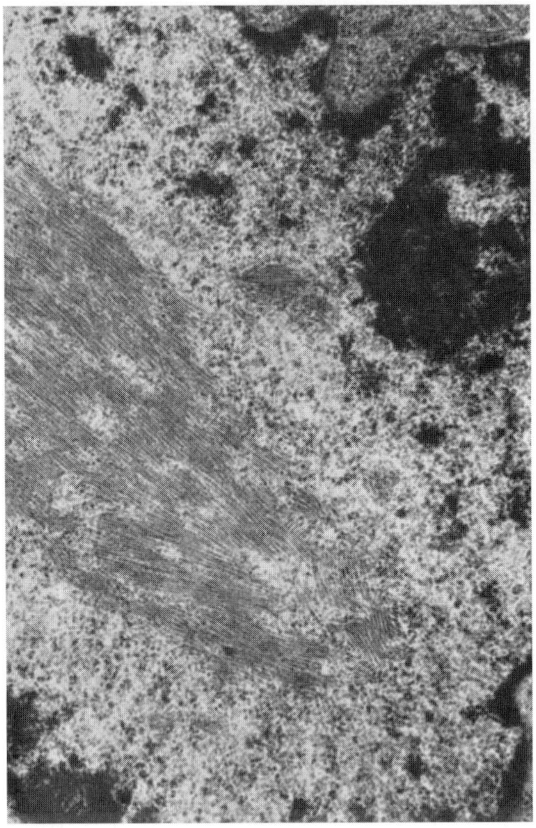

FIGURE 23-15. Characteristic microfibrillar nuclear inclusion found in osteoclasts of patients with Paget's disease.

virus infections, which share many clinical and pathologic features with Paget's disease.[397] These shared features include involvement of a single organ, a prolonged latent period, absence of fever and an acute inflammatory process, giant cells, and intracellular inclusions. Immunocytologic evidence indicates that measles and/or respiratory syncytial virus antigens are present in the osteoclasts of Paget's disease.[398,399] Viral mRNA sequences of measles virus or canine distemper virus have been detected in bone or marrow mononuclear cells of pagetic patients by some but not all investigators.[396] The reasons for the differences in the results of these molecular studies are unknown, but the ultrastructural, immunohistologic, and positive molecular studies taken together strongly implicates a viral presence in Paget's disease. Considerable new insights into the pathogenesis of Paget's disease should emerge when further progress has been made in better defining the osteoclast inclusions and the nature of the gene abnormalities in families with 18q linkage.

Drug Treatment

A variety of medications can now be offered to patients with Paget's disease who previously would have had little chance for relief of their symptoms.

Indications for Drug Treatment

The indications for treatment have evolved during the past 25 years as new and increasingly more effective drugs have become available. Some reasons to prescribe drug therapy are listed in Table 23-6. Bone pain is one of the most common indications. If the pain is adjacent to a joint, bone pain may be difficult to distinguish from joint pain. In this situation treating Paget's disease may clarify the origin of the pain since arthritic pain is not relieved by specific therapy for Paget's disease. In preparation for elective orthopaedic surgery on pagetic bone or after emergency surgery for a fracture it seems appropriate to institute therapy in order to prevent acceleration of the osteolytic process, reduce bleeding, and prevent hypercalcemia. If hypercalcemia occurs as a consequence of immobilization, drug therapy should reverse this promptly. Recurrent urinary calculi associated with hypercalciuria should be prevented by therapy. Neurological syndromes associated with the spinal cord or nerves may occasionally be reversed by drugs. Drug therapy can reduce increased cardiac output and may benefit patients with underlying heart disease. Prevention of complications in patients with skull, vertebral, pelvic, and lower extremity disease may be a major benefit of treatment, but has not been proven in long-term clinical trials.

TABLE 23-6. Indications for Drug Treatment of Paget's Disease

1. Bone pain
2. Orthopaedic Surgery
   A. Preoperative
   B. After emergency surgery for fracture
3. Hypercalcemia associated with immobilization
4. Recurrent urinary calculi associated with hypercalciuria
5. Neurological deficits associated with spinal disease
6. Increased cardiac output
7. Prevention of complications

Calcitonin

In 1975, salmon calcitonin became the first drug approved for Paget's disease in the United States. It was evaluated in this disorder because in animal studies it was found to be effective in suppressing the activity and numbers of osteoclasts, the cells believed to be the primary mediators of the disease. Treatment was instituted by subcutaneous injections, of 50–100 units, usually on a daily basis. The first day a decrease in urinary hydroxyproline excretion and mild hypocalcemia and hypophosphatemia could be seen, signifying a reduction of bone resorption.[382] The serum alkaline phosphatase activity usually decreased two to four weeks later, indicating that a fall in bone formation was a secondary effect in response to reduced bone resorption.[382] During a period of months of continued treatment urinary hydroxyproline excretion and serum alkaline phosphatase activity decreased on the average by 50 percent whether there were modest or quite high levels of these biochemical indices.[382] If treatment was continued for years the majority of patients remained at a plateau of biochemical responsiveness, in the normal range if the baseline tests were elevated twofold or less, or at much higher levels if the disease was more extensive. In up to 25 percent of patients, the biochemical indices returned to baseline levels despite continuous treatment. These patients nearly always developed high titers of antisalmon calcitonin antibodies in the circulation.[382] These patients could be successfully treated again if human calcitonin was administered, demonstrating the specificity of the antibodies toward blocking the biological activity of salmon calcitonin.[382]

Coincident with lowering of the biochemical indices of Paget's disease, salmon calcitonin produced the following effects: (1) relief of bone pain usually within one to two weeks, (2) reduction of increased skin temperature over affected extremities, (3) healing of osteolytic lesions seen in x-rays, (4) reduction of bone cell activity and woven bone in bone biopsies, (5) reduction of elevated cardiac output, (6) improvement of neurologic deficits, and (7) stabilization of decreased auditory acuity.

Side effects occurred in up to 20 percent of patients treated with subcutaneous salmon calcitonin but often did not result in discontinuation of treatment. The more common were nausea, facial flushing, and a metallic taste sensation. Abdominal pain and diarrhea were rare as were tetany and allergic reactions. Although acute increases in serum parathyroid hormone could be measured in response to acute hypocalcemia, secondary hyperparathyroidism did not become a clinical problem.[382]

Salmon calcitonin is now infrequently used in the treatment of Paget's disease for a variety of reasons. Frequent injections are required, while newer agents can be taken by mouth or be given intravenously infrequently. There are considerably more potent drugs available that can reduce the disease activity of more severely affected patients much better than salmon calcitonin. The hormone also lost effectiveness in a significant number of patients, as previously discussed. It should be noted that the nasal spray form of salmon calcitonin is not approved for Paget's disease because of its relatively low bioavailability in most patients, and that human calcitonin is no longer commercially available.

Bisphosphonates

Although the bisphosphonates are prescribed for greater numbers of patients with osteoporosis than Paget's disease, it is of interest that most of these agents were initially tested in patients with Paget's disease and that in the United States five bisphosphonates are approved for Paget's disease and two for osteoporosis. The approved bisphosphonates and their recommended dose schedules are summarized in Table 23-7.

Etidronate was initially approved for treatment of Paget's disease in 1977. It is administered orally at a dose of about 5 mg/kg body weight daily for 6 months.[382] The drug must be taken with water only and no food or other pills should be taken for at least 2 hours before or after etidronate. The drug produces a gradual decrease in biochemical indices that average 50 percent of baseline, the same as seen with calcitonin treatment. After 6 months of treatment biochemical remission may persist for months or occasionally years. Higher doses or more prolonged therapy may decrease the biochemical indices greater than 50 percent, but there is a risk of inducing osteomalacia due to impaired mineralization in these patients.[382] This could result in pathologic fractures of pagetic bone. In patients treated with the standard dose the clinical benefits are similar to those produced by salmon calcitonin with two exceptions. Bone pain may be transiently increased by etidronate as well as other bisphosphonates, but usually there is later pain relief. Osteolytic lesions usually do not improve and may even worsen after etidronate therapy.[382] Calcitonin therapy has improved the lesions in such instances. Because of the fear of inducing osteomalacia it has been advised to wait at least six months before repeating a course of treatment. This can be effective, but about 30 percent of patients become unresponsive to etidronate during the second or third treatment cycle.[400] These patients are responsive to other bisphosphonates. Etidronate is generally well tolerated. Some patients may develop loose stools. This is more likely in patients with intestinal disorders.

A group of bisphosphonates with greater potency than etidronate and less potential for producing osteomalacia have become available for treatment of Paget's disease since 1994. Pamidronate, alendronate, and risedronate are aminobisphosphonates with far greater potencies than etidronate. Tiludronate has a chlorophenyl side chain that confers only a modest increase in potency. Most of these agents have been compared to etidronate in clinical trials but not with each other.

Pamidronate is the only approved bisphosphonate (1994) used intravenously. A single infusion of 60 mg can reduce serum alkaline phosphatase activity and urinary hydroxyproline excretion to the normal range for one year or more in patients whose baseline indices are two to three times normal.[401] (Fig. 23-16). Patients with more severe disease may require additional infusions to bring the biochemical parameters into or near the normal range. It appears that pamidronate cannot completely suppress disease activity in all patients even if more than one gram is given during a period of one year.[402] The reason for this is unknown.

Intravenous pamidronate generally produces early relief of bone pain, although there may be a transient increase in pain. Improvement of osteolytic disease has also been described.

TABLE 23-7. Bisphosphonates Approved for Paget's Disease in the United States

Drug	Dosage and Administration Commonly Used
Etidronate disodium (Didronel®)	• 5 mg/kg BW/day for 6 months—tablet • No food or pills 2 h before or after • Can repeat, but preferably after at least 6 months of no drug
Pamidronate disodium (Aredia®)	• 60 or 90 mg intravenously over 2 h • May be repeated depending on biochemical response • More severely affected patients may require several infusions
Alendronate sodium (Fosamax®)	• 40-mg tablet daily for 6 months • Take in morning at least 30 min before breakfast with large glass of water. Do not lie down • May be repeated
Tiludronate disodium (Skelid®)	• 400-mg tablet daily for 3 months • No food or pills 2 h before or after • May be repeated
Risedronate sodium (Actonel®)	• 30-mg tablet daily for 2 months • Take in morning at least 30 min before breakfast or pills with water • May be repeated

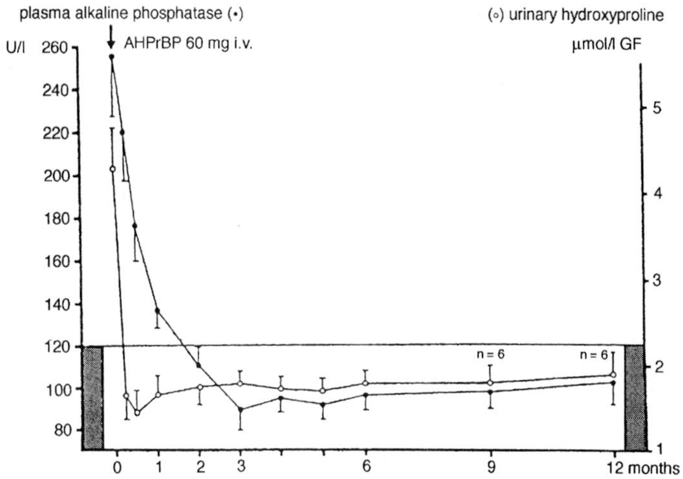

FIGURE 23-16. Plasma alkaline phosphatase (•) and urinary hydroxyproline (○) excretion (mean ± SEM) in 11 patients (n = 6 at 9 and 12 months) with Paget's disease before and up to one year after a single intravenous infusion of 60 mg pamidronate. (*From Thiebaud D et al: Am J Med 85:207, 1988.*)

In about 30 percent of patients treated with the initial infusion of pamidronate an acute phase reaction occurs, manifested by fever, chills, and myalgia. A similar response occurs with the dimethyl form of pamidronate and is associated with an acute rise in serum interleukin-6, which precedes the onset of symptoms.[403] This usually begins 8–12 h after the end of the infusion and seldom lasts more than 48 h. Rarely allergic reactions of the eye have occurred. Asymptomatic hypocalcemia is common. It is generally felt that calcium intake should be maintained at 1,000–1,500 mg daily to lessen the degree of hypocalcemia. A very small percentage of patients are nonresponsive to pamidronate,[404] and some patients who have received multiple infusions of pamidronate appear to become resistant to further treatment. Another bisphosphonate may prove effective.

In 1995 oral alendronate was approved for treatment of Paget's disease in addition to osteoporosis. A 40-mg daily dose over six months was established as very effective in suppressing bone turnover in Paget's diasease[405,406] as compared to 5–10 mg in postmenopausal osteoporosis. Serum alkaline phosphatase activity was reduced by 73 and 79 percent, and urinary collagen crosslink excretion by 86 percent and 75 percent in the two studies.[405,406] The serum alkaline phosphatase activity became normal in 48 and 63 percent of the patients and there was improvement in radiologic abnormalities in 48 percent of patients as compared to 4 percent in placebo-treated patients.[405] No defects in mineralization were found in bone biopsies and no serious gastrointestinal complications were noted. In the great majority of patients whose serum alkaline phosphatase activity was reduced to normal, this parameter remained suppressed for at least one year.

The most potent bisphosphonate available for treatment of Paget's disease, risedronate, was approved in 1998. A 30-mg tablet taken daily for two[407] or three[408] months produces an excellent biochemical remission. The 2-month course in 62 patients whose mean serum alkaline phosphatase activity was four times normal reduced enzyme activity by 69 percent and resulted in a normal level in 73 percent of patients by month 12 (Fig. 23-17). At month 18, 53 percent of the patients were still in biochemical remission. In a trial of risedronate in patients with more severe disease (mean alkaline phosphatase activity about seven times normal), 84 days of a daily 30-mg tablet was repeated 112 days later if enzyme activity was not normal.[408] Overall, nearly 54 percent of the patients had normal enzyme activity by the end of their followup. Bone pain was reduced significantly and the drug was well tolerated.

Tiludronate, approved in 1997, is somewhat more potent than etidronate, as a three month course of treatment with 400 mg tablets daily is more effective in reducing serum alkaline phosphatase activity than 6 months' treatment with etidronate.[409] Tiludronate also has been demonstrated to be effective in healing osteolytic lesions[410] and does not cause a mineralization defect. Although there are no comparative trials the aminobisphosphonates appear to be more effective in inducing full biochemical remissions than does tiludronate.

Miscellaneous Drugs

Plicamycin (mithramycin), calcium supplementation with chlorothalidone, and gallium nitrate have all been demonstrated to suppress disease activity with varying degrees of effectiveness.[302] None have become standard therapy, either because of considerations of relative toxicity to other therapy or because of the small numbers of patients evaluated.

Clodronate, an earlier bisphosphonate, is approved for treatment of Paget's disease in some countries.[382] Ibandronate and

FIGURE 23-17. Change from baseline in serum alkaline phosphatase concentrations in patients receiving risedronate 30 mg daily for 2 months (n = 62) or etidronate 400 mg daily for 6 months (n = 61). Data are means ± SEM. The biochemical improvement was significantly better for risedronate-treated patients at each time point. (*From Miller PD et al: A randomized, double-blind comparison of risedronate and etidronate in the treatment of Paget's disease of bone. Am J Med 106:513, 1999.*)

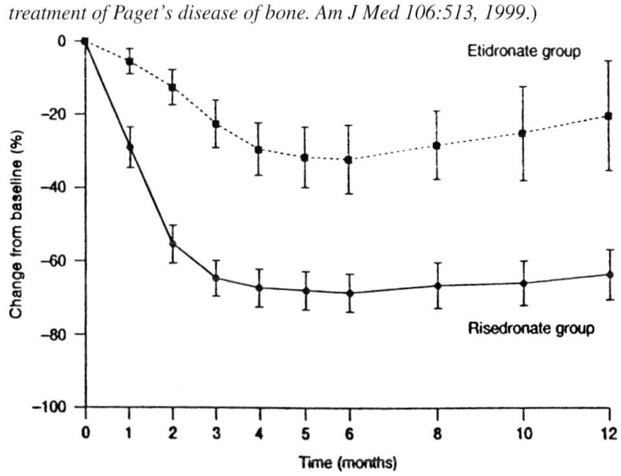

zoledronate are powerful newer aminobisphosphonates under study that can be safely administered intravenously over minutes.

Choice of Drug

Any of the available drugs is likely to be effective in suppressing disease activity in patients with mild disease (alkaline phosphatase activity up to twice normal). Because treatment with salmon calcitonin requires nearly continuous administration and etidronate often loses effectiveness with time, these drugs should no longer be considered first-line therapy.

For patients with severe disease the aminobisphosphonates are highly effective. The choice of drug needs to be individualized according to the patient's desire for oral or intravenous therapy and the cost of treatment. Patients with preexisting esophageal or intestinal disease should tolerate intravenous therapy better than oral therapy.

Biochemical and Radiological Monitoring of Therapy

Measurement of total serum alkaline phosphatase activity appears to be sufficient for pretreatment and followup evaluation of disease activity in most patients. To determine the effect of therapy the test can be done every one to two months until a plateau is reached (preferably in the normal range). Then evaluation could be every three to four months. This allows early determination of reactivation of disease activity.

In patients with discernible osteolytic lesions a follow-up radiograph one year after initiating therapy is useful in assessing the efficacy of treatment. If improvement is noted the radiograph could be repeated biannually or more frequently if biochemical suppression is not optimal. There appears to be no advantage in performing serial bone scans in most patients.

Surgery

Elective surgery is required in the management of certain patients with Paget's disease and may produce benefits which cannot be achieved by medical means.[382] Occipital decompression may be needed in patients with neurologic deficits secondary to basilar impression. Neurosurgery also may be necessary in patients with vertebral disease. Total hip replacement in patients with severe degenerative arthritis may permit pain-free normal ambulation. Patients with severe bowing of the tibia may have difficulty in ambulation not only because of deformity, but also because of painful degenerative arthritis of the knee. Tibial osteotomy can correct the anatomic abnormality as well as reduce the pain resulting from the arthritis, greatly improving ambulation. Total knee replacement is infrequently needed by patients with tibial deformities.

In a series of patients undergoing tibial osteotomy, treatment with calcitonin appeared to prevent excessive hemorrhage and postoperative hypercalcemia.[411] It is likely that any patient with Paget's disease requiring orthopedic surgery can benefit from treatment with a drug which suppresses the activity of the disease. Ideally, the treatment should be administered a minimum of 2 to 3 months before surgery.

REFERENCES

1. Albright FA, Reifenstein EC Jr: *The Parathyroid Glands and Metabolic Bone Disease*. Baltimore, Williams & Wilkins, 1948, p 81.
2. Endres DB, Villanueva R, Sharp CF Jr, Singer FR: Immunochemiluminometric and immunoradiometric determinations of intact and total immunoreactive parathyrin: Performance in the differential diagnosis of hypercalcemia and hypoparathyroidism. *Clin Chem* 37:162, 1991.
3. Calvo MS, Eyre DR, Gundberg CM: Molecular basis and clinical application of biological markers of bone turnover. *Endocr Rev* 17:333, 1996.
4. Uffmann M, Fuerst TP, Jergas M, Genant HK: Noninvasive assessment of bone, in Avioli LV, Krane SM (eds): Metabolic Bone Disease and Clinically Related Disorders, 3rd ed. San Diego, Academic Press, 1998, p 275.
5. Grampp S, Genant HK, Mathur A, Lang P, Jergas M, Takada M, Glüer C-C, Lu Y, Chavez M: Comparisons of non-invasive bone mineral measurements in assessing age-related loss, fracture discrimination, and diagnostic classification. *J Bone Miner Res* 12:697, 1997.
6. Bordier P, Matrajt H, Miravet L, Hioco D: Mésure histologique de la masse et de la résorption des travées osseuses. *Pathol Biol (Paris)* 12:1238, 1964.
7. Parfitt AM, Drezner MK, Glorieux FH, Kanis JA, Malluche H, Meunier PJ, Ott SM, Recker RR: Bone histomorphometry: Standardization of nomenclature, symbols, and units. *J Bone Miner Res* 2:595, 1987.
8. Harris WH, Jackson RH, Jowsey J: The in vivo distributions of tetracyclines in canine bone. *J Bone Joint Surg* [*Am*] 44A:1308, 1962.
9. Epker BN, Hattner R, Frost HM: Radial sites of osteon closure. *J Lab Clin Med* 64:643, 1964.
10. Glorieux FH, Karsenty G, Thakker RV: Metabolic bone disease in children, in Avioli LV, Krane SM (eds): *Metabolic Bone Disease and Clinically Related Disorders*, 3rd ed. San Diego, Academic Press, 1998, p 759.
11. Mankin H: Rickets, osteomalacia and renal osteodystrophy. *J Bone Joint Surg* [*Am*] 56A:101, 1974.
12. Fraser D, Kooh SW, Scriver CR: Hyperparathyroidism as the cause of hyperaminoaciduria and phosphaturia in human vitamin D deficiency. *Pediatr Res* 1:425, 1967.
13. Fraser D, Kooh SW, Kind HP, Holick MF, Tanaka Y, DeLuca HF: Pathogenesis of hereditary vitamin D dependent rickets: An inborn error of vitamin D metabolism involving defective conversion of 25-hydroxyvitamin D to 1α,25-dihydroxyvitamin D. *N Engl J Med* 289:817, 1973.
14. Brooks MH, Bell NH, Love L, Stern PH, Orfei E, Queener SF, Hamstra AJ, DeLuca HF: Vitamin D dependent rickets type II: Resistance of target organs to 1,25-dihydroxyvitamin D. *N Engl J Med* 298:996, 1978.
15. Arnaud CD, Glorieux F, Scriver CR: Serum parathyroid hormone levels in acquired vitamin D deficiency. *Pediatrics* 49:837, 1972.
16. Vainsel M, Manderlier T, Otten J: Urinary excretion of adenosine 3′,5′-monophosphate in vitamin D deficiency. *Eur J Clin Invest* 6:127, 1976.
17. Robins SP, Black D, Paterson CR, Reid DM, Duncan A, Seibel MJ: Evaluation of urinary hydroxypyridinium crosslink measurements as resorption markers in metabolic bone diseases. *Eur J Clin Invest* 21:310, 1991.
18. Haussler MR, McCain TA: Basic and clinical concepts related to vitamin D metabolism and action. *N Engl J Med* 297:1041, 1977.
19. Eastwood JB, DeWardener HE, Gray RW, Lemann JL Jr: Normal plasma 1,25-(OH)2-vitamin D concentrations in nutritional osteomalacia. *Lancet* 1:1377, 1979.
20. Parfitt AM: Osteomalacia and related disorders, in Avioli LV, Krane SM (eds): *Metabolic Bone Disease and Clinically Related Disorders*, 3rd ed. San Diego, Academic Press, 1998, p 328.
21. Marie PJ, Glorieux FH: Relation between hypomineralized periosteocytic lesions and bone mineralization in vitamin D resistant rickets. *Calcif Tissue Int* 35:443, 1983.
22. Loomis WF: Rickets. *Sci Am* 223:77, 1970.
23. Bachrach S, Fisher J, Parks JS: An outbreak of vitamin D deficiency rickets in a susceptible population. *Pediatrics* 64:871, 1979.
24. Dwyer JT, Dietz WH Jr, Hass G, Suskind R: Risk of nutritional rickets among vegetarian children. *Am J Dis Child* 133:134, 1979.
25. Thompson GR, Lewis B, Booth CC: Absorption of vitamin D_3-^3H in control subjects and patients with intestinal malabsorption. *J Clin Invest* 45:94, 1966.

26. Arnaud SB, Goldsmith RS, Lambert PW, Go VLW: 25-Hydroxyvitamin D_3: Evidence of an enterohepatic circulation in man. *Proc Soc Exp Biol Med* 149:570, 1975.
27. Parfitt AM, Podenphant J, Villanueva AR, Frame B: Metabolic bone disease with and without osteomalacia after intestinal bypass surgery: A bone histomorphometric study. *Bone* 6:211, 1985.
28. Stellon AJ, Webb A, Compston J, Williams R: Lack of osteomalacia in chronic cholestatic liver disease. *Bone* 7:181, 1986.
29. Bikle DD, Halloran BP, Gee E, Ryzen E, Haddad JG: Free 25-hydroxyvitamin D levels are normal in subjects with liver disease and reduced total 25-hydroxyvitamin D levels. *J Clin Invest* 78:748, 1986.
30. Horst RL, Jorgensen NA, DeLuca HF: The determination of 24,25-dihydroxyvitamin D and 25,26-dihydroxyvitamin D in plasma from normal and nephrectomized man. *J Lab Clin Med* 93:277, 1979.
31. Richens A, Rowe DJF: Disturbance of calcium metabolism by anticonvulsant drugs. *Br Med J* 4:73, 1970.
32. Hahn TJ: Drug-induced disorders of vitamin D and mineral metabolism. *Clin Endocrinol Metab* 9:107, 1980.
33. Nuovo MA, Dorfman HD, Sun CJ, Chalew SA: Tumor-induced osteomalacia and rickets. *Am J Surg Pathol* 13:588, 1989.
34. Lyles KW, Berry WR, Haussler M, Harrelson JM, Drezner MK: Hypophosphatemic osteomalacia: Association with prostatic carcinoma. *Ann Intern Med* 93:275, 1980.
35. Wang JT, Lin CJ, Burridge SM, Fu GK, Labuda M, Portale AA, Miller WL: Genetics of vitamin D 1alpha-hydroxylase deficiency in 17 families. *Am J Hum Genet* 63:1694, 1998.
36. Schmidt-Gayk H, Schmitt W, Grawunder C, Ritz E, Tschoepe W, Pietsch V, Andrassy K, Bouillon R: 25-Hydroxy-vitamin D in nephrotic syndrome. *Lancet* 2:105, 1977.
37. Malluche HH, Goldstein DA, Massry SG: Osteomalacia and hyperparathyroid bone disease in patients with nephrotic syndrome. *J Clin Invest* 63:494, 1979.
38. Mittal SK, Dash SC, Tiwari SC, Agarwal SK, Saxena S, Fishbane S: Bone histology in patients with nephrotic syndrome and normal renal function. *Kidney Int* 55:1912, 1999.
39. Liberman UA, Samuel R, Halabe A, Kauli R, Edelstein S, Weisman Y, Papapoulos SE, Clemens TL, et al: End-organ resistance to 1,25-dihydroxycholecalciferol. *Lancet* 1:504, 1980.
40. Marx SJ, Bliziotes MM, Nanes M: Analysis of the relation between alopecia and resistance to 1,25-dihydroxyvitamin D. *Clin Endocrinol (Oxf)* 25:373, 1986.
41. Haussler MR, Haussler CA, Jurutka PW, Thompson PD, Hsieh JC, Remus LS, Selznick SH, Whitfield GK: The vitamin D hormone and its nuclear receptor: molecular actions and disease states. *J Endocrinol* 154:S57, 1997.
42. Brickman AS, Coburn JW, Massry SG: 1,25-Dihydroxyvitamin D_3 in normal man and patients with renal failure. *Ann Intern Med* 80:161, 1974.
43. Albright F, Butler AM, Bloomberg E: Rickets resistant to vitamin D therapy. *Am J Dis Child* 54:529, 1937.
44. The HYP Consortium: A gene (PEX) with homologies to endopeptidases is mutated in patients with x-linked hypophosphatemic rickets. *Nat Genet* 11:130, 1995.
45. Dixon PH, Christie PT, Wooding C, Trump D, Grieff M, Holm I, Gertner JM, Schmidtke J, Shah B, Shaw N, Smith C, Tau C, Schlessinger D, Whyte MP, Thakker RV: Mutational analysis in x-linked hypophosphatemia. *J Clin Endocrinol Metab* 83:3615, 1998.
46. Winters RW, Graham JB, Williams TF, McFalls VW, Burnett CH: A genetic study of familial hypophosphatemia and vitamin D resistant rickets with a review of the literature. *Medicine (Baltimore)* 37:97, 1958.
47. Adams JE, Davies M: Intra-spinal new bone formation and spinal cord compression in familial hypophosphatemic vitamin D resistant osteomalacia. *Q J Med* (new series) 61:117, 1986.
48. Reitz R, Weinstein RL: Parathyroid hormone seretion in familial vitamin-D-resistant rickets. *N Engl J Med* 289:941, 1973.
49. Short E, Morris RC Jr, Sebastian A, Spencer M: Exaggerated phosphaturic response to circulating parathyroid hormone in patients with familial X-linked hypophosphatemic rickets. *J Clin Invest* 58:152, 1976.
50. Lyles KW, Burkes EJ Jr, McNamara CR, Harrelson JM, Pickett JP, Drezner MK: The concurrence of hypoparathyroidism provides new insights to the pathophysiology of X-linked hypophosphatemic rickets. *J Clin Endocrinol Metab* 60:711, 1985.
51. Condon JR, Nassim JR, Rutter A: Defective intestinal phosphate absorption in familial and non-familial hypophosphatemia. *Br Med J* 3:138, 1970.
52. Chesney RW, Mazess RB, Rose P, Hamstra AJ, DeLuca HF: Supranormal 25-hydroxyvitamin D and subnormal 1,25-dihydroxyvitamin D: Their role in X-linked hypophosphatemic rickets. *Am J Dis Child* 134:140, 1980.
53. Seino Y, Shimotsuji T, Ishii T, Ishida M, Ikehara C, Yamaoka K, Yabwichi H, Dokoh S: Treatment of hypophosphatemic vitamin D resistant rickets with massive dose of 1α-hydroxyvitamin D_3 during childhood. *Arch Dis Child* 55:49, 1980.
54. Delvin EE, Glorieux FH: Serum 1,25-dihydroxyvitamin D concentration in hypophosphatemic vitamin D resistant rickets. *Calif Tissue Int* 33:173, 1981.
55. Lyles KW, Drezner MK: Parathyroid hormone effects on serum 1,25-dihydroxyvitamin D levels in patients with X-linked hypophosphatemic rickets: Evidence for abnormal 25-hydroxyvitamin D 1-hydroxylase activity. *J Clin Endocrinol Metab* 54:638, 1982.
56. Brickman AS, Coburn JW, Kurokawa K, Bethune JE, Harrison HE, Norman AW: Actions of 1,25-dihydroxycholecalciferol in patients with hypophosphatemic, vitamin D resistant rickets. *N Engl J Med* 289:495, 1973.
57. Stamp TCB, Baker LRI: Recessive hypophosphatemic rickets, and possible etiology of the "vitamin D resistant" syndrome. *Arch Dis Child* 51:360, 1976.
58. Perry W, Stamp TCB: Hereditary hypophosphatemic rickets with autosomal recessive inheritance and severe osteosclerosis. *J Bone Joint Surg [Br]* 60B:430, 1978.
59. Tieder M, Modai D, Shaked U, Samuel R, Arie R, Halabe A, Maor J, Weissgarten J, et al: "Idiopathic" hypercalciuria and hereditary hypophosphatemic rickets. *N Engl J Med* 316:125, 1987.
60. Econs MJ, McEnery PT: Autosomal dominant hypophosphatemic rickets/osteomalacia: Clinical characterization of a novel renal wasting disorder. *J Clin Endocrinol Metab* 82:674, 1997.
61. Econs MJ, McEnery PT, Lennon F, Speer MC: Autosomal dominant hypophosphatemic rickets is linked to chromosome 12p13. *J Clin Invest* 100:2653, 1997.
62. Nagant de Deuxchaisnes C, Krane SM: The treatment of adult phosphate diabetes and Fanconi syndrome with neutral sodium phosphate. *Am J Med* 43:508, 1967.
63. Frymoyer JW, Hodgkin W: Adult-onset vitamin D resistant hypophosphatemic osteomalacia: A possible variant of vitamin D resistant rickets. *J Bone Joint Surg [Am]* 59A:101, 1977.
64. Econs MJ, Friedman NE, Rowe PSN, Speer MC, Francis F, Strom TM, Oudet C, Smith JA, Ninomiya JT, Lee BE, Bergen H: A PHEX gene mutation is responsible for adult-onset vitamin D–resistant hypophosphatemic osteomalacia: evidence that the disorder is not a distinct entity from x-linked hypophosphatemic rickets. *J Clin Endocrinol Metab* 83:3459, 1998.
65. Minari M, Castellani A, Garella S: Renal tubular acidosis associated with vitamin D resistant rickets: Role of phosphate depletion. *Miner Electrolyte Metab* 10:371, 1984.
66. Dent CE, Gertner JM: Hypophosphatemic osetomalacia in fibrous dysplasia. *Q J Med* 45:411, 1976.
67. McArthur RG, Hayles AB, Lambert PW: Albright's syndrome with rickets. *Mayo Clin Proc* 54:313, 1979.
68. Aschinberg LC, Solomon LM, Zeis PM, Justice P, Rosenthal IM: Vitamin D resistant rickets associated with epidermal nevus syndrome: Demonstration of a phosphaturic substance in the dermal lesions. *J Pediatr* 91:56, 1977.
69. Wilkins GE, Granleese S, Hegele RG, Holden J, Anderson DW, Bondy GP: Oncogenic osteomalacia: Evidence for a humoral phosphaturic factor. *J Clin Endocrinol Metab* 80:1628, 1995.
70. Takeda E, Taketani Y, Morita K, Miyamoto K: Sodium-dependent phosphate co-transporters. *Int J Biochem Cell Biol* 31:377, 1999.
71. Bressot C, Courpron P, Edouard C, Meunier P: *Histomorphometrie des ostéopathies endocriniennes*. Lyon, Association Corporative des Étudiants en Médecine de Lyon, 1976, p 117.
72. Dent CE, Winter CE: Osteomalacia due to phosphate depletion from excessive aluminum hydroxide ingestion. *Br Med J* 1:551, 1974.
73. Ahmed KY, Varghese Z, Wills MR, Meinhard E, Skinner RK, Baillod RA, Moorhead JE: Persistent hypophosphatemia and

osteomalacia in dialysis patients not on oral phosphate binders: Response to dihydrotachysterol therapy. *Lancet* 2:439, 1976.
74. Teotia SPS, Teotioa M: Secondary hyperparathyroidism in patients with endemic skeletal fluorosis. *Br Med J* 1:637, 1973.
75. Balena R, Kleerekoper M, Foldes JA, Shih MS, Rao DS, Schober HC, Parfitt AM: Effects of different regimens of sodium fluoride treatment for osteoporosis on the structure, remodeling and mineralization of bone. *Osteoporosis Int* 8:428, 1998.
76. Khairi MRA, Altman RD, DeRosa GP, Zimmerman J, Schenk RK, Johnston CC: Sodium etidronate in the treatment of Paget's disease of bone: A study of long-term results. *Ann Intern Med* 87:656, 1977.
77. Boyce BF, Smith L, Fogelman I, Johnston E, Ralston S, Boyle IT: Focal osteomalacia due to low dose diphosphonate therapy in Paget's disease. *Lancet* 1:821, 1984.
78. Adamson BB, Gallacher SJ, Byars J, Ralston SH, Boyle IT, Boyce BF: Mineralisation defects with pamidronate therapy for Paget's disease. *Lancet* 342:1459, 1993.
79. Kooh SW, Fraser D, Reilly BJ, Hamilton JR, Gall DG, Bell L: Rickets due to calcium deficiency. *N Engl J Med* 297:1264, 1977.
80. Pettifor JM, Ross FP, Travers R, Glorieux FH, DeLuca HF: Dietary calcium deficiency: A syndrome associated with bone deformities and elevated serum 1,25-dihydroxyvitamin D concentrations. *Metab Bone Dis Rel Res* 2:301, 1981.
81. Marie PJ, Pettifor JM, Ross FP, Glorieux FH: Histological osteomalacia due to dietary calcium deficiency in children. *N Engl J Med* 307:584, 1982.
82. Legius E, Proesmans W, Eggermont E, Vandamme-Lombaerts R, Bouillon R, Smet M: Rickets due to dietary calcium deficiency. *Eur J Pediatr* 148:784, 1989.
83. Albright F: Hypoparathyroidism as a cause of osteomalacia. *J Clin Endocrinol Metab* 16:419, 1956.
84. Schutt-Aine JC, Young MA, Pescovitz OH, Chrousos GP, Marx SJ: Hypoparathyroidism: A possible cause of rickets. *J Pediatr* 106:255, 1985.
85. Hanukoglu A, Chalew S, Sowarski AA: Late-onset hypocalcemia, rickets, and hypoparathyroidism in an infant of a mother with hyperparathyroidism. *J Pediatr* 112:751, 1988.
86. Lamm CI, Norton KI, Murphy RJC, Wilkins IA, Rabinowitz JG: Congenital rickets associated with magnesium sulfate infusion for tocolysis. *J Pediatr* 113:1078, 1988.
87. Wilson JD, Hadden DR: Pseudohypoparathyroidism presenting with rickets. *J Clin Endocrinol Metab* 51:1184, 1980.
88. Whyte MP: Hypophosphatasia, in Scriver CR, Beaudet AL, Sly WS, Valle D (eds): The Metabolic and Molecular Bases of Inherited Disease, 7th ed. New York, McGraw-Hill, 1995, p 4095.
89. Whyte MP, Teitelbaum SL, Murphy WA, Bergfeld MA, Avioli LV: Adult hypophosphatasia: Clinical, laboratory, and genetic investigation of a large kindred with review of the literature. *Medicine (Baltimore)* 58:329, 1979.
90. Frame B, Frost HM, Pak CYC, Reynolds W, Argen RJ: Fibrogenesis imperfecta ossium: A collagen defect causing osteomalacia. *N Engl J Med* 285:769, 1971.
91. Carr AJ, Smith R, Athanasou N, Woods DG: Fibrogenesis imperfecta ossium. *J Bone Joint Surg [Br]* 77:820, 1995.
92. Chesney RW, Kaplan BS, Phelps M, DeLuca HF: Renal tubular acidosis does not alter circulating values of calcitriol. *J Pediatr* 104:51, 1984.
93. Kraut JA, Gordon EM, Ransom JC, Horst R, Slatopolsky E, Coburn JW, Kurokawa K: Effect of chronic metabolic acidosis on vitamin D metabolism in humans. *Kidney Int* 24:644, 1983.
94. Phelps KR, Einhorn TA, Vigorita VJ, Lieberman RL, Uribarri J: Acidosis-induced osteomalacia: Metabolic studies and skeletal histomorphometry. *Bone* 79:171, 1986.
95. Shike M, Harrison JE, Sturtridge WC, Tam CS, Bobechko PE, Jones G, Murray TM, Jeejeebhoy KN: Metabolic bone disease in patients receiving long-term total parenteral nutrition. *Ann Intern Med* 92:343, 1980.
96. Klein GL, Targoff CM, Ament ME, Sherrard DJ, Bluestone R, Young JH, Norman AW, Coburn JW: Bone disease associated with total parenteral nutrition. *Lancet* 2:1041, 1980.
97. Ott SM, Maloney NA, Klein GL, Alfrey AC, Ament ME, Coburn JW, Sherrard DJ: Aluminum is associated with low bone formation in patients receiving chronic parenteral nutrition. *Ann Intern Med* 98:910, 1983.
98. Stamp TCB, Round MM, Rowe DJF, Haddad JG: Plasma levels and therapeutic effect of 25-hydroxycholecalciferol in epileptic patients taking anticonvulsant drugs. *Br Med J* 4:9, 1972.
99. Balsan S, Garabedian M, Larchet M, Gorski AM, Cournot G, Tau C, Bourdeau A, Silve C, Ricour C: Long-term nocturnal calcium infusions can cure rickets and promote normal mineralization in hereditary resistance to 1,25-dihydroxyvitamin D. *J Clin Invest* 77:1661, 1986.
100. Sakati N, Woodhouse NJY, Niles N, Harfi H, de Grange DA, Marx S: Hereditary resistance to 1,25-dihydroxyvitamin D: Clinical and radiological improvement during high-dose oral calcium therapy. *Horm Res* 24:280, 1986.
101. Glorieux FH, Scriver CR, Reade TM, Goldman H, Roseborough A: Use of phosphate and vitamin D to prevent dwarfism and rickets in X-linked hypophosphatemia. *N Engl J Med* 287:481, 1972.
102. Lyles KW, Harrelson JM, Drezner MK: The efficacy of vitamin D and oral phosphorus therapy in X-linked hypophosphatemic rickets and osteomalacia. *J Clin Endocrinol Metab* 54:307, 1982.
103. Kirschman GH, DeLuca HF, Chan JCM: Hypophosphatemic vitamin D resistant rickets: Metabolic balance studies in a child receiving 1,25-dihydroxyvitamin D_3, phosphate, and ascorbic acid. *Pediatrics* 61:451, 1978.
104. Glorieux FH, Marie PJ, Pettifor JM, Delvin EE: Bone response to phosphate salts, ergocalciferol, and calcitriol in hypophosphatemic rickets. *N Engl J Med* 303:1023, 1980.
105. Harrell RM, Lyles KW, Harrelson JM, Friedman NE, Drezner MK: Healing of bone disease in X-linked hypophosphatemic rickets/osteomalacia: Induction and maintenance with phosphorus and calcitriol. *J Clin Invest* 75:1858, 1985.
106. Firth RG, Grant CS, Riggs BL: Development of hypercalcemic hyperparathyroidism after long-term phosphate supplementation in hypophoshatemic osteomalacia. *Am J Med* 78:669, 1985.
107. Carpenter TO, Keller M, Schwartz D, Mitnick M, Smith C, Ellison A, Carey D, Comite F, Horst R, Travers R, Glorieux FH, Gundberg CM, Poole AR, Insogna KL: 24,25 dihydroxyvitamin D supplementation corrects hyperparathyroidism and improves skeletal abnormalities in x-linked hypophosphatemic rickets—A clinical research center study. *J Clin Endocrinol Metab* 81:2381, 1996.
108. Goodyer PR, Kronick JB, Jequier S, Reade TM, Scriver CR: Nephrocalcinosis and its relationship to treatment of hereditary rickets. *J Pediatr* 3:700, 1986.
109. Stickler GB, Morgenstern BZ: Hypophosphatemic rickets: Final height and clinical symptoms in adults. *Lancet* 2:902, 1989.
110. Balsan SB, Tieder M: Linear growth in patients with hypophosphatemic vitamin D resistant rickets: Influence of treatment regimen and parental height. *J Pediatr* 116:365, 1990.
111. Scriver CR, Tenenhouse HS, Glorieux FH: X-linked hypophosphatemia: An appreciation of a classic paper and a survey of progress since 1958. *Medicine (Baltimore)* 70:218, 1991.
112. Verge CF, Lam A, Simpson JM, Cowell CT, Howard NJ, Silink M: Effects of therapy in X-linked hypophosphatemic rickets. *N Engl J Med* 325:1843, 1991.
113. Saggese G, Baroncelli GI, Bertelloni S, Perri G: Long-term growth hormone treatment in children with renal hypophosphatemic rickets: effects on growth, mineral metabolism, and bone density. J Pediatr 127:395, 1995.
114. Marie PJ, Glorieux FH: Bone histomorphometry in asymptomatic adults with hereditary hypophosphatemic vitamin D resistant osteomalacia. *Metab Bone Dis Rel Res* 4:249, 1982.
115. Rubinovitch M, Said SE, Glorieux FH, Cruess RL, Rogala E: Principles and results of corrective lower limb osteotomies for patients with vitamin D resistant hypophosphatemic rickets. *Clin Orthop* 237:264, 1988.
116. Whyte MP, McAlister WH, Patton LS, Magill HL, Fallon MD, Lorentz WB Jr, Herrod HG: Enzyme replacement therapy for infantile hypophosphatasia attempted by intravenous infusions of alkaline phosphatase rich Paget plasma: Results in three additional patients. *J Pediatr* 105:926, 1984.
117. Thomson DL, Frame B: Involutional osteopenia: Current concepts. *Ann Intern Med* 85:789, 1976.
118. Meunier PJ, Bianchi GGS, Edouard CM, Bernard JC, Coupron P, Vignon GE: Bony manifestations of thyrotoxicosis. *Orthop Clin North Am* 3:745, 1975.
119. Ebeling PR, Atley LM, Guthrie JR, Burger HG, Dennerstein L,

Hopper JL, Wark JD: Bone turnover markers and bone density across the menopausal transition. *J Clin Endocrinol Metab* 81:3366, 1996.
120. LeBoff MS, Kohlmeier L, Hurwitz S, Franklin J, Wright J, Glowacki J: Occult vitamin D deficiency in postmenopausal women with acute hip fracture. *JAMA* 281:1505, 1999.
121. Avioli LV, McDonald JE, Lee SW: The influence of age on the intestinal absorption of 47Ca absorption in postmenopausal osteoporosis. *J Clin Invest* 44:1960, 1965.
122. Gallagher JC, Riggs BL, Eisman J, Hamstra A, Arnaud SB, De Luca HF: Intestinal calcium absorption and serum vitamin D metabolites in normal subjects and osteoporotic patients: Effect of age and dietary calcium. *J Clin Invest* 64:729, 1979.
123. Morris HA, Need AG, Horowitz M, O'Loughlin PD, Nordin BEC: Calcium absorption in normal and osteoporotic postmenopausal women. *Calcif Tissue Int* 49:240, 1991.
124. Gallagher JC, Nordin BEC: Oestrogens and calcium metabolism. *Front Horm Res* 2:98, 1973.
125. Heshmati HM, Khosla S, Burritt MF, O'Fallon WM, Riggs BL: A defect in renal calcium conservation may contribute to the pathogenesis of postmenopausal osteoporosis. *J Clin Endocrinol Metab* 83:1916, 1998.
126. Heath H, Sizemore GW: Plasma calcitonin in normal man: Differences between men and women. *J Clin Invest* 60:1135, 1977.
127. Shamonki IM, Frumar AM, Tataryn IV, Meldrum DR, Davidson BH, Parthemore JG, Judd HL, Deftos LJ: Age-related changes of calcitonin secretion in females. *J Clin Endocrinol Metab* 50:437, 1980.
128. Milhaud G, Benezech-Leferre M, Moukhtar MS: Deficiency of calcitonin in age related osteoporosis. *Biomedicine* 29:272, 1978.
129. Chestnut CH III, Baylink DJ, Sisom K, Nelp WB, Roos BA: Basal plasma immunoreactive calcitonin in postmenopausal osteoporosis. *Metabolism* 29:559, 1980.
130. Taggart HM, Chestnut CH III, Ivey JL, Baylink DJ, Sisom K, Huber MB, Roos BA: Deficient calcitonin response to calcium stimulation in postmenopausal osteoporosis. *Lancet* 1:475, 1982.
131. Reginster JY, Deroisy R, Albert A, Denis D, Lecart MP, Collette J, Franchimont P: Relationship between whole plasma calcitonin levels, calcitonin secretory capacity, and plasma levels of estrone in healthy women and postmenopausal osteoporotics. *J Clin Invest* 83:1073, 1989.
132. Sjoberg HE, Torring O, Granberg B, Ehrnsten U, Bucht E: Postmenopausal osteoporosis: Response of immunoextracted calcitonin to a calcium clamp. *Bone* 10:15, 1989.
133. Tiegs RD, Body JJ, Wahner HW, Barta J, Riggs BL, Heath H III: Calcitonin secretion in postmenopausal osteoporosis. *N Engl J Med* 312:1097, 1985.
134. Morimoto S, Tsuji M, Okada Y, Omishi T, Kumahara Y: The effect of oestrogens on human calcitonin secretion after calcium infusion in elderly female subjects. *Clin Endocrinol (Oxf)* 13:135, 1980.
135. Stevenson JC, Abeyasekera G, Hillyard CJ, Phang KG, McIntyre I, Campbell S, Lane G, Townsend PT, et al: Regulation of calcium-regulating hormones by exogenous sex steroids in early postmenopause. *Eur J Clin Invest* 13:481, 1983.
136. Leggate J, Farish E, Fletcher CD, McIntosh W, Hart DM, Sommerville JM: Calcitonin and postmenopausal osteoporosis. *Clin Endocrinol (Oxf)* 20:85, 1984.
137. Selby PL, Peacock M, Barkworth SA, Brown WB, Taylor GA: Early effects of ethinyloestradiol and norethisterone treatment in postmenopausal women on bone resorption and calcium regulating hormones. *Clin Sci* 69:265, 1985.
138. Lobo RA, Roy S, Shoupe D, Endres DB, Adams JS, Rude RK, Singer FR: Estrogen and progestin effects on urinary calcium and calciotropic hormones in surgically-induced postmenopausal women. *Horm Metab Res* 17:370, 1985.
139. Body JJ, Heath H III: Estimates of circulating monomeric calcitonin: Physiologic studies in normal and thyroidectomized man. *J Clin Endocrinol Metab* 57:897, 1983.
140. Monier-Faugere MC, Langub MC, Malluche HM: Bone biopsies: A modern approach, in Avioli LV, Krane SM (eds): *Metabolic Bone Disease and Clinically Related Disorders*, 3rd ed. San Diego, Academic Press, 1998, p 237.
141. Darby AJ, Meunier PJ: Mean wall thickness and formation periods of trabecular bone packets in idiopathic osteoporosis. *Calcif Tissue Int* 33:199, 1981.
142. Seeman E, Wahner HW, Offord KP, Kumar R, Johnson WJ, Riggs BL: Differential effects of endocrine dysfunction on the axial and appendicular skeleton. *J Clin Invest* 69:1302, 1982.
143. Riggs BL, Jowsey J, Kelly PJ: Quantitative microradiographic study of bone remodeling in Cushing's syndrome. *Metabolism* 15:773, 1966.
144. Jowsey J, Riggs BL: Bone formation in hypercortisonism. *Acta Endocrinol (Copenh)* 63:21, 1970.
145. Bressot C, Meunier PJ, Chapuy MC, Le jeune E, Edouard C, Darby AJ: Histomorphometric profile, pathophysiology and reversibility of corticosteroid-induced osteoporosis. *Metab Bone Dis Relat Res* 1:303, 1979.
146. Aaron JE, Francis RM, Peacock M, Makins NB: Contrasting microanatomy of idiopathic and corticosteroid-induced osteoporosis. *Clin Orthop* 243:294, 1989.
147. Minaire P, Meunier P, Edouard C, Bernard J, Courpron P, Bouret J: Quantitative histological data on disuse osteoporosis: Comparison with biological data. *Calcif Tissue Res* 17:57, 1974.
148. Jowsey J, Johnson KA: Juvenile osteoporosis: Bone findings in seven patients. *J Pediatr* 81:511, 1972.
149. Smith R: Idiopathic osteoporosis in the young. *J Bone Joint Surg [Br]* 62-B:417, 1980.
150. Rauch G, Travers R, Norman ME, Taylor A, Parfitt AM, Glorieux FH: Deficient bone formation in idioopathic juvenile osteoporosis. *J Bone Miner Res* 15:957, 2000.
151. Jaffe HL: *Metabolic, Degenerative, and Inflammatory Diseases of Bones and Joints*. Philadelphia, Lea & Febiger, 1972, p 162.
152. Smith DM, Nance WE, Kang KW, Christian JC, Johnston CC Jr: Genetic factors in determining bone mass. *J Clin Invest* 52:2800, 1973.
153. Seeman E, Hopper JL, Bach LA, Cooper ME, Parkinson E, McKay J, Jerums G: Reduced bone mass in daughters of women with osteoporosis. *N Engl J Med* 320:554, 1989.
154. Cohen-Solal ME, Baudoin C, Omouri M, Kuntz D, De Vernejoul MC: Bone mass in middle-aged osteoporotic men and their relatives: Familial effect. *J Bone Miner Res* 13:1909,1998.
155. Uitterlinden AG, Burger H, Huang Q, Yue F, McGuigan FEA, Grant SFA, Hofman A, van Leeuwen JPTM, Pols HAP, Ralston SH: Relation of alleles of the collagen type $1\alpha1$ gene to bone density and the risk of osteoporotic fractures in postmenopausal women. *N Engl J Med* 338:1016, 1998.
156. Gueguen R, Joanny P, Guillemin F, Kuntz C, Pourel J, Siest G: Segregation analysis and variance components analysis of bone mineral density in healthy families. *J Bone Miner Res* 10:2017, 1995.
157. Riggs BL, Khasla S, Melton LJ III: A unitary model for involutional osteoporosis: Estrogen deficiency causes both type I and type II osteoporosis postmenopausal women and contributes to bone loss in aging men. *J Bone Miner Res* 13:763, 1998.
158. Daniell HW: Osteoporosis of the slender smoker: Vertebral compression fractures and loss of metacarpal cortex in relation to postmenopausal cigarette smoking and lack of obesity. *Arch Intern Med* 136:298, 1976.
159. Seeman E, Melton LJ III, O'Fallon WA, Riggs BL: Risk factors for spinal osteoporosis in men. *Am J Med* 75:977, 1983.
160. Aloia JF, Cohn SH, Vaswani A, Yeh JK, Yuen K, Ellis K: Risk factors for postmenopausal osteoporosis. *Am J Med* 78:95, 1985.
161. Melton LJ, Riggs BL: Epidemiology of age-related fractures, in Avioli LV (ed): *The Osteoporotic Syndrome: Detection, Prevention and Treatment*. New York, Grune & Stratton, 1983, p 45.
162. Ettinger B, Pressman A, Sklarin P, Bauer DC, Cauley JA, Cummings SR: Association between low levels of serum estradiol, bone density, and fractures among elderly women: The study of osteoporotic fractures. *J Clin Endocrinol Metab* 83:2239, 1998.
163. Eriksen EFL, Colvard DS, Berg NJ, Graham ML, Mann KG, Spelsberg TC, Riggs BL: Evidence of estrogen receptors in normal human osteoblast-like cells. *Science* 241:84, 1988.
164. Oursler MJ, Osdoby P, Pyfferoen J, Figgs BL, Spelsberg TC: Avian osteoclasts as estrogen target cells. *Proc Natl Acad Sci USA* 88: 6613, 991.
165. Cosman F, Shen V, Xie F, Seibel M, Ratclife A, Lindsay R: Estrogen protection against bone resorbing effects of parathyroid hormone infusion. *Ann Intern Med* 118:337, 1993.
166. Manolagas SC, Jilka RL: Bone marrow cytokines and bone remodeling: Emerging insights into the pathophysiology of osteoporosis. *N Engl J Med* 332:305, 1995.

167. Kawaguchi H, Pilbeam CC, Vargas SJ, Morse EE, Lorenzo JA, Raisz LG: Ovariectomy enhances and estrogen replacement inhibits the activity of bone marrow factors that stimulate prostaglandin production in cultured mouse calvariae. *J Clin Invest* 96:539, 1995.
168. Suda T, Takahashi N, Udagawa N, Jimi E, Gillespie MT, Martin TJ: Modulation of osteoclast differentiation and function by the new members of the tumor necrosis factor receptor and ligand families. *Endocr Rev* 20:345, 1999.
169. Gallagher JC, Riggs BL, DeLuca HF: Effect of estrogen on calcium absorption and serum vitamin D metabolites in postmenopausal osteoporosis. *J Clin Endocrinol Metab* 51:1359, 1980.
170. Cheema C, Grant BF, Marcus R: Effects of estrogen on circulating "free" and total 1,25-dihydroxyvitamin D and on the parathyroid vitamin D axis in postmenopausal women. *J Clin Invest* 83:537, 1989.
171. Longcope C, Baker RS, Hui SL, Johnston CC Jr: Androgen and estrogen dynamics in women with vertebral crush fractures. *Maturitas* 6:309, 1984.
172. Nordin BEC, Robertson A, Semark RF, Bridges A, Philcox JC, Need AG, Horowitz M, Morris HA, Deam S: The relation between calcium absorption, serum dehydroepiandrosterone, and vertebral mineral density in postmenopausal women. *J Clin Endocrinol Metab* 60:651, 1985.
173. Devogelaer JP, Crabbe J, Nagant de Deuxchaishes C: Bone mineral density in Addison's disease: Evidence for an effect of adrenal androgens on bone mass. *Br Med J* 294:798, 1987.
174. Forbes AP: Fuller Albright: His concept of postmenopausal osteoporosis and what's come of it. *Clin Orthop* 269:128, 1991.
175. Garnero P, Sornay-Rendu E, Chapuy M, Delmas PD: Increased bone turnover in late postmenopausal women is a determinant of osteoporosis. *J Bone Miner Res* 11:337, 1996.
176. Drinkwater BL, Bruemner B, Chestnut CS III: Menstrual history as a determinant of current bone density in young athletes. *JAMA* 263:545, 1990.
177. Biller BMK, Saxe V, Herzog DB, Rosenthal DI, Holzman S, Klibanski A: Mechanisms of osteoporosis in adult and adolescent women with anorexia nervosa. *J Clin Endocrinol Metab* 68:548, 1989.
178. Seeman E, Szmukler GI, Formica C, Tsalamandris C, Mestrovic R: Osteoporosis in anorexia nervosa: The influence of peak bone density, bone loss, oral contraceptive use, and exercise. *J Bone Miner Res* 7:1467, 1992.
179. Klibanski A, Biller BMK, Rosenthal DI, Schoenfeld DA, Saxe V: Effects of prolactin and estrogen deficiency in amenorrheic bone loss. *J Clin Endocrinol Metab* 67:124, 1988.
180. Johansen JS, Riis BJ, Hassager C, Moen M, Jacobson J, Christiansen C: The effect of a gonadotropin-releasing hormone agonist analog (Nafarelin) on bone metabolism. *J Clin Endocrinol Metab* 67:701, 1988.
181. Grinspoon S, Miller K, Coyle C, Krempin J, Armstrong C, Pitts S, Herzog D, Klibanski A: Severity of osteopenia in estrogen-deficient women with anorexia nervosa and hypothalamic amenorrhea. *J Clin Endocrinol Metab* 84:2049, 1999.
182. Davis SR, Dalais FS, Simpson ER, Murkies AL: Phytoestrogens in health and disease. *Recent Prog Horm Res* 54:185, 1999.
183. Prior JC: Progesterone as a bone-trophic hormone. *Endocr Rev* 11:386, 1990.
184. Daniell HW: Osteoporosis after orchiectomy for prostate cancer. *J Urol* 157:439, 1997.
185. Diamond T, Campbell J, Bryant C, Lynch W: The effect of combined androgen blockade on bone turnover and bone mineral densities in men treated for prostate carcinoma: longitudinal evaluation and response to intermittent cyclic etidronate therapy. *Cancer* 83:1561, 1998.
186. Maillefert JF, Sibilia J, Michel F, Saussine C, Javier RM, Tavernier C: Bone mineral density in men treated with synthetic gonadotropin-releasing hormone agonists for prostatic carcinoma. *J Urol* 161: 1219, 1999.
187. Francis RM, Peacock M, Aaron JE, Selby PL, Taylor GA, Thompson J, Marshall DH, Horsman A: Osteoporosis in hypogonadal men: Role of decreased plasma 1,25-dihydroxyvitamin D, calcium malabsorption, and low bone formation. *Bone* 7:261, 1986.
188. Jackson JA, Kleerekoper M, Parfitt AM, Rao DS, Villanueva AR, Frame B: Bone histomorphometry in hypogonadal and eugonadal men with spinal osteoporosis. *J Clin Endocrinol Metab* 65:53, 1987.
189. Finkelstein JS, Neer RM, Biller BMK, Crawford JD, Klibanski A: Osteopenia in men with a history of delayed puberty. *N Engl J Med* 326:600, 1992.
190. Colvard DS, Eriksen EF, Keeting PE, Wilson EM, Lubahn DB, French FS, Riggs BL, Spelsberg TC: Identification of androgen receptors in normal human osteoblast-like cells. *Proc Natl Acad Sci USA* 86:854, 1989.
191. Pederson L, Kremer M, Judd J, Pascoe D, Spelsberg TC, Riggs BL, Oursler MJ: Androgens regulate bone resorption activity of isolated osteoclasts in vitro. *Proc Natl Acad Sci USA* 96:505, 1999.
192. Peris P, Guanabens N, Monegal A, Suris X, Alvarez L, Martinez de Osaba MJ, Hernandez MV, Munoz-Gomez J: Aetiology and presenting symptoms in male osteoporosis. *Br J Rheumatol* 34:936, 1995.
193. Francis RM, Peacock M, Marshall DH, Horsman A, Aaron JE: Spinal osteoporosis in men. *Bone Miner* 5:347, 1989.
194. Richardson ML, Genant HK, Cann CE, Ettinger B, Gordan GS, Kolb FO, Reiser UJ: Assessment of metabolic bone diseases by quantitative computed tomography. *Clin Orthop* 195:224, 1985.
195. Khosla S, Melton LJ III, Atkinson EJ, O'Fallon WM, Klee GG, Riggs BL: Relationship of serum sex steroid levels and bone turnover markers with bone mineral density in men and women: a key role for bioavailable estrogen. *J Clin Endocrinol Metab* 83:2266, 1998.
196. Clarke BL, Ebeling PR, Jones JA, Wahner HW, O'Fallon WM, Riggs BL, Fitzpatrick LA: Changes in quantitative bone histomorphometry in aging healthy men. *J Clin Endocrinol Metab* 81:2264, 1996.
197. Orwoll ES, Bell NH, Nanes MS, Flessland-Pettinger MB, Mallinak NJS, Cain DF: Collagen N-telopeptide excretion in men: The effects of age and intrasubject variability. *J Clin Endrinol Metab* 83:3930, 1998.
198. Bilezikian JP, Morishima A, Bell J, Grumbach MM: Increased bone mass as a result of estrogen therapy in a man with aromatase deficiency. *N Engl J Med* 339:599, 1998.
199. Reid IR: Glucocorticoid osteoporosis-mechanism and management. *Eur J Endocrinol* 137:209, 1997.
200. Weinstein RS, Jilka RL, Parfitt AM, Manolagas SC: Inhibition of osteoblastogenesis and promotion of apoptosis of osteoblasts and osteocytes by glucocorticoids. Potential mechanisms of their deleterious effects on bone. *J Clin Invest* 102:274, 1998.
201. Ebeling PR, Erbas B, Hopper JL, Wark JD, Rubinfeld AR: Bone mineral density and bone turnover in asthmatics treated with long-term inhaled or oral glucocorticoids. *J Bone Miner Res* 13:1283, 1998.
202. Fucik RF, Kukreja SC, Hargis GK, Bowser EN, Henderson WJ, Williams GA: Effects of glucocorticoids on function of the parathyroid glands in man. *J Clin Endocrinol Metab* 49:152, 1975.
203. Lukert BP, Adams JS: Calcium and phosphorus homeostasis in man. *Arch Intern Med* 136:1249, 1976.
204. Slovik DM, Neer RM, Ohman JL, Lowell FC, Clark MB, Segre GV, Potts JT Jr: Parathyroid hormone and 25-hydroxyvitamin D levels in glucocorticoid-treated patients. *Clin Endocrinol (Oxf)* 12:243, 1980.
205. Findling JW, Adams ND, Lemann J Jr, Gray RW, Thomas CJ, Tyrell BJ: Vitamin D metabolites and parathyroid hormone in Cushing's syndrome: Relationship to calcium and phosphorus homeostasis. *J Clin Endocrinol Metab* 54:1039, 1982.
206. Harrison HE, Harrison HC: Transfer of Ca^{45} across intestinal wall in vitro in relation to action of vitamin D and cortisol. *Am J Physiol* 199:265, 1960.
207. Klein RG, Arnaud SB, Gallagher JC, DeLuca HF, Riggs BL: Intestinal calcium absorption in exogenous hypercortisonism. *J Clin Invest* 60:253, 1977.
208. Stoll GM, Harris S, Sokoll LJ, Dawson-Hughes B: Accelerated bone loss in hypothyroid patients overtreated with L-thyroxine. *Ann Intern Med* 113:265, 1990.
209. Mundy GR, Shapiro JL, Bardelin JG, Canalis EM, Raisz LG: Direct stimulation of bone resorption by thyroid hormones. *J Clin Invest* 58:529, 1976.
210. Krane SM, Brownell GL, Stanbury JB, Corrigan H: The effect of thyroid disease on calcium metabolism in man. *J Clin Invest* 35:874, 1956.
211. Singhelakis P, Alevizaka CC, Ikkos DG: Intestinal calcium absorption in hyperthyroidism. *Metabolism* 23:311, 1974.
212. Bouillon R, Muls E, DeMoor P: Influence of thyroid function on the serum concentration of 1,25-dihydroxyvitamin D_3. *J Clin Endocrinol Metab* 51:793, 1980.
213. Silverberg SJ, Locker FG, Bilezikian JP: Vertebral osteopenia: a new indication for surgery in primary hyperparathyroidism. *J Clin Endocrinol Metab* 81:4007, 1996.

214. Melton LJ III, Atkinson EJ, O'Fallon WM, Heath H III: Risk of age-related fractures in patients with primary hyperparathyroidism. *Arch Intern Med* 152:2269, 1992.
215. McNair P, Madsbad S, Chistensen MS, Christiansen C, Faber OK, Binder C, Transbol I: Bone mineral loss in insulin-treated diabetes mellitus. Studies on pathogenesis. *Acta Endocrinol (Copenh)* 90:463, 1979.
216. Heath H III, Melton LJ III, Chu CP: Diabetes mellitus and risk of skeletal fracture. *N Engl J Med* 303:567, 1980.
217. Raskin P, Stevenson MRM, Barilla DE, Pak CYC: The hypercalciuria of diabetes mellitus: Its amelioration with insulin. *Clin Endocrinol (Oxf)* 9:329, 1978.
218. Schneider LE, Schedl HP, McCain T, Haussler MR: Experimental diabetes reduces circulating 1,25-dihydroxyvitamin D in the rat. *Science* 196:1452, 1977.
219. Heath H III, Lambert PW, Service FJ, Arnaud SB: Calcium homeostasis in diabetes mellitus. *J Clin Endocrinol Metab* 49:462, 1979.
220. Frazer TE, White NH, Hough S, Santiago JV, McGee BR, Bryce G, Mallon J, Avioli LV: Alterations in circulating vitamin D metabolites in the young insulin-dependent diabetic. *J Clin Endocrinol Metab* 53:1154, 1981.
221. Storm TL, Sorensen OH, Lund B, Lund B, Christiansen JS, Andersen AR, Lumholtz IB, Parving HH: Vitamin D metabolism in insulin-dependent diabetes mellitus. *Metab Bone Dis Rel Res* 5:107, 1983.
222. Prockop DJ, Kivirikko KK: Heritable diseases of collagen. *N Engl J Med* 311:376, 1984.
223. Rowe DW, Shapiro JR: Osteogenesis imperfecta, in Avioli LV, Krane SM (eds): *Metabolic Bone Disease and Clinically Related Disorders*, 3rd ed. Philadelphia, Saunders, 1998, p 651.
224. Smith R: Idiopathic juvenile osteoporosis. *Am J Dis Child* 133:889, 1979.
225. Smith R: Idiopathic juvenile osteoporosis: experience of twenty-one patients. *Br J Rheumatol* 34:68, 1995.
226. Saggese G, Bertelloni S, Baroncelli GI, Perri G, Calderazzi A: Mineral metabolism and calcitriol therapy in idiopathic juvenile osteoporosis. *Am J Dis Child* 145:457, 1991.
227. de Vernejoul MC, Marie P, Kuntz D, Gueris J, Miravet L, Ryckewaert A: Non-osteomalacic osteopathy associated with chronic hypophosphatemia. *Calcif Tissue Int* 34:219, 1982.
228. Lawoyin S, Sismilich S, Browne R, Pak CYC: Bone mineral content in patients with calcium urolithiasis. *Metabolism* 28:1250, 1979.
229. Pacifici R, Rothstein M, Rifas L, Lau KH, Baylink DJ, Avioli LV, Hruska K: Increased monocyte interleukin-1 activity and decreased vertebral bone density in patients with fasting idiopathic hypercalciuria. *J Clin Endocrinol Metab* 71:138, 1990.
230. Bikle DD, Genant HK, Cann C, Recker RR, Halloran BP, Strewler GJ: Bone disease in alcohol abuse. *Ann Intern Med* 103:42, 1985.
231. Diamond T, Stiel D, Lunzer M, Wilkinson M, Posen S: Ethanol reduces bone formation and may cause osteoporosis. *Am J Med* 86:282, 1989.
232. Giuliani N, Girasole G, Vescovi PP, Passeri G, Pedrazzoni M: Ethanol and acetaldehyde inhibit the formation of early osteoblast precursors in murine and human bone marrow cultures. *Alcohol Clin Exp Res* 23:381, 1999.
233. Rodino MA, Shane E: Osteoporosis after organ transplantation. *Am J Med* 104:459, 1998.
234. Ebeling PR, Thomas DM, Erbas B, Hopper JL, Szer J, Grigg AP: Mechanisms of bone loss following allogeneic and autologous hemopoietic stem cell transplantation. *J Bone Miner Res* 14:342, 1999.
235. Selby PL, Davies M, Adams JE, Mawer EB: Bone loss in celiac disease is related to secondary hyperparathyroidism. *J Bone Miner Res* 14:652, 1999.
236. Valentine JF, Sninsky CA: Prevention and treatment of osteoporosis in patients with inflammatory bowel disease. *Am J Gastroenterol* 94:878, 1999.
237. Slemenda CW, Hui SL, Longcope C, Johnston CC Jr: Cigarette smoking, obesity, and bone mass. *J Bone Miner Res* 4:737, 1989.
238. Krall EA, Dawson-Hughes B: Smoking increases bone loss and decreases intestinal calcium absorption. *J Bone Miner Res* 14:215, 1999.
239. Baron JA, La Vecchia C, Levi F: The antiestrogenic effect of cigarette smoking in women. *Am J Obstet Gynecol* 162:502, 1990.
240. Matkovic V, Fontana D, Tominac C, Goel P, Chesnut CH III: Factors that influence peak bone mass formation: A study of calcium balance and the inheritance of bone mass in adolescent females. *Am J Clin Nutr* 52:878, 1990.
241. Griffith GC, Nichols G, Asher JD, Flanagan B: Heparin osteoporosis. *JAMA* 193:91, 1965.
242. Weinstein RS, Bryce GF, Sappington LJ, King DW, Gallagher BB: Decreased serum ionized calcium and normal vitamin D metabolite levels with anticonvulsant drug treatment. *J Clin Endocrinol Metab* 58:1003, 1984.
243. Stanisavljevic S, Babcock AL: Fractures in children treated with methotrexate for leukemia. *Clin Orthop* 125:139, 1977.
244. Zonneveld IM, Bakker WK, Dijkstra PF, Bos JD, van Soesbergen RM, Dinant HJ: Methotrexate osteopathy in long-term, low-dose methotrexate treatment for psoriasis and rheumatoid arthritis. *Arch Dermatol* 132:184, 1996.
245. Gough AK, Lilley J, Eyre S, Holder RL, Emery P: Generalised bone loss in patients with early rheumatoid arthritis. *Lancet* 344:23, 1994.
246. McCaughan GW, Feller RB: Osteoporosis in chronic liver disease: pathogenesis, risk factors, and management. *Dig Dis* 12:223, 1994.
247. Chines A, Pacifici R, Avioli LV, Teitelbaum SL, Korenblat PE: Systemic mastocytosis presenting as osteoporosis: A clinical and histomorphometric study. *J Clin Endocrinol Metab* 72:140, 1991.
248. Resnick D, Niwayama G: *Diagnosis of Bone and Joint Disorders*, 2nd ed. Philadelphia, Saunders, 1988.
249. Phillips AJ, Ostlere SJ, Smith R: Pregnancy-associated osteoporosis: Does the skeleton recover? *Osteoporosis Int* 11:449, 2000.
250. Meema S, Bunker ML, Meema HE: Preventive effect of estrogen on postmenopausal bone loss. *Arch Intern Med* 135:1436, 1975.
251. Aitken JM, Hart DM, Lindsay R: Oestrogen replacement therapy for prevention of osteoporosis after oophorectomy. *Br Med J* 3:515, 1973.
252. Ettinger B, Genant HK, Cann CE: Long-term estrogen replacement therapy prevents bone loss and fractures. *Ann Intern Med* 102:319, 1985.
253. Stevenson JC, Cost MP, Gangor KF, Hillard TC, Lees B, Whitehead MI: Effects of transdermal versus oral hormone replacement therapy on bone density in spine and proximal femur in postmenopausal women. *Lancet* 335:265, 1990.
254. The Writing Group for the PEPI: Effects of hormone therapy on bone mineral density: results from the postmenopausal estrogen/progestin interventions (PEPI) trial. *JAMA* 276:1389, 1996.
255. Lufkin EG, Wahner HW, O'Fallon WM, Hodgson SF, Kotowicz MA, Lane AW, Judd HL, Caplan RH, Riggs BL: Treatment of postmenopausal osteoporosis with transdermal estrogen. *Ann Intern Med* 117:1, 1992.
256. Genant HK, Lucas J, Weiss S, Akin M, Emkey R, McNaney-Flint H, Downs R, Mortola J, Watts N, Yang HM, Banav N, Brennan JJ, Nolan JC: Low dose esterified estrogen therapy: Effects on bone, plasma estradiol concentrations, endometrium, and lipid levels. *Arch Int Med* 157:2609, 1997.
257. Chestnut CH III, Bell NH, Clark GS, Drinkwater BL, English SC, Johnston CC Jr, Notelovitz M, Rosen C, Cain DF, Flessland KA, Mallinak NJS: Hormone replacement therapy in postmenopausal women: Urinary N-telopeptide of type I collagen monitors therapeutic effect and predicts response of bone mineral density. *Am J Med* 102:29, 1997.
258. Weiss NS, Ure CL, Ballard JH, Williams AR, Daling JR: Decreased risk of fractures of the hip and lower forearm with postmenopausal use of estrogen. *N Engl J Med* 303:1195, 1980.
259. Nieves JW, Komar L, Cosman F, Lindsay R: Calcium potentiates the effect of estrogen on bone mass: review and analysis. *Am J Clin Nutr* 67:18, 1998.
260. Barrett-Connor E, Young R, Notelovitz M, Sullivan J, Wiita B, Yang HM, Nolan J: A two-year, double-blind comparison of estrogen-androgen and conjugated estrogens in surgically menopausal women. Effects on bone mineral density, symptoms and lipid profiles. *J Reprod Med* 44:1012, 1999.
261. Ward RL, Morgan G, Dalley D, Kelley PJ: Tamoxifen reduces bone turnover and prevents lumbar spine and proximal femoral bone loss in early postmenopausal women. *Bone Miner* 22:87, 1993.
262. Khovidhunkit W, Shoback DM: Clinical effects of raloxifene hydrochloride in women. *Ann Intern Med* 130:431, 1999.
263. Delmas PD, Bjarnson NH, Mitlak BH, Ravoux AC, Shah AS, Huster WJ, Draper M, Christiansen C: Effects of raloxifene on bone mineral density, serum cholesterol concentrations, and uterine endometrium in postmenopausal women. *N Engl J Med* 337:1641, 1997.

264. Rogers MJ, Gordon S, Benford HL, Coxon FP, Luckman SP, Monkkonen, Frith JC: Cellular and molecular mechanisms of action of bisphosphonates. *Cancer* 88 (Suppl) 2891,2000.
265. Meunier PJ, Confovreux E, Tupinon I, Hardouin C, Delmas PD, Balena R: Prevention of early postmenopausal bone loss with cyclical etidronate therapy (A double-blind, placebo controlled study and 1-year followup). *J Clin Endocrinol Metab* 82:2784, 1997.
266. Hosking D, Chilvers CE, Christiansen C, Ravn P, Wasnich R, Ross P, McClung M, Balske A, Thompson D, Daley M, Yates AJ: Prevention of bone loss with alendronate in postmenopausal women under 60 years of age. Early Postmenopausal Intervention Cohort Study Group. *N Engl J Med* 338:L 485, 1998.
267. Fogelman I, Ribot C, Smith R, Ethgen D, Sod E, Reginster J-Y: Risedronate reverses bone loss in post-menopausal women with low bone mass: Results from a multinational double-blind, placebo-controlled trial. *J Clin Endrocrinol Metab* 85:1895, 2000.
268. Gruber HE, Ivey JL, Baylink DJ, Matthews M, Nelp WB, Sisom K, Chestnut CH III: Long-term calcitonin therapy in postmenopausal osteoporosis. *Metabolism* 33:295, 1984.
269. Civitelli R, Gonnelli S, Zacchei F, Bigazzi S, Vattimo A, Avioli LV, Gennari C: Bone turnover in postmenopausal osteoporosis: Effect of calcitonin treatment. *J Clin Invest* 82:1268, 1988.
270. Hosking DJ, Ross PD, Thompson DE, Wasnich RD, McClung M, Bjarnason NH, Ravn P, Cizza G, Daley M, Yates AJ: Evidence that increased calcium intake does not prevent early postmenopausal bone loss. *Clin Ther* 20:933, 1998.
271. Dawson-Hughes B, Harris SS, Krall EA, Dallal GE: Effect of calcium and vitamin D supplementation on bone density in men and women 65 years of age or older. *N Engl J Med* 337:670, 1997.
272. Riggs BL, O'Fallon WM, Muhs J, O'Connor MK, Kumar R, Melton LJ III: Long-term effects of calcium supplementation on serum parathyroid hormone level, bone turnover, and bone loss in elderly women. *J Bone Miner Res* 13:168, 1998.
273. Need AG, Horowitz M, Philcox JC, Nordin BEC: 1,25-dihydroxycholecalciferol and calcium therapy in osteoporosis with calcium malabsorption. *Miner Electrolyte Metab* 11:35, 1985.
274. Riggs BL, Nelson KI: Effect of long term treatment with calcitriol on calcium absorption and mineral metabolism in postmenopausal osteoporosis. *J Clin Endocrinol Metab* 61:457, 1985.
275. Christiansen C, Christensen MS, Rodbro P, Hagen C, Transbol I: Effect of 1,25-dihydroxyvitamin D_3 in itself or combined with hormone treatment in preventing postmenopausal osteoporosis. *Eur J Clin Invest* 11:305, 1981.
276. Katznelson L: Therapeutic role of androgens in the treatment of osteoporosis in men. *Baillieres Clin Endocrinol Metab* 12:453, 1998.
277. Katznelson L, Finkelstein JS, Schoenfeld DA, Rosenthal DI, Anderson EJ. Klibanski A: Increase in bone density and lean body mass during testosterone administration in men with acquired hypogonadism. *J Clin Endocrinol Metab* 81:4358, 1996.
278. Snyder PJ, Peachey H, Berlin JA, Hannoush P, Haddad G, Dlewati A, Santanna J, Loh L, Lenrow DA, Holmes JH, Kapoor SC, Atkinson LE, Strom BL: Effects of testosterone replacement in hypogonadal men. *J Clin Endocrinol Metab* 85:2670, 2000.
279. Orwoll E, Ettinger M, Weiss S, Miller P, Kendler D, Graham J, Adami S, Weber K, Lorenc R, Pietschmann P: Alendronate treatment of osteoporosis in men. *J Bone Miner Res* 14:S184, 1999.
280. Adachi JD, Bensen WG, Brown J, Hanley D, Hodsman A, Josse R, Kendler DL, Lentle B, Olszynski W, Ste-Marie LG, Tenenhouse A, Chines AA: Intermittent etidronate therapy to prevent corticosteroid-induced osteoporosis. *N Engl J Med* 337:382, 1997.
281. Saag KG, Emkey R, Schnitzer TJ, Brown JP, Hawkins F, Goemaere S, Thamsborg G, Liberman UA, Delmas PD, Malice MP, Czachur M, Daifotis AG: Alendronate for prevention and treatment of glucocorticoid-induced osteoporosis. Glucocorticoid-Induced Osteoporosis Intervention Study Group. *N Engl J Med* 339:292, 1998.
282. Boutsen Y, Jamart J, Esselinckx W, Stoffel M, Devogelaer FP: Primary prevention of glucocorticoid-induced osteoporosis with intermittent intravenous pamidronate: A randomized trial. *Calcif Tissue Int* 61:266, 1997.
283. Cohen S, Levy RM, Keller M, Boling M, Emkey RD, Greenwald M, Zizic TM, Wallach S, Sewell KL, Lukert BP, Axelord DW, Chines AA: Risedronate therapy prevents corticosteroid-induced bone loss. A twelve-month, multi-center, randomized, double-blinded, palcebo-controlled, parallel-group study. *Arthritis Rheum* 42:2309, 1999.
284. Hahn TJ, Halstead LR, Teitelbaum SL, Hahn BH: Altered mineral metabolism in glucocorticoid-induced osteopenia: Effect of 25-hydroxyvitamin D administration. *J Clin Invest* 64:655, 1979.
285. Sambrook P, Birmingham J, Kelly P, Kempler S, Nguyen T, Pocock N, Eisman J: Prevention of corticosteroid osteoporosis. A comparison of calcium, calcitriol, and calcitonin. *N Engl J Med* 328:1747, 1993.
286. Nagant de Deuxchaisnes C, Devogelaer JP, Esselinck W, Bouchez B, Depresseux G, Rombouts-Lindemans C, Huaux JP: The effect of low dosage glucocorticoids on bone mass in rheumatoid arthritis: A cross-sectional and a longitudinal study using single photon absorptiometry. *Adv Exp Med Biol* 171:209, 1984.
287. Reid IR, Wattie DJ, Evans MC, Stapleton JP: Testosterone therapy in glucocorticoid-treated men. *Arch Int Med* 156:1173, 1996.
288. Ringe JD, Welzel D: Salmon calcitonin in the therapy of corticoid-induced osteoporosis. *Eur J Clin Pharmacol* 33:35, 1987.
289. Reeves HL, Francis RM, Manas DM, Hudson M, Day CP: Intravenous bisphosphonate prevents symptomatic osteoporotic vertebral collapse in patients after liver transplantation. *Liver Transpl Surg* 4:404, 1998.
290. Frost HM: Personal experience in managing acute compression fractures, their aftermath, and the bone pain syndrome, in osteoporosis. *Osteoporos Int* 8:13, 1998.
291. Punk KK, Chan KWL: Analgesic effect of intranasal salmon calcitonin in the treatment of osteoporotic vertebral fractures. *Clin Ther* 11:205, 1989.
292. Murray TM, Singer FR (eds): Proceedings of the International Workshop on Fluoride and Bone. *J Bone Miner Res* 5:1990.
293. Pak CYC, Sakhaee K, Bell NH, Licata A, Johnston C, Rubin B, Bonnick S, Piziak V, Graham H, Ballard J, Berger R, Fears W, Breslau N, Rubin C, Adams-Huet B: Comparison of nonrandomized trials with slow-release sodium fluoride with a randomized placebo-controlled trial in postmenopausal osteoporosis. *J Bone Miner Res* 11:160, 1996.
294. Lindsay R, Nieves J, Formica C, Henneman E, Woelfert L, Shen V, Dempster F, Cosman F: Randomised controlled study of effect of parathyroid hormone on vertebral-bone mass and fracture incidence among postmenopausal women on oestrogen with osteoporosis. *Lancet* 350:550, 1997.
295. Rittmaster RS, Bolognese M, Ettinger MP, Hanley DA, Hodsman AB, Kendler DL, Rosen CJ: Enhancement of bone mass in osteoporotic women with parathyroid hormone followed by alendronate. *J Clin Endocrinol* 85:2129, 2000.
296. Chestnut CH III, McClung MR, Ensrud KE, Bell NH, Genant HK, Harris ST, Singer FR, Stock JL, Yood RA, Delmas PD, Kher MS, Pryor-Tillotson S, Santoro AC II: Alendronate treatment of the postmenopausal osteoporotic woman: Effect of multiple dosages on bone mass and bone remodeling. *Am J Med* 99:144, 1995.
297. Liberman UA, Weiss SR, Broll J, Minne HW, Quan H, Bell NH, Rodriguez-Portales J, Down RW Jr, Dequeker J, Favus M, Seeman E, Recker RR, Capizzi T, Santora AC II, Lombardi A, Shah RV, Hirsch LJ, Karpf DB: Effect of oral alendronate on bone mineral density and the incidence of fractures in postmenopausal osteoporosis. *N Engl J Med* 333:1437, 1995.
298. Black DM, Cummings SR, Karpf DB, Cauley JA, Thompson DE, Nevitt MW, Bauer DC, Genant HK, Haskell WL, Marcus R, Ott SM, Torner JC, Quandt SA, Reiss TF, Ensrud KE: Randomised trial of effect of alendronate on risk of fracture in women with existing fractures. *Lancet* 348:1535, 1996.
299. Greenspan SL, Parker RA, Ferguson L, Rosen HN, Maitland-Ramsey L, Karpf D: Early changes in biochemical markers of bone turnover predict the long-term response to alendronate therapy in representative elderly women: A randomized clinical trial. *J Bone Miner Res* 13:1431, 1998.
300. de Groen PC, Lubbe DF, Hirsch LJ, Daifotis A, Stephenson W, Freedholm D, Pryor-Tillotson S, Seleznick MJ, Pinkas H, Wang KK: Esophagitis associated with the use of alendronate. *N Engl J Med* 335:1016, 1996.
301. Stock JL, Bell NH, Chestnut CH III, Ensrud KE, Genant HK, Harris ST, McClung MR, Singer FR, Yood RA, Pryor-Tillotson S, Wei L, Santora AC II: Increments in bone mineral density of the lumbar spine and hip and suppression of bone turnover are maintained after discontinuation of alendronate in postmenopausal women. *Am J Med* 103:291, 1997.

302. Harris ST, Watts NB, Genant HK, McKeever CD, Hangartner T, Keller M, Chestnut CH III, Brown J, Eerickson EF, Hoseyni MS, Axelrod DW, Miller PD: Effects of risedronate treatment on vertebral and non-vertebral fractures in women with postmenopausal osteoporosis. A randomized controlled trial. *JAMA* 282:1344, 1999.
303. Miller PD, Watts NB, Licata AA, Harris ST, Genant HK, Wasnich RD, Ross PD, Jackson RD, Hoseyni MS, Schoenfeld SL, Valent DJ, Chestnut CH III: Cyclical etidronate in the treatment of postmenopausal osteoporosis: efficacy and safety after seven years of treatment. *Am J Med* 103:468, 1997.
304. Wimalawansa SJ: Combined therapy with estrogen and etidronate has an additive effect on bone mineral density in the hip and vertebrae: Four-year randomized study. *Am J Med* 99:36, 1995.
305. Bone HG, Greenspan SL, McKeever C, Bell N, Davidson M, Downs RW, Emkey R, Meunier PJ, Miller SS, Mulloy AL, Recker RR, Weiss SR, Heyden N, Musliner T, Suryawanshi S, Yates AJ, Lombardi A: Alendronate and estrogen effects in postmenopausal women with low bone density. Alendronate/Estrogen Study Group. *J Clin Endocrinol Metab* 85:720, 2000.
306. Thiebaud D, Burckhardt P, Kriegbaum H, Huss H, Mulder H, Juttmann JR, Schoter KH: Three monthly intravenous injections of ibandronate in the treatment of postmenopausal osteoporosis. *Am J Med* 103:298, 1997.
307. Schnitzer T, Bone HG, Crepaldi G, Adami S, McClung M, Kiel D, Felsenberg D, Recker RR, Tonino RP, Roux C, Pinchera A, Folder AJ, Greenspan SL, Levine MA, Emkey R, Santora AC II, Kaur A, Thompson DE, Yates J, Orloff JJ: Therapeutic equivalence of alendronate 70 mg once-weekly and alendronate 10 mg daily in the treatment of osteoporosis. Alendronate Once-Weekly Study Group. *Aging (Milano)* 12:1,2000.
308. Silverman SL, Chestnut C, Andriano K, Genant H, Gimona A, Maricic M, Stock J, Baylink D: Salmon calcitonin nasal spray reduces risk of vertebral fracture(s) in established osteoporosis and has continuous efficacy with prolonged treatment: Accrued 5 year worldwide data of the PROOF study. *Bone* 23:S174, 1998.
309. Langlois JA, Rosen CJ, Visser M, Hannan MT, Harris T, Wilson PW, Kiel DP: Association between insulin-like growth factor I and bone mineral density in older women and men: The Framingham Heart Study. *J Clin Endocrinol Metab* 83:4257, 1998.
310. Marcus R: Recombinant human growth hormone as potential therapy for osteoporosis. *Baillieres Clin Endocrinol Metab* 12:251, 1998.
311. Cummings SR, Bauer DC: Do statins prevent bone cardiovascular disease and fracture? *JAMA* 283:3255, 2000.
312. Lane NE, Sanchez S, Modin GW, Genant HK, Ini E, Arnaud DC: Parathyroid hormone treatment can reverse corticosteroid-induced osteoporosis. Results of a randomized controlled clinical trial. *J Clin Invest* 102:1627, 1998.
313. Jones G, Nguyen T, Sambrook PN, Eisman JA: Thiazide diuretics and fractures: can meta-analysis help? *J Bone Miner Res* 10:106, 1995.
314. Mosekilde L, Melsen F: Effect of antithyroid treatment on calcium-phosphorus metabolism in hyperthyroidism: II. Bone histomorphometry. *Acta Endocrinol (Copenh)* 87:751, 1978.
315. Glorieux FH, Bishop NJ, Plotkin H, Chabot G, Lanque G, Travers R: Cyclic administration of pamidronate in children with severe osteogenesis imperfecta. *N Engl J Med* 339:947, 1998.
316. Hoekman K, Papapoulos SE, Peters ACB, Bijvoet OLM: Characteristics and bisphosphonate treatment of a patient with juvenile osteoporosis. *J Clin Endocrinol Metab* 61:952, 1985.
317. Whyte MP: Skeletal disorders characterized by osteosclerosis or hyperostosis, in Avioli LV, Krane SM (eds): *Metabolic Bone Disease and Clinically Related Disorders*, 3rd ed. San Diego, Academic Press, 1998, p 697.
318. Sly WS, Whyte MP, Sundaram V, Tashian RE, Hewett-Emmett D, Geribaud P, Vainsel M, Baluarte HJ, et al: Carbonic anhydrase II deficiency in 12 families with the autosomal recessive syndrome of osteopetrosis with renal tubular acidosis and cerebral calcification. *N Engl J Med* 313:139, 1985.
319. Jagadha V, Halliday WC, Becker LE, Hinton D: The association of infantile osteopetrosis and neuronal storage disease in two brothers. *Acta Neuropathol* 75:233, 1998.
320. Frattini A, Orchard PJ, Sobacchi C, Giliani S, Abinun M, Mattsson JP, Keeling DJ, Andersson AK, Wallbrandt P, Zecca L, Notarangelo LD, Vezzoni P, Villa A: Defects in TCIRG1 sub-unit of the vacuolar proton pump are responsible for a subset of human autosomal recessive osteopetrosis. *Nat Genet* 25:343, 2000.
321. Bollerslev J: Autosomal dominant osteopetrosis: Bone metabolism and epidemiological, clinical, and hormonal aspects. *Endocr Rev* 10:45, 1989.
322. Van Hul W, Bollerslev J, Gram J, Van Hul E, Wuyts W, Benichou O, Vonhoenocker F, Willems PJ: Localization of a gene for autosomal dominant osteopetrosis (Albers-Schonberg disease to chromosome 1p21. *Am Hum Genet* 61:363, 1997.
323. Shapiro F, Glimcher MJ, Holtrop ME, Tashjian AH Jr, Brickley-Parsons D, Kenzora JE: Human osteopetrosis: A histological, ultrastructural and biochemical study. *J Bone Joint Surg [Am]* 62-A:384, 1980.
324. Milgram JW, Jasty M: Osteopetrosis: A morphological study of twenty-one cases. *J Bone Joint Surg [Am]* 64-A:912, 1982.
325. Walker DG: Bone resorption restored in osteopetrotic mice by transplants of normal bone marrow and spleen cells. *Science* 190:784, 1975.
326. Coccia PF, Krivit W, Cervenka J, Clawson C, Kersey J, Kim TH, Nesbit ME, Ramsay NKC, et al: Successful bone-marrow transplantation for infantile malignant osteopetrosis. *N Engl J Med* 302:701, 1980.
327. Eapen M, Davies SM, Ramsay NK, Orchard PJ: Hematopoietic stem cell transplantation for infantile osteopetrosis. *Bone Marrow Transplant* 22:941, 1998.
328. Key L, Carnes D, Cole S, Holtrop M, Bar-Shavit Z, Shapiro F, Arceci R, Steinberg J, Gundberg C, Kahn A, Teitelbaum S, Anast C: Treatment of congenital osteopetrosis with high-dose calcitriol. *N Eng J Med* 310:409, 1984.
329. Key LL Jr, Rodriguiz RM, Willi SM, Wright NM, Hatcher HC, Eyre DR, Cure JK, Griffin PP, Ries WL: Long-term treatment of osteopetrosis with recombinant human interferon gamma. *N Engl J Med* 332:1594, 1995.
330. Slatopolsky E, Delmez JA: Renal osteodystrophy, in Avioli LV, Krane SM (eds): *Metabolic Bone Disease and Clinically Related Disorders*, 3rd ed. San Diego, Academic Press, 1998, p 443.
331. Hodsman AB, Sherrard DJ, Wong EGC, Brickman AS, Lee DBN, Alfrey AC, Singer FR, Norman AW, Coburn JW: Vitamin D resistant osteomalacia in hemodialysis patients lacking secondary hyperparathyroidism. *Ann Intern Med* 94:629, 1981.
332. Eastwood JB, Harris E, Stamp TCB, DeWardener HE: Vitamin D deficiency in the osteomalacia of chronic renal failure. *Lancet* 2:1209, 1976.
333. Sherrard DJ, Baylink DJ, Wergedahl JE, Maloney N: Quantitative histological studies on the pathogenesis of uremic bone disease. *J Clin Endocrinol Metab* 39:119, 1974.
334. Bressot C, Courpron P, Edouard C, Meunier P: *Histomorphométrie des ostéopathies endocriniennes*. Lyon, Association Corporative des Etudiants en Médecine de Lyon, 1976, p 85.
335. Hercz G, Pei Y, Greenwood C, Manuel A, Saiphoo C, Goodman WG, Segre GV, Fenton S, Sherrard DJ: Aplastic osteodystrophy without aluminum: The role of suppressed parathyroid function. *Kidney Int* 44:860, 1993.
336. Mason RS, Lissner D, Wilkinson M, Posen S: Vitamin D metabolites and their relationship to azotaemic osteodystrophy. *Clin Endocrinol (Oxf)* 13:375, 1980.
337. Portale AA, Booth BE, Tsai HC, Morris RC Jr: Reduced plasma concentration of 1,25-dihydroxyvitamin D in children with moderate renal insufficiency. *Kidney Int* 21:627, 1982.
338. Hodsman AB, Sherrard DJ, Alfrey AC, Ott S, Brickman AS, Miller NL, Maloney NA, Coburn JW: Bone aluminum and histomorphometric features of renal osteodystrophy. *J Clin Endocrinol Metab* 54:539, 1982.
339. Teitelbaum SL, Bergfeld MA, Freitag J, Hruska KA, Slatopolsky E: Do parathyroid hormone and 1,25-dihydroxyvitamin D modulate bone formation in uremia? *J Clin Endocrinol Metab* 51:247, 1980.
340. Weinstein RS: Decreased mineralization in hemodialysis patients after subtotal parathyroidectomy. *Calcif Tissue Int* 34:16, 1982.
341. Sherrard DJ, Ott SM, Andress DL: Pseudohyperparathyroidism: Syndrome associated with aluminum intoxication in patients with renal failure. *Am J Med* 79:127, 1985.
342. Slatopolsky E, Delmez J: Bone disease in chronic renal failure and after renal transplantation, in Coe FL, Favus MJ (eds): *Disorders of Bone and Mineral Metabolism*. New York, Raven Press, 1991, p 905.

343. Wilson L, Felsenfeld A, Drezner MK, Llach F: Altered divalent ion metabolism in early renal failure: Role of 1,25$(OH)_2D$. *Kidney Int* 27:565, 1985.
344. Brickman AS, Sherrard DJ, Jowsey J, Singer FR, Baylink DJ, Maloney N, Massry SG, Norman AW, Coburn JW: 1,25-Dihydroxy-cholecalciferol: Effect on skeletal lesions and plasma parathyroid hormone levels in uremic osteodystrophy. *Arch Intern Med* 134:883, 1974.
345. Masry SG: Requirements of vitamin D metabolites in patients with renal disease. *Am J Clin Nutr* 33:1530, 1980.
346. Bordier P, Zingraff J, Gueris J, Jungers P, Marie P, Pechet M, Rasmussen H: The effect of $1\alpha(OH)D_3$ and $1\alpha,25(OH)_2D_3$ on the bone in patients with renal osteodystrophy. *Am J Med* 64:101, 1978.
347. Eastwood JB, Stamp TCB, DeWardener HE, Bordier PJ, Arnaud CD: The effect of 25-hydroxyvitamin D_3 in the osteomalacia of chronic renal failure. *Clin Sci Mol Med* 52:499, 1977.
348. Wells SA Jr, Ross AJ III, Dale JK, Gray RS: Transplantation of the parathyroid glands: Current status. *Surg Clin North Am* 59:167, 1979.
349. Andress DL, Norris KC, Coburn JW, Slatopolsky EA, Sherrard DJ: Intravenous calcitriol in the treatment of refractory osteitis fibrosa of chronic renal failure. *N Engl J Med* 321:274, 1989.
350. Tsukamoto Y, Nomura M, Takahashi Y: The "oral 1,25 $(OH)_2$ D_3 pulse therapy" in hemodialysis patients with severe secondary hyperparathyroidism. *Nephrology* 57:23, 1991.
351. Goldenberg MM: Paricalcitol, a new agent for the management of secondary hyperparathyroidism in patients undergoing chronic renal dialysis. *Clin Ther* 21:432, 1999.
352. Malluche HH, Smith AJ, Abreo K, Faugere MC: The use of deferoxamine in the management of aluminum accumulation in bone in patients with renal failure. *N Engl J Med* 311:140, 1984.
353. Thompson RC Jr, Gaull GE, Horwitz SJ, Schenk RK: Hereditary hyperphosphatasia: Studies of three siblings. *Am J Med* 47:209, 1969.
354. Whalen JP, Horwith M, Krook L, McIntyre I, Mena A, Viteri F, Town B, Nunez EA: Calcitonin treatment in hereditary bone dysplasia with hyperphosphatasemia: A radiographic and histologic study of bone. *AJR* 129:29, 1977.
355. Nunez EA, Horwith M, Krook L, Whalen JP: An electron microscopic investigation of human familial bone dysplasia: Inhibition of osteocytic osteolysis and induction of osteocytic formation of elastic fibers following calcitonin treatment. *Am J Pathol* 94:1, 1979.
356. Doyle FH, Woodhouse NJY, Glen CA, Joplin CF, MacIntyre I: Healing of the bones in juvenile Paget's disease treated by human calcitonin. *Br J Radiol* 47:9, 1974.
357. Blanco O, Stivel M, Mautalen C, Schajowicz F: Familial idiopathic hyperphosphatasia. A study of two siblings treated with porcine calcitonin. *J Bone Joint Surg* [*Br*] 59B:421, 1977.
358. Dunn V, Condon VR, Rallison ML: Familial hyperphosphatasemia: Diagnosis in early infancy and response to human thyrocalcitonin therapy. *AJR* 132:541, 1979.
359. Cassinelli HR, Mautalen CA, Heinrich JJ, Miglietta A, Bergada C: Familial idiopathic hyperphosphatasia (FIH): Response to long-term treatment with pamidronate (APD). *Bone Miner* 19:175, 1992.
360. Albright F, Butler AM, Hampton AO, Smith P: Syndrome characterized by osteitis fibrosa disseminata, areas of pigmentation and endocrine dysfunction, with precocious puberty in females: Report of five cases. *N Engl J Med* 216:727, 1937.
361. Albright F: Polyostotic fibrous dysplasia: A defense of the entity. *J Clin Endocrinol* 7:307, 1947.
362. Von Recklinghausen F: Die Fibrose oder deformirende Ostitis, die Osteomalacie und die osteoplastische Carcinose in ihren gegenseitigen Beziehungen, in *Festschrift für Rudolf Virchow*. Berlin, G Reimer, 1891.
363. Harris WH, Dudley HR Jr, Barry RJ: The natural history of fibrous dysplasia: An orthopaedic, pathological and roentgenographic study. *J Bone Joint Surg* [*Am*] 44A:207, 1962.
364. Schwartz DT, Alpert M: The malignant transformation of fibrous dysplasia. *Am J Med Sci* 247:35, 1964.
365. Gianoutsos MP, Thompson JF, Marsden FW: Mazabraud's syndrome: Intramuscular myxoma associated with fibrous dysplasia of bone. *Aust N J Surg* 60:825, 1960.
366. Benedict PH: Endocrine features in Albright's syndrome (fibrous dysplasia of bone). *Metabolism* 11:30, 1962.
367. McArthur RG, Hayles AB, Lambert PW: Albright's syndrome with rickets. *Mayo Clin Proc* 54:313, 1979.
368. Shires R, Whyte MP, Avioli LV: Idiopathic hypothalamic hypogonadotropic hypogonadism with polyostotic fibrous dysplasia. *Arch Intern Med* 139:1187, 1979.
369. Cuttler L, Jackson JA, Saeed uz-Zafar M, Levitsky LL, Mellinger RC, Frohman LA: Hypersecretion of growth hormone and prolactin in McCune-Albright syndrome. *J Clin Endocrinol Metab* 68:1148, 1989.
370. Shenker A, Weinstein RS, Moran A, Pescovitz OH, Charest NJ, Feuillan PP, Spiegel AM: Severe endocrine and nonendocrine manifestations of the McCune-Albright syndrome associated with activating mutations of stimulatory G protein G_s. *J Pediatr* 123:509, 1993.
371. Marie PJ, de Pollak C, Chanson P, Lomri A: Increased proliferation of osteoblastic cells expressing the activating G_s α mutation in monostotic and polyostotic fibrous dysplasia. *Am J Pathol* 150:1059, 1997.
372. Riminucci M, Fisher LW, Shenker A, Spiegel AM, Bianco P, Robey PG: Fibrous dysplasia of bone in the McCune-Albright syndrome: Abnormalities in bone formation. *Am J Pathol* 151:1587, 1997.
373. Weinstein LS, Shenker A, Gejman PV, Merino MJ, Friedman E, Spiegel AM: Activating mutations of the stimulatory G protein in the McCune-Albright syndrome. *N Engl J Med* 325:1688, 1991.
374. Yamamoto T, Ozono K, Kasayama S, Yoh K, Hiroshima K, Takagi M, Matsumoto S, Michigami T, Yamaoka K, Kishimoto T, Okada S: Increased IL-6 production by cells isolated from the fibrous bone dysplasia tissues in patients with McCune-Albright syndrome. *J Clin Invest* 98:30, 1996.
375. Singer FR: Fibrous dysplasia of bone. The bone lesion unmasked. *Am J Pathol* 151:1511, 1997.
376. Liens D, Delmas PD, Meunier PJ: Long-term effects of intravenous pamidronate in fibrous dysplasia of bone. *Lancet* 343:953, 1994.
377. Weinstein RS: Long-term aminobisphosphonate treatment of fibrous dysplasia. Spectacular increase in bone density. *J Bone Miner Res* 12:1314, 1997.
378. Chapurlat RD, Delmas PD, Liens D, Meunier PJ: Long-term effects of intravenous pamidronate in fibrous dysplasia of bone. *J Bone Miner Res* 12:1746, 1997.
379. Feuillan PP, Foster CM, Pecovitz OH, Hench KD, Shawker T, Dwyer A, Malley JD, Barnes K, Loriaux DL, Cutler GB Jr: Treatment of precocious puberty in the McCune-Albright syndrome with the aromatase inhibitor testolactone. *N Engl J Med* 315:1115, 1986.
380. Stephenson RB, London MD, Hankin FM, Kaufer H: Fibrous dysplasia: An analysis of options for treatment. *J Bone Joint Surg* 69-A:400, 1987.
381. Paget J: On a form of chronic inflammmation of bones (osteitis deformans). *Med Chir Trans* 60:27, 1877.
382. Singer FR, Krane SM: Paget's disease of bone, in Avioli LV, Krane SM (eds): *Metabolic Bone Disease and Clinically Related Disorders*, 3rd ed. San Diego, Academic Press, 1998, p 545.
383. Singer FR, Leach RJ: Genetics of Paget's disease, in Econs MJ (ed): *The Genetics of Osteoporosis and Metabolic Bone Disease,* Totowa, NJ, The Humana Press, 2000, p 309.
384. Hughes AE, Ralston SH, Marken J, Bell C, MacPherson H, Wallace RGH, van Hul W, Whyte MP, Nakatsuka K, Hovy L, Anderson DM: Mutations in TNFSF11A, affecting the signal peptide of RANK, cause familial expansile osteolysis. *Nat Genet* 24:45, 2000.
385. Franck WA, Bress NM, Singer FR, Krane SM: Rheumatic manifestations of Paget's disease of bone. *Am J Med* 56:592, 1974.
386. Heistad DD, Abboud FM, Schmid PG, Mark AL, Wilson WR: Regulation of blood flow in Paget's disease of bone. *J Clin Invest* 55:69, 1975.
387. Barry HC: *Paget's Disease of Bone*. Baltimore, Williams & Wilkins, 1969.
388. Arnalich F, Plaza I, Sobrino JA, Oliver J, Barbado J, Pena JM, Vazquez JJ: Cardiac size and function in Paget's disease of bone. *Int J Cardiol* 5:491, 1984.
389. Waxman AD, Ducker S, McKee D, Siemsen JK, Singer FR: Evaluation of ^{99m}Tc diphosphonate kinetics and bone scans in patients with Paget's disease before and after calcitonin treatment. *Radiology* 125:761, 1977.
390. Khairi MRA, Wellman HN, Robb JA, Johnston CC Jr: Paget's disease of bone (osteitis deformans): Symptomatic lesions and bone scan. *Ann Intern Med* 79:348, 1973.
391. Waxman AD, McKee D, Siemsen JK, Singer FR: Gallium scanning in Paget's disease of bone: The effects of calcitonin. *AJR* 134:303, 1980.

392. Nagant de Deuxchaisnes C, Krane SM: Paget's disease of bone: Clinical and metabolic observations. *Medicine (Baltimore)* 43:233, 1964.
393. Posen S, Clifton-Bligh P, Wilkinson M: Paget's disease of bone and hyperparathyroidism: Coincidence or causal relationship? *Calcif Tissue Res* 26:107, 1978.
394. Rebel A, Malkani K, Baslé M, Bregeon C: Osteoclast ultrastructure in Paget's disease. *Calcif Tissue Res* 20:187, 1976.
395. Mills BG, Singer FR: Nuclear inclusions in Paget's disease of bone. *Science* 194:201, 1976.
396. Singer FR: Update on viral etiology of Paget's disease of bone. *J Bone Miner Res* (Suppl 2)14:29, 1999.
397. Singer FR: Paget's disease of bone: A slow virus infection? *Calcif Tissue Int* 31:185, 1980.
398. Rebel A, Baslé M, Pouplard A, Kouyoumdjian S, Filon R, Lepatezour A: Viral antigens in osteoclasts from Paget's disease of bone. *Lancet* 2:344, 1980.
399. Mills BG, Singer FR, Weiner LP, Suffin SC, Stabile E, Holst P: Evidence for both respiratory syncytial virus and measles virus antigens in the osteoclasts of patients with Paget's disease of bone. *Clin Orthop* 183:303, 1984.
400. Meunier PJ, Ravault A: Treatment of Paget's disease with etidronate disodium, in Singer FR, Wallach S (eds): *Paget's Disease of Bone, Clinical Assessment, Present and Future Therapy*. New York, Elsevier, 1991, p 176.
401. Thiebaud D, Jaeger P, Gobelet C, Jacquet AF, Burckhardt P: A single infusion of the bisphosphonate AHPrBP (A PD) as treatment of Paget's disease of bone. *Am J Med* 85:207, 1988.
402. Cundy T, Wattie D, King AR: High-dose pamidronate in the management of resistant Paget's disease. *Calcif Tissue Int* 58:6, 1996.
403. Schweitzer DH, Oostendorp-van de Ruit M,Van der Plujim G, Lowik CW, Papapoulos SE: Interleukin-6 and the acute phase response during treatment of patients with Paget's disease with the nitrogen-containing bisphosphonate dimethylaminohydroxypropylidene bisphosphonate. *J Bone Miner Res* 10:956, 1995.
404. Harinck HIJ, Bijvoet OLM, Blanksma HJ, Dahlinghaus-Nienhuys PJ: Efficacious management with APD in Paget's disease of bone. *Clin Orthop Rel Res* 217:79, 1987.
405. Reid IR, Nicholson GC, Weinstein RS, Hosking DJ, Cundy T, Kotowicz MA, Murphy WA Jr, Yeap S, Dufresne S, Lombardi A, Musliner TA, Thompson DE, Yates AJ: Biochemical and radiologic improvement in Paget's disease of bone treated with alendronate: A randomized placebo-controlled trial. *Am J Med* 171:341, 1996.
406. Siris E, Weinstein RS, Altman R, Conte JM, Favus M, Lombardi A, Lyles K, Mc Ilwain H, Murphy WA Jr, Reda C, Rude R, Seton M, Tiegs R, Thompson D, Tucci JR, Yates AJ, Zimering M: Comparative study of alendronate versus etidronate for the treatment of Paget's disease of bone. *J Clin Endocrinol Metab* 81:961, 1996.
407. Miller PD, Brown JP, Siris ES, Hoseyni MS, Axelrod DW, Bekker PJ: A randomized, double-blind comparison of risedronate and etidronate in the treatment of Paget's disease of bone. *Am J Med* 106:513, 1999.
408. Siris ES, Chines AA, Altman RD, Brown JP, Johnston CC Jr, Lang R, McClung MR, Mallette LE, Miller PD, Ryan WG, Singer FR, Tucci JR, Eusebio RA, Bekker PJ: Risedronate in the treatment of Paget's disease of bone: an open label, multicenter study. *J Bone Miner Res* 13:1032, 1998.
409. Reginster JY, Colson F, Morlock G, Combe B, Ethgen D, Geusens P: Evaluation of the efficacy and safety of oral tiludronate in Paget's disease of bone. *Arthritis Rheum* 35:967, 1992.
410. Devogelaer JP, Malghem J, Stasse P, Nagant de Deuxchaisnes C: Biological and radiological responses to oral etidronate and tiludronate in Paget's disease of bone. *Bone* 20:259, 1997.
411. Meyers M, Singer FR: Osteotomy for tibia vara in Paget's disease under cover of calcitonin. *J Bone Joint Surg* [*Am*] 60A:810, 1978.

CHAPTER 24

Nephrolithiasis

Bruce Ettinger

INTRODUCTION

Epidemiology

About 10–12 percent of men and 3–5 percent of women in the United States have *urolithiasis* during their lifetimes.[1] The incidence in men is about 1.3 in 1,000 yearly and is apparently increasing.[1] Stones are the cause of 1 in every 1,000 hospital admissions in the United States, or about 200,000 admissions yearly. Patients with calcium stone disease or magnesium ammonium phosphate (MAP) (struvite) stones typically show clinical evidence of disease during midlife, whereas patients with uric acid stones tend to be older and patients with cystine stones tend to be younger (Fig. 24-1).[2]

Kidney stone prevalence varies widely, both throughout the world and within countries. The concept of high-prevalence "stone belts" in the United States derives largely from a nationwide survey of U.S. hospital admissions for stone disease between 1948 and 1952[3] in which the prevalence of stone disease in the southeastern United States was 65 percent higher than nationally. A similar study of hospital admissions yielded a different distribution of high-prevalence regions[4] but also found that the southeastern part of the country had 35 percent more stone disease. These studies fostered the concept of a stone belt and prompted investigations of soil, water, and food in these regions. More recently, the stone belt concept has been disproven. First, a large epidemiologic study based on self-reports of stone disease from more than a million men and women showed an increasing prevalence from north to south and from west to east, and found that temperature, sunlight, and beverage consumption accounted for nearly all these regional differences.[5] Another large survey based on self-reports of 45,289 male physicians aged ≥40 years did not find regional differences in kidney stone incidence.[6]

Classification of Calculi by Clinical Presentation

The term *nephrolithiasis* refers specifically to stones that form in the renal pelvis or calices. Such stones, which represent 90–95 percent of the urinary tract calculi encountered in industrialized countries, are responsible for the ureteral colic with which stone disease is associated. Stones in the upper tract that grow or coalesce to mold the collecting system of the kidney are appropriately termed *staghorn calculi*. Staghorn stones usually result from infection and are most often composed of struvite or magnesium ammonium phosphate (MAP), but are occasionally composed of uric acid or cystine. In cases of extreme supersaturation, copious amorphous, semisolid precipitates may be formed by uric acid, cystine, or calcium phosphate crystals; these precipitates produce bilateral intrarenal or extrarenal obstruction, either of which may cause acute renal failure.

Nephrocalcinosis, or calcification within the renal parenchyma, is an uncommon radiologic finding and is usually bilateral, affecting the medullary or corticomedullary areas of the kidneys. *Cortical* nephrocalcinosis (e.g., in acute cortical necrosis of chronic glomerulonephritis) is rare. *Medullary* nephrocalcinosis is often due to dystrophic calcification related to local tissue injury; examples are renal tuberculosis, infarction, mercury poisoning, and tumor. Nephrocalcinosis and nephrolithiasis coexist in only a few conditions, including medullary sponge kidney, renal tubular acidosis (RTA), primary hyperparathyroidism, and other hypercalcemic conditions. Nephrocalcinosis in a patient with nephrolithiasis strongly suggests one of these conditions.

Bladder stones, which account for ≤5 percent of urinary tract stones in the United States, occur principally in elderly men with prostatic obstruction. About 60 percent of bladder stones are composed of calcium salts, 40 percent of struvite, and <10 percent of uric acid. In a few rare cases these patients also have nephrolithiasis. Bladder stones are endemic among children in southern Asia, southern Europe, and the Middle East. These stones are composed predominantly of ammonium acid urate admixed with various proportions of calcium oxalate, a stone composition almost never found in industrialized nations. Although the pathogenesis of endemic bladder stones is unknown, diet apparently plays a major role: Such stones are sometimes referred to as *malnutrition stones*. The same stones were common in young boys in the western world a century ago but became rare after industrialization.[7]

Classification of Calculi by Crystalline Structure

Stones are classified into five major types on the basis of their crystalline components. The term *mixed* is used when the second largest crystalline component contributes >15 percent of stone mass. Based on the results from three large stone analysis centers, the data in Table 24-1 give the relative frequencies of the five stone types.[8–11] Almost all the stones reported in these three series were composed of calcium oxalate; the other principal stone types occur rarely.

Crystallographic analysis of urinary calculi is a key diagnostic step. Classification by crystallographic type (1) provides information about stone pathogenesis, (2) provides the diagnosis in some cases, and (3) defines general or specific approaches (or both) to medical or surgical therapy. Stone analysis is diagnostically useful when it reveals one of the less common stone types, in which case analysis either makes the diagnosis obvious (struvite, cystine, or

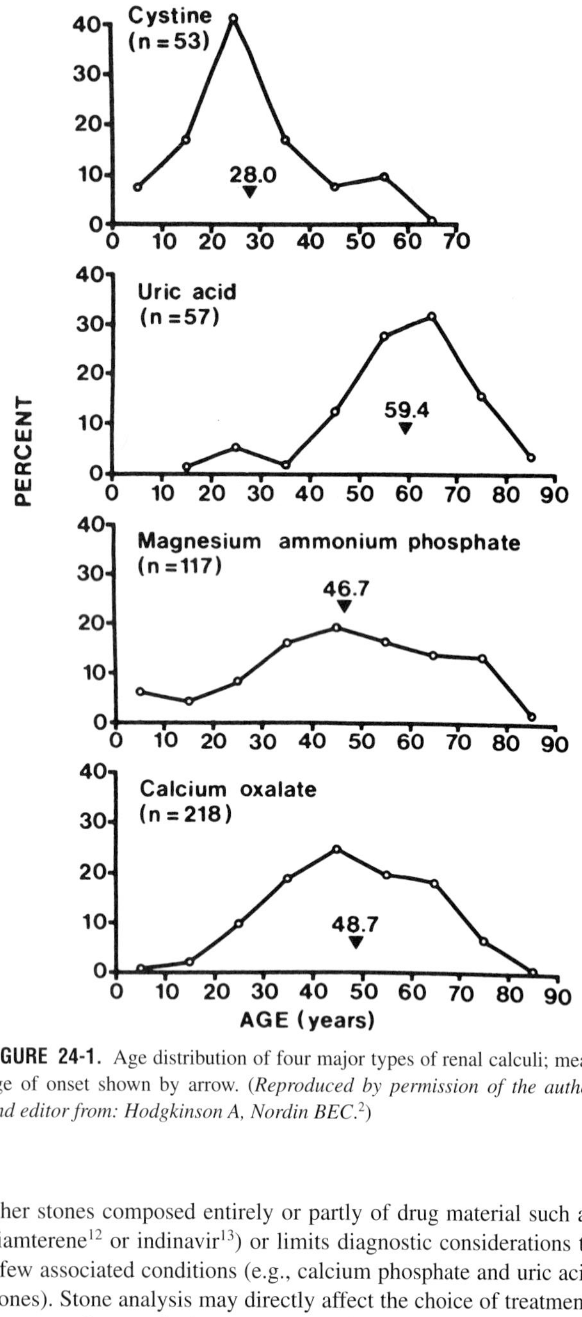

FIGURE 24-1. Age distribution of four major types of renal calculi; mean age of onset shown by arrow. (*Reproduced by permission of the author and editor from: Hodgkinson A, Nordin BEC.*[2])

other stones composed entirely or partly of drug material such as triamterene[12] or indinavir[13]) or limits diagnostic considerations to a few associated conditions (e.g., calcium phosphate and uric acid stones). Stone analysis may directly affect the choice of treatment. For example, a calculus composed of a uric acid nucleus surrounded by calcium oxalate crystals indicates a different mechanism and mandates different therapy than would be the case if the components were reversed. Because calculi of different crystalline structures respond differently to shock-wave lithotripsy, knowledge of stone analysis may facilitate the determination of specific therapy.

Quantitating Clinical Stone Events

Numerous terms and concepts have been introduced in an attempt to clarify and standardize the assessment of the morbidity of stone disease. The Mayo Clinic group[14] uses the term *metabolic activity* to define clinical or radiographic evidence (or both) of new stone formation or stone growth; a patient who shows no such evidence during a 12-month period is considered to have metabolically inactive stone disease. Similarly, the term *surgical activity* describes urologic surgical intervention as a function of time. Coe and associates[7,15] described five interrelated characteristics of stone disease which together define stone morbidity: (1) stone "burden," or the number of stones seen on x-ray films, (2) the rate of formation of new stones, (3) the rate of growth of existing stones, (4) the number and extent of clinical events (infections, surgical procedures, and hospitalizations), and (5) the extent of renal damage caused by stones.

Theories of Stone Pathogenesis

Three theories have been proposed for stone pathogenesis: the matrix theory, the inhibitor theory, and the crystalloid theory. Each has been modified since it was first proposed, and each has current proponents; none of these theories, however, is exclusive of the others.

The *matrix theory* holds that the organic matrix in all stones is critical to stone formation. The process is considered analogous to mineralization of the *osteoid*, the organized organic matrix of bone. Matrix proteins (mostly mucoproteins) in urine and stone material were studied most extensively by Boyce.[16] Critics of this theory note that the matrix substance is similar or identical in stones of all crystalline types as well as in concretions artificially precipitated from urine, suggesting that the material is trapped as an "innocent bystander" instead of causing stone formation. The authors of the most recent comprehensive review of urinary stone matrix commented on the paucity of new research in this area.[17]

The *inhibitor theory* maintains that stone formation results from a deficiency of urinary substances which normally inhibit crystallization and crystal growth or aggregation. This theory became attractive more than three decades ago, when Thomas and Howard[18] found that urine from stone patients readily calcified rachitic rat cartilage, whereas urine from normal subjects did not. The authors introduced the terms *good urine* and *evil urine*, attributing their findings to the relative absence of inhibitor substances in evil urine, which were first identified as low-molecular-weight peptides. The alternative view—that evil urine might be more supersaturated by mineralizing substances—was not critically tested. Other natural inhibitors of crystallization and crystal

TABLE 24-1. Approximate Prevalence Rates of Five Major Stone Types Reported by Four Large Stone Analysis Centers

	Investigator			
	Prien[8]	Herring[9]	Smith[10]	Mandel*
Total number of stones	24,000	10,000	4,525	28,900
Stone type:				
Calcium oxalate	80–84†	72	70	60
Calcium phosphate	1–2	2	9	13
MAP-struvite	6–9	16	9	11
Uric acid	6–10	7	10	13
Cystine	1–2	0.9	0.7	0.6

Note: In cases of mixed composition, the predominant crystal form is reported.

MAP = magnesium ammonium phosphate.

*Personal communication, Gretchen S. Mandel, PhD, September 1991.

†Ranges of annual prevalence data during years 1952–1961.

Source: Adapted and reproduced with permission of the editor and publisher from: Ettinger B, Insogna KL: Nephrolithiasis, in Felig P, Baxter JD, Frohman LA (eds): *Endocrinology and Metabolism*, 3rd ed. New York, McGraw-Hill, 1995, p. 1597.[11a]

growth—including pyrophosphate, citrate, magnesium, and other poorly defined substances—have been implicated by various investigators.[7,15,19] Such substances may be more important in preventing crystals from growing and aggregating into clinically significant stone masses than in preventing crystallization. However, stone pathogenesis is probably not promoted by deficiency of one or more of these substances. A comparison of urinary inhibitors in 25 patients who each had formed more than 10 stones failed to show any lower inhibitory activity than healthy controls.[20]

The *crystalloid* (or precipitation-crystallization) *theory* considers stone formation in strictly physical chemical terms. This theory relates crystallization and the growth of calculi in urine to supersaturation by stone-forming constituents. Of the three classic theories of stone pathogenesis, this theory has the most experimental support and also provides a conceptual framework on which a clinical approach to stone disease can be based.

Physicochemical Aspects of Stone Formation

Fig. 24-2 shows the relative zones and ranges of saturation of the five major stone-forming constituents in normal urine.[2] The three zones of saturation—undersaturated, metastably supersaturated, and oversaturated—are segregated by two limits: the solubility product and the formation product. These terms may be better understood by using several examples. If excess solid material such as calcium oxalate is added to distilled water and left to dissolve for a prolonged period, the solution and the remaining solid phase eventually reach a stable equilibrium. This equilibrium defines the solubility of the material in aqueous solution; to determine the *solubility product*, the concentration of calcium is multiplied by oxalate ions in solution. The solid material is then removed, leaving a saturated solution of calcium oxalate with no solid phase. If a concentrated calcium or oxalate solution is added to the saturated solution, it remains clear and free of solid phase to a critical concentration: the *formation product*. The solution then clouds as solid calcium oxalate crystals form and begin to grow. The zone between the solubility product and the formation product defines a metastable, saturated solution in which spontaneous precipitation does not occur (the metastably supersaturated zone shown in Fig. 24-2). A metastable solution can lead to crystallization and support crystal growth. At and above the formation product, spontaneous nucleation inevitably occurs (the labile, or oversaturated, zone shown in Fig. 24-2). A supersaturated solution produces both spontaneous nucleation and crystal growth.

The term *nucleation* (instead of *precipitation*) is used to define the initiation of a crystalline solid phase in aqueous solution. Crystal nuclei contain only about 100 atoms and are of no clinical consequence; enlargement of these nascent particles into a solid phase of substantial mass produces clinical consequences. Although related, crystal nucleation and crystal growth must be considered separately. Urinary calculi occur through the combined processes of homogeneous crystal growth, epitaxial crystal growth, and crystal aggregation. The first two processes require that crystals be laid on a lattice structure. Homogeneous crystallization occurs when crystals are laid on the surface of an identical crystal lattice; epitaxial crystallization occurs when a crystal lattice provides an acceptable fit for the crystalline and atomic structure of added nonidentical crystals. Aggregation, or agglomeration, depends on crystals adhering to each other to form large clusters. The binding forces bringing about aggregation may be promoted or inhibited by substances which affect neither nucleation nor other processes of crystal growth.

The crystalloid theory can readily explain the four "minor" types of stones: cystine, uric acid, struvite, and pure calcium phosphate. Each stone type can be understood in relatively straightforward terms of supersaturation with respect to the ionic constituents of urine. In contrast, understanding calcium oxalate stone disease in terms of crystalloid theory is complicated by the interaction of numerous other ions that can alter the solubility of calcium oxalate (see Calcium Oxalate and Mixed Calcium Stones).

Evaluation and Treatment

The Role of the Internist

The internist is usually expected to identify, interpret, and treat metabolic abnormalities that lead to stone formation. Patients referred for medical management often have had multiple stone

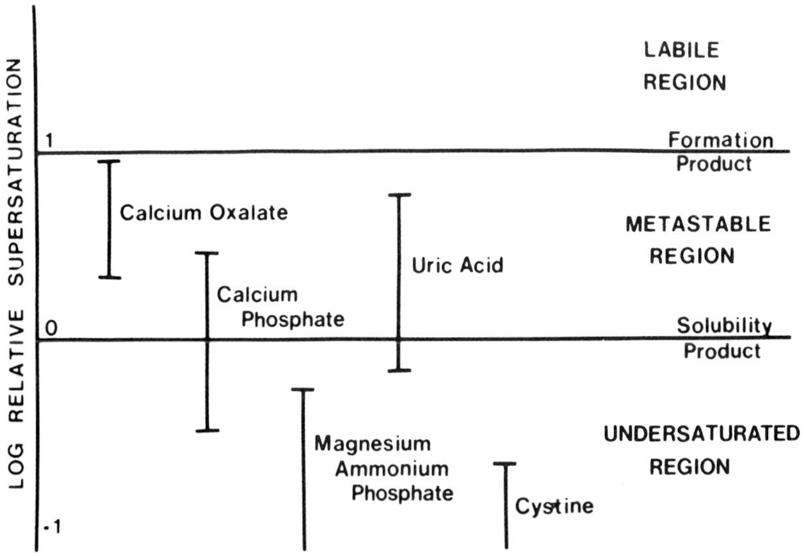

FIGURE 24-2. Three zones of saturation in urine: undersaturation, metastable, saturation, and oversaturation (labile region). Ranges of saturation of five major crystalline stone constituents in normal urine are shown. (*Adapted and reproduced by permission of the author and editor from Hodgkinson A, Nordin BEC.*[2])

events or surgical procedures. The finding of an unusual stone type (e.g., cystine) sometimes prompts a referral. The internist is rarely asked to help make decisions involving urologic surgery. However, anyone providing medical care to patients with nephrolithiasis should be aware of the latest advances in the urologic management of this disease.

Clinical Presentation

The principal clinical consequences of renal stones are pain, hematuria, obstruction, and infection. Impaired renal function is not a natural or predictable outcome of stone disease but results from stone-related complications such as chronic obstruction, infection, postoperative scarring, and surgical removal of renal tissue.

Ureteral colic produces pain of extreme intensity. The term *colic* is a misnomer because the pain typically begins as vague discomfort and increases gradually, reaching maximum intensity about an hour after onset and rendering the patient incapable of lying down or sitting still. Obstruction of the ureteropelvic junction produces pain in the flank and is often associated with nausea and vomiting. A stone too large to negotiate the ureteropelvic junction may produce intermittent obstruction in a ball-valve fashion. Obstruction lower in the ureter causes pain that radiates from the flank toward the anterior pelvis. Obstruction of the ureterovesical junction produces pain that radiates to the ipsilateral testicle or labium; stones in this region that have passed into the bladder often cause urgency and dysuria, symptoms that mimic cystitis. Staghorn stones or other stones that remain adherent to the renal papillae usually do not produce symptoms, although microscopic or gross hematuria often occurs. Few of these patients experience nagging, chronic flank discomfort.

Surgical Management of Nephrolithiasis

In the past 25 years, considerable improvements have been made in basic kidney surgery; new techniques include anatrophic nephrolithotomy and coagulum pyelolithotomy. However, urologic treatment of stones has been revolutionized by two less invasive techniques: percutaneous nephrolithotomy and lithotripsy. *Lithotripsy*, or stone smashing, is now routinely accomplished through percutaneous nephrostomy or by focusing high-energy waves produced by external devices (extracorporeal shock-wave lithotripsy [ESWL]). Estimates indicate that percutaneous lithotripsy is associated with one-tenth the morbidity of surgical nephrolithotomy and that ESWL is associated with one-tenth the morbidity of percutaneous lithotripsy.[21]

Although the urologist chooses the stone removal procedure, the internist should have a basic knowledge of shock-wave principles, the effects of shock waves in tissue and animal studies, and the clinical results obtained with ESWL therapy. Overall, ESWL is 80 percent successful in completely eliminating stones; however, its effectiveness in eliminating large stones (2.5–3.0 cm) is <50 percent, particularly for stones in the lower renal calices. In such cases, urologists thus use percutaneous lithotripsy as the initial treatment. For patients in whom stone material is still evident after percutaneous lithotripsy or ESWL, current practice now is to give ESWL immediately. Complete elimination of stones is imperative for reducing the likelihood of stone recurrence.

The immediate complications of ESWL include severe pain (sometimes requiring hospitalization), hematuria, perinephric hematoma, obstruction by large stone fragments or by minute stone fragments filling the ureter (*steinstrasse*), and, rarely, hemorrhage or septicemia. About 5 percent of patients receiving ESWL must be hospitalized as a result of these complications. ESWL traumatizes the kidney in a way analogous to the pounding it might receive in a boxing match. Subcapsular and intrarenal hematomas as well as less dramatic signs of renal injury occur in most patients who receive ESWL.[22] The long-term effects of such injury are not known, but the incidence of initial hypertension occurring within a few years ranges from <1 to 9 percent.[23]

Much still must be learned about the biological effects of ESWL. The efficacy and safety of ESWL depend largely on the way in which the shock-wave energy is generated (spark-gap, piezoelectric crystals, lasers, ultrasound), wave power (total number and kilovoltage of shocks delivered), and the amount of energy transferred to the stone and surrounding tissue. ESWL technology in clinical use today is much different from that used in the 1980s because of new devices that have numerous advantages: No anesthesia is required, the patient need not be immersed in a water bath, and renal trauma is reduced by improved methods of delivering the energy to the stone.[24]

Medical Management of Nephrolithiasis

Medical management of patients with stone disease can be subdivided into several phases. In phase I, risk factors that predispose to stone formation are identified. This evaluation includes careful radiologic identification of the number, location, and size of preexisting stones. In phase II, therapy is begun and elimination or amelioration of the risk factors associated with stone formation is documented. The end result of this phase is the choice of a final regimen for long-term treatment. For some patients, this regimen includes only increased fluid intake and restricted dietary intake; for others, it also includes an agent chosen to reduce excretion or enhance the solubility of a stone-forming constituent. In phase III, the results of long-term treatment are monitored. For patients with preexisting stones, clinical stone events must be differentiated in terms of old vs. new stones; this differentiation requires radiologic assessment either after each symptomatic stone event or, if no symptoms have occurred, yearly. In phase IV, all or part of a therapeutic regimen is discontinued in a patient determined to no longer need it.

Evaluation: Phase I

In working with patients, internists should clarify from the outset that their role in care differs from the role of urologists and that patients should maintain continuity of care with the referring urologist. Patients should be made aware that they are important participants in their own care. Empirical therapy should be discontinued several weeks before analytic screening. Collapsible 24-hour urine collection containers and instructions for urine collection may be mailed to patients so that they can bring to the first visit an initial urine specimen collected while they were on a customary (or so-called free or usual) diet. The history and physical examination should be complete; particular care should be given to history of stone events, family history of stones, medications, and diet. The number, composition, and location of stones as well as the outcome of stone events (e.g., stones passed, nephrolithotomy) should be chronologically recorded to serve as the basis for determining stone morbidity. A brief dietary history, focusing particularly on the consumption of animal protein, dairy products, foods rich in oxalate, and salt, should be obtained; obtaining a detailed, quantitative dietary history is not essential.

When stones are radiopaque, their number, size, and location should be documented on plain x-ray films. A plain x-ray film

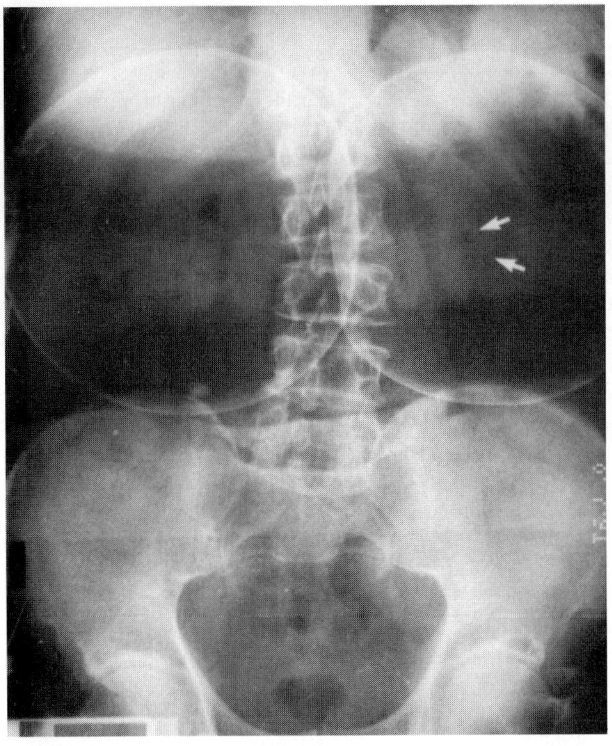

FIGURE 24-3. X-ray film showing coned-down view of kidneys done using a balloon device to enhance imaging of renal calculi. (*Reproduced by permission of the editor and publisher from Ettinger B, Insogna KL.*[11a])

obtained before an intravenous pyelogram (IVP) is usually unacceptable for diagnostic purposes; most are not done with the care necessary to delineate clearly the number, size, and location of existing stones and are thus a notorious source of misinformation. Patients should be prepared with diet instruction and laxatives as for an IVP, and a coned-down view of the kidneys should be obtained instead of a kidney, ureter, and bladder (KUB) view. Because it includes the lower pelvis, the KUB view usually does not show the upper poles of the kidneys clearly. We prefer to use the balloon device originally designed to apply ureteral compression during an IVP. Placing the balloon device over the upper abdomen and then inflating the device (Fig. 24-3) moves intestinal gas as well as gastric and colonic contents away from the kidneys, improving the diagnostic quality of the x-ray films. The IVP should have no role in defining stone burden or response to therapy; serial IVPs are commonly misused to monitor stone disease and expose the patient to an unacceptable dose of radiation.

Ultrasonography should be used to image nonopaque calculi. Ultrasonography can also be used for imaging opaque stones, but we do not recommend its routine use for this purpose, because ultrasonography is expensive, is less sensitive, and does not define stone size as well as x-ray films do. All calculi produce a similar ultrasonographic picture: an echogenic focus with posterior acoustic shadowing. Ultrasonography easily distinguishes nonopaque stones (e.g., those composed of uric acid) from masses such as tumor or blood clot. Among 64 patients evaluated after lithotripsy for residual stone fragments, abdominal x-ray films and sonography both showed stones in 53 percent, sonography alone showed stones in 16 percent, and x-ray films alone showed stones in 31 percent.[25]

Computed tomography (CT) is also an excellent method for imaging nonopaque renal calculi: All calculi appear as bright objects on CT. Some researchers have suggested that the CT number can be used to distinguish stone composition, but technical problems such as partial volume effects make this distinction impractical. The current clinical practice in diagnosing nonopaque calculi is to use ultrasound first and to reserve CT for selected patients. CT has the advantage of being more reproducible and less operator-dependent; moreover, if contrast material is used, CT can more accurately define renal collecting structures and obstruction. Disadvantages of CT include higher cost and radiation exposure.

The results of previous stone analyses should be examined, and a recent stone, if available, should be sent to a reference laboratory for crystallographic analysis; simple chemical stone analysis is inadequate. An initial fasting serum autochemistry panel should include calcium, phosphorus, bicarbonate, chloride, creatinine, uric acid, and albumin concentrations. If a stone is unobtainable for analysis, a urine sample should be screened for cystine (see Cystinuria, Laboratory Evaluation). A 24-h urine specimen collected while the patient is on a free diet should be analyzed for creatinine, sodium, calcium, oxalate, uric acid, and citrate. Urine volume should be noted. Excretion of creatinine serves as an index of completeness of the collection. We recommend that no preservative be added to the 24-h urine container; instead, the aliquot used for measuring calcium, oxalate, and cystine is acidified with 6 *N* hydrochloric acid, and the remainder of the sample is frozen until analyzed.

A clean, voided, fasting urine sample should be obtained in the early morning for culture and pH determination by nitrazine paper or pH meter. If cystinuria is suspected or if stone analysis is unavailable, a nitroprusside test for cystine should be done on this specimen; cystine crystals can be seen if the specimen is acidified by adding a few drops of glacial acetic acid and is then cooled.

If the initial early-morning urinary pH is extreme (<6.0 or >7.0), serum electrolyte concentrations should be remeasured and the patient should be given a roll of nitrazine paper to record variations in urinary pH for several days by making pH measurements upon arising and after meals; such measurements should show normal pH variability. If uric acid stone disease is suspected, serial monitoring of urinary pH is indicated to search for the low, relatively fixed pH seen in many such patients.

When making biochemical determinations for patients with urolithiasis, remember: in stone disease, measurement is most important. What the laboratory cannot determine will not be known; what it reports in error will not be corrected by using instinct, medical experience, or art; the information taken from the measurements will direct treatment. When measurements vary, seem ambiguous, or raise suspicion of error, they must be repeated. No expense is as unreasonable as years of misdirected treatment or as great as the cost of treating the urologic consequences of preventable stones.[26]

Evaluation of Patients Who Have a Single Stone Event As is universally agreed, patients in whom even one cystine, uric acid, calcium phosphate, or magnesium ammonium phosphate stone has formed should be considered as having a chronic disease that requires extensive evaluation and aggressive medical management. For patients who have a single calcium oxalate stone, no clear and accepted rules exist to guide evaluation or treatment. Some researchers view the first calcium oxalate stone as an indication for extensive evaluation and suggest that treatment for any risk factors identified during the evaluation will be cost-effective. These researchers argue that risk factors are found as frequently in patients with a single stone as in patients with recurrent stone disease and believe that patients with one stone are simply at the beginning of a chronic process.[27,28] In contrast, some researchers quote reports of relatively low recurrence rates, low morbidity, and relatively low success rates for medical treatments[29] and thus advise minimal evaluation. On the basis of 6 clinical trials of patients who had passed a single stone and who were stone-free at the outset, the risk of recurrent stones was 5–8 percent per year among subjects receiving no treatment.[29–34]

The author recommends that minimal evaluation include coned-down x-ray films of the kidneys to detect additional "silent" stones, crystallographic stone analysis, and chemical screening, including a serum autochemistry panel, determination of urinary pH, and collection of a 24-h urine specimen on a free diet. Urinary chemical analysis should include total volume, calcium, uric acid, oxalate, and citrate. When ordered together as a panel, the entire chemistry evaluation costs about $200 at most commercial laboratories.

Extensive Metabolic Evaluations Within the biomedical literature, opinion varies widely about which tests are needed, particularly in evaluating calcium oxalate lithiasis, in which the extremes are a simple serum biochemical panel and a 3-day hospital stay for extensive measurement of serum and urinary response to manipulation of diet and calcium intake.

A tiered approach may be the most appropriate. Today, experts favor simple, empiric, nonselective therapy for uncomplicated calcium oxalate lithiasis.[35] Patients without complications are stone-free, have no infection or bowel disease, and are normocalcemic. Decisions about initial clinical management can be made without an extensive metabolic evaluation. For patients in whom stone disease remains active after treatment, more extensive studies can be done to help guide further management.

Therapy: Phase II

The therapeutic program usually consists of forced hydration, dietary moderation, and drug therapy.

Forced Hydration Water, as a universal solvent, should be the mainstay of therapy for all types of nephrolithiasis. The desirable daily urine output is 2 L, for which daily intake of 3 L of fluid is necessary, provided that fluid loss via the skin or gastrointestinal tract is not accelerated. In a 5-year study of 199 patients who passed their first calcium oxalate stone, Borgi and coworkers[34] found that patients randomly assigned to receive high levels of fluid intake increased their mean 24-h urine volume output from about 1–2.5 L; and for patients assigned to receive high levels of fluid intake, stones recurred less than half as often as in untreated controls.

A definite plan of forced fluids should be designed. Patients should drink a glass of water at bedtime, refill the glass, and keep it near the lavatory. Patients who follow this regimen will invariably awaken early in the morning and can then drink the waiting glass of water; they should drink another glass of water immediately upon arising. When setting a goal for daily urine volume, physicians should emphasize nocturnal hydration. The choice of fluids other than water requires understanding the contribution of beverages to the urinary excretion of various metabolites. For example, hypocitraturic stone formers who ingested 1.2 L of orange juice per day excreted 40 percent more urinary citrate but also excreted 36 percent more urinary oxalate without a change in calcium excretion.[36] In a similar group of patients, ingestion of 2 L of lemonade per day nearly tripled the excretion of citrate without changing oxalate or calcium excretion.[37] In healthy subjects, drinking a large volume of cola (3 qt per day) reduced urinary excretion of citrate 24 percent while increasing urinary oxalate by about 50 percent.[38] Epidemiologic studies of beverage intake indicate that the risk of stone formation for men and for women is decreased with higher intake of coffee, tea, beer, and wine, whereas the risk is increased with higher intake of grapefruit juice.[39,40] A randomized trial of 1,009 stone-forming men showed that those assigned to avoid soft drinks had an overall 6.4 percent lower risk of stone recurrence after 3 years of follow-up[41]; interestingly, the group most likely to benefit from this dietary advice were those initially consuming soft drinks acidified with phosphoric acid instead of citric acid—those avoiding phosphoric acid drinks reduced their recurrence rate by 15 percent compared with controls.

Restriction of Animal Protein in the Diet Epidemiologic studies have shown that high intake of animal protein increases the risk of kidney stone development for men[42] and for women.[43] However, a randomized clinical trial in which subjects combined low intake of animal protein with intake of fiber failed to reduce the frequency of calcium stone recurrence.[32] Nevertheless, all patients with nephrolithiasis should be advised to moderate their intake of animal protein. On average, American men consume 108 g of protein daily—54 percent more than the Recommended Daily Allowance (RDA); about half this protein intake comes from animal flesh. Reducing the intake of animal protein may help reduce the excretion of cystine, uric acid, calcium, oxalate, and phosphorus. A reduced intake of animal protein can also reduce the load of nonvolatile (fixed) acid, thus limiting excessive urinary acidity.

Because many patients are unable or unwilling to change their lifelong practice of eating meat, a rigid diet is often impractical and unacceptable. Table 24-2 shows a sample diet that provides 97 g of total protein but limits protein from animal flesh to 35 g; additional protein must come from cereals, vegetables, and legumes. This diet conforms with cholesterol-lowering guidelines, which recommend that fat contribute no more than 30 percent to total caloric intake.

Avoidance of Dietary Calcium Restriction Epidemiologic studies indicate that the higher the calcium intake, the lower the risk of having a first stone[42,43]; among 45,619 male physicians, those in the highest quartile for calcium intake had 34 percent lower risk of having a first stone event than those in the lowest quartile for calcium intake. Because severe restriction of dairy products also does not prevent recurrence of calculi[44] and increases the risk for developing osteoporosis, two low-fat dairy portions should be encouraged for patients with nephrolithiasis.

Reduced Sodium Intake High sodium intake increases cystine excretion in patients with cystinuria[45] and may cause hypercalciuria or augment the hypercalciuria caused by other mechanisms.[46] High sodium excretion reduces urinary citrate, a substance important in solubilizing calcium and inhibiting calcium oxalate crystal agglomeration.[46] The adverse effects of a high intake of salt and animal protein are apparently additive.[45] Salt intake can be reasonably moderated by avoiding obviously salty foods and by not salting food at the table. Salt may be used lightly in cooking. By

TABLE 24-2. Mean U.S. Dietary Protein Intake vs. Reduced Animal Protein Diet Prescribed for Patients with Kidney Stones (g)

	Sources of Protein					
	Red Meat, Fish, Poultry	Cereal Products	Dairy Products	Egg Products	Other Protein	Total Protein
U.S. diet	52 (7.5 oz)	22	18	4	12	108
Stone diet	35 (5.0 oz)	26	15	4	18	97

Note: Both diets are calculated to provide 2,400 kcal/day, sufficient for a moderately active 80-kg man. The following food allocations are offered to illustrate a diet that provides 16 percent of calories in the form of protein and 30 percent in the form of fat: Meat, 5 oz; cheese, 1 slice; milk, 1 cup; egg, half; bread, 6 slices; cereal, 1–1/2 cups; starches, 2–1/2 cups; beans, 1/2 cup; vegetables, 3 servings; fruit, 5 servings; fat, 6 tsp.

Source: Reproduced by permission of the editor and publisher from: Ettinger B, Insogna KL.[11a]

following these simple suggestions, patients can conveniently reduce their daily salt intake to the range of 4–5 g, reducing daily sodium excretion to <100 mEq.

What Can Be Expected from Medical Treatment? Most medical treatments for nephrolithiasis have been accepted without definitive and critical experimental studies. When evaluating a clinical trial, the reader should look for the following design criteria: (1) adequate number of treated subjects and controls (a minimum of 20 subjects receiving active treatment), (2) adequate characterization of subjects, including pretreatment stone rate, stone burden, and metabolic profile, (3) adequate follow-up (a minimum of 2 years and preferably 3 years), and (4) objectively measured and impartially determined end points, including the growth of preexisting stones, the appearance of new stones on x-ray films, and the passage of new stones.

Referral bias may complicate the evaluation of clinical trial results. Many patients seek care and are thus entered into treatment programs soon after one stone event or a cluster of events. Such early treatment, however, creates a substantial bias toward the apparent efficacy of treatment, given that stone events are usually plotted before and after therapy is initiated (i.e., stones per patient-year). This bias, statistically termed *regression to the mean*, is a problem, particularly when follow-up is short.

Cointervention may also obscure the meaning of clinical trials. Patients typically begin a program of fluids, dietary control, and a therapeutic agent simultaneously, but the drug is usually credited with reducing stone events and often with reducing biochemical abnormalities.[47]

Careful, regular radiologic assessment of stone burden and the differentiation of new and old stones are critical in determining the efficacy of therapy. Greater credence should be given to reports of clinical trials in which regular radiologic follow-up is part of the outcome assessment.

What criteria can be used to determine the adequacy and scientific validity of such trials? Certainly, a trial showing nearly total stone prevention in 30 patients with recurrent stones during a 3-year period cannot be disputed even if a double-blind randomized design was not used. In this hypothetical trial, about 11 failures would be predicted if treatment were ineffective. However, few therapies yield such convincing results. In clinical trials of patients with recurrent calcium oxalate stones, mean stone event risk among placebo-treated subjects is usually 10–15 percent per year.[47,48] A convenient guideline is that effective treatment halves the odds of stone recurrence or reduces recurrence to 5 percent per year.

If a treatment produces salutary changes in either the urinary biochemical profile or in vitro tests of crystallization, is its efficacy sufficiently established? For nephrolithiasis caused by cystine or uric acid, urinary biochemical analysis provides reliable indicators of stone risk that may be considered surrogates for stone events. However, this is not true for calcium oxalate stones.[48]

Phase III: Long-Term Follow-Up

After the initial therapeutic period, the patient is seen at 6-month or 1-year intervals, depending on preexisting activity of stone disease, presence of stones on x-ray films, and perceived need for supervision, reinforcement of the program, or both. Appropriate analyses and plain x-ray films are obtained at least yearly.

Phase IV: Discontinuation of Treatment

Patients are best advised that the first goal of therapy is to control stone formation for a few years. Assuming that this has been achieved, for which patients should drug treatment be stopped? The following risk factors contribute strongly to recurrence: previous rate of stone events, stone burden, and extreme deviation in the urinary biochemical profile. We recommend discontinuing part or all of the therapeutic program after 3 years of successful treatment if the pretreatment stone event rate during that period was <0.5 stone yearly and if no stones are visible on x-ray films.

CYSTINURIA

Although nephrolithiasis is rarely caused by cystinuria, we describe cystinuria first because we understand its heredity and metabolic basis as well as why calculi develop and how they can be diagnosed, dissolved, and prevented.

History

Cystine stones were recognized as a distinctive stone type in 1810, and their familial occurrence was described shortly afterward.[49,50] The relation between excessive cystine excretion and cystine stones was recognized as early as 1855. However, nearly a century passed before reports of increased orthinine, lysine, and arginine excretion enabled Dent and Rose[51] to synthesize the classic transport hypothesis. They noted that each contributing amino acid had two amino or guanidine groups and suggested that these structurally related amino acids share a common resorptive mechanism located in the renal tubule and defective in patients with cystinuria.

Genetics

Cystinuria is a classic example of simple autosomal-recessive inheritance. In homozygotes, cystinuria increases excretion rates of cystine and the dibasic amino acids markedly, and the incidence of cystine stones is extremely high. Heterozygotes, however, are at almost no risk for developing cystine stones; such patients can be identified biochemically by their slightly increased excretion of cystine and the dibasic amino acids.[52] Three distinct genetic patterns can be identified by studying both intestinal transport and urinary amino acid excretion in cystinuric pedigrees. These patterns differ according to the presence or degree (or both) of abnormal transport of the four amino acids in the intestine and the presence or absence of abnormal amino acid excretion rates in heterozygotes.[49] Some apparently homozygous patients are "double heterozygotes" in that they have two different allelic mutations instead of a double mutation of a single gene. Double heterozygotes cannot be clinically distinguished from homozygotes. Homozygous cystinuria affects about 1 in 18,000 people, indicating that 1 in 60 or 70 persons is heterozygous.[49]

Pathophysiology

Five group-specific amino acid transport systems have been recognized; each system mediates the transport of a group of structurally related amino acids. The SLC3A1 gene on chromosome 2 has been shown to code for a 79 kDa protein responsible for the transport of the dibasic amino acids cystine, ornithine, lysine, and arginine (COLA). To date, 21 different mutations and 9 polymorphisms have been reported in the SLC3A1 gene in cystinuria. Readers interested in the molecular genetics of cystinuria are referred to the comprehensive review by Gitomer and Pak.[53]

Cystine is not an essential amino acid. Cystinuric patients, who cannot absorb cystine, produce it endogenously from methionine. Loss of amino acids into the urine in cystinuria is not nutritionally meaningful. Children with cystinuria have normal intellectual and physical development.

Amino acids in plasma are freely filtered at the glomerulus. Normally, 97–99 percent of the filtered amino acid load is resorbed by specific transport systems in the proximal tubule. The system in the luminal brush border is shared by all four dibasic amino acids and is normally responsible for their nearly quantitative resorption. This system is defective in patients with cystinuria.

The entire load of filtered cystine may be spilled by patients with homozygous cystinuria. The daily cystine excretion rate in these patients is >400 mg (1,664 μmol) and is usually in the range of 600–1,300 mg (2,497–5,399 μmol). Because maximum cystine solubility at usual urinary pH is 300 mg/L (1,248 μmol/L), predisposition of cystinuric patients to the formation of cystine stones is self-evident.

One or more cystine stones develop in almost all patients with cystinuria; for unknown reasons, about 10 percent have no stones. Cystine stones may first occur any time from infancy to the eighth decade,[52] but mean age at onset is about 20 years (Fig. 24-1). Although men and women are affected equally, morbidity is greater in men for unexplained reasons.[25]

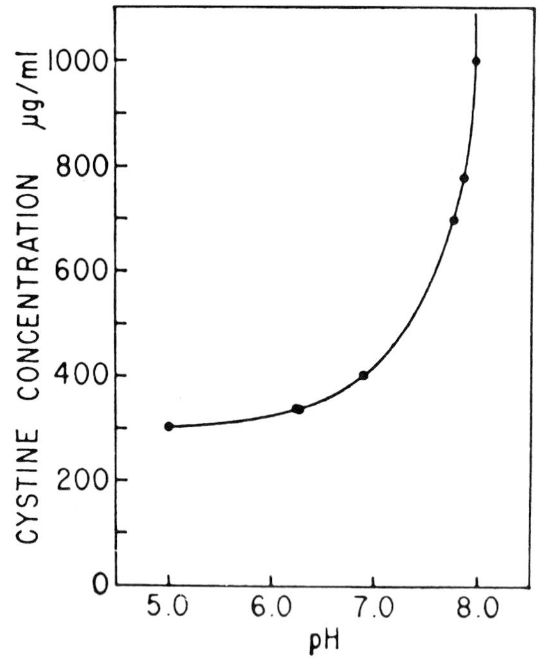

FIGURE 24-4. Effect of urinary pH on solubility of cystine. Number of subjects is shown above bars. (*Adapted and reproduced by permission of the author and publisher from Dent CE, Senior B.*[54])

Dependence of Cystine Solubility on Urinary pH

Figure 24-4 shows the slope of the curve of cystine ionization and solubility as a function of pH; because the pK_a of cystine is 8.4, variations in urinary pH within the usual physiologic range (pH 5.0–7.0) have little influence on cystine solubility, but maximal urine alkalinization (pH 7.8–8.0) increases cystine solubility by a factor of 2–3.[54]

Dependence of Cystine Excretion on Salt Intake

The dependence of cystine excretion on sodium intake was recognized during a study of the effect of glutamine on cystine excretion.[55] Glutamine administration was reported to reduce cystine excretion in one patient,[56] but this result was not confirmed in other patients.[57] Jaeger and coworkers[55] found that glutamine reduced cystine excretion only in subjects whose sodium intake was high (150–300 mEq/day); these investigators also showed that simply reducing salt intake can lower cystine excretion profoundly. These observations were confirmed by Norman and Manette,[45] who found that reducing the mean daily sodium intake of five cystinuric patients from 184–87 mEq reduced urinary cystine excretion by 46 percent.

Effect of Cysteine-Complexing Agents

D-Penicillamine (β,β-dimethylcysteine) is the prototype of a group of sulfhydryl compounds used as cysteine-complexing agents. When these agents are present, cysteine combines with the complexing agent to form a mixed disulfide instead of forming a sulfhydryl linkage with another cysteine (Fig. 24-5). The cysteine-penicillamine disulfide is about 50 times more soluble than

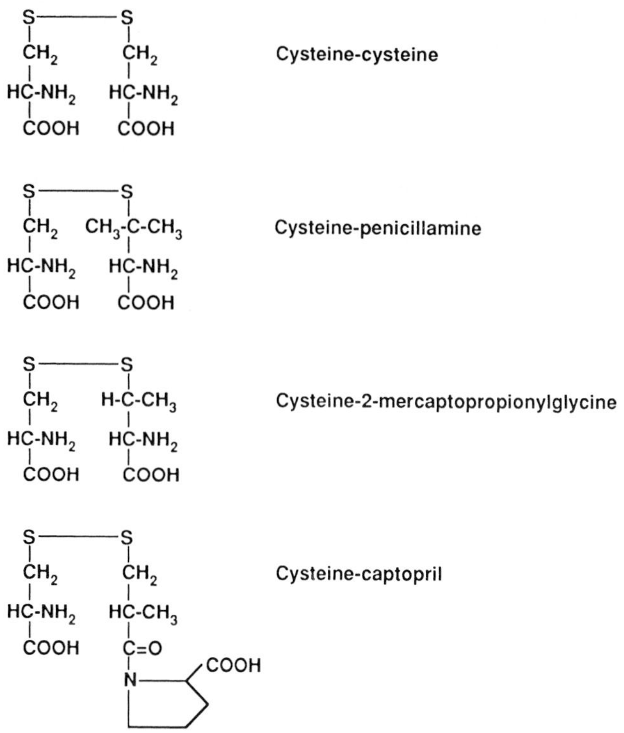

FIGURE 24-5. Chemical structures of cystine and related cysteine disulfides. (*Revised and reproduced by permission of the editor and publisher from Ettinger B, Insogna KL.*[11a])

cystine. Penicillamine not only prevents cystine stones but can dissolve preexisting stones.[49,50,58]

Clinical Findings

In cystinuric patients, stones are usually multiple and bilateral. A particularly characteristic pattern is a staghorn calculus with multiple small "satellite" stones (Fig. 24-6). A few patients with cystinuria have stones of mixed composition or may alternatively have cystine stones and either calcium oxalate, pure calcium phosphate, or MAP stones.[49,58,59] This observation is explained by the occasional coincidence of cystinuria with other stone risk factors, the adverse influence of alkali treatment on calcium phosphate solubility, and chronic infection resulting from urologic instrumentation.

Extracorporeal shock-wave lithotripsy and other stone-fragmenting techniques are only marginally effective in breaking large cystine stones into particles small enough to be passed spontaneously. Further information about urologic procedures specific to cystine stones is available.[60,61] Percutaneous irrigation chemolysis using n-acetyl cysteine at pH 9 has dissolved cystine stone remnants within a few days, but this material can be quite irritating.[61] Renal transplantation (from a noncystinuric donor) has been successful in patients with cystinuria. This procedure "cures" cystinuria but is used only in patients with end-stage renal failure.

Clinical Evaluation

Clinical Diagnosis

Cystinuria should be considered in any patient with recurrent renal calculi. The diagnosis is suggested by an early onset of stone disease or by a characteristic radiologic stone pattern. Because of their sulfur content, cystine stones are radiopaque, but they are less dense than calcium stones. A family history of stones is common in patients with stone disease and thus is not a useful diagnostic clue. However, cystinuria is improbable if the family history is negative.

Laboratory Evaluation

Cystinuria is diagnosed by stone analysis, demonstrated cystine crystalluria, urinary cystine screening, and (ultimately) quantitative urinary amino acid analysis. Cystine forms unmistakable flat, hexagonal ("benzene ring") crystals in urine that are best observed in cooled, concentrated specimens allowed to stand overnight. The specimen should be acidified to a pH of 4–5 by adding a few drops of glacial acetic acid to enhance formation of cystine crystals. Demonstration of cystine crystals is pathognomonic, but they may not be detectable in a dilute, fresh urine specimen.

The cyanide-nitroprusside test is the simplest and most useful chemical screen for cystinuria. The test is based on alkaline reduction of cystine to cysteine and a colorimetric reaction of free sulfhydryl groups with nitroprusside. The test is positive (the solution turns purple) when the cystine concentration reaches 150 mg/dL (6,242 μmol/L); a positive result is occasionally seen in heterozygotes and is rarely seen in dehydrated normal persons.[62] A simplified screening test takes advantage of the impregnation of ketone test strips with nitroprusside[63]; after the absence of ketones

FIGURE 24-6. Multiple cystine stones assuming a characteristic pattern of a staghorn calculus and multiple satellite stones. (*Adapted and reproduced by permission of the author, editor, and publisher from Insogna KL, Broadus AE.*[11b])

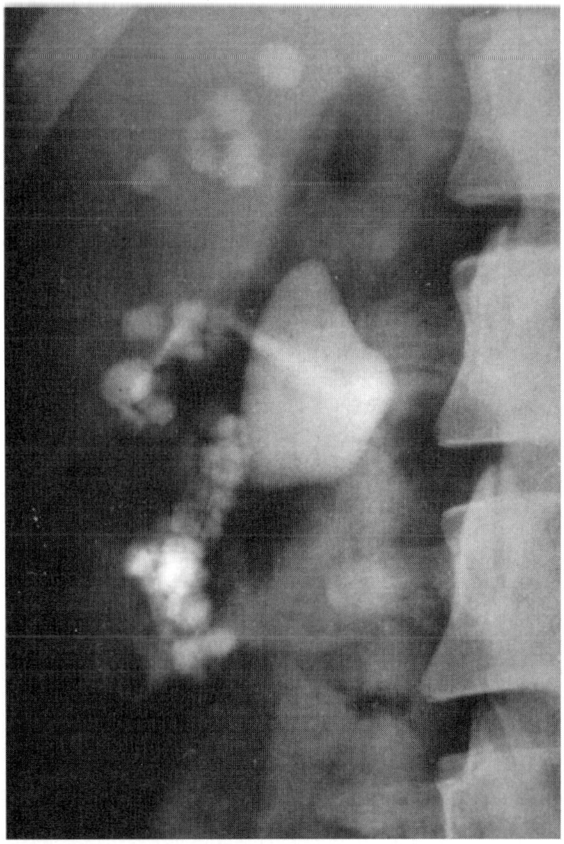

TABLE 24-3. Alkali Therapy: Drug Formulations, Daily Doses, and Costs

				To Provide 60 mEq Base/day	
Drug	**Supplier**	**Dose Form**	**Salts(s)**	**Total Dose**	**Mean Cost Wholesale, $**
Sodium bicarbonate	Lilly	Tablet (648 mg)	Sodium	8 tablets	0.58
Bicitra	Willen	Solution: citrate	Sodium	4 tbsp	1.42
Polycitra	Willen	Solution: citrate	Sodium, potassium	2 tbsp	1.17
Polycitra K	Willen	Solution: citrate	Potassium	2 tbsp	1.16
Polycitra K	Willen	Crystals: citrate	Potassium	2 packages	1.18
Urocit-K	Mission	Tablet (wax matrix): citrate	Potassium	6 tablets	1.56
K-lyte	Bristol	Tablet (effervescent): citrate	Potassium	2 tablets*	2.20
Effer-K	Nomax	Tablet (effervescent): bicarbonate	Potassium	2 tablets*	0.35

*Dose provides only 50 mEq daily.

Source: Reproduced by permission of the editor and publisher from Ettinger B, Insogna KL.[11a]

in the specimen is confirmed, two drops of 1 *M* sodium cyanide are added to six drops of urine. A ketone test strip wetted with this solution turns purple in the presence of elevated levels of urine cystine.

A positive nitroprusside test should be followed by quantitation of 24-h urinary cystine excretion. Amino acid column chromatography can quantitate each of the four related amino acids but is expensive ($250–$300). Because only cystine excretion is clinically important, simpler and less expensive techniques are preferred. When monitoring the effects of penicillamine and other cysteine-complexing agents (see Cystinuria, Treatment), a quantitative technique should be used to distinguish cystine from the mixed cysteine–penicillamine disulfide should be used. We prefer the anion-exchange, high-performance liquid chromatography method employing an abbreviated amino acid column analysis optimized for cystine; its upper limit of normal is 31 mg (130 μmol) daily. This analysis is commercially available from several reference laboratories.

Screening for Other Types of Stones

Stones formed by cystinuric patients may be composed entirely of calcium salts or may be admixtures of cystine and calcium salts. The prevalence of mixed stone diathesis was 15 percent[58] in one series and 30 percent in another.[59] Screening cystinuric patients for calcium stone risk factors (hypercalciuria, hyperuricosuria, and hypocitraturia) yields about the same prevalence of these abnormalities as would be expected in patients with calcium stones.[60]

Treatment

The treatment of cystinuria is guided by urinary cystine concentration and by awareness that the maximum solubility of cystine within the physiologic pH range is 300 mg/L (1,248 μmol/L). Therapeutic measures include hydration, sodium restriction, alkalinization, and cysteine-complexing drugs.

Forced Hydration

Forced hydration is important in treating all stone disease but is the cornerstone of treatment in cystinuria. Urine volume should be sufficient to ensure a cystine concentration <250 mg/L (1,040 μmol/L).

Alkalinization of the Urine

Alkali must be given in a daily dose of 60–100 mEq, an amount sufficient to buffer the acid production rate and produce a urinary pH of 7.5–8.0. This dose is given as bicarbonate or citrate salts in four divided doses; many physicians prefer citrate because it is metabolized to bicarbonate in the liver, producing more prolonged and constant alkalinization. Some physicians advocate a single dose of acetazolamide (350–500 mg) at bedtime, but we discourage this approach because the induced RTA may further increase the risk of calcium phosphate stones or cause deposition of calcium phosphate salts on preexisting cystine stones.[35] Table 24-3 lists some commonly used alkali preparations.

Dietary Advice

Daily salt intake should be restricted to <100 mEq. We thus encourage the use of alkali preparations that contain potassium instead of sodium. In addition, patients should be instructed to moderate animal protein intake to reduce the fixed acid load. Diets sufficiently restricted in methionine to substantially reduce cystine excretion are unpalatable and thus are not recommended.

Cysteine-Complexing Drugs

Penicillamine

Given in four divided doses, usually 1,500 mg daily, penicillamine reduces the excretion of cystine to about 300 mg (1,248 μmol) daily.[52,58,64,65] In a daily urine volume of 2 L, cystine concentration of about 600 μmol/L provides a good therapeutic effect (Fig. 24-7).[65] Intestinal absorption may be enhanced by taking penicillamine before meals, and use of alkali therapy enhances formation of the cysteine-penicillamine complex. In about two-thirds of patients who follow this regimen, stone burden is diminished or eliminated within about 12 months.[58]

Penicillamine causes side effects in about half the patient population.[52,58,64] The most common serious toxicity is a hypersensitivity syndrome characterized by fever and rash that typically occurs within the first few weeks of treatment. Lymphadenopathy, arthralgia, thrombocytopenia, and granulocytopenia may accompany these symptoms. In addition, long-term treatment is associated with a risk of loss of skin turgor, especially in the intertriginous areas, resulting in disfiguring cosmetic changes. Penicillamine is also associated with a rare but serious skin

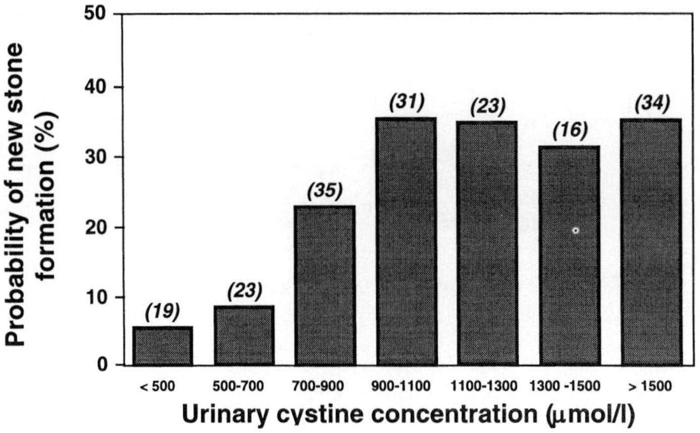

FIGURE 24-7. Probability of new stone formation at different levels of urinary cystine concentration. (*Adapted and reproduced by permission of the author and publisher from Lindell Å, Denneberg T, Hellgren E, et al.*[65])

disease, elastosis perforans serpiginosa. Other, relatively minor side effects of long-term treatment include minor gastrointestinal distress, malodorous breath and urine, and loss of taste. Potentially serious renal toxicity has been reported in about 10 percent of cases. This toxicity is heralded by proteinuria and may progress to frank nephrotic syndrome; renal biopsy specimens show membranous glomerulonephritis. Because this side effect may occur even after many months with no apparent toxicity, patients should monitor urine protein weekly using urinary test strips. Penicillamine may antagonize the effect of vitamin B_6; pyridoxine in daily doses of 50 mg should thus be prescribed. Penicillamine should be avoided in pregnancy because of reported fetal scalp anomalies.

In some patients, side effects are clearly dose-related, resolve rapidly after penicillamine is discontinued, and may not reappear when the drug is reintroduced at a lower dose. In cases of hypersensitivity reaction, desensitization is readily accomplished; once the reaction has subsided, the drug is started again at a daily dose of 125 mg, which is increased gradually over a few weeks. We give a glucocorticoid when a penicillamine rash first occurs and continue the glucocorticoid at a low dose during the period of drug desensitization.

Because of its toxicity and cost, penicillamine should be used selectively in patients with cystinuria. A regimen of vigorous hydration and alkalinization prevents stone recurrence in about 30–50 percent of patients and diminishes rates of stone complications in many others. Indications for penicillamine include (1) inability to control stones with conservative measures (such patients frequently excrete >1,000 mg of cystine daily), (2) cystine stones in a single functioning kidney, and (3) a large stone burden. For most patients who have been rendered free of stones, we recommend stopping penicillamine therapy. The rare patient who shows a severe cystine stone diathesis may be maintained on long-term penicillamine therapy at a reduced level; half the usual dose is generally used, an amount sufficient to maintain a 24-h urinary cystine concentration of about 800 μmol/L in 2 L of urine.

Other Cysteine-Complexing Drugs

Because of the frequent side effects of penicillamine, other sulfhydryl compounds have attracted interest (Fig. 24-5). Mercaptopropionylglycine (MPG), which has a higher oxidation-reduction potential than penicillamine and is thus more efficient in binding to cysteine, is usually given at two-thirds the dose of penicillamine.[66,67] Early use suggested that MPG was associated with fewer serious side effects than penicillamine, but more widespread experience has shown that the two drugs have a similar potential for causing serious reactions.[66] In a multicenter trial, MPG toxicity developed in 35 percent of patients who had previously reacted to penicillamine. In this study, among 49 patients treated first with penicillamine and subsequently with MPG, fewer instances of rash and gastrointestinal reactions were observed in patients taking MPG. However, clinically significant proteinuria developed in 12.2 percent of patients taking penicillamine and in 10.2 percent of patients taking MPG. Renal glomerular damage is apparently an autoimmune reaction, and IgG antinuclear antibodies were found in 22 percent of patients who took MPG for a mean of 6 years.[68] The cost of prescribing 1,500 mg daily of penicillamine or 1,000 mg daily of MPG is about $2,500 per year. *N*-acetyl-D-penicillamine has been reported to be effective in reducing cystine concentration in patients with cystinuria and may have fewer side effects than penicillamine. However, experience with this drug is limited,[49] and 1,600 mg daily costs about $8,500 a year.

A mixed disulfide also forms between cysteine and the antihypertensive drug captopril. The effect of captopril on cystine excretion is probably mediated by the formation of a cysteine-captopril disulfide (Fig. 24-5), but because small doses occasionally have profound effects on cystine excretion, some researchers have hypothesized that captopril also affects renal tubular amino acid transport.[69] Although initial reports indicated a profound reduction in cystine excretion in patients who were given 75–150 mg of captopril daily,[70,71] other studies did not show any benefit.[72,73] Several clinical studies indicate that captopril therapy is not as effective as penicillamine or MPG in reducing calculous events[69,74] and that adding captopril to either of these treatments does not enhance their effectiveness.[75] We do not recommend captopril use for treating cystinuria unless it is also prescribed for cardiac or hypertensive effects. Perhaps further study of this drug's mechanism of action will lead to development of safer, better-tolerated therapy for cystinuria.

URIC ACID STONES

Epidemiology

The prevalence of uric acid stones in the United States is estimated to be about 1 in 1,000 persons.[76–78] Uric acid stones are

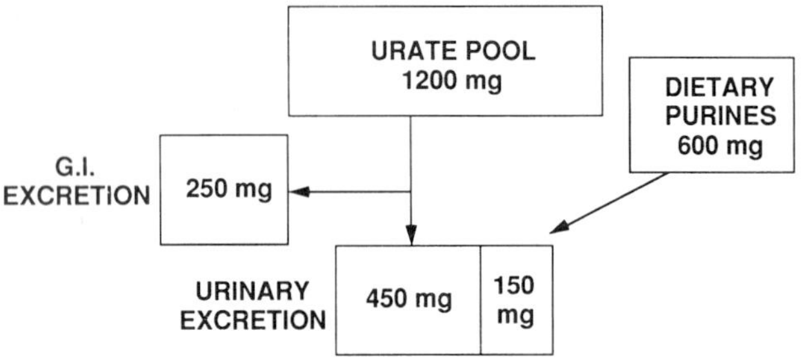

FIGURE 24-8. Fate of urate in an average 70-kg man. *(Adapted and reproduced by permission of the editor and publisher from Ettinger B.*[81]*)*

usually pure, affect predominantly middle-aged and older men (Fig. 24-1),[2] and represent only 5 percent of stone disease in western countries. In some countries, such as Israel, uric acid stones are more common, accounting for 40 percent of all stones.

The pathogenesis of uric acid stones is well understood, and preventive treatment is highly effective.[79,80] The relations among hyperuricosuria, uric acid, and calcium oxalate stone formation are described later in this chapter (see Calcium Oxalate and Mixed Calcium Stones).

Purine Metabolism and Uric Acid Excretion

In humans, uric acid is the end product of purine catabolism. Dietary and endogenous purines both contribute to the metabolic pool (Fig. 24-8).[81] About half the nucleic acid purines in the diet can be recovered as urinary uric acid.[76] Endogenous purines are usually metabolized at a constant rate; purine intake therefore accounts for much of the variation in rates of uric acid production. Uric acid is eliminated by two routes: About a quarter to a third of the uric acid produced daily enters enteric secretions and is destroyed by intestinal flora (*intestinal uricolysis*); the remaining two-thirds to three-quarters is excreted in urine.

Uric Acid Solubility in Urine

Uric acid stones form when urine is oversaturated by undissociated uric acid; this oversaturation occurs at a concentration of 100 mg/L (0.6 mmol/L). Urinary pH is a major determinant of uric acid saturation. At pH 5.5 (the pK_a of uric acid), half the total urate is in the form of insoluble undissociated uric acid, and half is in the form of soluble urate salt (Fig. 24-9).[81] A small change in pH has a dramatic effect. For example, increasing urinary pH from 5.2 to 5.8 halves the amount of undissociated uric acid; increasing urinary pH from 5.2 to 6.4 reduces the amount of undissociated uric acid by 84 percent.

Risk Factors for Uric Acid Stones

Risk factors for uric acid stones are hyperuricosuria, acidic urine, and low urine volume. Of these, persistently acidic urine is the most important and may be the only abnormality in some patients with uric acid stones.

Effect of Diet on Urinary pH and Uric Acid Excretion

Altering the intake of dietary animal protein causes major changes in urinary excretion of uric acid. For example, consuming 140 g of

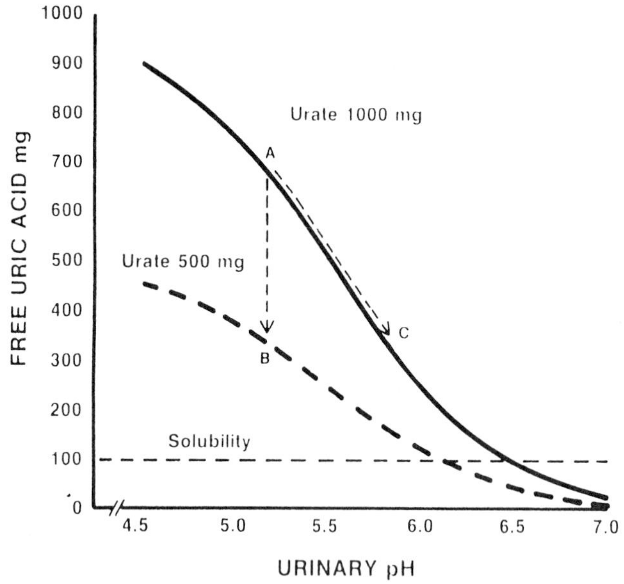

FIGURE 24-9. Effect of urinary pH on free uric acid at two levels of total urate excretion (500 and 1,000 mg). Increasing urinary pH from 5.2 to 5.8 (A → C) has the same effect as halving total urate excretion (A → B). *(Adapted and reproduced by permission of the editor and publisher from Ettinger B.*[81]*)*

protein daily (instead of 70 g) may double the body's total uric acid excretion.[82] This additional 70-g protein load contributes fixed acid sufficient to lower urinary pH by 0.5–1.0, shifting the equilibrium between urate and undissociated uric acid toward the latter. Dietary excess may thus quadruple excretion of the insoluble undissociated uric acid moiety.

Gout and Uric Acid Stones

Uric acid stones form in about 20 percent of patients with primary gout, that is, 1,000 times more often than in the general population.[76–78] In half the affected patients, stone disease is recurrent. Stone symptoms precede articular symptoms (occasionally by many years) in 40 percent of these patients.[76]

The gouty population usually has two combined risk factors for uric acid stone formation: hyperuricosuria and excessive urine acidity. A strong correlation exists between the excretion rate of uric acid and the frequency of uric acid stones (Table 24-4)[76]; uric acid stones form in almost half of gouty patients who excrete >1,000 mg (5.9 mmol) daily.[83] About 20 percent of the gouty population in whom uric acid stones form do not have hyperuricosuria;

TABLE 24-4. Relation between Rate of Uric Acid Excretion and Frequency of Uric Acid Stones in 1,319 Patients with Primary Gout

Urinary Uric Acid (mg)	Percentage of Gouty Population	Percentage of Patients with Stones
<400	12	24
400–599	36	24
600–799	30	32
800–999	16	31
1,000–1,600	6	49

Source: Adapted by permission of the author, editor, and publisher from Yü TF.[76]

the sole cause of stone diathesis in such patients is excessive urinary acidity. In fasting morning specimens, urinary pH is ≤5.0 in about half these patients compared with 15 percent of normal subjects.[78] The abnormality is also manifested by lower gastrointestinal absorption of alkali[84] and by absence of the normal postprandial alkaline tide.

In spite of numerous investigations, the reason for excessively acidic urine among patients with uric acid lithiasis is still unknown. Patients with gout excrete relatively more titratable acid and relatively less ammonia than do normal subjects. The defect in ammonia production may be primary or may be secondary to an abnormality in the excretion of titratable acid, or both abnormalities may reflect an unknown fundamental defect in acid-base regulation.

Other Clinical Disorders Associated with Uric Acid Stones

Several rare inborn metabolic defects are associated with marked overproduction of uric acid and with a particularly fulminant diathesis of articular gout and uric acid stone disease. These defects include hypoxanthine-guanine pyrophosphoribosyl transferase (HPRT) deficiency (Lesch-Nyhan syndrome), phosphoribosyl pyrophosphate (PRPP) synthetase overactivity, and glucose-6-phosphatase deficiency (type 1 glycogen storage disease). Affected patients have extreme uric acid overproduction rates and usually have a serum uric acid concentration exceeding 10 mg/dl (6 mmol/L) as well as daily uric acid excretion rates >1,000 mg. Uric acid stones form in about three-quarters of such patients, often before age 20 years.[76–78]

Patients with polycythemia vera, myeloid metaplasia, and myelocytic leukemia frequently have hyperuricemia and hyperuricosuria because of increased nucleic acid turnover rates. Gouty arthritis occurs in only 10 percent of patients with myeloproliferative disorders, but uric acid stones form in up to half of such patients. The stones tend to recur and are occasionally the first clinical manifestation leading to a diagnosis of the underlying disorder. Such patients are also at risk for acute uric acid nephropathy.

Numerous drugs (such as probenecid, salicylates, ascorbic acid, and x-ray contrast agents) produce acute uricosuria by inhibiting net uric acid resorption. Continued therapy with these agents, however, results in a new steady state in which uric acid excretion rates should be no greater than pretreatment rates. Nevertheless, probenecid treatment is associated with apparent increased frequency of stone formation in patients with primary gout.[76] Clearly, uricosuric drugs should not be used to treat patients with uric acid overproduction.

The frequency of uric acid stones is increased in patients with inflammatory bowel disease.[76,78] The association is particularly strong in patients who have had ileostomy; in these patients, loss of both bicarbonate and volume as a result of the ileostomy leads to persistently acidic, concentrated urine. Uric acid excretion rates are usually normal in such patients.

Differentiating Uric Acid from Other Purine-Related Stones

Other purine bases or metabolites are sparingly soluble in urine and can form stones in unusual circumstances. Xanthine stones occur in patients with xanthinuria, a rare autosomal-recessive disorder caused by deficiency of xanthine oxidase; xanthinuria is associated with hypouricemia and hypouricosuria. Xanthine stones occasionally develop in patients with rare inborn errors of urate metabolism who are given allopurinol.[14,77,78] Stones composed of 2,8-dihydroxyadenine have been found in a few patients with deficient adenine phosphoribosyl transferase activity.[76] A specific diagnosis of these rare disorders depends on crystallographic analysis of stones.

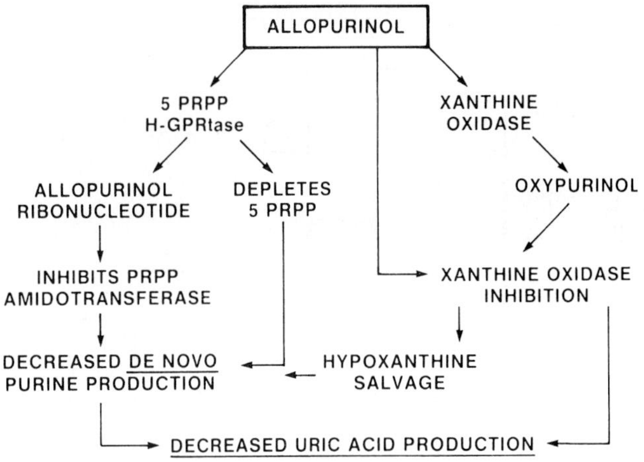

FIGURE 24-10. Ways in which allopurinol reduces uric acid production. PRPP = phosphoribosyl pyrophosphate; H-Gprtase = hypoxanthine-guanine phosphoribosyl transferase. (*Adapted 1999 and reproduced by permission of the author and publisher from: Rastegar A, Thier SO. Copyright © 1972 Massachusetts Medical Society. All rights reserved.*[85])

Mechanisms of the Effect of Allopurinol on Uric Acid

Allopurinol is an analog of hypoxanthine, and both allopurinol and its principal metabolite, oxypurinol, are competitive inhibitors of xanthine oxidase. If this were the only metabolic effect of the drug, xanthine and hypoxanthine would accumulate and might precipitate in urine. However, two metabolic processes prevent this result (Fig. 24-10).[85] First, hypoxanthine is recycled via a "salvage pathway"; this process lets hypoxanthine be reincorporated into nucleic acid production. The enzyme hypoxanthine guanine phosphoribosyltransferase (HGPRtase) directs this salvage process. Second, the adenylic and guanylic acids formed from hypoxanthine salvage inhibit de novo purine synthesis by blocking glutamine phosphoribosylpyrophosphate amidotransferase, the enzyme that directs the first step in purine synthesis.[86]

Absorption of dietary purine is decreased by allopurinol.[87,88] Consequently, its ability to reduce total oxypurine and urate excretion is far greater in subjects whose dietary purine intake is high (Fig. 24-11). This effect has been confirmed by in vitro studies using the rat jejunum.[89]

Efficacy of Medical Treatment of Uric Acid Lithiasis

Medical treatment of uric acid lithiasis is highly successful in controlling stone diathesis. Uric acid stones should dissolve within several weeks of treatment. If not dissolved after 3 months, calculi must be suspected of being admixed or covered with calcium salts or possibly misdiagnosed cystine, triamterene, or some other rare, nonopaque calculi.

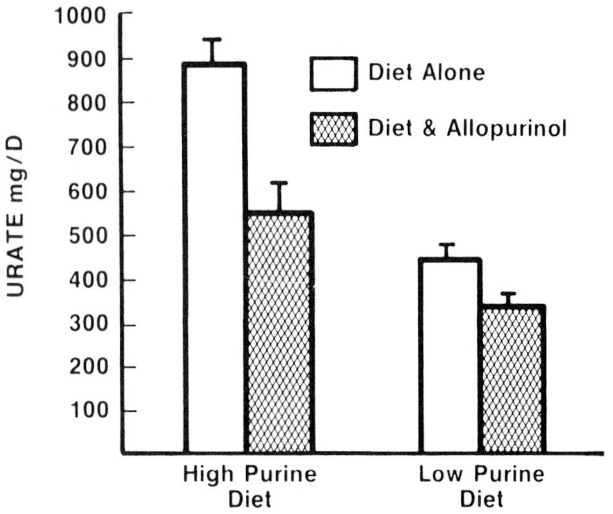

FIGURE 24-11. Reduction of urinary urate excretion in subjects receiving high- or low-purine diet with and without allopurinol therapy. (*Adapted and reproduced by permission of the author and publisher from Pak CYC, Barilla DE, Holt K, et al.*[87])

The efficacy of allopurinol in treating uric acid lithiasis has never been evaluated in a controlled trial and has never been compared with diet or alkali therapy. The results of two prospective studies of medical treatment[90,91] have a bearing on this question. Using only potassium citrate (75 mEq/day), Hosking[90] dissolved uric acid calculi in 75 percent of patients. Using potassium citrate (90 mEq/day) combined with allopurinol, Erickson and coworkers[91] dissolved uric acid stones in 71 percent of patients.

Evaluation

Imaging Uric Acid Stones

Uric acid stones are radiolucent and are identified on x-ray films only by the "filling defect" seen after introduction of a contrast agent. Renal ultrasound and CT are both useful in establishing an accurate diagnosis. Both methods help distinguish uric acid stones from other lesions of the collecting system (e.g., clot; tumor; or, rarely, sloughed renal papilla).

Urinary Collection

All patients with uric acid stones should be screened for the three risk factors that predispose to uric acid stone formation: low urine volume, excessively acidic urine, and hyperuricosuria. This screening requires that patients collect a 24-h urine specimen while on a free diet.

The collection container should be free of acid. The uricase method is the most reliable for measuring the concentration of uric acid in serum and urine. Recent use of uricosuric agents may invalidate the urine test; the most common collection error is collecting urine samples shortly after administration of contrast material, which produces uricosuria.

Researchers do not agree about what constitutes hyperuricosuria. Most consider the upper limit to be 750 mg (4.5 mmol) for women and 800 mg (4.8 mmol) for men. Total urate excretion is not as meaningful as concentration of undissociated uric acid, which can be estimated from urine volume, total uric acid excretion, and mean urinary pH.

Measuring Urinary Acidity

Nitrazine paper provides an accurate measure of urinary pH within the physiologic range and is convenient for determining urinary pH during outpatient visits and at home. When we screen patients for excessively acidic urine, we instruct them to test the pH of urine voided throughout the day, particularly upon arising and after meals. Normal subjects show peaks and troughs of urinary pH with at least some values >6.0.

Therapy

Correction of Aciduria

Moderation of the intake of animal protein is crucial in a therapeutic program. A diet rigidly restricted in purines and protein is unpalatable, but patients who reduce the total ingestion of meat, poultry, and fish from 8 oz (56 g) to 5 oz (35 g) daily (a realistic goal) derive two benefits: Less total uric acid is excreted, and reduced urine acidity reduces undissociated and insoluble uric acid.[82]

The use of alkali (Table 24-3) is an integral part of therapy, especially for patients whose urine is persistently acidic. Using nitrazine paper, patients can adjust the dose of alkali to maintain a urinary pH between 6.0 and 6.5. Because of the solubility characteristics of uric acid, the goal of alkali therapy is different for patients with uric acid stones than for patients with cystinuria (compare Figs. 24-4 and 24-9).[54,79] A dose of alkali prescribed to patients with uric acid lithiasis must not cause urinary pH to exceed 7.0. This degree of alkalinization not only is unnecessary but is potentially dangerous because it increases the risk of formation of calcium phosphate stones. Because of its longer action and possible protection against calcium stone formation, potassium citrate may be preferred to sodium-containing alkali.[92,93]

Treatment with Allopurinol

Indications for Allopurinol Therapy

Because it is effective and easy to use, allopurinol has become a popular agent for treating uric acid stones. However, treatment using only diet modification and alkali is preferred in many cases.

Although the half-life of allopurinol is only a few hours, its metabolite, oxypurinol, has a half-life of 15–20 hours, extending the biological effects of the drug and enabling effectiveness with a single daily dose, usually 300 mg. This dose reduces uric acid excretion a mean 30–40 percent; the hypouricosuric effect may increase slightly during the first few weeks of use. Many physicians do not recognize that the concentration of undissociated uric acid can be reduced much more substantially using diet modification and alkali. Allopurinol is sometimes inappropriately given to patients with uric acid lithiasis who do not excrete excessive uric acid.

Indications for allopurinol therapy include one or all of the following: hyperuricemia, gouty arthritis, recurrent uric acid stone disease, and substantial overproduction [>800 mg/day (>4.8 mmol/day)] of uric acid. Patients with a single uric acid stone in whom overproduction of uric acid is not marked and articular symptoms are not present should be managed conservatively.

Hazards of Allopurinol Therapy

Allopurinol is usually well tolerated and is relatively nontoxic. Gastrointestinal intolerance occurs in about 1 percent of cases, and hypersensitivity reactions occur in about 2 percent. The first sign of a hypersensitivity reaction is pruritus, which nearly always develops during the first few weeks of treatment. If treatment is not stopped, the reaction progresses to a rash, usually maculopapular. Again, prompt discontinuation of the drug prevents a potentially life-threatening hypersensitivity reaction, which occurs in about 1 in 1,000 patients. This advanced phase of the reaction is preceded by fever, chills, and an extensive skin rash and may progress to nephritis and hepatitis, resulting in death in 20 percent of cases.[94] When initiating allopurinol therapy, physicians should always advise patients that at the first signs of itching or rash, use of the drug should be discontinued.

CALCIUM PHOSPHATE STONES

Although calcium phosphate in the form of hydroxyapatite may be admixed in typical calcium oxalate stones, pure calcium phosphate stones are rare (Table 24-1). Calcium phosphate stones are given separate status to emphasize the unique aspects of their pathogenesis and because their presence is often an important diagnostic clue to the basis of stone formation.

Crystalline Forms of Calcium Phosphate

Pure calcium phosphate stones form in sterile, alkaline urine. The major crystalline form of calcium phosphate is hydroxyapatite $[Ca_{10}(PO_4)_6(OH)_2]$. Brushite $(CaHPO_4 \cdot 2H_2O)$ is not commonly identified in calculi but may form a nidus that later develops into the more mature hydroxyapatite crystalline form.

Effect of pH on Solubility of Calcium Phosphate

HPO_4^{2-} concentration increases markedly as pH increases; the solubility and formation products for calcium phosphate are both reduced. Pure calcium phosphate stones suggest an underlying disorder of urine acidification manifested by persistently alkaline urine. This scenario is illustrated by a study[95] that compared 15 patients with calcium phosphate stones and 15 patients with calcium oxalate stones. In contrast to patients with calcium oxalate stones, patients with phosphate stones had higher fasting urinary pH; and whereas no patients with calcium oxalate stones had an abnormal response to ammonium chloride loading, one-third of the calcium phosphate group responded abnormally by not manifesting sufficiently low (<5.3) urinary pH.

Renal Tubular Acidosis

The process of renal acidification normally maintains the pH of extracellular fluids in two ways: by reclaiming filtered bicarbonate and by excreting a quantity of acid equal to the daily systemic production of fixed acid.[7,96] The proximal tubular resorptive mechanism is a high-capacity system that resorbs 90 percent of filtered bicarbonate. The distal tubular mechanism is a low-capacity, high-gradient system that resorbs the remaining bicarbonate and sets the final urinary pH. The gradient of the distal process is sufficient to produce pH ≤5.0 and enables the kidney to excrete ammonium and titratable acid in quantities sufficient to balance systemic acid production and to regenerate the bicarbonate consumed in buffering the daily production of acid.

Renal tubular acidosis (RTA) is a rare but important cause of calcium phosphate stones.[7,96,97] Several types of RTA have been identified, but only patients with the distal (classic, or type 1) form are at risk for development of calcium phosphate stones. Patients with complete distal RTA typically have systemic hyperchloremic acidosis and persistently alkaline urine. The exact nature of the defect in distal tubular acidification is unknown, but affected patients are only rarely capable of generating urinary pH <5.5. Calcium phosphate nephrolithiasis or nephrocalcinosis (or both) has been reported in more than half of such patients[97]; nephrocalcinosis is more common than nephrolithiasis.

The pathogenesis of distal RTA is largely unknown. A familial form associated with an autosomal-dominant pattern of inheritance causes growth retardation, rickets, and nephrocalcinosis or nephrolithiasis during childhood. Eighth-nerve deafness and RTA associated with an autosomal-recessive pattern of inheritance have also been reported. Sjögren's syndrome and other hyperglobulinemic states cause acquired distal RTA in adults. Rare causes of distal RTA include medullary sponge kidney, amphotericin B administration, and obstructive uropathy.[7] No pathogenetic unifying link has been found between these disorders and the distal acidification defect.

Patients with proximal (type 2, or bicarbonate-losing) RTA typically have systemic hyperchloremic acidosis and osteopenia. The distal acidification mechanism is normal in these patients, and stones do not occur. Proximal RTA is also frequently associated with aminoaciduria, glycosuria, and other elements of Fanconi's syndrome; these features are not found in patients with distal RTA.

Pathophysiology of Stone Disease in Renal Tubular Acidosis

Patients with distal RTA usually have multiple risk factors for calcium phosphate stone formation. The most consistent abnormality is alkaline urine, usually fixed at pH ≥6.5. Acidosis inhibits production of citrate in the renal cortex; accordingly, citrate excretion is reduced in patients with RTA.[98] Citrate is normally responsible for binding and solubilizing urinary calcium. Most patients also have hypercalciuria; at least two mechanisms contribute to it. Systemic acidosis is buffered to some extent by bone mineral dissolution that releases both calcium and phosphate for eventual renal excretion. In addition, renal calcium resorption is reduced, possibly because of an acidosis-induced defect in calcium resorption in the distal nephron.[7] Intestinal calcium absorption is usually normal or decreased in patients with RTA. The principal risk factors for stone formation in distal RTA are thus alkaline urine, reduced citrate excretion, and hypercalciuria.

Incomplete Renal Tubular Acidosis

RTA is considered complete when systemic acidosis accompanies the acidification defect and incomplete when the process is not severe enough to produce systemic acidosis. Incomplete distal RTA is far more common than complete RTA among stone-forming patients and can be identified by acid-loading studies in about 5 percent of patients affected with recurrent calcium stones. Among 518 consecutive patients with stone disease, the prevalence of incomplete distal RTA was 7 percent.[99] Several other small series emphasized the association between incomplete distal RTA and recurrent formation of calcium phosphate stones.[100–102] In some patients, the defect apparently results from tubular damage caused by severe stone disease, medullary sponge kidney, staghorn calculi, or associated pyelonephritis. In other patients, the acidification defect is the apparent primary cause of renal stone formation.[99,103]

The mechanisms by which this partial defect contributes to formation of kidney stones are apparently similar to, although less severe than, the mechanisms observed in patients who have complete RTA syndrome. Relatively alkaline urine, hypercalciuria, and hypocitraturia are thus all seen in patients with incomplete RTA.[99–104]

Acetazolamide is a noncompetitive carbonic anhydrase inhibitor used primarily in treating glaucoma. Although inhibition of bicarbonate resorption in the proximal tubule is the principal action of this drug, it also inhibits citrate production, decreases excretion of ammonia as well as titratable acid, and raises urinary pH, in essence producing iatrogenic RTA.[105] Pure calcium phosphate stones develop in about 5–10 percent of patients receiving acetazolamide.

Patients with primary hyperparathyroidism, sarcoidosis, and vitamin D intoxication may also have pure calcium phosphate stones. Although the stones that form in patients with primary hyperparathyroidism as a group appear to have increased calcium phosphate content, calcium oxalate and mixed stones are most commonly found.[106] Parathyroid hormone (PTH) may cause renal bicarbonate wasting and may predispose a patient to formation of calcium phosphate stones (see Chap. 22).

Evaluation

Identification

Calcium phosphate stones can be identified only by crystallographic analysis and should be suspected in patients with coincident nephrocalcinosis or specific diseases known to cause RTA. The medication history of patients with stone disease should always include information about acetazolamide or antacid intake.

Renal Acidification Tests

The presence of calcium phosphate stones mandates extensive evaluation of renal acidification. When a urea-splitting infection is present, urinary pH results are uninterpretable. If urinary pH is $\leq$5.5 when checked early in the morning, complete RTA can be ruled out. Patients with pH $\geq$6.0 at initial evaluation may be given a roll of nitrazine paper to record first early-morning urinary pH for a few days. This simple maneuver documents normal acidification capability in almost all patients and precludes acid-loading studies in all but a small percentage of cases. Patients who have urinary pH $\geq$6.1 on 2 fasting morning specimens have a 90 percent likelihood of failing an ammonium chloride test and should be further evaluated for RTA.[107]

Equivocal laboratory results indicate acid-loading studies for clarification. In the "acute" acid-loading study, which is used most commonly, 0.1 g of oral ammonium chloride is given per kilogram of body weight; urinary pH, venous blood pH, and P_{CO_2} are then measured at baseline and hourly for 6 h.[3] Although this study is convenient, the results may be uninterpretable because the medication causes vomiting; a nonabsorbable antacid should be given with the drug to help prevent gastric irritation and vomiting. The normal renal response to the induced acidosis is manifested by urinary pH <5.3. Incomplete RTA is diagnosed on the basis of normal serum electrolyte concentrations and nonmaximal acidification of urine. If test results are equivocal or a patient has gastric intolerance, a "long" acid-loading test lasting 3 consecutive days may be done.[103]

Treatment

Complete Distal RTA

Patients with complete distal RTA are treated with alkali in quantities sufficient to normalize serum bicarbonate concentration. In adults, this amount is usually 1 mEq per kilogram of body weight daily. In children, acid production rates and dose per kilogram are several times higher.[108] The alkali is given daily in four to six divided doses. Sodium bicarbonate tablets are inexpensive and effective, but many physicians and some patients prefer citrate preparations (Table 24-3).

Alkalinization has a dramatic effect on the skeletal manifestation of RTA and can restore normal growth rates in children.[108] Any hypercalciuria is reduced or eliminated, and excretion of citrate is normalized.

Incomplete Distal RTA

The preferred treatment is potassium citrate because it corrects the hypercalciuria and hypocitraturia which occur in patients with incomplete distal RTA. In an uncontrolled trial of such patients, oral potassium citrate therapy prevented formation of new stones during a 34-month period.[102]

MAGNESIUM AMMONIUM PHOSPHATE STONES

Terminology

Various synonymous terms, including *struvite stone*, *infection stone*, and *triple phosphate stone*, are used to describe MAP stones. Struvite stones are composed of MAP ($MgNH_4PO_4 \cdot 6H_2O$) admixed with minor amounts of carbonate-apatite [$Ca_{10}(PO_4)_6 \cdot CO_3$]. Triple phosphate refers to the three different cations (magnesium, ammonium, and calcium) found with the phosphate anion. Urologists use the term *infection stone* to distinguish such stones from metabolic stones.

History and Epidemiology

MAP stones are an ancient disease manifestation. Before surgery or antibiotics were available, the outlook for affected patients was bleak. Surgical and medical advances have dramatically altered this outlook, and rates of both prevalence and recurrence of MAP stones have clearly decreased in the past two decades, perhaps by as much as 75 percent.[109,110]

The peak prevalence of MAP stones occurs in three sectors of the population: young boys, middle-aged women, and elderly patients of both sexes. MAP stones represent only a small percentage of total stones (Table 24-1). Nevertheless, because of the high morbidity as well as the difficulty of medical and surgical management, their importance far outweighs their frequency.

Pathophysiology

The formation of MAP stones results from supersaturation of urine with magnesium ammonium phosphate and carbonate-apatite. Such supersaturation occurs only when infection with urea-splitting bacteria is present. MAP stone formation can be

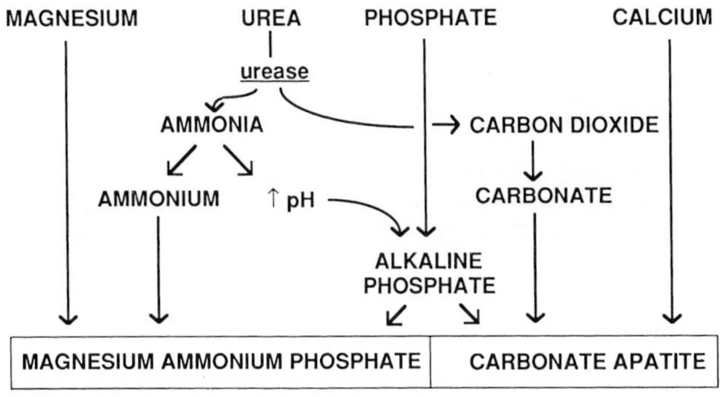

FIGURE 24-12. Biochemical steps leading to formation of magnesium ammonium phosphate (MAP) stones in urine. (*Reproduced by permission of the editor and publisher from Ettinger B, Insogna KL.*[11a])

reproduced in vitro simply by adding purified urease to normal urine[109]; urease initiates the sequence of reactions shown in Fig. 24-12. Increased concentration of ammonium, carbonate, and alkaline pH that changes PO_{4-1} into PO_{4-2} oversaturates the urine with both MAP and carbonate-apatite.

An in vitro model has been suggested in which urease-producing bacteria, such as *Proteus* species, adhere to renal epithelial cells and form small colonies enclosed in a glycocalix coat secreted by the bacteria.[111] The glycocalix may protect the bacteria from antibiotic action and also traps struvite and apatite crystals. These crystal-encrusted microcolonies then combine with inflammatory cells, debris, and urinary mucoproteins to form a stone matrix. The matrix of MAP stones may have an important role in calculus growth. The large, soft, gel-like matrix may mineralize rapidly and assumes a classic staghorn calculous appearance within weeks.[112]

Bacteriology

About 90 percent of clinical isolates of *Proteus* species, *Staphylococcus aureus*, and *Bacteroides* species produce urease. About 30 percent of *Klebsiella* and *Pseudomonas* isolates are urease-positive. In contrast, *Escherichia coli* rarely, if ever, produce urease. Although all urea-splitting bacterial strains have been implicated, *Proteus* species are identified in almost 90 percent of these patients.[105] Colony counts are frequently <100,000/mL, a finding important for proper diagnosis and management.

Clinical Risk Factors

Two major categories of patients are at risk for MAP stones: (1) patients with anatomic or functional abnormalities of the urinary tract (or both), which predispose to infection, and (2) patients with antecedent metabolic stones in whom infection introduced by urologic procedures is established at the stone site. The first category includes patients with megaloureter, ureteral reflux or obstruction, ileal conduits, nephrostomy drainage, or bladder outlet obstruction necessitating either intermittent catheterization or an indwelling catheter. The second category includes patients with metabolic stones, particularly patients who need frequent instrumentation for stones. Stone disease in such patients ultimately becomes self-perpetuating; stones predispose to infection, and infection predisposes to stone formation.

Serious Morbidity from MAP Stones

Untreated staghorn calculi can grow and invade locally in a way similar to a neoplasm. Untreated patients have about a 50 percent chance of losing the affected kidney within 5 years. Renal impairment associated with a unilateral staghorn stone is usually insufficient to greatly alter renal function tests; the condition can be identified by visualizing a shrunken or scarred cortical outline (or both) during the nephrogram phase of the IVP. Patients with staghorn calculi in a single functioning kidney or with bilateral staghorn stones may have azotemia. About 25 percent of patients with bilateral staghorn stones die within 5 yr.[111]

Evaluation

Identifying MAP stones is usually not difficult. Such stones are diagnosed by the characteristic staghorn configuration of the stone, by crystallographic analysis, or by both. The apatite content confers radiopacity on MAP stones, which are less dense than oxalate stones but—except for occasional matrix concretions—are readily seen on plain x-ray films.

The bacteriologic aspect of diagnosis is less straightforward. The colony count of urease-producing bacteria is <100,000/mL in half and <10,000/mL in 20 percent of patients. Mixed infections are common, and a tendency exists to neglect the importance of the urea-splitting organisms when they are overshadowed by larger numbers of other organisms (e.g., *E. coli*). Thus, for patients suspected of having MAP stones, obtaining colony counts of all gram-negative organisms in the urine culture is important. Moreover, regardless of the colony count or presence of mixed infection, urease-producing organisms can be cultured from stone material. Surgical specimens should thus be cultured to establish a clear bacteriologic diagnosis.

Other aspects of diagnosis relate to metabolic screening and the search for structural or functional abnormalities of the urinary tract. A carefully obtained IVP is essential. Cystoscopy and retrograde pyelography may be indicated. Patients with MAP stones should have a careful and complete urinary biochemical evaluation. Smith reported that more than 60 percent of patients with MAP stones have urinary biochemical abnormalities which predispose to metabolic stone formation.[105] For such patients, it may be possible to document a historical sequence of stones with differing composition.

Treatment

The prognosis for patients with MAP stones has improved considerably as medical and surgical approaches to the disease have become better coordinated and more sophisticated.[113] In a series of patients monitored for 7 yr, a meticulous medical-surgical approach rendered >90 percent of patients free of both stones and infection.[114] This optimistic report is tempered by general experience showing a mean 30 percent stone recurrence rate and a mean 40 percent infection recurrence rate.[109]

For patients in whom metabolic stone diathesis is complicated by MAP stones, fewer specific data are available. In Smith's experience,[110] when all stone material was removed at surgery, the prognosis was good; 81 percent of such patients remained stone-free.

Antibiotic Therapy

The approach to antimicrobial therapy differs at different times in a patient's course. Short-term administration of antibiotics almost never eliminates infection when a MAP stone is present. Culture-specific bactericidal drugs are given 24–48 hours before surgery and are continued for 10–14 days after all urologic devices have been removed. Patients considered free of stones and infection after surgery are usually maintained on either low-dosage bactericidal agents or broad-spectrum drugs for 6–12 months, with serial urine cultures taken every 1–3 months during treatment. However, in one series of stone-free patients, stopping antibiotics after only 2 weeks had no adverse consequences.[114]

Patients in whom stones remain after surgery and patients in whom surgery cannot be attempted are treated with long-term antibiotic therapy. Low-dose, culture-specific bactericidal agents are preferred to broad-spectrum agents.[109,112] The goal in these patients is to render the urine sterile during therapy and to limit both stone growth and the frequency of infection symptoms; therapy is continued indefinitely. Most reports suggest that if the urine is successfully and permanently sterilized, a patient's condition will remain stable.[115,116] Long-term antimicrobial treatment is occasionally associated with reduced stone mass.[109,112]

Complete removal of all stone material is the goal of surgical therapy and represents the only reliable method of cure in patients with MAP stones. The success of this approach depends on meticulous attention to detail during surgery and in the periods immediately before and after surgery. Complete removal of MAP stones is hampered by their friability and by their tendency to mold to inaccessible areas of the collecting system. These difficulties led to development of various surgical techniques, including coagulum lithotomy, irrigation of the renal pelvis and collecting system, and nephroscopy. Percutaneous and extracorporeal lithotripsy of staghorn calculi may substantially simplify MAP stone surgery. These two procedures combined are likely to become the preferred treatment because they can eliminate all stone material in about three-quarters of these patients. Urologic treatment of MAP stones has been reviewed comprehensively.[113]

Urease Inhibitors

Because production of urease by an organism is the main pathogenic event in MAP stone formation, enzyme-specific inhibitors have been developed. Acetohydroxamic acid, a potent urease inhibitor, has been approved for this use. In a recent review of three randomized, double-blind trials using 341 patients, those who took acetohydroxamic acid up to 2 yr had about half the prevalence of stone growth as patients taking placebo.[113] In about 20 percent of patients, the drug caused serious side effects, including rash, headache, phlebitis, thromboembolism, hemolytic anemia, and iron deficiency anemia. The usual dose of acetohydroxamic acid is 10 to 15 mg per kilogram of body weight divided into three or four oral doses; the maximal daily dose is 1.5 g. Patients with moderate renal insufficiency require lower doses; patients with substantial renal failure should not receive this drug. Acetohydroxamic acid should be prescribed by physicians experienced in its use and competent to integrate it into a comprehensive urologic treatment program.

CALCIUM OXALATE AND MIXED CALCIUM STONES

Epidemiology

Calcium stone disease predominantly affects persons living in industrialized nations and accounts for 75 percent of all cases of nephrolithiasis (Table 24-1). The incidence of calcium stone disease has steadily increased during the last few decades.[1,117] This increase has occurred mostly in men: the men-to-women ratio increased from 1.8:1.0 in 1954 to 3.8:1.0 in 1970.[1] The incidence of calcium stones peaks for an extended period during the middle four decades of life.[1]

About half these stones are composed of pure calcium oxalate, and half are admixtures of calcium oxalate and calcium phosphate. Calcium oxalate crystals may exist as either the monohydrate (whewellite) or dihydrate (weddellite) species; an admixture of the two is most common. We do not know whether the presence of calcium phosphate in mixed stones is important for crystal nucleation or growth, but the calcium phosphate content of these stones apparently reflects urinary pH.[7,118] The percentages of pure calcium phosphate stones and of stones composed of calcium phosphate admixed with calcium oxalate have decreased in recent years[119]; the apparent decreases have been attributed to altered diet, particularly to decreased animal protein intake.[117]

Evidence shows that diet plays a major role in the increasing incidence of calcium stones. Surveys in the United Kingdom found that intake of animal protein (meat, poultry, and fish) is the primary dietary variable associated with an increased incidence of calcium oxalate stones; intake of calcium, oxalate, magnesium, and carbohydrate is relatively unimportant.[117] Increased dietary protein adds to urinary excretion of calcium, uric acid, and oxalate and reduces urinary pH; all these factors predispose to calcium oxalate stones instead of to other types.[46,117]

Physical Chemistry

The concepts of saturation chemistry apply to calcium stone formation, but a single discrete biochemical abnormality, such as that which defines cystine stone disease or cystinuria, is not seen in patients with calcium stone disease.

The complex solution chemistry of calcium oxalate is illustrated by the activity of calcium ions in a solution such as urine. At a given pH, calcium can form soluble complexes with the anions citrate, oxalate, sulfate; and with four species of phosphate ions. These anions can also form soluble complexes with other cations besides calcium. Computing calcium ion activity in such a system necessitates solving about a dozen simultaneous equations.

Although techniques and interpretations differ, the findings from several laboratories have had similar implications with regard to saturation and predisposition to crystal formation and growth in stone-forming urine.[120–122] The *activity product ratio* (*APR*) describes the saturation of urine by calcium oxalate. An APR of unity indicates that urine is saturated, a value less than unity indicates undersaturation, and values progressively greater than unity define increasing degrees of supersaturation. The APR in patients with recurrent calcium stones is typically higher than in normal persons. These results can usually be attributed to increased calcium concentration in the urine of stone-forming patients and to a variable tendency toward increased oxalate concentration. Similar observations have been made about brushite, suggesting that the calcium phosphate system may be an important crystal nidus, particularly in alkaline urine.

The *formation product ratio* (*FPR*) is a measurement of the minimum supersaturation needed to cause spontaneous nucleation. The measurement is made by adding calcium to urine and noting the activity product at which cloudiness appears. The FPR is normally 8–10 times the APR of calcium oxalate.[120–122] The FPR (or an equivalent parameter) in patients with recurrent calcium stones is often less than normal, indicating an unexplained predisposition to crystallization in stone-forming urine.

This predisposition has been attributed to the process of heterogeneous nucleation (e.g., of crystals of calcium oxalate and either monosodium urate or uric acid), a deficiency of unidentified inhibitors in stone-forming urine, and the presence of "promoters" of crystallization in stone-forming urine. Stone formation apparently results from an imbalance of forces that cause or prevent crystallization and growth of calcium salts in urine.

Natural History of Calcium Oxalate Lithiasis

In quantitating the risk of stone recurrence, epidemiologists have relied on three methods of data acquisition: retrospective, retrolective, and prospective. A *retrospective*, or population-based, study either asks all subjects to recall previous stone events or reviews health records and other data bases. Although limited by the accuracy of a person's recall and the incompleteness of medical data collection, this method is less biased than a *retrolective* study, which relies on data collection from stone clinic patients. When such patients are asked to recall initial and subsequent stone events, recurrence rates and risk of stone morbidity are exaggerated. Bek-Jensen and Tiselius quantitated the bias introduced in this manner.[123] Among patients seen at a stone clinic, the annual stone event rate was 0.19 stone per patient-year for 3 yr after the first stone event but was 0.66 stone per patient-year during the 3 yr just before the stone clinic visit. Using the retrolective method, others[124] have concluded that the interval between stone events shortens with time. Among six retrospective and retrolective studies recently reviewed,[29] mean cumulative recurrence reached 25 percent after 5 yr and 52 percent after 10 yr.[1,30,31,125–127] Recurrence rates were predictably lower by about half in the population-based studies. For example, Marshall and associates,[125] analyzing stone clinic patients, reported an 8 percent annual recurrence rate in men after the first stone event. In contrast, Johnson and associates,[1] studying the population of Rochester, Minnesota, found a recurrence rate of <4 percent annually for men. Both groups of investigators found relatively low annual recurrence rates for women: 6 percent in the stone clinic study and 2 percent in the population-based study.

Estimates of stone morbidity from stone treatment centers also tend to exaggerate rates of hospitalization and urologic surgery. For example, a history of hospitalization was positive for 90 percent of patients seen at a stone evaluation center after the first stone[27] but for only 23–45 percent of such patients identified by population surveys.[6,128] Among patients referred to two centers for stone evaluation, 38 percent[21] and 74 percent[19] had a history of surgical removal. In contrast, a population-based study found that only 5 percent of stone patients needed surgery.[129]

Ideally, *prospective* studies are used to define the natural history of calcium stone disease. To conduct such a study, however, new patients with single stones must be identified soon after the clinical event, patients with additional existing stones must be identified and excluded, and a sufficient number of subjects must be monitored long enough to obtain sufficiently robust statistics for recurrence. Ljunghall and Danielson[130] identified 54 such patients who were seen at emergency departments. Figure 24-13[130] shows that the annual recurrence rate in this study was about 10 percent during the first 4 yr of follow-up; recurrence was less frequent thereafter, and recurrence was three times as probable in men as in women. Patients seen at the Mayo Clinic for evaluation of a first[131,132] stone received fluid and diet advice and were then monitored for 5 yr; the annual recurrence rate was about 5 percent. In a prospective trial of single-stone patients who were health plan members of the Kaiser Permanente Medical Care Program in Northern California, the annual recurrence rate was about 4 percent during a mean 3.4-yr period among 99 patients who were given general dietary advice.[32]

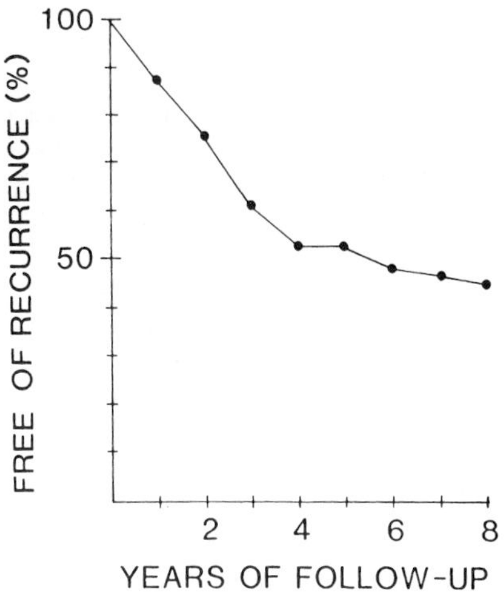

FIGURE 24-13. Percentage of untreated patients free of recurrence after a single renal stone in relation to time of follow-up. (*Reproduced by permission of the author and publisher from Ljunghall S, Danielson BG.*[130])

The risk of subsequent recurrence is about two to three times greater in patients who have had two or more stone events compared with single-stone patients. Stone patients who have had a relapse may be expected to have stones frequently. These aspects of risk determination are germane to (1) consideration of metabolic screening in patients who have had a single stone event, (2) initiation of treatment in patients who have had one or more stone events, and (3) proposed duration of therapy (see Evaluation of Calcium Oxalate Stones and Treatment of Calcium Oxalate Nephrolithiasis).

Risk Factors

The risk factors that predispose to calcium stone formation can be separated into two categories (Table 24-5): (1) general risk factors (e.g., a family history) and (2) specific, treatable metabolic risk factors (e.g., hypercalciuria).[11b]

Family History

A family history of renal stones in one or more first-degree relatives is found in 35–50 percent of patients with calcium stone disease.[132–134] The most commonly found association is between the patient (male or female) and male first-degree relatives, in whom the risk for stone formation may be 5–10 times the risk in

TABLE 24-5. Risk Factors for Calcium Stone Formation

General	Specific
Family history	Low urine volume
Medications	Hypercalciuria
Urinary pH	Hyperoxaluria
Diet	Hyperuricosuria
	Hypocitraturia

Source: Adapted by permission of the author, editor, and publisher from Insogna KL, Broadus AE: Nephrolithiasis, in Felig P, Baxter JD, Broadus AE, Frohman LA (eds): *Endocrinology and Metabolism,* 2d ed. New York, McGraw-Hill, 1987, p 1557.[11b]

the general population. The lifetime risk for brothers of index case patients is nearly 50 percent.[132] The severity of calcium stone disease is not different in these kindreds than in other stone patients.

Coe and associates[133] examined the familial association between hypercalciuria and calcium stone disease. Among 44 first-degree relatives, 43 percent were hypercalciuric, suggesting an autosomal-dominant mode of inheritance. A history of renal stones was also common in these first-degree relatives, but a history of stone disease and the presence of hypercalciuria were unrelated; equal percentages of normocalciuric and hypercalciuric relatives reported a history of stones.

Family history information was evaluated for 206 patients seen at the Yale Renal Stone Clinic for common calcium stones (K.L. Insogna, M.D., unpublished data).* A history of stone disease in one or more first-degree relatives was found for half these patients. Familial patterns of identified risk factors—low urine volume, hyperuricosuria, and hypercalciuria—were analyzed by isolating patients with only one risk factor and excluding patients with combined risk factors. Family history was positive in 71 percent of patients with low urine volume, 62 percent of hyperuricosuric patients, 50 percent of hypercalciuric patients, and 41 percent of patients in whom no risk factor was identified; inherited risks, environmental risks, or a combination were not explained by a simple metabolic pattern.

The marked familial tendency toward calcium stone formation is unexplained. Specific, rare disorders with an autosomal-dominant or autosomal-recessive inheritance pattern, such as RTA, familial forms of hyperparathyroidism, and primary hyperoxaluria, account for only a small percentage of affected family members. In recent years, despite extensive search for genetic disorders linked to abnormalities of calcium absorption or vitamin D metabolism, hypercalciuric patients have not been found to have any of the known gene mutations of vitamin D metabolism or its receptors.[135]

Medication

Vitamin A and vitamin D intoxication as well as the milk-alkali syndrome are described in detail in Chap. 22. All three conditions are characterized by hypercalcemia, nephrocalcinosis, and azotemia and are only rarely associated with renal stone formation. Large doses of ascorbic acid (≥4 g/day) have been reported to lead to increased urinary oxalate excretion, although considerable disagreement exists about both reproducibility and clinical significance of this effect.[136,137] Little evidence exists to show that vitamin C intake predisposes to formation of calcium oxalate stones in persons with no history of stone disease,[138] but exacerbation of calcium oxalate stone disease in patients with a history of stones has been reported.

Urinary pH

Solubility of calcium oxalate in aqueous solution is not influenced by alteration in pH within the limits of the physiologic range. However, concentration of urinary citrate is dependent on urinary pH, and citrate has an important role in complexing and solubilizing calcium (see Hypocitraturia).

Low Urine Volume

Initial urine volume of <1 L daily is observed in about 25 percent of patients with common calcium stones who are screened.[124,139] Pak and associates[140] showed that dilution not only reduces the concentration of calcium and oxalate but enhances the solubility of calcium oxalate. Failure to increase urine volume has been associated with stone recurrence,[132,141] and a 5-yr randomized study[34] showed that high fluid intake reduces stone recurrence by 15 percent in patients who had a first calcium stone event. In that study,[34] subjects were instructed to measure urine volume at home every 2–3 months and to maintain urine volume at ≥2 L per day.

Hypercalciuria

The term *idiopathic hypercalciuria* was introduced in 1953 by Albright and colleagues[142] and was further defined in 1958 by Henneman and coworkers[143]; this group both defined idiopathic hypercalciuria and introduced the question of its pathogenesis, initiating a controversy which still persists. The term idiopathic hypercalciuria encompassed three apparent abnormalities: normocalcemic hypercalciuria, a tendency toward hypophosphatemia, and frequent infection of the urinary tract. The investigators reasoned that the primary abnormality in their patients was a pyelonephritis-induced defect in renal calcium resorption which led to hypercalciuria, secondary hyperparathyroidism, and a consequent tendency toward hypophosphatemia. The finding of bacteriuria was spurious (*Staphylococcus albus* was the organism frequently identified) but was a central feature of their hypothesis. The same investigators presented evidence for increased intestinal calcium absorption in these patients but interpreted this finding as a secondary response to the renal calcium "leak." This study introduced the key elements of the controversy about the diagnosis and pathogenetic importance of "renal" hypercalciuria, "absorptive" hypercalciuria, and subtle ("normocalcemic") primary hyperparathyroidism.

Hypercalciuria is a difficult subject: the biomedical literature cannot be summarized easily, reflecting in part the complexity of the putative pathogenetic mechanisms responsible for hypercalciuria and in part the fact that many published series have been flawed in design, methodology, interpretation, or all these. Readers should pay particular attention to (1) the limits used in defining hypercalciuria in view of established calcium excretion limits expressed on an absolute basis (milligrams per day), which are not necessarily interchangeable with limits expressed on a weight basis (miligrams per kilogram of body weight daily); (2) the impact of dietary influences on both detection and definition of hypercalciuria, particularly calcium and sodium; (3) the shortcomings of certain widely used diagnostic criteria (e.g., classification on the basis of results of fasting calcium excretion); and (4) the importance of study conditions in collecting and interpreting metabolic data. These four points explain much of the controversy.

*Department of Medicine, Yale School of Medicine, New Haven, CT 06520-8020.

Investigators find even the simple issues of defining hypercalciuria and estimating its frequency problematic; the many problems and variables include (1) use of multiple definitions of hypercalciuria, (2) differences in patterns of calcium excretion in different populations, (3) influence of dietary factors besides calcium on calcium excretion, and (4) the difficulty of assigning a statistical upper limit of calcium excretion in the normal population because of the apparent upwardly skewed values in this population.[7,14,15,119,144–147] Among these issues, dietary influences are by far the most important.

The biomedical literature contains reports of two main types of metabolic studies: those using groups of outpatients, almost all of whom were on an unrestricted diet for metabolic screening, and those using groups of inpatients given rigidly defined "metabolic" diets. Each approach reflects a bias. The unrestricted-diet approach seems relevant, because stone disease develops in patients on habitual diets and because dietary factors may play a role in causing hypercalciuria, stones, or both. Investigators using metabolic diets in predominantly inpatient studies note that only controlled studies are likely to generate consistent data. A clear understanding of hypercalciuria may require that elements of both approaches be used; patients should be screened both while on an unrestricted diet as well as under more defined conditions. Moreover, research studies aimed at elucidating the details of pathogenesis must be done under carefully controlled conditions.

At the Yale Renal Stone Clinic (Karl L. Insogna, MD, unpublished data), results of metabolic screening of outpatients on unrestricted diets were systematically compared with the results for patients given a defined metabolic diet containing 1 g calcium, 1 g protein per kilogram of body weight, and 100 mEq sodium daily. The defined diet (see Evaluating Dietary Hypercalciuria) is designed to facilitate detection of hypercalciuria in patients who have a true underlying defect in calcium metabolism and to minimize other dietary influences.

As shown in Table 24-6,[11b] some patients were hypercalciuric only when on the unrestricted diet (group A); some were hypercalciuric while on either the unrestricted or defined diet but showed moderate to marked reduction in calcium excretion on a restricted diet, even though calcium intake had increased in patients on this diet (group B); some had a comparable degree of hypercalciuria on either diet (group C); and some were hypercalciuric only on the defined diet (group D). In the first two groups, dietary factors besides calcium must have at least contributed to hypercalciuria in patients on the unrestricted diet. Conversely, hypercalciuria in group D patients would have been missed entirely if they had not also been screened after being given the defined diet with unrestricted calcium.

Hypercalciuria in patients given the defined diet was highly correlated with underlying alteration in calcium metabolism. About 80 percent of these patients clearly had abnormalities.[144,148,149] In contrast, detailed investigation showed that <20 percent of patients found to be hypercalciuric on only the unrestricted diet had true abnormalities of mineral metabolism.

To maximize detection of hypercalciuria associated with calcium stone disease, patients must be screened while on an unrestricted diet and while on a defined diet containing high-normal calcium content. The unrestricted intake specimen is critical in assessing numerous risk factors for calcium stone formation, including low urine volume, hyperuricosuria, and hypercalciuria.[144] This specimen allows detection of dietary hypercalciuria in patients (22 percent in Table 24-6) who are not hypercalciuric while following a defined diet.[11b] The defined 1,000-mg (25-mmol) calcium diet specimen maximizes detection of true underlying defects in calcium metabolism and minimizes dietary influences besides calcium. Hypercalciuria would not have been detected in 30 percent of the patients listed in Table 24-6 if they had been screened on only an unrestricted diet, because calcium intake was restricted at screening.[11b] When patients are screened for hypercalciuria, the circumstances should be such that the abnormality in patients is expressed.

In normal persons, increasing calcium intake from low normal (400 mg/day) to high normal (1,000 mg/day) has a moderate impact on calcium excretion, increasing it a mean 6 mg per 100-mg increase in dietary calcium intake. In contrast, in most patients with hypercalciuria and stone disease, the calculated upward slope of calcium excretion vs. calcium intake is steep (about 20 percent) Evaluating patients whose calcium intake is increased distinguishes them further from normal subjects (Fig. 24-14).[144,146,147,149]

The defined high-normal calcium diet used for screening outpatients has been used in inpatient studies and gives equivalent results. Given these findings and the ease with which this diet can be used by outpatients, a sophisticated metabolic testing facility is unnecessary for identifying hypercalciuric patients.

What Is the Clinical Utility of Diagnosing Hypercalciuria?

Although hypercalciuria is the most common risk factor identified in patients with calcium stone disease, the statistical relation between calcium excretion and calcium stone formation is weak.

TABLE 24-6. Results of Screening for Hypercalciuria in 122 Hypercalciuric Patients on an Unrestricted or Defined Diet

Diet Being Followed When Hypercalciuria Was Detected	*Mean Calcium Excretion per Day (mg)* Unrestricted Diet*	Defined Diet†	No. of Patients
A. Unrestricted diet only	334	236	27
B. Unrestricted and defined diets: calcium excretion decreased >50 mg/day on defined diet	422	331	17
C. Unrestricted and defined diets	354	365	41
D. Defined diet only	224	328	37

*Mean values for daily sodium excretion on the unrestricted diet in the four groups were 190, 214, 172, and 121 mEq, respectively.

†Defined diet contained 100 mg calcium, 100 mEq sodium, and 1 g protein per kilogram of body weight daily.

Source: Adapted and reproduced by permission of the author, editor, and publisher from Insogna KL, Broadus AE.[11b]

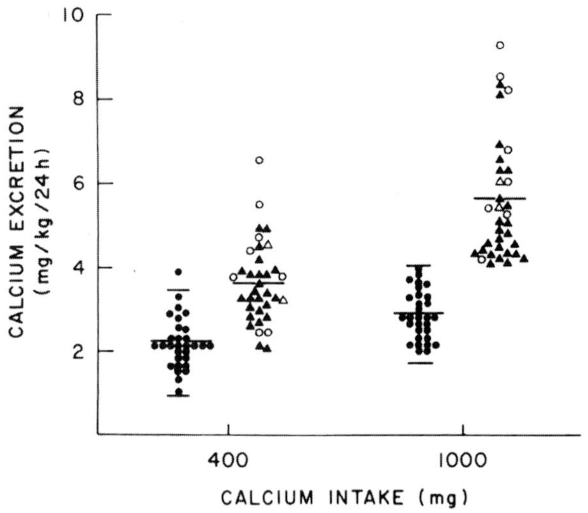

FIGURE 24-14. Urinary calcium excretion determined on both 400-mg and 1,000-mg calcium diets; 30 normal subjects (closed circles), 25 patients with absorptive hypercalciuria (closed triangles), 2 patients with renal hypercalciuria (open triangles), and 8 patients with subtle primary hyperparathyroidism (open circles). Diets were identical except for calcium intake. *(Adapted 1999 and reproduced by permission of the author and publisher from: Broadus AE, Thier SO.[131] Copyright © 1979 Massachusetts Medical Society. All rights reserved.)*

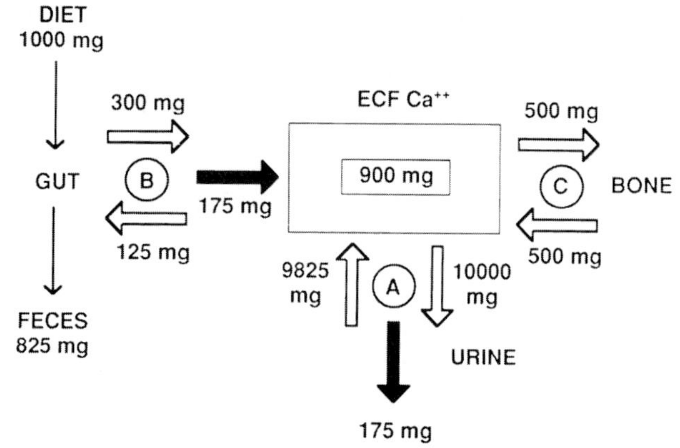

FIGURE 24-15. Schema of calcium metabolism in normal subject in calcium balance. Open arrows denote unidirectional fluxes; solid arrows denote net fluxes. Three mechanisms that can lead to hypercalciuria are denoted A, B, and C (see text). *(Adapted and reproduced by permission of the author, editor, and publisher from Insogna KL, Broadus AE.[11b])*

Many patients with calcium stone disease are not hypercalciuric. Moderate hypercalciuria imparts some risk; however, the risk that stone disease will develop increases markedly at daily excretion rates ≥400 mg (≥10 mmol/day).[98]

Calcium Homeostasis and Mechanisms for Hypercalciuria

Readers should review the discussion of calcium and phosphorus homeostasis in Chap. 22, particularly the sections on control of bone mineral exchange, proximal and distal processes of calcium resorption in the renal tubule, sequence of activation and metabolism of vitamin D, mechanisms and control of intestinal calcium absorption, and calcium and phosphorus homeostasis and balance.

Figure 24-15 illustrates calcium homeostasis in a normal person in calcium balance.[11b] Hypercalciuria can be produced by three mechanisms individually or in some combination: (1) defective renal tubular calcium resorption, (2) increased net calcium absorption, and (3) increased bone resorption. Regardless of the cause, calcium excreted in the urine must ultimately be derived from dietary calcium, bone mineral, or both. Subtle abnormalities are sufficient to produce hypercalciuria. For example, a 1–2 percent error in renal tubular handling of calcium results in clinically significant hypercalciuria.

Classification of Forms of Hypercalciuria

Secondary Hypercalciuria Among the secondary forms of hypercalciuria listed in Table 24-7,[11b] only the first four are encountered with any frequency in an adult population with stone disease. The most important form of secondary hypercalciuria is primary hyperparathyroidism, which was identified in a mean 7.2 percent of 3,084 patients with calcium stone disease in eight large series.[106] The "subtle" variety of this disease can easily be overlooked and requires special diagnostic attention. Among patients seen at the Yale Renal Stone Clinic (Karl L. Insogna, M.D., unpublished data) for calcium oxalate or calcium phosphate stones, 5 percent had primary hyperparathyroidism, 2 percent had complete RTA, and 5 percent had sarcoidosis.

Constitutional Hypercalciuria The term *constitutional hypercalciuria* refers to patients of large size who appear to be hypercalciuric in absolute terms but are not hypercalciuric relative to weight and who appear to be metabolically normal as determined by detailed evaluation. Expressing calcium excretion on a weight-adjusted basis is the only way to normalize for the wide range of body sizes in the patient population, particularly the size dif-

TABLE 24-7. Classification of Hypercalciuria

Secondary hypercalciuria due to
Primary hyperparathyroidism
Sarcoidosis
Distal renal tubular acidosis
Vitamin D excess
Immobilization, rapidly progressive osteoporosis
Uncontrolled diabetes mellitus
Glucocorticoid excess
Thyrotoxicosis
Acromegaly
Furosemide administration
Constitutional hypercalciuria
Dietary hypercalciuria
Idiopathic hypercalciuria
Resorptive
Subtle primary hyperparathyroidism
Renal
Absorptive

Source: Reproduced by permission of the author, editor, and publisher from Insogna KL, Broadus AE.[11b]

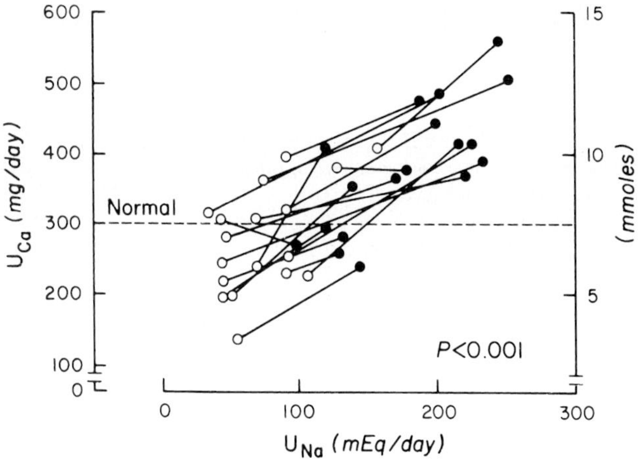

FIGURE 24-16. Twenty-four-hour calcium excretion plotted as a function of sodium excretion in 18 patients first identified as hypercalciuric while on a free unrestricted diet. Patients were allowed 500–700 mg of calcium daily; daily sodium intake varied from 80 mEq (open circles) to 200 mEq (closed circles). (*Reproduced by permission of the author and publisher from Muldowney FP, Freaney R, Moloney MF.*[152])

ference between the sexes. In persons whose diets include a 1,000-mg daily calcium intake, hypercalciuria exists if daily calcium excretion exceeds 4 mg (0.1 mmol) per kilogram of body weight. When calcium excretion is adjusted for body weight, metabolic evaluation may allow better discrimination. If absolute hyperexcretion of calcium is used as the criterion for metabolic evaluation (groups B, C, and D in Table 24-6), 78 percent of patients meeting that criterion had absorptive hypercalciuria, 14 percent had constitutional hypercalciuria, and 8 percent could not be classified. If daily calcium excretion >4 mg (0.1 mmol) per kilogram of body weight on the defined diet were the only criterion for hypercalciuria, about 90 percent of patients meeting that criterion would clearly have absorptive hypercalciuria.[11b,148,149]

Like any other type of hypercalciuria, constitutional hypercalciuria is a risk factor for calcium stone formation. The volume of urine excreted by patients of large body size is not proportionately larger than that excreted by patients of small size. Thus, like other stone patients, patients with constitutional hypercalciuria should be considered for medical treatment.

Dietary Hypercalciuria The 44 patients in groups A and B in Table 24-6[11b] show that hypercalciuria can be profoundly affected by dietary factors other than calcium intake. Although daily calcium intake was several hundred milligrams higher on the defined diet than on the unrestricted diet, mean daily calcium excretion in these 44 patients decreased almost 100 mg on the defined diet.[143] Calcium excretion can be increased by dietary protein, sodium, and carbohydrate and can be decreased by dietary oxalate and phosphate,[7,14,15,19,147–149] although carbohydrate, oxalate, and phosphate appear to be relatively unimportant.

Of the dietary constituents (calcium, protein, and sodium) considered to possibly account for dietary hypercalciuria, sodium is the most strongly correlated with calcium excretion.[150] Sodium inhibits the resorption of calcium in the proximal tubule and possibly in more distal segments of the nephron; available evidence suggests that sodium-induced hypercalciuria is renal in origin.[151–153] Hypercalciuric patients studied while following a low-calcium, high-sodium diet are in negative calcium balance, and imposition of high sodium intake increases fasting calcium excretion.[152] Uncontrolled sodium intake frequently leads to misclassification of patients as having renal hypercalciuria (i.e., as having a primary renal calcium leak).

Increasing sodium intake increases calcium excretion, although the medical literature shows some disagreement about the magnitude of this effect.[152–154] The best estimates available from the medical literature are that every 100 mmol (2.3 g) of dietary sodium is associated with a 1-mmol (40-mg) increase in urinary calcium excretion in normal persons and a 2-mmol (80-mg) increase in urinary calcium excretion among hypercalciuric patients with recurrent calcium nephrolithiasis.[155] Further, several investigators have reported that appearance and disappearance of hypercalciuria depended on sodium intake.[150,153,154] In one such study (the results of which are shown in Fig. 24-16), 18 patients previously defined as hypercalciuric on an unrestricted diet were instructed to use a diet containing 500–700 mg (12.5–17.5 mmol) of calcium and 80–200 mEq of sodium.[151,152] About half the patients were normocalciuric on the 80-mEq-sodium diet. Higher sodium intake caused calcium excretion to increase by a mean of about 100 mg (2.5 mmol) daily.

Some researchers have suggested that idiopathic hypercalciuria results from disordered proximal tubular function. Defects have been shown in proximal tubular resorption of multiple ions, including sodium and calcium.[156,157] Such patients may be more sensitive than normal persons to variation in sodium intake. Whether the calculated upward slope of calcium excretion vs. sodium intake is steeper in patients who are considered hypercalciuric than in nonhypercalciuric patients with stone disease, normal persons, or both is unclear.

Protein ingestion profoundly influences urinary calcium levels: increasing protein ingestion from 0.5 g per kilogram of body weight daily (a restricted intake) to 2 g per kilogram daily (a liberal intake) can double calcium excretion in normal persons.[147] In a study of normal persons, daily dietary protein in the form of red meat was increased from 1 to 2 g per kilogram of body weight.[28] In addition, the effect of increasing the sodium intake from 100 to 310 mEq was measured. Increasing the intake of dietary protein or sodium raised urinary calcium levels by 33 percent; increasing the intake of both raised urinary calcium levels by 73 percent. These dietary manipulations also reduced citrate excretion by 29 percent and increased the tendency for calcium oxalate crystal agglomeration. Breslau and coworkers[158] found that when dietary protein was changed from vegetable sources to animal sources while total dietary protein was kept constant at 75 g/day, urinary calcium levels increased by half. These investigators postulated that the higher sulfur content of the animal protein diet increased the load of fixed acid and thus caused bone dissolution. This interpretation was supported by reduced levels of urinary cAMP, serum immunoreactive PTH, and 1,25-$(OH)_2D$ as well as by failure to find a compensatory increase in intestinal calcium absorption.

Idiopathic Hypercalciuria As shown in Table 24-7,[11b] patients can be subdivided by mechanisms responsible for hypercalciuria. The four subtypes of idiopathic hypercalciuria described here are somewhat unconventional and are outlined to encourage consideration of physiologic mechanisms.

Resorptive Hypercalciuria Resorptive hypercalciuria is a primary disorder in which increased resorption of bone mineral results in secondary hypercalciuria. Skeletal calcium mobilization increases the ambient concentration of calcium in extracellular fluids, thus suppressing parathyroid function, 1,25-$(OH)_2D$ synthesis, and intestinal calcium absorption while increasing the filtered load of calcium; this process is associated with increased fractional calcium excretion resulting from suppression of PTH. The best-studied example of resorptive hypercalciuria is the immobilization syndrome.[159] Other examples of resorptive hypercalciuria are rapidly progressive osteoporosis, cancer-associated osteolysis, and hyperthyroidism. Hypercalciuria observed in patients with complete distal RTA, primary hyperparathyroidism, glucocorticoid excess, sarcoidosis, and (possibly) absorptive or renal hypercalciuria (or both) may have a resorptive component (as noted later).

TABLE 24-8. Pathophysiologic Features in Three Patients with Primary Hyperparathyroidism

	Patient		
Feature	**A**	**B**	**C**
Fasting serum calcium concentration (mg/dL)	11.0	11.3	10.2
24-h calcium excretion (mg)	439	275	452
History of renal stones	Yes	No	Yes
Plasma 1,25-$(OH)_2D$ concentration (pg/mL)	90	57	90

Values shown are mean data from Broadus et al.[160,163]

Source: Adapted and reproduced by permission of the author and publishers from Broadus AE, Horst RL, Littledike ET, Mahaffey JE, Rasmussen H;[160] adapted 1999 and reproduced by permission of the author and publisher from: Broadus AE, Horst RL, Lang R, Littledike ET, Rasmussen H.[163]

Subtle Primary Hyperparathyroidism The term *subtle primary hyperparathyroidism* describes a disorder consisting of slightly abnormal serum calcium concentration, marked hypercalciuria, and stone disease. The term *normocalcemic primary hyperparathyroidism* was previously used in describing such patients, but this term should be avoided because these patients usually have a characteristic pattern of intermittent hypercalcemia that deviates 0.5 mg/dL above and below the upper normal limit and have a mean fasting serum calcium concentration of about 10.2–10.3 mg/dl.[106,160–162] A mean serum calcium concentration in this range should not be considered normal in ambulatory, healthy young adults, especially those affected with hypercalciuria and stone disease.

Studies have clarified the pathophysiologic features leading to hypercalciuria in patients with primary hyperparathyroidism, particularly those with subtle primary hyperparathyroidism.[160,163] As shown in Table 24-8,[81] the fasting serum calcium concentration in patients A and B was nearly identical, but marked hypercalciuria was present in patient A, who was following an unrestricted-calcium diet and had a history of stones, whereas patient B was normocalciuric and had no stones. The disproportionate hypercalciuria in patient A resulted from the markedly elevated circulating concentration of 1,25-$(OH)_2D$; in contrast, the 1,25-$(OH)_2D$ level was within the normal range in patient B. The disproportionate hypercalciuria in patient A was thus predominantly absorptive in nature and was markedly similar to that observed in patients with absorptive hypercalciuria syndrome, except that the primary pathogenetic abnormality in patient A was parathyroid hyperfunction.

Patient C (Table 24-8) was similar to patient A except that the mean fasting serum calcium concentration was 10.2 mg/dL. Representative measurements of fasting serum calcium concentration during several months were 10.1, 10.3, 10.7, 10.1, and 10.0 mg/dL. Like patient A, patient C had a marked increase in circulating 1,25-$(OH)_2D$ concentration, had excessive gastrointestinal tract absorption of calcium, and was hypercalciuric on this basis. Patient C had an extreme case of the disproportionate hypercalciuria that characterizes some patients with primary hyperparathyroidism.[157,163,164]

Subtle primary hyperparathyroidism should be strongly suspected in any hypercalciuric patient with a mean fasting serum calcium concentration >10 mg/dL.

Renal Calcium Leak Patients diagnosed with a renal leak of calcium (renal hypercalciuria) are considered to have a primary tubular defect in calcium absorption. The increase in fractional calcium excretion in these patients reduces the ambient concentration of ionized calcium, leading to secondary hyperparathyroidism, reduced renal tubular phosphate resorption and serum phosphorus concentration, stimulated 1,25-$(OH)_2D$ synthesis, increased intestinal calcium absorption, and increased mineral resorption from bone (Fig. 24-17). Total hypercalciuria in patients with renal hypercalciuria thus has both renal absorptive and bone resorptive components.

The renal leak hypothesis dates from the 1950s and was the pathogenetic formulation then favored by Henneman and associates.[143] Studies done in the mid-1970s generated considerable evidence to support this hypothesis.[165–167] The most important of these studies historically is that of Coe and associates,[167] who reported increased circulating immunoreactive PTH in two-thirds of hypercalciuric patients and showed that both hypercalciuria and secondary hyperparathyroidism can be reversed by using a thiazide diuretic. The same investigators created a model of renal hypercalciuria in normal subjects by giving them furosemide.[167] Pak and coworkers[166,168,169] introduced additional diagnostic criteria for renal hypercalciuria, including increased fasting calcium excretion with abnormal or inappropriate values for serum immunoreactive PTH, total cAMP excretion, or both; these investigators also reported that such abnormalities can be partially reversed using a thiazide diuretic.

Frequency of renal hypercalciuria and validity of the criteria for diagnosis remain controversial. What the diagnostic criteria should be is rarely debated. Patients should have both decreased renal calcium absorption and secondary hyperparathyroidism. In practice, this debate focuses mainly on interpretation of fasting calcium excretion values in hypercalciuric patients.

Most researchers agree that hypercalciuric patients have higher calcium excretion rates than do normal subjects at all levels of calcium intake, including the fasting state.[148,154,157,168] Two laboratories have reported increased fasting fractional calcium excretion in hypercalciuric patients, providing conclusive evidence for a renal calcium leak.[149,170] However, whether such a "calcium leak" is of primary or secondary pathogenetic importance is unclear.

Four points bear on this controversy. First, a renal calcium leak can be induced in normal subjects by administration of 1,25-$(OH)_2D$. The sequence of events in this model is 1,25-$(OH)_2D$-induced hyperabsorption of calcium from the intestine, parathyroid

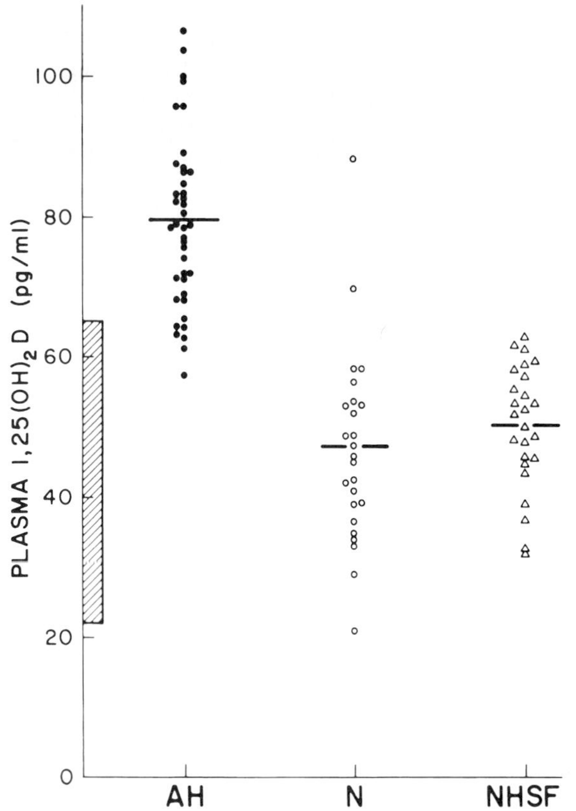

FIGURE 24-17. Plasma 1,25-$(OH)_2D$ concentrations in 50 patients with absorptive hypercalciuria (AH), 25 normal subjects (N), and 25 nonhypercalciuric stone-forming patients (NHSF). All samples were obtained after patients had been restricted to 400 mg/day, calcium and ≅100 mEq/day for at least 10 days. Horizontal bars represent mean values; hatched bar represents normal range for plasma 1,25-$(OH)_2D$ concentration. (*Reproduced by permission of the author and publisher from Broadus AE, Insogna KL, Lang R, et al.*[149])

suppression, and a resultant increase in fasting fractional calcium excretion.[171,172] Second, identical results were observed in 45 patients diagnosed with absorptive hypercalciuria.[159] In these patients, a strong correlation was found between degree of parathyroid suppression in the fasting state and fasting fractional calcium excretion. Third, although fasting calcium excretion was excessive in about half the hypercalciuric patients studied whose calcium intake was restricted, immunoreactive PTH was normal[149,156,157,173–175] or reduced[170,176–178] in almost all cases. Given the sensitivity of modern parathyroid function tests, it is irrational to regard such patients as having a primary renal calcium leak. Fourth, increased sodium intake was reported to increase fasting excretion,[152] yet sodium intake was controlled in only a few published series.[149,169]

Although renal tubular calcium resorption is often reduced in hypercalciuric patients, a renal calcium leak is only rarely of primary pathogenetic importance. The terms *fasting hypercalciuria* and *unclassifiable hypercalciuria* are thus used in describing such patients.[149,169] Using both increased fasting calcium excretion and evidence of secondary hyperparathyroidism as required criteria, one group estimated that renal hypercalciuria accounts for about 5–10 percent of hypercalciuric patients and that unclassifiable hypercalciuria accounts for about 15 percent.[156,157,179] At the Yale Renal Stone Clinic, patients who fulfill the criteria for primary renal hypercalciuria are exceedingly rare.[149]

Absorptive Hypercalciuria In absorptive hypercalciuria, excessive intestinal absorption of calcium leads to a postprandial increase in extracellular calcium concentration, which both increases the filtered load of calcium and suppresses parathyroid function (the absorbed calcium load is spilled directly into the urine). Suppression of parathyroid function adds a secondary renal component to hypercalciuria in these patients. In patients who have severe absorptive hypercalciuria[149] or who are given a rigidly calcium-restricted diet,[180] a bone-resorptive component also may exist, but this component is considered neither quantitatively important nor a particular threat to skeletal health.

Postulated mechanisms of absorptive hypercalciuria include (1) hyperabsorption of calcium resulting from a primary intestinal defect, (2) increased circulating 1,25-$(OH)_2D$ concentration resulting from a primary renal phosphate leak, and (3) increased circulating 1,25-$(OH)_2D$ concentration resulting from disordered control of its production. Some patients in whom production of 1,25-$(OH)_2D$ is disordered may have a fundamental proximal tubular abnormality, which results in several presumably related abnormalities, including decreased resorption of phosphate and other ions and increased 1,25-$(OH)_2D$ production. These hypotheses may not be mutually exclusive.

Most of the evidence supporting a primary intestinal abnormality in calcium absorption in patients with absorptive hypercalciuria was found by Pak and coworkers.[166,181–184] Their intestinal perfusion studies revealed selective jejunal hyperabsorption of calcium.[182] In contrast, exogenous 1,25-$(OH)_2D$ increases calcium absorption in both the jejunum and the ileum and stimulates jejunal uptake of magnesium as well as calcium. The intestinal hyperabsorption hypothesis predicts that affected patients should have low circulating 1,25-$(OH)_2D$ values. Although a spectrum of circulating 1,25-$(OH)_2D$ values has been reported in hypercalciuric patients, a subpopulation with low or low-normal values has not been identified.

The frequency with which increased plasma concentration of 1,25-$(OH)_2D$ is observed in patients in whom hypercalciuria has not been classified by metabolic subtype and in patients who are thought to have absorptive hypercalciuria is somewhat controversial.[149,174,175,177,178,184,185] More than 80 percent of patients with absorptive hypercalciuria have frank elevation of circulating 1,25-$(OH)_2D$ concentration; high-normal values are seen in the remaining 20 percent of patients (Fig. 24-17).[186] Issues of patient selection and study conditions generate the most disagreement about the role of 1,25-$(OH)_2D$ in hypercalciuria. In most studies, patients were both selected and studied while on a free diet. These series reported increased circulating 1,25-$(OH)_2D$ concentrations in about 40–50 percent of the patients studied. A study population selected on the basis of calcium excretion while on a free diet would include many patients with dietary and constitutional hypercalciuria; while the population of patients with true idiopathic hypercalciuria would thus be considerably diluted. In the series conducted at Yale, the criteria for inclusion were (1) hypercalciuria on a defined high-normal calcium intake, (2) hyperabsorption of calcium as shown by calcium tolerance testing, and (3) normal or low concentration of serum immunoreactive PTH and nephrogenous cAMP.[149] These criteria should substantially increase the number of patients with true "metabolic" idiopathic hypercalciuria in a study population and should distinguish clear from borderline cases.

The studies described reveal the importance of dietary calcium as a determinant of circulating 1,25-$(OH)_2D$ concentration (Fig. 24-18).[187] On a low-calcium diet, most hypercalciuric patients had elevated levels of 1,25-$(OH)_2D$, and segregation of plasma 1,25-$(OH)_2D$ values in hypercalciuric and nonhypercalciuric patients was nearly complete. In contrast, the 1,25-$(OH)_2D$ levels of hypercalciuric patients on the high-normal, 1,000-mg (25-mmol) calcium diet were reduced into the normal range, and overlap of values between hypercalciuric and nonhypercalciuric was nearly complete. Thus, although these short-term studies do not necessarily reflect steady-state conditions,[187] such studies emphasize the need to study patients in defined conditions.

Absorptive hypercalciuria in most cases may be viewed as a 1,25-$(OH)_2D$-mediated syndrome. Increased circulating 1,25-$(OH)_2D$ concentrations in these patients have also been shown to result from increased production of the hormone,[186] and blockage of calcitriol synthesis with ketoconazole reduces the intestinal calcium absorption and urinary calcium hyperexcretion in these patients.[188] What mechanisms lead to increased 1,25-$(OH)_2D$ production?

FIGURE 24-18. Values for plasma 1,25-$(OH)_2D$ concentrations in 15 patients with absorptive hypercalciuria (AH) (circles) and in 10 nonhypercalciuric stone-forming patients (NHSF) (triangles) studied while they were receiving 400 mg calcium daily and again 3 days after beginning a diet containing 1,000 mg calcium daily. Daily sodium intake was controlled at about 100 mEq. Horizontal bars represent mean values, and cross-hatched bar represents normal range for plasma 1,25-$(OH)_2D$ concentration. Note marked suppressibility of plasma 1,25-$(OH)_2D$ concentrations in patients with absorptive hypercalciuria as well as extensive overlap between the values for the two groups on receiving 100 mg calcium daily. *(Reproduced by permission of the author and publisher from Broadus AE, Insogna KL, Lang R, et al.[187] Copyright © 1984 Massachusetts Medical Society. All rights reserved.)*

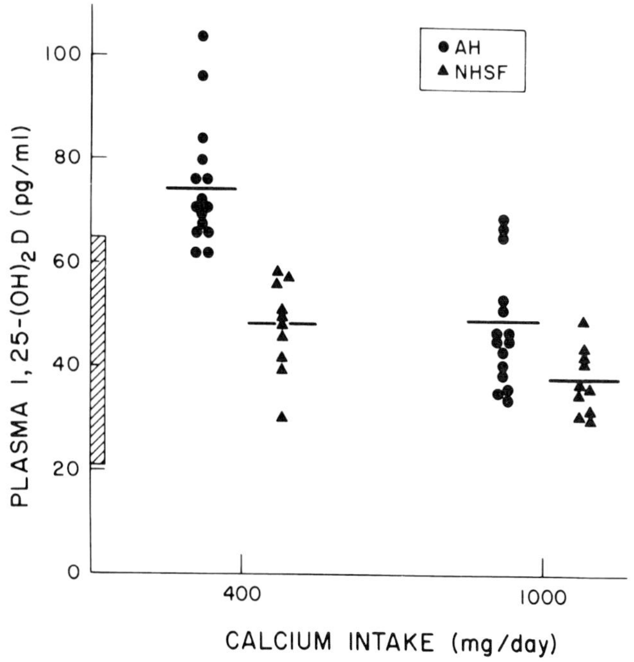

The phosphate leak hypothesis holds that the primary pathogenetic abnormality in patients with absorptive hypercalciuria is a renal tubular leak of phosphate; the resultant hypophosphatemia stimulates 1-hydroxylase activity and thus stimulates 1,25-$(OH)_2D$ synthesis.[189]

Evidence supporting the phosphate leak hypothesis includes (1) a tendency toward hypophosphatemia in some hypercalciuric patients,[143,156,175,185] (2) inappropriately high levels of excreted urinary phosphate for any given serum calcium level,[190] (3) a statistically significant inverse correlation between plasma concentration of 1,25-$(OH)_2D$ and serum phosphorus concentration in hypercalciuric patients compared with normal subjects,[175,178,185] and (4) partial reversal of elements of the syndrome in patients treated with oral phosphate.[174,178,191] A phosphate leak in such patients is apparently not a fixed abnormality, because the serum phosphorus concentration has normal diurnal variation; in the early afternoon, values approach those found in normal subjects.[192]

Evidence against the phosphate leak hypothesis includes (1) the comparative rarity with which hypophosphatemia is observed in hypercalciuric patients,[157,177,191,193] (2) a tendency of stone patients to manifest hypophosphatemia without hypercalciuria,[149,183,192,194] and (3) the hypocalciuric response to phosphate treatment, which is not proportional to pretreatment serum phosphorus concentration.[174,178,194]

The aggregate data can be interpreted in three ways. First, the relation of serum phosphorus concentration to hypercalciuria (and, specifically, to 1,25-$(OH)_2D$ production) is a classic example of "guilt by association" in that no direct pathogenic link exists between these abnormalities. Second, absorptive hypercalciuria is pathogenetically heterogeneous; certain patients have hypophosphatemic absorptive hypercalciuria, whereas 1,25-$(OH)_2D$ production is increased in others on some other basis. Third, phosphate loss and disordered control of 1,25-$(OH)_2D$ may be due to a fundamental proximal tubular lesion.

The disordered-control hypothesis has received attention only recently and is suggested by the extreme sensitivity of circulating 1,25-$(OH)_2D$ concentration to variation in calcium intake among patients with absorptive hypercalciuria. More direct evidence is provided by the response in these patients when a high-normal calcium diet is continued for several weeks: an apparent "escape" phenomenon is observed, with a rebound increase in circulating 1,25-$(OH)_2D$ level and a pronounced decrease in the tubular maximum for phosphate/glomerular filtration rate (TmP/GFR).[187] Hypercalciuric patients may have numerous abnormalities in proximal tubular function, including defective resorption of calcium, phosphate, sodium, magnesium, and fluid.[156,157,195] However, debate remains as to the specificity of these findings in hypercalciuric vs. nonhypercalciuric patients.

A hypothesis that would explain the increased 1,25-$(OH)_2D$ production, the tendency toward hypophosphatemia, and the marked sensitivity to dietary calcium intake in hypercalciuric patients is that such patients are hypersensitive to the proximal tubular effects of PTH.[187] However, no direct evidence supports this hypothesis.

The disordered-control hypothesis for absorptive hypercalciuria pathogenesis is suggested by numerous observations and is favored, in various forms, by several current investigators. The evidence is insufficient to substantiate this hypothesis.

Bone Effects in Hypercalciuria

In the 1970s, attention was first focused on bone density in patients with recurrent calcium nephrolithiasis.[196] The working hypotheses were that calcium stone-forming patients would have lower bone density than those not affected and that low bone density would be most prevalent among hypercalciuric stone-forming patients, particularly those with fasting hypercalciuria ("renal calcium leak"). These predictions have not been substantiated. The only consistent pattern found was that patients with recurrent calcium nephrolithiasis who were treated by long-term dietary calcium restriction were more likely to have reduced bone density.[197–199] Biochemical tests in patients with recurrent calcium nephrolithiasis have shown no differences in calcium metabolism between patients with low bone density and patients with normal bone density, but patients with low bone density consume, on average, about 300 mg less calcium daily.[199] With or without hypercalciuria, therefore, a history of calcium nephrolithiasis is not a risk factor for low bone density or osteoporotic fractures[200] and does not require bone mineral assessment.

TABLE 24-9. Some Common Foods Rich in Oxalate

Vegetables	Fruits	Starches	Miscellaneous
Beans, green	Blackberries	Fruit cake	Chocolate
Beans, dried	Blueberries	Grits, corn	Cocoa
Beets	Currants, red	Soy crackers	Peanuts
Eggplant	Grapes, Concord	Wheat bran	Pecans
Green pepper	Peels, citrus		Tofu (soy curd)
Greens*	Raspberries		Almonds
Okra	Rhubarb		Tea
Parsley	Strawberries		Cola
Potato, sweet	Tangerines		
Rutabagas			
Squash, summer			
Watercress			

Underlined items have proved to substantially increase urinary oxalate excretion.

*Dark green leafy vegetables such as chard, kale, spinach, beet greens, and collard greens.

Source: Adapted and reproduced with permission of the editor and publisher from: Ettinger B, Insogna KL.[11a]

Hyperoxaluria

Although oxalate is the major anionic constituent of calcium stones, patients rarely manifest disorders of oxalate metabolism. However, until recently, relatively subtle abnormalities in oxalate metabolism could easily pass undetected because methods for measuring urinary oxalate were inaccurate. Subtle abnormalities could have a major impact on the tendency for calcium stone formation because of the extreme insolubility of oxalate in aqueous solution. Calcium stone disease could be better controlled if oxalate production could be inhibited in a way analogous to the inhibition of uric acid synthesis by allopurinol or if oxalate could be complexed in a way analogous to how penicillamine-cysteine disulfide forms (see Treatment of Hyperoxaluria).

Oxalate Metabolism

Oxalate is a metabolic end product and serves no known function. Although it forms numerous complexes and salts in urine, oxalate is clinically relevant because of the insolubility of its calcium salt. The metabolic pool of oxalate is derived from intes-tinal absorption and endogenous production.[201,202] Oxalate is absorbed throughout the small intestine and large intestine by diffusion.[201–204] This process, which was first considered simple, passive diffusion, occurs via a facilitated anion exchange mechanism.[204] When a simple isotopic solution of oxalate is given to a patient in the fasting state, about 15 percent is absorbed. However, only 5–10 percent is absorbed from foods. We lack good methods for measuring oxalate in food, and our knowledge of dietary oxalate content is limited. Depending on dietary habits and the particular food table used, estimates of typical adult daily intake of oxalate vary from 100 to 900 mg (1,111 to 9,999 μmol).[201] Table 24-9 lists foods believed to have high oxalate content. Even less is known about bioavailability of oxalate in foods and beverages.

The two main metabolic sources of oxalate are ascorbic acid and glyoxylate (Fig. 24-19).[201–203,205] The metabolism of ascorbic acid accounts for about 30 percent of daily oxalate production and excretion, but the exact metabolic pathway responsible for ascorbic acid oxidation is unknown. Glyoxylate oxidation accounts for most other oxalate production. Lactic dehydrogenase is the most important enzyme in conversion of glyoxylate to oxalate. Much of the metabolic pool of glyoxylate is also transaminated to glycine by alanine-glyoxylate aminotransferase (AGT), a hepatic peroxi-

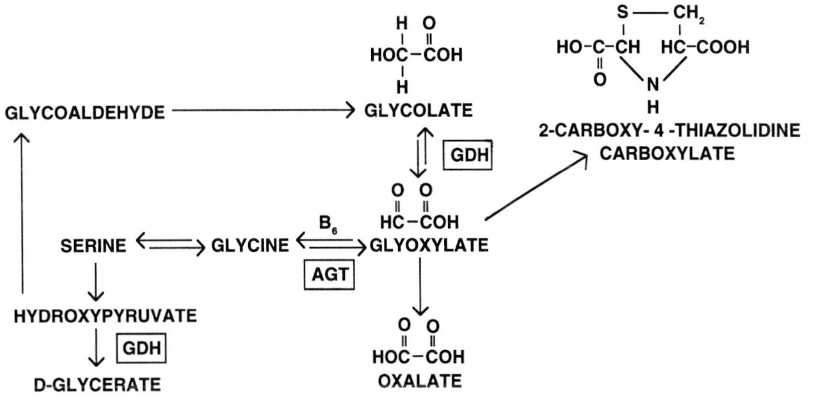

FIGURE 24-19. Pathways of oxalate metabolism. (*Adapted and reproduced by permission of the author and publisher from Dobbins JW, Binder HJ.*[203])

TABLE 24-10. Classification and Causes of Hyperoxaluria

Increased Endogenous Oxalate Production
Primary hyperoxaluria, types 1 and 2
Administration or increased intake of oxalate precursors
Ethylene glycol
Methoxyflurane
Ascorbic acid
Pyridoxylate
Pyridoxine deficiency
Increased oxalate intake or absorption (or both)
Excessive dietary oxalate
Enteric hyperoxaluria
Low calcium intake
Hyperabsorption of calcium

Source: Modified and reproduced by permission of the author, editor, and publisher from Insogna KL, Broadus AE.[11b]

somal enzyme that requires pyridoxine (vitamin B_6) as a cofactor. Another important enzyme, glyoxylate reductase (GDH), converts glyoxylate to glycolate and directs its metabolism away from oxalate. This same enzyme acts as D-glycerate reductase, directing the metabolism of hydroxypyruvate to D-glycerate instead of allowing it to enter the pathway to oxalate via glycoaldehyde.

Classification of Hyperoxaluric States

Hyperoxaluria is conventionally classified as a disorder associated with either increased endogenous oxalate production or increased oxalate absorption (Table 24-10).[11b]

All forms of primary hyperoxaluria are rare inborn errors of oxalate metabolism and are the most malignant crystal deposition diseases known.[201,202,205] Type 1 hyperoxaluria (glycolic aciduria), inherited as an autosomal-recessive trait, results from AGT deficiency, which converts glyoxylate to glycine (Fig. 24-19).[203] This deficiency results in accumulation of glyoxylate and increased production and excretion of glyoxylate, oxalate, and glycolate. Type 1 primary hyperoxaluria can be explained either by complete absence of AGT or by a trafficking abnormality which places this enzyme in the mitochondrion instead of the peroxisome.[206] The distinction may have great clinical relevance, because patients with the trafficking defect appear to have less severe stone disease and may respond to pyridoxine therapy.[207] Heterozygotes are clinically unaffected and cannot be identified by chemical screening. Type 2 hyperoxaluria (L-glyceric aciduria) results from a GDH deficiency,[201,202,206] which leads to preferential production of oxalate from glyoxylate as well as to an increase in oxalate synthesis as a result of hydroxypyruvate shunting to glycolate via glycoaldehyde. In addition, absence of GDH causes production of L-glyceric acid, the unusual form that is the hallmark of type 2 hyperoxaluria. Few patients with the type 2 syndrome have been described; the mechanism of inheritance is unknown but is presumed to be autosomal-recessive.

Patients with type 1 hyperoxaluria typically have calcium oxalate stones in early childhood, usually before age 6 yr. In addition to particularly virulent, recurrent stone formation, deposits of oxalate (oxalosis) also usually develop in soft tissue, including the heart, blood vessels, central nervous system, bone marrow, and kidney. Most untreated patients die before age 20 yr as a result of renal insufficiency produced by stone complications, infections, and oxalosis-induced interstitial nephritis. Patients with type 2 hyperoxaluria have recurrent calcium oxalate stones at an early age, but soft tissue oxalosis does not occur. Hyperoxaluric patients who are seen for calcium oxalate stones in adulthood are described occasionally; some researchers speculate that such patients may have a mild form of primary hyperoxaluria.

The enzyme alcohol dehydrogenase initiates conversion of ethylene glycol to oxalate. A common ingredient in automotive antifreeze preparations and industrial solvents, ethylene glycol is a rare cause of poisoning from accidental or intentional ingestion. Poisoning produces massive hyperoxaluria and oxalosis, commonly resulting in acute renal failure and death.

The anesthetic agent methoxyflurane is partially metabolized to oxalate in the liver. Acute renal failure after methoxyflurane anesthesia is occasionally reported and apparently results from hyperoxaluria and renal oxalosis.[201,202]

Oxidation of ascorbic acid normally accounts for much of the endogenous production of oxalate. "Megadoses" of ascorbic acid increase endogenous oxalate production and excretion, although such an increase may have no clinical effect.[136] Ingestion of vitamin C has been reported to possibly exacerbate stone disease, and its use is discouraged in stone patients.[137] Whether taking megadoses of ascorbic acid increases the prevalence of stone disease in the general population is unclear.

Pyridoxine is a cofactor in transamination of glyoxylate to glycine (Fig. 24-19),[203] and pyridoxine deficiency has been reported to increase oxalate production and excretion in humans and in experimental animals.[201,207] Clinical examples of this association, however, are rare. Pharmacologic doses of pyridoxine are used as therapy in patients with calcium stone disease in an attempt to force the transamination reaction toward glycine, thus reducing the conversion of glyoxylate to oxalate. Pyridoxylate, a drug combination containing glyoxylate and pyridoxine, was used in some European countries for treating coronary heart disease until calcium oxalate lithiasis developed in some of the patients receiving this drug.[208] Although 435 mg of pyridoxine was included in the daily dose of the drug, patients excreted twice as much oxalate when taking the drug than they did when it was withdrawn.

Because of poor total intestinal absorption of oxalate from foods, frank hyperoxaluria rarely results solely from excessive oxalate intake. Massive ingestion of one or more of the foods considered high in oxalate content (Table 24-9) occurs only in persons with unusual dietary habits and is usually readily identified by dietary history. High consumption of rhubarb is often cited as causing dietary hyperoxaluria.[174]

Enteric hyperoxaluria, by far the most common and clinically important hyperoxaluric state, is identified in 2–5 percent of patients seen for calcium oxalate stones.[7,15,16,201–203] The frequency of stone disease in patients with chronic inflammatory bowel disease is estimated to be about double the frequency in the general population. Enteric hyperoxaluria was described as a distinct entity in the early 1970s.[209] Hyperoxaluria and a predisposition to calcium stone disease were associated with various gastrointestinal conditions, including regional enteritis, nontropical sprue, chronic pancreatic and biliary tract disease, blind loop syndrome, and ileal resection or jejunoileal bypass.[201–203,210] Calcium oxalate stones were particularly common in patients after jejunoileal bypass surgery for obesity: the reported frequency was 17–32 percent. Ulcerative colitis is not associated with enteric hyperoxaluria.

The main abnormality seen in affected patients is increased intestinal oxalate absorption[210] related directly to fat malabsorption and steatorrhea. The colon is the major site of oxalate absorption[201–203]; enteric hyperoxaluria is found in jejunoileal bypass patients in whom only a small percentage of the small intestine's absorptive surface is functional.[203] The terms *colonic hyperoxaluria* and *absorptive hyperoxaluria* are thus equally descriptive synonyms for this disorder.

Two hypotheses may explain increased colonic oxalate absorption in patients with enteric hyperoxaluria. The *solubility theory* holds that malabsorbed fatty acids bind calcium and keep it within the intestine, decreasing the quantity of calcium oxalate formed and freeing more oxalate for passive absorption. The *permeability theory* holds that exposure of the colonic mucosa to unabsorbed bile acids and fatty acids produces a nonspecific increase in diffusion of oxalate across the mucosa. Considerable evidence supports each of these hypotheses, and both mechanisms probably apply.[201–203] In addition, patients with enteric disorders may have other stone risk factors, including intestinal fluid loss and low urine volume, malabsorption of magnesium with hypomagnesuria, reduced pyrophosphate excretion, and hypocitraturia.[201,211]

Moderately increased oxalate excretion is observed in patients with calcium stone disease who show no evidence of primary or enteric hyperoxaluria.[201,212–214] Reported daily excretion rates in these patients are only slightly elevated, in the range of 50–80 mg (556–889 μmol). Nevertheless, oxalate is believed to have a relatively greater impact than calcium on urine supersaturation; moderate increases in oxalate excretion could thus represent an im-portant risk factor for stone formation. Several mechanisms might explain the observed variable and moderate increases in oxalate excretion. First, increased oxalate absorption and excretion are particularly evident in hypercalciuric patients who follow a calcium-restricted diet[186–189] or who are treated with calcium-binding agents (e.g., cellulose phosphate).[215,216] Until recently, patients with recurrent calcium stone disease were almost always instructed to avoid dietary calcium, and reduced calcium in the intestinal lumen may enable more oxalate absorption. Second, patients with increased intestinal calcium absorption and hypercalciuria show a coincident increase in oxalate absorption.[214,217] This mechanism was shown directly in normal subjects in whom absorptive hypercalciuria was created by the administration of 1,25-$(OH)_2D$.[218]

Hyperuricosuria

Identification of Hyperuricosuric Calcium Oxalate Lithiasis

Syndrome An apparent association between calcium stone disease and clinical gout, hyperuricemia, or both was first reported in the late 1960s.[83,219] In 1968, Gutman and Yü[83] reported that subjects with gouty arthritis tended to form calcium-containing calculi; in that series, 8 percent of calculi were composed of calcium oxalate, 4 percent were composed of calcium phosphate, and 4 percent were admixtures of calcium and uric acid. Hyperuricosuria, not hyperuricemia, was subsequently recognized as a risk factor for calcium stone formation; this clinical syndrome was termed *hyperuricosuric calcium oxalate nephrolithiasis*.[7,15,220,221]

Crystallographic identification of mixed calcium-uric acid stones is unusual; 4–8 percent of patients with clinical stone disease have mixed stones or have a history of passing both calcium oxalate and uric acid stones.[222] Patients in whom mixed calculi form resemble patients with uric acid lithiasis but usually are older, are often Asian, and excrete acidic urine.[223]

The strongest evidence for the role of uric acid in calcium oxalate lithiasis is the effectiveness of allopurinol in preventing calcium oxalate stones among the subset of patients with isolated hyperuricosuria.[224–228] Numerous hypotheses are reviewed here, but none of them adequately explain why hyperuricosuria is a risk factor for calcium oxalate stone lithiasis.

Definition and Prevalence of Hyperuricosuria About a third of patients with calcium stones are hyperuricosuric.[7,15,221] About half also have hypercalciuria. In most hyperuricosuric patients with calcium stone disease, hyperuricosuria is mild; only about 15 percent of patients excrete >1,000 mg (5.9 mmol) daily. In addition, mild hyperuricosuria is frequently intermittent, presumably because of dietary variation.

Two mechanisms may account for hyperuricosuria in patients with calcium stone disease: (1) uric acid overproduction and (2) consumption of a purine-rich diet. Coe[7,221] emphasized the clinical significance of excessive purine intake by such patients. He found by diet survey that purine intake was about 70 percent higher in hyperuricosuric calcium stone patients than in a control population. In addition, restricting purine intake eliminated hyperuricosuria in 70 percent of these patients, suggesting that only 30 percent had true overproduction of uric acid.

Most epidemiologic studies have found no higher prevalence of hyperuricosuria in patients with calcium oxalate nephrolithiasis than in normal patients.[80,141,229–232] However, by examining urinary uric acid saturation of urine specimens passed in the early morning, Tiselius and Larsson[233] found that 63 percent of patients with calcium oxalate nephrolithiasis had uric acid supersaturation. This highly unstable situation resulted mainly from transient decrease in urinary pH and partly from higher concentration of urine in the early morning.

Does hyperuricosuria increase the severity of calcium oxalate nephrolithiasis? Stone recurrence rates of hyperuricosuric patients are not higher than rates observed in stone-forming patients with other metabolic profiles.[223,229,234] Whereas some researchers have found that hyperuricosuria is frequently associated with past calculus surgery,[229,234] others have reported the opposite.[223] Although hyperuricosuric patients may have one or more additional risk factors for calcium stone formation, combined abnormalities do not influence the severity of stone disease.[7,221,223]

Several hypotheses could explain the pathogenetic relation between hyperuricosuria and formation of calcium stones. Lonsdale[235] first reported similar lattice structure among crystals of calcium oxalate monohydrate, calcium oxalate dihydrate, uric acid, and monosodium urate and then suggested that epitaxy may occur between any of these crystal pairs. Investigators have induced heterogeneous nucleation and crystal growth of calcium oxalate by both uric acid and monosodium urate.[7,15,221,236–238]

An alternative hypothesis is that crystals of uric acid or monosodium urate may adsorb normally occurring macromolecular inhibitors of calcium oxalate crystallization.[239–242] Microcrystalline or colloidal urates have not been found in urine, and more recent experiments thus refute this hypothesis.[243,244]

The most probable cause of the observed interaction between uric acid and calcium oxalate is a simple "salting-out" effect. Pak and associates[87] reported that oral purine loading is associated

TABLE 24-11. Outcomes of Clinical Trials Using Allopurinol Unselectively or Selectively

Reference	No. of Patients Treated with Allopurinol	Annual Rate of Stone Treated with Therapy*	Selective Recurrence (percent)
Ahmad and associates[245]	24	No	Placebo†
Fellström and associates[246]	31	No	28
Marangella and associates[247]	34	No	Advice†
Robertson and associates[248]	12	No	Advice†
Scott and associates[249]	33	No	17
Smith[250]	49	No	20
Sonoda and associates[251]	134	No	30
Tiselius and associates[252]	99	No	15
Ulshöfer and associates[253]	70	No	9
Wilson and associates[254]	17	No	25
Coe[225]	48	Yes	4
Ettinger and associates[224]	29	Yes	11
Oka and associates[227]	44	Yes	20
Okada and associates[226]	15	Yes	12
Pak[228]	21	Yes	8

* Allopurinol was given selectively (i.e., only to patients who had hyperuricosuria without hypercalciuria).

† Data are insufficient for calculations of rate, but no differences were noted between allopurinol treatment and placebo or general advice.

Source: Adapted and reproduced by permission of the publisher from Ettinger B: Does hyperuricosuria play a role in calcium oxalate lithiasis? *J Urol* 141:738–741, 1989.[223]

with a reduction of the calcium oxalate formation product. In the same study,[87] allopurinol treatment slowed calcium oxalate crystallization and crystal growth. Ryall and coworkers[243] showed that uric acid in solution reduces the calcium oxalate formation product. Increasing urinary urate by 3–4 mmol/L doubled calcium oxalate crystal volume and created a marked tendency for these crystals to aggregate into large masses.

Allopurinol is effective for reducing stone recurrence only in calcium oxalate stone-forming patients in whom hyperuricosuria is the only metabolic abnormality. In four of five trials in which allopurinol was given to such patients,[224–228] recurrence rates were low (Table 24-11).[87] In a double-blind, placebo-controlled study, subjects receiving allopurinol at 300 mg daily had 51 percent fewer recurrences than subjects treated with placebo (Fig. 24-20),[224] and the growth of preexisting calculi was 39 percent less frequent in patients receiving allopurinol. In 10 other clinical trials,[245–254] allopurinol was given to patients with calcium oxalate lithiasis regardless of the urinary metabolic profile; 9 of 10 trials showed no benefit (Table 24-11).[87] Allopurinol and its metabolites do not affect calcium oxalate crystallization or solubility in vitro.[86,247,252,255–257] Laboratory and clinical trial results provide compelling evidence for a specific metabolic effect mediated through uric acid.

FIGURE 24-20. Life-table plot showing proportion of patients with no calculus events during treatment with allopurinol or placebo. (*Reproduced by permission of the publisher from Ettinger B, Tang A, Citron JT, et al.*[224] *Copyright © 1986 Massachusetts Medical Society. All rights reserved.*)

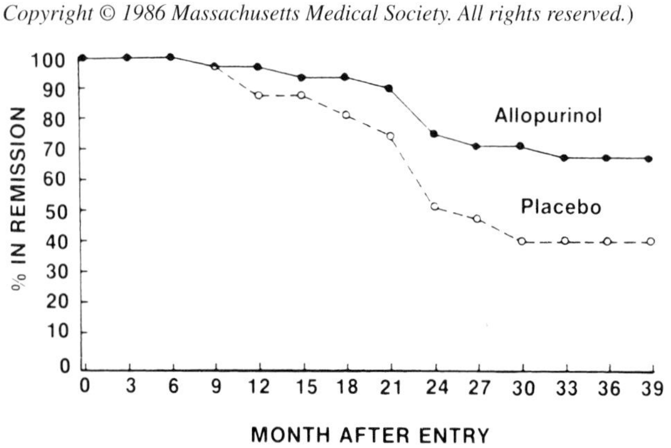

Hypocitraturia

Various conditions associated with disturbance in acid-base balance are accompanied by hypocitraturia. Among these conditions, distal RTA and enteric hyperoxaluria have received the most attention.

In distal RTA, renal tubular dysfunction leads to systemic acidosis and hypocitraturia.[258] In enteric hyperoxaluria, multiple factors have been implicated in contributing to hypocitraturia. In many patients, metabolic acidosis is caused by bicarbonate losses from the gastrointestinal tract. In other patients, a combination of factors, including hypocitratemia, a reduced renal filtered load, and increased renal citrate resorption due to hypomagnesuria, may contribute to hypocitraturia.[211]

Acetazolamide induces exogenous RTA accompanied by hypocitraturia (see Calcium Phosphate Stones).[259] Potassium depletion causes intracellular metabolic acidosis in the renal cortex and is also associated with hypocitraturia.[260]

Many reports describe hypocitraturia in patients with calcium oxalate nephrolithiasis who have normal acid-base status and no gastrointestinal disease; prevalence estimates range from 15–40 percent.[261–264] In the largest series to date, which studied both men and women, no relation was found between severity of stone disease and 24-h excretion of citrate, calcium, or both combined.[262] In contrast, Parks and Coe[264] found that compared with normal women, those with stones excreted about 25 percent less citrate. Such differences were not found between normal men and men with calcium stones. Using discriminant analysis, the investigators found that stone risk depended more on the excess of calcium over citrate content than on absolute calcium and citrate concentrations. This "imbalance" theory, though provocative, remains untested.

A major difficulty in assessing the importance of hypocitraturia in calcium stone formation is that most studies do not control for the many dietary factors which may influence citrate excretion. Urinary citrate excretion may vary considerably; in one study, the citrate level was elevated on one occasion but normal on another in about two-thirds of the subjects.[262]

Metabolism of Citrate

Although the average American diet contains about 4 g of citrate daily, dietary citrate appears to have little influence on final urinary citrate content.

Both filtered at the glomerulus and extracted from peritubular blood, citrate is the most abundant organic acid found in urine. Citrate is metabolized extensively by the kidneys. Metabolic alkalosis induces a prompt, dramatic increase in citrate excretion. Although several processes contribute to this effect, the primary mechanism appears to be inhibition of citrate metabolism in renal tubular cells. Conversely, systemic acidosis is associated with decreased citrate excretion, which results partly from an increased rate of renal citrate metabolism.[265]

Effect of Citrate on Urinary Crystallization

By complexing about half the total urinary calcium, citrate reduces saturation of urine by calcium oxalate and brushite. Citrate also increases the limits of metastability for these two salts, tending to decrease their tendency to nucleate spontaneously.[266] Citrate may have other salutary effects on one or more steps in crystal growth. Using an artificial-crystal growth system, Kok and associates[267] found that citrate therapy doubled both urinary excretion of citrate and ability of urine to inhibit crystal agglomeration.

Clinical Trials of Citrate Therapy

In one study, treatment with potassium citrate for periods ranging from 1 to 4 years decreased the stone formation rate in almost all the 89 patients studied.[268] These patients were heterogeneous, and hypocitraturic calcium oxalate stone disease was associated with various metabolic abnormalities; even in patients with no diarrheal syndromes or RTA, response to treatment was impressive. In another study, 13 patients with hypercalciuria that was apparently refractory to thiazide therapy were found to be hypocitraturic; stone disease in these patients responded clinically to potassium citrate supplementation.[269] However, neither of these trials compared citrate therapy with placebo.

No Metabolic Abnormality: Idiopathic Calcium Oxalate Stones

In the older biomedical literature, the term *idiopathic calcium oxalate stone disease* was used frequently as a synonym for calcium stone disease in general, presumably because stone pathogenesis was viewed as enigmatic in all patients. However, meticulous evaluation should identify one or more risk factors for stone formation in about 80–90 percent of patients with recurrent calcium stone disease. The term *idiopathic calcium stone disease* now is used to describe only cases in which no clinical risk factors for stone formation can be identified.

In patients with idiopathic calcium stone disease, the natural history and morbidity of stone formation do not differ from those observed in patients who have well-recognized risk factors for stone formation.

Evaluation of Calcium Oxalate Stones

The first section of this chapter gives recommendations for urine collection and biochemical tests; the next section discusses evaluation of calcium oxalate and citrate abnormalities.

Evaluating Hypercalciuria

Hypercalciuria in patients on an unrestricted calcium diet is usually defined as a calcium excretion rate exceeding 300 mg (7.5 mmol) daily in men and 250 mg (6.2 mmol) daily in women.[147–149] By these criteria, hypercalciuria is found in about 40 percent of patients with calcium nephrolithiasis.[7,14,15,129,134] Calcium excretion can be expressed on a weight-adjusted basis as well; hypercalciuria is defined as calcium exceeding 4 mg (0.1 mmol) per kilogram of body weight daily in men, women, and children. We recommend using both absolute and weight-adjusted limits and considering a patient hypercalciuric if either limit is exceeded. The most useful definition is calcium exceeding 4 mg (0.1 mmol) per kilogram of body weight daily; in patients in whom this limit is exceeded on a defined high-normal calcium diet, a true disorder of calcium metabolism is highly probable.

According to investigators who continue to use a calcium-restricted diet in screening patients for hypercalciuria, a daily calcium excretion rate >200 mg in a patient on a 400-mg calcium diet is considered abnormal.[18,165,166,168] We do not recommend that 24-h urine samples be collected for patients on either a restricted- or an unrestricted-calcium diet to measure the impact of calcium intake on calcium excretion or to assess the potential benefit of therapeutic restriction of dietary calcium. Such an approach does not optimize either specificity or sensitivity (Fig. 24-14).

Evaluating Subtle Hyperparathyroidism

An essential goal of diagnosis is to identify patients with subtle primary hyperparathyroidism. This diagnosis (see Chap. 22) should be considered if mean total fasting serum calcium concentration exceeds 10 mg/dl (2.5 mmol/L) on more than one occasion. In most clinical laboratories, serum calcium is determined by using an autochemistry method; the usual upper limits are 10.2–10.3 mg/dL (2.54–2.57 mmol/L). The borderline-to-elevated serum calcium level should be confirmed by measurement of the ionized calcium in serum. The diagnosis of primary hyperparathyroidism in these patients depends on the simultaneous finding of intermittent hypercalcemia and elevated or clearly inappropriate serum PTH levels determined by a sensitive PTH assay. Recently improved immunoreactive PTH assays have eliminated many of the problems encountered with older assays. The calcium tolerance test is rarely necessary, and the thiazide challenge test is unpredictable and nonspecific. Parathyroid ultrasound, venous sampling, and other such techniques are useful for localization but not for diagnosis. The data must be interpreted with great care; needless and inappropriate neck explorations should not be done in patients in whom hyperparathyroidism is suspected but not confirmed by biochemical evidence.

Evaluating Dietary Hypercalciuria

Dietary hypercalciuria is most easily detected by having patients collect specimens while on an unrestricted diet and while on a defined diet. Sodium should be measured in the free intake specimen; excretion >100 mEq daily is considered excessive. Dietary hypercalciuria may account for the wide swings in calcium excretion observed in some "hypercalciuric" patients.

Evaluating Subtypes of Hypercalciuria

After secondary forms of hypercalciuria, dietary hypercalciuria, and subtle primary hyperparathyroidism have been excluded, are further diagnostic measures warranted to distinguish renal from absorptive hypercalciuria? Although the literature reflects disagreement on this point, the pragmatic answer is probably no. Absorptive hypercalciuria is the most common subtype of idiopathic hypercalciuria, primary renal hypercalciuria is rare, and clinical bone disease does not appear to result from either renal or absorptive hypercalciuria. The differential diagnosis is extremely subtle and may necessitate use of techniques that are not usually available. Empirical therapy with a thiazide is equally effective in each hypercalciuric subtype.

Evaluating Hyperoxaluria

The available methods for measuring oxalate concentration include colorimetric, isotope dilution, and enzymatic techniques.[270] The outmoded, inaccurate precipitation method should be avoided. The most difficult and demanding aspect of measurement is sample extraction. The normal range for daily oxalate excretion is usually 15–40 mg per day (167–444 μmol/day).[209] A difference in oxalate excretion between men and women has not been observed. Daily oxalate excretion among consecutive calcium stone patients exceeded 40 mg (444 μmol) in 8 percent[271] but rarely exceeded 80 mg (888 μmol). Oxalate excretion correlates closely with urine volume, body mass index, and calcium excretion.[86,271,272]

Daily excretion of >100 mg (1,111 μmol) indicates probable primary hyperoxaluria.[201,202,205] Primary hyperoxaluria should be considered in any child who is seen for calcium stones. Siblings of affected patients should be screened routinely. Type 1 and type 2 syndromes can be distinguished by the different patterns of excretion of glyoxylate, glycolate, and L-glyceric acid.

Enteric hyperoxaluria should be suspected in stone patients who have a characteristic, chronic enteric disorder and can be confirmed by a demonstrated increase in oxalate excretion. In these patients, daily urinary excretion rates depend greatly on oxalate intake but usually exceed 60 mg (667 μmol).[201–203] In addition to measurement of oxalate excretion, patients should be completely screened for other risk factors for stone formation. Patients with enteric hyperoxaluria are often relatively hypocalciuric, and this clue may be important for accurate diagnosis if the manifestations of intestinal disease are subtle. If not previously documented and quantified, steatorrhea should be assessed by fecal fat determination.

Evaluating Hyperuricosuria

Hyperuricosuria is best shown in an outpatient setting while patients are on their usual diets. Coincident fasting, hyperuricemia, and hyperuricosuria suggest overproduction of uric acid, whereas concurrent normouricemia and hyperuricosuria suggest that the patient consumes large quantities of purines. A thorough dietary history can help identify patients whose diet is too rich in purine because of overconsumption of animal protein and may provide a basis for subsequent instructions to moderate purine intake.

Suggested daily upper-normal limits for uric acid excretion are 800 mg (4.8 mmol) for men and 750 mg (4.5 mmol) for women.[82,220,221] By these criteria, 10 percent of normal men and 5 percent of normal women are hyperuricosuric.[221] Pak and coworkers[183] used an upper limit of 600 mg (3.6 mmol) daily for both sexes and considered this limit a "functional definition" of hyperuricosuria on the basis of the quantity of uric acid usually needed to supersaturate urine with monosodium urate. This definition, however, is unusually permissive, classifying 60 percent of normal men as hyperuricosuric; in addition, monosodium is not the uric acid moiety responsible for increasing calcium stone formation.

Evaluating Hypocitraturia

Citrate is measured enzymatically using the citrate lyase method, which is available in commercial laboratories. The excretion of citrate varies widely from day to day, depending on diet. About a third of patients who form calcium oxalate stones excrete less than the lower limit of normal, which is 320 mg (1,666 μmol) daily. Urinary citrate excretion in normal subjects is reported to increase with age (i.e., about 70 mg (364 μmol) per decade); data are scarce, however, and an age-related increase in citrate excretion was not seen in patients with stone disease.[262] In most studies, citrate excretion is about 20 percent higher in women than in men, regardless of age.[261–264]

Evaluating Combinations of Metabolic Risk Factors

Because stone formation is believed to result when forces promoting crystallization overcome those preventing it, some researchers have suggested the use of a saturation-inhibition index that quantifies these forces.[121] The usefulness of a stone probability index has been challenged on theoretical and practical grounds.[139] Because most of the variables measured are closely correlated with at least two other variables, a multiplicative model is inappropriate. Moreover, Ryall and coworkers[139] showed considerable overlap between stone-forming patients and normal subjects for urinary volume, pH, calcium, oxalate, uric acid, and glycosaminoglycan. The predictive value of these biochemical tests, alone or in combination, has never been validated.

Treatment of Calcium Oxalate Nephrolithiasis

Is Treatment Needed?

Treating patients with any form of stone disease is a program, not simply a pill. This treatment program consists of (1) specific instructions to force fluids,[273,274] (2) guidelines for dietary moderation,[273–275] and, for some patients, (3) an agent to reduce stone recurrence.

When trying to predict the future risk of stone formation in a person who has recurrent stone events, physicians should remember that the most important predictors of stone events are the number and frequency of past events. Among 155 patients with a history of recurrent calcium oxalate stones who received either placebo or no medication, each increment of 0.5 stone yearly in the previous stone event rate was associated with a 36 percent increase in subsequent recurrence rates.[276] Similarly, for each additional stone seen on baseline kidney x-ray films, subsequent annual rates of recurrence doubled. In these patients, none of the usual urinary biochemical tests helped to predict recurrence.

Treatment Goals

What constitutes an effective response to treatment? In most clinical trials of calcium oxalate lithiasis, recurrence rates are about 20–30 percent in subjects assigned to placebo or "no active treatment."[48] These rates are about half those calculated from reports by these patients describing stone activity before entering the trial. Readers should thus be skeptical of the purported clinical benefits of specific therapy unless treatment reduces yearly stone recurrence rates to between 5 and 10 percent, about half the rates observed with placebo.

Choosing a Treatment

After deciding to add medication to the stone prevention program, the physician must choose between correcting one or all metabolic deviations and giving empirical therapy. This issue is controversial, and clinical investigations have not compared these two approaches. Gaining extensive clinical experience with one or two types of therapy may be wiser than using many kinds of treatment without fully understanding their risks and benefits. Readers should remember that the success of medical treatment of calcium oxalate lithiasis must be measured by prevention of stone events, not by alterations in urinary biochemistry.

Treatment of Subtle Hyperparathyroidism Associated with Nephrolithiasis

Patients with both subtle primary hyperparathyroidism and nephrolithiasis should have a neck exploration. They should be treated by an experienced surgeon, because about 80 percent of such patients have a single, small parathyroid adenoma, consistent with the view that the disorder is simply a mild form of primary hyperparathyroidism.[277] In a series reported in 1980, before improved PTH assays were available,[278] 17 of 52 surgical patients presumed to have subtle hyperparathyroidism and recurrent calcium lithiasis had normal parathyroid glands, 14 had hyperplasia, and 12 had a single adenoma. After about 5 yr, stone disease remission occurred only in the 12 in whom adenomas were removed; stones recurred in 61 percent of the patients with hyperplasia. These poor results dampened enthusiasm about an aggressive approach to subtle hyperparathyroidism. However, improved diagnostic methods, particularly measurement of plasma immunoreactive PTH, justify reevaluation.

Patients who are not considered good candidates for neck exploration or who have persistent hyperparathyroidism after exploration can be managed successfully with oral neutral phosphate sufficient to provide 1,500 mg of daily elemental phosphorus. This phosphate intake level has been shown in short-term studies to reduce circulating 1,25-$(OH)_2D$, calcium absorption and excretion, and stone formation rates.[279] This therapy is basically antihypercalciuric instead of antihypercalcemic and is not recommended for patients with moderate to severe hypercalcemia.

Treatment of Hypercalciuria

Dietary Hypercalciuria

Patients with dietary hypercalciuria are managed with a program of forced fluids as well as moderation of sodium intake (about 100 mEq/day), calcium intake (about 400–600 mg/day [10–15 mmol/day]), and animal protein intake (about 35 g daily) (Table 24-2). The effects of fluid and dietary therapy can be monitored by 24-h urine collection; measurement of sodium excretion monitors compliance.

Renal Hypercalciuria

Given adequate grounds for a diagnosis of primary renal hypercalciuria, the preferred agents are thiazide-like diuretics.[225,280] Thiazides are also preferred in treating hypercalciuric patients with coincident hypertension. Conventional antihypertensive doses of thiazides are used in treating stone disease. Their hypocalciuric effect results from both volume contraction and direct action to increase calcium resorption in the distal nephron.[281] This effect is shared by all thiazide congeners and related diuretics (e.g., chlorthalidone, indapamide); no single agent is preferred. Giving single daily doses improves compliance. On average, thiazides halve calcium excretion rates.[225,280,282] High salt intake can usually overcome the antihypercalciuric effect of the drug. The most common side effect is a feeling of lassitude, which is usually transient and apparently is unrelated to hypokalemia. Triamterene-containing diuretic agents are not used in patients with urolithiasis, because triamterene and its products have been identified in kidney stones.[12]

Absorptive Hypercalciuria

Patients with absorptive hypercalciuria are instructed to follow a program of forced fluids and dietary moderation (Table 24-2). Additional measures may include the administration of either neutral phosphates or a thiazide diuretic, which appear to have an equivalent antihypercalciuric effect in such patients.[194,225,273,279–281] Neutral phosphate sufficient to provide 1,500 to 2,000 mg of daily elemental phosphorus is given in three or four divided doses. This treatment has never been rigorously evaluated in a randomized, double-blind clinical trial. Acidic phosphate preparations are ineffective.[283] Patients tend to prefer phosphate salt tablets to liquid forms. All phosphate salts are cathartic, and this side effect may reduce compliance and often necessitates limiting the dose; beginning with a small dose and slowly increasing to tolerance may help overcome this problem.

Sodium cellulose phosphate is a nonabsorbable cation exchange resin that binds to calcium and prevents its absorption from the intestine.[215,216] This substance is specifically intended for patients with absorptive hypercalciuria.[216] Magnesium supplements must also be taken, and calcium and oxalate intake must be restricted. Backman and coworkers[216] reported side effects—mainly gastrointestinal discomfort and synovitis—in 9 of 35 patients. In contrast, Pak[215] noted that the drug was "well tolerated" by 18 patients. The question of cellulose phosphate's efficacy is unresolved. Stones recurred in 22 percent of Pak's patients[215] during a mean 2.4-yr follow-up and in 47 percent of patients studied by Backman and coworkers[216] in a 2-yr trial. The marked difference in efficacy might have resulted because Backman and coworkers[216] neither gave magnesium supplements nor restricted the diets of their subjects. The effects and required dose of sodium cellulose phosphate must be monitored by serial measurement of urinary calcium excretion to avoid creating calcium malabsorption, secondary hyperparathyroidism, or a negative calcium balance. Cellulose phosphate is expensive: 15 g of the drug plus 116 mg of magnesium daily costs more than $1,500 per year. In addition, the drug must be taken three times daily, mixed in water, taken with or just after each meal, and the magnesium supplements (a mandatory part of the regimen) must be taken separately three times daily. We suggest that the drug be used only in rare cases of severe absorptive hypercalciuria which cannot be managed by other means.

Empirical Therapy for Hypercalciuria

By far the most extensive experience with either thiazides or phosphate therapy is in empirical treatment of hypercalciuric patients who are not classified by metabolic subtype. Each form of treatment appears to result in a roughly equivalent decrease in rates of calcium excretion, and each has been reported to reduce stone formation.[7,14,15,225,280,282–287] Given the simplicity, high patient acceptance, low cost, and more extensive documentation of the efficacy of thiazide therapy,[288] we prefer it to phosphate therapy.

Although about 10 percent of patients treated with either thiazides or phosphates do not have the anticipated hypocalciuric response, the dose need not be increased or the treatment altered immediately. Biochemical changes correlate poorly, if at all, with the success or failure of treatment.[48,273]

Treatment of Hyperoxaluria

Primary Hyperoxaluria

Like patients with cystinuria, patients with primary hyperoxaluria should be given particularly detailed instructions about hydration. In addition, these patients are usually placed on a low-oxalate diet, even though little urinary oxalate excretion is derived from this diet. Large doses of pyridoxine (200–400 mg/day) can be expected to normalize oxalate excretion in about 20 percent of patients and can reduce its excretion in about 30 percent.[289] In rare cases, much smaller doses of pyridoxine (as little as 2 mg/day) have been effective.[290] Treatment with a combination of orthophosphate (35 mg/kg body weight) and pyridoxine (3 mg/kg body weight) was effective in preventing new stones and in slowing the progression of renal failure (only 5 of 25 patients had progression to end-stage renal disease) in a group of 25 young patients with primary hyperoxaluria.[290] Pyridoxine in daily doses of 500–2,000 mg may cause sensory ataxia as a result of neuropathy affecting the peripheral nerves responsible for vibration and position sense.[292,293] Magnesium supplements and phosphate have been reported to reduce stone formation in uncontrolled studies,[201,205] but both agents should be used cautiously, if at all, in patients with moderate or advanced renal insufficiency. Dialysis does not effectively control progressive systemic oxalosis, and primary hyperoxaluria is currently considered a contraindication for renal transplantation without concomitant liver transplantation.

Enteric Hyperoxaluria

Treatment of patients with enteric hyperoxaluria is multifaceted; general measures include hydration, control of steatorrhea, and prescription of an oxalate-restricted diet.[201–203,294] Patients with a short bowel have difficulty consuming large quantities of fluid and maintaining adequate urine output. A low-fat diet may improve steatorrhea, but a diet rigidly restricted in fat is unpalatable, and many patients prefer to use medium-chain triglycerides.[295] For many patients, these measures suffice; for others, hyperoxaluria and other risk factors cannot be controlled and other measures are required.

Numerous agents have been used in attempts to bind oxalate in the intestinal contents and limit its bioavailability. These agents include calcium, magnesium, aluminum, cholestyramine, and colestipol.[294] Many such agents also bind bile acids and fatty acids. Calcium 1,000–2,000 mg (25–50 mmol) daily is probably the best choice. A considerable margin of safety in calcium dosage exists because many patients absorb calcium poorly and are relatively hypocalciuric before therapy. The antacid Camalox is a useful combination agent because it contains calcium carbonate, aluminum hydroxide, and magnesium hydroxide; a typical daily starting dose of 900 mg (22.5 mmol) is provided by 15 mL (or 3 tablets) taken three times daily with meals. Long-term trials of such binding agents have not been reported. Major stone complications are considered an indication for restoring intestinal continuity in patients with a jejunoileal bypass.[201]

Oxalate Complexation by Cysteine

Recent reports indicate progress in the search for an oxalate-complexing agent.[295] In rats poisoned with ethylene glycol, excessive urinary oxalate was dramatically reduced by giving cysteine, which apparently forms an adduct with glyoxylate between its sulfhydryl and amino nitrogen groups (Fig. 24-19).[203] A promising new drug, (L)-2-oxothiazolidine-4-carboxylate (OTZ), is converted to cysteine in the liver and has proved to reduce oxalate excretion by 30 percent in normal subjects.[296] The effectiveness of this drug is hoped to be even greater in subjects with primary hyperoxaluria, because they would have high concentrations of glyoxylate available for binding to cysteine in the liver. Inhibition of hepatic aldehyde dehydrogenase and glycolate oxidase have been suggested as possible types of therapy for primary hyperoxaluria[297] and should be further studied.

Treatment of Hyperuricosuria

Patients with hyperuricosuric calcium oxalate nephrolithiasis are treated with a program of high fluid intake, moderation of purine and animal protein, and, often, allopurinol. The principle of dietary moderation instead of restriction is emphasized because of poor compliance with a diet low in animal protein. Sodium restriction is also advised for patients who have coincident dietary hypercalciuria.

Allopurinol is effective in preventing stone recurrence in patients with hyperuricosuric calcium oxalate stone disease (Fig. 24-20).[224–228] (The mechanism of action, dosage, and toxicity of allopurinol are described in detail in Uric Acid Stones.) When 300 mg of the drug is given daily, uric acid excretion may be reduced by 40 percent, a reduction that should suffice to reduce daily uric acid excretion to about 500 mg (3 mmol). A single daily dose of allopurinol is adequate and enhances compliance.

Thiazides are effective in patients with hyperuricosuric calcium oxalate nephrolithiasis.[48,298] Using thiazides in such patients, Lærum and Larsen[298] reported an annual stone recurrence rate of 6 percent, and Ettinger and coworkers[48] reported a recurrence rate of 9 percent. Allopurinol has far fewer minor side effects but is associated with a risk of developing rare serious allergic reactions. About half of patients with hyperuricosuria also have hypercalciuria. In patients with such combined overexcretion, allopurinol alone clearly does not stop stone recurrence.[223] In a few patients, combined allopurinol and thiazide therapy was evaluated; stone recurrence was reduced substantially.[221,281] Because addition of allopurinol does not add to the stone prevention afforded by indapamide[282] and because the risk of serious allergic reactions increases when thiazides are used with allopurinol,[299] beginning treatment with thiazide alone is wise.

Whether careful use of alkali would also be beneficial is unknown. As additional therapy, a single dose of 30 mEq at bedtime to offset early-morning urine acidity can be considered; this dose could reduce saturation of urine by uric acid and inhibit growth of calcium oxalate crystals.[300] In a preliminary report, administration of 60–80 mmol daily of potassium citrate to hyperuricosuric nephrolithiasis patients was associated with an 8 percent annual rate of stone recurrence.[301] Several factors limit applicability of these results: hyperuricosuria was liberally defined as citrate excretion exceeding 600 mg (3.6 mmol) daily; citrate excretion was low in two thirds of subjects, about twice the usual prevalence expected; only 14 subjects were monitored for ≥2 years; and three subjects also received thiazide.

Treatment of Hypocitraturia

Numerous citrate-containing drugs are available (Table 24-3). Potassium citrate embedded in a wax matrix tablet may produce a more sustained increase in citrate excretion than other forms of oral alkali do. Potassium is more useful than sodium citrate for correcting thiazide-induced potassium depletion. Among 72 patients monitored for a mean of 3.5 years, a mixture of sodium and potassium citrate taken in daily doses of 18.5–28 mmol was associated with an 8 percent annual rate of stone recurrence.[302] More recently, potassium citrate was rigorously evaluated in 2 double-blind, randomized, placebo-controlled clinical trials.[303,304] Both studies monitored patients for a mean of 3 years, and both showed similar and striking benefits of citrate over placebo: the study by Barcelo and coworkers[303] showed stone recurrence in 80 percent of subjects receiving placebo compared with only 28 percent of subjects receiving potassium citrate; and Ettinger and coworkers[304] showed formation of new calculi in 64 percent of patients receiving placebo compared with 13 percent of those taking potassium magnesium citrate.

Treatment of Patients Free of Metabolic Abnormalities

Idiopathic calcium stone disease is diagnosed by exclusion. The decision to treat this condition is made, as for any patient with stone disease, by assessing stone-related morbidity. Almost all agents used to treat patients with calcium stones were first introduced on empirical grounds and were reported to be beneficial in patients with no obvious risk factors for stone formation. Although uncontrolled studies have reported the efficacy of oral phosphates[285–287] and thiazides,[47,226,280] more credence should be given to the results of adequate double-blind controlled studies using thiazides and citrates (Fig. 24-21).[48,282,298,303,304]

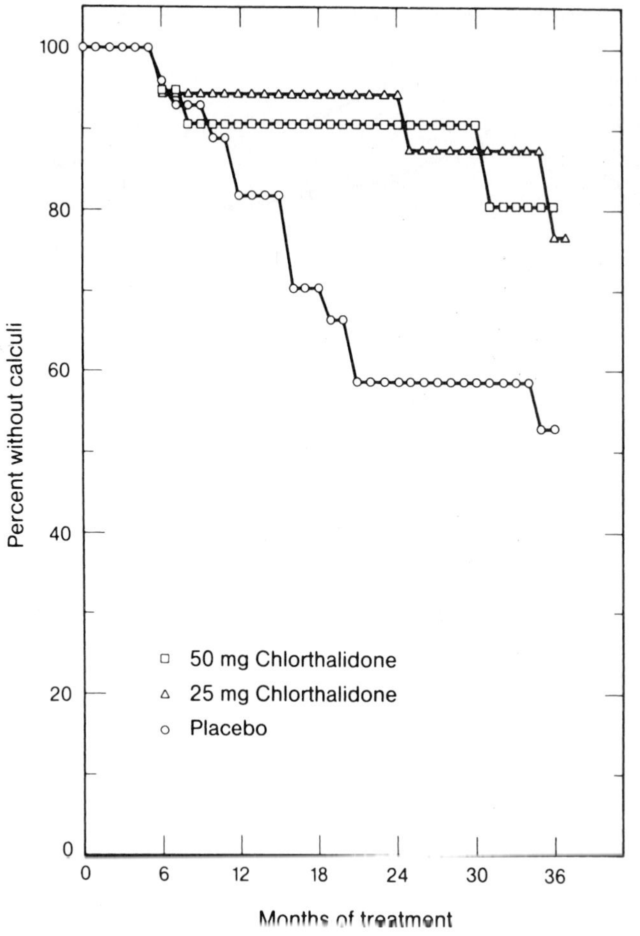

FIGURE 24-21. Life-table plot showing percentage of patients with no calculus events during treatment with 25 mg chlorthalidone, 50 mg chlorthalidone, or placebo. (*Reproduced by permission of the editor and publisher from Ettinger B, Insogna KL.*[11a])

Discontinuing Treatment

The decision to stop medical therapy for calcium oxalate stones is often made by the patient. After a few symptom-free years, patients appear to forget past pain and may come to consider medication an unnecessary nuisance. Joost and Putz[305] reported 5-yr follow-up of 26 patients with recurrent stone disease who had been prescribed thiazides, allopurinol, or magnesium hydroxide; 80 percent had stopped treatment after 2–3 years. Nevertheless, the annual recurrence rate among these patients was only about 7 percent. Mean urine volume in this cohort was 600 ml higher during follow-up, which may account for the low recurrence rate. Another posttreatment follow-up study also showed a high remission rate.[306] After 3 years of receiving ineffective treatment (potassium acid phosphate), placebo, or diet advice, 71 patients with recurrent stone disease were followed for 3 more years while receiving no treatment (Fig. 24-22). Recurrence was rare, and only one lithotomy was necessary. Residual stones were associated with a higher risk of recurrence. On the basis of these studies, for the average calcium oxalate stone patient, we usually recommend stopping medication after 3 yr, provided that no residual stones remain in the kidneys. Because residual stones and a history of frequent stone events both portend much higher recurrence rates, we suggest continuing therapy in such cases for 5 yr or longer. After stopping treatment, patients should be recalled for annual follow-up radiographic evaluation.

CLOSING COMMENTS

We close this chapter with the words of Lynwood H. Smith, who contributed much to our understanding and treatment of nephrolithiasis:

> [W]e have gone through several phases in our studies of idiopathic calcium urolithiasis. In the 1970s, it seemed that this was a syndrome made up of precise conditions. With further study it is clear that multiple abnormalities often may be present with significant overlap of risk factors. This situation suggests that we do not as yet understand basic pathophysiology in

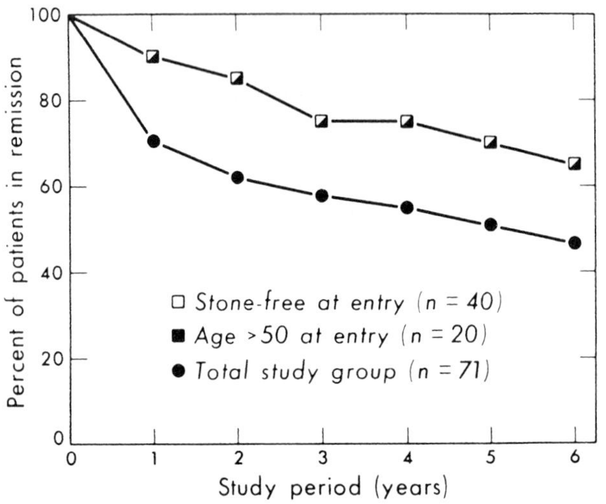

FIGURE 24-22. Life-table plot showing percentage of 71 patients with no calculus events during 3-yr treatment with acid phosphate, calcium restriction, or placebo and 3 additional years of follow-up with no treatment. About 45 percent of the entire group remained stone-free after 6 yr. Patients who were older at the start or who were free of stones at the start were less likely to have recurrence of stones. (*Adapted and reproduced by permission of the publisher from Ettinger B.*[306])

many patients who are believed to have this syndrome. Fresh approaches with new ideas challenging former concepts clearly are needed.[10]

Acknowledgments

Karl L. Insogna, MD, a coauthor of this chapter in the previous edition, kindly allowed me to republish his cogent arguments on mechanisms and evaluation of the hypercalciurias.

The Medical Editing Department of Kaiser Foundation Hospitals provided editorial assistance.

REFERENCES

1. Johnson CM, Wilson DM, O'Fallon WM, et al: Renal stone epidemiology: A 25-year study in Rochester, Minnesota. *Kidney Int* 16:624, 1979.
2. Hodgkinson A, Nordin BEC: Prevention of urolithiasis, in Coggins CH, Cummings NB (eds): *Prevention of Kidney and Urinary Tract Diseases.* Washington, DC, USGPO, 1978, pp 195–224.
3. Boyce WH, Garvey FK, Strawcutter HE: Incidence of urinary calculi among patients in general hospitals, 1948 to 1952. *JAMA* 161:1437, 1956.
4. Sierakowski R, Finlayson B, Landes RR, et al: The frequency of urolithiasis in hospital discharge diagnoses in the United States. *Invest Urol* 15:438, 1978.
5. Soucie JM, Coates RJ, McClellan W, et al: Relation between geographic variability in kidney stones prevalence and risk factors for stones. *Am J Epidemiol* 143:487, 1996.
6. Curhan GC, Rimm EB, Willett WC, et al: Regional variation in nephrolithiasis incidence and prevalence among United States men. *J Urol* 151:838, 1994.
7. Coe FL: *Nephrolithiasis: Pathogenesis and Treatment.* Chicago, Year Book, 1978.
8. Prien EL: Crystallographic analysis of urinary calculi: A 23-year survey study. *J Urol* 89:917, 1963.
9. Herring LC: Observations on the analysis of ten thousand urinary calculi. *J Urol* 88:545, 1962.
10. Smith LH: The medical aspects of urolithiasis: An overview. *J Urol* 141:707, 1989.
11. a. Ettinger B, Insogna KL: Nephrolithiasis, in Felig P, Baxter JD, Frohman LA (eds): *Endocrinology and Metabolism*, 3rd ed. New York, McGraw-Hill, 1995, pp 1565–1615. b. Insogna KL, Broadus AE: Nephrolithiasis, in Felig P, Baxter JD, Broadus AE, Frohman LA (eds): *Endocrinology and Metabolism*, 2nd ed. New York, McGraw-Hill, 1987, pp 1500–1577.
12. Ettinger B, Oldroyd NO, Sörgel F: Triamterene nephrolithiasis. *JAMA* 244:2443, 1980.
13. Bruce RG, Munch LC, Hoven AD, et al: Urolithiasis associated with the protease inhibitor indinavir. *Urology* 50:513, 1997.
14. Smith LH: Urolithiasis, in Schrier RW, Gottschalk CW (eds): *Diseases of the Kidney*, 4th ed. Boston, Little, Brown, 1988, pp 785–813.
15. Coe FL, ed: *Nephrolithiasis.* New York, Churchill Livingstone, 1980.
16. Boyce WH: Organic matrix of human urinary concretions. *Am J Med* 45:673, 1968.
17. Morse RM, Resnick MI: Urinary stone matrix. *J Urol* 139:602, 1988.
18. Thomas WC Jr, Howard JE: Studies in the mineralizing propensity of urine from patients with and without renal calculi. *Trans Assoc Am Physicians* 72:181, 1959.
19. Pak CYC: *Calcium Urolithiasis: Pathogenesis, Diagnosis, and Management.* New York, Plenum, 1978.
20. Porile JL, Asplin JR, Parks JH, et al: Normal calcium oxalate crystal growth inhibition in severe calcium oxalate nephrolithiasis. *J Am Soc Nephrol* 7:602, 1996.
21. Drach GW: Surgical overview of urolithiasis. *J Urol* 141:711, 1989.
22. Kelley JM: Extracorporeal shock wave lithotripsy of urinary calculi: Theory, efficacy, and adverse effects. *West J Med* 153:165, 1990.
23. Lingeman JE, Woods JR, Toth PD: Blood pressure changes following extracorporeal shock wave lithotripsy and other forms of treatment for nephrolithiasis. *JAMA* 263:1789, 1990.
24. Miller HC, Collins LA, Turbow AM, et al: Initial EDAP LT-01 lithotripsy group experience in the United States. *J Urol* 142:1412, 1989.
25. Coughlin BF, Risius B, Streem SB, et al: Abdominal radiograph and renal ultrasound versus excretory urography in the evaluation of asymptomatic patients after extracorporeal shock wave lithotripsy. *J Urol* 142:1419, 1989.
26. Coe FL, Parks JH: Pathophysiology of kidney stones and strategies for treatment. *Hosp Pract* 23:185, 1988.
27. Strauss AL, Coe FL, Parks JH: Formation of a single calcium stone of renal origin: Clinical and laboratory characteristics of patients. *Arch Intern Med* 142:504, 1982.
28. Pak CYC: Should patients with single renal stone occurrence undergo diagnostic evaluation? *J Urol* 127:855, 1982.
29. Uribarri J, Oh MS, Carroll HJ: The first kidney stone. *Ann Intern Med* 111:1006, 1989.
30. Ljunghall S, Christensson T, Wengle B: Prevalence and incidence of renal stone disease in a health-screening programme. *Scand J Urol Nephrol [Suppl]* 41:39, 1977.
31. Sutherland JW, Parks JH, Coe FL: Recurrence after a single renal stone in a community practice. *Miner Electrolyte Metab* 11:267, 1985.
32. Hiatt RA, Ettinger B, Caan B, et al: Randomized controlled trial of a low animal protein, high fiber diet in the prevention of recurrent calcium oxalate kidney stones. *Am J Epidemiol* 144:25, 1996.
33. Ahlstrand C, Tiselius HG: Recurrences during a 10-year follow-up after first renal stone episode. *Urol Res* 18:397, 1990.
34. Borghi L, Meschi T, Amato F, et al: Urinary volume, water and recurrences in idiopathic calcium nephrolithiasis. *J Urol* 155:838, 1996.
35. Pak CYC: Southwestern Internal Medicine Conference: Medical management of nephrolithiasis—a new, simplified approach for general practice. *Am J Med Sci* 313:215, 1997.
36. Wabner CL, Pak CY: Effect of orange juice consumption on urinary stone risk factors. *J Urol* 149:1405, 1993.
37. Seltzer MA, Low RK, McDonald M, et al: Dietary manipulation with lemonade to treat hypocitraturic calcium nephrolithiasis. *J Urol* 156:907, 1996.
38. Weiss GH, Sluss PM, Linke CA: Changes in urinary magnesium citrate, and oxalate levels due to cola consumption. *Urology* 39:331, 1992.
39. Curhan GC, Willett WC, Rimm EB, et al: Prospective study of beverage use and the risk of kidney stones. *Am J Epidemiol* 143:240, 1996.
40. Curhan GC, Willett WC, Speizer FE, et al: Beverage use and risk for kidney stones in women. *Ann Intern Med* 128:534, 1998.

41. Shuster J, Jenkins A, Logan C, et al: Soft drink consumption and urinary stone recurrence: A randomized prevention trial. *J Clin Epidemiol* 45:911, 1992.
42. Curhan GC, Willett WC, Rimm EB, et al: A prospective study of dietary calcium and other nutrients and the risk of symptomatic kidney stones. *N Engl J Med* 328:833, 1993.
43. Curhan GC, Willett WC, Speizer FE, et al: Comparison of dietary calcium with supplemental calcium and other nutrients as factors affecting the risk for kidney stones in women. *Ann Intern Med* 126:497, 1997.
44. Nordin BEC, Barry H, Bulusu L, et al: Dietary treatment of recurrent calcium stone disease, in Cifuentes Delatte L, Rapado A, Hodgkinson A (eds): *Urinary Calculi: Recent Advances in Aetiology, Stone Structure, and Treatment.* International Symposium on Renal Stone Research, Madrid, 1972. Basel, Karger, 1973, pp 170–176.
45. Norman RW, Manette WA: Dietary restriction of sodium as a means of reducing urinary cystine. *J Urol* 143:1193, 1990.
46. Kok DJ, Iestra JA, Doorenbos CJ, et al: The effects of dietary excesses in animal protein and in sodium on the composition and the crystallization kinetics of calcium oxalate monohydrate in urines of healthy men. *J Clin Endocrinol Metab* 71:861, 1990.
47. Churchill DN: Medical treatment to prevent recurrent calcium urolithiasis: A guide to critical appraisal. *Miner Electrolyte Metab* 13:294, 1987.
48. Ettinger B, Citron JT, Livermore B, et al: Chlorthalidone reduces calcium oxalate calculus recurrence but magnesium hydroxide does not. *J Urol* 139:679, 1988.
49. Rosenberg LE, Scriver CR: Disorders of amino acid metabolism, in Bondy PK, Rosenberg LE (eds): *Metabolic Control and Disease.* Philadelphia, Saunders, 1980, pp 73–102.
50. Segal S, Thier SO: Cystinuria, in Scriver CR, Beaudet AL, Sly WS, Valle D (eds): *The Metabolic Basis of Inherited Disease*, 6th ed. New York, McGraw-Hill, 1989, pp 2479–2496.
51. Dent CE, Rose GA: Amino acid metabolism in cystinuria. *Q J Med* 20:205, 1951.
52. Crawhall JC, Purkiss P, Watts RW, et al: The excretion of amino acids by cystinuric patients and their relatives. *Ann Hum Genet* 33:149, 1969.
53. Gitomer WL, Pak CYC: Recent advances in the biochemical and molecular biological basis of cystinuria. *J Urol* 156:1907, 1996.
54. Dent CE, Senior B: Studies on the treatment of cystinuria. *Br J Urol* 27:317, 1955.
55. Jaeger P, Portmann L, Saunders A, et al: Anticystinuric effects of glutamine and of dietary sodium restriction. *N Engl J Med* 315:1120, 1986.
56. Miyagi K, Nakada F, Ohshiro S: Effect of glutamine on cystine excretion in a patient with cystinuria. *N Engl J Med* 301:196, 1979.
57. Van Den Berg CJ, Jones JD, Wilson DM, et al: Glutamine therapy of cystinuria. *Invest Urol* 18:155, 1980.
58. Dahlberg PJ, Van Den Berg CJ, Kurtz SB, et al: Clinical features and management of cystinuria. *Mayo Clin Proc* 52:533, 1977.
59. Sakhaee K, Poindexter JR, Pak CYC: The spectrum of metabolic abnormalities in patients with cystine nephrolithiasis. *J Urol* 141:819, 1989.
60. Singer A, Das S: Cystinuria: A review of the pathophysiology and management. *J Urol* 142:669, 1989.
61. Aabech J, Andersen JT: Treatment of cystine stones: Combined approach using open pyelolithotomy, percutaneous pyelolithotripsy, extracorporeal shock wave lithotripsy and chemolysis. *Scand J Urol Nephrol* 27:415, 1993.
62. Smith A: Evaluation of the nitroprusside test for the diagnosis of cystinuria. *Med J Aust* 2:153, 1977.
63. David RM, Shihabi ZK, O'Connor ML: Simplified method for cystinuria screening. *Clin Chem* 32:1417, 1986.
64. Halperin EC, Thier SO, Rosenberg LE: The use of D-penicillamine in cystinuria: Efficacy and untoward reactions. *Yale J Biol Med* 54:439, 1981.
65. Lindell A, Denneberg T, Hellgren E, et al: Clinical course and cystine stone formation during tiopronin treatment. *Urol Res* 23:111, 1995.
66. Denneberg T, Jeppsson JO, Stenberg P: Alternative treatment of cystinuria with alpha-merkaptopropionylglycine, Thiola. *Proc Eur Dial Transplant Assoc* 20:427, 1983.
67. Harbar JA, Cusworth DC, Lawes LC, et al: Comparison of 2-mercaptopropionylglycine and D-penicillamine in the treatment of cystinuria. *J Urol* 136:146, 1986.
68. Lindell Å, Denneberg T, Eneström S, et al: Membranous glomerulonephritis induced by 2-mercaptopropionylglycine (2-MPG). *Clin Nephrol* 34:108, 1990.
69. Streem SB, Hall P: Effect of captopril on urinary cystine excretion in homozygous cystinuria. *J Urol* 142:1522, 1989.
70. Sloand JA, Izzo JL Jr: Captopril reduces urinary cystine excretion in cystinuria. *Arch Intern Med* 147:1409, 1987.
71. Sandroni S, Stevens P, Barraza M, et al: Captopril therapy of recurrent nephrolithiasis in a child with cystinuria. *Child Nephrol Urol* 9:347, 1988.
72. Aunsholt NA, Ahlbom G: Lack of effect of captopril in cystinuria (letter). *Clin Nephrol* 34:92, 1990.
73. Dahlberg PJ, Jones JD: Cystinuria: Failure of captopril to reduce cystine excretion (letter). *Arch Intern Med* 149:713, 1989.
74. Cohen TD, Streem SB, Hall P: Clinical effect of captopril on the formation and growth of cystine calculi. *J Urol* 154:164, 1995.
75. Chow GK, Streem SB: Medical treatment of cystinuria: Results of contemporary clinical practice. *J Urol* 156:1576, 1996.
76. Yü TF: Uric acid nephrolithiasis, in Kelley WN, Weiner IM (eds): *Uric Acid.* New York, Springer-Verlag, 1978, pp 397–422. (Handbook of Experimental Pharmacology; v. 51)
77. Levinson DJ, Sorensen LB: Uric acid stones, in Coe FL (ed): *Nephrolithiasis: Pathogenesis and Treatment.* Chicago, Year Book, 1978, pp 172–202.
78. Holmes EW: Uric acid nephrolithiasis, in Coe FL (ed): *Nephrolithiasis.* New York, Churchill Livingstone, 1980, pp 188–207.
79. Preminger GM: Pharmacologic treatment of uric acid calculi. *Urol Clin North Am* 14:335, 1987.
80. Wilson DM: Uric acid lithiasis, in Rous SN (ed): *Stone Disease: Diagnosis and Management.* Orlando, Grune & Stratton, 1987, pp 109–123.
81. Ettinger B: Allopurinol for the treatment of uric acid and calcium calculi, in Pak CYC (ed): *Pharmacologic Treatment of Endocrinopathies.* Basel, S. Karger, 1991, pp 16–36.
82. Fellström B, Danielson RG, Karlström B, et al: The influence of a high dietary intake of purine-rich animal protein on urinary urate excretion and supersaturation in renal stone disease. *Clin Sci* 64:399, 1983.
83. Gutman AB, Yü TF: Uric acid nephrolithiasis. *Am J Med* 45:756, 1968.
84. Khatchadourian J, Preminger GM, Whitson PA, et al: Clinical and biochemical presentation of gouty diathesis: Comparison of uric acid versus pure calcium stone formation. *J Urol* 154:1665, 1995.
85. Rastegar A, Thier SO: The physiologic approach to hyperuricemia. *N Engl J Med* 286:470, 1972.
86. Elion GB: Allopurinol and other inhibitors of urate synthesis, in Kelley WN, Weiner IM (eds): *Uric Acid.* Berlin, Springer-Verlag, 1978, vol 51, pp 485–514.
87. Pak CYC, Barilla DE, Holt K, et al: Effect of oral purine load and allopurinol on the crystallization of calcium salts in urine of patients with hyperuricosuric calcium urolithiasis. *Am J Med* 65:593, 1978.
88. Morris GS, Simmonds HA, Toseland PA, et al: Urinary oxalate levels are not affected by dietary purine intake or allopurinol. *Br J Urol* 60:292, 1987.
89. Shaw MI, Parsons DS: Absorption and metabolism of allopurinol and oxypurinol by rat jejunum in vitro: Effects on uric acid transport. *Clin Sci* 66:257, 1984.
90. Hosking DH: The use of K-Lyte (potassium citrate) in uric acid lithiasis, in Walker VR, Sutton RAL, Cameron ECB, Pak CYC, Robertson WG (eds): *Urolithiasis.* Proceedings of the 6th International Symposium on Urolithiasis and Related Clinical Research, Vancouver, Canada, July 24–28, 1988. New York, Plenum, 1989, pp 809–812.
91. Erickson SB, Wilson DM, Smith LH: Dissolution of uric acid stones, in Walker VR, Sutton RAL, Cameron ECB, Pak CYC, Robertson WG (eds): *Urolithiasis.* Proceedings of the 6th International Symposium on Urolithiasis and Related Clinical Research, Vancouver, Canada, July 24–28, 1988. New York, Plenum, 1989, pp 821–823.
92. Sakhaee K, Nicar M, Hill K, et al: Contrasting effects of potassium citrate and sodium citrate therapies on urinary chemistries and crystallization of stone-forming salts. *Kidney Int* 24:348, 1983.

93. Pak CYC, Sakhaee K, Fuller C: Successful management of uric acid nephrolithiasis with potassium citrate. *Kidney Int* 30:422, 1986.
94. Hande KR, Noone RM, Stone WJ: Severe allopurinol toxicity: Description and guidelines for prevention in patients with renal insufficiency. *Am J Med* 76:47, 1984.
95. Gault MH, Parfrey PS, Robertson WG: Idiopathic calcium phosphate nephrolithiasis. *Nephron* 48:265, 1988.
96. Cogan MG, Rector FC Jr: Acid-base disorders, in Brenner BM, Rector FC Jr (eds): *The Kidney*, 3rd ed. Philadelphia, Saunders, 1986, pp 457–517.
97. Brenner RJ, Spring DB, Sebastian A, et al: Incidence of radiographically evident bone disease, nephrocalcinosis, and nephrolithiasis in various types of renal tubular acidosis. *N Engl J Med* 307:217, 1982.
98. Simpson DP: Regulation of renal citrate metabolism by bicarbonate ion and pH: Observations in tissue slices and mitochondria. *J Clin Invest* 46:225, 1967.
99. Danielson BG, Backman U, Fellström B, et al: Experience with the short ammonium chloride test, in Smith LH, Robertson WG, Finlayson B (eds): *Urolithiasis: Clinical and Basic Research*. New York, Plenum, 1981, pp 71–76.
100. Tannen RL, Falls WF Jr, Brackett NC Jr: Incomplete renal tubular acidosis: Some clinical and physiological features. *Nephron* 15:111, 1975.
101. Konnak JW, Kogan BA, Lau K: Renal calculi associated with incomplete distal renal tubular acidosis. *J Urol* 128:900, 1982.
102. Preminger GM, Sakhaee K, Skurla C, et al: Prevention of recurrent calcium stone formation with potassium citrate therapy in patients with distal renal tubular acidosis. *J Urol* 134:20, 1985.
103. Batlle DC, Kurtzman NA: Distal renal tubular acidosis, in Coe FL (ed): *Hypercalciuric States: Pathogenesis, Consequences, and Treatment*. Orlando, Grune & Stratton, 1984, pp 239–274.
104. Backman U, Danielson BG, Fellström B, et al: The clinical importance of renal tubular acidosis in recurrent renal stone formers, in Smith LH, Robertson WG, Finlayson B (eds): *Urolithiasis: Clinical and Basic Research*. New York, Plenum, 1981, pp 67–69.
105. Parfitt AM: Acetazolamide and sodium bicarbonate induced nephrocalcinosis and nephrolithiasis: Relationship to citrate and calcium excretion. *Arch Intern Med* 124:736, 1969.
106. Broadus AE: Nephrolithiasis in primary hyperparathyroidism, in Coe FL (ed): *Nephrolithiasis*. New York, Churchill Livingstone, 1980, pp 59–85.
107. Chafe L, Gault MH: First morning urine pH in the diagnosis of renal tubular acidosis with nephrolithiasis. *Clin Nephrol* 41:159, 1994.
108. McSherry E, Morris RC Jr: Attainment and maintenance of normal stature with alkali therapy in infants and children with classic renal tubular acidosis. *J Clin Invest* 61:509, 1978.
109. Griffith DP: Struvite stones. *Kidney Int* 13:372, 1978.
110. Smith LH: Renal lithiasis and infection, in Thomas WC Jr (ed): *Renal Calculi: A Guide to Management*. Springfield, IL, Thomas, 1976, pp 77–96.
111. McLean RJ, Nickel JC, Noakes VC, et al: An in vitro ultrastructural study of infectious kidney stone genesis. *Infect Immun* 49:805, 1985.
112. Griffith DP, Bruce RR, Fishbein WN: Infection (urease)-induced stones, in Coe FL (ed): *Nephrolithiasis*. New York, Churchill Livingstone, 1980, pp 231–260.
113. Lerner SP, Gleeson MJ, Griffith DP: Infection stones. *J Urol* 141:753, 1989.
114. Silverman DE, Stamey TA: Management of infection stones: The Stanford experience. *Medicine (Baltimore)* 62:44, 1983.
115. Chinn RH, Maskell R, Mead JA, et al: Renal stones and urinary infection: A study of antibiotic treatment. *Br Med J* 2:1411, 1976.
116. Feit RM, Fair WR: The treatment of infection stones with penicillin. *J Urol* 122:592, 1979.
117. Robertson WG, Peacock M: The pattern of urinary stone disease in Leeds and in the United Kingdom in relation to animal protein intake during the period 1960–1980. *Urol Int* 37:394, 1982.
118. Robertson WG, Peacock M, Heyburn PJ, et al: Risk factors in calcium stone disease of the urinary tract. *Br J Urol* 50:449, 1978.
119. Hodgkinson A, Marshall RW: Changes in the composition of urinary tract stones. *Invest Urol* 13:131, 1975.
120. Pak CYC, Holt K: Nucleation and growth of brushite and calcium oxalate in urine of stone-formers. *Metabolism* 25:665, 1976.
121. Robertson WG, Peacock M, Marshall RW, et al: Saturation-inhibition index as a measure of the risk of calcium oxalate stone formation in the urinary tract. *N Engl J Med* 294:249, 1976.
122. Finlayson B: Physicochemical aspects of urolithiasis. *Kidney Int* 13:344, 1978.
123. Bek-Jensen H, Tiselius HG: Stone formation and urine composition in calcium stone formers without medical treatment. *Eur Urol* 16:144, 1989.
124. Coe FL, Keck J, Norton ER: The natural history of calcium urolithiasis. *JAMA* 238:1519, 1977.
125. Marshall V, White RH, Chaput de Saintonge M, et al: The natural history of renal and ureteric calculi. *Br J Urol* 47:117, 1975.
126. Blacklock NJ: The pattern of urolithiasis in the Royal Navy, in Hodgkinson A, Nordin BEC (eds): *Renal Stone Research Symposium*, 1968, Leeds, England. London, Churchill, 1969, pp 33–47.
127. Williams RE: Long-term survey of 538 patients with upper urinary tract stone. *Br J Urol* 35:416, 1963.
128. Ljunghall S, Hedstrand H: Epidemiology of renal stones in a middle-aged male population. *Acta Med Scand* 197:439, 1975.
129. Ljunghall S: Incidence and natural history of renal stone disease and its relationship to calcium metabolism. *Eur Urol* 4:424, 1978.
130. Ljunghall S, Danielson BG: A prospective study of renal stone recurrences. *Br J Urol* 56:122, 1984.
131. Wilson DM: Clinical and laboratory approaches for evaluation of nephrolithiasis. *J Urol* 141:770, 1989.
132. Resnick M, Pridgen DB, Goodman HO: Genetic predisposition to formation of calcium oxalate renal calculi. *N Engl J Med* 278:1313, 1968.
133. Coe FL, Parks JH, Moore ES: Familial idiopathic hypercalciuria. *N Engl J Med* 300:337, 1979.
134. Ljunghall S, Backman U, Danielson BG, et al: Epidemiological aspects of renal stone disease in Scandinavia. *Scand J Urol Nephrol [Suppl]* 53:31, 1979.
135. Zerwekh JE, Hughes MR, Reed BY, et al: Evidence for normal vitamin D receptor messenger ribonucleic acid and genotype in absorptive hypercalciuria. *J Clin Endocrinol Metab* 80:2960, 1995.
136. Sestili MA: Possible adverse health effects of vitamin C and ascorbic acid. *Semin Oncol* 10:299, 1983.
137. Smith LH: Risk of oxalate stone from large doses of vitamin C. *N Engl J Med* 298:856, 1978.
138. Curhan GC, Willett WC, Rimm EB, et al: A prospective study of the intake of vitamins C and B6, and the risk of kidney stones in men. *J Urol* 155:1847, 1996.
139. Ryall RL, Darroch JN, Marshall VR: The evaluation of risk factors in male stone-formers attending a general hospital out-patient clinic. *Br J Urol* 56:116, 1984.
140. Pak CYC, Sakhaee K, Crowther C, et al: Evidence justifying a high fluid intake in treatment of nephrolithiasis. *Ann Intern Med* 93:36, 1980.
141. Strauss AL, Coe FL, Deutsch L, et al: Factors that predict relapse of calcium nephrolithiasis during treatment: A prospective study. *Am J Med* 72:17, 1982.
142. Albright F, Henneman P, Benedict PH, et al: Idiopathic hypercalciuria: A preliminary report. *Proc R Soc Med* 46:1077, 1953.
143. Henneman PH, Benedict PH, Forbes AP, et al: Idiopathic hypercalciuria. *N Engl J Med* 259:802, 1958.
144. Broadus AE, Thier SO: Metabolic basis of renal-stone disease. *N Engl J Med* 300:839, 1979.
145. Nordin BEC, Peacock M, Wilkinson R: Hypercalciuria and calcium stone disease. *Clin Endocrinol Metab* 1:169, 1972.
146. Peacock M, Hodgkinson A, Nordin BEC: Importance of dietary calcium in the definition of hypercalciuria. *Br Med J* 3:469, 1967.
147. Lemann J Jr, Adams ND, Gray RW: Urinary calcium excretion in human beings. *N Engl J Med* 301:535, 1979.
148. Broadus AE, Dominguez M, Bartter FC: Pathophysiological studies in idiopathic hypercalciuria: Use of an oral calcium tolerance test to characterize distinctive hypercalciuric subgroups. *J Clin Endocrinol Metab* 47:751, 1978.
149. Broadus AE, Insogna KL, Lang R, et al: A consideration of the hormonal basis and phosphate leak hypothesis of absorptive hypercalciuria. *J Clin Endocrinol Metab* 58:161, 1984.
150. Burtis WJ, Gay L, Insogna KL, et al: Dietary hypercalciuria in patients with calcium oxalate kidney stones. *Am J Clin Nutr* 60:424, 1994.
151. Breslau NA, McGuire JL, Zerwekh JE, et al: The role of dietary sodium on renal excretion and intestinal absorption of calcium and on vitamin D metabolism. *J Clin Endocrinol Metab* 55:369, 1982.

152. Muldowney FP, Freaney R, Moloney MF: Importance of dietary sodium in the hypercalciuria syndrome. *Kidney Int* 22:292, 1982.
153. Sabto J, Powell MJ, Breidahl MJ, et al: Influence of urinary sodium on calcium excretion in normal individuals: A redefinition of calciuria. *Med J Aust* 140:354, 1984.
154. Silver J, Rubinger D, Friedlaender MM, et al: Sodium-dependent idiopathic hypercalciuria in renal stone formers. *Lancet* 2:484, 1983.
155. Massey LK, Whiting SJ: Dietary salt, urinary calcium, and kidney stone risk. *Nutr Rev* 53:131, 1995.
156. Lau YK, Wasserstein A, Westby GR, et al: Proximal tubular defects in idiopathic hypercalciuria: Resistance to phosphate administration. *Miner Electrolyte Metab* 7:237, 1982.
157. Sutton RAL, Walker VR: Responses to hydrochlorothiazide and acetazolamide in patients with calcium stones. *N Engl J Med* 302: 709, 1980.
158. Breslau NA, Brinkley L, Hill KD, et al: Relationship of animal protein-rich diet to kidney stone formation and calcium metabolism. *J Clin Endocrinol Metab* 66:140, 1988.
159. Stewart AF, Adler M, Byers CM, et al: Calcium homeostasis in immobilization: An example of resorptive hypercalciuria. *N Engl J Med* 306:1136, 1982.
160. Broadus AE, Horst RL, Littledike ET, et al: Primary hyperparathyroidism with intermittent hypercalcaemia: Serial observations and simple diagnosis by means of an oral calcium tolerance test. *Clin Endocrinol (Oxf)* 12:225, 1980.
161. Yendt ER, Gagne RJA: Detection of primary hyperparathyroidism, with special reference to its occurrence in hypercalciuric females with "normal" or borderline serum calcium. *Can Med Assoc J* 98:331, 1968.
162. Muldowney FP, Freaney R, McMullin JP, et al: Serum ionized calcium and parathyroid hormone in renal stone disease. *Q J Med* 45:75, 1976.
163. Broadus AE, Horst RL, Lang R, et al: The importance of circulating 1,25-dihydroxyvitamin D in the pathogenesis of hypercalciuria and renal stone formation in primary hyperparathyroidism. *N Engl J Med* 302:421, 1980.
164. Parks J, Coe F, Favus M: Hyperparathyroidism in nephrolithiasis. *Arch Intern Med* 140:1479, 1980.
165. Bordier P, Ryckewart A, Gueris J, et al: On the pathogenesis of so called idiopathic hypercalciuria. *Am J Med* 63:398, 1977.
166. Pak CYC: Physiological basis for absorptive and renal hypercalciurias. *Am J Physiol* 237:F415, 1979.
167. Coe FL, Canterbury JM, Firpo JJ, et al: Evidence for secondary hyperparathyroidism in idiopathic hypercalciuria. *J Clin Invest* 52:134, 1973.
168. Pak CYC, Galosy RA: Fasting urinary calcium and adenosine 3′5′-monophosphate: A discriminant analysis for the identification of renal and absorptive hypercalciurias. *J Clin Endocrinol Metab* 48:260, 1979.
169. Pak CYC, Kaplan R, Bone H, et al: A simple test for the diagnosis of absorptive, resorptive and renal hypercalciurias. *N Engl J Med* 292:497, 1975.
170. Muldowney FP, Freaney R, Ryan JG: The pathogenesis of idiopathic hypercalciuria: Evidence for renal tubular calcium leak. *Q J Med* 49:87, 1980.
171. Broadus AE, Erickson SB, Gertner JM, et al: An experimental human model of 1,25-dihydroxyvitamin D-mediated hypercalciuria. *J Clin Endocrinol Metab* 59:202, 1984.
172. Adams ND, Gray RW, Lemann J Jr, et al: Effects of calcitriol administration on calcium metabolism in healthy men. *Kidney Int* 21:90, 1982.
173. Von Lilienfeld-Toal H, Bach D, Hesse A, et al: Parathyroid hormone is normal in renal stone patients with idiopathic hypercalciuria and high fasting urinary calcium. *Urol Res* 10:205, 1982.
174. Van Den Berg CJ, Kumar R, Wilson DM, et al: Orthophosphate therapy decreases urinary calcium excretion and serum 1,25-dihydroxyvitamin D concentrations in idiopathic hypercalciuria. *J Clin Endocrinol Metab* 51:998, 1980.
175. Gray RW, Wilz DR, Caldas AE, et al: The importance of phosphate in regulating plasma 1,25-$(OH)_2$-vitamin D levels in humans: Studies in healthy subjects, in calcium-stone formers and in patients with primary hyperparathyroidism. *J Clin Endocrinol Metab* 45:299, 1977.
176. Burckhardt P, Jaeger P: Secondary hyperparathyroidism in idiopathic hypercalciuria: Fact or theory? *J Clin Endocrinol Metab* 53:550, 1981.
177. Coe FL, Favus MJ, Crockett T, et al: Effects of low-calcium diet on urine calcium excretion, parathyroid function and serum $1,25(OH)_2D_3$ levels in patients with idiopathic hypercalciuria and in normal subjects. *Am J Med* 72:25, 1982.
178. Shen FH, Ivey JL, Sherrard DJ, et al: Further evidence supporting the phosphate leak hypothesis of idiopathic hypercalciuria. *Adv Exp Med Biol* 103:217, 1978.
179. Pak CYC: Pathogenesis, consequences, and treatment of the hypercalciuric states. *Semin Nephrol* 1:356, 1981.
180. Maierhofer WJ, Gray RW, Cheung HS, et al: Bone resorption stimulated by elevated serum 1,25-$(OH)_2$-vitamin D concentrations in healthy men. *Kidney Int* 24:555, 1983.
181. Brannan PG, Morawski S, Pak CYC, et al: Selective jejunal hyperabsorption of calcium in absorptive hypercalciuria. *Am J Med* 66:425, 1979.
182. Krejs GJ, Nicar MJ, Zerwekh JE, et al: Effect of 1,25-dihydroxyvitamin D_3 on calcium and magnesium absorption in the healthy human jejunum and ileum. *Am J Med* 75:973, 1983.
183. Pak CYC, Britton F, Peterson R, et al: Ambulatory evaluation of nephrolithiasis: Classification, clinical presentation and diagnostic criteria. *Am J Med* 69:19, 1980.
184. Kaplan RA, Haussler MR, Deftos LJ, et al: The role of 1 alpha, 25-dihydroxyvitamin D in the mediation of intestinal hyperabsorption of calcium in primary hyperparathyroidism and absorptive hypercalciuria. *J Clin Invest* 59:756, 1977.
185. Shen FH, Baylink DJ, Nielsen RL, et al: Increased serum 1,25-dihydroxyvitamin D in idiopathic hypercalciuria. *J Lab Clin Med* 90:955, 1977.
186. Insogna KL, Broadus AE, Dreyer BE, et al: Elevated production rate of 1,25-dihydroxyvitamin D in patients with absorptive hypercalciuria. *J Clin Endocrinol Metab* 61:490, 1985.
187. Broadus AE, Insogna KL, Lang R, et al: Evidence for disordered control of 1,25-dihydroxyvitamin D production in absorptive hypercalciuria. *N Engl J Med* 311:73, 1984.
188. Breslau NA, Preminger GM, Adams BV, et al: Use of ketoconazole to probe the pathogenetic importance of 1,25-dihydroxyvitamin D in absorptive hypercalciuria. *J Clin Endocrinol Metab* 75:1446, 1992.
189. Tanaka Y, Deluca HF: The control of 25-hydroxyvitamin D metabolism by inorganic phosphorus. *Arch Biochem Biophys* 154:566, 1973.
190. Williams CP, Child DF, Hudson PR, et al: Inappropriate phosphate excretion in idiopathic hypercalciuria: The key to a common cause and future treatment? *J Clin Pathol* 49:881, 1996.
191. Barilla DE, Zerwekh JE, Pak CYC: A critical evaluation of the role of phosphate in the pathogenesis of absorptive hypercalciuria. *Miner Electrolyte Metab* 2:302, 1979.
192. Tschöpe W, Ritz E, Schmidt-Gayk H: Is there a renal phosphorus leak in recurrent renal stone formers with absorptive hypercalciuria? *Eur J Clin Invest* 10:381, 1980.
193. Edwards NA, Hodgkinson A: Phosphate metabolism in patients with renal calculus. *Clin Sci* 29:93, 1965.
194. Insogna KL, Ellison AS, Burtis WJ, et al: Trichlormethiazide and oral phosphate therapy in patients with absorptive hypercalciuria. *J Urol* 141:269, 1989.
195. Lemann J Jr, Gray RW, Wilz DR: Evidence for a renal PO_4 leak in patients with calcium nephrolithiasis. *Adv Exp Med Biol* 103:225, 1978.
196. Alhava EM, Juuti M, Karjalainen P: Bone mineral density in patients with urolithiasis: A preliminary report. *Scand J Urol Nephrol* 10:154, 1976.
197. Hess B, Casez JP, Takkinen R, et al: Relative hypoparathyroidism and calcitriol up-regulation in hypercalciuric calcium renal stone formers—impact of nutrition. *Am J Nephrol* 13:18, 1993.
198. Jaeger P, Lippuner K, Casez JP, et al: Low bone mass in idiopathic renal stone formers: Magnitude and significance. *J Bone Miner Res* 9:1525, 1994.
199. Trinchieri A, Nespoli R, Ostini F, et al: A study of dietary calcium and other nutrients in idiopathic renal calcium stone formers with low bone mineral content. *J Urol* 159:654, 1998.
200. Sowers MR, Jannausch M, Wood C, et al: Prevalence of renal stones in a population-based study with dietary calcium, oxalate, and medication exposures. *Am J Epidemiol* 147:914, 1998.
201. Smith LH: Enteric hyperoxaluria and other hyperoxaluric states, in Coe JL (ed): *Nephrolithiasis*. New York, Churchill Livingstone, 1980, pp 136–164.

202. Williams HE: Oxalic acid and the hyperoxaluric syndromes. *Kidney Int* 13:410, 1978.
203. Dobbins JW, Binder HJ: Derangements of oxalate metabolism in gastrointestinal disease and their mechanisms, in Glass GBJ (ed): *Progress in Gastroenterology*. New York, Grune & Stratton, vol 3, 1977, pp 505–518.
204. Knickelbein RG, Aronson PS, Dobbins JW: Oxalate transport by anion exchange across rabbit ileal brush border. *J Clin Invest* 77:170, 1986.
205. Hillman RE: Primary hyperoxaluria, in Scriver CR, Beaudet AL, Sly WS, Valle D (eds): *The Metabolic Basis of Inherited Disease*, 6th ed. New York, McGraw-Hill, 1989; pp 933–944.
206. Danpure CJ, Smith LH: The Primary Hyperoxalurias, in Coe FL, Favus MJ, Pak CYC, Parks JH, Preminger GM (eds): *Kidney Stones: Medical and Surgical Management*. Philadelphia, Lippincott-Raven, 1996, pp 859–881.
207. Scheinman JI: Primary hyperoxaluria. *Miner Electrolyte Metab* 20:340, 1994.
208. Daudon M, Reveillaud RJ, Normand M, et al: Piridoxilate-induced calcium oxalate calculi: A new drug-induced metabolic nephrolithiasis. *J Urol* 138:258, 1987.
209. Smith LH, Fromm H, Hofmann AF: Acquired hyperoxaluria, nephrolithiasis, and intestinal disease: Description of a syndrome. *N Engl J Med* 286:1371, 1972.
210. Chadwick VS, Modha K, Dowling RH: Mechanism for hyperoxaluria in patients with ileal dysfunction. *N Engl J Med* 289:172, 1973.
211. Rudman D, Dedonis JL, Fountain MT, et al: Hypocitraturia in patients with gastrointestinal malabsorption. *N Engl J Med* 303:657, 1980.
212. Hodgkinson A: Evidence of increased oxalate absorption in patients with calcium-containing renal stones. *Clin Sci Mol Med* 54:291, 1978.
213. Galosy R, Clarke L, Ward DL, et al: Renal oxalate excretion in calcium urolithiasis. *J Urol* 123:320, 1980.
214. Marangella M, Fruttero B, Bruno M, et al: Hyperoxaluria in idiopathic calcium stone disease: Further evidence of intestinal hyperabsorption of oxalate. *Clin Sci* 63:381, 1982.
215. Pak CYC: A cautious use of sodium cellulose phosphate in the management of calcium nephrolithiasis. *Invest Urol* 19:187, 1981.
216. Backman U, Danielson BG, Johansson G, et al: Treatment of recurrent calcium stone formation with cellulose phosphate. *J Urol* 123:9, 1980.
217. Jaeger P, Portmann L, Jacquet AF, et al: Influence of the calcium content of the diet on the incidence of mild hyperoxaluria in idiopathic renal stone formers. *Am J Nephrol* 5:40, 1985.
218. Erickson SB, Cooper K, Broadus AE, et al: Oxalate absorption and postprandial urine supersaturation in an experimental human model of absorptive hypercalciuria. *Clin Sci* 67:131, 1984.
219. Smith MJV, Hunt LD, King JS Jr, et al: Uricemia and urolithiasis. *J Urol* 101:637, 1969.
220. Coe FL, Raisen L: Allopurinol treatment of uric-acid disorders in calcium-stone formers. *Lancet* 1:129, 1973.
221. Coe FL: Hyperuricosuric calcium oxalate nephrolithiasis. *Kidney Int* 13:418, 1978.
222. Coe FL: Uric acid and calcium oxalate nephrolithiasis. *Kidney Int* 24:392, 1983.
223. Ettinger B: Does hyperuricosuria play a role in calcium oxalate lithiasis? *J Urol* 141:738, 1989.
224. Ettinger B, Tang A, Citron JT, et al: Randomized trial of allopurinol in the prevention of calcium oxalate calculi. *N Engl J Med* 315:1386, 1986.
225. Coe FL: Treated and untreated recurrent calcium nephrolithiasis in patients with idiopathic hypercalciuria, hyperuricosuria, or no metabolic disorder. *Ann Intern Med* 87:404, 1977.
226. Okada Y, Nonomura M, Takeuchi H, et al: Experimental and clinical studies on calcium lithiasis: II. Prevention of recurrent calcium stones with thiazides and allopurinol. *Hinyokika Kiyo* 32:1247, 1986.
227. Oka T, Koide T, Sonoda T: A study on the effect of the treatment for idiopathic calcium urolithiasis on the prevention of recurrence: Estimation of stone episodes and clinical effect. *Nippon Hinyokika Gakkai Zasshi* 76:65, 1985.
228. Pak CYC: Medical management of nephrolithiasis. *J Urol* 128: 1157, 1982.
229. Fellström B, Backman U, Danielson BG, et al: Urinary excretion of urate in renal calcium stone disease and in renal tubular acidification disturbances. *J Urol* 127:589, 1982.
230. Hodgkinson A: Uric acid disorders in patients with calcium stones. *Br J Urol* 48:1, 1976.
231. Schwille P, Samburger N, Wach B: Fasting uric acid and phosphate in urine and plasma of renal calcium-stone formers. *Nephron* 16:116, 1976.
232. Pylypchuk G, Ehrig U, Wilson DR: Idiopathic calcium nephrolithiasis: I. Differences in urine crystalloids, urine saturation with brushite and urine inhibitors of calcification between persons with and persons without recurrent kidney stone formation. *Can Med Assoc J* 120:658, 1979.
233. Tiselius HG, Larsson L: Urinary excretion of urate in patients with calcium oxalate stone disease. *Urol Res* 11:279, 1983.
234. Coe FL, Kavalach AG: Hypercalciuria and hyperuricosuria in patients with calcium nephrolithiasis. *N Engl J Med* 291:1344, 1974.
235. Lonsdale K: Epitaxy as a growth factor in urinary calculi and gallstones. *Nature* 217:56, 1968.
236. Meyer JL, Bergert JH, Smith LH: The epitaxially induced crystal growth of calcium oxalate by crystalline uric acid. *Invest Urol* 14:115, 1976.
237. Pak CYC, Arnold LH: Heterogeneous nucleation of calcium oxalate by seeds of monosodium urate. *Proc Soc Exp Biol Med* 149:930, 1975.
238. Coe FL, Lawton RL, Goldstein RB, et al: Sodium urate accelerates precipitation of calcium oxalate in vitro. *Proc Soc Exp Biol Med* 149:926, 1975.
239. Robertson WG, Knowles F, Peacock M: Urinary acid mucopolysaccharide inhibitors of calcium oxalate crystallisation, in Fleish H, Robertson WG, Smith LH, Vahlensieck W (eds): *Urolithiasis Research*. New York, Plenum, 1976, pp 331–335.
240. Tiselius HG: Effects of sodium urate and uric acid crystals on the crystallization of calcium oxalate. *Urol Res* 12:11, 1984.
241. Fellström B, Backman U, Danielson BG, et al: Inhibitory activity of human urine on calcium oxalate crystal growth: Effects of sodium urate and uric acid. *Clin Sci* 62:509, 1982.
242. Pak CYC, Holt K, Zerwekh JE: Attenuation by monosodium urate of the inhibitory effect of glycosaminoglycans on calcium oxalate nucleation. *Invest Urol* 17:138, 1979.
243. Ryall RL, Hibberd CM, Marshall VR: The effect of crystalline monosodium urate on the crystallisation of calcium oxalate in whole human urine. *Urol Res* 14:63, 1986.
244. Goldwasser B, Sarig S, Azoury R, et al: Hyperuricosuria and calcium oxalate stone formation, in Schwille PO, Smith LH, Robertson WG, Vahlensieck W (eds): *Urolithiasis and Related Clinical Research*. New York, Plenum, 1985, pp 859–862.
245. Ahmad R, Goldsmith HJ, Lovatt G: Allopurinol and recurrent renal stone formation, in *Abstracts of the 20th Congress of the European Dialysis and Transplant Association*, 12th Annual Conference of the European Dialysis and Transplant Nurses Association, London, June 19–22, 1983, p 2.
246. Fellström B, Backman U, Danielson BG, et al: Allopurinol treatment of renal calcium stone disease. *Br J Urol* 57:375, 1985.
247. Marangella M, Tricerri A, Ronzani M, et al: The relationship between clinical outcome and urine biochemistry during various forms of therapy for idiopathic calcium stone disease, in Schwille PO, Smith LH, Robertson WG, Vahlensieck W (eds): *Urolithiasis and Related Clinical Research*. New York, Plenum, 1985, pp 561–564.
248. Robertson WG, Peacock M, Selby PL, et al: A multicentre trial to evaluate three treatments for recurrent idiopathic calcium stone disease: A preliminary report, in Schwille PO, Smith LH, Robertson WG, Vahlensieck W (eds): *Urolithiasis and Related Clinical Research*. New York, Plenum, 1985, pp 545–548.
249. Scott R, Mathieson A, McLelland A: The reduction in stone recurrence and oxalate excretion by allopurinol, in Rose GA, Robertson WG, Watts RWE (eds): *Oxalate in Human Biochemistry and Clinical Pathology*. Proceedings of an international meeting in London, October 26–27, 1979. London, Wellcome Foundation, 1979; pp 191–197.
250. Smith MJV: Placebo versus allopurinol for renal calculi. *J Urol* 117:690, 1977.
251. Sonoda T, Koide T, Oka T, et al: A study of allopurinol in the prevention of recurrent calcium oxalate stones. *Hinyokika Kiyo* 31:2071, 1985.

252. Tiselius HG, Larsson L, Hellgren E: Clinical results of allopurinol treatment in prevention of calcium oxalate stone formation. *J Urol* 136:50, 1986.
253. Ulshöfer B, Zenke J, Achilles W, et al: The effect of long-term treatment with allopurinol on stone recurrence in calcium urolithiasis, in Schwille PO, Smith LH, Robertson WG, Vahlensieck W (eds): *Urolithiasis and Related Clinical Research.* New York, Plenum, 1985, pp 517–519.
254. Wilson DR, Strauss AL, Manuel MA: Comparison of medical treatments for the prevention of recurrent calcium nephrolithiasis. *Urol Res* 12:39, 1984.
255. Finlayson B, Reid F: The effect of allopurinol on calcium oxalate (whewellite) precipitation. *Invest Urol* 15:489, 1978.
256. Finlayson B, Burns J, Smith A, et al: Effect of oxipurinol and allopurinol riboside on whewellite crystallization: In vitro and in vivo observations. *Invest Urol* 17:227, 1979.
257. Baggio B, Gambaro G, Paleari C, et al: Hydrochlorothiazide and allopurinol vs. placebo on urinary excretion of stone promoters and inhibitors. *Curr Ther Res* 34:145, 1983.
258. Morrissey JF, Ochoa M Jr, Lotspeich WO, et al: Citrate excretion in renal tubular acidosis. *Ann Intern Med* 58:159, 1963.
259. Gordon EE, Sheps SG: Effect of acetazolamide on citrate excretion and formation of renal calculi: Report of a case and study of five normal subjects. *N Engl J Med* 256:1215, 1957.
260. Fourman P, Robinson JR: Diminished urinary excretion of citrate during deficiencies of potassium in man: A preliminary communication. *Lancet* 2:656 1953.
261. Menon M, Mahle CJ: Urinary citrate excretion in patients with renal calculi. *J Urol* 129:1158, 1983.
262. Hosking DH, Wilson JWL, Liedtke RR, et al: Urinary citrate excretion in normal persons and patients with idiopathic calcium nephrolithiasis. *J Lab Clin Med* 106:682, 1985.
263. Nicar MJ, Skurla C, Sakhaee K, et al: Low urinary citrate excretion in nephrolithiasis. *Urology* 21:8, 1983.
264. Parks JH, Coe FL: A urinary calcium-citrate index for the evaluation of nephrolithiasis. *Kidney Int* 30:85, 1986.
265. Simpson DP: Citrate excretion: A window on renal metabolism. *Am J Physiol* 244:F223, 1983.
266. Nicar MJ, Hill K, Pak CYC: Inhibition by citrate of spontaneous precipitation of calcium oxalate *in vitro. J Bone Miner Res* 2:215, 1987.
267. Kok DJ, Papapoulos SE, Bijvoet OLM: Excessive crystal agglomeration with low citrate excretion in recurrent stone formers. *Lancet* 1:1056, 1986.
268. Pak CYC, Fuller C, Sakhaee K, et al: Long-term treatment of calcium nephrolithiasis with potassium citrate. *J Urol* 134:11, 1985.
269. Pak CYC, Peterson R, Sakhaee K, et al: Correction of hypocitraturia and prevention of stone formation by combined thiazide and potassium citrate therapy in thiazide-unresponsive hypercalciuric nephrolithiasis. *Am J Med* 79:284, 1985.
270. Barlow IM, Harrison SP: Improved urinary oxalate kit (letter). *Clin Chem* 36:1523, 1990.
271. Trinchieri A, Ostini F, Nespoli R, et al: Hyperoxaluria in patients with idiopathic calcium nephrolithiasis. *J Nephrol* 11 Suppl 1:70, 1998.
272. Yendt ER: Hyperoxaluria in idiopathic calcium oxalate nephrolithiasis. *Md Med J* 37:857, 1988.
273. Hosking DH, Erickson SB, Van Den Berg CJ, et al: The stone clinic effect in patients with idiopathic calcium urolithiasis. *J Urol* 130:1115, 1983.
274. Insogna KL, Broadus AE: Nephrolithiasis, in Krieger DT, Bardin CW (eds): *Current Therapy in Endocrinology and Metabolism, 1985–1986.* St. Louis, Mosby, 1985, pp 353–363.
275. Pak CYC, Smith LH, Resnick MI, et al: Dietary management of idiopathic calcium urolithiasis. *J Urol* 131:850, 1984.
276. Citron J, Tang A, Ettinger B: A model for predicting stone recurrences (abstract). *Urol Res* 12:97, 1984.
277. Yendt ER, Cohanim M: Clinical and laboratory approaches for evaluation of nephrolithiasis. *J Urol* 141:764, 1989.
278. Ljunghall S, Källsen R, Backman U, et al: Clinical effects of parathyroid surgery in normocalcaemic patients with recurrent renal stones. *Acta Chir Scand* 146:161, 1980.
279. Broadus AE, Magee JS, Mallette LE, et al: A detailed evaluation of oral phosphate therapy in selected patients with primary hyperparathyroidism. *J Clin Endocrinol Metab* 56:953, 1983.
280. Yendt ER, Cohanim M: Prevention of calcium stones with thiazides. *Kidney Int* 13:397, 1978.
281. Costanzo LS, Windhager EE: Calcium and sodium transport by the distal convoluted tubule of the rat. *Am J Physiol* 235:F492, 1978.
282. Borghi L, Meschi T, Guerra A, et al: Randomized prospective study of a nonthiazide diuretic, indapamide, in preventing calcium stone recurrences. *J Cardiovasc Pharmacol* 22:S78, 1993.
283. Ettinger B: Recurrent nephrolithiasis: Natural history and effect of phosphate therapy: A double-blind controlled study. *Am J Med* 61:200, 1976.
284. Thomas WC Jr: Use of phosphates in patients with calcareous renal calculi. *Kidney Int* 13:390, 1978.
285. Wikström B, Backman U, Danielson BG, et al: Phosphate treatment of calcium urolithiasis, in Schwille PO, Smith LH, Robertson WG, Vahlensieck W (eds): *Urolithiasis and Related Clinical Research.* New York, Plenum, 1985, pp 495–498.
286. Heyburn PJ, Robertson WG, Peacock M: Phosphate treatment of recurrent calcium stone disease. *Nephron* 32:314, 1982.
287. Smith LH, Thomas WC Jr, Arnaud CD: Orthophosphate therapy in calcium renal lithiasis, in Cifuentes Delatte L, Rapado A, Hodgkinson A (eds): *Urinary Calculi: Recent Advances in Aetiology, Stone Structure, and Treatment.* International Symposium on Renal Stone Research, Madrid, 1972. Basel, Karger, 1973, pp 188–197.
288. Ettinger B: Thiazide treatment of recurrent calcium stones, in Drach GW (ed): *Common Problems in Infections and Stones.* Chicago, Mosby-Year Book, 1991, pp 191–204.
289. Mitwalli A, Ayiomamitis A, Grass L, et al: Control of hyperoxaluria with large doses of pyridoxine in patients with kidney stones. *Int Urol Nephrol* 20:353, 1988.
290. Yendt ER, Cohanim M: Response to a physiologic dose of pyridoxine in type I primary hyperoxaluria. *N Engl J Med* 312:953, 1985.
291. Milliner DS, Eickholt JT, Bergstralh EJ, et al: Results of long-term treatment with orthophosphate and pyridoxine in patients with primary hyperoxaluria. *N Engl J Med* 331:1553, 1994.
292. Schaumburg H, Kaplan J, Windebank A, et al: Sensory neuropathy from pyridoxine abuse: A new megavitamin syndrome. *N Engl J Med* 309:445, 1983.
293. Berger A, Schaumburg HH: More on neuropathy from pyridoxine abuse (letter). *N Engl J Med* 311:986, 1984.
294. Dobbins JW: Nephrolithiasis and intestinal disease. *J Clin Gastroenterol* 7:21, 1985.
295. Bais R, Rofe AM, Conyers RAJ: The inhibition of metabolic oxalate production by sulfhydryl compounds. *J Urol* 145:1302, 1991.
296. Holmes RP, Assimos DG, Leaf CD, Whalen JJ: The effects of (L)-2-oxothiazolidine-4-carboxylate on urinary oxalate excretion. *J Urol* 158:34, 1997.
297. Holmes RP: Pharmacological approaches in the treatment of primary hyperoxaluria. *J Nephrol* 11 Suppl 1:32, 1998.
298. Laerum E, Larsen S: Thiazide prophylaxis of urolithiasis: A double blind study in general practice. *Acta Med Scand* 215:383, 1984.
299. Young JL Jr, Boswell RB, Nies AS: Severe allopurinol hypersensitivity: Association with thiazides and prior renal compromise. *Arch Intern Med* 134:553, 1974.
300. Tiselius HG: The effect of pH on the urinary inhibition of calcium oxalate crystal growth. *Br J Urol* 53:470, 1981.
301. Pak CYC, Peterson R: Successful treatment of hyperuricosuric calcium oxalate nephrolithiasis with potassium citrate. *Arch Intern Med* 146:863, 1986.
302. Berg C, Larsson L, Tiselius HG: The effects of a single evening dose of alkaline citrate on urine composition and calcium stone formation. *J Urol* 148:979, 1992.
303. Barcelo P, Wuhl O, Servitge E, et al: Randomized double-blind study of potassium citrate in idiopathic hypocitraturic calcium nephrolithiasis. *J Urol* 150:1761, 1993.
304. Ettinger B, Pak CYC, Citron JT, et al: Potassium-magnesium citrate is an effective prophylaxis against recurrent calcium oxalate nephrolithiasis. *J Urol* 158:2069, 1997.
305. Joost J, Putz A: Calcium oxalate stone formers five years later, in Schwille PO, Smith LH, Robertson WG, Vahlensieck W (eds): *Urolithiasis and Related Clinical Research.* New York, Plenum, 1985, pp 557–560.
306. Ettinger B: Recurrence of nephrolithiasis: A six-year prospective study. *Am J Med* 67:245, 1979.

PART VIII

Miscellaneous Disorders

CHAPTER 25

Disorders of Growth and Development

Margaret H. MacGillivray

The growth of the human organism from the zygote stage to its culmination in adult stature is a complex phenomenon involving a multitude of regulatory mechanisms that control tissue differentiation, generation, and maturation. In practical terms, growth is the net of mass produced and retained minus that destroyed or lost. Terminal or mature size represents an equilibrium between the incremental and decremental processes, while aging signifies an imbalance in which more tissue is lost than is replaced. Tissue differentiation and maturation, although not explicit in this definition, are essential components of growth.

Throughout childhood and adolescence, gains in height and weight are sensitive and reasonably accurate indexes of the health and well-being of an individual. In general, stature or height is a more accurate basis for evaluating the overall growth process because healthy children show wide variability in weight. However, in chronically malnourished children weight is the more sensitive indicator of disease; linear growth is disturbed to a lesser degree.

This chapter discusses the mechanisms that control the overall growth processes of healthy children as well as the many factors that disturb or enhance growth and provides criteria for differentiating children with pathologic growth from those with short or tall stature at either limit of the normal growth channels. Practical information on diagnostic procedures and therapy is also given.

BIOLOGICAL STAGES OF GROWTH

The growth of all tissues consists of an initial, critical phase of rapid cell division (*hyperplasia*). During this period, diseases that interfere with DNA replication may have a permanent stunting effect because tissues are denied their full complement of cells. The second phase is attributable to both hyperplasia and increased cell size (*hypertrophy*). In the final stage, cellular enlargement is responsible for the attainment of full organ size.[1,2] Maturity is a period of equilibrium. It is followed by the process of aging, which is characterized by more tissue degeneration than regeneration (Fig. 25-1). Most studies support the hypothesis that tissues grow first by cellular multiplication and later by cellular size increase; a notable exception is the report by Sands and colleagues,[3] who observed that cell size increased during the early phase of tissue growth and that cellular multiplication continued throughout all the stages.

The phases of cellular hyperplasia, hyperplasia plus hypertrophy, and hypertrophy alone do not occur simultaneously in all organs; also, the length of time spent in each of these stages varies from one tissue to another (Fig. 25-2). Hence, growth in terms of cellular behavior is not the homogeneous process suggested by external body measurements.[1,4] Nevertheless, the adult state is achieved by virtue of smooth integration of these growth phenomena.

A comparison of brain growth with musculoskeletal growth illustrates the individualistic growth characteristics of different tissues. The greatest rates of DNA synthesis in the brain take place before birth. After birth, there is a gradual reduction in mitotic rates; by 6 to 8 months of life, the critical period of brain growth is completed and the infant possesses the total number of brain cells needed for the remainder of its life. In contrast, the critical phase of growth for the musculoskeletal system lasts 15 to 20 years and extends from fetal life to early adulthood.

The long-range impact of disease on the growth process depends on the timing, duration, and severity of the insult. In general, the prognosis for recovery is better if the injury occurs during the stage of hypertrophy rather than that of hyperplasia. The risk of irreparable damage to the growth process is especially high if prolonged injury occurs during both stages, e.g., microcephaly due to fetal alcohol syndrome and viral infections of the central nervous system (CNS).

CONTROL OF GROWTH PROCESSES

Normal growth is controlled by a number of interacting forces, including genetic mechanisms, tissue-specific factors, hormone regulators, the responsiveness of tissues, and nutritional influences.

Genetic Factors

Two aspects of growth are influenced by genetic mechanisms that are polygenic in nature: the first is regulation of the rate of cellular multiplication and therefore overall size, and the second is control of the pace of maturation. Studies indicate that birth size does not correlate with midparental height (mean height of parents) or with paternal size or subsequent adult stature but does correlate with maternal size (prepregnancy weight of the mother). On this basis, it has been concluded that genetic factors may not play a dominant role in the growth of the fetus.[5] However, during the first 12 to 18 months of postnatal life, genetic influences become increasingly apparent. In this period the linear growth curves of two-thirds of infants shift; the direction of the change correlates best with the mean height of the parents. Approximately one-half drift upward and the remainder downward in growth percentile. From age 2 years to adulthood, genetic mechanisms play a dominant role; thus, a close correlation exists between midparental height and the child's stature.[6] Opinions differ as to the constancy of the

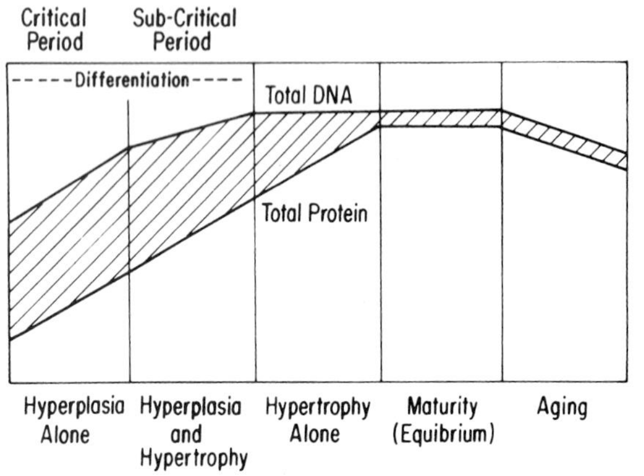

FIGURE 25-1. Representation of the various stages of organ growth and differentiation. During the phase of hyperplasia, growth is due entirely to cellular multiplication, which is represented by the steepness of the DNA slope. In the next phase, the rate of DNA synthesis is less rapid but the rate of protein synthesis is unchanged; consequently, tissue growth is now the result of both cellular multiplication and cellular enlargement. This is followed by a stage of growth due to hypertrophy alone as DNA synthesis plateaus but protein synthesis persists at its previous rate. At maturity, constancy of size is due to equilibrium between tissue gained and tissue lost. During the aging process, tissue loss exceeds replacement. (*From Weiss and Kavanau.*[2])

linear growth rate during childhood. One group has proposed that growth occurs in brief spurts alternating with longer periods of growth cessation (i.e., saltation and stasis) while another has reported that human growth occurs continuously.[7,8] Regardless, an individual child shows remarkable adherence to his/her growth percentile throughout childhood—so much so that deviation upward or downward on the height centiles after the age of 3 years is a prompt to closely monitor the child for a growth abnormality. Genetic controls also regulate the pace of biological maturation in children, which is best illustrated by familial patterns of delayed or early sexual maturation and age of attainment of adult stature.

Both the X and Y chromosomes contain growth-regulating genes. The special influence of the X chromosome is inferred from growth studies in females. As a rule, girls develop 2 years earlier than boys do, and sisters are more similar in pattern of osseous maturation than are brothers. Recently, a growth regulating gene has been identified in the pseudoautosomal region (PAR 1) of the X and Y chromosomes (Xp 22 or Yp 11.3). This novel homeobox-containing gene has been called SHOX by one group and PHOG by another.[9,10] The term SHOX is derived from short stature homeobox X-containing gene and the name PHOG from pseudoautosomal homeobox-containing osteogenic gene. The gene has 6 exons, giving rise to 2 mRNAs (SHOXa, SHOXb), and is highly conserved across species (mammals, fish, flies). The SHOXb gene is expressed in bone marrow fibroblasts and its absence is believed to be responsible for the short stature of Turner Syndrome as well as the poor growth of some children with idiopathic growth failure. Interestingly, the mouse homologue OG-12a is not on the X chromosome, and this may explain why XO mice are not short. This discovery is likely to lead to the development of a novel therapy that is more specific than the one currently approved (growth hormone). The mechanism is believed to involve haploinsufficiency.

FIGURE 25-2. Critical periods of high mitotic rate with increasing cell number for various tissues. By 6 to 8 months of postnatal life, cellular multiplication in the brain is completed. In contrast, rapid rates of DNA synthesis persist for years in muscle, skeleton, and adipose tissues. (*From Smith and Bierman.*[4])

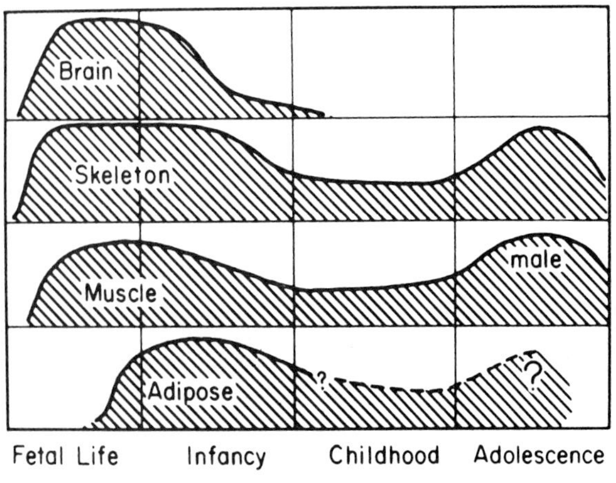

Genetic factors are also known to influence size by race. Although black infants at birth are smaller than white infants, their stature and pace of osseous maturation during the childhood years are equal to or even a little ahead of those of white children from families of comparable income.[11] Japanese children raised in the United States and Chinese children raised in the United Kingdom are taller than are Japanese and Chinese children raised in Japan and Hong Kong, respectively. However, final heights of the Asian emigrés are somewhat lower than those of adult Americans and Europeans.[12]

Peptide Growth Factors and Hormonal Influences

The early concept of the endocrine system consisted of an organized network of ductless glands that secreted the classical hormones into the bloodstream; these chemical messengers traveled to distal organs and enhanced their growth and activity. Currently, the endocrine system is viewed in a much broader context that includes the classical network of ductless glands as well as a large number of peptide growth factors produced in many tissues. These factors may work locally on the cells from which they originate via *autocrine mechanisms* or may influence adjacent tissues via *paracrine mechanisms.* Alternatively, peptide growth factors may be transported through the bloodstream like classical hormones and work through endocrine mechanisms.

In many instances, the classical hormones regulate the production of specific peptide growth factors that control cell proliferation; as such, these growth factors are the mediators or proximal effectors by which the classical hormones control the growth of tissues. A good example of this type of interaction is the one exhibited by growth hormone (GH) on insulin-like growth factor-I (IGF-I) production and somatic growth.

Insulin-Like Growth Factors

In the late 1950s, Daughaday and Salmon observed that GH administration to hypophysectomized rats resulted in increased incorporation of sulfate and thymidine into cartilage in vivo. In subsequent experiments, GH itself did not produce these effects in vitro, whereas serum from GH-treated hypophysectomized rats did. They concluded that the enhanced uptake of sulfate and thymidine was due to a substance in serum that was GH-dependent, which they called sulfation factor.[13] Subsequently, other names were given to this serum factor—i.e., nonsuppressible insulin-like growth factor (NSILA), somatomedin C (Sm C), and insulin-like growth factor (IGF). The data derived from many pioneering investigations formed the basis for the somatomedin hypothesis of GH action, which proposed that GH regulates the growth of skeletal and extraskeletal tissues through its ability to control the production of IGF-I.

Isaakson and colleagues have reported that GH and IGF-I stimulate chondrocytes at different stages of maturation.[14] They observed that isolated epiphyseal chondrocytes suspended in culture contain chondrocyte progenitor cells which form large colonies, while more differentiated chondrocytes form small colonies. GH selectively stimulated the formation of large colonies, whereas IGF-I promoted the formation of small or normal-sized colonies. As a result of these observations with prechondrocytes and somewhat similar effects of GH on preadipocytes, the dual effector theory of GH action was proposed. It states that GH directly stimulates the differentiation of chondrocyte and adipocyte progenitor cells; and also stimulates local production of IGF-I, which enhances the proliferation of the differentiating cells via autocrine/paracrine mechanisms.

Historically, the term *somatomedin* ("mediator of growth") was proposed by investigators whose research focus was somatic growth. By contrast, the name *IGF* was used by researchers working in the field of insulin physiology. Although early studies showed that IGFs are biologically and structurally related to proinsulin, the insulin-like properties of these peptides were not neutralized in the presence of excess anti-insulin antibodies; hence, the origin of the term NSILA (non-suppressible insulin-like activity).

The IGFs (IGF-I, IGF-II) belong to a family of soluble peptide growth factors that circulate primarily bound to one of six IGF binding proteins (IGFBP). They act as autocrine and paracrine growth factors in many tissues where they control mitosis, differentiation, chemotaxis, and programmed cell death (apoptosis). They also have an endocrine mode of action on somatic growth that is dependent on GH-controlled hepatic production of IGF. Most of their actions are determined by free IGFs interacting with the IGF receptors; less than 1 percent of circulating IGFs are in free form and have a short half-life of 10 minutes, whereas IGFs bound to the 150 kd circulating complex have a half-life of approximately 12 hours (Fig. 25-3).[15–18]

The main IGFs in human serum are IGF-I, a 70-amino acid (molecular weight of 7,647) simple chain, basic peptide (isoelectric point 8.1–8.5) that has greater GH dependency than does IGF-II, a slightly acidic peptide (molecular weight of 7,471) containing 67 amino acids. The latter has structural homology with rat multiplication stimulating activity (MSA) isolated from rat hepatocytes. MSA is now referred to as rIGF-II. The two peptides are homologous to each other (45 of 73 aa) and to proinsulin (approximately 50 percent). Like proinsulin, both IGFs have A & B chains connected by disulfide bands, but their C peptide regions have no homology to that of proinsulin. The structural similarities between IGFs and insulin permit them to bind (albeit with much lower affinity) to the insulin receptor and explain why insulin is able to bind to IGF-I receptor. IGFs also bind with high affinity to IGFBPs while insulin cannot.[16,18]

During fetal life, the IGFs are local growth factors acting independently of GH via paracrine and autocrine mechanisms to stimulate growth in a tissue-specific manner. Although circulating levels of IGF-I are low in fetal life, there is a positive correlation between serum IGF-I levels and birth size. It is generally agreed that fetal growth occurs in an environment of relative GH resistance based on the following evidence: (1) GH levels are very high in mid- and late gestation, (2) GH receptors are scarce during fetal life, and (3) serum levels of IGF-I, IGFBP-3, and ALS in the fetus are very low. In postnatal life, the local tissue actions of IGFs persist while the IGFs increasingly assume an endocrine mode of action under the control of GH. The importance of insulin in fetal growth is evident from studies documenting stunted growth in infants with pancreatic agenesis or insulin receptor dysfunction (leprechaunism) while overgrowth was observed in hyperinsulinemic infants of diabetic mothers.[19,20]

Evidence confirming the essential roles of the IGFs in fetal and postnatal growth was obtained from studies of mice with null mutations in the IGF and IGF receptor genes. It is now clear that IGF-I is essential to fetal as well as postnatal growth whereas IGF-II has a major influence on fetal and placental growth. The IGF-I

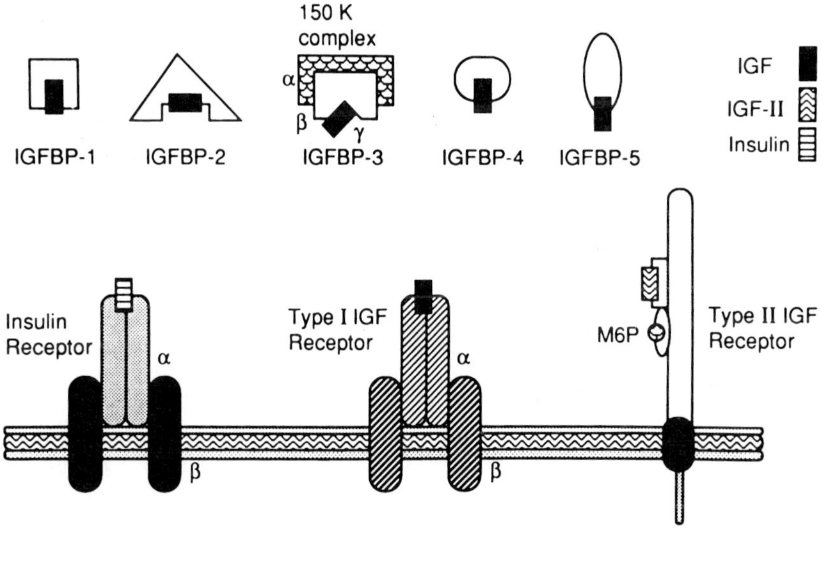

FIGURE 25-3. Schematic representation of IGF binding proteins and IGF receptors on the cell surface. The type I IGF receptor and the insulin receptor share structural and functional properties. The postnatal growth-promoting actions of the IGFs are mediated through the type I IGF receptor, while the hypoglycemic actions of the IGFs are exerted through the insulin receptor. The type II IGF receptor is identical to the mannose-6-phosphate receptor; it has not been linked to the growth-promoting effects of the IGFs. (*From Pinchas et al.*[17])

receptor (Type 1 IGF receptor) is critical to the anabolic actions of IGF-I and IGF-II while the IGF-II receptor (Type 2 IGF receptor) enhances IGF-II turnover and regulates the movement of lysosomal enzymes. Nullification of either IGF-I or IGF-II genes results in mice having low birth weights (60 percent of controls) but normal morphogenesis. Death from respiratory failure was very high in the IGF-I knockout mice (50–95 percent). Survivors continued to exhibit growth failure postnatally and were infertile. Placental growth was not abnormal in IGF-I knockout mice. Nullification of both IGF-I and IGF-II genes resulted in even lower birth weights (30 percent of controls) as well as perinatal death in all animals from respiratory failure due to muscle hypoplasia.[18,21,22]

Knockout mice lacking a functional IGF-I receptor were also underweight (45 percent of controls) and all died after birth. Simultaneous nullification of the IGF-I gene and IGF-I receptor gene did not cause more severe growth retardation than loss of only the IGF-I receptor. These findings suggest that both IGFs work through the IGF-I receptor in fetal life.[23]

Mice with simultaneous knockouts of the IGF-II gene and IGF-I receptor gene have extreme growth retardation equal to that seen in mice lacking both IGF-I and IGF-II functional genes (30 percent of controls). Hence, the IGF-II receptor does not appear to be involved in the anabolic actions of either IGF-I or IGF-II because an intact IGF-I gene did not lessen the growth insult in the mice lacking functional IGF-II and IGF-I receptor.

Surprisingly, nullification of only the IGF-II receptor gene resulted in increased fetal growth but all mice died close to or after birth. Hence, the IGF-II receptor regulates IGF-II turnover and prevents the accumulation of excess IGF-II. A nonfunctional IGF-II receptor leads to high levels of IGF-II, which work through the IGF-I receptor. Concurrent knockouts of the IGF-II gene and the IGF-II receptor gene resulted in reduced birth weights (60 percent of controls) but all mice survived. Though fascinating, the relevance of these mouse knockout studies to human somatic growth is presently unknown.[18]

In contrast to mice with null mutations of the IGFs or IGF receptor genes, transgene mice overexpressing IGF-I are larger than controls by 4 weeks of age and adults weigh 30 percent more than controls. Excess growth was seen in skeletal, connective, and adipose tissues and muscle, but no convincing increase occurred in linear growth. The degree of overgrowth is less than that of mice overexpressing the GH gene. The difference may relate to the somewhat modest overexpression of IGF-I in the transgene mouse combined with reduced expression of pituitary GH. In contrast, transgene mice overexpressing IGF-II have reduced fat mass but do not have enhanced somatic growth; only the thymus, which expressed the transgene, was overgrown. Because these animals had very high levels of circulating IGF-II, it would appear that IGF-II does not have an endocrine mode of action on somatic growth but acts in an autocrine-paracrine manner because overgrowth was observed only in those tissues that overexpressed the IGF-II transgene locally.[24–26]

Genomic imprinting plays an important role in the action of IGF in mice and humans. This phenomenon involves variable DNA methylation of one of the two alleles of autosomal genes leading to gene expression which is controlled by parent of origin, i.e., IGF-II gene knockout causes fetal growth retardation only when the disrupted gene is inherited from the father because the maternally derived IGF-II gene (normal or mutated) is imprinted and not expressed in the offspring. Conversely, the IGF-II receptor gene is paternally imprinted (i.e., not expressed in offspring); hence, the only active IGF-II receptor gene is of maternal origin. Consequently, fetal growth is potentially regulated by both paternal and maternal influences on the IGF-II system.[27–31]

IGFs and the Type 1 IGF receptor (IGF-I receptor) have been linked to tumorigenesis. Transgene mice overexpressing IGF-II in pancreatic beta cells have an increased risk of pancreatic tumors. In humans, overexpression of IGF-II and the type 1 IGF receptor are associated with development of Wilms' tumor. Mutation of WT1, a tumor suppressor gene, is often present in patients with Wilms' tumor. WT1 is known to repress IGF-II and type 1 IGF receptor gene transcription; null mutation of WT1 results in overexpression of these genes such that excess production of IGF-II working through the IGF-I receptor stimulates uncontrolled growth. Overexpression of the Type 1 IGF receptor has been found in some human cancers involving lung and breast. Also, transgene mice overexpressing IGF-II in mammary tissue have an increased incidence of breast tumors.[18,32,33]

In theory, measurement of circulating IGF-I levels in well-nourished subjects should reflect the 24-hr secretion of GH from the pituitary gland; the latter is difficult to quantitate because of its pulsatile secretion. The liver is the main source of circulating IGFs (hepatocytes) as well as IGFBP-3 (hepatic endothelial and Kupffer cells) and ALS (hepatocytes). All three components of the IGF-I 150-kDa complex are regulated by GH; hence, they are predicted to be low in GH-deficient or GH-resistant states and high in acromegaly. In practice, very severely GH-deficient children (93 percent of subjects with peak GH <5 ng/ml) have low levels of IGF-I and IGFBP-3 while reduced values are seen in only 43 percent of less severely GH-deficient children (peak GH 5–10 ng/ml). Surprisingly, low IGF-I and IGFBP-3 also are seen in some "GH-sufficient" children with idiopathic growth failure. Whether these children have a subtle defect in GH secretion or action remains to be determined. Care must be taken in the interpretation of low IGF-I levels because they are also found in malnourished children slowly growing; IGFBP-3 may be more clinically relevant because it is less dependent on nutrition as a rule (Fig. 25-4). Measurement of IGF-I and IGFBP-3 are clues to GH deficiency but normal values have been observed in some well-nourished GH-deficient children (20 percent) as well as in "GH sufficient" growth-retarded children who have an excellent growth response to GH therapy. Hence, measurements of IGF-I and IGFBP-3 are helpful in the overall evaluation of pathologically short, slowly-growing children, but they are not the gold standard for deciding which child should receive GH treatment. Nor are these tests predictive of the magnitude of the growth response in children undergoing GH treatment. Patients with GH resistance more consistently have low levels of IGF-I and IGFBP-3 than do GH deficient subjects.[34–38]

Circulating levels of IGF-I are age-dependent. The lowest values are seen before 5 years of age and then rise. Peak concentrations of IGF-I occur during the most rapid growth phase of puberty. Gonadal steroid production appears to be directly responsible for the pubertal rise of IGF-I because the increase also occurs in children with GH resistance. Following puberty, the IGF-I levels decline to adult values. Elderly adults have low IGF-I levels because GH production falls. Previous studies have shown that IGF-I levels in childhood correlate better with bone age and Tanner stage than with chronologic age.[38–40]

During starvation, nutritional factors override the control of GH on IGF-I. Fasting lowers IGF-I levels to approximately 10 percent of basal values, and refeeding restores concentrations

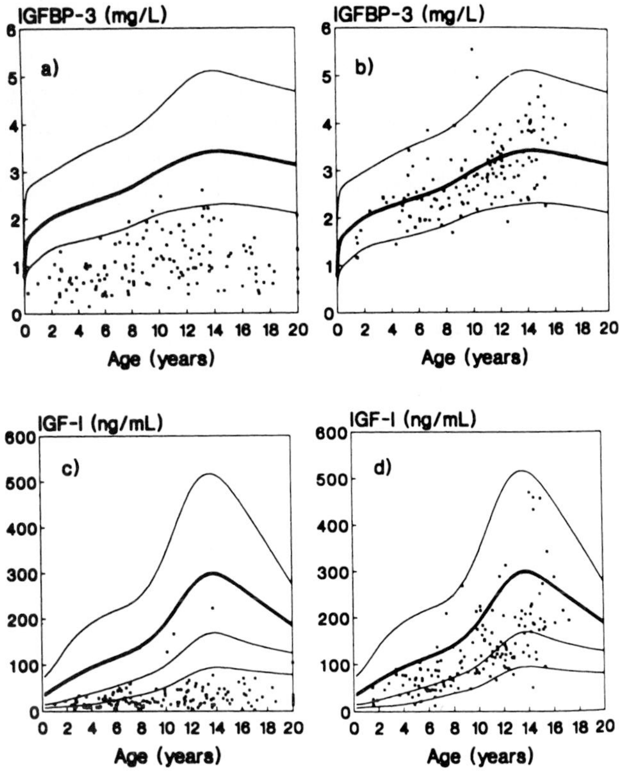

FIGURE 25-4. The normal range (5th to 95th percentiles) for plasma concentrations of IGFBP-III are shown for chronologic age in *A* and *B*. *C* and *D* depict the normal range (1st to 95th percentiles) of IGF-I plasma concentrations. IGFBP-3 and IGF-I measurements from growth hormone–deficient children are displayed in *A* and *C*, respectively, while IGFBP-3 and IGF-I levels from short children with normal GH secretion are depicted in *B* and *D*, respectively. Note the similarity of IGFBP-3 and IGF-I profiles based on chronologic age in normal children. (*From Blum and Ranke.*[38])

toward normal. Studies have shown that food-deprived animals develop a state of GH resistance which leads to low IGF-I levels because the number of GH receptors decreases. Animals experiencing milder forms of nutritional deprivation (i.e., reduced-protein diets) also develop GH resistance and low IGF-I levels, but this occurs without a significant fall in GH receptor number; presumably, the mechanism is a post-GH receptor defect.[41–43]

Diet-restricted rats also exhibit IGF-I resistance because infusions of IGF-I fail to increase weight gain and linear growth. Nevertheless, when IGF-I was administered to diet-restricted human volunteers, it appeared to have some beneficial effects because the protein losses due to nutritional deprivation were reduced.

Low serum IGF-I levels are observed in patients with GH deficiency, GH resistance (Laron syndrome), hypothyroidism, malnutrition, and hepatic failure; in infancy and old age; and in many children with idiopathic growth failure (neurosecretory defect, bioinactive GH, normal-variant short stature [NVSS], idiopathic short stature, etc.).[44]

High serum IGF-I levels are present in acromegaly, pituitary gigantism, and IGF-I resistance syndrome. Transient physiologic elevations also occur during the adolescent growth spurt. The interpretation of IGF-I levels must be based on the normal range for age. For example, a 70-year-old individual with a value that is normal for a 20-year-old may have excess GH secretion.[45]

Measurement of serum IGF-I is difficult because it is contained within the 150-kDa IGFBP complex which interferes with the interaction between IGF-I and the antisera used in radioimmunoassays (RIAs) (see Chap. 5). Current technical improvements include treatment of serum to separate IGFs from the IGFBPs (acid-gel chromatography, acid-ethanol extraction, and Sep-pak chromatography); use of antibodies that are specific for IGF-I and IGF-II C-peptide regions; and use of a biosynthetic radiolabeled IGF-I analog with reduced affinity for IGFBPs. In contrast to IGF-I assays, measurement of IGFBP-3 is technically simple and does not require its separation from IGF peptides. Also, it is less age- and nutrition-dependent while still being GH-dependent. Normal serum levels of IGFBP-3 are relatively high (1–5 mg/L) and permit discrimination of low from normal values even in young infants.

The IGF-I and IGF-II genes are large and complex; the organization of each is remarkably well conserved among the mammalian species, suggesting that the two growth factors diverged from a common ancestral gene.[15,16] These genes belong to the insulin-IGF gene family. The human IGF-I gene spans 80 Kb on chromosome 12 q and contains 6 exons. The human IGF-II gene contains 10 exons and is approximately 35 Kb; it is located on chromosome 11 p 15.5 contiguous with and just 3′ to the insulin gene. IGF-I and IGF-II peptides are small, 70- and 67-amino acid single chain molecules, respectively. These molecules consist of four contiguous domains named B, C, A, and D and resemble proinsulin structurally. The IGF peptides differ from insulin as follows: insulin lacks the D domain and loses the C domain (C-peptide) during posttranslational processing of proinsulin to insulin; the final insulin product contains B and A chains joined by disulfide bonds. The D domain is unique to the IGFs, which do not undergo a posttranslational processing step similar to insulin. Similarities of amino acid structure between insulin and IGFs are restricted to domains B and A of these peptides. Multiple forms of IGF mRNAs are produced in all species through use of different promotors (mammals); variable transcription initiation sites (mammals and chickens); differential RNA splicing (all species); alternative RNA polyadenylation (mammals and chickens); and endonucleocytic cleavage (IGF-II). The ontogeny of IGF-I and IGF-II mRNA expression indicates they are regulated by developmental factors as well as tissue specific determinants. The functional significance of the various transcripts has not been fully defined. The main IGF-I transcripts resulting from alternative mRNA splicing generate two precursor molecules (IGF-1A and IGF-1B) with 153 and 195 amino acids, respectively, which contain the active 70-amino acid IGF-I peptide. Like IGF-I, IGF-II is synthesized as a precursor molecule containing the active 67-amino acid peptide. In humans, IGF-II is expressed at relatively high levels throughout life, whereas, IGF-II production in rodents falls markedly after birth in most tissues. It is hypothesized that the continued activity of promotor I in the liver maintains IGF-II expression in humans postnatally. Unlike classical endocrine peptides, the IGF genes are expressed in multiple tissues and their products, the IGFs, are not stored in secretory granules before secretion.[46]

IGF-I gene expression is controlled by multiple factors.[46] Postnatally, GH and nutrition are the major regulators of IGF-I and, to a lesser extent, IGF-II. GH predominantly controls the transcription of IGF-I in the liver and thus is the major influence on the endocrine mechanism of IGF-I action. Malnutrition due to protein or caloric deficiency suppresses IGF-I production in the

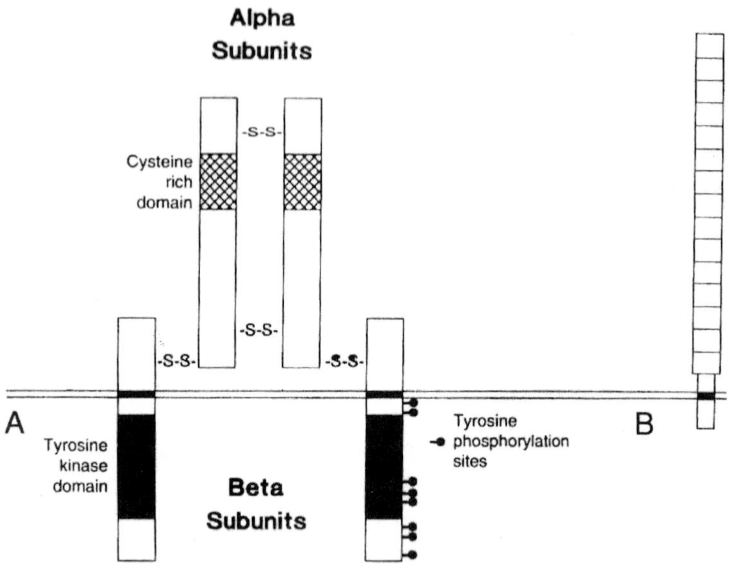

FIGURE 25-5. The Type I IGF receptor (*A*) and the Type II IGF/mannose-6-phosphate receptor (*B*). The insulin is also a heterotetramer with a structure very similar to that of the Type I IGF receptor. The Type II IGF receptor is identical to the mannose-6-phosphate receptor; it translocates mannose-6-phosphate moieties and IGF-II to the lysosomes for degradation. A signaling function has not been identified for this receptor and it does not mediate the growth promoting actions of the IGFs. (*From D'Ercole AJ.*[18])

liver as well as in other tissues while also causing GH resistance. The factors that control the paracrine-autocrine actions of IGFs in tissues are tissue-specific, e.g., sex steroid influences in the gonads, parathyroid hormone effects in bone, estrogen actions in the uterus, and thyroid hormone influences in the thyroid gland. In fetal life, the control of IGF gene expression has not been defined but the pattern suggests that developmental regulation and tissue specificity are important influences. The control of IGF-II gene expression is less well understood; in the rat, high levels of transcription occur in fetal life followed by a postnatal decline of IGF-II mRNA in most tissues except the adult rat brain. A variety of mesenchymal and embryonic tumors overexpress IGF-II mRNA (Wilms' tumor, rhabdomyosarcoma, neuroblastoma, pheochromocytoma, hepatoblastoma, leiomyoma, leiomyosarcoma, liposarcoma, and colon carcinoma). Some of these tumors produce "big" IGF-II that binds less well to IGFBPs and causes non-islet–cell tumor hypoglycemia. The embryonal tumors of Beckwith Wiedemann Syndrome may overexpress IGF-II because of paternal isodisomy or absence of maternal imprinting of the IGF-II gene.[28,32]

The IGFs exert their growth promoting effects through the type 1 IGF receptor (commonly referred to as the IGF-I receptor), which has a high degree of structural and functional similarity to the insulin receptor.[18,47–49] The receptors for insulin and IGF-I are composed of two extracellular α subunits that bind the ligand with high affinity and two β subunits that anchor the receptor in the membrane (Fig. 25-3). The subunits are linked to each other by disulfide bonds to form an $\alpha 2$ $\beta 2$ heterotetromeric complex; the α subunits are actually joined by two disulfide bonds while the alpha beta subunits are joined by one disulfide bond (Fig. 25-5). The β subunits of the Type 1 IGF receptor and insulin receptor have similar signal transduction mechanisms (i.e., both possess tyrosine kinase activities and adenosine-triphosphate binding sites in their intracellular cytoplasmic domains). Binding of IGFs to the alpha subunits of the Type 1 IGF receptor induces a conformational change in the receptor that leads to autophosphorylation of the beta subunit. The activated Type 1 IGF receptor phosphorylates other tyrosine containing substrates such as (1) IRS-I (insulin receptor substrate I, a 185-kd protein that is the predominant substrate of insulin receptor kinase), which contains phosphotyrosine motifs that can associate with SH2, Grb2, Syp, and Nck, and (2) Shc (Src homology domain-containing protein), which then associates with Grb2 and activates Ras leading to a cascade of protein kinases (Raf and MAP kinase) (Fig. 25-6). We lack information on how the cell distinguishes between the IGFs and insulin when the signal transduction pathways appear to be similar if not identical. There may be divergence in the downstream pathways for the two ligands that have not been identified. The gene for the Type 1 IGF receptor is on chromosome 15, while the gene for the insulin receptor is on chromosome 11. It is believed that these two genes evolved from a common ancestral gene.

The type 2 IGF receptor (commonly called the IGF-II receptor) is identical to the mannose-6-phosphate receptor and has no homology to either the type 1 IGF receptor or the insulin receptor. It has no intrinsic tyrosine kinase domain or other known signal transduction mechanism (Fig. 25-3). Type 2 IGF receptors are located on intracellular membranes in equilibrium with plasma membrane receptors and bind both IGF-II and mannose-6-phosphate-containing lysosomal enzymes. It appears that this receptor is bifunctional only in mammals, that is, it facilitates translocation of lysosomal enzymes to lysosomes and it also binds IGF-II. Thus, it facilitates IGF-II biological effects and enhances the degradation of IGF-II by receptor-mediated internalization. Knockout mice lacking type 2 IGF receptors are large because the excess accumulation of IGF-II stimulates overgrowth through the IGF-I receptor. The type 2 IGF receptor binds IGF-II with high affinity, IGF-I with lower affinity, and does not bind insulin at all. In contrast, the type 1 IGF receptor binds both IGF-I and IGF-II with high affinity and binds insulin with 100-fold less affinity. The hypoglycemic properties of the IGFs are mediated by free IGFs working through the insulin receptor because this effect can be blocked by the presence of antibody to the insulin receptor but not by antibody to the Type 1 IGF receptor.[18]

The bioavailability of IGFs is regulated by IGF binding proteins (IGFBPs) that confine the peptides to the intravascular space, prolong their half-life, and allow for steady delivery of IGF-I in contrast to the pulsatile nature of GH in circulation.[50–54] In addition, IGFBPs interact with their own receptors and bind to IGFs with an affinity that exceeds the type 1 IGF receptor. The functions of the IGFBPs include (1) prevention of hypoglycemia, (2)

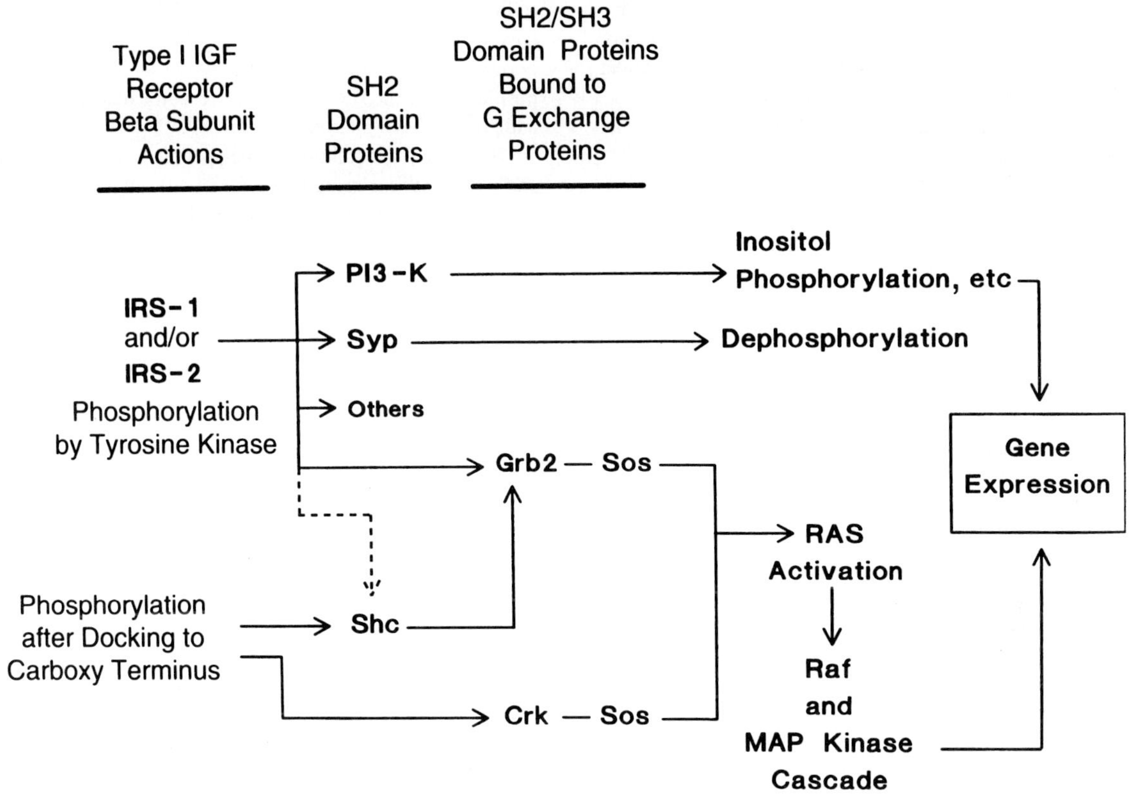

FIGURE 25-6. IGF signaling is mediated by the Type I IGF receptor. The theoretical pathways are depicted. Docking of Shc and Crk to the β subunit has not been proven. The lines from IRS 1 and IRS-2 indicate binding of phosphorylated IRS to the SH2 domains of these proteins. The dashed line from IRS to Shc indicates that IRS may bind to Shc, which permits binding to the Grb2/Sos complex. (*From D'Ercole AJ.*[18])

prolongation of IGF half-life in circulation, (3) control of IGF passage to extravascular space, (4) regulation of IGF interaction with IGF receptors, (5) possible enhancement of IGF action in certain tissues, (6) direct interactions with cells by interacting with IGFBP receptors independent of IGFs, (7) regulation of cell growth and survival (apoptosis, antiapoptosis), and (8) protection of circulating IGFs from enzyme degradation. Six IGFBPs have been identified to date. They have a highly conserved set of 16 or more cysteines that shape their secondary structure, which is also conserved. They share 50 percent homology among themselves (in N and C terminals mainly) and 80 percent homology between other species. The IGFBP genes and the homeobox gene clusters (Hox A to D) are in close proximity and may have evolved together. The Hox genes are DNA binding proteins that are regulated by retinoic acid, like some of the IGFBP genes. The IGFBPs (1 through 6) are located on chromosomes 7, 2, 7, 17, 2 and 12 respectively; Hox A is on chromosome 7, Hox B on chromosome 17, Hox C on chromosome 12, and Hox D on chromosome 2.

Most of the IGF-I and IGF-II circulate in a ternary IGFBP-3 150-kDa complex composed of an λ subunit (IGF); the glycosylated 40–44 kDa β subunit (IGFBP-3); and a glycosylated 85-kDa α subunit (ALS).[18,50–54] Interaction between the α and β subunits largely depends on the presence of IGFs. The 150-kDa complex prevents IGFs from crossing the capillary barriers (Fig. 25-3). However, IGF peptides in complexes of 40–50 kDa may exit the vascular compartment and act on tissues. Very little free IGFs exist in circulation though they predominate in saliva, which has low levels of IGFBPs. IGFs bound to the 150-kDa IGFBP-3 complex are unable to exert insulin-like effects, whereas free IGFs possess 5 to 10 percent of the hypoglycemia potency of insulin. The total circulating IGF concentration is approximately 100 nmol/L compared to the usual insulin concentration of 100 pmol/L. If the circulating IGFs were not complexed, their hypoglycemic potential would be 50- to 100-fold more than that of insulin. High-dose IGF-I infusions have caused hypoglycemia because of elevated free IGF-I levels.

Low levels of IGFBP-3 have been observed in some patients with non-islet–cell tumor hypoglycemia due to overproduction of IGF-II by mesenchymal tumors (Wilms' tumor, neuroblastoma, leiomyoma, leiomyosarcoma, fibrosarcoma). Expression of the IGF-II gene by the tumors yields a high molecular weight peptide (10–15 kDa); in serum this IGF-II is contained in a 60-kDa complex rather than a 150-kDa complex. Defective binding of the abnormal IGF-II–IGFBP-3 complex to the alpha subunit of the ternary complex (ALS) results in a reduced level of circulating 150-kDa IGFBP-3 and allows IGF-II to exert its hypoglycemic effects.[32]

Measurement of IGFBP-3 is influenced by the presence of IGFBP proteases (kallikreins, cathepsins, and matrix metalloproteinases) which degrade IGFBPs by proteolysis. Proteases for IGFBP-3 were first identified in serum of pregnant women; subsequently, proteases for IGFBP-2, -3, -4, -5 were found in serum, seminal plasma, cerebrospinal fluid, and urine. Proteases break down the circulating IGFBPs and the fragments lose their high affinity for IGFs; the liberation of free IGFs permits them to exit the vascular space and exert mitogenic and anabolic effects. This phenomenon occurs during the latter stages of pregnancy. Proteases also act locally in the extravascular space where they promote IGF release at the tissue level. IGFBPs may exert direct stimulatory as well as inhibitory effects at the cell level.[51–54]

IGFBP-1, a 25-kDa protein, is produced in the liver, decidua, and kidneys; it is the most abundant IGFBP in amniotic fluid.[54] The levels are regulated by metabolic factors; low concentrations are seen (1) after meals, (2) during hyperinsulinemic hypoglycemia, (3) in obese subjects, and (4) in large-for-gestation infants. Insulin suppresses IGFBP-1 gene expression. Elevated IGFBP-1 levels are observed in hypoinsulinemic states (intrauterine growth retardation, fasting, poorly-controlled Type 1 diabetes mellitus) and in chronic renal failure, where they may lower free IGFs and play a role in the growth deceleration of these children. IGFBP-1 contains a recognition sequence that permits it to interact with integrin receptors. Other names for IGFBP-1 include Hep G2 (human hepatoma cell line), PP12 (placental protein 12), and AFBP (amniotic fluid binding protein). IGFBP-1 binds equally to IGF-I and to IGF-II with an affinity that is fivefold less than IGFBP-3. IGFBP-1 has a diurnal pattern; i.e., high at night and in early morning hours followed by a decline. Unlike IGFBP-3, GH does not regulate serum IGFBP-1 levels.

IGFBP-2, a 31-kDa protein is neither phosphorylated or glycosylated.[54] It also possesses a recognition sequence for membrane integrin receptors. Levels of IGFBP-2 are age-dependent, being high in young infants and older subjects and low in young adults. IGFBP-2 is the major IGFBP in cerebrospinal fluid because it is produced by many neural tissues. The concentration of IGFBP-2 in seminal fluid is remarkably high, in the range of 10,000 ng/ml. Metabolic influences on IGFBP-2 are similar to those seen with IGFBP-1 but to a lesser extent; protein restriction elevates IGFBP-2 levels more than does caloric restriction.

IGFBP-4, a 24-kDa protein, is produced in fibroblasts, neuroblastoma cells, prostate cells, and bone cells.[54] It is regulated by vitamin D and PTH in bone and by retinoic acid inhibition in neuroblastoma cells. IGFBP-4 occurs mainly as an extracellular soluble protein and its functions are not well defined.

IGFBP-5, a 29-kDa protein, occurs in several glycosylated forms. High tissue levels are seen in the rapidly growing fetus; after puberty, the levels decline. Unlike the other IGFBPs, IGFBP-5 binds to bone cells and to the extracellular matrix. Bone cells produce large amounts of IGFBP-5. IGFBP-5 is also found in CSF, connective tissue, and kidneys. Production of IGFBP-5 by osteoblasts is increased by IGF-I and retinoic acid and decreased by FGF, TGF-B, and platelet-derived growth factor BB. Knowledge about the mechanisms regulating IGFBP-5 production is still incomplete.[54]

IGFBP-6, a 34-kDa O-glycosylated protein, is found mainly in CSF and serum and is regulated by IGF-II and other hormones. It is the only IGFBP that preferentially binds IGF-II (more than 2-fold) as compared to IGF-I. Excess concentrations inhibit IGF-II gene expression in osteoblasts while having little effect on IGF-I actions. The IGFBP-6 gene is expressed in ovary, prostate, and fibroblasts. Estrogen-receptor negative breast cancer cell lines produce IGFBP-6, which is enhanced by retinoic acid but not by IGF-I. Retinoic acid also increases IGFBP-6 expression in osteoblasts by 1000 percent.[54]

In summary, the IGFs are essential for fetal and postnatal growth. During organogenesis, the IGFs and IGFBPs seem to act by autocrine/paracrine mechanisms because they are expressed in a tissue-specific and developmentally-specific manner. Postnatally, IGF-I takes on endocrine functions, while IGF-II may continue to have only local growth-promoting actions. Although IGFs are important regulators of fetal growth, IGF-1 is the major stimulator of postnatal growth. The Type 1 IGF receptor mediates most prenatal and postnatal IGF actions in humans.[16–18]

The factors regulating tissue-specific expression of the IGF-I and IGF-II genes during fetal life are not fully understood. Placental somatomammotropin (CS, placental lactogen) appears to stimulate IGF-I and IGF-II synthesis, while nutrition affects IGF-I but not IGF-II production. Nutritional influences and GH have fewer effects in fetal life than in postnatal life.

Hormonal Regulation

In infancy growth is primarily dependent on nutrition, whereas during childhood GH is the major determinant of growth. Sex hormones and GH control the adolescent growth spurt. Normal thyroid function is essential to each of these stages of growth. Insulin and glucocorticoids influence carbohydrate, fat, and protein metabolism; provide sources of energy needed for growth; and exert a permissive influence on the anabolic actions of GH. Whether insulin acts only permissively or whether it also functions as a growth factor is still unsolved because of the inseparable link between insulin and nutrition. The growth excess of hyperinsulinemic obese children appears to result from increased insulin concentration coupled with increased nutrient intake. Conversely, poor growth in insulin-deficient (type 1) diabetic youngsters is associated with intracellular undernutrition. Skeletal growth and ossification are dependent on PTH, the vitamin D metabolites, and, possibly, calcitonin.

Growth Hormone

The growth hormone molecule secreted by the somatotropes of the anterior pituitary gland is a single-chain polypeptide (molecular weight of 22,000) containing 191 amino acid residues with two intrachain disulfide bridges. A form with a molecular weight of 20,000 is produced in lower abundance by means of alternative splicing of GH mRNA. Approximately 4 to 10 percent of the wet weight of the pituitary gland consists of GH (5 to 15 mg per gland). Although GH shares structural homology with prolactin and chorionic somatomammotropin, it is the only member of this family of peptides that exhibits postnatal growth-promoting activity in humans.

Synthesis of GH by the somatotrope is genetically controlled by the GH N gene, one of five genes in the GH gene cluster located on the long arm of chromosome 17.[55,56] The genes in the cluster from 5′ to 3′ are hGH-N, human chorionic somatomammotropin-L (hCS-L), hCS-A, hGH-V, and hCS-B (Fig. 25-7). A closely related gene which codes for prolactin is located on chromosome 6.[57] The hGH-N gene is expressed only in the somatotropes of the pituitary gland, while the other genes—hCS-A, hCS-B, and hGH-V—are expressed in the syncytiotrophoblastic epithelial cells of the placenta. Little is known about the hCS-L gene. The major product of the GH-V gene is a 22-kDa basic peptide (GH variant, GH-V, or placental GH) that differs from GH-N by only 13 amino acids (Fig. 25-8). The second product of the GH-V gene is a membrane-bound 26-kDa peptide (GH-V2) that contains 104 carboxyterminal amino acids. GH-V2 derives from an alternatively spliced GH-V transcript that retains intron 4 of the GH-V gene. The GH-V gene is developmentally regulated, and the ratio of GH-V2 to GH-V is higher in late pregnancy than in

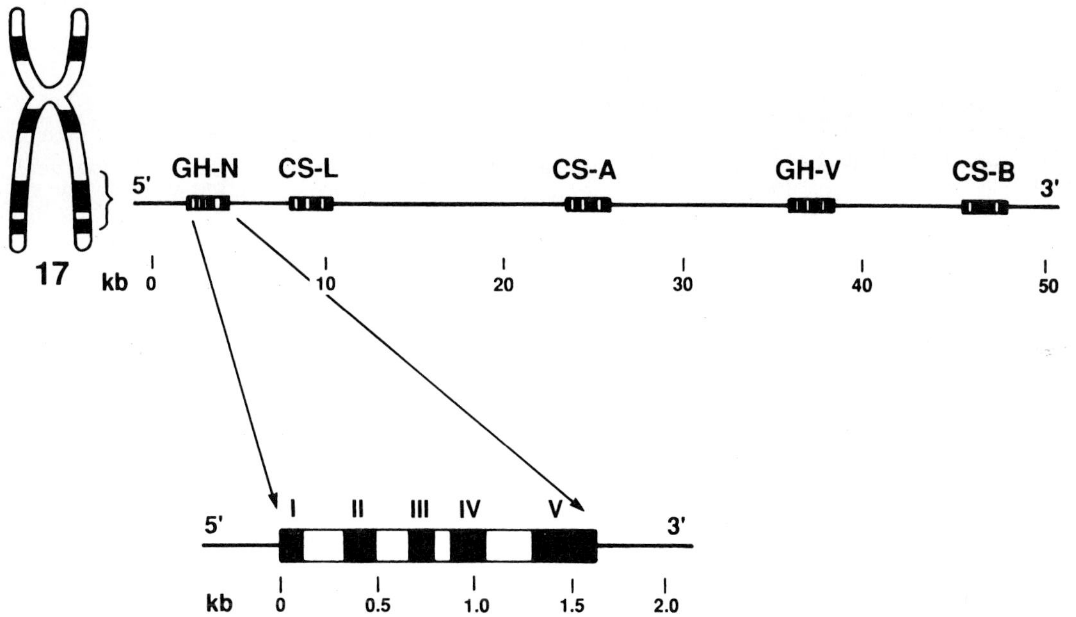

FIGURE 25-7. The five genes in the human GH gene cluster on the long arm of chromosome 17. From 5′ to 3′, the genes in the cluster are GH-N, CS-L, CS-A, GH-V, and CS-B. The GH-N gene is expressed only in the pituitary gland, whereas the remaining genes are active only in the placenta. The five genes have extensive DNA sequence homology, and each is composed of five coding regions or exons (I–V) and four introns. (*From Phillips and Venencak-Jones.*[55])

early pregnancy. GH-V is a biologically active somatogen and lactogen; it binds more efficiently to somatogenic than to lactogenic receptors and is equal to GH-N in stimulating weight gain in hypophysectomized rats.[58–60] Serum levels of GH-V rise in pregnancy and are presumed to play a role in suppressing maternal pituitary production of GH-N late in gestation. Based on numerous studies, it would appear that GH-V gene serves an important function in pregnancy, but its specific contribution has not been defined.[61] The assumption has been made that GH-V regulates placental and fetal growth, but this seems unlikely because

FIGURE 25-8. The products of the GH-N and GH-V genes. The major products of the GH-N gene, which is expressed in the pituitary gland, are 22- and 20-kDa peptides. The latter are derived from alternative splicing of the GH-N mRNA, which results in omission of the amino acids shown in solid circles (d). The product of the GH-V gene, which is expressed exclusively in the syncytiotrophoblastic cells of the placenta, is a 22-kDa peptide that differs from GH-N by only 13 amino acid substitutions, which are shown as solid circles (d). By alternative splicing of the GH-V mRNA, intron 4 of the GH-V gene is retained and the product is predicted to be a 26-kDa peptide. Unlike GH-V, which is secreted, the GH-V2 product is membrane-bound. (*From Cooke et al.*[57])

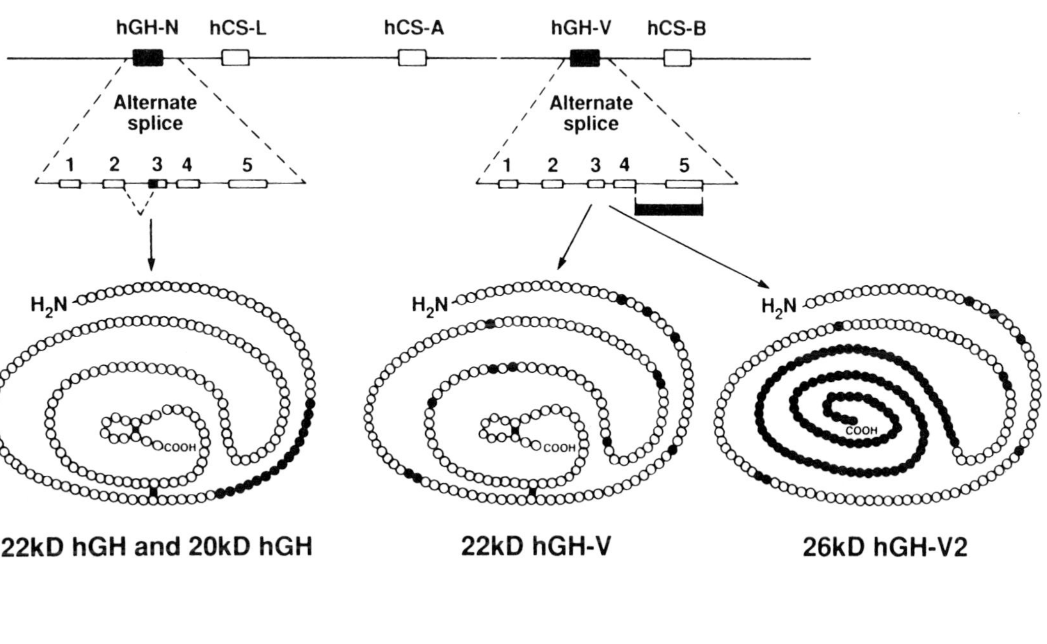

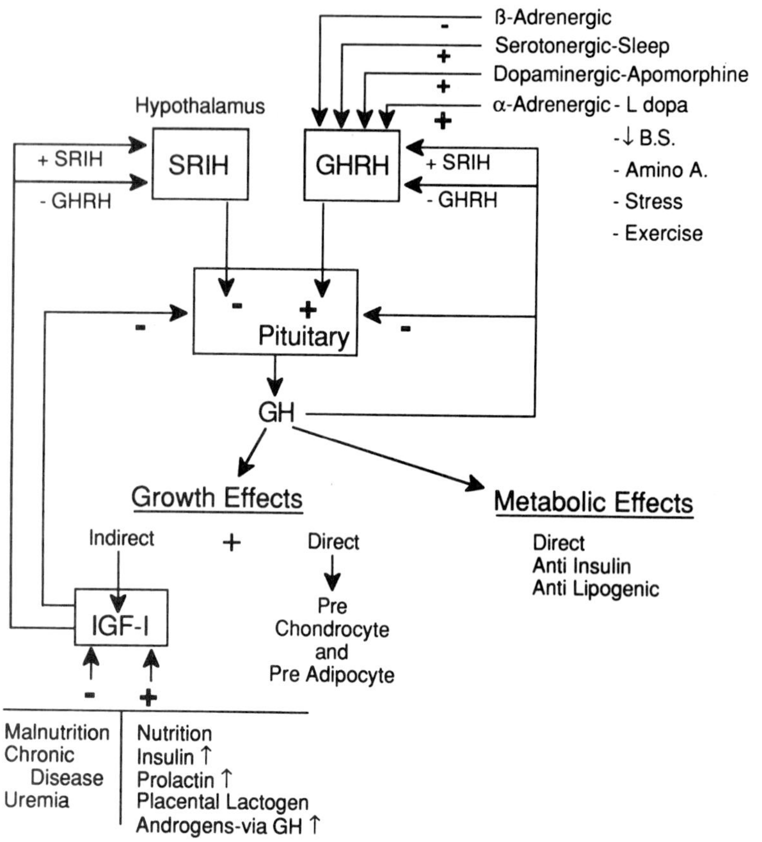

FIGURE 25-9. GH secretion is regulated by hypothalamic hormones: somatostatin inhibits and growth hormone releasing hormone (GHRH) stimulates GH secretion. GHRH production is enhanced by α-adrenergic, dopaminergic, and serotoninergic neurons and suppressed by β-adrenergic neurons. GH and IGF-I inhibit GHRH secretion and enhance somatostatin production. These phenomena indirectly suppress GH secretion. GH production at the pituitary level is directly suppressed by the negative feedback effects of IGF-I and GH. GH acts directly on carbohydrate and lipid metabolism and directly and indirectly on growth. IGF-I production is enhanced by nutrition, insulin, prolactin, placental lactogen, and androgens. IGF-I production is suppressed by malnutrition, chronic diseases, glucocorticoids, and high doses of estrogen.

deletions of GH-V with or without deletions of the hCS genes do not compromise placental and fetal development. It is possible that redundancy within the robust GH gene family provides backup mechanisms for such gene deletions.[62–64]

GH secretion is regulated primarily by two hypothalamic hormones; *somatostatin* (SRIH), which inhibits, and *growth hormone releasing hormone* (GHRH), which stimulates GH secretion. Each pulse of GH is generated by a combination of a rise in GHRH and a decline in SRIH. Current hypotheses concerning the mechanisms that regulate GH secretion are illustrated in Fig. 25-9. Somatostatin, a tetradecapeptide, is present in high concentrations in the preoptic basal area of the hypothalamus, CNS, and GI tract, particularly the pancreas.[65,66] In humans, SRIH is initially produced as a large precursor which is processed to 14- and 28-amino acid peptides. SRIH is secreted episodically into the portal circulation and acts on the somatrope to suppress basal and stimulated GH secretion while having no effect on GH synthesis. Somatostatin suppresses the GH response to insulin hypoglycemia, arginine infusion, levodopa ingestion, and deep sleep. Somatostatin also blocks thyrotropin releasing hormone (TRH)-induced thyroid stimulating hormone (TSH) release but does not block the prolactin rise following TRH stimulation. The extrapituitary effects of somatostatin include suppression of glucagon and insulin secretion by the pancreas. GH secretion is also inhibited by IGF-I and by GH itself; IGF-I acts directly on the pituitary gland, and both GH and IGF-I act on hypothalamic regulatory centers (i.e., by stimulating somatostatin production and suppressing GHRH release) (Fig. 25-9).

GHRH cell bodies in the arcuate nucleus and adjacent ventromedial nucleus are the site of GHRH production. The axons of the GHRH neurons extend to the median eminence and terminate on the capillaries of the portal circulation. GHRH is secreted episodically and stimulates GH transcription and secretion by the somatotrope in a species-specific and pulsatile fashion. The cellular components involved in GH secretion include GHRH receptors, cyclic AMP (cAMP), and free cytosolic Ca^{2+}. Extrahypothalamic sources of GHRH include placenta, ovary, testis, lymphocytes, and pancreas but its function in these tissues is not fully defined. Final proof of the existence of GHRH was provided when the hormone was isolated from the pancreatic tumors of two patients who had developed acromegaly as a result of tumor-derived GHRH.[67,68] The structure of human hypothalamic GHRH is identical to GHRH isolated from pancreatic tumors.[69–71] Isolation of GHRH from the pancreatic tumors culminated many years of frustrating research. Its existence had been suggested by animal studies carried out more than two decades ago and later by clinical and laboratory documentation of acromegaly due to hypersecretion of biologically active GHRH from pancreatic tumors.[72] Synthetic GHRH administration to normal subjects [1 to 10 μg per kilogram of body weight intravenously (IV)] results in rapid and large increments in serum GH concentration; peak GH concentrations occur 15 to 30 min after IV bolus injection. Synthetic GHRH also stimulates modest elevations of serum GH and IGF-I concentrations in many patients with idiopathic hypopituitarism. Accelerated growth rates have been reported in GH-deficient children treated with GHRH.[73] Synthetic human GHRH appears to be relatively specific for the somatotrope: No change has been observed in serum concentrations of glucose, gonadotropins [follicle stimulating hormone (FSH) or luteinizing hormone (LH)], TSH, or hydrocortisone. A modest rise in prolactin has been reported after

GHRH administration. The only side effect observed to date has been slight facial flushing.

Release of the hypothalamic hormones GHRH and somatostatin is in turn regulated by biogenic amines derived from neurosecretory neurons in the CNS. Somatostatin secretion is regulated primarily by cholinergic mechanisms (i.e., agonists inhibit and antagonists stimulate SRIH production). In contrast, secretion of GHRH is enhanced by alpha-adrenergic, dopaminergic, and serotoninergic neurons and suppressed by β-adrenergic tracts. Presumably, β-adrenergic agonists stimulate SRIH and thereby inhibit GH secretion. Alpha-adrenergic pathways (norepinephrine and α-adrenergic receptors) are primary regulators of GHRH release. Drugs that mimic the action of norepinephrine (α-adrenergic agonists, e.g., clonidine) enhance GHRH production; those that block the alpha receptors (e.g., phentolamine) inhibit GHRH release. Dopaminergic receptor stimulation (e.g., by apomorphine) also enhances GHRH release. However, oral administration of levodopa appears to enhance GHRH release via α-adrenergic rather than dopaminergic pathways. Evidence for this was derived from studies reporting that phentolamine prevents levodopa-induced GH release. The normal somatotrope has no demonstrable dopamine receptor. However, GH-secreting pituitary adenomas paradoxically have a dopamine receptor that inhibits GH secretion when stimulated. This accounts for the suppression of plasma GH levels in approximately 80 percent of acromegalic patients treated with either levodopa or the dopaminergic agent bromocriptine. The actual significance of the serotoninergic pathways in the control of GH is less well understood. Administration of 5-hydroxytryptophan, a serotonin precursor, enhances GH release, and cyproheptadine, a serotonin antagonist, decreases GH responses to exercise, hypoglycemia, and 5-hydroxytryptophan. Beta-adrenergic blocking agents (e.g., propranolol) augment GH responses to levodopa, glucagon, and antidiuretic hormone (ADH), and the β-adrenergic agonist isoproterenol inhibits GH release.

Synthetic hexapeptides that stimulate GH secretion by a pathway distinct from that of GHRH have been classified as GH-releasing peptides (GHRP). They are not homologous to GHRH and work through their own tissue receptors; this suggests the existence of endogenous ligands. The GHRPs stimulate GH secretion by an intact pituitary gland and enhance the GH response to GHRH. Their action is not blocked by SRIH.[74–76]

Galanin, a naturally occurring neuropeptide that is present in the median eminence, has been shown to enhance GH responses to GHRH. The physiologic significance of galanin is poorly understood; it may influence pulsatile GH secretion by lowering the inhibitory effects of SRIH, but it does not appear to be as important as GHRH.[77]

PACAP is a pituitary adenylate cyclase-activating peptide that is a member of the secretin-glucagon-vasoactive intestinal peptide family. PACAP was isolated from the hypothalamus and has receptors in the hypothalamus and pituitary gland. Binding of PACAP increases cAMP, alters calcium levels in somatotropes, and stimulates GH release. The clinical significance of PACAP is being determined.[78]

The gut-brain peptide family has been found in the hypothalamus and several of its members stimulate GH secretion. They include galanin, substance P, cholecystokinin, VIP, motilin, neurotensin, and peptide histidine isoleucine amide (PHI). Their precise contribution to the control of GH secretion is uncertain.[79]

Under physiologic conditions, the pituitary gland secretes approximately eight discrete peaks of GH each day, with very low basal levels between the episodic bursts. In children and young adults, approximately 50 to 75 percent of the daily production of GH occurs during the early nighttime hours that follow the onset of deep sleep; in contrast, prolactin and cortisol concentrations rise progressively during the later hours of sleep. GH secretion is stimulated by exercise, emotional stress, high-protein meals, rapid onset of hypoglycemia, and prolonged fasting; it is suppressed by elevated glucose levels in healthy nondiabetic subjects.

Sex steroids increase GH production twofold or threefold during puberty. This increase in GH secretion results from greater pulse amplitude, not from an increased frequency of GH peaks.[80,81]

Approximately 50 percent of GH in circulation is bound to a high-affinity GH binding protein (GHBP), which is identical to the extracellular domain of the GH receptor (Fig. 25-10).[82,83] Most of the remaining GH in circulation is free except for the 5 percent that is bound to a low-affinity 100-kDa GHBP. The main GH in circulation has a molecular mass of 22-kDa. Less abundant is the 20-kDa GH, which retains growth-promoting activity. Larger forms of GH (45-kDa) represent aggregations of 22-kDa molecules.

In general terms, GH is an anabolic hormone that stimulates postnatal growth, antagonizes the action of insulin, and possesses lipolytic activity. Direct influences of GH on isolated extraskeletal tissues (e.g., heart muscle, diaphragm, adipocytes, hematopoietic cells, and hepatocytes) and on perfused organs (e.g., liver) have been documented. GH also plays an important role in carbohydrate, fat, protein, and mineral metabolism (Table 25-1).

The GH receptor is primarily somatogenic and has 30 percent sequence identity with the prolactin receptor. Both of these hormone receptors belong to the cytokine receptor superfamily. The GH receptor is a single-chain polypeptide that contains a signal peptide of 12 to 24 amino acids and a mature protein of 614 to 626 amino acids. The mature protein contains an extracellular hormone-binding domain of about 250 amino acids, a single membrane-spanning domain, and an intracellular domain of about 350 amino acids (Fig. 25-10). The extracellular domain of the GH receptor is identical to the soluble GHBP found in circulation. Multiple membrane-associated GH receptors have been identified; at least three have been shown to be immunologically distinct, but their roles have not been defined. Analysis of GH mRNA by Northern blot hybridization has revealed at least two transcripts that correspond to the smaller soluble and larger membrane-associated GH receptors. This observation suggests that soluble GHBP in circulation is derived from alternative splicing of GH receptor mRNA but does not exclude the possibility that it is also generated by proteolysis of the membrane receptor.[83,84] Most children with GH resistance syndrome (Laron-type) have a deficiency of the GH receptor and lack soluble GHBP in circulation. Some of these patients have extensive deletions of the GH receptor gene, and this eliminates large portions of the GH binding domain; thus cells are unable to bind and respond to GH.[85–86]

The human GH receptor gene spans 87 kb on chromosome 5 and consists of 9 coding exons and several 5′ noncoding exons. GH signal transduction requires the binding of a single GH molecule to two molecules of the GH receptor (GHR); this event enhances dimerization of the GH receptor and a conformational change which produces an increased binding and activation of JAK2 (Fig. 25-11). The activated JAK2 autophosphorylates and also phosphorylates tyrosines within the GHR.[87] These phosphorylated tyrosines within GHR and JAK2 recruit various signaling

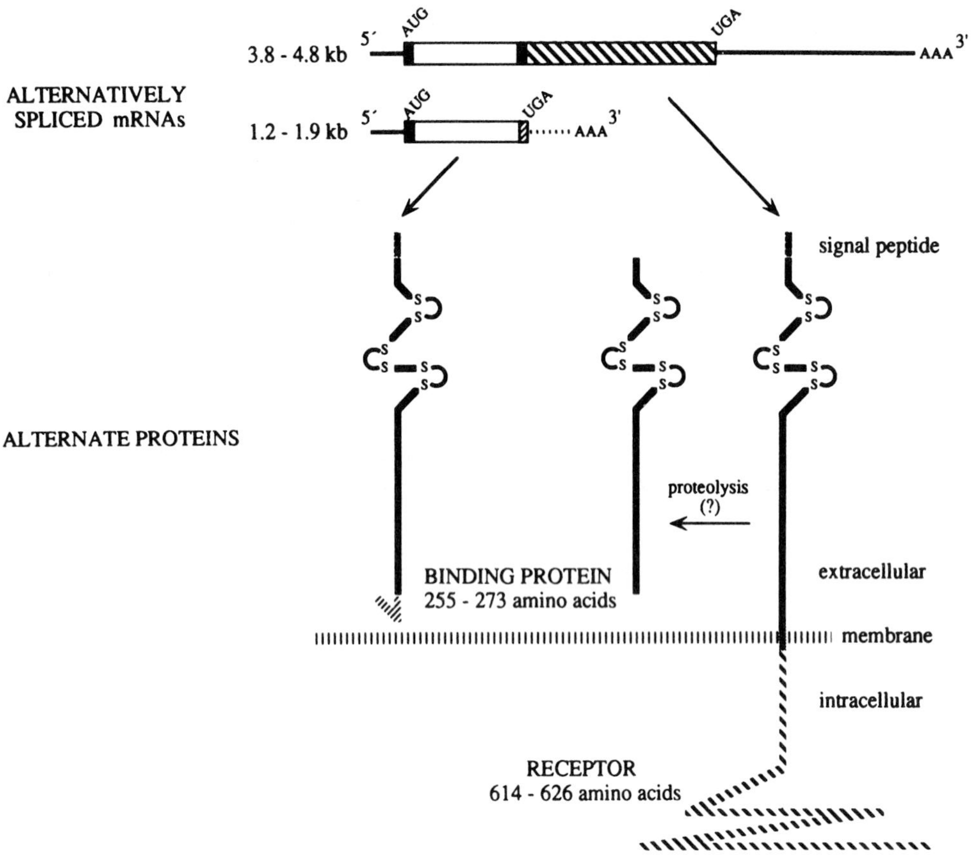

FIGURE 25-10. Schematic representation of GH receptor mRNAs and the GH receptor. Circulating GH binding protein is derived from either alternative splicing of the GH receptor mRNA as shown or from proteolytic cleavage of the extracellular domain of the GH receptor. The GH receptor consists of an extracellular domain, a membrane-spanning domain, and an intracellular domain. (*From Matthews.*[83])

proteins that contain domains that bind to phosphorylated tyrosines with high affinity (e.g., SH2, etc.). Binding of these signaling proteins to the phosphorylated tyrosines permits the following: (1) activation of the signaling proteins (P13 and SHP2), (2) translocation of the signaling protein to a site that allows it to be phosphorylated and activated by JAK2 (e.g., Stat proteins), and (3) recruitment of signaling molecules (e.g., Shc-Grb2-SOS) that initiate a variety of cellular responses. The activated pathways include (1) Stat proteins (1, 3, and 5), which appear to regulate GH-responsive genes (e.g., Spi 2.1 and c-fos), (2) IRS proteins (including IRSI and IRS2), which activate PI3 kinase, most likely SHP2, and initiate metabolic and nuclear events, and (3) the RAS-MAP pathway, which appears to regulate gene transcription and metabolic actions. All of the pathways activated by GH are also used by many cytokines that activate JAK kinases. Specificity of response likely depends on multiple factors, i.e., essential differences in receptor expression, availability of JAK kinases, differences in response kinetics, variability of high-affinity binding sites for signaling molecules, individual differences in the cellular environment after receptor activation, and intricate regulatory mechanisms of each of the signaling pathways.

GHBP is the extracellular domain of the GHR; it serves to prolong the half-life of GH and modulates GH binding to the GHR. In most children with GH resistance (Laron Syndrome), the levels are very low; hence, GHBP levels provide information about the GHR. In a minority of subjects with GH resistance, GHBP levels may be normal if the GHR mutation is located in the intracellular domain. The levels of GHBP are lowest in the young rapidly growing child. Subsequently, the levels rise in childhood and plateau in puberty and adulthood. In addition to GH resistance, low GHBP levels are seen in patients with malnutrition, diabetes mellitus, hypothyroidism, and chronic liver disease. Elevated GHBP levels occur in obesity, early pregnancy, and with estrogen treatment. The ligand-mediated immunofunctional assay (LIFA) is the most accurate method for quantitating GHBP.

TABLE 25-1. Metabolic Effects of Growth Hormone

Increases DNA, RNA, protein synthesis; mitosis; sulfate incorporation
Lowers urinary nitrogen concentration and blood urea nitrogen
Raises urinary hydroxyproline cencentration
Fat: stimulates lipolysis, liberates free fatty acids
Carbohydrate
Early: insulin-like effect
Late: insulin antagonism
Prolonged GH excess causes carbohydrate intolerance and diabetes mellitus
Mineral: decreases urinary phosphorus excretion, increases urinary calcium excretion
Electrolyte: permits retention of potassium, sodium, chloride, and magnesium

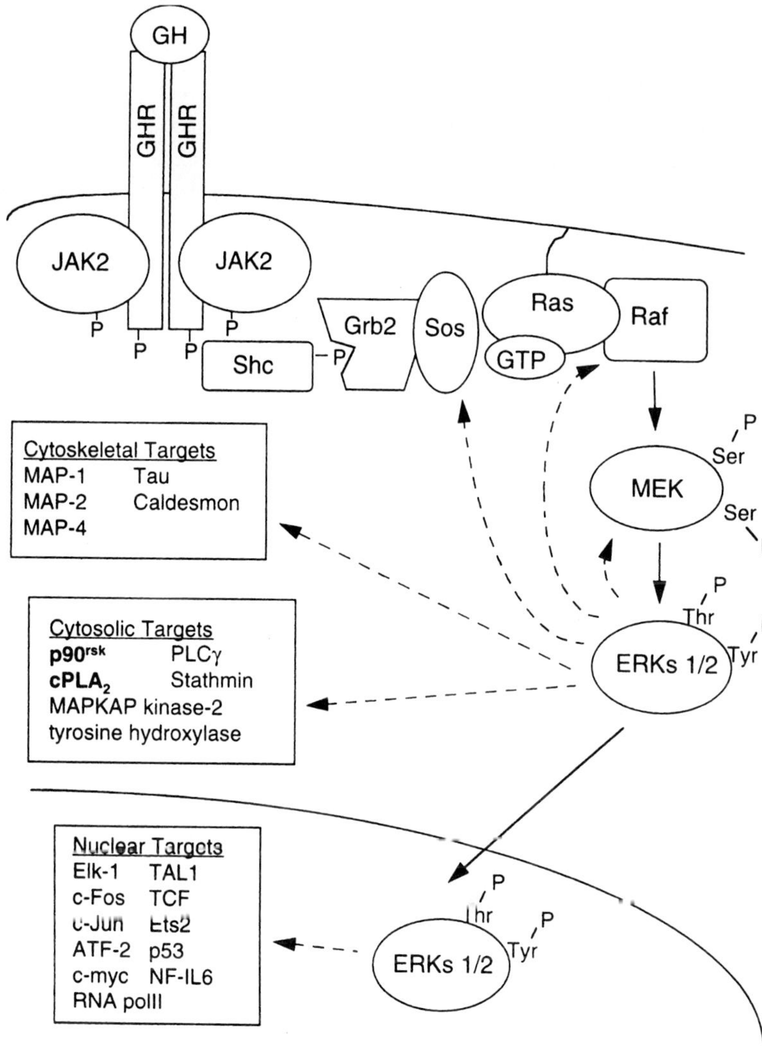

FIGURE 25-11. Growth hormone receptor (GHR) signaling via the MAP kinase ERKs 1 and 2. A signaling cascade leading from GHR to the MAP kinase and activation of subsequent targets is shown. Pathways and proteins regulated by GH are depicted by solid arrows and signaling molecules and by bolded targets. The dotted arrows and the targets in plain text have not been shown to be involved in GH signal transduction but are utilized in cells treated with other cytokines. (*From Carter-Su.*[87])

Thyroid Hormone

Thyroid hormone by itself does not fulfill the criteria needed to classify it as a true growth-promoting hormone because it is unable to stimulate cellular multiplication in the absence of GH. Nevertheless, the importance of the synergism between these hormones has been demonstrated in studies which showed that maximal GH stimulation of tissues requires the presence of T_4. Furthermore, primary hypothyroidism causes a reduction in both the number of somatotrophs and the GH content of the anterior pituitary; it also leads to GH unresponsiveness to stimulation by insulin hypoglycemia or L-arginine. The growth spurt that follows thyroid replacement therapy is accompanied by a return of normal pituitary gland GH content and response to stimuli.

It has been suggested that during fetal life, somatic growth is not dependent on T_4 because infants with congenital hypothyroidism due to thyroid dysfunction or pituitary-hypothalamic disorders are of normal body size at birth. This conclusion requires reexamination, as a majority of congenitally hypothyroid infants have lingual or hypoplastic thyroid glands and those with anencephaly or other types of hypopituitarism have variable degrees of thyroid function. Evidence that thyroid hormone may influence fetal somatic growth is derived from experiments documenting that growth in three animal species (rat, sheep, and monkey) is impaired after fetal thyroidectomy.[88]

In contrast to the uncertainties about the role of T_4 in fetal somatic growth, it is evident that T_4 is essential for normal brain development, specifically neuronal and neuroglial cell growth in the cerebrum and cerebellum, nerve terminal maturation, axonal and dendritic proliferation, and normal myelinization. Studies suggest that T_4 increases the production of nerve growth factor, which stimulates axon outgrowth and increased neuron cell size and plays a crucial role in the development and survival of sympathetic and sensory neurons. If these data are confirmed, thyroid hormone may have an indirect rather than a direct influence on brain development.[89]

Acquired hypothyroidism in childhood usually delays puberty, but rarely, a child exhibits precocious sexual development, ovarian cysts, galactorrhea, diabetes insipidus, and a large sella without bony erosion; all these abnormalities regress with thyroid replacement.

Gonadal Steroids: Androgens, Estrogens, and the Pubertal Growth Spurt

The growth spurt of puberty is dependent mainly on gonadal steroids and GH; adrenal steroids are probably not essential.

Studies indicate that males experience rapid growth during puberty because of sex steroid–mediated enhancement of GH secretion; this in turn stimulates increased production of IGF-I and accounts for the elevated levels observed in adolescence.[38,39,90] Growth rates in males with isolated GH deficiency do not accelerate sufficiently during puberty, yet osseous maturation progresses and epiphyseal fusion occurs. Consequently, their adult height is compromised. Treatment of these individuals with GH during puberty is essential. Normal thyroid function is a fundamental requirement of the pubertal growth process. Hypothyroid children usually have delayed adolescence; those who experience puberty do not exhibit a growth spurt.

The precise mechanisms that control the onset of puberty have not been fully defined. In human and nonhuman primates, the pituitary gland releases increased quantities of FSH and LH at three periods of life: during fetal life, during the first 6 months of infancy, and during adolescence and adulthood. Suppression of gonadotropin production during the decade of "childhood," between infancy and adolescence, has been attributed to two mechanisms: (1) intrinsic CNS inhibitory influences operating independently of sex steroids (this accounts for the diphasic pattern of gonadotropin secretion seen during childhood in patients with gonadal dysgenesis) and (2) increased sensitivity of the hypothalamic-pituitary regulatory centers (the "gonadostat") to the negative feedback effects of low childhood levels of gonadal steroids.[91] Coincident with the onset of puberty, the arcuate nucleus of the hypothalamus becomes progressively less sensitive to the inhibitory effects of the sex steroids and the intrinsic CNS inhibitory influences gradually are suppressed. Removal of these restraints on gonadotropin releasing hormone (GnRH) secretion allows the pulsatile production of GnRH in increasing amounts, which in turn stimulates augmented secretion of pituitary gonadotropins.[91–96] A model of the mechanisms that control gonadal sex steroid production is shown in Fig. 25-12.

Two separate processes—*gonadarche* and *adrenarche*—account for the increased production of sex steroids in the peripubertal and pubertal periods. Gonadarche, the final activation and maturation of the hypothalamic-pituitary-gonadal axis, is the sine qua non of puberty. It is responsible for the adolescent growth spurt, development of secondary sexual characteristics, and eventual attainment of fertility. Adrenarche signifies increased androgen production from the zona reticularis of the adrenal gland; it occurs about 2 years before gonadarche. Serum concentration of dehydroepiandrosterone (DHEA) usually begins to increase by 8 years of age in boys and girls; this serves as a biochemical marker of adrenal androgenesis. The temporal relation between adrenarche and gonadarche initially suggested that adrenal androgen may have a regulatory influence on the timing of puberty. However, it is now evident that adrenarche is not essential for the onset of gonadarche and that the two events are independent processes. The mechanisms responsible for adrenarche have not been fully defined; hypotheses include (1) an intrinsic alteration in the activity of the enzymes involved in adrenal androgen synthesis (*"escalator" theory*), (2) the production of a pituitary androgen stimulating hormone (ASH), although as ASH has yet to be isolated (*zonal theory*), and (3) an extrapituitary stimulating factor such as estrogen.[91,97] The role of adrenal androgens in puberty is not clearly understood aside from the stimulation of sexual hair growth in females.

During puberty the Leydig cells of the testes secrete increasing amounts of testosterone, which circulates either bound to protein (i.e., sex hormone–binding globulin, SHBG) or in a biologically

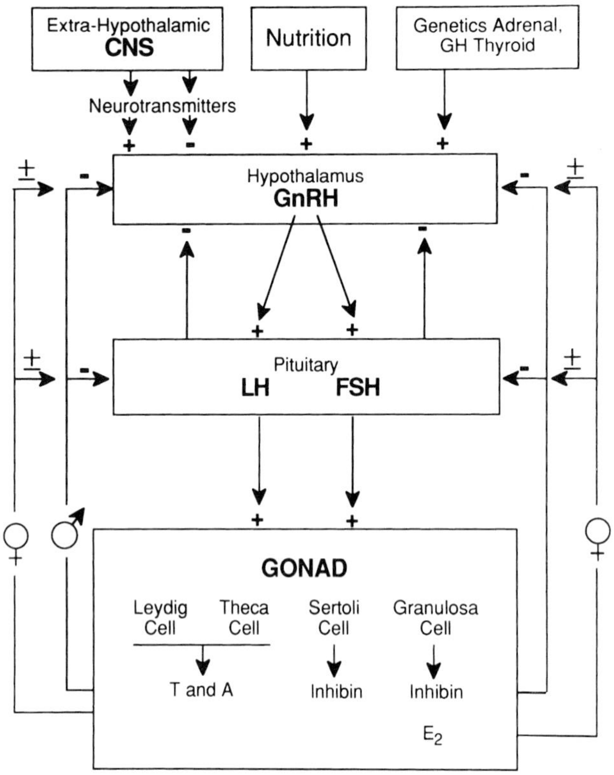

FIGURE 25-12. Schematic representation of the CNS-hypothalamic-pituitary-gonadal axis in males and females. Stimulatory effects are represented by +, and inhibition is shown by −. Gonadotropin releasing hormone (GnRH) stimulates secretion of luteinizing hormone (LH) and follicle stimulating hormone (FSH), which have negative feedback effects on GnRH via a short-loop mechanism. In males, LH stimulates the Leydig cells to produce testosterone (T) and androstenedione (A), which inhibit hypothalamic and pituitary production of GnRH and LH, respectively. In females, LH stimulates the production of testosterone and androstenedione from the theca and interstitial cells. The granulosa cells aromatize these androgens to form E_2, which has a biphasic effect on the mature female pituitary-hypothalamic centers. Testosterone appears to exert a minor influence on female gonadotropin production. FSH stimulation of inhibin production by Sertoli's cells in males and granulosa cells in females results in a suppression of FSH production. In females, FSH stimulates E_2 production by granulosa cells. In the preantral follicle, theca cells with LH receptors encircle granulosa cells with FSH receptors. LH stimulates theca cell development and enhances 17α-hydroxylase activity and lyase activity, which are necessary for androgen production; the latter becomes the substrate for E_2 production in granulosa cells. The rising E_2 levels in the late follicular phase augment LH responsiveness to (GnRH), which causes further androgen production by the theca cells. Early in the gonadotropin surge, FSH induces LH receptors on the granulosa cells, which have been primed by E_2; with luteinization of the granulosa cell, progesterone and E_2 production is enhanced by LH as well as FSH. The increasing progesterone production synergizes with the rising E_2 production to stimulate a further surge in pituitary gonadotropin production, leading to ovulation.

active free form. Testosterone stimulation of DNA, RNA, and protein synthesis and cell mitosis requires the entrance of free hormone into the cytoplasm of androgen-sensitive cells, where it is metabolized to either 5α- or 5β-dihydrotestosterone (DHT) by 5α- or 5β-reductase. Both testosterone and DHT form complexes with the cytoplasmic receptor that enter the nucleus. There they interact with nuclear acceptor sites and stimulate cellular multiplication. In adult males and females, DHT is not present in skeletal muscle. It thus appears that testosterone may directly promote muscular growth during sexual maturation.[98–100]

During early fetal life in males, conversion of testosterone to DHT via the action of 5α-reductase in the external genital tissues is essential for the complete sexual differentiation of the external genitalia. The wolffian duct system develops normally in XY individuals who lack 5α-reductase. Therefore, it can be concluded that the internal genital duct system is testosterone- rather than DHT-dependent. During adolescence, XY subjects with 5α-reductase deficiency develop muscular, virile physiques even though they were phenotypic females during their prepubertal years.[100]

Our understanding of the actions of androgens on skeletal growth and epiphyseal maturation has been revolutionized by the pivotal studies of patients with homozygous mutations in the genes for the aromatase enzyme and the estrogen receptor. Men with profound estrogen deficiency due either to absence of the aromatase enzyme or to estrogen resistance do not fuse their epiphyses and continue to grow into the third decade. Adult heights far exceed genetic target height. Increased bone turnover, osteoporosis, joint pains, and skeletal deformities are the major abnormalities even though these men have androgen levels that are normal or above normal. There appears to be an absence or blunting of the male pubertal growth spurt. High gonadotropins, insulin resistance, and lipid derangements are other features. These findings suggest that estrogen, not androgen, controls the integrity of bone, the pubertal growth spurt, and epiphyseal fusion. Also, estrogen influences the regulation of gonadotropins, insulin action, and lipid homeostasis. Pubertal growth also requires augmented GH because patients with isolated GH deficiency grow suboptimally during puberty.[101–113]

The preceding discussion applies also to the female adolescent growth spurt. Estrogen production in females as well as males depends entirely on the conversion of androgens to estrogens by the aromatase enzyme. Females lacking aromatase in utero will experience fetal virilization of the external genitalia because the high levels of fetal and placental androgens are not aromatized to estrogens. Their mothers also became transiently virilized during pregnancy. When these girls enter puberty, aromatase deficiency causes them to develop hirsutism and clitoromegaly. They also have osteoporosis and absence of a growth spurt and fail to develop breasts and menstruation. Their epiphyses remain unfused.[101–106] Whether estrogens are the only sex steroids that are totally responsible for the growth spurt is uncertain. In females, the onset of the adolescent growth spurt coincides with breast development and ovarian production of estrogens. The magnitude of the growth spurt is less than in males. Estrogens increase the width of the pelvic bones and hips, which are characteristic features of sexually mature women. Increased adiposity, weight gain, and pace of bone maturation in pubertal girls are estrogen-mediated.

Nutrition

The rate of growth and sexual maturation in children is influenced by their nutritional state. Frisch and McArthur have proposed that the onset of menses in healthy girls occurs at a critical weight that approximates the 10th percentile. Improved nutrition and freedom from chronic infections are factors that have contributed to the taller stature and earlier puberty of European and American children. In countries where malnutrition is prevalent, poor linear growth and delayed adolescence are common. In this country, anorexia nervosa, chronic disease, and malnutrition slow growth by causing negative energy balance and suppression of gonadotropins and IGF-I production. Recommended nutrient intake based on age are given in Table 25-2.

TABLE 25-2. Daily Requirement of Nutrients

	Energy, kcal	Protein, g
Infants		
<6 months	117 × kg	2.2
6–12 months	108 × kg	2.0
Children		
1–3 years	1,360	16
4–6 years	1,830	20
7–9 years	2,190	25
Male adolescents		
10–12 years	2,600	30
13–15 years	2,900	37
16–19 years	3,070	38
Female adolescents		
10–12 years	2,350	29
13–15 years	2,490	31
16–19 years	2,310	30

Source: *WHO Monograph Series*, no. 61, 1974.

PHYSIOLOGY OF SKELETAL GROWTH

In long bones, growth occurs at the cartilaginous growth plate, which is organized into three functionally and structurally distinct layers: (1) the resting zone nearest the epiphysis where rarely dividing chondrocytes are arranged irregularly in a bed of cartilage matrix, (2) the proliferative zone nearer the metaphysis where the chondrocytes show a flatter shape and are arranged in columns parallel to the long axis of bone, daughter cells from proliferative zone chondrocytes line up along the long axis of bone, and (3) the hypertrophic zone, where the proliferative zone chondrocytes farthest from the epiphysis stop replicating and become the terminally differentiated hypertrophic chrondrocytes. These terminally differentiated cells form a layer adjacent to the metaphysis. The mechanism of endochondral ossification involves a two-step process of chondrogenesis and ossification, which are tightly coupled to keep the growth plate width constant while new bone is formed at the junction of the growth plate and the metaphyseal bone. Chondrogenesis (i.e., new cartilage formation) involves growth plate chondrocyte proliferation, hypertrophy, and extracellular matrix secretion (consisting of type 2 collagen, mucopolysaccharides, and core proteins). Ossification depends on blood vessels and bone cell precursors from the metaphysis invading the growth plate and remodeling newly-formed cartilage into bone. The rate of bone growth is determined by chondrogenesis.[114] The growth plate exhibits spatial polarities in that the proliferative chondrocytes undergo terminal differentiation near the metaphyseal but not near the epiphyseal border of the growth plate. Metaphyseal but not epiphyseal blood vessels invade the growth plate, remodeling it into bone. Consequently, the metaphysis but not the epiphysis elongates as growth ensues. When rabbit distal ulnar growth plates were inverted in their original beds, blood vessel and bone cell invasion ceased in the metaphysis and arose in the epiphysis. Longitudinal bone growth also occurred in the epiphyseal but not the metaphyseal surface of the growth plate. These findings indicate that intrinsic factors control the polarity of the growth plate which in turn, controls the polarity of adjacent longitudinal bone. Fibroblast growth factors (FGFs) and their receptors (FGFRs) negatively regulate longitudinal bone growth. Activating FGFR 3 mutations impair growth causing skeletal dysplasias (e.g., achondroplasia and hypochondroplasia). Inactivating FGFR 3 mutations stimulate growth. FGF 2 infusions have paradoxical effects; stimulatory at low dose and inhibitory at high dose.[115,116]

Endochondrial ossification is hormonally controlled. An excess of glucocorticoids disturbs the protein matrix and causes osteoporosis. Vitamin D deficiency or PTH excess leads to abnormalities in mineralization and osteomalacia. Bone width is determined by the thickness of the diaphyseal cortex, which is formed by membranous ossification directly from the periosteum.

The fetus develops primary centers of ossification in the cartilaginous anlage of long bones at 7 weeks. By the third fetal month, the process of ossification extends to the metaphyses and the growth plate begins to contain chondrocytes. In early fetal life, the epiphyseal ends of long bones exist mainly as cartilage. Later in gestation, secondary centers of ossification convert the cartilaginous epiphyses to bone. Bone age or biological age is defined by the size and appearance of these secondary centers of epiphyseal ossification.

Osteocalcin (bone Gla protein), which is secreted by osteoblasts, is an important noncollagenous protein that is contained in the bone matrix and also circulates in blood. The serum concentration is believed to reflect the rate of bone formation and osteoblast activity. In healthy children, osteocalcin levels vary with age and sex and parallel the growth velocity curve. A sharp increase in serum osteocalcin concentrations occurs during the growth spurt of normal as well as precocious puberty. Growth hormone–deficient children have low serum levels of osteocalcin which rise after GH therapy. Presumably, GH therapy stimulates IGF-I production in bone, increasing the number of functional osteoblasts as well as bone mineralization. Osteocalcin levels are reliable biochemical markers of altered bone metabolism. Levels are low in patients with type I diabetes mellitus and in children receiving glucocorticoid therapy. The rise in serum osteocalcin after GH therapy correlates with the linear growth response and may predict which children are likely to benefit from GH administration.

DEVELOPMENTAL STAGES

Intrauterine Life

The initial growth period of the fetus is one of rapid cellular generation, differentiation, and organogenesis. During this embryonic period, the fetus grows primarily by a process of cellular multiplication. Extraordinary linear growth rates are observed during fetal life. Peak velocities of 10 to 11 cm/month occur at 4 to 5 months gestation; the growth rate gradually declines during the last trimester as uterine constraints become a limiting force. However, even this growth rate is spectacular: 2 cm/month (Fig. 25-13). In the last trimester, adipose tissue is formed at an increasing rate; fetal weight doubles during the last 2 months of pregnancy.

The size of a full-term newborn is mainly dependent on the size of the mother, not the father. In controlled animal studies, the offspring of large mothers and small fathers are larger than the products of matings between small mothers and large fathers.[117]

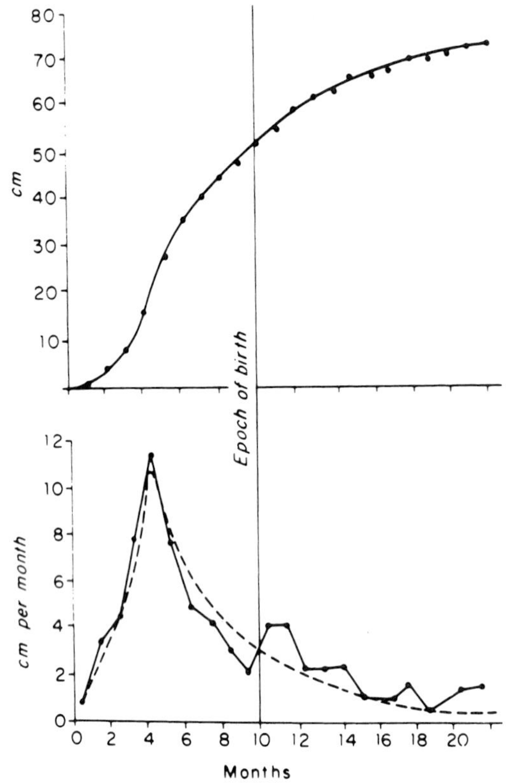

FIGURE 25-13. Linear growth by lunar months during fetal life and in the first postnatal year. The slowing of the late fetal growth rate is compatible with the concept of constraints to growth by the uterus and is followed postnatally by a brief period of accelerated "catch-up" growth. (*From Smith.*[118])

This observation indicates that lifelong adequate nutrition is essential for girls in order to enhance their adult height and the size of their offspring.

An additional factor that influences fetal growth is uterine size in the late gestational period. In women with twins or triplets, uterine constraints may limit fetal size.

The placenta is yet another determinant of fetal growth and well-being because it is the portal for the delivery of nutrients and the removal of metabolic wastes. The placenta is a fetal organ that grows by cellular multiplication until the 35th week of gestation. Thereafter, it enlarges by cellular hypertrophy until full size is achieved at the 38th to 40th week. Any disturbance of early placental growth due to embryologic abnormalities, infections, or vascular insults may cause permanent growth retardation.[1]

Gender plays a minor role in determining fetal growth rate. Males grow faster after 32 weeks gestation and at birth are more muscular and have less adipose tissue than females. Newborn boys have a slightly larger head circumference and are, on average, 0.9 cm longer and 150 g heavier than girls.[118] However, osseous maturation is more rapid in girls than in boys after 30 weeks gestation. At birth, bone age in females is 2 weeks ahead of that in males; by 1 year, this difference has increased to 8 weeks.

Infancy: Birth to 2 Years of Age

In the first year of life, linear growth and weight gain continue at a rate that is still remarkable although less spectacular than during

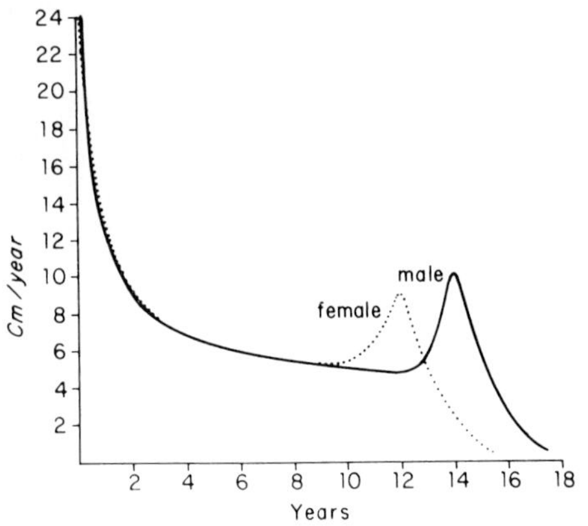

FIGURE 25-14. Velocity curves for length (<2 years) and height (2 to 18 years) for females and males show deceleration of the growth rate from infancy until the onset of adolescence. (*From Smith*[118] *and Tanner et al.*[127])

fetal life. The fastest gains in length occur in the first months after birth, when uterine constraints are no longer present. By 1 year, the infant has accumulated generous stores of adipose tissue, has tripled its birth weight, and has grown 25 additional cm (an increase of 50 percent of birth length). Male infants continue to grow slightly faster in length, weight, and head circumference during the first 3 to 6 months after birth. These phenomena have been attributed to increased testosterone production in males, which gradually diminishes by 6 months of postnatal age.[119] In the second year, there is continued deceleration of linear growth rates. By the age of 2 years, linear growth has stabilized at a rate that is characteristic of the childhood years (Fig. 25-13).

Childhood

The period of childhood, which extends from age 2 years to the onset of puberty, is characterized by relatively stable rates of gain in height (5 to 7.5 cm/year) and weight (2 to 2.5 kg/year). Throughout these years, there is a slight deceleration in the linear growth rate (Fig. 25-14) and an acceleration in weight gain (Fig. 25-15). The major period of brain growth has already been completed, and cellular multiplication in the musculoskeletal and adipose systems continues at a slower pace than is evident during infancy or adolescence. In the years before puberty, there is an increased gain in adipose tissue. During this period, lymphoid tissue reaches its maximum size relative to body size.

FIGURE 25-15. Growth velocity curves for females and males show gradual increases in rates of weight gain from 2 years until adolescence. (*From Smith*[118] *and Tanner et al.*[127])

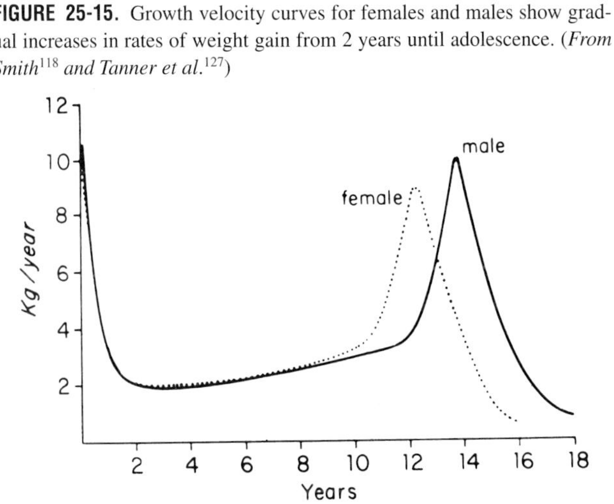

Adolescence

Adolescence is the last period of major growth. During this period, there is attainment of adult stature, sexual maturation, and reproductive function.

Among healthy children, chronologic age at the onset of puberty and the rate of sexual maturation are highly variable. These differences are largely dependent on genetic factors. The individual's sex also plays a role; the average girl enters and completes pubertal development 1 to 2 years ahead of the average boy. The most accurate criterion for the assessment of adolescence is not chronologic age but the individual's biological age (bone age) and physical stage of sexual maturation, based on Tanner's criteria.[120]

The sequence of physiologic and hormonal events during adolescence in girls is shown in Fig. 25-16. The first signs of puberty in females are the appearance of breast buds and the beginning of the adolescent growth spurt; for the average girl, these events occur at 11 years of age. They are followed by the appearance of pubic hair at 11.5 years, peak growth rates (approximately 9 cm/year) at 12 years, the appearance of axillary hair at 12.5 to 13 years, and menarche at 12.5 years. Almost invariably, menarche occurs after the attainment of peak growth velocity. Slower rates of linear growth continue after menarche until age 16 to 17 years, when epiphyseal fusion occurs; this information has relevance to the management of girls who are concerned about genetic tall stature. Adolescence in females is also associated with widening hips due to fat deposition and a general increase in body adipose tissue. The normal ranges in chronologic age for each pubertal event in girls are listed in Table 25-3.

In boys, the first signs of adolescence are axillary sweat, body odor, testicular enlargement, and thinning of the scrotal skin. The average boy gains 25 cm and 20 kg during adolescence.[120] FSH is primarily responsible for growth of the seminiferous tubules and thus for increments in testes size in addition to sperm development. LH is the regulator of androgen, primarily testosterone, production by the Leydig cells. Evidence suggests that optimal sexual maturation depends on the interaction of FSH and LH in the testes.[96]

The sequence of physiologic events and their relation to the hormonal changes in adolescent boys are depicted in Fig. 25-17. Unlike girls, who simultaneously exhibit increased growth velocity and breast buds at the outset of puberty, boys begin their growth spurt approximately 1 year after the first signs of testicular enlargement and achieve greater peak rates of linear growth (mean 10.3 cm/year) at age 14, compared to age 12 in girls. The male adolescent growth spurt is largely due to the increased secretion of sex steroids, which enhances the production of GH. Deficiencies of either of these hormones or a lack of T_4 will impair the adolescent growth spurt. Males achieve greater growth velocities, muscular development, and statural height than do females because of augmented androgen production. The essential roles of the aromatase enzyme, estrogens, and the estrogen receptor were previously discussed.

In the average male, testicular size increases at age 12 years. This is followed 1 year later by the onset of penis enlargement.

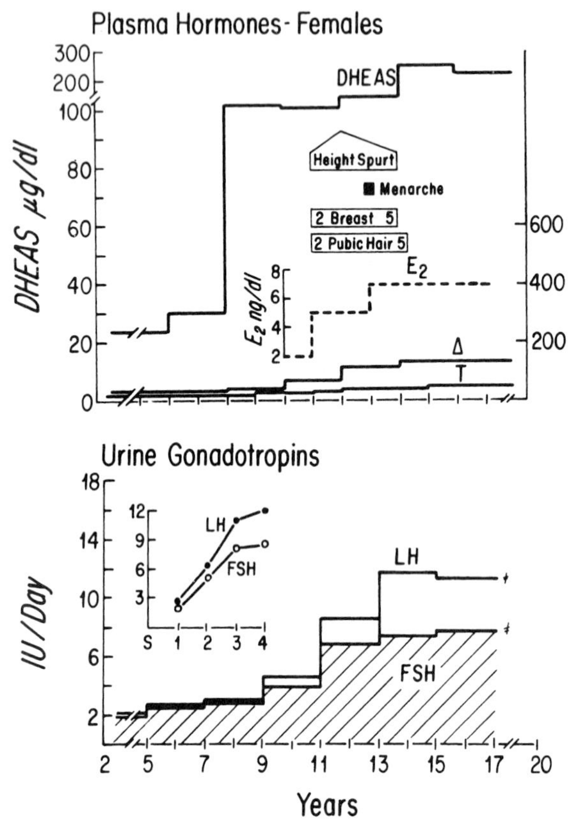

	FSH Excretion, IU/day	LH Excretion, IU/day
S1 (completely prepubertal, t1)	1–5	1–5
S2 (only breast tissue, t2 or t3)	4–9	4–9
S3 (breasts and sexual hair, t3 to t4)	5–11	6–16
S4 adult breasts and hair, t4 to t5)	5–12	7–28
Midcycle peak	39–49	108–122

Not shown in the diagram is the sleep-associated increase in LH secretion during early and midpuberty. (*Tanner criteria from Tanner*[95]; *hormonal events of puberty from Grumbach et al,*[81] *Kelch et al,*[86] *Penny et al.*[196])

FIGURE 25-16. Relation between the stages of pubertal development in girls based on Tanner (t) criteria and the hormonal events of puberty. Increased plasma levels of DHEA sulfate from the adrenal gland (adrenarche) are detected before increased secretion of gonadotropins or gonadal steroids (gonadarche). E_2 = estradiol, Δ = androstenedione, T = testosterone. Based on chronologic age, urinary gonadotropin levels appear to increase before the average age of breast development. However, when urinary gonadotropin excretion is based on stage of sexual maturation (S), a positive correlation exists with stages 2 and 3.

The first ejaculation of seminal fluid and nocturnal emissions occur at approximately 14 years of age. Pubic hair growth begins at approximately 12.5 to 13 years; the first signs of axillary and facial hair occur 2 years later (i.e., 14.5 to 15 years). Acne and apocrine sweat are characteristic features of adolescence. The male physique undergoes striking changes as a result of androgen action: shoulder width increases, facial bone structure enlarges, vocal cords expand to deepen the voice, muscle cell number doubles, and muscle mass and strength show striking gains. Early developers are athletically superior with regard to strength and coordination compared to late developers. However, the later onset of adolescence may contribute to the tall stature seen in some adult males.[120]

TABLE 25-3. Range of Chronologic Ages for Pubertal Events in Healthy Girls

Event	Age, Years: Onset	Completion
Height spurt	9½–14½	12–17½
Breast bud*	8–13	10½–16
Pubic hair	8–14	11–17½
Menarche	10–16	

*Asymmetry when breast = Tanner 5; will not resolve spontaneously: Nine to 16 years in other series.

Source: Based on Tanner.

Approximately one-half of boys develop a small amount of breast tissue (2 to 3 cm in diameter) midway through adolescence. Usually this lasts for 12 to 18 months and resolves completely. Progressive breast enlargement over a period of 1 to 2 years is not likely to resolve spontaneously, and mastectomy via a periareolar incision should be considered before excessive stretching of breast skin occurs. In most instances, these boys have idiopathic gynecomastia. However, the possibility of Klinefelter's syndrome, true hermaphroditism, choriocarcinoma, or estrogen-producing lesions must be considered.

Adult height in males is usually attained by age 18. Growth cessation occurs first in the hands and feet, followed by the legs, trunk, and shoulder girdle. The ranges in age for the events of male adolescence are shown in Table 25-4.

SHORT STATURE

Clinical Approach to Short Stature

It is important to emphasize that many healthy children who are growing along a normal lower growth channel (3rd to 10th percentile) and whose size is compatible with their genetic endowment have innocent short stature that requires reassurance but no medical treatment.

The care of children with short stature has become controversial because questions have been raised about the validity of the traditional GH provocative tests and because more physicians are willing to prescribe GH treatment for "short children" because they believe that such therapy has long-term benefits. Also, some of the current disagreement is due to confusion about the precise meaning of the term *short stature* when it is applied to heterogeneous populations of children receiving empiric GH treatment.

The problem with nomenclature arose when the term *short stature* was used increasingly to describe children with pathologic heights or growth rates when in fact they could be described more accurately as having growth failure. Examples of the innocent-sounding terminology that was used to describe these children in-

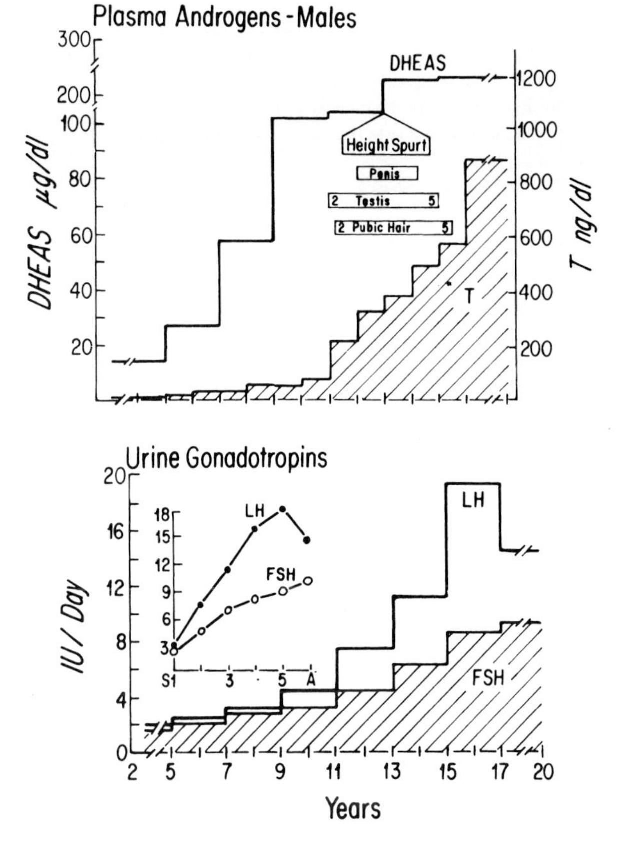

	FSH Excretion, IU/day	LH Excretion, IU/day
S1 (prepubertal)	0.5–5	0.5–6
S2 (testes ⩾ 2 cm, scrotal changes)	2–9	2–13
S3 (penis > 7 cm)	3–12	5–23
S4 (further penis and testes growth)	3–14	9–29
S5 (prostate palpable, sexual hair)	5–16	9–39
SA [adult testes (> 4cm) and penis (> 13 cm stretched)]	5–16	8–24

Sleep-associated increases in LH secretion have been documented in early and midpuberty. After adolescence, daytime and nighttime excretion of LH are equal. (*From Grumbach et al,*[81] *Tanner,*[95] *Reiter et al*[95] *Penny et al.*[197])

FIGURE 25-17. Relation between the stages of pubertal development in boys and the hormonal events during adolescence. As noted in girls, DHEA sulfate levels are increased before any evidence of sexual maturation. Based on chronologic age, increased gonadotropin excretion appears to precede the onset of testicular enlargement. However, when gonadotropin excretion is related to stages of sexual maturation (S), there is a positive correlation between increased gonadotropin output and stages 2, 3, and 4. Positive correlations also exist for increases in LH excretion, testes enlargement, and testosterone concentration (T).

TABLE 25-4. Range of Chronologic Ages for Pubertal Events in Healthy Boys

	Age, Years	
Event	**Onset**	**Completion**
Testes enlargement	10–13½	14½–18
Height spurt	10½–16	2½–3*
Penis enlargement	11–14½	13½–17
Pubic hair	10–15	14–18

* Years after onset.

Source: Based on Tanner.

clude normal variant short stature (NVSS), idiopathic short stature (ISS), and constitutional short stature (CSS).[122–124]

Most physicians try to avoid using stigmatizing names for children with growth problems. Therefore, terms such as *dwarf* and *midget* are seldom used now. However, there is a clear need for language that conveys whether a child has innocent short stature in contrast to growth failure due to an idiopathic cause or other entity.

The following is a practical approach to the management of children with a growth disorder. There is general agreement that an abnormally low growth rate for chronologic age with abnormal or normal height is a warning sign of growth failure which requires investigation. When first seen, children whose heights are 2 to 3 SD below the mean should be remeasured at 6-month intervals to determine the growth velocity. If it is pathologic for chronologic age, the child should be thoroughly evaluated. Children with more severe growth failure (i.e., height more than 3 SD below the mean and abnormal or normal growth velocity) require prompt and thorough investigation. The causes of short stature and growth failure are shown in Table 25-5.

Before the first examination, it is advisable to ask parents to send in previous heights and weights obtained from school health records, personal physicians, or clinics. Annual school photographs are particularly valuable in growth problems that are associated with changing facial appearance, e.g., hypothyroidism and Cushing's syndrome. The initial medical evaluation involves taking the patient's history and performing a physical examination and laboratory and radiographic studies.

History

A complete history includes details of the child's health from conception to the time of examination; specifics of maternal health, including drug use and diseases before and during the pregnancy; information on height, weight, rate of maturation, and health of family members; and assessment of emotional stresses within the family. Questions should focus on the presence and location of headaches, visual problems, frequency of respiratory or other infections, presence of chronic disease, use of medications, character of stools, frequency of urination, and details of nutritional intake.

Physical Examination

A thorough examination either indicates excellent health or provides clues to an endocrinopathy or an underlying chronic disease in a major organ (GI tract, kidney, heart, lungs, or CNS) or stigmata of one of the many growth-deficiency syndromes.[125] Malnutrition due to inadequate food intake, malabsorption, or underlying chronic disease tends to disturb weight gain more severely than it affects linear growth.

TABLE 25-5. Differential Diagnosis of Short Stature

- Causes of normal short stature
  - Genetic or familial short stature
  - Constitutional delay with or without delayed adolescence
  - Genetic short stature
- Pathologic growth
  - Intrauterine disturbances
  - Placental dysfunction
    - *Maternal factors*
      - Malnutrition
      - Diseases
      - Drug use
    - *Fetal disease*
      - Infections
      - Congenital abnormalities
      - Chromosomal abnormalities
  - Premature delivery
  - Genetic syndromes: Bloom, Hallerman-Streiff-François Russell-Silver, Seckel's, Donahue's, Dubowitz, progeria, DeLange's, Williams
  - Postnatal malnutrition
    - Poverty, ignorance neglect
    - Mechanical gastrointestinal disorders
      - Esophageal stenosis, web, reflux,
      - Pyloric stenosis
      - Duodenal atresia, stenosis, bands, annular pancreas
      - Malrotation, volvulus
      - Foreign body
      - Aganglionosis (Hirschsprung's)
      - Short bowel syndrome
  - Digestive diseases
    - Enzyme deficiencies
      - Proteolytic enzymes: trypsin, cystic fibrosis
      - Disaccharidases: sucrase, isomaltase, lactase α-antitrypsin: liver cirrhosis
    - Intolerance: milk protein allergy
  - Chronic infection: *Escherichia coli*, salmonella, Giardiasis, shigella, staphylococcus, etc.
  - Inflammatory bowel disease: ulcerative colitis Granulomatous ileocolitis
  - Tumor: neural crest tumors
  - Miscellaneous: celiac disease, gluten sensitivity, immunologic disorders, acrodermatitis
  - Endocrine Causes
    - Hypothyroidism: congenital or acquired: primary, secondary (TSH) or tertiary (TRH)
    - GH deficiency (also assess anterior pituitary function: TSH, ACTH, prolactin, FSH-LH) (see Table 25-13)
    - Cushing's syndrome: glucocorticoid excess
    - Short adult stature due to precocious sexual maturation
  - Metabolic disorders
    - Glycogen storage disease
    - Cystinosis
    - Fructose intolerance
    - Galactosemia
    - Mucopolysaccharidoses
    - Diabetes insipidus: vasopressin-resistant Vasopressin-sensitive
  - Bone disorders (skeletal dysplasias)
    - Chondrodystrophies: achondroplasia hypochondroplasia
    - Rickets: hypophosphatemia, vitamin D deficiency or resistance
    - Epiphyseal dysplasia
    - Metaphyseal dysplasia
    - Spondyloepiphyseal dysplasia
    - Osteogenesis imperfecta
    - Multiple exostoses syndrome
  - Chromosome abnormalities
    - X chromosome abnormalities: gonadal dysgenesis Turner syndrome
    - Trisomy syndromes
  - Environmental deprivation syndrome: emotional (?), parental (?), nutritional (?)
  - Anoxemia
    - Pulmonary disease: cystic fibrosis, hypoplastic lung, fibrous dysplasia (?)
    - Hemoglobinopathies
    - Cardiovascular disease
  - Chronic disease in a major organ
    - Kidney: renal insufficiency, acidosis
    - Neurologic system: microcephaly, hydrocephalus diencephalic syndrome, degenerative disease, neurofibromatosis
    - Hepatic cirrhosis
    - Malignancy
  - Primordial dwarfism
  - Drugs: daily cortisone therapy for asthma, collagen disease, nephrotic syndrome, rheumatoid arthritis aplastic anemia, malignancy (leukemia, Hodgkin's etc

Measurements

Carefully maintained growth records (accurate measurements displayed on standard growth charts) are essential for the early detection of growth problems due to nutritional inadequacies, endocrine disorders, or the onset of an underlying chronic disease.[126] The presence of disproportionate short stature points to problems in bone growth (e.g., chondrodystrophies or other skeletal dysplasias), while normal body proportions are characteristic of most of the remaining growth disorders (Table 25-5).

1. Length: From birth to 1 1/2 to 2 years, measure infant on a flat, horizontal board that has one vertical, immovable end to brace the head; the other vertical end slides along a track until it touches the soles of the feet. Place the infant supine and hold the knees flat.[118]
2. Height: For children > age 2, stand child with buttocks and heels (remove shoes and socks) against a vertical rule that has a movable device at right angles to the rule that can be lowered until it touches the top of the cranium.
3. Weight: Measure with a minimum of clothing.
4. Head circumference: Place nonstretchable tape over maximal occipital prominence and just above eyebrows.
5. Body proportions:
   a. Lower segment length (L) is the distance from the upper level of the pubic bone to the point where the medial aspect of the heel touches the floor.
   b. Derive upper segment length (U) by subtracting L from height (H); i.e., $U = H - L$.
   c. Calculate the U/L ratio. At birth, $U/L = 1.7$; it decreases as leg length increases until it equals 1.0 at 7 to 10 years of age. The U/L ratio for adult white males (0.95) is greater than that for adult black males (0.85), who tend to have longer leg length. The current standards for U/L ratio have many deficiencies.

6. Span: Stand patient flat against wall with arms outstretched at shoulder height. With nonstretchable tape held against wall (i.e., behind patient), measure the widest distance between extended fingers. Usually, span and height measurements are similar. Marked discrepancies point to disproportionate growth of limb versus trunk.
7. Other measurements include: *sitting height* measures trunk length; *triceps skin fold thickness* estimates subcutaneous adipose tissue (use calipers and measure at midpoint between shoulder and elbow posteriorly); *testis length* and *width* or *volume* (latter measured with a Prader orchidometer); and *penis* stretched *length, width,* and *circumference.*

Plotting Growth Data on Standard Growth Curves

The most recently developed growth curves for American children are based on cross-sectional measurements of a nationally representative sample; they do not make allowances for genetic and ethnic influences on height or for the variability of age of onset of adolescence in normal children. The Tanner-Whitehouse growth charts,[127] based on data collected in English children, are the ones most widely used internationally. The disadvantages of the available charts are not serious if the physician is aware that children whose growth follows the 3rd percentile and whose parents are short are growing normally based on midparental height. Growth curves that are adjusted to correct for parental height have been developed by Tanner et al.[127] Standardized growth charts for specific growth disorders such as Turner's syndrome, Noonan's syndrome, achondroplasia, Marfan syndrome, and Down syndrome have also become available.[128–130]

The physical measurements (height, weight, etc.) of an individual can be expressed either in terms of percentiles for chronologic age, with the range of normal being the 3rd to 97th percentiles, or in terms of standard deviations (SD) above or below the mean. One SD extends from the 16th to the 84th percentile; 2 SD extends from the 2 1/2th to the 97 1/2 percentile, approximating the 3rd and 97th percentiles on the growth curve. Data have been collected that give the SD in centimeters for each age and sex. Thus, a child's height can be given an SD score or a Z score by performing the following calculations. Subtract the child's height (cm) from the mean height (cm) for chronologic age and divide the difference by the SD (in cm) for chronologic age. A child with a Z score of -3 has a height 3 SD below the mean for chronologic age. This approach provides a method for comparing heights of children with diverse ages and a means of assessing the effects of a particular therapy on the growth process.

The growth curves also allow for the expression of an individual's size in terms of height age (HA) and weight age (WA). HA is defined as the chronologic age at which the patient's height would fall at the 50th percentile. This is calculated by drawing a horizontal line from the patient's position on the growth curve to the 50th percentile and dropping a vertical line to age in years. It does not take into account genetic influences on stature and pace of maturation. Nevertheless, it is extremely valuable when used to compare an individual's stature with his or her biological age (i.e., bone age). For example, a healthy 15-year-old male with delayed adolescence and a height age of 11 and bone age of 11 has a much better prognosis for adult height than does a 15-year-old sexually maturing young man with genetic short stature whose height age is 13 and whose bone age is 15.

The method for calculating WA is similar to that for HA but is more subject to error. The relation among chronologic age, HA, WA, and bone age in a patient helps delineate the etiology of the growth disorder; e.g., a 2-year-old with HA = 18 months and WA = 6 months is likely to have a nutritional problem that impairs weight gain more seriously than it impairs linear growth. Conversely, a 6-year-old child with HA = 3, WA = 4, and a bone age of 3 may have GH or thyroid deficiency.

Radiographic Studies

Skeletal maturation (bone age) is based on the size, shape, and number of the secondary centers of ossification. To minimize x-ray exposure, the left hand and wrist, and occasionally the knee, are most commonly used for radiographic study. The carpal, metacarpal, and phalangeal epiphyses are compared with standards obtained on healthy children at different ages. When there is variation in the maturation of these epiphyses more weight is given to the metacarpal and phalangeal centers than to the carpal epiphyses. The standard in the Greulich and Pyle *Radiographic Atlas* that most closely approximates that of the child indicates his or her bone age.[131] Bone age is of great value in children with significant growth disorders due to endocrine disturbances. In situations where a problem in mineralization exists or bone growth is disordered (skeletal dysplasia), cautious interpretation of bone age is advisable.

Prediction of estimated adult height based on present height and bone age can be made from the Bayley and Pinneau predictive tables[132] in the Greulich and Pyle atlas. This requires consideration of midparental height. Height prediction cannot be made accurately in children with pathologic growth but is useful in healthy children with normal types of short stature. However, patients must be advised that these estimations do not make allowances for rapid progress in sexual maturation, which may accelerate bone age disproportionately to height gain and result in stature that is lower than predicted.

Laboratory Studies

Additional laboratory tests may be ordered on the basis of evidence obtained during the history, physical, growth-curve, and radiographic evaluations. Further information concerning hormone determinations, hematologic tests, chromosome analyses, blood chemistry determinations, and elaborate radiologic procedures (e.g., CT scan and MRI) is discussed in the sections to follow dealing with specific growth disorders.

Causes of Short Stature

Introduction

Two examples of normal short stature discussed in this section are genetic short stature and constitutional growth delay. In both entities, growth rate is normal, height is within 2 SD of the mean, body proportions are normal, and general health is good. These children are different from the subgroups of pathologically short patients who have been classified as having NVSS or simple "short stature."[122–124] The characteristics of the children in the latter subgroups are heights greater than 2 SD from the mean and abnormally low growth rates. GH responses to provocative stimuli are normal and IGF-I levels are low or normal in many. GH treatment is beneficial for a majority. There is disagreement over whether these children have atypical forms of GH deficiency or

GH resistance. They represent a heterogeneous group of children who have growth failure of varying etiologies.[133,134]

Causes of Normal Short Stature

Genetic or Familial Short Stature

Throughout childhood and adolescence, growth in children with genetic short stature remains consistently at lower percentiles, with rates equal to or greater than 5 cm/year. These children's heights are in the normal range based on midparental stature, and they are healthy, well-proportioned young individuals. Bone age based on radiologic examination of the left wrist is usually within 2 SD of chronologic age. Occasionally, a child inherits both short stature and constitutional growth delay (Table 25-5). This combination increases the severity of the growth problem. The greatest burden to some families is the emotional stress which results from teasing, feelings of inadequacy, and parental guilt. Diagnostic studies can usually be kept to a minimum (bone age determination, T_4 assay) if the history and physical and growth data implicate genetic short stature.

The ultimate height of these children can be estimated directly from midparental height or calculated using either predictive data that include allowances for midparental height or the unadjusted predictive tables of Bayley and Pinneau.[132] A simple way of determining whether a short child with short parents is growing normally is to calculate midparental height by averaging the parents' heights and adding 6.5 cm if the child is a boy and subtracting 6.5 cm if the child is a girl. Then the percentile on which the midparental height falls is determined. The child's growth curve followed to adult height should fall within ± 5 cm of midparental height after skeletal age has been taken into account. There is no effective treatment for genetic short stature. Androgen therapy is contraindicated because of the risk of acceleration in bone maturation, which further compromises adult height. Oxandrolone, a synthetic androgen, when given during adolescence, has not enhanced the ultimate heights of genetically short boys. There is no evidence to suggest that use of pharmacologic doses of GH would increase the adult height of genetically short children. At present, the management of genetic short stature consists mainly of supportive counseling, career planning, and encouraging the child to engage in appropriate physical activities which build self-confidence.

Constitutional Growth Delay with or without Delayed Adolescence

Children with constitutional growth delay have a more gradual rate of biological aging. The slow growth pattern starts at about 2 years of age. By kindergarten, the child is shorter and younger-appearing than the majority of his or her schoolmates, although health is good and body proportions are normal. Bone age is lower than chronologic age and is equal or close to height age. Growth rates are 5 cm or more per year; linear growth, with height at a lower percentile, is a characteristic feature. A dip in the growth rate before the start of puberty is usually seen. The family has a history of slow maturation and delayed onset of adolescence. Parental heights are average to tall, although an occasional family with genetic short stature has the added burden of familial slow maturation. Males are affected more often than females; most such boys are also delayed in sexual maturation, although an occasional patient enters puberty at age 12 years. Those with delayed adolescence continue to grow at approximately 5 cm/year and do not have a growth spurt until age 15 to 16. In contrast, the average boy's growth velocity accelerates at 13 years. This is the chronologic age when all growth charts show a steeper slope representative of the mean increase in growth velocity during puberty. Consequently, the growth curve of the delayed developer often falls below the 5th percentile around age 13 and steepens later as puberty begins. As long as the prepubertal linear growth rate is more than 5 cm/year, there is usually no need for concern. These young men reach their adult height at 20 to 21 years of age instead of the usual 18 years. They may not begin shaving regularly until age 20 years or more.

The diagnostic criteria for delayed adolescence include absence of testicular enlargement and other signs of secondary sexual maturation in a boy who is 14 years of age.[120]

The management of delayed adolescence in a boy depends on his chronologic age when first seen and his history and physical characteristics. If a young man of 14 to 15 is healthy but has no evidence of testicular enlargement or sexual hair, the management can be limited to determining his bone age, plotting his growth curve, and giving him reassurance. Alternatively, the assessment may be extended to include a complete blood count (CBC) and sedimentation rate, biochemical profile, T_4 assay, and urinalysis. These tests exclude the possibility that chronic diseases such as renal insufficiency, hypothyroidism, and chronic inflammatory bowel disease are present. If the data support the clinical diagnosis of delayed adolescence, the patient is reassured and examined every 6 months. Most boys enter puberty within the following 12 to 18 months and agree to allow sexual maturation to proceed without androgen supplementation. If, however, the patient is very emotionally distressed, modest doses of androgens may be used for 3 to 6 months in conjunction with psychological counseling.[135]

A patient who presents at age 16 years without any evidence of puberty may still have an innocent delay of adolescence. However, a search for organic disease is indicated before this diagnosis is made. Boys who grow less than 5.0 cm/year or who have an abnormal physical sign or symptom (small penis, hypoplastic testes, pallor, dry skin, cushingoid features, headaches, visual disturbances, or anosmia) require thorough investigation. The differential diagnosis of delayed adolescence includes (1) gonadotropin deficiency (either idiopathic or due to organic disease in the hypothalamus or pituitary, i.e., GnRH or FSH-LH deficiency, respectively), (2) primary testicular disease (hypoplastic testes, Leydig cell deficiency or dysfunction), (3) sex chromosome defects (Klinefelter's syndrome), (4) hypothyroidism (primary hypothyroidism or TSH or TRH deficiency), (5) Cushing's syndrome or disease (glucocorticoid treatment of asthma, rheumatoid arthritis, etc., or lesions in the hypothalamus, pituitary, or adrenal gland), and (6) chronic disease (chronic inflammatory bowel disease, cystic fibrosis, cardiac disease, CNS lesions, renal insufficiency, etc.).

The extent of the diagnostic evaluation must be individualized for each patient. The following are diagnostic procedures which aid in confirming or excluding diseases listed in the differential diagnosis:

1. CBC, sedimentation rate, biochemical profile
2. Assays for TSH, T_4 (RIA), T_3 (RIA), free T_4; TRH stimulation test (optional)
3. Assays of urine and/or plasma FSH and LH concentrations
4. GnRH testing (optional; may not differentiate hypothalamic from pituitary dysfunction with a single injection or infusion)
5. Measurement of plasma GH and cortisol responses to insulin hypoglycemia and L-arginine infusion (other provocative tests may be substituted)

6. Plasma testosterone and DHEA sulfate assays, serum prolactin
7. Determinations of diurnal patterns of plasma cortisol and 24-h urinary 17-ketosteroid, 17-hydroxycorticosteroid, and cortisol output before and after low- and high-dose dexamethasone administration for suspected Cushing's syndrome
8. Chromosome analysis for Klinefelter's syndrome or Kallmann's Syndrome
9. hCG stimulation to test Leydig cell function
10. Radiologic studies: bone age, skull x-rays (optional: CT scan or MRI of head, skeletal survey for bone disease, GI series, chest x-ray for heart or lung disease, kidney studies)
11. Visual acuity, fields, and funduscopic examinations for suspected organic lesions in the hypothalamic-pituitary axis

One of the following treatment programs may be used in healthy boys with delayed adolescence who need treatment for psychological reasons. If chronic disease (e.g., Crohn's disease) is discovered to be the cause of delayed adolescence, these treatment programs are not applicable because they may advance bone age without promoting linear growth or sexual maturation.

1. Testosterone enanthate 75 to 100 mg every 3 to 4 weeks for 3 to 6 months. If a permanent lack of androgens exists and satisfactory height has been achieved, the full virilizing dose is 200 mg intramuscularly (IM) every 2 to 3 weeks. Bone age is measured at the beginning and every 6 months if the effect of therapy on osseous maturation is an important factor.
2. Oxandrolone 0.05 to 0.1 mg per kilogram of body weight per day for 3 to 6 months (oxandrolone is an oral synthetic nonaromatized androgen with potent anabolic and weak androgenic properties). Oxandrolone is used in situations in which the priority is linear growth and sexual maturation can be postponed.
3. Human chorionic gonadotropin (hCG) 500 to 1,000 units (U) IM three times weekly for 1 to 2 months; plasma testosterone concentration is monitored, and the dose is adjusted accordingly. hCG is useful only if Leydig cell function is intact.

Delayed adolescence in girls is present when breast tissue and/or sexual hair have not appeared by 14 years of age. Usually, menarche occurs 2.3 years after the onset of breast development, but it can occur as late as 4.5 years after breast budding.[120]

The differential diagnoses of delayed menarche in girls include (1) emotional disorders (e.g., anorexia nervosa), (2) gonadotropin deficiency, (3) primary ovarian disease (embryologic defects or acquired disease, e.g., agenesis, polycystic ovarian disease, or torsion of the ovary), (4) chronic disease, (5) absence of the uterus, (6) X chromosome abnormalities (Turner's syndrome), (7) XY male pseudohermaphrodism (androgen insensitivity, 17α-hydroxylase deficiency, embryologic defects in the testes, e.g., agenesis or absence of Leydig cells) and (8) absence of aromatase.

On the initial evaluation, the history and physical examination guide the extent to which the patient is investigated. A healthy-appearing girl who presents at age 15 years without breast tissue and with a normal height and growth rate probably will begin puberty in the following 6 to 12 months and needs only reexamination and reassurance. However, if she is short or if her growth rate is 4.5 cm or less per year, a search must be initiated for chromosomal abnormalities, pituitary-hypothalamic disorders, and chronic diseases. On rare occasions, girls have presented with excellent breast growth, normal sexual hair, and primary amenorrhea due to congenital absence of the uterus; the vaginal examination shows an absence of the cervix. Pelvic sonography and peritoneoscopic examination are indicated if a normal female karyotype and elevated gonadotropin concentrations are discovered or if absence of the uterus is suspected. Gonadectomy must be performed in females who possess a Y chromosome because of the increased risk of gonadal malignancy. Estrogen therapy for simple delayed adolescence in girls is unnecessary except for psychological reasons.

Pathologic Short Stature (Table 25-5)

Intrauterine Growth Disturbances

Abnormal intrauterine growth must be considered in any newborn whose birth weight is inappropriately low for gestational age. These babies are usually referred to as small-for-date infants; the prognosis for their recovery depends on the timing, severity, and duration of the intrauterine insult. As a rule, small-for-date infants whose growth accelerates and achieves a normal channel by 6 months postnatal age grow normally thereafter. If they show persistence of an abnormal growth rate at 2 years of age, they are likely to be short throughout childhood and adulthood. In contrast, the growth prognosis for prematurely born infants with appropriate weight for gestational age is more favorable, with a majority having catch-up growth during the first two years of life. A careful evaluation of the health of the mother, the placenta, and the fetus is needed to determine the likely cause of the fetal growth abnormality.

Maternal and Placental Disorders Fetal growth is influenced adversely by maternal malnutrition and poor health. Toxemia, hypertension, cardiac disease, and renal insufficiency may impair growth of the fetus either directly or by causing placental dysfunction.

Drugs ingested by pregnant women are a potential hazard to fetal growth and well-being. The teratogenic effects to the fetus of excessive alcohol ingestion (*fetal alcohol syndrome*)[136] include (1) intrauterine growth failure, (2) microcephaly (and possibly hydrocephalus), (3) mental retardation, which may be mild or severe (IQ range 15 to 105; in 16 of 20 infants the IQ was <80), (4) facial abnormalities, including small midface, strabismus, ptosis, short palpebral fissures, epicanthal folds, thin upper lip, short nose, micrognathia, and maxillary hypoplasia, (5) minor joint and limb abnormalities, including limited range of movement and altered palm creases, and (6) behavioral problems, mainly hyperactivity, short attention span, and learning difficulties, but not rebelliousness, negativism, or psychosis.[136] Narcotic (heroin and morphine) addiction during pregnancy causes intrauterine growth failure in half the offspring and also increases the risk of prematurity and intrauterine infection. Anticoagulants (e.g., warfarin) used in mothers with prosthetic mitral valves have resulted in infants with mental retardation, hypotonia, seizures, optic atrophy, flat facies, hypoplastic nose, and stippled epiphyses. Anticonvulsants (e.g., phenytoin) have caused intrauterine growth failure, mental retardation, hypertelorism, cleft lip and palate, and hypoplastic distal phalanges with small nails. Aminopterin used for abortion in the first trimester causes poor fetal growth, microcephaly, craniofacial abnormalities, and shortness of limbs. Heavy cigarette smoking is associated with an increased incidence of prematurity as well as smaller-sized offspring.

Fetal Disorders The fetal diseases that interfere most frequently with growth are intrauterine infections which are maternally transmitted, congenital abnormalities of major organ systems, chromosomal defects, and a variety of growth-deficiency syndromes of genetic or unknown origin.

Maternally transmitted infections include (1) rubella, which causes microcephaly, mental retardation, deafness, cataracts, chorioretinitis, microphthalmus, congenital heart disease (patent ductus arteriosus, pulmonary stenosis, septal defects, etc.); (2) toxoplasmosis, caused by a protozoan agent, which causes fetal growth retardation, hepatosplenomegaly, microcephaly or hydrocephalus, retinal pigmentation, mental retardation, and intracranial calcification; (3) cytomegalovirus, which causes poor fetal growth, hepatosplenomegaly, jaundice, retinopathy, mental retardation, and intracranial calcification; and (4) syphilis, which is associated with small fetal size, brain and bone abnormalities, and nasal mucous membrane lesions.

Congenital malformations of the brain, lung, etc., may interfere with fetal growth. Many chromosomal defects cause intrauterine growth failure: trisomy 18, trisomy 13, Down syndrome (trisomy 21), etc. Children who began life with IUGR resulting from intrinsic fetal disease and who continue to exhibit permanent postnatal growth retardation have been given the designation of primordial growth failure. The endocrine system is not likely to be a contributing factor because birth size is normal in infants with congenital deficiencies of GH, thyroid, and gonadal hormones. Nevertheless, there is evidence that inactivating mutations of the GHR and deletion of the IGF-I gene cause small birth size.[137–139] The phenotypic characteristics of various syndromes with IUGR and short stature are fully described in *Smith's Recognizable Patterns of Human Malformation*.[140]

Postnatal Malnutrition

Malnutrition due to inadequate food supplies is the major cause worldwide of poor growth in infancy and childhood. In this country, poverty and parental neglect or ignorance are the usual reasons for growth failure due to malnutrition. Poor weight gain and sometimes actual weight loss are the main findings. A careful history with particular emphasis on caloric intake and a thorough physical examination are essential. Characteristically, these infants are hungry and have very little subcutaneous fat and muscle mass. They are prone to develop gastroenteritis and dehydration, which further compromise their nutritional state. The cachexia, dehydration, and electrolyte abnormalities in these infants may mimic salt loss due to Addison's disease or adrenogenital syndrome, but can be easily differentiated from those disorders by documenting stress elevations of plasma cortisol and aldosterone concentrations.

Management consists of hospitalizing the child in a clean area, avoiding unnecessary diagnostic tests, and providing optimal nutrition. Weight gain on this simple regimen provides adequate proof of the diagnosis. The need for cultures, blood chemistry studies, and hormone determinations (plasma cortisol and 17-hydroxyprogesterone and urinary 17-ketosteroid, allopregnanetriol, aldosterone, etc., concentrations) must be individualized. Dietary counseling and psychological support for the mother, plus home supervision after discharge by a visiting nurse, suffice if the mother-child relation is a healthy one. The prognosis for catch-up growth and subsequent normal stature is good if the duration and severity of the period of malnutrition are not excessive. If parental neglect has placed the infant in jeopardy, removal to a good foster home is advisable.

Gastrointestinal diseases that compromise growth in infants and young children include esophageal reflux, obstructive lesions of the bowel, and deficiencies of the digestive enzymes. Cystic fibrosis of the pancreas produces malabsorption due to insufficiency of pancreatic enzymes (trypsin, lipase, amylase). It also causes chronic pulmonary disease because of airway obstruction from abnormally thick mucus, combined with bacterial superinfection. Persistent elevation of sweat sodium concentration above 70 mEq/L is diagnostic for this disorder. Concentrations above 50 mEq/L should elicit suspicion. Children with disaccharidase enzyme abnormalities need the expertise of a pediatric gastroenterologist who is skilled in performing endoscopic biopsies of the proximal small bowel for histology and quantitative enzyme determinations. Diarrheal stools that are acidic ($pH < 6$) and contain reducing substance by Clinitest Reagent tablet (>0.25 percent) strongly suggest this disorder.

Chronic inflammatory bowel disease (Crohn's disease) occurs most frequently (78 percent of cases) between the ages of 10 and 29 years. Growth failure and delayed sexual maturation result from decreased caloric intake and increased losses of nutrients. Hypoalbuminemia occurs in 50 percent of patients; anemia (iron and folate deficiencies) is also a frequent complication. Improved growth has occurred in prepubertal children treated with nutritional support or by surgical resection of the diseased bowel. If bone age is >13 years, surgery may not result in catch-up growth. Androgens should be used with extreme caution because they do not enhance growth in the absence of adequate protein and caloric intake and may compromise adult height.

Endocrine Causes of Short Stature

Hypothyroidism *Congenital Hypothyroidism* Congenital hypothyroidism occurs in approximately 1 of 4,000 newborns with a female/male ratio of 4:1. Data from screening programs indicate that 84 percent of congenitally hypothyroid infants have thyroid dysgenesis or agenesis, 8 percent have enzymatic defects in hormonogenesis, and 8 percent have either TSH or TRH deficiency. Early recognition and treatment afford the best hope of ameliorating or reversing the harmful effects of hypothyroidism on the brain. The placenta is relatively impermeable to maternal thyroid hormones; thus, the factors that influence the infant's prognosis for intelligence are the severity of intrauterine hypothyroidism, postnatal age at diagnosis, and adequacy of treatment.

After birth, linear growth is poor in hypothyroid infants. The diagnosis of congenital primary hypothyroidism is confirmed by low serum T_4, low free T_4, and high TSH concentrations. Additional criteria include absence or dysgenesis of the tibial epiphysis on knee x-ray and absence, hypoplasia, or maldescent of the thyroid gland by technetium scan. Breast-fed infants were once believed to be partially protected by breast milk because of its thyroid hormone content. This concept is no longer considered valid because breast milk contains insignificant amounts of thyroid hormone.

Early signs of congenital hypothyroidism include a large posterior fontanel, suture separation, feeding difficulties, prolonged unconjugated hyperbilirubinemia, and hypothermia. These subtle features usually go unnoticed by most physicians. Therefore, the advantage of screening is detection of these infants before the development of obvious signs such as cretinous facies, myxedematous protruding tongue, hypotonia, umbilical hernia, mottling, lethargy, and constipation. The benefits of early detection and treatment justify the approximate cost of $5,000 per case identified. Approximately 80 percent of congenitally hypothyroid infants treated before 3 months of age have IQs > 90, whereas only 45 percent of infants treated before 6 months have IQs > 90.[141–143] Recent studies indicate that the mean IQ of congenitally hypothyroid children identified by neonatal screening programs is similar to that of the general population. However, about 15 percent of these children have IQ scores below the normal range.

Management consists of administering L-thyroxine 10 to 15 μg per kilogram of body weight per day for the first year.[144,145] The thyroxine tablet is crushed and mixed in a teaspoon of formula or cereal. The criteria for judging response to treatment include improvements in the infant's behavior and appearance, increased growth rate, assessment of developmental milestones, and serum T_4 and TSH concentrations. In a few infants, TSH elevations have persisted even though the clinical response was excellent and the serum T_4 concentration was normal for age. Therefore, TSH concentrations have not been relied on exclusively.[146] Initially, these infants must be seen every 4 to 6 weeks to monitor growth and T_4 levels and adjust the thyroid hormone dose. From age 6 months to 1 year, they are examined at 2- to 3-month intervals and then every 6 months until the age of 4 to 5 years. Thereafter, yearly examinations are sufficient to monitor progress and adjust the dose. Assessment of developmental progress and intelligence must be made before the child's entry into kindergarten to determine whether there is a need for special educational support.

Acquired Hypothyroidism The onset of acquired hypothyroidism in childhood can be readily diagnosed from the linear growth curve. Deceleration or complete cessation of growth is the earliest sign. The myxedematous physical findings seen in adults are usually absent. Features of acquired hypothyroidism include pallor, stocky physique, coarseness of facial features and puffiness about the eyes, delayed dental development, cool hands and feet, constipation, sluggish behavior, and occasionally, muscle hypertrophy. Scalp hair may be normal or sparse and dry. Rarely, children with hypothyroidism exhibit precocious sexual development, ovarian cysts, hyperprolactinemia, and diabetes insipidus, which regress after thyroid replacement is begun. A goiter, usually due to thyroiditis, may be present, or there may be no palpable thyroid tissue. These children tend to socialize with inappropriately young playmates and by nature are quiet and studious. School performance is usually satisfactory until thyroid hormone is prescribed, after which there is frequently an adjustment period characterized by deterioration in school performance, rebelliousness, and "acting-out" behavior. Gradual increments in thyroid dosage have been tried but have not significantly altered this difficult transition period. Family members and school authorities should be informed of the changes in personality which follow the patient's discovery of new energies and interests. With time, there is a return to behavior patterns that are appropriate for chronologic age. The intelligence of these children is not adversely affected by the period of hypothyroidism.

The possible etiologies of acquired hypothyroidism include embryologic defects (thyroid hypoplasia), maldescent (lingual thyroid), chronic lymphocytic thyroiditis (Hashimoto's disease), acute and subacute thyroiditis, and pituitary hypothalamic disease. Lingual thyroid, when present, may be seen as a mass in the midline posterior portion of the extended tongue. Hypothyroidism develops in 40 to 50 percent of children who clinically have a goiter due to chronic lymphocytic thyroiditis. Primary hypothyroidism is characterized by elevated serum concentrations of TSH and low serum T_4, free T_4, and T_3 levels. In secondary hypothyroidism, the TSH concentration is low or normal and fails to increase after TRH stimulation. In tertiary hypothyroidism, the disease is in the hypothalamus; TRH stimulation elevates serum TSH levels.

The thoroughness of the diagnostic evaluation depends on the suspected etiology. It should include construction of a growth curve, measurement of serum T_4, free T_4, T_3, and TSH concentrations, and determinations of thyroid antibody titers against thyroglobulin and peroxidase enzyme. Thyroid scans (^{99m}Tc or ^{123}I) or thyroid ultrasound exams are occasionally needed. Measurement of bone age gives valuable data concerning the patient's biological age, the estimated age of onset of disease, and remaining growth potential. Skull x-rays (anteroposterior and lateral views) are useful for evaluating sella size and detecting bony erosion. Long-standing primary hypothryoidism may result in pituitary hypertrophy and sellar enlargement. The sella is free of erosion and returns to normal size with thyroid replacement. Electrocardiograms show low voltage but are not essential for the diagnosis. Anemia is a common finding that disappears with thyroid medication. Pituitary function tests (e.g., TRH stimulation and GH responses) and special radiologic (CT or MRI of the pituitary and hypothalamus), neurologic, and ophthalmologic studies must be considered in children with hypothyroidism and low serum TSH concentrations.

Treatment consists of oral L-thyroxine, 0.1 mg per square meter of body surface (3 to 4 μg per kilogram of body weight) per day, given as a single dose. The dose must be individualized because absorption and metabolism vary among patients.

The clinical response to treatment in primary hypothyroidism consists of a catch up growth spurt, disappearance of the abnormal physical stigmata, and improvement in facial features, including a loss of puffiness and pallor. The most valuable laboratory data are serum T_4, TSH, and hemoglobin concentrations and hematocrit. These indices should be monitored every 2 months for the first 6 months. Bone age x-rays (at 6 to 12 months) are optional during the growth spurt and are not needed after the patient resumes growth at a normal percentile. After the patient is stabilized, the growth response and serum T_4 and TSH concentrations can be evaluated every 6 to 12 months to be certain of compliance. The prognosis for adult height is excellent if the patient is compliant and if the bone age is not advanced. In cases where noncompliance is persistent, the entire weekly dose can be administered by a visiting nurse or school nurse once a week.[147] This therapy cannot safely be used in adults or in children with compromised cardiac or adrenal function. Excessive daily doses of thyroid should be avoided because that protocol causes disproportionate acceleration of bone maturation and aggravates behavioral problems.

The thyroid treatment doses for patients with secondary or tertiary hypothyroidism are slightly lower than those for primary hypothyroidism. Usually, two-thirds or even one-half of the normal dose provides satisfactory serum thyroxine concentrations. It is especially important to avoid overtreatment in these children because undue acceleration of osseous maturation shortens the period of responsiveness if GH therapy is also needed. The prognosis for normal intelligence is excellent in children who acquire hypothyroidism after 1 to 2 years of age.

GH Deficiency The clinical features of patients with GH deficiency vary with the etiology, age at onset, and severity of the disorder. Those with congenital GH deficiency have characteristic growth patterns that distinguish them from children with acquired disease. In general, the idiopathic form is more common than the organic variety (disease due to tumor, trauma, embryologic defect, etc.). However, this may change because the MRI is now detecting structural defects in the hypothalamic-pituitary area in many children with presumed idiopathic disease.

The prevalence of GH deficiency was estimated to be as low as 1 in 30,000 births and as high as 1 in 4,018 in two studies carried out in Great Britain.[148,149] In the United States the estimated incidence of GH is 1 in 3,480 live births.[150]

A classification of the causes of GH deficiency and GH resistance is outlined in Table 25-6. No attempt is made to distinguish whether the defect in GH secretion is due to disease in the hypothalamus or the pituitary gland.

Congenital GH Deficiency Infants with congenital GH deficiency usually have normal birth length and weight. They grow normally for 3 to 6 months, but linear growth rates decelerate thereafter. Their linear growth curves deviate progressively from the mean. The severity of the growth disorder is not usually appreciated until the child is 2 to 5 years of age, at which time it is obvious that a marked height discrepancy exists between the patient and his or her peers. After 3 years of age, growth rates in affected children are almost always <5 cm/year. Characteristically, these patients have normal body proportions for chronologic age. Most but not all children with GH deficiency are overweight for height and some are frankly obese. Excessive accumulation of fat occurs predominantly in the chest and abdominal areas, and the overlying skin has a grossly ripply or bosselated appearance. The general appearance of the child is always younger than is appropriate for chronologic age. In early childhood, the faces are frequently cherubic, infantile, or doll-like and the voice may be high-pitched. Frontal bossing, a common feature, is due to undergrowth of facial bones. Eruption and shedding of primary teeth usually are delayed. The permanent teeth also may appear late and are often crowded and irregularly positioned. Muscle mass is diminished, hair is thin, and nail growth is poor. Skeletal age in a prepubertal hypopituitary patient is always delayed, and the degree of retardation of bone maturation is proportional to that of height age. Head circumference is within the normal range for age, but the sella turcica is often small. Closure of the anterior fontanel is usually very much delayed.

During early infancy and childhood, patients with GH deficiency may experience recurring episodes of fasting hypoglycemia and convulsions which, if untreated, may result in mental retardation, a seizure disorder, and even death. Therapy with GH is highly effective. Some of these infants have a concomitant deficiency of ACTH and their treatment includes maintenance doses of hydrocortisone (10 to 15 mg per square meter of surface per day in two or three divided doses PO) in addition to GH (0.18 to 0.3 mg per kilogram of body weight per week divided and given daily SC). During illnesses, stress doses of hydrocortisone given orally (60 mg/m^2 per day in three divided doses) or parenterally (60 mg/m^2 IM or IV in two or three divided doses) are required. Glucose-containing electrolyte solutions must frequently be used IV when oral intake is curtailed in these children. The tendency to fasting hypoglycemia usually disappears by 5 years of age but may reappear if severe illnesses prevent oral intake for prolonged periods. Apart from the problems of hypoglycemia and seizures during the early childhood years, children with idiopathic GH deficiency are generally healthy and have normal intelligence. Emotional problems are more frequent, however, in this popula-

TABLE 25-6. Causes of GH Deficiency or Defective GH Action

Congenital GH Deficiency
Decreased GH secretion
Idiopathic
Genetic
Prop-1 or Pit-1 mutation
GH gene deletion type 1A
Types IB, II, III
Abnormal GH peptide
GHRH-R mutation
IGF gene mutation
Embryologic defects
Aplasia, hypoplasia, ectopia
Anencephaly, arhinencephalia
Septo-optic dysplasia
Midline facial dysplasia
Empty sella syndrome
Miscellaneous syndromes
Biologically inactive GH
Neurosecretory defects
GH resistance
Laron dwarfism
Pygmy
Acquired GH Deficiency
Idiopathic
Neurosecretory defects
CNS tumors
Craniopharyngioma
Optic glioma
Dysgerminoma
Hamartoma
Trauma
Perinatal insult: breech deliveries, hypoxemia, asphyxia, difficult forceps delivery, intracranial hemorrhage, precipitate or prolonged delivery, twin pregnancy
Child abuse
Accidental trauma
Inflammatory diseases
Viral encephalitis
Fungal
Unknown etiology
Bacteria, group B streptococcal meningitis, etc.
Granulomatous: tuberculosis, syphilis, sarcoidosis
Autoimmunity: lymphocytic hypophysitis
Irradiation: CNS radiation for brain tumors, leukemia
Vascular lesions
Aneurysms, pituitary vessels
Infarction
Hematologic disorders
Hemochromatosis
Sickle cell disease
Thalassemia
Histiocytosis
Transient defects in GH secretion or action
Peripuberty (secretion)
Psychosocial stress (secretion, action)
Glucocorticoid excess (?)
Primary hypothyroidism (secretion, action)
Malnutrition
Drug use

tion, because patients are perceived to be much younger than their chronologic age and are treated accordingly. Excessive teasing and social isolation are common complaints in older untreated patients.

GH-deficient boys with microphallus and hypoplastic testes are likely to also have gonadotropin deficiency, which may be partial or complete. The gonadotropin status usually cannot be accurately assessed until their adolescent years. Small doses of androgen should be prescribed during infancy and early childhood to bring the penis size into the normal range for age. During the adolescent and adult years, testicular growth and enhanced virilization can be facilitated in gonadotropin-deficient hypopituitary males through the use of hCG in combination with human menopausal gonadotropin (hMG).[151] In children with isolated idiopathic GH deficiency who are treated with GH from an early age, pubertal maturation is likely to begin normally, whereas puberty is often delayed in those who begin treatment late in childhood. Hypopituitarism of organic origin (birth trauma, embryologic brain defects, etc.) carries a high risk of multiple pituitary hormone deficiencies.

There are several causes of congenital GH deficiency (Table 25-6). *Idiopathic hypopituitarism* is the most common type of hypopituitarism, but this is likely to change. By definition, no organic lesion or etiologic factor can be identified. Males are affected more frequently than are females. The disorder may involve only GH (*isolated GH deficiency*) or may be associated with deficiencies of TSH and/or gonadotropins and/or ACTH (*idiopathic multiple primary deficiencies*). Prepubertal children with GH plus TSH or ACTH deficiency are likely to exhibit gonadotropin deficiency (partial or complete) in their adolescent years.

Magnetic resonance imaging (MRI) studies of the hypothalamus and pituitary gland in patients with idiopathic GH deficiency have shown that the sella volume tends to be small and that stalk abnormalities are most frequent in children with multiple pituitary hormone deficiencies. Those with diabetes insipidus frequently have an absent or ectopic posterior pituitary gland, and the bright spot indicating the neurohypophyses is absent. Imaging studies are indicated in all children with isolated idiopathic GH deficiency as well as in subjects with multiple hormone deficiencies.

Genetic transmission of GH deficiency is found in 3 to 30 percent of affected children. Some families are distinguished by the presence of GHD in a parent or sibling and by the presence of consanguinity. Isolated GHD (IGHD) has been caused by 4 known mendelian defects within the GH gene itself or within a regulatory locus that is essential for normal GH production. Type 1 A IGHD, the most severe, is an autosomal recessive condition resulting from homozygous deletions of the GH N gene, which leads to absence of GH production in fetal life. Affected infants are short at birth and experience severe hypoglycemia. Response to GH is initially good but then treatment failure occurs because of resistance due to development of GH antibodies. Type 1 B IGHD is also caused by an autosomal recessive mechanism, but the defect causes GH deficiency rather than absence and the response to GH treatment is good. No mutations in the GH N gene have been identified and hence, the abnormality appears to involve genes that control GH production, possibly those regulating GHRH production. Type 2 IGHD is caused by an autosomal dominant disorder in families with an affected parent and occasionally an affected sib. Male to male transmission excludes X-linked inheritance. In one family, a mutation of the GH N gene resulted in a mutant GH product which may have interfered with secretion of the normal GH molecule by a dominant negative effect. Type 3 IGHD is an X-linked disorder that has been associated with immunoglobulin deficiencies in 4 affected males. GH treatment improves height as well as serum immunoglobulin levels. The gene locus is presumed to be adjacent to the gene necessary for normal immunoglobulin synthesis.[152–158]

Familial occurrences of combined pituitary hormone deficiencies (CPHD) are caused by mutations in pituitary-specific homeodomain transcription factor genes which are essential in embryologic life for several anterior pituitary cell lineages. At least five DNA-binding transcription factors are known to control the ontogeny of pituitary cells (Rpx, Ptx-1, Ptx-2, Prop-1, and Pit-1).[159–167] In the mouse pituitary gland, Rpx is the earliest active transcription factor (8.5 days). Expression of Prop-1 follows soon after and appears to suppress Rpx. Absence of Prop-1 leads to continued expression of Rpx and results in deficiencies of GH, Prl, TSH, LH, and FSH. A similar pituitary disorder occurs in humans with loss of function mutations in Prop-1. This suggests that suppression of Rpx is necessary for progression of pituitary development. Paradoxically, however, absence or continued production of Rpx causes multiple pituitary hormone deficiencies, with the former being associated with septooptic dysplasia in the mouse, though this may not be the case in humans. The Ptx genes (Ptx-1 and Ptx-2) influence the differentiation and function of all anterior pituitary cell types including corticotrophs, thyrotrophs, gonadotrophs, somatotrophs, and lactotrophs. Mutation of Ptx-1 may be a cause of Treacher-Collins Franceschetti Syndrome and mutation of Ptx-2 may cause Rieger syndrome (coloboma, glaucoma, anal stenosis, umbilical hernia, and partial pituitary hormone deficiencies). The temporal influences of these transcription factors on pituitary development are given in Table 25-7. A more detailed discussion of the importance of Pit-1 and Prop-1 follows.

Pit-1 (GHF-I or POU 1F1) is a member of the POU family of transcription factors, which are part of the helix-turn-helix super family of proteins. Pit 1 has two protein domains, POU-S (POU-specific) and POU-HD (POU-homeo), which are necessary for high-affinity DNA binding on the promoter regions of the GH, Prl, and βTSH genes. At least nine point mutations have been documented in the Pit-1 gene of subjects with familial combined pituitary hormone deficiency involving GH, Prl, and TSH. All children with Pit-1 gene mutations have GH deficiency and variable onset and severity of thyrotropin deficiency. Basal prolactin levels may be normal, but usually there is no prolactin rise after TRH. The pituitary gland is hypoplastic in many patients while in others it is of normal size. Inheritance may be sporadic or due to an autosomal dominant mechanism. Corticotropin and gonadotropin levels are normal in individuals with Pit-1 gene mutations; hence, spontaneous puberty and fertility are preserved. The Snell dwarf mouse and the Snell-Jackson dwarf mouse have mutations or rearrangements of the Pit-1 gene.[164–167]

Prop-1 gene (prophet of Pit-1) controls the expression of Pit-1 during embryonic life. It encodes a homeodomain transcription protein that is essential for differentiation of gonadotrophs, somatotrophs, thyrotrophs, and lactotrophs. Sporadic or familial mutations in the Prop-1 gene causes deficiencies of gonadotropins, GH, TSH, and Prl. The phenotype includes remarkable short stature, sexual immaturity, normal hand and foot size, variable sella turcica enlargement, and low levels of GH, IGF-I, IGFBP-3, gonadotropins, sex hormones, thyroxine, and Prl with normal serum levels of corticotropin, cortisol, TSH, IGFBP-1, and IGFBP-2.[162]

Mutations in the GHRH receptor gene on chromosome 7 have been described in families with isolated GHD. The abnormal

TABLE 25-7. Temporal Relationships between Transcription Factors and Pituitary Development

Transcription Factors	Rpx, Ptx-1[a]	Prop-1, Ptx-1[b]	Pit-1[c]
Pituitary function	POMC (ACTH, MSH)	FSH, LH	GH
	αGSU (α subunits for FSH, LH, TSH)	GH	TSH
		TSH	Prl
		Prl	

[a]Rpx and Ptx-1 influence the development of embryonic pituitary cells, which will subsequently differentiate further depending on the actions of other transcription factors such as Prop-1 and Pit-1.

[b]Prop-1 and Ptx-1 influence the futher differentiation of precursor pituitary cells into gonadotropes and to the precursor cells for GH TSH, Prl (Pit-1 dependent cell).

[c]Pit-1 is the essential final transcription factor that is needed for development of somatotropes, thyrotropes and lactotropes.

GHRH R gene produces a nonfunctional GHRH R protein that lacks the membrane spanning and the G protein-binding site. Affected children fail to release GH after standard provocative tests and after GHRH administration. They respond well to GH treatment. A homozygous nonsense mutation in exon 3 of the GHRH R gene was recently documented in 17 growth-retarded adults in two villages in Pakistan (Dwarfs of Sindh). Consanguinity was prevalent among this population with many first-cousin marriages. Adult heights were approximately 130 cm for men and 114 cm for women. Fertility was intact in affected individuals. None were dysmorphic and males had normal-sized genitalia. Hypoglycemia was not a feature. A GHRH R mutation is responsible for the growth failure seen in the little mouse (lit). Somatotroph differentiation is intact and appears to be independent of GHRH.[168,169]

Recently a missense mutation in the GH N gene was reported in an extremely short boy with bioinactive GH. Serum GH levels were high and serum IGF-I levels were low. The mutant GH is biologically inert because it cannot activate the GH receptor. Also, it has a high affinity for GHBP and GHR and prevents exogenous GH from interacting with the GH R. The action appears to be dominant-negative in that the mutant GH interfered with receptor dimerization and tyrosine phosphorylation.[158] Interruptions in the ontogeny of pituitary cells lead to multiple pituitary hormone deficiencies depending on where the defect occurs. For example, (1) absence of Rpx or Ptx will prevent the differentiation of cell types needed for ACTH, MSH, FSH, LH, GH, TSH, Prl; (2) absence of Prop-1 leads to deficiencies of FSH, LH, GH, TSH, Prl; (3) absence of Pit-1 leads to deficiencies of GH, TSH, Prl; and (4) absence of GSU leads to absence of subunits for glycoprotein hormones—FSH, LH, and TSH.

Embryologic defects include aplasia, hypoplasia, and ectopic location of the pituitary. They may occur as isolated, congenital defects or in association with anencephaly or arhinencephalia. The latter comprises a spectrum of embryologic abnormalities that interfere with midline cleavage of the forebrain and cause midline dysplasia of the face.[170–172]

The syndrome of septo-optic dysplasia (De Morsier's syndrome) consists of optic nerve and optic disk hypoplasia with or without abnormalities of the septum pellucidum and corpus callosum. Growth failure and hypopituitarism occur in 60 percent of cases. Other features include median facial cleft, hyperprolactinemia, and diabetes insipidus. Septo-optic dysplasia may represent a mild form of arhinencephalia.[170,171]

An increased incidence of hypopituitarism has been documented in patients with cleft lip and palate.[173]

Extension of the subarachnoid space into the sella turcica is responsible for the *empty sella syndrome.* It is presumed to result from an incompetent sella diaphragm and an increase in CSF pressure.[174–176] In the absence of surgery or radiation, the condition is called *primary* empty sella syndrome. Familial cases are rare. In most patients, pituitary function is normal and the sella turcica is diffusely enlarged. Empty sella syndrome is seen most frequently in obese middle-aged women; it is rarely recognized during childhood. The disorder can be readily distinguished from pituitary tumor by CT or MRI studies of the hypothalamus and pituitary gland. Most of the reported cases have associated cranial defects. One kindred has been described in which empty sella syndrome was transmitted as an autosomal dominant trait in association with Rieger's anomaly of the anterior chamber of the eye.[177]

Children with *biologically inactive GH* present with growth failure and have the following characteristics: height that is below the mean by >3 SD, abnormal growth rate (<4 cm/year), apparent good health, normal body proportions, normal plasma GH responses by RIA but abnormally low ratios of radioreceptor-measured/RIA-measured GH concentrations, low serum IGF-I concentrations which improve after 3 to 10 daily injections of GH, and improvement of linear growth with GH therapy.[133] The assumption is made that the endogenous GH in these children has reduced biological activity but is immunologically reactive. Biologically inactive GH is thought to be one of the etiologic factors in NVSS.[122]

GH neurosecretory dysfunction was first described in children who had received prior cranial radiation and in very short children with unexplained poor growth (i.e., growth velocity < 4 cm/year, peak GH concentration > 10 ng/mL after provocative testing, low serum IGF-I levels, and abnormally low diurnal frequency and amplitude of GH pulses).[134,178] Spontaneous GH secretion in these children was found to be lower than in controls but higher than in patients with classical GH deficiency. The data suggested that these children have a subtle deficiency of GH as a result of defective neuroregulation of GH secretion. Treatment with exogenous GH enhanced linear growth velocity in the majority. Assessment of spontaneous GH secretion is labor-intensive because serum samples for GH measurement must be obtained at 15- to 20-min intervals, or alternatively, a plasma sample can be collected by means of a constant withdrawal portable pump for an integrated GH concentration. These studies cannot be carried out safely in small children.

Recently, the validity of spontaneous GH secretion studies has been questioned because additional investigations have shown that mean GH levels in very short children are not significantly different from those of control subjects matched for age and pubertal stage.[179,180] The use of both IGF-I and IGFBP-3 measurements in these children may better distinguish them from normally growing subjects.[181]

GH Resistance or Laron Syndrome Children with GH resistance resemble congenitally GH deficient subjects except they are small at birth and have high serum levels of GH, exaggerated GH responses to provocative tests, and low serum levels of IGF-I and IGFBP-3.[182–190] Affected children do not grow when treated with rGH, nor do they have a rise in IGF-I or IGFBP-3. Hypoglycemia is a frequent problem in the early years. The endogenous GH produced by these children is biologically active and binds normally in standard GH receptor assays. Adults with GH resistance seldom exceed 130 cm in height and are usually fertile. This entity is seen most commonly in offspring of consanguinous marriages involving Jewish parents of middle Eastern extraction. Another large population has been identified in Equador (possibly of Jewish ancestry). The remaining affected individuals are distributed worldwide. Inheritance is autosomal recessive. A variety of genetic defects have been identified in the GH receptor gene i.e., gene deletions and point mutations (missense, nonsense, and abnormal splicing). Most of the mutations occur in the extracellular GH-binding domain of the GH receptor and lead to an absence of serum GHBP and lack of GH binding and signaling through the GHR. Measurement of serum GHBP is an important diagnostic test. Less frequently, GH resistance is caused by mutations in the intracellular domains of the GHR. In such subjects, serum levels of GHBP are either normal or increased. The fundamental cause of GH resistance is either failure of GH binding or an abnormality of receptor dimerization and signal transduction. Inheritance is autosomal recessive and the female to male ratio is one except in Equador, where females outnumber males 19:1. The latter has not been explained.

Recently, GH resistance was reported in a subject with a mutation in only one GHR gene. Presumably, the abnormality had a dominant negative effect by preventing GH receptor dimerization.[191]

Many investigators have hypothesized that heterozygosity for mutations in the GH receptor gene may explain the growth abnormality seen in some children with idiopathic short stature (idiopathic growth failure). These children have relative (partial) GH resistance which allows them to benefit from exogenous GH treatment.[192–194]

A highly unusual cause of GH resistance was a partial deletion of the IGF-I gene reported in a 15-year-old boy who had prenatal and postnatal growth retardation, microcephaly, sensorineural hearing loss, and mental retardation. Serum IGF-I level was low but IGFBP-3 and GHBP levels were normal.[139]

Human recombinant IGF-I is the only effective treatment for GH resistance. Growth rates increase significantly (8 to 13 cm/yr) on IGF-I treatment (120 μg/kg daily given subcutaneously). Potential adverse effects include hypoglycemia, headaches, papilledema, seizures, and altered facial features. Access to IGF-I treatment depends on the patient participating in approved research protocol.[195,196]

Acquired GH Deficiency Children with acquired GH deficiency by definition grow normally during early childhood and then fail to grow because they develop GH deficiency. It is essential that organic disease be excluded. The causes of acquired GH deficiency are discussed briefly here.

Craniopharyngioma is the most common *CNS tumor* that causes GH deficiency in childhood. The tumor is believed to rise from embryonic squamous cell rests located at the junction of the adenohypophysis and neurohypophysis. Because of its location, expansion may cause permanent injury to the hypothalamus, optic nerves, and pituitary gland. The only complaint may be growth failure. Other clinical features include visual field defects, signs and symptoms of increased intracranial pressure, and multiple pituitary endocrine deficiencies. After surgical extirpation of the tumor, a majority of children have panhypopituitarism. Destruction of the satiety center may result in uncontrolled hyperphagia and obesity. Normal or excessive growth has been observed after surgery in some hyperphagic patients who have abnormally low GH responses and normal somatomedin levels.[197] Recent studies suggest that hyperprolactinemia or hyperinsulinism may account for the normal IGF-I levels and sustained growth in these children.[198,199] Other CNS tumors that cause hypopituitarism in childhood are optic gliomas, germinomas, ependymomas, meningiomas, colloid cysts of the third ventricle, and, rarely, chromophobe adenomas.

Trauma may also produce GH deficiency. Perinatal injury to the pituitary and/or hypothalamus may account for a significant number of childhood cases of presumed congenital idiopathic GH deficiency. A careful review of the birth histories of these children has shown that 50 to 65 percent of patients had one or more significant perinatal insults. Birth size is generally normal. The male/female ratio is 4:1. Perinatal risk factors include intrapartum hypoxemia or asphyxia, breech deliveries, difficult forceps deliveries, intracranial hemorrhage, precipitate or prolonged labor, twin pregnancies, and postnatal seizures. Other risk factors include bleeding during pregnancy and toxemia.[200,201] Throughout childhood, accidental head trauma or child abuse may result in hypopituitarism.

Inflammatory diseases, including bacterial meningitis, viral encephalitis, and fungal infections of the CNS, may cause permanent injury to the pituitary and hypothalamus. Giant cell granuloma of the pituitary gland is a rare cause of hypopituitarism. Its presentation may be indistinguishable from that of pituitary adenoma[202]; the diagnosis is usually made at autopsy or by obtaining pituitary tissue for histologic examination. The disease is usually of unknown etiology, but has been seen in association with tuberculosis, syphilis, and sarcoidosis.

Lymphocytic hypophysitis is considered an *autoimmune disorder,* the clinical characteristics of which resemble those of pituitary tumors. Hypopituitarism is frequently present. The disease has been described most frequently in women who are pregnant or were recently pregnant.[203–205]

Irradiation for tumors of the head and neck carries a high risk for impaired hypothalamic-pituitary function.[206–208] The doses of radiation usually exceed 4,000 rads. GH deficiency is the most common abnormality; TSH and ACTH secretion usually are preserved. Less is known about the gonadotropin status of these children. Primary thyroid dysfunction due to radiation injury of the thyroid gland is not uncommon. Usually, the patient appears euthyroid and has an elevated TSH level with normal T_4 and T_3 concentrations. Clinical hypothyroidism with low T_4 and T_3 levels has also been observed in these children. In the early stages after cranial radiation, GH responses to pharmacologic stimulation may be normal, but spontaneous GH secretion is low.

Aneurysms of the pituitary vessels and infarction of the pituitary gland due to vascular malformations are extremely rare causes of hypopituitarism in childhood.[209]

Impaired hypothalamic-pituitary function may be observed in patients with *thalassemia major* who have iron overload. Normal GH responses and low somatomedin levels have been documented.[210–212]

Permanent vasopressin deficiency and diabetes insipidus are the most common CNS complications of *disseminated histiocytosis.* Most affected children have inadequate GH responses to provocative tests but grow satisfactorily and do not require treatment. Those with growth failure and abnormal GH responses benefit from GH therapy. Usually TSH, ACTH, FSH, and LH secretion remain normal.[213]

Transient Defects in GH Secretion or Action Transient or functional hypopituitarism has been documented in prepubertal males and has been called the "lazy pituitary syndrome."[214] Therapy with GH or androgens accelerates growth velocity. Normal GH responses to provocative stimuli have been observed after the onset of puberty.[215,216]

Hypopituitarism has been documented in young children with growth failure who come from hostile home environments. Psychological stress and nutritional factors are the probable causes of the entity known as *psychosocial dwarfism.* These patients have delayed onset of speech, are withdrawn, and have abnormal sleep patterns and bizarre eating habits. After these children are placed in foster homes or after the home stresses are resolved, pituitary function returns to normal, growth accelerates, and they exhibit improved behavior and normal dietary habits.[217–220]

Transient GH deficiency due to depletion of pituitary GH has been documented in primary hypothyroidism. Treatment with thyroid hormone is associated with catch-up growth and normal GH responses to provocative stimuli.

Diagnosis of GH Deficiency The diagnostic evaluation and treatment of GH deficiency depends on the age of the child and the presence or absence of hypoglycemia. Small infants with hypoglycemia require immediate evaluation and treatment but are able to undergo only limited diagnostic studies. The most practical test involves measurement of glucose, plasma cortisol, GH, and insulin concentrations during a documented episode of spontaneous hypoglycemia. Serum T_4 and TSH concentrations should also be determined. Insulin-induced hypoglycemia is a hazardous diagnostic test in small infants. L-Arginine stimulation is safe but requires an infusion and six or more blood samples. The diagnosis of GH and ACTH deficiency in the neonatal period is based on a plasma GH level <10 ng/ml and a plasma cortisol concentration <5 μg/dL during fasting hypoglycemia or L-arginine challenge. Frequent feedings at 3- to 4-h intervals coupled with GH and hydrocortisone treatment usually restore carbohydrate homeostasis. With advancing age, the tendency to hypoglycemia lessens. During illness, therapy with stress doses of hydrocortisone (see previous discussion) may be needed to protect the patient from hypoglycemia and seizures. Parents can also be taught to give rectal glucose (25 mL of 50 percent glucose diluted in equal parts with tap water and dispensed from a pediatric Fleet's enema container that has been emptied of enema solution).

Opinions differ concerning the appropriate age for conducting pituitary function tests beyond infancy. If growth failure is the child's only problem, it may be preferable to wait until 3 or 4 years of age; however, diagnostic evaluation can be performed at an earlier age depending on the circumstances. No child should undergo GH testing while hypothyroid because the results are unreliable. Treatment with T_4 for 1 or 2 months prior to assessment of GH responsiveness is recommended.

The usual indications for the evaluation of GH deficiency include (1) pathologic short stature in a child with normal body proportions (height >2 SD below the mean), (2) abnormal growth rate for chronologic age (<7 cm/year prior to age 3, <5 cm/year from age 3 to onset of puberty, and <6 cm/year during the pubertal years), (3) delayed skeletal maturation (bone age >2 SD below the mean for chronologic age), and (4) special clinical considerations (e.g., microgenitalia, prior hypoglycemia, history of head trauma, CNS tumor, hypoxemia, or intracranial hemorrhage). In addition, tests of pituitary function are necessary when linear growth in children with suspected acquired hypopituitarism decelerates or ceases, even if height is within the normal range.

Valuable information is obtained from the following: construction of growth curves, serum T_4 and TSH assays (T_3 and TRH stimulation tests are optional), insulin hypoglycemia challenge for GH and cortisol secretion (if severe GH deficiency is suspected, use only 0.05 U regular insulin per kilogram of body weight as an IV bolus and take the precautions noted in Table 25-13), L-arginine stimulation test for GH, prolactin determination, urine specific gravity and/or osmolality (on the second voided urine after an overnight water-deprivation test to assess vasopressin secretion), CBC, urinalysis, biochemical profile, bone age determination, anteroposterior and lateral skull x-rays for sella size and shape, examinations of visual fields and acuity, funduscopic examination, and CT scan or MRI of hypothalamus and pituitary (in selected cases only). GHRH stimulation tests are not routinely performed in pathologically short children because a majority of these patients have excellent reserves of pituitary GH. Only children with severe classical GH deficiency show poor GH responses to GHRH.

The diagnosis of classical GH deficiency is based on a peak GH of <8 to 10 ng/mL after two provocative stimuli. Severe GH deficiency is present when the peak GH level is <4 ng/mL. Because monoclonal IRMA GH assays give lower concentrations than do standard polyclonal GH RIAs, the diagnostic criteria must be adjusted in accordance with the GH assay used. Many studies have suggested that GH treatment should not be confined exclusively to children with classical GH deficiency as a majority of subjects with severe idiopathic growth failure will benefit from GH treatment. Characteristically, this group has normal GH responses to provocative tests, low IGF-1 and IGFBP-3 levels, and pathologic height, growth rate, and bone age for chronologic age.

Treatment Recombinant human GH (rGH) is the approved treatment for both childhood onset GHD (COGHD) and adult onset GHD (AOGHD).[221] Children require higher doses of rGH than do adults; 0.18 to 0.3 mg/kg per week divided and given subsequently daily or 3 to 6 times weekly. Daily therapy yields greater growth velocities and cumulative height gains in prepubertal children. Four pharmaceutical companies have received FDA approval to market somatropin (rGH, 191 amino acids) and their products are equally efficacious and have similar safety profiles. Somatrem (rGH 192 amino acids) is still available but is being used less frequently. The product choices include a lyophylized or aqueous rGH and pen delivery systems are available. A sustained release depot rGH formulation is now available. The biopotency of rGH is 3 IU per mg and dosing is done exclusively by weight in the United States, whereas, in Europe, unit dosing is still being used. The rGH dose for AOGHD is very low because adults are more prone to develop arthralgias, weight gain, sodium and water retention, swollen fingers and ankles, and carpal tunnel syndrome. Blood pressure has not increased on rGH treatment. The starting dose in adults should be very small (e.g., 3 μg/kg daily in adults compared to children, who receive 26 to 43 μg/kg daily based on the 0.18 to 0.3 mg/kg per week dose). Depending on tolerance, the adult dose can be increased gradually to approximately 6 μg/kg daily given subcutaneously. Compliance with rGH treatment in adults is largely dependent on selecting a dose that does not cause discomfort, yet is therapeutic (see Chap. 7).

The frequency of side effects from rGH treatment in childhood is remarkably low but careful monitoring and reporting is an essential of good medical care.[222] Adverse events include: (1) Pseudotumor cerebri or benign intracranial hypertension, which has been reported in about 30 children receiving rGH. More frequently it occurs in patients with renal failure or Turner syndrome. Careful ophthalmologic and neurologic examinations are indicated if the patient complains of headaches, nausea, dizziness, ataxia, or vision changes after starting rGH treatment. These problems subside when rGH treatment is temporarily stopped or the rGH dose is halved. No permanent sequelae has been reported. (2) Slipped capital femoral epiphysis (SCFE) is a rare occurrence in obese children with hypopituitarism or hypothyroidism prior to and during treatment. Pain in the hip, knee, or ankle is a complaint that warrants hip X-rays. (3) Miscellaneous reports of pancreatitis, increased number of nevi, scoliosis, and prepubertal gynecomastia may or may not have a direct relationship to rGH treatment. Antibodies to GH are almost never seen currently. Leukemia is not believed to occur more frequently during or following GH treatment in childhood if the patient is free of known risk factors. Worldwide, approximately 50 children have developed leukemia during and after rGH treatment. Fewer than 20 were from the United States and most of these had other risk factors (prior malignancies, chemotherapy, radiation treatment, and syndromes or chromosomal abnormalities with a known increased risk for malignancy, e.g., Bloom syndrome, Down Syndrome, Fanconi anemia). In the United States, there is a twofold or fourfold increased risk of leukemia in the at-risk population. Hence, children with a prior history of malignancy need to have this issue disclosed prior to receiving rGH therapy, and their oncologists should also give approval for this treatment. The database of rGH experience in more than 30,000 children documents that the risk of neoplasm is not increased in rGH treated subjects.

Prior to 1985, the standard GH used for treatment was purified GH extracted from human pituitary glands. This preparation was withdrawn from human use in 1985 because four young adults who had received GH in the late 1960s and early 1970s died of Creutzfeldt-Jakob disease (CJD).[223–225] CJD is a slow degenerative disease of the central nervous system caused by a transmissible unconventional prion. It has been classified as one of the subacute spongiform encephalopathies. Clinically, the disease is characterized by progressive truncal ataxia, tremors of the head and extremities, speech disturbances, involuntary movements, dementia, and death. Seldom is CJD seen in patients before age 30 years unless there is a genetic or infectious etiology.

In the first year of rGH treatment, children with GHD grow 9 to 12 cm/yr if compliance is good. Subsequently, growth rates decline to 7 to 8 cm/yr. Appetite improves and loss of subcutaneous tissue leads to a more mature appearance. Until recently, rGH therapy in COGHD was discontinued when the epiphyses fused, but this is no longer the standard of care because GH is important in adulthood for bone mineral density, control of body weight and fat mass distribution as well as possible protection against fractures, cardiac morbidity, and mortality. There is a general agreement about administering rGH treatment to adults who developed panhypopituitarism after hypophysectomy for a pituitary tumor (AOGHD). This opinion is also true for childhood-onset panhypopituitarism due to a tumor or congenital anomaly in the hypothalamic-pituitary area. We lack information about the need for adult rGH treatment in children who had isolated GH deficiency and completed their therapy. A significant number of these children (25–40 percent) have normal GH levels when provocative tests are repeated in adulthood and many express disinterest in resuming rGH therapy. The current criteria for diagnosing GH deficiency in adulthood was based on subjects with severe disease, i.e., peak GH (after insulin hypoglycemia or arginine) <5 ng/ml (polyclonal assay) or 3 ng/ml (monoclonal assay). Whether these criteria are valid in younger adults with less severe disease is unknown. Among those retested in adulthood, the likelihood of confirming persistent GHD was highest in the group with original peak GH <5 ng/ml and in those with craniopharyngioma or anatomic abnormalities in the pituitary hypothalamic region. Patients with isolated COGHD and peak GH between 5 to 10 ng/ml were more likely to have normal GH peaks in adulthood. In control subjects, GH production is highest in the second decade and declines by 14 percent for each subsequent 10 years of adult life. Hence, the diagnostic cut off for GHD in 20-year-old subjects should be higher than the one for 40- to 50-year-old adults. This fact is not taken into consideration at present.[227,228]

Guidelines for prescribing rGH in children have been prepared by the Lawson Wilkins Pediatric Endocrine Society.[229] Marked improvement in adult height outcomes are being seen in children receiving rGH therapy. Age at onset of treatment and duration of therapy correlate directly with outcome. The best adult heights were observed in individuals who started rGH therapy at a young age. The mean adult height standard deviation scores now range from −0.7 SD to −1.3 SD in published studies. These are significantly greater than the adult heights seen in the pituitary GH era, when most adult heights were between −3 SD and −2 SD depending on dose and duration of treatment.[230,231]

Human GH releasing hormone (GHRH) is also an approved treatment for GHD but it is only used in a very small number of patients. Its efficacy is less than rGH and should be used only in patients with functional pituitary glands. No adult heights are available.

Small doses of androgens given simultaneously with GH during the prepubertal years enhance linear growth responses.[232,233] A regimen of oxandrolone, 0.05 to 0.1 mg per kilogram of body weight per day PO, plus GH increases growth rates without significant enlargement of the phallus. When microphallus is present, GH treatment can be combined with a small dose of depot testosterone (25 mg IM monthly for 2 or 3 months). Androgen therapy should never be used without concurrent GH administration because bone maturation usually accelerates without compensatory increases in height and ultimate stature may be compromised. Bone age must be evaluated at both the start and the completion of each treatment period to assess the effects of therapy on bone maturation relative to height gain. Lastly, androgens should not be combined with GH if bone age has moved significantly ahead of height age during the previous treatment period. In these circumstances, it is safer to use only GH treatment. Thyroid hormone determination should be performed at 6- to 12-month intervals because hypopituitary children with previously normal serum T_4 levels have been known to develop hypothyroidism during GH treatment. This may be due to a stimulation of somatostatin release by GH which in turn suppresses TSH secretion. In this situation, thyroid replacement must be administered concurrently to ensure an optimal growth response to administered GH. At present, GH therapy should be continued until the epiphyses close to obtain maximal growth.

Assessment of gonadotropin secretion is usually postponed until the adolescent years. In a male who has reached age 14 years and has no increase in testicular size, 24-h urinary FSH and LH excretion (by RIA) and plasma testosterone concentration should be determined. Stimulation of pituitary FSH and LH by GnRH is now being standardized. Unfortunately, a single GnRH injection may not indicate whether dysfunction exists in the pituitary or the hypothalamus. Absence of a rise in plasma and/or urinary FSH and LH concentration is indicative of either pituitary disease or prolonged endogenous lack of GnRH. Repeated GnRH stimulation has been used to differentiate pituitary from hypothalamic dysfunction.

The treatment of gonadotropin deficiency depends on the height and bone age of the patient. If the patient is 14 years old, bone age is $<$14 years, and height is approximately 5 ft, GH plus testosterone 17β-cypionate or testosterone enanthate (50 to 100 mg every 3 to 4 weeks) results in increased growth velocity as well as penis and sexual hair growth. After the patient has achieved a height of 5 ft 4 in. or has begun epiphyseal fusion (bone age = 16 years), larger doses of testosterone (200 mg every 2 to 3 weeks IM) are needed to promote sexual maturation. Transdermal testosterone treatment is becoming increasingly popular but is more expensive. For reasons that are poorly understood, many gonadotropin-deficient hypopituitary males do not achieve satisfactory beard growth or muscular development. An alternative treatment program for gonadotropin-deficient males involves simultaneous administration of hMG and hCG to promote testicular maturation, virilization, and fertility. The treatment of pituitary hormone deficits is summarized in Table 25-8.

Cushing's Syndrome Obesity, linear growth failure, and delayed adolescence may be the only signs of Cushing's syndrome in childhood. In contrast to obese normal children who grow rapidly, those with Cushing's syndrome exhibit linear growth deceleration and subtle or obvious cushingoid facial features. Annual school photographs often document the onset of a cushingoid facial appearance. The diagnostic protocol includes measurement of diurnal plasma cortisol concentrations; plasma ACTH concentration; 24-h excretion of 17-hydroxycorticosteroids, 17-ketosteroids, and cortisol; low-dose dexamethasone suppression test (20 μg per kilogram of body weight per day divided into four doses and given at 6-h intervals); high-dose dexamethasone suppression test (80 μg/kg per day given in four doses); ACTH stimulation test; skeletal x-rays for osteoporosis and bone age; and CT scans of the head and abdomen. Abdominal ultrasonography may also aid in the detection of an adrenal lesion. These less invasive diagnostic tests have almost entirely replaced adrenal arteriography and/or angiography, which were once the only means for localizing an adrenal tumor.

The treatment of Cushing's syndrome due to adrenal adenoma or carcinoma is unilateral adrenalectomy and supportive glucocorticoid therapy during and after surgery until function is restored in the contralateral adrenal gland. Bilateral adrenalectomy is necessary for Cushing's syndrome due to micronodular adrenal disease, a non-ACTH-dependent form of glucocorticoid excess. The choices of therapy for bilateral adrenal hyperplasia (Cushing's disease) include (1) transsphenoidal pituitary microadenectomy, (2) pituitary irradiation, and (3) bilateral adrenalectomy. One study has documented the presence of pituitary microadenomas in 14 of 15 children with Cushing's disease.[234] In the hands of an experienced neurosurgeon, pituitary microadenectomy leads to rapid amelioration of glucocorticoid excess, resumption of growth, and progression through puberty; other pituitary functions generally improve or remain unchanged. Jennings and coworkers reported favorable results after cranial irradiation for childhood Cushing's disease.[235] However, the long-range impact of cranial irradiation on pituitary function and behavior is unknown. Bilateral adrenalectomy has been widely used as therapy in children

TABLE 25-8. Treatment of Hormone Deficits and Monitoring Schedule for Childhood Onset Hypopituitarism

Hormone Deficit	Treatment	Monitoring Criteria
TRH-TSH	L-Thyroxine 2 μg/kg per day PO	Growth rate, serum T_4 concentration
GH	0.04 mg/kg/day SC (range = 0.18–0.3 mg/kg per week)	Linear growth rate, bone age, clinical appearance, T_4, IGF-1
ACTH	Oral hydrocortisone or cortisone acetate, 10–15 mg/m^2 per day divided into 2 or 3 doses; triple dose during stress	Fasting blood sugar, plasma cortisol concentrations
FSH-LH	**Males**	
	1. Depot-testosterone 100–200 mg IM every 2–4 weeks	Dose depends on age
	2. Transdermal testosterone Testodermal 5 mg Androderm 2.5, 5 mg	
	3. hCG 1,000–2,000 U in 0.2–0.4 mL diluent IM three times weekly; Pergonal menotropins, one vial in 1 mL diluent, IM three times weekly; hCG and Pergonal menotropins may be combined in single syringe.	HCG/Pergonal are used mainly to enhance virilization, testes volume and sperm formation
	Females	
	1. Ethinyl estradiol or Premarin PO	Dose varies with age -small doses are used initially. The Vivele patch may be cut in half
	2. Transderm β Estradiol Vivele 0.0375, 0.05, 0.075, 0.1 mg/day Estraderm 0.05 mg/day Apply twice weekly to skin	
Vasopressin	DDAVP Rhinal tube or nasal spray DDAVP tablet 0.1, 0.2 mg tablets Dose varies with age and patient response	Seldom used in young infants

with Cushing's disease. Unfortunately, 25 to 45 percent of patients develop hyperpigmentation and enlargement of the sella turcica due to Nelson's syndrome. Glucocorticoid (hydrocortisone, 12 to 15 mg per square meter of body surface per day PO, or cortisone acetate, 30 mg/m^2 per day PO) and mineralocorticoid replacement (9α-fluorocortisone, 0.1 mg/day PO) also are needed after bilateral adrenalectomy. These patients also require stress doses of hydrocortisone (60 to 75 mg per square meter of body surface per day) with febrile illness, trauma, anesthesia, etc. Careful periodic evaluation for Nelson's syndrome is mandatory. Cyproheptadine, bromocriptine, metyrapone, and mitotane are seldom used in childhood Cushing's disease.

Short Adult Stature Due to Precocious Sexual Maturation

During the early childhood years, children with precocious puberty or who secrete excessive amounts of androgens, as in non-salt-losing congenital adrenal hyperplasia (CAH), are at risk for short stature in their adult years. Before epiphyseal fusion, these children are tall, but their markedly accelerated pace of bone maturation without compensatory increases in height results in epiphyseal fusion and growth cessation at an inappropriately young age.

Bone Disorders (Chondrodysplasias or Skeletal Dysplasias)

Disproportionate short stature is the distinguishing characteristic of the chondrodysplasias, a clinically and genetically heterogeneous group of bone diseases that disturb to varying degrees the length and shape of long bones, trunk, and skull. They are caused by gene mutations that interfere with endochondral ossification; i.e., either abnormal growth plate chondrocyte differentiation and proliferation or defective bone matrix production. Table 25-9 lists the human chondrodysplasia mutations. Defects in the COL2A1 and FGFR3 genes account for the great majority of patients with chondrodysplasias.[236,237]

The Type 2 collagen gene (COL2A1) mutations now exceed 30 in number. All involve one of the two COL2A1 genes (alleles) and the defects are located in the triple helical domain of the molecule. The gene defect either promotes accumulation of mutant collagen molecules in the extracellular matrix of cartilage or diminishes the quantity of normal cartilage matrix. Genetic transmission is autosomal dominant and the mutant gene either has a dominant negative mode of action (mutant gene product interferes with the function of the product of the normal gene) or causes haploinsufficiency (loss of the product of one allele causes a quantitative reduction of Type 2 collagen). The severity ranges from achondrogenesis Type 2 and hypochondrogenesis to milder disorders such as spondyloepiphysial osteoarthritis (often called late onset SED). Intermediate forms include SED congenita and KNIEST dysplasia. The most common COL2A1 mutations cause a substitution of the glycine residues that normally occupy every third position in the collagen triple helix and thereby interfere with the normal assembly of the helix. Type 2 collagen is the major structural protein of cartilage and qualitative or quantitative changes in Type 2 collagen interfere with endochondral ossification. However, the precise mechanisms involved have not defined.

Achondroplasia (most common chondrodysplasia), hypochondroplasia, and thanotropic dwarfism (TD) are caused by activating mutations in the FGFR3 gene located on chromosome 4 p 16.3 near the Huntington disease gene locus. The FGFR3 protein is a membrane-spanning tyrosine kinase receptor composed of an extracellular ligand-binding domain (with 3 linked immunoglobulin subdomains), a transmembrane domain, and a split intracellular tyrosine kinase domain. Achondroplasia maps to the transmembrane domain, hypochondroplasia to the proximal tyrosine kinase domain, and TD to the distal tyrosine domain. The FGFR3 in these disorders is constitutively activated. Hence signal transduction proceeds in the absence of ligand and the rate of endochondral bone growth is slowed by mechanisms which are under investigation.

One clinical classification divides the chondrodystrophies into those with predominantly short limbs (e.g., achondroplasia) and those with predominantly short trunk (e.g., spondyloepiphyseal dysplasia). Other clinical features used to classify these patients include age of onset, location of the defect, i.e., in proximal, medial, or distal segments of limbs, and presence of associated physical abnormalities, e.g., polydactylism in Ellis–van Creveld syndrome (chondroectodermal dysplasia) or fine hair in cartilage-hair hypoplasia.

The radiographic classifications are based on the location of the abnormality in the long bones, e.g., epiphyses (epiphyseal dysplasia), metaphyses (metaphyseal dysplasia), or diaphysis (Fig. 25-18). When both the spine and the long bones have disordered growth, the terms *spondyloepiphyseal* and *spondylometaphyseal* dysplasia have been used. Further subdivision of these groups has been based on other distinguishing abnormalities. The clinical and radiographic classifications are descriptive and do not provide information on the cellular abnormalities responsible for abnormal bone growth.

The pathophysiologic classification is based on the histochemical and ultrastructural characteristics of cartilage and bone. It thus gives more detailed information on the possible pathogenesis of many of these disorders. Examples include abnormal chondrocyte metabolism (mucopolysaccharidoses), chondrocyte proliferation (achondroplasia), chondrocyte maturation and degeneration (metaphyseal dysplasia), and epiphyseal ossification (epiphyseal dysplasia).[238]

This group of disorders is characterized by poor linear growth from early life, abnormal body proportions, distinguishing physical and radiographic data, bone age close to chronologic age (and ahead of height age), normal sexual maturation, and appropriate age of epiphyseal fusion. Detailed endocrine evaluation is seldom needed. The genetic implications must be shared with patients as adulthood approaches.

Achondroplasia/Hypochondroplasia Two treatments for achondroplasia have become available. The first involves the use of GH administration, which improves growth velocity mainly in the first year, with fewer effects in the second and third years of treatment. It appears that modest gains in final height can be achieved with GH therapy, but the evidence is inconclusive. The second approach involves limb-lengthening operations using small percutaneous incisions through which the long bones of the extremities are broken.[239] The method developed by Villarubias in Barcelona involves the use of one externally fixated bar that controls the gradual distraction of the callus. This device allows for limb stretching at a rate of 1.2 mm/day. Bilateral tibial lengthening is done first. Subsequently, the femurs are lengthened, along with percutaneous tenotomies of the adductors and the internal rectorus. The Villarubias technique does not permit weight bearing, so that after a brief hospitalization of 3 to 5 days the patient must

TABLE 25-9. Summary of Human Chondrodysplasia Mutations

Locus	Chromosomal Location	Gene Product Function	Clinical Phenotype	Inheritance Pattern	Proposed Effect of Mutation
COL2A1	12q13.11	Extracellular matrix protein	Achondrogenesis type II	AD	Dominant negative
			Hypochondrogenesis	AD	Dominant negative
			SED congenita	AD	Dominant negative
			Kniest dysplasia	AD	Dominant negative
			Last-onset SED	AD	Dominant negative
			Stickler dysplasia	AD	Haploinsufficiency
COL9A2	1p33-p32.3	Extracellular matrix protein	MED	AD	Dominant negative
COL10A1	6q21-q22	Extracellular matrix protein hypertrophic cartilage	Schmid-type metaphyseal chrondrodysplasia	AD	Haploinsufficiency
COL11A2	6p21.3	Extracellular matrix protein	Stickler-like dysplasia	AD	Dominant negative
				AR	Loss of function
COMP	19p12-13.1	Extracellular matrix protein	Psuedoachondroplasia	AD	Dominant negative
			MED Fairbanks	AD	Dominant negative
			MED Ribbing	AD	Dominant negative
FGFR3	4p16.3	Tyrosine kinase transmembrance receptor for FGFs	Thanatophoric dysplasia	AD	Gain of function
			Achondroplasia	AD	Gain of function
			Hypochondroplasia	AD	Gain of function
PTHrPR	3p21-p22	G protein transmembrane receptor for PTH and PTHrP	Jansen-type metaphyseal chondrodysplasia	AD	Gain of function
DTDST	5q31-q34	Transmembrane sulfate transporter	Diatrophic dysplasia	AR	Loss of function
			Atelosteogenesis type II	AR	Loss of function
			Achondrogenesis type IB	AR	Loss of function
ARSE	Xp22.3	Arylsulfatase enzyme	Chondrodysplasia punctata	XLR	Loss of function
SOX9	17q24.1-q25.1	Transcription factor	Campomelic dysplasia	AD	Haploinsufficiency

SED: Spondyloepiphyseal dysplasia; MED: Multiple epiphyseal dysplasia; AD: Autosomal dominant; AR: Autosomal recessive; XLR: Sex-linked recessive.

spend many months in a wheelchair. This approach is said to be associated with less pain and discomfort than alternative approaches. Prophylactic tenotomies prevent the contractures encountered with other techniques. Care must be taken to preserve the blood supply, which is essential for good callus healing. Complications include muscle contractions, stretching of nerves, joint stiffness, vascular complications, problems at the pin site, and various psychological difficulties. This procedure has yielded as much as 12 in. of height and has corrected the lordosis that is a constant feature of achondroplasia. Expert care by skilled orthopedists, geneticists, psychologists, and physical therapists is required for a successful outcome. Most importantly, the patient should be the individual who makes the decision. Emotional maturity and stability are prerequisites. It has been recommended that surgery be postponed until children reach the age of 14 to 20 years. Finally, it is important to inform patients and their families that experience with these procedures is still limited and that the risks are significant (Fig. 25-19).

FIGURE 25-18. Classification of the chondrodystrophies based on radiographic abnormalities in the long bones. (*From Rimoin DL: The Chondrodystrophies. Adv Hum Genet 5:1, 1975.*)

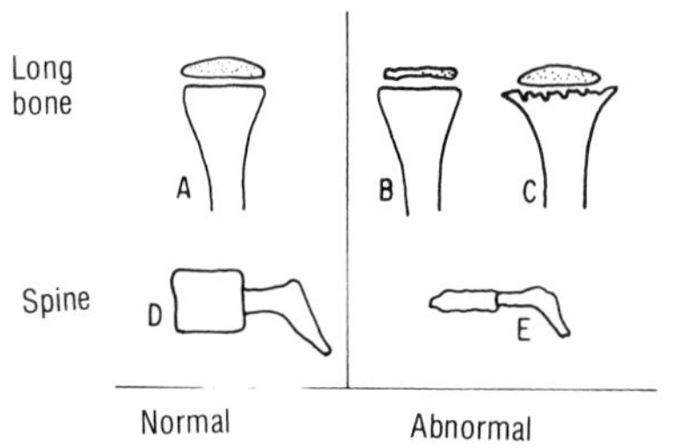

Involvement	Classification
A + D	Normal
B + D	Epiphyseal dysplasia
C + D	Metaphyseal dysplasia
B + E	Spondyloepiphyseal dysplasia
C + E	Spondylometaphyseal dysplasia

Hypochondroplasia is an autosomal dominant disorder that differs from but resembles a mild form of achondroplasia. Poor growth starts after 2 years of age and adult heights are 120 to 150 cm compared to 120 to 130 cm for adult achondroplasia patients. The facial features of achondroplasia are absent. Head size is moderately large. Rhizomelia is less striking than in achondroplasia. Skeletal X-rays confirm the diagnosis and should be performed in short children with the phenotypic characteristics of hypochondroplasia. The treatment options are similar to those for achondroplasia.

Chromosome Abnormalities: Turner's Syndrome

Turner's syndrome occurs in approximately 1 in 2,500 to 5,000 female live births. The frequency in female fetuses is as high as 3 percent, but most are lost through spontaneous abortion.[240] Monosomy X (45,X) accounts for 90 percent of affected fetuses, whereas liveborn girls with Turner's syndrome have a wide variety of karyotypes (50 percent are 45,X, and the remainder may have isochromosomes of the long arm of X, ring X, deletions of the short arm of X, or various mosaicisms).

The phenotype of Turner's syndrome is diverse; most girls have easily recognizable physical characteristics, while in some the fetuses may consist only of short stature and absence of sexual

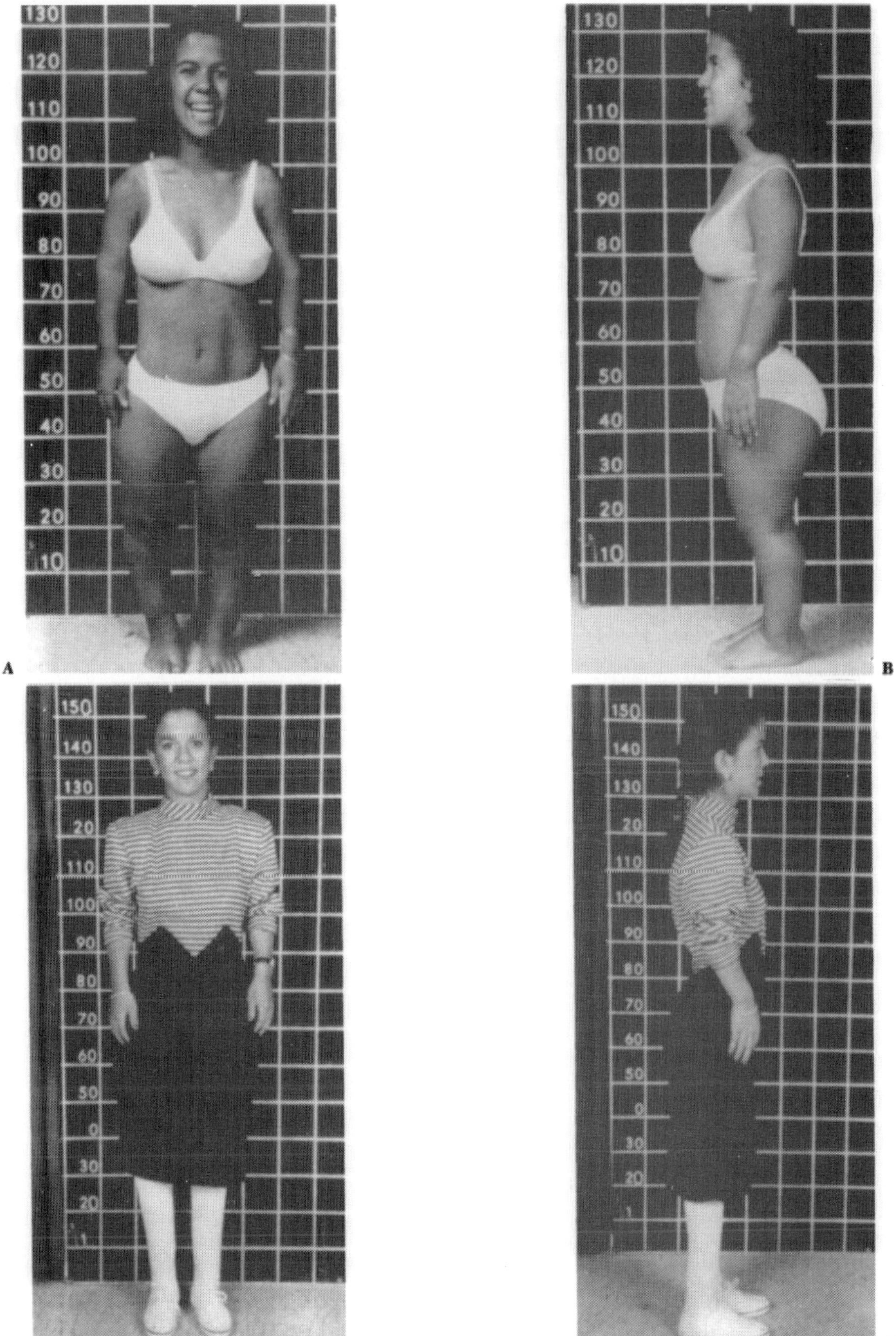

FIGURE 25-19. A young woman with achondroplasia is shown before (*A* and *B*) and after (*C* and *D*) leg lengthening. Final height (61.5 inches) was increased by approximately 12 in. (*From Rimoin.*[239])

maturation in adolescence. For this reason, it is advisable to perform a karyotype in all girls with unexplained growth failure. In infancy, the usual clues are loose skin folds in the posterior neck region (Bonnevie-Ullrich syndrome), which later form the pterygium colli (webbed neck); lymphedema of the dorsum of the feet and hands; increased carrying angles and various nail abnormalities, such as rudimentary, dysplastic, or hyperconvex nails surrounded by abundant soft tissue. In childhood and adolescence, the most constant feature is short stature, which may be accompanied by some of the well-recognized features of Turner's syndrome. Characteristically, the facial appearance is triangular in shape with midfacial hypoplasia, micrognathia, epicanthal folds, ptosis, prominent low set, rotated or malformed ears, and a short, broad webbed neck with a low posterior hairline. The webbed neck is a residual of intrauterine edema, which is presumed to result from failure to open lymphatic channels. Other features include a broad or shieldlike chest with widely set nipples, increased carrying angles, numerous pigmented nevi, bicuspid aortic valve, wide aortic root diameter, and coarctation of the aorta. The renal anomalies are malrotation, horseshoe-shaped kidney, duplication of renal pelvis and ureter, and hydronephrosis from ureteropelvic obstruction. Numerous skeletal abnormalities have been described, including bone rarefaction of the hands, elbows, and feet; vertebral hypoplasia; osteochondrosis-like changes in the spine; angular configuration of proximal carpal bones described by Kosowicz; short fourth metacarpals and metatarsals; bayonet or Madelung's deformity of the radius; and deformities of medial tibial and femoral condyles. The main health problems result from recurrent otitis media and conductive hearing loss, hypertension (coarctation of the aorta or renal arteries or idiopathic), autoimmune diseases (type 1 diabetes mellitus and Hashimoto's thyroiditis), and rarely GI hemorrhage from intestinal telangiectasia. Intelligence is normal in girls with Turner's syndrome. However, mean performance IQ is lower than that of the general population because space-form perception is deficient while verbal IQ abilities are normal. Poor performance in mathematics is a common complaint. Difficulty in socializing is common, but the incidence of psychopathology is not greater in girls with Turner's syndrome.

In a fetus with X chromosomal abnormalities, ovarian differentiation and function appear to be normal until 14 to 18 weeks gestation. Thereafter, oocytes are lost at a rapid rate and the streak gonad develops through a process of accelerated stromal fibrosis. Oocyte loss and stromal fibrosis are not absolute in all girls with Turner's syndrome. It has been estimated that 5 percent of these girls will have spontaneous puberty, but the actual incidence of transient ovarian function may be higher. Maintenance of ovarian function is more frequent in patients with mosaic karyotypes but also is seen in 45,X individuals. In most instances, ovarian function will fail over time. However, a few women with Turner's syndrome have experienced persistence of ovulatory menses and successful pregnancies.

The diagnosis of Turner's syndrome is confirmed by chromosomal analysis of peripheral leukocytes. The presence of Y chromosome material is likely if clitoromegaly or posterior labial fusion is seen in a girl with Turner's syndrome. The risk of gonadoblastoma is as high as 25 percent in Y-bearing dysgenetic gonads. Examination of the patient's DNA with Y-specific probes is necessary. In girls with a Y fragment, ultrasound examination of the pelvis can be used to monitor gonadal size, but early prophylactic gonadectomy is strongly recommended by most endocrinologists. Selection of other laboratory tests is individualized on the basis of age and therapeutic goals. Plasma gonadotropins, especially FSH, are high in the first years of life, return to normal values until about 10 years of age, and then become elevated again. This pattern of FSH secretion has been described as diphasic. Other diagnostic studies include thyroid function tests, echocardiography, renal ultrasound, bone age determination, and hearing tests.

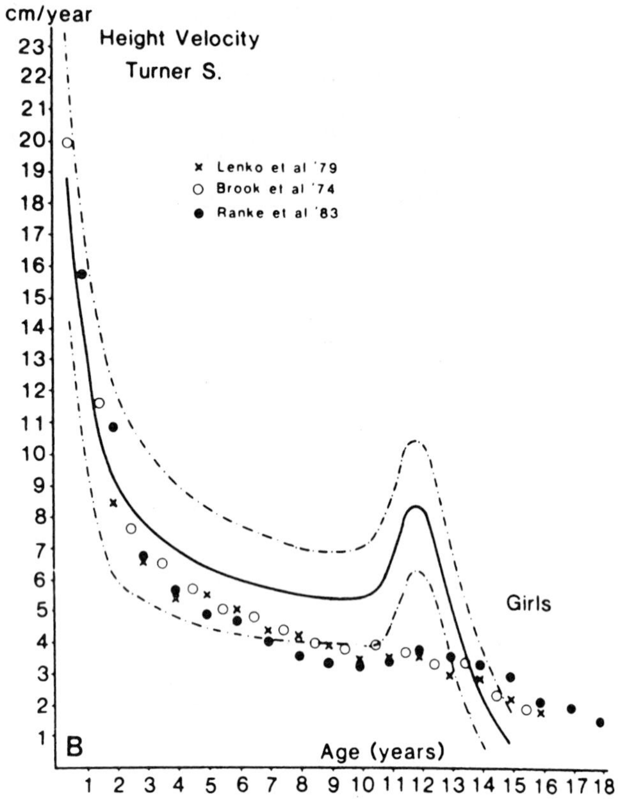

FIGURE 25-20. Depicted on the normal female height velocity curve are the mean growth velocities of untreated girls with Turner's syndrome. The data were obtained from three growth studies of patients with Turner's syndrome. Note the normal growth velocity in Turner's syndrome during the first 3 years of life, followed by declining growth rates in childhood and absence of a pubertal growth spurt in adolescence. (*From Neely and Rosenfeld*[241] *and Ranke et al.*[242])

Short stature is the most constant feature of Turner's syndrome. Moderate intrauterine growth retardation is usually the rule, with birth length and weight falling below the 10th percentile for full-term infants. Birth length is reduced 2.8 cm below the mean. Growth rates may be normal or reduced, in the first 3 years after which gradual deceleration in growth velocity occurs. Without treatment, there is no pubertal growth spurt and the epiphyses remain open, permitting a prolonged period of slow growth (Fig. 25-20). Greater retardation of leg growth is responsible for the disproportionate ratio of upper limbs to lower limbs. Skeletal maturation remains normal or slightly delayed during childhood but falls increasingly behind in adolescence unless sex steroids are administered. The growth disorder in Turner's syndrome is likely caused by absence of the SHOX gene. Spontaneous GH secretion and GH responses to provocative stimuli are normal in childhood, but during the pubertal years are lower than in sexually maturing adolescents in whom GH production is increased. Serum IGF-I levels follow a similar pattern. Deficiencies of gonadal or adrenal

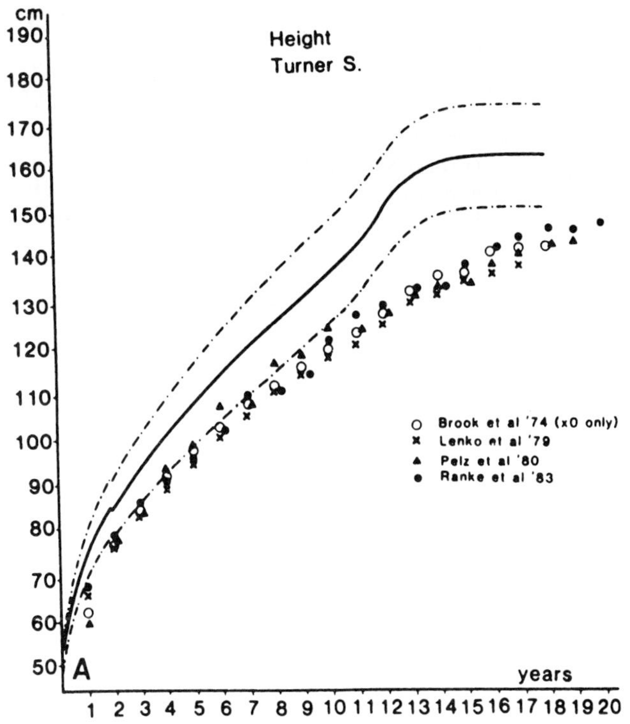

FIGURE 25-21. The mean heights of untreated girls with Turner's syndrome are placed on the normal female growth curve. The data were derived from four European studies.[242] Note the progressive decline in growth velocity during childhood and the absence of a pubertal growth spurt. (*From Lyon et al.*[128]) Growth curves based on these studies are used to project adult height of girls with Turner's syndrome and to estimate the effect of various therapies on final height.

steroids are also not the explanation, as linear growth is preserved in children who lack these hormones and have normal chromosomes. It is possible that tissue responses to trophic stimuli are suboptimal in Turner's syndrome because decreased cell turnover has been observed in patients with aneuploidy. Also, the long-range adverse effects of intrauterine edema on growing fetal tissues are unknown.

The mean adult height of 366 girls with Turner's syndrome was 144 cm, with a range of 136 to 147 cm.[241] In 1983, Ranke and colleagues described the growth patterns of 150 untreated German girls with Turner's syndrome.[242] This information and data from three other growth studies were used by Lyon and associates to construct normative growth velocity curves for untreated girls with Turner's syndrome[128] (Fig. 25-21). They determined that a strong correlation (0.95) existed between the height centile of a girl in childhood and her final height centile on the Turner curves and that the accuracy of the prediction was not influenced by prior estrogen treatment or initial bone age. They concluded that it is possible to predict or project the adult height of a girl with Turner's syndrome and to use that information to evaluate the efficacy of current hormonal treatment.

Growth hormone (0.375 mg/kg/wk) has been approved for treatment of Turner syndrome based on efficacy data from historical controls and from an open-label controlled study. The mean ± SD adult height after GH alone was 150.4 ± 5.5 cm, which represented an 8.4 cm gain over the mean projected adult height at enrollment. Treatment with GH plus oxandrolone resulted in a mean adult height of 152.1 ± 5.9 cm, which amounted to a gain of 10.3 cm over the projected adult height. In contrast, untreated controls had a mean adult height of 144.6, which matched the adult heights from the historical database. Combination treatment with GH plus oxandrolone was associated with higher insulin levels (insulin resistance) and more weight gain than was observed when only GH was given. These adverse effects might be avoided if a reduced dose of oxandrolone (0.05 mg/kg/day or less) is used instead of the original dose given in combination treatment trial (0.125 mg/kg/day per os of oxandrolone).[243,244]

The use of low-dose estrogen treatment to promote growth acceleration in patients with Turner's syndrome is controversial. Ethinyl estradiol has been administered in doses ranging from 25 to 125 ng/kg per day. When given alone, ethinyl estradiol treatment (100 ng/kg per day) has yielded short-term modest improvements in growth velocity followed by declining responsiveness. Potentially adverse effects on bone maturation and final height have been observed. Lower doses (25 to 50 ng/kg per day) do not improve growth velocity. When it is given in combination with GH, the growth response is not greater than the response to GH alone.

Replacement therapy with estrogen and progesterone for breast development and menstruation is usually started between ages 12 and 14 years. Usually the dose of estrogen is low initially and is increased gradually to promote breast growth. The choices for low-dose initial estrogen treatment include either an oral estrogen [ethinyl estradiol (10 mcg) or premarin (0.3 mg) every other day] or transdermal estrogen (half of 0.0375 mg Vivelle patch twice weekly). After 6 to 9 months, the dose is gradually increased and Provera is used cyclically, e.g., daily estrogen for 24 days and Provera, 5 to 10 mg on the last 7 to 10 days of estrogen treatment. On rare occasions breast development is poor because of possible injury to the breast primordium in utero. In such patients, the option of undergoing breast augmentation in late adolescence can be reviewed.

Sex education should be started at age 8 years. These girls need to be told that a majority of individuals with Turner's syndrome have underdeveloped ovaries and that they will need hormone therapy for breast development and menstruation. Also, information about adoption and in vitro fertilization procedures with a donor egg should be provided. In the rare patient with functioning ovaries, genetic transmission is possible and genetic counseling is advisable.

Many of the phenotypic abnormalities that characterize Turner's syndrome are present also in Noonan's syndrome, a familial growth disorder with an autosomal dominant mode of inheritance.[245,246] Approximately 70 percent of males with Noonan's syndrome have cryptorchism and hypogonadism, whereas gonadal function tends to be normal in affected females. Hence, transmission usually occurs through the affected female. The cardiovascular defects include pulmonary stenosis, peripheral branch stenosis, and asymmetric septal hypertrophy. In contrast, the cardiovascular lesions of Turner's syndrome are extracardiac, mainly coarctation of the aorta or renal arteries. The main features of Noonan's syndrome are short stature; triangular facies with micrognathia; prominent, low-set ears; hypertelorism; ptosis; epicanthal folds; antimongoloid slant of eyes; low posterior hairline; pterygium colli; shield-shaped chest with hypoplastic, widely spaced nipples; cubitus valgus; lymphedema of the dorsum of hands and feet; clinodactylism; scoliosis; kyphosis; pectus excavatum (funnel chest); pigmented nevi; dystrophic nails; a tendency to keloid formation, and a varied incidence of mental retardation. The karyotype is normal in affected individuals. Genetic counseling is essential because this is a heritable growth disorder.

Environmental Deprivation Syndrome (Psychosocial Dwarfism and Emotional, Maternal, and Parental Deprivation Syndromes)

Environmental deprivation syndrome is a growth disorder that occurs in young infants and children from infancy to early childhood whose family life is filled with turmoil. Usually, one child exhibits "psychosocial dwarfism" and the others are not affected. Previous studies implicated disturbed mother-child interaction, but the problem may result from conflict between the child and either or both parents or be due to entire family pathology. The importance of emotional stress vs. malnutrition in a particular child with deprivation syndrome is not readily evident from the history. These children are said to have large appetites, and their eating behavior is abnormal; e.g., they may have pica, eat from garbage cans or the toilet bowl, or eat animal food. Foul, bulky stools may occur. Restless sleep patterns have been described. These children are developmentally delayed and frequently display temper tantrums. The physical features resemble those seen in hypopituitarism and some patients actually have laboratory evidence of GH, TSH, and ACTH deficiencies. In addition, they exhibit abdominal protuberance, body hypertrichosis, and sparse scalp hair, all signs of long-standing malnutrition.[217–220]

The management of these children consists of placing them in a happy environment and providing optimal nutrition, which leads to improvement in growth and behavior. Usually, this can be achieved with hospitalization, but the child should be protected from infection, and diagnostic studies should be avoided or postponed in order to minimize stress during this recuperative period. Blood count, serum T_4 determination, biochemical profile, and urinalysis are usually adequate at the start. The behavioral changes in the child should be recorded along with the daily caloric intake and changes in stool character. At the outset, a psychologist or health worker should follow the child and work with the parents. If the child is sent home, home visits should be regularly carried out and the growth progress of the child should be monitored every 1 to 2 months. If weight loss or lack of progress in growth is observed, attempts should be made to move the child to a secure and supportive foster home.

Anoxemia

Optimal cellular growth requires an adequate supply of oxygen. Poor linear growth, weight gain, and delayed adolescence are frequently seen in patients who have severe anoxemia due to chronic pulmonary disorders (cystic fibrosis of pancreas), cardiovascular deficits (right-to-left shunts), or red blood cell diseases (hemoglobinopathies, sickle cell or Cooley's anemia, aplastic anemia, etc.). Marked improvement in growth has resulted from prolonged transfusion programs aimed at correcting anemia in children with sickle cell disease or Cooley's anemia. Unfortunately, the risk of hemosiderosis due to iron overload limits the length of time during which transfusion programs can be used at present.

GROWTH EXCESS

The normal and abnormal causes of excessive growth during childhood and adolescence are listed in Table 25-10. An extensive review of overgrowth disorders has been written by Juan Sotos.[247–252]

TABLE 25-10. Causes of Growth Excess in Childhood and Adolescence

Normal variants
Familial, genetic, constitutional tall stature
Familial early maturation
Overnutrition/obesity
Abnormal
Endocrine causes
Pituitary gigantism/acromegaly
Congenital adrenal hyperplasia
Precocious sexual maturation
Hyperthyroidism
Hyperinsulinism
Excess sex hormone–tumors
Chromosomal abnormalities
XXY, XXYY
XYY
Trisomy X (XXX females)
Fragile X syndrome
Trisomy 8p
Genetic Disorders–Syndromes
Marfan syndrome
Beals syndrome
Homocystinuria
Sotos syndrome (Cerebral gigantism)
Weaver syndrome
Beckwith–Wiedemann syndrome
Miscellaneous
Infant of diabetic mother
Gigantism and lipodystrophy

Normal Variants

Familial, Genetic, or Constitutional Tall Stature

Healthy girls and boys with extremely tall predicted adult height may seek medical help to slow or arrest linear growth. The only treatment available at present is sex steroids. This presents a dilemma for the physician, who must decide whether the risks of treatment with high-dose estrogens or androgens are greater or lesser than the psychosocial trauma of very tall stature. These hormones can suppress the hypothalamic-pituitary-gonadal axis and have carcinogenic potential. In addition, there is always the possibility of error in height prediction. Some children show extremely rapid bone maturation as they go through puberty and have adult heights that are shorter than predicted. Despite these shortcomings, useful information can be obtained from the patient's growth curve and from estimations of bone age and adult height.

The indications for treating genetic tall stature in healthy girls [predicted height >183 cm (6 ft)] are psychosocial only. Treatment is nonphysiologic and should be undertaken only after careful estimation of predicted final height and evaluation of the physical and mental health of the patient. Girls exposed to stilbestrol during fetal life must not be placed at risk with pharmacologic doses of sex steroids. Mean height reduction is 6 cm if treatment is begun when the chronologic and bone ages are <13 years; the earlier treatment is begun, the greater is the curtailment of predicted adult stature. Treatment schedules vary considerably; ethinyl estradiol, 0.15 to 0.3 mg/day continuously, and 10 mg of medroxyprogesterone or 5 mg of norethindrone on the first 7 to 10 days of each calendar month are examples. Curtailment of adult height is due to estrogen-mediated reduction of somatomedin concentration and growth velocity coupled with acceleration of bone maturation. Hormone therapy is usually prescribed for 18 months to 2 years and is discontinued after linear growth has ceased for three consecutive monthly measurements. Careful follow-up of these patients includes menstrual history and determination of reproductive capacity and changes in vaginal cytology. If a young woman is postmenarchal and has a bone age of 14 years, estrogen treatment provides negligible benefits and should not be used.[253]

Similarly, in tall boys whose predicted adult height is 195 to 200 cm (approximately 6 ft 6 in.), testosterone treatment (500 mg per square meter of body surface of long-acting testosterone per month IM given at 2- to 3-week intervals) reduces estimated adult stature by about 8 cm if the starting bone age is 12 to 14 years. At a later bone age, the benefits of treatment are insufficient to justify the risks. Normal testicular function has been reported in a series of 29 boys after cessation of treatment.[254]

In summary, reduction in adult height can be accomplished only if pharmacologic doses of sex hormones are used to promote early adolescence and rapid maturation of bone age. Physicians who prescribe these steroids must advise parents that the long-term effects on patients and their offspring are unknown.

Familial Early Maturation

Children with familial early maturation are different from patients with genetic tall stature because they grow physically and biologically at a rapid pace during childhood and achieve adolescence and adult height at the earliest limits of normal. During childhood, they are tall and look more mature than their chronologic age; unfortunately, they are expected to behave accordingly. Their bone age and height age are proportionately advanced ahead of their chronologic age. Usually their parents are of average height, and there is a family history of early development. The predicted adult height is compatible with parental height, and medical therapy is not needed. Psychological support and sex education should be offered to these children and their families to help them understand and accept the psychosocial stresses that accompany early development.

Pathologic Overgrowth

Congenital Adrenal Hyperplasia

CAH is an inherited disorder of adrenal steroidogenesis. The most common form of the disease is due to a deficiency of the enzyme 21-hydroxylase with or without salt loss. Molecular genetic studies have identified an active CYP21 gene that encodes the enzyme 21 hydroxylase (microsomal P450C21) and an inactive homologous pseudogene (CYP2IP) that is located 30 Kb away from the active gene. The CYP genes are contained in the HLA complex on chromosome 6 p 21.3 adjacent to and alternating with genes encoding the fourth component of complement (C4B and C4A). CYP21 and CYP 21P have 98 percent identity but multiple mutations render CYP21P completely inactive. Mutations that cause 21-hydroxylase deficiency usually result from recombinations between CYP21 and CYP 21P (either deletions or gene conversions.[255] Less common defects are deficiencies of 11β-hydroxylase or 3β-hydroxysteroid dehydrogenase. In patients with deficient cortisol synthesis there is overproduction of ACTH, adrenal cortical hyperplasia, and excessive production of intermediary steroid metabolites with androgenic activity. In the rare patients with 17α-hydroxylase deficiency, gonadal and adrenal sex steroids cannot be synthesized. Thus, genetic males have a female phenotype and genetic females do not become sexually mature. The disease follows an autosomal recessive pattern of inheritance (see Chap. 11).

Exposure of the female fetus to excessive amounts of adrenal androgens results in varying degrees of masculinization of the external genitalia, manifested by labioscrotal fusion, a urogenital sinus, and clitoral hypertrophy. Because müllerian duct development is not suppressed by excesses of adrenal androgen, the ovaries, fallopian tubes, uterus, and upper vagina are normal.

The external genitalia of the male fetus are not affected significantly by the overproduction of adrenal androgens and are structurally normal, but scrotal hyperpigmentation may be present. There are exceptions: in boys born with 3β-hydroxysteroid dehydrogenase deficiency, synthesis of fetal testicular hormones is defective; they cannot achieve full virilization of the external genitalia. XY male pseudohermaphrodites with a 17α-hydroxylase deficiency totally lack sex steroid production and are hypertensive, phenotypic females with no müllerian structures.

Females with non-salt-losing CAH usually are diagnosed and treated in the newborn period because of their genital abnormalities. Failure to make an early diagnosis and provide cortisone therapy results in excessive androgen production, which causes heterosexual precocious development with masculinization and clitoromegaly. The problem is often not suspected in boys with the non-salt-losing form of the disease until several years have passed because their genitalia are normal at birth. By then, the continued overproduction of androgens has caused acceleration in the rate of somatic growth, accompanied by even more rapid osseous maturation, virilization with acne, deepening of the voice, increased musculature, growth of sexual hair, and enlargement of the penis. The testes usually remain prepubertal in size, however, because of the absence of gonadotropin stimulation.

Both males and females with the classic salt-losing variety of CAH have a normal early neonatal course, but after 7 days of age are at risk for developing vomiting, diarrhea, severe dehydration, and shock, with the clinical and biochemical features of classic addisonian crisis. Patients with the 11β-hydroxylase defect develop hypertension as a result of overproduction of deoxycorticosterone.

A nonclassical or late-onset form of adrenal hyperplasia due to 21-hydroxylase deficiency has been identified. It is inherited by an autosomal recessive mode of transmission. The clinical manifestations include virilization in late childhood or adolescence and even postpubertally. Initially, the presentation in childhood resembles premature pubarche, while in adolescent or adult females the picture resembles that of polycystic ovarian disease. At birth, affected females have normal external genitalia. During the adolescent years, affected girls are likely to develop hirsutism, severe acne, menstrual irregularities, and later, infertility. The diagnosis is confirmed by elevated 17-hydroxyprogesterone (17-OHP) levels before and after ACTH stimulation. Low-dose glucocorticoid therapy is necessary to correct the hyperandrogenic state and restore normal menstrual cycles.

Diagnosis

The biochemical abnormalities in CAH are determined by the position of the deficient enzyme in the biosynthetic pathways involving cortisol, aldosterone, and androgen production. In the newborn period, elevated serum 17-OHP and Δ^4-androstenedione in the presence of reduced serum cortisol levels are diagnostic of classic CAH due to a deficiency of 21-hydroxylase enzyme. Increased serum testosterone is present in genetic females, but the level may not reach diagnostic significance in genetic males. Urine 17-ketosteroid and pregnanetriol measurements are used less frequently now because serum assays are more practical. Hyponatremia, hyperkalemia, metabolic acidosis, and high plasma renin levels are indicators of mineralocorticoid deficiency. Plasma renin measurements are helpful in screening for hypovolemia due to subtle defects in aldosterone biosynthesis. In different forms of CAH, the hormone profiles needed for diagnosis vary with the enzyme abnormality.

Newborn screening for 21-hydroxylase deficiency has been carried out in selected geographic areas using RIA measurement of 17-OHP concentrations in a drop of blood deposited on microfilter paper.[256,257] When the diagnosis of classic CAH is made by means of neonatal screening, the incidence of affected males is equal to that of females; a majority (75 percent) are salt wasters. When the diagnosis is made by case detection, females outnumber males. This observation indicates that many males die undiagnosed in infancy. The incidence worldwide varies from 1 in 5,000 to 1 in 15,000. The Yupik Eskimos in Alaska have the highest frequency, approximately 1 in 500.

Prenatal diagnosis of CAH can be made as early as 8 to 11 weeks gestation using chorionic villus tissue for HLA typing by standard means or molecular genetics techniques. Later in gestation, prenatal diagnosis is made by HLA genotyping of amniocytes and measurement of amniotic fluid 17-OHP and Δ^4-androstenedione levels.[257]

Prenatal treatment with dexamethasone, 0.5 mg tid, should be initiated as soon as pregnancy is diagnosed in a woman at risk of transmitting CAH to her offspring. After the diagnostic studies are completed, treatment can be discontinued if the fetus is a male or an unaffected female. This treatment has prevented or lessened the masculinization of the external genitalia in affected female infants. The maximum daily dose of dexamethasone should not exceed 20 μg/kg of maternal prepregnancy weight per day. To date, no fetus exposed to dexamethasone has died or has developed cleft palate or placental degeneration. However, the sample size is very small, and further assessment is essential.[257]

Treatment

The treatment of CAH involves the replacement of deficient hormones. Children with 21-OH deficiency and salt wasting require hydrocortisone and mineralocorticoid therapy. Although aldosterone deficiency is not obvious in the simple form of 21-OH deficiency, many of these children have elevated plasma renin levels that respond favorably to 9α-fludrocortisone treatment. Combined hormone treatment frequently makes it possible to reduce the glucocorticoid dose, which improves linear growth. Androgen levels also fall on this regimen. The daily dose of oral hydrocortisone now used (10 to 15 mg/m^2 in two or three divided doses) is lower than the one previously administered. During stress, the glucocorticoid dose must be increased. Mineralocorticoid therapy consists of 9α-fludrocortisone 0.15 to 0.2 mg/day in infancy and 0.05 to 0.1 mg/day in childhood. Blood pressure is monitored at each visit. Longer-acting glucocorticoid preparations such as prednisone may be used at bedtime instead of hydrocortisone on an intermittent basis. However, this treatment may cause abnormally slow linear growth.

Measurement of serum 17-OHP, Δ^4-androstenedione, testosterone, and plasma renin are performed at approximately 3- to 4-month intervals to monitor biochemical control and compliance. Linear growth, bone maturation, and pubertal development are also regularly assessed because this clinical information and the biochemical monitors form the basis for decisions concerning adjustments in medication.

A sodium supplement (2 to 4 g/day of sodium chloride) is frequently provided to salt wasters in the first 6 to 12 months of life. In early childhood, the risk of hypoglycemia is significant during periods of severe illness and curtailed food intake. Intravenous therapy with glucose containing electrolyte solution (5 to 10 percent in half-normal saline) will protect these children from developing hypoglycemia. Within the first 6 months of life, the clitoris is usually recessed and the vaginal orifice is exteriorized. Additional reconstructive surgery may be needed in adolescence if the size of the vaginal orifice cannot be adequately enlarged by means of dilators.

Psychological support, sex education, and personalized medical care in an atmosphere of privacy are essential to the emotional well-being of young women with CAH.

Precocious Sexual Maturation

A classification of the causes of sexual precocity is given in Table 25-11. *True precocious puberty* or *gonadotropin–dependent precocious puberty* is defined as activation of the hypothalamic-pituitary-gonadal axis at an abnormally early age. In girls, breast enlargement, sexual hair, accelerated rates of linear growth, and menstruation before the age of 8 years are seen. Boys with precocious puberty exhibit progessive enlargement of the testes and penis, development of sexual hair, and growth spurt before age 10 years. Early onset of acne is common. Precocious puberty occurs more frequently in girls than in boys. Seventy-five percent of these females have no identifiable organic lesion and are classified as having idiopathic or constitutional precocious puberty. The long-range prognosis for health is good. Fertility and age of menopause are normal. The major physical abnormality is eventual short stature. The prognosis for adult height is especially poor if precocious puberty begins in the first years of life and if bone age advances rapidly without compensatory gains in height.[258]

In contrast to girls, boys are at greater risk of having a space-occupying CNS and lesion (>50 percent of boys in some series are thus affected). Careful neuroradiologic and endocrine evaluation is required to rule out CNS tumors, especially in boys. The most common CNS tumors are hamartomas, germinomas, teratomas, ependymomas, and, less frequently, optic gliomas, astrocytomas, chorioepitheliomas, and neurofibromas. These tumors tend to be located in the posterior hypothalamus, pineal gland, median eminence, or floor of the third ventricle. Conditions that may be associated with true precocious puberty include prenatal anoxia, microcephaly, hydrocephalus, head trauma, CNS infections, severe primary hypothyroidism, poorly controlled CAH, and androgen producing tumors outside the CNS. Precocious puberty also may be transmitted by either autosomal recessive or autosomal dominant inheritance. The latter occurs only in males and may be transmitted by an affected father or an unaffected mother.[258]

Incomplete or partial precocious puberty is the early appearance of one of the characteristics of complete puberty, e.g., isolated breast development (premature thelarche), isolated sexual hair growth (premature pubarche or adrenarche), or isolated premature menarche.

TABLE 25-11. Classification of Precocious Sexual Maturation

True precocious puberty or gonadotropin-dependent
- Complete
  - Idiopathic
    - Sporadic (more common in females)
  - Familial
    - Autosomal recessive
    - Autosomal dominant (males)
  - Organic lesions of the hypothalamic-pituitary region
    - Congenital: hydrocephalus, cysts
    - Acquired
      - Tumors: pinealoma, glioma, hamartoma, teratoma, ependymoma, chorioepithelioma
      - Trauma
      - Inflammation: meningitis, encephalitis
      - Hydrocephalus
  - Associated with other conditions
    - Neurofibromatosis
    - McCune-Albright syndrome
    - Primary hypothyroidism
- Incomplete
  - Premature thelarche
  - Premature adrenarche (pubarche)
  - Premature menarche

Precocious pseudopuberty or gonadotropin-independent
- Isosexual
  - Ectopic gonadotropin production: hepatoblastoma, choriocarcinoma, dysgerminoma
  - Ovarian tumors, testicular tumors
  - Boys with non-salt-losing congenital adrenal hyperplasia or virilizing tumors
  - McCune-Albright syndrome
  - Iatrogenic
  - Familial male precocious puberty (testitoxicosis)
- Heterosexual
  - Girls with congenital adrenal hyperplasia, adrenal virilizing tumors, ovarian virilizing tumors
  - Boys with feminizing tumors (adrenal or testicular), gynecomastia
  - Iatrogenic

Premature thelarche is seen only in girls, is usually bilateral, and is not accompanied by estrogenization of the vaginal mucosa, growth of pubic or axillary hair, or acceleration of linear growth or bone maturation. Most commonly, it presents in the second year of life, persists for a variable period, and regresses within 2 years. Subsequently, puberty occurs at the appropriate age in a majority of cases. These children and their families need reassurance and psychological support; medications should be avoided. Careful follow-up every 6 months by a single observer is advisable because early breast development may be the first sign of complete puberty. When this occurs, the child will exhibit progressive changes, including appearance of sexual hair and rapid linear growth. Premature thelarche is presumed to result from a transient elevation of gonadotropin concentrations, the precise etiology of which is unknown.

Premature adrenarche (or pubarche) is the isolated early appearance of sexual hair. Pubic hair alone may appear (pubarche), or hair in both the pubic and axillary areas may appear. It occurs more frequently in healthy girls than in boys and also is seen with severe CNS dysfunction. Increased production of adrenal androgens (e.g., DHEA, DHEA sulfate) from the zona reticularis has been reported in these children. Linear growth and bone maturation may accelerate slightly in some children though, they never exhibit the features of intense androgen stimulation. In affected children, height age and hormone levels (plasma DHEA sulfate, testosterone, 17-hydroxyprogesterone, urinary 17-ketosteroids) are appropriate for bone age. Management consists of reassurance and psychological support. Careful follow-up examinations every 4 to 6 months are advisable because premature pubarche may be the first sign of precocious puberty, androgen-producing tumors, or adrenal dysfunction (late-onset congenital adrenal hyperplasia).

Isolated premature menarche presents as vaginal spotting or frank menstruation without other signs of sexual maturation. The phenomenon is poorly understood. It is more frequently seen in children with McCune-Albright syndrome and may precede the appearance of the bony lesions. An ultrasound examination of the pelvis may document the presence of an ovarian cyst.

Precocious pseudopuberty or *gonadotropin–independent precocious puberty* is characterized by sexual maturation due to autonomous production of sex steroids (ovarian, testicular, or adrenal hormones) or to ectopic gonadotropin-like hormones (e.g., hCG). The hypothalamic-pituitary axis is suppressed as LH and FSH are in the prepubertal range and have a negligible response to GnRH stimulation. In patients who have ectopic production of hCG, care must be taken to use specific antisera which distinguish hCG from LH. The antisera used in routine RIAs cross-react with hCG and give falsely elevated levels of LH.[258]

In girls, the ovarian lesions include granulosa cell tumors, thecal lipoid tumors, and functional ovarian cysts. The mass is frequently palpable by abdominal and rectal examination and is readily confirmed by pelvic ultrasound. In boys with autonomously functioning testicular tumors (embryonal testicular carcinomas) or ectopic tumors that secrete androgens or hCG (dysgerminomas, hepatoblastomas), the clinical picture mimics true puberty. Testicular tumors usually cause unilateral testicular enlargement. Boys with untreated or poorly managed CAH exhibit sexual precocity; their testes remain prepubertal in size, in contrast to the greater testicular volumes observed in boys with true puberty.

Precocious pseudopuberty is also observed in McCune-Albright syndrome, characterized by large areas of skin hyperpigmentation (café au lait spots), bony lesions (polyostotic fibrous dysplasia), and sexual precocity.[258,259] Gonadotropin production is suppressed in a majority of these patients, who usually have autonomously functioning ovarian follicular cysts. Rarely, a child with McCune-Albright syndrome may present with isolated menses before the appearance of skin or bone lesions. The syndrome also includes abnormalities of the thyroid gland (autonomous multinodular goiter), pituitary (acromegaly, hyperprolactinemia), and adrenal gland (non-ACTH-dependent Cushing's syndrome). The variable presentation of patients with McCune-Albright syndrome requires that this diagnosis be considered in all children with atypical sexual precocity and that careful physical examinations, cranial and skeletal x-rays, and endocrine diagnostic tests be repeated at regular intervals. In the McCune-Albright syndrome the Gs α subunit is mutated at position 201 as a post-zygotic somatic event. This causes a deficiency of intrinsic guanosine triphosphatase leading to persistent activation of adenyl cyclase and cAMP production resulting in precocious sex hormone production. McCune-Albright syndrome results from a postzygotic somatic mutation of Gs α. Early mutations give global manifestations and later mutations result in more focal disease.

Familial male precocious puberty is a unique example of gonadotropin-independent sexual precocity (other names include testitoxicosis and Familial Leydig Cell Hyperplasia). It is inherited by an autosomal-dominant mechanism that affects only males. Carrier females can transmit the disease but are asymptomatic. Affected boys have testicular enlargement, sperm production, axillary and pubic hair development, large penis, increased muscle development, acne, and rapid growth. Onset of symptoms is between one to four years of age and compromised adult height is the main adverse consequence. The disease is caused by a constitutive activation of the LH receptor, which leads to continuous activation of the G proteins and sex hormone production. In childhood, the gonadotropins remain suppressed after GnRH stimulation but a normal response is seen in adult men. At least 11 missense mutations in the LH receptor have been identified. Females with the abnormal LH receptor do not develop precocious puberty because both LH and FSH are required for ovarian steroidogenesis. The treatment regimens vary. Testosterone and spironolactone have proven to be effective. Ketoconazole also works by blunting sex hormone production, but the benefits may not last because of an escape phenomenon characterized by increased LH and FSH. If early activation of the GnRH mechanism develops, GnRH analog treatment is added to the therapy being used.

Children who exhibit precocious sexual maturation that is not compatible with their phenotype are said to have *heterosexual precocity.* Examples include girls who are masculinized because of CAH (noncompliance or untreated non-salt losers) or because they develop androgen-producing tumors. Feminizing tumors may similarly cause heterosexual precocity in boys. Heterosexual precocity is pathologic and requires immediate investigation and treatment.

The diagnostic approach to precocious puberty should be individualized. In general, a personal and family history should be obtained for each patient, with previous and current growth data and each child should undergo ophthalmologic examination, complete physical examination, bone age determination, and (in females) vaginal cytology for maturation index. The diagnosis of central precocious puberty is confirmed by documentation of an exaggerated LH response to exogenous GnRH stimulation and increased frequency and amplitude of spontaneous secretory gonadotropin pulses. Selection of other tests will depend on the patient's presentation, i.e., serum hCG, FSH, LH, alpha fetoprotein, prolactin, estradiol and testosterone, MRI of the hypothalamus and pituitary, CT of abdomen, and ultrasound of pelvis. The extent of the diagnostic evaluation depends on the nature of the clinical problem. For example, a 3-year-old girl with a 1-year history of isolated, nonprogressive breast enlargement probably needs minimal testing, e.g., bone age determination and vaginal cytology for maturation index. The same holds true for an 8-year-old girl with a 6-month history of breast enlargement, growth of sexual hair, and accelerated linear growth. However, patients with rapid appearance of complete puberty in the first years of life should have a thorough endocrine and radiologic evaluation, especially boys. The diagnosis of idiopathic constitutional precocious puberty can be made only after a thorough evaluation has excluded the presence of organic disease.

The treatment of precocious sexual maturation depends on the etiology of the disorder. Surgery with or without radiation and chemotherapy may be required if a tumor is found. Precocious thelarche or adrenarche does not require treatment. The aims of treatment for idiopathic precocious puberty are suppression of sexual maturation (in girls: regression of breast size, cessation of menses, return to normal rate of linear growth and bone maturation; in boys: cessation of erections, curtailment of phallic growth, reduction of testicular volume, return to normal rate of linear growth and bone maturation).

The long-acting depot GnRH agonist (leuprolide) is the approved therapy for gonadotropin dependent precocious puberty. Prolonged use of this drug causes down regulation of GnRH receptors leading to decreased LH and FSH secretion. Lupron depot Ped is administered every 28 days intramuscularly (0.3 mg/kg per dose, maximum dose is 15 mg). Serum gonadotropin and sex steroid levels as well as LH responses to GnRH stimulation should return to the prepubertal range within 1 month of the initial depot injection. Clinically, the treatments lead to regression of breast size in girls and of testis volume of boys along with reduction of the growth rate and bone maturation. Final heights appear to be increased over the pretreatment height estimate if bone age is young when treatment is started. Approximately one-quarter of patients receiving GnRH agonist therapy grow at a pathologically slow rate, prompting concern that the predicted height gains may not be attained in some subjects. Apart from an occasional skin reaction and a single report of an anaphylactic reaction, the GnRH agonists appear to provide a relatively safe means of achieving reversible suppression of gonadotropin production. However, the long-range safety of these agents has not been proved conclusively.[260,261]

Prior to the availability of GnRH analogs, the most widely used treatment for precocious puberty was medroxyprogesterone acetate, 100 to 300 mg IM every 2 weeks. Medroxyprogesterone acetate administration usually suppresses menstruation and curtails breast growth. However, its effects on linear growth, bone maturation, and adult height are variable and controversial.

Outside of the United States, cyproterone acetate (70 to 150 mg per square meter of body surface per day PO) has been widely used as treatment for precocious puberty. In children whose bone age was <11 years, the drug reduced both growth velocity and the rate of osseous maturation. Among the potential side effects of medroxyprogesterone and cyproterone acetate is mild adrenal suppression. The long-term effects of these agents have also not been carefully evaluated.

Children with precocious puberty need supportive counseling and sex education in order to adjust to the extra demands encountered because of their mature appearance. The emotional and social development of these children has been reported to be between the chronologic age and the physical age, depending on the patient's range of experience. Their emotional adjustment is generally satisfactory, and their verbal IQs are higher than their performance IQs, which tend to be average.[262]

Acromegaly and Gigantism

Gigantism in childhood is a rare disease that is characterized by rapid linear growth in the presence of normal rates of osseous maturation. Therefore, the patient is at risk for extraordinarily tall stature in adulthood (7 ft or more).[263] Acromegalic features usually accompany the excessive growth velocity. Extremely large hands and feet, overgrowth of the mandible and supraorbital ridges, coarse facies, splanchnomegaly, joint discomfort, and weakness are common features. Radiologic examination of the skull may reveal thick calvaria, enlargement of the sella with erosion, and increased size of the sinuses. Cortical thickening of bones with tufting of the terminal phalanges and overgrowth of soft tissues are additional characteristic radiologic findings. Longstanding active acromegaly may cause diabetes mellitus and cardiac decompensation. In most patients, excessive GH secretion can be demonstrated. Fasting GH levels may be elevated and nonsuppressible, or GH concentration may paradoxically increase during a glucose tolerance test. However, deficiencies of other pituitary hormones may result from intrasellar pressure from the tumor. In rare cases, all the clinical features of acromegaly are present and the GH concentration is normal or low. The IGF-I concentration is elevated in active acromegaly. The usual lesion is a GH-secreting pituitary adenoma or, less commonly, somatotroph hyperplasia. Rare causes include pancreatic malignancies, which produce ectopic GHRH or ectopic GH.[264] Treatment consists mainly of surgical removal of the tumor. Radiation and/or chemotherapy may also be necessary. Pharmacologic doses of estrogen are palliative. The somatostatin analog octreotide is an effective medical therapy if GH excess persists after surgery. A long-acting preparation is now available.[265]

Hyperthyroidism

Hyperthyroidism during fetal life and in early childhood causes acceleration in linear growth and osseous maturation. Early closure of the fontanels and craniosynostosis have been reported in young infants. However, hyperthyroidism in late childhood is not likely to compromise adult stature because there is proportional advancement of height and osseous maturation, which return to normal after therapy has been initiated.[266]

Chromosome Abnormalities

XYY Genotype

The distinguishing feature of adult males with XYY syndrome is their tendency to have tall stature that is not caused by overproduction of androgens. Chromosome analysis confirms the diagnosis so that endocrine testing and therapy usually are not needed. Surprisingly, during childhood, boys with XYY genotype are not taller than their XY peers.[247–252,267] A recent evaluation of XYY males in a general population has shown that they are not more aggressive than height-matched XY males although, as a group, they have slightly lower mean intelligence scores. The increased crime rate previously reported for the XYY population was mainly accounted for by property offenses rather than acts of violence. Criminal behavior by this group correlates only with low intelligence and not with height or an inherent tendency toward overaggressiveness. A similar explanation has been offered for the increased frequency of XYY individuals in penal mental institutions. Psychological support and career counseling should be offered to these patients.

Klinefelter's Syndrome

The XXY genotype is associated with tall stature, eunuchoid appearance, and arm span greater than height.[247–252] Gynecomastia during the adolescent and adult years often is present. If Leydig cell function is intact, phallic size is normal. However, in patients with a deficiency of testosterone, penile growth is inadequate. The testes are small because of tubular dysgenesis, and facial and body hair are sparse. Infertility is almost always present. Confirmation of the diagnosis depends on chromosome analysis. Elevated plasma and urinary concentrations of the gonadotropins and low to normal levels of plasma testosterone are characteristic. During adolescence, especially after age 14, boys with high gonadotropin and low plasma testosterone levels should receive long-acting testosterone preparations (testosterone enanthate or testosterone 17β-cypionate, 200 to 400 mg/month, given at 2- or 4-week intervals) to increase penis size, sexual hair growth, and muscle mass and to enhance psychosocial well-being. The newer transdermal testosterone patches are an effective alternative to injectable testosterone. Androgen treatment for emotionally disturbed patients with personality disorders should be undertaken only if approved by the patient's psychotherapist and under close supervision.

In the general population, young men with the XXY genotype have mean intelligence scores that are substantially lower than those of height-matched XY controls. The increased frequency of XXY males in penal mental institutions is attributable to psychosocial pathology, which correlates with low intelligence in specific patients, not to a genotypic or height-determined tendency toward criminality or overaggressiveness in the group as a whole.[267]

Miscellaneous Syndromes

Marfan Syndrome and Homocystinuria

The tall, slender stature that characterizes both Marfan syndrome and the homocystinuria syndrome is associated with a generalized disease of connective tissue which involves the eye, cardiovascular system, and skeletal system. The etiology of Marfan syndrome is a defective fibrillin gene (FBN 1) mapped to chromosome 15 q 21.1. Fibrillin is a connective tissue protein found in microfibrils and elastic tissue.

In homocystinuria, the enzyme activity of cystathionine synthase is decreased, causing an accumulation of homocystine and methionine and a deficiency of cystathionine and cystine. Vitamin B_6 treatment is beneficial in most patients with residual cystathionine β synthase activity. Mental retardation is present in more than 50 percent of patients with homocystinuria, whereas normal intelligence is characteristic of patients with Marfan syndrome. The similarities and differences of these two phenotypically similar diseases are listed in Table 25-12.

Skovby and McKusick[268] have reported impressive benefits from the use of conjugated estrogens (Premarin 10 mg/day) or ethinyl estradiol 0.15 mg/day in young girls with Marfan syndrome age 4 1/2 to 9 1/2 years. The final height ranged from 156 to 165 cm, a reduction of 12.5 to 17 cm of predicted height. Treatment lasted from 33 to 78 months and was not discontinued until bone age was 16 and growth had ceased for 12 months. There was no benefit of estrogen treatment in girls with Marfan syndrome after spontaneous menarche had occurred. The authors concluded that estrogen treatment must be started before or early in the growth spurt, preferably when the bone age is <10 years.

Cerebral Gigantism (Sotos' Syndrome)

Children with Sotos's syndrome are large from birth and have accelerated osseous maturation. The most common findings are gigantism, prominent forehead, hypertelorism, dolichocephalus, large hands and feet, pointed chin, poor coordination, delayed development early in infancy, and mental retardation in 85 percent of cases (IQ range 18 to 119, mean 72). No chromo-

TABLE 25-12. Comparison of Marfan Syndrome with Homocystinuria

	Marfan Syndrome	Homocystinuria
Intelligence	Normal	60 percent of patients retarded
Skeletal	Tall, slender stature Long limbs, arachnodactyly Span > height Scoliosis, kyphosis Pectus excavatum or carinatum Hypotonic muscles	Tall slender stature Osteoporosis, collapsed vertebrae Scoliosis (variable present) Pectus excavatum or carinatum Increased fractures
Joints	Hyperextensible	Asymmetric spasticity (variable)
Eye	Lens subluxation—upward Myopia, blue sclerae	Lens subluxation—downward Myopia, occasional cataracts Retinal detachment (variable)
Cardiovascular	Dilation of ascending aorta with or without dissecting aneurysm Aortic regurgitation	Medial degeneration of aorta Irregular inner surface of vessels due to fibrosis and hyperplasia Frequent thromboses
Other	Hernias	Hernias
Inheritance	Autosomal dominant (1 in 20,000)	Autosomal recessive (1 in 200,000)
Biochemical defect	Defective fibrillin in connective tissue due to mutation of fibrillin gene on 15q21.1	Connective tissue disease due to cystathionine β synthase deficiency—some respond to vitamin B6

somal abnormalities have been found, and numerous investigations have failed to show any endocrine abnormalities (GH and somatomedin levels are normal). Glucose intolerance is found in 14 percent of affected children, which is more frequent than in healthy children. At birth, these children are large (mean weight 3,400 g, 75th percentile) and long (55.2 cm, 97th percentile). Growth is most rapid in the first 3 to 4 years, followed by normal rates during childhood and stature in adulthood is variably tall. The major handicaps are intellectual retardation and emotional disorders (temper tantrums, aggressive behavior, hitting and pushing occur mainly in childhood from frustrations resulting from communication problems). Excessive sweating and whining are also present. Genetic transmission is autosomal dominant in some families but most cases are sporadic in nature. An autosomal recessive inheritance is also possible but rare.[247–252,269]

Obesity

Obese boys and girls are taller by 6 cm or more than normal-weight children of comparable age and have a larger bony frame.[270] Bone age, height age, and dental maturation are advanced during childhood. Usually, obese children reach adolescence early and are of average height as adults. Occasionally, the diagnosis of Cushing's syndrome is considered, but it can be readily disproved because these children are tall and have normal growth rates and pubertal development, features that are not seen in states of glucocorticoid excess. Psychological stress, especially in late childhood and adolescence, is the main problem of obese children; as a rule, they are otherwise healthy. Metabolic and endocrine testing may cause unnecessary concern. Glucose intolerance with elevated insulin levels may be a result of the obesity. They usually return to normal with weight reduction. Increased urinary 17-hydroxycorticosteroid excretion and poor GH responses to stimulation tests have been reported in obese subjects. Treatment consists of restricted caloric intake and vigorous physical activities. Only highly motivated patients have long-term success in controlling their weight.

Beckwith-Wiedemann Syndrome

Beckwith-Wiedemann Syndrome is associated with prenatal and postnatal overgrowth. First described in 1963, this disorder is characterized by omphalocele or umbilical defects, macroglossia, gigantism, ear lobe malformation, and port wine nevus (nevus flammeus) in the central forehead and eyelid area. Persistent hypoglycemia from hyperinsulinism occurs in 30 to 50 percent of babies in the first days of life. Usually hypoglycemia resolves by four months of age. Prominent eyes, prognathism, visceromegaly (liver, kidneys, heart), gastrointestinal malrotation, and cryptorchidism are other features. Hemihypertrophy is present in 12 percent of cases. There is an increased incidence (7.4 percent) of malignant tumors in these children; i.e., Wilms' tumor, adrenal cortical carcinoma, nephroblastoma, hepatoblastoma, and rhabdomyosarcoma. Neoplasms were associated with hemihypertrophy. Growth is above the 90th percentile until age 4 years and normal thereafter. Adult heights are usually taller than parental heights. The syndrome has been genetically linked to the chromosome 11 p 15 region but the precise gene has not been isolated. Autosomal dominant inheritance with variable penetrance has been observed. Paternal duplication of the 11 p 15 region may cause this disorder. The IGF-2 gene is normally imprinted in the mother and is located at 11 p 15.5; it is overexpressed in Wilms' tumor. Genetic studies suggest that Beckwith-Wiedemann Syndrome may result from loss of normal suppression of the maternally inherited IGF-2 gene.[247–252,271]

Infant of a Diabetic Mother

Gigantism is a common finding in infants born of mothers with poorly controlled diabetes and in some infants born many years before a diagnosis of maternal diabetes. The excess tissue is mostly fat resulting from increased fetal adipogenesis. Hypoglycemia due to hyperinsulinism and respiratory disease are commonly found in the newborn period.

Gigantism and Lipodystrophy

Total and partial lipodystrophy have been reported in children. In addition to partial or generalized fat loss, affected individuals may have increased height, advanced bone age, hirsutism, muscle hypertrophy, abdominal protuberance, penile or clitoral enlargement, liver and renal disease, hyperglycemia, hyperlipemia, and hypermetabolism. No specific treatment is available.[272]

APPENDIX: DETAILS OF TESTING PROCEDURES IN CHILDREN

Pituitary-Hypothalamic Evaluation

Growth Hormone

Preparation of Patient

Do not evaluate GH responses to stimuli while patient is hypothyroid. Administer L-thyroxine, 3 to 4 μg per kilogram of body weight per day PO, 1 to 2 months before performing GH stimulation tests if patient is hypothyroid.
Nothing by mouth after 10 P.M.
Keep patient at rest and fasting except for water throughout test. Insert a no. 21 butterfly needle which is kept patent by flushing with dilute heparinized saline (0.1 mL heparin added to 30 mL saline) after each sample is obtained, or use a slow saline infusion to prevent the needle from clogging.

Diagnostic Tests for GH

See Table 25-13.

Interpretation of GH Tests

Severe GH deficiency: peak GH concentration <4 ng/mL on two of the above tests
Normal response: peak GH concentration >10 ng/mL on any test at any time (polyclonal RIA)

Factors Which Modify GH Stimulation Tests

Food (suppresses)
Obesity (suppresses)
Hypothyroidism (suppresses)
Glucocorticoids (suppress)
Puberty (enhances)
Estrogens (enhance)
Androgens (enhance)

ACTH Reserve

See Table 25-14.

TSH Reserve

See Table 25-15.

FSH and LH Concentrations

The reported plasma FSH and LH concentrations in normal children and adolescents vary greatly depending on the source of the standards [Second International Reference Preparation/Human Menopausal Gonadotropin (IRP/HMG) or pituitary FSH LH] and the definition of international unit (IU). The normal range for the laboratory performing the assay must be the basis for interpreting basal gonadotropin values in plasma or urine and for evaluating FSH and LH responses to GnRH (Figs. 25-16 and 25-17).

TABLE 25-13. Diagnostic Tests for Growth Hormone

Test	Method	Comment
Insulin hypoglycemia	Give regular insulin 0.05–0.1 U/kg IV; glucose nadir <40 mg/dL at 20–30 minutes; take samples at 0, +30, +45, +60, +90 minutes	Peak GH concentration at 45–75 minutes; peak cortisol >15 μg/dL; requires constant supervision
Arginine	L-arginine monohydrochloride (10 percent), 0.5 g/kg IV over 30 minutes; same sampling times for insulin;	No discomfort; may cause hypoglycemia in hypopituitary children
Arginine-insulin	Same doses as in above two tests; give arginine over 30 minutes; give insulin at +90 minutes	Same precautions as insulin hypoglycemia test
Clonidine	0.075–0.15 mg/m² PO take samples at 0, +30, +60, +90, and +120 minutes (25 μg PO also used)	Peak GH concentrations at 60–90 minutes; somnolence and fall in blood pressure result; dose-related side effects
Levodopa	10 mg/kg PO maximum dose = 500 mg; take samples at 0, +30, +60, +90, +120 minutes; crush tablets or open capsule	Keep patients recumbent; nausea, vomiting result; peak GH concentration at 45–120 minutes
Propranolol	Give 0.75 mg/kg PO 30–60 minutes before glucagon, insulin or arginine (20 mg for patients who weigh <20 kg; 40 mg for all others)	Do not use in asthmatic or cardiac patients; weakness, pallor, sweating, confusion result
Glucagon	Give 0.03 mg/kg IM or subcutaneously; sample times same as for insulin, +150 and 180 minutes	Nausea, vomiting result; peak GH at 45–120 minutes
Sleep	Take samples at 60 and 90 minutes after onset of deep sleep	Questionable reliability
Exercise	Have patients exercise strenuously for 20 minutes; take samples at 0, +20, +40, and +60 minutes	Questionable reliability
Diurnal GH profile	Take samples at 20-minute intervals over 24 hours	Requires special staff and diagnostic unit; interpretation based on number and amplitude of GH pulses; questionable reliability

TABLE 25-14. Test for ACTH Reserve

Test	Dose and Sampling Times	Comments and Results
Insulin hypoglycemia	Give insulin dose (see Table 25-13) Measure plasma cortisol concentration at 0, 30, 60, 90, and 120 minutes	Normal response Basal cortisol concentration 10–25 μg/dl Peak concentration >15 μg/dl

LH and FSH Levels: Responses to GnRH Stimulation

Spontaneous LH pulse amplitude increases progressively throughout puberty, whereas FSH pulse amplitude does not change significantly. Nocturnal increases in mean plasma LH levels and LH pulse amplitude and frequency are characteristic of pubertal stages 1 through 4. In stage 5 of puberty, gonadotropin pulses are similar throughout the day and night.

The pubertal gonadotropin response to GnRH stimulation (100 μg IV) is defined as a peak LH level which is at least twice the baseline concentration (i.e., an LH-predominant response). During childhood, the peak LH to FSH ratio is characteristically below 1. The ratio of peak LH to peak FSH increases progressively during puberty in both boys and girls.

Prolactin Concentration

Basal prolactin concentration <20 ng/mL

Peak prolactin concentration after TRH administration = 10 to 150 ng/mL in prepubertal child

Vasopressin

See Table 25-16.

Adrenal Function Tests

Basal Hormone Levels

Plasma Cortisol Concentration

8 A.M.: 10 to 25 μg/dL
8 P.M.: 1 to 8 μg/dL

ACTH Suppression Tests

1. Days 1 and 2: obtain control 24-h urine collections.
2. Days 3 and 4 (and possibly day 5): give low-dose dexamethasone, 20 μg per kilogram of body weight per day (in four doses per day, every 6 h).
3. Days 6 and 7 (and possibly day 8): give high-dose dexamethasone, 80 μg/kg per day (in four doses per day, every 6 h).
4. Obtain 24-h urine collection on days 1, 2, 4 (possibly day 5), 6, 7 (and possibly day 8) for 17-hydroxycorticosteroids and creatinine determinations (17-ketosteroids and free cortisol determinations optional).
5. Measure plasma cortisol concentration every 12–24 h on days 1, 4, and 7.

Normal response: by day 4, plasma cortisol concentration is <5 μg/dL and urinary 17-hydroxycorticosteroid excretion is <2 mg/24 h or <1 mg per gram of creatinine.

Abnormal values: Cushing's syndrome is diagnosed if 17-hydroxycorticosteroid excretion is >2 mg/24 h on days 4 and 5. If Cushing's syndrome is due to bilateral adrenal hyperplasia, urinary 17-hydroxycorticosteroid excretion is <2 mg/24 h by days 7 and 8, except if hyperplasia is due to an autonomous ACTH-producing tumor or to adrenal carcinoma; then urinary 17-hydroxycorticosteroid excretion exceeds 2 mg/24 h on days 7 and 8. Rarely, a hypothalamic tumor is not suppressed.

ACTH Stimulation Tests

Intravenous Synthetic ACTH (Cosyntropin) Bolus

1. High Dose ACTH Test
   Dose: 0.25 mg IV.
   Measure plasma cortisol concentration at 0, 30, 60, and 90 min. A normal response is a peak plasma cortisol concentration exceeding 20 μg/dL.
2. Low Dose ACTH Test[273]
   Dose: 1 μg/M^2 IV.
   Dilute 250 μg cosyntropin in 10 ml normal saline at patient's bedside. Use 30 unit insulin syringe to promptly measure 4 units (0.04 ml = 1 μg) and give IV immediately to prevent loss on glass or tubing.
   Collect blood sample at 0 and 20 min.
   Normal cortisol response = 18 μg/dl or more.

The low dose test is believed to be a more accurate and sensitive screening test for ACTH deficiency.[273]

IV Infusion of ACTH

Administer 0.25 mg cosyntropin in 250 mL saline over 6 h. Measure plasma cortisol concentration at 0 and 6 h. A normal response is a plasma cortisol concentration exceeding 30 μg/dL at 6 h.

TABLE 25-15. Test for TSH Reserve

Test	Dose and Sampling Times	Comments and Results
TRH	Give 10 μg/kg IV or 200 μg/1.7 m^2 IV Measure plasma TSH concentration at 0, 30, and 60 minutes	Normal response Basal = 4.5 ± 3.6 μU/ml (varies with assay) Peak TSH = 20–40 μU/ml (increment in TSH exceeds 10 μU/ml Peak at 15–30 minutes

TABLE 25-16. Vasopressin Tests

Test	Dose and Sampling Times	Comments and Results
Water deprivation: overnight 8 P.M.–8 A.M.	Void and discard 7:00 A.M. urine, void and record 8:00 A.M. specific gravity	Use if no history of polydipsia or polyuria Normal response: specific gravity >1.020
Daytime	At 0 time Record body weight; Obtain serum sodium, chloride, and osmolality Obtain urine sample and record specific gravity and volume Recheck these indices every 2 hours	Use when polydipsia or polyuria present; criteria for vasopressin-sensitive diabetes insipidus: Weight loss >5 percent of body weight Serum osmolality >290 mOsm Serum sodium >150 mEq/l Urine specific gravity <1.005 Plasma vasopressin <2 pg/ml Positive response to vasopressin Constant supervision necessary especially for infants and small children Stop test if weight loss exceeds 5 percent

Unresponsiveness occurs in patients with Addison's disease or Cushing's syndrome due to adrenal carcinoma. The test is unreliable in patients with prolonged adrenal suppression.

REFERENCES

1. Winik M: Nutrition, growth, and development, in Freinkel N (ed): *The Year in Metabolism*. New York, Plenum, 1977, p 379.
2. Weiss P, Kavanau JL: A model of growth and growth control in mathematical terms. *J Gen Physiol* 41:1, 1957.
3. Sands J, Dobbing J, Gratrix C: Cell number and cell size: Organ growth and development and the control catch-up growth in rats. *Lancet* 2:503, 1979.
4. Smith DW, Bierman EL: *The Biologic Ages of Man*. Philadelphia, Saunders, 1973.
5. Garn SM, Pesick SD; Relationship between various maternal body mass measures and size of the newborn. *Am J Clin Nutr* 36:664, 1982.
6. Smith DW, Truog W, Rogers JE, Greitzer LJ, Skinner AL, McCann JJ, Harvey MS: Shifting linear growth during infancy: Illustration of genetic factors in growth from fetal life through infancy. *J Pediatr* 89:225, 1976.
7. Lampl M, Veldhuis JD, Johnson ML: Saltation and stasis: A model of human growth. *Science* 258:801, 1992.
8. Munson PJ, Counts DR, Cutler GB, Baron J, Heinrichs C, Lampl M, et al: Patterns of human growth. *Science* 268:442, 1995.
9. Rao E, Weiss B, Fukami M, Rump A, Niesler B, Mertz A, et al: Pseudoautosomal deletions encompassing a novel homeobox gene cause growth failure in idiopathic short stature and Turner Syndrome. *Nat Genet* 16:54, 1997.
10. Ellison JW, Wardak Z, Young MF, Robey PG, Webster M, Chiong W: PHOG, a candidate gene for involvement in the short stature of Turner Syndrome. *Hum Mol Genet* 6:1341, 1997.
11. Wingerd J, Solomon IL, Schoen EJ: Parent-specific height standards for preadolescent children of three racial groups. *Pediatrics* 52:555, 1973.
12. Wheeler E, Tan SP: Trends in the growth of ethnic Chinese children living in London. *Ann Hum Biol* 10:441, 1983.
13. Daughaday WH: Growth hormone and the somatomedins, in Daughaday WN (ed): *Endocrine Control of Growth*. New York, Elsevier, 1981, p 1.
14. Isaksson OGP, Lindahl A, Isgaard J, Nilsson JT, Carlsson B: Dual regulation of cartilage growth, in Spencer EM (ed): *Modern Concepts of Insulin-Like Growth Factors*. New York, Elsevier, 1991, p 121.
15. Daughaday WH, Rotwein P: Insulin-like growth factors I and II, peptide, messenger ribonucleic acid and gene structures, serum and tissue concentrations. *Endocr Rev* 10:68, 1989.
16. Rotwein P: Molecular Biology of IGF-I and IGF-II, in Rosenfeld R and Roberts C Jr (eds): *Contemporary Endocrinology* in press. Torowa, NJ, Humana Press Inc, 1999, p 19.
17. Pinchas C, Fielder PJ, Yukihuro H, Frisch H, Guidiec LC, Rosenfeld RG: Clinical aspects of insulin-like growth factor binding proteins. *Acta Endcrinol (Copenh)* 124:72, 1991.
18. D'Ercole AJ: Insulin-like growth factors and their receptors in growth. *Endocrinol Metab Clin North Am* 25:573, 1996.
19. D'Ercole AJ: The insulin-growth factors and fetal growth, in Spencer EM (ed): *Modern Concepts of Insulin-Like Growth Factors*. New York, Elsevier, 1991, p 9.
20. Menon RK, Sperling MA: Insulin as a growth factor. *Endocrinol Metab Clin North Am* 25:633, 1996.
21. DeChiara TM, Efstratiadis A, Robertson EJ: A growth-deficiency phenotype in heterozygous mice carrying an insulin-like growth factor II gene disrupted by targeting. *Nature* 345:78, 1990.
22. Filson AJ, Louvi A, Efstratiadis A, Robertson EJ: Rescue of the T-associated maternal effect in mice carrying null mutation in IgF-2 and IgF-2r, two reciprocally imprinted genes. *Development* 118:731, 1993.
23. Liu JP, Baker J, Perkins AS, Robertson EJ, Efstratiadis A: Mice carrying null mutations of the genes encoding insulin-like growth factor I (IgF-1) and type 1 IgF receptor (IgF1r). *Cell* 75:73, 1999.
24. Matthews LS, Hammer RE, Behringer RR, D'Ercole AJ, Bell GI, Brinster RL, Palmeter RD: Growth enhancement of transgenic mice expressing human insulin-like growth factor I. *Endocrinology* 123:2827, 1988.
25. Rogler CE, Yang D, Rosetti L, Donohoe J, Alt E, Chang CJ, et al: Altered body composition and increased frequency of diverse malignancies in insulin-like growth factor-II transgenic mice. *J Biol Chem* 269:13779, 1994.
26. van Buul-Offers SC, de Haan K, Reijnen-Gresnigt MG, Meinsma D, Jansen M, Oei SL, Bonte EJ, et al: Over expression of human insulin-like growth factor-II in transgenic mice causes increased growth of the thymus. *J Endocrinol* 144:491, 1995.
27. Barlow DP, Stoger R, Herrmann BG, Saito K, Schweifer N: The mouse insulin-like growth factor type-2 receptor is imprinted and closely linked to the Tme locus. *Nature* 349:84, 1991.
28. Ohlsson R, Nystrom A, Pfeifer-Ohlsson S, Tohonen V, Hedborg F, Schofield P, et al: IGF2 is parentally imprinted during human embryogenesis and in the Beckwith-Wiedemann syndrome. *Nat Genet* 4:94, 1993.
29. Giannoukakis N, Deal C, Paquette J, Goodyer CG, Polychronakos C: Parental genomic imprinting of the human IGF2 gene. *Nat Genet* 4:98, 1993.
30. Steenman MJ, Rainier S, Dobry CJ, Grundy P, Horon IL, Feinberg AP: Loss of imprinting of IGF2 is linked to reduced expression and abnormal methylation of H19 in Wilms' tumor patients. *Nat Genet* 7:433, 1994.
31. Deal CL: Parental genomic imprinting. *Curr Opin Pediatr* 4:445, 1995.
32. Daughaday WH, Emanuele MA, Brooks MH, Barbato AL, Kapadia M, Rotwein P: Synthesis and secretion of insulin-like growth factor II by a leiomyosarcoma with associated hypoglycemia. *N Engl J Med* 319:1434, 1988.
33. Drummond IA, Madden SL, Rohwer-Nutter P, Bell GI, Sukhatme VP, Rauscher FJ 3rd: Repression of the insulin-like growth factor II gene by the Wilms Tumor suppressor WT1. *Science* 257:674, 1992.
34. Underwood LE, D'Ercole AJ, Van Wyk JJ: Somatomedin-C and the assessment of growth. *Pediatr Clin North Am* 27:771, 1980.

35. Clemmons DR, Van Wyk JJ: Factors controlling blood concentrations of somatomedin-C. *J Clin Endocrinol Metab* 13:113, 1984.
36. Rosenfeld RG, Wilson DM, Lee PD, Hintz RL: Insulin-like growth factors I and II in evaluation of growth retardation. *J Pediatr* 109:428, 1986.
37. Spagnoli A, Rosenfeld RG: The mechanisms by which growth hormones brings about growth. *Endocrinol Metab Clin North Am* 25:615, 1996.
38. Blum WF, Ranke MB: Plasma IGFBP3 levels as clinical indicators, in Spencer EM (ed): *Modern Concepts of Insulin-Like Growth Factors*. New York, Elsevier, 1991, p 381.
39. Cara JF, Rosenfield RF, Furlanetto RW: A longitudinal study of the relationship of plasma somatomedin-C concentration to the pubertal growth spurt. *Am J Dis Child* 141:562, 1987.
40. Vaccarello MA, Diamond FB Jr, Guevara-Aguirre J, Rosenbloom AL, Fielder PJ, Gargosky S, et al: Hormonal and metabolic effects and pharmcokinetics of recombinant insulin-like growth factor-I in growth hormone receptor deficiency/Laron syndrome. *J Clin Endocrinol Metab* 77:273, 1993.
41. Underwood LE, Clemmons DR, Maes M, D'Ercole AJ, Ketelslegers JM: Regulation of somatomedin-C/insulin-like growth factor I by nutrients. *Horm Res* 24:166, 1986.
42. Davenport ML, D'Ercole AJ, Underwood LE: Effect of maternal fasting on fetal serum insulin-like growth factors (IGFs) and tissue IGF messenger ribonucleic acids. *Endocrinology* 126:2062, 1990.
43. Underwood LE, Thissen JP, Moats-Staats BM, Bruton E, Maes M, Ketelslegers JM: Nutritional regulation of IGF-I and post-natal growth, in Spencer EM (ed): *Modern Concepts of Insulin-Like Growth Factors*. New York, Elsevier, 1991, p 37.
44. Chernausek SD, Underwood LE, Utiger RD, Van Wyk JJ: Growth hormone secretion and plasma somatomedin-C in primary hypothyroidism. *Clin Endocrinol (Oxf)* 19:337, 1983.
45. Parker MW, Johanson AJ, Rogol AD, Kaiser DL, Blizzard RM: Effect of testosterone on somatomedin-C concentrations in prepubertal boys. *J Clin Endocrinol Metab* 58:87, 1984.
46. Rotwein P: Structure, evolution, expression and regulation of insulin-like growth factors I and II. *Growth Factors* 5:31, 1999.
47. LeRoith D, Werner H, Beitner-Johnson D, Roberts CT Jr: Molecular and cellular aspects of the insulin-like growth factor I receptor. *Endocr Rev* 16:143, 1995.
48. Bulter AA, Yakar S, Gewolb IH, Karas M, Okubo Y, LeRoith D: Insulin-like growth factor-I receptor signal transduction: At the interface between physiology and cell biology. *Comparative Biochemistry and Physiology Part B* 121:19, 1998.
49. Rechler MM, Nissley SP: Insulin-like growth factor (IGF)/somatomedin receptor subtypes: Structure, function, and relationships to insulin receptors and IGF carrier proteins. *Horm Res* 24:152, 1986.
50. Baxter RC: Physiological roles of the IGF binding proteins, in Spencer EM (ed): *Modern Concepts of Insulin-Like Growth Factors*. New York, Elsevier, 1999, p 371.
51. Drop SLS, Brinkman A, Kortleve DJ, Groffen CAH, Schuller A, Swarthoff EC: The evolution of the insulin-like growth factor binding protein family, in Spencer EM (ed): *Modern Concepts of Insulin-Like Growth Factors*. New York, Elsevier, 1991, p 311.
52. Baxter RC, Martin JL: Binding proteins for the insulin-like growth factors: Structure, regulation and function. *Prog Growth Factor Res* 1:49, 1989.
53. Guidice LC, Farrel EM, Pham H, Lamson G, Rosenfeld RG: Insulin-like growth factor binding proteins in maternal serum throughout gestation and in the puerperium effects of a pregnancy-associated serum protease activity. *J Clin Endocrinol Metab* 71:806, 1990.
54. Collet-Solberg PF, Cohen P: The role of insulin-like growth factor binding proteins and the IGFBP proteases in modulating IGF action. *Endocrinol Metab Clin North Am* 25:591, 1996.
55. Phillips JA, Venencak-Jones CL: Genetics of growth hormone and its disorders. *Adv Hum Genet* 18:305, 1989.
56. Chen EY, Liao YC, Smith DH, Barrera-Saldana HA, Gelinas RE, Seeburg PH: The human growth hormone locus: Nucleotide sequence biology and evolution. *Genomics* 4:479, 1989.
57. Cooke NE, Emery JG, Ray J, Urbanek M, Estes PA, Liebhaber SA: Placental expression of the human growth hormone-variant gene. *Trophoblast Res* 5:61, 1991.
58. Liebhaber SA, Urbanek M, Ray J, Tuan R, Cooke NE: Characterization and histologic localization of human growth hormone-variant gene expression in the placenta. *J Clin Invest* 83:1985, 1989.
59. Cooke NE, Ray J, Watson MA, Kuo BA, Liebhaber SA: The human growth hormone gene and the highly homologous growth hormone variant gene display different splicing patterns. *J Clin Invest* 82:270, 1988.
60. Cooke NE, Ray J, Emery JG, Liebhaber SA: Two distinct species of human growth hormone-variant mRNA in the human placenta predict the expression of novel growth hormone proteins. *J Biol Chem* 263:9001, 1988.
61. Frankenne F, Closset J, Gomez F, Scippo ML, Smal J, Hennen G: The physiology of growth hormones (GH) in pregnant women and partial characterization of the placental GH variant. *J Clin Endocrinol Metab* 66:1171, 1988.
62. Goossens M, Brauner R, Czernichow P, Duquesnoy P, Rappaport R: Isolated growth hormone (GH) deficiency Type 1A associated with double deletion in the human GH gene cluster. *J Clin Endocrinol Metab* 62:712, 1986.
63. Parks JS, Nielsen PV, Sexton LA, Jorgensen EH: An effect of gene dosage on production of human chorionic somatomammotropin. *J Clin Endocrinol Metab* 60:994, 1985.
64. Simon P, Decoster C, Brocas H, Schwers J, Vassart G: Absence of human chorionic somatomammotropin during pregnancy associated with two types of gene deletion. *Hum Genet* 74:235, 1986.
65. Guillemin R, Gerich JE: Somatostatin: Physiological and clinical significance. *Annu Rev Med* 27:379, 1976.
66. Brazeau P, Vale W, Burgus R, Ling N, Butcher M, Rivier J, Guillemin R: Hypothalamic peptide that inhibits the secretion of immunoreactive pituitary growth hormone. *Science* 179:77, 1973.
67. Rivier J, Spress J, Thorner M, Vale W: Characterization of a growth hormone releasing factor from a human pancreatic islet tumor. *Nature* 300:276, 1982.
68. Guillemin R, Brazeau P, Bohlen P, Esch F, Ling N, Wehrenberg W: Growth hormone releasing factor from a human pancreatic tumor that caused acromegaly. *Science* 218:585, 1982.
69. Bloch B, Brazeau P, Ling N, Bohlen P, Esch F, Wehrenberg WB, Benoit R, Bloom F, Guilleman R: Immunochemical detection of growth hormone releasing factor in brain. *Nature* 301:607, 1983.
70. Barinaga M, Yamonoto G, Rivier C, Vale W, Evans R, Rosenfeld MG: Transcriptional regulation of growth hormone gene expression by growth hormone-releasing factor. *Nature* 306:84, 1983.
71. Bohlen P, Brazeau P, Bloch B, Ling N, Gaillard R, Guilleman R: Human hypothalamic growth hormone releasing factor (GRF): Evidence for two forms identical to tumor derived GRF-44-NHz and GRF 40. *Biochem Biophys Res Commun* 114:930, 1983.
72. Frohman LA, Szabo M, Berelowitz M, Stachura ME: Partial purification and characterization of a peptide with growth hormone releasing activity from extrapituitary tumors in patients with acromegaly. *J Clin Invest* 65:43, 1980.
73. Thorner MO, Reschke J, Chitwood J, Rogol AD, Furlanetto RW, Rivier J, Vale J, Blizzard RM: Acceleration of growth in two children treated with human growth hormone releasing factor. *N Engl J Med* 312:4, 1985.
74. Bowers CY, Momany FA, Reynolds GA, Hong A: On the in vitro and in vivo activity of a new synthetic hexapeptide that acts on the pituitary to specifically release growth hormone. *Endocrinology* 114:1537, 1984.
75. Bowers CY, Reynolds GA, Durham D, Barrera CM, Pezzole SS, Thorner MO: Growth hormone releasing peptide stimulates GH release in normal men and acts synergistically with GH releasing hormone. *J Clin Endocrinol Metab* 70:975, 1990.
76. Bowers CY: On a peptidomimetric growth hormone-releasing peptide. *J Clin Endocrinol Metab* 79:940, 1994.
77. Ottlecz A, Snyder GD, McCann SM: Regulatory role of galanine in control of hypothalamic anterior pituitary function. *Proc Natl Acad Sci USA* 85:9861, 1988.
78. Goth MI, Lyons CE, Canny BJ, Thorner MO: Pituitary adenylate cyclase activating polypeptides, growth hormone (GH) releasing peptide and GH releasing hormone stimulate GH release through distinct pituitary receptors. *Endocrinology* 130:939, 1992.
79. Cutler L: The regulation of growth hormone secretion. *Endocrinol Metab Clin North Am* 25:241, 1996.
80. Link K, Blizzard RM, Evans WS, Kaiser DL, Parker MW, Rogol AD: The effect of androgens on the pulsatile release and twenty-four-hr mean concentration of growth hormone in peripubertal males. *J Clin Endocrinol Metab* 62:159, 1986.
81. Martha PM Jr, Rogol AD, Veldhuis JD, Kerrigan JR, Goodman DW, Blizzard RM: Alterations in the pulsatile properties of circulating

growth hormone concentrations during puberty in boys. *J Clin Endocrinol Metab* 69:563, 1989.
82. Baumman G, Amburn K, Shaw MA: The circulating growth hormone (GH)-binding protein complex: a major constituent of plasma GH in man. *Endocrinology* 122:976, 1988.
83. Matthews LS: Molecular biology of growth hormone receptors. *Trends in Endocrinol Metab* 2:176, 1991.
84. Daughaday WH, Trivedi B: Absence of serum growth hormone binding protein in patients with growth hormone receptor deficiency (Laron Dwarfism). *Proc Natl Acad Sci USA* 84:4636, 1987.
85. Leung DW, Spencer SA, Cachianes G, Hammonds RG, Collins C, Henzel WJ, Barnard R, Waters MJ, Wood WI: Growth hormone receptor and serum binding protein: Purification, cloning, expression. *Nature* 330:537, 1987.
86. Baumann G, Shaw MA, Winter RJ: Absence of plasma growth hormone-binding protein in Laron type dwarfism. *J Clin Endocrinol Metab* 65:814, 1987.
87. Carter-Su C, Smit LS: Signaling via JAK tyrosine kinases; growth hormone receptor as a model system. *Recent Progr Horm Res* 53:61, 1998.
88. Kerr GK, Tyson IB, Allen JR, Wallace JH, Scheffler G: Deficiency of thyroid hormone and development of the fetal rhesus monkey. *Biol Neonate* 21:282, 1972.
89. Walker P, Weichel ME, Fisher DA, Guo SM: Thyroxine increases nerve growth factor concentration in adult mouse brain. *Science* 204:427, 1979.
90. Kerrigan JR, Rogol AD: The impact of gonadal steroid hormone on growth hormone secretion during childhood and adolescence. *Endocr Rev* 13:281, 1992.
91. Reiter EO, Grumbach MM: Neuroendocrine control mechanisms and the onset of puberty. *Annu Rev Physiol* 44:595, 1982.
92. Ducharme JR, Collu R: Puberty development: Normal, precocious, and delayed. *J Clin Endocrinol Metab* 11:57, 1982.
93. Ducharme JR, Forest MG, De Peretti E, Sempe M, Collu R, Bertrand J: Plasma adrenal and gonadal sex steroids in human pubertal development. *J Clin Endocrinol Metab* 42:468, 1976.
94. Grumbach MM, Roth JC, Kaplan SL, Kelch RP: Hypothalamic pituitary regulation of puberty: Evidence and concepts derived from clinical research, in Grumabach MM et al (eds): *The Control of the Onset of Puberty*. New York, Wiley, 1974, p 115.
95. Lee PA, Jaffe RB, Midgley AR Jr: Serum gonadotropin, testosterone and prolactin concentrations throughout puberty in boys: A longitudinal study. *J Clin Endocrinol Metab* 39:664, 1974.
96. Lee PA, Xenakis T, Winer J, Matsenbaugh S: Puberty in girls; correlation of serum levels of gonadotropins, prolactin, androgens, estrogens, and progestins with physical changes. *J Clin Endocrinol Metab* 43:775, 1976.
97. Anderson DC: The adrenal androgen-stimulating hormone does not exist. *Lancet* 2:454, 1980.
98. Mainwaring WIP: The mechanism of action of androgens, in *Monographs on Endocrinology*. New York, Springer-Verlag, 1977, p vol 10.
99. Kelch RP, Lindholm UB, Jaffe RB: Testosterone metabolism in target tissues: II. Human fetal and adult reproductive tissues, perineal skin and skeletal muscle. *J Clin Endocrinol Metab* 32:449, 1971.
100. Peterson RE, Imperato-McGinley, Gautier T, Sturla E: Male pseudohermaphroditism due to steroid 5 alpha reductase deficiency. *Am J Med* 62:170, 1977.
101. Shozu M, Akasofu K, Harada T, Kubota Y: A new cause of female pseudohermaphroditism: placental aromatase deficiency. *J Clin Endocrinol Metab* 72:560, 1991.
102. Harada N, Ogawa H, Shozu M, Yamada K, Suhara K, Nishida E, Takagi Y: Biochemical and molecular genetic analyses on placental aromatase (P450AROM) deficiency. *J Biol Chem* 267:4781, 1992.
103. Conte FA, Grumbach MM, Ito Y, Fisher CR, Simpson ER: A syndrome of female pseudohermaphrodism, hypergonadotropic hypogonadism, and multicystic ovaries associated with missence mutations in the gene encoding aromatase (P450 arom). *J Clin Endocrinol Metab* 78:1287, 1994.
104. Ito Y, Fisher CR, Conte FA, Grumbach MM, Simpson ER: Molecular basis of aromastase deficiency in an adult female with sexual infantilism and polycistic ovaries. *Proc Natl Acad Sci USA* 90:11673, 1993.
105. Morishima A, Grumbach MM, Simpson ER, Fisher C, Kenan Q: Aromatase deficiency in male and female siblings caused by a novel mutation and the physiological role of estrogens. *J Clin Endocrinol Metab* 80:3689, 1995.
106. Morishima A: Aromatase deficiency in the male: The physiologic role of estrogens. *Clin Endocrinol, Japan* 44:65, 1996.
107. Smith EP, Boyd J, Frank GR, Takahashi H, Cohen RM, Specker B, Williams TC, Lubahn DB, Korach KS: Estrogen resistance caused by a mutation in the estrogen-receptor gene in a man. *N Engl J Med* 331:1056, 1994.
108. Mango D, Montemuno A, Scirpa P, Bompiani A, Menini E: Four cases of pregnancy with low estrogen production due to placental enzymatic deficiency. *Eur J Obstet Gynecol Reprod Biol* 2:63, 1978.
109. Simpson ER, Mahendroo MS, Means GD, Kilgore MW, Hinshelwood MM, Graham-Lorence S, Amarneh B, Ito Y, Fisher CR, Micheal MD, Mendelson CR, Bulun SE: Aromatase cytochrome P450, the enzyme responsible for estrogen biosynthesis. *Endocr Rev* 15:342, 1994.
110. Bulun SE: Aromatase deficiency in women and men: Would you have predicted the phenotypes? *J Clin Endocrinol Metab* 81:867, 1996.
111. Ho KY, Evans WS, Blizzard RM, Veldhuis JD, Merriam GR, Samojlik E, et al: Effects of sex and age on the 24-h profile of growth hormone secretion in man: Importance of endogenous estradiol concentrations. *J Clin Endocrinol Metab* 64:51, 1987.
112. Sharpe RM: Roles of Oestrogen in the male. *Trends in Endocrinol and Metab* 9:371, 1998.
113. Martin LG, Clark JW, Conner TB: Growth hormone secretion enhanced by androgens. *J Clin Endocrinol Metab* 28:425, 1968.
114. DeLuca F, Baron J: Control of bone growth by fibroblast growth factors. *Trends in Endocrinol* 10:61, 1999.
115. Abad V, Uyeda JA, Temple HT, DeLuca F, Baron J: Determinants of spatial polarity in the growth plate. *Endocrinology* 140:1, 1999.
116. Mancila EE, DeLuca F, Uyeda JA, Czerwiec FS, Baron J: Effects of fibroblast growth factor-2 on longitudinal bone growth. *Endocrinology* 139:2900, 1998.
117. Walton A, Hammond J: The maternal effects of growth and conformation in shire-horse-Shetland pony crosses. *Proc R Soc London (Biol)* 125:311, 1938.
118. Smith DW: Growth and its disorders, in *Major Problems in Clinical Pediatrics*. Philadelphia, Saunders, 1977, p vol 15.
119. Forest MG: Plasma androgens in normal and premature newborns and infants: Evidence for maturation of the gonadostat's regulation. *Proceedings of the Fourteenth International Gonadostat's Congress of Pediatrics*, Buenos Aires, 1974.
120. Tanner JM: Growth at Adolescence, 2nd ed. Oxford, Blackwell, 1955.
121. Odell WD, Swerdloff RS: Etiologies of sexual maturation. A model system based on the sexually maturing rat. *Recent Prog Horm Res* 32:245, 1976.
122. Rudman D, Kutner MH, Blackston RD, Cushman RA, Bain RP, Patterson JH: Children with normal-variant short stature: Treatment with human growth hormone for six months. *N Engl J Med* 305:123, 1981.
123. Van Vliet G, Styne DM, Kaplan SL, Grumbach MM: Growth hormone treatment for short stature. *N Engl J Med* 309:1016, 1983.
124. Gertner JM, Genel M, Granfredi SP, Hintz RL, Rosenfeld RG, Tamborlane WV, Wilson DM: Prospective clinical trial of human growth hormone in short children without growth hormone deficiency. *J Pediatr* 104:172, 1984.
125. Jones KL: *Smith's Recognizable Patterns of Human Malformations*, 4th ed. Philadelphia, Saunders, 1988.
126. Brunner KM, Recker B: Reference charts used frequently by endocrinologists in assessing the growth and development of children, in Lifshitz (ed): *Pediatric Endocrinology*, 2nd ed. New York, Marcel Dekker, 1990, p 983.
127. Tanner JM, Whitehouse RH, Marshall WA, Carter BS: Prediction of adult height, from height, bone age, and occurrence of menarche at ages 4 to 16 with allowance for mid parent height. *Arch Dis Child* 50:14, 1975.
128. Lyon AL, Preece MA, Grant DB: Growth curve for girls with Turner syndrome. *Arch Dis Child* 60:932, 1985.
129. Horton WA, Rotter JI, Rimoin DL, Scott CI, Hall JG: Standard growth curves for achondroplasia. *J Pediatr* 93:435, 1978.
130. Cronk C, Crocker AC, Pueschel SM, Shea AM, Zackai E, Pickens G, et al: Growth charts for children with Down syndrome: 1 month to 18 y of age. *Pediatrics* 81:102, 1988.

131. Greulich WW, Pyle SE: *Radiographic Atlas of Skeletal Development of the Hand and Wrist*, 2nd ed. Stanford, Stanford University Press, 1959.
132. Bayley N, Pinneau S: Tables for predicting adult height from skeletal age. *J Pediatr* 40:432, 1952.
133. Kowarski AA, Schneider J, Ben-Galim E, Weldon VV, Daughaday WH: Growth failure with normal serum RIA-GH and low somatomedin activity: Somatomedin restoration and growth acceleration after exogenous GH. *J Clin Endocrinol Metab* 47:461, 1978.
134. Spiliotis BE, August GP, Hung W, Sonis W, Mendelson W, Bercu BB: Growth hormone neurosecretory dysfunction. *JAMA* 251:2223, 1984.
135. Rosenfeld RG, Northcraft GB, Hintz RL: A prospective, randomized study of testosterone treatment of constitutional delay of growth and development in male adolescents. *Pediatrics* 69:681, 1982.
136. Clarren SK, Smith DW: The fetal alcohol syndrome. *N Engl J Med* 298:1063, 1978.
137. Laron Z, Blum W, Chatelain P, Ranke M, Rosenfeld R, Savage M, et al: Classification of growth hormone insensitivity syndrome. *J Pediatr* 122:241, 1993.
138. Woods KA, Camacho-Hubner C, Savage MO, Clark AJ: Intrauterine growth retardation and postnatal growth failure associated with deletion of the insulin-like growth factor I gene. *N Engl J Med* 335:1342, 1996.
139. Woods KA, Camacho-Hubner C, Barter D, Clark AJL, Savage MO: Insulin-like growth factor I gene deletion causing intrauterine growth retardation and severe short stature. *Acta Paediatr Suppl* 423:39, 1997.
140. Jones KL: *Smith's Recognizable Patterns of Human Malformations*, 5th ed. Philadelphia, Saunders, 1997.
141. Glorieux J, Dussault JH, Letarte J, Guyda H, Morissette J: Preliminary results on the mental development of hypothyroid infants detected by the Quebec Screening program. *J Pediatr* 102:19, 1983.
142. New England Congential Hypothyroidism Collaborative. Characteristics of infantile hypothyroidism discovered on neonatal screening. *J Pediatr* 104:539, 1984.
143. Smith DW, Blizzard RM, Wilkins L: The mental prognosis in hypothyroidism of infancy and childhood. *Pediatrics* 19:1011, 1957.
144. Abbassi V, Aldige C: Evaluation of sodium L-thyroxine (T_4) requirement in replacement therapy of hypothyroidism. *J Pediatr* 90:298, 1977.
145. Rezvani I, DiGeorge AM: Reassessment of the daily dose of oral thyroxine for replacement therapy in hypothyroid children. *J Pediatr* 90:291, 1977.
146. Schultz RM, Glassman MS, MacGillivray MH: Elevated threshold for thyrotropin suppression in congenital hypothryroidism. *Am J Dis Child* 134:19, 1980.
147. Sekadde CB, Slaunwhite WR Jr, Aceto T Jr, Murray KA: Administration of thyroxine once a week. *J Clin Endocrinol Metab* 39:759, 1974.
148. Vimpani GV, Vimpani AF, Lidgard GP, Cameron EHD, Farquhar JW: Prevalence of severe growth hormone deficiency. *Br Med J* 2:427, 1977.
149. Parkin JM: Incidence of growth hormone deficiency. *Arch Dis Child* 49:905, 1974.
150. Lindsay R, Feldkamp M, Harris D, Robertson J, Rallison M: Utah Growth Study: Growth standards and the prevalence of growth hormone deficiency. *J Pediatr* 125:29, 1994.
151. Clopper RR, Mazur T, MacGillivray MH, Peterson RE, Voorhess ML: Data on virilization and erotosexual behavior in male hypopituitarism during gonadotropin and androgen treatment. *J Androl* 4:303, 1983.
152. Illig R, Prader A, Ferrandez A: Hereditary prenatal growth hormone deficiency with increased tendency to growth hormone antibody formation ("A-type" of isolated growth hormone deficiency). *Acta Paediatr Scand* 60:607, 1971.
153. Phillips JA: Genetic defects in processing growth hormone, in Bercu BB (ed): *Basic and Clinical Aspects of Growth Hormone*. New York, Plenum, 1988, p 57.
154. Parks JS, Pfaffle RW, Brown MR, et al: Growth hormone deficiency, in Weintraub (ed): *Molecular Endocrinology: Basic Concepts and Clinical Correlations*. New York, Raven, 1995, p 473.
155. Perez Juarado LA, Argente J: Molecular basis of familial growth hormone deficiency. *Horm Res* 42:189, 1994.
156. Phillips JA, Cogan JD: Molecular basis of familial human growth hormone deficiency. *J Clin Endocrinol Metab* 76:11, 1994.
157. Cogan JD, Phillips JA III, Sakati N, Frisch H, Schober E, Milner RD: Heterogeneous growth hormone (GH) gene mutations in familial GH deficiency. *J Clin Endocrinol Metab* 76:1224, 1993.
158. Takahashi Y, Kaji H, Okimura Y, Goji K, Abe H, Chihara K: Short stature caused by a mutant growth hormone. *N Engl J Med* 334:432, 1996.
159. Cogan JD, Wu W, Phillips JA III, Arnhold IJP, Agapito A, Fofanova OV, et al: The Prop 1 2-Base pair deletion is a common cause of combined pituitary hormone deficiency. *J Clin Endocrinol Metab* 83:3346, 1998.
160. Tremblay JJ, Lanetot C, Drouin J: The pan-pituitary activator of transcription, Ptx1 (pituitary homeobox 1) acts in synergy with SF-1 and Pit 1 and is an upstream regulator of the Lim-homeodomain gene Lim 3/Lhx3. *Mol Endocrinol* 12:428, 1998.
161. Fofanova O, Takamura N, Kinoshita E, Parks JS, Brown MR, Peterkova VA, et al: Compound heterozygous deletion of the Prop-1 gene in children with combined pituitary hormone deficiency. *J Clin Endocrinol Metab* 83:2601, 1998.
162. Rosenbloom AL, Almonte AS, Brown MR, Fisher DA, Baumbach L, Parks JS: Clinical and biochemical phenotype of familial anterior hypopituitarism from mutation the Prop 1 gene. *J Clin Endocrinol Metab* 84:50, 1999.
163. Parks JS, Adess ME, Brown MR: Genes regulating hypothalamic and pituitary development. *Acta Paediatr Suppl* 423:28, 1997.
164. Radovick S, Nations M, Du Y, Berg LA, Weintraub BD, Wondisford FE: A mutation in the POU-homeodomain of pit-1 responsible for combined pituitary hormone deficiency. *Science* 257:1115, 1992.
165. Cohen LE, Wondisford FE, Salvatoni A, Maghnie M, Brucker-Davis F, Weintraub BD, et al: A "hot spot" in the Pit-1 gene responsible for combined pituitary hormone deficiency: Clinical and molecular correlates. *J Clin Endocrinol Metab* 80:679, 1995.
166. Anderson B, Rosenfeld MG: Pit 1 determines cell types during development of the anterior pituitary gland. *J Biol Chem* 269:29335, 1994.
167. Cohen LE, Wondisford FE, Radovick S: Role of Pit-1 in the gene expression of the growth hormone prolactin and thyrotropin. *Endocrinol Metab Clin North Am* 25:523, 1996.
168. Wajnrajch MP, Gertner JM, Harbison MD, Chua SC Jr, Leibel RL: Nonsense mutations of the human growth hormone releasing hormone receptor causes growth failure analogous to that of the little (lit) mouse. *Nat Genet* 12:88, 1996.
169. Baumann G, Maheshwari H: The dwarfs of Sindh: Severe growth hormone (GH) deficiency caused by a mutation in the GH-releasing hormone receptor gene. *Acta Paediatr Suppl* 423:33, 1997.
170. Kaplan SL, Grumbach MM, Hoyt WF: A syndrome of hypopituitary dwarfism, hypoplasia of optic nerves and malformation of the prosencephalon. *Pediatr Res* 4:480, 1970.
171. Stewart C, Castro-Magana M, Sherman J, Angulo M, Collipp PJ: Septo-optic dysplasia and median cleft face syndrome in a patient with isolated growth hormone deficiency and hyperprolactinemia. *Am J Dis Child* 137:484, 1983.
172. Patel H, Tze WJ, Crichton JU, McCormick AQ, Robinson GC, Dolman CL: Optic nerve hypoplasia with hypopituitarism. *Am J Dis Child* 129:175, 1975.
173. Rudman D, Davis GT, Priest JH, Patterson JH, Kutner MH, Heymsfield SB, Bethel RA: Prevalence of growth hormone deficiency in children with cleft lip or palate. *J Pediatr* 93:378, 1978.
174. Berke JP, Buxton LF, Kokmen E: The empty sella. *Neurology* 25:1137, 1975.
175. Jordan RM, Kendall JW, Kerber CW: The primary empty sella syndrome; analysis of the clinical characteristics, radiographic features, pituitary function and cerebrospinal fluid adenohypophysial hormone concentrations. *Am J Med* 62:569, 1977.
176. Onur K, Lala V, Zimmer J, Juan CS, AvRuskin TW: The primary empty sella syndrome in a child. *J Pediatr* 90:425, 1977.
177. Kleinmann RE, Kazarian EL, Raptopoulos V, Braverman LE: Primary empty sella and Rieger's anomaly of the anterior chamber of the eye. *N Engl J Med* 304:90, 1981.
178. Bercu BB, Shulman D, Root AW, Spiliotis BE: Growth hormone (GH) provocative testing frequently does not reflect endogenous GH secretion. *J Clin Endocrinol Metab* 63:709, 1986.
179. Rose SR, Ross JL, Uriarte M, Barnes KM, Cassorla FG, Cutler GB Jr: The advantage of measuring stimulated as compared with sponta-

neous growth hormone levels in the diagnosis of growth hormone deficiency. *N Engl J Med* 319:201, 1988.
180. Rose SR, Municchi G, Barnes KM, Cutler GB Jr: Overnight growth hormone concentrations are usually normal in pubertal children with idiopathic short stature—a clinical research center study. *J Clin Endocrinol Metab* 81:1063, 1996.
181. Rosenfeld RG, Albertsson-Wikland K, Cassorla F, Frasier SD, Hasegawa Y, Hintz RL, et al: Diagnostic controversy: The diagnosis of childhood growth hormone deficiency revisited. *J Clin Endocrinol Metab* 80:1532, 1995.
182. Godowski P, Leung DW, Meachaem LR, Galgani JP, Hellmiss R, Keret R, et al: Characterization of human growth hormone receptor gene and demonstration of a partial gene deletion in two patients with Laron-type dwarfism. *Proc Natl Acad Sci USA* 86:8083, 1989.
183. Amselem S, Duquesnoy P, Attree O, Novelli G, Bousnina S, Postal-Vinay MC, Goossens M: Laron dwarfism and mutations of the growth hormone receptor gene. *N Engl J Med* 321:989, 1989.
184. Rosenbloom AL, Guevara-Aguirre J, Rosenfeld RG, Fielder PJ: The little women of Loja—Growth hormone receptor deficiency in an inbred population of Southern Equador. *N Engl J Med* 323:1367, 1990.
185. Rosenbloom AL, Guevara-Aguirre J, Vaccarello MA, Rosenfeld RG, Fielder PJ, Diamond FB: Growth hormone receptor deficiency (Laron syndrome), in Spencer EM (ed): *Modern Concepts of Insulin-Like Growth Factors*. New York, Elsevier, 1991, p 49.
186. Rosenbloom AL, Rosenfeld RG, Guevara-Aguirre J: Growth hormone (GH) insensitivity due to primary GH receptor deficiency. *Endocr Rev* 15:369, 1994.
187. Berg MA, Guevara-Aguirre J, Rosenbloom AL, Rosenfeld RG, Francke U: Mutation creating a new splice site in growth hormone receptor genes of 37 Ecuadorean patients with Laron syndrome. *Human Mutat* 1:24, 1992.
188. Kou K, Lajara R, Rotwein P: Amino acid substitutions in the intracellular part of the growth hormone receptor in a patient with Laron syndrome. *J Clin Endocrinol Metab* 76:54, 1993.
189. Duquesnoy P, Sobrier ML, Duriez B: A single amino acid substitution in the exoplasmic domain of the human growth hormone (GH) receptor confers familial GH resistance (Laron syndrome) with positive GH-binding activity by abolishing receptor homodimerization. *EMBO J* 13:1386, 1994.
190. Woods KA, Fraser NC, Postel-Vinay MC, Savage MO, Clark AJ: A homozygous splice site mutation affecting the intracellular domain of the growth hormone (GH) receptor resulting in Laron syndrome with elevated GH-binding protein. *J Clin Endocrinol Metab* 81:1686, 1996.
191. Ayling RM, Ross R, Towner P, Von Laue S, Finidori J, Moutoussamy S, et al: A dominant negative mutation of the growth hormone receptor causes familial short stature. *Nat Genet* 16:13, 1997.
192. Attie KM: Mutations of the growth hormone receptor-widening the search. *J Clin Endocrinol Metab* 81:1683, 1996.
193. Goddard AD, Covello R, Luoh SM, Clackson T, Attie KM, Gesundheit N, et al: Mutation of the growth hormone receptor in children with idiopathic short stature. *N Engl J Med* 333:1093, 1995.
194. Rosenfeld RG: Broadening the growth hormone insensitivity syndrome. *N Engl J Med* 333:1145, 1995.
195. Rosenbloom AL, Rosenfeld RG, Guevara-Aguirre J: Growth hormone insensitivity. *Pediatr Clin North Am* 44:423, 1997.
196. Carel JC, Chaussain JL, Chatelain P, Savage MO: Growth hormone insensitivity syndrome (Laron syndrome): Main characteristics and effects of IGF1 treatment. *Diabetes and Metabolism* 22:251, 1996.
197. Thomsett MJ, Conte FA, Kaplan SL, Grumbach MM: Endocrine and neurologic outcome in childhood craniopharyngioma: Review of effect of treatment in 42 patients. *J Pediatr* 97:728, 1980.
198. Blethen SL, White NH, Santiago JV, Daughaday WH: Plasma somatomedins in children with hyperinsulinism. *J Clin Endocrinol Metab* 52:748, 1981.
199. Bucher J, Zapf J, Torresani T, Prader A, Froesch ER, Illig R: Insulin-like growth factors I and II, prolactin, and insulin in 19 growth hormone-deficient children with excessive, normal, or decreased longitudinal growth after operation for craniopharyngioma. *N Engl J Med* 309:1142, 1983.
200. Rona RJ, Tanner JM: Aetiology of idiopathic growth hormone deficiency in England and Wales. *Arch Dis Child* 52:197, 1977.
201. Craft WH, Underwood LE, Van Wyk JJ: High incidence of perinatal insult in children with idiopathic hypopituitarism. *J Pediatr* 96:397, 1980.
202. Del Pozo JM, Roda JE, Montoya JG, Iglesias JR, Hurtado A: Intrasellar granuloma. *J Neurosurg* 53:717, 1980.
203. Bottazzo GF, McIntosh C, Stanford W, Preece M: Growth hormone cell antibodies and partial growth hormone deficiency in a girl with Turner's syndrome. *Clin Endocrinol (Oxf)* 12:1, 1980.
204. Portocarrero CJ, Robinson AG, Taylor AL, Klein I: Lymphoid hypophysitis. *JAMA* 246:1811, 1981.
205. Asa SL, Bilbao JM, Kovacs K, Josse RG, Kreines K: Lymphocytic hypophysitis of pregnancy resulting in hypopituitarism: A distinct clinicopathologic entity. *Ann Intern Med* 95:166, 1981.
206. Richard GE, Wara WM, Grumbach MM, Kaplan SL, Sheline GE, Conte FA: Delayed onset of hypopituitarism: Sequelae of therapeutic irradiation of central nervous system, eye, and middle ear tumors. *J Pediatr* 89:553, 1976.
207. Samaan NA, Bakdash MM, Caderao JB, Cangir A, Jesse RH, Ballantyne AJ: Hypopituitarism after external irradiation: Evidence for both hypothalamic and pituitary origin. *Ann Intern Med* 83:771, 1975.
208. Duffner PK, Cohen ME, Anderson SW, Voorhess ML, MacGillivray MH, Panahon A, Brecher ML: Long-term effects of treatment on endocrine function in children with brain tumors. *Ann Neurol* 14:528, 1983.
209. Russell JD, Wise PH, Rischbieth HG: Vascular malformation of the hypothalamus: A cause of isolated growth hormone deficiency. *Pediatrics* 66:306, 1980.
210. Saenger P, Schwartz E, Markenson AL, Graziano JH, Levine LS, New MI, Hilgartner MW: Depressed serum somatomedin activity in beta-thalasemia. *J Pediatr* 96:214, 1980.
211. Costin G, Kogut MD, Hyman CB, Ortega JA: Endocrine abnormalities in thalssemia major. *Am J Dis Child* 133:497, 1979.
212. McIntosh N: Endocrinopathy in thalassaemia major. *Arch Dis Child* 51:195, 1976.
213. Braunstein GD, Kohler PO: Pituitary function in Hand-Schuller-Christian disease: Evidence for deficient growth hormone release in patients with short stature. *N Engl J Med* 286:1225, 1972.
214. Underwood LE, Van Wyk JJ: Hormones in normal and aberrant growth, in Williams RH (ed): *Textbook of Endocrinology*. Philadelphia, Saunders, 1981, p 1177.
215. Penny R, Blizzard RM: The possible influence of puberty on the release of growth hormone in 3 males with apparent growth hormone deficiency. *J Clin Endocrinol Metab* 34:82, 1972.
216. Gourmelen M, Phan-Huu-Trung MT, Girard F: Transient partial hGH deficiency in prepubertal children with delay of growth. *Pediatr Res* 13:221, 1979.
217. Patton RG, Gardner LI: Influence of family environment on growth: The syndrome of "maternal deprivation." *Pediatrics* 30:957, 1962.
218. Powell GF, Brasel JA, Blizzard RM: Emotional deprivation and growth retardation simulating idiopathic hypopituitarism. I. Clinical evaluation of the syndrome. *N Engl J Med* 276:1271, 1967.
219. Powell GF, Brasel JA, Raiti S, Blizzard RM: Emotional deprivation and growth retardation simulating idiopathic hypopituitarism: II. Endocrinologic evaluation of the syndrome. *N Engl J Med* 276:1279, 1967.
220. Krieger I, Mellinger RC: Pituitary function in the deprivation syndrome. *J Pediatr* 79:216, 1971.
221. Carroll PV, Christ ER, and the members of Growth Hormone Research Scientific Committee: Growth hormone deficiency in adulthood and the effects of growth hormone replacement: A review. *J Clin Endocrinol Metab* 83:382, 1998.
222. Allen DB: Safety of growth hormone therapy: Current topics. *J Pediatr* 128:58, Supplement 5, 1996.
223. Gibbs CJ Jr, Joy A, Heffner R, Franko M, Miyazaki M, Asher DM, Parisi JE, Brown PW, Gajdusek DC: Clinical and pathological features and laboratory confirmation of Creutzfeldt-Jakob disease in a recipient of pituitary-derived human growth hormone. *N Engl J Med* 313:734, 1985.
224. Johnson RT, Gibbs CJ: Creutzfeldt-Jakob disease and related transmissible spongiform encephalopathies. *N Engl J Med* 339:1994, 1998.
225. Powell-Jackson J, Kennedy P, Whitcombe EM, Weller RO, Preece MA, Newsom-Davis J: Creutzfeldt-Jakob disease after administration of human growth hormone. *Lancet* 3:244, 1985.
226. MacGillivray MH, Blethen SL, Buchlis JG, Clopper RR, Sandberg DE, Conboy DE: Current dosing of growth hormone in children with growth hormone deficiency: How physiologic. *Pediatrics* 102:527, 1998.

227. de Boer H, van der Veen EA: Why retest young adults with childhood onset growth hormone deficiency. *J Clin Endocrinol Metab* 82:2032, 1997.
228. Toogood AA, Shalet SM: Diagnosis of severe growth hormone (GH) deficiency in young adults who received GH replacement therapy during childhood. *Acta Paediatr Suppl* 423:117, 1997.
229. Drug and Therapeutics Committee of the Lawson Wilkins Pediatric Endocrine Society: Guidelines for the use growth hormone in children with short stature. *J Pediatr* 127:857, 1995.
230. Blethen SL, Baptista J, Kuntze J, Foley T, La Franchi S, Johanson A: Adult height in growth hormone deficient children treated with biosynthetic GH. *J Clin Endocrinol Metab* 82:418, 1997.
231. Buchlis JG, Irizarry L, Crotzer BC, Shine BJ, Allen L, MacGillvray MH: Comparison of final heights of growth hormone treated versus untreated children with idiopathic growth failure. *J Clin Endocrinol Metab* 83:1075, 1998.
232. Raiti S, Trias E, Levitsky L, Grossman MS: Oxandrolone and human growth hormone: Comparison of growth stimulating effects in short children. *Am J Dis Child* 126:597, 1973.
233. MacGillivray MH, Kolotkin M, Munschauer RW: Enhanced linear growth hormone responses in hypopituitary dwarfs treated with growth hormone plus androgen versus growth hormone alone. *Pediatr Res* 8:103, 1974.
234. Styne DM, Grumbach MM, Kaplan SL, Wilson CB, Conte FA: Treatment of Cushing's disease in childhood and adolescence by transsphenoidal microdenomectomy. *N Engl J Med* 310:899, 1984.
235. Jennings AS, Liddle GW, Orth DN: Results of treating childhood Cushing's disease with pituitary irradiation. *N Engl J Med* 297:957, 1977.
236. Horton WA: Molecular genetics of human chondrodysplasias. *Eur J Hum Genet* 3:357, 1995.
237. Horton WA: Molecular genetics of human chondrodysplasias. *Growth, Genet Horm* 13:49, 1997.
238. Shohat M, Remoin DL: The skeletal dysplasias, in Lifshitz F (ed): *Pediatric Endocrinology*, 2nd ed. New York, Marcel Dekker, 1990, p 147.
239. Rimoin DL: Limb lengthening: Past, present, future. *Growth Genet Horm* 7:1, 1991.
240. Lippe B: Turner syndrome. *Endocrinol Metab Clin North Am* 20:121, 1991.
241. Neely EK, Rosenfeld RG: Growth in Turner syndrome. *Endocrinologist* 1:313, 1991.
242. Ranke MB, Pfluger H, Rosendahl W, Stubbe P, Enders H, Bierich JR, Majewski F: Turner syndrome: Spontaneous growth in 150 cases and review of the literature. *Eur J Pediatr* 141:81, 1983.
243. Nilsson KO, Albertsson-Wikland K, Alm J, Aronson S, Gustafsson J, Hagenas L, et al: Improved female height in girls with Turner's syndrome treated with growth hormone and oxandralone. *J Clin Endocrinol Metab* 81:635, 1996.
244. Rosenfeld RG, Attie KM, Frane J, Brasel JA, Burstein S, Cara JF: Growth hormone therapy of Turner's syndrome: Beneficial effect on adult height. *J Pediatr* 132:319, 1998.
245. Collins E, Turner G: The Noonan syndrome—a review of the clinical and genetic features of 27 cases. *J Pediatr* 83:941, 1973.
246. Romano AA, Blethen SL, Dana K, Noto RA: Growth hormone treatment in Noonan syndrome—The National Cooperative Growth Study Experience. *J Pediatr* 128(5):18, 1996.
247. Sotos JF: Overgrowth disorders. *Clin Pediatr* 35:517, 1996.
248. Sotos JF: Overgrowth. Section II, Hormonal Causes. *Clin Pediatr* 35:579, 1996.
249. Sotos JF: Overgrowth. Section III, Other hormonal causes. *Clin Pediatr* 35:637, 1996.
250. Sotos JF: Overgrowth. Section IV, Genetic disorders associated with overgrowth. *Clin Pediatr* 36:39, 1997.
251. Sotos JF: Overgrowth. Section V, Syndromes and other disorders associated with overgrowth. *Clin Pediatr* 36:89, 1997.
252. Sotos JF: Overgrowth. Section VI, Genetic syndromes and other disorders associated with overgrowth. *Clin Pediatr* 36:157, 1997.
253. Frasier SD: Tall stature and excessive growth syndrome, in Lifshitz F (ed): *Pediatric Endocrinology*, 2nd ed. New York, Marcel Dekker, 1990, p 197.
254. Zachman M, Ferrandez A, Murset G, Guehn HG, Prader A: Testosterone treatment of excessively tall boys. *J Pediatr* 88:116, 1976.
255. Speiser PW, White PC: Congenital adrenal hyperplasia due to steroid 21-hydroxylase deficiency. *Clin Endocrinol* 49:411, 1998.
256. Pang S, Wallace MA, Hofman L, Thuline HC, Dorche C, Lyon ICT, et al: Worldwide experience in newborn screening for classical congenital adrenal hyperplasia due to 21 hydroxylase deficiency. *Pediatrics* 81:866, 1988.
257. Speiser PW, Laforgia N, Kato K, Pareira J, Khan R, Yang SY, et al: First trimester prenatal treatment and molecular genetic diagnosis of congenital adrenal hyperplasia (21 hydroxylase deficiency). *J Clin Endocrinol Metab* 70:838, 1990.
258. Shankar RR, Pescovitz OH: Precocious puberty. *Adv Endocinol Metab* 6:55, 1995.
259. Holland FJ: Gonadotropin-independent precocious puberty. *Endocrinol Metab Clin North Am* 20:191, 1991.
260. Manasco PK, Pescovitz OH, Hill SC, Jones JM, Barnes RM, Hench KD, Loriaux DL, Cutler GB: Six-year results of luteinizing hormone releasing hormone (LHRH) agonist treatment in children with LHRH-dependent precocious puberty. *J Pediatr* 115:105, 1989.
261. Wheeler MD, Styne DM: The treatment of precocious puberty. *Endocrinol Metab Clin North Am* 20:183, 1991.
262. Solyom AE, Austad CC, Sherick I, Bacon GG: Precocious sexual development in girls: The emotional impact on the child and her parents. *J Pediatr Psychol* 5:385, 1980.
263. Spence HJ, Trias EP, Raiti S: Acromegaly in a 9 1/2 year old boy. *Am J Dis Child* 123:504, 1972.
264. Melmed S: Acromegaly. *N Engl J Med* 322:966, 1990.
265. Barkan AL, Kelch RP, Hopwood NJ, Beitins IZ: Treatment of acromegaly with the long-acting somatostatin analogue SMS 201-999. *J Clin Endocrinol Metab* 66:16, 1988.
266. Schlesinger S, MacGillivray MH, Munschauer RW: Acceleration of growth and bone maturation in childhood thyrotoxicoses. *J Pediatr* 83:233, 1973.
267. Watkin HA, Mednick LSA, Schulsinger F, Bakkestrom E, Christensen KO: Criminality of XYY and XXY men. *Science* 193:547, 1976.
268. Skovby F, McKusick VA: Estrogen treatment of tall stature in girls with Marfan's syndrome. *Birth Defects: Original Article Series*, vol 13. New York, Alan R. Liss, 1977, p 155.
269. Sotos JF: Cerebral gigantism. *Am J Dis Child* 131:625, 1977.
270. Garn SM, Clark DC: Nutrition, growth, development and maturation. Findings from the ten state nutrition survey of 1968–1970. *Pediatrics* 56:306, 1975.
271. Filippi G, McKusick VA: The Beckwith-Wiedemann syndrome. *Medicine (Baltimore)* 49:279, 1970.
272. Senior B, Gellis SS: The syndrome of total lipodystrophy and of partial lipodystrophy. *Pediatrics* 33:593, 1964.
273. Rose SR, Lusting RH, Burghen GA, Burstein S, Pitukcheewanont P, Broome D: Diagnosis of ACTH deficiency: Low dose and one hour ACTH test versus overnight metyrapone. *Pediatr Res* 43:83A, 1998.
274. Penny R, Goldstein IP, Frasier SD: Overnight follicle stimulating hormone (FSH) and luteinizing hormone (LH) excretion in normal males. *J Clin Endocrinol* 43:1394, 1976.
275. Penny R, Goldstein IP, Frasier SD: Overnight gonadotropin excretion in normal females. *J Clin Endocrinol* 44:780, 1977.

CHAPTER 26

Gastrointestinal Hormones and Carcinoid Syndrome

Pradip K. Ghosh
Thomas M. O'Dorisio

In the beginning of the twentieth century, Bayliss and Starling discovered the first gastrointestinal (GI) peptide hormone, secretin, in the extracts of intestinal mucosa.[1] Shortly thereafter, this blood borne chemical messenger was termed a "hormone" from the Greek military word meaning "arouse to activity." Since the discovery of secretin in 1902 and gastrin in 1905, scientists have been trying to search for new "hormones" in GI extracts. The number of putative GI regulatory substances has increased rapidly, especially during the past two decades. More than 45 peptides have, thus far, been identified. Unlike endocrine glands, the neuroendocrine cells in GI tract are not grouped together; rather they are dispersed.

It was originally thought that GI peptides were secreted from only neuroendocrine cells; however, subsequent studies indicated that most of them are also present in the brain and enteric nerves. The endocrine-paracrine cell secretory products exert modulatory effects on neighboring exocrine and endocrine cells of gut through cell-to-cell contact and by diffusion. These substances may diffuse to the lamina propria and exert paracrine action on nerve terminals, blood vessels, and smooth muscle, or circulate through the blood stream to perform an endocrine activity on distant target organs.

The mechanisms of action of these peptides are similar to other peptide hormones. They first attach to specific cell membrane receptors and produce changes in ion channels with subsequent changes in cyclic nucleotide levels, intracellular calcium concentrations, and associated phosphatidyl ionositol pathways. Our understanding of the biochemistry, physiology, and clinical significance of gut hormones continues to grow at a remarkable rate. During the period 1986–1999, there have been nearly 20,000 publications on GI peptides. It is clear from the literature that these peptides play a role in a wide variety of absorptive, secretory, digestive, motor, and trophic actions on the GI tract and also modulate other endocrine and nonendocrine organ systems.[2–4]

In light of their wide-ranging biological effects, it is not surprising that several GI peptides have found application in clinical diagnostic settings. These peptides have been utilized in the evaluation of the secretory functions of the stomach and pancreas, as localizing tools in both radiologic and endoscopic evaluations of the GI tract, and as diagnostic probes for the presence of endocrine tumors.[2] Although useful in diagnostic evaluations, GI peptides have not been extensively used as therapeutic agents. Somatostatin and its clinically approved synthetic analog, octreotide acetate, have clearly shown usefulness in the treatment of a variety of clinical abnormalities, including endocrine tumors and various secretory diarrhea.[5]

The hyposecretion and hypersecretion of several GI neuropeptides are associated with a variety of disease states. Several clinical syndromes have been described in which tumors of neuroendocrine cell origin elaborate specific tumor products that give rise to distinctive clinical features.[2,6] For example, carcinoid tumors, one of the most frequently occurring and well-known primary neuroendocrine tumors of the small intestine (enterochromaffinic cell origin), secrete several peptide substances [e.g., substance P, motilin, neurotensin, growth hormone releasing hormone (GHRH), and corticotropin releasing hormone (CRH)] and amines [5-hydroxytryptamine (serotonin) and histamine].[7–12] These secretory products collectively give rise to the carcinoid syndrome, which is characterized clinically by diarrhea, flushing, hypotension, and metastases to the liver (described later).[7–9]

This chapter reviews the cellular localization and distribution of GI peptides and, where established, summarizes their biological effects, clinical significance, and potential diagnostic and therapeutic uses in disease states. The final section focuses on the clinical presentation, diagnosis, pathophysiology, and treatment of carcinoid tumors, the most common adult neuroendocrine tumor (greater than 50 percent) of the gastroenteropancreatic system.

LOCALIZATION AND DISTRIBUTION OF GI PEPTIDES

Identifying the cellular location of GI peptides is important for understanding their physiologic and pathophysiologic roles in regulating gastrointestinal functions.[13,14] A variety of immunohistochemical and radioimmunologic methodologies have permitted a detailed analysis of the cellular and subcellular localization of GI peptides and regional differences in the distribution of peptides in the GI tract and other tissues.[15,16] Using these techniques, several peptides, such as vasoactive intestinal polypeptide (VIP), substance P, neuropeptide Y (NPY), calcitonin gene-related peptide (CGRP), and galanin, has been colocalized in nerve fibers, ganglion cells that originate in the submucosal (Meissner's) plexus and the myenteric (Auerbach's) plexus, both of which constitute the intrinsic nervous system (Table 26-1).[13] Indeed, most enteric nerve cells appear to contain one or more peptides, which may

TABLE 26-1. Predominant Cellular Distribution of Gastrointestinal Peptides

Nerve Fibers and Ganglion Cells	Endocrine Cells in the GI Tract	Pancreatic Islets
Calcitonin gene-related peptide	Calcitonin gene-related peptide	Glucagon
Cholecystokinin	Cholecystokinin	Insulin
Galanin	Gastrin	Pancreatic polypeptide
Met-enkephalin	Glucose-dependent insulinotropic peptide	Somatostatin
Neurotensin	Motilin	
Neuropeptide Y (NPY)	Neurotensin	
Peptide histidine isoleucine (PHI)	PYY	
Somatostatin	Secretin	
Substance P	Somatostatin	
Vasoactive intestinal polypeptide	Substance P	

Source: Modified from Go and Koch with permission.[13]

coexist with nonpeptide neurotransmitters such as acetylcholine and norepinephrine.[3]

Other GI peptides have been localized in endocrine cells of the GI mucosal layer [e.g., glucose-dependent insulinotropic polypeptide (GIP)], in pancreatic islet cells (insulin and somatostatin), or in both sites (e.g., glucagon) (Table 26-1).[15–17] In the small and large intestine of human, approximately 3 billion endocrine cells are present, with the greatest density occurring in the proximal duodenum and the lowest density occurring in the distal colon.[18]

Ultrastructural and immunohistochemical studies of endocrine cells in the GI tract and pancreas [collectively termed the Gastro-Entero-Pancreatic (GEP) system] have revealed the existence of at least 15 different cell types.[17] According to the APUD (amine precursor uptake and decarboxylation) concept proposed by A. G. E. Pearse, the endocrine cells of the gut and pancreas belong to a larger group of cells which have a similar neuroectodermal origin (neural crest tissue) and share a number of cytochemical (cholinesterase positivity), ultrastructural (amine storage), and functional characteristics.[19,20] However, the neuroectodermal origin of gut and pancreatic endocrine cells is controversial, and a number of investigators have presented evidence refuting this hypothesis.[21–23] Pancreatic endocrine cells are now believed to have an endodermal rather than neuroectodermal origin.

Many of the individual endocrine cell types are confined to a specific region of the GI tract or pancreas (Fig. 26-1).[2] For example, G endocrine cells containing gastrin occur principally in the stomach, whereas S, CCK, M, and GIP endocrine cells (containing secretin, cholecystokinin, motilin, and GIP respectively) occur only in the duodenum and jejunum.[17] Somatostatin is unusual in that the cells producing this pivotal regulatory peptide are localized in stomach, pancreas, upper and lower intestine, and colon.[24–26] Its wide distribution in the GEP system implies a pivotal regulatory role for this peptide.

Based on the cellular location of GI peptides (nerve fibers/ganglion cells or endocrine cells) and the manner in which peptides are delivered from their storage sites to their target cells, GI peptides can be broadly classified into several functional (regulating) groups: endocrine, paracrine, neurocrine, and autocrine (Table 26-2).[14] Endocrine peptides such as gastrin, CCK, secretin, GIP, and possibly motilin achieve their biological effects on target tissues through circulation.

In contrast, other peptides, such as somatostatin and probably motilin, function in a local (paracrine) manner and achieve their

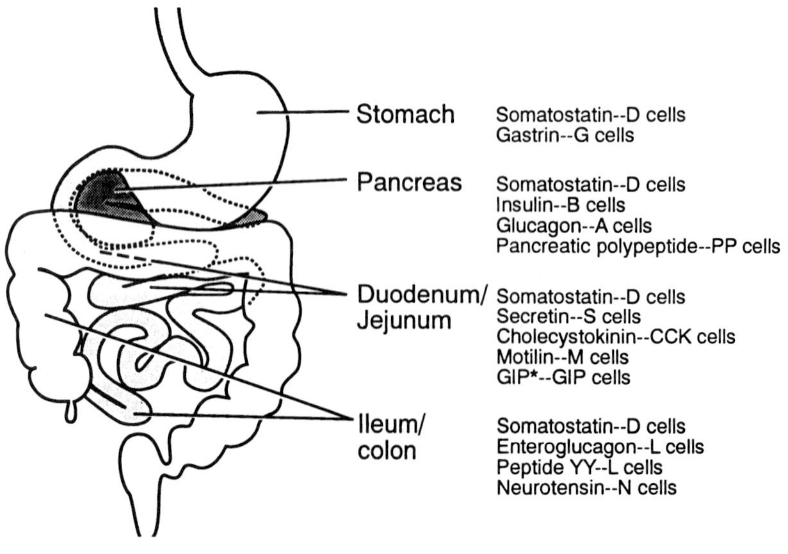

FIGURE 26-1. Distribution of gastrointestinal peptides and corresponding endocrine cells. GIP = gastric inhibitory peptide or glucose-dependent insulinotropic peptide. (*Adapted from Walsh with permission.*[2])

TABLE 26-2. Functional Classification of GI Regulatory Peptides

Peptide	Endocrine	Paracrine	Neurocrine	Autocrine
Bombesins (GRP, NB)			+	
CCK	+		+	
CGRP			+	
Galanin			+	
Gastrin	+			
Motilin	+			
Neurotensin	+		+	
NPY			+	
Opioids (dynorphin, Met-enk)			+	
PP, PYY	+			
Somatostatin	+	+	+	+
Secretin	+			
Tachykinins (SP, SK, NK)			+	
VIP/PHI			+	

CCK = cholecystokinin; CGRP = calcitonin gene-related peptide; GRP = gastrin-releasing peptide; met-enk = methionine-enkephalin-Arg-Gly-Leu; NB = neuromedin B; NK = neuromedin K; NPY = neuropeptide Y; PHI = peptide histidine isoleucine; PP = pancreatic polypeptide; PYY = peptide YY; SK = substance K; SP = substance P; VIP = vasoactive intestinal polypeptide.

Source: Modified from Makhlouf et al. with permission.[14]

regulatory effects on target cells after release into the interstitial space rather than into the general circulation. Neurocrine peptides such as VIP, neuropeptide Y, and substance P influence the postsynaptic membranes on their target cells following release into the synaptic cleft. Finally, some peptides may inhibit their own release through an ultra short feedback loop. For example, somatostatin congeners [(D-Trp8-D/Cys14)-somatostatin and des-Asn5-(D-Try8)-somatostatin] block/CCK- and arginine-induced release of somatostatin from pancreatic D cells, suggesting that somatostatin is able to regulate its own secretion (autocrine effect).[27]

To date, somatostatin is the only GI peptide known to function as an endocrine, neurotransmitter, paracrine, and autocrine substance (depending on the tissue in which it is located).[5] In addition, somatostatin occurs in numerous hypothalamic nuclei, especially in the anterior paraventricular region, and may also be classified as a neuroendocrine substance.[28] The cell bodies of neurons in this hypothalamic region synthesize somatostatin, which then passes down the axons as far as the median eminence. Depolarization of the axonal terminal in the median eminence releases somatostatin into the capillary plexus of the superior hypophyseal artery, which then travels through the hypothalamo-hypophyseal portal system to the anterior pituitary and executes its function on anterior pituitary cells in controlling growth hormone release.

REGULATION, BIOLOGICAL ACTIONS AND CLINICAL APPLICATIONS

Somatostatin

Somatostatin (SS) was first isolated from sheep hypothalamus[29] and later found in the GI tract and pancreas.[30–32] SS is secreted from the delta (D) cells located in the mucosa of the gastric antrum and found from the cardia to the rectum of the GI tract, in the pancreatic islets, in myenteric plexus, and in the abdominal portion of the vagus nerve.[33] The peptide exists in two active forms: somatostatin-14 (SS-14) and somatostatin-28 (SS-28). SS-14 is a 14-amino acid peptide with a cyclic molecular structure,[34] while SS-28, a 28-amino acid peptide, is identical to SS-14 from the carboxy terminus, and has 14 additional amino acids attached to the amino terminal end.[35] Recombinant DNA technology has revealed another larger somatostatin prohormone, pre-prosomatostatin,[36] in which the active peptide resides at the carboxyl terminal end of the prohormone. Both SS-14 and SS-28 are derived from preprosomatostatin through posttranslational processing. Both of them are found in the gut mucosa, though SS-14 is predominantly located in the gut nerves.[37,38] In humans, both SS-14 and SS-28 appear in the circulation, while SS-14 is the principal circulating somatostatin in dogs.[39–41]

Regulation

Antidromic release of several peptides, especially gastrin releasing peptide (GRP), bombesin (BN), and vasoactive intestinal polypeptide (VIP), stimulate SS release from D cells, while substance P inhibits it.[42–44] In the stomach, both corpus and antrum contain D cells, and the control mechanisms of these cells are different between cephalic and gastric phase. Cephalic phase of gastric function is characterized by distension of stomach with subsequent activation of vagal pathways resulting in inhibition of SS-14 release, but this function is reversed by atropine.[44–47] In the gastric phase, several food materials and luminal pH influence the secretion of somatostatin. Several reports indicate that mixed meals stimulate SS release from stomach and pancreas.[48,49] Low luminal pH stimulates, while high pH inhibits, SS secretions. Moreover, several other peptides such as gastric inhibitory peptide [(GIP), also termed glucose-dependent insulinotropic peptide], secretin, calcitonin gene-related peptide (CGRP), cholecystokinin (CCK), and gastrin also stimulate SS secretion from D cells. Acetylcholine that is released from postganglionic nerve terminals stimulates somatostatin release in dogs, pigs and humans.[50,51–54]

Biological Actions

Somatostatin is a potent inhibitor of gastric acid secretion. Several studies have indicated that somatostatin possesses a wide

TABLE 26-3. Summary of the Effects of Somatostatin

System	Effect Product/Function	Affected
Anterior pituitary		
Endocrine	Inhibition of secretion	Growth hormone Thyrotropin
Gastrointestinal tract		
Endocrine	Inhibition of gut hormone secretion	Gastrin Cholecystokinin Secretin Enteroglucagon Neurotensin Gastric inhibitory peptide Vasoactive intestinal polypeptide Motilin
Exocrine	Inhibition of secretion	Acid Pepsin Fluid/electrolytes
Absorption	Inhibition	Glucose Amino acids Triglycerides Calcium
Motility	Inhibition	Gastric emptying Small bowel transit time
Mucosal protection	Cytoprotection	Stomach, and duodenum
Hemodynamics	Decrease in blood flow	Mesenteric and celiac arteries
Gut Immunity	Inhibition	Immune cells of gut tissue Peyer's patches
Pancreas		
Exocrine	Inhibition of secretion	Electrolytes Digestive enzymes
Endocrine	Inhibition of secretion	Insulin from β cells Glucagon from α cells Pancreatic polypeptide
Liver		
Hemodynamics	Decrease in blood flow	Portal vein
Exocrine	Inhibition of secretion	Bile acid
Kidney		
Homeostasis	Fluid/electrolyte balance	Diuresis
Spleen		
Lymphocytes	Inhibition	DNA, IgM, and IgA

Source: From O'Dorisio and Redfern with permission.[5]

range of functions on the brain, pituitary gland, and GI tract. The diverse effects of somatostatin are depicted in Table 26-3.

In the anterior pituitary, somatostatin plays an integral physiologic role in regulating the release of growth hormone and, possibly, thyroid hormone.[55–59] Five different subtypes of somatostatin receptors, designated as SSTR1-SSTR5, have been identified.[60,61] Both native somatostatin and its congeners appear to exert their regulatory functions through binding to somatostatin receptors on the target cell membrane.[5]

In the stomach, somatostatin inhibits gastric acid and pepsin responses to gastrin. It also inhibits basal and food-stimulated acid secretion[62,63] and protects gastroduodenal mucosa against injury independently of the inhibition of acid secretion.[64,65] The stomach has high sensitivity for SS-14 versus SS-28.[66–68] In the small intestine, somatostatin inhibits absorption (glucose, triglycerides, amino acids, and calcium) and suppresses fluid and electrolyte secretion induced by secretagogues such as VIP and prostaglandins.[69–73] Somatostatin also affects the motor activity of stomach and intestine. It inhibits the cyclic interdigestive motor and electrical activity in the stomach and small intestine.[74,75]

Somatostatin inhibits both the exocrine and endocrine secretory functions of the pancreas. Both SS-14 and SS-28 are equally potent in inhibiting pancreatic exocrine secretion.[76] They inhibit the secretion of electrolytes and enzymes stimulated by a meal or by administration of exogenous secretin, CCK, or a combination of the two.[77,78] Somatostatin also has profound effects on insulin secretion from beta cells, glucagon secretion from alpha cells, and on its own secretion from delta cells.[27,77,79–81] It has been observed that chronic infusion of somatostatin causes pancreatic hypoplasia due to inhibition of DNA, RNA, and protein synthesis.[82]

Several studies have also shown that somatostatin inhibits release of most gastrointestinal peptides. These include gastrin, CCK, secretin, GIP, VIP, motilin, and enteroglucagon.[83] Gastrin-induced stimulation of histamine release from ECL cells is inhibited by somatostatin in stomach through SS receptors (SSTR2) subtypes.[84,85]

Somatostatin is considered to be one of several neuropeptides capable of regulating immune function. Electron microscopic and immunocytochemical investigations demonstrate that SS immunoreactive nerve terminals are very close to the immune structures, Peyer's patches of intestine, and in close contact with lymphocytes in the submucosa of small intestine.[86] Somatostatin may also exert inhibitory action on immune cells in the gut tissue. Somatostatin significantly inhibits the synthesis of DNA, IgA, and IgM in lymphocytes isolated from spleen, Peyer's patches, and mesenteric lymph nodes.[87]

Clinical Relevance and Applications

We have been able to extrapolate normal physiology from the very rare cases of somatostatin-secreting tumors. Excess secretions of somatostatin resulting from somatostatinoma tumors have been carefully described.[88–90] Somatostatinomas usually occur in the pancreas but may also occur in the small intestine.[91] The major clinical manifestations of somatostatin hypersecretion include diabetes mellitus (Type 2), steatorrhoea, cholelithiasis, hypochlorhydria, and achlorhydria.[92,93]

Hyposomatostatinemic states are not easily detectable, and no disease has been attributed to a deficiency of somatostatin secretion. However, patients with duodenal ulcers have been shown to have lower levels of somatostatin in the antral mucosa.[94,95] It is intriguing to speculate that diseases such as diabetic retinopathy, with its attendant neovascularization, may be related in part to a loss of somatostatin nerve fibers that are known to innervate the retina.[5] A very recent report suggests that somatostatin congeners may delay the occurrence of diabetic retinopathy.[96]

Somatostatin exhibits a wide range of inhibitory functions that have important clinical applications in the treatment of acromegaly,[97] endocrine tumors,[98] secretory diarrhea,[99–103] dumping syndrome,[104–106] pancreatitis, and solid tumors.[97] However, the short half-lives of SS-14 (1–2 min) and SS-28 (2–3 min) limit their clinical usefulness.[107–109] Chemical synthesis of a number of potent congeners of native somatostatin with longer half-lives have been developed. These peptides include octreotide, BIM-23014C (somatuline), RC-160, MK-678, and several other congeners. Of these, octreotide [half-life of 60 min (IV), 60–120 min (SC)] is being used widely as it exhibits a broad spectrum of biologic actions similar to native somatostatin.

The ability of somatostatin and its congener, octreotide acetate, to inhibit growth hormone and thyrotropin secretion has been successfully applied in the treatment of acromegaly and some forms of hyperthyroidism.[110,111] Both conditions can result from peptide-secreting tumors. Excess production of growth hormone results in stimulation of hepatic somatomedin-C (now termed "insulin-like growth factor-1" or IGF-1), which in turn acts at the tissue level to produce the characteristic clinical features of acromegaly.[112] Long-term octreotide acetate treatment of acromegaly patients who are resistant to surgery or radiation results in marked reduction of growth hormone and IGF-1 levels (many GH and IGF-1 levels return to normal) with significant improvement in symptoms (Fig. 26-2).[113] Octreotide acetate is FDA approved for treatment of GH-secreting tumors and lanreotide is presently being studied in patients with acromegaly.

Somatostatin or octreotide administration has been shown to reduce both the early and late symptoms of dumping syndrome.[114–116] Dumping syndrome is a collective term for the symptoms associated with rapid gastric emptying that typically

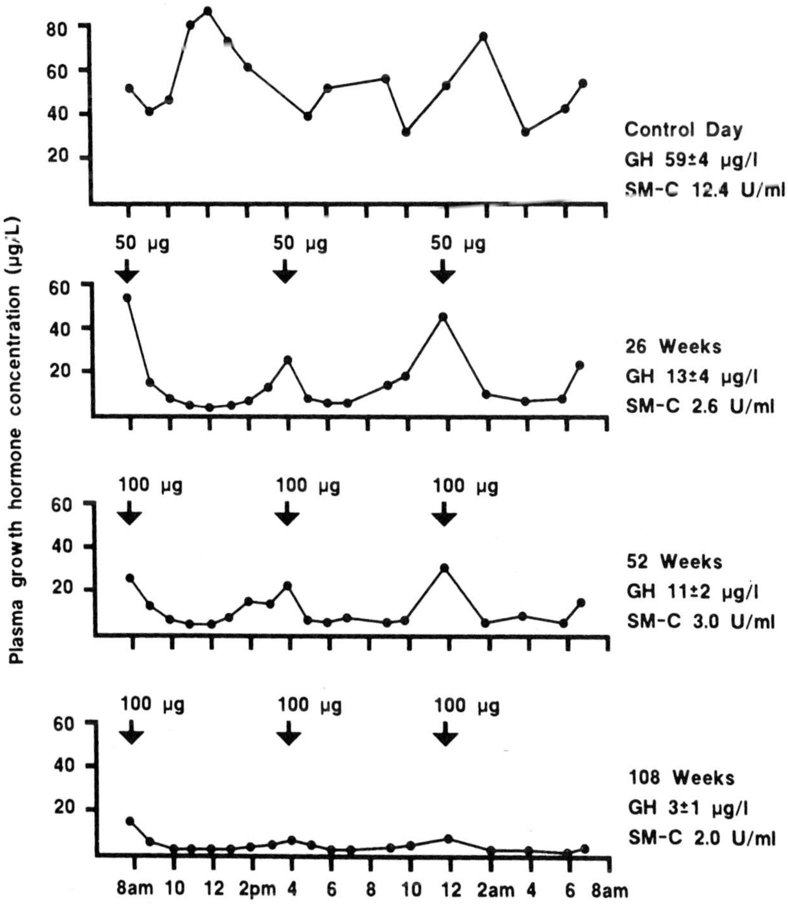

FIGURE 26-2. Plasma growth hormone levels measured over 24 h in an acromegalic patient at baseline and after 26, 52, and 108 weeks of octreotide therapy. Margin: mean 24-h plasma growth hormone and somatomedin-C levels. (*From Lamberts et al. with permission.*[113])

occurs in patients with gastric surgery. However, more commonly, there also appears to be "functional" form of rapid gastric emptying associated with hyper/hypoglycemia that is not associated with gastric surgery. The mechanism by which somatostatin or octrotide reduces the symptoms of dumping syndrome is unclear, although it may involve decreasing gastric emptying, intestinal motility, and gut peptide secretion [e.g. VIP, peptide YY (PYY), neurotensin, insulin, glucagon, motilin, and bradykinin].[117–119]

The inhibitory action of somatostatin and octreotide on pancreatic exocrine secretions are also being clinically applied to prevent pancreatitis after pancreatic surgery and following transplantation of pancreas.[97] In addition, octreotide has been used in controlling migraine headache in some patients[97] and in reducing gastrointestinal bleeding.[120,121]

The intestinal antisecretory effect of somatostatin and octreotide has clinical implications in the control of secretory diarrhea (Table 26-4). It has been observed that octreotide is useful in patients who exhibit severe diarrhea, flushing, and electrolyte imbalance associated with carcinoid syndrome and vasoactive intestinal polypeptide-secreting tumors, and in some patients with AIDS (cryptosporidial diarrhea).[122–127] In addition, there have been reports of octreotide being used successfully in the treatment of infants with idiopathic secretory diarrhea.[128,129]

Somatostatin and octreotide have the ability to prevent neoplastic changes in tissue and inhibit growth of tumor by inhibiting the release of growth factors. This function of somatostatin provides the potential to study octreotide in a clinical setting for the management of patients with solid tumor such as tumors of breast, pancreas, ovary, kidney, and colon.[64] The function may be dependent on presence of SST2 receptors, either on tumor blood vessels or tumor itself. The inhibition of tumor growth may be due to reduction of blood supply to the tumor tissue as it has been observed in chick chorioallantoic membrane model.[130] In addition, octreotide has applications in the treatment of several neuroendocrine tumors of GI tract, including carcinoid tumors, VIPomas, gastrinomas, glucagonomas, and insulinomas (Table 26-5) and their target organ manifestations (e.g., secretory diarrhea, gastric acid hypersecretion, and skin rash).

Because of the excellent safety profile and virtual lack of significant dose-limiting side effects of octreotide, it will undoubtedly continue to be clinically useful for many endocrine tumors and antagonism at the tumor's target tissue.

Gastrin

The existence of a substance released by the stomach in response to digested food components that subsequently stimulates gastric acid secretion was first postulated by J. S. Edkins in 1905.[144] Later it was termed "gastrin." Its isolation and characterization was done by Gregory and Tracy in 1961.[145,146] Gastrin and cholecystokinin (CCK) belongs to the same peptide family, which is characterized by the presence of a common amino acid sequence (Gly-Trp-Met-Asp-Phe amide) at the carboxy-terminal end.[147] It is thought that gastrin probably develops from CCK in the evolution of gene duplication. The biological activity of all peptides in this family is believed to reside in the C-terminal sequence[2] that results in some degree of overlap in biological actions of these peptides and the ability of cholecystokinin (CCK) to prevent gastrin's interaction with its receptor.[148] Multiple molecular forms of biologically active gastrin have been identified in mucosal extracts. They are G-17 ("little" gastrin), G-34 ("big" gastrin), and G-14 (minigastrin).[149] The amino acid sequence of G-14 is identical to the first 14 amino acids of G-17 from the C-terminal end while the amino acid sequence of G-17 is identical to G-34 for the first 16 amino acids from the C-terminal end. G-34 and G-17 are the most abundant circulating gastrin species, followed by smaller amounts of G-14.[150] A larger precursor, termed "preprogastrin" (101 amino acid residues) also exists in circulation and gives rise to smaller gastrin after posttranslational enzymatic cleavage.[151] The distribution of gastrin is age-dependent. In adults, it is produced and secreted by antral G cells of stomach and small amounts by duodenum. It has also been established that gastrin- secreting cells also contain VIP, PYY, ACTH, and TRH.[152–154] In the GI tract, G-17 is most abundant in antrum and G-34 is mostly located in duodenum.[155] All gastrin species exist in both nonsulfated (gastrin I) and sulfated (gastrin II) forms.[150] Biological potency of gastrin does not depend on sulfation of the molecule.[150] G-17 is about five times more potent than G-34[156] and the half-life of G-34 (38 min) is longer than that of G-17 (6 min).

Regulations

Gastrin secretion is influenced by: (1) peptides and amino acids in the gastric lumen; (2) pH of antral mucosa; (3) circulating catecholamines; and (4) neural reflexes. The small peptide and amino acid fragments, derived from protein digestion in GI tract, stimulate gastrin release.[157] Not all amino acids are equipotent in releasing gastrin. When in contact with antral mucosa, the aromatic amino acids, such as phenylalanine and tryptophan, stimulate gastrin release.[158] The pH of gastric luminal contents also controls the release of gastrin. Its secretion is inhibited by acidification of antral mucosa (below pH 3) and thus provides a negative feedback mechanism of gastrin secretion in response to gastrin-induced release of HCl.[159,160] This loss of HCl feedback inhibition of gastrin most often occurs in patients with pernicious anemia. Gastrin release is also increased by epinephrine and is blocked by β-adrenergic "blockers".[161] The cholinergic mechanism in controlling gastrin secretion is complex. In dog, insulin induced hypoglycemia stimulates gastrin release through activation of vagal-cholinergic reflexes and is blocked by administration of atropine or antral denervation.[162,163] Antral mucosa also contains somatostatin, which inhibits gastrin release in a probable paracrine manner. Studies indicate that administration of somatostatin or its congeners to patients with Zollinger-Ellison-syndrome inhibits gastrin release.[164]

Biological Actions

Gastrin has a wide range of biological effects on the epithelium and smooth muscle of the GI tract. Many of these actions are pharmacologic rather than physiologic (Table 26-6).[149,150,165] Protein meal increases gastric acid secretion and this response is mediated through secretion of gastrin during the gastric phase of acid secretion.[159,166,167] All three types of gastrin (G-34, G-17, and G-14) stimulate acid secretion, possibly due to presence of identical C-terminal tetrapeptide.[168,169] Gastrin plays a major role in mediating the acid secretory response to gastric distension but only a minor role in mediating the cephalic phase of gastric acid secretion.[2]

In addition to stimulating acid secretion, gastrin also exerts some action on gastric motility (emptying) and trophic effects on mucosal growth, especially on the acid secreting pyloric gastric mucosa[170] the latter via stimulating DNA, RNA, and protein synthesis.[149,171] The gastrin mediated gastric acid secretion is

TABLE 26-4. Use of Octreotide Acetate in Controlling Secretory Diarrhea

Condition	Dose/Route	Comments	Reference
Carcinoid syndrome	50–150 mg SC bid	25 patients: 72 percent had decreased 5-HIAA in urine and 88 percent had symptomatic improvement	131
	100 mg SC bid, increased to 1,000 mg/day	Diarrhea reduced in 83 percent of 12 patients; treatment up to 4 years slowed tumor growth in 67 percent of cases.	132
VIPoma (pancreatic Cholera syndrome)	100 mg SC bid	65-year-old female; reduced K+, HCO3- Water loss; also lowered plasma levels of neurotensin, motilin, VIP, PP, GIP, glucagons	133
	100 mg SC bid	72-year-old female; decreased stool weight and plasma VIP	134
	50 mg SC bid	43-year-old male; possible shrinkage of tumor; diarrhea controlled for 14 months	135
	50 mg SC bid	2 patients; decreased hormone release with symptomatic improvement	136
	50 mg SC bid	5 patients; 4 patients had decreased VIP concentrations, and all showed symptomatic improvement	137
	50 mg/h IV	1 patient; male, 5 months; ganglioneuroblastoma; NPY also present; administration of up to 300 mg SC ineffective	138
	50 mg SC bid increased to tid	44-year-old female; reduction in jejunal and ileal secretion of fluid in perfusion study; decrease in stool output	139
	100–600 mg SC daily	4 patients; suppressed release of peptides with symptomatic improvements	140
	50–1,000 mg daily	86 percent of patients improved or completely resolved diarrhea in 3 months	127
Gastrinoma	220–675 mg SC daily	25 patients; 60 percent improved, 30 percent unchanged, 10% worse	127
	1,500 mg daily	9 patients with metastatic disease, 6 had reduction in symptoms; in 2, dose of H2 blockers could be reduced	141
AIDS	100–300 mg SC, tid	1 patient; maintained 8 months 300 mg/kg tid without diarrhea; eats normal diet	122
	50 mg SC bid, increased to 200 mg SC, tid	1 patient; no demonstrable cryptosporidial infection; stopped diarrhea, and patient gained weight	123
	10–100 mg/hr IV	1 patient, cryptosporidiosis-positive; maintained on 75 mg/h for 9 months with a reduced severity of diarrhea	124
	100 mg SC bid	2 patients with cryptosporidiosis responded with reduced diarrhea; 2 patients with concomitant CMV infection did not respond well	142
Idiopathic diarrhea of infancy	1.9 mg/kg SC bid	1 patient; 60 percent decrease in stool output; possible tolerance at 26 weeks	129

SC = subcutaneous; bid = 2 times daily; tid = 3 times daily; 5-HIAA = 5-hydroxyindoleacetic acid; VIP = Vasoactive intestinal polypeptide; IV = intravenous; GIP = gastric inhibitory peptide; PP = pancreatic polypeptide; NPY = neuropeptide Y; AIDS = acquired immunodeficiency syndrome; CMV = cytomegalovirus.

Source: Modified from Redfern et al. with permission.[143]

dependent on interaction among gastrin, acetylcholine, and histamine.[172,173] Cephalic vagal stimulation enhances gastrin-induced acid secretion while vagotomy or anticholinergic agents decrease this response. Similarly, H2 receptor antagonists inhibit gastrin-induced gastric acid secretion indicating that histamine could be a final mediator for gastrin-induced acid secretion.

Gastrin also appears to play a role in carcinogenesis of gastric tissue, particularly in rats treated with omeprazole (acid-reducing

TABLE 26-5. Efficacy of Octreotide Acetate (Sandostatin) on GEP Peptide-Producing Tumors

Tumor	Sign/Symptoms	Dose	Clinical Response (1–10)*	Comment
Gastrinoma	Zollinger-Ellison syndrome	220–675 mg daily	6	Diarrhea, abdominal pain improved, very high dose may be needed
Carcinoid syndrome	Carcinoid syndrome Flushing/diarrhea	150–450 mg tid	9.5	Flushing and wheezing most responsive; tumor shrinkage (>50 percent) at very high doses noted in 17 percent of patients
VIPomas	Watery diarrhea	250 mg daily	8	Excellent correlation between somatostatin receptors and clinical response to octreotide
Glucagonoma	Glucagonoma syndrome	200–300 mg daily	8, rash 10, diarrhea	Rash responds over time Diarrhea responds Diabetes mellitus improves in 50 percent of patients
Insulinoma	Hypoglycemia	200–675 mg	4.5	Must watch for worsening of hypoglycemia
PPoma	Asymptomatic or diarrhea	250–320 mg	10	Diarrhea, when present, resolves

*1 = poor response; 10 = best response; PP = pancreatic polypeptide.

Source: Modified from O'Dorisio and Redfern with permission.[5]

medication).[174] In humans, only rare carcinoids have been observed after prolonged administration of this drug.[175] Of particular therapeutic importance, gastrin stimulates the in vivo growth of colon cancer in rodents and humans that possess gastrin receptors.[176–179] The relevance of chronically elevated gastrin, as seen in pernicious anemia, and its trophic action on colonic mucosa remains to be elucidated.

TABLE 26-6. Actions of Gastrin

Functions	Involved Organs/Tissues
1. Trophic action	Gastric mucosa Small intestinal mucosa
2. Water and electrolyte secretion	Pancreas Stomach Small intestine Brunner's glands Liver Pancreas
3. Acid secretion	Stomach
4. Digestive enzyme secretion	Stomach Small intestine Pancreas
5. Inhibition of water/salt/glucose absorption	Small intestine
6. Stimulation of smooth muscle	Lower esophageal sphincter Stomach Small intestine Colon Gallbladder
7. Inhibition of smooth muscle	Pyloric sphincter Ileocecal sphincter
8. Increase in blood flow	Stomach Small intestine Pancreas
9. Release of hormones	Insulin from pancreas Calcitonin from thyroid gland

Clinical Relevance and Application

Excess secretion of gastrin is associated with a number of disease states, the best known being the Zollinger-Ellison (gastrinoma) syndrome.[180] This syndrome is characterized by hypergastrinaemia, mucosal hyperplasia of the gastric fundus, severe peptic ulcer disease, and profuse diarrhea. These findings occur as a consequence of gastrin producing non-beta-islet cell tumors or "gastrinoma" located extrapancreatically.[91] Hypergastrinemia is also associated with antral G-cell hyperfunction,[181,182] isolated retained antrum (after a Billroth II gastrectomy),[183] atrophic gastritis,[184] pernicious anemia,[185] vagotomy,[186] uremia,[2] and antisecretory drugs.[187,188] Gastrinomas are often referred to as "pancreatic islet tumors," although there are no gastrin-secreting cells in normal adult pancreas.[189,190] In patients with sporadic Zollinger-Ellison syndrome, gastrinomas originating in the pancreas may be due to involvement of adjacent lymph nodes.[191,192]

Gastrin, per se, has no clinical therapeutic applications. However, pentagastrin, a synthetic short acting analog of the C-terminal pentapeptide, has been used diagnostically to identify patients with achlorhydria and to evaluate gastric acid secretion in patients with peptic ulcer disease who are undergoing vagotomy.[2] With the advent of the very powerful proton-pump inhibitors, vagotomy is rarely performed for peptic ulcer disease. Pentagastrin is also useful in the diagnosis of medullary carcinoma of the thyroid. A circulating calcitonin concentration of >400 pg/ml after intravenous infusion of pentagastrin (0.5 μg/kg body wt) is highly suggestive of medullary thyroid carcinoma. Intravenous pentagastrin has become commercially unavailable. A promising provocative test utilizes a proton-pump inhibitor, omeprazole, to stimulate endogenous gastrin and abnormal levels of calcitonin in patients with medullary thyroid cancer.[193] Pentagastrin has been used clinically to assess the severity of symptoms (especially flushing attacks induced by eating) associated with both carcinoid tumor and medullary carcinoma of the thyroid.[194]

Cholecystokinin

Cholecystokinin (CCK) is one of the oldest gastrointestinal hormones, originally purified from porcine intestine as a 33-amino acid peptide, CCK-33. CCK exists in a variety of biologically active molecular forms, each of which is derived from prepro-CCK (a 114-amino acid peptide). These are CCK-58, CCK-39, CCK-33, CCK-22, CCK-8, CCK-5, and CCK-4.[195] The amidated carboxy terminal pentapeptide of CCK that possesses biological activity is identical to that of gastrin. CCK is produced and secreted by mucosal endocrine cells (I cells) of the duodenum and proximal jejunum.[196,197] CCK has also been localized in a subpopulation of pituitary and adrenal medullary cells,[198,199] in cerebral cortex,[200–202] in dopaminergic neurons of the mesencephalon,[203] and in peripheral nerves of the GI tract.[204] In small intestine, some CCK neurons are colocalized with galanin, neuropeptide Y (NPY), substance P, somatostatin, calcitonin gene related peptide (CGRP), and VIP.[205,206] In contrast to gastrin, which naturally exists in both sulfated and nonsulfated forms, all circulating molecular forms of CCK are sulfated.[148] Indeed, sulfation of tyrosine residue at position 7 (from the C-terminal end) is critical for full biological potency.[150]

TABLE 26-7. Biological Effects of CCK

Organs/Tissues	Functions
Stomach	Stimulates acid secretion (weak)
	Decreases gastric emptying rate
	Decreases LES* pressure
Small intestine	Increases small intestinal motility
	Decreases intestinal transit time
	Releases intestinal peptidases
	Increases intestinal lymph flow
	Increases secretion of gastric inhibitory peptide
Large intestine	Increases colonic motility
Pancreas	Induces hypertrophy and hyperplasia of pancreas
	Stimulates synthesis and release of pancreatic amylase
	Increases secretion of bicarbonate
	Enhances insulin release
	Increases secretion of somatostatin
	Increases secretion of pancreatic polypeptide
Liver	Stimulates hepatic secretion of bicarbonate into bile
Gallbladder	Stimulates gallbladder contraction
	Induces relaxation of sphincter of Oddi
Thyroid gland	Increases secretion of calcitonin

*LES = lower esophageal sphincter.

Source: Modified from Walsh with permission.[150]

Release

Several nutrients influence the release of CCK, which appears to be species-specific. In humans and several other mammalian species, intragastric or intraintestinal administration of mixed meals cause an elevation of plasma CCK levels.[207] It has been established that fatty acids, amino acids, and protein stimulate CCK release in dog and human when administered into the duodenum through perfusion.[208,209] In the rat, only protein is effective in releasing CCK, while amino acids and lipids are ineffective when administered intragastrically.[210] In general, carbohydrate is a weak stimulant of CCK.[207] In humans, the principal circulating molecular species after the ingestion of a meal are CCK-8, CCK-22, and CCK-33.[207] Inhibition of gut proteases by trypsin inhibitors in rats increases pancreatic exocrine secretion[211] through release of CCK.[212,213] Thus active proteases in the gut control CCK release through a negative feedback mechanism. In humans, the existence of similar feedback mechanisms in controlling CCK has been debated. Several studies indicate that pancreatic juice and bile in the intestine appear to modify CCK secretion through a feedback mechanism.[214–217]

Biological Actions

CCK was discovered and named on the basis of its ability to stimulate gallbladder contraction. Several studies indicate that CCK is the most important regulator of gallbladder function, predominantly contraction.[207,214,218–220] The action of CCK in gallbladder is mediated through interaction with type A CCK receptors.[221,222] Blockage of CCK receptors by selective antagonists inhibits CCK-induced gallbladder contraction.[214,218,223] In addition to gallbladder contraction, CCK has the ability to stimulate hepatic secretion of bicarbonate into bile and to induce relaxation of the sphincter of Oddi (Table 26-7).[224–226] Pancreatic exocrine secretion is also influenced by circulating CCK. It increases both synthesis and secretion of pancreatic amylase,[227–229] while it is a weak stimulant of water and bicarbonate secretion.[230,231] In humans CCK acts synergistically with secretin to secrete bicarbonate.[232] Pancreatic function of CCK is mediated through mobilization of calcium and turnover of phosphoionositol,[233] that in turn changes the K^+ conductance pathway of acinar cells leading to hyperpolarization.[234] This stimulus-secretion coupling is the major mechanism of CCK in secreting pancreatic enzymes from acinar cells. CCK also stimulates growth of pancreatic tissue[235,236] as evidenced by atrophy of pancreas following treatment of animals with CCK receptor antagonists.[237] The action of CCK in pancreatic growth is mediated through inducing ornithine decarboxylase, a rate-limiting enzyme, responsible for biosynthesis of polyamines that in turn facilitate synthesis of DNA, RNA, and protein in the pancreas.[238] CCK is also known to stimulate the release of insulin[239–244] and pancreatic polypeptide (PP)[245–249] in several animal species as well as in humans. CCK has effects on gastrointestinal motility and is mediated through relaxation of lower esophageal sphincter[250–254] and by reducing gastric emptying through relaxation of proximal part of stomach and constriction of pyloric sphincter.[255–260] CCK also affects bowel motility either directly by stimulating smooth muscle contraction of the intestine[258] or through release of acetylcholine from postganglionic parasympathetic neurons.[261]

Clinical Relevance and Applications

No recognized disease states to date are associated with hypersecretion or hyposecretion of CCK. Because of its extensive biological effects, CCK has a number of potential clinical applications.[2] The action of CCK in stimulating gallbladder contraction is used in radiographic and ultrasonic assessment of gallbladder emptying.[262] CCK has also been used in testing exocrine function of pancreas by measuring the amount of fluid, bicarbonate, and pancreatic enzymes in pancreatic juice collected following infusion of CCK along with secretin.[263,264] In addition to the use of CCK for diagnostic purposes, it can be used therapeutically. Patients who receive intravenous alimentation (total parenteral nutrition) tend to develop gallstones due to stasis of the gallbladder.[265,266] Gallstone formation in these patients can be prevented by administration of CCK.[267] CCK may also have potential clinical use in the treatment of obesity (by suppressing appetite) and the treatment of exocrine pancreatic insufficiency (by increasing the size of the pancreas).[2]

Secretin

The secretin family of peptides is the largest group of GI hormones and includes vasoactive intestinal polypeptide (VIP), gastric inhibitory polypeptide (GIP), glucagon, glucagon-like peptides 1 and 2 (GLP-I and GLP-II), pituitary adenylyl cyclase activating peptide (PACAP), peptide histidine isoleucine (PHI) [or peptide histidine methionine (PHM)], growth hormone releasing factor (GHRF), and oxyntomodulin.

Secretin, a basic linear 27-amino acid peptide, was discovered in 1902 by Bayliss and Starling and represents the first GI hormone described.[1] Secretin-producing endocrine cells in the intestine have been characterized primarily on the basis of the production of secretin and their morphological properties.[268–270] The majority of secretin-producing cells, known as S-cells, appear to be localized to the villi of the proximal small intestine.[271] In most mammalian species including human, secretin immunoreactivity is highest in duodenum and lowest in the ileum. Recent observations indicate that substance P is coexpressed in some duodenal S-cells.[272] Extraintestinal sources of secretin are the subject of controversy. It has been reported that secretin can be produced from gastric antrum,[273] β-cells of the pancreatic islets of developing rats,[274] and from thalamus, hypothalamus, and olfactory lobe.[275]

Release

Secretin is released into the circulation and/or intestinal lumen from upper small intestinal mucosal S-cells in response to ingestion of a mixed meal. The endogenous acid that enters the duodenum is the major stimulant for the release of secretin.[276,277] The pH of proximal duodenum ranges from 3.0 to 5.0 and the threshold for secretin release from duodenum ranges betwen 4 and 4.5 depending on species. Secretin release can be abolished by administration of H2 receptor antagonists, which increase the duodenal pH by reducing gastric acid secretion.[278] Secretin release is also stimulated by bile salts and fatty acids.[279,280] Several other factors also influence the release of secretin. Studies indicated that gamma-amino butyric acid (GABA) stimulates both basal and acid-induced release of secretin.[281] The factors that inhibit secretin release include somatostatin,[282,283] and Met-enkephalin.[284]

It is known that pancreatic exocrine secretion is inhibited in the interdigestive phase by pancreatic proteases excreted into the proximal small intestine.[285–289] This inhibition is mediated through suppression of both secretin and CCK.[286–291] Recent studies indicate that secretin release induced by duodenal acidification in rats is mediated through the release of secretin-releasing peptide by acid.[292] Thus, there exists a feedback control of secretin by pancreatic secretion. Secretin stimulates pancreatic juice secretion and proteases in the juice inactivate the secretin-releasing peptide in the lumen of small intestine that, in turn, inhibits further release of secretin. It has been observed that secretin action is mediated through cAMP, Ca^{++} and protein kinase C.[293]

Biological Actions

The primary physiologic action of circulating secretin is stimulation of pancreatic water and bicarbonate secretion.[294,295] Immunoneutralization of endogenous secretin in rats and dogs after ingestion of a meal resulted in inhibition of pancreatic secretion of water and bicarbonate indicating that secretin is involved in the secretion of water and bicarbonate from pancreas. On the other hand, pancreatic actions of secretin can be potentiated by CCK in dogs and humans.[232,296] Secretin is also known to inhibit gastrin release and gastric acid secretion.[150,297] In humans, physiological doses of secretin inhibited pentagastrin-stimulated acid secretion.[298] In several mammalian species including dogs, cats, and humans, secretin can stimulate pepsin secretion.[299–302] Secretin also has a wide range of pharmacological effects. It increases bile flow and bicarbonate concentration of bile,[303–305] delays gastric emptying,[306,307] inhibits contraction of small intestine and colon,[308] relaxes the lower esophageal sphincter, increases gastric mucous, and induces adipose tissue lipolysis (Table 26-8).[297] In addition to inhibition of gastrin secretion, pharmacological dose of secretin also stimulates release of insulin, glucagon, somatostatin, and pancreatic polypeptide.[309–312]

Clinical Relevance and Applications

Hypersecretinemia has been reported to be associated with Zollinger-Ellison syndrome, duodenal ulcer disease (in combination with gastric acid hypersecretion), and chronic renal failure.[313]

TABLE 26-8. Biological Effects of Secretin

Organs/Tissues/Systems	Functions
Stomach	Decreases growth of gastric mucosa
	Inhibits acid secretion
	Stimulates pepsin secretion
	Decreases smooth muscle contraction of stomach
	Delays gastric emptying
	Decreases LES pressure
	Decreases blood flow in gastric mucosal artery
	Inhibits gastrin secretion
Intestine	Increases water and electrolyte secretion from Brunner's gland
	Inhibits smooth muscle contraction of small and large intestine
	Increases blood flow in small intestinal artery
Pancreas	Increases water and bicarbonate secretion
	Enhances blood flow in pancreatic artery
	Increases insulin secretion
	Stimulates glucagons release
	Increases pancreatic polypeptide release
	Enhances somatostatin secretion
Liver	Increases water and electrolyte secretion
	Decreases blood flow in hepatic artery
Gallbladder	Increases gallbladder contraction
	Inhibits sphincter of Oddi
Adipose tissue	Induces adipose tissue lipolysis
Cardiovascular function	Increases heart rate
	Enhances stroke volume

The underlying cause of increased circulating levels of secretin in these disease states is unclear, although decreased renal clearance of secretin may contribute to hypersecretinemia in renal failure.[314] This supposition is strengthened by the prolonged $t_{1/2}$ of secretin in azotemic patients compared to normal subjects (6 min vs. 2.4 min).[313] Furthermore, elevation of circulating secretin levels (in addition to gastrin) in gastrinoma patients may produce mild antagonism of endogenous gastrin, since secretin is known to inhibit gastric acid secretion (probably by inhibition of gastrin).

Hyposecretinemia occurs in some patients with celiac disease and achlorhydria.[315,316] Malabsorption in patients with celiac disease may be a consequence of a diminished pancreatic secretory response to the ingestion of a meal as well as the marked loss of intestinal absorptive area associated with denudation of the villi.[2] Patients with celiac sprue exhibit a markedly attenuated secretin response to acidification of the duodenum, an observation that may explain the poor meal-stimulated pancreatic secretory output.[315]

Secretin has two principal diagnostic uses in the gut endocrine field: evaluation of the secretory function of the exocrine pancreas and identification of patients with gastrin-secreting tumors (gastrinomas).[2] Typically, pancreatic secretory testing is performed in duodenally intubated patients by means of intravenous secretin administration in a dose of 2 U/kg, alone or in combination with CCK.[317] The volume, electrolyte composition, and amylase output of pancreatic juices secreted into the duodenum are subsequently determined. This approach is useful in evaluating the involvement of the pancreas in patients who exhibit intestinal malabsorption and helping to identifying patients with pancreatic cancer or chronic pancreatitis.

In the majority of patients with gastrinoma, the condition may be diagnosed by the prompt increase in circulating gastrin concentrations after the intravenous administration of secretin (Fig. 26-3).[318,319] The mechanism for this is unknown and considered paradoxic. In normal subjects, secretin produces a minimal effect on basal gastrin concentrations, and actually inhibits gastrin release induced by ingestion of a meal. An absolute gastrin rise of 200 pg/mL above basal, following a 2 U/kg secretin bolus, is considered diagnostic of gastrinoma.[320]

FIGURE 26-3. Rapid increase in serum gastrin concentrations in response to secretin in patients with gastrinoma. Note that an absolute increase of 200 pg/ml over basal values is very suggestive of gastrinoma. (*From McGuigan with permission.*[320])

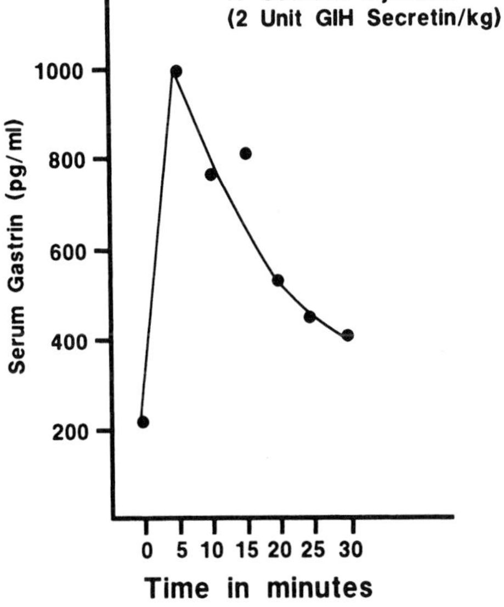

By increasing pancreatic blood flow, secretin may also be helpful in localizing vascular or endocrine tumors by angiography.[321] Secretin has become commercially unavailable and a useful diagnostic screening test, like that for medullary thyroid carcinoma, is now lacking.

Vasoactive Intestinal Polypeptide

Vasoactive intestinal polypeptide (VIP) was first isolated from porcine intestine as a potent vasodilating agent and later its sequence was established.[322–325] VIP is a basic single-chain linear peptide containing 28 amino acid residues and is a part of a large family of related peptides that include secretin, glucagon, GIP, PHI, PACAP, and GHRH.[325] Immunocytochemical studies revealed that VIP is widely distributed in nerve cell bodies located in both myenteric and submucous plexuses in stomach, and in both small and large intestine. In some neurons, VIP is colocalized with CGRP,[326] CCK, GRP, dynorphine, NPY, and galanin.[327,328]

Release

Pancreatic cholera or watery diarrhea-hypokalaemia-achlorhydria (WDHA) syndrome is a life-threatening disease associated with elevation of plasma VIP.[329] Studies indicate that esophageal and gastric distension stimulate the release of VIP.[330,331] VIP release from the peripheral nervous system is also increased by stimulation of preganglionic parasympathetic nerve fibers or by stimulation of local electrical field.[332] Amino acids, glucose, and a mixed meal do not affect VIP release while fat and ethanol in the duodenum increases VIP release.[333] It has been suggested that the appearance of VIP in the circulation represents a spillover phenomenon resulting from the release of neural VIP and failure to degrade VIP intravascularly.[4,332]

Biological Actions

The physiological function of VIP has not been completely established. The biological effects of VIP, thus far established in different mammalian species, include stimulation of water and electrolyte secretion from pancreas; intestine, and gallbladder; enzyme secretion from pancreas; mucous secretion from intestine; increased bile flow; inhibition of acid and pepsin secretion from stomach; and inhibition of intestinal absorption. It also causes both contraction and relaxation of smooth muscles in GI tract.[334–336] In addition, VIP also regulates enterocytic carbohydrate metabolism through inhibition of glycolysis and glucose oxidation.

While VIP has a limited known physiologic role, its pharmacological effects are diverse (Table 26-9). The relaxation of GI smooth muscles caused by VIP may be direct as effects are observed in isolated muscle cells.[337] Electrical stimulation of gastric neurons produces relaxation of gastric smooth muscles in association with release of VIP from VIP containing neurons.[330,338] Blockage of endogenous VIP through immunoneutralization reduces gastric smooth muscle relaxation in response to electrical stimulation of gastric neurons.[339,340]

Vagus nerve stimulation causes an increased release of VIP and the pattern of VIP release parallels the flow of pancreatic juice.[341,342] The flow of pancreatic juice in response to vagal

TABLE 26-9. Pharmacologic Actions of VIP

System/Organ/Tissue	Functions
Digestive system	
Esophagus	Relaxation of LES*
	Contraction in body
Stomach	Inhibition of acid/pepsin secretion
	Relaxation of antral/fundic smooth muscle
	Relaxation of muscularis mucosa
Small intestine	Stimulation of water and electrolytes secretion
	Stimulation of secretion from Bruner's gland
	Contraction/relaxation of circular smooth muscle
	Contraction of longitudinal smooth muscle
Large intestine	Relaxation of smooth muscle
	Water and chloride secretion
Liver	Stimulation of biliary secretion
Pancreas	Stimulation of water and bicarbonate secretion
Gallbladder	Relaxation of smooth muscle
	Inhibition of fluid and NaCl absorption
Cardiovascular system	Chronotropic effect on heart
	Inotropic effect on heart
	Vasodilatation
Endocrine system	
Pituitary-hypothalamus	Stimulation of prolactin release
	Inhibition of somatostatin release
Pancreas	Release of insulin, glucagons, somatostatin, PP**
Thyroid gland	Release of thyroid hormone
Adrenal gland	Steroid hormone production
Kidney	Stimulation of rennin secretion
Respiratory system	Bronchodilation
	Stimulation of submucosal gland secretion
Urogenital system	Inhibition of myoelectrical and smooth muscle activity
	Potentiation of electrically induced and pilocarpine-induced prostatic secretion
	Erection
Metabolism	Lipolysis
	Glycogenolysis

*LES = Lower esophageal sphincter; **PP = Pancreatic polypeptide.

Source: Modified from Fahrenkrug with permission.[332]

stimulation is reduced by VIP antiserum, indicating that VIP may have some role in pancreatic secretion.[342] It is well known that VIP is a strong stimulant for intestinal secretion of water and electrolytes in animals and humans.[343,344]

Clinical Relevance and Applications

No clinical abnormality of the GI tract has been attributed to a deficiency of VIP. However, some studies indicated a deficiency of VIP-containing neurons in the lungs of patients with asthma.[345] Low levels of VIP in asthmatic patients may contribute to the bronchial smooth muscle hyperactivity in the disease.[346,347] VIP also acts as neurotransmitter in controlling penile erection. Studies indicated that intracavernous injection of VIP in patient with impotence induces penile erection.[348]

Excess secretion of VIP occurs as a result of non-beta-cell pancreatic tumors (VIPomas).[91] Short "bursts" of VIP are associated with transient yet profound episodes of hypotension. Prolonged hypersecretion of VIP can produce severe watery diarrhea, profound hypokalemia, hypochlorhydria (rarely), hypercalcemia, and flushing.[349,350] Octreotide acetate, a synthetic congener of somatostatin, is effective in controlling these symptoms, (Table 26-4). Other tumors including ganglioneuroblastoma and pheochromocytoma are also associated with increased levels of VIP.

Currently, VIP has no therapeutic applications, and its clinical usefulness is limited to serving as a functional marker for VIP-producing tumors.

Gastric Inhibitory Polypeptide (Glucose-Dependent Insulinotropic Peptide)

Gastric inhibitory polypeptide (GIP) was first detected as a contaminant of partially purified porcine CCK.[351] The peptide was named "GIP" because of its ability to inhibit gastric acid secretion. It is now better known as glucose-dependent insulinotropic peptide (GIP) as it accelerates the release of insulin from pancreas. GIP is a linear peptide consisting of 42 amino acid residues and is produced by K cells of duodenum and jejunum.[352] There are at least two molecular forms of circulating GIP. They are GIP_{1-42} with a molecular weight of 5 kDa, and pro-GIP, with a molecular weight of 8 kDa.[353]

Release

It is generally agreed that plasma levels of GIP increase in response to a mixed meal. Most specifically, carbohydrates and fat are the major stimuli for GIP release.[354–358] Fatty acids and glucose, digested products of fat, and carbohydrates, respectively, in

TABLE 26-10. Biological Effects of GIP*

System/Organs	Effects
Gastrointestinal system	
Stomach	Inhibits acid secretion
	Decreases pepsin secretion
	Reduces gastrin secretion
	Inhibits contraction of smooth muscle
Small intestine	Inhibits motility
	Increases secretion
	Inhibits water and electrolyte absorption
Pancreas	Stimulates pancreatic secretion (in vitro)
	Augments insulin secretion in the presence of glucose or amino acids
Liver metabolism	Augmentation of insulin mediated inhibition of glucose formation
	Inhibition of glucagon induced glycogenolysis
Adipose tissue	Stimulates fatty acid synthesis

*GIP = gastric acid inhibitory peptide or glucose-dependent insulinotropic peptide.

the intestinal lumen stimulate the secretion of GIP. Among fatty acids, long-chain fatty acids are most effective.[359,360] It has been observed that GIP response to fats is greater and more prolonged than to carbohydrate.[358] This may be due to the fact that slowing of gastric emptying by fat exposes the intestinal lumen for a prolonged time and thus exerts long lasting GIP secretion. Moreover, GIP release in response to fatty acids is secreted mainly from the jejunum, whereas duodenal GIP release is stimulated by glucose.[361] Some amino acids, specially arginine, histidine, isoleucine, lysine, and threonine in the intestinal lumen also stimulate GIP release.[361,362] Typically, circulating GIP remains elevated for approximately 6 h postprandially, and peak levels may be up to six times the basal values.

Biological Actions

GIP has diverse actions on the GI tract, pancreas, and other organ systems (Table 26-10).[363] The major actions of GIP are stimulation of intestinal secretion and inhibition of gastric secretion. GIP inhibits pentagastrin-stimulated acid secretion in dogs in a dose-dependent manner.[364] In the dog, meal-stimulated gastric acid and gastrin secretions are increased by intravenous administration of anti-GIP serum, suggesting that GIP may mediate its action on gastric acid secretions through inhibiting gastrin secretions.[365] In humans, a supraphysiological dose of GIP is a weak inhibitor of gastric acid secretion.[366,367] Studies indicate that somatostatin may be the final mediator of the action of GIP. In isolated perfused stomach preparation, infusion of GIP increases somatostatin secretion.[368] GIP also inhibits water and electrolyte absorption in the small intestine.[369] Administration of GIP inhibits gastric motor activity in dogs[370] and reduces Na^+ movement from lumen to interstitium in rabbit salivary glands.[371] The most important biological effect of GIP is the augmentation of pancreatic insulin release in response to orally or intraduodenally administered glucose or amino acids.[4,150,363]

In most animals, and even in humans, GIP is most effective as an insulinotropic agent only in the presence of elevated glucose.[358,372,373] GIP also exerts effects on glucose and fat metabolism. The peptide augments insulin-mediated inhibition of hepatic glucose production and inhibits glucagons-stimulated glycogenolysis.[374] GIP alters fat metabolism by stimulating fatty acid synthesis in adipose tissue.

Clinical Relevance and Applications

Clearly defined clinical syndromes associated with excess or deficiency of GIP have not been described. However, exaggerated release of GIP in response to glucose and fat has been observed in patients with diabetes mellitus,[370,375] chronic pancreatitis,[376,377] duodenal ulcers,[378] and obesity.[379] Food restriction in obese patients causes reversal of GIP response to glucose and fat. In patients with celiac disease, GIP release is blunted, which is not associated with decrease in insulin release.[380] The clinical significance of these observations remains to be established.

Motilin

Motilin, a linear peptide containing 22 amino acids, was originally isolated from hog small intestine in 1971[381] and later its sequence was established by Brown et al. in 1973.[382] Based on its ability to stimulate gastric motor activity, it was termed "motilin." Immunohistochemical studies indicate that motilin is secreted from specialized cells of small intestine known as M cells. In dogs, monkeys, and humans, the M cells are abundant in the duodenum and the jejunum, while the ileum contains very few motilin-secreting cells. This is supported by the evidence of marked decrease in plasma motilin in dogs following surgical removal of duodenum.[383,384] It has been observed that some motilin-secreting cells also contain serotonin.[385] Several studies also indicate the presence of motilin in the brain and peripheral nerves, but those studies have been strongly debated. As with members of the secretin family, the biological activity of motilin is attributed to the amino-terminal sequence rather than the carboxy-terminal sequence.[386]

Release

Motilin is released during the fasting (interdigestive) state and its secretion varies across individuals in different animal species including humans.[387,388] In dogs, the increase in motilin secretion is synchronized with the onset of the interdigestive myoelectric complex in the duodenum.[387,389] Involvement of the sympathetic system in the control of motilin secretion is minimal, although the parasympathetic nerve plays some role in the secretion of motilin in some animal species. It has been demonstrated that stimulation of vagus nerve increases plasma levels of motilin.[390] In fasting period, intake of food inhibits cyclical release of motilin. It was speculated that some hormones and neuropeptides influence the release of motilin. Insulin abolished the cyclic elevation of plasma motilin[391] while corticotropin-releasing factor inhibited basal release of motilin.[392] Bombesin is a potent stimulant of motilin release[393] while somatostatin inhibits the secretion of motilin.[394] It has been suggested that motilin secretion from M cells is also influenced by exogenous motilin through positive feedback mechanism.[395] In humans, cyclic variations in the plasma concentration of motilin are abolished by atropine, pancreatic polypeptide, and calcitonin.[396–398]

Biological Actions

Motilin primarily affects the GI tract (Table 26-11).[386] The most important action of motilin is to induce activity "fronts" and thus mimic phase III of the MMC in dogs and humans.[399,400] The induction of activity "fronts" can also be achieved by alkalinization or acidification of the duodenum.[401] In this experimental situation, fluctuations in migrating motor complexes correlate closely with increases in circulating motilin concentrations, suggesting that motilin is intimately involved in the regulation of

TABLE 26-11. Biological Effects of Motilin

System/Organ/Tissue	Effects
Gastrointestinal system	
Esophagus	Stimulates contraction of LES*
Stomach	Increases pepsin secretion
	Induction of activity fronts and mimic Phase III of MMC**
	Accelerates gastric emptying of liquid in dogs
	Delays gastric emptying in humans
Small intestine	Accelerates the migration of phase III MMC*
	Reduces absorption of water and electrolytes
Large intestine	Stimulates electrical activity of the sigmoid colon
Pancreas	Increases water and bicarbonate secretion (weak)
Gallbladder	Induces tonic contraction of gallbladder in dog but not in humans
	Increases electrical activity of the sphincter of Oddi
GI peptides	Increases release of PP***
	Increases secretion of somatostatin

*LES = Lower esophageal sphincter; **MMC = Migrating motor complex; ***PP = Pancreatic polypeptide.

interdigestive motility.[401] Immunoneutralization of endogenous motilin by administration of specific motilin antisera inhibits activity fronts in the proximal intestine but not in the distal intestine, indicating that circulating motilin is involved in the motor control of proximal intestine.[402] The effect of motilin on interdigestive motility is inhibited by a meal,[403,404] duodenal acidification,[405] pentagastrin,[403,404] and somatostatin.[406] In dogs and humans, administration of exogenous motilin stimulates contraction of the lower esopha-geal sphincter[407,408] and increases the output of pepsin from the stomach.[409] The effect of motilin on gastric emptying is still controversial. Administration of exogenous motilin in dogs accelerates gastric emptying of liquid solution but not the solid food,[410] while in humans it accelerates the gastric emptying of the meal.[411]

Motilin is a weak stimulant of pancreatic secretion. Exogenous motilin stimulates pancreatic secretion of water, bicarbonate, and protein in dogs.[412] Motilin also exhibits function on the gallbladder. Motilin infusion induces gall bladder contraction in dogs[413] but not in humans.[414,415] Motilin also alters secretion of some GI hormones. Administration of motilin increases the release of PP and somatostatin in dogs,[416,417] and in man it increases PP secretion.[397]

Clinical Relevance and Applications

Several disease states have been associated with hyper- or hypomotilinemia, but the clinical significance of this association has not been elucidated. Hypermotilinemia has been found in some patients with Zollinger Ellison syndrome,[418] with pheochromocytomas,[419] and mostly in patients with small cell carcinoma of the lung.[420] Although specific endocrine tumors that secrete motilin have not been identified, elevated circulating motilin concentrations (fasting) have been reported in patients with diabetes and patients with diarrhea associated with carcinoid syndrome, inflammatory bowel disease, infectious diarrhea, tropical malabsorption, and small bowel resection.[421,422] Reduced circulating motilin levels are associated with hyperthyroidism and pregnancy.[423,424] Motilin may have therapeutic potential in restoring normal intestinal motility patterns after abdominal surgery, although some results have been disappointing.[425] It has been demonstrated that erythromycin, an antibiotic, stimulates GI motor activity by interacting with motilin receptors.[426,427]

Pancreatic Polypeptide Family

Pancreatic polypeptide (PP) was initially recognized as a contaminant of insulin preparation from avian pancreas[428] and later it became apparent that PP is a separate peptide secreted from pancreas. Immunohistochemical studies using antisera raised against bovine PP indicate that PP is localized not only in pancreas but also in other other organs such as in the endocrine cell of the ileum and the colon and in nervous system.[429,430] The discovery of two separate structurally related peptides from porcine brain and duodenum by Tatemoto and his colleagues[431,432] provides a clear picture about the existence of a "PP family" in different organs. These structurally homologous peptides are termed as neuropeptide-Y (NPY) and peptide YY (PYY). In almost all species, each member consists of a 36-amino acid linear peptide with a carboxy-terminal tyrosine amide.[4]

PP is the most extensively studied peptide in this family and is predominantly located in the islets of the pancreas and, to a lesser extent, in the exocrine parenchyma and in the epithelium of the pancreatic ducts.[433] In the pancreas, PP cell density decreases from head to tail and is just opposite to the glucagons cell density.[434] PYY, which originally was isolated from duodenum, is primarily localized in the hindgut (terminal ileum, colon, and rectum).[435,436] Two major forms of PYY (PYY 1-36 and PYY 3-36) exist in both tissue and in the circulation. It has been observed that PYY colocalizes with enteroglucagon in L cells of rats, pigs, and in humans.[437,438]

The neurotransmitter NPY, which was identified initially in extracts of porcine brain, is widely distributed in the central nervous system (e.g., frontal, parietal, and temporal lobes of cerebral hemisphere; hypothalamus; caudate nucleus of basal ganglia; median eminence of hypothalamus; and pineal gland), the peripheral nervous system, and notably in the GI tract, respiratory tract, reproductive tract, heart, peripheral blood vessels, kidney, and spleen.[433,439]

Release

The release of PP into the circulation occurs in a biphasic manner after a meal.[433] This pattern of meal-induced PP secretion may represent the overall effects of three phases of PP release: cephalic-vagal, gastric, and intestinal. In the cephalic-vagal phase, the release of PP occurs as a result of the sight, smell, and taste of food.[440] The cephalic phase of PP secretion is blocked by anticholinergics and by truncal vagotomy indicating the dependence on vagal-cholinergic system.[440] In the gastric phase, PP release is induced by gastric distension caused by a meal, possibly through vagovagal or gastropancreatic reflexes and by direct interaction of food components (e.g., amino acids) with receptors within the gastric mucosa.[433] In the intestinal phase, PP release results from the presence of fat, amino acids, and glucose in the proximal small intestine.[441] The intestinal phase of PP secretion is not mediated by neural reflexes due to distension of the small intestine. It remains unclear whether the intestinal phase of PP release is an

TABLE 26-12. Biological Effects of Pancreatic Polypeptide Family

Polypeptide Type	System/Organ/Tissue	Effect
Pancreatic polypeptide	Esophagus	Increases LES* activity
	Stomach	Increases basal gastric acid secretion
		Increases basal secretion of pepsin
		Inhibits pentagastrin-stimulated acid secretion in dogs
		Stimulates gastric emptying
	Intestine	Induces fluid and electrolyte secretion (from small/large intestine)
		Increases transit time
	Pancreas	Inhibits fluid, bicarbonate, and protein secretions
	Gallbladder	Relaxes gallbladder smooth muscle
	Endocrine	Decreases plasma motilin and somatostatin
Peptide YY	Stomach	Inhibits gastric acid secretion
	Small intestine	Regulates motility
		Inhibits fluid and electrolyte secretion
		Trophic effects on intestinal development and dietary adaptation
	Pancreas	Inhibits secretin stimulated pancreatic secretion in cat
		Inhibits meal stimulated pancreatic secretion in dog
NPY**	Esophagus	Causes contraction and relaxation of LES
	Small intestine	Inhibits fluid and electrolyte secretion
	Pancreas	Inhibits pancreatic protein secretion
	Cardiovascular	Vasoconstriction and reduction of blood flow
	Feeding	Stimulates feeding

*LES = Lower esophageal sphincter; **NPY = Neuropeptide Y.

indirect result of the release of other GI peptides (e.g., CCK) that subsequently induce the release of PP from the pancreas, or a direct result of absorbed nutrients stimulating the pancreas to release PP.[433] The effects of a meal on the release of PYY are controversial. Initial studies in rats and humans did not indicate any rise in plasma PYY in response to a meal,[442,443] but other studies in dogs[444] and humans[445] have indicated that PYY is released into circulation in response to fat components of meal. In the GI tract, NPY is released from the nerve endings following sympathetic stimulation and by enteral feedings. It also may be involved in vasoconstriction after erection, leading to loss of erection.

Biological Actions

The biological actions of PP are varied and include alterations in gastric, intestinal, and pancreatic secretion; GI and gallbladder motility; and hormone release (Table 26-12). The actions of PP vary considerably among species, and whether they are inhibitory or stimulatory often depends on the experimental conditions. For example, in humans PP produced no effect on basal or pentagastrin-stimulated gastric acid and pepsin secretion, whereas in dogs, PP stimulated basal gastric acid secretion but inhibited pentagastrin-stimulated gastric acid secretion.[446,447] The physiological significance of PP secretions in humans remains to be elucidated.

PYY inhibits secretin-stimulated pancreatic secretion in cats[435] and meal-stimulated pancreatic secretion in dogs.[448] In humans, PYY has no effects on pancreatic secretion.[449] PYY also inhibits gastric acid secretion in dogs[450] and humans,[449] and gastric emptying in dogs, and humans.[451,452]

NPY has diverse effects that include regulation of cardiovascular functions,[453] release of pituitary hormones,[454] and influence feeding.[455] It is a potent inhibitor of intestinal fluid and electrolyte secretion. NPY also influences gut motility and causes contraction and relaxation of the lower esophageal sphincter.

Clinical Relevance and Applications

Several endocrine tumors may be associated with excess secretion of PP, including carcinoid tumors, VIPomas, glucagonomas, gastrinomas, insulinomas, and multiple endocrine adenomatosis type I (MEAI).[456–458] Elevated circulating levels of PP are frequently observed in patients with VIPomas, and PP is thought to contribute to the clinical diarrheal symptoms of the VIPoma syndrome.[433,459] Elevated circulating concentrations of PP have also been reported in patients with juvenile and maturity-onset diabetes mellitus and renal disease.[460,461]

Clinical conditions associated with decreased secretion of PP include cystic fibrosis, obesity, and acute pancreatitis, especially in patients who exhibit steatorrhea and pancreatic calcification.[462–464] Indeed, several animal studies have indicated that PP may have potential in the treatment of acute pancreatitis.[465] However, clinical studies of the therapeutic potential of PP in treating pancreatitis have not been reported. Patients with idiopathic chronic autonomic failure exhibit decreased PP responses and these changes are not correlated with changes in plasma catecholamines.[466] Diminished PP responses are also observed in patients with diabetes with autonomic neuropathy.[467]

Neurotensin

The existence of neurotensin (NT) with potent vasodilatory and cyanotic functions was first discovered by Carraway and Leeman

TABLE 26-13. Gastrointestinal Actions of Neurotensin

Stomach
Decrease in gastric acid and pepsin secretion
Decrease in gastric motility and gastric emptying
Reduction in gastric blood flow
Alteration in antroduodenal motor activity
Small intestine
Increase in intestinal fluid secretion and blood flow
Increase in intestinal capillary permeability
Inhibition of intestinal absorption of water and electrolytes
Decrease in motility
Pancreas
Stimulation of pancreatic exocrine secretion
Release of insulin, glucagons, pancreatic polypeptide

in 1973 during isolation of substance P from bovine hypothalamus.[468] These investigators later isolated and sequenced the peptide and established that NT is a 13-amino acid peptide.[469] NT has also been found in the bovine and human intestines.[470,471] Neuromedin N, a NT-like peptide, is also found in porcine spinal cord.[472] NT is localized in specific endocrine cells of GI tract, termed N-cells.[473] NT is more localized in the ileum than in the duodenum and jejunum.[474,475] The functional properties of neurotensin reside in the carboxy-terminal region, as indicated by full intrinsic biological activity of the peptide $NT_{8\text{-}13}$.[476]

Release

Neurotensin is released into the circulation after ingestion of a mixed meal or fat but not in response to isocaloric amino acid and glucose solutions.[477,478] Infusion of fat into the jejunum of humans and dogs increases NT release.[479] Resection of ileum following fat infusion into the jejunum decreases this fat-induced release of NT.[479] In humans, NT is rapidly increased following intake of food and the response is blocked by administration of atropine, indicating the involvement of neural pathway.[480] In addition to neural involvement in the release of NT, several neuropeptides including substance P, bombesin, and gastrin-releasing peptide induce release of NT in humans.[481,482]

Biological Actions

NT produces a wide variety of effects on the GI system (Table 26-13). These include inhibition of gastric acid secretion, motility, and gastric emptying; alterations in intestinal blood flow; stimulation of pancreatic and intestinal secretions; GI motility; and modulation of exocrine and endocrine functions of the pancreas.[483] The combination of NT with secretin causes potentiation of protein output from pancreas, while combination of NT with CCK potentiates pancreatic bicarbonate secretion.[484] Infusion of NT also decreases the lower esophageal sphincter, decreases gastric emptying, and inhibits the interdigestive migrating complex.[485,486] It has also been observed that NT induces the release of histamine from mast cells, increases vascular permeability, and stimulates an inflammatory reaction.[487–489]

Clinical Relevance and Applications

Disease states correlated with a deficiency of NT have not been described. Although NT-producing tumors are very rare, some neuroendocrine neoplasm shows an elevation of NT secretion along with other peptides, particularly VIP.[490,491] About 12 percent of patients with VIPomas and watery diarrhea exhibit high plasma levels of NT.[491] Meal-stimulated release of NT is enhanced in patients with dumping syndrome.[492] Elevated circulating levels of neurotensin may occur in some patients with pancreatic endocrine tumors and carcinoid tumors.[493] Specific symptoms attributed to hypersecretion of neurotensin have not been defined. Currently, neurotensin has no clinical therapeutic application.

Substance P

Substance P, a tachykinin family member, was first discovered by von Euler and Gaddum from extracts of equine intestine in 1931.[494] Along with substance P, bombesin, substance K, neuromedin K, neuromedin B, and gastrin-releasing peptide also belong to the tachykinin family.[495] It is an 11-amino acid oligopeptide and is distributed widely in the GI tract with the highest concentrations found in the proximal small intestine.[496,497] Most of the substance P in the GI tract is located in the myenteric and submucosal plexuses, but small amounts are also present in the endocrine cells.[4,498] Substance P is also found in the spinal cord, vagus nerves, and other peripheral nerves.[150] It has been documented that substance P is also present in the lower esophageal sphincter, pylorus,[498,499] and pancreas.[500] Although functioning primarily as a neurotransmitter or neuromodulator in the central and peripheral nervous systems, substance P appears in the vasculature of the small intestine during peristalsis, suggesting a physiologic role.[501,502]

Release

Several pharmacological evidences indicate that serotonin, neurotensin, and CCK-8 withdrawal releases substance P from myenteric plexus of guinea-pig.[503–505] The release of substance P is influenced by intraluminal pressure. The pressure rise that causes peristalsis also increases release of substance P. This pressure-induced increase in substance P release can be stimulated by a ganglion stimulant, indicating the involvement of cholinergic nicotine control on substance P neurons.[506]

Biological Actions

Substance P has a wide variety of actions on the GI system. It increases GI motility and blood flow to the gut; stimulates secretion from the small intestine, pancreas, and salivary glands; and inhibits gastric acid secretion.[507–510] The most striking effect of substance P is its potent spasmogenic effect on GI smooth muscle.[495] Whether this spasmogenic response represents a direct action on smooth muscle or an indirect effect via myenteric neurons is unclear. Substance P also exerts some function on intestinal mucosa. It has been observed that substance P increases short circuit current in mucosa of guinea pig ileum, indicating stimulation of chloride secretion.[511] The role of substance P on pancreatic secretion is not well established. In guinea pigs, the peptide increases the amylase secretion from pancreas.[512] Substance P also exhibits vasodilator activity, especially in splanchnic bed. In guinea pig ileum, stimulation of submucosal ganglia causes vasodilation due to cholinergic mechanism. This cholinergic mechanism abolishes following extrinsic denervation and noncholinergic mechanism develops through release of substance P.

Substance P also plays a role in inflammation and modulation of the immune response[513] through specific receptors such as neurokinin-1 receptor (NK-1R), NK-2R AND NK-3R.

Clinical Relevance and Applications

Clinical conditions associated with decreased tissue content of substance P include Hirschsprung's disease and Huntington's chorea.[514] Hirschsprung's disease (congenital megalocolon) is characterized by a narrowing of the rectosigmoid colon caused by the congenital absence of ganglion cells from the myenteric and submucosal plexuses (aganglionosis). Decreased content of substance P has been observed in aganglionic segments of the large intestine, suggesting the involvement of substance P in the pathophysiology of this disease.[515]

Elevated tissue content and significantly increased circulating concentrations of substance P have been noted in patients with carcinoid tumors, suggesting that substance P contributes to the clinical features of the carcinoid syndrome.[8] Studies from several laboratories indicate that tachykinin is present in gut carcinoids,[516,517] and some symptoms of carcinoid patients, especially flushing, are associated with release of tachykinin.

Galanin

Galanin, a 29-amino acid peptide, was first isolated from porcine small intestine in 1983.[518] The peptide was named due to the presence of glycine and alanine in the N-terminal and the C-terminal of the peptide, respectively. In galanin, the C-terminal peptide, alanine, is amidated and is variable (several amino acid substitutions depending on species of animal) while the N-terminal part of galanin molecule (1–15 amino acid) is highly conserved between species. The structure of human galanin was first determined in 1991 by molecular cloning and by other molecular methods.[519–521] It has been established that human galanin is nonamidated and has an additional amino acid, serine, at the N-terminal of the peptide (30-amino acid peptide).[522] The peptide is found both in the central and peripheral nervous system. Moreover, galanin-containing nerve fibers are also present in the muscle layers of GI tract and pancreas.[523,524] In some myenteric neurons, galanin coexists with VIP.[525] Galanin is also present in the sensory areas of the dorsal horn of the spinal cord, indicating some sensory function.[526]

Release

The information so far available regarding release of galanin is not clear and concise. The release of galanin from different tissues requires different stimulus. In pigs, basal release of galanin-like immunoreactivity is increased by distension of gut, instillation of bile, and amino acids in the gut.[527] Pancreatic release of galanin is influenced by activity of pancreatic nerves.[528]

Biological Actions

The biological function of galanin varies, as the structure of the peptide is different in different animal species. The peptide has wide varieties of effect on the gastrointestinal system, the neuroendocrine system, and the nervous system, and on food intake. It may cause excitation in some gut smooth muscles and inhibition in others. In the GI tract, galanin influences the motility, luminal secretion, and other GI peptide release. It also inhibits insulin secretion from the pancreas. One of the important functions of galanin is to inhibit gastrin and gastric acid secretion.[529–532] This inhibition of gastric acid secretion by galanin may be either direct through inhibition on parietal cells or indirect through modifying the release of gastrin. In humans, galanin causes hypersecretion of saliva with increased bicarbonate and electrolyte output.[533]

Galanin also exerts some function on GI motility. It increases the lower esophageal sphincter pressure in porcine intestine and thus affects intestinal motility.[534] Galanin also increases GI motility by acting on the smooth muscle of the GI tract in rats[535,536] and humans.[537] The galanin-induced contraction of GI tract cannot be blocked by tetrodotoxin or atropine, indicating that this peptide may act directly on the smooth muscles of the GI tract. It has also been observed that galanin plays a role in neuromodulation in the enteric nervous system as evidenced by inhibition of neuronally evoked acetylcholine release from myenteric plexus.[538] Moreover, acetylcholine release induced by VIP and substance P is suppressed by galanin. The actions of galanin in GI motility are region/tissue specific. It is also evident that some of the actions are dependent on the N-terminal part while others are dependent on C-terminal part. In both cases, the whole molecule seems to be required for full biological potency. There are two possible mechanisms by which galanin exerts its effect on myenteric neurons: (1) it opens K^+ channels that lead to hyperpolarization; or (2) it blocks the voltage sensitive Ca^{++} channels leading to decrease afterhyperpolarization.[539–541]

In the pancreas, galanin can influence both exocrine and endocrine functions. It has been observed that galanin increases blood glucose in dogs,[518] possibly by inhibiting insulin release from the pancreas.[542] Studies on most mammalian species indicate that galanin inhibits basal as well as stimulated insulin (by glucose, and neurotransmitters) and somatostatin secretion from pancreas.[542,543] Galanin also affects somatostatin release, although this function is controversial. Some studies showed that galanin inhibits somatostatin release while other studies did not support this effect.[544] Pancreatic enzyme (e.g., amylase) secretion is also suppressed by galanin in rats and pigs.[545–548] In humans, galanin inhibits the postprandial rise in glucose, insulin, PYY, neurotensin, pancreatic polypeptide, and somatostatin.[532] The effect of galanin on secretion of pancreatic polypeptide is controversial. Pancreatic polypeptide release is suppressed by galanin in humans but not in pigs.[532]

Galanin increases fat intake and plays some role in obesity, especially in postmenopausal women.[549] The peptide also increases heart rate[550] and modulates several physiological functions including cognition, learning, feeding behavior, and depression. Studies in rat showed that galanin could inhibit acetylcholine release in the hippocampus.[551] Recent studies using galanin knockout mice revealed that galanin has some antinociceptive function[552] and is possibly mediated through opoid mechanism.[553]

CARCINOID SYNDROME

The GI tract is considered to be the largest endocrine organ because neuroendocrine (NE) cells are interspersed throughout its length. These cells sometimes exhibit neoplastic change leading to the development of NE tumors. Although NE tumors in the GI tract are unusual, they frequently express clinical syndrome due to the effects of their elevated circulating secretory products. Classification of NE tumors can be categorized according to their embryologic origin, staining characteristics, and clinical features, and are referred to as islet cell tumors (pancreatic location), carcinoids, and argentaffinomas (when tumors are positive with silver stain). The NE tumors of GI tract are indolent in their growth, leading to the term, "carcinoid" that are between indolent carcinomas and more aggressive adenomas. Carcinoid tumors were first identified as a specific, distinct type of growth and the name "carcinoid" was first applied by Oberndofger in 1907.[554]

The first description of a tumor with the morphological characteristics of carcinoid tumors appeared in 1838,[555] but it was not until 1907 that the name "Karzinoide" (carcinoid) was used.[554] The collection of symptoms and physical findings now termed "carcinoid syndrome" was first described in 1954 by Thorson and associates, who observed right-sided valvular disease, asthma, cyanosis, and peripheral vascular disease in a series of patients with small intestinal primary carcinoids and liver metastases.[556]

Carcinoid syndrome represents a constellation of symptoms and physical findings resulting from the release of potent biologically active products from primary carcinoid tumors and their associated metastases. The typical symptoms of the carcinoid syndrome are diarrhea, flushing, perspiration, cardiac insufficiency, and asthma. They are usually slow-growing neoplasms that originate from the ubiquitous Kulchitsky's or enterochromaffin cells, which in turn are part of the APUD system.[557] These tumors constitute a relentlessly progressive type of cancer and represent well the indolent, episodic, clinically expressed behavior of endocrine cancers of the gastroenteropancreatic (GEP) system.

Carcinoid tumors are the most frequently occurring primary APUD tumor of the small intestine and, for that matter, of the whole GEP endocrine system. They are characterized by a relatively slow rate of growth, local spread, and distant metastases as compared with other malignant tumors. The carcinoid syndrome appears in less than 10 percent of patients with carcinoid tumors and liver metastases.[558] Approximately 25 percent of all small bowel tumors and 46 percent of all malignant tumors of the small bowel are attributable to carcinoid tumors.[10–12] Although the incidence of carcinoid tumors is relatively low (estimated incidence of 4–8 cases per million persons per year), these neoplasms are among the best-known tumors of the GI tract, partly because of their dramatic symptoms when they metastasize to the liver.[10]

Although once exclusively attributed to secretion of biogenic amines, notably 5-hydroxytryptamine (5-HT), the symptoms that often accompany carcinoid tumors are now believed to result from secretion of additional substances such as motilin, neuropeptide K (NPK), kinins, and prostaglandins.[7–9] It has been observed that NPK is elevated more frequently in carcinoids from the midgut than the foregut.[559] Carcinoids contain numerous neurosecretory granules composed of serotonin, CRH, GHRH, and neurotensin.

Pathology

Typically, primary carcinoid tumors develop in the GI tract, especially in the appendix, terminal ileum, and rectum.[7] Other GI sites include the colon, stomach, duodenum, and Meckel's diverticulum. In rare instances, primary carcinoid tumors may also occur in the biliary tract, pancreatic duct, bronchus, esophagus, thymus, ovary, and testis.[9,91] Recent studies indicated that carcinoid syndrome can be caused by a atypical carcinoid of the uterine cervix.[560]

Carcinoid tumors in the GI tract are classified as foregut, midgut, and hindgut based on their anatomic location.[561] In a recent 40-year review by Modlin and Sandor of 8,350 cases from the National Cancer Data Registry, 74 percent of all carcinoids were noted to be from the gut and 25 percent from the tracheobroncho-pulmonary system.[562] The small intestine comprises 51 percent of all gut carcinoids with 15 percent to ileum (high malignancy) and 19 percent to appendix (low malignancy). Foregut carcinoid tumors are located in the stomach and proximal duodenum; midgut tumors are located in the distal duodenum, small intestine, ascending colon, and proximal transverse colon; and hindgut tumors are located in the distal transverse colon, descending colon, and rectum. Midgut tumors, which are associated most frequently with carcinoid syndrome, are described as classical carcinoids, whereas foregut and hindgut tumors are described as atypical carcinoids.[7]

Primary tumors are usually small (<1 cm in diameter) and are rarely identified during routine radiologic procedures. Furthermore, primary tumors are usually asymptomatic. It has been documented that only 3.7 percent of patients of 3,718 carcinoid tumor cases exhibit signs and symptoms of carcinoid syndrome.[563] Carcinoid syndrome is frequently associated with primary tumors of the ileum and jejunum but not usually with tumors of the stomach, duodenum, and ovary. Bronchial carcinoid tumors can often give rise to the most severe clinical features of carcinoid syndrome, including prolonged flushing attacks, disorientation, anxiety, rhinorrhea, bronchospasm, and fever.[9]

Large primary tumors (>2 cm in diameter), especially of the midgut, frequently metastasize, whereas smaller tumors (<1 cm) metastasize in only 2 percent of patients.[10,11,563] Mesenteric lymph nodes, liver, and peritoneum represent the principal metastatic sites, but the tumor may also spread to the lung, bone, skin, ovary, brain, mediastinum, and spleen.[7] Mesenteric lymphatic metastases may induce abnormal bowel distension, fixation, or filling patterns that may become visible with barium contrast radiography.[9]

Histologically, carcinoid tumor cells from the midgut, appendix, and colon are monomorphous with small, dark oval nuclei; they display few mitotic figures. Tumors in the small intestine take the form of insular-like tumor buds that occasionally anastomose.[7] Tumor cells from these locations show an argentaffin reaction with silver stains, whereas tumor cells from bronchial, gastric, and pancreatic carcinoids exhibit an argyrophilic reaction.[7]

Immunohistochemical studies of carcinoid tumor tissue from the stomach, small and large intestines, liver, lung, ovary, prostate, and thymus reveal the presence of chromogranin A and synaptophysin.[564–567] Chromogranin A belongs to a family of proteins (the chromatogranins/secretogranins) that are stored in peptide hormones and neuropeptides in secretory granules of endocrine cells and neurons.[564–567] The presence of chromogranin A in carcinoid tumors (together with neuron-specific enolase) suggests that these tumors are derived from neuroendocrine tissue. Interestingly, chromogranin A is a precursor for pancreastatin, a 49-amino acid peptide that is capable of inhibiting glucose-stimulated insulin release and acid secretion in rats.[567] Synaptophysin, which originally was isolated from neuronal presynaptic vesicles, is an integral membrane protein of small vesicular organelles in both endocrine cells and neurons.[564]

Although their precise biological function is unclear, chromogranin A, pancreastatin, and synaptophysin may serve as useful markers for both normal and neoplastic neuroendocrine cells and tissues.[564] Indeed, immunohistochemical localization of chromogranin A is becoming an established technique to help identify a variety of endocrine and neuroendocrine tumors, including carcinoid tumors.[566] Further, chromogranin A levels are elevated in the plasma of patients with endocrine tumors such as carcinoid (most likely a consequence of increased secretion of peptides costored with chromogranin A).[567] Thus, measurement of plasma chromo-

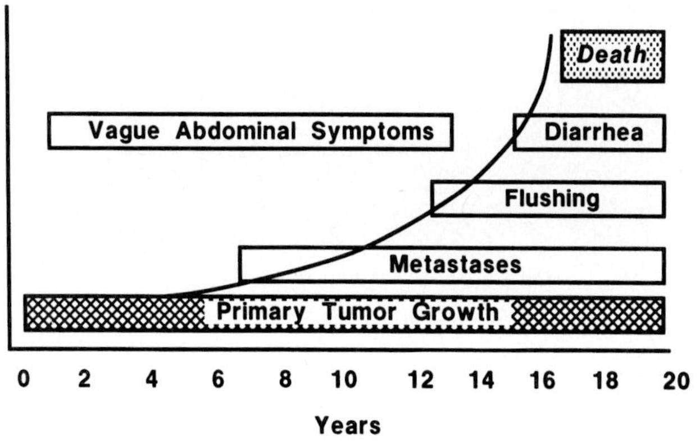

FIGURE 26-4. Natural history of carcinoid tumor growth and associated symptom complex. (*From Vinik and Moattari with permission.*[132])

granin A levels may be of clinical benefit in the early diagnosis of some endocrine tumors.[567,568] Our experience during the past three years suggest that pancreastatin may be more helpful than chromogranin A in defining tumor burden and therapeutic efficacity.

Symptoms

In the early stages of growth (typically for the first 6 to 12 years), primary carcinoid tumors are often accompanied by vague abdominal symptoms and consequently are frequently not recognized.[132] Overt, sustained clinical symptoms such as flushing and diarrhea do not usually develop until the primary tumor metastasizes to the liver, mesenteric lymph nodes, or other regions (Fig. 26-4).[132]

The principal symptoms of carcinoid syndrome include flushing (precipitated by stress, alcohol, and/or food and epinephrine congeners used in decongestants), diarrhea (secretory, malabsorptive, colicky, and hypermotile in nature), cramping, abdominal pain (colicky and often partially obstructive), cardiac fibrosis, peptic ulcer disease (rate, possibly resulting from the production of gastrin by some tumors and local release of histamine or other undetermined acid-producing substances), and pellagra (Table 26-14).[12,557,569] The chronologic sequence of clinical manifestations of carcinoid tumors shows considerable heterogeneity. Flushing may develop with or without diarrhea; this suggests that a combination of secretagogues is required for the expression of the complete syndrome.[5] Recently, it has been observed that

TABLE 26-15. Secretory Products of Carcinoid Tumors

Peptides	Amines	Other
Bradykinin, lysyl-bradykinin	Serotonin	$PGE_{2\alpha}$, PGE_2
Substance P	Dopamine	
Neurotensin	Histamine	
Motilin	5-hydroxyindoleacetic acid	
VIP		
Neuropeptide K		
GRP		
Calcitonin		
Somatostatin		

VIP = vasoactive intestinal polypeptide; GRP = gastrin-releasing peptide; PG = prostaglandin.

intestinal absorption of Cl^-, Na^+, K^+, and water decreases in patients with carcinoid tumors.[570] They also observed that luminal content of non-substance P, tachykinin, and PGE2 increases in patients with carcinoid tumors and contributed to secretory diarrhea.[570]

The symptoms of carcinoid syndrome vary according to the regional location of the carcinoid tumor.[7] For example, the carcinoid syndrome associated with bronchial carcinoid tumors exhibits the most severe clinical features. Flushing attacks are usually severe and protracted (lasting up to 4 days) and often are accompanied by facial edema, anxiety, tremulousness, agitation, lacrimation, sweating, salivation, nausea, vomiting, fever, and explosive diarrhea.[9]

The carcinoid syndrome associated with gastric carcinoid tumors is unique in that the flushes may start as bright red erythematous patches that eventually coalesce.[9] The flushes may be triggered by spicy foods, cheese, and low doses of pentagastrin.[9]

Pathophysiology and Mediators of the Carcinoid Syndrome

The full spectrum of clinical features associated with carcinoid syndrome results from the secretion of a wide variety of biologically active peptides, amines, and prostaglandins (Table 26-15) Most of them are found to increase with the flares of symptoms and following provocative testing with epinephrine-, pentagastrin-, and tyramine-containing food.[571] However, the rarity of carcinoid tumors that produce the recognized syndrome, combined with

TABLE 26-14. Principal Clinical Signs and Symptoms of the Carcinoid Syndrome

Clinical Signs/Symptom	Frequency, %	Comments
Flushing	80	Episodic; precipitated by stress, associated with hypotension
Diarrhea	76	Secretory, malabsorptive, obstructive, hypermotile
Pain	70	Dull or aching, midepigastric location, partial obstruction
Wheezing	10–20	May be asthmatic, bronchospasm
Cardiac fibrosis	50	Serotonin implicated in pathogenesis
Peptic ulcers	Rare	Thought to be due to gastrin-producing tumors
Pellagra	Rare	Thought to be due to niacin deficiency caused by diarrhea

Source: From O'Dorisio and O'Dorisio with permission.[91] Data incorporated from refs. 12, 132, 569.

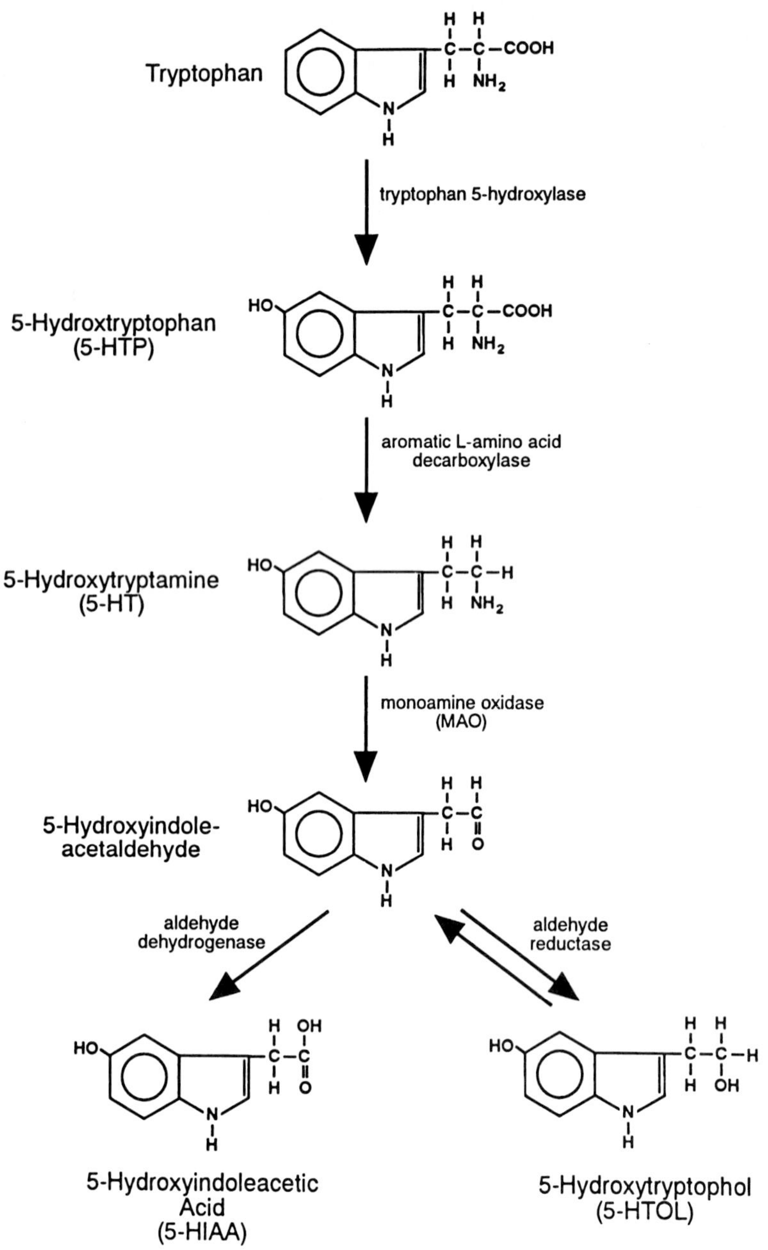

FIGURE 26-5. Synthesis and catabolism of 5-hydroxytryptamine. (*From Douglas with permission.*[572])

incomplete information regarding peptide tumor secretagogues, precludes full identification of carcinoid tumor pathophysiology.

Serotonin (5-hydroxy-tryptamine) is produced from dietary tryptophan in carcinoid tumors originating from midgut.[7] Initially, tryptophan is hydroxylated to form 5-hydroxytryptophan (5-HTP) by the influence of an enzyme 5-hydroxylase (a rate-limiting enzyme). It is then decarboxylated to produce 5-hydroxytryptamine (5-HT) by decarboxylase in the tumor (Fig. 26-5).[572] Following synthesis, 5-HT is released into the circulation. It is taken up by the platelets and stored in the secretory granules or catabolized by aldehyde dehydrogenase to 5-hydroxyindole acetic acid (5-HIAA) and subsequently excreted in the urine. Thus, excessive secretion of 5-HT from carcinoid tumors leads to elevated urinary concentrations of 5-HIAA in the majority of carcinoid patients.[7,8,557] 5-HIAA is usually not elevated unless there is metastasis to the liver.[573]

Urinary 5-HT secretion may be within the normal range or only slightly increased because of extensive renal catabolism of 5-HT to 5-HIAA. However, in a small number of carcinoid patients, typically those with foregut tumors (e.g., foregut tumors of bronchus, pancreas, and stomach), urinary levels of 5-HT and 5-HTP may be markedly elevated whereas levels of 5-HIAA may be only modestly increased.[7,8,557] One explanation for this change in 5-HT excretory products is that some carcinoid tumors lack decarboxylase enzyme and therefore are unable to synthesize 5-HT from 5-HTP. In these patients, the 5-HTP enters the circulation and is excreted by the kidney. Some 5-HTP is converted to 5-HT by the kidney, leading to elevated urinary excretion of 5-HT.

5-HT has a wide variety of physiologic effects that can give rise to the flushing, diarrhea, malabsorption, intestinal hypermotility, abdominal cramps, nausea, and vomiting associated with carcinoid syndrome.[574] Both in vivo and in vitro (using isolated muscle strip) studies indicate that 5-HT alters the GI motility. It has been observed that 5-HT increases small intestinal motility but decreases gastric and colonic motility.[559] Administration of 5-HT blocker in patients with carcinoid syndrome decreases the diarrhea but not the flushing symptoms,[575] indicating that flushing in carcinoid patients may not be related to the elevation of 5-HT. Serotonin is also believed to be involved in the etiology of the cardiac fibrosis (tricuspid valve involvement) commonly seen in carcinoid syndrome.[12]

Flushing in carcinoid syndrome may result not only from 5-HT release but also from the actions of a plethora of other vasoactive agents, including histamine, bradykinin, substance P (SP), neurotensin, motilin, somatostatin, prostaglandins, neuropeptide K, gastrin-releasing peptide, and VIP (unusual).[8] However, the involvement of many of these peptides has not been completely delineated. Studies indicate that a high blood level of bradykinin is associated with flushing episodes of carcinoid patients. Vasoactive tachykinins including substance P, neuropeptide K, and neurokinin A are also important mediators associated with carcinoid syndromes. Norheim and his associates observed about 100 percent increases in tachykinin levels in 9 out of 13 patients with pentagastrin-induced flushing.[576] Carcinoid tumor is also associated with release of SP. Immunocytochemical studies indicate that high levels of immunoreactive SP (ISP) are present in the general circulation, in tumor extracts, and in venous effluents from tumors in patient with carcinoid syndrome. Several lines of evidence indicate the presence of SP immunoreactivity in enterochromaffin cells that store 5-HT. Thus intestinal carcinoid tumors may produce not only 5-HT but also SP, and both of them are stored within the secretory granules. Feldman and O'Dorisio measured SP and neurotensin levels in patients with carcinoid syndrome before and after a flushing attack induced by alcohol (30 mL of dry sherry).[577] The development of facial flushing 1.5 to 5.0 min after the ingestion of alcohol was not preceded by an elevation in the plasma concentration of SP or neurotensin.

Diagnosis

Nonfunctioning carcinoid tumors are so slow growing that the diagnosis and its syndrome may not be made unequivocally for several years. They can cause an intermittent abdominal pain leading to a change in bowel habits due to partial bowel obstruction in the intestine. Thus, early primary carcinoid tumors are especially difficult to diagnose because the associated symptoms are vague and mimic other GI complaints (e.g., irritable bowel syndrome and spastic colon).[8] Carcinoid syndrome is more easily diagnosed when episodes of flushing, diarrhea, and wheezing are experienced by a patient with evidence of tumor metastasis. An accurate diagnosis usually hinges on the results of specific diagnostic tests for tumor markers and the results of imaging techniques such as computerized tomography and scintigraphy (OctreoScan^R) (Table 26-16).

TABLE 26-16. Diagnostic Approaches in Suspected Carcinoid Syndrome

Determine 5-HIAA and 5-HT levels
Measure fasting peptide profile, including substance P, neurotensin, and pancreastatin
Localize tumor with venous catheterization—measure arterial-venous gradients of peptides (e.g., substance P)
Examine patient for curable ovarian testicular, or bronchial primary carcinoid tumors if 5-HIAA/5-HT levels are elevated
Consider surgical exploration in any symptomatic patient if metastases are detected by CT, scintillation scanning, arteriography, or ultrasonography
Consider surgical resection of hepatic metastases after
  Evaluation of hepatic/cardiac function
  Identification of possible extrahepatic metastases (e.g., bone)
Evaluate possible nutrient malabsorption in patients with severe diarrhea
All patients suspected of carcinoid syndrome should have ^{111}In-octreotide scan (when available in the United States)

5-HIAA = 5-hydroxyindoleacetic acid; 5-HT = 5-hydroxytryptamine; CT = computed tomography.

Source: Adapted from Oates and Roberts with permission.[581]

Laboratory Diagnostic Tests

The presence of a variety of tumor markers in urine, plasma, or serum may be indicative of carcinoid tumor, although the diagnostic usefulness of each tumor marker varies with the location of the carcinoid tumor (Table 26-17).[7] No single marker is capable of identifying early all patients with carcinoid tumors. However, the most widely used, inexpensive, and effective screening procedure is measurement of urinary 5-HIAA.[578] This test is positive in 93 percent of patients with carcinoid tumors along with liver metastases.[579] Urinary excretion of 5-HIAA and plasma serotonin

TABLE 26-17. Usefulness of Tumor Markers in Diagnosing Carcinoid Syndrome

Tumor Marker	Specimen	Foregut	Midgut	Hindgut
5-HIAA	Urine	+	+++	—
Chromogranin A (pancreastatin)	Plasma	+++	+++	+++
APGP (IR-7B2)	Plasma	++	+++	++
NPK	Plasma	—	++	—
PP	Serum	++	+	+
HCG_α	Serum	++	+	+
HCG_β	Serum	+	+	+
Gastrin	Serum	++	—	—
Neurotensin	Plasma	+	—	—

Foregut = stomach and proximal duodenum; midgut = distal duodenum, small intestine, ascending colon, and proximal transverse colon; hindgut = distal transverse colon, descending colon, and rectum; 5-HIAA = 5-hydroxyindoleacetic acid; APGP (IR-7B2) = immunoreactive pituitary protein 7B2; NPK = neuropeptide K; PP = pancreatic polypeptide; $hCG_{\alpha/\beta}$ = human chorionic gonadotropin; +++ = very useful; ++ = useful; + = may be useful; — = not useful.

Source: From Wilander et al. with permission.[7]

should be measured in all patients suspected of having carcinoid tumor or syndrome. Urinary excretion of >30 mg 5-HIAA during a 24-h period is considered a positive result (normal range, 2 to 8 mg/24 h); some patients may excrete as much as 1,000 mg/24 h.[9] However, these values may vary according to the analytic procedure used (e.g., radioenzymatic assay or high-pressure liquid chromatography). Certain foods (e.g., bananas, pineapple, red plums, walnuts, tomatos) and medicines (e.g., cough medicines, muscle relaxant, acetaminophen, caffeine, certain antidepressant drugs containing MAO inhibitors) must be avoided for a day or two before the test as those foods and medicines can contribute to the increase in 5-HIAA in the urine. In a study of 75 patients with carcinoid syndrome, urinary and platelet 5-HIAA concentrations were elevated in 64 patients.[580] Similarly, Wilander and his associates found that 88 percent of patients with carcinoid tumors (most of whom had carcinoid syndrome) had increased levels of 5-HIAA; the degree of increase was associated with the size of the tumor mass in midgut carcinoid tumors.[7] Clinically relevant elevations of 5-HIAA are usually present when carcinoid tumor has metastasized to the liver.

In addition to 5-HIAA, some investigators measured fasting, whole-blood concentrations of 5-HT in patients with suspected carcinoid tumors.[9] Measurement of 5-HT is especially valuable because the consumption of foods containing large amounts of this amine does not influence the results (in contrast to 5-HIAA levels, which increase after consumption of 5-HT rich foods as a result of catabolism during intestinal absorption) and because this method rarely detects anything but carcinoid tumors.[557] 5-HT concentrations in whole blood (or plasma prepared from blood collected in ascorbic acid tubes) from carcinoid patients range from 790 to 4,500 ng/dL (normal range, 71 to 310 ng/dL).[9] However, as in the case of urinary 5-HIAA measurements, 5-HT values in blood may vary according to the method used (HPLC or enzymatic).

A high percentage of patients with carcinoid tumors also have elevated plasma or serum concentrations of neuropeptide Y (66 percent), pancreatic polypeptide (60 percent), human chorionic gonadotropin-α (69 percent), a novel anterior pituitary gland protein (APPG) or IR-7B2 (64 percent), chromogranin A, and motilin (52 percent).[582–588] Plasma levels of PP are especially elevated in patients with bronchial and midgut carcinoids.[584] Plasma concentrations of other GI peptides, such as SP and neurotensin, are also elevated in carcinoid patients.[577] However, these peptides are of limited diagnostic value in confirming the presence of carcinoid tumors.[577] If these tests are negative, pentagastrin-induced flushing is a sensitive and specific sign of the carcinoid syndrome.[570]

Diagnostic Imaging Techniques

A variety of diagnostic imaging techniques are available to identify primary and secondary carcinoid tumor sites and determine the extent of disease.[8] These techniques include CT, ultrasound (US), magnetic resonance imaging (MRI), radiography, hepatic and mesenteric artery angiography, endoscopy, barium contrast studies, and ^{131}I-metaiodobenzylguanidine (^{131}I-MIBG) or ^{99m}Tc Scintigraphy.[12,557,589–591] Another convincing technique, somatostatin receptor scintigraphy, has been used to effectively localize carcinoid tumors and may be supplemented by ultrasonography for liver metastases.[592] This approach exploits the propensity of most endocrine tumors to express high-affinity receptors (predominately subtype 2, SST2) for somatostatin as surgically excised carcinoid tumor tissue has been shown to bind somatostatin analogs in vitro.[593] This imaging method involves the intravenous administration of ^{111}Indium-DOTA-octreotide (OctreoScan^{R}) followed by gamma camera scintigraphy.[594] Although this procedure is costly, it is successful in almost 92 percent of carcinoids.[595] Somatostatin receptor-positive tumors in the abdomen as small as 1 cm in diameter can be visualized safely and quickly (within 30 min after isotope administration) using this technique. There are some cases with all the symptoms and chemical findings of carcinoid syndrome but standard tests fail to detect the presence of tumor. In these cases, OctreoScan^{R} can be a great help in confirming the diagnosis of carcinoid tumor. Additionally, a positive OctreoScan generally predicts a good response to octreotide (somatostatin congener).

Many of these imaging techniques are particularly applicable to tumor identification in specific locations.[8] Small bowel tumors can occassionally be identified by a barium contrast series, a method that may reveal abnormal bowel distension, fixation, or filling defects associated with mesenteric lymph node metastatic tumors.[589] Liver metastases (>2 cm) may be identified using hepatic angiography, but can also be evaluated using ^{99m}Tc liver-spleen scintiscan or CT or MRI scan of the abdomen.[8] When routine procedures are not successful, tumor localization with venous catheterization and measurement of blood levels, especially arterial-venous gradients of peptides (e.g., substance P), may be a useful alternative diagnosic approach. These techniques are not widely available. Somatostatin receptor imaging (Octreoscan^{R}) in a practiced medical center may be considered the best initial diagnostic procedure when clinical suspicion is high and, especially, when biochemical evidence also present.

Differential Diagnosis

Patients with systemic mastocytosis may also develop attacks of flushing, hepatomegaly, and diarrhea that are very similar to those of symptoms in carcinoid syndrome. Panic attacks, menopause, medullary carcinoma of the thyroid, and the rare VIPoma syndrome may also be accompanied by flushing attacks (Table 26-18). Occasionally, patients with pheochromocytoma (a catecholamine-secreting tumor) may also exhibit flushing attacks, although this is a rare occurrence and is seen when epinephrine is the predominant catecholamine. These diseases can be differentiated from carcinoid tumors by the absence of elevated levels of 5-HIAA or 5-HT and the lack of a flushing response to the intravenous administration of epinephrine.[8] However, the flushing response to epinephrine is not always a reliable diagnostic test.

Treatment

It is well known that carcinoid tumors vary in their size, growth rate, and location and in exhibiting symptoms. Therefore, the treatment should be individualized depending on the condition of patient. In patients with carcinoid tumor who develop carcinoid syndrome, the principal clinical manifestations that require therapy include flushing, diarrhea, cardiac disease (e.g., congestive heart failure, fibrotic valvular lesions, or carcinoid tumor involvement of myocardium or pericardium), bronchospasm, and painful enlargemnt of the liver.[596] In a small percentage of patients, development of peptic ulcer disease, severe hypoalbuminemia, pellagra, muscle wasting, myopathy, arthropathy, retroperitoneal fibrosis, edema, hypertension, and hyperglycemia may also necessitate therapeutic intervention.

TABLE 26-18. Differential Diagnosis of Flushing Syndromes

Flushing Syndrome	Features	Hormone Assay
Carcinoid	Diarrhea, wheezing, myopathy	Urinary 5-HIAA, substance P, NKA
Medullary carcinoma, thyroid	Mass in neck, familial	TCT (pentagastrin provocative test)
Pheochromocytoma	Paroxysmal hypertension, tachycardia	Urine VMA
Menopause		FSH
Panic attacks	Phobias, anxiety	
Mastocytosis	Dyspepsia, ulcer disease, dermatographia	Histamine
Idiopathic	—	—

5-HIAA = 5-hydroxyindoleacetic acid; NKA = neuropeptide K; TCT = thyrocalcitonin; VMA = vanillylmandelic acid; FSH = follicle stimulating hormone.

Source: Adapted from Vinik et al. with permission.[8]

The therapeutic options for treating carcinoid tumors include surgical removal of the tumor, embolization, tumor-targeted radiotherapy, antineoplastic chemotherapy to decrease tumor size, and pharmacologic therapy to block the actions of secretagogues (e.g., most prominently octreotide acetate as well and antagonists of alpha-adrenergic, 5-HT, H1 and H2 histamine receptors).[132,592,597–601]

Surgery

Surgical extirpation and tumor debulking may be appropriate in any patient in whom the primary carcinoid tumor can be localized. If the primary carcinoid tumor is detected in an early stage, surgical removal is usually curative. Debulking (removal of large portion of tumor) can effectively diminish the amount of harmful hormones/peptides being produced and flooding the circulation. Cryoablation, a new experimental technique using a freezing probe, has been used in some hospitals in destroying carcinoid tumor metastases in the liver when it is unresectable surgically. However, surgical removal of carcinoid tumors in patients who exhibit the carcinoid syndrome can be associated with initial risk of carcinoid crisis during surgery. This can be available with pre-, peri-, and postoperative use of octreotide acetate. These complications which are due to inherent properties of the carcinoid tumor rather than the surgical procedure, may include adhesion formation and development of short bowel syndrome.[9] It has been proposed that primary treatment for a carcinoid tumor, located anywhere in the gut, is surgical. Those who exhibit widely metastatic disease or who are not resectable may be the candidate for cryoreduction, surgical debulking, and hepatic arterial embolization followed by octreotide treatment for palliation of symptoms.[602]

Antitumor Chemotherapy

Chemotherapy for treatment of carcinoid tumor has been in use for more than 20 years. Several cytotoxic agents (such as 5-fluorouracil, streptozotocin, lomustine, Adriamycin, cisplatin, carmustine, and etoposide) and their combinations are available. Individual agents used alone have been disappointing, though a combination of agents (such as leucovorin-fluorouracil and streptozotocin, 5-fluorouracil and lomustine, Adriamycin and cisplatin, and carmustine and etoposide) has been frequently used in the treatment of carcinoid tumor patients.[603] Each combination has produced good response in only 20–30 percent of the cases. However, some patients who exhibit severe carcinoid symptoms may experience a paradoxic aggravation of their symptoms in response to chemotherapy. The potential for an adverse response to chemotherapy in some patients necessitates a reduction in the usual chemotherapeutic dose and pretreatment with agents such as octreotide acetate to lessen the severity of carcinoid symptoms.[596]

Antineoplastic chemotherapy is generally not recommended unless the patient's daily activities are impaired, the tumor is growing rapidly, or the tumor becomes life-threatening.[557] We reserve the use of aggressive chemotherapy for patients with malignant carcinoid syndrome in whom no somatostatin receptors can be demonstrated by OctreoScan[R] imaging. Further, the risks of chemotherapy-induced renal toxicity preclude the chronic use of such agents as streptozotocin.

Pharmacologic Therapy

A wide variety of pharmacologic agents have been proposed to alleviate the symptoms of carcinoid syndrome, including somatostatin and octreotide acetate, 5-HT receptor antagonists, synthetic antiestrogen (tamoxifen), steroids, methyldopa, human leukocyte interferon, and cholestyramine.[600,601,604] H1 and H2 receptor antagonists are especially effective in preventing the patchy, bright red flushing attacks that occur postprandially in patients with gastric carcinoids.[605] 5-HT receptor antagonists such as methysergide maleate and cyproheptadine ameliorate the flushing associated with carcinoid tumors but are rarely effective in decreasing the often-severe diarrhea.[9] However, ketanserin A, another antagonist of the 5-HT-M receptor, decreases the volume of diarrhea induced by carcinoid tumors.[606] A very selective serotonin receptor antagonist, ondansetron, can cause improvement of GI symptoms in carcinoid patients possibly by decreasing gastric emptying.[607]

Octreotide, a long-acting synthetic analog of naturally occurring somatostatin, provides the most dramatic and effective control of symptoms of carcinoid syndrome.[132,597,598,608] Octreotide administration markedly inhibits diarrhea, flushing, wheezing, myopathy, and secretion of gut hormones associated with carcinoid tumors.[132,598,609] Octreotide injections not only "squelch" the symptoms of carcinoid syndrome but also are now believed to retard and, sometimes, decrease the growth of tumors. Octreotide acetate is becoming the mainstay of treatment for patients with advanced carcinoid tumors, with or without the carcinoid syndrome. In addition to therapeutic use, octreotide acetate can also be used for diagnostic purpose. Octreotide treatment is expensive and needs to be injected subcutaneously 2–4 times a day. To minimize the inconvenient multiple daily injection, a long-acting preparation of octreotide is now available in Europe and the United State

TABLE 26-19. Clinical and Biochemical Effects of Octreotide in 14 Patients with Carcinoid Syndrome

Response to Octreotide	Diarrhea %	Flushing %	Wheezing %	Urinary 5-HIAA, %	Blood 5-HT, %
Positive responders*	58	89	67	63	10
Partial responders**	17	11	33	12	10
Negative responders***	0	0	0	0	10

*Positive responders: 75% drop in intensity or frequency of symptom or level of biochemical marker.

**Partial responders: 25 to 75% improvement.

***Negative responders: clinical and/or biochemical values increased by more than 25% of initial values.

5-HIAA = 5-hydroxyindoleacetic acid; 5-HT = 5-hydroxytryptamine.

Source: From Vinik et al. with permission.[578]

as Sandostatin–LAR (Long Acting Release). It is given intramuscularly, every 28 days.

Sandostatin[R] is useful in the symptomatic therapy of the carcinoid syndrome and VIPoma. It has been recently approved for pituitary GH-secreting tumors clinically expressing with acromegaly. The majority of patients with carcinoid syndrome will have a complete symptomatic remission following treatment with Sandostatin[610,611] as this drug reduces the serum levels of mediators such as serotonin and its urinary metabolite, 5-HIAA.[612] Vinik and his colleagues investigated the clinical and biochemical effects of octreotide in 14 patients with histologically proven carcinoid tumors.[578] Patients initially received octreotide acetate at a dose of 100 μg subcutaneously, every 12 h; this was later increased to 375 μg every 6 h. Octreotide acetate treatment abolished or significantly improved diarrhea (75 percent of patients), flushing (100 percent of patients), and wheezing (100 percent of patients) (Table 26-19).

In a similar study involving 53 malignant carcinoid patients, Kvols reported that octreotide (450 μg/day subcutaneously) resolved both flushing and diarrhea (89 percent of patients) and urinary output of 5-HIAA (≥50 percent) (72 percent of patients).[600] Hepatic pain, impairment of liver function, and tumor mass also decreased during octreotide therapy. Kvols also reported that octreotide was dramatically effective in reducing the symptoms of carcinoid crisis. Carcinoid crisis, which usually occurs in carcinoid patients during the induction of anesthesia before surgery, is characterized by abrupt severe hypotension, prolonged cutaneous flushing, confusion, and sometimes death. Octreotide is used for intravenous delivery or kept available during surgery involving any patient with known carcinoid. Somatostatin mediates its action via five different receptors that are present in normal tissue as well as in neuroendocrine gastroenteropancreatic tumors. The two subtypes type II and type V can recognize both lanreotide and octreotide.[613]

Interferon, a natural substance originally derived from white blood cells, has potent inhibitory effect on the growth of carcinoid tumors. Of the several varieties of interferon, only interferon-α has been used in treating patients with carcinoid tumors.[614] Although interferon has beneficial effects in suppressing tumor growth of carcinoid syndrome, it often produces unpleasant side effects including extreme fatigue and flu-like symptoms.

Prognosis

The prognosis of carcinoid tumor patients is generally good, with an overall survival of 82 percent.[132,601] Histopathologically determined "typical" carcinoids grow slowly. Data on survival of patients with small tumor size without spread, treated by surgical removal, reveals a complete cure of patients. A 20-year retrospective study with 150 patients with GI tract carcinoid tumors indicated that surgically treated patients with carcinoid tumors have overall 83 percent 5-year survival rate.[615] However, the 5-year survival appears to be directly related to the size and the location of the tumor at the time of surgery. Five-year survival is greater than 95 percent if the tumor that is found is less than 2 cm in size, but drops to 64 percent if an ileal or jejunal tumor greater than 2 cm is found at time of surgery and is accompanied by regional lymph node involvement. The 5-year survival is only 18 percent if a distant metastasis (especially to the liver) is found at the time of surgery. The overall 5-year survival is excellent for carcinoids of the appendix (86 percent) and rectum (72 percent), while small intestinal (55 percent), gastric (49 percent) and colonic carcinoids (42 percent) exhibit a poor prognosis.[616] A sharp increase in the natural course of the carcinoid syndrome symptom complex occurs during the 7-year period from the first appearance of sustained symptoms (diarrhea and flushing) to death. Mean survival time from the occurrence of the initial flushing episode has been estimated to be 38 months, with approximately 25 percent of patients living longer than 6 years.[617] In the early decades, when effective treatment was unavailable, the average survival from the onset of flushing in patients with carcinoid syndrome was 3 years and, from the onset of diagnosis, 2 years. Now, with the advent of new drugs (especially octreotide acetate), the range has extended to more than 10 years. Most of the patients (about 75 percent) would die due to the harmful effects of excessive hormones released by the tumors. In the last decades, the survival time has increased to 5 years or more because of the effective combinations of treatment including octreotide, chemotherapy, surgery, and biological response mediators.

Acknowledgment

The authors wish to recognize Jan Redfern, Ph.D., for both creative and constructive contributions toward this manuscript.

REFERENCES

1. Bayliss WM, Starling EH: The mechanism of pancreatic secretion. *J Physiol* (*Lond*) 28:325, 1902.
2. Walsh JH: Gastrointestinal peptide hormones, in Sleisenger MH, Fordtran JS (eds): *Gastrointestinal Disease: Pathophysiology, Diagnosis, Management,* 4th ed. Philadelphia, Saunders and Harcourt Brace Jovanovich, 1989, pp 78–107.

3. Sundler F, Bottcher E, Ekblad E, Hakanson R: The neuroendocrine system of the gut. *Acta Oncol* 28:303, 1989.
4. Green DW, Gomez G, Greeley GH Jr: Gastrointestinal peptides. *Gastroenterol Clin North Am* 18:695, 1989.
5. O'Dorisio TM, Redfern JS: Somatostatin and somatostatin-like peptides: Clinical research and clinical applications, in Mazzaferri EL (ed): *Advances in Endocrinology and Metabolism,* vol 1. Chicago, Mosby Year Book, 1990, pp 175–230.
6. Bloom SR: Clinical syndromes of gut hormones, in Thompson JC, Cooper CW, Rayford PL, Greeley GH Jr, Singh P, Townsend CM Jr (eds): *Gastrointestinal Endocrinology: Receptors and Post-Receptor Mechanisms.* San Diego, Academic Press, 1990, pp 479–490.
7. Wilander E, Lundqvist M, Oberg K: Gastrointestinal carcinoid tumors: Histogenic, histochemical, immunohistochemical, clinical and therapeutic aspects. *Prog Histochem Cytochem* 19:S1, 1989.
8. Vinik Al, McLeod MK, Fig LM, Shapiro B, et al: Clinical features, diagnosis, and localization of carconoid tumors and their management. *Gastroenterol Clin North Am* 18:865, 1989.
9. Kowlessar OD: The carcinoid syndrome, in Sleisenger MH, Fordtran JS (eds): *Gastrointestinal Disease: Pathophysiology, Diagnosis, Management,* 4th ed. Philadelphia, Saunders. 1989, pp 1560–1570.
10. Godwin JD II: Carcinoid tumors: An analysis of 2837 cases. *Cancer* 36:560, 1975.
11. Beaton HL: Carcinoid tumors of the alimentary tract. *CA* 32:92, 1982.
12. Strodel WE, Vinik AI, Thompson NW, Eckhauser FE, Talpos GB: Small bowel carcinoid tumors and the carcinoid syndrome, in Thompson NW, Vinik AI (eds): *Endocrine Surgery Update.* New York, Grune & Stratton, 1983, pp 277–291.
13. Go VLW, Koch TR: Distribution of gut peptides, in Schultz SG, Makhlouf GM (eds): *Handbook of Physiology: The Gastrointestinal System II.* Bethesda, MD, American Physiological Society, 1989, pp 111–122.
14. Makhlouf GM, Grider JR, Schubert ML: Identification of physiological function of gut peptides, in Schultz SG, Makhlouf GM (eds): *Handbook of Physiology: The Gastrointestinal System II.* Bethesda, MD, American Physiological Society, 1989, pp 123–131.
15. Polak JM: Endocrine cells of the gut, in Schultz SG, Makhlouf GM (eds): *Handbook of Physiology: The Gastrointestinal System II.* Bethesda, MD, American Physiological Society, 1989, pp 79–96.
16. Solcia E, Capella C, Buffa R, Usellini L, et al: Endocrine cells of the digestive system, in Johnson LR (ed): *Physiology of the Gastrointestinal Tract.* New York, Raven Press, 1981, pp 39–58.
17. Solcia E, Capella C, Fiocca R, Cornaggia M, Bosi F: The gastroenteropancreatic endocrine system and related tumors. *Gastroenterol Clin North Am* 18:671, 1989.
18. Sjölund K, Sandén G, Håkanson R, Sundler F: Endocrine cells in human intestine: An immunocytochemical study. *Gastroenterology* 85:1120, 1983.
19. Pearse AGE: The APUD concept and hormone production. *Clin Endocrinol Metab* 9:211, 1980.
20. Pearse AGE: Common cytochemical properties of cells producing polypeptide hormones, with particular reference to calcitonin and the thyroid C-cells. *Vet Rec* 79:587, 1966.
21. Le Douarin N: A biological cell labeling technique and its use in experimental embryology. *Dev Biol* 30:217, 1973.
22. Andrew A: Further evidence that enterochromaffin cells are not derived from the neural crest. *J Embryol Exp Morphol* 31:589, 1974.
23. Like AA, Orci L: Embryogenesis of the human pancreatic islets: A light and electron microscopic study. *Diabetes* 21(Suppl 2):511, 1972.
24. Baldissera FG, Holst JJ, Jensen SL, Krarup T: Distribution and molecular forms of peptides containing somatostain immunodeterminants in extracts from the entire gastrointestinal tract of man and pig. *Biochim Biophys Acta* 838:132, 1985.
25. Polak JM, Pearse AGE, Grimelius L, Bloom SR, Arimura A: Growth-hormone release-inhibiting hormone in gastrointestinal and pancreatic D cells. *Lancet* 1:1220, 1975.
26. Yamada T, Chiba T: Somatostatin, in Schultz SG, Makhlouf G (eds): *Handbook of Physiology: The Gastrointestinal System II.* Bethesda, MD, American Physiology Association, 1989, pp 431–453.
27. Ipp E, Rivier J, Dobbs RE, Brown M, et al: Somatostatin analogs inhibit somatostatin release. *Endocrinology* 104: 1270, 1979.
28. Sagar SM, Martin JB: Hypothalamohypophysiotropic peptide system, in Bloom FE (ed): *Handbook of Physiology: The Nervous System IV.* Bethesda, MD, American Physiological Society, 1986, pp 413–462.
29. Brazeau P, Vale W, Burgus R, Ling N, et al: Hypothalamic polypeptide that inhibits the secretion of immunoreactive pituitary growth hormone. *Science* 179:77, 1973.
30. Arimura A, Sato H, Dupont A, Nishi N, Schally AV: Somatostatin: Abundance of immunoreactive hormone in rat stomach and pancreas. *Science* 189:1007, 1975.
31. Dubois MP: Presence of immunoreactive somatostatin in discrete cells of the endocrine pancreas. *Proc Natl Acad Sci USA* 72:1340, 1975.
32. Hokfelt T, Efendic S, Hellerstrom C, Johansson O, et al: Cellular localization of somatostatin in endocrine-like cells and neurons of the rat with special reference to the A1-cells of the pancreatic islets and to the hypothalamus. *Acta Endocrinol Suppl* 1, 1975.
33. Blasi A, Mangiameli A: The role of gastrointestinal hormones in the control of gastric secretory and motor functions, in Cheli R (ed): *Gastric Secretion.* New York, Raven Press, 1986, pp 41–47.
34. Brazeau P, Vale W, Burgus R, Ling N, et al: Hypothalamic polypeptide that inhibits the secretion of immunoreactive pituitary growth hormone. *Science* 179:77, 1973.
35. Pradayrol L, Jörnvall H, Mutt V, Ribet A: N-terminally extended somatostatin: The primary structure of somatostatin-28. *FEBS Lett* 109:55, 1980.
36. Shen LU, Pictet RL, Rutter WJ: Human somatostatin: I. Sequence of the cDNA. *Proc Natl Acad Sci USA* 79:4575, 1982.
37. Keast JR, Furness JB, Costa M: Somatostatin in human enteric nerves: Distribution and characterization. *Cell Tissue Res* 237:299, 1984.
38. Penman E, Wass JAH, Butler MG, Penny ES, et al: Distribution and characterization of immunoreactive somatostatin in human gastrointestinal tract. *Regul Pept* 7:53, 1983.
39. Kronheim S, Berelowitz M, Pimstone BL: The characterization of somatostatin-like immunoreactivity in human serum. *Diabetes* 27: 523, 1978.
40. Baldissera FG, Munoz-Perez MA, Holst JJ: Somatostatin 1-28 circulates in human plasma. *Regul Pept* 6:63, 1983.
41. Conlon JM, Srikant CB, Ipp E, Schusdziarra V, et al: Properties of endogenous somatostatin-like immunoreactivity and synthetic somatostatin in dog plasma. *J Clin Invest* 62:1187, 1978.
42. Inui T, Kinoshita Y, Yamaguchi A, Yamatani T, Chiba T: Linkage between capsaicin-stimulated calcitonin gene related peptide and somatostatin release in rat stomach. *Am J Physiol* 261:G770, 1991.
43. Kwok YN, Mcintosh CHS, Pederson RA, Brown JC: Effect of substance P on somatostatin release from the isolated perfused rat stomach. *Gastroenterol* 88:90, 1985.
44. Holst JJ, Skak-Nielsen T, Orskov C, Seier-Poulsen S: Vagal control of the release of somatostatin, vasoactive intestinal polypeptide, gastrin-releasing peptide and HCI from porcine non-antral stomach. *Scand J Gastroenterol* 27:677, 1992.
45. Schubert ML, Saffouri B, Makhlouf GM: Identical patterns of somatostatin secretion from isolated antrum and fundus of rat stomach. *Am J Physiol* 254:G20, 1988.
46. Olesen M, Holst JJ, Sottimano C, Nielsen OV: Autonomic nervous control of fundic secretion of somatostatin and antral secretion of gastrin and somatostatin in pigs. *Digestion* 36:24, 1987.
47. McIntosh CHS, Pederson RA, Mueller MK, Brown JC: Autonomic nervous control of gastric somatostatin secretion from the perfused rat stomach. *Life Sciences* 29:1477, 1981.
48. Beylot M, Chayvialle JA, Riou JP, Souquet JC, et al: Regulation of somatostatin secretion in man: Study of the role of free fatty acids and ketone bodies. *Metabolism* 33:988, 1984.
49. Penman E, Wass JAH, Medbak S, Morgan L, et al: Response of circulating immunoreactive somatostain to nutritional stimuli in normal subjects. *Gastroenterology* 81:692, 1981.
50. Weigert N, Schaffer K, Wegner U, Schusdiziarra V, et al: Functional characterization of a muscarinic receptor stimulating gastrin release from rabbit antral G cells in primary culture. *Eur J Pharmacol* 264:337, 1994.
51. Buchan AMJ, Macleod MD, Meloche RM, Kwok YN: Muscarinic regulation of somatostatin from primary cultures of human antral epithelial cells. *Pharmacology* 44:33, 1992.
52. Park J, Takeda H, DelValle J, Yamada T: Differential response of D-cells from the canine gastric antrum and fundus to stimulants of somatostatin release. *Gastroenterology* 106:A831 (Abstract), 1994.

53. Holst JJ, Jorgensen PN, Rasmussen TN, Schmidt P: Somatostatin restraint of gastrin secretion in pigs revealed by monoclonal antibody immunoneutralization. *Am J Physiol* 263:G908, 1992.
54. Kajimura M, Reuben MA, Sachs G: The muscarinic receptor gene expressed in rabbit parietal cells is the m3 subtype. *Gastroenterology* 103:870, 1992.
55. Patel YC, Srikant CB: Somatostatin mediation of adenohypophysial secretion. *Annu Rev Physiol* 48:551, 1986.
56. Arimura A, Fishback JB: Somatostatin: Regulation of secretion. *Neuroendocrinology* 33:246, 1981.
57. Delitala G, Tomasi P, Virdis R: Neuroendocrine regulation of human growth hormone secretion: Diagnostic and clinical applications. *J Endocrinol Invest* 11:441, 1988.
58. Reichlin S: Somatostatin: I. *N Engl J Med* 309:1495, 1983.
59. Reichlin S: Somatostain: II. *N Engl J Med* 309:1556, 1983.
60. Hoyer D, Bell GI, Berelowitz M, Epelbaum J, et al: Classification and nomenclature of somatostain receptors. *Trends Pharmacol Sci* 16:86, 1995.
61. Hoyer D, Lubbert H, Bruns C: Molecular pharmacology of somatostain receptors. *Naunyn Schmiedebergs Arch Pharmacol* 350: 441, 1994.
62. Colturi TJ, Unger RH, Feldman M: Role of circulating somatostatin in regulation of gastric acid secretion, gastrin release, and islet cell function: Studies in healthy subjects and duodenal ulcer patients. *J Clin Invest* 74:417, 1984.
63. Konturek SJ, Tasler J, Cieszkowski M, Coy DH, Schally AV: Effect of growth hormone release-inhibiting hormone on gastric secretion, mucosal blood flow, and serum gastrin. *Gastroenterology* 70:737, 1976.
64. Szabo S, Usadel KH: Cytoprotection-organoprotection by somatostatin: Gastric and hepatic lesions. *Experientia* 38:254, 1982.
65. Palitzsch KD, Schuler H, Schwedes U, Usadel KH: Protection against duodenal ulceration by somatostatins. *Klin Wochenschr* 64(Suppl 7): 93, 1986.
66. Hirst B, Conlon J, Coy D, Holland J, Shaw B: Comparison of the gastric exocrine inhibitory activities and plasma kinetics of somatostatin-28 and somatostatin-14 in cats. *Regul Peptides* 4:227, 1982.
67. Konturek S, Kwiecien N, Obtulowicz W, Bielanski W, et al: Effects of somatostatin-14 and somatostatin-28 on plasma hormonal and gastric secretory responses to cephalic and gastrointestinal stimulation in man. *Scand J Gastroenterol* 20, 31, 1985.
68. Seal A, Yamada T, Debas H, Hollinshead J, et al: Somatostatin-14 and -28 clearance and potency on gastric function in dogs. *Am J Physiol* 243:G97, 1982.
69. Lucey MR: Endogenous somatostatin and the gut. *Gut* 27:457, 1986.
70. Dueno MI, Bai JC, Santangelo WC, Krejs GJ: Effect of somatostatin analog on water and electrolyte transport and transit time in human small bowel. *Dig Dis Sci* 32:1092, 1987.
71. Carter RF, Bitar KN, Zfass AM, Makhlouf GM: Inhibition of VIP-stimulated intestinal secretion and cyclic AMP production by somatostatin in the rat. *Gastroenterology* 74:726, 1978.
72. Krejs GJ: Effect of somatostatin infusion on VIP-induced transport changes in the human jejunum. *Peptides* 5:271, 1984.
73. Dharmsathaphorn K, Sherwin RS, Dobbins JW: Somatostatin inhibits fluid secretion in the rat jejunum. *Gastroenterology* 78:1554, 1980.
74. Ormsbee HS, Koehler SL, Telford GL: Somatostatin inhibits motilin-induced interdigestive contractile activity in the dog. *Dig Dis* 23:781, 1978.
75. Poitras P, Steinbach JH, Van Deventer G, Code CF, Walsh JH: Motilin independent ectopic fronts of the interdigestive myoelectric complex in dogs. *Am J Physiol* 239:G215, 1980.
76. Vaysse N, Chayvialle J, Pradayrol L, Esteve J, et al: Somatostatin 28: Comparison with somatostatin 14 for plasma kinetics and low-dose effects on the exocrine pancreas in dogs. *Gastroenterology* 81:700, 1981.
77. Walsh JH: Gastrointestinal hormones, in Johnson LR (ed): *Physiology of the Gastrointestinal Tract*, 2nd ed. New York, Raven Press, 1987, pp 181–253.
78. Solomon TE: Control of exocrine pancreatic secretion, in Johnson LR (ed): *Physiology of the Gastrointestinal Tract*, 2nd ed. New York, Raven Press, 1987, pp 1173–1207.
79. Moreau JP, DeFeudis FV: Pharmacological studies of somatostatin and somatostatin-analogues: Therapeutic advances and perspectives. *Life Sci* 40:419, 1987.
80. Koerker DJ, Ruch W, Chideckel E, Palmer J, et al: Somatostatin: Hypothalamic inhibitor of the endocrine pancreas. *Science* 184:482, 1974.
81. Unger RH, Dobbs RE, Orci L: Insulin, glucagon, and somatostatin secretion in the regulation of metabolism. *Annu Rev Physiol* 40:307, 1978.
82. Morisset J, Genik P, Lord A, Solomon T: Effects of chronic administration of somatostatin on rat exocrine pancreas. *Reg Peptides* 4:49, 1982.
83. Reichlin S: Somatostatin: Historical aspects. *Scand J Gastroenterol* 21:1, 1986.
84. Prinz C, Sachs G, Walsh J, Wu V: The somatostatin receptor subtype in rat enterochromaffin-like cells. *Gastroenterology* 107:1067, 1994.
85. Zaki M, Harrington L, McCuen R, Coy DH, et al: Somatostatin receptor subtype 2 mediates inhibition of gastrin and histamine secretion from human, dog, and rat antrum. *Gastroenterology* 111:919, 1996.
86. Feher E, Fodor M, Burnstock G: Distribution of somatostatin-immunoreactive nerve fibers in Peyer's patches. *Gut* 33:1195, 1992.
87. Stanisz AM, Befus D, Bienenstock J: Differential effects of vasoactive intestinal peptide, substance P, and somatostatin on immunoglobulin synthesis and proliferations by lymphocytes from Peyer's patches, mesenteric lymph nodes, and spleen. *J Immunol* 136:152, 1986.
88. Larsson LI, Hirsch MA, Holst JJ, Ingemansson S, et al: Pancreatic somatostatinoma: Clinical features and physiological implications. *Lancet* 1:666, 1977.
89. Ganda OP, Weir GC, Soeldner JS, Legg MA, et al: "Somatostatinoma": A somatostatin-containing tumor of the endocrine pancreas. *N Engl J Med* 296:963, 1977.
90. Krejs GJ, Orci L, Conlon JM, Ravazzola M, et al: Somatostatinoma syndrome: Biochemical, morphologic and clinical features. *N Engl J Med* 301:285, 1979.
91. O'Dorisio TM, O'Dorisio MS: Endocrine tumors of the gastroenteropancreatic (GEP) axis, in Mazzaferri EL (ed): *Textbook of Endocrinology*, 3rd ed. New York, Elsevier, 1986, pp 764–817.
92. O'Dorisio TM, Vinik AI: Pancreatic polypeptide and mixed hormone producing tumors of the gastrointestinal tract, in Cohen S, Soloway RD (eds): *Contemporary Issues in Gastroenterology*. Edinburgh, Churchill-Livingstone, 1984, pp 117–128.
93. Kelly TR: Pancreatic somatostatinoma. *Am J Surg* 146:671, 1983.
94. Chayvialle JAP, Descos F, Bernard C, Martin A, Barbe C, Partensky C: Somatostatin in mucosa of stomach and duodenum in gastroduodenal disease. *Gastroenterology* 75:13, 1978.
95. Sumii K, Fukushima T, Hirata K, Matsumoto Y, et al: Antral gastrin and somatostatin concentrations in peptic ulcer patients. *Peptides* 2(Suppl 2):281, 1981.
96. Grant MB, Mames RN, Fitzgerald KM et al: The efficacy of octreotide in the therapy of severe nonproliferative and early proliferative diabetic retinopathy. *Diabetes Care* 23:504, 2000.
97. Harris AG: Future medical prospects for Sandostatin. *Z Gastroenterol* 28(Suppl 2):55, 1990.
98. Battershill PE, Clissold SP: Octreotide. A review of its pharmacodynamic and pharmacokinetic properties, and therapeutic potential in conditions associated with excessive peptide secretion. *Drugs* 38:658, 1989.
99. Cook DJ, Kelton JG, Stanisz AM, et al: Somatostatin treatment for cryptosporidial diarrhea in a patient with the acquired immunodeficiency syndrome (AIDS). *Ann Intern Med* 108:708, 1988.
100. Dunne MJ, Elton R, Fletcher T, et al: Sandostatin and gastroenteropancreatic endocrine tumors-therapeutic characteristics, in O'Dorisio TM (ed): *Sandostatin in the Treatment of Gastroenteropancreatic Endocrine Tumors*. New York, Springer-Verlag, 1987, pp 93–114.
101. Katz MD, Erstad BL, Rose C: Treatment of severe cryptosporidium-related diarrhea with octreotide in a patient with AIDS. *Drug Intell Clin Pharm* 22:134, 1988.
102. Kvols LK: Therapy of the malignant carcinoid syndrome and metastatic islet cell carcinoma, in O'Dorisio TM (ed): *Sandostatin in the Treatment of Gastroenteropancreatic Endocrine Tumors*. New York, Springer-Verlag, 1987, pp 65–82.
103. Robinson ENJ, Fogel R: SMS 201-995, a somatostatin analogue, and diarrhea in the acquired immunodeficiency syndrome (AIDS). *Ann Intern Med* 109:680, 1988.

104. Hopman WPM, Wolberink RGJ, Lamers CBHW, van Tongeren JHM: Treatment of the dumping syndrome with the somatostatin analogue SMS 201-995. *Ann Surg* 207:155, 1988.
105. Primrose JN, Johnston D: Somatostatin analogue SMS 201-995 (octreotide) as a possible solution to the dumping syndrome after gastrectomy or vagotomy. *Br J Surg* 76:140, 1989.
106. Woltering E, O'Dorisio T, Williams S, et al: Treatment of nonendocrine gastrointestinal disorders with octreotide acetate. *Metabolism* 39:176, 1990.
107. Patel YC, Wheatley T: In vivo and in vitro plasma disappearance and metabolism of somatostatin-28 and somatostatin-14 in the rat. *Endocrinology* 112:220, 1983.
108. Polonsky K, Jaspan J, Berelowitz M, Pugh W, et al: The in vivo metabolism of somatostatin-28; Possible relationship between diminished metabolism and enhanced biological action. *Endocrinology* 111:1698, 1982.
109. Seal A, Yamada T, Debas HT, Debas H, et al: Somatostatin-14 and -28: Clearance and potency on gastric function in dogs. *Am J Physiol* 243:G97, 1982.
110. Battershill PE, Clissold SP: Octreotide: A review of its pharmacodynamic and pharmacokinetic properties, and therapeutic potential in conditions associated with excessive peptide secretion. *Drugs* 38:658, 1989.
111. Katz MD, Erstad BL: Octreotide, a new somatostatin analogue. *Clin Pharmacol* 8:255, 1989.
112. Daughaday WH: The anterior pituitary, in Wilson JD, Foster DW (eds): *Williams Textbook of Endocrinology*. Philadelphia, Saunders, 1985, pp 568–613.
113. Lamberts SWJ, Uitterlinden P, Del Pozo E: SMS 201-995 induces a continuous decline in circulating growth hormone and somatomedin-C levels during therapy of acromegalic patients for over two years. *J Clin Endocrinol Metab* 65:703, 1987.
114. Hopman WPM, Wolberink RGJ, Lamers CBHW, Van Tongeren JHM: Treatment of the dumping syndrome with the somatostatin analogue SMS 201 995. *Ann Surg* 207:155, 1982.
115. Primrose JN, Johnston D: Somatostatin analogue SMS 201-995 (octreotide) as a possible solution to the dumping syndrome after gastrectomy or vagotomy. *Br J Surg* 76:140, 1989.
116. Woltering E, O'Dorisio T, Williams ST, Lebrado L, Fletcher WS: Treatment of nonendocrine gastrointestinal disorders with octreotide acetate. *Metabolism* 39:176, 1990.
117. Thrilby RC: Somatostatin and postgastrectomy dumping. *Gastroenterology* 97:1344, 1989.
118. Richards WO, Geer R, O'Dorisio TM, Robarts T, et al: Octreotide acetate induces fasting small bowel motility in patients with dumping syndrome. *J Surg Res* 49:483, 1990.
119. Geer RJ, Richards WO, O'Dorisio TM, Woltering EO, et al: Efficacy of octreotide acetate in treatment of severe postgastrectomy dumping syndrome. *Ann Surg* 212:678, 1990.
120. Burroughs AK, McCormick PA: Somatostatin and octreotide in gastroenterology. *Aliment Pharmacol Ther* 5:331, 1991.
121. Grosman I, Simon D: Potential gastrointestinal uses of somatostatin and its synthetic analogue octreotide. *Am J Gastroenterol* 85:1061, 1990.
122. Cook DJ, Kelton JG, Stanisz AM, Collins SM: Somatostatin treatment for cryptosporidial diarrhea in a patient with the acquired immunodeficiency syndrome (AIDS). *Ann Intern Med* 108:708, 1988.
123. Robinson EN Jr, Fogel R: SMS 201-995, a somatostatin analogue, and diarrhea in the acquired immunodeficiency syndrome (AIDS). *Ann Intern Med* 109:680, 1988.
124. Katz MD, Erstad BL, Rose C: Treatment of severe cryptosporidium-related diarrhea with octreotide in a patient with AIDS. *Drug Intell Clin Pharm* 22:134, 1988.
125. Kvols LK: Therapy of the malignant carcinoid syndrome and metastatic islet cell carcinoma, in O'Dorisio TM (ed): *Sandostatin in the Treatment of Gastroenteropancreatic Endocrine Tumors*. New York, Springer-Verlag, 1989, pp 65–82.
126. Maton PN, O'Dorisio TM, O'Dorisio MS, Malarkey WB, et al: Successful therapy of pancreatic cholera with the long-acting somatostatin analogue SMS 201-995: Relation between plasma concentrations of drug and clinical and biochemical responses. *Scand J Gastroenterol* 21(Suppl 119):181, 1986.
127. Dunne MJ, Elton R, Fletcher T, Hofker P, Shui J: Sandostatin and gastroenteropancreatic endocrine tumors: Therapeutic characteristics, in O'Dorisio TM (ed): *Sandostatin in the Treatment of Gastroenteropancreatic Endocrine Tumors*. New York, Springer-Verlag, 1987, pp 93–114.
128. Smith SS, Shulman DI, O'Dorisio TM, McClenathan DT, et al: Watery diarrhea, hypokalemia, achlorhydria syndrome in an infant: Effect of the long-acting somatostatin analogue SMS 201-995 on the disease and linear growth. *J Pediatr Gastroenterol Nutr* 6:710, 1987.
129. Jaros W, Biller J, Greer S, O'Dorisio TM, Grand R: Successful treatment of idiopathic secretory diarrhea of infancy with the somatostatin analogue SMS 201-995. *Gastroenterology* 94:189, 1988.
130. Woltering EA, Barrie R, O'Dorisio TM, Arce D, et al: Somatostatin analogues inhibit angiogenesis in the chick chorioallantoic membrane. *J Surg Res* 50:245, 1991.
131. Kvols LK, Moertel CG, O'Connell MJ, Schutt AJ, et al: Treatment of the malignant carcinoid syndrome: Evaluation of a long-acting somatostatin analogue. *N Eng J Med* 315:663, 1986.
132. Vinik A, Moattari AR: Use of somatostatin analog in management of carcinoid syndrome. *Dig Dis Sci* 34:14S, 1989.
133. Maton PN, O'Dorisio TM, Howe BA, McArthur KE, et al: Effect of a long-acting somatostatin analogue (SMS 201-995) in a patient with pancreatic cholera. *N Eng J Med* 312:17, 1985.
134. Santangelo WC, O'Dorisio TM, Kim JG, Severino G, Krejs GJ: Pancreatic cholera syndrome: Effect of a synthetic somatostatin analog on intestinal water and ion transport. *Ann Intern Med* 103:363, 1985.
135. Kraenzlin ME, Ch'ng JLC, Wood SM, Carr DH, Bloom SR: Long-term treatment of a VIPoma with somatostatin analogue resulting in remission of symptoms and possible shrinkage of metastases. *Gastroenterology* 88:185, 1985.
136. Wood SM, Kraenzlin ME, Adrian TE, Bloom SR: Treatment of patients with pancreatic endocrine tumors using a new long-acting somatostatin analogue: Symptomatic and peptide responses. *Gut* 26: 438, 1985.
137. Ch'ng JLC, Anderson JV, Williams SJ, Carr DH, Bloom SR: Remission of symptoms during long term treatment of metastatic pancreatic endocrine tumours with long acting somatostatin analogue. *Br Med J* 292:981, 1986.
138. Oberg K, Jakobsson A, Gustafsson G, Willander E, et al: WDHA syndrome caused by a ganglioneuroblastoma producing vasoactive intestinal polypeptide and neuropeptide Y: Treatment with SMS 201-995, a somatostatin analogue. *Scand J Gastroenterol* 21(Suppl 119): 228, 1986.
139. Edwards CA, Cann PA, Read NW, Holdsworth CD: The effect of somatostatin analogue SMS 201-995 on fluid and electrolyte transport in a patient with secretory diarrhoea. *Scand J Gastroenterol* 21(Suppl 119):259, 1986.
140. Anderson JV, Bloom SR: Neuroendocrine tumours of the gut: Long-term therapy with the somatostatin analogue SMS 201-995. *Scand J Gastroenterol* 21(Suppl 119):115, 1986.
141. Kvols LK, Buck M, Moertel CG, Schutt AJ, et al: Treatment of metastatic islet cell carcinoma with a somatostatin analogue (SMS 201-995). *Ann Intern Med* 107:162, 1987.
142. Rene E, Regnier B, Laine MJ, Bonfils S: Somatostatin and cryptosporidial diarrhea during AIDS. *Can J Physiol Pharmacol* 64:70, 1986.
143. Redfern JS, Mekhjian HS, O'Dorisio TM: Use of somatostatin-like peptides in the treatment of diarrhea, in Lebenthal E, Duffey M (eds): *Textbook of Secretory Diarrhea*. New York, Raven Press, 1990, pp 421–428.
144. Edkins JS: On the chemical mechanism of gastric secretion. *Proc R Soc Lond (Biol)* 76:376, 1905.
145. Gregory PA, Tracy HJ: The preparation and properties of gastrin. *J Physiol (Lond)* 156:523, 1961.
146. Gregory PA, Tracy HJ: The constitution and properties of two gastrins extracted from hog antral mucosa. Gut 5:103, 1964.
147. Gregory RA: A review of some recent developments in the chemistry of the gastrins. *Bioorg Chem* 8:497, 1979.
148. O'Dorisio TM: Gastrointestinal hormones, in Mazzaferri EL (ed): *Endocrinology: A Clinical Review of Endocrinology*, 2nd ed. Flushing, NY, Medical Examination Publishing Co, 1980, pp 772–807.
149. Dockray GJ, Gregory RA: Gastrin, in Schultz SG, Makhlouf GM (eds): *Handbook of Physiology: The Gastrointestinal System II*. Bethesda, MD, American Physiological Society, 1989, pp 311–336.
150. Walsh JH: Gastrointestinal hormones and peptides, in Johnson LR (ed): *Physiology of the Gastrointestinal Tract*. New York, Raven Press, 1981, pp 59–144.

151. Boel E, Vuust J, Norris F, Norris K, et al: Molecular cloning of human gastrin cDNA: Evidence for evolution of gastrin by gene duplication. *Proc Natl Acad Sci USA* 80:2866, 1983.
152. Sundler F, Hakanson R: Gastric endocrine cell typing at the light microscopic level, in Hakanson R, Sundler F (eds): *The Stomach as an Endocrine Organ*. Amsterdam, Elsevier, 1991, pp 9–26.
153. Larsson LI: ACTH-like immunoreactivity in the gastrin cell. Independent changes in gastrin and ACTH-like immunoreactivity during ontogeny. *Histochemistry* 56:245, 1978.
154. Tsuruo Y, Hokfelt T, Visser TJ, Kimmel JR, et al: TRH-like immunoreactivity in endocrine cells and neurons in the gastrointestinal tract of the rat and guinea pig. *Cell Tissue Res* 253:347, 1988.
155. Lamers C, Walsh J, Jansen J, Harrison A, et al: Evidence that gastrin 34 is preferentially released from the human duodenum. *Gastroenterology* 83:233, 1982.
156. Walsh JH, Isenberg JI, Arnfield J, Maxwell V: Clearance and acid-stimulating action of human big and little gastrin in duodenal ulcer subjects. *J Clin Invest* 57:1125, 1976.
157. Elwin CE: Gastric acids responses to antral application of some amino acids, peptides, and isolated fractions of a protein hydrolysate. *Scand J Gastroenterol* 9:239, 1974.
158. Taylor I, Byrne W, Christie D, Ament M, Walsh J: Effect of individual L-amino acids on gastric acid secretion and serum gastrin and pancreatic polypeptide release in humans. *Gastroenterology* 83:273, 1982.
159. Walsh J, Grossman M: Medical progress; Gastrin. *N Engl J Med* 292:1324, 1975.
160. Walsh J, Richardson C, Fordtran J: pH dependence of acid secretion and gastrin release in normal and ulcer patients. *J Clin Invest* 55:462, 1975.
161. Stadil F, Rehfeld J: Release of gastrin by epinephrine in man. *Gastroenterology* 65:210, 1973.
162. Csendes A, Walsh J, Grossman M: Effects of atropine and of antral acidification of gastrin release and acid secretion in response to insulin and feeding in dogs. *Gastroenterology* 63:257, 1972.
163. Nilsson G, Simon J, Yalow R, Berson S: Plasma gastrin and gastric acid responses to sham feeding and feeding in dogs. *Gastroenterology* 63:51, 1972.
164. Raptis S, Dollinger HC, Berger L, Schlegel W, et al: Effects of somatostatin on gastric secretion and gastrin release in man. *Digestion* 13:15, 1975.
165. Mulholland MW, Debas HT: Physiology and pathophysiology of gastrin: Review. *Surgery* 103:135, 1988.
166. Feldman M, Walsh JH, Wong HC, Richardson CT: Role of gastrin heptadecapeptide in the acid secretory response to amino acids in man. *J Clin Invest* 61:308, 1978.
167. McGuigan J, Isaza J, Landor J: Relationships of gastrin dose, serum gastrin, and acid secretion. *Gastroenterology* 61:659, 1971.
168. Carter D, Taylor I, Elashoff J, Grossman M: Reappraisal of the secretory potency and disappearance rate of pure human minigastrin. *Gut* 20:705, 1979.
169. Eysselein V, Maxwell V, Reedy T, Wunsch E, Walsh J: Similar acid stimulatory potencies of synthetic human big and little gastrins in man. *J Clin Invest* 73:1284, 1984.
170. Johnson LR: The trophic action of gastrointestinal hormones. *Gastroenterology* 70:278, 1976.
171. Johnson LR: Regulation of gastrointestinal growth, in Johnson LR (ed): *Physiology of the Gastrointestinal Tract*. New York, Raven Press, 1981, pp 169–196.
172. Soll A: Potentiating interactions of gastric stimulants on [^{14}C] aminopyrine accumulation by isolated canine parietal cells. *Gastroenterology* 83:216, 1982.
173. Soll A, Walsh J: Regulation of gastric acid secretion. *Ann Rev Physiol* 41:35, 1979.
174. Ekman L, Hansson E, Havu N, Carlsson E, Lundberg C: Toxicological studies on omeprazole. *Scand J Gastroenterol* 108:53, 1985.
175. Solcia E, Rindi G, Havu N, Elm G: Qualitative studies of gastric endocrine cells in patients treated long-term with omeprazole. *Scand J Gastroenterol* 166:129, 1989.
176. Winsett OE, Townsend CM Jr, Glass EJ, Thompson JC: Gastrin stimulates growth of colon cancer. *Surgery* 99:302, 1986.
177. Lamote J, Willems G: Stimulating effect of pentagastrin on cancer cell proliferation kinetics in chemically induced colon cancer in rats. *Regul Pept* 20:1, 1988.
178. McGregor DB, Morriss LL, Manalo PB, Bomberger RA, Pardini RS: Pentagastrin stimulation of human colon carcinoma. *Arch Surg* 124:470, 1989.
179. Smith JP, Solomon TE: Effects of gastrin, proglumide, and somatostatin on growth of human colon cancer. *Gastroenterology* 95:1541, 1988.
180. Zollinger RM, Ellison EH: Primary peptide ulcerations of the jejunum associated with islet cell tumors of the pancreas. *Ann Surg* 142:709, 1955.
181. Lewin KJ, Yang K, Ulrich T, Elashoff JD, Walsh JH: Primary gastrin cell hyperplasia: Report of five cases and a review of the literature. *Am J Surg Pathol* 8:821, 1984.
182. Keuppens F, Willems G, De Graef J, Woussen-Colle MC: Antral gastrin cell hyperplasia in patients with peptic ulcer. *Ann Surg* 191:276, 1980.
183. Webster MW, Barnes EL, Stremple JF: Serum gastrin levels in the differential diagnosis of recurrent peptic ulceration due to retained gastric antrum. *Am J Surg* 135:248, 1978.
184. Strickland RG, Bhathal PS, Korman MG, Hansky J: Serum gastrin and the antral mucosa in atrophic gastritis. *Br Med J* 4:451, 1971.
185. McGuigan JE, Trudeau WL: Serum gastrin concentrations in pernicious anemia. *N Engl J Med* 282:358, 1970.
186. Becker HD, Reeder DD, Thompson JC: Effect of truncal vagotomy with pyloroplasty or with antrectomy on food-stimulated gastrin values in patients with duodenal ulcer. *Surgery* 74:580, 1973.
187. Gehling N, Lawson MJ, Alp MH, Rofe SB, Butler RN: Antral gastrin concentrations in duodenal ulcer patients after cimetidine and highly selective vagotomy. *Aust NZ J Surg* 56:793, 1986.
188. Festen HPM, Thijs JC, Lamers CBHW, Jansen JMBJ, et al: Effect of oral omeprazole on serum gastrin and serum pepsinogen I levels. *Gastroenterology* 87:1030, 1984.
189. Dockray GJ, Gregory RA: Gastrin, in Schultz SG, Makhlouf GM (eds): *Handbook of Physiology: The Gastrointestinal System II*. Bethesda, MD, American Physiological Society, 1989, pp 311–336.
190. Walsh JH: Gastrointestinal hormones, in Johnson LR (ed): *Physiology of the Gastrointestinal Tract I*, 2nd ed. New York, Raven Press, 1987, pp 181–254.
191. Norton JA, Doppman JL, Collen MJ, Harmon JW, et al: Prospective study of gastrinoma localization and resection in patients with Zollinger-Ellison syndrome. *Am J Surg* 204:468, 1988.
192. Stabile BE, Morrow DJ, Passaro E Jr: The gastrinoma triangle: Operative implications. *Am J Surg* 147:25, 1984.
193. Erdogan MF, Gullu S, Baskal N, Uysal AR, et al: Omeprazole: Calcitonin stimulation test for the diagnosis follow-up and family screening in medullary thyroid carcinoma. *J Clin Endocrinol Metab* 82:897, 1997
194. Ahlman H, Dahlström A, Grönstad K, Tisell LE, et al: The pentagastrin test in the diagnosis of the carcinoid syndrome: Blockade of gastrointestinal symptoms by ketanserin. *Ann Surg* 201:81, 1985.
195. Rehfeld JF: Cholecystokinin, in Schultz SG, Makhlouf GM (eds): *Handbook of Physiology: The Gastrointestinal System II*. Bethesda, MD, American Physiological Society, 1989, pp 337–358.
196. Buffa R, Solcia E, Go VLW: Immunohistochemical identification of the cholecystokinin cell in the intestinal mucosa. *Gastroenterology* 70:528, 1976.
197. Polak J, Pearse A, Bloom S, Buchan A, et al: Identification of cholecystokinin-secreting cells. *Lancet* 2:1016, 1975.
198. Rehfeld JF, Hansen HF, Larsson LI, Stengaard-Pedersen K, Thorn NA: Gastrin and cholecystokinin in pituitary neurons. *Proc Natl Acad Sci USA* 81:1902, 1984.
199. Bardram L, Hilsted L, Rehfeld JF: Cholecystokinin, gastrin and their precursors in pheochromocytomas. *Acta Endocrinol* (copenh) 120:479, 1989.
200. Rehfeld JF: Immunochemical studies on cholecystokinin II. Distribution and molecular heterogeneity in the central nervous system and small intestine of man and hog. *J Biol Chem* 253:4022, 1978.
201. Crawley JN: Comparative distribution of cholecystokinin and other neuropeptides: Why is this peptide different from all other peptides? *Ann NY Acad Sci* 448:1, 1985.
202. Fallon JH, Seroogy KB: The distribution and some connections of cholecystokinin neurons in the rat brain. *Ann NY Acad Sci* 448:121, 1985.
203. Stevens J: An anatomy of Schizophrenia. *Arch Gen Psych* 29:177, 1973.
204. Larsson LI, Rehfeld JF: Localization and molecular heterogeneity of cholecystokinin in the central and peripheral nervous system. *Brain Res* 165:201, 1979.

205. Furness JB, Costa M, Rokaeus A, Mcdonald TJ, Brooks B: Galanin-immunoreactive neurons in the guinea-pig small intestine: their projections and relationship to other enteric neurons. *Cell Tissue Res* 250:607, 1987.
206. Furness JB, Pompolo S, Murphy R, Giraud A: Projections of neurous with neuromedin U-like immunoreactivity in the small intestine of the guinea pig. *Cell Tissue Res* 257:415, 1989.
207. Liddle RA, Goldfine ID, Rosen MS, Taplitz RA, Williams JA: Cholecystokinin bioactivity in human plasma. Molecular forms, responses to feeding, and relationship to gallbladder contraction. *J Clin Invest* 75:1144, 1985.
208. Kleibeuker JH, Beekhuis H, Jansen JB, Piers DA, Lamers CB: Cholecystokinin is a physiological hormonal mediator of fat-induced inhibition of gastric emptying in man. *Eur J Clin Invest* 18:173, 1988.
209. Watanabe SW, Chey WY, Lee KY, Chang TM: Importance of pancreatic enzyme secretion in response to fat in dog. *Gastroenterology* 86:1293, 1984.
210. Liddle RA, Green GM, Conrad CK, Williams JA: Proteins but not amino acids, carbohydrates, or fats stimulate cholecystokinin secretion in the rat. *Am J Physiol* 251:G243, 1986.
211. Green GM, Lyman RL: Feedback regulation of pancreatic enzyme secretion as a mechanism for trypsin inhibitor-induced hypersecretion in rats. *Proc Soc Exp Biol Med* 140:6, 1972.
212. Liddle RA, Goldfine ID, Williams JA: Bioassay of plasma cholecystokinin in rats: effects of food, trypsin inhibitor, and alcohol. *Gastroenterology* 87:542, 1984.
213. Owyang C, May D, Louie DS: Trypsin suppression of pancreatic enzyme secretion. *Gastroenterology* 91:637, 1986.
214. Liddle RA, Gertz BJ, Kanayama S, Beccaria L, et al: Effects of a novel cholecystokinin (CCK) receptor antagonist, MK-329, on gallbladder contraction and gastric emptying in humans: implications for the physiology of CCK. *J Clin Invest* 84:1220, 1989.
215. Hildebrand P, Beglinger C, Gyr K, Jansen JBMJ, et al: Effects of a cholecystokinin receptor antagonist on intestinal phase of pancreatic and biliary responses in man. *J Clin Invest* 85:640, 1990.
216. Jansen JBMJ, Jebbink MCW, Douglas BR, Lamers CBHW: Effect of loxiglumide (CR-1505) on bombesin- and meal-stimulated plasma cholecystokinin in man. *Eur J Clin Pharmacol* 38:367, 1990.
217. Gomez G, Upp JR Jr, Lluis F, Alexander RW, et al: Regulation of the release of chlecystokinin by bile salts in dogs and humans. *Gastroenterology* 94:1036, 1988.
218. Niederau C, Heintges T, Rovati L, Strohmeyer G: Effects of loxiglumide on gallbladder emptying in healthy volunteers. *Gastroenterology* 97:1331, 1989.
219. Pendleton RG, Bendesky RJ, Schaffer L, Nolan TE, et al: Roles of endogenous cholecystokinin in biliary, pancreatic and gastric function: studies with L-364, 718, a specific cholecystokinin receptor antagonist. *J Pharmacol Exp Ther* 241:110, 1987.
220. Meyer BM, Werth BA, Beglinger C, Hildebrand P, et al: Role of cholecystokinin in regulation of gastrointestinal motor functions. *Lancet* 2:12, 1989.
221. Schjoldager B, Molero X, Miller LJ: Functional and biochemical characterization of the human gallbladder muscularis cholecystokinin receptor. *Gastroenterology* 96:1119, 1989.
222. Schjoldager B, Shaw MJ, Powers SP, Schmalz PF, et al: Bovine gallbladder muscularis: Source of a myogenic receptor for cholecystokinin. *Am J Physiol* 254:G294, 1988.
223. Douglas BR, Jebbink MC, Tjon a Tham RT, Jansen JB, Lamers CB: The effect of loxiglumide (CR-1505) on basal and bombesin-stimulated gallbladder volume in man. *Eur J Pharm* 166:307, 1989.
224. Sarles JC, Bidart JM, Devaux MA, Echinard C, Castagnini A: Action of cholecystokinin and caerulein on the rabbit sphincter of Oddi. *Digestion* 14:415, 1976.
225. Toouli J, Watts JM: Actions of cholecystokinin-pancreozymin, secretin, and gastrin on extra-hepatic billiary tract motility in vitro. *Ann Surg* 175:439, 1972.
226. Behar J, Biancani P: Pharmacologic characterization of excitatory and inhibitory cholecystokinin receptors of the cat gallbladder and sphincter of Oddi. *Gastroenterology* 92:764, 1987.
227. Leroy J, Morrisset JA, Webster PD: Dose-related response of pancreatic synthesis and secretion to cholecystokinin-pancreozymin. *J Lab Clin Med* 78:149, 1971.
228. Rothman SS, Wells H: Enhancement of pancreatic enzyme synthesis by pancreozymin. *Am J Physiol* 213:215, 1971.
229. Schick J, Kern H, Scheele G: Hormonal stimulation in the exocrine pancreas results in coordinate and anti-coordinate regulation of protein synthesis. *J Cell Biol* 99:1569, 1984.
230. Debas HT, Grossman MI: Pure cholecystokinin: Pancreatic protein and bicarbonate responses. *Digestion* 9:469, 1978.
231. Henriksen FW, Worming H: The interaction of secretin and pancreozymin on the exocrine pancreatic secretion in dogs. *Acta Physiol Scand* 70:241, 1967.
232. You C, Rominger J, Chey W: Potentiation effect of cholecystokinin-octapeptide on pancreatic bicarbonate secretion stimulated by a physiologic dose of secretin in humans. *Gastroenterology* 85:40, 1983.
233. Calderon P, Furnelle J, Christophe J: Phosphatidylinositol turnover and calcium movement in the rat pancreas. *Am J Physiol* 238:G247, 1980.
234. Maruyama Y, Peterson O, Flanagan P, Pearson G: Quantification of Ca^{2+}-activated K^{+} channels under hormonal control in pig pancreas acinar cells. *Nature* 305:228, 1983.
235. Brants F, Morriset J: Trophic effect of cholecystokinin-pancreozymin on pancreatic acinar cells from rats of different ages. *Proc Soc Exp Biol Med* 153:523, 1976.
236. Folsch UR, Winckler K, Wormsley KG: Influence of repeated administration of cholecystokinin and secretin on the pancreas of the rat. *Scand J Gastroenterol* 13:663, 1978.
237. Niederau C, Liddle RA, Williams JA, Grendell JH: Pancreatic growth: Interaction of exogenous cholecystokinin, a protease inhibitor, and a cholecystokinin receptor antagonist in mice. *Gut* 28:63, 1987.
238. Rosewicz S, Lewis LD, Liddle RA, Logsdon CD: Effects of chlecystokinin on pancreatic ornithine decarboxylase gene expression. *Am J Physiol* 255:G818, 1988.
239. Verspoh EJ, Ammon HPT, Williams JA, Goldfine ID: Evidence that cholecystokinin interacts with specific receptors and regulates insulin release in isolated rat islets of Langerhans. *Diabetes* 35:38, 1986.
240. Otsuki M, Sakamoto C, Maeda M, Yuu H, et al: Effect of caerulein on exocrine and endocrine pancreas in the rat. *Endocrinlogy* 105:1396, 1979.
241. Rushakoff RJ, Goldfine ID, Carter JD, Liddle RA: Physiological concentrations of cholecystokinin stimulate amino acid-induced insulin release in humans. *J Clin Endocrinol Metab* 65:395, 1987.
242. Hermansen K: Effects of cholecystokinin (CCK)-4, nonsulfated CCK-8, and sulfated CCK-8 on pancreatic somatostatin, insulin, and glucagons secretion in the dog: Studies in vitro. *Endocrinology* 114:1770, 1984.
243. Dupre J, Curtis JD, Unger RH, Waddell RW, Beck JC: Effects of secretin, pancreozymin, or gastrin on the response of the endocrine pancreas to administration of glucose or arginine in man. *J Clin Invest* 48:747, 1969.
244. Zawalich WS: Synergistic impact of cholecystokinin and gastric inhibitory polypeptide on the regulation of insulin secretion. *Metabolism* 37:778, 1988.
245. Liddle RA, Gertz BJ, Kanayama S, Beccaria L, et al: Regulation of pancreatic endocrine function by chlecystokinin: Studies with MK-329, a nonpeptide cholecystokinin receptor antagonist. *J Clin Endocrinol Metab* 70:1312, 1990.
246. Hildebrand P, Ensinck JW, Ketterer S, Delco F, et al: Effect of a cholecystokinin antagonist on meal-stimulated insulin and pancreatic polypeptide release in humans. *J Clin Endocrinol Metab* 72:1123, 1991.
247. Beglinger C, Meyer F, Hacki W, Gyr K: The release of pancreatic polypeptide by exogenous CCK in man and dog. *Digestion* 22:225, 1981.
248. Meyer FD, Gyr K, Hacki WH, Beglinger C, et al: The release of pancreatic polypeptide by CCK-octapeptide and some analogues in the dog. *Gastroenterology* 80:742, 1981.
249. Schmid R, Schusdziarra V, Schulte-Frohlinde E, Maier V, Classen M: Effect of CCK on insulin, glucagons, and pancreatic polypeptide levels in humans. *Pancreas* 4:653, 1989.
250. Resin H, Stern DH, Sturdevant RAL, Isenberg JI: Effect of C-terminal octapeptide of cholecystokinin on lower esophageal sphincter pressure in man. *Gastroenterology* 64:946, 1973.
251. Fisher RS, DiMarino AJ, Cohen S: Mechanism of cholecystokinin inhibition of lower esophageal sphincter pressure. *Am J Physiol* 228:1469, 1975.

252. Domschke W, Lux G, Domschke S, Strunz V, Bloom SR, Wunsch E: Effects of vasoactive intestinal polypeptide on resting and pentagastrin-stimulated lower esophageal sphincter pressure. *Gastroenterology* 75:9, 1978.
253. Siegel SR, Brown FC, Castell DO, Johnson LF, Said SI: Effects of vasoactive intestinal popypeptide (VIP) on lower esophageal sphincter pressure in awake baboons: comparison with glucagons and secretin. *Dig Dis Sci* 24:345, 1979.
254. Rattan S, Said SI, Goyal RK: Effect of vasoactive intestinal polypeptide (VIP) on the lower esophageal sphincter pressure. *Proc Soc Exp Biol Med* 155:40, 1977.
255. Anuras S, Cooke AR, Christensen J: An inhibitory innervation of the gastroduodenal junction. *J Clin Invest* 54:529, 1974.
256. Chey WY, Hitanant S, Hendricks J, Lorber SH: Effect of secretin and cholecystokinin on gastric emptying and gastric secretion in man. *Gastroenterology* 58:820, 1970.
257. Fisher RS, Lipshuls W, Cohen S: The hormonal regulation of pyloric sphincter function. *J Clin Invest* 52:1289, 1973.
258. Yamagishi T, Debas HT: Cholecystokinin inhibits gastric emptying by acting on both proximal stomach and pylorus. *Am J Physiol* 234:E375, 1978.
259. Isenberg JI, Csendes A: Effect of octapeptide of cholecystokinin on canine pyloric pressure. *Am J Physiol* 222:428, 1972.
260. Valenzuela JE: Effect of intestinal hormones and peptides on intragastric pressure in dogs. *Gastroenterology* 71:766, 1976.
261. Vizi SE, Bertaccini G, Impicciatore M, Knoll J: Evidence that acetylcholine released by gastrin and related polypeptides contributes to their effect on gastrointestinal motility. *Gastroenterology* 64:268, 1973.
262. Hopman WPM, Rosenbusch G, Jansen JBMJ, de Jong AJL, Lamers CBHW: Gallbladder contraction: Effects of fatty meals and cholecystokinin. *Radiology* 157:37, 1985.
263. Burton P, Evans DG, Harper AA, Howat HT, et al: A test of pancreatic function in man based on the analysis of duodenal contents after administration of secretin and pancreozymin. *Gut* 1:111, 1960.
264. Sun DCH, Shay H: Pancreozymin-secretin test: The combined study of serum enzmymes and duodenal contents in the diagnosis of pancreatic disease. *Gastroenterology* 38:570, 1960.
265. Messing B, Bories C, Kunstlinger F, Bernier JJ: Does total parenteral nutrition induce gallbladder sludge formation and lithiasis. *Gastroenterology* 84:1012, 1983.
266. Roslyn JJ, Pitt HA, Mann LL, Ament ME, Denbesten L: Gallbladder disease in patients on long-term parenteral nutrition. Gastroenterology 84:148, 1983.
267. Doty JE, Pitt HA, Porter-Fink V, Denbesten L: Cholecystokinin prophylaxis of parenteral nutrition-induced gallbladder disease. *Ann Surg* 201:76, 1985.
268. Polak J, Bloom S, Colling I, Pearse AGE: Immunofluorescent localization of secretin in the canine duodenum. *Gut* 12:605, 1971.
269. Polak J, Colling I, Bloom S, Pearse A: Immunofluorescent localization of secretin and enteroglucagon in human intestinal mucosa. *Scand J Gastroenterol* 6:739, 1971.
270. Bussolati G, Capella C, Solcia E, Vassallo G, Vezzadini P: Ultrastructural and immunofluorescent investigations on the secretin cell in the dog intestinal mucosa. *Histochemie* 26:218, 1971.
271. Inokuchi H, Fujimoto S, Hattori T, Kawai K: Tritiated thymidine radioautographic study on the origin and renewal of secretin cells in the rat duodenum. *Gastroenterology* 89:1014, 1985.
272. Roth KA, Gordon JI: Spatial differentiation of the intestinal epithelium: analysis of enteroendocrine cells containing immunoreactive serotonin, secretin, and substance P in normal and transgenic mice. *Proc Natl Acad Sci USA* 87:6408, 1990.
273. Chey WY, Chang TM, Park HJ, Lee KY, Escoffery R: Secretin-like immunoreactivity and biological activity in the antral mucosa. *Endocrinology* 113:651, 1983.
274. Wheeler MB, Nishitani J, Buchan AMJ, Kopin AS, et al: Identification of a transcriptional enhancer important for enteroendocrine and pancreatic islet cell-specific expression of the secretin gene. *Mol Cell Biol* 12:3531, 1992.
275. O'Donohue TL, Charlton CG, Miller RL, Boden G, Jacobowitz DM: Identification, characterization, and distribution of secretin immunoreactivity in rat and pig brain. *Proc Natl Acad Sci USA* 78:5221, 1981.
276. Chey WY, Lee KY, Hendricks RA, Rhodes RA, Tai HH: Plasma secretin concentration in fasting and postprandial state in man. *Am J Dig Dis* 23:981, 1978.
277. Schaffalitzky de Muckadell OB, Fahrenkrug J: Secretin pattern of secretin in man. Regulation of gastric acid. *Gut* 19:812, 1978.
278. Rominger JM, Chey WY, Chang TM: Plasma secretin concentrations and gastric pH in healthy subjects and patients with digestive disease. *Dig Dis Sci* 26:591, 1981.
279. Osnes M, Hanssen LE, Flaten O, Myren J: Exogenous pancreatic secretion and immunoreactive secetin (IRS) release after intraduodenal instillation of bile in man. *Gut* 19:180, 1978.
280. Watanabe S, Chey WY, Lee KY, Chang TM: Secretin is relased by digestive products of fat in dogs. *Gastroenterology* 90:1008, 1986.
281. Murthy SNS, Lavy A, Morgantini DS, Chey WY: Neurohumoral regulation of secretin secretions in canine duodenal mucosa in vitro. *Peptides* 7:229, 1986.
282. Boden G, Sivitz MC, Owen OE, Essa-Koumar N, Landor HJ: Somatostatin suppresses secretin and pancreatic exocrine secretin. *Science*. Washington, DC, 190:163, 1975.
283. Hanssen LE, Kanssen KF, Myren J: Inhibition of secretin release and pancreatic bicarbonate secretion by somatostatin infusion in man. *Scand J Gastroenterol* 12:391, 1977.
284. Chey WY, Konturek SH, Schally AV, Tsasler J: Enkephalin inhibits the release and action of secretin on pancreatic secretion in dog. *J Physiol Lond* 298:429, 1980.
285. Green GM, Lynn RL: Feedback regulation of pancreatic enzyme secretion as a mechanism for trypsin inhibitor-induced hypersecretion in rats. *Proc Soc Exp Biol Med* 140:6, 1972.
286. Liddle RA, Goldfine ID, Williams JA: Bioassay of plasma cholecystokinin in rats: effects of food, trypsin and alcohol. *Gastroenterology* 87:542, 1984.
287. Louie DS, May D, Miller P, Owyang C: Cholecysokinin mediates feedback regulation of pancreatic enzyme secretion in rats. *Am J Physiol* 250:G252, 1986.
288. Li P, Ren XS, Chang TM, Chey WY: Effect of pancreatic proteases on plasma cholecystokinin, secretin and pancreatic exocrine secretion in response to sodium oleate. *Gastroenterology* 98:1642, 1990.
289. Shiratori K, Jo YH, Lee KY, Chang TM, Chey WY: Effect of pancreatic juice and trypsin on oleic acid-stimulated pancreatic secretion in dogs. *Gastroenterology* 96:1330, 1989.
290. Lu L, Louie D, Owyang C: A cholecystokinin releasing peptide mediates feedback regulation of pancreatic secretion. *Am J Physiol* 19:G430, 1989.
291. Miyasaka K, Guan D, Liddle RA, Green GM: Feedback regulation by trypsin: Evidence for intraluminal CCK-releasing peptide. *Am J Physiol* 257:G175, 1989.
292. Li P, Lee KY, Chang TM, Chey WY: Mechanism of acid-induced release of secretin in rats: Presence of a secretin releasing factor. *J Clin Invest* 86:1474, 1990.
293. Xue W, Chang TM, Chey WY: Cyclic adenosine monophosphate — and — Ca^{2+}-dependent release of secretin from isolated secretin-enriched cells of canine duodenal mucosa. *Gastroenterology* 98:A532, 1990.
294. Hubel KA: Secretin: A long progress note. *Gastroenterology* 62:318, 1972.
295. Chey WY, Kim MS, Lee KY, Chang TM: Effects of rabbit anti-secretin serum on postprandial pancreatic secretion in dogs. *Gastroenterology* 77:1268, 1979.
296. Chey WY, Lee KY, Chang TM, Chen YF, Millikan L: Potentiation effect of secretin on cholecystokinin-stimulated pancreatic secretion in dogs. *Am J Physiol* 246:G248, 1984.
297. Chey WY, Chang TM: Secretin, in Schultz SG, Makhlouf GM (eds): *Handbook of Physiology: The Gastrointestinal System II*. Bethesda, MD, American Physiological Society, 1989, pp 359–402.
298. You CH, Chey WY: Secretin is an enterogastrone in humans. *Dig Dis Sci* 32:466, 1987.
299. Magee DF, Nakajima S: Stimulatory action of secretin on gastric pepsin secretion. *Experientia* 24:689, 1968.
300. Stening GF, Johnson LR, Grossman MI: Effect of secretin on acid and pepsin secretion in cat and dog. *Gastroenterology* 56:468, 1969.
301. Berstad A: Stimulation of gastric secretion of pepsin by secretin in man. *Scand J Gastroenterol* 4:617, 1969.
302. Berstad A, Petersen H: Dose-related relationship of the effect of secretin on acid and pepsin secretion in man. *Scand J Gastroenterol* 5:647, 1970.
303. Wheeler HO, Ross E, Bradley S: Canalicular bile production in dogs. *Am J Physiol* 214:866, 1968.

304. Soloway RD, Clark ML, Powell KM, Senior JR, Brooks FP: Effects of secretin and bile infusions on canine bile composition and flow. *Am J Physiol* 222:681, 1972.
305. Boyer JL, Bloomer JR: Canalicular bile secretion in man. Studies utilizing the biliary clearance of [^{14}C] mannitol. *J Clin Invest* 54:773, 1974.
306. Jim HO, Lee KY, Chang TM, Chey WY, Dubois A: Is secretin an enterogastrone? It is the dog. *Gastroenterology* 5:A93, 1991.
307. Valenzuela JE, Difillippi C: Inhibition of gastric emptying in humans by secretin, the octapeptide of cholecystokinin and intraduodenal fat. *Gastroenterology* 81:898, 1981.
308. Dinoso VP, Meshkinpour H, Lorber SH, Gutierrez JG, Chey WY: Motor responses of the sigmoid colon and rectum to exogenous cholecystokinin and secretin. *Gastroenterology* 65:434, 1973.
309. Brodows RG, Chey WY: Physiological doses of secretin do not stimulate acute insulin release. *J Clin Endocrinol Metab* 50:603, 1980.
310. Otsuki M, Sakamoto C, Ohki A, Yuu H, et al: Effects of porcine secretin on exocrine and endocrine function in the isolated perfused rat pancreas. *Am J Physiol* 241:G43, 1981.
311. Ipp E, Dobbs RE, Harris V, Arimura A, et al: The effects of gastrin, gastric inhibitory polypeptide, secretin and octapeptide of cholecystokinin upon immunoreactive somatostatin release by the perfused canine pancreas. *J Clin Invest* 60:1216, 1977.
312. Glaser B, Vilnik AI, Sive AA, Floyd JC Jr: Plasma human pancreatic polypeptide response to administered secretin: Effects of surgical vagotomy, cholinergic blockage, and chronic pancreatitis. *J Clin Endocrinol Metab* 50:1094, 1980.
313. Chey WY, Rhodes RA, Tai HH: Role of secretin in man, in Bloom SR (ed): *Gut Hormones*. Edinburgh, Churchill-Livingstone, 1978, pp 183–196.
314. Thompson JC, Llanos OL, Schafmayer A, Teichmann RK, Rayford PL: Mechanism of release and catabolism of secretin, in Bloom SR (ed): *Gut Hormones*. Edinburgh, Churchill-Livingstone, 1978, pp 176–181.
315. Rhodes RA, Tai HH, Chey WY: Impairment of secretin release in celiac sprue. *Dig Dis Sci* 23:833, 1978.
316. Rominger JM, Chey WY, Chang TM: Plasma secretin concentrations and gastric pH in healthy subjects and patients with digestive diseases. *Dig Dis Sci* 26:591, 1981.
317. Meyer JH: Pancreatic physiology, in Sleisenger MH, Fordtran JS (eds). *Gastrointestinal Disease: Pathophysiology, Diagnosis, Management*, 4th ed. Philadelphia, Saunders, 1989, pp 1777–1788.
318. Mignon M, Rigaud D, Cambray S, Chayvialle JA, et al: A comparative evaluation of secretin bolus and secretin infusion as secretin provocation tests in the Zollinger-Ellison syndrome. *Scand J Gastroenterol* 20:791, 1985.
319. Lamers CBH, Van Tongeren JHM: Comparative study of the value of the calcium, secretin, and meal stimulated increase in serum gastrin to the diagnosis of the Zollinger-Ellison syndrome. *Gut* 18:128, 1977.
320. McGuigan JE: The Zollinger-Ellison syndrome, in Sleisenger MH, Fordtran JS (eds): *Gastrointestinal Disease: Pathophysiology, Diagnosis, Management*, 4th ed. Philadelphia, Saunders, 1989, pp 909–925.
321. Debas HT, Soon-Shiong P, McKenzie AD, Bogoch A, et al: Use of secretin in the roentgenologic and biochemical diagnosis of duodenal gastrinoma. *Am J Surg* 145:408, 1983.
322. Said SI, Mutt V: Long-acting vasodilator peptide from lung tissue. *Nature* 224:699, 1969.
323. Said SI, Mutt V: Polypeptide with broad biological activity: Isolation from small intestine. *Science* 169:1217, 1970.
324. Said SI, Mutt V: A peptide fraction from lung tissue with prolonged peripheral vasodilator activity. *Scand J Clin Lab Invest* 24(Suppl 107):51, 1969.
325. Mutt V, Said SI: Structure of the procine vasoactive intestinal octacosapeptide: The amino-acid sequence: Use of kallikrein in its determination. *Eur J Biochem* 42:581, 1974.
326. Ekblad E, Ekman R, Hakanson R, Sundler F: Projections of peptide-containing neurons in rat colon. *Neuroscience* 27:655, 1988.
327. Melander T, Hokfelt T, Rokaeus A, Fahrenkrug J, et al: Distriution of galanin-like immunoreactivity in the gastro-intestinal tract of several vertebrate species. *Cell Tissue Res* 239:253, 1985.
328. Kuwahara A, Mikami S, Yanaihara N: Coexistence of immunoreactive gastrin-releasing peptide and substance P in the myenteric plexus of rat stomach. *Biomed Res* 6:443, 1985.
329. Bloom SR: Vasoactive intestinal peptide, the major mediator of the WDHA (pancreatic cholera) syndrome: Value of measurement in diagnosis and treatment. *Am J Dig Dis* 23:373, 1978.
330. Fehrenkrug J, Haglund U, Jodal Lundgren O, Olbe L, Schaffalitzky de Muckadell OB: Nervous release of vasoactive intestinal polypeptide in the gastrointestinal tract of cats: Possible physiological implications. *J Physiol* 284:291, 1978.
331. Schubert ML, Makhlouf GM: Gastrin secretion induced by distension is mediated by gastric cholinergic and vasoactive intestinal peptide neurons in rats. *Gastroenterology* 104:834, 1993.
332. Fahrenkrug J: Vasoactive intestinal peptide, in Schultz SG, Makhlouf GM (eds): *Handbook of Physiology: The Gastrointestinal System II*. Bethesda, MD, American Physiological Society, 1989, pp 611–629.
333. Schaffalitzky de Muckadell OB, Fahrenkrug J, Holst JJ, Lauritsen KB: Release of vasoactive intestinal polypeptide (VIP) by intraduodenal stimuli. *Scand J Gastroenterol* 12:793, 1977.
334. Fahrenkurg J: Vasoactive intestinal peptide, in Makhlouf GM (ed): *Handbook of Physiology: The Gastrointestinal System II*. Bethesda, MD, American Physiological Society, 1989, pp 611–629.
335. Laburthe M, Amiranoff B: Peptide receptors in intestinal epithelium, in Makhlouf GM (ed): *Handbook of Physiology: The Gastrointestinal System II*. Bethesda, MD, American Physiological Society, 1989, pp 215–243.
336. Said SI: Vasoactive intestinal peptide. *J Endocrinol Inves* 9:191, 1986.
337. Binder HJ, Lemp GF, Gardner JD: Receptors for vasoactive intestinal peptide and secretin on small intestinal epithelial cells. *Am J Physiol* 238:G190, 1980.
338. Ito S, Ohga A, Ohta T: Gastric vasodilatation and vasoactive intestinal peptide output in response to vagal stimulation in the dog. *J Physiol* 404:669, 1988.
339. Grider JR, Cable MB, Said SI, Makhlouf GM: Vasoactive intestinal peptide as a neural mediator of gastric relaxation. *Am J Physiol* 248:G73, 1985.
340. De Beurme FA, Lefebvre RA: Vasoactive intestinal polypeptide as possible mediator of relaxation in the rat gastric fundus. *J Pharm Pharmacol* 40:711, 1988.
341. Fahrenkrug J, Schaffalitzky de Muckadell OB, Holst JJ, Jensen SL: Vasoactive intestinal polypeptide in vegally-mediated pancreatic secretion of fluid and HCO_3. *Am J Physiol* 237:E535, 1979.
342. Holst JJ, Fahrenkrug J, Knuhtsen S, Jensen SL, et al: Vasoactive intestinal polypeptide (VIP) in the pig pancreas: Role of VIPergic nerves in control of fluid and bicarbonate secretion. *Reg Peptides* 8:245, 1984.
343. Waldman DB, Gardner JD, Zfass AM, Makhlouf GM: Effects of vasoactive intestinal peptide, secretin, and related peptides on rat colonic transport and adenylate cyclase activity. *Gastroenterology* 73:518, 1977.
344. Krejs GJ, Fordtran JS, Bloom SR, Fahrenkrug J, et al: Effect of VIP infusion on water and ion transport in the human jejunum. *Gastroenterology* 78:722, 1980.
345. Ollerenshaw S, Jarvis D, Woolcock A, Sullivan C, Scheibner T: Absence of immunoreactive vasoactive intestinal polypeptide in tissue from the lungs of patients with asthma. *N Engl J Med* 320:1244, 1989.
346. Said S: Vasoactive intestinal polypeptide (VIP) in asthma. *Ann NY Acad Sci* 629:305, 1991.
347. Said SI: Vasoactive intestinal polypeptide and asthma. *N Engl J Med* 320:1271, 1989.
348. Roy JB: Petrone RL, Said SI: A clinical trial of intracavernous vasoactive intestinal peptide to induce penile erection. *J Urol* 143:302, 1990.
349. O'Dorisio TM, Mekhjian HS: VIPoma syndrome, in Cohen S, Soloway RD (eds): *Contemporary Issue in Gastroenterology*. Edinburgh, Churchill Livingstone, 1984, pp 101–116.
350. Bloom SR, Polak JM: VIPomas, in Said SI (ed): *Vasoactive Intestinal Peptide*. New York, Raven Press, 1982, p 457.
351. Castresana M, Lee K, Chey W, Yajima H: Effects of motilin and octapeptide on cholecystokinin on antral and duodenal myoelectric activity in the interdigestive state and during inhibition by secretin and gastric inhibitory polypeptide. *Digestion* 17:300, 1978.
352. Buchan AMJ, Polak JM, Capella C, Solcia E, Pearse AGE: Electron-immunocytochemical evidence for the K cell localization of gastric inhibitory polypeptide (GIP) in man. *Histochem* 56:37, 1978.

353. Karup T, Holst JJ: The heterogeneity of gastric inhibitory polypeptide in porcine and human gastrointestinal mucosa evaluated with fiver different antisera. *Regul Pept* 9:35, 1984.
354. Cataland S, Crockett SE, Brown JC, Mazzaferri EL: Gastric inhibitory polypeptide (GIP) stimulation by oral glucose in man. *J Clin Endocrinol Metab* 39:223, 1974.
355. Falco JM, Crockett SE, Cataland S, Mazzaferri EL: Gastric inhibitory polypeptide (GIP) stimulation by oral glucose in man. *J Clin Endocrinol Metab* 41:260, 1976.
356. Thomas FB, Mazzaferri EL, Crockett SE, Makhjian HS, et al: Stimulation of secretion of gastric inhibitory polypeptide and insulin by intraduodenal amino acid perfusion. *Gastroenterology* 70:523, 1976.
357. Sykes S, Morgan J, English J, Marks V: Evidence for preferential stimulation of gastric inhibitory polypeptide secretion in the rat by actively transported carbohydrates and their analogues. *J Endocrinol* 5:210, 1980.
358. Pederson RA, Schubert HE, Brown JC: Gastric inhibitory polypeptide—its physiological release and insulinotropic action in the dog. *Diabetes* 24:1050, 1975.
359. Ohmeda A, Kobayashi T, Nihei J: Effect of endogenous gastric inhibitory polypeptide (GIP) on the removal of triacylglycerol in dogs. *Regul Pept* 6:25, 1983.
360. Ross SA, Shaffer ES: The importance of triglyceride hydrolysis for the release of gastric inhibitory polypeptide. *Gastroenterology* 80:108, 1981.
361. Thomas FB, Shook DF, O'Dorisio TM, Cataland S, et al: Localization of gastric inhibitory polypeptide release by intestinal glucose perfusion in man. *Gastroenterology* 72:49, 1977.
362. Thomas FB, Sinar D, Mazzaferri EL, Cataland S, et al: Selective release of gastric inhibitory polypeptide by intraduodenal amino acid perfusion in man. *Gastroenterology* 74:1261, 1978.
363. Brown JC, Buchan AMJ, McIntosh CHS, Pederson RA: Gastric inhibitory polypeptide, in Schultz SG, Makhlouf GM (eds): *Handbook of Physiology: The Gastrointestinal System II.* Bethesda, MD, American Physiological Society, 1989, pp 403–430.
364. Pederson RA, Brown JC: Inhibition of histamine-pentagastrin-, and insulin-stimulated canine gastric secretion by pure "gastric inhibitory polypeptide." *Gastroenterology* 62:393, 1972.
365. Wolfe MM, Hocking MP, Maico DG, McGuigan JE: Effects of antibodies to gastric inhibitory peptide on gastric acid secretion and gastrin release in the dog. *Gastroenterology* 84:941, 1983.
366. Anderson DK, Elahi D, Brown JC, Tobin JD, Andres R: Oral glucose augmentation of insulin secretion. Interactions of gastric inhibitory polypeptide with ambient glucose and insulin levels. *J Clin Invest* 62:152, 1978.
367. Arnold R, Creutzfeldt W, Ebert R, Becker HD, et al: Serum gastric inhibitory polypeptide (GIP) in duodenal ulcer disease: relationship to glucose tolerance, insulin and gastrin release. *Scand J Gastroenterol* 13:41, 1978.
368. McIntosh CHS, Pederson RA, Koop H, Brown JC: Gastric inhibitory polypeptide stimulated secretion of somatostatin-like immunoreactivity from the stomach: inhibition by acetylcholine or vagal stimulation. *Can J Physiol Pharmacol* 59:468, 1981.
369. Helman C, Barbezat G: The effect of gastric inhibitory polypeptide on human jejunal water and electrolyte transport. *Gastroenterology* 72:376, 1977.
370. Brown J, Dryburgh J, Ross S, Dupre J: Identification and actions of gastric inhibitory polypeptide. *Recent Prog Horm Res* 31:487, 1975.
371. Denniss A, Young J: Modification of salivary duct electrolyte transport in rat and rabbit by physalaemin, VIP, GIP and other enterohormones. *Pflugers Arch* 376:73, 1978.
372. Elahi D, Anderson DK, Brown JC: Pancreatic α- and β-cell responses to GIP infusion in normal man. *Am J Physiol* 237:E185, 1979.
373. Pederson RA, Brown JC: The insulinotropic action of gastric inhibitory polypeptide in the perfused isolated rat pancreas. *Endocrinology* 99;780, 1976.
374. Anderson DK, Sun YS, Bruncardi FC, Berlin SA, et al: Regulation of hepatic glucose production by gastric inhibitory polypeptide (GIP), insulin (INS), and glucagons (GLUC). *Dig Dis Sci* 29:A5 (abst) 1984.
375. Creutzfeldt W, Ebert R: GIP in obesity, diabetes and hyperlipoproteinemia, in Hessel LW, Krans HMJ (eds): *Lipoprotein Metabolism and Endocrine Regulation.* 1979, pp 65–73.
376. Botha J, Vinik A, Brown J: Gastric inhibitory polypeptide (GIP) in chronic pancreatitis. *J Clin Endocrinol Metab* 42:791, 1976.
377. Ebert R, Creutzfeldt W, Brown J, Frerichs H, Arnold R: Response of gastric inhibitory polypeptide (GIP) to test meal in chronic pancreatitis-relationship to endocrine and exocrine insufficiency. *Diabetologia* 12:609, 1976.
378. Arnold R, Creutzfeldt W, Ebert R, Becker H, et al: Serum gastric inhibitory polypeptide (GIP) in duodenal ulcer disease: Relationship to glucose tolerance, insulin, and gastric release. *Scand J Gastroenterol* 13:41, 1978.
379. Creutzfeldt W, Ebert R, Willms B, Frerichs H, Brown J: Gastric inhibitory polypeptide (GIP) and insulin in obesity: Increased response to stimulation and defective feedback control of serum levels. *Diabetologia* 14:15, 1978.
380. Lauritsen K, Lauritzen J, Christensen K: Gastric inhibitory polypeptide and insulin release in response to oral and intravenous glucose in celiac disease. *Scand J Gastroenterol* 17:241, 1982.
381. Brown JC, Mutt V, Dryburgh JR: The further purification of motilin, a gastric motor activity stimulating polypeptide from the mucosa of the small intestine of hogs. *Can J Physiol Pharmacol* 49:399, 1971.
382. Brown JC, Cook MA, Dryburgh JR: Motilin, a gastric motor activity stimulating polypeptide: The complete amino acid sequence. *Can J Biochem* 51:533, 1973.
383. Tanaka M, Sarr MG: Total duodenectomy: Effect on canine gastrointestinal motility. *J Surg Res* 42:483, 1987.
384. Tanaka M, Sarr MG: Role of the duodenum in the control of canine gastrointestinal motility. *Gastroenterology* 94:622, 1988.
385. Polak JM: Motilin immunocytochemical localization indicates possible molecular heterogeneity or the existence of a motilin family. *Gastroenterology* 76:1065, 1979.
386. Vantrappen G, Peeters TL; Motilin, in Schultz SG, Makhlouf GM (eds): *Handbook of Physiology: The Gastrointestinal System II.* Bethesda, MD, American Physiological Society, 1989, pp 545–558.
387. Itoh Z, Takeuchi S, Aizawa I, Mori K, et al: Changes in plasma motilin concentration and gastrointestinal contractile activity in conscious dogs. *Dig Dis* 23:929, 1978.
388. You CH, Chey WY, Lee KY: Studies on plasma motilin concentration and interdigestive motility of the duodenum in humans. *Gastroenterology* 79:62, 1980.
389. Poitras P, Steinbach J, Van Deventer G, Code C, Walsh J: Motilin independent ectopic fronts of the interdigestive myoelectric complex in dogs. *Am J Physiol* 239:G215, 1980.
390. Lee KY, Chang T, Chey WY: Effect of electrical stimulation of the vagus on plasma motilin concentraion in dog. *Life Sciences* 29;1093, 1981.
391. Lemoyne M, Wassef R, Tasse D, Trudel L, Poitras P: Motilin and the vagus in dog. *Can J Physiol Pharmacol* 62:1092, 1984.
392. Bueno L, Fargeas MJ, Gue M, Peeters TL, et al: Effects of corticotropin-releasing factor on plasma motilin and somatostatin levels and gastrointestinal motility in dogs. *Gastroenterology* 91:884, 1986.
393. Poitras P, Tasse D, Leprise P: Stimulation of motilin release by bombesin in dogs. *Am J Physiol* 245:G249, 1983.
394. Misumi A, Shiratori K, Lee KY, Barkin JS, Chey WY: Effects of SMS 201-995, a somatostatin analogue, on the exocrine pancreatic secretion and gut hormone release in dogs. *Surgery* 103:450, 1987.
395. Hall KE, Greenberg GR, El-Sharkawy TY: Diamant NE: Relationship between porcine motilin induced migrating motor complex-like activity, vagal integrity, and endogenous motilin release in dogs. *Gastroenterology* 87:76, 1984.
396. Svenberg T, Christofides D, Fitzpatric ML, Areola-Ortiz F, et al: Interdigestive biliary output in man: Relationship to fluctuations in plasma motilin and effect of atropine. *Gut* 23:1024, 1982.
397. Janssens J, Hellemans J, Adrian TE, Bloom SR, et al: Pancreatic polypeptide is not involved in the regulation of the migrating motor complex in man. *Reg Peptides* 3:41, 1982.
398. Demol P, Hotz J, Muller MK, Trompeter R, et al: Effect of calcitonin on the interdigestive motility and on gastric and pancreatic secretion in humans. *Arch Internationales Physiol Bioch* 94:331, 1986.
399. Itoh Z, Honda R, Hiwatashi K, Takeuchi S, et al: Motilin-induced mechanical activity in the canine alimentary tract. *Scand J Gastroent* [Suppl]39:93, 1976.
400. Vantrappen G, Janssens J, Peeters TL, Bloom SR, et al: Motilin and the interdigestive migrating motor complex in man. *Dig Dis Sci* 24:497, 1979.

401. Fox JET, Track NS, Daniel EE: Relationship of plasma motilin concentration to fat ingestion, duodenal acidification and alkalinization and migrating motor complexes in dogs. *Can J Physiol Pharmacol* 59:180, 1981.
402. Lee KY, Chang T, Chey WY: Effect of rabbit antimotilin serum on myoelectric activity and plasma motilin concentration in fasting dog. *Am J Physiol* 245:G547, 1983.
403. Tioh Z, Takeuchi S, Aizawa I, Takayanagi R: Effect of synthetic motilin on gastric motor activity in conscious dogs. *Dig Dis* 22:813, 1977.
404. Itoh Z, Honda R, Hiwatashi K, Takeuchi S, et al: Motilin-induced mechanical activity in the canine alimentary tract. *Scand J Gastroenterol* 11:93, 1976.
405. Itoh Z, Aizawa I, Honda R, Takeuchi S, Mori K: Regular and irregular cycles of interdigestive contractions in the stomach. *Am J Physiol* 238:G85, 1980.
406. Poitras P, Steinbach JH, Vandevener G, Code CF, Walsh JH: Effect of somatostatin on plasma level of motilin and the IDMC in dogs. *Endocrinol Jpn* SR1:163, 1980.
407. Itoh Z, Aizawa I, Honda R, Hiwatashi K, Couch EF: Control of lower-esophageal-sphincter contractile activity by motilin in conscious dogs. *Dig Dis* 23:341, 1978.
408. Lux G, Rosch W, Domschke S, Domschke W, et al: Intravenous 13-Nle-motilin increases the human lower esophageal sphincter pressure. *Scand J Gastroenterol* 11:75, 1976.
409. Konturek SJ, Dembinski A, Krol R, Wunsch E: Effect of 13-NLE-motilin on gastric secretion, serum gastrin level and mucosal blood flows in dogs. *J Physiol* 264:665, 1977.
410. Debas HT, Yamagishi T, Dryburgh JR: Motilin enhances gastric emptying of liquids in dogs. *Gastroenterology* 73:777, 1977.
411. Christofides ND, Modlin IM, Fitzpatrick ML, Bloom SR: Effect of motilin on the rate of gastric emptying and gut hormone release during breakfast. *Gastroenterology* 76:903, 1979.
412. Magee DF, Naruse S: The role of motilin in periodic interdigestive pancreatic secretion in dogs. *J Physiol* 355:441, 1984.
413. Tanaka M, Sarr MG, Miller LJ, Malagelada JR: Changes in tone of canine gallbladder measured by an electronic pneumatic barostat. *Am J Physiol* 259:G314, 1990.
414. Svenberg T, Christofides ND, Fitzpatrick ML, Bloom SR, Welbourn RB: Oral water causes emptying of the human gallbladder through actions of vagal stimuli rather than motilin. *Scand J Gastroenterol* 20:775, 1985.
415. Pomeranz IS, Davison JS, Shaffer EA: In vitro effects of pancreatic polypeptide and motilin on contractility of human gallbladder. *Dig Dis Sci* 28:539, 1983.
416. Aizawa I, Itoh Z, Harris V, Unger RH: Plasma somatostatin-like immunoreactivity during the interdigestive period in the dog. *J Clin Invest* 68:206, 1981.
417. Schick R, Schusdziarra V: Modulation of motilin-induced somatostatin release in dogs by naloxone. *Peptides* 6:861, 1985.
418. Chiang HCV, O'Dorisio TM, Huang SC, Maton PN, et al: Multiple hormone elevations in ZE syndrome. *Gastroenterology* 99:1565, 1990.
419. Vinik AI, Shapiro B, Thompson NW: Plasma gut hormone levels in 37 patients with pheochromocytomas. *World J Surg* 10:593, 1986.
420. Noseda A, Peeters TL, Delhaye M: Increased plasma motilin concentrations in small cell carcinoma of the lung. *Thorax* 42:784, 1987.
421. Besterman HS, Bloom SR, Christofides ND, Mallinson CN, et al: Gut hormone profile in inflammatory bowel disease. *Gut* 19:A988, 1978.
422. Besterman HS, Adrian TE, Mallinson CN, Christofides ND, et al: Gut hormone release after intestinal resection. *Gut* 23:854, 1982.
423. Aoyagi K, Mishima Y, Murakami S, Ito K: Serum gastrin and motilin in treated and untreated hyperthyroidism. *Bull Tokyo Med Dent Univ* 29:153, 1982.
424. Christofides ND, Ghatei MA, Bloom SR, Borberg C, Gillmer MDG: Decreased plasma motilin concentrations in pregnancy. *Br Med J* 285:1453, 1982.
425. Ruppin H, Kirndörfer D, Domschke S, Domschke W, et al: Effect of 13-Nle-motilin in postoperative ileus patients: A double-blind trial. *Scand J Gastroenterol* [Suppl]39:89, 1976.
426. Depoortere I, Peeters TL, Vantrappen G: The erythromycin derivative EM-523 is a potent motilin agonist in man and in rabbit. *Peptides* 11:515, 1990.
427. Inatomi N, Satoh H, Maki Y, Hashimoto N, et al: An erythromycin derivative, EM-523, induces motilin-like gastrointestinal motility in dogs. *J Pharmacol Exp Ther* 251:707, 1989.
428. Kimmel JR, Hayden LJ, Pollock HG: Isolation and characterization of a new pancreatic polypeptie hormone. *J Biol Chem* 250:9369, 1975.
429. Buffa R, Capella C, Fontana P: Types of endocrine cells in the human colon and rectum. *Cell Tissue Res* 182:227, 1978.
430. Leduque P, Paulin C, Dubois PM: Immunocytochemical evidence for substance related to the bovine pancreatic polypeptide peptide YY group of peptides in the human fetal gastrointestinal tract. *Regul Pept* 6:219, 1983.
431. Tatemoto K: Neuropeptide Y: Complete amino acid sequence of the brain peptide. *Proc Soc Natl Acad Sci USA* 79:5485, 1982.
432. Tatemoto K, Carlquist M, Mutt V: Neuropeptide Y–a novel brain peptide with structural similarities to peptide YY and pancreatic polypeptide. *Nature* 296:659, 1982.
433. Taylor IL: Pancreatic polypeptide family: Pancreatic polypeptide, neuropeptide Y, and peptide YY, in Schultz SG, Makhlouf GM (eds): *Handbook of Physiology: The Gastrointestinal System II.* Bethesda, MD, American Physiological Society, 1989, pp 475–543.
434. Orci L, Baetens D, Ravazzola M: Pancreatic polypeptide and glucagons: Non-random distribution in pancreatic islets. *Life Sci* 19:1811, 1976.
435. Tatemoto K: Isolation and characterization of peptide YY (PYY), a candidate gut hormone that inhibits pancreatic exocrine secretion. *Proc Natl Acad Sci USA* 79:2514, 1982.
436. Jeng YJ, Hill FLC, Luis F, Gomez G, et al: Peptide YY release and actions, in Thompson JC, Cooper CW, Rayford PL, Greeley GH Jr, Singh P, Townsend CM Jr (eds): *Gastrointestinal Endocrinology: Receptors and Post-Receptor Mechanisms.* San Diego, Academic Press, 1990, pp 371–386.
437. Aponte G, Fink AS, Meyer JH: Regional distribtion and release of peptide YY with fatty acids of different chain length. *Am J Physiol* 12:G745, 1985.
438. Solcia E, Riocca R, Capella C: Glucagon and PP-related peptides in intestinal L cells and pancreatic/gastric A or PP cells. Possible interrelationships of peptides and cells during evolution, fetal development and tumor growth. *Peptides* 6:233, 1985.
439. Tatemoto K, Mutt V: Isolation of two novel candidate hormones using a chemical method for finding natural occurring polypeptides. *Nature* 285:417, 1980.
440. Taylor IL, Feldman M, Richardson CT, Walsh JH: Gastric and cephalic stimulation of pancreatic polypeptide release. *Gastroenterology* 75:432, 1978.
441. Scarpello JH, Vinik AI, Owyang C: The intestinal phase of pancreatic polypeptide release. *Gastroenterology* 82:406, 1982.
442. Lundberg JM, Tatemoto K, Terenius LPM: Localization of peptide YY (PYY) in gastrointestinal endocrine cells and effects on intestinal blood flow and motility. *Proc Natl Acad Sci USA* 79:4471, 1982.
443. Chen MH, Balasubramanian A, Murphy RF: Sensitive radioimmunoassay for measurement of circulating peptide YY. *Gastroenterology* 87:1332, 1984.
444. Taylor IL: Distribution and release of peptide YY in dog measured by specific radioimmunoassay. *Gastroenterology* 88:731, 1985.
445. Adrian TE, Ferrai GL, Bacaresse-Hamilton A: Human distribution and release of PYY, a putative new gut hormone. *Gastroenterology* 89:1070, 1985.
446. Greenberg GR, McCloy RF, Adrian TE, Boron JH, Bloom SR: Effect of bovine pancreatic polypeptide on gastric acid and pepsin output in man. *Acta Hepatogastroenterol* 25:384, 1978.
447. Lin TM, Evans DC, Chance RE, Spray GF: Bovine pancreatic peptide: Action on gastric and pancreatic secretion in dogs. *Am J Physiol* 232:E311, 1977.
448. Pappas TN, Debas HT, Goto Y: Peptide YY inhibits meal-stimulated pancreatic and gastric secretion. *Am J Physiol* 245:G118, 1985.
449. Adrian TE, Savage AP, Sagor GR: Effect of peptide YY on gastric pancreatic, and biliary function in humans. *Gastroenterology* 89:484, 1985.
450. Pappas TN, Debas HT, Taylor IL: The enterogastrone-like effect of peptide YY is vagally mediated in the dog. *J Clin Invest* 77:49, 1986.
451. Pappas TN, Chang AM, Debas HT: Peptide YY release by fatty acids is sufficient to inhibit gastric emptying in dog. *Gastroenterology* 91:1386, 1986.

452. Allen JM, Fitzpatric ML, Yeats JC: Effects of peptide YY and neuropeptide Y on gastric emptying in man. *Digestion* 30:255, 1984.
453. Wahlestedt C, Wohlfart B, Hakanson R: Effects of neuropeptide Y (NPY) on isolated guinea-pig heart. *Acta Physiol Scand* 129:307, 1987.
454. McDonald JK, Lumpkin MD, Samson WK, McCann SM: Neuuropeptide Y affects secretion of luteinizing hormone and growth hormone in ovariectomized rats. *Proc Natl Acad Sci USA* 82:561, 1985.
455. Levine AS, Morley JE: Neuropeptide Y: a potent inducer of consummatory behavior in rats. *Peptides* 5:1025, 1984.
456. Friesen SR, Tomita T, Kimmel JR: Pancreatic polypeptide update: Its roles in detection of the trait for multiple endocrine adenopathy syndrome, type I and pancreatic polypeptide-secreting tumors. *Surgery* 94:1028, 1983.
457. Lamers CBH, Diemel J, Roeffen W: Serum levels of pancreatic polypeptide in Zollinger-Ellison syndrome, and hyperparathyroidism from families with multiple endocrine adenomatosis type I. *Digestion* 18:297, 1978.
458. Polak JM, Bloom SR, Adrian TE, Heitz P, et al: Pancreatic polypeptide in insulinomas, gastrinomas, VIPomas and glucagonomas. *Lancet* 1:328, 1976.
459. Schwartz TW: Pancreatic-polypeptide (PP) and endocrine tumours of the pancreas. *Scand J Gastroenterol* 14(Suppl 53):93, 1979.
460. Floyd JC, Fajans SS, Pek S, Chance RE: Regulations in healthy subjects of the secretion of human pancreatic polypeptide, a newly recognized pancreatic islet polypeptide. *Trans Assoc Am Physicians* 89:146, 1976.
461. Hållgren R, Lundqvist G, Chance RE: Serum levels of human pancreatic polypeptide in renal disease. *Scand J Gastroenterol* 12:923, 1977.
462. Adrian TE, McKiernan J, Johnstone DI, Hiller EJ, et al: Hormonal abnormalities of the pancreas and gut in cystic fibrosis. *Gastroenterology* 79:460, 1980.
463. Lassmann V, Vague P, Vialettes B, Simon MC: Low plasma levels of pancreatic polypeptide in obesity. *Diabetes* 29:428, 1980.
464. Lassmann V, Cabrerizzo Garcia L, Vialettes B, Vague P: Impaired pancreatic polypeptide response to insulin hypoglycemia in obese subjects. *Horm Metab Res* 17:663, 1985.
465. Coelle EF, Taylor IL, Lewin K, Adham N: Beneficial effect of pancreatic polypeptide in experimental pancreatitis. *Dig Dis Sci* 28:1083, 1983.
466. Polinsky R, Taylor I, Chew P, Weise V, Kopin I: Pancreatic polypeptide responses to hypoglycemia in chronic autonomic failure. *J Clin Endocrinol Metab* 54:48, 1982.
467. Bysschaert M, Donckier J, Dive A, Ketelslegers J, Lambert A: Gastric acid and pancreatic polypeptide responses to sham feeding are impaired in diabetic subjects with autonomic neuropathy. *Diabetes* 34:1181, 1985.
468. Carraway R, Leeman SE: The isolation of a new hypotensive peptide, neurotensin, from bovine hypothalami. *J Biol Chem* 248:6854, 1973.
469. Carraway R, Leeman SE: The amino acid sequence of a hypothalamic peptide, neurotensin. *J Biol Chem* 250:1907, 1975.
470. Kitabgi P, Carraway R, Leeman SE: Isolation of tridecapeptide from bovine intestine tissue and its partial characterization as neurotensin. *J Biol Chem* 251:7053, 1976.
471. Hammer RA, Leeman SE, Carraway R, Williams RH: Isolation of human intestinal neurotensin. *J Biol Chem* 225:2476, 1980.
472. Minamino N, Kanagawa K, Matsuo H: Neuromedin N: A novel neurotensin-like peptide identified in porcine spinal cord. *Biochim Biophys Res Commun* 122:542, 1984.
473. Sundler F, Hakanson R, Leander S, Uddman R: Light and electron microscopic localization of neurotensin in the gastrointestinal tract. *Ann NY Acad Sci* 400:94, 1982.
474. Carraway RE, Mitra SP: The use of radioimmunoassay to compare the tissue and subcellular distributions of neurotensin and neuromedin N in the cat. *Endocrinology* 120:2092, 1987.
475. Yamashita Y, Holst Pederson J, Palnaes Hansen C: Distribution of neurotensin-like immunoreactivities in porcine and human gut. *Scand J Gastroenterol* 25:481, 1990.
476. Granier C, Van Rietschoten J, Kitabgi P, Poustis C, Freychet P: Synthesis and characterization of neurotensin analogues for structure/activity relationship studies: Acetyl-neurotensin-(8-13) is the shortest analogue with full binding and pharmacological activities. *Eur J Biochem* 124:117, 1982.
477. Go VLW, Demol P: Role of nutrients in the gastrointestinal release of immunoreactive neurotensin. *Peptides* 2(Suppl 2):267, 1981.
478. Rosell S, Rökaeus A: The effect of ingestion of amino acids, glucose and fat on circulating neurotensin-like immunoreactivity (NTLI) in man. *Acta Physiol Scand* 107:263, 1979.
479. Eaves ER, Korman MG, Mercuri J, Ward F, Hansky J: The localization of the site(s) of neurotensin release in man and dog. *J Gastroenterol Hepatol* 3:83, 1988.
480. Shaw C, Buchanan KD: Intact neurotensin (NT) in human plasma: Response to oral feeding. *Regul Pept* 7:145, 1983.
481. Fletcher DR, Shulkes A, Bladin PH, Hardy KJ: The effect of atropine on bombesin and gastrin releasing peptide stimulated gastrin, pancreatic polypeptide and neurotensin release in man. *Regul Pept* 7:31, 1983.
482. Yanaihara N, Sato H, Inoue A, Sakura N, et al: Comparative study on distribution of bombesin-, neurotensin-, and α-endorphin-like immunoreactivities in canine tissues. *Adv Exp Med Biol* 120A:29, 1979.
483. Ferris CF: Neurotensin, in Schultz SG, Makhlouf GM (eds): *Handbook of Physiology: The Gastrointestinal System II*. Bethesda, MD, American Physiological Society, 1989, pp 559–586.
484. Baca I, Feurle GE, Haas M, Mernitz T: Interaction of neurotensin, cholecystokinin, and secretin in the stimulation of the exocrine pancreas in the dog. *Gastroenterology* 84:556, 1983.
485. Keinke O, Wulschke S, Ehrlein HJ: Neurotensin slows gastric emptying by a transient inhibition of gastric and prolonged inhibition of duodenal motility. *Digestion* 34:281, 1986.
486. Thor K, Rosell S, Rokaeus A, Kager L: (Gln)4–neurotensin changes the motility pattern of the duodenum and proximal jejunum from a fasting-type to a fed-type. *Gastroenterology* 83:569, 1982.
487. Carraway RE, Cochrane DE, Salmonsen R, Muraki K, Boucher W: Neurotensin elevates hematocrit and plasma levels of the leukotrienes, LTB4, LTC4, LTD4 and LTE4, in anesthetized rats. *Peptides* 12:1105, 1991.
488. Harper SL, Barrowman JA, Kvietys PR, Granger DN: Effect of neurotensin on intestinal capillary permeability and blood flow. *Am J Physiol* 247:G161, 1984.
489. Bar-Shavit Z, Terry S, Blumberg S, Goldman R: Neurotensin-macrophage interaction: Specific binding and augmentation of phagocytosis. *Neuropeptides* 2:325, 1982.
490. Shulkes A, Boden R, Cook I, Gallagher N, Furness JB: Characterization of a pancreatic tumor containing vasoactive intestinal peptide, neurotensin and pancreatic polypeptide. *J Clin Endocrinol Metab* 58:41, 1984.
491. Blackburn AM, Bryant MG, Adrian TE, Bloom SR: Pancreatic tumors produce neurotensin. *J Clin Endocrinol Metab* 52:820, 1981.
492. Blackburn AM, Lawaetz O, Bloom SR: Plasma neurotensin release and gastric emptying in the dumping syndrome. *Life Sci* 32:833, 1983.
493. Theodorsson-Norheim E, Öberg K, Rosell S, Boström H: Neurotensin-like immunoreactivity in plasma and tumor tissue from patients with endocrine tumors of the pancreas and gut. *Gastroenterology* 85:881, 1983.
494. Von Euler US, Gaddum JH: An unidentified depressor substance in certain tissue extracts. *J Physiol (Lond)* 72:74, 1931.
495. Maggio JE, Mantyh PW: Gut tachykinins, in Schultz SG, Makhlouf GM (eds): *Handbook of Physiology: The Gastrointestinal System II*. Bethesda, MD, American Physiological Society, 1989, pp 661–690.
496. Pearse AGE, Polak JM: Immunocytochemical localization of substance P in mammalian intestine. *Histochemistry* 41:373, 1975.
497. Holzer P, Bucsics A, Saria A, Lembeck F: A study of the concentrations of substance P and neurotensin in the gastrointestinal tract of various mammals. *Neuroscience* 7:2919, 1982.
498. Wattchow DA, Furness JB, Costa M: Distribution and coexistence of peptides in nerve fibers of the external muscle of the human gastrointestinal tract. *Gastroenterology* 95:32, 1988.
499. Ferri GL, Adrian TE, Allen JM, Soimero L, et al: Intramural distribution of regulatory peptides in the sigmoid-recto-anal region of the human gut. *Gut* 29:762, 1988.
500. Larson LI: Innervation of the pancreas by substance P, enkephalin, vasoactive intestinal polypeptide and gastrin/CCK immunoreactive nerves. *J Histochem Cytochem* 27:1283, 1979.
501. Hökfelt T, Johansson O, Ljungdahl A, Lundberg JM, Schultzberg M: Peptidergic neurons. *Nature* 284:515, 1980.
502. Donnerer J, Barthó L, Holzer P, Lembeck F: Intestinal peristalsis associated with release of immunoreactive substance P. *Neuroscience* 11:913, 1984.
503. Gintzler AR: Substance P involvement in the expression of gut dependence on opiates. *Brain Res* 182:224, 1980.

504. Hutchison JB, Dockray GJ: Evidence that the action of cholecystokinin octapeptide on the guinea-pig ileum longitudinal muscle is mediated in part by substance P release from the myenteric plexus. *Eur J Pharmacol* 69:87, 1981.
505. Wiley J, Owyang C: Participation of serotonin and substance P in the action of cholecystokinin on colonic motility. *Am J Physiol* 252: G431, 1987.
506. Donnerer J, Bartho L, Holzer P, Lembeck F: Intestinal peristalsis associated with release of immunoreactive substance P. *Neuroscience* 11:913, 1984.
507. Bury RW, Mashford ML: Substance P–its pharmacology and physiological roles. *Aust J Exp Biol* 55:671, 1977.
508. Bartho L, Holzer P: Search for a physiological role of substance P in gastrointestinal motility. *Neuroscience* 16:1, 1985.
509. Keast JR: Mucosal innervation and control of water and ion transport in the intestine. *Rev Physiol Biochem Pharmacol* 109:1, 1987.
510. McFadden D, Zinner MJ, Jaffe BM: Substance P-induced intestinal secretion of water and electrolytes. *Gut* 27:267, 1986.
511. Kachur JF, Miller RJ, Field M, Rivier J: Neurohumoral control of ileal electrolyte transport. II Neurotensin and substance P. *J Pharmacol Exp Ther* 220:456, 1982.
512. Jensen RT, Gardner JD: Interaction of physalaemin, substance P and eledoisin with specific membrane receptors on pancreatic acinar cells. *Proc Natl Acad Sci USA* 76:5679, 1979.
513. Payan DG: Neuropeptides and inflammation: The role of substance P. *Annu Rev Med* 40:341, 1989.
514. Powell D, Cannon P, Skrabanek P, Kirrane J: The pathophysiology of substance P in man, in Bloom SR (ed): *Gut Hormones*. Edinburgh, Churchill Livingstone, 1978, pp 524–529.
515. Phillips SF: Megacolon: Congenital and acquired, in Sleisenger MH, Fordtran JS (eds): *Gastrointestinal Disease: Pathophysiology, Diagnosis, Management*, 4th ed. Philadelphia, Saunders, 1989, pp 1389–1402.
516. Roth KA, Makk G, Beck O: Isolation and characterization of substance P, substance P 5-11, and substance K from two metastatic ileal carcinoids. *Regul Pept* 12:185, 1985.
517. Conlon JM, Deacon CF, Richter G, Schmidt WE, Creutzfeldt W: Measurement and partial characterization of the multiple forms of neurokinin A-like immunoreactivity in carcinoid tumors. *Regul Pept* 13:183, 1986.
518. Tatemoto K, Rokaeus A, Jornvall H, McDonald TJ, Mutt V: Galanin—a novel biologically active peptide from porcine intestine. *Febs Lett* 164:124, 1983.
519. Evans HF, Shine J: Human galanin: Molecular cloning reveals a unique structure. *Endocrinology* 129:1682, 1991.
520. Strauss RM, Kaplan LM: Molecular analysis of human galanin: Peptide structure and species-specific regulation of gene expression. *Gastroenterology* 100:A669, 1991.
521. Bersani M, Johnsen AH, Hojrup P, Dunning BE, et al: Human galanin: Primary structure and identification of two molecular forms. *Febs Lett* 283:189, 1991.
522. Bradbury AF, Smyth DG: Peptide amidation. *TIBS* 16:112, 1991.
523. Rattan S: Role of galanin in the gut. *Gastroenterology* 100:1762, 1991.
524. Myojin T, Kitamura N, Hondo E, Baltazar ET, et al: Immunohistochemical localization of neuropeptides in bovine pancreas. *Anat Histol Embryol* 29:167, 2000.
525. Bishop AE, Polak JM, Bauer FE, Chistofides ND, et al: Occurrence and distribution of a newly discovered peptide, galanin, in the mammalian enteric nervous system. *Gut* 27:849, 1986.
526. Chang JLC, Christofides ND, Anand P, Gibson SJ, et al: Distribution of galanin immunoreactivity in the central nervous system and the response of galanin-containing neuronal pathways to injury. *Neuroscience* 16:343, 1985.
527. Harling H, Messell T, Poulsen SS, Rasmussen TN, Holst JJ: Galanin and vasoactive intestinal polypeptide—coexistence and corelease from the vascularity perfused pig ileum during distension and chemical stimulation of the mucosa. *Digestion* 50:61, 1991.
528. Dunning BE, Taborsky GJ Jr: Galanin release during pancreatic nerve stimulation is sufficient to influence islet function. *Am J Physiol* 256:E191, 1989.
529. Yagchi RV, Alptekin N, Rossowski WJ, Brown A, et al: Inhibitory effect of galanin on basal and pentagastrin-stimulated gastric acid secretion in rats. *Scand J Gastroenterol* 25:853, 1990.
530. Soldani G, Mengozzi G, Della Longa A, Intorre L, et al: An analysis of the effects of galanin on gastric acid secretion and plasma levels of gastrin in the dog. *Eur J Pharmacol* 154:313, 1988.
531. Madaus S, Schusdziarra V, Seufferlein T, Classen M: Effect of galanin on gastrin and somatostatin release from the rat stomach. *Life Sci* 42:2381, 1988.
532. Bauer FE, Zintel A, Kenny MJ, Calder D, et al: Inhibitory effect of galanin on postprandial gastrointestinal motility and gut hormone release in humans. *Gastroenterology* 97:260, 1989.
533. Bauer FE, Ghatei MA, Zintel A, Bloom SR: Galanin: Hydrokinetic action on salivary glands in man. *Aliment Pharmacol Therap* 3:591, 1989.
534. Harling H, Messell T, Jensen SL, Holst JJ, Poulsen SS: Occurrence, distribution and motor effects of galanin in the porcine lower esophageal sphincter. *Digestion* 42:151, 1989.
535. Ekblad E, Hakanson R, Sundler F, Wahlestedt C: Galanin neuromodulatory and direct contractile effects on smooth muscle preparations. *Br J Pharamacol* 86:241, 1985.
536. Fox JET, Brooks B, McDonald TJ: Actions of galanin fragments on rat, guinea-pig, and canine intestinal motility. *Peptides* 9:1183, 1988.
537. Maggi CA, Patacchini R, Santicioli P: Human isolated small intestine: Motor responses of the longitudinal muscle to field stimulation and exogenous neuropeptides. *Naunyn Schmiedebergs Arch Pharmacol* 339:415, 1989.
538. Yau WM, Dorsett JA, Youther ML: Evidence for galanin as an inhibitory neuropeptide on myenteric cholinergic neurons in the guinea pig small intestine. *Neurosci Lett* 72:305, 1986.
539. Palmer JM, Schemann M, Tamura K, Wood JD: Galanin mimics slow synaptic inhibition in myenteric neurons. *Eur J Pharmacol* 124:379, 1986.
540. Tamura K, Palmer JM, Wood JD: Galanin suppresses nicotinic synaptic transmission in the myenteric plexus of guinea pig small intestine. *Eur J Pharmacol* 136:445, 1987.
541. Tamura K, Palmer JM, Winkelmann CK, Wood JD: Mechanism of action of galanin on myenteric neurons. *J Neurophysiol* 60:966, 1988.
542. McDonald TJ, Dupre J, Tatemoto K, Greenberg GR, et al: Galanin inhibits insulin secretion and induces hyperglycemia in dogs. *Diabetes* 34:192, 1985.
543. Amiranoff B, Lorinet AM, Laburthe M: Galanin inhibits somatostatin release by the rat islet cell tumor in culture, Rin-m. *Eur J Pharmacol* 191:401, 1990.
544. Kwok YN, Verchere CB, McIntosh CH, Brown JC: Effect of galanin on endocrine secretions from isolated perfused rat stomach and pancreas. *Eur J Pharmacol* 145:49, 1988.
545. Ahren B, Andren-Sandberg A, Nilsson A: Galanin inhibits amylase secretion from isolated rat pancreatic acini. *Pancreas* 3:559, 1988.
546. Powers MA, Pappas TN: Galanin is a potent inhibitor of pancreatic exocrine secretion. *Gastroenterology* 96:A398, 1989.
547. Yagci RV, Alptekin N, Zacharia S, Coy DH, et al: Galanin inhibits pancreatic amylase secretion in the pentobarbital-anesthetized rat. *Regul Pep* 34:275, 1991.
548. Takacs T, Hegyi P, Czako L, Balaspiri L, Lonovics J: Effects of galanin(1-16) on pancreatic secretion in anesthetized and conscious rats. *Res Exp Med (Berl)* 199:275, 2000.
549. Milewicz A, Bidzinska B, Mikulski E, Demissie M, Tworowska U: Influence of obesity and menopausal status on serum leptin, cholecystokinin, galanin and neuropeptide Y levels. *Gynecol Endocrinol* 14:196, 2000.
550. Narvaez JA, Diaz-Cabiale Z, Hedlund PB, Aguirre JA, et al: The galanin receptor antagonist M40 blocks the central cardiovascular actions of the galanin N-terminal fragment (1-15). *Eur J Pharmacol* 399:197, 2000.
551. Scott MK, Ross TM, Lee DH, Wang HY, et al: 2,3-Dihysro-dithin and–dithiepine-1,1,4,4-tetroxides: Small molecule non-peptide antagonists of the human galanin hGAL-1 receptor. *Bioorg Med Chem* 8:1383, 2000.
552. Kerr BJ, Cafferty WB, Gupta YK, Bacon A, et al: Galanin knockout mice reveal nociceptive deficits following peripheral nerve injury. *Eur J Neurosci* 12:793, 2000.
553. Wang D, Lundeberg T, Yu LC: Antinociceptive role of galanin in periaqueductal grey of rats with experimentally induced mononeuropathy. *Neuroscience* 96:767, 2000.
554. Oberndorfer S: Karzinoede Tumoren des Dunndarms. *Frankf Z Path (Wiesbaden)* 1:426, 1907.

555. Rosenberg JM, Welch JP: Ileal tumor causing carcinoid syndrome without hepatic metastases. *Arch Surg* 119:485, 1984.
556. Thorson A, Biorck G, Björkman G, Waldenström J: Malignant carcinoid of the small intestine with metasteses to the liver, valvular disease of the right side of the heart (pulmonary stenosis and tricuspid regurgitation with septal defects), peripheral vasomotor symptoms, bronchoconstrictions and an unusual type of cyanosis: A clinical and pathological syndrome. *Am Heart J* 47:795, 1954.
557. Feldman JM: Carcinoid tumors and the carcinoid syndrome. *Curr Probl Surg* 26:829, 1989.
558. Tomassetti P: Clinical aspects of carcinoid tumors. *Ital J Gastroenterol Hepatol* 2:S143, 1999.
559. Sandler M, Snow PJ: An atypical carcinoid tumour secreting 5-hydroxytryptophan. *Lancet* 1:137, 1958.
560. Koch CA, Azumi N, Furlong MA, Jha RC, et al: Carcinoid syndrome caused by an atypical carcinoid of the uterine cervix. *J Clin Endocrinol Metab* 84:4209, 1999.
561. Williams ED, Sandler M: The classification of carcinoid tumours. *Lancet* 1:238, 1963.
562. Modlin IM, Sandor A: An analysis of 8305 cases of carcinoid tumors. *Cancer* 79:813, 1997.
563. Cheek RC, Wilson H: Carcinoid tumors. *Curr Probl Surg* Nov:4, 1970.
564. Wiedenmann B, Huttner WB: Synaptophysin and chromogranins/secretogranins—widespread constituents of distinct types of neuroendocrine vesicles and new tools in tumor diagnosis. *Virchows Arch [B]* 58:95, 1989.
565. Huttner WB, Gerdes HH, Rosa P: The granin (chromogranin/secretogranin) family. *Trends Biochem Sci* 16:27, 1994.
566. Deftos LJ: Chromogranin A: Its role in endocrine function and as an endocrine and neuroendocrine tumor marker. *Endocr Rev* 12:181, 1991.
567. Simon JP, Aunis D: Biochemistry of the chromogranin A protein family. *Biochem J* 262:1, 1989.
568. O'Connor DT, Takiyyuddin MA, Cervenka JH, Parmer RJ, et al: Circulating chromogranin A as a diagnostic tool in clinical chemistry. *Acta Histochem* 38:27, 1990.
569. Woods HF, Bax HDS, Thorpe JAC, Smith JAR: Carcinoid tumors and the carcinoid syndrome, in O'Dorisio TM (ed): *Sandostatin in the Treatment of GEP Endocrine Tumors*. Berlin, Springer-Verlag, 1989, pp 15–22.
570. Makridis C, Theodorsson E, Akerstrom G, Oberg K, Knutson L: Increased intestinal non-substance P tachykinin concentrations in malignant midgut carcinoid disease. *J Gastroenterol Hepatol* 14:500, 1999.
571. Vinik AI, McLeod MK, Gig LM, Shapiro B, et al: Clinical features, diagnosis and localization of carcinoid tumors and their management. *Gastro Clin N Am* 18:865, 1989.
572. Douglas WW: Histamine and 5-hydroxytryptamine (serotonin) and their antagonists, in Gilman AG, Goodman LS, Gilman A (eds): *The Pharmacological Basis of Therapeutics*, 6th ed. New York, Macmillan, 1980, pp 609–646.
573. Nuttall KL, Pingree SS: The incidence of elevations in urine 5-hydroxyindoleacetic acid. *Ani Clin Lab Sci* 28:167, 1998.
574. Sjoerdsma A, Weissbach H, Terry LL, Udenfriend S: Further observations on patients with malignant carcinoid. *Am J Med* 23:5, 1957.
575. Sandler M, Scheuer P, Watt PJ: 5-hydroxytryptophan-secreting bronchial carcinoid tumor. *Lancet* 2:1067, 1961.
576. Norheim I, Theodorsson-Norheim LS, Brodin E, Oberg K: Tachykinins in carcinoid tumors: Their use as a tumor marker and possible role in the carcinoid flush. *J Clin Endocrinol Metab* 63:605, 1986.
577. Feldman JM, O'Dorisio TM: Role of neuropeptides and serotonin in the diagnosis of carcinoid tumors. *Am J Med* 81(Suppl 6B):41, 1986.
578. Vinik AI, Thompson N, Eckhauser F, Moattari AR: Clinical features of carcinoid syndrome and the use of somatostatin analogue in its management. *Acta Oncol* 28:389, 1989.
579. Norheim I, Oberg K, Theodorsson-Magnusson A, Wide L, Wilander E: Malignant carcinoid tumors. *An Surg* 206:115, 1987.
580. Feldman JM: Urinary serotonin in the diagnosis of carcinoid tumors. *Clin Chem* 32:840, 1986.
581. Oates JA, Roberts LJ II: Carcinoid syndrome, in Braunwald E, Isselbacher KJ, Petersdorf RJ, Wilson JD, Martin JB, Fauci AS (eds): *Harrison's Principles of Internal Medicine*, 11th ed. New York, McGraw-Hill, 1987, pp 1585–1588.
582. Norheim I, Theodorsson-Norheim E, Brodin E, Öberg K: Tachykinins in carcinoid tumors: Their use as a tumor marker and possible role in the carcinoid flush. *J Clin Endocrinol Metab* 63:605, 1986.
583. Norheim I, Theodorsson-Norheim E, Brodin E, Öberg K, et al: Antisera raised against eledoisin and kassinin detect elevated levels of immunoreactive material in plasma and tumor tissue from patients with carcinoid tumors. *Regul Pept* 9:245, 1984.
584. Öberg K, Grimelius L, Lundqvist G, Lörelius LE: Update on pancreatic polypeptide as a specific marker for endocrine tumors of the pancreas and gut. *Acta Med Scand* 210:145, 1981.
585. Öberg K, Wide L: hCG and hCG subunits as tumor markers in patients with endocrine pancreatic tumors and carcinoids. *Acta Endocrinol (Copenh)* 98:256, 1981.
586. Suzuki H, Ghatei MA, Williams SJ, Uttenthal LO, et al: Production of pituitary protein 7B2 immunoreactivity by endocrine tumors and its possible diagnostic value. *J Clin Endocrinol Metab* 63:758, 1986.
587. O'Connor DT, Deftos LJ: Secretion of chromogranin A by peptide-producing endocrine neoplasms. *N Engl J Med* 314:1145, 1986.
588. Öberg K, Theodorsson-Norheim E, Norheim I: Motilin in plasma and tumor tissues from patients with carcinoid syndrome. *Scand J Gastroenterol* 22:1041, 1987.
589. Bancks NH, Goldstein HM, Dodd GD: The roentgenologic spectrum of small intestinal carcinoid tumors. *AJR* 123:274, 1975.
590. Hulnick DH: Small intestine, in Megibow AJ, Balthazar EJ (eds): *Computed Tomography of the Gastrointestinal Tract*. St. Louis, Mosby, 1986, pp 257–259.
591. Kressel HY: Strategies for magnetic resonance imaging of focal liver disease. *Radiol Clin North Am* 26:607, 1988.
592. Oberg K: Carcinoid tumors: Current concepts in diagnosis and treatment. *Oncologist* 3:339, 1998.
593. Reubi JC, Maurer R, von Werder K, Torhorst J, et al: Somatostatin receptors in human endocrine tumors. *Cancer Res* 47:551, 1987.
594. Lamberts SWJ, Bakker WH, Reubi JC, Krenning EP: Somatostatin-receptor imaging in the localization of endocrine tumors. *N Engl J Med* 323:1246, 1990.
595. Patel YC: Somatostatin-receptor imaging for the detection of tumors. *N Engl J Med* 323:1274, 1990.
596. Warner RRP: Carcinoid, in Bardin CW (ed): *Current Therapy in Endocrinology and Metabolism*, 4th ed. Philadelphia, Decker, 1991, pp 491–496.
597. Arnold R: Therapeutic strategies in the management of endocrine GEP tumors. *Eur J Clin Invest* 20(Suppl 1):S82, 1990.
598. Gorden P: NIH Conference: Somatostatin and somatostatin analogue (SMS 201-995) in treatment of hormone-secreting tumors of the pituitary and gastrointestinal tract and non-neoplastic diseases of the gut. *Ann Intern Med* 110:35, 1989.
599. Ahlman H, Scherstén T, Tisell LE: Surgical treatment of patients with the carcinoid syndrome. *Acta Oncol* 28:403, 1989.
600. Kvols LK: Therapeutic considerations for the malignant carcinoid syndrome. *Acta Oncol* 28:433, 1989.
601. Moertel CG: Treatment of the carcinoid tumor and the malignant carcinoid syndrome. *J Clin Oncol* 1:727, 1983.
602. Sweeney JF, Rosemurgy AS: Carcinoid tumors of the gut. *Cancer Control* 4:18, 1997.
603. Kvols LK: Metastatic carcinoid tumors and the carcinoid syndrome: A selective review of chemotherapy and hormonal therapy. *Am J Med* 81(Suppl 6B):49, 1986.
604. Nobin A, Lindblom B, Månsson B, Sundberg M: Interferon treatment in patients with malignant carcinoids. *Acta Oncol* 28:445, 1989.
605. Roberts LJ II, Marney SR Jr, Oates JA: Blockade of the flush associated with metastatic gastric carcinoid by combined histamine H_1 and H_2 receptor antagonists: Evidence for an important role of H_2 receptors in human vasculature. *N Engl J Med* 300:236, 1979.
606. Antonsen S, Hansen MGJ, Bukhave K, Rask-Madsen J: Influence of a new selective 5-HT_2 receptor antagonist (ketanserin) on jejunal PGE_2 release and ion secretion due to malignant carcinoid syndrome. *Gut* 23:A887, 1982.
607. Wymenga AN, de Vries EG, Leijsma MK, Kema IP, Kleibeuker JH: Effects of ondansetron on gastrointestinal symptoms in carcinoid syndrome. *Eur J Cancer* 34:1293, 1998.
608. Oates JA: The carcinoid syndrome. *N Engl J Med* 315:702, 1986.
609. Saslow SB, O'Brien MD, Camilleri M, von der Ohe M, et al: Octreotide inhibition of flushing and colonic motor dysfunction in carcinoid syndrome. *Am J Gastroenterol* 92:2250, 1997.

610. Bakker WH, Krenning EP, Breeman WA: Receptor scintigraphy with a readioiodinated somatostatin, analog: Radiolabeling, purification, biological activity and in vivo application in animals. *J Nucl Med* 31:1501, 1990.
611. Maton PN: The use of the long-acting somatostatin analog, octreotide acetate, in patients with islet cell tumors. *Gastro Clin North Am* 18:897, 1989.
612. Oberg K, Norheim I, Theodorsson E: Treatment of malignant midgut carcinoid tumors with a long-acting somatostatin analogue octreotide. *Acta Oncologica* 30:503, 1991.
613. Fehmann HC, Wulbrand U, Arnold R: Treatment of endocrine gastroenteropancreatic tumors with somatostatin analogues. Recent Results. *Cancer Res* 153:15, 2000.
614. Oberg K, Erickson B: The role of interferons in the management of carcinoid tumors. *Acta Oncol* 30:519, 1991.
615. Shebani KO, Souba WW, Finkelstein DM, Stark PC, Elgadi KM, Tanabe KK, Ott MJ: Prognosis and survival in patients with gastrointestinal tract carcinoid tumors. *Ann Surg* 229:815, 1999.
616. Lauffer JM, Zhang T, Modlin IM: Review article: Current status of gastrointestinal carcinoids. *Aliment Pharmacol Ther* 13:271, 1999.
617. Davis Z, Moertel CG, McIlrath DC: The malignant carcinoid syndrome. *Surg Gynecol Obstet* 137:637, 1973.

CHAPTER 27

Multiglandular Endocrine Disorders

Leonard J. Deftos
Stephen I. Sherman
Robert F. Gagel

MULTIPLE ENDOCRINE NEOPLASIA TYPE 1 (MEN 1)

Definition and History

Since the first decade in this century, individuals have been recognized with tumors affecting multiple glands in various combinations.[1] Over time, consistent patterns of such tumors were found to occur in several members of affected families. From these observations, certain widely recognized hereditary syndromes of multiglandular endocrine neoplasia have emerged. These include multiple endocrine neoplasia type 1 (MEN 1), also known as the multiple endocrine adenomatosis (MEA)—peptic ulcer syndrome or Wermer's syndrome—and the two variants of multiple endocrine neoplasia type 2 (MEN 2), 2A and 2B, which are described later. It should be understood that not every example of polyglandular endocrine neoplasia fits one of these well-defined hereditary syndromes. As knowledge advances, it has been possible to delineate additional distinct genetic disorders manifested by various combinations of tumors of endocrine glands beyond the classic syndromes described in this chapter.

MEN 1 is an autosomal dominant disorder with a high degree of penetrance and some variability of expression. Affected individuals typically have tumors of the parathyroid and pituitary glands and enteropancreatic and carcinoid tumors; they may have other nonendocrine tumors as well.[1,2]

The recent identification of the MEN 1 gene has provided new insight into the molecular events leading to this syndrome and has made it possible to more clearly define the clinical features associated with a molecular defect of menin, the protein encoded by the *MEN 1* gene. MEN 1 will be defined as the clinical syndrome associated with loss of function mutations of the *MEN 1* gene.

The tissues involved in MEN 1 are summarized in Table 27-1. The early reports, which led to the recognition of this syndrome, were based on autopsy studies. Erdheim appears to have been the first to describe the appearance of more than one endocrine tumor in a single individual in his report of autopsy studies published in 1903.[3] In a subsequent autopsy study, Cushing and Davidoff reported thyroid, parathyroid, and adrenal hyperplasia in four acromegalic patients.[4] Lloyd described a case of "hypophyseo-parathyreo-insular syndrome" in 1929.[5] An early premortem description of patients with what would probably now be recognized as MEN 1 was published by Rossier and Dressler in 1939.[6] They reported sisters with multiple endocrine disorders whose brothers had peptic ulcer disease. These authors were apparently the first to recognize the familial nature of multiple endocrine neoplasia. The specific association among adenomas of the parathyroid glands, the pituitary, and the pancreatic islets was recognized by Underdahl et al.[7] in 1953 and by Moldawer et al.[8] in 1954. Current understanding of the syndrome is largely attributable to Wermer,[8] who in 1954 described the familial aggregation of multiple adenomas of these glands and proposed that they constituted a distinct syndrome inherited as an autosomal dominant disorder. He noted the association with peptic ulcer disease in these patients and suggested the possibility of a genetic relationship between the ulcer disease and the endocrine adenomatosis. In 1955, an independent investigation led Zollinger and Ellison to the recognition of the syndrome that bears their names.[9] They described the association of severe peptic ulcer disease and gastric hypersecretion with non-insulin–producing islet-cell tumors of the pancreas. It was subsequently recognized that the same syndrome may also be manifested by malabsorption or watery diarrhea.[10] It was gradually appreciated that the Zollinger-Ellison syndrome is produced by gastrin-secreting pancreatic neoplasms and can occur as a component of MEN syndrome along with insulinomas and parathyroid and pituitary tumors.[11–13]

The causative gene for this autosomal dominant syndrome was first mapped in 1988. Larsson and her colleagues mapped the gene to chromosome 11q and provided initial evidence for the tumor suppressor nature of the *MEN 1* gene.[14] Subsequent mapping studies by several groups refined the locus and the *MEN 1* gene was identified in 1997,[15] a finding subsequently confirmed by a second consortium.[16]

The clinical features of MEN 1 may be due to either the hypersecretion by one (or more) particular tumor or to the tumor mass and its infringement on adjacent tissues. In general, the tumors are small and benign and hormone hypersecretion accounts for the clinical syndrome, as exemplified by hyperparathyroidism. However, pituitary and pancreatic tumors, especially the former, can become clinically manifest through a mass effect. Those tumors with a substantial malignant potential, such as gastrinomas and certain carcinoids, account for one-third of the deaths in MEN 1.[17]

Components of the Syndrome

The approximate relative frequencies of the various glandular tumors constituting the MEN 1 syndrome are indicated in Table 27-2. This table is based on a large number of reports and reviews; it should be understood that generally uncommon associations may occur quite

TABLE 27-1. Major Components of MEN 1

Parathyroid tumors
Pituitary tumors
Enteropancreatic tumors
Adrenal cortical adenomas
Other tumors
Endocrine tumors
Nonendocrine tumors

frequently within particular pedigrees. As shown in the table, primary hyperparathyroidism is the most common manifestation of the syndrome, occurring in as many as 100 percent of affected individuals in some series.[18–20] The next most common site of involvement is the pancreatic islets. Several kinds of enteropancreatic lesions are generally recognized in this syndrome. They include insulinomas arising from the beta cells of the islets of Langerhans and gastrinomas of delta cell origin, which produce the Zollinger-Ellison syndrome. The pancreatic tumors are most often multifocal; they may appear as areas of hyperplasia rather than well-localized nodular adenomas, and either may become malignant. Pituitary adenomas are less common and include nonfunctional, prolactin, growth hormone, and ACTH-producing tumors. The pituitary tumors are rarely malignant.[1,2,21–24] The fourth major component of this syndrome are adrenal cortical adenomas.[25,26] In most cases these are nonfunctional and rarely become carcinomatous. As Table 27–2 indicates, adenomas of the other endocrine glands are much less common.

TABLE 27-2. Approximate Relative Frequencies of Components of the MEN 1 Syndrome[1,2]

	Frequency, Percent of Patients
Hyperparathyroidism	>87
Enteropancreatic tumors	
Gastrinomas	54
Benign	20
Malignant	30
Insulinomas	21
Benign	20
Malignant	5
Nonfunctioning	
Benign	<5
Malignant	<5
Other	
Endocrine	2
Nonendocrine	10
Pituitary tumors	
Chromophobe or nonfunctioning	
Benign	40
Malignant	<5
Eosinophilic or acromegalic (benign)	15
Cushing's disease, basophilic	5
Mixed and other types (benign)	<5
Prolactin-secreting	15
Other tumors	
Carcinoid and bronchial adenoma	<5
Lipoma/liposarcoma	5
Adrenal cortical adenoma	20–40
Thyroid adenomas	5
Angiofibromas of skin	88
Collagenomas of skin	72

Nonendocrine tumors can be a component of MEN 1, with lipomas, angiofibromas, and collagenomas occurring regularly in the affected members of most pedigrees.[27,28] The majority of MEN 1 cases are familial, but *de novo* mutations and coincidental occurrence of two sporadic tumors may also occur [1,29]

Primary Hyperparathyroidism

Primary hyperparathyroidism is the single most common feature of MEN 1, occurring in >90 percent of gene carriers.[30] It has become clear that although one or more of the parathyroid glands may appear at surgery to be normal, all these glands have the potential for neoplastic enlargement. If only one or two enlarged glands are removed at the time of the original operation, the likelihood of persistent or recurrent hyperparathyroidism is great.[30,31] Two treatment recommendations have evolved: subtotal parathyroidectomy[31] and total parathyroidectomy with autotransplantation.[32] Regardless of the approach there is a high probability of recurrent hyperparathyroidism; the major advantage of autotransplantation to the nondominant arm is the ease of removal of additional parathyroid tissue.

There has been considerable difference of opinion about the proper description of the pathologic process in these parathyroid glands. Although the contemporaneous enlargement of multiple glands has prompted some authors to use the term hyperplasia, others have preferred to use the term multiple adenomas. The latter term carries the implication that the neoplastic changes are primary processes which may arise concurrently but independently in the different glands; it is more in keeping with current theories of pathogenesis. From a pragmatic standpoint, the use of the term multiglandular primary hyperparathyroidism has considerable appeal.[2,33] Histologically, these glands are usually dominated by chief cells, but clear-cell dominance may be seen, as well as a mixed picture. Parathyroid carcinoma is uncommon. Patients with primary multiglandular hyperparathyroidism are fairly often found to have relatives with either familial primary hyperparathyroidism or MEN 1, but other conditions such as sporadic isolated primary multiglandular parathyroid disease,[34] the hyperparathyroidism-jaw tumor syndrome, or familial hypocalciuric hypercalcemia[35,36] may present with hypercalcemia.

Evidence has recently been reported of a circulating factor in the plasma of MEN 1 patients that acts as a mitogen on parathyroid cells.[37] This factor resembles basic fibroblast growth factor (bFGF).[38,39] There is also evidence for a clonal origin of neoplastic parathyroid cells in MEN 1.[40]

Many of the clinical features of primary hyperparathyroidism in MEN 1 are similar to those of the nonfamilial disease.[1] However, the genetic basis of the hyperparathyroidism in MEN 1 does present clinical differences.[1,2] Primary hyperparathyroidism has an earlier onset in MEN 1. Although sporadic hyperparathyroidism is a disease of the 5th to 7th decades, half of MEN 1 carriers manifest the disease by ages 18–25 and 90 percent by age 50.[30,41,42] Some carriers may not express the disease,[43] while others do by age 8.[41] Hyperparathyroidism in MEN 1 occurs equally in genders, while the sporadic disease occurs 2–3 times more commonly in females.

One example of interaction between separate components of the MEN 1 syndrome is the relationship between hyperparathyroidism and gastrinoma. It has been known for a number of years that calcium is a potent stimulus for gastrin secretion[44] and that hypergastrinemia associated with early Zollinger-Ellison syndrome in MEN 1 can be reversed by correction of hyperparathyroidism.[45]

The likely explanation for this observation became clear only recently when the calcium sensing receptor (CaR) was identified on the gastrin producing cell and shown to be linked to gastrin secretion.[46] More importantly, the recent linkage of the CaR to growth regulatory pathways in other cell types raises the possibility that the hypercalcemia may be a factor in stimulation of G cell neoplastic transformation.[47]

Enteropancreatic Tumors—Overview

Like parathyroid tumors, enteropancreatic neuroendocrine tumors develop at younger ages and in more sites in MEN 1 than in sporadic cases.[41,42] The enteropancreatic tumors in MEN 1 are usually multiple at the time of surgery.[48] Although primary hyperparathyroidism is often present when the enteropancreatic tumor becomes manifest in some cases of the Zollinger-Ellison syndrome, an insulinoma can be expressed first in MEN 1,[49] but not during childhood.

These enteropancreatic tumors may be too small to be imaged and thus present with symptoms of hormone excess rather than mass effects[50] Gastrinoma is the most common among the enteropancreatic tumors, with prevalence of up to 54 percent.[1,51] Insulinoma is second at 21 percent.[1,51] Glucagonoma, VIPoma, growth hormone releasing factor-secreting tumor, intestinal carcinoid, and somatostatinoma are less frequent.[52] MEN 1 patients can have more than one enteropancreatic neuroendocrine tumor. MEN 1 is found in approximately one-fifth of cases with Z-E syndrome, while 4 percent of patients have an insulinoma. Other hormone-producing tumors occur with a lower frequency.[51–53]

Nonfunctional pancreatic tumors are a major component of MEN 1. Nonfunctional is a misnomer because most produce pancreatic polypeptide.[54] Approximately 50 percent of MEN 1 pancreatic surgical specimens have multiple tumors,[48,55] and diffuse micronodules are usually present.[50] In one immunohistologic study of macro- and micro-nodules, positive staining was: pancreatic polypeptide, 26 percent; glucagon, 24 percent; insulin, 23 percent; gastrin, 4 percent; somatostatin, 4 percent; VIP, 0.5 percent; neurotensin, 0.5 percent; and no hormone, 18 percent.[56] The importance of diffuse islet hyperplasia or nesidioblastosis (islets budding from ducts) in the MEN 1 pancreas is unclear.[1]

Malignant Potential

The pancreatic tumors differ markedly from the other elements of the MEN 1 syndrome in that both functional and nonfunctional tumors may take a malignant course, with invasion and metastasis in as many as half of affected individuals in some series.[12,13,57]

Insulinoma

Insulinoma is a fairly common and often clinically striking feature of the MEN 1 syndrome, manifest in 10–20 percent of cases.[58] The mean age of onset is 30 years in MEN 1 compared to age 45 in sporadic cases.[2,58] This tumor arises from the beta cells of the islets of Langerhans; it secretes excessive amounts of insulin. Although there are multiple islet tumors, the insulinoma syndrome is usually caused by one hypersecreting adenoma, often the largest islet tumor.[59] The clinical presentation is similar to that seen with sporadic insulinomas; the principal features are hypoglycemia and its associated neuroglycopenic symptoms.[2,58] These symptoms may include seizures, loss of consciousness, and symptoms associated with the counter-regulatory response. Typically, patients have a constant sensation of hunger, and the hypoglycemia may be masked by a constant carbohydrate intake. These patients often have nightmares or other nocturnal symptoms when their carbohydrate intake is interrupted by sleep. They are frequently affected by marked weight gain and may have hypoglycemic symptoms when they attempt to restrict their caloric intake in order to lose weight. Insulinomas may be single or multiple and may be poorly demarcated.[60] The common occurrence of multiple insulinomas or nodular hyperplasia of the beta cells makes selective resection extremely difficult, and a subtotal pancreatectomy is frequently required.[61] Of all the components of the MEN 1 syndrome, insulinoma probably constitutes the most severe hazard to the patient because of the neurologic effects of hypoglycemia.[2]

The most reliable test for insulinoma is a monitored fast. Most patients will become symptomatically hypoglycemic by 48 hours with a glucose of 40 mg/dl; negative tests should be carried to 72 hours.[1] Insulin mediation of hypoglycemia is established by an insulin concentration above 6 μU/ml at the time of hypoglycemia.[1]

Insulinomas in MEN 1 are usually benign. Preoperative location can be done by selective arteriography with calcium infusion[60] or transhepatic venous sampling.[62,63] Small tumors are best localized by intraoperative ultrasound.[64–66] Octreotide radionuclide scanning has low sensitivity for insulinomas.[62] Approximately 15 percent of MEN 1 insulinomas recur late after surgery; this could be due to malignancy, incomplete resection, or a new insulinoma.

Gastrinoma

Gastrin-producing tumors, which are derived from the delta cells of the islets of Langerhans, may occur in patients with insulin-producing tumors; more often, though, patients are afflicted with only one or the other type of pancreatic tumor.[67] Although for some time the Zollinger-Ellison syndrome was treated as a completely separate entity, it is now recognized that individual patients may have the gastrinoma syndrome alone or as a feature of MEN 1.[2] The Zollinger-Ellison syndrome is likely to be diagnosed because of the severe symptoms of the ulcer diathesis, with gastric hypersecretion and/or secretory diarrhea and malabsorption. For this reason, it is often the presenting complaint of the index case in an affected family. It should be borne in mind that hyperparathyroidism may mimic or unmask the Zollinger-Ellison syndrome.[45,67,68]

The Zollinger-Ellison syndrome was initially described as a triad of (1) nonbeta islet cell tumor of the pancreas, (2) gastric acid hypersecretion, and (3) severe peptic ulcers of the stomach and small intestine, but the disease is now seen in milder forms.[1,9] The usual features of Zollinger-Ellison syndrome are due to gastrin's stimulation of acid secretion by the stomach. Gastrinomas are concentrated in the duodenum of MEN 1 patients, while 40 percent–80 percent of sporadic gastrinomas occur in the pancreas.[1] Additionally, most sporadic gastrinomas are solitary and large, while those in MEN 1 are multiple, small, and submucosal. MEN 1 gastrinomas may have lesser or similar malignant propensity than do sporadic tumors, but metastases can occur, and they can dominate the clinical picture.[1,69,70]

Glucagonomas

Glucagonomas are rare in MEN 1 (3 percent), with most cases occurring after age 40. They are often large and metastatic at presentation.[71] There have been several reports of pancreatic alpha cell tumors that secrete glucagon, usually in association with a distinctive rash, termed migratory necrolytic erytema.[1,72,73] A kindred has been reported with glucagonoma and MEN 1.[74] There have also been reports of pancreatic tumors that secrete somatostatin as well as glucagon.[1,74]

Vipoma

Pancreatic tumors secreting vasoactive intestinal peptide, also called vipomas, have been reported with MEN 1. Such tumors produce a clinical picture of pancreatic cholera,[75] sometimes called the Verner-Morrison syndrome or WDHA syndrome for watery diarrhea, hypokalemia, and achlorhydria.[10] Most tumors are pancreatic, but they can also occur in association with intestinal carcinoids or pheochromocytomas.[76] Like glucagonomas, VIPomas usually present after age 40 and are large and metastatic. Hypercalcemia, whose etiology is unclear, may occur in up to 50 percent of cases.[76]

GRFoma

GRFoma is a rare tumor producing growth hormone-releasing factor (GRF or GHRH) that stimulates the pituitary to release excessive growth hormone.[77] Approximately one-third of GRFomas are associated with MEN 1.[78] GRFomas occur in the lung (53 percent), pancreas (30 percent), or small intestine (10 percent), and are often large and metastatic at presentation.[1,77,78] The diagnosis of GRFoma is made by demonstrating an increased serum GH and GHRH.[1,52,78]

Somatostatinomas

Somatostatin-secreting pancreatic tumors produce mild diabetes mellitus, gall bladder disease, weight loss, and anemia, because of somatostatin's respective inhibition of bile flow and gall bladder contractility, pancreatic secretion, and absorption of lipids, vitamin B12, and folate.[74,79] Although associated with MEN 1 (or with MEN 2), their prevalence in an MEN 1 population is very low.[1,55,79]

Ppomas and Nonfunctional Pancreatic Endocrine Tumors

Ppomas are pancreatic tumors that oversecrete pancreatic polypeptide.[80] Although they are common in MEN 1[54,81,82] they do not cause a recognizable endocrine syndrome. Nonfunctional tumors either do not produce a hormonal peptide or do not secrete enough to cause a recognizable syndrome.[79,81,83] However, these tumors can cause symptoms by local or metastatic growth.

Pituitary Tumors

Pituitary tumors are manifest in 10–30 percent of MEN 1 patients.[1] They can be functioning or nonfunctioning.

Chromophobe Adenomas

A variety of functional and histologic types of pituitary tumors have been described in association with multiple endocrine neoplasia. Historically, the most commonly described tumor type appears to be the nonfunctioning chromophobe adenoma.[1,2] Although these tumors do not produce hormones, they may cause significant endocrine effects when their mass impinges on normal pituitary cells and interferes with the hypothalamic-pituitary axis. It now appears that a number of the reported "nonfunctional" tumors may well have been prolactinomas.[84,85] In fact, patients from the family originally studied by Wermer were reevaluated and were found to have evidence of prolactinomas.[85]

Functioning Pituitary Adenomas

In addition to reports of chromophobe adenomas, there have been a substantial number of reports of acromegaly caused by eosinophilic pituitary adenomas.[1,86] There have also been reports of Cushing's syndrome in MEN 1, most caused by pituitary tumors, although pancreatic tumor cells also may secrete adrenocorticotropic hormone (ACTH).[87] Although precocious puberty has been described in endocrine polyneoplasia,[88] gonadotropin-secreting pituitary adenomas have not been demonstrated in the MEN 1 syndrome.[1]

The majority of pituitary tumors are prolactinomas (40–75 percent) with approximately 10 percent secreting prolactin and growth hormone, 10 percent growth hormone only, and 5 percent ACTH.[86,87] Numerous series document that prolactinomas are the most common pituitary tumor in the MEN 1 syndrome.[84–86] The possibility that hyperprolactinemia was caused by the tumor mass interfering with the transfer of hypothalamic prolactin inhibitory factor to the appropriate pituitary cells has not been rigorously excluded in every case. In several cases, however, it has been demonstrated by immunohistolochemistry and electron microscopy that the pituitary tumor cells contain prolactin.[23,89]

Other Associations

Lipomas

Lipomas seem especially common in MEN 1 involving 20–35 percent of cases.[27] They can be single or multiple and occur anywhere, including large visceral lipomas. In certain kindreds[13] lipomas are closely associated with the more typical features of parathyroid, pituitary, and pancreatic tumors. The lipomas may be small and few in number or may be large and quite prominent.[27,28] In kindreds in which lipomas occur, they are often a useful sign, indicating which members will be affected.[88] Recent studies have demonstrated loss of heterozygosity at the MEN 1 locus in lipomas (likely loss of the normal MEN 1 allele), indicating that lipomas have a similar method of tumor formation as do other components of the MEN 1 syndrome.[90,91]

Bronchial Adenomas and Carcinoid Tumors

Several types of carcinoid tumors are associated with MEN 1. Thymic and bronchial carcinoid tumors are uncommon and have a later age of onset than other manifestations of this syndrome. The improved management of other components of this clinical syndrome and attendant improvement in longevity has made these tumors more of a clinical problem than was reported 2 decades ago.[92,93] Thymic carcinoids are uncommon and approximately 25 percent of all reported cases are associated with MEN 1.[94,95] There is increasing concern about thymic malignancy, particularly in males, in the context of MEN 1, and some recommend thymectomy at the time of parathyroid surgery.[96,97] Allelic loss at the MEN 1 locus has been identified in a high percentage of MEN 1-related carcinoid tumors.[94,98] The third type of carcinoid tumor is a gastric or duodenal wall gastrin-producing carcinoid tumor that is the most common cause of Zollinger-Ellison syndrome in MEN 1. This carcinoid variant was discussed in an earlier section.

Adrenal Cortical Adenomas

Adrenocortical nodules may be found in half of MEN 1 gene carriers.[25,26] Generally, they are nonfunctional and do not appear to cause any clinical symptoms. There have been rare case reports of cortisol and aldosterone-producing adrenocortical adenomas and hyperplasia in association with the MEN 1 syndrome.[13]

Thyroid Adenomas

Some patients with MEN 1 have been noted to have thyroid hyperplasia or follicular adenomas.[4,12,13] These are nonfunctioning lesions that may occur in as many as 50 percent of carefully examined autopsy specimens from unselected subjects.[99] Therefore, the significance of these findings in MEN 1 is questionable. Hyperthyroidism has only rarely been associated with cases of MEN, and its etiologic relationship to MEN 1 is uncertain.[2]

Other Associated Tumors

Renal adenomas or carcinomas, and leiomyomas have been reported as incidental findings in patients with other endocrine tumors.[13,100] It is particularly important to interpret the older reports with care because of the uncertain relationship of many of those cases to what is now recognized as the MEN 1 syndrome. Unilateral pheochromocytoma has been reported in at least 10 cases of familial MEN 1[1,29] and this possibility should be considered in the differential diagnosis of an adrenal nodule. Several types of skin lesions have been reported in MEN 1, including multiple facial angiofibromas in 88 percent, collagenomas in 72 percent, confetti-like hypopigmented macules in 6 percent, and multiple gingival papules in 6 percent.[1,27] These latter have findings been reported with tuberous sclerosis.[1]

Clinical Evaluation

Patient Evaluation

There are two principal settings in which diagnostic studies are likely to be undertaken.[1,2] A patient may appear with the clinical features of one or more of the component disorders and therefore be evaluated for other features of the syndrome, or asymptomatic subjects may be investigated because of their familial relationship to a patient with the disorder.

Patients may present with common problems such as nephrolithiasis or other features of hyperparathyroidism, peptic ulcer disease, or symptoms of hypoglycemia. They may have manifestations of pituitary tumors as headaches, visual field disturbances, amenorrhea, impotence, secondary hypothyroidism, or evidence of pituitary hyperfunction as in acromegaly. In the absence of suggestive clinical signs or symptoms or a suspicious family history, patients with typical primary hyperparathyroidism have a very low risk of developing MEN 1.[29,101]

In patients with positive family histories, multiglandular parathyroid involvement, or symptoms or signs of other glandular tumors, the risk is greater.[29] In such cases, the diagnostic yield is great enough to justify investigation to determine whether other components of the MEN 1 syndrome are present. Fortunately, such an assessment is fairly easily carried out. Determination of the serum calcium level should be made in order to detect hyperparathyroidism. Hypergastrinemia is usually symptomatic, and determination of the serum gastrin level or gastric acid secretion, perhaps employing a calcium or secretin stimulation test,[44] (secretin is no longer available in the U.S.) helps exclude or confirm the diagnosis of Zollinger-Ellison syndrome. The diagnosis of Zollinger-Ellison syndrome can be problematic in patients with hyperparathyroidism because hypercalcemia may cause hypergastrinemia and increased gastric acid secretion, mimicking gastrinoma (see Chap. 26). For this reason, it has been recommended that definitive evaluation for gastrinoma be carried out after parathyroidectomy in such cases. Some investigators have found that a calcium stimulation or secretin test generally provides adequate discrimination between gastrinoma and the effects of hyperparathyroidism,[102] although others have disagreed.[40] Most reports indicate that extremely high gastrin levels can usually be attributed to a gastrinoma, although hypercalcemia causes amplification of gastrin secretion. The use of a standard test meal, with pancreatic polypeptide levels determined before and during the meal, has reportedly been useful in diagnosing pancreatic tumors in patients with MEN 1.[54]

Although x-ray examination of the sella turcica may be a generally satisfactory method of ascertaining whether pituitary enlargement has occurred, this methodology has been replaced by MRI.[1] Imaging procedures of the sella for screening purposes are necessary only if there is other evidence of pituitary dysfunction or if the patient or a relative is known to have MEN 1. Serum prolactin levels should be measured in both men and women. Evaluation of the adrenal glands is indicated only in rare cases in which there appears to be abnormal adrenal function. Thyroid nodules may be detected by means of palpation of the gland. The benign nature of the thyroid lesions reported with MEN 1 should not distract the physician from proper evaluation of any thyroid nodule for possible malignancy. It is generally not necessary to screen patients or relatives for disorders only rarely associated with this syndrome unless there is a specific reason for suspecting such abnormalities.

Family Evaluation

Initial Evaluation

Once it has been determined that the proband has two or more of the typical components of the MEN syndrome, family studies should be carried out; such studies may also be indicated in patients with multiglandular parathyroid disease alone or a multifocal insulinoma.[2] It should be realized that a family evaluation is a detailed and often difficult process.

There is currently disagreement about the role of genetic testing for screening of potential MEN 1 kindreds. In kindreds where there is a family history of endocrine neoplasms, genetic analysis is likely to identify a mutation of the MEN 1 gene. In such kindreds subsequent screening of the kindred will be greatly facilitated by this information.[29] In contrast, analysis for germline MEN 1 mutations in a kindred with no family history is less likely to be fruitful and may not be cost-effective. There are currently few commercial sources for MEN 1 genetic testing because of its rarity and the necessity to screen the entire gene for inactivating mutations. Nonetheless, identification of a specific MEN 1 gene mutation in a kindred greatly simplifies subsequent screening efforts because 50 percent of kindred members can be excluded from biochemical testing on the basis of a negative genetic test. In the remaining family members, repeated evaluation is required because individuals may appear to be normal when first studied but develop abnormalities some years later.

The first step is a meticulous review of the family members' medical histories, searching for manifestations that the family may be able to recall, such as kidney stones, peptic ulcers, low blood sugar, and premature menopause. Considerations of compliance, time, and cost require that screening be performed simply, quickly, and cheaply. Physical examination, determinations of serum calcium and prolactin concentrations and fasting blood sugar level, and x-ray examination of the sella turcica, together with the review of the medical history, generally constitute an adequate screening examination. In most reported kindreds, primary hyperparathyroidism has been a consistent feature of MEN 1, found in 90–100 percent of gene carriers by the age of 40.[18–20] Therefore, measurement of the serum calcium concentration in first degree relatives of the affected patient, particularly those over the age of 20 years, will generally provide a sufficient level of screening. There are rare kindreds in which prolactinoma is the primary clinical manifestation; if this variant is suspected, the addition of a serum prolactin to the screening protocol may be indicated.[103] More distant relatives require investigation if there are historical or clinical findings suggestive of the disorder or if findings indicating MEN 1 are present in intermediate relatives.

Further Evaluation

Once the diagnosis of MEN 1 has been established in a family, the occurrence of any one feature of this disorder in an individual family member provides presumptive evidence of the genetic disease. It is important that relatives of the propositus understand that negative tests at the initial evaluation do not exclude the possibility of future development of features of the disease. Furthermore, members of such families should understand that often the tumors do not develop concurrently and that another organ may be affected years after the treatment of the initial tumor.

Differential Diagnosis

In addition to MEN type 2, discussed subsequently, the other disorders that should be considered in the differential diagnosis are summarized in Table 27-3. They are discussed in detail elsewhere.[1]

Epidemiology

Inheritance of MEN 1 follows an autosomal dominant pattern; thus, approximately equal numbers of males and females are affected.[1,2] The degree of penetrance is quite high, although the expression is variable; the pattern, or combination, of adenomas may differ between family members. Therefore, the family history is usually strongly positive, and screening of the relatives of affected individuals is highly productive. This disorder has been found in both white and black families in North America and in families from Europe and Central America as well.[1]

The prevalence of MEN 1 in the general population is estimated at 2.5 per 1,000 by autopsy studies and 0.01–0.175 by biochemical tests.[1,86,104] Its apparent prevalence has been steadily increasing owing to the increased awareness of this syndrome and the improvement in diagnostic methods. The frequency of MEN 1 appears to be sufficient to warrant a screening investigation in patients who present with any of the typical features.

TABLE 27-3. Other Disorders Affecting Multiple Endocrine Glands

McCune-Albright syndrome
Sexual precocity
Hyperthyroidism
Growth hormone oversecretion
Adrenal hyperfunction
Carney complex
Bilateral adrenal hypersecretion
Acromegaly
Testicular tumors
Thyroid tumors
Von Hippel-Lindau syndrome
Pheochromocytoma
Pancreatic tumors and cysts
Prolactinomas
Carcinoid tumors
Medullary thyroid carcinoma
Neurofibromatosis type 1
Pheochromocytoma
Hyperparathyroidism
Adrenal adenoma
Radiation-induced parathyroid and thyroid tumors
MEN 1 and MEN 2 in a single patient[1,104]

Familial diseases that affect a single gland are less likely to be a diagnostic problem.

MEN in Other Species

Endocrine polyneoplasia with a pattern similar to that of MEN 1 in humans has been observed in a variety of species, but spontaneously occurring examples are extremely rare.[105] Quite a high incidence has been observed in irradiated rats,[106] suggesting that multiple somatic mutations are present in irradiated animals.

Pathogenesis

In his landmark paper in 1954, Wermer[107] demonstrated the autosomal dominant inheritance of this syndrome. He postulated that the heritable abnormality is in a gene responsible for regulation of the growth of the affected glands. The gene for MEN 1 was localized to chromosome 11 in 1988 and shown to be a tumor suppressor gene.[14] In MEN 1 there is most commonly a germline inactivating mutation of the allele inherited from the affected parent (Fig. 27-1). Transformation occurs somatically when the normal copy is inactivated in a single cell through deletion or inactivation (Fig. 27-1).

Continuous refinement of the chromosomal region containing the MEN 1 gnee led to its identification in 1997.[15] It is a 9kb gene containing 10 exons that encodes a 610-amino acid protein named "menin" (Fig. 27-2).[15] The protein does not have other known human homologies. Menin has two nuclear localization domains near its carboxyterminus and recent studies have shown that it interacts with Jun D, a nuclear trancription factor.[108] Members of this class of transcription factor are important in the regulation of transcription of many genes and interaction of menin with Jun D suppressed its transcriptional activity in an in vitro transcription model.[109] It is currently unclear how inactivation of menin leads to unregulated and specific growth of certain types of neuroendocrine cells.

Sporadic tumors of the type found in MEN 1 may also have mutations of the MEN 1 gene. Two-thirds of menin germline and somatic mutations predict protein truncation and are likely inactivating mutations (Fig. 27-3). Only one large deletion has been reported to date,[110] excluding menin function as a dominant negative.

More than 100 different germline MEN 1 mutations are spread over 9 coding exons (Fig. 27-2),[1] and there is only limited clustering of mutations.[16,111–114] Thus testing is complex because it cannot be directed at several bases or several exons and requires sequencing or other screening approaches that analyze the entire gene (Fig. 27-3). Within a family or in a population with a founder effect, identification of the specific mutation will greatly simplify

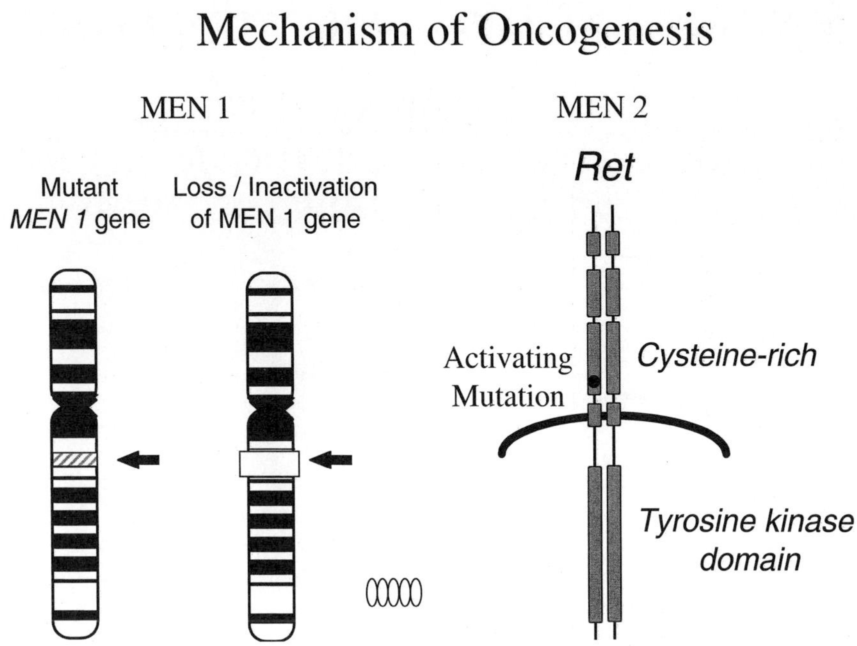

FIGURE 27-1. Mechanisms of transformation in multiple endocrine neoplasia types 1 (MEN 1) and 2 (MEN 2). In MEN 1 there is a germline mutation of the MEN 1 gene inherited from the affected parent. Loss of the normal MEN 1 allele occurs in a single cell somatically and generally results from either a large deletion or loss of part or all of a chromosome during mitosis. In contrast the mutations of the *RET* proto-oncogene found in MEN 2 activate the mitogen-activated protein kinase pathways that regulate cell growth.

screening because restriction analysis, denaturing gradient gel electrophoresis, or sequencing of a single exon provide more direct screening approaches.[15,108,110,112] Genetic testing is currently available only in academic research laboratories, but it seems likely that this type of testing will become available commercially as the technology for analysis of large genes improves.

Diagnosis

Members of MEN 1 kindreds with a positive genetic test or those who have not received genetic testing should undergo periodic biochemical testing, beginning by age 15 or as early as age 8.[1] Individuals with a negative genetic test can be excluded from further screening, although it is prudent to repeat the genetic test twice to exclude sample mix-up or technical error. Testing is dictated by clinical importance, cost, and local availability. A practical panel would include serum calcium, parathyroid hormone, and prolactin, repeated approximately every two years.[1] Although a patient who does not convert to a positive test by age 30 has about a 10 percent likelihood of being a gene carrier, testing should be continued indefinitely until a maximal age for conversion to a positive test has been determined.[43] Patients with established MEN 1

FIGURE 27-2. Mutations of the MEN 1 gene. The MEN 1 gene maps to chromosome 11q13. More than 100 mutations, mostly inactivating, have been identified in kindreds with MEN 1.

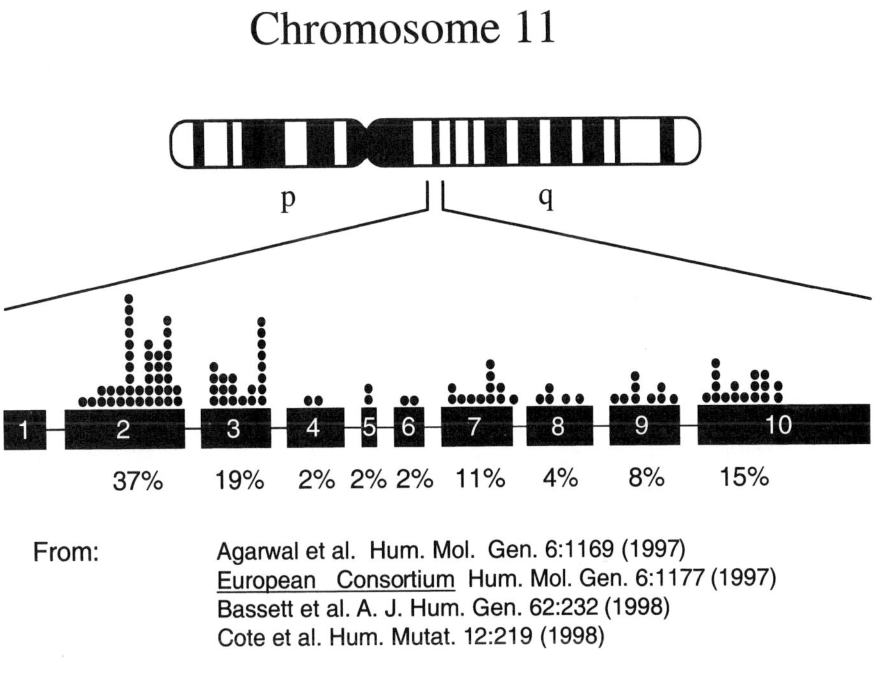

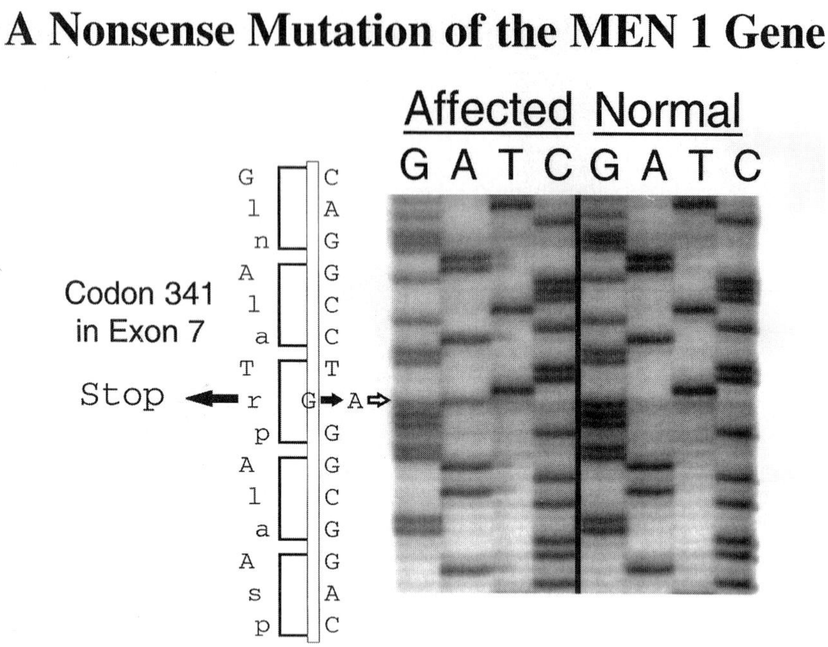

FIGURE 27-3. Detection of a mutation of the MEN 1 gene. DNA sequence shows normal exon 7 (right sequencing panel) and sequence from normal and mutant allele (left sequencing panel). The mutant DNA sequence changes a tryptophan to a stop codon, thereby creating an inactive protein. Other members of this kindred with MEN 1 were also found to harbor this mutant sequence.

should undergo periodic testing to monitor for the development of new endocrinopathies and the recurrence of treated disorders.[1,86]

Relation to Other Syndromes

A small number of cases have been reported in which patients had elements associated with MEN 1 and other elements associated with MEN 2.[86,115–120] In some of these cases, the findings reported were not diagnostic for the syndrome to which they were ascribed. In other cases, certain major features of both categories of MEN were present. However, these reports do not describe co-occurrence of two or more of the distinguishing diagnostic features of each syndrome (e.g., a patient with medullary thyroid carcinoma and pheochromocytoma as well as an islet cell tumor and a pituitary adenoma). The lack of evidence for inheritance of these atypical combinations is consistent with sporadic occurrence. A kindred with islet cell tumors and pheochromocytoma has, on more careful evaluations, been found to have von Hippel Lindau syndrome.[121]

Management

The management of the component disorders of MEN is presented in detail in other chapters. There are, however, some special considerations when these disorders occur in cases of MEN 1. In general, surgical treatment is the basis of management.[1,86]

Parathyroid

When parathyroidectomy is undertaken, it must be borne in mind that the patient has (or will have) multiglandular involvement. Subtotal parathyroidectomy (3½ glands) is one of the preferred surgical procedures,[31,122] even though gross enlargement may not be obvious in all parathyroid glands.[31] Recurrent hyperparathyroidism occurs in more than 60 percent of patients treated by this method. If a less extensive procedure is performed, the likelihood of persistence or recurrence of hyperparathyroidism approaches 100 percent. If a patient with a small remnant of one gland again develops hyperparathyroidism, completion of a total parathyroidectomy and autotransplantation to the nondominant arm should be considered. Total parathyroidectomy and autografting of parathyroid tissue (e.g., to the forearm) is a useful procedure for primary managment of hyperparathyroidism in MEN 1.[32] Total parathyroidectomy and autotransplantation is associated with a lower incidence of recurrent hyperparathyroidism and the operative procedure for recurrent disease, removal of a portion of the transplanted tissue, is much easier. The incidence of permanent hypoparathyroidism for subtotal parathyroidectomy is as high as 24 percent[31] and as high as 36 percent for total parathyroidectomy with autotransplantation.[122] A second indication for parathyroid surgery, hypergastrinemia, or Zollinger-Ellison Syndrome, will be discussed later in the section on gastrinoma.

Pituitary

The most common pituitary tumor in MEN 1 is a prolactinoma. Current managment approaches for prolactinoma in MEN 1 do not differ from recommendations for sporadic prolactinomas (see Chapter 7). Dopamine agonist therapy remains the primary therapeutic modality. Long-term experience shows that prolactinomas can be controlled successfully with first- or second-generation dopaminergic agents. Unresponsive tumors may contain elements that are derived from other cell lineages besides the lactotropic cells.

Transsphenoidal hypophysectomy advances have improved steadily during the past 2 decades and have made the management of pituitary neoplasms by an experienced neurosurgeon much safer and more reliable than was previously the case.[2] In patients with minimal suprasellar extension of a pituitary tumor, a trial of dopamine agonist therapy may result in a significant reduction or disappearance of the pitutiary tumor. In patients with visual field abnormalities, it may be appropriate to try a short-term course of dopamine agonist therapy, but in most cases a surgical approach should be considered.

Acromegaly is the second most common clinical pituitary tumor syndrome associated with MEN 1. In cases where there is a high probability of surgical cure, transsphenoidal surgery is the preferred surgical approach. Primary therapy with octreotide or lanreotide with or without surgery or radiotherapy is being debated for treatment of large growth hormone secreting tumors where the probability of surgical cure is low (see Chap. 7). There is general agreement that normalization of the IGF-1 level is desirable because of the potential that elevated levels of this growth factor could contribute to tumor development in other organs.

The differential diagnosis of acromegaly in the context of MEN 1 should include a growth hormone-releasing hormone producing tumor, most commonly carcinoid or pancreatic islet cell tumors.[123] Although such tumors are uncommon causes of sporadic acromegaly,[52] it is relatively more common in the context of MEN 1 and provides another example of how a hormonal product produced by one tumor can stimulate growth of another manifestation.

Cushing's syndrome caused by an ACTH producing pituitary tumor is the third most common pituitary-related clinical syndrome. Management of pituitary Cushing's disease in the context of MEN 1 does not differ from that described for the sporadic variety (see Chapter 7).

Finally, nonfunctional pituitary tumors, those most commonly producing the alpha subunit of the glycoprotein hormones, are managed by a combination of surgery and radiotherapy.

Gastrinoma

There has been an evolution in thought regarding management of Zollinger-Ellison syndrome in the context of MEN 1. Following the identification of this clinical syndome in the 1950s management of the Zollinger-Ellison syndrome was largely based on total gastrectomy.[9] Subsequently attempts were made to resect gastrinomas,[124] efforts that were associated with low success rates.[125,126] The combination of low surgical success rates and the development of pharmacologic therapy to reduce gastric acid secretion (H_2 receptor antagonists and proton pump inhibitors) resulted in a recommendation for medical treatment of gastrinoma.[127] The subsequent recognition that the majority of MEN 1 Zollinger-Ellison cases were caused by duodenal wall carcinoid-like tumors[128–130] has led to operative strategies for resection of both duodenal wall and pancreatic islet tumors,[131–133] although the long-term impact of these approaches on cure and survival remain controversial.[69]

Gastrinoma should be considered in any MEN 1 patient with consistent symptoms, and fasting gastrin should be measured periodically in asymptomatic MEN 1 patients older than age 20. Fasting and stimulated gastrin are the most useful test.[51,53] Documentation of fasting gastric pH above 3.0 in a patient not taking acid blocking medications can exclude Zollinger-Ellison syndrome. Virtually all cases have high fasting gastrin,[2] and acid-blocking drugs with drug-induced hypergastrinemia should be excluded.[69] The Zollinger-Ellison syndrome can be attenuated by successful parathyroidectomy, although it is not known if the growth of the gastrinomas slows.[134]

Most patients have a gastrin above 1,000 pg/ml. If gastric acid is below pH 3.0, the diagnosis is established. Provocative testing for hypergastrinemia can be used in uncertain cases. Stimulants have included secretin, calcium infusion, and a standardized meal, with the most effective being secretin (no longer commercially available in the United States). An increase of serum gastrin greater than 200 pg/ml is considered diagnostic.[53,135] Management combines acid control and tumor evaluation best by imaging with radioactive pentetreotide, which can be useful to distinguish local from metastatic gastrinoma.[136]

Insulinoma

Insulinomas are often multiple in the MEN 1 syndrome, usually requiring a subtotal or nearly total pancreatectomy for adequate resection.[1,86] In cases of metastatic insulinomas and other instances in which adequate resection is not possible, or for interim management, diazoxide,[137] glucagon,[138] octreotide, or chemotherapy with streptozotocin[139] or other combinations[140,141] may be helpful. In both gastrinoma and insulinoma, resection of the tumor is important, if it can be accomplished, because of the malignant potential of the pancreatic tumors as well as their endocrine effects.

Although there are multiple islet tumors, the insulinoma syndrome is usually due to one hypersecreting adenoma, often the largest islet tumor.[59] The most reliable test is a monitored fast. Most patients will become symptomatically hypoglycemic by 48 hours with a glucose of 40 mg/dl; negative tests should be carried to 72 hours.[1,59,86] Insulin mediation of hypoglycemia is established by an insulin concentration above 6 μU/ml at the time of hypoglycemia.[142]

The most important general considerations in the management of MEN 1 are recognition of other elements of the syndrome in patients who present with one of its components and awareness of the implications for the families of patients with this heritable disease.[1,86,143]

MULTIPLE ENDOCRINE NEOPLASIA TYPE 2 (MEN 2)

Multiple endocrine neoplasia type 2 (MEN 2) is a second autosomal dominant hereditary syndrome, clearly separable from MEN 1. Medullary thyroid carcinoma (MTC), a neoplasm derived from calcitonin producing or C cells, is found in more than 90 percent of gene carriers, pheochromocytoma in approximately one-half, and hyperparathyroidism in 10–20 percent. This syndrome was first identified in 1961 when Sipple presented evidence for an association between pheochromocytoma and thyroid tumor.[144] He reported the case of a 33-year-old male with bilateral pheochromocytomas and a poorly differentiated invasive thyroid tumor thought to be a follicular adenocarcinoma. Sipple reviewed the literature and presented five other patients with pheochromocytoma and thyroid tumor. The pheochromocytomas were bilateral in four of the patients. The thyroid tumors were variously described as follicular adenocarcinoma, papillary adenocarcinoma, adenocarcinoma, and anaplastic carcinoma.

In the early 1960s there were additional case reports of the simultaneous occurrence of pheochromocytomas and thyroid carcinomas (reviewed by Deftos[86]). In 1967 Williams reported 2 cases of pheochromocytomas and thyroid cancer; he reviewed 15 others.[145] He was able to establish that at least 11 of the total of 17 cases of thyroid tumor actually were MTC. In the same year Schimke and Hartmann[146] also reviewed the previous reports of the simultaneous occurrence of pheochromocytoma and MTC and added their own studies of two families in which these two tumors occurred simultaneously in each of five patients.[146]

Since Sipple's original description <40 years ago this syndrome has received disproportionate attention because of the fascinating clinical presentations and its genetic underpinnings. Studies that have defined its natural history, strategies for early detection and treatment, and more recently the successful effort to

TABLE 27-4. Multiple Endocrine Neoplasia Type 2 (MEN 2)

Multiple endocrine neoplasia type 2A (MEN 2A)
Medullary thyroid carcinoma (100 percent)
Pheochromocytoma (50 percent)
Parathyroid neoplasia (10–20 percent)
Variants of MEN 2A
MEN 2A with cutaneous lichen amyloidosis (MEN 2A/CLA)
MEN 2A with Hirschsprung disease
Familial medullary thyroid carcinoma (FMTC)
Multiple endocrine neoplasia type 2B
Medullary thyroid carcinoma (100 percent)
Pheochromocytoma (50 percent)
No parathyroid disease
Marfanoid habitus (nearly 100 percent)
Intestinal ganglioneuromatosis and mucosal neuromas (nearly 100 percent)

identify the causative gene have not only led to the elucidation of several new biological pathways, but have improved outcomes.

The current categorization of MEN 2 is shown in Table 27-4. There are three broad categories of MEN 2: MEN 2A, Familial MTC, and MEN 2B. Medullary thyroid carcinoma is the unifying feature of these subtypes and is seen in all forms.

MEN 2A or Sipple's syndrome is the association of MTC, pheochromocytomas (50 percent), and hyperparathyroidism (10–20 percent). Several rare variants of MEN 2A have been described: MEN 2A with Hirschsprung's disease[147] and MEN 2A with cutaneous lichen amyloidosis, a pruritic skin lesion located on the upper back.[148,149] MEN 2B is the association of medullary thyroid carcinoma, unilateral or bilateral pheochromocytomas, oral and gastrointestinal neuromas, and features of Marfan's syndrome such as pectus abnormalities, long and thin digits, and long arms and legs.[150] Familial medullary thyroid carcinoma (FMTC) is a clinical syndrome in which gene carriers develop only medullary thyroid carcinoma without other manifestations of MEN 2.[151] MEN 2A and FMTC most often occur in the context of a kindred, although clearly defined *de novo* mutations have been described.[152,153] In contrast, MEN 2B most often occurs as a *de novo* mutation, although a number of kindreds exhibit autosomal dominant transmission.[154–156]

The availability of large and well-defined families with hereditary MTC made this disorder an early target for gene mapping studies. The causative gene was mapped to chromosome 10q in 1987[157,158] and mutations of the *RET* proto-oncogene were identified in 1993 (Fig. 27-4).[159,160] The *RET* proto-oncogene encodes a tyrosine kinase receptor and in combination with a second extracellular protein (GFR-α)[161] forms a receptor for a small peptide important for neuronal survival, glial cell-derived neurotrophic factor (GDNF) (Fig. 27-4).[162]

RET mutations affect two broad regions of the tyrosine kinase receptor. The most common affect a cysteine-rich extracellular domain important for dimerization of the receptor and change a cysteine to another amino acid at codons 609, 611, 618, 620, 630, or 634 (Fig. 27-4).[159,160] Intracellular mutations affect codons 768,[163] 790, 791,[164] 804,[165] 883,[166,167] 891,[168,169] 918,[170] and 922 (Fig. 27-4). Approximately 80 percent of all mutations occur at codon 634 and a substitution of cysteine to arginine accounts for approximately 50 percent of all mutations.[171] Mutations at codons 609, 611, 618, and 620 account for 10–15 percent of all mutations and a met 918 thr substitution accounts for 3–5 percent.[171]

The RET mutations differ from the mutations associated with the MEN 1 gene in that they activate the receptor (Fig. 27-1). Mutations of the extracellular domain cause dimerization of the receptor (Fig. 27-1) and activation of mitogen-activated kinase pathways linked to cell growth (Fig. 27-4). The codon 918 mutation does not cause dimerization of the receptor, but does cause activation of downstream signaling pathways (Fig. 28-4).

There is substantial genotype-phenotype correlation. Codon 634 mutations are most commonly associated with classic MEN 2A whereas mutations of codons 609, 611, 618, and 620 are more

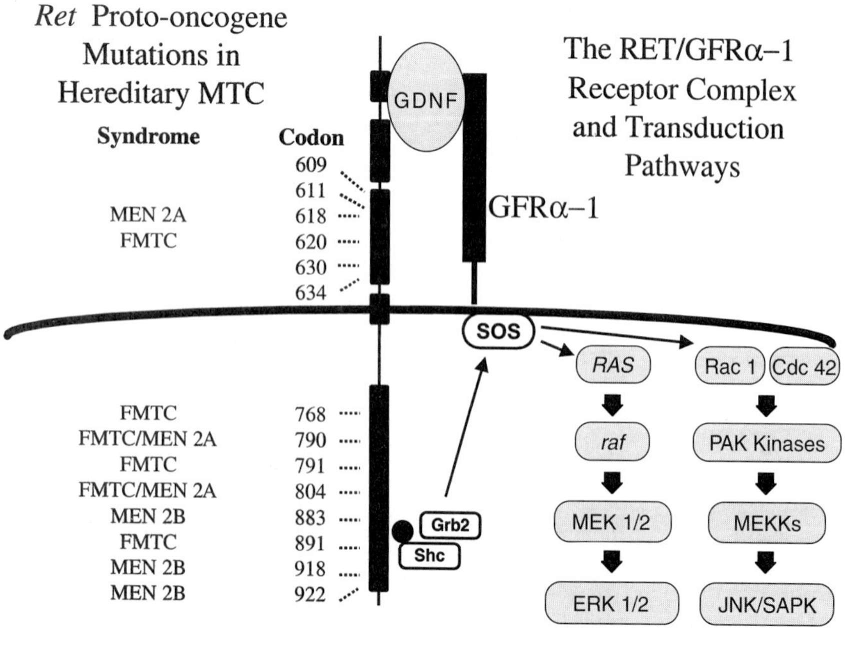

FIGURE 27-4. *RET* Proto-oncogene mutations and the *RET* signal transduction pathways. The *RET*/GFRa-1 signaling complex forms a recepor for glial cell-derived neurotrophic factor (GDNF). The left panel shows genotype-phenotype correlations for mutations at specific codons. It is important to recognize that some of these correlations are based on small sample size and should be considered preliminary, particularly those affecting the intracellular domain. In the right panel is shown the tyrosine kinase signaling pathways activated by the mutant *RET*.

commonly associated with FMTC, although there is overlap (Fig. 27-4).[171] Clearly defined phenotypes have been found for several of the intracellular domain mutations. Codon 768, 791, and 891 mutations have been associated only with FMTC and codon 883, 918, and 922 mutations have been identified only in patients or kindreds with MEN 2B. The other intracellular domain mutations have been associated with either FMTC or MEN 2A (Fig. 27-4).

It is important to recognize that information regarding genotype-phenotype correlation is still being assembled and that a careful family history for pheochromocytoma should be obtained from all patients regardless of the mutation. Pheochromocytoma occurs in approximately 50 percent of MEN 2A gene carriers, but kindreds with a codon 634 mutation have been described in which only 1 in 10 gene carriers developed pheochromocytoma.[148] Clinicians should be cautious about classifying a kindred as FMTC unless there is detailed multigenerational information.

In a small percentage of FMTC or MEN 2A kindreds (estimated to be 1–3 percent) no *RET* mutation has been identified. The *RET* gene containing 21 exons and only 4–6 exons are routinely screened for mutations. It is possible that *RET* mutations will be subsequently be identified or a second gene in the *RET* signal transduction pathway may harbor mutations. In the absence of a clearly defined genetic defect in these kindreds, screening by more traditional methods (described later) should be continued.

INDIVIDUAL COMPONENTS OF THE MEN 2A SYNDROME AND THEIR MANAGEMENT

Medullary Thyroid Carcinoma

The parafollicular cell comprises <1 percent of the thyroidal cell population and attracted little attention until the discovery of (thyro)calcitonin (CT) in the early 1960s. Although MTC was characterized as a distinct tumor type by Hazard in the late 1950s, it was Williams who first suggested that MTC was a neoplasm composed of C cells.[172] The identification of CT production by MTC[173,174] and subsequent studies in hereditary MTC,[175] showing progression from normal to C cell hyperplasia to MTC,[176] proved his hypothesis and led to the designation of the parafollicular cell as the C or calcitonin-producing cell. In addition to CT production, MTC produces a broad spectrum of ectopic cellular proteins (carcinoembryonic antigen and histaminase)[177,178] and peptide hormones (neurotensin,[179] vasoactive intestinal peptide, proopiomelanocortin products, and others).[86]

Embryology

Thyroidal C cells are now generally accepted to be of neural crest origin.[180,181] These cells migrate from the neural crest during embryonic life to form the ultimobranchial organ in nonmammalian species and are incorporated into the developing thyroid gland in mammals. The neural crest origin of C cells offers a potential explanation for the association of MTC with other tumors of neural crest origin; it also appears to explain production of a wide variety of bioactive substances by these tumors.[182] Because these cells do not participate in iodine metabolism, they do not concentrate iodide or produce thyroglobulin.[183]

Pathology

An MTC is usually a firm, rounded tumor located most commonly at the juncture of the upper one-third and lower two-thirds of each thyroid lobe along superior–inferior central axis.[184] It is commonly bilateral and multifocal in familial cases. The cells are usually polyhedral or polygonal in shape and are arranged in a variety of patterns.[185] The arrangement of the cells can be influenced by the distribution of stromal elements, which can be scanty or predominant. Calcification is commonly found in the tumor; the calcifications are more dense and irregular than the homogeneous psammoma bodies that occur in other thyroid cancers. Dense calcifications may be visible on x-ray. A common feature of MTC is the presence of amyloid. The amyloid has the histochemical characteristics of the immune amyloids, but immunochemical and immunohistologic studies suggest that it is also secreted by the C cells and is structurally related to calcitonin.[186] Although the presence of amyloid has long been considered to be important in the diagnosis of medullary thyroid carcinoma, the diagnosis is best established through the use of specific immunohistochemical procedures for calcitonin which demonstrate the abnormal C cells.[178,187] The histologic features of the tumor vary and in general cannot be used for prognosis. However, immunohistochemical studies suggest that cellular heterogeneity of calcitonin production may indicate a grave prognosis.[188]

The diagnosis of MTC can be made by fine needle aspiration when positive immunohistochemical staining for CT or the presence of amyloid is detected,[189,190] although consideration should be give to metastasis of another CT producing tumor such as breast or small cell lung carcinoma occur but mixed tumors containing malignant elements of thyroid follicles are rare.[191–194]

C Cell Hyperplasia

C cell hyperplasia has emerged as a distinct pathologic entity.[176] Wolfe and colleagues demonstrated C cell hyperplasia as an early histologic lesion in individuals subsequently shown to be gene carriers. These patients had small but progressive increases in plasma calcitonin concentration during calcium infusion and consequently underwent thyroidectomy. The thyroid glands removed did not display the presence of MTC but did show clusters of hyperplastic parafollicular cells, which were calcitonin-positive on immunohistologic studies. The presence of increased calcitonin levels in these cells was confirmed by means of bioassay and immunoassay. These hyperplastic parafollicular cells were localized to the areas where C cells are usually most prominent: the upper and middle portions of the lateral thyroid lobes.[195] These cells exhibited no nuclear atypia or invasive tendencies. These observations suggest that, at least in familial cases of MTC, the true malignancy is preceded by progressive hyperplasia of C cells. It is unclear whether C cell hyperplasia precedes sporadic MTC, although diffuse C cell hyperplasia is found in approximately a third of cases of sporadic MTC.[196]

This predecessor of MTC can become manifest in early childhood or as late as the second decade.[176,197,198] The identification of these putative premalignant lesions raised the possibility that the MTC could be cured if it could be detected at this early stage and led to the development of several provocative tests for CT release. The cumbersome 4-hour calcium infusion utilized in these early studies[175] has been replaced by a short calcium infusion,[199] a bolus injection of pentagastrin (0.4 micrograms/kg body weight over 10–15 seconds),[200,201] or a combined calcium and pentagastrin test (discussed later).[202] Application of provocative CT testing in kindreds with MEN 2A and FMTC led to the consistent identification of C cell hyperplasia or microscopic MTC without evidence of extrathyroidal metastasis. The mean age of detection of CT abnormalities using these approaches is 10–13 years of age.[203]

Occurrence

MTC is a rare neoplasm, accounting for 4 to 12 percent of all thyroid cancer.[204] The ratio of affected females to males is closer to unity than in other thyroid tumors. Although the majority of cases reported in the earlier literature appeared to occur sporadically, an appreciation of the familial incidence of the tumor has resulted in an increasing identification of inherited cases.[205] In cases of apparent sporadic MTC where there is no family history, approximately 6 percent are found by genetic testing to harbor a causative germline *RET* mutation.[153,206–208] Despite its rarity, the tumor has acquired a clinical importance that far outweighs its prevalence because of the potential for using biochemical and molecular techniques to identify and cure MTC before it has metastasized.

C Cell Adenoma

Several instances of C cell adenoma have been reported.[209,210] These tumors are rare and there are no definitive criteria to separate these tumors from low grade MTC.

Natural History

The natural history of MTC can vary greatly; this may make decisions regarding therapy difficult. The tumor is generally regarded as intermediate between the aggressive behavior of anaplastic thyroid carcinoma and the more indolent behavior of papillary and follicular thyroid carcinoma. However, it can be rapidly progressive and widely metastatic and can lead to death within months of diagnosis. By contrast, it can be indolent and compatible with decades of life.[211,212] In patients with extrathyroidal metastasis approximately one-half will die from a tumor 10–15 years after diagnosis. One predictor of aggressive behavior is the presence of either a germline or somatic RET proto-oncogene codon 918 mutation (Fig. 27-4).[213] Patients with MEN 2B or the 25 percent of patients with a sporadic MTC with a codon 918 mutation have more extensive metastasis and generally die at a younger age than do those without this specific mutation.[213] Although rare, somatic codon 918 RET mutations have been described in MTCs from patients with germline RET mutations causing MEN 2A[214] and somatic codon 634 mutations have been identified in patients with sporadic MTC.[215] Medullary thyroid carcinoma commonly spreads via regional lymphatics; local metastases have been present in the majority of tumors reported. Distant metastases can involve any organ; lung, liver, bone, and adrenal gland are relatively common sites.[211] The most common presentation is a thyroid nodule, and the most common symptom is diarrhea.

Calcitonin Gene Products and Screening for the Tumor

Calcitonin Gene Products

Calcitonin is a 32-amino acid polypeptide that is one of two secretory peptides derived from alternative RNA processing of the CT gene (*CALC I*). This gene is expressed in a variety of neuroendocrine and neuronal cells. In the C cell, some other neuroendocrine cell types in the lung, breast, prostate, pituitary, and other cell types, the primary RNA transcript is processed to include CT coding exon 4; in neuronal cell types the primary transcript is processed to exclude CT exon 4 by splicing exon 3 to 5, producing an mRNA coding for a second peptide, calcitonin gene-related peptide (CGRP). Medullary thyroid carcinomas most commonly produce both CT and CGRP, indicating an aberrant splicing pattern, although CT production most commonly dominates and is therefore the better tumor marker.

Calcitonin is a useful and relatively specific marker of MTC. It is measured by either radioimmunoassay (RIA)[216] or 2-site immunoassay.[217,218] Most radioimmunoassays for CT utilize polyclonal antibodies and therefore detect CT monomer (32-amino acid peptide) as well as higher molecular weight forms that include dimers and precursor forms. In 1–5 per 1,000 samples there is a nonspecific form of immunoreactivity. Two-site assays for CT monomer are generally more sensitive (routinely provide sensitivity to 1–5 pg/ml) and do not detect this interfering substance. In clinical situations where there are low-level elevations of serum calcitonin (usually <100 pg/ml) that do not increase after pentagastrin or calcium stimulation, it is important to perform a measurement with a 2-site assay to eliminate the possibility of a nonspecific elevation.

Although it is difficult to make direct correlations, basal calcitonin values less than 200 pg/ml are most commonly associated with intrathyroidal C cell hyperplasia or carcinoma; basal values between 200 and 1,000 may be associated with intrathyroidal disease with or without local metastasis, and for values greater than 1,000 pg/ml, distant metastasis should be sought. These values are intended to provide only a general guide for extent of disease; microscopic carcinomas may be associated with nodal or distant metastasis. Other neuroendocrine carcinomas of lung (Kulchitsky cell), breast, prostate, or other sites may also produce CT and these possibilities should be considered in the differential diagnosis, although most commonly values greater than 1,000 pg/ml are associated with MTC.

C cells also secrete chromogranin A (CgA), a high-molecular-weight protein originally discovered in the secretory granules of pheochromocytomas and now known to be present in other endocrine tissues, among them the parathyroid, pancreas, and pituitary.[219] This protein could thus be a marker for each of the endocrine neoplasias of both MEN 1 and MEN 2.[219] CgA has also been reported to be produced by CT-negative MTC[220] and may be produced by a variety of neuroendocrine carcinomas. Finally, MTC commonly produces carcinoembryonic antigen, a marker that is relatively insensitive for early diagnosis, but is useful for long-term follow-up because there is less minute-to-minute variability of plasma levels than is observed for calcitonin.

Calcitonin Screening for Medullary Thyroid Carcinoma

Calcium stimulates release of CT from the C cell through interaction with the calcium sensing receptor, a G protein-coupled receptor that is activated by an increasing calcium concentration. Activation of this receptor stimulates an increase in cytosolic calcium concentration leading to release of CT (and most other secretory products of the C cell) from cytoplasmic secretory granules. Although a 4-hour calcium infusion was originally used to stimulate CT release, this test has been replaced by shorter and equally effective approaches. One approach utilizes a short calcium infusion that raises the serum calcium concentration by approximately 1 mg/dl and induces reliable stimulation of CT release.[205] A second approach utilizes pentagastrin, the terminal 5 amino acids of gastrin, to stimulate CT release. Pentagastrin is normally administered intravenously (0.5 micrograms/kg body weight) over 10–15 seconds with measurement of the serum CT basally and at 2, 5, and 10 minutes. Peak plasma levels of CT occur within 2–5 minutes after administration and decline thereafter. The mechanism by which pentagastrin stimulates CT release has not been defined. Although an effective secretagogue, pentagastrin can causes significant symptoms that include epigastric burning and pressure, nausea, flushing, and, hypotension. The hypotensive effect is rare and occurs predominantly in patients with large MTCs and is presumably related to the release of a vasodilatory substance, perhaps calcitonin gene-related peptide, from the tumor. Finally, a combination of a short calcium infusion followed by pentagastrin is generally considered to be the most effective stimulus for CT release. Use of the pentagastrin will become more difficult in the future because the manufacturer in the United States has discontinued production, in part as a result in the decline of pentagastrin testing that has resulted from the use of genetic testing for RET mutations (discussed later).

Other Provocative Agents

Several other agents have been reported to be useful in the diagnosis of MTC. They include the oral administration of whiskey and use of omeprazole to stimulate endogenous gastrin secretion. These agents have not been widely used, and their clinical value has not been established.[86,201,221,222]

Calcitonin Measurements in the Evaluation of Therapy

The effectiveness of therapy in patients with CT-producing tumors can be monitored by means of serial measurements of plasma CT concentration before and following therapy.[86] There are several important points regarding the use of CT measurements for this purpose. The first is the misconception that patients who have a normal (hence detectable) basal CT value following surgery are cured. Normal basal CT values in thyroidectomized patients are most commonly less than 5 pg/ml, whereas the normal range for a patient with an intact thyroid may range between 15–30 pg/ml. A CT value greater than 10 pg/ml, measured in a specific 2-site immunoassay, is suspicious for persistent MTC. The second is that clinicians should be suspicious of residual MTC in patients with a normal basal but abnormal calcium-stimulated CT values. A question that often arises is how often provocative calcium testing should be performed following surgical cure of a MTC. There are no prospective data to address this question, but most clinicians perform a calcium stimulation test 6–12 months following surgery and then every 2–4 years thereafter for a period of 8–12 years. If serum CT values remain undetectable a decade following surgery, it is likely the patient is cured.

Other Tumor Products

Prostaglandins

Abnormal concentrations of prostaglandins (PGs) are present in the tumor and blood of some patients with MTC. These excess PGs have been implicated in the pathogenesis of the diarrhea commonly seen in patients with this tumor. It is known that PGs can stimulate intestinal smooth muscle, and diarrhea seems to be a more prominent symptom in patients with an extensive tumor burden. Furthermore, diarrhea may be decreased by surgical removal of the tumor and treatment with PG inhibitors. However, patients with diarrhea and MTC may have normal PG levels, and patients with elevated PG levels may not have diarrhea. Furthermore, excess PG production occurs in a variety of other tumors that are not associated with diarrhea.[223]

Serotonin

MTC can be associated with abnormal serotonin production and a carcinoid-like syndrome that includes flushing. In some patients, the carcinoid-like syndrome is uncovered by procedures, such as calcium infusion, that stimulate the secretory activity of MTC. The tumor can also produce peptides such as bradykinin and kallikrein, which are integral to the carcinoid syndrome. As with prostaglandins, serotonin and its metabolites may contribute to the diarrhea commonly seen in patients with MTC.[223]

Histaminase

Elevated levels of histaminase, an enzyme that catalyzes the deamination of histamine, are commonly found in the tumor and serum of patients with MTC. This may play a role in the abnormal result of a histaminase test observed in some patients with this tumor, although alternative explanations are possible. Unlike PGs and serotonin and like calcitonin, abnormal histaminase production seems to be somewhat specific for MTC as opposed to other tumors. Thus, the measurement of histaminase level may have some clinical value in the diagnosis and management of a patient with MTC. Although histaminase is generally not as sensitive a marker for MTC as is calcitonin, it may be useful in identifying patients with metastatic MTC.[224]

Peptide Hormones

In addition to calcitonin and the other products of the CT gene, MTC can produce a variety of other peptide hormones, including ACTH, melanocyte stimulating hormone (MSH), somatostatin, and β-endorphin.[224]

This group of peptides, including calcitonin, is also commonly represented in other tumors of neural crest origin, notably oat-cell carcinoma of the lung. It has also been reported that pituitary cells produce calcitonin or a substance immunochemically related to calcitonin. The concurrent production of this variety of peptide hormones may represent an independent expression of the malignant state. However, it has been postulated that the production of some of these peptide hormones may be regulated by closely related genes and that there may even be a precursor molecule common to some of them.[223]

Genetic Testing for Multiple Endocrine Neoplasia Type 2A or Familial Medullary Thyroid Carcinoma

A consensus has developed among clinicians caring for large MEN 2A or FMTC kindreds that routine genetic testing should be performed prior to the age of 5 years in all children at hereditary risk for development of MTC. These tests are commercially available from several sources.* The first step in this process is to determine the specific RET proto-oncogene mutation in the family by obtaining a RET proto-oncogene analysis on a family member with known MEN 2A. The molecular diagnostic laboratory will focus on the most common extracellular domain mutations

*Information on genetic testing can be obtained from the University of Texas M.D. Anderson Web site at: http://endocrine.mdacc.tmc.edu

initially (codons 609, 611, 618, 620, 630, and 634) and the intracellular codon 918 (Fig. 27-4). If no mutation is found at these sites, *some* laboratories will examine for the presence of the rarer intracellular domain mutations (codons 768, 790, 791, 804, or 891). In the rare member of a family with hereditary MTC in whom no mutation is identified, it is important to inquire whether the laboratory has analyzed for the less common intracellular domain mutations and to send a sample to a laboratory that analyzes for these mutations in the event it has not been performed. Once the specific mutation in the kindred has been identified, DNA from other family members at genetic risk should also be analyzed. It is important that clinicians be aware that molecular analysis for DNA abnormalities, like other laboratory testing, may have an error rate of 5 percent or more. Causes for false-positive test results include sample mix-up, contamination of the assay tube with DNA from an individual with the same mutation, or the rare artifactual mutation created during the polymerase chain reaction. Polymerase chain reaction is so sensitive that airborne laboratory contamination by a single DNA molecule from an affected individual can create a false-positive test result. False-negative test results occur most commonly as a result of sample mix-up or a failure of adequate amplification of the mutant allele of the RET gene. The important point is that clinicians should repeat the test result twice, preferably in a different laboratory, before concluding that a test result is either positive or negative.

Clinical Use of Genetic Information

There is general consensus that gene carriers with extracellular domain mutations (codons 609, 611, 618, 620, and 634) should have a thyroidectomy performed sometime between 3 and 7 years and that the decision to perform a thyroidectomy should not await an abnormal calcium or pentagastrin test. There is abundant evidence that microscopic MTC occurs in MEN 2A in children as young as 3 years of age and that 50 percent of gene carriers with normal pentagastrin test results were found to have MTC at the time of thyroidectomy, leading to the possibility that metastasis could have occurred.

There is less certainty about the appropriate course of action in kindreds with the rarer intracellular domain mutations associated with FMTC including codon 768, 804, 790, 791, and 891. In some kindreds with these mutations the clinical course of MTC is benign, and there are some kindreds in which no deaths can be attributed to MTC. It may be appropriate in such kindreds to delay thyroidectomy until there is clear-cut evidence of CT abnormalities, although such a decision should be based on an unambiguous family history of benign MTC behavior over several generations. In collecting such family history it is important to recognize that MTC as a clinical entity was not identified until 1959 and that individuals, particularly those who presented with widespread metastasis where the thyroid was not identified as the primary neoplasm, may have been given a different diagnosis.

Identification of Germline RET Protooncogene Mutations in Apparent Sporadic MTC

A recent finding has been the recognition that 6–7 percent of patients with apparent sporadic MTC and no identifiable family history for MTC have germline RET mutations. Although surprising, studies from multiple referral centers, those most likely to obtain a careful family history, have confirmed these observations (reviewed in Wohllk[153]). These observations suggest that individuals with sporadic MTC should have a routine germline (peripheral blood) analysis of the RET gene performed and, if positive, mutational analysis should be extended to first degree relatives to determine whether this individual represents the rare de novo mutation or is a member of a larger kindred.

It is important to recognize that a negative genetic test result in an individual with apparent sporadic MTC does not exclude hereditary disease with 100 percent certainty. One to three percent of kindreds with proven hereditary MTC do not have an identifiable mutation of the RET gene and it is possible that the patient with apparent sporadic MTC could belong to one of these kindreds. However, the calculated probability (using Bayes theorem) of a first-degree relative being a gene carrier is extremely low (<0.1 percent), providing reassurance to most patients. When patients are not reassured by this type of analysis, continued CT testing is required.[153]

Clinical Outcome of Prospective Screening for Hereditary MTC

Prospective screening studies initiated in the 1970s, based on annual pentagastrin testing, led to thyroidectomy with normalization of basal CT values.[225] Subsequent follow-up, averaging more than 25 years, has demonstrated several important points. First, there were a number of false-positive pentagastrin tests when these individuals were subsequently tested by molecular analysis of the RET gene. Second, most of these patients remain without evidence of MTC or CT abnormalities. Finally, one patient has developed localized metastatic MTC and several have elevated serum CT values. These findings reaffirm the validity of early screening and thyroidectomy. However, the finding of at least one case of metastatic disease provides a cautionary note: either microscopic MTC metastasizes earlier than previously suspected or a few residual C cells became transformed during the 20 years since thyroidectomy. Similar findings have been reported by others, suggesting that either thyroidectomy should be performed earlier or that the completeness of thyroidectomy must be improved. The community of clinicians caring for these families have responded to this type of information by recommending earlier thyroidectomy, although proof that earlier intervention will improve the long-term outcome is not available and will require long-term follow-up.

Pheochromocytoma

Unilateral or bilateral pheochromocytomas occur in approximately 50 percent of gene carriers with Sipple's syndrome or MEN 2A and in MEN 2B. Familial MTC is defined by the absence of pheochromocytomas (Table 27-4). Prospective screening studies performed during past 25 years have provided considerable information regarding the features of these tumors and their natural history. There are several distinct features of pheochromocytomas in MEN 2 that separate them from sporadic pheochromocytomas. First, they are most commonly bilateral and multicentric. Second, bilateral pheochromocytomas may develop asynchronously, their detection separated by as much as 10 years. Finally, the pheochromocytomas in MEN 2 have a characteristic pattern of catecholamine secretion that separates them from sporadic pheochromocytoma and at least one other major cause of hereditary pheochromocytoma, von Hippel Lindau Syndrome (VHL).[226]

Adrenal Medullary Hyperplasia

Adrenal medullary hyperplasia is a predecessor of the pheochromocytomas seen in MEN 2, just as C cell hyperplasia is a predecessor of MTC.[227,228] Although cases of adrenal medullary hyperplasia had been reported previously in the literature, none of them occurred in patients with MTC.[86] DeLellis and colleagues described the adrenal glands of 10 patients from a large kindred with familial MTC.[229] There was an increase in the medullary volume of adrenal glands compared with controls. The increase in medullary mass resulted from diffuse and/or multifocal proliferation of the adrenal medulla. Multifocal proliferation can produce an adenomatous appearance. In addition, the ratio of epinephrine to norepinephrine was increased in the tumor,[229] findings that have been confirmed in subsequent analyses. These findings suggest that a sequence of events similar to that postulated for MTC and hyperparathyroidism takes place in the development of pheochromocytomas: hypertrophy develops into hyperplasia, multifocal hyperplasia develops into nodularity, and nodularity undergoes neoplastic transformation to pheochromocytomas. This transformation is the final stage of the sequence in most tumors, but malignant transformation can also be seen.[229]

Natural History of Pheochromocytoma in MEN 2

Prospective screening studies in MEN 2A kindreds have more clearly defined the clinical events in the development of pheochromocytoma in MEN 2A. The first symptoms may include intermittent palpitations, headaches, and tremulousness. Unlike sporadic pheochromocytomas or pheochromocytomas associated with VHL, hypertension is rare early in the course of the disease. The clinical features are attributable to a disproportionate production of epinephrine by these tumors, a feature that differentiates them from the pattern of predominate norepinephrine production by sporadic or VHL pheochromocytomas (Fig. 27-5).[226] Early in the course of pheochromocytoma development plasma and urinary catecholamines may be normal unless obtained during or shortly after an attack. CT or MRI evaluation (greater anatomical resolution is generally offered by CT) may show only slight enlargement of one or both adrenal glands. Prospective studies have shown that the transition from infrequent to frequent symptoms is associated with measurable catecholamine abnormalities. Measurement of both metanephrines and fractionated catecholamines provide the greatest sensitivity for detection of medullary abnormalities. A recent report indicates the usefulness of plasma metanephrines for early diagnosis of pheochromocytoma. Abnormal urine metanephrine or catecholamine values are generally associated with a radiographic abnormality. There have been rare descriptions of extra-adrenal pheochromocytomas in MEN 2. In a patient with clearly abnormal catecholamine or metanephrine values and no imageable abnormalities, scanning with radiolabeled metaiodobenzyl guanidine or pentetreotide may provide localization information, although neither of these procedures are required in a patient with an adrenal abnormality.

Patients who do not undergo routine annual screening may present at a later point with large pheochromocytomas and clinical findings that include hypertension, tachycardia, ventricular arrhythmias, headache, and weight loss.

The goal of prospective screening for pheochromocytoma is to detect pheochromocytomas when they are small and easily managed. The sudden death associated with the undetected and unsuspected pheochromocytoma in a patient with MEN 2 is currently uncommon because of the combination of prospective screening and early detection, the use of adrenergic antagonists, and improved surgical and anesthetic techniques. Deaths from pheochromocytoma most commonly occur in patients who eschew routine screening or in patients with undetected MEN 2. Women of childbearing age should be evaluated on a regular basis. Labor and delivery is a stressful period and several deaths related to pheochromocytomas have been reported. It is useful to have a discussion with newly-married couples about the necessity for screening prior to consideration of pregnancy.

Treatment

Individuals with abnormal catecholamines or symptoms thought to be caused by abnormal catecholamines should be treated with combined alpha- and beta-adrenergic antagonists in preparation for surgical removal of an abnormal adrenal gland. Alternatively treated with alpha methytyrosine, a competitive inhibitor of tyrosine hydroxylase, can reduce symptoms and the risk of cardiac arrhythmias or hypertension; it is frequently used in combination with adrenergic antagonist therapy. The length of pretreatment required depends upon the presence or absence of hypertension. In individuals without hypertension, a shorter period of pretreatment may suffice, whereas patients with hypertension may have intravascular volume depletion and require 7–14 days of treatment to normalize intravascular volume, thereby reducing the probability of hypotension following removal of the pheochromocytoma. A more detailed discussion of pheochromocytoma management can be found in Chap. 12

Surgical management has evolved rapidly over the past 5 years. Endoscopic adrenalectomy through a flank approach is currently the most commonly used approach for a unilateral small pheochromocytoma because of the low morbidity associated with the procedure. In individuals with bilateral pheochromocytomas or a large unilateral tumor, an anterior approach may be indicated. Adrenal insufficiency leading to the deaths of at least two patients has been reported in patients receiving bilateral adrenalectomy. This has led to greater interest in cortical sparing adrenalectomy, a technique that has been used with success to manage MEN 2- and VHL-related pheochromocytomas.[230,231]

Individuals with a surgically excised unilateral pheochromocytoma should have urine catecholamines and metanephrine measurements performed annually thereafter because of the 50 percent probability of development of pheochromocytoma in the contralateral adrenal gland during the next 8–10 years. Even after bilateral adrenalectomy there is small, perhaps 1–3 percent probability of recurrence, thought to be related to either an adrenal rest, incomplete removal of the adrenal gland, or seeding by chromaffin cells from the pheochromocytoma. In rare MEN 2A families with malignant pheochromocytoma, prophylactic bilateral adrenalectomy early in life may be indicated.

Hyperparathyroidism

Occurrence

Hyperparathyroidism occurs in 10–20 percent of patients with MEN 2A or one of its variants.[147,232,233] The hyperparathyroidism initially described was characterized by multiglandular hyperplasia or multiple adenomas. Since the onset of prospective screening and early thyroidectomy, hyperparathyroidism has become an uncommon event. In one kindred with MEN 2A and a prior history of hyperparathyroidism of 15–20 percent, none of the children or young adults in whom thyroidectomy was performed (average age 13) has developed hyperparathyroidism during a follow-up period that is now approaching 25 years.[225]

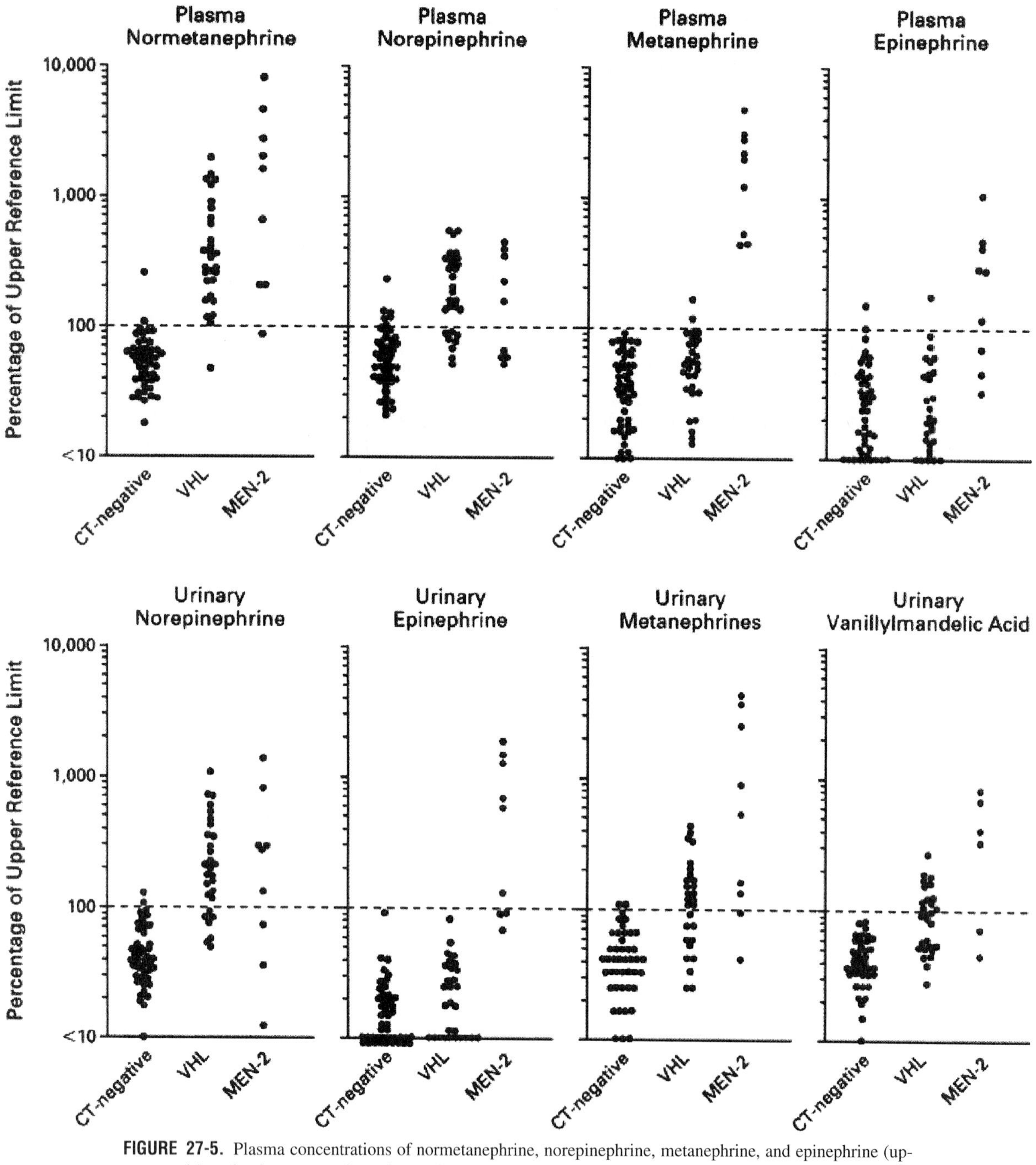

FIGURE 27-5. Plasma concentrations of normetanephrine, norepinephrine, metanephrine, and epinephrine (upper panels) and urinary excretion of norepinephrine, epinephrine, metanephrines, and vanillylmandelic acid (lower panels).

The values are expressed as percentages of the upper reference limit for each test. Data on individual patients are shown for three groups of patients with von Hippel-Lindau disease and multiple endocrine neoplasia type 2 (MEN 2), as follows: patients with von Hippel-Lindau disease or MEN 2 in whom a pheochromocytoma was ruled out on the basis of normal computed tomography (CT-negative), patients with von Hippel-Lindau disease who had histologically verified pheochromocytomas (VHL), and patients with MEN 2 who had histologically verified pheochromocytomas. The values for patients with pheochromocytoma were determined when the tumors were first identified by computed tomography. The dotted horizontal line represents the upper reference limit for each test. The scales are logarithmic. (*Reprinted with permission from the New England Journal of Medicine 340:1872, 1999*).

Whether this kindred is representative of all kindreds is not clear. The prevalence of hyperparathyroidism and the probability of recurrence is higher in selected but uncommon MEN 2A kindreds.[233]

Hyperparathyroidism is seen most commonly in kindreds with any codon 634 amino acid substitution and less commonly with exon 10 mutations (codon 609, 611, 618, and 620).[171] Hyperparathyroidism has not been reported in kindreds with intracellular domain mutations at codons 768, 791, and 891 and is uncommon in kindreds with codon 790 and 804 mutations.[164,171]

Pathology

Steiner and colleagues reviewed the literature on MEN 2A in 1968 and recorded 10 cases with parathyroid adenoma and 3 cases with parathyroid hyperplasia.[147] In later reports the prevalence of parathyroid hyperplasia in patients with MTC has increased and has even approached 100 percent, although clinically relevant hyperparathyroidism with hypercalcemia is far less common.[198,234]

Etiology of Hyperparathyroidism

The identification of RET expression in MEN 2A parathyroid adenomas provides a compelling argument for involvement of RET in the genesis of parathyroid disease in MEN 2A.[235] However, if this were the only factor involved in the development of parathyroid adenomas, one would expect that gene carriers in the New England kindred (cys634gly *RET* mutation) that had a significant rate of hyperparathyroidism in the first generation[175] would develop this disorder in the next generation. Yet none of the approximately 30 children who had a thyroidectomy performed for early C cell abnormalities diagnosed by prospective CT screening have developed hyperparathyroidism, although one case of hypercalcemia in this group was attributable to a pheochromocytoma.[225] The possibility that the thyroidectomy in these young patients modified the clinical course of hyperparathyroidism is an attractive but as yet unproven hypothesis that will be clarified by continued observation.

Multiple Endocrine Neoplasia Type 2A with Cutaneous Lichen Amyloidosis

The description in the late 1980s of two MEN 2A kindreds with a pruritic cutaneous lesion located on the upper back with histologic features of cutaneous lichen amyloidosis (CLA)[148,149] has led to the identification of at least 15 kindreds with this variant.[236–240] Another characteristic of the MEN 2A/CLA variant is the low penetrance of hyperparathyroidism. Patients with CLA complain of intense pruritis on the upper back leading to scratching and excoriation. Most commonly the cutaneous lesion develops in the early 20s and enlarges thereafter. There is a direct correlation between the age of the patient and the size of the lesion.[240] All reported kindreds with this variant have a codon 634 mutation. A puzzle that has not been completely resolved is why the penetrance of this particular manifestation is so low (15–20 of approximately 500 reported kindreds). Attempts to find other mutations or polymorphisms within the RET gene have identified no other abnormalities and sequencing of the GDNF gene in several patients has identified no mutations.

The likely explanation for the pruritus is the expression of RET in the dorsal spinal ganglia of the spinal cord.[241] Excessive sensory neuronal firing, caused by the RET mutation, provides a potential explanation for the sensory abnormalities. The phenomenon in MEN 2 patients may actually be more common than previously suspected. Careful questioning will frequently elicit the history, particularly from children of parents with MEN 2A, that mom or dad frequently requests a "back scratch" on the upper back.

MEN 2A with Hirschsprung Disease

Although the molecular abnormalities (codon 609, 618, and 620 RET mutations) place this variant as a subgroup of MEN 2A, the gastrointestinal manifestations will be discussed later in the section on gastrointestinal abnormalities in MEN 2B.

Multiple Endocrine Neoplasia Type 2B

In 1966 Williams and Pollock described two patients with MTC and pheochromocytomas who had neuromas involving the mucous membranes of the lips, tongue, and eyes.[150] In 1968 Schimke and colleagues described three additional patients with this syndrome; they recorded the presence of megacolon in each patient.[242] In one patient rectal biopsy was consistent with ganglioneuromatosis of the submucous and myenteric plexuses. In the same year Gorlin and coworkers reemphasized the association between neuromas, pheochromocytomas, and MTC by reviewing 17 published cases.[243] In several patients the neuromas were congenital or were noticed within the first few years of life, thus becoming manifest before the other features of the syndrome. These authors also commented on the presence of a marfanoid habitus, intestinal ganglioneuromatosis, and medullated corneal nerve fibers in this group of patients and thus articulated the features of this syndrome as it is currently appreciated: MTC, pheochromocytomas, diffuse neuroganglionatosis involving the mucosa of the gastrointestinal tract, and a marfanoid habitus.[244]

Mucosal Neuromas

The presence of neuromas with a centrofacial distribution is the most consistent component of the MEN 2B syndrome.[244] The most prominent microscopic feature of the neuromas is an increase in the size and number of nerves. The nerves are tortuous and highly branched and are often surrounded by a thickened perineurium; both medullated and unmedullated fibers are involved. Ganglion cells and connective tissue may be present, but the connective tissue often is not prominent. This latter feature usually distinguishes these neuromas from the neurofibromas of von Recklinghausen's neurofibromatosis.[223]

The neuromas are most noticeable in the oral cavity. The lips, tongue, and buccal mucosa are common sites. The oral lesions usually are the first components of the syndrome to appear. They are almost invariably present by the first decade and can even be present at birth.[244] The mucosal neuromas, along with the ocular findings described later, give the affected patients a very characteristic facial appearance (Fig. 27-6). Because of this, there is a striking similarity in the appearance of different subjects with the syndrome, even though they may be unrelated and of the opposite sex.

Mucosal neuromas can be present in the eyelids, conjunctiva, and cornea. The tarsal neuromas result in thickened eyelids and retracted eyelashes, which give the eye a hooded, sleepy look. In addition to the neuromas, a variety of other ocular abnormalities have been reported. The medullated corneal nerves are thickened; they traverse the cornea and anastomose in the pupillary area.

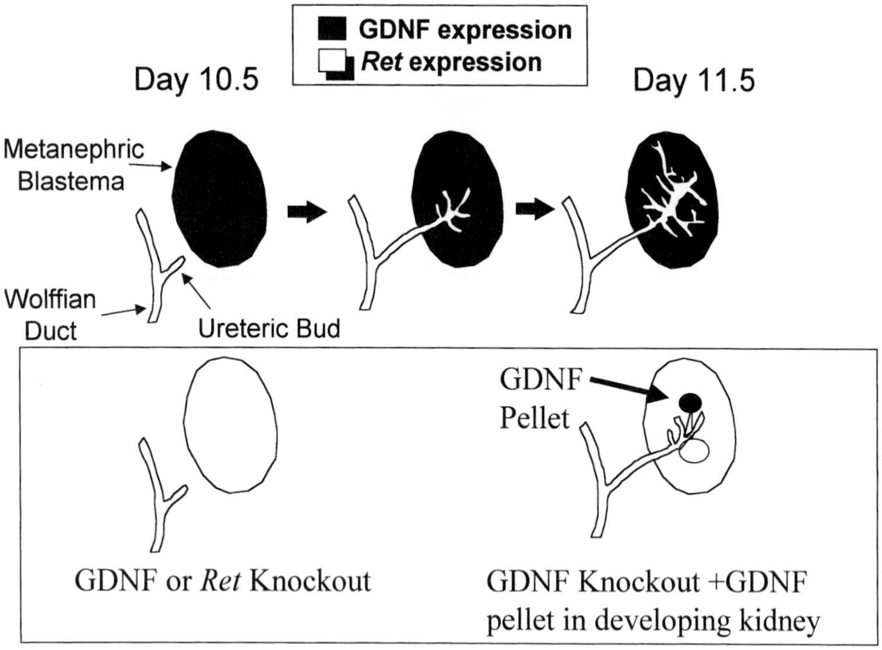

FIGURE 27-6. Mucosal neuromas associated with multiple endocrine neoplasia type 2B.

These hypertrophied nerve fibers are seen readily with the slit lamp but occasionally may be evident on direct funduscopic examination.[244]

Gastrointestinal Abnormalities Associated with MEN 2B

One of the most prominent features of MTC is the presence of gastrointestinal (GI) abnormalities.[197,204] Diarrhea is a common symptom in affected patients.[204] The etiology of the diarrhea seen in these patients is unclear, but is likely to be related to a humoral factor because of its disappearance when tumor mass (and hence plasma levels of CT) is decreased or completely removed.[205] A number of agents have been utilized to manage the diarrhea. Most effective are loperamide, diphenoxylate with atropine, dilenoxin with atropine, or tincture of opium. Agents that have been used with mixed success include nutmeg[245] or cimetidine. Octreotide reduces flushes associated with MTC, but is rarely effective for controlling diarrhea, and may worsen it.[246]

In patients with MEN 2B, there is in addition to the humoral factor produced by MTC, disordered gastrointestinal motility caused by ganglioneuromatosis that is distributed throughout the small and large intestine and in the esophagus and stomach.[197] There is a proliferation of the neural elements of the myenteric and submucosal plexuses. The vagus nerve, derived from the neural crest of the first 5 somites where *RET* is expressed, has also been noted to be enlarged.

Children with MEN 2B will frequently come to attention because of GI symptoms rather than MTC or pheochromocytoma.[247] Functional difficulties in swallowing, megacolon, diarrhea, and constipation characterize the early years of many of these children. Obstruction or pseudo-obstruction is an occasional presentation. It is important to decompress the gastrointestinal tract and observe MEN 2B patients who present with obstructive signs because the problem may be caused by disordered peristalisis rather than a true obstruction. Superimposition of the humorally-caused diarrhea onto the disordered gastrointestinal function caused by neuronal disorganization can lead to almost continuous GI symptoms in MEN 2B patients with metastatic MTC. The usual measures for managing diarrhea in the context of MTC mentioned previsusly may be insufficient in this group of patients.

Molecular Abnormalities in MEN 2B

Almost all patients with MEN 2B have a codon met918thr RET mutation. A handful of patients have been described with codon 883[166,167] or 922 mutations. The met918thr substitution activates the tyrosine kinase domain and causes autophosphorylation of the receptor in the absence of dimerization. There is subsequent activation of mitogen activated protein kinase pathways leading to transformation.

The role of the GDNF/GFRα-1/RET receptor system in the normal development of the gastrointestinal neuronal system has been clearly delineated. Mice in which any component of this system has been deleted or inactivated develop profound gastrointestinal neuronal abnormalities.[248–251] In the developing embryo RET expression progresses from the neural crest into the developing gastrointestinal tract and is enticed into the developing gastrointestinal anlage by GDNF expression.[252,253] It is therefore not surprising that approximately one-half of patients with Hirschsprung disease are found to have abnormalities of this receptor complex, most defined as loss of function mutations.[254–257] Gain of function mutations may also cause gastrointestinal abnormalities. The germline codon 918 mutation causes ganglioneuromatosis and a number of kindreds with MEN 2A and Hirschsprung disease have been found to have codon 609, 618, and 620 mutations of the RET gene.[153,258,259]

Despite the fact that *RET* is expressed extensively during renal development, the presence of activating mutations does not cause any significant developmental or neoplastic effect. There have been occasional MEN 2A patients described with prominent renal collecting systems and one patient who developed a renal cell carcinoma.

Marfanoid Habitus

A marfanoid habitus is seen commonly in MEN 2B.[244,260] The marfanoid habitus refers to a tall, slender body with an abnormal upper- to lower-body-segment size ratio and poor muscle development. The extremities are thin and long; there may be lax joints and hypotonic muscles. Associated with the marfanoid habitus may be dorsal kyphosis, pectus excavatum (funnel chest), pectus carinatum (pigeon breast), pes cavus, and a high-arched palate. In contrast to patients with true Marfan syndrome, no patients with MEN 2B have been reported to have aortic abnormalities, ectopia lentis, homocystinuria, or mucopolysaccharide abnormalities.

Treatment of MTC and Pheochromocytoma in MEN 2B

MTC

There is consensus that all patients with MEN 2B should have a total thyroidectomy performed during the first year of life,[261] preferably during the first few months because of early development of metastasis.[262] Cure is difficult, in part because these children frequently do not come to attention until after the development of metastasis. The MTC is almost always bilateral. In addition to a total thyroidectomy, regional lymph node dissection should be performed.

Pheochromocytoma

Approximately one-half of patients with MEN 2B will develop unilateral or bilateral pheochromocytomas. Screening and clinical management do not differ from that described for MEN 2A.

Clinical Outcome in Multiple Endocrine Neoplasia Type 2

The introduction of prospective screening techniques for MTC and pheochromocytoma and improved management techniques has markedly improved the outcome for MEN 2 gene carriers. It seems likely that earlier diagnosis by genetic testing can only improve the outcome, making it reasonable to believe that in the future most MEN 2A gene carriers will live a normal life span. The future for those affected with MEN 2B is less clear because of the complex gastrointestinal issues in addition to the MTC and pheochromocytoma. However, the identification of the molecular cause for this variant holds the promise that strategies will be developed to address these issues.

POLYGLANDULAR ENDOCRINE INSUFFICIENCY SYNDROMES

When immune dysfunction affects two or more endocrine glands and other nonendocrine immune disorders are seen, the polyglandular autoimmune (PGA) syndromes should be considered. The coincidence of diabetes mellitus and Addison's disease in the same patient had been noticed since the nineteenth century.[263] The combination of lymphocytic thyroiditis and Addison's disease in the absence of infectious adrenalitis in two patients was reported by Schmidt in 1926.[264] However, an autoimmune basis for polyendocrinopathy syndromes was advanced by Blizzard and Kyle in 1963, supported by evidence of anti-adrenal antibodies in half and antithyroid antibodies in one-third of patients with both thyroiditis and Addison's disease.[265] Subsequent reports have identified a heterogeneous collection of autoimmune endocrinopathies that could coexist within individual patients, including dysfunction of adrenals, thyroid, parathyroids, ovaries, testes, and adenohypophysis, along with nonendocrine manifestations such as pernicious anemia, mucocutaneous candidiasis, and vitiligo.[266]

TABLE 27-5. Disease Associations in Polyglandular Autoimmune Syndromes (PGA)

PGA I	PGA II	PGA III
Mucocutaneous candidiasis	Addison's	Type I diabetes and autoimmune thyroid disease, or Addison's and autoimmune thyroid disease
Hypoparathyroidism	Hypothyroidism	
Addison's	Graves' disease	
Hypogonadism	Type I diabetes	
Alopecia	Hypogonadism	
Hypothyroidism	Myasthenia gravis	
Malabsorption	Vitiligo	
Chronic active hepatitis	Alopecia	
Vitiligo	Pernicious anemia	
Pernicious anemia	Celiac disease	

The polyglandular autoimmune syndromes are designated PGA types I, II, III, and IV (Table 27-5). The type I syndrome usually starts in childhood and is characterized by mucocutaneous candidiasis, hypoparathyroidism, and adrenal insufficiency. Patients with the type II (or Schmidt) syndrome are more likely to present as adults, and typically have autoimmune dysfunction of the adrenal glands along with thyroiditis and type I diabetes mellitus. The type III syndrome is more heterogeneous, consisting of autoimmune thyroid disease combined with any autoimmune glandular dysfunction other than adrenal insufficiency, and the type IV syndrome combines autoimmune endocrinopathies with nonendocrine autoimmune diseases.

Clinical Manifestations

Polyglandular Autoimmune Syndrome Type I

PGA type I, usually diagnosed during the first decade of life, requires two of three components for diagnosis: chronic mucocutaneous candidiasis, chronic hypoparathyroidism, and Addison's disease.[266,267] This disorder is also called autoimmune polyendocrinopathy-candidiasis-ectodermal dystrophy (APECED), emphasizing the three major disease components. The endocrine components of PGA type I, including Addison's disease or hypoparathyroidism, may not develop until the fourth decade of life, necessitating continued surveillance. Other autoimmune glandular defects can include gonadal failure, hypothyroidism, anterior hypophysitis, and pernicious anemia. Pancreatic beta cell destruction with type I diabetes mellitus is rare. Other features can include dental enamel hypoplasia, ungual dystrophy, tympanic membrane sclerosis, vitiligo, renal insufficiency due to tubulointerstitial disease, and keratoconjunctivitis. Patients commonly develop autoimmune hepatitis, and other gastrointestinal manifestations include malabsorption (variably attributed to intestinal lymphangiectasia, IgA deficiency, bacterial overgrowth, or hypoparathyroidism), asplenism, achalasia, and cholelithiasis. At the outset only one organ system may be involved, but this number increases as time passes; eventually patients usually manifest between two and five components of the syndrome. Although fewer than half of patients develop all three primary components, those who present at an earlier age appear more likely to acquire the complete syndrome. Of the patients described in three large series, 57 percent were female, 15 percent had a family history of the syndrome, and 7 percent died from complications.[266–268]

Mucocutaneous candidiasis typically presents first, before age 5 years.[266–269] The candidiasis is poorly responsive to treatment, with frequent relapses, and it occurs at some time in most patients with PGA type I. Sites most commonly affected include oral, vaginal, and esophageal mucous membranes, along with the dermis and skin appendages. Rare complications can include esophageal stricture and systemic infection. Systemic antifungal therapy can be attempted periodically but results are variable.[270–272]

Chronic hypoparathyroidism develops before age 10 and eventually involves at least 80 percent of patients. In one variant, seen primarily among Iranian Jews, hypoparathyroidism occurs more commonly than the other syndrome components.[273,274] When presenting during infancy, the autoimmune failure of parathyroid function along with candidiasis must be distinguished from the congenital dysfunction associated with DiGeorge's syndrome. Parathyroid autoantibodies can be detected by indirect immunofluorescence in up to 40 percent of patients, a frequency similar to that in patients with idiopathic hypoparathyroidism in the absence of polyglandular disorders.[275] Recently, the extracellular domain of the calcium-sensing receptor has been implicated as a parathyroid autoantigen in half of patients, but the resultant antibodies may only be secondary markers of the disease rather than etiologic.[276,277]

In PGA type I, autoimmune adrenal insufficiency commonly occurs by age 15, and eventually affects nearly 100 percent of patients.[266–268] Typical symptoms include lassitude, malaise, anorexia, abdominal pain, nausea, weakness, and myalgias; physical findings include hypotension, mucocutaneous hyperpigmentation, and loss of axillary and pubic hair in postpubertal women. Weight loss, a prominent symptom in adult-onset adrenal insufficiency, is usually muted in children.[278] Laboratory findings include hyponatremia, hyperkalemia, hypoglycemia, and eosinophilia. Histologically, the adrenal glands are usually atrophic, with extensive infiltration with small lymphocytes, monocytes, plasma cells, and macrophages. Autoimmune adrenalitis can be easily distinguished from tuberculous Addison's disease when there is no evidence of pulmonary tuberculosis and absence of adrenal calcifications. However, age of onset does not permit distinction between the two etiologies except that tuberculous Addison's is rare before age 10. Similarly, existence of other autoimmune endocrinopathies may be helpful in the setting of hypoparathyroidism, but diabetes and thyroid disease have been frequently reported in patients with tuberculous Addison's disease. In autoimmune adrenal insufficiency, mineralocorticoid and glucocorticoid function can be lost simultaneously or sequentially. Occasionally, mineralocorticoid deficiency, due to zona glomerulosa involvement, can develop years before glucocorticoid deficiency from zona fasciculata involvement, leading to misdiagnosis as isolated primary hypoaldosteronism.[279] Patients with autoimmune Addison's generally demonstrate a variety of autoantibodies directed against adrenal-specific antigens. Some of the antibodies recognize cytoplasmic components of cells of the dysfunctional gland, e.g., antibodies directed against adrenal side chain cleavage enzyme (P450scc), steroid 21-hydroxylase (P450c21), and steroid 17-alpha hydroxylase (P450c17). Disagreement exists, however, about the relative frequency with which these autoantibodies may be detected.[280–282] Adrenal cortex autoantibodies can be identified in 40–50 percent of PGA type I patients who have not yet developed clinical evidence of adrenal insufficiency, but their presence in children with the syndrome indicates a high risk of subsequent glucocorticoid deficiency within 10 years.[283,284]

Up to half of PGA type I patients develop hypergonadotropic hypogonadism. Gonadal failure is associated with detectable serum autoantibodies with cytotoxic effects on multiple steroid-producing cells, including Leydig cells of the theca interna, corpus luteum, and placenta.[285,286] In addition, these autoantibodies commonly react with adrenal cortical cells. Clinically, hypogonadism can present in females as either primary or secondary amenorrhea.[268] In men, however, hypogonadism is uncommon.[287]

Type I diabetes mellitus occurs in up to 10 percent of PGA type I patients.[266–269] Serologically, autoantibodies against numerous pancreatic antigens have been detected in PGA type I patients, including glutamic acid decarboxylase and L-amino acid decarboxylase. However, a clear association between such autoantibodies and either abnormal glucose tolerance or frank diabetes in PGA type I patients remains elusive.[288–290]

Hashimoto's thyroiditis, anterior hypophysitis, and pernicious anemia due to parietal cell dysfunction have all been described in PGA type I patients. Although the frequency of Hashimoto's thyroiditis may not be much greater than that reported in non-PGA patients, hypothyroidism develops at an earlier age, generally before age 20.[266–268] In addition, antithyroid antibodies are found more commonly in PGA type I patients who do not develop hypothyroidism. Isolated deficiencies of growth hormone, adrenocorticotrophic hormone, and prolactin have been reported in occasional patients, and others have been described with pituitary autoantibodies.[268,291] Intrinsic factor autoantibodies, when found in PGA type I patients, are strongly associated with either clinical or latent pernicious anemia.[268] Autoimmune hepatitis, which occurs in 15 percent of PGA type I patients, may be associated with autoantibodies directed against either hepatic cytochromes P450c1A2 or P450c2A6.[292,293]

Polyglandular Autoimmune Syndrome Type II

Autoimmune adrenalitis in association with either autoimmune thyroid disease or type I diabetes mellitus are the clinical features of PGA type II or Schmidt's syndrome.[294–296] The prevalence of this rare combination is estimated at only 15–45 cases per million persons.[296] PGA type II has a predominantly adult age of onset and a 2:1 female predominance. By definition, Addison's disease occurs in 100 percent of these cases, along with all varieties of autoimmune thyroid disease (70 percent), type I diabetes (50 percent), and rarely vitiligo, hypergonadotropic hypogonadism, alopecia, hypophysitis, myasthenia gravis, chronic active hepatitis, atrophic gastritis, and pernicious anemia.

As in PGA type I, adrenal insufficiency in Schmidt's syndrome is associated with autoantibodies directed against adrenal cortical antigens, particularly steroid 21-hydroxylase (P450c21).[281] Mineralocorticoid deficiency can predate glucocorticoid deficiency, with elevations in plasma renin activity as evidence of zona glomerulosa involvement.[297] Either simultaneously or up to several years later, increased ACTH levels can be detected and eventually deficient cortisol levels are seen.

The spectrum of autoimmune thyroid disease seen in PGA type II includes goitrous hypothyroidism, atrophic hypothyroidism, hyperthyroid Graves' disease, silent lymphocytic thyroiditis, and euthyroid Graves' ophthalmopathy.[298] In half of cases, thyroid disease is detected simultaneously with adrenal insufficiency, whereas the thyroid disease may either precede (25 percent) or follow (25 percent) the adrenal involvement.[296] Antibodies directed against thyroid peroxidase and thyroglobulin are common but do not necessarily predict eventual thyroid dysfunction.

Type I diabetes mellitus occurs in approximately half the affected individuals. Although some patients develop diabetes in childhood, adult-onset insulin-dependent diabetes is more commonly seen in PGA type II. Antibodies directed against pancreatic islet cells can be detected in up to half of patients within one year of diagnosis, and may persist for a longer period of time than is typical in isolated type I diabetes. Among patients in whom anti-islet cell antibodies persist for up to 5 years, another autoimmune disease occurs in nearly 30 percent, and 67 percent have antithyroid or antiparietal cell antibodies.[299,300]

Dermatologic manifestations include vitiligo, caused by antibodies against the melanocyte, and alopecia and are less common than in the type I syndrome. Mucocutaneous candidiasis is not seen in PGA type II. A few patients develop a late onset form of transient hypoparathyroidism, caused by antibodies that inhibit the interaction of parathyroid hormone with its receptor. PGA type II is seen in approximately 25 percent of myasthenic patients and in a higher percentage of patients with thymoma. Megaesophagus, associated with isolated adrenal insufficiency in Allgrove's syndrome, has also been described as a cause of persistent dysphagia and vomiting in PGA II.

Incomplete forms of PGA type II have been described, including type I diabetes and autoimmune thyroid disease in a patient with a sibling who has complete PGA type II.[266] Other possible incomplete forms can include the presence of adrenal cortical autoantibodies combined with either type I diabetes, autoimmune thyroid disease, or autoantibodies directed against thyroid or islet cell antigens.[296]

Other Polyglandular Autoimmune Syndromes

In the absence of either adrenal insufficiency or hypoparathyroidism, the coexistence of autoimmune thyroid disease with another autoimmune disease is defined as PGA type III.[296] Common "other" conditions include type I diabetes mellitus, atrophic gastritis, pernicious anemia, vitiligo, alopecia, hypergonadotropic hypogonadism, and arthridities such as systemic lupus erythematosis and rheumatoid arthritis. Of particular note is the combination of thyroid disease and myasthenia gravis. Of all patients with myasthenia, 6 percent have overt thyrotoxicosis, 10 percent subclinical hyperthyroidism, and 6 percent various degrees of thyroid failure.[301] Finally, PGA type IV may be diagnosed in the presence of any autoimmune endocrinopathy associated with any other autoimmune disease.

Genetics and Pathogenesis

The underlying mechanisms resulting in autoimmune endocrinopathies remain elusive, but probably include inherited as well as acquired components. The PGA type I syndrome shows no human leukocyte antigen (HLA) associations and, when familial, appears to be inherited in an autosomal recessive manner. The Finnish variant of PGA type I was linked to chromosome 21q22.3, and mapped to a 500-kb segment. In 1997, the responsible gene was identified, called either APECED (autoimmune polyendocrinopathy-candidiasis-ectodermal dystrophy) or AIRE (autoimmune regulator), that appears to code for a transcription factor that is expressed in the thymus, lymph nodes, pancreas, adrenal cortex, and fetal liver.[302–304] At least nine mutations have been identified in this gene, including point deletions, missense and nonsense base pair substitutions, and multinucleotide deletions.[305] In the Finnish population, the most common mutation has been a C-to-T substitution in codon 257, introducing a premature stop codon (R257X) in exon 6.[302] Although this mutation is also seen in North American patients, another common allele is a 13 base pair deletion in exon 8 (1094-1106del) that has also been reported in an Italian study.[304,305] Most patients have been homozygotes, but compound heterozygotes have been reported as well.[302,306]

The type II and III syndromes are usually associated with the DR3 or DR4 HLA haplotypes in North America, or both, and are inherited in an incompletely penetrant autosomal dominant manner suggestive of polygenic inheritance.[307,308] In both British and German cohorts, DR3 but not DR4 was associated with PGA type II.[309,310] Epidemiologic studies of twins with isolated forms of either type I diabetes or Graves' disease show development of disease in both twins in only 50 percent of cases. Additional factors must therefore contribute to development of the immune dysregulation. Animal models of PGA type II may exist. Following a cytomegalovirus infection, certain mice strains develop lymphocytic adrenalitis, insulitis, hepatitis, myocarditis, and sialoadenitis.[311] Treatment of newborn BALB/c mice with cyclosporin A followed by thymectomy, which may yield a permanent deficiency of certain regulatory T cells, leads to acquisition of autoimmune disease of many organs, including thyroiditis, adrenalitis, orchitis/oophoritis, and insulitis.[312]

Diagnosis and Treatment

The clinical manifestations of Addison disease often develop slowly, may be difficult to detect, and can be fatal if not diagnosed and treated. Thus, prospective screening of PGA types I and II should be routinely performed. The most effective screening test for adrenal insufficiency is a rapid Cortrosyn stimulation test. This test is often performed in the fasting state so that a fasting blood glucose can also be obtained to screen for hyperglycemia. Other screening tests include a basal thyroid stimulating hormone, luteinizing hormone (LH), follicle stimulating hormone (FSH), and testosterone in males, and LH, FSH, and estradiol in females. Measurement of pituitary hormones are necessary to avoid misdiagnosis of hypopituitarism, although failure to find appropriate elevations of relevant pituitary hormones may lead one to suspect hypophysitis. A serum calcium and phosphorus measurement should be added in families with suspected PGA type I. These studies are performed every one to two years up to about age 50 in families with PGA type II and III syndrome and until about age 40 in patients with type I syndrome. Screening studies for autoantibodies directed against potentially affected endocrine organs may be appropriate, although their prognostic values are quite variable. Considerations within the differential diagnosis of polyglandular failure include DiGeorge syndrome (hypoparathyroidism due to glandular agenesis and mucocutaneous candidiasis), Kearns-Sayre syndrome (hypoparathyroidism, primary hypogonadism, type I diabetes, and hypopituitarism), Wolfram syndrome (congenital diabetes insipidus and diabetes mellitus), and congenital rubella (type I diabetes and hypothyroidism).

With the exception of Graves' disease, the management of each of the endocrine components of the PGA syndromes involves hormone replacement and is covered in detail in the chapters on adrenal (Chap. 11), thyroid (Chap. 9), gonadal (Chaps. 15 and 16), and parathyroid (Chap. 22) disease. Several points deserve emphasis. Primary hypothyroidism can mask adrenal insufficiency by prolonging the half-life of cortisol. Therefore, thyroid hormone treatment in a patient with unsuspected adrenal insufficiency can precipitate adrenal crisis. All patients with hypothyroidism within the context of a PGA syndrome should be screened for adrenal insufficiency and, if present, have concomitant therapy initiated with corticoids and thyroid hormone. Other interactions of potential therapeutic importance include antagonism of the intestinal effects of vitamin D by cortisol and thyroid hormone, exaggeration of complications of type I diabetes mellitus with concurrent untreated hypothyroidism and/or adrenal insufficiency, and difficulty in diagnosing primary thyroid and adrenal disease in the setting of coexisting hypophysitis.

NONAUTOIMMUNE POLYGLANDULAR DEFICIENCY SYNDROMES

Crow-Fukase Syndrome

The clinical characteristics of Crow-Fukase syndrome are highlighted by an acronym that emphasizes its cardinal components: polyneuropathy (P), organomegaly (O), endocrinopathy (E), M-proteins (M), and skin changes (S).[313,314] The most important feature of the disease is a severe, progressive sensorimotor polyneuropathy that is associated with a plasma cell dyscrasia. Localized collections of plasma cells (plasmacytomas) can cause sclerotic bone lesions and produce monoclonal IgG or IgA proteins. Endocrine manifestations include male gynecomastia, hypogonadism (both hypergonadotropic and hypogonadotropic), hyperprolactinemia, type II diabetes, primary hypothyroidism, hypoparathyroidism, and Addison disease. Dramatic skin changes occur, including hyperpigmentation, thickening of the dermis, hirsutism and hypertrichosis, angiomas, and hyperhidrosis.[315] Organomegaly with hepatomegaly and lymphadenopathy have been reported in about two-thirds of the cases, and splenomegaly is seen in about one-third of these individuals. Other manifestations include increased central nervous system pressure with papilledema, peripheral edema, ascites, pleural effusions, glomerulonephritis, fever, and arterial thrombosis. Five-year survival is estimated at about 60 percent.

The widespread systemic nature of the disorder may cause confusion with connective tissue diseases. The endocrine manifestations suggest an autoimmune basis of the disorder, but most patients who have been studied do not have circulating antibodies against endocrine cells. Increased serum and tissue levels of interleukin 1 beta, interleukin 6, vascular endothelial growth factor/vascular permeability factor, and tumor necrosis factor alpha have been documented, but the exact pathophysiologic basis for the POEMS syndrome remains uncertain.[316–319] Therapy directed against the plasma cell dyscrasia, such as local radiation of bony lesions or chemotherapy, may result in endocrine improvement. Recent reports suggest a possible role for either plasmapheresis or all-*trans* retinoic acid in treating the syndrome based on reduction of levels of potentially pathogenetic cytokines.[320,321]

REFERENCES

1. Marx SJ: Multiple endocrine neoplasia type 1, in Scriver CS, et al. (eds): *Metabolic Basis of Inherited Disease.* New York, McGraw Hill, in press.
2. Deftos LJ, Catherwood BD, Bone HG: Multiglandular endocrine disorders, in Felig PL, Baxter J, Broadus AE, Frohman LA (eds): *Endocrinology and Metabolism.* New York, McGraw Hill, 1995; pp 1703–1732.
3. Erdheim J: Zur normalen und pathologischen Histologie der Glandula Thyreoidea, Parathyreoidea und Hypophysis. *Beitr Pathol Anat* 33:158, 1903.
4. Cushing H, Davidoff LM: The pathological findings in four autopsied cases of acromegaly with a discussion of their significance. The Rockefeller Institute of Medical Research, 1927.
5. Lloyd PC: Hypophyseo-patathyreo-insular syndrome. *Bull Johns Hopkins Hospital*, Vol. 45, 1929.
6. Rossier PH, Dressler M: Familare ErkrankunginnersekRETorischer Drusen kombiniert mit Ulcuskrankheit. *Schweiz Med Wochenschr* 20:985, 1939.
7. Underdahl LO, Woolner LB, Black BM: Multiple endocrine adenomas: report of 8 cases in which the parathyroids, pituitary and pancreatic islets were involved. *J Clin Endocrinol* 13:20, 1953.
8. Moldawer MP, Nardi GL, Raker JW: Concomitance of multiple adenomas of parathyroids and pancreatic islets with tumor of pituitary: syndrome with familial incidence. *Am J Med Sci* 228:190, 1954.
9. Zollinger R, Ellison E: Primary peptic ulcerations of the jejunum associated with iselt cell tumors of the pancreas. *Ann Surg* 142:709, 1955.
10. Verner JV, Morrison AB: Islet cell tumor and a syndrome of refractory watery diarrhea and hypokalemia. *Am J Med* 25:374, 1958.
11. Schmid JR, Labhart A, Rossier PH: Relationship of multiple endocrine adenomas to syndrome of ulcerogenic islet cell adenomas (Zollinger-Ellison): Occurence of both syndromes in one family. *Am J Med* 31:313, 1961.
12. Huizenga KA, Goodrick WIM, Sunnerskill WHJ: Peptic ulcer with islet cell tumor. *Am J Med* 37:564, 1964.
13. Ballard HS, Frame B, Hartsock RJ: Familial multiple endocrine adenoma-peptic ulcer complex. *Medicine* 43:481, 1964.
14. Larsson C, Skogseid B, Oberg K, et al: Multiple endocrine neoplasia type 1 gene maps to chromosome 11 and is lost in insulinoma. *Nature* 332:85, 1988.
15. Chandrasekharappa SC, Guru SC, Manickam P, et al: Positional cloning of the gene for multiple endocrine neoplasia-type 1. *Science* 276:404, 1997.
16. Bassett JH, Forbes SA, Pannett AA, et al: Characterization of mutations in patients with multiple endocrine neoplasia type 1. *Am J Hum Genet* 62:232, 1998.
17. Doherty GM, Olson JA, Frisella MM, et al: Lethality of multiple endocrine neoplasia type I. *World J Surg* 22:581, discussion 586, 1998.
18. Benson L, Ljunghall S, Akerstrom G, et al: Hyperparathyroidism presenting as the first lesion in multiple endocrine neoplasia type 1. *Am J Med* 82:731, 1987.
19. Marx SJ, Vinik AI, Santen RJ, et al: Multiple endocrine neoplasia type I: Assessment of laboratory tests to screen for the gene in a large kindred. *Medicine (Baltimore)* 65:226, 1986.
20. Lamers CB, Froeling PG: Clinical significance of hyperparathyroidism in familial multiple endocrine adenomatosis type I (MEA I). *Am J Med* 66:422, 1979.
21. Vanderweghe M, Schutyser J, Braxer K, et al: A case of multiple endocrine adenomatosis with primary amenorrhea. *Postgrad Med*: 618, 1978.
22. Carlson HE, Levine GA, Goldberg NJ, et al: Hyperprolactinemia in multiple endocrine adenomatosis, type 1. *Arch Intern Med* 138:1807, 1978.
23. Tourniaire J, Trouillas J, Maillet P, et al: Polyadenomatose endocrinienne associant un adenome hypophysaire a prolactine et un adenome parathyroidien intrathyroidien. *Ann Endocrinol* 38:1, 1977.
24. Levine JH, Sagel J, Rosebrock GL, et al: Hyperprolactinemia and the multiple endocrine adenomatosis type 1 (MEA-1) syndrome [editorial]. *Arch Intern Med* 138:1777, 1978.
25. Skogseid B, Rastad J, Gobl A, et al: Adrenal lesion in multiple endocrine neoplasia type 1. *Surgery* 118:1077, 1995.
26. Burgess JR, Harle RA, Tucker P, et al: Adrenal lesions in a large kindred with multiple endocrine neoplasia type I. *Arch Surg* 131:699, 1996.
27. Darling TN, Skarulis MC, Steinberg SM, et al: Multiple facial angiofibromas and collagenomas in patients with multiple endocrine neoplasia type 1. *Arch Dermatol* 133:853, 1997.

28. Wermer P: Endocrine adenomatosis and peptic ulcer in a large kindred: Inherited multiple tumors and mosaic pleotropism in man. *Am J Med* 35:205, 1963.
29. Dackiw APB, Cote GJ, Fleming JB, et al: Screening for MEN 1 mutations in patients with atypical endocrine neoplasia. *Ann Surg* In press, 1999.
30. Rizzoli R, Green J III, Marx SJ: Primary hyperparathyroidism in familial multiple endocrine neoplasia type I. Long-term follow-up of serum calcium levels after parathyroidectomy. *Am J Med* 78:467, 1985.
31. Burgess JR, David R, Parameswaran V, et al: The outcome of subtotal parathyroidectomy for the treatment of hyperparathyroidism in multiple endocrine neoplasia type 1. *Arch Surg* 133:126, 1998.
32. Wells SA Jr., Ellis GJ, Gunnells JC, et al: Parathyroid autotransplantation in primary parathyroid hyperplasia. *N Engl J Med* 195:57, 1976.
33. Paloyan E, Lawrence AM: Laboratory diagnosis of parathyroid tumors. *Ann Clin Lab Sci* 4:241, 1974.
34. Scholz DA, Purnell DC, Edis AJ, et al: Primary hyperparathyroidism with multiple parathyroid gland enlargement: review of 53 cases. *Mayo Clin Proc* 53:792, 1978.
35. Chou YH, Pollak MR, Brandi ML, et al: Mutations in the human Ca(2+)-sensing-receptor gene that cause familial hypocalciuric hypercalcemia. *Am J Hum Genet* 56:1075, 1995.
36. Pearce SH, Trump D, Wooding C, et al: Calcium-sensing receptor mutations in familial benign hypercalcemia and neonatal hyperparathyroidism. *J Clin Invest* 96:2683, 1995.
37. Marx SJ, Sakaguchi K, Green J III, et al: Mitogenic activity on parathyroid cells in plasma from members of a large kindred with multiple endocrine neoplasia type 1. *J Clin Endocrinol Metab* 67:149, 1988.
38. Zimering MB, Brandi ML, de Grange DA, et al: Circulating fibroblast growth factor-like substance in familial multiple endocrine neoplasia type 1. *J Clin Endocrinol Metab* 70:149, 1990.
39. Zimering MB, Katsumata N, Friesen HG, et al: Fibroblast growth factor-like autoantibodies in plasma from patients with multiple endocrine neoplasia type 1 and prolactinoma. *Ann NY Acad Sci* 815:520, 1997.
40. Friedman E, Sakaguchi K, Bale AE, et al: Clonality of parathyroid tumors in familial multiple endocrine neoplasia type 1. *N Engl J Med* 321:213, 1989.
41. Trump D, Farren B, Wooding C, et al: Clinical studies of multiple endocrine neoplasia type 1 (MEN 1). *Q J Med* 89:653, 1996.
42. Marx S, Spiegel AM, Skarulis MC, et al: Multiple endocrine neoplasia type 1: Clinical and genetic topics. *Ann Intern Med* 129:484, 1998.
43. Giraud S, Choplin H, Teh BT, et al: A large multiple endocrine neoplasia type 1 family with clinical expression suggestive of anticipation. *J Clin Endocrinol Metab* 82:3487, 1997.
44. Deveney CW, Deveney KS, Way LW: The Zollinger-Ellison syndrome—23 years later. *Ann Surg* 188:384, 1978.
45. Norton JA, Cornelius MJ, Doppman JL, et al: Effect of parathyroidectomy in patients with hyperparathyroidism, Zollinger-Ellison syndrome, and multiple endocrine neoplasia type I: A prospective study. *Surgery* 102:958, 1987.
46. Ray JM, Squires PE, Curtis SB, et al: Expression of the calcium-sensing receptor on human antral gastrin cells in culture. *J Clin Invest* 99:2328, 1997.
47. McNeil L, Hobson S, Nipper V, et al: Functional calcium-sensing receptor expression in ovarian surface epithelial cells. *Am J Obstet Gynecol* 178:305, 1998.
48. Le Bodic MF, Heymann MF, Lecompte M, et al: Immunohistochemical study of 100 pancreatic tumors in 28 patients with multiple endocrine neoplasia, type 1. *Am J Surg Pathol* 20:1378, 1996.
49. Benya RV, Metz DC, Venzon DJ, et al: Zollinger-Ellison syndrome can be the initial endocrine manifestation in patients with multiple endocrine neoplasia-type I. *Am J Med* 97:436, 1994.
50. Skogseid B, Oberg K, Akerstrom G, et al: Limited tumor involvement found at multiple endocrine neoplasia type I pancreatic exploration: can it be predicted by preoperative tumor localization? *World J Surg* 22:673, discussion 667, 1998.
51. Metz DC, Jensen RT: Endocrine tumors of the pancreas, in Haubrich WB, Berk JE, Schaffner F (eds): *Bockus Gastroenterology*. Philadelphia, WB Saunders Publishing Company, 1994, p 3002.
52. Thorner MO, Frohman LA, Leong DA, et al: Extrahypothalamic growth-hormone-releasing factor (GRF) secretion is a rare cause of acromegaly: Plasma GRF levels in 177 acromegalic patients. *J Clin Endocrinol Metab* 59:846, 1984.
53. Jensen RT, Gardner JD: Gastrinoma, in Brooks FP, DiMagno EP, (eds): *The Exocrine Pancreas*. New York, Raven Press, 1993, pp. 931–972.
54. Skogseid B, Oberg K, Benson L, et al: A standardized meal stimulation test of the endocrine pancreas for early detection of pancreatic endocrine tumors in multiple endocrine neoplasia type 1 syndrome: Five years experience. *J Clin Endocrinol Metab* 64:1233, 1987.
55. Kloppel G, Willemer S, Stamm B, et al: Pancreatic lesions and hormonal profile of pancreatic tumors in multiple endocrine neoplasia type I. An immunocytochemical study of nine patients. *Cancer* 57:1824, 1986.
56. Marx SJ, Menczel J, Campbell G, et al: Heterogeneous size of the parathyroid glands in familial multiple endocrine neoplasia type 1. *Clin Endocrinol* 35:521, 1991.
57. Isenberg JI, Walsch JH, Grossman MI: Zollinger-Ellison syndrome. *Gastroenterology* 65:140, 1973.
58. Galbut DL, Markowitz AM: Insulinoma: Diagnosis, surgical management, and long-term follow-up. Review of 41 cases. *Am J Surg* 139:682, 1980.
59. Rasbach DA, van Heerden JA, Telander RL, et al: Surgical management of hyperinsulinism in the multiple endocrine neoplasia, type 1 syndrome. *Arch Surg* 120:584, 1985.
60. Doppman JL, Miller DL, Chang R: Insulinomas: Localization with selective intraarterial injection of calcium. *Radiology* 178:237, 1991.
61. Lo CY, Lam KY, Fan ST: Surgical strategy for insulinomas in multiple endocrine neoplasia type I. *Am J Surg* 175:305, 1998.
62. Doherty GM, Doppman JL, Shawker TH, et al: Results of a prospective strategy to diagnose, localizer and resect insulinomas. *Surgery* 110:989, 1991.
63. Sheppard BC, Norton JA, Doppman JL, et al: Management of islet cell tumors in patients with multiple endocrine neoplasia: a prospective study. *Surgery* 106:1108, 1989.
64. Norton JA, Gromack DT, Shawter TA, et al: Intraoperative ultrasonographic localization of islet cell tumors. A prospective comparison to palpation. *Ann Surg* 207:160, 1988.
65. Service FJ, Dale AJ, Elveback LR, et al: Insulinoma: Clinical and diagnostic features of 60 consecutive cases. *Mayo Clin Proc* 51:417, 1976.
66. Service FJ, McMahon MM, O'Brien PC, et al: Functioning insulinoma—incidence, recurrence, and long-term survival of patients: A 60-year study. *Mayo Clin Proc* 66:711, 1991.
67. Gogel HK, Buckman MT, Cadieux D, et al: Gastric secretion and hormonal interactions in multiple endocrine neoplasia type I. *Arch Intern Med* 145:855, 1985.
68. Zaniewski M, Jordan PH Jr., Yip B, et al: Serum gastrin level is increased by chronic hypercalcemia of parathyroid or nonparathyroid origin. *Arch Intern Med* 146:478, 1986.
69. Jensen RT: Management of the Zollinger-Ellison syndrome in patients with multiple endocrine neoplasia type 1. *J Intern Med* 243:477, 1998.
70. Wever HC, Benson DJ, Lin JT, et al: Determinants of metastatic rate and survival in patients with Zollinger-Ellison syndrome: A prospective long-term study. *Gastroenterology* 108:1637, 1995.
71. Leichter SB: Clinical and metabolic aspects of glucagonoma. *Medicine* 59:100, 1980.
72. Wilkinson DS: Necrolytic migratory erythena with carcinoma of the pancreas. *Trans St John's Hosp Dermatol Soc* 59:244, 1973.
73. Assaad SN, Carrasco CH, Vassilopoulou SR, et al: Glucagonoma syndrome. Rapid response following arterial embolization of glucagonoma metastatic to the liver. *Am J Med* 82:533, 1987.
74. Krejs GJ, Orci L, Conlon JM, et al: Somatostatinoma syndrome. *N Engl J Med* 301:285, 1979.
75. Namihira Y, Achord JL, Subramony C: Multiple endocrine neoplasia, type 1, with pancreatic cholera. *Am J Gastroenterol* 82:794, 1987.
76. Capella C, Polak JM, Butta R: Morphologic patterns and diagnostic criteria of VIP-producing endocrine tumors. A histologic, histochemical, ultrastructural, and biochemical study of 32 cases. *Cancer* 52:1860, 1983.
77. Rivier J, Spress J, Thorner M, et al: Characterization of a growth-hormone releasing factor from a human pancreatic islet cell tumor. *Nature* 300:276, 1982.

78. Asa SL, Singer W, Kovacs K, et al: Pancreatic endocrine tumour producing growth hormone-releasing hormone associated with multiple endocrine neoplasia type I syndrome. *Acta Endocrinol (Copenh)* 115:331, 1987.
79. Vinik AI, Strodel WE, Eckhauser FE, et al: Somatostatinomas, ppomas and neurotensinomas. *Semin Oncol* 14:263, 1987.
80. Friesen SR, Kimmel JR, Tomita T: Pancreatic polypeptide as screening marker for pancreatic polypeptide apudomas in multiple endocrinopathies. *Am J Surg* 139:61, 1980.
81. Takahashi H, Nakano K, Adachi Y, et al: Multiple nonfunctional pancreatic islet cell tumor in multiple endocrine neoplasia type I. A case report. *Acta Pathol Jpn* 38:667, 1988.
82. Skogseid B, Eriksson B, Lundqvist G, et al: Multiple endocrine neoplasia type 1: A 10-year prospective screening study in four kindreds. *J Clin Endocrinol Metab* 73:281, 1991.
83. Eckhauser FE, Cheung PS, Vinik, et al: Nonfunctioning malignant neuroendocrine tumors of the pancreas. *Surgery* 100:978, 1986.
84. Farid NR, Buehler S, Russell NA, et al: Prolactinomas in familial multiple endocrine neoplasia syndrome type 1. *Am J Med* 69:874, 1980.
85. Goldman M, Holub D: Prolactinomas and the multiple endocrine adenomatosis type-1 complex [letter]. *Ann Intern Med* 91:791, 1979.
86. Deftos LJ: *Medullary Thyroid Carcinoma*. Karger, Basel, 1983, pp 1–114.
87. O'Neal LW, Kipnis DM, Luse SA, et al: SecRETion of various endocrine substances by ACTH-secRETing tumors—gastrin, melanotropin, norepinephrine, serotonin, parathormone, vasopressin, glucagon. *Cancer* 21:1219, 1968.
88. Snyder N III, Scurry MT, Deiss WP: Five families with multiple endocrine adenomatosis. *Ann Intern Med* 76:53, 1972.
89. Levine JH, Sagel J, Rosebrock GL, et al: Hyperprolactinemia in the multiple endocrine adenomatosis type 1 (MEA-1) syndrome. *Arch Intern Med* 38:1777, 1977.
90. Pack S, Turner ML, Zhuang Z, et al: Cutaneous tumors in patients with multiple endocrine neoplasia type 1 show allelic deletion of the MEN1 gene. *J Invest Dermatol* 110:438, 1998.
91. Vortmeyer AO, Boni R, Pak E, et al: Multiple endocrine neoplasia 1 gene alterations in MEN 1-associated and sporadic lipomas [letter]. *J N C I* 90:398, 1998.
92. Burgess JR, Greenaway TM, Parameswaran V, et al: Enteropancreatic malignancy associated with multiple endocrine neoplasia type 1: Risk factors and pathogenesis. *Cancer* 83:428, 1998.
93. Zahner J, Borchard F, Schmitz U, et al: [Thymus carcinoid in multiple endocrine neoplasms type I]. *Dtsch Med Wochenschr* 119:135, 1994.
94. Teh BT, Zedenius J, Kytola S, et al: Thymic carcinoids in multiple endocrine neoplasia type 1. *Ann Surg* 228:99, 1998.
95. Manes JL, Taylor HB: Thymic carcinoid in familial multiple endocrine adenomatosis. *Arch Pathol* 95:252, 1973.
96. Burgess JR, Greenaway TM, Shepherd JJ: Expression of the MEN-1 gene in a large kindred with multiple endocrine neoplasia type 1. *J Intern Med* 243:465, 1998.
97. Thompson NW: The surgical management of hyperparathyroidism and endocrine disease of the pancreas in the multiple endocrine neoplasia type 1 patient. *J Intern Med* 238:269, 1995.
98. Bale AE, Norton JA, Wong EL, et al: Allelic loss on chromosome 11 in hereditary and sporadic tumors related to familial multiple endocrine neoplasia type 1. *Cancer Res* 51:1154, 1991.
99. Mortensen JD, Woolner LB, Bennett WA: Gross and microscopic findings in clinically normal thyroid glands. *J Clin Endocrinol Metab* 15:1270, 1955.
100. Mallek R, Mostbeck G, Walter RM, et al: Contrast MRI in multiple endocrine neoplasia type 1 (MEN) associated with renal cell carcinoma. *Eur J Radiol* 10:105, 1990.
101. Muhr C, Ljunghall S, Akerstrom G, et al: Screening for multiple endocrine neoplasia syndrome (type 1) in patients with primary hyperparathyroidism. *Clin Endocrinol (Oxf)* 20:153, 1984.
102. Lamers CB, Buis JT, van Tongeren J: Secretin-stimulated serum gastrin levels in hyperparathyroid patients from families with multiple endocrine adenomatosis type I. *Ann Intern Med* 86:719, 1977.
103. Olufemi SE, Green JS, Manickam P, et al: Common ancestral mutation in the MEN1 gene is likely responsible for the prolactinoma variant of MEN1 (MEN1Burin) in four kindreds from Newfoundland. *Hum Mutat* 11:264, 1998.
104. Lips CJ, Vasen HF, Lamers CB: Multiple endocrine neoplasia syndromes. *Crc Crit Rev Oncol Hematol* 2:117, 1984.
105. Effron M, Griner L, Benirschke K: Nature and rate of neoplasia found in captive wild mammals, birds, and reptiles at necropsy. *J Natl Cancer Inst* 59:185, 1977.
106. Berdjis CC: Pluriglandular syndrome: I. Multiple endocrine adenomas in irradiated rats. *Oncologia* 13:441, 1960.
107. Wermer P: Genetic aspects of adenomatosis of endocrine glands. *Am J Med* 16:363, 1954.
108. Guru SC, Goldsmith PK, Burns AL, et al: Menin, the product of the MEN1 gene, is a nuclear protein. *Proc Nat Acad Sci USA* 95:1630, 1998.
109. Agarwal SK, Guru SC, Heppner C, et al: Menin interacts with the AP1 transcription factor JunD and represses JunD-activated transcription. *Cell* 96:143, 1999.
110. Kishi M, Tsukada T, Shimizu S, et al: A large germline deletion of the MEN1 gene in a family with multiple endocrine neoplasia type 1. *Jpn J Cancer Res* 89:1, 1998.
111. Agarwal SK, Kester MB, Debelenko LV, et al: Germline mutations of the MEN1 gene in familial multiple endocrine neoplasia type 1 and related states. *Hum Mol Genet* 6:1169, 1997.
112. Teh BT, Kytola S, Farnebo F, et al: Mutation analysis of the MEN1 gene in multiple endocrine neoplasia type 1, familial acromegaly and familial isolated hyperparathyroidism [see comments]. *J Clin Endocrinol Metab* 83:2621, 1998.
113. Giraud S, Zhang CX, Serova-Sinilnikova O, et al: Germ-line mutation analysis in patients with multiple endocrine neoplasia type 1 and related disorders. *Am J Hum Genet* 63:455, 1998.
114. Cote GJ, Lee JE, Evans DB, et al: Five novel mutations in the familial multiple endocrine neoplasia, type 1 (MEN 1) gene. *Hum Mutat* 12:219, 1998.
115. Hansen OP, Hansen M, Hansen HH, et al: Multiple endocrine adenomatosis of mixed type. *Acta Med Scand* 200:327, 1976.
116. Duh QY, Hybarger CP, Geist R, et al: Carcinoids associated with multiple endocrine neoplasia syndrome. *Am J Surg* 154:142, 1987.
117. Anderson RJ, Lufkin EG, Sizemore GW, et al: Acromegaly and pituitary adenoma with phaeochromocytoma: A variant of multiple endocrine neoplasia. *Clin Endocrinol (Oxf)* 14:605, 1981.
118. Cameron D, Spiro HM, Landsberg L: Zollinger-Ellison syndrome with multiple endocrine adenomatosis type II [letter]. *N Engl J Med* 299:152, 1978.
119. Tuch BE, Carter JN, Armellin GM, et al: The association of a tumour of the posterior pituitary gland with multiple endocrine neoplasia type 1. *Aust N Z J Med* 12:179, 1982.
120. O'Halloran DJ, Shalet SM: A family pedigree exhibiting features of both multiple endocrine neoplasia type 1 and McCune-Albright syndromes. *J Clin Endocrinol Metab* 78:523, 1994.
121. Carney JA, Go VLW, Gordon H, et al: Familial pheochromocytoma and islet cell tumor of the pancreas. *Am J Med* 68:515, 1980.
122. Hellman P, Skogseid B, Oberg K, et al: Primary and reoperative parathyroid operations in hyperparathyroidism of multiple endocrine neoplasia type 1. *Surgery* 124:993, 1998.
123. Melmed S: Extrapituitary acromegaly. *Endocrinol Metab Clin North Am* 20:507, 1991.
124. Norton JA, Doppman JL, Collen MJ, et al: Prospective study of gastrinoma localization and resection in patients with Zollinger-Ellison syndrome. *Ann Surg* 204:468, 1986.
125. Jensen RT, Doppman JL, Gardner JD: Gastrinoma, in Go VLW, Gardner JD, Brooks FP, Lebenthal E, DiMagno EP, Scheele GA (eds): *The Exocrine Pancreas*. New York, Raven Press, 1986, pp 727–745.
126. Jensen RT, Fraker DL: Zollinger-Ellison syndrome. Advances in treatment of gastric hypersecretion and the gastrinoma [clinical conference]. *Jama* 271:1429, 1994.
127. McArthur KE, Collen MJ, Maton PN, et al: Omeprazole: Effective, convenient therapy for Zollinger-Ellison syndrome. *Gastroenterology* 88:939, 1985.
128. DeLellis RA, Gagel RF, Kaplan MM, et al: Gastrinoma of duodenal G-cell origin. *Cancer* 38:201, 1976.
129. Pipeleers-Marichal M, Somers G, Willems G, et al: Gastrinomas in the duodenums of patients with multiple endocrine neoplasia type 1 and the Zollinger-Ellison syndrome. *N Engl J Med* 322:723, 1990.
130. Modlin IM, Lawton GP: Duodenal gastrinoma: The solution to the pancreatic paradox [editorial]. *J Clin Gastroenterol* 19:184, 1994.

131. Norton JA: Gastrinoma: Advances in localization and treatment. *Surg Onc Clin North Am* 7:845, 1998.
132. Thompson NW, Pasieka J, Fukuuchi A: Duodenal gastrinomas, duodenotomy, and duodenal exploration in the surgical management of Zollinger-Ellison syndrome. *World J Surg* 17:455, 1993.
133. Thompson NW: Current concepts in the surgical management of multiple endocrine neoplasia type 1 pancreatic-duodenal disease. Results in the treatment of 40 patients with Zollinger-Ellison syndrome, hypoglycaemia or both. *J Intern Med* 243:495, 1998.
134. Metz DC, Pisegna JR, Fishbeyn VA, et al: Current maintenance doses of omeprazole in Zollinger-Ellison syndrome are too high. *Gastroenterology* 103:1498, 1992.
135. Frucht H, Howard JM, Slaff JE: Secretin and calcium provocative tests in patients with Zollinger-Ellison syndrome: A prospective study. *Ann Intern Med* 111:713, 1989.
136. Termanini B, Gibril F, Reynolds JC, et al: Value of somatostatin receptor scintigraphy: A prospective study in gastrinoma of its effect on clincial management. *Gastroenterol* 112:335, 1997.
137. Graber AL, Porte DJ, Williams RH: Clinical use of diazoxide and mechanism for its hyperglycemic effects. *Diabetes* 15:143, 1966.
138. Hoff AO, Vassilopoulou-Sellin R: The role of glucagon administration in the diagnosis and treatment of patients with tumor hypoglycemia. *Cancer* 82:1585, 1998.
139. Schein PS: Chemotherapeutic, management of the hormone-secreting malignancies. *Cancer* 30:1616, 1972.
140. Moertel CG, Kvols LK, O'Connell MJ, et al: Treatment of neuroendocrine carcinomas with combined etoposide and cisplatin. Evidence of major therapeutic activity in the anaplastic variants of these neoplasms. *Cancer* 68:227, 1991.
141. Moertel CG, Johnson CM, McKusick MA, et al: The management of patients with advanced carcinoid tumors and islet cell carcinomas. *Ann Intern Med* 120:302, 1994.
142. Service FJ, O'Brien PC, McMahon MM, et al: C-peptide during the prolonged fast in insulinoma. *J Clin Endocrinol Metab* 76:655, 1993.
143. Deftos LJ: Clinical essentials of calcium and skeletal disorders, *Multiple Endocrine Neoplasia*, Professional Communications, 1998; pp 137–151.
144. Sipple JH: The association of pheochromocytoma with carcinoma of the thyroid gland. *Am J Med* 31:163, 1961.
145. Williams ED: Medullary carcinoma of the thyroid. *J Clin Pathol* 20:395, 1967.
146. Schimke RN, Hartmann WH: Familial amyloid-producing medullary thyroid carcinoma and pheochromocytoma: a distinct genetic entity. *Ann Intern Med* 63:1027, 1965.
147. Steiner AL, Goodman AD, Powers SR: Study of a kindred with pheochromocytoma, medullary carcinoma, hyperparathyroidism and Cushing's disease: Multiple endocrine neoplasia, type 2. *Medicine* 47:371, 1968.
148. Gagel RF, Levy ML, Donovan DT, et al: Multiple endocrine neoplasia type 2a associated with cutaneous lichen amyloidosis. *Ann Intern Med* 111:802, 1989.
149. Nunziata V, Giannattasio R, di Giovanni G, et al: Hereditary localized pruritus in affected members of a kindred with multiple endocrine neoplasia type 2A (Sipple's syndrome). *Clin Endocrinol* 30:57, 1989.
150. Williams ED, Pollock DJ: Multiple mucosal neuromata with endocrine tumours: A syndrome allied to Von Recklinghausen's disease. *J Pathol Bacteriol* 91:71, 1966.
151. Farndon JR, Leight GS, Dilley WG, et al: Familial medullary thyroid carcinoma without associated endocrinopathies: A distinct clinical entity. *Br J Surg* 73:278, 1986.
152. Mulligan LM, Eng C, Healey CS, et al: A de novo mutation of the RET proto-oncogene in a patient with MEN 2A. *Hum Mol Genet* 3:1007, 1994.
153. Wohllk N, Cote GJ, Bugalho MM, et al: Relevance of RET proto-oncogene mutations in sporadic medullary thyroid carcinoma. *J Clin Endocrinol Metab* 81:3740, 1996.
154. Vasen HFA, van der Feltz M, Raue F, et al: The natural course of multiple endocrine neoplasia type IIb: A study of 18 cases. *Arch Intern Med* 152:1250, 1992.
155. Sizemore GW, Carney JA, Gharib H, et al: Multiple endocrine neoplasia type 2B: Eighteen-year follow-up of a four-generation family. *Henry Ford Hosp J* 40:236, 1992.
156. Goodfellow PJ: Mapping the inherited defects associated with multiple endocrine neoplasia type 2A, multiple endocrine neoplasia type 2B, and familial medullary thyroid carcinoma to chromosome 10 by linkage analysis. *Endocrinol Metab Clin North Am* 23:177, 1994.
157. Mathew CG, Chin KS, Easton DF, et al: A linked genetic marker for multiple endocrine neoplasia type 2A on chromosome 10. *Nature* 328:527, 1987.
158. Simpson NE, Kidd KK, Goodfellow PJ, et al: Assignment of multiple endocrine neoplasia type 2A to chromosome 10 by linkage. *Nature* 328:528, 1987.
159. Mulligan LM, Kwok JB, Healey CS, et al: Germ-line mutations of the RET proto-oncogene in multiple endocrine neoplasia type 2A. *Nature* 363:458, 1993.
160. Donis-Keller H, Dou S, Chi D, et al: Mutations in the RET proto-oncogene are associated with MEN 2A and FMTC. *Hum Mol Genet* 2:851, 1993.
161. GFRa Nomenclature Committee: Nomenclature of GPI-linked receptors for the GDNF ligand family. *Neuron* 19:485, 1997.
162. Lin LF, Doherty DH, Lile JD, et al: GDNF: A glial cell line-derived neurotrophic factor for midbrain dopaminergic neurons. *Science* 260:1130, 1993.
163. Eng C, Smith DP, Mulligan LM, et al: A novel point mutation in the tyrosine kinase domain of the RET proto-oncogene in sporadic medullary thyroid carcinoma and in a family with FMTC. *Oncogene* 10:509, 1995.
164. Berndt I, Reuter M, Saller B, et al: A new hot spot for mutations in the ret protooncogene causing familial medullary thyroid carcinoma and multiple endocrine neoplasia type 2A. *J Clin Endocrinol Metab* 83:770, 1998.
165. Bolino A, Schuffenecker I, Luo Y, et al: RET mutations in exons 13 and 14 of FMTC patients. *Oncogene* 10:2415, 1995.
166. Gimm O, Marsh DJ, Andrew SD, et al: Germline dinucleotide mutation in codon 883 of the RET proto-oncogene in multiple endocrine neoplasia type 2B without codon 918 mutation. *J Clin Endocrinol Metab* 82:3902, 1997.
167. Smith DP, Houghton C, Ponder BA: Germline mutation of RET codon 883 in two cases of de novo MEN 2B. *Oncogene* 15:1213, 1997.
168. Hofstra RM, Fattoruso O, Quadro L, et al: A novel point mutation in the intracellular domain of the ret protooncogene in a family with medullary thyroid carcinoma. *J Clin Endocrinol Metab* 82:4176, 1997.
169. Dang GT, Cote GJ, Schultz PN, et al: A codon 891 exon 15 RET proto-oncogene mutation in familial medullary thyroid carcinoma: A detection strategy. *Mol Cell Probes* 13:77, 1999.
170. Hofstra RM, Landsvater RM, Ceccherini I, et al: A mutation in the RET proto-oncogene associated with multiple endocrine neoplasia type 2B and sporadic medullary thyroid carcinoma [see comments]. *Nature* 367:375, 1994.
171. Eng C, Clayton D, Schuffenecker I, et al: The relationship between specific RET proto-oncogene mutations and disease phenotype in multiple endocrine neoplasia type 2. International RET mutation consortium analysis. *JAMA* 276:1575, 1996.
172. Williams ED: Histogenesis of medullary carcinoma of the thyroid. *J Clin Pathol* 19:114, 1966.
173. Melvin KEW, Tashjian AH Jr: The syndrome of excessive thyrocalcitonin produced by medullary carcinoma of the thyroid. *Proc Natl Acad Sci USA* 59:1216, 1968.
174. Deftos LJ, Goodman AD, Engelman K, et al: Suppression and stimulation of calcitonin secretion in medullary thyroid carcinoma. *Metabolism* 20:428, 1971.
175. Melvin KEW, Tashjian AH Jr, Miller HH: Studies in familial (medullary) thyroid carcinoma. *Recent Prog Horm Res* 28:399, 1972.
176. Wolfe HJ, Melvin KEW, Cervi-Skinner SJ, et al: C-cell hyperplasia preceding medullary thyroid carcinoma. *N Engl J Med* 289:437, 1973.
177. Baylin SB, Mendelsohn G, Weisburger WR, et al: Levels of histaminase and L-dopa decarboxylase activity in the transition from C-cell hyperplasia to familial medullary thyroid carcinoma. *Cancer* 44:1315, 1979.
178. DeLellis RA, Rule AH, Spiler I, et al: Calcitonin and carcinoembryonic antigen as tumor markers in medullary thyroid carcinoma. *Am J Clin Pathol* 70:587, 1978.
179. Zeytinoglu FN, Gagel RF, Tashjian AHJ, et al: Characterization of neurotensin production by a line of rat medullary thyroid carcinoma cells. *Proc Natl Acad Sci USA* 77:3741, 1980.

180. Le Douarin N, Le Lievre C: Demonstration de l'origine neurales des cellules a calcitonine du corps ultimobranchial chez l'embryon de poulet. *Compt Rend* 270:2857, 1970.
181. Le Douarin N: *The neural crest: Developmental and cell biology series*. Vol. 12. Cambridge, Cambridge University Press, 1982, p 259.
182. Pearse AG, Takor TT: Neuroendocrine embryology and the APUD concept. *Clin Endocrinol* 5:229S, 1976.
183. Holm R, Sobrinho-Simoes M, Nesland JM, et al: Medullary thyroid carcinoma with thyroglobulin immunoreactivity. A special entity? *Lab Invest* 57:258, 1987.
184. Williams ED, Brown CL, Doniach I: Pathological and clinical findings in a series of 67 cases of medullary carcinoma of the thyroid. *J Clin Pathol* 19:103, 1966.
185. Hazard JB: The C-cells (parafollicular cells) of the thyroid gland and medullary thyroid carcinoma: A review. *Am J Pathol* 88:214, 1977.
186. Liu FS: Immunohistochemical and ultrastructural study on medullary carcinoma of the thyroid. *Chung Hua Chung Liu Tsa Chih* 12:213, 1990.
187. Deftos LJ, Bone HGd, Parthemore JG: Immunohistological studies of medullary thyroid carcinoma and C cell hyperplasia. *J Clin Endocrinol Metab* 51:857, 1980.
188. Lippman SM, Mendelson G, Trump DL, et al: The prognostic and biological significance of cellular heterogeneity in medullary thyroid carcinoma: A study of calcitonin, L-dopa decarboxylase, and histaminase. *J. Clin Endocrinol Metab* 54:233, 1982.
189. Walts AE, Said JW: Specific tumor markers in diagnostic cytology. Immunoperoxidase studies of carcinoembryonic antigen, lysozyme and other tissue antigens in effusions, washes and aspirates. *Acta Cytol* 27:408, 1983.
190. Travis WD, Wold LE: Immunoperoxidase staining of fine needle aspiration specimens previously stained by the Papanicolaou technique. *Acta Cytol* 31:517, 1987.
191. Kobayashi K, Teramoto S, Maeta H, et al: Simultaneous occurrence of medullary carcinoma and papillary carcinoma of the thyroid. *J Surg Oncol* 59:276, 1995.
192. Kovacs CS, Mase RM, Kovacs K, et al: Thyroid medullary carcinoma with thyroglobulin immunoreactivity in sporadic multiple endocrine neoplasia type 2-B. *Cancer* 74:928, 1994.
193. Parker LN, Kollin J, Wu SY, et al: Carcinoma of the thyroid with a mixed medullary, papillary, follicular, and undifferentiated pattern. *Arch Intern Med* 145:1507, 1985.
194. Pastolero GC, Coire CI, Asa SL: Concurrent medullary and papillary carcinomas of thyroid with lymph node metastases. A collision phenomenon. *Am J Surg Pathol* 20:245, 1996.
195. Wolfe HJ, DeLellis RA: Familial medullary thyroid carcinoma and C-cell hyperplasia. *Clin Endocrinol Metab* 10:351, 1981.
196. Ekblom M, Valimaki M, Pelkonen R, et al: Familial and sporadic medullary thyroid carcinoma: Clinical and immunohistological findings. *Q J Med* 65:899, 1987.
197. Carney JA, Sizemore GW, Lovestedt SA: Mucosal ganglioneuromatosis, medullary thyroid carcinoma, and pheochromocytoma: Multiple endocrine neoplasia, type 2b. *Oral Surg Oral Med Oral Pathol* 41:739, 1976.
198. Keiser JR, Beaven MA, Doppman J, et al: Sipple's syndrome: Medullary thryoid carcinoma, pheochromocytoma, and parathyroid disease. *Ann Intern Med* 78:561, 1973.
199. Parthemore JG, Bronzert D, Roberts G, et al: A short calcium infusion in the diagnosis of medullary thyroid carcinoma. *J Clin Endocrinol Metab* 39:108, 1974.
200. Hennessey JF, Gray TK, Cooper CW, et al: Stimulation of thyrocalcitonin secretion by pentagastrin and calcium in 2 patients with medullary thyroid carcinoma of the thyroid. *J Clin Endocrinol Metab* 36:200, 1973.
201. Hennessey JF, Wells SA, Ontjes DA, et al: A comparison of pentagastrin injections and calcium infusion as provocative agents for the detection of medullary carcinoma of the thyroid. *J Clin Endocrinol Metab* 39:487, 1974.
202. Wells SA Jr, Ontjes DA, Cooper CW, et al: The early diagnosis of medullary carcinoma of the thyroid gland in patients with multiple endocrine neoplasia type II. *Ann Surg* 182:362, 1975.
203. Gagel RF, Jackson CE, Block MA, et al: Age-related probability of development of hereditary medullary thyroid carcinoma. *J Pediatr* 101:941, 1982.
204. Hill CSJ, Ibanez ML, Samaan NA, et al: Medullary (solid) carcinoma of the thyroid gland: An analysis of the M. D. Anderson hospital experience with patients with the tumor, its special features, and its histogenesis. *Medicine (Baltimore)* 52:141, 1973.
205. Deftos LJ: Calcitonin in clinical medicine. *Adv Intern Med* 23:159, 1978.
206. Komminoth P, Kunz EK, Matias-Guiu X, et al: Analysis of RET proto-oncogene point mutations distinguishes heritable from nonheritable medullary thyroid carcinomas. *Cancer* 76:479, 1995.
207. Decker RA, Peacock ML, Borst MJ, et al: Progress in genetic screening of multiple endocrine neoplasia type 2A: Is calcitonin testing obsolete? *Surgery* 118:257, 1995.
208. Eng C, Mulligan LM, Smith DP, et al: Low frequency of germline mutations in the RET proto-oncogene in patients with apparently sporadic medullary thyroid carcinoma. *Clin Endocrinol* 43:123, 1995.
209. Beskid M: Thyroid C-cells in normal and goitrous gland: A histochemical study. *Acta Histochem* 54:313, 1975.
210. Milhaud G, Calmettes C, Jullienne A, et al: A new chapter in human pathology: Calcitonin disorders and therapeutic use, in Talmage RV, Munson PL (eds): *Calcium, Parathyroid Hormone, and the Calcitonins*. Amsterdam, Excerpta Medica, 1972, pp 56–70.
211. Saad MF, Ordonez NG, Rashid RK, et al: Medullary carcinoma of the thyroid: A study of the clinical features and prognostic factors in 161 patients. *Medicine* 63:319, 1984.
212. Sizemore GW, Carney JA, Heath H III: Epidemiology of medullary carcinoma of the thyroid gland: A 5-year experience (1971–1976). *Surg Clin North Am* 57:633, 1977.
213. Zedenius J, Larsson C, Bergholm U, et al: Mutations of codon 918 in the RET proto-oncogene correlate to poor prognosis in sporadic medullary thyroid carcinomas. *J Clin Endocrinol Metab* 80:3088, 1995.
214. Eng C, Mulligan LM, Healey CS, et al: Heterogeneous mutation of the RET proto-oncogene in subpopulations of medullary thyroid carcinoma. *Cancer Res* 56:2167, 1996.
215. Kimura T, Yoshimoto K, Yokogoshi Y, et al: Mutations in the cysteine-rich region of the RET proto-oncogene in patients diagnosed as having sporadic medullary thyroid carcinoma. *Endocrine J* 42:517, 1995.
216. Deftos LJ: Radioimmunoassay for calcitonin in medullary thyroid carcinoma. *JAMA* 227:403, 1974.
217. Motte P, Vauzelle P, Gardet P, et al: Construction and clinical validation of a sensitive and specific assay for serum mature calcitonin using monoclonal anti-peptide antibodies. *Clin Chim Acta* 174:35, 1988.
218. Seth R, Motte P, Kehely A, et al: A sensitive and specific two-site enzyme-immunoassay for human calcitonin using monoclonal antibodies. *J Endocrinol* 119:351, 1988.
219. O'Connor DT, Burton D, Deftos LJ: Immunoreactive human chromagranin A in diverse polypeptide hormone producing human tumors and normal endocrine tissues. *J Clin Endocrinol Metab* 57:1084, 1983.
220. Sobol RE, Memoli V, Deftos LJ: Hormone-negative, chromogranin A-positive endocrine tumors. *N Engl J Med* 320:444, 1989.
221. Dymling JF, Ljungberg O, Hillyard CJ, et al: Whisky: A new provacative test for calcitonin secretion. *Acta Endocrinol (Copenh)* 82:500, 1976.
222. Anast C, David L, Winnacker J, et al: Serum calcitonin-lowering effect of magnesium in patients with medullary thyroid carcinoma. *J Clin Invest* 56:1615, 1975.
223. Deftos LJ, Roos B: Medullary thyroid carcinoma and calcitonin gene expression, in Peck WA (ed): *Bone and Mineral Research*. New York, Elsevier, pp 267–316.
224. Deftos LJ: Calcitonin and medullary thyroid carcinoma, in Wyngaarden JB, Smith LH, Bennett JC, Plum F (eds): *Cecil Textbook of Medicine*. Philadelphia, Saunders, 1991, pp 1420–1423.
225. Gagel RF, Tashjian AH Jr, Cummings T, et al: The clinical outcome of prospective screening for multiple endocrine neoplasia type 2a: An 18-year experience. *N Engl J Med* 318:478, 1988.
226. Eisenhofer G, Lenders JW, Linehan WM, et al: Plasma normetanephrine and metanephrine for detecting pheochromocytoma in von Hippel-Lindau disease and multiple endocrine neoplasia type 2. *N Engl J Med* 340:1872, 1999.
227. Ljungberg O: On medullary carcinoma of the thyroid. *Acta Pathol Microbiol Scand* [A] 231:1, 1972.

228. Carney JA, Sizemore GW, Tyce GM: Bilateral adrenal medullary hyperplasia in multiple endocrine neoplasia, type 2: The precursor of bilateral pheochromocytoma. *Mayo Clin Proc* 50:3, 1975.
229. DeLellis RA, Wolfe HJ, Gagel RF, et al: Adrenal medullary hyperplasia. A morphometric analysis in patients with familial medullary thyroid carcinoma. *Am J Pathol* 83:177, 1976.
230. Neumann HP, Bender BU, Reincke M, et al: Adrenal-sparing surgery for phaeochromocytoma. *Br J Surg* 86:94, 1999.
231. Lee JE, Curley SA, Gagel RF, et al: Cortical-sparing adrenalectomy for patients with bilateral pheochromocytoma. *Surgery* 120:1064, discussion 1070, 1996.
232. Cushman P Jr: Familial endocrine tumors: Report of two unrelated kindred affected with pheochromocytomas, one also with multiple thyroid carcinomas. *Am J Med* 32:352, 1962.
233. Howe JR, Norton JA, Wells SA Jr: Prevalence of pheochromocytoma and hyperparathyroidism in multiple endocrine neoplasia type 2A: Results of long-term follow-up. *Surgery* 114:1070, 1993.
234. Melvin KEW, Miller HH, Tashjian AH Jr: Early diagnosis of medullary carcinoma of the thyroid gland by means of calcitonin assay. *N Engl J Med* 285:1115, 1971.
235. Pausova Z, Soliman E, Amizuka N, et al: Role of the RET proto-oncogene in sporadic hyperparathyroidism and in hyperparathyroidism of multiple endocrine neoplasia type 2. *J Clin Endocrinol Metab* 81:2711, 1996.
236. Chabre O, Labat F, Pinel N, et al: Cutaneous lesion associated with multiple endocrine neoplasia type 2A: Lichen amyloidosis or notalgia paresthetica. *Henry Ford Hosp J* 40:245, 1992.
237. Chabre O, Labat-Moleur F, Berthod F, et al: Cutaneous lesion asociated with multiple endocrine neoplasia type 2A-an early clinical marker. *Presse Med* 21:299, 1992.
238. Kousseff BG, Espinoza C, Zamore GA: Sipple syndrome with lichen amyloidosis as a paracrinopathy: Pleiotropy, heterogeneity, or a contiguous gene? *J Am Acad Dermatol* 25:651, 1991.
239. Hofstra RM, Sijmons RH, Stelwagen T, et al: RET mutation screening in familial cutaneous lichen amyloidosis and in skin amyloidosis associated with multiple endocrine neoplasia. *J Invest Derm* 107:215, 1996.
240. Robinson MF, Furst EJ, Nunziata V, et al: Characterization of the clinical features of five families with hereditary primary cutaneous lichen amyloidosis and multiple endocrine neoplasia type 2. *Henry Ford Hosp J* 40:249, 1992.
241. Tsuzuki T, Takahashi M, Asai N, et al: Spatial and temporal expression of the *ret* proto-oncogene product in embryonic, infant and adult rat tissues. *Oncogene* 10:191, 1995.
242. Schimke RN, Hartmann WH, Prout TE, et al: Syndrome of bilateral pheochromocytoma, medullary thyroid carcinoma and multiple neuromas: A possible regulatory defect in the differentiation of chromaffin tissue. *N Engl J Med* 279:1, 1968.
243. Gorlin RJ, Sedano HO, Vickers RA, et al: Multiple mucosal neuromas, pheochromocytoma and medullary carcinoma of the thyroid-a syndrome. *Cancer* 22:293, 1968.
244. Rashid M, Khairi MR, Dexter RN, et al: Mucosal neuroma, pheochromocytoma and medullary thyroid carcinoma: Multiple endocrine neoplasia type 3. *Medicine (Baltimore)* 54:89, 1975.
245. Fawell WN, Thompson G: Nutmeg for diarrhea of medullary carcinoma of thyroid. *N Engl J Med* 289:106, 1973.
246. Modigliani E, Guliana JM, Maroni M, et al: [Effects of subcutaneous administration of sandostatine (SMS 201.995) in 18 cases of thyroid medullary cancer]. *Ann Endocrinol (Paris)* 50:483, 1989.
247. Carney JA, Go VL, Sizemore GW, et al: Alimentary-tract ganglioneuromatosis. A major component of the syndrome of multiple endocrine neoplasia, type 2b. *N Engl J Med* 295:1287, 1976.
248. Schuchardt A, D'Agati V, Larsson-Blomberg L, et al: Defects in the kidney and enteric nervous system of mice lacking the tyrosine kinase receptor Ret [see comments]. *Nature* 367:380, 1994.
249. Treanor JJS, Goodman L, de Sauvage F, et al: Characterization of a multicomponent receptor for GDNF. *Nature* 382:80, 1996.
250. Durbec P, Marcos-Gutierrez CV, Kilkenny C, et al: GDNF signalling through the ret receptor tyrosine kinase. *Nature* 381:789, 1996.
251. Trupp M, Arenas E, Falnzilber M, et al: Functional receptor for GDNF encoded by the c-ret proto-oncogene. *Nature* 381:785, 1996.
252. Durbec PL, Larsson-Blomberg LB, Schuchardt A, et al: Common origin and developmental dependence on c-ret of subsets of enteric and sympathetic neuroblasts. *Development* 122:349, 1996.
253. Pichel JG, Shen L, Sheng HZ, et al: Defects in enteric innervation and kidney development in mice lacking GDNF. *Nature* 382:73, 1996.
254. Edery P, Lyonnet S, Mulligan LM, et al: Mutations of the RET proto-oncogene in Hirschsprung's disease [see comments]. *Nature* 367:378, 1994.
255. Angrist M, Bolk S, Thiel B, et al: Mutation analysis of the RET receptor tyrosine kinase in Hirschsprung's disease. *Hum Mol Genet* 4:821, 1995.
256. Angrist M, Bolk S, Halushka M, et al: Germline mutations in glial cell-derived neurotrophic factor (GDNF) and RET in a Hirschsprung disease patient. *Nat Genet* 14:341, 1996.
257. Attie T, Pelet A, Edery P, et al: Diversity of RET proto-oncogene mutations in familial and sporadic Hirschsprung disease. *Hum Mol Genet* 4:1381, 1995.
258. Decker RA, Peacock ML: Occurrence of MEN 2a in familial Hirschsprung's disease: A new indication for genetic testing of the RET proto-oncogene. *J Ped Surg* 33:207, 1998.
259. Mulligan LM, Eng C, Attie T, et al: Diverse phenotypes associated with exon 10 mutations of the RET proto-oncogene. *Hum Mol Genet* 3:2163, 1994.
260. Dyck PJ, Carney JA, Sizemore GW, et al: Multiple endocrine neoplasia, type 2b: Phenotype recognition; neurological features and their pathological basis. *Ann Neurol* 6:302, 1979.
261. Samaan NA, Draznin MB, Halpin RE, et al: Multiple endocrine syndrome type IIb in early childhood. *Cancer* 68:1832, 1991.
262. Stjernholm MR, Freudenbourg JC, Mooney HS, et al: Medullary carcinoma of the thyroid before age 2 years. *J Clin Endocrinol Metab* 51:252, 1980.
263. Ogle JW: Brain disease from diabetes mellitus. *St. George's Hosp Rep* 1:178, 1866.
264. Schmidt MB: Eine biglandulare Erkrankung (Nebennieren und Schilddrüse) bei Morbus Addisonii. *Verh Dtsch Ges Pathol* 21:212, 1926.
265. Blizzard RM, Kyle MA: Studies of the adrenal antigens and antibodies in Addison's disease. *J Clin Invest* 42:1653, 1963.
266. Neufeld M, MacLaren NK, Blizzard R: Two types of autoimmune Addison's disease associated with different polyglandular autoimmune (PGA) syndromes. *Medicine* 60:355, 1981.
267. Ahonen P, Myllarniemi S, Sipila I, Perheentupa J: Clinical variation of autoimmune polyendocrinopathy-candidiasis-ectodermal dystrophy (APECED) in a series of 68 patients. *N Engl J Med* 322:1829, 1990.
268. Betterle C, Greggio NA, Volpato M: Clinical review 93: Autoimmune polyglandular syndrome type I. *J Clin Endocrinol Metab* 83: 1049, 1998.
269. Brun JM: Juvenile autoimmune polyendocrinopathy. *Horm Res* 16:308, 1982.
270. Appleboom TM, Flowers FP: Ketoconazole in the treatment of chronic mucocutaneous candidiasis secondary to autoimmune polyendocrinopathy-candidiasis syndrome. *Cutis* 30:71, 1982.
271. Proto G, Leoni S, Torossi I, et al: Autoimmune polyendocrinopathy and chronic mucocutaneous candidiasis. *Minerva Med* 83:475, 1992.
272. DePadova-Elder SM, Ditre CM, Kantor GR, Koblenzer PJ: Candidiasis endocrinopathy syndrome. Treatment with itraconazole. *Arch Dermatol* 130:19, 1994.
273. Zlotogora J, Shapiro MS: Polyglandular autoimmune syndrome type I among Iranian Jews. *J Med Genet* 29:824, 1992.
274. Bjorses P, Aaltonen J, Vikman A, et al. Genetic homogeneity of autoimmune polyglandular disease type I. *Am J Hum Genet* 59:879, 1996.
275. Blizzard RM, Chee D, Davis W: The incidence of parathyroid and other antibodies in the sera of patients with idiopathic hypoparathyroidism. *Clin Exp Immunol* 1:119, 1966.
276. Li Y, Song YH, Rais N, et al: Autoantibodies to the extracellular domain of the calcium sensing receptor in patients with acquired hypoparathyroidism. *J Clin Invest* 97:910, 1996.
277. Rose NR: Is idiopathic hypoparathyroidism an autoimmune disease. *J Clin Invest* 97:899, 1996.
278. Grant DB, Barnes ND, Moncrieff MW, Savage MO: Clinical presentation, growth, and pubertal development in Addison's disease. *Arch Dis Child* 60:925, 1985.
279. Saenger P, Levine LS, Irvine WJ, et al: Progressive adrenal failure in polyglandular autoimmune disease. *J Clin Endocrinol Metab* 54:863, 1982.

280. Uibo R, Aavik E, Peterson P, et al: Autoantibodies to cytochrome P450 enzymes P450scc, P450c17, and P450c21 in autoimmune polyglandular disease types I and II and in isolated Addison's disease. *J Clin Endocrinol Metab* 78:323, 1994.
281. Chen S, Sawicka J, Betterle C, et al: Autoantibodies to steroidogenic enzymes in autoimmune polyglandular syndrome, Addison's disease, and premature ovarian failure. *J Clin Endocrinol Metab* 81:1871, 1996.
282. Peterson P, Uibo R, Peranen J, Krohn K: Immunoprecipitation of steroidogenic enzyme autoantigens with autoimmune polyglandular syndrome type I (APS I) sera; further evidence for independent humoral immunity to P450c17 and P450c21. *Clin Exp Immunol* 107:335, 1997.
283. Betterle C, Volpato M, Rees Smith B, et al: I. Adrenal cortex and steroid 21-hydroxylase autoantibodies in adult patients with organ-specific autoimmune diseases: Markers of low progression to clinical Addison's disease. *J Clin Endocrinol Metab* 82:932, 1997.
284. Betterle C, Volpato M, Rees Smith B, et al: II. Adrenal cortex and steroid 21-hydroxylase autoantibodies in children with organ-specific autoimmune diseases: Markers of high progression to clinical Addison's disease. *J Clin Endocrinol Metab* 82:939, 1997.
285. Irvine WJ, Chan MM, Scarth L, et al: Immunological aspects of premature ovarian failure associated with idiopathic Addison's disease. *Lancet* 2:883, 1968.
286. McNatty KP, Short RV, Barnes EW, Irvine WJ: The cytotoxic effect of serum from patients with Addison's disease and autoimmune ovarian failure on human granulosa cells in culture. *Clin Exp Immunol* 22:378, 1975.
287. Weinberg U, Kraemer FB, Kammerman S: Coexistence of primary endocrine deficiencies: A unique case of male hypergonadism associated with hypoparathyroidism, hypoadrenocorticism, and hypothyroidism. *Am J Med Sci* 272:215, 1976.
288. Tuomi T, Bjorses P, Falorni A, et al: Antibodies to glutamic acid decarboxylase and insulin-dependent diabetes in patients with autoimmune polyendocrine syndrome type I. *J Clin Endocrinol Metab* 81:1488, 1996.
289. Husebye ES, Gebre-Medhin G, Tuomi T, et al: Autoantibodies against aromatic L-amino acid decarboxylase in autoimmune polyendocrine syndrome type I. *J Clin Endocrinol Metab* 82:147, 1997.
290. Davenport C, Radford PM, Al-Bukhari TA, et al: Heterogeneity in the occurrence of a subset of autoantibodies to glutamic acid decarboxylase in autoimmune polyendocrine patients with islet cell antibodies. *Clin Exp Immunol* 111:497, 1998.
291. Arvanitakis C, Knouss RF: Selective hypopituitarism. Impaired cell-mediated immunity and chronic mucocutaneous candidiasis. *JAMA* 225:1492, 1973.
292. Clemente MG, Obermayer-Straub P, Meloni A, et al: Cytochrome P450 1A2 is a hepatic autoantigen in autoimmune polyglandular syndrome type 1. *J Clin Endocrinol Metab* 82:1353, 1997.
293. Clemente MG, Meloni A, Obermayer-Straub P, et al: Two cytochromes P450 are major hepatocellular autoantigens in autoimmune polyglandular syndrome type 1. *Gastroenterology* 114:324, 1998.
294. Carpenter CCJ, Solomon N, Silverberg SG, et al: Schmidt's syndrome (thyroid and adrenal insufficiency): A review of the literature and a report of fifteen new cases including ten instances of coexistent diabetes mellitus. *Medicine* 43:153, 1964.
295. Lechuga-Gomez Ee, Meyerson J, Bigazzi PE, Walfish PG: Polyglandular autoimmune syndrome type II. *Can Med Assoc J* 138:632, 1988.
296. Betterle C, Volpato M, Greggio AN, Presotto F: Type 2 polyglandular autoimmune disease (Schmidt's syndrome). *J Ped Endocrinol Metab* 9:113, 1996.
297. Betterle C, Scalici C, Presotto F, et al: The natural history of adrenal function in autoimmune patients with adrenal autoantibodies. *J Endocrinol* 117:467, 1988.
298. Doniach D, Bottazzo GF: Polyendocrine autoimmunity, in Franklin EC (ed): *Clinical Immunology Update*. Amsterdam, Elsevier North Holland, 1981, pp 95–121.
299. Irvine WJ, McCallum CJ, Gray RS, et al: Pancreatic islet-cell antibodies in diabetes mellitus correlated with the duration and type of diabetes, coexistent autoimmune disease, and HLA type. *Diabetes* 26:138, 1977.
300. Bottazzo GF, Mann JI, Thorogood M, et al: Autoimmunity in juvenile diabetics and their families. *Br Med J* 2:165, 1978.
301. Kiessling WR, Pflughaupt KW, Ricker K, et al: Thyroid function and circulating antithyroid antibodies in myasthenia gravis. *Neurology* 31:771, 1981.
302. Nagamine K, Peterson P, Scott HS, et al: Positional cloning of the APECED gene. *Nat Genet* 17:393, 1997.
303. The Finnish-German APECED Consortium: An autoimmune disease, APECED, caused by mutations in a novel gene featuring two PHD-type zinc-finger domains. *Nat Genet* 17:399, 1997.
304. Rosatelli MC, Meloni A, Devoto M, et al: A common mutation in Sardinian autoimmune polyendocrinopathy-candidiasis-ectodermal dystrophy patients. *Hum Genet* 103:428, 1998.
305. Heino M, Scott HS, Chen Q, et al: Mutation analyses of North American APS-1 patients. *Hum Mutat* 13:69, 1999.
306. Wang CY, Davoodi-Semiromi A, Huang W, et al: Characterization of mutations in patients with autoimmune polyglandular syndrome type 1 (APS1). *Hum Genet* 103:681, 1998.
307. Maclaren NK, Riley WJ: Inherited susceptibility to autoimmune Addison's disease is linked to human leukocyte antigens-DR3 and/or DR4, except when associated with type I autoimmune polyglandular syndrome. *J Clin Endocrinol Metab* 62:455, 1986.
308. Latinne D, Vandeput Y, De Bruyere M, et al: Addison's disease: Immunological aspects. *Tissue Antigens* 30:23, 1987.
309. Boehm BO, Manfras B, Seidl S, et al: The HLA-DQ beta non-Asp-57 allele: A predictor of future insulin-dependent diabetes mellitus in patients with autoimmune Addison's disease. *Tissue Antigens* 37:130, 1991.
310. Weetman AP, Zhang L, Tandon N, Edwards OM: HLA associations with autoimmune Addison's disease. *Tissue Antigens* 38:31, 1991.
311. Bartholomaeus WN, O'Donoghue H, Foti D, et al: Multiple autoantibodies following cytomegalovirus infection: Virus distribution and specificity of autoantibodies. *Immunology* 64:397, 1988.
312. Sakaguchi S, Sakaguchi N: Organ-specific autoimmune disease induced in mice by elimination of T cell subsets. V. Neonatal administration of cyclosporin A causes autoimmune disease. *J Immunol* 142:471, 1989.
313. Bardwick PA, Zvaifler NJ, Gill GN, et al: Plasma cell dyscrasia with polyneuropathy, organomegaly, endocrinopathy, M protein, and skin changes: The POEMS syndrome. Report on two cases and a review of the literature. *Medicine (Baltimore)* 59:311, 1980.
314. Soubrier MJ, Dubost JJ, Sauvezie BJ: POEMS syndrome: A study of 25 cases and a review of the literature. French Study Group on POEMS Syndrome. *Am J Med* 97:543, 1994.
315. Longo G, Emilia G, Torelli U: Skin changes in POEMS syndrome. *Haematologica* 84:86, 1999.
316. Rose C, Zandecki M, Copin MC, et al: POEMS syndrome: Report on six patients with unusual clinical signs, elevated levels of cytokines, macrophage involvement and chromosomal aberrations of bone marrow plasma cells. *Leukemia* 11:1318, 1997.
317. Bova G, Pasqui AL, Saletti M, et al: POEMS syndrome with vascular lesions: A role for interleukin-1beta and interleukin-6 increase—a case report. *Angiology* 49:937, 1998.
318. Lesprit P, Godeau B, Authier FJ, et al: Pulmonary hypertension in POEMS syndrome: A new feature mediated by cytokines. *Am J Respir Crit Care Med* 157:907, 1998.
319. Watanabe O, Maruyama I, Arimura K, et al: Overproduction of vascular endothelial growth factor/vascular permeability factor is causative in Crow-Fukase (POEMS) syndrome. *Muscle Nerve* 21:1390, 1998.
320. Authier FJ, Belec L, Levy Y, et al: All-trans-retinoic acid in POEMS syndrome. Therapeutic effect associated with decreased circulating levels of proinflammatory cytokines. *Arthritis Rheum* 39:1423, 1996.
321. Ako S, Kaneko Y, Higuchi M, et al: Crow-Fukase syndrome—immunoadsorption plasmapheresis effectively lowers elevated interleukin-6 concentration. *Nephrol Dial Transplant* 14:419, 1999.

CHAPTER 28

Ectopic Hormone Production

Glenn D. Braunstein

GENERAL PRINCIPLES

Paraneoplastic Syndromes

Most clinical abnormalities found in patients with cancer are directly related to the growth of the primary tumor and to metastases, infections, or therapy. In addition, these patients may exhibit one or more remote effects of cancer. Such remote effects, or *paraneoplastic syndromes,* include the signs, symptoms, and biochemical abnormalities that occur in patients as a result of cancer which are not due to the mass effects of the primary neoplasm or its metastases. The spectrum of paraneoplastic syndromes is large and covers every organ system (Table 28-1). Paraneoplastic syndromes are relatively common in patients with cancer, being found in approximately 7–10 percent of patients at the time of diagnosis, 20 percent at any time period, and in up to 50 percent at some time during the course of disease.[1,2] The most common paraneoplastic syndromes involve ectopic hormone production, neurologic dysfunction, and hematologic abnormalities.

Many of the nonendocrine paraneoplastic syndromes result from immunologic abnormalities. Some syndromes are associated with the production of site-specific antibodies. Examples include subacute cerebellar degeneration, which is associated with anti-Purkinje cell cytoplasmic antibodies (anti-Yo antibody), the Lambert-Eaton syndrome with antibodies directed against the voltage-gated calcium channels, the antiacetylcholine receptor antibodies found in patients with myasthenia gravis associated with thymomas, and autoantibodies to desmoplakin I and other skin antigens in paraneoplastic pemphigus.[3,4] Circulating antibodies may also cause a paraneoplastic syndrome through the formation of immune complexes. The deposition of an immune complex composed of carcinoembryonic antigen and anticarcinoembryonic antigen has been described in patients with nephrotic syndrome associated with cancer.[5] Similarly, glomerular membrane deposition of IgG and IgM in patients with the nephrotic syndrome and lung carcinoma has been noted.[6,7] Cell-mediated immune dysfunction in patients with cancer is well known and accounts for the anergy found with late-stage disease. Lymphocytes that are cytotoxic for muscle cells have been found in patients with cancer-associated dermatomyositis.[8] The alterations in normal immunity found in cancer patients also account for some of the unusual infections encountered. For many years the syndrome of progressive multifocal leukoencephalopathy was thought to be a paraneoplastic syndrome primarily found in lymphoproliferative and myoproliferative neoplasms. However, it is now known that this syndrome is the consequence of central nervous system (CNS) infection with a papovavirus (JC virus or SV40-PML virus).[9]

Another mechanism by which tumors may give rise to a paraneoplastic syndrome is through the depletion of substrates. Examples include a pellagra-like dermatitis secondary to the niacin deficiency found in some patients with carcinoid tumors and the necrolytic migratory erythema from amino acid depletion in the hypercatabolic state induced by glucagon-secreting tumors. Also, the hypoglycemia found in markedly cachectic patients may result from a lack of sufficient quantities of gluconeogenic amino acids to allow the liver to synthesize adequate quantities of glucose during fasting.[10]

Tumors also may secrete excessive quantities of normally occurring proteins. A number of growth factors that are considered to be local or paracrine regulators of cell function may be secreted in sufficient quantities to act systemically. Eosinophilopoietin production in lymphoproliferative disorders may be responsible for the eosinophilia associated with these tumors.[11] Disseminated intravascular coagulation has been associated with mucin-producing adenocarcinomas in which the mucin appears to activate factor X.[12] These examples illustrate the wide range of pathophysiologic mechanisms that may give rise to nonendocrine paraneoplastic syndromes.

Eutopic versus Ectopic Hormone Production

Until recently, the definition of eutopic and ectopic hormone production was relatively straightforward. *Eutopic hormone production* referred to the secretion of a hormone by a neoplasm derived from a tissue or organ that normally produces the hormone, while *ectopic hormone production* was defined as the secretion of a hormone by a neoplasm derived from a tissue or organ that does not normally produce that hormone. Using these definitions, excessive production of adrenocorticotropin (ACTH) by a corticotrope adenoma of the pituitary represents eutopic production of ACTH, while Cushing's syndrome resulting from production of ACTH by a small cell carcinoma of the lung represents ectopic production. However, many normal tissues, including lung, contain small amounts of immunoreactive ACTH or pro-opiomelanocortin (POMC).[13] This finding has resulted in the hypothesis that the elevated serum and tumor levels of immunoreactive ACTH or POMC are due to a quantitative difference in the amounts of ACTH/POMC synthesized by tumor cells in contrast to normal cells. In addition, if cancer cells contain the enzymes that process the biologically inactive POMC to the biologically active ACTH molecule, Cushing's syndrome may result.[13] Growth hormone, prolactin, insulin, corticotropin releasing factor (CRF), human chorionic gonadotropin (hCG), somatostatin, calcitonin, vasoactive intestinal peptide (VIP), and parathyroid hormone-related

TABLE 28-1. Spectrum of Paraneoplastic Syndromes

Ectopic hormone syndromes (see Table 28-2)	Secondary amyloidosis
Neurologic syndromes	Dermatologic syndromes
Dementia	Acanthosis nigricans
Dermatomyositis-polymyositis	Acquired icthyosis
Lambert-Eaton syndrome	Acquired tylosis
Limbic encephlalitis	Bazex's syndrome
Myesthenia gravis	Bowen's disease
Necrotizing myelopathy	Dermatitis herpetiformis
Opsoclonus-myoclonus	Erythemia annulare centrifugum
Paraneoplastic retinopathy	Erythemia gryatum repens
Peripheral neuropathies	Erythromelalgia
Stiff-man syndrome	Exfoliative dermatitis
Subacute cerebellar degeneration	Extramammary Paget's disease
Subacute sensory neuropathy	Hypertrichosis lanuginosa
Myopathies	Leser-Trelat sign
Acute necrotizing myopathy	Melanosis
Carcinomatous neuromyopathy	Pachydermoperiostosis
Dermatomyositis-polymyositis	Pemphigoid
Hematologic syndromes	Pityriasis rotunda
Acquired von Willebrand disease	Pruritis
Autoimmune hemolytic anemia	Pyoderma gangrenosum
Circulating anticoagulant	Sweet's syndrome
Cold hemagglutinin disease	Tripe palms
Cryoglobulinemia	Gastrointestinal syndromes
Disseminated intravascular coagulation	Anorexia-cachexia
Eosinophilia	Dysguesia/hypogeusia
Erythrocytosis	Protein-losing enteropathy
Granulocytopenia	Rheumatologic syndromes
Granulocytosis	Hypertrophic pulmonary osteoarthropathy
Hyperviscosity syndrome	Polyarteritis
Hypogammaglobulinemia	Rheumatoid arthritis-like arthropathy
Megaloblastic anemia	Secondary gout
Microangiopathic hemolytic anemia	Vascular syndromes
Red cell aplasia	Nonbacterial thrombotic endocarditis
T- and B-cell dysfunction	Venous thrombosis
Thrombocytopenia	Miscellaneous syndromes
Thromobocytosis	Fever
Renal syndromes	Hyperlipidemia
Glomerulonephritis	Lactic acidosis
Nephrotic syndrome	Porphyria cutanea tarda
Renal tubular acidosis	

protein (PTH-rp) have also been demonstrated in normal nonendocrine tissues.[14–22] In an effort to maintain the concept of ectopic hormone production while recognizing the possibility that all normal tissues may secrete small quantities of at least immunoreactive forms of peptide hormones, ectopic hormone production may be redefined as the excessive secretion of a hormone by a neoplasm derived from a tissue or organ that is not the known *physiologic* source of that hormone. This definition is not wholly satisfactory because the small quantities of peptide hormones that are secreted by normal tissues may have a physiologic autocrine or paracrine function. Nevertheless, this is a satisfactory working definition that encompasses the current state of knowledge.

A large number of hormones are produced ectopically, although not all are associated with clinical syndromes (Table 28-2). It is of interest that neither the thyronines nor the steroid hormones are on this list. Presumably, the synthesis of these classes of hormones requires orderly enzymatic steps absent in tumors that are not derived from the thyroid, adrenals, or steroid-secreting gonadal cells. Although nonendocrine tumors do not synthesize steroid hormones from cholesterol, they may have enzyme systems that convert one steroid hormone to another. Indeed, the gynecomastia found in some males with lung, gastric, and hepatic carcinomas is caused by the conversion of dehydroepiandosterone to estrone and estradiol by the tumors.[23,24]

Importance of Ectopic Hormone Production

Consideration of ectopic hormone production is important for several reasons. First, the recognition of the syndrome may lead to the diagnosis of the tumor. Although most patients are known to harbor a tumor when the ectopic hormone syndrome is diagnosed, there are many examples of ectopic hormone syndromes occurring months to years before the diagnosis of a tumor. This is most commonly seen in patients who have slowly growing neoplasms such as bronchial carcinoids, malignant thymomas, or islet-cell carcinomas. With these tumors, Cushing's syndrome from ectopic production of ACTH or CRF or acromegaly from secretion of growth hormone releasing factor (GHRF) commonly antedates the

TABLE 28-2. Hormones Produced Ectopically and Their Associated Clinical Syndromes

Eutopic Source of Hormone	Hormone	Syndrome
Hypothalamus	Corticotropin releasing factor	Cushing's syndrome
	Growth hormone releasing hormone	Acromegaly
	Somatostatin	None
	Gonadotropin releasing hormone	None
	Thyrotropin releasing hormone	None
	Antidiuretic hormone	SIAD
	Oxytocin	None
Pituitary	Pro-opiomelanocortin/ACTH	Cushing's syndrome
	Growth hormone	Acromegaly
	Prolactin	Galactorrhea
Placenta	Human chorionic gonadotropin	Precocious puberty (childhood) Gynecomastia (adults)
	Placental lactogen	None
Heart	Atrial natriuretic factor	Hyponatremia
Gastrointestinal tract	Gastrin	Zollinger-Ellison syndrome
	Glucagon	Glucagonoma syndrome
	Vasoactive intestinal peptide	Diarrhea, hypokalemia
	Cholecystokinin	None
	Bombesin/gastrin-releasing peptide	Cushing's syndrome
	Secretin	None
Kidney	Erythropoietin	Polycythemia
	Prorenin/renin	Hypertension, hypokalemia
Parathyroid	Parathormone	Hypercalcemia
Parafollicular cells	Calcitonin	None
Liver	Insulin-like growth factors	Hypoglycemia
Multiple sites	Parathyroid hormone-releated peptide	Hypercalcemia
	Transforming growth factor	?Hypercalcemia
	Epidermal growth factor	?Hypercalcemia
	Platelet-derived growth factor	?Hypercalcemia
	Tumor necrosis factor	?Hypercalcemia
	Interleukins	?Hypercalcemia
Unknown	Phosphatonin	Oncogenic osteomalacia

other manifestations of the underlying malignancy, and it is during the evaluation of these patients for this syndrome that the underlying tumor is discovered. In some patients, the tumor may be discovered at such an early stage that the patient can be cured through surgical resection.

Ectopic hormone production is also important because the patient may succumb to the metabolic effects of the hormone rather than to the direct effects of the neoplasm. The intense catabolic state induced by the full-blown ectopic ACTH syndrome, the severe hyponatremia that may occur with the syndrome of inappropriate antidiuresis (SIAD), and the hypercalcemic crisis that occurs with excessive production of PTH-rp are examples. Prompt treatment of these metabolic abnormalities can be expected to prolong survival, assuming that the patient is not preterminal from the other effects of the neoplasm.

Aditionally an understanding of ectopic hormone syndromes is important because failure to recognize the presence of a syndrome may lead to an erroneous diagnosis in a patient with known cancer. The hypercortisolemia found with ectopic ACTH production, the hyponatremia found with SIAD, and humoral hypercalcemia are each associated with neurologic abnormalities, including behavioral disorders and alterations of consciousness. These conditions may be mistaken for the presence of CNS metastases or infections that in turn may result in inappropriate therapy.

Furthermore, the hormone itself may serve as a tumor marker for localizing the neoplasm, monitoring the effects of therapy, and detecting a recurrence. For example, approximately 70 percent of tumors associated with the clinical ectopic ACTH syndrome are located between the jaw and the diaphragm. The finding of an elevated, nonsuppressible ACTH level in such a patient should lead to a careful search for a lung, thymic, or thyroid tumor. Once a tumor is identified, serial measurements of the ectopic hormone may provide objective evidence of the effects of therapy. In many instances, the changes in the serum or plasma concentrations of a hormone accurately reflect changes in the mass of the tumor. Although a persistently elevated hormone level is indicative of a persistent tumor, the reverse is not always true, as the ectopically produced hormone may decrease at a time when the tumor mass is increasing. Immunohistologic staining for hormone-secreting cells in tumor tissues has demonstrated that most tumors are quite heterogeneous, with much variability in the proportion of cells that synthesize the hormone.[25] Either selective loss of the hormone-producing cells from overgrowth by more rapidly dividing cells that do not secrete the hormone or selective destruction of hormone-producing cells by chemotherapy or radiotherapy may account for the discordance between changes in the marker levels and tumor growth.[26] This phenomenon is also illustrated by studies in which multiple tumor markers were measured.[27,28] Indeed, it is the exception rather than the rule that all tumor markers and tumor growth remain concordant throughout the course of disease. Nevertheless, a rising level of the ectopically produced hormone is almost always indicative of recurrence or progression of the disease. The only exception occurs immediately after surgical manipulation of the tumor or shortly after radiation therapy or induction chemotherapy. In these situations, necrosis of tumor tissue may lead to the release of preformed hormone into the circulation, which may result in a transient increase in the hormone level.

The presence of an ectopic hormone syndrome may provide prognostic information. Patients with hypercalcemia associated with cancer and PTH-rp have a shorter life expectancy than patients without elevations of serum calcium or elevated PTH-rp concentrations.[29,30] Similarly, paraneoplastic Cushing's syndrome in patients with small cell lung cancer is associated with a shorter survival than in patients without ectopic ACTH production.[31]

Finally, ectopic hormone syndromes are important because their study may lead to the discovery of new hormones. The discovery, purification, and structural characterization of GHRF and PTH-rp are recent examples of hormones that were initially isolated from cancers causing acromegaly and hypercalcemia, respectively. The humoral factor responsible for oncogenic osteomalacia has not yet been identified, but the existence of this phospaturetic hormone, termed phosphatonin, is clearly predicted from the studies carried out with tumor extracts from patients with this syndrome.[32,33]

TABLE 28-3. Criteria for Ectopic Hormone Production

1. Presence of an endocrine syndrome associated with a neoplasm derived from a tissue that is not the physiologic source of the hormone known to cause the syndrome
2. Disapperance of the endocrine syndrome after removal or effective treatment of the tumor recurrence of syndrome with relapse of tumor
3. Excessive quantities of circulating hormone associated with a neoplasm derived from a tissue that is not the physiologic source of the hormone
4. Return of circulating hormone to normal or subnormal levels after removal or effective treatment of the tumor; recurrence of elevated hormone levels with relapse of tumor
5. Persistence of syndrome or excesssive hormone production after removal or suppression of the normal physiologic endocrine source of the hormone
6. Extraction of the hormone from the tumor tissue in quantities greater than expected from blood contamination
7. Greater concentration of the hormone in the tumor than in the surrounding nonneoplastic tissue
8. Immunochemical or histochemical localization of the hormone in the tumor cells, especially in secretory granules
9. Arteriovenous hormone concentration difference across the tumor, with higher levels in the venous effluent
10. Detection of messenger RNA for the hormone in the tumor tissue by Northern analysis, in situ hybridization, or in vitro cell-free translation systems
11. In vitro synthesis and secretion of the hormone by the tumor, especially with incorporation of radiolabeled precursors into the hormone
12. Demonstration of in vivo hormone production after tumor transplantation into an animal model

Criteria for Ectopic Hormone Production

Multiple criteria have been developed to establish ectopic hormone production (Table 28-3). Most of the clinical criteria are sufficient to lead to a presumptive diagnosis of ectopic hormone production but not to an unequivocal diagnosis. Both the presence of an endocrine syndrome associated with a nonendocrine neoplasm and the finding of increased quantities of a circulating hormone associated with a neoplasm derived from the tissue that is not the physiologic source of the hormone are not definitive because of the possibility of coexistence of an endocrine neoplasm with a nonendocrine cancer. For example, several studies have shown that hyperparathyroidism due to parathyroid adenomas or hyperplasia occurs with a greater than expected frequency in patients with cancer.[34–37] A patient with an ectopic CRF-producing neoplasm will present with Cushing's syndrome associated with elevated plasma ACTH. In this situation, it may be erroneously concluded that the tumor was secreting ACTH when in fact the source of the ACTH was actually the anterior pituitary corticotropes responding to the ectopic CRF. A third example of how an erroneous conclusion may be reached utilizing clinical criteria alone is seen in the case of the SIAD in association with some neoplasms. Chemotherapeutic drugs such as cyclophosphamide and vincristine may cause hyponatremia, which could be mistakenly attributed to the secretion of antidiuretic hormone (ADH) by the tumor. A lung tumor associated with SIAD may actually not be secreting ADH but may have so altered intrathoracic pressure that the stretch receptors present in the great pulmonary veins and left atrium may be inappropriately stimulated, which in turn may lead to the release of ADH from the hypothalamus and posterior pituitary. Removal of the lung tumor may reestablish normal intrathoracic pressure, and the excessive ADH release will cease. Recurrence of the tumor may again alter intrathoracic pressure in such a manner that ADH release from the hypothalamus and posterior pituitary is again stimulated. Thus, recurrence of the syndrome or an elevation of ADH levels cannot be used as evidence that the tumor is secreting the hormone directly.

Although persistence of a syndrome of excessive hormone production after the removal or suppression of the normal physiologic endocrine source of that hormone is indicative of ectopic production of the hormone in most instances, there are exceptions. The most frequent exceptions are seen in some patients with Cushing's disease in whom ACTH is not suppressed after the administration of even very high doses of dexamethasone. Another example is the presence of hyperparathyroidism due to a parathyroid adenoma in an accessory parathyroid gland in a patient who also harbors a cancer. A neck exploration may reveal four suppressed parathyroid glands, and it may be erroneously concluded that the cancer is responsible for elaborating the parathyroid hormone.

If the tumor contains a greater concentration of the hormone than does the surrounding normal tissue or than can be accounted for by the amount of contaminating blood, a stronger case can be made for ectopic production of the hormone by the tumor. However, there are potential exceptions. Several tumors have been shown to possess receptors for hormones, and it is conceivable that some concentrate hormones from the circulation.[38,39] A much stronger criterion is the specific localization of the hormone in secretory granules within the tumor tissue. Although the presence of a hormone in such secretory granules does not necessarily indicate that the hormone is secreted, a reasonable cause-and-effect relation may be assumed if the tumor contains the hormone in the secretory granules and the patient exhibits the appropriate clinical syndrome with an elevation of the same hormone in the blood.

The last four criteria for ectopic hormone production in Table 28-3 unequivocally establish the production of the hormone by the tumor. Of course, each criterion assumes that the methods used for detecting the hormone or its messenger RNA are specific.

An example of how these various criteria may be used to establish the presence of an ectopic hormone syndrome is provided in the reports of Melmed and colleagues, who described a 60-year-old male with acromegaly and elevated serum growth hormone and insulin-like growth factor-I (IGF-I) concentrations.[40,41] The finding of a normal pituitary on high-resolution CT scan prompted a search for a possible GHRF-producing neoplasm. A CT scan of the abdomen (Fig. 28-1) revealed a large mass in the region of the head of the pancreas, which at surgery was found to be a partially cystic vascular mass consistent with an intramesenteric pancreatic islet cell tumor. At the time of surgery, an arteriovenous gradient of growth hormone was present across the tumor; the growth hormone concentration in a peripheral artery was 34 ng/ml, and that in a tumor vein was 368 ng/ml. Postoperatively, the serum growth hormone levels rapidly fell from 34 to 2 ng/ml over the expected rate of disappearance based on the half-life of growth hormone (Fig. 28-2). GHRF was not detected in the peripheral blood or in a tumor vein. Elevated levels of immunoreactive growth hormone were found in the tumor tissue, and immunoreactive growth hormone was localized in juxtanuclear granules in the tumor cells by both immunohistochemistry and immunoelectron microscopy (Fig. 28-3). The tumor growth hormone comigrated with pituitary growth hormone on Sephadex column chromatography. In addition, dispersed tumor cells secreted immunoreactive growth hormone into tissue culture medium for several weeks, and the tumor cells were able to synthesize growth hormone. Finally, messenger RNA extracted from the tumor cells hybridized with a cDNA probe for human growth hormone and migrated as a 0.9 Kb transcript on Northern gel electrophoresis, consistent with the size of pituitary growth hormone mRNA. Six months postoperatively, the acromegaly had remitted, the serum growth hormone was 1.4 ng/ml, the serum IGF-I was normal, and dynamic growth hormone response to glucose normalized. One year after tumor resection, the patient had the return of the clinical features of acromegaly associated with a rising growth hormone and IGF-I level, coinciding with the presence of multiple intraperitoneal and liver metastasis. Injection of GHRF or TRH did not stimulate growth hormone secretion as is often seen in patients with eutopic growth hormone hypersecretion from a pituitary somatotrope adenoma.[41] Thus, virtually all the criteria for ectopic hormone production outlined in Table 28-3 were satisfied in this case study.

Frequency of Ectopic Hormone Production

The frequency of ectopic hormone production varies considerably, depending to a great extent on the population of patients studied and whether clinical or biochemical criteria are utilized for making the diagnosis. Table 28-4 summarizes a number of studies that have examined the frequency of the most common paraneoplastic endocrine syndromes.[42–65] Hypercalcemia is the most frequently recognized syndrome, being found in 10–14 percent of patients with cancer. However, the frequency among the different types of cancer varies considerably. Thus, patients with multiple myeloma and breast carcinoma tend to have a higher incidence of hypercalcemia than do patients with lung carcinoma. Even among patients with lung carcinoma, there is substantial variability in the frequency of hypercalcemia; patients harboring squamous cell carcinomas have a much higher frequency than do patients with small cell carcinoma. If the incidence of hypercalcemia in carcinoma patients is assessed in a population in which breast carcinoma is overrepresented, the incidence of hypercalcemia will be higher than that in a population in which breast carcinoma is underrepresented. Thus, the incidence figures are heavily prone to ascertain-

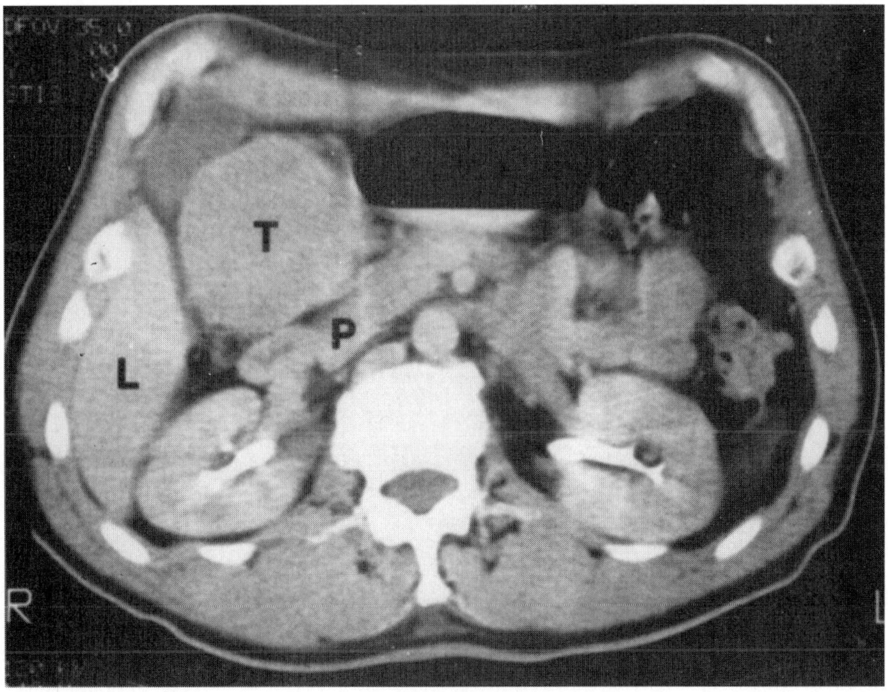

FIGURE 28-1. Abdominal CT scan of the acromegalic male described in the text showing an 8.1 × 6.6-cm mass adjacent to the liver. T = tumor mass; L = liver; P = pancreas. (*Reprinted from Melmed and coworkers,*[40] *with permission.*)

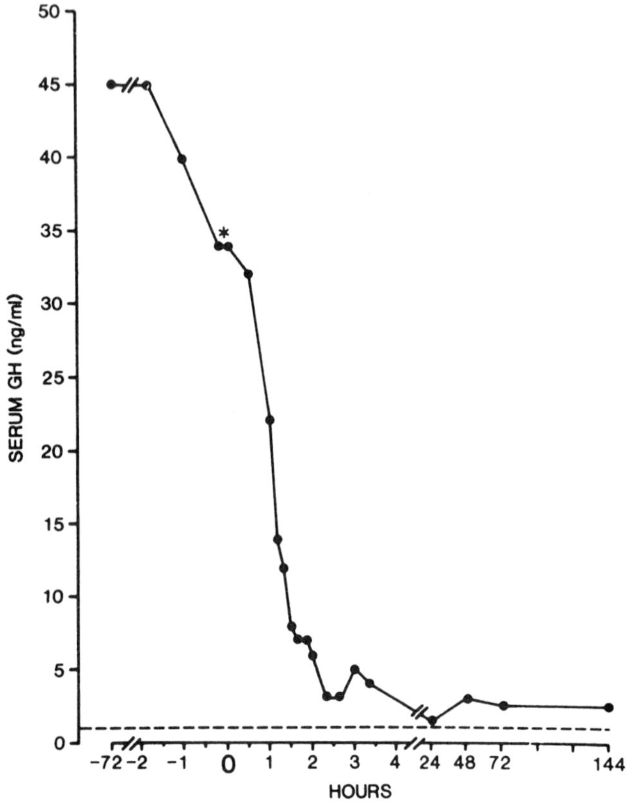

FIGURE 28-2. Serum growth hormone levels in the patient with a growth hormone-secreting islet-cell tumor described in the text. Preoperative growth hormone levels varied between 25 and 60 ng/ml. Abdominal surgery was begun at −2 h and just before tumor removal at 0 h (*), blood was drawn from a tumor vein and peripheral artery for growth hormone measurements. The simultaneous arteriovenous gradient of GH levels across the tumor: peripheral artery, 34 ng/ml; tumor vein, 368 ng/ml. (*Reprinted from Melmed and coworkers,*[40] *with permission.*)

ment bias. In addition, the various reported frequencies are dependent on the criteria used to diagnose ectopic hormone production. Incidence figures based on clinical criteria are uniformly lower than are those based on biochemical criteria. For example, less than 5 percent of patients with small cell carcinoma of the lung have clinically recognizable Cushing's syndrome.[45,53,57,58] In contrast, between 24 and 78 percent of patients with small cell carcinoma of the lung have elevated ACTH levels, and between one-quarter and one-half of these patients have elevated serum cortisol concentrations that do not suppress appropriately after dexamethasone administration.[45,53,54,66–70] The same phenomenon is also true in regard to SIAD in patients with small cell carcinoma of the lung. Approximately 10–15 percent of patients with this tumor

FIGURE 28-3. Immunoelectron micrographs of a growth hormone-secreting islet cell tumor demonstrating the presence of cytoplasmic growth hormone in secretory granules (arrow) (×40,800). (*Reprinted from Melmed and coworkers,*[40] *with permission.*)

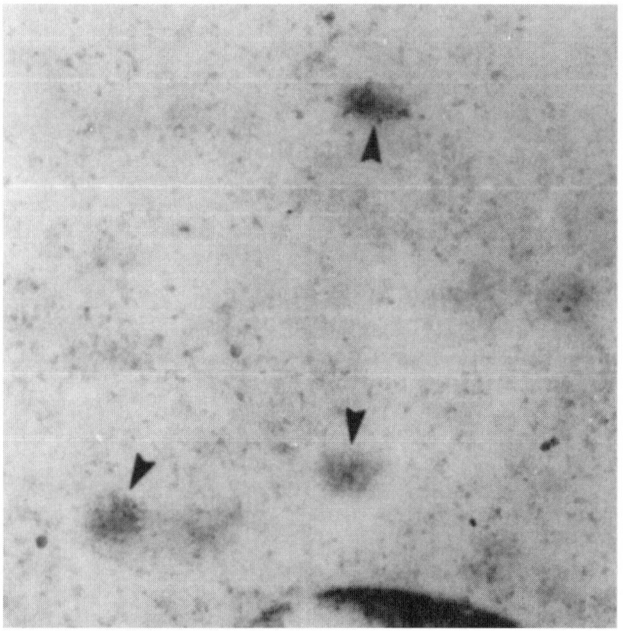

TABLE 28-4. Frequency of Paraneoplastic Endocrine Syndromes

Syndrome	Tumor	Frequency %
Cushing's syndrome	Small cell lung carcinoma	1.3–4.8
	Squamous cell lung carcinoma	0
	Adenocarcinoma of lung	0
SIAD	Small cell lung carcinoma	9.5–14
	Lung carcinoma (all)	1.6
	Head and neck cancers	3%
Hypercalcemia	Carcinomas in general	10–14
	Breast carcinoma	7.2–22.8
	Multiple myeloma	21.2–28.1
	Renal cell carcinoma	5–12.7
	Lung cancer (all)	6.8–12.5
	Squamous cell carcinoma	24
	Small cell carcinoma	1
	Adenocarcinoma	3
	Large cell carcinoma	8
	Lymphoma	9.8
	Leukemia	11.5
Polycythemia	Renal cell carcinoma	0.9–3.5
	Cerebellar hemangioblastoma	9–20

Source: From references 42–65.

TABLE 28-5. Factors Responsible for the Low Frequency of Diagnosis of Ectopic Hormone Production

Low index of clinical suspicion
Minimal clinical expression
Ectopic hormone replaces eutopic hormone
Syndrome obscured by other effects of cancer
Inadequate long-term follow-up of patient
Periodic hormonogenesis
Hormone production without clinical expression
Hormone excess not associated with clinical syndromes
Secretion of hormone precursor without processing to active hormone
Secretion of hormone subunits
Secretion of hormone fragments
Ectopic secretion of unidentified hormones
Hormone assay factors
Insensitive assay
Assay specificity issues
Presence of interfering substances

Source: Adapted from references 73–75.

have symptomatic or asymptomatic hyponatremia.[50,55,57,59] However, 40–68 percent fail to excrete a standardized water load appropriately,[55,64,70] and close to half of these patients have elevated plasma or urinary ADH or neurophysin levels.[52–54,58,64,66–71] Thus, reliance only on the presence or absence of a clinical syndrome will give a spuriously low frequency of ectopic hormone production.

Several other factors are responsible for the low frequency of diagnosis of ectopic hormone production (Table 28-5).[72–75] The physician caring for the patient may have a low index of clinical suspicion that an ectopic hormone syndrome is present. Patients with the ectopic ACTH syndrome, SIAD, or hypercalcemia may complain of weakness and anorexia that may be attributable to other effects of cancer or therapy rather than to the hypokalemic alkalosis and catabolic effects of large amounts of circulating cortisol seen with the ectopic ACTH syndrome, the hyponatremia seen with excessive ADH, or the direct effects of an increase in serum calcium. Early in the course of ectopic hormone production, the ectopic hormone may actually replace the eutopic hormone, and therefore a hormone excess syndrome may not be clinically apparent. Low levels of ACTH from a tumor may stimulate cortisol production from the adrenals, and the cortisol will suppress pituitary ACTH production. The patient will not exhibit the signs or symptoms of Cushing's syndrome until the cortisol production rate rises above normal for several weeks or months. In addition, the clinical features of an ectopic hormone syndrome may actually be obscured by other manifestations of the neoplasm. One reason why patients with the ectopic ACTH syndrome associated with small cell carcinoma of the lung generally do not have cushingoid features with centripetal redistribution of fat may be the coexistence of cancer cachexia. Also, some paraneoplastic endocrine syndromes occur as a late manifestation of the neoplasm and therefore may not be apparent to the clinician unless the patient is followed over a long period. The phenomenon of periodic hormonogenesis may account for an underdiagnosis of ectopic hormone production. Bailey originally described this phenomenon in which some neoplasms secrete excessive quantities of their hormones intermittently and in an autonomous fashion.[76] This has been well described for the ectopic ACTH syndrome. Biochemical testing during the intervals between excessive hormone production may give normal results.

There are many situations in which hormones are produced ectopically without clinical expression, and a diagnosis of ectopic hormone production will thus be missed unless a battery of hormone determinations are made in blood or urine samples from such patients. In some instances, the hormone excess may not be associated with a clinical syndrome. Mild hypercalcemia is usually asymptomatic and is detected as part of a multiphasic panel of tests run on a blood sample. In addition, there may be situations in which the body's homeostatic mechanisms are able to compensate for the excessive concentration of the ectopic hormone. For instance, prolonged elevation of human chorionic gonadotropin (hCG) may lead to down regulation of testicular Leydig cell receptors, which in turn may lead to a decrease in the Leydig cells' responsiveness to the effects of hormones.[77] There are numerous examples of tumors that secrete hormone precursors that do not undergo processing to the active hormone. One of the best studied examples concerns the ectopic ACTH syndrome, in which the major form of the hormone circulating in the blood and present in the tumor tissue is a large molecular form ("big" ACTH; proACTH, POMC) that is immunologically active but biologically inactive. This precursor of ACTH may be converted into biologically active ACTH by trypsin exposure. Indeed, a high frequency (17–88 percent) of elevated concentrations of immunoreactive ACTH has been found in the circulation of patients with all types of lung cancer.[54,67,69,78–81] This is in contrast to the low (<5 percent) prevalence of clinical Cushing's syndrome in such patients. It has been proposed that this difference is due to the inability of the majority of lung cancers to convert POMC to ACTH. In addition to hormone precursor molecules, some tumors secrete biologically inactive hormone subunits, such as the α and β subunits of hCG, or biologically inactive fragments of hormones.

Ectopic hormone production may be undiagnosed if the tumor secretes an unidentified hormone. For instance, before the discovery of PTH-rp, ectopic production of the PTH-like hormone was diagnosed only when the patient developed hypercalcemia. Since the advent of immunoassays for measuring PTH-rp, it has been found that some patients with cancer but without hypercalcemia also have elevated levels of this hormone.[20] Alternatively, the patient may exhibit a full-blown syndrome from the ectopic production of an unidentified hormone. In this situation, the fact that the syndrome is actually a paraneoplastic syndrome may not be appreciated. This was the case with the description of the first patient with a hypoglycemia-inducing mesenchymal tumor who had an intrathoracic fibrosarcoma associated with neuroglucopenic symptoms that responded to a rectal glucose drip.[82] The symptoms were attributed to the mechanical displacement of the heart and blood vessels by the tumor, which resulted in "lack of nourishment to the brain and accumulation of toxemia in the brain [which] could induce mental disturbance."[82] Another theory stated that such tumors, being quite large, consume more glucose than the body's homeostatic mechanisms can cope with.[83] It is now recognized that the hypoglycemia occurring with these non-islet cell tumors is primarly due to excessive production of insulin-like growth factors, especially insulin-like growth factor-II.[84]

Hormone assay factors may also be responsible for the low frequency of diagnosis of ectopic hormone production. Some assays may be too insensitive to detect ectopic hormone production, especially when the hormone levels are too low to elicit a clinical syndrome. Thus, before the advent of a sensitive and relatively specific RIA for hCG based on antibodies generated against the β subunit of the hormone, hCG RIAs exhibited substantial cross-reaction with human luteinizing hormone. Therefore, hCG could not be measured with confidence until the quantities measured exceeded the normal physiologic levels of luteinizing hormone. This resulted in the development of pregnancy tests that required that 500 mIU of hCG/ml of urine or serum be reached or exceeded before the test would become positive. The beta-hCG RIA allowed the detection of 5 mIU/ml of hCG in the presence of physiologic concentrations of luteinizing hormone, a 100-fold increase in sensitivity over the earlier pregnancy tests.[85] Because most patients with ectopic hCG production have levels under 15 mIU/ml of blood, the earlier urinary pregnancy tests would not have been sufficiently sensitive to detect the ectopic production of this hormone.[86] Assay specificity issues may also result in low detection of ectopic hormone secretion. Thus, two-site immunomimetric assays that are highly specific for biologically active ACTH may fail to recognize the large molecular weight pro-ACTH molecule that is the predominant form of ACTH present in the circulation of patients with the ectopic ACTH syndrome.[87,88] Another problem with immunomimetric assays is their susceptibility to interference by many different substances, including proteases, circulating binding proteins for the ligand, heterophilic antibodies, hyperlipidemia, contaminant radioactivity in serum, and other nonspecific serum factors.

Etiology of Ectopic Hormone Production

Any etiologic theory of the mechanisms of ectopic hormone production must provide an adequate explanation for two observations. First, the ectopically produced hormones closely resemble the eutopic hormone, at least in their amino acid sequences. Some tumors produce prohormones, hormone subunits, or fragments of hormones. When analyzed, these proteins are structurally identical to the analogous sequence in the native hormone or prohormone. Alterations in the carbohydrate composition of several ectopically produced glycoproteins have been noted.[89–91] These findings indicate that the translation of the RNA sequence into the protein proceeds normally and that the differences between ectopically and eutopically produced hormones relate to posttranslational modifications such as glycosylation and enzymatic modification of prohormones or of the hormone itself.

Second, ectopic hormone production is not random. Certain tumor types are associated with specific clinical syndromes and hormone production. Even within the same organ system, different histologic varieties of a tumor give rise to different syndromes. Thus, hypercalcemia is found with squamous cell carcinoma of the lung, while Cushing's syndrome is associated primarily with small cell carcinoma of the lung (Table 28-4). In a thorough analysis of the literature, Levine and Metz concluded that the majority of the ectopic hormone-producing tumors could be segregated into two main groups (Table 28-6).[74] The tumors in each group share embryologic, morphologic, and hormone-producing capabilities. Each of the group I tumors is capable of secreting any of the hormones characteristic of that group, and several have been shown to secrete multiple hormones.[49] The group I tumors are derived from neuroectoderm cells, which constitute the APUD system of Pearse (see later discussion). The group II tumors are derived from endoderm and mesoderm and primarily secrete glycoprotein hormones, peptides, and growth factors. A small group of tumors of neural crest origin that embryologically and histologically resemble group I tumors are associated with the secretion of hormones of groups I and II and therefore constitute a transitional group. Although the Levine-Metz classification is reasonably accurate for the association between tumor types and clinical syndromes, it is not as useful when ectopic hormone production per se is considered. Thus, hCG or its β-subunit is produced by a wide variety of neoplasms, not just those associated with group II, even though the clinical syndromes of gynecomastia in adults and precocious puberty in children are seen only with group II tumors. Similarly, elevated concentrations of proACTH are found in patients with squamous cell carcinoma of the lung (a group II tu-

TABLE 28-6. Levine-Metz Classification of Tumors Producing Ectopic Hormones

	Group I (APUD)	Group II	Transitional
Tumors	Foregut carcinoid	Hepatoma	Pheochromocytoma
	Small cell carcinoma	Cholangioma	Melanoma
	Pancreatic islet-cell tumors	Wilms' tumor	
	Some tumors of pancreatic and biliary ducts	Hypernephroma	
		Adrenocortical carcinoma	
	Thyroid medullary carcinoma	Nongerminal gonadal tumors	
	Malignant epithelial thymomas	Vascular tumors	
		Connective tissue and mesodermal tumors	
		Reticuloendothelial tumors	
		Non-small-cell lung carcinoma	
		GI tumors (except APUD)	
		Melanoma	
Hormones	Insulin	PTH-rp	Biogenic amines
	Calcitonin	Erythropoietin	ACTH
	ACTH/POMC	hCG	Calcitonin
	ADH	hPL	Glucagon
	Gastrin	PRL	Secretin
	Glucagon	GH	hPL
	Secretin	IGF	PTH-rp
	Biogenic amines	Renin	Erythropoietin

Source: Adapted from Levine and Metz.[74]

mor) as well as small cell carcinoma of the lung (a group I tumor), although clinical Cushing's syndrome is seen primarily in association with group I tumors.

De Novo Synthesis from Gene Mutation

According to this theory, the process of oncogenesis involves a variety of gene mutations. The resulting alterations in the DNA may then lead to the synthesis of new proteins, some of which may possess biological activity resembling that found with hormones. Because hormone production is not entirely random and the tumor hormones, prohormones, fragments, and subunits that are produced ectopically are identical to the eutopic hormones, at least in regard to the translated protein, this theory cannot explain ectopic hormone production.

Sponge Theory

In 1964, Unger and colleagues suggested that some tumors concentrate hormones from the circulation and release them at the time of cell death.[38] Support for this hypothesis includes the observation that some adrenocortical carcinomas apparently develop "ectopic" receptors for gonadotropins and beta-adrenergic hormones.[39,92] As virtually all the ectopically produced hormones described to date have been shown to be synthesized and secreted by tumor cells in culture, this hypothesis cannot account for ectopic hormone production.

Endocrine Cell Hypothesis

In a series of studies, Pearse and colleagues showed the wide distribution of cells of neuroectodermal origin that have the properties of concentrating amine precursors such as dopa and 5-hydroxy tryptophan, decarboxylating them, and converting them into biogenic amines.[93,94] These APUD (*a*mine *p*recursor *u*ptake and *d*ecarboxylation) cells contain multiple decarboxylating enzymes and chromogranin A.[93–95] Histologically, these cells exhibit secretory granules, a prominent rough endoplasmic reticulum, and a Golgi apparatus indicating active peptide synthesis. As was noted above, these cells are widely distributed throughout the body (Table 28-7), and all neoplasms of these cells can produce a variety of polypeptides, primarily those associated with group I tumors of the Levine-Metz classification (Table 28-6), as well as biogenic amines. A substantial amount of experimental evidence indicates that APUD cells are derived from the neural crest.[96] However, some studies suggest that the gastrointestinal (GI) tract and pancreatic APUD cells, and possibly those found in the respiratory tract, may be of endodermal origin.[97,98] In addition, the finding that thyroid C cells contain immunoreactive thyroglobulin[99] and that both islet cell β granules and zymogen granules may coexist in the same pancreatic cell[100,101] raises the possibility that cells may develop APUD characteristics through cellular differentiation of totipotential local tissue progenitor cells rather than through migration of cells from the neural crest.

It has been hypothesized that ectopic hormone production is a result of secretion of the hormones by APUD cells in tumors.[96] Certainly this is a viable hypothesis for the group I tumors of the Levine-Metz classification (Table 28-6) and the tumors listed in Table 28-7. However, this theory cannot account for the production of the hormones by the Levine-Metz group II tumors, which do not have APUD cell characteristics, or explain the ectopic production of APUD (group I) hormones by group II tumors. The APUD cells contain convertases and other processing enzymes that allow the secretion of biologically active hormones. This may explain why clinical syndromes due to the ectopic secretion of group I hormones are seen more frequently with tumors that have APUD characteristics than with group II tumors, which may not be capable of appropriately processing group I prohormones.

A variation of the APUD hypothesis of ectopic hormone production is the cell hybridization hypothesis of Warner[102] who proposed that ectopic hormone production represents the fusion of a malignant cell with an APUD-type "bystander" cell, which results in the malignant cell secreting the polypeptide that APUD-type cells can secrete. Warner further suggested that the production of the hormones by these fused cells may give the clone of hormone-producing cells a survival advantage. Support for this theory is circumstantial and based on histologic and histochemical findings such as the demonstration of mucin-secreting carcinoid tumors, the presence of argentophil cells in some adenocarcinomas of the GI tract, and the existence of carcinosarcomas and adenocanthomas. There is no direct evidence that such cell hybridization takes place in vivo; even if it did, the same criticisms that have been used to discount the APUD theory as a unifying hypothesis for ectopic hormone production would apply to the cell hybridization theory.

TABLE 28-7. APUD Cell Distribution

APUD Cell Type	Tumor
Thyroid parafollicular cells	Medullary carcinoma of the thyroid
Adrenal medullary cells	Pheochromocytoma
Gastrointestinal neuroendocrine cells	Gastrointestinal carcinoids
Pancreatic neuroendocrine cells	Islet-cell tumors
Respiratory tract Kultschitsky's cells	Small cell carcinoma; bronchial carcinoid
Argyrophil cells of the thymus	Thymomas
Anterior pituitary cells	Pituitary adenomas
Carotid body and sympathetic ganglia cells	Paragangliomas; neuroblastoma
Melanocytes	Melanomas
Urogenital neuroendocrine cells	Prostate carcinoma
?Parathyroid chief cell	Parathyroid adenoma

Gene Derepression

All nucleated diploid cells in any individual contain the same genetic information that was initially present in the zygote. During the process of cellular differentiation and specialization, portions of the genome become repressed and are no longer expressed. It has been estimated that the average cell expresses <10 percent of its genetic information.[103] According to the derepression hypothesis, portions of the tumor cell's DNA become derepressed during the process of neoplastic transformation allowing the gene to be expressed. If the derepressed portion of the genome normally codes for a hormone, that tumor may express the hormone ectopically. The possibility of derepression has clearly been shown in the frog experiments of Gurdon, who transplanted the nucleus from a differentiated adult frog cell into an enucleated frog egg which subsequently developed into an adult frog.[104] Similarly, when the nucleus from a frog kidney carcinoma is placed into an enucleated frog ovum, differentiation to the tadpole stage occurs.[105] Derepression is an attractive concept because it could account for the production of hormones by nonendocrine tumors that are structurally identical to the hormone secreted by the normal endocrine gland and could also account for the production of prohormones, fragments, and subunits. The production of prohormones could reflect the lack of derepression of the genes responsible for directing the synthesis of the cytoplasmic hormone-processing enzymes. However, this hypothesis does not account for the nonrandom association of certain tumors with specific hormones or explain why polypeptide hormones such as calcitonin, ACTH, and hCG are more frequently produced than are hormones such as growth hormone and placental lactogen.

Cellular Dedifferentiation

The cellular dedifferentiation hypothesis is an extension of the gene derepression hypothesis. This theory suggests that tumor tissues regress from a differentiated state to an undifferentiated state.[106,107] At each step in this process, the dedifferentiated cell resembles a stage in normal cell development during the process of differentiation. The dedifferentiated cell will have the ability to make all the products normal for that particular stage of differentiation. The nonrandom nature of ectopic hormone production provides strong evidence against this hypothesis.

Dysdifferentiation or Blocked Ontogenesis

According to this theory, every tissue in the body contains stem or renewal cells that are either totipotential or relatively undifferentiated. These cells are normally responsible for replenishing cells that are lost through disease or injury. The genome of these cells is either unrepressed or not fully repressed. During the process of differentiation, the genome of the stem cells undergoes progressive repression until the adult, specialized state is reached. At each stage, the differentiating cell may express a variety of proteins specific for that stage. Thus, a stem cell in the skin may be capable of secreting fetal and placental proteins, while in the adult state these cells are not able to produce these proteins. According to this theory, neoplasia takes place in these progenitor cells and the morphologic and functional characteristics of the tumor depend on the stage of the differentiation process in which oncogenesis occurs.[108,109] This theory differs from the dedifferentiation theory in that the neoplasm is derived from cells that have not fully differentiated rather than from cells that have gone from a differentiated state to a less differentiated state.

This theory is attractive because it accounts for several phenomena that are observed with cancer. It is well established that tumor populations are heterogeneous, and immunohistochemical studies have shown that different tumors contain variable numbers of hormone-secreting cells.[25] This theory also accounts for the phenomenon of hormone production by granulomas and inflammatory lesions.[110,111] It also provides a possible explanation for the nonrandom association of certain hormones with specific tumors. Local factors such as cell surface contact and the presence of growth factors or other paracrine substances may modulate the proliferation and differentiation of the stem cells in a particular organ. The experimental work with small cell carcinoma carried out by Baylin and colleagues has shown how the dysdifferentiation theory can account for the APUD characteristics of tumor cells. This does not necessarily indicate that the tumor originated from a neuroectodermal cell but rather that APUD characteristics may be a feature of the degree of cell differentiation.[112]

Excessive Expression of Normal Genes

As was previously noted, many immunoreactive polypeptide hormones have been detected in normal nonendocrine tissues using sensitive immunoassay techniques. The low levels of these hormones may represent incomplete repression of the portion of the genome that is responsible for the hormone production (gene leakage) or may reflect the production of the hormones from the stem cells present in the tissues. If the process of repression is incomplete, ectopic hormone production may merely represent excessive expression of normal genes and may be directly related to proliferation of the neoplastic cells and tumor mass. If this is correct, ectopic peptide synthesis may be a "universal concomitant of neoplasia," as suggested by Odell and colleagues.[72] Clinical syndromes occur only when tumors elaborate bioactive forms of hormones.

Therapy

Specific therapies have been devised for the treatment of each of the ectopic hormone syndromes and will be discussed later under the specific syndromes. In general, several therapeutic approaches may be used for the treatment of ectopic hormone syndromes. The first approach is to remove the tumor, if possible. If the primary neoplasm is unresectable or if metastases are present, hormone production may be inhibited through the use of chemotherapy or radiation therapy. If these approaches are unsuccessful and the metabolic derangements from the ectopic hormone syndrome substantially contribute to morbidity, therapy directed at the target organ or target organ products may be instituted. Using the ectopic ACTH syndrome as an example, Cushing's syndrome may be reversed through bilateral adrenalectomy and the administration of physiologic doses of glucocorticoids and mineralocorticoids. In some patients, a medical adrenalectomy may be accomplished through the use of mitotane (o,p′-DDD). Alternatively, the function of the target organ, in this case the adrenal, may be blocked. The block may take place at the target organ receptor or at an intracellular step in target organ activity. In some tissues, it is possible to block the cell membrane receptors for hormones through hormone antagonists or agonists, with the agonists causing down regulation of the receptor. In the case of the ectopic ACTH syndrome, there are no clinically effective ACTH agonists or antagonists that are useful for the treatment of Cushing's syndrome. Instead, target organ activity is blocked through the use of inhibitors of the enzymatic pathways required for steroid hormone production. Such inhibitors include aminoglutethimide, ketoconazole, and metyrapone. Finally, if the metabolic derangements are due to overproduction of a target organ product, this product may be antagonized. For the ectopic ACTH syndrome, mifepristone (RU-486) is an effective glucocorticoid antagonist and has been useful in the treatment of some patients with Cushing's syndrome.[113] As we gain further insight into the biochemical mediators of hormone action, it is likely that additional approaches to therapy will be forthcoming.

Hormones as Tumor Markers

The experience gained from the use of hCG as a tumor marker in patients with gestational and nongestational trophoblastic disease served as a major impetus for the search for hormones, enzymes, oncofetal proteins, and other cellular components that could be used as markers of neoplasms. In fact, in patients with gestational trophoblastic disease, hCG measurements fulfill virtually all the criteria for an ideal tumor marker (Table 28-8). hCG may be measured in the blood or urine through rapidly performed, technically simple, and inexpensive immunomimetric assays. If one uses a

TABLE 28-8. The Ideal Tumor Marker

1. Present in blood or urine
2. No false positives (specific)
3. No false negatives (sensitive)
4. Levels fluctuate appropriately with changes in tumor growth
5. Rapid half-life in blood
6. Rapidly performed
7. Technically simple
8. Inexpensive

cutoff level of 25 mIU/ml of serum, only pregnancy and an occasional nontrophoblastic neoplasm will be positive and virtually all patients with trophoblastic disease will have measurable quantities of hCG (no false negatives). The levels of hCG in the serum and urine accurately reflect tumor burden and fluctuate concordantly with changes in tumor growth. In addition, the approximately 24-h half-life of hCG allows for an assessment of the efficacy of therapy within a few days of the initiation of treatment. After the initial disappearance of the hormone, an early recurrence of the tro phoblast disease may be detected through serial measurements of hCG levels.[114]

Unfortunately, the excellent experience with the use of hCG as a marker of gestational trophoblastic disease has not been duplicated for most other tumor markers, including carcinoembryonic antigen, alpha-fetoprotein, CA-125, and prostate-specific antigen. The major limitations to the use of tumor markers involve *sensitivity* and *specificity*. To detect as many cancers as possible, the method of measuring the tumor marker should be highly sensitive. However, as the sensitivity of the test increases, the number of patients without cancer who are either normal or have benign disease processes and test positive increases. Therefore, the test loses its specificity, or the ability to rule out disease when none is present. In fact, the sensitivity and specificity of a test, along with the prevalence of the disease in the population being studied, determine the utility of that test as a screen for cancer.

The interaction of test sensitivity and specificity and cancer prevalence can be illustrated by examining the experience with the use of measurements of immunoreactive hCG (or its β-subunit) in the sera of patients with nontrophoblastic neoplasms. The combined data from 66 published studies are shown in Tables 28-9 and 28-10 for patients with and without cancer, respectively.[114] Overall, approximately 18 percent of patients with cancer are found to have immunoreactive hCG in circulation, while 2.4 percent of control patients without cancer have circulating immunoreactive hCG by assays that have a sensitivity of 5 mIU/ml. Thus, the sensitivity of hCG measurements as a tumor marker is 18 percent, while the specificity is 97.6 percent (100 percent − 2.4 percent). Table 28-11 illustrates the effect of cancer prevalence on the diagnostic accuracy of hCG measurements. If we assume that the prevalence of cancer in the population being examined is 1 percent (Table 28-11, top), we find that for every 100,000 patients screened, 1,000 will have cancer. Of this 1,000, 18 percent (180) will have immunoreactive hCG present in the circulation (true positives), while 820 patients with cancer will not have immunoreactive hCG detected by these tests (false negatives). Of the 99,000 patients without cancer, 96,624 (99,000 × 97.6 percent) will not have hCG detected in their circulation (true negatives), while 2,376 patients without cancer (99,000 × 2.4 percent) will have hCG detected (false positives). In this situation, the predictive value of a positive test—that is, the percentage of patients who have immunoreactive hCG in the circulation who actually have cancer—is 7 percent, while the false-positive rate (100 percent − 7 percent) is 93 percent. The predictive value of a negative test (the percentage of noncancerous patients with negative hCG results) is 99 percent with only 1 per cent false negatives. Thus, in this population, the number of false

TABLE 28-9. Immunoreactive hCG or hCGβ-Subunit in Sera of Patients with Cancer

Tumor or Site	*N*		Percent Positive	
Islet cell	104		39.4	
Gynecologic	2,010		28.6	
Ovary		633		28.6
Endometrium		348		16.7
Cervix		976		33.8
Vulva/vagina		37		27.0
Carcinoid	41		26.8	
Gastrointestinal	2,165		18.0	
Oropharynx		298		14.8
Esophagus		124		17.7
Gastric		232		20.7
Small intestine		24		16.7
Colon/rectum		693		9.8
Hepatic		281		22.1
Biliary		26		30.7
Pancreatic		200		20.0
Lung	1,365		17.4	
Breast	3,031		16.8	
Melanoma	244		13.9	
Genitourinary	658		11.8	
Renal		119		6.7
Bladder		176		23.3
Prostate		363		8.0
Sarcoma	136		11.8	
Hemopoietic	544		6.1	
Lymphoma	399		5.3	
Miscellaneous	576		10.4	
Total	11,213		18.0	

Source: From Braunstein,[114] with permission.

TABLE 28-10. Immunoreactive hCG or hCGβ-Subunit in Sera of Control Patients without Cancer

Type of Control	*N*		Percent Positive	
Premenopausal females	430		0.7	
Postmenopausal females	242		0	
Normal males	438		0.2	
Castrate males	4		0	
Blood donors	165		2.4	
Benign disease	1,963		3.6	
Gynecologic		528		6.6
Gastrointestinal		318		6.0
Breast		254		4.3
Lung		174		2.9
Genitourinary		84		0
Neurologic		10		0
Hypothyroid		10		0
Unspecified		650		0
Other normal	172		0	
Miscellaneous	691		2.7	
Total	4,105		2.4	

Source: From Braunstein,[114] with permission.

TABLE 28-11. Predictive Value of hCG Measurements for Cancer Screening

Sensitivity of test: 18 percent (105)
Specificity of test: 97.6 percent (105)
Example 1
Assumed prevalence of cancer: 1 percent

	Test Result		
	Positive	*Negative*	*Total*
Cancer	180 (TP)	820 (FN)	1000
Benign disorders	2376 (FP)	96,624 (TN)	99,000
Total	2556	97,444	100,000

Predictive value of a positive test $\left(\frac{TP}{TP + FP} \times 100\right)$: 7 percent
False positives: 93 percent
Predictive value of a negative test $\left(\frac{TN}{TN + FN} \times 100\right)$: 99 percent
False negatives: 1 percent
Example 2
Assumed prevalence of cancer: 10 percent

	Test Result		
	Positive	*Negative*	*Total*
Cancer	1800	8200	10,000
Benign disorders	2160	87,840	90,000
Total	3960	96,040	100,000

Predictive value of a positive test: 45 percent
False positives: 55 percent
Predictive value of a negative test: 91 percent
False negatives: 9 percent

TP = true positives; FP = false positives; FN = false negatives; TN = true negatives.

positives markedly exceeds the number of true positives; therefore, approximately 9 of every 10 patients with detectable immunoreactive hCG in the circulation will undergo unnecessary further diagnostic evaluation.

If the prevalence of cancer in the population being evaluated is 10-fold higher (10 percent) (Table 28-11, bottom), the predictive value of a positive test rises to 45 percent and the number of false positives decreases to 55 percent. However, the number of false negatives rises dramatically to 9 percent. In this population, a patient with a positive test result is more likely to harbor a neoplasm than is the case in a population with a 1 percent prevalence of cancer, but almost 10 percent of patients with a negative test will have cancer.

These calculations suggest that hCG measurements are not particularly useful as a screening test for nontrophoblastic cancer. In actuality, hCG and other potential tumor markers generally perform worse in a screening situation than is suggested in much of the medical literature. This occurs because of biases in the ascertainment of many of the patient populations that have been the subject of reports. To establish the value of a tumor marker, investigators usually measure the marker in the blood or urine of patients with well-established neoplasms. Most markers are more likely to be positive in patients with advanced disease than in patients with minimal disease. Therefore, the sensitivity of the test established in research laboratories with well-defined populations often overestimates the actual sensitivity of the test in terms of detection of early cancer, a stage when the disease is potentially curable and not diagnosable with other screening tests. Some investigators have tried to increase the sensitivity of tumor marker tests by measuring multiple markers in the blood and evaluating patients further if any of the markers are positive. This strategy (parallel testing) increases the sensitivity of the test but markedly decreases the specificity because each test will give false-positive results. Another strategy is to measure a tumor marker and subject all samples that give positive test results to measurements of a different tumor marker and to consider a combined test positive only if both are positive (serial testing). This increases the specificity of tumor marker testing but reduces the sensitivity. Indeed, for any test that is <100 percent sensitive or 100 percent specific, an increase in sensitivity of the testing strategy will lead to a decrease in specificity and vice versa.[115]

SPECIFIC SYNDROMES

Hypercalcemia of Malignancy

Hypercalcemia is the most frequently encountered paraneoplastic endocrine abnormality, being found in 10 to 14 percent of patients with cancer (Table 28-4). A wide spectrum of neoplasms are associated with hypercalcemia (Table 28-12).[29,116–122] Metastatic adenocarcinoma of the breast and squamous cell carcinoma of the lung and head and neck region account for more than half the patients with tumor-associated hypercalcemia. If patients with documented bony metastases are excluded, approximately half of patients with tumor-associated hypercalcemia have a squamous cell carcinoma of the lung or clear cell carcinoma of the kidney.[123–125]

Pathophysiology of Hypercalcemia
(Table 28-13)

Bony Metastases

The idea that osseous metastases are directly associated with calcium abnormalities was first suggested by Virchow, who in 1855 described three patients with bone metastases who had ectopic calcification in various tissues.[125] The association of hypercalcemia with tumor types such as breast carcinoma and multiple myeloma, almost exclusively when the tumors involve the bone, led to the hypothesis that direct tumor-induced osteolysis can account for the hypercalcemia.[126] Indeed, various tumor cells have been shown to release prostaglandins, epidermal growth factor, lymphotoxins, PTH-rp, and other substances that are capable of

TABLE 28-12. Tumor Types Associated with Hypercalcemia

Tumor Type	Percent
Breast	36
Lung	15
Head and neck	8
Lymphoma	7
Multiple myeloma	7
Kidney	6
Gastrointestinal tract	4
Leukemia	2
Ovary	1
Miscellaneous*	15

*Carcinomas of the endometrium, cervix, vagina, vulva, penis, testis, adrenal, and prostate; pheochromocytoma; neuroblastoma; melanoma; thymoma; osteogenic sarcoma; lymphosarcoma; reticulum cell sarcoma; hemangiosarcoma; fibrosarcoma; rhabdomyosarcoma; leiomyosarcoma.

Source: Based on data on 1055 patients from eight series of patients.[29,116–122]

TABLE 28-13. Pathophysiologic Mechanisms of Hypercalcemia in Cancer

Bony metastasis
Elaboration of humoral substances
Parathyroid hormone
Parathyroid hormone-related protein
Prostaglandins
Cytokines
Conversion of 25(OH)-vitamin D to $1,25(OH)_2$-vitamin D
Coexistence of cancer and another disease
Primary hyperparathyroidism
Other causes of hypercalcemia

stimulating osteoclastic bone resorption.[20,118,127,128] Thus, some tumor cells may directly stimulate osteoclastic bone resorption and lead to an uncoupling of bone resorption and formation characteristic of the hypercalcemia of malignancy.[129] In addition, monocytes and lymphocytes in close proximity to the tumor cells may be responsible for the release of bone-resorbing cytokines.

It is clear that the presence of tumor cells in bone alone is not sufficient to cause hypercalcemia. Some tumors, such as small cell carcinoma of the lung, adenocarcinoma of the colon, and adenocarcinoma of the prostate, metastasize to the bone and are only rarely associated with hypercalcemia (Table 28-4),[125] indicating that the tumor cell type is an important factor determining whether the patient will develop hypercalcemia with bone metastases. Ralston and coworkers demonstrated that there was no association between the presence or extent of osseous metastases and the frequency or severity of hypercalcemia in a large group of cancer patients assessed by bone scan.[126] In fact, patients with a light bone tumor load had a higher mean serum calcium level than did those with a heavy bone tumor load. When analysis was restricted to patients who had hypercalcemia, the highest mean serum calcium levels were found in patients without evidence of metastatic bone disease. These data indicate that although 60–80 percent of patients with hypercalcemia and cancer have skeletal metastases,[118,126] the cause of the hypercalcemia is probably multifactorial and includes both direct and indirect local production of stimulators of osteoclastic bone resorption, including prostaglandins and cytokines, as well as the secretion of PTH-rp, the substance responsible for the majority of cases of humoral hypercalcemia in patients with nonmetastatic solid tumors (see later discussion).

Systemic Elaboration of Humoral Substances

Historical Perspective The development of our understanding of the humoral hypercalcemia of cancer and the mediators involved parallels the history of endocrinology. The early studies were observational. In 1924, Zondek and coworkers described a patient with hypercalcemia who at autopsy was found to have normal parathyroid glands and carcinoma of the gallbladder.[130] In 1936, Gutman and associates described a patient with symptomatic hypercalcemia and bronchogenic carcinoma who had normal parathyroid glands, no skeletal metastases, and a small focus of monostotic Paget disease.[131] The next major step was conceptual and was provided by Albright in his discussion of a 51-year-old man with a renal cell carcinoma that was metastatic to the ilium.[132] Because of the presence of hypophosphatemia associated with the hypercalcemia, this patient underwent a parathyroid exploration with a finding of three normal parathyroid glands. Subsequently, the patient's tumor and iliac metastases were treated with radiation therapy, which led to a concomitant decrease in the serum calcium concentration and a rise in the serum phosphate concentration. A normal fourth parathyroid gland was found at necropsy. Albright hypothesized that the tumor was secreting a parahormone (PTH)-like substance, as hypercalcemia resulting from osteolysis alone would be expected to be associated with hyperphosphatemia. However, bioassay of the tumor tissue for the presence of PTH was negative. In 1956, two groups reported several patients with malignancies, normal bone x-rays, hypercalcemia, and hypophosphatemia whose biochemical abnormalities normalized after surgical resection of the tumors. With tumor recurrence, there was a temporally associated increase in serum calcium.[133,134] No parathyroid bone or renal abnormalities were found at surgery or autopsy in the patients studied. These observations supported Albright's contention that the tumors were producing a PTH-like substance that was responsible for the hypercalcemia. As additional patients with the syndrome were reported, the term *pseudohyperparathyroidism* was applied to this condition.[135] After the purification of PTH, immunoassays were developed, and in 1964 the presence of a material immunologically similar to bovine PTH was extracted from several tumor tissues.[123,136,137]

With the advent of RIAs, there was initial support for the concept that the PTH-like substance is actually PTH. One study found that 95 percent of patients with hypercalcemia associated with cancer had inappropriately high PTH levels as measured by an RIA directed against the carboxy-terminal portion of the molecule.[138] Sherwood and colleagues demonstrated immunoreactive PTH in several tumor extracts, and other investigators showed arteriovenous differences in PTH concentrations across tumors.[139–141] However, several investigators found that there were differences between the immunoreactive PTH-like substances in the sera of patients with cancer and hypercalcemia and in the sera of patients with hypercalcemia from primary hyperparathyroidism.[142,143] Because both amino- and carboxy-terminal fragments of PTH were known to be present in circulation, it was conceivable that the differences between pseudohyperparathyroidism and hyperparathyroidism reflected differences in the processing of the hormone at the time of or after secretion. The difficulties in interpreting RIA data were highlighted by the study of Raisz and colleagues, who had the same serum samples from patients with primary hyperparathyroidism and humoral hypercalcemia of cancer measured for immunoreactive PTH by four different laboratories.[144] There were marked differences in the results. However, it was generally found that PTH assays that used antisera generated against amino-terminal portions of the molecule gave lower serum concentrations of PTH than did RIAs that used antisera against the carboxy-terminal portion of the molecule. Because the carboxy-terminal fragment of PTH is elevated in patients with renal insufficiency and also appears to be released continuously even when the amino-terminal fragment of PTH release is suppressed, it is understandable how some of these immunoassay discrepancies could occur.

An important study was reported in 1973 by Powell and coworkers who described 11 patients with nonparathyroid neoplasms associated with hypercalcemia and hypophosphatemia in the absence of bony metastases.[145] Remission of biochemical abnormalities occurred in nine patients after antitumor therapy. These investigators were unable to demonstrate PTH in the patients' blood or the tumor tissue despite using three different

RIAs that covered virtually all regions of the PTH molecule. However, the tumor extracts did cause bone resorption by bioassay, leading to the conclusion that the humoral hypercalcemia factor was not PTH. During the 1970s a variety of other substances were found to stimulate osteoclastic bone resorption in vitro, and this fueled the effort to determine whether one or more of these substances could be the humoral hypercalcemic factor produced by cancers. The two substances that received the most attention were prostaglandins of the E series and "osteoclastic activating factor."[146–148]

Major strides in unraveling the pathogenesis of humoral hypercalcemia of malignancy were made during the 1980s through the use of molecular biological tools. Early studies showed the absence of PTH messenger RNA by in situ hybridization in tumors associated with nonmetastatic hypercalcemia.[149] Subsequently, several tumor cell lines derived from patients with this syndrome were established and secreted a biologically active bone-resorbing factor.[150,151] This led to purification and sequencing of the PTH-rp protein and the cloning of the gene.[152] Synthetic peptides based on the structure of the PTH-rp protein were used as immunogens for the development of immunoassays to measure the concentrations of the protein in body fluids and tissues. The use of these assays has established the fact that the majority of patients with humoral hypercalcemia of malignancy have elevated levels of PTH-rp, establishing this factor as Albright's predicted PTH-like substance that is responsible for the syndrome.

Parathyroid Hormone As was noted earlier, the majority of patients who had been diagnosed as having "pseudohyperparathyroidism" due to the ectopic production of PTH most likely had the syndrome on the basis of excessive production of PTH-rp. The close homology between the PTH and PTH-rp molecules in their first 13 amino acids might have accounted for some of the positive results reported in early PTH immunoassays. In addition, the presence of renal insufficiency in some patients and the inability to completely shut off the release of the carboxy-terminal fragments of PTH even in the face of hypercalcemia might have been important factors in accounting for the spurious diagnosis of ectopic PTH production by tumors.[118] Finally, the coexistence of hyperparathyroidism and cancer may have accounted for some of the examples of "pseudohyperparathyroidism."

Although the bona fide ectopic production of PTH appears to be exceedingly rare, it does occur. For instance, Yoshimoto and associates described a 70-year-old man with a small cell carcinoma of the lung, multiple metastases, and normal parathyroid glands at autopsy. He had markedly elevated serum PTH levels by three separate assays as well as high concentrations of PTH in a tumor extract that cochromatographed with human PTH on gel filtration chromatography. Northern blot analysis also showed the presence of PTH mRNA in the tumor.[153] Similarly, authentic ectopic PTH secretion has been reported in patients with ovarian carcinoma, a primitive neuroectodermal tumor, squamous cell carcinoma of the lung, and thymoma.[154–157]

Parathyroid Hormone–Related Protein After the 1973 report of Powell and colleagues,[145] which demonstrated that the syndrome of humoral hypercalcemia of malignancy is not due to the production of immunoreactive PTH, several groups of investigators sought the putative PTH-like factor. In 1980, Stewart and associates examined 50 consecutive patients with humoral hypercalcemia of malignancy and found that they segregated into two groups that were distinguishable primarily on the basis of nephrogenous cyclic AMP excretion.[119] More than 80 percent of these patients had elevated nephrogenous cyclic AMP and harbored squamous cell carcinomas of the head and neck, lung, esophagus, and vulva; squamous metaplasia; renal cell carcinomas; or transitional cell carcinomas. The patients with low cyclic AMP excretion had hematologic malignancies including myeloma and lymphoma as well as breast carcinoma. The patients with elevated nephrogenous cyclic AMP excretion exhibited hypercalcemia, hypophosphatemia, decreased tubular reabsorption of phosphate, increased fasting calcium excretion for a given level of serum calcium and low $1,25(OH)_2D_3$ serum concentrations compared with patients with primary hyperparathyroidism, and undetectable serum immunoreactive PTH levels.[119,158] The sera from patients in this group were active in a kidney cortex cytochemical bioassay for PTH, and the biological activity could not be completely inhibited by preincubation with antiserum against PTH.[159] Several tumor cell lines elaborating the PTH-like substance were established.[150,151] One such line, when transplanted into nude mice, led to the development of hypercalcemia, hypophosphatemia, and elevation of $1,25(OH)_3D_3$ serum concentrations.[160] The biochemical abnormalities were inhibited by analogs to PTH that also inhibited PTH activity in vitro and in vivo. The biologically active components of these cell lines were purified and found to reside in a protein with a molecular mass of 17–18 kDa. Amino-terminal sequence analysis demonstrated significant homology with the first 13 amino acids of PTH and also allowed the preparation of synthetic oligonucleotides which were used to isolate the cDNA for PTH-rp.[152] The full-length DNA coding for the protein was isolated, and the amino acid structure was predicted.[151]

PTH-rp has been found to exist in three isoforms of 139, 141, and 173 amino acids resulting from alternate splicing of exons. There is a 36-amino acid prepropeptide. Eight of the first 13 amino-terminal amino acids are homologous with those found in PTH, and this accounts for the PTH-like biological activity both in vivo and in vitro. The amino acid sequence of PTH and PTH-rp diverges completely after the first 13 amino acids. It is likely that the genes for both PTH and PTH-rp are derived from a common ancestral gene. Synthetic amino-terminal peptides containing the first 34 amino acids retain full biological activity, while no biological activity has been demonstrated for the carboxy-terminal fragments.[20,151,161]

PTH-rp fulfills the criteria for the humoral hypercalcemic factor for the majority of nonmetastatic solid tumors. First, serum immunoreactive PTH-rp is elevated in 53–83 percent of patients with nonmetastatic hypercalcemia,[120–122,162] and serum concentrations of PTH-rp have been correlated with total serum calcium concentrations.[120,163] Second, therapy for tumors associated with hypercalcemia has led to a decrease in serum calcium and a parallel reduction in PTH-rp levels.[122,162] Third, serum PTH-rp concentrations have been correlated with nephrogenous cyclic AMP excretion in patients with this syndrome.[162] Fourth, PTH-rp has been isolated from tumors associated with this syndrome, and the tumors contain PTH-rp mRNA.[164,165] Fifth, the infusion of PTH-rp into animals leads to the development of hypercalcemia, and the administration of anti-PTH-rp antibodies reverses the hypercalcemia in animal models.[166–168] Finally, infusion of PTH-rp (1-36) into human volunteers increased serum ionized calcium, decreased serum phosphorous, increased the fractional excretion of phosphorous, increased nephrogenous cAMP excretion, increased plasma 1,25-dihydroxy vitamin D levels, and suppressed endogenous PTH (1-84).[169]

PTH-rp production by tumors is not limited to nonmetastatic solid neoplasms, and elevated levels have been found in patients with metastases to the bone as well as in one-third to one-half of patients with hematologic malignancies.[120–122,170]

Depending on the assay utilized, between 5 and 90 percent of normal individuals have detectable concentrations of immunoreactive PTH-rp in their blood.[171] Normal concentrations are generally below 2.5 pmol/L with assays based on antisera to the 1-34 fragment of PTH-rp, and below 2.1 pmol/L for carboxy-terminal assays (amino acids 109–138).[120–122,162] PTH-rp is widely distributed throughout the body as assessed by immunoassay, immunohistochemistry, and mRNA determinations. Thus, it is present in keratinocytes of the epidermis, pancreatic islet cells, stomach, adrenal cortex and medulla, hypothalamus, pituitary, brain, thyroid, bone marrow, myometrium, placenta, and lactating mammary glands.[172–175] In fact, the highest concentrations of the protein are found in milk.[162,174] Although the physiologic functions of PTH-rp are unknown, it has been speculated that it may play a role in calcium transport in the breast, where the production of PTH-rp is under the control of prolactin, and in transplacental calcium transport.[175–177] PTH-rp may also have an important autocrine function. The protein has been shown to be produced by lectin-stimulated T lymphocytes. Incubation of lymphocytes with synthetic PTH-rp (1-34) led to suppression of DNA synthesis.[178] The widespread distribution of PTH-rp raises the possibility that production of the hormone by neoplasms is not strictly ectopic but may represent excessive eutopic production.

Prostaglandins In 1970, prostaglandins of the E series (PGEs) were found to stimulate osteoclastic bone resorption and increase cyclic AMP in vitro.[179,180] A few years later, Tashjian and associates studied mouse $HSDM_1$ fibrosarcoma and rabbit VX_2 carcinoma tumors, which are associated with nonmetastatic hypercalcemia.[181,182] The tumor tissues from these animals contain high quantities of PGE_2, and the tumor cells secrete the prostaglandin in vitro and stimulate osteoclastic bone resorption. Arteriovenous concentration differences of PGE_2 across the tumor confirm the in vivo production, and the administration of an inhibitor of prostaglandin synthesis—indomethacin—to tumor-bearing animals lowers the elevated serum calcium and plasma PGE_2 levels in a parallel fashion.[183] Indomethacin also inhibits PGE_2 and bone resorption–stimulating activity produced by tumor cells grown in vitro. Finally, infusion of PGE_2 into rats was found to produce hypercalcemia.[184] These studies provided strong support for the concept that some tumors may cause hypercalcemia through osteoclastic bone resorption stimulated by the excessive production by prostaglandins.

The first study in humans appeared in 1974 with the description of a hypercalcemic patient with a renal cell carcinoma associated with a high concentration of E-type prostaglandin in liver metastases and a low plasma prostaglandin level.[185] The administration of indomethacin was associated with a decline in serum calcium, which again rose after the cessation of the medication. Additional cases of patients with renal cell carcinoma and hypercalcemia who were responsive to indomethacin were reported[147,186] In 1975, Seyberth and colleagues studied 29 patients with solid tumors, including 14 with hypercalcemia.[146] They evaluated prostaglandin production in these patients by measuring the urinary excretion of the major urinary metabolite of PGE_1 and PGE_2, 7 alpha-hydroxy-5,11-diketotetranorprostane-1,16-dioic acid (PGE-M). They found that 12 of the 14 patients with humoral hypercalcemia associated with solid tumors had elevations of urinary PGE-M, as did 2 patients who were normocalcemic at the time of study but subsequently developed hypercalcemia. Patients who were hypercalcemic as a result of hyperparathyroidism or hematologic malignancies had normal urine concentrations of PGE-M. Five of 13 normocalcemic patients who had solid tumors also had elevations of this urinary metabolite. Six hypercalcemic patients with solid tumors received inhibitors of prostaglandin synthesis and had a concomitant decrease in serum calcium and urinary PGE-M levels. These investigators subsequently found that urinary cyclic AMP excretion was normal in patients with elevated PGE-M levels, in contrast to patients who had nonmetastatic hypercalcemia with normal PGE-M levels, who demonstrated elevated urinary cyclic AMP concentrations.[187]

Despite this initial positive report, relatively few hypercalcemic patients with neoplasms have been found to have a reduction in serum calcium with the use of inhibitors of prostaglandin synthesis.[188,189] In addition, it has been noted that there is no correlation between PGE levels and the degree of hypercalcemia or the presence or absence of metastases.[125,190] It is of interest that indomethacin may lower the urinary excretion of PGE without consistently altering plasma PGE levels or serum calcium.[190] Because PGE is extensively metabolized during the first pass through the lungs and liver, it has been calculated that the venous blood concentration of PGE_2 would need to be greater than 10 times the upper limit of normal to result in an arterial PGE_2 blood concentration that is the minimal effective concentration required to increase bone resorption in vitro.[190] Concentrations of that magnitude have not been found in patients with hypercalcemia associated with nonmetastatic solid tumors.

As noted earlier, prostaglandin production by tumor cells is probably most important in inducing osteolysis in the region surrounding osseous tumor deposits. It is clear that tumors do synthesize and secrete prostaglandins, as do monocytes and macrophages, which are also found in the area of bone metastases.[118] In this regard, it has long been known that after the initial administration of estrogens or antiestrogens, patients with breast cancer metastatic to the bone may develop acute, severe hypercalcemia. Breast cancer cells have been shown to release E-series prostaglandins after exposure to estrogens in vitro, and there is a concomitant increase in bone resorbing activity, which can be inhibited by indomethacin and flufenamic acid.[191] Unfortunately, the administration of prostaglandin synthesis inhibitors has not been shown to be effective in lowering serum calcium in hypercalcemic patients with metastatic breast cancer. Although the reasons for this are unclear, concentrations of the prostaglandin synthesis inhibitors in the area of the bone metastases that can be achieved after oral administration may be insufficient to inhibit prostaglandin synthesis in vivo. Alternatively, because elevated concentrations of PTH-rp have been found in some patients with metastatic breast cancer, the hypercalcemia associated with such tumors may be multifactorial.

Cytokines Interest in cytokines as potential mediators of hypercalcemia in patients with cancer began in 1974, when Mundy and associates described the production of an osteoclast-activating factor produced in vitro by multiple myeloma cells.[148] This substance was similar to a material produced by phytohemagglutinin-transformed normal lymphocytes. Similar osteoclast-activating-factor activity was found in cells derived from hypercalcemic patients with Burkitt's lymphoma, T-cell lymphoma, and some leukemias. Subsequent work has indicated that the osteoclast-activating-factor activity can be accounted for by a group of cytokines and growth factors including interleukin-Iα, interleukin-Iβ, intraleukin-6, transforming growth factor-α, transforming growth factor-β, tumor necrosis factor-β (lymphotoxin), colony-stimulating factors, and epidermal growth factor.[20,127] These cytokines may be produced by the tumor cells or by transformed lymphocytes, monocytes, or macrophages in the vicinity of the tumor cells. Several different mechanisms for stimulation of bone reabsorption by the cytokines have been described, including the activation of preexisting osteoclasts, stimulation of the proliferation of osteoclast progenitor cells without activation of preexisting osteoclasts, and stimulation of PGE_2 synthesis in the bone.[192] Thus, as is the case with prostaglandins, cytokines appear to be local mediators of bone resorption in patients with metastatic solid tumors associated with hypercalcemia as well as in patients with hematologic and lymphoproliferative disorders involving the bone.

Conversion of 25(OH)-vitamin D to 1,25(OH)$_2$-vitamin D

In addition to renal tubular cells, the vitamin-D-1α-hydroxylase enzyme is present in keratinocytes, fibroblasts, trophoblasts, alveolar macrophages, and lymphocytes. Several tumors, including HIV-I–associated and unassociated lymphomas, HTLV-I–mediated adult T-cell leukemia/lymphoma, small cell carcinoma of the lung, and melanoma, have been found to be associated with elevated 1,25(OH)$_2$-vitamin D levels with dysregulated 25(OH)-1α-vitamin D hydroxylase activity.[193–198] High levels of 1,25(OH)$_2$-vitamin D have been found in more than half of patients with lymphomas.[198,199] In patients with lymphomas associated with elevated 1,25-dihydroxy vitamin D levels and hypercalcemia, therapy with glucocorticoids reduces both the serum calcium and 1,25-dihydroxy vitamin D concentrations in a parallel fashion.[193]

Coexistence of Cancer and Primary Hyperparathyroidism

The association of hyperparathyroidism and nonparathyroid malignancies is well established in patients with both type I and type II multiple endocrine neoplasia syndromes. Additionally, numerous investigators have reported an increased incidence of malignant breast, thyroid, GI, genitourinary, and pulmonary neoplasms in patients with hyperparathyroidism.[34–37,200–203] These studies have suggested that between 34 and 42 percent of patients with parathyroid adenomas or hyperplasia have an associated neoplasm, raising the possibility that hypercalcemia or hyperparathyroidism predisposes a patient to neoplasia. Alternatively, neoplasms may produce a parathyrotropic substance that leads to the development of parathyroid hyperplasia or adenoma(s).

However, caution should be exercised in interpreting the literature because of three considerations. First, both hyperparathyroidism and neoplasms are relatively common, and the frequency of both increases with age.[204] This, coupled with the increased scrutiny that a patient undergoes during an evaluation for one of the conditions which incidentally could uncover the other, may account for the apparent association. Second, some of these studies utilized histologic criteria for the diagnosis of parathyroid hyperplasia or adenoma in patients with cancer. One of the major criteria for parathyroid chief cell hyperplasia is a reduction in stromal fat. In a study of hypercalcemic patients with nonmetastatic tumors and undetectable parathyroid hormone who exhibited the clinical features of the humoral hypercalcemia of cancer syndrome, 70 percent had markedly reduced amounts of parathyroid stromal fat, giving a histologic appearance that was indistinguishable from that of chief cell hyperplasia. Similar data were found in 20 percent of normocalcemic cancer patients.[129] These histologic findings undoubtedly represent the effects of weight loss and cachexia on the parathyroid glands rather than functional parathyroid abnormalities. Third, the association between well-differentiated thyroid cancer and hyperparathyroidism in some of these series may have been due to the inclusion of patients who received head and neck irradiation for benign disorders during childhood and adolescence, a known risk factor for both problems.[205,206]

Clinical Manifestations and Diagnosis

Hypercalcemia is generally a late and often preterminal manifestation of malignancy, with death usually occurring within 3 months of the diagnosis.[29,30,37,207–209]

The signs and symptoms of hypercalcemia fall into four groups. Nonspecific general complaints of fatigue, weakness, headaches, behavioral abnormalities, and malaise are present in more than half the patients and are an especially prominent complaint in individuals with calcium concentrations below 14 mg/dl.[29] Gastrointestinal manifestations include anorexia, nausea, vomiting, constipation, and abdominal discomfort and are present in one-half to three-quarters of patients at the time of presentation.[29,117] Neurologic abnormalities are also prominent, especially in patients with serum calcium above 14 mg/dl.[29,117] Patients often complain of drowsiness, visual abnormalities, confusion, and memory impairment and are frequently found to be lethargic, confused, stuporous, or comatose. There are usually no localizing signs. Finally, the hypercalcemia may lead to a nephrogenic diabetes insipidus resulting in polyuria, thirst, and polydipsia. If fluid intake is insufficient, findings of dehydration may be present.

Patients who have humoral hypercalcemia of malignancy share many of the clinical and biochemical findings of primary hyperparathyroidism, although there are clinical and biochemical differences between these diseases (Table 28-14).[123,210–212] Considering the close biochemical similarity in the actions of PTH and PTH-rp, it is of interest that three laboratory abnormalities cannot be explained on the basis of the direct biochemical effects of these two hormones.[213] Patients with hyperparathyroidism generally have hyperchloremic acidosis, while individuals with humoral hypercalcemia of malignancy have hypochloremic alkalosis and do not exhibit the renal bicarbonate wasting found with primary hyperparathyroidism. Although in vitro both PTH and PTH-rp stimulate renal 25(OH)-vitamin D1α-hydroxylase activity, clinically patients with primary hyperparathyroidism have elevated levels of 1,25(OH)$_2$ vitamin D while patients with the humoral hypercalcemia of malignancy generally have normal or low levels. Finally, patients with malignancy-associated hypercalcemia exhibit uncoupling of bone resorption and bone formation as assessed through histomorphometric evaluation, while patients with primary hyperparathyroidism usually demonstrate coupling of the resorption and formation activity. Thus, some of the clinical manifestations of humoral hypercalcemia of malignancy may not be explained by simply implicating excessive production of PTH-rp. Instead, it is likely that other humoral factors, nutritional deficiencies, and metabolic abnormalities contribute to the observed differences between the two diseases.

Figure 28-4 provides an algorithm for evaluating patients with hypercalcemia and cancer. A bone scan is the most sensitive screening test for detecting osteolytic metastases. If lytic lesions are found, the hypercalcemia may be due to local prostaglandin or

TABLE 28-14. Comparison of Primary Hyperparathyroidism and Humoral Hypercalcemia of Malignancy

Feature	Primary Hyperparathyroidism	Humoral Hypercalcemia of Malignancy
History	Long, indolent course (1–25 years)	Short, rapidly progressive course (weeks to months)
Sex	60 percent female	75 percent male
Major symptoms	None; renal stones, peptic ulcer, pancreatitis, bone pain, memory impairment	Weight loss, lethargy, obtundation, polyuria, nocturia, nausea, vomiting
Serum calcium	Rarely >14 mg/dl	Often >14 mg/dl
Urine calcium/ serum calcium	Lower	Higher
Serum phosphate	Normal or decreased	Normal or decreased
Serum chloride	Often >102 mEq/L	Often ≤102 mEq/L
Serum HCO_3	Normal or low	Elevated
Serum Cl/PO_4	Usually >35	Usually <35
Alkaline phosphatase	Usually normal	Often elevated
Nephrogenous cAMP	Elevated	Elevated
$1,25(OH)_2D_3$	Normal to elevated	Normal to low
Hematocrit	>38 percent in 90 percent	<38 percent in 75 percent
Serum PTH	Normal to elevated	Low
Serum PTH-rp	Low	High
Bone biopsy	Elevated osteoclastic bone resorption and osteoblastic bone formation (coupled resorption formation)	Elevated osteoclastic bone resorption, depressed bone formation (uncoupled resorption formation)

Source: From references 123 and 210–212.

cytokine production or may represent osteoclastic reabsorption from secretion of PTH-rp. If the bone scan is normal, a determination of serum concentrations of PTH and PTH-rp should be performed. Elevated levels of PTH are almost always due to the coexistence of primary hyperparathyroidism, while elevations of PTH-rp point to the neoplastic production of PTH-rp as the etiology of the hypercalcemia.[30,37] If the PTH and PTH-rp concentrations are normal or low, a measurement of $1,25(OH)_2$ vitamin D should be performed; if it is elevated, this suggests the presence of lymphoma or leukemia or the possibility of an associated granulomatous disease or vitamin D intoxication. If the $1,25(OH)_2$ vitamin D levels are normal, a therapeutic trial of indomethacin or another prostaglandin synthesis inhibitor may be given. A decrease in calcium provides presumptive evidence of prostaglandin-mediated hypercalcemia. An absence of change in the calcium concentration suggests the presence of bony micrometastases that are too small to be seen by bone scan or the coexistence of another cause of hypercalcemia.

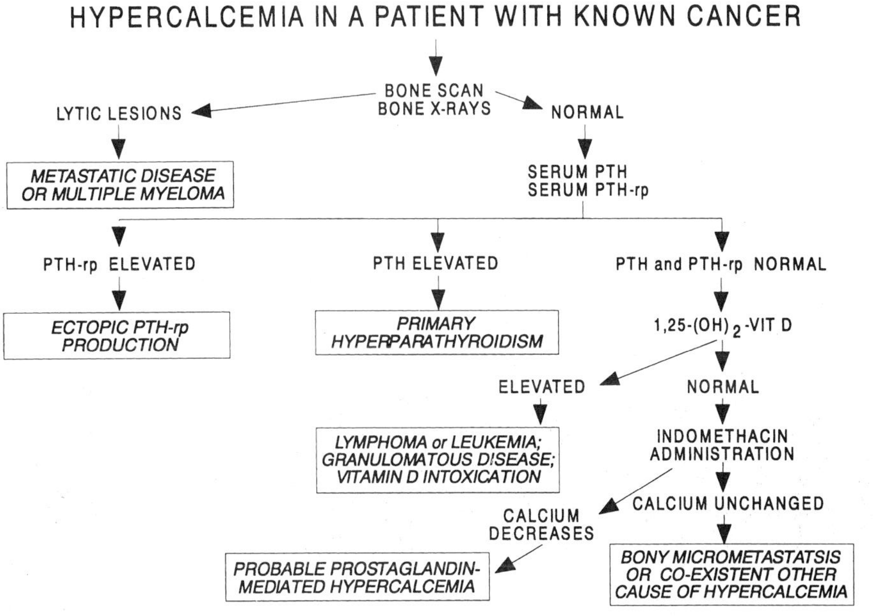

FIGURE 28-4. Algorithm for evaluating patients with cancer and hypercalcemia. See text for details.

Therapy

The mainstays of therapy for humoral hypercalcemia include the treatment of the underlying tumor and therapies directed toward directly reducing serum calcium. Hydration with normal saline not only expands intravascular fluid volume, which decreases the serum calcium, but also promotes urinary calcium excretion. The rate of urine flow may be enhanced with diuretics such as furosemide or ethacrynic acid with careful attention to and replacement of the potassium lost in urine. Concurrently, medications may be administered to inhibit bone resorption. Glucocorticoids are effective in patients with prostaglandin-mediated hypercalcemia and patients with hematologic and lymphoproliferative neoplasms with cytokine production or enhanced conversion of 25(OH)-vitamin D to 1,25$(OH)_2$ vitamin D. Calcitonin, mithramycin, bisphosphonates, and gallium nitrate are medications that inhibit osteoclastic bone resorption. Finally, if these measures are not effective, a dangerously elevated serum calcium may be reduced through peritoneal dialysis or hemodialysis using a calcium-free dialysis solution.[214–218]

Once the acute hypercalcemia has been effectively treated, further exacerbations of hypercalcemia may be prevented through the maintenance of adequate hydration, ambulation, and exercise and the administration of oral bisphosphonates or phosphates. In the rare patient with prostaglandin-mediated hypercalcemia due to systemic overproduction of prostaglandin, indomethacin or another prostaglandin synthesis inhibitor may be effective.

Ectopic POMC/ACTH Syndrome

The first recorded example of the ectopic POMC/ACTH syndrome was reported in 1928 by Brown, 4 years before Cushing's classic paper describing the syndrome which bears his name.[219] Brown's patient was a 45-year-old obese female with hyperpigmentation, glucose intolerance, hypertension, hirsutism, weakness, and plethora who was found to have bilateral adrenal hyperplasia associated with a small cell carcinoma of the lung. In 1961, Christy demonstrated the presence of an adrenal weight-maintaining factor in the plasma of two patients with neoplasms and this syndrome.[220] This was followed shortly by the demonstration of immunoreactive ACTH in tumor tissue and plasma.[221,222] Subsequent studies by Liddle and colleagues showed that the ACTH present in tumors from patients with Cushing's syndrome closely resembled the biologically active hormone in the pituitary.[223]

Prevalence and Tumor Types

Cushing's syndrome is a relatively uncommon paraneoplastic syndrome associated with cancer. The ectopic production of POMC/ACTH accounts for 15–20 percent of patients with Cushing's syndrome.[125,224] Close to half the patients with this syndrome have a small cell carcinoma of the lung, while an additional 11 percent harbor a bronchial carcinoid and 13 percent have an epithelial thymic neoplasm or thymic carcinoid (Table 28-15).[225–228] Thus, close to 70 percent of patients presenting with this syndrome have a tumor between the clavicles and the diaphragm. Islet cell tumors of the pancreas, carcinoid tumors arising from sites other than the lung, pheochromocytomas and other tumors of chromaffin tissue, ovarian neoplasms, and medullary carcinoma of the thyroid account for the majority of the remaining 30 percent of tumor types associated with this syndrome.[225–228] Altogether, 84 percent of the tumor types have APUD characteristics, while the remaining 16 percent are squamous cell tumors, adenocarcinomas, or hepatomas.[226]

TABLE 28-15. Tumors Associated with the Ectopic POMC/ACTH Syndrome (*N* = 220)

Tumor	Percent
Small cell carcinoma of lung	45
Thymic carcinoma/carcinoid	13
Bronchial carcinoid	11
Islet-cell tumor	10
Other carcinoid	4
Pheochromocytoma	2
Ovarian carcinoma	2
Other*	13

*Esophageal, gastric, ileal, appendicular, colonic, cervical, breast, prostate, and laryngeal carcinoma; medullary carcinoma of the thyroid; acute myelogenous leukemia.

Source: From references 225–228.

Between 1.3 and 4.8 percent of patients with small cell carcinoma of the lung have clinically recognizable ectopic POMC/ACTH syndrome (Table 28-4).[43,53,54,57,58] In contrast, 19 percent of patients with small cell carcinoma of the lung examined at autopsy have unequivocal pathologic evidence of ACTH excess as reflected by bilateral adrenal hyperplasia and the presence of Crooke's hyaline changes in the pituitary.[229] Using biochemical criteria, between one-fourth and one-half of patients with small cell carcinoma of the lung have elevations of plasma or urine cortisol and do not show appropriate suppression of plasma cortisol after an overnight dexamethasone suppression test.[43,53,70,230] In addition, between 24 and 78 percent of patients with small cell carcinoma have elevated concentrations of immunoreactive POMC/ACTH in the serum or plasma.[54,66,67,69,72,78,90,231] The dichotomy between the high prevalence of elevated blood immunoreactive ACTH concentrations and the low frequency of the clinical ectopic POMC/ACTH syndrome is due to the secretion by these tumors of immunologically active forms of POMC/ACTH with little or no biological activity (see later).

POMC Products Produced by Tumors

In the anterior pituitary, the 1,200-base POMC mRNA encodes for the pre-POMC protein, which contains a 26-amino acid signal peptide along with the 241-amino acid POMC protein (Fig. 28-5). POMC is glycosylated and has a molecular mass of approximately 31 kDa. In the anterior pituitary it undergoes post-translational processing through convertases, with the generation of ACTH, N-terminal fragment, joining peptide, and beta-lipotropin (β-LPH). β-LPH is further processed to γ-LPH and β-endorphin.[90,224] A small quantity of pro-ACTH, a 22-kDa glycosylated form of ACTH, has also been detected in pituitary extracts.[90,232] In the human fetal pituitary intermediate lobe, the amino-terminal peptide is further processed to generate gamma melanocyte stimulating hormone (γ-MSH), and ACTH is cleaved to form α-MSH [N-α-acetyl-($ACTH^{1\text{-}13}$)-NH_2] and corticotropin-like intermediate peptide (CLIP). γ-LPH is also cleaved to form the 18-residue β-MSH (Fig. 28-5).

Each of the POMC-derived peptide produced by the normal anterior pituitary and the fetal intermediate lobe has been found in extracts of tumors removed from patients with the ectopic PMOC/ACTH syndrome.[91,224,233–239] Met-enkephalin has also been found in tumor extracts.[240,241] Although this molecule was originally thought to be derived from β-lipotropin molecules since it shares a common amino acid sequence with the C-terminal

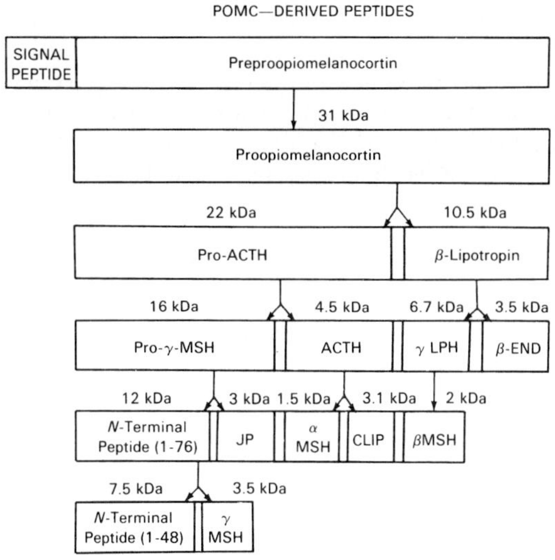

FIGURE 28-5. Proopiomelanocortin-derived peptides. JP = joining peptide; CLIP = corticotropin-like intermediate peptide; MSH = melanocyte stimulating hormone; β-END = β-endorphin.

portion of β-LPH, met-enkephalin is actually derived from a separate precursor, pro-enkephalin.

In patients with the clinical syndrome, both the biologically active nonglycosylated 39-amino acid ACTH moiety and ACTH precursors are present in the tumor and circulation.[87] As has been noted previously, a number of investigations have found that the majority of patients with lung cancer of any histologic type have elevations of immunoreactive ACTH in the circulation but do not exhibit any clinical syndrome. In addition, the majority of extracts derived from lung cancers of all histologic types, including squamous cell carcinoma, adenocarcinoma, small cell carcinoma, and poorly differentiated carcinoma, have been found to contain immunoreactive ACTH, and over one-third also contain immunoreactive β LPH.[68] The immunoreactive ACTH in the tumors and blood of patients without the clinical syndrome lacks biological activity, as reflected by absent or reduced binding in a radioreceptor assay.[67] This form of ACTH represents the glycosylated 22,000-dalton pro-ACTH molecule initially described by Yalow as "big ACTH."[90,231] Digestion of this intermediate form of ACTH with trypsin generates biologically active ACTH.

It is of interest that POMC mRNA has been found to be widely distributed in normal tissues, including the stomach, pancreas, brain, placenta, adrenal medulla, and testis.[242] In addition, POMC peptides have been found in many normal tissues.[68,72,243,244] In this regard, Odell and colleagues hypothesized that all normal tissues produce small amounts of the ACTH precursor and carcinomas produce increased quantities of this material. Selected carcinomas are capable of converting this ACTH precursor into biologically active ACTH, thereby producing the ectopic POMC/ACTH syndrome.[72,245] However, recent studies suggest an alternative mechanism. The POMC mRNA in nonpituitary tissues and tumors that is not associated with the ectopic POMC/ACTH syndrome is smaller (approximately 800 bases) than the 1,200-base POMC mRNA present in the pituitary.[242,246–248] In contrast, the 1,200-base POMC mRNA has been found in tumors associated with the clinical syndrome.[249] This, together with the observation that the ratio of POMC mRNA to POMC peptides present in nonpituitary tissues is much greater than that in the pituitary, suggests that POMC gene expression in normal tissues and tumors not associated with the clinical syndrome is inefficient or defective.[224]

Clinical Manifestations

There are two major modes of presentation of patients with the ectopic PMOC/ACTH syndrome. The first is found in individuals with clinically apparent neoplasms, especially small cell carcinoma of the lung, in which there is rapid onset of clinical and biochemical aberrations. The usual patient is a male 45–60 years old, often with a cigarette smoking history of multiple packs over many years, who has the acute onset of profound proximal muscle weakness; pitting edema of the lower extremities; neuropsychiatric symptoms such as mood change, mania, depression, and obtundation; and hypertension. Either weight loss from the underlying neoplasm or weight gain may be present. Polyuria and polydipsia may also be present as a result of glucose intolerance. Women may note the onset of acne and hirsutism. Biochemically, these patients generally exhibit a profound hypokalemic ($K < 3$ mEq/L) alkalosis ($HCO_3 > 28$ mEq/L) due to a combination of increase secretion of cortisol, corticosterone, and 11-deoxycorticosterone, all of which interact with the mineralocorticoid receptor. In addition, the inactivation of cortisol is reduced because of an ACTH-induced inhibition of 11β-hydroxysteroid dehydrogenase, which converts cortisol to cortisone, the latter being devoid of mineralocorticoid activity.[250] The patients usually have either overt diabetes mellitus or glucose intolerance. Although some patients may appear to be cushingoid, most presenting in this manner do not, presumably because they have not had enough time to develop the centripetal fat redistribution and moon facies characteristic of Cushing's disease. Alternatively, the highly malignant nature of the underlying neoplasm in these patients, along with the attendant weight loss and cachexia, may obscure the more typical cushingoid features. The average survival of patients presenting in this manner is 4 months or less.[31,227–229,251]

The second major mode of presentation is seen primarily in patients with occult tumors, especially pulmonary and thymic carcinoids.[228] These patients usually harbor small neoplasms, some of which may be benign, and generally present with signs and symptoms closely mimicking Cushing's disease. Thus, typical cushingoid features are common, with centripetal obesity, moon facies, buffalo hump, increased supraclavicular fat pads, thinning of the skin with purplish stria, easy bruising, plethora, hirsutism, acne, psychiatric symptoms, polydipsia, polyuria, and hypertension. Virtually all these patients have significant proximal muscle weakness, and approximately one-half exhibit hyperpigmentation. Hypokalemic alkalosis may also be present, but it is generally of a milder degree than in patients with more overt neoplasms.[227,228,252] This group of patients is most difficult to differentiate clinically and biochemically from patients with Cushing's disease.

The Ectopic Corticotropin Releasing Hormone Syndrome

In 1971, Upton and Amatruda described two patients, one with a pancreatic tumor and the other with a small cell carcinoma of the lung, who exhibited the clinical ectopic POMC/ACTH syndrome but whose tumors contained bioactive corticotropin releasing hormone (CRH).[253] Subsequently, several additional patients have been reported with the spectrum of tumors including bronchial carcinoid, prostatic carcinoma, medullary carcinoma of the thyroid, and intrasellar gangliocytoma.[254–260] Both the rapid-onset and slow-onset types of presentation described above have been noted in these patients. Some but not all of these tumors also contain POMC and related peptides, including biologically active ACTH. The pituitary in these patients demonstrates corticotroph hyperplasia, indicating that the CRH is biologically active.[254,255,261] It appears that the clinical features of Cushing's syndrome result from CRH stimulation of pituitary ACTH secretion with or without concomitant secretion of biologically active ACTH from the tumor. It is also of interest that materials closely related immunologically to CRH have been found in normal stomach, pancreas, and adrenal glands, along with various tumors, including those not associated with Cushing's syndrome.[262]

Diagnosis

In patients with overt neoplasms and a rapid onset of the ectopic POMC/ACTH syndrome, the biochemical diagnosis does not present difficulties (Fig. 28-6). The 24-h urine free cortisol concentration is generally four or more times above the upper limit of normal, and these patients fail to demonstrate a 50 percent or greater suppression of serum or urine cortisol concentrations after the administration of either low-dose (1 mg overnight; 0.5 mg orally every 6 h for eight doses) or high-dose (2 mg orally every 6 h for eight doses) dexamethasone because of the autonomous secretion of ACTH from the tumor. Measurement of plasma ACTH can differentiate between the ectopic POMC/ACTH syndrome and the presence of an adrenal adenoma or carcinoma that autonomously secretes excessive quantities of cortisol. In the latter group of patients, plasma ACTH levels are suppressed, while in patients with the ectopic POMC/ACTH syndrome, the levels usually exceed 200 pg/ml.[125,227]

Unfortunately, not all patients with the ectopic POMC/ACTH syndrome follow this classical scheme. Close to 80 percent of patients with pituitary-dependent Cushing's disease have more than 50 percent suppression of plasma or 24-h urine cortisol levels

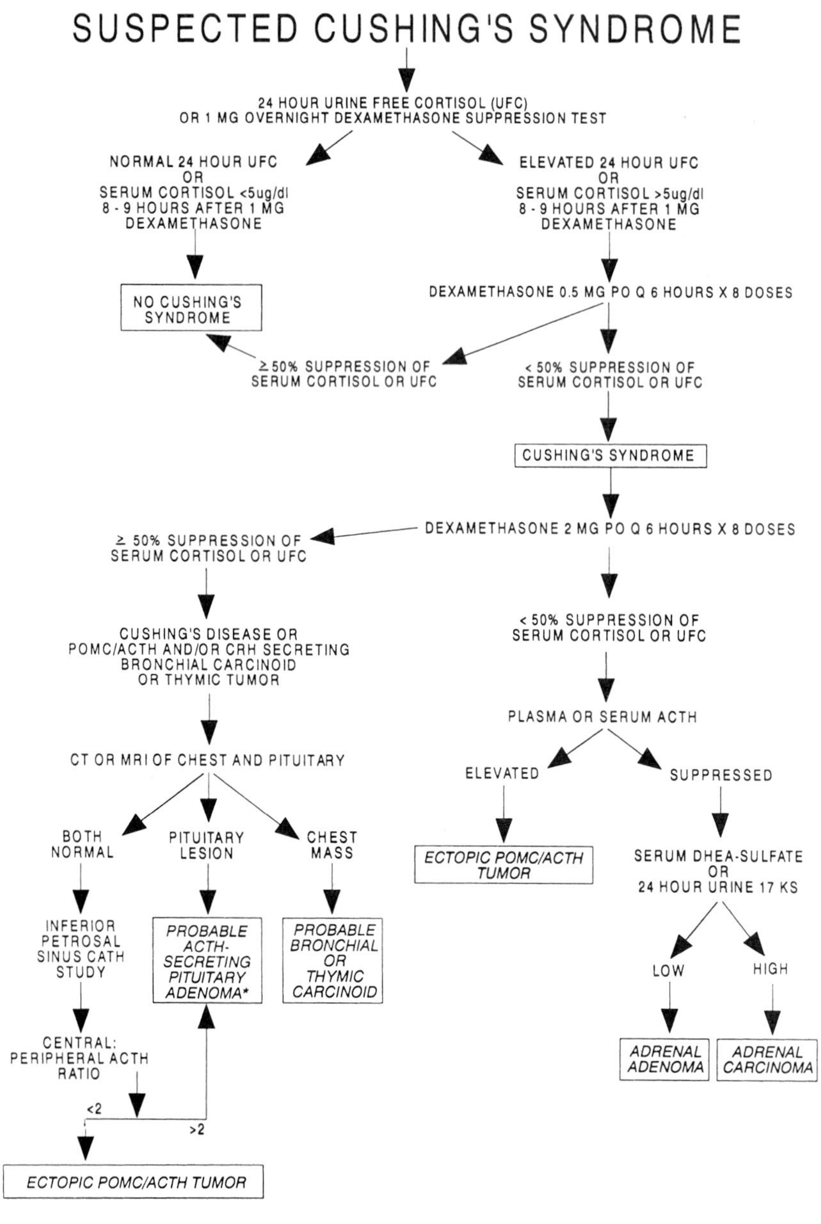

FIGURE 28-6. Algorithm for the evaluation of a patient with suspected Cushing's syndrome. See text for details. (*The rare pure CRH-secreting tumor potentially may give similar results. Plasma CRH levels should help differentiate these entities.)

after 2 days of ingesting 8 mg of dexamethasone each day, while 11 percent of patients with the ectopic POMC/ACTH syndrome also show such suppression.[228] Similarly, close to 90 percent of patients with Cushing's disease and 63 percent of patients with ectopic POMC/ACTH syndrome demonstrate a 100 percent or greater rise in either plasma ACTH or urinary 17-hydroxysteroids after metyrapone administration.[228] This overlap in biochemical responses between patients who have Cushing's disease and those with the ectopic POMC/ACTH syndrome is seen primarily in individuals who have occult neoplasms as well as patients with the ectopic CRH syndrome. Indeed, in the group of patients with occult tumors and Cushing's syndrome, an incorrect diagnosis is initially made in approximately 70 percent.[263]

When CRH is administered as an intravenous bolus over 30 s at a dose of 1 μg/kg, normal individuals show a prompt rise in ACTH followed by an increase in plasma cortisol (Fig. 28-7).[264] As expected, patients with ACTH-independent Cushing's syndrome resulting from primary adrenocortical disease demonstrate little or no rise in either ACTH or cortisol. In contrast, individuals with pituitary ACTH-dependent Cushing's disease have elevations of basal ACTH and cortisol concentrations and exhibit an exuberant rise in both hormones after CRH administration. Patients with ectopic POMC/ACTH Cushing's syndrome also have elevated plasma ACTH and cortisol concentrations but demonstrate no further increase after receiving CRH. Unfortunately, only 90 percent of patients with pituitary ACTH-dependent Cushing's disease show a rise in ACTH, while 8 percent of patients with the ectopic POMC/ACTH syndrome show a similar rise. Because of the four- to six-fold greater prevalence of pituitary ACTH-dependent Cushing's disease, the predictive value of a positive CRH test in identifying Cushing's disease is 99 percent, but the predictive value of a negative test (with an insufficient rise in ACTH) is only 63 percent.[265] Thus, this test is not as useful in differentiating between the two diseases as the initial reports suggested. It is of interest that CRH has been found in tumors from patients with the ectopic POMC/ACTH syndrome who have an increase in ACTH after a CRH test, suggesting that the false-positive responses in this syndrome are due to the ectopic production of CRH by the tumor, which leads to hyperplasia of the pituitary corticotrophs which are responsive to exogenous CRH.[258]

Another technique developed to differentiate eutopic pituitary ACTH-dependent Cushing's syndrome from ectopic POMC/ACTH Cushing's syndrome is selective venous blood sampling from multiple sites with measurement of ACTH. Because the pituitary venous effluent drains into the inferior petrosal sinuses, catheterization of the sinuses with simultaneous blood sampling of both sinuses and a peripheral vein will show a gradient of 2 or greater in the unstimulated state or 3 or greater during a simultaneous infusion of CRH in patients with an ACTH-secreting pituitary adenoma.[265–267] In contrast, patients with the ectopic POMC/ACTH syndrome have a gradient below 2 in the basal state or during CRH infusion. The localization of the tumor producing the syndrome may be accomplished through sampling of blood from a variety of other sites throughout the venous vascular tree. Because of the potential for microsecretory bursts of ACTH secretion, it is important to carry out the procedure as rapidly as possible.[266,268]

Serum serotonin or urine 5-hydroxyindolacetic acid measurements are occasionally useful in patients with the ectopic POMC/ACTH syndrome due to carcinoid tumors or small cell carcinoma of the lung.[269] Because the majority of patients with this syndrome harbor a neoplasm within the chest, a CT or MRI scan of the chest and mediastinum should be performed on all patients who do not have an overt tumor but fulfill the biochemical criteria for the ectopic POMC/ACTH syndrome. Similarly, patients who appear to have classical Cushing's disease should also have a CT or MRI scan of the chest unless radiographic procedures or inferior petrosal sinus studies have clearly demonstrated the presence of an ACTH-secreting pituitary adenoma.

Treatment

Slow-growing, well-localized bronchial or thymic carcinoids may be successfully removed surgically. However, between one-quarter and one-half of the patients will have lymph node metastasis and thus will not be cured unless a lymph node dissection is carried out and/or postoperative mediastinal irradiation given.[252] Bilateral

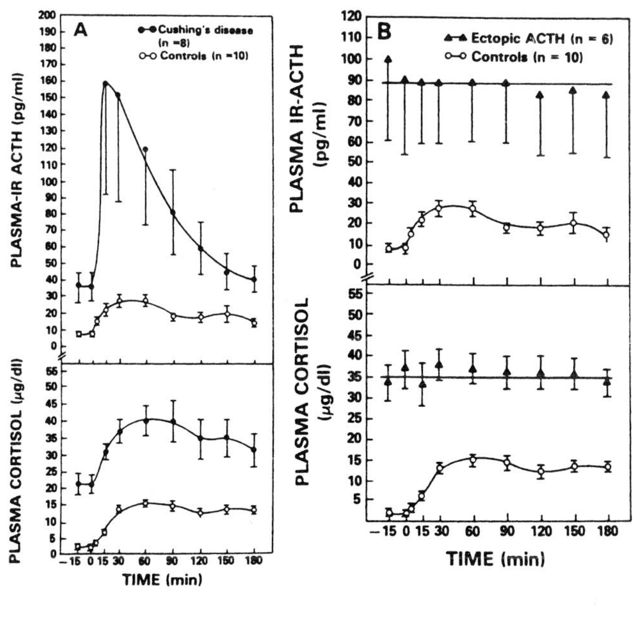

FIGURE 28-7. Plasma ACTH and cortisol responses to the administration of CRH in 8 patients with untreated Cushing's disease, 6 patients with ectopic POMC/ACTH secretion, and 10 control patients. (*Reprinted from Chrousos and colleagues,[264] with permission.*)

adrenalectomy is certainly effective in reversing the metabolic abnormalities but may be inappropriate in a patient with a highly malignant neoplasm such as small cell carcinoma of the lung. Inhibitors of glucocorticoid synthesis including aminoglutethimide, metyrapone, and ketoconazole have been used successfully in treating some, but not all, patients with this syndrome.[224,270–272] Combinations of inhibitors and the adrenlytic agent o,p′-DDD have also been used.[273] Similarly, glucocorticoid receptor blockade with the glucocorticoid antagonist RU-486 has been effective in a limited number of patients.[113] Finally, octreotide, a long-acting somatostatin analog has been used in patients with the ectopic POMC/ACTH syndrome and led to the rapid correction of the hypercortisolemia in less than half of the subjects.[274]

TABLE 28-16. Tumor Types Associated with SIAD

	Cases,	Percent
Bronchogenic carcinoma	83	
Small cell carcinoma		59
Non-small-cell carcinoma		24
Lymphoma	3	
Pancreatic carcinoma	2	
Laryngeal carcinoma	1	
Duodenal carcinoma	1	
Miscellaneous tumors*	10	

*Prostate (small cell), cervical (small cell), bladder, colon, thymoma, mesothelioma, olfactory neuroblastoma, sarcoma, lymphosarcoma, reticulum cell sarcoma, Ewing's sarcoma, malignant histiocytosis.

Source: From references 226 and 284–287.

Syndrome of Inappropriate Antidiuresis in Cancer

The first description of the syndrome of inappropriate antidiuresis (SIAD) in patients with cancer appeared in 1938.[275] In 1957, Schwartz and coworkers published the classic description of two patients with bronchogenic carcinoma who exhibited hyponatremia, continual loss of sodium in urine, and an impaired ability to dilute their urine.[276] Recognizing the similarity in the biochemical features between the two patients with lung cancer and normal subjects given injections of pitressin tannate-in-oil and free access to fluid, Schwartz et al. proposed that the syndrome is due to the inappropriate secretion of antidiuretic hormone [arginine vasopressin (AVP)].[277] In 1963, an increased concentration of antidiuretic hormone was found to be present in the urine of a patient with a lung tumor and this syndrome[278] and in tumor tissue by bioassay.[279] That a tumor could be the source of AVP was suggested by the finding in 1964 of increased concentrations of AVP in the plasma and tumor tissue of a patient with a bronchogenic carcinoma who also exhibited destruction of the posterior pituitary from a metastatic lesion.[280] More direct evidence of tumor production was provided by the studies of George et al., who demonstrated the incorporation of radiolabeled amino acids into AVP by lung tumor cells in vitro.[281] The similarity of the biosynthetic pathway for tumor and hypothalamic production of AVP was shown by Yamaji and colleagues in 1981 with the in vitro production of provasopressin by a small cell carcinoma of the lung maintained in vitro.[282] In the same year, a nude mouse bearing a small cell carcinoma of the lung derived from a patient with SIAD exhibited increased blood and tumor levels of AVP, excessive sodium loss in the urine, and decreased free water clearance, mimicking the human syndrome.[283]

Prevalence and Tumor Types

Between one-half and two-thirds of patients in reported series of SIAD have an underlying malignancy as the etiology.[284,285] This undoubtedly represents a reporting bias, as transient SIAD is frequently seen in patients with conditions such as meningitis and head trauma. The vast majority of patients with SIAD associated with cancer have a bronchogenic carcinoma, especially small cell carcinoma, which accounts for three-quarters of the patients with cancer-associated SIAD (Table 28-16).[226,284–287] Other histologic types of lung tumors, lymphomas, and an array of different types of tumors account for the remaining cases.

The prevalence of SIAD depends on how the condition is defined. The clinical syndrome associated with small cell carcinoma of the lung occurs in 7–14 percent of patients.[50,53–55,64,288] Even within this group, the patients may be asymptomatic and merely demonstrate hyponatremia and a urinary concentrating defect. On the basis of an abnormal water load test, between 35 and 66 percent of patients with small cell carcinoma of the lung are classified as having SIAD.[55,64,70,284] However, close to 70 percent of patients with other malignancies also exhibit abnormalities in the ability to excrete a water load, raising the possibility that this test gives nonspecific results in all patients.[70] Increased concentrations of plasma or urinary AVP levels are found in 33–71 percent of these patients.[52–55,64,72] Elevated AVP levels have also been noted in 43 percent of patients with colon carcinoma who do not exhibit clinical SIAD.[72] Using immunoassays for neurophysins, North and colleagues found that approximately 65 percent of patients with small cell carcinoma of the lung have elevated concentrations of neurophysins in the circulation.[71,289] Close to one-third have increased quantities of vasopressin-associated neurophysin alone, 12 percent have elevations of oxytocin-associated neurophysin alone, and 22 percent have elevations of both neurophysins.[71] Approximately 20 percent of patients with non-small-cell carcinoma of the lung also have elevations of neurophysins in the serum. Because AVP and AVP-associated neurophysin are synthesized together, along with a glycopeptide as provasopressin, and are normally secreted in equimolar amounts, it is not surprising that both are elevated in about half the patients with small cell carcinoma of the lung. Immunohistologic staining for AVP-associated neurophysin in small cell carcinoma of the lung has shown the presence of the antigen in 72 percent of the tissue specimens examined.[290] Thus, it appears that many patients with small cell carcinoma of the lung have a propensity for developing SIAD, although only a minority exhibit the clinical syndrome.

Tumor Peptides and Pathophysiology

Early studies demonstrated that the substance with antidiuretic activity extracted from tumors closely resembles that extracted from the posterior pituitary in terms of the dose-response effect in bioassay and inactivation by thioglycolate, vasopressinase, and vasopressin antibodies.[286,291,292] In addition, these materials appear to be identical to AVP immunologically and physicochemically. Direct evidence of in vitro synthesis was provided through immunoassay measurements of AVP production in vitro and through the incorporation of tritiated phenylalanine into a peptide resembling AVP.[281,293–295] Finally, in carefully performed pulse-chase experiments using labeled cysteine and glucosamine, Yamaji and associates found a small cell carcinoma of the lung that synthesized and secreted a 20,000-dalton glycosylated provasopressin which could be cleaved by trypsin to yield neurophysin, AVP, and a glycopeptide.[282,296] The mRNA for preprovasopressin also has been demonstrated in small cell carcinoma of the lung.[297]

Although it is clear that some lung tumors are capable of synthesizing and secreting AVP, it is safe to conclude that many cases of SIAD cannot be accounted for by ectopic production of AVP by these tumors, because only three-fourths of patients with SIAD associated with lung cancer have been found to have inappropriately elevated concentrations of AVP.[298] Also, some patients with typical SIAD actually have resetting of the hypothalamic osmostat, as manifested by a lowered osmotic threshold for the release of AVP from the hypothalamus.[299] In the latter situation, the rise of AVP with increasing plasma osmolality during a hypertonic saline infusion has a normal slope, but the entire curve is shifted to the left.

Because the normal physiologic regulation of AVP secretion from the hypothalamus and posterior pituitary is mediated through baroreceptors as well as osmoreceptors, there are multiple situations in which neoplasms may lead to a release of hypothalamic-pituitary AVP as opposed to ectopic production of the hormone by the tumor. Such mechanisms include obstruction of the vena cava, infiltration of the vagus nerve leading to baroreceptor denervation, hypothalamic metastases, carcinomatous neuropathy, CNS or pulmonary infections, pain, and alterations of intrathoracic pressure sufficient to stimulate the baroreceptors in the left atrium and great veins.[125,299,300] Similarly, a number of medications used in patients with cancer may be associated with hyponatremia. These drugs include cyclophosphamide, vincristine, cisplatin, doxorubicin, vinblastine, and bleomycin.[301,302]

It has also been proposed that some tumors may synthesize an AVP-releasing factor.[299] In patients who have SIAD without measurable levels of AVP, another antidiuretic substance may be produced by the tumor. One candidate substance is arginine vasotocin, a fetal peptide related to AVP, which may be produced by some tumors.[72] The natriuresis found in this syndrome may be due in part to the secretion of atrial natriuretic peptide (ANP), as plasma levels of this hormone are elevated in some patients with SIAD[303–306] and the mRNA for ANP has been isolated from small cell carcinomas associated with hyponatremia.[307]

Criteria for SIAD and Clinical Features

Vasopressin acts on the renal collecting tubule by binding with the AVP V_2 receptor, an interaction that stimulates adenylyl cyclase activity and ultimately allows the collecting ducts to become permeable to water. This results in the reabsorption of water from the hypotonic urine entering the collecting ducts that pass through the hypertonic renal medullary region. The net effect is the excretion of more concentrated urine and the delivery of the reabsorbed water to the intravascular and extravascular spaces. Normally, the secretion of AVP by the hypothalamus and posterior pituitary is tightly regulated through osmolar and volume mechanisms. With inappropriate secretion of AVP, inappropriate water retention and a reduction of body tonicity occur. The cardinal features of SIAD include the following:

1. Dilutional hyponatremia ($Na^+ < 130$ mEq/L), hypoosmolality (<280 mOsmol/kg), and low serum blood urea nitrogen (BUN), creatinine, uric acid, and albumin.
2. The presence of a urine osmolality that is inappropriately high for the serum hypoosmolality. This does not imply that urine osmolality must always be greater than serum osmolality in patients with SIAD, although it usually is; it implies only that the urine is not maximally dilute (50–60 mOsmol/kg), which it should be when AVP is suppressed. This criterion is reflected in the inability of patients with SIAD to excrete a water load normally.
3. The presence of continued natriuresis with a urine sodium concentration greater than 20 mEq/L despite the hyponatremia. The urine sodium excretion reflects sodium intake so that the administration of increasing quantities of sodium results in an equivalent loss of sodium in the urine. The natriuresis may be absent if the patient's sodium intake is severely restricted. The cause of the natriuresis is multifactorial and includes an increase in the glomerular filtration rate from the expanded extracellular fluid space, which in turn results in an increased filtered load of sodium. Additionally, serum aldosterone levels are either normal or low but are inappropriately low relative to the hyponatremia, which is a stimulus for aldosterone secretion. In the face of extracellular volume expansion, there is a decrease in the proximal tubular sodium reabsorption because of factors that are incompletely understood. Finally, atrial natriuretic factor levels are increased in these patients, and this may also enhance the natriuresis.[300]
4. Little or no edema despite the approximately 4–5 liters of water retention. There is an escape from the effects of the ADH that ultimately occurs in these patients. The reasons include a decrease in the tonicity of the normally hypertonic renal medullary interstitial space as a result of the dilutional effects, an increase in the water delivered to the distal nephron from the elevated glomerular filtration rate, and the hypokalemia that is present in approximately half the patients, which antagonizes the effect of AVP at the renal tubular level.[286]
5. The absence of a condition that results in a reduced effective vascular volume, including dehydration, congestive heart failure, and liver disease associated with ascites. These conditions are associated with an appropriate increase in hypothalamic and posterior pituitary secretion of AVP.
6. Normal renal, adrenal, thyroid, and anterior pituitary function.

The clinical manifestations of SIAD depend on the rate of development of hyponatremia and hypoosmolality as well as the actual level of serum sodium. Only a quarter of patients with SIAD exhibit clinical symptoms.[287] Symptoms may be precipitated through the ingestion of a thiazide diuretic, the administration of excessive oral or intravenous fluids during chemotherapy, or acutely as a result of tumor lysis with release of stored AVP. Also, water intoxication in predisposed patients may theoretically be precipitated by the ingestion of nonsteroidal analgesics that potentiate the antidiuretic effect of AVP by blocking PGE_2, an inhibitor of AVP action.[300]

It is uncommon for symptoms other than nonspecific malaise to occur above a serum sodium of 120 mEq/L. Between 115 and 120 mEq/L, the signs and symptoms of water intoxication include anorexia, nausea, vomiting, abdominal cramps, bloating, ileus, myoclonus, muscle weakness, restlessness, irritability, hostility, withdrawal, confusion, and headache. Serum sodium levels below 110 mEq/L are associated with severe muscle weakness, hyporeflexia, ataxia, extrapyramidal signs such as rigidity, bulbar or pseudobulbar palsies, positive Babinski signs, hemiparesis, stupor, coma, and seizures.

The diagnosis of SIAD is rarely difficult in patients with symptoms that fulfill the classical criteria. Secondary causes of

ADH secretion from volume depletion due to adrenal insufficiency, diuretic use, diarrhea, or hemorrhage are associated with typical signs and symptoms, including orthostatic hypotension and tachycardia, dry mucous membranes, and decreased skin turgor. In addition, dehydration leads to a low urinary sodium concentration, as do the conditions associated with volume overload and decreased effective vascular volume, such as congestive heart failure, cirrhosis of the liver, and the nephrotic syndrome. Pseudohyponatremia from elevations of serum glucose, lipids, or proteins is excluded through the measurement of plasma osmolality, which is normal rather than decreased, or correction of the serum sodium concentration for the level of glucose, triglycerides, or protein. Patients with primary polydipsia may have a low plasma osmolality but uniformly have a low urine osmolality and thus may be easily differentiated from patients with SIAD.

Plasma AVP measurements are of interest but add little to the management of these patients. The presence of an inappropriately elevated plasma AVP concentration in a patient with a neoplasm does not in itself indicate that the neoplasm is secreting the hormone ectopically. Tumors may be associated with SIAD through multiple mechanisms, as outlined previously.

In small cell carcinoma of the lung, there is a tendency for patients with more extensive disease to have a higher prevalence of an inability to excrete a water load than is seen in patients with limited disease.[55] However, taking into account the stage of the disease, there is no difference in the survival of patients who have SIAD vs. those who do not.[55,70,287,288] The abnormalities in water load tests, as well as the concentrations of AVP and neurophysins, reasonably parallel the clinical course of patients with small cell carcinoma of the lung and therefore may be used as markers of the disease.[55,289,290]

Therapy

Mild water intoxication is treated with fluid restriction to 800 ml per day or less. This reduces intravascular volume, resulting in a lowering of the glomerular filtration rate and a decrease in renal sodium loss.

For severe water intoxication, especially in patients with serum sodium levels below 110 mEq/L, a combination of 3 percent hypertonic sodium chloride with a loop diuretic such as furosemide or ethacrynic acid with replacement of urine sodium and potassium losses usually increases the serum sodium effectively. Because individuals with SIAD are fluid overloaded to begin with, the administration of hypertonic saline alone may result in congestive heart failure and hypertension. Also, because these patients excrete an amount of sodium in their urine equivalent to their sodium intake, hypertonic saline alone rarely leads to a sustained increase in serum sodium. The loop diuretics increase free water clearance and, together with the hypertonic saline, result in a rise in the sodium concentration.[300,301,308]

When one is using hypertonic saline and a loop diuretic, it is important to monitor the rate of rise of serum sodium. Overzealous correction of hyponatremia in severely debilitated patients has been associated with central pontine myelinosis. This problem can be avoided if the rate of rise of serum sodium is kept at <2 mEq/L per h until a level of serum sodium of 120 mEq/L is achieved, at which time the rate should be reduced. This therapy should be discontinued before the sodium reaches 130 mEq/L in order to avoid hypernatremia and hyperchloremia.[309]

For patients who are mildly symptomatic or exhibit chronic SIAD, three drugs are currently available. The first is demeclocycline, a tetracycline antibiotic that induces a nephrogenic diabetes insipidus by inhibiting the formation and action of cyclic AMP in the collecting ducts of the renal tubules. This drug may be initiated at a dose of 1,200 mg a day in divided doses. Urine osmolality decreases in 3–6 days, at which time the dose may be gradually decreased to a maintenance level of 300–900 mg/day. The goal is to maintain serum sodium within the normal range while the patient has free access to fluid. The side effects of this medication include nausea, vomiting, diarrhea, photosensitivity dermatitis, a dose-related rise in BUN without renal dysfunction, and nephrotoxicity, especially in patients with hepatic insufficiency.

Another drug that induces a nephrogenic diabetes insipidus is lithium carbonate in doses of 900–2,100 mg/day. The CNS, renal, and cardiac toxicities of this drug render it inferior to demeclocycline as a treatment for SIAD.[310]

Oral urea acts as an osmotic diuretic and enhances water clearance. Thirty grams of urea are dissolved in 100 ml of water or juice and are administered with 15 g of magnesium and aluminum hydroxide once a day.[301] The only adverse reaction to this medication is the potential for hypernatremic dehydration if the patient does not drink enough fluid. This therapy is reasonable to use if demeclocycline is not tolerated.

Finally, with small cell carcinoma of the lung, chemotherapy is effective in resolving SIAD in the majority of patients at the time of initial presentation.[59] Indeed, Hainsworth and colleagues found that 16 of 17 patients with small cell carcinoma had resolution of their SIAD between 8 and 26 days after the institution of chemotherapy.[59] Unfortunately, the majority have a return of SIAD at the time of progression, and one of the other therapies must be administered.

Hypoglycemia Associated with Malignancy

The first reports of hypoglycemia associated with a neoplasm were published in 1929 when Nadler and Wolfer[311] and Elliot[312] described a patient with a hepatoma who had neuroglucopenic symptoms and a blood sugar as low as 13 mg/dl. The following year, Doege and Potter independently described a patient with low-grade fibrosarcoma and hypoglycemia, whose hypoglycemia remitted after removal of the tumor, only to return with the recurrence of the malignancy.[82,313]

In the same year, Anderson described the association of hypoglycemia and adrenocortical carcinoma.[314] Since that time, hundreds of patients with the association have been reported and extensively reviewed.[315,316] Several eponyms have been used to describe specific associations, including Doege-Potter syndrome (mesenchymal tumors), Nadler-Wolfer-Elliot syndrome (hepatoma), Anderson's syndrome (adrenocortical tumors), and Rosenfeldt's syndrome (pseudomyxoma).[315]

Incidence and Tumor Types

Paraneoplastic hypoglycemia is rare. Hypoglycemia was found to occur in 1.2 percent of hospitalized patients, most often as a result of complications of diabetes mellitus, renal insufficiency, malnutrition, liver disease, infection, and shock.[317] In the few patients who had an underlying malignancy, hypoglycemia was associated with insulin therapy, extensive liver metastases, and malnutrition.[317] Despite its low prevalence, hypoglycemia is associated relatively frequently with some tumor types.

Approximately half the patients with tumor-associated hypoglycemia harbor neoplasms of mesenchymal origin, which include

TABLE 28-17. Tumor Types Associated with Hypoglycemia ($N = 246$)

	Patients, Percent	
Sarcoma	46	
Fibrosarcoma		24
Mesothelioma		9
Leiomyosarcoma/rhabdomyosarcoma		6
Hemangiopericytoma		4
Other		3
Hepatoma	19	
Adrenocortical carcinoma	10	
Lymphoma	6	
Neuroectodermal tumors	2	
Gastric carcinoma	2	
Colon carcinoma	1	
Other*	14	

*Cholangiocarcinoma, teratomas, pseudomyxoma, Wilms' tumor, lung carcinoma, melanoma.

Source: From references 315 and 318–320.

fibrosarcomas, mesotheliomas, leiomyosarcomas, rhabdomyosarcomas, and hemangiopericytomas, as well as a variety of other histologic types (Table 28-17).[315,318–320] Approximately 10 percent are benign tumors or of very low grade malignancy.[315,318] Many of these tumors have a spindle cell morphology.[315] They tend to be large neoplasms, ranging from 310 g to 20 kg.[316,319] A third of these tumors are located within the thorax, one-half in the retroperitoneal area, 11 percent intra-abdominally, and approximately 6 percent in unique sites.[321] The sex distribution is equal.[315]

Hepatocellular carcinoma is the second most common tumor associated with hypoglycemia. Approximately 1–2 percent of hepatocellular carcinomas are associated with hypoglycemia, although the incidence is as high as 26 percent in hepatocellular carcinomas in Asian patients.[322–325] Males are affected approximately four times more frequently than are females. McFadzean and Yueng divided these patients into two groups.[325] The first group consisted of 87 percent of the patients, who had rapidly growing, poorly differentiated hepatomas with marked replacement of the liver parenchyma. These patients experienced muscle weakness and wasting, and hypoglycemia was found in the terminal or preterminal state and could easily be controlled with glucose infusions. In contrast, the second group, composed of 13 percent of the patients, had slow-growing, well-differentiated neoplasms without evidence of substantial cachexia or muscle weakness when the hypoglycemia appeared. In this group, death occurred 2–10 months after the onset of hypoglycemia, whereas in the other group, death generally occurred within 2 weeks.[325]

Adrenocortical carcinoma accounts for approximately 10 percent of patients with tumor-associated hypoglycemia. The tumors generally are highly malignant and are associated with metastases at the time of diagnosis. Both sexes are affected equally, and survival is generally <6 months from diagnosis. The tumors may be otherwise functional or nonfunctional; when they are functional, about half are associated with Cushing's syndrome and half with virilization.[315]

Pathophysiology

Abnormalities of glucose metabolism have been noted in patients with malignancy-associated hypoglycemia. Tumor cells exhibit a high rate of glycolysis, and it was proposed that large mesenchymally derived tumors weighing multiple kilograms may consume enough glucose to overwhelm the body's conterregulatory mechanisms.[315,326] However, calculations based on an arterial-venous glucose difference across a tumor and in vitro glucose uptake studies suggest that even tumors in the range of 1.4–6.0 kg consume less than 400 g of glucose per day, while the liver is capable of producing more than 800 g of glucose per day.[326,327] Thus, overutilization of glucose by the tumor is insufficient to account for the hypoglycemia. These patients also exhibit an increase in glucose utilization by peripheral tissues, as shown by the large amount of glucose that must be infused to keep the blood glucose within the normal range.[326] Of interest in this regard, Stuart and coworkers demonstrated insulin receptor proliferation in the liver and muscle of a patient with a hypoglycemia-producing colon carcinoma that metastasized to the liver.[327] The threefold to fivefold increase in insulin receptors associated with elevations of IGF-II, which can act through insulin receptors, may account for the high total body glucose utilization.

In addition to overutilization of glucose by tumor and peripheral tissues, there is evidence of deficient hepatic glucose production in these patients.[318,326,328–330] With the exception of patients with slow-growing hepatomas that extensively replace the normal liver parenchyma, most patients with tumor-associated hypoglycemia do not exhibit sufficient destruction of the normal liver to account for the deficient hepatic glucose production, as experimental studies have shown that more than 75 percent of the liver must be destroyed before hypoglycemia ensues.[331] A problem in glycogenolysis is present, as histologic studies have shown that glycogen is present in the livers of these patients and the administration of glucagon and epinephrine to some patients results in an increase in hepatic glucose output.[331,332] Also, there is an inadequate amount of gluconeogenesis, as reflected in increased blood lactate levels and possible reductions in gluconeogenic amino acids.[318,326,333] Part of the reduction in hepatic glucose production may reflect an absent or sluggish response to the hypoglycemia of the insulin counterregulatory hormones. Indeed, growth hormone, ACTH, cortisol, and glucagon may be inappropriately low considering the level of the blood sugar in these patients, a response that may be due to a slow decrease in blood sugar which does not activate the sympathetic nervous system and stress-induced release of the counterregulatory hormones.[331] Also, the low levels of growth hormone noted in the basal state in these patients as well as after arginine infusion may reflect suppression of growth hormone secretion directly by IGF-II.[330,333–335]

Several different humoral factors secreted by these tumors have been implicated in the pathogenesis of the disorder. In 1962, after the development of the insulin immunoassay, Olefesky and associates reported elevated serum insulin levels in a patient with a fibrosarcoma.[336] During the next two decades, >100 patients were described as having elevated concentrations of bioactive or immunoactive insulin or insulin-like activity in blood or tumor tissue. An in-depth analysis of the data by Skrabanek and Powell suggested that insulin production by non-islet-cell tumors is rarely, if ever, responsible for the hypoglycemia.[316] Occasional carcinoid tumors that resemble islet cell tumors have been associated with excessive insulin secretion.[337] More recently, a neuroectodermal pelvic tumor was shown to contain insulin, proinsulin, and secretory granules and to be responsible for elevated insulin levels and hypoglycemia in a patient.[338] Nevertheless, ectopic insulin production is exceedingly rare, and in most series immunoreactive insulin levels are low and insulin mRNA is absent from tumor tissue.[335] Although there have been occasional suggestions that tumors may release a pancreatic beta-cytotropic substance that stimulates insulin secretion, no such substance has been identified in these tumors, and pancreatic hyperplasia has not been found at autopsy.[315,316,339]

Before the development of insulin RIAs, insulin biological activity was divided into that which could be suppressed with insulin antibodies, which represented the true insulin activity, and that which could not be suppressed by these antibodies, designated nonsuppressible insulin-like activity (NSILA). Subsequently, NSILA was fractionated by acid-ethanol, which separated the activity into high-molecular-weight proteins, NSILA-p or NSILAP, and a soluble fraction containing low-molecular-weight proteins, NSILA-s.[331,340] NSILA-s was found to consist of several peptides, including IGF-I and IGF-II, with molecular masses of approximately 7,650 and 7,500 dalton, respectively.[331] In 1974, Megyesi and coworkers used a radioreceptor assay for NSILA-s that was primarily responsive to IGF-II and noted that three of seven patients with non-islet cell tumors associated with hypoglycemia had elevated serum concentrations of IGF-II.[341] Further studies by this group indicated that nearly 40 percent of patients with the syndrome had elevated serum IGF-II-like activity.[322,331] Daughaday and coworkers, using a different radioreceptor assay, found that more than 90 percent of patients had elevated IGF-II concentrations in their serum.[84] However, Zapf and colleagues were unable to demonstrate elevated IGF-II concentrations using a different radioreceptor assay or an RIA.[320,342] These discrepancies were partially explained by Merimee, who noted elevated serum IGF-II concentrations in two patients with non-islet-cell tumors as measured by a radioreceptor assay; however, 2–4 months later, when the sera were remeasured in the same assay, the activity was lost, indicating that the IGF-II molecule produced by these tumors was unstable during storage.[334]

Chromatography of serum and tumor extracts from these patients has revealed that 60 percent exhibit an increased proportion of a high-molecular-weight precursor of IGF-II compared to that in normal serum, and in some patients virtually all the IGF-II is in the "big" 10- to 15-kDa fraction.[333,343,344] Finally, several investigators have shown that tumors contain IGF-II mRNA.[333,335,343,344] Although it has been suggested that NSILP may be responsible for the hypoglycemia found in some patients, levels of this protein have been inconsistently elevated and have been noted to increase in some patients after the removal of hypoglycemia-producing tumors at a time when the blood sugar levels have returned to normal.[340,343]

From the available data, it would appear that the pathogenesis of non-islet-cell-tumor-associated hypoglycemia is multifactorial. These tumors produce an increased quantity of a high-molecular-weight form of IGF-II, probably as a result of incomplete processing of the protein.[333,344] This 10- to 15-kDa IGF-II binds poorly to the circulating IGF-binding proteins.[344,345] In contrast, approximately 99 percent of normal 7.5-kDa IGF-II binds avidly to IGF-binding proteins, forming a 140-150 kD ternary complex consisting of IGF-II, IGF-Binding Protein-3 and an acid-labile complexing component.[344,346,347] This complex does not cross the capillary membrane easily. With less protein binding, the high-molecular-weight IGF-II traverses the capillaries readily and is free to interact with IGF receptors or insulin receptors present throughout the body, leading to an increase in glucose uptake by both the tumor and peripheral tissues. In contrast to proACTH (POMC), the high-molecular-weight form of IGF-II retains receptor-binding activity.[343] The elevated IGF-II probably inhibits pituitary growth hormone secretion in a manner analogous to the inhibition observed with IGF-I and insulin that is mediated through IGF-I receptors.[348] This would account for the observed reduction in serum growth hormone levels during periods of hypoglycemia or after arginine infusion and would also account for the lowered concentrations of IGF-I in patients with this syndrome.[349] The decreased growth hormone also lowers some of the species of IGF-binding proteins, and this would further account for an increase in free IGF-II in the circulation. Finally, the elevated IGF-II concentrations may lead to an inhibition of the release of gluconeogenic amino acids from muscle tissue, accounting for some of the decrease in hepatic glucose output observed with this syndrome.[333]

Clinical Manifestations and Diagnosis

In general, hypoglycemic symptoms may be divided into the sympathomimetic types of symptoms, such as tachycardia, diaphoresis, piloerection, and tremulousness, which reflect a relatively rapid rate of fall of blood sugar, and the CNS symptoms, which reflect the actual level of blood sugar. In patients with non-islet cell-tumor hypoglycemia, the neuroglucopenic symptoms predominate because the rate of fall of blood sugar is generally slow.[84,315,318,331] Thus, episodes of behavioral abnormalities, obtundation, seizures, or coma, especially in the early morning or after fasting, are commonly observed. The symptoms are usually insidious and may be intermittently present for weeks, months, or years before the diagnosis of the underlying neoplasm.

Other symptoms are related to the location and size of the neoplasm. Mesenchymal tumors are usually located in the retroperitoneal, intra-abdominal, or thoracic regions and are associated with pain, abdominal fullness, cough, dyspnea, or peripheral neurologic symptoms. When they are located within the abdomen or retroperitoneal space, a mass is often palpable. Hepatomegaly, jaundice, fever, abdominal pain, and nonspecific symptoms including malaise, weakness, anorexia, and weight loss are commonly seen in patients with hepatocellular carcinoma. The other large group of non-islet-cell tumors associated with hypoglycemia—adrenocortical carcinomas—may have associated clinical findings of excessive glucocorticoids, mineralocorticoids, or adrenal androgens.

The diagnosis of this syndrome requires the demonstration of fasting hypoglycemia with suppressed serum insulin concentrations in association with the presence of a non-islet-cell neoplasm. It is important to keep in mind that during a 72-h fast, normal men generally maintain a plasma glucose above 55 mg/dl, while normal women may have plasma glucose levels of 30 mg/dl or less.[350] The other causes of fasting hypoglycemia with suppressed insulin levels must be ruled out. These include fulminant liver failure, chronic renal failure, severe malnutrition, adrenal insufficiency, alcohol use, and the ingestion of drugs that interfere with gluconeogenesis. Measurements of IGF-II may be helpful if the levels are elevated but are not useful in the differential diagnosis if they are normal, since some patients with this syndrome have normal total levels of IGF-II with an elevated proportion of high-molecular-weight IGF-II, which binds poorly to the IGF-binding proteins.

Therapy

The only therapy that is uniformly effective in this syndrome is that directed at the primary tumor. Surgical extirpation, radiation therapy, or chemotherapy may be effective in reducing the tumor bulk to the extent that the hypoglycemia disappears. If such therapy is ineffective, frequent carbohydrate feedings and the administration of glucocorticoids, growth hormone, or glucagon may ameliorate the symptoms. Diazoxide, phenytoin, and somatostatin are rarely effective.[330,331,351]

The prognosis depends to a great extent on the underlying disease. In a review of mesenchymal tumors associated with hypoglycemia, Anderson and Lokich noted that approximately 20 percent of the tumors are inoperable and that those which are operable generally recur locally rather than with distant metastases.[321] Most recurrences occur within 2 years of the primary surgery. A little more than a third of patients with resected thoracic tumors exhibit a recurrence, while close to two-thirds of abdominal lesions recur locally after the initial surgery. Approximately 25 percent of patients with thoracic tumors die of the disease, while almost half with abdominal tumors die as a direct result of the neoplasm. The prognosis for patients with primary hepatocellular carcinomas and malignant adrenocortical carcinomas associated with hypoglycemia is poor, with the majority of patients succumbing within 1 year of diagnosis.

Oncogenic Osteomalacia

In 1947, McCance described a teenage female with an osteoid tumor of the femur associated with osteomalacia that improved after removal of the tumor.[352] However, it was Prader and coworkers who suggested a cause-and-effect relation while describing an 11-year-old girl with osteomalacia associated with a giant cell reparative granuloma of a rib.[353] The osteomalacia improved after removal of the granuloma.[353] Subsequently, approximately 85 cases of oncogenic osteomalacia have been reported in the literature.[354]

Incidence and Tumor Types

Oncogenic osteomalacia appears to be rare, although it is likely that the association is underreported because these tumors are often small, usually measuring 1–4 cm in diameter, and are often located in unusual areas.[354] Because these tumors may be quite indolent, it is likely that many patients with mild "idiopathic hypophosphatemic osteomalacia" may actually have this syndrome. Indeed, this syndrome may occur relatively frequently with tumors such as prostatic carcinoma. Lyles and associates studied in detail two hypophosphatemic patients with prostatic carcinoma who had the typical clinical and biochemical findings of oncogenic osteomalacia.[355] They noted that 21 percent of the patients they studied with prostatic carcinoma had hypophosphatemia, raising the possibility that they also suffered from a milder form of oncogenic osteomalacia.[355]

The vast majority of tumors associated with this syndrome are mesenchymal-derived neoplasms that contain multinucleated giant cells, extensive vascularity, fibrous tissue, and often osteoid formation. The spectrum of tumors includes giant cell granulomas and tumors, hemangiomas, fibromas, hemangiopericytomas, fibroangiomas, osteoblastomas, chondromas or chondroblastomas, and fibrous xanthanomas.[356,357] Weidner and Santa Cruz classified the majority of these tumors into four groups: mixed connective tissue tumors in soft tissue with prominent vascularity and osteoclast-like giant cells, osteoblastoma-like tumors in the bone, nonossifying fibroma-like tumors in the bone, and ossifying fibroma-like tumors in the bone.[358] Most but not all tumors fit this classification. Tumors such as prostatic carcinoma are of endodermal origin, and oat cell carcinoma, which has also been associated with this syndrome, is of neuroectodermal origin.[359] Other tumors associated with this syndrome include sarcoma, multiple myeloma, fibrous malignant histocytoma, neurofibromatosis, and neurinomas.[360–363] Electron microscopic studies of these tumors have not shown the presence of secretory granules.[354,362]

Approximately 10 percent of these tumors are malignant, and 5 percent are multiple.[356] Fifty-five percent are located in bone, approximately half of which are found in the long bones, including the femur and tibia.[354,364] Another common site of involvement is the head, with lesions being noted in the mandible, maxilla, skull, and ethmoid regions. Approximately 45 percent of these tumors are found in soft tissues including skin, with two-thirds of the soft tissue tumors being located in the legs.[354] The nasopharyngeal region is another site of soft tissue involvement.

Clinical Features and Biochemical Abnormalities

More than 90 percent of patients present with generalized bone pain, especially involving the weight-bearing bones of the legs, ankles, hips, and lower back. Profound muscle weakness is present in two-thirds, with approximately 40 percent exhibiting abnormal gait or being bedridden. Fatigue, myalgias, and multiple fractures are also common complaints.[354,356,357,364] The average age at onset is 33 years and at the time of diagnosis is 38 years, with a range of 7–73 years, and symptoms are present for an average of 5 years, with a range of 3 months–17 years.[356,357,364,365] Males and females are affected equally.

Hypophosphatemia is uniformly present, with a mean phosphate level of approximately 1.5 mg/dl.[354,356,357] Serum calcium concentrations are generally normal, and alkaline phosphatase levels are elevated. Virtually all patients have a marked decrease in the renal tubular reabsorption of phosphate with phosphaturia. Calcium and phosphorus balance studies have also demonstrated a decrease in GI tract absorption of both minerals.[366] Parathyroid hormone and calcitonin levels are normal,[356,367] as are serum 25(OH)-vitamin D and 24,25(OH)$_2$ vitamin D levels.[356] 1,25(OH)$_2$-vitamin D levels are undetectable or low (mean level of 13.4 pg/ml with the normal range of 19–50 pg/ml) in more than 80 percent of the patients in whom this metabolite has been measured.[354,356,365,366] One-third of patients have aminoaciduria, and nearly half have glycosuria.[356,357,366,368]

Pathophysiology

These patients exhibit an acquired Fanconi-like proximal renal tubular reabsorption dysfunction manifested by phosphaturia, glycosuria, and aminoaciduria. In addition, they have a defect in the conversion of 25(OH)-vitamin D levels to 1,25(OH)$_2$-vitamin D in the proximal tubules, suggesting an inhibition of 25(OH)-vitamin D-1α-hydroxylase enzyme.

The etiology of the proximal tubular defect in these patients is unknown but is clearly humoral in nature and is associated with an underlying neoplasm. The evidence includes the association of the syndrome with the neoplasms, most of which are very similar pathologically; the disappearance of the syndrome after removal of the tumor; and the recurrence of the syndrome with recurrence of the neoplasm. The most convincing data come from experimental studies with tumor extracts and heterotransplantation. Saline extracts of tumors have been shown to induce phosphaturia and decrease tubular reabsorption of phosphate in puppies, rats, and mice.[369–373] Tumors propagated in nude mice have resulted in hypophosphatemia, hyperphosphaturia, and a defect in the conversion of 25(OH)-vitamin D to 1,25(OH)-vitamin D.[374–376] Cell culture medium from two tumors associated with the syndrome inhibited sodium-dependent phosphate transport in cultured renal cells without stimulating cAMP.[377,378] The factor, termed phosphatonin, is heat labile and lipid insoluble with a mass between 8 and 25 kD.[32,33] One study showed that the activity was destroyed by trypsin.[379] Fukumoto and coworkers pointed out the similarity between this syndrome and the features of maleic acid-induced proximal tubular dysfunction but were unable to demonstrate the presence of maleic acid in the serum or urine of the patient they studied.[368] The syndrome shares many similarities with x-linked hypophosphatemic rickets, which may also represent overproduction of phosphatonin.[32,33,378,379]

The clinical features clearly reflect the profound hypophosphatemia and reduced $1,25(OH)_2$-vitamin D levels. Bone biopsies demonstrate osteomalacia with increased osteoclastic bone resorption, which probably accounts for the maintenance of the normal serum calcium and normal parathyroid hormone level.[380] The decrease or inhibition of the 25(OH)-vitamin D-1α-hydroxylase enzyme is all the more striking considering the profound degree of hypophosphatemia, which should be a potent stimulus for the conversion of 25(OH)-vitamin D to $1,25(OH)_2$-vitamin D.

Differential Diagnosis

A number of conditions that result in osteomalacia and hypophosphatemia must be considered. These include nutritional deficiency in elderly house-bound individuals, adult-onset hypophosphatasia, intestinal malabsorption, renal tubular acidosis, vitamin D-resistant rickets, chronic renal failure, phosphate-binding antacids, familial or acquired defects of renal tubular phosphate transport seen with X-linked hypophosphatemic rickets, Fanconi's syndrome, heavy metal poisoning, and cystinosis.[354,356,358]

These conditions can usually be eliminated from consideration through a careful family history, occupational and drug history, consideration of the age at onset, and performance of tests for urinary phosphoethanolamine and serum alkaline phosphatase to rule out adult-onset hypophosphatasia; fecal fat and D-xylose excretion for the evaluation of steatorrhea; ability of the urine to be acidified after ammonium chloride administration; and a screen for heavy metal poisoning by cadmium, lead, or copper.[366,381]

Therapy

More than 80 percent of patients are cured with removal of the tumor.[354] If one considers only symptomatic patients, more than 90 percent have a complete disappearance of symptoms between 1 day and 1 year after total removal of the tumor. Within 1–2 days, the serum phosphate usually increases, the tubular reabsorption of phosphate returns to normal, and the phosphaturia ceases.[357] If the tumor recurs, the syndrome generally also recurs.[354]

Massive doses of vitamin D, 1-α-(OH)-D_3, and dihydrotachysterol have rarely been effective. Similarly, the administration of phosphate (2 gm/day) alone has not induced symptomatic remissions, although 15–30 percent of patients show some degree of improvement with the combination of phosphate and vitamin D administration.[354,356] The most effective medical therapy is supplementation with $1,25(OH)_2$-vitamin D (2–4 μg), which has led to improvement in up to 70 percent of the patients in whom it has been tried.[354,356] However, $1,25(OH)_2$-vitamin D alone rarely completely corrects the syndrome. The prognosis for these patients is excellent, reflecting the generally benign nature of the majority of the underlying neoplasms.

Ectopic Growth Hormone and Growth Hormone Releasing Hormone Production

Ectopic Growth Hormone Production

In 1968, Steiner and associates described a patient with hypertrophic osteoarthropathy, adenocarcinoma of the lung, and elevated serum levels of growth hormone, which reverted to normal after removal of the tumor.[382] The following year, Cameron and coworkers described a similar patient with normal serum concentrations of growth hormone (GH) but elevated concentrations in the lung tumor in comparison to the surrounding normal lung tissue.[383] Subsequently, Greenberg and coworkers demonstrated the synthesis and release of GH from a poorly differentiated lung carcinoma associated with hypertrophic osteoarthropathy maintained in tissue culture for 4 months.[384] The tumor incorporated [^{14}C]leucine into growth hormone that comigrated with monomeric pituitary GH on both paper and Sephadex chromatography.

Immunoreactive GH has been found in 39 percent of bronchogenic carcinomas, including adenocarcinoma, large cell carcinomas, and small cell carcinoma, although no arterial-venous difference in GH concentrations across the tumors were found.[385] Close to two-thirds of gastric carcinomas have also been found to contain immunoreactive GH,[385] and all 12 breast carcinomas studied through immunohistochemistry by Ghosh and colleagues showed the presence of growth hormone-containing tumor cells.[386] The significance of these findings is open to question in view of the presence of both immunoreactive GH and receptor-assayable GH-like material that is present in a number of normal tissues including the liver, kidney, lung, muscle, colon, stomach, and brain.[17] In addition, the possibility that proteolytic enzymes present in tissues may degrade the radiolabeled GH used in the RIAs must be kept in mind. This possibility was illustrated by Caplan and associates, who described a young woman with acromegaly associated with a cystic beta cell adenoma of the pancreas.[387] The tumor tissue extract contained immunoreactive GH, which comigrated with GH extracted from normal human pituitary, and serial dilutions of the tumor extract also demonstrated parallelism to the reference GH. However, further investigation showed that the GH activity was spurious and was due to proteolytic enzyme damage of the tracer used in the RIA. The acromegaly in that patient was subsequently shown to be due to the secretion of growth hormone releasing hormone (GHRH) rather than GH.[388]

The clinical significance of the presence of GH in tumors is unclear. Many patients with lung cancer, carcinoids, and endometrial carcinoma either fail to suppress serum GH after a glucose load or show a paradoxic increase.[389–391] For a time, GH was considered a prime candidate for the humoral mediator of hypertrophic pulmonary osteoarthropathy. However, growth hormone is not uniformly elevated in patients with osteoarthropathy.[382,390] Full-blown acromegaly would be anticipated to be the consequence of the ectopic secretion of growth hormone. However, to date, only the patient described by Melmed and colleagues with acromegaly and an intramesenteric pancreatic islet cell tumor fulfills the criteria for ectopic growth hormone production, attesting to its varity.[40,41] Also, some of the abnormalities in GH secretion in patients with tumors may be due to the secretion of GHRH, somatostatin, or other substances.

Ectopic Production of Growth Hormone Releasing Hormone

In 1959, Altmann and Schutz described a patient who had acromegaly that did not respond to pituitary radiotherapy but remitted after the removal of a pulmonary carcinoid tumor.[392] In 1976, Sonksen and coworkers reported a patient with acromegaly whose hormonal abnormalities remitted after the removal of a bronchial carcinoid tumor that did not contain immunoreactive GH.[393] Subsequently, Shalet and colleagues described a similar patient and showed that the tumor cells grown in culture released a substance that stimulated GH secretion from rat pituitary cells.[394] Partial purification and characterization of GHRH was described by Frohman and associates in 1980, and in 1982 both Rivier and coworkers and Guillemin and colleagues independently isolated and clinically characterized GHRH from patients with GHRH-secreting pancreatic islet cell tumors associated with acromegaly.[388,395–397]

Tumor Types

To date, there have been 41 well-described patients with ectopic GHRH production associated with clinical acromegaly (Table 28-18).[398–402] Most of these patients harbor a carcinoid, especially a bronchial carcinoid, or a pancreatic islet cell tumor. Elevations of plasma GHRH without acromegaly or marked elevations of growth hormone have been found in 15 of 44 (34 percent) patients with small cell carcinoma of the lung, 2 of 28 (7 percent) patients with non-small cell lung carcinoma and 1 of 10 (10 percent) patients, with nonmalignant lung disease.[403] The absence of acromegaly in these patients probably reflects the relatively low concentration of GHRH in their sera.

Immunoreactive GHRH is present in a large proportion of carcinoids, islet cell tumors, small cell carcinomas of the lung, pheochromocytomas, endometrial carcinomas, and medullary carcinomas of the thyroid tumor tissue extracts.[399,400–402] GHRH has been localized immunohistochemically in islet cell tumors; carcinoid tumors of the lung, thymus, appendix, and cecum; medullary carcinoma of the thyroid; small cell carcinoma of the lung; and pheochromocytoma.[404–407]

Many of these tumors contain other hormones as assessed by immunohistochemical means. Thus, somatostatin, gastrin, gastrin-releasing peptide, calcitonin, insulin, glucagon, vasoactive intestinal peptide, pancreatic polypeptide, and ACTH have been described in association with GHRH-secreting tumors.[399,400]

There is molecular heterogeneity of the GHRH produced by tumors. The predominant forms are GHRH (1-40)OH and GHRH (1-44)NH_2, with lesser amounts of GHRH (1-37)OH.[399,400] Additionally, a single patient was found to have the biologically inactive GHRH (3-40)OH in his serum.[399] These findings suggest that variable posttranslation proteolysis occurs to modify the forms of GHRH produced by the tumors.

Clinical Features

Patients with GHRH-secreting tumors associated with acromegaly present at an average age of approximately 40 years with typical acromegalic features. The diagnosis is made approximately 6 years after the onset of the disease and is somewhat shorter in patients with pancreatic islet cell tumors and longer in patients with pulmonary carcinoid neoplasms. There is a female predominance, with a female to male ratio of 2.7:1. In addition to the acromegalic features, other endocrine abnormalities may coexist. These include the Zollinger-Ellison syndrome, insulin-induced hypoglycemia, galactorrhea, and hyperparathyroidism with pancreatic islet cell tumors; galactorrhea, Cushing's syndrome, and carcinoid syndrome with carcinoid tumors; and catecholamine excess with pheochromocytomas.[400] GHRH-secreting tumors may also be present as part of the multiple endocrine neoplasia 1 (MEN 1) syndrome. Symptoms from the mass effects of the underlying neoplasm also may be present and are especially apparent with the bronchial carcinoids, which may produce cough, hemoptysis, atelectasis, and recurrent pneumonias that follow obstructive pulmonary infections. Slightly more than one-third of these tumors are malignant, although most are slow-growing.

Diagnosis

The diagnosis of GHRH-secreting tumors is often made serendipitously after an attempt at neurosurgical removal of a

TABLE 28-18. Tumors Associated with Ectopic GHRH Production

		Immunochemical Studies			
	Clinical Acromegaly	*Immunohistochemical Presence of GHRH in Tumor*		*Immunoreactive GHRH in Tumors*	
Tumor Type	Total (Malignant)	*N*	Positive, Percent	*N*	Positive, Percent
Carcinoid	27 (13)	92	17	15	87
Bronchial	21 (8)	10	10		10
Intestinal	3 (2)	82	18		18
Other	3 (3)				
Pancreatic islet-cell	9 (3)	81	17	49	37
Small cell carcinoma of lung	2 (2)			13	69
Sympathetic neural tumors	2 (0)	13	15	38	53
Adrenal adenoma	1 (0)	—	—	—	—
Medullary carcinoma of thyroid		—	—	8	50

Source: From references 398–402.

suspected growth hormone-secreting pituitary adenoma, at which time somatotrope hyperplasia is found rather than a pituitary adenoma (with one exception in a patient with MEN).[408,409] Because somatotrope hyperplasia and the excessive secretion of GH from the hyperplastic somatotropes are direct results of excessive GHRH stimulation, a search for a source of GHRH may then uncover the neoplasm. In addition to peripheral sources of ectopic GHRH secretion, the possibility that the GHRH excess is due to eutopic secretion from a hypothalamic hamartoma, choristoma, glioma, or gangliocytoma must be considered.[410]

The standard diagnostic tests for acromegaly do not differentiate GH-secreting pituitary adenomas from GHRH-secreting tumors. In both conditions, the sella turcica may be enlarged and there may appear to be an intrasellar tumor. Similarly, with both conditions, GH does not suppress appropriately after the administration of glucose, immunoreactive GH in the serum may rise after a bolus injection of thyrotropin releasing hormone (TRH) of insulin-induced hypoglycemia, and either no response or a rise in serum GH may occur after the administration of exogenous GHRH.[400-402,410] A higher percentage of patients with ectopic acromegaly have elevated prolactin levels than in acromegalic patients with pituitary adenomas (71 vs. 29 percent, $p < 0.01$).[402] The only test that clearly differentiates the two conditions is measurement of peripheral levels of GHRH. Normal individuals generally have GHRH levels of 10 pg/ml or less, while patients with GHRH-secreting tumors have levels that range between 300 pg/ml and 50 ng/ml.[400]

Therapy

The most effective therapy for these patients is removal of the neoplasm. When this is accomplished, the acromegaly in virtually all patients remits and the GH secretory dynamics return to normal. Even after partial debulking of tumors in the presence of metastatic disease, there may be improvement in the acromegaly.[400] In patients with persistent disease, the somatostatin analog octreotide has led to clinical and biochemical improvement in the acromegaly as well as reduction in GH and GHRH levels, indicating that the drug has a peripheral effect on the tumor as well as its known effect on the pituitary somatotropes.[401,410] Dopamine agonists are not useful. The long-term prognosis of these patients is unclear, although only approximately 10–15 percent have died directly from the disease.[400]

Ectopic Production of Placental Proteins

Human Chorionic Gonadotropin

Human chorionic gonadotropin is a eutopic product of gestational and nongestational trophoblastic disease. Before the development of the β-hCG RIA, several case reports described patients with the ectopic production of hCG. The associated tumors were bronchogenic carcinoma, hepatoma or hepatoblastoma, adrenocortical carcinoma, melanoma, undifferentiated retroperitoneal carcinoma, breast carcinoma, and renal cell carcinoma.[411] Two clinical syndromes were present in most of the patients reported. Adult males exhibited gynecomastia and occasionally other signs of feminization, and isosexual precocious puberty was present in young boys with hCG-secreting hepatoblastomas.[411,412] After the development of sensitive and specific hCG RIAs, immunoreactive hCG was found to be present in approximately 18 percent of patients with a wide variety of nontrophoblastic neoplasms (Table 28-9).[114] Most of these patients do not have clinical symptoms attributable to the hCG primarily because the quantities of hCG are quite low in all but a fraction of them. Also, the majority of the hCG assays used in these studies measure both intact hCG and its biologically inactive β-subunit. Recent studies with specific assays have shown that it is the free hCGβ-subunit that is present in the circulation of patients with hCG-secreting nontrophoblastic neoplasms.[413] Because an hCG-like substance is present in the blood of normal individuals and patients with a variety of benign diseases (Table 28-10), hCG measurements are not useful as a screening test for nontrophoblastic neoplasms. In addition, the presence or absence of hCG and the quantitative levels generally show poor correlation with the stage of disease, may not show concordant changes with disease progression or regression, and have little or no prognostic value.[114] Recently, there has been interest in the measurement of a fragment of the β subunit of hCG, the β-core fragment, which is present in the urine of one-half to three-quarters of patients with cancer and 6 percent of nonpregnant healthy individuals.[414]

Human Placental Lactogen

Human placental lactogen (hPL), which, like hCG, is normally secreted by the syncytiotrophoblast of the placenta during pregnancy, is also found in patients with gestational and nongestational trophoblastic disease. However, unlike hCG, serial measurements of hPL in those conditions are not useful for monitoring the effects of therapy because the concentrations of this hormone are generally low. hPL has also been noted to be produced ectopically by nontrophoblastic neoplasms, especially those of gynecologic or GI tract origin (Table 28-19).[114] Although overall approximately 14 percent of patients with cancers may have small quantities of immunoreactive hPL in their sera, close to half the tumor specimens that have been examined immunohistochemically for the presence

TABLE 28-19. Immunoreactive hPL in Sera of Patients with Cancer and Control Patients

Tumor or Site	N		Positive, Percent	
Patients with cancer				
Gynecologic	344		30.8	
Ovary		219		38.4
Cervix		125		17.6
Gastrointestinal	274		13.5	
Esophagus		16		0
Gastric		46		26.1
Colon/rectum		174		9.2
Hepatic		24		29.2
Biliary		13		15.4
Leukemia	13		7.7	
Lung	64		4.7	
Prostate	57		0	
Miscellaneous	60		15	
Total	812		14.3	
Controls	**N**		**Positive, Percent**	
Normal volunteers	455		0	
Benign disease	180		0	
Breast		57		0
Gastrointestinal		54		0
Genitourinary		19		0
Other		50		0
Total	630		0	

Source: From Braunstein,[114] with permission.

TABLE 28-20. Paraneoplastic Erythrocytosis Associated with Neoplasms and Other Pathologic Conditions in 340 Patients

Site of Pathology	Percent of Total	
Kidney	52.6	
Hypernephroma		35.3
Cystic kidney		10.3
Hydronephrosis		4.1
Wilms' tumor		0.9
Hemangioma		0.9
Adenoma		0.6
Sarcoma		0.6
Liver (primarily hepatoma)	18.8	
Central nervous system (cerebellar hemangioblastoma)	14.7	
Uterus (fibromyoma)	7.4	
Adrenal (adrenocortical adenoma, carcinoma; pheochromocytoma)	3.2	
Ovary	2.1	
Lung	0.9	
Thymus	0.3	

Source: From Hammond and Winnick,[422] with permission. Also noted with leiomyoma of esophagus and skin,[423] fibrous histiocytoma of parotid,[424] hepatic hemangioma,[425] and breast cancer.[426]

of hPL have been found to contain cells that stain positively for this hormone.[415–418] However, hPL has also been detected by immunohistochemical techniques in approximately 13 percent of benign breast disease, and the specificity of hPL as a tumor marker thus is questionable.[417,418] As with hCG, hPL measurements do not consistently correlate with disease stage or changes in tumor mass or provide prognostic information.[27,419–421]

Paraneoplastic Erythrocytosis

Polycythemia is associated with benign and malignant lesions of the kidney as well as neoplasms of the liver, cerebellum, uterus, and adrenal (Table 28-20).[422–426] In the majority of the patients studied with erythrocytosis, elevations of the serum or tissue levels of erythropoietin have been noted (Table 28-21).[422,427–432] Approximately 3–4 percent of patients with hypernephroma, 3–12 percent of patients with hepatocellular carcinoma, and 9–20 percent of patients with cerebellar hemangioblastoma exhibit erythrocytosis.[51,423,433,434] Serum erythropoietin levels are increased in up to one-third of patients wih renal cell carcinoma and 23 percent of individuals with hepatocellular carcinoma, although the majority of patients in these studies did not have erythrocytosis.[435,436] This discrepancy may relate to the conteracting effects of the inhibition of erythrocytosis by malignancy or to the secretion of a biologically inactive form of erythropoietin. Alternatively, the anemia that often accompanies malignancy may result in tissue hypoxia that serves as a potent stimulus for physiologic erythropoietin production.[437]

Because erythropoietin is normally produced by the kidney and liver, the production of excessive quantities of this hormone in benign and malignant renal and hepatic disorders probably represents eutopic production. Most of the data concerning erythropoietin production by tumors have come from studies of renal cell carcinoma. Several investigators have demonstrated the secretion of erythropoietin by tumor cells in vitro[438–440] as well as the presence of erythropoietin mRNA by in situ hybridization in several hypernephromas with an absence of the mRNA in adjacent normal kidney cells.[432] The erythropoietin from a cerebellar cyst was physiochemically similar to erythropoietin derived from anemic patients.[441] In addition to the eutopic or ectopic production of erythropoietin, other mechanisms may be responsible for erythrocytosis. Thus, virilizing ovarian or adrenal tumors that secrete androgens may lead to the stimulation of erythropoiesis. Glucocorticoid-producing adrenal tumors may result in "stress polycythemia," and excessive production of prostaglandin A or E may stimulate erythropoiesis through enhancement of erythropoietin action on the erythrocyte progenitor cells in the marrow.[422]

The diagnosis of polycythemia is generally made fortuitously when a serum hematocrit is found to be elevated above 55 percent in a male and 50 percent in a female, reflecting the increase in total red cell mass. In most instances, the erythrocytosis is asymptomatic, although venous thrombosis may occur as an unusual complication.[429] Paraneoplastic erythrocytosis may be differentiated from dehydration with hemoconcentration and stress polycythemia through the absence of clinical findings of dehydration and the presence of an increase in the total red cell mass, which is elevated in paraneoplastic erythrocytosis but normal in stress polycythemia. Measurements of the partial pressure of oxygen in arterial blood and hemoglobin electrophoresis allow differentiation from secondary polycythemia due to hypoxia or the presence of a hemoglobinopathy. Erythrocytosis is a prominent feature of

TABLE 28-21. Proportion of Patients with Paraneoplastic Erythrocytosis Who Exhibit Elevations of Serum and Tissue Erythropoietin Concentrations

	Increased Serum Erythropoietin		*Increased Tissue Erythropoietin*	
Condition	*N* Total	*N* Elevated (Percent)	*N* Total	*N* Elevated (Percent)
Cystic kidney	11	5 (45)	12	10 (83)
Hypernephroma	10	9 (90)	13	11 (85)
Hepatoma	9	6 (67)	8	2 (25)
Cerebellar hemangioblastoma	10	6 (60)	6	6 (100)
Uterine fibromyoma	6	0 (0)	6	2 (33)
Hydronephrosis	5	4 (80)	2	0 (0)
Pheochromocytoma	2	2	1	1
Wilms' tumor	2	2	2	2

Source: From references 422 and 427–432.

polycythemia vera, but these patients also exhibit pancytosis with elevations of the white cell and platelet counts as well as splenomegaly. Elevated serum erythropoietin concentrations are found in patients with paraneoplastic erythrocytosis as well as other secondary causes of polycythemia, while the levels tend to be normal or low in patients with polycythemia vera.[428]

Successful removal of the erythropoietin-producing tumor is associated with a decrease in erythropoietin levels and a decrease in the erythrocytosis.[422] If tumor removal is not possible and the patient develops the symptomatic form of polycythemia, phlebotomy may relieve the symptoms.[429]

Ectopic Production of Calcitonin

Serum calcitonin measurements are useful for the diagnosis and monitoring of therapy in patients with medullary carcinoma of the thyroid or C cell hyperplasia. In 1970, Milhaud and coworkers described a patient with hypercalcitonemia associated with a bronchial carcinoid tumor.[442] Since then, several investigators have measured calcitonin in the serum of patients with neoplasms and overall have found elevations in approximately half the patients studied and 6.7 percent of patients with benign disorders (Table 28-22).[443–454] Many of the tumors associated with hypercalcitonemia have APUD characteristics and include small cell carcinoma of the lung, carcinoid tumors, pheochromocytomas, melanoma, and islet cell tumors. Elevated tissue calcitonin concentrations have been found in 95 percent of APUD-type tumors and close to 40 percent of tumors without APUD characteristics.[455] Although some investigators have been unable to detect calcitonin in normal tissues,[449,455] others have been able to extract calcitonin from a variety of normal tissues or demonstrate calcitonin by immunohistochemical techniques in normal tissues.[456,457] Between 16 and 38 percent of the patients studied have had a rise in serum calcitonin levels after pentagastrin administration, although the increase is proportionally less than that found in patients with medullary carcinoma of the thyroid.[447,448,545]

TABLE 28-22. Serum Immunoreactive Calcitonin Levels in Patients with Malignancies and Benign Diseases

Tumor	Number Positive/ Total Number		Positive, Percent	
Lung	127/257		49.4	
Small cell		91/147		61.9
Squamous		15/55		27.3
Adenocarcinoma		16/38		42.1
Anaplastic/ large cell		4/13		30.8
Alveolar		1/4		25.0
Carcinoid	5/11		45.5	
Breast	36/73		49.3	
Colon	8/30		26.7	
Stomach	4/11		36.4	
Esophagus	0/2		0	
Pancreatic	6/15		40	
Melanoma	4/10		40	
Leukemia	48/57		84.2	
CGL		32/33		97
AML		8/8		100
Other myeloproliferative		8/11		72.7
CLL		0/10		0
ALL		0/2		0
Miscellaneous	3/10		30	
Total	289/540		52.0	
Benign				
Normal and miscellaneous controls	2/100		2	
Benign breast	0/75		0	
GI	13/59		22	
Benign pulmonary	5/65		7.7	
Total	20/299		6.7	

Source: From references 443–454.

The source of the calcitonin excess in patients with nonmedullary cancers is unclear, as a catheterization study in such patients demonstrated that four of six patients had elevated calcitonin levels emanating from the thyroid rather than from the tumor.[446,458] The apparent high frequency of hypercalcitonemia in patients with neoplasms may actually be an artifact in some assays. Roos and colleagues showed that heating of serum from patients with squamous cell carcinoma and hypercalcitonemia abolished the elevated immunoreactive calcitonin but did not alter the immunoreactive calcitonin present in patients with small cell carcinoma of the lung or adenocarcinoma of the lung.[459] Nevertheless, it is clear that some tumors are capable of synthesizing and secreting calcitonin. Tumor cells derived from squamous cell carcinoma of the lung, small cell carcinoma of the lung, and breast carcinoma have been shown to produce immunoreactive calcitonin in vitro.[445,460–462] A calcitonin-producing breast carcinoma was propagated in nude mice and continued to proliferate and secrete calcitonin.[445]

In culture, several of these tumors produce high-molecular-mass species of calcitonin including 40-, 13-, and 10-kDa proteins.[445,462,463] In the BEN squamous cell carcinoma of the lung cell line, both high-molecular-mass species and biologically active 3,500-dalton calcitonin are secreted.[461] A greater proportion of the immunoreactive calcitonin present in the circulation of patients with nonthyroid tumors exists in large-molecular-weight forms than is found in the plasma of patients with medullary carcinoma of the thyroid.[459] The calcitonin mRNA from the BEN cell line closely resembles the calcitonin mRNA from medullary carcinoma of the thyroid, as do the translation products produced in a wheat germ system. However, other human lung tumor cell lines that contain mRNA for both calcitonin and calcitonin gene-related product have calcitonin mRNA that is larger than that found in medullary thyroid carcinoma.[464] Thus, as is the case with ectopic ACTH-secreting tumors, some calcitonin-secreting neoplasms may exhibit abnormalities in transcription of calcitonin mRNA or posttranslational processing of synthesized preprocalcitonin or procalcitonin.

There are no clinical manifestations of calcitonin excess in patients with nonthyroid neoplasms. The differential diagnosis of hypercalcitonemia in these patients includes the presence of chronic renal failure, acute pancreatitis, sepsis, hypercalcemia, and pernicious anemia.[112,465]

Other Hormones Produced by Tumors

Prolactin

In 1971, Turkington described a 53-year-old male with an undifferentiated bronchogenic carcinoma who exhibited hyperprolactinemia, which decreased after a course of radiation therapy to the tumor.[466] He also described a 49-year-old woman with hypernephroma, hyperprolactinemia, and galactorrhea who exhibited a return of prolactin to the normal range after surgical resection of the tumor. The hypernephroma was grown in culture and continued to release prolactin over a 2-week period.[466] Turkington noted that only 1 of 21 patients with lung cancer had hyperprolactinemia. In contrast, one-third of 21 patients with lung cancer studied by Davis and colleagues had hyperprolactinemia, although none exhibited gynecomastia, galactorrhea, or hypogonadism.[467] In patients who were tested, there was a normal prolactin response to L-dopa and TRH. There was no correlation with the presence or absence of hyperprolactinemia or the quantitative level of the prolactin elevation and the histology or tumor burden in these patients.[467] In a larger study, Molitch and coworkers examined 215 patients with cancer and found that 15 (7 percent) had hyperprolactinemia.[468] However, 12 of these 15 patients were receiving phenothiazines or opiates or had undergone prior radiation therapy to the chest wall or brain, which could account for the prolactin elevation. In fact, only two patients (1 percent) had hyperprolactinemia without another known cause being present. Elevated serum prolactin levels were found in 31 percent (229/743) of patients with uterine cervical carcinoma.[469] The authors did not note whether the patients were taking medications that could lead to hyperprolactinemia or control their assay for protease activity that can artifically elevate prolactin levels by degrading the radioiodinated prolactin tracer in the RIA.[13] Thus, the true prevalence of ectopic prolactin secretion in their study is not known. They also found immunohistochemical localization of prolactin in 22 or 49 (41 percent) cervical carcinoma specimens and evidence of prolactin secretion into the medium of 5 of 8 primary cervical carcinoma tissue cultures.[469] Immunoreactive prolactin has been found in a variety of other tumor tissues and cell lines.[470–472]

Vasoactive Intestinal Peptide

The syndrome of "pancreatic cholera," also referred to as the WDHA syndrome (*w*atery *d*iarrhea, *h*ypokalemia, and *a*chlorhydria) or Wermer-Morrison syndrome, is associated with excessive production of VIP and is usually associated with a non-β-cell tumor of the pancreatic islets. Using a sensitive RIA, Said and Faloona found elevated VIP concentrations in five of six patients with lung carcinoma and in a patient with a ganglioneuroblastoma of the adrenal and another patient with a pheochromocytoma.[473] Elevated levels of VIP were also present in the tumor tissue.[473] Subsequent studies demonstrated an arterial-venous gradient in VIP concentration across a malignant renal APUDoma associated with this syndrome[474] and the presence of VIP by immunoperoxidase staining in ganglioneuromas, ganglioneuroblastomas, and neuroblastomas.[475,476] Removal of the tumor is effective in lowering plasma VIP concentrations and reversing the syndrome. For tumors that are nonresectable, the long-acting somatostatin analog octreotide may be effective in suppressing VIP production by these tumors, as has been shown in patients with VIP-secreting non-β-islet-cell tumors of the pancreas.[477]

Somatostatin

Elevated concentrations of plasma immunoreactive somatostatin have been identified in patients with small cell carcinoma of the lung and carcinoid tumors, often in association with the ectopic production of ACTH.[455,478] Elevated concentrations of somatostatin have also been identified in tumor extracts from carcinoids and small cell cancer of the lung as well as in small cell cancer of the lung cell lines.[455,478,479] There is substantial heterogeneity in the somatostatin molecules that have been extracted from tumor tissues, with species 13,3–4, and 1.6 kDas being noted.[478] No clinical manifestations have been described from the excessive production of somatostatin by these tumors, probably because the actual concentrations of somatostatin in plasma are rather low in comparison to the concentrations in patients with pancreatic somatostatinomas.[478]

Other Gastrointestinal Hormones

Ectopic gastrin production associated with the Zollinger-Ellison syndrome has been reported with an ovarian cystadenoma and a pancreatic cystadenocarcinoma.[480,481]

Glucagon secretion has been described in a patient with a renal endocrine tumor who exhibited edema, rash, malabsorption, villous hypertrophy of the small intestine, and decreased motility of the jejunum and colon, which reversed after removal of the tumor.[482] Hunstein and coworkers reported a 76-year-old male with a glucagon-secreting large cell carcinoma of the lung who exhibited a typical glucagonoma syndrome with necrolytic migratory erythema, glucose intolerance, and weight loss.[483] Elevated glucagon levels were present in the patient's plasma, and immunoreactive glucagon was found in the carcinoma cells, with no abnormalities noted in the pancreas.[483] Immunoreactive glucagon also has been found in lung carcinoma and ovarian carcinoid tumors.[483,484]

Immunoreactive bombesin-like peptide, which probably represents its mammalian counterpart, gastrin-releasing peptide, has been found in a variety of tumors, including lung cancers associated with ectopic ACTH, carcinoid tumors, medullary carcinoma of the thyroid, and pheochromocytoma. Increased levels have also been found in the peripheral circulation of two patients with bronchial carcinoids and one with medullary carcinoma of the thyroid.[485] No clinical symptoms have been attributed to excessive production of this peptide.

Renin

Renin production has been associated with several tumors, including Wilms' tumor (nephroblastoma), juxtaglomerular cell tumors (hemangiopericytomas), and hypernephroma, which may be considered to be eutopic sources of the hormone.[486–491] Ectopic production has been found in ovarian carcinomas, pancreatic adenocarcinomas, lung tumors, acute myeloid leukemia, and an adrenal paraganglioma.[492–497] Some of the renin-producing tumors are associated with hypokalemic alkalosis and hypertension, while others are not. In addition to renin, prorenin may be secreted by these tumors.[492,495] Removal of the tumors cures the hypertension and hypokalemia. Unresectable lesions may be treated with inhibitors of angiotensin-converting enzyme.[494]

REFERENCES

1. Nathanson L, Hall TC: Introduction: Paraneoplastic syndromes. *Semin Oncol* 24:265, 1997.
2. Naschitz JE, Abrahamson J, Yeshurun D: Clinical significance of paraneoplastic syndrome. *Oncology* 46:40, 1989.
3. Dropcho EJ: Neurologic paraneoplastic syndromes. *J Neuro Sci* 153:264, 1998.
4. Cohen PR, Kurzrock R: Mucocutaneous paraneoplastic syndromes. *Semin Oncol* 24:334, 1997.
5. Costanza ME, Perin V, Schwartz RS, Nathansen L: Carcinoembryonic antigen-antibody complexes in a patient with colonic carcinoma and nephrotic syndrome. *N Engl J Med* 289:520, 1973.

6. Richard-Mendes da Costa C, Dupont E, Hamers R, Hooghe R, Dupuis F, Potuliege R: Nephrotic syndrome in bronchogenic carcinoma: Report of two cases with immunochemical studies. *Clin Nephrol* 2:245, 1974.
7. Maesaka JK, Mittal SK, Fishbane S: Paraneoplastic syndromes of the kidney. *Semin Oncol* 24:373, 1997.
8. Friou GJ: Current knowledge and concepts of the relationship of malignancy, autoimmunity, and immunologic disease. *Ann NY Acad Sci* 230:23, 1974.
9. Richardson EP Jr: Our evolving understanding of progressive multifocal leukoencephalopathy. *Ann NY Acad Sci* 230:358, 1974.
10. Marks LJ, Steinke J, Podolsky S, Egdahl RH: Hypoglycemia associated with neoplasia. *Ann NY Acad Sci* 230:147, 1974.
11. Miller AM, McGarry MP: A diffusible stimulator of eosinophilopoiesis produced by lymphoid cells as demonstrated with diffusion chambers. *Blood* 48:293, 1976.
12. Pineo GF, Brain MC, Gallus AS, Hirsch J, Hatton MWC, Regoeczi E: Tumors, mucus production, and hypercoagulability. *Ann NY Acad Sci* 230:262, 1984.
13. Odell WD: Endocrine/metabolic syndromes of cancer. *Semin Oncol* 24:299, 1997.
14. Braunstein GD: Production of human chorionic gonadotropin by nontrophoblastic tumors and tissues, in Tomoda Y, Mitzutani S, Narita O, Klopper A (eds): *Placental and Endometrial Proteins: Basic and Clinical Aspects.* Utrecht, The Netherlands, VNU Science Press, 1988, pp 493–502.
15. Pellegrini I, Lebrun JJ, Ali S, Kelly PA: Expression of prolactin and its receptor in human lymphoid cells. *Mol Endocrinol* 6:1023, 1992.
16. Rosenzweig JL, Havrankova J, Lesniak MA, Brownstein M, Roth J: Insulin is ubiquitous in extra pancreatic tissues of rats and humans. *Proc Natl Acad Sci USA* 77:572, 1980.
17. Kyle CV, Evans MC, Odell WD: Growth hormone-like material in normal human tissues. *J Clin Endocrinol Metab* 53:1138, 1981.
18. Saito E, Iwasa S, Odell WD: Widespread presence of large molecular weight adrenocorticotropin-like substances in normal rat extrapituitary tissues. *Endocrinology* 113:1010, 1983.
19. Suda T, Tomori N, Tozawa F, Demura H, Shizume K, Mouri T, Miura Y, Sasano N: Immunoreactive corticotropin and corticotropin-releasing factor in human hypothalamus, adrenal, lung cancer and pheochromocytoma. *J Clin Endocrinol Metab* 58:919, 1984.
20. Strewler GJ, Nissenson RA: Hypercalcemia in malignancy. *West J Med* 153:635, 1990.
21. Said SI, Rosenberg RN: Vasoactive intestinal polypeptide: Abundant immunoreactivity in neural cell lines and normal nervous tissue. *Science* 192:907, 1976.
22. Fischer JA, Tobler PH, Kaufmann M, Born W, Henke H, Copper PE, Sagar SM, Martin JB: Calcitonin: Regional distribution of the hormone and its binding sites in the human brain pituitary. *Proc Natl Acad Sci USA* 78:7801, 1981.
23. Kew MC, Kirschner MA, Abrahams GE, Katz M: Mechanism of feminization in primary liver cancer. *N Engl J Med* 296:1084, 1977.
24. Kirschner MA, Lippman A, Berkowitz R, Mayrer E, Drejka M: Estrogen production as a tumor marker in patients with gonadotropin-producing neoplasms. *Cancer Res* 41:1447, 1981.
25. Kuida CA, Braunstein GD, Shintaku P, Said JW: Human chorionic gonadotropin expression in lung, breast, and renal carcinoma. *Arch Pathol Lab Med* 112:282, 1987.
26. Braunstein GD, McIntire KR, Waldmann TA: Discordance of human chorionic gonadotropin and alpha-fetoprotein in testicular teratocarcinomas. *Cancer* 31:1065, 1973.
27. Samaan NA, Smith JP, Rutledge FN, Schultz PN: The significance of measurement of human placental lactogen, human chorionic gonadotropin, and carcinoembryonic antigen in patients with ovarian carcinoma. *Am J Obstet Gynecol* 126:186, 1976.
28. Sussman HH, Weintraub BD, Rosen SW: Relationship of ectopic placental alkaline phosphatase to ectopic chorionic gonadotropin and placental lactogen: Discordance of three "markers" for cancer. *Cancer* 33:820, 1974.
29. Ralston SH, Gallacher SJ, Patel U, Campbell J, Boyle IT: Cancer-associated hypercalcemia: Morbidity and mortality: Clinical experience in 126 treated patients. *Ann Intern Med* 112:499, 1990.
30. Hutchesson ACJ, Bundred NJ, Ratcliffe WA: Survival in hypercalcaemic patients with cancer and co-existing primary hyperparathyroidism. *Postgrad Med J* 71:28, 1995.
31. Dimopoulos MA, Fernandez JF, Samaan NA, Holoye PY, Vassilopoulou-Sellin R: Paraneoplastic Cushing's syndrome as an adverse prognostic factor in patients who die early with small cell cancer. *Cancer* 69:66, 1992.
32. Econs MJ, Drezner MK: Tumor-induced osteomalacia—unveiling a new hormone. *N Engl J Med* 330:1679, 1994.
33. Kumar R: Phosphatonin—a new phosphaturetic hormone? (Lessons from tumour-induced osteomalacia and X-linked hypophataemia). *Nephrol Dial Transplant* 12:11, 1997.
34. Samaan NA, Hickey RC, Hill CS Jr, Medellin H, Gates RB: Parathyroid tumors: Preoperative localization and association with other tumors. *Cancer* 33:933, 1974.
35. Farr HW, Fahey TJ Jr, Nash AG, Farr CM: Primary hyperparathyroidism and cancer. *Am J Surg* 126:539, 1973.
36. Drezner MK, Lebovitz HE: Primary hyperparathyroidism in paraneoplastic hypercalcemia. *Lancet* 1:1004, 1977.
37. Walls J, Ratcliffe WA, Howell A, Bundred NJ: Parathyroid hormone and parathyroid hormone-related protein in the investigation of hypercalcemia in two hospital populations. *Clin Endocrinol* 41:407, 1994.
38. Unger RH, Lochner J de V, Eisentraut AM: Identification of insulin and glucagon in a bronchogenic metastasis. *J Clin Endocrinol Metab* 24:823, 1964.
39. Schorr I, Rathnam P, Saxena BB, Ney RL: Multiple specific hormone receptors in the adenylate cyclase of an adrenocortical carcinoma. *J Biol Chem* 246:5806, 1971.
40. Melmed S, Ezrin C, Kovacs K, Goodman RS, Frohman LA: Acromegaly due to secretion of growth hormone by an ectopic pancreatic islet-cell tumor. *N Engl J Med* 312:9, 1985.
41. Ezzat S, Ezrin C, Yamashita S, Melmed S: Recurrent acromegaly resulting from ectopic growth hormone gene expression by a metastatic pancreatic tumor. *Cancer* 71:66, 1993.
42. Woodard HQ: Changes in blood chemistry associated with carcinoma metastatic to bone. *Cancer* 6:1219, 1953.
43. Jessiman AG, Emerson K Jr, Shah RC, Moore FD: Hypercalcemia in carcinoma of the breast. *Ann Surg* 157:377, 1963.
44. Galasko CSB, Burn JI: Hypercalcemia in patients with advanced mammary cancer. *Br Med J* 2:573, 1971.
45. Kato Y, Ferguson TB, Bennett DE, Burford TH: Oat cell carcinoma of the lung: A review of 138 cases. *Cancer* 23:517, 1969.
46. Warren MM, Utz DG, Kelalis PP: Concurrence of hypernephroma and hypercalcemia. *Ann Surg* 174:863, 1971.
47. Davis HL Jr, Wiseley AN, Ramirez G, Ansfield FJ: Hypercalcemia complicating breast cancer: Clinical features and management. *Oncology* 28:126, 1973.
48. Bender RA, Hansen H: Hypercalcemia in bronchogenic carcinoma: A prospective study of 200 patients. *Ann Intern Med* 80:205, 1974.
49. Rees LH, Ratcliffe JG: Ectopic hormone production by nonendocrine tumours. *Clin Endocrinol (Oxf)* 2:263, 1974.
50. Eagan RT, Maurer LH, Forcier RJ, Tulloh M: Small cell carcinoma of the lung: Staging, paraneoplastic syndromes, treatment and survival. *Cancer* 33:527, 1974.
51. Chisholm GD: Nephrogenic ridge tumors and their syndromes. *Ann NY Acad Sci* 230:403, 1974.
52. Richardson RL, Greco FA, Oldham RK, Liddle GW: Tumor products and potential markers in small cell lung cancer. *Semin Oncol* 5:253, 1978.
53. Hansen M, Hammer M, Hummer L: Diagnostic and therapeutic implications of ectopic hormone production in small cell carcinoma of the lung. *Thorax* 35:101, 1980.
54. Hansen M, Hansen HH, Hirsch FR, Arends J, Christensen JD, Christensen JM, Hummer L, Kuhl C: Hormonal polypeptides and amine metabolites in small cell carcinoma of the lung, with special reference to stage and subtypes. *Cancer* 45:1432, 1980.
55. Comis RL, Miller M, Ginsberg SJ: Abnormalities in water homeostasis in small cell anaplastic lung cancer. *Cancer* 45:2414, 1980.
56. Burt ME, Brennan MF: Incidence of hypercalcemia and malignant neoplasm. *Arch Surg* 115:704, 1980.
57. Lokich J: The frequency and clinical biology of the ectopic hormone syndromes of small cell carcinoma. *Cancer* 50:2111, 1982.
58. Merrill WW, Bondy PK: Production of biochemical marker substances by bronchogenic carcinomas. *Clin Chest Med* 3:307, 1982.
59. Hainsworth JD, Workman R, Greco FA: Management of the syndrome of inappropriate antidiuretic hormone secretion in small cell lung cancer. *Cancer* 51:161, 1983.

60. De la Monte SM, Hutchins GM, Moore GW: Paraneoplastic syndromes and constitutional symptoms in prediction of metastatic behavior of small cell carcinoma of the lung. *Am J Med* 77:851, 1984.
61. Laski ME, Vugrin D: Paraneoplastic syndromes in hypernephroma. *Semin Nephrol* 7:123, 1987.
62. Amatruda TT Jr, Upton GV: Hyperadrenocorticism and ACTH-releasing factor. *Ann NY Acad Sci* 230:168, 1974.
63. Canellos GP: Hypercalcemia in malignant lymphoma and leukemia. *Ann NY Acad Sci* 230:240, 1974.
64. Gilbey ED, Bondy PK, Fosling M: Impaired water excretion in oat cell lung cancer. *Br J Cancer* 34:323, 1976.
65. Ferlito A, Rinaldo A, Devaney KO: Clinicopathological consultation. Syndrome of inappropriate antidiuretic hormone secretion associated with head and neck cancers: Review of the literature. *Ann Otol Rhinol Laryngol* 106:878, 1997.
66. Gewirtz G, Yalow RS: Ectopic ACTH production in carcinoma of the lung. *J Clin Invest* 53:1022, 1974.
67. Wolfsen AR, Odell WD: ProACTH: Use for early detection of lung cancer. *Am J Med* 66:765, 1979.
68. Odell WD, Wolfsen AR, Bachelot I, Hirose F: Ectopic production of lipotropin by cancer. *Am J Med* 66:631, 1979.
69. Ratcliffe JG, Podmore J, Stack BHR, et al: Circulating ACTH and related peptides in lung cancer. *Br J Cancer* 45:230, 1982.
70. Trump DL, Abeloff MD, Hsu TH: Frequency of abnormalities of cortisol secretion and water metabolism in patients with small cell carcinoma of the lung and other malignancies. *Chest* 81:576, 1982.
71. Maurer LH, O'Donnell JF, Kennedy S, Faulkner CS, Rist K, North WG: Human neurophysins in carcinoma of the lung: Relation to histology, disease stage, response rate, survival, and syndrome of inappropriate antidiuretic hormone secretion. *Cancer Treat Rep* 67:971, 1983.
72. Odell WD, Wolfsen AR, Yoshimoto Y, Weitzman R, Fisher D, Hirose FM: Ectopic peptide synthesis: A universal concomitant of neoplasia. *Trans Assoc Am Physicians* 90:204, 1977.
73. Rees LH: Concepts in ectopic hormone production. *Clin Endocrinol (Oxf)* 5:363s, 1976.
74. Levine RJ, Metz SA: A classification of ectopic hormone-producing tumors. *Ann NY Acad Sci* 230:533, 1974.
75. Orth DN: Ectopic hormone production, in Felig P, Baxter JD, Broadus AE, Frohman LA (eds): *Endocrinology and Metabolism,* 2nd ed. New York, McGraw-Hill, 1987, pp 1692–1735.
76. Bailey RE: Periodic hormonogenesis—a new phenomenon: Periodicity in function of a hormone-producing tumour in man. *J Clin Endocrinol Metab* 32:317, 1971.
77. Kirschner MA, Wider JA, Ross GT: Leydig cell function in men with gonadotrophin producing testicular tumors. *J Clin Endocrinol Metab* 30:504, 1970.
78. Gropp C, Havemann K, Scheuer A: Ectopic hormones in lung cancer patients at diagnosis and during therapy. *Cancer* 46:347, 1980.
79. Yalow RS, Eastridge CE, Higgins G, Wolf J: Plasma and tumour ACTH in carcinoma of the lung. *Cancer* 44:1789, 1979.
80. Ayvazian LF, Schneider B, Gewirtz G, Yalow RS: Ectopic production of big ACTH in carcinoma of the lung. *Am Rev Respir Dis* 111:279, 1975.
81. Torstensson S, Thoren M, Hall K: Plasma ACTH in patients with bronchogenic carcinoma. *Acta Med Scand* 207:353, 1980.
82. Doege DW: Fibrosarcoma of the mediastinum. *Ann Surg* 92:955, 1930.
83. Landau BR, Wills N, Craig JW, Leonards JR, Moriwaki T: The mechanism of hepatoma-induced hypoglycemia. *Cancer* 15:1188, 1962.
84. Daughaday WH: Hypoglycemia in patients with non-islet cell tumors. *Endocrinol Metab Clin North Am* 18:91, 1989.
85. Vaitukaitis JL, Braunstein GD, Ross GT: A radioimmunoassay which specifically measures human chorionic gonadotropin in the presence of human luteinizing hormone. *Am J Obstet Gynecol* 113:751, 1972.
86. Braunstein GD, Rasor J, Thompson R, Van Scoy-Mosher M, Wade ME: Prospective evaluation of serum chorionic gonadotropin measurements for the immunodiagnosis of cancer. *Clin Res* 29:98A, 1981.
87. Stewart PM, Gibson S, Crosby SR, et al: ACTH precursors characterize the ectopic ACTH syndrome. *Clin Endocrinol* 40:199, 1994.
88. Findling JW: Eutopic or ectopic adrenocorticotropic hormone-dependent Cushing's syndrome: A diagnostic dilemma. *Mayo Clin Proc* 65:1314, 1990.
89. Fein HG, Rosen SW, Weinstraub DB: Increased glycosylation of serum human chorionic gonadotropin and subunits from eutopic and ectopic sources: Comparison with placental and urinary forms. *J Clin Endocrinol Metab* 50:1111, 1980.
90. Orth DN, Nicholson WE: Different molecular forms of ACTH. *Ann NY Acad Sci* 297:27, 1977.
91. Tanaka I, Nakai Y, Nakao K, Oki S, Fukata J, Imura H: γ-melanotrophin-like immunoreactivities in human pituitaries, ACTH-producing pituitary adenomas, and ectopic ACTH-producing tumours: Evidence for an abnormality in glycosylation in ectopic ACTH-producing tumours. *Clin Endocrinol (Oxf)* 15:353, 1981.
92. Katz MS, Kelley TM, Dax EM, Pineyro MA, Partilla JS, Gregerman RI: Ectopic β-adrenergic receptors coupled to adenylate cyclase in human adrenocortical carcinomas. *J Clin Endocrinol Metab* 60:900, 1985.
93. Pearse AGE: The cytochemistry and ultrastructure of polypeptide hormone-producing cells of the APUD series and the embryologic, physiologic and pathologic implications of the concept. *J Histochem Cytochem* 17:303, 1969.
94. Smith LH: The APUD cell concept. *J Surg Oncol* 8:137, 1976.
95. O'Connor DT, Deftos LJ: Secretion of chromogranin A by peptide-producing endocrine neoplasms. *N Engl J Med* 314:1145, 1986.
96. Weichert AF III: The neural ectodermal origin of the peptide-secreting endocrine glands: Unifying concept for the etiology of multiple endocrine adenomatosis and the inappropriate secretion of peptide hormones by nonendocrine tumors. *Am J Med* 49:232, 1970.
97. Sidhu GS: The endodermal origin of digestive and respiratory tract APUD cells: Histopathologic evidence and a review of the literature. *Am J Pathol* 96:5, 1979.
98. Baylin SB: "APUD" cells: Fact and fiction. *Trends Endocrinol Metab* 1:198, 1990.
99. Kameda Y, Ikeda A: Immunochemical and immunohistochemical studies on the 27S iodoprotein of dog thyroid with reference to thyroglobulin-like reaction of the parafollicular cells. *Biochim Biophys Acta* 577:241, 1979.
100. Melmed RN, Turner RC, Holt SJ: Intermediate cells of the pancreas: II. The effects of dietary soybean trypsin inhibitor on acinar-β cell structure and function in the rat. *J Cell Sci* 13:279, 1973.
101. Melmed RN, Benitez CJ, Holt SJ: Intermediate cells of the pancreas: III. Selective autophagy and destruction of β-granules in intermediate cells of the rat pancreas induced by alloxan and streptozotocin. *J Cell Sci* 13:297, 1973.
102. Warner TFCS: Cell hybridisation in the genesis of ectopic hormone-secreting tumours. *Lancet* 1:1259, 1974.
103. Tagnon HJ, Hildebrand J: Paraneoplastic syndromes. *Eur J Cancer Clin Oncol* 17:969, 1981.
104. Gurdon JB: Adult frogs derived from the nuclei of single somatic cells. *Dev Biol* 4:256, 1962.
105. King TJ, DiBerardino MA: Transplantation of nuclei from the frog renal adenocarcinoma: I. Development of tumor nuclear-transplant embryos. *Ann NY Acad Sci* 126:115, 1965.
106. Uriel J: Cancer, retrodifferentiation, and the myth of Faust. *Cancer Res* 36:4269, 1976.
107. Shields R: Gene derepression in tumours. *Nature* 269:752, 1977.
108. Pierce GB: Neoplasms, differentiations and mutations. *Am J Pathol* 77:103, 1974.
109. Anderson NG, Coggin JH Jr: Molecular mechanisms in blocked ontogeny and retrogenesis. *Ann NY Acad Sci* 230:508, 1974.
110. Vorherr H, Massry SG, Fallet R, Kaplan L, Kleeman CR: Antidiuretic principle in tuberculous lung tissue of a patient with pulmonary tuberculosis and hyponatremia. *Ann Intern Med* 72:383, 1970.
111. Dupont AG, Somers G, Van Steirteghem AC, Warson F, Vanhaelst L: Ectopic andrenocorticotropin productions: Disappearance after removal of inflammatory tissue. *J Clin Endocrinol Metab* 58:654, 1984.
112. De Bustros A, Baylin SB: Hormone production by tumours: Biological and clinical aspects. *Clin Endocrinol Metab* 14:221, 1985.
113. Nieman LK, Chrousos GP, Kellner C, et al: Successful treatment of Cushing's syndrome with the glucocorticoid antagonist RU 486. *J Clin Endocrinol Metab* 61:536, 1985.
114. Braunstein GD: Placental proteins as tumor markers, in Herberman RB, Mercer DW (eds): *Immunodiagnosis of Cancer,* 2nd ed. New York, Marcel Dekker, 1991, pp 673–701.

115. Galen RS: Predictive value of immunodiagnostic cancer tests, in Herberman RB, Mercer DW (eds): *Immunodiagnosis of Cancer,* 2nd ed. New York, Marcel Dekker, 1991, pp 3–11.
116. Myers WPL: Hypercalcemia in neoplastic disease. *AMA Arch Surg* 80:140, 1960.
117. Warwick OH, Yendt ER, Olin JS: The clinical features of hypercalcemia associated with malignant disease. *Can Med Assoc J* 85:719, 1961.
118. Singer FR, Sharp CF Jr, Rude RK: Pathogenesis of hypercalcemia in malignancy. *Miner Electrolyte Metab* 2:161, 1979.
119. Stewart AF, Horst R, Deftos LJ, Cadman EC, Lang R, Broadus AE: Biochemical evaluation of patients with cancer-associated hypercalcemia: Evidence for humoral and nonhumoral groups. *N Engl J Med* 303:1377, 1980.
120. Budayr AA, Nissenson RA, Klein RF, Pun KK, Clark OH, Diep D, Arnaud CD, Strewler GJ: Increased serum levels of a parathyroid hormone-like protein in malignancy-associated hypercalcemia. *Ann Intern Med* 111:807, 1989.
121. Kao PC, Klee GG, Taylor RL, Heath H III: Parathyroid hormone-related peptide in plasma of patients with hypercalcemia and malignant lesions. *Mayo Clin Proc* 65:1399, 1990.
122. Henderson JE, Shustik C, Kremer R, Rabbani SA, Hendy GN, Goltzman D: Circulating concentrations of parathyroid hormone-like peptide in malignancy and in hyperparathyroidism. *J Bone Miner Res* 5:105, 1990.
123. Lafferty FW: Pseudohyperparathyroidism. *Medicine (Baltimore)* 45:247, 1966.
124. Skrabanek P, McPartlin J, Powell D: Tumor hypercalcemia and "ectopic hyperparathyroidism." *Medicine (Baltimore)* 59:262, 1980.
125. Howlett TA, Rees LH. Ectopic hormones: *Spec Topics Endocrinol Metab* 7:1, 1985.
126. Ralston S, Fogelman I, Gardner MD, Boyle IT: Hypercalcaemia and metastatic bone disease: Is there a causal link? *Lancet* 2:903, 1982.
127. Guise TA, Mundy GR: Cancer and Bone. *Endocrinol Rev* 19:18, 1998.
128. Bujndred NJ, Ratcliffe WA, Walker RA, Coley S, Morrison JM, Ratcliffe JG: Parathyroid hormone related protein and hypercalcaemia in breast cancer. *Br Med J* 303:1506, 1991.
129. Sharp CF Jr, Rude RJ, Terry R, Singer FR: Abnormal bone and parathyroid histology in carcinoma patients with pseudohyperparathyroidism. *Cancer* 49:1449, 1982.
130. Zondek H, Petow H, Siebert W: Bie Bedeutung der Kalzium Bestimmung im Blut fur diagnose der Niereninsuffizienz. *Z Klin Med* 99:129, 1924.
131. Gutman AB, Tyson TL, Gutman EB: Serum calcium, inorganic phosphorous and phosphatase activity in hyperparathyroidism, Paget's disease, multiple myeloma, and neoplastic disease of the bones. *Arch Intern Med* 57:379, 1936.
132. Case records of the Massachusetts General Hospital. *N Engl J Med* 225:789, 1941.
133. Connor TB, Thomas WC Jr, Howard JE: Etiology of hypercalcemia associated with lung carcinoma. *J Clin Invest* 35:697, 1956.
134. Plimpton CH, Gellhorn A: Hypercalcemia in malignant disease without evidence of bone destruction. *Am J Med* 21:750, 1956.
135. Fry L: Pseudohyperparathyroidism with carcinoma of bronchus. *Br Med J* 1:301, 1962.
136. Tashjian AH Jr, Levine L, Munson PL: Immunochemical identification of parathyroid hormone in non-parathyroid neoplasms associated with hypercalcemia. *J Exp Med* 119:467, 1964.
137. Goldberg MF, Tashjian AH Jr, Order SE, Dammin GJ: Renal adenocarcinoma containing a parathyroid hormone-like substance and associated with marked hypercalcemia. *Am J Med* 36:805, 1964.
138. Benson RC Jr, Riggs BL, Pickard BM, Arnaud CD: Radioimmunoassay of parathyroid hormone in hypercalcemic patients with malignant disease. *Am J Med* 56:821, 1974.
139. Sherwood LM, O'Riordan JLH, Aurbach GD, Potts JT Jr: Production of parathyroid hormone by nonparathyroid tumors. *J Clin Endocrinol Metab* 27:140, 1967.
140. Knill-Jones RP, Buckle RM, Parson V, Calne RY, Williams R: Hypercalcemia and increased parathyroid-hormone activity in a primary hepatoma: Studies before and after hepatic transplantation. *N Engl J Med* 282:704, 1970.
141. Buckle RM, McMillan M, Mallinson C: Ectopic secretion of parathyroid hormone by a renal adenocarcinoma in a patient with hypercalcaemia. *Br Med J* 4:724, 1970.
142. Roof BS, Carpenter B, Fink DJ, Gordan GS: Some thoughts on the nature of ectopic parathyroid hormones. *Am J Med* 50:686, 1971.
143. Riggs BL, Arnaud CD, Reynolds JC, Smith LH: Immunologic differentiation of primary hyperparathyroidism from hyperparathyroidism due to nonparathyroid cancer. *J Clin Invest* 50:2079, 1971.
144. Raisz LG, Yajnik CH, Bockman RS, Bower BF: Comparison of commercially available parathyroid hormone immunoassays in the differential diagnosis of hypercalcemia due to hyperparathyroidism or malignancy. *Ann Intern Med* 91:739, 1979.
145. Powell D, Singer FR, Murray TM, Minkin C, Potts JT Jr: Nonparathyroid humoral hypercalcemia in patients with neoplastic diseases. *N Engl J Med* 289:176, 1973.
146. Seyberth HW, Segre GV, Morgan JL, Sweetman BJ, Potts JT Jr, Oates JA: Prostaglandins as mediators of hypercalcemia associated with certain types of cancer. *N Engl J Med* 293:1278, 1975.
147. Robertson RP, Baylink DJ, Marini JJ, Adkison HW: Elevated prostaglandins and suppressed parathyroid hormone associated with hypercalcemia and renal cell carcinoma. *J Clin Endocrinol Metab* 41:164, 1975.
148. Mundy GR, Raisz LG, Cooper RA, Schechter GP, Salmon SE: Evidence for the secretion of an osteoclast stimulating factor in myeloma. *N Engl J Med* 291:1041, 1974.
149. Simpson EL, Mundy GR, D'Souza SM, Ibbotson KJ, Bockman R, Jacobs JW: Absence of parathyroid hormone messenger RNA in nonparathyroid tumors associated with hypercalcemia. *N Engl J Med* 309:325, 1983.
150. Strewler GJ, Williams RD, Nissenson RA: Human renal carcinoma cells produce hypercalcemia in the nude mouse and a novel protein recognized by parathyroid hormone receptors. *J Clin Invest* 71:769, 1983.
151. Martin TJ, Ebeling PR, Rodda CP, Kemp BE: Humoral hypercalcemia of malignancy: Involvement of a novel hormone. *Aust N Z J Med* 18:287, 1988.
152. Suva LJ, Winslow GA, Wettenhall REH, et al: A parathyroid hormone-related protein implicated in malignant hypercalcemia: Cloning and expression. *Science* 237:893, 1987.
153. Yoshimoto K, Yamasaki R, Sakai H, Tezuka U, Takahashi M, Iizuka M, Sekiya T, Saito S: Ectopic production of parathyroid hormone by small cell lung cancer in a patient with hypercalcemia. *J Clin Endocrinol Metab* 68:976, 1989.
154. Nussbaum S, Gaz R, Arnold A: Ectopic secretion of parathyroid hormone from an ovarian cancer with DNA rearrangement of the 5′ regulatory region of the PTH gene. *Clin Res* 38:462A, 1990.
155. Strewler GJ, Budayr AA, Bruce RJ, Clark OH, Nissenson RA: Secretion of authentic parathyroid hormone by a malignant tumor. *Clin Res* 38:462A, 1990.
156. Rizzoli R, Pache J-C, Didierjean L, Burger A, Bonjour JP: A thymoma as a cause of true ectopic hyperparathyroidism. *J Clin Endocrinol Metab* 79:912, 1994.
157. Nielsen PK, Rasmussen AK, Feldt-Rasmussen U, Brandt M, Christensen L, Olgaard K: Ectopic production of intact parathyroid hormone by a squamous cell lung carcinoma in vivo and in vitro. *J Clin Endocrinol Metab* 81:3793, 1996.
158. Rude RK, Sharp CF Jr, Fredericks RS, Oldham SB, Elbaum N, Link J, Irwin L, Singer FR: Urinary and nephrogenous adenosine 3′,5′-monophosphate in the hypercalcemia of malignancy. *J Clin Endocrinol Metab* 52:765, 1981.
159. Goltzman D, Stewart AF, Broadus AE: Malignancy-associated hypercalcemia: Evaluation with a cytochemical bioassay for parathyroid hormone. *J Clin Endocrinol Metab* 53:899, 1981.
160. Strewler GJ, Wronski TJ, Halloran BP, Miller SC, Leung SC, Williams RD, Nissenson RA: Pathogenesis of hypercalcemia in nude mice bearing a human renal carcinoma. *Endocrinology* 119:303, 1986.
161. Goltzman D, Hendy GN, Banville D: Parathyroid hormone-like peptide: Molecular characterization and biological properties. *Trends Endocrinol Metab* 1:39, 1989.
162. Burtis WJ, Brady TG, Orloff JJ, et al: Immunochemical characterization of circulating parathyroid hormone-related protein in patients with humoral hypercalcemia of cancer. *N Engl J Med* 322:1106, 1990.
163. Ratcliffe WA, Hutchesson ACJ, Bundred NJ, Ratcliffe JG: Role of assays for parathyroid-hormone-related protein in investigation of hypercalcaemia. *Lancet* 339:164, 1992.

164. Honda S, Yamaguchi K, Suzuki M, Sato Y, Adachi I, Kimura S, Abe K: Expression of parathyroid hormone-related protein mRNA in tumors obtained from patients with humoral hypercalcemia of malignancy. *Jpn J Cancer Res* 79:677, 1988.
165. Ikeda K, Mangin M, Dreyer BE, et al: Identification of transcripts encoding a parathyroid hormone-like peptide in messenger RNAs from a variety of human and animal tumors associated with humoral hypercalcemia of malignancy. *J Clin Invest* 81:2010, 1988.
166. Stewart AF, Mangin M, Wu T, Goumas D, Insogna KL, Burtis WJ, Broadus AE: Synthetic human parathyroid hormone-like protein stimulates bone resorption and causes hypercalcemia in rats. *J Clin Invest* 81:596, 1988.
167. Rabbani SA, Mitchell J, Roy DR, Hendy GN, Goltzman D: Influence of the amino-terminus on in vitro and in vivo biological activity of synthetic parathyroid hormone-like peptides of malignancy. *Endocrinology* 123:2709, 1988.
168. Kukreja SC, Shevrin DH, Wimbiscus SA, Ebeling PR, Danks JA, Rodda CP, Wood WI, Martin TJ: Antibodies to parathyroid hormone-related protein lower serum calcium in athymic mouse models of malignancy-associated hypercalcemia due to human tumors. *J Clin Invest* 82:1798, 1988.
169. Everhart-Caye M, Inzucchi SE, Guinness-Henry J, Mitnick MA, Stewart AF: Parathyroid hormone (PTH)-related protein(1-36) is equipotent to PTH(1-34) in humans. *J Clin Endocrinol Metab* 81:199, 1996.
170. Kremer R, Shustik C, Tabak T, Papavasiliou V, Golotzman D: Parathyroid-hormone-related peptide in hematologic malignancies. *Am J Med* 100:406, 1996.
171. Bilezikian JP: Measurement of parathyroid hormone-related peptide in the circulation. *Trends Endocrinol Metab* 2:1, 1991.
172. Ikeda K, Weir EC, Mangin M, Dannies PS, Kinder B, Deftos LJ, Brown EM, Broadus AE: Expression of messenger ribonucleic acids encoding a parathyroid hormone-like peptide in normal human and animal tissues with abnormal expression in human parathyroid adenomas. *Mol Endocrinol* 2:1230, 1988.
173. Thiede MA, Rodan GA: Expression of a calcium-mobilizing parathyroid hormone-like peptide in lactating mammary tissue. *Science* 242:278, 1988.
174. Budayr AA, Halloran BP, King JC, Diep D, Nissenson RA, Strewler GJ: High levels of a parathyroid hormone-like protein in milk. *Proc Natl Acad Sci USA* 86:7183, 1989.
175. Thiede MA: The mRNA encoding a parathyroid hormone-like peptide is produced in mammary tissue in response to elevations in serum prolactin. *Mol Endocrinol* 3:1443, 1989.
176. Rodda CP, Kubota M, Heath JA, Ebeling PR, Moseley JM, Care AD, Caple IW, Martin TJ: Evidence for a novel parathyroid hormone-related protein in fetal lamb parathyroid glands and sheep placenta: Comparisons with a similar protein implicated in humoral hypercalcaemia of malignancy. *J Endocrinol* 117:261, 1988.
177. Abbas SK, Pickard DW, Rodda CP, Heath JA, Hammonds RG, Wood WI, Caple IW, Martin TJ, Care AD: Stimulation of ovine placental calcium transport by purified natural and recombinant parathyroid hormone-related protein (PTHrP) preparations. *Q J Exp Physiol* 74:549, 1989.
178. Adachi N, Yamaguchi K, Miyake Y, Honda S, Nagasaki K, Akiyama Y, Adachi I, Abe K: Parathyroid hormone-related protein is a possible autocrine growth inhibitor for lymphocytes. *Biochem Biophys Res Commun* 166:1088, 1990.
179. Klein DC, Raisz LG: Prostaglandins: Stimulation of bone resorption in tissue culture. *Endocrinology* 86:1436, 1970.
180. Chase LR, Aurbach GD: The effect of parathyroid hormone on the concentration of adenosine 3′,5′-monophosphate in skeletal tissue in vitro. *J Biol Chem* 245:1520, 1970.
181. Tashjian AH Jr, Voelkel EF, Levine L, Goldhaber P: Evidence that the bone resorption-stimulating factor produced by mouse fibrosarcoma cells is prostaglandin E_2: A new model for the hypercalcemia of cancer. *J Exp Med* 136:1329, 1972.
182. Voelkel EF, Tashjian AH Jr, Franklin R, Wasserman E, Levine L: Hypercalcemia and tumor-prostaglandins: The VX_2 carcinoma model in the rabbit. *Metabolism* 24:973, 1975.
183. Flower RJ: Drugs which inhibit prostaglandin biosynthesis. *Pharmacol Rev* 26:33, 1974.
184. Franklin RB, Tashjian AH Jr: Intravenous infusion of prostaglandin E_2 raises plasma calcium concentration in the rat. *Endocrinology* 97:240, 1975.
185. Brereton HD, Halushka PV, Alexander RW, Mason DM, Keiser HR, DeVita VT: Indomethacin-responsive hypercalcemia in a patient with renal-cell adenocarcinoma. *N Engl J Med* 291:83, 1974.
186. Ito H, Sanada T, Katayama T, Shimazaki J: Indomethacin-responsive hypercalcemia. *N Engl J Med* 293:558, 1975.
187. Seyberth HW, Segre GV, Hamet P, Sweetman BJ, Potts JT Jr, Oates JA: Characterization of the group of patients with the hypercalcemia of cancer who respond to treatment with prostaglandin synthesis inhibitors. *Trans Assoc Am Physicians* 89:92, 1976.
188. Tashjian AH Jr: Prostaglandin, hypercalcemia and cancer. *N Engl J Med* 293:1317, 1975.
189. Coombes RC, Neville AM, Bondy PK, Powles TJ: Failure of indomethacin to reduce hydroxyproline excretion of hypercalcemia in patients with breast cancer. *Prostaglandins* 12:1027, 1976.
190. Caro JF, Besarab A, Flynn JT: Prostaglandin E and hypercalcemia in breast carcinoma: Only a tumor marker? *Am J Med* 66:337, 1979.
191. Valentin-Opran A, Eilon G, Saez S, Mundy GR: Estrogens and antiestrogens stimulate release of bone resorbing activity by cultured human breast cancer cells. *J Clin Invest* 75:726, 1985.
192. Tashjian AH Jr, Voelkel EF, Lazzaro M, Singer FR, Roberts AB, Derynck R, Winkler ME, Levine L: Alpha and β human transforming growth factors stimulate prostaglandin production and bone resorption in cultured mouse calvaria. *Proc Natl Acad Sci USA* 82:4535, 1985.
193. Breslau NA, McGuire JL, Zerwekh JE, Frenkel EP, Pak CYC: Hypercalcemia associated with increased serum calcitriol levels in three patients with lymphoma. *Ann Intern Med* 100:1, 1984.
194. Rosenthal LN, Insogna KL, Godsall JW, Smaldone L, Waldron JA, Stewart AF: Elevations in circulating 1,25-dihydroxyvitamin D in three patients with lymphoma-associated hypercalcemia. *J Clin Endocrinol Metab* 60:29, 1985.
195. Zaloga GPL, Eil C, Medbery CA: Humoral hypercalcemia in Hodgkin's disease. *Arch Intern Med* 145:155, 1985.
196. Davies M, Hayes ME, Mawer EB, Lumb GA: Abnormal vitamin D metabolism in Hodgkin's lymphoma. *Lancet* 1:1186, 1985.
197. Schaefer K, Saupe J, Pauls A, von Herrath D: Hypercalcemia and elevated serum $1,25\text{-}(OH)_2\text{-}D_3$ in a patient with Hodgkin's lymphoma. *Klin Wochenschr* 64:89, 1986.
198. Adams JS, Fernandez M, Gacad MA, Gill PS, Endres DB, Rasheed S, Singer FR: Vitamin D metabolite-mediated hypercalcemia and hypercalciuria patients with AIDS- and non-AIDS-associated lymphoma. *Blood* 73:235, 1989.
199. Seymour JF, Gagel RF, Hagemeister FB, Dimopoulos MA, Cabanillas F: Calcitriol production in hypercalcemic and normocalcemic patients with non-Hodgkin lymphoma. *Ann Intern Med* 121:633, 1994.
200. Katz A, Kaplan L, Massry SG, Heller R, Plotkin D, Knight I: Primary hyperparathyroidism in patients with breast carcinoma. *Arch Surg* 101:582, 1970.
201. Kaplan L, Katz AD, Ben-Isaac C, Massry SG: Malignant neoplasms and parathyroid adenoma. *Cancer* 28:401, 1971.
202. Petro AB, Hardy JD: The association of parathyroid adenoma and non-medullary carcinoma of the thyroid. *Ann Surg* 181:118, 1975.
203. Newman HK, Plucinski TE: Unsuspected nonmedullary carcinoma of the thyroid in patients with hyperparathyroidism. *Am J Surg* 134:799, 1977.
204. Heath H, Hodgson SF, Kennedy MA: Primary hyperparathyroidism: Incidence, morbidity and potential economic impact in a community. *N Engl J Med* 302:189, 1980.
205. Rao SD, Frame B, Miller MJ, Kleerekoper M, Block MA, Parfitt AM: Hyperparathyroidism following head and neck irradiation. *Arch Intern Med* 140:205, 1980.
206. Katz A, Braunstein GD: Clinical biochemical and pathologic features of patients with radiation-associated hyperparathyroidism. *Arch Intern Med* 143:79, 1983.
207. Fisken RA, Heath DA, Bold AM: Hypercalcaemia—a hospital survey. *Q J Med* 49:405, 1980.
208. Blomqvist CP: Malignant hypercalcaemia—a hospital survey. *Acta Med Scand* 220:455, 1986.
209. Warrell RP Jr, Israel R, Frisone M, Snyder T, Gaynor JJ, Bockman RS: Gallium nitrate for acute treatment of cancer-related hypercalcemia: A randomized, double-blind comparison to calcitonin. *Ann Intern Med* 108:669, 1988.
210. Buckle RM: Ectopic PTH syndrome, pseudohyperparathyroidism; hypercalcemia of malignancy. *J Clin Endocrinol Metab* 3:237, 1974.

211. Burtis WJ, Wu TL, Insogna KL, Stewart AF: Humoral hypercalcemia of malignancy. *Ann Intern Med* 108:454, 1988.
212. Boyd JC, Ladenson JH: Value of laboratory tests in the differential diagnosis of hypercalcemia. *Am J Med* 77:863, 1984.
213. Ikeda K, Ogata E: Humoral hypercalcemia of malignancy: Some enigmas on the clinical features. *J Cell Biochem* 57:384, 1995.
214. Ebie N, Ryan W, Harris J: Metabolic emergencies in cancer medicine. *Med Clin North Am* 70:1151, 1986.
215. Singer FR, Fernandez M: Therapy of hypercalcemia of malignancy. *Am J Med* 82(suppl 2A):34, 1987.
216. Schaiff RA, Hall TG, Bar RS: Medical treatment of hypercalcemia. *Clin Pharm* 8:108, 1989.
217. Siris ES, Hyman GA, Canfield RE: Effects of dichloromethylene diphosphonate in women with breast carcinoma metastatic to the skeleton. *Am J Med* 74:401, 1983.
218. Elomaa I, Blomqvist C, Grohn P, Porkka L, Kairento AL, Selander K, Lamberg-Allardt C, Holmstrom T: Long-term controlled trial with diphosphonate in patients with osteolytic bone metastases. *Lancet* 1:146, 1983.
219. Brown WH: A case of pluriglandular syndrome: "Diabetes of bearded woman." *Lancet* 2:1022, 1928.
220. Christy NP: Adrenocorticotrophic activity in the plasma of patients with Cushing's syndrome associated with pulmonary neoplasms. *Lancet* 1:85, 1961.
221. Holub DA, Katz FH: A possible etiological link between Cushing's syndrome and visceral malignancy. *Clin Res* 9:194, 1961.
222. Meador CK, Liddle GW, Island DP, Nicholson WE, Lucas CP, Nockton JG, Luetscher JA: Cause of Cushing's syndrome in patients with tumors arising from nonendocrine tissue. *J Clin Endocrinol Metab* 22:693, 1962.
223. Liddle GW, Nicholson WE, Island DP, Orth DN, Abe K, Lowder SC: Clinical and laboratory studies of ectopic humoral syndromes. *Recent Prog Horm Res* 25:283, 1969.
224. Schteingart DE: Ectopic secretion of peptides of the proopiomelanocortin family. *Endocrinol Metab Clin North Am* 20:453, 1991.
225. Azzopardi JG, Williams ED: Pathology of 'nonendocrine' tumors associated with Cushing's syndrome. *Cancer* 22:274, 1968.
226. Imura H, Matsukura S, Yamamoto H, Hirata Y, Nakai Y, Eno J, Tanaka A, Nakamura M: Studies on ectopic ACTH-producing tumors: II. Clinical and biochemical features of 30 cases. *Cancer* 35:1430, 1975.
227. Jex RK, van Heerden JA, Carpenter PC, Grant CS: Ectopic ACTH syndrome: Diagnostic and therapeutic aspects. *Am J Surg* 149:276, 1985.
228. Howlett TA, Drury PL, Perry L, Doniach I, Rees LH, Besser GM: Diagnosis and management of ACTH-dependent Cushing's syndrome: Comparison of the features in ectopic and pituitary ACTH production. *Clin Endocrinol (Oxf)* 24:699, 1986.
229. Singer W, Kovacs K, Ryan N, Horvath E: Ectopic ACTH syndrome: Clinicopathological correlations. *J Clin Pathol* 31:591, 1978.
230. Kohler PC, Trump DL: Ectopic hormone syndromes. *Cancer Invest* 4:543, 1986.
231. Yalow RS: Big ACTH and bronchogenic carcinoma. *Annu Rev Med* 30:241, 1979.
232. Ratter SJ, Gillies G, Hope J, et al: Pro-opiocortin related peptides in human pituitary and ectopic ACTH secreting tumours. *Clin Endocrinol (Oxf)* 18:211, 1983.
233. Jeffcoate WJ, Rees LH, Lowry PJ, Besser GM: A specific radioimmunoassay for human β-lipotropin. *J Clin Endocrinol Metab* 47:160, 1978.
234. Ueda M, Takeuchi T, Abe K, Miyakawa S, Ohnami S, Yanaihara N: β-melanocyte-stimulating hormone immunoreactivity in human pituitaries and ectopic adrenocorticotropin-producing tumors. *J Clin Endocrinol Metab* 50:550, 1980.
235. Kleber G, Hollt V, Oelkers W, Quabbe HJ: Elevated plasma and tissue concentrations of β-endorphin and β-lipotropin associated with an ectopic ACTH-producing lung tumor. *Horm Metab Res* 12:385, 1980.
236. Pullan PT, Clement-Jones V, Corder R, Lowry PJ, Besser GM, Rees LH: ACTH, LPH and related peptides in the ectopic ACTH syndrome. *Clin Endocrinol (Oxf)* 13:437, 1980.
237. Baker J, Holdaway IM, Jagusch M, Kerr AR, Donald RA, Pullan PT: Ectopic secretion of ACTH and met-enkephalin from a thymic carcinoid. *J Endocrinol Invest* 5:33, 1982.
238. Sheng SL, Seurin D, Bertagna X, Girard F: Molecular forms of beta-endorphin in ACTH/LPH hypersecretion syndromes in man. *Horm Res* 20:95, 1984.
239. Hale AC, Besser GM, Rees LH: Characterization of pro-opiomelanocortin-derived peptides in pituitary and ectopic adrenocorticotropin-secreting tumours. *J Endocrinol* 108:49, 1986.
240. Pullan PT, Clement-Jones V, Corder R, Lowry PJ, Rees GM, Rees LH, Besser GM, Macedo MM, Galvao-Teles A: Ectopic production of methionine enkephalin and beta-endorphin. *Br Med J* 1:758, 1980.
241. Lundberg JM, Hamberger B, Schultzberg M, et al: Enkephalin- and somatostatin-like immunoreactivities in human adrenal medulla and pheochromocytoma. *Proc Natl Acad Sci USA* 76:4079, 1979.
242. DeBold CR, Menefee JK, Nicholson WE, Orth DN: Proopiomelanocortin gene is expressed in many normal tissues and in tumors not associated with ectopic adrenocorticotropin syndrome. *Mol Endocrinol* 2:862, 1988.
243. Odell WD, Saito E: Protein hormone-like materials from normal and cancer cells: "Ectopic" hormone production. *Proc 13th Int Cancer Congress,* Part E: *Cancer Management.* New York, Liss, 1983, p 247.
244. Orwoll ES, Kendall JW: β-endorphin and adrenocorticotropin in extrapituitary sites: Gastrointestinal tract. *Endocrinology* 107:438, 1980.
245. Odell WD: Ectopic ACTH secretion. *Endocrinol Metab Clin North Am* 20:371, 1991.
246. Bardin CW, Shaha C, Mather J, Salomon Y, Margioris AN, Liotta AS, Gerendai I, Chen CL, Krieger DT: Identification and possible function of proopiomelanocortin derived peptides in the testis. *Ann NY Acad Sci* 438:346, 1984.
247. Chen CLC, Chang CC, Krieger DT, Bardin WC: Expression and regulation of proopiomelanocortin-like gene in the ovary and placenta: Comparison with the testis. *Endocrinology* 118:2382, 1986.
248. Jingami H, Nakanishi S, Imura I, Numa S: Tissue distribution of messenger RNAs coding for opioid peptide precursors and related RNA. *Eur J Biochem* 142:441, 1984.
249. DeKeyzer Y, Rousseau-Merck MF, Luton JP, Girard F, Kahn A, Bertagna X: Pro-opiomelanocortin gene expression in human phaeochromocytomas. *J Mol Endocrinol* 2:175, 1989.
250. Walker BR, Campbell JC, Fraxer R, Stewart PM, Edwards CRW: Mineralocorticoid excess and inhibition of 11β-hydroxysteroid dehydrogenase in patients with ectopic ACTH syndrome. *Clin Endocrinol* 37:483, 1992.
251. Abeloff MD, Trump DL, Baylin SB: Ectopic adrenocorticotrophic (ACTH) syndrome and small cell carcinoma of the lung—assessment of clinical implications in patients on combination chemotherapy. *Cancer* 48:1082, 1981.
252. Pass HI, Doppman JL, Nieman L, et al: Management of the ectopic ACTH syndrome due to thoracic carcinoids. *Ann Thorac Surg* 50:52, 1990.
253. Upton GV, Amatruda TT Jr: Evidence for the presence of tumor peptides with corticotropin-releasing-factor-like activity in the ectopic ACTH syndrome. *N Engl J Med* 285:419, 1971.
254. Carey RM, Varma SK, Drake CR Jr, Thorner MO, Kovacs K, Rivier J, Vale W: Ectopic secretion of corticotropin-releasing factor as a cause of Cushing's syndrome: A clinical, morphologic, and biochemical study. *N Engl J Med* 311:12, 1984.
255. Asa S, Kovacs K, Tindal GT, Barrow DL, Horvath E, Vecsei P: Cushing's disease associated with an intraseller gangliocytoma producing corticotropin-releasing factor. *Ann Intern Med* 101:789, 1984.
256. Belsky JL, Cuello B, Swanson LW, Simmons DM, Jarrett RM, Braza F: Cushing's syndrome due to ectopic production of corticotropin-releasing factor. *J Clin Endocrinol Metab* 60:496, 1985.
257. Schteingart DE, Lloyd RV, Akil H, Chandler WF, Ibarra-Perez G, Rosen SG, Olgetree R: Cushing's syndrome secondary to ectopic CRH-ACTH secretion. *J Clin Endocrinol Metab* 63:770, 1986.
258. Suda T, Kondo M, Totani R, et al: Ectopic adrenocorticotropin syndrome caused by lung cancer that responded to corticotropin-releasing hormone. *J Clin Endocrinol Metab* 63:1047, 1986.
259. Fjellestad-Paulsen A, Abrahamsson P-A, Bjartell A, Grino M, Grimelius L, Hedeland H, Falkmer S: Carcinoma of the prostate with Cushing's syndrome. *Acta Endocrinol (Copenh)* 119:506, 1988.
260. Tourniaire J, Rebattu B, Conte-Devolk B, Trouillas J, Grino M, Berger-Dutrieux N, Peix JL, Pugeat M: Syndrome de Cushing secondaire à la production ectopique de CRF par un carcinome medullaire ducorps thyroide. *Ann d'Endocrinol (Paris)* 4:61, 1988.

261. Adams EF, Skrabal F, Carroll D, Loizou M, White MC, Biggins JA, Mashiter K: Ectopic corticotrophin-releasing-factor and growth hormone releasing factor secretion: Diagnosis using human pituitary cell culture. *Horm Res* 25:80, 1987.
262. Wakabayashi I, Ihara T, Hattori M, Tonegawa Y, Shibasaki T, Hashimoto K: Presence of corticotropin-releasing factor-like immunoreactivity in human tumors. *Cancer* 55:995, 1985.
263. Findling JW, Tyrrell JB: Occult ectopic secretion of corticotropin. *Arch Intern Med* 146:929, 1986.
264. Chrousos GP, Schulte HM, Oldfield EH, Gold PW, Cutler GB Jr, Loriaux DL: The corticotropin-releasing factor stimulation test: An aid in the evaluation of patients with Cushing's syndrome. *N Engl J Med* 310:622, 1984.
265. Loriaux DL, Nieman L: Corticotropin-releasing hormone testing in pituitary disease. *Endocrinol Metab Clin North Am* 20:363, 1991.
266. Findling JW, Aron DC, Tyrrell JB, Shinsako JH, Fitzgerald PA, Norman D, Wilson CB, Forsham PH: Selective venous sampling for ACTH in Cushing's syndrome: Differentiation between Cushing's disease and the ectopic ACTH syndrome. *Ann Intern Med* 94:647, 1981.
267. Oldfield EH, Doppman JL, Nieman LK, Chrousos GP, Miller DL, Katz DA, Cutler GB Jr, Loriaux DL: Petrosal sinus sampling with and without corticotropin-releasing hormone for the differential diagnosis of Cushing's syndrome. *N Engl J Med* 325:897, 1991.
268. Drury PL, Ratter S, Tomlin S, Williams J, Dacie JE, Rees LH, Besser GM: Experience with selective venous sampling in diagnosis of ACTH-dependent Cushing's syndrome. *Br Med J* 284:9, 1982.
269. Horai T, Nishihara H, Tateishi R, Matsuda M, Hattori S: Oat-cell carcinoma of the lung simultaneously producing ACTH and serotonin. *J Clin Endocrinol Metab* 37:212, 1973.
270. Sonino N, Boscaro M, Merola G, Mantero F: Prolonged treatment of Cushing's disease by ketoconazole. *J Clin Endocrinol Metab* 61:718, 1985.
271. Jeffcoate WJ, Rees LH, Tomlin S, Jones AE, Edwards CRW, Besser GM: Metyrapone in long-term management of Cushing's disease. *Br Med J* 2:215, 1977.
272. Tabarin A, Navarranne A, Guerin J, Corcuff JB, Parneix M, Roger P: Use of ketoconazole in the treatment of Cushing's disease and ectopic ACTH syndrome. *Clin Endocrinol* 34:63, 1991.
273. Carey RM, Orth DN, Hartmann WH: Malignant melanoma with ectopic production of adrenocorticotropic hormone: Palliative treatment with inhibitors of adrenal steroid biosynthesis. *J Clin Endocrinol Metab* 36:482, 1973.
274. Cheung NW, Boyages SC: Failure of somatostatin analogue to control Cushing's syndrome in two cases of ACTH-producing carcinoid tumours. *Clin Endocrinol* 36:361, 1992.
275. Winkler AW, Cranshaw OS: Chloride depletion conditions other than Addison's disease. *J Clin Invest* 17:1, 1938.
276. Schwartz WB, Bennett W, Curelop S, Bartter FC: A syndrome of renal sodium loss and hyponatremia probably resulting from inappropriate secretion of antidiuretic hormone. *Am J Med* 23:529, 1957.
277. Leaf A, Bartter FC, Santos RF, Wrong O: Evidence in man that urinary electrolyte loss induced by pitressin is a function of water retention. *J Clin Invest* 32:868, 1953.
278. Thorn NA, Transbol I: Hyponatremia and bronchogenic carcinoma associated with renal excretion of large amounts of antidiuretic material. *Am J Med* 35:257, 1963.
279. Amatruda TT, Mulrow PJ, Gallagher JC, Sawyer WH: Carcinoma of the lung with inappropriate antidiuresis: Demonstration of antidiuretic-hormone-like activity in tumor extract. *N Engl J Med* 269:544, 1963.
280. Bower BF, Mason DM, Forsham PH: Bronchogenic carcinoma with inappropriate antidiuretic activity in plasma and tumor. *N Engl J Med* 271:934, 1964.
281. George JM, Capen CC, Phillips AS: Biosynthesis of vasopressin in vitro and ultrastructure of a bronchogenic carcinoma. *J Clin Invest* 51:141, 1972.
282. Yamaji T, Ishibashi M, Katayama S, Itabashi A, Ohsawa N, Kondo Y, Mizumoto Y, Kosaka K: Neurophysin biosynthesis in vitro in oat cell carcinoma of the lung with ectopic vasopressin production. *J Clin Invest* 69:1441, 1981.
283. Kondo Y, Mizumoto Y, Katayama S, Murase T, Yamaji T, Ohsawa N, Kosaka K: Inappropriate secretion of antidiuretic hormone in nude mice bearing a human bronchogenic oat cell carcinoma. *Cancer Res* 41:1545, 1981.
284. Moses AM, Miller M, Streeten DHP: Pathophysiologic and pharmacologic alterations in the release and action of ADH. *Metabolism* 25:697, 1976.
285. DeTroyer A, Demanet JC: Clinical, biological and pathogenic features of the syndrome of inappropriate secretion of antidiuretic hormone: A review of 26 cases with marked hyponatraemia. *Q J Med* 45:521, 1976.
286. Bartter FC, Schwartz WB: The syndrome of inappropriate secretion of antidiuretic hormone. *Am J Med* 42:790, 1967.
287. Vorherr H: Para-endocrine tumor activity with emphasis on ectopic ADH secretion: Genetic, diagnostic, prognostic and therapeutic aspects. *Oncology* 29:382, 1974.
288. Lockton JA, Thatcher N: A retrospective study of thirty-two patients with small-cell bronchogenic carcinoma and inappropriate secretion of antidiuretic hormone. *Clin Radiol* 37:47, 1986.
289. North WG, Maurer LH, Valtin H, O'Donnell JF: Human neurophysins as potential tumor markers for small cell carcinoma of the lung: Application of specific radioimmunoassays. *J Clin Endocrinol Metab* 51:892, 1980.
290. Memoli VA, North WG: A monoclonal antibody to human neurophysin recognizes pulmonary neuroendocrine carcinomas. *Lab Invest* 56:50a, 1987.
291. Edwards CRW: Vasopressin and oxytocin in health and disease. *Clin Endocrinol Metab* 6:223, 1977.
292. Baumann G, Lopez-Amor E, Dingman JF: Plasma arginine vasopressin in the syndrome of inappropriate antidiuretic hormone secretion. *Am J Med* 52:19, 1972.
293. Rees LH, Bloomfield GA, Rees GM, Corrin B, Franks LM, Ratcliffe JB: Mutiple hormones in a bronchial tumour. *J Clin Endocrinol Metab* 38:1090, 1974.
294. Pettengill OS, Faulkner CS, Wurster-Hill DH, Maurer LH, Sorenson GD, Robinson AG, Zimmerman EA: Isolation and characterization of a hormone-producing cell line from human small cell anaplastic carcinoma of the lung. *J Natl Cancer Inst* 58:511, 1977.
295. Martin TJ, Greenberg PB, Beck C, Johnston CI: Synthesis of peptide hormones by human tumours in cell culture, in Scow RO (ed): *Endocrinology.* Amsterdam, Excerpta Medica, 1973, p 1198.
296. Yamaji T, Ishibashi M, Katayama S: Nature of the immunoreactive neurophysins in ectopic vasopressin-producing oat cell carcinomas of the lung: Demonstration of a putative common precursor to vasopressin and neurophysin. *J Clin Invest* 68:388, 1981.
297. Sausville E, Carney D, Battey J: The human vasopressin gene is linked to the oxytocin gene and is selectively expressed in a cultured lung cancer cell line. *J Biol Chem* 260:10236, 1985.
298. Padfield PL, Morton JJ, Brown JJ, Lever AF, Robertson JIS, Wood M, Fox R: Plasma arginine vasopressin in the syndrome of antidiuretic hormone excess associated with bronchogenic carcinoma. *Am J Med* 61:825, 1976.
299. Zerbe R, Stropes L, Robertson G: Vasopressin function in the syndrome of inappropriate antidiuresis. *Annu Rev Med* 31:315, 1980.
300. Moses AM, Scheinman SJ: Ectopic secretion of neurohypophyseal peptides in patients with malignancy. *Endocrinol Metab Clin North Am* 20:489, 1991.
301. Kinzie BJ: Management of the syndrome of inappropriate secretion of antidiuretic hormone. *Clin Pharm* 6:625, 1987.
302. Sorensen JB, Kristjansen PEG, Osterlind K, Hammer M, Hansen M: Syndrome of inappropriate antidiuresis in small-cell lung cancer: Classification and effect of tumor regression. *Acta Med Scand* 222:155, 1987.
303. Cogan E, DeBieve MF, Pepersack T, Abramow M: Natriuresis and atrial natriuretic factor secretion during inappropriate antidiuresis. *Am J Med* 84:409, 1988.
304. Kothe MJC, Prins JM, DeWit R, Velden KVD, Schellekens PTA: Small-cell carcinoma of the cervix with inappropriate antidiuretic-hormone secretion: Case report. *Br J Obstet Gynaecol* 97: 647, 1990.
305. Manoogian C, Pandian M, Ehrlich L, Fisher D, Horton R: Plasma atrial natriuretic hormone levels in patients with the syndrome of inappropriate antidiuretic hormone secretion. *J Clin Endocrinol Metab* 67:571, 1988.
306. Shimizu K, Nakano S, Nakano Y, Ando M, Seki K, Kameda N: Ectopic atrial natriuretic peptide production in small cell lung cancer with the syndrome of inappropriate antidiuretic hormone secretion. *Cancer* 68:2284, 1991.

307. Bliss DP Jr, Battey JF, Linnoila RI, Birrer MJ, Gazdar AF, Johnson BE: Expression of the atrial natriuretic factor gene in small cell lung cancer tumors and tumor cell lines. *J Natl Cancer Inst* 82:305, 1990.
308. Hantman D, Rossier B, Zohlman R, Schrier R: Rapid correction of hyponatremia in the syndrome of inappropriate secretion of antidiuretic hormone: An alternative treatment to hypertonic saline. *Ann Intern Med* 78:870, 1973.
309. Ayus JC, Krothapalli RK, Arieff AI: Changing concepts in treatment of severe symptomatic hyponatremia. *Am J Med* 78:897, 1985.
310. Forrest JN Jr, Cox M, Hong C, Morrison G, Bia M, Singer I: Superiority of demeclocycline over lithium in the treatment of chronic syndrome of inappropriate secretion of antidiuretic hormone. *N Engl J Med* 298:173, 1978.
311. Nadler WH, Wolfer JA: Hepatogenic hypoglycemia associated with primary liver cell carcinoma. *Arch Intern Med* 44:700, 1929.
312. Elliott CA: Hepatic hypoglycemia associated with primary liver cell carcinoma. *Trans Assoc Am Physicians* 44:121, 1929.
313. Potter RP: Intrathoracic tumors. *Radiology* 14:60, 1930.
314. Anderson HB: Tumor of adrenal gland with fatal hypoglycemia. *Am J Med Sci* 180:71, 1930.
315. Laurent J, Debry G, Floquet J: *Hypoglycemia Tumors.* Amsterdam, Excerpta Medica, 1971.
316. Skrabanek P, Powell D: Ectopic insulin and Occam's razor: Reappraisal of the riddle of tumour hypoglycaemia. *Clin Endocrinol (Oxf)* 9:141, 1978.
317. Fischer KF, Lees JA, Newman JH: Hypoglycemia in hospitalized patients: Causes and outcomes. *N Engl J Med* 315:1245, 1986.
318. Marks V: Hypoglycaemia: II. Other causes. *Clin Endocrinol Metab* 5:769, 1976.
319. Gorden P, Hendricks CM, Kahn CR, Megyesi K, Roth J: Hypoglycemia associated with non-islet-cell tumor and insulin-like growth factors: A study of the tumor types. *N Engl J Med* 305:1452, 1981.
320. Widmer U, Zapf J, Froesch ER: Is extrapancreatic tumor hypoglycemia associated with elevated levels of insulin-like growth factor II? *J Clin Endocrinol Metab* 55:833, 1982.
321. Anderson N, Lokich JJ: Mesenchymal tumors associated with hypoglycemia: Case report and review of the literature. *Cancer* 44:785, 1979.
322. Edmondson HA, Steiner PE: Primary carcinoma of the liver. *Cancer* 7:462, 1954.
323. McDonald RA: Primary carcinoma of liver: *Arch Intern Med* 99:266, 1957.
324. Anderson IF, Webster AL, Wypkema W: Primary malignant hepatoma associated with hypoglycaemia. *S Afr Med J* 41:505, 1967.
325. McFadzean AJS, Yeung RTT: Further observations on hypoglycemia in hepatocellular carcinoma. *Am J Med* 47:220, 1969.
326. Unger RH: The riddle of tumor hypoglycemia. *Am J Med* 40:325, 1966.
327. Stuart CA, Prince MJ, Peters EJ, Smith FE, Townsend CM III, Poffenbarger PL: Insulin receptor proliferation: A mechanism for tumor-associated hypoglycemia. *J Clin Endocrinol Metab* 63:879, 1986.
328. Butterfield WJH, Kinder CH, Mahler RF: Hypoglycemia associated with sarcoma. *Lancet* 1:703, 1960.
329. Landau BR, Wills N, Craig JW, Leonards JR, Moriwakis A: The mechanism of hepatoma-induced hypoglycemia. *Cancer* 15:1188, 1962.
330. Chung J, Henry RR: Mechanisms of tumor-induced hypoglycemia with intraabdominal hemangiopericytoma. *J Clin Endocrinol Metab* 81:919, 1996.
331. Kahn CR: The riddle of tumour hypoglycaemia revisited. *Clin Endocrinol Metab* 9:335, 1980.
332. Volpe R, Evans J, Clarke DW, Forbath N, Ehrlich R: Evidence favoring the sarcomatous origin of an insulin-like substance in a case of fibrosarcoma with hypoglycemia. *Am J Med* 38:540, 1965.
333. Daughaday WH, Deuel TF: Tumor secretion of growth factors. *Endocrinol Clin North Am* 20:539, 1991.
334. Merimee TJ: Insulin-like growth factors in patients with nonislet cell tumors and hypoglycemia. *Metabolism* 35:360, 1986.
335. Ron D, Powers AC, Pandian MR, Godine JE, Axelrod L: Increased insulin-like growth factor II production and consequent suppression of growth hormone secretion: A dual mechanism for tumor-induced hypoglycemia. *J Clin Endocrinol Metab* 68:701, 1989.
336. Olefesky S, Bailey I, Samols E, Bilkus D: A fibrosarcoma with hypoglycaemia and a high serum-insulin level. *Lancet* 2:378, 1962.
337. Shames JM, Dhurandhar NR, Blackard WG: Insulin-secreting bronchial carcinoid tumor with widespread metastases. *Am J Med* 44:632, 1968.
338. Shetty MR, Boghossian HM, Duffell D, Freel R, Gonzales JC: Tumor-induced hypoglycemia: A result of ectopic insulin production. *Cancer* 49:1920, 1982.
339. Lyall SS, Marieb NJ, Wise JK, Cornog JL, Neville EC, Felig P: Hyperinsulinemic hypoglycemia associated with a neurofibrosarcoma. *Arch Intern Med* 135:865, 1975.
340. Plovnick H, Ruderman NB, Aoki T, Chideckel EW, Poffenbarger PL: Non-β-cell tumor hypoglycemia associated with increased nonsuppressible insulin-like protein (NSILP). *Am J Med* 66:154, 1979.
341. Megyesi K, Kahn CR, Roth J, Gorden P: Hypoglycemia in association with extrapancreatic tumors: Demonstration of elevated plasma NSILA-s by a new radioreceptor assay. *J Clin Endocrinol Metab* 38:931, 1974.
342. Zapf J, Rinderknecht E, Humbel RE, Froesch ER: Nonsuppressible insulin-like activity (NSILA) from human serum: Recent accomplishments and their physiologic implications. *Metabolism* 27:1803, 1978.
343. Daughaday WH, Emanuele MA, Brooks MH, Barbato AL, Kapadia M, Rotwein P: Synthesis and secretion of insulin-like growth factor II by a leiomyosarcoma and associated hypoglycemia. *N Engl J Med* 319:1434, 1988.
344. Shapiro ET, Bell GI, Polonsky KS, Rubenstein AH, Kew MC, Tager HS: Tumor hypoglycemia: Relationship to high molecular weight insulin-like growth factor II. *J Clin Invest* 85:1672, 1990.
345. Daughaday WH, Kapadia M: Significance of abnormal serum binding of insulin-like growth factor II in the development of hypoglycemia in patients with non-islet-cell tumors. *Proc Natl Acad Sci USA* 86:6778, 1989.
346. Daughaday WH, Deuel TF: Tumor secretion of growth factors. *Endo Clin N Amer* 20:539, 1991.
347. Baxter RC: The role of insulin-like growth factors and their binding proteins in tumor hypoglycemia. *Horm Res* 46:195, 1996.
348. Weber MM, Melmed S, Rosenbloom J, Yamasaki H, Prager D: Insulin-like growth factor 2 action in rat somatotrophs is mediated by the insulin-like growth factor I receptor. *Clin Res* 40:24A, 1992.
349. Teale JD, Marks V: Inappropriately elevated plasma insulin-like growth factor II in relation to suppressed insulin-like growth factor I in the diagnosis of non-islet cell tumour hypoglycemia. *Clin Endocrinol (Oxf)* 33:87, 1990.
350. Merimee TJ, Tyson JE: Stabilization of plasma glucose during fasting: Normal variations in two separate studies. *N Engl J Med* 291:1275, 1974.
351. Frizelle FA, Pfiefer MV: Paraneoplastic hypoglycaemia treated with somatostatin analoogue SMS 201-995. *Eur J Surg Oncol* 22:546, 1996.
352. McCance RA: Osteomalacia with Losser's nodes (Milkman's syndrome) due to a raise resistance to vitamin D acquired about the age of 15 years. *Q J Med* 16:33, 1947.
353. Prader VA, Illig R, Vehlinger E, Stalder G: Rachitis infolge Knochentumors. *Helv Paediatr Acta* 14:554, 1959.
354. Nuovo MA, Dorfman HD, Sun CCJ, Chalew SA: Tumor-induced osteomalacia and rickets. *Am J Surg Pathol* 13:588, 1989.
355. Lyles KW, Berry WR, Haussler M, Harrelson JM, Drezner MK: Hypophosphatemic osteomalacia: Association with prostatic carcinoma. *Ann Intern Med* 93:275, 1980.
356. Ryan EA, Reiss E: Oncogenous osteomalacia: Review of the world literature of 42 cases and report to two new cases. *Am J Med* 77:501, 1984.
357. Cotton GE, Van Puffelen P: Hypophosphatemic osteomalacia secondary to neoplasia. *J Bone Joint Surg* 68A:129, 1986.
358. Weidner N, Santa Cruz D: Phosphaturic mesenchymal tumors: A polymorphous group causing osteomalacia or rickets. *Cancer* 59:1442, 1987.
359. Taylor HC, Fallon MD, Velasco ME: Oncogenic osteomalacia and inappropriate antidiuretic hormone secretion due to oat-cell carcinoma. *Ann Intern Med* 101:786, 1984.
360. Stanbury SW: Tumour-associated hypophosphataemic osteomalacia and rickets. *Clin Endocrinol (Oxf)* 1:256, 1972.
361. Sirota JH, Hamerman D: Renal function studies in an adult subject with Fanconi syndrome. *Am J Med* 16:138, 1954.
362. Rico H, Fernandez-Miranda E, Sanz J, Gomez-Castresana F, Escriba A, Hernandez ER, Krsnik I: Oncogenous osteomalacia: A new case secondary to a malignant tumor. *Bone* 7:325, 1986.
363. Hauge BN: Vitamin D resistant osteomalacia. *Acta Med Scand* 153:271, 1956.

364. Weidner N, Bar RS, Weiss D, Strottmann MP: Neoplastic pathology of oncogenic osteomalacia/rickets. *Cancer* 55:1691, 1985.
365. Weider N: Review and update: Oncogenic osteomalacia-rickets. *Ultrastruct Pathol* 15:317, 1991.
366. Drezner MK, Feinglos MN: Osteomalacia due to 1α,25-dihydroxycholecalciferol deficiency: Association with a giant cell tumor of bone. *J Clin Invest* 60:1046, 1977.
367. Parker MS, Klein I, Haussler MR, Mintz DH: Tumor-induced osteomalacia: Evidence of a surgically correctable alteration in vitamin D metabolism. *JAMA* 245:492, 1981.
368. Fukumoto Y, Tarui S, Tsukiyama K, et al: Tumor-induced vitamin D-resistant hypophosphatemic osteomalacia associated with proximal renal tubular dysfunction and 1,25-dihydroxyvitamin D deficiency. *J Clin Endocrinol Metab* 49:873, 1979.
369. Aschinberg LC, Solomon LM, Zeis PM, Justice P, Rosenthal IM: Vitamin D-resistant rickets associated with epidermal nevus syndrome: Demonstration of a phosphaturic substance in the dermal lesions. *J Pediatr* 91:56, 1977.
370. Jefferis AF, Taylor PCA, Walsh-Waring GP: Tumour-associated hypophosphataemic osteomalacia occurring in a patient with an odontogenic tumour of the maxilla. *J Laryngol Otol* 99:1011, 1985.
371. Yoshikawa S, Nakamura T, Takagi M, Imamura T, Okano K, Sasaki S: Benign osteoblastoma as a cause of osteomalacia. *J Bone Joint Surg* 59:279, 1977.
372. Lau K, Stom MC, Goldberg M, Goldfarb S, Gray RW, Lemann J Jr, Agus ZS: Evidence for a humoral phosphaturic factor in oncogenic hypophosphatemic osteomalacia. *Clin Res* 27:421A, 1979.
373. Popovtzer MM: Tumor-induced hypophosphatemic osteomalacia (TUO): Evidence for a phosphaturic cyclic AMP-independent action of tumor extract. *Clin Res* 29:418A, 1981.
374. Lyles KW, Lobaugh B, Paulson DF, Drezner MK: Heterotransplantation of prostatic cancer from an affected patient creates an animal model for tumor-induced osteomalacia (TIO) in the athymic nude mouse. *Calcif Tissue Int* 34:533, 1982.
375. Gitelis S, Ryan WG, Rosenberg AG, Templeton AC: Adult onset hypophosphatemic osteomalacia secondary to neoplasm: A case report and review of the pathophysiology. *J Bone Joint Surg* 68A:134, 1986.
376. Miyauchi A, Fukase M, Tsutsumi M, Fujita T. Hemangiopericytoma-induced osteomalacia: Tumor transplantation in nude mice causes hypophosphatemia and tumor extracts inhibit renal 25-hydroxyvitamin D-1-hydroxylase activity. *J Clin Endocrinol Metab* 67:46, 1988.
377. Cai Q, Hodgson SF, Kao PC, Lennon VA, Klee GG, Zinsmiester AR, Kumar R: Brief report: Inhibition of renal phosphate transport by a tumor product in a patient with oncogenic osteomalacia. *N Engl J Med* 330:1645, 1994.
378. Wilkins, GE, Granleese S, Hegele RG, Holden J, Anderson DW, Bondy GP: Oncogenic osteomalacia: Evidence for a humoral phosphaturic factor. *J Clin Endocrinol Metab* 80:1628, 1995.
379. Nelson AE, Robinson BG, Mason RS: Oncogenic osteomalacia: Is there a new phosphate regulating hormone? *Clin Endocrinol* 47:635, 1997.
380. Siris ES, Clemens TL, Dempster DW, Shane E, Segre GV, Lindsay R, Bilezikian JP: Tumor-induced osteomalacia: Kinetics of calcium, phosphorus, and vitamin D metabolism and characteristics of bone histomorphometry. *Am J Med* 82:307, 1987.
381. Case records of the Massachusetts General Hospital: Case 52–1989. *N Engl J Med* 321:1812, 1989.
382. Steiner H, Dahlback O, Waldenstrom J: Ectopic growth hormone production and osteoarthropathy in carcinoma of the bronchus. *Lancet* 1:783, 1968.
383. Cameron DP, Burger HD, DeKretzer DM, Catt KJ, Best JB: On the presence of immunoreactive growth hormone in a bronchogenic carcinoma. *Aust Ann Med* 18:143, 1969.
384. Greenberg PB, Beck C, Martin TJ, Burger HG: Synthesis and release of human growth hormone from lung carcinoma in cell culture. *Lancet* 1:350, 1972.
385. Beck C, Burger HG: Evidence for the presence of immunoreactive growth hormone in cancers of the lung and stomach. *Cancer* 30:75, 1972.
386. Ghosh L, Ghosh BC, Gupta TKD: Intracellular demonstration of growth hormone in human mammary carcinoma cells. *Am J Surg* 135:215, 1978.
387. Caplan RH, Koob L, Abellera RM, Pagliara AS, Kovacs K, Randall RV: Cure of acromegaly by operative removal of an islet cell tumor of the pancreas. *Am J Med* 64:874, 1978.
388. Frohman LA, Szabo M, Berelowitz M, Stachura ME: Partial purification and characterization of a peptide with growth hormone-releasing activity from extrapituitary tumors in patients with acromegaly. *J Clin Invest* 65:43, 1980.
389. Benjamin F, Casper DJ, Sherman L, Kolodny HD: Growth-hormone secretion in patients with endometrial carcinoma. *N Engl J Med* 281:1448, 1969.
390. Sparagana M, Phillips G, Hoffman C, Kucera L: Ectopic growth hormone syndrome associated with lung cancer. *Metabolism* 20:730, 1971.
391. Oberg K, Norheim I, Wide L: Serum growth hormone in patients with carcinoid tumours: Basal levels and response to glucose and thyrotrophin releasing hormone. *Acta Endocrinol (Copenh)* 109:13, 1985.
392. Altmann HW, Schutz W: Uber ein Knochenhaltiges Bronchuscarcinoid. *Beitr Pathol Anat* 120:455, 1959.
393. Sonksen PH, Ayres AB, Braimbridge M, et al: Acromegaly caused by pulmonary carcinoid tumours. *Clin Endocrinol (Oxf)* 5:503, 1976.
394. Shalet SM, Beardwell CG, MacFarlane IA, Ellison ML, Norman CM, Rees LH, Hughes M: Acromegaly due to production of a growth hormone releasing factor by a bronchial carcinoid tumour. *Clin Endocrinol (Oxf)* 10:61, 1979.
395. Cronin MJ, Rogol AD, Dabney LG, Thorner MO: Selective growth hormone and cyclic AMP stimulating activity is present in a human pancreatic islet cell tumor. *J Clin Endocrinol Metab* 55:381, 1982.
396. Rivier J, Spiess J, Thorner MO, Vale W: Characterization of a growth hormone-releasing factor from a human pancreatic islet tumor. *Nature* 300:276, 1982.
397. Guillemin R, Brazeau P, Bohlen P, Esch F, Ling N, Wehrenberg WB: Growth hormone-releasing factor from a human pancreatic tumor that caused acromegaly. *Science* 218:585, 1982.
398. Scheithauer BW, Carpenter PC, Bloch B, Brazeau P: Ectopic secretion of a growth hormone-releasing factor: Report of a case of acromegaly with bronchial carcinoid tumor. *Am J Med* 76:605, 1984.
399. Frohman LA, Downs TR: Ectopic GRH syndromes, in Robbins RJ, Melmed S (eds): *Acromegaly: A Century of Scientific and Clinical Progress.* New York, Plenum, 1987, pp 115–125.
400. Sano T, Asa SL, Kovacs K: Growth hormone-releasing hormone-producing tumors: Clinical, biochemical, and morphological manifestations. *Endocr Rev* 9:357, 1988.
401. Faglia G, Arosio M, Bazzoni N: Ectopic acromegaly. *Endo Metab Clin N Amer* 21:575, 1992.
402. Losa M, Schopohl J, von Werder K: Ectopic secretion of growth hormone-releasing hormone in man. *J Endocrinol Invest* 16:69, 1993.
403. Schopohl J, Losa M, Frey C, Wolfram G, Huber R, Permanetter W, von Pawel J, Muller OA, von Werder K: Plasma growth hormone (GH)-releasing hormone levels in patients with lung carcinoma. *Clin Endocrinol* 34:463, 1991.
404. Asa Sl, Kovacs K, Thorner MO, Leong DA, Rivier J, Vale W: Immunohistochemical localization of growth hormone-releasing hormone in human tumors. *J Clin Endocrinol Metab* 60:423, 1985.
405. Bostwick DG, Quan R, Hoffman AR, Webber RJ, Chang JK, Bensch KG: Growth hormone-releasing factor immunoreactivity in human endocrine tumors. *Am J Pathol* 117:167, 1984.
406. Christofides ND, Stephanou A, Suzuki H, Yiangou Y, Bloom SR: Distribution of immunoreactive growth hormone-releasing hormone in the human brain and intestine and its production by tumors. *J Clin Endocrinol Metab* 59:747, 1984.
407. Dayal L, Lin HD, Tallberg K, Reichlin S, DeLellis RA, Wolfe HJ: Immunocytochemical demonstration of growth hormone-releasing factor in gastrointestinal and pancreatic endocrine tumors. *Am J Clin Pathol* 85:13, 1986.
408. Thorner MO, Perryman RL, Cronin MJ, et al: Somatotroph hyperplasia: Successful treatment of acromegaly by removal of a pancreatic islet tumor secreting a growth hormone-releasing factor. *J Clin Invest* 70:965, 1982.
409. Aida M, Furukawa Y, Hanyu K, et al: Familial multiple endocrine neoplasia with a pancreatic carcinoid tumor. *J Clin Exp Med* 101:152, 1977.
410. Melmed S: Extrapituitary acromegaly. *Endocrinol Metab Clin North Am* 20:507, 1991.
411. Braunstein GD, Vaitukaitis JL, Carbone PP, Ross GT: Ectopic production of human chorionic gonadotropin by neoplasms. *Ann Intern Med* 78:39, 1973.

412. Braunstein GD, Bridson WE, Glass A, Hull EW, McIntire WR: *In vivo* and *in vitro* production of human chorionic gonadotropin and alpha-fetoprotein by a virilizing hepatoblastoma. *J Clin Endocrinol Metab* 35:857, 1972.
413. Bellet D, Rouas N, Marcillac I, Housseau F, Cottu P, Troalen F, Bidart JM: Free hCGβ and nongonadal neoplasms, in Lustbader JW, Puett D, Ruddon RW (eds): *Glycoprotein Hormones. Structure, Function, and Clinical Implications,* New York, Springer-Verlag, 1994, pp 264–280.
414. Braunstein GD: β-core fragment: Structure, production, metabolism, and clinical utility, in Lustbader JW, Puett D, Ruddon RW (eds): *Glycoprotein Hormones. Structure, Function, and Clinical Implications.* New York, Springer-Verlag, 1994, pp 293–320.
415. Horne CHW, Reid IN, Milne GD: Prognostic significance of inappropriate production of pregnancy proteins by breast cancers. *Lancet* 2:279, 1976.
416. Harach HR, Skinner M, Gibbs AR: Biological markers in human lung carcinoma: An immunopathological study of six antigens. *Thorax* 38:937, 1983.
417. Eiermann W, Brutting G, Prechtel K: Detection of pregnancy specific proteins β1-(SP1) glycoprotein and human placental lactogen in benign breast disease, in Lehmann FG (ed): *Carcino-Embryonic Proteins,* vol II. Amsterdam, Elsevier/North Holland, 1979, pp 477–480.
418. Prechtel K, Eiermann W, Groh M, Brutting G, Hogel B: Ein Beitrag zur Bewertung des Nachweises von schwangerschaftsspezifischen Hormonen (Human placental lactogen and beta-1-glycoprotein) in Brustdrusenexzidaten bei Mastopathie und mammacarcinom. *Pathologe* 4:12, 1983.
419. Muggia FM, Rosen SW, Weintraub BD, Hansen HH: Ectopic placental proteins in nontrophoblastic tumors. *Cancer* 36:1327, 1975.
420. Stanhope CR, Smith JP, Britton JC, Crosley PK: Serial determination of marker substances in ovarian cancer. *Gynecol Oncol* 8:284, 1979.
421. Szymendera JJ, Kaminska JA, Nowacki MP, Szawlowski A, Gadek A: The serum levels of human α-fetoprotein, AFP, choriogonadotropin, hCG, placental lactogen, hPL, and pregnancy-specific β_1-glycoprotein, SP_1, are of no clinical significance in colorectal carcinoma. *Eur J Cancer Clin Oncol* 17:1047, 1981.
422. Hammond D, Winnick S: Paraneoplastic erythrocytosis and ectopic erythropoietins. *Ann NY Acad Sci* 230:219, 1974.
423. Doll DC, Weiss RB: Neoplasia and the erythron. *J Clin Oncol* 3:429, 1985.
424. VanWingerden JJ, VanRensburg PG, Coetzee BP: Malignant fibrous histiocytoma of the parotid gland associated with polycythemia. *Head Neck Surg* 8:218, 1986.
425. Taillan B, Sanderson F, Fuzibet JG, Vinti H, Pesce A, Dujardin P: Polycythemia secondary to hepatic hemangioma with abnormal secretion of erythropoietin. *Am J Med* 87:700, 1989.
426. Bohnen RF, Banisadre M, Gulbrandson RN, Zanjani ED: Erythrocytosis caused by an erythropoietin-producing breast adenocarcinoma. *West J Med* 152:417, 1990.
427. Anagnostou A, Chawla MS, Pololi L, Fried W: Determination of plasma erythropoietin levels: An early marker of tumor activity. *Cancer* 44:1014, 1979.
428. Koeffler HP, Goldwasser E: Erythropoietin radioimmunoassay in evaluating patients with polycythemia. *Ann Intern Med* 94:44, 1981.
429. Shulkin BL, Shapiro B, Sisson JC: Pheochromocytoma, polycythemia, and venous thrombosis. *Am J Med* 83:773, 1987.
430. Nielsen OJ, Jespersen FF, Hilden M: Erythropoietin-induced secondary polycythemia in a patient with a renal cell carcinoma: A case report. *APMIS (Copenh)* 96:688, 1988.
431. Rigatti P, Montorsi F, Guazzoni G, Viale G, Bulfamante G, Coggi G: Adult nephroblastoma induced erythrocytosis: Report of a case and review of the literature. *Scand J Urol Nephrol* 24:159, 1990.
432. DaSilva JL, Lacombe C, Bruneval P, et al: Tumor cells are the site of erythropoietin synthesis in human renal cancers associated with polycythemia. *Blood* 75:577, 1990.
433. Thorling EB: Paraneoplastic erythrocytosis and inappropriate erythropoietin production. *Scand J Hematol* [*Suppl*] 17:1, 1972.
434. Hwang SJ, Lee SD, Wu JC, Chang CF, Lu CL, Tsay SH, Lo KJ: Clinical evaluation of erythrocytosis in patients with hepatocellular carcinoma. *Chin Med J (Taipei)* 53:262, 1994.
435. Kew MC, Fisher JW: Serum erythropoietin concentrations in patients with hepatocellular carcinoma. *Cancer* 58:2485, 1986.
436. Ljungberg B, Rasmuson T, Grankvist K: Erythropoietin in renal cell carcinoma: Evaluation of its usefulness as a tumor marker. *Eur Urol* 21:160, 1992.
437. Gross AJ, Wolff M, Fandrey J, Miersch WD, Dieckmann, KP, Jelkmann W: Prevalence of paraneoplastic erythropoietin production by renal cell carcinomas. *Clin Invest* 72:337, 1994.
438. Sherwood JB, Goldwasser E: Erythropoietin production by human renal carcinoma cells in culture. *Endocrinology* 99:504, 1976.
439. Sytkowski AJ, Richie WR, Bicknell KA: New human renal carcinoma cell line established from a patient with erythrocytosis. *Cancer Res* 43:1415, 1983.
440. Sytkowski AJ, Bicknell KA, Smith GM, Garcia JF: Secretion of erythropoietin-like activity by clones of human renal carcinoma cell line GKA. *Cancer Res* 44:51, 1984.
441. Waldmann TA, Rosse WF: Tumors producing erythropoiesis-stimulating factors, in Sundermann FW, Sundermann FW Jr (eds): *Hemoglobin: Its Precursors and Metabolism.* Philadelphia, Lippincott, 1964, pp 276–280.
442. Milhaud G, Calmette C, Raymond JP, Bignon J, Moukhtar MS: Carcinoid secretant de la thyrocalcitonin. *Compte Rendu Hebdomadaire des Séances de l'Academie des Sciences,* Series D, 270:2192, 1970.
443. Milhaud G, Calmette C, Taboulet J, Julienne A, Moukhtar MS: Hypersecretion of calcitonin in neoplastic conditions. *Lancet* 1:462, 1974.
444. Coombes RC, Hillyard C, Greenberg PB, MacIntyre I: Plasma-immunoreactive-calcitonin in patients with non-thyroid tumours. *Lancet* 1:1080, 1974.
445. Coombes RC, Ellison ML, Easty GC, Hillyard CJ, James R, Galante L, Girgis S, Heywood L, et al: The ectopic secretion of calcitonin by lung and breast carcinomas. *Clin Endocrinol (Oxf)* 5:387s, 1976.
446. Silva OL, Becker KL, Primack A, Doppman JL, Snider RH: Increased serum calcitonin levels in bronchogenic cancer. *Chest* 69:495, 1976.
447. Hansen M, Hansen HH, Tryding N: Small cell carcinoma of the lung: Serum calcitonin and serum histaminase (diamine oxidase) at basal levels and stimulated by pentagastrin. *Acta Med Scand* 204:257, 1978.
448. Mulder H, Hackeng WHL: Ectopic secretion of calcitonin. *Acta Med Scand* 204:253, 1978.
449. Schwartz KE, Wolfsen AR, Forster B, Odell WD: Calcitonin in nonthyroidal cancer. *J Clin Endocrinol Metab* 49:438, 1979.
450. Silva OL, Broder LE, Doppman JL, Snider RH, Moore CF, Cohen MH, Becker KL: Calcitonin as a marker for bronchogenic cancer: A prospective study. *Cancer* 44:680, 1979.
451. Hillyard CJ, Oscier DG, Foa R, Catovsky D, Goldman JM: Immunoreactive calcitonin in leukaemia. *Br Med J* 2:1392, 1979.
452. Becker KL, Nash DR, Silva OL, Snider RH, Moore CF: Urine calcitonin levels in patients with bronchogenic carcinoma. *JAMA* 243:670, 1980.
453. Mulder H, Silberbusch J, Hackeng WHL, VanDerMeer C, DenOttolander GJH: Hypercalcitoninaemia in patients with chronic inflammatory disease. *Neth J Med* 23:129, 1980.
454. Samaan NA, Castillo S, Schultz PN, Khalil KG, Johnston DA: Serum calcitonin after pentagastrin stimulation in patients with bronchogenic and breast cancer compared to that in patients with medullary thyroid carcinoma. *J Clin Endocrinol Metab* 51:237, 1980.
455. Abe K, Adachi I, Miyakawa S, Tanaka M, Yamaguchi K, Tanaka N, Kameya T, Shimosato Y: Production of calcitonin, adrenocorticotropic hormone, and β-melanocyte-stimulating hormone in tumors derived from amine precursor uptake and decarboxylation cells. *Cancer Res* 37:4190, 1977.
456. Becker KL, Snider RH, Moore CF, Monaghan KG, Silva OL: Calcitonin in extrathyroidal tissues of man. *Acta Endocrinol (Copenh)* 92:746, 1979.
457. Becker KL, Monaghan KG, Silva OL: Immunocytochemical localization of calcitonin in Kulchitsky cells of human lung. *Arch Pathol Lab Med* 104:196, 1980.
458. Silva OL, Becker KL, Primack A, Doppman JL, Snider RH: Hypercalcitonemia in bronchogenic cancer: Evidence for thyroid origin of the hormone. *JAMA* 234:183, 1975.
459. Roos BA, Lindall AW, Baylin SB, O'Neil JA, Frelinger AL, Birnbaum RS, Lambert PW: Plasma immunoreactive calcitonin in lung cancer. *J Clin Endocrinol Metab* 50:659, 1980.

460. Ellison M, Woodhouse D, Hillyard C, Dowsett M, Coombes RC, Gilby ED, Greenberg PB, Neville AM: Immunoreactive calcitonin production by human lung carcinoma cells in culture. *Br J Cancer* 32:3731, 1975.
461. Zajac JD, Martin TJ, Hudson P, Niall H, Jacobs JW: Biosynthesis of calcitonin by human lung cancer cells. *Endocrinology* 116:749, 1985.
462. Lumsden J, Ham J, Ellison ML: Purification and partial characterization of high-molecular-weight forms of ectopic calcitonin from a human bronchial carcinoma cell line. *Biochem J* 191:239, 1980.
463. Bertagna XY, Nicholson WE, Pettengill OS, Sorenson GD, Mount CD, Orth DN: Ectopic production of high molecular weight calcitonin and corticotropin by human small cell carcinoma cells in tissue culture: Evidence for separate precursors. *J Clin Endocrinol Metab* 47:1390, 1978.
464. Nelkin BD, Rosenfeld KI, deBustros A, Leong SS, Roos BA, Baylin SB: Structure and expression of a gene encoding human calcitonin and calcitonin gene related peptide. *Biochem Biophys Res Commun* 123:648, 1984.
465. Mulder H: Ectopic secretion of calcitonin as a tumor marker. *Anticancer Res* 3:247, 1983.
466. Turkington RW: Ectopic production of prolactin. *N Engl J Med* 285:1455, 1971.
467. Davis S, Proper S, May PB, Ertel NH: Elevated prolactin levels in bronchogenic carcinoma. *Cancer* 44:676, 1979.
468. Molitch ME, Schwartz S, Mukherji B: Is prolactin secreted ectopically? *Am J Med* 70:803, 1981.
469. Hsu CT, Yu MH, Lee CYG, Jong HL, Yeh MY: Ectopic production of prolactin in uterine cervical carcinoma. *Gynecol Oncol* 44:166, 1992.
470. Podmore J, Wilson B, Cowden EA, Beastall GH, Ratcliffe JG: Multiple hormones in human tumors, in Lehman GF (ed): *Carcino-Embryonic Proteins*, vol 1. New York, Elsevier/North Holland, 1979, pp 457–463.
471. Rosen SW, Weintraub BD, Aaronson SA: Non random ectopic protein production by malignant cells: Direct evidence in vitro. *J Clin Endocrinol Metab* 50:834, 1980.
472. Ginsburg E, Vonderhaar BK: Prolactin synthesis and secretion by human breast cancer cells. *Cancer Res* 55:2591, 1995.
473. Said SI, Faloona GR: Elevated plasma and tissue levels of vasoactive intestinal polypeptide in the watery-diarrhea syndrome due to pancreatic bronchogenic and other tumors. *N Engl J Med* 293:155, 1975.
474. Hamilton I, Reis L, Bilimoria S, Long RG: A renal vipoma. *Br Med J* 281:1323, 1980.
475. Mendelsohn G, Eggleston JC, Olson JL, Said SI, Baylin SB: Vasoactive intestinal peptide and its relationship to ganglion cell differentiation in neuroblastic tumors. *Lab Invest* 41:144, 1979.
476. Cooney DR, Voorhess ML, Fisher JE, Brecher M, Karp MP, Jewett TC: Vasoactive intestinal peptide producing neuroblastoma. *J Pediatr Surg* 17:821, 1982.
477. Maton PN, O'Dorisio TM, Howe BA, et al: Effect of a long-acting somatostatin analogue (SMS 201-995) in a patient with pancreatic cholera. *N Engl J Med* 312:17, 1985.
478. Penman E, Wass JAH, Besser GM, Rees LH: Somatostatin secretion by lung and thymic tumours. *Clin Endocrinol (Oxf)* 13:613, 1980.
479. Szabo M, Berelowitz M, Pettengill OS, Sorenson GD, Frohman LA: Ectopic production of somatostatin-like immuno- and bioactivity by cultured human pulmonary small cell carcinoma. *J Clin Endocrinol Metab* 51:978, 1980.
480. Long TT III, Barton TK, Draffin R, Reeves WJ, McCarty KS Jr: Conservative management of Zollinger-Ellison syndrome: Ectopic gastrin production by an ovarian cystadenoma. *JAMA* 243:1837, 1980.
481. Margolis RM, Jang N: Zollinger-Ellison syndrome associated with pancreatic cystadenocarcinoma. *N Engl J Med* 311:1380, 1984.
482. Gleeson MH, Bloom SR, Polak JM, Henry K, Dowling RH: Endocrine tumour in kidney affecting small bowel structure, motility, and absorptive function. *Gut* 12:773, 1971.
483. Hunstein W, Trumper LH, Dummer R, Schwechheimer K: Glucagonoma syndrome and bronchial carcinoma. *Ann Intern Med* 109:920, 1988.
484. Sakura H, Hamada Y, Tsuruta S, Okamoto K, Nakamura S: Large glucagon-like immunoreactivity in a primary ovarian carcinoid. *Cancer* 55:1001, 1985.
485. Price J, Nieuwenhuijzen-Kruseman AC, Doniach I, Howlett TA, Besser GM, Rees LH: Bombesin-like peptides in human endocrine tumors: Quantitation, biochemical characterization, and secretion. *J Clin Endocrinol Metab* 60:1097, 1985.
486. Ganguly A, Gribble J, Tune B, Kempson RL, Luetscher JA: Renin-secreting Wilms' tumor with severe hypertension: Report of a case and brief review of renin-secreting tumors. *Ann Intern Med* 79:835, 1973.
487. Mitchell JD, Baxter TJ, Blair-West JR, McCredie DA: Renin levels in nephroblastoma (Wilms' tumour): Report of a renin secreting tumour. *Arch Dis Child* 45:376, 1970.
488. Sheth KJ, Tang TT, Blaedel ME, Good TA: Polydipsia, polyuria, and hypertension associated with renin-secreting Wilms' tumor. *J Pediatr* 92:921, 1978.
489. Spahr J, Demers LM, Shochat SJ: Renin producing Wilms' tumor. *J Pediatr Surg* 16:32, 1981.
490. Kihara I, Kitamura S, Hashimo T, Seida H, Watanabe T: A hitherto unreported vascular tumor of the kidney: A proposal of juxtaglomerular cell tumor. *Acta Pathol Jpn* 18:197, 1968.
491. Hollifield JW, Page DL, Smith C, Michelakis AM, Staab E, Rhamy R: Renin-secreting clear cell carcinoma of the kidney. *Arch Intern Med* 135:859, 1975.
492. Ruddy MC, Atlas SA, Salerno FG: Hypertension associated with a renin-secreting adenocarcinoma of the pancreas. *N Engl J Med* 307:993, 1982.
493. Hauger-Klevene JH: High plasma renin activity in an oat cell carcinoma: A renin-secreting carcinoma? *Cancer* 26:1112, 1970.
494. Aurell M, Rudin A, Tisell LE, Kindblom LG, Sandberg G: Captopril effect on hypertension in patient with renin-producing tumour. *Lancet* 2:149, 1979.
495. Atlas SA, Hesson TE, Sealey JE, Dharmgrongartama B, Laragh JH, Ruddy MC, Aurell M: Characterization of inactive renin ("Prorenin") from renin-secreting tumors of nonrenal origin: Similarity to inactive renin from kidney and normal plasma. *J Clin Invest* 73:437, 1984.
496. Wulf GG, Jahns-Streubel G, Strutz F, Basenau D, Hufner M, Buske C, Wormann B, Hiddemann W: Paraneoplastic hypokalemia in acute myeloid leukemia: A case of renin activity in AML blast cells. *Ann Hematol* 73:139, 1996.
497. Fried G, Wikstrom LM, Hoog A, Arver S, Cedermark B, Hamberger B, Grimelius L, Meister B: Multiple neuropeptide immunoreactivities in a renin-producing human paraganglioma. *Cancer* 74:142, 1994.

CHAPTER 29

Hormone-Responsive Tumors

Andrea Manni

Steroid and polypeptide hormones stimulate the growth of a large variety of target tissues either directly or through the elaboration of growth factors acting in an intracrine, autocrine, or paracrine fashion. Hormones are also known to exert a profound influence on differentiation as well as the expression and activity of several genes controlling programmed cell death or apoptosis. Preservation of a normal phenotype is highly dependent upon the maintenance of a delicate balance between proliferative, differentiated, and apoptotic events. Whenever, as a result of genetic aberrations and epigenetic events, these highly regulated processes are disrupted in favor of uncontrolled tissue growth, carcinogenesis will occur. If the cellular mechanisms underlying autonomous tissue growth are linked to the growth-promoting effects of hormones, the clinical result is a hormone-responsive tumor.

Hormonally responsive tumors are quite prevalent. They account for 20 percent of all newly diagnosed male cancers and 40 percent of all newly diagnosed female cancers and are best represented by breast, endometrial, and prostate adenocarcinomas. These three particular forms of cancer arise in the target organs that are most responsive to the growth regulatory influences of estrogens, progestins, and androgens. The early observations of Bitter, Huggins, Furth, and others first established the association between sex steroids and these target gland tumors.[1–6] The early theory that hormones influence the growth of some human cancers has been extended by Henderson and colleagues[7] who have suggested that sex steroids play a pathogenic role in about 30 percent of all human cancers in the United States.

In addition to breast, endometrial, and prostate cancer, well-differentiated thyroid cancers (i.e., papillary, follicular, and mixed papillary-follicular tumors) are truly hormone-responsive neoplasms (Table 29-1). Their dependency on TSH is well documented and is exploited both diagnostically when performing a total body scan and therapeutically with radioactive iodine treatment and administration of suppressive doses of thyroid hormones. Table 29-1 also provides a noninclusive list of tumors variously linked to the endocrine system but without a rigorous demonstration of true hormone dependency. Some of these (e.g., melanomas and meningiomas) manifest a marked discrepancy in male–female incidence and prognosis and occasionally possess steroid receptors, thus suggesting the possibility of hormonally regulated growth.[8] Glucocorticoids have been shown to induce cytolytic effects in the treatment of leukemia and lymphomas.[9,10] Thus, some clinicians consider these hematologic malignancies to be hormonally responsive. Epidemiologic data indicate that 10 years of oral contraceptive use can reduce the risk of developing ovarian cancer by about 50 percent,[11] yet mechanisms directly linking hormones with the growth control of ovarian cancer have not been firmly established. Both pancreatic cancers and melanomas have been shown at times to possess estrogen receptors.[12,13] While controlled trials have demonstrated minimal benefit from tamoxifen therapy in pancreatic cancer,[14,15] a randomized trial has shown significant prolongation of survival with the addition of tamoxifen to chemotherapy in patients with melanoma.[16] Finally, experimental models of pancreatic cancer have been shown to be growth inhibited by the administration of an LHRH superagonist.[17] However, there is no evidence at present that this therapy is beneficial in humans.

This chapter will focus on hormonal issues related to sex-steroid–responsive breast, endometrial, and prostate cancers. Among these, breast cancer will be discussed in the greatest detail because it is the most extensively studied tumor at the basic level. Therefore, it provides a rich source of examples to illustrate concepts that are likely to be applicable to other hormone-responsive tumors.

HORMONAL INFLUENCE ON NORMAL BREAST DEVELOPMENT AND MAMMARY CARCINOGENESIS

Postnatal growth of the mammary gland can be divided into two major phases; ductal growth that is initiated with puberty and alveolar differentiation which occurs during pregnancy. Estrogen,[18] possibly in concert with growth hormone,[19] is the principal hormone stimulating ductal growth that leads to ductal elongation and branching and the formation of the immature structures called type I terminal duct lobular units (TDLUs). Evidence supporting the effect of estrogen is provided by the presence of the estrogen receptor in ductal epithelium[20] and the observation that local implants of antiestrogens block ductal growth during puberty.[21] In addition, transgenic mice lacking the expression of the estrogen receptor gene demonstrate only rudimentary ductal growth.[22] In the human breast, the type I TDLUs are the least differentiated structures with the highest proliferative capacity.[23,24] In addition, they are the most common sites of breast cancer development in women. Collectively, these data indicate that estrogen-induced proliferation of these ductal structures makes them highly susceptible to transformation.

Considerable evidence points to the importance of local estrogen production in the process of mammary carcinogenesis. The finding of high tumor estrogen concentrations has been felt to reflect, at least in part, the in situ estradiol production from plasma estrogen precursors.[25,26] In support of this contention, numerous studies have, indeed, demonstrated aromatase expression in

TABLE 29-1. Classification of Hormone Responsive Tumors

	Hormone Dependency		
	Sex Steroids	**Glucocorticoids**	**Polypeptides**
Proven hormone responsive			
Breast cancer	×		
Endometrial cancer	×		
Prostate cancer	×		
Thyroid cancer			×
Putative hormone responsive			
Leukemia/lymphoma		×	
Ovarian cancer	×		×
Renal cell carcinoma	×		
Melanoma	×		
Pancreatic cancer	×		×
Vaginal cancer	×		
Meningiomas	×		

malignant breast tissues, although no consensus has yet been reached regarding the relative importance of stromal versus tumor epithelial sources of the enzyme.[27–29] Particularly relevant to the role of aromatase in mammary carcinogenesis is the report by Bulun et al.,[30] who measured aromatase in benign breast tissue obtained from women without breast cancer. These investigators observed that the highest aromatase transcript levels were detected in the upper outer quadrant of the breast, the region in which breast tumors most commonly develop. Finally, aromatase transgenic mice models have shown that overexpression of this estrogen biosynthetic enzyme leads to the development of various preneoplastic histopathologic changes.[31] Furthermore, in response to carcinogen administration such as DMBA, these transgenic animals almost uniformly develop breast neoplasms compared with the absence of neoplastic changes observed in nontransgenic wild-type mice.[32]

Two general but not exclusive mechanisms have been proposed for explaining estrogen-induced neoplasia. The first involves receptor-mediated nongenotoxic promoting effects. In this case, physiologic concentrations of estradiol bind to the estrogen receptor, enhance the mitotic rate, and in this manner increase the number of genetic mutations expected. The second mechanism, on the other hand, involves a direct nonreceptor-mediated genotoxic action. Estradiol is metabolically transformed to catecholestrogens and quinones that directly or indirectly may cause DNA damage and resultant mutations. This mechanism could take place at concentrations similar to those required for receptor binding but would be expected to be augmented with increasing estradiol concentrations in tissue. It is conceivable that the two mechanisms could work in an additive or synergistic fashion because DNA damage induced by a direct genotoxic action would be expected to be more harmful in rapidly growing cells due to inadequate DNA repair mechanisms.

The role of progesterone in breast cell proliferation still remains somewhat controversial. Although the antiestrogenic activity of progesterone is well documented for the endometrium,[33,34] fewer data are available regarding the human mammary gland. A few studies have shown a higher mitotic activity of epithelial cells in the luteal phase of normally cycling women than in the early follicular phase.[35,36] These results have been interpreted as evidence supporting a role of progesterone in the promotion of breast epithelial cell mitosis that could have carcinogenic implications. This interpretation, however, is not shared by other investigators. Also, local application of progesterone to women undergoing surgery for benign breast disease was found to decrease the mitotic activity of the normal lobular epithelial cells.[37,38] In contrast, estradiol treatment produced the expected stimulatory effect on mitosis. Studies conducted in cultures of normal human breast cells have shown that progesterone has an antiproliferative and antiestrogenic effect.[39] The antiestrogenic action of progesterone is mediated by its ability to decrease the estrogen receptor level[40] and to stimulate the enzyme 17-beta-hydroxysteroid-dehydrogenase that converts estradiol, the active estrogen, into estrone, its less active metabolite.[41] On the other hand, it should be noted that, in a variety of experimental breast cancer models in culture, progestins have been found to have both proliferative and antiproliferative effects.[42–45] Although the influence of progesterone on breast cell proliferation is not totally defined, its role in alveolar differentiation is well-established. Progesterone plays a clear role in the development of alveolar buds, which begins at the time of puberty. It appears that alveolar differentiation requires the coordinated action of estradiol, prolactin, and progesterone.[18] Estrogen controls alveolar development indirectly by stimulating prolactin secretion from the pituitary and inducing progesterone receptor synthesis. The essential role of progesterone receptors for alveolar development is demonstrated in mice carrying a null mutation for this gene, which have severely reduced alveolar development.[46,48] Of interest, mice carrying a deletion in the prolactin receptor gene have a similar phenotype.[48] This differentiating effect of progesterone has been shown to have a protective effect on experimentally induced mammary carcinogenesis by either chemical carcinogens and radiation.[49] These observations have raised concerns that an unopposed estrogen effect due to a defect in progesterone secretion during the luteal phase might be a promoting factor in human breast cancer development.

Role of Growth Factors and Stromal/Epithelial Interactions

Normal mammary epithelial growth is dependent on the local production of peptide growth factors. Modern techniques of genetic manipulations in transgenic mice have provided direct evidence supporting the role of these growth factors in normal breast physiology. EGF and TGF-α, which signal through the same receptor, are positive effectors of both ductal and alveolar growth.[50,51] Transgenic mice carrying a point mutation in the kinase domain of the EGF receptor have defects both in ductal growth and alveolar development during pregnancy.[52] In contrast, TGF-β isoforms have consistently been found to have antiproliferative actions.[53] Transgenic mice overexpressing TGF-β1 under the control of the whey acidic protein promoter failed to develop alveoli and lobules during pregnancy.[54] The FGF growth factor family also appears to have a prominent role in alveolar development. Transgenic mice carrying the dominant negative form of the FGF-R2 receptor have significant deficits in lobular alveolar development.[55] Finally, insulin-like growth factors and the type I IGF receptor have been shown to be highly expressed in mammary epithelium and exert a positive effect on both ductal and alveolar growth.[56,57] In addition, the IGFs may also play an important role in mammary epithelial cell survival by blocking involution of the mammary gland.[58] The effects of IGF-I and IGF-II are likely to be strongly influenced by the different IGF binding proteins, which have been shown to be variably expressed in the mammary epithelium and stroma.[59] The biological role of these binding proteins, however, still remains to be elucidated.

Within the context of growth factor regulation of normal breast physiology, it is important to emphasize the critical role of stromal epithelial interactions in normal breast function and mammary carcinogenesis. Although malignant transformation occurs within the epithelial elements of the breast, no breast cancer would become clinically significant without interaction with the surrounding stroma. The extracellular matrix produced by breast stromal cells provides more than a simple passive scaffolding for epithelial cells. Early experiments in rodents emphasized the importance of the interaction with a specific breast stromal matrix for normal mammary epithelium development.[60] Subsequent coculture experiments have demonstrated that mammary epithelial cells undergo significant morphologic and functional differentiation when grown in contact with the appropriate matrix.[61] Clearly, stromal epithelial interactions are altered in breast cancer. When cultured on an artificial extracellular matrix construct, malignant breast epithelium loses most of the differentiation responses to extracellular matrix components that characterize normal breast epithelium.[62] Furthermore, strong evidence suggests that distinct populations of fibroblasts exist in normal as opposed to malignant breasts. Fibroblasts isolated from the stroma of breast cancer specimens manifest fetal-like features as opposed to fibroblasts surrounding normal breast epithelium. This consists of the coexpression of IGF-II instead of IGF-I and stromelysin-3, a protease which is absent in the stroma surrounding normal mammary epithelium.[63,64] These data provide strong evidence supporting a tumor specific stromal cell phenotype in breast cancer.

The role of androgens is well-established in prostatic development as well as in function and proliferation of normal and malignant prostatic tissue. As in the case of estrogens in the breast, it is now recognized that many of the androgenic actions in the prostate are mediated through the elaboration of polypeptide growth factors acting in an autocrine/paracrine fashion (for review, see Reference 65). As an example, it has been shown in the developing rat prostate that the proliferative effect of testosterone could be abolished by an antibody against keratinocyte growth factor (KGF) and that KGF administration was able to mimic the effect of testosterone.[66] Similarly, TGF-β, which is negatively regulated by androgens, has been shown to be responsible for the massive apoptosis in the prostate induced by androgen deprivation.[67] Additional growth factors possibly involved in the mediation of androgen action in the prostate include EGF,[68] TGF-α,[69] IGFs,[70] fibroblast growth factors,[71] and nerve growth factors.[72] Elegant tissue recombination experiments have shown that stromal epithelial interactions, under the control of androgens, play a fundamental role in prostatic development, function of the adult normal prostate, and prostatic carcinogenesis (summarized in Reference 73). According to this concept, androgens act upon androgen receptor-positive prostatic smooth muscle cells to induce development, growth, and maintenance of differentiation in adulthood. Through paracrine mechanisms, smooth muscle acting under the influence of androgens maintains prostatic epithelial structure and function, while prostatic epithelium in turn maintains smooth muscle differentiation. Thus, complex reciprocal smooth muscle-epithelial cell interactions, mediated by the local synthesis of paracrine factors under the influence of androgens, play a critical role in the development and function of the normal prostate. Sequential disruption in these reciprocal homeostatic interactions between the epithelium and the stroma are considered to be important in prostatic carcinogenesis. It is postulated that as a result of genetic damage to prostate epithelium, this cellular compartment loses its normal phenotype and sends aberrant signaling to smooth muscle. As a result, prostatic smooth muscle cells begin to dedifferentiate, resulting in abnormal smooth muscle to epithelial signaling. The result is a vicious cycle of sequential loss of differentiation in both epithelial and smooth muscle compartments leading to the promotion and progression of prostate cancer. This hypothesis is supported by several observations which have been summarized in a recent review.[73] This hypothesis also emphasizes the concept of "tumor stroma" as an essential component of the carcinogenic process similar to that discussed earlier for breast cancer.

Genetic Changes in Hormone-Responsive Tumors

Hereditary Tumors

Five to 10 percent of human breast cancers are hereditary. Of these, a still undefined fraction can be accounted for by mutations in the two recently identified susceptibility genes, BRCA1 and BRCA2. BRCA1, mapped to chromosome 17q21, contains 22 exons and encodes a protein of 1,863 amino acids. BRCA2, linked to chromosome 13q12-13, is an even larger gene composed of 27 exons that encode a protein of 3,418 amino acids. The normal function of these two tumor suppressor genes remains to be fully elucidated. Their expression is coordinately regulated and cell-cycle dependent, suggesting that they may function in overlapping regulatory pathways involved in the control of cell proliferation and differentiation.[74] Both BRCA1 and BRCA2 have been found to interact physically with Rad51, which implies a role for these genes in DNA repair.[75,76] One hundred and thirty-two distinct mutations of BRCA1 have been identified throughout the gene. Most of them produce truncated proteins varying in length from 5 percent to 99 percent of the complete protein. Similarly, all the mutations found in BRCA2 cause premature termination of the encoded protein and are distributed evenly throughout the gene. Women who inherit a mutated copy of either gene have a similarly high risk of developing breast cancer, which has been estimated up to 85 percent by age 70 years.[77,78] However, as more population-based studies emerge, the actual risk may be significantly lower. An important issue that needs to be addressed with regard to the penetrance of these mutations is the interaction of BRCA mutations with other known risk factors for breast cancer. BRCA1 is also associated with an increased risk of ovarian cancer, which has been estimated to range between 26 percent and 85 percent by age 70 years.[77–80] The risk of prostate cancer is estimated to be threefold higher in male mutation carriers,[79] while the risk of colon cancer is fourfold higher in both male and female mutation carriers.[79] Mutations in the BRCA2 gene have been associated with a much lower risk of ovarian cancer (<10 percent by age 70 years) but with an increased risk of male breast cancer.[78]

Initial studies performed in families with large numbers of breast and ovarian cancers indicated that nearly half of the tumors were due to BRCA1 mutations.[80] More recent studies performed in less selected but still high-risk families (≥3 cases of breast and/or ovarian cancer) indicated that the prevalence of BRCA1 mutations was between 12.8 percent and 16 percent.[81,82] Much lower prevalence was reported in recent population-based series of women unselected for family history with a diagnosis of breast cancer before age 35 years (6.2 percent) and women with breast cancer before age 45 who had at least a mother or sister with breast cancer (7.2 percent).[83] Overall, these and other studies point to a number of characteristics that are helpful in predicting the presence of a BRCA1 mutation. They include early age of diagnosis, increased number of relatives with ovarian cancer or both breast and ovarian cancer, Ashkenazi ancestry, and a total of four or more relatives with breast cancer.[81–84] The commercial introduction of genetic testing for cancer predisposition has raised a number of issues that are only beginning to be addressed. One must weigh the potential benefits of BRCA1 and BRCA2 testing against several limitations and possible risks. They include still undefined cancer risk figures, the absence of proven chemopreventive strategies in carriers, the possibility of discrimination in employment or in obtaining insurance, and the potential for adverse psychological effects of learning the results. Because of all of these concerns, current guidelines indicate that genetic testing should be provided only as part of a carefully monitored research protocol that includes pretest education and genetic counseling. A recent study conducted in high-risk families following these guidelines has found no adverse psychological effects from genetic testing for BRCA1 and actually demonstrated a statistically significant benefit for noncarriers.[85] Recently, a task force of the Cancer Genetics Studies Consortium (CGSC) sponsored by the National Human Genome Research Institute convened to identify appropriate follow-up for individuals found to be carriers of BRCA1 and BRCA2 mutations.[86] These are provided in Table 29-2. As can be seen, these recommendations are tentative in the absence of solid information and are likely to be modified as more pertinent data become available.

A fraction of hereditary breast cancers is not due to mutations of the BRCA1 and BRCA2 genes. A number of rare hereditary diseases have been found to be associated with an increased risk of breast cancer. The clinical manifestations, genetic mutation and mode of inheritance of these conditions are summarized in Table 29-3.

TABLE 29-2. Options for Surveillance for Carriers of BRCA1 and BRCA2 Mutations

Intervention	Provisional Recommendation	Quality of Evidence*	Cautionary Issues
Breast cancer			
Breast self-examination	Education regarding monthly self-examination	III Expert opinion only	Benefit not proven
Clinician breast examination	Annually or semi-annually, beginning at age 25–35 yr	III Expert opinion only	Benefit not proven
Mammography	Annually, beginning at age 25–35 yr	III Expert opinion only (I Randomized trial, average-risk women aged 50–69 yr)	Risks and benefits not established for women under age 50 yr
Ovarian cancer Transvaginal ultrasound with color Doppler and CA-125 level	Annually or semi-annually, beginning at age 25–35 yr	III Expert opinion only	Benefit not proven; level of ovarian cancer risk estimated to be lower in BRCA2 mutation carriers
Prostate cancer Prostate cancer surveillance (BRCA1 mutation carriers only)	Inform regarding options for screening involving rectal examination and prostate-specific antigen level, annually, beginning at age 50 yr	III Expert opinion only	Benefit not proven; many agencies do not recommend screening due to uncertainty of benefit from early detection
Colon cancer Colon cancer surveillance	Follow recommendations for general population: fecal occult blood test annually and flexible sigmoidoscopy every 3–5 yr, beginning at age 50 yr	Evidence from average risk populations: I randomized trial (fecal occult blood test); II-2 case control study (sigmoidoscopy)	Relevance of population-based data uncertain

*I = highest quality (randomized controlled trials); II = intermediate quality (nonrandomized trials and observational studies [II-2 indicates case-control study]); and III = lowest quality (expert opinion and case reports).

Source: Reproduced with permission from Burke W., et al.[86]

TABLE 29-3. Rare Genetic Conditions Associated with Increased Breast Cancer Risk

Condition	Clinical Manifestations	Genetic Mutation	Mode of Inheritance
Li-Fraumeni syndrome	Breast cancer, sarcoma, brain tumors, leukemia, adrenocortical carcinoma	p53	Autosomal dominant
Cowden's disease	Multiple mucocutaneous lesions, vitiligo, angiomas, benign proliferative disease of multiple organ systems, breast cancer, thyroid cancer, colonic neoplasms	PTEN	Autosomal dominant
Muir-Torre syndrome	Cancers of the GI tract, skin, and GU system; and breast benign and malignant tumors	MSH2 MLH1	Autosomal dominant
Peutz-Jeghers syndrome	Abnormal melanin deposits, GI polyposis, cancers of the GI tract, breast, uterus, ovary and testis	Unknown	Autosomal dominant
Ataxia-telangiectasia	Cerebellar ataxia, oculocutaneous telangiectasias, radiation hypersensitivity, leukemia, lymphoma, and numerous solid tumors, including breast	ATM	Autosomal recessive

Source: Adapted from Hoskins KF, et al.[87]

Several studies have indicated a familial clustering for prostate cancer. An increased risk for developing this tumor has consistently been observed in members of families containing probands. A distinct true hereditary form of prostate cancer has also been identified using segregation analysis.[88,89] This is a rare disorder that accounts for approximately 9 percent of all prostate cancer. It follows a dominant Mendelian form of inheritance with high penetrance. The criteria for diagnosis are that there are more than three affected family members, that it occurs in three successive generations, or that two family members have developed the disease before age 55.[88] Twin studies have also supported a genetic component for prostate cancer by demonstrating a concordance rate among heterozygotic twins of 0.043 versus 0.192 for monozygotic twins.[90] Major research effort is being placed to find specific predisposition genes which, at present, have not been identified.

Sporadic Tumors

Although most of the hereditary breast cancer susceptibility genes have been identified, the genetic changes responsible for the occurrence of sporadic tumors, which constitute at least 90 percent of all breast cancers, remain to be elucidated. The current view is that multiple somatic mutations leading to activation of oncogenes and deletion of tumor suppressor genes act in concert to promote the development and the progression of sporadic human breast cancers. Typical oncogenes found to be amplified and/or overexpressed in breast cancer code for molecules such as growth factors, growth factor receptors, signal transducers, transcription factors, cell cycle proteins, and regulators of apoptosis. The net effect resulting from activation of these oncogenic products is disregulated cell proliferation leading to transformation and subsequent progression to an aggressive phenotype.

The EGF receptor superfamily, which includes the EGF receptor itself or erbB-1/HER-1, erbB-2/HER-2/neu, erbB-3/HER-3, and erbB-4/HER-4, is involved mammary tumorigenesis through amplification and overexpression. The protein products of these genes are transmembrane tyrosine kinases which, following ligand binding (or as a result of overexpression per se), dimerize, auto and transphosphorylate, and activate ras signalling through interaction with the Grb2/SOS complex. Activated ras induces a series of phosphorylation steps involving Raf-1, MEK, and MAPK/ERK that ultimately activate a variety of nuclear transcription factors involved in tumor initiation and progression (Fig. 29-1) Although several members of the EGF receptor family appear to be overexpressed in breast cancer, amplification and overexpression of the HER-2/neu gene has been studied most extensively. HER-2/neu is amplified and/or overexpressed in approximately 20 percent of human tumors.[91] Although the ligand for this receptor remains unknown, its activation results from heterodimerization with HER-3 or HER-4 following binding of these two latter receptors to heregulin or the neu differentiation factor (NDF) family of peptides. HER-2/neu amplification has been observed in ductal carcinoma in situ, predominantly in the comedo type, and invasive carcinomas of high histologic grade, but not in benign lesions such as ductal hyperplasia and atypical ductal hyperplasia.[92] These findings indicate that HER-2/neu amplification is an important event in the development of high-grade ductal malignancies but not in the genesis of earlier benign proliferative lesions. The importance of HER-2/neu in mammary carcinogenesis is emphasized by several mouse models that have been engineered to overexpress either the activated neu oncogene or the unactivated neu protooncogene in the mammary gland.[93,94] These models show that overexpression of either gene results in breast cancer development with a latency period which is dependent upon the genetic background of the mouse.[93,94] HER-2/neu overexpression is also involved in tumor progression as evidenced by its association with poor prognosis and poor response to some chemotherapeutic and anti-hormonal agents.[95–97] Overexpression of HER-2/neu is currently exploited therapeutically with the introduction of monoclonal antibodies directed to the extracellular domain of the receptor, which have been found to reduce cell proliferation and to sensitize breast cancer cells to chemotherapeutic agents.[98,99] Encouraging preliminary results have been recently reported in Phase II[100] and III[101] clinical trials testing a recombinant humanized monoclonal antibody either alone or in combination with chemotherapeutic drugs in patients with HER-2/neu overexpressing metastatic breast cancer.

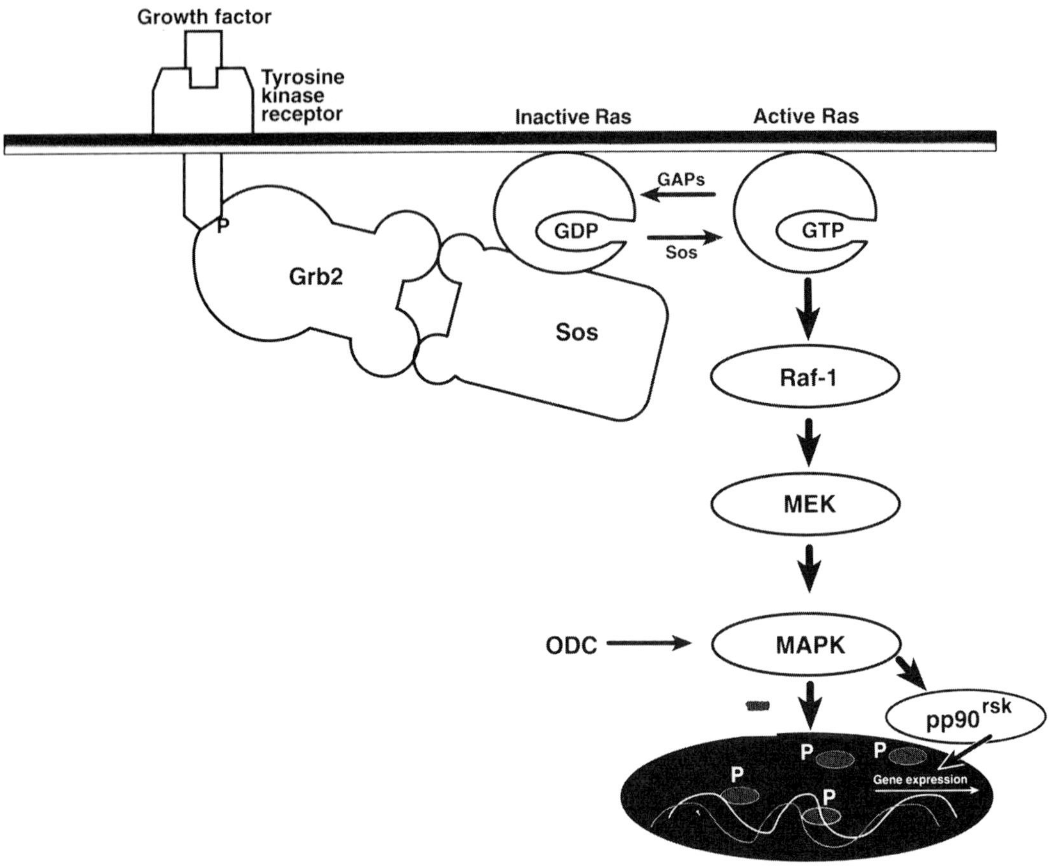

FIGURE 29-1. Simplified scheme illustrating activation of the MAPK cascade by growth factor receptor tyrosine kinases. Abbreviations are as follows: SOS, son of sevenless; GAP, GTPase activating protein; MAPK, mitogen activated protein kinase; MEK, MAPK/extracellular signal-regulated kinase; ODC, ornithine decarboxylase; $pp90^{rsk}$, pp90 ribosomal S6 kinase; Grb2, growth factor receptor binding protein.

Although the frequency of ras mutations in human breast cancer is less than 5 percent, deregulation of the ras signalling pathway, through mechanisms that do not necessarily involve mutation of ras itself, is likely to play an important role in breast cancer development.[102] Overexpression of normal H-ras protein has been reported in 20–60 percent of human breast cancers,[103] although its clinical importance remains unclear. Recent data point to the potential critical role of MAPK, a central element of the ras signalling pathway (Fig. 29-1), in human breast cancer development. Sivaraman et al.[104] reported that MAPK expression and activity is elevated 5- to 20-fold in breast cancer specimens over benign conditions such as fibroadenoma and fibrocystic disease. Using in situ reverse transcription-polymerase chain reaction, these authors demonstrated that MAPK overexpression was localized to malignant epithelial cells and metastatic cells within involved lymph nodes. These findings indicate that increased MAPK expression and activity may be a critical element in the initiation as well as metastatic potential of some human breast cancers. Further support for the importance of MAPK is provided by recent reports by Manni et al.[105,106] who observed increased activity of this enzyme in human breast epithelial cells partially transformed by induction of overexpression of ornithine decarboxylase, the first rate-limiting enzyme in polyamine biosynthesis. These investigators reported cooperativity between activation of the polyamine pathway and HER-2/neu signalling in inducing transformation of mammary epithelial cells, which may be mediated through stimulation of the MAPK cascade (Fig. 29-1).

c-Myc is a nuclear phosphoprotein that functions as a transcription factor. c-Myc dimerizes with a helix-loop-helix protein named Max and the heterodimeric complex binds specifically to E box DNA sequences (CACGTG), resulting in transcriptional activation of target genes. Some of these target genes, such as ornithine decarboxylase, CAD, p53, ECA 39, and cdc25A, are believed to play important roles in cellular proliferation and/or apoptosis (see Reference 107 for review). c-Myc expression is also highly regulated by estrogen and other mitogenic growth factors known to be expressed by breast tissues.[107] Given this physiologic context, it is not surprising that c-Myc disregulation may contribute to malignant transformation of breast epithelium. c-Myc overexpression alone, however, is not sufficient to induce a fully transformed phenotype. In vitro data indicate that transformation of normal cells by c-Myc requires coactivation or overexpression of additional oncogenic proteins.[107] Also, transgenic mice with targeted c-Myc overexpression to the mammary gland develop mammary tumors with a relatively long latency after multiple pregnancies.[107] This finding indicates that, in addition to c-Myc overexpression, additional genetic changes must occur prior to tumor development. The fact that double transgenic mice in which c-Myc is co-overexpressed with other oncogenes develop breast tumors with a short latency also supports this view.[107] Overall, the c-Myc gene is amplified in approximately 20 percent of human breast cancers. Despite considerable variability in the literature, c-Myc amplification has been generally found to correlate with adverse pathological, biochemical, kinetic, and clinical features of human breast cancer (see Reference 107 for detailed review).

Amplification of the chromosome 11q13 region has been detected in 15–20 percent of human breast cancers.[108,109] Interest in this region was driven by the finding that its mouse homologue is a frequent integration site by MMTV. The search for candidate genes within this amplicon first focused on FGF-3 and FGF-4 because mouse breast carcinogenesis is promoted by an MMTV insertional activation of these genes. However, neither FGF3 or FGF4 has been found to be overexpressed in human mammary tumors. In contrast, amplification of this chromosomal region is consistently accompanied by overexpression of cyclin D1.[110] Cyclin D1 plays a critical role in cell-cycle control through complex formation with cyclin-dependent kinases 4 and 6 leading to RB phosphorylation. Therefore, it is not surprising that increased cyclin D1 expression may cause disregulation in cell division, thus leading to transformation. Support for this contention is provided by the finding that transgenic mice overexpressing cyclin D1 in breast tissues under the control of the MMTV promoter develop mammary hyperplasia and neoplasia.[111]

As in most human cancers, the most common genetic abnormality in breast cancer is loss of specific chromosome arms. Loss of heterozygosity points to regions of chromosomes likely to harbor tumor suppressor genes.[112,113] At present, 12 chromosome arms have been shown to be frequently affected by loss of heterozygosity in primary breast tumors. They include chromosomes 1p, 1q, 3p, 6q, 7q, 11p, 8p, 13q, 16q, 17p, 17q, and 18q.[112,113] The identification of the target genes affected by loss of heterozygosity is only in its infancy. Among the hereditary breast cancer susceptibility genes, only p53 has been shown to be frequently mutated (25–45 percent) in nonfamilial or sporadic breast carcinomas.[114]

Epidemiology of Hormone-Responsive Tumors

Age and Hormones

Age is the predominant determinant of overall cancer risk in the general population, with most life-threatening cancers occurring in people over 65.[115] The explanation for this age-related increase in incidence is believed to be multifactorial, including a natural decline in immune and mesenchymal tissue function, impaired subcellular repair mechanisms, and accumulated damage from oxidation and environmental carcinogens combined with the prolonged effects of endogenous risk factors such as obesity and exposure to sex steroids. Figure 29-2 compares the age-specific incidence rates of breast, endometrial, and prostate cancers relative to cancers of all sites in men and women. For breast and endometrial cancers, the incidence curves begin to plateau or decline by age 65, presumably as a delayed response to the decline in ovarian sex steroid levels occurring with menopause.

The role of unopposed estrogen effect on endometrial carcinogenesis is very well established. The risk of endometrial cancer is significantly increased in hyperestrogenic states such as obesity, polycystic ovary syndrome, and the presence of granulosa-theca cell tumors of the ovary. Postmenopausal estrogen replacement therapy is also clearly associated with an increased risk for endometrial cancer.[11] Furthermore, an increased incidence of this malignancy has been observed with chronic tamoxifen administration, an antiestrogen with estrogen agonistic activity in the uterus, either in the setting of adjuvant therapy[116] or chemoprevention of breast cancer.[117] Progestins, on the other hand, appear to have a protective effect. The 50 percent reduction in the risk of endometrial cancer reported with the use of oral contraceptive has been attributed to the progestational component of these drugs.[118] Also, administration of progesterone simultaneously with estrogen in postmenopausal women appears to have a protective effect, although it may not eliminate completely the increased risk associated with estrogen use.[11]

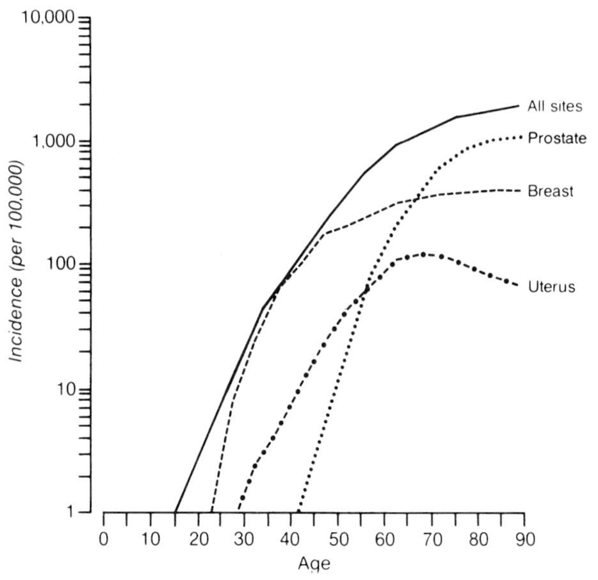

FIGURE 29-2. Age-specific incidence rates of individual hormone-responsive cancers (breast, uterine/endometrial, prostate) in comparison to the combined incidence of cancers from all sites in men and women. (*Reproduced with permission from Fraumeni et al.,*[117] *originally derived from NCI/SEER program data on US white population, 1981–1985.*)

Several breast cancer risk factors such as early menarche, late menopause, and postmenopausal obesity point to the importance of cumulative estrogen exposure as a determinant of mammary carcinogenesis. Numerous studies have been conducted to compare serum hormone levels in patients and healthy women to determine whether breast cancer risk is associated with higher estrogen levels. A recently published meta-analysis of 29 epidemiologic studies has, indeed, shown a positive association between serum estradiol concentration and breast cancer risk in postmenopausal women, thus providing support for the theory that endogenous estrogens play a crucial role in human mammary carcinogenesis.[119] A recent nested case-control study within the Prospective Nurses Health Study Cohort has reported a positive correlation between circulating IGF-I levels and breast cancer development in premenopausal but not postmenopausal women.[120] If confirmed, this finding would provide additional rationale for the use of tamoxifen as a chemopreventive agent, as this antiestrogen has been shown to reduce circulating IGF-I levels.

Exogenous estrogen administration has been shown to confer a modest but definite increased breast cancer risk. A recent meta-analysis of 54 different studies that included a total of 53,297 women with breast cancer and 100,239 controls has reviewed the influence of oral contraceptives.[121] This meta-analysis found that increased risk of breast cancer was associated with current (relative risk: 1.24) and recent (relative risk: 1.16) (as defined by use 1–4 years prior to diagnosis of breast cancer) oral contraceptive use. Within the latter group, the risk was greatest for those women who began oral contraceptives before the age of 20. However, this excess risk does not persist because there is no evidence of increased risk of breast cancer 10 or more years after cessation of oral contraceptives. An additional significant finding of this study was that breast cancers diagnosed in women who had ever used oral contraceptive tended to be more localized to the breast. Another recent meta-analysis has addressed the relationship between postmenopausal hormone replacement and breast cancer in 52,505 patients and 108,411 controls from 51 studies.[122] The main finding of the meta-analysis is that for current or recent users of hormone replacement therapy, the risk for breast cancer increases in relation to increasing duration of use. The risk increased by 2.3 percent for each year of use. Following discontinuation of hormone replacement therapy for five years or more, there was no longer a significant increased risk of breast cancer. As in the case of oral contraceptives, tumors diagnosed in every user of hormone replacement therapy were less likely to be metastatic to either regional lymph nodes or to distant sites. At present, it remains unclear whether the addition of progesterone alters the risk of developing breast cancer associated with postmenopausal estrogen replacement.

Compared to breast and endometrial cancer, prostate cancer shows an even more marked and steadily rising incidence associated with age, as shown in Fig. 29-2. This may reflect the relative lack of change in circulating androgen levels in men over age 50, thus allowing the tumor promoting effect of androgens to accumulate with advancing age. Black males have a higher incidence of prostate cancer than whites, perhaps as a result of their higher circulating level of testosterone. A recent prospective case control study of men participating in the Physicians Health Study has evaluated the relationship between plasma IGF-I and prostate cancer incidence.[123] This study found that men in the highest quartile of IGF-I levels had a relative risk of 4.3 (95 percent CI 1.8–10.6) compared with men in the lowest quartile. This association is stronger than that of any previously reported risk factor such as androgen levels or anthropomorphic variables. However, this observation needs to be confirmed by additional studies before plasma IGF-I measurement can be introduced in clinical practice for prostate cancer screening.

Geography and Diet

A compelling body of evidence indicates that Western style diets, along with a more sedentary and stress-filled lifestyle, account for the increased obesity, earlier maturity, and greater amount of cardiovascular disease and cancer that were uncommon even in the eighteenth and nineteenth centuries.[124] In particular, it is now accepted that the worldwide geographic variations in organ-specific and age-specific cancer rates are attributable less to genetic and ethnic differences than to environmental influences, of which diet must be considered the most prominent. This is certainly true for the most common epithelial malignancies including breast, prostate, and endometrial cancers.

The observed shifts in ethnic incidence of breast, prostate, and gastrointestinal cancers occurring within two generations of immigrants from low-incidence areas (Japan, Poland) living in high-incidence regions (Hawaii, California) are generally attributable to changes in dietary habits.[115,124] Figure 29-3 shows the strong linear correlation that exists between per capita dietary fat consumption and breast cancer mortality in many different nations.[124,125] As economic advances affect low cancer incidence countries such as Japan, Iceland, Italy, and Greece, dietary shifts toward more fat and higher total caloric consumption (with a lower intake of fiber and complex carbohydrates), occur in parallel with rising breast, prostate, and colon cancer rates.

The majority of animal experiments and human population data studies indicate strong positive correlations between breast and prostate cancer incidence and total dietary fat intake.[126–132] However, some studies do not directly support the fat hypothesis but indicate that specific types of fat, total caloric intake, and/or obesity are more important links to cancer.[115] An important hormonal connection is found in the close association between obesity and breast and endometrial cancer incidences, generally attributable to the increased conversion of circulating androstenedione to estrogen within excess adipose tissue.[115] Putative associations between the incidence of hormone-responsive cancers and specific dietary components have been proposed.[125] Of this, phytoestrogens have received considerable attention. These compounds, which fall under the two main categories of isoflavons and ligands, have both estrogenic and antiestrogenic properties, and are found in a wide range of commonly consumed foods such as soy and flax products. Accumulating evidence indicates that phytoestrogens may provide health benefits in the area of cardiovascular diseases, cancer, osteoporosis, and menopausal symptoms. Specifically, diets rich in phytoestrogens may reduce the risk of breast, endometrial, and prostate cancer (see Reference 133 for a detailed recent review).

Endocrine Mechanisms Controlling the Growth of Hormone-Dependent Tumors

Although steroid hormones have long been known to influence the growth of hormone-dependent tumors such as breast, prostate, and endometrial cancers, the precise cellular mechanisms subserving these effects still remain to be fully elucidated. Although nongenomic effects may very well have important phenotypic manifestations, this section will focus on steroid hormone actions that are receptor-mediated and will concentrate on estrogen receptors and breast cancer as a paradigm because considerably more information is available on this subject.

Steroid hormone receptors are members of the nuclear receptor family, which also includes receptors for retinoids, thyroid hormone, fatty acids, and prostaglandins and a number of so-called orphan receptors, the ligands of which have yet to be identified. A detailed review of basic aspects of receptor structure and function is covered elsewhere (see Chap. 4) The primary focus of attention will be on recent developments that are germane to hormonal control of tumor growth. The reader is referred to recently published reviews on this topic for detailed information.[134,135]

A major advance in the understanding of nuclear receptor physiology has been derived from the determination of models for the ligand binding domain based on crystal structures of three different receptors (e.g., RXRα, RARγ, and Trα).[136–139] It appears that a major consequence of ligand binding is the induction of an alteration in the conformation of the ligand binding domain. This conformational change is ligand-specific and has important physiologic consequences. For instance, when the antiestrogen raloxifene binds to the estrogen receptor, the ligand-estrogen receptor complex does not bind to estrogen response elements but instead

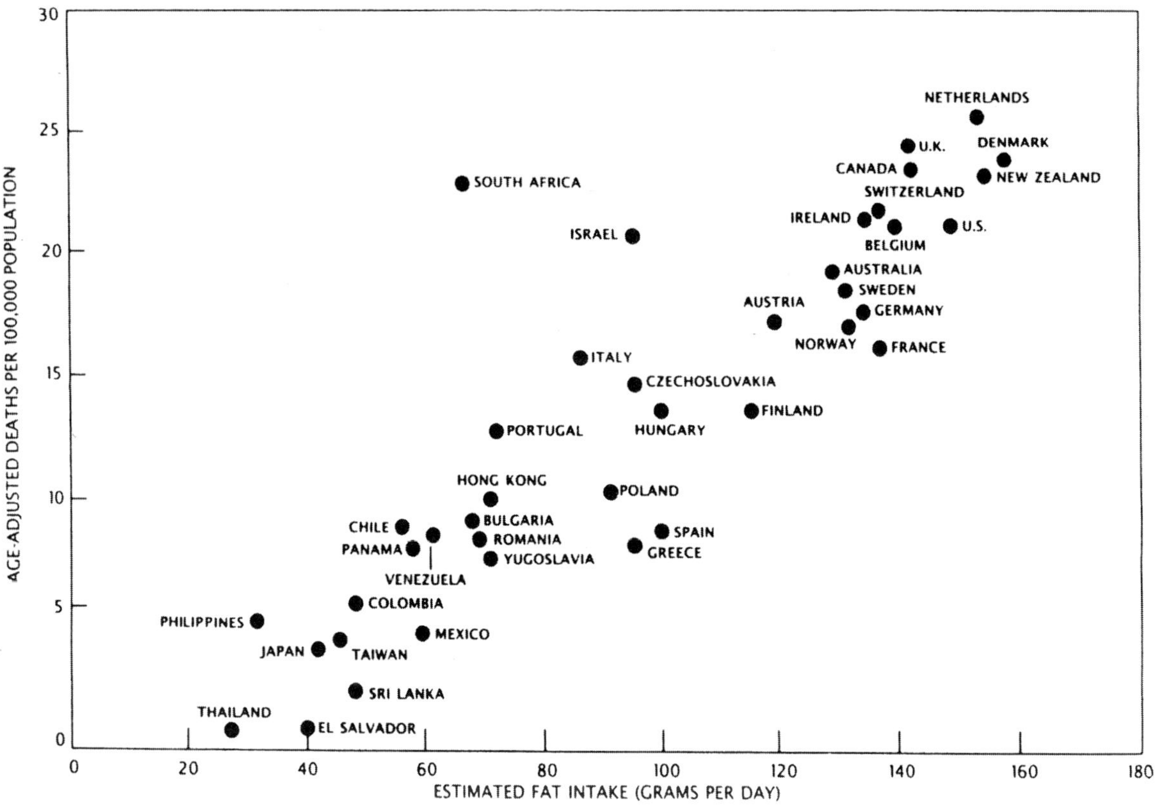

FIGURE 29-3 Correlation between per capita dietary fat consumption and reported breast cancer mortality in different nations. (*Reproduced from Cohen,[126] previously published in Carroll KK, Cancer Res 35:3374–3383, 1975.*)

to unique DNA sequences called raloxifene-response elements that produce an estrogen agonistic effect in some tissues and estrogen antagonistic effects in others.[140] Therefore, based on improved knowledge of structure-function relationships, it is possible to develop optimal compounds called selective estrogen receptor modulators (SERM) that behave as antiestrogens in the uterus and breast but exert estrogen agonistic activity on bone, lipids, and the cardiovascular system.

Another important consequence of the ligand-induced conformational change in the ligand binding domain of the receptor is the formation of a novel surface that allows the recruitment of coactivators and corepressors that have profound influences on the transcriptional activity of the activation function-2 (AF-2) (see Reference 134 for review). At present, it appears that the p160 proteins and CBP/p300 are the most important receptor interacting proteins with regard to their ability to potentiate receptor mediated transcription. Their influence on transcription is likely to occur through different mechanisms, which are outlined and summarized in Fig. 29-4. Pure antiestrogens, such as ICI-182780, and nonsteroidal antiestrogens with mixed agonistic/agonistic activity, such as tamoxifen, inhibit binding of these coactivator proteins and thus block AF-2 induced transcription.[141] These two classes of hormone antagonists, however, differ with regard to their influence on the activity of the activation function-1 (AF-1) located in the N-terminal or A/B domain of the receptor. Pure antiestrogens inhibit AF-1 activity, primarily by inducing estrogen receptor degradation.[142,143] Based on in vitro studies, it has also been suggested that ICI-182780 blocks receptor dimerization and DNA binding.[144] However, subsequent in vivo studies have challenged this conclusion.[145,146] The antiestrogen tamoxifen, on the other hand, clearly allows receptor dimerization and DNA binding with preservation of AF-1 activity, which accounts for the agonistic action of the compound. Because the relative importance of AF-1 and AF-2 is promoter- and cell type-specific, tamoxifen has mixed agonistic/antagonistic activity depending upon the specific target gene and tissue.

The mechanisms by which estradiol • estrogen receptor complex stimulate breast cancer cell proliferation are complex and multifaceted. Estrogen could stimulate growth directly by activating cell cycle-related proteins such as cyclin D1, B1, and E[147,148] or through induction of certain protooncogenes such as *myc* and *fos*[149,150] that are closely linked to proliferation. An additional mechanism by which estrogens stimulate breast cancer cell proliferation is by inducing the synthesis of polypeptide growth factors acting in an autocrine/paracrine fashion (see Reference 151 for review). These findings have again emphasized the importance of stromal epithelial interactions in the hormonal control of breast cancer growth. For instance, ovarian hormones have been shown to regulate in vivo the expression of stromal IGF-II,[152] which exerts its mitogenic effect through binding to the type I IGF-I receptor present on the membrane of epithelial cancer cells. Conversely, estrogens can stimulate the production of growth factors such as PDGF[153] by epithelial cells, which exert their effect on the surrounding stroma. Estrogen has also been found to inhibit the production of the bifunctional growth factor TGFβ,[154] which has an antiproliferative effect on epithelial cells but a stimulatory

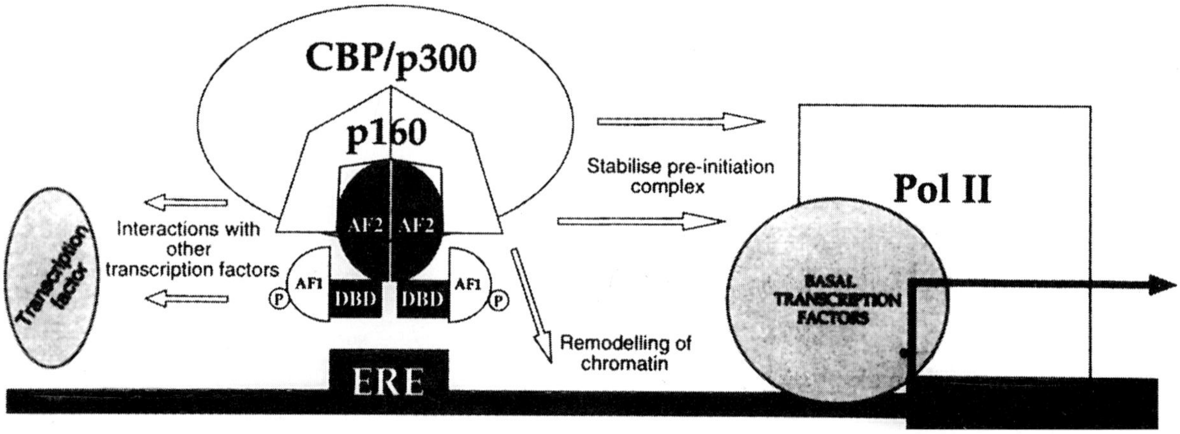

FIGURE 29-4. Interactions between receptors and coactivator proteins. Activated receptors bind p160 proteins and proteins of the CBP/p300 family in a ligand-dependent manner. This DNA-bound complex may then stimulate the expression of hormone-responsive genes by a number of possible mechanisms including the remodeling of chromatin, interaction with other transcription factors, and the stabilization of the preinitiation complex, which consists of DNA polymerase and basal transcription factors. Abbreviations are as follows: AF_1, activation function 1; AF_2, activation function 2; DBD, DNA binding domain; CBP, cAMP response element binding protein; ERE, estrogen response element; Pol II, polymerase II. (*Reproduced from White and Parker.*[136])

effect on the stroma. Demonstration, however, of the role of growth factors as essential mediators of hormone action has been difficult because targeted antigrowth factor treatment has not consistently been shown to inhibit hormonally stimulated growth.[155–158] The complexity of the interaction between estrogens and growth factor is further highlighted by the recent appreciation of the crosstalk between the classic estrogen receptor pathway and growth factor signalling involving different protein kinase cascades. EGF has been shown to increase ER transcriptional activity by phosphorylation of serine residue 118 in the AF-1 domain induced by activation of the MAPK kinase pathway.[157,160] Kato et al.[161] demonstrated that overexpression of either ras or MAPK kinase, both of which activate MAPK, stimulated serine 118 phosphorylation and transcriptional activity of the estrogen receptor in COS cells. Serine 118, however, is not the only residue in the estrogen receptor molecule to be phosphorylated by growth factor signalling. Activation of HER-2/neu by heregulin in breast cancer cells has been shown to result in direct and rapid phosphorylation of estrogen receptor on tyrosine residues followed by ER • ERE interaction and production of an estrogen induced protein (i.e., progesterone receptor).[162] Agents working through the cyclic AMP pathway such as the neurotransmitter dopamine have also been shown to activate the estrogen receptor.[163] However, it is not known whether this is achieved by phosphorylation of the receptor itself or other proteins involved in transcriptional activation. A simplified scheme of the influence of growth factors, estrogens, and antiestrogens on estrogen receptor phosphorylation and activation is shown in Fig. 29-5. Conversely, the estrogen receptor pathway has been shown to potentiate the stimulatory effects of growth factors on the activity of the AP-1 transcription factor family (fos-jun heterodimers and jun-jun homodimers).[164] Along this line, estrogens have been shown to stimulate the expression of genes that lack ERE sequences but contain AP-1 responsive elements by enhancing AP-1 mediated transcription.[165] Several alternative mechanisms may explain how nuclear receptors influence the activity of other transcription factors. One may involve binding of the receptor and other factors at composite response elements in the DNA.[166,167] Another may be through the recently discovered CBP/p300 proteins, which have the potential for making multiple contacts with other transcription factors (Fig. 29-4).

Although estrogens increase cell proliferation in ER positive breast cancer cells, it should be noted that estrogens can also promote negative regulatory mechanisms of tumor growth. They include stimulation of the retinoic acid receptor alpha[168] and increased expression of the tumor suppressor genes p53[169] and BRCA1.[170] As discussed in a recent review,[135] it is possible that when the tumor cells lose a functional estrogen receptor, these breaks are no longer operative, thus facilitating accelerated cell proliferation now driven by constitutively active regulatory pathways which have bypassed the need for estrogen stimulation.

Mechanisms of Tumor Progression

Breast and prostate cancer share a similar natural history. Although estrogens and androgens are involved in the development of virtually all breast and prostate cancers respectively, at the time of clinical presentation, approximately one-third of breast cancers and up to 90 percent of prostate cancers are still hormone-dependent. Hormone-dependent tumors exhibit a relatively indolent clinical course and are amenable to endocrine therapy, which allows long-term remissions with only modest toxicity. Unfortunately, however, progression to a hormone-independent aggressive phenotype eventually occurs in every case of breast and prostate cancer, resulting in the patients demise. Interestingly, during this transition from hormone-dependence to hormone-independence, breast and prostate tumors may go through an intermediate phase of hormone supersensitivity. This possibility is suggested by the clinical observation that breast cancers relapsing from an initial response to ovariectomy frequently respond to second line therapy with aromatase inhibitors.[171] This finding indicates that such tumors have not become hormone-resistant but instead have adapted to grow in response to castrate levels of estrogens, as they regress upon further reduction in serum estrogen levels induced by aromatase inhibitor therapy.

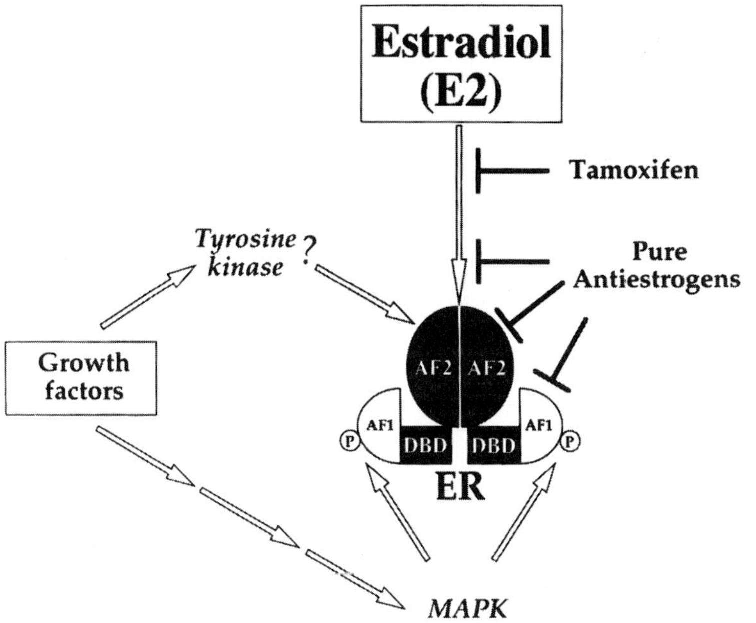

FIGURE 29-5. Activation of the estrogen receptor. The receptor may be activated by ligand binding and, in addition, by stimulation with growth factors acting via MAPK to phosphorylate AF-1. The receptor may also be target for tyrosine kinase(s) resulting in activation of AF-2. Partial antagonists such as tamoxifen block ligand-dependent activity but not growth factor stimulation of AF-1. Pure antagonists, on the other hand, prevent both modalities of receptor activation (*Reproduced from White and Parker.*[136])

Considerable research emphasis is being placed on elucidating the molecular events mediating the transition of breast and prostate cancers through these various phases of hormone responsiveness. Identification of such steps can unveil critical targets for therapeutic intervention and possibly chemoprevention.

An obvious possibility for the development of hormone independence is the loss of receptors for estrogens or androgens by breast and prostate cancer cells, respectively. However, it is clear that this does not frequently occur because expression of hormone receptors is relatively well-preserved during breast and prostate cancer progression.[172,173] An alternative hypothesis that is still being pursued is that mutations in hormone receptors resulting in proteins with altered function may be responsible for transition to hormone independence. It is clear that it is possible to induce mutations in nearly all of the functional domains of the estrogen receptor, resulting in a variety of proteins exhibiting multiple phenotypes both dominant negative and dominant positive with constitutive activity (see References 174 and 175 for review). However, mutations of the estrogen receptor have been found very infrequently in breast cancer specimens[176] and their presence does not correlate with either hormone responsiveness or hormone receptor status.[177] In contrast, multiple ER mRNA variants derived from alternative splicing have been identified that have the potential to provide estrogen receptor proteins with a dominant positive or negative phenotype (Table 29-4).[178–182] However, their role in the development of hormone independence remains unproven because they are similarly expressed in normal and neoplastic breast tissue,[183–186] and the corresponding variant proteins have not been convincingly demonstrated in tumor tissue.

With regard to prostate cancer, amplification and increased protein expression of the wild type androgen receptor has been shown in 30 percent of recurrent tumors but not in primary cancers.[187] This finding indicates that some recurrent tumors may not be androgen-independent but may have actually acquired increased sensitivity and capacity to grow in the presence of a reduced androgen milieu. Several mutations of the androgen receptor have been identified in clinical specimens (Table 29-5).[188–198] Of interest, many can lead to altered proteins that are transcriptionally activated when bound to hormones other than androgens such as estrogen, progesterone, or even antiandrogens (Table 29-5). However, the exact frequency of these mutations and their association with progressive stages of prostate cancer remains controversial and deserves further attention.

It is quite clear that neither loss nor mutations of the receptors can account for all cases of hormone independence. Hence, additional mechanisms need to be invoked (see References 174 and 175 for review). It should be kept in mind that hormone action does not take place in isolation but occurs within a very complex cellular milieu characterized by interaction of the receptor with other transcription factors and crosstalk of the hormone receptor pathway with classic growth factor signalling. It is possible, for instance, that altered expression and/or activity of coactivators and corepressors could have major influence on hormone action and convert a negative signal (e.g., tamoxifen

TABLE 29-4. Examples of Exon Deletions of the Estrogen Receptor and the Corresponding Phenotype

	Dominant Negative	
Mutation	Potential Protein Product[a]	Reference
In-frame exon 3 deletion	61.2 kDa ER	[178]
In-frame exon 4 deletion	53.7 kDa ER	[179]
Out-of-frame exon 7 deletion	51.3 kDa ER	[178]
		[180]
Exon 6,7 duplication	77 kDa ER	[181]
	Dominant positive	
Out-of-frame exon 5 deletion	42 kDa ER	[183]

[a] All protein products are based on hypothetical protein production in the original samples except the 77 kDa ER, which has been identified as a unique product of MCF-7 cells, and the 42 kDa ER, which has been detected in BT-20 human breast cancer cells.

Source: Reproduced from Tonetti DA and Jordan VC.[175]

Table 29-5. Androgen Receptor Gene Mutations Detected in Clinical Prostate Cancers[1]

Tumor Characteristics	n	Exons Studied	Mutations Found	Exons	Comments	Ref.
Untreated stage B prostate cancers	26	Exons E-H	1/26 (4 percent)	Exon E	No data from activational properties	188
Metastatic hormone-refractory prostate cancers	7	Exons B-H	1/7 (14 percent)	Exon D	Activated by adrenal androgens and progesterone	189
Untreated stage B primary tumors (7), endocrine-therapy-resistance autopsy samples (8)	15	Exons B-H	1/8 (13 percent) hormone-therapy-resistant patients showed one mutation in 1) prostate and one in the corresponding 2) metastasis	1) Exon D 2) Exon H	No data from activational properties	190
Transurethral resection specimens from advanced prostate cancers	24	Exons D-H	6/24 (25 percent)	Exon H	No data from activational properties	191
Hormone-refractory local recurrences	18	Exons B-H	No mutations			173
Untreated prostate cancers	40	CAG repeats	1/40 (3 percent)	Exon A	Activated by flutamide	192
Hormone refractory metastases: bone marrow (8), pleural fluid (1), and skin nodule (1)	10	Exons B-H	Mutations in 5/10 (50 percent) of cases	1) Exon H 2) Exon H 3) Exon H 4) Exon D 5) Exon D Exon E Exon H Exon H	Mutations in cases 1 and 2 were activated by estrogen and progesterone	193
Hormone-refractory local recurrences	7	Exon H (codon 877)	No mutations			194
Hormone-refractory local recurrences	13	Exons B-H	1/13 (8 percent)	Exon D	No abnormal activation	187
Untreated primary tumors	25	Exons A-H	11/25 (44 percent)	1) Exon A 2) Exon B 3) Exon D 4) Exon F 5) Exon G 6) Exon H	No data from activational properties	195
Untreated primary tumors (23), hormone-refractory local recurrences (6)	29	Exons B-H	1/29 (3 percent) germ-line mutation	Exon E	Mutated receptor was activated by estradiol	196
Untreated primary tumors (31), hormone-refractory recurrences (13)	44	Exons A-H	1/44 (2 percent) primary tumors	Exon F	No data from activational properties	197
Untreated primary stage B and C tumors (30), hormone-refractory recurrences obtained from autopsy (22)	52	Exons B-H	0/30 3/22 (14 percent)	1) Exon H 2) Exon H 3) Exons D and H	No data from activational properties	198

Source: Reproduced from Koivisto P, et al.[199]

inhibition of tumor cell proliferation) to a positive signal (e.g., tamoxifen-stimulated growth).[200,201] Constitutive overexpression of estrogen-regulated polypeptide growth factors or estrogen-stimulated genes involved in cell cycle control, such as cyclin D and E, could result in estrogen-independent and antiestrogen-resistant proliferation of breast cancer cells.[202–204] Several studies have provided evidence supporting estrogen independent activation of the estrogen receptor by growth factor[159,160] or growth factor receptors such as HER-2/neu[162] through stimulation of estrogen receptor phosphorylation with consequent increase in transcriptional activity. Such effect could be mediated, at least in some cases, by growth factor induced activation of MAPK, which has been shown to directly phosphorylate the estrogen receptor on serine 118 on the AF-1 domain.[161] Ligand-independent, growth factor-induced stimulation of the androgen receptor has also been observed in prostate cancer.[205–207] Hence, similar mechanisms of tumor progression are likely to occur in this malignancy. Obviously, both in the case of breast and prostate cancer, constitutive activation of alternative growth factor/oncogene signalling mechanisms could completely bypass the hormone receptor pathway and lead to hormone independence by activation of critical downstream target genes.

CLINICAL CHARACTERISTICS OF HORMONE-RESPONSIVE CANCERS

Breast Cancer

Breast cancer is a major worldwide health problem. It is the most common of all life-threatening malignancies in western countries and represents about a third of all female cancers. Approximately 185,000 new cases are diagnosed yearly in the United States alone. More than 45,000 American women die yearly from this malignancy, second only to lung cancer deaths. Breast cancer in men is an uncommon disease with an incidence rate less than 1 percent that of females. Of interest, approximately 80 percent of male breast tumors are initially hormone-dependent (in contrast to only 30 percent of female breast cancers) and respond to hormonal therapies such as tamoxifen or orchiectomy. In general, however, the natural history of male breast cancer closely resembles that of its female counterpart, with nearly a third of male breast cancer patients dying of the disease.[208]

Risk Factors

The major risk factors for breast cancer are listed in Table 29-6. Several of these, like family history, geographic and ethnic differences, endogenous hormone levels, exogenous hormone use, and dietary factors, have been discussed in previous sections of this chapter. Overall, exposure of the breast ductal epithelium to estrogen constitutes the major known risk factor for breast cancer with the total duration of a woman's menstrual history correlating positively with the risk of developing the disease. A woman who experiences menopause after age 55 has twice the risk of developing breast cancer that a woman who undergoes menopause before age 45 has. Likewise, an artificial and/or premature menopause resulting from surgery, radiation, or drugs confers some protection against breast cancer. Obesity is a risk factor only in postmenopausal women because adipose tissue represents the major source of estrogens after the menopause due to its high content of the enzyme aromatase. Early pregnancy exerts a protective effect against breast cancer, presumably as a result of its differentiating action on the mammary gland, which makes it less susceptible to oncogenic insults. In contrast, a delay in first pregnancy (i.e., beyond age 30) represents a risk factor presumably because of the presence of already-initiated mammary epithelial cells, which are promoted and expanded by the hormonal surge of pregnancy.

Radiation exposure, particularly during youth, is an environmental risk factor for breast cancer. This risk has been identified by studies including atomic bomb survivors in Hiroshima and Nagasaki, women who received radiotherapy for mastitis or Hodgkin's disease, and women subjected to repeated diagnostic radiologic studies for scoliosis or tuberculosis. Of note, radiation exposure beyond age 40 does not seem to pose additional risk, and present-day diagnostic chest radiographs and mammography screening constitute no significant risk for developing radiation-induced breast cancer.

Benign breast disease comprises a mixture of heterogeneous lesions associated with no or varying degrees of malignant potential (Table 29-7).[209] It should be noted that since the introduction of mammographic screening programs, the diagnosis of ductal carcinoma in situ has become much more frequent (15–20 percent of all breast cancers versus 0–5 percent in the premammographic era). Ductal carcinoma in situ is still considered to be a premalignant lesion because the proliferating cells have not yet invaded the basement membrane of the ductal-lobular unit. However, if left untreated, there is a high probability that development of invasive cancer will occur. Lobular carcinoma in situ carries the same risk for subsequent development of invasive cancer. However, this risk is not restricted to the area of the lesion, but is nearly equally divided between each breast. Therefore, lobular carcinoma in situ is not considered to be a premalignant lesion per se but rather a high risk marker for the subsequent development of invasive breast cancer.

Diagnosis

Breast cancer commonly presents as a palpable mass. However, nonpalpable mammographic abnormalities are increasingly more common presentations now that screening mammography is recommended for all women age 40 years or older. A mammographically detectable mass or clustering of micro calcifications that leads to a suspicion of carcinoma frequently occurs in the absence of any palpable breast abnormality. Conversely, up to 10–15 percent of palpable breast lesions may not be detectable by mammography. A palpable mass, an ill-defined thickening of the

TABLE 29-6. Risk Factors for Breast Cancer

Family history (genetics)
Number of ovulatory cycles (early menarche, late menopause)
Parity and age of first full-term pregnancy
Endogenous hormone levels
Exogenous hormone use
Benign breast disease (see Table 29-7 for details)
Obesity (postmenopausal women)
Diet (high fat, alcohol ingestion)
Exposure to ionizing radiation in youth
Prior history of breast, endometrial, or ovarian cancer

TABLE 29-7. Benign Breast Disease Associated with Increased Risk of Invasive Breast Cancer

A.	No risk lesions
	Cysts
	Apocrine change
B.	Minimal risk lesions (1.5–2.0-fold)
	Florid hyperplasia
	Sclerosing adenosis
	Intraductal papilloma
	Fibroadenoma (certain histologic subtypes)
C.	Intermediate risk lesions (4.0–5.0-fold)
	Atypical ductal hyperplasia
	Atypical lobular hyperplasia
D.	High risk lesions (10.0–11.0-fold)
	Ductal carcinoma in situ
	Lobular carcinoma in situ

Source: This table has been compiled based on a recent review by Jensen RA.[209]

breast, and a bloody nipple discharge are worrisome clinical signs that should prompt further medical evaluation. The palpable mass or mammographic area of suspicion can be biopsied by fine needle aspiration (FNA) or surgical excision. FNA is a quick, simple, and accurate office procedure without significant complications. When cancer is discovered by means of FNA or surgical biopsy, a staging evaluation is undertaken before the start of definitive treatment.

Pathology and Prognosis

The most common type of breast cancer is infiltrating ductal carcinoma (70 percent). Lobular (5–10 percent), medullary (5 percent), colloid (3 percent), and tubular (1 percent) types are much less prevalent. Paget's disease of the breast accounts for 3 percent of all breast cancers; it presents as an erythematous, scaling, weeping lesion of the nipple that is associated with an underlying cancer in at least 60 percent of cases. Inflammatory breast carcinoma is an uncommon but particularly lethal form of breast cancer that presents with skin inflammation (often mistaken for infection), edema, warmth, erythema, and induration. The characteristic pathologic finding underlying inflammatory breast cancer is tumor cells infiltrating throughout the dermal lymphatic vessels.

Human breast cancer is a highly heterogeneous disease whose clinical outcome is determined by a very complex interplay of several patient- and tumor-related prognostic factors (Table 29-8) (see Reference 210 for detailed review). Knowledge of these prognostic factors is at times important in the selection of the most appropriate type of therapy. Axillary lymph node involvement still remains the most powerful prognostic factor in determining the clinical outcome of patients with apparently localized disease. Recurrence rates and the subsequent mortality from metastatic breast cancer are positively related to the extent of lymph node involvement at the time of diagnosis. Estrogen and progesterone receptors are routinely measured because their presence imparts a relatively favorably prognosis and predicts responsiveness to hormonal therapy both in the adjuvant and metastatic setting. An increasing number of additional prognostic factors (selected examples are listed in Table 29-8) have been reported. They are particularly useful in identifying, among patients with node negative tumors, the relatively small subgroup (approximately 30 percent) with aggressive disease who are likely to relapse and who should be targeted for intensive adjuvant therapy.

TABLE 29-8. Selected List of Adverse Prognostic Factors in Breast Cancer

Patient characteristics
Young, premenopausal
Black race
Tumor characteristics
Stage
Large size
Positive lymph nodes
Bone marrow micrometastasis
Distant metastasis
Histologic features*
Microvessel density
Negative estrogen/progesterone receptors
Presence of EGF receptors†
High proliferative activity‡
HER-2neu amplification/overexpression
c-myc amplification
p53 mutations/overexpression
Increased expression of the components of urokinase system of plasminogen activation (uPA, PA1-1)

Source: A detailed discussion of each of the listed prognostic factors with pertinent references can be found in a recent review by Klijn JGM et al.[210]

*Tubular, cribriform, mucinous type cancers carry better prognosis than ductal carcinoma not otherwise specified (NOS).

†An inverse relationship has been observed between expression of EGF receptors and estrogen receptors.

‡As determined by a variety of techniques including mitotic index (MI), thymidine labelling index (TLI), bromodeoxyuridine labelling, S-phase fraction (SPF), expression of Ki67, PCNA nuclear protein, and mitosin.

Treatment

Surgical treatment of breast cancer has evolved from a radical Halstedian approach to a more limited, breast-preserving surgery in conjunction with local radiotherapy. Axillary lymph nodes are still usually removed for prognostic purposes. The recognition that human breast cancer is frequently a systemic disease from its outset has prompted this drastic change in surgical treatment with more emphasis being placed on adjuvant therapy in the attempt to eradicate micrometastasis, which are ultimately responsible for tumor relapse and patient death.

Current evidence indicates that endocrine treatment has a definite role in the adjuvant therapy of breast cancer. An overview published by the Early Breast Cancer Trialists Collaborative Group has shown that for women less than 50 years of age, ovarian ablation was associated with an approximate 25 percent reduction in the annual odds of recurrence and death.[211] Because the patients were not selected based on hormone receptor status, it is likely that the benefit of ovarian ablation is greater in women with estrogen receptor positive tumors. Most of the information available on hormonal adjuvant therapy of breast cancer is related to the use of tamoxifen. The Early Breast Cancer Trialists Collaborative Group has recently updated the overview of 55 randomized trials begun before 1990, which included a total of 37,000 women.[116] Estrogen receptor status was positive in 18,000, unknown in 12,000, and negative in 8,000 patients. This updated analysis provided some important conclusions. First, women with estrogen receptor negative tumors receive minimal, if any, benefit from adjuvant tamoxifen treatment. Tamoxifen, on the other hand, substantially improves the 10-year survival of women with estrogen receptor positive tumors and that of women whose tumors are of unknown estrogen receptor status. The overview also confirmed that five-year duration of treatment is clearly superior to just one or two years of therapy. Of importance is that the beneficial effect of tamoxifen was found to be independent of nodal status, age, menopausal status, and administration of chemotherapy. Therefore, these updated findings do not confirm the data from previous overviews, which indicated that adjuvant tamoxifen is not particularly effective in young, premenopausal women. Finally, the overview shows that five years of tamoxifen treatment reduces the incidence of contralateral breast cancer by half. Although the incidence of endometrial cancer is confirmed to be increased, the absolute decrease in contralateral breast cancer was about twice as large as the absolute increase in the incidence of endometrial cancer. In summary, this updated overview suggests that adjuvant therapy with tamoxifen for five years is indicated in virtually every woman with localized breast cancer unless the tumor is estrogen receptor negative. However, this conclusion cannot be generalized to women with very small tumors (<1 cm, usually detected by screening mammograms) because no definitive data are available on adjuvant therapy in this group of patients who enjoy an excellent prognosis with local therapy alone.

Hormonal therapy induces objective tumor regression in approximately one-third of unselected patients with metastatic breast cancer. The introduction of estrogen and progesterone receptor measurements has significantly increased our ability to predict hormone responsiveness. Patients with tumors positive for both estrogen and progesterone receptors have a 70 percent response rate to endocrine treatment, whereas patients with tumors negative for both receptors have less than 10 percent probability of response. Tumors positive for one receptor exhibit an intermediate response rate (25–30 percent if ER positive, PR negative and 40–45 percent if ER negative, PR positive).[212,213] All available endocrine therapies produce similar objective response rates (for a detailed review, see Reference 214). Therefore, the current approach is to use them sequentially, with the least toxic therapy given first, as illustrated in Fig. 29-6.[215] Tamoxifen (10 mg twice a day, orally) still represents the initial endocrine treatment of choice in postmenopausal women. The newer, nonsteroidal, antiestrogen toremifene (60 mg daily, orally), has been approved by the Food and Drug Administation (FDA) for use in advanced breast cancer. However, it is unlikely that this drug will introduce a significant advance because it has a very similar profile to tamoxifen. Not surprisingly, major crossresistance has been observed between the two agents.[216,217] In contrast, the pure steroidal antiestrogen ICI 182780 (Faslodex) offers more therapeutic promise. This compound has been shown to have a very different mechanism of antiestrogenic action from tamoxifen and in a phase I trial, has been shown to induce objective remissions in patients who had become resistant to tamoxifen.[218] Following the demonstration of the antitumor action of the aromatase inhibitor aminoglutethamide in the treatment of metastatic breast cancer, newer compounds have been generated with increased selectivity and reduced toxicity (see Reference 219 for updated review). Two of them, e.g. anastrozole (Arimidex) (1 mg daily, orally) and letrozole (Fermara) (2.5 mg daily, orally) have been approved by the FDA and are available for routine clinical use in the United States. Both nonsteroidal competitive aromatase inhibitors have been compared with megestrol in phase III, randomized clinical trials involving women with metastatic disease progressive on tamoxifen.[220,221] Overall, the aromatase inhibitors seem to have a better toxicity profile and, at times, superior antitumor efficacy. Therefore, as shown in Fig. 29-6, these compounds have replaced megestrol as second-line endocrine therapy. In the case of premenopausal women, the standard initial endocrine therapy is ovarian ablation, either surgical or medical with LHRH superagonists. Analog of LHRH produce a paradoxic inhibition of pituitary gonadotropin secretion and, consequently, gonadal steroidogenesis. The endocrine and clinical effects observed with these drugs have indeed been found to be comparable to those reported with surgical ovariectomy. The development of long-acting preparations (Gosorelin acetate implant, Zoladex 3.6 mg subcutaneously, monthly) has greatly facilitated the clinical applicability of this

FIGURE 29-6 Outline of sequential endocrine therapies for postmenopausal and premenopausal women with metastatic breast cancer. (*Modified from Buzdar and Hortobagyi.*[217])

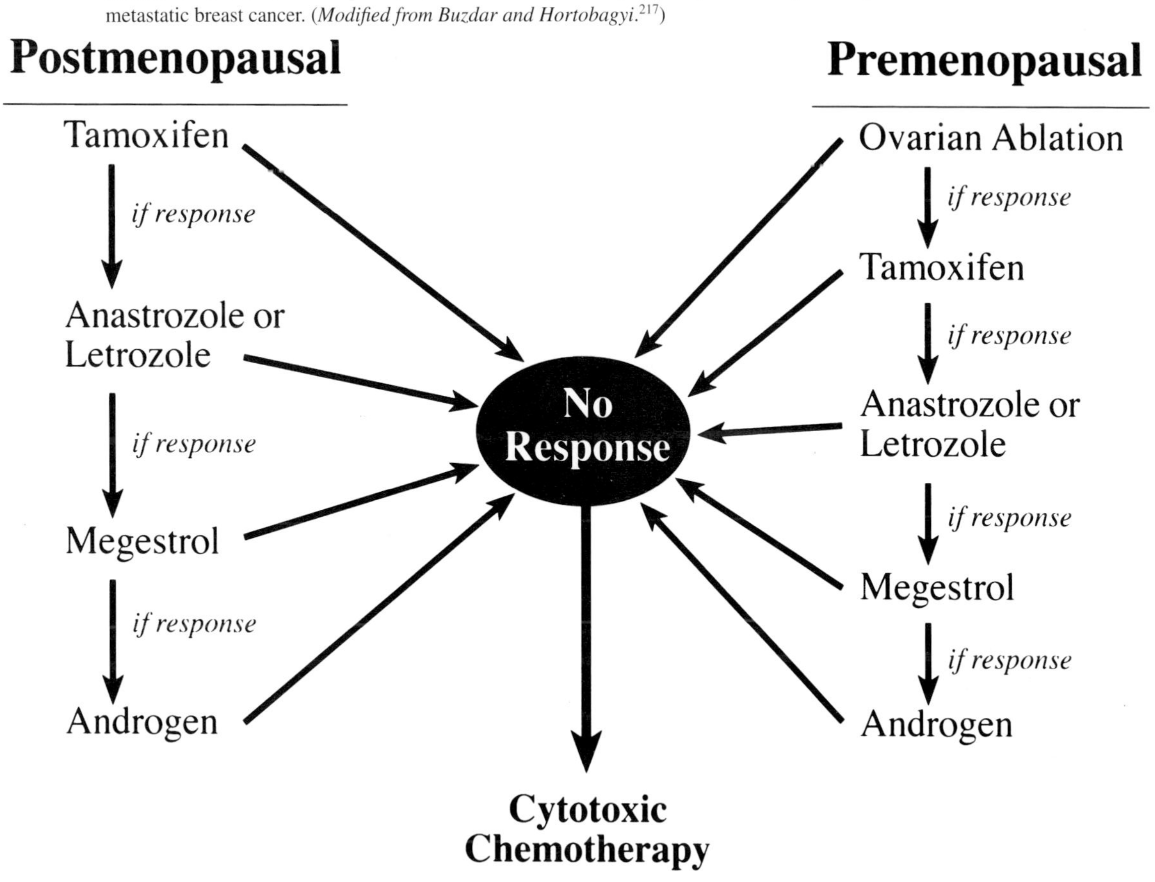

form of therapy. Tamoxifen has also been shown to be effective, with a response rate similar to that of ovariectomy.[222,223] At the time of relapse, the sequence of endocrine therapy is the same as for postmenopausal women (Fig. 29-6). In view of its greater toxicity, cytotoxic chemotherapy is reserved for patients whose disease has become hormone-resistant.

Newer promising therapies are being developed based on improved understanding of tumor biology at the cellular and molecular level. For instance, bisphosphonates, known inhibitors of osteoclast mediated bone resorption, have been demonstrated to have antiosteolytic effect in patients with breast cancer, resulting in reduction of the frequency of skeletal complications.[224] More importantly, the bisphosphonate clodronate (1,600 mg daily orally for two years), has recently been shown to reduce the incidence and number of bony metastasis in patients with primary breast cancer at high risk of relapse due to the presence of micrometastasis in the bone marrow.[225] It is likely that inhibition of osteoclast-induced degradation of bone matrix by bisphosphonates causes a reduction in the local release of bone-derived growth factors (e.g., IGF-I and TGF-β), which results in inhibition of tumor cell proliferation and diminished release of bone resorbing substances such as PTH-rP.[226] These alterations in the bone environment would be expected to create an unfavorable milieu for the formation of metastatic deposits. Surprisingly, administration of clodronate was also found to reduce the development of visceral metastasis in the same group of patients.[225] It is possible that bisphosphonates may directly influence the survival as well as adhesiveness and invasiveness of tumor cells, thus reducing their metastatic potential in general.

During the last few years, the adverse influence of HER-2/neu overexpression on breast cancer biologic behavior has been firmly established. Based on these findings, HER-2/neu targeted therapy has been introduced with the development of the humanized monoclonal antibody Herceptin. In a recent phase III clinical trial involving 469 women with metastatic breast cancer, the combination of Herceptin (loading dose 4 mg/kg IV followed by 2 mg/kg IV weekly) plus chemotherapy was found to be superior to chemotherapy alone, both with regard to response rate (62 percent versus 36 percent) and median time to disease progression (8.6 months versus 5.5 months).[103] Herceptin (same dose as noted earlier) was also found to be effective as a single agent in an additional study involving 222 women who had relapsed after previous chemotherapy for metastatic disease. The overall response rate was 15 percent with a median duration of response of 8.4 months.[227] These encouraging results demonstrate the successful application of basic laboratory observations to the clinical setting.

Treatment of Estrogen Deficiency in Women Surviving Breast Cancer

Earlier diagnosis of breast cancer with improved probability of long-term survival and the ovarian failure induced by routine use of adjuvant chemotherapy in young women have contributed to the expanding pool of postmenopausal breast cancer survivors. It is now clear that hormone replacement therapy not only ameliorates symptoms of estrogen deficiency but also improves quality of life and survival of postmenopausal women by reducing cardiovascular morbidity and mortality and by decreasing the risk of osteoporosis. In breast cancer survivors, however, these beneficial effects are counterbalanced by the serious concern of estrogen-induced reactivation of micrometastasis. To address this important issue, a consensus conference, which included patient advocates and a multidisciplinary panel of experts, was held in 1997 and resulted in a Consensus Statement.[228] Although there was significant diversity of opinions, some general trends emerged that can be summarized as follows. Despite small observational studies showing no increased risk of recurrence in women with breast cancer receiving estrogen replacement, both physicians and patients remain very skeptical about the routine clinical use of hormone replacement therapy in breast cancer survivors. As much as possible, alternative methods should be used to reduce the risk of morbidity and mortality associated with menopause. The introduction of effective lipid-lowering drugs such as the "statins" has been shown to decrease cardiovascular events and mortality. Newer bisphosphonates such as alendronate are also effective drugs for the prevention and treatment of osteoporosis. Selective estrogen receptor modulators (SERMs) such as raloxifene are viewed as promising new agents because they appear to have an estrogen-like effect on bone and lipids while exhibiting an antiestrogenic action on the breast and uterus. Phytoestrogens (as discussed earlier) are another potentially useful class of compounds. SERMs and phytoestrogens, however, will not be useful to relieve acute symptoms of menopause such as those of vasomotor instability or symptoms of urogenital atrophy. Furthermore, additional studies are still necessary to fully appreciate the impact of SERMs and phytoestrogens on morbidity and mortality. The participants of this Consensus Conference felt that clinical trials should probably be conducted to evaluate the use of estrogen in selected groups of women at very low risk of relapse based on tumor characteristics. It would be of particular interest to study the combined use of tamoxifen and hormone replacement therapy to determine whether the use of this antiestrogen reduces the risk of estrogen-induced reactivation of micrometastasis without adversely affecting the benefit of hormone replacement therapy. In the absence of these trials, the use of estrogen in women with a history of breast cancer should only be considered as the last resource in highly selected patients who are fully informed about its possible adverse consequences.

Chemoprevention

The reduction in the incidence of contralateral breast cancer observed in the adjuvant tamoxifen trials[116] has stimulated interest in testing the potential role of tamoxifen as a chemopreventive agent. Preliminary results of the National Surgical Adjuvant Breast and Bowel Project (NSABP) Protocol P1, involving 13,388 pre- and postmenopausal women at high risk of breast cancer, has shown a 45 percent reduction in the incidence of invasive breast cancer in the tamoxifen group compared to the placebo group.[117] This beneficial effect seems to be restricted to estrogen receptor positive tumors because no change was observed in the incidence of estrogen receptor negative breast cancers. In support of these findings, the Multiple Outcomes of Raloxifene Evaluation (MORE) trial, which included 7,704 postmenopausal women with osteoporosis (i.e., not at increased risk of breast cancer) has shown a decrease in the incidence of breast cancer among women in the raloxifene arm (60–120 mg orally daily) compared to the placebo group.[229] Although encouraging, these results need to be viewed with caution because the duration of follow-up is short and neither study has yet shown any effect on breast cancer mortality. It is still possible that tamoxifen and raloxifene may simply treat subclinical breast cancers and postpone their development rather than preventing them. Caution in interpreting the results of the NSABP-P1 and MORE trials is further dictated by the failure of preliminary analysis of the Royal Marsden Hospital Chemoprevention Trial (which included women at high risk of breast cancer based on family history)[230] and the Italian Tamoxifen Prevention Study (which included women at slightly reduced risk)[231] to demonstrate any reduction in breast cancer incidence by tamoxifen. Multiple factors such as the characteristics of the population under study, duration of treatment, and duration of follow-up are likely to play an important role in accounting for these early discrepant results. It is clear that we need to wait for these trials to mature before the possible value of tamoxifen as a chemopreventive agent in breast cancer can be rigorously defined.

TABLE 29-9. Risk Factors for Endometrial Cancer

Obesity
Nulliparity
Early menarche
Late menopause
Exogenous estrogens
Tamoxifen
Polycystic ovarian disease
Estrogen-secreting tumors
Hereditary nonpolyposis
Colorectal cancer syndrome
Hypertension
Diabetes mellitus

Endometrial Cancer

The most common pelvic malignancy in women is endometrial cancer, which accounts for 9 percent of all female cancers, amounting to more than 30,000 cases and 6,000 deaths in the United States yearly. Although this represents nearly half of all gynecologic malignancies, endometrial cancer accounts for only 13 percent of gynecologic cancer deaths and 4 percent of total female cancer deaths. Despite the relatively high prevalence of this form of uterine cancer, there has been a steady decline in deaths from endometrial cancer during the past 50 years. The median age at diagnosis is 63 years, with 75–80 percent of patients diagnosed after menopause.

Risk Factors

The risk factors for endometrial cancer are listed in Table 29-9. More so than for breast cancer, long-term exposure to unopposed estrogen effect is the common denominator for most of the risk factors.[11] Unlike the findings in breast cancer, progestins appear to have a protective effect. When used as part of postmenopausal hormone replacement, they reduce, although not completely eliminate, the risk of endometrial cancer associated with estrogen use.[11] Progesterone is the dominant component of current combination oral contraceptives, which have been shown to lower the risk of endometrial cancer by 50 percent.[118] Polycystic ovarian disease serves as the risk factor for the majority of endometrial carcinomas diagnosed in premenopausal women as a result of unopposed estrogen exposure due to chronic anovulation.[232,233] Endometrial cancer is also the most common extracolonic cancer in women with hereditary nonpolyposis colorectal cancer syndrome.[234,235] Of interest, endometrial cancers associated with estrogen-related risk factors such as obesity, and unopposed estrogen therapy appear to have a more favorable prognosis as a result of their better differentiated histologic grade, more superficial extent of myometrial invasion, presence of steroid receptors, and increased sensitivity to endocrine therapy.[236]

Diagnosis

Endometrial cancer usually presents with postmenopausal bleeding. The likelihood that postmenopausal vaginal bleeding is due to endometrial cancer increases with age, ranging from 9 percent for women in their 50s to 60 percent for those in their 80s.[237] Definitive diagnosis is based upon adequate endometrial sampling, which can either be performed in the office or in the operating room under anesthesia (dilatation and curettage). Once the diagnosis is established, a full surgical staging (as introduced by the International Federation of Gynecology and Obstetrics in 1988) is performed to rule out metastatic disease and determine the extent of pelvic invasion by the tumor (Table 29-10).[238]

Pathology and Prognosis

Eighty to 95 percent of endometrial cancers are classic endometrioid adenocarcinomas. The remainder are composed of more rare histologic types such as papillary serous and clear cell carcinomas, which carry a much worse prognosis. As expected, prognosis is highly influenced by surgical staging (Table 29-10) with a five-year survival of 83 percent in Stage I, 73 percent in

TABLE 29-10. 1988 System for Surgical Staging of Carcinoma of the Uterus

Stage and Grade*	Features
Stage IA; grade 1, 2, or 3	Tumor limited to endometrium
Stage IB; grade 1, 2, or 3	Invasion of less than half the myometrium
Stage IC; grade 1, 2, or 3	Invasion of more than half the myometrium
Stage IIA; grade 1, 2, or 3	Endocervical glandular involvement only
Stage IIB; grade 1, 2, or 3	Cervical stromal invasion
Stage IIIA; grade 1, 2, or 3	Tumor invading serosa or adnexa, or malignant peritoneal cytology
Stage IIIB; grade 1, 2, or 3	Vaginal metastasis
Stage IIIC; grade 1, 2, or 3	Metastasis to pelvic or para-aortic lymph nodes
Stage IVA; grade 1, 2, or 3	Tumor invasion of the bladder or bowel mucosa
Stage IVB	Distant metastasis including intra-abdominal or inguinal lymph nodes

*Grade reflects the amount of nongland forming tumor (i.e., solid growth pattern). Grade I: $\leq$5 percent; Grade II: 6–50 percent; Grade III: >50 percent.

Source: Reproduced from Rose PG.[238]

TABLE 29-11. Prognostic Factors in Endometrial Cancer

Histologic type
Grade
Tumor size
Myometrial invasion
Capillary-lymphatic space invasion
Positive peritoneal cytology
Hormone receptor status
Aneuploidy
High S-phase
HER-2neu (overexpressed in 10 percent)
p53 mutations (present in 10–20 percent)

Stage II, 52 percent in Stage III, and 27 percent in Stage IV disease.[239] The major prognostic factors in endometrial cancer are summarized in Table 29-11. The presence of estrogen and progesterone receptors directly correlates with better tumor differentiation, less myometrial invasion, a lower incidence of nodal metastasis, and improved survival.[240,241]

Treatment

Approximately 90 percent of endometrial cancers present with early stage disease that can be treated with surgical resection of all tumor-bearing tissue. This usually involves a total abdominal hysterectomy and bilateral salpingo oophorectomy. Alternatively, radical hysterectomy and pelvic and periaortic lymph node resection is indicated for more locally advanced disease. Although no definite survival improvement has been demonstrated, postoperative adjuvant radiation therapy is frequently administered except for low-risk Stage I cancers. Based on the extent of disease, adjuvant radiation therapy can be tailored to treat the pelvis, the pelvis and the periaortic region, or the whole abdomen (for detailed review of surgical treatment and radiation therapy of endometrial cancer, see References 238 and 242).

Women with metastatic disease are usually treated with hormone therapy or chemotherapy. Because of its lower toxicity, hormone therapy is usually employed first. Progestins were first reported to cause regression of endometrial cancer 30 years ago. Response to progestin does not appear to depend upon the specific agent used, dose, or route of administration (see Reference 242 for review). In contrast, clinical response is clearly dependent on the tumor histologic grade and receptor (ER/PR) status as shown in Table 29-12.[236,243–246] In particular, the presence of progesterone receptors within the tumor tissue is essential for eliciting a clinical response to progestins. Although there is generally a good (>80 percent) concordance between biochemical and immunohistochemical determination of PR in endometrial tumors, immunohistochemical determination has provided important data regarding tumor heterogeneity, PR expression, and endocrine response. Tumors with abundant PR content (800–2,000 fmol/mg of protein) can show intratumor proportions of PR positive immunostaining cells that range from 20–90 percent.[247] Immunohistochemical studies also indicate that the failure of some PR positive endometrial cancers to respond to progestin therapy is due to PR negative tumors that were falsely designated as PR positive by biochemical assays, contamination with receptor-positive nonneoplastic endometrium and myometrium, or tumors with endocrine unresponsive PR negative tumor cell populations admixed with PR positive tumor cells.

TABLE 29-12. Endometrial Cancer: Characteristics and Response to Progestins

Tumor Characteristic	Clinical Response Rate, Percent
Tumor Grade	
Well differentiated	52
Poorly differentiated	16
Tumor Receptor Status	
ER^+/PR^+	77
ER^-/PR^-	9

Source: Adapted from references 236 and 243–246.

The antiestrogen tamoxifen is the only other form of hormonal manipulation that has been evaluated and found to be effective in treating endometrial cancer. At doses of 20–40 mg a day, tamoxifen has been reported to induce response rates ranging from 0 percent to 53 percent with an overall average of 22 percent.[248–250] Not unlike the progestins, it appears that tamoxifen is more likely to be effective in patients with well-differentiated receptor positive tumors. The antitumor efficacy of tamoxifen in women with metastatic endometrial cancer contrasts with its tumor-promoting effect when administered for adjuvant therapy or chemoprevention of breast cancer. These discrepant effects are likely to be related to the mixed agonistic/antagonistic properties of tamoxifen with one prevailing over the other under different biologic and clinical settings.

Cytotoxic chemotherapy is often used for advanced or recurrent endometrial carcinoma when hormonal therapy is ineffective. Agents found to be effective include cyclophosphamide, 5-fluorouracil, doxorubicin, cis-platin, carboplatin, and more recently, paclitaxel. When used alone, these agents produce response rates between 20 and 35 percent. When used in combination, objective responses are observed in 40–60 percent of patients (see Reference 242 for review). At present, there is no compelling evidence that either hormonal therapy or chemotherapy prolongs survival when given to patients with high-risk tumors in an adjuvant setting.

Prostate Cancer

There are large geographic and racial differences in the incidence of clinically diagnosed prostate cancer; these differences range over 100-fold when one compares low incidence populations such as those in Shanghai, China, with high incidence populations such as African-Americans in Alameda, California. Cancer of the prostate is now the most common malignancy in American males, with 184,500 new cases expected to be diagnosed in the United States in 1998. Prostate cancer is now second only to lung cancer as a cause of cancer-related deaths in the United States. Pathologists find microscopic foci of well-differentiated adenocarcinomas in clinically normal autopsied prostate glands with an incidence ranging from 10 (in 50-year-old men) to 70 percent (in men over 80 years of age). Because there is approximately an 8 percent lifetime chance of being diagnosed with prostate cancer, it is possible that 90 percent of all prostate cancers are "latent" or incidental, remaining undetected and clinically unimportant for decades. Despite this apparent indolent growth rate, less than half of all clinically diagnosed prostate cancers are detected early enough to achieve complete tumor resection before there has been tumor spread beyond the prostate gland. Problems associated with prostate cancer can be expected to increase. As the average life ex-

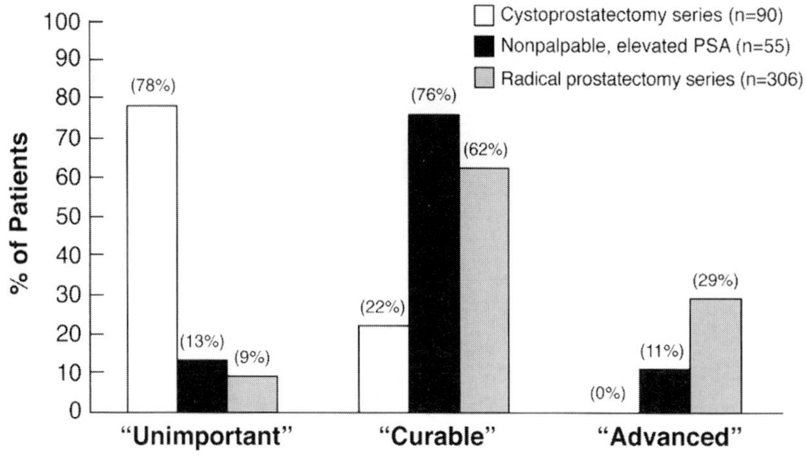

FIGURE 29-7. Comparison of the prognostic categories of prostate cancer detected in the cytoprostatectomy specimens (similar to autopsy discovered cancer), radical prostatectomy specimens (cancer discovered by digital rectal exam) and the nonpalpable cancers detected because of PSA elevation. (*Reproduced from Trump et al.,*[257] *modified from Ohori et al.*[256])

pectancy is prolonged, the proportion of elderly people in the population will increase (the population over age 60 will increase more than 60 percent during the next 30 years), as will the incidence rate of this age-related malignancy. Uncontrolled carcinoma of the prostate has a major impact on the quality and duration of life, although many men with prostate cancer die from other comorbid illnesses rather than from this malignancy.

Risk Factors

Though prostatic cancer and BPH are often found concurrently in older men, BPH is not a proven risk factor for the development of prostate cancer.[251,252] As was discussed earlier, increasing age, dietary factors, and hormones all appear to play a significant role in the etiology of prostate cancer. An etiological association between hormones and prostate cancer is supported by the clinical observations that prostatic cancer does not develop in eunuchs, and that latent prostate cancer is lower than expected in cirrhotic males who have elevated blood levels of endogenously produced estrogens.[251,252] Of interest, cigarette smoking, alcohol use, height, weight, blood group, body hair distribution, urban versus rural site of residence, have not been found to be associated with an increased risk of prostate cancer.

Diagnosis

Cancer of the prostate does not cause any symptoms until it is locally advanced or metastatic. Patients with locally advanced disease experience symptoms of bladder outlet obstruction such as hesitancy, nocturia, incomplete bladder emptying, and diminished urinary stream. Additional symptoms indicative of local invasion include perineal pain, sudden development of erectile dysfunction, or hematuria. Twenty to 30 percent of patients with prostate cancer present with symptoms related to metastatic disease such as bone pain and fatigue.

Because symptomatic prostate cancer is virtually always incurable, considerable emphasis has recently been placed on early diagnosis through regular screening consisting of digital rectal exam (DRE) and prostate specific antigen (PSA) measurement. In case that the DRE is abnormal and/or the PSA is elevated (above 4 ng/ml), a transrectal ultrasound with guided biopsies is recommended. There is no question that the introduction of screening has significantly increased the proportion of prostate cancers that are pathologically confined to the prostate.[253] Because of the high frequency of "latent" cancers found at autopsy or in cystoprostatectomy specimens removed for the treatment of bladder cancer, some authorities have questioned the clinical significance of nonpalpable cancers detected because of an elevated PSA. As can be seen in Fig. 29-7, however, this category of tumors more closely resembles clinical cancers than incidentally discovered tumors.[254,255] Only 13 percent of nonpalpable, PSA-detected tumors exhibited "unimportant" pathologic features (based on volume and grade). This percentage is only slightly higher than that of tumors detected by DRE (9 percent) and substantially lower than that of incidentally discovered tumors (78 percent). Figure 29-7 also shows that a larger fraction of PSA detected cancers are curable compared to tumors discovered by DRE (76 versus 62 percent). In support of these findings are the recent data from the first prospective, randomized study of prostate cancer screening conducted by Labrie.[256] This trial, which included more than 46,000 men, has revealed an almost threefold decrease in annual death rate from prostate cancer among the screened men. Although these data will need confirmation, in the aggregate, current evidence indicates that screening identifies clinically significant disease and can have an impact on prostate cancer mortality. At present, both the American Urological Association and the American Cancer Society recommend that men over age 50 who have a life expectancy of at least 10 years have an annual DRE and PSA measurement. Men at high risk for developing prostate cancer, such as African Americans and those with a positive family history, should begin screening at age 40.

Pathology and Prognosis

The most common tumor arising in the prostate is adenocarcinoma originating from the peripheral acinar glands. The degree of differentiation has major prognostic importance. Most commonly, this is determined using the histologic criteria developed by Gleeson, which include the degree of glandular differentiation and structure of architecture viewed at low-power magnification. Both the dominant morphology of the specimen and the secondary pattern (i.e., the next, most common pattern) are assigned a grade ranging from 1 (most differentiated) to 5 (least differentiated). The two grades are arithmetically added to provide a final Gleeson score, which spans from 2 to 10.[257] A clear association has been demonstrated between a higher Gleeson score and a higher mortality.[257] As expected, tumor stage is another critical prognostic factor. As shown in Table 29-13, a new TNM system (based on *T*umor size, *N*odal status, and presence of distant *M*etastasis) was

TABLE 29-13. Comparison of the ASCC/VICC 1992 TNM Staging System and Whitemore-Jewett Staging System

Whitemore-Jewett	TNM
A Nonpalpable, diagnosed after TURP	
A1 <5 percent resected specimen	T1 Clinical inapparent tumor not palpable or visible by imaging
	T1a Tumor incidental histologic finding in 5 percent or less of tissue resected
	T1b Tumor incidental histologic finding in more than 5 percent of tissue resected
	T1c Tumor identified by needle biopsy (e.g., because of elevated PSA)
A2 >5 percent resected specimen	
B Palpable	T2 Tumor confined within prostate
	T2a Tumor involves half of a lobe or less
	T2b Tumor involves more than half of a lobe but not both lobes
	T2c Tumor involves both lobes
B1 One lobe	
B2 Both lobes	
C Capsular penetration	T3 Tumor extends through the prostatic capsule
	T3a Unilateral extracapsular extension
	T3b Bilateral extracapsular extension
	T3c Tumor invades seminal vesicle(s)
	T4 Tumor is fixed or invades adjacent structures other than seminal vesicles
	T4a Tumor invades any of bladder neck, external sphincter, rectum
	T4b Tumor invades levator muscles and/or is fixed to pelvic wall
D	
D1 Regional nodes	N
D2 Beyond regional nodes	M M/a Nonregional nodes
	M/b Bones
	M/c Other sites

Source: Reproduced from Trump DL.[255]

introduced in 1992 to replace the old Whitemore/Jewett (ABCD) scheme. Advantages of the TNM system include its greater detail and the inclusion of a new category, T_{1C}, for nonpalpable tumors detected because of an elevated PSA. Moreover, this classification accommodates those tumors that are not palpable but visible by an imaging study in the T2–T4 categories, as appropriate. Clearly, survival is inversely related to tumor stage.

Aside from histologic grade, tumor stage, and PSA level,[254,258,259] there are no well-established prognostic markers in prostate cancer. Potentially promising markers include DNA ploidy,[260] nuclear morphometry,[261] apoptotic index,[262] and p53.[263] However, their practical usefulness in the clinical management of prostate cancer remains to be determined. In contrast to breast cancer, measurement of hormone receptors (e.g., androgen receptors) has not proven to be particularly useful either prognostically or therapeutically. Because 80 percent of prostate cancers are initially hormone-responsive, it is accepted common practice to treat all patients with androgen ablation.

Treatment

The choices of treatment of prostate cancer depend upon the stage of the disease at the time of diagnosis. Watchful waiting may be a reasonable option for men with a life expectancy of <10 years for a clinically localized prostate cancer (T1) with a favorable grade (i.e., grade 1 or 2).[264] A typical example may be a tumor classified as T1a (i.e., comprising <5 percent of a pathologic specimen obtained by transurethral resection for presumed benign prostatic hypertrophy). When discussing this option with the patient, it should be made clear, however, that a small fraction of these tumors with overall favorable prognosis will progress locally or metastasize.[264] All other patients with cancer confined to the prostate (T1 and T2) need to undergo definitive therapy. The choice between radical prostatectomy and radiation therapy remains a controversial issue that is beyond the scope of this review. Patients with clinical stage T3 prostate cancer are rarely cured by either radical prostatectomy or radiotherapy because they already have occult metastasis at the time of diagnosis. In this setting, adjuvant hormonal therapy with androgen ablation has been frequently used with improved short-term local control, longer progression-free survival, and recently increased overall survival.[265,266] An alternative approach currently under scrutiny is to use neoadjuvant hormonal therapy with the goal of downstaging the tumor prior to definitive treatment. In the first randomized and prospective trial testing this approach, Labrie et al.[267] reported an increase in organ-confined disease and negativity of surgical margins in the group of patients treated with hormone ablation for three months before radical prostatectomy compared to radical prostatectomy alone.

Treatment of disseminated prostate cancer has traditionally consisted of medical or surgical castration. Because of its associated cardiovascular toxicity, estrogen therapy has been largely abandoned and has been replaced by treatment with GnRH analogs (see References 268 and 269 for detailed review). These compounds have been found to be highly effective in reducing circulating testosterone and dihydrotestosterone levels to the same extent as observed with surgical orchiectomy. Furthermore, the introduction of once-monthly preparations (Leupron depot 7.5 mg IM) has significantly increased the practical applicability of this form of therapy. Frequency of tumor regression or stabilization does not differ between patients treated with orchiectomy or long-acting GnRH analogues. A potential drawback associated with the use of these compounds is the initial (1–2 weeks upon initiation of therapy) rise in testosterone, which causes a transient disease flare in 5–10 percent of patients. In occasional patients, severe reactions with spinal cord compression or death have been observed. However, this complication can be prevented with the concomitant use of antiandrogen therapy. Future use of GnRH antagonists will also obviate this problem, as these compounds are devoid of the initial agonistic effect observed with GnRH superagonists. Although approximately 80 percent of patients with metastatic prostate cancer respond to either medical or surgical castration, disease progression inevitably occurs following a median duration of response of 12–18 months.[268,269] In order to improve the efficacy of androgen ablation, Labrie and his collaborators have introduced the strategy of "complete androgen blockade."[270] The rationale for this approach is based on the observation that the adrenal glands contribute to 5 percent of the total androgen pool and that following surgical orchiectomy, the concentration of dihydrotestosterone in prostate cancer tissue only falls by 50–80 percent.[271] Therefore, in order to completely abolish androgenic stimulation of prostate cancer, it may be necessary to combine medical or surgical castration with antiandrogen therapy aimed at eliminating the effects of these residual androgens of adrenal origin. Several randomized studies have tested the validity of this therapeutic approach. One of the largest has been conducted by the Southwest Oncology Group in conjunction with the Eastern Cooperative Oncology Group (i.e., Inter-group study).[272] This trial, which enrolled 603 patients, compared the GnRH analogue leuprolide plus the antiandrogen flutamide to leuprolide alone. The results of this study demonstrated a small but significant survival advantage for patients receiving complete androgen deprivation (median survival 35.1 months in the leuprolide/flutamide arm compared to 29.3 months in the leuprolide/placebo arm). Of interest, this study demonstrated that the most striking benefit from complete androgen blockade occurred in the subgroup of patients with minimal metastatic disease (e.g., only axial skeletal metastasis and good performance status). Some,[273,274] but not all studies,[275,276] have confirmed the advantages of combination versus single modality therapy. Of particular concern are the results of a recent large trial testing orchiectomy plus antiandrogen therapy versus orchiectomy alone, which failed to demonstrate a significant advantage from complete androgen blockade.[277] Therefore, this therapeutic approach still remains somewhat controversial and its potential superior antitumor effect needs to be weighed against its higher cost and greater toxicity (e.g., diarrhea).

Upon disease progression following androgen ablation, limited therapeutic options are available. For patients treated with medical or surgical castration alone, treatment modalities aimed at inhibiting adrenal androgen secretion/action can be employed. These include medical adrenalectomy with aminoglutethamide (250 mg four times daily) plus hydrocortisone (20 mg twice daily), the androgen biosynthetic inhibitor ketoconazole (400 mg three times daily), or the use of antiandrogens such as flutamide 250 mg three times daily). Unfortunately, however, objective tumor regression is observed in only 10–20 percent of patients with a median duration of only 6 months. Similarly modest results have been reported with cytotoxic chemotherapy in patients with tumors that have become hormone refractory (see Reference 255 for review).

Chemoprevention

In the United States, the National Cancer Institute has initiated a large scale clinical trial for chemoprevention of prostate cancer conducted by the Southwest Oncology Group. More than 18,000 healthy men over the age of 55 with a life expectancy >10 years have been randomized to a seven-year treatment with either placebo or the 5α-reductase inhibitor finasteride, which is currently approved as a treatment for benign prostatic hyperplasia. All men will be subjected to annual DRE and PSA measurement, and prostate biopsy will be recommended in case of abnormal DRE or elevated PSA. Finally, all participants will undergo prostatic biopsy at the end of the trial to determine the influence of finasteride treatment on prostate cancer development at least at the pathological level.

REFERENCES

1. Bittner JJ: The causes of mammary cancer in mice. *Harvey Lect* 42:221, 1947.
2. Huggins C: Endocrine-induced regression of cancers. *Science* 156:1050, 1967.
3. Furth J: Hormones as etiological agents in neoplasia, in Becker FF (ed): *Cancer: A Comprehensive Treatise*, vol 1. New York, Plenum, 1975, p 75.
4. Miller AB: An overview of hormone associate cancer. *Cancer Res* 38:3985, 1978.
5. Thomas DB: Do hormones cause breast cancer? *Cancer* 53:595, 1984.
6. Hawkins RA, Miller WR: What is the role of sex hormones in cancer development? *Rev Endocr Related Cancer* 30:13, 1988.
7. Henderson BE, Ross RK, Pike MC, Casagrande JT: Endogenous hormones as a major factor in human cancer. *Cancer Res* 42:3232, 1982.
8. Benz CC, Lewis BJ: Hormones and cancer, in Greenspan FJ, Baxter JD (eds): *Basic and Clinical Endocrinology*, 4th ed. San Mateo, California, Appleton and Lange, 1993.
9. Claman HN: Corticoids and lymphoid cells. *N Engl J Med* 287:388, 1972.
10. Baxter JD, Forsham PH: Tissue effects of glucocorticoids. *Am J Med* 53:573, 1972.
11. Bernstein L, Ross RK, Henderson BE: Relationship of hormone use to cancer risk. *J Natl Cancer Inst Monogr* 12:137, 1992.
12. Greenway B, Igbal MJ, Johnson PJ, et al: Estrogen receptor proteins in malignant and fetal pancreas. *Br Med J* 238:751, 1981.
13. Fisher RI, Neifeld JP, Lippman ME: Oestrogen receptors in human malignant melanoma. *Lancet* 2:337, 1976.
14. Keating JJ, Johnson PJ, Cochrane AMG, Gazzard BG, Krasner N, Smith PM, et al: A prospective randomized controlled trial of tamoxifen and cyproterone acetate in pancreatic carcinoma. *Br J Cancer* 60:789, 1989.
15. Bakkevold KE, Pettersen A, Arnesjo B, Espehaug B: Tamoxifen therapy in unresectable adenocarcinoma of the pancreas and the papilla of Vater. *Br J Surg* 77:725, 1990.
16. Cocconi G, Bella M, Calabresi F, Tonato M, Canaletti R, Boni C, Buzzi F, Ceci G, Corgna E, Costa P, Lottici R, Papadia F, Sofra MC, Bacchi M: Treatment of metastatic malignant melanoma with dacarbazine plus tamoxifen. *N Engl J Med* 327:516, 1992.

17. Szende B, Srkalovic G, Groot K, Lapis K, Schally AV: Regression of nitrosamine-induced pancreatic cancers in hamsters treated with luteinizing hormone-releasing hormone antagonists or agonists. *Cancer Res* 50:3716, 1990.
18. Imagawa W, Yang J, Guzman R, Nandi S: Control of mammary gland development, in Knobil E, Neill JD (eds): *The Physiology of Reproduction*, 2nd ed. New York, Raven Press, 1994, p 1033.
19. Kleinberg D, Ruan W, Catanese B, Newman C, Feldman F: Non-lactogenic effects of growth hormone on growth and insulin-like growth factor-I messenger ribonucleic acid of rat mammary gland. *Endocrinology* 126:3274, 1990.
20. Haslam S, Nummy K: The ontogeny and cellular distribution of estrogen receptors in normal mouse mammary gland. *J Steroid Biochem Mol Biol* 42:589, 1992.
21. Silberstein G, Van Horn K, Shyamala G, Daniel C: Essential role of endogenous estrogen in directly stimulating mammary growth demonstrated by implants containing pure antiestrogens. *Endocrinology* 134:84, 1994.
22. Lubahn DB, Moyer JS, Golding TS, Couse JF, Korach KS, Smithies O: Alteration of reproductive function but not prenatal sexual development after insertional disruption of the mouse estrogen receptor gene. *Proc Natl Acad Sci USA* 90:11162, 1993.
23. Russo J, Gusterson B, Rogers A, Russo I, Wellings S, van Zweiten M: Biology of disease: Comparative study of human and rat mammary tumorigenesis. *Lab Invest* 62:244, 1990.
24. Russo I, Russo J: Mammary gland neoplasia in long-term rodent studies. *Environ Health Perspect* 104:938, 1996.
25. Vermeulen A, Deslypere JP, Paridaens R, Leclercq G, Roy F, Heuson JC: Aromatase, 17β-hydroxysteroid dehydrogenase and intra-tissular sex hormone concentrations in cancerous and normal glandular breast tissue in postmenopausal women. *Eur J Cancer Oncol* 22:515, 1986.
26. Mehta RR, Valcourt L, Graves J, Green R, Das Gupta TK: Subcellular concentration of estrone, estradiol, androstenedione and 17β-hydroxysteroid dehydrogenase (17-β-OH-SDH) activity in malignant and non-malignant human breast tissues. *Int J Cancer* 40:305, 1987.
27. Lipton A, Santner SJ, Santen RJ, Harvey HA, Deil PD, White-Hershey D, et al: Aromatase activity in primary and metastatic human breast cancer. *Cancer* 59:779, 1987.
28. Silva MC, Rowlands MG, Dowsett M, Gusterson B, McKinna JA, Fryatt I, et al: Intratumoral aromatase as prognostic factor in human breast carcinoma. *Cancer Res* 49:2588, 1989.
29. Santner SJ, Pauley RL, Tait L, Kaseta J, Santen RJ: Aromatase activity and expression in breast cancer and benign breast tissue stromal cells. *J Clin Endocrinol Metab* 82:200, 1997.
30. Bulun SE, Sharda G, Rink J, Sharma S, Simpson ER: Distribution of aromatase P450 transcripts and adipose fibroblasts in the human breast. *J Clin Endocrinol Metab* 81:1273, 1996.
31. Tekmal RR, Ramachandra N, Gubba S, Durgam VR, Mantione J, Toda K, et al: Overexpression of *int-5/aronzatase* in mammary glands of transgenic mice results in the induction of hyperplasia and nuclear abnormalities. *Cancer Res* 56:3180, 1996.
32. Keshava N, Fang C, Bhalla KN, Tekmal RR: Environmental mutagen (DMBA) acts synergistically in *int-5/aromatase* transgenic mice that have increased mammary estrogen activity. *Mutat Res* 379:S151, 1997.
33. Bayard F, Damilano S, Robel P, Baulieu EE: Cytoplasmic and nuclear estradiol and progesterone receptors in human endometrium. *J Clin Endocrinol Metab* 46:635, 1978.
34. Clarke CL, Sutherland RL: Progestin regulation of cellular proliferation. *Endocr Rev* 2:266, 1990.
35. Meyer JS: Cell proliferation in normal human breast ducts, fibroadenomas, and other ductal hyperplasias measured by nuclear labeling with tritriated thymidine. Effects of menstrual phase, age and oral contraception. *Hum Pathol* 8:67, 1977.
36. Masters JRW, Drife JO, Scarisbrick JJ: Cyclic variation of DNA synthesis in human breast epithelium. *J Natl Cancer Inst* 58:163, 1977.
37. Barrat J, Lignieres B de, Marpeau L, Larue L, Fournier S, Nahoul K, et al: Effet in vivo de l'adminstration locale de progesterone sur l'activite mitotique des galactophores humains. *J Gynecol Obstet Biol Reprod* 19:269, 1990.
38. Chang KJ, Lee TT, Linares-Cruz G, Fournier S, de Lignieres B: Influence of percutaneous administration of estradiol and progesterone on human breast epithelial cell in vivo. *Fertil Steril* 63:785, 1995.
39. Gompel A, Malet C, Spritzer P, Kuttenn F, Mauvais-Jarvis P: Progestin effect on cell proliferation and 17β-hydroxysteroid dehydrogenase activity in normal human beast cells in culture. *J Clin Endocrinol Metab* 63:1174, 1986.
40. Gill PG, Vignon F, Bardon S, Derocq D, Rochefort H: Difference between R5020 and the antiprogestin RU486 in antiproliferative effects on human breast cancer cells. *Breast Cancer Res Treat* 10:37, 1987.
41. Prudhomme JF, Malet C, Gompel A, Lalardrie JP, Ochoa C, Boue A, et al: 17β-Hydroxysteroid dehydrogenase activity in human breast epithelial cell and fibroblast cultures. *Endocrinology* 114:1483, 1984.
42. Horwitz KB, Freidenberg GR: Growth inhibition and increase of insulin receptors in antiestrogen-resistant T47DCO human breast cancer cells by progestins: Implications for endocrine therapies. *Cancer Res* 45:167, 1985.
43. Braunsberg H, Coldham NG, Leake RE, Cowan SK, Wong W: Actions of a progestogen on human breast cancer cells: Mechanisms of growth stimulation and inhibition. *Eur J Cancer Clin Oncol* 23:563, 1987.
44. Vignon F, Bardon S, Chalbos D, Rochefort H: Antiestrogenic effect of R5020, a synthetic progestin in human breast cancer cells in culture. *J Clin Endocrinol Metab* 56:1124, 1983.
45. Sutherland RL, Hall RE, Pang GYN, Musgrove EA, Clarke CL: Effect of medroxyprogesterone acetate on proliferation and cell cycle kinetics of human mammary carcinoma cells. *Cancer Res* 48:5084, 1988.
46. Lydon J, DeMayo F, Funk C, Mani S, Hughes A, Montgomery J, et al: Mice lacking progesterone receptor exhibit pleiotropic reproductive abnormalities. *Genes Dev* 9:2266, 1995.
47. Lydon JP, DeMayo FJ, Conneely OM, O'Malley BW: Reproductive phenotypes of the progesterone receptor null mutant mouse. *J Steroid Biochem Mol Biol* 56:67, 1996.
48. Ormandy CJ, Camus A, Barra J, Damotte D, Lucas B, Buteau H, et al: Null mutation of the prolactin receptor gene produces multiple reproductive defects in the mouse. *Genes Dev* 11:167, 1997.
49. Segaloff A: Inhibition by progesterone of radiation-estrogen-induced mammary cancer in rat. *Cancer Res* 33:1136, 1973.
50. Snedeker S, Brown C, DiAugustine R: Expression and functional properties of transforming growth factor α and epidermal growth factor during mouse mammary gland ductal morphogenesis. *Dev Biol* 88:276, 1991.
51. Vonderhaar B: Local effects of EGF, alpha-TGF, and EGF-like growth factor on lobuloalveolar development of the mouse mammary gland in vivo. *J Cell Physiol* 132:581, 1987.
52. Fowler K, Walker F, Alexander W, Hibbs M, Nice E, Bohmer R, et al: A mutation in the epidermal growth factor receptor in waved-2 mice has a profound effect on receptor biochemistry that results in impaired lactation. *Proc Natl Acad Sci USA* 92:1465, 1995.
53. Silberstein G, Daniel C: Reversible inhibition of mammary gland growth by transforming growth factor-β. *Science* 237:291, 1987.
54. Jhappan C, Geiser A, Kordon E, Bagheri D, Henninghausen L, Roberts A, et al: Targeting of a transforming growth factor β1 transgene to the pregnant mammary gland inhibits alveolar development and lactation. *EMBO J* 12:1835, 1995.
55. Jackson D, Bresnick J, Dickson C: A role for fibroblast growth factor signaling in the lobuloalveolar development of the mammary gland. *J Mam Gland Biol Neoplasia* 2:385, 1997.
56. Richert M, Wood T: Role for the insulin-like growth factors in postnatal growth of marine mammary gland. *Endocrinology*, in press, January, 1999.
57. Ruan W, Newman C, Kleinberg D: Intact and amino-terminally shortened forms of insulin-like growth factor I induce mammary gland differentiation and development. *Proc Natl Acad Sci USA* 89:10872, 1992.
58. Neuenschwander S, Schwartz A, Wood T, Roberts J, Henninghausen L, LeRoith D: Involution of the lactating mammary gland is inhibited by the IGF system in a transgenic mouse model. *J Clin Invest* 97:2225, 1996.
59. Richert MM, Wood TL: Expression and regulation of insulin-like growth factors and their binding proteins in the normal breast, in Manni A (ed): *Contemporary Endocrinology: Endocrinology of Breast Cancer*. New Jersey, Humana Press, in press.

60. Sakakura T, Nishizuka Y, Dawe CJ: Capacity of mammary fat pads of adult C3H/HeMs mice to interact morphogenetically with fetal mammary epithelium. *J Natl Cancer Inst* 63:733, 1979.
61. Wicha MS, Lowrie G, Kohn E, Bagavandoss P, Mahn T: Extracellular matrix promotes mammary epithelial growth and differentiation in vitro. *Proc Natl Acad Sci USA* 79:3213, 1982.
62. Petersen OW, Ronnov-Jessen L, Howlett AR, Bissell MJ: Interaction with basement membrane serves to rapidly distinguish growth and differentiation pattern of normal and malignant human breast epithelial cells [published erratum appears in *Proc Natl Acad Sci USA* 1993; 90:2556]. *Proc Natl Acad Sci USA* 89:9064, 1992.
63. Basset P, Bellocq JP, Wolf C, Stoll I, Hutin P, Limacher JM, et al: A novel metalloproteinase gene specifically expressed in stromal cells of breast carcinomas. *Nature* 348:699, 1990.
64. Cullen KJ, Smith HS, Hill S, Rosen N, Lippman ME: Growth factor messenger RNA expression by human breast fibroblasts from benign and malignant lesions. *Cancer Res* 51:4978, 1991.
65. Lee C: Cellular interactions in prostate cancer. *Br J Urol* 79:21, 1997.
66. Sugimura Y, Cunha GR, Hayward S, et al: Keratinocyte growth factor (KGF) is a mediator of testosterone-induced prostatic development. *Mol Cell Differ* 1:423, 1993.
67. Kim IY, Ahn HJ, Zelner DJ, Park L, Sensibar JA, Lee C: Expression and localization of transforming growth factor-β receptors type I and type II in the rat ventral prostate during regression. *Mol Endocrinol* 10:107, 1996.
68. Hiramatsu M, Kashimata M, Minami N, Sato A, Muragama M, Minami N: Androgenic regulation of EGF in the mouse ventral prostate. *Biochem Int* 17:311, 1988.
69. Hofer D, Sherwood E, Bromberg W, Mendelsohn J, Lee C, Kozlowski JM: Autonomous growth of androgen-independent prostatic carcinoma cells: Role of TGF-α. *Cancer Res* 51:2780, 1991.
70. Peehl DM, Cohen P, Rosenfeld RG: The insulin-like growth factor system in the prostate. *World J Urol* 13:306, 1996.
71. Sherwood ER, Fong CJ, Lee C, Kozlowski JM: Basic fibroblast growth factor: A potential mediator of stromal growth in the human prostate. *Endocrinology* 130:2955, 1992.
72. Djakiew D: Role of nerve growth factor-like protein in the paracrine regulation of prostate growth. *J Androl* 13:476, 1992.
73. Hayward SW, Rosen MA, Cunha GR: Stromal-epithelial interactions in the normal and neoplastic prostate. *Br J Urol* 79:18, 1997.
74. Rajan JV, Wang M, Marquis ST, Chodosh LA: Brca2 is coordinately regulated with Brca1 during proliferation and differentiation in mammary epithelial cells. *Proc Natl Acad Sci USA* 93:13078, 1996.
75. Scully R, Chen J, Plug A, Xiao Y, Weaver D, Feunteun J, et al: Association of BRCA1 with Rad51 in mitotic and meiotic cells. *Cell* 88:265, 1997.
76. Mizuta R, LaSalle JM, Cheng HL, Shinohara A, Ogawa H, Copeland N, et al: RAB22 and RAB163/mouse BRCA2: Proteins that specifically interact with the RAD51 protein. *Proc Natl Acad Sci USA* 94:6927, 1997.
77. Easton DF, Ford D, Bishop DT, and the Breast Cancer Linkage Consortium: Breast and ovarian cancer incidence in BRCA1-mutation carriers. *Am J Hum Genet* 56:265, 1995.
78. Ford D, Easton DF: The genetics of breast and ovarian cancer. *Br J Cancer* 72:805, 1995.
79. Ford D, Easton DF, Bishop DT, Narod SA, Goldgar DE, and the Breast Cancer Linkage Consortium: Risks of cancer in BRCA1-mutation carriers. *Lancet* 343:692, 1994.
80. Easton DF, Bishop DT, Fod D, Crockford GP, and the Breast Cancer Linkage Consortium: Genetic linkage analysis in familial breast and ovarian cancer. *Am J Hum Genet* 52:678, 1993.
81. Shattuck-Eidens D, Oliphant A, McClure M, et al: BRCA1 sequence analysis in women at high risk for susceptibility mutations: Risk factor analysis and implications for genetic testing. *JAMA* 278:1242, 1997.
82. Couch FJ, DeShano ML, Blackwood MA, et al: BRCA1 mutations in women attending clinics that evaluate the risk of breast cancer. *N Engl J Med* 336:1409, 1997.
83. Malone KE, Daling JR, Thompson JD, O'Brien CA, Francisco LV, Ostrander EA: BRCA1 mutations and breast cancer in the general population. Analyses in women before age 35 years and in women before age 45 years with first-degree family history. *JAMA* 279:922, 1998.
84. Berry DA, Parmigiani G, Sanchez J, Schildkraut J, Winer E: Probability of carrying a mutation of breast-ovarian cancer gene BRCA1 based on family history. *J Natl Cancer Inst* 89:227, 1997.
85. Lerman C, Narod S, Schulman K, Hughes C, Gomez-Caminero A, Bonney G, Gold K, Trock B, Main D, Lynch J, Fulmore C, Snyder C, Lemon SJ, Conway T, Tonin P, Lenoir G, Lynch H: BRCA1 testing in families with hereditary breast-ovarian cancer: A prospective study of patient decision making and outcomes. *JAMA* 275:1885, 1996.
86. Burke W, Daly M, Garber J, Botkin J, Ellis Kahn MJ, Lynch P, McTiernan A, Offit K, Perlman J, Petersen G, Thomson E, Varricchio C, for the Cancer Genetics Studies Consortium: Recommendations for follow-up care of individuals with an inherited predisposition to cancer. *JAMA* 277:997, 1997.
87. Hoskins KF, Stopfer JE, Calzone KA, Merajver SD, Rebbeck TR, Garber JE, Weber BL: Assessment and counseling for women with a family history of breast cancer. *JAMA* 273:577, 1995.
88. Carter BS, Beaty TH, Steinberg GD, et al: Mendelian inheritance of familial prostate cancer. *Proc Natl Acad Sci* 89:3367, 1992.
89. Bastacky SI, Wojno KJ, Walsh PC, et al: Pathological features of hereditary prostate cancer. *J Urol* 153:987, 1995.
90. Grönberg H, Damber L, Damber JE: Studies of genetic factors in prostate cancer in a twin population. *J Urol* 152:1484, 1994.
91. Slamon DJ, Godolphin W, Jones LA, Holt JA, Wong SG, Keith DE, Levin WJ, Stuart SG, Udove J, Ullrich A, Press MF: Studies of the HER-2/neu proto-oncogene in human breast and ovarian cancer. *Science* 244:707, 1989.
92. Pauletti G, Dandekar S, Smith K, Robbins P, Dawkins H, Papadimitriou J, et al: Chronology of HER-2/neu gene amplification in proliferative and malignant ductal lesions of the breast as determined by fluorescence in situ hybridization (FISH). *Proc Am Assoc Cancer Res* 38:414, 1997.
93. Muller WJ, Sinn E, Pattengale PK, Wallace R, Leder P: Single-step induction of mammary adenocarcinoma in transgenic mice bearing the activated c-neu oncogene. *Cell* 54:105, 1988.
94. Rowse GJ, Ritland SR, Gendler SJ: Genetic modulation of neu proto-oncogene-induced mammary tumorigenesis. *Cancer Res* 58:2675, 1998.
95. Slamon DJ, Clark GM, Wong SG, et al: Human breast cancer: Correlation of relapse and survival with amplification of the HER-2/neu oncogene. *Science* 235:177, 1987.
96. Muss HB, Thor AD, Berry D, Kute T, Liu ET, Koerner F, et al: c-erbB2 expression and response to adjuvant therapy in women with node-positive early breast cancer. *N Engl J Med* 330:1260, 1994.
97. Wright C, Nicholson S, Angus B, Sainsbury JR, Farndon J, Cairns J, et al: Relationship between c-erbB-2 protein product expression and response to endocrine therapy in advanced breast cancer. *Br J Cancer* 65:118, 1992.
98. Pietras RJ, Fendly BM, Chazin VR, Pegram MD, Howell SB, Slamon DJ: Antibody to HER-2/neu receptor blocks DNA repair after cisplatin in human breast and ovarian cancer cells. *Oncogene* 9:1829, 1994.
99. Arteaga C, Winnier A, Poirer M, Lopez-Larraza D, Shawver L, Hurd S, et al: p185c-erbB-2 signaling enhances cisplatin-induced cytotoxicity in human breast carcinoma cells: Association between an oncogenic receptor tyrosine kinase and drug-induced DNA repair. *Cancer Res* 54:3758, 1994.
100. Pegram MD, Lipton A, Hayes DF, Weber BL, Baselga JM, Tripathy D, Baly D, Baughman SA, Twaddel T, Glaspy JA, Slamon DJ: Phase II study of receptor-enhanced chemosensitivity using recombinant humanized anti-p185$^{HER2/neu}$ monoclonal antibody plus cisplatin in patients with HER2/neu-overexpressing metastatic breast cancer refractory to chemotherapy treatment. *J Clin Oncol* 16:2659, 1998.
101. Slamon D, Leyland-Jones B, Shak S, Paton V, Bajamonde A, Fleming T, Eiermann W, Wolter J, Baselga J, Norton L: Addition of Herceptin™ (humanized anti-HER2 antibody) to first line chemotherapy for HER2 overexpressing metastatic breast cancer (HER2 + /MBC) markedly increases anticancer activity: A randomized, multinational controlled phase III trial. *Proceedings of the American Society of Clinical Oncology*, Thirty-Fourth Annual Meeting, May 16–19, 1998, Los Angeles, California, pp 98a, Abstract #377.
102. Clark GJ, Der CJ: Aberrant function of the Ras signal transduction pathway in human breast cancer. *Breast Cancer Res Treat* 35:133, 1995.

103. Hand PH, Vilasi V, Thor A, Ohuchi N, Schlom J: Quantitation of Harvey ras p21 enhanced expression in human breast and colon carcinomas. *J Natl Cancer Inst* 79:59, 1987.
104. Sivaraman VS, Wang HY, Nuovo GJ, Malbon CC: Hyperexpression of mitogen-activated protein kinase in human breast cancer. *J Clin Invest* 99:1478, 1997.
105. Manni A, Wechter R, Gilmour S, Verderame MF, Mauger D, Demers LM: Ornithine decarboxylase over-expression stimulates mitogen-activated protein kinase and anchorage-dependent growth of human breast epithelial cells. *Int J Cancer* 70:175, 1997.
106. Manni A, Wechter R, Verderame MF, Mauger D: Cooperativity between the polyamine pathway and HER-2neu in transformation of human mammary epithelial cells in culture: Role of the MAPK pathway. *Int J Cancer* 76:563, 1998.
107. Nass SJ, Dickson RB: Defining a role for c-Myc in breast tumorigenesis. *Breast Cancer Res Treat* 44:1, 1997.
108. Bieche I, Liderau R: Genetic alterations in breast cancer. *Genes Chromosomes Cancer* 14:227, 1995.
109. Devilee P, Schuuring E, van de Vijver MJ, Cornelisse CJ: Recent developments in the molecular genetic understanding of breast cancer. *Crit Rev Oncog* 5:247, 1994.
110. Schuuring F Involvement of the chromosome 11q13 region in human malignancy: Cyclin D1 and EMS1 are two new candidate oncogenes—a review. *Gene* 159:83, 1995.
111. Wang T, Cardiff R, Zukerberg L, Lees E, Arnold A, Schmidt E: Mammary hyperplasia and carcinoma in MMTV-cyclin D1 transgenic mice. *Nature* 369:669, 1994.
112. Bieche I, Lidereau R: Genetic alterations in breast cancer. *Genes Chromosome Cancer* 14:227, 1995.
113. Brenner AJ, Aldaz CM: The genetics of sporadic breast cancer, in *Etiology of Breast and Gynecological Cancers*. New York, Wiley-Liss, 1997, p 63.
114. Osborne RJ, Merlo GR, Mitudomi T, Venesio T, Liscia DS, Cappa APM, et al: Mutations in the p53 gene in primary human breast cancer. *Cancer Res* 51:6194, 1991.
115. Fraumeni JF Jr, Hoover RN, Devesa SS, Kinlen LJ: Epidemiology of cancer, in DeVita VT Jr, Hellman S, Rosenberg SA (eds): *Cancer: Principles and Practice of Oncology*. Philadelphia, Lippincott, 1989, p 196.
116. Early Breast Cancer Trialists' Collaborative Group: Tamoxifen for early breast cancer: An overview of the randomised trials. *Lancet* 351:1451, 1998.
117. Fisher B, Costantino JP, Wickerham DL, Redmond CK, Kavanah M, Cronin WM, Vogel V, Robidoux A, Dimitrov N, Atkins J, Daly M, Wieand S, Tan-Chiu E, Ford L, Wolmark N, and other National Surgical Adjuvant Breast and Bowel Project Investigators. *J Natl Cancer Inst* 90:1371, 1998.
118. Oral contraceptives use and the risk of endometrial cancer: The Centers for Disease Control Cancer and Steroid Hormone Study. *JAMA* 249:1600, 1983.
119. Thomas HV, Reeves GK, Key TJA: Endogenous estrogen and postmenopausal breast cancer: A quantitative review. *Cancer Causes Control* 8:922, 1997.
120. Hankinson SE, Willett WC, Colditz GA, Hunter DJ, Michaud DS, Deroo B, Rosner B, Speizer FE, Pollak M: Circulating concentrations of insulin-like growth factor-I and risk of breast cancer. *Lancet* 351:1393, 1998.
121. Collaborative Group on Hormonal Factors in Breast Cancer: Breast cancer and hormonal contraceptives: Collaborative reanalysis of individual data on 53,297 women with breast cancer and 100,239 women without breast cancer from 54 epidemiological studies. *Lancet* 347:1713, 1996.
122. Collaborative Group on Hormonal Factors in Breast Cancer: Breast cancer and hormone replacement therapy: Collaborative reanalysis of data from 51 epidemiological studies of 52,705 women with breast cancer and 108,411 women without breast cancer. *Lancet* 350:1047, 1997.
123. Chan JM, Stampfer MJ, Giovannucci E, Gann PH, Ma J, Wilkinson P, Hennekens CH, Pollak M: Plasma insulin-like growth factor-I and prostate cancer risk: A prospective study. *Science* 279:563, 1998.
124. Cohen LA: Diet and Cancer. *Sci Am* 257:42, 1987.
125. Willet W, London S: Dietary factors and the etiology of breast cancer, in Harris JR, Hellman S, Henderson IC, Kinne DW (eds): *Breast Diseases*, 2nd ed., Philadelphia, Lippincott, 1991, p 136.
126. Freedman LS, Clifford C, Messina M: Analysis of dietary fat, calories, body weight, and the development of mammary tumors in rats and mice: A review. *Cancer Res* 50:5710, 1990.
127. National Academy of Sciences, National Research Council, Committee on Diet, Nutrition and Cancer: *Diet, Nutrition, and Cancer*. Assembly of Life Sciences. National Academy Press, Washington, DC, 1982.
128. National Academy of Sciences, National Research Council, Food and Nutrition Board: *Diet and Health: Implications for Reducing Chronic Disease Risk*. Council on Life Sciences. National Academy Press, Washington, DC, 1989.
129. U.S. Department of Health and Human Services, Public Health Service: *The Surgeon General's Report on Nutrition and Health*. DHHS (PHS) publication no. 88-50211, US Government Printing Office, Washington, DC, 1988.
130. Schatzkin A, Greenwald P, Byar DP, Clifford CK: The dietary fat-breast cancer hypothesis is alive. *JAMA* 261:3284, 1989.
131. Prentice RL, Kakar F, Hursting S, et al: Aspects of the rationale for the Women's Health Trial. *J Natl Cancer Inst* 80:802, 1988.
132. Boyd NF, Cousins M, Beaton M, et al: Clinical trial of low-fat, high carbohydrate diet in subjects with mammographic dysplasia: Report of early outcomes. *J Natl Cancer Inst* 80:1244, 1988.
133. Tham DT, Gardner CD, Haskell WL: Potential health benefits of dietary phytoestrogens: A review of the clinical epidemiological, and mechanistic evidence. *J Clin Endocrinol Metab* 83:2223, 1998.
134. White R, Parker MG: Molecular mechanisms of steroid hormone action. *Endocrine-Related Cancer* 5:1, 1998.
135. Ciocca DR, Fanelli MA: Estrogen receptors and cell proliferation in breast cancer. *TEM* 8:313, 1997.
136. Bourguet W, Ruff M, Chambon P, Gronemeyer H, Moras D: Crystal-structure of the ligand-binding domain of the human nuclear receptor RXR-alpha. *Nature* 375:377, 1995.
137. Renaud JP, Rochel N, Ruff M, Vivat V, Chambon P, Gronemeyer H, Moras D: Crystal structure of the RAR-γ ligand-binding domain bound to all-trans retinoic acid. *Nature* 378:681, 1995.
138. Wagner RL, Apriletti JW, McGrath ME, West BL, Baxter JD, Fletterick RJ: A structural role for hormone in the thyroid hormone receptor. *Nature* 378:690, 1995.
139. Brzozowski AM, Pike ACW, Dauter Z, Hubbard RE, Bonn T, Engstrom O, Ohman L, Greene GL, Gustafson J-A, Carlquist M: Molecular basis of agonism and antagonism in the oestrogen receptor. *Nature* 389:753, 1997.
140. Yang NN, Venugopalan M, Hardikar S, Glasebrook A: Identification of an estrogen response element activated by metabolites of 17β-estradiol and raloxifene. *Science* 273:1222, 1996.
141. Dauvois S, Parker MG: Mechanism of action of hormone antagonists, in Parker M (ed): *Steroid Hormone Action*. Oxford, IRL Press, 1993, p 161.
142. Gibson MK, Nemmers LA, Beckman WC Jr, Davis VL, Curtis SW, Korach KS: The mechanism of ICI 164,384 antiestrogenicity involves rapid loss of estrogen receptor in uterine tissue. *Endocrinology* 129:2000, 1991.
143. Dauvois S, Danielian PS, White R, Parker MG: Antiestrogen ICI 164,384 reduces cellular estrogen receptor content by increasing its turnover. *Proc Natl Acad Sci USA* 89:4037, 1992.
144. Fawell SE, White R, Hoare S, Sydenham M, Page M, Parker MG: Inhibition of estrogen receptor-DNA binding by the "pure" antiestrogen ICI 164,384 appears to be mediated by impaired receptor dimerization. *Proc Natl Acad Sci USA* 87:6883, 1990.
145. Reese JC, Katzenellenbogen BS: Differential DNA-binding abilities of estrogen receptor occupied with two classes of antiestrogens: Studies using human estrogen receptor overexpressed in mammalian cells. *Nucleic Acids Res* 19:6595, 1991.
146. Metzger D, Berry M, Ali S, Chambon P: Effect of antagonists on DNA-binding properties of the human estrogen-receptor *in vitro* and *in vivo*. *Mol Endocrinol* 9:579, 1995.
147. Thomas T, Thomas TJ: Regulation of cyclin B1 by estradiol and polyamines in MCF-7 breast cancer cells. *Cancer Res* 55:2487, 1994.
148. Foster JS, Wimalasena J: Estrogen regulates activity of cyclin-dependent kinases and retinoblastoma protein phosphorylation in breast cancer cells. *Mol Endocrinol* 10:488, 1996.
149. van der Burg B, van Selm-Miltenburg AJP, de Laat SW, van Zoelen EJJ: Direct effects of estrogen on c-fos and c-myc protooncogene

expression and cellular proliferation in human breast cancer cells. *Mol Cell Endocrinol* 64:223, 1989.

150. Dubik D, Shiu RPC: Mechanism of estrogen activation of c-myc oncogene expression. *Oncogene* 7:1587, 1992.
151. Dickson RB, Lippman ME: Growth factors in breast cancer. *Endocr Rev* 16:559, 1995.
152. Manni A, Badger B, Wei L, Zaenglein A, Grove R, Khin S, Heitjan D, Shimasaki S, Ling N: Hormonal regulation of insulin-like growth factor II and insulin-like growth factor binding protein expression by breast cancer cells in vivo: Evidence for stromal epithelial interactions. *Cancer Res* 54:2934, 1994.
153. Bronzert DA, Pantazis P, Antoniades HN, Kasid A, Davidson N, Dickson RB, Lippman ME: Synthesis and secretion of platelet-derived growth factor by human breast cancer cell lines. *Proc Natl Acad Sci USA* 85:5763, 1987.
154. Knabbe C, Lippman ME, Wakefield L, Flanders K, Kasid A, Derynck R, Dickson RB: Evidence that TGFβ is a hormonally regulated negative growth factor in human breast cancer. *Cell* 48:417, 1987.
155. Arteaga CL, Osborne CK: Growth inhibition of human breast cancer cells in vitro with an antibody against the type I somatomedin receptor. *Cancer Res* 49:6237, 1989.
156. Van der Burg B, Isbrucker L, van Selm-Miltenburg AJP, de Laat SW, van Zoelen EJJ: Role of estrogen-induced insulin-like growth factors in the proliferation of human breast cancer cells. *Cancer Res* 50:7770, 1990.
157. Glickman PL, Manni A, Bartholomew M, Demers L: Polyamine involvement in basal and estradiol-stimulated insulin-like growth factor I secretion and action in breast cancer cells in culture. *J Steroid Biochem Mol* 37:1, 1990.
158. Stewart AJ, Johnson MD, May FEB, Westley BR: Role of insulin-like growth factors and the type I insulin-like growth factor receptor in the estrogen-stimulated proliferation of human breast cancer cells. *J Biol Chem* 265:21172, 1990.
159. Ignar-Trowbridge DM, Teng CT, Ross KA, Parker MG, Korach KS, McLachlan JA: Peptide growth factors elicit estrogen receptor-dependent transcriptional activation of an estrogen-responsive element. *Mol Endocrinol* 7:992, 1993.
160. Ignar-Trowbridge DM, Pimentel M, Parker MG, McLachlan JA, Korach KS: Peptide growth factor cross-talk with the estrogen receptor requires the A/B domain and occurs independently of protein kinase C or estradiol. *Endocrinology* 137:1735, 1996.
161. Kato S, Endoh H, Masuhiro Y, Kitamoto T, Uchiyama S, Sasaki H, Masushige S, Gotoh Y, Nishida E, Kawashima H, Metzger D, Chambon P: Activation of the estrogen receptor through phosphorylation by mitogen-activated protein kinase. *Science* 270:1491, 1995.
162. Pietras RJ, Arboleda J, Reese DM, Wongvipat N, Pegram MD, Ramos L, Gorman CM, Parker MG, Sliwkowski MX, Slamon DJ: HER-2 tyrosine kinase pathway targets estrogen receptor and promotes hormone-independent growth in human breast cancer cells. *Oncogene* 10:2435, 1995.
163. Power RF, Mani SK, Codina J, Conneely OM, O'Malley BW: Dopaminergic and ligand-independent activation of steroid hormone receptors. *Science* 254:1636, 1991.
164. Philips A, Chalbos D, Rochefort H: Estradiol increases and anti-estrogen antagonize the growth factor-induced activation protein-1 activity in MCF-7 breast cancer cells without affecting c-fos and c-jun synthesis. *J Biol Chem* 268:14103, 1993.
165. Umayahara Y, Kawamori R, Watada H, Imano E, Iwama N, Morishima T, Yamasaki Y, Kajimoto Y, Kamada T: Estrogen regulation of the insulin-like growth factor I gene transcription involves an AP-1 enhancer. *J Biol Chem* 269:16433, 1994.
166. Diamond MI, Miner JN, Yoshinaga SK, Yamamoto KR: Transcription factor interactions: Selectors of positive or negative regulation from a single DNA element. *Science* 249:1266, 1990.
167. Gaub M-P, Bellard M, Scheuer I, Chambon P, Sassone-Corsi P: Activation of the ovalbumin gene by the estrogen receptor involves the Fos-Jun complex. *Cell* 63:1267, 1990.
168. Rishi AK, Shao ZM, Baumann RG, et al: Estradiol regulation of the human retinoic acid receptor a gene in human breast carcinoma cells is mediated via an imperfect half-palindromic estrogen response element and Sp1 motifs. *Cancer Res* 55:5999, 1995.
169. Dinda S, Khattree N, Hurd C, Jhanwar SC, Moudgil VK: Estradiol regulation of proliferation of T47D breast cancer cells: alterations in p53 tumor suppressor protein and mRNA levels [abst no. A1970]. *Proc Am Assoc Cancer Res* 38:294, 1997.
170. Marks JR, Huper G, Vaughn JP, et al: BRCA1 expression is not directly responsive to estrogen. *Oncogene* 14:115, 1997.
171. Santen RJ, Worgul TJ, Lipton A, Harvey H, Boucher A, Samojlik E, Wells SA: Aminoglutethimide as treatment of postmenopausal women with advanced breast carcinoma. *Ann Intern Med* 96:94, 1982.
172. Robertson J: Oestrogen receptor: A stable phenotype in breast cancer. *Br J Cancer* 73:5, 1996.
173. Ruizeveld de Winter JA, Janssen PJ, Sleddens HM, Verleun-Mooijman MC, Trapman J, Brinkmann AO, Santerse AB, Schroder FH, van der Kwast TH: Androgen receptor status in localized and locally progressive hormone refractory human prostate cancer. *Am J Pathol* 144:735, 1994.
174. Murphy LC: Mechanisms of hormone independence in human breast cancer. *In Vivo* 12:95, 1998.
175. Tonetti DA, Jordan VC: The role of estrogen receptor mutations in Tamoxifen-stimulated breast cancer. *J Steroid Biochem Mol Biol* 62:119, 1997.
176. McGuire WL, Chamness GC, Fuqua SA: Estrogen receptor variants in clinical breast cancer. *Mol Endocrinol* 5:1571, 1991.
177. Karnik PS, Klukarni S, Liu XP, Budd GT, Bukowski RM: Estrogen receptor mutations in tamoxifen-resistant breast cancer. *Cancer Res* 54:349, 1994.
178. Wang Y, Miksicek RJ: identification of a dominant negative form of the human estrogen receptor. *Mol Endocrinol* 5:1707, 1991.
179. Pfeffer U, Fecarotta E, Castagnetta L, Vidali G: Estrogen receptor variant messenger RNA lacking exon 4 in estrogen-responsive human breast cancer cell lines. *Cancer Res* 53:741, 1993.
180. Fuqua SAW, Fitzgerald SD, Allred DC, Elledge RM, Nawaz Z, McDonnell DP, O'Malley BW, Greene GL, McGuire WL: Inhibition of estrogen receptor action by a naturally occurring variant in human breast tumors. *Cancer Res* 52:483, 1992.
181. Pink JJ, Wu SQ, Wolf DM, Bilimoria MM, Jordan VC: A novel 80 kDa human estrogen receptor containing a duplication of exons 6 and 7. *Nucleic Acids Res* 24:962, 1996.
182. Fuqua SAW, Fitzgerald SD, Chamness GC, Tandon AK, McDonnell DP, Nawaz Z, O'Malley BW, McGuire WL: Variant human breast tumor estrogen receptor with constitutive transcriptional activity. *Cancer Res* 51:105, 1991.
183. Pfeffer U, Fecarotta E, Vidali G: Coexpression of multiple estrogen receptor variant messenger RNAs in normal and neoplastic breast tissues and in MCF-7 cells. *Cancer Res* 55:2158, 1995.
184. Pfeffer U, Fecarotta E, Arena G, Forlani A, Vidali G: Alternative splicing of the estrogen receptor primary transcript normally occurs in estrogen receptor positive tissues and cell lines. *J Steroid Biochem Mol Biol* 56:99, 1996.
185. Leygue ER, Watson PH, Murphy LC: Estrogen receptor variants in normal human mammary tissue. *J Natl Cancer Inst* 88:284, 1996.
186. Skipper JK, Young LJ, Bergeron JM, Tetzlaff MT, Osborn CT, Crews D: Identification of an isoform of the estrogen receptor messenger RNA lacking exon four and present in the brain. *Proc Natl Acad Sci USA* 90:7172, 1993.
187. Koivisto P, Kononen J, Palmberg C, Hyytinen E, Tammela T, Trapman J, Isola J, Visakorpi T, Kallioniemi OP: Androgen receptor gene amplification: A possible molecular mechanism for failure of androgen deprivation therapy in prostate cancer. *Cancer Res* 57:314, 1997.
188. Newmark JR, Hardy DO, Tonb DC, Carter BS, Epstein JI, Isaacs WB, Brown TR, Barrack ER: Androgen receptor gene mutations in human prostate cancer. *Proc Natl Acad Sci USA* 89:6319, 1992.
189. Culig Z, Hobisch A, Cronauer MV, Cato AC, Hittmair A, Radmayr C, Eberle J, Bartsch G, Klocker H: Mutant androgen receptor detected in an advanced-stage prostatic carcinoma is activated by adrenal androgens and progesterone. *Mol Endocrinol* 7:1541, 1993.
190. Suzuki H, Sato N, Watabe Y, Masai M, Seino S, Shimazaki J: Androgen receptor gene mutations in human prostate cancer. *J Steroid Biochem Mole Biol* 46:759, 1993.
191. Gaddipati JP, McLeod DG, Heidenberg HB, Sesterhenn IA, Finger MJ, Moul JW, Srivastava S: Frequent detection of codon 877 mutation in the androgen receptor gene in advanced prostate cancers. *Cancer Res* 54:2861, 1994.
192. Schoenberg MP, Hakimi JM, Wang S, Bova GS, Epstein JI, Fischbeck KH, Isaacs WB, Walsh PC, Barrack ER: Microsatellite mutation

(CAG_{24-18}) in the androgen receptor gene in human prostate cancer. *Biochem Biophys Res Commun* 198:74, 1994.
193. Taplin ME, Bubley GJ, Shuster TD, Frantz ME, Spooner AE, Ogata GK, Keer HN, Balk SP: Mutation of the androgen-receptor gene in metastatic androgen-independent prostate cancer. *N Engl J Med* 332:1393, 1995.
194. Visakorpi T, Hyytinen E, Koivisto P, Tanner M, Keinänen R, Palmberg C, Palotie A, Tammela T, Isola J, Kallioniemi OP: In vivo amplification of the androgen receptor gene and progression of human prostate cancer. *Nat Genet* 9:401, 1995.
195. Tilley WD, Buchanan G, Hickey TE, Bentel JM: Mutations in the androgen receptor gene are associated with progression of human prostate cancer to androgen independence. *Clin Cancer Res* 2:277, 1996.
196. Elo JP, Kvist L, Leinonen K, Isomaa V, Henttu P, Lukkarinen O, Vihko P: Mutated human androgen receptor gene detected in prostatic cancer patients is also activated by estradiol. *J Clin Endocrinol Metab* 80:3494, 1995.
197. Evans BAJ, Harper ME, Daniels CE, Watts CE, Matenheila S, Green J, Griffiths K: Low incidence of androgen receptor gene mutations in human prostatic tumors using single strand conformation polymorphism analysis. *Prostate* 28:162, 1996.
198. Suzuki H, Akakura K, Komiya A, Aida S, Akimoto S, Shimazaki J: Codon 877 mutation in the androgen receptor gene in advanced prostate cancer: Relation to antiandrogen withdrawal syndrome. *Prostate* 29:153, 1996.
199. Koivisto P, Kolmer M, Visakorpi T, Kallioniemi OP: Androgen receptor gene and hormonal therapy failure of prostate cancer. *Am J Pathol* 152:1, 1998.
200. Jackson T, Richer J, Bain D, Takimoto G, Tung L, Horwitz K: The partial agonist activity of antagonist occupied steroid receptors is controlled by a novel hinge domain binding coactivator L7/SPA and the corepressors N- CoR or SMRT. *Mol Endocrinol* 11:693, 1997.
201. Smith C, Nawaz Z, O'Malley B: Coactivator and corepressor regulation of the agonist/antagonist activity of the mixed antiestrogen, 4-hydroxytamoxifen. *Mol Endocrinol* 11:657, 1997.
202. Clarke R, Brunner N, Katz D, PPG, Dickson R, Lippman M, Kern F: The effects of a constitutive expression of transforming growth factor-α on the growth of MCF-7 human breast cancer cells in vitro and in vivo. *Mol Endocrinol* 3:372, 1989.
203. Wang T, Cardiff R, Zucherberg L, Lees E, Arnold A, Schmidt E: Mammary hyperplasia and carcinoma in MMTV-cyclin D1 transgenic mice. *Nature* 369:669, 1994.
204. Wilcken N, Prall O, Musgrove E, Sutherland R: Inducible overexpression of cyclin D1 in breast cancer cells reverses the growth inhibitory effects of antiestrogens. *Clin Cancer Res* 3:849, 1997.
205. Culig Z, Hobisch A, Cronauer MV, Radmayr C, Trapman J, Hittmair A, Bartsch G, Klocker H: Androgen receptor activation in prostatic tumor cell lines by insulin-like growth factor-I, keratinocyte growth factor and epidermal growth factor. *Cancer Res* 54:5475, 1994.
206. Culig Z, Hobisch A, Radmayr C, Hittmair A, Cronauer MV, Bartsch G, Klocker H: Regulation of androgen receptor-mediated transcription in DU-145 cells in response to insulin-like growth factor-I, cyclic adenosine monophosphate, phorbol ester and retinoic acid. *Proc Am Assoc Cancer Res* 36:271 (abst), 1995.
207. Nazareth LV, Weigel NL: Activation of the human androgen receptor through a protein kinase A signaling pathway. *J Biol Chem* 271:19900, 1996.
208. Donegan WL, Redlich PH, Lang PJ, Gall MT: Carcinoma of the breast in males: A multiinstitutional study. *Cancer* 83:498, 1998.
209. Jensen RA: Benign breast lesions: Pathologic classification and risk potential, in *Contemporary Endocrinology: Endocrinology of Breast Cancer*. Totowa, New Jersey, Humana Press, Inc., in press.
210. Klijn JGM, Berns EMJJ, Foekens JA: Prognostic and predictive factors in breast cancer, in *Contemporary Endocrinology: Endocrinology of Breast Cancer*. Totowa, New Jersey, Humana Press, Inc., in press.
211. Early Breast Cancer Trialists' Collaborative Group: Systemic treatment of early breast cancer by hormonal, cytotoxic, or immune therapy. *Lancet* 339:1, 1992.
212. Wittliff JL: Steroid-hormone receptors in breast cancer. *Cancer* 53:630, 1984.
213. McGuire WL, Chamness GC, Fuqua SAW: Mini-review—estrogen receptor variants in clinical breast cancer. *Mol Endocrinol* 5:1571, 1991.
214. Santen RJ, Manni A, Harvey H, Redmond C: Endocrine treatment of breast cancer in women. *Endocrine Rev* 11:1, 1990.
215. Buzdar AU, Hortobagyi G: Update on endocrine therapy for breast cancer. *Clin Cancer Res* 4:527, 1998.
216. Vogel CL, Shemano I, Schoenfelder J, Gams RA, Green MR: Multicenter phase II efficacy trial of toremifene in tamoxifen-refractory patients with advanced breast cancer. *J Clin Oncol* 11:345, 1993.
217. Stenbygaard LE, Herrstedt J, Thomsen JF, Svendsen KR, Engelholm SA, Dombernowsky P: Toremifene and tamoxifen in advanced breast cancer—a double-blind, cross-over trial. *Breast Cancer Res Treat* 25:57, 1993.
218. Howell A, Robertson J: Response to a specific antioestrogen (ICI 182780) in tamoxifen-resistant breast cancer. *Lancet* 345:989, 1995.
219. Harvey HA: Aromatase inhibitors in breast carcinoma, in *Contemporary Endocrinology: Endocrinology of Breast Cancer*. Totowa, New Jersey, Humana Press, Inc., in press.
220. Buzdar AU, Jonat W, Howell A, Jones SE, Blomqvist C, Vogel CL, Eiermann W, Wolter JM, Azab M, Webster A, Plourde PV, on behalf of the Arimidex Study Group: Anastrozole, a potent and selective aromatase inhibitor, versus megestrol acetate in postmenopausal women with advanced breast cancer: Results of an overview analysis of two phase III trials. *J Clin Oncol* 14:2000, 1996.
221. Dombernowsky P, Smith I, Falkson G, et al: Letrozole, a new oral aromatase inhibitor for advanced breast cancer: Double-blind randomized trial showing a dose effect and improved efficacy and tolerability compared with megestrol acetate. *J Clin Oncol* 16:453, 1998.
222. Ingle JN, Krook JE, Green SJ, Kubista TP, Everson KL, Ahmann DL, Chang MN, Bisel HF, Windschit HE, Twito DL: Randomized trial of bilateral oophorectomy versus Tamoxifen in premenopausal women with metastatic breast cancer. *J Clin Oncol* 4:178, 1986.
223. Buchanan RB, Blamey RW, Durrant KR, Howell A, Paterson AG, Preece PE, Smith DC, Williams CJ, Wilson RG: A randomized comparison of tamoxifen with surgical oophorectomy in premenopausal patients with advanced breast cancer. *J Clin Oncol* 4:1326, 1986.
224. Hortobagyi GN, Theriault RL, Porter L, et al: Efficacy of pamidronate in reducing skeletal complications in patients with breast cancer and lytic bone metastases. *N Engl J Med* 335:1785, 1996.
225. Diel IJ, Solomayer EF, Costa SD, Gollan C, Goerner R, Wallwiener D, Kaufmann M, Bastert G: Reduction in new metastases in breast cancer with adjuvant clodronate treatment. *N Engl J Med* 339:357, 1998.
226. Mundy GR, Yoneda T: Bisphosphonates as anticancer drugs. *N Engl J Med* 339:398, 1998.
227. Cobleigh MA, Vogel CL, Tripathy D, Robert NJ, Scholl S, Fehrenbacher L, Paton V, Shak S, Lieberman G, Slamon D: Efficacy and safety of Herceptin™ (humanized anti-HER2 antibody as a single agent in 222 women with HER2 overexpression who relapsed following chemotherapy for metastatic breast cancer. *Proceedings of the American Society of Clinical Oncology*, Thirty-Fourth Annual Meeting, May 16–19, 1998, Los Angeles, California, p 97a, Abstract #376.
228. Boar's Head Workshop Conference: Consensus Statement: Treatment of estrogen deficiency symptoms in women surviving breast cancer. *J Clin Endocrinol Metab* 83:1993, 1998.
229. Cummings SR, Norton L, Eckert S, Grady D, Cauley J, Knickerbocker R, Black DM, Nickelsen T, Glusman J, Krueger K for the MORE Investigators: Raloxifene reduces the risk of breast cancer and may decrease the risk of endometrial cancer in post-menopausal women. Two-year findings from the multiple outcomes of raloxifene evaluation (MORE) trial. *Proceedings of the American Society of Clinical Oncology*, Thirty-Fourth Annual Meeting, May 16–19, 1998, Los Angeles, California, p 2a, Abstract #3.
230. Powles T, Eeles R, Ashley S, Easton D, Chang J, Dowsett M, Tidy A, Viggers J, Davey J: Interim analysis of the incidence of breast cancer in the Royal Marsden Hospital tamoxifen randomised chemoprevention trial. *Lancet* 352:98, 1998.
231. Veronesi U, Maisonneuve P, Costa A, Sacchini V, Maltoni C, Robertson C, Rotmensz N, Boyle P on behalf of the Italian Tamoxifen Prevention Study: Prevention of breast cancer with tamoxifen: Preliminary findings from the Italian randomised trial among hysterectomised women. *Lancet* 352:93, 1998.
232. Jackson RL, Dockerty MB: The Stein-Leventhal syndrome. Analysis of 43 cases with special reference to endometrial carcinoma. *Am J Obstet Gynecol* 73:161, 1957.

233. Gallup DG, Stock RJ: Adenocarcinoma of the endometrium in women 40 years of age or younger. *Obstet Gynecol* 64:117, 1984.
234. Mecklin JP, Jarvinen JH: Tumor spectrum in cancer family syndrome (hereditary nonpolyposis colorectal cancer). *Cancer* 68:1109, 1991.
235. Watson P, Lynch HT: Extracolonic cancer in hereditary nonpolyposis colorectal cancer. *Cancer* 71:677, 1993.
236. Barrett RJ, Geisinger KR, McCarty KS Jr: Endometrial carcinoma: Prognostic factors. *Rev Endocr Related Cancer* 32:11, 1990.
237. Hawwa ZM, Nahhas WA, Copenhaver EH: Postemenopausal bleeding. *Lahey Clin Found Bull* 19:61, 1970.
238. Rose PG: Endometrial carcinoma. *N Engl J Med* 335:640, 1996.
239. Abeler VM, Kjorstad KE: Endometrial adenocarcinoma in Norway: A study of a total population. *Cancer* 67:3093, 1991.
240. Zaino RJ, Satyaswaroop PG, Mortel R: The relationship of histologic and histochemical parameters to progesterone receptor status in endometrial adenocarcinoma. *Gynecol Oncol* 16:196, 1983.
241. Creasman WT: Prognostic significance of hormone receptors in endometrial cancer. *Cancer* 71:1467, 1993.
242. Cohen CJ and Thomas GM: Endometrial Cancer, in Holland JF, Bast Jr RC, Morton DL, Frei III E, Kufe DW, Weichselbaum RR (eds): *Cancer Medicine*, 4th ed. Baltimore, Maryland, Williams and Wilkins, 1997, p 2263.
243. DiSaia PJ, Cressman WT: Adenocarcinoma of the uterus, in: *Clinical Gynecologic Oncology*. St. Louis, Mosby, 1989, p 161.
244. Thigpen T: Systemic therapy with single agents for advanced or recurrent endometrial carcinoma, in Surwit EA, Alberts DS (eds): *Endometrial Cancer*. Boston, Kluwer, 1989, p 93.
245. Merkel DE, Osborne CK: Use of steroid receptor assay in cancer management. *Rev Endocr Related Cancer* 30:5, 1988.
246. Surwit EA, Alberts DS (eds): *Endometrial Cancer*. Boston, Kluwer, 1989, p 1.
247. Satyaswaroop PG, Zaino RJ, Mortel R: Carcinoma of the endometrium and hormonal receptors, in Surwit EA, Alberts DS (eds): *Endometrial Cancer*. Boston, Kluwer, 1989, pp 71–92.
248. Moore TD, Phillips PH, Nerenstone SR, et al: Systemic treatment of advanced and recurrent endometrial carcinoma—current and future directions. *J Clin Oncol* 9:1071, 1991.
249. Bonte J, Ide P, Billiet G, et al: Tamoxifen as a possible chemotherapeutic agent in endometrial adenocarcinoma. *Gynecol Oncol* 11:140, 1981.
250. Slavik M, Petty WM, Blessing JA, et al: Phase II clinical study of tamoxifen in advanced endometrial carcinoma. A GOG Study. *Cancer Treat Rep* 70:1019, 1986.
251. Perez CA, Fair WR, Ihde DC: Carcinoma of the prostate, in DeVita VT Jr, Hellman S, Rosenberg SA (eds): *Cancer: Principles and Practice of Oncology*. Philadelphia, Lippincott, 1989, p 1023.
252. Gittes RF: Carcinoma of the prostate. *N Engl J Med* 324:236, 1991.
253. Catalona WJ, Smith DS, Ratliff TL, Basler JW: Detection of organ-confined prostate cancer is increased through prostate-specific antigen-based screening. *JAMA* 270:948, 1993.
254. Ohori M, Wheeler TM, Dunn JK, Stamey TA, Scardino PT: The pathologic features and prognosis of prostate cancers detectable with current diagnostic tests. *J Urol* 152:1714, 1994.
255. Trump DL, Shipley WU, Dillioglugil O, Scardino PT: Neoplasms of the Prostate, in Holland JF, Bast RC Jr, Morton DL, Frei E III, Kufe DW, Weichselbaum RR (eds): *Cancer Medicine* 4th ed. Williams and Wilkins, Baltimore, Maryland, 1997, p 2125.
256. Labrie F, Dupont A, Candas B, Cusan L, Gomez JL, Diamond P, Bélanger A, Brousseau G, Lévesque J: Decrease of prostate cancer death by screening: First data from the Quebec Prospective and Randomized Study. *Proceedings of the American Society of Clinical Oncology*, Thirty-Fourth Annual Meeting, May 16–19, 1998, Los Angeles, California, p 2a, Abstract #4.
257. Gleason DF, Mellinger GT: The Veterans Administration Cooperative Urological Research Group Prediction of prognosis for prostatic adenocarcinoma by combined histological grading and clinical staging. *J Urol* 111:58, 1974.
258. Catalona WJ: Drug therapy: Management and treatment of cancer of the prostate. *N Engl J Med* 331:994, 1994.
259. Ohori M, Goad JR, Wheeler TM, Eastham JA, Thompson TC, Scardino PT: Can radical prostatectomy alter the progression of poorly differentiated prostate cancer? *J Urol* 152:1843, 1994.
260. Lieber MM: DNA content/ploidy as prognostic factors in prostate cancer. *Prostate* 4:119, 1992.
261. Diamond DA, Berry SJ, Umbricht C, Jewett HJ, Coffey DS: Computerized image analysis of nuclear shape as a prognostic factor for prostatic cancer. *Prostate* 3:321, 1982.
262. Aihara M, Scardino PT, Truong LD, Wheeler TM, Goad JR, Thompson TC: The frequency of apoptosis correlates with the prognosis of Gleason Grade 3 adenocarcinoma of the prostate. *Cancer* 75:522, 1995.
263. Effert PJ, McCoy RH, Walther PJ, Lui ET: p53 gene alterations in human prostate carcinoma. *J Urol* 150:257, 1993.
264. Chodak GW, Thisted RA, Gerber GS, Johansson JE, Adolfsson J, Jones GW, Chisholm GD, Moskovitz B, Livne PM, Warner J: Results of conservative management of clinically localized prostate cancer. *N Engl J Med* 330:242, 1994.
265. Pilepich MV, Krall JM, Al-Sarraf M, Madhu MJ, Doggett RL, Sause WT, Lawton CA, Abrams RA, Rotman M, Rubin P, Shipley WU, Grignon D, Caplan R, Cox JD: Androgen suppression with radiation therapy compared with radiation therapy alone for locally advanced prostatic carcinoma—a randomized comparative trial of the Radiation Therapy Oncology Group. *Urology* 45:616, 1995.
266. Bolla M, Gonzalez D, Warde P, Dubois JB, Mirimanoff R-O, Storme G, Bernier J, Kuten A, Sternberg C, Gil T, Collette L, Pierart M: Improved survival in patients with locally advanced prostate cancer treated with radiotherapy and goserelin. *N Engl J Med* 337:295, 1997.
267. Labrie F, Cusan L, Gomez JL, Diamond P, Suburu R, Lemay M, Tetu B, Fradet Y, Candas B: Down-staging of early stage prostate cancer before radical prostatectomy: the first randomize trial of neoadjuvant combination therapy with flutamide and a luteinizing hormone-releasing hormone agonist. *Urology* 44:29, 1994.
268. Santen RJ: Endocrine treatment of prostate cancer. *J Clin Endocrinol Metab* 75:685, 1992.
269. Manni A, Santen RJ: Endocrine aspects of prostate cancer, in Becker KL, Bilezikian JP, Bremner WJ, Hung W, Kahn CR, Loriaux DL, Nylén ES, Rebar RW, Robertson GL, Wartofsky L (eds): *Principles and Practice of Endocrinology and Metabolism*, 2nd ed. Philadelphia, Lippincott, 1995, p 1875.
270. Emond JP, Fazekas AT, Raynaud JP, Husson JM: New hormonal therapy in prostatic carcinoma: Combined treatment with an LHRH agonist and an antiandrogen. *Clin Invest Med* 5:267, 1982.
271. Geller J: Overview of enzyme inhibitors and anti-androgens in prostatic cancer. *J Androl* 12:364, 1991.
272. Crawford ED, Eisenberger MA, McLeod DG, Spaulding JT, Benson R, Dorr FA, Blumenstein BA, David MA, Goodman PJ: A controlled trial of leuprolide with and without flutamide in prostatic carcinoma. *N Engl J Med* 321:419, 1989.
273. Janknegt RA, Abbou CC, Bartoletti R, et al: Orchiectomy and nilutamide or placebo as treatment of metastatic prostatic cancer in a multinational double-blind randomized trial. *J Urol* 149:77, 1993.
274. Denis LJ, Carneiro de Moura JL, Bono A, et al: Goserelin acetate and flutamide versus bilateral orchiectomy: A phase III EORTC trial (30853). *Urology* 42:119, 1993.
275. Beland G, Elhilali M, Fradet Y, Laroche B, Ramsey EW, Trachtenberg J, Venner PM, Tewari HD: Total androgen ablation: Canadian experience. *Urol Clin North Am* 18:75, 1991.
276. DiSilverio F, Serio M, Costantini A: The use of the LHRH analogue goserelin alone or in combination with the antiandrogen cyproterone acetate in the treatment of advanced prostatic carcinoma: An Italian multicenter trial. *J Urol* 143:308A, 1990.
277. Eisenberger MA, Blumenstein BA, Crawford ED, Miller G, McLeod DG, Loehrer PJ, Wilding G, Sears K, Culkin DJ, Thompson IM, Bueschen AJ, Lowe BA: Bilateral orchiectomy with or without flutamide for metastatic prostate cancer. *N Engl J Med* 339:1036, 1998.

CHAPTER 30

Hormones, Aging, and Endocrine Disorders in the Elderly

John E. Morley

The human population is growing progressively older (Fig. 30-1). In ancient Rome the average human being could expect to live 22 years. In the Middle Ages life expectancy was 33 years, and in 1900 it had risen to 40 years. At the end of World War II life expectancy for whites in the United States was 66.7 years, and by 1998 it was 74 years for males and 80 years for females. At present the Japanese are the most long-lived population, with an average life expectancy at birth of 77 years for males and 83 years for females. In contrast, life expectancy in both Zambia and Malawi today is 36 years for males and 37 years for females. Increasing life expectancy has led to an increase in the percentage of the population over 65 years old such that in 1900, 4 percent of the U.S. population was over 65 years old, while by 1990, this proportion was 12.7 percent; it is projected to rise to 21.2 percent by 2030. Although the largest proportion of persons over 60 years of age live in the developed nations, by the year 2000 almost two-thirds of the world's 600 million older persons will be living in developing countries, making aging a truly international issue. Finally, it should be recognized that a female who reaches 65 years still has 20 years on average to live, and a male has 14.5 years. This extended longevity of those who reach old age is particularly important in light of the potential for the development of microvascular complications in older persons with diabetes mellitus.

The demographic aging imperative has resulted in an increasing awareness of the importance of the interaction of aging and a variety of disease processes. With advancing age there is often a blurring of the distinctions between health and disease, with the two existing as extremes on a continuum rather than as static, distinct entities. This is particularly true in regard to endocrine disorders, where the age-related decline in glandular function often results in an older person having hormonal values which would be considered borderline abnormal in a young person. This can lead to diagnostic dilemmas and results in an increasing frequency of endocrine deficiency diseases such as hypothyroidism, diabetes mellitus, and hypogonadism. Table 30-1 lists the putative effects of aging on endocrine disorders.

In addition to the decreased functional reserve, aging is also associated with decreased T-suppressor lymphocytes and increased circulating autoantibodies; this increases the propensity to develop an autoimmune disease and further increases the prevalence of hypoendocrine disease with advancing age. It also increases the likelihood of more than one endocrine disorder occurring in the same person (polyglandular failure syndromes).[1] Increased visceral adipose tissue that occurs in middle age and in the young leads to increased production of tumor necrosis factor-alpha, which plays a role in the increased insulin resistance associated with aging.[2,3] Altered receptor and postreceptor responsiveness leads to an increased prevalence of diabetes mellitus and can also result in atypical presentations (e.g., apathetic thyrotoxicosis). The atypical presentation of excessive thyroid hormone secretion in older persons results in part from the decrease in adrenergic β-receptors and postreceptor responsiveness.[4] Table 30-2 compares the differences in the presentation of hyperthyroidism in young and old persons. One study found that older persons with thyrotoxicosis had approximately 5 fewer clinical signs than did younger persons.[5]

Older persons can have nonspecific presenting symptoms of disease (e.g., weight loss, delirium, dementia, depression, and fatigue). This often leads to delays in seeing a physician or missed diagnoses. Table 30-3 lists the endocrine and metabolic causes of dementia, delirium, and depression in older persons.

Most normal laboratory test values have been established using young, healthy persons, and abnormal results may reflect the aging process (e.g., low IGF-I or a diminished thyroid stimulating hormone (TSH) response to thyrotropin releasing hormone (TRH) in older males). This can be further complicated by the presence of an intercurrent disease, such as euthyroid sick syndrome, which can also alter basal and stimulated hormone levels.

Malignant neoplasia are more prevalent with advancing age, and ectopic hormone production from neoplasms can mimic endocrine diseases. Consideration of ectopic hormone production in older persons can result in the early diagnosis of an occult cancer or the solution of a clinical problem. It can help prevent an inadequate or incorrect treatment of an endocrinopathy. The effectiveness of therapy or the demonstration of a recurrence of a cancer may be facilitated by the monitoring of ectopic hormone production. Cancer anorexia may be due to the production of ectopic hormones such as bombesin and calcitonin.[6] The presence of hypersecretory endocrine disease in older persons, especially when the biochemical parameters are out of proportion to the clinical presentation, should suggest the possibility of ectopic hormone secretion.

Changes due to aging may mimic endocrine disease. In 1886 Victor Horsley suggested that older persons resembled myxedematous monkeys and that thyroid deficiency could result in "mere senility." Table 30-4 summarizes the similarities between hypothyroidism and the aging process. Despite these similarities, there is little evidence that the aging process is related to thyroid deficiency, and an excess of thyroid hormone may in fact aggravate the aging process, for example, by producing accelerated osteoporosis or catabolism leading to severe weight loss. However, there is a selective age-related decrease in the T_3 responsiveness to certain biomarkers of thyroid hormone action (Table 30-5).[7–9] The major defect appears to occur at the pretranslational level. There is

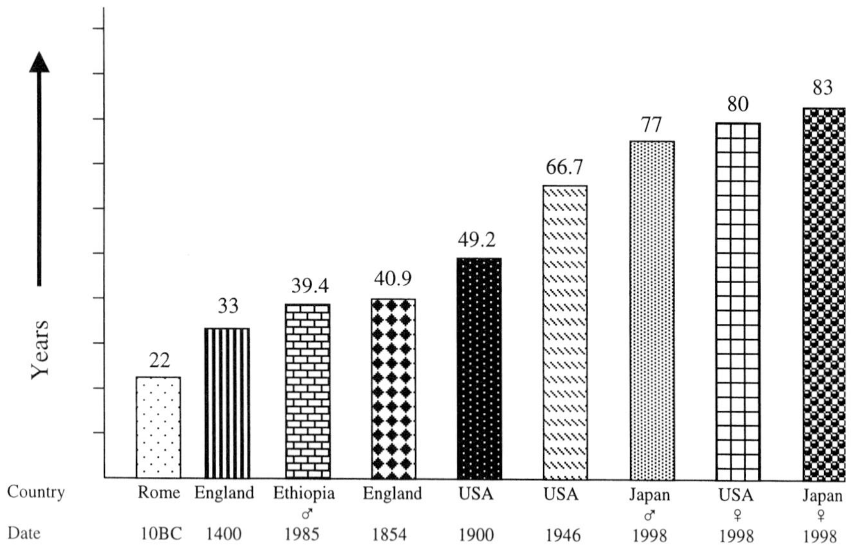

FIGURE 30-1. The aging of the human population. Shown are examples of life expectancy from Roman times to the present.

also an in vivo decrease in plasma membrane T_3 transport with advancing age.[10] The thyroid hormone resistance syndrome of aging is highly selective. The failure to see marked increases in TSH with aging in the face of relative thyroid hormone resistance appears to be due to both an increase in pituitary nuclear receptors[11] and decreased hypothalamic secretion of TRH.[12]

Older persons often have a decreased functional reserve of endocrine target organs as a result of aging per se or secondary to an intercurrent disease. This can lead to a need for lower than normal replacement doses of hormones in older persons.

If an older person has chronic obstructive pulmonary disease or angina, keeping the replacement dose of thyroid hormone at a level that just restores the circulating hormonal values to normal may ameliorate the symptoms of the disease and improve the functional quality of life. Similarly, an older person with osteopenia may develop worsening bone disease if the thyroid replacement dose results in hormonal levels in the upper half of the normal range. Calcitonin therapy for Paget disease may result in severe anorexia and weight loss in older persons.[13]

Persons over 65 years take, on the average, four to six prescription drugs and three to four nonprescription drugs a day.[14] This can result in altered circulating hormone levels (e.g., phenytoin and thyroid hormone levels) and decreased hormone responsiveness (e.g., cimetidine and testosterone). Drugs such as rifampin and phenytoin increase thyroid hormone turnover and thus may result in a requirement for a relatively higher replacement

TABLE 30-1. Effects of Aging and Related Diseases on Endocrine Disorders

Effect	Consequence
Decreased functional reserve of endocrine organs	Increased prevalence of endocrine deficiency diseases
Decreased T-suppressor lymphocytes increased circulating autoantibodies	Increased autoimmune endocrine diseases
Increased visceral adipose tissue associated with increased tumor necrosis-alpha production	Increased insulin resistance
Decreased receptor and postreceptor responsiveness	Atypical presentations; delayed diagnosis, increased prevalence of diabetes mellitus
Nonspecific response to hormonal imbalance (e.g., weight loss, fatigue, delirium, depression, and dementia)	Delayed or missed diagnosis
Altered normal ranges	Inappropriate diagnosis
Intercurrent disease	Diagnostic dilemma
Increased prevalence of neoplasia	Ectopic hormone production
Aging changes mimicking endocrine deficiency disease	Delayed or missed diagnosis or inappropriate diagnosis
Decreased functional reserve of target organs	Decreased replacement dose of hormones
	Increased propensity to develop untoward effects from hormone replacement
Polypharmacy	Interference with hormonal measurement
	Altered circulating hormones
	Decreased hormonal responsiveness
	Increased or decreased replacement dose
	Poor compliance
	Adverse drug reactions

TABLE 30-2. Differences in the Presentation of Hyperthyroidism between Young and Old Persons

	Signs and Symptoms, Percent						
	Nordyke et al.*				Tibaldi et al.†	Davis et al.‡	Martin and Deam**
Age range	20–40	60	70	80	75–95	60–82	70–101
Appetite increased	50–61	31	10	36	—	11	—
Appetite decreased	5–9	14	21	27	—	36	—
Weight loss	29–52	76	78	82	44	69	83
Palpitations	58–67	58	52	45	36	63	37
Tachycardia	83–84	79	76	70	28§	11¶	50§
Nervousness	59–73	64	69	55	20	55	—
Dizziness/syncope	—	—	—	—	20	—	—
Memory loss	—	—	—	—	8	—	51
Tremor	69	62	67	73	36	89	53
Atrial fibrillation	0–1	1	8	17	32	39	60
Eyelid lag	19	18	17	0	12	35	—
Thyroid enlargement	97–99	84	83	73	32	63	48
Muscle weakness	—	—	—	—	—	—	55
Apathy/depression	—	—	—	—	—	—	15

*Nordyke RA, Gilbert FI, Harada ASM: Influence of age on clinical findings. *Arch Intern Med* 148:626, 1988.

†Tibaldi JM, Barzel US, Albin J, Surks M: Thyrotoxicosis in the very old. *Am J Med* 81:619, 1986.

‡Davis PJ, Davis FB: Hyperthyroidism in patients over the age of 60 years. *Medicine* 53:161, 1974.

**Martin FIR, Deacon DR: Hyperthyroidism in elderly hospitalized patients: Clinical features and outcomes. *Med J Aust* 164:200, 1996.

§>90/min.

¶>120/min.

dose. Patients on β blockers may have elevated thyroid hormone levels, resulting in inappropriate treatment for hyperthyroidism.[15] Nonprescription cough mixtures containing iodine may precipitate thyroid disorders or interfere with the uptake of radioactive iodine. The Genon metabolic "anticancer" diet includes taking a large supplement of thyroid extract with iodine. Vitamin ingestion in a megadosage may mimic endocrine disease; for example, vitamin A may produce hypercalcemia by activating cathepsin D in the parathyroid gland, resulting in increased circulating parathyroid hormone (PTH). Megadoses of vitamin C interfere with the ability to measure glucose in the blood. Ginseng tea used as a health food may produce hypertension secondary to its ability to increase the hypothalamic-pituitary-adrenal axis.[16] Theophylline may interact with thyroid hormones to produce tachycardia and weight loss. Multiple drugs may interact with oral hypoglycemic agents to precipitate hypoglycemia.

Noncompliance with prescription medications is common in older persons and increases with the number of medications. Special care needs to be paid to improving compliance to hormone replacement therapy in older persons with memory problems and dementia (e.g., through the use of calendar pillboxes and by writing down medication instructions).

Certain endocrine disorders are peculiar to older persons or are most common in older persons; examples include type II (age-related) osteopenia, Paget's disease, and hypertension due to an endothelinoma.

TABLE 30-3. Metabolic Causes of Psychiatric Disturbances in Older Persons

Delirium	Dementia
Hypoxemia	Hypoxemia
Electrolyte disturbances	Electrolyte disturbances
Acid-base abnormalities	Hyperlipidemia
Uremia	Hypothyroidism
Hepatic failure	Hypoglycemia
Thyroid disorders	Diabetes mellitus
Hypoglycemia	Hypoparathyroidism
Hypoparathyroidism	Hyperparathyroidism
Hyperparathyroidism	Hypoadrenalism
Hypoadrenalism	Malnutrition
Hypopituitarism	Pernicious anemia
Isolated ACTH deficiency	Folate deficiency
Exogenous corticosteroids	Dehydration
Thiamine deficiency	
Pellagra	
Porphyria	
Depression	
Hypokalemia	
Apathetic thyrotoxicosis	
Hypothyroidism	
Diabetes mellitus	
Hyperparathyroidism	
Cushing disease	
Addison disease	
Malnutrition	
Pernicious anemia	
Folate deficiency	
Impotence	

TABLE 30-4. Similarities between Hypothyroidism and the Aging Process

Bradycardia	Muscular weakness
Hypertension	Lethargy
Hypercholesterolemia	Cognitive dysfunction
Weight gain	Impotence
Cold intolerance	Dry skin
Constipation	Decreased hearing
Dry, brittle hair	Decreased dark adaptation

TABLE 30-5. Biochemical Alterations in Response to Triiodothyronine with Age

Decreased	No Change	Increased
Malate dehydrogenase	Angiotensin	Cerebral GLUT-1
Apolipoprotein A(1)	Converting enzyme	
Na^+K^+ATPase	α-Glycerophosphate	
Spot 14	Dehydrogenase	
Ca^{24}ATPase		

Source: (Based on Mooradian et al.[7–9])

THEORIES OF AGING

The major theories of aging are summarized in Table 30-6. No single theory adequately describes all the features of aging. In the last few years numerous genetic mutations have been identified that extend cell and animal lifespan.[17–23]

System-based theories of aging suggest that alteration of the endocrine system or immune system with advancing age leads to deterioration of the organism and the aging process. Neuroendocrine theories of aging suggest that a central pacemaker results in endocrine organ failure, which leads to the aging process. The finding by Snowdon that the age of menopause predicts the age of death provides support for this theory.[24] Denckla found that hypophysectomy and hormone replacement lead to life extension. This prompted him to suggest the presence of a "death hormone" that decreases oxygen consumption and accelerates the aging process.[25] The failure of Denckla to ascertain the adequacy of hypophysectomy and the possibility that hypophysectomy had merely removed pituitary tumors have cast doubt on this possibility. The role of a multiple hormone lack in the aging process remains to be determined (*vide infra*).

TABLE 30-6. Theories of Aging

Genetic Theories
Human fibroblasts: TERT is a gene controlling a catalytic unit of telomerase that extends replicative ability of cells in culture
Nematode: AGE1 (phosphatidylinositol-3-kinase) and DAF2 (insulin receptor) extend lifespan by 40–100 percent
Fruit fly: METHUSELAH (mth: GTP-binding protein) and SOD-1 (Cu/Zn-superoxide dismutase) extend lifespan by 40–100 percent
Environmental Theories
Background radiation producing genetic mutations
Error catastrophe theory
Large molecule cross-linking (glucose-driven)
Dietary restriction theory
System-Based Theories
Hormonal decline ("Hormonal Fountain of Youth")
Neuroendocrine pacemaker
"Death" hormone
Glucocorticoid cascade hypothesis
Immune theory
Thymic failure
NO (nitric oxide) cytokine theory of aging
Cellular Theories
Free radical theory
Oncogene theory
Mitochondrial DNA theory
DNA and RNA based theories

It is now well established that some normal human cells have a fixed number of population doublings in vitro after which they cease dividing—the "Hayflick limit."[26] The linkage of this in vitro phenomenon to whole organism aging is suggested by two lines of evidence. Firstly, there is a decrease in the number of doublings when cells are obtained from older donors.[27] Secondly, the longer the species lives, the more population doublings can be derived from its cells in vitro.[26] CD_{28ds}, a cell surface marker related to proliferation, is expressed at a lower rate in T cells from old humans.[28] With cellular aging, there is a decrease in the repetitive DNA sequences (TTA GGG) called telomeres.[29] Telomeres can be synthesized by an RNA-associated enzyme called telomerase, whose activity is reduced with aging but markedly increased in immortal cancer cells. Telomeres shorten over the lifespan during population doublings and telomere shortening is seen in fibroblasts and lymphocytes from older individuals.[29] Regulation of the G1 cell cycle requires activity of the cyclin dependent kinases.[30] The cyclin E/-cdk2/PCNA complex phosphorylates the retinoblastoma protein allowing E2F, a transcription factor, to be released. E2F then activates gene transcription allowing DNA synthesis. Cellular senescence is associated with the induction of a protein, p21, that combines with the cyclin complex inhibiting retinoblastoma protein phosphorylation.[31] This then results in growth arrest and cell death. While the activity of genes such as p21 increase, those of genes for other proteins such as cfos and p53 decrease with cellular aging.[32,33] Conditions that cause accelerated aging, such as diabetes mellitus, cause a reduction in the capacity of cells to continue to divide.

A number of molecular theories of aging have been developed. The best known of these is the free radical theory. This theory suggests that the generation of reactive oxygen species, such as superoxide, the hydroxyl radical, hydrogen peroxide, and nitric oxide result in permanent damage to DNA and cellular proteins.[34] There has been particular interest in the role of free radical damage in producing damage to mitochondrial DNA. mtDNA shows an exponential increase in deletions and mutations with aging.[35] Levels of 8-hydroxydeoxyguanosine, a byproduct of free radical damage, rise with age in a number of tissues.[36] Iron stimulates free radical formation, while a number of intracellular substances such as superoxide dismutaces, catalases, glutathione peroxidase, and antioxidant vitamins protect against free radical damage. High levels of superoxidase dismutase activity correlate with lifespan.[35] Dietary restriction reduces free radical production and results in life extension.[37] Flies bred selectively for high levels of antioxidant activity and transgenic flies with transgenic expression of superoxide dismutase have enhanced survival.[18] Despite this impressive body of evidence supporting the free radical theory of aging, it has been difficult to clearly demonstrate enhancement of lifespan in humans or animals ingesting high levels of antioxidants. It would appear that free radical activity explains some but not all of the inter- and intraspecies differences in aging.

A key aging theory concerns damage to DNA and its ability to be repaired. This theory suggests that aging is associated with an increase in oncogene production (such as the BCLZ gene) and a decrease in the ability of cells to undergo excision—repair of DNA.[39] If repair processes are impaired, then random background radiation damage would have a greater propensity to produce genetic mutations that shorten maximum lifespan.[38] There is some evidence that excision repair capacity of DNA correlates with maximal lifespan of different species.[29]

Increasing glucose levels with age leads to the glycation of long-lived proteins.[40] These modified, cross-linked proteins interact with free radicals to produce so-called advanced glycation end (AGE) products. Glycation of lipoproteins leads to cross-linking with protein molecules in the arterial wall, resulting in atherosclerosis, an almost universal pathologic concomitant of aging.[41] Glycation of DNA can lead to a slowing in its unwinding rate.[42] Binding of AGE products to macrophages results in the production of multiple cytokines.[43] Persons with diabetes die on the average one-third earlier than do nondiabetics. The glycation theory of aging is intriguing but requires further evidence.

There is increasing knowledge concerning the role of genes in organismic aging. Studies in human twins have suggested that approximately 26 percent of the life span is hereditable.[44] The importance of hereditability has been highlighted by the studies in fruit flies demonstrating the ability to select for longer or shorter life spans[45] and the studies in mice by Takeda et al.[46] resulting in the production of a variety of senescence accelerated mice (SAM). Human centenarians have a greater frequency of the apolipoprotein E_2 gene than of the E_4 gene.[47] E_4 genotypes have higher levels of vascular disease and Alzheimer's disease. Two genes in the nematode (aenorhabdites elegans) markedly extend lifespan.[19,20] They are age-1, which produces a phosphadidylinositol 3-kinase, and daf-2, an insulin-receptor like gene. These genes are considered to be "candidate longevity genes" for humans.

Persons with Werner syndrome age at an accelerated rate. The patients have a defective WRN gene, which codes for a protein with helicase and exonuclease activity. This gene appears to alter DNA replication and repair and be related to a greater rate of loss of DNA telomene activity. Polymorphism of the WRN-DNA has been shown to be a risk factor for myocardial infarction.[48]

In 1969, Muhlen and Ockenfels[49] showed that glucocorticoids damaged the hippocampus. This finding was confirmed by Landfield et al.[50] in 1981. Since then, a variety of anatomical and biochemical studies have demonstrated that the hippocampus is particularly vulnerable to glucocorticoid damage.[51] This has led to the formulation of the glucocorticoid cascade hypothesis of aging. This hypothesis suggests that over the life-span, there is failure of adrenal glucocorticoid regulation resulting in accelerated hippocampal damage with aging (Fig. 30-2). Against this hypothesis is that caloric-restricted rats who live long have elevated cortisol levels and there is little evidence of cortisol dysregulation with aging.[52]

It has been suggested that multiple age-related changes in the immune system accelerate the aging process. In this model, the thymus and thymic hormones play a major role in leading to

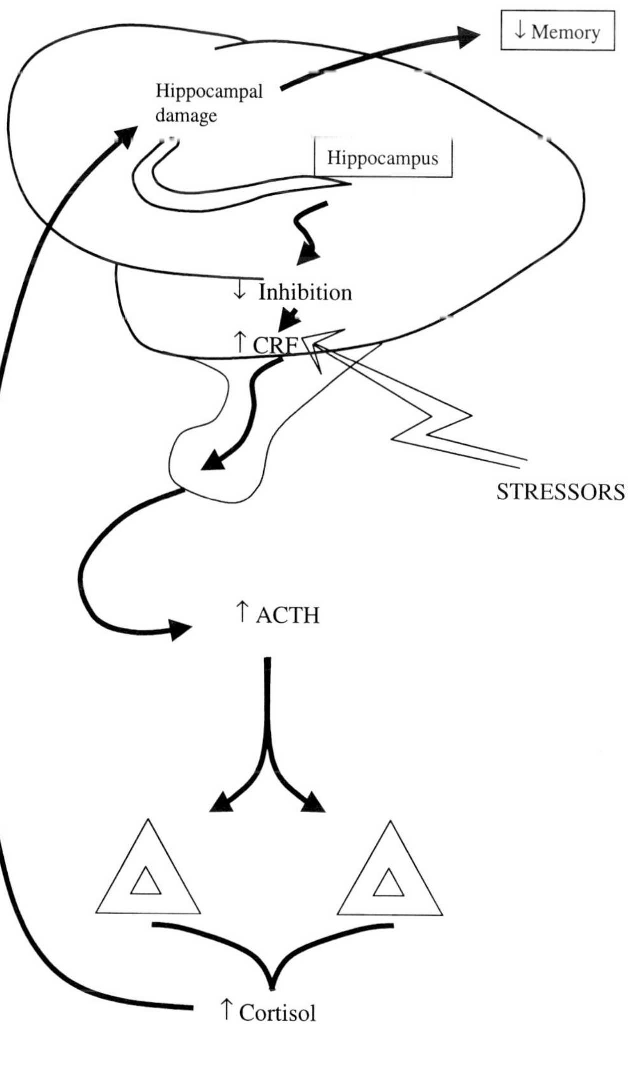

FIGURE 30-2. Theoretical mechanism by which stress and glucocorticoids produce hippocampal aging.

the deterioration of T-cell function with aging.[53] Thymic hormones produce a partial restoration of immunity both in vivo and in vitro.[54] Walford has suggested that these immune changes with aging are related to genes of the major histocompatibility complex.[55] Congenic animals differing only at the major histocompatibility locus have different life spans. This locus also regulates the superoxide dismutase enzyme, linking the immune theory of aging to the free radical theory of aging. In addition, the production of interleukin-1α accelerates senescence in cellular systems.[56]

The role of cytokine overproduction with aging—in particular overproduction of tumor necrosis factor–alpha (TNFα) has become an increasingly exciting possible cause of aging changes. The middle age increase in adipose tissue results in an increase in TNFα production.[3] Increased intestinal permeability with aging leads to bacterial translocation and increased cytokine activation. Chronic inflammatory conditions, such as arthritis, can also increase cytokine production. Increased cytokine production will result in increased free radical production, including activation of nitric oxide synthase (NOS). Not only does this produce tissue damage, but NOS activation leads to insulin resistance[57,58 (and unpublished observations)] with the development of hyperglycemia, hypertriglyceridemia, and hypertension. The hyperglycemia results in increased tissue glycation. This comprehensive theory of aging is called the NO (nitric oxide) Cytokine Theory of Aging (Fig. 30-3). Although this theory remains speculative, it has sufficient experimental basis to make it an attractive holistic theory.

Overall, it appears that the regulation of aging is a complex process that involves both genetic and environmental components. It seems likely that different aspects of aging are regulated by different processes. Alterations in the endocrine system with aging may play an important role in coordinating the aging process in different organs.

HORMONAL CHANGES

Table 30-7 summarizes the major hormonal changes associated with the aging process.

Growth Hormone and IGF-I

There is an age-related decline in growth hormone pulses in older persons.[59] This is associated with an age-related decrease in the number and size of somatotrophs.[60] The growth hormone response to growth hormone releasing hormone is attenuated with advancing age.[61,62] The major decrease in the growth hormone response in males occurs at about 40 years of age,[61] explaining the failure of Pavlov et al., who utilized controls up to 49 years of age, to find a significant decrease in the growth hormone response to growth hormone releasing hormone.[63] The decrease in the growth hormone response in the female appears to occur approximately a decade later.[64] In postmenopausal females estrogen

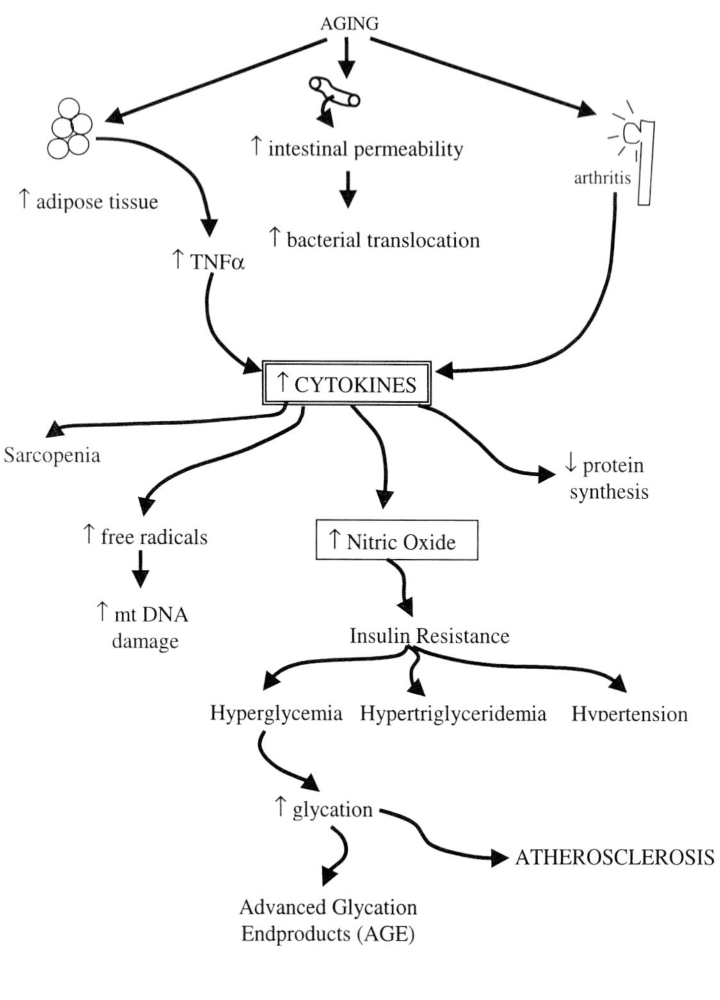

FIGURE 30-3. The nitric oxide cytokine theory of aging.

TABLE 30-7. Major Changes Associated with the Aging Process

Hormone	Effect of Aging
Pituitary hormones	
Growth hormone	
24-h secretion	Decreased
Response to GHRH	Decreased
Response to repetitive GHRH	Restored
Response to arginine	Unchanged
Prolactin	
TSH	
Basal	Normal
Response to TRH	Decreased (males)
ACTH	
Basal	Normal
Response to CRF	Mild increase
β-endorphin	Blunting of circadian rhythm
Gonadotropins	
Males	Inappropriately low (LH) and increased (FSH)
Females	Increased
Thyroid hormones	
Thyroxine	Normal
Triiodothyronine	Mild decrease
Adrenal hormones	
Cortisol, basal	Normal or mild increase
Dexamethasone suppression	Less efficient
Aldosterone	Decreased
Dehydroepiandrosterone sulfate	Decreased
Epinephrine	Unchanged/Increased in old-old
Calcitropic hormones	
PTH	Increased
Calcitonin	Decreased
25(OH) Vitamin D	Decreased
1,25$(OH)_2$ Vitamin D	Normal or decreased
Pancreatic hormones	
Insulin	Increased
Amylin	Increased
Glucagon	Unchanged
Pancreatic polypeptide	Increased
Sex hormones:	
Males Testosterone	Normal or decreased
Bioavailable testosterone	Decreased
Dehydrotestosterone	Decreased
Sex hormone-binding globulin	Normal or increased
Estradiol	Normal
Inhibin	Decreased
Activin	Increased
Females Estradiol	Decreased
Estrone	Decreased
Androstenedione	Decreased
Testosterone	Decreased
Miscellaneous	
Norepinephrine	Increased
Renin	Decreased
Gastric inhibitory polypeptide	Unchanged
Glucagon-like peptide	Unchanged
Cholecystokinin	Increased
Vasoactive intestinal peptide	Increased; loss of circadian rhythm
Atrial natriuretic factor	Increased
Arginine vasopressin	Increased, loss of circadian rhythm

administration can restore the growth hormone response to growth hormone releasing hormone.[65] Repeated administration of growth hormone releasing hormone results in an increased response to the releasing hormone after a number of days of administration. The growth hormone response to insulin hypoglycemia is diminished with the decreased responsiveness, again starting at middle age.[66,67] There is also a decrease in the response to apomorphine with advancing age.[68]

Animal studies have strongly supported the concept that increased somatostatin secretion is responsible for the diminished secretion of growth hormone seen with advancing age.[59] Somatostatin produces this effect both by inhibiting the effect of growth hormone releasing hormone on the pituitary and by decreasing the secretion of growth hormone releasing hormone. In humans, arginine increases growth hormone secretion by inhibiting hypothalamic somatostatin release.[69] Arginine administration in older humans results in a growth hormone response equivalent to that seen in younger persons.[70,71] However, a somatostatin infusion study found that growth hormone in old and young persons was equally suppressed by somatostatin casting some doubt on the concept of excess somatostatin release.[72]

IGF-I levels are reduced in older males and females, and this reduction is correlated with 24-h growth hormone release.[73–76] In institutionalized malnourished older persons IGF-I levels are even further reduced compared with age-matched controls.[77] A severely malnourished 87-year-old male with hypoglycemia was demonstrated to have very low levels of circulating growth hormone binding protein and decreased expression of growth hormone receptor messenger ribonucleic acid, which was thought to be responsible for his growth hormone resistance.[78]

The alterations in the hypothalamic pituitary liver growth hormone axis with aging are summarized in Fig. 30-4.

Prolactin

There appears to be a mild but significant increase in prolactin levels with advancing age.[79] This parallels the decrease in dopaminergic activity seen with aging. Older persons with diabetes mellitus have been reported to have even greater increases in prolactin levels.[80]

Hypothalamic-Pituitary-Thyroid Axis

Overall there are no major age-related daytime changes in basal TSH levels with aging, though 2.7–3.5 percent of older men and 7.1–17.4 percent of older women may have elevated serum TSH levels, representing incipient hypothyroidism in many older persons.[81–83] Careful circadian sampling demonstrated that TSH was suppressed by 50 percent over the 24-h period in old compared to young persons.[84] This is predominantly due to a blunting of the nocturnal TSH amplitude increase present in young persons.[84] The TSH response to TRH is suppressed in elderly men but not in older women.[85] Centenarians have suppressed basal TSH levels compared to persons <80 years of age.[86] A number of studies have found a subset of older persons with suppressed TSH values in the hyperthyroid range.[87] While it would appear that in most cases these are spurious values unrelated to thyroid hormone excess, Sawin et al.[88] reported that older persons with low serum TSH levels were a risk factor for subsequent development of atrial fibrillation in older persons.

With advancing age there is a decrease in the thyroxine pro-

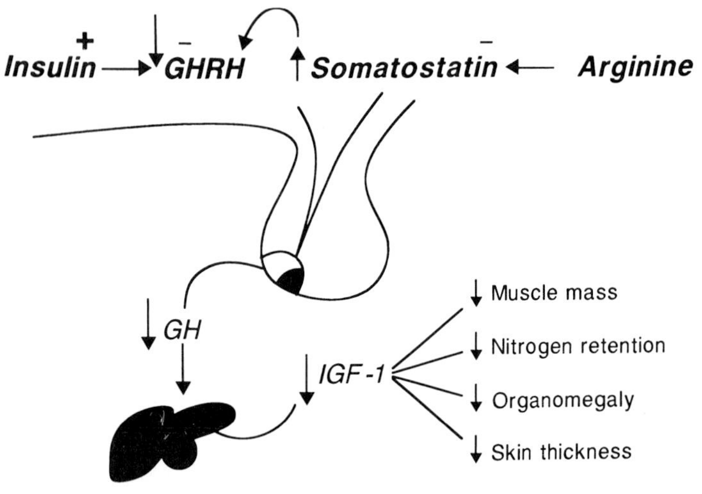

FIGURE 30-4. Alterations in the hypothalamic-pituitary-liver growth hormone axis with aging.

duction rate from 80 to 60 μg per day.[89] This is balanced by a decrease in the metabolic clearance rate of thyroxine with aging.[90] Free thyroxine levels are not altered with aging. Triiodothyronine levels decrease with advancing age as a result of the decreased production rate and no change in the metabolic clearance rate.[91,92] There is a progressive decline in radioactive iodine uptake in the thyroid gland from middle age to 90 years of age.[93] Antibodies to thyroid peroxidase are significantly more prevalent in persons 60–85 years of age than in those under 50 years of age; but less prevalent in centenarians.[94] A combination of borderline elevated TSH and high antithyroid peroxidase antibodies (1:64 or greater) is highly predictive of the subsequent development of clinically significant hypothyroidism.[95]

It should also be remembered that many older persons may have marked changes in thyroid hormone levels because of an intercurrent illness that results in the development of the euthyroid sick syndrome (Table 30-8).

Hypothalamic-Pituitary-Adrenal Axis

With advancing age there is a reduction in the secretion rate of cortisol and a decrease in the metabolic clearance rate, resulting in plasma levels of cortisol that remain unchanged with aging.[96–98] The cortisol acrophase tends to occur earlier with aging.[99] The adrenal maintains its ability to produce cortisol in response to exogenous ACTH administration throughout life, though in view of the decreased plasma clearance of cortisol, this is suggestive of a decreased adrenal responsiveness.[100] There is a tendency for ACTH levels to be greater in response to corticotropin releasing factor (CRF), insulin, hypoglycemia, metyrapone, and surgical stress.[101] Older persons often fail to appropriately suppress the hypothalamic-pituitary-adrenal axis after the administration of dexamethasone, though this may result from dementia, depression, or an intercurrent illness.[16]

Older persons have a blunting of the circadian rhythm of β-endorphin secretion compared with younger persons.[102] β-endorphin levels in the cerebrospinal fluid (CSF) are reduced in older persons compared with younger persons.[103] Age-related differences in β-endorphin to exercise[104] and the cold pressor test[105] have not been demonstrated.

Basal aldosterone levels, 24-h urinary aldosterone excretion, and the aldosterone plasma clearance rate decrease with aging.[9] Aldosterone and plasma renin activity levels show diminished responses with advancing age.[106] These changes tend to increase the propensity of older persons to develop hyporeninemic hypoaldosteronism.

The secretion of dehydroepiandrosterone (DHEA) declines linearly from 20 to 96 years of age.[107,108] DHEA sulfate has been

TABLE 30-8. Comparison between the Changes in Aging and Changes Due to the Euthyroid Sick Syndrome

	Aging	Euthyroid Sick Syndrome
Thyroxine (T4) level	Normal	Normal or decreased
Thyroxine production rate	Decreased	Decreased
Thyroxine clearance rate	Decreased	Decreased
T4 binding to TBG	Unchanged	Decreased
Triiodothyronine (T3) level	Decreased	Markedly decreased
Triiodothyronine production rate	Decreased	Decreased
Triiodothyronine clearance rate	Unchanged	Decreased
Reverse T3 levels	Unchanged	Increased
TSH	Decreased, unchanged, or increased*	Normal, decreased, or increased
TSH response to TRH (males)	Decreased	Decreased
TSH response to TRH (females)	Unchanged	Decreased

*Increase is due to incipient hypothyroidism, which occurs with increasing frequency in old age.

associated inversely with future mortality, especially from coronary heart disease,[109] but this has not been confirmed in other studies. In experimental animals, DHEA exerts a protective effect against tumorigenesis, immune disorders, and diabetes mellitus.[110]

A number of studies have examined the effect of DHEA replacement in older persons. High doses of DHEA (100 mg) have been reported to increase strength and muscle mass in older males but not in females.[111] DHEA has had variable effects on immune function.[112] There is little evidence that DHEA improves mood or enhances cognitive function in humans.[113] Despite the large amount of enthusiasm in the lay press and some scientific journals for DHEA replacement therapy in older persons, there is little evidence to support its use.

Pregnenolone levels also decline with aging.[114] Pregnenolone is an extremely potent memory-enhancing agent in mice.[115] Sih et al.,[116] however, failed to find any effects on strength, function, or cognition of 50 mg pregnenolone replacement in a double blind crossover trial. Pregnenolone may have a small effect on improving quality of sleep.[117]

The overall consensus is that there is an age-related increase in systemic sympathetic nervous system activity. There is also some evidence for a regional increase in norepinephrine release in the heart but not in the kidney.[118] Norepinephrine levels increase with advancing age, while circulating epinephrine levels are unchanged[16] except in the very old where they may be elevated.[119] The increase in norepinephrine levels parallels the increase in systolic blood pressure seen in older persons.[120] There is both an increase in norepinephrine appearance in plasma and a decrease in the norepinephrine clearance rate.[121,122] Stepwise multiple linear regression analysis suggests that norepinephrine appearance rates play a more important role in increasing norepinephrine levels than does the decrease in clearance rates,[123] and compartment analysis has suggested that the increased appearance rate occurs mainly in the extravascular space, suggesting an increased tone of the sympathetic nervous system.[123] Both age and percentage of body fat play an important role in producing the increased norepinephrine appearance rate. Older persons have increased norepinephrine responsiveness to both upright posture and oral glucose ingestion.[16]

Isoproterenol produces less of an increase in the heart rate in older persons, suggesting a decrease in adrenergic responsiveness with advancing age.[9] There is a small decrease in the proportion of β-adrenergic receptors in the high-affinity state, a reduction in receptor affinity, and a reduced activity of the catalytic unit of adenylyl cyclase.[124] α-adrenergic receptor function is altered less with advancing age, with only a mild decrease in the affinity for agonist binding[125] and a reduction in epinephrine-mediated inhibition of NaF-stimulated platelet membrane adenylyl cyclase activity in elderly persons.[126] These findings are compatible with an uncoupling of the platelet α_2-adrenergic receptor adenylyl cyclase complex with advancing age. However, this is not due to a reduction in the guanine nucleotide binding protein Giα_2.[127] Preliminary studies have suggested that the changes in α_2-adrenergic receptor activity is due to appropriate down regulation of the receptor in response to the increased circulatory levels of catecholamines.[128]

Sex Hormones

Male

Although the effects of aging on testosterone levels in males were once controversial, it is now clear that testosterone levels decrease with age. A longitudinal study following healthy males over the age of 60 years for 14 years demonstrated a fall in testosterone in every male.[129] The rate of decline in testosterone levels is between 1 and 2 percent per year. This is seen even more dramatically in the decrease in bioavailable testosterone that occurs with advancing age (Fig. 30-5).[130] The circadian rhythm of testosterone is also lost with advancing age.[131]

Dihydrotestosterone is decreased in older persons unless there

FIGURE 30-5. Comparison of luteinizing hormone (LH) and bioavailable testosterone (BT) levels with aging. Demonstrates the failure of LH to rise appropriately in response to the falling BT levels seen with aging. (*Data from Korenman et al.*[79])

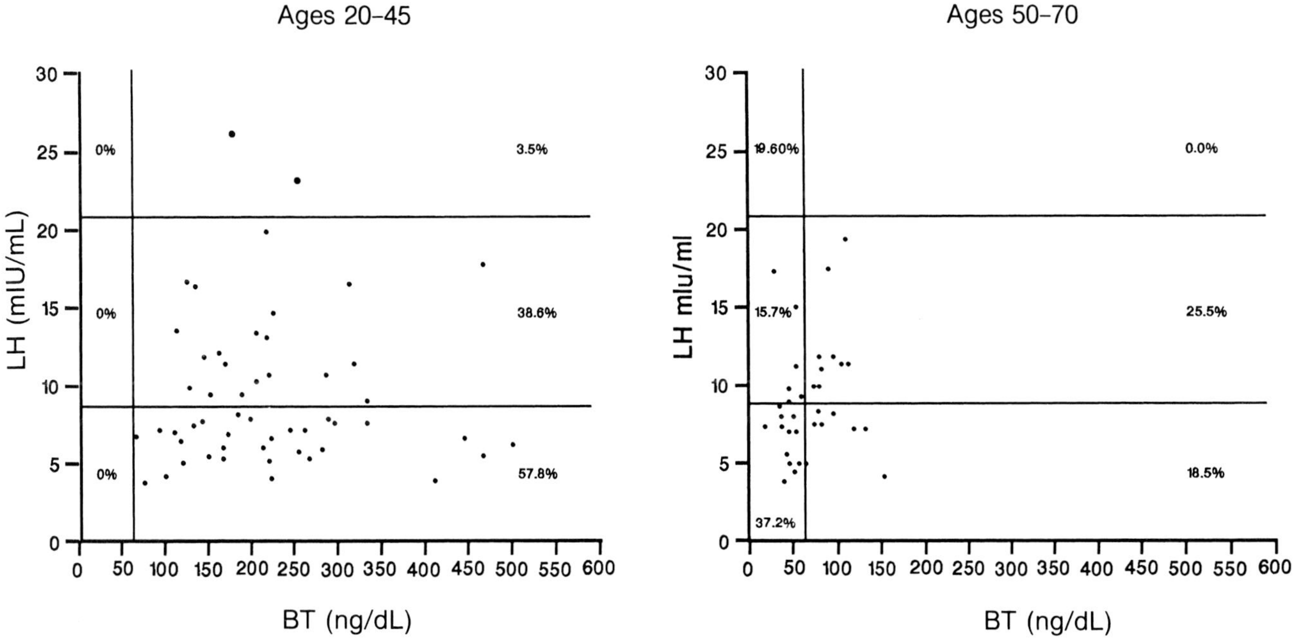

is significant prostatic hypertrophy, in which case it may be increased.[132] The testosterone production rate is decreased in subjects >70 years of age (mean 4.0 mg/24 h) compared to subjects under <50 years of age (mean 6.6 mg/24 h).[133] The decreased production rate is partially balanced by a decrease in the plasma clearance rate of testosterone in older adults (530 ± 35 mg/liter per 24 h). The plasma clearance rate of testosterone is directly proportional to the free testosterone level. There is a decrease in testicular weight and the total number of Leydig cells with advancing age.[134] There is an impaired testosterone response to exogenous human chorionic gonadotropin (hCG) with advancing age, though whether this is secondary to the decrease in basal testosterone production or is due to refractoriness to gonadotropin stimulation is uncertain.[135]

Estradiol levels are unchanged with age, resulting in an increase in the ratio of estradiol to testosterone.[134] However, there is a decline in free and bioavailable estradiol levels with aging. Estradiol production rates are unchanged with age, but there is a decrease in the clearance rates.[136] Peripheral conversion of testosterone to estradiol and androstenedione to estrone increases with aging.[136] This increased aromatization is presumably secondary to the increased obesity seen in old males. Sex hormone-binding globulin (SHBG) levels are unchanged or slightly increased with aging.[129,137] As testosterone is bound with greater avidity to SHBG than is estradiol, the ratio of free estradiol to bioavailable testosterone is greatly increased.

Though it has been stated that luteinizing hormone (LH) levels increase with age,[138,139] recent studies have reevaluated this issue. As can be seen in Fig. 30-5, older persons with markedly depressed bioavailable testosterone levels fail to show the expected increase in LH levels.[130] A longitudinal study demonstrated that LH levels do increase above the normal range in the old-old (i.e., those older than 80 years).[129] There is a decrease in LH amplitude with aging without a change in the pulse frequency, suggesting a hypothalamic defect.[140,141] There is also a decreased response to naloxone, suggesting increased opioid tone in older males.[142] Furthermore, there is a blunted response to gonadotropin releasing hormone (GnRH) in older compared with younger men[143] and a mild age-related decline in the ratio of LH bioactivity to immunoreactivity,[144] suggesting a pituitary defect. Testosterone is less effective at inhibiting LH in older males than in younger males.[145,146] Thus, it appears that with advancing age there is a defect in the testicular secretion of testosterone (primary hypogonadism) coupled with a failure of the hypothalamic-pituitary axis to sense the falling testosterone level (secondary hypogonadism). This central failure results in only a minority of older men having elevated LH levels, while the majority have inappropriately normal LH levels for the decreased levels of circulating testosterone (Fig. 30-6).

Testes from older men histologically show thickening of the basement membrane, peritubular fibrosis, and impaired spermatogenic maturation. The areas of testicular degeneration are patchy in distribution, allowing normal spermatogenesis to occur in more than half of males >70 years of age.[147] Sperm counts tend to decrease with advancing age, and there is diminished sperm motility and altered morphology in older men.[148] Increased follicle stimulating hormone (FSH) levels with advancing age are inversely correlated with daily sperm production.[136] Inhibin levels appear to decrease with advancing age.[147] Activin levels increase in males at 50 years of age.[149] This increase appears to be partly responsible for the increase in FSH.

Female

The average age at menopause in the United States is 51 years, with the majority of women experiencing menopause between 45 and 55 years. Cigarette smoking results in menopause occurring 1–2 years earlier than might be predicted. With the onset of menopause, estrone replaces estradiol as the major circulating estrogen.[150] After menopause, estradiol levels decrease by 35-fold, estrone levels by 20-fold, testosterone levels by 1.5-fold, and androstenedione levels by 1.5-fold. Progesterone levels are not altered with advancing age. After menopause, the estradiol production rate is 12 μg/24 h and the plasma clearance rate is reduced by 30 percent.[151] Estrone production rates are 55 μg/24 h, and there is a 20 percent reduction in the clearance rate. Postmenopausally, the major source of estrogens is the adrenal gland, with most estrone

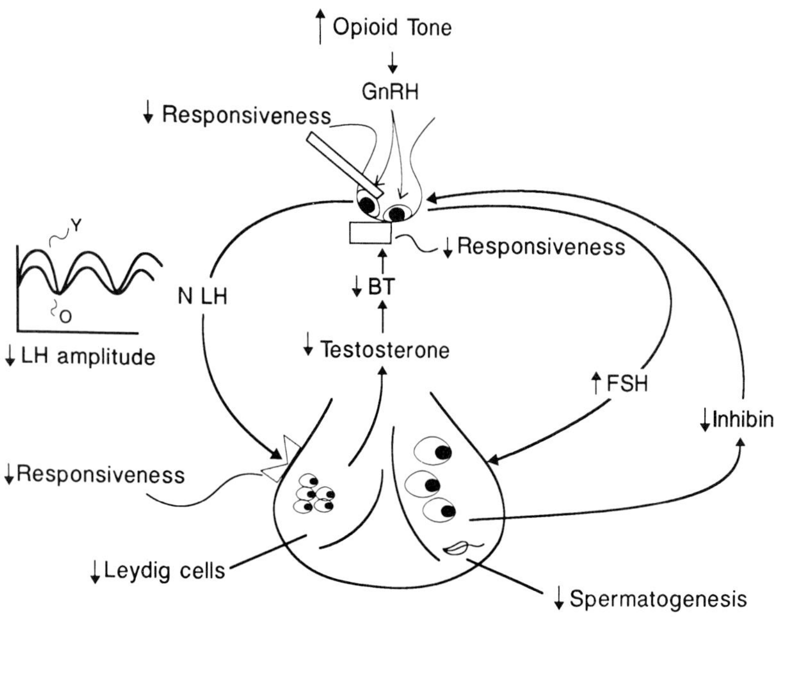

FIGURE 30-6. Major changes in the hypothalamic-pituitary-gonadal axis that occur with aging. BT = bioavailable testosterone; LH = luteinizing hormone; FSH = follicle stimulating hormone; GnRH = gonadotropin releasing hormone.

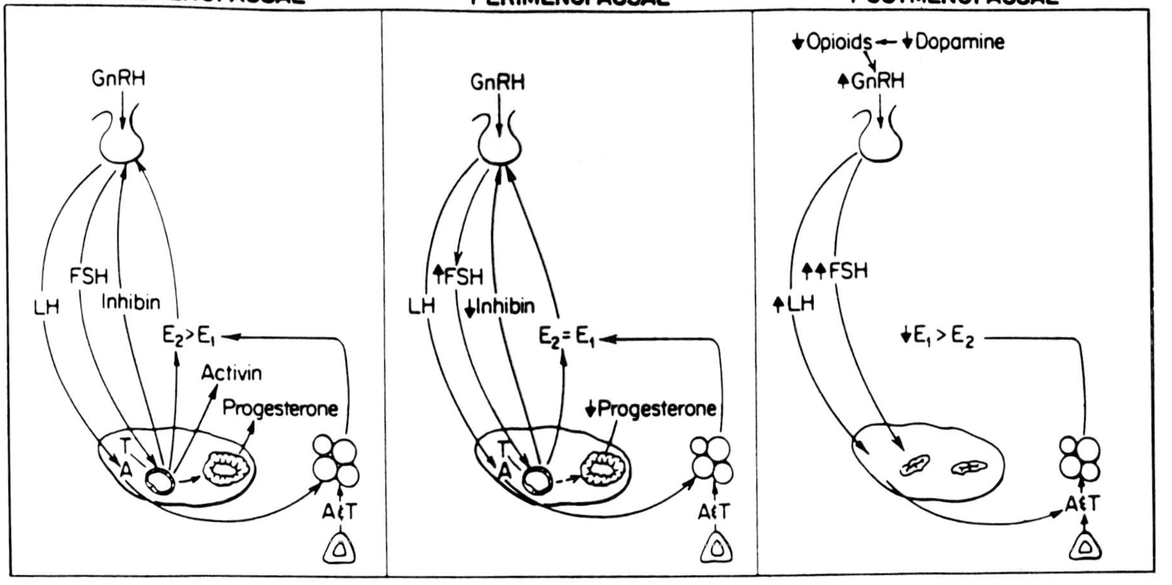

FIGURE 30-7. Alterations in the hypothalamic-pituitary-ovarian axis with aging.

being produced by peripheral aromatization of androstenedione.[151] The rate of peripheral conversion in postmenopausal women is double that in premenopausal women.

The changes in the hypothalamic-pituitary-ovarian axis with aging are delineated in Fig. 30-7. Postmenopausally, both LH and FSH levels are increased, with FSH levels increasing to a greater extent.[150] These increases represent alterations in production rates, as gonadotropin clearance rates are not altered postmenopausally.[151] The relatively higher FSH levels may be secondary to the slower clearance rate of FSH. After menopause, there appears to be no alteration in LH and FSH levels.[152]

The lack of estrogen postmenopausally results in a decrease in the opioid inhibitory tone of GnRH secretion.[153] This effect of estrogen appears to be mediated through a decrease in central nervous system (CNS) dopaminergic activity.[154]

Hormones Associated with Water Metabolism

Older persons with loss of the activities of daily living are at major risk of developing either dehydration or hyponatremia. Older persons also have an impaired thirst response to dehydration.[155] Both animal[156] and human[157] studies have suggested that this is due to a failure of the opioid drinking drive. There is also evidence that the impaired release of peripheral angiotensin II, a potent dipsogen in animals, may play a role in the development of dehydration in older persons.[158]

Basal arginine vasopressin (AVP) levels tend to be increased in older subjects at any level of osmolality.[159] Older persons fail to show the normal nocturnal increase in vasopressin, and this may explain the nocturnal diuresis seen in older persons.[160] They also fail to show prolonged inhibition of AVP after an ethanol infusion.[161] By contrast, the volume-pressure (baroreceptor)–mediated release of AVP is impaired in older humans.[159] The borderline vasopressin excess provides a partial explanation for the fact that 53 percent of patients >60 years of age in a nursing home develop hyponatremia at least once a year.[162] The majority of these older persons who develop hyponatremia have evidence of the syndrome of inappropriate antidiuretic hormone (ADH). Other causes of hyponatremia in institutionalized patients include tube feeding with insufficient salt in the supplements and malnutrition.[163]

Atrial natriuretic hormone (ANH) levels are increased in older persons.[164] The increased levels are much lower than are those seen in patients with cardiac failure.[165] There is an attenuation of the cAMP response to ANH with advancing age, suggesting a reduction in the ability of ANH to activate its receptors with advancing age.[164]

FRAILTY, HORMONES, AND AGING

With advancing age there is an increase in functional dependence as well as an increased propensity to fall and suffer injuries. Four major factors appear to be involved in the development of frailty syndromes in older persons: (1) a decrease in muscle mass, (2) a decrease in bone mass, (3) a decrease in the ability to maintain balance coupled with an increased reliance on visual cues, and (4) a decrease in cognitive processing. Four hormonal systems whose function is often decreased with aging play an important role in maintaining the integrity of muscle and bone mass: the growth hormone–IGF-1 system, testosterone, estradiol, and vitamin D. A cross-sectional study found that the major factors predicting loss of muscle mass with aging were calculated free testosterone and IGF-1 levels as well as physical activity.[166] Another study has shown that testosterone is correlated with strength and a variety of measures of functional status.[167] The physiologic changes seen with aging and the effects of those hormones on these systems are described in Table 30-9. In addition, low levels of DHEA in older institutional subjects have been correlated with a loss in the ability of these persons to carry out the activities of daily living,[168] and DHEA has been shown to improve cognitive function in old animals.[169] Alterations in balance in older persons and animals appear to be related predominantly to a decreased input of

TABLE 30-9. A Comparison of the Effects of Aging and Growth Hormone, Testosterone in Males, Estrogen in Females, and Vitamin D

Author	Sex	GH Dose (μg/kg/d)	Duration (months)	Lean Mass	Fat Mass	Muscle Strength	*BMD* Hip	*BMD* Spine	Resting Energy Expenditure
Cohn et al. (1993)	m	12.9+	12	+6 percent	−16 percent	—	—	—	—
Papadakis (1996)	m	12.9+	6	+4.3 percent	−13.1 percent	0	0	+0.9 percent	—
Welle (1996)	m	12.9+	3	+8.8 percent	0	↑ in 1/4 groups	—	—	—
Holloway (1996)	f	20	6	—	−4.5 percent	—	0	0	—
Thompson (1995)	f	25	1	+3.5 percent	−2.5 percent	—	—	—	+7 percent
Erdsieck (1995)	f	145*	6	±2.5 percent	−6.0 percent	—	—	—	—
Taaffe (1994)	m	20	2.5	0	0	0	—	—	—
Yarasheski (1995)	m	12.5	4	+4.6 percent	0	0	—	—	—

*Administered 3 times/week.

BMD = bone mineral density; m = male; f = female.

β-adrenergic tone from the locus ceruleus to the cerebellum as a result of a decrease in β receptor and postreceptor function.[170] This loss of β-adrenergic tone results in an inability to appropriately regulate the flow of neuronal messages in the cerebellum.

Growth Hormone

In 1990, Rudman et al.[171] published their study on pharmacological growth hormone replacement for 6 months in males over 60 years of age with low plasma IGF-1 levels. In this study, IGF-1 levels rose to the normal range for young men and there was a 14.4 percent increase in lean body mass, an 8.8 percent decrease in adipose tissue mass, 1.6 percent increase in bone mass, and a tendency for skin thickness to increase. This led to much enthusiasm for the concept of the somatopause and a putative rejuvenating effect of growth hormone. Cautionary tales of the Snell dwarf mouse, which is growth hormone-deficient, living longer than its normal-sized control[172] and the early mortality of Parisian men with higher normal growth hormone levels[173] have failed to stem the tide of enthusiasm for growth hormone replacement therapy in older man. In addition, in Rudman's study, year-long treatment resulted in side effects such as carpal tunnel syndrome and arthralgias, which necessitated terminating the study in many of the subjects.[174]

Since the original study, a number of other studies have examined the effect of growth hormone in older persons (Table 30-10). Overall these studies have demonstrated an increase in lean body mass, a decrease in adipose mass, an increase in total body water, minimal or no change in muscle strength, no change in V_{O_2}, an increase in resting energy expenditure, no change in glucose metabolism or cholesterol, and no change in hip bone mineral density with perhaps a mild increase in spine bone mineral density.[174–183] A number of adverse effects have been noted including water retention, carpal tunnel syndrome, malaise, and joint stiffness. Overall growth hormone replacement for the somatopause has failed to show functional benefits, while producing side effects. The long-term safety of growth hormone is untested. Exercise appears to be more efficacious than growth hormone in improving functional status. There is some evidence that in malnourished older persons, growth hormone may reverse the catabolic state.[184,185]

Recently peptide and nonpeptide growth hormone secretagogues have been developed. These agents increase growth hormone and IGF-1 in older persons. Whether they will lead to a physiological replacement of growth hormone in older persons and improve functional status remains to be determined.

Testosterone

Hypogonadism occurs in 4 percent of males by 40 and 70 percent by 70 years of age.[186] Testosterone produces important effects on muscle strength.[187] Three studies have demonstrated an increase in muscle strength during testosterone treatment in older males.[188–190] Testosterone replacement has also been shown to increase bone mineral density in older males with low testosterone levels.[191] In one study the increases were only seen in the lumbar spine, but in this study, most of the men also received calcium and vitamin D.[192] These studies are in keeping with the findings in 3 studies that have shown low testosterone to be a risk factor for minimal trauma hip fracture.[193–195] The mechanism by which testosterone improves bone density is uncertain. While one study found an increase in $1,25(OH)_2$ vitamin D and intestinal calcium absorption,[196] other studies have failed to find changes in vitamin D or $1,25(OH)_2$ vitamin D with testosterone replacement.[188,189] It is possible that testosterone produces its effects on bone secondarily to aromatization to estradiol. Hypogonadal males have an increase in osteoclastic activity similar to that seen in postmenopausal females.[197] Testosterone replacement decreased body fat and leptin levels (*vide infra*).[188]

TABLE 30-10. Effects of Growth Hormone in Older Persons

Body composition	No change in weight Increase in lean body mass (2.5–11.9%) Decrease in body fat (0–14.5%) Mild decrease in extracellular fluid Mild increase in intracellular fluid
Muscle strength	No change
Aerobic capacity	No change
Resting energy expenditure	Increased (+7%)
Metabolic parameters	Total cholesterol and LDL—no change or mild decrease HDL cholesterol—no change Triglycerides—no change Fasting insulin—no change
Bone mineral density	Spine—no change or mild increase Hip—no change
Quality of life	No effects on mood, cognition and attention span
Adverse effects	Arthralgia Carpal tunnel syndrome Fatigue Gynecomastia

With aging, males, but not females, decrease their hemoglobin by 1–2 g/dl. Testosterone replacement restores the hemoglobin to normal levels.[189] Animal studies have shown that testosterone plays a role in cognitive function.[187] The SAMP8 mouse, an animal model of Alzheimer's disease, overproduces β-amyloid protein and has low testosterone levels.[198] Testosterone replacement in this mouse enhanced memory and inhibited amyloid precursor protein overproduction.[199] Bioavailable testosterone is strongly negatively correlated with memory decline in older males.[114] Two studies in older males have demonstrated that testosterone can restore cognitive function.[200,201]

Testosterone replacement decreased angina[202] and decreased the degree of ST depression[203–205] in older males. Acutely administered testosterone improves myocardial function, possibly by releasing nitric oxide and producing coronary vasodilatation.[206] In older men, epidemiological studies have shown that low testosterone levels are associated with an increased risk of coronary artery disease.[207] Testosterone replacement in older males either has no effect on or decreases LDL cholesterol.[208]

Testosterone replacement produces either no effect or a small increase on prostate specific antigen levels.[209] Two retrospective studies have failed to demonstrate any negative effects of testosterone replacement on benign prostatic hypertrophy[210,211] and a prospective study showed no effects on urinary symptoms.[212]

Overall, these studies support the concept that low testosterone levels may play an important role in the pathogenesis of frailty syndromes. The Saint Louis University Androgen Deficiency in Aging Males questionnaire has been demonstrated to have excellent sensitivity and specificity to identify males with low bioavailable testosterone levels (Table 30-11). Persons who score positively for the questionnaire but have normal testosterone levels often are depressed. Testosterone replacement reverses the majority of symptoms.[213]

Estrogens

The utility of estrogen therapy in white females in the 10 years after menopause has been clearly established. Estrogen decreases overall mortality and the death rate from cardiovascular disease.[214] The HERS study has suggested that cardiovascular mortality increased for the first two years after introduction of estrogen before declining.[215] Estrogens decrease the levels of high-density lipoprotein$_2$ (HDL_2) and apoprotein AI and AII.[216] It should be noted that the addition of progesterone to estrogen negates the beneficial effects of estrogen on HDL and HDL_2 levels.[217] Numerous studies have demonstrated that estrogens slow the rate of bone loss in postmenopausal women for at least the first 10 years after menopause and reduce the future risk of fracture by at least 50 percent.[218] Estrogen therapy may also increase muscle strength and enhance cognitive function even in older females,[219] though these effects are controversial. Estrogen does increase dendritic spines, the function of nerve growth factor, and memory retention in rodents.[220] Prolonged use of estrogen increases the propensity to develop breast cancer.

TABLE 30-11. The Saint Louis University Androgen Deficiency in Aging Males (ADAM) Questionnaire

1. Do you have a decrease in libido (sex drive)?
2. Do you have a lack of energy?
3. Do you have a decrease in strength and/or endurance?
4. Have you lost height?
5. Have you noticed a decreased "enjoyment of life"?
6. Are you sad and/or grumpy?
7. Are your erections less strong?
8. Have you noted a recent deterioration in your ability to play sports?
9. Are you falling asleep after dinner?
10. Has there been a recent deterioration in your work performance?

A "yes" answer to #1 or #7 or any three other questions represents a positive test.

Vitamin D, Type II (Age-Related) Osteopenia, and Hip Fracture

Hip fracture represents a major cause of morbidity and mortality in older persons.[221] There is a 20 percent excess mortality in the first year after a hip fracture. One-half of older whites and one-third of older blacks suffering from a hip fracture will be discharged to a nursing home.[221] Approximately one-half of persons who suffer a hip fracture require significant assistance with the activities of daily living for a short period, and one-quarter require long-term assistance. The incidence of hip fractures in the United States in persons over 65 years of age is 6.63 fractures per 1,000 per year, with the peak incidence of 35.4 per 1,000 per year occurring in 95-year-old white females. Two-thirds of all hip fractures occur in those over the age of 75 years. While hip fractures occur most commonly in older white women (80.7 per 1,000 per year), appreciable numbers of hip fractures occur in white men (4.28 per 1,000), black women (3.06 per 1,000), and black men (2.38 per 1,000). The rate of hip fracture in nursing home residents is 3 to 11 times higher than community age-matched older persons.[222] Osteoporosis is percent in 63.5 percent of white female nursing home residents aged 65–74 years and 85.8 percent >85 years.[222] In white males over 85 years residing in nursing homes, the prevalence of osteoporosis was 79.6 percent and in black women 56 percent and in black men, 47.1 percent.

The major factors in hip fracture are osteopenia, falls, and the mechanics of landing (Fig. 30-8). In three quarters of women with hip fractures, the bone density is 3 or more SD below the young normal mean.[223] However, bone mass does not decrease as rapidly as hip fractures increase, and the rate of Colles' fracture remains relatively stable with advancing age. This suggests the importance of other factors in the pathogenesis of hip fractures. With advancing age, a number of factors make people more vulnerable to falling when they encounter simple environmental hazards such as a throw rug. These factors include drugs (especially barbiturates, selective serotonin reuptake inhibitors, and psychotropics, and polypharmacy),[223–226] visual disturbances, poor balance (related to altered neuronal input to the cerebellum, such as decreased β-adrenergic activity), cognitive dysfunction, muscle weakness, and postural and meal-associated hypotension. Meal-associated hypotension appears to be related to the release of the vasodilatory peptide hormone, calcitonin gene-related peptide.[227] Another important factor in the pathogenesis of hip fracture is the mechanics of the fall. Older persons often react more slowly than do younger persons and fail to protect themselves with their hands. Older persons also often fall sideways rather than forward or backward, increasing the mechanical stress on the femur. Decreased muscle strength also leads to a decrease in protection of the femur and an increase in hip fractures.[228] Wearing hip protectors in the nursing home decreased the incidence of hip fractures.[229]

Vitamin D deficiency may play a crucial role in the pathogenesis of many hip fractures and of frailty in general. A number of studies have suggested that vitamin D deficiency plays a role in up to 40 percent of hip fractures.[222] However, these studies did not utilize tetracycline labeling techniques, making the diagnosis suspect. Vitamin D deficiency not only predisposes to osteomalacia but also may result in decreased muscle strength. Numerous studies have suggested that a number of older persons have decreased 25(OH) vitamin D levels and, in a lower number of cases, a decrease in its active metabolite $1,25(OH)_2$ vitamin D.[222] A recent longitudinal study in New Mexico demonstrated that highly healthy older persons have a decline in vitamin D levels with aging.[230] This appears to be particularly true of the institutionalized elderly, who are at greater risk of suffering a hip fracture. A number of studies have found osteoporosis to be present in the majority of females (70–85 percent) and males (50–60 percent) living in nursing homes. The major factor correlating with decreased bone density was low body weight, suggesting a role for malnutrition in the development of decreased bone density in this population. Factors associated with hip fracture in this population include IGF-I, 25(OH) vitamin D, and $1,25(OH)_2$ vitamin D levels,[231,232] as well as low testosterone levels in the aging male (*vide supra*).

The reasons for declining vitamin D levels with aging are multifactorial (Fig. 30-9). The major source of vitamin D is synthesis in the skin of cholecalciferol after exposure to ultraviolet light. Some older persons are housebound and do not go out into the sun, and others who do often bundle themselves to such an extent that they receive no sun exposure. Other older persons with skin cancer apply sun block to prevent further cancers, leading to a decrease in vitamin D levels.[233] Older skin has been demonstrated to be less capable of synthesizing cholecalciferol on exposure to ultraviolet light compared with young skin.[234] Armbrecht et al. have shown that older kidneys fail to synthesize $1,25(OH)_2$ vitamin D as well as do younger kidneys do because of a defect in 1 α-hydroxylase activity with advancing age.[235] Finally, older persons with a poor nutritional intake may further compromise their vitamin D status by decreasing their intake of vitamin D. In addition, Horst et al.[236] found a reduction in calcitriol receptors in both bone and intestine. Chapuy et al.[237] showed that 800 IU of vitamin D and calcium supplementation daily reduced hip fractures in female nursing home residents. A similar replacement regimen improved bone mineral density in free-living older persons in Boston[238] but failed to be effective in older persons in Holland. The high daily milk product intake in Holland presumably explained this discrepancy. For these reasons, it is recommended that the majority of older persons take a 400 IU vitamin D supplement daily.[239] Clinically, vitamin D deficiency can be suspected when an older person has a low or low-normal calcium level and a raised alkaline phosphatase level.

An approach to the prevention of hip fractures in nursing home residents is presented in Fig. 30-10.

SEXUALITY AND AGING

The full expression of sexuality involves a delicate balance of social, cultural, psychological, hormonal, and physical factors. For many people, sexuality is considered a proclamation of life while aging is a herald of approaching death.[134] For this reason, sexuality plays an important role in the quality of life of many older persons. A number of studies have documented a decrease in sexual activity with advancing age. These changes are due to a variety of factors, including the development of disease and frailty, a decrease in available partners, social and cultural beliefs, psychological factors, hormonal changes, and the development of impotence.

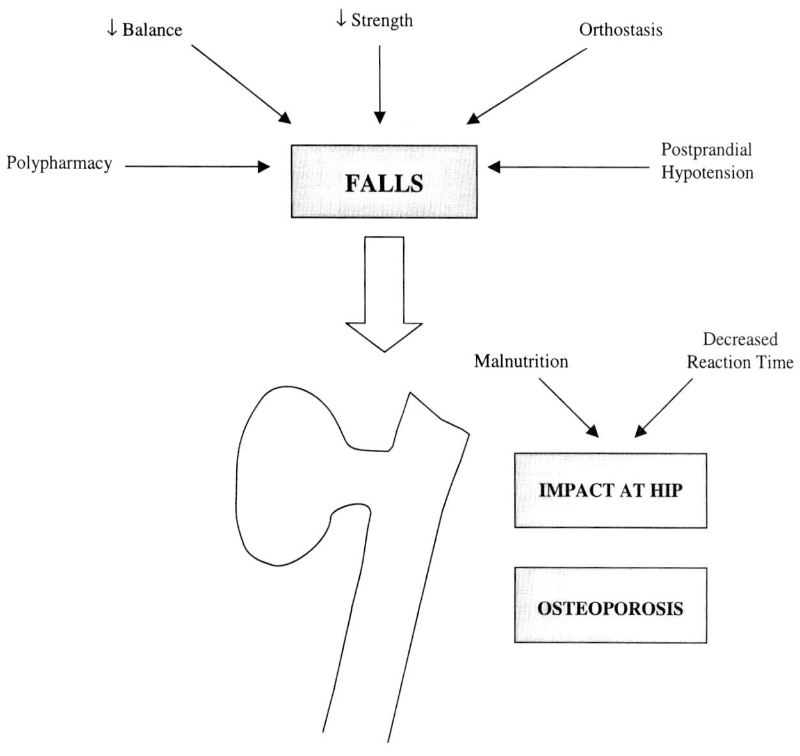

FIGURE 30-8. Causes of hip fracture in older persons.

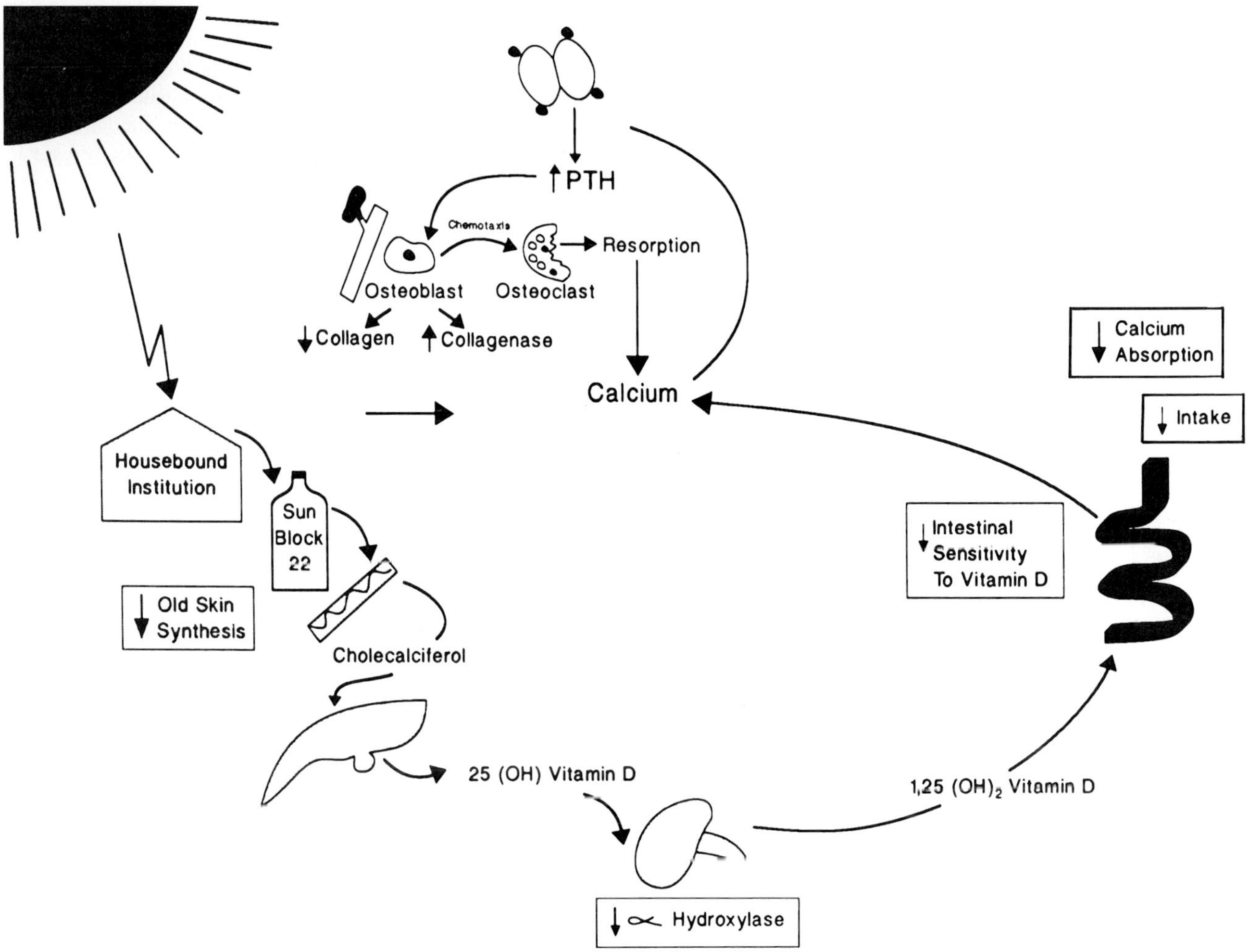

FIGURE 30-9. The major factors responsible for the decline in vitamin D levels with age.

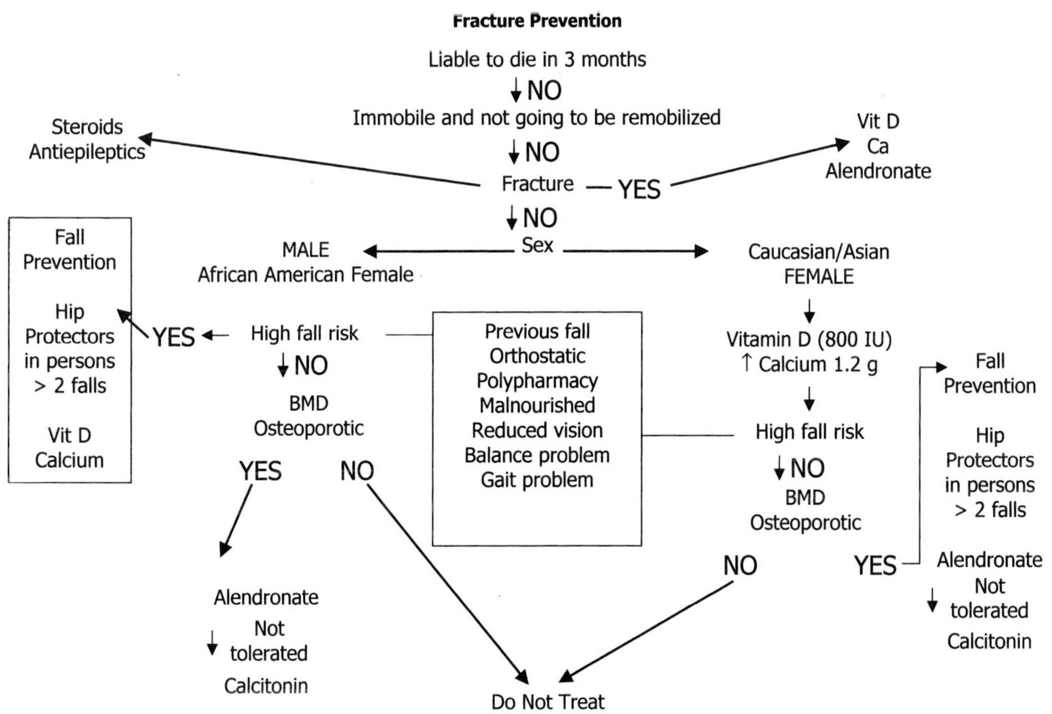

FIGURE 30-10. Approach to the prevention of hip fractures in nursing homes.

Males

Dionko et al. found that 73.8 percent of married men in the United States over 60 years of age are sexually active.[240] In contrast, only 10 percent of males of a similar age in Japan are still sexually active.[241] In apparently healthy males between the ages of 50–70 years, 20 percent were unable to obtain or sustain an erection adequate for intercourse. Slag et al. found that one in three persons over 50 years of age who had at least one illness also had erectile dysfunction.[242] In contrast, a survey of healthy 80-year-old Californians found that 63 percent were still having intercourse "at least several times a year."[243]

Sexual activity in males consists of both libido and potency. *Libido* refers to the sexual desire and drive, thoughts and fantasies, and satisfaction and pleasure associated with sexual activity. Libido is predominantly driven by sex hormones, as was first noted in the fourteenth century B.C. in Assyria when castration was used as a treatment for sexual offenders. *Potency* consists of the ability to obtain and maintain an erection and to ejaculate. Potency and libido are to some extent interdependent.

The major causes of impotence or erectile dysfunction are listed in Table 30-12. Nearly half of older males are impotent as a result of atherosclerotic vascular disease impeding blood flow in the penile artery.[244] In some of these males, blockage of the penile artery is only partial and the person needs to exercise his buttocks to demonstrate the fall in penile blood flow (i.e., the "pelvic steal" syndrome). A rare cause of obstructed arterial blood flow is penile Raynaud's phenomenon, which is seen in some persons with vasculitides.[245] The diagnosis of penile arterial disease is made by measuring the penile blood pressure and comparing it with the brachial blood pressure (penile-brachial pressure index) or by utilizing duplex ultrasonography, which can demonstrate penile blood flow and more accurately delineates the state of the deep penile vessels. Older persons with vascular impotence have a 23 percent greater chance of developing a myocardial infarction or a stroke over the subsequent 2–3 years than do impotent persons with normal penile blood pressure.[246] Impotent males with low penile brachial pressure indexes are more likely to have abnormal electrocardiographic stress or dipyridamole thallium testing than are those with normal pressures.[247] These findings strongly suggest that arterial vascular impotence is closely correlated with atherosclerotic disease in other parts of the body.

TABLE 30-12. Causes of Impotence in Older Males

Vascular	Endocrine disorders
Arterial	Increased prolactin
Penile Raynaud's phenomenon	Thyroid disease
Venous leakage	Hypogonadism
Medications	Cushing disease
Diuretics	Neuropathy
Antihypertensive medications	Autonomic
Tranquilizers	Sensory
Antidepressants	Nutritional
H_2 receptor antagonists	Zinc deficiency
Cytotoxic agents	Protein-energy malnutrition
Nonsteroidal anti-inflammatory agents	Peyronie's disease
Estrogens	Psychiatric disorders
Digoxin	Depression
Anticonvulsants	Widower's syndrome
Carbonic anhydrase inhibitors	Performance anxiety
Metoclopramide	Spinal cord damage
Baclofen	Tumor
Disopyramide	Trauma
Street drugs	Central nervous system
Tobacco	Multiple sclerosis
Alcohol	Temporal lobe epilepsy
Opiates	Stroke
Diabetes mellitus	

Venous leakage from the corpora cavernosa causes from 14 to 54 percent of all cases of impotence and is increasingly common with advancing age because of age-related alterations in the tunica albuginea.[248,249] These patients cannot maintain an erection after obtaining an adequate response to intracorporeal papaverine injection.[250] The diagnosis is confirmed by cavernosography.[251]

Elevated prolactin levels have been clearly associated with impotence, but hyperprolactinemia in unselected series of impotent male occurs in <5 percent.[253] Most of these prolactin elevations are drug-related, and only 0.5–1 percent of impotent males have prolactinomas.

Depression results in decreased nocturnal penile tumescence, decreased testosterone levels, and impotence.[134] These changes may be due to increased levels of CRF in many depressed patients, resulting in suppression of LH release and altered autonomic nervous system tone.[253]

Approximately 10 percent of all older impotent males have a psychological problem as the primary cause of their impotence, and nearly half of these men have some degree of performance anxiety (i.e., inability to obtain an adequate erection related to anxiety because of a previous failure) associated with their organic impotence.[252] Widower's syndrome occurs in older males who develop impotence to protect them from amorous advances while still grieving for the former spouse.[254]

Medications play a role in 25 percent of all cases of impotence in older persons.[253] Impotence in older persons is often multifactorial, with two-thirds of impotent patients having more than one contributory factor.[253]

The major treatment modalities available for the management of impotence are outlined in Table 30-13. After excluding treatable causes of impotence such as depression and endocrine disorders, the majority of older persons have five options for the treatment of impotence: sildenafil (Viagra), a penile prosthesis, a vacuum tumescence device, intracavernosal injection therapy, or a urethral suppository. The decision about which therapy to use is based on the patient's needs (e.g., daily versus weekly intercourse, his preference, and the stability of his relationship).

Sildenafil (Viagra) has revolutionized the management of erectile dysfunction. This drug blocks phosphodiesterase 5 and increases cyclic GMP resulting in smooth muscle relaxation and thus, erections. It is effective in approximately 80 percent of persons.[255] It is less efficacious in diabetics.[256] In hypogonadal males, better results are obtained when testosterone is replaced first. This drug cannot be used with nitrates as this has resulted in sudden death. Other side effects are minor and include flushing, dizziness, dyspepsia, and mild visual disturbances. A slow release phentolamine is under development to enhance erections by blocking the α-adrenergic constriction of smooth muscle.

Penile prostheses are the gold standard for the treatment of impotence. The satisfaction rate with penile prostheses is around 80 percent provided that adequate counseling is carried out before the operation. There are two types of prostheses: semi-rigid (or malleable) and inflatable. The inflatable penile prosthesis may be self-contained within the penis or may have parts in the abdomen and scrotum as well. Inflatable prostheses have a 5-year half-life,

TABLE 30-13. Modalities Available for the Treatment of Impotence in Older Men

1. Vacuum tumescence devices (external suction devices)
2. Penile prosthesis
3. Sildenafil
4. Intracavernosal injections
Papaverine
Phentolamine
Prostaglandin E_1
5. Surgery
Arterial revascularization*
Venous leakage ligation
6. Psychological treatments
Treatment of depression
Psychotherapy
7. Hormonal treatments
Testosterone
Bromocriptine
Treatment of thyroid disease
8. Medications*
Yohimbine
Pentoxifylline
Slow release dopamine
Oral phentolamine
Isoxsuprine
Zinc
Transdermal nitroglycerine
Opioid antagonists
9. Adjust medications to those less likely to cause impotence or, when possible, discontinue medication

*Experimental.

are much more expensive than the semi-rigid form, and require manual dexterity, limiting their use in persons with arthritis or frailty syndromes. Overall, semi-rigid prostheses are usually the best choice for older persons.

Smooth muscle contraction is produced by norepinephrine. A slow release oral phentolamine (alpha blocker) is under study as another oral agent to increase potency. Slow release apomorphine is also under consideration as an agent to produce erections.

Direct injections of either papaverine (with or without phentolamine) or prostaglandin E_1 into the corpora cavernosa produce good-quality erections in most persons.[254] Patients can self-inject at home with good success. Side effects include bruising pain on injection, induration, urethral bleeding, and priapism, and long-term use may result in scarring or fibrosis. Urethral insertion of a suppository containing prostaglandin E_1 will also produce erections. It is much less effective than direct intracavernosal injections.[257]

Vacuum tumescence devices are clear cylinders that can be placed over the penis. Through a connection with a hand-operated suction pump, they produce external negative pressure around the penis, resulting in an erection. The erection is maintained by slipping a rubber band or ring over the base of the penis. These devices have a high satisfaction rate and can produce erections in some patients who have had penile prostheses removed.[258] Side effects include premature loss of penile rigidity, failure to ejaculate, pain or discomfort, inconvenience, and occasional bruising. They are particularly useful in older persons who are in a well-bonded relationship and wish to have intercourse no more frequently than once or twice a week.

Testosterone therapy has been clearly demonstrated to enhance normal sexual drive, ejaculation, and spontaneous erections in young hypogonadal males.[259] In eugonadal males, testosterone has been shown to produce an increase in sexual interest.[260] In a single-blind crossover study, testosterone therapy increased sexual activity and nocturnal penile tumescence in eugonadal men.[261] Morales et al.,[262] utilizing testosterone undeconate absorbed through the lymphatic system, found improvement in sexual function in two-thirds of subjects. However, in older persons this improvement is often short-lived.

In the last decade there has been dramatic improvement in the understanding of the pathophysiology of impotence. This has been accompanied by major advances in the ability to treat impotence. Impotence has clearly become a major medical disease whose diagnostic work-up and treatment can be undertaken by an endocrinologist. Appropriate management of sexual dysfunction in older males is an important quality of life issue.

Females

Females have been shown in survey studies to have an increased prevalence of sexual dysfunction at the time of menopause.[134] Coital frequency and sexual thoughts decline significantly after menopause.[263] This decline in sexuality is more closely related to the decrease in testosterone than to estradiol levels. Libido and sexual response after bilateral salpingoophorectomy was substantially enhanced by ethinyl estradiol treatment.[264] Estrogen replacement therapy in postmenopausal women enhances vaginal expansion and lubrication after sexual arousal. Estrogens also enhance vaginal blood flow and vaginal electropotential difference.[265]

Testosterone was first shown to enhance libido in females in 1943.[266] The antiandrogen cyproterone acetate, which is used to treat hirsutism, decreases libido in 60 percent of females.[267] Two studies have suggested that a combination of testosterone and estradiol is superior to estradiol alone in enhancing libido.[268,269] One study demonstrated improved bone mineral density and muscle mass in postmenopausal women receiving testosterone with estrogen compared to estrogen alone.[270]

In women over age 80, the following were the major sexual problems reported: anorgasmia (30 percent), partner's impotence (30 percent), poor vaginal lubrication (30 percent), and decreased libido (23 percent).[243] The Starr-Weiner report found that 23 percent of women over 60 had anorgasmia and that 17.6 percent had dyspareunia.[271] Treatment with estrogen or estrogen cream and treatment of depression are important therapeutic modalities for the management of sexual difficulties in older women.

DIABETES MELLITUS

Diabetes mellitus is present in nearly 18 percent of persons between 65 and 74 years of age.[272] Diabetes mellitus is particularly prevalent in African-Americans, occurring in 25.9 percent between 65 and 74 years of age.[273] Older African-Americans with diabetes mellitus have retinopathy twice as often as do whites, have renal disease three times as often, and are two and a half times more likely to have an amputation. Of the 6.5 million type II diabetics in the United States, 3.1 million are over the age of 65 years.[274] Older diabetics are more likely to be institutionalized, have a greater risk of suffering a disability, and have a greater risk of premature death.[275,276] Many older diabetics with Type II diabetes are not obese.[277] In these diabetics, there is a decrease in insulin production that is coupled with the increased insulin resistance of aging to produce hyperglycemia.[278]

TABLE 30-14. Reasons for Glucose Control in Older Individuals with Diabetes Mellitus

Prevention of hyperglycemic coma	Management of glucose toxicity
Hyperosmolar coma	Pain
Ketoacidosis	Incontinence
Lactic acidosis	Dehydration
Prevention of long-term complications	Increased platelet adhesiveness
Nephropathy	Myocardial infarction
Neuropathy	Stroke
Visual disturbances	Infection
Retinopathy	Poor red cell deformability
Cataracts	Peripheral vascular disease
	Poor recovery from stroke
	Accelerated atherosclerosis
	Trace minimal deficiency
	Accelerated aging

TABLE 30-15. Some Similarities between Diabetes Mellitus and the Aging Process

Decreased DNA unwinding rate
Increased basement membrane thickness
Increased tissue glycolation
Memory problems
Osteopenia
Accelerated atherosclerosis
Decreased renal function
Increased cataracts
Increased propensity to develop incontinence
Increased propensity to develop unusual infection

Hyperglycemia of Aging

Blood glucose levels tend to increase with advancing age.[279] The reasons for this are multifactorial. Older persons tend to have a defect in both insulin receptors and postreceptor responsiveness.[280,281] Noninsulin-mediated glucose transport into cells is also impaired with aging.[282] Aging is associated with a decrease in the mRNA and protein concentrations of the GLUT-4 glucose transporter in muscle.[283] In addition, the second phase of insulin secretion is somewhat attenuated in older persons.[284] Approximately 80 percent of the hyperglycemia of aging can be attributed to environmental factors such as obesity and physical inactivity, with <20 percent being due to age per se.[285,286] Amylin is a peptide hormone produced by the islets of Langerhan and cosecreted with insulin.[287] The possible role of amylin in the hyperglycemia of aging remains to be determined. A single study has shown that amylin levels decline in middle age and increase again in older persons.[288] This study found a correlation between the increase in amylin and the delayed return of glucose to baseline in older persons.

Should Blood Glucose Be Controlled in Older Individuals?

There are numerous reasons for regulating blood glucose in older persons (Table 30-14).[289] Blood glucose control will prevent the development of diabetic hyperglycemia comas, which are often fatal in older persons.[279] There is evidence that age interacts with hyperglycemia to accelerate the development of retinopathy, nephropathy, and neuropathy.[290] A Japanese study demonstrated that tight control of glucose for 5 years in persons over the age of 65 years markedly delayed the progression of retinopathy.[291] The increased urination produced by the osmolar effect of hyperglycemia is a major reason for controlling glucose levels in older persons.[289] Increased urination results in nocturia, with the need to get up more frequently at night and therefore, poor sleep and an increased risk of falling. This osmotic diuresis can also result in incontinence in older persons. Finally, older persons fail to have a normal recognition of thirst, resulting in the osmotic diuresis that leads to mild dehydration associated with fatigue.

Hyperglycemia is associated with an increased perception of pain caused by a decreased responsiveness to endogenous opioids.[292] This results in older diabetics complaining of pain more often than do age- and disease-matched controls.

Older diabetic patients with hyperglycemia have been demonstrated to have problems of memory retention to a greater extent than do matched controls.[293] These memory problems appear to play a role in reducing compliance in this population.[294] Animal studies have demonstrated that normalization of glucose can reverse the effects of hyperglycemia on memory dysfunction.[295] Studies in older humans have demonstrated that improved glucose control improves cognitive performance.[296,297]

Retrospective studies have suggested that hyperglycemia is associated with a poor outcome after a stroke.[283] Older diabetics who have had a stroke are more likely to have a second stroke than are nondiabetics who have had a stroke, and older diabetics also die sooner.[298]

Diabetes has been associated with pressure ulcer development.[299] Older persons with diabetes have poorer functional status than other older persons.[277,300] Diabetes in older persons is associated with a greater rate of falling and more injurious falls.

Diabetes mellitus can be considered a form of accelerated aging, with persons who have diabetes appearing to be 5–10 years older than are those who do not have diabetes.[279] Hyperglycemia has been suggested to play a role in producing this premature aging. Table 30-15 lists a number of similarities between diabetes mellitus and the aging process.

Special Features in the Management of Older Diabetics

There are a number of special problems seen typically in older persons. These problems may modulate the approach to older diabetics (Table 30-16).

Of particular concern is the development of depression, which may be more common in older persons with diabetes mellitus.[289] Depression is highly correlated with increased hospital admissions and mortality in older diabetics.[301] All older diabetics should be screened for depression, utilizing the Geriatric Depression Scale.[302] When this scale suggests depression, intervention with low-dose antidepressants is appropriate.[303]

Diet in Older Diabetics

Generally, major dietary changes are not recommended for diabetics >70 years of age. The majority of diabetics >70 years of age are not overweight; they are usually underweight. Thus, care should be taken to prescribe weight-reducing diets only when such diets are appropriate. Because of their increased propensity

TABLE 30-16. Special Problems That Commonly Interfere with the Management of Older Persons with Diabetes Mellitus

Problem	Outcome	Management
Hypodipsia	Dehydration: hyperosmolar coma	Drink 4–8 glasses of water daily
Anorexia	Hypoglycemia	Early detection of weight loss; adjust hypoglycemic agents, diagnose cause, and manage appropriately
Visual disturbance	Inadequate insulin dosing; hyper- or hypoglycemia	Predraw insulin syringes; insulin syringe magnifier
Decreased activities of daily living	Decreased food intake; hypoglycemia	Adaptive devices; Meals on Wheels
Decreased physical activity	Obesity; hyperglycemia	Exercise program
Altered renal and hepatic function	Hypoglycemia	Decreased dose of hypoglycemics
Cognitive impairment	Poor compliance	Memory aids
Depression	Poor compliance; death; suicide	Early detection and management of depression
Impaired baroreceptor response	Orthostatic hypotension made worse by diabetic autonomic neuropathy and dehydration	Detection; adequate fluid intake; nonpharmacologic and pharmacologic management
Multiple medications	Drug interactions; hypoglycemia	Be aware of potential interactions; limit drugs where possible
Multiple disease processes	Multiple medications; anorexia; dehydration; amputations; infection	Treat where appropriate; create priority list for management decisions
Poverty	Poor dietary intake; cannot afford specialized diets	Recognize; advise social worker; realistic management plan

to develop hypoglycemia, all older diabetics on oral hypoglycemic agents or insulin should eat a bedtime snack. Some older diabetics have large variations of glucose immediately after a meal, and this may be associated with symptoms. Under these circumstances, the addition of fiber to the diet may greatly improve a diabetic's quality of life. Glucose is also responsible for meal-associated hypotension in older persons.[304] This drop in blood pressure may be associated with falls and syncope after the meal in older individuals.[305] Symptoms 2 or 3 h after a meal often mean that an older diabetic has gastroparesis. Metoclopramide, while improving the gastroparesis, crosses the blood brain barrier and can result in CNS symptoms such as delirium and parkinsonism. Erythromycin, which activates the motilin receptor, may be an alternative in some older diabetics. Cisapride has fewer CNS effects and is as effective as metoclopromide in the treatment of gastroparesis.

Oral Hypoglycemia Agents

A number of age-associated changes may modulate the action of oral sulfonylureas in older persons. These changes include decreases in hepatic blood flow, hepatic oxidative metabolism, serum albumin, and renal function.[289] Finally, hypoglycemic counterregulatory hormones, specifically growth hormone and cortisol responses, are reduced in older persons.[306] The end result of these changes is to increase the propensity of older persons to develop hypoglycemia when they take sulfonylureas. The increased occurrence of hypoglycemia in older compared with younger subjects has been clearly demonstrated by the Swedish Spontaneous Adverse Drug Reporting System.[307] Hypoglycemia has been shown to be more common in extreme old age, in association with insulin use, in persons with polypharmacy, and in those discharged from hospital in the last 30 days.[308] Chlorpropramide should be used with caution in older diabetics because of the prolonged hypoglycemia and hyponatremia it produces.[289] The second-generation oral agents, glipizide, glyburide, or glynase, and glimepride, are generally preferred in older persons because their nonionic binding to albumin reduces their propensity to produce drug-drug interactions in a population that is likely to be on multiple medications.[289] However, in some diabetics >80 years of age, tolbutamide in a single daily dose may be an excellent therapeutic modality.[289] Repaglinide has been tested in persons over the age of 65 years, has similar efficacy to that seen in younger persons, and produces the same degree of hypoglycemia.[309]

Metformin, a biguanide, has been shown to produce lactic acidosis in <1 in 10,000 patients per year.[307] A number of the patients in this study were >75 years of age. Other side effects of metformin that can be worrisome in older persons include gastrointestinal discomfort, anorexia, weight loss, and interference with the absorption of vitamin B_{12} and folate.[310,311] Over the age of 80 years, it is recommended that a creatinine clearance is obtained before using metformin. For practical purposes, this limits the use of metformin to persons <80 years of age.

Thiazolidonediones appear to be particularly appropriate agents for older persons as they decrease insulin resistance and do not cause hypoglycemia.[312] Troglitazone was tested in older persons as monotherapy and produced excellent results.[313] No data on ronsigletazone and proglitzaone has been published.

Insulin

Older diabetics, especially those with visual disturbances, have been shown to make errors between 10 and 20 percent when drawing up insulin.[289] All older diabetics should have their ability to draw up insulin in the correct amount checked at each visit. If the patient is shown to be incapable of doing this, it is usually best to have the pharmacist supply the patient with predrawn insulin syringes, one week at a time. A syringe magnifier may help some older diabetics. Older diabetics with tremors, arthritis, or muscle weakness may benefit from utilizing needle guides and vial holders, which allow them to place the insulin syringe directly into the vial, eliminating the risk of jabbing themselves during the process.

Monitoring Treatment

Older diabetics adapt well to self-monitoring of blood glucose without negatively altering their perception of the quality of life.[314] Glycosylated hemoglobin levels may be falsely elevated in some older diabetics.[315] Fructosamine has been demonstrated to be a highly effective, cost-effective means of monitoring intermediate diabetic control in older diabetics.[316] The development of a fingerstick fructosamine monitor by the LNX Company, San Diego, CA, represents a major advance for monitoring older persons in the office practice.

TABLE 30-17. Comparison of Diabetics and Nondiabetics in the Nursing Home

	Diabetics	Nondiabetics
Age (years)	80	80.1
Overweight (percent)	21	25
Underweight (percent)	9	0
Cataracts (percent)	51	51
Retinopathy (percent)	7	2
Renal failure (percent)	30	10
Proteinuria (percent)	32	0
Nephropathy (percent)	28	10
Urinary tract infection (percent)	55	30
Skin infections (percent)	34	18
Amputations (percent)	13	6
Stroke (percent)	32	34
Angina/myocardial infarction (percent)	60	48
Peripheral vascular disease	26	12

Source: Adapted from Mooradian et al.[199]

Diabetes in Nursing Home Residents

There are 190,000 diabetics in nursing homes, with 75 percent being over 75 years of age. Among diabetics in nursing homes, 9 percent are overweight and 21 percent are underweight.[317] The American Diabetic Association diet has been shown to be ineffective at altering glycemic control in nursing homes.[318] Diabetic diets can lead to malnutrition and should be avoided in nursing homes. Diabetics in nursing homes are more likely to have retinopathy, neuropathy, renal failure, amputations, atherosclerotic cardiovascular disease, peripheral vascular disease, and infections than are nondiabetics in nursing homes (Table 30-17). Thus, overall, diabetics in nursing homes are sicker than nondiabetic residents.

Mooradian et al. demonstrated that acceptable glucose control can be obtained in most nursing home residents, with minimal episodes of hypoglycemia.[317] This was in contrast to the extremely poor control of diabetes in Welsh nursing homes.[319] All nursing home residents with diabetes mellitus who are receiving either oral sulfonylureas or insulin should have a prescription for 1 mg glucagon intramuscularly when hypoglycemia occurs and oral glucose cannot be given. When a diabetic nursing home resident misses a meal, the insulin dose should be halved and chemstrips should be checked every 6 h until the resident begins to eat again. The rapid acting (Lys-Pro) insulin needs to be utilized with caution in the nursing home.

Summary

Diabetes mellitus is commonly not diagnosed in older persons; more than half the persons over 65 years of age with this disorder may not have the diagnosis made.[310] Older diabetics have a number of unique features to which endocrinologists need to pay careful attention in order to optimize diabetic management. Much evidence supports the use of blood glucose control in older diabetics.

Leptin

Leptin is a peptide hormone produced in adipose tissue. In animals, leptin decreases food intake and increases the resting metabolic rate. In postmenopausal women, leptin levels are related to food intake.[320] In females, leptin levels increase at middle age along with fat mass and decrease beyond the age of 70 years as fat mass declines.[321]

In older men, leptin levels continue to increase as fat mass decreases and this is related to the fall in testosterone levels in both cross-sectional and longitudinal studies.[322,323] Testosterone replacement therapy in older males results in a decrease in leptin levels.[189] Within the hypothalamus, leptin levels decrease neuropeptide Y and nitric oxide resulting in a decrease in food intake.[324] Thus, the fall in testosterone with age results in an increase in leptin production which leads to a decrease in food intake (Fig. 30-11).

NUTRITIONAL DISORDERS

In older persons, the major nutritional problem is protein-energy malnutrition, which is present in 9–12 percent of older outpatients, 17–65 percent of older hospitalized patients, and between 26 and 59 percent of nursing home residents.[325] An underweight state is much more highly correlated with mortality in older persons than is being overweight.[326] Undernutrition in older persons is associated with a decline in CD_4+T-lymphocytes, increased infection, anemia, hip fractures, impaired cognition, and pressure ulcers. Most older persons with protein-energy malnutrition ingest sufficient calories to maintain their serum albumin at the cost of muscle protein. This results in older persons presenting with a picture where weight loss predominates (i.e., a marasmic picture). When an older person has an infection, cytokines are released and albumin levels fall, resulting in a kwashiorkor-type picture.

Weight loss in older persons has multiple causes, many of which are treatable (Table 30-18).[327] Recent studies have suggested that depression is the most common cause of weight loss in older persons.[328,329] Endocrine causes of weight loss include hyperthyroidism, hypoadrenalism, and pheochromocytoma. In addition, there is an anorexia of aging that appears to occur in response to the decrease in metabolic rate and the reduced physical activity that occur with advancing age.[327] The decrease in food intake in older persons is in part due to a decrease in the ability to appreciate the hedonic qualities of food because of the alterations in taste and smell that occur with advancing age. Older persons demonstrate early satiatiety because of a decrease in fundic compliance and more rapid filling of the antrum.[330] The decrease in fundic adaptive relaxation with aging is due to a decline in nitric oxide synthase activity.[331] Older persons also have higher basal levels of cholecystokinin (a satiety hormone) and a greater increase in response to fat.[332] Cholecystokinin decreases food intake more potently in older than in younger persons. Animal studies have shown that with aging there are decreases in the endogenous opioid (dynorphin) and neuropeptide Y feeding drives in the hypothalamus.[325] Medroxyprogesterone acetate has been demonstrated to increase food intake in older persons with cancer.[325] Growth hormone has been utilized to treat severe protein-energy malnutrition in older persons because of its anabolic effects.

Obesity is associated with only a minimal increase in mortality in older persons, and with advancing age it appears to be a problem only when it interferes with carrying out the activities of daily living (e.g., in persons with osteoarthritis) or when it is associated with a specific obesity-associated disease such as diabetes mellitus or hypertension.[333] Older persons are at increased risk for developing obesity because of a decrease in the resting metabolic rate, a decrease in the thermic effect of feeding, and a

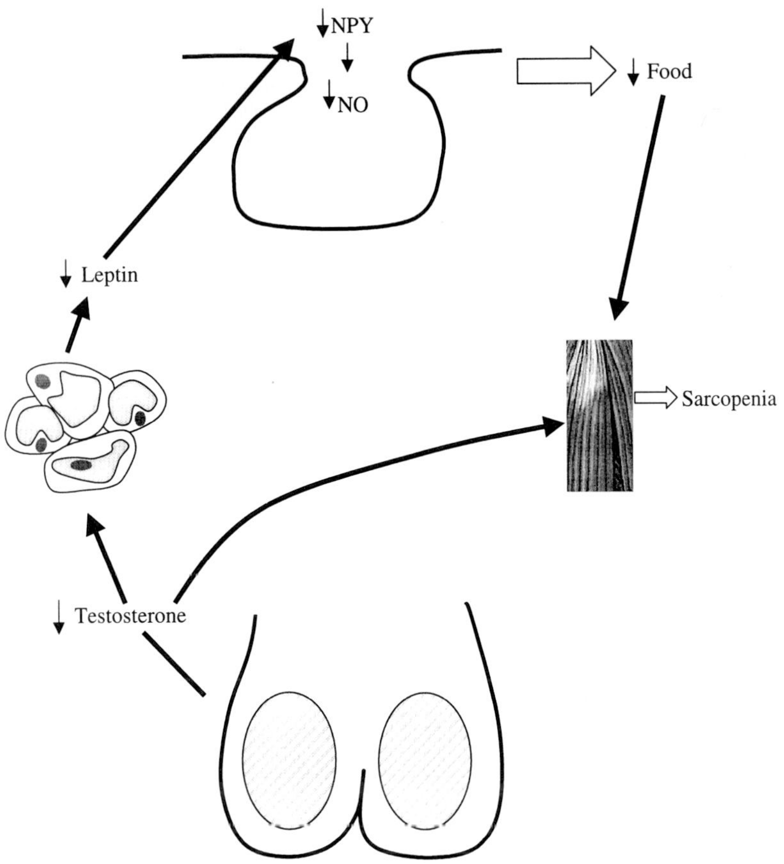

FIGURE 30-11 Relationship of the decrease in testosterone with aging to anorexia and sarcopenia.

TABLE 30-18. Causes of Weight Loss in Older Persons

I. Social
  - A. Poverty
  - B. Problems with shopping
  - C. Problems with food preparation

II. Psychosocial
  - A. Depression
  - B. Dementia
  - C. Late-life paranoia
  - D. Anorexia nervosa (tardive)
  - E. Manipulative behaviors
  - F. Excessive burden of life

III. Medical
  - A. Hypermetabolism
    1. Hyperthyroidism
    2. Pheochromocytoma
    3. Parkinson's disease
  - B. Anorexia
    1. Hyperparathyroidism
    2. Candidal esophagitis
    3. *Helicobacter pylori*
    4. Medications, e.g., digoxin, theophylline
    5. Cancer
    6. Unpalatable diets, e.g., low-cholesterol, low-salt
    7. Infections (interleukins, cachectin)
    8. Hypoadrenalism
  - C. Mixed
    1. Chronic obstructive pulmonary disease
    2. Cardiac cachexia

IV. Malabsorption
  - A. Gluten enteropathy
  - B. Lactose deficiency

decrease in habitual physical activity. Despite this, most obesity is seen in middle age in males rather than in old age; 30.5 percent of men aged 45–54 are obese, while only 25.8 percent aged 65–74 years are obese.[333] Obesity in females shows a continuous increase to the age of 74, after which the prevalence tends to decrease. Changes in body adipose tissue follow a similar pattern, with a marked increase in the early forties and a decline after age 75 years.[333] Fat distribution changes with age, with the waist–hip ratio increasing in both sexes over the ages of 17–96 years.[333]

The decreased risks associated with obesity in advancing age suggest that management intervention should be limited to those who are >130 percent of average body weight unless they have a specific obesity-associated disease. The utility of different weight-loss methods in older persons is described in Table 30-19.

Cholesterol levels tend to rise with age to a plateau by 55 years in males and 60 years in females.[334] Total cholesterol levels are less predictive of new-onset coronary heart disease in older adults.[335] HDL cholesterol appears to be a better predictor than total cholesterol for coronary heart disease in young-old subjects but not in old-old subjects.[336]

A number of studies have suggested that low cholesterol levels predict total mortality in older persons, particularly those residing in institutions.[337] This appears to be related to the fact that low cholesterol levels are a marker for protein-energy malnutrition[338] and possibly for cytokine activity that results from underlying infections or neoplasms.[338] Major dietary alterations in older persons can be hazardous.[339,340] For these reasons, it would appear inappropriate to recommend cholesterol-lowering diets in persons >75 years of age.

TABLE 30-19. Utility of Weight-Loss Methods in Older Persons

Method	Utility in older persons
Exercise	Mall walking programs, swimming, tai chi; chair exercises are primary modality
Diet	Only if more than 130 percent of average weight, associated with diabetes mellitus, or interferes with activities of daily living
Behavior modification	Yes
Low-calorie and very-low-calorie diets	Should be avoided
Drugs	
Anorectic agents	Rarely indicated
Thermogenic agents	Potentially dangerous
Fat absorption inhibitor (Orlistat)	Little data; give with fat soluble vitamins
Gastric balloon	Not useful
Surgery	
Gastric restriction	Only when massive obesity is associated with sleep apnea
Jejunoileal bypass	Never used

CONCLUSION

As an individual ages, a panoply of hormonal changes occur. Many of these changes are first evident in the early forties. The role of these hormonal changes in the expression of the phenotypic changes seen with aging is uncertain. However, it appears that hormones may play a role in preventing or treating the frailty syndromes seen in older persons. Atypical presentations of endocrine disorders in older persons often create a diagnostic challenge for the endocrinologist.

REFERENCES

1. Trence DL, Morley JE, Handwerger BS: Polyglandular autoimmune syndromes. *Am J Med* 77:107, 1984.
2. Katsuki A, Sumida Y, Murashima S, Murata K, Takarada Y, Ito K, Fujii M, Tsuchihashi K, Goto H, Nakatani K, Yano Y: Serum levels of tumor necrosis factor-alpha are increased in obese patients with noninsulin-dependent diabetes mellitus. *J Clin Endocrinol Metab* 83:859, 1998.
3. Pfeiffer A, Janott J, Mohlig M, Ristow M, Rochlitz H, Busch K, Schatz H, Schifferdecker E: Circulating tumor necrosis factor alpha is elevated in male but not in female patients with type II diabetes mellitus. *Horm Metab Res* 29:111, 1997.
4. Mooradian AD, Scarpace PJ: The response of isoproterenol-stimulated adenylate cyclase activity after administration of L-triiodothyronine is reduced in aged rats. *Horm Metab Res* 21:638, 1989.
5. Trivalle C, Doucet J, Chassagne P, Landrin I, Kadri N, Menard JF, Bercoff E: Differences in the signs and symptoms of hyperthyroidism in older and younger patients. *J Am Geriatr Soc* 44:50, 1996.
6. Morley JE, Levine AS: Pharmacology of eating behavior. *Ann Rev Pharmacol Toxicol* 25:127, 1985.
7. Mooradian AD, Wong NCW: Age-related changes in thyroid hormone action. *Eur J Endocrinol* 131:451, 1994.
8. Mooradian AD, Girgis W, Shah GN: Thyroid hormone-induced GLUT-1 expression in rat cerebral tissue-effect of age. *Brain Res* 747:144, 1997.
9. Mooradian AD, Wong NCW, Shah GN: Age-related changes in the responsiveness of apolipoprotein A(1) to thyroid hormone. *Am J Physiol-Regulatory Integrative & Comparative Physiology* 40: R1602, 1996.
10. Mooradian AD: The hepatic transcellular transport of 3-5-3′ triiodothyronine is reduced in aged rats. *Biochim Biophys Acta* 1054:1, 1990.
11. Donda A, Reymond MJ, Zurich MG, Lemarchand-Beraud T: Influence of sex and age on T3 receptors and T3 concentration in the pituitary gland of the rat: Consequences on TSH secretion. *Mol Cell Endocrinol* 54:29, 1987.
12. Cizza G, Brady LS, Calogero AE, Bagdy G, Lynn AB, Kling M, Blackman MR, Chrousos GP, Gold PW: Central hypothyroidism is associated with advanced age in male Fischer 344/N rats: In vivo and in vitro studies. *Endocrinology* 131:2672, 1992.
13. Morley JE, Krahn DD, Gosnell BA, Billington CJ, Levine AS: Interrelationships between calcitonin and other modulators of feeding behavior. *Psychopharmacol Bull* 20:463, 1984.
14. Solomon DM, Judd HL, Sur MC, Rubenstein LZ, Morley JE: New issues in geriatric care. *Ann Intern Med* 108:718, 1988.
15. Morley JE, Shafer RB: Thyroid function screening in new psychiatric admissions. *Arch Intern Med* 42:591, 1982.
16. Mooradian AD, Morley JE, Korenman SG: Endocrinology in aging. *Dis Mon* 34:398, 1988.
17. Lin YJ, Seroude L, Benzer S: Extended lifespan and stress resistance in the *Drosophila mutant methuselah. Science* 282:943, 1998.
18. Ailion M, Inoue T, Weaver CI, Holdcraft RW, Thomas JH: Neurosecretory control of aging in Caenorhabditis elegans. *Proc Natl Acad Sci* 96:7394, 1999.
19. Hsin H, Kenyon C: Signals from the reproductive system regulate the lifespan of C-elegans. *Nature* 399:362, 1999.
20. Kimura KD, Tissenbaum, HA, Liu Y, Ruvkun G: *daf*-2 An insulin receptor like gene that regulates longevity and diapause in *Caemorhabditis elegans. Science* 277:942, 1997.
21. Yodoi J, Hirota K, Oono T, et al: Redox regulation of signal transduction pathways by thioredoxin superfamily. *1999 World Congress on Oxidants and Antioxidants in Biology*, p 45, 1999.
22. Bodnar AG, Ouellete M, Frolkis M, et al: Extension of lifespan by introduction of telomerase into normal human cells. *Science* 279:349, 1998.
23. Jiang XR, Jimenez G, Chang E, et al: Telomerase expression in human somatic cells does not induce changes associated with a transformed phenotype. *Nat Genet* 21:111, 1999.
24. Snowdon DA: Early natural menopause and the duration of post menopausal life: Findings from a mathematical model of life expectancy. *J Am Geriatr Soc* 38:402, 1990.
25. Denckla WD: Role of the pituitary and thyroid glands in the decline of minimal O_2 consumption with age. *J Clin Invest* 53:572,1974.
26. Effros RB: Replicative senescence in the immune system: Impact of the Hayflice limit on T-cell function in the elderly. *Am J Hum Genet* 62:1003, 1998.
27. Hayflick L: Recent advances in the cell biology of aging. *Mech Ageing Dev* 14:59, 1980.
28. Effros RB, Boucher N, Porter V, Zhu X, Spaulding C, Walford RL, Kronenberg M, Cohen D, Schachter F: Decline in CD28 + T cells in centenarians and in long-term T cell cultures: A possible cause for both in vivo and in vitro immunosenescence. *Exp Gerontol* 29:601, 1994.
29. Johnson FB, Marciniak RA, Ruarente L: Telomeres, the nucleolus and aging. *Curr Opin Cell Biol* 10:332, 1998.
30. Stein GH, Drullinger LF, Soulard A, Dulic V: Differential roles for cyclin-dependent kinase inhibitors p21 and p16 in the mechanisms of senescence and differentiation in human fibroblasts. *Mol Cell Biol* 19:2109, 1999.
31. Steen GM, Beeson M, Gordon L: Failure to phosphorylate the retinoblastoma gene product in senescent human fibroblasts. *Science* 249:666, 1990.
32. Pereira-Smith OM, Smith JR: Genetic analysis of indefinite division in human cells: Identification of four complementation groups. *Proc Natl Acad Sci* 85:6042, 1988.
33. Seshadri T, Campizi J: Repression of c-fos transcription and an altered genetic program in senescent human fibroblasts. *Science* 247:205, 1990.
34. Beckman KB, Ames BN: Mitrochondrial aging: Open questions. *Ann NY Acad Sci* 854:118, 1998.
35. Beckman KB, Ames BN: The free radical theory of aging matures. *Physiol Rev* 78:547, 1998.
36. Helbock JH, Beckman KB, Ames BN: 8-Hydroxydeoxyguanosine and 8-hydroxyguanine as biomarkers of oxidative DNA damage. *Methods Enzymol* 300:156, 1999.
37. Harman D: Free radical theory of aging. *Mutat Res* 275:257, 1992.
38. Wei Q: Effect of aging on DNA repair and skin carcinogenesis: A

minireview of population-based studies. *J Invest Dermatol Symp Proc* 3:19, 1998.
39. Clark AM, Rubin MA: The modification by x-irradiation of the life span of haploid and diploid. *Habrobracon Radiat Res* 15:244, 1961.
40. Brownlee M, Cerami A, Vlassarci M: Advanced glycosylation end products in tissue and the biochemical bases of diabetic complications. *N Engl J Med* 318:1315, 1988.
41. Wautier JL, Guillausseau PJ: Diabetes, advanced glycation end products and vascular disease. *Vasc Med* 3:131, 1998.
42. Hartnell JM, Morley JE, Mooradian AD: Reduction of alkali-induced white blood cell DNA unwinding rate: A potential biomarker of aging. *J Gerontol* 44:B125, 1989.
43. Lopes-Virella MF, Virella G: Modified lipoproteins, cytokines and macrovascular disease in non-insulin-dependent diabetes mellitus. *Ann Med* 28:347, 1996.
44. Herskind AM, McGue M, Holm NV, Sorensen TI, Harvald B, Vaupel JW: The heritability of human longevity: A population-based study of 2872 Danish twin pairs born 1870–1900. *Hum Genet* 97:319, 1996.
45. Martin GM: Genetics and the pathobiology of ageing. *Philos Trans R Soc Lond B Biol Sci* 352:1773, 1997.
46. Takeda T, Hosokawa M, Higuchi K: Senescence-accelerated mouse (SAM): A novel murine model of accelerated senescence. *J Am Geriatr Soc* 39:911, 1991.
47. Louhija J, Miettinen HE, Kontula K, Tikkanen MJ, Miettinen TA, Tilvis RS: Aging and genetic variation of plasma apolipoproteins. Relative loss of the apolipoprotein E4 phenotype in centenarians. *Arterioscler Thromb* 14:1084, 1994.
48. Ye L, Miki T, Nakura J, et al: Association of a polymorphic variant of the Werner helicase gene with myocardial infarction in a Japanese population. *Am J Med Genet* 68:494, 1997.
49. Muehlen K aus der, Ockenfels H: [Morphological alterations in the diencephalon and telencephalon following disturbances to the feedback mechanism adenohypophysis-adrenal cortex. Studies on the guinea pig after administration of cortisone and hydrocortisone] [German]. *Z Zellforsch Mikrosk Anat* 93:126, 1969.
50. Porter NM, Landfield PW: Stress hormones and brain aging: Adding injury to insult? *Nat Neurosci* 1:3, 1998.
51. McEwen BS: Stress and the aging hippocampus. *Front Neuroendocrinol* 20:49, 1999.
52. Nelson JF, Karelus K, Bergman MD, Felicio LS: Neuroendocrine involvement in aging: Evidence from studies of reproductive aging and caloric restriction. *Neurobiol Aging* 16:837 discussion 855, 1995.
53. Goya RG, Brown OA, Bolognani F: The thymus-pituitary axis and its changes during aging. *Neuroimmunomodulation* 6:137, 1999.
54. Hirokawa K: Reversing and restoring immune functions. *Mech Ageing Dev* 93:119, 1997.
55. Walford RL: Multigene families, histocompatibility system, transformation meiosis, stem cells and DNA repair. *Mech Ageing Dev* 9:19, 1979.
56. Maier JAM, Voculalas P, Roeder D, Maciaq T: Extension of the life span of human endothelial cells by an interleukin-1a antisense oligomer. *Science* 249:1570, 1990.
57. Morley JE: An overview of diabetes mellitus in older persons. *Clin Geriatr Med* 15:211, 1999.
58. Honing MLH, Morrison PJ, Banga JD, Stroes ESG, Rabelink TJ: Nitric oxide availability in diabetes mellitus. *Diab Metab Rev* 14:241, 1998.
59. Kelijman M: Age-related alterations of the growth hormone/insulin-like-growth factor I axis. *J Am Geriatr Soc* 39:295, 1991.
60. Sun YK, Xi XP, Fenoglio CM, et al: The effect of age on the number of pituitary cells immunoreactive to growth hormone and prolactin. *Hum Pathol* 15:169,1984.
61. Shilaski T, Shizume K, Nakahara M, et al: Age-related changes in plasma growth hormone response to growth hormone-releasing factor in man. *J Clin Endocrinol Metab* 58:212, 1984.
62. Giusti M, Lomeo A, Marini G, et al: Role of aging on growth hormone and prolactin release after growth hormone releasing hormone and domperidone in man. *Horm Res* 27:134, 1987.
63. Pavlov EP, Harmon SM, Merriam GR, et al: Responses of growth hormone (GH) and somatomedin C to GH-releasing hormone in healthy aging men. *J Clin Endocrinol Metab* 62:595, 1986.
64. Lang I, Schernthaner G, Pietschmann P, et al: Effects of sex and age on growth hormone response to growth hormone-releasing hormone in healthy individuals. *J Clin Endocrinol Metab* 65:53, 1987.
65. Dawson-Hughes B, Stern D, Goldman J, et al: Regulation of growth hormone and somatomedin C secretion in postmenopausal women: Effect of physiological estrogen replacement. *J Clin Endocrinol Metab* 63:424, 1986.
66. Kalk WJ, Vinik AI, Pimstone BL, et al: Growth hormone response to insulin hypoglycemia in the elderly. *J Gerontol* 28:431,1973.
67. Muggeo M, Fedele D, Tiengo A, et al: Human growth hormone and cortisol response to insulin stimulation in aging. *J Gerontol* 39:546, 1991.
68. Lal S, Nair NPV, Thavundagil JX, et al: Growth hormone response to apomorphine, a dopamine receptor agonist, in normal aging and in dementia of the Alzheimer type. *Neurobiol Aging* 10:227, 1989.
69. Alba-Roth J, Muller OA, Schopohl J, et al: Arginine stimulates growth hormone secretion by suppressing endogenous somatostatin secretion. *J Clin Endocrinol Metab* 67:1186, 1988.
70. Dudl RJ, Ensinek JW, Palmer HE, et al: Effect of age on growth hormone secretion in man. *J Clin Endocrinol Metab* 67:11, 1973.
71. Blichert-Toft M: Stimulation of the release of corticotrophen and sommatotrophin by metyrapone and arginine. *Acta Endocrinol [Suppl](Copenh)* 195:65, 1975.
72. Mulligan T, Vinaules AJ, Godschalk M, Iranmerh A, Veldhues JD: Synthetic somatostatin analog supresses daytime growth hormone secration equivolently in young and older men. *J Am Geriatr Soc.* In press, 1999.
73. Rudman D, Kutner MH, Rogers CM, et al: Impaired growth hormone secretion in the adult population: Relation to age and adiposity. *J Clin Invest* 67:1361, 1981.
74. Vermeulen A: Nyctohemeral growth hormone profiles in young and aged men: Correlation with somatomedin C levels. *J Clin Endocrinol Metab* 64:884, 1987.
75. Tan K, Baxter RC: Serum insulin-like growth factor I levels in adult diabetic patients: The effect of age. *J Clin Endocrinol Metab* 63:651, 1986.
76. Bennett AE, Wahner MW, Riggs BL, et al: Insulin-like growth factors I and II: Aging and bone density in women. *J Clin Endocrinol Metab* 59:7012, 1984.
77. Rudman D, Nagraj HS, Mattson DE, et al: Hyposommatomedinemia in the nursing home patient. *J Am Geriatr Soc* 34:427, 1986.
78. Shuto Y, Nakano T, Sanno N, Domoto H, Sugihara H, Domoto H, Wakabayashi I: Reduced growth hormone receptor messenger ribonucleic acid in an aged man with chronic malnutrition and growth hormone resistance. *J Clin Endocrinol Metab* 84:2320, 1999.
79. Sawin CT, Carlson HE, Geller A, Castelli WP, Bacharach P: Serum prolactin and aging: Basal values and changes with estrogen use and hypothyroidism. *J Gerontol* 44:131, 1989.
80. Mooradian AD, Morley JE, Billington CJ, Slag MF, Elson MK, Shafer RB: Hyperprolactinemia in male diabetics. *Postgrad Med J* 61:11, 1985.
81. Sawin CT, Chopra D, Azizi F, Mannix JE, Bacharach P: The aging thyroid: Increased prevalence of elevated serum thyrotropin in the elderly. *JAMA* 242:247, 1979.
82. Jeffreys PM, Farran MEA, Hoffenberg R, Fraser PM, Hodkinson HM: Thyroid function tests in the elderly. *Lancet* i:924, 1972.
83. Rosenthal MJ, Hun WC, Garry PJ, Goodwin JS: Thyroid function in the elderly: Microsomal antibodies as a discriminant for therapy. *JAMA* 258:209, 1987.
84. Greenspan SL, Klibanski A, Rowe JW, Elahi D: Age-related alterations in pulsatile secretion of TSH: Role of dopaminergic regulation. *Am J Physiol* 260:E486, 1991.
85. Kaiser FE: Variability of responses to TRH in normal elderly. *Age Ageing* 16:345, 1987.
86. Mariotti S, Barbesino G, Catuegli P, Bartalena L, Sansoni P, Fagnoni F, Monti D, Fagiolo U, Franceschi C, Pinchera A: Complex alteration of thyroid function in healthy centenarians. *J Clin Endocrinol Metab* 77:1130, 1993.
87. Drinka PJ, Siebers M, Voeks SK: Poor positive predictive value of low sensitive thyrotropin assay levels for hyperthyroidism in nursing home residents. *South Med J* 86:1004, 1993.
88. Sawin CT, Geller A, Wolf PA, Belanger AJ, Baker E, Bacharach P, Wilson PW, Benjamin EJ, D'Agostino RB: Low serum thyrotropin concentrations as a risk factor for atrial fibrillation in older persons. *N Engl J Med* 331:1249, 1994.
89. Spaulding SW: Age and the thyroid. *Endocrinol Clin North Am* 16:1013, 1987.
90. Gregerman RI, Gaffney GW, Shock NW: Thyroxine turnover in eu-

thyroid man with special reference to changes in age. *J Clin Invest* 41:2065, 1962.
91. Herrmann J, Heinen E, Kroll MJ, Rodoff KM, Kruskemper ML: Thyroid function and thyroid hormone metabolism in elderly people: Low T3-syndrome in old age. *Klin Wochenschr* 59:315, 1981.
92. Burrows AE, Shakespear RA, Mesch RD, Cooper E, Aickin EM, Burke CW: Thyroid hormones in the elderly sick: T_4 euthyroidism. *Br Med J* 4:437, 1975.
93. Gaffney GW, Gregerman RI, Shock NW: Relationship of age to the thyroidal accumulation, renal excretion and distribution of radioiodide in euthyroid man. *J Clin Endocrinol Metab* 22:786, 1962.
94. Mariotti S, Sansoni P, Barbesino G, Caturegli P, Monti D, Cossarizza A, Giacomelli T, Passeri G, Fagiolo U, Pinchera A, et al: Thyroid and other organ-specific autoantibodies in healthy centenarians. *Lancet* 339:1506, 1992.
95. Rosenthal MJ, Hunt WC, Garry PJ, Goodwin JS: Thyroid failure in the elderly. Microsomal antibodies as discriminant for therapy. *JAMA* 258:209, 1987.
96. Samuels LT: Factors affecting the metabolism and distribution of cortisol as measured by levels of 17-hydroxycorticosteroids in blood. *Cancer* 10:746, 1957.
97. West CD, Brown H, Simmons EL, Carter DB, Kumage LF, Engelbert EL: Adrenocortical function and cortisol metabolism in old age. *J Clin Endocrinol Metab* 21:1197, 1961.
98. Romanoff LP, Morris CW, Welch P, Rodriguez RM, Pincus G: The metabolism of cortisol ^{4}C-14 in young and elderly men: I. Secretion rate of cortisol and daily excretion of tetrahydrocortisone and cortalone (20 alpha and 20 beta). *J Clin Endocrinol Metab* 21:1413, 1961.
99. Touitou Y, Salon J, Bogdan A, Touitou C, Reinberg A, Beck M, Sodiyez JC, Demey-Ponsort E, Van Couwenberge M: Adrenal circadian system in young and elderly human subjects: A comparative study. *J Endocrinol* 93:201, 1982.
100. Friedman M, Green MF, Shrland DG: Assessment of hypothalamic-pituitary-adrenal function in the geriatric age group. *J Gerontol* 24:292, 1969.
101. Pavlov EP, Hrman SM, Chrousos GP, Lourizux DL, Blackman MR: Responses of plasma adrenocorticotrophin, cortisol, and dehydroepiandrosterone to avine corticotrophin-releasing hormone in healthy aging men. *J Clin Endocrinol Metab* 62:767, 1986.
102. Rolandi E, Franceschini R, Marabini A, et al: Twenty-four hour beta-endorphin secretory pattern in the elderly. *Acta Endocrinol (Copenh)* 115:441, 1987.
103. Facchinetti G, Petraglia F, Nappi G, et al: Different patterns of central and peripheral beta-endorphin, beta lipoprotein and ACTM throughout life. *Peptides* 4:469, 1983.
104. Hatfield BD, Goldfarb AM, Sforzo GA, et al: Serum beta-endorphin and affective responses to graded exercise in young and elderly men. *J Gerontol* 42:429, 1987.
105. Casale G, Pecorini M, Cuzzoni G, de Nicola P: Beta endorphin and cold pressor test in the aged. *Gerontology* 31:101, 1985.
106. Tsunoda K, Abe K, Goto T, Yasujima M, Sato M, Omata K, Seino M, Yoshinaga K: Effect of age on the renin-angiotensin aldosterone system in normal subjects: Simultaneous measurement of active and inactive renin, renin substrate and aldosterone in plasma. *J Clin Endocrinol Metab* 62:384, 1986.
107. Yamaji T, Ibayashi H: Plasma dehydroepiandrosterone sulfate in normal and pathological conditions. *J Clin Endocrinol Metab* 29:273, 1969.
108. Oventreich N, Brind JC, Rizer RL, Vogelman JM: Age changes in sex differences in serum dehydroepiandrosterone sulfate concentrations throughout adulthood. *J Clin Endocrinol Metab* 59:531, 1984.
109. Barrett-Connor E, Khaw KT, Yen SCC: A prospective study of dehydroepiandrosterone sulfate, mortality and cardiovascular disease. *N Engl J Med* 315:1519, 1986.
110. Pashko LL, Schwartz AG: Effect of food restriction, dehydroepiandrosterone or obesity on the binding of 3H-7,12-dimethylbenz(a) anthracene to mouse skin DNA. *J Gerontol* 38:8, 1983.
111. Morales AJ, Haubrich RH, Hwang JY, Asakura H, Yen SS: The effect of six months treatment with a 100 mg daily dose of dehydroepiandrosterone (DHEA) on circulating sex steroids, body composition and muscle strength in age-advanced men and women. *Clin Endocrinol* 49:421, 1998.
112. Yen SS, Morales AJ, Khorram O: Replacement of DHEA in aging men and women. Potential remedial effects. *Ann NY Acad Sci* 774:128, 1995.
113. Wolkowitz OM, Reus VI, Roberts E, Manfredi F, Chan T, Ormiston S, Johnson R, Canick J, Brizendine L, Weingartner H: Antidepressant and cognition-enhancing effects of DHEA in major depression. *Ann NY Acad Sci* 774:337, 1995.
114. Morley JE, Kaiser FE, Raum WJ, Perry HM III, Flood JF, Jensen J, Silver AJ, Roberts E: Potentially predictive and manipulable blood serum correlates of aging in the healthy human male: Progressive decreases in bioavailable testosterone, dehydroepiandrosterone sulfate, and the ratio of insulin-like growth factor 1 to growth hormone. *Proc Natl Acad Sci* 94:7537, 1997.
115. Flood JF, Morley JE, Roberts E: Memory-enhancing effects in male mice of pregnenolone and steroids metabolically derived from it. *Proc Natl Acad Sci* 89:1567, 1992.
116. Sih R, Kamel H, Horani M, Morley JE: Dehydroepiandrosterone and pregnenolone. *Hormone Replacement Therapy* 13:241, 1999.
117. Steiger A, Trachsel L, Guldner J, Hemmeter U, Rothe B, Rupprecht R, Vedder H, Holsboer F: Neurosteroid pregnenolone induces sleep-EEG changes in man compatible with inverse agonistic GABAA-receptor modulation. *Brain Res* 615:267, 1993.
118. Esler MD, Turner AG, Kaye DM, Thompson JM, Kingwell BA, Morris M, Lambert GW, Jennings GL, Cox HS, Seals DR: Aging effects on human sympathetic neural function. *Am J Physiol* 268:R278, 1995.
119. Blandini F, Martignoni E, Melzi d'Eril GV, Biasio L, Sances G, Lucarelli C, Rizzo V, Costa A, Nappi G: Free plasma catecholamine levels in healthy subjects: A basal and dynamic study. The influence of age. *Scand J Clin Lab Invest* 52:9, 1992.
120. Tuck ML, Griffiths RF, Johnson L, Stern N, Morley JE: Hypertension in the elderly. *J Am Geriatr Soc* 36:630, 1988.
121. Linares OA, Halter JB: Sympathochromaffin system activity in the elderly. *J Am Geriatr Soc* 35:448, 1987.
122. Hoeldtke RD, Cilmi KM: Effects of aging on catecholamine metabolism. *J Clin Endocrinol Metab* 60:479,1985.
123. Linares OA, Supiano MA, Morrow LA, Halter JB: Norepinephrine release and metabolism in the elderly by compartmental analysis: Relationship to dietary salt. *Clin Res* 34:950A, 1986.
124. Scarpace PJ: Decreased beta-adrenergic responsiveness during senescence. *Fed Proc* 45:51, 1986.
125. Hyland L, Docherty JR: An investigation of age-related change in pre- and post-functional alpha-adrenoreceptors in human saphenous vein. *Eur J Pharmacol* 114:361, 1985.
126. Supiano MA, Linares OA, Halter JB, Reno KM, Rosen SG: Functional uncoupling of the platelet $alpha_2$-adrenergic receptor-adenylate cyclase complex in the elderly. *J Clin Endocrinol Metab* 64:1160, 1987.
127. Supiano MA, Hogikyan RV: High affinity platelet α_2-adrenergic receptor density is decreased in older humans. *J Gerontol* 48:B173, 1993.
128. Hogikyan RV, Supiano MA: Arterial α-adrenergic responsiveness is decreased and sympathetic nervous system activity is increased in older humans. *Am J Physiol* 266:E717, 1995.
129. Morley JE, Kaiser FE, Perry HM III, Patrick P, Morley PM, Stauber PM, Vellas B, Baumgartner RN, Garry PJ: Longitudinal changes in testosterone, luteinizing hormone, and follicle-stimulating hormone in healthy older men. *Metabolism: Clinical and Experimental* 46:410, 1997.
130. Korenman SG, Morley JE, Mooradian AD, Davis SS, Kaiser FE, Silver AJ, Viosca SP, Garza D: Secondary hypogonadism in older men: Its relationship to impotence. *J Clin Endocrinol Metab* 71:963, 1990.
131. Zumoff B, Strain GW, Kream J, et al: Age variation of the 24-hour plasma concentrations of androgens, estrogens and gonadotropins in normal adult men. *J Clin Endocrinol Metab* 54:534, 1982.
132. Pirke KM, Doerr P: Age-related changes in free plasma testosterone, dihydrotestosterone and estradiol. *Acta Endocrinol (Copenh)* 80:171, 1975.
133. Vermeulen A, Reubens R, Verdonck L: Testosterone secretion and metabolism in male senescence. *J Clin Endocrinol Metab* 34:730, 1972.
134. Morley JE: Endocrine factors in geriatric sexuality clinics. *Geriatr Med* 7:85, 1991.
135. Harman SM, Tsitouras PD: Reproductive hormones in aging men, in Measurement of sex steroids, basal luteinizing hormone and Leydig cell response to human chorionic gonadotropin. *J Clin Endocrinol Metab* 51:35, 1980.
136. Morley JE, Kaiser FE: Testicular function in the aging male, in Arm-

brecht HJ, Coe RM, Wongsurawat N (eds): *Endocrine Function and Aging*. New York, Springer-Verlag, 1990, pp 94–114.
137. Vermeulen A, Verdonck L: Some studies on the biological significance of free testosterone. *J Steroid Biochem* 3:421, 1972.
138. Deslypere JP, Vermeulen A: Leydig cell function in normal men: Effect of age, lifestyle, residence, diet and activity. *J Clin Endocrinol Metab* 59:955, 1984.
139. Baker HWG, Burges HG, DeKretser DM, et al: Changes in the pituitary-testicular system with age. *Clin Endocrinol (Oxf)* 5:349, 1976.
140. Tenover JS, Matsumoto AM, Clifton DK, Bremner WJ: Age-related alterations in the circadian rhythms of pulsatile luteinizing hormone and testosterone secretion in healthy men. *J Gerontol* 43:163, 1988.
141. Kaiser FE, Viosca SP, Mooradian AD, Morley JE, Korenman SG: Impotence and aging: Alterations in hormonal secretory patterns. *Endo Soc Abstr* 70:778A, 1988.
142. Vermeulen A, Deslypere JP, Kaufman JM: Influence of antiopioids on luteinizing hormone pulsatility in aging men. *J Clin Endocrinol Metab* 68:68, 1989.
143. Harman SM, Tsitouras PD, Costa PT, et al: Reproductive hormones in aging men: II. Basal pituitary gonadotropins and gonadotropin responses to luteinizing hormone-releasing hormone. *J Clin Endocrinol Metab* 54:547, 1982.
144. Tenover JS, Matsumoto AM, Plymate SR, et al: The effects of aging in normal men on bioavailable testosterone and luteinizing hormone secretion: Response to clomiphene citrate. *J Clin Endocrinol Metab* 65:1118, 1987.
145. Winters SJ, Sherins RJ, Troen P: The gonadotropin-suppressive activity of androgen is increased in elderly men. *Metabolism* 33:1052, 1984.
146. Winters SJ, Atkinson L: Serum LH concentrations in hypogonadal men during transdermal testosterone replacement through scrotal skin: Further evidence that ageing enhances testosterone negative feedback. The Testoderm Study Group. *Clin Endocrinol (Oxf)* 47:317, 1997.
147. Engle ET: The male reproductive system, in Lansing AI (ed): *Cowdry's Problems of Aging*, 3rd ed. Baltimore, Williams & Wilkins, 1952, pp 708–729.
148. Natoli A, Riondino G, Brancati A: Studio delta funizone gonadale ammonia e spermatogenetica nel corso della senescenza muschille. *G Gerontol* 20:1103, 1972.
149. Loria P, Petraglia F, Concari M, Bertolotti M, Martella P, Luisi S, Grisolia C, Foresta C, Volpe A, Genazzani AR, Carulli N: Influence of age and sex on serum concentrations of total dimeric activin A. *Eur J Endocrinol* 139:487, 1998.
150. Jiroutek MR, Chen MH, Johnston CC, Longcope C: Changes in reproductive hormones and sex hormone-binding globulin in a group of postmenopausal women measured over 10 years. *Menopause* 5:90, 1998.
151. Judd HL, Korenman SG: Effects of aging on reproductive function in women, in Korenman SG (ed): *Endocrine Aspects of Aging*. New York, Elsevier, 1982, pp 163–197.
152. Scalgia H, Medina M, Pinto-Ferreira AI, et al: Pituitary LH and FSH secretion and responsiveness in women of old age. *Acta Endocrinol (Copenh)* 81:673, 1976.
153. Petraglia A, Porro C, Facchinetti R, et al: Opioid control of LH secretion in humans: Menstrual cycle, menopause and aging reduce effect of naloxone but not of morphine. *Life Sci* 38:2103, 1986.
154. Melis GB, Cagnacci A, Gambacciani M, et al: Chronic bromocriptine administration restores luteinizing hormone response to naloxone in post-menopausal women. *Neuroendocrinology* 47:159, 1988.
155. Phillips PA, Rollo BJ, Ledingham JCG, et al: Reduced thirst after water deprivation in healthy elderly men. *N Engl J Med* 311:753, 1984.
156. Silver AJ, Flood JF, Morley JE: Effect of aging on fluid ingestion in mice. *J Gerontol* 46:B117, 1991.
157. Silver AJ, Morley JE: The role of the opioid system in the hypodysia associated with aging. *J Am Geriatr Soc* (in press).
158. Yanamoto T, Harada H, Fukuyama J, et al: Impaired arginine-vasopressin secretion associated with hypoangiotensinemia in hypernatremic dehydrated elderly patients. *JAMA* 259:1039, 1988.
159. Helderman JH: The impact of normal aging on the hypothalamic-neurohypophyseal-renal axis, in Korenman SG (ed): *Endocrine Aspects of Aging*. New York, Elsevier, 1982, pp 9–32.
160. Asplund R, Aberg H: Diumal variation in the levels of antidiuretic hormone in the elderly. *J Intern Med* 229:131, 1991.
161. Helderman JH, Vestal RE, Rowe JW, et al: The response of arginine vasopressin to intravenous ethanol and hypertonic saline in man: The impact of aging. *J Gerontol* 33:39, 1978.
162. Miller M, Morley JE, Rubenstein LZ: Hyponatremia in a nursing home population. *J Am Geriatr Soc* 43:1410, 1995.
163. Rudman D, Rachette D, Rudman IW, Mattson DE, Erve PR: Hyponatremia in tube-fed elderly men. *J Chronic Dis* 39:73, 1986.
164. Knight EL, Fish LC, Kiely DK, Marcantonio ER, Davis KM, Minaker KL: Atrial natriuretic peptide and the development of congestive heart failure in the oldest old: A seven-year prospective study. *J Am Geriatr Soc* 47:407, 1999.
165. Ohashi M, Fujia N, Nawata M, et al: High plasma concentrations of human atrial natriuretic polypeptide in aged men. *J Clin Endocrinol Metab* 64:81, 1987.
166. Baumgartner RN, Waters DL, Gallagher D, Morley JE, Garry PJ: Predictors of skeletal muscle mass in elderly men and women. *Mech Age Develop* 107:123, 1999.
167. Morley JE, Kaiser FE, Raum WJ, Perry HM III, Flood JF, Jensen J, Silver AJ, Roberts E: Potentially predictive and manipulable blood serum correlates of aging in the healthy human male: Progressive decreases in bioavailable testosterone, dehydroepiandrosterone sulfate, and the ratio of insulin-like growth factor 1 to growth hormone. *Proc Natl Acad Sci* 94:7537, 1997.
168. Rudman D, Shetty KR, Mattson DE: Plasma dehydroepiandrosterone sulfate in nursing home men. *J Am Geriatr Soc* 38:421, 1990.
169. Flood JF, Roberts E: Dehydroepiandrosterone sulfate improves memory in aging mice. *Brain Res* 448:178, 1988.
170. Rosenthal MJ, Morley JE, Flood JF, Scarpace PJ: Relationship between behavioral and motor responses of mature and old mice and cerebellar adrenergic receptor density. *Mech Ageing Dev* 45:231, 1988.
171. Rudman D, Feller AG, Nagraj HS, et al: Effects of human growth hormone in men over 60 years old. *N Engl J Med* 323:1, 1990.
172. Eicher EM, Beamer WG: New mouse dw allele: Genetic location and effects on lifespan and growth hormone levels. *J Hered* 71:187, 1980.
173. Maison P, Balkau B, Simon D, Chanson P, Rosselin G, Eschwege E: Growth hormone as a risk for premature mortality in healthy subjects: Data from the Paris prospective study. *Br Med J* 316:1132, 1998.
174. Cohn L, Feller AG, Draper MW, Rudman IW, Rudman D: Carpal tunnel syndrome and gynaecomastia during growth hormone treatment of elderly men with low circulating IGF-1 concentrations. *Clin Endocrinol* 39:417, 1993.
175. Papadakis MA, Grady D, Black D, et al: Growth hormone replacement in healthy older men improves body composition but not functional ability. *Ann Intern Med* 124:708, 1996.
176. Wells S, Thornton C, Statt M, et al: Growth hormone increases muscle mass and strength but does not rejuvenate myofibrillar protein synthesis in healthy subjects over 60 years old. *J Clin Endocrinol Metab* 81:3239, 1996.
177. Holloway L, Butterfield G, Hintz RL, et al: Effects of recombinant human growth hormone on metabolic indices, body composition, and bone turnover in healthy elderly women. *J Clin Endocrinol Metab* 79:470, 1994.
178. Thompson JL, Butterfield GE, Marcus R, et al: The effects of recombinant human insulin-like growth factor 1 and growth hormone on body composition in elderly women. *J Clin Endocrinol Metab* 80:1845, 1995.
179. Erdsieck R, Pols H, Valk N, et al: Treatment of post-menopausal osteoporosis with a combination of growth hormone and pamidronate: A placebo controlled trial. *Clin Endocrinol* 43:557, 1995.
180. Taaffe DR, Pruitt L, Reim J, et al: Effect of recombinant human growth hormone on the muscle strength response to resistance exercise in elderly men. *J Clin Endocrinol Metab* 79:1361, 1994.
181. Yarasheski KE, Zachwieja JJ, Campbell JA, et al: Effect of growth hormone and resistance exercise on muscle growth and strength in older men. *Am J Physiol* 268:E268, 1995.
182. Lieberman SA, Hoffman AR: The somatopause: Should growth hormone deficiency in older people be treated? *Clin Geriatr Med* 13:671, 1997.
183. Marcus R, Butterfield G, Holloway L, et al: Effects of short term administration of recombinant human growth hormone to elderly people. *J Clin Endocrinol Metab* 70:519, 1990.
184. Binnerts A, Wilson JH, Lamberts SW: The effects of human growth hormone administration in elderly men with recent weight loss. *J Clin Endocrinol Metab* 67:1312, 1988.
185. Kaiser FE, Silver AJ, Morley JE: The effect of recombinant human

growth hormone on malnourished older individuals. *J Am Geriatr Soc* 39:235, 1991.
186. Morley JE, Kaiser FE: Sexual function with advancing age. *Med Clin North Am* 73:1483, 1989.
187. Mooradian AD, Morley JE, Korenman SG: Biological action of androgens. *Endocr Rev* 8:1, 1987.
188. Morley JE, Perry HM III, Kaiser FE, Kraenzle D, Jensen J, Houston K, Mattammal M, Perry HM Jr: Effects of testosterone replacement therapy in old hypogonadal males: A preliminary study. *J Am Geriatr Soc* 41:149, 1993.
189. Sih R, Morley JE, Kaiser FE, Perry HM III, Patrick P, Ross C: Testosterone replacement in older hypogonadal men: A 12-month randomized controlled trial. *J Clin Endocrinol Metab* 82:1661, 1997.
190. Urban RJ, Bodenburg YH, Gilkison C, Foxworth J, Coggan AR, Wolfe RR, Ferrando A: Testosterone administration to elderly men increases skeletal muscle strength and protein synthesis. *Am J Physiol* 269:E820, 1995.
191. Reid IR, Wattie DJ, Evans MC, Stapleton JP: Testosterone therapy in glucocorticoid-treated men. *Arch Int Med* 156:1173, 1996.
192. Snyder PJ, Peachey H, Hannoush P, Berlin JA, Loh L, Holmes JH, Dlewati A, Staley J, Santanna J, Kapoor SC, Attie MF, Haddad JG, Strom BL: Effect of testosterone treatment on bone mineral density in men over 65 years of age. *J Clin Endocrinol Metab* 84:1966, 1999.
193. Abassi AA, Rudman D, Wilson CR, Drinka PJ, Basu SN, Mattson DE, Richardson TJ: Observations on nursing home residents with a history of hip fracture. *Am J Med Sci* 310:229, 1995.
194. Jackson JA, Riggs MW, Spiekerman AM: Testosterone deficiency as a risk factor for hip fractures in men: A case-control study. *Am J Med Sci* 304:4, 1992.
195. Stanley HL, Schmitt BP, Poses RM, Deiss WP: Does hypogonadism contribute to the occurrence of a minimal trauma hip fracture in elderly men? *J Am Geriatr Soc* 39:766, 1991.
196. Francis RM, Peacock M, Aaron JE, et al: Osteoporosis in hypogonadal men: Role of decreased plasma, 1,25 dihydroxy vitamin D, calcium malabsorption and low bone formation. *Bone* 7:261, 1986.
197. Vanderschueren D, Bouillon R: Androgens and bone. *Calcified Tissue Int* 56:341, 1995.
198. Flood JF, Morley JE: Age-related changes in footshock avoidance acquisition and retention in senescence accelerated mouse (SAM). *Neurobiol Aging* 14:153, 1993.
199. Flood JF, Farr SA, Kaiser FE, LaRegina M, Morley JE: Age-related decrease of plasma testosterone in SAMP8 mice: Replacement improves age-related impairment of learning and memory. *Physiol Behav* 57:669, 1995.
200. Janowsky JS, Oviatt SK, Orwoll ES: Testosterone influences spatial cognition in older men. *Behav Neurosci* 108:325, 1994.
201. Herbst KL, Anawalt BD, Cherrier M, Craft S, Matsumoto AM, Bremner WJ: Testosterone administration improves spatial and verbal memory in normal men. *J Invest Med* 47:23A, 1999.
202. Wu SZ, Weng XZ: Therapeutic effects of an androgenic preparation on myocardial ischemia and cardiac function in 62 elderly male coronary heart disease patients. *Chin Med J* 106:415, 1993.
203. Jaffe MD: Effect of testosterone cypionate on postexercise ST segment depression. *Br Heart J* 39:1217, 1977.
204. Webb CM, Adamson DL, deZeigler D, Collins P: Effect of acute testosterone on myocardial ischemia in men with coronary artery disease. *Am J Cardiol* 83:437, 1999.
205. Rosano GM, Leonardo F, Pagnotta P, Pelliccia F, Panina G, Cerquetani E, della Monica PL, Bonfigli B, Volpe M, Chierchia SL: Acute anti-ischemic effect of testosterone in men with coronary artery disease. *Circulation* 99:1666, 1999.
206. Chou TM, Sudhir K, Hutchison SJ, Ko E, Amidon TM, Collins P, Chatterjee K: Testosterone induces dilation of canine coronary conductance and resistance arteries *in vivo*. *Circulation* 94:2614, 1996.
207. Barrett-Connor EL: Testosterone and risk factors for cardiovascular disease in men. *Diabete et Metabolisme* 21:156, 1995.
208. Uyanik BS, Ari Z, Bumus B, Yigitoglu MR, Arslan T: Beneficial effects of testosterone undecanoate on the lipoprotein profiles in healthy elderly men. A placebo-controlled study. *Jpn Heart J* 38:73, 1997.
209. Cooper CS, Perry PJ, Sparks AE, MacIndoe JH, Yates WR, Williams RD: Effect of exogenous testosterone on prostate volume, serum and semen prostate specific antigen levels in healthy young men. *J Urol* 159:441, 1998.
210. Hartnell J, Korenman SG, Ciosca SP: Results of testosterone enanthate therapy for hypogonadism in older men. *Endocrine Soc Abstr*, No 428, Atlanta, 1990.
211. Hajjar RR, Kaiser FE, Morley JE: Outcomes of long-term testosterone replacement in older hypogonadal males: A retrospective analysis. *J Clin Endocrinol Metab* 82:3793, 1997.
212. Gooren LJ: A ten-year safety study of the oral androgen testosterone undecanoate. *J Androl* 15:212, 1994.
213. Morley JE, Kaiser FE, Sih R, Hajjar R, Perry HM III: Testosterone and frailty. *Clin Geriatr Med* 13:685, 1997.
214. Bush TL, Cowan LD, Barrett-Connor E, et al: Estrogen use and all-cause mortality. *JAMA* 249:903, 1983.
215. Hulley S, Grady D, Bush T, Furbert C, Herrington D, Riggs B, Vittinghoff E: Randomized trial of estrogen plus progestin for secondary prevention of coronary heart disease in postmenopausal women. Heart and Estrogen/progestin Replacement Study (HERS) Research Group. *JAMA* 280:605, 1998.
216. Chetkowski RJ, Meldrum DR, Steingold KA, et al: Biologic effects of transdermal estradiol. *N Engl J Med* 314:1615, 1986.
217. Hirvonen E, Malkonen M, Manninen V: Effects of different progestogens on lipoproteins during postmenopausal replacement therapy. *N Engl J Med* 304:560, 1981.
218. Pierron RL, Perry HM II, Grossberg G, et al: The aging hip. *J Am Geriatr Soc* 38:1339, 1990.
219. Birge S, Price S, McGee S, et al: The role of estrogen in the prevention of hip fracture in women over age 69, in Chirstensen C, Overguard K (eds): *3rd International Symposium on Osteoporosis*. Copenhagen, Abstracts, 1990, pp 1196–1197.
220. Birge SJ: Is there a role for estrogen replacement therapy in the prevention and treatment of dementia? *J Am Geriatr Soc* 44:865, 1996.
221. Kellie SE, Brody JA: Sex-specific and race-specific hip fracture rates. *Am J Public Health* 80:326, 1990.
222. Zimmerman SI, Girman CJ, Buie VC, Chandler J, Hawkes W, Martin A, Holder L, Hebel JR, Sloane PD, Magaziner J: The prevalence of osteoporosis in nursing home residents. *Osteoporosis Int* 9:151, 1999.
223. Morley JE, Gorbien MJ, Mooradian AD, et al: UCLA Geriatric Grand Rounds: Osteoporosis. *J Am Geriatr Soc* 36:845, 1988.
224. Ray WA, Griffen MR, Schaffner W, et al: Psychotropic drug use and risk of hip fracture. *N Engl J Med* 316:363, 1987.
225. Taggart H, McA: Do drugs affect the risk of hip fracture? *J Am Geriatr Soc* 36:1006, 1988.
226. Liu B, Anderson G, Mittmann N, To T, Axcell T, Shear N: Use of selective serotonin-reuptake inhibitors or tricyclic antidepressants and risk of hip fractures in elderly people. *Lancet* 351:1303, 1998.
227. Edwards BJ, Perry HM III, Kaiser FE, Morley JE, Kraenzle D, Stevenson R, Kreutter D: Relationship of age and calcitonin gene-related peptide to postprandial hypotension. *Mech Ageing Dev* 87:61, 1996.
228. Frontera WR, Meredith CN, O'Reilly KP, Knuttgen MG, Evans WJ: Strength conditioning in older men: Skeletal muscle hypertrophy and improved function. *J Appl Physiol* 64:1038, 1988.
229. Greenspan SL, Myers ER, Kiel DP, Parker RA, Hayes WC, Resnick NM: Fall direction, bone mineral density, and function: Risk factors for hip fracture in frail nursing home elderly. *Am J Med* 104:539, 1998.
230. Perry HM III, Horowitz M, Morley JE, Patrick P, Vellas B, Baumgartner R, Garry PJ: Longitudinal changes in serum 25-hydroxyvitamin D in older people. *Metabolism* In press, 1999.
231. Nagraj MS, Gregans GA, Mattson DE, Rudman IW, Rudman D: Osteopenia in the men of a veterans administration nursing home. *Am J Clin Nutr* 51:100, 1990.
232. Rudman D, Rudman IW, Mattson DE, et al: Fractures in the men of a veterans administration nursing home: Relation to 1,25 dihydroxyvitamin D. *J Am Coll Nutr* 8:324, 1989.
233. Matsuoka LY, Wortsman J, Hanifan N, Holick MF: Chronic sunscreen use decreases circulating concentrations of 25 hydroxyvitamin D. *Arch Dermatol* 124:1802, 1988.
234. McLaughlin J, Holick MF: Aging decreases the capacity of human skin to produce vitamin D_3. *J Clin Invest* 76:1536, 1985.
235. Armbrecht HJ, Zenser TV, Davis BB: Effect of age on the conversion of 25-hydroxyvitamin D_3 to 1,25 dihydroxyvitamin D by kidney of rat. *J Clin Invest* 66:1118, 1980.
236. Horst RL, Goff JP, Reinhardt TA: Advancing age results in a reduction of intestinal and bone 1,25 dihydroxyvitamin D receptor. *Endocrinology* 126:1053, 1990.

237. Chapuy MC, Arlot ME, Delmas PD, Meunier PJ: Effect of calcium and cholecalciferol treatment for three years on hip fractures in elderly women. *Br Med J* 308:1081, 1994.
238. Dawson-Hughes B, Harris SS, Krall EA, Dallal GE: Effect of calcium and vitamin D supplementation on bone density in men and women 65 years of age or older. *N Engl J Med* 337:670, 1997.
239. Morley JE: A place in the sun does not guarantee adequate vitamin D. *J Am Geriatr Soc* 37:663, 1989.
240. Dionko AC, Brown MB, Herzog AR: Sexual function in the elderly. *Arch Intern Med* 150:197, 1990.
241. Aoki M, Kumcemoto Y, Mori K: Studies on sexual activity in Japanese males based on inquiry about sexual behavior. *Hinyokika Kiyo* 33:1623, 1987.
242. Slag MF, Morley JE, Elson MK, et al: Impotence in medical clinic outpatients. *JAMA* 249:1736, 1983.
243. Bretschneider JG, McCoy NL: Sexual interest and behavior in healthy 80 to 102-year olds. *Arch Sex Behav* 17:109, 1988.
244. Kaiser FE, Viosca SP, Morley JE, et al: Impotence and aging: Clinical and hormonal factors. *J Am Geriatr Soc* 36:511, 1988.
245. Mooradian AD, Viosca SP, Kaiser FE, Morley JE, Korenman SG: Penile Raynaud's phenomenon: A possible cause of erectile failure. *Am J Med* 85:748, 1988.
246. Morley JE, Korenman SG, Kaiser FE, et al: Relationship of penile brachial pressure index to myocardial infarction and cerebrovascular accidents in older males. *Am J Med* 84:445, 1988.
247. Kaiser FE, Udhoji V, Ciosca SP, et al: Cardiovascular stress tests in patients with vascular impotence. *Clin Res* 37:89A, 1989.
248. Shabsighi R, Fishman IJ, Quesada ET, et al: Evaluation of vasculogenic erectile impotence using penile duplex ultrasonography. *J Urol* 142:1469, 1989.
249. Tudoriu T: My views about the applied anatomy on the penis and the physiopathology of erection. *Arch Intern Urol* 61:249, 1989.
250. Williams G, Mulachy J, Harnell G, Keely E: Diagnosis and treatment of venous leakage: A curable cause of impotence. *Br J Urol* 61:151, 1988.
251. Stig CG, Welterauer U, Sommerkamp H: Intra-individual comparative study of dynamic and pharmacocavernography. *Br J Urol* 64:93, 1989.
252. Morley JE: Impotence. *Am J Med* 80:L897, 1986.
253. Ono N, Lumpkin MD, Samson WK, et al: Intrahypothalamic action of corticotropin-releasing factor to inhibit growth hormone and LH release in the rat. *Life Sci* 35:1117, 1984.
254. Morley JE, Kaiser FE: Impotence in elderly men. *Drugs Aging* (in press).
255. Goldstein I, Luc TF, Padma-Nathan H, Rosen RC, Steers WD, Wicker PA: Oral sildenafil in the treatment of erectile dysfunction. Sildenafil Study Group *N Engl J Med* 338:1397, 1998 [published erratum appears in *N Engl J Med* 339:59, 1998].
256. Rendell MS, Rajfer J, Wicker PA, Smith MD: Sildenafil for treatment of erectile dysfunction in men with diabetes: A randomized controlled trial. Sildenafil Diabetes Study Group. *JAMA* 281:421, 1999.
257. Padma-Nathan H, Hellstrom WJ, Kaiser FE, Labasky RF, Lue TF, Nolten WE, Norwood PC, Peterson CA, Shabsigh R, Tam PY: Treatment of men with erectile dysfunction with transurethral alprostadil. Medicated Urethral System for Erection (MUSE) Study Group. *N Engl J Med* 336:1, 1997.
258. Korenman SG, Viosca SP, Kaiser FE, Mooradian AD, Morley JE: Use of a vacuum tumescence device in the management of impotence. *J Am Geriatr Soc* 38:217, 1990.
259. Davidson JM, Camargo CA, Smith ER: Effects of androgen on sexual behavior in hypogonadal men. *J Clin Endocrinol Metab* 48:955, 1979.
260. O'Carrol R, Bancroft J: Testosterone therapy for low sexual interest and erectile dysfunction in men: A controlled study. *Br J Psychiatry* 145:146, 1986.
261. Billington CJ, Mooradian AD, Duffy L, et al: Testosterone therapy in impotent patients with normal testosterone. *Clin Res* 31:718A, 1983.
262. Morales A, Johnston B, Heaton JW, Clark A: Oral androgens in the treatment of hypogonadal impotent men. *J Urol* 152:1115, 1994.
263. McCoy NC, Davidson JM: A longitudinal study of the effects of menopause on sexuality. *Maturitas* 7:203, 1985.
264. Dennerstein L, Burrows GD, Wood C, et al: Hormones and sexuality: Effect of estrogen and progestogen. *Obstet Gynecol* 56:316, 1980.
265. Stemmens JP, Tsai CL, Semmens EC, et al: The effects of estrogen therapy on vaginal physiology during menopause. *Obstet Gynecol* 66:15, 1985.
266. Salmon TJ, Gast SH: Effect of androgens in libido in women. *J Clin Endocrinol Metab* 3:235, 1943.
267. Mazenod B, Pugeat M, Forest MG: Hormones, sexual function and erotic behavior in women, in Sitsen JMA (ed): *Handbook of Sexology, vol 6*. Amsterdam, Elsevier, 1988, pp 316–351.
268. Burger H, Hailes J, Nelson J, et al: Effect of combined implants of estradiol and testosterone on libido in post menopausal women, in Campbell S (ed): *Management of Menopause and Postmenopause Years*. Lancaster Time Press, Lancaster, UK, 1976, p 149.
269. Sherwin BB, Gelfand MM: The role of androgen in maintenance of sexual functioning in oophorectomized women. *Psychosom Med* 49:397, 1987.
270. Davis SR, McCloud P, Strauss BJ, Burger H: Testosterone enhances estradiol's effects on postmenopausal bone density and sexuality. *Maturitas* 21:227, 1995.
271. Starr B, Weiner M: *The Starr-Weiner Report on Sex and Sexuality in the Mature Years*. New York, McGraw-Hill, 1981.
272. Harris MI, Flegal KM, Cowie CC, Eberhardt MS, Goldstein DE, Little RR, Wiedmeyer HM, Byrd-Holt DD: Prevalence of diabetes, impaired fasting glucose, and impaired glucose tolerance in U.S. adults. The Third National Health and Nutrition Examination Survey, 1988–1994. *Diabetes Care* 21:518, 1998.
273. Lieberman LS: Diabetes and obesity in elderly black Americans, in Jackson JS (ed): *The Black American Elderly*. New York, Springer, 1988, pp 130–189.
274. Huse DM, Oster G, Kellen AR, et al: The economic costs of non-insulin dependent diabetes mellitus. *JAMA* 262:2708, 1989.
275. Waugh NR, Dallas JM, Jung RT, Newton RW: Mortality in a cohort of diabetic patients. *Diabetologia* 32:103, 1989.
276. Sinclair AJ, Robert IE, Croxson SC: Mortality in older people with diabetes mellitus. *Diabet Med* 14:639, 1997.
277. Miller DK, Lui LYL, Perry HM III, Kaiser FE, Morley JE: Reported and measured physical functioning in older inner city diabetic African Americans. *J Gerontol* 54:M230, 1999.
278. Meneilly GS, Ryan AS, Minaker KL, Elahi D: The effect of age and glycemic level on the response of the beta-cell to glucose-dependent insulinotropic polypeptide and peripheral tissue sensitivity to endogenously released insulin. *J Clin Endocrinol Metab* 83:2925, 1998.
279. Morley JE, Mooradian AD, Rosenthal MJ, Kaiser FK: Diabetes in elderly persons: Is it different? *Am J Med* 83:533, 1987.
280. Bolinder J, Ostman J, Arner P: Influence of aging on insulin receptor binding and metabolic effects of insulin on human adipose tissue. *Diabetes* 32:959, 1983.
281. Pogano G, Cassander M, Diana A, et al: Insulin resistance in the aged: The role of peripheral insulin receptors. *Metabolism* 30:46, 1981.
282. Forbes A, Elliott T, Tildesley H, Finegood D, Meneilly GS: Alterations in non-insulin-mediated glucose uptake in the elderly patient with diabetes. *Diabetes* 47:1915, 1998.
283. Shepherd PR, Katz BB: Glucose transporters and insulin action. *N Engl J Med* 341:248, 1999.
284. Chen M, Bergman RN, Pauni G, Porte D Jr: Pathogenesis of age-related glucose intolerance in man: Insulin resistance and decreased B-cell function. *J Clin Endocrinol Metab* 60:13, 1985.
285. Zavaroni I, Dall'Aglio E, Bruschi F, et al: Effect of age and environmental factors on glucose tolerance and insulin secretion in a worker population. *J Am Geriatr Soc* 34:271, 1986.
286. Shimokata H, Muller DC, Fleg JL, et al: Age as independent determinant of glucose tolerance. *Diabetes* 40:44, 1991.
287. Cooper GJS, Willis AC, Clark A, et al: Purification and characterization of a peptide from amyloid-rich pancreases of type 2 diabetic patients. *Proc Natl Acad Sci USA* 84:8628, 1987.
288. Edwards BJ, Perry HM, Kaiser FE, Morley JE, Kraenzle D, Kreutter DK, Stevenson RW: Age-related changes in amylin secretion. *Mech Ageing Dev* 86:39, 1996.
289. Morley JE, Perry HM III: The management of diabetes mellitus in older individuals. *Drugs* 41:548, 1991.
290. Naliboff BD, Rosenthal M: Effects of age on complications in adult onset diabetes. *J Am Geriatr Soc* 37:838, 1989.
291. Morisaki N, Watanabe S, Kobayashi J, Kanzaki T, Takahashi K, Yokote K, Tezuka M, Tashiro J, Inadera H, Saito Y, et al: Diabetic control and progression of retinopathy in elderly patients: Five year follow-up study. *J Am Geriatr Soc* 42:142, 1994.

292. Morley GK, Mooradian AD, Levine AS, Morley JE: Why is diabetic peripheral neuropathy painful? The effect of glucose on pain perception in humans. *Am J Med* 77:79, 1984.
293. Mooradian AD, Perryman K, Fitten LJ, et al: Cortical function in elderly non-insulin dependent diabetic patients. *Arch Intern Med* 148:2369, 1988.
294. Rost K, Rotes D, Quill T, et al: Recall of prescription medication changes. *Diabetes* 38(Suppl 2): 40A, 1989.
295. Flood JF, Mooradian AD, Morley JE: Characteristics of learning and memory in streptozocin-induced diabetic mice. *Diabetes* 39:1391, 1990.
296. Meneilly GS, Cheung E, Tessier D, Yakura C, Tuokko H: The effect of improved glycemic control on cognitive functions in the elderly patient with diabetes. *J Gerontol* 48:M117, 1993.
297. Gradman TJ, Laws A, Thompson LW, Reaven GM: Verbal learning and/or memory improves with glycemic control in older subjects with non-insulin-dependent diabetes mellitus. *J Am Geriatr Soc* 41:1305, 1993.
298. Olson T, Vutanen M, Asplund K, et al: Prognosis after stroke in diabetic patients: A controlled prospective study. *Diabetologia* 33:244, 1990.
299. Brandeis GH, Berlowitz DR, Hossain M, Morris JN: Pressure ulcers: The Minimum Data Set and the Resident Assignment Protocol *Adv Wound Care* 8:18, 1995.
300. Bourdel-Marchasson I, Dubroca B, Manciet G, Decamps A, Emeriau JP, Dartigues JF: Prevalence of diabetes and effect on quality of life in older French living in the community: The PAQUID Epidemiological Survey. *J Am Geriatr Soc* 45:295, 1997.
301. Rosenthal MJ, Fajardo M, Gilmore S, Morley JE, Naliboff BD: Hospitalization and mortality of diabetes in older adults. A 3-year prospective study. *Diabetes Care* 21:231, 1998.
302. Yesavage JA, Brink TL, Rose TL, et al: Development and validation of a geriatric depression screening scale: A preliminary report. *J Psychiatr Res* 17:37, 1983.
303. Fitten LJ, Morley JE, Gross PL, et al: UCLA geriatric grand rounds: Depression. *J Am Geriatr Soc* 37:459, 1989.
304. Jansen RWMM, Peeters TL: The effect of oral glucose, protein, fat and water loading on blood pressure and the gastrointestinal peptides VIP and somatostatin in hypertensive elderly subjects. *Eur J Clin Invest* 20:192, 1990.
305. Aronow WS, Ahn C: Association of postprandial hypotension with incidence of falls, syncope, coronary events, stroke, and total mortality at 29-month follow-up in 599 older nursing home residents. *J Am Geriatr Soc* 45:1051, 1997.
306. Rosenthal MJ, Hartnell JM, Morley JE, et al: Diabetes in the elderly. *J Am Geriatr Soc* 35:435, 1987.
307. Wilholm BE, Westerholm B: Drug utilization and morbidity statistics for the evaluation of drug safety in Sweden. *Acta Med Scand* [*Suppl*] 683:107, 1984.
308. Shorr RI, Ray WA, Daugherty JR, Griffin MR: Incidence and risk factors for serious hypoglycemia in older persons using insulin or sulfonylureas. *Arch Intern Med* 157:1681, 1997.
309. Hatorp V, Huant WC, Strange P: Pharmacokinetic profiles of repaglinide in elderly subjects with type 2 diabetes. *J Clin Endocrinol Metab* 84:1475, 1999.
310. Morley JE: An overview of diabetes mellitus in older persons. *Clin Geriatr Med* 15:211, 1999.
311. Lee A, Morley JE: Metformin decreases food consumption and induces weight loss in subjects with obesity with type II non-insulin-dependent diabetes. *Obesity Res* 6:47, 1998.
312. Santiago JV: Troglitazone. *Compr Ther* 23:560, 1997.
313. Kumar S, Prange A, Schulze J, Lettis S, Barnett AH: Troglitazone, an insulin action enhancer, improves glycaemic control and insulin sensitivity in elderly type 2 diabetic patients. *Diabet Med* 15:772, 1998.
314. Gilden JL, Casia C, Hendryx M, et al: Effects of self-monitoring of blood glucose on quality of life in elderly diabetic patients. *J Am Geriatr Soc* 38:511, 1990.
315. Arnetz BB, Kallner A, Theorell T: The influence of aging on hemoglobin Ajc. *J Gerontol* 37:648, 1982.
316. Negro H, Morley JE, Rosenthal MJ: Utility of serum fructosamine as a measure of glycemia in young and old diabetic and non-diabetic subjects. *Am J Med* 85:360, 1988.
317. Mooradian AD, Osterweil D, Petrasek D, Morley JE: Diabetes mellitus in elderly nursing home patients: A survey of clinical characteristics and management. *J Am Geriatr Soc* 36:391, 1988.
318. Coulston AM, Mandelbaum D, Reaven GM: Dietary management of nursing home residents with non-insulin diabetes mellitus. *Am J Clin Nutr* 51:67, 1990.
319. Sinclair AJ, Allard I, Bayer A: Observations of diabetes care in long-term institutional settings with measures of cognitive function and dependency. *Diabetes Care* 20:778, 1997.
320. Morley JE, Perry HM, Baumgartner RP, Garry PJ: Commentary: Leptin, adipose tissue and aging—Is there a role for testosterone? *J Gerontol* 54:B108, 1999.
321. Larsson H, Elmstahl S, Berglund G, Ahren B: Evidence for leptin regulation of food intake in humans. *J Clin Endocrinol Metab* 83:4382, 1998.
322. Perry HM, Morley JE, Horowitz M, Kaiser FE, Miller DK, Wittert G: Body composition and age in African American and Caucasian women—relationship to plasma leptin levels. *Metab Clin Exp* 46:1399, 1997.
323. Baumgartner RN, Ross RR, Waters DL, Brooks WM, Morley JE, Montoya GD, Garry PJ: Serum leptin in elderly people: Associations with sex hormones, insulin, and adipose tissue volumes. *Obes Res* 7:141, 1999.
324. Baumgartner RN, Waters DL, Morley JE, Patrick P, Montoya GD, Garry PJ: Age-related changes in sex hormones affect the sex difference in serum leptin independently of changes in body fat. *Metab Clin Exp* 48:378, 1999.
325. Morley JE: Anorexia of aging: Physiologic and pathologic. *Am J Clin Nutr* 66:760, 1997.
326. Morley JE: Nutritional status of the elderly. *Am J Med* 81:679, 1986.
327. Morley JE, Silver AJ: Anorexia of aging. *Neurobiol Aging* 9:9, 1988.
328. Morley JE, Kraenzle D: Causes of weight loss in a community nursing home. *J Am Geriatr Soc* 42:583, 1994.
329. Wilson MM, Vaswani S, Liu D, Morley JE, Miller DK: Prevalence and causes of undernutrition in medical outpatients. *Am J Med* 104:56, 1998.
330. Morley JE, Thomas DR: Anorexia and aging: Pathophysiology. *Nutrition* 15:499, 1999.
331. Morley JE, Kumar VB, Mattammal MB, Farr S, Morley PM, Flood JF: Inhibition of feeding by a nitric oxide synthase inhibitor: Effects of aging. *Eur J Pharmacol* 311:15, 1996.
332. MacIntosh CG, Andrews JM, Jones KL, Wishart JM, Morris HA, Jansen JBMJ, Morley JE, Horowitz M, Chapman IM: Effects of age on concentrations of plasma cholecystokinin, glucagon-like peptide 1, and peptide YY and their relation to appetite and pyloric motility. *Am J Clin Nutr* 69:999, 1999.
333. Morley JE, Glick Z: Obesity, in Morley JE, Glick Z, Rubenstein LZ (eds): *Geriatric Nutrition*. New York, Raven Press, 1990, pp 293–306.
334. Miller NE: Aging and plasma lipoproteins, in Hazzard WR, Andres R, Bierman EL, Blass JP (eds): *Principles of Geriatric Medicine and Gerontology*, 2nd ed. New York, McGraw-Hill, 1990, pp 767–776.
335. Anderson KM, Castelli WP, Levy D: Cholesterol and mortality: 30 years of follow-up from the Framingham study. *JAMA* 257:2176, 1987.
336. Castelli WP, Garrison RJ, Wilson PWF, et al: Incidence of coronary heart disease and lipoprotein cholesterol levels: The Framingham study. *JAMA* 256:2835, 1986.
337. Foretta B, Tortsat D, Wolmark Y: Cholesterol as a risk factor for mortality in elderly women. *Lancet* 1:868, 1989.
338. Kaiser FE, Morley JE: Cholesterol can be lowered in older persons: Should we care? *J Am Geriatr Soc* 38:8, 1990.
339. Noel MA, Smith TK, Ettinger WH: Characteristics and outcomes of hospitalized older patients who develop hypocholesterolemia. *J Am Geriatr Soc* 39:455, 1991.
340. Buckler DA, Kelber ST, Goodwin JS: The use of dietary restrictions in malnourished nursing home patients. *J Am Geriatr Soc* 42:1100, 1994.

CHAPTER 31

Hormones and Athletic Performance

David C. Cumming

ENERGY SUPPLY AND PHYSICAL WORK

The endocrine system at rest is characterized by endogenous rhythmic fluctuations in hormone levels. Superimposed on these internal rhythms is the capacity to respond to changes in the external environment. Thus, stress, feeding, trauma, and other stimuli are followed by adjustments of hormonal control. Physical activity, both short-term acute activity and repeated exertion during a longer interval, may induce changes in the circulating levels of a number of hormones. Although much information about endocrine responses to physical exertion has come from investigations of exercise, such research also has important applications in industrial, military, and other forms of work as well as in recreational and competitive sports.

For optimal physical work to be carried out, nervous, cardiac, vascular, pulmonary, and metabolic functions must be coordinated and adjusted. The detailed mechanisms of control of this coordination are unclear, but the central role of the endocrine system in the regulation of fluid and electrolyte balance, energy metabolism, and cardiac and vascular function, together with neuroendocrine influences on other systems, indicates the importance of the endocrine system in exercise and the capacity for physical work.

Muscular work is dependent on the supply of energy and oxygen. The basic fuel for muscular work is adenosine triphosphate (ATP). Enough ATP is stored for direct use in muscle for less than 1 s of activity. Creatine phosphate can supply ATP for a further 15 to 30 s; after that, stored carbohydrates and fats must be metabolized to supply continuing energy needs.

Oxygen consumption increases substantially during the first few minutes of exercise until the demands of active tissues are met and a steady state is reached in which oxygen uptake and demand are balanced. In light exercise (10 to 40 percent of maximal oxygen consumption), the demand for oxygen from energy output during the initial 2 to 4 min can be met aerobically by both stored myoglobin and the blood perfusing the muscle. During severe exercise (70 to 90 percent of maximal oxygen consumption), the energy demands cannot be totally accounted for by the aerobic process even in early exercise; therefore, anaerobic sources must contribute so that lactic acid is produced. The point at which this process begins is the *anaerobic threshold*. Maximal aerobic capacity or maximal oxygen consumption ($V_{O_{2max}}$) can be defined as the point at which no further increase in oxygen uptake occurs with an increase in energy demand, i.e., the exercise workload. $V_{O_{2max}}$ is used as a measure of fitness by which comparisons of workload are made among individuals of differing fitness.

$V_{O_{2max}}$ can be determined by means of various tests, such as continuous versus discontinuous exercise, bicycle versus treadmill or other form of exercise, and arm versus leg exercise. The duration of the test may also vary. The criteria used to determine $V_{O_{2max}}$ include (1) no further increase in oxygen consumption despite increasing workload (plateau phenomenon), (2) blood lactate levels greater than 80 mg/ml of blood, (3) heart rate greater than 190 beats per minute, and (4) respiratory quotient greater than unity. Determination of $V_{O_{2max}}$ therefore does not provide a specific measure but varies in accordance with the kind of test used. Nevertheless, it is the best single measure of fitness.

Exercise cannot be described as a single entity, as the characteristics of different activities place different demands on the body. The way in which energy is handled varies with exercise load, type, and duration and the fitness of the individual. Energy consumption at strenuous workloads can be 120 times basal levels; at less intense but sustained activity such as distance running, energy utilization is about 23 to 30 times basal levels. The ability to sustain a maximal load is limited, while less strenuous loads can be sustained for longer periods.

EVALUATING HORMONAL RESPONSE TO EXERCISE AND TRAINING

There are many experimental protocols and subjects involved in research on physical activity. Comparisons among investigations are therefore difficult, if not impossible, even when the comparisons are based on $V_{O_{2max}}$. A comparison of the effects of a weightlifting experiment with the responses to an endurance activity may produce different results, and a comparison of exhaustive exercise for 15 min with 4 hr of submaximal exercise or a 1,000-km race spanning several days is clearly meaningless.

Nevertheless, exercise in many forms can produce changes in a range of hormonal systems. The variables that determine the response include fitness of the individual, aptitude for the exercise, type of exercise, duration, percentage of maximal aerobic capacity, and workload. The hormonal influences on physical activity are complex, and measurement of responses can be influenced by a large number of variables (Table 31-1). In addition, it is generally assumed that changes in hemoconcentration are, at least in part, responsible for the observed changes in serum hormone levels. Blanket acceptance of this assumption as applicable to all hormones in all circumstances is clearly an inappropriate oversimiplification worthy of further research. This chapter will review current knowledge about the effects of exercise and training on the endocrine system and will examine the role of endogenous and exogenous hormones in modifing an athlete's ability to perform.

TABLE 31-1. Hormonal Responses to Exercise and Training: Modifying Factors

1. Characteristics of the exercise activity
   a. Intensity of the exercise
   b. Duration of the activity
   c. Type of exercise—e.g., running, cycling, swimming
      Hemoconcentration
      Muscle groups involved
      Posture during exercise
   d. Special effects, e.g., immersion, high altitude
2. Fitness of the individual
   a. Cardiopulmonary fitness
   b. Strength and flexibility
   c. Familiarity of subject with specific activity
   d. Training during previous 24 hours
3. Baseline endocrine function
   a. Age-related differences
   b. Sex-related differences
   c. Effects of biological rhythms
      Circadian, Menstrual, Lifetime,
      Maturational, Circhoral
   d. Stress—Physical and Psychological
   e. Metabolic—glucose, salt and fluid loads
   f. Endocrine disorders
4. Methods of sampling the hormones
   a Blood versus urine
   b. Indwelling cannula versus repeated stabs
   c. Length of presampling baseline
   d. Sampling frequency and duration
   e. Fluids maintaining IV patency
5. Biochemistry of the hormones
   a. Blood production rates—direct and indirect
   b. Protein binding—specific and nonspecific
   c. Clearance rates and systems—target tissues/metabolism and excretion in liver and/or kidney
6. Ambient conditions
   a. Temperature, humidity, altitude, pO2
   b. Laboratory versus free range
   c. Competitive versus noncompetitive

EFFECTS OF PHYSICAL ACTIVITY AND TRAINING ON ENDOCRINE FUNCTION

Endocrine Regulation of Fluid Balance during Physical Work

During strenous or prolonged physical work there is a considerable loss of water and electrolytes in sweat, as evaporation is the main means for dissipating heat generated from the inefficient muscular use of chemical energy. Substantial changes occur in serum electrolytes with increased levels of K^+ and Na^+.[1] Blood flow is diverted to working muscle and away from the kidneys. To minimize the loss through normal endocrine mechanisms, increases in aldosterone and arginine vasopressin (AVP) would be anticipated. The decreased plasma volume, increased serum sodium and potassium levels, and fluid loss during exercise, together with the activation of the ACTH-adrenal axis, could increase aldosterone and AVP levels through their individual mechanisms. One might expect that as part of training for endurance activity fluid balance is more carefully controlled as part of a physiologic adaptation to fitness. This appears to be the case. In addition, it is generally believed that changes in hemoconcentration are, in part, responsible for the measured changes in hormones.[2]

Arginine Vasopressin, Exercise, and Training

It was recognized many years ago that exercise inhibits the diuresis induced by water loading and bioassay evidence of the presence of a humoral factor found in the blood was assumed to explain the exercise-associated antidiuresis.[3] Antidiuretic hormone or arginine vasopressin was found to be increased when specific assay systems became available.[4–6] Subsequent studies have generally but not universally concluded that AVP increases with physical exertion.[7,8] The increase is progressive with increasing intensity and duration and correlates with increasing plasma osmolality in submaximal exercise but not high intensity short term exercise.[9–12] The response is not modified by gender[13] or training, [14–16] although as may be anticipated with increased fitness, the response to the same absolute workload is diminished.[17] The return to basal levels after exercise is quite rapid, occurring within 1 h of ending the activity despite continuing hemoconcentration.[9,18] AVP has also been implicated in the increase in plasma volume that occurs with training.[14]

Various factors have been implicated in the increase in AVP with exercise, including high plasma osmolality, extracellular fluid volume contraction, hydration, body temperature, angiotensin II, psychological factors, altered metabolism, and peripheral nerve stimulation.[9,18,19] The change in response to exercise is greater than would be anticipated from a comparable change if hypertonic fluids were given and from a comparable heat stress.[9] The involvement of angiotensin is unclear because converting enzyme inhibition has been reported to diminish or have no effect on the vasopressin response.[20,21] Dehydration and fluid loading both diminish the response.[22–25] Predictability of exercise reduces the response while unpredictability enhances it, suggesting a significant psychological component.[26] The response is not changed by posture, hypoxia, or opiate inhibitors.[20,26] A direct afferent arc from the muscle may induce the release of AVP from neurosecretory cells in the supraoptic nucleus.[27] Melatonin and GABA but not opioids exert at least partial control over the AVP response.[28–30]

Aldosterone, Exercise, and Training

Acute exercise significantly changes the functioning of the renin-angiotensin-aldosterone axis. A sixfold increase in aldosterone levels was observed after a marathon run, a change that was entirely prevented by adequate fluid replacement.[31,32] The increment is workload-related and is mediated at least in part by plasma volume, sodium levels, pH and hypoxemia.[5,9,10,16,18,19,33–39] Blockade of aldosterone activity with spironolactone reduces plasma volume increase by 40 percent.[40] The onset is rapid, but the levels return to normal more slowly, depending on the initial exercise load. Plasma renin activity increases two- to fivefold as a result of exercise, and the changes appear to be in direct proportion to the workload. Angiotensinogen levels decrease with exercise, presumably as a result of conversion to angiotensin II. The level of angiotensin II increases with exercise and appears to be at least partly responsible for the increased aldosterone levels. The increase in angiotensin II but not aldosterone can be blocked by the β-blocker propranolol.[41] Other factors are involved in the activation of aldosterone production, including the ACTH-adrenal axis.[15] Energy deprivation has no effect, but manipulation of physiologic saline to minimize fluid loss modulates the changes.[42] A psychological component is present because hypnotic suggestion of running activates the axis.[43] Basal levels of active hormones in the axis and responses are reduced for maximal workloads in trained individuals.[27,34,42,43] Prolonged, repeated competitive exercise does not result in continued activation of the axis, and basal values were regained each day within 12 hr of competition during a 20-day race despite continuing fluid loss.[44] Trained athletes also have a greater tolerance to a fluid load without suppressing their hormonal response.[45] These changes might be expected to improve endurance performance. The American College of Sports Medicine has some detailed recommendations to minimize risk of dehydration and hyperthermia in individuals participating in regular physical activity.[46] The recommendations include increased fluid intake in the 24 hours prior to and during physical activity, together with recommendations to improve palatability of the fluid and its electrolyte content.

GASTROINTESTINAL HORMONES IN TRAINING AND EXERCISE

"Runner's trots" is a phenomenon well recognized by endurance athletes. There are descriptive reports concerning exercise-induced gastrointestinal distress, but the role of gastrointestinal hormones and/or enzymes is not definitively established. Almost half of the individuals completing a 67-km race complained of intestinal cramps.[47] Although intensity dependant increases in esophageal contractions and gastroesophageal reflux have been described in both trained and untrained subjects,[48,49] strenuous exercise seems to have little effect on postprandial gastric secretory or motor function.[50] Others have reported decreased orocecal transit time in women during mild exercise but without change in either gastrin or motilin.[51] In contrast, epidemiological evidence suggests that physical activity may reduce the risk of gall bladder disease.[52]

Gastrin, vasoactive intestinal peptide, secretin, pancreatic polypeptide, neurokinin A, pancreastatin glucagon-like peptide I, and cholecystokinin have been reported to increase and pepsinogen decreases with endurance running.[53–56] If the exercise is sufficiently prolonged the levels of gastrin appears to decrease.[57] The effect on other peptides is unclear. Vasointestinal peptide, secretin, and pancreatic polypeptide increase with prolonged mild bicycle riding.[58,59] Although gastric inhibitory polypeptide increases with exercise it is not affected by training,[60,61] and there was no difference in exercise associated increases in gastrin and vasointestinal peptide between endurance trained runners and field hockey players.[62] Vasoactive intestinal peptide response appears to be extinguished by glucose ingestion suggesting a metabolic role.[63]

It is clear that the levels of most gastrointestinal hormones change with physical activity and perhaps training. There is little understanding of the importance of these changes in athletic performance, metabolic regulation, and gastrointestinal function.

METABOLIC CONTROL IN EXERCISE AND TRAINING (TSH-THYROID AXIS)

The role of thyroxine (T_4), triiodothyronine (T_3), and reverse triodothyronine (rT_3) in modulating the rate of metabolic processes suggests that the thyroid axis may be responsive to changes in energy balance associated with physical work. As discussed later, repeated physical work accompanied by energy deficiency results in partial shutdown of the thyroid and the reproductive axes. The thyroid axis is, however, substantially buffered against sudden change, although disturbance of circadian variation is apparent.

Acute Responses

Most studies have found no change in thyroid stimulating hormone (TSH) levels with acute exercise.[4,64–69] Some authors have reported a slight fall.[70,71] Increased TSH levels were reported with acute exercise in untrained subjects[66] and after prolonged and strenuous exercise,[72–74] but the increment is minute compared with the response to TRH stimulation. Response seems to vary with time of day, being maximal at night.[75] Diurnal variation of TSH is also altered.[76]

Levels of total T_4, total T_3, and their free moieties generally increase slightly with acute exercise, but the increase is usually small.[65,67,71,74,77–80] Because less than 0.05 percent of circulating T_4 is unbound, it is not surprising that changes in total hormone do not exceed the exercise-induced hemoconcentration. Individual studies have observed a decrease in T_4[81] or T_3[82]. The latter may result from alterations in peripheral conversion to favor the production of rT_3.[74] The different individual responses with acute exercise have been related to fitness and workload by means of measurement of the "double product" (heart rate in beats per minute multiplied by systolic blood pressure in mmHg); fitter individuals have an increase, and the less fit have a decrease.[82] Other researchers have suggested a biphasic response based on the fitness of athletes running marathons and ultramarathons.[83]

Effect of Training

Alterations in thyroid function may occur with repeated exercise, temperature, diet, and season.[84] Thyroxine degradation has been estimated to be 75 percent higher in athletes than in nonathletes and approaches levels found in hyperthyroidism, but reverts to normal quickly.[85,86] Short-term endurance and strength training induced a reduction in thyroid hormones[87,88] that subsequently was no longer seen after prolonged training. The effect was no longer seen when the training load was increased by 50 mi per week.[89,90] There is a small increase in the resting metabolic rate in endurance-trained athletes when this rate is determined per kilogram of fat-free weight.[91] Basal thyroid hormones were not related to fitness (as assessed by maximal oxygen consumption) or percentage of body fat. Deficient energy intake in experimental conditions and in amenorrheic runners, bulimia, and anorexia results in decreases in resting metabolic rate.[92–99] Impaired muscle function is reported in women athletes with lowered thyroid levels.[98,99] The changes in RMR are generally ascribed to the alterations in thyroid function, although some have suggested that catecholamines play a significant role at least in the short term.[100]

There is little information about physical activity in athletes with hypothyroidism treated with hormone replacement. A case report suggests that TSH and PRL responses to TRH may be increased by training even in nonendurance-trained hypothyroid athletes despite apparently normal thyroid function.[101] Lactate levels for a specific workload are increased suggesting impaired muscle function.[102] Careful monitoring may be advisable in hypothyroid athletes, although the changes are unlikely to be sufficient to produce clinical symptoms. Hyperthyroid individuals have impaired exercise tolerance, which should be respected during treatment.[103]

GLUCOREGULATION IN TRAINING AND EXERCISE: INSULIN AND GLUCAGON IN EXERCISE

The supply of fuel to exercising and nonexercising tissues during physical activity is one of the crucial factors that determine performance of a task. The responses of the glucoregulatory system vary with load. In mild to moderate exercise, the glucoregulatory response resembles that in the basal state, with glucose levels tightly controlled by insulin and glucagon. In high-intensity exercise, the catecholamine response increases and glucose is less tightly regulated and may even increase. Regulation of fatty acids is generally less tightly controlled because there are no mechanisms to effect such control.[104]

Increased glucose utilization by working muscles would lead to hypoglycemia if hepatic glucose production were not increased. Glucagon stimulates both glycogenolysis and gluconeogenesis, resulting in elevated glucose levels. Insulin facilitates glucose transport through cell membranes and increases glycogen synthetase activity, promoting glycogen storage. Because the supply of glucose to working muscle is one of the prime limiting factors in physical activity and because even mild exercise increases glucose uptake from the circulation,[104,105] it can be expected that both insulin and glucagon are responsive to an increased metabolic load and are likely to be changed with physical activity and training. Training induces an increase in responsiveness of muscle uptake to insulin through increase in GLUT4 glucose transporters. Such effects improve glucoregulation and reduce the risk of developing noninsulin dependant diabetes mellitus.[105]

Insulin and Exercise

During moderate exercise, insulin levels remain unchanged during the first 40 to 60 min of exercise. More prolonged or strenuous exercise induces a decline in insulin levels.[104–109] The insulin decline may not be essential to maintain glucose homeostasis.[110] Counterregulatory hormones, catecholamines, glucagon, GH, and cortisol tend to increase with more strenuous activity, inducing hepatic glycogenolysis, gluconeogenesis, and lipolysis to provide increased FFA for use as a metabolic fuel.[111] Further modulation is through neuropeptide Y increasing and endothelin-1 decreasing splanchnic gluconeogenesis.[112,113] During short-term strenuous exercise, when the counterregulatory hormones increase rapidly, glucose levels may transiently increase.[114] After exercise, insulin levels rapidly return to baseline. The changes in insulin during and after exercise seem to be related to the intensity of the activity and muscle mass involved rather than the exercise energy requirements.[115,116]

Prior carbohydrate intake may increase preexercise insulin levels and prevent insulin decline, maintaining circulating glucose as the substrate used in exercise until supplies decline and extending exercise tolerance.[117–119] Fasting induces a reduced insulin response and glucose levels are maintained even with prolonged fasting by hepatic gluconeogenesis.[120–122] The remarkable increase in glucose uptake by exercising muscles (30-fold) can result from increased insulin action on the muscles through increased receptor content[123] as well as non-insulin-mediated uptake by muscle.[124] It appears that the muscle glucose uptake, which is not directly mediated by insulin, still requires at least basal insulin levels to occur.[125] Increased insulin availability above basal levels has little effect on glucose transport, and the supply of glucose to the muscle is maintained during exercise despite decreased insulin.[126,127] The decline in insulin with exercise can be prevented by α-adrenergic blockade but not β-blockade.[128,129] Insulin also plays a role in controlling the sensitivity of hepatic glucose production.[130,131] Glycogen recovery in muscle can be facilitated by consumption of food with a high glycemic index.[132] As discussed later, endurance training can modify the responses reducing hepatic glycogenolysis and gluconeogenesis.[133,134]

Glucagon and Exercise

Glucagon levels increase during strenuous exercise, but the response is variable at lesser intensities.[109,128,135–138] However, the rise in glucagon is not necessarily linear with duration or intensity of exercise. Decreasing blood glucose levels stimulate glucagon,[109] and preloading with glucose generally blunts the glucagon response.[118,139] Fasting and hypoglycemia have been reported to produce a variable effect on glucagon response, depending on the blood glucose level attained.[120,121] The increase in glucagon can occur without a prior fall in glucose levels.[140] In general, levels of glucagon correspond significantly with epinephrine and norepinephrine levels,[141] although β-blockade with propranolol has little, if any, inhibitory effect on the glucagon response to moderate exercise.[129] Opiate blockade reduces glucagon response to exercise, suggesting that the release of endogenous opiates may be related, at least in part, to the increase in glucagon.[142]

The response of glucagon and other counterregulatory hormones is usually adequate to maintain glucose levels during exercise, although asymptomatic and symptomatic hypoglycemia can occur with prolonged and strenuous exercise in nondiabetic individuals.[143–144] This emphasizes the importance of maintaining glucose intake during prolonged exercise such as marathon running.

Effects of Training

Training induces a reduction in basal insulin levels and in the exercise-associated changes in both glucagon and insulin, including changes in insulin pulsatile release.[106,107,128,133,134,137,145–148] The decline in glucose with exercise may decrease or even be reversed.[149] There are gender differences in the relative importance of sources of nutrient; women use lipids to a greater degree than do men, who use more carbohydrate and protein.[150] Neither gender nor menstrual cycle has an important effect on glucoregulatory hormones during exercise.[151,152]

Training also increases sensitivity to insulin at rest and in response to a glucose load.[153–157] The increase in insulin sensitivity changes by 20 to 30 percent when maximal oxygen consumption is increased by 15 to 20 percent. These changes probably relate to increased tissue binding of insulin.[158] Insulin decline with activity is also reduced during acute exercise in trained individuals. The long-term significance of enhanced insulin sensitivity has been questioned.[159] It appears to be very rapidly reversed on refraining from exercise even for a few days and is not modified by acute exercise.[160–163] The benefits may not be seen in obese hypertriglyceridemic men with impaired carbohydrate tolerance.[164]

Growth Hormone in Exercise

The Effect of Exercise and Training

The release of growth hormone (GH) is controlled by the interplay of GH releasing factor and somatostatin, which inhibits the effect of GH releasing factor. Many other hormones and substances influence GH release (Table 31-2) and also can modulate the effect of physical activi\ty on GH levels. In exercise and

TABLE 31-2. A Partial List of Factors that Influence Growth Hormone Secretion

Increase GH levels	Decrease GH levels
Stress	
Stage III and IV sleep	REM sleep
Alpha-adrenergic agonists	Alpha-adrenergic antagonists
Beta-adrenergic antagonists	Beta-adrenergic agonists
Hypoglycemia	Hyperglycemia
Low free fatty acids	High free fatty acids
Some forms of diabetes mellitus	Obesity
Glucagon	High glucocorticoid levels
Androgens	Hypothyroidism
Estrogens	IGF-I
Opiates	Substance P
VIP	Neurotensin
Bombesin	
Motilin	

training, growth hormone is involved in the metabolic fuel adaptation and probably tissue repair postexercise. Basal release of GH is ultradian and pulsatile, with low levels of GH occurring as a result of an increased influence of somatostatin.[165,166] Training tends to reduce basal GH levels in men,[167–169] but not in women, in whom increased basal GH levels have been observed.[170] Training at altitude produces no further change in trained runners.[169] The influence of training on physiologic rhythms has not been studied, but it may influence responses to pharmacologic stimulation.[151,171]

The observation that GH increases during strenuous exercise in most individuals was among the earliest identified endocrine responses to exercise and exercise-associated GH changes have been extensively investigated.[172] The effect has been used clinically to examine GH release, particularly in children, but with variable results.[173] The GH response to physical activity has been shown to be influenced by a number of factors, including fitness, fatness, prior feeding, and age. Gender differences have been reported to have no effect on response.[151,174] Manipulating androgen levels in men[175] has no effect, but similar manipulation with estrogen in women does modify the response.[176,177] Priming children with sex steroids fails to increase sensitivity.[178] The menstrual cycle may or may not influence the response.[179,180] Increasing age influences the GH response to exercise, which can be reversed by training.[151,181,182] Type of activity, fitness, fatness, maturation, food intake, training, time of day, oxygen avaiability, acid-base status, and recent exercise patterns can all modify the response range of physical activities increase GH levels.[64,183–195] Release is not consistent until at least 30 to 40 percent of maximal oxygen consumption, although prolonged exercise even at 10 percent of maximal oxygen consumption may release GH.[196] Serum GH levels increase progressively with an increasing load until the maximal load is reached, at which time the response, may decrease.[64,106,107,197–199] The effect of training on GH response to exercise is unclear.[106,107,186,200,201]

The Effect of Metabolic and Pharmacologic Manipulations

The control of GH release during exercise has been further examined by means of metabolic and pharmacologic manipulations. Hypoinsulinemia associated with fasting or lowered blood glucose may be a stimulus to exaggerated GH secretion with exercise in normal humans.[202] Hyperglycemia induced in normal subjects preceding exercise decreases the normal GH increment during intense exercise and eliminates the normal GH response to mild exercise.[203,204] This blunted GH response to exercise may be due to hyperinsulinemia, as diabetic subjects do not show the same reduction in GH response.[203–205] Obese women with higher insulin levels also have a substantially reduced GH response to exercise.[206] Free fatty acids (FFA) elevated above 3 mEq/liter induced by an infusion of soybean oil emulsion and heparin can completely block the GH increase seen during exercise.[207] The effects of nonphysiologic levels of FFA, glucose, and possibly insulin are probably mediated at the hypothalamic level.[208,209]

Neuroendocrine Control of GH Release with Exercise

There is considerable and conflicting evidence regarding the neuroendocrine pathways that regulate GH secretion during exercise. Mechanisms involving cholinergic, serotoninergic, α-adrenergic, dopaminergic, and opioidergic pathways have been proposed.[210–215] There may be interactions among the pathways, and they may operate at different exercise intensities.

Relatively light exercise and insulin-induced hypoglycemia increased GH levels in one study, but not through GH releasing hormone; it was postulated that the mechanism involves the inhibition of somatostatin.[216] A somatostatin analog eliminates the exercise-associated GH increment.[217] Exercise elevated GH even when levels were increased during the infusion of GH releasing hormone, again suggesting that exercise influences GH levels through the inhibition of somatostatin.[214]

Atropine reduced the normal GH response to cycle ergometer work at moderate intensity, suggesting involvement of cholinergic pathways, but failed to affect GH increments during high-intensity work.[210] Specific muscarinic receptor blockade also inhibits the exercise-induced GH response.[218] The γ-aminobutyric acid (GABA) receptor agonist sodium valproate also inhibits exercise-associated GH responses.[219,220] Opoid inhibition does not change this effect.[221]

Pharmacologic agents that affect central serotoninergic pathways have been shown to modify GH secretion in many circumstances.[222,223] Cyproheptadine blunts GH responses by approximately 50 percent during exercise at a moderate work rate (600 kpm/min), but its effects at higher intensities have not been tested.[211] This suppression of the normal GH increment could be due to the anticholinergic properties of cyproheptadine,[210] but this is unlikely because cyproheptadine reduces the increment induced by the serotonin precursor 5-hydroxytryptophan and suppresses GH in a manner similar to that of other serotonin antagonists, such as methysergide and melatonin, during insulin-induced hypoglycemia (IIH).[211,224] GH levels are increased by α-adrenergic[225,226] and decreased by β-adrenergic[227] stimulation. Dopaminergic agents, L-dopa,[228] apomorphine,[229] and bromocriptine[230] can also increase GH levels. As the dopamine-induced GH response can be inhibited by phentolamine,[231] this action may be mediated through an α-adrenergic receptor or a neuronal intermediary with α-adrenergic activity. The involvement of dopaminergic and adrenergic mechanisms in exercise-induced GH increments is shown by the potentiation of GH responses to exercise with L-dopa,[232] bromocriptine,[233] pyridoxine hydrochloride,[234] and propranolol,[235,236] and suppression of exercise-induced GH increases after pimozide and clonidine.[210,237] In contrast, α_2-adrenergic blockade by idazoxan augments the GH response to exercise.[238]

The release of GH and prolactin (PRL) after the administration of a met-enkephalin analog can be blocked by naloxone,[239] suggesting that opioid peptides modulate the secretion of these hormones. Naloxone is ineffective in reducing GH responses to moderate exercise,[240–242] but high doses of naloxone and naltrexone obliterate GH and PRL increases even with high-intensity exercise.[20,214] Opiate receptors may therefore mediate GH and PRL increments during intense exercise, inducing peripheral elevations in peripheral levels of β-endorphin.[243–245]

The mechanisms of GH release at different exercise rates are unclear, as is the relation of these mechanisms to the mechanisms that cause GH secretion in other circumstances. A model for GH control in exercise can be postulated as follows: during moderate exercise, increases in GH levels can be modified by drugs affecting dopaminergic, α-adrenergic, β-adrenergic, cholinergic, and serotoninergic pathways.[210,231–234] Stress-induced GH release due to IIH is mediated by a serotoninergic pathway.[224] This increment is accompanied by a synchronous cortisol elevation[246] that could also be mediated by serotoninergic neurons. Although GH increases with exercise up to the anaerobic threshold may occur in the absence of a cortisol increment,[210,247] these increases are still inhibited by serotonin antagonism.

Simultaneous increases in GH, PRL, and cortisol during intense exercise may be due to the concomitant increase of ACTH and β-endorphin because naloxone suppresses exercise-induced GH and PRL increases.[214,245,246] Pyridoxine, a coenzyme involved in the conversion of L-dopa to dopamine, enhances the GH increase that occurs with intense exercise.[234] The dopaminergic influence on GH release in this situation may involve a final serotoninergic mechanism, as cyproheptadine reduces the GH response to L-dopa without altering PRL suppression and because serotonin depletion follows the administration of dopamine or L-dopa.[248–250]

The GH increase at high work rates represents a stress similar to IIH as synchronous GH and cortisol increases occur.[246] Both conditions may be similarly mediated by serotonin neurons because serotonin antagonists reduce GH responses to both in exercise and IIH. However, the basic peripheral stimulus is different. Hypoglycemia stimulates GH by means of a direct action at the hypothalamus,[209] whereas the exercise stimulus remains to be elucidated but seems to interact to some degree only with the altered blood glucose mechanism. Opioid peptides do not mediate GH release due to IIH but seem to play a role in the exercise-induced GH rise.[251]

Effects of Increased GH with Exercise

The role for increased GH during exercise has been suggested to be that of mobilizing FFA for fuel.[252] This seems exaggerated because the FFA response to infused or injected GH is slower than lipolysis during short-term exercise[253,254] and FFA and glucose levels are not reduced when GH increments are pharmacologically blocked.[210] Norepinephrine is probably more important in this role.[255] The specific functions of GH increments with exercise remain unknown but probably represent a generalized stress response. The anabolic properties of GH may also be important during the recovery phase that follows stress.

ACTH-CORTISOL AXIS

Exercise and the ACTH-Cortisol Axis

The ACTH-adrenal axis is primarily involved in glucoregulation, physiological stress, and immune responses to exercise and training, but changes in basal and exercise-related increases may also reflect psychological well-being. The ACTH-cortisol response to acute physical activity depends on the relative intensity of the workload and duration of the activity. Levels of cortisol may increase in anticipation of exercise.[106] Early studies of low-intensity exercise (less than 50 percent of maximal oxygen consumption) found that cortisol levels usually decrease, probably as a result of increased removal from the circulation.[256] With prolonged or more intense exercise, circulating cortisol levels increase in proportion to the workload in laboratory settings [12,64,191,197,257–261] and in free exercise studies.[4,31,79,262–265] This increase occurs despite a decrease in the half-life of cortisol and increased tissue uptake.[258,266] The cortisol increase is ACTH-mediated.[243–245,267] The cortisol response peaks about 30 minutes after that of ACTH and the degree of change may be dissassociated from that of ACTH suggesting that other factors may be involved in the control of cortisol.[268] The change in ACTH is driven by CRH.[268] The critical value that results in an increase in circulating cortisol levels is 60 to 70 percent of maximal oxygen consumption, and the response increases with greater exercise intensity.[196,269] In contrast, exercise for 30 min at 80 percent of maximal heart rate produced no change in either cortisol or ACTH,[270] emphasizing the need for optimal respiratory measures of exercise load. Very prolonged racing (six-day ski race) produced very complex changes at various stages of the race and abolished the circadian variation of ACTH and cortisol.[271]

A number of metabolic, psychological, and other variables alter the cortisol response to a given workload. Early studies have suggested that altitude and hypoxia increase the cortisol response to any workload[256,272–274]: more recent and perhaps better-performed studies have supported this finding.[189,275] The cortisol response parallels lactic acid production,[258,276] and glucose loading and high ketogenic diet modify the exercise associated changes.[277–280] Psychological factors such as level of competition, level of the athlete, degree of success, stress, mood, and music can all influence the cortisol behavior responses.[281–289] Ambient temperature may modify the response through mechanisms that may be perhaps psychological as much as physiological.[290] Single leg working produces a greater increase than exercise with two legs, probably because of a greater metabolic response from harder-working muscles.[291] Cortisol levels may decline with exhaustive exercise. The increase to exhaustion is not linear, perhaps because of negative feedback of high cortisol levels, depletion or near depletion of the adrenals, or a defense mechanism to avoid total cortisol depletion.[292,293]

There is inconsistency in the results of studies of the effects of circadian and menstrual rhythms on ACTH-adrenal response to exercise.[294–297] Age influences the response more by restricting the level of performance in older individuals than the adrenal response.[298] Gender has complex effects on both basal and exercise-induced changes, which is interactive with training.

The Effect of Physical Training

The response of basal cortisol levels to training seems to depend on the training load. Cortisol has been implicated as one of the markers for a poorly delineated phenomenon variously described as overtraining, overreaching, or overloading.[299] The phenomenon is described in more detail in a subsequent section. Some but not all reports suggest that highly trained male athletes have higher basal cortisol and ACTH levels, perhaps as a result of increased rates of production.[300–305] A sudden increase in the intensity of training produces a further increase in cortisol levels over several days.[306] Serum ACTH and cortisol levels appear to be elevated in women with normal menstruation, and exercise-associated oligoamenorrhea, persisting into the off season.[307–318] A somewhat unexpected finding is that although ACTH is elevated in amenorrheic athletes, corticotropin releasing hormone (CRH) is not similarly increased.[319] The relationship between alteration of the ACTH-adrenal axis and menstrual dysfunction is dealt with in the subsequent section. In men, the effects of training are much more variable and alterations do not generally persist beyond the end of the season.[308] Training programs have been reported to decrease basal ACTH levels even as arguably more accurate but cross-sectional 24-h frequent sampling pulse studies have shown no difference between athletes and nonathletes.[309,310]

ACTH and cortisol responses to CRF are blunted in both male and female athletes.[301,302,320] The relative cortisol response (increase from the baseline of cortisol versus increase from the baseline of ACTH) is enhanced in runners, yet the cortisol response to ACTH does not appear to be enhanced.[320]

Cortisol and ACTH responses to the same absolute workload fall with training.[321] However, in response to the same relative intensity, well-controlled studies have shown clear potentiation of the cortisol response[273] or no change.[106,107] The response to marathon running appears to be proportional to individual fitness, whereas other field and laboratory studies have shown no cortisol response to intense exercise in endurance-trained athletes.[4,197] Training may enhance ACTH response to short-term supramaximal exercise.[267] Many of these investigations have used endurance training as the investigative regime. The response to a maximal treadmill test may differ depending on the training regime used; sprint interval training but not endurance training was shown to induce an increased cortisol response to a maximal load.[322] There was no increase in basal cortisol levels during the course of this study.

Physiologic Significance

The physiologic significance of the cortisol response to activity is unclear; possible explanations include defense of fluid volume and blood pressure, catabolic effect of labile protein stores to generate amino acids and energy for the healing of damaged tissues *after* exercise, and psychogenic effects. A training effect is seen as cortisol response to ACTH diminishes, but ACTH and cortisol responses to CRH have been reported to increase.[323] Abolition of the cortisol response using metapyrone decreases insulin levels, and increases growth hormone, epinephrine, and norepinephrine.[324] Immediate physiologic requirements therefore appear to metabolic. Glucocorticoid deficiency and short-term administration may, respectively, inhibit and enhance physical activity in animals; ACTH has no effect in humans.[256,325–327] Although athletes may have high-normal or supraphysiologic basal cortisol levels, they are not cushingoid in appearance. The significance of high glucocorticoid levels in loss of muscle in overtrained athletes is unknown. Regular physical activity protects against the muscle atrophy usually induced by glucocorticoids in rats, but changes in the testosterone/cortisol ratio are regarded as significant in muscle loss in overtrained athletes.[328,329] The interrelationship of increased cortisol levels with effects on the immune system has received much attention. Concern that there might be an immune suppressive effect rather than direct evidence of such an effect has been expressed in the various studies.[330–333]

Control Mechanisms

Exercise induces an increase in cortisol beyond the maximal induced by ACTH, suggesting other factors may be present in the control of exercise-induced changes in cortisol.[334] The inhibition of ACTH and cortisol induced by dexamethasone may be overcome by high-intensity exercise.[335] Increases and no change have been reported with naloxone.[336,337] ACTH cortisol response may be reduced or eliminated by arginine-glutamine salts, phosphatidylserine, and benzodiazepine.[338,339–340]

Finally a matter of concern is the accuracy of all of the measurements of cortisol. Free cortisol measures are substantially different from total cortisol and the circadian variations in cortisol levels have lead to suggestions that urinary free cortisol may be most appropriate sampling methodology for investigations of long term influences.[341,342]

CATECHOLAMINES IN EXERCISE

"Getting the adrenaline going" is synonymous with the excitement of sports but the emotional component is but one of the several important effects associated with exercise and training-associated changes in catecholamines. During exercise both circulating epinephrine and norepinephrine levels increase. This is to be expected, as these hormones are involved in inotropic and chronotropic effects on the heart, redistribution of blood flow, substrate mobilization through the promotion of glycogenolysis and lipolysis, psychological effects, and immune response. The differential responses of epinephrine and norepinephrine suggest that there is also some difference in function. Norepinephrine is related to hemodynamic changes, whereas epinephrine is more clearly related to sympathetic activity and blood glucose levels.[343]

Epinephrine and Norepinephrine

The responses of epinephrine and norepinephrine to physical activity are not necessarily the same for a given exercise intensity. Mild exercise produces little or no response in either hormone, but at moderate exercise levels significant norepinephrine release occurs with minimal change in circulating epinephrine.[136,140,344] The increase in norepinephrine is probably a consequence of release from sympathetic postganglionic neurons. At intense or prolonged exercise levels both hormones increase significantly.[136,140,345,346] Graded exercise produces a lower response than continuous prolonged exercise.[141] The responses are directly related to workload and oxygen uptake and are greater with small muscle groups than with large muscle groups.[107,140,347,348] The increase in epinephrine is abrupt in onset at strenuous workloads, whereas prolonged work to the point of exhaustion induces a progressive increase in epinephrine.[106,140] These increases in catecholamines involve both conjugated and free hormone and may be higher in capillary blood than in venous blood.[349–351] The changes persist for 24 h after prolonged exercise.[352] The determining factor in catecholamine release may be reaching the anaerobic threshold; beyond this point circulating epinephrine and norepinephrine levels increase out of proportion to the increasing workload.[353]

Control of Catecholamine Release

The factors responsible for hormone release are not clear. In one study, the response during exercise occurred approximately at the time of reaching the anaerobic threshold, suggesting that the production of lactate may influence the initiation of catecholamine response to exercise.[354] Fasting enhances the catecholamine response to activity, but glucose loading seems to have little effect.[121,355–357] Hypoxia enhances the response in trained subjects but not in untrained subjects.[358] The exercise load is much more of a determining factor than is the psychological state, negating the concept of "getting the adrenaline pumping" before exercise.[359] The menstrual cycle does not influence response, but men show a slightly different pattern of epinephrine release with a similar pattern of norepinephrine release.[360]

Endogenous opiate inhibition was reported to have no influence on catecholamine release, but β blockade with timolol augmented basal and maximal exercise-stimulated epinephrine levels.[361,362] Other researchers disagree, suggesting that opioid inhibition may influence catecholamine response during exercise.[33,242] The basal levels of norepinephrine were increased, whereas the response to maximal exercise was blunted. Although the immediate effect of β-blockade during exercise is contradictory,[363–365] propranolol and other β-blockers may enhance exercise-induced catecholamine increase after exercise.[366]

Dopamine Responses to Exercise

The relationship of dopamine to modulation of hypothalamic-pituitary function is well established and increasing importance is being given to dopamine as part of the exercise-associated catecholamine response. Dopamine increases during exercise in a manner similar to that of epinephrine and norepinephrine, although the elevation may persist longer after exercise than that of the other catecholamines.[348,350,352,367–369] There is no dopamine response to exercise that involves small muscle groups; this is in contrast to the responses of other catecholamines.[370] Dopamine levels may also be chronically elevated in highly trained athletes.[371] Elevations in dopamine β-hydroxylase suggest that dopamine may act as a precursor for other catecholamines.[372] In one study, no differences were found in the dopamine responses to physical activity in eumenorrheic, oligomenorrheic, and amenorrheic runners.[373]

Effects of Training

Training results in a diminished catecholamine response to the same absolute level of physical activity, but paradoxically may actually increase the ability to secrete epinephrine in response to other stimuli.[107,373–378] The response is probably unchanged at the same relative workload.[107,376] Platelet assays of catecholamines, considered as a measure of long-term catecholamine concentration in the circulation, respond little to acute exercise, but basal levels are substantially elevated in athletes.[367] Very prolonged exercise leads to substantial elevations of free catecholamines; levels may also be chronically elevated in highly trained athletes.[352,379]

Effects of Catecholamine Release

The effects of catecholamine release include increased glycogenolysis and increased FFA concentrations.[352] Epinephrine enhances muscular glycogen utilization, glycolysis, and carbohydrate utilization.[380] Although similar glucagon and epinephrine changes are observed, catecholamines are unlikely to be entirely responsible for the increase in glucagon, as decreased glucose availability enhances glucagon and epinephrine secretion during prolonged exercise.[373] The lipase response to circulating epinephrine levels may increase with training.[381,382] Cardiovascular but not respiratory adaptations to exercise are mediated at least in part by catecholamines.[383,384] Redistribution of circulation to working muscles and to the skin for heat loss and sweating is mediated through changes in catecholamines directly or indirectly via other intermediate hormones.[385] Training and exercise lower blood pressure by 6–10 mm Hg through increased levels of dopamine, prostalandin E, and taurine; decreased levels of norepinephrine and endogenous ouabain-like substance; and a lower Na^+/K^+ ratio.[386] There is also decreased tissue sensitivity to norepinephrine and epinephrine.[387,388] Training appears to enhance central and peripheral dopaminergic tone at the expense of the noradrenergic: this produces alterations in many aspects of motor function including control of vascular flows, muscle tone, visual processing, protein and calcium homeostasis, and perhaps optimal utilization of food intake.[389] Several of the suggested dopamine related benefits remain to be proven. Evidence has also suggested that mental performance and psycholgical well-being may be improved through exercise; this improvement may be mediated through catecholamines.[390,391]

ENDOGENOUS OPIATES IN EXERCISE AND TRAINING

The wide range of possible effects of endogenous opiates (EO) has encouraged research into their role in exercise performance, their psychological and behavioral effects (including mood, appetite changes, exercise addiction, and pain perception), and their role in a variety of hormonal changes, including exercise-associated reproductive dysfunction.

Response to Acute Physical Activity

In most physiologic situations, β-END and ACTH are released concurrently from the pituitary and have a common precursor, pro-opiomelanocortin (POMC). Strenuous physical activity is consistently accompanied by an increase in EO, but lesser activity produces an inconsistent response. Investigations have generally supported the simultaneous release of β-END and ACTH.[244,265,392–398] Resistance exercise has generally not produced an increase in β-END except when the program is very strenuous.[399–403] The disassociation of cortisol and β-END in at least some exercise protocols suggested that the control mechanisms may not be identical. Several investigators have suggested that the trigger for β-END release is anaerobiosis.[394] Although an increase in lactate levels is consistently found when β-END is released, lactate formation alone does not seem sufficient to trigger release.[399,404,405] Change in pH has also been suggested as a trigger.[406] Below the anaerobic threshold, responses are individual and varied. Increases above baseline were lower at the end of a 100-mi supermarathon than at 60 mi, suggesting that, like glucocorticoids, EO tend to be depleted with extremely strenuous exercise.[293,407] The return to baseline values after exercise is quite rapid.[408]

The response of β-END to exercise shows a circadian variation.[232,409] Neither β-END nor met-enkephalin are released in synchrony with catecholamines.[271,410] The increased physical stress of a hot ambient temperature and dehydration progressively enhance the exercise-associated opiate response.[411] There is no effect of the menstrual cycle and no gender differences in response.[412] Hypoxia, hyperoxia, and altitude have no effect on exercise release.[413,414] Psychological stress does augment release, and other psychological variables that influence ACTH also affect β-END response.[281,285] The β-endorphin response to maximal intensity exercise decreased with training in one study,[316] but other investigations have provided variable results.[270,322,415,416] Negative energy balance over several days induces an enhanced opiate response to exercise, suggesting that the prime mover in prompting endorphin release during exercise is indeed metabolic.[417]

Physiologic Significance of the Exercise-Associated Opiate Increase

Endogeous opiates are messengers in a number of systems. The relationship of central and peripheral opiate systems remains unclear, but there is better understanding of the effects of opiate peptides in relation to exercise. Most studies of the functional importance of EO in exercise have employed the opiate antagonist naloxone although longer-acting oral preparations such a naltrexone are also useful tools in the investigation of opiate effects.

The Influence of Endogenous Opiates on Exercise Performance

Many investigations of the effect of opioids on cardiopulmonary function in exercise in physiologic and pathologic states have been carried out with entirely negative or physiologically insignificant results.[33,242,361,418–422] The time to exhaustion in both graded, maximal-intensity exercise and prolonged submaximal exercise depends on a number of physiologic factors, e.g., cardiopulmonary fitness and muscle glycogen stores, as well as determination and pain perception. Opiate receptor blockade does not have a significant effect on the time to exhaustion or other variables of performance.[33,418,419,421,422]

Endogenous Opiates, Analgesia, and Exercise

Exercise-associated analgesia[281] has been described in humans[423] but is more clearly demonstrated in animals,[424] and is generally regarded as similar to other forms of stress-induced opioid-mediated analgesia.[425] Opioid-induced analgesia by prolonged swimming and nonopioid-induced analgesia by short activity have been described.[426] What appears to be nonopioid (naloxone resistant) analgesia is found with exercise in the human.[427] "Negative addiction" was described in runners who continued to exercise against medical advice after being injured.[428] Tolerance of pain may be as great a factor in these circumstances as is a psychological dependency on running. The increasing frequency of running-associated injuries may also reflect analgesic effects as runners try to push themselves beyond their physiologic capacity.

Endogenous Opiates, Food Intake, and Exercise

It has been suggested that self-starvation, exacerbated by excessive exercise, is itself an addiction to the body's endogenous opioids.[429] Several lines of human and animal research have supported the idea that exercise and training may influence appetite and caloric intake and that the control of food and water intake may be mediated, at least in part, through endogenous opiates.[430] In humans, palatable food induces no change in endogenous opiates, but unpalatable food induces a stress response with increased β-END and ACTH levels.[431] Accurate human studies of dietary intake, endogeous opioids, and exercise are much more difficult because measurements of caloric intake and energy expenditure are relatively imprecise. In a now venerable study, caloric intake corresponded with physical activity only within the normal activity range, and sedentary individuals did not decrease intake to suit their relatively low energy expenditure.[432] When studies have examined caloric intake in response to an exercise program, the energy intake has in some cases decreased, or, where an increase was found, the change did not correspond to the energy requirements of the increased physical activity.[433–435] Acute exercise may also influence appetite in humans.[436]

Excessive physical activity, often described as purposeless, is a common feature of anorexia nervosa.[437] In such patients, obsessional personality characteristics are linked to high level exercising and that exercising is associated with a greater degree of obsessive-compulsive symptomatology.[438] Running is a socially acceptable way of expressing a drive to burn calories, so that at least some patients who present with exercise-associated amenorrhea may in fact have anorexia nervosa. The increased prevalence of anorexia nervosa, "cosmetic emaciation," and habitual exercise may be more than coincidental.[439] One-third of 182 women athletes practiced "pathogenic weight control behavior" and one-fifth of elite Norwegian athletes had eating disorders.[440,441] Similarities in personalities and behaviors have been described in habitual male athletes and teenage patients with anorexia nervosa; others have found few similarities.[442,443] Subtle changes in body image and eating attitudes do occur.[444] A particularly important observation was that animals that were allowed free access to a treadmill but were kept on a food schedule tended to increase their activity, self starve, and die.[445] The parallels with strict dieting and intense exercise in humans are obvious and triggers for the development of eating disorders in athletes have been defined as including prolonged periods of dieting, frequent weight fluctuations, a sudden increase in training volume, and traumatic events such as injury or loss of a coach.[446] Some view sports and exercise as an integral part of the pathogenesis and progression in self-starvation.[447]

Endogenous opioids have been popularly linked to what has come to be called "anorexia athletica." CSF total opioid activity is elevated in patients with anorexia nervosa, although β-END levels may be normal.[448] Naloxone administration stimulates weight gain in patients with anorexia nervosa, suggesting that EO may have an appetite-inhibitory effect in anorectic patients, in contrast to the findings in animal studies.[449,450] Naltrexone, a long-acting orally effective opioid blocker, has reported as effective in treating anorexia nervosa and bulimia.[451] The chronic elevation of peripheral β-END found in many women exercisers[452] may be related to the pathologic eating behavior common in women athletes. This important area should be studied further, perhaps with a more critical diagnostic appraisal.

Exercise Addiction and Opiates

The "positive addiction" of running, described many years ago, has maintained credibility despite a lack of systematic evidence.[452–454] For running or another activity to be considered addictive, three criteria must be established: pleasurable reward of the activity, tolerance requiring increasing activity to maintain the reward, and withdrawal symptoms if the activity is stopped.[455] Runners who discontinued their activity voluntarily or through injury experienced changes in sleep patterns, increased sexual tension, and other effects, but most information is anecdotal rather than scientific.[456] Evidence of exercise dependence has been reported in power lifters and competitive and recreational runners.[457–460] Direct human evidence of an opiate involvement is tenuous at best.[461]

Exercise and Mood

Psychologic advantages associated with running and other forms of exercise include reduced anxiety, better stress management, reduction of depression, improved self-esteem, an improved feeling of well-being, and a heightened sense of personal control.[462,463] Acute exercise, particularly running, is associated with a transient elevation in mood,[464,465] so that the "runners' high" has become an accepted part of the folklore of running and is popularly associated with altered EO levels induced by running. The evidence for the runner's high is almost entirely anecdotal, e.g., the account of Mandell,[466] with little objective psychometric data.

In human research, at least four variables have to be considered in the investigation of mood changes with acute exercise: the fitness of the subjects, the exercise activity, the dose of antagonist, and the means of measuring affect. The methodology of the studies has varied and therefore there is some discrepancy among the results. Most investigators have discounted EO involvement in exercise-associated mood changes.[467–469] Studies do support the concept that exercise has an acute effect on mood, but the changes do not measure up to the powerful images created by Mandell.

Reproductive Dysfunction and Endogenous Opiates

The role of endogenous opiates in exercise-associated reproductive dysfunction has been intensively investigated. This will be dealt with in the sections on the reproductive effects of exercise.

Endogenous Opiates in Acute Exercise-Induced Hormonal Change

The involvement of EO in controlling peripheral hormone levels led to investigations of their importance in exercise-induced hormonal changes, generally looking at acute change and using naloxone as the investigative probe. Unfortunately, the results have been inconsistent. Differences in subjects, fitness, exercise load, and dosage of naloxone make comparison among the studies very difficult. Growth hormone and PRL responses to exercise have been reported to be reduced[214,240] or unchanged[33,241] by naloxone in doses varying from 0.4 to 15 mg. Plasma catecholamines, norepinephrine, and epinephrine have been reported to be enhanced by high-dose naloxone (12.2 mg)[33] and unchanged with a 10-fold lower dose.[470] Similarly, exercise-induced increases in plasma renin activity and aldosterone were increased with high-dose naloxone and were not changed with lower doses of this opiate antagonist. An infusion of β-END induced changes in insulin and glucagon, suggesting possible physiologically significant involvement.[471] These various findings suggest that EO are involved in the hormonal response to stressful exercise but that their physiologic importance remains to be clarified.

Summary

Physical exercise involves a complex interrelation of cardiac, pulmonary, vascular, metabolic, hormonal, psychological, neurologic, and biochemical functions. It is perhaps the most physiologic stimulus that can be used to "stress" the organism. The involvement of endorphins and other opiates in many of these areas has justifiably stimulated research interest. Such work has clearly shown that endorphins are involved in exercise-associated analgesia and are clearly not involved to a significant degree in determining exercise performance. Involvement in mood alteration and at least some hormonal changes seem likely, but further work is required to demonstrate EO involvement in reproductive dysfunction and exercise addiction. We can only guess at the importance of EO in other areas, such as metabolism and even bowel function, where "runners' trots" are an interesting but poorly explained phenomenon.

It is important that approaches to the problems be multidisciplinary and that subjects' fitness and training, the exercise methodology, and the method of administering antagonists used in acute studies be given careful consideration in designing studies. The emotional responses to impending exercise may vary depending on the familiarity of the subject with physical activity.

The psychological and physiologic responses to exercise are different between habitual exercisers and untrained individuals. Investigations should control for fitness and attempt to diminish stress as a component in the response to exercise. This is also important in animal experiments, where investigators take little account of the stress in animals forced to exercise. It is possible to train animals to run spontaneously and to quantitate such activity. However, it is naive to believe that opiates work in isolation without interaction with other hormones and neuromodulators. Before full understanding can be achieved, the role of many other similarly active substances must be clarified.

PROLACTIN AND EXERCISE

Prolactin has received much attention in regard to exercise because increased levels of PRL are associated with menstrual dysfunction in women and impaired spermatogenesis and decreased libido in men. No teleologically satisfactory explanation for the exercise-associated changes in PRL has been suggested. The transient effects of exercise are comparable to other physiologic stimuli on PRL except in extreme situations.[263] Levels increase with exercise in sedentary controls[20,64,202,241,251,258,310,472–474] and in recreational and competitive runners.[183,214,262,309,407,425,475,476] Levels rapidly normalize even after very strenuous activity.[477] The effects of training appear minimal, as equivalent exercise loads produce generally similar serum PRL increases in trained and untrained individuals.[301,478–480] Some researchers have suggested that the PRL response occurs only in trained individuals[183,481] and differs according to the degree of training.[482] Serum PRL may not increase after a typical daily training session[483] or even during intensive exercise in amenorrheic runners.[257,310] This is not solely because of the hypoestrinism, as PRL levels increase in agonadal women in response to exercise.[183] Dopamine agonists are capable of suppressing the prolactin-induced increase associated with exercise;[484] the lack of response in amenorrheic athletes suggests that an increased tonic dopaminergic tone may be present. This could contribute to exercise-associated dysfunction. Levels are elevated after participation in competitive team sports and normalize within 3 to 4 h after the competition.[485,486]

Effects of Training on Prolactin

Basal PRL levels have been described as being reduced in trained male runners and in women runners with an increased training load[300,487,488] but not in swimmers, in whom PRL levels increase with heavier training.[452] It is unclear whether the increase persists when training loads are kept constant for a long period. Relatively light training in previously sedentary individuals and weight training are not sufficient to suppress PRL levels.[169,489,490] Nocturnal secretion is augmented on days when endurance training takes place.[491] Even with lower basal prolactin levels, exercise can induce a larger prolactin increase in trained runners than in untrained individuals.[492]

Mechanisms

The mechanisms of PRL increase with exercise are unclear. The response to stimulation with metoclopramide is reduced,[480] and domperidone increases the prolactin response to exercise.[493] Clonidine, an α_2-adrenergic agonist, has no effect on exercise-associated changes in prolactin.[494] Buspirone and valproate increase basal and exercise-stimulated levels.[221,495] Neither hormone replacement therapy nor birth control pills altered prolactin response.[176,496]

Hyperoxia and hypoxia have no consistent effect on timing of prolactin release.[189,478,497–499] Prolactin levels may increase when the anaerobic threshold is reached, perhaps synchronously with a GH increase.[500] Even prolonged (90-min) exercise below this threshold fails to elicit any response.[501] Treatment with a base and with lactic acid both induce a response, but glucose loading or depletion has no effect.[501–503] Prolactin response to exercise may be changed by environmental heat and changes in body temperature but not acute changes in fluid balance,[504–510] is reduced by facial cooling[505,511]; and is exaggerated by stress and reduced with habituation.[202,512]

Prolactin increments with exercise appear to be correlated with pro-opiomelanocortin derivatives, ACTH, and beta-endorphins.[513] Inconsistent effects of naloxone have been reported.[20,33,470,514,515] The response to thyrotropin releasing hormone (TRH) may be decreased in trained female subjects[480] and augmented in male subjects.[70] Serotonin may also be a controlling factor.[516] The control of and effects of exercise-associated PRL responses remain enigmatic. It is possible that mildly elevated prolactin levels induced by physiological events such as exercise may be overinterpreted in clinical situations.

EXERCISE, TRAINING, AND THE HYPOTHALAMIC-PITUITARY-GONADAL AXIS

One area that has long been considered an exception to the rule that exercise is good for you involves the reproductive response to training, particularly in young women. The effects of strenuous physical activity on the reproductive system in women have gained widespread recognition: delayed menarche, oligoamenorrhea, inadequate luteal phase, and anovulatory cycles occur, although probably not with the frequency that was originally suggested. Research on the effects of exercise on the hypothalamic-pituitary-gonadal (HPG) axis in men has been performed for a considerably longer time, but without the publicity given to studies in women. Attention was focused on the effects of physical activity on men when it became apparent that parallels exist between the sexes in terms of the chronic reproductive effects of exercise. This section will review the acute and chronic effects of strenuous physical activity on the HPG axis in men and women and examine mechanisms that may be involved in those changes.

TABLE 31-3. Factors Determining Exercise Associated Changes in Serum Testosterone Levels

Synthesis/secretion	Gonadotropin mediated (LH and FSH) Other (prolactin, catecholamines)
Testicular blood flow	
Protein binding	Specific, high affinity (SHBG, CBG) Non-specific, low affinity (albumin)
Clearance	Target tissue uptake and metabolism Hepatic metabolism

Acute Exercise and the HPG Axis in Men

Serum testosterone levels at any particular time depend on a number of factors (Table 31-3), some of which can be altered by acute exercise or training. It is important to note that luteinizing hormone (LH) pulses or acute LH increments do not produce a testosterone increment in less than 20 to 30 min.[517] An exercise-associated increase in serum testosterone levels occurring with exercise before this time cannot be the result of an LH effect. Testosterone is bound in circulation to a specific high-affinity plasma protein, sex hormone–binding globulin (SHBG), and to albumin, which has a large capacity but low affinity. Substantial changes in albumin can occur without significant effects on the levels of total testosterone. A small amount (less than 2 percent) of testosterone circulates as the free steroid. The binding of testosterone to SHGB reduces its clearance. It seems likely that the biologically active portion of the hormone is bound to albumin and the small unbound fraction,[518,519] which together amount to approximately 35 percent of the total levels. The majority (>95 percent) of testosterone (4 to 10 mg daily) is secreted directly from the testes. In males, approximately half the testosterone produced is cleared through the liver and the remainder is cleared through extrahepatic metabolism.[520] The androgen target organs, including muscle, are responsible for extrahepatic clearance. It is apparent that along with changes in synthesis and secretion, modifications of binding or clearance could play significant roles in changes in circulating testosterone in response to physical activity. As with other hormonal systems, acute exercise-associated responses of the male HPG axis depend on the intensity and duration of the activity and the fitness of the individual.

Short-Term Exercise and the HPG Axis

The first paper on the effects of short-term strenuous physical activity on testicular androgens, which was published in 1973, summarized most of the questions and problems that still remain to be explained.[522] Increases in circulating total and biologically active testosterone levels have been reported during free and treadmill running, weight training, resistance exercise, and ergometer cycling and have ranged from 13 percent to 185 percent.[73,258,522–529] The testosterone response has been reported to increase with increased exercise load.[530,531] Similar workloads produce similar responses regardless of whether the load is aerobic or anaerobic.[532] In this situation the response seems to differ from that of cortisol, in which the increase begins at the anaerobic threshold. Dietary intake may modify basal levels of testosterone but not the exercise response to high-intensity resistance exercise.[533] Increased and decreased ambient temperature, altitude, hypoxia, and dehydration similarly have no effect on testosterone responses to intense exercise.[189,534–536] Acute exercise-induced testosterone increments are also seen in older men, despite their very different hormonal milieu (higher estradiol, higher SHBG, and lower free testosterone.).[537–539]

Although a 120-min swim terminating in a maximal effort induced a clear increase in circulating testosterone,[522] a consistent decrease in serum testosterone levels was seen in elite swimmers undertaking a tethered swim graded to maximum during approximately 14 min.[540] There is no clear reason for this unexpected finding. Increases in androstenedione and estrogens have also been reported.[257] Conflicting evidence exists with regard to gonadotropin response: LH and FSH levels have been reported as unchanged,[73,524] increased,[258,541] and decreased.[525]

Mechanism of Exercise-Associated Testosterone Increase

Problems arise in trying to explain the exercise-associated increase in serum testosterone levels because of the inconsistent LH response to short-term intense exercise and because serum testosterone levels increase more quickly than would be anticipated from an increase in serum LH. A variety of mechanisms have been proposed. Nonspecific mechanisms associated with short-term exercise-induced serum testosterone elevations include a decreased metabolic clearance rate (MCR) and decreased plasma volume. Testosterone is cleared via hepatic and extrahepatic mechanisms. Hepatic blood flow approximates 1,250 liters/m^2 per day; the MCR of testosterone through the liver is approximately half this value. This implies that the 50 percent reduction in hepatic blood flow that is observed during strenuous exercise[542] should have little effect on the MCR of testosterone. However, clearance through the liver depends on protein binding and hepatic blood flow. Binding to a specific protein such as SHBG inhibits hepatic metabolism, whereas albumin binding does not. Thus the splanchnic extraction of testosterone approximates 50 percent. The real hepatic reserve may therefore be smaller than would be anticipated from blood flow and clearance rate figures. The metabolic clearance rate of testosterone has been described as being reduced during physical activity.[543,544] Exercise rates in both studies were moderate, and the time course of clearance changes seems to occur after the testosterone increments reported elsewhere.[258,523] Suitable markers for extrahepatic clearance have not been described. Measurement of 3 alpha-androstanediol glucuronide may provide a marker for clearance through tissues that convert testosterone to dihydrotestosterone prior to use. Although this excludes the liver, it also excludes muscle, which uses testosterone directly.

Changes in hemoconcentration were considered important in some[514,528,529] but by no means all studies.[258,525–527,541,543] The assumptions are that measured components such as hematocrit and hemoglobin accurately reflect the degree of fluid loss, that changes are not influenced by the differential binding of the steroid, and that physiologic changes such as increased temperature do not affect binding. The association constants of testosterone with SHBG (1.6 to 1.9 $\times$ 10^9 liters/mol) and albumin (4 $\times$ 10^4 liters/mol) are very different.[545] Because of the characteristics of testosterone binding, even substantial changes in albumin have little influence on circulating testosterone levels. Based on the association constants, it can be calculated that if the serum albumin doubled without a change in SHBG, the increase in total testosterone would approximate 6 percent. Although variable hemoconcentration has been reported with different forms of exercise, circulating SHBG changes little with short-term or longer-term running, and increases in the testosterone/SHBG ratio suggest that hemoconcentration does not play a significant role. A confusing study reports an increase in testosterone that exceeds that of SHBG, yet free testosterone also increases.[79]

For nonspecific mechanisms to be responsible for the acute exercise-induced rise in serum testosterone, we would expect all circulating steroids to be affected in the same manner given that MCR and hemoconcentration do not differentiate between hormones. The temporal patterns of change among the various steroid hormones does not provide this picture.[258] In one study, the testosterone increase was distinct from those of androstenedione and dehydroepiandrosterone (DHEA), adrenal androgens whose increments were simultaneous with that of cortisol.[258] The clear difference in responses among the hormones suggests that specific mechanisms are involved.

What mechanism could exist independent of gonadotropin stimulation of testosterone? The involvement of the sympathetic system in testicular testosterone production has suggested that a direct neural pathway may stimulate testosterone production during exercise in some species.[522,546] As discussed earlier, circulating catecholamine levels also increase substantially during exercise. β-blockade inhibits testosterone responses to exercise, whereas L-dopa, phentolamine, and clonidine have no effect.[524,547] It remains unclear exactly what mechanisms may be operative in increasing circulating testosterone levels in any exercise protocol, and it is possible that the mechanisms responsible early in exercise differ from those observed subsequently. As a consistent increase in testosterone was observed prior to cycle ergometry[258] and testosterone levels were proportional to anticipated workload,[523] there is an anticipatory rise that is presumably independent of hepatic perfusion or hemoconcentration.

The Effects of Prolonged Exercise on the HPG Axis in Men

Prolonged acute submaximal exercise bouts (exceeding 2 h) may be associated with complex changes in circulating androgen. Responses have been examined under laboratory conditions and during free activity such as marathon and ultramarathon races as well as in cross-country skiing. Several studies have reported an initial testosterone increase with exercise, followed by a decline to or below baseline values.[68,265,477,485–525,548–552] The decrease appears to be proportional to the preceding workload.[553] Lowered testosterone levels may follow even relatively short-term but strenuous physical activity.[73] Stresses such as surgery, myocardial infarction, and simulated warfare training also result in decreased testosterone levels. Several mechanisms may be important in decreasing circulating testosterone levels during and after prolonged exercise, including suppressed gonadotropin release and a more direct effect by elevated prolactin, cortisol, or catecholamine levels. Alterations in β-endorphin have been popularly blamed for acute exercise-associated suppression of the HPG axis in both men and women, although this has been difficult to prove as opiate antagonism does not prevent the exercise-induced decrease in LH that has been observed by some but by no means all investigators.[488,507,548,550,554] Response to gonadotropin releasing hormone (GnRH) has been reduced[555] and increased[477] after prolonged, exhaustive exercise. Pulsatile LH release does not decrease after 60 and 120 min of treadmill running in men, although the area under the multiple sample curve is decreased after exercise.[548,554] The response of testosterone levels to stimulation with HCG has also been described as being reduced.[555]

We are again faced with the difficulty of explaining a change in serum testosterone levels that does not appear to be mediated by alterations in central control. Prolactin responses to intense or prolonged exertion are transient and unlikely to influence postexercise testosterone levels. In one study, decreases in serum testosterone followed increments in cortisol levels induced by insulin hypoglycemia or injection of hydrocortisone hemisuccinate.[556] As described earlier, increases in serum cortisol accompany prolonged or intense exercise; therefore, a similar mechanism may be operative. A decline in serum testosterone levels was observed accompanying an exercise-induced cortisol increment.[258] A persistent increase in catecholamines accompanies and follows physical activity; this may be related to testicular resistance to endogenous gonadotropins.[477] The exercise-associated decline in serum testosterone levels remains unclear. It is possible that the decline results from subtle interference at either the hypothalamic or the gonadal level or because of increased androgen consumption after strenuous exercise to repair structural and metabolic injury to the tissues.

Effect of Endurance Training on the HPG Axis in Men

The consistent testosterone decline that follows prolonged submaximal exercise suggests that there may be a continuing suppression of circulating testosterone associated with chronic involvement in endurance training. A recent review determined that there was a consistent range of alterations in gonadal hormones and semen profile even leading to clinical oligospermia.[557] Several cross-sectional and prospective studies have supported this idea. In contrast, military training including a heavy physical exercise component resulted in an increase in mean plasma testosterone, androstenedione, and LH with no significant change in SHBG.[558] Prospective studies using two relatively light training regimes also found increased levels of testosterone.[559,560] Some cross-sectional studies have reported no change in serum testosterone even with heavy training.[561]

Symptomatic Impairment of the HPG Axis in Men

In contrast to cyclic endocrine control of reproduction in women, endocrine control of the male reproductive system is steady state with a typical endocrine servomechanism. Symptomatic changes in testicular androgenesis and spermatogenesis are slower and less clearly definable. There is some evidence that males with a high level of physical activity may have some impairment of fertility.[557,562] Normal sperm counts are generally found in runners even with very strenuous training regimes.[561] Anecdotal information has also suggested that libido may be impaired in some runners during periods of intense endurance training.[300,563] Reduced testosterone levels may play a role in this, but chronic fatigue could also be significant. Predicting the athlete with problems is not easy; only body mass index and exercise load have been able to predict.[564,565] Although osteoporotic fractures in a hypogonadal marathoner with anorexia nervosa have been described in a case report,[566] fears about widespread effects on bone loss in men do not appear to have been justified.[567] There are two anecdotal accounts of symptomatic hypogonadal male runners being treated successfully with estrogen receptor antoganists (clomiphene and tamoxifen),[568,569] but the more general approach to review with an athlete is the possibility of decreasing the exercise load. For addicted athletes, this is very often not a option they are willing to adopt. In the latter case, recurrent muscle injury was relieved by tamoxifen.[569]

Androgen-dependent skeletal muscle hypertrophy and synergism with GH are well accepted. Increased utilization of testosterone may be needed to maintain muscle in chronic exercisers, and so basal testosterone or testosterone/cortisol ratios may be important.[570] The problem of "overtraining"[299] is discussed in a subsequent section. A consequence of severe training regimes could be to reduce the repair of muscle damage because of lowered circulating testosterone levels. As testosterone and GH also interact in stimulating cardiac muscle hypertrophy, it is possible that significant lowering of testosterone levels influences the repair of cardiac muscle.

The aerobic capacity of runners is dependent on central and peripheral factors. There is a correlation between fitness as judged by maximal oxygen consumption and exercise-associated decreases in testosterone.[558] Testosterone increases the synthesis of erythropoietin, which stimulates erythropoiesis; lowered testosterone levels could be related to exercise-associated anemia, which has been described in endurance-trained athletes. It is, however, difficult to believe that the reductions in serum testosterone levels generally observed in endurance-trained athletes could affect erythropoiesis.

Physical inactivity, male gender, and elevated blood lipids are among the well-recognized risk factors for atherosclerotic heart disease. Androgens are important in regulating blood lipid levels: The levels of high-density lipoprotein cholesterol (HDLC) in the blood of men are significantly lower than values in women. Because HDLC has a cardioprotective effect, the risk of atherosclerosis is increased in men. In contrast, endurance training has been associated with lower overall cholesterol, lower low-density lipoprotein cholesterol (LDLC), and higher HDLC.[571,572] This change in pattern may contribute to the beneficial effects of exercise on atherosclerotic heart disease. It is unclear whether the physiologic reductions in androgens could play a significant role in these changes. Androgens may also be important in hepatic and renal function; in the brain, including effects on aggression; and in the immune system. Although there has been concern about the normal functioning of the immune system in endurance-trained athletes, any effect of lowered but still physiologic serum testosterone levels on the immune system and on hepatic and renal function remains speculative. Social and other pressures influence aggression, so that any short-term increases or longer-term reductions in testosterone would be likely to have little influence.

Mechanisms of Long-Term Activity-Associated Suppression of Circulating Testosterone Levels

The fall in serum testosterone levels must result from decreased production rates, decreased binding, or increased clearance. There is scant evidence of decreased binding.[300] No studies have shown long-term increases in hepatic or extrahepatic clearance of testosterone in endurance-trained or other athletes, although basal estradiol clearance is increased in women athletes, presumably through increased hepatic metabolism.[573] Evidence of an altered LH pulsatile release in male runners[548,554] has been disputed.[574,575] LH pulse frequency is not significantly altered in runners with acute exercise.[548,554] The GnRH-induced LH response appears to be impaired.[548] No evidence has supported increased opioidergic tone as being important in the generation of GnRH-LH suppression in athletes, and the effects of catecholamines have received little attention.[407,575] Chronic elevation of serum cortisol levels has been associated with overtraining or a shift in cortisol/testosterone ratios associated with strenuous exercise.[329] It is possible but unlikely that such a change could exert a direct effect on testicular testosterone production. Serum PRL levels are chronically depressed rather than elevated and are therefore not likely to be involved in the fall in testosterone in highly trained male runners.[574]

Suppression of the HPG axis in men is associated with starvation, a vegetarian diet, and a low-fat, high-fiber diet.[576,577] An anorectic subgroup with reduced total and free testosterone and a preoccupation with caloric intake and lean body mass was described among a group of 20 high-mileage runners.[563] Significant reductions in total and free testosterone in wrestlers were associated with their practices in trying to "make weight."[578] The possibility of an association between exercise and anorexia nervosa has been raised, but the reliability of human data has been criticized. Although there were significant correlations among total and free testosterone and body weight and body fat in young male wrestlers, no correlation was observed between physiologic reductions in serum testosterone levels and body fat in cross-sectional studies of runners and controls.[300,444,578] Leptin, an appetite-suppressing hormone secreted by fat cells, has been associated with hypogonadism in women but circulates in normal levels in endurance trained men.[579]

In summary, it seems likely that the chronic suppressive effects of endurance training on the HPG axis in men result from a mechanism of inhibition that is central and is analogous to that described in women, perhaps involving a nutritional-metabolic influence. The possibility of peripheral effects of increased utilization of steroids is worthy of further investigation. It is unlikely that clinical manifestations of reproductive suppression with training are common in men. Further investigation is essential to provide continuing reassurance that "exercise is good for you" and to define the physiologic boundaries and the effects of overstepping them. As a final comment on male reproductive function, evidence suggests that contrary to widely held belief, abstaining from sex does not improve athletic performance.[580]

EXERCISE AND THE REPRODUCTIVE SYSTEM IN WOMEN

Acute Exercise-Associated Changes in Reproductive Hormones

There have been few studies of hormonal responses to acute exercise in women.[183,258,259,263,264,475,549,581–583] In general, these studies reflect the problems in explaining the responses of male reproductive hormones to acute exercise. Variable responses of LH, follicle stimulating hormone (FSH), estradiol, progesterone, and testosterone have been described. Some studies[183,257] have also addressed the question of how acute responses to exercise might be involved in the genesis of exercise-associated amenorrhea by examining differences in the responses to exercise in normally menstruating and amenorrheic runners. Such differences as there are tend to reflect the chronic suppression of the HPG axis rather than provide a reason for the amenorrhea; there is scant evidence that acute exercise-induced hormonal responses play a significant role in the genesis of reproductive dysfunction.[183]

Reproductive Effects of Exercise in Women

A popular picture has emerged in which thin high-mileage runners commonly have reproductive problems. Endurance training, particularly distance running, has become associated with an increased frequency of reproductive dysfunction in women; delayed menarche, an inadequate luteal phase, anovulatory cycles, and oligoamenorrhea have all been reported as being more common in women athletes. The significance of physical activity alone in generating exercise-associated reproductive dysfunction has been increasingly questioned.[584] Prospective studies attempting to reproduce changes have shown little effect.[585] It seems likely that "runner's amenorrhea" or any other overt reproductive dysfunction usually blamed on endurance training occurs only in individuals in whom another factor is compromising the normal functioning of the HPG-axis. In this section we will examine the accuracy of the runner's amenorrhea stereotype and consider mechanisms that might be responsible for reproductive dysfunction and subclinical changes.

Pubertal development and menarche are delayed in competitive athletes and ballet dancers.[584] This delay appears to reflect the level of competition but not the individual sports activity. There was no difference in age of menarche among groups of athletes from various sports disciplines or between swimmers and runners, although both groups differed from unathletic girls. Menarche is delayed in ballet dancers to a much greater degree than it is in Olympic athletes.[586] Some authors have offered explanations for the delay in menarche that are unrelated to physical activity. Relatively low body fat gives prepubertal individuals a greater strength/weight ratio, a benefit in sports such as gymnastics. A somatotype with increased height, longer legs, narrower hips, and better neuromuscular coordination occurs more frequently with delayed puberty; this may result in better athletic performance. Early maturers may socialize away from sports activity. Factors related to physical activity and nutritional status are, however, more likely to be involved.

Some aspect of physical activity appears important as only premenarcheally trained athletes have a significant delay in the onset of menses, proportional to the time in training.[587] Advancement of pubertal stages and/or resumption of menses occurred in ballet dancers during inactivity, suggesting that energy balance might be involved.[588] However, a genetic component may also be present, so that the resolution of the question is very difficult even with studies designed to control for all these factors. In dancers, leanness is the best predictor of menarche and is superior in this regard to activity level and maternal age of menarche.[589]

Subclinical luteal-phase abnormalities and anovulatory cycles are relatively common. Reduced luteal phase length and midluteal progesterone levels in runners and teenage swimmers, abnormalities of basal body temperature graphs, delayed endometrial maturation in runners, and decreased salivary progesterone levels in recreational runners have all been reported.[590] The frequency of secondary amenorrhea/oligomenorrhea in runners was examined in a study based on replies received from 128 women not taking birth control pills out of 400 members of U.S. collegiate track and field and cross-country teams.[591] The frequency of amenorrhea (defined as three periods or less in the previous year) varied from 6 to 43 percent depending on weekly mileage. The prevalence of menstrual dysfunction has been considerably lower in subsequent investigations.[592–596] Such surveys are not based on true epidemiologic principles and may be biased because runners with problems

TABLE 31-4. Pathophysiologic Factors of Exercise-Induced Changes in Reproductive Function

Stress of training and/or competing
Physical stresses
Emotional stresses
Nutritional and metabolic
Abnormalities of nutrition and energy drain
Altered lean-fat ratio
Loss of weight
Predisposition
Immature hypothalamus—young gynecological age
History of menstrual irregularity
Hormonal changes with exertion
Repeated acute changes
Chronic changes

are more likely to respond; some researchers have suggested that there is not a significant increase in exercise-associated amenorrhea.[594]

Reproductive dysfunction has been associated mostly with runners, with little investigation of other forms of activity. Swimmers and cyclists have a lower frequency of reproductive dysfunction than do runners.[597] The relatively greater frequency in the runners correlated with body build. Similarly, there is a lower prevalence of oligoamenorrhea in racquet players and sprinters than there is in middle-distance runners (800 to 5,000 m).[598] This also correlated with a more linear physique. Surprisingly, ball players were not very different from distance runners despite being clearly different in physique.

Factors Involved in the Genesis of Exercise-Associated Menstrual Dysfunction (Table 31-4)

Functional abnormalities of the HPG axis have been associated with the extremes of reproductive life, abnormal dietary practices, extremes of body fat content, psychological stress, and pathologic conditions including androgen excess, hyperprolactinemia, hypothyroidism, and ovarian failure. Although acute exercise-induced elevations in serum testosterone and prolactin levels occur, they have generally been considered insignificant and, together with psychological stress, have been abandoned as possible causes for exercise-associated reproductive dysfunction.[584] The endocrine, neuroendocrine, and metabolic characteristics of oligoamenorrheic runners has, as described later, been well characterized and a consensus has formed that exercise-associated reproductive dysfunction is caused by a nutritional deficit. The "messenger" linking the nutritional distress and the reproductive system remains to clarified. A further evolution has been the recognition that athletic amenorrhea is not a single entity but may encompass patients with anorexia nervosa, with the female athlete triad, and exercise-related menstrual irregularity.[599] The three groups are clearly related, overlapping but distinguishable. The roles of psychological stress, physical stress, and predisposition are considered of little importance and are reviewed elsewhere.

The Endocrinology of Exercise-Associated Reproductive Dysfunction

The female athlete triad consists of amenorrhea, anorexia, and osteoporosis: it can perhaps be distinguished from exercise-associated reproductive dysfunction in the matter of degree. "Athletic amenorrhea" has generally been considered as hypothalamic with low or normal gonadotropins and estradiol; occasional patients have a more clearly pathologic cause for their amenorrhea.[584] Abnormalities in several systems are now recognized. There are disturbances of varying severity in the pulsatile release of GnRH with abnormalities of pituitary release of LH and FSH and abnormal ovarian function.[600–602] Accompanying the reproductive changes are activation of the CRH-ACTH-cortisol axis,[310,311–314,320,602–604] suppression of the TRH-TSH-thyroid axis,[87,89,602] and metabolic abnormalities including hypoinsulinemia, lower glucose levels, elevated IGFBP-1, reduced IGF-1/IGFBP-1 ratio, and elevated growth hormone and GHBP. Some have interpreted the metabolic changes as a physiological adaptation to maintain adequate blood glucose levels in a state of energy deficiency.[604]

Chronically altered frequency and amplitude of LH pulsatile release have been observed in the early follicular phase in normally menstruating and frequently in amenorrheic runners.[602,605–607] It is generally inferred that an inhibitory mechanism is responsible for the reduction in LH pulsatile release. Neurotransmitter control of the cycle is complex and involves catecholamines, catechol estrogens, EO, and probably other neuromodulators. For normal GnRH pulses to occur, two events are necessary: first, the individual GnRH neurons must release their product in a cyclic fashion, and second, that cyclic release must be made synchronous. It is likely that these two events require different stimulatory neurotransmitters. Norepinephrine and GABA may be involved in stimulation. Evidence strongly suggests that dopamine and EO inhibit the GnRH-LH axis physiologically through the menstrual cycle and inappropriately in women with hypothalamic amenorrhea.[608] Circulating β-endorphin levels are higher in amenorrheic than in eumenorrheic runners,[312] but the administration of opiate antagonists to amenorrheic runners has not confirmed the popular view that EO suppress the GnRH-LH axis[609,610]; however, increases in pulse amplitude were reported in some subjects with naloxone and an orally active analog, nalmefene.[611,612] Melatonin, norepinephrine, dopamine, and catechol estrogens have also been linked to exercise associated oligoamenorrhea.[309,452,613–617]

Body Composition and Nutrition

Body fat has been suggested as a trigger for the onset of menarche and the maintenance of normal cycles.[618] Low body weight, dieting, weight loss, and reduced body fat are associated with primary and secondary amenorrhea. Some studies have supported an association of low body fat with amenorrhea in women who exercise.[584] Amenorrheic athletes were lighter and leaner and had lost more weight after the onset of running than were their normally menstruating counterparts in some studies, but several large-scale studies have failed to find an association between lower body fat and amenorrhea.[584] Some authors suggested that the linear physique of runners is more likely to be associated with amenorrhea but failed to find a correlation within this group.[619,620] The variability of findings suggests that methodologic considerations may influence the conclusions. There are method-specific differences in body fat estimates, and differing conclusions can be drawn from the same population depending on the means of calculation.[621]

One study utilizing the hydrostatic method, the "gold standard," suggested that menstrual irregularity in exercise is more frequent in runners with a low percentage of body fat.[622] Arguably the most accurate means of measuring fat and its component parts is MRI. Decreased subcutaneous fat and internal depots were observed.[623,624]

However, in the final analysis, low body fat is not invariably associated with menstrual irregularity, and menstrual irregularity is not invariably associated with reduced body fat. A further argument against the critical body fat has been the lack of an explanation of how fat depots could communicate with the hypothalamus.

A possible answer to this has been found in the discovery of leptin. Leptin is a secretory product of adipocytes and appears to act as a satiety agent to the brain specifically modulating the expression of neuropeptide Y, an orexigenic peptide. Although body mass does correlate with leptin and low fat mass,[625] there remain some questions. Leptins are low in normal-weight women with hypothalamic amenorrhea and weight-restored amenorrheic women with anorexia nervosa.[626,627] Levels in men are lower than in women with smaller body mass.[626,628] Leptin levels correlate with glucose, insulin, and glucagon and may occur with fasting or exercise without change in body weight.[626,629–633] Finally, it appears that granulosa and cumulus cells can manufacture leptin,[634] raising the possible question of whether normal leptin levels are a reflection of ovarian function rather than a required factor.

Dietary restriction without a change in body fat has been the other major hypothesis; this too shares the difficulty in explaining exactly what the messenger might be.[635] Malnutrition reduces gonadotropin levels before puberty and in adults.[635–639] Injuries preventing exercise in amenorrheic young ballet dancers precipitated menarche or were followed by the resumption of menses with no weight change.[588] It was postulated that an "energy drain" of exercise may delay menarche or result in amenorrhea without alteration of body composition. A relatively small change in weight of 1 to 2 kg around the critical level can regulate menstruation in some athletes.[311,587] Cross-sectional studies of diet have provided conflicting evidence of macronutrient deficiencies in amenorrheic athletes,[311,317,626,640–648] although the most consistent finding has been that amenorrheic runners have a caloric deficit compared with their normally menstruating peers. Dietary intake even in normally menstruating runners does not seem to match the increase in energy output that their activity requires.[584] The long-held belief that if dietary intake is constant and energy output is increased, weight will be progressively lost is open to question. Malnutrition is capable of altering the metabolic cost of exercise,[646] and it is possible that the "relative malnutrition" of physical activity can have the same effect.[649] Runners have a consistently superior food efficiency compared with nonrunners.[606] As the requirements for the body to remain efficient become more stringent, reproductive function may be initially compromised and later sacrificed to minimize energy loss, together with steps to reduce glucose utilization and lower metabolism.[630] The thermal readjustment with luteal levels of progesterone requires an increase of a mean 500 calories per cycle.[647] A teleological hypothesis would suggest that reproductive shutdown to save the energy cost of the menstrual cycle is a more immediate goal than preventing pregnancy, although the long-term effects are the same. Amenorrheic runners have been shown to have a decrease in the metabolic rate, supporting the concept that energy balance is critical in the development of reproductive dysfunction and that there appears to be a relationship between energy balance and estradiol levels.[648,650] Short-term aggressive refeeding, however, has produced mixed results.

Consequences and Management

Other than transient impairment of fertility, loss of bone has become the major concern of athletic amenorrhea. Bone density is lowered in amenorrheic athletes.[651] Estrogen status and heredity are major determinants of bone mass and together with diet probably explain most of the variance in bone mineral density seen in amenorrheic athletes.[652,653] There is conflicting evidence about whether luteal phase abnormalities can cause problems with loss of bone.[654–657] Hormone replacement therapy has been recommended as appropriate in amenorrheic young women with evidence of bone loss or even for prophylaxis, but there is limited evidence of an effectiveness.[658]

Management of exercise-associated reproductive dysfunction remains a matter of debate. Estrogen therapy will reverse many of the metabolic changes alone,[659] but the usual advice provided is to reverse the physiological abnormalities that caused the problem, i.e., to reduce exercise load and increase dietary intake. Anecdotal information only suggests that this might be effective.[660] In a survey of physicians' self-reported treatments, hormone replacement was offered by 92 percent, calcium by 87 percent, vitamins by 26 percent, advice concerning increased calories by 64 percent, decreased workload by 57 percent, and weight gain by 43 percent.[661]

Summary

Prospective studies make it clear that oligoamenorrhea does not occur in healthy, normally menstruating women runners when their exercise load is increased. Nonetheless, there are changes in the function of the hypothalamic-pituitary axis. The changes that occur with training would progressively reduce the luteal phase and its accompanying caloric "waste" resulting from preparations for pregnancy. When nutrition is in question or when another factor is present, the need to conserve calories may be sufficient to stop menstruation altogether. Amenorrheic runners have a greater need to preserve calories through progressive reduction in the resting metabolic rate, but other messengers may be important. Pos-sible signals could include deficiencies of neurotransmitter pre-cursors, alteration in thyroid function, activation of "stress" hormones, alterations in glucoregulatory and other metabolic hormones, changes in steroid metabolism in fat tissue, changes in hepatic metabolism of binding proteins, and an exaggerated peripheral response to exercise in a nutritionally stressed subject. Bone health remains an issue for amenorrheic athletes, and individuals with prolonged amenorrhea should be monitored for changes in bone mineral density.

OVERTRAINING

Exercise training is designed to consistently upgrade physiological and metabolic variables. At an imprecisely defined and probably very individual threshold, a series of changes occurs that results in poorer performance despite increasing workload. This condition, poorly defined but well recognized by athletes, is usually called overtraining. Other terms that have been used with some shades of meaning include overload and overreaching. Overtraining is perhaps another example of a volume threshold effect in exercise.

The symptoms of overtraining are nonspecific. There may be fatigue, "banal illness," mood disturbance, frequent upper respiratory tract infections, and frequent minor injury, together with a decrease in performance.[662,663] The hypothesized causes for overtraining include amino acid imbalance, autonomic imbalance, and glycogen depletion.[664–666]

Several biological markers for recognizing overtraining have been suggested without universal acceptance. These include physiological performance, cortisol, cortisol to testosterone ratios, catecholamines, evidence of immune suppression, and psychological tests.[662,663,667–671] Management of the problem is rest, which may need to be prolonged, and training with a more individualized set of goals. The best management is clearly preventive.[672]

USE OF PERFORMANCE-ENHANCING ENDOCRINE DRUGS (DOPING) IN COMPETITIVE AND RECREATIONAL SPORTS ACTIVITY

The use of drugs and practices to enhance athletic performance is as old as organized competition. It is, however, now more scientific and widespread at all levels of sport. A universally acceptable definition of *doping* in sport remains elusive, although in a general sense it refers to using an artificial method to gain an unfair advantage in competition. The International Olympic Committee chose not to define doping per se but has banned specific substances or groups of substances and certain physical methods. Groups of drugs that they have banned include stimulants, narcotics, anabolic steroids, β-blockers, diuretics, and peptide hormones and their analogs. Physical methods also banned include blood doping (autotransfusion) and any chemical, pharmacologic, or physical manipulation such as urine substitution. Drugs such as alcohol, marijuana, local anesthetics, and corticosteroids are subject to restrictions. The banned drugs and practices are summarized in detail on the Olympic Organizations Web site (www.olympic.org) and were last updated in January 1998 (Table 31-5). More than 1 million individuals in the United States, including a quarter of a million adolescents, use or have used anabolic steroids in an industry whose annual receipts exceed $100 million more than 10 years ago.[672]

Since 1976 two-thirds of the infractions at the Olympic Games have been for the use of anabolic steroids. These drugs are used frequently without detection provided that they are discontinued early enough to allow elimination from the body and are perhaps masked by other substances. They are, therefore, particularly important in sport. Other drug usage relevant to endocrinology includes the use of human growth hormone and, more recently, erythropoietin to enhance muscle size and red blood cell mass, respectively. An international conference on Doping in Sport has provided a consensus statement termed the Lausanne statement that is available on the Internet (www.nodoping.org/Declaration_e.html). There is little that is new in this area: anecdotes continue to accumulate and, because it is unethical to take anabolic steroids for and to provide high doeses of drugs for research, we will probably not have any scientific evidence to indicate the effectiveness of the drugs and their dangers.

TABLE 31-5. Anabolic Steroids Banned by the International Olympic Committee

Bolasterone
Boldenone
Clostebol
Dihydrochlormethlytestosterone
Fluoxymesterone
Mesterolone
Metandienone
Methyltestosterone
Nandrolone
Norethandrolone
Oxandrolone
Oxymesterone
Oxymetholone
Stanozol
Testosterone and related compounds

Mens Sana in Corpore Sano: Ethical Aspects of Doping in Sports

Sport has meaning, purpose, and values that surpass the physical experience, including self-discipline, dedication, perseverence, and endurance. The sporting ideal is that individuals compete against each other based on their talent and training. Sport is also a focus for local, regional, and national pride. Governments recognize the nation-building role of sport and provide facilities and funding so that individuals can compete optimally in international competitions.

The Canadian Task Force on National Sport Policy established a long-term goal in the area of high-performance sport, attempting to "develop a Canadian Sport system which will provide opportunities to enable athletes with talent and dedication to *win* [emphasis added] at the highest levels of international competition."[673] It tied funding to international success. The task force report was published in 1988, the year in which a Canadian sprinter was deprived of the Olympic 100-m gold medal because his urine was found to contain traces of stanozolol. Although there is no direct link between sport policy and the use of anabolic steroids, the atmosphere fostered makes governments that fail to enforce the regulations of the International Olympic Committee at least as culpable as the athletes involved. Suspicions concerning the extent of doping in East Germany (because of the astounding success of the athletes) were proven when the political climate changed after the reunification of the two Germanies.[674] It is difficult to believe that other governments are not at least tacitly supporting doping programs. Some have suggested that national in-season testing protocols are designed to find out about clearance and masking of drugs rather than to find athletes breaking rules.

Winning at all costs becomes acceptable because of national and personal pride, media pressure to win, and the large financial rewards in some sports for the few who are very successful. When factors other than talent and training, such as the use of banned drugs and practices, enter into the results of competition, this is considered unfair and constitutes cheating. The use of doping—more euphemistic terms include *ergogenic aids* and *performance-enhancing drugs*—is considered to be cheating. There is in sport a moral climate in which such practices are acceptable if the risk of detection is low. Athletes no longer regard striving to win as important; winning even by risking the life or health of the athletes is the only acceptable outcome. Some may argue that the rules should be changed to permit individuals who wish to use anabolic steroids and other drugs to do so. These drugs could be viewed as just another aid, like complex machinery, efficient organization, and good training. Permitting the use of drugs may endanger the health of the athletes involved, but sport itself may be dangerous. We do not ban hang gliding or motorcycle racing; therefore, it may be argued, we have no right to interfere with an individual's choice. A physiologic rationale can be used that suggests that strenuous sports activity invariably places the participants in a catabolic state. Providing anabolic steroids merely returns the athlete to physiologic norms.

This question goes beyond the danger of steroids. Pressure to compete on an even basis demands that athletes who wish to compete must take performance-enhancing drugs or remain second class, a situation many people would regard as unfair. Winning should remain a triumph of talent, training, dedication, and character, not a triumph of chemistry. As Thomas Murray says, "If I said that I could put the shot 90 ft with the aid of a sling or 2 mi with a cannon, you would rightly tell me that I had missed the point of the sport."[675]

Physicians must also answer the specific ethical questions that apply to them. Should physicians refuse to provide anabolic steroids to athletes, or should they consider circumstances under which these drugs can be provided? Should doctors consider anabolic steroids as forbidden drugs in the sense of narcotic drugs? Because athletes seem to obtain adequate supplies of drugs from unofficial sources, should physicians refuse to monitor the health of individuals who are self-prescribing anabolic steroids? It is clearly unethical and unacceptable to provide a drug solely for the purpose of enhancing sports performance, but refusal to monitor a patient is less clear from an ethical point of view. Refusing to monitor patients may be a greater evil. Physicians should warn individuals in a nonjudgmental way about the known and possible dangers of steroids but should consider monitoring these patients for several reasons, including the health of the individual, the need for even anecdotal information about people taking these drugs, and because refusal by physicians to become involved, overestimating the benefits and understating the side effects, has probably increased the utilization of anabolic steroids. As care givers, physicians must ask themselves whether individuals taking these drugs are better off unsupervised. Would we abandon those who abuse narcotics or alcohol or prescription drugs?

Androgenic-Anabolic Steroids

Anabolic steroids are the most widely abused performance-enhancing drugs. The recognition that humoral factors, notably testosterone, are responsible for many of the visible differences in secondary sex characteristics and for gender differences in muscle mass and strength led to the attempted development of compounds that could differentially influence the androgenic and anabolic effects of testosterone. Such a disassociation has not been convincingly achieved, and particularly in high doses these drugs have strong androgenic effects. The medical indications for the use of anabolic steroids are relatively few. Use of anabolic steroids to enhance sport performance is not recognized; therefore, for physicians to prescribe them is at best unethical and at worst illegal.

Medical Indications for Anabolic Steroids

Generally accepted uses for anabolic-androgenic steroids include testosterone deficiency such as that resulting from bilateral orchidectomy, cryptorchidism, bilateral torsion, orchitis, vanishing testis syndrome, gonadotropin deficiency, and GnRH deficiency resulting from congenital absence or injury secondary to tumors, trauma, or irradiation.[676] Drugs can also be used with well-characterized pubertal delay. Indications for use in women include metastatic breast cancer and, for some anabolic steroids in low doses, as part of a hormone replacement program for postmenopausal women. In Canada, the problems of anabolic steroid abuse by athletes has led to restrictions on all androgen replacement, including that in postmenopausal women. Anabolic steroids have also been used in other conditions, including aplastic and hypoplastic anemias, debilitating disease (e.g., burns), and hereditary angioneurotic edema. These drugs have also been used for the promotion of growth and for osteoporosis. Their use in debilitating conditions, promotion of growth, and osteoporosis remains controversial. Some researchers have suggested that these drugs may be effective in speeding the healing of injured tissues, but this is of doubtful validity. There is no other medical reason for their use in sports medicine, where they are being used not to treat illness but to enhance performance in healthy young men and women.

Extent of the Use of Anabolic Steroids in Various Populations

Evidence on the extent of anabolic steroid use is elusive and consists largely of rumor and speculation. Medical authorities associated with the U.S. Olympic squad have identified a relatively small number of athletes but believe that the usage is widespread, particularly among athletes involved in weight lifting and track and field.[677] Other sources of information include the results of drug testing during training and at the time of competition and necessarily incomplete voluntary surveys of athletes at various levels admitting to steroid use. It is, however, apparent that the use of the drugs is frequent and extensive, especially at national and international levels of competition and in sports where a premium is placed on large body size and strength.

Judicial and other official inquiries have been held in Canada, the United States, Australia, and the United Kingdom. These inquiries generally focused on steroid use in athletes at the highest levels of national and international competition. Testimony was heard that suggested that up to 80 percent of male athletes at international levels use steroids at some time during their training. An Australian senate standing committee heard evidence that 70 percent of Australian athletes competing internationally had used performance-enhancing drugs.

Robert Kerr of San Gabriel, California, testified before the Dubin Commission in Canada that he prescribed anabolic steroids to approximately 20 medalists in the 1984 Olympic Games and had also prescribed steroids to several thousand athletes in various sports, including track and field, baseball, ice hockey, roller hockey, cycling, and swimming.[678] Other steroid-prescribing physicians gave similar testimony. The Australian committee heard testimony that children as young as 10 years of age were given steroids to enhance performance.[679] Most countries now have clear antidoping legislation, yet the public perception persists that it is perhaps impossible to do well in sport without artificial aids. The admitted use of androstenedione, a drug banned by the U.S. Olympic committee but permitted in baseball, by a high-achieving baseball player tends to support the public view. Recent estimates of anabolic steroid use are hard to find, perhaps because of decreasing interest. Pat Connolly estimated that 30 percent and 40 percent of the U.S. womens' track and field teams at the 1984 and 1988 Olympic Games, respectively, had used anabolic steroids.[678] At collegiate levels of sport, 17 to 20 percent of collegiate athletes from seven universities in the United States who responded to a survey reported that they used anabolic steroids.[680] Use in adolescent boys is between 4 and 12 percent and between 0.5 and 2 percent in girls.[681] It has been suggested that at least in high school athletes illegal drug use is commoner in those who use anabolic steroids.[682] A small proportion of nonathletes (1 to 2 percent), both men and women, admit to using anabolic steroids merely to enhance appearance or to improve physique for occupations where this is important (e.g., police, security guards, and fire fighters).[680]

Sources of Illicit Anabolic Steroids

These drugs are provided in high school predominantly by illicit sources (95 percent). Other sources of illicit anabolic steroids may include physicians, veterinarians, other countries, mail order, and drugs manufactured in the Third World and smuggled in. There is little doubt that black market drugs are readily available through gymnasiums.[683] Analysis of drugs purchased on the black market in Germany reveals that the labelling is frequently unrelated to the contents.[684]

The Use of Anabolic Steroids by Athletes

Alkylation of testosterone at the 17-alpha position produced orally active derivatives resistant to hepatic degradation, and esterification of the 17 beta-hydroxy group with a range of carboxylic acids produced a range of lipid-soluble, slow-release injectable derivatives.[655] Testosterone is produced in adult males at the rate of 4 to 10 mg daily. Oral replacement dosage using methandrostenolone is 35 to 70 mg per week. Athletes using anabolic steroids report doses of 250–3,200 mg/week with "stacking" and "pyramiding" to minimize the health risk and chance of detection and to maximize the anabolic effects.[685] The cycles are characteristically 6 to 12 weeks in length and involve a progressive increase (pyramiding) of several oral and injectable steroids (stacking) to a peak followed by a reduction prior to competition. The dose of each drug is severalfold higher than that recommended by the manufacturers and may involve different drugs for different parts of the cycle. This is done to avoid the effects of receptor down regulation by using just one drug and to obtain a balance of anabolic and androgenic effects.[686]

There is no scientific evidence that stacking is more effective than single drug regimens and certainly no evidence that it is safer. It is possible that unknown interactions among the various drugs have a greater potential for more adverse effects than does the use of a single preparation. Because anabolic steroids are obtained by athletes from black market sources, the nature and quantity of the drugs are open to question. The lack of monitoring by physicians also means that little scientific data are available on the potential side effects of these drugs. Human chorionic gonadotropin (hCG) is sometimes combined with anabolic steroid regimens to prevent the testicular atrophy, reduction of spermatogenesis, and decline in endogenous testosterone production that accompany anabolic steroid use.[683] Dose response relationships of anabolic actions versus potentially serious side effects is unknown.[687] The frequency of acute life-threatening side effects is low but the risk may be underrecognized or underreported.[687] In contrast, some have suggested that the risks are insignificant and exaggerated.[688]

Anabolic Steroids and Athletic Performance

Mode of Action of Anabolic Steroids

Potential mechanisms of action for supraphysiologic doses of testosterone and other anabolic steroids include action via the receptor with or without an increase in receptor number, an anabolic effect on cellular activity independent of the receptor, and an antagonistic effect on catabolic hormones, particularly glucocorticoids. It has also been suggested that the response of muscles to anabolic steroids may be genetically different in elite athletes.[689] In a rat model, training alone increased RNA polymerase activity by 50 percent and specific cytoplasmic binding by 90 percent.[690] The additional use of nandrolone decanoate (Retabolil) (0.1 mg/100 g) induced a further increase in RNA polymerase activity but reduced androgen receptor activity by 21 percent.[690] This supports the concept both of increased receptor effects and of an effect that is independent of the number of available receptors.

It is accepted that anabolic steroids have an anticatabolic effect mediated through antagonistic effects on glucocorticoids, but the exact mechanism through which this occurs is unclear. Binding to the glucocorticoid receptor is low, and androgens have little direct effect on receptor number.[691] Androgens do, however, block the glucocorticoid-induced induction of glutamine synthetase.[692] Some evidence does, however, support a direct anticatabolic effect of anabolic steroids via the glucocorticoid receptor.[693]

The relation between testosterone levels and aggression and the supposed role of testosterone in determining social rank in nonhuman primates has led to suggestions that the psychological effects of testosterone may be important.[694,695] The relation in these situations is by association, which does not prove causality. Athletes feel that steroids give them the ability to train with greater intensity and for longer periods.[696,697] The importance of psychological effects remains questionable.[698]

Effectiveness of Anabolic Steroids as Ergogenic Aids

Athletes and coaches with personal experience of anabolic steroids are convinced of the effectiveness of these drugs in improving performance.[678,699–701] Several possible benefits are claimed (Table 31-6). Physicians and scientists have generally taken the conservative view that there is no consistent scientific proof that anabolic steroids enhance performance. The differences between the medical and scientific views of the effectiveness of the drugs and the coaches' and athletes' views support the view that physicians do not understand the use of steroids. The Council on Scientific Affairs of the American Medical Association agreed in 1988 that improvement in muscular strength may occur with anabolic steroids used in conjunction with strenuous training and a high-protein diet.[698]

Anabolic steroids have been used by athletes in two ways. First, they have been used to increase muscle bulk, strength, and power when combined with increased dietary protein intake. Strenuous exercise induces a catabolic state, and this can be reversed by using anabolic steroids. The steroids permit training at levels which would otherwise induce catabolism. They have also been used in lower doses to enhance athletic performance yet do not have a significant effect on aerobic metabolism or maximal oxygen consumption. There is also speculation that the androgenic action may have psychological benefits by making athletes more aggressive and competitive in both training and competition.[702] Other researchers have suggested that this contributes to an imagined effect of steroids.[703]

Because of the inconsistency in results, several metaanalytic papers have tried to reconcile differences in steroid dose, training, fitness, and dietary intake among athletes. Although some investigators disagree,[703] the evidence suggests that a combination of

TABLE 31-6. Possible Benefits of Anabolic Steroids

Increase muscle bulk and strength
More aggressive approach to competition
Muscle damage repair facilitated?
Change in reaction times?
Better tolerance to training

anabolic steroids, intensive strength training, and a protein-rich diet leads to gain in strength, body weight, and lean body mass.[700] Haupt and Rovere, in perhaps the best metaanalysis of the literature,[704] examined 20 variables in 24 studies published prior to 1984 and found 14 that suggested an increase in strength and 10 in which no improvement was found. They concluded that anabolic steroids will consistently result in significant strength increases when given to athletes who have been intensively trained in weight lifting immediately before the start of the steroid regimen and who continue intensive weight training during the steroid regimen, when the athletes maintain a high-protein diet, and when the changes in athletes' strength are measured by the single repetition-maximal weight technique for those exercises with which the athlete trains.[704] It seems likely that anabolic steroids alone are ineffective and that concomitant with heavy training in a previously well-trained individual and taken for at least 3 to 4 months, they may play a significant role in enhancing certain types of athletic performance.[700]

Anabolic Steroid Abuse in Women

There is little information on the effects of the drugs in women. Strauss and colleagues described 10 women athletes who reported a significant increase in muscle size, muscle strength, and performance.[683] In a recent review Honour points out that it remains difficult to address the questions in a scientific forum.[701]

Problems with Assessing Benefits to Athletes

The published studies are confusing because the dosage, type, and duration of steroid use; the status of training before beginning steroids; and the method of evaluation of strength and body composition differ among studies. The scientific investigations may not be relevant to the issue because they do not encompass the variety of agents, patterns of self-medication, or dosage levels commonly used. The difference between winning and losing at a high-performance sport is relatively small, measured in the 100 m dash, for example, in hundredths of a second. Even minor improvement may substantially improve the performance of an athlete. It is questionable whether appropriate studies to resolve the issue can even be completed or should be undertaken. Certainly they cannot be performed in the normal manner of investigative studies. Regardless of any ability of the medical and scientific world to demonstrate an effect of steroids, their value is accepted within the sports world. They are believed to augment and facilitate but not replace training. The testimony from athletes at the Dubin Enquiry is compelling.[678]

Adverse Effects of Anabolic Steroids in Athletes

Most of the adverse effects of anabolic steroids (Table 31-7) are based on studies at doses substantially below those used to enhance athletic performance. There is little evidence of long-term harmful effects of steroids in the athletic population,[705] but physicians continue to caution against interpreting the lack of evidence as indicating that these drugs are safe to use. Other health risk behaviors are widespread in users of anabolic steroids,[705] which may interact with steroids to produce unrecognized effects. Neither the medical community nor the pharmaceutical industry has good reason to study the effects of supraphysiologic doses of anabolic steroids. The effects of duration of treatment, patterns of administration, and drug-drug interactions have never been systematically explored. The descriptions of life-threatening side effects tend to be anecdotal. Accounts of liver cancer, stroke, myocardial infarction and cardiomyopathy, suicide, and homicidal and nearly homicidal range[700,706–709] have been published. The frequency of these problems in relation to that in the general population is not known. The side effects are frequently disregarded by athletes to some degree because of the "immortality of the young," the need to win regardless of health risks, and to some degree because of the credibility gap that has emerged on the efficacy of anabolic steroids. The lack of trust in physicians has been recognized for many years.[710] If physicians and scientists cannot accept the fact that these drugs are effective, can athletes trust their judgment about side effects?

TABLE 31-7. Side Effects of Anabolic Steroids

Stunting of growth in children and adolescents
Changes in blood lipids to an atherogenic pattern
Adverse psychological effects including aggressive behavior and acute psychosis
Effects on HPG axis in women (changes are generally reversible when the drugs are discontinued)
Increased facial and body hair, acne
Deepening of the voice
Male pattern baldness
Clitorimegaly
Decreased breast size
Alterations in libido
Male musculature
Amenorrhea, oligomenorrhea, anovulation, infertility
Effects on HPG axis in men
Acne
Gynecomastia
Changes in libido
Testicular atrophy
Infertility
Impaired liver function and biochemical changes
Benign and malignant tumors of the liver, hepatoma, peliosis hepatis
Fluid retention with occasional hypertension

The cardiac effects of anabolic steroids have been recently reviewed.[708,709] Hypertension, ventricular remodeling, myocardial ischemia, and sudden cardiac death have each been temporally and causally associated with anabolic steroid use in humans. These effects persist long after use has been discontinued and have significant impact on subsequent morbidity and mortality. Diet is of minimal importance in determining the lipid response to steroids.[712] Sudden death in athletes is not rare,[708] but the importance of the atherogenic effects of anabolic steroids is unclear.

Anabolic steroid use is associated with several behavioral effects and psychological symptoms.[706–708] Dissatisfaction with existing body morphology may lead to continuing problems after initiating use of anabolic steroids. Occasional anecdotes about various psychiatric episodes must be evaluated aginst a background of more than 1,000,000 individuals in the United States being exposed to anabolic steroids. It appears that an extremely small percentage of individuals using anabolic-androgenic steroids appear to experience mental disturbances severe enough to result in clinical treatment and medical case reports. Even among those so affected, the roles of previous psychiatric history, genetic susceptibility to addictions or mental disorders, environmental and peer influences, and individual expectations remain unclear.[702]

Reported side effects of anabolic steroids in women include increased facial and body hair, acne, deepening of the voice, male pattern baldness, clitoromegaly, decreased breast size, alterations in libido, male musculature, amenorrhea, oligomenorrhea, anovulation, and infertility.[696] Some changes (e.g., facial hair growth, clitoromegaly, laryngeal enlargement, and deepening of the voice) are not reversible when the drugs are discontinued.

Few specific studies have been performed in women athletes. A study of 10 weight-trained women athletes taking doses of anabolic steroids approximately ninefold higher than recommended confirmed these effects.[683] The drugs were taken in 9-week cycles, and the users averaged about three cycles per year. The majority of these women had facial hair growth, clitoromegaly, increased libido, decreased or absent menstruation, acne, and decreased body fat. The side effects described by some of these women included loss of scalp hair, increased body hair, decreased breast size, and aggressiveness.

A long list of reproductive side effects occur in men, including acne, changes in libido, testicular atrophy, and a dose-dependent effect on sperm production.[685,712,713] Serum testosterone levels are suppressed during steroid use and remain suppressed to half their initial values for 3 to 4 months after high-dose anabolic steroid administration. The frequency of side effects include testicular atrophy in 56 percent of men using anabolic steroids and gynecomastia in 52 percent.[714] Azoospermia appears reversible with gonadotropins.[714] Attempts to self-treat gynecomastia with tamoxifen, an antiestrogen, have been unsuccessful,[715] but surgery has been successful.[716]

Other Endocrine Changes

The levels of TSH, total and free thyroxine, triiodothyronine, and TBG are all decreased while growth hormone is increased.[717] Although there is probably little effect on the ACTH-cortisol axis and no effect on cortisol-binding globulin, adrenal androgens are suppressed with reduced levels of DHEA and its sulfate.[718] Insulin resistance and diminished glucose tolerance have also been observed.[719]

Impaired Liver Function and Liver Disease

Changes in hepatic function and liver damage including tumors are well described and are mostly found with the orally active 17-α alkylated testosterone derivatives.[720] Liver damage can result from intrahepatic cholestasis but is rarely fatal.[696] Evidence of liver damage from injectable anabolic steroids is rare but can persist for several months after the drugs have been discontinued.[696] Some biochemical changes (e.g., elevated AST and ALT levels) probably reflect muscle damage rather than hepatic dysfunction.[683] It is suggested that liver-specific enzymes (e.g., LDH and alkaline phosphatase) should be used to monitor hepatic function.[683] When this was done, fewer than 10 percent of athletes appeared to have abnormal liver function tests.[701] Peliosis hepatis, the occurrence of blood-filled cysts in the liver, has been reported in a body builder receiving anabolic steroids.[721] Liver cancer has also been reported in a small number of athletes who used anabolic steroids.[722]

As was indicated earlier, muscle enzymes are substantially higher in athletes using steroids than in nonusers. Creatinine kinase is also elevated.[723–725] This could reflect an effect of these drugs on the muscles or, more likely, the consequences of pushing muscles harder than would be normally possible. It is not clear what effect the presumed muscle damage might have in the long term. Massive rhabdomyolysis has been described in a weight lifter taking anabolic steroids,[726] but this effect is far more common in marathoners and ultramarathoners.[727]

Miscellaneous and Anecdotal Accounts

Wilms' tumor has been reported in association with anabolic steroid use,[728] and adenocarcinoma of the prostate has been described in a 40-year-old body builder using anabolic steroid drugs.[729] Fluid retention is not uncommon with steroid use.[724] The occasional occurrence of hypertension is probably idiosyncratic, as with other sex steroids, although some researchers have observed an elevation of mean systolic blood pressure.[704]

The use of anabolic steroids to stimulate red blood cell production has been recognized and used clinically for many years.[730] It is not surprising that substantial evidence shows that athletes using anabolic steroids also increase their hematocrit. Some evidence suggests that humoral immunity may be impaired by anabolic steroid use. IgG, IgM, and IgA are significantly lower in anabolic steroid users than in controls.[731,732] The number and relative distribution of T cells was unchanged, but the response to a β-cell mitogen, *Staphylococcus aureus* Cowan Strain I, was enhanced. Natural killer cell activity was also significantly greater in anabolic steroid users.[732] Four of 13 steroid-using body builders and 3 of 8 nonsteroid-using body builders had positive antinuclear antibodies.[732] Occasional rare neuropathies have been reported in body builders and severe sepsis has been reported also on an occasional basis.[733,734] HIV transmission has probably occurred through sharing needles.[735]

Detection of Anabolic Steroids

The focus in detecting banned drugs is on the major games. Widespread press coverage was devoted to disqualifications (and desertions) from the 1983 Pan American Games and the 1984 and 1988 Olympic Games, but this was less apparent at the recent Olympic Games in Atlanta. A World Anti-doping Agency (WADA) has recently been founded as part of the struggle to "think positive, test negative" (www.wada-ama.org). Although it is possible to detect anabolic steroids at picomolar levels using gas chromatography/mass spectrophotometry the suspicions remain that the athletes are eluding capture rather than competing clean. Metabolites of all banned anabolic steroids are readily detected in the urine of tested athletes with less than 30 min of testing using gas chromatography/mass spectrophotometry.[736–738] Particularly important is the security used in the collection, labeling, and handling of the samples.

The problem, however, does not lie in detecting the drugs at major competitions. The value of anabolic steroids is almost entirely during the training period. Clearance times for water-soluble and fat-soluble drugs are recognized, and it should be impossible to detect the drugs in urine when the drugs are stopped at an appropriate time before the likely time of testing. This is likely to be a problem only when the elimination time is prolonged, as in the oil-based depot preparations. Nandrolone, for example, may take up to 9 months to be eliminated from the urine.

Breakdowns in regimes for avoiding detection should occur only on isolated occasions, but the problem of black market drugs that are often unlabeled or mislabeled means that athletes may not know what they are taking. The individual variation in clearance times means that some way of defining the clearance for each individual athlete would be useful. The very high number of positive tests found in athletes during training[739] suggests that testing facilities have been used by athletes with this purpose in mind. The problem of controlling steroid abuse, therefore, does not lie in the laboratory at the major games.

Controlling the Steroid Epidemic

Approaches to controlling the "steroid epidemic" have included identification of users by testing at competition and during training, control of the manufacture and distribution of steroids, banning possession of these drugs, and education of users and potential users.[739,740] Mandatory random drug testing has been suggested as the only method to control steroid use, but its acceptability remains limited by law courts and in the case of professional sports by player-management agreements. Getting caught at the games remains only a slight deterrent.

Warnings of harmful side effects tend to be unheeded.[741,742] Knowledge and acceptance of the benefits is quite high among athletes, while knowledge and acceptance of significant side effects is low. Educational interventions at the high school level have had little effect on intent to take steroids, and some researchers have suggested that education would need to occur in the preteen or early teen years. Practical recommendations for teaching have been made but seem inadequate in view of failures.[743]

The use of the drugs may be proscribed and control of the anabolic steroids may be transferred from the U.S. Food and Drug Administration to the Drug Enforcement Agency. This may not have the desired effect if the policing of anabolic steroids has to compete with the problem of policing hard and soft ilicit recreational drugs as well as alcohol and tobacco.[681,744,745] Many would consider that the use of alcohol by 45 percent of teenagers and the use of amphetamines by 8.5 percent are significantly greater social problems.[715] Controlling prescribing by the few physicians involved is not worthwhile because most of these drugs come from the black market.[746] It is unlikely in the absence of an international will to control anabolic steroids and other ergogenic aids that attempts to reduce anabolic steroid use will be effective. Winning remains too important. Anabolic steroids only transiently become important at the times of major sports events and when things go dramatically wrong. The recent Lausanne Conference reaffirms the principles but it is unlikely that much will change.

OTHER ERGOGENIC AIDS

Growth Hormone

The extent of use and effectiveness of GH is not known.[747] Until the advent of recombinant human GH, its use was restricted by the availability of the drug. Interest has, however, increased in its use.[748] There are animal data that suggest that it may produce some muscle hypertrophy. The adverse effect of persistent high GH levels in patients with acromegaly suggests that supraphysiologic doses may be counterproductive. To date, there remain few human data. Decrease in fat mass and an increase in lean body mass were observed with 6 weeks of GH administration in supraphysiologic doses during training in highly trained athletes.[749] It remains unclear how this might translate into enhanced performance. Although there are some obvious concerns related to health, nothing is known about complications of its use in athletes.

Erythropoietin

Blood doping has been banned by the International Olympic Committee but is difficult to detect other than by suppression of erythropoietin levels in the circulation.[750] Animal experimentation has suggested some physiological benefit.[751] The availability of recombinant erythropoietin has had a profound effect on some patients with chronic renal failure but there have been problems with hypertension and coagulation of vascular access.[752] There have been few studies of the effects of erythropoietin in athletes. Endurance runners with low-normal hematologic parameters were unchanged by erythropoietin, but exercise performance does not appear to increase, perhaps because of an effect on erythrocyte turnover.[753,754] These drugs are being used,[755] but the extent of use is unknown. This use has been associated with deaths.[756] Because, like growth hormone, there are no urine tests for this drug, athletes may be able to continue its use for the present without detection. The use of this drug does, however, seem rather more dangerous than that of GH or anabolic steroids. The combination of an elevated hematocrit in the resting state with the hemoconcentration associated with prolonged exercise may result in a dangerous increase in blood viscosity in athletes taking erythropoietin.

REFERENCES

1. Rose LI, Carroll DR, Lowe SL, Peterson EW, Cooper KH: Serum electrolyte changes after marathon running. *J Appl Physiol* 29:449, 1970.
2. Kargotich S, Goodman C, Keast D, Morton AR: The influence of exercise-induced plasma volume changes on the interpretation of biochemical parameters used for monitoring exercise, training and sport. *Sports Med* 26:101, 1998.
3. Vera R, Croxatto H: Muscular work and antidiuretic substance in the blood. *J Appl Physiol* 7:172, 1954.
4. Dessypris A, Wagar G, Fyhrquist F, Makinen T, Welin WG, Lamberg BA: Marathon run: Effects on blood cortisol-ACTH, iodothyronine-TSH, and vasopressin. *Acta Endocrinol (Copenh)* 95:151, 1980.
5. Beardwell CG, Geleen G, Palmer HM, Roberts D, Salamonson L: Radioimmunoassay of plasma vasopressin in physiological and pathological states in man. *J Endocrinol* 67:189, 1975.
6. Baylis PH, Heath DA: The development of a radioimmunoassay for the measurement of human arginine vasopressin. *Clin Endocrinol (Oxf)* 7:91, 1977.
7. Viti A, Lupo C, Lodi L, Bonifazi M, Martelli G: Hormonal changes after supine posture, immersion, and swimming. *Int J Sports Med* 10:402, 1989.
8. Lenz T, Weiss M, Werle E, Walz U, Kohler U, Pinther J, Weicker H: Influence of exercise in water on hormonal, metabolic and adrenergic receptor changes in man. *Int J Sports Med* 9(suppl 2):S125, 1988.
9. Wade CE, Claybaugh J: Plasma renin activity, vasopressin concentration and urinary excretory responses to exercise in man. *J Appl Physiol* 49:930, 1980.
10. Convertino VA, Keil LC, Bernauer EM: Plasma volume, osmolality, vasopressin, and renin activity during exercise in man. *J Appl Physiol* 50:123, 1981.
11. Nazar K, Jezova D, Kowalik-Borowka E: Plasma vasopressin, growth hormone and ACTH responses to static handgrip in healthy subjects. *Eur J Appl Physiol* 58:400, 1989.
12. Inder WJ, Hellemans J, Swanney MP, Prickett TC, Donald RA: Prolonged exercise increases peripheral plasma ACTH, CRH, and AVP in male athletes. *J Appl Physiol* 85:835, 1998.
13. Maresh CM, Wang BC, Goetz KL: Plasma vasopressin, renin activity, and aldosterone responses to maximal exercise in active college females. *Eur J Appl Physiol* 54:398, 1985.
14. Convertino VA, Brock PJ, Keil LC, Bernauer EM, Greenleaf JE: Exercise induced hypervolemia: Role of plasma albumin, renin and vasopressin. *J Appl Physiol* 48:665, 1980.
15. Melin B, Eclache JP, Geelen G, Annat G, Allevard AM, et al: Plasma AVP, neurophysin, renin activity, and aldosterone during submaximal exercise performed to exhaustion in trained and untrained men. *Eur J Appl Physiol* 44:141, 1980.
16. Shoemaker JK, Green HJ, Ball-Burnett M, Grant S: Relationships between fluid and electrolyte hormones and plasma volume during exercise with training and detraining. *Med Sci Sports Exerc* 30:497, 1998.

17. Convertino VA, Keil LC, Greenleaf JE: Plasma volume, renin, and vasopressin responses to graded exercise after training. *J Appl Physiol* 54:508, 1983.
18. Rocker L, Kirsch KA, Heyduck B, Altenkirch HU: Influence of prolonged physical exercise on plasma volume, plasma proteins, electrolytes, and fluid-regulating hormones. *Int J Sports Med* 10:270, 1989.
19. Montain SJ, Laird JE, Latzka WA, Sawka MN: Aldosterone and vasopressin responses in the heat: Hydration level and exercise intensity effects. *Med Sci Sports Exerc* 29:661, 1997.
20. Farrell PA, Gustafson AB, Garthwaite TL, Kalkhoff RK, Cowley AW Jr, Morgan WP: Influence of endogenous opioids on the response of selected hormones to exercise in humans. *J Appl Physiol* 61:1051, 1986.
21. Khokhar AM, De Silva P, Harvard CWH, Bird R, Forsling ML, Slater JDH: The mechanism of exercise mediated vasopressin release in man (abstract). *Eur J Clin Invest* 9:111, 1979.
22. Viinamaki O: The effect of hydration status on plasma vasopressin release during physical exercise in man. *Acta Physiol Scand* 139:133, 1990.
23. Viinamaki O, Heinonen OJ, Kujala UM, Alen M: Glucose polymer syrup attenuates prolonged endurance exercise-induced vasopressin release. *Acta Physiol Scand* 136:69, 1989.
24. Brandenberger G, Candas V, Follenius M, Kahn JM: The influence of the initial state of hydration on endocrine responses to exercise in the heat. *Eur J Appl Physiol* 58:674, 1989.
25. Brandenberger G, Candas V, Follenius M, Libert JP, Kahn JM: Vascular fluid shifts and endocrine responses to exercise in the heat: Effect of rehydration: *Eur J Appl Physiol* 55:123, 1986.
26. Perrault H, Cantin M, Thibault G, Brisson GR, Brisson G, Beland M: Plasma and atrial natriuretic peptide during brief upright and supine exercise in humans. *J Appl Physiol* 66:2159, 1989.
27. Koizumi K, Ishikawa T, McBrooks C: Control of activity neurons in the supraoptic nucleus. *Neurophysiology* 27:878, 1964.
28. Meehan RT: Renin, aldosterone, and vasopressin responses to hypoxia during 6 hours of mild exercise. *Aviat Space Environ Med* 57:960, 1986.
29. Chiodera P, Volpi R, Capretti L, Giuliani N, Maffei ML, Coiro V: Effect of melatonin on arginine vasopressin secretion stimulated by physical exercise or angiotensin II in normal men. *Neuropeptides.* 32:125, 1998.
30. Chiodera P, Coiro V, Volpi R, Maffei ML, Caiazza A, et al: Role of GABA and opioids in the regulation of the vasopressin response to physical exercise in normal men. *Reg Peptid* 49:57, 1993.
31. Newmark SR, Himathongkam T, Martin RP, Cooper KH, Rose LI: Adrenocortical response to marathon running. *J Clin Endocrinol Metab* 42:393, 1976.
32. Newmark SR, Toppo FR, Adams G: Fluid and electrolyte replacement in the ultramarathon runner. *Am J Sports Med* 19:389, 1991.
33. Grossman A, Bouloux P, Price P, Drury PL, Lam KS, et al: The role of opioid peptides in the hormonal responses to acute exercise in man. *Clin Sci* 67:483, 1984.
34. Luger A, Deuster PA, Debolt JE, Loriaux DL, Chrousos GP: Acute exercise stimulates the renin-angiotensin-aldosterone axis: Adaptive changes in runners. *Horm Res* 30:5, 1988.
35. Lijnen P, Hespel P, Vanden Eynde E, Amery A: Urinary excretion of electrolytes during prolonged physical activity in normal man. *Eur J Appl Physiol* 53:317, 1985.
36. Freund BJ, Claybaugh JR, Dice MS, Hashiro GM: Hormonal and vascular fluid responses to maximal exercise in trained and untrained males. *J Appl Physiol* 63:669, 1987.
37. Hespel P, Lijnen P, Van Hoof R, Fagard R, Goossens W, et al: Effects of physical endurance training on the plasma renin-angiotensin-aldosterone system in normal man. *J Endocrinol* 116:443, 1988.
38. Yamauchi T, Harada T, Kurono M, Matsui N: Effect of exercise-induced acidosis on aldosterone secretion in men. *Eur J Appl Physiol* 77:409, 1998.
39. Cargill RI, McFarlane LC, Coutie WJ, Lipworth BJ: Acute neurohormonal responses to hypoxaemia in man. *Eur J Appl Physiol* 72:256, 1996.
40. Luetkemeier MJ, Flowers KM, Lamb DR: Spironolactone administration and training-induced hypervolemia. *Int J Sports Med* 15:295, 1994.
41. Bonelli J, Waldhausl W, Magometschnigg D, SchwarzMeier J, Korn A, Hitzenberger G: Effect of exercise and prolonged oral administration of propranolol on haemodynamic variables, plasma renin concentration, plasma aldosterone and c-AMP. *Eur J Clin Invest* 7:337, 1977.
42. Opstad PK, Oktedalen O, Aakvaag A, Fonnum F, Lund PK: Plasma renin activity and serum aldosterone during prolonged physical strain: The significance of sleep and energy deprivation. *Eur J Appl Physiol* 54:1, 1985.
43. Kosunen KJ, Kuopposalmi K, Naveri H, Rehunen S, Narvanen S, Adlercreutz H: Plasma renin activity, angiotensin II, and aldosterone during hypnotic suggestion of running. *Scand J Clin Lab Invest* 37:99, 1988.
44. Wade CE, Dressendorfer RH, O'Brien JC, Claybaugh JR: Renal function, aldosterone, and vasopressin secretion following repeated long distance running. *J Appl Physiol* 50:709, 1981.
45. Freund BJ, Claybaugh JR, Hashiro GM, Dice MS: Hormonal and renal responses to water drinking in moderately trained and untrained humans. *Am J Physiol* 254:R417, 1988.
46. Convertino VA, Armstrong LE, Coyle EF, Mack GW, Sawka MN, et al: American College of Sports Medicine position stand. Exercise and fluid replacement. *Med Sci Sports Exerc* 28:i, 1996.
47. Rehrer NJ, Brouns F, Beckers EJ, Frey WO, Villiger B, et al: Physiological changes and gastro-intestinal symptoms as a result of ultra-endurance running. *Eur J Appl Physiol* 64:1, 1992.
48. Soffer EE, Merchant RK, Duethman G, Launspach J, Gisolfi C, Adrian TE: Effect of graded exercise on esophageal motility and gastroesophageal reflux in trained athletes. *Dig Dis Sci* 38:220, 1993.
49. Soffer EE, Wilson J, Duethman G, Launspach J, Adrian TE: Effect of graded exercise on esophageal motility and gastroesophageal reflux in nontrained subjects. *Dig Dis Sci* 39:193, 1994.
50. Feldman M, Nixon JV: Effect of exercise on postprandial gastric secretion and emptying in humans: *J Appl Physiol* 53:851, 1982.
51. Keeling WF, Harris A, Martin BJ: Orocecal transit during mild exercise in women. *J Appl Physiol* 68:1350, 1990.
52. Utter A, Goss F: Exercise and gall bladder function: *Sports Med* 23:218, 1997.
53. Banfi G, Marinelli M, Bonini P, Gritti I, Roi GS: Pepsinogens and gastrointestinal symptoms in mountain marathon runners. *Int J Sports Med* 17:554, 1996.
54. O'Connor AM, Johnston CF, Buchanan KD, Boreham C, Trinick TR, Riddoch CJ: Circulating gastrointestinal hormone changes in marathon running. *Int J Sports Med* 16:283, 1995.
55. Oktedalen O, Opstad PK, Schaffalitzky de Muckadell OB: The plasma concentrations of secretin and vasoactive intestinal polypeptide (VIP) after long-term, strenuous exercise. *Eur J Appl Physiol* 52:5, 1983.
56. Philipp E, Wilckens T, Friess E, Platte P, Pirke KM: Cholecystokinin, gastrin and stress hormone responses in marathon runners. *Peptides* 13:125, 1992.
57. Dessypris A, Kangas S, Chatzikonstantinou KS, Xirogiannis I, Chatzikonstantinou S: The super-marathon run (Spartathlon, 248 km): variations in blood gastrin. *Ann Gastroenterol Hepatol* 27:13, 1991.
58. Galbo H, Hilsted J, Fahrenkrug J, Schaffalitzky de Muckadell OB: Fasting and prolonged exercise increase vasoactive intestinal polypeptide (VIP) in plasma. *Acta Physiol Scand* 105:374, 1979.
59. Hilsted J, Galbo H, Sonne B, Schwartz T, Fahrenkrug J, et al: Gastroenteropancreatic hormonal changes during exercise. *Am J Physiol* 239:G136, 1980.
60. Hurley RS, Bossetti BM, O'Dorisio TM, Tenison EB, Welch MA, Rice RR: The effect of exercise training on body weight and peptide hormone patterns in normal weight college-age men. *J Sports Med Phys Fit* 31:52, 1991.
61. Krotkiewski M, Bjorntorp P, Holm G, Marks V, Morgan L, et al: Effects of physical training on insulin, connecting peptide (C-peptide), gastric inhibitory polypeptide (GIP) and pancreatic polypeptide (PP) levels in obese subjects. *Int J Obesity* 8:193, 1984.
62. MacLaren DP, Raine NM, O'Connor AM, Buchanan KD: Human gastrin and vasoactive intestinal polypeptide responses to endurance running in relation to training status and fluid ingested. *Clin Sci* 89:137, 1995.
63. Opstad PK: The plasma vasoactive intestinal peptide (VIP) response to exercise is increased after prolonged strain, sleep and energy deficiency and extinguished by glucose infusion. *Peptides* 8:175, 1987.
64. Gawel MJ, Park DM, Alaghband-Zadeh J, Rose FC: Exercise and hormonal secretion. *Postgrad Med J* 55:373, 1979.

65. Terjung RL, Tipton CM: Plasma thyroxine and thyroid stimulating hormone levels during submaximal exercise in humans. *Am J Physiol* 220:1840, 1971.
66. Mason JW, Hartley LH, Kotchen TA, Wherry FE, Pennington LL, Jones LG: Plasma thyroid stimulating hormone response in anticipation of muscular exercise in the human. *J Clin Endocrinol Metab* 37:403, 1979.
67. Stock MJ, Chapman C, Stirling JL, Campbell IT: Effects of exercise, altitude and food on blood hormone and metabolite levels. *J Appl Physiol* 45:350, 1978.
68. Berchtold P, Berger M, Cuppers HJ, Herrmann J, Nieschlag E, et al: Non-glucoregulatory hormones (T4, T3, rT3, TSH, testosterone) during physical exercise in juvenile-type diabetics. *Horm Metab Res* 10:269, 1978.
69. Federspil G, Franchimont P, Hazee-Hagelstein MT: Serum TSH and prolactin levels during prolonged muscular exercise in man. *Horm Metab Res* 8:323, 1977.
70. Smallridge RC, Whorton NE, Burman KD, Ferguson EW: Effects of exercise and physical fitness on the pituitary-thyroid axis and on prolactin secretion in male runners. *Metabolism* 34:949, 1985.
71. Opstad PK, Falch D, Oktedalen O, Fonnum F, Wergeland R: The thyroid function in young men during prolonged exercise and the effect of energy and sleep deprivation. *Clin Endocrinol (Oxf)* 20:657, 1984.
72. Refsum HE, Stromme SB: Serum thyroxine, tri-iodothyronine and thyroid stimulating hormone after prolonged heavy exercise. *Scand J Clin Lab Invest* 39:455, 1979.
73. Galbo H, Hummer L, Petersen IB, Christensen NJ, Bie N: Thyroid and testicular hormone responses to graded and prolonged exercise in man. *Eur J Appl Physiol* 36:101, 1977.
74. Sander M, Rocker L: Influence of marathon running on thyroid hormones. *Int J Sports Med* 9:123, 1988.
75. Scheen AJ, Buxton OM, Jison M, Van Reeth O, Leproult R, et al: Effects of exercise on neuroendocrine secretions and glucose regulation at different times of day. *Am J Physiol* 274:E1040, 1998.
76. Van Reeth O, Sturis J, Byrne MM, Blackman JD, L'Hermite-Baleriaux M, et al: Nocturnal exercise phase delays circadian rhythms of melatonin and thyrotropin secretion in normal men *Am J Physiol* 266:E964, 1994.
77. Kirkeby K, Stromme SB, Bjerkedahl I, Hertzenberg L, Refsum HE: Effects of prolonged, strenuous exercise on lipids and thyroxine in serum. *Acta Med Scand* 202:463, 1977.
78. DeNayer P, Malvaux P, Ostyn M, Vand Den Schreick HG, Beckers C, De Visscher M: Serum free thyroxine and binding proteins after muscular exercise. *J Clin Endocrinol Metab* 28:714, 1968.
79. Bosco C, Tihanyl J, Rivalta L, Parlato G, Tranquilli C, et al: Hormonal responses in strenuous jumping effort. *Jap J Physiol* 46:93, 1996.
80. Kraemer RR, Blair MS, McCaferty R, Castracane VD: Running-induced alterations in growth hormone, prolactin, triiodothyronine, and thyroxine concentrations in trained and untrained men and women. *Res Q Exer Sport* 64:69, 1993.
81. O'Connell M, Robbins DC, Horton ES, Sims EAH, Danforth E Jr: Changes in serum concentration of 3,5,3_-triiodothyronine during prolonged moderate exercise. *J Clin Endocrinol Metab* 49:242, 1979.
82. Caralis DG, Edwards L, David PJ: Serum total and free thyroxine and triiodothyronine during dynamic muscular exercise in man. *Am J Physiol* 233:E115, 1977.
83. Hesse V, Vilser C, Scheibe J, Jahreis G, Foley T: Thyroid hormone metabolism under extreme body exercises. *Exp Clin Endocrinol* 94:82, 1989.
84. Tomasi TE: Utilization rates of thyroid hormones in mammals. *Comp Biochem Physio A-Comp Physiol* 100:503, 1991.
85. Irvine CHG: Effect of exercise on thyroxine degradation in athletes and non-athletes. *J Clin Endocrinol Metab* 28:942, 1968.
86. Balsam A, Leppo E: Effect of physical training on the metabolism of thyroid hormones in man. *J Appl Physiol* 38:212, 1975.
87. Boyden TW, Parmenter RW, Stanforth P, Rotkin T, Wilmore JH: Evidence for mild thyroidal impairment in women undergoing endurance training. *J Clin Endocrinol Metab* 53:53, 1982.
88. Pakarinen A, Alen M, Hakkinen K, Komi P: Serum thyroid hormones, thyrotropin and thyroxine binding globulin during prolonged strength training. *Eur J Appl Physiol* 57:394, 1988.
89. Boyden TW, Parmenter RW, Rotkis TC, Stanforth P, Wilmore JH: Thyroidal changes associated with endurance training. *Med Sci Sports Exerc* 16:243, 1984.
90. Alen M, Pakarinen A, Hakkinen K: Effects of prolonged training on serum thyrotropin and thyroid hormones in elite strength athletes. *J Sports Sci* 11:493, 1993.
91. Poehlman ET, Tremblay A, Nadeau A, Dussault J, Theriault G, Bouchard C: Heredity and changes in hormones and metabolic rates with short-term training. *Am J Physiol* 250:E711, 1986.
92. Loucks AB, Verdun M: Slow restoration of LH pulsatility by refeeding in energetically disrupted women. *Am J Physiol* 275:R1218, 1998.
93. Loucks AB, Callister R: Induction and prevention of low-T3 syndrome in exercising women. *Am J Physiol* 264:R924, 1993.
94. McCargar LJ, Simmons D, Craton N, Taunton JE, Birmingham CL: Physiological effects of weight cycling in female lightweight rowers. *Can J Appl Physiol* 18:291, 1993.
95. McCargar LJ, Crawford SM: Metabolic and anthropometric changes with weight cycling in wrestlers. *Med Sci Sports Exerc* 24:1270, 1992.
96. Obarzanek E, Lesem MD, Goldstein DS, Jimerson DC: Reduced resting metabolic rate in patients with bulimia nervosa. *Arch Gen Psychiatr* 48:456, 1991.
97. Loucks AB, Laughlin GA, Mortola JF, Girton L, Nelson JC, Yen SS: Hypothalamic-pituitary-thyroidal function in eumenorrheic and amenorrheic athletes. *J Clin Endocrinol Metab* 75:514, 1992.
98. Harber VJ, Petersen SR, Chilibeck PD: Thyroid hormone concentrations and muscle metabolism in amenorrheic and eumenorrheic athletes. *Can J Appl Physiol* 23:293, 1998.
99. Harber VJ, Petersen SR, Chilibeck PD: Thyroid hormone concentrations and skeletal muscle metabolism during exercise in anorexic females. *Can J Appl Physiol* 75:1197, 1997.
100. Herring JL, Mole PA, Meredith CN, Stern JS: Effect of suspending exercise training on resting metabolic rate in women. *Med Sci Sports Exerc* 24:59, 1992.
101. Cumming DC, Grainger JA, Campbell LG, Wall SR: TSH and prolactin responses to TRH in a treated hypothyroid athlete: Effect of activity and rest. *J Sports Med Phys Fitness* 25:243, 1985.
102. Monzani F, Caraccio N, Siciliano G, Manca L, Murri L, Ferrannini E: Clinical and biochemical features of muscle dysfunction in subclinical hypothyroidism. *J Clin Endocrinol Metab* 82:3315, 1997.
103. Kimura H, Kawagoe Y, Kaneko N, Fessler HE, Hosoda S: Low efficiency of oxygen utilization during exercise in hyperthyroidism. *Chest* 110:1264, 1996.
104. Holloszy JO, Kohrt WM, Hansen PA: The regulation of carbohydrate and fat metabolism during and after exercise. *Front Biosci* 3:D1010, 1998.
105. Goodyear LJ, Kahn BB: Exercise, glucose transport, and insulin sensitivity. *Ann Rev Med* 49:235, 1998.
106. Hartley LH, Mason JW, Hogan RP, Jones LG, Kotchen TA, et al: Multiple hormonal responses to prolonged exercise in relation to physical training. *J Appl Physiol* 33:602, 1972.
107. Hartley LH, Mason JW, Hogan RP, Jones LG, Kotchen TA, et al: Multiple hormonal responses to graded exercise in relation to physical training. *J Appl Physiol* 33:607, 1972.
108. Benadé AJS, Wyndham CH, Jansen CR, Rogers GG, de Bruin EJP: Plasma insulin and carbohydrate metabolism after rest and during prolonged aerobic exercise. *Pflug Arch* 342:207, 1973.
109. Galbo H, Christensen NJ, Holst JJ: Glucose induced decrease in glucagon and epinephrine responses to exercise in man. *J Appl Physiol* 42:525, 1977.
110. Tuttle KR, Marker JC, Dalsky GP, Schwartz NS, Shah SD, et al: Glucagon, not insulin, may play a secondary role in defense against hypoglycemia during exercise. *Am J Physiol* 254:E713, 1988.
111. Rodgers CD, Vranic M: Mediation of glucoregulation at rest and during exercise by the glucose-fatty acid cycle in vivo and in vitro studies. *Can J Appl Physiol* 23:534, 1998.
112. Ahlborg G, Lundberg JM: Inhibitory effects of neuropeptide Y on splanchnic glycogenolysis and renin release in humans. *Clin Physiol* 14:187, 1994.
113. Ahlborg G, Weitzberg E, Lundberg JM: Endothelin-1 infusion reduces splanchnic glucose production in humans. *J Appl Physiol* 77:121, 1994.
114. Mitchell TH, Abraham G, Schiffrin A, Leiter LA, Marliss E: Hyperglycemia after intense exercise in IDDM during continuous insulin infusion. *Diabetes Care* 11:311, 1988.

115. Ben-Ezra V, Jankowski C, Kendrick K, Nichols D: Effect of intensity and energy expenditure on postexercise insulin responses in women. *J Appl Physiol* 79:2029, 1995.
116. Brambrink JK, Fluckey JD, Hickey MS, Craig BW: Influence of muscle mass and work on post-exercise glucose and insulin responses in young untrained subjects. *Acta Physiol Scand* 161:371, 1997.
117. Mikines KJ, Farrell PA, Sonne B, Tronier B, Galbo H: Post-exercise dose-response relationship between plasma glucose and insulin secretion. *J Appl Physiol* 64:988, 1988.
118. Jenkins AB, Chisholm DJ, James DE, Ho KY, Kraegen EW: Exercise-induced hepatic glucose output is precisely sensitive to the rate of systemic glucose supply. *Metabolism* 34:431, 1985.
119. Burke LM, Claassen A, Hawley JA, Noakes TD: Carbohydrate intake during prolonged cycling minimizes effect of glycemic index of preexercise meal. *J Appl Physiol* 85:2220, 1998.
120. Sotsky MJ, Shilo S, Shamoon H: Regulation of counterregulatory hormone secretion in man during exercise and hypoglycemia. *J Clin Endocrinol Metab* 68:9, 1989.
121. Nieman DC, Carlson KA, Brandstater ME, Naegele RT, Blankenship JW: Running endurance in 27-h-fasted humans. *J Appl Physiol* 63:2502, 1987.
122. Burstein R, Shpilberg O, Rubinstein A, Bashan N, Falk B, Epstein Y: The effect of prolonged intermittent exercise, combined with food deprivation, on plasma metabolite concentration. *Aviat Space Environ Med* 62:555, 1991.
123. Okuno Y, Fuji S, Okada K, Tabata T, Tanaka S, Wada M: Effects of acute exercise on insulin binding to erythrocytes in normal men. *Horm Metab Res* 15:366, 1983.
124. Bonen A, Tan MH, Clune P, Kirby RL: Effects of exercise on insulin binding to human muscle. *Am J Physiol* 248:E403, 1985.
125. DeFronzo RA, Ferrannini E, Sato Y, Felig P: Synergistic interaction between exercise and insulin on peripheral glucose uptake. *J Clin Invest* 68:1468, 1981.
126. Felig P, Wahren J, Hendler R, Ahlborg G: Plasma glucagon levels in exercising man. *N Engl J Med* 287:184, 1972.
127. Araujo-Vilar D, Osifo E, Kirk M, Garcia-Estevez DA, Cabezas-Cerrato J, Hockaday TD: Influence of moderate physical exercise on insulin-mediated and non-insulin-mediated glucose uptake in healthy subjects. *Metab Clin Exp* 46:203, 1997.
128. Galbo H, Christensen NJ, Holst JJ: Catecholamines and pancreatic hormones during autonomic blockade in exercising man. *Acta Physiol Scand* 101:428, 1977.
129. Adams JH, Irving G, Koeslag JH, Lochner JD, Sandell RC, Wilkinson C: Beta-adrenergic blockade restores glucose's antiketogenic activity after exercise in carbohydrate-depleted athletes. *J Physiol* 386:439, 1987.
130. Jenkins AB, Furler SM, Chisholm DJ, Kraegen EW: Regulation of hepatic glucose output during exercise by circulating glucose and insulin in humans. *Am J Physiol* 250:R411, 1986.
131. Wolfe RR, Nadel ER, Shaw JH, Stephenson LA, Wolfe MH: Role of changes in insulin and glucagon in glucose homeostasis in exercise. *J Clin Invest* 77:900, 1986.
132. Burke LM, Collier GR, Hargreaves M: Muscle glycogen storage after prolonged exercise: Effect of the glycemic index of carbohydrate feedings. *J Appl Physiol* 75:1019, 1993.
133. Coggan AR, Kohrt WM, Spina RJ, Kirwan JP, Bier DM, Holloszy JO: Plasma glucose kinetics during exercise in subjects with high and low lactate thresholds. *J Appl Physiol* 73:1873, 1982.
134. Coggan AR, Swanson SC, Mendenhall LA, Habash DL, Kien CL: Effect of endurance training on hepatic glycogenolysis and gluconeogenesis during prolonged exercise in men. *Am J Physiol* 268:E375, 1995.
135. Bloom SR, Johnson RH, Park DM, Rennie MJ, Sulaimen WR: Differences in the metabolic and hormonal responses to exercise between racing cyclists and untrained individuals. *J Physiol* 258:1, 1976.
135a. Naveri H, Kuoppasalmi K, Harkonen M: Metabolic and hormonal changes in moderate and intense long-term running exercises. *Int J Sports Med* 6:276, 1985.
136. Galbo H, Holst JJ, Christensen NJ, Hilsted J: Glucagon and plasma catecholamines during beta-receptor blockade in exercising man. *J Appl Physiol* 42:855, 1976.
137. Gyntelberg F, Rennie MJ, Hickson RC, Holloszy JO: Effect of training on the response of plasma glucagon to exercise. *J Appl Physiol* 43:302, 1976.
138. Vanhelder WP, Radomski MW, Goode RC, Casey K: Hormonal and metabolic response to three types of exercise of equal duration and external work output. *Eur J Appl Physiol* 54:337, 1985.
139. Felig P, Wahren J: Role of insulin and glucose in the regulation of hepatic glucose production during exercise. *Diabetes* 28(Suppl 1):71, 1979.
140. Terjung R: Endocrine response to exercise. *Exerc Sport Sci Rev* 7:153, 1979.
141. Galbo H, Holst JJ, Christensen NJ: Glucagon and plasma catecholamine responses to graded and prolonged exercise in man. *J Appl Physiol* 38:70, 1975.
142. Angelopoulos TJ, Robertson RJ, Goss FL, Utter A: Insulin and glucagon immunoreactivity during high-intensity exercise under opiate blockade. *Eur J Appl Physiol* 75:132, 1997.
143. Felig P, Cherif A, Minagawa A, Wahren J: Hypoglycemia during prolonged exercise in normal men. *N Engl J Med* 306:895, 1982.
144. Sutton J, Coleman MJ, Millar AP, Lazarus L, Russo P: The medical problems of mass participation in athletic competition: The "City-to-Surf" Race. *Med J Aus* 2:127, 1972.
145. Hartung GH, Myhre LG, Tucker DM, Burns JW: Hormone and energy substrate changes during prolonged exercise in the heat. *Aviat Space Environ Med* 58:24, 1987.
146. Naveri H: Blood hormone and metabolite levels during graded cycle ergometer exercise. *Scand J Clin Lab Invest* 45:599, 1985.
147. Drouin R, Lavoie C, Bourque J, Ducros F, Poisson D, Chiasson JL: Increased hepatic glucose production response to glucagon in trained subjects. *Am J Physiol* 274:E23, 1998.
148. Engdahl JH, Veldhuis JD, Farrell PA: Altered pulsatile insulin secretion associated with endurance training. *J Appl Physiol* 79:1977, 1995.
149. Koivisto V, Hendler R, Nadel E, Felig P: Influence of physical training on the fuel-hormone response to prolonged low intensity exercise. *Metabolism* 31:192, 1982.
150. Tarnopolsky LJ, MacDougall JD, Atkinson SA, Tarnopolsky MA, Sutton JR: Gender differences in substrate for endurance exercise. *J Appl Physiol* 68:302, 1990.
151. Friedmann B, Kindermann W: Energy metabolism and regulatory hormones in women and men during endurance exercise. *Eur J Appl Physiol* 59:1, 1989.
152. Lavoie JM, Dionne N, Helie R, Brisson GR: Menstrual cycle phase dissociation of blood glucose homeostasis during exercise. *J Appl Physiol* 62:1084, 1987.
153. Dela F, Mikines KJ, Von Linstow M, Galbo H: Effect of training on response to a glucose load adjusted for daily carbohydrate intake. *Am J Physiol* 260:E14, 1991.
154. Oshida Y, Yamanouchi K, Hayamizu S, Sato Y: Long-term mild jogging increases insulin action despite no influence on body mass index or $V_{O_{2max}}$. *J Appl Physiol* 66:2206, 1989.
155. O'Rahilly SO, Hosker JP, Rudenski AS, Matthews DR, Burnett MA, Turner RC: The glucose stimulus-response curve of the beta-cell in physically trained humans, assessed by hyperglycemia clamps. *Metabolism* 37:919, 1988.
156. Tremblay A, Nadeau A, Despres JP, St-Jean L, Theriault G, Bouchard C: Long-term exercise training with constant energy intake: II. Effect on glucose metabolism and resting energy expenditures. *Int J Obes* 14:75, 1990.
157. Krzentowski G, Pirnay F, Luyckx AS, Lacroix M, Mosora F, Lefebvre PJ: Effect of physical training on utilization of a glucose load given orally during exercise. *Am J Physiol* 246:E412, 1984.
158. Cortright RN, Dohm GL: Mechanisms by which insulin and muscle contraction stimulate glucose transport. *Can J Appl Physiol* 22:519, 1997.
159. Lavoie JM, Helie R, Peronnet F, Cousineau D, Provencher PJ: Effects of muscle CHO-loading manipulations on hormonal responses during prolonged exercise. *Int J Sports Med* 6:95, 1985.
160. Young JC, Enslin J, Kuca B: Exercise intensity and glucose tolerance in trained and nontrained subjects. *J Appl Physiol* 67:39, 1989.
161. Tremblay A, Nadeau A, Fournier G, Bouchard C: Effect of a three-day interruption of exercise-training on resting metabolic rats and glucose-induced thermogenesis in training individuals. *Int J Obes* 12:163, 1988.
162. King DS, Dalsky GP, Clutter WE, Young DA, Staten MA, et al: Effects of lack of exercise on insulin secretion and action in trained subjects. *Am J Physiol* 254:E537, 1988.

163. Mikines KJ, Sonne B, Tronier B, Galbo H: Effects of acute exercise and detraining on insulin action in trained men. *J Appl Physiol* 66:704, 1989.
164. Lampman RM, Schteingart DE, Santinga JT, Savage PJ, Hydrick CR, et al: The influence of physical training on glucose tolerance, insulin sensitivity, and lipid and lipoprotein concentrations in middle-aged hypertriglyceridaemic, carbohydrate intolerant men. *Diabetologia* 30:380, 1987.
165. Tannenbaum GS, Ling N: The interrelationship of growth hormone (GH)–releasing factor and somatostatin in the generation of ultradian rhythm of GH secretion. *Endocrinology* 115:1952, 1984.
166. Vance ML, Kaiser DL, Evans WS, Furlanetto R, Vale W, et al: Pulsatile growth hormone secretion in normal man during a continuous 24 hour infusion of human growth hormone releasing factor (1–40): Evidence for intermittent somatostatin excretion. *J Clin Invest* 75:1584, 1985.
167. Tremblay A, Pinsard D, Coveney S, Catellier C, Laferriere G, et al: Counterregulatory response to insulin-induced hypoglycemia in trained and nontrained humans. *Metabolism* 39:1138, 1990.
168. Hackney AC, Ness RJ, Schrieber A: Effects of endurance exercise on nocturnal hormone concentrations in males. *Chronobiol Int* 6:341, 1989.
169. Hurley RS, Bossetti BM, O'Dorisio TM, Welch MA, Rice RR, et al: The response of serum growth hormone and prolactin to training in weight-maintaining healthy males. *J Sports Med Phys Fitness* 30:45, 1990.
170. Rogol AD, Weltman JY, Evans WS, Veldhuis JD, Weltman AL: Long-term endurance training alters the hypothalamic-pituitary axes for gonadotropins and growth hormone. *Endocrinol Metab Clin North Am* 21:817, 1992.
171. Dela F, Mikines KJ, Tronier B, Galbo H: Diminished arginine-stimulated insulin secretion in trained men. *J Appl Physiol* 69:261, 1990.
172. Hunter WM, Greenwood FC: Studies on the secretion of pituitary growth hormone. *Br Med J* i:804, 1964.
173. Seip RL, Weltman A, Goodman D, Rogol AD: Clinical utility of cycle exercise for the physiologic assessment of growth hormone release in children. *Am J Dis Child* 144:998, 1990.
174. Kraemer WJ, Staron RS, Hagerman FC, Hildika RS, Fry AC, et al: The effects of short-term resistance training on endocrine function in men and women. *Eur J Appl Physiol* 78:69, 1998.
175. Fryburg DA, Weltman A, Jahn LA, Weltman JY, Samojlik E, et al: Short-term modulation of the androgen milieu alters pulsatile, but not exercise- or growth hormone (GH)-releasing hormone-stimulated GH secretion in healthy men: Impact of gonadal steroid and GH secretory changes on metabolic outcomes. *J Clin Endocrinol Metab* 82:3710, 1997.
176. Kraemer RR, Johnson LG, Haltom R, Hikida RS, Fry AC, et al: Effects of hormone replacement on growth hormone and prolactin exercise responses in postmenopausal women. *J Appl Physiol* 84:703, 1998.
177. Dawson-Hughes B, Stern D, Goldman J, Reichlin S: Regulation of growth hormone and somatomedin-C secretion in postmenopausal women: Effect of physiological estrogen replacement. *J Clin Endocrinol Metab* 63:424, 1986.
178. Lanes R, Lifshitz F, Sekaran C, Fort P, Recker B: Premarin priming does not alter growth hormone release following exercise. *J Endocrinol Invest* 9:443, 1986.
179. Hornum M, Cooper DM, Brasel JA, Bueno A, Sietsema KE: Exercise-induced changes in circulating growth factors with cyclic variation in plasma estradiol in women. *J Appl Physiol* 82:1946, 1997.
180. Kanaley JA, Boileau RA, Bahr JA, Misner JE, Nelson RA: Substrate oxidation and GH responses to exercise are independent of menstrual phase and status. *Med Sci Sports Exerc* 24:873, 1992.
181. Kraemer WJ, Hakkinen K, Newton RU, McCormick M, Nindl BC, et al: Acute hormonal responses to heavy resistance exercise in younger and older men. *Eur J Appl Physiol* 77:206, 1998.
182. Deuschle M, Blum WF, Frystyk J, Orskov H, Schweiger U, et al: Endurance training and its effect upon the activity of the GH-IGFs system in the elderly. *Int J Sports Med* 19:250, 1998.
183. Cumming DC, Rebar RW, Stern B, Brunsting LA III, Strich G, et al: The effects of acute exercise on endocrine homeostasis, in Laron Z, Rogol AD (eds): *Hormones and Sport.* Proceedings of Serono Symposium, vol. 55. New York, Raven Press, pp 73–87, 1989.
184. Fahey TD, Del Valle-Zuris A, Oehlson G, Trieb M, Seymour J: Pubertal stage differences in hormonal and hematological responses to maximal exercise in males. *J Appl Physiol* 46:823, 1979.
185. Vahl N, Jorgensen JO, Jurik AG, Christiansen JS: Abdominal adiposity and physical fitness are major determinants of the age associated decline in stimulated GH secretion in healthy adults. *J Clin Endocrinol Metab* 81:2209, 1996.
186. Weltman A, Weltman JY, Womack CJ, Davis SE, Blumer JL, et al: Exercise training decreases the growth hormone (GH) response to acute constant-load exercise. *Med Sci Sports Exerc* 29:669, 1997.
187. Nevill ME, Holmyard DJ, Hall GM, Allsop P, van Oosterhout A, Burrin JM, Nevill AM: Growth hormone responses to treadmill sprinting in sprint- and endurance-trained athletes. *Eur J Appl Physiol* 72:460, 1996.
188. Roemmich JN, Sinning WE: Weight loss and wrestling training: Effects on growth-related hormones. *J Appl Physiol* 82:1760, 1997.
189. Struder HK, Hollmann W, Donike M, Platen P, Weber K: Effect of O2 availability on neuroendocrine variables at rest and during exercise: O2 breathing increases plasma prolactin. *Eur J Appl Physiol* 74:443, 1996.
190. Smith JA, Gray AB, Pyne DB, Baker MS, Telford RD, Weidemann MJ: Moderate exercise triggers both priming and activation of neutrophil subpopulations. *Am J Appl Physiol* 270:R838, 1996.
191. Gotshalk LA, Loebel CC, Nindl BC, Putukian M, Sebastianelli WJ, et al: Hormonal responses of multiset versus single-set heavy-resistance exercise protocols. *Can J Appl Physiol* 22:244, 1997.
192. Struder HK, Hollmann W, Donike M, Platen P, Weber K: Effect of O2 availability on neuroendocrine variables at rest and during exercise: O2 breathing increases plasma prolactin. *Eur J Appl Physiol* 74:443, 1996.
193. Keim NL, Anderson BL, Barbieri TF, Wu MM: Moderate diet restriction alters the substrate and hormone response to exercise. *Med Sci Sports Exerc* 26:599, 1994.
194. Gordon SE, Kraemer WJ, Vos NH, Lynch JM, Knuttgen HG: Effect of acid-base balance on the growth hormone response to acute high-intensity cycle exercise. *J Appl Physiol* 76:821, 1994.
195. Cappon JP, Ipp E, Brasel JA, Cooper DM: Acute effects of high fat and high glucose meals on the growth hormone response to exercise. *J Clin Endocrinol Metab* 76:1418, 1993.
196. Galbo H: Endocrinology and metabolism in exercise. *Int J Sports Med* 2:203, 1981.
197. Farrel PA, Garthwaite TL, Gustafson AB: Plasma adrenocorticotropin and cortisol responses to submaximal and exhaustive exercise. *J Appl Physiol* 55:1441, 1983.
198. Karagiorgios A, Garcia JF, Brooks GA: Growth hormone response to continuous and intermittent exercise. *Med Sci Sports* 11:302, 1979.
199. Snegovskaya V, Viru A: Steroid and pituitary hormone responses to rowing: relative significance of exercise intensity and duration and performance level. *Eur J Appl Physiol* 67:59, 1993.
200. Bullen BA, Skrinar GS, Beitins IZ, Carr DB, Reppert SM, et al: Endurance training effects on plasma hormonal responsiveness and sex hormone secretion. *J Appl Physiol* 56:1453, 1984.
201. Bonifazi M, Bela E, Lupo C, Martelli G, Zhu B, Carli G: Influence of training on the response to exercise of adrenocorticotropin and growth hormone plasma concentrations in human swimmers. *Eur J Appl Physiol* 78:394, 1998.
202. Galbo H, Christansen NJ, Mikines KJ, Sonne B, Hilsted J, Fahrenkrug J: The effect of fasting on the hormonal response to graded exercise. *J Clin Endocrinol Metab* 52:1106, 1981.
203. Bonen A, Belcastro AN, MacIntyre K, Gardner I: Hormonal responses during intense exercise preceded by glucose ingestion. *Can J Appl Sport Sci* 5:85, 1980.
204. Hansen P: The effect of intravenous glucose infusion on the exercise induced serum growth hormone rise in normals and juvenile diabetics. *Scand J Clin Lab Invest* 28:195, 1971.
205. Rennie MJ, Johnson RH: Effect of an exercise diet program on metabolic changes in runners. *J Appl Physiol* 231:967, 1974.
206. Gustafson AB, Farrell PA, Kalkhoff RK: Impaired plasma catecholamine response to submaximal treadmill exercise in obese women. *Metabolism* 39:410, 1990.
207. Casanueva F, Villanueva L, Penalva A, Vila T, Cabezas-Cerato J: Free fatty acid inhibition of exercise induced growth hormone. *Horm Metab Res* 13:348, 1981.
208. Taylor LM, Blockard WG: Effects of lipids on growth hormone synthesis by isolated pituitaries. *Proc Soc Exp Biol Med* 137:1026, 1971.
209. Aizawa T, Yasuda N, Greer MA: Hypoglycemia stimulates ACTH secretion through a direct effect on the basal hypothalamus. *Metabolism* 30:996, 1981.

210. Few JD, Davies CTM: The inhibiting effect of atropine on growth hormone release during exercise. *Eur J Appl Physiol* 43:221, 1980.
211. Smythe GA, Lazarus L: Suppression of human growth hormone secretion by melatonin and cyproheptadine. *J Clin Invest* 54:116, 1974.
212. Hansen AP: The effect of adrenergic receptor blockade on the exercise induced growth hormone rise in normals and juvenile diabetics. *J Clin Endocrinol Metab* 33:807, 1971.
213. Schwinn G, Schwarck H, McIntosh C, Milstrey HR, Willms B, Kobberlin J: Effect of dopamine receptor blocking agent, pimozide, on the growth hormone response to arginine and exercise and on the spontaneous growth hormone fluctuations. *J Clin Endocrinol Metab* 43:1183, 1976.
214. Moretti C, Fabbri A, Gnessi L, Cappa M, Calzolari A, et al: Naloxone inhibits exercise induced release of prolactin and GH in athletes. *Clin Endocrinol* 18:135, 1983.
215. Cappa M, Grossi A, Benedetti S, Drago F, Loche S, Ghigo E: Effect of the enhancement of the cholinergic tone by pyridostigmine on the exercise-induced growth hormone release in man. *J Endocrinol Invest* 16:421, 1993.
216. Gil-Ad I, Leibowitch N, Josefsberg Z, Wasserman M, Laron Z: Effect of oral clonidine, insulin-induced hypoglycemia and exercise on plasma GHRH levels in short-stature children. *Acta Endocrinol (Copenh)* 122:89, 1990.
217. Di Luigi L, Conti FG, Casini A, Guidetti L, Zezze G, et al: Growth hormone and insulin-like growth factor I responses to moderate submaximal acute physical exercise in man: Effects of octreotide, a somatostatin analogue, administration. *Int J Sports Med* 18:257, 1997.
218. Arends J, Wagner ML, Willms BL: Cholinergic muscarinic receptor blockade suppresses arginine- and exercise-induced growth hormone secretion in type I diabetic subjects. *J Clin Endocrinol Metab* 66:389, 1988.
219. Steardo L, Iovino M, Monteleone P, Agrusta M, Orio F: Pharmacological evidence for a dual GABAergic regulation of growth hormone release in humans. *Life Sci* 39:979, 1986.
220. Steardo L, Iovino M, Monteleone P, Agrusta M, Orio F: Evidence for a GABAergic control of the exercise-induced rise in GH in man. *Eur J Clin Pharmacol* 28:607, 1985.
221. Coiro V, Volpi R, Maffei ML, Caiazza A, Caffarri G, et al: Opioid modulation of the gamma-aminobutyric acid-controlled inhibition of exercise-stimulated growth hormone and prolactin secretion in normal men. *Eur J Endocrinol* 131:50, 1994.
222. Smythe GA: The role of serotonin and dopamine in hypothalamic-pituitary function. *Clin Endocrinol (Oxf)* 7:325, 1977.
223. Smythe GA, Duncan MW, Bradshaw JE, Cai WY: Serotoninergic control of growth hormone secretion: Hypothalamic dopamine, norepinephrine and serotonin levels and metabolism in three hyposomatotropic rat models and normal rats. *Endocrinology* 110:376, 1982.
224. Bivens CH, Lebovitz HE, Feldman JM: Inhibition of hypoglycemia induced growth hormone secretion by the serotonin antagonists cyproheptadine and methysergide. *N Engl J Med* 289:236, 1973.
225. Blockard WG, Heidnigsfelder SA: Adrenergic receptor control mechanism for growth hormone secretion. *J Clin Invest* 47:1407, 1968.
226. Lal S, Tolis G, Martin JB, Brown GM, Guyda H: Effect of clonidine on growth hormone, prolactin, luteinizing hormone, follicle stimulating hormone and thyroid stimulating hormone in the serum of normal men. *J Clin Endocrinol Metab* 41:827, 1975.
227. Parra A, Schultz RB, Foley TP Jr, Blizard RM: Influence of epinephrine-propranolol infusion on growth hormone release in normal and hypopituitary patients. *J Clin Endocrinol Metab* 30:134, 1970.
228. Boyd AE, Lebovitz HE, Pfeiffer JB: Stimulation of human growth hormone secretion by l-dopa. *N Engl J Med* 283:1425, 1970.
229. Maany I, Fraser A, Mandels J: Apomorphine: Effect on GH. *J Clin Endocrinol Metab* 40:162, 1975.
230. Camanni F, Massara F, Belforte L, Molinatti GM: Changes in plasma growth hormone levels in normal and acromegalic subjects following administration of an infusion of 2-bromo-alpha-ergocryptine. *J Clin Endocrinol Metab* 40:363, 1975.
231. Massara F, Camanni F: Effects of various adrenergic receptor stimulating and blocking agents on HGH secretion. *J Endocrinol* 54:195, 1972.
232. Liberman B, Cesar FP, Wajchenberg BL: Human growth hormone (hGH) stimulation tests: The sequential exercise and l-dopa procedure. *Clin Endocrinol (Oxf)* 10:649, 1979.
233. Mayer G, Schwinn G: Human growth hormone release: Suppression by TRH and augmentation by bromocryptine (abstract). *Acta Endocrinol (Copenh)* 87:10, 1978.
234. Moretti C, Fabbri A, Gnessi L, Bonifacio V, Fraioli F: Pyridoxine (B6) suppresses the rise in prolactin and increases the rise in growth hormone induced by exercise. *N Engl J Med* 307:444, 1982.
235. McClaren NK, Taylor GE, Raiti S: Propranolol augmented, exercise induced human growth hormone release. *Pediatrics* 56:804, 1975.
236. Shanis BS, Moshang T: Propranolol and exercise as a screening test for growth hormone deficiency. *Paediatrics* 57:712, 1976.
237. Joffe BI, Haitas B, Edelstein D, Panz V, Lamprey JM, et al: Clonidine and the hormonal responses to graded exercise in healthy subjects. *Horm Res* 23:136, 1986.
238. Struthers AD, Burrin JM, Brown MJ: Exercise-induced increases in plasma catecholamines and growth hormone are augmented by selective alpha-2-adrenoceptor blockade in man. *Neuroendocrinology* 44:22, 1986.
239. Stubbs WA, Delitala G, Jones A, Jeffcoate WL, Edwards CRW, Ratter SJ, Besser GM: Hormonal and metabolic responses to an enkephalin analogue in normal man. *Lancet* 2:1225, 1978.
240. Spiler IJ, Molitch ME: Lack of modulation of pituitary hormone stress response by neural pathways involving opiate receptors. *J Clin Endocrinol Metab* 50:516, 1980.
241. Mayer G, Wessel J, Kobberling J: Failure of naloxone to alter exercise-induced growth hormone and prolactin release in normal men. *Clin Endocrinol (Oxf)* 13:413, 1980.
242. Staessen J, Fiocchi R, Bouillon R, Fagard R, Hespel P, et al: Effects of opioid antagonism on the haemodynamic and hormonal responses to exercise. *Clin Sci* 75:293, 1988.
243. Carr DB, Bullen BA, Skrinar GS, Arnold MA, Rosenblatt M, et al: Physical conditioning facilitates the exercise-induced secretion of beta-endorphin and beta-lipotropin. *N Engl J Med* 305:560, 1981.
244. Fraioli F, Moretti C, Paolucci D, Aliciccio E, Crescenzi F, Fortunio G: Physical exercise stimulates marked concomitant release of beta-endorphin and adrenocorticotropic hormone (ACTH) in peripheral blood in man. *Experientia* 36:987, 1981.
245. Gambert SR, Garthwaite TL, Pontzer CH, Cook EE, Tristani FE, et al: Running elevates plasma beta-endorphin immunoreactivity and ACTH in untrained human subjects. *Proc Soc Exp Biol Med* 168:1, 1981.
246. Rosak C, Vogel D, Althoff PH, Neubauer M, Brecht HM, Schoffling K: Hormonal and metabolic parameters following insulin-induced hypoglycemia. *Endokrinologie* 79:337, 1982.
247. Schnabel A, Kinderman W, Schmitt WM, Biro G, Stegman H: Hormonal and metabolic consequences of prolonged running at the individual anaerobic threshold. *Int J Sports Med* 3:163, 1982.
248. Koenig J, Mayfield MA, McCann SM, Krulich L: Stimulation of prolactin secretion by morphine: Role of the central serotoninergic system. *Life Sci* 25:853, 1979.
249. Karebath M, Doaz JL, Huttunen M: Serotonin synthesis by brain synaptosomes, effect of L-dopa, 1-3-methoxytyrosine, and catecholamines. *Biochem Pharmacol* 21:1245, 1972.
250. Goodwin FK, Dunner DL, Gershon ES: Effect of L-dopa treatment on brain serotonin metabolism in depressed patients. *Life Sci* 10:751, 1971.
251. Grossman A, Stubbs WA, Gaillard RC, Delitala G, Rees LH, Besser GM: Studies of the opiate control of prolactin, GH and TSH. *Clin Endocrinol (Oxf)* 14:381, 1981.
252. Hunter WM, Fonseke CC, Passmore R: The role of growth hormone in the mobilization of fuel for muscular exercise. *Q J Physiol Cogn Med Sci* 50:406, 1965.
253. Raben MS, Hollenberg CH: Effect of growth hormone on plasma fatty acids. *J Clin Invest* 59:484, 1965.
254. Daughaday WH, Kipnis DM: The growth promoting actions of somatotropin. *Recent Prog Horm Res* 22:49, 1966.
255. Galbo H: *Hormonal and Metabolic Adaptations to Exercise.* New York, Springer-Verlag, 1983.
256. Davies CTM, Few JD: Effects of exercise on adrenocortical function. *J Appl Physiol* 35:887, 1973.
257. Loucks AB, Horvath SM: Exercise induced stress responses of amenorrheic and eumenorrheic runners. *J Clin Endocrinol Metab* 59:1109, 1984.
258. Cumming DC, Brunsting LA III, Strich G, Greenberg L, Ries AL, Rebar RW: Reproductive hormone increases in response to acute exercise in men. *Med Sci Sports Exerc* 18:369, 1986.
259. Cumming DC, Wall SR, Galbraith MA, Belcastro AN: Reproductive hormone responses to resistance exercise. *Med Sci Sports Exerc* 9:234, 1987.

358. Kjaer M, Bangsbo J, Lortie G, Galbo H: Hormonal response to exercise in humans: Influence of hypoxia and physical training. *Am J Physiol* 254:R197, 1988.
359. Hyyppa MT, Aunola S, Kuusela V: Psychoendocrine responses to bicycle exercise in healthy men in good physical condition. *Int J Sports Med* 7:89, 1986.
360. Tarnopolsky LJ, MacDougall JD, Atkinson SA, Tarnopolsky MA, Sutton JR: Gender differences in substrate for endurance exercise. *J Appl Physiol* 68:302, 1990.
361. Bramnert M, Hokfelt B: Lack of effect of naloxone in a moderate dosage on the exercise induced increase in blood pressure, heart rate, plasma catecholamines, plasma renin activity and plasma aldosterone in healthy males. *Clin Sci* 68:185, 1984.
362. Gullestad L, Dolva LO, Kjeldsen SE, Eide I, Kjekshus J: The effects of naloxone and timolol on plasma catecholamine levels during short-term dynamic exercise. *Scand J Clin Lab Invest* 47:847, 1987.
363. Schnabel A, Kindermann W, Salas-Fraire O, Cassens J, Steinkraus V: Effect of beta-adrenergic blockade on supramaximal exercise capacity. *Int J Sports Med* 4:278, 1983.
364. Erisksen J, Thaulow E, Mundal R, Opstad P: Comparison of beta-adrenergic receptor blockers under maximal exercise. *Br J Clin Pharmacol* 13:209S, 1982.
365. Irving MH, Britton BJ, Wood WG, Padgham C, Caruthers M: Effects of beta adrenergic blockade on plasma catecholamines in exercise. *Nature* 248:531, 1974.
366. Planz G, Planz R: Influence of propranolol on catecholamine concentration in blood of normotensive man during physical exercise and depending of the drug effect on dosage intervals. *Arch Int Pharmacodyn Ther* 1(suppl):58, 1980.
367. Chamberlain KG, Pestell RG, Best JD: Platelet catecholamine contents are cumulative indexes of sympathoadrenal activity. *Am J Physiol* 259:E141, 1990.
368. Van Loon GR, Schwartz L, Sole MJ: Plasma dopamine responses to standing and exercise in man. *Life Sci* 24:2273, 1979.
369. Musso NR, Gianrossi R, Pende A, Vergassola C, Lotti G: Plasma dopamine response to sympathetic activation in man: A biphasic pattern. *Life Sci* 47:619, 1990.
370. Hartling OJ, Kelbaek H, Gjorup T, Nielsen MD, Trap-Jensen J: Plasma concentrations of adrenaline, noradrenaline and dopamine during forearm dynamic exercise. *Clin Physiol* 9:399, 1989.
371. Imai N, Stone CK, Woolf PD, Liang CS: Effects of naloxone on systemic and regional hemodynamic responses to exercise in dogs. *J Appl Physiol* 64:1493, 1988.
372. Peronnet F, Cleroux J, Perrault H, Thibault G, Cousineau D, de Champlain J, Guilland JC, Klepping J: Plasma norepinephrine, epinephrine, and dopamine beta-hydroxylase activity during exercise in man. *Med Sci Sports Exerc* 17:683, 1985.
373. Chin NW, Chang FE, Dodds WG, Kim MH, Malarkey WB: Acute effects of exercise on plasma catecholamines in sedentary and athletic women with normal and abnormal menses. *Am J Obstet Gynecol* 157:938, 1987.
374. Cousineau D, Ferguson RJ, de Champlain J, Gauthier P, Cote P, Baourassa M: Catecholamines in coronary sinus during exercise in man before and after training. *J Appl Physiol* 43:801, 1977.
375. Hickson RC, Hagberg JM, Coulee RK, Jones DA, Ehsairi AA, Winder WW: Effects of training on hormonal response to exercise in competitive swimmers. *Eur J Appl Physiol* 41:211, 1979.
376. Peronnet F, Cléroux J, Perrault H, Cousineau D, de Champlain J, Nadeau R: Plasma norepinephrine response to exercise before and after training in humans. *J Appl Physiol* 51:812, 1981.
377. Kjaer M, Galbo H: Effect of physical training on the capacity to secrete epinephrine. *J Appl Physiol* 64:11, 1988.
378. Mazzeo RS: Catecholamine responses to acute and chronic exercise. *Med Sci Sports Exerc* 23:839, 1991.
379. Pestell RG, Hurley DM, Vandongen R: Biochemical and hormonal changes during a 1000 km ultramarathon. *Clin Exp Pharmacol Physiol* 16:353, 1989.
380. McAllister RM: Adaptations in control of blood flow with training: Splanchnic and renal blood flows. *Med Sci Sports Exerc* 30:375, 1998.
381. Crampes F, Beauville M, Riviere D, Garrigues M: Effect of physical training in humans on the response of isolated fat cells to epinephrine. *J Appl Physiol* 61:25, 1986.
382. Riviere D, Crampes F, Beauville M, Garrigues M: Lipolytic response of fat cells to catecholamines in sedentary and exercise-trained women. *J Appl Physiol* 66:330, 1989.
383. Christensen NJ, Galbo H: Sympathetic nervous activity during exercise. Annu Rev Physiol 45:139, 1983.
384. Folgering H, Th M, Borm JFE, van Haaren RHLM: Metabolic aspects of maximal exercise performance after slow release metoprolol and after atenolol. *Eur J Clin Pharmacol* 23:283, 1982.
385. McAllister RM: Endothelial-mediated control of coronary and skeletal muscle blood flow during exercise: Introduction. *Med Sci Sports Exerc* 27:1122, 1997.
386. Kjaer M: Adrenal medulla and exercise training. *Eur J Appl Physiol* 77:195, 1998.
387. Lash JM: Training-induced alterations in contractile function and excitation-contraction coupling in vascular smooth muscle. *Med Sci Sports Exerc* 30:60, 1998.
388. McAllister RM: Adaptations in control of blood flow with training: splanchnic and renal blood flows. *Med Sci Sports Exerc* 30:375, 1998.
389. Gilbert C: Optimal physical performance in athletes: Key roles of dopamine in a specific neurotransmitter/hormonal mechanism. *Mechs Ageing Det* 84:83, 1995.
390. van Zijderveld GA, van Doornen LJ, van Faassen I, Orlebeke JF, van Dyck R, Tilders FJ: Adrenaline and the relationship between neurosomatism, aerobic fitness and mental task. *Biol Psychol* 36:157, 1993.
391. Peyrin L, Pequignot JM, Lacour JR, Fourcade J: Relationships between catecholamine or 3-methoxy 4-hydroxy phenylglycol changes and the mental performance under submaximal exercise in man. *Psychopharmacology* 93:188, 1987.
392. Eipper BA, Mains RE: Structure and biosynthesis of proadrenocorticotropin/endorphin and related peptides. *Endocr Rev* 1:1, 1980.
393. Kjaer M, Secher NH, Bach FW, Sheikh S, Galbo H: Hormonal and metabolic responses to exercise in humans: Effect of sensory nervous blockade. *Am J Physiol* 257:E95, 1989.
394. De Meirleir K, Naaktgeboren N, Van Steirteghem A, Gorus F, Olbrecht J, Block P: Beta-endorphin and ACTH levels in peripheral blood during and after aerobic and anaerobic exercise. *Eur J Appl Physiol* 55:5, 1986.
395. Oltras CM, Mora F, Vives F: Beta-endorphin and ACTH in plasma: Effects of physical and psychological stress. *Life Sci* 40:1683, 1987.
396. Kraemer WJ, Patton JF, Knuttgen HG, Marchitelli LJ, Cruthirds C, et al: Hypothalamic-pituitary-adrenal responses to short-duration high-intensity cycle exercise. *J Appl Physiol* 66:161, 1986.
397. Heitkamp HC, Schmid K, Scheib K: Beta-endorphin and adrenocorticotropic hormone production during marathon and incremental exercise. *Eur J Appl Physiol* 66:269 1993.
398. Kraemer RR, Dzewaltowski DA, Blair MS, Rinehardt KF, Castracane VD: Mood alteration from treadmill running and its relationship to beta-endorphin, corticotropin, and growth hormone. *J Sports Med Phys Fit* 30:241, 1990.
399. Kraemer RR, Acevedo EO, Dzewaltowski D, Kilgore JL, Kraemer GR, Castracane VD: Effects of low-volume resistive exercise on beta-endorphin and cortisol concentrations. *Int J Sports Med* 17:12, 1996.
400. Kraemer WJ, Dziados JE, Marchitelli LJ, Gordon SE, Harman EA, et al: Effects of different heavy-resistance exercise protocols on plasma beta-endorphin concentrations. *J Appl Physiol* 74:450, 1993.
401. McGowan RW, Pierce EF, Eastman N, Tripathi HL, Dewey T, Olson K: Beta-endorphins and mood states during resistance exercise. *Percept Mot Skills* 76:376, 1993.
402. Pierce EF, Eastman NW, Tripathi HT, Olson KG, Dewey WL: Plasma beta-endorphin immunoreactivity: Response to resistance exercise. *J Sports Sci* 11:499, 1993.
403. Kraemer WJ, Fry AC, Warren BJ, Stone MH, Fleck SJ, et al: Acute hormonal responses in elite junior weightlifters. *Int J Sports Med* 13:103, 1992.
404. Goldfarb AH, Hatfield BD, Armstrong D, Potts J: Plasma beta-endorphin concentration: Response to intensity and duration of exercise. *Med Sci Sports Exerc* 22:241, 1990.
405. Schwarz L, Kindermann W: Beta-endorphin, adrenocorticotropic hormone, cortisol and catecholamines during aerobic and anaerobic exercise. *Eur J Appl Physiol* 61:165, 1990.
406. Taylor DV, Boyajian JG, James N: Acidosis stimulates beta-endorphin release during exercise. *J Appl Physiol* 77:1913, 1994.
407. Bortz WM II, Angwin P, Mefford IN, Boarder MR, Noyce N, Barachas JD: Catecholamines, dopamine and endorphin levels during extreme exercise (letter). *N Engl J Med* 305:466, 1981.

408. Elias AN, Fairshter R, Pandian MR, Domurat E, Kayaleh R: Beta-endorphin/beta-lipotropin release and gonadotropin secretion after acute exercise in physically conditioned males. *Eur J Appl Physiol* 58:522, 1989.
409. McMurray RG, Hill D, Field KM: Diurnal variations of beta-endorphin at rest and after moderate intensity exercise. *Chronobiol Int* 7:135, 1990.
410. Boone JB Jr., Sherraden T, Pierzchala K, Berger R, Van Loon GR: Plasma Met-enkephalin and catecholamine responses to intense exercise in humans. *J Appl Physiol* 73:388, 1992.
411. Kelso TB, Herbert WG, Gwazdauskas FC, Goss FL, Hess JL: Exercise, themoregulatory stress and increased plasma β-endorphin/β-lipotropin in humans. *J Appl Physiol* 57:444, 1984.
412. Goldfarb AH, Jamurtas AZ, Kamimori GH, Hegde S, Otterstetter R, Brown DA: Gender effect on beta-fendorphin response to exercise. *Med Sci Sports Exerc* 30:1672, 1998.
413. Casti A, Orlandini G, Troglio MG, Bacciottini F, Michelini M, et al: Acute and chronic hyperbaric oxygen exposure in humans: Effects on blood polyamines, adrenocorticotropin and beta-endorphin. *Acta Endocrinologica* 129:436, 1993.
414. Appenzeller O, Wood SC: Peptides and exercise at high and low altitudes. *Int J Sports Med* 13 Suppl 1:S135, 1992.
415. Farrell PA, Kjaer M, Bach FW, Galbo H: Beta-endorphin and adrenocorticotropin response to supramaximal treadmill exercise in trained and untrained males. *Acta Physiol Scand* 130:619, 1987.
416. Lobstein DD, Ismail AH: Decreases in resting plasma beta-endorphin/-lipotropin after endurance training. *Med Sci Sports Exerc* 21:161, 1989.
417. Walberg-Rankin J, Franke WD, Gwazdauskas FC: Response of beta-endorphin and estradiol to resistance exercise in females during energy balance and energy restriction. *Int J Sports Med* 13:542, 1992.
418. Surbey GS, Andrew GM, Cervenko FW, Hamilton PP: Effects of naloxone on exercise performance. *J Appl Physiol* 57:674, 1984.
419. McMurray RG, Sheps DS, Guinan DM: Effects of naloxone on maximal stress testing in females. *J Appl Physiol* 56:436, 1984
420. Mahler DA, Cunningham LN, Skrinar GS, Kraemer WJ, Colice GL: Beta-endorphin activity and hypercapnic ventilatory responsiveness after marathon running. *J Appl Physiol* 66:2131, 1989.
421. Gordon NF, Duncan JJ, Kohl HW: Effect of opioid antagonism on the ability to tolerate maximal anaerobic exercise. *S Afr Med J* 76:268, 1989.
422. Strassman RJ, Appenzeller O, Lewy AJ, Qualls CR, Peake GT: Increase in plasma melatonin, beta-endorphin, and cortisol after a 28.5-mile mountain race: Relationship to performance and lack of effect of naltrexone. *J Clin Endocrinol Metab* 69:540, 1989.
423. Black J, Chesher JB, Starmer GA, Egger G: The painlessness of the long distance runners. *Med J Aust* 1:522, 1979.
424. Mogil JS, Sternberg WF, Balian H, Liebeskind JC, Sadowski B: Opioid and nonopioid swim stress-induced analgesia: A parametric analysis in mice. *Physiol Behav* 59:123, 1996.
425. Janal MN, Colt EWD, Clarke WC, Glusman M: Pain sensitivity, mood and plasma endocrine levels in man following long distance running: Effects of naloxone. *Pain* 19:13, 1984.
426. Tierney G, Carmody J, Jamieson D: Stress analgesia: The opioid analgesia of long swims suppresses the non-opioid analgesia induced by short swims in mice. *Pain* 46:89, 1991.
427. Droste C, Greenlee MW, Schreck M, Roskamm H: Experimental pain thresholds and plasma beta-endorphin levels during exercise. *Med Sci Sports Exerc* 23:334, 1991.
428. Morgan WP: Negative addiction in runners. *Exerc Med Sci Sport* 7:52, 1979.
429. Davis C, Claridge G: The eating disorders as addiction: A psychobiological perspective. *Addict Behav* 23:463, 1998.
430. Epling F, Pierce D, (eds), Activity anorexia: Theory, Research and Treatment. Hillsdale, NJ, Lawrence Ehrlbaum, 1996.
431. Melchior JC, Rigaud D, Chayvialle JA, Colas-Linhart N, Laforest MD, et al: Palatability of a meal influences release of beta-endorphin, and of potential regulators of food intake in healthy human subjects. *Appetite* 22:233, 1994.
432. Mayer J, Roy P, Mitra KP: Relation between caloric intake, body weight and physical work: Studies in an industrial population in West Bengal. *Am J Clin Nutr* 4:169, 1956.
433. Watt EW, Wiley J, Fletcher G: Effect of dietary control and exercise training on daily food intake and serum lipids in postmyocardial infarction patients. *Am J Clin Nutr* 29:900, 1976.
434. Katch FI, Michael ED, Jones EM: Effect of physical training on the body composition and diet of females. *Res Quart* 40:99, 1969.
435. Johnson RE, Mastropoulos JA, Wharton MA: Exercise dietary intake and body composition. *J Am Diet Assoc* 61:399, 1972.
436. Edholm OG, Fletcher JG, Widdowson EM, McCance RA: Energy expenditure and food intake of individual men. *Br J Nutr* 9:286, 1955.
437. Feighner JP, Robins E, Guze SB, Woodruff RA, Winokur G, Munoz R: Diagnostic criteria for use in psychiatric research. *Arch Gen Psychiatry* 26:57, 1972.
438. Davis C, Kaptein S, Kaplan AS, Olmsted MP, Woodside DB: Obsessionality in anorexia nervosa: The moderating influence of exercise. *Psychosom Med* 60:192, 1998.
439. Diehl NS Johnson CE, Rogers RL, Petrie TA: Social physique anxiety and disordered eating: What's the connection? *Addict Behav* 23:1, 1998.
440. Sundgot-Borgen J: Prevalence of eating disorders in elite female athletes. *Int J Sport Nutr* 3:29, 1993.
441. Rosen LW, McKeag DB, Hough DO, Curley V: Pathogenic weight control behaviour in female athletes. *Phys Sports Med* 14:79, 1986.
442. Yates A, Leehay K, Shisslak CM: Running an analogue of anorexia nervosa. *N Engl J Med* 308:251, 1983.
443. Powers PS, Schocken DD, Boyd FR: Comparison of habitual runners and anorexia nervosa patients. *Int J Eat Dis* 23:133, 1998.
444. Wheeler GD, Wall SR, Belcastro AN, Conger P, Gumming DC: Are anorexic tendencies prevalent in the habitual runner? *Br J Sports Med* 20:77, 1986.
445. Epling WF, Pierce WD, Stefan L: Schedule induced self starvation: Possible implications for anorexia nervosa, in Bradshaw CM, Szabadi E, Lowe CF (eds): *Quantification of Steady State Operant Behaviour.* Amsterdam, Elsevier, 1981, pp 393–397.
446. Sundgot-Borgen J: Risk and trigger factors for the development of eating disorders in female elite athletes. *Med Sci Sports Exerc* 26:414, 1994.
447. Davis C, Kennedy SH, Ravelski E, Dionne M: The role of physical activity in the development and maintenance of eating disorders. *Psychol Med* 24:957, 1994.
448. Kaye WH, Pickar D, Naber D, Ebert MH: Cerebrospinal fluid opioid activity in anorexia nervosa. *Am J Psychiatry* 139:643, 1982.
449. Moore R, Mills IH, Forster A: Naloxone in the treatment of anorexia nervosa: Effect on weight gain and lipolysis. *J R Soc Med* 74:129, 1981.
450. Mills IH: The neuronal basic of compulsive behaviour in anorexia nervosa. *J Psychiatr Res* 19:231, 1985.
451. Marrazzi MA, Bacon JP, Kinzie J, Luby ED: Naltrexone use in the treatment of anorexia nervosa. In Clin Psychopharmacol 10:163, 1995.
452. Russell JB, Mitchell D, Musey PI, Collins DC: The role of β-endorphins and catechol-estrogens on the hypothalamic-pituitary axis in female athletes. *Fertil Steril* 42:690, 1984.
453. Glasser W: *Positive Addiction.* New York, Harper & Row, 1976.
454. Sachs ML: Running addiction, in Sachs MH, Sachs ML (eds): *The Psychology of Running.* Champaign, IL, Human Kinetics, 1981, pp 116–126.
455. Steinberg H, Sykes EA: Introduction to symposium on endorphins and behavioural processes: Review of literature on endorphins and exercise. *Pharmacol Biochem Behav* 23:857, 1985.
456. Szabo A: The impact of exercise deprivation on well-being of habitual exercises. *Austral J Sci Med Sport.* 27:68, 1995.
457. Pierce EF, McGowan RW, Lynn TD: Exercise dependence in relation to competitive orientation of runners. *J Sportsmed Phys Fit* 33:189, 1993.
458. Furst DM, Germone K: Negative addiction in male and female runners and exercisers. *Percept Motor Skills* 77:192, 1993.
459. Pierce EF, Morris JT: Exercise dependence among competitive power lifters. *Percept Motor Skills* 86:1097, 1997.
460. Pierce EF, Rohaly KA, Fritchley B: Sex differences on exercise dependence for men and women in a marathon road race. *Percept Motor Skills* 84:991, 1997.
461. Pierce EF, Eastman NW, Tripathi HL, Olson KG, Dewey WL: Beta-endorphin response to endurance exercise: Relationship to exercise dependence. *Percept Motor Skills* 77:767, 1993.
462. McCann IL, Holmes DS: Influence of aerobic exercise on depression. *J Pers Soc Psychol* 46:1142, 1984.
463. Morgan WP: Affective beneficence of vigorous physical activity. *Med Sci Sports Exerc* 17:94, 1985.

464. DeVries HA, Wiswell RA, Bulbulian R, Moritani T: Tranquilizer effect of exercise. *Am J Phys Med* 60:57, 1981.
465. Morgan WP: Anxiety reduction following acute physical activity. *Psychiatr Ann* 9:36, 1979.
466. Mandell AJ: The second second wind. *Psychiatr Am* 9:57, 1979.
467. Markoff RA, Ryan P, Young T: Endorphins and mood changes in long distance running. *Med Sci Sports Exerc* 14:11, 1982.
468. Kraemer RR, Dzewaltowski DA, Blair MS, Rinehardt KF, Castracane VD: Mood alteration from treadmill running and its relationship to beta-endorphin, corticotropin, and growth hormone. *J Sports Med Phys Fitness* 30:241, 1990.
469. McGowan RW, Pierce EF, Eastman N, Tripathi HL, Dewey T, Olson K: Beta-endorphins and mood states during resistance exercise. *Percept Motor Skills* 76:376, 1993.
470. Bramnert M, Hokfelt B: The influence of naloxone on exercise-induced increase in plasma pituitary hormones and the subjectively experienced level of exhaustion in healthy males. *Acta Endocrinol (Copenh)* 115:125, 1987.
471. Inder WJ, Livesey JH, Donald RA: Peripheral plasma levels of beta-endorphin in alcoholics and highly trained athletes and the relationship to a measure of central opioid tone. *Horm Metab Res* 30:523, 1998.
472. Zaworonok ME, Hudson RW, Orban WA: The prolactin response of males to a standard MVO2 treadmill test. *J Androl* 8:378, 1987.
473. Keizer HA, Kuipers H, de Haan J, Beckers E, Habets L: Multiple hormonal responses to physical exercise in eumenorrheic trained and untrained women. *Int J Sports Med* 8(Suppl 3):139, 1987.
474. Hashimoto T, Migita S, Matsubara F: Response of thyrotropin, prolactin and free thyroid hormones to graded exercise in normal male subjects. *Endocrinol Jpn* 33:735, 1986.
475. Shangold MM, Gatz JM, Thysen B: Acute effects of exercise on plasma concentrations of prolactin and testosterone in recreational women runners: *Fertil Steril* 35:699, 1981.
476. Chang FE, Dodds WG, Sullivan M, Kim MH, Malarkey WB: The acute effects of exercise on prolactin and growth hormone secretion: Comparison between sedentary women and women runners with normal and abnormal cycles. *J Clin Endocrinol Metab* 62:551, 1986.
477. Tanaka H, Cleroux J, de Champlain J, Ducharme JR, Collu RJ: Persistent effects of a marathon run on the pituitary-testicular axis. *Endocrinol Invest* 9:97, 1986.
478. Bouissou P, Brisson GR, Peronnet F, Helie R, Ledoux M: Inhibition of exercise-induced blood prolactin response by acute hypoxia. *Can J Sport Sci* 12:49, 1987.
479. Odink J, Van der Beek EJ, Van den Berg H, Bogaards JJ, Thissen JT: Effect of work load on free and sulfate-conjugated plasma catecholamines, prolactin, and cortisol. *Int J Sports Med* 7:352, 1986.
480. Ronkainen H: Depressed follicle-stimulating hormone, luteinizing hormone, and prolactin responses to the luteinizing hormone-releasing hormone, thyrotropin-releasing hormone, and metoclopramide test in endurance runners in the hard-training season. *Fertil Steril* 44:755, 1985.
481. Brisson GR, Volle MA, De Carufel D, Desharnais M, Tanaka M: Exercise induced dissassociation of the blood prolactin response in young women according to their sports habits. *Horm Metab Res* 12:201, 1980.
482. Mougin C, Henriet MT, Baulay A, Haton D, Berthelay S, Gaillard RC: Plasma levels of beta-endorphin, prolactin and gonadrotropins in male athletes after an international nordic ski race. *Eur J Appl Physiol* 57:425, 1988.
483. Chang FE, Richards SR, Kim MH, Malarkey WB: Twentyfour hour prolactin profiles and prolactin responses to dopamine in long distance running women. *J Clin Endocrinol Metab* 59:631, 1984.
484. De Meirleir K, Baeyens L, L'Hermite M, L'Hermite-Baleriaux M, Olbrecht J, Holmann W: Pergolide mesylate inhibits exercise-induced prolactin release in man. *Fertil Steril* 43:628, 1985.
485. Tegelman R, Carlstrom K, Pousette A: Hormone levels in male ice hockey players during the night after a 26-hour cup tournament. *Andrologia* 22:261, 1990.
486. Carli G, Bonifazi M, Lodi L, Lupo C, Martelli G, Viti A: Hormonal and metabolic effects following a football match. *Int J Sports Med* 7:36, 1986.
487. Hackney AC, Sinning WE, Bruot BC: Hypothalamic-pituitary-testicular axis function in endurance-trained males. *Int J Sports Med* 11:98, 1990.
488. Boyden TW, Pamenter RW, Grosso D, Stanforth P, Rotkis T, Wilmore JH: Prolactin responses, menstrual cycles and body composition of women runners. *J Clin Endocrinol Metab.* 54:711, 1982.
489. Hakkinen K, Pakarinen A, Alen M, Komi PV: Serum hormones during prolonged training of neuromuscular performance. *Eur J Appl Physiol* 53:287, 1985.
490. Hurley RS, Bossetti BM, O'Dorisio TM, Welch MA, Rice RR, et al: The response of serum growth hormone and prolactin to training in weight-maintaining healthy males. *J Sportsmed Phys Fit* 30:45, 1990.
491. Hackney AC, Ness RJ, Schrieber A: Effects of endurance exercise on nocturnal hormone concentrations in males. *Chronobiol Int* 6:341, 1989.
492. Hackney AC, Fahrner CL, Stupnicki R: Reproductive hormonal responses to maximal exercise in endurance-trained men with low resting testosterone levels. *Exp Clin Endocrinol Diabet* 105:291, 1997.
493. Mannelli M, Pupilli C, Fabbri G, Musante R, De Feo ML, et al: Endogenous dopamine (DA) and DA2 receptors: A mechanism limiting excessive sympathetic-adrenal discharge in humans. *J Clin Endocrinol Metab* 66:626, 1988.
494. Rahkila P, Hakala E, Alen M, Salminen K, Laatikainen T: Beta-endorphin and corticotropin release is dependent on a threshold intensity of running exercise in male endurance athletes. *Life Sci* 43:551, 1988.
495. Marvin G, Sharma A, Aston W, Field C, Kendall MJ, Jones DA: The effects of buspirone on perceived exertion and time to fatigue in man. *Exp Physiol* 82:1057, 1997.
496. Bemben DA, Boileau RA, Bahr JM, Nelson RA, Misner JE: Effects of oral contraceptives on hormonal and metabolic responses during exercise. *Med Sci Sports Exerc* 24:434, 1992.
497. Struder HK, Hollmann W, Donike M, Platen P, Weber K: Effect of O_2 availability on neuroendocrine variables at rest and during exercise: O_2 breathing increases plasma prolactin. *Eur J Appl Physiol* 74:443, 1996.
498. Knudtzon J, Bogsnes A, Norman N: Changes in prolactin and growth hormone levels during hypoxia and exercise. *Horm Metab Res* 21:453, 1989.
499. Utsunomiya T, Kadota T, Yanaga T: Pituitary hormone responses to exercise at high altitudes. *Nippon Naibunpi Gakkai Zasshi* 60:1214, 1984.
500. De Meirleir KL, Baeyens L, L'Hermite-Baleriaux M, L'Hermite M, Hollmann W: Exercise-induced prolactin release is related to anaerobiosis. *J Clin Endocrinol Metab* 60:1250, 1985.
501. Mastrogiacomo I, Toderini D, Bonanni G, Bordin D: Gonadotropin decrease induced by prolonged exercise at about 55% of the VO2max in different phases of the menstrual cycle. *Int J Sports Med* 11:198, 1990.
502. Luger A, Watschinger B, Deuster P, Svoboda T, Clodi M, Chrousos GP: Plasma growth hormone and prolactin responses to graded levels of acute exercise and to a lactate infusion. *Neuroendocrinology.* 56:112, 1992.
503. Elias AN, Wilson AF, Naqvi S, Pandian MR: Effects of blood pH and blood lactate on growth hormone, prolactin, and gonadotropin release after acute exercise in male volunteers. *Proc Soc Exp Biol* 214:156, 1997.
503. Vigas M, Jezova D: Glucose administration does not modulate prolactin response to exercise, TRH or haloperidol injection. *Physiol Res* 43:293, 1994.
504. Melin B, Cure M, Pequignot JM, Bittel J: Body temperature and plasma prolactin and norepinephrine relationships during exercise in a warm environment: Effect of dehydration. *Eur J Appl Physiol* 58:146, 1988.
505. Brisson GR, Bouchard J, Peronnet F, Boisvert P, Garceau F: Evidence for an interference of selective face ventilation on hyperprolactinemia induced by hyperthermic treadmill running. *Int J Sports Med* 8:387, 1987.
506. Brisson GR, Peronnet F, Ledoux M, Pellerin-Massicotte J, Matton P, et al: Temperature-induced hyperprolactinemia during exercise. *Horm Metab Res* 18:283, 1986.
507. Brisson GR, Audet A, Ledoux M, Matton P, Pellerin-Massicotte J, Peronnet F: Exercise-induced blood prolactin variations in trained adult males: A thermic stress more than an osmotic stress. *Horm Res* 23:200, 1985.
508. Christensen SE, Jorgensen O, Moller J, Moller N, Orskov H: Body temperature elevation, exercise and serum prolactin concentrations. *Acta Endocrinol (Copenh)* 109:458, 1985.

509. Ronnemaa T, Marniemi J, Leino A, Karanko H, Puukka P, Koivisto VA: Hormone response of diabetic patients to exercise at cool and warm temperatures. *Eur J Appl Physiol* 62:109, 1991.
510. Saini J, Bothorel B, Brandenberger G, Candas V, Follenius M: Growth hormone and prolactin response to rehydration during exercise: effect of water and carbohydrate solutions. *Eur J Appl Physiol* 61:61, 1990.
511. Brisson GR, Boisvert P, Peronnet F, Quirion A, Senecal L: Face cooling-induced reduction of plasma prolactin response to exercise as part of an integrated response to thermal stress. *Eur J Appl Physiol* 58:816, 1989.
512. Voigt K, Ziegler M, Grunert-Fuchs M, Bickel U, Fehm-Wolfsdorf G: Hormonal responses to exhausting physical exercise: The role of predictability and controllability of the situation. *Psychoneuroendocrinology* 15:173, 1990.
513. Oleshansky MA, Zoltick JM, Herman RH, Mougey EH, Meyerhoff JL: The influence of fitness on neuroendocrine responses to exhaustive treadmill exercise. *Eur J Appl Physiol* 59:405, 1990.
514. Mesaki N, Sasaki J, Motobu M, Nabeshima Y, Shoji M, et al: Effect of naloxone on hormonal changes during exercise. *Nippon Sanka Fujinka Gakkai Zasshi* 41:1991, 1989.
515. Coiro V, Passeri M, Davoli C, Bacchi-Modena A, Bianconi L, et al: Oxytocin reduces exercise-induced ACTH and cortisol rise in man. *Acta Endocrinol (Copenh)* 119:405, 1988.
516. De Meirleir K, L'Hermite Baleriaux M, L'Hermite M, Rost R, Hollmann W: Evidence for serotoninergic control of exercise-induced prolactin secretion. *Horm Metab Res* 17:380, 1985.
517. Baker HWG, Santen RJ, Berger HG, de Kretser DM, Hudson B, et al: Rhythms in the secretion of gonadotropins and gonadal steroids. *J Steroid Biochem* 6:793, 1975.
518. Pardridge WM: Transport of protein bound hormones into tissues in vivo. *Endocr Rev* 2:103, 1981.
519. Vermeulen A, Verdonck L, Van Der Straeten M, Orie N: Capacity of testosterone binding globulin in human plasma and its influence on specific binding of testosterone and its clearance rate. *J Clin Endocrinol Metab* 29:1470, 1969.
520. Baird DT, Horton R, Longcope C, Tait JF: Steroid dynamics under steady state conditions. *Recent Prog Horm Res* 25: 611, 1969.
522. Sutton JR, Coleman MJ, Casey J, Lazarus L: Androgen responses during physical exercise. *Br Med J* i:520, 1973.
523. Wilkerson JE, Horvath SM, Gutin B: Plasma testosterone during treadmill exercise. *J Appl Physiol* 49:249, 1980.
524. Jezova D, Vigas M: Testosterone response to exercise during blockade and stimulation of adrenergic receptors in man. *Horm Res* 15:141, 1981.
525. Schmid P, Pusch PP, Wolf WW, Pilger E, Pessenhofer H, et al: Serum FSH, LH and testosterone in humans after physical exercise. *Int J Sports Med* 3:84, 1982.
526. Mathur DN, Toriola AL, Dada OA: Serum cortisol and testosterone levels in conditioned male distance runners and non-athletes after maximal exercise. *J Sports Med Phys Fitness* 26:245, 1986.
527. Vogel RB, Books CA, Ketchum C, Zauner CW, Murray FT: Increase of free and total testosterone during submaximal exercise in normal males. *Med Sci Sports Exerc* 17:119, 1984.
528. Kraemer WJ, Marchitelli L, Gordon SE, Harman E, Dziados JE, et al: Hormonal and growth factor responses to heavy resistance exercise protocols. *J Appl Physiol* 69:1442, 1990.
529. Metivier G, Gauthier R, de la Chevotriere J, Grymala D: The effect of acute exercise on the serum levels of testosterone and luteinizing (LH) hormone in human male athletes. *J Sports Med Phys Fitness* 20:235, 1980.
530. Gotshalk LA, Loebel CC, Nindl BC, Putukian M, Sebastianelli WJ, et al: Hormonal responses of multiset versus single-set heavy-resistance exercise protocols. *Can J Appl Physiol* 22:244, 1997.
531. Duclos M, Corcuff JB, Rashedi M, Fougere V, Manier G: Does functional alteration of the gonadotropic axis occur in endurance trained athletes during and after exercise? A preliminary study. *Eur J Appl Physiol* 73:427, 1996.
532. Hackney AC, Prem, MC, McMurray RG: Influence of aerobic versus anaerobic exercise on the relationship between reproductive hormones in men. *J Sports Sci* 13:305, 1995.
533. Volek JS, Kraemer WJ, Bush JA, Incledon T, Boetes M: Testosterone and cortisol in relationship to dietary nutrients and resistance exercise. *J Appl Physiol* 82:49, 1997.
534. Hoffman JR, Falk B, Radom-Isaac S, Weinstein Y, Magazanik A, et al: The effect of environmental temperature on testosterone and cortisol responses to high intensity, intermittent exercise in humans. *Eur J Appl Physiol* 75:83, 1997.
535. Sakamoto K, Wakabayashi I, Yoshimoto S, Masui H, Katsuno S: Effects of physical exercise and cold stimulation on serum testosterone level in men. *Jap J Hyg* 46:635, 1991.
536. Hoffman JR, Maresh CM, Armstrong LE, Gabaree CL, Bergeron MF, et al: Effects of hydration state on plasma testosterone, cortisol and catecholamine concentrations before and during mild exercise at elevated temperature. *Eur J Appl Physiol Occup Physiol* 69:294, 1994.
537. Zmuda JM, Thompson PD, Winters SJ: Exercise increases serum testosterone and sex hormone-binding globulin levels in older men. *Metab Clin Exp* 45:935, 1996.
538. Hakkinen K, Pakarinen A: Acute hormonal responses to heavy resistance exercise in men and women at different ages. *Int J Sports Med* 16:507, 1995.
539. Nicklas BJ, Ryan AJ, Treuth MM, Harman SM, Blackman MR, Hurley BF: Testosterone, growth hormone and IGF-I responses to acute and chronic resistive exercise in men aged 55–70 years. *Int J Sports Med* 16:445, 1995.
540. Cumming DC, Wall SR, Quinney HA, Belcastro AN: Decrease in serum testosterone levels with maximal intensity swimming exercise in trained male and female swimmers. *Endocr Res* 13:31, 1987.
541. Kuopposalmi K: Plasma testosterone and sex-hormone-binding capacity in physical exercise. *Scand J Clin Lab Invest* 40:411, 1980.
542. Rowell LB: Human cardiovascular adjustments to exercise and thermal stress. *Physiol Rev* 53:75, 1974.
543. Sutton JR, Coleman MJ, Casey JH: Testosterone production rate during exercise, in Landry F, Orban WAR (eds): *3rd International Symposium on Biochemistry of Exercise*. Miami, Symposium Specialists, 1978, pp 227–234.
544. Cadoux-Hudson TA, Few JD, Imms FJ: The effect of exercise on the production and clearance of testosterone in well trained young men. *Eur J Appl Physiol* 54:321, 1985.
545. Burke CW, Anderson DC: Sex hormone binding globulin is an estrogen amplifier. *Nature* 240:38, 1972.
546. Levin J, Lloyd CW, Lobotsky J, Friedrich EH: The effect of epinephrine on testosterone production. *Acta Endocrinol (Copenh)* 55:184, 1967.
547. Kindermann W, Schnabel A, Schmitt A, Biro G, Hippchen M: Catecholamine, STH, cortisol, glucagon, insulin und sexual hormone bei korperlicher belastung und betal-blockade. *Klin Wohenschr* 60:505, 1982.
548. MacConnie SE, Barkan A, Lampman RM, Schork MA, Beitins IZ: Decreased hypothalamic gonadotropin releasing hormone secretion in male marathon runners. *N Engl J Med* 315:411, 1986.
549. Webb ML, Wallace JP, Hamill C, Hodgson JL, Mashaly MM: Serum testosterone concentration during two hours of moderate intensity treadmill running in trained men and women. *Endocr Res* 10:27, 1984.
550. Schurmeyer T, Jung K, Nieschlag E: The effects of an 1100 kilometer run on testicular adrenal and thyroid hormones. *Int J Androl* 7:276, 1984.
551. Urhausen A, Kinderman W: Behaviour of testosterone, sex hormone binding globulin (SHBG) and cortisol before and after a triathlon. *Int J Sports Med* 8:305, 1987.
552. Johansson C, Tsai L, Hultman E, Tegelman R, Pousette A: Restoration of anabolic deficit and muscle glycogen consumption in competitive orienteering. *Int J Sports* 11:204, 1990.
553. Keizer H, Janssen GM, Menheere P, Kranenburg G: Changes in basal plasma testosterone, cortisol, and dehydroepiandrosterone sulfate in previously untrained males and females preparing for a marathon. *Int J Sports Med* 10(Suppl 3):S139, 1989.
554. McColl EM, Wheeler GD, Gomes P, Bhambhani Y, Cumming DC: The effects of acute exercise on LH pulsatile release in high mileage male runners. *Clin Endocrinol (Oxf)* 31:617, 1989.
555. Kujala UM, Alen M, Huhtaniemi IT: Gonadotrophin-releasing hormone and human chorionic gonadotrophin tests reveal that both hypothalamic and testicular endocrine functions are suppressed during acute prolonged physical exercise. *Clin Endocrinol (Oxf)* 33:219, 1990.
556. Cumming DC, Quigley ME, Yen SSC: Acute suppression of circulating testosterone levels by cortisol in man. *J Clin Endocrinol Metab* 57:671, 1983.

557. De Souza MJ, Miller BE: The effect of endurance training on reproductive function in male runners. A 'volume threshold' hypothesis. *Sports Med* 23:357, 1997.
558. Remes K, Kuopposalmi K, Adlercreutz H: Effects of longterm physical training on plasma testosterone, androstenedione, luteinizing hormone, sex hormone binding globulin capacity. *Scand J Lab Invest* 39:743, 1979.
559. Johnson CC, Stone MH, Byrd RJ, Lopez SA: The response of serum lipids and plasma androgens to weight training exercise in sedentary males. *J Sports Med Phys Fitness* 23:39, 1983.
560. Peltonen P, Marniemi J, Hietanen E, Vuori I, Enholm C: Changes in serum lipids, lipoproteins and heparin releasable lipolytic enzymes during moderate physical training in man: A longitudinal study. *Metabolism* 30:518, 1981.
561. Bagatell CJ, Bremner WJ: Sperm counts and reproductive hormones in male marathoners and lean controls. *Fertil Steril* 53:688, 1990.
562. Jensen CE, Wiswedel K, McLoughlin J, van der Spuy Z: Prospective study of hormonal and semen profiles in marathon runners [see comments]. *Fertil Steril* 64:1189, 1995.
563. Ayers JWT, Komesu Y, Romain T, Ansbacher RA: Anthropometric, hormonal and psychologic correlates of semen quality in endurance trained male athletes. *Fertil Steril* 43:917, 1985.
564. Mantzoros CS, Georgiadis EI: Body mass and physical activity are important predictors of serum androgen concentrations in young healthy men. *Epidemiology* 6:432, 1995.
565. Skarda ST, Burge MR: Prospective evaluation of risk factors for exercise-induced hypogonadism in male runners. *West J Med* 169:9, 1998.
566. Aloia JF, Cohn SH, Babu T, Abesamic C, Kalici N, Ellis K: Skeletal mass and body composition in marathon runners. *Metabolism* 27:1793, 1978.
567. Bennell KL, Brukner PD, Malcolm SA: Effect of altered reproductive function and lowered testosterone levels on bone density in male endurance athletes. *Br J Sports Med* 30:205, 1996.
568. Burge MR, Lanzi RA, Skarda ST, Eaton RP: Idiopathic hypogonadotropic hypogonadism in a male runner is reversed by clomiphene citrate *Fertil Steril* 67:783, 1997.
569. Naessens G, De Slypere JP, Dijs H, Driessens M: Hypogonadism as a cause of recurrent muscle injury in a high level soccer player. A case report. *Int J Sports Med* 16:413, 1995.
570. Hakkinen K: Neuromuscular and hormonal adaptations during strength and power training: A review. *J Sports Med Phys Fitness* 29:9, 1989.
571. Hartung GH, Foreyt JP, Mitchell RE, Vlasek I, Gotto AM: Relation of diet to high-density-lipoprotein cholesterol in middle aged marathon runners, joggers and inactive men. *N Engl J Med* 302:357, 1980.
572. Kantor MA, Cullinane EM, Herbert PN, Thompson PD: Acute increase in lipoprotein lipase following prolonged exercise. *Metabolism* 33:454, 1984.
573. Keizer HA, Doorfman J, Bunnik GSJ: Influence of physical exercise on sex hormone metabolism. *Med Sci Sports Exerc* 48:765, 1980.
574. Wheeler GD, Singh M, Pierce WD, Epling WF, Cumming DC: Endurance training decreases serum testosterone levels in men without change in LH pulsatile release. *J Clin Endocrinol Metab* 72:422, 1991.
575. Rogol AD, Veldhuis JD, Williams FA, Johnson ML: Pulsatile secretion of gonadotropins and prolactin in male marathon runners: Relation to the endogenous opiate system. *J Androl* 5:21, 1984.
576. Hamalainen EK, Adlercreutz H, Puska P, Pietinen P: Decrease of serum total and free testosterone during a low-fat high fibre diet. *J Steroid Biochem* 18:369, 1983.
577. Zubiran S, Gomez-Mont F: Endocrine disturbance in chronic human malnutrition. *Vitam Horm* 11:97, 1952.
578. Strauss RH, Lanese RR, Malarkey WB: Weight loss in amateur wrestlers and its effect on testosterone levels. *JAMA* 254:3337, 1985.
579. Hickey MS, Houmard JA, Considine RV, Tyndall GL, Midgette JB, et al: Gender-dependent effects of exercise training on serum leptin levels in humans. *Am J Physiol* 272: E562, 1997.
580. Boone T, Gilmore S: Effects of sexual intercourse on maximal aerobic power, oxygen pulse, and double product in male sedentary subjects. *J Sportsmed Phys Fit I* 35:214, 1995.
581. Bonen A, Ling WY, MacIntyre KP, Neil R, McGrail JC, Belcastro AN: Effects of exercise on the serum concentrations of FSH, LH, progesterone and estradiol. *Eur J Appl Physiol* 42:15, 1979.
582. Jurkowski JE, Jones NL, Walker WC, Younglai EV, Sutton JR: Ovarian hormone response to exercise. *J Appl Physiol* 44:109, 1978.
583. Mastrogiacomo I, Toderini D, Bonanni G, Bordin D: Gonadotropin decrease induced by prolonged exercise at about 55% of the VO2max in different phases of the menstrual cycle. *Int J Sports Med* 11:198, 1990.
584. Cumming, DC, Wheeler GD, Harber VJ: Physical activity, nutrition, and reproduction, in Campbell KL, Wood JW (eds): *Human Reproductive Ecology, Interactions of Environment, Fertility, and Behavior Ann NY Acad Sci* 709:55, 1994.
585. Rogol AD, Weltman A, Weltman JY, Seip RL, Snead DB, et al: Durability of the reproductive axis in eumenorrheic women during 1 yr of endurance training. *J Appl Physiol* 72:1571, 1992.
586. Frisch RE, Wishak G, Vincent L: Delayed menarche and amenorrhea in ballet dancers. *N Engl J Med* 303:17, 1980.
587. Frisch RE, Gotz-Welbergen AV, McArthur JV, Albright T, Witschi J, et al: Delayed menarche and amenorrhea of college athletes in relation to age of onset of training. *JAMA* 246:1559, 1981.
588. Warren MP: The effects of exercise on pubertal progression and reproductive function in girls. *J Clin Endocrinol Metab* 51:1150, 1980.
589. Brooks-Gunn J, Warren MP: Mother-daughter differences in menarcheal age in adolescent girls attending national dance company schools and non-dancers. *Ann Hum Biol* 15:35, 1988.
590. Ellison PT, Lager C: Exercise-induced menstrual disorders. *N Engl J Med* 313:825, 1985.
591. Feicht CB, Johnson TS, Martin BJ, Sparkes KE, Wagner WW Jr: Secondary amenorrhoea in athletes. *Lancet* 2:1145, 1978.
592. Speroff L, Redwine DB: Exercise and menstrual dysfunction. *Phys Sports Med* 8:42, 1979.
593. Dale E, Gerlach DH, Wilhite AL: Menstrual dysfunction in distance runners. *Obstet Gynecol* 54:47, 1979.
594. Shangold MM, Levine HS: The effect of marathon training on menstrual function. *Am J Obstet Gynecol* 143:862, 1982.
595. Lutter JM, Cushman S: Menstrual patterns in female runners. *Phys Sports Med* 10:60, 1983.
596. Glass AR, Yahiro JA, Deuster PA, Ferguson EW, Vigersky RA: Amenorrhea in Olympic marathon runners. *Fertil Steril* 48:740, 1987.
597. Sanborn CF, Martin BJ, Wagner WW: Is athletic amenorrhea specific to runners? *Am J Obstet Gynecol* 143:859, 1982.
598. Toriola AL: Survey of menstrual function in young Nigerian athletes. *Int J Sports Med* 9:29, 1988.
599. De Cree C: Sex steroid metabolism and menstrual irregularities in the exercising female. A review. *Sports Med* 25:369, 1998.
600. Baer JT: Endocrine parameters in amenorrheic and eumenorrheic adolescent female runners. *Int J Sports Med* 14:191, 1993.
601. De Souza MJ, Miller BE, Loucks AB, Luciano AA, Pescatello LS, et al: High frequency of luteal phase deficiency and anovulation in recreational women runners: Blunted elevation in follicle-stimulating hormone observed during luteal-follicular transition. *J Clin Endocrinol Metab* 83:4220, 1998.
602. Laughlin GA, Yen SS: Nutritional and endocrine-metabolic aberrations in amenorrheic athletes. *J Clin Endocrinol Metab* 81:4301, 1996.
603. Jahreis G, Kauf E, Frohner G, Schmidt HE: Influence of intensive exercise on insulin-like growth factor I, thyroid and steroid hormones in female gymnasts. *Growth Reg* 1:95, 1991.
604. Lindholm C, Hirschberg AL, Carlstrom K, von Schoultz B: Altered adrenal steroid metabolism underlying hypercortisolism in female endurance athletes. *Fertil Steril* 63:1190, 1190.
605. Cumming DC, Vickovic MM, Wall SR, Fluker MR: Defects in pulsatile LH release in normally menstruating runners. *J Clin Endocrinol Metab* 60:810, 1985.
606. Cumming DC, Vickovic MM, Wall SR, Fluker MR, Belcastro AN: The effects of acute exercise on pulsatile release of luteinizing hormone in women runners. *Am J Obstet Gynecol* 153:482, 1985.
607. Veldhuis JD, Evans WS, Demers LM, Thorner MO, Wakat D, Rogol AD: Altered neuroendocrine regulation of gonadotropin secretion in women distance runners. *J Clin Endocrinol Metab* 61:557, 1985.
608. Quigley ME, Sheehan KL, Casper RF, Yen SSC: Evidence for increased dopaminergic and opioid activity in patients with hypothalamic hypogonadotropic amenorrhea. *J Clin Endocrinol Metab* 50:949, 1980.
609. Dixon G, Eurman P, Stern B, Schwartz B, Rebar RW: Hypothalamic function in amenorrheic runners. *Fertil Steril* 42:377, 1984.

610. Samuels MH, Sanborn CF, Hofeldt F, Robbins R: The role of endogenous opiates in athletic amenorrhea. *Fertil Steril* 55:507, 1991.
611. McArthur JW, Turnbull BA, Pehrson J, Bauman M, Henley K, et al: Nalmefene enhances LH secretion in a proportion of oligo-amenorrheic athletes. *Acta Endocrinologica* 128:325, 1993.
612. McArthur JW, Bullen BH, Beitins IZ, Pagano M, Badger TM, Klibanski A: Hypothalamic amenorrhea in runners of normal body composition. *Endocr Res Commun* 7:13, 1980.
613. Berga SL, Loucks AB, Rossmanith WG, Kettel LM, Laughlin GA, Yen SS: Acceleration of luteinizing hormone pulse frequency in functional hypothalamic amenorrhea by dopaminergic blockade. *J Clin Endocrinol Metab* 72:151, 1991.
614. De Cree C: The possible involvement of endogenous opioid peptides and catecholestrogens in provoking menstrual irregularities in women athletes. *Int J Sports Med* 11:329, 1990.
615. De Cree C, Ball P, Seidlitz B, Van Kranenburg G, Geurten P, Keizer HA: Responses of catecholestrogen metabolism to acute graded exercise in normal menstruating women before and after training. *J Clin Endocrinol Metab* 82:3342, 1997.
616. De Cree C, Van Kranenburg G, Geurten P, Fujimori Y, Keizer HA: 4-Hydroxycatecholestrogen metabolism responses to exercise and training: Possible implications for menstrual cycle irregularities and breast cancer. *Fertil Steril* 67:505, 1997.
617. Diaz B, Garcia R, Colmenero MD, Terrados N, Fernandez B, Marin B: Melatonin and gonadotropin hormones in pubertal sportsgirls. *Rev Espan Fisiol* 49:17, 1993.
618. Frisch RE: Body fat, menarche and reproductive ability. *Semin Reprod Endocrinol* 3:45, 1985.
619. Sanborn CF, Martin BJ, Wagner WW: Is athletic amenorrhea specific to runners? *Am J Obstet Gynecol* 143:859, 1982.
620. Sanborn CF, Albrecht BH, Wagner WW: Athletic amenorrhea: Lack of association with body fat. *Med Sci Sports Exerc* 19:207, 1987.
621. Cumming DC, Rebar RW: Lack of consistency in the indirect methods of estimating body fat. *Fertil Steril* 41:739, 1984.
622. Carlberg KA, Buckman MT, Peake GT, Riedesel ML: Body composition of oligo/amenorrheic athletes. *Med Sci Sports Exerc* 15:215, 1983.
623. Frisch RE, Snow R, Gerard EL, Johnson L, Kennedy D, et al: Magnetic resonance imaging of body fat of athletes compared with controls, and the oxidative metabolism of estradiol. *Metab Clin Exp* 41:191, 1992.
624. Frisch RE, Snow RC, Johnson LA, Gerard B, Barbieri R, Rosen B: Magnetic resonance imaging of overall and regional body fat, estrogen metabolism, and ovulation of athletes compared to controls. *J Clin Endocrinol Metab* 77:471, 1993.
625. Montague CT, Prins JB, Sanders L, Digby JE, O'Rahilly S: Depot- and sex specific differences in human leptin mRNA expression: Implications for the control of regional fat distribution. *Diabetes* 46:342, 1997.
626. Macut D, Micic D, Pralong FP, Bischof P, Campana A: Is there a role for leptin in human reproduction? *Gynecol Endocrinol* 12:321, 1998.
627. Audi L, Mantzoros CS, Vidal-Puig A, Vargas D, Gussinye M, Carrascosa A: Leptin in relation to resumption of menses in women with anorexia nervosa [see comments]. *Mol Psychiatr* 3:544, 1998.
628. Licinio J, Negrao AB, Mantzoros C, Kaklamani V, Wong ML, et al: Sex differences in circulating human leptin pulse amplitude: Clinical implications. *J Clin Endocrinol Metab* 83:4140, 1998.
629. De Silva A, De Courten M, Zimmet P, Nicholson G, Kotowicz M, et al: Lifestyle factors fail to explain the variation in plasma leptin concentrations in women. *Nutrition* 14:653, 1998.
630. Judd SJ: Disturbance of the reproductive axis induced by negative energy balance *Reprod Fertil Devel* 10:65, 1998.
631. Ahren B, Larsson H: Leptin—a regulator of islet function? Its plasma levels correlate with glucagon and insulin secretion in healthy women. *Metab Clin Exp* 46:1477, 1997.
632. Schwartz MW, Prigeon RL, Kahn SE, Nicolson M, Moore J, et al: Evidence that plasma leptin and insulin levels are associated with body adiposity via different mechanisms. *Diab Care* 20:1476, 1996.
633. Widjaja A, Levy JC, Morris RJ, Frayn KN, Humphreys SM, et al: Determinants of within subject variation of testing serum leptin concentrations in healthy subjects. *Exp Clin Endocrinol Diabetes* 108:208, 2000.
634. Cioffi JA, Van Blerkom J, Antczak M, Shafer A, Wittmer S, Snodgrass HR: The expression of leptin and its receptors in pre-ovulatory human follicles. *Mol Hum Reprod* 3:467, 1997.
635. Steiner RA: Nutritional and metabolic factors in the regulation of reproductive hormone secretion in the primate. *Proc Nutr Soc* 46:159, 1987.
636. Kulin HE, Bwibo N, Mutie D, Santner SJ: Gonadotropin excretion during puberty in malnourished children. *J Pediatr* 105:325, 1984.
637. Vigersky RA, Andersen AE, Thompson RH, Loriaux DL: Hypothalamic dysfunction in secondry amenorrhea associated with simple weight loss. *N Engl J Med* 297:1141, 1977.
638. Beumont PJV, George GCW, Pimstone BL, Vinik AI: Body weight and the pituitary response to hypothalamic releasing hormones. *J Clin Endocrinol Metab* 43:487, 1976.
639. Chakravarty I, Sreedhar R, Ghosh KK, Bulusu S: Circulating gonadotropin profile in severe cases of protein calorie malnutrition. *Fertil Steril* 37:650, 1982.
640. Drinkwater BL, Nilson K, Chesnut CH III, Bremner WJ, Shainoltz S, Southworth M: Bone mineral content of amenorrheic and eumenorrheic athletes. *N Engl J Med* 311:277, 1984.
641. Marcus R, Cann C, Madvig P, Minkoff J, Goddard M, et al: Menstrual function and bone mass in elite women distance runners. *Ann Intern Med* 102:158, 1985.
642. Nelson ME, Fisher EC, Catsos PD, Meredith CN, Turksoy RN, Evans WJ: Diet and bone status in amenorrheic runners. *Am J Clin Nutr* 43:910, 1986.
643. Lloyd T, Buchanan JR, Bitzer S, Waldman CJ, Myers C, Ford BG: Interrelationships of diet, athletic activity, menstrual status and bone density among collegiate women. *Am J Clin Nutr* 46:681, 1987.
644. Schweiger UF, Herman R, Laessle W, Riedel M, Schweiger R, Pirke KM: Caloric intake, stress and menstrual function in athletes. *Fertil Steril* 49:447, 1988.
645. Brooks SM, Sanborn CF, Albrecht BH, Wagner WW: Diet in athletic amenorrhea (letters). *Lancet* 1:559, 1984.
646. Bruce V, Crosby LO, Reicheck N, Pertschuk M, Lusk E, Mullen JL: Energy expenditure in primary malnutrition during standardized exercise. *Am J Phys Med* 63:165, 1984.
647. Dalvit SP: The effect of the menstrual cycle on patterns of food intake. *Am J Clin Nutr* 34:1811, 1981.
648. Myerson M, Gutin B, Warren MP, May MT, Contento I, et al: Resting metabolic rate and energy balance in amenorrheic and eumenorrheic runners. *Med Sci Sports Exerc* 23:15, 1990.
649. Brownell KD, Steen SN, Wilmore JH: Weight regulation practices in athletes: Analysis of metabolic and health effects. *Med Sci Sports Exerc* 19:546, 1987.
650. Zanker CL, Swaine IL: The relationship between serum oestradiol concentration and energy balance in young women distance runners. *Int J Sports Med* 19:104, 1998.
651. Drinkwater BL, Nilson K, Ott S, Chesnut CH III, Bremner WJ, et al: Bone mineral density after resumption of menses in amenorrheic athletes. *JAMA* 256:380, 1986.
652. Armamento-Villareal R, Villareal DT, Avioli LV, Civitelli R: Estrogen status and heredity are major determinants of premenopausal bone mass. *J Clin Invest* 90:2464, 1992.
653. Baer JT, Taper LJ, Gwazdauskas FG, Walberg JL, Novascone MA, et al: Diet, hormonal, and metabolic factors affecting bone mineral density in adolescent amenorrheic and eumenorrheic female runners. *J Sports Med Phys Fit* 32:51, 1992.
654. De Souza MJ, Miller BE, Sequenzia LC, Luciano AA, Ulreich S, et al: Bone health is not affected by luteal phase abnormalities and decreased ovarian progesterone production in female runners. *J Clin Endocrinol Metab* 82:2867, 1997.
655. Hetland ML, Haarbo J, Christiansen C, Larsen T: Running induces menstrual disturbances but bone mass is unaffected, except in amenorrheic women. *Am J Med* 95:53, 1993.
656. Prior JC, Vigna YM, Schechter MT, Burgess AE: Spinal bone loss and ovulatory. *N Eng J Med* 323:1221, 1221.
657. Winters KM, Adams WC, Meredith CN, Loan MD, Lasley BL: Bone density and cyclic ovarian function in trained runners and active controls. *Med Sci Sports Exerc* 28:776, 1996.
658. Cumming DC: Exercise associated amenorrhea, low bone density, and estrogen replacement therapy. *Arch Int Med* 156:2213, 1996.
659. Ruby BC, Robergs RA, Waters DL, Burge M, Mermier C, Stolarczyk L: Effects of estradiol on substrate turnover during exercise in amenorrheic females. *Med Sci Sports Exerc* 29:1160, 1997.
660. Dueck CA, Matt KS, Manore MM, Skinner JS: Treatment of athletic amenorrhea with a diet and training intervention program. *Int J Sport Nutr* 6:24, 1996.

661. Haberland CA, Seddick D, Marcus R, Bachrach LK: A physician survey of therapy for exercise-associated amenorrhea: A brief report. *Clin J Sport Med* 5:246, 1995.
662. McKenzie DC: Markers of excessive exercise. *Can J Appl Physiol* 24:66, 1999.
663. Foster C: Monitoring training in athletes with reference to overtraining syndrome. *Med Sci Sports Exerc* 30:1164, 1998.
664. Gastmann UA, Lehmann MJ: Overtraining and the BCAA hypothesis. *Med Sci Sports Exerc* 30:1173, 1998.
665. Lehmann M, Foster C, Dickhuth HH, Gastmann U: Autonomic imbalance hypothesis and overtraining syndrome. *Med Sci Sports Exerc* 30:1140, 1998.
666. Snyder AC: Overtraining and glycogen depletion hypothesis. *Med Sci Sports Exerc* 30:1146, 1998.
667. Fry AC, Kraemer WJ, Ramsey LT: Pituitary-adrenal-gonadal responses to high-intensity resistance exercise overtraining. *J Appl Physiol* 85:2352, 1998.
668. Kentta G, Hassmen P: Overtraining and recovery. A conceptual model. [Review] [53 refs]. *Sports Medicine* 26:1, 1998.
669. Uusitalo AL, Huttunen P, Hanin Y, Uusitalo AJ, Rusko HK: Hormonal responses to endurance training and overtraining in female athletes. *Clin J Sport Med* 8:178, 1998.
670. Urhausen A, Gabriel H, Kindermann W: Blood hormones as markers of training stress and overtraining. *Sports Med* 20:251, 1995.
671. Hooper SL, MacKinnon LT, Gordon RD, Bachmann AW: Hormonal responses of elite swimmers to overtraining. *Med Sci Sports Exerc* 25:741, 1993.
672. Steinacker JM, Lormes W, Lehmann M, Altenburg D: Training of rowers before world championships. *Med Sci Sports Exerc* 30:1158, 1998.
673. Canada: *Report of the Task Force on National Sport Policy Building Canada's Sport System*. Ottawa, Fitness and Amateur Sport, 1988.
674. Franke WW, Berendonk B: Hormonal doping and androgenization of athletes: A secret program of the German Democratic Republic government. *Clin Chem* 43:1262, 1997.
675. Berger A, Murray TH, Fost N: Comments from the lay press: Excerpts from three newspaper editorials and commentaries. *Phys Sports Med* 12:187, 1984.
676. Wilson JD: Androgens, in Gilman AG, Rall TW, Nies AS, Taylor P (eds): *The Pharmacological Basis of Therapeutics*, 8th ed. New York, Pergamon, 1990, pp 1413–1430.
677. Cowart VS: Issues of drugs and sports gain attention as Olympic Games open in South Korea. *JAMA* 260:1513, 1988.
678. United States Congress, Senate Judiciary Committee: Hearing on Steroid Abuse in America, April 3, 1989, testimony of Pat Connolly.
679. Australia, Parliament: *Drugs in Sport: An Interim Report of the Senate Standing Committee on Environment, Recreation and the Arts.* Commonwealth of Australia, 1989, p 75.
680. Pope HG, Katz DL, Champoux R: Anabolic steroid use among 1010 college men. *Phys Sports Med* 16:75, 1988.
681. Bahrke MS, Yesalis CE, Brower KJ: Anabolic-androgenic steroid abuse and performance-enhancing drugs among adolescents. *Child Adolesc Psychiatr Clin North Am* 7:821, 1998.
682. Ewing BT: High school athletes and marijuana use. *J Drug Educ* 28:147, 1998.
683. Strauss RH, Wright JE, Finerman GAM, Catlin DH: Side effects of anabolic steroids in weight trained men. *Phys Sports Med* 11:87, 1983.
684. Musshoff F, Daldrup T, Ritsch M: Anabolic steroids on the German black market. *Archiv fur Kriminologie* 199:152, 1997.
685. Evans NA: Gym and tonic: A profile of 100 male steroids users. *Br J Sports Med* 31:54, 1997.
686. Friedl KE, Yesalis CE: Self-treatment of gynecomastia in bodybuilders who use anabolic steroids. *Phys Sports Med* 17:67, 1989.
687. Wu FC: Endocrine aspects of anabolic steroids. *Clinical Chemistry* 43:1289, 1997.
688. Street C, Antonio J, Cudlipp D: Androgen use by athletes: A reevaluation of the health risks. *Can J Appl Physiol* 21:421, 1996.
689. Wilson JD: Androgen abuse by athletes. *Endocr Rev* 9:181, 1988.
690. Rogozkin VA: Anabolic steroid metabolism in skeletal muscle. *J Steroid Biochem* 11:923, 1979.
691. Hickson RC, Czerwinski SM, Falduto MT, Young AP: Glucocorticoid antagonism by exercise and androgenic-anabolic steroid. *Med Sci Sports Exerc* 22:331, 1990.
692. Tanaka H, Gibb W, Ducharme JR, Collu R: Influence of compensatory overload on glucocorticoid receptors in rat skeletal muscle. *Steroids* 51:115, 1988.
693. Max SR: Glucocorticoid-mediated induction of glutamine synthetase in skeletal muscle. *Med Sci Sports Exerc* 22:325, 1990.
694. Olweus D, Mattson A, Schalling D, Low H: Testosterone, aggression, physical, and personality dimensions in normal adolescent males. *Psychosom Med* 42:253, 1980.
695. Rose RM, Holaday JW, Bernstein IS: Plasma testosterone, dominance rank and aggressive behaviour in male Rhesus monkeys. *Nature* 231:366, 1971.
696. Wilson JD, Griffin JE: The use and misuse of androgens. *Metabolism* 29:1278, 1980.
697. Hervey GR: Are athletes wrong about anabolic steroids? *Br J Sports Med* 9:74, 1975.
698. Council on Scientific Affairs: Drug abuse in athletes: Anabolic steroids and human growth hormone. *JAMA* 259:1703, 1988.
699. Wade NA: Doctors denounce them but athletes aren't listening. *Science* 176:1399, 1972.
700. Sturmi JE, Diorio DJ: Anabolic agents. *Clin Sports Med* 17:261, 1998.
701. Honour JW: Steroid abuse in female athletes. *Curr Opin Obstet Gynecol* 9:181, 1997.
702. Bahrke MS, Yesalis CE 3rd, Wright JE: Psychological and behavioural effects of endogenous testosterone and anabolic-androgenic steroids. An update. *Sports Medicine* 22:367, 1996.
703. Crist DM, Stackpole PJ, Peake GT: Effects of androgenic substances on neuromuscular power and body composition. *J Appl Physiol* 54:366, 1983.
704. Haupt HA, Rovere GD: Anabolic steroids: A review of the literature. *Am J Sports Med* 12:469, 1984.
705. Middleman AB, DuRant RH: Anabolic steroid use and associated health risk behaviours. *Sports Med* 21:251, 1996.
706. Rubinow DR, Schmidt PJ: Androgens, brain, and behavior. *Am J Psychiatr* 153:974, 1996.
707. Porcerelli JH, Sandler BA: Anabolic-androgenic steroid abuse and psychopathology. *Psychiatr Clin N Am* 21:829, 1998.
708. Hausmann R, Hammer S, Betz P: Performance enhancing drugs (doping agents) and sudden death—a case report and review of the literature. *Int J Legal Med* 111:261, 1998.
709. Sullivan ML, Martinez CM, Gennis P, Gallagher EJ: The cardiac toxicity of anabolic steroids. *Prog Cardiovasc Dis* 41:1, 1998.
710. Hearing before the Senate Subcommittee to Investigate Juvenile Delinquency of the Committee on the Judiciary: *Proper and Improper Use of Drugs by Athletes*. United States Senate, 93rd Congress. Washington, DC, U.S. Government Printing Office, 1973.
711. Kleiner SM, Calabrese LH, Fieldler KM, Naito HK, Skibinski CI, Fieldler KM: Dietary influences on cardiovascular disease risk in anabolic steroid-using and nonusing bodybuilders. *J Am Coll Nutr* 8:109, 1989.
712. Rogol AD: Drugs to enhance performance in the adolescent. *Semin Adolesc Med* 1:317, 1985.
713. Wroblewska AM: Androgenic—anabolic steroids and body dysmorphia in young men. *J Psychosom Res* 42:225, 1997.
714. Korkia P, Stimson GV: Indications of prevalence, practice and effects of anabolic steroid use in Great Britain. *Int J Sports Med* 18:557, 1997.
715. Friedl KE, Yesalis CE: Self-treatment of gynecomastia in bodybuilders who use anabolic steroids. *Phys Sports Med* 17:67, 1989.
716. Reyes RJ, Zicchi S, Hamed H, Chaudary MA, Fentiman IS: Surgical correction of gynaecomastia in bodybuilders [see comments]. *Br J Clin Pract* 49:177, 1995.
717. Alen M, Rahkila P, Reinila M, Vihko R: Androgenic-anabolic steroid effects on serum thyroid, pituitary and steroid hormones in athletes. *Am J Sports Med* 15:357, 1987.
718. Ruokonen A, Alen M, Bolton N, Vihko R: Response of serum testosterone and its precursor steroids, SHBG and CBG, to anabolic steroid and testosterone self administration in man. *J Steroid Biochem* 23:33, 1985.
719. Cohen JC, Hickman RJ: Insulin resistance and diminished glucose tolerance in powerlifters ingesting anabolic steroids. *J Clin Endocrinol Metab* 64:960, 1987.
720. Hartgens F, Kuipers H, Wijnen JA, Keizer HA: Body composition, cardiovascular risk factors and liver function in long-term andro-

genic-anabolic steroids using bodybuilders three months after drug withdrawal. *Int J Sports Med* 17:429, 1996.
721. Cabasso A: Peliosis hepatis in a young adult bodybuilder. *Med Sci Sports Exerc* 26:2, 1994.
722. Kosaka A, Takahashi H, Yajima Y, Tanaka M, Okamura K, et al: Hepatocellular carcinoma associated with anabolic steroid therapy: Report of a case and review of the Japanese literature. *J Gastroenterol* 31:450, 1996.
723. Hakkinen K, Alen M: Training volume, androgen use and serum creatine kinase activity. *Br J Sports Med* 23:188, 1989.
724. McKillop G, Ballantyne FC, Borland W, Ballantyne D: Acute metabolic effects of exercise in bodybuilders using anabolic steroids. *Br J Sports Med* 23:186, 1989.
725. Boone JB, Lambert CP, Flynn MG, Michaud TJ, Rodriguez-Zayas JA, Andres FF: Resistance exercise effects on plasma cortisol, testosterone and creatine kinase activity in anabolic-androgenic steroid users. *Int J Sports Med* 4:293, 1990.
727. Milne CJ: Rhabdomyolysis, myoglobinuria and exercise. *Sports Med* 6:93, 1988.
728. Prat J, Gray GF, Stolley PD, Coleman JW: Wilms tumor in an adult associated with androgen abuse. *JAMA* 237:2322, 1977.
729. Roberts JT, Essenhigh DM: Adenocarcinoma of prostate in a forty-year old body builder. *Lancet* 2:742, 1986.
730. Shahidi NT: Androgens and erythropoiesis. *N Engl J Med* 289:72, 1973.
731. Duda M: Steroids lower immunity, lipids. *Phys Sports Med* 16:56, 1988.
732. Calabrese LH, Kleiner SM, Barna BP, Skibinski CI, Kirkendall DT, Lahita RG, Lombardo JA: The effects of anabolic steroids and strength training on the human immune response. *Med Sci Sports Exerc* 21:386, 1989.
733. Mondelli M, Cioni R, Federico A: Rare mononeuropathies of the upper limb in bodybuilders. *Muscle & Nerve* 21:809, 1998.
734. Evans NA: Local complications of self administered anabolic steroid injections. *Brit J Sports Med* 31:349, 1997.
735. Sklarek HM, Mantovani RP, Erens E, Heisler D, Niederman MS, Fein AM: AIDS in a body builder using anabolic steroid drugs (letter). *N Engl J Med* 311:1701, 1984
736. Bowers LD, Segura J: Anabolic steroids, athletic drug testing, and the Olympic Games *Clin Chem* 42:999, 1996.
737. Catlin DH, Hatton CK, Starcevic SH: Issues in detecting abuse of xenobiotic anabolic steroids and testosterone by analysis of athletes' urine. *Clin Chem* 43:1280, 1997.
738. Bowers LD: Analytical advances in detection of performance-enhancing compounds. *Clinical Chemistry* 43:1299, 1997.
739. Hallagan JB, Hallagan LF, Snyder MB: Anabolic-androgenic steroid use by athletes. *N Engl J Med* 321:1042, 1989.
740. Cowart VS: Blunting "steroid epidemic" requires alternatives, innovative education. *JAMA* 264:1641, 1990.
741. Ryan AJ: Anabolic steroids are fools gold. *Fed Proc* 40:2682, 1981.
742. Goldberg L, Bosworth EE, Bents RT, Trevisan L: Effect of an anabolic steroid education program on knowledge and attitudes of high school football players. *J Adolesc Health Care* 11:210, 1990.
743. Isetts BJ: Preparing community educational presentations on ergogenic drug use. *Am J Hosp Pharm* 46:2028, 1989.
744. Cowart V: Classifying steroids as controlled substances suggested to decrease athletes' supply, but enforcement could be a major problem (news). *JAMA* 257:3029, 1987.
745. Shroyer JA: Getting tough on steroids: Can we win the battle? *Phys Sports Med* 18:106, 1990.
746. Hallagan JB, Hallagan LF, Snyder MB: Anabolic-androgenic steroid use by athletes. *N Engl J Med* 321:1042, 1989.
747. Smith DA, Perry PJ: The efficacy of ergogenic agents in athletic competition. Part II: Other performance-enhancing agents. *Ann Pharmacother* 26:653, 1992.
748. Cowart VJ: Human growth hormone: The latest ergogenic aid? *Phys Sports Med* 16:175, 1988.
749. Crist DM, Peake GT, Egan PA, Walters DL: Body composition response to exogenous GH during training in highly conditioned adults. *J Appl Physiol* 65:579, 1988.
750. Berglund B: Development of techniques for detection of blood doping in sport. *Sports Med* 5:27, 1988.
751. Lavoie C, Diguet A, Milot M, Gareau R: Erythropoietin (rHuEPO) doping: Effects of exercise on anaerobic metabolism in rats. *Int J Sports Med* 19:281, 1998.
752. Canadian Erythropoietin Study Group: Association between recombinant human erythropoietin and quality of life and exercise capacity of patients receiving haemodialysis. *Br Med J* i:573, 1990.
753. Ricci G, Masotti M, De Paoli Vitali E, Vedovato M, Zanotti G: Effects of exercise on haematologic parameters, serum iron, serum ferritin, red cell 2,3-diphosphoglycerate and creatine contents, and serum erythropoietin in long-distance runners during basal training. *Acta Haematol (Basel)* 80:95, 1988.
754. Schmidt W, Maassen N, Trost F, Boning D: Training induced effects on blood volume, erythrocyte turnover and haemoglobin oxygen binding properties. *Eur J Appl Physiol* 57:490, 1988.
755. Albert K: A bad boost (erythropoietin, genetically engineered hormone being abused by athletes). *Sports Illustrated* 73:29, 1990.
756. Ramotar JE: Cyclists' deaths linked to erythropoietin? *Phys Sports Med* 18:48, 1990.

Index

Adrenal gland(s), 385–632
activity of, rhythmicity of, 409–410
blood supply of, *389*
disorders of, hypertension from, 588–593
fetal, 403–404
function of
in hypothyroidism, 324
tests of, in children, 1310
in thyrotoxicosis, 301
hemorrhage in
Addison's disease from, 464
clinical features of, 468, 468t
hyperplasia of, congenital, hypogonadism from, 682
pharmacologic actions of VIP on, 1328t
tumors of, adrenal hyperfunction from, 480–491
Adrenal hyperplasia:
congenital, hypertension in, 590–591
congenital lipoid, 460–461
virilizing, 449
Adrenal hypoplasia congenita, 465
Adrenal insufficiency:
hypercalcemia in, 1137
hypovolemic hyponatremia in, 245
metyrapone testing for, 443–444
Adrenal medulla:
glucocorticoids and, 431–432
hyperplasia of, in pheochromocytoma of MEN 2, 1368–1369
Adrenal sex steroids, ovarian sex steroids versus, 414
Adrenal steroids, obesity and, 974
Adrenalectomy:
bilateral, for Cushing's disease, 489
for corticotroph adenoma, 200
for Cushing's syndrome, 1296–1297
Adrenalitis, diffuse lymphocytic, 463
Adrenarche, 413–414, 1278
premature, 1305
Adrenergic antagonist drugs, thyroid function and, 288
Adrenergic axon terminals, physiology of, 527–528
Adrenergic receptors, 529t, 529–530
Adrenocortical insufficiency, 461–475
causes of, *461*
hypoaldosteronism and, 474–475
primary, 461–469; *See also* Addison's disease
secondary, 469–470
clinical features of, 470
diagnosis of, *470,* 470–472
etiology of, 469
isolated adrenocorticotropic hormone deficiency in, 469
laboratory features of, 470
pathophysiology of, 469–470
prognosis for, 474
survival in, 474
treatment of, 472–473
Adrenocorticotropic hormone (ACTH):
actions of, 177, 406–408
deficiency of, 204–205
hypothalamic, 153
isolated, 469
ectopic, syndrome involving, 479, 480
features of, 482
Adrenocorticotropic hormone (ACTH) *(continued)*
treatment of, 490
tumors causing, 479t
excessive cortisol secretion dependent on, 199
in glucocorticoid regulation, 405–410
in mineralocorticoid regulation, 413
plasma
assays of, 439
levels of, in children, 447
preparations of, 619–620
regulation of, 114
corticotropin releasing hormone in, 130–131
release of
direct patterns of, 408–410
glucocorticoid feedback on, 410–411
vasopressin and, 225
reserve of, test for, in children, 1310t
rhythmic secretion of, 144
secretion of, 177, *178*
stimulation tests with
in children, 447, 1310–1311
in 21-hydroxylase deficiency, *810*
rapid, 442–443
for adrenocortical insufficiency, 471, *471*
suppression tests with, in children, 1310
synthesis of, 177, *178*
direct patterns of, 408–410
Adrenocorticotropic hormone-cortisol axis, exercise and, 1488–1489
Adrenodoxin, in transport of electrons to P450scc, 398
Adrenodoxin reductase, in transport of electrons to P450scc, 397–398
Adreno-genital syndrome, 449
Adrenoleukodystrophy, 465
Age:
adrenal steroidogenesis and, 403–404, *404*
Cushing's syndrome distribution by, 476
growth hormone secretion and, 176
hormone-responsive tumors and, *1433,* 1433–1434
insulin-like growth factor levels and, 1268, *1269*
ovarian activity and, 736–739
in fetal period, 736
menarche and, 737, *737*
menopause and, 738–739
postmenarche, 737–738, *738*
premenarche and, 736, *736*
plasma concentrations of cholesterol based on, *1011*
sporadic goiter and, 354
testicular function and, 672
thyroid cancer and, 360
thyroid function and, 281
Aging; *See also* Elderly
endocrine disorders and, 1456t
hormones and, 1455–1476
changes in, 1460–1465, 1461t
frailty and, 1465–1468
hyperglycemia of, 1471
hypothyroidism compared with, 1457t
nutritional disorders and, 1474–1476
sexuality and, 1468–1471
female, 1471
male, 1469–1471
Aging *(continued)*
theories of, 1458t, 1458–1460
trends in, 1455, *1456*
Agonadism, true, 800, 800t
Agonists:
activation of G protein-coupled receptors by, confirmation changes and, 63–64
inverse, 64
Albers-Schönberg disease, 1198–1199
Albright-McCune-Sternberg syndrome, 1202–1203
Albright's syndrome, 1202–1203
Albumin:
in plasma, physical state of, 416–417
relative affinities of steroids for, 417t
in thyroxine binding, 272
Albuminuria, monitoring for, in diabetes management, 868
Alcohol; *See* Ethanol
Alcoholic ketoacidosis, 890
Alcoholism, chronic, osteoporosis in, 1194
Aldosterone:
changes in, during menstrual cycle and pregnancy, 491–492
for congenital adrenal hyperplasia, 457t, 812
exercise and training and, 1484–1485
as glucocorticoid agonist, 422–423
levels of, in aging, 1462
metabolism of, 420
as mineralocorticoid, 567
in plasma
concentrations of, 415t
physical state of, 418
secretion rate of, 415t
Aldosteronism:
primary
hypertension in, 588–590
treatment of, 590
primary idiopathic hyperplasia differentiated from, 589–590
Alendronate sodium (Fosamax):
for osteoporosis, 1197, *1197, 1198*
in osteoporosis prevention, 1196
for Paget's disease of bone, 1208t, 1209
Alkali therapy:
for calcium phosphate stones, 1236
for cystinuria, 1230, 1230t
for hyperuricosuria, 1254–1255
Alkalosis:
metabolic, in malignancy-associated hypercalcemia, 1127
respiratory, hypophosphatemia from, 1155–1156
Allergy, insulin, 894
Allopurinol:
effect of, on uric acid, mechanisms of, 1233
for hyperuricosuria, 1250, *1250,* 1250t, 1254
for uric acid stones, 1234–1235
Allstrom-Hallgren syndrome, 155t
Alopecia, in endocrine disorders, 21
Alpha$_1$ antitrypsin deficiency, hyperlipidemias secondary to, 1014
Alstrom syndrome, 671
Amenorrhea:
clinical approach to, 817, 819
in endocrine disorders, 23–24
exercise-related, 754

Amenorrhea *(continued)*
nutritional, 753–754
primary, 745–749
clinical classification of, 747t
definition of, 745
with normal stature
and no/minimal pubertal development, 747–748, *748*
and normal pubertal development, 748–749
with short stature and no pubertal development, 745–747
secondary, 750–754
clinical classification of, 750t
dysmenorrhea and, 763–766
exercise and, 1496–1497
female infertility and, 759–763
from galactorrhea, 752
hirsutism and, 757–759
from hyperprolactinemia, 751–753
menorrhagia and, 763–766
nutritional, 753–754
from polycystic ovary syndrome, 754–757
from premature ovarian failure, 750–751
virilization and, 757–759
Amiloride, for nephrogenic diabetes insipidus, 239
Amino acid analogs, as hormones, 5
Amino acid neurotransmitters, 137–138
Aminoglutethimide:
in adrenal steroid biosynthesis inhibition, 414–415
for corticotroph adenoma, 200
for Cushing's disease, 489
Amiodarone:
thyroid function and, 288–289
thyrotoxicosis induced by, 296
Amplitude-modulated enzyme assays, 100
Anabolic steroids:
abuse of, in women, 1502
athletic performance and, 1501–1502
banned by International Olympic Committee, 1499t
benefits of, possible, 1501t
detection of, 1503
as ergogenic aids, effectiveness of, 1501–1502
illicit, sources of, 1501
medical indications for, 1500
mode of action of, 1501
side effects of, 1502t
use of
by athletes, 1501
adverse effects of, 1502–1503
benefits of, assessing, problems with, 1502
controlling, 1504
in various populations, extent of, 1500
Analgesia, exercise-induced, 1491
Analyte, labeled, hormone immunoassays using, 93
Anaplastic carcinoma, of thyroid, *370*, 370–371
Anastrozole (Arimidex), for breast cancer, 1441
Androgen(s):
abuse of, 686
action of, 648–649
Androgen(s) *(continued)*
adrenal
actions of, 437
measurement of, in adrenocortical function evaluation, 444–445
in plasma, physical state of, 418
regulation of, 413–414
blockade of, for prostate cancer, 1447
deficiency of, 654–655
gynecomastia from, 663
in Klinefelter syndrome, 668
primary hypogonadism and, 668–673
in acquired disorders, 672–673
in aging men, 672
from congenital/developmental disorders, 668–672
in systemic illness, 673
excess of
functional, 758
hypogonadism from, 682
for gonadotropin deficiency in women, 207
hypertension and, 569
in male contraception, 686
in menopausal hormone therapy, 771
metabolism of, 420–421
defective, genital virilization defects from, 805
production of
deficient, secondary hypogonadism and, 678–682
by ovarian interstitial cells, 726
in prostatic development, 1429
in pubertal growth spurt, 1277–1279
replacement
for constitutional delayed puberty, 678
for erectile dysfunction, 661
for Kallmann syndrome, 680
for male hypogonadism, 682–686
preparations and regimens for, 682–685, 683t
risks and side effects of, 685–686
secretion, abnormal, in polycystic ovary syndrome, 756
target tissues, defects in, genital virilization defects from, 804–806
Androgen insensitivity syndrome, 805–806
Androgen resistance:
hypogonadism and, 666–667, *667*
molecular basis for, 677
syndromes involving, 676–678
Androstenedione:
levels of, in aging, 1464
plasma concentrations of, 415t
secretion rate of, 415t
Anemia:
in Addison's disease, 469, 469t
in endocrine disorders, 22
in hypothyroidism, 323
Aneuploidy, 780
Aneurysms:
in hypothalamic area, 148
pituitary vessel, growth hormone deficiency from, 1293
Angina pectoris, hypothyroidism and, 323
Angiography:
computed tomography, in renovascular hypertension diagnosis, 585–586
Angiography *(continued)*
renal, in renovascular hypertension diagnosis, 585–586
Angioplasty, for renovascular hypertension, 588
Angiotensin, responsiveness to, regulation of, 563
Angiotensin II:
in blood pressure regulation, 557
in mineralocorticoid regulation, 411–412
Angiotensin II receptor antagonists, 563
Angiotensin-converting enzyme (ACE), 561
Angiotensin-converting enzyme (ACE) gene, hypertension and, 557
Angiotensinogen, 561
Angiotensinogen (AGT) gene polymorphisms, hypertension and, 556–557
Angiotensins:
actions of, 561–563
in blood pressure maintenance, 563–564
formation and metabolism of, *558*
mechanism of action of, 563
production of, 51
Anorchia, congenital, 671, 800, 800t
Anorexia:
in endocrine disorders, 21
hypothalamic, 154–155
Anorexia athletica, 1491
Anorexia nervosa:
amenorrhea in, 754
endogenous opiates and, 1491
hyperlipidemias secondary to, 1015
pubertal delay from, 748
Anosomia, in endocrine disorders, 21
Anoxemia, short stature from, 1302
Antiandrogens, 686–687
for prostate cancer, 1447
Antibiotics, in magnesium ammonium phosphate stone management, 1238
Antibody(ies):
antithyroid
in Graves' disease and autoimmune thyroiditis, 291t
in thyrotoxicosis diagnosis, 302
heterophilic, in hormone assays, 102
monoclonal, 97
nature of, 95–96
polyclonal, 96
production of, 95–97
structure of, 95–96
Anticonvulsants:
androgen deficiency from, 672
vitamin D metabolism abnormalities from, 1185
Antioxidants:
lipid metabolism and, 1047
lipid/lipoprotein metabolism and, 1048
Antithyroid antibodies in serum, tests for, 278
Antithyroid drugs:
for Graves' thyrotoxicosis, 303–304, 304t
hypothyroidism from, 320
for thyrotoxicosis, 304–307
for thyrotroph adenoma, 203–204
Antral follicles, 713–715
Apnea, sleep, in acromegaly, 190
Apolipoprotein B-100, familial defective, 1021–1023
Apolipoproteins, deficiencies of, familial, 1031–1032, 1032t

Apoplexy, pituitary, 183
Apoprotein C-II deficiency, familial, 1027–1029
Apoproteins:
biosynthesis of, 996
function of, 996–997, 997t
in lipoproteins, 994t, 994–995
metabolic functions of, 997t
structure of, 996
Apparent mineralocorticoid excess, 591
Appendages:
in hypothyroidism, 321–322
in thyrotoxicosis, 298
Appetite; *See also* Anorexia; Satiety
disorders of, in endocrine disorders, 21
Arachidonate metabolism, *70*
Arginine vasopressin:
exercise and training and, 1484
in glucocorticoid regulation, 405
levels of, in elderly, 1465
Aromatase:
deficiency of, virilization due to, 815
inhibitors of, for breast cancer, 1441
peripheral, increased, gynecomastia from, 664
Arteries, of ovary, 707, *708*
Arteriosclerosis, in diabetic nephropathy, 901, *902*
Arteriovenous fistula, of cavernous sinus, 182
Arthritis, in acromegaly, 190
Ascorbic acid, hyperoxaluria and, 1248
Aspiration cytology, fine needle, in thyroid nodule evaluation, 361–362, *362*
Ataxia-telangiectasia:
breast cancer risk and, 1431t
primary hypogonadism and, 671
Atherosclerosis, 1037–1038
complicating hypertension, 556
in diabetic nephropathy, 901, *902*
in familial hypercholesterolemia, 1028, 1028t
in iatrogenic Cushing's syndrome, 614
renovascular hypertension from, 582
in type V hyperlipidemia, 1028, 1028t
Atherosclerotic cardiovascular disease, postmenopausal, 768–769
Athletic performance; *See also* Exercise and training
hormones and, 1483–1504
Atorvastatin (Lipitor):
dosage of, 1057, 1058t
for hyperlipoproteinemia, 1056–1057
indications for, 1057–1058
Atresia, in follicular development, 732
Atretic follicles, 715, *715*
Atrial fibrillation, in thyrotoxicosis, 299
Atrial natriuretic hormone (ANH), levels of, in aging, 1465
Atrial natriuretic peptide (ANP):
hypertension and, 572–573
in mineralocorticoid regulation, 413
neurologic effects of, 140
Atropine, growth hormone response to exercise and, 1487
Autocrine effects, on vasopressin secretion, 223
Autocrine mechanisms, of peptide growth factors, 1266
Autocrine regulation, 4
of testis function, 646
Autoimmune adrenocortical insufficiency, 462–463
Autoimmune disease:
endocrine excess syndromes from, 14
growth hormone deficiency from, 1293
polyglandular, 671
Autoimmune syndromes, polyglandular, 1373–1376
Autoimmune thyroiditis:
chronic, hypothyroidism from, 316–317
transient hypothyroidism in, 317–318
Autoimmunity:
in diabetes etiology, 849–850
premature ovarian failure and, 751
Autonomic failure:
generalized, 540–543
classification of, 541t
hypoglycemia-associated, 544–545, *545*
Autonomic function, indirect tests of, in sympathochromaffin system disease diagnosis, 546–547, 547t
Autonomic nervous system:
hypertension and, 573
in insulin secretion regulation, 835
obesity and, 974–975
peripheral, disorders of, erectile dysfunction from, 660
Autonomic neuropathy:
acute, 542t
diabetic, 25–26
classical, 544–545
Autosomal dominant hypocalcemia, 1147–1148
Autosomal dominant thyrotoxicosis, 296–297
Avascular necrosis of bone in iatrogenic Cushing's syndrome, 613
Avidin, in molecular recognition, 97–99
Axoneme complex, 640
Azospermia, 655, 666
in cryptorchidism, 674
evaluation of, 662
idiopathic, 676, 677
in Klinefelter syndrome, 670

Babinski-Froehlich syndrome, 155t
Band keratopathy:
in endocrine disorders, 27
in primary hyperparathyroidism, 1120, *1120*
Bardet-Biedl syndrome, 155t
Barr body, 668
Bartter's syndrome, 492
Beckwith-Wiedmann syndrome, excess growth in, 1308
Beclomethasone dipropionate, structure of, *611*
Behavioral effects of anabolic steroids, 1502
Behavioral modification, in obesity management, 978
Behavioral symptoms of hypothyroidism, 322
"Benecol," 1047
Beta-adrenergic antagonists:
for pheochromocytoma, 539
for thyrotoxicosis, 307
Betamethasone:
for congenital adrenal hyperplasia, 457t
structure of, *611*
Bile acid sequestrants, for hyperlipoproteinemia, 1054–1055
Bile acid-binding resins:
for familial defective apolipoprotein B-100, 1022–1023
in familial hypercholesterolemia management, 1020
Biliary obstruction, hyperlipidemias secondary to, 1014
Binding proteins, in immunoassays, 95–96
Bioamines, as neurotransmitters, 111
Bioassays, of hormones, 91–93
Biogenic amines, receptors for, 62, *62*
Biological rhythms, pineal gland and, 143
Biopsy:
bone, in bone metabolic disease evaluation, 1181–1182
needle, in thyroid function evaluation, 279
Biotin, in molecular recognition, 97–99
Bisphosphonate bone scan, technetium-labeled, 1181, *1181*
Bisphosphonates:
for bone tumors, 1136
for breast cancer, 1442
for hypercalcemia, 1125
for hypercalcemia of malignancy, 1130
for myeloma bone disease, 1134–1135
for osteolytic lesions due to malignancy, 1135–1136
in osteoporosis prevention, 1196
for Paget's disease of bone, 1208t, 1208–1209, *1209*
Bitemporal hemianopsia, in anterior pituitary disease, 183, *183*
Bladder neuropathy, 907
therapy for, 908
Bladder stones, 1221
Bleeding, postmenopausal, 771
Blood pressure:
actions of insulin influencing, 574–575
classification of, 554t
elevation of; *See also* Hypertension
mineralocorticoid, mechanisms of, 568
hormonal modifiers of, 557–579
renin-angiotensin system as, 557–566
low; *See* Hypotension
maintenance of, angiotensins in, 563–564
regulation of, 555–556
renin-angiotensin system in, 564–566
vasopressin and, 220–221, 225
Blood vessels:
actions of insulin on, influencing blood pressure, 574
of ovary, 707, *708*
peripheral, disorders of, erectile dysfunction from, 660
structure of, actions of insulin influencing, 575
Blood volume, vasopressin and, 220–221
Body composition:
fuel reserves and, 842t
measurement techniques for, 954t
Body fat:
distribution of, 960–962, *961*
low, athletic amenorrhea and, 1497–1498
Body mass index (BMI), 953, 955–956
diabetes risk and, 962t
mortality risk and, *958*, 959t
Body temperature, variations of, in endocrine disorders, 20

Bone(s):
avascular necrosis of, in iatrogenic Cushing's syndrome, 613
biopsy of, in bone metabolic disease evaluation, 1181–1182
disease of, hyperparathyroid, 1115–1116, *1116, 1117, 1118, 1119*
disorders of, short stature from, 1297–1298
in endocrine disorders, 24–25
glucocorticoids and, 430
growth hormone actions on, 177
hypercalciuria and, 1247
in hypothyroidism, 325
loss of, in thyrotoxicosis, 301
metabolic disease of, 1179–1210
clinical evaluation of, 1179–1182
biochemical markers of bone turnover in, 1180
clinical chemistry in, 1179–1180
history in, 1179
nuclear medicine in, 1180–1181
physical examination in, 1179
radiology in, 1180–1181
fibrous dysplasia as, 1202–1203, *1203*
hereditary hyperphosphatasia as, 1201–1202
osteomalacia as, 1182–1189; *See also* Osteomalacia
osteopetrosis as, 1198–1199, *1199*
osteoporosis as, 1189–1198; *See also* Osteoporosis
Paget's disease of bone as, 1203–1210; *See also* Paget's disease of bone
renal osteodystrophy as, 1199–1201
rickets as, 1182–1189; *See also* Rickets
metastases to, 1131–1136; *See also* Osteolysis, localized
hypercalcemia and, 1394–1395
Paget's disease of, 1203–1210; *See also* Paget's disease of bone
calcitonin for, 1098
parathyroid hormone actions on, 1090–1093
remodeling of, *1091*
resorption of, hypercalcemia from, 1111–1112
tumors of, bisphosphonates for, 1136
turnover of, biochemical markers of, 1180, 1180t
vitamin D actions in, 1107–1108
Bone scans:
in bone metabolic disease evaluation, 1181, *1181*
in Paget's disease of bone, 1205, *1206*
Bone turnover, 1090, *1091*
Bonnevie-Ullrich syndrome, 671
Borjeson-Forssman-Lehman syndrome, hypogonadotropic hypogonadism in, 681t
Brain:
as endocrine gland, 3
in gonadotropin releasing hormone secretion regulation, 642–643
Brain natriuretic peptide, neurologic effects of, 140
Breast:
cancer of
chemoprevention of, 1442–1443
diagnosis of, 1439–1440
hereditary, 1429–1431
Breast *(continued)*
hormone replacement therapy and, 770
hypercalcemia associated with, parathyroid hormone-related protein in, 1128
oral contraceptives and, 771–772
osteolysis mediated by, parathyroid hormone-related protein in, 1133
pathology of, 1440
prognosis of, 1440, 1440t
progression of, mechanisms of, 1436–1439
risk factors for, 1433, 1439, 1439t
risk for, genetic conditions associated with, 1431t
sporadic, genetic changes responsible for, 1431–1433
treatment of, 1440–1442
development of, normal, hormonal influence on, 1427–1429
male, enlargement of; *See* Gynecomastia
oxytocin and, 225
BRL 26830A, in obesity management, 985
Bromocriptine:
for acromegaly, 193
for hyperprolactinemia, 753
for lactotroph adenoma, 196
Bronchial adenomas, in MEN 1 syndrome, 1358
"Brown tumors" in hyperparathyroidism, 1115, *1117*
Brownian motion, 100
Buserelin, in ovulation induction, *761*
Bypass, gastric, for morbid obesity, 986–987

C cell adenoma, in MEN 2A syndrome, 1366
C cell hyperplasia:
in medullary thyroid cancer, 372, *372*
in MEN 2A syndrome, 1365–1366
Cabergoline:
for hyperprolactinemia, 753
for lactotroph adenoma, 197
Calcifediol, pharmacology of, 1149t
Calciferol, pharmacology of, 1149t
Calcification, inhibitors of, rickets and osteomalacia from, 1187
Calcitonin, 1093–1098
biochemistry of, 1095–1098, *1096, 1097*
biological effects of, 1094–1095
biosynthesis of, 1097, *1097*
ectopic production of, 1414
gene for, RNA processing pathways for, *1097*
gene products of, 1366
for hereditary hyperphosphatasia, 1202
historical notes on, 1093–1094
homologue sequences of, from various species, *1096*
for hypercalcemia of malignancy, 1130
measurements of, in evaluation of medullary thyroid carcinoma therapy, 1367
mechanism of action of, 1094–1095
molecular biology of, 1095–1098, *1096,* 1097
phosphate reabsorption and, 1154
receptor for, alignment of, vs. PTH/PTHrP receptor, *1095*
salmon
for osteoporosis, 1197, 1198
in osteoporosis prevention, 1196
Calcitonin *(continued)*
for Paget's disease of bone, 1207–1208
in screening for medullary thyroid carcinoma, 1366–1367
sequence of, *1093*
as therapeutic agent, 1098
Calcitonin gene-related peptide, hypertension and, 570
Calcitriol, pharmacology of, 1149t
Calcium:
in cellular regulation of PTH secretion, 1084–1085, *1085*
channels for, intracellular, 74
deficiency of, rickets from, 1187
dietary, in nephrolithiasis management, 1226
intake of, adaptation to, 1107
intestinal transport of, 1105–1107, *1106*
intracellular
changes in, 74
vitamin D activation and, 1102
kidney stones containing, in hyperparathyroidism, 1116
metabolism of
cellular and extracellular, 1079–1081
glucocorticoids and, 430–431
oral, for hypoparathyroidism, 1142–1143
protein kinases dependent on, 75
receptors for, 63
renal leak of, hypercalciuria from, 1244–1245
serum levels of
elevated; *See* Hypercalcemia
serum concentration of parathyroid hormone and, *1082*
vitamin D activation and, 1102
Calcium carbonate, for hypocalcemia, 1152
Calcium channels, G protein-activated, 70–71
Calcium chloride, for hypocalcemia, 1151
Calcium gluconate, for hypocalcemia, 1151
Calcium oxalate stones, 1238–1255
epidemiology of, 1238
evaluation of, 1251–1252
idiopathic, 1251
natural history of, 1239
physical chemistry of, 1238–1239
risk factors for, 1239–1251, 1240t
family history as, 1239–1240
hypercalciuria as, 1240–1247
hyperoxaluria as, 1247–1249
hyperuricosuria as, 1249–1250
hypocitraturia as, 1250–1251
low urine volume as, 1240
medication as, 1240
urinary pH as, 1240
treatment of, 1252–1255
discontinuing, 1255
goals of, 1252–1253
need for, 1252
selection of, 1253
Calcium phosphate:
crystalline forms of, 1235
solubility of, pH and, 1235
Calcium phosphate stones, 1235–1236
Calculi; *See* Nephrolithiasis
Call-Exner bodies in secondary follicle, 712, *712*
Calmodulin, 75
protein kinases dependent on, 75

Caloric restriction, thyroid function and, 287
Calories:
  lipid metabolism and, 1046
  lipoprotein metabolism and, 1046
Cancer:
  in acromegaly, 190
  adrenal
    Cushing's syndrome from, 478
    features of, 482
    treatment of, 490
  androgen deficiency in, 673
  breast; *See* Breast, cancer of
  endometrial, 1443–1444
    hormone replacement therapy and, 770
  germ cell, 689–690
  hypercalcemia associated with, 1109–1110, 1110t; *See also* Hypercalcemia, malignancy-associated
  hypocalcemia associated with, 1149–1150
  hypoglycemia associated with, 1406–1409
  obesity and, 964
  parathyroid, surgery for, 1122
  primary hyperparathyroidism coexistent with, 1398
  prostate; *See also* Prostate cancer
  risk of, in multinodular goiter, 356–357
  syndrome of inappropriate antidiuresis in, 1404–1406
  thyroid, 297, 366–378; *See also* Thyroid gland, cancer of
Capping, in messenger RNA biosynthesis, 29
Captopril, for cystinuria, 1231
Carbamazepine (Tegretol):
  for pituitary diabetes insipidus, 237–238
  thyroid function and, 289
Carbohydrates:
  lipid metabolism and, 1046
  lipoprotein metabolism and, 1046
  metabolism of
    glucocorticoid actions on, 424–425, *425*
    growth hormone actions on, 177
    thyroid hormone effects on, 274
Carbon monoxide (CO), as neurotransmitter, 141
Carcinoid syndrome, 1333–1340
  diagnosis of, 1337t, 1337–1338
  differential diagnosis of, 1338, 1339t
  laboratory diagnostic tests in, 1337–1338
  mediators of, 1335–1337
  octreotide acetate efficacy on, 1324t
  pathology of, 1334–1335
  pathophysiology of, 1335–1337
  prognosis of, 1340
  secretory diarrhea in, octreotide acetate for, 1323t
  secretory products in, 1335t
  symptoms of, 1335, *1335*, 1335t
  treatment of, 1338–1340
Carcinoid tumors:
  in MEN 1 syndrome, 1358
  secretory products of, 1335t
Carcinoma; *See* Cancer
Cardiac arrest, thyroid function and, 287
Cardiac autonomic neuropathy, 907–908
Cardiovascular disease:
  in acromegaly, 190
  atherosclerotic, postmenopausal, 768–769
Cardiovascular disease *(continued)*
  in diabetes, 908–912
    diagnosis of, 910
    incidence of, 909
    pathogenesis of, 909–910
    prevalence of, 909
    risk factors for, 909t, *910*
    screening for, 910
    therapy of, 910–912, *911*
  obesity and, 958–960, *959*, 960
Cardiovascular system:
  actions of thyroid hormones on, 274
  alcohol and, 1047–1048
  disease of; *See* Cardiovascular disease
  glucocorticoids and, 429–430
  hormone actions on, 12
  in hypocalcemia, 1141
  in hypothyroidism, 322–323
  oral contraceptives and, 771
  pharmacologic actions of VIP on, 1328t
  secretin effects on, 1326t
  in thyrotoxicosis, 299
Carpal tunnel syndrome:
  in acromegaly, 190
  in endocrine disorders, 26
Castrate syndrome, functional prepubertal, 671
Castration, bilateral, surgical or traumatic, 672
Cataracts, in endocrine disorders, 26
Catecholamines:
  biochemistry of, 525–527
  biological effects of, 531–532
  biological inactivation of, 528–529
  biosynthesis of, 525–526, *526*
  circulating, in insulin secretion regulation, 835
  degradation of, 526–527, *527*
  energy expenditure and, 974–975
  in exercise, 1489–1490
  formation of, 528
  hypertension and, 573
  kinetics of, 532–533
  measurement of, 532–533
    potential sources of error in, 546t
    in sympathochromaffin system disease diagnosis, 545–546
  parathyroid hormone secretion and, 1085–1086
  release of, 528
  storage of, 528
  thyroid hormone interactions with, 274
  venous plasma concentrations of, physiologic adaptation of, 533–535, *534*
Catechol-*O*-methyl transferase (COMT), in catecholamine degradation, 526–527, *527*
Cavernous sinus, arteriovenous fistula of, 182
Cavitation, in tertiary follicle, *709*, 712–713
Celiac disease, hypersecretinemia in, 1327
Cell structure, G proteins and, 71
Cells, growth of, kinase cascades promoting, 81–82
Cellular communication methods, 49, *50*
Cellular dedifferentiation, in ectopic hormone production, 1392
Cellular signaling, second messenger systems in, 71–78
Central nervous system (CNS):
  disorders of
    erectile dysfunction from, 659
    in neuroendocrine disease, 158–159
  in endocrine disorders, 25
  glucocorticoids and, 431
  in hypocalcemia, 1140–1141
  hypothalamic-pituitary axis and, 635–636
  rhythms of, neuroendocrine function and, 143–145
  tumors of, growth hormone deficiency from, 1293
Cerebral gigantism, 159, 1307–1308
Cerebrospinal fluid rhinorrhea, in anterior pituitary disease, 184
Cerebrotendinous xanthomatosis, 1039–1040
Cerivastatin (Baycol), for hyperlipoproteinemia, 1056–1058, 1058t
Chaperone proteins, 60
CHARGE syndrome, hypogonadotropic hypogonadism in, 681t
Chemical goitrogens, 356, 356t
Chemiluminescence in immunoassays, 98
Chemotherapy:
  antitumor, for carcinoid syndrome, 1339
  for endometrial cancer, 1444
Child(ren):
  adrenal function tests in, 1310
  adrenocortical function in, 445–447
  dexamethasone suppression tests in, 445–447
  glucocorticoid therapy in, 624
  growth of, 1281, *1281*
  hyperlipidemia in, treatment of, 1063
  hypothyroidism in, 328
  low-fat, high-complex-carbohydrate diet for, 1053
  pituitary-hypothalamic evaluation in, 1309–1311
  sex steroid concentrations in, 446t
  thyroid function in, 281
  virilization in, clinical approach to, 817, *818*
Chlorpropamide (Diabinese), for pituitary diabetes insipidus, 236–237, *237*
Cholecalciferol; *See* Vitamin D3
Cholecystokinin (CCK), 1325–1326
  endogenous, in obesity management, 986
  neurologic effects of, 138
Cholesterol:
  absorption of, inhibitors of, for hyperlipoproteinemia, 1062
  in atherosclerotic plaques, 1037
  balance of, in body, 998t
  biosynthesis of, agents reducing, for hyperlipoproteinemia, 1061–1062
  conversion of, to pregnenolone, 395–398
  dietary
    in hyperlipidemia management, 1048–1049
    lipid metabolism and, 1042–1043
    lipoprotein metabolism and, 1042–1043
    plasma cholesterol levels and, *1011*
  HDL
    concentrations of, factors influencing, 1031t
    deficiency of, with planar xanthomas, 1032, 1032t

Cholesterol *(continued)*
disorders of, 1030–1034, 1032t
plasma concentrations of, age-related changes in, *1011*
intracellular storage and transport of, 393–394
intracellular transport of, in steroidogenesis, 722
LDL
classification of, 1009t
plasma concentrations of, age-related changes in, *1011*
treatment decisions based on, 1009t
levels of, in elderly, 1475–1476
serum concentrations of, death from coronary artery disease and, *1008*
as steroid hormone precursor, 392–395
synthesis and catabolism of, 997–998
synthesis of, 392–393
total
classification of, 1009t
plasma concentrations of, age-related changes in, *1011*
uptake of, 392–393, *393*
Cholesterol gallstones, obesity and, 963–964
Cholesterol saturated fat index of foods, 1050, 1051t
Cholesterol side-chain cleavage, in steroidogenesis, 722
Cholesterol substrate of ovarian steroids, 721–722, *722*
Cholesteryl ester storage disease, 1039
Cholesteryl ester transfer protein, in lipoprotein metabolism, 1000
Cholestyramine (Questran):
in familial hypercholesterolemia management, 1020, 1021t
for hyperlipoproteinemia, 1054–1055
for thyrotoxicosis, 306
Chondrodysplasia:
Jansen's metaphyseal, 1139
mutations causing, summary of, 1298t
short stature from, 1297–1298
Chondrodystrophies, classification of, *1298*
Choriocarcinomas, thyrotoxicosis in, 297
Chromaffin cells, physiology of, 527–528
Chromatographic assays, 101
Chromatography, liquid, in plasma cortisol determinations, 438
Chromophobe adenomas, in MEN 1 syndrome, 1358
Chromosome(s):
abnormalities of
causing growth excess, 1307
premature ovarian failure from, 750–751
short stature from, 1298, 1300–1302
errors in, 780
sex; *See* Sex chromosomes
structural anomalies in, 7780
X, *782,* 782–783
Y, 781–782, *782*
structural anomalies of, 795–796
Chvostek's sign, in hypocalcemia, 1140
Chylomicron retention disease, 1036
Chylomicrons, 993, *994,* 994t
composition of, 994–995, 995t
increased, dietary factors in causation and correction of, 1049t
metabolism of, 1000
Cigarette smoking; *See* Smoking
Cimetidine, androgen deficiency from, 672
Circadian rhythms, 143
Circulation, fetal, sex steroids in, 787–788
Cirrhosis:
hepatic
androgen deficiency in, 673
gynecomastia and, 664
neuroendocrine alterations in, 157
Citrate, metabolism of, 1251
Climacteric, 766
symptoms of, 767–768
Clinidine, for postural hypotension, 543
Clodronate:
for breast cancer, 1442
for Paget's disease of bone, 1209–1210
Clofibrate (Atromid-S):
in familial hypercholesterolemia management, 1020
for hyperlipoproteinemia, 1059
for pituitary diabetes insipidus, 237
Clomiphene citrate:
in ovulation induction, 760
in polycystic ovary syndrome management, 757
"Codfish" deformities, in osteoporosis, 1190, *1190*
Coffee, lipid/lipoprotein metabolism and, 1048
Colesevelam (WelCol), for hyperlipoproteinemia, 1054–1055
Colestipol (Colestid):
in familial hypercholesterolemia management, 1020, 1021t
for hyperlipoproteinemia, 1054–1055
Coma:
in diabetic ketoacidosis, 890
hyperosmolar hyperglycemic nonketotic, 892
myxedema, 328–329
Communication, cellular, 49, *50*
Competitive protein-binding radioassay, in plasma cortisol determinations, 438
Complement factors, in immunoassays, 103
Computed tomography angiography, helical, in renovascular hypertension diagnosis, 585–586
Computed tomography (CT):
in nephrolithiasis evaluation, 1225
in pheochromocytoma localization, 538–539
quantitative, in bone metabolic disease evaluation, 1180–1181
Congenital adrenal hyperplasia (CAH), 447–449
clinical and laboratory findings in, 448t
diagnosis of
hormone values used for, 811t
prenatal, 455–456
growth excess in, 1303–1304
hypertension in, 590–591
hypogonadism from, 682
management of, hormone values used for, 811t
nonclassic, 451
missense mutations causing, 455
P450c21 gene mapping in, 453
point mutations causing, 454, 454t
salt-wasting, 450
simple virilizing, 450–451
missense mutations causing, 455
Congenital adrenal hyperplasia (CAH) *(continued)*
treatment of, 812–813, *814*
prenatal, 455–456
virilizing syndromes of, 807–815
from 3βHSD deficiency, 815
from 11β-hydroxylase deficiency, 813–815
from 21-hydroxylase deficiency, 808–813
Congenital anorchia, 671
Congenital embryopathic disorders, 145–147
congenital hypothyroidism, 318, 319
Congenital lipoid adrenal hyperplasia, 460–461, 801
Congestive heart failure:
obesity and, 960
thyroid function and, 287
from thyrotoxicosis, 299
Connexins, 713, *713*
Constipation, in endocrine disorders, 22
Constitutional growth delay, 1286–1287
Contraception, chemical, 771–772
Contraceptives, oral, 771–772
benefits and risks of, 771t, 771–772
breast cancer risk and, 1433–1434
for hirsutism, 758–759
for menarcheal menorrhagia, 749
Contragestion, 771–772
Contrast agents, radiographic, iodinated, thyroid function and, 289
Converting enzyme inhibitors, 561
Convulsions, in endocrine disorders, 25
Copeptin, neurophysins and, 226
Coronary artery disease:
death from, serum cholesterol concentrations and, *1008*
in familial hypercholesterolemia, 1016–1017, 1017t
obesity and, 958–960, *960*
thyroid function and, 287
Coronary heart disease:
alcohol consumption and, 1047–1048
coffee and, 1048
Corpora lutea, 718–720, *719, 721*
Corpus albicans, *708,* 720
Corpus luteum, 718–720, *719,* 721, 727, 727–728
Cortex, ovarian, 707, *708*
Cortical nephrocalcinosis, 1221
Corticosteroid-binding globulin, 416
properties of, 416t
relative affinities of steroids for, 417t
Corticosteroids:
inhaled, 619
urinary, measurement of, 439–440
Corticosterone:
as glucocorticoid agonist, 422
metabolism of, 420
plasma concentrations of, 415t
secretion rate of, 415t
Corticosterone methyl oxidase deficiencies, 459–460
Corticotroph adenoma, 198–200
Corticotroph cells, 173
hormones secreted by, 173, 174t

Corticotropin releasing hormone (CRH), 130–132
ACTH stimulation by, 405
in glucocorticoid regulation, 405
hypothalamic, rhythmicity of, 408–409
testing of, in adrenocortical function evaluation, 444
Cortisol:
for adrenal crisis, 472
for chronic adrenal insufficiency, 472–473
for congenital adrenal hyperplasia, 457t
deficiency of, 204–205
diurnal rhythm of, changes in, 410
as glucocorticoid agonist, 422
levels of
in aging, 1462
exercise and, 1488–1489
metabolism of, 418–420
pathways of, *419*
mineralocorticoid actions of, 567
in plasma
distribution of, *416*
physical state of, 415–416
plasma concentrations of, 415t
determination of, 438
production rate for, 440
radioactive, intravenously administered, urinary steroid metabolites of, 417t
release of, direct patterns of, 408–410
salivary, measurement of, 438
secretion of
rate of, 415t
stress and, 427
structure of, *611*
synthesis of, direct patterns of, 408–410
urinary free, measurement of, 439–440
Cortisol-binding proteins, 416–417
Cortisone:
metabolism of, pathways of, *419*
secretion of, excessive, 198–200
structure of, *611*
Cortisone acetate, for congenital adrenal hyperplasia, 457t
Cortrosyn stimulation test, rapid, for polyglandular autoimmune syndromes, 1375
Cosyntropin; *See* Adrenocorticotropic hormone (ACTH)
Cowden's disease, breast cancer risk and, 1431t
Craniopharyngioma(s), 147, 181–182
growth hormone deficiency from, 1293
Cretinism:
endemic goiter and, 352
etiology of, iodine deficiency and, 353
historical overview of, 349
hypothyroidism in, 320
nongoitrous, 318
Crow-Fukase syndrome, 1376
Cryptorchidism, 636, 655, 673–674
Cryptorchism, 807
Crystalloid theory, of stone pathogenesis, 1223
Crystalloids of Reinke, 718, *719*
Cushing's disease, 198–200
age distribution of, 476
definition of, 476
endocrine abnormalities in, 478t
etiology of, 478–479
Cushing's disease *(continued)*
hypertension in, 591
hypothalamus and, 153
occurrence of, 476
pathogenesis of, 478–479
pathology of, 476–478
pathophysiology of, 479–480
sex distribution of, 476
treatment of, 487–489
Cushing's syndrome, 476–480
age distribution of, 476
classification of, 476, 476t
clinical features of, 480t
CT scans in, *488*
definition of, 476
dexamethasone suppression tests for, 440–441, *442*
evaluation algorithm for, *1402*
glucocorticoids and, 610–611, 612–615
gynecomastia and, 664
hypogonadism in, 682
iatrogenic
atherosclerosis in, 614
avascular necrosis of bone in, 613
diagnosis of, 615
glucocorticoid dose- and time-dependency of, 614–615
infections in, 614
manifestations of, 612–615
myopathy in, 614
ocular changes in, 613
osteoporosis in, *613,* 613–614, *614*
in MEN 1 syndrome, management of, 1363
occurrence of, 476
osteoporosis in, 1193–1194
pathology of, 476–478
pathophysiology of, 479–480
prognosis for, 491
sex distribution of, 476
short stature in, 1296–1297
spontaneous, iatrogenic Cushing's syndrome compared with, 612
treatment of, 487–491
Cutaneous lichen amyloidosis, multiple endocrine neoplasia type 2A with, 1371
Cyanoketone, in adrenal steroid biosynthesis inhibition, 415
Cyclic adenosine monophosphate (cAMP):
calcium/calmodulin interplay with, 77
in cellular signaling, 71–72
effects of, on gene transcription, 83–84
ion channels regulated by, 83
nephrogenous, 1088
urinary, response of, to parathyroid hormone in pseudohypoparathyroidism, *1144*
Cyclic guanosine monophosphate (cGMP), ion channels regulated by, 83
Cyclic nucleotide phosphodiesterase, in cellular signaling, 71–72
Cyclic nucleotides, kinase-independent actions of, 83–84
Cyclosporine, androgen deficiency from, 672
Cyproheptadine, growth hormone response to exercise and, 1487
Cyproterone acetate:
as antiandrogen, 687
for hirsutism, 759
Cysteine, oxalate complexation by, treatment of, 1254
Cysteine-complexing agents:
for cystinuria, 1230–1231
effect of, 1228–1229
Cystic fibrosis, infertility and, 662
Cystine:
chemical structure of, *1229*
excretion of, salt intake and, 1228
solubility of, urinary pH and, 1228
urinary concentration of, new stone formation and, *1231*
Cystine stones, 1227
multiple, *1229*
Cystinuria, 1227–1231
clinical diagnosis of, 1229
clinical evaluation of, 1229–1230
clinical findings in, 1229, *1229*
genetics of, 1228
history of, 1227–1228
laboratory evaluation of, 1229–1230
pathophysiology of, 1228
treatment of, 1230–1231
Cysts, of anterior pituitary, 182
Cytochemical assays, of hormones, 92–93
Cytochrome P450, in steroidogenesis, 395, *396*
Cytokines:
hypercalcemia of malignancy and, 1397–1398
in myeloma bone disease, 1133–1134
thyrotoxicosis induced by, 296
Cytology, aspiration, fine needle, in thyroid nodule evaluation, 361–362, *362*
Cytoplasmic glucocorticoid receptor, relative affinities of steroids for, 417t
Cytoskeleton, G proteins and, 71
Cytotoxic drugs:
androgen deficiency from, 672
sperm production impairment by, 676

Dawn phenomenon, 870
Decidua basalis, 762
Decidua capsularis, 762
Decidua parietalis, 762
Dehydration:
in diabetic ketoacidosis, 889
in elderly, 1465
Dehydroepiandrosterone (DHEA) secretion, in aging, 1462–1463
Deiodinases:
iodothyronine, activity of, conditions/drugs altering, 270t
iodotyrosine, defect in, hypothyroidism from, 319
Demeclocycline, for syndrome of inappropriate antidiuresis in cancer, 1406
Deoxycorticosterone:
as mineralocorticoid, 567
in plasma, physical state of, 418
11-Deoxycorticosterone:
metabolism of, 420
plasma concentrations of, 415t
secretion rate of, 415t
Deoxycorticosterone acetate, for congenital adrenal hyperplasia, 812
11-Deoxycortisol:
metabolism of, 420
plasma concentrations of, 415t
secretion rate of, 415t

Depression, in endocrine disorders, 25
Desensitization, adrenergic receptor, 530
17,20-Desmolase deficiency, 804
Desmopressin (DDAVP):
  for diabetes insipidus
    dipsogenic, 238, *239*
    gestational, 238
    pituitary, 235–236, *236*, 237
  for enuresis/nocturia, 240
  for nocturnal polyuria, 238
Desogestrel, 772
Detumescence, physiology of, 654
Development:
  disorders of, 1265–1311
  glucocorticoids and, 432–433
  hormone actions on, 12
  stages of, 1280–1282
Dexamethasone:
  for congenital adrenal hyperplasia, prenatal, 456
  structure of, *611*
Dexamethasone suppression tests, 440–441, *442*
  in children, 445–447
  low-dose, for Cushing's syndrome, *483*, 483–484
Dexfenfluramine, in obesity management, 985
DHEA:
  metabolism of, 420
  in plasma, physical state of, 418
  plasma concentrations of, 415t
  secretion rate of, 415t
DHEA-S:
  metabolism of, 420
  in plasma, physical state of, 418
  plasma concentrations of, 415t
  secretion rate of, 415t
Diabetes Control and Complications Trial, 861–865
  cohorts of patients in
    baseline characteristics of, 861t
    follow-up of, 864t
  design of, 861
  intensive therapy in, 862t
    effects of, 864t
  intensive treatment and metabolic goals of, 861
  results of, 861–865
  treatment recommendations from, 865, 866t
Diabetes insipidus (DI), 228–239
  differential diagnosis of, 233–235
  dipsogenic, 232
    management of, 238–239
  gestational, 232
    management of, 238
  management of, 235–239
  nephrogenic, 233, 233t
    management of, 239
  pituitary, 228–232
    causes of, 228t
    management of, 235–238
  primary polydipsia and, 232, 232t
Diabetes mellitus, 827–912
  in acromegaly, 190
  in Addison's disease, 463
  aging process compared with, 1472t
  classification of, 845–846, 846t
Diabetes mellitus *(continued)*
  clinical, 845–912
  coexisting genetic hyperlipidemia in, 1012–1013
  complications of, long-term, 894–912
    cardiovascular disease as, 908–912, 909t, *910*, 911, 912
    nephropathy as, *898*, 900–903, 901, 902, 903, 904
    neuropathy as, 904–908, *905*, 905t
    pathophysiology of, 895–896, *896*
    retinopathy as, 896–900, *897, 898, 899, 900*
  definition of, 845
  diabetic ketoacidosis in, 887–892; *See also* Diabetic ketoacidosis (DKA)
  diagnosis of, 857–858
    criteria for, 847t
  diet-induced hyperlipidemia in, 1012
  in elderly, 1471–1474
    diet and, 1472–1473
    insulin for, 1473
    management of, 1472, 1472t
    monitoring treatment in, 1473
    oral hypoglycemics for, 1473
  endocrine pancreas and, 828–842; *See also* Pancreas, endocrine
  fuel homeostasis and, 842–845
  gestational, 856
    therapy of, 887
  glucocorticoid therapy and, 623
  history of, 827–828
  hyperlipidemia in patients with, 1063–1064
  hyperosmolar hyperglycemic nonketotic coma in, 892
  hypertension and, 578
  hypoglycemia in, 543–545
  impact of, on cardiovascular disease, 909t
  infant of mother with, gigantism in, 1308–1309
  insulin-dependent, with ketoacidosis, 1010–1012
  ion transport abnormalities in, 575–576
  islet amyloid polypeptide and, 841–842
  low-fat, high-complex-carbohydrate diet in, 1052
  management of, laboratory tests and examinations in, 868t
  metabolic emergencies in, 887–892
  neuroendocrine alterations in, 157
  in nursing home residents, 1473t, 1473–1474
  obesity and, 962t, 962–963
  osteoporosis in, 1194
  polyneuropathy in, 25
  poorly controlled, without ketoacidosis, 1012
  risk of developing, family history and, 848t
  screening for, 858
    recommendations for, 847t
  secondary hyperlipidemia from, 1010–1013
  therapy of, 858–887
    Diabetes Control and Complications Trial in, 861–865; *See also* Diabetes Control and Complications Trial
    history of, *858*, 859–860
    metabolic, elements of, 865, 867–869
    for Type 1, 860–875
Diabetes mellitus *(continued)*
  Type 1, 846–851
    clinical presentation of, 850–851, *851*
    epidemiology of, 847
    incidence of, worldwide, *848*
    with ketoacidosis, 1010–1012
    pathoetiology of, 847–850
      autoimmunity in, 849–850, *850*
      genes in, 847–849, *849*
    prevention of, 875
    therapy of, 860–875
      diet in, 871
      exercise in, 871–872, *872*
      future, 873–875
      insulin in, 869–871
      regimens for, 866t
      whole organ pancreas transplantation in, 827–873, *873*
  Type 2, 851–856
    cardiovascular disease with, risk factors for, 909t
    clinical presentation of, 856
    development of, timeline for, *849*
    epidemiology of, 851–853
    genetics of, 854–856
    pathoetiology of, 853–854, *854*
    prevalence of
      by gender and ethnic group, *853*
      worldwide, *852*
    screening for, 853
    therapy of, 875–887
      alternative, 887
      combination, 885–886
      comparison of methods in, 880t
      diet in, 878–879, 879t
      exercise in, 878–879
      future of, 887
      medications in, 879–885, *881*, 881t, *882*, 882t, *883, 884, 885*, 885t, *886*
      metabolic goals of, 876–877
      monitoring in, 886
      options in, 877–886
      pathophysiology relevant to, *875*, 875–876
      United Kingdom Prospective Diabetes Study (UKPDS) in, 876t, 876–877, *877, 878*, 878t
  urinary tract disorders in, 23
  well-controlled, 1012
Diabetic ketoacidosis (DKA), 887–892
  clinical characteristics of, 889t, 889–890
  diagnosis of, 890
  hypophosphatemia in, 1156, *1156*
  insulin dependent diabetes and, 1010–1012
  laboratory findings in, 889t
  pathogenesis of, *888*, 888–889
  treatment of, 890–892, 891t
Diacylglycerol in protein kinase C activation, 75–76
Dialysis:
  chronic, hypophosphatemia from, 1187
  for end-stage renal disease in diabetic nephropathy, 902
Diarrhea:
  diabetic, 907
    therapy for, 908
  in endocrine disorders, 22

Diarrhea *(continued)*
in MEN 2B syndrome, 1372
secretory
octreotide acetate in, 1322, 1323t
somatostatin for, 1322
Diencephalic syndrome, 155
Diet(s):
for abetalipoproteinemia, 1035
in cystinuria management, 1230
fad, in obesity management, 984
in familial hypercholesterolemia management, 1019
in gestational diabetes management, 887
goiter and
endemic, 351
sporadic, 355
hormone-responsive tumors and, 1434, *1435*
in hyperlipidemia management, 1042–1053
drug therapy related to, 1053
low-fat, high-complex-carbohydrate
chemical composition of, 1052
for children, 1053
in diabetes, 1052
in hypertension, 1053
predicted plasma cholesterol lowering from, 1052
in pregnancy, 1052–1053
in obesity management, 978–984
in older diabetics, 1472–1473
plasma lipids and, 1042t, 1042–1050
plasma lipoproteins and, 1042t, 1042–1050
in Type 1 diabetes management, 871
in Type 2 diabetes management, 878–879, 879t
in type III hyperlipoproteinemia management, 1026–1027
for type IV hyperlipoproteinemia, 1030
uric acid excretion and, 1232
urinary pH and, 1232
very-low-energy, 979–983
Diffuse lymphocytic adrenalitis, 463
Digoxin, androgen deficiency from, 672
Dihydrotachysterol, pharmacology of, 1149t
Dihydrotestosterone, levels of, in aging, 1463–1464
1,25-Dihydroxycholecalciferol (1,25$(OH)_2D_3$), in malignancy-associated hypercalcemia, 1128–1129
1α,25-Dihydroxyvitamin D (1α-25-$(OH)_2$D):
circulating and extrarenal, 1103
mechanism of action of, in intestine, *1106*
metabolism of, further, 1103–1104, *1104*
1α,25-Dihydroxyvitamin D_3 (1α-25-$(OH)_2$D):
for renal osteodystrophy, 1201
for rickets and osteomalacia, 1188–1189
24, 25-Dihydroxyvitamin D (24,25-$(OH)_2$D), role of, 1103
Diltiazem, for thyrotoxicosis, 307
Diodothyronines:
metabolism of, 266
production of, 266t
Diplopia, in anterior pituitary disease, 184
Dipsogenesis, 226
Disordered-control hypothesis, of absorptive hypercalciuria, 1246
Distal ileal bypass surgery, in familial hypercholesterolemia management, 1020
Diuresis, water, 224
Diuretics, thiazide; *See* Thiazide diuretics
hypercalcemia induced by, 1137
DNA binding, of nuclear receptors, 57–58
DNA-based theories, of aging, 1458, 1458t
DOC acetate, for congenital adrenal hyperplasia, 457t
Donor oocyte in vitro fertilization, in Turner's syndrome, 747
Dopamine (DA):
anatomic pathways of, 135
biological effects of, 531
dopaminergic receptors and, 530
in prolactin inhibition, 134
response of, to exercise, 1490
thyroid function and, 288
thyrotropin secretion and, 269
Dopamine agonists:
for acromegaly, 193
for gonadotroph adenoma, 202
for hyperprolactinemia, 753
for lactotroph adenomas, 188, 196–197
for prolactinoma in MEN 1 syndrome, 1362
Doping in sports, 1499–1504; *See also* Anabolic steroids
Down syndrome:
sperm production impairment in, 675
testicular dysfunction in, 672
Drug(s):
altering iodothyronine deiodinase activity, 270t
ameliorating thyroid hormone action, 307
androgen deficiency from, 672
antithyroid
for Graves' thyrotoxicosis, 303–304, 304t
for thyrotoxicosis, 304–307
calcium oxalate stone risk and, 1240
for carcinoid syndrome, 1339
endocrine, performance-enhancing, in sports, 1499–1504; *See also* Anabolic steroids
erectile dysfunction and, 661t
glucocorticoid interactions with, 624, 624t
hypercalcemia induced by, 1137–1138
for hyperlipidemia, dietary therapy related to, 1053
hyperlipidemias induced by, 1015, 1015t
in hyperlipoproteinemia management, 1053–1062
hyperprolactinemia related to, 752
hypomagnesemia from, 1158
inhibiting extrathyroidal T3 production, 307
metabolism of
in hypothyroidism, 323–324
in thyrotoxicosis, 301
in obesity management, 984–986
in renovascular hypertension management, 586
thyroid function and, 288–289
thyrotoxicosis induced by, 296
in Type 2 diabetes management, 879–885, *881*, 881t, *882*, 882t, *883, 884, 885,* 885t, *886*
uric acid stones associated with, 1233
vasopressin secretion and, 223
Drug interference with immunoassays, 103
Dual x-ray absorptiometry (DXA), in bone metabolic disease evaluation, 1180–1181
Dual-energy absorption techniques, in body composition assessment, 953
Dumping syndrome, somatostatin for, 1321–1322
Duodenal ulcer disease, hypersecretinemia in, 1326
Duplex Doppler imaging in renovascular hypertension diagnosis, 585
Dwarf, 1283; *See also* Short stature
Dwarfism, psychosocial, 1294
Dysdifferentiation, in ectopic hormone production, 1392
Dysgerminomas, suprasellar, 147–148
Dysmenorrhea, 763–766
operative hysteroscopy for, 765
Dysphagia, oropharyngeal, in endocrine disorders, 21

Ears, in endocrine disorders, 21
Ectopic ACTH syndrome, 479, 480
features of, 482
treatment of, 490
tumors causing, 479t
Ectopic corticotropin releasing hormone syndrome, 1401–1402
Ectopic growth hormone production, 1410
Ectopic hormone production:
clinical syndromes associated with, 1385t
criteria for, 1386t, 1386–1387, *1388*
in elderly, 1455
etiology of, 1390–1392
eutopic production versus, 1383–1384
frequency of, 1387–1390, 1388t, 1389t
in hypercalcemia of malignancy, 1394–1400
importance of, 1384–1386
therapy for, 1392
Ectopic POMC/ACTH syndrome, 1400–1404
clinical manifestations of, 1401
diagnosis of, 1402–1403
POMC products produced by tumors in, 1400–1404
prevalence of, 1400
treatment of, 1403–1404
tumor types in, 1400
Ectopic production, of calcitonin, 1414
Ectopic testes, 673
Ectopic thyrotoxicosis, 297
Edwards syndrome, 155t
Eicosanoids, 764
Ejaculation:
physiology of, 653
premature, 653
retarded, 653
retrograde, 653
Ejaculatory dysfunction, infertility from, 663
Elderly; *See also* Aging
diabetes in, 1471–1474
endocrine disorders of, 1455–1476
growth hormone levels in, 1460–1461, *1462*
hormonal changes in, 1460–1465, 1461t
hyperlipidemia in, treatment of, 1063
hyperthyroidism in, presentation of, 1457t
hypothalamic-pituitary-adrenal axis in, 1462–1643
hypothalamic-pituitary-thyroid axis in, 1461–1462
insulin-like growth factor-1 levels in, 1461, *1462*

Elderly; *See also* Aging *(continued)*
nutritional disorders in, 1474–1476
osteoporosis in, 1191–1192
psychiatric disturbances in, metabolic causes of, 1457t
sex hormones in, 1463–1465
sexuality in, 1468–1471
female, 1471
male, 1469–1471
water metabolism disorders in, 1465
Electrolyte metabolism:
in hypothyroidism, 323
in thyrotoxicosis, 300
Electrolytes, loss of, renal, abnormal, in hyperaldosteronism, 492
Embryopathic disorders, congenital, 145–147
Emetic effects, on vasopressin secretion, 221, *222*
Empty sella, 183
Endocrine, definition of, 3
Endocrine cell hypothesis, of ectopic hormone production, 1391
Endocrine disorders:
clinical manifestations of, 19–27
auditory, 21
body temperature variations as, 20
cardiovascular, 23
central nervous system, 25
cutaneous, 20–21
fatigue as, 19–20
gastrointestinal, 21–22
hemopoietic, 22–23
nasal, 21
neuromuscular, 25–26
ophthalmic, 26–27
sexual, 23–24
tongue and, 21
urinary tract, 23
vocal, 21
weakness as, 19–20
multiglandular, 1355–1376; *See also* Multiglandular endocrine disorders
musculoskeletal, 24–25
obesity and, 964–965
treatment of, 17
Endocrine glands:
abnormalities of, without hormonal imbalance, 15
evolution of, 10
hyperfunction of, *12,* 14
hypofunction of, *12,* 12–13
Endocrine pancreas, 828–842; *See also* Pancreas, endocrine
Endocrine system:
disorders of, 12–15; *See* Endocrine disorders
multiple syndromes involving, 14–15
evolution of, *5,* 8–10
in hypothyroidism, 324–325
integration of, 10–11
nervous system distinguished from, 3–4, *4*
obesity and, 974–975
pharmacologic actions of VIP on, 1328t
regulatory ligands of, origin of, 8–9
reproductive, perinatal adaptations of, 791
status of, clinical assessment of, 15–17
history in, 15
laboratory testing in, 15–17
physical examination in, 15
Endocrinology, definitions and scope of, 3–5
Endocrinopathies, hypercalcemia in, 1136–1137
Endocytosis:
in peptide hormone metabolism, 36, *36*
receptor-mediated, *65*
Endogenous opiates, in exercise and training, 1490–1492
Endogenous opioid peptides, neurologic effects of, 138–140
Endometrium:
anatomy of, 763–764
cancer of, 1443–1444
diagnosis of, 1443
hormone replacement therapy and, 770
pathology of, 1443–1444
prognosis of, 1443–1444, 1444t
risk factors for, 1443, 1443t
surgical staging of, 1443t
treatment of, 1444
physiology of, *762, 763,* 763–764
prostaglandins, *764,* 764–765
β Endorphin, levels of, in aging, 1462
Endothelial lipase, in lipoprotein metabolism, 999–1000
Endothelins:
hypertension and, 570
neurologic effects of, 140
Endothelium-derived releasing factor, hypertension and, 570–571
Energy:
expenditure of, obesity and, 968–971, *969*
in hypothyroidism, 323–324
supply of, physical work and, 1483
in thyrotoxicosis, 300
Enhanced dissociation hypothesis, 94
Enuresis, 239–240
Environmental factors:
in hypertension, 556–557
in obesity, 968
thyroid function and, 281
Environmental goitrogens, 356
Environmental hormones, prenatal virilization by, 816
Enzyme(s):
active in lipoprotein metabolism, 998–1000
in hormone action, 7–8
nonrenin renin-like, 559
steroidogenic, nomenclature for, 37, 39t
Enzyme assays, amplitude-modulated, 100
Enzyme contaminants with immunoassays, 103
Enzyme immunoassays (EIA), 98
Epinephrine:
anatomic pathways of, 135
biological effects of, 531
biological roles of, 535
energy expenditure and, 974–975
in exercise, 1489
hyperglycemic action of, 531–532
plasma concentrations of
in pheochromocytoma, 537–538, *538*
venous, 533t
for metabolic effects, 532t
physiologic adaptation of, 533–535, *534*
Epithelial growth factor, in mammary tumorigenesis, 1431
Epithelial tissues, glucocorticoids and, 429
Erectile dysfunction, 653, 658–662
causes of, 659–661, 661t
definition of, 658
drugs associated with, 661t
evaluation of, 660–661
infertility from, 662
treatment of, 661–662
Erection:
physiology of, 652–653
psychogenic, 652–653
reflexogenic, 652
Ergocalciferol; *See* Vitamin D2
Erythrocytosis, paraneoplastic, 1413–1414
Erythroid cells, glucocorticoids and, 429
Erythropoietin:
as ergogenic aid for athletes, 1504
hypertension and, 569–570
Escalator theory, of adrenarche, 1278
Esophagus:
motilin effects on, 1330t
pharmacologic actions of VIP on, 1328t
Estradiol, levels of, in aging, 1464
Estrogen(s):
actions of, 437
aging and, 1464–1465
frailty and, 1467
breast development and, 1427
deficiency of
in breast cancer survivors, treatment of, 1442
osteoporosis in, 1192–1193
excess of
gynecomastia from, 663–664
increased serum thyroxine-binding globulin concentrations and, 282
in men, hypogonadism from, 682
for gonadotropin deficiency in women, 207
gonadotropin releasing hormone regulation and, 125–126
for hyperlipoproteinemia, 1060–1061
in hyperprolactinemia management, 198
hypertension and, 569
mammary carcinogenesis and, 1427–1428, 1435–1436
metabolism of, 420–421
oral, preparations and doses of, 769t
in plasma, physical state of, 418
in pubertal growth spurt, 1277–1279
replacement
breast cancer risk and, 1434
for osteoporosis, 1197–1198
for premature ovarian failure, 751
for Turner's syndrome, 798–799
in Turner's syndrome, 745–747
for type III hyperlipoproteinemia, 1026
tumors secreting, gynecomastia from, 664
types of, for therapeutic use, 769t
vitamin D activation and, 1102
Estrogen synthesis aromatase deficiency, virilization due to, 815
Estrone, levels of, in aging, 1464
Ethanol:
abuse of
chronic, osteoporosis in, 1194
hyperlipidemias secondary to, 1014–1015
hypophosphatemia from, 1156
androgen deficiency from, 672

Ethanol *(continued)*
injection of, for thyrotoxicosis from thyroid adenoma, 309
lipid/lipoprotein metabolism and, 1047–1048
Ethical aspects of doping in sports, 1499–1500
Ethinyl estradiol, for Turner's syndrome, 798–799
Ethylene glycol, hyperoxaluria and, 1248
Etidronate (Didronel):
for hypercalcemia of malignancy, 1130
for osteoporosis, 1197–1198
in osteoporosis prevention, 1196
for Paget's disease of bone, 1208t
Etiocholanolone glucuronide, plasma concentrations and secretion rate of, 415t
Etiocholanolone sulfate, plasma concentrations and secretion rate of, 415t
Etomidate, in adrenal steroid biosynthesis inhibition, 415
Eugonadotropic hypogonadism, 666
Eunuchoidism, 655, *655*
hypogonadotropic, 678–680
in Klinefelter syndrome, 668, *669*
Euthyroid sick syndrome, 1462, 1462t
Exchange lists in dietary diabetes management, 871
Exercise:
ACTH-cortisol axis and, 1488–1489
acute, hypothalamic-pituitary-gonadal axis in men and, 1493
addiction to, opiates and, 1491–1492
amenorrhea related to, 754
analgesia induced by, 1491
catecholamines in, 1489–1490
fuel homeostasis and, 844, *845*
in gestational diabetes management, 887
glucagon and, 1486
growth hormone in, 1486–1488
increased growth hormone with, effects of, 1488
insulin and, 1486
intensive, pubertal delay from, 748
mood and, 1492
in obesity management, 976–978, 977t, *978*
prolactin and, 1492–1493
prolonged, hypothalamic-pituitary-gonadal axis in men and, 1494–1495
reproductive system and, in women, 1496–1498
short-term, hypothalamic-pituitary-gonadal axis and, 1493–1494
and training
aldosterone and, 1484–1485
arginine vasopressin and, 1484
endocrine regulation of fluid balance during, 1484–1485
endogenous opiates in, 1490–1492
gastrointestinal hormones in, 1485
glucoregulation and, 1486–1488
growth hormone release and, 1486–1487
hormonal response to, evaluating, 1483, 1484t
hypothalamic-pituitary-gonadal axis and, 1493–1496
metabolic control in, 1485
thyroid function and, 1485
in Type 1 diabetes management, 871–872, *872*
in Type 2 diabetes management, 878–879
Exocrine, definition of, 3
Exons, 29
Expansion, in ovulation, 735, *735*
Extracellular signals, intracellular amplification of, 72
Extraglandular disorders, hormone deficiency secondary to, 13
Extrahypophyseal neurons, 224
Extrathyroidal hormonogenesis, 265
Exudates, hard, in diabetic retinopathy, *897,* 898
Eye(s):
glucocorticoids and, 432
in iatrogenic Cushing's syndrome, 613
in thyrotoxicosis, 298

Fad diets, in obesity management, 984
Familial Apo-A-1, C-III, A-IV deficiency, 1031–1032, 1032t
Familial Apo-A-1 variants, 1032, 1032t
Familial apolipoprotein A-I and C-III deficiency, 1031, 1032t
Familial apoprotein C-II deficiency, 1027–1029
Familial defective apolipoprotein B-100, 1021–1023
Familial diseases with storage of sterols, 1039–1042
Familial early maturation, 1303
Familial glucocorticoid deficiency, 465
Familial hyperalphalipoproteinemia, 1034
Familial hypoalphalipoproteinemia, 1032–1033
Familial hypocalciuric hypercalcemia, 1119–1120, *1120,* 1139
Familial hypoparathyroidism, 1142–1143
Familial lecithin cholesterol acyltransferase deficiency, 1036
Familial medullary thyroid carcinoma, 1364, *1364*
genetic testing for, 1367–1368
Familial short stature, 1286
Familial tall stature, 1302–1303
Familial X-linked hypophosphatemic rickets, 1186
Family history, calcium oxalate stone risk and, 1239–1240
Fanconi's syndrome, osteomalacia and rickets in, 1187
Fasting:
neuroendocrine alterations from, 156–157
thyroid function and, 287
Fasting hypercalciuria, 1245
Fat:
body
distribution of, 960–962, *961*
low, athletic amenorrhea and, 1497–1498
dietary
hormone-responsive tumors and, 1434, *1435*
in hyperlipidemia management, 1049
intake of, spontaneous food intake and, 968, 968t
lipid metabolism and, 1043–1046
lipoprotein metabolism and, 1043–1046
as energy reservoir, 842
metabolism of, growth hormone actions on, 177
saturated, in hyperlipidemia management, 1050
Fatigue, in endocrine disorders, 19–20
Fatty acids:
free, metabolism of, 1003–1004
monounsaturated, 1044
omega-3, 1044–1046
in hyperlipidemia management, 1049–1050
polyunsaturated, 1044, 1045
saturated, 1043
Feedback inhibition, in cholesterol synthesis, 998
Feedback loops, in neuroendocrine system, 113–115, *114*
Feedback regulation:
glucocorticoid, of ACTH release, 410–411
of gonadotropin releasing hormone, 125–127
of gonadotropin secretion, 651–652
Feeding cycles, ACTH and cortisol diurnal patterns and, 409
Female pseudohermaphroditism, 807–816; *See also* Virilization of genetic female
Feminization, testicular:
primary amenorrhea from, 748–749, *749*
syndromes involving, 676
Fenfluramine, in obesity management, 985
Fenofibrate (Tricor):
for hyperlipoproteinemia, 1060
for type III hyperlipoproteinemia, 1026
"Fertile" eunuch syndrome, 680
Fertility:
premature ovarian failure and, 751
Turner's syndrome and, 747
Fertilization, in vitro:
with donor oocyte, for premature ovarian failure, 751
donor oocyte, in Turner's syndrome, 747
Fetal alcohol syndrome, growth in, 1287
Fetus:
adrenal steroidogenesis in, 403–404
circulation of, sex steroids in, 787–788
disorders of, fetal growth and, 1287–1288
gonadal function in, control of, 789–791, *790*
growth of, 1280, *1280*
risk of lactotroph adenoma to, 198
testicular development in, 641–642
thyroid function in, *280,* 280–281
Fiber, lipid metabolism and, 1047
Fibric acid derivatives:
for hyperlipoproteinemia, 1061
for type III hyperlipoproteinemia, 1026
Fibrillation, atrial, in thyrotoxicosis, 299
Fibroblastic tissues, glucocorticoids and, 429
Fibrogenesis imperfecta ossium, bone metabolic disease in, 1188
Fibromuscular dysplasia, renovascular hypertension from, 582
Fibrous dysplasia, 1202–1203, *1203*
Finasteride:
for hirsutism, 759
in prostate cancer prevention, 1447
Fine needle aspiration cytology, in thyroid nodule evaluation, 361–362, *362*
Fish eye disease, 1032, 1032t
Fish oils:
for type III hyperlipoproteinemia, 1026
for types I and V hyperlipoproteinemia, 1029
Fistula, arteriovenous, of cavernous sinus, 182

9α-Fludrocortisone, for congenital adrenal hyperplasia, 1304
Fludrocortisone (Florinef):
  for congenital adrenal hyperplasia, 457, 457t
  for postural hypotension, 542
Fluid and electrolyte balance:
  glucocorticoids and, 429–430
  during physical work, endocrine regulation of, 1484–1485
Fluid metabolism:
  in hypothyroidism, 323
  in thyrotoxicosis, 300
Fluocinoone acetonide, structure of, *611*
Fluorescence, in immunoassays, 98
Fluorescence polarization, in homogenous assay systems, 99–100
Fluorescence spectroscopy, phase-modulation, 100
9α-Fluorocortisol:
  for chronic adrenal insufficiency, 473
  for hyporeninemic hypoaldosteronism, 475
9α-Fluorohydrocortisone, for congenital adrenal hyperplasia, 813
Flushing syndromes, differential diagnosis of, 1339t
Flutamide, for hirsutism, 759
Fluvastatin (Lescol):
  dosage of, 1057, 1058t
  for hyperlipoproteinemia, 1056–1057
  indications for, 1057–1058
Follicle(s):
  antral, 713–715
  atretic, 715, *715*
  development of
    atresia in, 732
    control mechanisms in, 731–735
    ovulation in, *734*, 734–735, *735*
    recruitment in, 731–732
    selection in, *732*, 732–734, *733*
  Graafian, 713–715, *714*, *715*
  growth factors acting on, 739
  ovarian, 709, *709*
  preantral, *709*, 709–715, *710*, *711*, *712*, *713*, *714*, *715*
  primary, *709*, 710–711
  primordial, *709*, 709–710, *710*, *711*
  secondary, *709*, *711*, 711–712
  tertiary, *709*, *712*, 712–713
Follicle stimulating hormone (FSH):
  actions of, 178
  assays for, 658t
  deficiency of, isolated, hypogonadism from, 682
  evaluation of, in children, 1309–1310
  regulation of, 114
  secretion of, 178, *179*
  in Sertoli cell function regulation, 645–646
  in spermatogenesis control, 649–651
  synthesis of, 178
Follicular carcinoma, of thyroid, 370, *370*
  radioactive iodine treatment of, 375–376
Follicular fluid, 713, *714*
Folliculogenesis, in polycystic ovary syndrome, 756
Folliculostellate cells, 174
Food(s):
  cholesterol-saturated fat index of, 1050, 1051t
  intake of
    alterations in, in hypothalamic disease, 153–155
    exercise and, endogenous opiates and, 1491
    obesity and, 971–974
  oxalate-rich, 1247t
  thermic effect of, 970
Formation product, in stone formation, 1223
Forskolin activation, of adenylyl cyclase, 68
Fracture(s):
  hip, osteopenia and, 1467–1468, *1468*
  Milkman, in osteomalacia, 1183
Frailty, hormones changes in elderly and, 1465–1468
Free radical theory, of aging, 1458, 1458t
Free thyroxine concentrations, serum, 278
Free thyroxine index, 278
  conditions altering, 277t
Fuel-hormone imbalance, 844–845
Fuels:
  availability or need for, hormonal responses to, 844t
  homeostasis of, 842–845
    basal state in, 843
    counterregulatory hormones in, 842
    energy stores in, 842–843
    exercise in, 844, *845*
    fed state in, 843–844
    fuel availability in, 843–844
    fuel need in, 844
    metabolism in, 842–843
    regulatory hormones in, 842
  metabolism of, 825–1075
    diabetes mellitus and, 827–912; *See also* Diabetes mellitus
  need for, 844
  reserves of, body composition and, 842t
Fungal infections, Addison's disease from, 464

G proteins:
  activation of, 67
  cell structure changes and, 71
  effectors of, 67–68
  hormone signals dependent on, phospholipid metabolism mediated by, 68–70, *69–70*
  ion channels activated by, 70–71
  Na/H exchange and, 71
  receptor affinity modulation by, 53
  receptors coupled to, 66–67; *See also* Receptor(s), G protein-coupled
  in signaling cascade, 64–65
GABA; *See* Gamma-aminobutyric acid (GABA)
Galactorrhea:
  amenorrhea in, 752
  in endocrine disorders, 24
Galanin, 1333
  neurologic effects of, 140
Gallbladder:
  cholecystokinin effects on, 1325, 1325t
  motilin effects on, 1330t
  pharmacologic actions of VIP on, 1328t
  secretin effects on, 1326t
Gallium nitrate, for hypercalcemia of malignancy, 1125, 1130
Gallstones:
  obesity and, 963–964
  very-low-energy diets and, 981, *982*
Gamma globulin, molecule of, schematic representation of, *95*
Gamma-aminobutyric acid (GABA):
  anatomic pathways of, 137
  in prolactin inhibition, 134
  receptors for, 63, 79
Gardner-Silengo-Wachtel syndrome, 807
Gaseous neurotransmitters, 140–141
Gastric bypass, for morbid obesity, 986–987
Gastric inhibitory polypeptide (GIP), 1328–1329
Gastrin:
  biological actions of, 1322–1324, 1324t
  clinical relevance and applications of, 1324–1325
  ectopic production of, in Zollinger-Ellision syndrome, 1415
  regulations of, 1322
Gastrinoma:
  hypergastrinemia in, 1324
  hypersecretinemia in, 1327
  in MEN 1 syndrome, 1357
    management of, 1363
  octreotide acetate efficacy on, 1324t
  secretory diarrhea in, octreotide acetate for, 1323t
Gastro-Entero-Pancreatic (GEP) peptide-producing tumors, octreotide acetate efficacy on, 1324t
Gastrointestinal peptide hormones, 1317–1340
  cholecystokinin as, 1325–1326
  distribution of, 1317–1319, *1318*
    cellular, 138t
  exercise and training and, 1485
  functional classification of, 1319t
  galanin as, 1333
  gastric inhibitory polypeptide as, 1328–1329
  gastrin as, 1322–1325
  localization of, 1317–1319
  motilin as, 1329–1330
  neurotensin as, 1331–1332
  pancreatic polypeptide family of, 1330–1331
  secretin as, 1326–1327
  somatostatin as, 1319–1322
  substance P as, 1332–1333
  vasoactive intestinal polypeptide as, 1327–1328
Gastrointestinal tract:
  abnormalities of, associated with MEN 2B syndrome, 1372
  galanin actions on, 1333
  gastric inhibitory polypeptide effects on, 1329t
  glucocorticoids and, 432
  in hypothyroidism, 323
  motilin effects on, 1330t
  neuroendocrine tumors of, 1333–1340; *See also* Carcinoid syndrome
  neurotensin actions on, 1332t
  pharmacologic actions of VIP on, 1328t
  somatostatin effects on, 1320t
  substance P actions on, 1332
  in thyrotoxicosis, 300
Gastroparesis, in autonomic neuropathy, 907
  therapy for, 908

Gastroplasty, vertical banded, for morbid obesity, 986–987
Gemfibrozil (Lopid):
for familial hypercholesterolemia, 1020
for hyperlipoproteinemia, 1060
for type III hyperlipoproteinemia, 1026
for type IV hyperlipoproteinemia, 1030
for type V hyperlipoproteinemia, 1029
Gender; *See* Sex
Gender role, psychosexual differentiation and, 791–792
Gene(s):
breast cancer susceptibility and, 1429–1430, 1430t
C4, 452
corticotropin releasing hormone, structures of, 130, *130*
derepression of, in ectopic hormone production, 1391–1392
in diabetes etiology, 847–849, *849*
gonadotropin releasing hormone, structures of, 124, *124*
growth hormone, 1272–1274, *1273*
growth hormone receptor, 1275–1276
growth hormone releasing hormone, structures of, 132, *132*
21-hydroxylase, 400, 451, *4552*
in 21-hydroxylase locus, 451–453
insulin-like growth factor, 1269–1270
MEN 1, 1355
mutations of, *1361, 1362*
mutation of, de novo synthesis from, in ectopic hormone production, 1391
normal, excessive expression of, in ectopic hormone production, 1392
P450c21, lesions of, causing 21-hydroxylase deficiency, 453–455
P450scc, in steroidogenesis, 397
regulating thyroid hormone, 274t
somatostatin, structures of, 127, *128*
SRY, 641
thyrotropin releasing hormone, structures of, 121, *122*
transcription of, cAMP effects on, 83–84
Wilm's tumor, in gonadal differentiation, 784
Gene conversions, causing 21-hydroxylase deficiency, 453–454, *454*
Gene regulation, by nuclear receptors, mechanism of, 59
Genetic changes, in hormone-responsive tumors, 1429–1433
Genetic diseases:
complex, with primary hypogonadism, 671
pituitary disorders from, 183
Genetic disorders, osteoporosis in, 1194
Genetic influences:
on abetalipoproteinemia, 1035
on autoimmune adrenocortical insufficiency, 462
in control of growth processes, 1265–1266
on cystinuria, 1228
on familial combined hyperlipidemia, 1023
on familial defective apolipoprotein B-100, 1021
on familial hypercholesterolemia, 1018–1019
on familial lecithin cholesterol acyltransferase deficiency, 1036
Genetic influences *(continued)*
on goiter formation, 354
on growth excess, 1302–1303
on growth hormone deficiency, 1291–1292
on hypertension, 556–557
on obesity, *966,* 966–968
on ovarian differentiation, 785–786
on polyglandular autoimmune syndromes, 1375
on premature ovarian failure, 750–751
on Tangier disease, 1033
on testicular differentiation, 785
on Type 2 diabetics, 854–856
on type III hyperlipoproteinemia, 1025
on type IV hyperlipoproteinemia, 1030
on types I and V hyperlipoproteinemia, 1028
Genetic polymorphisms, osteoporosis in, 1191
Genetic sex, 779–783
Genetic short stature, 1286
Genetic syndromes associated with obesity, 975
Genetic testing:
for familial medullary thyroid carcinoma, 1367–1368
for multiple endocrine neoplasia type 2A, 1367–1368
Genetic theories, of aging, 1458t, 1459
Genital blastema, 641
Genital ducts, differentiation of, 786–787
Genital tract, obstruction of, infertility from, 662
Genital virilization, defective, 801–807
Genitalia:
abnormal, newborn with, clinical approach to, 816–817, *817*
anomalous, primary amenorrhea and, 749
external
differentiation of, 787
female
in 21-hydroxylase deficiency, *809*
teratologic malformations of, 816
feminization of, 787
masculinization of, 787
internal
female, development of, 786, *786*
male, development of, *786,* 786–787
male, in 17-hydroxylase deficiency, *803*
sex steroid actions on, 788–789
Genito-palato-cardiac syndrome, 807
Genitourinary symptoms in autonomic neuropathy, 907
Genomic imprinting, action of insulin-like growth factor and, 1268
Geography:
goiter and, endemic, 351
hormone-responsive tumors and, 1434
Germ cell aplasia, infertility in, 675
Germ cells:
cancers of, 689–690
degeneration of, 639
development of, 638–641
meiotic phase of, 638–639, *639*
proliferative phase of, 638
spermiogenesis in, 639
primordial, 728
types of, in spermatogenic cycle, *640*
Gestational diabetes, 856
therapy of, 887
Gestational diabetes insipidus, 232
management of, 238
Gestational thyrotoxicosis, 297
Gestodene, 772
Gigantism, 150, 1306–1307
cerebral, 159, 1307–1308
lipodystrophy and, 1309
Gland(s):
endocrine
abnormalities of, without hormonal imbalance, 15
evolution of, 10
hyperfunction of, *12,* 14
hypofunction of, *12,* 12–13
mammary; *See* Breast
pineal, 141–143; *See also* Pineal gland
pituitary, 173–258; *See also* Pituitary gland
sexual, accessory, dysfunction of, infertility from, 663
thyroid, 259–383; *See also* Thyroid gland
Glaucoma, in endocrine disorders, 27
Globulin:
corticosteroid-binding, 416, 416t
thyroxine-binding, 271
Glomerulosclerosis, nodular, Kimmellstein-Wilson, in diabetic nephropathy, 901, *903*
Glucagon:
actions of, 839–841
biosynthesis of, 838–839
chemistry of, 838–839
ectopic production of, 1415
exercise and, 1486
in insulin secretion regulation, 834, *834*
secretion of, 839
Glucagonomas:
in MEN 1 syndrome, 1357–1358
octreotide acetate efficacy on, 1324t
Glucocorticoid cascade hypothesis, of aging, 1458t, 1459, *1459*
Glucocorticoid-remediable hyperaldosteronism, 590
Glucocorticoids:
actions of, 423–433
on adrenal medulla, 431–432
on bone, 430–431
on calcium metabolism, 430–431, *431*
on carbohydrate metabolism, 424–425, *425*
on cardiovascular system, *429,* 429–430
on central nervous system, 431
on development, 432–433
on eye, 432
on fluid and electrolyte balance, 429–430
on gastrointestinal tract, 432
on glycogen metabolism, 425, *426*
on growth, 432
on hormone production and clearance, 433
on intermediary metabolism, 423, *424*
on lipid metabolism, 426
molecular mechanisms of, 421–422
on nucleic acid metabolism, 426–429
on protein metabolism, 426–429
on reproductive function, 433
for adrenal crisis, 472
adverse influences of, 610–611
agonist activity of, 617

Glucocorticoids *(continued)*
  agonists and antagonists of, 422–423
  bioavailability of, 615–616
  for chronic adrenal insufficiency, 472–473
  clearance of, 616–617
  clinical conditions responding to, 610t
  concentration at sites of action of, 617
  for congenital adrenal hyperplasia, 812–813
  Cushing's syndrome and, 610–611, 612–615
  deficiency of, familial, 465
  definition of, 421
  distribution of, 616
  drug interactions with, 624, 624t
  excess of, hypogonadism from, 682
  in feedback regulation of ACTH, 410–411
  glucocorticoid potencies of, 616t
  for hypercalcemia of malignancy, 1130
  hypertension and, 568–569
  interrelations of, with other hormones, 433
  kinetic considerations on, 612
  metabolism of, 616–617
  mineralocorticoid potencies of, 616t
  phosphate reabsorption and, 1154
  in plasma, physical state of, 415–416
  plasma concentrations of, in children, 445, 446t
  plasma half-life of, 616t
  potency of
    determinants of, 615–618
    overall estimation of, 617
  preparations of, 618–620
    inhaled, 619
    intraarticular, 618–619
    orally active, 618
    parenterally active, 618, 618t
    topical, 618t, 619
  regulation of, 405–411
    hypothalamic-pituitary-adrenal axis in, 405
    hypothalamus in, 405
    pituitary in, 405–410
  resistance to, 617–618
  sensitivity to, variations in, 617–618
  stress and, 433–434
  structure-activity relations of, 423–434
  structures of, *611*
  therapeutic influences of, 609–610
    molecular mechanisms for, 611–612
  therapy with, 609–629
    adjunctive, 621
    alternate day, 622–623
    in children, 624
    circadian rhythm and, 621
    in diabetic, 623
    dosage adjustment in, 621–622
    dose-response considerations on, 620–621
    empirical data on, need for, 620
    Kaposi's sarcoma and, 624
    objective criteria for, cognizance of, 621
    patient selection for, 620
    peptic ulcer and, 623–624
    in pregnancy, 623
    psychiatry and, 623
    sensitivity to, testing for, 620
    short-term versus long-term, 620
    side effects of, measures to reduce, 621
    surgery and, 623
  thyroid function and, 288

Glucocorticoids *(continued)*
  for thyrotoxicosis from thyroiditis, 308
  thyrotropin secretion and, 269
  urinary concentrations of, in children, 445, 446t
  withdrawal of, 625–629
    indications in, for steroid coverage, 628–629
    protocols for, 628–629
    syndromes associated with, 627–628
Glucopenic effects, on vasopressin secretion, 222
Glucose:
  control of, in elderly, rationale for, 1471t, 1471–1472
  counterregulation of
    pathophysiology of, in type I diabetes mellitus, 544–545
    physiology of, 543, *544*
  in feeding regulation, 972
  glucagon secretion and, 839, 840, *840*
  homeostasis of, physiology of, exercise and, *872*
  insulin gene expression and, 832
  metabolism of, in insulin secretion regulation, 832–834, *834*
  transporters of, 837t, 837–838
  turnover of, in postabsorptive and postprandial states, *843*
Glucose-dependent insulinotropic peptide, 1328–1329
Glucotoxicity, in Type 2 diabetes, 875–876
Glutamate receptors, 63, 79
Glycation, diabetes-specific complications and, 895–896, *896*
Glycation theory, of aging, 1459
Glycemia:
  in diabetes diagnosis, 857
  diabetes-specific complications and, 895
  retinopathy risk and, *857*
  in Type 1 diabetes
    acute, monitoring of, 865
    chronic, monitoring of, 865, 867–868
Glycine receptors, 80
Glycogen, metabolism of, glucocorticoid actions on, 425, *426*
Glycoprotein hormones, receptors for, 63
α-Glycosidase inhibitors, for Type 2 diabetes, *881,* 882–883
Glycosylated hemoglobin:
  assays for, 868, 869t
  in glycemia monitoring, 867–868
Goiter, 349–359
  classification of, 349, 350t
  definition of, 349
  endemic, 351–353
    causes of, 353
    clinical findings in, 352
    cretinism and, 352
    development of, 352
    prophylaxis of, 353
    thyroid cancer related to, 352
    thyroid gland hyperfunction and, 352
  etiology of, 349–351
  historical overview of, 349
  nontoxic, 356–359
    complications of, 356
    incidence of, 356

Goiter *(continued)*
    laboratory evaluation of, 357
    medical therapy of, 357
      results of, 357–358
    multinodular, carcinoma risk in, 356–357
    presentations of, 356
    radioiodine therapy of, 358
    surgical treatment of, 358–359
  sporadic, 353–356
    age and, 354
    genetic influences on, 354
    inherited thyroid hormone biosynthesis defects and, 354–355, *355*
    in pregnancy, 354
    sex and, 354
  toxic multinodular, 296
    thyrotoxicosis from, treatment of, 309
  toxic uninodular, 296
Goitrogens, 355–356
Gonadal disease, 633–824
  ovary in, 707–778; *See also* Ovary(ies)
  testis in, 635–690; *See also* Testis
Gonadal dysgenesis, 745–747
  XX, 799
  XY, 799–800, 800t
Gonadal function:
  in Cushing's syndrome, 481
  in hypothyroidism, 324
  in thyrotoxicosis, 301
Gonadal sex, 783–786
Gonadal steroids, in pubertal growth spurt, 1277–1279
Gonadarche, 1278
Gonadogenesis anomalies without chromosomal abnormality, 799–800
Gonadotroph adenoma, 200–202
Gonadotroph cells, hormones secreted by, 174, 174t
Gonadotropin(s):
  assays for, 658t
  chorionic; *See* Human chorionic gonadotropin (hCG)
  deficiency of
    in men, 205–206
    in women, 206–207
  disorders of, hypothalamic disease and, 150–152
  human chorionic; *See* Human chorionic gonadotropin (hCG)
  for hypogonadism, 687–688
  in ovarian hormone biosynthesis control, 723
  in ovulation induction, *760,* 760–761, *761,* 761t
  pituitary, in fetal gonadal function control, 789–791, *790*
  secretion of
    cyclical changes in, 144–145
    feedback regulation of, 651–652
    gonadotropin releasing hormone regulation of, 643–644
  for spermatogenesis induction in Kallmann syndrome, 680
  in testicular function control, 644–649
Gonadotropin releasing hormone (GnRH), 124–127
  agonists of
    as antiandrogens, 686
    hypogonadism from, 682

Gonadotropin releasing hormone (GnRH) *(continued)*
analogs of
for gonadotroph adenoma, 202
for prostate cancer, 1447
for cryptorchidism, 674
functions of, 124–125
in gonadotropin secretion regulation, 643–44
for hypogonadism, 687–688
neurons containing, 124
pulsatile
in ovulation induction, 761–763
for spermatogenesis induction in Kallmann syndrome, 680, 688
secretion of
brain regulation of, 642–643
feedback regulation of, 125–127
Gonadotropin releasing hormone (GnRH) neurons, hypothalamic, 635–636
Gonads:
dysgenesis of, mixed, 796
dysgenetic, sex chromosome anomalies associated with, 795–799
fetal, function of, control of, 789–791, *790*
steroidal production by, 787
steroidogenesis in, pathways of, *802*
Gout, uric acid stones and, 1232t, 1232–1233
Graafian follicles, 713–715, *714, 715*
Granulomatous disorders, hypercalcemia in, 1136
Granulomatous hypophysitis, 182
Granulosa cells, *709,* 709–710, *710, 714*
cytodifferentiation of, 723–726
first level of, 724, *724*
fourth level of, 725–726
second level of, 724
third level of, 724–725, *725*
growth factors acting on, 739
heterogeneity of, 726
oocyte growth and, 729–730
Graves' disease, 291–294
euthyroid, 312–313
extrathyroidal manifestations of, 311–315
infiltrative ophthalmopathy in, 311–314, *312,* 312t, *313*
myxedema in, 314–315
pathogenesis of, 294
neonatal, 311
ophthalmopathy in, pathogenesis of, 294
pathogenesis of, 292–293
thyroid acropachy in, 314–315
thyroid autoantibodies in patients with, 291t
thyrotropin receptor-stimulating antibodies in, 291
Graves' thyrotoxicosis:
development of, hypothetical scheme for, *292*
natural history of, *293,* 293–294
pathogenesis of, 292–293
risk factors for, 293
treatment of, 303–304
GRFoma, in MEN 1 syndrome, 1358
Growth:
in adolescence, 1281–1282, *1282,* 1282t
biological stages of, 1265
cell, kinase cascades promoting, 81–82
in childhood, 1281, *1281*
delay of, constitutional, 1286–1287
disorders of, 1265–1311

Growth *(continued)*
excess, 1302–1309
in acromegaly, 1306–1307
in Beckwith-Wiedemann syndrome, 1308
causes of, 1302t
in cerebral gigantism, 1307–1308
chromosome abnormalities causing, 1308
in congenital adrenal hyperplasia, 1303–1304
familial/genetic, 1302–1303
in gigantism, 1306–1307
in homocystinuria, 1307
in hyperthyroidism, 1308
in infant of diabetic mother, 1308–1309
in Klinefelter's syndrome, 1307
in Marfan syndrome, 1307
in obesity, 1308
pathologic, 1303–1309
fetal, 1280, *1280*
glucocorticoids and, 432
of hormone-dependent tumors, endocrine mechanisms controlling, 1434–1436
in infancy, *1280,* 1280–1281
intermediary metabolism and, 11
intrauterine
disturbances of, 1287–1288
retardation of, in Turner's syndrome, 1300
oocyte, 729–731
processes of, control of, 1265–1279
genetic factors in, 1265–1266
gonadal steroids in, 1277–1279
growth hormone in, 1272–1276, *1277*
hormones in, 1272–1279
nutrition in, 1279
thyroid hormone in, 1277
short stature and, 1282–1302; *See also* Short stature
skeletal, physiology of, 1279–1280
Growth curves, standard, plotting growth data on, 1285
Growth factor signaling, 80–82
Growth factors:
in breast physiology, 1428–1429
epithelial, in mammary tumorigenesis, 1431
insulin-like, 1266–1272
in mammary carcinogenesis, 1435–1436, *1437*
ovarian, 739
peptide, hormonal influences and, 1266
Growth hormone (GH):
actions of, 177, 1275
transient defects in, 1294
aging and, 1460–1461, *1462*
frailty and, 1466
biologically inactive, 1292
deficiency of, 207–208
acquired, 1293–1294
causes of, 1290t
congenital, 1290–1293
diagnosis of, 1294
embryologic defects in, 1292
hypothalamic disease and, 150
in obesity, 964–965
short stature from, 1289–1296
treatment of, 1294–1296
diagnostic tests for, 1309t
effects of, in older persons, 1466t

Growth hormone (GH) *(continued)*
as ergogenic aid for athletes, 1504
evaluation of, in children, 1309
excess of, hypothalamic disease and, 150
in growth regulation, 1272–1276, *1277*
hypertension and, 570
metabolic effects of, 1275, 1276t
neurosecretory dysfunction of, 1292
in obesity management, 986
phosphate reabsorption and, 1154
production of, ectopic, 1410
recombinant human, for growth hormone deficiency, 1294–1295
regulation of, 114–115
resistance to, 1293
secretion of, 176, *176,* 176t
circadian rhythm and, 145
excessive
acromegaly from, 188–194; *See also* Acromegaly
demonstration of, 191–192
determining consequences of, 192
establishing cause of, 192
with exercise
increased, effects of, 1488
neuroendocrine control of, 1487–1488
factors influencing, 1487t
regulation of, *1274,* 1274–1275
transient defects in, 1294
synthesis of, 175–177
control of, 1272
transport of, 17–177
for Turner's syndrome, 1301
Growth hormone releasing hormone (GHRH), 132–133
axon terminals containing, immunocytochemical distribution of, *121*
ectopic production of, 1411–1412
in growth hormone secretion regulation, *1274,* 1274–1275
human, for growth hormone deficiency, 1295
GTP hydrolysis, 65, *66*
Guanosine monophosphate (GMP), cyclic:
protein kinases dependent on, 73
signaling with, nitric oxide and, 73–74
Guanosine triphosphate (GTP) hydrolysis, 65, *66*
Guanylyl cyclase activity, receptors with, 77–78
Gynecomastia, 663–665
causes of, 663–665, 664t
in endocrine disorders, 24
evaluation of, 665
familial, 664
palpation for, 656, *656*
pathological, 663–665
physiological, 663
refeeding, 664
treatment of, 665

[3H] labeling, in immunoassays, 98
Hamartomas, hypothalamic, 148
Harris lines, in rickets, 1182–1183
Head, irradiation of, thyroid cancer and, *360,* 360–361
Headache(s):
in acromegaly, 190
in anterior pituitary disease, 183
in endocrine disorders, 25

Heart:
alcohol and, 1047–1048
disease of
obesity and, 958–960, *960*
thyroid function and, 287
effects of anabolic steroids on, 1502
failure of
congestive, obesity and, 960
in hypothyroidism, 322
size of, in endocrine disorders, 23
Height-weight tables, in fatness assessment, 954–956
Hematologic malignancy(ies), 1133–1135
hypercalcemia associated with, parathyroid hormone-related protein in, 1128
Hematopoietic system:
in hypothyroidism, 323
in thyrotoxicosis, 300
Hemianopsia, bitemporal, in anterior pituitary disease, 183, *183*
Hemochromatosis:
hypogonadism from, 680
pituitary disorders from, 182
Hemodynamic effects:
on thirst, 226
on vasopressin secretion, 220–221
Hemodynamic effects in immunoassays, 103
Hemoglobin, glycosylated:
assays for, 868, 869t
in glycemia monitoring, 867–868
Hemopoietic system, in endocrine disorders, 22–23
Hemorrhage(s):
adrenal
Addison's disease from, 464
clinical features of, 468, 468t
dot and blot, in diabetic retinopathy, 897, *897*
in thyroid nodule, 329–330
Hepatic cirrhosis:
androgen deficiency in, 673
gynecomastia and, 664
Hepatic lipase:
deficiency of, 1027
in lipoprotein metabolism, 999
Hepatitis, thyroid function and, 287
Hepatocellular carcinoma, hypoglycemia and, 1407
Herceptin, for breast cancer, 1442
Hereditary hyperphosphatasia, 1201–1202
Hereditary medullary thyroid carcinoma, 1364, *1364*
Hermaphroditism, true, 795
Hernia uteri inguinalis, 801
Heterophilic antibodies, in hormone assays, 102
Heterosexual precocity, 1306
Hexahistidine tagged peptides, 97
High-pressure liquid chromatography, 101
Hill plots, in ligand binding kinetics determination, 52, *52*
Hilus cells, 718, *719*
Hirsutism:
amenorrhea and, 757–759
in endocrine disorders, 21
management of, 758–759
in polycystic ovary syndrome, 755
Hisrchsprung disease, multiple endocrine neoplasia type 2A with, 1371
Histaminase, in medullary thyroid carcinoma, 1367
Histamine, anatomic pathways of, 137
Histiocytosis, disseminated, growth hormone deficiency in, 1294
Histiocytosis X, hypothalamic infiltration with, 148, *149*
HLA linkage, in 21-hydroxylase deficiency, 451–452, *452*
Homocystinuria:
growth excess in, 1307
Marfan syndrome compared with, 1308t
Homogeneous assay systems, 99–100
Hormonal sex, 787–792
Hormone(s):
actions of, 11–12
classification of, 8
integrated, 10
in adjuvant therapy of breast cancer, 1440–1441, *1441*
administration of, hormone excess states from, 14
aging and, 1455–1476
changes in, 1460–1465, 1461t
frailty and, 1465–1468
amino acid analogs as, 5
antagonism of, 11
antagonists of, abnormal production or administration of, 13
assays of, 91–104
chromatographic, 101
in endocrine status assessment, 15
future trends in, 104
interference with, 102–103
nomenclature for, 93
quality control of, 103–104
receptor assays in, 100
separation systems in, 99
associated with water metabolism in elderly, 1456
athletic performance and, 1483–1504
bioassays of, 91–93
biosynthetic defects, hormonal overproduction and, 14
breast development and, normal, 1427–1429
circulation of, 5–6
classification of, 49
corticotropin releasing, 130–132
counterregulatory, in fuel homeostasis, 842
crosstalk among, 84
cytochemical assays of, 92–93
deficiency of, syndromes involving, 12–13
definition of, 3
ectopic production of, 14
for endometrial cancer, 1444
environmental, prenatal virilization by, 816
epinephrine and norepinephrine as, 535
evaluation of, in anterior pituitary lesion evaluation, 184
excess of, syndromes involving, 13–14
families of, diversification of, 10
free
levels of, in endocrine status assessment, 15–16
measurements of, 94–95
gastrointestinal, 1317–1340; *See also* Gastrointestinal peptide hormones
Hormone(s) *(continued)*
glycoprotein, receptors for, 63
gonadotropin releasing, 124–127; *See also* Gonadotropin releasing hormone (GnRH)
growth hormone releasing, 132–133
axon terminals containing, immunocytochemical distribution of, *121*
ectopic production of, 1411–1412
hypersecretion of, secondary, 14
hypophysiotropic, 112–113
structures of, *122*
hyporesponsiveness to, 13
hypothalamic, in growth hormone secretion regulation, *1274,* 1274–1275
immunoassays of, types of, 93–95
in insulin secretion regulation, 834
internalization of, 7
levels of, regulation of, 6–7, *7*
mechanisms of action of, 7–8
metabolism of, 6
defects of, hormonal excess from, 14
fine-tuning, 11
modifying blood pressure, 557–579
multiple, recruitment of, for coordinated responses, 10–11
for nonendocrine diseases, 17
origin of, 8–9
ovarian, biogenesis of, 720–723
pancreatic, 830–842; *See also* Pancreatic hormones
parathyroid, 1081–1093; *See also* Parathyroid hormone (PTH)
peptide, 5, 29–37; *See also* Peptide(s)
in peptide growth factor regulation, 1266
pineal, 142–143
pituitary; *See* Pituitary hormones
production of, ectopic, 1383–1415; *See also* Ectopic hormone production
for prostate cancer, 1446, 1447
regulatory, in fuel homeostasis, 842
release of, 5
reproductive, acute exercise-associated changes in, 1496–1497
response of, to exercise and training, 1483, 1484t
responses to, mechanisms for attenuating or terminating, 11
responsiveness of, regulation of, 8
sensitivity of target cells to, evaluation of, 17
sex; *See* Sex steroids
signaling mechanisms of, *50*
steroid, 5, 37–43; *See also* Steroid hormones
synergisms among, 10–11
synthesis of, 5
thyroid, 43–46, 262–330; *See also* Thyroid hormones
thyrotropin releasing, 121–124; *See also* Thyrotropin-releasing hormone (TRH)
total, measurements of, 94–95
tropic, 11
as tumor markers, 1392–1394
tumors responsive to, 1427–1447; *See also* Tumor(s), hormone-responsive
types of, 5, 51t
uptake of, 7

Hormone(s) *(continued)*
in vitro assays of, 91–92
complementarity of in vivo assays with, 93
in vivo assays of, 91
complementarity of in vitro assays with, 93
Hormone replacement therapy (HRT):
long-term, 769–771
administration modes for, 769–770
benefits and risks of, 770–771
for menopause, 767–768
in postmenopausal osteoporosis prevention, 768
Hormone response elements (HREs), 422
Hot flush/flash, in menopause, 767
Howship lacuna, 1092
3βHSD deficiency, 815
in congenital adrenal hyperplasia, 448t
Human chorionic gonadotropin (hCG):
for cryptorchidism, 674
ectopic production of, 1412
in fetal gonadal function control, 789
for spermatogenesis initiation, 683t, 687–688
as tumor marker, 1392–1394, 1393t, 1394t
tumors secreting, gynecomastia from, 664
Human immunodeficiency virus (HIV):
hyperlipidemias secondary to, 1013–1014
infection with, thyroid function and, 287
Human placental lactogen, ectopic production of, 1412–113
Humoral hypercalcemia of malignancy, primary hyperparathyroidism versus, 1127
Humoral substances, systemic elaboration of, in hypercalcemia of malignancy, 1395–1398
"Hungry bone" syndrome, 1141
Hydatidiform mole, thyrotoxicosis in, 297
Hydration, forced:
for cystinuria, 1230
for nephrolithiasis, 1226
Hydrocortisone, for congenital adrenal hyperplasia, 1304
Hydrocortisone hemisuccinate:
for congenital adrenal hyperplasia, 812
effect of, on pulmonary function in acute asthma, *611*
1α-Hydroxycholecalciferol, pharmacology of, 1149t
17-Hydroxycorticosteroids, measurement of, 440
1α-Hydroxylase activity, renal, factors influencing, 1101t
17α-Hydroxylase deficiency, 803–804
21-Hydroxylase deficiency
clinical forms of, 450–451
CYP21 mutations causing, 808t
diagnosis of, 811t, 811–812
HLA typing applied to, *809*
incidence of, 451
pathophysiology of, 449–450
salt wasting in, 808, 808t
pathogenesis of, *809*
treatment of, 812–813, *814*
virilization of genetic female in, 808–813
pathogenesis of, *809*
11β-Hydroxylase deficiency, virilization in, 459, 813–815
21-Hydroxylase locus, genetics of, 451–455
Hydroxy-3-methylglutaryl coenzyme A reductase (HMG CoA reductase) inhibitors:
in familial hypercholesterolemia management, 1019–1020, 1021t
for hyperlipoproteinemia, 1056–1058
side effects of, 1057
structure of, *1057*
17α-Hydroxyprogesterone:
plasma concentrations of, 415t
secretion rate of, 415t
17-Hydroxyprogesterone (17-OHP):
concentrations of, in 21-hydroxylase deficiency, 811, *812*
measurement of, in congenital adrenal hyperplasia diagnosis, 456
3β-Hydroxysteroid dehydrogenase:
deficiency of, 457–458
in steroidogenesis, 398
17β-Hydroxysteroid dehydrogenase:
deficiency of, 804
in steroidogenesis, 401–402
3β-Hydroxysteroid dehydrogenase deficiency, 801, 803
11β-Hydroxysteroid dehydrogenase in steroidogenesis, 403
5-Hydroxytryptamine, synthesis and catabolism of, *1336*
1α-Hydroxyvitamin D3, for renal osteodystrophy, 1201
25-Hydroxyvitamin D3, for renal osteodystrophy, 1201
Hyperaldosteronism, 491–493
glucocorticoid-remediable, 590
primary, 491
secondary, 491–493
classification of, 491t
Hyperalphalipoproteinemia, familial, 1034
Hypercalcemia, 1109–1139
approach to patient with, 1111–1112
causes of, 1109t
clinical features of, 1109, 1110t
defense against, 1109–1110
drug-induced, 1137–1138
familial hypocalciuric, 1119–1120, *1120,* 1139
in granulomatous disorders, 1136
ICU, 1138
immobilization and, 1138
of infancy, idiopathic, 1138–1139
malignancy-associated, 1109–1110, 1110t, 1394–1400
calcitonin for, 1098
clinical manifestations of, 1398–1399
diagnosis of, 1398–1399, *1399*
humoral, 1395–1398
primary hyperparathyroidism compared with, 1399t
primary hyperparathyroidism versus, 1127
incidence of, 1111
medical management of, 1125
parathyroid hormone-related protein in, 1125–1127
prevalence of, 1111
therapy for, 1400
treatment of, 1129–1131
Hypercalcemia *(continued)*
pathophysiology of, 1394–1398, 1395t
renal phosphate handling in, 1154
in sarcoidosis, 1136
signs and symptoms of, 1109, *1110*
Hypercalcemic crisis, medical management of, 1124–1125
Hypercalciuria:
absorptive, *1245,* 1245–1246
treatment of, 1253
bone effects in, 1247
calcium oxalate stone risk and, 1240–1247
classification of forms of, 1242t, 1242–1247
constitutional, 1242–1243
diagnosis of, clinical utility of, 1241–1242
dietary, 1243, *1243*
evaluation of, in calcium oxalate stone evaluation, 1251–1252
treatment of, 1253
empirical therapy for, 1253–1254
evaluation of, in calcium oxalate stone evaluation, 1251
fasting, 1245
idiopathic, 1243–1244
osteoporosis in, 1194
mechanisms for, calcium homeostasis and, 1242
renal, 1244–1245
treatment of, 1253
screening for, results of, 1241t
secondary, 1242
subtypes of, evaluation of, in calcium oxalate stone evaluation, 1252
unclassifiable, 1245
Hypercapnia, vasopressin secretion and, 222
Hypercholesterolemia, 1015–1030
familial, 1015–1021
clinical characteristics of, *1016,* 1016–1017, *1017*
coronary artery disease in, 1016–1017, 1017t
definition of, 1015–1016
diagnostic laboratory features of, 1017
genetics of, 1018–1019
pathophysiology of, 1017–1018
treatment of, 1019–1021, 1021t
hypertriglyceridemia combined with, 1023–1027
Hyperchylomicronemia, 1027–1029
Hyperglycemia:
of aging, 1471
epinephrine and, 531–532
in hypothalamic disease, 155
stress, fuel-hormone imbalance in, 844–845
Hypergonadism, hypothalamic, 152
Hypergonadotropic hypogonadism, 665–666
in occult ovarian failure, 751
Hyperinsulinemia:
hypertension, insulin resistance, and obesity related to, 577
obesity and, 962
Hyperkalemia:
in Addison's disease, 468–469, 469t
in hyporeninemic hypoaldosteronism, 474, 475
Hyperlipidemia(s), 993, 1006–1015
in children, treatment of, 1063
classification of, 1006t, 1006–1007

Hyperlipidemia(s) *(continued)*
in diabetic patient, treatment of, 1063–1064
diagnosis of, laboratory tests in, 1064–1065
dietary, 1009–1010
diet-induced, in diabetes, 1012
drug-induced, 1015, 1015t
in elderly, treatment of, 1063
familial combined, 1023–1024
genetic, coexisting with diabetes, 1012–1013
lipoprotein(a), 1039
primary, versus secondary, 1010t
secondary, 1009–1015
to acquired immunodeficiency syndrome, 1013–1014
to alcohol, 1014–1015
to alpha1 antitrypsin deficiency, 1014
to anorexia nervosa, 1015
to biliary obstruction, 1014
to diabetes, 1010–1013
to human immunodeficiency virus, 1013–1014
to hypothyroidism, 1013
versus primary, 1010t
to renal disease, 1013
treatment of
dietary, 1042–1053
pharmaceutical therapy related to, 1053
phased approach to, 1050, 1052–1053
single-diet concept for, 1048–1050
in women, treatment of, 1062–1063
Hyperlipoproteinemia:
bile acid sequestrants for, 1054–1055
clofibrate for, 1059
diagnosis of, criteria for, 1007–1009
estrogens for, 1060–1061
fenofibrate for, 1060
future advances in treatment of, 1061–1062
gemfibrozil for, 1060
HMG CoA reductase inhibitors for, 1056–1058
nicotinic acid for, 1055–1056
orlistat for, 1061
pharmaceutical agents for, 1053–1062
primary type III, 1024–1027
for probucol, 1059
treatment of
in special patient populations, 1062–1064
surgical, 1062
type IV, 1029–1030
types I and V, 1027–1029
Hypermagnesemia, 1159
Hypernatremia:
adipsic, 240–242
causes of, 241t
differential diagnosis of, 242t
essential, 241
from thirst deficiency, 240
Hyperosmolar hyperglycemic nonketotic coma, 892
Hyperoxaluria:
calcium oxalate stone risk and, 1247–1249
classification and causes of, 1248t, 1248–1249
evaluation of, in calcium oxalate stone evaluation, 1252
treatment of, 1254
Hyperparathyroidism:
bone mineral density decrease in, *1119*
etiology of, 1113–1114
familial hypocalciuric hypercalcemia in, 1119–1120, *1120*
in Men 2A syndrome, management of, 1369, 1371
in multiple endocrine neoplasia type 2, 1363, 1364
parathyroid hormone levels in, *1087*
primary (1° HPT), 1112–1125
asymptomatic, diagnosis and management of, 1123–1124
bone disease in, 1115–1116, *1116, 1117, 1118, 1119*
bone mineral density index in, *1118*
cancer coexistent with, 1398
clinical presentation of, 1114–1115, *1115*
definitive diagnosis of, 1121
history of, 1112–1113
humoral hypercalcemia of malignancy compared with, 1399t
humoral hypercalcemia of malignancy versus, 1127
kidney disease in, 1116
laboratory findings in, 1121
medical management of, 1124–1125
multiple endocrine neoplasia and, 1118–1119, 1119t
in multiple endocrine neoplasia type 1, 1356–1357
nonspecific features of, 1116–1118
osteoporosis in, 1194
parathyroid surgery for, 1122–1123
pathophysiologic features of, 1244t
physical findings in, 1120, *1120*
preoperative localization studies in, 1121–1122
subtle
hypercalciuria in, 1244
with nephrolithiasis
evaluation of, 1251
treatment of, 1253
in renal osteodystrophy, 1200
serum and urinary calcium and, *1111*
Hyperphosphatasia, hereditary, 1201–1202
Hyperphosphatemia, disorders causing, 1156–1157
Hyperpigmentation:
in Addison's disease, 466, *467*
of skin, in Addison's disease, 20–21
Hyperplasia, in tissue growth, 1265, *1266*
Hyperprebetalipoproteinemia, 1029
Hyperprolactinemia, 152–153, 194–198
amenorrhea in, 751–753
causes of, 194t, 194–195, 752
clinical features of, 195
diagnosis of, 195–196
hypogonadism and, 681, 682
idiopathic, 752–753
in renal failure, 158
treatment of, 196–198, 753
Hypersensitization, adrenergic receptor, 530
Hypertension:
accelerated, 564
adrenal disorders and, 588–593
androgens and, 569
Hypertension *(continued)*
atrial natriuretic peptides and, 572–573
autonomic nervous system and, 573
benign intracranial, 158
body fat distribution and, *961*
calcitonin gene-related peptide and, 570
catecholamines and, 573
classification of, 554
complications of, 556
in congenital adrenal hyperplasia, 590–591
in Cushing's disease, 591
in Cushing's syndrome, 481
definition of, 553
diabetes mellitus and, 578
endocrinology of, 553–593
endothelin and, 570
endothelium-drived hyperpolarizing factor and, 571
environmental influences on, 556–557
epidemiology of, 555, *555*
erythropoietin and, 569–570
essential, 564–566, *565*
estrogens and, 569
evaluation of patient with, 579–581
experimental, 564
genetic influences on, 556–557
glucocorticoids and, 568–569
growth hormone and, 570
human renovascular, 564
insulin and, 573–579, *574*
insulin resistance and, 573–579, *574*
hyperinsulinemia and obesity related to, 577
therapeutic implications and, 578–579
low-fat, high-complex-carbohydrate diet in, 1053
mineralocorticoids and, *566*, 566–568
nitric oxide and, 570–571, *571*
obesity and, 963
in pheochromocytomas, 536–537, 591–593, *592, 593*
pregnancy-associated, obesity and, 966
progestins and, 569
relative weight and, *961*
renovascular, 581–588; *See also* Renovascular hypertension
secondary
findings on physical examination suggestive of, 579t
history features suggestive of, 579t
thyroid hormone and, 569
types of, 554t
vasopressin and, 569
Hyperthyroidism:
definition of, 289
endemic goiter and, 352
in Graves' disease, 291
growth excess in, 1307
gynecomastia and, 664
hypercalcemia in, 1136–1137
presentation of, in young and elderly, 1457t
somatostatin for, 1321
thyrotoxicosis differentiated from, 289
Hyperthyroxinemia, 276, 282–283
causes of, 282t

Hypertriglyceridemia, 1027–1030
  alcohol consumption and, 1047
  hypercholesterolemia combined with, 1023–1027
  obesity and, 963
  in pregnancy, 1029
Hypertrophy, in tissue growth, 1265, *1266*
Hyperuricosuria:
  calcium oxalate stone risk and, 1249–1250
  evaluation of, in calcium oxalate stone evaluation, 1252
  treatment of, 1254–1255
Hyperventilation, tetany and, 1140
Hypervolemic hyponatremia, 246
  therapy for, 247
Hypoaldosteronism:
  hyperreninemic, 475
  hyporeninemic, 474–475
  normoreninemic, 475
Hypoalphalipoproteinemia, familial, 1032–1033
Hypobetalipoproteinemia, 1035–1036
Hypocalcemia, 1139–1152
  approach to patient with, 1150–1152
  autosomal dominant, 1147–1148
  biochemical findings in, 1147t
  causes of, 1139t
  clinical features of, 1140t, 1140–1141
  defenses against, 1139
  diagnostic evaluation of, 1150–1151
  hypoparathyroidism and, 1141–1143
  malignancy-associated, 1149–1150
  medications causing, 1149
  neonatal, 1150
  treatment of, 1151–1152
  vitamin D abnormalities causing, 1148–1149
Hypocalciuric hypercalcemia, familial, 1119–1120, *1120*, 1139
Hypochloremic acidosis, in hyporeninemic hypoaldosteronism, 474
Hypocholesterolemia, omega-3 fatty acids and, 1045, *1045*
Hypochondroplasia, short stature from, 1297–1298
Hypocitraturia:
  calcium oxalate stone risk and, 1250–1251
  evaluation of, in calcium oxalate stone evaluation, 1252
  treatment of, 1255
Hypoglycemia, 543–545
  autonomic failure associated with, 544–545, *545*
  fuel-hormone imbalance in, 844
  glucagon secretion and, 839
  in insulin therapy, 892–893
  insulin-induced, in adrenocortical function evaluation, 444
  malignancy-associated, 1406–1409
  vasopressin secretion and, 222
Hypoglycemics, oral:
  for diabetes in elderly, 1473
  for Type 2 diabetes, 879–880, *881*, 881t
Hypogonadism:
  hypergonadotropic, in occult ovarian failure, 751
  hypogonadotropic, 747–748, *748*
  hypothalamic, 150–152
Hypogonadism *(continued)*
  male, 654–688
    adult, 655
    androgen therapy for, 682–686
    antiandrogens for, 686–687
    causes of, 665–667
    clinical manifestations of, 654t, 654–658
    differential diagnosis of, 658–665
      erectile dysfunction in, 658–662
      gynecomastia in, 663–665
      infertility in, 662–663
    evaluation of, 654–658
      seminal fluid analysis in, 658
      serum testosterone measurement in, 656–658, 657–658t
    gonadotropin releasing hormones for, 687–688
    gonadotropins for, 687–688
    history of, 656
    hypergonadotropic, 665–666
    hypogonadotropic, 666
      idiopathic, 678–680
    osteoporosis in, 1193
    physical examination in, 656, *656*
    prepubertal, 655
      treatment of, 683t, 683–684
    primary, 665, *665, 666*, 668–678
      androgen deficiency in, 668–673
      androgen resistance syndromes in, 676–678
      causes of, 667t
      sperm production deficiency in, 668–673
        isolated, 673–676
    secondary, 666, *666*, 678–682
      in acquired disorders, 680–682
      in aging men, 680
      androgen production deficiency in, 678–682
      causes of, 668t
      complex genetic syndromes and, 680, 681t
      constitutional delayed puberty and, 678–680, *679*
      drugs causing, 682
      estrogen excess and, 682
      hemochromatosis and, 680
      hyperprolactinemia and, 681
      hypopituitarism and, 680–681
      sperm deficiency in, 678–682
    serum testosterone measurement in, 656–658, 657–658t
    treatment of, 682–688, 683t
Hypogonadotropic eunuchoidism, 678–680
Hypogonadotropic hypogonadism, 666, 747–748, *748*
  idiopathic, 678–680
Hypomagnesemia, 1158–1159
  causes of, 1159t
  hypoparathyroidism and, 1142
Hyponatremia:
  in Addison's disease, 468–469, 469t
  in elderly, 1465
  hypervolemic, 245–246
    therapy for, 247
  hypovolemic, 245–246
    therapy for, 247
Hypoparathyroidism, 1141–1143
  familial, 1142–1143
  postsurgical, 1131
  rickets and/or osteomalacia in, 1188
  serum and urinary calcium and, *1111*
Hypophosphatasia, rickets and/or osteomalacia in, 1188
Hypophosphatemia:
  causes of, 1155t
  chronic, osteoporosis in, 1194
  disorders causing, 1154–1156
  metabolic bone disease in, 1186–1187
Hypophysiotropic hormones, 112–113, 119–121
  structures of, *122*
Hypophysiotropic neurons, organization of, *119*
Hypophysitis:
  granulomatous, 182
  lymphocytic, 182
Hypopituitarism:
  childhood onset, treatment of, 1296t
  hypogonadism and, 680–681
  idiopathic, growth hormone deficiency from, 1291
  primary amenorrhea in, 747
Hyporeninemic hypoaldosteronism, 474–475
Hypospadias:
  isolated, 807
  pseudovaginal perineoscrotal, 805
Hypotension:
  postural
    in generalized autonomic failure, 540–543
    mechanisms of, 541t, 541–542
    treatment of, 542–543
  thirst and, 226
Hypothalamic anorexia, 154–155
Hypothalamic hypergonadism, 152
Hypothalamic hyperprolactinemia, 152
Hypothalamic hypogonadism, 150–152
Hypothalamic hypothyroidism, 153, 321
Hypothalamic obesity, 154, 155t
Hypothalamic-pituitary axis, central nervous system and, 635–636
Hypothalamic-pituitary portal system, median eminence and, 118
Hypothalamic-pituitary-adrenal axis:
  aging and, 1462–1463
  function of, evaluation of, 628
  suppression of
    glucocorticoid kinetics and dosage required for, 625–626, *625–626*
    glucocorticoid withdrawal and, 625–629
    return to normal function after, kinetics of, 626–627, *626–627*
  tests to evaluate, *437*
Hypothalamic-pituitary-gonadal axis:
  in aging, 1464, *1464*
  differentiation of, 787–792
  exercise and training and, 1493–1496
Hypothalamic-pituitary-ovarian axis, in aging, 1465, *1465*
Hypothalamic-pituitary-testicular axis, 642–652
  alterations in
    with androgen resistance, *667*
    with primary hypogonadism, *665, 666*
    with secondary hypogonadism, *666*
  schematic diagram of, *643*

Hypothalamic-pituitary-thyroid axis, aging and, 1461–1462
Hypothalamus:
anatomic relations of, *115*
congenital embryopathic disorders affecting, 145–147
coronal sections through, *117*
diseases of, 145–156
etiology of, 146t
neurometabolic functions and, 153–156
pituitary function and, 149–153
disorders of, hyperprolactinemia from, 752
in feedback regulation of gonadotropin secretion, 651–652
functional defects in, in polycystic ovary syndrome, 756
in glucocorticoid regulation, 405
hamartomas of, 148
in hormone regulation, 112–113
inflammatory disorders of, 148–149
irradiation of, 149
in neuroendocrine organization, *112*
pharmacologic actions of VIP on, 1328t
polyostotic fibrous dysplasia involving, 149
trauma to, 148–149
tuber cinereum of, *116*
tumors of, 147–148
vascular disorders involving, 148
Hypothyroidism, 315–329
adaptive, 315
adrenal function in, 324
after radioiodine therapy, 318
aging process compared with, 1457t
appearance in, general, 321
appendages in, 321–322
cardiovascular system in, 322–323
causes of, 316t, 316–321
central, 320–321
thyrotropin secretion in, 321
in children, 328
from chronic autoimmune thyroiditis, 316–317
clinical manifestations of, 321–325
congenital, 318, 319
defenses against, 315–316
drug metabolism in, 323–324
endocrine system in, 324–325
energy in, 323–324
fluid and electrolyte metabolism in, 323
gastrointestinal system in, 323
gonadal function in, 324
hematopoietic system in, 323
hereditary, 318–320
hyperlipidemias secondary to, 1013
hyperprolactinemia from, 752
hypothalamic, 153, 321
illness-related, 315, 325
from infiltrative thyroid disease, 318
laboratory diagnosis of, 325–326, *326*
musculoskeletal system in, 322
nervous system in, 322
in newborn infants, 328
nutrient metabolism in, 323–324
overt, 315
pathophysiology of, 315–316
pituitary, 320–321
pituitary function in, 324
Hypothyroidism *(continued)*
postoperative, 318
pregnancy in, 325
pulmonary system in, 322–323
from radioactive iodine therapy, 307–308
renal function in, 323
short stature in, 1288–1289
skin in, 321–322
subclinical, 315, 327
surgery and, 325
thyroid gland in, 322
from thyroid hormone synthesis defects
acquired, 320
inherited, 318–319
transient, in autoimmune thyroiditis, 317–318
treatment of, 326–327
Hypothyrotropic hypothyroidism, 320–321
Hypothyroxinemia, 276, 283
causes of, 282t
Hypotriglyceridemia, omega-3 fatty acids and, 1045, *1045*
Hypoventilation syndrome, obesity, 965
Hypovolemic, thirst and, 226
Hypovolemic hyponatremia, 245–246
therapy for, 247
Hypoxia, vasopressin secretion and, 222
Hysteroscopy, operative, 765

ICI 182780 (Faslodex), for breast cancer, 1441
Illness, steroid coverage for adrenocortical insufficiency patient during, 473
Immobilization:
hypercalcemia from, 1138
osteoporosis and, 1194
Immotile cilia syndrome, 675
Immune responses, glucocorticoids and, 426–427
Immune system, vitamin D actions in, 1108
Immune theory, of aging, 1458t, 1459–1460
Immunoassays:
enzyme, 98
optimization and validation of, 101–102
radioactive tracers for, 97–98
reagents for, 95–99
Immunochemiluminometric assay, 98
Immunoelectrochemiluminometric assay, 98
Immunosuppressive therapy, postorgan transplantation, osteoporosis and, 1194–1195
Impotence:
in autonomic neuropathy, 907
therapy for, 908
in endocrine disorders, 23
in older males
causes of, 1469t
treatment modalities for, 1470t, 1470–1471
In vitro fertilization:
with donor oocyte, for premature ovarian failure, 751
donor oocyte, in Turner's syndrome, 747
Incontinence, in autonomic neuropathy, 907
Infant(s); *See also* Newborn
of diabetic mother, excess growth in, 1308–1309
Infant(s)*(continued)*
diarrhea in, idiopathic, octreotide acetate for, 1323t
Graves' disease in, 311
growth of, *1280,* 1280–1281
hypercalcemia in, idiopathic, 1138–1139
hypothyroidism in, 328
sex steroid concentrations in, 446t
thyroid function in, 281
Infarction, pituitary:
growth hormone deficiency from, 1293
pituitary disorders from, 182–183
Infection stone, 1236
Infection(s):
HIV, thyroid function and, 287
in iatrogenic Cushing's syndrome, 614
magnesium ammonium phosphate stones and, 1237
Infertility:
clinical approach to, 817, 819
definition of, 662
in endocrine disorders, 24
female, 759–763
male, 662–663
causes of, 662t
in polycystic ovary syndrome, management of, 757
varicocele and, 674
Inflammatory bowel disease, uric acid stones in, 1233
Inflammatory disease, growth hormone deficiency from, 1293
Inflammatory responses, glucocorticoids and, 426–427
Infradian rhythm, 144
Infundibular process, 217
Infundibulum, 217
Inhibin B, 638
Inhibitor theory, of stone pathogenesis, 1222–1223
Inorganic iodine, for thyrotoxicosis, 306
Inositol-1-4-5-triphosphate (IP3 receptor), 74, *75*
Insulin, 830–838
actions of, 835t, 835–838
influencing blood pressure, *574,* 574–575
allergy to, 894
amino acid sequence of, 830, *830*
biosynthesis of, 830–831, *831*
chemistry of, *830,* 830–831
for diabetes, in elderly, 1473
for diabetic ketoacidosis, 890–891
exercise and, 1486
in food intake regulation, 973
formulations of, available, 860t
for gestational diabetes, 887
for hyperosmolar hyperglycemic nonketotic coma, 892
hypertension and, 573–579
hypoglycemia used by, in adrenocortical function evaluation, 444
implantable pumps for, in diabetes management, 874
lipodystrophy from, 893–894, *894*
lispro, for diabetes, 873
phosphate reabsorption and, 1154
preparations of, development of, 860–861

Insulin *(continued)*
receptors for, structure of, *836*
secretion of, 831–835, *833*
failure of, in Type 2 diabetes, 854, *855*
in vivo, regulation of, 832, 832t
structure of, *33*
therapy with, complications of, 892–894
for Type 1 diabetes, 869–871
regimens for, 870, *870*
for Type 2 diabetes, *883,* 884–885, *885,* 885t
Insulin analogs, for diabetes, 873
Insulin resistance:
hypertension and, 573–579
hyperinsulinemia, and obesity related to, 577
in obesity, 963
therapeutic implications of, 578–579
ion transport abnormalities in, 575–576
obesity and, 962–963
overlapping domains of, 855
in polycystic ovary syndrome, 756–757
renal sodium handling in, 577
sympathetic nervous system in, 577
in Type 2 diabetes, 853–854
Insulin-like growth factors (IGFs), 1266–1272
aging and, 1460–1461, *1462*
bioavailability of, 1270–1271
fetal growth and, 1267–1268
receptors for, 1270, *1270*
Insulinoma:
in MEN 1 syndrome, 1357
management of, 1363
octreotide acetate efficacy on, 1324t
Integrins, 1092
Intensive care unit (ICU), hypercalcemia and, 1138
Interferon, for carcinoid syndrome, 1340
Interferon-alfa:
thyroid function and, 289
thyrotoxicosis induced by, 296
Interleukin 1 (IL-1), tumor-associated, hypercalcemia and, 1129
Interleukin 1α, in myeloma bone disease, 1134
Interleukin 2, thyrotoxicosis induced by, 296
Interleukin 6 (IL-6):
in myeloma bone disease, 1134
tumor-associated, hypercalcemia and, 1129
Interstitial cells, ovarian, 715–718, *716, 717, 718, 719, 726,* 726–731, *727, 729*
Interstitium, testicular, 636–637, *637*
Intestine:
calcium transport in, 1105–1107, *1106*
cholecystokinin effects on, 1325t
disease of, osteoporosis and, 1195
gastric inhibitory polypeptide effects on, 1329t
motilin effects on, 1330t
neurotensin actions on, 1332t
pharmacologic actions of VIP on, 1328t
phosphate absorption in, 1152–1153
secretin effects on, 1326t
vitamin D actions in, 1105–1107
Intravenous pyelography, in renovascular hypertension diagnosis, 584
Introns, 29
Iodide:
cellular uptake of, regulation of, 44
thyroid, transport of, 263–264
Iodide *(continued)*
defect in, hypothyroidism from, 319
in thyroid secretion regulation, 270
Iodide organification defects, hypothyroidism from, 319
Iodinated radiographic contrast agents, thyroid function and, 289
Iodination, in immunoassays, 98
Iodine:
abundance of, goiter and, 351
deficiency of
etiology of cretinism and, 353
hypothyroidism from, 320
excess of
hypothyroidism from, 320
thyroid function and, 288
inorganic, for thyrotoxicosis, 306
metabolism of, 43–44, *44*
radioactive
for follicular carcinoma of thyroid, 375–376
for Graves' thyrotoxicosis, 303, 304, 304t
for hypothyroidism, thyroiditis from, 330
for nontoxic goiter, 358
for thyrotoxicosis, 307–308
hypothyroidism after, 318
from thyroid adenoma, 308
in thyroid hormone biosynthesis, 262–263
thyrotoxicosis induced by, 295–296
Iodothyronine analogs, structural formulas of, *263*
Iodothyronine deiodinase, activity of, conditions/drugs altering, 270t
Iodothyronines:
production rates of, 266t
serum concentrations of, 266t
structural formulas of, *263*
Iodotyrosine deiodinase, defect in, hypothyroidism from, 319
Ion channel receptors, 78–80
Ion channels:
G protein-activated, 70–71
regulated by cAMP and cGMP, 83
Ion transport abnormalities in diabetes and insulin resistance, 575–576
Ionizing radiation:
androgen deficiency and, 672–673
sperm production impairment by, 675–676
Iopanoic acid, for thyrotoxicosis, 306
Irradiation:
cranial, for Cushing's disease, 1296
external beam, for thyroid carcinomas, 376
external neck, hypothyroidism after, 318
head and neck
growth hormone deficiency from, 1293
thyroid cancer and, *360,* 360–361
hypothalamic, 149
Ischemic nephropathy, in renovascular hypertension, 583
Islet amyloid polypeptide, 841–842
Islets of Langerhans, 828
cell types in, 828, 828t, *829*
electron micrograph of, *829*
transplantation of, whole organ transplantation versus, for Type 1 diabetes, 874t, 874–875
Isoproterenol, response to, in aging, 1463
Jansen's metaphyseal chondrodysplasia, 1139
Joint(s):
in endocrine disorders, 24–25
glucocorticoids for injection into, 618–619

Kallmann syndrome, 636, 678–680, 747–748, *748*
gonadotropin releasing hormone for, 688
testis size in, *656*
Kaposi's sarcoma, glucocorticoid therapy and, 624
Karyotype, 779, *781*
Kennedy's disease, 677
Keratopathy, band:
in endocrine disorders, 27
in primary hyperparathyroidism, 1120, *1120*
Ketoacidosis:
alcoholic, 890
diabetic, 887–892; *See also* Diabetic ketoacidosis (DKA)
Ketoconazole:
in adrenal steroid biosynthesis inhibition, 415
androgen deficiency from, 672
as antiandrogen, 687
for corticotroph adenoma, 200
for Cushing's disease, 489
Ketogenesis, biochemical pathway of, *888*
17-Ketogenic steroids, measurement of, 440
Ketones, monitoring of, in diabetes management, 868
17-Ketosteroid reductase in steroidogenesis, 401–402
Kidney(s):
actions of insulin on, influencing blood pressure, 574
complication of hypertension involving, 556
disease of
end-stage, in diabetic nephropathy, 902–903
hyperlipidemias secondary to, 1013
hyperparathyroid, 1116
thyroid function and, 287
failure of
acute, hypercalcemia and, 1138
chronic
androgen deficiency in, 673
hyperphosphatemia in, 1156–1157
hypersecretinemia in, 1326
renal osteodystrophy in, 1199–1201
vitamin D metabolism abnormalities in, 1185
gynecomastia and, 664
neuroendocrine alterations in, 157–158
function of
in hypothyroidism, 323
in thyrotoxicosis, 300
in glucagon degradation, 841
insufficiency of
chronic, hypocalcemia in, 1150
hyperphosphatemia from, 1156
mineralocorticoid actions on, 436–437
parathyroid hormone effects on, 1090
pharmacologic actions of VIP on, 1328t
phosphate excretion by, increased, hypophosphatemia from, 1155
phosphate handling by, 1153–1154

Kidney(s) *(continued)*
as renin source, 559
sodium handling by, insulin resistance and, 577
somatostatin effects on, 1320t
stones in, 1221–1256; *See also* Nephrolithiasis
transplantation of
in diabetic nephropathy, 902, 903
for renal osteodystrophy, 1201
vasopressin actions on, 224–225
vitamin D actions in, 1108
vitamin D loss through, 1186
Kimmellstein-Wilson nodular glomerulosclerosis, in diabetic nephropathy, 901, *903*
Kinase cascades:
hormone signal amplification in, 60, *60*
promoting cell growth, 81–82
Kinases, cyclic nucleotide actions independent of, 83–84
Kleine-Levin syndrome, 155t
Klinefelter syndrome, 668–670, 792–794, *794*
features of, 669t
growth excess in, 1307
mosaic, 669–670
mutant phenocopy of, 670
serum FSH, LH and total testosterone in, *670*
Kyphoscoliosis, in rickets, 1183

Lability of mood, in thyrotoxicosis, 299
Lactogen, human placental, ectopic production of, 1412–1413
Lactotroph adenoma, 194–198
diagnosis of, 195–196
pathology of, 195
pregnancy and, 198
treatment of, 196–198
Lactotroph cells, 173
hormones secreted by, 173, 174t
Lagophthalmos, in endocrine disorders, 27
Lamellae, 1091
Langerhans-cell histiocytosis, hypothalamic infiltration with, 148, *149*
Laron syndrome, 1293
Laser therapy for diabetic retinopathy, *899*, 899–900, *900*
Latex particle agglutination assays, 99
Laurence-Moon syndrome, 155t
Laurence-Moon-Biedl syndrome, hypogonadotropic hypogonadism in, 681t
Lauric acid, 1044
"Lazy pituitary syndrome," 1294
Lecithin, lipid/lipoprotein metabolism and, 1048
Lecithin cholesterol acyltransferase:
deficiency of, familial, 1036
in lipoprotein metabolism, 999
Lentigines, multiple, hypogonadotropic hypogonadism and, 681t
Leopard syndrome, hypogonadotropic hypogonadism in, 681t
Leptin:
athletic amenorrhea and, 1498
levels of, in elderly, 1474
resistance to, in obesity, 971–972
Leriche's syndrome, 660
Letrozole (Fermara), for breast cancer, 1441
Leukocytes:
function of, glucocorticoids and, 428
movement of, glucocorticoids and, 427t, 427–428
Leukopenia, in endocrine disorders, 22–23
Leukotrienes, 764
Leuprolide, for prostate cancer, 1447
Levine-Metz classification, of tumors producing ectopic hormones, 1390, 1390t
Leydig cells, 636, *637*
hypoplasia of, 801
luteinizing hormone in regulation of, 643–645
tumors of, 690
LH resistance, 671–672
Libido:
changes in
in endocrine disorders, 23
in menopause, 767
male, physiology of, 652
in older males, 1469
Liddle's syndrome, 557
Li-Fraumeni syndrome, breast cancer risk and, 1431t
Light/dark cycles, ACTH and cortisol circadian rhythms and, 409
Lipase:
endothelial, in lipoprotein metabolism, 999–1000
hepatic
deficiency of, 1027
in lipoprotein metabolism, 999
lipoprotein, in lipoprotein metabolism, 999
Lipemia retinalis in hyperchylomicronemia, 1027
Lipid(s):
abnormalities of, obesity and, 963
average values for, 1008t
determinations of, in hyperlipidemia diagnosis, 1064
metabolism of
disorders of, 993–1065
glucocorticoid actions on, 426
monitoring of, in Type 2 diabetes, 886
synthesis and catabolism of, 997–998
Lipid goals for diabetic patient, 871t
Lipodystrophy:
gigantism and, 1309
insulin, 893–894, *894*
Lipogenesis, thyroid hormones stimulating, 274
Lipoid adrenal hyperplasia, congenital, 460–461
Lipolysis, thyroid hormones stimulating, 274
Lipomas, in MEN 1 syndrome, 1358
Lipoprotein(s):
abnormal, composition of, 996
abnormalities of, dietary factors in causation and correction of, 1049t
average values for, 1008t
classification of, 993–994, *994*
composition of, 994–996, 995t
high-density, 993, *994*, 994t
alcohol consumption and, 1047
composition of, 995, 995t
decreased, dietary factors in causation and correction of, 1049t
Lipoprotein(s) *(continued)*
disorders of, 1030–1034
metabolism of, 1001–1003, *1002*
low-density, 993, *994*, 994t
composition of, 995, 995t
increased, dietary factors in causation and correction of, 1049t
metabolism of, 1001, *1002*
structure of, *997*
metabolism of, 1000–1004
enzymes and transfer proteins active in, 998–1000
particles of, atherogenicity of, 1006, 1006t
plasma, 993–997
apoprotein content of, 994t
receptors for, *1004*, 1004–1006, *1005*
separations of, in hyperlipidemia diagnosis, 1064–1065
structure of, 997, *997*
in thyroid hormone binding, 272
very low density, 993, *994*, 994t
composition of, 995, 995t
increased, dietary factors in causation and correction of, 1049t
metabolism of, 1000–1001, *1001*
β-Lipoprotein, assays of, 439
Lipoprotein lipase, in lipoprotein metabolism, 999
Lipoprotein X, composition of, 996
Lipoprotein(a):
composition of, 994t, 995
hyperlipidemia associated with, 1039
metabolism of, 1003
Liquid chromatography, in plasma cortisol determinations, 438
Liquid-phase precipitation, 99
Liquor folliculi, 713
Lispro insulin, for diabetes, 873
Lithium carbonate:
hypercalcemia induced by, 1138
hypothyroidism from, 320
for syndrome of inappropriate antidiuresis in cancer, 1406
thyroid function and, 289
for thyrotoxicosis, 306
Lithotripsy, 1224
Liver:
cholecystokinin effects on, 1325t
disease of
chronic, androgen deficiency in, 673
increased serum thyroxine-binding globulin concentrations and, 282
thyroid function and, 287
effects of anabolic steroids on, 1503
gastric inhibitory polypeptide effects on, 1329t
glucagon action on, 840–841
insulin actions on, 835t
pharmacologic actions of VIP on, 1328t
protein/nucleic acid metabolism in, glucocorticoid actions on, 426
secretin effects on, 1326t
somatostatin effects on, 1320t
Looser zones, in osteomalacia, 1183
Lovastatin (Mevacor):
dosage of, 1057, 1058t
for familial defective apolipoprotein B-100, 1022

Lovastatin (Mevacor) *(continued)*
for familial hypercholesterolemia, 1019–1020, 1021t
for hyperlipoproteinemia, 1054t
mechanism of action of, 1056–1057
indications for, 1057–1058
side effects of, 1057
structure of, *1057*
Lowe syndrome, hypogonadotropic hypogonadism in, 681t
Luminescence, in immunoassays, 98–99
Lung(s):
disorders of, in obesity, 965
in hypothyroidism, 323
Luteinization, *727,* 727–728
Luteinizing hormone (LH):
actions of, 178, *179*
deficiency of, isolated, 680
endogenous, in idiopathic hypogonadotropic hypogonadism, *679*
evaluation of, in children, 1309–1310
in interstitial androgen production, *726,* 726–727
levels of, in aging, *1463,* 1464
in Leydig cell regulation, 643–645
regulation of, 114
secretion of, 178
in spermatogenesis control, 649–651
synthesis of, 178
Luteolysis, 720, 728
Lymphocytes, function of, glucocorticoids and, 428
Lymphocytic hypophysitis, 182
Lymphoma, thyroid, 373
Lymphotoxin, in myeloma bone disease, 1133–1134

Macroadenomas, pituitary:
discovering consequences of, 192
transsphenoidal surgery for, efficacy of, 186t
Macromastia, pubertal, persistent, 665
Macrophages, function of, glucocorticoids and, 428
Macular edema, in diabetic retinopathy, 899–900, 900t
Magnesium:
balance of, 1158
deficiency of, hypoparathyroidism and, 1142
depletion of, causes of, 1159t
metabolism of, disorders of, 1157–1159
parathyroid hormone secretion and, 1085
supplemental, for absorptive hypercalciuria, 1253
Magnesium ammonium phosphate stones, 1236–1238
Magnesium sulfate, for hypocalcemia, 1151
Magnetic resonance angiography in renovascular hypertension diagnosis, 585
Magnetic resonance imaging (MRI):
in anterior pituitary lesion evaluation, 184, *185*
in diabetes insipidus diagnosis, 234, *235*
Malabsorption, hypophosphatemia from, 1187
Malabsorption syndrome, pseudofractures in, 1183, *1183*
Male pseudohermaphroditism, 801–807; *See also* Virilization, genital, defective
Malignancy; *See also* Cancer
hypercalcemia of, 1109–1110, 1110t, 1125–1136, 1394–1400; *See also* Hypercalcemia, malignancy-associated
Malnutrition:
hypophosphatemia from, 1187
neuroendocrine alterations in, 156–157
postnatal, growth and, 1288
pubertal delay from, 748
reproductive dysfunction and, 1498
Malnutrition stones, 1221
Mammary gland; *See* Breast
Mannitol, for hypervolemia hyponatremia, 247
Marble bone disease, 1198–1199
Marfan syndrome:
growth excess in, 1307
homocystinuria compared with, 1308t
Marfanoid habitus, in MEN 2B syndrome, 1373
Marijuana, androgen deficiency from, 672
Martsolf syndrome, hypogonadotropic hypogonadism in, 681t
Maternal disorders, fetal growth and, 1287
Matrix theory, of stone pathogenesis, 1222
Maturity onset diabetes of youth, 855, 856–857
McCune-Albright syndrome, 149, 1305
Median eminence, 217
anatomy of, 118
diagram of, *120*
hypothalamic-pituitary portal system and, 118
Medications; *See* Drug(s)
Medulla, ovarian, 707, *708*
Medullary nephrocalcinosis, 1221
Medullary thyroid carcinoma, *371,* 371–373
calcitonin screening for, 1366–1367
familial, 1364, *1364*
genetic testing for, 1367–1368
follow-up of patients with, 378
in MEN 2A syndrome, 1365–1367
in MEN 2B syndrome, treatment of, 1373
in multiple endocrine neoplasia type 2, 1363–1364
Megestrol acetate, as antiandrogen, 686–687
Meiotic maturation, in oocyte growth, *730,* 730–731, *731*
Melatonin, 142–143
synthesis of, stages of, *142*
Membrane proteins, transport of, subcellular, 34, *35*
Men:
gonadotropin deficiency in, 205–206
hyperprolactinemia in, clinical features of, 195
Menarche, 737, *737*
delayed, exercise and, 1496
time of, 745
Menarcheal menorrhagia, 749–750
Meningiomas, 182
Menopause, 738–739, 1464
endocrinology of, 766–767
problems after, 768–769
sexuality after, 1471
Menorrhagia, 763–766
menarcheal, 749–750
operative hysteroscopy for, 765
Menstrual cycle, 737–738, *738*
aldosterone changes during, 491–492
Menstrual cycle *(continued)*
disturbances of
in endocrine disorders, 23–24
exercise-induced, 1497
in polycystic ovary syndrome, 755
endometrium during, 763, *763*
morphology of, *762*
regulation of, in polycystic ovary syndrome, 757
Mercaptopropionylglycine (MPG), for cystinuria, 1231
Messenger RNA, biosynthesis of, 29–31
Metabolic alkalosis, in malignancy-associated hypercalcemia, 1127
Metabolic disorders:
neuroendocrine alterations from, 156–158
obesity and, 962–963
Metabolism:
of adrenocortical steroids, 418–421
calcium, cellular and extracellular, 1079–1081
carbohydrate, thyroid hormone effects on, 274
drug
in hypothyroidism, 323–324
in thyrotoxicosis, 301
fuel, 825–1075; *See also* Fuel metabolism
hormone, 6
inborn errors of, uric acid stones and, 1233
intermediary, 11
iodine, 43–44, *44*
mineral, 1079–1159
nutrient
in hypothyroidism, 323–324
in thyrotoxicosis, 300–301
of ovarian steroid hormones, 722–723
pharmacologic actions of VIP on, 1328t
Metaphyseal chondrodysplasia, Jansen's, 1139
Metastasis(es):
to adrenal, 464
to anterior pituitary, 182
bony, hypercalcemia and, 1394–1395
osteoblastic, hypocalcemia with, 1149
osteolytic, pathophysiology of, 1131–1132
Metformin:
in obesity management, 986
for Type 2 diabetes, *881,* 881–882, *882,* 882t, *883*
Methimazole:
thyroid function and, 288
for thyrotoxicosis, 304–306, *305*
for thyrotroph adenoma, 203–204
Methylprednisolone:
for congenital adrenal hyperplasia, 457t
structure of, *611*
Metrorrhagia, in endocrine disorders, 24
Metyrapone:
in adrenal steroid biosynthesis inhibition, 414
for corticotroph adenoma, 200
for Cushing's disease, 489
Metyrapone testing, 443–444
in children, 447
Mevastatin, structure of, *1057*
Microadenectomy, for Cushing's disease, 1296
Microaneurysms, in diabetic retinopathy, 897, *897*
Microconversions, causing congenital adrenal hyperplasia, 454, 454t

Midget, 1283; *See also* Short stature
Midodrine, for postural hypotension, 542–543
Mifepristone, 772
Milk-alkali syndrome, 1138
Milkman fractures, in osteomalacia, 1183
Mineralocorticoids:
  actions of
    molecular mechanisms of, 434–435
    steps in, *434*
  agonists and antagonists of, 435
  in blood pressure elevation, mechanisms of, 568
  for chronic adrenal insufficiency, 472–473
  for congenital adrenal hyperplasia, 812–813, 1304
  definition of, 434
  excess of, apparent, 591
  hypertension and, *566,* 566–568
  measurement of, in adrenocortical function evaluation, 444
  physiologic actions of, 435–437
  plasma concentrations of, in children, 445, 446t
  regulation of, 411–413
  urinary concentrations of, in children, 445, 446t
Minerals:
  lipid/lipoprotein metabolism and, 1048
  metabolism of, 1079–1159
    hormone actions in, 11–12
Mithramycin, for hypercalcemia of malignancy, 1130
Mitotane:
  in adrenal steroid biosynthesis inhibition, 414
  for Cushing's disease, 489
Mixed gonadal dysgenesis, 796
Möbius syndrome, hypogonadotropic hypogonadism in, 681t
Molecular abnormalities in MEN 2B syndrome, 1372
Molecular theories, of aging, 1458, 1458t
Monoclonal antibodies, 97
Mononeuritis multiplex, 907
  in diabetes, 25
Mononeuropathy, in endocrine disorders, 26
Monounsaturated fatty acids, 1044
Mood:
  exercise and, 1492
  lability of, in thyrotoxicosis, 299
Morbid obesity, surgery for, 986–987
Mortality:
  in acromegaly, 190–191, 191t
  obesity and, 956–958, *957, 958, 959*
Mosaic pattern, in Paget's disease of bone, 1206
Mosaicism, 747
Motilin, 1329–1330
MTP, inhibitors of, for hyperlipoproteinemia, 1062
Mucification, in ovulation, 735, *735*
Mucosal neuromas, in multiple endocrine neoplasia type 2B, 1371–1372, *1372*
Muir-Torre syndrome, breast cancer risk and, 1431t
Müllerian ducts:
  abnormalities of, primary amenorrhea in, 748
  persistent, 800–801
Müllerian inhibiting substance, 786–787
Multianalyte assays, 99
Multiglandular endocrine disorders, 1355–1376
  multiple endocrine neoplasia type 1 as, 1355–1363; *See also* Multiple endocrine neoplasia type 1 (MEN 1)
  multiple endocrine neoplasia type 2 as, 1363–135, 1364t
Multiple antigenic peptides (MAPs), 96–97
Multiple endocrine neoplasia (MEN), *372,* 372–373, 1118–1119, 1119t
Multiple endocrine neoplasia type 1 (MEN 1), 1355–1363
  adrenal cortical adenomas in, 1358–1359
  bronchial adenomas in, 1358
  carcinoid tumors in, 1358
  chromophobe adenomas in, 1358
  clinical evaluation of, 1359–1360
  components of, 1355–1359, 1356t
  definition of, 1355
  diagnosis of, 1361–1362
  differential diagnosis of, 1360, 1360t
  enteropancreatic tumors in, 1357–1358
  gastrinoma in, 1357
  glucagonomas in, 1357–1358
  GRFoma in, 1358
  history of, 1355
  insulinoma in, 1357
  lipomas in, 1358
  management of, 1362–1363
  in other species, 1360
  pancreatic endocrine tumors in, 1358
  pathogenesis of, 1360–1361, *1361, 1362*
  pituitary adenomas in, functioning, 1358
  pituitary tumors in, 1358
  ppomas in, 1358
  primary hyperparathyroidism in, 1356–1357
  relation of, to other syndromes, 1362
  somatostatinomas in, 1358
  thyroid adenomas in, 1359
  vipoma in, 1358
Multiple endocrine neoplasia type 2 (MEN 2), 1363–1365, 1364t
  clinical outcome of, 1373
Multiple endocrine neoplasia type 2A (MEN 2A), 1364
  with cutaneous lichen amyloidosis, 1371
  genetic testing for, 1367–1368
  with Hirschsprung disease, 1371
  hyperparathyroidism in, 1369, 1371
  medullary thyroid carcinoma in, 1365–1367
  pheochromocytoma in, 1368–1369, *1370*
Multiple endocrine neoplasia type 2B (MEN 2B), 1371–1373
Multiple myeloma, osteolysis and, 1133–1134
Mumps orchitis:
  androgen deficiency and, 673
  sperm production impairment in, 675
Muscle(s):
  in acromegaly, 190
  atrophy of, spinal bulbar, 677
  as body protein reservoir, 842
  growth hormone actions on, 177
  insulin actions on, 835t, 837, 838
  protein/nucleic acid metabolism in, glucocorticoid actions on, 426
  in thyrotoxicosis, 299
Muscle(s) *(continued)*
  weakness of
    in Cushing's syndrome, 482
    in thyrotoxicosis, 299
Musculoskeletal system, in hypothyroidism, 322
Mutant phenocopy, of Klinefelter syndrome, 670
Mutations:
  missense
    causing nonclassic congenital adrenal hyperplasia, 455
    causing simple virilizing congenital adrenal hyperplasia, 455
  point
    causing congenital adrenal hyperplasia, 454, 454t
    known, effects of, on 21-hydroxylase activity, 454–455
Myocardial infarction:
  in endocrine disorders, 23
  thyroid function and, 287
Myopathy:
  in endocrine disorders, 26
  in iatrogenic Cushing's syndrome, 614
Myotonic dystrophy, 670
  spermatogenesis impairment in, 675
Myristic acid, 1044
Myxedema, in Graves' disease, 314–315
  localized, *315*
  pathogenesis of, 294
Myxedema coma, 328–329

Najjar syndrome, 807
Naloxone, growth hormone response to exercise and, 1487–1488
Nausea, vasopressin secretion and, 221, *222*
Neck:
  irradiation of, thyroid cancer and, *360,* 360–361
  masses in, differential diagnosis of, 262t
Needle biopsy, in thyroid function valuation, 279
Nelson's syndrome, treatment of, 490–491
Neonatal Graves' disease, 311
Neonatal hypocalcemia, 1150
Nephrectomy, for renovascular hypertension, 588
Nephrocalcinosis, 1221
  in endocrine disorders, 23
Nephrogenic diabetes insipidus, 233, 233t
  management of, 239
Nephrogenous cAMP, 1088
Nephrolithiasis, 1221–1256
  age distribution of, by type, 1222
  calcium oxalate, 1238–1255; *See also* Calcium oxalate stones
  calcium phosphate, 1235–1236
  classification of
    by clinical presentation, 1221
    by crystalline structure, 1221
  clinical events involving, quantitating, 1222
  clinical presentation of, 1224
  cystinuria causing, 1227–1231; *See also* Cystinuria
  in endocrine disorders, 23
  evaluation of, 1223–1227
    internist in, 1223–1224
  formation of, physicochemical aspects of, 1223, *1223*

Nephrolithiasis *(continued)*
in hyperparathyroidism, 1116
magnesium ammonium phosphate, 1236–1238
medical management of, 1224–1227
metabolic activity involving, 1222
pathogenesis of, theories of, 1222–1223
prevalence of, 1221
by type, 1222t
surgical activity involving, 1222
surgical management of, 1224
treatment of, 1223–1227
internist in, 1223–1224
uric acid, 1231–1235; *See also* Uric acid stones
Nephropathy:
assessment of, in Diabetes Control and Complications Trial, 862–864, *863*
diabetic, 900–903
clinical characteristics of, 900–901, *901, 902, 903*
course of, *901*
incidence of, 901
pathogenesis of, 901–902
prevalence of, 901
risk factors for, 901–902
screening for, 902
treatment of, 902–903
ischemic, in renovascular hypertension, 583
Nephrotic syndrome, thyroid function and, 287
Nerves, of ovary, 707–709
Nervous system:
autonomic
hypertension and, 573
in insulin secretion regulation, 835
obesity and, 974–975
peripheral, disorders of, erectile dysfunction from, 660
central; *See* Central nervous system (CNS)
endocrine system distinguished from, 3–4, *4*
in hypothyroidism, 322
sympathetic, insulin resistance and, 577
in thyrotoxicosis, 299
Neuroactive substances, in periventricular and arcuate nucleus neurons, 118t
Neuroblastomas, sympathochromaffin, 540
Neuroendocrine control of growth hormone release with exercise, 1487–1488
Neuroendocrine system:
anatomic aspects of, 115–119
diseases of, 145–159
CNS disorders in, 158–159
hypothalamic, 145–156; *See also* Hypothalamus, diseases of
feedback loops in, 113–115, *114,* 114t
function of, CNS rhythms and, 143–145
systemic disease and, 156–158
tumors of, 1333
of gastrointestinal tract, 1333–1340; *See also* Carcinoid syndrome
Neuroendocrinology, 111–159
brain-hypothalamic-pituitary-target organ regulation in, 111–115
definition of, 111
general concepts in, 111
pineal gland in, 141–143
Neurohypophysis, 217–247; *See also* Pituitary gland, posterior
ectopic, 146, *147*
Neurological symptoms, in acromegaly, 190
Neuromas, mucosal, in multiple endocrine neoplasia type 2B, 1371–1372, *1372*
Neuromodulation, 112
Neuromuscular abnormalities, in endocrine disorders, 25–26
Neuron(s):
arcuate nucleus, neuroactive substances in, 118t
extrahypophyseal
oxytocin-producing, 224
vasopressin-producing, 224
gonadotropin releasing hormone, hypothalamic, 635–636
hypophysiotropic, 119–121
organization of, *119*
to neuron interactions, 111–112
paraventricular, neuroactive substances in, 118t
schematic diagram of, *113*
Neuropathy:
in acromegaly, 190
autonomic
acute, 542t
diabetic, classical, 544–545
in Diabetes Control and Complications Trial, 864
diabetic, 904–908
autonomic, 907–908
classification of, 905t
compression, 907
distal sensorimotor, 905–907
motor, 907
in endocrine disorders, 25–26
Neuropeptide Y (NPY), 1330
biologic effects of, 1331t
neurologic effects of, 140
Neuropeptides, 138
affecting hunger/satiety, 973
Neurophysins, 217
copeptin and, 226
Neurotensin, 1331–1332
neurologic effects of, 138
Neurotransmitter(s), 3, 111, 135–141
amino acid, 137–138
bioaminergic
anatomic pathways of, 135–137
biosynthesis of, 135
metabolism of, 135
neuropharmacology of, 137
crosstalk among, 84
enzymes associated with, *136*
epinephrine and norepinephrine as, 535
function of, drugs altering, *137*
gaseous, 140–141
in gonadotropin releasing hormone regulation, 127
major brain metabolites associated with, *136*
neuropeptides as, 138
pineal, 142–143
in pituitary hormone secretion regulation, 137t
signaling mechanisms of, *50*
types of, 51t
Newborn; *See also* Infant(s)
with abnormal genitalia, clinical approach to, 816–817, *817*
Niacin; *See* Nicotinic acid (niacin)
Nicotinic acetylcholine receptor, 78
Nicotinic acid (niacin):
derivatives of, for hyperlipoproteinemia, 1061
for familial combined hyperlipidemia, 1024
for familial hypercholesterolemia, 1020, 1021t
for hyperlipoproteinemia, 1055–1056
type III, 1026
type IV, 1030
Nitric oxide cytokine theory, of aging, 1460, *1460*
Nitric oxide (NO):
cGMP signaling and, 73–74
hypertension and, 570–571, *571*
as neurotransmitter, 140–141
Nocturia, 239–240
Nonimmunologic molecular recognition systems, 97–99
Nonradioactive tracers, for immunoassays, 98–99
Nonsteroidal androgen receptor antagonists, as antiandrogens, 687
Noonan syndrome, 671
short stature in, 1301–1302
19–Nor-deoxycorticosterone, as mineralocorticoid, 567
Norepinephrine:
anatomic pathways of, 135
biological effects of, 531
biological roles of, 535
energy expenditure and, 974–975
in exercise, 1489
levels of, in aging, 1463
plasma concentrations of
in pheochromocytoma, 537–538, *538*
venous, 533t
physiologic adaptation of, 533–535, *534*
Normocalcemic primary hyperparathyroidism, 1244
Nose, in endocrine disorders, 21
Nuclear hormone receptors, ligands for, structure of, 55t
Nuclear medicine, in bone metabolic disease evaluation, 1180–1181
Nuclear receptor proteins, structural organization of, 57–59, *58, 59*
Nuclear receptor signaling, 53–60
Nuclear receptor superfamily, human:
DNA binding domain of, alignment of, *57*
evolution of, *56*
Nuclear receptors:
activity of, modification of, by phosphorylation, 59–60
DNA binding of, 57–58
gene regulation by, mechanism of, 59
intracellular localization of, 59
knockout studies of, 56–57
ligand independent activation of, 59
for triiodothyronine, 272–273
Nucleation, in stone formation, 1223
Nuclei, hypothalamic, 116, 118
Nucleic acid, metabolism of, glucocorticoid actions on, 426–429
Nursing home residents, diabetes in, 1473t, 1473–1474

Nutrient metabolism:
in hypothyroidism, 323–324
in thyrotoxicosis, 300–301
Nutrition:
disorders of, in elderly, 1474–1476
exercise-associated reproductive dysfunction and, 1497–1498
growth and, 1279
total parenteral, osteomalacia from, 1188
Nutritional amenorrhea, 753–754
Nutritional deficiency, hypogonadism from, 682
Nutritional recovery, hypophosphatemia from, 1156
Nutritional status, insulin-like growth factor levels and, 1268–1269

Obesity, 953–987
body fat distribution and, 960–962, *961*
cancer and, 964
cardiovascular disease and, 958–960, *959, 960*
in Cushing's syndrome, 480–481, *481*
definition of, 953
diabetes and, 962t, 962–963
economic costs of, 956
in elderly, 1475
endocrine disorders and, 964–965
etiology of, 966–975
autonomic nervous system in, 974–975
endocrine systems in, 974–975
energy expenditure in, 968–971, *969*
environmental factors in, 968
food intake in, 971–974
genetic factors in, *966*, 966–968
excess growth in, 1308
gallstones and, 963–964
hypertension and, 963
insulin resistance and hyperinsulinemia related to, 577
hypothalamic, 154, 155t
lipid abnormalities and, 963
lipid metabolism and, 1046
lipoprotein metabolism and, 1046
massive, hypogonadism from, 682
medical complications of, 956t, 956–966
metabolic disorders and, 962–963
morbid, surgery for, 986–987
mortality and, 956–958, *957, 958, 959*
neuroendocrine alterations in, 157
in polycystic ovary syndrome, 755
prevalence of, 956
prevention of, 975–976
pulmonary disorders and, 965
skeletal disorders and, 965
treatment of, 975–987
behavioral modification in, 978
diet in, 978–984; *See also* Diet(s)
exercise in, 976–978, 977t, *978*
fad diets in, 984
pharmacological treatment in, 984–986
Obstructive sleep apnea syndrome, obesity and, 965
Occupation theory, 52
Octreotide acetate (Sandostatin):
for acromegaly, 193–194, *194*
applications of, 1321–1322
Octreotide acetate (Sandostatin) *(continued)*
for carcinoid syndrome, 1339–1340
for GEP peptide-producing tumors, efficacy of, 1324t
for postural hypotension, 543
for thyrotroph adenoma, 203, 204t
Oligomenorrhea, in endocrine disorders, 23–24
Oligozoospermia, 655
idiopathic, 676, 677
Omega-3 fatty acids, 1044–1046
in hyperlipidemia management, 1049–1050
Oncogenic osteomalacia, 1409–1410
Ontogenesis, blocked, in ectopic hormone production, 1392
Oocyte meiotic inhibitor, 731, *731*
Oocytes, 707, 728–731, *729, 730, 731*
donor
for in vitro fertilization, in Turner's syndrome, 747
in vitro fertilization with, for premature ovarian failure, 751
growth of, 729–731
Oogonia, 728–729
Ophthalmic abnormalities, in endocrine disorders, 26–27
Ophthalmopathy:
in Graves' disease, pathogenesis of, 294
infiltrative, in Graves' disease, 311–314, *312*, 312t, *313*
Ophthalmoplegia, in endocrine disorders, 26–27
Opiates:
endogenous, in exercise and training, 1490–1492
hypogonadism from, 682
Opioids, endogenous, in food intake regulation, 973
Optic nerve, atrophy of, in endocrine disorders, 26
Oral contraceptives, 771–772
breast cancer risk and, 1433–1434
for hirsutism, 758–759
for menarcheal menorrhagia, 749
Orchiopexy, for cryptorchidism, 674
Orchitis:
androgen deficiency and, 673
sperm production impairment in, 675
Orgasm, male, physiology of, 653–654
Orlistat (Xenical), for hyperlipoproteinemia, 1061
Oropharyngeal dysphagia, in endocrine disorders, 21
Oropharyngeal effects, on vasopressin secretion, 220
Orphan receptors, 56
Orthostatic hypotension, in generalized autonomic failure, 540–543
Osmolality:
plasma, diabetes insipidus and, *230*, 230–231
urine, diabetes insipidus and, *230*, 231, *231*
Osmoreceptors, 218, 220
Osmotic effects:
on thirst, 226
on vasopressin secretion, 218–220, *219, 220*
Osteitis deformans, 1203, 1206; *See also* Paget's disease of bone
Osteitis fibrosa, in hyperparathyroidism, 1115, *1116*
Osteitis fibrosa cystica, in hyperparathyroidism, 1115, *1117*
Osteoarthritis:
in acromegaly, 190
in obesity, 965
Osteoblast, 1091
Osteoblastic metastases, hypocalcemia with, 1149
Osteoclast, 1091–1092
differentiation, fusion and survival mechanisms of, 1092, *1093*
Osteocytes, 1091
Osteodystropy, renal, 1199–1201
Osteolysis, localized, 1131–1136
bone microenvironment as "soil" for, 1132–1133
breast cancer-mediated, parathyroid hormone-related protein in, 1133
clinical manifestations of, 1131
from malignancy, therapy of, 1135–1136
pathophysiology of, 1131–1132
Osteomalacia, 1182–1189
bone pathology in, 1184
classification of, 1184, 1185t
clinical presentation of, 1182–1184
in endocrine disorders, 25
hypophosphatemic, 1187
laboratory findings in, 1183–1184
oncogenic, 1409–1410
pathogenesis of, 1184
radiologic features of, 1182–1183, *1183*
in renal osteodystrophy, 1200
symptoms and signs of, 1182
treatment of, 1188–1189
vitamin D deficiency in, 1184–1185
vitamin D malabsorption and, 1185
vitamin D metabolism abnormalities and, 1185–1186
Osteopenia, 1189
age-related, 1467–1468
in endocrine disorders, 24–25
Osteopetrosis, 1198–1199, *1199*
Osteoporosis, 1189–1198
aging and, 1191–1192
bone pathology in, 1191
calcitonin for, 1098
in chronic alcoholism, 1194
in chronic hypophosphatemia, 1194
classification of, 1191, 1192t
clinical presentation of, 1189–1191
in Cushing's syndrome, 482, 1193–1194
diabetes mellitus and, 1194
in endocrine disorders, 24–25
established, treatment of, 1196–1198
estrogen deficiency and, 1192–1193
genetic disorders and, 1194
genetic polymorphisms and, 1191
in iatrogenic Cushing's syndrome, *613*, 613–614, *614*
in idiopathic hypercalciuria, 1194
immobilization and, 1194
immunosuppressive therapy and, 1194–1195
intestinal disease and, 1195
juvenile, 1194
laboratory findings in, 1190–1191
obesity and, 965
pathogenesis of, 1191–1195

Osteoporosis *(continued)*
postmenopausal, 768
prevention of, hormone replacement therapy in, 770
prevention of, 1195t, 1195–1196
in breast cancer survivors, 1442
primary hyperparathyroidism and, 1194
radiologic features of, 1190, *1190*
symptoms and signs of, 1189–1190
testosterone deficiency and, 1193
thyroid replacement and, 1456
thyrotoxicosis and, 1194
weightlessness and, 1194
Osteoporosis circumscripta, 1204, *1204*
Osteosclerosis:
myeloma and, 1133
in renal osteodystrophy, 1200
Osteosclerosis fragilis generalisata, 1198–1199
Ovarian growth factors, 739
Ovarian hyperstimulation syndrome (OHSS), 760
Ovarian sex steroids, adrenal sex steroids versus, 414
Ovary(ies), 707–778
activity of, physiologic correlates of, with aging, 736–739
anatomy of, 707–709
blood vessels of, 707, *708*
cytodifferentiation of, 723–731
differentiation of, 785–786
disorders of
in middle age, 766–771
in teenagers, 745–750
in young adults, 750–766
failure of
occult, 751
premature, 750–751
follicles of, 709, *709*
formation of, defective, 799
functional defects in, in polycystic ovary syndrome, 756
histology of, 709–720
hormones of, biogenesis of, 720–723
innervation of, 707–709
interstitial cells of, 715–718, *716, 717, 718, 719*
morphology of, 707, *708*
physiology of, 707–739
polycystic, 754–757
hyperprolactinemia from, 752
obesity and, 964
Overtraining, 1488, 1498–1499
Overweight; *See also* Obesity
definition of, 953
Ovulation, *734,* 734–735, *735*
dysfunctional, diagnosis of, 759–763
induction of
agents in, 759t
anti-estrogen, 760
gonadotropins in, *760,* 760–761, *761,* 761t
pulsatile gonadotropin releasing hormone in, 761–763
stimulation of, in gonadotropin deficiency, 207
Oxalate:
complexation of, by cysteine, treatment of, 1254
foods rich in, 1247t
metabolism of, *1247,* 1247–1248
Oxidases, mixed-function, 721
Oxytocin:
amino acid sequence of, *218*
biologic actions of, 225–226
biosynthesis of, 217–218
chemistry of, 217
clearance of, 224
distribution of, 224
release of, 217–218
secretion of, 223

Paget's disease of bone, 1203–1210
bone pathology in, 1205–1206
calcitonin for, 1098
clinical presentation of, 1204–1205
drug treatment of, 1207–1210
laboratory findings in, 1205
pathogenesis of, 1206–1207
radiologic features of, *1204,* 1204–1205, *1205*
surgery for, 1210
symptoms and signs of, 1204
therapy of, biochemical and radiological monitoring of, 1210
Pain, abdominal, in endocrine disorders, 22
Palmitic acid, 1044
Pamidronate disodium (Aredia):
for fibrous dysplasia, 1203
for hypercalcemia of malignancy, 1130
for myeloma bone disease, 1134
for osteolytic lesions due to malignancy, 1135
for Paget's disease of bone, 1208t, 1208–1209, *1209*
Pancreas:
cholecystokinin effects on, 1325t, 1325–1326
endocrine, 828–842
anatomy of, 828
development of, 828–830
gene knockout experiments and, 830t
hormones of, 830–842; *See also* Pancreatic hormones
islet-cell types in, 828, 828t
galanin actions on, 1333
gastric inhibitory polypeptide effects on, 1329t
motilin effects on, 1330t
neurotensin actions on, 1332t
pharmacologic actions of VIP on, 1328t
secretin effects on, 1326t
somatostatin effects on, 1320t
transplantation of, for Type 1 diabetes, 872–873, *873*
islet transplantation versus, 874t, 874–875
tumors of, in MEN 1 syndrome, 1358
Pancreatic cholera syndrome, secretory diarrhea in, octreotide acetate for, 1323t
Pancreatic hormones:
glucagon as, 838–841; *See also* Glucagon
insulin as, 830–838; *See also* Insulin
islet amyloid polypeptide as, 841–842
pancreatic polypeptide as, 841
somatostatin as, 841
Pancreatic polypeptide, 841
Pancreatic polypeptides, 1330–1331
Pancreatitis:
hypocalcemia in, 1150
postsurgical prevention of, somatostatin in, 1322
Papaverine:
for erectile dysfunction, 661
injections of, for impotence in older men, 1470
Papillary carcinoma, of thyroid, 368–370, *369*
recurrence and survival in, influence of initial treatment on, 373t
Papilledema, in endocrine disorders, 27
Paracrine mechanisms, of peptide growth factors, 1266
Paracrine regulation, 4
of testis function, 646
Paramesonephric ducts, persistent, 800–801
Paramethasone, structure of, *611*
Paraneoplastic erythrocytosis, 1413–1414
Paraneoplastic syndromes, 1383
frequency of, 1388t
spectrum of, 1384t
Parathyroid glands:
adenomas of, hyperparathyroidism from, 1113–1114
anatomy of, 1081
embryology of, 1081
in hypothyroidism, 325
surgery of, for primary hyperparathyroidism, 1122–1123
in thyrotoxicosis, 301
Parathyroid hormone (PTH), 1081–1093
actions of, on bone, 1090–1093
assay of, 1086–1088, *1087, 1088*
biological effects of, 1088–1093
biosynthesis of, 1082–1084, *1083*
regulation of, 1084
chemistry of, *1082,* 1082–1083
circulating fragments of, origins of, 1086, *1086*
clearance of, from plasma, 1086
effects of, on kidney, 1090
elevated, in obesity, 965
hypercalcemia of malignancy and, 1129, 1396
mechanism of action of, 1088–1093
metabolism of, 1086, *1086*
pathophysiology of, 1114–1115, *1115*
processing of, 1083–1084
receptors for, 1088–1090
molecular defects in, disorders resulting from, 1093
secretagogues of, 1085–1086
secretion of
cellular regulation of, by calcium, 1084–1085, *1085*
physiology of, 1081–1082
serum concentration of, serum calcium levels and, *1082*
structure of, *1082*
in vitamin D activation, 1101
Parathyroid hormone-related protein (PTHrP):
in breast cancer-mediated osteolysis, 1133
effects of, modulation of, by tumor-associated factors, 1128
in hypercalcemia
associated with breast cancer, 1128
associated with hematologic malignancies, 1128
in malignancy-associated hypercalcemia, 1125–1127
osteoclastic bone resorption in metastatic bone cancer and, 1131–1132

Parathyroid storm, medical management of, 1124–1125
Parathyroidectomy, in multiple endocrine neoplasia type 1, 1362
Paresthesias:
in distal sensorimotor neuropathy, 905
in hypothyroidism, 322
P450aro, in steroidogenesis, 402
Pars nervosa, 217
Particle assays, 99
P45011AS, disorders of, 459–460
P450c11β:
deficiency of, 459
in congenital adrenal hyperplasia, 448t
in steroidogenesis, 401
P450c17:
deficiency of, 458–459
in congenital adrenal hyperplasia, 448t
in steroidogenesis, 398–400
P450c21:
deficiency of, in congenital adrenal hyperplasia, 448t
in steroidogenesis, 400–401
P450c11AS:
deficiency of, in congenital adrenal hyperplasia, 448t
in steroidogenesis, 401
Pendred's syndrome, 319
Penicillamine:
as cysteine-complexing agent, 1228–1229
for cystinuria, 1230–1231
Penis:
abnormalities of, erectile dysfunction from, 660
prosthesis for, for impotence in older men, 1470
Pentagastrin, clinical applications of, 1324–1325
Peptic ulcer, glucocorticoid therapy and, 623–624
Peptide(s), 5, 29–37
atrial natriuretic
hypertension and, 572–573
neurologic effects of, 140
biosynthesis of, 31–35
calcitonin gene-related, hypertension and, 570
commercial assays of, 95t
endogenous opioid, neurologic effects of, 138–140
gastrointestinal, 1317–1340; *See also* Gastrointestinal peptide hormones
growth hormone releasing, 133
hexahistidine tagged, 97
in medullary thyroid carcinoma, 1367
metabolism of, 36–37
multiple antigenic, 96–97
as neurotransmitters, 111
plasma, assays of, 439
in prolactin release, 134–135
propiomelanocortin-derived, 1400, *1401*
receptors for, *62,* 62–63
secretion of, 35
transport of, 35
tumor, in syndrome of inappropriate antidiuresis, 1404–1405
vasoactive intestinal
neurologic effects of, 138
production of, by tumors, 1415
Peptide YY, 1330
biologic effects of, 1331t
Perchlorate, for thyrotoxicosis, 307
Perimenopause, 766
Perineoscrotal hypospadias, pseudovaginal, 805
Periorbital edema, in endocrine disorders, 26
Peripheral vascular disease, erectile dysfunction from, 660
Peroxisome proliferator activated receptor gamma, insulin resistance and, 575
Peutz-Jeghers syndrome, breast cancer risk and, 1431t
Pharmacologic effects, on vasopressin secretion, 223
Pharmacotherapy:
for corticotroph adenoma, 200
for somatotroph adenoma, 193–194, *194*
Phase-modulation fluorescence spectroscopy, 100
Phenothiazines, hyperprolactinemia related to, 752
Phenoxybenzamine hydrochloride (Dibenzyline), for pheochromocytoma, 539
Phentermine, in obesity management, 985
Phentolamine, for erectile dysfunction, 661
Phenytoin, thyroid function and, 289
Pheochromocytoma(s), 536–540
clinical manifestations of, 536–537, 591–592, 592t
diagnosis of, 537–539
distribution of, 536
hypercalcemia in, 1137
hypertension in, 591–593, *592, 593*
malignant, 539
in MEN 2 syndrome, 1363
management of, 1368–1369, *1370*
in MEN 2B syndrome, treatment of, 1373
origin of, 536
screening for, 539
treatment of, 539–540
Phosphatase signaling, localization of, 77
Phosphatases:
phosphoprotein, 76–77
protein tyrosine, 82
serine/threonine, 76–77
Phosphate:
absorption of, decreased, hypophosphatemia from, 1155
extracellular, 1152
homeostasis of, 1152–1154
for hypophosphatemic rickets, 1189
intestinal absorption of, 1107, 1152–1153
intracellular, 1152
metabolism of, disorders of, 1152–1157
neutral, for absorptive hypercalciuria, 1253
parathyroid hormone secretion and, 1086
preparations of, 1157t
renal handling of, 1153–1154
sodium cellulose, for absorptive hypercalciuria, 1253
Phosphate leak hypothesis, of absorptive hypercalciuria, 1246
Phosphatidylinositol 3 (PI-3) kinase, metabolic effects of insulin and, 836–837
Phosphodiesterase (PDE), in cellular signaling, 71–72
Phospholipase A2:
metabolism of, *70*
responsiveness of, to G proteins, 68
Phospholipase C:
activation of, *70*
responsiveness of, to G proteins, 68–69
Phospholipase D, responsiveness of, to G proteins, 69–70
Phospholipid transfer protein, in lipoprotein metabolism, 1000
Phospholipids, synthesis and catabolism of, 998
Phosphoprotein phosphatases, 76–77
Phosphorus:
elemental, for hypophosphatemia, 1156
in vitamin D activation, 1101–1102
Phosphorylation, nuclear receptor activity modification by, 59–60
Photocoagulation, laser, for diabetic retinopathy, *899,* 899–900, *900*
Physical activity; *See* Exercise and training
Physical activity counseling, guidelines for, 977t
Pineal gland, 141–143
anatomy of, 141–142
biological rhythms and, 143
hormones of, 142–143
neural innervation of, *141*
neurotransmitters from, 142–143
region of, tumors in, 158
Pinealocyte, 142
Pinealoma, 158
Pioglitazone, for Type 2 diabetes, *881,* 883
Pituitary adenomas, 147, *180,* 180–181
of Cushing's disease, 476–477, *477*
hormonal hypersecretion from, 188–204
radiation therapy for, 187–188
Pituitary diabetes insipidus, 228–232
management of, 235–238
Pituitary function tests in growth hormone deficiency diagnosis, 1294
Pituitary gland:
anatomy of, 118–119, 173–175
anterior
cells of, differentiation of, 174–175
diseases of, 173–208, 180–208
causes of, 180–183
clinical presentation of, 183–184
hormonal hypersecretion in, 188–204
hormonal hyposecretion in, 204–208
hormones of, physiology of, 175–177
mass lesions causing, 180–182
mass lesions of
evaluation and treatment of, 184–188
radiation therapy for, 187–188
treatment of, 184–188
origin of, 174
somatostatin effects on, 1320, 1320t
development of
earliest, 175
transcription factors and, temporal relationship between, 1292t
embryology of, 174–175, *175*
enlargement of
causes of, 180t
physiologic, 181
in feedback regulation of gonadotropin secretion, 652

Pituitary gland *(continued)*
function of
defects in, in polycystic ovary syndrome, 756
hypothalamic disease and, 149–153
in hypothyroidism, 324
in glucocorticoid regulation, 405–410
in hormone regulation, 112–113
infarction of, growth hormone deficiency from, 1293
macroadenomas of, transsphenoidal surgery for, efficacy of, 186t
in neuroendocrine organization, *112*
pharmacologic actions of VIP on, 1328t
posterior, 217–247
anatomy of, 217
chemistry of, 217
hormones of; *See* Oxytocin; Vasopressin
pathology of, 228–247
thirst deficiency as, 240–242
vasopressin deficiencies as, 228–240; *See also* Vasopressin, deficiencies of
vasopressin excess as, 242–247; *See also* Vasopressin, excess of
tumors of, in MEN 1 syndrome, 1358
management of, 1362–1363
Pituitary gonadotropins, in fetal gonadal function control, 789–791, *790*
Pituitary hormones:
abnormalities of, signs and symptoms of, 184
anterior, physiology of, 175–177
congenital deficiencies of, 183
feedback loops for, components of, 114t
hypersecretion of, 188–204
posterior; *See* Oxytocin; Vasopressin
secretion of
neurotransmitter regulation of, 137t
in thyrotoxicosis, 301
Pituitary hypothyroidism, 320–321
Pituitary incidentaloma, 184
Pituitary-adrenal reserve, tests of, 441–443
Placental disorders, fetal growth and, 1287
Placental lactogen, human, ectopic production of, 1412–1413
Placental proteins, ectopic production of, 1412–1413
Plant sterols:
lipid metabolism and, 1047
storage diseases involving, 1041–1042
Plasma:
binding of steroids to, physiologic role of, 417–418
testosterone transport in, 646–647
Plasma renin activity:
in hypertension evaluation, 580–581
peripheral, in renovascular hypertension diagnosis, 584
Plasminogen, in ovulation, 735
Pleurihormonal cells, 174
Plicamycin (mitramycin):
for hypercalcemia of malignancy, 1125, 1130
for Paget's disease of bone, 1209
Pneumocystic carinii infections, thyroid function and, 287
Point mutations:
causing congenital adrenal hyperplasia, 454, 454t
Point mutations *(continued)*
known, effects of, on 21-hydroxylase activity, 454–455
Polycystic ovary syndrome (PCOS), 754–757
androgen secretion abnormality in, 756
clinical features of, 755, 755t
hyperprolactinemia from, 752
hypothalamic-pituitary function defects in, 756–757
insulin resistance in, 756–757
management of, 757
obesity and, 964
pathophysiology of, *755,* 755–756
Polydipsia, primary:
causes of, 232t
diabetes insipidus from, 232
management of, 238–239
Polyglandular autoimmune disease, 671
Polyglandular autoimmune (PGA) syndromes, 1373–1376
clinical manifestations of, 1373–1375
diagnosis of, 1375–1376
disease associations in, 1373t
genetics of, 1375
hypoparathyroidism associated with, 1141
pathogenesis of, 1375
treatment of, 1375–1376
Polyglandular deficiency syndromes, nonautoimmune, 1376
Polyglandular endocrine insufficiency syndromes, 1373–1376
Polyglandular failure syndromes, 463, 463t
Polyneuropathy, diabetic, 25
Polyostotic fibrous dysplasia, 149
Polypeptide(s):
gastric inhibitory, 1328–1329
islet amyloid, 841–842
pancreatic, 841, 1330–1331
vasoactive intestinal, 1327–1328
Polyunsaturated fatty acids, 1044, 1045
POMC peptides, in mineralocorticoid regulation, 413
Postmenopausal bleeding, 771
Postpartum thyroiditis, 294–295, *295*
transient hypothyroidism in, 317–318
Postpartum thyrotoxicosis, 311
Postural hypotension:
in generalized autonomic failure, 540–543
mechanisms of, 541t, 541–542
treatment of, 542–543
Potassium channels, G protein-activated, 70
Potassium ion in mineralocorticoid regulation, 412–413
Potency, in older males, 1469–1471
Ppomas:
in MEN 1 syndrome, 1358
octreotide acetate efficacy on, 1324t
Prader-Willi syndrome, 154, 155t
Prader-Willi-Labhart syndrome, hypogonadotropic hypogonadism in, 681t
Pravastatin (Pravachol):
for hyperlipoproteinemia, 1054t
mechanism of action of, 1056–1057
indications for, 1057–1058
side effects of, 1057
structure of, *1057*
"Prayer sign" in diabetes, 912, *912*
Prazosin hydrochloride (Minipress), for pheochromocytoma, 539
Precocious pseudopuberty, 689, 1305
Precocious puberty, 152, 688–689
in endocrine disorders, 24
Precocious sexual maturation:
adult short stature from, 1297
classification of, 1305t
growth excess from, 1304–1306
Prednisolone, structure of, *611*
Prednisone:
for congenital adrenal hyperplasia, 457t
structure of, *611*
Pregnancy:
aldosterone changes during, 491–492
diabetes in, 856
diabetes insipidus in, 234
GH-V gene in, 1273–1274
glucocorticoid therapy in, 623
goiter during, 354
hypertension associated with, obesity and, 966
hypertriglyceridemia in, 1029
in hypothyroidism, 325
lactotroph adenoma and, 198
low-fat, high-complex-carbohydrate diet in, 1052–1053
thyroid hormone concentrations in, 280, *280*
thyrotoxicosis in, 297, 310–311
Pregnenolone:
conversion of cholesterol to, 395–398
levels of, in aging, 1463
as steroid hormone precursor, 722
steroid hormones derived from, 390
structure of, *390*
Premature ovarian failure, 750–751
Premature thelarche, benign, 791
Premenstrual syndrome, 766
Prepo-opiomelanocortin, structure of, *406*
Primordial follicle, *709,* 709–710, *710, 711*
Primordial germ cells, 728
Probucol (Loerlco):
in familial hypercholesterolemia management, 1020
for hyperlipoproteinemia, 1059
Progestagens, hypogonadism from, 682
Progesterone:
alveolar development and, 1428
breast development and, 1428
cyclic, for premature ovarian failure, 751
in gonadotropin releasing hormone regulation, 126
plasma concentrations of, 415t
secretion rate of, 415t
Progesterone receptor antagonists, 772
Progestins:
for endometrial cancer, 1444
hypertension and, 569
Progestogens:
for menarcheal menorrhagia, 749
new, 772
Prolactin inhibiting factor, 133–134
Prolactin (PRL):
actions of, 177
aging and, 1461
concentration of, evaluation of, in children, 1310

Prolactin (PRL) *(continued)*
deficiency of, 208
disorders of, hypothalamic disease and, 152–153
levels of, exercise and, 1492–1493
production of, by tumors, 1414–1415
regulation of, 114–115
secretion of, 177
diurnal variation in, 145
synthesis of, 177
Prolactin releasing factor, 134–135
Prolactinoma:
hyperprolactinemia from, 752
in MEN 1 syndrome, management of, 1362
Pro-opiomelanocortin (POMC)/adrenocorticotropin (ACTH) syndrome, ectopic, 1400–1404
Proopiomelanocortin products:
actions of, 177
secretion of, 177
synthesis of, 177, *178*
Prophylthiouracil, for thyrotoxicosis, 304–306
Propranolol, for thyrotoxicosis, 307
Proptosis, in Graves' disease, 312, *313*
Propylthiouracil:
thyroid function and, 288
for thyrotroph adenoma, 203–204
Prorenin, 558–559
Prostaglandin E1 (Alprostadil):
for erectile dysfunction, 661
injections of, for impotence in older men, 1470
Prostaglandins:
E series, hypercalcemia and, 1129
endometrial, *764,* 764–765
hypercalcemia of malignancy and, 1397
in medullary thyroid carcinoma, 1367
Prostate cancer, 1444–1447
age and, *1433,* 1434
androgen receptor mutations in, 1437, 1438t
chemoprevention of, 1447
diagnosis of, 1445
genetic factors in, 1431
hormonal therapies for, *686*
pathology of, 1445–1446
prognosis of, *1445,* 1445–1446
progression of, mechanisms of, 1436–1439
risk factors for, 1445
staging of, 1445–1446, 1446t
treatment of, 1446–1447
Prostate specific antigen (PSA), 1445
Prostatectomy, radical, for prostate cancer, 1446
Protein(s):
animal, dietary, restriction of, for nephrolithiasis, 1226, 1227t
binding, in immunoassays, 95–96
calcium binding, 74–75
chaperone, 60
cortisol-binding, 416–417
G; *See* G proteins
in insulin secretion regulation, 834
insulin-like growth factor binding, 1270–1272
lipid/lipoprotein metabolism and, 1048
membrane, transport of, subcellular, 34, *35*
metabolism of, glucocorticoid actions on, 426–429

Protein(s) *(continued)*
nuclear receptor, structural organization of, 57–59, *58, 59*
parathyroid hormone-related; *See also* Parathyroid hormone-related protein (PTHrP)
hypercalcemia of malignancy and, 1396–1397
phosphorylation of, regulation of, *72*
placental, ectopic production of, 1412–1413
RGS, 66
secretory
synthesis of, 31, *32*
transport of, subcellular, 34, *35*
serum, disorders of, hypercalcemia and, 1139
serum thyroid hormone-binding, 271–272
steroidogenic acute regulatory, deficiency of
in congenital adrenal hyperplasia, 448t
in testosterone biosynthesis errors, 801
synthesis of, thyroid hormone effects on, 274
transfer, active in lipoprotein metabolism, 1000
transport, 3
Protein hormones, receptors for, 63
Protein kinase A, in insulin secretion, 833
Protein kinase C, 75–76
in insulin secretion, 833
Protein kinases:
calcium/calmodulin dependent, 75, *76*
cAMP interplay with, 77
classification of, 73t
cyclic GMP dependent, 73
second messenger-activated, 72–73
subcellular localization of, 73
Protein tyrosine phosphatase, 82
P450scc:
in conversion of cholesterol to pregnenolone, 395–398
transport of electrons to, 397–398
Pseudofractures, in osteomalacia, 1183, *1183*
Pseudohermaphroditism, 651
dysgenetic male, 800
female, 807–816; *See also* Virilization of genetic female
male, 801–807; *See also* Virilization, genital, defective
Pseudohyperparathyroidism, 1395
Pseudohypoaldosteronism, 475
Pseudohypoparathyroidism, 1143–1147
biochemical features of, 1144–1145
clinical features of, 1144–1145
diagnosis of, 1147
pathogenesis of, 1145–1147
phenotypic abnormalities in, *1143*
symptoms and signs in, 1144t
type IA, 1145–1146
type IB, 1146–1147
type II, 1147
Pseudotumor cerebri, 158–159
Pseudovaginal perineoscrotal hypospadias, 805
Psychiatric disease, thyroid function and, 287–288
Psychiatry, in glucocorticoid therapy, 623
Psychogenic erection, 652–653
Psychological disturbances, in Cushing's syndrome, 481–482
Psychological factors, in obesity, 968

Psychological symptoms:
of anabolic steroids, 1502
of hypothyroidism, 322
in menopause, 767
Psychosexual differentiation, gender role and, 791–792
Psychosocial dwarfism, 1294
Pubertal macromastia, persistent, 665
Puberty:
constitutional delayed, 678
delayed
clinical approach to, 817, *818,* 819
in women, exercise and, 1496
disorders of, 745–748
events in, chronologic age ranges for, 1283t
genital changes during, *650*
growth spurt in, 1277–1279
idiopathic delayed, 748
precocious, 152, 688–689
classification of, 689t
in endocrine disorders, 24
growth excess from, 1304–1306
true, 688–689
pseudo, precocious, 689
stages of, *746*
Pulmonary system, in hypothyroidism, 322–323
Purine, stones related to, uric acid stones differentiated from, 1233
Purine metabolism, uric acid excretion and, 1232, *1232*
Pyelography, intravenous, in renovascular hypertension diagnosis, 584
Pyridoxine:
growth hormone response to exercise and, 1488
hyperoxaluria and, 1248

Quality control, of hormone assays, 103–104
Quantitative computerized tomography (QCT), in bone metabolic disease evaluation, 1180–1181

Radiation, ionizing:
androgen deficiency and, 672–673
sperm production impairment by, 675–676
Radiation therapy:
for corticotroph adenoma, 200
cranial, for Cushing's disease, 1296
for Cushing's syndrome, 489
for endometrial cancer, 1444
external neck
hypoparathyroidism after, 1142
hypothyroidism after, 318
head and neck, growth hormone deficiency from, 1293
for lactotroph adenoma, 197–198
for pituitary adenoma, pituitary disorders from, 182
for somatotroph adenoma, 193, *193*
for thyrotroph adenoma, 203
Radioactive iodine, for thyrotoxicosis, 307–308
from thyroid adenoma, 308
Radioactive tracers, for immunoassays, 97–98
Radioassay, competitive protein-binding, in plasma cortisol determinations, 438

Radiographic contrast agents, iodinated, thyroid function and, 289
Radioimmunoassay:
of β-lipoproein, 439
of plasma ACTH, 439
in plasma cortisol determinations, 438
Radioiodine therapy:
for follicular carcinoma of thyroid, 375–376
for Graves' thyrotoxicosis, 303, 304, 304t
for hypothyroidism, thyroiditis from, 330
for nontoxic goiter, 358
for thyrotoxicosis, 307–308
hypothyroidism after, 318
Radioiodine uptake, thyroid, in thyrotoxicosis diagnosis, 302
Radioisotopic scan, of thyroid in thyroid nodule evaluation, 362–364
Radioligand binding, 50
Radiology:
in anterior pituitary lesion evaluation, 184
in bone metabolic disease evaluation, 1180–1181
in osteomalacia, 1182–1183, *1183*
in osteoporosis evaluation, 1190
in Paget's disease of bone evaluation, *1204,* 1204–1205, *1205*
in renal osteodystrophy evaluation, 1199–1200
in rickets, 1182–1183, *1183*
in short stature evaluation, 1285
Radionuclide tests, thyroid, 279
radiation exposure from, 279t
Raloxifene:
in breast cancer prevention, 1442
in osteoporosis prevention, 1195
Ramus ovaricus artery, 707
Rathke's pouch, 174
Receptor(s), 49–53
for acetylcholine, 62
adrenergic, 529t, 529–530
affinity of, modulation of, by G protein, 53
analysis of, methods of, 50
androgen, mutations of, in prostate cancer, 1437, 1438t
binding of, kinetics of, 51–53
for biogenic amines, 62, *62*
calcitonin, alignment of, vs. PTH/PTHrP receptor, *1095*
for calcium, 63
coupling of, to G protein, 66–67
cytoplasmic glucocorticoid, relative affinities of steroids for, 417t
estrogen
activation of, 1436, *1437*
exon deletions of, phenotypes corresponding to, 1437t
G protein-coupled
changes in confirmation of, upon agonist activation, 63–64
classes of, *62*
"classic," model of, *61*
desensitization of, 64, *65*
ligand binding by, 63
mutated, *63*
sensitivity of, regulation of, 64
signaling through, 60–71
structure of, 61–63
Receptor(s) *(continued)*
GABA, 79
for GABA, 63
glutamate, 79
for glutamate, 63
glycine, 80
for glycoprotein hormones, 63
hormone
definition of, 3
origin of, 9
5HT3 serotonin, 80
insulin, structure of, *836*
insulin-like growth factor, 1270, *1270*
ion channel, 78–80
lipoprotein, *1004,* 1004–1006, *1005*
nicotinic acetylcholine, 78
nuclear
DNA binding of, 57–58
for triiodothyronine, 272–273
nuclear hormone, ligands for, structure of, 55t
orphan, 56
parathyroid hormone, 1088–1090, *1089*
molecular defects in, disorders resulting from, 1033
for peptide hormones, *62,* 62–63
for protein hormones, 63
quantitation of, 51, *51*
radioligand binding and, 50
for retinoic acid, 56
with serine kinase activity, 80–81
spare, 52, *53*
steroid hormone, mechanism of action of, 53, 55, *55*
thrombin, 63
for thyroid hormones, 55
with treonine kinase activity, 80–81
with tyrosine kinase activity, 80–82
Receptor assays, 100
Recruitment, in follicular development, 731–732
5α-Reductase:
deficiency of, 805
androgen resistance in, 677–678
in steroidogenesis, 402
Reflexes, in endocrine disorders, 26
Reflexogenic erection, 652
Regulatory ligands, of endocrine system:
actions of, receptors and mediators of, 9
origin of, 8–9
Reifenstein syndrome, 806
Renal angiography in renovascular hypertension diagnosis, 585–586
Renal arteriography in renovascular hypertension diagnosis, 585
Renal hypercalciuria, 1244–1245
treatment of, 1253
Renal osteodystrophy, 1199–1201
Renal scintigraphy, in renovascular hypertension diagnosis, 584–585
Renal tubular acidosis, calcium phosphate stones and, 1235–1236
Renin, 558–560
ectopic production of, 1415
in plasma, activity of, in hypertension evaluation, 580–581
plasma activity of, peripheral, in renovascular hypertension diagnosis, 584
Renin *(continued)*
renal, regulation of, 559–560
sources of, 559
substrate for, 561
tumors secreting
hypertension and, 564
management of, 588
Renin-angiotensin system:
in blood pressure, 564–566
in blood pressure regulation, 557–566
components of, 558–564
in mineralocorticoid regulation, 411–412
neurologic effects of, 138
vasopressin secretion and, 222
Renovascular hypertension, 581–588
causes of, 581–582, 582t
clinical features of, 583
diagnostic studies for, 583–586
evaluation for, 583
management of, 586–588
prevalence of, 581
screening for, 583–586
signs and symptoms of, 583t
Repaglinide, for Type 2 diabetes, 880–881, *881*
Reproductive system:
dysfunction of, exercise-induced, endogenous opiates and, 1492
endocrine, perinatal adaptations of, 791
glucocorticoids and, 433
hormone actions on, 12
side effects of anabolic steroids involving, 1502–1503
in women, exercise and, 1496–1498
Respiratory alkalosis, hypophosphatemia from, 1155–1156
Respiratory function, in thyrotoxicosis, 300
Respiratory system, pharmacologic actions of VIP on, 1328t
RET proto-oncogene mutations:
in apparent sporadic medullary thyroid carcinoma, identification of, 1368
in hereditary medullary thyroid carcinoma, 1364, *1364*
Retinal changes, in endocrine disorders, 27
Retinoic acid:
mechanism of action of, 55
receptors for, 56
Retinoids, hormone binding domains for, 58–59
Retinopathy:
diabetic, 896–900
clinical characteristics of, 896–898, *897*
epidemiology of, 898, *898*
incidence of, 898, *898*
pathogenesis of, 898–899
prevalence of, 898
proliferative, high risk characteristics for, 898t
risk factors for, 898–899
risk of, glycemia and, *857*
screening for, 899
therapy for, *899,* 899–900, *900*
evaluation of, in Diabetes Control and Complications Trial, 862, *863*
Retractile testes, 673
Revascularization, surgical, for renovascular hypertension, 586–588
RGS proteins, 66
Rhabdomyolysis, hyperphosphatemia with, 1157

Rheumatoid factors, in immunoassays, 103
Rhinorrhea, cerebrospinal fluid, in anterior pituitary disease, 184
Rhodopsin, as G protein-coupled receptor, 61–62
Rhythms:
biological, pineal gland and, 143
CNS, neuroendocrine function and, 143–145
Ribonucleic acid (RNA), messenger, biosynthesis of, 29–31
Rickets, 1182–1189
bone pathology in, 1184
calcium deficiency and, 1187
classification of, 1184, 1185t
clinical presentation of, 1182–1184
hypophosphatemic, 1186–1187
laboratory findings in, 1183–1184
pathogenesis of, 1184
radiologic features of, 1182–1183, *1183*
symptoms and signs of, 1182, *1182*
treatment of, 1188–1189
vitamin D deficiency in, 1184–1185
vitamin D malabsorption and, 1185
vitamin D metabolism abnormalities and, 1185–1186
vitamin D-dependent, 1186
vitamin D-resistant, 1186
Rifampin, thyroid function and, 289
Risedronate sodium (Actonel):
in osteoporosis prevention, 1196
for Paget's disease of bone, 1208t, 1209, *1209*
Rosiglitazone, for Type 2 diabetes, *881*, 883
Rothmund-Thompson syndrome, hypogonadotropic hypogonadism in, 681t
RUD syndrome, hypogonadotropic hypogonadism in, 681t
Ruffled border, 1092

Salivary cortisol measurement, 438
Salt wasting, in 21-hydroxylase deficiency, 808, 808t
pathogenesis of, *809*
Sandostatin, for carcinoid syndrome, 1340
"Sandwich" assay methodology, 93–94
Saponins, lipid metabolism and, 1047
Sarcoidosis:
hypercalcemia in, 1136
hypothalamic involvement in, 148
pituitary disorders from, 182
Sarcoma, Kaposi's, glucocorticoid therapy and, 624
Satiety, mediators of, 973–974
Saturated fatty acids, 1043
Scatchard analysis, of receptor binding, 52, *52*
Schmidt's syndrome, 463
Schmorl's node in osteoporosis, 1190
Scintigraphy, renal, in renovascular hypertension diagnosis, 584–585
Second messenger systems, in cellular signaling, 71–78
protein kinases in, 72–73
Second messengers, in hormone action, 7
Secretin, 1326–1327
Secretory proteins:
synthesis of, 31, *32*
transport of, subcellular, 34, *35*
Sella turcica:
empty, 183
mass lesions of, surgery for, 184–187; *See also* Transsphenoidal surgery
Seminal fluid, analysis of, 658
normal values for, 659t
Seminiferous cords, 641
Seminiferous tubule, *637*, 637–638
Serine kinase activity, receptors with, 80–81
Serine/threonine phosphatases, 76–77
Serotonin:
anatomic pathways of, 135–136
circadian rhythms and, 136
in medullary thyroid carcinoma, 1367
Serotonin receptor, 5HT3, 80
Sertoli cell-only syndrome, 675
Sertoli cells:
function of, follicle stimulating hormone regulation of, 645–646
tumors of, 680
Set point theory, of obesity, 971–972
Sex:
Cushing's syndrome distribution by, 476
determination of
normal, 779–792
primary, errors of, 792–800
fetal growth and, 1280
genetic, 779–783
gonadal, 783–786
hormonal, 787–792
sporadic goiter and, 354
thyroid cancer and, 360
thyroid function and, 281
Sex chromosomes:
anomalies of
associated with bisexual gonadal development, 795
associated with dysgenetic gonads, 795–799
associated with functional testes and male phenotype, 792–795
associated with ovaries and female phenotype, 795
properties and function of, 780–783
Sex cords, 641
Sex steroids:
actions of, on genitalia, 788–789
adrenal versus ovarian, 414
in aging, 1463–1465
concentration of, in infants and children, 446t
disorders of, hypogonadism from, 682
exogenous, defective virilization due to, 806–807
in fetal circulation, 787–788
secretion of, in polycystic ovary syndrome, 756
Sexual differentiation, 779–819
disorders of, 792–819
classification of, 793t
clinical approach to, 816–819, *817, 818*
clinical features suggestive of, 792t
primary sex determination errors as, 792–800
errors of, 800–816
normal sex determination and, 779–792
Sexual dimorphism, parameters of, 780t
Sexual glands, accessory, dysfunction of, infertility from, 663
Sexual maturation, precocious:
adult short stature from, 1297
growth excess from, 1304–1306
Sexual response, male, physiology of, 652–654
Sexuality, aging and, 1468–1471
in females, 1471
in males, 1469–1471
Short stature, 1282–1302
adult, from precocious sexual maturation, 1297
from anoxemia, 1302
causes of, 1285–1302
in chondrodysplasias, 1297–1298, *1299*
clinical approach to, 1282–1285
history in, 1283
laboratory studies in, 1285
physical examination in, 1283–1285
radiographic studies in, 1285
constitutional, 1286–1287
in Cushing's syndrome, 1296–1297
differential diagnosis of, 1284t
endocrine causes of, 1288–1297
familial, 1286
genetic, 1286
growth hormone deficiency causing, 1289–1296
hypothyroidism and, 1288–1289
normal, causes of, 1286–1287
pathologic, 1287–1302
in Turner's syndrome, 1298, 1300–1302
Sibutramine, in obesity management, 985
Sickle cell disease, androgen deficiency in, 673
Signal recognition particle receptor, 31
Signal transduction:
biology of, 49–84
G protein-mediated, 60–71
Sildenafil (Viagra):
for erectile dysfunction, 661–662
for impotence in older men, 1470
Silosterolemia, 1041–1042
Simvastatin (Zocor):
dosage of, 1057, 1058t
for familial defective apolipoprotein B-100, 1022
for hyperlipoproteinemia, 1054t, 1056–1057
indications for, 1057–1058
side effects of, 1057
structure of, *1057*
Sipple's syndrome, 372, 1364
Sitostanol, lipid metabolism and, 1047
Sitosterol, lipid metabolism and, 1047
Sitosterolemia, 1040–1042
Situs inversus, 636
in immotile cilia syndrome, 675
in varicocele, 674
Skeletal disorders, in obesity, 965
Skeletal dysplasias, short stature from, 1297–1298
Skeletal growth, physiology of, 1279–1280
Skin:
in acromegaly, 190
in Cushing's syndrome, 481, *481*
in endocrine disorders, 20–21
hyperpigmentation of, in Addison's disease, 466, *467*
in hypothyroidism, 321–322
in menopause, 768

Skin *(continued)*
in thyrotoxicosis, 298
vitamin D actions in, 1108
Skin fold measurements, in fatness assessment, 953
Sleep apnea, in acromegaly, 190
Sleep apnea syndrome, obesity and, 965
Sleep-wake cycle, 144, *144*
Smith-Lemli-Opitz syndrome, 807, 1037
Smoking:
body weight and, mortality and, 956–958, *957*
menopause and, 766
thyroid function and, 281
Sodium:
excess of, abnormal distribution of, in hyperaldosteronism, 492
intake of, reduced, in nephrolithiasis management, 1226–1227
loss of, extrarenal, in hyperaldosteronism, 491
renal handling of, insulin resistance and, 577
restriction of, in hyperaldosteronism, 491
Sodium channels, G protein-activated, 71
Sodium ion, in mineralocorticoid regulation, 413
Sodium ipodate, for thyrotoxicosis, 306
Sohval-Soffer syndrome, 671
Solid-phase adsorption, 99
Solid-phase precipitation, 99
Solubility product, in stone formation, 1223
Somatomedin, 1267
Somatostatin, 127–130, 841
biological actions of, 1319–1321, 1320t
clinical relevance and applications of, 1321–1322
distribution of, 127–128
functions of, 130
in growth hormone secretion regulation, *1274,* 1274–1275
neuroendocrine function of, 128–129
production of, by tumors, 1415
regulation of, 1319
secretion of, 128–129
aging and, 1461
thyrotropin secretion and, 269
Somatostatin analogs:
for acromegaly, 193–194, *194*
for gonadotroph adenoma, 202
for thyrotroph adenoma, 203, 204t
Somatostatinomas, in MEN 1 syndrome, 1358
Somatotroph adenoma:
acromegaly and, 188–194
pathology of, 188
Somatotroph cells, 173
hormones secreted by, 173, 174t
Sorbitol accumulation, diabetes-specific complications and, 896
Sotos' syndrome, 1307–1308
Spectroscopy, fluorescence, phase-modulation, 100
Sperm:
deficiency of, secondary hypogonadism and, 678–682
morphology and motility of, 640–641, *641*
Sperm *(continued)*
production of, 654–655
deficient
isolated disorders causing, 673–676
primary hypogonadism and, 668–673
in acquired disorders, 672–673
in aging men, 672
from congenital/developmental disorders, 668–672
in systemic illness, 673
impaired, isolated, hypogonadism from, 682
isolated impairment in, 655
transport of, 640
impaired, infertility from, 662
Spermatogenesis:
hormonal control of, 649–651
initiation of, 650–651
gonadotropin therapy in, 687–688
maintenance of, 651
gonadotropin therapy in, 688
organization of, 639–640
phases of, schematic diagram of, *638*
stimulation of, in gonadotropin deficiency, 206
Spermatogonia, 637, 638
Spermatozoa:
classification of, 638
structure of, *641*
Spinal bulbar muscular atrophy, 677
Spinal cord:
injury to
androgen deficiency from, 673
sperm production impairment by, 676
lesions of, erectile dysfunction from, 659–660
Spironolactone:
androgen deficiency from, 672
as antiandrogen, 687
for hirsutism, 759
Spleen, somatostatin effects on, 1320t
Spondyloepiphyseal dysplasia, short stature from, 1297
Spondylometaphyseal dysplasia, short stature form, 1297
Sponge theory, of ectopic hormone production, 1391
Sporadic nonautoimmune thyrotoxicosis, 296–297
Sports, performance-enhancing endocrine drugs in, 1499–1504; *See also* Anabolic steroids
SRY gene, 641
Staghorn calculi, 1221, *1229*
Starvation, 844
pubertal delay from, 748
Stearic acid, 1044
Steatorrhea, in abetalipoproteinemia, 1034
Steroid hormone receptor superfamily, 53, *54*
Steroid hormones, 5, 37–43
adrenal
biosynthesis of, 389–404
acute regulation of, 394–395
cholesterol in, 392–395
cytochrome P450 in, 395, *396*
cytochrome P450C11β and P450c11AS in, 401
Steroid hormones *(continued)*
cytochrome P450c17 in, 398–400
cytochrome P450c21 in, 400–401
developmental aspects of, 403–404
3β-Hydroxysteroid dehydrogenase in, 398
11β-hydroxysteroid dehydrogenase in, 403
17β-hydroxysteroid dehydrogenase in, 401–402
inhibitors of, 414–415
17-ketosteroid reductase in, 401–402
P450aro in, 402
pathways of, *802*
principal pathways of, *396*
5α-reductase in, 402
regulation of, 404–414
steroid sulfatase in, 402
steroid sulfotransferase in, 402
chemistry of, *390,* 390–392, *391*
cholesterol as precursor of, 392–395
metabolism of, 418–421
variations in, 421
in plasma
concentrations of, 414–421
physical state of, 415–418
relative affinities of, for CBG, cytoplasmic glucocorticoid receptor, and albumin, 417t
trivial and systematic names of, 391, 392t
anabolic, in sports, 1499–1504; *See also* Anabolic steroids
commercial assays of, 95t
formation of, cholesterol substrate for, 37, *37, 38*
with glucocorticoid activity, 567
gonadal
production of, 787
in pubertal growth spurt, 1277–1279
synthesis of, pathways of, *802*
in gonadotropin releasing hormone regulation, 125–126
hormone binding domains for, 58–59
hormone-dependent tumor growth and, 1434–1436
mechanism of action of, 53, 55, *55*
metabolism of, 42–43
with mineralocorticoid activity, 567–568
ovarian, 720–723
metabolism of, 722–723
sex; *See* Sex steroids
synthesis of
disorders of, 447–461
congenital lipoid adrenal hyperplasia as, 460–461
11β-hydroxylase deficiency as, 459
21-hydroxylase deficiency as, 449–457
3β-hydroxysteroid dehydrogenase deficiency as, 457–458
P450c17 deficiency as, 458–459
P450c11AS disorders as, 459–460
pathway of, 39–41, *40*
rate-controlling step in, 37–39, *38*
trophic regulation of, 41–42
transport of, 42–43
Steroid receptors:
biochemistry of, 55
molecular biology of, 55

Steroid sulfatase:
deficiency of, hypogonadotropic hypogonadism in, 681t
in steroidogenesis, 402
Steroid sulfotransferase in steroidogenesis, 402
Steroid withdrawal syndromes, 627–628
Steroidogenic acute regulatory protein (StAR), 394–395
deficiency of
in congenital adrenal hyperplasia, 448t
in testosterone biosynthesis errors, 801
Sterol storage diseases, 1037–1039
Sterols, plant:
lipid metabolism and, 1047
storage disease involving, 1041–1042
Stomach:
cholecystokinin effects on, 1325t
gastric inhibitory polypeptide effects on, 1329t
motilin effects on, 1330t
neurotensin actions on, 1332t
pharmacologic actions of VIP on, 1328t
secretin effects on, 1326t
somatostatin effects on, 1320
Stones; *See* Nephrolithiasis
kidney, in hyperparathyroidism, 1116
Stress:
cortisol secretion and, 427
glucocorticoids and, 433–434
neuroendocrine alterations from, 156
vasopressin secretion and, 222
Stress hyperglycemia, fuel-hormone imbalance in, 844–845
Stroke, in endocrine disorders, 23
Stromal epithelial interactions, in breast function and mammary carcinogenesis, 1429, 1435–1436
Struma ovarii, 297
Struvite stone, 1236
Substance P, 1332–1333
neurologic effects of, 138
Sulfonylureas:
for diabetes in elderly, 1473
for Type 2 diabetes, 879–880, *881*, 881t
Suppository, urethral, for impotence in older men, 1470–1471
Suppurative thyroiditis, 330
Suprasellar dysgerminomas, 147–148
Surgery:
for breast cancer, 1440
for carcinoid syndrome, 1339
for corticotroph adenoma, 199–200
for endometrial cancer, 1444
for familial hypercholesterolemia, 1020
glucocorticoid therapy and, 623
for hyperlipoproteinemia, 1062
for hyperprolactinemia, 753
hypoparathyroidism after, 1141
in hypothyroid patient, 325
for lactotroph adenoma, 197
for morbid obesity, 986–987
for nephrolithiasis, 1224
for Paget's disease of bone, 1210
for pheochromocytoma, 539, 593
for pheochromocytoma of Men 2, 1369
pituitary, pituitary disorders from, 182
for pituitary mass lesions, 184–187; *See also* Transsphenoidal surgery
Surgery *(continued)*
for primary aldosteronism, 590
for prostate cancer, 1446
for renovascular hypertension, 586–588
for somatotroph adenoma, 192–193, 193t
steroid coverage for adrenocortical insufficiency patient during, 473, 473t
for thyroid carcinoma, 373–375
for thyrotoxicosis from thyroid adenoma, 308–309
for thyrotroph adenoma, 203
transsphenoidal, for Cushing's disease, 487–488
Sweating, excessive, in endocrine disorders, 21
Swyer syndrome, 799–800
Sympathetic nervous system, insulin resistance and, 577
Sympathochromaffin system, 525–547; *See also* Catecholamines
diseases of, diagnostic testing for, 545–547
organization of, 527–528
pathophysiology of, 536–545
generalized autonomic failure in, 540–543
hypoglycemia in, 543–545
neuroblastomas in, 540
pheochromocytoma in, 536–540
physiology of, 525–535
integrated, 532–535
Synapse, 111
Syndrome of inappropriate antidiuresis (SIAD) in cancer, 1404–1406
Syndrome of inappropriate antidiuretic hormone (SIADH), 243–245
causes of, 243t
therapy for, 246–247
System-based theories, of aging, 1458, 1458t

Tachycardia, in endocrine disorders, 23
"Take Control," 1047
Tamoxifen:
for breast cancer, 1440–1441, *1441*, 1442
in breast cancer prevention, 1442–1443
for endometrial cancer, 1444
in osteoporosis prevention, 1195
Tangier disease, 1032t, 1033–1033
Tea, lipid/lipoprotein metabolism and, 1048
Technetium-labeled bisphosphonate bone scan, 1181, *1181*
Teenagers, ovarian disorders in, 745–750
Telangiectasia, ataxia, primary hypogonadism and, 671
Temperature:
environmental, vasopressin secretion and, 222
regulation of, hypothalamic disease and, 155–156
Tendon xanthomas in familial hypercholesterolemia, 1016, *1016*
Teratologic malformations of external genitalia, 816
Testicular dysgenesis syndromes, 800t
Testicular feminization, primary amenorrhea from, 748–749, *749*
Testicular feminization syndrome, 676
Testicular regression syndromes, 800
Testis, 635–690
anatomy of, 635, 636–638
descent of, 642
Testis *(continued)*
development of, 641–642
fetal, 641–642
neonatal, 642
pubertal, 642
differentiation of, 784–785
ectopic, 673
in elderly, 1464
formation of, defective, 799–800
function of
autocrine regulation of, 646
gonadotropin control of, 644–649
paracrine regulation of, 646
in Klinefelter syndrome, 668
male hypogonadism and, 654–688; *See also* Hypogonadism, male
physiology of, 642–654
retractile, 673
rudimentary, 800t
size of, assessment of, 656, *656*, 656t
tumors of, 689–690
Testosterone:
assays for, 657–658t
bioavailable, 646
biosynthesis of, inborn errors of, 801, *802*
clinical actions of, 649t
deficiency of, osteoporosis in, 1193
gel, transdermal, 684
for gonadotropin deficiency in men, 205–206
for gynecomastia, 665
levels of
in aging
in female, 1464
in male, *1463*, 1463–1464
in males, frailty and, 1466–1467
low
in aging men, 672
in obesity, 964
in male internal genital development, 787
metabolism of, 647–648, *648*
non-permeation-enhanced nonscrotal patch, 684
oral preparations of, 684–685
permeation-enhanced nonscrotal patch, 684
plasma concentrations of, 415t
replacement
for Klinefelter syndrome, 670
for male hypogonadism
preparations and regimens for, 682–685, 683t
risks and side effects of, 685–686
scrotal patch, 684
secretion rate of, 415t
serum levels of
exercise-associated changes in
factors determining, 1493t
mechanism of, 1494
long-term activity-associated suppression of, mechanisms of, 1495–1496
serum measurement of, 656–658, 657–658t
therapy with, for impotence in older men, 1471
transdermal, 684
transport of, in plasma, 646–647
Testosterone biosynthetic enzyme defects, 671
Testosterone cypionate, for male hypogonadism, 682–683, 683t

Testosterone enenthate, for male hypogonadism, 682–683, 683t
Tetany, carpal spasm in, *1140*
Tetrahydrocannabinol, androgen deficiency from, 672
Tetrahydrolipstatin, in obesity management, 985–986
Thalassemia major, growth hormone deficiency in, 1293
Theca interstitial cells, *709,* 713
  ovarian, 716, *717*
Theca lutein cells, 720, *721*
Thelarche, premature, 1305
  benign, 791
Thermic effect of food, 970
Thermogenic actions, of thyroid hormones, 274
Thiazide diuretics:
  for absorptive hypercalciuria, 1253
  hypercalcemia induced by, 1137
  for hyperuricosuria, 1254
  hyponatremia induced by, 245–246
  for nephrogenic diabetes insipidus, 239
  for pituitary diabetes insipidus, 238
Thiazolidinediones, for Type 2 diabetes, *881,* 883, *884*
Thirst, 226
  deficiency of, 240–242
Thrombin receptors, 63
Thrombocytes, glucocorticoids and, 429
Thyroglobulin:
  biosynthesis of, defects in, hypothyroidism from, 319
  serum concentrations of, 278
  synthesis of, in thyroid hormonogenesis, *264,* 264–265
  in thyroid hormone synthesis, 45
Thyroid acropachy in Graves' disease, 314–315
Thyroid gland, 259–383
  adenomas of, in MEN 1 syndrome, 1359
  agenesis/dysgenesis of, hypothyroidism from, 318
  anatomy of, 261–262, *262*
  cancer of, 297, 366–378
    anaplastic, *370,* 370–371
    clinical staging of, 366, 366t, *367–368*
    endemic goiter related to, 352
    external beam irradiation for, 376
    follicular, 370, *370*
      radioactive iodine treatment of, 375–376
    follow-up of patients with, 377–378
    histologic classification of, 366, 366t
    medullary, *371,* 371–373; *See also* Medullary thyroid carcinoma
    molecular biology of, 366–368
    papillary, 368–370, *369*
      recurrence and survival in, influence of initial treatment on, 373t
    poorly differentiated, 370
    primary, 368–373
    secondary, 373
    surgical treatment of, 373–375
    thyroid hormones for, 376, *376*
    treatment of, molecular biology in, 376–377
  cholecystokinin effects on, 1325t
  disorders of, in Addison's disease, 463
  enlarged; *See* Goiter
Thyroid gland *(continued)*
  function of
    age and, 281
    caloric restriction and, 287
    cardiac disease and, 287
    in children, 281
    daily variations in, 279–280
    environmental factors affecting, 281
    evaluation of, 274–279
      free thyroxine index in, 278
      needle biopsy in, 279
      serum thyroid hormone-binding capacity in, 277–278
      serum thyrotropin concentrations in, *275,* 275–276, *276*
      serum thyroxine concentrations in, 276–277, 277t
      ultrasonography in, 279
    fasting and, 287
    fetal, *280,* 280–281
    human immunodeficiency virus infection and, 287
    in infants, 281
    liver disease and, 287
    nonthyroidal illness and, 283–287
    physiological variables affecting, 279–281
    pregnancy and, 280
    psychiatric disease and, 287–288
    radionuclide tests of, 279
    renal disease and, 287
    sex and, 281
    smoking and, 281
    testing strategies for, 275t
  function of, exercise and training and, 1485
  histology of, 262
  in hypothyroidism, 322
  imaging of, in thyrotoxicosis diagnosis, 302
  lymphoma of, 373
  nodule(s) of
    evaluation of, 361–364
      fine needle aspiration cytology in, 361–362, *362*
      laboratory diagnosis in, 361
      physical characteristics in, 361
      radioisotopic scan of thyroid in, 362–364
      ultrasound in, 362, *363*
    hemorrhage in, 329–330
    solitary, 359–366
      management of, 364–366
  painful, 329–330
  pharmacologic actions of VIP on, 1328t
  physical examination of, 261
  physiology of, 262–289
  radioiodine uptake by, in thyrotoxicosis diagnosis, 302
  radioisotopic scan of, in thyroid nodule evaluation, 362–364
  in thyrotoxicosis, 299
  TSH stimulation of, 350–351
  tumors of, in multiple endocrine neoplasia type 2, 1363–1364
Thyroid hormone(s), 43–46
  actions of, 272–274
    drugs ameliorating, 307
    inherited defects in, hypothyroidism from, 319–320
    in tissues, tests of, 279
Thyroid hormone(s) *(continued)*
  autoantibodies stimulating, in Graves' disease and autoimmune thyroiditis, 291t
  biosynthesis of, 262–265
    acquired defects in, hypothyroidism from, 320
    colloid endocytosis in, 265
    defects in, inherited biosynthetic, 318–319
    hormone release in, 265
    inherited defects in, goiter and, 354–355, *355*
    iodine in, 262–263
    thyroglobulin synthesis in, *264,* 264–265
    thyroid iodide transport in, 263–264
    tyrosyl iodination and coupling in, 264
  biosynthetic pathway for, distinctive, anatomy of, 44–45, *45*
  cellular binding of, 271–272
  cellular uptake and binding of, 272
  chemistry of, 262, *263*
  commercial assays of, 95t
  concentrations of, in pregnancy, 280, *280*
  deficiency of, delayed puberty from, 678
  degradation of, increased, hypothyroidism from, 320
  in elderly, 1455–1456
    drug interactions with, 1456–1457
  energy expenditure and, 974
  free, measurements of, 94–95
  in growth regulation, 1277
  hormone binding domains for, 58–59
  hypertension and, 569
  iodine metabolism and, 43–44, *44*
  major circulating, 43, *44*
  mechanism of action of, 55
  metabolism of, 265–266, *267*
  production of, 265–269, *266,* 266t
    decreased; *See* Hypothyroidism
    regulation of, 266–269, *267*
      thyrotropin-releasing hormone in, 268–269
  receptors for, 55
  regulation of, genes in, 274t
  replacement, for hypothyroidism, 326
  resistance to, hypothyroidism from, 319–320
  secretion of, regulation of, by iodide, 270
  serum binding of, alterations in, 281–283
  serum concentrations of, in hypothyroidism diagnosis, 325
  suppression of, in solitary thyroid nodule management, 364–366
  for thyroid carcinomas, 376, *376*
  thyrotoxicosis induced by, 295
  in thyrotropin secretion regulation, *267,* 267–268, *268*
  tissue responses to, 273–274
  total, measurements of, 94–95
  transport of, 271–272
  withdrawal of, 327–328
Thyroid hormone-binding capacity, serum, 277–278
Thyroid hormone-binding ratios, conditions altering, 277t
Thyroid stimulating hormone (TSH):
  release of, glucocorticoids and, 433
  reserve of, test for, in children, 1310t
  secretion of, goiter and, 350

Thyroid stimulating hormone (TSH) *(continued)*
- serum levels of, aging and, 1461, 1462, 1462t
- thyroid gland stimulation by, 350–351

Thyroid storm, 309–310
Thyroidectomy, subtotal, for thyrotoxicosis, 308
Thyroiditis, 294–295
- autoimmune
  - chronic, hypothyroidism from, 316–317
  - thyroid autoantibodies in patients with, 291t
  - transient hypothyroidism in, 317–318
- painless, 294–295, *295*
  - with thyrotoxicosis, transient hypothyroidism in, 317–318
- postpartum, 294–295, *295,* 311
  - transient hypothyroidism in, 317–318
- radiation, 330
- silent, 294–295, *295*
- subacute, 294, *295,* 329
- suppurative, 330

Thyrotoxicosis, 289–315
- adrenal function in, 301
- apathetic, 298
- appearance in, general, 298, *298*
- appendages in, 298
- autosomal dominant, 296–297
- bone-parathyroid-vitamin D system in, 301
- cardiovascular system in, 299
- causes of, 290t, 290–297
- cholestyramine for, 306
- clinical manifestations of, 297–301
- cytokine-induced, 296
- definition of, 289
- drug metabolism in, 301
- drug-induced, 296
- ectopic, 297
- electrolyte metabolism in, 300
- endocrine system in, 301
- energy in, 300
- exogenous, 295–296
- eyes in, 298
- fluid metabolism in, 300
- gastrointestinal system in, 300
- gestational, 297
- gonadal function in, 301
- Graves', 291–294
  - development of, hypothetical scheme for, *292*
  - natural history of, *293,* 293–294
  - pathogenesis of, 292–293
  - risk factors for, 293
  - treatment of, 303–304
- hematopoietic system in, 300
- hypercalcemia in, 1136–1137
- hyperthyroidism differentiated from, 289
- inorganic iodine for, 306
- iodine-induced, 295–296
- iopanoic acid for, 306
- laboratory diagnosis of, 301–303, *303*
- lithium carbonate for, 306
- masked, 298
- methimaxole for, 304–306, *305*
- muscle in, 299
- nervous system in, 299
- nutrient metabolism in, 300–301
- osteoporosis in, 1194

Thyrotoxicosis *(continued)*
- overt, 289
- painless thyroiditis with, transient hypothyroidism in, 317–318
- pathophysiology of, 290
- perchlorate for, 307
- pituitary hormone secretion in, 301
- postpartum, 311
- in pregnancy, 310–311
- pregnancy-related, 297
- prophylthiouracil, 304–306
- radioactive iodine therapy for, 307–308
- renal function in, 300
- respiratory function in, 300
- skin in, 298
- sodium ipodate for, 306
- sporadic nonautoimmune, 296–297
- subclinical, 289, 309
- subtotal thyroidectomy for, 308
- symptoms and signs of, 298t
- from thyroid adenoma, treatment of, 308–309
- thyroid gland in, 299
- thyroid hormone-induced, 295
- in thyroiditis, 294–295
  - treatment of, 308
- thyrotropin-dependent, 297
- from toxic multinodular goiter, treatment of, 309
- treatment of, 303–309

Thyrotroph adenoma, 202–204
Thyrotroph cells, hormones secreted by, 174, 174t
Thyrotropin receptor-stimulating antibodies:
- in Graves' disease, 291
- in thyrotoxicosis diagnosis, 302

Thyrotropin (TSH):
- actions of, 180
- circadian rhythm and, 144, *144*
- deficiency of, 205
- disorders of, hypothalamic disease and, 153
- mechanism of action of, 269–270
- secretion of, *179,* 179–180
  - in central hypothyroidism, 321
  - daily variations in, 279–280
  - regulation of, 266–269
    - dopamine in, 269
    - glucocorticoids in, 269
    - somatostatin in, 269
    - thyroid hormones in, *267,* 267–268, *268*
    - thyrotropin-releasing hormone in, 268–269
- serum concentrations of
  - in hypothyroidism diagnosis, 325
  - in thyroid function evaluation, *275,* 275–276, *276*
  - in thyrotoxicosis diagnosis, 301
- synthesis of, 179
- thyrotoxicosis dependent on, 297

Thyrotropin-releasing hormone stimulation test, in thyrotoxicosis diagnosis, 302
Thyrotropin-releasing hormone (TRH), 121–124
- effects of, 123–124
- location of, 121
- metabolism of, 121
- neuroendocrine function of, 123

Thyrotropin-releasing hormone (TRH) *(continued)*
- physiologic role of, 123
- receptors for, 121
- stimulation test of, 278–279
- in thyroid hormone production regulation, 268–269

Thyroxine (T4), 43, *44*
- globulin binding, 271
- metabolism of, glucocorticoids and, 433
- production of, 265, *266,* 266t
  - aging and, 1461–1462, 1462t
- serum concentrations of
  - conditions altering, 277t
  - high, in nonthyroidal illness, 286–287
  - low, in nonthyroidal illness, 286
  - in thyroid function evaluation, 276–277, 277t
  - in thyrotoxicosis diagnosis, 301–302
- for solitary thyroid nodules, 365t
- in thyrotropin secretion regulation, *267,* 267–268, *268*
- transport of, 45–46
- for TSH deficiency, 205

L-Thyroxine (T4):
- for hypothyroidism, 326–327, 1289
  - dosage of, factors altering, 327t

Tiludronate disodium (Skelid), for Paget's disease of bone, 1208t
Tissue(s):
- epithelial, glucocorticoids and, 429
- fibroblastic, glucocorticoids and, 429
- hypersensitivity to, endocrine excess syndromes from, 14
- responses of, to thyroid hormones, 273–274
- thyroid hormone action in, tests of, 279

Tongue, in endocrine disorders, 21
Tonsils, in Tangier disease, 1033
Toremifene, for breast cancer, 1441
Total parenteral nutrition (TPN), osteomalacia from, 1188
Toxic multinodular goiter, 296
- thyrotoxicosis from, treatment of, 309

Toxic thyroid adenoma, 296
Toxic uninodular goiter, 296
Training; *See also* Exercise and training
- ACTH-cortisol axis in exercise and, 1488–1489
- catecholamine response to exercise and, 1490
- endurance, hypothalamic-pituitary-gonadal axis in men and, 1495
- glucagon response to exercise and, 1486
- prolactin response to exercise and, 1492–1493
- thyroid function and, 1485

Tranexamic acid, for menarcheal menorrhagia, 749
Transcription, in messenger RNA biosynthesis, 29–31
Transfer proteins, active in lipoprotein metabolism, 1000
Transforming growth factor-α (TGF-α), tumor-associated, hypercalcemia and, 1129
Transforming growth factor-β (TGF-β), in breast cancer metastasis to bone, 1132–1133

Transplantation:
organ, immunosuppressive therapy after, osteoporosis and, 1194–1195
pancreatic, for Type 1 diabetes, 872–873, *873*
islet transplantation versus, 874t, 874–875
renal
in diabetic nephropathy, 902, 903
for renal osteodystrophy, 1201
Transport proteins, 3
Transsphenoidal hypophysectomy, for pituitary tumor in MEN 1 syndrome, 1362
Transsphenoidal microsurgery, for Cushing's disease, 487–488
Transsphenoidal surgery:
for acromegaly in MEN 1 syndrome, 1363
complications of, 186, 186t
for corticotroph adenoma, 199–200
efficacy of, 186, 186t
for lactotroph adenoma, 197
postoperative management of, 187
preoperative management of, 186–187
for somatotroph adenoma, 192–193, 193t
Transthyretin (TTR):
thyroid hormone binding alterations and, 283
in thyroxine binding, 272
Trauma:
growth hormone deficiency from, 1293
head, hypothalamic involvement in, 148–149
steroid coverage for adrenocortical insufficiency patient during, 473
Tremor, in thyrotoxicosis, 299
Treonine kinase activity, receptors with, 80–81
Triamcinolone:
for congenital adrenal hyperplasia, 457t
structure of, *611*
Triamcinolone acetonide, structure of, *611*
Triglyceride, synthesis and catabolism of, 998
Triiodothyronine (T3):
levels of, in aging, 1462, 1462t
nuclear receptors for, 272–273
production of, 265–266, *266*, 266t
extrathyroidal
drugs inhibiting, 307
regulation of, 270–271
serum concentrations of, 278
low, in nonthyroidal illness, 285–286
reverse, 278
in thyrotoxicosis diagnosis, 301–302
in thyrotropin secretion regulation, *267*, 267–268, *268*
3,3′,5′-Triiodothyronine (reverse T3), 43, *44*
3,5,3′-Triiodothyronine (T3), 43, *44*
Trilostane, in adrenal steroid biosynthesis inhibition, 415
Triple phosphate stone, 1236
Troglitazone, for Type 2 diabetes, *881*, 883, *884*
Trophic regulation, of steroid hormone synthesis, 41–42
Trophoblastic tumors, thyrotoxicosis related to, 297
Tropic hormones, 11
Trousseau's sign, in hypocalcemia, 1140
Tryptophan, brain uptake of, appetite and, 972
Tuberculosis, Addison's disease from, 436–464, 462
Tuberoeruptive xanthomas, in type III hyperlipoproteinemia, *1024*, 1024–1025, *1025*
Tumor(s):
adrenal
adrenal hyperfunction from, 480–491
clinical features of, 480–482
etiology of, 485–487
features of, suggesting specific etiology, 482
laboratory features of, 482
localization of, 485, 487, *488*
treatment of, 490
adrenocortical, Cushing's syndrome from, 478
associated with ectopic GHRH production, 1411t
associated with hypoglycemia, 1406–1407, 1407t
associated with oncogenic osteomalacia, 1409
associated with syndrome of inappropriate antidiuresis, 1404, 1404t
bone, bisphosphonates for, 1136
breast, hereditary, 1429–1431
brown, in hyperparathyroidism, 1115, *1117*
carcinoid
in MEN 1 syndrome, 1358
secretory products of, 1335t
causing ectopic ACTH syndrome, 479t
CNS, growth hormone deficiency from, 1293
ectopic hormone production by, 1386
Levine-Metz classification of, 1390, 1390t
ectopic POMC/ACTH syndrome associated, 1400t
estrogen-secreting, gynecomastia from, 664
GEP peptide-producing, octreotide acetate efficacy on, 1324t
hormone-responsive, 1427–1447
classification of, 1428t
clinical characteristics of, 1439–1447
epidemiology of, 1433–1434
genetic changes in, 1429–1433
growth of, endocrine mechanisms controlling, 1434–1436
progression of, mechanisms of, 1436–1439
human chorionic gonadotropin-secreting, gynecomastia from, 664
hypercalcemia-associated, 1394t
of hypothalamus, 147–148
in Nelson's syndrome, treatment of, 490
neuroendocrine, 1333
of gastrointestinal tract, 1333–1340; *See also* Carcinoid syndrome
non-germ cell, 690
pancreatic, in MEN 1 syndrome, 1358
paraneoplastic erythrocytosis and, 1413–1414
pineal region, 158
pituitary, in MEN 1 syndrome, 1358
POMC products produced by, 1400–1401
prolactin produced by, 1414–1415
renin-secreting
hypertension and, 564
management of, 588
of testis, 689–690
thyroid, in multiple endocrine neoplasia type 2, 1363–1364
Tumor(s) *(continued)*
trophoblastic, thyrotoxicosis related to, 297
vitamin D metabolism abnormalities from, 185–186
Tumor marker(s):
hormones as, 1392–1394
ideal, 1393t
Tumor necrosis factor (TNF), hypercalcemia and, 1129
Tumoral calcinosis syndrome, hyperphosphatemia in, 1156
Tunica albuginea, 636
Turner's syndrome, 745–747, 796–799
clinical features of, 796–797, *797*
diagnosis of, 798–799, *799*
phenotype-karyotype correlations in, 797–798
short stature in, 1298, 1300–1302
treatment of, 798–799
Tyrosine, brain uptake of, appetite and, 972
Tyrosine kinase activity, receptors with, 80–82
Tyrosyl iodination and coupling, in thyroid hormonogenesis, 264

Ulcer, peptic, glucocorticoid therapy and, 623–624
Ultradian rhythms, 143
Ultrasonography:
in nephrolithiasis evaluation, 1225
in thyroid function evaluation, 279
in thyroid nodule evaluation, 362, *363*
United Kingdom Prospective Diabetes Study (UKPDS), 876t, 876–877, *877*, *878*, 878t
Urea, oral, for syndrome of inappropriate antidiuresis in cancer, 1406
Urease inhibitors, in magnesium ammonium phosphate stone management, 1238
Urethral suppository, for impotence in older men, 1470–1471
Uric acid:
allopurinol effect on, mechanisms of, 1233
excretion of
diet and, 1232
purine metabolism and, 1232, *1232*
solubility of, in urine, 1232, *1232*
Uric acid stones, 1231–1235
clinical disorders associated with, 1233
epidemiology of, 1231–1232
evaluation of, 1234
gout and, 1232t, 1232–1233
imaging of, 1234
medical treatment of, efficacy of, 1233–1234
purine-related stones differentiated from, 1233
risk factors for, 1232
therapy of, 1234–1235
Urinary corticosteroids, measurement of, 439–440
Urinary tract, stones in, 1221–1256; *See also* Nephrolithiasis
Urine:
acidity of, measuring, 1234
pH of
calcium oxalate stone risk and, 1240
cystine solubility and, 1228
diet and, 1232

Urine *(continued)*
saturation zones and ranges in, 1223, *1223*
uric acid solubility in, 1232, *1232*
volume of, low, calcium oxalate stone risk and, 1240
Urogenital sinus, differentiation of, 787
Urogenital system, pharmacologic actions of VIP on, 1328t
Urolithiasis, 1221
Uterus:
cancer of, 1443–1444
hormone replacement therapy and, 770
oxytocin and, 225

Vacuum tumescence devices, for impotence in older men, 1471
Vanishing testis syndrome, 671
Varicocele, 636, 655, 674
Vasculitis, androgen deficiency and, 673
Vasoactive agents, glucocorticoids and, 427
Vasoactive intestinal peptide (VIP):
neurologic effects of, 138
production of, by tumors, 1415
Vasoactive intestinal polypeptide (VIP), 1327–1328
in prolactin release, 134–135
Vasopressin:
amino acid sequence of, *218*
biologic actions of, 224–225
biosynthesis of, 217–218
chemistry of, 217
clearance of, 223–224
deficiencies of, 228–240
diabetes insipidus from, 228–239; *See also* Diabetes insipidus (DI)
enuresis from, 239–240
nocturia from, 239–240
postural hypotension from, 240
disorders of, hypothalamic disease and, 153
distribution of, 223–224
excess of, 242–247
differential diagnosis of, 246
in hypervolemic hyponatremia, 246
in hypovolemia hyponatremia, 245–246
in syndrome of inappropriate antidiuresis, 243t, 243–245, *244*
therapy for, 246–247
exercise and training and, 1484
hypertension and, 569
levels of, in elderly, 1465
release of, 217–218
secretion of, 218–223
autocrine effects on, 223
emetic effects on, 221, *222*
glucopenic effects on, 222
hemodynamic effects on, 220–221
hypoxia-hypercapnia and, 222
oropharyngeal effects on, 220
osmotic effects on, 218–220, *219, 220*
pharmacologic effects on, 223
renin-angiotensin and, 222
stress and, 222
temperature and, 222
thirst and, 226
Vasopressin tests in children, 1311t
Ventricular hypertrophy, left, complicating hypertension, 556
Verapamil, for thyrotoxicosis, 307
Vertical banded gastroplasty, for morbid obesity, 986–987
Vesicle assays, 99
Vipoma:
hypercalcemia in, 1137
in MEN 1 syndrome, 1358
VIPomas:
octreotide acetate efficacy on, 1324t
pancreatic polypeptide oversecretion in, 1331
secretory diarrhea in, octreotide acetate for, 1323t
Virilization:
amenorrhea and, 757–759
in endocrine disorders, 24
of genetic female, 807–816
from congenital adrenal hyperplasia, 807–815
from defective estrogen synthesis aromatase deficiency, 815
prenatal, by environmental hormones, 816
genital, defective, 801–807
from 17α-hydroxylase deficiency, 803–804
from androgen target tissue defects, 804–806
from 3β-hydroxysteroid dehydrogenase deficiency, 801, 803
from 17β-hydroxysteroid dehydrogenase deficiency, 804
from 17,20-desmolase deficiency, 804
from exogenous sex steroids, 806–807
from Leydig cell hypoplasia, 801
from testosterone biosynthesis errors, 801, *802*
of unknown etiology, 807
primary amenorrhea from, 749
Virilizing adrenal hyperplasia, 449
simple, 450–451
missense mutations causing, 455
Viscera, in acromegaly, 190
Vision:
evaluation of, in anterior pituitary lesion evaluation, 184
impairment of, in anterior pituitary diseases, 183, *183*
Vitamin(s), lipid/lipoprotein metabolism and, 1048
Vitamin A:
for abetalipoproteinemia, 1035
hypercalcemia induced by, 1137–1138
Vitamin C, calcium oxalate stone risk and, 1240
Vitamin D, 1098–1109
absorption of, 1100
actions of
in bone, 1107–1108
cellular basis of, 1105
in immune system, 1108
in intestine, 1105–1107
in kidney, 1108
mechanism of, 55
in skin, 1108
activation of, 1100–1103
Vitamin D *(continued)*
biosynthesis of, 1099–1100
chemical structure of, *1099*
chemistry of, 1099–1100
deficiency of
hip fracture in elderly and, 1467–1468
hypocalcemia from, 1148–1149
in osteoporosis, 1190
in rickets, 1184–1185
historical information on, 1098–1099
hormone binding domains for, 58–59
hypercalcemia induced by, 1137
for hypocalcemia, 1151–1152
for hypoparathyroidism, 1142–1143
in hypothyroidism, 325
levels of, in aging, factors responsible for, *1469*
malabsorption of
osteomalacia from, 1185
rickets from, 1185
metabolism of, abnormal
osteomalacia from, 1185–1186
rickets from, 1185–1186
metabolites of
assay of, 1108–1109
transport of, 1103
nutrition and, 1104–1105
for oncogenic osteomalacia, 1409
peripheral resistance to, 1186
pharmacology of, 1149t
phosphate reabsorption and, 1154
renal loss of, 1186
serum concentrations of, ultraviolet radiation and, *1101*
status of, 1102
in thyrotoxicosis, 301
transport of, 1103
Vitamin D2:
biosynthesis of, 1099–1100
chemical structure of, *1099*
chemistry of, 1099–1100
for rickets and osteomalacia, 1188, 1189
Vitamin D3:
absorption of, 1100
biosynthesis of, 1099–1100
chemical structure of, *1099*
Vitamin E:
for abetalipoproteinemia, 1035
deficiency of, in abetalipoproteinemia, 1034
Vitamin K, for abetalipoproteinemia, 1035
Voice, in endocrine disorders, 21

Water:
composition of, 226–227
distribution of, 226
intake of, vasopressin secretion and, 220
metabolism of
hormone actions in, 11–12
hormones associated with, in elderly, 1465
turnover of, *227*, 227–228
Water balance, regulation of, 226–228
Water diuresis, 224
Water intoxication, from DDAVP for primary polydipsia, 238
Weakness:
in Cushing's syndrome, 482
in endocrine disorders, 19–20, 26

Weight gain:
in acromegaly, 190
in endocrine disorders, 20
Weight loss:
amenorrhea from, 753–754
in elderly, 1474, 1475t
in endocrine disorders, 20
methods to achieve, in elderly, 1476t
for obstructive sleep apnea syndrome, 965
Weightlessness, osteoporosis and, 1194
Weight-management strategy, selection criteria for, 979t
Weinstein syndrome, 671
Werner syndrome, 671
Wilm's tumor gene, in gonadal differentiation, 784
Wolman disease, 465, 1038–1039
Women:
gonadotropin deficiency in, 206–207
hyperlipidemia in, treatment of, 1062–1063
hyperprolactinemia in, clinical features of, 195
Women *(continued)*
reproductive system in, exercise and, 1496–1498
Work, physical; *See* Exercise and training

X chromosome, *782,* 782–783
Xanthoma tuberosum, in type III hyperlipoproteinemia, *1024,* 1024–1025, *1025*
Xanthomas, 1038
eruptive, in hyperchylomicronemia, 1027, *1028*
planar, HDL deficiency with, 1032, 1032t
tendon, in familial hypercholesterolemia, 1016, *1016, 1017*
Xanthomatosis, 1040–1042, 1041–1042
cerebrotendinous, 1039–1040
X-ray absorptiometry, dual, in bone metabolic disease evaluation, 1180–1181
XX males, 794–795
XY gonadal dysgenesis, 799–800, 800t
XYY genotype, growth excess in, 1307
XYY males, 794
XYY syndrome, 670

Y chromosome, 781–782, *782*
structural anomalies of, 795–796
Y chromosome microdeletions, 675, *675*
Yohimbine, for postural hypotension, 543
Young syndrome, infertility in, 662

Zeitgeber, 143, 144
Zollinger-Ellison syndrome:
hypergastrinemia in, 1324
hypersecretinemia in, 1326–1327
in MEN 1 syndrome, 1357
Zona fasciculata, 389, *390*
Zona glomerulosa, 389, *390*
Zona pellucida, *709,* 711, *714*
in oocyte growth, 730
Zona reticularis, 389, *390*
Zonal theory, of adrenarche, 1278

NOTES

NOTES

NOTES

NOTES

NOTES

NOTES

NOTES

NOTES

NOTES

NOTES

NOTES

ISBN 0-07-022001-8
90000
9 780070 220010
FELIG/ ENDOCRIN METABOL